Ingle's
ENDODONTICS 6

Ingle's ENDODONTICS 6

JOHN I. INGLE, DDS, MSD
Lecturer
Loma Linda University
School of Dentistry
Loma Linda, California

LEIF K. BAKLAND, DDS
Professor and Chair
Department of Endodontics
School of Dentistry
Loma Linda University
Loma Linda, California

J. CRAIG BAUMGARTNER, MS, DDS, PHD
Professor and Chairman
Department of Endodontology
Oregon Health & Sciences University
Portland, Oregon

2008
PEOPLE'S MEDICAL PUBLISHING HOUSE
SHELTON, CONNECTICUT

People's Medical Publishing House
2 Enterprise Drive, Suite 509
Shelton, CT 06484
Tel: 203-402-0646
Fax: 203-402-0854
E-mail: info@pmph-usa.com

© 2008 PMPH-USA.

All rights reserved. Without limiting the rights under copyright reserved above, no part of this publication may be reproduced, stored in or introduced into a retrieval system, or transmitted, in any form or by any means (electronic, mechanical, photocopying, recording, or otherwise), without the prior written permission of the copyright holder.

09 10 11 12 / PMPH / 9 8 7 6 5 4 3 2

ISBN 978-1-55009-333-9
Printed in China by People's Medical Publishing House
Production Editor: Patricia Bindner; Typesetter: Integra; Cover Design: Norm Reid

---

Sales and Distribution

Canada
McGraw-Hill Ryerson Education
Customer Care
300 Water St
Whitby, Ontario L1N 9B6
Canada
Tel: 1-800-565-5758
Fax: 1-800-463-5885
www.mcgrawhill.ca

Foreign Rights
John Scott & Company
International Publisher's Agency
P.O. Box 878
Kimberton, PA 19442
USA
Tel: 610-827-1640
Fax: 610-827-1671

Japan
United Publishers Services Limited
1-32-5 Higashi-Shinagawa
Shinagawa-ku, Tokyo 140-0002
Japan
Tel: 03-5479-7251
Fax: 03-5479-7307
Email: kakimoto@ups.co.jp

United Kingdom, Europe,
Middle East, Africa
McGraw Hill Education
Shoppenhangers Road
Maidenhead
Berkshire, SL6 2QL
England
Tel: 44-0-1628-502500
Fax: 44-0-1628-635895
www.mcgraw-hill.co.uk

Singapore, Thailand, Philippines,
Indonesia, Vietnam, Pacific Rim, Korea
McGraw-Hill Education
60 Tuas Basin Link
Singapore 638775
Tel: 65-6863-1580
Fax: 65-6862-3354
www.mcgraw-hill.com.sg

Australia, New Zealand
Elsevier Australia
Tower 1, 475 Victoria Avenue
Chatswood NSW 2067
Australia
Tel: 0-9422-8553
Fax: 0-9422-8562
www.elsevier.com.au

Brazil
Tecmedd Importadora e Distribuidora
de Livros Ltda.
Avenida Maurilio Biagi 2850
City Ribeirao, Rebeirao, Preto SP
Brazil
CEP: 14021-000
Tel: 0800-992236
Fax: 16-3993-9000
Email: tecmedd@tecmedd.com.br

India, Bangladesh, Pakistan,
Sri Lanka, Malaysia
CBS Publishers
4819/X1 Prahlad Street 24
Ansari Road, Darya, New Delhi-110002
India
Tel: 91-11-23266861/67
Fax: 91-11-23266818
Email: cbspubs@vsnl.com

People's Republic of China
PMPH
Bldg 3, 3rd District
Fangqunyuan, Fangzhuang
Beijing 100078
P.R. China
Tel: 8610-67653342
Fax: 8610-67691034
www.pmph.com

Notice: The authors and publisher have made every effort to ensure that the patient care recommended herein, including choice of drugs and drug dosages, is in accord with the accepted standard and practice at the time of publication. However, since research and regulation constantly change clinical standards, the reader is urged to check the product information sheet included in the package of each drug, which includes recommended doses, warnings, and contraindications. This is particularly important with new or infrequently used drugs. Any treatment regimen, particularly one involving medication, involves inherent risk that must be weighed on a case-by-case basis against the benefits anticipated. The reader is cautioned that the purpose of this book is to inform and enlighten; the information contained herein is not intended as, and should not be employed as, a substitute for individual diagnosis and treatment.

Dedication

The editors of Ingle's *ENDODONTICS* are proud to dedicate this edition to two of the most inspired and beloved teachers and practitioners of endodontics during our generation: Dr. Dudley H. Glick and Dr. Alfred L. Frank. True gentlemen, world famous, innovators, and the closest of friends. So close, Al and Dudley were often referred to as Al Glick and Dudley Frank. Both practiced in Beverly Hills, both with a bevy of famous patients, they could have been long time competitors. Instead, they were inseparable - Damon and Pythias - professionally, academically, and socially. Their wives, Ellie Glick and Teri Frank, are the very best of friends. Between them they have eight sons.

Both were born, raised and educated in Ohio; they served with honor and decoration in World War II and following the war Dudley and Al were both graduated in dentistry from the University of Southern California. As predoctoral dental students they were infamous for their unusual interest in endodontics, in a school famous for its restorative dentistry. Upon graduation they both started general practices in the Los Angeles area and were soon noted for their superb restorative dentistry. They joined the endodontic faculty at USC and when word of their endodontic skills spread, referrals started to pour in. After consulting a number of endodontic friends, they "took the leap," and announced they were limiting themselves to endodontics, among the first really fulltime endodontists in Southern California.

They were the last of the "self-trained" endodontists. Self trained, that is, by taking every postgraduate endodontic course and attending available meetings, and visiting professionally with the nation's best known endodontists; first on the West Coast and then nationwide.

Over the years they became the endodontist's endodontists. If we, ourselves, needed root canal treatment, we would travel cross country to have either Al or Dudley perform the treatment. There was never a fee! They were proud of the trust placed in them by other skilled professionals. In fact, dentists, physicians and the clergy were rarely charged in their offices. That was their strong belief in professional courtesy. And everyone else paid the same fee, whether you were Cary Grant, Nancy Regan, Mae West or Joe the plumber. Except teachers who received a reduced fee.

As they gained in renown, both Al and Dudley, were inundated with requests to speak to national and foreign audiences. No one made and retained so many devoted friends around the world. Their homes in Beverly Hills became a haven for the famous and students alike, sometimes for weeks at a time, as young people came to learn from the masters.

They never ceased their dedication to teaching, at USC, at UCLA, at Loma Linda, and at Cedars-Sinai Hospital. Both Dudley and Al were honored over and over by societies and universities alike.

They became famous locally, nationally internationally, yet remained the same modest, generous, considerate, literally lovable gentlemen they always were, brimming with integrity and honesty. This is what endeared them to those of us fortunate to have been their friends and disciples, students, employees and patients. We only wish the entire specialty profession had had the same opportunity.

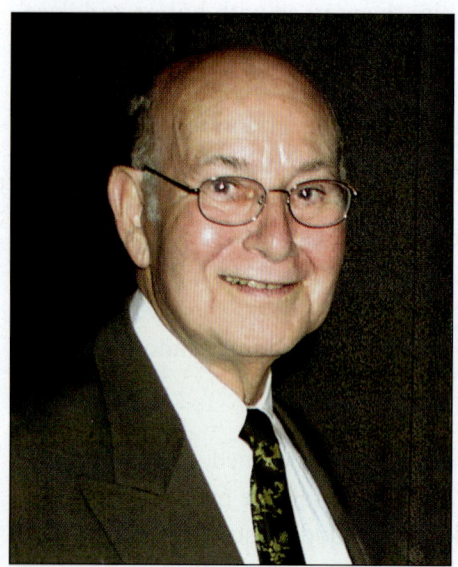

Dr. Dudley H. Glick

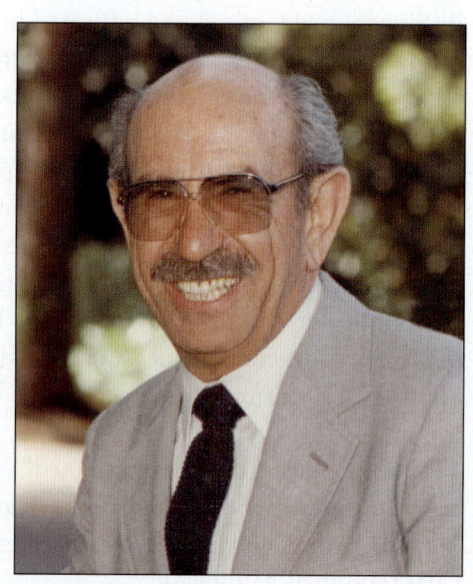

Dr. Alfred L. Frank

Preface to the First Edition of Endodontics 1965 "Pull and be Damned Road"

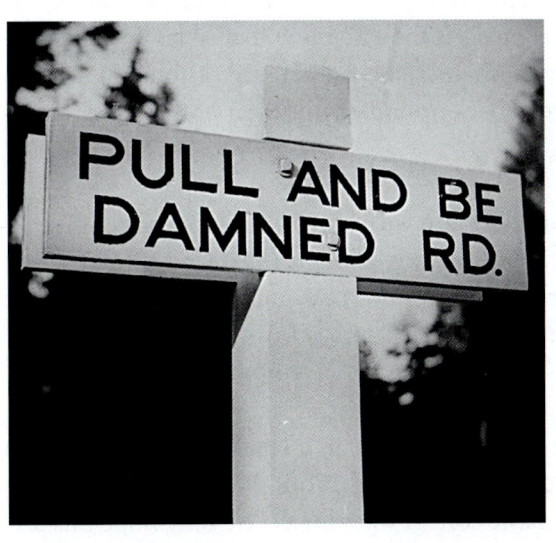

This book was begun at Sne-oosh Beach, a quiet retreat overlooking Puget Sound and the San Juan Islands. At Sne-oosh it is possible to escape from complex civilization, and concentrate on the job at hand—writing an endodontic text.

Hard by Sne-oosh is an old Indian trail called PULL AND BE DAMNED ROAD. One could hardly imagine a more fitting location while writing a text on the pulpless tooth than nearby PULL AND BE DAMNED ROAD, for "Pull and be damned" could well be the motto of the dental profession from its inception.

PULL AND BE DAMNED ROAD goes down to the shores of Skagit Bay, an inside passage of the gentle Pacific leading ominously to DECEPTION PASS. This delusive inlet, which so easily deceived the early explorers, reminds us of how our profession has practiced self-deception over the years. Unfortunately, many pass into the "pull and be damned" deceptive phase of dental practice, never to return.

Inside DECEPTION PASS, however, lies HOPE ISLAND, our symbol of the future. HOPE we must have, coupled with resolve. HOPE that the future of dentistry will noticeably improve. HOPE that an enlightened profession will be guided by the concept of retention and rehabilitation of the dental apparatus. HOPE for the rejection of "oral amputation."

In this new text we hope to inspire dentists to consider root canal treatment as an integral part of their practice. We discuss in great detail the operative aspects of endodontic therapy: cavity preparation, canal débridement and filling. We leave to others the detailed discussion of anti-infectives, local anesthesia, oral microbiology, although these subjects are dealt with in this text, brief and to the point. We have spent, however, and unusual amount of space and time in developing the chapter on DIFFERENTIAL DIAGNOSIS OF ORAL AND PERIORAL PAIN, so necessary in arriving at a proper diagnosis. Diagnosis of pain is falling more and more in the province of endodontics. Proper diagnosis is the discipline that separates the really competent dentist from the merely mechanical. So a great deal of thought and talent has gone into developing the four background chapters on normal and pathologic pulp and periapical tissues.

Snee-oosh Beach is no Walden Pond, nor are we Thoreau for that matter. But we may learn from Walden. "Simplify, Simplify!" was Thoreau's text, and simplification we have taken to heart. We have removed the "mumbo-jumbo" from endodontic treatment, a significant factor that discouraged dentists from including endodontics in their practice.

We have attempted to present the subject, not only in a simplified form, but in a systematic manner leading to success, pleasure and profit. We have attempted to remove the mystery and retain the basic core of the subject. We only hope this text succeeds in bringing some order out of the present chaos.

John I. Ingle
Seattle, Washington
1964

Preface
"Pull and be Damned Road" Revisited

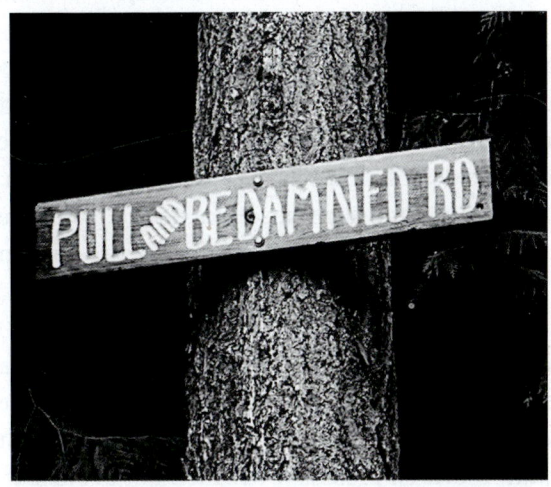

The original sign for Pull and be Damned Road has been pilfered so many times the authorities have had to place a new sign over 20 feet above the ground. (Courtesy of Dr. James Stephens.)

Over 40 years ago the preface to the first edition of *Endodontics* featured "**Pull And Be Damned Road.**" Nothing from the first edition left such a lasting impression as that saying. Even today, "old timers" come up to me at meetings to reminisce about this preface. They may not remember the details of endodontic cavity preparation or the chapter on pain first expressed in that edition. Those features have become an integral part of any endodontic practice. But they do remember "Pull and Be Damned Road." And for good reason.

Forty years ago it was more prevalent to extract teeth than to save them by root canal therapy. A plea was made in this preface to trust endodontic treatment and to reverse this trend toward "oral amputation." Gradually this became a fact, as endodontics spurred ahead and full dentures declined.

And this brings to mind an incident I long have savored. I was a speaker at the Hinman Dental Meeting in Atlanta. Joining me as a headliner was Dr. Will Menninger, head of the famous Menninger Psychiatric Clinic, then based in Topeka, Kansas. Dr. Menninger and his brother Karl were unquestionably the world's most famous psychiatrists. Dr. Will had been a brigadier general in World War II, head of all the army's psychiatrists. In 1948 he was the first psychiatrist on the cover of *TIME* magazine. It was an honor for me to be on the same program with him, and I eagerly attended his first lecture that preceded mine.

When I began my lecture, there was Dr. Menninger seated in the front row. I considered it professional courtesy on his part, but I did notice him taking notes.

The Hinman had a format wherein each lecturer would repeat his same lecture the next day. I didn't attend Dr. Menninger's second lecture but he attended mine. There he was again, seated in the front row. I was flattered beyond measure. At the end of the lecture I asked him why his sudden interest in endodontics. His reply was startling.

"Dr. Ingle," he said, "I was so impressed with your lecture, but I was also terribly embarrassed. On behalf of my profession I must apologize to you for my past behavior. When I think of how many patients I have recommended that they have their teeth extracted, I am appalled at the destruction I have caused. I had no idea. Now I find these teeth could have been saved and their abscesses healed. You have no idea how thankful I am to you, for directing me from my past behavior." Spoken like a psychiatrist!

We've come a long way since those days, a time of wholesale extractions. But we face a new challenge today; not wholesale extractions but **selective extractions;** for the sole purpose of placing an implant. Once again, dentists are urging patients to have teeth extracted, ignoring the fact that a healthy root is far preferable to a mechanical implant; less costly, less painful, less time consuming, and above all, more biological.

Now I'm not saying implants are unhealthy or less successful. What I am expressing is my concern that many salvable teeth are being sacrificed on the altar of insatiability. Back to pull and be damned. I'm not against implants! As a matter of fact, implant therapy is now being taught in a number of endodontic post doctoral programs. The thesis being, however, that teeth that cannot or should not be saved by endodontics may well be extracted and replaced by an implant rather than a bridge. And who better to place that implant than a well-trained endodontist who has just made that judgment?

The 6th edition of *Endodontics* is replete with new innovations and knowledge. Now, more than ever, it remains the "Bible of Endodontics" a name long applied by others to the previous editions.

I feel most comfortable as I "pass the torch" to the new editors, Leif Bakland and Craig Baumgartner. And I have a feeling the profession will come to its senses; veering off "Pull and Be Damned Road" and onto the "Road Best Traveled."

John I. Ingle
December 2007

▼ Acknowledgements

Once again, I am particularly indebted to my wife Joyce and my son Geoffrey, who were so helpful in manuscript preparation and computer utilization. And speaking of computers, I am especially indebted to my computer "maven", Lynda Arnett, who frequently spent hours "setting me straight and bailing me out" of trouble.

Being isolated in a city without a school of dentistry presents a problem in literature search. Dr. Robert Bravin of El Cajon CA, who has a nearly complete library of the *Journal of Endodontics*, was especially helpful in providing back issues of JOE. In addition, I received a great deal of help from the dental school library at the University of Southern California and Chief Librarian, Professor Frank Mason, as well as Librarian John Glueckert. And at the University of Washington, in the Department of Dental Health Sciences, Dr. Peter Milgrom, chairman, and Janessa M. Stream Graves, Research Coordinator, were most helpful with trends and statistics. I received similar help from Jill Cochran at the American Association of Endodontists.

Finally, I must acknowledge the advice and counseling I received from my dear friend the late Dr. Dudley Glick. But most of all, I acknowledge, with pride and admiration, my coeditors, Dr. Leif K. Bakland and Dr J. Craig Baumgartner. They have carried the major load in producing this edition of *Endodontics*, tireless hours, hundreds of emails, phone calls and faxes. I leave this text in the good hands of these skilled and highly knowledgeable individuals.

John I. Ingle

A textbook with the scope and format of this, the 6th edition of *Ingle's Endodontics*, would not be possible but for the tremendous effort by numerous individuals. Each contributor to this book devoted considerable time to research, preparation, and writing. To them I express much gratitude for their efforts, but also for putting up with my deadline prodding. My hope is that this collaborative effort makes them as proud as it makes me.

Editing manuscripts from around the world (Europe, Asia, and the Americas) would be impossible but for the expert secretarial support provided by Luci Denger and Shannon Kokanour in the Department of Endodontics at Loma Linda University. These capable coworkers skillfully completed in a timely fashion all the requests for changes, corrections, formatting and interactions with authors and publisher. To both Luci and Shannon – your contributions are most appreciated.

Anyone who takes on the job of editing a major text book knows that it will have an impact on the "day job" that each of us has. Were it not for an understanding dean, Dr. Charles Goodacre, and a cooperative department faculty, Drs. Mahmoud Torabinejad, Robert Handysides, and David Jaramillo, there would neither be the time nor the energy to complete this task. To them I say a heartfelt "Thank you."

This grand textbook is not the result of any single individual, a fact that is true with regards to the editing as well as the writing and publishing. This was truly a team effort by John I. Ingle, J. Craig Baumgartner and me. We were in contact with each other, often daily, and I appreciate so many aspects of that interaction. John continues to teach me grammar and style, and Craig has a way of seeing through problems with humor and clarity. John and Craig, you have truly enriched my life.

Producing a textbook is more than writing – to reach you, the reader, it needs to be assembled, printed and distributed. My appreciation for making this possible goes to:

Brian Decker, who enthusiastically supported the notion of a textbook dedicated to the specialty of endodontics; Tricia Bindner, who served as production manager and who prodded when necessary and was always available for help and advice; and the support staff at BC Decker. Thank you all.

Looking back at the past several months of intense effort and the setting aside of other activities, it is clear to me that one person in my life made it possible, namely my wife Grete. Understanding when pressures mounted, re-assuring when doubts occurred, Grete unfailingly supported my efforts. Without her selfless partnership, my work could not have been completed on time. From my heart, thank you Grete.

Leif K. Bakland

I want to acknowledge and thank my dear wife Teddi, for her loving support of my academic endeavors. In addition, I especially want to thank John Ingle for the honor of being asked to participate in the editing of the 6th edition of *Ingle's Endodontics*. Also thanks to our co-editor, Leif Bakland, for his enthusiastic encouragement on virtually a daily basis during the long process of editing a text of this enormity. And finally a hearty thanks to all the contributors for their expertise and the tireless effort required to make this text the very best it can be.

J. Craig Baumgartner

Figure Acknowledgements

▼ Chapter 1

Figure 2:	Ingle JI, PDQ Endodontics 2005, Figure 5-4
Figure 15:	Ingle JI, Bakland L, Endodontics 5th ed.2002, Fig 1-6
Figure 16:	Ingle JI, Bakland L, Endodontics 5th ed.2002, Fig 1-7
Figure 18:	Ingle JI, Bakland L, Endodontics 5th ed.2002, Fig 1-9
Figure 19:	Ingle JI, Bakland L, Endodontics 5th ed.2002, Fig 1-10
Figure 20:	Ingle JI, Bakland L, Endodontics 5th ed.2002, Fig 1-11
Figure 23	Ingle JI, PDQ Endodontics 2005, Figure 7-38
Figure 24	Ingle JI, Bakland L, Endodontics 5th ed.2002, Fig 1-15
Figure 25:	Ingle JI, Bakland L, Endodontics 5th ed.2002, Fig 1-16
Figure 26:	Ingle JI, Bakland L, Endodontics 5th ed.2002, Fig 1-17
Figure 28	Ingle JI, PDQ Endodontics 2005, Figure 11-6

▼ Chapter 11

Figure 3:	Modified from Ingle-Bakland, Endodontics; 2002
Figure 8:	Modified from Ingle-Bakland, Endodontics; 2002
Figure 21:	Modified from Ingle-Bakland, Endodontics; 2002

▼ Chapter 22

Figure 3:	Ingle JI, PDQ Endodontics 2005, Figure 3-4

▼ Chapter 26C

Figure 2:	Ingle JI, Bakland L, Endodontics 5th ed.2002, p476
Figure 3:	Ingle JI, Bakland L, Endodontics 5th ed.2002, p477
Figure 4:	Ingle JI, Bakland L, Endodontics 5th ed.2002, p 479
Figure 5:	Ingle JI, Bakland L, Endodontics 5th ed.2002, p 480

▼ Chapter 38

Figure 2:	Ingle JI, PDQ Endodontics 2005, Figure 11-3 A,B
Figure 3:	Ingle JI, PDQ Endodontics 2005, Figure 11-3 C
Figure 5:	Ingle JI, PDQ Endodontics 2005, Figure 11-5
Figure 9:	Ingle JI, PDQ Endodontics 2005, Figure 11-8

Contents

Preface to First Edition vii
Preface to Sixth Edition ix

▼ THE DISCIPLINE OF ENDODONTICS

1 Modern Endodontic Therapy; Past, Present and Future
   John I. Ingle, Harold C. Slavkin 1

2 History of Endodontics
   James L. Gutmann 36

3 Ethics, Morals, the Law and Endodontics
   Bruce H. Seidberg 86

4 Effects of Dental Implants on Treatment Planning for Prosthodontics, Periodontics and Endodontics
   Mahmoud Torabinejad 105

▼ PATHOBIOLOGY

5 Structure and Function of the Dentin-Pulp Complex
   Syngcuk Kim, Karin J. Heyeraas, Sivakami R. Haug 118

6 Morphology of Teeth and Their Root Canal Systems
   Blaine M. Cleghorn, Charles J. Goodacre, William H. Christie 151

7 Microbiology of Endodontic Disease
   J. Craig Baumgartner, José F. Siqueira Jr., Christine M. Sedgley, Anil Kishen 221

8 Non-Microbial Endodontic Disease
   P.N. R. Nair 309

9 Inflammation and Immunological Responses
   Ashraf F. Fouad, George T.-J. Huang 343

10 Mechanisms of Odontogenic and Non-Odontogenic Pain
   Jennifer L. Gibbs, Kenneth M. Hargreaves 376

11 Non-Odontogenic Toothache and Chronic Head and Neck Pain
   Bernadette Jaeger, Marcela Romero Reyes 392

12 Pulpal Pathosis
   G. R. Holland, Stephen B. Davis 468

13 Periapical Lesions of Endodontic Origin
   Zvi Metzger, Itzhak Abramovitz 494

▼ EXAMINATION, EVALUATION, DIAGNOSIS, AND TREATMENT PLANNING

14 Diagnosis of Endodontic Disease
- A Endodontic Examination
  Robert A. Handysides, David E. Jaramillo, John I. Ingle 520
- B Diagnostic Testing
  James C. Kulild 532
- C Laser Doppler Flowmetry
  Asgeir Sigurdsson 547

15 Diagnostic Imaging
- A Endodontic Radiography
  Richard E. Walton 554
- B Digital Imaging for Endodontics
  Allan G. Farman, Ramya Ramamurthy, Lars G. Hollender 573
- C Ultrasonic Imaging
  Elisabetta Cotti 590

16 Radiographic Interpretation
Dag Ørstavik, Tore Arne Larheim 600

17 Rhinosinusitis and Endodontic Disease
Roderick W. Tataryn 626

18 Endodontic-Periodontal Interrelationships
Ilan Rotstein, James H.S. Simon 638

19 Tooth Infractions
Leif K. Bakland 660

20 Vertical Root Fractures of Endodontically Treated Teeth
Aviad Tamse 676

▼ MANAGEMENT

21 Treatment of Endodontic Infections, Cysts, and Flare-Ups
J. Craig Baumgartner, Paul A. Rosenberg, Michael M. Hoen, Louis M. Lin 690

22 Pharmacologic Management of Endodontic Pain
Kenneth M. Hargreaves, Al Reader, John M. Nusstein, J. Gordon Marshall, Jennifer L. Gibbs 713

23 Anxiety and Fear in the Endodontic Patient
Stanley F. Malamed 737

24 The Medically Complex Endodontic Patient
Bradford R. Johnson, Dena J. Fischer, Joel B. Epstein 749

25 Drug Interactions and Laboratory Tests
Paul D. Eleazer 780

26		**Endodontics Instruments and Armamentarium**	
	A	Dental Dam and Its Application William G. Schindler	791
	B	Introduction of Nickel-Titanium Alloy to Endodontics William A. Brantley	800
	C	Instruments for Cleaning and Shaping Timothy A. Svec	813
	D	Electronic Apex Locators Adam Lloyd, John I. Ingle	848
	E	Lasers in Endodontics Adam Stabholz, Joshua Moshonov, Sharonit Sahar-Helft, Jean-Paul Rocca	857
	F	Visual Enhancement James K. Bahcall	870
27		**Preparation of Coronal and Radicular Spaces** Ove A. Peters, Ravi S. Koka	877
28		**Irrigants and Intracanal Medicaments** Markus Haapasalo, Wei Qian	992
29		**Root Canal Filling Materials** James David Johnson	1019
30		**Obturation of the Radicular Space** Fred W. Benenati	1053
31		**Retreatment of Non-Healing Endodontic Therapy and Management of Mishaps** Alan H. Gluskin, Christine I. Peters, Ralan Dai Ming Wong, Clifford J. Ruddle	1088
32		**Treatment Outcome: The Potential for Healing and Retained Function** Shimon Friedman	1162

▼ **SURGICAL PROCEDURES IN ENDODONTICS**

33	**Endodontic Surgery** Gerald N. Glickman, Gary R. Hartwell	1233
34	**Osseointegrated Dental Implants** Jaime L. Lozada, Alejandro Kleinman	1295

▼ **RELATED ENDODONTIC TREATMENT**

35	**Vital Pulp Therapy** George Bogen, Nicholas P. Chandler	1310
36	**Endodontic Considerations in Dental Trauma** Martin Trope	1330
37	**Pathologic Tooth Resorption** Jens Ove Andreasen, Leif K. Bakland	1358

38	**Tooth Discoloration and Bleaching** Ilan Rotstein, Yiming Li	1383
39	**Endodontic Therapy for Primary Teeth** J. Todd Milledge	1400
40	**Restoration of Endodontically Treated Teeth** Charles J. Goodacre, Nadim Z. Baba	1431
41	**Operations Management in Endodontic Practice** Martin D. Levin	1474
Index		1513

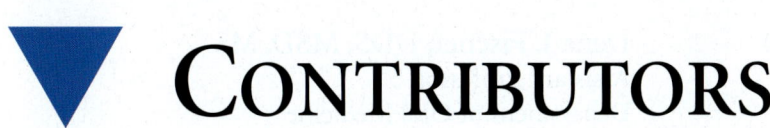

CONTRIBUTORS

Itzhak Abramovitz, DMD
Department of Endodontics
Hadassah School of Dental Medicine
Hebrew University
Jerusalem, Israel

Jens Ove Andreasen, DDS, Odont. Dr.
Associate Professor
Department of Oral and Maxillofacial Surgery
University Hospital
Copenhagen, Denmark

Nadim Z. Baba, DMD, MSD
Associate Professor
Department of Restorative Dentistry
Loma Linda University
Loma Linda, California

James K. Bahcall, DMD, MS
Associate Professor and Chairman
Department of Surgical Sciences and
Director of the Postgraduate Program in Endodontics
Marquette University School of Dentistry
Milwaukee, Wisconsin

Leif K. Bakland, DDS
Professor and Chair
Department of Endodontics
School of Dentistry
Loma Linda University
Loma Linda, California

J. Craig Baumgartner, MS, DDS, PhD
Professor and Chairman
Department of Endodontology
Oregon Health & Sciences University
Portland, Oregon

Fred W. Benenati, DDS, MEd
Clinical Professor Emeritus
Department of Endodontics
University of Oklahoma
College of Dentistry
Oklahoma City, Oklahoma

George Bogen, DDS
Private Practice in Endodontics
Los Angeles, California

William A. Brantley, MS, PhD
Professor and Director of Graduate Program
in Dental Materials Science
College of Dentistry
The Ohio State University
Columbus, Ohio

L. Stephen Buchanan, DDS, FICD, FACD
Private Practice Limited to Endodontics and
    Implant Surgery
Santa Barbara, California
Assistant Clinical Professor
University of Southern California and
UCLA School of Dentistry
Los Angeles, California

**Nicholas P. Chandler, BDS, MSc, PhD,
    LDSRCS(Eng), FDSRCPS(Glas),
    FDSRCS(Ed), FFDRCSI**
Associate Professor
Department of Oral Rehabilitation
School of Dentistry
University of Otago
Dunedin, New Zealand

William H. Christie, DMD, MS, FRCD (C)
Professor, Division Head
Endodontology
University of Manitoba
Winnipeg, Manitoba, Canada

Blaine M. Cleghorn, DMD, MSc
Associate Professor
Director, Clinical Affairs
Dalhousie University
Halifax, Nova Scotia, Canada

Elisabetta Cotti, DDS, MS
Professor and Chair
Department of Conservative Dentistry and
 Endodontics
University of Cagliari
Cagliari, Italy

Stephen B. Davis, DDS
Director, Endodontic Residency Program
Veteran Affairs Long Beach Healthcare System
Long Beach, California

Paul D. Eleazer, DDS, MS
Chair, Professor
Department of Endodontics and Pulp Biology
University of Alabama at Birmingham
Birmingham, Alabama

Joel B. Epstein, DMD, MSD, FRCD(C)
Professor and Head
Department of Oral Medicine and Diagnostic Sciences
College of Dentistry
University of Illinois at Chicago
Chicago, Illinois

**Allan G. Farman, BDS, LDSRCS, PhD, EdS,
 MBA, DSc**
Professor of Radiology and Imaging Science
Department of Surgical and Hospital Dentistry
The University of Louisville
School of Dentistry
Louisville, Kentucky

Dena J. Fischer, DDS, MSD, MS
Assistant Professor
Department of Oral Medicine
College of Dentistry
University of Illinois at Chicago
Chicago, Illinois

Ashraf F. Fouad, BDS, DDS, MS
Associate Professor and Chairman
Department of Endodontics, Prosthodontics
and Operative Dentistry
Baltimore College of Dentistry
University of Maryland
Baltimore, Maryland

Shimon Friedman, DMD
Professor, Head, Discipline of Endodontics
Director, MSc Endodontics Program
Faculty of Dentistry
University of Toronto
Toronto, Ontario, Canada

Jennifer L. Gibbs, DDS, PhD
Endodontic Resident / Post Doctoral Fellow
University of California at San Francisco
San Francisco, California

Gerald N. Glickman, DDS, MS, MBA, JD
Professor and Chair
Department of Endodontics
Director of Graduate Endodontics
Texas A & M Health Science Center
Baylor College of Dentistry
Dallas, Texas

Alan H. Gluskin, DDS
Professor and Chair
Department of Endodontics
Arthur A. Dugoni School of Dentistry
University of the Pacific
San Francisco, California

Charles J. Goodacre, DDS, MSD
Dean and Professor of Prosthodontics
Department of Restorative Dentistry
Loma Linda University School of Dentistry
Loma Linda, California

Contributors

James L. Gutmann, DDS, PhD (hc), FICD, FACD, FADI
Honorary Professor
Wuhan University
Wuhan, China

Markus Haapasalo, Dr Odont (PhD)
Professor, Head of Division of Endodontics
Acting Head of the Department of Oral
Biological and Medical Sciences
Faculty of Dentistry
University of British Columbia
Vancouver, British Columbia, Canada

Robert A. Handysides, DDS
Assistant Professor
Department of Endodontics
School of Dentistry
Loma Linda University
Loma Linda, California

Kenneth M. Hargreaves, DDS, PhD
Professor and Chair
Department of Endodontics
President's Council Endowed Chair in Research
University of Texas at San Antonio
San Antonio, Texas

Gary R. Hartwell, DDS, MS
Professor and Chair
Department of Endodontics
University of Medicine and Dentistry of New Jersey
New Jersey Dental School
Newark, New Jersey

Sivakami R. Haug, BDS, Dr. Odont
Post-doctorate, Department of Biomedicine
Section for Physiology, Faculty of Medicine
University of Bergen
Bergen, Norway

Karin J. Heyeraas, Dr. Odont
Professor of Physiology
Department of Biomedicine
Section for Physiology, Faculty of Medicine
University of Bergen
Bergen, Norway

Michael M. Hoen, DDS
Associate Professor
Department of Endodontics
Director of Graduate Endodontics
University of Detroit
Mercy School of Dentistry
Detroit, Michigan

G. R. Holland, BSC (Hons), BDS (Hons), PhD
Professor
Department of Cariology, Restorative Sciences and Endodontics
School of Dentistry
Professor
Department of Cell and Development Biology
Faculty of Medicine
University of Michigan
Ann Arbor, Michigan

Lars G. Hollender, DDS, PhD
Professor Emeritus
Department of Oral Medicine
School of Dentistry
University of Washington
Seattle, Washington

George T.-J. Huang, DDS, MSD, DSc
Associate Professor
Department of Endodontics
Baltimore College of Dentistry
University of Maryland
Baltimore, Maryland

John I. Ingle, DDS, MSD
Lecturer
Loma Linda University
School of Dentistry
Loma Linda, California

Bernadette Jaeger, DDS
Associate Professor of Oral Medicine and Orofacial Pain
University of Southern California
School of Dentistry
Los Angeles, California

David E. Jaramillo, DDS
Assistant Professor
Department of Endodontics
School of Dentistry
Loma Linda University
Loma Linda, California

Bradford R. Johnson, DDS, MHPE
Associate Professor and Director of
Postdoctoral Endodontics
Department of Endodontics
School of Dentistry
University of Illinois at Chicago
Chicago, Illinois

James David Johnson, DDS, MS
Chair and Clinical Associate Professor
Program Director, Advanced Education
Program in Endodontics
Department of Endodontics
School of Dentistry
University of Washington
Seattle, Washington

Wm. Ben Johnson, DDS
Associate Clinical Professor
Nova Southeastern University
Ft. Lauderdale, Florida
Louisiana State University
New Orleans, Louisiana
Baylor College of Dentistry
Dallas, Texas

Syngcuk Kim, DDS, MPh, PhD
Louis I. Grossman Professor and Chair
Department of Endodontics
School of Dental Medicine
University of Pennsylvania
Philadelphia, Pennsylvania

Anil Kishen, BDS, MDS, PhD
Assistant Professor
Department of Restorative Dentistry
National University of Singapore
Singapore, Republic of Singapore

Alejandro Kleinman, DDS
Associate Professor
Restorative Department
Coordinator, Internship Program in Implant Dentistry
School of Dentistry
Loma Linda University
Loma Linda, California

Ravi S. Koka, DDS, MS
Assistant Professor
Arthur A. Dugoni School of Dentistry
University of the Pacific
San Francisco, California

James C. Kulild, DDS, MS
Professor and Director
Advanced Specialty Education Program
in Endodontics
UMKC School of Dentistry
Kansas City, Missouri

Tore Arne Larheim, DDS, PhD
Professor
Institute of Clinical Dentistry
Faculty of Dentistry
University of Oslo
Oslo, Norway

Martin D. Levin, DMD
Adjunct Assistant Professor, Postgraduate Endodontics
College of Dental Medicine
Nova Southeastern University
Fort Lauderdale, Florida

Yiming Li, DDS, MSD, PhD
Professor and Director
Center for Dental Research
School of Dentistry
Loma Linda University
Loma Linda, California

Louis M. Lin, BDS, DMD, PhD
Professor and Director
Advanced Education Program in Endodontics
College of Dentistry
New York University
New York, New York

Contributors

Adam Lloyd, BDS, MS
Assistant Professor
Department of Endodontics
Nova Southeastern University
Fort Lauderdale, Florida

Jaime L. Lozada, DDS
Professor and Director
Graduate Program in Implant Dentistry
School of Dentistry
Loma Linda University
Loma Linda, California

Stanley F. Malamed, DDS
Professor of Anesthesia & Medicine
School of Dentistry
University of Southern California
Los Angeles, California

J. Gordon Marshall, DMD
Associate Professor
Department of Endodontology
OHSU School of Dentistry
Portland, Oregon

Zvi Metzger, DMD
Director of Research Laboratories
The Goldschleger School of Dental Medicine
Tel-Aviv University
Tel-Aviv, Israel

J. Todd Milledge, DDS
Clinical Associate Professor of Pediatric Dentistry
School of Dentistry
Loma Linda University
Loma Linda, California

Joshua Moshonov, DMD
Clinical Associate Professor, Acting Chair
Department of Endodontics
Hadassah School of Dental Medicine
Hebrew University
Jerusalem, Israel

P.N.R. Nair, BVSc, DVM, PhD (hc)
Senior Scientist
Institute of Oral Biology
Centre of Dental & Oral Medicine
University of Zurich
Zurich, Switzerland

John M. Nusstein, DDS, MS
Associate Professor
Section Head of Endodontics
Director, Graduate Endodontic Clinic
College of Dentistry
The Ohio State University
Columbus, Ohio

Dag Ørstavik, Cand Odont, Dr Odont
Professor and Head
Department of Endodontics
Institute of Clinical Dentistry
Faculty of Dentistry
University of Oslo
Oslo, Norway

Christine I. Peters, Dr Med Dent
Assistant Professor
Department of Endodontics
Arthur A. Dugoni School of Dentistry
University of the Pacific
San Francisco, California

Ove A. Peters, DMD, MS, PhD
Professor of Endodontics
Arthur A. Dugoni School of Dentistry
University of the Pacific
San Francisco, California

Wei Qian, DMD, PhD
Research Associate
Department of Oral Biological and
Medical Sciences
Faculty of Dentistry
University of British Columbia
Vancouver, British Columbia

Ramya Ramamurthy, BDS, MS
Fourth Year International DDS Student
University of California
San Francisco, California

Al Reader, DDS, MS
Professor and Program Director of Endodontics
College of Dentistry
The Ohio State University
Columbus, Ohio

Jean-Paul Rocca, DDS, PhD
Professor and Head
Clinical Research Unit
Dental Faculty
University of Nice
Nice, France

Marcela Romero Reyes, DDS, PhD
Lecturer, Section of Orofacial Pain and Medicine
University of California at Los Angeles
School of Dentistry
Post Doctoral Fellow
Department of Neurology
Headache Research and Treatment Program
University of California at Los Angeles
School of Medicine
Los Angeles, California

Paul A. Rosenberg, DDS
Professor and Chair, Ignatius N. Sally Quartaro
Department of Endodontics
College of Dentistry
New York University
New York, New York

Ilan Rotstein, DDS
Chair, Surgical Therapeutic and Bioengineering Sciences
Associate Dean, Continuing Oral Health Professional Education
University of Southern California
School of Dentistry
Los Angeles, California

Clifford J. Ruddle, DDS, FACD, FICD
Assistant Professor of Endodontics
School of Dentistry
Loma Linda University
Loma Linda, California
Associate Clinical Professor
School of Dentistry
University of California Los Angeles and
University of California San Francisco

Sharonit Sahar-Helft, DMD
Clinical Instructor
Department of Endodontics
Hebrew University
Hadassah School of Dental Medicine
Jerusalem, Israel

William G. Schindler, DDS, MS
Clinical Professor
Department of Endodontics
University of Texas Health Science Center
San Antonio, Texas

Christine M. Sedgley, BDS, MDSc, MDS, FRACDS, PhD
Assistant Professor
Cariology, Restorative Sciences & Endodontics
School of Dentistry
University of Michigan
Ann Arbor, Michigan

Bruce H. Seidberg, DDS, MScD, JD, DABE, FCLM, FACD, FAAHD, FPFA
Chief of Dentistry
Crouse Hospital
Senior Attending Endodontist
St. Joseph's Hospital
Syracuse, New York

E. Steve Senia
Former Director, Postdoctoral Endodontics
University of Texas at San Antonio
San Antonio, Texas

Contributors

Asgeir Sigurdsson, Cand Odont, MS
Adjunct Associate Professor
Department of Endodontics
University of North Carolina
School of Dentistry
Chapel Hill, North Carolina

James H. S. Simon, DDS
Director
Advanced Education Program in Endodontics and
Wayne G. and Margaret L. Bemis Endowed Professor
of Endodontics
School of Dentistry
University of Southern California
Los Angeles, California

José F. Siqueira Jr, DDS, MSc, PhD
Chairman and Professor
Department of Endodontics
Estácio de Sá University
Rio de Janeiro, RJ, Brazil

Harold C. Slavkin, BS, DDS
Dean and G. Donald and Marian James Montgomery
Professor of Dentistry
School of Dentistry
University of Southern California
Los Angeles, California

Adam Stabholz, DMD
Dean and Chairman
Department of Endodontics
Hadassah School of Dental Medicine
Hebrew University
Jerusalem, Israel

Timothy A. Svec, DDS, MS
Associate Professor and Director
Advanced Education Program in Endodontics
University of Texas Dental Branch
Houston, Texas

Aviad Tamse, DMD
Professor and Chair
Director of Graduate Endodontic Program
Department of Endodontology
Goldchlager School of Dental Medicine
Tel-Aviv University
Tel-Aviv, Israel

Roderick W. Tataryn, DDS, MS
Private Practice, Endodontics
Spokane, Washington

Mahmoud Torabinejad, DMD, MDS, PhD
Professor of Endodontics, Director of the Advanced
 Education Program in Endodontics
School of Dentistry
Loma Linda University
Loma Linda, California

Martin Trope, DMD
Professor and Chair
Department of Endodontics
School of Dentistry
University of North Carolina
Chapel Hill, North Carolina

Richard E. Walton, DMD, MS
Professor of Endodontics
College of Dentistry
University of Iowa
Iowa City, Iowa

Ralan Dai Ming Wong, DDS, MS
Associate Professor
Department of Endodontics
Arthur A. Dugoni School of Dentistry
University of the Pacific
San Francisco, California

# THE DISCIPLINE OF ENDODONTICS

CHAPTER 1

MODERN ENDODONTIC THERAPY: PAST, PRESENT AND FUTURE

JOHN I. INGLE, HAROLD C. SLAVKIN

Because I'll have you know, Sancho, that a mouth without teeth is like a mill without its stone and you must value a tooth more than a diamond.

Miguel de Cervantes, Don Quixote

"Through shifting times there passed—those little bands of struggling beings who someday would be men. They survived through plasticity,—through a growing capacity to recognize, in changing times, that today is different than yesterday, and tomorrow from today. Many—most without doubt—were conservative creatures. These died by dry, unanticipated stream beds, or numbed and froze in unanticipated storms. Those, quite obviously, were not your ancestors. It was the others—the witty, sensitive, the flexible, the ones who could recognize a changing environment—these were the ones to assemble a new and most remarkable genetic package: Ourselves."

Robert Ardrey, The Territorial Imperative

Change

It was Benjamin Franklin (not Mark Twain) who said, "The only two certainties in life are death and taxes." Change has been the one constant of history. The challenge is not to avoid change, but to manage it. But change can be "for better or for worse."

Fortunately, or unfortunately, we have experienced both in endodontics. The disappointment in root canal filling materials such as silver points, numerous intracanal disinfectants, and several sealers is an example of the failures we have endured. The move from film to digital radiographs, more profound local anesthetics, standardization of endodontic instruments, and new instrument alloys with novel geometric designs are only a few of the advances over the years. There are now many exciting developments to improve the quality and the output of our endeavors; some of them will be "winners" and some will be losers. Time and experimentation will determine which is which.

In Chapter 2, Dr. James Gutmann presents an historical chronicle of endodontics, so there is no need to repeat it here. But it might be interesting (as well as educational) to follow through on two early changes in endodontics that still affect us today—nomenclature and instrument design and standardization.

NOMENCLATURE

During World War II, Dr. Balint Orban was asked by the federal government to solve the problem of high altitude toothache being suffered by a number of Army Air Corps Pilots. This experience renewed his interest in pulp pathology. Dr. Orban, a famous physician, psychiatrist, dentist, periodontist, author and a superb histopathologist, was then asked to modernize endodontic nomenclature, which he did.[1]

He first tackled the pulpal conditions and defined the various stages of pulpitis, wisely basing a classification on the symptoms of pulpalgia facing any dentist diagnosing painful toothache. He matched these symptoms with what he knew was happening pathologically in the pulp. They ranged from *reversible* incipient pulpalgia, through *irreversible* advanced pulpalgia with its excruciating pain, to the painless *necrosis* of the pulp. "Reversible" pulps can be saved, but most really painful pulps are inflamed and/or infected beyond redemption.

Before this time we spoke of "hyperemia of the pulp" with no proof that hyperemia occurred. It was not until 1965 that Beveridge and Brown[2] followed by Van Hassel[3] demonstrated changes in intrapulpal pressures that were related to a number of clinical variables, including inflammation.

Orban also changed the nomenclature for *periapical* disease, basing it on his classification of *periodontitis* for periodontal disease. "Inflammation of the periodontium anywhere is periodontitis" he would say. "It's **apical periodontitis** at the apex of the tooth – just as it is **marginal periodontitis** at the alveolar crest".[4] Before Orban, we spoke of pyorrhea and trench mouth or Vincent's disease.

So changes in nomenclature, informed by critical observation, helped to form a background for an avalanche of research efforts that placed endodontics on a much more scientific footing.

INSTRUMENT DESIGN AND STANDARDIZATION

Until 1957, most endodontic instruments came in 6 sizes – 1 through 6. There were *files* that were to be used in a push–pull rasping motion and **reamers** that were to be used in a rotary motion. There was no standardization within a size or between sizes, or among manufacturers. The design of most files and reamers was based on the original design developed by Kerr Co. in 1904, more than a half century before (Figure 1). Hence, the designation K files and K reamers. The only variation was the Swedish Hedström file shaped like a wood screw. And of course, there was also the ubiquitous broach that came in small, medium, and large sizes. Change was called for!

In 1957, a plea went out to the profession and the manufacturers to standardize endodontic instruments.[5] It was answered by a Swiss company, and a study was undertaken to develop a standard that all manufacturers would adhere to and that would be accepted by the profession.

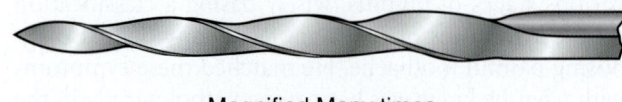

Magnified Many times.
Note the triple cutting edge

Figure 1 The original Kerr reamer, ca. 1904 (titled a broach at that time), is the origin of today's K-style instruments. Reproduced with permission from Kerr Dental Manufacturing Co. 1904 catalog.

In 1958, a proposal was introduced to standardize the taper of instruments as well as the length. In addition, based on the metric system, a formula for a graduated increment in size from one instrument to the next was developed.[6,7] The new numbering system allowed for numbers from 10 to 100 based on the tip diameter, #10 for a tip size of 0.1 mm to #100 for a tip size of 1.0 mm. The cutting blades were to extend up the shaft for 16 mm and the advance in taper was to be a gain of 0.3 mm, which figured out to be an increase of 0.01875 mm/mm (Figure 2). This figure soon became clumsy for manufacturing and was changed to 0.02 mm/mm. Hence these new standardized instruments came to be known as 0.02 instruments.

At first, most companies were unwilling to junk all their overage machines that produced instruments, while one Swiss company that backed the change began to capture the market. When the newly designed instruments were designated as the "International Standard" by the International Standards Organization, all the companies, worldwide, changed their manufacture to the new standard that remains the standard today.[8]

For a number of years there was not much movement in instrument design. And then it blossomed! Today there is a plethora of design changes as well as

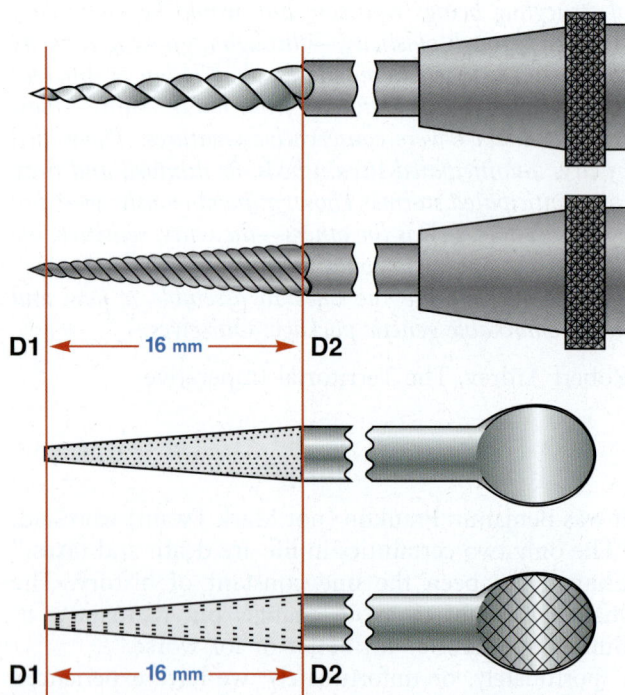

Figure 2 Original recommendation for standardized instruments. The number of the instrument is determined by the diameter size at D1 in hundredths of millimeters. Diameter 2 (D2) is uniformly 0.32 mm greater than D1, a gain of 0.02 mm/1 mm of cutting blades.

size changes. The standard .02 taper instrument has now been joined by .04, .06, .08, even up to .12 mm/mm tapers. The original K style instruments have been joined by a colony of other designs; a few proved impractical and have disappeared from the market. Carbon steel gave way to stainless steel that is now being challenged by nickel/titanium, with probably more to come.

"Finger-powered" instruments, although they still have their place, are slowly being overtaken by electric-powered rotary instruments. According to an anonymous industry representative, in 1996 less than 1 million nickel–titanium (NiTi) rotary instruments were sold in the United States, compared to 20 million stainless steel instruments. In 8 years, by 2004, sales of NiTi rotary files had jumped from 1 million to 11.4 million, and by 2006 to 13.4 million. At the same time, 2004 and 2006, sales of stainless instruments reached a plateau of 23.5 and 24 million, respectively. With these two examples of **change** that has taken place in endodontics, it is obvious that there will be more in the future.

PRESENT STANDING OF ENDODONTICS

Speaking of change, what has been the impact on endodontics from the present rush toward implants? At a time when successful outcome in endodontics has vastly improved, when the stigma of painful root canal therapy is disappearing, when treatment time has been shortened, and when endodontic fees compare so favorably to implant and prosthetic fees, one wonders why this move toward implants. Conversations among endodontists often include comments about situations in which patients have been advised by general dentists or specialists, in for example, periodontics, that a tooth an endodontist might consider suitable for treatment should instead be replaced with an implant.

This has become a disturbing trend and the specialty of endodontics faces a challenge to educate both colleagues in dentistry and patients about the demonstrated benefits in maintaining the natural teeth. In Chapter 4, Dr. Mahmoud Torabinejad addresses this controversy that highlights the importance of involvement by the endodontic community. Such involvement also includes incorporating the area of implant dentistry into the scope of practice for endodontists. In Chapter 33, Drs. Jaime Lozada and Alejandro Kleinman describe the procedures involved in replacing a tooth that cannot be retained (e.g., due to a vertical root fracture); many endodontists are beginning to incorporate implant dentistry in their practices. What then is the present standing of endodontics? With the profession? With the public? Let us look at some interesting facts.

DEFINITION OF ENDODONTICS

First, we had better define endodontics—what is endodontology or what encompasses the practice of endodontics? The best definition may be modified from the definition by the American Association of Endodontists.[9]

"Endodontics is that branch of dentistry that is concerned with the morphology, physiology and pathology of the human dental pulp and periradicular tissues. Its study and practice encompass the basic clinical sciences including biology of the normal pulp; the etiology, diagnosis, prevention and treatment of diseases and injuries of the pulp; and associated periradicular conditions.

The scope of endodontics includes, but is not limited to, the differential diagnosis and the treatment of oral pain of pulpal or periradicular origin; vital pulp therapy, such as pulp capping and pulpotomy; nonsurgical treatment of root canal systems with or without periradicular pathosis of pulpal origin and the obturation of these root canal systems; selective surgical removal of pathological tissues resulting from pulpal pathosis; repair procedures related to such surgical removal of pathological tissues; intentional replantation and replantation of avulsed teeth; surgical removal of tooth structure, such as root-end resection and root-end filling; hemisection, bicuspidization and root resection; endodontic implants; bleaching of discolored dentin and enamel; retreatment of teeth previously treated endodontically; and treatment procedures related to coronal restorations by means of post and/or cores involving the root canal space.

The endodontic specialist is responsible for the advancement of endodontic knowledge through research; the transmission of information concerning the most recent advances in biologically acceptable procedures and materials; and the education of the public as to the importance of endodontics in keeping the dentition in a physiologically functional state for the maintenance of oral and systemic health."

To this one might add: the diagnosis of extraoral referred pain; the management of traumatic injuries to the teeth; the biopsy of pathological tissue, and the growing recognition of pathological conditions between the maxillary posterior teeth and the maxillary sinus.

RECENT ATTITUDES TOWARD DENTISTRY AND ENDODONTIC THERAPY

Increasingly, the term "root canal" has become fashionable and generally known. In conversation, people proudly proclaim that they have had a "root canal." The stigmata of fear and pain are fast disappearing.

Another impressive factor in the acceptance of endodontics is television. Countless advertisements emphasize a beautiful smile—not just toothpaste advertisements, but commercials in every field, from Buicks to beer. At the same time, the constant barrage of denture adhesives and cleanser advertisements produces a chilling effect. The public sees the problems that develop from the loss of teeth. Obvious missing teeth are anathema.

There is no question that the public's acceptance of endodontic treatment is on the rise. In 1969, for example, the American Dental Association (ADA) estimated that 6 million teeth were treated endodontically each year. By 1990, the ADA reported 20,754,000 endodontic procedures, or 2.1% of all dental procedures. By 1999, they reported that total endodontic activity had increased to 21,932,800 procedures, but now accounted for only 1.7% of the total dental procedures that numbered 1 billion 250,000 procedures.[10,11]

This upward trend was also documented by the Public Affairs Committee of the AAE. Reporting on the surveys of the general public made by the Opinion Research Institute in 1984 and 1986, the Committee noted that 28% of 1,000 telephone respondents reported that they had had root canal therapy by 1986, an increase of 5% points over the 23% reported in 1984.[12] Also, in 1986, 62% said that they would choose root canal therapy over extraction, an increase of 10% points over the 52% in 1984. More than half the respondents (53%) believed that an endodontically treated tooth would last a lifetime.[12]

Twenty years later, in 2006, the AAE was reporting similar positive figures.[13] On the other hand, 63% of the respondents described root canal therapy as "painful." It turned out, however, that the respondents who had had root canal therapy were 6 times more likely to describe the procedure as "painless" than the cohort who had never had root canal treatment.[13] In other words, patients have been shown to anticipate more pain than they will actually experience during endodontic treatment.[14] Clearly, the profession has a mission to continue educating the public to reverse its image of endodontics and promote the value of an endodontically treated tooth.

The rate of the use of endodontic services similar to the rate in the United States (28%) was reported from Norway also, where 27% of an older age group (66–75 years) had had root canal therapy, as had 12% of a younger age group (26–35 years). Incidentally, 100% of the root-filled teeth in the younger group were still present 10–17 years later, a remarkable achievement.[15]

The growth in endodontic services is also reflected in the sales of endodontic equipments, supplies, and instruments. In 1984, according to an anonymous industry representative, endodontics was a $20 million market, growing at a rate of 4% per year.[16] By 1997, 13 years later, the endodontic market, through dental dealer retail stores alone, was $72 million, up from $65.6 million in 1996, a growth of nearly 10%. One must add to these sales another 10% to account for mail order/telephone sales, a grand total of nearly $80 million in 1997. Worldwide sales were probably double this figure![17] In the year 2005, it was revealed that total endodontic sales exceeded $200 million in the USA alone and $400 million worldwide.

Future of Endodontics as a Speciality

Every 4 years the American Dental Association Survey Center publishes a review of all aspects of dentistry including a report entitled "The Economics of Endodontics". In this report, the Survey Center covers endodontic services and utilization, growth of the specialty, location of endodontists, characteristics of endodontists, finances, referrals, and "A Look at the Future." The latest report was published in 2003 covering the years through 1999 with a few references in the years 2000 and 2001.[10] Portions of the report were published in the *Journal of Endodontics* in 2006.[11]

The report paints a rather pleasant picture of the present but voices some concerns about the distant future. Some concerns had not developed by 1999, such as the impact implants would have on the practice of endodontics. The report also predicted that the population of the United States would not reach 300 million until 2010 when in reality this figure was reached in October of 2006. On the whole, however, their concerns for the future bear review and attention.

One changing relationship arising is between the specialty and general practitioners. For instance, the ratio between general dentists and endodontists is dropping; in 1982, there were 50.3 possible referring general dentists to each endodontist. But by 2002, the

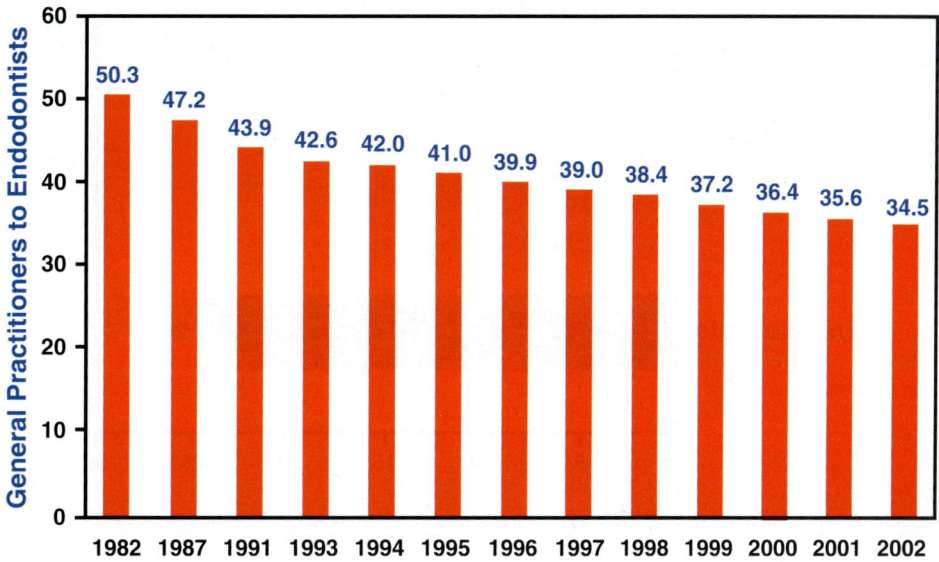

Figure 3 Ratio of general practitioners to endodontists, 1982–2002. Source: American Dental Association Survey Center, 1982–2002 Distribution of dentists in the United States by region and state.

ratio was down to 34.5 and falling (Figure 3). Although general dentists perform about 75% of all endodontic procedures, they still refer 25% to endodontists; whether this will change is open to speculation.

The number of endodontists has grown at a faster rate than any other dental specialty. Between 1982 and 2002 "the number of professionally active endodontists had increased by 85%." In contrast, "[g]eneral practitioners grew at a rate of 33% from 1982 to 2002."[10,11] In 1989, there were 2,500 endodontic specialists in the United States.[18] By the year 2003, the number had risen to 4258 practicing endodontists.[19] Between 1982 and 2003, the number of endodontists grew 107.9%, faster than any other specialty, well exceeding the rate of the growth of general practitioners (38.4%).[20] By November of 2006, according to the AAE, the specialty had grown to 4,859 endodontist members (personal communication, AAE).

There is no question that the greatest share of endodontic procedures is carried out by America's general practitioners (Table 1). On the other hand, the specialty of endodontics is growing as well. For example, only 5% of those patients who had had root canal therapy in 1986 were treated by a specialist.[12] By 1999, however, endodontists were providing 4.4 million procedures, which was 20.3% of the 21.9 million total endodontic procedures provided by all dentists, endodontists included (see Table 1).[10]

In 1999, there were over 1 billion dental services rendered. Only 1.7% of these procedures were endodontic. It is interesting to note, however, that while

Table 1 Distribution of Endodontic Procedures by Specialty, 1990 and 1999				
Type of Dentist	1990		1999	
General practitioners	15,758,100	76.1%	16,493,200	75.2%
Endodontists	3,860,700	18.6%	4,459,900	20.3%
Pediatric dentists	942,200	4.5%	721,300	3.3%
Oral and maxillofacial surgeons	108,800	0.5%	188,900	0.9%
Orthodontic and dentofacial Orthopedists	0	0.0%	0	0.0%
Periodontists	31,800	0.2%	50,700	0.2%
Prosthodontists	25,400	0.1%	18,800	0.1%
Total	20,754,000	100.0%	21,932,800	100.0%

Source: American Dental Association Survey Center, 1990 and 1999 Surveys of Dental Services Rendered.

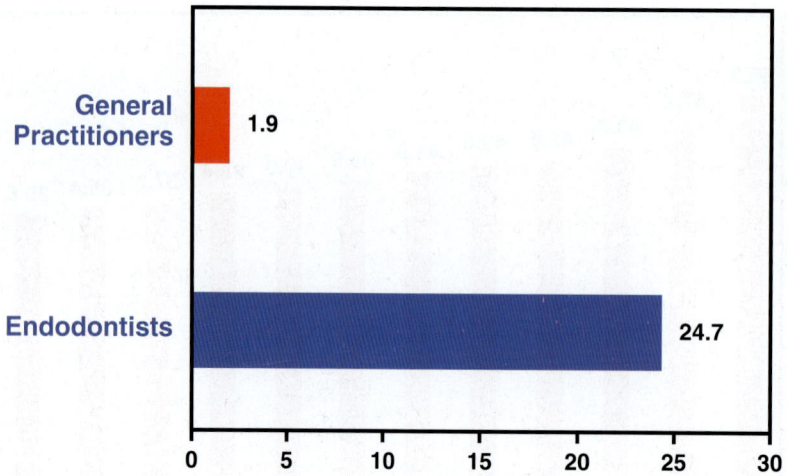

Figure 4 Total root canal treatments per week per dentist, 1999. Source: American Dental Association Survey Center. 1999 Survey of Dental Services Rendered.

<2% of the total services were endodontic, 15% of the total dental expenditures in 1999 went for endodontic treatment at a cost of 8.2 billion dollars.[10]

On a *per capita basis*, 6% of the total population received endodontic services in 1999. On the other hand, 9% of all dental patients received some form of endodontic treatment. In this same vein, general practitioners performed 16.5 million root canal procedures in 1999 compared to 4.5 million by endodontic specialists (see Table 1). However, endodontists performed 24.7 procedures a week compared to only 1.9 by general practitioners (Figure 4). The average number of endodontic procedures in 1999 by a general practitioner (94.6) versus each endodontic specialist (1263.3) is striking (Figure 5).[10]

It is interesting to note the differences in the type of procedures performed by specialists versus general dentists. Endodontists performed 61.9% of the molar root canal treatments and general practitioners did 29.6% of the molars—less than half. The remainder was probably done by oral surgeons. By the same token, general dentists did 20.1% of the anterior root canal procedures

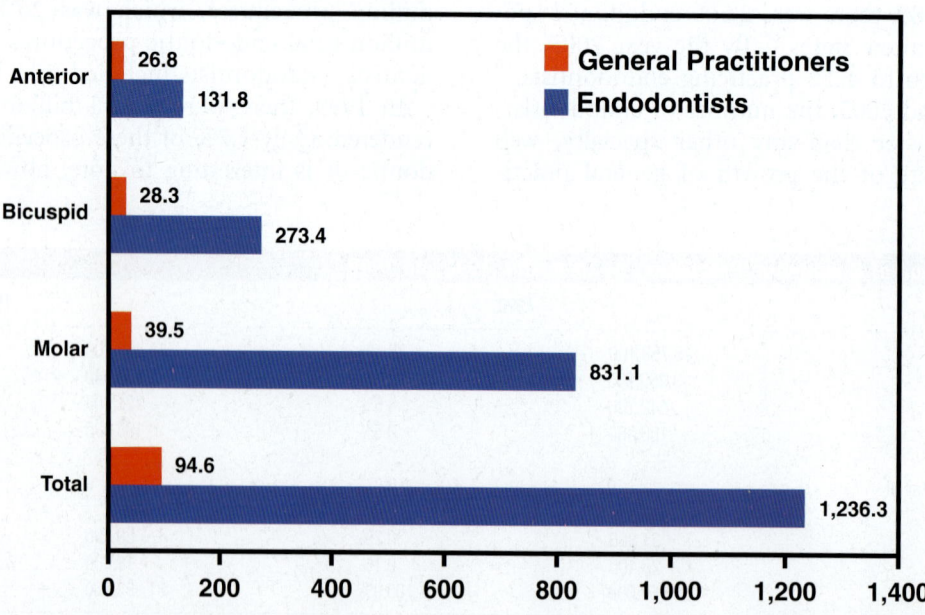

Figure 5 Root canal treatments per dentist, 1999. Source: American Dental Association, Survey Center. 1999 Survey of Dental Services Rendered.

Table 2 Endodontic Procedures Completed by General Practitioners and Endodontists, 1999

Endodontic Procedures	General Practitioners		Endodontists	
Molar root canals	4,887,500	29.6%	2,761,900	61.9%
Biscuspid root canals	3,501,600	21.2%	908,500	20.4%
Anterior root canals	3,317,600	20.1%	438,000	9.8%
Pulpotomy	1,802,800	10.9%	158,700	3.6%
Pulp cap	1,609,200	9.8%	16,400	0.4%
Bleaching	1,237,600	7.6%	23,900	0.5%
Apicoectomy	136,900	0.8%	152,500	3.4%
Root amputation	0	0.0%	0	0.0%
Total	16,493,200	100%	4,459,000	100%

Source: American Dental Association, Survey Center, 1990 and 1999 Surveys of Dental Services Rendered.

and 9.8% of the pulp cappings, whereas the specialists treated only half as many anterior teeth and performed only 0.4% of the pulp cappings (Table 2).[10,11] Molar endodontics fairly well defines the difference in endodontic treatment performed between general dentists and endodontists.

Another consideration by the ADA survey group concerned amalgam versus resin restorations being placed, particularly in the posterior teeth. They pointed out the age old record of amalgams protecting the pulp over long periods of time. In the year 2000, the jury was still out on the life span of posterior resins, so they were speculating on how failing resins in the future would impact the amount of endodontics to be done. They pointed out that amalgam restorations had declined from 100 million to 80 million between 1990 and 1999, a 20% decline, whereas resin restorations increased from 47.7 million in 1990 to 85.8 million in 1999, an 80% increase (Figure 6).[10]

Failing resins impacting an increase in endodontics may not be predictable at this time, whereas the age of patients in the future is predictable. Most root canal treatment is performed for patients between the ages of 25 and 64, particularly molar endodontics, done mostly by endodontists (Figure 7). Unfortunately, projected future change in the US population shows a severe drop off in the very age groups most prone to endodontic therapy (Figure 8). So this population shift may reduce the number of patients seeking endodontic services; at the same time the number of referring general dentists is decreasing.[10,11] It is possible that the aging population (<64) will provide an increasing pool of patients needing endodontic services.

The present good news is that in the years 1997–1998, endodontists enjoyed an average net income of $230,000, second only to oral surgeons, a surprising figure considering average gross

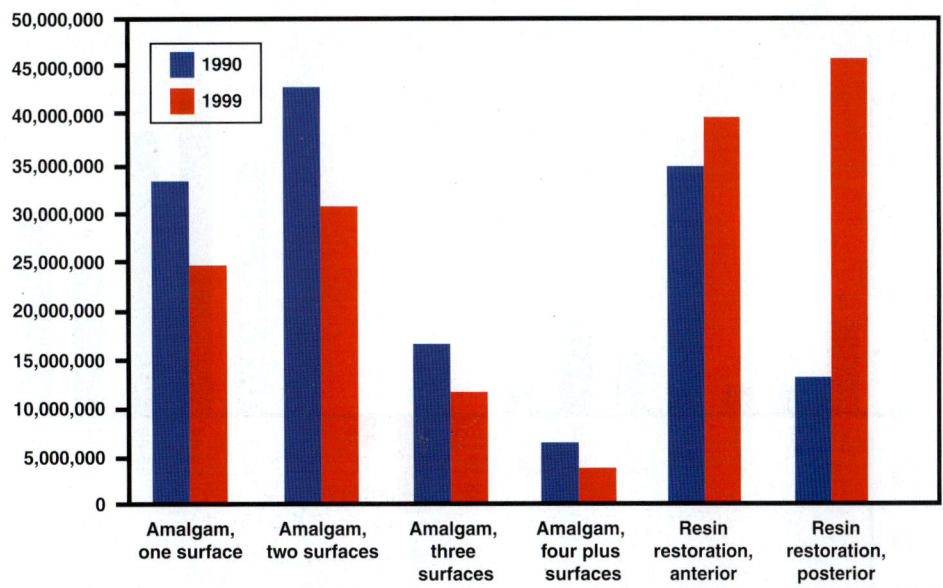

Figure 6 Number of amalgams and resins, 1990 (blue) and 1999 (red). Source: American Dental Association, Survey Center. 1990 and 1999 Surveys of Dental Services Rendered.

8 / Endodontics

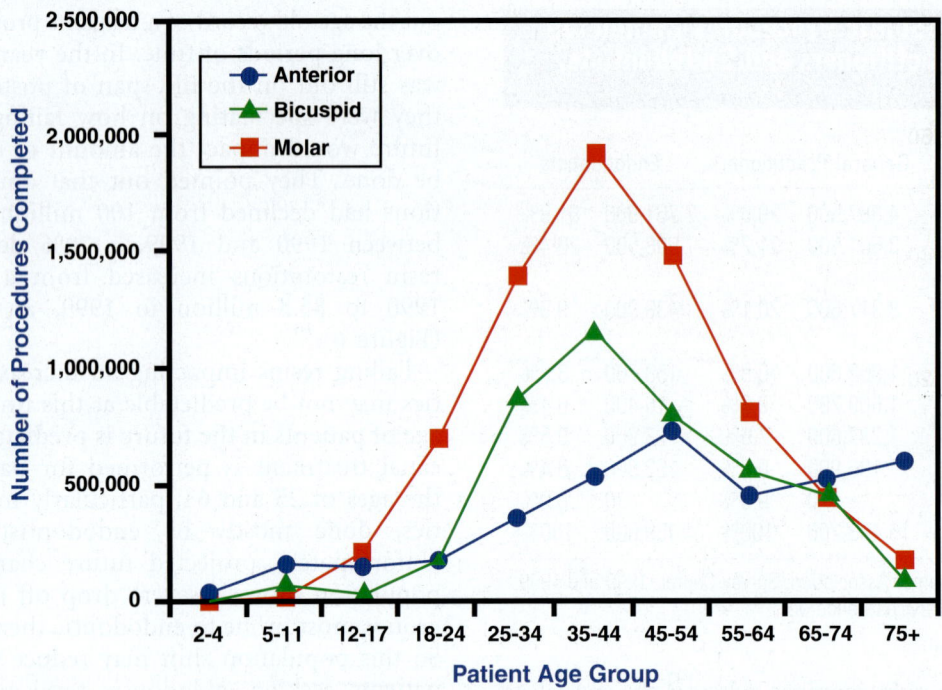

Figure 7 Root canal treatments by age. Source: American Dental Association, Survey Center. 1999 Survey of Dental Services Rendered.

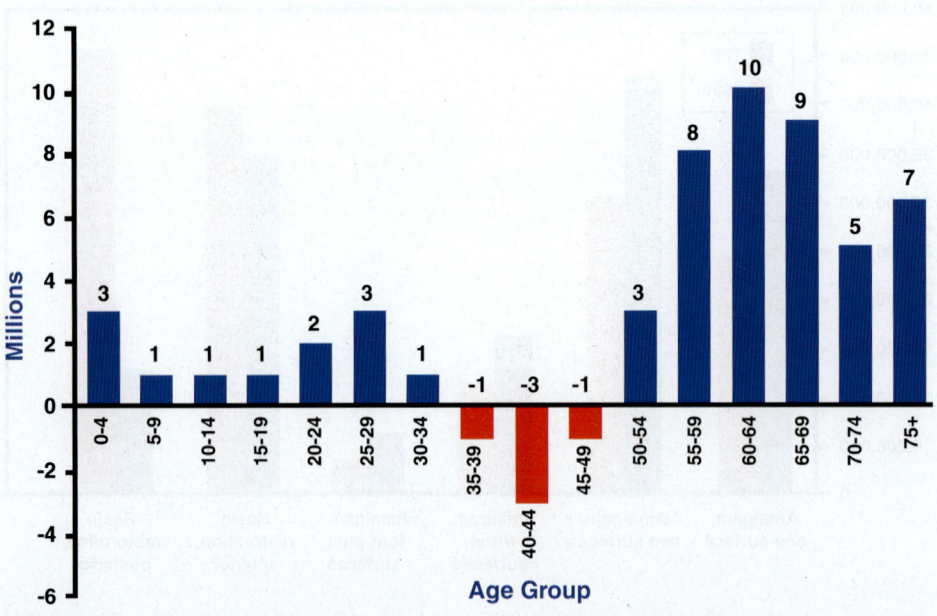

Figure 8 Projected change in the US population from 2000 to 2020. Source: American Dental Association, Survey Center.

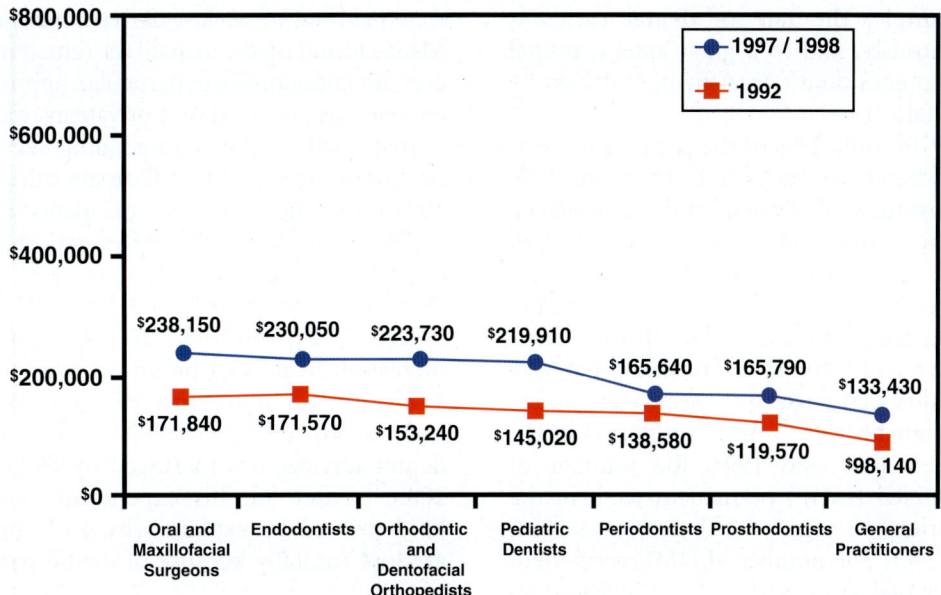

Figure 9 Average net income of specialists, 1990 and 1997–1998. Source: American Dental Association Survey Center. 1993 Survey of Dental Practice Specialists in Private Practice and 1998/1999 Survey of Dental Practice.

endodontist billings of $491,550 (Figure 9). Only general practitioners and pediatric dentists reported lower billings. The reason is endodontic office expenses were exceptionally low—$237,320, lowest of all dentists. The average endodontic office employs only 5.6 nondentist staff (Figure 10).[10] But remember, these figures, even though they are the latest available, are nearly 10 years old.

In spite of many encouraging figures for the present practice of endodontics, the future may not be as

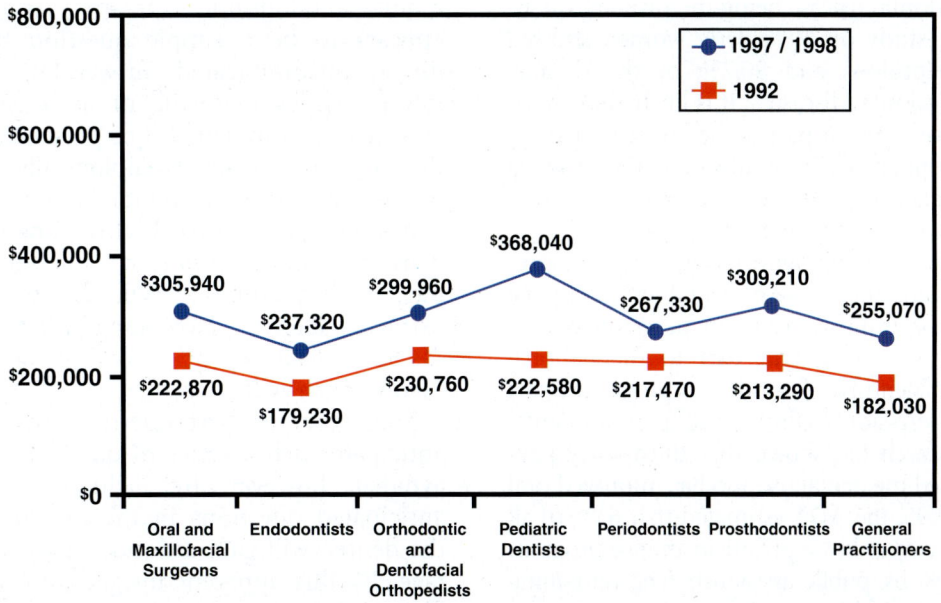

Figure 10 Average Practice Expenses per Owner, 1992 and 1997/1998. Source: American Dental Association Survey Center. 1993 Survey of Dental Practice Specialists in Private Practice and 1998/1999 Survey of Dental Practice.

"rosy." For example, the rate of dental caries is declining precipitously, and to a great extent, pulpal disease, leading to endodontic treatment, is driven by the index of dental caries.

Early in the 1970s, only 28% of the permanent teeth of American children were caries-free. Then, in 1988, the National Institute of Dental and Craniofacial Research (NIDCR) proudly announced that half of all children in the United States aged 5–17 years had no decay in their permanent teeth. None![21] Then again, between 1999 and 2002 the National Health and Nutrition Examination Survey (NHANES) reported that 62% of children and adolescents aged 6–19 years were caries-free in their permanent teeth.[22] And as reported in the NHANES between 1974 and 1994, the number of decayed-missing-filled (DMF) permanent teeth in the children, not caries-free (aged 6–18) decreased from 4.44 to 1.90 (57.2%). The number of DMF permanent surfaces also decreased, from 8.64 to 3.56 (58.8%) during this period.[23] In the year 2003, however, tooth decay was rising, reported as 78% of adolescents, perhaps indicating an emerging problem for older children consuming "junk food" and sugary drinks.[24]

As far as older adults are concerned, the NIDCR reported a remarkable decline in edentulism as well, particularly in the middle-aged, a group in which "total tooth loss has been practically eliminated."[25] Indeed, during the 1999–2002 survey, adults older than 20 years retained an average of 24 of 28 natural teeth, and only 8% were edentulous.[22] The elderly (age 65 and older), however, "are still in serious trouble," root caries and periodontal disease being the primary offenders.[25] A recent study of 398 elderly women showed 36.4% were edentulous and 80.7% of the dentate women had periodontal disease.[26] It is likely that endodontists will share a greater part of the burden, carrying for our aging population. In addition, as the growing immigrant population in the United States becomes more affluent, it will increasingly seek care.

All of these encouraging figures suggest greater preventive measures and higher use of dental services by the public. Part of the improvement can be credited to a healthier economy and lifestyle, part to the national water supply and dentifrice fluoridation programs, part to the dental profession's efforts, and part to dental insurance. A research has shown that third-party payment has increased the dental use and has improved oral health.[27–29] By 1995, the ADA estimated that 63% of all US citizens were covered by a private insurance program and another 5.3% by public assistance. The remaining 31.4% were not covered by any insurance program.[30]

Regardless, costs are high: in 2003, 43.1% of dental expenditures were paid by private insurance and 48.2% were paid out of pocket. Government programs such as Medicaid and Medicare paid the remaining 8.2%.[30] However, for endodontics in particular, approximately 70% of patients were covered by a private insurance program.[31]

In providing these burgeoning services, the dental profession has fared well financially. From 1986 to 1995, the net income of dentists increased by 30.7%.[32] In 2003, the ADA reported that dentists annually averaged $177,340 net, a 31% increase from 1986 (when adjusted for 2003 dollars).[33]

Dental expenditures by the public have also increased, from $3.4 billion in 1967 to $10 billion in 1977, to $25.3 billion in 1987, to $47.5 billion in 1996, and to $67 billion in 2003.[30] The expenditure for dental services has increased by 509% from 1975 to 2005.[34] After all this expenditure and care, one is hard-pressed to explain why 15.1 million workdays are lost annually because of dental pain.[35]

ENDODONTICS CASE PRESENTATION

All of these improvements notwithstanding, many patients still must be convinced that root canal therapy is an intelligent, practical solution to an age-old problem—the loss of teeth. The "case for endodontic treatment" must be presented to the patient in a straightforward manner. The patient with the correct "oral image" will be anxious to proceed with therapy.

"Is this tooth worth saving, doctor?" This sentiment is voiced more often than not by the patient who has been informed that his or her tooth will require endodontic therapy. Superficially, this appears to be a simple question that requires a direct, uncomplicated answer. It should not be interpreted as a hostile or as a challenge to the treatment recommendations presented for the retention of the tooth. Psychologically, however, this initial question is a prelude to a Pandora's box of additional queries that disclose doubts, fears, apprehensions, and economic considerations: for example, "Is it painful?" "Will this tooth have to be extracted later?" "How long will this tooth last?" "Is it a dead tooth?" "Will it turn black?" and "How much will it cost?"

Following the first question, the dentist should anticipate such a series of questions. These may be avoided, however, by including the answers to anticipated questions in the presentation. In turn, the dentist will gain a decided psychological advantage. By this apparent insight into his or her problems, the patient is assured that the dentist is cognizant of the very questions the patient was about to raise or possibly was too reticent to ask.

Most of the patient's fear and doubts can be allayed by giving a concise answer to each question.

In today's world, the patient may have been offered the choice between saving the tooth by root canal treatment and extracting the tooth and replacing it with an implant. Unless the tooth is hopeless, the dedicated dentist, one who believes in root canal therapy, should be able to make a positive case for retaining the tooth.

To answer patients' questions, the ADA has produced two inexpensive pamphlets entitled: *Root Canal Treatment—Following up on your dentist's recommendations* and *Understanding Root Canal Treatment**. The AAE also publishes a number of pamphlets for patients: the *Your Guide To* series: *Endodontic Treatment, Dental Symptoms, Cracked Teeth, Endodontic Retreatment, Endodontic Surgery, Endodontic Post-Treatment Care, and Dental Symptoms*†. Although this approach is somewhat impersonal, it is a tangible reference, particularly when the patient returns home and tries to explain to an interested spouse what endodontic therapy involves.

Based on previous experiences in the office, the average patient has sufficient confidence in the dentist's ability to help. The patient is ready to accept the professional knowledge and advice offered but likes to have some part in evaluating the reasonableness of treatment. The professional person and the staff must spend time and thought necessary to understand the patient's initial resistance, which is sometimes based on false assumptions and beliefs in matters dealing with pulpless teeth. However, once the patient is secure in the thought that this is the correct treatment, most of the fears and apprehensions related to unfamiliarity with endodontic therapy will be dissipated.

A dental appointment is still associated with fear in the minds of many people (Figure 11).[36–38] The mere thought of treating the "nerve" of a tooth implies pain. Patients require reassurance, supported by all available psychological and therapeutic methods of relaxation and pain control. The patient must be reassured that endodontic therapy need not be painful and usually requires no more than a local anesthetic.

All too often we hear negative remarks about root canal therapy: "Trying to do anything positive in Tacoma is akin to getting a *root canal* without Novocain." Or, "Whew! What you just heard was a collective

---

*American Dental Association, 211 E. Chicago Ave. Chicago IL 60611

†American Association of Endodontists 211 E. Chicago Ave. Suite 1100, Chicago, IL 60611

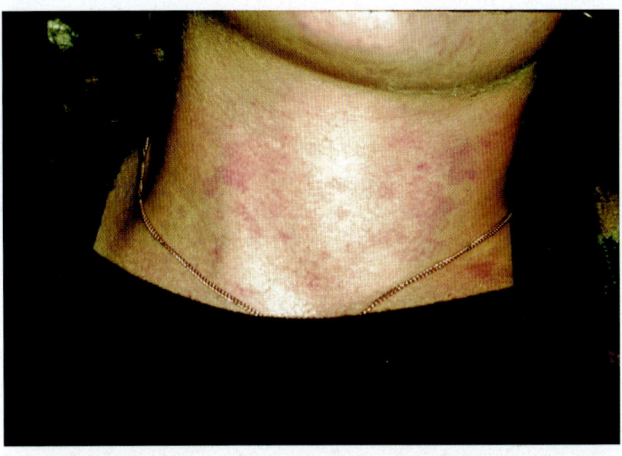

Figure 11 Rash (possibly hives) occurred in this terrified patient who was merely sitting in the dental chair prior to root canal treatment. The patient's apprehension was allayed by sympathetic management, allowing successful completion in a four canal molar. Courtesy of Dr. Norbert Hertl.

sigh of relief following *7 months of agonizing root canal*"—remarks made following President Clinton's "confession" on television. In contrast to these commonly heard excoriations, LeClaire et al.[38] reported that 43.9% of endodontic patients reported a decrease in fearfulness after having root canal therapy. Furthermore, 96.3% said that "they would have root canal therapy again to save a tooth". It should be explained to the concerned patient that root canal therapy is a specialized form of dental procedure designed to retain a tooth safely and comfortably. The tooth, when properly treated and restored, can be retained as long as any other tooth. It is not a "dead tooth" as long as the roots of the tooth are embedded in healthy surrounding tissues. Although teeth do not turn "black" following root canal therapy, a slight change in color owing to reduced translucency may occur. Discoloration associated with pulp necrosis and leakage around restorations can be managed successfully (see Chapter 38). Most often, retention of the tooth and bleaching, veneering, or crowning (Figure 12) are preferable to extraction and/or an implant and replacement with a prosthetic appliance.[12]

There is a little doubt that economic considerations play an important role (and for some a supreme role) in the final decision. Some patients "think financially," and even though they are able to afford treatment, they allow financial considerations to govern decisions that should logically be made on a physiological basis only. It is necessary to point out to these people the financial advantage of retaining a tooth by endodontic therapy rather than by extraction and prosthetic or implant replacement. In addition, it

12 / Endodontics

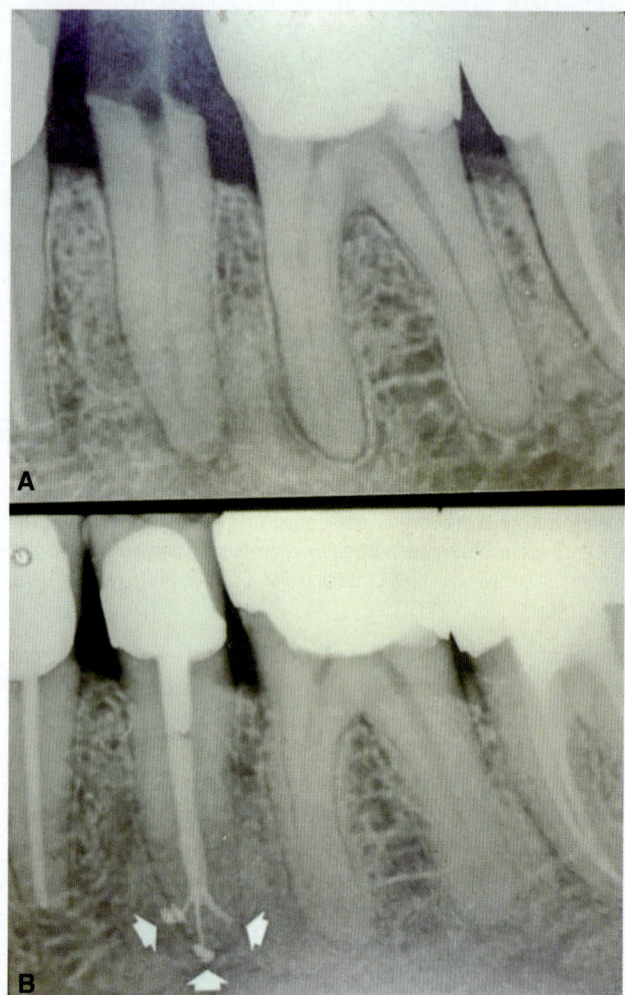

Figure 12 Fractured premolar restored by endodontics and post and core crown. ***A***, Tooth immediately following fracture. ***B***, Restoration and periapical healing at 3-year recall. Note spectacular filling at trifurcation and apex (arrows). Courtesy of Dr. Clifford J. Ruddle.

should be mentioned in all honesty that any vital tooth prepared for a bridge abutment might eventually become a possible candidate for future endodontic therapy.

Also, the patient who says "Pull it out" should be informed of the problems that will arise if a space is left unfilled, that is, tilting, reduced masticatory efficiency, future periodontal problems, root caries, and cosmetic effects. Another commonly heard statement by the patient is, "It's only a back tooth, anyway," or "If it were a front tooth I would save it, but no one sees it in back." This patient thinks cosmetically. The disadvantages of the loss of any tooth, let alone a posterior one, so essential for mastication, must be explained.

Fortunately, today's patient is becoming more sophisticated, too "tooth conscious" to permit indiscriminate extraction without asking whether there is an alternative. Extraction contributes to a crippling aberration from the normal dentition. There is no doubt that a normally functioning, endodontically treated, and well-restored natural tooth is vastly superior to the best prosthetic or implant replacement.

INDICATIONS

The indications for endodontic therapy are legion. Every tooth, from central incisor to third molar, is a potential candidate for treatment. Far too often the expedient measure of extracting a pulpless tooth is a short-sighted attempt at solving a dental problem. Endodontic therapy, on the other hand, extends to the dentist and the patient the opportunity to save teeth.

The concept of retaining every possible tooth, and even the healthy roots of periodontally involved teeth, is based on the even distribution of the forces of mastication. The final success of any extensive restorative procedure depends on the root surface area attached through the periodontal ligaments to the alveolar bone. Like the proverbial "horseshoe nail," root-filled teeth may often be the salvation of an otherwise hopeless case.

To carry this concept one step further, the importance of retaining even endodontically treated *roots*, over which a full denture may be constructed, the so-called *overdenture*, is recognized.[39] On some occasions, attachments may be added to these roots to provide additional retention for the denture above (Figure 13). At other times, the treated roots are

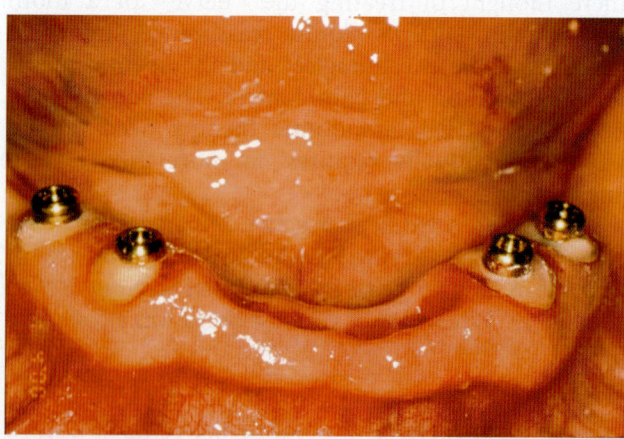

Figure 13 Four locator overdenture attachments (Zest anchors) ensure adequate retention for mandibular full denture. Courtesy of Dr. A.L. Schneider.

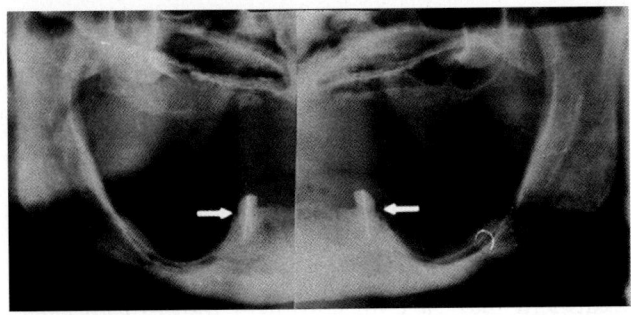

Figure 14 Dramatic demonstration of alveolar bone remaining around retained canines, but badly resorbed under maxillary full and mandibular partial dentures. Courtesy of Drs. J.L. Lord and S. Teel.

merely left in place on the assumption that the alveolar process will be retained around roots, and there will not be the usual ridge resorption so commonly seen under full or even partial dentures (Figure 14).

Modern dentistry incorporates endodontics as an integral part of restorative and prosthetic treatment. Any tooth with pulpal involvement, provided that it has adequate periodontal support, can be a candidate for root canal treatment. Even severely broken-down teeth and potential and actual abutment teeth can be candidates for the tooth-saving procedures of endodontics, provided all options with benefits and disadvantages are explained to the patient.

One of the greatest services rendered by the profession is the retention of the first permanent molar (Figure 15). In contrast, the long-range consequences

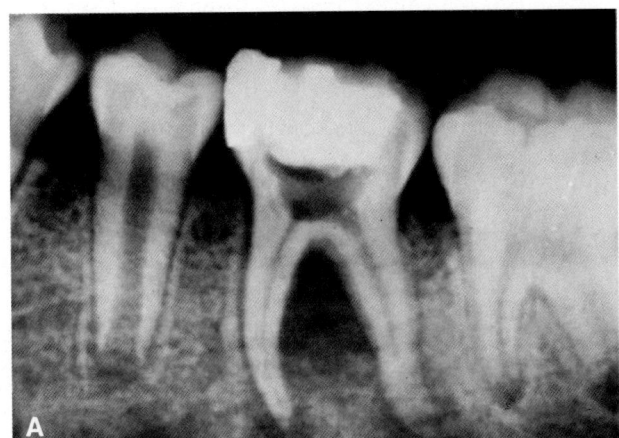
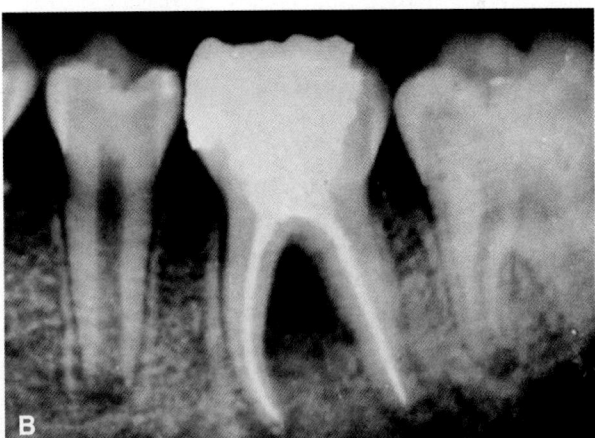
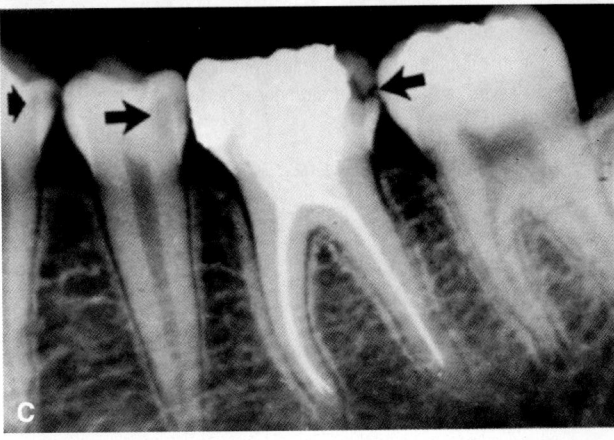

Figure 15 ***A,*** Pulpless first molar following failure of pulpotomy. Note two periapical lesions and complete loss of intraradicular bone. Draining sinus track opposite furcation is also present. ***B,*** Completion of endodontic treatment without surgery. ***C,*** Two-year recall radiograph. Total healing was complete in 6 months. New carious lesions now involve each interproximal surface.

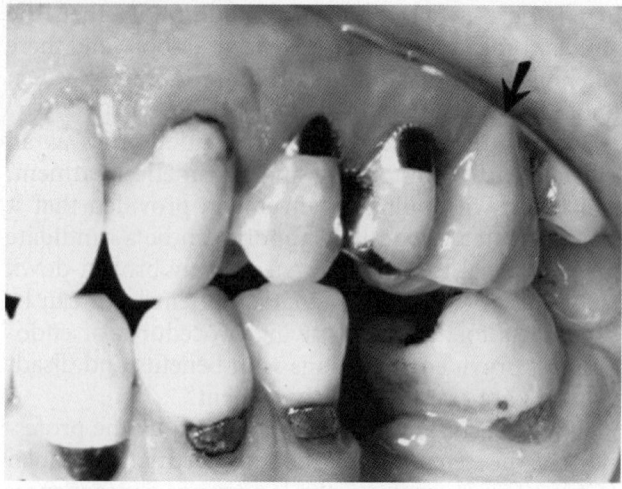

Figure 16 Extrusion, recession (arrow), tipping, malocclusion, rotation, and gingival cemental caries are only a few of the long-range consequences following early extraction of a permanent first molar.

of breaking the continuity of either arch are also well known (Figure 16). Root canal therapy often provides the only opportunity for saving first molars with pulp involvement.

In addition to saving molars for children, saving posterior teeth for adults is also highly desirable. Retaining a root-filled terminal molar, for example, means saving two teeth—the molar's opposite tooth as well (Figure 17A). Moreover, root canal treatment may save an abutment tooth of an existing fixed prosthesis. The gain is doubled if the salvaged abutment is also the terminal posterior tooth in the arch and has a viable opponent (see Figure 17B).

Another candidate for endodontic therapy is the adolescent who arrives in the office with a grossly

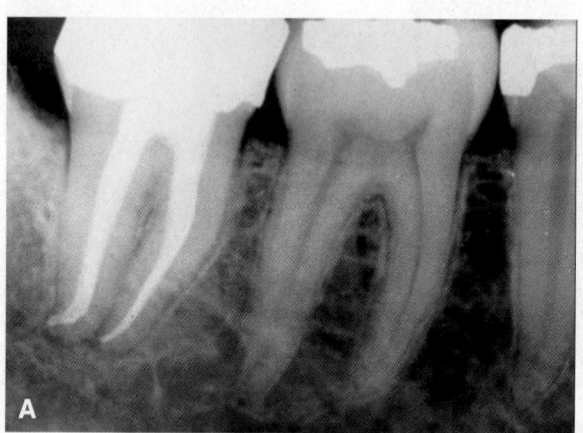 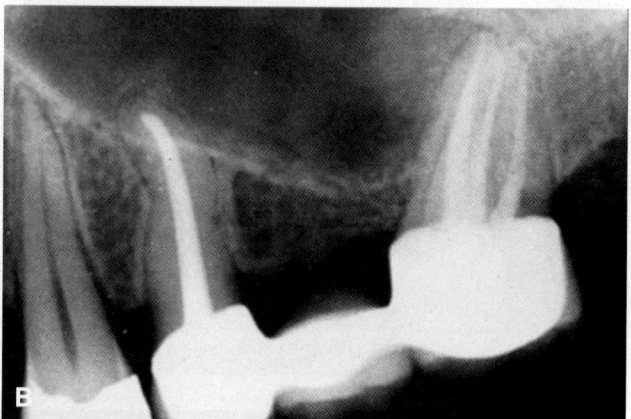

Figure 17 *A,* Terminal molar retained by endodontic treatment saves opposing molar as well. Courtesy of Dr. L. Stephen Buchanan. *B,* Fixed partial denture possible only because abutment teeth are saved by root canal treatment. Courtesy of Dr. Norbert Hertl.

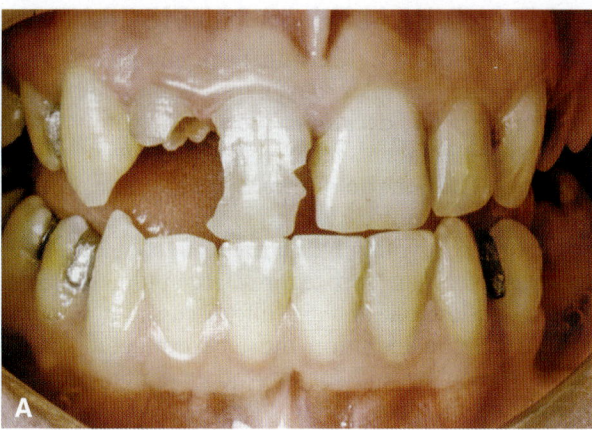 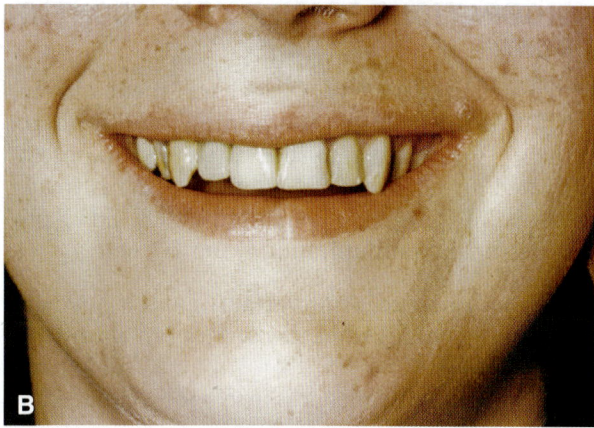

Figure 18 A, Caries decimated dentition in a 14-year-old girl. Personality problems had developed in this youngster related to her pain and embarrassing appearance. **B,** Restoration following endodontic therapy has restored cosmetic appearance and confidence so necessary for an adolescent.

damaged dentition and is faced with multiple extractions and dentures (Figure 18). Many of these children are mortified by their appearance. It is gratifying to see the blossoming personality when an esthetic improvement has been achieved. The end result in these cases would not be possible without root canal therapy (Figure 19).

A growing area in which endodontics plays an important role is dental trauma (see Chapter 36). Advances have been made in the understanding of dental trauma, and endodontics as a discipline has played an important role in developing treatment approaches. This is understandable considering the importance that the pulp plays in traumatic dental injuries.

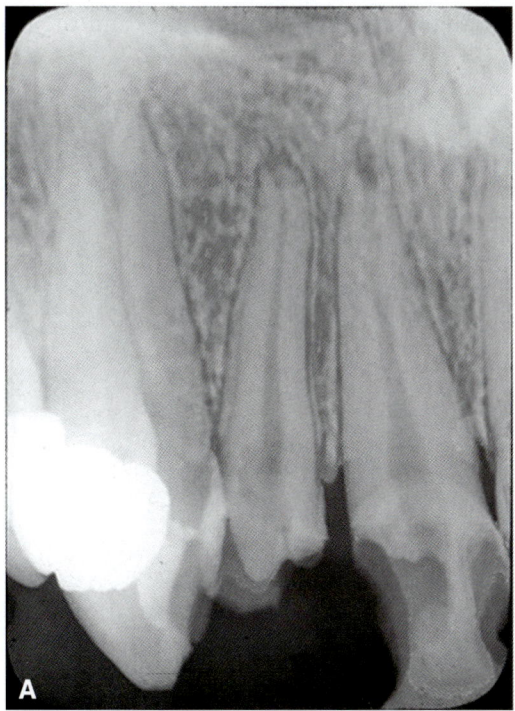 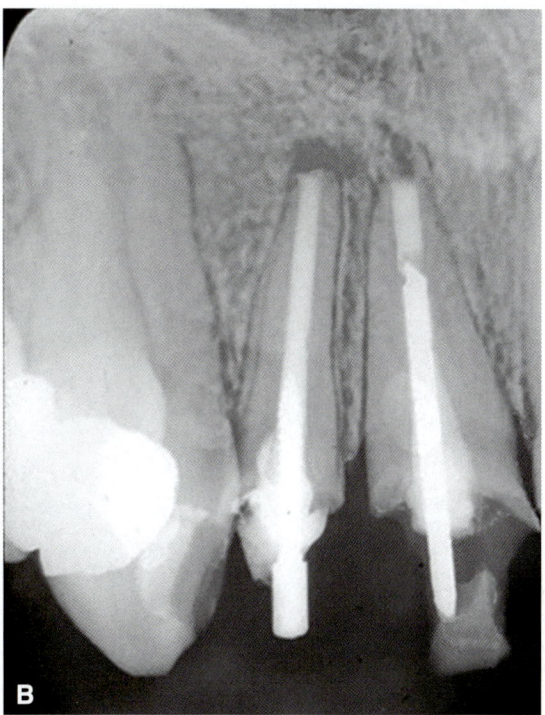

Figure 19 A, Obvious pulp involvement of incisors shown in Figure 18. **B,** Root canal treatment of these incisors makes possible post restoration followed by cosmetic provisional crowns.

CONSIDERATIONS PRIOR TO ENDODONTIC THERAPY

Although it is true that root canal treatment can be performed on virtually any tooth in the mouth, there are some important considerations that must be evaluated prior to recommending root canal treatment. Some of these were delineated by Dr. Ed Beveridge (personal communication, June 1971):

1. Is the tooth needed or important? Does it have an opponent? Could it some day serve as an abutment for prosthesis?
2. Is the tooth salvageable, or is it so badly damaged it cannot be restored?
3. Is the entire dentition so completely broken down it would be virtually impossible to restore?
4. Is the tooth serving esthetically, or would the patient be better served by its extraction and a more cosmetic replacement?
5. Is the tooth so severely involved periodontally that it would be lost soon for this reason?
6. Is the practitioner capable of performing the needed endodontic procedures?

Endodontists wish that patients are referred to them before procedural mishaps, such as root perforations, occur; if a mishap does occur during treatment by a general dentist, the patient is entitled to be given the option of care by a specialist.

AGE AND HEALTH AS CONSIDERATIONS

Age need not be a determinant in endodontic therapy. Simple and complex dental procedures are routinely performed on deciduous teeth in young children and on permanent teeth in patients well into their nineties. The same holds true for endodontic procedures. It should be noted, however, that complete removal of the pulp in young immature teeth should be avoided if possible. The procedures for pulp preservation are more desirable and are fully discussed in Chapter 34.

Health consideration must be evaluated for endodontics as it would for any other dental procedures. Most often, root canal therapy will be preferable to extraction. In severe cases of heart disease, diabetes, or radiation necrosis, root canal treatment is far less traumatic than extraction, for example.[40] Even in patients with terminal cancer, leukemia, or AIDS, endodontics is often preferred over extraction. Pregnancy, particularly in the second trimester, is usually a safe time for treatment. In all of these situations, however, endodontic surgery is likely to be as traumatic as extraction.

STATUS OF THE ORAL CONDITION

Pulpally involved teeth may simultaneously have periodontal lesions and be associated with other dental problems such as rampant decay, orthodontic misalignment, root resorption, and/or a history of traumatic injuries. Often the treatment of such teeth requires a team effort of dental specialists along with the patient's general dentist.

The presence of *periodontal lesions* must be evaluated with respect to the correct diagnosis: Is the lesion of periodontal or endodontic origin, or is it a combined situation? The answer to this question will determine the treatment approach and the outcome; generally, lesions of endodontic origin will respond satisfactorily to endodontic treatment alone (Figure 20), whereas those of periodontal origin will not be affected simply by endodontic

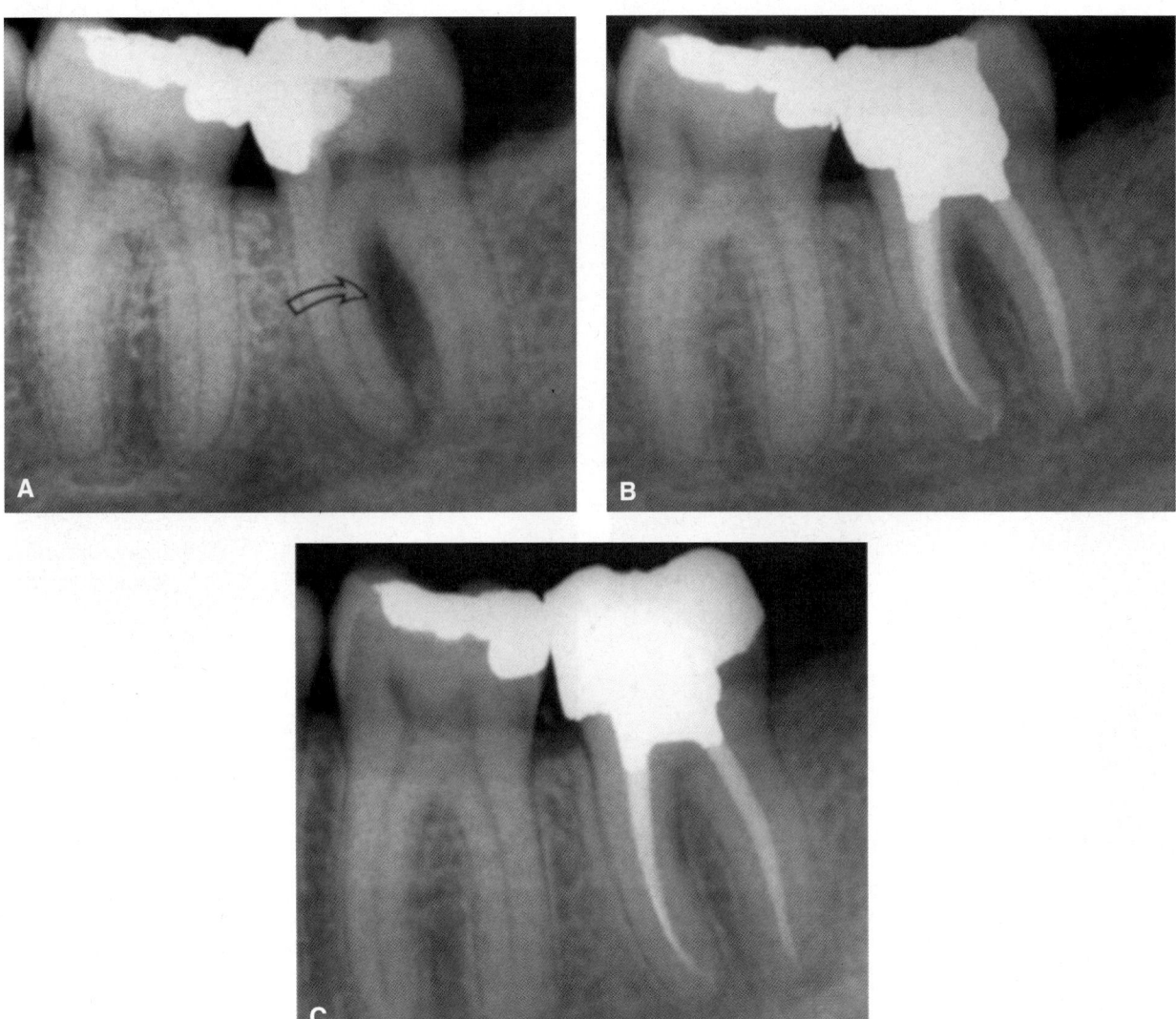

Figure 20 ***A****,* Mandibular molar with furcal bone loss (arrow) from endodontic infection and not from periodontal disease. ***B****,* Root canal treatment completed with no periodontal intervention. ***C****,* One-year control shows recovery of furcal lesion by endodontic treatment alone.

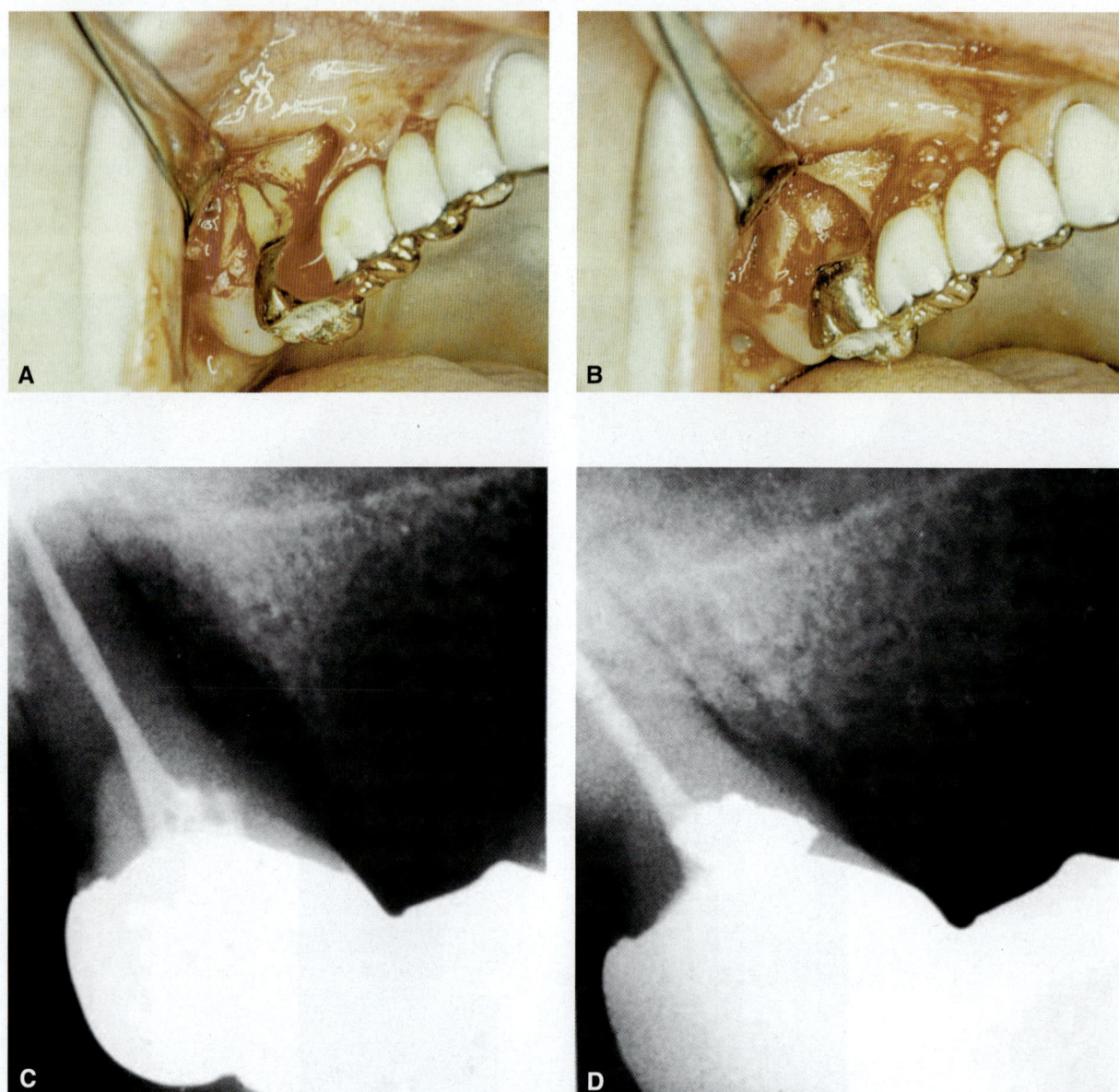

Figure 21 ***A***, Retraction of surgical flap reveals the extent of periodontal lesion completely involving buccal roots of second molar abutment of full arch periodontal prosthesis. ***B***, Total amputation of buccal roots reveals cavernous periodontal bone loss. ***C***, Extensive bone loss seen in ***A*** and ***B*** is apparent in radiograph taken at the time of treatment. ***D***, Osseous repair, 1 year following buccal root amputation. Solidly supported palatal root serves as adequate terminal abutment for full arch prosthesis. Courtesy of Dr. Dudley H. Glick.

procedures (Figure 21).[41] Combined lesions—those that develop as a result of both pulpal infection and periodontal disease—respond to a combined treatment approach in which endodontic intervention precedes, or is done simultaneously with, periodontal treatment (Figure 22).[42] Even teeth with apparently hopeless root support can be saved by endodontic treatment and root amputation (Figure 23).

Today many teeth with necrotic pulps, once condemned to extraction, are saved by root canal therapy, as are teeth with large periapical lesions or apical cysts (Figure 24),[43–47] teeth with perforations or internal or cervical resorption (Figure 25). Teeth badly fractured by trauma

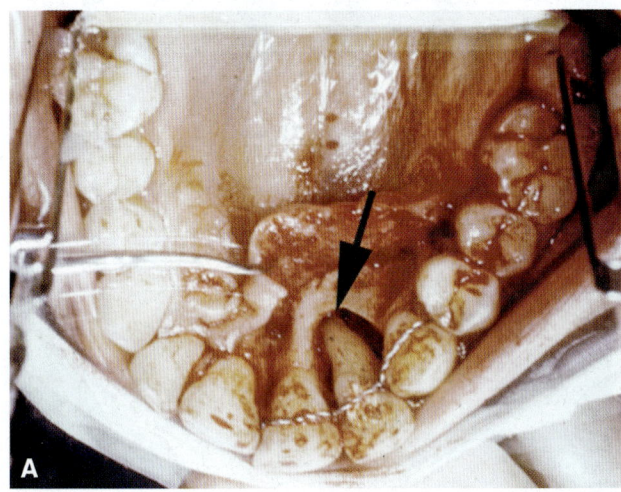
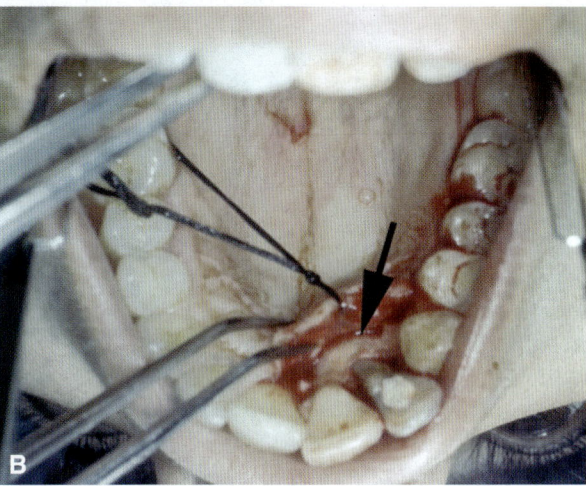

Figure 22 ***A,*** Periodontal/endodontic lesion (arrow) resulting in deep bony pocket palatal to maxillary lateral incisor. Endodontic treatment has been completed. The pocket and the root have been thoroughly curetted and the flap will be repositioned. ***B,*** "Re-entry," 2 years later showing complete repair (arrow). Courtesy of anonymous Latin American endodontist.

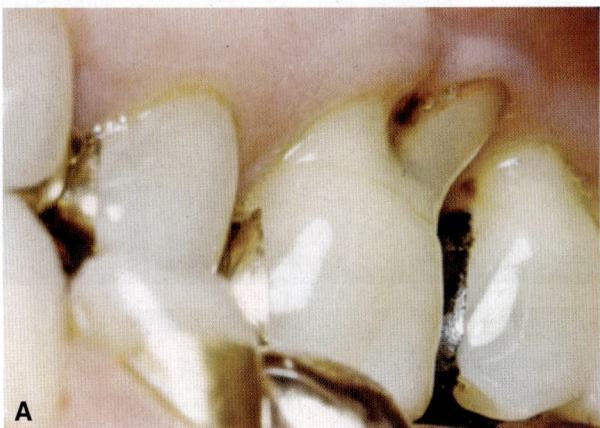
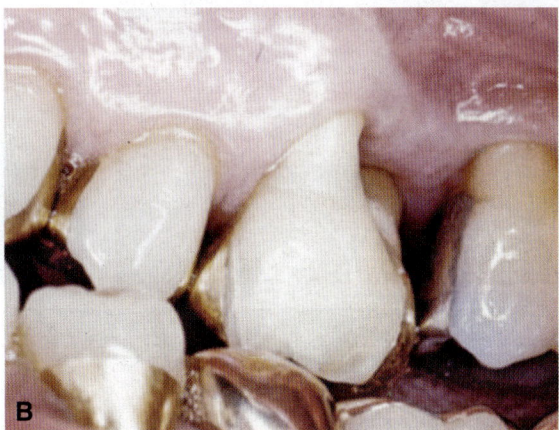

Figure 23 Amputation of periodontally involved distobuccal root allows retention of restored maxillary first molar. Root canal treatment in two remaining roots is necessary.

20 / Endodontics

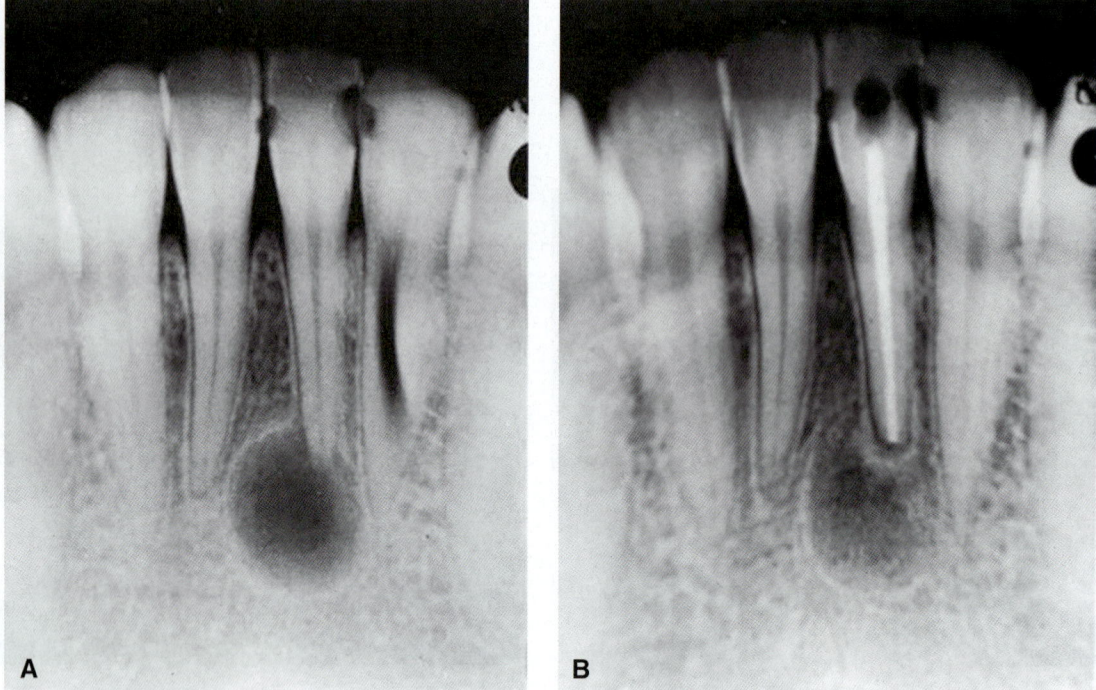

Figure 24 ***A,*** Radiographic appearance of an apical cyst (left) apparent in pretreatment radiograph. ***B,*** Total repair of cystic cavity in 6-month recall film is signaled by complete lamina dura that has developed periapically. Biopsy confirmed the initial diagnosis of an apical cyst.

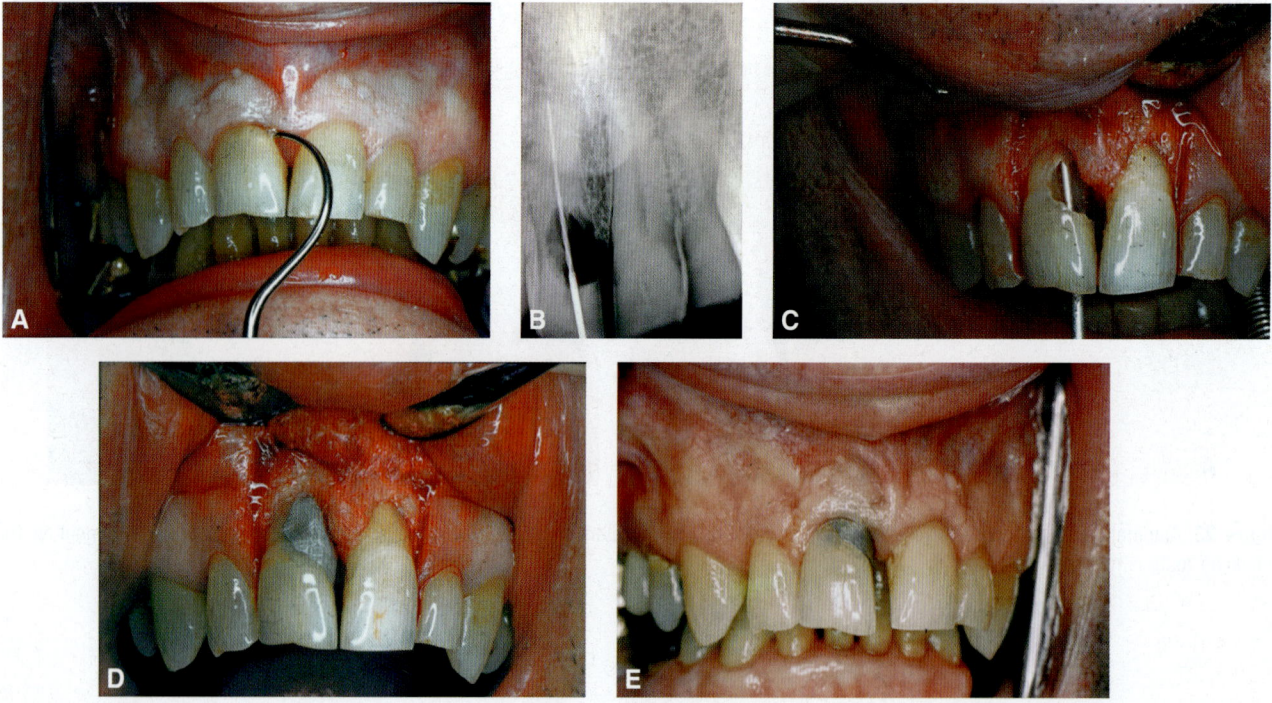

Figure 25 ***A,*** Exploration of deep cervical resorptive defect, source of constant discomfort. ***B,*** Resorption was the result of an attack by sled dog on a 67-year-old Alaskan. ***C,*** Following pulpectomy and curettage of lesion, a silver point is placed to act as an internal matrix and preserve the canal space. ***D,*** Restoration restores contour and seals the chamber. The silver point is withdrawn and the root canal is obturated. The flap is repositioned. ***E,*** Recall 5 years later showing complete healing and retention of tooth badly damaged by cervical resorption. Today, resin materials would be used instead of amalgam.

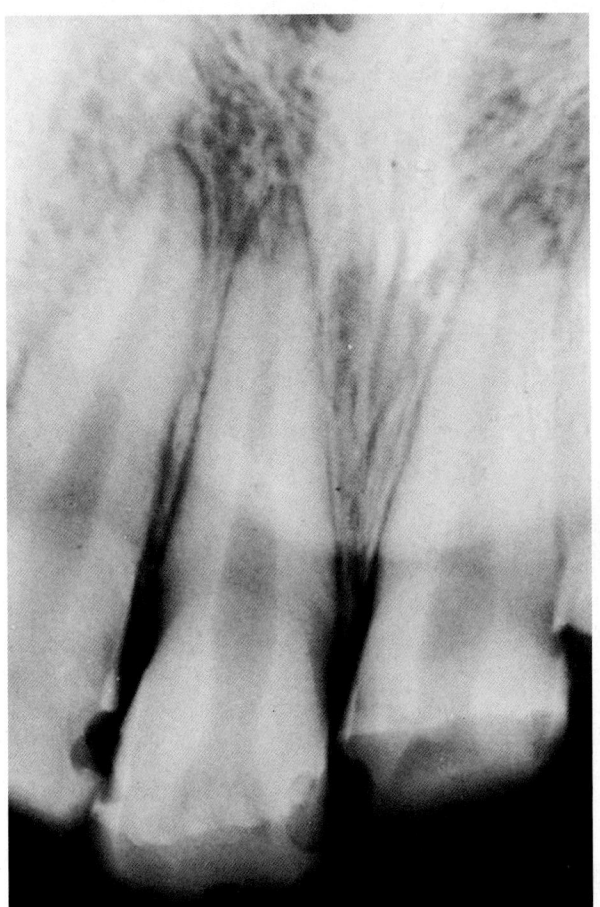

Figure 26 Maxillary incisors fractured into the pulp and also cariously involved. Endodontics can play an important role in the management of such situations.

(Figure 26), and pulpally involved teeth with tortuous or apparently obstructed canals or instruments separated within, teeth with flaring open apices (Figure 27), teeth that are hopelessly discolored (Figure 28), and traumatically injured teeth.

Most of these complicated dental situations can be managed, often by a team approach involving various specialists along with the patient's general dentist. In all instances, the anticipated outcome must be discussed with the patient who should decide which treatment option to choose.

Controversies in Endodontics

There have been a number of controversies in endodontics, some solved, some abandoned, some remaining. Dr. Mahmoud Torabinejad will address some in Chapter 4. One controversy that comes to mind is the theory of focal infection and selective localization. This is also covered in Chapter 7. Another is the problem of flare-ups that will be thoroughly discussed in Chapter 21.

There are two controversies, however, that deserve our present and continued attention. The first deals with the efficacy of single-appointment therapy, and the second is the determination of where the apical terminus of the root canal should be, both for cleaning and shaping and for obturating the canal. A good deal of research and cognition has been expended in their behalf, but no universal agreements have been reached.

SINGLE-APPOINTMENT THERAPY

Single-appointment root canal therapy has become a common practice. When questioned, however, most general dentists reply that they reserve one-appointment treatment for vital pulp cases and immediate periapical surgery cases. In 1982, only 12.8% of dentists queried thought that necrotic teeth would be successfully treated

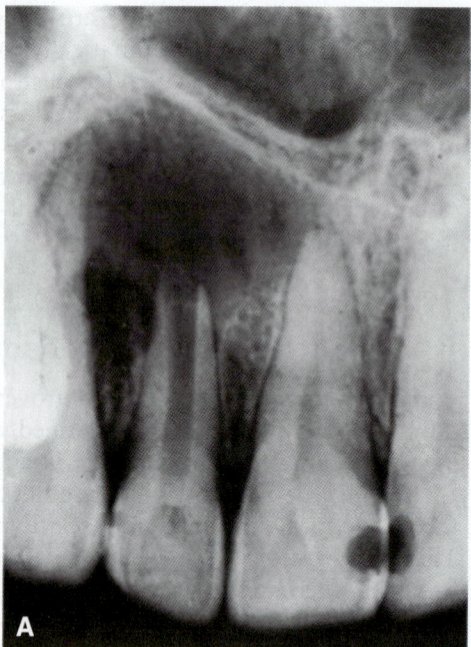 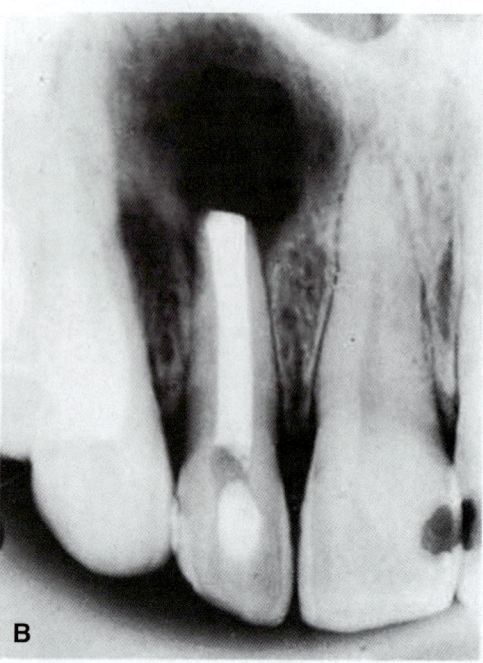

Figure 27 *A,* Flaring apex of incompletely formed root follows pulpal death caused by impact trauma at an early age. *B,* Obturation of "blunderbuss" canal is accomplished by retrofilling from a surgical approach. Historically, this was a common procedure. Today, such teeth are managed more conservatively without surgery. Ingle JI. Dental Digest 1956;62:410.

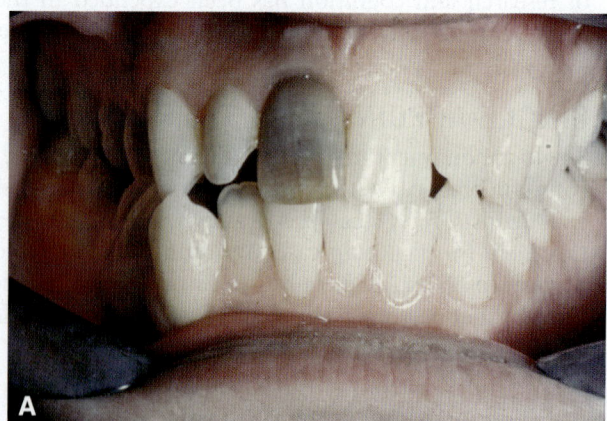 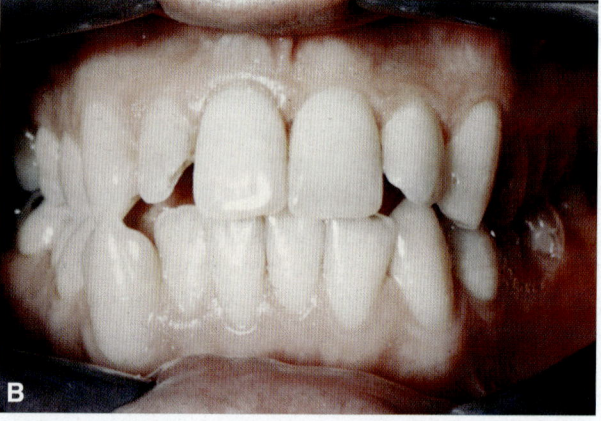

Figure 28 "Before" *A* and "after" *B,* photos demonstrating results of one internal bleaching treatment with Superoxol. The patient, a young medical student, recognized that the discolored tooth was off-putting and was overjoyed with the result. This is also an historical illustration; today, bleaching agents such as Superoxol are not used due to the risk of cervical resorption.

in one appointment.[48] On the other hand, endodontists have been treating patients in one-appointment visits for some time. At one time, 86% of the directors of postgraduate endodontic programs, when surveyed, reported that nonsurgical one-visit treatment was part of their program.[49] Today it is universal.

What are the advantages and disadvantages of single-visit endodontics?

Advantages:

1. Immediate familiarity with the internal anatomy, canal shape, and contour facilitates obturation

2. No risk of bacterial leakage beyond a temporary coronal seal between appointments
3. Reduction of clinic time
4. Patient convenience—no additional appointment or travel
5. Low cost

Perceived Disadvantages:
1. No easy access to the apical canal if there is a flare-up
2. Clinician fatigue with extended one-appointment operating time
3. Patient fatigue and discomfort with extended operating time
4. No opportunity to place an intracanal disinfectant (other than allowing NaOCl to disinfect during treatment)

What has held back one-appointment endodontics? The major consideration has been the concern about postoperative pain and failure.

POSTOPERATIVE PAIN

The fear that patients will probably develop postoperative pain and that the canal has been irretrievably sealed has probably been the greatest deterrent to single-visit therapy. Yet the literature shows no real difference in pain experienced by patients treated with multiple appointments.[48–65] In spite of this evidence, 40% of the endodontic course directors surveyed were of the opinion that necrotic cases treated in one visit have more flare-ups.[48] The University of Iowa group,[50] however, found this not to be true—3.2 flare-ups for two-appointment cases versus 2.6 for one-treatment cases. Nor did Galberry find this to be true in Louisiana,[57] nor did Nakamuta and Nagasawa[58] in Japan, who had only 7.5% pain incidence after treating 106 infected cases in single appointments. More to the point, the symptoms experienced by the Japanese patients were not flare-ups, but mild pain, and needed no drugs or emergency treatment.

Oliet[56] reported that only 3% of his cohort of 264 patients receiving single-appointment treatment had severe pain, compared with 2.4% of the 123 patients treated in two visits. Wolch's[52] records of over 2,000 cases treated at a single appointment showed that <1% of patients indicated any severe reaction. Pekruhn[55] reported no statistically significant difference between his two groups. Mulhern et al.[59] reported no significant difference in the incidence of pain between 30 single-rooted teeth with necrotic pulps treated in one appointment and 30 similar teeth treated in three appointments. At the University of Oklahoma, however, Roane et al.[60] found a "two to one higher frequency of pain following multiple visit treatment when compared to those completed in one visit." More recent reports from Brazil,[61] and Fava[62–64], from the Netherlands found no difference in the incidence of pain between one- and two-visit cases, and Trope[65] reported no flare-ups in one-appointment cases with no apical lesions.

However, retreatment of failed cases with apical periodontitis made the difference. These cases suffered a 13.6% flare-up rate.[65] One might expect pain from any case, as reported by Harrison et al.[66] Of 229 patients treated twice, 55.5% had no interappointment pain, 28.8% had slight pain, and 15.7% had moderate to severe pain. Eleazer and Eleazer[67] compared the flare-up rate between one and two appointments in treating necrotic canal molars. In the two-visit cohort, there was a 16% flare-up rate, whereas in the one-visit group, there was only a 3% flare-up experience, which proved to be significant. Ørstavik et al.[68] also reported fewer flare-ups following single-appointment therapy. And even more recently, 2006, Al-Negrish and Habahbeh[69] reported from Jordan on 112 cases of asymptomatic, necrotic pulp central incisors, half treated in one appointment and half treated in two appointments. "...more flare-ups occurred in the two appointment group 13.8% than in the single visit group 9.2%. Flare-ups occurred after 2 days and after 7 days, 5.2% and 1.8% respectively." They further stated, "This should draw the attention of dentists not to over-react to early postobturation symptoms by immediately initiating root canal retreatment or extracting the involved tooth." In light of these studies, neither pain nor flare-ups appear to be valid reasons to avoid single-appointment root canal therapy.

SUCCESS VERSUS FAILURE

If pain is not a deterrent, how about fear of failure? Pekruhn[70] has published a definitive evaluation of single-visit endodontics. From the clinics of the Arabian–American Oil Company, he reported a 1-year recall of 925 root-filled teeth of 1,140 possible cases. His failure rate was 5.2%, very comparable to many multiple-visit studies. Pekruhn was surprised to learn that his rate of failure was higher (15.3%) in teeth with periradicular lesions that had had no prior access opening. If this type of case had been previously opened, the incidence of failure would drop to 6.5%. The highest failure rate (16.6%) was in endodontic retreatment cases. Symptomatic cases were twice as likely to fail as were asymptomatic cases (10.6% versus 5.0%).

A Japanese study followed *one-visit cases* for as long as 40 months and reported an 86% success rate.[58] Oliet[56] again found no statistical significance between his two groups. The majority of the postgraduate directors of endodontics also felt that the chance of successful healing was equal for either type of therapy.[49] The original investigators in this field, Fox et al.,[51] Wolch,[52] Soltanoff,[53] and Ether et al.,[54] were convinced that single-visit root canal therapy could be just as successful as multiple-visit therapy. None, however, treated the acutely infected or abscess case in a single visit.

In marked contrast to these positive reports, Sjögren and his associates in Sweden sounded a word of caution.[71] At *a single appointment*, they cleaned and obturated 55 single-rooted teeth with apical periodontitis. All of the teeth were initially infected. After cleaning and irrigating with sodium hypochlorite and just before obturation, they cultured the canals. Using advanced *anaerobic* bacteriologic techniques, they found that 22 (40%) of the 55 canals tested positive and the other 33 (60%) tested negative. Periapical healing was then followed for *5 years*. Complete periapical healing occurred in 94% of the 33 cases that yielded *negative* cultures! But in those 22 cases in which the canals tested positive prior to root canal filling, "the success rate of healing had *fallen to just 68%*," a statistically significant difference.[71] In other words, if a canal is still infected at the time of filling at a single dental appointment, there may be a 26% greater chance of failure than if the canal is disinfected. Their conclusions emphasized the importance of eliminating bacteria from the canal system before obturation, and this objective could not be achieved reliably without an effective intracanal medicament. This is one limited study, but it was done carefully and provided the evidence correlating the presence of bacteria to longer-term outcomes.

Ørstavik colleagues[72] faced up to this problem and studied 23 teeth with apical periodontitis, all but one infected initially. At the end of each sitting, apical dentin samples were cultured anaerobically. No chemical irrigants were used during cleaning and shaping, and at the end of the first appointment, 14 of the 23 canals were still infected. At an earlier time, Ingle and Zeldow,[73,74] using aerobic culturing, found much the same. Ørstavik et al.[72] then sealed calcium hydroxide in the canal. In 1 week, at the start of the second appointment, only one root canal had sufficient numbers of bacteria "for quantification"—the calcium hydroxide was that effective! They also found "a tendency for teeth causing symptoms to harbor more bacteria than symptomless teeth."

In a follow-up study, Trope et al.[75] treated teeth with apical periodontitis, with and without calcium hydroxide, in one or two visits. They reached a number of conclusions that are as follows:

1. "[C]alcium hydroxide disinfection after chemomechanical cleaning will result in negative cultures in most cases."
2. "[I]nstrumentation and irrigation alone decrease the number of bacteria in the canal 1000-fold; however the canals cannot be rendered free of bacteria by this method alone."
3. "[T]he additional disinfecting action of calcium hydroxide before obturation resulted in a 10% increase in healing rates. This difference should be considered clinically important."

In another 52-week comparative study in North Carolina of the "periapical healing of infected roots [in dogs] obturated in one step or with prior calcium hydroxide disinfection," the researchers concluded that "$Ca(OH)_2$ disinfection before obturation of infected root canals results in significantly less periapical inflammation than obturation alone."[76]

One has to ask, therefore, wouldn't it be better to extend one more appointment, properly medicate the canal between appointments, and improve the patient's chances by filling a bacteria-free canal? Unfortunately, there is a widely held but anecdotal opinion that current chemomechanical cleaning techniques are superior, predictably removing the entire bacterial flora. If this is so, single-visit treatment of necrotic pulp cases would definitely be indicated. However, research has yet to be published to corroborate these opinions. Until then, it may be more prudent to use an intracanal medicament such as calcium hydroxide or povidone iodine within a multiple-visit regimen, for cases in which a mature bacterial flora is present within the canal system prior to treatment.

Although single appointments would be very appropriate in *cases with vital pulps*, on the other hand, for symptomatic teeth with necrotic pulps and apical periodontitis and for failed cases requiring retreatment, there may be a risk of lower success rates in the long term. To date, the evidence for recommending either one- or multiple-visit endodontics is not consistent. The prudent practitioner needs to make decisions carefully as new evidence becomes available.

Wolch[52] said it best: "In the treatment of any disease, a cure can only be affected if the cause is removed. Since endodontic diseases originate from an infected or affected pulp, it is axiomatic that the root canal must be thoroughly and carefully debrided and obturated" (personal communication, 1983).

DETERMINATION OF THE APICAL TERMINUS AND CLEANING THE APICAL PATENCY

The second controversy to be discussed surrounds the determination of an accurate *working length*, one of the most critical steps of endodontic therapy. The cleaning, shaping, and obturation of the root canal system cannot be accomplished accurately unless the working length is determined precisely.[77–79] And if the working length is to be established slightly short of the apical foramen, what of that tiny space that lies beyond the constriction—the *apical patency area*? What if this space contains toxic debris and harmful bacteria that could prevent future healing and repair? Simon[80] has stressed the need for clarification and consistency in the use of terms relating to working length determination. Working length (Figure 29) is defined in the endodontic glossary as "the distance from the coronal reference point to the point at which canal preparation and obturation should terminate."[81]

The *anatomic apex* is the tip or the end of the root determined morphologically, whereas the *radiographic apex* is the tip or the end of the root determined radiographically.[81] Root morphology and radiographic distortion may cause the location of the radiographic apex to vary from the anatomic apex.

The *apical foramen* is the main apical opening (entrance/exit) of the root canal. It is frequently eccentrically located well away from the anatomic or the radiographic apex[82–84] (Figure 30). Palmer[84] investigation showed that this deviation occurred in 68–80% of the teeth in his study.

An accessory foramen is an orifice on the surface of the root communicating with a lateral or an accessory canal.[81] They may exist as a single foramen or as multiple foramina.

The *apical constriction* (minor apical diameter) (Figure 31) is the apical portion of the root canal having the narrowest diameter. This position may vary but is usually 0.5–1.0 mm short of the center of the apical foramen.[81–83] The *minor diameter* widens apically toward the foramen (*major diameter*) and assumes a funnel shape. This is the area of "apical patency" that will be discussed later.

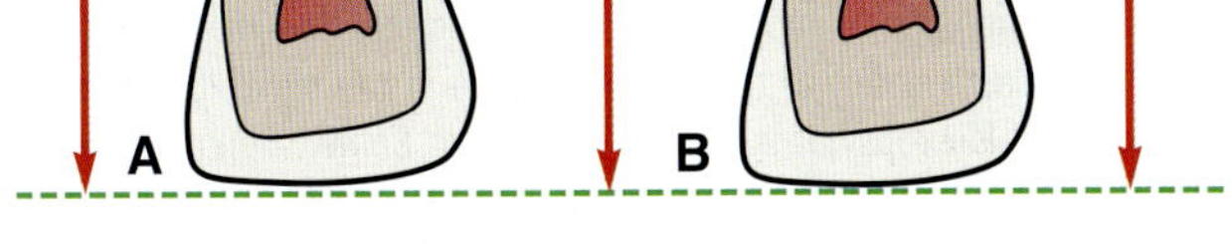

Figure 29 Care should be exercised to establish the position of the foramen. Hopefully, it appears at the apex **A** and 0.5–1.0 mm is simply subtracted from the tooth length as a "safety factor." The lateral exit of the canal **B** is sometimes seen in the radiograph or discovered by instrument placement and re-examined radiographically. Today, electronic apex locators are important instruments for determining the apical exit of root canals. Reproduced with permission from Serene T, Krasny R, Ziegler P, et al. Principles of Preclinical Endodontics. Dubuque, IA: Kendall/Hunt Publishing; 1974.

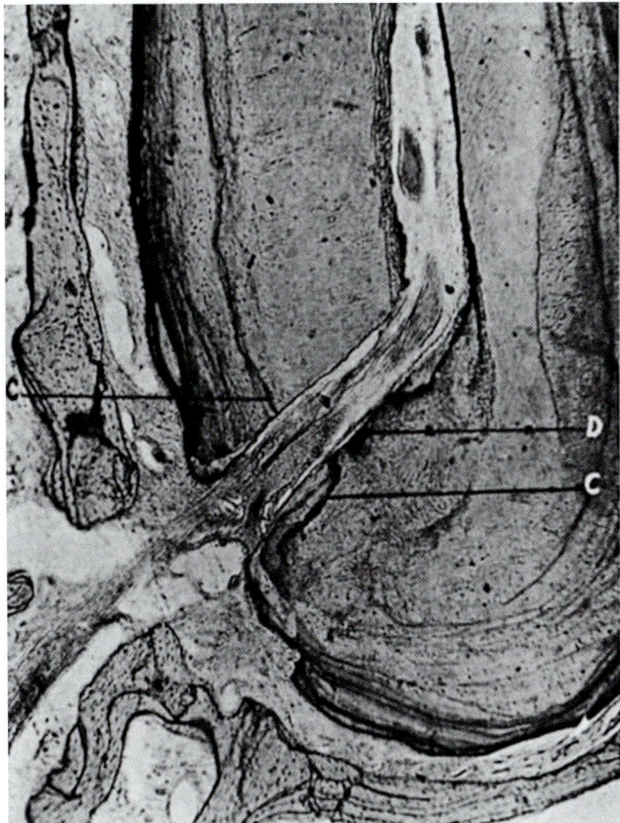

Figure 30 The apical foramen, some distance from the radiographic apex, stresses the importance of finding the actual orifice by electric apex locator (EAL). D, Dentin; C, Cementum. Reproduced with permission from Skillen WG. J Am Dent Assoc 1930;17:2082.

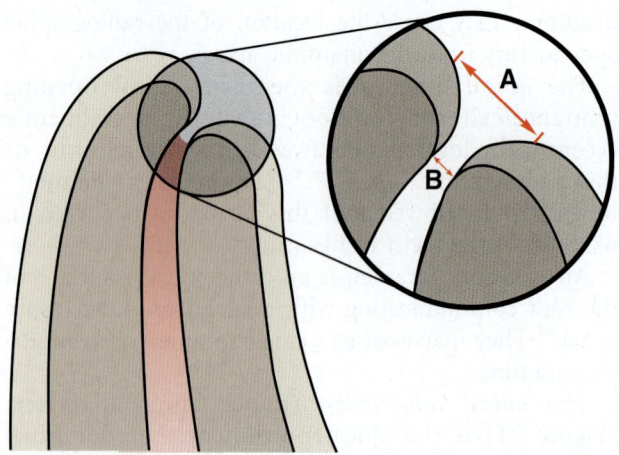

Figure 31 Diagrammatic view of the root apex. The importance of differentiating between the *minor diameter* **B** and the *major diameter* (radiographic apex) **A** is apparent. Courtesy of Dr. Stephen Weeks.

The apical third is the most studied region of the root canal.[82,83,85–90] Dummer[83] and his associates reported many variations in the apical constriction. In 6% of cases, the constriction may be blocked by the cementum.

The *cementodentinal junction* is the region where the dentin and the cementum are united, the point at which the cemental surface terminates at or near the apex of the tooth.[81] It must be pointed out, however, that the cementodentinal junction is a histological landmark that cannot be located clinically or radiographically. Langeland[91] has reported that the cementodentinal junction does not always coincide with the apical constriction. The location of the cementodentinal junction also ranges from 0.5 to 3.0 mm short of the apical constriction.[81–88, 92–96]

Therefore, it is generally accepted that the apical constriction is most frequently located 0.5–1.0 mm short of the apical foramen, but with variations. These variations may be revealed by the patient's reaction to an overextended instrument or by an electric apex locator (EAL).

Now to complicate matters further, Brynolf[97] (Figure 32) has pointed out that the apical constriction may disappear completely when apical disease destroys, by resorption, the entire apical structure.

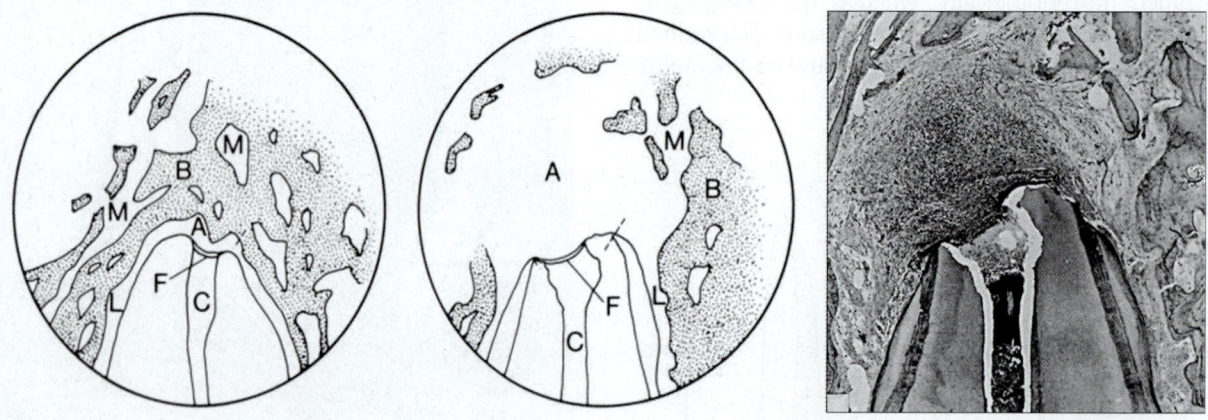

Figure 32 Brynolf's interpretation of the normal and resorbed *lamina dura*. *Left*, Radiographic appearance of the normal lamina dura under magnification. *Center*, Loss of lamina dura at the apex along with inflammatory resorption as a result of the necrotic tissue in the canal (C). **A**, apical soft tissue; **B**, bone trabeculae; **C**, root canal; **F**, foramen; **L**, PDL; **M**, medullary space. *Right*, Necropsy of specimen detailed in *Center*. Reproduced with permission from Brynolf I, Odontologisk Revy 1967;18 Suppl 11:27.

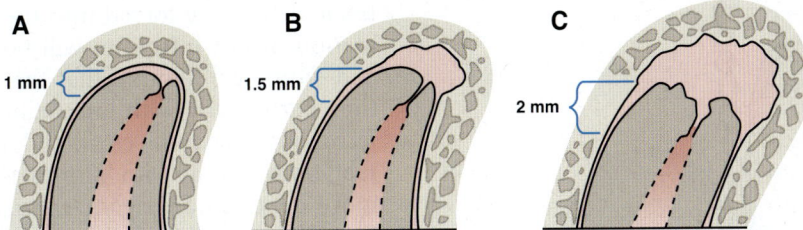

Figure 33 Weine's recommendations for determining the working length based on radiographic evidence of root/bone resorption. ***A***, If no root or bone resorption is evident, preparation should terminate 1.0 mm from the apical foramen. ***B***, If bone resorption is apparent but there is no root resorption, shorten the working length by 1.5 mm. ***C***, If both root and bone resorption are apparent, shorten the length by 2.0 mm. Courtesy of Dr. Franklin Weine.

Weine[98] (Figure 33) faced this complication early on and recommended a compromise based on the radiographic evidence. If in the radiograph there appears to be a normal periodontal ligament width, that is, no bone or tooth resorption is evident, the working length should terminate 1.0 mm, "safety allowance," from the apical foramen. If there appears to be bony resorption but no apparent tooth resorption, the working length should be shortened by 1.5 mm. On the other hand, if both bone and tooth resorption is apparent radiographically, the length of the tooth measurement should be shortened by 2.0 mm. This should "draw back" the point of apical constriction far enough in the canal to establish an apical stop. Enlarging instruments and obturation should not proceed beyond this point. In 1922, Davis[99] was the "first to suggest that careful treatment of the apical tissue was a requirement for success in root canal treatment."[100]

Weine's recommendation, however, is not infallible! Take the case exhibited by Brynolf (see Figure 32) in which the entire apical structure has been destroyed. In these cases and in youngsters where the canal is wide open, the so-called "blunderbuss" canal, the primary filling point will have to be adjusted—cut back—until it fits tightly at the apex and exhibits "tugback."

Another variation involves canal preparation following the so-called partial pulpectomy. Nygaard-Ostby showed in the case of pulpectomy of a vital, yet inflamed, pulp that it was wise to retain a portion of the pulp at the apex to assure periapical healing.[101] Careful cleaning, shaping, and obturation to this pulpal "stump" allow this tiny segment of tissue to continue producing dentin and cementum (Figure 34).

In marked contrast, three endodontic programs in the United States, in 1997, were teaching "penetration of the foramen, to or beyond the radiographic apex."[102] Schilder[103–105] declared "his aim was to debride and to fill to the apex…" He further admitted

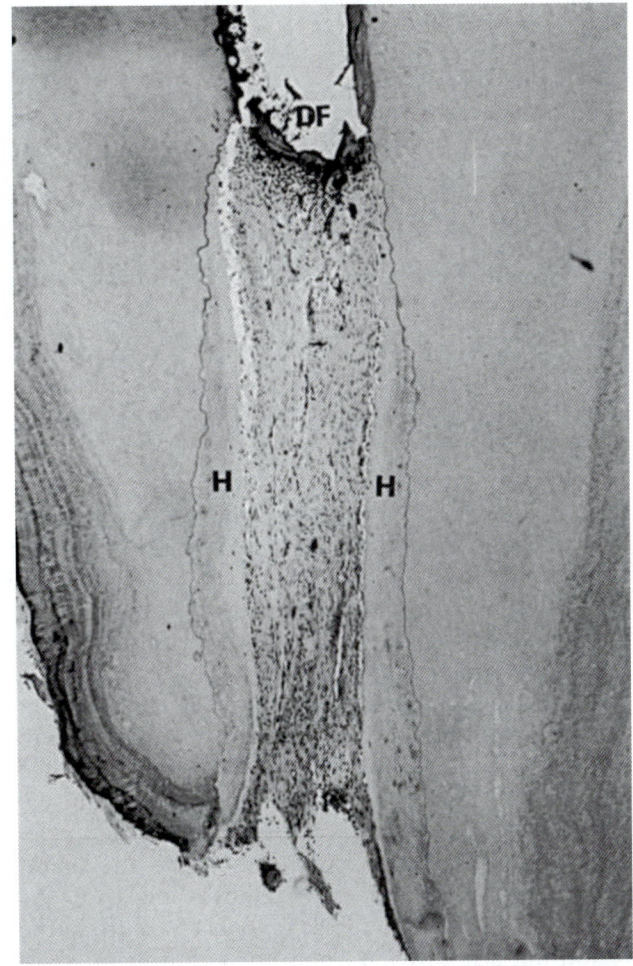

Figure 34 Partial pulpectomy. Observation period of 6 months. Only slight accumulation of lymphocytes adjacent to the plug of dentin particles and remnants of Kloropercha (DF at top). Cell-rich fibrous connective tissue occupies the residual pulp canal. Large deposits of hard tissue (H) along the walls. Reproduced with permission from Hörstad P, Nygaard-Østby B. Oral Surg Oral Path Oral Med Oral Radiol Endod 1978;46:275.

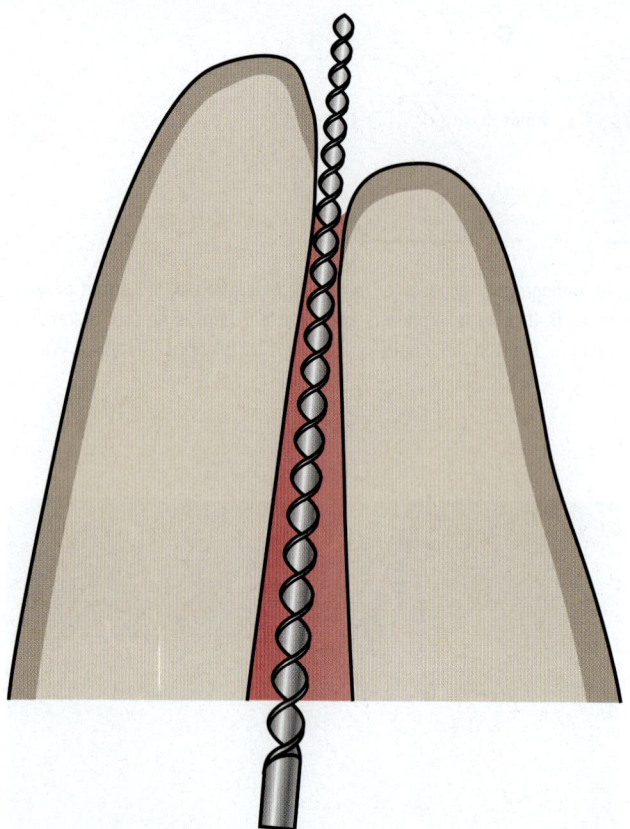

Figure 35 Overextension of root canal instrument, beyond the minor diameter to the radiographic apex, traumatizes periodontal soft tissue and may deposit toxic canal debris and bacteria periapically.

that "his procedure in most cases involved instrumentation beyond the root canal limit, inside the adjacent periodontal ligament" (Figure 35).

In addition to the concern with the extent of the working length measurement, one must also be concerned with the breadth of preparation in the apical one-third of the canal. Initially it was thought that cleansing with a No. 25 instrument was adequate in most cases. Today, however, with the advent of the nickel–titanium rotary instruments, it is not unusual to use a No. 60 or a LightSpeed instrument in an attempt to thoroughly clean and shape the apical preparation. This not only removes most of the packed tissue, dentin filings, and bacteria from the region but also provides room for a thorough irrigation with NaOCl and EDTA to remove the smear layer as well.[106] The importance of thoroughly cleansing and disinfecting this area was emphasized by Baumgartner and Falkler[107] when they disclosed the presence of 50 different strains of bacteria in the apical 5.0 mm of infected root canals, 68% of which were strict anaerobes. If these bacteria, along with tissue debris, are forced into the apical tissue, inflammation, if not infection, will be the result. Al-Omari and Dummer[108] found that this occurred 81% of the time particularly with linear filing as in the step-back technique. Hartwell et al.[109] found much the same; that linear filing with K files produced significantly more debris and irrigant extrusion than with rotary file preparation. So how can this be prevented or at least minimized?

APICAL PATENCY AND ITS PREPARATION

"Apical patency is leaving the apical foramen accessible, free from dentin chips, pulp fragments, and other debris," as well as bacteria.[110] In an excellent review of the subject entitled *The Importance of Apical Patency and Cleaning the Apical Foramen in Root Canal Preparation*, Sousa[110] points out that maintaining apical patency does not necessarily clean the foramen but avoids apical blockage by dentin chips and debris, thus retaining true working length. "The apical foramen should be instrumented to be cleaned." In 1997, a survey of 53 university endodontic departments revealed that 50% were teaching "the concept of patency to their undergraduates or graduates or both."[102] Far earlier, Buchanan and Ruddle[111,112] were advocates of maintaining apical patency, depending to a great extent on NaOCl presence and irrigation to clean the apical foramen space. Patency files passing through the NaOCl tend to be sterile.[113] Both Buchanan and Ruddle prefer to recapitulate, beyond the working length, to the foramen with a No. 10 or No. 15 0.02 file after each enlarging instrument is used. They also suggest that fresh NaOCl is to be left in the canal for another 5 min or so. Sousa[110] also recommends using a file, one or two sizes beyond the last enlarging instrument to clean the remaining space to the foramen. Remember the 50 strains of bacteria that may be lurking there!

So what does this all "boil down to?" It boils down to success versus failure, healing versus disease. In the final analysis, where should the preparation and the obturation terminate? As far as preparation is concerned, a good case has been made that the apical constriction, 0.5–1.0 mm short of the apical foramen, is the best point for termination. This should be followed by maintaining apical patency and then cleaning and disinfecting the tiny area to the apical foramen.

As far as obturation is concerned, "[I]n terms of percentage rates of success, metaanalysis showed that obturation 0 to 1.0 mm short of the apex (group A) was better than obturation 1 to 3 mm short of the apex (group B); both [groups] were superior to obturation beyond the apex (group C)."[114] "This finding is not surprising; it has been shown that obturating materials in periradicular tissues are an irritant and they adversely impact healing".[100]

Modern endodontics, therefore, extends from efforts to save the pulp—pulp capping—to implants. To be proficient as a specialist, one must be knowledgeable as well as skillful. That should not be asking too much! After all we are dealing with the smallest organ in the body.

A case for change has been made in this chapter; change that has affected our past, change that is presently occurring, and changes that will undoubtedly affect our future. But we may be in for a big surprise. Already underway, our scientists are plotting to grow human teeth in the laboratory that could then be implanted in place of their diseased or damaged precursors. Who is to say they will not succeed? At least we should start considering the possibility.

Anticipating the Future

The opportunities for oral health care in the twenty-first century are enormous. Perhaps foremost is the realization of comprehensive oral health care, and this will require health literacy, health promotion, risk assessment, and advances in disease and disorder prevention. The profession still faces an enormous backlog of dental disease and must make every effort and employ all our skills and knowledge to improve the nation's oral health. "More than 51 million school hours are lost each year because of dental illness. Dental disease is the single most common chronic childhood disease—five times more common than asthma."[115]

The twenty-first century also promises remarkable advances and transformations by the convergence of six major determinants, any one of which might be sufficient to profoundly transform well-being and quality of life for many, many millions of people:

1. The biological and biotechnological revolutions
2. A major redistribution and increase in global population
3. Changing demographics in industrialized as well as developing nations
4. Changing patterns of diseases and disorders, including the emergence and re-emergence of infectious diseases (often with unique pathogens), and changes in the organization and the management of health care
5. Instant global communication systems through the Internet, cable, satellite, and wireless technologies
6. A continuing exponential rate of growth in information technology, especially driven by bioinformatics and nanotechnology that will advance computer speed, memory, and complexity.

These global six determinants are already changing the way we live now and they will continue to have profound implications for the future of health care, oral health care, endodontics and well-being of all people.[115]

The Past and Present as Prologue for the Future

The intellectual activity and contributions from the eighteenth, nineteenth, and twentieth centuries have provided the foundations for present-day science and technology. Moreover, more has been learned and implemented in the last 100 years than in the past 5,000 years. The rate and magnitude of scientific discovery, the fuel for the engine of technology, continues to accelerate. The convergence of the biological and digital revolutions with clinical dentistry and medicine is changing and transforming diagnostics, treatment planning, procedures, techniques, therapeutics, biomaterials, and predictable outcomes of therapy.[116-134] We have come a long way since Pasteur, Koch, Ehrlich, and Vannevar Bush established the foundations for the emerging fields of microbiology, immunology, and computer sciences during the last century. In tandem, dental and medical education were transformed vis-à-vis the Flexner and Gies Reports from the 1920s in America, and today we are anticipating another level of major transformation in health professional education.[135]

The seeds were sown for the convergence of chemistry, physics, and biology into molecular biology, as well as the convergence of Charles Darwin's theories of evolution with fruit fly genetics, population genetics and DNA sequencing of 38,000-year-old bones of Neanderthal into the synthesis of evolutionary biology. These enormous efforts have produced a foundation that enabled the Human Genome Project to be completed by October 2004 and further to acquire a molecular genetic data base for many viral, bacterial, yeast, plant, invertebrate, vertebrate, primate, and human genomes.[136-139] These efforts further established the foundations for bioinformatics, tissue engineering, nanobiotechnology, stem cell biology, and tissue and organ regenerations.[116–134] Our future perspective is filled with enthusiasm.

Transforming Advances

Three transforming advances will be highlighted: (1) saliva as a diagnostic and informative fluid, (2) tissue engineering, and (3) tooth regeneration.

SALIVA AS A DIAGNOSTIC AND INFORMATIVE FLUID

During the last decade, enormous progress has been made in identifying informative biomarkers found in saliva, and also in identifying oral buccal epithelial cells from which DNA can be extracted for human genomic studies and diagnostics.

Today, saliva is being used to harvest oral buccal epithelial cells and to thereby isolate genomic DNA representing 23,000 human genes and to be able to ascertain single nucleotide polymorphisms informative for complex human diseases. Beyond genomics, saliva is also informative for biomarkers that indicate viral infections such as measles, mumps, rubella, hepatitis A and B and, of course, HIV-1 and -2. Direct antigen detection is also available for influenza A and B, streptococcus group A (N-acetylglucosamine), salivary estradiol, several breast cancer biomarkers (e.g., CA-15, epidermal growth factor receptor (EGFR), cathepsin-D and Waf 1), zinc-binding cystic fibrosis antigen, and several markers for type 2 diabetes. Beyond the hundreds of different types of oral bacteria species as well as yeast organisms, many hormones and drugs such as aldosterone, cortisol, estrogens, insulin, melatonin, progesterone, testosterone, carbamazepine, lithium, methadone, phenytoin antipyrine, threohilline, caffeine, cocaine, continine, ethanol, marijuana, and various opiates are now identified and measured in saliva. And the list continues with the addition of informative messenger RNAs (so-called "transcriptome" representing human saliva).

Further, miniature devices for "point-of-care" are being developed for salivary diagnostics using microfluidics, microcapillary electrophoresis, and other nanobiotechnology advances.

TISSUE ENGINEERING

As clinicians, it is our opportunity to translate the fundamental discoveries of science and technology, as are now rapidly occurring in stem cell biology, molecular biology, genomics, functional genomics, and biomaterials/biotechnology/information technology, into concrete advancements for our patients and communities. This approach provides a bridge over which clinicians can traverse to learn how to apply scientific advances in tissue engineering and regeneration to their clinical practices.

The convergence between stem cells and biotechnology has made it possible to envision the design and fabrication of biological tissues applicable to a large number of human diseases and disorders. Three decades ago, the first tissue engineering proof of principle was established with bone marrow transplantation for myelogenous leukemia. Less than 10 years ago, the first cartilage tissue engineering product was approved by the FDA and is being used for a variety of knee applications.

Tissue engineering is a contemporary field of biomedical therapy focused at developing and improving procedures and complementary biomaterials for the design and fabrication of new tissues to replace damaged tissues and is based upon the principles of cell biology, developmental biology, molecular biology, and bioengineering. Tissue engineering is presently focused on tissue replacements such as bone, cementum, dentin and enamel as well as periodontal ligament, oral mucosa, muscle and nerves. Recent progress has literally been astonishing.[116–136, 139–143]

TOOTH REGENERATION

The prospects for tooth regeneration are enormously promising.[144] During the past 50 years, a foundation has been provided for understanding the evolution, developmental biology, histogenesis and differentiation, and extracellular matrix-mediated biomineralization of vertebrate tooth organs. Based upon the knowledge of biological principles, it is becoming readily feasible to design and fabricate tooth organs in the not too distant future.[144]

Is the knowledge base and techniques presently available sufficient to design and fabricate tooth organs for tooth replacement applications in clinical dentistry? Does the knowledge gained from experimental embryology, autotransplantation of teeth, human genetics, adult stem cell biology, and the identification of human and mouse morphoregulatory genes for tooth morphogenesis lead to biomimetic designs and fabrication for tooth regeneration?

The answer to these questions would appear to be affirmative. For example, the National Institutes of Health recently released a Request for Applications to establish Centers for Excellence in Regenerative Medicine with tooth organ regeneration being one of the suggested models. It is becoming readily apparent that despite many of the recent clinical advances in mechanical solutions to tooth restoration and dental implants, or the advancements of autotransplantation of human teeth for tooth replacement, the twenty-first century provides a number of unique opportunities to enable biological solutions to biological problems including tooth organ regeneration. The recent convergence of the human genome completion,[136–138] scientific advances toward understanding the molecular regulation of tooth morphogenesis,[144] stem cell biology,[125,126,140,141] nanotechnology, and biotechnology offer unprecedented opportunities to realize tooth regeneration. One of the next critical steps will be to apply the knowledge of molecular regulation of tooth morphogenesis to manipulate adult stem cells in becoming odontogenic phenotypes.

Significant progresses have been made in stem cell biological research, which has advanced our understanding in the area of hematopoiesis, tissue engineering (e.g., bone, cartilage, and muscle), and biomaterials. Recently, studies have shown that adult stem cells have a much higher degree of developmental potential than previously thought, and this has prompted considerations to explore the potential of stem cell-mediated muscle, bone, cartilage, and dentin regeneration.

Stem cells are truly remarkable. They have the potential to grow into an array of specialized cells and hold great promise for treating medical and dental conditions, such as missing teeth. Conventionally, these pluripotent cells are divided into embryonic and adult stem cells. The difference is mainly in the number of types of differentiated cells that can be produced by the stem cell. When exploring the potential of stem cell-mediated tissue regeneration, recent studies have focused on the application of adult bone marrow because it is readily accessible and contains both hematopoietic and stromal fibroblast stem cells.[120–129] Systemically injected mouse bone marrow-derived cells have given rise to muscle, cartilage, bone, liver, heart, brain, lung alveolar epithelium, intestine, and, of course, hematocytes. Although most of these animal studies now serve as precursors for future human clinical trials in treating certain medical and dental conditions, the basic scientific principles learned from these current analyses have certainly advanced our understanding of the biological regulation of tissue engineering. In contrast to previous paradigms, postnatal stem cells have a much greater potential when it comes to tissue regeneration.

To date, there is no study demonstrating bone marrow-mediated tooth regeneration. This might be attributed to an as yet incomplete understanding of proper manipulation of adult somatic stem cells and several other confounding issues. The knowledge of molecular regulation of tooth morphogenesis will significantly enhance the focus on the importance of signaling pathways when studies begin to explore the regulatory issues of progenitor cell differentiation.[144–147] Accordingly, as studies begin to discover the precise molecular regulation of stem cell proliferation and differentiation, bone marrow-derived progenitors hold great promise in tooth regeneration.[116]

Meanwhile, odontogenic stem cells have been identified, isolated, and tested from adult dental pulp tissue.[117,130,133,148] After being transplanted into immunocompromised mice, dental pulp stem cells regenerate dentin-like tissue; curiously, the quantity of regenerated dentin tissue appears to far exceed the dentin tissue generated in situ during the lifetime of a particular tooth organ. Thus, odontogenic stem cells isolated from adult dental pulp can serve as a resource to regenerate large amount of dentin tissue that can be used in tooth repair.

Collectively, a new paradigm is emerging, which suggests an understanding of common mechanisms that are critical in regulating the fate of stem cells. These discoveries also reveal several signaling networks that underlie the specific regulatory properties of tooth morphogenesis. Indeed, there remain many questions and technical obstacles before stem cells will be used to regenerate teeth. However, there are several significant lines of evidence to consider, which are as follows:

1. Enamel organ epithelia and dental papilla mesenchymal tissues contain stem cells during postnatal stages of life
2. Late cap stage and bell stage tooth organs contain stem cells
3. Odontogenic adult stem cells respond to mechanical as well as chemical "signals".
4. Presumably, adult bone marrow as well as dental pulp tissues contain "odontogenic" stem cells
5. Epithelial–mesenchymal interactions are prerequisite for tooth regeneration.

The authors express "guarded enthusiasm," yet there is a little doubt that adult stem cell-mediated tooth regeneration will be realized in the not too distant future. The advances in basic, translational, and pre-phase 1 clinical trials are impressive. In tandem, the changing demographics within industrial nations indicate an increasing societal demand for "body parts" to address the quality of life issues for aging populations. The prospects for tooth regeneration could be realized in the next few decades and could be rapidly utilized to improve the quality of human life in many nations around the world.

References

1. Ingle JI. A suggested nomenclature for pulpal and periapical pathosis. J Seattle Dist Dent Soc 1963;1:11.

2. Beveridge EE. The measurement of human dental intrapulpal pressure and its response to clinical variables. Oral Surg Oral Med Oral Pathol Oral Radiol Endod 1965;19:655.

3. Van Hassel HJ. Physiology of the human dental pulp. Oral Surg Oral Med Oral Pathol Oral Radiol Endod 1971;32:126.

4. Orban B. Classification and nomenclature of periodontal diseases. J Periodont 1942;13:88.

5. Ingle JI. The need for endodontic instrument standardization. Oral Surg Oral Med Oral Pathol Oral Radiol Endod 1955;8:1211.

6. Ingle JI, Levine M. The need for uniformity of endodontic instruments, equipment and filling materials. In: Grossman, LI editor. Transactions of the Second International Conference on Endodontics. Philadelphia, PA: University of Penn; 1958. p.123.

7. Ingle JI. A standardized endodontic technique utilizing newly designed instruments and filling materials. Oral Surg Oral Med Oral Pathol Oral Radiol Endod 1961;14:83.

8. Revised ANSI/ADA specification N0. 28 for root canal files and reamers Type K. American Dental Association Council on Dental Materials, Instruments & Equipment. Chicago. J Am Dent Assoc Press 2002.

9. American Association of Endodontists. Definition of Endodontics. AAE Membership Roster; 2005–2006.

10. Brown JL, Nash KD, Warren M. The economics of endodontics. Draft 8/12/2003, American Dental Association, Survey Center, 1999 Survey of Dental Services Rendered.

11. Johns BA, Brown LJ, Nash KD, Warren M. The endodontic workforce. J Endod 2006;32(9):838.

12. Burns, R. Survey documents more people choosing root canal therapy over extractions. Report of the Public Affairs Committee of the American Association of Endodontists. Public education report. April 1987.

13. American Association of Endodontists press release March 29, 2000. Pain jokes no laughing matter to root canal specialists. http//www.aae.org/pressroom/ releases/newspain.htm.

14. Watkins CA. Anticipated and experienced pain associated with endodontic therapy. J Am Dent Assoc 2002;133:45.

15. Molven O, Halse A, Riordan PJ. Prevalence and distribution of root filled teeth in former dental school patients: follow-up after 10–17 years. Int Endod J 1985;18:247.

16. Torrey Report. American Dental Trade Association; 1984.

17. Dental products marketing strategic survey—1997: Strategic Dental Marketing.

18. American Dental Association. The Economics of Endodontics; 2005.

19. American Association of Endodontists recertification document; 1989.

20. American Dental Association, Survey Center, 1982–2003. Distribution of Dentists in the United States by Region & State.

21. National Institute of Dental Research. Dental caries continues downward trend in children. J Am Dent Assoc 1988;117:625.

22. Beltran-Aguilar ED, Barker LK, Teresa Canto M, et al. Surveillance for dental caries, dental sealants, tooth retention, edentulism, and enamel fluorosis—United States, 1988–1994 and 1999–2002. MMWR Surveill Summ 2005;54(3):1–43.

23. Brown LJ, Wall TP, Lazar V. Trends in total caries experience: permanent and primary teeth. J Am Dent Assoc 2000;131(2):223–31.

24. Brown E. Children's dental visits and expenses, United States, 2003 Statistical brief #117. March 2006 Agency for Healthcare Research and Quality, Rockville, MD. http//www.Meps.ahrq.gov/papers/st117/stat118.pdf.

25. National Institute of Dental Research. Survey of adult dental health. J Am Dent Assoc 1987;114:829

26. Famili P, Cauley J, Suzuki JB, Weyant R. Longitudinal study of periodontal disease and edentulism with rates of bone loss in older women. J Periodontol 2005;76(1):11–15.

27. Bailit H, Newhouse J, Brook R, et al. Does more generous dental insurance coverage improve oral health? J Am Dent Assoc 1985;110:701.

28. Manski RJ, Edelstein BL, Moeller JF. The impact of insurance coverage on children's dental visits and expenditures 1996. J Am Dent Assoc 2001;132(8):1137–45.

29. Wall TP, Brown LJ. Recent trends in dental visits and private dental insurance, 1988 & 1999. J Am Dent Assoc 2003;134(5):621–7.

30. Sommers JP. Dental expenditures in the 10 largest states, 2003. Statistical brief #112, Jan. 2006. Agency for Healthcare Research & Quality, Rockville, MD. http/www.meps.ahrq.gov/papers/st112stat112.pdf.

31. American Dental Association. 2002 Survey of Dental Practice. Endodontists in private practice; 2004.

32. Brown LJ. Net income, gross billings and practice expenditures of independent dentists. J Am Dent Assoc 1998;129(7):1031–5.

33. American Dental Association. 2004 Survey of Dental Practice—Income from the Private Practice of Dentistry (January 2006).

34. American Dental Association. Consumer Price Index for Dental Services, 1970–2005. Published 2006.

35. US Dept of Human Services. Oral health in America: a report of the Surgeon General. Rockville, MD: US Dept. of Health & Human Services, National Institute of Dental & Craniofacial Research; National Institutes of Health; 2000. http/www2.nidcr.nih.gov/sgr/execsuum.htm.

36. Milgrom P, Fiset L, Melnick S, Weinstein P. The prevalence and practice management consequences of dental fear in a major US city. J Am Dent Assoc 1988;116:641.

37. Gatchel RJ. The prevalence of dental fear and avoidance: expanded adult and recent adolescent surveys. J Am Dent Assoc 1989;118:591.

38. LeClaire AJ, Skidmore AE, Griffin JA Jr, Balaban FS. Endodontic fear survey. J Endod 1988;14:560.

39. Lord J, Teel S. The overdenture: patient selection, use of copings. J Prosthet Dent 1974;32:41

40. Hayward JR, Kerr DA, Jesse RH, Ingle JI. The management of teeth related to the treatment of oral cancer. CA Cancer J Clin 1969;19:98.

41. Hiatt WH. Regeneration of the periodontium after endodontic therapy and flap operation. Oral Surg Oral Med Oral Pathol Oral Radiol Endod 1959;12:1471.

42. Prichard J. The intrabony technique as a predictable procedure. J Periodontol 1957;28:202.

43. Sommer RF, Ostrander FD, Crowley MC. Clinical endodontics. 2nd ed. Philadelphia, PA: WB Saunders; 1961.

44. Grossman LI, Rossman SR. Correlation of clinical diagnosis and histopathologic findings in 101 pulpless teeth with areas of rarefaction [abstract]. J Dent Res 1955;34:692.

45. Priebe WA, Lazansky JP, Wuehrmann AH. The value of roentgenographic film in the differential diagnosis of periradicular lesions. Oral Surg Oral Med Oral Pathol Oral Radiol Endod 1954;7:979.

46. Bhaskar SN. Synopsis of oral pathology. 7th ed. St. Louis, MO: CV Mosby; 1986.

47. Crump MC, Natkin E. Relationship of broken root canal instruments to endodontic case prognosis: a clinical investigation. J Am Dent Assoc 1970;80:1341.

48. Calhoun RL, Landers RR. One-appointment endodontic therapy: a nationwide survey of endodontists. J Endod 1982;8:35.

49. Landers RR, Calhoun RL. One-appointment endodontic therapy: an opinion survey. J Endod. 1980;6:799.

50. Walton R, Fouad A. Endodontic interappointment flare-ups: a prospective study of incidence and related factors. J Endod 1992;18:172.

51. Fox JL, Atkinson JS, Dinin PA. Incidence of pain following one-visit endodontic treatment. Oral Surg Oral Med Oral Pathol Oral Radiol Endod 1970;30:123.

52. Wolch I. The one-appointment endodontic technique. J Can Dent Assoc 1975;41:613.

53. Soltanoff W. Comparative study of the single visit and multiple visit endodontic procedure. J Endod 1978;4:278.

54. Ether S, et al. A comparison of one and two visit endodontics. J Farmacia Odontol New Orleans, Louisiana State Univ 1978;8:215.

55. Pekruhn RB. Single-visit endodontic therapy: a preliminary clinical study. J Am Dent Assoc 1981;103:875.

56. Oliet S. Single-visit endodontic therapy: a preliminary clinical study. J Am Dent Assoc 1981;103:873.

57. Galberry JH. Incidence of post-operative pain in one appointment and multi-appointment endodontic treatment: a pilot study [thesis]. Louisiana State University, Baton Rouge, LA; 1983.

58. Nakamuta H, Nagasawa H. Study on endodontic treatment of infected root canals in one visit. Personal communication; 1983.

59. Mulhern JM, Patterson SS, Newton CW, Ringel AM. Incidence of postoperative pain after one appointment endodontic treatment of asymptomatic pulpal necrosis in single-rooted teeth. J Endod 1982;8:370.

60. Roane JB, Dryden JA, Grimes EW. Incidence of post-operative pain after single- and multiple-visit endodontic procedures. Oral Surg Oral Med Oral Pathol Oral Radiol Endod 1983;55:68.

61. Genet J. Factors determining the incidence of post-operative pain in endodontic therapy. J Endod 1986;12:126.

62. Fava L. A comparison of one versus two appointment endodontic therapy in teeth with non-vital pulps. Int Endod J 1979;22:179.

63. Fava L. One appointment root canal treatment: incidence of post-operative pain using a modified double flared technique. Int Endod J 1991;24:258.

64. Fava L. A clinical evaluation of one and two-appointment root canal therapy using calcium hydroxide. Int Endod J 1994;27.

65. Trope M. Flare-up rate of single-visit endodontics. Int Endod J 1991;24:24.

66. Harrison JW, Baumgartner JC, Svec TA. Incidence of pain associated with clinical factors during and after root canal therapy. Part I. Interappointment pain. J Endod 1983;9:384.

67. Eleazer PD, Eleazer KR. Flare-up rate in pulpally necrotic molars in one-visit versus two-visit endodontic treatment. J Endod 1998;24:614.

68. Ørstavik O, Sigurdsson A, Moiseiwitsch J, et al. Sensory and affective characteristics of pain following treatment of chronic apical periodontitis [abstract]. J Dent Res 1996;75:373.

69. Al-Negrish A, Habahbeh R. Flare-up rate related to root canal treatment of asymptomatic pulpally necrotic central incisor teeth in patients attending a military hospital. J Dent 2006;34:635

70. Pekruhn R. The incidence in failure following single-visit endodontic therapy. J Endod 1986;12:68.

71. Sjögren U, Figdor D, Persson S, Sundqvist G. Influence of infection at the time of root filling on the outcome of the endodontic treatment of teeth with apical periodontitis. Int Endod J 1997;30:297.

72. Ørstavik D, Kerekes K, Molven O. Effects of apical reaming and calcium hydroxide dressing on bacterial infection during treatment of apical periodontitis. Int Endod J 1991;24:1.

73. Ingle JI, Zeldow BJ. An evaluation of mechanical instrumentation and the negative culture in endodontic therapy. J Am Dent Assoc 1958;57:471.
74. Zeldow BJ, Ingle JI. Correlation of the positive culture to the prognosis of endodontically treated teeth. J Am Dent Assoc 1963;66:23.
75. Trope M, Delano EO, Orstavik D. Endodontic treatment of teeth with apical periodontitis: single vs. multivisit treatment. J Endod 1999;25:345.
76. Katebzadeh N, Hupp J, Trope M. Histological periapical repair after obturation of infected canals in dogs. J Endod 1999;25:364.
77. Inoue N, Skinner DH. A simple and accurate way of measuring root canal length. J Endod 1985;11:421.
78. Bramante CM, Berbert A. A critical evaluation of some methods of determining tooth length. Oral Surg Oral Med Oral Pathol Oral Radiol Endod 1974;37:463.
79. Seidberg BH, Alibrandi BU, Fine H, Logue B. Clinical investigation of measuring working length of root canals with an electronic device and with digital-tactile sense. J Am Dent Assoc 1975;90:379.
80. Simon JHS. The apex: how critical is it? Gen Dent 1994;42:330.
81. American Association of Endodontists. Glossary: contemporary terminology for endodontics. 6th ed. Chicago, IL: American Association of Endodontists; 1998.
82. Kuttler Y. Microscopic investigation of root apexes. J Am Dent Assoc 1955;50:544.
83. Dummer PMH, McGinn JH, Ree DG. The position and topography of the apical constriction and apical foramen. Int Endod J 1984;17:192.
84. Palmer MJ, Weine FS, Healey HJ. Position of the apical foramen in relation to endodontic therapy. J Can Dent Assoc 1971;8:305.
85. Green D. A stereomicroscopic study of the root apicies of 400 maxillary and mandibular teeth. Oral Surg Oral Med Oral Pathol Oral Radiol Endod 1956;9:249.
86. Green FN. Microscopic investigation of root canal diameters. J Am Dent Assoc 1958;57:636.
87. Green D. Stereomicroscopic study of 700 root apices of maxillary and mandibular teeth. Oral Surg Oral Med Oral Pathol Oral Radiol Endod 1960;13:728.
88. Chapman CE. A microscopic study of the apical region of human anterior teeth. J Br Endod Soc 1969;3:52.
89. Morfis A, Sylaras SN, Georgopoulou M, et al. Study of the apices of human permanent teeth with the use of a scanning electron microscope. Oral Surg Oral Med Oral Pathol Oral Radiol Endod 1994;77:172.
90. Guiterrez G, Aguayo P. Apical foraminal openings in human teeth. Number and location. Oral Surg Oral Med Oral Pathol Oral Radiol Endod 1995;79:769.
91. Langeland K, cited in Riccuci D. Apical limit of root canal instrumentation and obturation. Int Endod J 1998;31:384.
92. Kuttler Y. A precision and biologic root canal filling technique. J Am Dent Assoc 1958;58:38.
93. Storms JL. Factors that influence success of endodontic treatment. J Can Dent Assoc 1969;35:83.
94. Levy AB, Glatt L. Deviation of the apical foramen from the radiographic apex. J NJ State Dent Soc 1970;41:12.
95. Burch JG, Hulen S. The relationship of the apical foramen to the anatomic apex of the tooth root. Oral Surg Oral Med Oral Pathol Oral Radiol Endod 1972;34:262.
96. Tamse A, Kaffe I, Fishel D. Zygomatic bone and interference with correct radiographic diagnosis in maxillary molar endodontics. Oral Surg Oral Med Oral Pathol Oral Radiol Endod 1980;50:563.
97. Brynolf I. Radiography of the periradicular region as a diagnostic aid. I. Diagnosis of marginal changes. Dent Radiogr Photogr 1978;51:21.
98. Weine FS. Endodontic therapy. St. Louis, MO: CV Mosby; 1982.
99. Davis WC. Pulpectomy versus pulp extirpation. Dent Items 1922;44:81–100.
100. Ricucci D, Langeland K. Apical limit of root canal instrumentation and obturation, part 2: a histologic study. Int Endod J 1998;31:394.
101. Horstad P, Nygaard-Ostby B. Partial pulpectomy. Oral Surg Oral Med Oral Pathol Oral Radiol Endod 1978;46:275.
102. Cailleteau JG, Mullaney TP. Prevalence of teaching patency and various instrumentation and obturation techniques in United States dental schools. J Endod 1997;23:394.
103. Schilder H. Filling root canals in three dimensions. Dent Clin North Am 1967;11:723–44.
104. Schilder H. Canal debridement and disinfection. In: Cohen S, Burns RC, editors. Pathways of the pulp. 2nd ed. St. Louis, MO: CV Mosby; 1976. p. 111.
105. Ricucci D. Apical limit of root canal instrumentation and obturation, part 1: Literature Review. Int Endod J 1998;31:384.
106. Khademi A, et al. Determination of the minimum instrumentation size for penetration of irrigants to the apical third of root canal systems. J Endod 2006;32:417.
107. Baumgartner JC, Falkler WA. Bacteria in the apical 5mm of infected root canals. J Endod 1991;17:380.
108. Al-Omari MAO, Dummer PMH. Canal blockage and debris extrusion with eight preparation techniques. J Endod 1995;21:154.
109. Beeson TJ, Hartwell GR. Comparison of debris extruded apically in straight canals: conventional filing versus 0.04 taper series 29. J Endod 1998;24:18.
110. Sousa RA. The importance of apical patency and cleaning of the apical foramen on root canal preparation. Braz Dent J 2006;17:6.

111. Buchanan S. Management of the curved root canal. J Calif Dent Assoc 1989;17:18.

112. Ruddle CJ. Alpha Omega Webcast, Oct. 19; 2006.

113. Izu KH, Thomas SJ, Zhang P, et al. Effectiveness of sodium hypochlorite in preventing inoculation of periapical tissues with contaminated patency files. J Endod 2004;30:92.

114. Schaeffer MA, White RR, Walton RE. Determining the optimum obturation length: a meta-analysis of literature. J Endod 2005;31:271.

115. United States. Dept. of Health and Human Services. National Institute of Dental and Craniofacial Research (US). Oral health in America: a report of the Surgeon General. Rockville, MD: US Public Health Service, Dept. of Health and Human Services; 2000.

116. Slavkin HC, Bartold PM. Challenges and potential in tissue engineering. Periodontology 2000–2006;41:9–15.

117. Bartold PM, Xiao Y, Lyngstaadas SP, et al. Principles and applications of cell delivery systems for periodontal regeneration. Periodontology 2000–2006;41:123–35.

118. Baum BJ, Tran SD. Synergy between genetic and tissue engineering: creating an artificial salivary gland. Periodontology 2000–2006;41:218–23.

119. Duailibi MT, Duailibi SE, Young CS, et al. Bioengineered teeth from cultured rat tooth bud cells. J Dent Res 2004;83:523–8.

120. Duailibi SE, Duailibi MT, Vacanti JP, Yelick PC. Prospects for tooth regeneration. Periodontology 2000–2006;41:177–87.

121. Ellingsen JE, Thomsen P, Lyngstadaas SP. Advances in dental implant materials and tissue regeneration. Periodontology 2000–2006;41:136–56.

122. Genco RJ, Scannapieco FA, Slavkin HC. Oral reports. The Sciences 2000;Nov/Dec:25–30.

123. Gronthos S, Akintoye SO, Wang CY, Shi S. Bone marrow stromal stem cells for tissue engineering. Periodontology 2000–2006;41:188–95.

124. Hsiong SX, Mooney DJ. Regeneration of vascularized bone. Periodontology 2000–2006;41:109–22.

125. Iohara K, Nakashima M, Ito M, et al. Dentin regeneration by dental pulp stem cell therapy with recombinant human bone morphogenetic protein 2. J Dent Res 2004;83:590–5.

126. Lavik E, Langer R. Tissue engineering: current state and perspectives. Appl Microbiol Biotechnol 2004;65:1–8.

127. Moradian-Oldak J, Wen HB, Schneider GB, Stanford CM. Tissue engineering strategies for the future generation of dental implants. Periodontology 2000–2006;41:157–76.

128. Ohazama A, Modino SA, Miletich I, Sharpe PT. Stem-cell-based tissue engineering of murine teeth. J Dent Res 2004;83(7):518–22.

129. Polimeni G, Xiropaidis AV, Wikesjo UM. Biology and principles of periodontal wound healing/regeneration. Periodontology 2000–2006;41:30–47.

130. Ripamonti U, Renton L. Bone morphogenetic proteins and the induction of periodontal tissue regeneration. Periodontology 2000–2006;41:73–87.

131. Slavkin HC. Applications of pharmacogenomics in general dental practice. Pharmacogenomics 2003;4:163–70.

132. Slavkin HC. Genomes, biofilms, and implications for oral health professionals. Dimens Dent Hyg 2003;1:16–20.

133. Srisuwan T, Tilkorn DJ, Wilson JL, et al. Molecular aspects of tissue engineering in the dental field. Periodontology 2000–2006;41:88–108.

134. Zeichner-David M. Regeneration of periodontal tissues: cementogenesis revisited. Periodontol 2000–2006;41:196–217.

135. DePaola DP, Slavkin HC. Reforming dental health professions education: a white paper. J Dent Educ 2004;68:1139–50.

136. International Human Genome Sequencing Consortium. Initial sequencing and analysis of the human genome. Nature 2001;409:860–921.

137. Human Genome Resources, National Center for Biotechnology Information, National Institutes of Health. 2005. http://www.ncbi.nlm.nih.gov/genome/guide/ (accessed January 2005).

138. International Human Genome Sequencing Consortium. Finishing the euchromatic sequence of the human genome. Nature 2004;431(7011):931–45.

139. McElheny V. Watson and DNA: making a scientific revolution. Hoboken, NJ: Perseus/Wiley; 2003.

140. Miura M, Gronthos S, Zhao M, et al. SHED: stem cells from human exfoliated deciduous teeth. Proc Natl Acad Sci USA 2003;100:5807–12.

141. Kaufman DS, Hanson ET, Lewis RL, et al. Hematopoietic colony-forming cells derived from human embryonic stem cells. Proc Natl Acad Sci USA 2001;98:10716–21.

142. Hughes FJ, Turner W, Belibasakis G, Martuscelli G. Effects of growth factors and cytokines on osteoblast differentiation. Periodontology 2000–2006;41:48–72.

143. Parsons AB. The proteus effect: stem cells and their promise for medicine. Washington, DC: National Academy of Sciences Press; 2004.

144. Chai Y, Slavkin HC. Prospects for tooth regeneration in the 21st century: a perspective. Microsc Res Tech 2003;60:469–79.

145. Bei M, Maas R. FGFs and BMP4 induce both Msx1-independent and Msx1-dependent signaling pathways in early tooth development. Development 1998;125:4325–33.

146. Jernvall J, Thesleff I. Reiterative signaling and patterning during mammalian tooth morphogenesis. Mech Dev 2000;92:19–29.

147. Shum L, Takahashi K, Takahashi I, et al. Embryogenesis and the classification of craniofacial dysmorphogenesis. In: Fonseca R, editor. Oral and maxillofacial surgery. Vol. 6. Philadelphia, PA: WB Saunders; 2000. pp. 149–94.

148. Gronthos S, Mankani M, Brahim J, et al. Postnatal human dental pulp stem cells (DPSCs) in vitro and in vivo. Proc Natl Acad Sci USA 2000;97:13625–30.

Chapter 2

History of Endodontics

James L. Gutmann

Endodontics is the branch of dentistry concerned with the morphology, physiology, and pathology of the human dental pulp and periapical tissues. Its study and practice encompass the basic clinical sciences including biology of the normal pulp; the etiology, diagnosis, prevention and treatment of diseases and injuries of the pulp; and associated periapical conditions.[1] However, while this represents the contemporary definition of endodontics, the true codification for the art and science of this discipline really did not occur until its recognition as a specialty and in fact it was not even until the first part of the twentieth century that the concept of "endodontics" began to take shape.

In the latter part of the nineteenth and the first part of the twentieth century, endodontics was referred to as root canal therapy or pathodontia.[2] Dr. Harry B. Johnston, of Atlanta, Georgia, a well-known lecturer and clinician in the early twentieth century coined the term endodontics from the Greek word "*en*," meaning in or within, and "*odous*," meaning tooth: the process of working within the tooth. In 1928, his practice was identified as the first practice to be "limited to endodontics."

In 1943 when a group of distinguished dental professionals met in Chicago to form an association of dental practitioners interested in root canal therapy, they used the term "endodontics" and called the organization the American Association of Endodontics. They envisioned endodontics as becoming a special area of dental practice. In an editorial that appeared in the first issue of the *Journal of Endodontia* in 1946, Dr. Balint Orban highlighted the need for the pursuit of quality within this emerging specialty.[3] "Today after much work and thought, things are looking brighter. The 'Endodontist' is not anymore a rebel against the ruling of 'science' but a recognized specialist of dentistry. The technique has been refined to such a degree that it gives standing to the dentist even in the eyes of the medical profession, and safety to the patient. Since root canal treatment has been elevated to the status of a specialty, those who intend to do this work must adequately prepare themselves for it."

The founding fathers of the American Association of Endodontists (AAE) responded to the call from three distinguished individuals as follows.[4] "On a call from Dr. W. Clyde Davis of Lincoln, Nebraska, Dr. John H. Hospers of Chicago and Dr. Louis I. Grossman of Philadelphia, a group of nineteen dentists whose names follow, met [on February 25] in Dining Room 4 at the Palmer House in Chicago for the purpose of organizing a society for the study of root canal therapy, with Dr. Hospers in the chair. The following were present: Dr. Charles M. White, Dr. G. L. Girardot, Dr. George C. Sharp, Dr. Saul Levy, Dr. Truman B. DeWitt, Dr. Douglas A. Meinig, Dr. T. C. Starshak, Dr. Henry Kahn, Dr. Sophia Bolotny, Dr. John H. Hospers, Dr. Harry B. Johnston, Dr. Edgar D. Coolidge, Dr. S.D. Green, Dr. Paul T. Dawson, Dr. George W. Meinig, Dr. J. W. Ritter, Dr. Vincent B. Milas, Dr. Arthur R. Sample and Dr. Clyde Davis."

By 1963, more than 200 dentists were limiting their practice to endodontics.[5]

Because of the remarkable growth and development of endodontics during the previous 25 years, and because of the untiring efforts of leaders in the AAE, the American Dental Association recognized "endodontists" as a special area of dentistry in 1963. The first examination and certification of diplomates occurred 2 years later in 1965.[4] As of this publication, there are about 6,600 members of the AAE and over 1300 certified diplomates.

In order to understand and appreciate the evolution of this dental specialty, a brief review of its historical roots is indicated. Because most of the elements of this evolution come from a rather diverse range of sources, the present codification of the definition and scope of this specialty will be used as a framework for this investigation.

The present definition of endodontics has been consolidated to focus on two areas[1]:

1. Morphology, physiology, and pathology of the human dental pulp and periapical tissues.
2. Etiology, diagnosis, prevention, and treatment of disease of the pulp and associated periapical conditions.

The present scope of endodontics has been distilled into the following outline, one that will be followed in this historical pursuit.

- Differential diagnosis and treatment of oral pain of pulpal and/or periapical origin, or referred pain.
- Vital pulp therapy (pulp capping, pulpotomy, apexogenesis, and apexification).
- Non-surgical treatment of root canal systems with or without periapical pathosis of pulpal origin, including obturation of these systems.
- Selective surgical removal of periapical pathosis resulting from the extension of pulpal pathosis including tooth structures: root-end resection, hemisection, bicuspidization, root resection, and root-end filling.
- Root repair procedures related to pathologic or odontiatrogenic pathosis/damage.
- Intentional replantation and replantation of avulsed teeth and management of other traumatic tooth injuries (luxations).
- Interrelationships between pulpal and periodontal disease.
- Endodontic endosseous implants (diodontic tooth implants).
- Bleaching of discolored dentin and enamel.
- Revision of previously treated root canal systems—both non-surgical and surgical.
- Coronal restorative procedures involving the root canal space and coronal access openings.

Definition

MORPHOLOGY, PHYSIOLOGY, AND PATHOLOGY OF THE HUMAN DENTAL PULP AND PERIAPICAL TISSUES

The dental pulp is the most unique organ and its relationship with both the tissues that it produces, dentin, and the associated surrounding tissues, enamel, cementum, periodontal ligament, and supporting bone is most interesting and challenging in terms of clinical assessments, diagnoses, and treatments. The study of the dental pulp, the adjacent dentin, and supporting oral structures has a long history of "discoveries and developments," and the history of endodontics would not be complete without first having an appreciation for the evolution of this chronology, as it reflects a true, global flavor. Table 1 provides a concise and impressionable listing of the chronology of discoveries in

Table 1 Chronology of Discoveries in Pulpodentinal Histology			
Author (place of activity)	Nationality	Year	Original Description
Van Leeuwenhoek (Delft)[329]	The Netherlands	1675	"Transparent pipes" in the tooth bone
Malpighi (Bologna)[330]	Italy	1686	"Substantia tubulosa" equal to dentine
De la Hire (Paris)[331]	France	1699	"Infinity of small fibrils," enamel rods
Hunter (London)[332]	Great Britain	1771	Madder refractive, avascular, different from other bones
Purkinje (Breslau)[333]	Germany	1835	Accurate description of tooth structures
Fränkel (Breslau)[334]	Germany	1835	Tubular dentine, contour lines
Raschkow (Breslau)[335]	Germany	1835	Cellular secretion theory of dentine; pulp innervation plexus (eponym)
Retzius (Stockholm)[336]	Sweden	1836	Tubular canal system in dentine
Müller (Berlin)[337]	Germany	1837	"Hollow fibrils in tubular tooth substance"
Linderer and Linderer (Berlin)[338]	Germany	1837	First (German) dental text including histology
Tomes (London)[339]	Great Britain	1838	Granular layer of dentine (eponym)
Schwann (Louvain)[340]	Belgium	1839	Cellular theory of vegetable and animal; "ivory cells with fibrous processes" in pig; nerve cells (eponym)
Nasmyth (London)[341]	Great Britain	1839	"Baccated fibrils" in dentine; pulp ossification theory
Henle (Zürich/Berlin)[342]	Switzerland	1841	"Ivory cells" with prolongation, "pulp conversion" into tubular dentine
Lintott (London)[343]	Great Britain	1841	Tubular fibrils filled with "calcareous substance"
Owen (London)[344]	Great Britain	1840–1845	Introduced terms of dentine, vasodentine and osteodentine (eponym:contour lines)
Tomes (London)[345]	Great Britain	1848	"Translucent dentine"; primary, "secondary dentine"
Czermak (Vienna)[346]	Austria	1850	"Interglovular spaces" in dentine (eponym)

Table 1 continued on page 38

Table 1 continued from page 37

Author	Country	Year	Contribution
Kölliker (Zürich, Würzburg)[347]	Switzerland/Germany	1852	"*Elfenbeinröhrchen*" (calcified pipes), first adequate description of pulp histology
Huxley (London)[348]	Great Britain	1853	"deposition" theory in dentinogenesis
Lent (Würzburg)[349] and Kölliker (Würzburg)[347]	Germany	1855	First correct description of odontoblast with its process and dentine formation
Tomes (London)[350]	Great Britain	1856	"Fibrillar" content of dentine tubes with sensory function *(eponym)*
Magitot (Paris)[351]	France	1858	Corroboration of odontoblastic layer
Harris (Baltimore)[352]	United States	1858	First American text including dental histology, 7th edition
Robin and Magitot (Paris)[353]	France	1860	"Tails of ivory cells" (odontoblastic processes) not related to tubuli
Neumann (Berlin)[354]	Germany	1863	Peritubular sheath *(eponym)*
Von Kölliker (Würzburg)[355]	Germany	1863	Epithelial and mesenchymal organization of dental organ
Waldeyer, (Breslau)[356,357]	Germany	1865	Coined term "*odontoblast*," odontoblastic conversion theory
Beale, (London)[358]	Great Britain	1865	Odontoblast-fiber-tubule relation
Hertz (Greifswald)[359]	Germany	1866	Odontoblastic intertubular substance
Boll (Bonn)[360]	Germany	1868	Evidence of dentine innervation
Legros and Magitot (Paris)[361]	France	1873	Histodifferentiation in odontogenesis
Hertwig (Berlin)[362]	Germany	1874	Epithelial root sheath *(eponym)*
Salter (London)[363]	Great Britain	1875	Classification secondary dentine
Von Ebner (Graz)[364]	Austria	1875	Collagen fibrils in dentine matrix
Salter (London)[363]	Great Britain	1875	First description of secondary dentine and pulpal diseases
Tomes (London)[365]	Great Britain	1876	Text on dental ontogeny and phylogeny
Baume (Berlin)[366]	Germany	1877	Atubular dentine formation in human tooth; coined term "denticle"
Hart (New York)[367]	United States	1878	First description of aurophilic interodontoblastic fibers and mantle dentine
Witzel (Essen)[368]	Germany	1879	Depiction of pulpoblasts forming atubular dentine; pulp capping
Bödecker (New York)[369]	United States	1879	Classification: primary and secondary dentine
Malassez (Paris)[370]	France	1885	Epithelial cell rests *(eponym)*
Von Brunn (Rostock)[371]	Germany	1887	Epithelial induction of root formation
Walkhoff (Munich)[372]	Germany	1888	Transparent dentine = odontoblastic fiber calcification
Weil (Munich)[373]	Germany	1888	Cell-free subodontoblastic layer *(eponym)*
Von Ebner (Vienna)[374]	Austria	1891	Incremental lines of dentine *(eponym)*
Röse (Freiburg)[375]	Germany	1891	Wax reconstruction of human, embryonic tooth formation dêntine taxonomy
Mummery (London)[376]	Great Britain	1892	Description of predentine layer
Bödecker (New York)[377]	United States	1894	American text dental histology and pathology
Gysi (Zürich) and Röse [378]	Switzerland	1894	First microphotographs of pulp and dentine
Höhl, Erwin (Leipzig)[379]	Germany	1896	Subdontoblastic cell-rich layer *(eponym)*
Röse, Carl (Munich)[380]	Germany	1898	Taxonomy of dentines
Von Korff, Karl (Kiel)[381]	Germany	1906	Interodontoblastic dentinogenetic fibrils *(eponym)*
Weidenreich, Franz (Heidelberg)[382]	Germany	1925	Mantle dentine, circumpulpal dentine

pulpodentinal histology (see the references cited in Table 1 for information on these early publications).[6] For today's student of pulpal histology and oral biology, this table represents an amazing codification of developments that have influenced current thought historically and provided contemporary clinical directives. Further information on the extensive contributions to the study of the entire oral biological complex of pertinence to endodontics can be found in the treatise on our pioneers in oral biology by Kremenak and Squier.[7] The true aficionado of pulp histology is directed to the most current publication on this topic[8] (Figure 1).

Extensive treatises on tooth morphology have existed for over 100 years,[9] with the major works in this area attributed to Hess[10] who made vulcanite corrosion preparations of almost 3000 permanent teeth. Additional historical contributions can be found in the studies of Barrett,[11] Pucci and Reig,[12] Skillen,[13] and Wheeler.[14] On the basis of the data recorded in these studies, Grossman[15] raised the following question; "One may well ask at this point if root canal work is justified in view of the complexity of the canals, since by no method can all the minute ramifications be filled." In rhetorical response to this query, Grossman indicated that Thomas[16] studied a large number of serial sections of root apices and found "that many canals seen in the apical region in individual sections, both ground and decalcified, do not communicate directly with the pulp. Many of them are imbedded vessels, their loopings being plainly demonstrated in serial sections. Sometimes such loopings arise from, and terminate in, the pulpal wall."

Kronfeld[17] responded more succinctly to Grossman's question in the following manner: "Microscopic findings

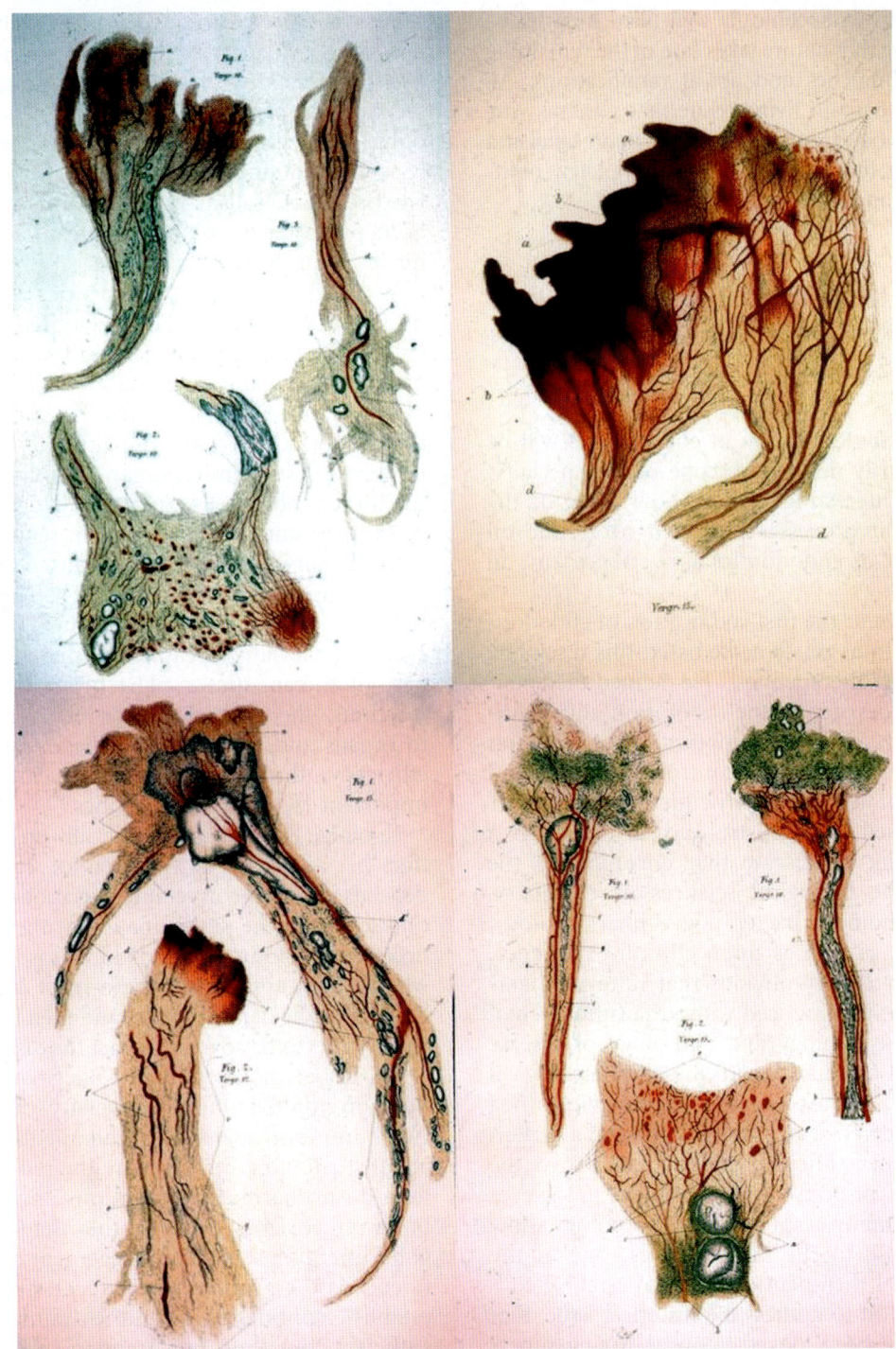

Figure 1 Photos of dental pulps that had either been diseased or challenged with various toxic chemicals, such as arsenic or phenoltannin that were used in pulp therapy in the late 1800s. This study represented one of the first extensive evaluations of pulp tissue in response to caries or medicinal treatment. Note the inflammation, presence of calcified material and fibrosis. From Witzel A. Die Antiseptische Behandlung der Pulpakrankheiten des Zahnes. Berlin: Commissionsverlag Von C. Ash & Sons; 1879. (See Table 3)

on extracted teeth with clinically well-filled, uninfected main canals prove that nature takes care of the remaining unfilled lateral branches and apical ramifications. All these fine canals contain living tissue that remains vital after the pulp has been removed from the main canal and forms cementum that eventually may completely obliterate the lateral canals."

ETIOLOGY, DIAGNOSIS, PREVENTION, AND TREATMENT OF DISEASE OF THE PULP AND ASSOCIATED PERIAPICAL CONDITIONS

This portion of the definition of endodontics will be addressed primarily under the scope of the specialty. However, it is interesting to note how some of the historical thought processes impacted over time on the development of endodontics as a science and an art.[1]

Coolidge[18] gave us the first codification of endodontics as a science in as much as he based this discipline on the concept of "therapeutics." He defined therapeutics as a science devoted to the restoration and maintenance of health. It was the application of remedies for the relief of suffering, the control of disease, and the restoration of adequate body function. He further defined it as used in dentistry and as based on a rational treatment of disease that encompasses the disciplines of the biological sciences of chemistry, physiology, pathology, bacteriology, pharmacology, and psychology, as well as upon clinical experience. Furthermore, "it is very obvious that rational therapeutics could not be practiced without a fundamental knowledge of the etiology and pathology of disease combined with a familiarity with the pharmacological action of drugs.... Just because improvement in a given case is observed after administration of a certain remedy, it is not sufficient evidence to prove the progress was in response to the remedy. However when a series of many cases of similar pathology show favorable response to the same remedy, one of the factors in rational therapeutics has been established."

Coolidge goes on to address the historical issue, that therapeutists have been looked upon as having superhuman powers, often with a mysterious or magical control over physical conditions. "The primitive belief that a deity or a demon is responsible for the cause of disease has been carried down through the ages, and occasional evidences of that belief are still found in the newspaper reports of sacrifice for atonement and persecution of persons suspected of witchcraft.... Not only are such practices to be found in the so-called backward countries, but in our own country, in isolated sections. Talismans and charms have not entirely been put aside even though great progress has been made in therapeutic procedure."

In his discussion of therapeutics and with a focus on pharmacology, Coolidge identifies an issue that is still prevalent and of concern today, including the use of N2 and its multiple variations, that are referred to as RC2B paste. "It has always been the desire of the therapeutist to find a drug with sufficient germicidal power to destroy microorganisms without damage to the human body cells. So far no drug has been developed that entirely meets such requirements, since some damage to tissue cells is caused by all drugs that have germicidal properties.... There are so very few conditions where drugs can be given the credit for the cure that alleviative treatment remains a very necessary part of therapeutics.... The promotion of beneficial reactions, the control of harmful reactions, the aid to organs and functions that have lost some of their efficiency, through disease or accident, and... very important factors in therapeutics."

Coolidge then focuses specifically on dental therapeutics: "... as in general therapeutics, curative treatment depends upon the correct interpretation of the symptoms of disease and the determination of their cause.... It is necessary to study each individual case in order to find what factors appear to be the most important in the etiology of the dental disease, and then to make an intelligent effort to remove or correct the disease."

Dr. Robert L. Levy of the College of Physicians and Surgeons of Columbia University calls attention to two important essentials of therapeutics[19]: "The therapeutist should always be sure the remedy used will at least do no harm. His intentions are to help Nature, but a remedy may hinder rather than help in spite of good intentions. In the management of patients, confidence is the great factor in successful treatment. To establish confidence, scientific training alone is not sufficient, but thorough training in the principles of therapeutics, combined with intellect and character that make up personality are all essential."

The issues of science do no harm, and rational therapeutics and all they espouse were to come crashing down on the dental professional in the early 1900s in the form of the focal infection theory. Apparently, the microbial populations in the oral cavity and the devastation that they rendered to patients globally in

---

[1] In the ensuing discussion, the reader is encouraged to substitute the word endodontics or endodontist for therapeutics or therapeutist where indicated to get the full flavor of content as it relates to the basis for the evolution for contemporary endodontics.

the form of caries and periodontal disease failed to gain the attention of the dentist who was concerned with restorations and esthetics. It took an earth-shaking presentation on the part of a British physician to bring the dental profession to it knees.

William Hunter[20] was a physician on staff at the Charing Cross Hospital in London, England in 1910. The focus of his interest in medicine was in the area of anemia and the sepsis producing such. He characterized the surgeon as having antisepsis, and Hunter felt that, although areas of surgery were immersed in antisepsis, the practice of medicine was often lapse and that "septic suppurations unfortunately occurred...as complications of various medical diseases." He ranked sepsis in medicine as "the most prevalent and potent infective disease in the body," focusing on the movement of staphylococcal and streptococcal organisms throughout the body, compromising specific regions or organ systems. When applying these principles to oral medicine, the physician was immune to the potential disease processes occurring in the oral cavity, regarding it as "matter of teeth and dentistry," with which he cannot deal. Hunter referred to these oral conditions as "oral sepsis," a topic he had lectured 10 years prior to his indictment. He claimed that all members of the medical profession had the responsibility to address "oral sepsis." "The matter of oral sepsis is, therefore, of urgent importance in relation to the whole multifarious and widespread group of affections—medical, surgical, and dental—caused by the actual presence or toxic action of pyogenic organisms (staphylococci and streptococci)." Hunter focused both on teeth and on supporting structures as being the seats of sepsis, especially in the poor patients who could not afford dental treatment.[20] "It is in poor patients that these septic conditions are most common. They have had 'no care' of their mouths; their fate is the relatively happier one of having their septic roots lying exposed in all their nakedness surrounded with tarter, overgrown it may be by foul, septic fungating gums. This sepsis is relatively open and above-board; it stares one in the face when it is looked for." Although displaying respect for the mechanical skills of the dentist, he voiced his contempt for the lack of awareness of the seat of oral sepsis, citing it as surgical malpractice.

In his presentation, Hunter cited systematic disease processes that he attributed to oral sepsis, such as gastritis, anemia, ulcers, colitis, and nephritis. He claimed that this "evil was so common and widespread that it is impossible to deal adequately with...." Needless to say, the dental profession would soon respond to this vehement indictment and succumb to the dictates of the medical profession.

In 1912, Rhein[21] was the first to respond intelligently to William Hunter's vicious attack on American dentistry. In doing so, Rhein directed the blame for the lack of concern for oral sepsis to the physicians. "It has been unfortunate that the insidious nature of this grave evil has been ignored by medical men for so many years. This apparent indifference of the physician to oral sepsis has unquestionably had an important bearing on the reckless indifference shown by so many dentists to the presence of septic foci in the alveolus." Additionally, he cites the low fees and the complaints of the dentists that they "cannot get paid for the time needed to remove pulps properly and to seal root canals aseptically," as causes for indifference on the part of the dentist.

In describing the presence of chronic apical periodontitis with a maxillary lateral incisor, Rhein labels it as a source of "septic poisoning," which many practicing dentists were treating with the approach of letting "sleeping dogs lie." In addition, he supports Hunter's accusation of the poor crown and bridge prostheses and chides the dental profession to realize that Hunter's observations are true. "If such be the facts, then let us acknowledge them honestly, and in attempting to drag ourselves from this quicksand of dishonor, let us not forget that instead of criticism we owe Dr. Hunter a debt of gratitude." Rhein urged the dentists to forget the "antique methods of preserving dead pulp tissue, and become familiar with a scientific method of obtaining strictly aseptic conditions."

In 1913, Logan[22] responded to overwhelming concepts of oral sepsis, addressing the treatment of chronic dentoalveolar abscesses, without extraction, to prevent the spread of sepsis. Hartzell,[23] in 1914, provided a discourse on oral bacteria, their role in secondary infections, and principles underlying their transmutation and their paths of entrance to the vital organs.

At the Panama Pacific Dental Congress in 1915, Buckley[24] echoed the words of Ulrich[25] that "... every tip of a devitalized tooth whether the root canal has been properly or improperly filled becomes a *locus resistancii minorii.*" In doing so, Buckley admitted that the removal of focal infection is appropriate but not to the extent of wholesale, unwarranted extraction[24]: "... the majority of teeth this involved, may be therapeutically or surgically treated so that they will not be a menace to the health of the individual."

During this time, Rosenow[26–29] and Billings[30] were rapidly clarifying and espousing the concept of focal infection and elective localization. They felt that bacteria had a predisposition to lodge in specific areas, producing a disease process remote from the original site of infection. Rosenow, working in an

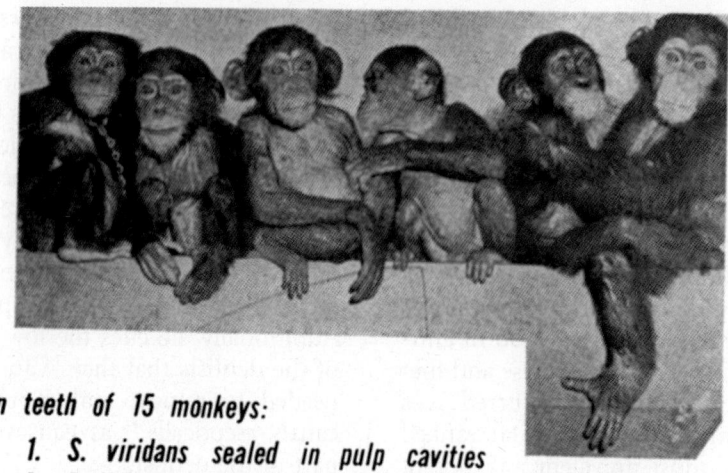

Figure 2 A study done in monkeys by Genvert H. et al. in 1941 as cited by Grossman L. Root Canal Therapy. 4th ed. Philadelphia: Lea & Febiger; 1955 that disputed the focal infection theory. Genvert had inoculated the periapical tissues creating a focus of infection at the root end of a number of teeth, but could not determine any systemic involvement resulting from such foci of infection.

area of immature bacteriology without thorough radiographic diagnosis and using extracted teeth dropped into tubes of media, secured mixed cultures of organisms from which he isolated *Streptococcus viridans*. He was concerned about this strain as being the organism of systemic infection. However, in 1917, Meyer[31] criticized the culturing of extracted teeth as a diagnostic technique and called attention to the possibility of culturing normal mouth organisms that contaminated the tooth during extraction. Grossman[32] pointed out that it was disconcerting, but true that practically every investigation dealing with the pulpless tooth made prior to 1936 was invalid (Figure 2). In 1928, Holman[33] reviewed the literature critically and commented on the theory of elective localization. "The specificity of the bacteria has not been proved and the theory of elective localization is so open to misinterpretation and so limited in its practical application that it cannot be considered as a help in the solution to the problem. A certain general bacterial adaptation to environment is conceded by everyone, but the factors on the side of the host are more variable and far more important."

However, the theories of focal infection and elective localization, when coupled, were to have a devastating effect on the dental profession, as not only pulpless teeth but also teeth with any possibility of chronic inflammation or infection, along with the surrounding periodontium, were considered as the primary source of systemic disease.

In 1918, Peak,[34] in a common sense approach to this problem, stated that all focal infection is not of dental origin and that even though the medical profession has indicted the dental profession "...we (dentists) are alive to the prevalence and importance of oral focal infection, and that we can be relied on to intelligently and conscientiously handle our end of the work." Even with this low key approach, Peak chose to land a "salvo" in the lap of the medical profession. "The ruthless extraction of teeth, as demanded by some of the physicians, is a crime against the patient, and indictment against the physician and the surgeon, and a sad commentary on the co-operation and understanding existing between the medical and dental professions."

Even Rosenow[27] deplored the thoughtless extraction of teeth; however, he did feel it necessary in the presence of systemic disease. "No one deplores more than I the ruthless extraction of teeth that has been practiced in some instances as a result of the work on focal infection. Vital teeth free from pyorrhea should never be extracted except as it becomes necessary for restorative work. The extraction of pulpless teeth seems to me to be indicated, regardless of the appearance of the radiograms, in cases of serious systemic diseases for which no other focus can be found." However, Rosenow[29] did not limit his directives to pulpless teeth. "Teeth, especially multi-rooted teeth, with deep fillings or caps, which manifest evidence of infection of the pulp, with or without pulp stones, and even symptomless teeth which react positively to vitality test and that have deep fillings, may be the source of systemic effects and may need to be removed." Even with these teeth, he felt "devitalization ... and the filling of root canal ... should cease."

Throughout the first half of the twentieth century, teeth and the seat of potential focal infection they represent have been implicated in multiple disease processes throughout the body, such as eye disease, arthritis, tonsillitis, stomach ulcers, cholecystitis, myositis, diabetes, and many more nondescript unexplained vague systemic conditions.[35–42] While there was an overwhelming tendency to radically eliminate the teeth in the hope of resolving these medical problems, some astute investigators attempted to dispel this irrational, irresponsible course of treatment. As a physician, Hatton[43] was one of the most vocal and sensible. "In all humbleness and as a physician, may I say a word to the physicians of this audience? The mouth and teeth, because of their position, are easily examined, yet the determination of the nature and extent of oral infection is a highly technical problem. It is true that any one can acquire much information from the study of dental roentgenograms, but to presume to arrive at a definite conclusion, solely from their examination, is a type of folly that no good physician would be guilty of in the study of any other part of the body. May I suggest that pulpless teeth are not dead teeth, that though the pulps are gone they are still embedded in a highly vascular fibrous membrane, and that the question of nutrition of hard parts of a tooth is still an open question, and that treatment and filling of the pulp canal can be accomplished even after infection has occurred."

An additional theory which emerged from the conflagrations of focal infection was the "hollow tube" theory. In their classic paper in 1931, Rickert and Dixon[44] demonstrated "halos of irritation" around the open ends of implanted platinum and steel hypodermic needles. For them, this finding "gave rather convincing evidence that the circulatory elements diffusing out of the openings of these tubes were not well tolerated by the vital tissues," and this was analogous to what occurs in the pulpless tooth. Therefore, root canal systems required a tight seal to prevent the irritation and inflammation of the periradicular tissues. In addition, the material used to fill the root canal or apical foramen could not irritate the tissues, and caution was expressed as to the use of these materials in root surgery, especially copper amalgam. While the need to prevent localized tissue irritation is valid, the hollow tube theory as promulgated by Rickert and Dixon was effectively disproved by Goldman and Pearson,[45] Torneck,[46,47] and Phillips[48] in the 1960s.

Focal infection is not dead, although its tenets have been severely dissembled over the years. There exist today professionals who will espouse one or more aspects of the focal infection theory when a diagnosis cannot be made or successful treatment achieved. The quality and success of both nonsurgical and surgical endodontics in contemporary practice, the control of microbiologic populations, and the present day etiology for endodontic therapy have all had a tremendous impact on lessening the intensity of the focal infection concept, and dispelling it as scientifically unsound.

Scope

DIFFERENTIAL DIAGNOSIS AND TREATMENT OF ORAL PAIN OF PULPAL AND/OR PERIAPICAL ORIGIN

Long before the beginning of the twentieth century, dental practitioners came to an agreement that the causes of pulpal injury are many and varied, and they were grouped as physical, chemical, and bacterial. Fish[49] in 1932 indicated that just cutting the dentinal fibrils, as in a cavity preparation, caused some degeneration of the elements of the pulp. Further and more deleterious damage was identified as being due to excessive heat generation during cavity preparation or the polishing of a restoration.[15] For completeness,

Table 2 Differential Diagnosis of Inflammatory Diseases of the Pulp	
The Pulp	The Periodontal Membrane
The pain is not always localized. Often difficult to locate	The pain is always localized. Easily located
The pain is sharp, lancinating, intermittent and throbbing. Usually worse during fatigue and at night when in reclining position	The pain is dull, steady, and continuous. It is not affected by position of body or time of day
The pulp is very sensitive to thermal changes and other irritants	The tooth is not affected by thermal changes or chemical irritants
The tooth is not tender to percussion	In early stages, pressure relieves and later intensifies the pain
The tooth does not seem elongated and does not interfere in occlusion	The tooth is raised in its socket and strikes first in occlusion
The tooth usually shows extensive caries or a large restoration	A sound unfilled tooth often develops periodontal pain
The regional lymph nodes in the submaxillary area are not affected	The regional lymph nodes are usually enlarged and tender to palpation
Body temperature is not affected	Body temperature is usually increased

Adapted from Prinz H[53].
The use of the term "periodontal membrane" was in vogue and used as such since the mid-1800s, as opposed to periodontal ligament. Even today, among periodontists, there is disagreement as to whether it is a membrane or ligament; however the perspective may be based on how the structure is viewed, that is, histologically or functionally.

even the potential for pressurized changes encountered at high altitudes was identified as a cause of pulpal problems in 1937.[50] While the possibility of "aerodontalgia" was of concern in the late 1930s and 1940s, Ritchey and Orban[51] indicated that high altitude itself would not cause pain in a tooth with a normal pulp. Kennon[52] observed that 65% of the aerodontalgic teeth had been restored with a period of 12 months or less prior to the onset of pain at high altitudes, but had been asymptomatic at ground level. This finding lent further support for the potential of immediate pulpal damage or degenerative changes that may occur following restorative dental procedures.

Regarding pulpal diagnosis and a reliable determination for such, Hermann Prinz[53] provided us with a detailed differential diagnostic scheme in 1937 (Table 2) to determine the difference between pulp and periapical pain. Codified pulp testing techniques in the 1800s to make this type of determination were almost nonexistent. In the early 1900s, the following tests were considered essential, as was a documented record of such, including an adamant dictate that "judgment must be exercised in the interpretation of the diagnostic symptoms".[54]

- Roentgenograms (in particular, bitewings for children's and young adult's teeth).
- Transillumination (noting the color changes between a tooth with a vital and non-vital pulp in addition to the labial and lingual soft tissues).
- Thermal vitality tests (use of ice or hot water).
- Electric pulp tester (the stalwart was the Burton pulp vitalometer) (Figure 3).
- Percussion and palpation.
- Mobility additional tests added by Grossman.[15]
- Test cavity additional tests added by Grossman.[15]
- Anesthetic test additional tests added by Grossman.[15]

In the early to mid-1900s, Grossman provided the dental community with a concise listing of diseases of the dental pulp and periapical tissues and diagnostic states.[15] These delineations and demarcations were carried forth well into the late 1900s in many countries and, while histopathologically sound, created confusion from a clinical diagnostic standpoint.

Diseases of the Pulp

The diseases of the pulp according to Grossman[15] are the following:

1. Pulpitis: (a) acute serous, (b) acute suppurative, (c) chronic ulcerative, (d) chronic hypertrophic.
2. Pulp degenerations: (a) calcific, (b) fibrous, (c) atrophic, (d) fatty.
3. Necrosis or gangrene of pulp.

Diseases of the Periapical Tissues

The diseases of the periapical tissues according to Grossman[15] are the following:

1. Acute apical periodontitis
2. Acute alveolar abscess
3. Chronic alveolar abscess
4. Subacute alveolar abscess
5. Granuloma
6. Cyst

With regard to these diagnostic states, two important issues were brought forth to the dental community that may still linger as controversial in some sectors even today: (1) are there bacteria in granulomas and (2) is the granuloma pathosis or a defense reaction? Kronfeld[17]

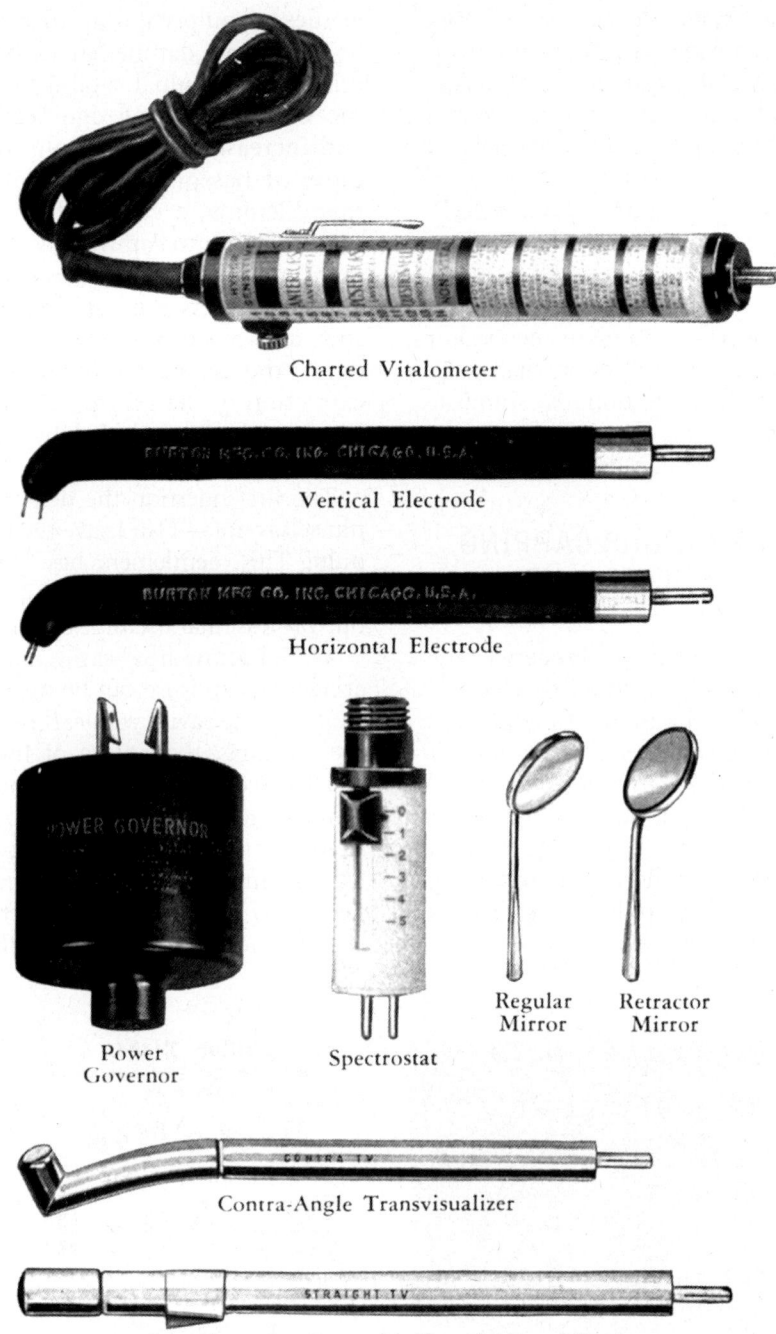

Figure 3 Burton vitalometer with attachments for determining the vitality of the pulp and transilluminator for further diagnostic use. From Coolidge ED. Endodontia—The Clinical Pathology and Treatment of the Dental Pulp and Pulpless Teeth. Philadelphia; Lea & Febiger: 1950.

in 1939 stated "While the bacteriologic method is a sensitive means for determining whether bacteria are present in a pulpless tooth, the histological method is useful in determining the location from which bacteria were obtained. For example, a tooth with a granuloma may have an infected root canal but a sterile periapical tissue.... The presence of bacteria can easily be demonstrated in smears from the root canal of an untreated pulpless tooth. It is not quite so simple to answer the questions as to whether or not bacteria are present in granulomas and radicular cysts, for the findings vary with the bacteriological technique used. A few investigators have reported bacteria in all granulomas. The majority of recent observers, however, agree that granulomas and cysts are found sterile in quite a large percentage of cases."

With regard to the second question, Schour stated[55] "...the formation of a granuloma is indicative of a defense reaction on the part of the periapical tissue. It may occur in the absence of infection. It has been shown that a granuloma may develop as a result of chemical or traumatic injury following removal of a vital pulp. Furthermore, although bacterial infection may stimulate the tissues to form a granuloma, the granuloma may persist even after removal of the infection."

VITAL PULP THERAPY (PULP CAPPING, PULPOTOMY, APEXOGENESIS, AND APEXIFICATION)

Phillip Pfaff, a German dentist to Frederick the Great, has been identified as being the first to mention pulp capping. He tailored a piece of metal, gold or lead, to "...*die Figur einer halben Hulse von einer Erbse, diren unterster Theil eine Vertiefung haben soll*" (...the shape of half a peapod, so that the lower surface should have a concavity) (Figure 4). In that way, the metal would be prevented from contacting the living, and therefore, sensible pulp.[56] Since then a multitude of publications have either extolled the virtues of pulp capping in retaining pulpal vitality, or they have damned it as being unreliable in the maintaining pulpal vitality, instead contributing to the development of significant pulpal calcification and increasing the difficulty of a root canal procedure, or has outright "killed" the dental pulp. To this dilemma, a careful delineation of when to cap and when not to cap was given to us in 1883 by W. E. Harding of Shrewsbury, England, as he astutely differentiated between capping of an accidental exposure and a carious exposure.[57] "In the 'good old days,' the treatment of an exposed pulp was the extraction of the tooth, but that mode of procedure has long been exploded by the progress of Dental Science.

The first question the dental surgeon of today asks himself is not,—Can I save the tooth, but can I save the pulp? This, gentlemen, has not added much or our labour and anxieties, but is also contributed much to our professional usefulness to mankind.

We all know how easily and successfully a case of accidental exposure can be treated. My usual plan is to swab out the cavity with carbolic acid, which will arrest the bleeding, then place of the point of exposure a small piece of court plaster, or blotting of Fletcher's artificial dentine. This can be applied in a more plastic state than the phosphate fillings, and unlike oxychloride of zinc it is non-irritant and easily removed if necessary. When this has hardened the permanent filling may be proceeded with at the same sitting.

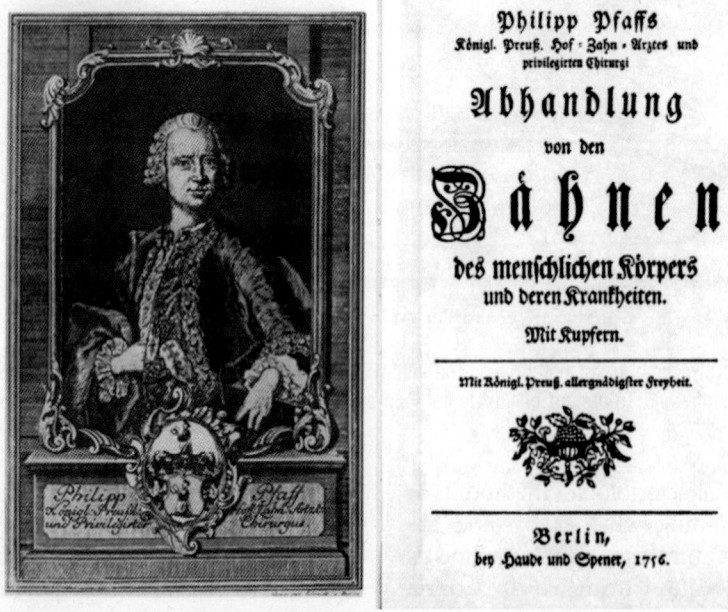

Figure 4 Frontispiece and Title page from Pfaff's original publication. (From author's collection).

The reason these cases are so easily dealt with is that the pulp is quite healthy, and if covered with a non-conductor at once, so as to exclude the germs of micro-organisms, it will heal by first intention.

But in those cases where the exposure results from caries the difficulties are vastly greater, as the pulp is almost sure to be inflamed, and probably suppurating. My experiences of these cases treated by capping is the reverse of satisfactory, the percentage of successful cases being small, and on this point I hope some of the gentlemen present will give us the benefit of experience.

The first point to determine is the condition of the pulp. The history of the case is often deceptive, for the cavity is in such a position as not to be exposed to the impact of food it may not have given much pain, and yet be suppurating; but in the odour we have a certain means of diagnosis. If that peculiar phosphatic odour is present, I very much doubt the possibility of saving the pulp, and think any attempt at capping will result in its death, and eventually in a chronic abscess; in such cases the destruction of the pulp is, I think, by far the best treatment. Should capping be determined upon, the application to the exposed surface of iodoform and eucalyptus oil has generally proved the most successful. It may then be covered with artificial dentine—and in these cases it is always safer to put in a temporary filling for a few weeks, which can be removed in case of pain. Hill's gutta percha over the artificial dentine answers very well."

The historical presentation by Harding highlights many key issues in the pulp capping controversy that has existed for decades. Firstly, the need to eliminate bacteria was highlighted, although it was not really taken into serious consideration regarding pulpal health until the publication by Kakehashi et al. in 1965.[58] Secondly, the need to establish a pulpal diagnosis was the key to choosing the right treatment; however, Harding could only identify two parameters, those being odor and the possibility of suppuration, for which the latter was guesswork at best. Thirdly, as with Harding, Seltzer and Bender discouraged the use of pulp capping on cariously exposed teeth.[59] As opposed to Harding, however, these latter authors were able to provide histological justification for their position.

While the contemporary use of pulp capping has been questioned, recent studies have endorsed this procedure in teeth with incompletely formed roots and exposed pulps. In particular, studies by Cvek and others have reported a high degree of success with pulp capping and partial pulpotomy in cases of teeth with traumatic pulp exposures of varying sizes and mature or immature root development (apexogenesis).[60,61]

Along with pulp capping, partial or full pulpotomies are considered within the realm of vital pulp therapy. Pulpotomies differ from pulp capping in the amount of tissue that is removed. From an historical viewpoint, it is possible that investigators and clinicians intermingled these procedures in their reports. However, a partial or full pulpotomy has been used with high degrees of success for carious, mechanical, and traumatic exposures of the pulp primarily in the presence of immature root development.

According to Hess, early attempts to preserve the vitality of an amputated pulp were made by Bodecker (1886), Prieiswerk (1900), and Fisher[15] (1912). In 1924, Leonard reported highly satisfactory results following pulpotomy in selected cases, using his techniques for over 20 years.[62] A few years later, Neuwirth experimented on teeth of dogs, the pulp of which had been amputated coronally and covered with non-irritating agents, including dentin dust. He found no pathological changes in any of the specimens examined.[15] His findings were confirmed by Hellner in 1930 and noted that dentin shavings dropped upon pulp tissue from the bur also produced a regional pulp calcification.[15] Similar findings were recorded by Pribyl in 1931.[15] On the other hand, Rebel observed secondary reparative dentin formation following pulpotomy but interpreted the presence of the osteoid due to metaplasia of the pulp.[63]

In 1933, Gottlieb, Orban, and Stein[64] obtained apical calcification in every case when, experimenting on animals, they incorporated up to 50% of dentin dust in an oxyphosphate cement and used it on contact with amputated pulp. In 1934, Loewenstein reported from 60 to 70% success in a series of 37 cases of pulp amputation,[15] while Novikoff in 1935 reported 16 cases of pulpotomy in children with age ranging from 7 to 10 years with only one failure.[65] In 1938, Hess, who had considerable experience with performing pulpotomies, reported that about 80% of cases showed complete walling off of the pulp stump with a calcific barrier.[15] Finally in 1938, Teuscher and Zander[66] provided us with experimental results on the use of a paste of calcium hydroxide to cover amputated pulps. Histological sections of selected cases showed formation of secondary reparative dentin over the pulp stump and maintenance of pulpal vitality. The actual reported technique of pulpotomy using calcium hydroxide was described by Zander and Law in 1942,[67] and histological evidence of repair with formation of a new layer of odontoblasts and a secondary irregular dentin barrier has been given by Zander and Glass in 1949.[68]

48 / Endodontics

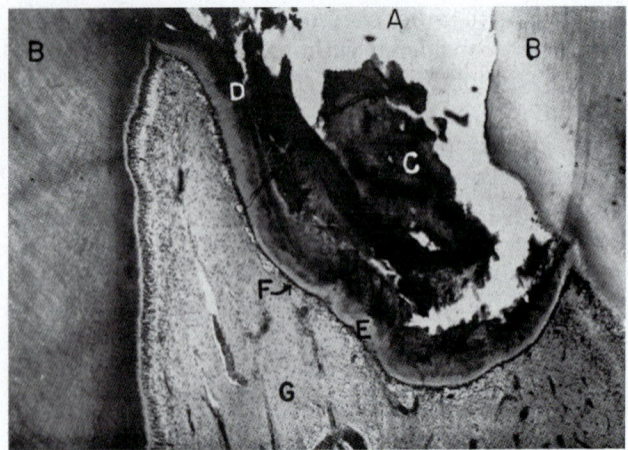

Figure 5 "Exposure eight weeks after capping with Ca(OH)$_2$. **A**, Site of exposure; **B**, Dentin walls; **C**, Remnant of necrotic area; **D**, Zone of demarcation and primitive dentin; **E**, New dentin barrier; **F**, Continuous odontoblastic layer and **G**, vital pulp." From Grossman L. Root Canal Therapy. 2nd ed. Philadelphia: Lea & Febiger; 1950.

The development of this material for routine use clinically, with substantial histologic data, is attributed to Hermann in 1930[70] and Zander in 1939.[71] Eastlick[72] recommended it for use with exposed pulps in teeth with immature apices in 1943 as Granath[73] did in 1959 for apexification procedures. The use of calcium hydroxide for apexification was popularized in the early 1960s by Dr. Alfred L. Frank in his presentation at the AAE meeting in 1964, and his detailed applications that became known as the "Frank Technique" were published in 1966.[74] Heithersay[75] has provided a rather extensive treatise on the wide range of applications for calcium hydroxide.

NON-SURGICAL TREATMENT OF ROOT CANAL SYSTEMS WITH OR WITHOUT PERIAPICAL PATHOSIS OF PULPAL ORIGIN, INCLUDING OBTURATION OF THESE SYSTEMS

The need for non-surgical root canal procedures and tooth retention was necessitated by the presence of the proverbial "toothache," a malady that has plagued man from time immemorial (Figure 6). Historically, many innovative

Historically, the most effective capping material has been calcium hydroxide (Figure 5). The earliest reference to this material is attributed to Nygren in 1838.[69]

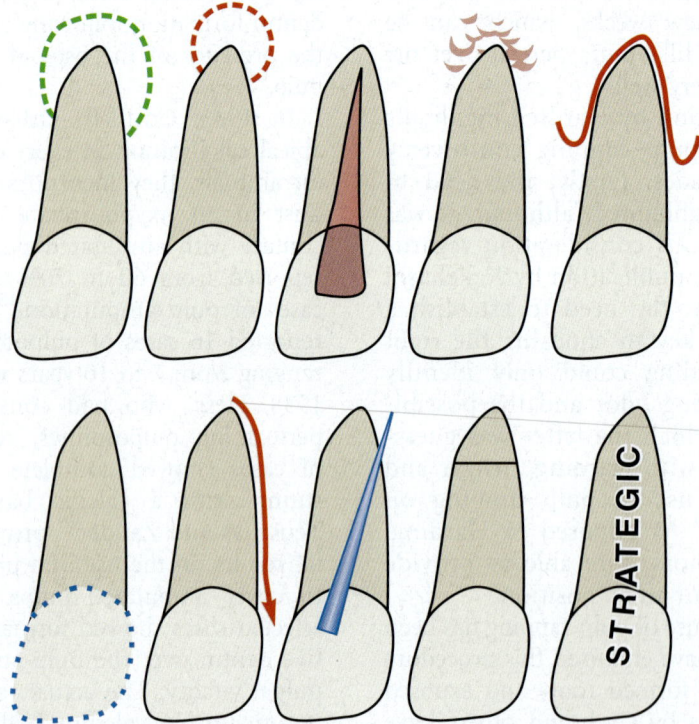

Figure 6 "Local contraindications to endodontic treatment" as cited by Grossman. 1, Large area of rarefaction; 2, cyst; 3, obstruction to apical foramen; 4, erosion of root apex; 5, loss of alveolar bone; 6, loss of crown preventing sterile field; 7, fistula discharging through gingival crevice; 8, lateral perforation; 9, fracture of root with death of pulp; 10, non-strategic tooth functionally and esthetically." From Grossman L. Root Canal Therapy. 2nd ed. Philadelphia: Lea & Febiger; 1950.

cures have been attempted with a wide range of fascinating outcomes.

Cure of the Toothache

As recorded in medical history, toothache has been the scourge of the ages. Many unusual remedies have been described; it is quite evident that necessity, instinct, and mere chance have taught civilizations the means to usual and unusual "cures." On Egyptian tablets, in Hebrew books, and from Chinese, Greek, and Roman medical writings are recorded descriptions and causes of this scourge. The Ebers papyrus[76] written about 1500 BC, contained the recipe for a medicament for "curing the gnawing of the blood in the tooth." The ingredients to be used included the following:

- The fruit of the Gebu plant—one thirty-second part
- Onion—one sixty-fourth part
- Cake—one sixteenth part
- Dough—one eighth part
- Anest plant—one thirty-second part
- Water—one-half part

This was left to stand and then chewed for 4 days.

Archigenes of Apamea (a Syrian city), who lived in Rome in the latter part of the first century, was well known as a physician and operator and distinguished himself with his daring trepanations.[73] He recommended various remedies for odontalgia, including a mouthwash made by boiling gallnuts and hallicacabum in vinegar and a concoction of roasted earthworms and spikenard ointment mixed with crushed eggs of spiders. His principal statement regarding dentistry was that odontalgia, in certain cases, was related to a disease in the anterior part of the tooth.

From the Middle Ages are recorded accounts of many "improved" methods of relieving the aching tooth. There was still a strong belief during this time that tooth decay was caused by presence of tooth "worms." The priest and physician Andrew Boorde,[77] who achieved fame in the late fifteenth century, described his own unique "deworming technique": "And if it (toothache) do come by worms, make a candle of wax with Henbane seeds and light it and let the perfume of the candle enter into the tooth and gape over a dish of cold water and then you may take the worms out of the water and kill them on your nail."

Abulcasis (1050–1122), known as abir-al-Qasim Khalaf ibu (Abbas al-Zahrowi), controlled toothaches through the use of cautery. He inserted a red-hot needle into the pulp through a tube which was designed to protect the surrounding structures[78]; Guy de Chauliac, a famous medieval surgeon, used a mixture of camphor, sulfur, myrrh, and asafetida as a filling material to cure toothache caused by worms.[79] In the later Middle Ages, French anatomist Ambrose Paré (1517–1592) wrote[73] "Toothache is, of all others, the most atrocious pain that can torment a man, being followed by death. Erosion (caries) is the effect of an acute and acrid humor. To combat this, one must recourse to cauterization ... By means of cauterization ... one burns the nerve, thus rendering it incapable of again feeling or causing pain."

The physician for the Imperial Baths at Calsbad, Johann Stephan Strabelbergen (1630), used oil of vitriol or a concoction made of a frog cooked in vinegar to kill worms in teeth. Lazarre Rivierre was the first to recommend a remedy that is still being used for toothache: placing a small piece of cotton moistened with oil of cloves in the cavity. He altered this with oil or camphor of oil or boxwood.[79] John Aubrey (1626–1697), in his book *Brief Lives*, reflects on bits of folklore designed to cure the toothache[80]: "To cure the Tooth-ach, Take a new Nail, and make the Gum bleed with it, and then drive it into an Oak. This did Cure William Neal, Sir William Neal's son, a very stout Gentleman, when he was almost Mad with the Pain, and had a mind to have Pistoll'd himself."

A history of the remedies used to combat toothache would be incomplete if it did not include the suggestions of the "founder of modern dentistry," Pierre Fauchard. Guerini translates from *Le Chirurgien Dentiste*, written in 1728 by Fauchard[73]

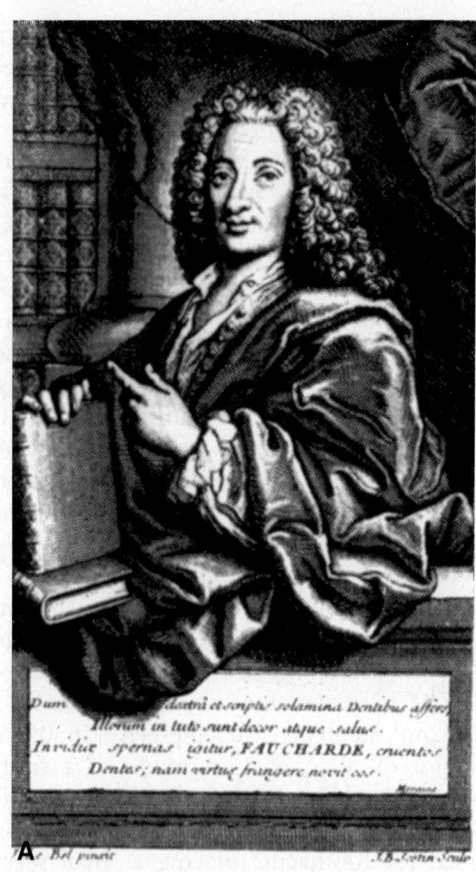

Figure 7 *A* & *B*. Frontispiece and Title page from Fauchard's original textbook. (From author's collection).

(Figure 7A,B): "Some pretend to cure toothache with an elixir of some special essence; others with plaster; others by means of prayers and signing of the cross; others with specifics for killing the worms which are supposed to gnaw the tooth and so cause pain; others pretend to be so clever that they can cure the most inveterate toothache by merely touching the tooth with a finger dipped into or washed with some rare and mysterious liquid; finally, they promise to cure every kind of toothache by scarifying the ears with a lancet or cauterizing them with a hot iron."

Finally, Fauchard speaks of another remedy, assuring his readers that with this remedy many persons who have had almost all of their teeth decayed and who suffered very often from toothache have found great relief: "It consists of rinsing the mouth every morning and also before going to bed with a spoonful of one's own rinse (urine) immediately after it has been emitted, always provided the individual be not ill. One is to hold it in the mouth for some time and the practice ought to be continued. This remedy is good, but undoubtedly not pleasant, except so far that it produced great relief. It is rather difficult in the beginning to accustom one's self to it. But what would not one do to secure his health and repose."

Fauchard goes on to speak of trepanation of the teeth when they are worn away or decayed and causing pain. He begins by saying: "Most of the varieties of pain caused by the canines and the incisors when worn away, or decayed cease after the use of the trepan." He uses the word trepan in a wide sense, meaning any instrument (even a needle or a pin) with which "one penetrates into the inner cavity of the teeth."

In 1756, L. B. Lenter, a German, wrote a pamphlet in which he recommended electricity as a means of curing toothache.[73] Other writers recommended the use of a magnet as an alternative. In 1770, Thomas Berdmore[81] published his *Treatise on the Disorders and Deformities of the Teeth and Gums*. In it, he addressed various causes of toothache and its cure. When the toothache was caused by "obstructions and inflammation of the nerves and vascular parts of the tooth," the treatment indicated was "counter-impression" and sedatives—primarily to divert the mind from the "disordered nerve." In practice, the burning of the ear with a hot iron was performed to serve as a "counter-impression." To Berdmore, however, this treatment was unacceptable.

In his book published in 1794, Raniere Gerbi, a professor at the University of Pisa, recommended a very singular cure for a violent toothache.[73] Under the name circulio anteodontalgicies [sic] he described an insect living habitually in the flowers of the *Cardisus spinosimus* that could be used as a remedy for a toothache. Other medical practitioners of this era in other countries described similar procedures using different types of insects.

Throughout the history, dental "scientists" were still pursuing the elusive "tooth worm." While no scientific accounts actually exist which support its presence, the Chinese dentists, especially, are said to understand how to make superstitions pay. When a patient with the toothache presents himself, they (the dentists) were in the habit of making an incision into the gums "to let the worms out." For this purpose, they used an instrument that had a hollow handle filled with artificial worms. When the incision was made, the operator, with a dexterous turn of the instrument, dropped the worms into the mouth, Generally, the excitement of the patient and the loss of blood caused at least a temporary relief. The worms were then collected, dried, and ready to be taken out of the next patient's gum[82] (Entrepreneurism at its finest!). In 1883, F. H. Balkwill of England in a bold exposé attempted to explain scientifically the causes of pain in teeth without pulps that exhibited "no evidence of pericemental irritation."[83]

Table 3 highlights a brief and concise listing of some of the major developments in the provision of "root

Table 3 Chronology of Important Developments in the "Roots" of Non-Surgical Endodontic Procedures to the Mid-Twentieth Century		
Clinician/Investigator	**Era or Year**	**Procedure, Technique, Instrument**
Fauchard[267]	18th century	Pulp extirpation, hole drilled into the tooth by file or drill held in a brace; roughened needle used to remove the pulp; cotton with essential oil placed; plug could be removed and replaced if pain present
Riviere[15]	1725	Used oil of clove for toothache; later used lint placed in the cavity that had been dampened with oil of cinnamon, clove, camphor or turpentine
Pfaff[268]	1756	Capping of the exposed pulp
Woofendale[383]	1783	Destroyed the pulp with cautery to alleviate pain; no pulp canal cavity filling
Longbothom[384]	1802	Recommended that root canals be filled when it was inadvisable to extract them
Hudson[15]	1809	Filled pulp cavity with gold; anterior teeth only, canal treatment not mentioned
Fitch[15]	1829	Formulas for toothache pills, opium, camphor, oil of clove and oil of cassia (from coarse cinnamon bark); laudanum (tincture of opium) also used
Koecker[385]	1826	Established criteria for pulp capping
Maynard[386]	1838	
Spooner[386]	1836	
Burdell[386]	1838	Condemned the use of arsenic for pulp destruction
Hill[386]	1847	Gutta-percha, "Hill's Stopping"
Arthur[386]	1852	Described the making of barbed broaches with handles
Shadoan[387]	1859	Used cobalt and creosote to destroy the nerve of the tooth
Barnum[386]	1862	Developed the dental rubber dam
Chase[388]	1866	Pulp mummification
Magitot[389] (see Figure 2-10)	1867	Suggested use of electric current for vitality testing
Bowman[15]	1867	Popularized the use of gutta-percha for filling root canals; introduced a solution of chloroform and gutta-percha in 1883; also tried the use of shellac with gutta-percha for tackiness and adherence; Bowman was also the co-inventor of the dental rubber dam clamp forceps with C. F. Allen
Keep[15]	1876	Oxychloride of zinc for capping and filling root canals
Witzel[390]	1879	Introduced phenol (initially in 1873)
Brophy[15]	1880	Used heat to evaluate the status of the pulp; traced sinus tracts; used test cavities to verify diagnosis
Allport[15]	1882	Used arsenic for short periods (24 h) on the pulp; reported on sloughing of a portion of the pulp while maintaining the rest for the pulp for years
Mills[391]	1883	Pulp knocking, popularized the removal of the pulp was by driving a slender wooden peg into the canal with a sharp blow from a mallet; technique had been used by some clinicians for over 20 years
Perry[327]	1883	Wrapped gutta-percha around a gold wire (roots of ThermaFil?); made gutta-percha points that were rolled in shellac (custom prepared cones?) and compacted them into the root canal
Evans[15]	1886	Developed an instrument to dry and disinfect the root canal

Table 3 continued on page 52

Table 3 continued from page 51

Register[392]	1888	Popularized Evans' technique of drying and sterilizing root canal with compressed air heated to 130°F
Rollins[386]	1889	Rubber dam clamps
Miller[82] (see Figure 2-11)	1890	Foundations of dental bacteriology; demonstrated the presence of bacteria in dead pulp tissue and in infected canal; emphasis on antisepsis
Gramm[393]	1890	Introduced copper points for filling root canals; later gold-plated them to prevent discoloration
Marshall[15]	1891	Popularized the use of the electric pulp tester
Schreier[15]	1883	Used sodium potassium alloy to destroy the pulp
Kirk[15]	1892	Used sodium dioxide for cleaning of the root canal and bleaching of discolored teeth
Breuer[15]	1893	"Ionization" treatment of pulpless teeth, empirical applications
Rollins[386]		Added vermillion to gutta-percha
Callahan[394]	1894	Used 40% sulfuric acid for the widening of root canals; claimed that the solution also removed pulp tissue and sterilized the canal
Brown[395]	1894	Claimed to diagnosed the "strangulation of a tooth nerve"; also detailed the use of hot, cold and percussion as diagnostic tests
Stevens[15]	1895	Marketed the wooden points for "pulp knocking"
Perry[396]	1895	"Tempered" Swiss watch broaches for better applications in the root canal; also used chloro-percha technique
Rhein[312]	1897	Popularized the use of ionization treatment for pulpless teeth in the USA, empirical applications
Tomes[15]	1897	Suggested paraffin for filling root canals
Rollins[386]	1898	Motorized root canal drill
Kells[397]	1899	Used x-rays for their diagnostic value; used first to assess root canal obturation
Gysi[15]	1899	Introduced trio paste for pulp mummification
Harlan[398]	1900	Used a solution of papain for digestion of dead pulp tissue
Price[399]	1901	Identified the value of x-rays in root canal work and the diagnosis of a non-vital pulp
Buest[15]	1901	Recommended that gutta-percha have a core of a silver wire to provide rigidity
Onderdonk[15]	1901	Called for bacteriologic examination of the root canal prior to obturation
Klotz[400]	1902	Detailed the use of a Morey nerve drill to enlarge the coronal orifice of the canal and enable the penetration of a nerve broach; identified need to know where root canal curvatures are located to prevent the formation of a "ledge" into the side of the canal
Myers[401]	1904	High pressure syringe for anesthetizing the pulp, "Myer Dental Obtunder" (intrapulpal anesthesia)
Vaughan[402]	1906	Infiltration anesthesia for anesthetizing the pulp
Buckley[403]	1906	Tricresol and formalin introduced
Prinz[404]	1912	Recommended a high melting-point paraffin for filling root canals
Callahan[394]	1914	Suggested a solution of varnish of chloroform and rosin for lining the root canals prior to obturation
Howe[15]	1917	Recommend ammoniacal silver nitrate for silver impregnation of the pulp tissue remnants to render them inert and sterilize the canal
Skillen[406] and Thomas[16]	1921	Detailed investigations into the development of the apices of teeth
Husband[407]	1925	Suggested copper amalgam for filling root canals
Grove[15]	1929	Made precision-fitting gold cones for obturation (canals were prepared with a special set of engine reamers)
Trebitsch[15]	1929	Introduced silver cones for root canal fillings
Stewart[408]	1930	Introduced a gold-tin amalgam for root canal filling
Jasper[195]	1933	Introduced silver points that had the same diameter and taper as the root canal instruments
Ross[409] and Grossman[411]	1935, 1935, 1936	Introduced a stable, organic clorin solution (azochloramid) for sterilization of root canals
Østby[412]	1944	Described in detail tissue reactions to root canal treatment procedures; described the "Østby Block Section" technique whereby the apical periodontium and root apex are removed intact following treatment procedures for the purpose of histological evaluation
Grossman[413]	1948	Introduced a penicillin suspension for root canals followed by a penicillin-streptomycin suspension; followed by a penicillin-streptomycin-bacitracin-sodium caprylate suspension (PBSC) in 1949
Kuttler[414]	1955	Defined the apical anatomy of the cemental-dentinal junction with regard to working length determination
Østby[415]	1961	Detailed description of the role of the blood clot in endodontic therapy
Sunada[416]	1962	Introduced the concept of the electronic apex locator

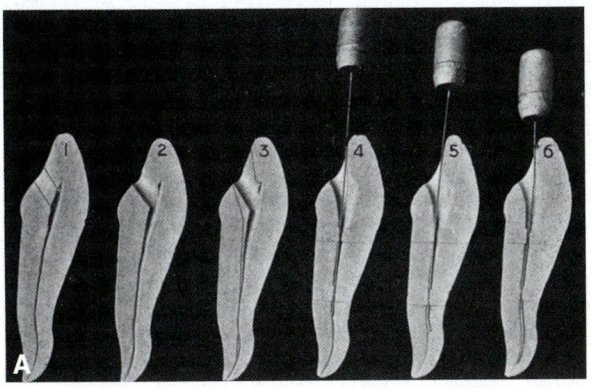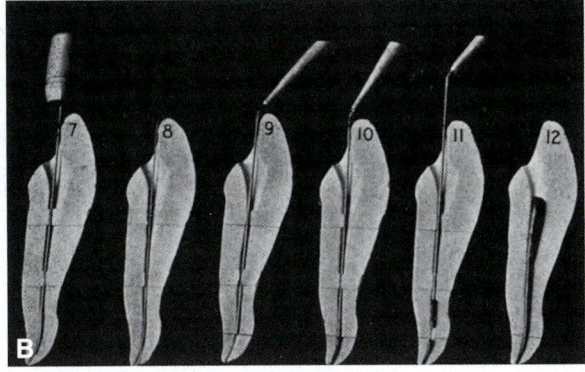

Figure 8 Root canal treatment procedures as described in 1936. **A,** "1, A plaster model of cuspid tooth enlarged 5 diameters. Outline drawn for opening into pulp chamber; 2 opening into pulp cavity but poor access to canal; 3, outline of desired opening to make a straight canal; 4, small file broach unable to pass curvature in canal; 5, small file broach bent at point to pass first curve; 6, small file broach bent and gently rotated to pass second curve. Repeated filing in and out from foramen gradually wears away the curves to compare with outline on model 3. **B,** "7, larger file broach slightly bent to continue enlarging canal to proper size for filling; 8, measuring wire inserted in canal and bent at right angles over incisal edge as measuring point; 9, root canal plugger No. 34 3 mm. shorter than measurement wire and inserted in canal to the bend; 10, plugger No. 34 carrying 3 mm piece of filling material (gutta-percha) into canal as far as the bend in plugger; 11, plugger No. 34 carrying second 3 mm. piece of filling material into place; 12, canal filled. (Berichten des IX. International Zahnörztekongresses Wien, Urban und Schwarzenberg, 1936.)" From Coolidge ED. Endodontia—The Clinical Pathology and Treatment of the Dental Pulp and Pulpless Teeth. Philadelphia; Lea & Febiger: 1950.

canal procedures and techniques" into the 1900s (Figure 8A,B). These developments laid the groundwork for the contemporary principles of root canal treatment. However, what may have impacted more on root canal therapy and its acceptance occurred in locations distant from each other in the mid-1900s. While in Montevideo, Uruguay, Dr. Francisco M. Pucci first pointed out the necessity for meticulous intracoronal preparation as the basis for ultimate success in intracanal preparation and obturation,[84] it was Dr. John I. Ingle in Seattle, Washington who gave us the standardized instruments to clean and shape canals properly[85] and Dr. Herbert S. Schilder in Boston, Massachusetts who provides us with many of the contemporary principles for successful canal obturation.[86]

SELECTIVE SURGICAL REMOVAL OF PERIAPICAL PATHOSIS RESULTING FROM THE EXTENSION OF PULPAL PATHOSIS INCLUDING TOOTH STRUCTURES: ROOT-END RESECTION, HEMISECTION, BICUSPIDIZATION, ROOT RESECTION, ROOT-END FILLING

Surgical endodontic procedures have a long history of trial and error with multiple authors and clinicians claiming revolutionary techniques. Table 4 provides a brief and concise listing of developments in this realm up to the beginning of the 1900s.

For the first half of the twentieth century, the development of endodontic surgery can be

Table 4 Chronology of Important Developments in the "Roots" of Surgical Endodontic Procedures to 1900		
Clinician/Investigator	**Era or Year**	**Procedure, Technique, Instrument**
Abulcasis[79]	11th century	Intentional replantation
Pare	1561	All provided detailed accounts of replantation citing multiple clinical situations; Hunter reached the conclusion that a vital periodontal ligament was a prerequisite for successful union of the tooth and the alveolus following replantation.
		Pfaff and Berdmore performed tore-end resections and placed root-end fillings of wax, lead or gold
Fauchard[267]	1712	
Pfaff[268]	1756	
Berdmore[417]	1768	
Hunter[269]	1778	

Table 4 continued on page 54

Table 4 continued from page 53

Heister[418]	1724	Managed chronic sinus tracts by opening them, cleaning them out or burning them out
Harris[419]	1839	Used a lancet or sharp bistory-pointed knife to puncture a tumor of the gums to release the pus
Desirabode[420] and Magitot[421]	1843 and 1860–1870	Claims made as to being the first to perform root-end resection
Hullihen	1845	Surgical trephination through the soft tissue, bone, and into the pulp chamber to alleviate a congested pulp—"Hullihen Operation"
Bronson[422]	1866	After applying carbolic acid to the gums, one perpendicular slit and one transverse slit was made in the overlying tissues and an engine drill was used to drill directly through to the end of the root to relieve congestion and effect a discharge of suppuration; this approach was labeled as "barbaric" by FY Clark; approach was also questioned by J. N. Farrar
Smith[423]	1871	Used root-end resection to manage a tooth with a necrotic pulp and surrounding alveolar abscess
Farrar[424]	1880	Performed a procedure on abscessed teeth referred to as an "apicotomy"
Martin	1881	Claimed by some to be the inventor of root-end resection to manage draining sinus tracts
Dunn[425]	1884	Amputated "fangs" using a tubular saw to enter the jaws removing the diseased soft tissue and root end
Farrar[229]	1884	Recommended the radical removal by amputation of any portion of roots of teeth that were of not further use
Black[230]	1886	Recommended the amputation of the apex of the root of any teeth in the case of long-neglected abscess
Younger[233]	1886	Reiterated Hunter's opinion on the need for a vital periodontal ligament following replantation
Grayston[426]	1887	Used cocaine anesthesia in the surgical management of an alveolar abscess
Fredel[274] and Sheff[275]	1887 and 1890	Initiated animal experiments to address the role of the periodontal ligament (referred to as the periosteum) in the resorptive process (referred to as adsorption)
Rhein[231]	1890	Recommended complete root amputation as a radical cure for a chronic alveolar abscess
Ottolingui[427]	1892	Presented a succinct technique for the immediate filling of a root canal followed by the resection of the root apex
Rhein[312]	1897	Describe surgical treatment for the management of the alveolar abscess, including marsupialization
Partsch[428–430]	1895–1900	Credited with the methodical development of "Wurzelspitzenresection" (root-end resection) first under chloroform anesthesia and later cocaine anesthesia; credited with packing the surgical cavity with iodoform gauze (Partsch I operation) and tissue reapproximation with suturing (Partsch II operation)

characterized as both progressive and regressive. While tremendous strides were being made by the European and American dental professionals in the enhancement and application of endodontic surgical techniques, in all areas of the oral cavity, the very roots of the focus of endodontics and its surgical component were being severely attacked from the ivory towers of the medical profession. William Hunter's classical presentation "An address on the role of sepsis and antisepsis in medicine," which was delivered to the Faculty of Medicine of McGill University in Montreal, in 1910, and published in London in 1911, initiated the conflagrations of "focal infection," a concept whose burning embers are still smoldering in multiple bastions around the world.[20] Before this indictment, however, surgical advances and diversified applications marked the entry of endodontics into the twentieth century.

On the heels of Partsch's achievements in the late 1800s and early 1900s (Figure 9), many European clinicians assumed the challenges of the *Wurzelspitzenresektion* procedure, and because of the clinical success attained, the concept of focal infection did not impact greatly on these surgical practices on the European Continent. German and Austrian authors such as Fischer, Mayhofer, Euler, Williger, Fryd, Kersting, Knoche, Witzel, Metz, and Hermann had a tremendous impact on the development of surgical endodontics. In 1908, Béal published a technique article on "*résection de l'apex*" (root-end resection) and, along with case reports, highlighted the

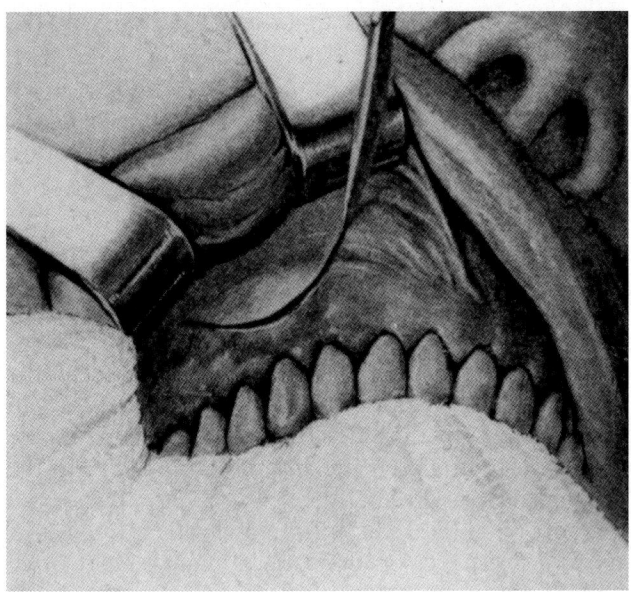

Figure 9 Semilunar incision on the buccal mucosa as promulgated by Partsch in the late 1800s. From Berger A. The Principles and techniques of Oral Surgery. Brooklyn: Dental Items of Interest Publishing Co.; 1930.

development of endodontic surgery in France.[87] Roy in 1925[88] and La Cronique in 1927[89] are often credited with the classic articles in France that addressed "*le curettage apical*" and "*amputation de l'apex.*" Both authors clearly presented detailed surgical indications and techniques to manage "*lesions radiculaires.*" In 1930, Duclos[90] compared techniques of simple drainage in the case of a periradicular abscess with those of complete root-end resection. In 1934, he presented detailed methods on the management of the apical portion of the canal following resection, favoring a circular preparation in the long axis of the root for the placement of amalgam.[91]

Some of the first and most important publications in Eastern Europe were from Czechoslovakia in 1913 by Bažant[92] entitled "*Resectioradicis,*" in which the indications for root-end resection are clearly outlined and detailed, and by Šmelhaus in 1916, who reported on his extensive experiences with periradicular surgery.[93] Later investigations by Kostečka[94] discussing causes of failure and the psychological aspects of the surgical procedure for the patient, and a text by Měštan in 1937, covering all aspects of periradicular surgery,[95] served as the benchmark for "*resekci kořenového hrotu*" (resection of the tip of the root) in Eastern Europe for the next 40 years.

The continued development of surgery on the European Continent led to the publication of some significant and detailed articles, monographs, and texts devoted to extensive coverage of all surgical concepts, especially molar surgery. The first of these was by Faulhaber and Neumann[96] in 1912, entitled *Die chirurgische Behandlung der Wurzelhauterkrankungen*, in which the authors combined both theoretical concepts and clinical techniques. They provided an extensive description of surgical armamentarium, anatomical considerations, and specific techniques used to gain surgical access to various portions of the oral cavity and a description of the use of amalgam as a root-end filling material.

In 1915, Neumann[97] focused strictly on lower molar surgery in his monograph entitled *Die Wurzelspitzenresektion an den unteren Molaren*. As today, there was considerable concern over the inferior alveolar canal, mental foramen, and their vital contents. Neumann provides the first detailed anatomical description of the relationships of the mandibular roots to both osseous and neurovascular structures and related these to periradicular surgical procedures. A uniting and expansion of these surgical concepts occurred in a 1921 publication of Faulhaber and Neumann's second edition of their 1912 text.[98] In 1926, Neumann published his *Atlas—der radikal chirurgischen Behandlung der Paradentosen*, which dealt primarily with the surgical management of periodontal disease.[99] However, he proposed a split thickness surgical flap, which in design is known as the modern day Oschenbein-Luebke flap used in root-end resection (Figure 10).

Otto Hofer, from Vienna, provided a thorough review of surgical flap designs in his 1935 extensive treatise entitled "*Wurzelspitzenresektion und Zystenoperationen,*" a paper he presented in Prague in 1934.[100] Hofer provided detailed descriptions of anterior surgical entries according to Csernyei,[101,102] Pichler,[103] and Wassmund,[104] which addressed not only root-end resection but also the Partsch I approach to soft tissue flap design and cyst management, as modified by the latter two clinicians into a "*periostalplastischen*" approach (split mucosa and periosteum). Once the cystic contents are removed and root ends managed, the flaps are split and layered into the osseous cavity with the anticipation of providing drainage and stimulating an internal to external granulation closure. While Pichler's and Wassmund's flap designs were "periostalplastischen" in concept, Csernyei's approach was considered as "*osteoplastischen*" in nature, in which the bone and periosteum are elevated intact and separate from the mucosa. In Csernyei's "*Operationsschema,*" which is a modified Partsch II procedure, a plate of bone is loosened

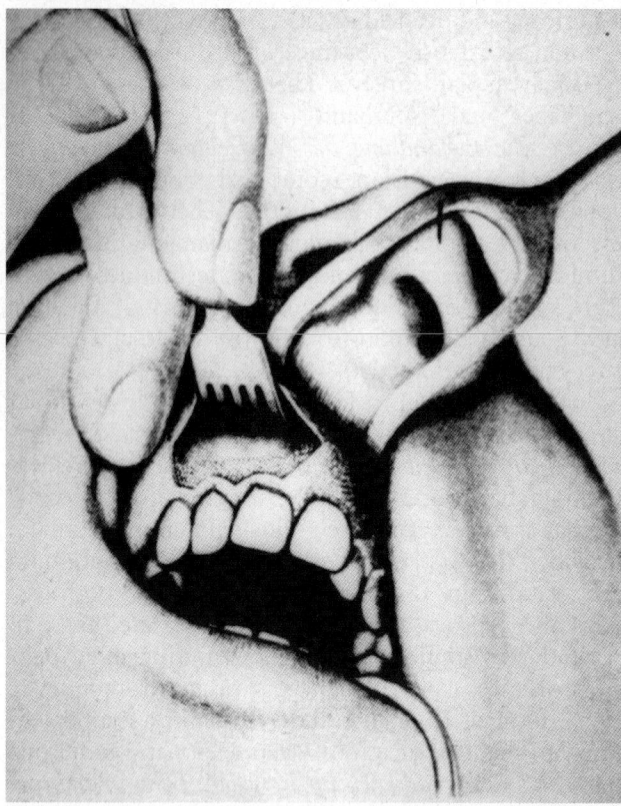

Figure 10 Neumann's depiction of a surgical flap in the attached gingiva that resembles the contemporary Oschenbein-Luebke flap. From Neumann R. Atlas—der radikal chirurgischen Behandlung der paradentosen. Berlin: Hermann Meusser; 1926.

intact, reflected, and replaced over the "*Wurzelspitzenresektion*" site. Csernyei's observations of healing with this flap design on dogs compared to Partsch's "semilunar" approach without regard to osseous integrity are quite interesting. Histological evaluations provided "a perfect ossification of the apical alveolus after 6 months" with the "*osteoplastischen*" method, whereas only scar tissue was formed with the Partsch technique. Contemporary endodontic surgery also cites scar tissue and healing by secondary intention as a disadvantage to the semilunar incision, *especially when the incision overlies the osseous defect.* Csernyei's flap design and osseous lid approach is presently in vogue for mandibular posterior teeth, having been further modified as a "bony lid only," and is espoused by Khoury as the "*Knochendeckelmethode.*"[105]

In 1936, Karl Peter from the University of Erlangen published his landmark text entitled *Die Wurzelspitzenresektion der Molaren*, which has served as the formative text for all contemporary endodontic surgical concepts.[106] Peter's text clearly outlined indications, providing a thorough literature review and historical development of periradicular surgery. Surgical flap designs for posterior teeth were detailed, and anatomical relationships of osseous and neurovascular structures were highlighted. Peter classified the position of the inferior alveolar canal relative to the molar roots, in addition to providing descriptive relationships of the maxillary sinus and its size and position relative to the roots of maxillary teeth.

Concomitantly, Held[107] from Switzerland published an extensive paper on the surgical management of all teeth in the mouth. He provided detailed anatomical considerations, both soft tissue and hard tissue, along with surgical techniques, principals of postoperative management, and guidelines for post-treatment evaluation. By this time, there had been so much input into the evaluation of various soft tissue incisions and flap designs by the multitude of European clinicians that the specific approaches had been labeled as to their inventors, advocators, or modifiers.

Surgical management of the resected root end was also detailed at this time, with the development of specific root-end preparation techniques. In 1914, von Hippel described the vertical slot root-end preparation referred to as the "*Slitsmethoden*," which was indicated to clean and seal the root canal when a post-core was present.[108] Ruud[109] modified this technique in 1947 adding retentive grooves, while Matsura[110] brought this technique to contemporary endodontic surgery in 1962. In the mid-1930s, Schupfer,[111,112] from the University of Innsbruck, detailed the transverse root-end preparation, which was perpetuated by Luks well into the 1970s.[113] However, either of these root-end preparation techniques may have been practiced prior to von Hippel or Schupfer by Schuster in 1913, with a vertical slot along the facial aspect of the root.[114] Variations in the techniques advocated for root-end preparation were necessitated by the difficulty encountered in gaining access to the resected root when only a small amount of bone or root was removed in the

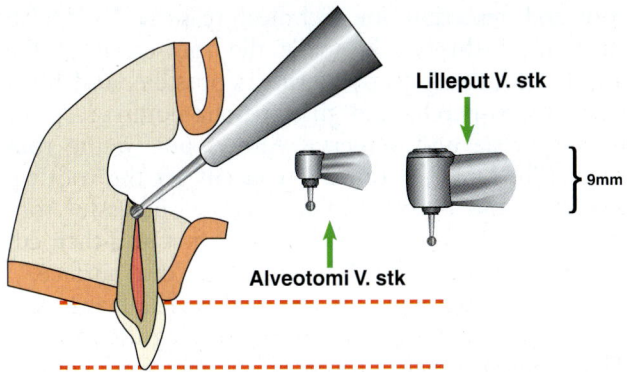

Figure 11 Drawing by Tangerud depicting miniature handpiece for root-end preparation as opposed to a straight handpiece. From Tangerud BJ. Den retrograde rotbehandling ved alveotomi. Nor Tannlìgeforen Tid 1939;49:170-175.

resection procedure. Tangerud[115] noted this problem in 1939 and developed a small (2.5mm high and 4mm broad) handpiece to facilitate root-end preparation (Figure 11).

In 1939, Castenfeldt,[116] from Stockholm, published a lengthy treatise on root-end filling and management of chronic apical periodontitis. He focused on residual infection in the resected dentinal tubules as being the major reason for surgical failure. A total seal of the root face with silver amalgam was recommended by removing all dentinal tubules at the resected root face (Figure 12). A bevel was cut in the dentin from the canal orifice to the cemental junction.

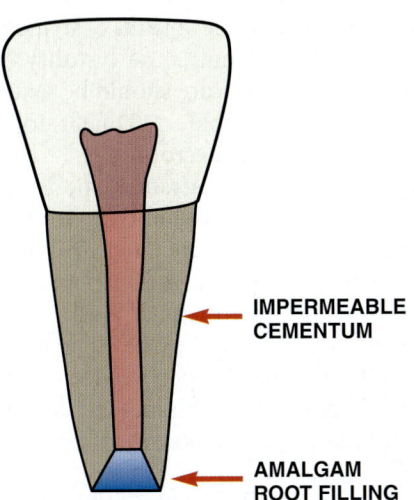

Figure 12 Complete covering of the resected root end as depicted by Castenfeld. From Castenfeldt T. Om retrograd rotfyllning vid radikaloperation av kronisk apical paradentit. Sven Tandlôk Tidskr 1939;32:227-260.

In the United Kingdom in 1927, Fawn from London had strong feelings about the "infection" present in the apical portion of the root with a nonvital pulp.[117] While Castenfeldt later indicated the need for a seal of the entire apical root face in these cases, Fawn felt that resection would remove the areas that harbor the bacteria. Fawn discussed the causes of failure of root-end resection and focused on diagnosis. In doing so, he identified a major problem that existed with the use of periradicular surgery and is still present today as the major cause of failure with surgical intervention. "For example, a great many men have grasped this operation as a means of avoiding an awkward situation. A tooth would be treated inadequately; after a lapse of time an abscess would develop. To cover up all possible reflection, root amputation is performed without proper diagnoses. Something of a surgical nature is done, which is eventually followed by failure."

Ross from England had recommended Castenfeldt's technique 4 years earlier for managing the exposed dentin.[118] His rationale for the complete amalgam closure was that success was to be measured by the "complete seal of the dentin." He frowned upon the use of silver nitrate to coat and impregnate the exposed dentinal tubules, which was a common practice in the United States at that time. "After removal of the apical third of the root, a rose head burr is inserted into the wound, and a cavity is cut into the exposed dentine in the root. As much dentine as possible is removed, and the root canal is then plugged with a solid coherent amalgam, which fills the canal and seals the end of the root. The operation should be done under strictly aseptic conditions, and the amalgam sterilized before being used...copper amalgam...has antiseptic properties, and further does not act as an irritant to the apical tissues."

Histological evaluation of root-end resections commenced with the studies of Bauer,[119,120] Euler,[121] and Kronfeld[122] in the 1920s. Cavina[123] from the Universities of Padua and Bologna in Italy published a lengthy paper on the indications, techniques, and results of "*l'amputazione degli apici delle radici dentali*" in 1930. In this paper, he was one of the first to discuss and relate to clinical procedures the histological findings of Bauer, Euler, and Kronfeld in the evaluation of healing of the periradicular tissues following surgery. Further studies at that time that addressed the healing of periradicular tissues and provided excellent histological data regarding the regeneration of the cementum and periodontal ligament were those of Gottlieb,[7,124] Steinhardt,[125] Häupl,[126] Takàcs,[127] and Herbert.[128] As stated by Gottlieb, "When a root end is amputated, we expose the surface of a transverse section of the root. The cavity caused by the operation is filled in with organized connective tissue and the root surface is embedded into this. As a rule, the wound caused by the operation heals... and it is likely that the exposed dentinal surface... may be covered, with or without resorption, by secondary cementum which may or may not unite with the surrounding bone; or the dentinal surface may be simply tolerated by the adjacent connective tissue, without having an influence of any consequence upon the environmental tissues."

From 1925 to 1935, there was a keen focus on the process and longitudinal evaluation of "Wurzelspitzenresektion" from the Ludwig-Maximilian University in Munich. Multiple university dissertations under the primary direction of Professor P. P. Kranz addressed all aspects of root-end surgical procedures.[129–134] Endodontic surgery on the European Continent had expanded, developed, and weathered the storm of focal infection that plagued the American dental profession. Not that the European community was immune to this concept, as focal infection was a serious focus of attention in the late 1930s and early 1940s relative to "Wurzelspitzenresektion." Fischer[135] and Wassmund[136] from Germany, Kostečka[137] from Czechoslovakia, and Gaerny[138] from Switzerland published key articles addressing the concepts of focal infection, relating them to the practice of surgical endodontics. Although mixed feelings prevailed, the use of periapical surgery continued as a major component of dental practice in Europe.

During these four decades, the development of periapical surgical concepts and techniques flourished and vacillated in the Americas. Early reports by Moorehead[139] in 1903 and Schamberg[140] in 1906 focused on the use of the Partsch I approach to root-end resection in which the "roughened" (resorbed) and associated periodontal membrane was removed with a bur (fissure, round, or rosehead), the root edges smoothed, and the cavity packed with iodoform or carbolated gauze for drainage. The patient would return for multiple visits until complete granulation of the cavity was observed. Schamberg provided a detailed, diagrammatic description of the technique used for root-end resection, errors commonly encountered in these procedures. "The operation that I advocate consists of a rapid ablation of the diseased area including the end of the root by means of a swiftly running bur." Ironically, the errors identified by Schamberg in resection are commonplace in contemporary surgical treatment. Schamberg also recommended root canal obturation subsequent to surgery, whereas Hartzell encouraged it prior to root-end resection for technical reasons.[141,142] "To succeed in this work, make the root-canal of the affected tooth as nearly sterile as possible, and fill it with chloro-percha and gutta-percha points... (prior to anesthesia and surgery). Always put in the root canal filling first, because if you cut off the root tip first it would be difficult to make a successful root filling; but if you fill the root canal first and then cut off the root tip, you will have a clean, oval surface."

Hartzell's technique for root-end resection was succinct, especially the procedure for locating the root tip. This approach was prompted by the high cost of radiographs that he felt precluded the advantage of the operation for many of his patients. "Now, you can judge where to make this opening by having explored your root canal with a slender instrument, and with the finger ends located the root end as nearly as you can, and then measured the depth of the root canal with your root canal plugger or broach. Then draw that out and lay it upon the tooth and estimate in the gum tissue about where the opening should be."

He also emphasized the need for a smooth root end to prevent future irritation in the surgical site. Hartzell's failures were "a trifle less than seven percent in three hundred and fifty-one cases treated in this way."[141] However, he only included teeth without "pyorrhea."

Buckley[143,144] indicated that surgical intervention was necessary for those teeth "where the medicinal treatment has failed." "The success of the operation depended on the thoroughness of the procedure. A vertical incision was used over the tooth, or a circular incision was indicated with two or more teeth... a vertical incision is made about one-half of three-fourths of an inch in length, direct over the affected root.... A bistoury (scalpel) is used for this purpose and care should be taken to make the incision as high as possible... so that it stops about on a line with the floor of the necrotic area."

In designing a surgical tissue flap, Brophy,[145] in 1915, cautioned the surgeon not to impinge on the free gingival margin, in essence negating the use of a full mucoperiosteal flap. "In the management of such an abscess, as in the treatment of all of the infectious diseases involving the gum tissue, it is essential that the continuity of the border of the gum be not divided. A division of the tissues at this point may lead to a recession and exposure of the neck of the tooth...."

Bone chisels and mallets were used by Buckley[144] to resect the root, which was a recent suggestion by Schamberg.[140] It was essential to remove the apex to the coronal depth of the periapical lesion. The root edges were smoothed and the cavity packed with iodoform gauze.

In 1913, Reid provided the dental literature with multiple articles on the trials and tribulations of root-end resection.[146–148] Techniques of resection with several burs were elucidated after root canal obturation. "...I would first use a diamond shaped drill, passing it through the root and succeed this with a fissure bur, cutting both ways until the end is severed from its parent. Final smoothing of the roughened end left by the bur can best be done with a fine Arkansas stone." He also cites root-end resection as the panacea for the fractured instrument beyond the root apex. "In glancing over the contents of one of our leading dental journals recent issue I came across a short article on root amputation, recommending the operation as a recourse for the removal of broken broaches or drills left protruding through the apical foramen. I prophesy that but few dentists have escaped this perplexing calamity, and those who have happened to meet with such a misfortune may possibly find this suggestion a panacea for such subsequent difficulties." Even though an advocate of this technique, Reid questioned the long-term success of his "partial root amputations," as he doubted the regeneration of the periodontal ligament. "So far as my knowledge goes, there is no evidence that the membrane is ever renewed, and if such as a fact, I feel confident we can never hope to be able to save partially amputated roots for any great length of time...."

For 6 years, from 1915 to 1920, the dental literature was besieged with articles written on root-end resection.[149–171] The use of the "crescent shaped" or semilunar incision was standard, as was sealing the gutta-percha at the root apex with a hot burnisher after resection on a root-filled tooth, or after resection and the pulling of a gutta-percha cone through the apical foramen. Zinc oxyphosphate was commonly used as a sealer with gutta-percha.

The placement of amalgam root-end fillings was becoming an acceptable procedure at that time. Garvin from Manitoba, Canada, "had the privilege" of seeing this technique performed by the Dean of the Dental School from Oslo, Norway, Dr. Immanuel Ottesen.[172] "An incision was made, the soft tissues were retracted, the alveolar bone over the apex removed with a chisel, the end of the root amputated and the area curetted, an amalgam filling inserted in the apex, an antiseptic placed in the wound and the tissues sutured at the line of incision."

In a series of articles from 1916 to 1919, Lucas indicated that he first polished the resected root end and then prepared a self-retentive cavity with a small bur in the root end for the placement of an amalgam.[151,157,167] In cases of the mandibular teeth, he had the referring dentist fill the entire canal with copper amalgam prior to surgical resection because "it is practically impossible to fill the remaining end of the canal after the apical end of the root is cut off." However, he did not recommend the use of copper amalgam in the maxillary teeth due to the potential of staining of the root structure.

In 1917, Ivy[152] and Howe[153] recommended the sealing of the apically resected tubules with silver nitrate. "By this means we believe the open tubuli of the bare root end are sealed, and any bacteria in them prevented from emerging."

In 1918, Prinz,[156] influenced significantly by Partsch and other European clinicians, presented a paper on the techniques of root-end resection. His procedures of incision, flap design, and management of presumed cystic lesions were reflections of the then advocated German techniques. His influence was to have a significant impact on the practice of endodontic surgery in the United States over the next 40 years (Figure 13).

In an attempt to disclose some of the problems perceived with the practice of root-end resection or apicoectomy and to highlight some personally advocated advantages of replantation, Edmund Kells, in 1918, lashed out at the perpetrators of sloppy techniques accompanying dramatic presentations of surgical expertise.[158] "It is undoubtedly safe to say that the operation of apicoectomy is quite 'the thing' nowadays, and is, in fact, a fad with many up-to-date operators. It is to be seen at clinics, in the 'movies,' and, taken all in all, is always most interesting to see, staged as it usually is with the accompanying dramatic accessories of *so called* asepsis. But, 'coming down from the clouds,' as it were, will the operation, as usually performed and as *invariably seen* by the writer, stand analysis, and how will it compare with the apparently neglected operation of replanting for the accomplishment of the same purpose?" Undoubtedly, Kells was influenced not only by the need for quality care and proper case management, but also by the pressures of the focal infection theory, which had gained significant momentum in the second decade of the twentieth century, and which was about to explode on the dental scene in the 1920s. After expounding on his technique of replantation, he arrives at two conclusions in his diatribe: "(1) The conditions to be found within the root-canal and beyond the root end must necessarily be and are infinitely better after replanting than after

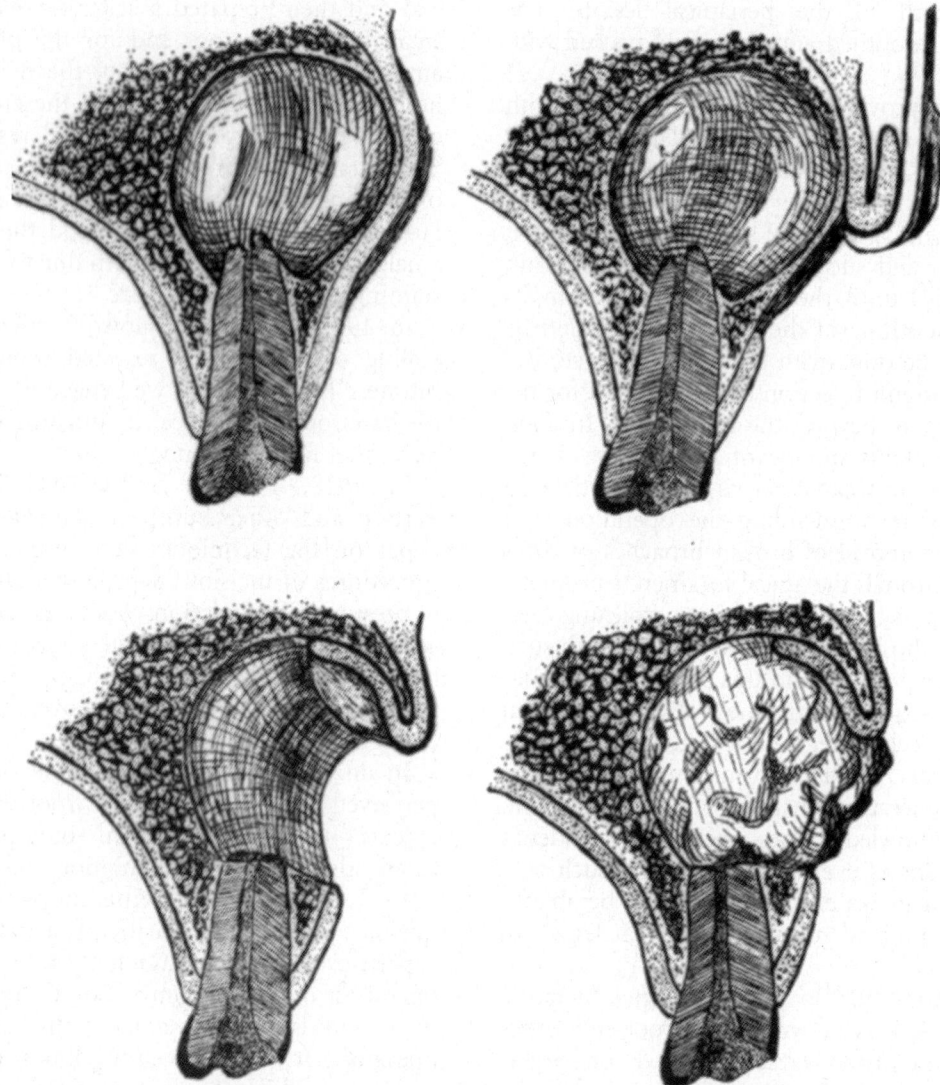

Figure 13 Schematic drawing of cyst management according to Prinz. Left to right upper diagrams, access is gained with tissue flap retracted; Lower left, the cyst is removed and the root end is resected to the base of the cavity; Lower right, the cavity is packed with iodoform gauze to stabilize the flap internally. From Prinz H. Diseases of the soft structures of the teeth and their treatment. Philadelphia: Lea & Febiger, 1928.

apicoectomy .... (2) That whenever a tooth or root can be extracted without injury to itself, there can be but one choice between the two operations."

At that same time, Arthur Smith of Rochester, New York, reported on a survey of eight questions on root-end amputation sent to prominent clinicians and authorities at that time.[160] On April 22, 1918, Dr. Carl Grove responded to Dr. Smith's first question thusly: (Question: Do you consider the root amputation in any case?) Dr. Grove's response was as follows: (author's entries in square brackets) "My dear doctor, As I am no longer a believer in apiectomy I do not think it is necessary for me to answer your questions, but I shall endeavor to state briefly why I believe these operations are a failure. In my opinion the percentage of successful cases of root amputations [apical resections] is extremely small. I question very much if there is ever a normal regeneration of bone following these operations; at least I am convinced from the investigations I have made that an attachment of tissue to the root end never takes place, which is, I believe, the chief cause for the failures. I do not regard radiographs as being conclusive evidence, as it is not possible to disclose minute changes or disease tissue that may exist, neither is it possible to determine by radiograph if there is a regeneration of bone in the rarefied area or if dense around the rarified area has resulted from the activity of the osteoblasts in the deposit of osseous tissue in the cancellous portion of the bone. These results can be produced by the stimulating of the osteoblasts by the use of certain remedies. Trusting this will explain my position regarding the question, and answer your inquiry, I am Yours very truly, Carl J, Grove." [The full concept of regeneration as we know it was not detailed[173]; however, the issue of attachment vis-à-vis Sharpey's fibers from the periodontal ligament into newly formed cementum does appear to be understood by Dr. Grove, along with bone regeneration.]

Controversies also existed at this time with the use of a chisel versus a bur to remove the root apex. Silverman was a major advocate of the chisel[159] as would be Mead in the 1930s and 1940s.[174] Silverman's rationale was as follows. Silverman referred to the chisel technique as "heat-less, quicker, cleaner and generally more convenient."

During this era, attention to surgical armamentarium was at its peak, with each surgeon or author advocating or inventing a "better mousetrap." However, one piece of equipment that was commonly used was the Killian headband, modified for root-end resection (Figure 14). This apparatus freed the operator to work in an unimpeded environment. Coupled with the "Schutzlaken" or surgical shield or drape as suggested by Witzel according to Partsch,[175] and demonstrated by Silverman in conjunction with the head band, the patient was "efficiently" treated in a "presumed" aseptic environment.[159]

At the beginning of the third decade of the twentieth century, the full impact of the focal infection theory had caught up with periapical surgery. Proper diagnosis and asepsis were demanded and more often than not extractions were the treatment of choice. However, a few brave surgeons persisted, focusing the objections to periradicular surgery on its use by the unqualified dentist, rather than on the merits of the surgical procedure. "Faulty dental work is very often traceable to the routine slovenly habits of the dentist who has no more than superficial smattering of science and art."[171]

Technique articles in the 1920s by Berger,[176] Ruggier,[177] Moorehead,[178] Kay,[179] Beavis,[180] and Posner[181] focused on similar techniques advocated from 1915 to 1920 with minor variations. Semilunar incisions were the *modus operandi* (Figures 15 and 16) although triangular flaps were beginning to appear; the use of the mallet and chisel to resect the apex was being replaced with the cross-cut fissure bur; root apices were cut to

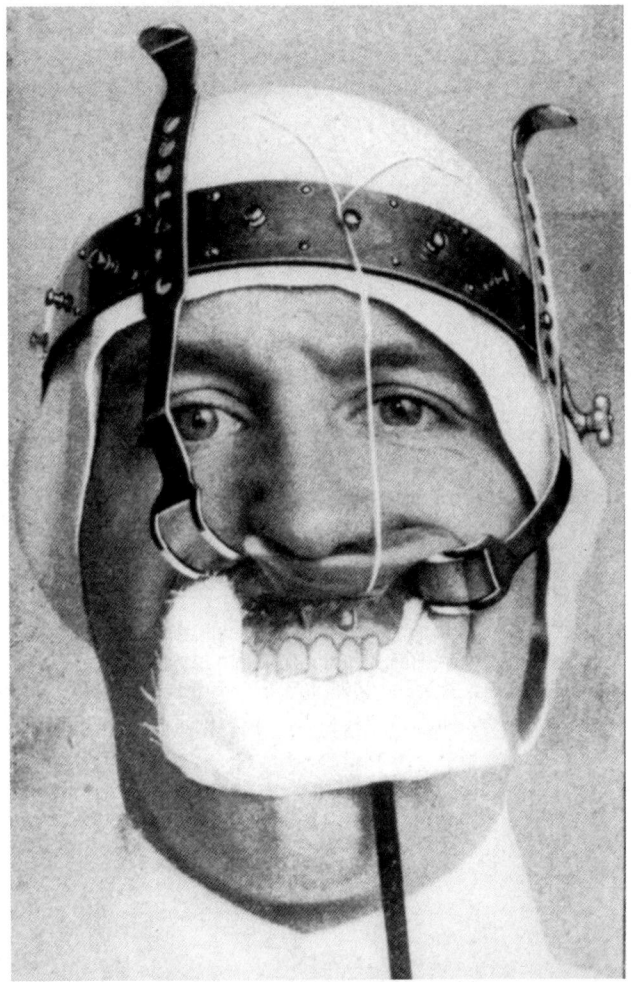

Figure 14 Patient wearing a *"Schutzlaken"* or surgical drape and Killian head band as depicted by Silverman. From Silverman SL. The status of apicoectomy. J Nat Dent Assoc 1918;5:255-263.

the base of the osseous lesion favoring a transverse cut as opposed to an angular cut; silver nitrate on the resected root surface had both proponents and opponents; the use of a hot burnisher at the apex was used sparingly; if any clinical evidence of "infection" was noticed a partial suturing technique with drain was advocated; and recall evaluation every 6 months was considered essential. Posner,[181] in an attempt to enhance the acceptance and practice of periapical surgery, even went to the extent of minimizing the perceived difficulty and need for special expertise required to efficiently and effectively perform these procedures.

In 1924, an article by Blayney and Wach[182] was published, which was "purely of academic interest," but it opened the doors for future investigation and challenge as to the exact nature of periradicular tissue repair following root-end curettage and resection. They showed that

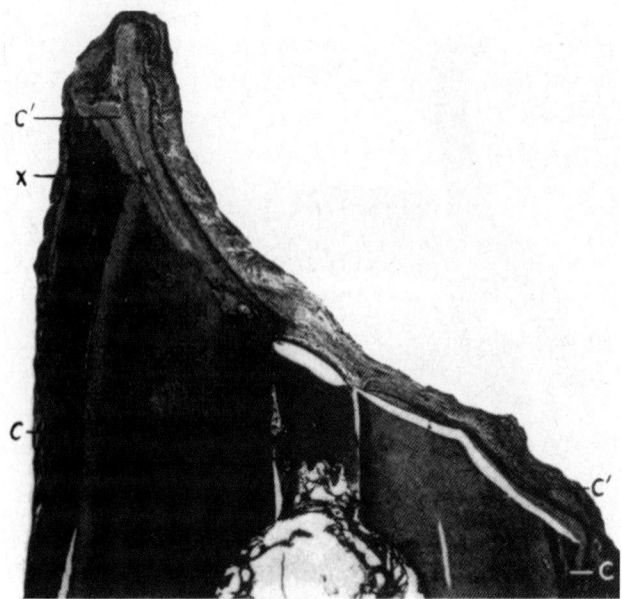

Figure 15 Successful healing with cemental apposition along the resected root surface. From Coolidge ED. Root resection as a cure for chronic periapical infection: a histologic report of a case showing complete repair. J Am Dent Assoc 1930;17:239-249.

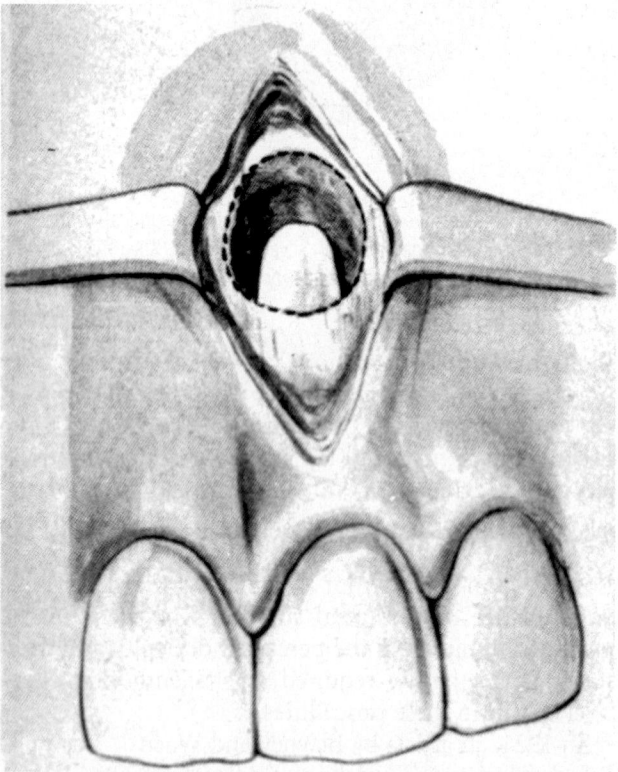

Figure 16 Weaver's "open window" surgical entry for periradicular curettage. From Weaver SM. Window method of periapical curettage. J Endodontia 1947; 2:4-5.

the periodontal ligament would heal and new cementum was deposited on the resected dentin. Boulger[183] later, in 1928, showed that healing can occur over fractured root ends and exposed dentin. These case reports paralleled the findings of Bauer,[119,120] Euler,[121] and Kronfeld[122] in Europe and led to closer scrutiny of healing responses as the next decade commenced.

Multiple investigations by Coolidge,[184] Blum,[185,186] Hill,[187] and Aisenberg[188] in North America and Garcia in South America[189] showed that healing will occur at the root apex with the layering of new cementum and the reestablishment of periodontal ligament fibers (see Figure 15). However, case numbers were few in these investigations and, while the impact of these on the concept of focal infection was initially minimal, it served as a continuing spark for those surgeons and academicians committed to total endodontic care and tooth maintenance.

Surgical practices in North America in the 1930s did not undergo major changes, and approaches to root apices, as outlined and depicted by Berger, were to be used routinely over the next 40–50 years.[190] Silver nitrate was commonly used and would be well into the 1940s, as was the iodoform gauze drain.[191,192] Gutta-percha was being placed with a sealer of zinc oxide-eugenol, and a hot burnisher was still the preferred treatment to smooth over the resected apex and perfect the seal.[193] However, a significant change in the root canal obturation technique in the 1930s was to have a lasting impact on not only non-surgical treatment but also surgical treatment and retreatment. While previous work had been done on the use of silver cones for root canal fillings in Germany, E. A. Jasper[194,195] introduced the use of standardized silver cones for canal obturation in 1931. This single event not only would polarize the dental profession, but also would lead to multiple controversies and misconceptions in treatment. Its impact on periapical surgery is still with us today and, with the advent of multiple retreatment procedures, there has been a renewed interest in developing a compatible root-end filling material that can be placed against those silver cones that cannot be non-surgically removed.

Surgical endodontics began to receive greater attention in the 1930s in the South American countries.[189,196–199] Coupled with input from Spain[200] and influenced heavily by the work of the Germans, the root-end resection technique had gained acceptance in multiple professional Latin American countries. However, some peculiar differences did exist in surgical management. For example, pastes made of zinc oxide were being placed in the bony cavity and left there while granulation and osseous fill occurred.[200]

In 1935, Ries Centeno and Gietz[197,198] published multiple articles on a comparative study of the methods of "*apicectomia*" as performed by leading professionals from South America and Spain. Questions to these leading authorities focused on types of anesthesia, flap design, methods of osseous entry, methods of root-end resection, pre-resection or post-resection canal obturation, materials used for obturation, experience with silver cone fillings, methods of obturation with canals presenting with posts, and the nature of surgical flap and cavity management after root-end resection. As would be expected, controversies existed in all areas of case management based upon the responses of the questioned individuals. Flap designs ranged from the semilunar to angled flaps in the attached tissue or at the free gingival margin, to an "S"-shaped flap design. Most clinicians had no experience with the filling of root canals "*con los conos de plata*" (with silver cones). Gutta-percha was the accepted canal filling material with some form of softening agent or paste, and amalgam was the apical filling of choice in properly prepared root-end cavity. "For the properly prepared retentive root-end cavity we use analgam only…in cases of canals that are obstructed amalgam is placed at the end of the root… for root amputation amalgam is used."

One of the contributors, Dr. Fernando Garcia from Buenos Aires, indicated an equal choice between amalgam and zinc oxide-eugenol.[189] This was one of the first indications of the use of zinc oxide-eugenol, by itself, as a root-end filling material. Interestingly, many of these same differences of opinion and controversies in practice exist today because the true biologic foundations of surgical endodontics are only now being explored with a serious purpose and intent.

Although small groups of surgical advocates and courageous individuals who believed in the tenets of quality endodontic therapy continued to pursue endodontic surgery, they did so under the shroud and pressure of the focal infection theory. Extractions were the treatment of choice for pulpless teeth. An editorial appeared in 1928[201] that was a stance adopted by a group of leading dental practitioners who believed that needless extractions were contraindicated and properly diagnosed, and executed root canal treatment would be as successful "as any other surgical procedures of similar exacting nature." The serious nature of this editorial highlights the impact that William Hunter's presentation in 1910 had upon the medical and dental profession.[44]

During the next 20 years, the dental literature produced a scant number of articles on endodontic surgery as compared to the previous two decades. Attention was focused on specific innovative or efficient techniques in case management because they facilitated the conservation of pulpless teeth during the exigencies of a period of world-wide aggression.

Between 1941 and 1950, Cyrus Jones from New York published multiple papers on the use of apical surgery in an expedient manner, primarily related to its use in the military setting.[202–204] "The present national emergency and the lack of spare time for the conscript patient and dentist lead us to present the following paper. Twenty-three years ago the writer was stationed in England at Codford Wilts on Salisbury Plains. Each day an aero squadron passed through that camp on its way to the front. It was the last stepping off place, and as such a critical inspection of all units was the order of the day. Examinations were made of the equipment of each individual, who also received a thorough medicodental examination. With the help of two sergeants, both dentists, an early morning examination was made of every mouth. Hopelessly diseased teeth and roots were marked for extraction. Sedative fillings with cement were later placed in teeth which had good potentialities. Amalgam fillings, where cavities were not too extensive, were also placed. Then came the problem of what to do with infected anterior teeth. Most of the men did not mind losing posterior teeth, but the thought of losing a front tooth was abhorrent for these young soldiers."

It was this set of circumstances that led Jones to recommend the one-visit root canal treatment followed by surgical curettage. He used chloroform at the apex to soften and dissolve the excess gutta-percha, "making a perfect joint and complete canal filling." Jones also advocated the use of antibiotics in the surgical site as would many other authors in the era. His rationale for this approach was "this technique is bold, unorthodox, and alien to all accepted procedures, but it works," especially in light of the frustration that plagued many unskilled dentists in their attempts to perform adequate non-surgical treatment. "In closing we will say that if a putrescent root canal may be filled perfectly at one sitting and the pathological effects of that tooth removed at the same time by means of a little oral surgery, why waste our time and energy and the patient's time by trying to treat an enormously infected area through at tiny apical foramen. It's like trying to put out a forest fire with a water pistol."

Later papers by Shapiro and Masters[205] in 1943 would also address the need for expediency in the management of infected anterior teeth in the military setting.

The post-resection filling technique, as described by Mead[174] in 1934 and Federspiel[206] in 1936, was an alternative and popular way of managing roots at this time and was supported by Phillips and Maxmen,[207]

Droba,[208] Wakefield,[209] Shapiro and Masters,[205] and Smith and Stevens.[210] Grossman[211] also provided details on this technique but he generally favored the technique of Jones. Droba performed surgical curettage followed by a through and through root canal obturation technique. He used eucalyptol, as did Shapiro and Masters, with the gutta-percha for better adaptation in the canal, followed by removal of the excess at the apex with a warm instrument. Eckes and Adams also supported this technique of filling through the root but, instead of eucalyptol, used zinc oxyphosphate cement as the sealer with gutta-percha.[212] Smith and Stevens used a zinc oxide-eugenol-iodoform injection filling technique.

During this period, more attention was focused on surgical curettement and total eradication of the soft tissues surrounding the root. Weaver developed his "open window apical curettage" method using a vertical incision down the long axis of the root[213,214] (see Figure 16). Root canals were obturated first so that more "collateral canals will...be filled." He emphasized thorough curettement, especially palatal to the root. The actual procedure of root-end resection in conjunction with curettage was frowned upon except when resorption was present. There were major concerns that root reduction would weaken the tooth and reduce the amount of viable periodontal ligament attachment.[213,215] Also, root-end resection may stimulate a resorptive process or create a source of continued periradicular irritation by opening the "infected dentinal tubules.[216]" "There is no supporting logic for resection or amputation of the root unless it shows signs of absorption. Amputation of the root is objectionable since it merely reduces the leverage and strength of the tooth and opens up fresh dentinal tubules."

However, Sommer was not as concerned with the exposed dentin, even if infected, but rather with the leakage from the root canal:[214] "...so long as the porous apical third is removed, the risk of future infection after a root resection lies much more in leakage from the root canal than in retained infected dentin."

When root-end resection was performed because of resorbed root ends[217] or blocked canals, they were often coated with silver nitrate to address the patent dentinal tubules.[218] Wedendal[219] recommended a vitallium-type cap that was fabricated to be cemented over the entire resected root surface. Other authors were beginning to alter previous opinions regarding the amount of root structure that should be removed. Instead of removing the root to the base of the osseous lesion, only a small portion of the root tip was removed. This was a revolutionary concept in periapical curettage and a smoothing over or rounding-off of the apex as a popular procedure. Eventually, curettage was to be considered as a terminal procedure, one that failed many times because the source of irritation in the poorly managed root canal system was not addressed.

An additional concern with the resection of the root end was the inability of the periapical tissues to form cementum over the exposed dentin. Even though this possibility had been shown in the 1920s, it still had a group of "doubting Thomases." However, histologic studies in the 1940s continued to show the presence of well-layered cementum on resected dentin with the formation of healthy connective tissue attachment.[217,220] Herbert's[221] observations on the reformation of cementum on resected dentin with chronic inflammation over the root canal filling material were especially pertinent to the concerns of many practitioners, who were so concerned about infected tubules that they may have missed the true essence of what is necessary to achieve success with root-end resection. "Such inflammatory reaction as remains in connection with these teeth is strictly limited to the tissues immediately adjacent to the apical end of the root canal filling and is not found in association with the cut surface of the dentine, which shows evidence of repair over most of its surface. This suggests that so long as the porous apical third is removed the risk of future infection after root resection lies much more in leakage from the root canal than in retained infected dentine."

The use of root-end preparations and root-end fills with amalgam was supported by Gaerny,[138] Garvin,[172] and Luks[222] as the most successful way to manage the end of the root canal system. "As stated in 1916, we are still of the opinion that root resection has a place in the general practice of dentistry and that in performing this operation it is preferable to place an amalgam filling in the apex of the tooth."[177]

In 1958, Messing[223] reintroduced the use of amalgam for the filling of the root canal prior to root-end resection, a technique reported by Lucas in 1916.[151] Messing was concerned with changes that occurred at the root apex when gutta-percha was resected and felt that a hot instrument was insufficient to rectify the aberrations of the gutta-percha dentin interface. "However, when the apex is resected one may be faced with a serious problem; the rotating blades of the bur tend to pull the gutta-percha away from the walls of the canal thus creating a defect. This has been found to occur when a mesio-distal cut is made, or when the apex is planed away in a coronal direction with a rosehead bur. It is not always possible to correct this defect by touching the end of the point with a hot instrument and compressing it into the canal." He also developed a specific amalgam carrier for the placement of the material deep into the apical third of the root. Ironically, this instrument has stood the test of time, known as the "Messing Gun" and is routinely used today for the placement of root-end amalgam fillings.

Sommer[218] and Eklof[224] advocated the use of a reverse silver cone placement if access to the canal could not be obtained through the crown and the canal had not been previously filled or was poorly filled.

In 1951, Everett[225] published a case report on the management of a non-vital maxillary lateral incisor. Root canal treatment and root-end resection were performed. Postoperative evaluation at 9 months revealed an asymptomatic tooth, with a relatively normal periodontal ligament space and nearly intact lamina dura. However, several millimeters apically there appeared a "well defined radiolucent area, giving the impression of a residual cyst." Three years later, the findings were similar and an exploratory surgical procedure was performed. As is commonly recognized today, Everett was describing the presence and persistence of scar tissue following periradicular surgery due to the position of the root apex of the lateral incisor relative to the palatal cortical plate of bone. This entity is of no clinical importance unless it is inflamed.[226] Previous identification of this type of lesion had been extremely limited[227] and it would be over 20 years before further in-depth investigations of this finding would appear in the literature.[226]

In 1959, Maxmen[228] published a lengthy paper entitled "The expanding scope of endodontics." This paper went far beyond previous publications in highlighting the full scope of periapical surgery, in addition to emphasizing the uniqueness of this aspect of dentistry. With great foresight and experience, Maxmen dispelled the concept that for so many years had been sacrosanct in the United States, but not necessarily in Europe: that apical surgery was limited to anterior teeth or maybe an occasional single-rooted premolar. However, he did caution those choosing to do posterior surgery. "These procedures should not be undertaken unless the operator is well trained in surgery, asepsis, and careful handling of tissue, and has a good working knowledge of the local structures." Not only is this paper to be considered as a classic article that would have a lasting impact on periapical surgery, but it also had an immediate impact on the solidification of the concepts of endodontic therapy, both non-surgical and surgical, that would in a few years serve as the basis for the approval of endodontics as a distinct specialty of dentistry.

With reference to surgical root or tooth resections, in 1884, Farrar[229] reports 9 years of successful "radical removal by amputation of any portions of teeth that can be of no further use" (Figures 17 and 18).

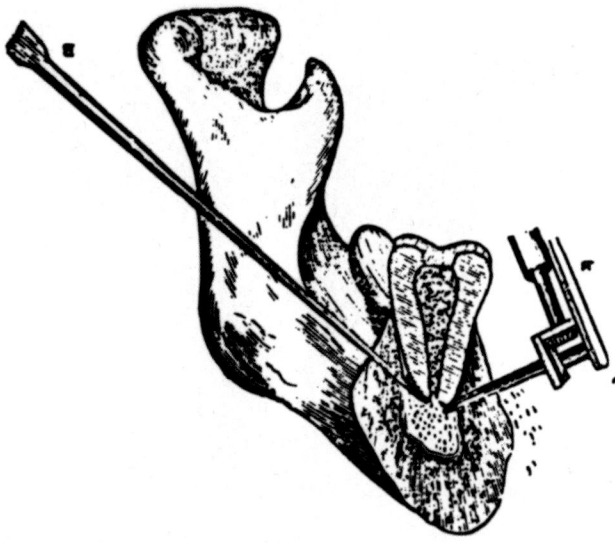

Figure 17 Farrar's initial description of managing an alveolar abscess by drilling through the cortical bone. If this were not possible, oftentimes a root would be resected as seen in Fig. 18. From Farrar JN. Radical treatment of alveolar abscess. Dent Cosmos 1880;22:376-383.

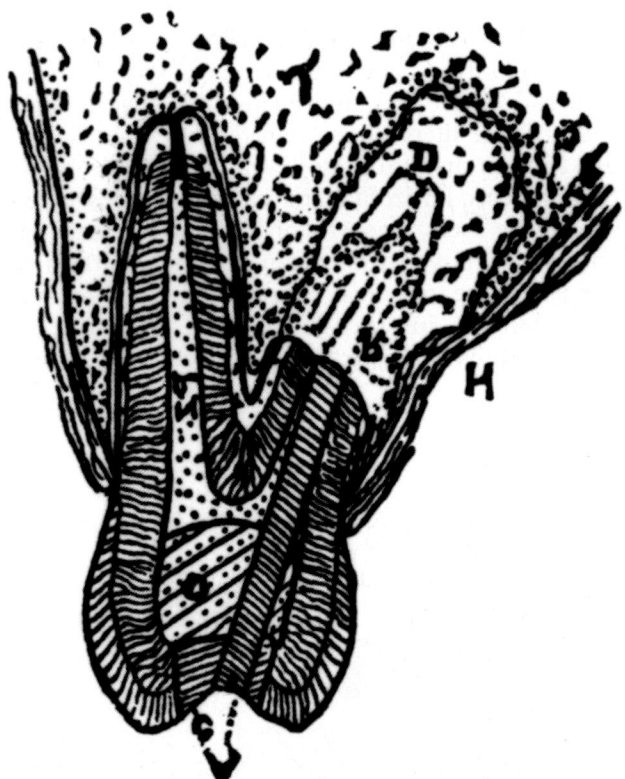

Figure 18 Farrar's diagram of root-end resection of a palatal root. From Farrar JN. Radical and heroic treatment of alveolar abscess by amputation of roots of teeth. Dent Cosmos 1884;26:79-81.

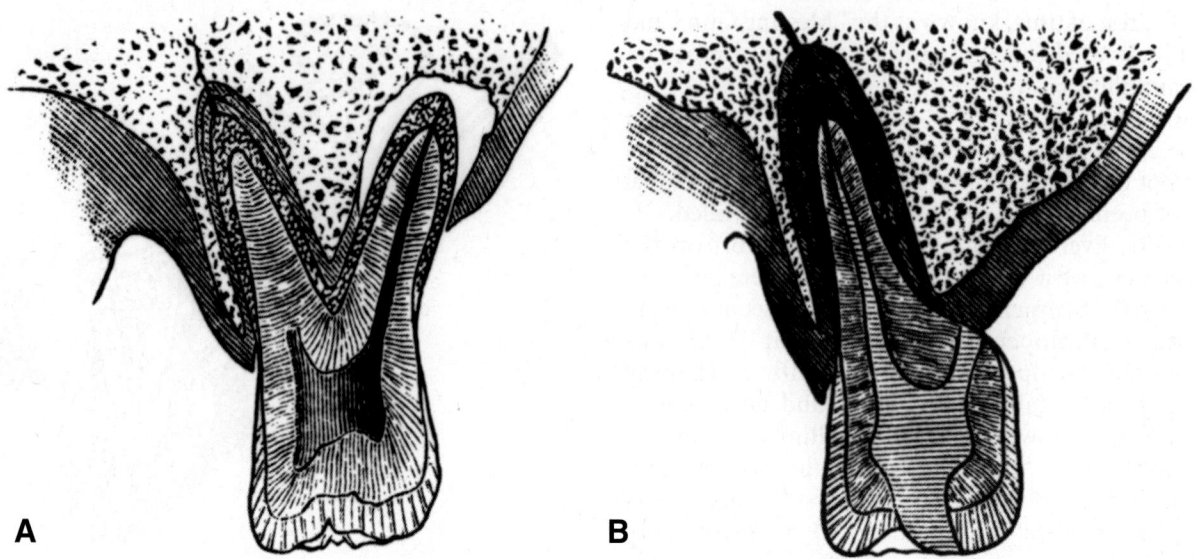

Figure 19 ***A,*** Diagram of palatal root exhibits extensive "pyorrhea alveolaris" or periodontal disease. ***B,*** Tooth following root resection and osseous repair. From Black GV. Amputation of the roots of teeth. In Litch WF. The American System of Dentistry. Philadelphia: Lea Brothers; 1886.

Black[230] in 1886 (Figures 19 and 20), Rhein[231] in 1890, White[232] in 1893, Younger[233] in 1894, and Walker in 1895[234] were also among the first to use this heroic procedure to eliminate roots chronically involved with "pyorrhea alveolaris" or "chronic abscess." Since then, the endodontic, periodontic, and surgical literature is replete with publications that support the use of resective procedures for furcation pathosis, horizontal and vertical fractures, excessive bone loss, non-restorable tooth structure, unfavorable root proximity, impaired endodontic management of the root canal, dehiscence, fenestration and root sensitivity, impaired prognosis of adjacent teeth, and resorptive and perforative defects. Historically, resections have received a wide range of creative and variable terminology, such as radisectomy, rhizectomy, odontic trisection, tooth separation, ampudontology, radectomy, root resection, odontosection, bisection, dissection, bicupidization, odontogenous resection, and tooth sectioning, with the commonly used terms of root amputation and tooth hemisection.[235]

One of the more interesting historical aspects of resections is the use of this procedure in teeth with vital pulps. This procedure was often used when the determination of the exact nature of the osseous destruction around a root could not be determined.[235] Sternlicht[236] is credited with initiating this approach to treatment, and other authors have reported on the use of this technique with long-term clinically successful follow-ups on both maxillary and mandibular teeth.[237–244] However, following vital root resections, internal resorption, pulpal inflammation, and pulp necrosis have been reported.[245–249] The long-term histological studies of Haskell,[237] Haskell and Stanley,[238,239,241,242] and Smuckler and Tagger[240] have however supported this technique in selected cases.

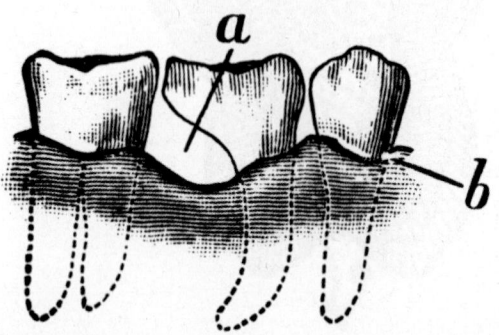

Figure 20 Diagram of root resection on a mandibular molar advocated by Black. From Black GV. Amputation of the roots of teeth. In Litch WF. The American System of Dentistry. Philadelphia: Lea Brothers; 1886.

ROOT REPAIR PROCEDURES RELATED TO PATHOLOGIC OR ODONTIATROGENIC PATHOSIS/DAMAGE

Radicular perforations have always been regarded as serious complications in the dental practice and from a historical perspective most likely resulted in tooth extractions in the majority of cases. These types of defects, whether of pathologic or mechanical origin, often required a creative approach to management.

In 1893, the problems of managing root perforations were being addressed.[250,251] Evans[252] discussed management of radicular perforations "below the line of the edge of the alveolar process" admitting that successful treatment is rare. In 1903, Peeso[253] recommended various treatment modalities for apical, middle, and coronal perforations.

1. Apical—fill as is and, if symptomatic, handle as an alveolar abscess, that is, root-end resection.
2. Middle—force a softened gutta-percha plug into the root and remove it to ascertain the extent and nature of the perforation; then fasten the plug to a condenser and pack it tightly into the perforation or use copper amalgam after the plug of gutta-percha show the amount of amalgam necessary, with "... care being used not to force it (amalgam) beyond the outer wall of the root."
3. Coronal—pack perforation in a similar manner to that for the middle, being careful not to force excess material into the tissues. In the furcation, a soft platinum or tin sheet was used to cover the perforation.

In 1912, Spaulding[250] claimed to have at least 36 years of experience in the treatment of perforations with lead. In this treatise, he identifies a perforation in the middle to apical third of the root as "... almost fatal; and the lead treatment I have described is the only one which gives almost sure hope of saving the tooth."

Since the late 1800s, many authors have recommended the sealing of root perforations with a multiplicity of materials, such as carbolic acid and tin foil, paraffin, gutta-percha, gold foil, zinc phosphate cement, formulations of calcium hydroxide, amalgam, iodoform, asbestos, Cavit, dentin chips, zinc oxide-eugenol, indium foil, Super-EBA cements, and Gelfoam, all with varying degrees of success.[235]

Prior to 1965, materials and techniques advocated in the non-surgical management of root perforations[254,255] were based upon the extensive animal and clinical studies of Euler[256] in 1925, Kubler[257] in 1934, Ruchenstein[258] in 1941, and Kaufmann[259] in 1944. Numerous studies from 1965 to 1972 by Taatz and Stiefel,[260] Lantz and Persson,[261-263] Seltzer and co-workers,[264] and Stromberg et al.[265] also evaluated the periodontal response from the furcation to the apex in both animal models and human subjects. These historical studies have provided the guidelines for the contemporary clinical management of root and tooth perforations.

INTENTIONAL REPLANTATION/ REPLANTATION OF AVULSED TEETH AND MANAGEMENT OF OTHER TRAUMATIC TOOTH INJURIES (LUXATIONS)

Replantation was a common operation ten centuries ago and was used primarily for odontalgia. Weinberger credits Abulcasis[79] with the first account of replantation in the eleventh century. Intentional replantation was recommended by Pare (cited by Lufkin)[266] in 1561 when a healthy tooth was extracted instead of a diseased one. In 1712, Pierre Fauchard[267] replanted a tooth 15 minutes after extraction, and subsequent observations of the patient revealed a stable tooth and oral environment.

In Prussia in 1756, Phillip Pfaff[268] described the use of tooth replantation and recommended root-end resection for long teeth, followed by root-end filling with wax or lead prior to replacement. In England, Thomas Berdmore[81] recommended replantations in 1768 with both immature teeth and teeth with fully formed roots. As with Pfaff, Berdmore performed root-end resection on teeth with fully formed roots followed by lead or gold as a root-end filling.

John Hunter[269] recommended the replantation procedure in 1778 when the crown was partially destroyed by caries (Figure 21). Once removed, the tooth was boiled to eradicate the disease process prior to replacement. Morrison[270] began the routine use of replantation in 1862 and reported his personal experiences with 300 cases over a 16-year period. Extractions were done carefully and the "amputation of the root or roots (was) generally not performed." The canals and pulp chamber were routinely filled prior to replantation. In 1876, Rabatz,[271] a court dentist in Vienna, presented 10 basic principles to be followed in transplanting and replanting teeth. All practitioners were cautioned to choose cases carefully and "never give our patient a decidedly favorable prognosis."

Taft[272] recommended the use of intentional replantation in 1877 when teeth exhibited a root abscess. All debris was scraped from the root and decay was excavated from the crown: "... this will occupy from thirty to sixty minutes." Following a new restoration, the tooth "should now be carefully replanted in its socket; the jaws should be closed firmly, which will carry the tooth to its precise position Ordinarily, no stays or ligatures will be required to hold it in position."

In 1881, Thompson[273] presented a lengthy treatise on replantation before the International Medical Congress. He focused on the pericemental tissues "as upon the condition of this tissue replantation is wholly dependent for its success." Further animal studies by

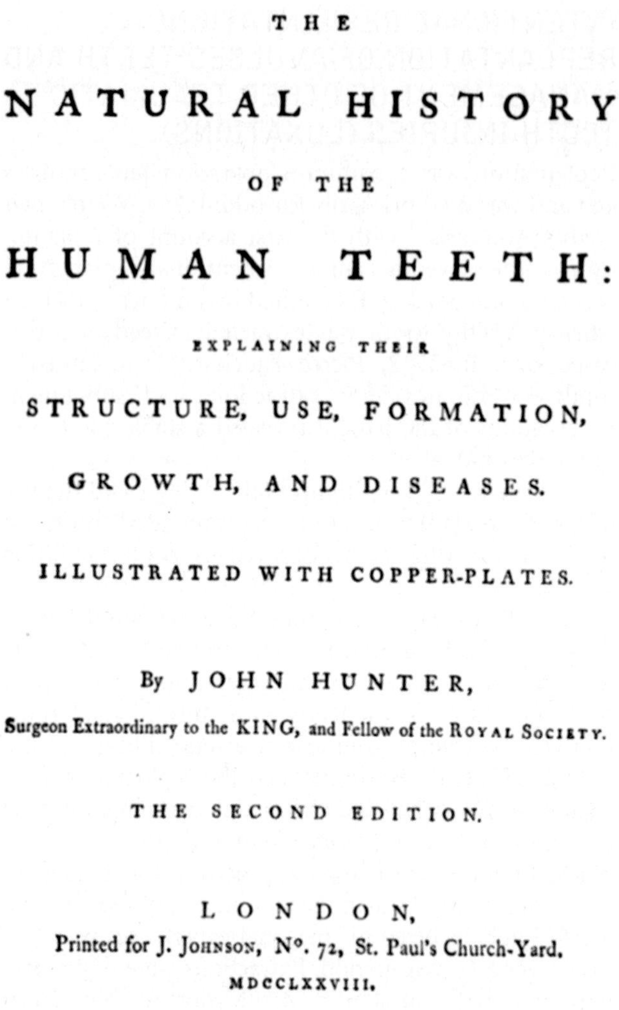

THE

NATURAL HISTORY

OF THE

HUMAN TEETH:

EXPLAINING THEIR

STRUCTURE, USE, FORMATION,

GROWTH, AND DISEASES.

ILLUSTRATED WITH COPPER-PLATES.

By JOHN HUNTER,

Surgeon Extraordinary to the KING, and Fellow of the ROYAL SOCIETY.

THE SECOND EDITION.

LONDON,
Printed for J. JOHNSON, N°. 72, St. Paul's Church-Yard.
MDCCLXXVIII.

Figure 21 Title page from Hunter's classic textbook. (From author's collection)

Fredel[274] in 1887 and Scheff[275] in 1890 began to address the role of the periodontal ligament in the success of replantation and the sequelae of the observed resorptive process following this procedure.

In the early 1900s, the use of replantation was minimal, having been partially replaced by the development of root-end resection techniques. However, for those who did practice the procedure of replantation, a controversy in technique and prognosis was evident at the Panama Pacific Dental Congress in 1915.[276] Opposing points of view on treatment addressed immediate versus delayed replantation, root canal obturation prior to or after replantation, removal or retention of the periodontal ligament, and the goal of ultimate healing—osseous union or ligament repair.

Regarding traumatic injuries and subsequent tooth management, there was little codification of diagnostic states and treatment regimes based on sound science until the later half of the twentieth century. This however does not negate the fact that history records many interesting aspects of the management of tooth trauma. For example, Abulcasis was known to use gold or silver wires to splint teeth loosened by trauma.[277] Berdmore[86] identified silk ligatures for tooth stabilization in addition to describing management of various types of luxation injuries based on patient age. "When a tooth is loosened by violence, but not moved out of its socket, ligature alone, and stringent washes to brace the gums, are sufficient for the cure.... When a tooth loses its natural position, without departing from the socket...the nerve of the tooth is, in this case, generally broken off, and the tooth-ache which attends it, is owing to the pressure point of the root on the lacerated nerve at bottom; it should be pressed on, therefore, as little as possible; and if the uneasiness continues after it becomes pretty firm in the socket, a little of the top should be filed off, that the opposite tooth may not bear on it at all ... the same may be said of teeth which are pushed inward, or outward or to a side, by violence ... by luxation of a tooth, I mean when it is raised or partially or totally from the bottom of the socket ... in young people a tooth which has been luxated, if instantly replaced, and forced quite to the bottom need only be secured by a ligature for some weeks... when the accident happens to a grown person, when the tooth is totally beat out, or when a surgeon is not at hand to reduce it in the very instant the swelling of the vessels, and extravasated blood prevent its sinking so deep as before; and as a prominence above the rest of the teeth would expose it to future injury and pain, it is found necessary to cut off a little piece of the point of the root, to smooth it well, to fill the hole in which the nerve formerly lodged with lead or gold; then to reduce it carefully and fasten it to the neighboring teeth...for people in advanced years, a hole should be drilled through the tooth sideways, close by the edge of the gums, before it is replaced; through which the gold wire or silken ligature should be passed, to secure the tooth more perfectly."

In the late 1930s, Zander and Law[67] were using the pulpotomy technique with calcium hydroxide on teeth that had suffered pulp exposures due to trauma. In 1945, Ellis[278] provided us with his classification and treatment of injuries to the teeth, and subsequently, Grossman[15] detailed these in his classical textbook citing many successful cases of managing apical root fracture management in the early 1930s. Even then, however, management of horizontal or diagonal root fractures in the middle or coronal third of the root was considered unfavorable. Management of luxation injuries dictated that the pulp always be removed prior to replantation, and the root tip may be removed prior to placement into the socket. If desired, a knob-like titanium or vitallium extension could be added to the root end to compensate for the portion removed.[15]

Interrelationships between Pulpal and Periodontal Diseases

Interrelationships between pulpal and periodontal diseases have been both confirmed and denied for over 100 years. During this time, little has been written concerning the diagnosis and management of these interrelated entities, other than indicating that teeth having these problems were often extracted based on a poor prognosis for retention. This was especially true if a periodontal pocket united with an apical lesion of pulpal origin. As a consequence, these interrelationships have posed significant diagnostic and treatment dilemmas for the clinician over the decades.

Historically, Dr. Lester Cahn[279] is often quoted as identifying a relationship between the presence of periodontal disease and its impact on pulpal demise, even though the literature is fraught with studies that claim that periodontal disease has no impact (Table 5). "... I have never found a pulp removed from a pyorrhetic tooth to be normal ... where a pathologic pulp is present, a pyorrhetic condition cannot be cured by treatment applied exclusively to the external surface of the root, with no treatment of the pulp itself."

From the opposite viewpoint, Seltzer et al.[280] provided significant support for the impact of pulp disease on the periodontium. "... interradicular periodontal lesions can be initiated and perpetuated by inflamed or necrotic pulps. Extension of the inflammatory lesions from the dental pulp apparently occurs through accessory or lateral canals situated in the furcation regions of premolars and molars ..."

As with many issues in dentistry, many remedies, techniques, processes, outcomes and classifications have been proposed to define the relationship between the pulp and the periodontium and to offer suggestions for treatment[281–283] (see Table 5).

Endodontic Endosseous Implants (Diodontic or through the Tooth Implants)

Little has been written about this treatment modality, and the contemporary use of endodontic endosseous implants is quite limited in light of advances in implant technology and techniques. Endodontic implant stabilizer can provide in some cases a sound physiologic procedure for stabilizing mobile teeth by increasing root length, altering root crown ratios, immobilizing fractured roots and periodontally compromised teeth, or supplying combinations of these benefits.[284–288] How will these be handled? The endodontic endosseous implant has an advantage in that it can be totally intraosseous without communication into the oral cavity.[284,287]

The use of metallic implant gain credibility in 1937 when Venable, et al.[289] determined the necessary characteristics of metallic substances to be used as intraosseous devices. They reported on the metal Vitallium that had been found to be completely inert in bodily fluids and consequently non-irritating to tissues. Recent studies, however, have questioned this outcome and newer alloys are being developed.[288]

Orlay[290] was one of the first almost 50 years ago to report on the use of this treatment modality to stabilize

Table 5 Classical and Contemporary Studies with Different Viewpoints on the Relationship of Pulp and Periodontal Diseases

Studies Supporting the Impact of Periodontal Disease on the Dental Pulp	Studies Questioning the Impact of Periodontal Disease on the Pulp	Studies Questioning the Impact of Periodontal Treatment Procedures on the Dental Pulp
Seltzer et al. (1963)[280]	Mazur and Massler (1964)[437]	Bergenholtz and Lindhe (1978)[444]
Stahl (1963, 1965)[431]	Hattler et al. (1977)[438]	Ross and Thompson (1978)[439]
Rubach and Mitchell (1965)[432]	Ross and Thompson (1978)[439]	Bergenholtz and Nyman (1984)[441]
Stallard (1972)[433]	Czarnecki and Schilder (1979)[440]	Jaoui et al. (1995)[445]
Bender and Seltzer (1972)[434]	Bergenholtz and Nyman (1984)[441]	Harrington et al. (2002)[443]
Sinai and Soltanoff (1973)[435]	Torabinejad and Kiger (1985)[442]	
Wang and Glickman (2002)[436]	Harrington et al. (2002)[443]	

periodontally compromised teeth. Technique articles on the placement of these types of implants are few but thorough in their description and details.[284,286] Prognosis has been reported to be over 90%; however, few if any extensive and meaningful studies are available in the last 30 years.[287,291]

Bleaching of Discolored Dentin and Enamel

The bleaching of non-vital teeth has had few "historical" publications, and the technique and materials were heavily, empirically driven. Most details on this process come to us from Grossman in his text entitled *Root Canal Therapy*.[15] In it, Dr. Grossman highlights the major causes for tooth discoloration:

- Decomposition of the pulp tissue
- Excessive hemorrhage following pulp removal
- Medicaments
- Filling materials
- General systemic conditions

Substances to reverse the stained tooth structure consisted of powerful oxidizing agents such as pyrozone (25% solution of hydrogen peroxide in ether), superoxol (30% solution of hydrogen peroxide), and sodium dioxide (yellowish amorphous powder). In an attempt to restore the translucency to the tooth, Renström (cited by Grossman)[15] recommended an 80% solution of chloral hydrate that had an index of refraction same as that enamel according to Cape and Kitchin.[292] The bleaching of teeth that are stained systemically or due to patient factors and that have vital pulps is more of a contemporary, aesthetic-driven modality and will therefore not be addressed here.

Pearson[293] brought a more contemporary perspective to bleaching almost 50 years ago, while Spasser,[294] in 1961, provided a simple bleaching technique for pulpless, darkened teeth that use sodium perborate, and Nutting and Poe,[295] in 1967, provided the dental profession with a more detailed treatise on the subject.

Revision of Previously Treated Root Canal Systems, Non-Surgical and Surgical

While surgical revision of less than ideal root canal treatment has a long and supportive history, routine application of non-surgical revision techniques had little emphasis historically. Much of the focus was on the removal of broken instruments in the root canal. Even in these cases, root-end resection was heavily favored based on the skill and experience of the clinician.

Furher (cited by Grossman)[15] in 1947 suggested a novel method of removing a broken instrument in the root canal. This consisted of inserting a broach alongside the broken fragment and attaching the broach to a spot-welding apparatus. The current was momentarily connected to spot-weld the broach to the fragment. When the broach was removed, the fragment attached to the broach was also removed. Unfortunately, there is no indication in his publication relation to the potential danger to the patient. Almost 30 years earlier, Waas[296] recommended the use of a 25% solution of iodo-trichlorid for dissolving the broken segment. The solution was pumped into the canal, carefully, for 3 to 5 minutes followed by a thorough rinsing of the canal with sterile water. Apparently after one or two applications of this corrosive solution, the segment could be rinsed, generally in pieces, from the canal in most cases. Some situations required multiple visits. Prinz[297] in 1922 recommended a similar solution called Lugol, which was made from 2 parts potassium iodide, 3 parts distilled water, and 2 parts iodine crystals. The solution was pumped into the canal to contact the fractured segment followed by the use of an explorer to pick around the segment. After several minutes, the solution was washed from the canal, the canal was dried, and the solution re-applied. After each application, the canal was rinsed with sterile water. If the segment could not be displaced, the Lugol solution was sealed in the canal for 2 to 3 days. However, because cotton fibers were dissolved by strong iodine solutions, asbestos fiber had to be placed in the canal and followed by a strong sealing cement.

G. R. Warner recommended that dialyzed iron be sealed in the root canal with a broken instrument fragment. The solution was changed every other day until the segment or its remnants could be rinsed from the canal.[298] In later years, a solution of strong acid (sulphuric 40% or nitric 50%) was recommended[54]; however, every few minutes after application, a solution of sodium bicarbonate was used to neutralize the acid. In doing so, the broken segment was often seen to rise from the canal within the resultant effervescence.

For the ready removal of gutta-percha, xylol or chloroform has been recommended[15,54]; however, the use was recommended in stages over a number of appointments to prevent the potential irritation of the tissues beyond the end of the canal.

Coronal Restorative Procedures Involving the Root Canal Space and Coronal Access Openings

The restoration of endodontically treated teeth did not receive any significant attention regarding alterations in the nature of the tooth structure or unique methods to replace the missing coronal tooth structure due to caries or endodontic access openings until the late 1950s and early 1960s. Up until that point and even to the present day, it was and is thought by many that all root-treated teeth were weakened, or better yet "brittle" due to moisture loss following the removal of the dental pulp,[299–302] even though G. V. Black[303] could not identify in 1895 any appreciably moisture loss in teeth during his investigation of the physical properties of dentin. "I have made a diligent search to find whether or not teeth from which the pulp had been removed, and the canals and pulp chamber filled without admitting the fluids of the mouth, were subject to a similar deterioration of strength. It is now well known that teeth treated in this way retain their color almost perfectly; and from my observation of the relation of color to strength of the teeth I am prepared to entertain the suppositions that they retain their strength also. Only one tooth came into my hands with a root-filling. It was a central incisor, and had not sufficient tissue for me to obtain a block; but it showed no undue percentage of water, and the color was good. Up to the present time I have been unable to obtain the history of the filling of this root."

However, the empirical concept of "brittleness" persisted and was further proffered by studies of Helfer et al.[304] in 1972. Twenty years later, in 1992, Gutmann[305] identified that potential changes in the strength of root-treated teeth reside in a multitude of factors that include a minimal but non-appreciable loss of moisture, alterations in the architectural changes of the coronal portion of the tooth subsequent to caries or endodontic access openings, the nature of collagen cross-linking in root-filled teeth versus normal vital teeth, the biomechanical behavior of the tooth structure of a root-treated tooth when placed under stress, and the nature of dentin toughness in pulpless teeth.

Present restorative challenges with root-treated teeth deal primarily with whether posts are necessary, the use of bonding agents and high compressive restorative materials. Here again, contemporary research efforts have shed light on historical dilemmas and have provided directions for present and future clinical considerations.[306–309] Further dilemmas within this scope of endodontics have resided in the possibility of coronal leakage through poor or faulty coronal restorations. While this latter dilemma began to surface in the 1980s, Dahlgren[310] in 1916 identified the problem of coronal leakage following the failure to restore root treated teeth properly.

Historical Faux Pas, Challenges, and Milestones

Throughout the history of endodontics, there have been many case reports or reviews or anecdotal observations that have impacted on our specialty and have led to significant changes in diagnostic and therapeutic patterns. Sadly, none of these were evidence based; however, clinicians and educators alike grasped onto the messages they provided and redirected courses of endodontic procedures, often in an erroneous manner and driven by sensationalism. The following represent only a few of these historical perspectives with comments regarding their possible role in our evolution over the years.

Tooth Resorption

Tooth/root resorption has been, for years, a difficult problem to prevent and manage. Historically, the destructive process was seen commonly with the use of intentional replantation in the eighteenth and nineteenth centuries.[86,267–269] The treatment of choice during this time frame was to either boil the tooth to eradicate any disease process in the tooth (caries)[269] or to scrape all the debris from the root (this will occupy from 30 to 60 min). Needless to say, these types of procedures encouraged the resorptive process. In the late 1800s, W. F. Thompson[273] presented a lengthy treatise on replantation before the International Medical Congress. He focused on the pericemental tissues "as upon the condition of this tissue replantation is wholly dependent for its success." Further studies by Fredel[274] in 1887 and Scheff[275] in 1890 began to address the role of the periodontal ligament in the success of replantation and the sequelae of the observed resorptive process following replantation. Certainly what is known today regarding the role of the periodontal ligament, inflammation, bacteria, and biofilms impacts greatly on the prevention and management of this process.[173,311] Sadly, however, there are many non-endodontic specialists and general dentists worldwide who believe that resorption is the malady and not a result of other insults. This has led to mismanagement of this destructive process, including multiple surgical procedures with ultimate failure and the wholesale extraction of teeth in many locations in favor of prosthetic replacement.

Surgical Root-End Filling Materials/ Procedures

For decades, amalgam was used as the main surgical root-end filling material. Farrar[229] is often credited with one of the first reports of placing a root-end amalgam filling subsequent to root-end resection. Rhein[312] used amalgams in 1887 to seal the pulp canal after complete root resection. Faulhaber and Neumann[96] in 1912 and von Hippel[108] in 1914 used amalgam to fill root canals from the resected root end when a post-core crown had been placed without proper non-surgical root canal treatment. Garvin[172] reported witnessing a root-end resection in 1915, which was followed by a root-end amalgam filling. Early reports in the twentieth century[151,155,161] indicated that amalgam was considered as a routine root-end filling material if the root canal filling material did not seal the canal at the newly formed apex. During that time and well into that century, amalgams contained high levels of copper or silver and definitely significant levels of zinc. The latter material was used primarily for its deoxidizing properties and for having an impact on the plasticity, retained mercury, dimensional change, compressive strength, and creep of the amalgam. However, in 1959, a single case report by Omnell,[313] which appeared in the dental literature, caused a significant change in the use of amalgam with zinc. In this case report, a zinc carbonate precipitate was identified as causing chronic inflammation at the resected root apex. This singular finding caused the endodontic profession to switch to the use of zinc-free amalgam for root-end filling, and a plethora of studies ensued that addressed the efficacy of zinc-free amalgams. Contemporary attempts to identify the presence and nature of this serendipitous finding have been unsuccessful.[314]

A technique that had been promulgated for a number of years for the sealing of the resected root end was the use of a heated instrument to burnish the resected gutta-percha root canal filling as an alternative to placing a root-end fill. This technique was often used when the root canal had been filled immediately prior to root-end resection or if the endodontist had treated the tooth previously. Burnishing was claimed to seal the margins of the gutta-percha and resected dentin and was often used when access to the resected root end was restricted or the endodontic surgeon did not have the necessary tools to achieve the task. However, in a publication by Tanzilli et al.,[315] extensive voids were noted on the resected root face between the gutta-percha and the dentin in a small group of specimens. This finding, presented in a case review format, caused the endodontist to abandon the use of heat burnishing the resected root end and encouraged the use of cold-burnishing, a technique that fared no better than did heat burnishing.

A similar impact on the endodontic profession occurred with the use of Super-EBA as a root-end filling material. In a single case report by Oynick and Oynick,[316] the presence of collagenous fibers was seen to be embedded in a Super-EBA root-end filling on an extracted tooth specimen. Endodontists were quick to adopt Super-EBA as the material of choice, with claims that the material would allow for a regenerative response (formation cementum, bone and periodontal ligament with insertion of Shapey's fibers)[173] on the resected root end, in particular on the root-end fill material. The same response was thought to occur with the use of immediate restorative material; however, in subsequent histological studies, regeneration could not be found. In all of the above cases, endodontists changed their clinical techniques and use of materials based heavily on empiricism and the desire to hope that the shortcomings of history could be transformed into future positive outcomes.

Within the realm of endodontics, and in particular surgical applications, many situations have arisen in which the course of history is repeated without regard for past achievements. For example, in 1962, Matsura published a technique article that described the use of a slot preparation in the root end when access was limited. This technique was rapidly labeled as the "Matsura" preparation.[110] However, evidence for this technique and approach to managing the root end was already evident in 1914[108,114] and with modifications purported in the mid-1930s.[111,112] Another example would be the nature of the angle of root-end resection and patent dentinal tubules as pathways for microorganisms. This issue was addressed contemporaneously by Vertucci and Beatty[317] and Tidmarsh and Arrowsmith[318] and reinforced by the proponents of flat resections and the use of ultrasonic root-end preparation. Concern for the angled, resected root ends, and exposed infected tubules was expressed by Ross[118] in 1935, and methods to manage were purported by both Ross, in 1939, and Castenfeldt.[116]

With regard to root-end cavity preparation, for almost 50 years the endodontic profession was limited to using miniature handpieces and burs or straight handpieces, depending on the surgical access. With the advent of ultrasonic root-end preparation, the profession was very quick to adopt this technology with little or no evidence-based information as to its efficacy or safety. Since its advent, over 20 published research endeavors have attempted to determine, with mixed results, the ability and predictability of this technique to result in no root fractures during cavity preparation.

Non-Surgical Management of Symptomatic Teeth with Necrotic Pulps

Possibly for clinical expediency or lack of understanding of microbial and immunological implications, clinicians have opted to manage patients who present in pain due to teeth with necrotic pulps, with or without periapical lesions, by gaining coronal access and leaving the tooth open for drainage. While many of these patients become symptom free, many do not and the ultimate ability to finally close these teeth to the oral cavity becomes a significant and controversial challenge. In 1936, Walker[319] indicated that leaving teeth open for drainage was a highly unscientific practice that had begun to permeate the profession. The challenge that this clinical situation posed led to a number of publications trying to answer the question, "to close or not to close."[320-324] Generally, this question was resolved with both retrospective studies and a better understanding of the biologic aspects of root canal procedures and their outcomes.[325,326] In the author's experience, this question has probably been the most frequently asked question in continuing education courses for 25 to 30 years and occasionally continues to surface.

In 1883, Dr. Safford G. Perry[327] wrapped gutta-percha around a gold wire and made gutta-percha points that were rolled in shellac and compacted into the root canal. In 1978, Dr. W. Ben Johnson[328] introduced to the dental community gutta-percha that was plasticized and wrapped around a K-file, which ultimate resulted in product called ThermaFil. Scientific advances allowed the use of high-tech plastic for future core materials. However, while highly successful, the introduction of this material and technique may have been premature relative to the need for properly shaped root canals for it to achieve its full impact in root canal obturation. While in some respects history has repeated itself with the development of this type of product, the adage of putting the cart before the horse may also have been an operative phenomenon.

Historical Stalwarts

The specialty of endodontics has had a long history of incorporating innovative materials, instruments, and techniques in order to remove offending etiologic factors and create the best possible environment for healing apically, following either non-surgical and/or surgical endodontic intervention. Historically, these entities served endodontics and its realm of applications quite well within a particular historical context. More often, however, their use or application was empirically based and would not necessarily pass the test of evidence-based contemporary directives. Furthermore, science has intervened and has dealt a blow to the continued use of many of these entities. The list below is only partial in nature as globally many other miracle cures, pastes, and mystery potions have existed but have never gained widespread use or endorsement.

1. Medicaments

    a. Formocreosol, camphorated or aqueous para-monochlorophenol, beechwood creosote, metacryslacetate, carbolic acid
    b. PBSN (Penicillin, bacitracin, streptomycin & nystatin); PBSC (Penicillin, bacitracin, streptromycin & sodium caprylate
    c. Microcide A
    d. SPAD
    e. Oil of cassia
    f. Iodoform
    g. Sulfathiozole
    h. Sulfanilamide
    i. Benzlog
    j. Arsenic trioxide
    k. Silver nitrate
    l. Mercuric chloride
    m. Azochloramid
    n. Serocalcium
    o. Dentinigine
    p. Calcium thymol
    q. Pulpatekt
    r. Citronellol
    s. Endoxyl

2. Irrigants

    a. Chloramine-T
    b. Hydrogen peroxide
    c. Anesthetic solutions
    d. Water

3. Surgical materials/instruments/techniques
   a. Horsehair sutures, silk sutures
   b. Root-end amalgams (zinc containing and zinc free)
   c. Miniature handpieces for root-end preparations
   d. Cold and warm burnishing of gutta-percha
   e. Coating of resected root ends with silver nitrate
   f. Curettage only procedures
   g. Chisels for root-end resection
   h. Canal preparation techniques/instruments/materials
   i. Carbon steel instruments
   j. Smooth broaches
   k. Metallic-handled test files
   l. Step-back instrumentation
   m. Electrosterilization of the canal
   n. Root canal culturing
4. Obturation materials/Techniques
   a. Formaldehyde or paraformaldehyde-containing pastes (SPAD, N2, RC2B)
   b. Mummification procedures
   c. Silver cones
   d. Oxychloride of zinc
   e. Kerr #3 spreader
   f. Chloroform-rosin (Johnson-Callahan) technique
   g. Hydron
5. Anesthetics
   a. Cocaine crystals
   b. Novocaine

Even with the justified abandonment of many historical techniques and materials in favor of more scientifically sound or clinically documented successful entities, there persists in some global markets the continued use of historical and empirical clinical "favorites," such as the following:

- Steroid creams and pastes as medicament
- Knockendeckel (bony lid) surgical methods
- Electrophoresis
- Surgical removal of sinus tracts
- Intracanal antibiotic pastes (using newer formulations)
- Cemented root canal files as filling materials
- Paste root canal fills (zinc phosphate and paraformadehyde-containing fillings)
- Placement of posts in every root-treated tooth
- Surgical trephination with overextended root canal fillings
- Non-surgical root canal treatment without aseptic (dental dam) isolation

History Admonishes the Future

History is so vast and its fleeting information so elusive that it is impossible to record all occurrences or developments in but a few pages. Regardless of this shortcoming, by addressing the history of this specialty in the manner presented, this chapter does not lay claim to any future developments and directions, for that is within the remaining chapters of this text. These chapters record the intense clarification and codification that endodontics has received in the past few decades based on extensive scientific research and clinical practice, some of which is evidence based. However, as it is known that history has a tendency to repeat itself, astute endodontists and future endodontists must gird themselves to prevent falling into the empirical abyss of personal favorites, untested remedies, and unscientific claims to success. It is within this framework that we must view history and learn from at least some of its lessons, lest we fall victim to its entrapments.

References

1. American Association of Endodontists. 2005–2006 Membership Directory, Chicago 2005.
2. Keane HC. A century of service to dentistry. Philadelphia: S. S. White Dental Manufacturing Co; 1944.
3. Orban B. Editorial. J Endod 1946;1:1.
4. Milas VB. A history of the American Association of Endodontists. Chicago: General Printing Co; 1968.
5. Ingle JI. Endodontics. Philadelphia: Lea & Febiger; 1965.
6. Baume LJ. The biology of pulp and dentine. A historic, terminologic–taxonomic, histologic–biochemical, embryonic and clinical survey. Monogr Oral Sci, Basel, S. Karger; 1980; 37–40.
7. Kremenak NW, Squier CA. Pioneers in oral biology: the stories of Gottlieb, Kronfeld, Orban, Weinmann, and Sicher and their Vienna-to-America migrations. Crit Rev Oral Biol Med 1997;8:108–28.
8. Hargreaves KM, Goodis HE, editors. Seltzer & Bender's Dental Pulp. Carol Stream IL: Quintessence; 2002.
9. Preiswerk G. Die Pulpa-Amputation, eine klinische, patho-histologische und bakteriologische Studie. Össterr.-Ungar. Vjschr. Zahnheilk; 1901.

10. Hess W, Zürcher E. The anatomy of the root canals of the teeth of the permanent and deciduous dentitions. New York: Wm Wood & Co.; 1925.
11. Barrett MT. The internal anatomy of the teeth with special reference to the pulp with its branches. Dent Cosmos 1925;67:581–92.
12. Pucci FM, Feig R. Conductos Radiculares. Buenos Aires: Editorial Medico-Quirurgica; 1944.
13. Skillen WG. Morphology of root canals. J Am Dent Assoc 1932;19:719–35.
14. Wheeler RC. Textbook of dental anatomy and physiology. Philadelphia: W. B. Saunders Co.; 1942.
15. Grossman LI. Root canal therapy. 3rd ed. Philadelphia: Lea & Febiger; 1950.
16. Thomas NG. Formation of the apices of teeth. J Natl Dent Assoc 1921;8:11–17.
17. Kronfeld R. Histopathology of the teeth. Philadelphia: Lea & Febiger; 1939.
18. Coolidge ED. Clinical pathology and treatment of the dental pulp and periodontal tissues. Philadelphia: Lea & Febiger; 1946.
19. Levy RL. Therapeutics and medicine. Chairman's Address. J Am Med Assoc 1932:99:355.
20. Hunter W. The role of sepsis and of antisepsis in medicine. Lancet (London) 1911;1:79–86; Dent Cosmos 1918; 60:585–602.
21. Rhein ML. Oral sepsis. Dent Cosmos 1912;54:529–34.
22. Logan WHG. Chronic oral infections associated with teeth and their treatment. Dent Rev 1913; 27:957–79.
23. Hartzell TB. Secondary infections having their primary origin in the oral cavity. J Allied Dent Soc 1914;9:166–85.
24. Buckley JP. Opening address. Trans Panama Pacific Dent Cong 1915;2:307–13.
25. Ulrich HL. Some medical aspects of certain mouth infections. Dent Rev 1914; 28:1135–44.
26. Rosenow EC. Studies on elective localization. Focal infection with special reference to oral sepsis. J Dent Res 1919;1:205–68.
27. Rosenow EC. Changing concepts in oral sepsis. J Natl Dent Assoc 1927;14:117–24.
28. Rosenow EC. Oral sepsis in its relationship to focal infection and elective localization. J Am Dent Assoc 1927;14:1417–38.
29. Rosenow EC. Studies on focal infection, elective localization and cataphoretic velocity of streptococci. Dent Cosmos 1934;76:721–44.
30. Billings F. Focal infection. New York: D Appleton & Co.; 1916.
31. Meyer FK. The present status of dental bacteriology. J Natl Dent Assoc 1917;4:966–96.
32. Grossman LI. Root canal therapy. Philadelphia: Lea & Febiger; 1940.
33. Holman WL. Focal infection and "elective localization"; a critical review. Arch Pathol Lab Med 1928;5:68–136.
34. Peak CA. Oral focal infection. Dent Summary 1918;38:430–8.
35. Goldberg HA. Pyorrhea alveolaris, alveolar abscess and their relations to arthritis. Trans Panama Pacific Dent Cong 1915;2:169–80.
36. Strietmann WH. Oral sepsis as related to systemic disease. Trans Panama Pacific Dent Cong 1915;2:147–53.
37. Rosenow EC. Oral sepsis in its relationship to focal infection and elective localization. Am Dent Surg 1927;47:101–2.
38. Lowrie WE. The relation of dental infection to eye disease. Am Dent Surg 1927;47:223–5.
39. Nodine AM. Focal infection from the stomatological point of view. Am Dent Surg 1927;47:266–70.
40. Hartzell TB. Review of the literature regarding infected teeth. J Am Dent Assoc 1926;13:441–71.
41. Leonard HJ. Indications for the removal of teeth from the standpoints of oral diagnosis and periodontia. Dent Cosmos 1931;73:390–6.
42. American Dental Association. Role of dental foci infection in specific types of body disease. J Am Dent Assoc 1951;42:655–86.
43. Hatton EH. Changes produced by disease in the pulp and periapical regions, and their relationship to pulp-canal treatment and to systemic disease. Dent Cosmos 1924;66:1183–9.
44. Rickert UG, Dixon CM. The controlling of root surgery. 8th Int Dent Cong 1931; Section 111:15–22.
45. Goldman M, Pearson AH. A preliminary investigation of the "hollow tube" theory in endodontics: studies with neotetrazolium. J Oral Ther Pharmacol 1965;1:616–26.
46. Torneck CD. Reaction of rat connective tissue to polyethylene tube implants. Part 1. Oral Surg Oral Med Oral Pathol 1966;21:379–87.
47. Torneck CD. Reaction of rat connective tissue to polyethylene tube implants. Part 2. Oral Surg Oral Med Oral Pathol 1967;24:674–83.
48. Phillips JM. Rat connective tissue response to hollow polyethylene tube implants. J Can Dent Assoc (Tor) 1967;33:59–64.
49. Fish EW. Experimental investigation of enamel, dentine, and the dental pulp. London: John Bale, Sons and Daniellson, Ltd; 1932.
50. Armstrong HG, Huber RE. Effect of high-altitude flying on human teeth and restorations. Dent Dig 1937;43:132–4.
51. Ritchey B, Orban B. Toothache at high altitudes. J Endod 1946;1:13–18.
52. Kennon RH. Dental problem concerning flying personnel. J Am Dent Assoc 1944;31:662–7.

53. Prinz H. Diseases of the soft structures of the teeth and their treatment. 2nd ed. Philadelphia: Lea & Febiger, Henry Kimpton; 1937.

54. Coolidge ED. Endodontia. The clinical pathology and treatment of the dental pulp and pulpless teeth. Philadelphia: Lea & Febiger; 1950.

55. Schour I. A review of Maximow's research on inflammatory reaction. J Am Dent Assoc 1930;17:1605–16.

56. Francke OC. Capping of the living pulp: from Phillip Pfaff to John Wessler. Bull Hist Dent 1971;19:17–31.

57. Harding WE. A few practical observations on the treatment of the pulp. J Brit Dent Assoc 1883;4:318–21.

58. Kakehashi S, Stanley HR, Fitzerald RT. The effects of surgical exposures of dental pulps in germ-free and conventional laboratory rats. Oral Surg Oral Med Oral Pathol 1965;20:340–9.

59. Seltzer S. Bender IB. The dental pulp. 3rd ed. Philadelphia: Lippincott; 1984.

60. Cvek M. Pulp reactions to exposure after experimental crown fracture or grinding in adult monkeys. J Endod 1982;8:391–7.

61. Cvek M, Lundberg M. Histological appearance of pulps after exposure by crown fracture, partial pulpotomy, and clinical diagnosis of healing. J Endod 1983;9:8–11.

62. Leonard NC. Partial pulp extirpation in children's teeth. J Am Dent Assoc 1924;11:221–6.

63. Rebel M. Partial amputation of dental pulp. Trans 8th Int Dent Congr. Gen Reports: 1931;210–42.

64. Gottlieb B, Orban B, Stein B. The root treatment in a case of a vital pulp. Aust J Dent 1933;37:422–7.

65. Novikoff J. Report on experiences with pulpotomy at the dental department of the Hebrew Orphan Asylum New York City. Dent Cosmos 1935;77:676–84.

66. Teuscher GW, Zander HA. A preliminary report on pulpotomy. Northwest Dent Res & Grad Quart Bull 1938;39:4–8.

67. Zander HA, Law DB. Pulp management in fractures of young permanent teeth. J Am Dent Assoc 1942;29:737–41.

68. Zander HA, Glass RL. Healing of phenolized pulp exposures. Oral Surg Oral Med Oral Pathol 1949;2:803–10.

69. Nygren JA. Rådigivare angående bästa sättet att vårda och bevara tåbderbas frusjget, Stockholm; 1838.

70. Hermann BW. Dentinobliteration der wurzelkanale nach der Behandlung mi Kalzium. Zahnaertzl Rund. 1930;39:888–99.

71. Zander HA. Reaction of pulp to calcium hydroxide. J Dent Res 1939;18:373–9.

72. Eastlick KA. Management of pulp exposures in the mixed dentition. J Am Dent Assoc 1943;30:179–87.

73. Guerini V. History of dentistry. Philadelphia: Lea & Febiger; 1909. Granath LE. Några Synpunkter på behandlinger av traumatiserade incisiver påbarm. Odontol Rev 1959;10:272–86.

74. Frank AL. Therapy for the divergent pulpless tooth by continued apical formation. J Am Dent Assoc 1966;72:87–93.

75. Heithersay GS. Calcium hydroxide in the treatment of pulpless teeth with associated pathology. J Br Endod Soc 1975;8:74–93.

76. Ebers GM. Ebers papyrus. Vol 2. Leipzig: Engleman; 1975.

77. Boorde A. The breviare of health. London: Thomas East Co; 1552.

78. Ring ME. Dentistry: an illustrated history. St. Louis: The C.V. Mosby Co; 1985.

79. Weinberger BW. An introduction to the history of dentistry. St. Louis: The C.V. Mosby Co; 1948.

80. Foley GH. Foley's footnotes. Wallingford PA: Washington Square East; 1972.

81. Berdmore T. Treatise on the disorders and deformities of the teeth and gums. London: B.White, J.Dodsley, T. Becket & P.A. de Hondt; 1770.

82. Miller WD. The microorganisms of the human mouth. Phildelphia: S.S. White Dental Manufacturing Co.; 1890.

83. Balkwill FH. On the treatment of pulpless teeth. Br Dent J 1883;4:588–92.

84. Pucci FM, Reig R. Conductos Radiculares. Montivideo: Casa a Barreiro y Ramos SA; 1946.

85. Ingle JI. A standardized endodontic technique utilizing newly designed instruments and filling materials. Oral Surg Oral Med Oral Pathol 1961;14:83–91.

86. Schilder H. Filling root canals in three dimensions. Dent Clin North Am 1967;11:723–44.

87. Béal M. De la Résection de l'apex. Rev Stomatol 1908;15:439–46.

88. Roy M. Le curettage apical. Odontologie 1925;43:5–29.

89. La Cronique GM. Faits cliniques à propos du curettage périapical avec amputation de l'apex. Rev Stomatol 1927;24:200–7.

90. Duclos J. A propos du ràpport sur le traitement chirurgical des affections apexiennes. Rev Stomatol (Paris) 1930;5:398–406.

91. Duclos J. Indications et techniques des diverse méthodes d' obturation des canauz par voie apicale. Rev Stomatol 1934;36:767–8.

92. Bažant F. Resectio radicis. Zubní Lék 1913;13:21–7.

93. Šmelhaus St. Maxillotomie, apiklnià lní resekce u zubů s neprůchodn?mi prudůchy kořenov?mi. Zubní Lék 1916;16:1–6.

94. Kostečka F. Nezdary při amputaci kořenového hrotu a jejich příčny. Zubní Lék 1924;24:239–43.

95. Měštan K. Resekce kořenového hrotu. Prague: Tožička; 1937.

96. Faulhaber B, Neumann R. Die chirurgischen Behandlung der Wurzelhauterkrankungen. Berlin: Hermann Meusser; 1912.

97. Neumann R, Die Wurzelspitzenresektion an den unteren Molaren. Berlin: Hermann Meusser; 1915.
98. Faulhaber B, Neumann R. Die chirurgische Behandlung der Wurzelhauterkrankungen. 2nd ed. Berlin: Hermann Meusser; 1921.
99. Neumann R. Atlas—der radikal chirurgischen Behandlung der Paradentosen. Berlin: Hermann Meusser; 1926.
100. Hofer O. Wurzelspitzenresektion und Zystenoperationen. Z Stomatol 1935;32:513–33.
101. Csernyei G. Il decorso della guarigione dopo l'amputazione dell' apice radicolare secondo Partsch e secondo la mia modificazione osteoplastica. La Stomatol 1930;28:1025–41.
102. Csernyei G. Die Heilungsvorgänge nach der Wurzelspitzenamputation bei der Partschschen periostalplastischen und bei der Cernyeischen osteoplastichen Methode. Zahnärztl Rdsch 1932;41:938–46.
103. Pichler H. Zur Frage der Wurzelspitzenresektion. Österr Z Stomatol 1921;19:15–26.
104. Wassmund M. Lehrbuch der praktischen Chirurgie des Mundes und der Kiefer. Leipzig: Hermann Meusser, 1935.
105. Khoury F. Moglichkeiten, Grenzen und Erfahrung mit der Knochendeckelmethode bei Wurzelspitzenresektionen im Molarenbereich des Unterkiefers. Dtsch Zahnärztl Z 1987;42:258–61.
106. Peter K. Die Wurzelspitzenresektion der Molaren. Leipzig: Hermann Meusser; 1936.
107. Held H. Contribution à l'étude de la resection apicale des dents antérieures, prémolaries et dents de six ans supérieures et inférieures. Schweiz Montasschr Zahnheilkd 1936;46:765–836.
108. von Hippel R. Zur Technik der Granulomoperation. Dtsch Monatsschr Zahnheilkd 1914;32:255–65.
109. Ruud AF. Slitsmethoden ved retrograk rotfylling. Nor Tannlægeforen Tid 1950;60:471–9.
110. Matsura SJ. A simplified root-end filling technique. J Mich State Dent Assoc 1962;44:40–1.
111. Schupfer C. Über ein neues Berfahren zur Abdichtung der Wurzelkanäle für Wurzelspitzenresektionen in besonderen Fällen. DZW 1935;38:741–2.
112. Schupfer C. A new method for dense closure of root canals during apical resection in difficult cases. Dent Items Interest 1936;58:367–70.
113. Luks S. Practical endodontics. Philadelphia: JB Lippincott Co; 1974; pp. 142–55.
114. Schuster E. Die Sektion der Zahnwurzel. Dtsch Monatsschr Zahnheilkd 1913;31:43–7.
115. Tangerud BJ. Den retrograde rotbehandling ved alveotomi Nor Tannlægeforen Tid 1939;49:170–5.
116. Castenfeldt T. Om retrograd rotfyllning vid radikaloperation av kronisk apical paradentit. Sven Tandlak Tidskr 1939;32:227–60.
117. Fawn GF. Root amputation. Br Dent J 1927;48:1025–32.
118. Ross WS. Apicectomy in the treatment of dead teeth. Br Dent J 1935;58:473–86.
119. Bauer W. Hitologische Befunde an Zähnen nach Wurzelspitzenamputation. Z Stomatol 1922;20:601–6.
120. Bauer W. Mikroskopische Befunde an Zähnen und Paradentien nach experimenteller Wurzelspitzenamputation unter besonderer. Berücksichtigung der Bedeutung funktioneller Auswirkungen. Z Stomatol 1925:23:122–35.
121. Euler H. Experimentelle Studien über den Heilverlauf. Dtsch Montasschr Zahnheilkd 1923;41:321–34.
122. Kronfeld R. Zur Frage der Wurzelspitzenamputation. Z Stomatol 1928;26:1105–22.
123. Cavina C. L'amputazione degli apici delle radici dentali. La Stomatol 1930;28:721–53.
124. Gottlieb B. Histological examination of united tooth fracture. Dent Items Interest 1926;48:877–95.
125. Steinhardt G. Pathologisch-anatomisch Befunde nach Wurzelspitzenresektionen und Wurzelfrakturen beim Menschen. DZW 1933;23:541–6.
126. Häupl K. Om rot-amputasjoner under saelig hensyntagen til rotfyllingssporsmålet og operasjonesteknikken. Nor Tannlaegeforen Tid 1932;42:37–51.
127. Takàcs S. Contributo sperimentale alla guarigione della ferita ossea da apicectomia dentaria. La Stomatol 1929;27:964–73.
128. Herbert WE. Cases treated by root resection. Br Dent J 1941;70:173–84.
129. Weisenbeck G. Probleme der Wurzelbehandlung spexiell der Amputation. Munich: Bayerischen Ludwig-Maximilins Universitat; 1926.
130. Schmidt E. Untersuchungen über Erfolge und Misserfolge der Wurzelspitzenresektionen, die am Zahnärztlichen Institut der Universität München in den Jahren 1908–1926 ausgeführt worden sind. Munich: Max Schick; 1927.
131. Kohlhagen E. Ein Beitrag zur Frage der Indikation für Wurzelspitzenresektionen an unteren Molaren. Munich: Schmidt & Erdel, Halle AS; 1932.
132. Hack H. Die Wurzelspitzenresektion mehrwurzeligen Zähnen. Munich: Bayerische Druckerei & Verlagsanstalt GmbH; 1934.
133. Moll A. Über die Wurzelspitzenresektion. Munich: Bayerische Druckerei & Verlagsanstalt GmbH; 1934.
134. Schmuck R. Über die gleichzeitige Wurzelspitzenresektion mehrerer nebeneinanderstehender Zähne. Munich: Universitäts-Buchdruckerei von Dr. C. Wolf & Sohn; 1935.
135. Fischer C-H. Die Wurzelspitzenresektion als Therapie bei der fokalen Infektion. Dtsch Zahn-, Mund- und Kieferheilkd 1938;5:624–31.
136. Wassmund M. Wurzelspitzenresektion und fokale Infection. Zahnärztl Rdsch 1942;51:1101–8.

137. Kostečka F. Fokální infekce a amputace kořenového hrotu. Cesk Stomatol 1936;36:13–21.
138. Gaerny A. Klinische und röntgenologische Resultate nach Wurzelspitzenresektion als Beitrag zu deren Indikationsstellung. Schweiz Monatsschr Zahnheilkd 1940;50:583–633.
139. Moorehead FR. Removal of roughened apex. Dent Cosmos 1903;45:163.
140. Schamberg ML. The surgical treatment of chronic alveolar abscess. Dent Cosmos 1906;48:15–24.
141. Hartzell TB. Root-tip amputation and external drainage for dental abscesses. Trans Natl Dent Assoc 1908;207–8.
142. Hartzell TB. Root tip amputation. Dominion Dent J 1911;23:473–82.
143. Buckley JP. The rational treatment of chronic dentoalveolar abscess, with root and bone complications. Dent Rev 1911;25:755–76.
144. Buckley JP. Root amputation. Dent Summary 1914;34:964–5.
145. Brophy TW. Oral surgery. A treatise on the diseases, injuries and malformations of the mouth and associated parts. Philadelphia: Blakiston's Son & Co.; 1915.
146. Reid JG. Amputations of roots of teeth. Dent Rev 1913;27:221–33.
147. Reid JG. Root Amputation. Dent Rev 1913;27:465.
148. Reid JG. Technique of root amputation. Dent Rev 1913;27:574–5.
149. Rasmussen AT. The rational treatment of chronic emphysema of the maxillary sinus. Dent Items Interest 1916;38:774–9.
150. Provan WF. Roots and their treatment. Dent Summary 1916;36:675–80.
151. Lucas CD. Root resection and apical canal filling after resection. Dent Summary 1916; 36:201–7.
152. Ivy RH. The aseptic transalveolar root resection operation. J Natl Dent Assoc 1917;4:553–64.
153. Howe PR. A method of sterilizing, and at the same time impregnating with a metal, affected dentinal tissue. Dent Cosmos 1917; 59:891–904.
154. Nodine AM. The technique of root resection and root amputation. Dent Cosmos 1917; 59:492–6.
155. Brooks E. Apiectomy. Dent Summary 1918;38:29–39.
156. Prinz H. The technique of root amputation. Dent Cosmos 1918;60:381–94.
157. Lucas CD. Indications and technic for root resection. Dent Summary 1918;38:39–42.
158. Kells CE. Replanting vs. apicoectomy. Dent Cosmos 1918;60:473–82.
159. Silverman SL. The status of apicoectomy. J Natl Dent Assoc 1918;5:255–63.
160. Smith AW. Root amputation. Dent Cosmos 1918;60:914–17.
161. Lyons CJ. Indication and contraindication for root resection. J Natl Dent Assoc 1919;6:790–3.
162. Gamin MH. Foci of infection in relation to non-vital teeth. J Natl Dent Assoc 1919;6:195–210.
163. Nodine AM. The radical treatment of focal infections from a military point of view. Dent Cosmos 1919;61:193–200.
164. Parker HJ. Root resection: a plea for a broader field. Dent Cosmos 1919;61:388–91.
165. Rickert UG. Advantages and disadvantages of reduced silver in dental therapeutics. J Natl Dent Assoc 1919;6:930–5.
166. Levy J. Root amputation. Dent Cosmos 1919;61:619–59.
167. Lucas CD. Technic of root resection. J Natl Dent Assoc 1919;6:793–800.
168. Nyman JE. The technique of root-resection. Dent Cosmos 1919;61:429.
169. Sausser ER. Root resection. Dent Cosmos 1919;61:41–51.
170. Lyons CJ. Surgical technic of apicoectomy. J Natl Dent Assoc 1920;7:700–4.
171. Gross SS. Apicoectomy - the culmination of perfect root canal operations. Dent Cosmos 1920;62:77–81.
172. Garvin MH. Root resection. J Can Dent Assoc (Tor.) 1942;8:126–9.
173. Andreasen JO, Munksgaard EC, Fredebo L, Rud J. Periodontal tissue regeneration including cementogenesis adjacent to dentin-bonded retrograde composite fillings in humans. J Endod 1993;19:151–3.
174. Mead SV. Oral surgery. St. Louis: The C.V. Mosby Co.; 1933.
175. Partsch C. Die chronische Wurzelhautenzundung. Leipzig: Georg Thieme; 1908.
176. Berger A. Indications for and limitations of apicoectomy. Dent Cosmos 1926;68:l200–2.
177. Ruggier JC. Apicoectomy and its advantages to prosthesis. Dent Dig 1926;32:166–9.
178. Moorehead FB. Root-end resection. Dent Cosmos 1927;69:463–7.
179. Kay AJ. Root amputation, etiology, selection of cases and surgical cases and surgical technique. Am Dent Surg 1927;47:666–8.
180. Beavis JO. Surgical modification of apicoectomy. Dent Cosmos 1928;70:699–703.
181. Posner JJ. Root amputation. Dent Cosmos 1928;701:158–64.
182. Blayney JR, Wach EC. A study of tissue repair around a resected root end. Dent Forum 1924;1:58–60.
183. Boulger EP. Histologic studies of a specimen of fractured roots. J Am Dent Assoc 1928;15:1778–89.
184. Coolidge ED. Root resection as a cure for chronic periapical infection: a histologic report of a case showing complete repair. J Am Dent Assoc 1930;17:239–49.

185. Blum T. Root amputation. A study of one hundred and fifty-nine cases. J Am Dent Assoc 1930;17:249–61.
186. Blum T. Additional notes on root amputation, including a study of thirty-eight new cases J Am Dent Assoc 1932;19:69–86.
187. Hill TJ. Regeneration of periodontal membrane after root curettement. Dent Cosmos 1931;73:799–801.
188. Aisenberg MS. Root resection after four years: report of a case. J Am Dent Assoc 1931;18:136–40.
189. Garcia GF. Apicectomia experimental. Rev Odontol 1937;25:145–60.
190. Berger A. The principles and technique of oral surgery. Brooklyn: Dental items of Interest Publishing Co.; 1930.
191. Prinz H. Diseases of the soft structures of the teeth and their treatment. Philadelphia: Lea & Febiger; 1928.
192. Levine JH. Surgical elimination of periapical pathosis without extraction of involved teeth. J Am Dent Assoc 1935;22:646–54.
193. Colton MB. A simple rational root-canal therapy employed in conjunction with apical resection and curettage. J Am Dent Assoc 1936;23:2128–32.
194. Jasper EA. The pulpless tooth. Dent Cosmos 1931;73:786–91.
195. Jasper EA. Root-canal therapy in modem dentistry. Dent Cosmos 1933;75:823–9.
196. Valenzuela Donoso M. Técnica del empaquetamiento en las apicectomias. La Odontol 1935;44:137–8.
197. Ries Centeno GA, Gietz E. Apicectomia—estudio comparative delos distintos pasos de la operacion. Prog Dent 1935;4:171–9.
198. Ries Centeno GA, Gietz E. Apicectomia—estudio comparative de los distintos pasos de la operacion. Prog Dent 1935;4:234–8.
199. Salles Cunha E. Observções esparsas sobre cirurga do penapice. Brasil Odontol 1939;15:341–6.
200. Arago L. Apicetomia. Nuestro procedimiento operatorio en tres tiempos. Rev Odontol 1931;19:286–7.
201. Kirk EC, editor. Root-canal surgery. Dent Cosmos 1928;70:454–6.
202. Jones CC. Periapical surgery in army life. Oral Health 1941;31:77–80.
203. Jones CC. Immediate root canal filling. Dent ltems Interest 1941;63:554–7.
204. Jones CC. Complicated endodontia and periapical curettage. Dent Items lnterest 1950;72:577–581.
205. Shapiro SS, Masters EB. A technique for apicoectomy with immediate root filling. Mil Surg 1943;93:368–72.
206. Federspiel MN. The indications for apicoectomy, with report of cases. Dent Cosmos 1936;78:726–31.
207. Phillips WA, Maxmen HA. A practical root resection technique for young permanent anterior teeth. Dent Dig 1941;47:60–4.
208. Droba HJ. Modified technique for treatment of periapically involved teeth. Dent Dig 1942;48:570–2.
209. Wakefield RG. Root canal therapy and resection technique. Oral Surg Oral Med Oral Pathol 1950;3:743–9.
210. Smith GL, Stevens FW. Use of sulfanilamide in surgical treatment of periapically infected anterior teeth. Mil Surg 1944;95:470–4.
211. Grossman LI. Immediate root resection. Br Dent J 1956;101:116–20.
212. Eckes HF, Adams FL. Combined root canal therapy and apicoectomy: a progress report. J Am Dent Assoc 1949;39:66–73.
213. Weaver SM. Root canal treatment with visual evidence of histologic repair. J Am Dent Assoc 1947;35:483–97.
214. Weaver SM. Window method of periapical curettage. J Endod 1947;2:4–5.
215. Berghagen N. Apicalcurettage. En metod for kirurgisk behandling av den kroniska periapikala ostiten. Sven Tandlak Tidskr 1954;47:163–73.
216. Barron SL, Crook JH, Gottlieb B. Periapical curettage or apicoectomy. Texas Dent J 1947;65:37–41.
217. Moen OH. Verification of results of root resection by photomicrographs. J Am Dent Assoc 1940;27:1071–9.
218. Sommer RF. Essentials for successful root resection. Am J Orthod Oral Surg 1946;32:76–100.
219. Wedendal PA. En ny metod for retrograde rotkanalsförslutning vid apicoectomia med samtidig överkapsling avsnittytan genom rotdentinet. Odontol Tid 1954;62:509–15.
220. Blum T. Life span of teeth whose roots have been resected. N.Y. J Dent 1945;15:60–2.
221. Herbert WE. Histological examination of two teeth treated by root resection. Br Dent J 1943;75:205–8.
222. Luks SJ. Root-end amalgam technique in the practice of endodontics. J Am Dent Assoc 1956;53:424–8.
223. Messing JJ. Obliteration of the apical third of the root canal with amalgam. Br Dent J 1958;104:125–8.
224. Eklof D. Retrograd rotbehandlung och rotyllning med silverstift. Sven Tandläk Tidskr 1955;48:81–2.
225. Everett RG. Apicoectomy followed by unusual radiologic finding. Oral Surg Oral Med Oral Pathol 1951;4:1531–3.
226. Rud J, Andreasen JO, Jensen JE. Radiographic criteria for the assessment of healing after endodontics surgery. Int J Oral Surg 1972;1:195–214.
227. Link KH. Klinische und röntgenologische Nachuntersuchungen bei Wurzelspitzenresektionen. Z Stomatol 1935;33:1217–26,1311–21.
228. Maxmen HA. The expanding scope of endodontics. J Mich State Dent Assoc 1959;41:25–40.

229. Farrar JN. Radical and heroic treatment of alveolar abscess by amputation of roots of teeth. Dent Cosmos 1884;26:79–81.

230. Black GV. Amputation of the roots of teeth. In: Litch WF, editor. The American Systemn of Dentistry. Philadelphia: Lea Brothers; 1886: pp. 990–2.

231. Rhein ML. Amputation of roots as a radical cure in chronic alveolar abscess. Dent Cosmos 1890;32:904–5.

232. White G. Treatment of chronic abscess caused by diseased roots. In: Trans Columbian Dent Congr. Chicago: Knight Leonard & Co.; 1893: pp. 623–6.

233. Younger WJ. Pyorrhea alveolaris. J Am Med Assoc 1894;23:790–6.

234. Walker WE. Amputation of tooth-roots. Dent Dig 1895;1:413–14.

235. Gutmann JL, Harrison JW. Surgical endodontics. Boston: Blackwell Scientific Publications; 1991.

236. Sternlicht HC. A new approach to the management of multirooted teeth with advanced periodontal diseased. J Periodontol 1963;34:150–8.

237. Haskell EW. Vital root resection. Oral Surg Oral Med Oral Pathol 1969;27:266–74.

238. Haskell EW, Stanley HR. Vital root resection on a maxillary first molar. Oral Surg Oral Med Oral Pathol 1972;33:92–100.

239. Haskell EW, Stanley HR. Resection of two vital roots. J Endod 1975;1:36–9.

240. Smuckler H, Tagger M. Vital root amputation: a clinical and histological study. J Periodontol 1976;47:324–30.

241. Haskell EW, Stanley HR. Vital hemisection of a mandibular second molar: a case report. J Am Dent Assoc 1981;102:503–6.

242. Haskell EW, Stanley HR. A review of vital root resection. Int J Periodontics Restorative Dent 1982;2(6):29–49.

243. Machtei EE, Vance M-G. Intentional and transitional vital root amputation. J Can Dent Assoc 1983;49:57–60.

244. Haskell EW, Stanley HR. Vital root resection: a conservative procedure for abutment teeth. Int J Prosthodont 1988;1:87–92.

245. Allen AL, Gutmann JL. Internal root resorption after vital root resection. J Endod 1977;3:438–40.

246. Haskell EW, Stanley HR, Goldman S. A new approach to vital root resection. J Periodontol 1980;51:217–24.

247. Tagger M, Smucker H. Microscopic study of the pulps of human teeth following vital root resection. Oral Surg Oral Med Oral Pathol 1977;4:96–105.

248. Filipowicz F, Umstott P, England M. Vital root resection in maxillary molar teeth: a longitudinal study. J Endod 1984;10:264–8.

249. Tagger M, Perlmutter S, Tagger E, Abrams M. Histological study of untreated pulps in hemisected teeth in baboons. J Endod 1988;14:288–92.

250. Spaulding JH. Thirty-six years' experience with lead in the treatment of perforated teeth, and teeth with enlarged foramina. Dent Rev 1912;26:986–93.

251. Parreidt R. Root-perforation and its treatment. Dent Cosmos 1903;45:580–1.

252. Evans G. A Practical teatise on artificial crown- and bridgework. 3rd ed. Philadelphia: The S.S. White Dental Manufacturing Co.; 1893.

253. Peeso FA. The "ABC" of crown and bridge work. Dent Cosmos 1903;45:274–9.

254. Wilkinson JE. Root perforation. Dent Summary 1903;23:407.

255. Brown SE. The treatment of perforated roots. Dent Summary 1905;25:53–9.

256. Euler H. Perforation iun Parodontium. Dtsch Monatsschr Zahnheilkd 1925;43:801–11.

257. Kubler A. Heilungsvorgänge nach Wurzelperforationen. Schweiz Monatsschr Zahnheilkd 1934;413–53.

258. Ruchenstein H. Les perforations radiculaires traitées au Calxyl. Schweiz Monatsschr Zahnheilkd 1941;51:685–719.

259. Kaufmann J Untersuchungen am Paradentium der traumatisch Perforierten Zahnwurzel. Schweiz Monatsschr Zahnheilkd 1944;54:387–447.

260. Taatz H, Stiefel A. Sur Therapie von Zahnperforationen. Zahnärztl Welt 1965;66:814–19.

261. Lantz B, Persson P-A. Experimental root perforation in dogs' teeth. A roentgen study. Odontol Revy 1965;16:238–57.

262. Lantz B, Persson P-A. Periodontal tissue reactions after root perforations in dogs' teeth. Odontol Tidskr 1967;75:209–20.

263. Lantz B, Persson P-A. Periodontal tissue reactions after surgical treatment of root perforations in dogs' teeth. Odontol Revy 1970;21:51–62.

264. Seltzer S, Sinai I, August D. Periodontal effects of root perforations before and during endodontic procedures. J Dent Res 1970;49:332–9.

265. Stromberg T, Hasselgren G, Bergstedt H. Endodontic treatment of traumatic root perforations in man. Swed Dent J 1972;65:457–66.

266. Lufkin AW. A history of dentistry. Philadelphia: Lea & Febiger; 1938.

267. Fauchard P. Le Chirurgien Dentiste ou Traité Des Dents. Paris: Chez Pierre-Jean Mariette; 1746.

268. Pfaff P. Abhandlungen von der Zahen des menschlichen Korpers un deren Erkrankungen. Berlin: Haude und Spencer; 1756.

269. Hunter J. A Practical treatise on the diseases of the teeth: intended as a supplement to the natural history of those parts. London: J. Johnson; 1778.

270. Morrison WH. Experience in the re-implantation of teeth. Dent Cosmos 1881;23:75–9.

271. Rabatz L. Trans- and replantation of teeth. Dent Cosmos 1876;18:442–3.
272. Taft J. Practrical treatise on operative dentistry. 3rd ed. Philadelphia: Lindsay & Blakiston; 1877.
273. Thompson WF. Replantation. Dent Cosmos 1881;23:561–71.
274. Fredel L. De la greffe dentaire. Rev et Arch Suisse d'Odontol 1887;1:201–18.
275. Scheff J. Die Replantation der Zahne. Ost Vjschr Zahnheilkd 19890;2:181–278.
276. Congdon MJ. The plantation of teeth. Trans Panama Pacific Dent Cong 1915;2:295–305.
277. Sklar G, Chernin D. A sourcebook of dental medicine. Waban, MA: Maro Publications; 2002.
278. Ellis RG. Classification and treatment of injuries to the teeth of children. Chicago: Year book Publishers; 1945.
279. Cahn LR. Pathology of pulps found in pyorrhetic teeth. Dent Items Interest 1927;49:598–617.
280. Seltzer S, Bender IB, Ziontz M. The inter-relationship of pulp and periodontal disease. Oral Surg Oral Med Oral Pathol 1963;16:1474–90.
281. Simon JHS, Glick DH, Frank AL. The relationship of endodontic-periodontic lesions. J Periodontol 1972;43:202–8.
282. Belk CE, Gutmann JL. Perspectives, controversies and directives on pulpal-periodontal relationships. Can Dent J 1990;56:1013–17.
283. Gutmann JL, Dumsha TC, Lovdahl PE. Problem solving in endodontics. St. Louis: Elsevier-Mosby; 2006.
284. Frank AL. Improvement of the crown-root ratio by endodontic endosseous implants. J Am Dent Assoc 1967;74:451–62.
285. Potashnick SR. Endodontic endosseous implants: review on a biological basis. N. Y. State Dent J 1976;42:30–5.
286. Silverbrand H, Rabkin M, Cranin AN. The uses of endodontic implant stabilizers in posttraumatic and periodontal disease. Oral Surg Oral Med Oral Pathol 1978;45:920–9.
287. Madison S, Bjorndal AM. Clinical application of endodontic implants. J Prosthet Dent 1988;59:603–8.
288. Larsen RM, Patten JR, Wayman BE. Endodontic endosseous implants: case reports and update of materials. J Endod 1989;15:496–500.
289. Venable C, Stuck W, Beach A. The effects on bone of the presence of metals based on electrolysis. Ann Surg 1937;105:917–38.
290. Orlay HG. Endodontic splinting treatment in periodontal disease. Br Dent J 1960;108:118–21.
291. Cranin AN, Rabkin MF, Garfinkel L. A statistical evaluation of 952 endosteal implants in humans. J Am Dent Assoc 1977;94:315–20.
292. Cape AT, Kitchin PC. Histologic phenomena of tooth tissues as observed under polarized light: with a not on the roentgen-ray spectra of enamel and dentin. J Am Dent Assoc 1930;19:193–227.
293. Pearson HH. Bleaching of the discolored pulpless tooth. J Am Dent Assoc 1958;56:64–8.
294. Spasser HF. A simple bleaching technique using sodium perborate. N. Y. State Dent J 1961;27:332–4.
295. Nutting EB, Poe GS. Chemical bleaching of discolored endodontically treated teeth. Dent Clin North Am 1967;11:655–62.
296. Waas MJ. Trichlorid of iodin in dentistry. Dent Cosmos 1918;60:908–10.
297. Prinz H. The removal of broken instruments from root canals. Br Dent J 1922;43:1167–9.
298. Warner GR. Broken root files. Oral Hyg 1929;19:1746.
299. Healey H. Coronal restoration of the treated pulpless tooth. Dent Clin North Am 1957;1:885–96.
300. Rosen H. Operative procedures on mutilated endodontically treated teeth. J Prosthet Dent 1961;11:973–86.
301. Baraban DJ. The restoration of pulpless teeth. Dent Clin North Am 1967;11:633–53.
302. Sokol DJ. Effective use of current core and post concepts. J Prosthet Dent 1984;52:231–4.
303. Black GV. An investigation of the physical characters of the human teeth in relation to their diseases and to practical dental operations, together with the physical characters of filling materials. Dent Cosmos 1895;37:353–421.
304. Helfer AR, Melnick S, Schilder H. Determination of the moisture content of vital and pulpless teeth. Oral Surg Oral Med Oral Pathol 1972;43:661–70.
305. Gutmann JL. The dentin-root complex: anatomic and biologic considerations in restoring endodontically treated teeth. J Prosthet Dent 1992;67:458–67.
306. Trautmann G, Gutmann JL, Nunn ME, et al. Restoring teeth endodontically treated through existing crowns. Part I. Survey of pulpal status upon access. Quintessence Int 2000;31:713–18.
307. Trautmann G, Gutmann JL, Nunn ME, et al. Restoring teeth endodontically treated through existing crowns. Part II. Survey of restorative materials commonly used. Quintessence Int 2000;31:719–28.
308. Trautmann G, Gutmann JL, Nunn ME, et al. Restoring teeth endodontically treated through existing crowns. Part III. Material usage and prevention of bacterial leakage. Quintessence Int 2001;32:27–32.
309. Trautmann G, Gutmann JL, Nunn ME, et al. Restoring teeth endodontically treated through existing crowns. Part IV. Material usage and prevention of dye leakage. Quintessence Int 2001;32:33–41.
310. Dahlgren BE. The root canal problem: asepsis and sterilization. Aust J Dent 1917;21:79–84.

311. Thomas JG, Nakaishi LA. Managing the complexity of a dynamic biofilm. J Am Dent Assoc 2006;137;10S–15S.

312. Rhein ML. Cure of acute and chronic alveolar abscess. Dent Items Interest 1897;19:688–702.

313. Omnell K-A. Electrolytic precipitation of zinc carbonate in the jaw. An unusual complication after root resection. Oral Surg Oral Med Oral Pathol 1959;12:846–52.

314. Kimura JT. A comparative analysis of zinc and non-zinc alloys used in retrograde endodontic surgery. Part 2. Optical emission spectographic analysis for zinc precipitation. J Endod 1982;8:407–9.

315. Tanzilli JP, Raphael D, Moodnik RM. A comparison of the marginal adaptation of retrograde techniques. A scanning electron microscopic study. Oral Surg Oral Med Oral Pathol 1980;50:74–80.

316. Oynick J, Oynick T. A study of a new material for retrograde fillings. J Endod 1978;4:203–6.

317. Vertucci F, Beatty RG. Apical leakage associated with retrofilling techniques: a dye study. J Endod 1986;12:331–6.

318. Tidmarsh BG, Arrowsmith MG. Dentinal tubules at the root ends of apicected teeth: a scanning electron microscopic study. Int Endod J 1989;22:184–9.

319. Walker A. Definite and dependable therapy for pulpless teeth. J Am Dent Assoc 1936;23:1418–24.

320. Weine FS, Healey HJ, Theiss EP. Endodontic emergency dilemma: leave tooth open or keep it closed? Oral Surg Oral Med Oral Pathol 1975;54:566–74.

321. August DS. Managing the abscessed tooth: instrument and close? J Endod 1977;3:316–18.

322. Bence R, Meyers RD, Knoff RV. Evaluation of 5,000 endodontic treatments: incidence of the opened tooth. Oral Surg Oral Med Oral Pathol 1980;49:82–4.

323. Goldman M. Endodontic first aid. Compend Contin Educ Dent 1981;2:129–34.

324. August DS. Managing the abscessed open tooth: Instrument and close part 2. J Endod 1982;8:364–6.

325. Balaban FS, Skidmore AE, Griffin JA. Acute exacerbations following initial treatment of necrotic pulps. J Endod 1984;10:78–81.

326. Tjäderhane LS, Pajari UH, Ahola RH, et al. Leaving the pulp chamber open for drainage has no effect on the complications of root canal therapy. Int Endod J 1995;28:82–5.

327. Perry SG. Preparing and filling the roots of teeth. Dent Cosmos 1883;25:185–94.

328. Johnson WB. A new gutta-percha technique. J Endod 1978;4:188–94.

329. Van Leeuwenhoek A. Microscopial observations of the structure of teeth and other bones. Phil Trans Martyn (London) 1675;10:1002–3.

330. Malpighi M. Opera Omnia (Scott, London 1686).

331. De la Hire P. Sur les dents. Histoire de l'Acadèmie Royale des Sciences. pp. 41–43 (Boudot, Paris, 1699–1701).

332. Hunter J. The natural history of the human teeth. 1st ed. London: Johnson; 1771, 2nd ed, 1778.

333. Purkinje JE. Der microtuomische Quetscher, lin bei microscopischen Unterscheengen unentberlliches Instrument. Arch Anat Physiol 1834; pp. 385–390.

334. Fränkel M. De penitiori dentium humanorum structura observationes; dissertatio inauguralis anatomico-physilogica. Vratislaviae (Breslau): Friedlaender; 1835.

335. Raschkow I. Meletemata circa mammalium dentium evolutionem; dissertatio inauguralis anatomico-physiologica. Vratislaviae (Breslau): Friedlaender; 1835.

336. Retzius AA. Mikroskopiska undersökningar öfver Tändernes, särdeles Tandbenets strucktur. Kongliga Vetenskapakademiens Handlingar; 1836. pp. 52–140.

337. Müller J. Handbuch der Physiologie des Menschen. Coblenz: Hölscher; 1837.

338. Linderer CJ, Linderer, J. Handbuch der Zahnheikunde. Berlin: Schlesinger'sche Buchhandlung; 1837, 2. Aufl. 1842.

339. Tomes J. On the structure of teeth, the vascularity of these organs, and their relations to bone. Proc Royal Soc Lond 1838.

340. Schwann T. Mikroskopische Versuchungen über die Übereinstimmung in der Struktur und dem Wachstum der Tiere und Pflanzen. Berlin: Reimer; 1839. pp. 117–32.

341. Nasmyth A. Researches on the development, structures and diseases of the teeth. London: Churchill; 1839.

342. Henle J. Von Zähnen; in Allgemeine Anatomie. Lehre von den Mischungs- und Formbestandtheilen des menschlichen Körpers. Leipzig: Boss; 1841. pp. 849–82.

343. Lintott W. On the structure, economy and pathology of the human teeth. London: Churchill; 1841.

344. Owen R. Odontography or a treatise on the comparative anatomy of the teeth; their physiological relations, mode of development, and microscopic structure, in the vertebrate animals, vol. I. London: Baillière; 1840–1845.

345. Tomes J. A course of lectures on dental physiology and surgery. London: Parker; 1848.

346. Czermak J. Beiträge zur mikroskopischen Anatomie der menschilichen Zähne. Z wiss Zool 1850;2:295–322.

347. Kölliker A. Handbuch der Gewebelehre des Menschen. Leipzig: Englmann; 1852; 2. Aufl. 1855; 3. Aufl. 1858;4. Aufl. 1863a;5 Aufl. 1867;6 Aufl. 1902.

348. Huxley TH. On the development of the teeth and on the nature and import of Nasmyth's 'persistent capsule'. Q J Microsc Sci 1853;1:149–64.

349. Lent, E.: Über die Entwicklung des Zahnbeins und des Schmelzes. Z wiss Zool 1855;6:121–34.

350. Tomes J. On the presence of soft tissue in the dentinal tubes. Philos Trans R Soc Lond 1856;146:515–22.

351. Magitot E. Développement et structure des dents humaines; thèse. Paris: Baillière; 1858.

352. Harris CA. The principles and practice of dental surgery. 7th ed. Philidephia: Lindsay & Blakiston; 1858.

353. Robin C, Magitot E. Mémoire sur la genèse et le développement des follicules dentaires jusqu'à l'époque de l'éruption des dents. J Physiol 1860;3:1–51, 300–22.

354. Neumann E. Ein Beitrag zur Kenntnis des normalen Zahnbein- und Knochengewebes. Leipzig: Vogel; 1863.

355. Von Kölliker A. Die Entwicklung der Zahnsäckchen der Wiederkäuer. Z. wiss. Zool. 1863;12:455–60.

356. Waldeyer W. Über den Ossifikationsprozess. Arch mikrosk Anat (Schultze) 1865;1:354–75.

357. Waldeyer W. Untersuchungen über die Entwicklung der Zähne. Z ration Med 1865;24:169–213.

358. Beale LS. New method of preparing the dental tissues for microscopical investigation. Arch Dent Lond 1864/1865;1:48–57.

359. Hertz H. Untersuchungen über den feineren Bau und die Entwicklung der Zähne. Arch Path Anat 1866;37:272–321.

360. Boll F. Untersuchungen über due Zahnpulpa. Arch mikrosk Anat EntwMech 1868;4:73–86.

361. Legros C, Magitot E. Origine et formation du follicule dentaire chez les mammifères. J Anat Physiol (Paris) 1873;9:449–503.

362. Hertwig O. Über das Zahnsystem der Amphibien und siene Bedeutung für die Genese des Skelets der Mundhöhle. Arch Mikrosk Anat, EntwMech 1874; 11 Suppl, 1–208.

363. Salter JS. Dental pathology and surgery. Philadelphia: Blakiston; 1875.

364. Von Ebner V. Über den feineren Bau der Knochensubstanz. Sber Akad Wiss Wien, Abt. III 1875;71:49–136.

365. Tomes CS. A manual of dental anatomy, human and comparative. London: Churchill; 1876, 2nd ed. 1878, 8th ed. 1923.

366. Baume R. Lehrbuch der Zahnheilkunde. Leipzig: Felix; 1877.

367. Hart JI. Minute structure of dentine. Dent Cosmos 1878;20:714–26.

368. Witzel A. Die antiseptische Behandlung der Pulpakrankheiten des Zahnes mit Beiträgen zur Lehre von den Neubildungen in der Pulpa. Berlin: Ash & Söhne; 1879.

369. Bödecker CFW. On secondary dentine. Dent Cosmos 1879;21:353–9, 409–16.

370. Malassez L. Sur le rôle des débris épithéliaux paradentaires. Arch Physiol Norm Pathol 1885;5:309–39.

371. Von Brunn A. Über die Ausdehnung des Schmelzorganes und seine Bedeutung für die Zahnbildung. Arch mikrosk Anat EntwMech 1887;29:367–83.

372. Walkhoff O. Die normale Entwicklung und die Physiologie des Zahnbeines in den verschiedenen Altersperioden des Menschen. Deutsch Mschr Zahnheilk 1887;5:246–314.

373. Weil A. Zur Histologie der Zahnpulpa. Deutsch Mschr Zahnheilk 1887;5:335–56; 1888;6:10–21, 403–13.

374. Von Ebner V. Histologie der Zähne mit Einschluss der Histogenese. In Scheff editor. Handbuch der Zahnheilkunde. Wien: Hölder; 1891. pp. 219–262.

375. Röse C. Über die Entwicklung der Zähne des Menschen. Arch mikrosk Anat EntwMech 1891;38:447–91.

376. Mummery JH. Some points in the structure and development of dentine. Philos Trans R Soc Lond 1892;182:527–45.

377. Bödecker CFW. Anatomy and pathology of the teeth. Philadelphia: White; 1894.

378. Gysi A, Röse C. Sammulung von Mikrophotographien zur Veranschaulichung der mikroskopischen Struktur der Zähne des Menschen. Zürich: Gysi; 1894.

379. Höhl E. Beitrag zur Histologie der Pulpa und des Dentins. Arch Anat Physiol 1896;32:31–54.

380. Röse C. Über die verschiedenen Abänderungen der Hartgewebe bei niedern Wirbeltieren. Anat Anz 1898;14:21–31, 33–69.

381. Von Korff K. Die Entwicklung der Zahnbeingrundsubstanz der Säugetiere. Arch mikrosk Anat EntwMech 1906;67:1–17.

382. Weidenreich F. Über den bau und die Entwicklung des Zahnbeins in der Reihe der Wirbeltiere (Knochenstudien IV, Teil). Z Anat EntwGesch 1925;76: 218–60.

383. Woofendale R. Practical observations on the human teeth. London: J. Johnson; 1783.

384. Longbothom BT. Treatise on dentistry. Baltimore: Prentiss & Cole; 1802.

385. Koecker L. Principles of dental surgery. London: T&G Underwood; 1826.

386. Gutmann JL. History. In: Cohen S, Burns RC, editors. Pathways of the pulp. 4th ed. St. Louis: The C. V. Mosby Co.; 1987.

387. Shadoan WH. Fang filling. Dent Registry West 1859;13:117–20.

388. Chase HS. Results of destroying pulps and plugging pulp cavities. Dent Cosmos 1866;7:464–5.

389. Magitot E. Ètudes sur les alterations de tissus dans la carie dentaire. Paris: Bailliere & fils; 1867.

390. Witzel A. Die Antiseptische Behandlung der Pulpakrankheiten des Zahnes. Berlin: Commissionsverlag Von C.Ash & Sons; 1879.

391. Mills GA. Removing pulp by driving a wooden plug into canal. Dent Cosmos 1883;25:447–8.

392. Register HC. Compressed and warm air as a germicide: pain obtunder and otherwise useful agents in dental practice. Dent Items Interest 1886;8:530–3.

393. Gramm CT. Filling of difficult root canals. Dent Cosmos 1890;32:751–2.

394. Callahan JR. Sulphuric acid in the treatment of opening root-canals. Dom Dent J 1896;8:297.

395. Brown AJ. Strangulated nerve. Dent Cosmos 1894;36:467–9.

396. Perry SG. Which method of root-canal filling will completely obliterate space? Western Dent J 1895;9:385–99.

397. Kells EC. Roentgen rays. Dent Cosmos 1899;41:1014–29.

398. Harlan AW. Pulp digestion. Dent Cosmos 1900;42:1272–4.

399. Price WA. The roentgen rays with associated phenomena and their applications to dentistry. Dent Cosmos 1900;42:117–29.

400. Klotz CE. Treatment of roots of teeth with putrescent pulps, and the filling thereof. Dom Dent J 1902:14:169–77.

401. Myers CG. Application of high pressure anaesthesia. Brit J Dent Sci 1907;50:1123–7.

402. Vaughan HS. The anesthetization of dental pulp by nerve blocking and pericemental injection. Dent Items Interest 1907;29:236–41.

403. Buckley JP. The rational treatment of putrescent pulps and their sequelae. Dent Cosmos 1906;48:537–44.

404. Prinz H. Filling root canals with an improved paraffin compound. Dent Cosmos 1912;54:1081–94.

405. Callahan JR. Rosin solution for the sealing of the dentinal tubuli and as an adjunct in the filling of root-canals. J Allied Dent Soc 1914;9:53–63.

406. Skillen WG. A report on the formation of dentin and cementum relative to the structure of the root end. J Natl Dent Assoc 1921;8:3–10.

407. Husband FC. Copper amalgam as a root filling material. Dom Dent J 1925;37:37–41.

408. Stewart HT. The pulpless tooth and its treatment. J Am Dent Assoc 1930;17:381–95.

409. Ross HJ. Azochloramid in root canal antisepsis. J Am Dent Assoc 1935;22:637–46.

410. Grossman LI. Root-canal therapy with azochloramid. Dent Cosmos 1935;77:598–600.

411. Grossman LI. A preliminary report on the use of azochloramid as a root canal disinfectant. J Am Dent Assoc 1936;23:774–81.

412. Østby BN. Om Vevsforandringer I Det Apikale Paradentium Hos Mennesket Ved Rotbehandling: Nye Klinisk-Røntgenologiske Og Histopathologiske Studier. Oslo: I Kommisjon Hos Jacob Dybwad; 1944.

413. Grossman LI. Treatment of infected pulpless teeth with penicillin. J Am Dent Assoc 1948;37:141–9.

414. Kuttler Y. Microscopic investigation of root apexes. J Am Dent Assoc 1955;50:544–52.

415. Østby BN. The role of the blood clot in endodontic therapy. Acta Odontol Scand 1961;19:323–421.

416. Sunada I. New method for measuring the length of the root canal. J Dent Res 1962;41:375–87.

417. Berdmore T. Treatise on the disorders and deformities of the teeth and gums. London: B.White, J.Dodsley, T. Becket & P.A. de Hondt; 1768.

418. Sazama L. Resekce korenovych hrotu. Prague: Avicenum; 1978.

419. Harris CA. The dental art, practical treatise of dental surgery. Baltimore: Armstrong & Berry; 1839.

420. Desirabode AM. Nouveaux elements compledts de la science et de l'art du dentiste. Paris: Labe; 1843.

421. American Academy of Dental Science. History of dental and oral science in America. S. S. White; 1876.

422. Bronson WA. Dead teeth. NY Odonto Soc Trans 1886;8–12.

423. Smith CS. Alveolar abscess. Am J Dent Sci 1871;5(third series);289–300.

424. Farrar JN. Radical treatment of alveolar abscess. Dent Cosmos 1880;22:376–83.

425. Dunn CW. Alveolar abscess treated by amputation of the fangs. Brit J Dent Sci 1884;27:237.

426. Grayston LDSI. On the treatment of alveolar abscess. Br Dent J 1887;8:10–14.

427. Ottolingui R. Methods of filling teeth. Dent Cosmos 1892;34:807–23.

428. Partsch C. Dritter Bericht der Poliklinik fur Sanh- und Mundkrankheiten des zahnärztlichen Instituts der Königl. Universität Breslau. Dtsch Monatsschr Zahnheilkd 1986;14:486–99.

429. Partsch C. Uber Wurzelresection. Dtsch Monatsschr Zahnheilkd 1989;16:80–6.

430. Partsch C. Uber Wurzelresection. Dtsch Monatsschr Zahnheilkd 1899;17:348–67.

431. Stahl SS. Pathogenesis of inflammatory lesions in pulp and periodontal tissues. Periodontics 1966;4:190–5.

432. Rubach WC, Mitchell DF. Periodontal disease, accessory canals and pulp pathosis. J Periodontol 1965;36:34–8.

433. Stallard RE. Periodontic-endodontic relationships. Oral Surg Oral Med Oral Pathol 1972;34:314–26.

434. Bender IB, Seltzer S. The effect of periodontal disease on the pulp. Oral Surg Oral Med Oral Pathol 1972;33:458–74.

435. Sinai I, Soltanoff W. The transmission of pathologic changes between the pulp and the periodontal structures. Oral Surg Oral Med Oral Pathol 1973;36:558–68.

436. Wang H-L, Glickman GN. Endodontic and periodontic interrelationships. In: Cohen S, Burns RC, editors. Pathways of the Pulp. St. Louis: Mosby; 2002.

437. Mazur B, Massler M. Influence of periodontal disease on the dental pulp. Oral Surg Oral Med Oral Pathol 1964;17:592–603.

438. Hattler AB, Snyder DE, Listgarten MA, Kemp W. The lack of pulpal pathosis in rice rats with the periodontal syndrome Oral Surg Oral Med Oral Pathol 1977;44:939–48.

439. Ross IF, Thompson RH. A long term study of root retention in the treatment of maxillary molars with furcation involvement. J Periodontol 1978;49:238–44.

440. Czarnecki RT, Schilder H. A histological evaluation of the human pulp in teeth with varying degrees of periodontal disease. J Endod 1979;5:242–53.

441. Bergenholtz G, Nyman S. Endodontic complications following periodontal and prosthetic treatment of patients with advanced periodontal disease. J Periodontol 1984;55:63–8.

442. Torabinejad M, Kiger RD. A histologic evaluation of dental pulp tissue of a patient with periodontal disease. Oral Surg Oral Med Oral Pathol. 1985;59:198–200.

443. Harrington GW. The perio-endo question: differential diagnosis. Dent Clin North Am 1979;23:673–90.

444. Bergenholtz G, Lindhe J. Effect of experimentally induced marginal periodontitis and periodontal scaling on the dental pulp. J Clin Periodontol 1978;5:59–73.

445. Jaoui L, Machtou P, Ouhayoun JP.Refer Long-term evaluation of endodontic and periodontic treatment. Int Endod J 1995;28:249–54.

Chapter 3

Ethics, Morals, the Law, and Endodontics

Bruce H. Seidberg

Introduction

In decades past, society held dentists in high esteem; however, the former maternalistic/paternalistic mindset has been replaced with suspicion, and inquiries of what is being told to the patient is often fueled by Internet surfing and false information. Today's patients are becoming more sophisticated about their dental needs; they are also becoming more sophisticated about their legal rights. Dentists are held to the same standard as physicians and other health providers with the tort of malpractice.[1] One does not have to be wrong to be sued. While providing a scientific and technological service, your patient may decide that your dental work is not meeting certain expectations. What may begin as a difference in opinion could turn into a costly and time-consuming lawsuit.[2]

Malpractice is the negligence arising out of the doctor–patient relationship (DPR), whereas negligence is the unreasonable act or omission by a provider that results in patient harm. To sustain a cause of action, the plaintiff patient must prove the four elements of malpractice: duty, breach of duty, proximate cause (departure from the standard of care), and damages. Patients are likely to bring legal action for a number of reasons, included, but not limited to those listed in Table 1.

Frequency of Claims

Endodontics had been identified as number one in dentistry in terms of the frequency of malpractice claims filed in California in 1985[3]; however, in 1987, Harman[4] reported that nationally, endodontic claims were the second most frequent producer of claims and dollar losses, with oral surgery being number one. There was an increase in the number of malpractice claims involving endodontics, primarily against general dentists, noted in 1998.[5] The American Association of Endodontists (AAE)[5] also recognized an increase in the number of malpractice claims involving endodontics. Since general practitioners are performing 75% or more of the endodontic procedures in America, it is implied that they would be involved in the majority of the malpractice cases. Insurance companies are no longer providing the percentage differences between generalists and specialists in their recent releases. Even if the perception is true, that the majority of the malpractice cases arise from general practice offices, one cannot preclude that endodontic specialists are without exposure.

The current frequency of endodontic claims has been relatively status quo when compared to national statistics. Between 2001 and 2005, endodontics was still number one in malpractice claims in California. There was a slight change in the year 2006, however, when

Table 1 Common Elements of Malpractice and Negligence

1. Failure to meet the standard of care
2. Practice beyond the scope of license
3. Perform procedures not competent to do
4. Delegate to a nonqualified person
5. Use materials not meeting standards
6. Insurance fraud
7. Failure to diagnose
8. Failure to refer

Table 2 Treatments Involved in Paid Claims; ADA Council on MI&RP Study 2005	
Crown and bridge	21.8%
Endodontics	20.0%
Simple extractions	13.6%
Dentures	6.7%
Surgical extractions	5.7%
Oral exams	5.1%
Implants	2.9%
Orthodontics	2.0%
Periodontal surgery	1.4%
Treatment of Temporal mandibular joint	0.2%
Other	20.6%
Total	100%

Table 3 Frequency of Dental Claims: MILMIC Insurance 2007		
	Frequency of Claims	Percent of Indemnity Payments
Crown and bridge/fillings	26.2	21.6
Endodontics	15.5	10
Oral surgery	7.9	13.5
Prosthodontics	4.2	1.0
Orthodontics	3.8	6.3
Periodontics	3.5	10.4
Implants	3.3	8.8
General negligence	20.6	6.3
Paresthesia	<1	7.6
All other	15.0	14.5
Total	100	100

endodontics slipped to second place after restorative dentistry.[6] The American Dental Association Council on Members Insurance and Retirement Plans (MI&RP)[7] undertook a study in 2005 involving 15 insurance companies that provide dental malpractice insurance to approximately 106,000 dentists. The focus of the study was to determine the frequency of claims for various phases of dentistry. Due to the involved time frame in the legal system method of scheduling and hearing cases, the 2005 study detailed statistics from 1999 only up to 2003. This national study indicated that endodontics was number two in claims for malpractice or negligence. The ADA study also indicated that the majority of the replying insurers did not differentiate between generalists and specialists, except for oral surgeons, which implies that there would be no difference in the final statistics, or minimal at best. The ADA study also categorized frequency by identifying paid claims provided by generalists (Table 2); they did not separate specialists. MILMIC, an insurance company from New York State, categorized the frequency differently, reporting similar results for similar categories in 2006[8] (Table 3). The MILMIC report also identified the percentage of indemnity for various claims, implying good news for endodontics, dropping to fourth place in the payment or settlement arena (see Table 3). The common areas of claims against endodontists are listed in Table 4.

Aside from the evidence-based scientific and technical methodologies, now known and available for patient care

Table 4 Alleged Errors in Claims against Endodontists
1. Treatment failure
2. Failure to meet the standard of care
3. "Broken instruments"
4. Treatment of the wrong tooth
5. Paresthesia
6. Inadequate precautions to prevent injury
7. Inappropriate procedures
8. Failure to warn (informed consent)

and endodontic therapy, and described elsewhere in this textbook, endodontists have to understand, and be concerned with, good risk management procedures, and have to improve communication skills with their referring dentists and patients. The major concerns affecting legal claims, as described by Seidberg, involve the DPR, informed consent, and good record keeping.[9] In addition, endodontists must be aware of what "standard of care" is, and what it means.

Ethics and Morals

Ethics, morals, and the law all intersect, influence, and impact each other. Ethical behavior encompasses rules and standards that govern members of a profession.

Table 5 Ethics
E = Expertise
T = Truthful
H = Honesty
I = Integrity
C = Compassion
S = Sagacity

Endodontists are guided by the Codes of Ethics of the American Dental Association, the AAE and those of the states in which they are licensed. Ethics is a systematic study of moral behavior of which actions must be supported by reason (Table 5).

The ethical basis for standard of care is to recommend the best therapy while minimizing potential harm, and to avoid placing a patient at an unreasonable risk of harm. Ethical concepts include patient autonomy (the right to understand and consent), nonmaleficence (from the Hippocratic Oath: "Do no harm"), beneficence (doing what is best for the patient), justice (fairness in allocation of services), and veracity (requires honesty in all dealings). It is an unethical conduct to refuse services to patients because of patient's race, creed, color, sex or national origin, or to deny care to patients based on a real or perceived disability. To do so violates the American Disablity Act.

Moral behavior is concerned with principles of right and wrong in relation to human action and character. It conforms to virtuous standards arising from conscience or sense of obligation and follows rules or habits of conduct from one's ingrained sense of what is right.

Standard of Care

As Milgrom and Ingle[10] have noted, dentists can no longer consider themselves immune to malpractice litigation by hiding behind a doctrine of "local community standards." Local community standards no longer have standing within the court systems.[11–13] Standard of care is in a constant state of change, vacillating between expert witnesses' testimony, new technology, and improved procedures. Local community standards have been replaced by national standards. The ease of availability to obtain continuing education from universities, professional journals, and local dental society-sponsored courses, and the mobility of dentists to travel to educational centers, implies an ease to develop a national standard. Today all dentists must meet the national standard of care.

The standard of care is defined as "that reasonable care and diligence ordinarily exercised by similar members of the profession in similar cases in like conditions given due regard for the state of the art."[9] Generalists are held to the standard of care of the specialist using the same degree of care and skill when acting in the same or similar circumstances.[14,15] Legal claims of malpractice and negligence will have the charge of a dentist's deviation from the standard of care as its primary focus. Along with authors who have alluded to the subject,[4,16,17] the AAE has issued guidelines that practicing endodontists are expected to adhere to and suggests a *national standard of care*. The *Appropriateness of Care and Quality Assurance Guidelines* can be obtained from the AAE.[5] It must be remembered that the guidelines are templates and not mandates. They do not *legally* set the standard of care. Contrary to belief, it is neither the specialists nor the national specialty organizations that set the standard. In the court system, the *plaintiff's dental expert witness* will define the standards and identify the deviation(s). The *defendant's dental expert witness* will counter with a different approach to the evidence, demonstrating that the standard of care has not been deviated from. The judge and/or the jury will then decide the case, and that will become the standard of care for that specific case. The prevailing party is usually one whose expert can be the most convincing.

Many dentists, including specialists, are willing to evaluate records and testify as an expert witness in court, supporting patients, who in their view have been treated below the standard of care. Most states require a certificate of merit authored by a dental expert witness before a lawsuit can go forward. *A word of caution*: there are many frivolous suits that can be discharged at the initial document review stage. If one is a willing expert, one must have a history for providing services for both sides of the aisle, for the plaintiff and/or for the defendant (not for the same case) at different times. One should not review cases all the time for only one side. One must be able to evaluate a case honestly and determine the merits to state whether or not the case is meritorious to go forward, or be able to declare that, in your opinion, no case exists.

Cohen and Schwartz[3] have stated that a meritorious claim by a patient is "any departure from the minimum quality of endodontic care." "Any departure" is rather broad and includes, but is not limited to, failure to properly diagnose, failure to perform comprehensive diagnostic tests, failure to properly document and record all findings and treatment, treatment of the wrong tooth, use of paraformaldehyde/steroid pastes such as N2 and other nonaccepted materials, root perforations, failure to obtain appropriate informed consent, failure to inform the patient of instrument separations in the canal, and failure to use a rubber dam.[18] The minimum quality is harder to define.

From the aforementioned list, "failure to use a rubber dam" is unconscionable and may result in the most disastrous consequences, namely swallowing or inhalation of an endodontic instrument (Figure 1) that may become lodged in a body cavity or an organ and may require a subsequent medical surgical procedure.

Instrument breakage or, as it is euphemistically referred to, "instrument separation" is a "disquieting event" and not necessarily a deviation from the standard of care or an actionable event. One must ask, "Did the file break because of overzealous use… or was it defectively manufactured?"[18] The unbroken end of the file should be saved in a coin envelope and placed in the patient's treatment record. If defective manufacturing can be proved, liability could shift to the manufacturer or be a shared responsibility. The root canal system is small and tortuous and the instruments very small and fragile. When in use, the instrument may bind and separate inadvertently. The act of separation can be argued as an unfortunate mishap and not negligence or malpractice. In any event, the patient should be informed promptly[18] and the mishap and fact that the patient has been informed is documented.

An example of a standard of care controversy, that has been the focus of a number of claims, is the *final terminus* of a root canal filling material. Charges have been made over the issue of *overfilling* through a normal apical exit or *overextending* the root canal filling because the apical foramen has been grossly enlarged or resorbed. "Normal" overfilling is often found defendable, whereas gross overextension is often not. There is a difference between the overfilled/overextended and underfilled/overextended terminus of filling materials. One could be hard-pressed in court to defend gross overextending, sometimes to the point of filling the

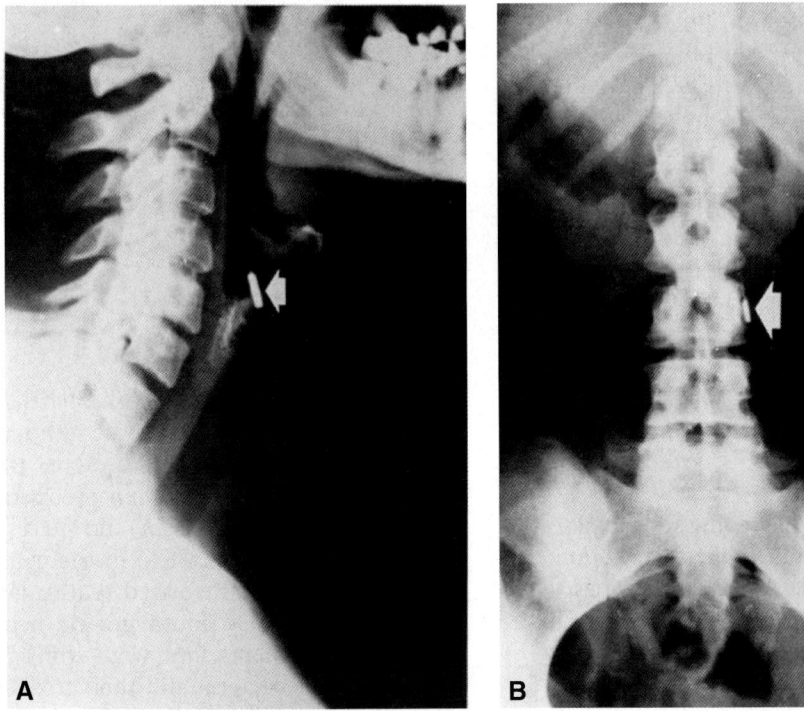

Figure 1 Two examples of swallowed endodontic instruments because a rubber dam was not used. ***A***, Radiograph taken 15 minutes after an endodontic broach (arrow) was swallowed. Reproduced with permission from Heling B., Heling J., Oral Surg Oral Med Oral Pathol Oral Radiol Endod 1977; 43:464. ***B***, Abdominal radiograph showing a broach in the duodenum (arrow). Reproduced with permission from Goultschin J. Heling B. Oral Surg Oral Med Oral Pathol Oral Radiol Endod 1971; 32:61.

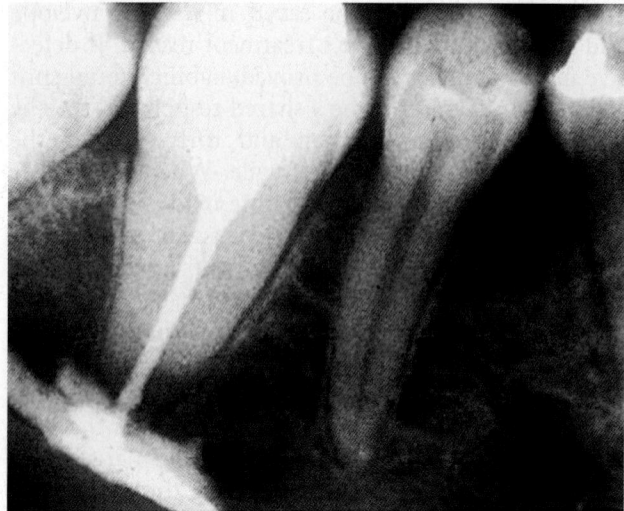

Figure 2 Massive overextension of RC2B (N2) into the inferior alveolar canal. The patient suffered permanent paresthesia. The lawsuit was settled out of court against the dentist and in favor of a 26-year-old secretary in Pennsylvania. Courtesy of Edwin J. Zeneman, DDS, JD.

mandibular canal (Figure 2). Both have been shown to heal; therefore, the onus would be on the expert witness of the defendant to demonstrate that healing of "overfilled" or "overextended" fillings can happen, and that is not necessarily negligence. On the one hand, filling "short" of the radiographic apex is still debatable. But on the other hand, a "puff" of cement from the apical constriction has become acceptable. Again, both have been shown to heal.

Filling just short of the radiographic apex (0.5 to 1.0 mm), at the apical constriction, is supported by several institutions and reports. By the same token, an inadequate root canal filling is hardly defensible as rising to the standard of care, even though the filling might appear radiographically to extend to the apex (Figure 3). Grossly underfilled canals, 3.0 to 6.0 mm short or more, are also hard to defend, particularly if an associated periapical lesion is radiographically apparent.

One must realize, however, that some root canals are so thoroughly calcified (obliterated) that penetration to the apex is virtually impossible. Root canal fillings that appear to be "underfilled" or "inadequate" and some that appear to be "grossly underfilled" have also been demonstrated to heal. Once again, the onus would be on the expert witnesses to demonstrate an adverse effect. In any event, informing the patient of the terminus filling complication and documenting it will reduce liability risks.

Swedish scientists analyzed 70 cases of "obliterated" canals over a recall period of 2 to 12 years.[19]

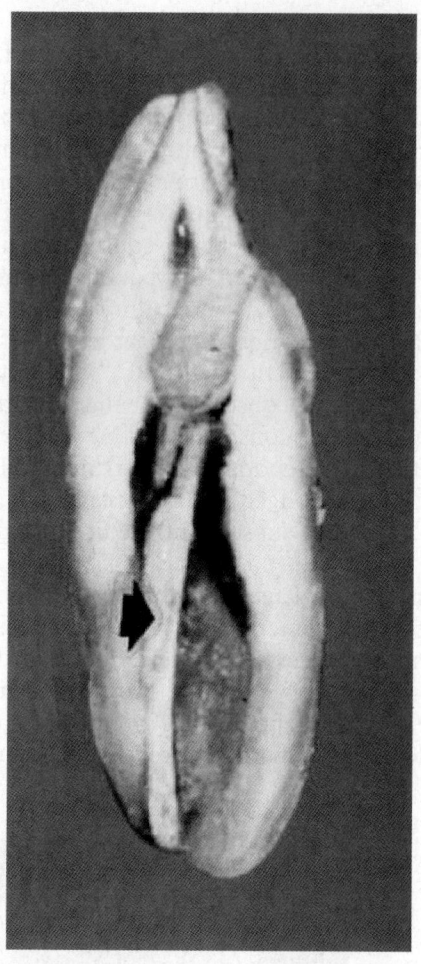

Figure 3 Lateral section of endodontic failure. Gutta-percha point (arrow) in no way obliterates the foramen. Radiographically, from the labial, the canal appears filled to the apex. Unfilled canal space contains necrotic and/or bacterial debris, a toxic irritant.

The overall success rate for the partially filled canals was 89%. When, in the initial radiograph, an intact periradicular contour was present, the success rate was an amazing 97.9%. When preoperative periapical radiolucencies were present, the success rate dropped to a disappointing 62.5%.[19] In the incompletely filled failure cases, it was theorized that canals were present but so narrow they could not be negotiated by the smallest instruments, but were still large enough for the passage of bacteria and their toxins.[19]

In the light of the low success rate (62.5%) of unfilled "obliterated" canals with apical radiolucencies, the dentist must seriously consider a surgical approach, and root end fillings would be within the standard of care if appropriately completed.

Paresthesia is another deviation claim from the standard of care in a patient's complaint following endodontic treatment or a surgical procedure. It has been identified with difficult extractions, improper injection techniques, or endodontic treatment mishaps. Numbness of the lip, chin, or cheek area affected is part of the claim that "the injection didn't wear off."[20] It may be caused by root canal sealers or cements that impinge on the inferior alveolar nerve when neurotoxic filling materials are used (e.g., N2, RC2B, Endomethazone, SPAD). It may also be caused by injections that separate the nerve bundle sheath, or extractions that adversely affect the mandibular nerve. Often, damage associated with alleged dental malpractice using paste fillings like N2 can result in complications seen with medical treatment, including death.[1,21]

Ørstavik et al.[20] surveyed the literature for reported cases of paresthesia related to endodontic treatment. They found 24 published cases; 86% of the patients were female, and usually where a paste-type filling had been used. Although five cases "healed in four months to two years, 14 showed no indication of the paresthesia healing...from 3 months up to 18 years." The remaining cases were resolved by surgical removal of the offending material. Ørstavik reported the 25th case, paresthesia following overfilling with Endomethazone. If the paresthesia persists for 3 years or more, the possibility of regeneration of the nerve must be considered negligible.[20] Others have reported the same or similar causes of nerve damage and paresthesia.[22–25]

Paladino et al.[26] have warned of the indefensibility of using the Sargenti endodontic technique (N2 or RC2B), informed consent or no informed consent: "A general dentist who performs a Sargenti root canal (sic) is going to have as an expert witness testifying against him, virtually every endodontist in town."[26] Further, "any patient who comes to a lawyer with a Sargenti-treated tooth has a prima facie case of negligence" against the dentist. "There is no way...a dentist can justify performing that procedure."[26]

Doctor–Patient Relationship

The DPR is the first of three primary concerns when thinking about risk management.[9] The question is: when does the relationship become legally binding? The DPR is a fiduciary one in which mutual trust and confidence are essential.[27] Theoretically, when a patient walks into an office and provides information to a providing doctor, the relationship begins. When there is only limited observation and suggestions made, however, no direct duty to the patient is attached.[28] Actually the relationship begins when the dentist examines the patient and gives advice about the care needed. In legal terms, this is referred to as *reliance*, and there is usually consideration in the form of a professional fee involved. There are circumstances, under the parameters of the American Disability Act, that supersede the preceding; a dentist cannot refuse dental care to any patient falling under the umbrella of that act of law. Good communication is critical for the DPR to reduce liability risk.[9]

Orr[1] reminds professionals that they be well advised to be very circumspect with regard to offering any criticism of a colleague, particularly without personally communicating with that colleague. A patient's subjective history and recollection of prior health professions interactions are notoriously inaccurate. There are many variables that interplay with bad experiences, including, but not limited to, a patient's difficulty to open wide enough for treatment, to comply with treatment, over anxiety reactions, medical compromises, and stress. The provider can also be having issues of being pressed for time, difficulty with the patient treatment, or just any other concern. Negative comments about previous providers or treatments should not be entered in patient documents.

Informed Consent

Informed consent is the second concern for risk management procedures.[9] It is the conversation a dentist has with a patient, prior to treatment, in which options and possible risks of the proposed treatment are explained and discussed. It is required by law in most states in one form or another. There are three sentinel legal cases that shaped the current concept of informed consent. In the 1914 case of *Schloendorff v Society of New York Hospital*,[29] Judge Benjamin Cardozo concluded that: "every human being of adult years and sound mind has a right to determine what shall be done with his own body; and a surgeon who performs an operation without his patient's consent commits an assault for which he is liable in damages." One of the first cases to label the lack of informed consent as professional negligence instead of assault and battery was *Nathanson v Kline*[30] in 1960. This case concluded that "the fundamental distinction between assault and battery on one hand, and negligence such as would constitute malpractice on the other, is that the former is intentional and the latter unintentional...." This was also the first case law to formalize the consent issue to dentists. The final distinctive case relative to informed consent was *Canterbury v Spence*[31] that refined the entire concept and established a new standard for information disclosure by concluding that "failure on the part of a health care provider to obtain a patient's informed consent before treatment constitutes professional negligence (substandard care) and not the intentional tort of assault or battery." Others have written extensively about informed consent.[26,32–35] Both Bailey[32] and Curley[33] have noted that informed consent was an outgrowth of assault and battery law, the unauthorized "offensive touching without consent." The practitioner must bear in mind that informed consent is the "*rule of law rather than just a standard of practice.*"[33] Bailey[32] has pointed out a variance among states in applying or interpreting the law. In the states of Alaska and Washington, for example, informed consent is not mandatory in severe emergencies. The Council on Insurance of the ADA noted that the issue of informed consent could be tried in court as a civil action where guilt is based on the "preponderance of evidence," that is easier to prove than "beyond a reasonable doubt," used in criminal cases.[34]

Informed consent is defined as the ongoing dialogue between a patient and a health care provider in which both parties exchange information, ask questions, and come to an agreement on the course of specific dental/medical treatment. It is based on a special fiduciary relationship between the doctor and the patient; a relationship of trust, confidence, and responsibility is formulated.[27] The elements of informed consent are listed in Table 6. Weichman[36] described the importance of the doctrine of informed consent, as well as other steps that must be taken by the dentist to maintain good patient relations. According to the doctrine of informed consent, a dentist must (1) describe the proposed treatment so that it is fully understood by the patient, (2) explain all risks attendant on such treatment, and (3) discuss alternative procedures or treatments that might apply to the patient's particular problem. To this should be added (4) the risks associated with doing nothing. Selbst[37] recommended that special care be taken to advise the retreatment patient of increased incidence of complications associated with retreatment cases, particularly the retreatment of paste fills.

Objective standards for informed consent are whether a reasonable or prudent person, in the patient's position, would have submitted to the dental procedure or the course of treatment if suitably informed of the risks. To sustain an informed consent lawsuit, a patient must prove that a reasonably prudent person (such as the patient) would not have undergone the treatment if

Table 6 Elements of Informed Consent Required by Law

The dentist *must* explain:
- The indicated procedure in understandable terms
- Reasons for the procedure
- Benefits of the procedure
- Alternatives and consequences of alternatives including no treatment at all
- Risks associated with the procedure

Sample Statement Of Consent For Endodontic Treatment

1. I hereby authorize Dr. _____, and any other agents or employees of _____ and such assistants as may be selected by any of them to treat the condition(s) described below:

   _____

   _____

2. The procedure(s) necessary to treat the condition(s) have been explained to me and I understand the nature of the procedure to be:

   _____

   _____

3. I have been informed of possible alternative methods of treatment including no treatment at all.
4. The doctor has explained to me that there are certain inherent and potential risks in any treatment plan or procedure.
5. It has been explained to me and I understand that a perfect result is not guaranteed or warranted and cannot be guaranteed or warranted.
6. I have been given the opportunity to question the doctor concerning the nature of the treatment, the inherent risks of the treatment, and the alternatives to this treatment.
7. This consent form does not encompass the entire discussion I had with the doctor regarding the proposed treatment.

Patient's signature

Figure 4 Informed consent form for endodontic procedures recommended by the American Association of Endodontists (AAE).

fully informed of the risks, benefits, and alternatives and that the lack of informed consent served as the proximate cause for the injury. This means that the failure of the dentist to warn the patient is what proximately caused the injury and that is a deviation from the standard of care. "Inform before you perform"[36] is the appropriate approach.

The AAE has suggested an informed consent form that will cover most situations (Figure 4). However, the AAE has stated that "a written consent form cannot be used as a substitute for the doctor's discussion with each individual patient."[38] A lack of a documented informed consent may be interpreted by a jury as evidence that such a discussion was never

CONSENT FOR LOCAL ANESTHETIC INJECTIONS
Please circle the appropriate response where indicated.

I, (print name) _____ , hereby authorize Dr. _____ to perform local anesthetic injections as necessary to perform the dental treatment for which I have been scheduled.

Very inflamed teeth may still have a sensation at the beginning of treatment due to the differences between the chemical makeup of the anesthetic agent and inflammation. If that occurs, additional anesthetic will be administered.

There are some risks in the administration of local anesthetics. Most risks are related to the position of the nerves under the tissue at the site of the injection which can not be determined prior to the administration of the anesthetic agent. Although the risks rarely occur, they might include, but are not limited to, loss of, or disturbed sensation of the tongue and lip on the side of the injection. If this occurs it is often temporary, and the normal sensation usually returns in several days. However, in very rare cases, the loss of sensation may extend for a longer period and may become permanent. In addition, injecting a foreign substance into the body such as an anesthetic may result in an allergic reaction, which is very rare, but may take place.

I further understand that individual reaction to treatment cannot be predicted, and that if I experience any unanticipated reactions following the injection(s), I agree to report them to the office as soon as possible.

The success of my dental treatment depends upon my cooperation in keeping scheduled appointments, following home care instruction, including oral hygiene and dietary instructions, taking prescribed medication and reporting to the office any change in my health status.

I acknowledge that no guarantees or assurances have been given by anyone as to the results that may be obtained. I have had an opportunity to discuss all of the above with the doctor, and have had all of my questions answered.

| I | have | (*have not*) | had local anesthetic injections in the past. |
| I | do | (*do not*) | have a problem with local anesthetics with epinephrine. |

_____   _____
Patient's Signature   If a Minor, Signature of Parent or Guardian

_____   _____   _____
Dental Assistant Signature   Dentist Signature   Date

Figure 5 Consent for Local Anesthetic Injections.

held.[1] Other samples of informed consent documents are in Figures 5–8.

Informed consent is the discussion and *not* the form. The purpose of the signed informed consent form is to provide evidence that the informed consent discussion took place. A document does not replace the verbal process of informed consent; it only acts to memorialize the process. It is the duty of the *dentist performing the procedure* to inform the patient. Obtaining informed consent cannot be delegated to

INFORMED REFUSAL FOR ENDODONTIC CONSULTATION, X-RAYS, DIAGNOSIS AND/OR TREATMENT (NON-SURGICAL OR SURGICAL ENDODONTICS)
PLEASE READ AND SIGN

I understand that the Endodontic therapy and/or other emergency care necessary for the relief of pain that has been explained to me. I prefer <u>not</u> to proceed with the recommended treatment at this time.

_____ I have decided to have the tooth removed

_____ I understand that the prognosis, if treated, is very guarded or unfavorable

_____ I wish to have a second opinion

_____ I want to think about the procedure and whether or not I will want to proceed; I will let your office know of my decision.

_____   Date _____
Patient's signature (If a Minor, Signature of Parent or Guardian)

_____
Relationship to the patient

_____   _____
Witness Signature   Doctor's Signature

Authorization must be signed by the patient, or by the nearest relative in case of a minor or when the patient is physically or mentally incompetent.

Figure 6 Informed Refusal for Treatment

CONSENT FOR ENDODONTIC CONSULTATION, X-RAYS, DIAGNOSIS AND/OR TREATMENT (NON-SURGICAL OR SURGICAL ENDODONTICS)

PLEASE READ AND SIGN

I hereby authorize **Dr.**_____ and/or to those in his employ: the charge for the care of the patient _____ and to administer any treatment, or to administer such anesthetics, and to perform such operations as may be deemed necessary or advisable in the diagnosis and the treatment of this patient.

I understand that the therapy, other than emergency care for the relief of pain, will not be started until the course of therapy has been explained to me, and once the nature and purpose of root canal treatment, and possible alternative methods of treatment have been explained to me, and the risks of not accepting the recommended therapy, I will verbally consent to accepting the therapy or request discharge from the doctor's care.

I do understand that during, or after, the treatment I may have periods of discomfort. I further understand that many factors contribute to the success or failure of root canal therapy which cannot be determined in advance. Therefore, in some cases treatment may have to be discontinued before it is completed, or may fail following treatment. Some of these factors include, but are not limited to, my resistance to infection, the location and shape of the root canal anatomy, my failure to keep scheduled appointments, the failure of my having the tooth restored following the treatment, periodontal (gum) involvement, or an undetected or after the fact caused split (crack) in the tooth.

I further understand that during and following treatment, I am to contact this Doctor's office if I have any additional questions, or I experience any unexpected reactions. I hereby give permission for the use of my x-rays and/or photographs taken during the course of treatment to be used in lectures, seminars and/or printed in journal format by the doctors.

I acknowledge that no guarantees or assurances have been given by anyone as to the results that may be obtained. I will not request or expect a refund of fees in the event that the treatment is not successful. It will be my responsibility to contact my family dentist within one week after treatment to have a cap/crown or other protective restoration placed on the tooth (teeth) and to phone this office for a recall appointment in one year for the evaluation of healing.

_____   Date _____
Patient's signature (If a Minor, Signature of Parent or Guardian)

_____
Relationship to the patient

_____   _____
Witness Signature   Doctor's Signature

Authorization must be signed by the patient, or by the nearest relative in case of a minor or when the patient is physically or mentally incompetent.

ADDITIONAL INFORMATION AS APPROPRIATE:

(This is the area where explanatory drawings may be made or additional comments relative to the specific case)

Figure 7 Consent for Endodontic Consultation

CONSENT FOR ENDODONTIC CONSULTATION, X-RAYS, DIAGNOSIS AND/OR TREATMENT (NON-SURGICAL OR SURGICAL ENDODONTICS)
PLEASE READ AND SIGN

I hereby authorize **Dr.**_____ and/or to those in his employ: to examine, consult and treat the patient _____ and to administer any treatment, or to administer such anesthetics, and to perform such operations as may be deemed necessary or advisable in the diagnosis and the treatment of this patient.

I understand that the therapy, other than emergency care for the relief of pain, will not be started until the course of therapy has been explained to me, and once the nature and purpose of root canal treatment, and possible alternative methods of treatment have been explained to me, and the risks of not accepting the recommended therapy, I will verbally consent to accepting the therapy or request discharge from the doctor's care.

The doctor(s) has explained to me that there are certain inherent and potential risks in any treatment plan or procedure. I understand general risks of treatment include, but are not limited to, complications resulting from the use of dental instruments, drugs, sedation, medicines, analgesics (pain killers), anesthetics and injections. These complications include, but are not limited to: swelling, sensitivity, bleeding, pain, infection, numbness and tingling sensation in the lip, tongue, chin, gums, cheeks, and teeth, which is transient but on infrequent occasions may be permanent; reactions to injections, changes in occlusion (biting); jaw muscle cramps and spasms, temporomandibular (jaw) joint difficulty, loosening of teeth, crowns or bridges; referred pain to ear, neck and head; nausea, vomiting, allergic reactions, delayed healing, sinus perforations and treatment failure. **Specific to the non-surgical endodontic therapy**, risks include, but are not limited to, the possibility of instruments separated and left within the root canals; perforations (extra openings) of the crown or root of the tooth; damage to bridges, existing fillings, crowns or porcelain veneers; loss of tooth structure in gaining access to canals, and cracked teeth. Fractures of the tooth (teeth) or crown(s) may occur during or after treatment. **Specific to the surgical endodontic therapy**, risks include, but are not limited to, the possibility of swelling, discoloration of the face, sensitivity, bleeding, pain, infection, numbness and tingling sensation (paresthesia) in the lip, tongue, chin, gums, cheeks, and teeth, which is transient but on infrequent occasions may be permanent; I further understand that prescribed medications and drugs may cause drowsiness and lack of awareness and coordination, which may be influenced by the use of alcohol, tranquilizers, sedatives or other drugs. It is not advisable to operate any vehicle or hazardous device until recovered from their effects. The use of the penicillin drugs may have an adverse effect on the use of birth control pills.

I do understand that during, or after, the treatment I may have periods of discomfort. I further understand that many factors contribute to the success or failure of root canal therapy which cannot be determined in advance. Therefore, in some cases treatment may have to be discontinued before it is completed, or may fail following treatment. Some of these factors include, but are not limited to, my resistance to infection, the location and shape of the canal anatomy, my failure to keep scheduled appointments, the failure of my having the tooth restored following the treatment, periodontal (gum) involvement, or an undetected or after the fact caused split (crack) in the tooth.

I further understand that during and following treatment, I am to contact this Doctor's office if I have any additional questions, or I experience any unexpected reactions. I hereby give permission for the use of my x-rays and/or photographs taken during the course of treatment to be used in lectures, seminars and/or printed in journal format by the doctors.

I acknowledge that no guarantees or assurances have been given by anyone as to the results that may be obtained. I will not request or expect a refund of fees in the event that the treatment is not successful. It will be my responsibility to contact my family dentist within one week after treatment to have a cap/crown or other

Figure 8 Consent for Endodontic Treatment. (Continued)

protective restoration placed on the tooth (teeth) and to phone this office for a recall appointment in one year for the evaluation of healing.

I understand that I am financially responsible for all charges whether or not paid by insurance. I hereby authorize release of all information necessary to secure payment. In the event this account is turned over for collection, I agree to pay all attorney's fees and court costs. All fees are due and will be paid by the time of completion, unless I contract for a specific payment plan that is agreeable to the doctor(s). Payment may be made by either cash, check, credit cards

_____ Date _____

Patient's signature (If a Minor, Signature of Parent or Guardian)

_____

Relationship to the patient

_____   _____

Witness Signature   Doctor's Signature

Authorization must be signed by the patient, or by the nearest relative in case of a minor or when the patient is physically or mentally incompetent.

ADDITIONAL INFORMATION AS APPROPRIATE:
(this is the place for drawings and or other appropriate comments)

Figure 8 (Continued)

a nonlicensed dental individual, like an assistant or a receptionist.[9]

When discussing consent with a patient, or designing the actual consent form, one must avoid a list of risks so specific that it can be deemed to exclude risks not mentioned. When in doubt as to how specific one should be in discussions and in the written form, use the following phrase: "Risks for this procedure include, but are not limited to risk x, risk y and risk z."[9]

Record Keeping

Maintaining a proper record is the primary dental defense in claims and the third concern for risk management procedures.[9] Good records are *accurate* (the information is true and correctly recorded), *complete* (all required information is included), and *authentic* (the information in the record is reliable and has not been altered). Dental records can be the most effective resource for the defense in a liability issue if written carefully.[1] The format of all records should follow the universally accepted medical/dental form that includes the patient's chief complaint, the dentist's findings (including but not limited to diagnostic tests radiographs, clinical examinations), the assessment or preliminary diagnosis, and the treatment plan. The format is commonly referred to as the SOAP. method (Table 7). Typical contents of a proper record are listed in Table 8. Careful writing, in the SOAP format, would most likely include some evidence of the thought process, including differential diagnosis,

Table 7 SOAP Record Documentation
S, Chief complaint: SUBJECTIVE findings
O, Clinical findings: OBJECTIVE findings
• Dental history
• Diagnostic testing
A, Diagnosis: ASSESSMENT
P, Treatment recommendation; PLAN

Table 8 Typical Contents of Proper Records
Demographics
SOAP diagnostic sheet
Radiographs and photographs
Copies of prescriptions
• Pharmacy
• Lab
Correspondence
• Patient
• Physician
• Referring dentist
Consultation and referral reports
Signed inform consent or refusal of treatment forms
Medical history (including physician's name/phone)
Dental history
Progress notes

Table 9 Additional Documented Items for Progress Notes
Cancellations/missed appointments
Patient comments and complaints
Referrals made
Referrals not followed or refused
Telephone conversations with the patient or physician
• Include date and time
Services provided
Date, time and initials for each entry
Instructions to the patient
Drugs administered/prescriptions
Unusual reactions
Patient refusal of recommended treatment plan or procedure

differing treatment options, and practitioner's and patient's preferences for treatment.[1] Weichman[36] and Hourigan[39] appropriately recommended that records should also consist, at a minimum, of good, well-processed, or digitalized radiographs; any variance at subsequent appointments; any objective findings made during treatment, such as the state of the pulp's vitality found on opening the chamber; any possible complications foreseen or encountered, such as curved roots, obliterated canals, postoperative problems, associated periodontal problems, anesthetics injected with a number of carpules; and full disclosure of any procedural accidents occurring during treatment, such as broken instruments, perforated or fractured roots. Additional items, listed in Table 9, should be entered in a patient's progress notes.

One must be careful not to enter derogatory or judgmental remarks about patients or former dentists in the records including infamous well-known coded descriptives. Juries quickly learn the meaning of the acronyms and find them offensive and unprofessional. Do not write, for example, "Patient SOB" as code for "Patient short of breath."

All financial records must be kept separate from treatment records. It is not prudent to have a clear link of financial arrangements and fees tied to patient's treatments. There are times when only treatment records may be requested by third parties, and the financial information should not accompany them.

Good risk management procedures include obtaining thorough and reliable medical and dental histories (Table 10). Failure to do so constitutes a departure

Table 10 Elements of a Basic Medical History
List of any systemic diseases (such as diabetes, hepatitis, rheumatic fever)
Medicines currently being taken including:
• Birth control pills
• Aspirin
• Any recreational drugs
Current treatments
Bleeding disorders or problems
Drug allergies
History of smoking, drinking, radiation and chemotherapy
Adverse reaction to dental anesthetics
Any prosthetic joint replacements
Dated signature of patient completing the form

from the standard of care. *Records should never be altered* because that would reduce authenticity and credibility. If corrections are necessary, they should be made with a single-line strikeout, the new entry made, dated, and initialed. All record entries must be initialed by the writer and all abbreviations must be understood by others. A list of office personnel abbreviations should be kept on file, including previous employees.

Referrals

Who among the many professionals caring for the patient shall assume responsibility? The referring dentist retains the responsibility for the directive care of the patient. "Who should be captain of the ship?" asked Beveridge (Beveridge EE, Personal communication to Ingle JI, 1971). "Let it become a mutual objective that no patient shall move from one practitioner to another without someone in command. Every patient deserves to have a clearly understood, readily identified, 'captain of his dental ship,'" he stated. Ideally, the dentist most responsible should be the general practitioner who has referred the patient to the endodontist, periodontist, or oral surgeon. His office should be the "clearinghouse" for central records and coordination of treatment. Howard[35] has also emphasized the importance of the general dentist being the "captain of the ship." This does not remove the actual treatment responsibilities and outcome of the actual treating dentist and should not interfere with the referral process. The failure to refer can be the basis for a negligent claim. But, just when should an endodontic patient be referred? The case described below suggests several deviations from the standard of care that must be understood and vividly demonstrates the old adage, "when in doubt, refer it out" should be done with knowledge and caution. The guidelines (Table 11) as to why generalists should consider referrals are the same that endodontists should consider. The decision to make a referral is a personal one based on an individual's own experience, an honest assessment of one's abil-

Table 11 Guidelines for Referral

Is the treatment technically beyond my capability?

Is there a high risk of complications for the indicated procedure?

Is the patient comfortable about my ability to perform the procedure?

Is this procedure in my repertoire?

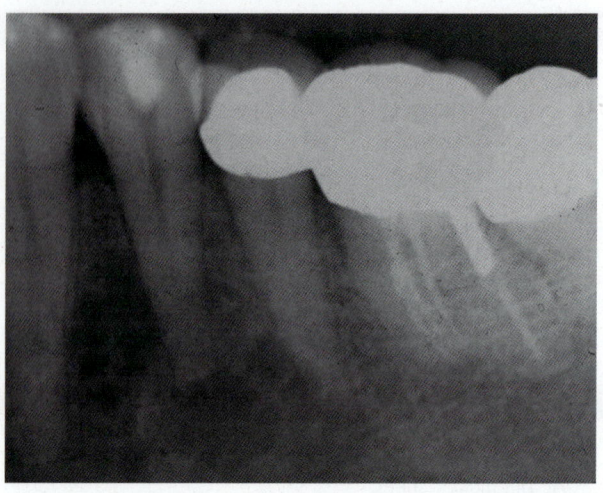

Figure 9 Early radiograph of ameloblastoma initially diagnosed as an apical abscess.

ities in particular areas, and where the comfort level is, drawing the line as to where one's expertise ends.

Case history of interest[44]: The patient in question is a 38-year-old female trial lawyer. She first reported to a general dentist who took full-mouth radiographs and developed a treatment plan. She was unhappy with the dentist and his diagnosis, and, asking around, transferred her appointment and her radiographs to a recommended prosthodontist. The original radiographs clearly showed a circular radiolucent lesion, about the size of a dime, in the left mandibular premolar area (Figure 9). The general dentist made no remark about this apparent lesion, nor was it included in his diagnosis or treatment plan. The prosthodontist, using only the original radiographs that were now over a year old, developed a treatment plan that did not include the lesion, but recommended root canal retreatment for the molar adjoining the lesion so that he could make a crown for the tooth. Only one root of the molar was treated by the endodontist referred to by the prosthodontist. The endodontist also ignored the lesion. The prosthodontist completed the molar crown and then began full-mouth restorative procedures by placing a maxillary bridge opposing the mandibular molar. By now nearly 2 years had passed and still no one had commented on the unusual bone trabeculation of the lesion, though buccal swelling had started in the left mandible.

A good deal of time was lost because the bridge made by the prosthodontist kept falling out and had to be recemented. Finally the patient pointed out the swelling in the mandible, but because she had no pain in the area the prosthodontist ignored her concern. After some time she insisted, so he referred her to the same endodontist who had treated her before. She did not remember being pulp tested, but his diagnosis was that she had an abscess from the first premolar and should have root canal treatment. He gave her an appointment, but when she arrived for treatment, his associate took over and did the treatment in one appointment. He also told her that he was treating an abscess, even though there was only bony swelling; no sinus tract, no discomfort or redness. He told her it would heal following the root canal treatment. He did not recommend a biopsy into the buccal lesion (Figure 10).

The lesion continued to noticeably swell to the buccal (but still no pain or sinus tract), and in disgust she went to another endodontist. He suggested root canal treatment for the second premolar, but by now she was disgusted and turned to the local university dental school for advice.

At the dental school clinic, the diagnosis was made that this was not a chronic apical abscess and sent her to oral and maxillofacial surgery where she had a biopsy taken and she was informed that she was suffering from an ameloblastoma that was not malignant but was destroying her jaw. By this time it had crossed the midline and was approaching the right first molar. They referred her to an oral and maxillofacial surgeon who specialized in such cases. He operated and excised her mandible from left second molar to right second premolar (Figure 11). He then implanted a section of one of her ribs and a metal device to maintain her jaw alignment (Figure 12).

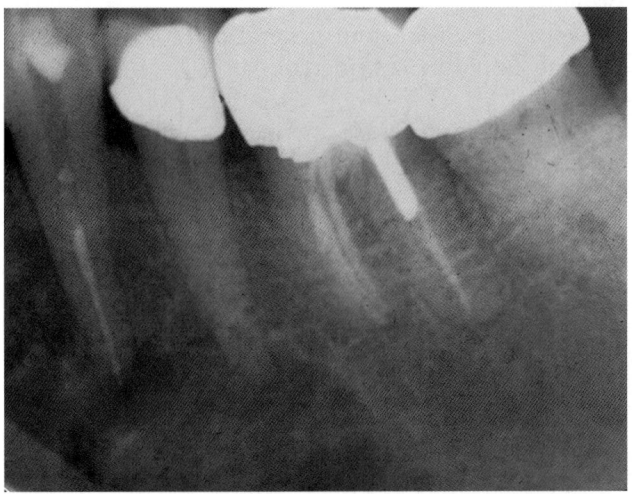

Figure 10 Later radiograph showing root canal filling placed in first premolar to treat what was thought to be an "apical abscess".

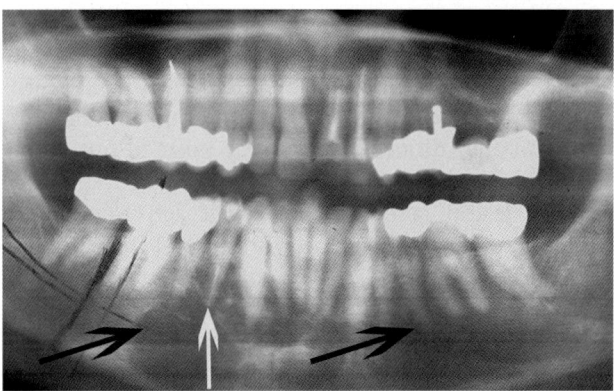

Figure 11 Presurgery panograph showing the extent of the growth of the ameloblastoma. Black arrow (left) marks the initial lesion. Black arrow (right) marks the extent of growth. White arrow marks second premolar with root canal filling shown in Figure 10. The pen marks are evidently the surgeon's mark for the left excision, and the parallel–diagonal marks are for the mandibular canal.

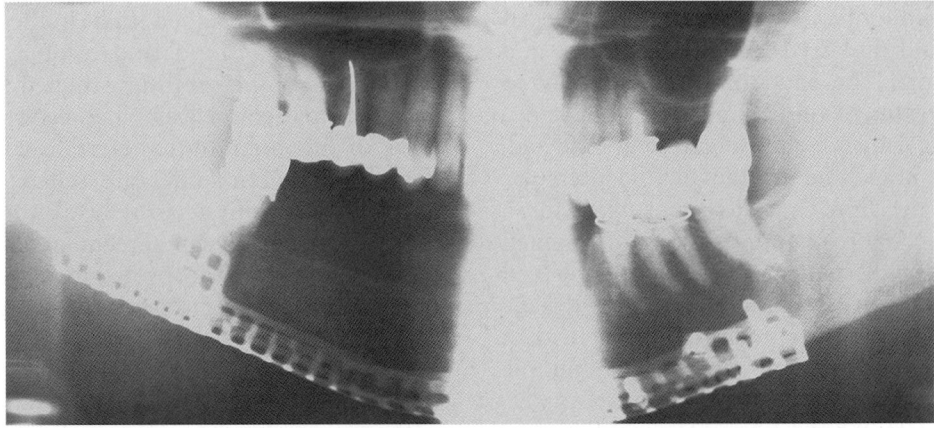

Figure 12 Postsurgical panograph shows the extent of excision of the mandible to remove the ameloblastoma—from left second molar to right second premolar. The metal framework holds the remaining mandible in position, while the implanted rib (vague image just above the metal) attaches and heals in place.

By now, over 6 years had elapsed, and she had been treated by a general dentist, a prosthodontist, three endodontists, an oral and maxillofacial surgeon in a dental school, and an oral and maxillofacial surgeon who had additional experience in such cases.

The patient lost over 2 years in her law practice, and even more when the word went out in the law community that she had "cancer" and would not live long enough to take on a new case.

She sued the original five dentists who all had the same insurance carrier. Expert witnesses testified about the lack of professional skill and their failure to meet the community standard of care. To protect their reputations they chose to settle out of court, and the insurance company paid over $1,000,000 to the plaintiff as well as her lawyer's fees. She eventually returned to her law practice.

The case history as reported above does not contain all of what is contained in the documents from all the providers to accurately comprehend and correlate the data and allegations. What can be pointed out is that the general dentist should have noted the radiographic lesion associated with the left mandibular premolars in his diagnostic workup and incorporated it in his treatment plan. He failed to make a proper diagnosis and recommendation. The patient left the general dentist prior to commencing treatment, and therefore he could have been dropped from the lawsuit. The prosthodontist should have taken new radiographs as he made a new treatment plan and he should have noted the lesion in question. He failed by requesting endodontic therapy on a tooth adjacent to the one with the alleged pathosis, and therefore he too failed to make a proper diagnosis. The first endodontist referred to should have seen the radiolucency in the premolar area on the radiograph when examining for the referred molar and should have pulp tested the premolars and discussed it with the patient and the prosthodontist. The endodontist had a duty to reevaluate his treatment on the molar since it had a complication and only one root was treated. If he had, he should have noted the changes in the premolar area. This was the third missed opportunity for a diagnosis. Had the prosthodontist initially listened to the concerns of the patient when she complained about the swelling in her mandible, he would have had another opportunity to redeem himself with a proper diagnosis or appropriate referral. The multiple failures of the bridge on the right side have no significance to the case at hand. The root canal filling by the first endodontist's associate was acceptable, except that the diagnostic procedures, more likely than not, failed to include all diagnostic tests to correlate clinical findings with radiographic findings—another failure to diagnose. The failure to not recommend a biopsy was not a deviation from the standard of care, unless there was more involvement than the case, as reported, states. The last endodontist failed to make a proper diagnosis and would have treated the second premolar unnecessarily had the patient agreed to his recommendation. Fortunately, the patient finally did receive a proper diagnostic evaluation in the dental school clinic that should have been made by all of the previous endodontists involved and by the prosthodontist. The patient suffered, due to the various deviations from the standard of care and from failure to be diagnosed and appropriately referred, as her case progressed with dental treatment through several providers.

Dietz[40] has listed four general categories in which referral should be considered.

(1) The complex case involving multiple, dilacerated, obstructed, or curved canals; malpositioned and malformed teeth; and complex root morphology. To this one might add unusual radiographic lesions that do not appear to be "standard" periapical lesions.
(2) Emergencies in which a patient needs immediate treatment for toothaches, broken crowns, clinical exposures, infection, or traumatically injured teeth.
(3) Medically compromised patients with cardiovascular conditions, diabetes, and blood disorders.
(4) Mentally compromised patients, those with a true mental disorder and those who have problems with dentistry.

Harman[41] has added that if the general dentist believes that a good and proper diagnosis goes beyond his or her abilities, then the dentist should refer the patient. Nash[42] has estimated that 85 to 90% of all endodontic referrals come from other dentists. The remainder are self-referrals, walk-ins, and patient or physician referrals.

Prearranged referral agreements are *not* appropriate. They violate the professional conduct rules of most State Education Departments as well as Codes of Ethics. It is not considered a prearranged referral to refer a patient to a plan participant in a managed care dental benefits plan or an employee dentist within a practice as long as she/he is a true specialist. It is *never* appropriate to give something of value in exchange for a referral.

The endodontist would much rather receive the patient at the beginning of treatment than become a "retreat-odontist." Failure to refer to a specialist when the generalist knew or should have known that the treatment was beyond his or her knowledge, technical skill, or ability to treat with a reasonable likelihood of success; failure to inform the patient of the reason for the referral, options, and risks; and failure to avoid referral to a specialist whom the referring dentist knew or should have known that he/she provided substandard care; and failure to keep accurate and complete documentation of the patient are all liability issues.

Summary

The primary line of defense is to avoid causing the patient to seek legal counsel by communicating properly when the DPR is established. The second line of defense is to avoid having an uninformed patient by having an appropriate consent for treatment. The third line of defense is to avoid creating damaging evidence by having a good record-keeping system. The umbrella of all defenses is to practice within the accepted standard of care and within one's capabilities.

References

1. Orr DL. Dentistry. In: Medical practice survival handbook, American College of Legal Medicine, Chap. 4. St. Louis, MO:Mosby/Elsevier;2007; pp. 489–99.
2. USAA Magazine; March 2003.
3. Cohen S, Schwartz S. Endodontics and the law. Calif Dent Assoc J 1985;13:97.
4. Harman B. A roundtable on referrals. Dent Econ 1987;77:44.
5. American Association of Endodontics. Appropriateness of care and quality assurance guidelines. 3rd ed. Chicago, IL:AAE; 1998.
6. Sievert K. Manager, risk Management. The California Dentists Insurance Co. (TDIC).
7. www/ada.org/prof/prac/liability (accessed September 6, 2007).
8. MILMIC of NYS. Underwriting Department; September 2007.
9. Seidberg BH. Dental litigation: triad of concerns in legal medicine, in the American College of Legal Medicine. 7th ed. St. Louis, MO: Mosby/Elsevier; 2007. pp. 499–506.
10. Milgrom P, Ingle JI. Consent procedures as a quality control. J Oral Surg 1975;33:115.
11. James AE, Perry S, Zaner RM, et al. The changing concept of standard of care and the development of medical imaging technology. Hum Med 1991;7(4).
12. Curley A. Standard of care definition varies. J Am Coll Dent Fall 1986;53(3):20–1.
13. Shandell R, Smith P. Standard of care: the preparation and trial of medical malpractice cases. Law Journal Press; 2000.
14. Weinstein B. Ethics and its role in dentistry. Gen Dent 1992;Sept–Oct:40(5):414–17.
15. *Taylor v. Robbins,* Tex., Harris County 281st Judicial District, No. 85-28095; May 4, 1988.
16. American Dental Association. Code on dental procedures and nomenclature. J Am Dent Assoc 1989;118:369.
17. American Association of Endodontists. Quality assurance guidelines. Chicago, IL:AAE; 1988.
18. Cohen S, Schwartz S. Endodontic complications and the law. J Endod 1987;13:191.
19. Åkerblom A, Hasselgren G. The prognosis for endodontic treatment of obliterated root canals. J Endod 1988;14:565.
20. Ørstavik D, Brodin P, Aas E. Paraesthesia following endodontic treatment: survey of the literature and report of a case. Int Endod J 1983;16:167–72.
21. Orr DL. Paresthesia of the trigeminal nerve secondary to endodontic manipulation with N2. Headache 1985;27(6):334–6.
22. Rowe AHR. Damage to the inferior alveolar nerve during or following endodontic treatment. Br Dent J 1983;153:306.
23. Cohenca C, Rotstein I. Mental nerve paresthesia associated with a non vital tooth. Endod Dent Traumatol 1996;12:298.
24. Reeh ES. Messer HH. Long term paresthesia following inadvertent forcing sodium hypochlorite through perforation in incisor. Endod Dent Traumatol 1989;5:200.
25. Joffe E. Complications during root canal therapy following accidental extrusion of sodium hypochlorite through the apical foramen. Gen Dent 1991;39:460.
26. Paladino T, Linoff K, Zinman E. Informed consent and record keeping. AGD Impact 1986;14:1.
27. Buckner F. The physician–patient relationship. Med Pract Mgmt 1994;Sept–Oct.
28. Liability arising from consultation. Medical legal lessons, ACLM, V8 #3; June 2000.
29. *Schloendorff v Society of New York Hospital.* 105 N.E. 92 (NY 1914).
30. *Nathanson v Kline,* 186 Kan. 393, 350 P.2nd 1093 (1960).
31. *Canterbury v Spence,* 464 F. 2d 772 (D.C. Cir. 1972) cert. denied, 409 US 1064 (1974).
32. Bailey B. Informed consent in dentistry. J Am Dent Assoc 1985;110:709.

33. Curley A. Informed consent, past, present and future. Sacramento, CA: The Dentists Insurance Co.;1989. p. 3.
34. American Dental Association. Council on Insurance Report. Informed consent: a risk management view. J Am Dent Assoc 1987;115:630.
35. Howard W. A roundtable on referrals. Dent Econ 1987;77:50.
36. Weichman JA. Malpractice prevention and defense. Calif Dent Assoc J 1975;3:58.
37. Selbst AG. Understanding informed consent and its relationship to the incidence of adverse treatment events in conventional endodontic therapy. J Endod 1990;16:387.
38. American Association of Endodontists. Informed consent. Communique 1986;3:4.
39. Hourigan MJ. Oral surgery for the general practitioner. Palm Springs Seminars; Mar. 1989.
40. Dietz G. A roundtable on referrals. Dent Econ 1987;77:51.
41. Harman B. A roundtable on referrals. Dent Econ 1987;77:72.
42. Nash K. Endodontic referrals. Calif Dent Assoc J 1987;15:47.
43. Seidberg BH. Advanced Endodontics, PC, Syracuse, NY; office records, 2000.
44. Ingle J. Personal communication 2007.

CHAPTER 4

Effects of Dental Implants on Treatment Planning for Prosthodontics, Periodontics, and Endodontics

MAHMOUD TORABINEJAD

After ascertaining the chief complaint, collecting pertinent information regarding the patient's medical and dental history, performing complete subjective as well as objective and radiographic tests, and analyzing the obtained data, the dentist should be able to come up with the right diagnosis. Once the nature of the problem is identified, proper treatment planning should be formulated for the patient. Treatment planning can sometimes become complicated and is affected by the views of the stakeholders (patients, insurance companies, dentists) who have different perspectives and expectations regarding the outcome of treatment. Patients are usually content as long as their treatment is functionally and esthetically pleasing. Insurance companies measure success by access to care, quality of care, and cost as well as survival rate of treatment. Dentists are usually concerned with the quality of delivery of provided care and fair compensation.[1]

In addition to general expectation of the stakeholders, a number of other factors can influence the treatment planning. These include procedure involved, the restorative material used, the influence of one treatment on another, the availability of specialized expertise, the projected longevity of treatment, the functional and psychological satisfaction achievable, the ability of the patient to maintain the results of treatment, the affordability of the services, and the individual clinician's skill and support.[2]

Treatment planning should be patient-centered, not based solely on dental insurance benefits or guided by the desires and clinical experience of the practitioner. It should be evidence based and ideally should preserve the biologic environment while maintaining or restoring esthetics, comfort, and function. The real art of dentistry is to coordinate and interface these perspectives and expectations among stakeholders, provide the best quality of care to the patient, and satisfy the needs of the other involved parties in most clinical situations.

The art and science of dentistry have been unitized to prevent oral diseases such as caries and inflammation of the periodontium, and restore function and esthetics to teeth affected by these diseases, using periodontal treatment, root canal therapy, and restorative procedures. Advances in both the biologic and technologic aspects of dentistry have resulted in the retention and rehabilitation of millions and millions of natural teeth, to the satisfaction of patients throughout the world. Despite these advances, many teeth develop decay, severe periodontal involvement, become fractured, and succumb to extraction. Traditionally, these teeth were treated endodontically or periodontally, or if not restorable, they were extracted and replaced with either fixed or removable prosthesis.

Introduction of cylindrical-style endosseous implants[3,4] to the dental profession, and their high survival rates, has significantly affected treatment planning in dentistry. The purpose of this chapter is to discuss the effects of dental implants on treatment planning for prosthodontics, periodontics, and endodontics.

Effects of Dental Implants on Prosthodontics

The benefits of extraction and replacement of a missing tooth with a fixed partial denture (FPD) are prevention of shifting of the adjacent teeth, improved chewing ability, and esthetics (Figure 1). Studies have shown no adverse effect on the surrounding alveolar bone[5] and attachment level between teeth supporting FPDs and a homologous tooth[6] and no difference in plaque index, gingival index, and probing depths between baselines.[7] It has also been found that if hygiene is maintained to a high level, no inflammation of the mucosa should be seen under the pontic, regardless of the pontic material used.[8]

Tooth preparation, impression, temporization, and cementation while fabricating an FPD can, however, all result in pulpal injury.[9] Endodontic treatment (Figure 2) is often needed in the years following crown cementation.[10] When examining teeth with advanced periodontal disease over an average period of 8.7 years, abutment teeth for bridges needed endodontic treatment five times more often (15% vs 3%) than non-abutment teeth. In a clinical study, Goodacre et al.[11]

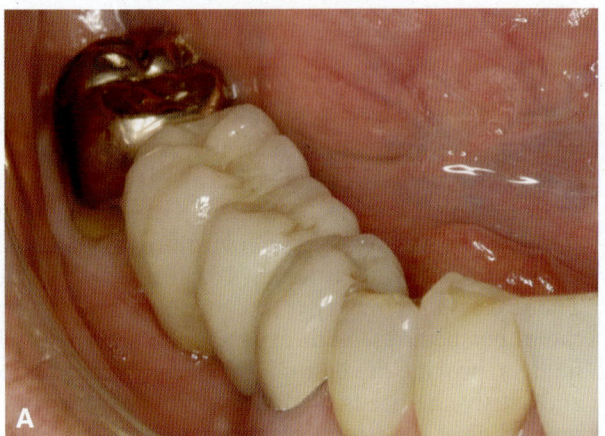 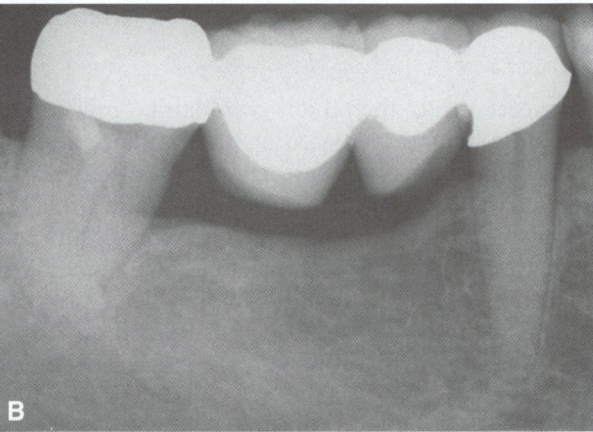

Figure 1 Replacement of missing teeth with a fixed partial denture can prevent shifting of the adjacent teeth. **A,** Clinical photo. **B,** Radiograph.

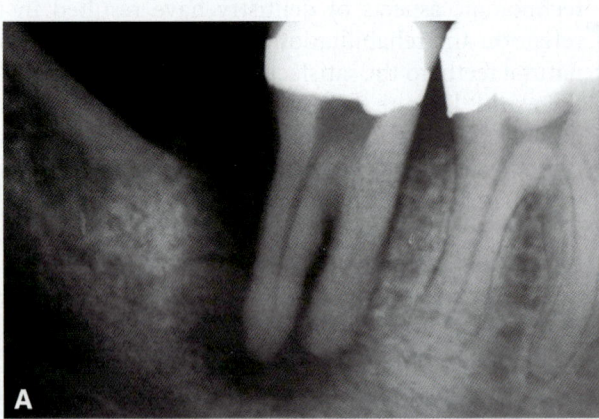 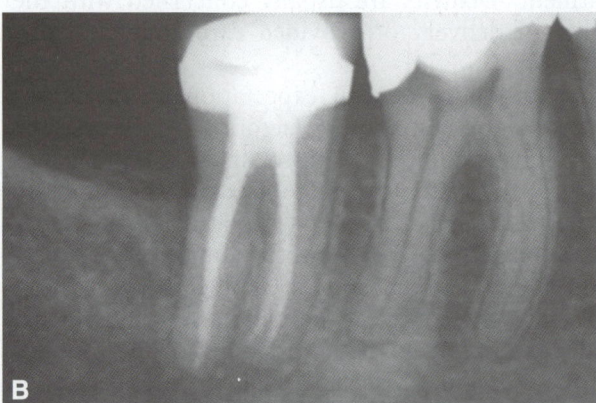

Figure 2 A, Pulpal necrosis occurred following tooth preparation and cementation of a crown resulting in a periapical lesion. **B,** Endodontic treatment resolved the extensive lesion. Photos courtesy of Dr. G.W. Harrington.

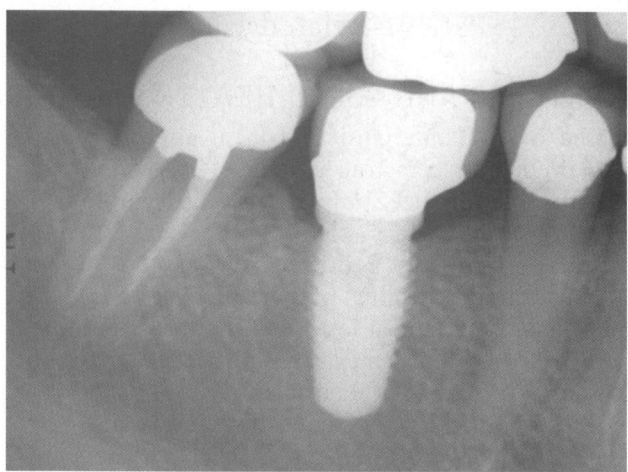

Figure 3 After 5 years of service, development of decay under crown margin of second mandibular molar.

report on the incidence of decay (0–27%) (Figure 3), pulpal problems (3–38%), and periodontal problems (4%), as well as technical complications such as porcelain fracture (2%), in patients who have had fixed prosthodontics for a 5-year period. The findings in these studies should be considered during treatment planning in light of recent reports on the high success rate for single-tooth implants.

Whereas previously, all efforts would have been made to extract hopeless teeth and place fixed or removable prostheses, the palpable benefits of implants have caused a paradigm shift in prosthetic and surgical dentistry. Clinicians are regularly confronted with difficult choices: Should a hopeless tooth be extracted and replaced with an FPD or single implant?

Placing a dental implant, rather than an FPD, provides a functional stimulus to help preserve the remaining bone, and prevent resorption, while preserving the enamel and dentin of the adjacent abutment teeth. Furthermore, this approach is less invasive to the pulp of the adjacent teeth. The biologic advantages over traditional prosthodontic methods include preservation of the natural dentition and supporting periodontium, improved esthetics, improved hygiene accessibility, and reduced future maintenance.[12,13] In a 3-year follow-up report of 78 single-tooth implants and 148 adjacent teeth, no adjacent teeth required extraction or endodontic treatment, and only 4 required restorations. Comparison of the periodontal status at crown placement and at follow-up revealed no differences for plaque and bleeding indices or for pocket probing depths of the adjacent teeth. There was, however, a significant influence of the horizontal distance on interproximal bone loss in closer distances of the anterior region, but not in the posterior region.[14] Peri-implant tissue differs from the gingiva surrounding natural teeth by having greater pocket depths and twice as much bleeding on probing.[15] The connective tissue portion around implants contains significantly more collagen (85% vs 60%) than around natural teeth, and fewer fibroblasts (1–3% vs 5–15%).[16] The majority of peri-implant tissue recession occurs during the first 3 months, with 80% showing buccal recession.[16] In patients with appropriate oral hygiene, however, the intra-crevicular position of the restoration margin does not appear to adversely affect peri-implant health and stability.[17]

Recently, Curtis et al.[2] discussed the impact of new scientific advances on treatment planning in dentistry. According to these authors, treatment planning in prosthodontics has changed significantly because of the recent advances in the success rate of single-tooth implants. In 1994, Creugers and associates[18] performed a meta-analysis on the dental literature since 1970, presenting clinical data regarding durability of conventional fixed bridges. These authors report an overall survival rate of 74.0 ± 2.1% after 15 years. Scurria et al.[19] in another meta-analysis of the literature reported an 87% 10-year survival rate for FPDs and a 69% 15-year survival rate. A recent systematic review[20] compared the outcomes of tooth-supported restorations with those of implant-supported restorations. The authors concluded that at 60 months, single-tooth replacements, supported by implants, had a higher survival rate than those supported by FPDs; however, if resin-bonded FPDs were excluded, no difference was found. They reported that FPD success rates continued to drop steadily beyond 60 months. These results are consistent with the results of another systematic review by Torabinejad et al.[21] that reported single-tooth implants, and endodontic treatments resulted in superior long-term survival, compared with FPDs.

Effects of Dental Implants on Periodontics

Previously, all efforts were made to save teeth with periodontal disease. Currently, the high success rates of implants have affected this concept, causing a paradigm shift in periodontics. Clinicians are asking:

Should a periodontally involved tooth be extracted and replaced with a dental implant?

The benefits of successful treatment of a tooth with periodontal disease include conservation of the crown and root structure, preservation of alveolar bone, and accompanying papillae, preservation of pressure perception, and lack of movement of the surrounding teeth. The harmful effects of extraction include bone resorption,[22] shifting of adjacent teeth,[23–25] and reduced esthetics and chewing ability.[26] Studies on long-term prognosis of teeth with periodontal disease show less than 10% tooth loss due to periodontal reasons.[27–29] Single-rooted teeth have better prognosis compared with molar teeth.[27–29] Presence of furcation involvement with or without surgical intervention is associated with poorer prognosis than those without furcation involvement.[30,31] As in prosthodontics, the new innovations in implant dentistry have also decreased reliance on high-risk periodontal procedures for tissue preservation and regeneration for teeth with moderate to sever periodontal disease.[2] This paradigm shift in periodontics is evident in recent surveys conducted by the American Academy of Periodontology, which show 63% of periodontists are placing their primary emphasis on periodontics and 27% are placing their primary emphasis on implants.[32]

Effects of Dental Implants on Endodontics

The high success rates of implants have also affected the thinking of clinicians for patients with pulpal and/or periapical diseases. Clinicians are asking: Should a pulpally/periapically-involved tooth be extracted and replaced with a dental implant? There are factors involved during decision-making in treatment planning, as to whether a tooth receives root canal treatment or is extracted and a dental implant placed. These factors can be divided into two broad categories: patient-related and treatment-related factors.[33]

Patient-Related Factors

SYSTEMIC AND LOCAL HEALTH FACTORS

Based on available clinical data, it appears most of the preoperative factors such as age, gender, tooth location, lesion size, pulp status, and symptoms do not affect outcomes of root canal treatment. A history of diabetes, however, may have a negative impact on the healing of periapical lesions.[34] The presence of periapical lesions is the major preoperative factor having a negative influence on the outcome of root canal therapy.[35–38]

Presence of some systemic disease can also affect the outcomes of implants.[39] Diabetic patients,[40] immune-suppressed individuals,[39] and patients who smoke[41–44] have a higher risk of complications following placement of implants.

PULP AND PERIODONTAL CONDITIONS

Indications for root canal therapy include teeth with irreversible pulpitis, necrotic pulps, restorable crowns, salvageable periodontal conditions, salvageable resorptive defects, and favorable crown-to-root ratio. Contraindications for root canal therapy are teeth without pulpal pathosis (except those done for prosthodontics reasons), with un-restorable crowns, with unsalvageable periodontal conditions, with unsalvageable resorptive or fracture defects, and with poor crown-to-root ratio. Root canal treatment is contraindicated when there is limited remaining tooth structure and the definitive crown will not be able to engage at least 1.5 to 2.0 mm of tooth structure with a cervical ferrule.[45,46] Bridge abutment teeth with root canal treatment fail more often than similar teeth with vital pulps.[47–49] On the other hand, crown placement has a significant positive effect on the survival of endodontically treated teeth.[50]

Indications for single-tooth implants are nonrestorable tooth, unsalvageable resorptive defects, poor crown–root ratio, unstable abutment, and single-rooted teeth with infractions or vertical root fractures (Figure 4). Other indications for the use of implants

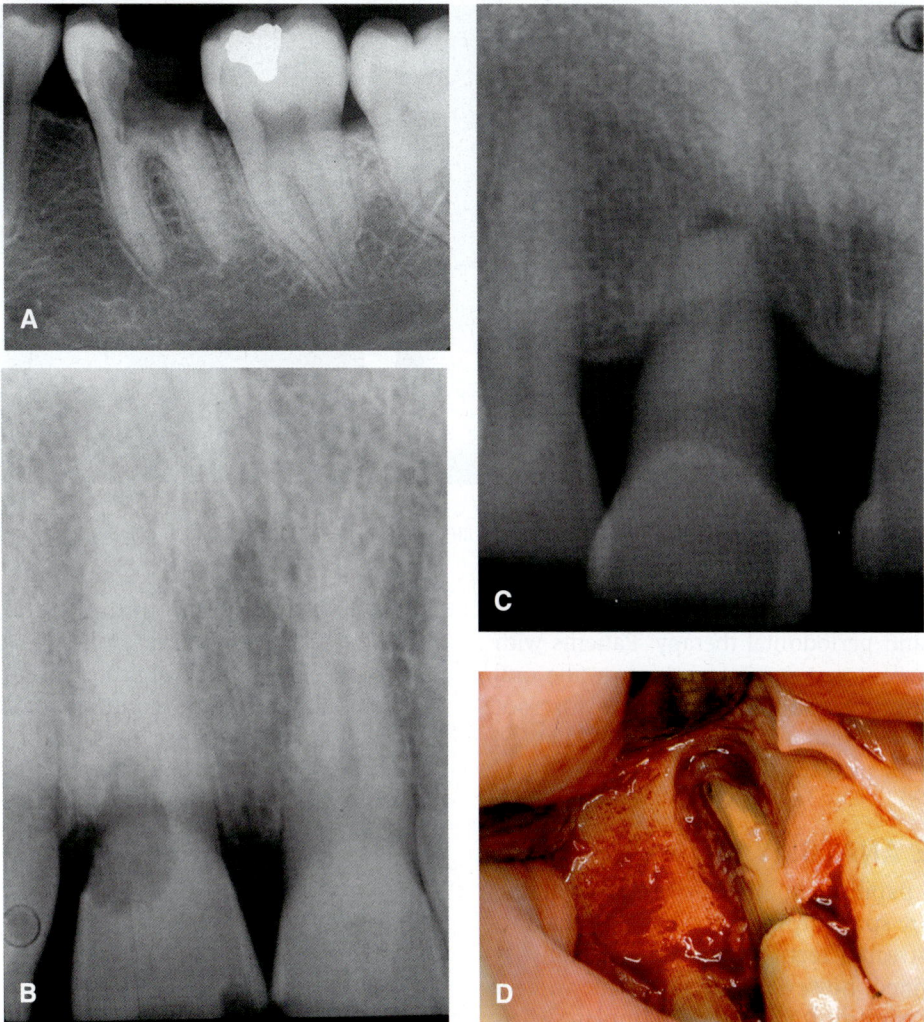

Figure 4 Root canal therapy is not indicated for teeth with **A**, un-restorable crowns; **B**, unsalvageable resorptive defects; **C**, poor crown–root ratio; or **D**, vertical root fractures.

include edentulous sites adjacent to teeth without restoration (Figure 5) or the need for restoration, abutment teeth with large pulp chambers, and abutment teeth with a history of avulsion or tooth luxation.[51] Single-tooth implants are contraindicated in patients who desire to keep their natural teeth, medically compromised patients, smokers, patients who are too old or too young, and patients with difficult surgical procedures.

BIOLOGIC ENVIRONMENTAL CONSIDERATIONS

Some patients are prone to recurrent caries or periodontal disease (Figure 6). Retaining teeth in such patients can be challenging and frustrating for the practitioner as well as the patients. Placement of implants

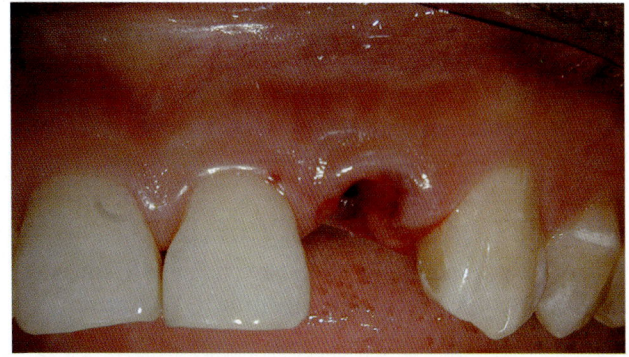

Figure 5 Single-tooth implants are a treatment option in edentulous sites adjacent to nonrestored teeth.

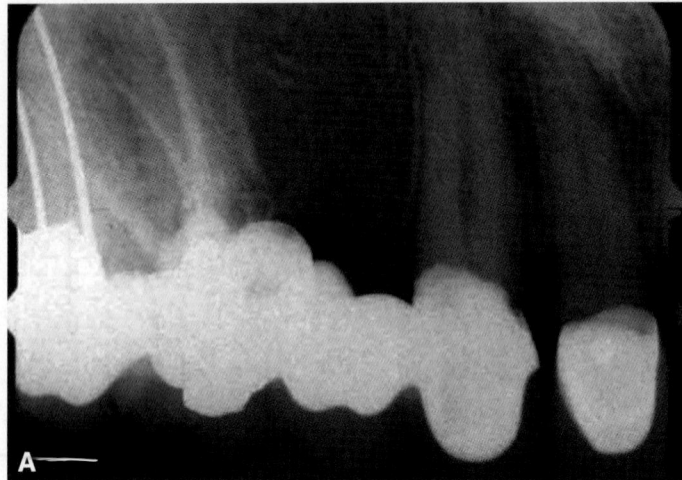
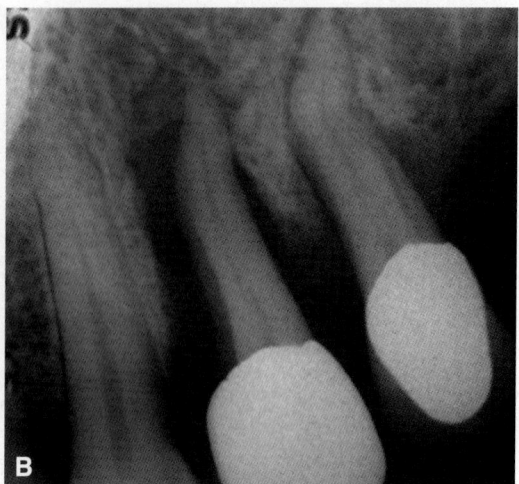

Figure 6 Patients prone to **A**, recurrent caries or **B**, periodontal disease are poor candidates for fixed partial dentures.

may be more prudent in patients needing both root canal treatment and periodontal therapy. Patients with limited abilities or interest in performing routine oral hygiene procedures are also poor candidates for root canal treatment or periodontal therapy, and may be better candidates for placement of implants.

SOFT TISSUE ANATOMY

The interdental papilla sometimes does not fill the cervical embrasure space around crowns that attach to both root-canal-treated teeth and dental implants. It has been determined, however, that soft tissue will fill the cervical embrasure around a crowned implant when the inciso–cervical distance from the proximal contact to the interproximal bone crest is 5 mm or less.[52]

Periodontal biotype (thick or thin) can affect the potential for soft tissue to fill the cervical embrasure space around implants (Figure 7). In a thin biotype, papillae adjacent to implants can seldom be recreated when the distance is more than 4 mm between the interproximal bone crest and the desired height of the interdental papillae.[53] Preservation of a tooth through root canal treatment may provide better soft tissue esthetics than extracting the tooth and placing a dental implant in a patient with thin biotype.

QUANTITY AND QUALITY OF BONE

Quantity and quality of bone have no significant effect on the outcome of root canal treatment. By contrast, the quantity of available bone affects the feasibility of placing implants without bone grafting. Bone quality also affects implant success with type IV bone (Figure 8), producing lower success compared with types I to III bone.[54] Retaining teeth, through root canal treatment, having a poor long-term prognosis, and performing high-risk endodontic surgical procedures as well, can substantially affect the amount of bone and prognosis of future implants in those sites. Early removal of teeth with poor prognosis and placement of dental implants may produce an environment more suitable for ideal implant positioning and optimal esthetics.[55]

TEETH WITH UNIQUE COLOR CHARACTERISTICS

Color matching in anterior teeth with unique dentin colorations can be a significant challenge for the practitioner. Retaining such teeth through root canal treatment (even with heroic efforts) without ceramic crowns may be esthetically advantageous to extracting them and placing implant crowns that do not match the surrounding environment (Figure 9).

Color-matching anterior teeth needing root canal treatment and a thick ceramic crown can sometimes be very difficult. Construction of a ceramic crown made for an implant usually produces a better color result because it can be fabricated with a greater thickness of porcelain that enhances the color-matching potential, particularly in esthetic regions of the mouth.

Treatment-Related Factors

ETHICAL CONSIDERATIONS

Dental practitioners have an obligation to provide the longest lasting, most cost-effective treatment that addresses the chief complaint of the patient and meets

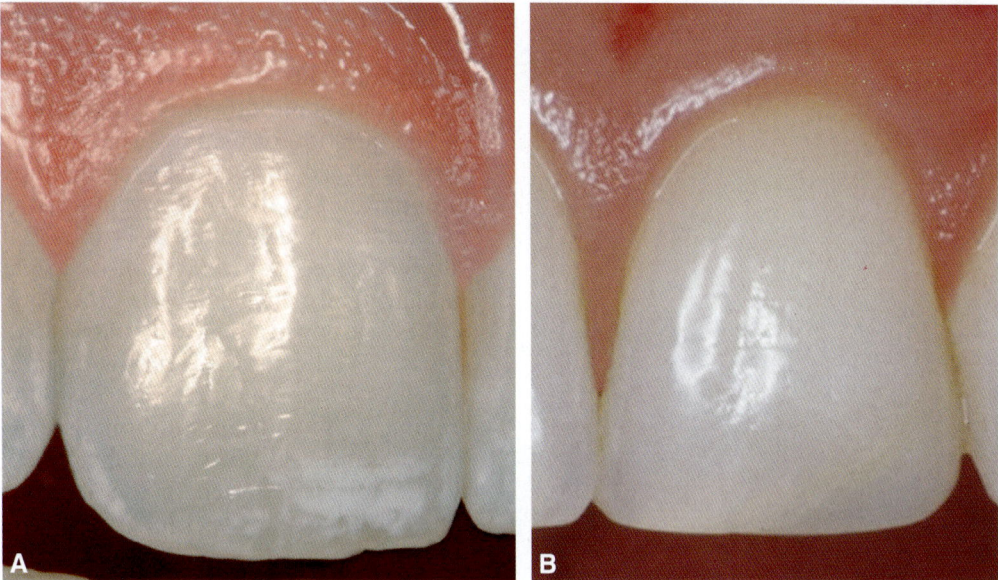

Figure 7 ***A,*** Patients with thick biotype gingiva and teeth in esthetic zones are good candidate for dental implants. ***B,*** Patients with thin biotype gingiva and teeth in esthetic zones are good candidate for root canal treatment.

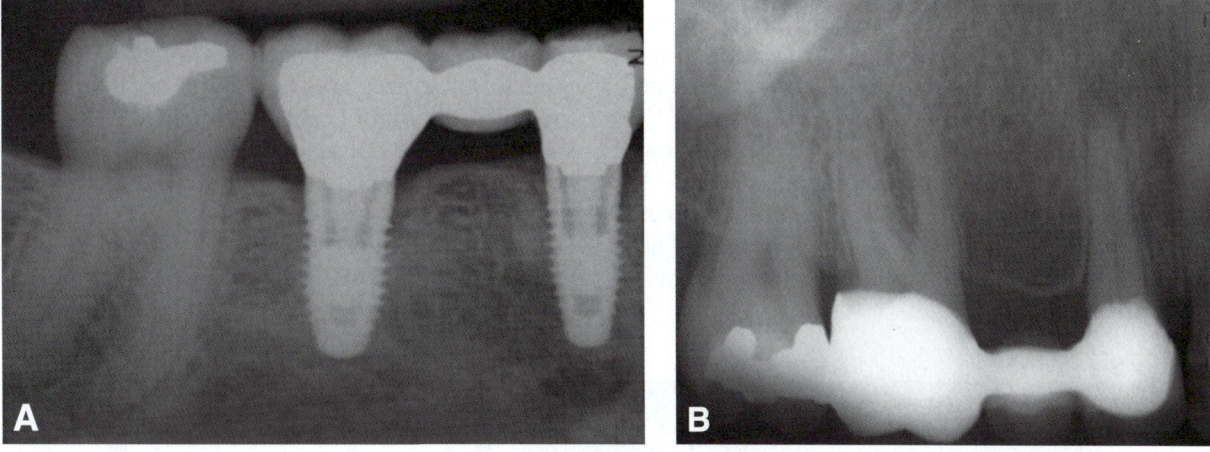

Figure 8 ***A,*** Mandibular molar region has good bone quality for implant placement. ***B,*** Maxillary molar region with poor quality bone is not ideal for dental implants.

or exceeds patient expectations whenever possible. Advice to the patient and the treatment provided should be patient-centered, not based solely on dental insurance benefits or guided by the desires and existing clinical experience of the practitioner. Practitioners should strive to present a balanced perspective regarding alternative treatments. The capacity to achieve balance requires practitioners to be familiar with both treatments. It is difficult to objectively present alternative treatment options when an individual has only substantive clinical experience with one option.

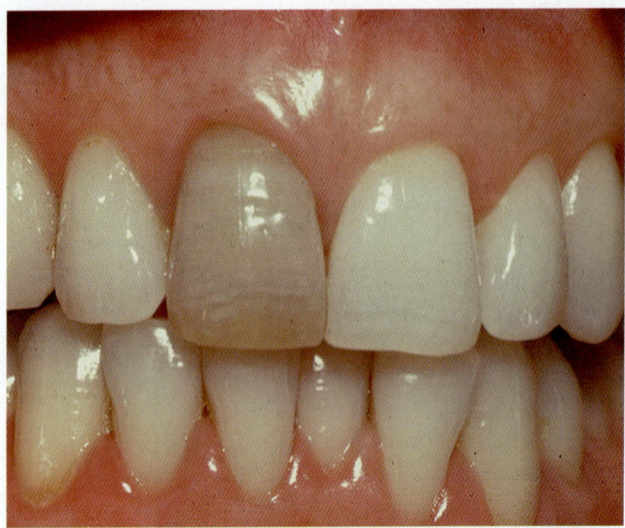

Figure 9 Retaining teeth through root canal treatment and bleaching without ceramic crowns in esthetic zones may be esthetically advantageous over placing implant crowns that are difficult to match to adjacent teeth.

PATIENT COMFORT AND PERCEPTIONS

The studies that have focused on the pretreatment anxiety of patients seeking root canal treatment are inconclusive. Whereas some note no difference between root canal treatment and extraction,[56,57] others[58] report higher anxiety levels in patients being considered for randomized controlled trial (RCT). A lack of data exists about examining pretreatment anxiety of patients seeking implant treatment. The most similar treatment that has been studied is extraction. However, patients presenting for extraction are often in pain, as are those presenting for root canal treatment. This may have the effect of raising the anxiety levels of both these patient populations.

The question of pain associated with treatment has been analyzed to some degree in implant literature, although not to the same extent as in the endodontic literature. Andersson et al.[59] found that 88.2% of subjects gave positive responses to the question of implant treatment being pain-free, with 70.6% giving a "Yes" response along with 17.6% stating, "Yes, with doubt." Watkins et al.,[60] on the other hand, observed a mean pain score of 22.7 out of 100 in 333 subjects seeking RCT, with an additional score of 19.9 noted "unpleasantness." Of significance, 20% of the endodontic cohort reported to the appointment in pain. One prospective study[61] focused on implant complications and found that 92% of the subjects felt the number of complications was acceptable. No endodontic study was found to have evaluated this question.

PROCEDURAL COMPLICATIONS

Root canal treatment can sometimes be associated with procedural accidents (Figure 10A). These mishaps can occur during different phases of root canal treatment.[62] Some of these accidents can have a negative impact on the outcomes of root canal treatment.[63–65] Studies have shown that the apical extension of root canal filling materials as well as quality of obturation can affect the prognosis of root canal treatment.[33,66]

As with root canal treatment, complications can occur with dental implants. Surgical implant complications

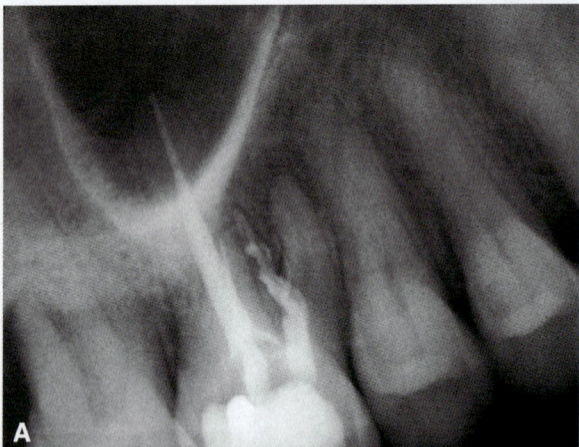 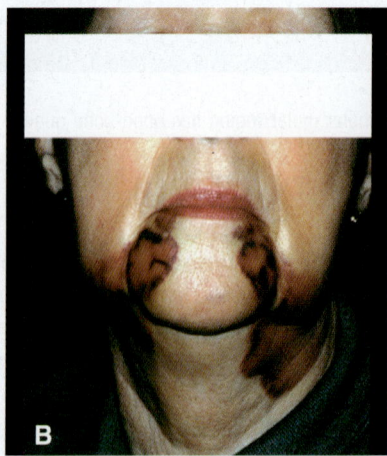

Figure 10 Root canal treatment or implant placement can sometimes be associated with procedural accidents. Examples are **A,** furcation perforation in a maxillary molar; **B,** a large hematoma following implant surgery.

include hematomas (Figure 10B), echymosis, and neurosensory disturbance.[54] Inflammation and/or proliferation of gingiva as well as soft tissue fenestration/dehiscence can occur following implant placement. Early implant loss can occur as a result of failure of the implant to integrate with the bone. Mechanical complications of implant placement include screw loosening, screw fracture, prosthesis fracture, and implant fracture.[54] Minor complications such as screw loosening are easily corrected, whereas major complications such as fenestration/dehiscence can result in clinical failure.

ADJUNCTIVE PROCEDURES REQUIRED

A number of adjunctive procedures can be performed in high-risk root canal treatment or placement of an implant and crown. Saving some teeth with significant decay or periodontal disease may require crown lengthening through surgery or orthodontic extrusion as well as periodontal disease therapy. In light of high success rates with dental implants, the value of such procedures needs to be reevaluated.

Lack of bone prior to placement of an implant may require bone grafting or distraction osteogenesis, sinus grafting, and ridge augmentation. These highly difficult technical procedures are expensive, unpleasant, and time consuming.

COST OF TREATMENT

According to the data collected by the American Dental Association (Jack Brown, personal communication) through its Services Rendered Survey that yield national and subnational estimates of fees for general practitioners (GPs) and specialists for each CDT4 code, the initial cost of an extraction, endosteal implant, abutment, and crown is approximately $2,850 and does not vary substantially whether a GP, an oral surgeon, or a periodontist provides the surgical care. On the other hand, the costs of an anterior root canal treatment provided by a GP with a resin-composite restoration, and a molar root canal treatment provided by an endodontist followed by an amalgam build-up and a porcelain fused to high noble metal crown are approximately $743 and $1,765, respectively. This simple analysis does not include consultation fees and pre-operative radiographs that may vary from simple periapical views to cone-beam tomography and CT scan for implant placement. Additional separately charged procedures such as surgical guides (stents) or provisional restorations may also be necessary. Retention of a periodontally sound tooth through root canal treatment clearly has tremendous cost benefit and cost-effectiveness in comparison with any alternative where the tooth is lost.

TREATMENT OUTCOMES

Clinical and radiographic examinations are the most common procedures used to determine outcomes of root canal therapy. Examination of the data regarding success and failure of root canal treatment shows significant variability in material composition, treatment procedures, and evaluation criteria. Some studies use recognized evaluation methods, such as the periapical index.[67] The periapical index relies on the comparison of the radiographs with a set of five radiographic images representing a radiographically healthy periapex (score 1) to a large periapical lesion (score 5). Another evaluation method that has been used in several studies is the system suggested by Halse and Molven,[68] who place radiographic findings in one of the following groups: (1) success, where there in no visible periapical lesion; (2) uncertain, where there is an uncertain finding such as an existing increased width of the periodontal ligament space; and (3) failure, where there is a pathologic finding such as a periapical radiolucency. The shortcomings of these methods of evaluation are that they determine "success" strictly on the basis of radiographic findings. As early as 1966, Bender and coworkers[69] noted that radiographic interpretation is often subject to personal bias and that a change in angulations can often give a completely different appearance to the lesion, making it appear either smaller or larger. It has also been shown that different observers may not agree on what they see in a radiograph, and in fact the same observer may disagree with himself if asked to review the same radiograph some time later.[70]

Based on the results of studies published since 1996, the American Dental Association Council on Scientific Affairs reports high implant survival rates for various clinical situations.[39] With regard to the single-tooth implant, the Council's evaluation of 10 studies involving over 1,400 implants shows survival rates (without giving length of time) ranging from 94.4% to 99%, with a mean survival rate of 96.7%. High mean survival rates were also reported for partially edentulous patients with implant FPDs. This report states that immediate loading of implants does not lower the survival rates, with three studies reporting survival rates ranging from 93.5% to 95.6%.[39] In a systematic review of clinical implant studies, Creugers and associates[71] predicted a 4-year survival rate of 97% for single implants. In another paper, Lindh et al.[72] performed a meta-analysis of implant studies involving partially edentulous patients. They reported a success rate of 97.5% after 6 to 7 years for a single-implant crown.

In a recent systematic review, Torabinejad et al.[21] compared the outcomes of endodontically treated teeth with those of single dental implant-supported crown, FPD, and no treatment following extraction. Success data in this review consistently ranked implant therapy as being superior to endodontic treatment, which in turn was ranked as being superior to fixed prosthodontic treatment (Table 1). At 97%, long-term survival was essentially the same for implant and endodontic treatments and was superior to extraction and replacement of the missing tooth with a FPD. Iqbal and Kim[73] have reported similar findings when they compared the survival of restored endontically treated teeth with implant-supported restorations.

ALTERNATIVE TREATMENTS

The treatment options following unsuccessful initial root canal treatment are re-treatment and/or endodontic surgery. In two separate searches, investigators at Loma Linda University searched for clinical articles pertaining to success and failure of nonsurgical and surgical re-treatment, and assigned levels of evidence to these studies. Their first search, related to nonsurgical re-treatment, resulted in the identification of 31 clinical studies and 6 review articles.[74] The success rate of non-surgical re-treatment ranged between 40% and 100%. Based on the literature, it appears that the success rate is very high in teeth without periapical lesions and when the cause of failure is identified and corrected properly.[74] Their second search, pertaining to success and failure of periapical surgery, located many clinical studies, most of which were case series.[75] The success rate of surgical endodontics varied from 31% to over 90%. The significant differences in the techniques, materials, and methods of evaluation make it very difficult to compare these studies. Most recent studies using new materials and techniques report high success rates for endodontic surgery.[76–79]

Considering factors involved in treatment planning for patients who have been afflicted by oral diseases or traumatic injuries, decision to keep a tooth through root canal treatment or periodontal therapy, or extraction and placement of a fixed or partial denture, or an implant supported restoration, should be based on scientific evidence. Ideally one should strive to preserve the biologic environment, while maintaining or restoring long-term esthetics, comfort, and function for the patient.

Table 1 Pooled and Weighted Survival and Success Rates of Dental Implants, Root Canal Treatment, and Three Unit Bridges 2–4, 4–6, and Over 6 Years

	Success	Survival
2–4 years		
Dental implant (pooled)	98 (95–99)	95 (93–97)
Dental implant (weighted)	99 (96–100)	96 (94–97)
Root canal treatment (pooled)	90 (88–92)	94
Root canal treatment (weighted)	89 (88–91)	–
Three unit bridge (pooled)	79 (69–87)	94
Three unit bridge (weighted)	78 (76–81)	–
4–6 years		
Dental implant (pooled)	97 (96–98)	97 (95–98)
Dental implant (weighted)	98 (97–99)	97 (95–98)
Root canal treatment (pooled)	93 (87–97)	94 (92–96)
Root canal treatment (weighted)	94 (92–96)	94 (91–96)
Three unit bridge (pooled)	82 (71–91)	93
Three unit bridge (weighted)	76 (74–79)	–
6+ years		
Dental implant (pooled)	95 (93–96)	97 (95–99)
Dental implant (weighted)	95 (93–97)	97 (96–98)
Root canal treatment (pooled)	84 (82–87)	92 (84–97)
Root canal treatment (weighted)	84 (81–87)	97 (97–97)
Three unit bridge (pooled)	81 (74–86)	82
Three unit bridge (weighted)	80 (79–82)	–

References

1. Torabinejad M, Bahjri K. Essential elements of evidenced-based endodontics: steps involved in conducting clinical research. J Endod 2005;31(8):563–9.
2. Curtis DA, Lacy A, Chu R, et al. Treatment planning in the 21st century: what's new? J Calif Dent Assoc 2002;30:503–10.
3. Brånemark PI, Zarb GA, Albrektsson T. Tissue-integrated prostheses: osseointegration in clinical dentistry. Chicago: Quintessence; 1985.
4. Schroeder A, Sutter F, Buser D, Krekeler G. Oral implantology. 2nd ed. New York: Thieme Medical Publishers; 1996.
5. Wyatt CC. The effect of prosthodontic treatment on alveolar bone loss: a review of the literature. J Prosthet Dent 1998;80(3):362–6.
6. Ericsson SG, Marken KE. Effect of fixed partial dentures on surrounding tissues. J Prosthet Dent 1968;20(6):517–25.
7. Silness J, Gustavsen F. Alveolar bone loss in bridge recipients after six and twelve years. Int Dent J 1985;35(4):297–300.
8. Tolboe H, Isidor F, Budtz-Jorgensen E, Kaaber S. Influence of pontic material on alveolar mucosal conditions. Scand J Dent Res 1988;96(5):442–7.
9. Langeland K, Langeland LK. Pulp reactions to crown preparation, impression, temporary crown fixation, and permanent cementation. J Prosthet Dent 1965;15:129–43.

10. Bergenholtz G, Nyman S. Endodontic complications following periodontal and prosthetic treatment of patients with advanced periodontal disease. J Periodontol 1984 Feb;55(2):63–8.
11. Goodacre CJ, Bernal G, Rungcharassaeng K, Kan JY. Clinical complications in fixed prosthodontics. J Prosthet Dent 2003;90:31–41.
12. Balshi TJ, Wolfinger GJ. Two-implant-supported single molar replacement: interdental space requirements and comparison to alternative options. Int J Periodontics Restorative Dent 1997;17(5):426–35.
13. Sharma P. 90% of fixed partial dentures survive 5 years. How long do conventional fixed partial dentures (FPDs) survive and how frequently do complications occur? Evid Based Dent 2005;6(3):74–5.
14. Krennmair G, Piehslinger E, Wagner H. Status of teeth adjacent to single-tooth implants. Int J Prosthodont 2003;16(5):524–8.
15. Brägger U, Burgin WB, Hammerle CH, Lang NP. Associations between clinical parameters assessed around implants and teeth. Clin Oral Implants Res 1997;8(5):412–21.
16. Small PN, Tarnow DP. Gingival recession around implants: a 1-year longitudinal prospective study. Int J Oral Maxillofac Implants 2000;15(4):527–32.
17. Giannopoulou C, Bernard JP, Buser D, et al. Effect of intracrevicular restoration margins on peri-implant health: clinical, biochemical, and microbiologic findings around esthetic implants up to 9 years. Int J Oral Maxillofac Implants 2003;18(2):173–81.
18. Creugers NH, Kayser AF, Van't Hof MA. A meta-analysis of durability data on conventional fixed bridges. Community Dent Oral Epidemiol 1994;22(6):448–52.
19. Scurria MS, Bader JD, Shugars DA. Meta-analysis of fixed partial denture survival: prostheses and abutments. J Prosthet Dent 1998;79:459–64.
20. Salinas TJ, Eckert SE. In patients requiring single-tooth replacement, what are the outcomes of implant—as compared to tooth-supported restorations? Int J Oral Maxillofac Implants 2007;22(Suppl):71–95.
21. Torabinejad M, Anderson P, Bader J, et al. The outcomes of endodontic treatment, single implant, fixed partial denture and no tooth replacement: a systematic review. J Prosthet Dent 2007;98(4):285–311.
22. Johnson K. A study of the dimensional changes occurring in the maxilla following tooth extraction. Aust Dent J 1969;14(4):241–4.
23. Love WD, Adams RL. Tooth movement into edentulous areas. J Prosthet Dent 1971;25(3):271–8.
24. Shugars DA, Bader JD, White BA, et al. Survival rates of teeth adjacent to treated and untreated posterior bounded edentulous spaces. J Am Dent Assoc 1998;129(8):1089–95.
25. Aquilino SA, Shugars DA, Bader JD, White BA. Ten-year survival rates of teeth adjacent to treated and untreated posterior bounded edentulous spaces. J Prosthet Dent 2001;85(5):455–60.
26. Oosterhaven SP, Westert GP, Schaub RM, van der Bilt A. Social and psychologic implications of missing teeth for chewing ability. Community Dent Oral Epidemiol 1988;16(2):79–82.
27. Hirschfeld L, Wasserman B. A long-term survey of tooth loss in 600 treated periodontal patients. J Periodontol 1978;49:225–37.
28. McFall WT, Jr. Tooth loss in 100 treated patients with periodontal disease. A long-term study. J Periodontol 1982;53:539–49.
29. Becker W, Berg L, Becker BE. The long term evaluation of periodontal treatment and maintenance in 95 patients. Int J Periodontics Restorative Dent 1984;4:54–71.
30. Wang HL, Burgett FG, Shyr Y, Ramfjord S. The influence of molar furcation involvement and mobility on future clinical periodontal attachment loss. J Periodontol 1994;65:25–9.
31. Langer B, Stein SD, Wagenberg B. An evaluation of root resections. A ten-year study. J Periodontol 1981;52:719–22.
32. American Academy of Periodontics. Characteristics and trends in private periodontal practice. Chicago: American Academy of Periodontics; 2004.
33. Torabinejad M, Goodacre C. Endodontic or dental implant therapy: the factors affecting treatment planning. J Am Dent Assoc 2006;137(7):973–7.
34. Fouad AF, Burleson J. The effect of diabetes mellitus on endodontic treatment outcome: data from an electronic patient record. J Am Dent Assoc 2003;134:43–51.
35. Matsumoto T, Nagai T, Ida K, et al. Factors affecting successful prognosis of root canal treatment. J Endod 1987;13:239–42.
36. Chugal NM, Clive JM, Spangberg LS. A prognostic model for assessment of the outcome of endodontic treatment: effect of biologic and diagnostic variables. Oral Surg Oral Med Oral Pathol Oral Radiol Endod 2001;91:342–52.
37. Friedman S, Abitbol S, Lawrence HP. Treatment outcome in endodontics: the Toronto Study. Phase 1: initial treatment. J Endod 2003;29:787–93.
38. Sjögren U, Hägglund B, Sundqvist G, Wing K. Factors affecting the long-term results of endodontic treatment. J Endod 1990;16:498–504.
39. ADA Council on Scientific Affairs. Dental endosseous implants: an update. J Am Dent Assoc 2004;135:92–7.
40. Fiorellini JP, Chen PK, Nevins M, Nevins ML. A retrospective study of dental implants in diabetic patients. Int J Periodontics Restorative Dent 2000;20:366–73.
41. Gorman LM, Lambert PM, Morris HF, et al. The effect of smoking on implant survival at second-stage surgery: DICRG Interim Report No. 5. Dental Implant Clinical Research Group. Implant Dent 1994;3:165–8.

42. Bain CA. Smoking and implant failure—benefits of a smoking cessation protocol. Int J Oral Maxillofac Implants 1996;11:756–9.

43. Kan JY, Rungcharassaeng K, Lozada JL, Goodacre CJ. Effects of smoking on implant success in grafted maxillary sinuses. J Prosthet Dent 1999;82:307–11.

44. Wallace RH. The relationship between cigarette smoking and dental implant failure. Eur J Prosthodont Restor Dent 2000;8:103–6.

45. Libman WJ, Nicholls JI. Load fatigue of teeth restored with cast posts and cores and complete crowns. Int J Prosthodont 1995;8:155–61.

46. Tan PL, Aquilino SA, Gratton DG, et al. In vitro fracture resistance of endodontically treated central incisors with varying ferrule heights and configurations. J Prosthet Dent 2005;93:331–6.

47. Eckerbom M, Magnusson T, Martinsson T. Reasons for and incidence of tooth mortality in a Swedish population. Endod Dent Traumatol 1992;8:230–4.

48. Randow K, Glantz PO, Zoger B. Technical failures and some related clinical complications in extensive fixed prosthodontics. An epidemiological study of long-term clinical quality. Acta Odontol Scand 1986;44:241–55.

49. Reuter JE, Brose MO. Failures in full crown retained dental bridges. Br Dent J 1984;157:61–3.

50. Aquilino SA, Caplan DJ. Relationship between crown placement and the survival of endodontically treated teeth. J Prosthet Dent 2002;87:256–63.

51. Salinas TJ, Block MS, Sadan A. Fixed partial denture or single-tooth implant restoration? Statistical considerations for sequencing and treatment. J Oral Maxillofac Surg 2004;62:2–16.

52. Choquet V, Hermans M, Adriaenssens P, et al. Clinical and radiographic evaluation of the papilla level adjacent to single-tooth dental implants. A retrospective study in the maxillary anterior region. J Periodontol 2001;72:1364–71.

53. Kan JY, Rungcharassaeng K, Umezu K, Kois JC. Dimensions of peri-implant mucosa: an evaluation of maxillary anterior single implants in humans. J Periodontol 2003;74:557–62.

54. Goodacre CJ, Bernal G, Rungcharassaeng K, Kan JY. Clinical complications with implants and implant prostheses. J Prosthet Dent 2003;90:121–32.

55. Rosenquist B, Grenthe B. Immediate placement of implants into extraction sockets: implant survival. Int J Oral Maxillofac Implants 1996;11:205–9.

56. Stabholz A, Peretz B. Dental anxiety among patients prior to different dental treatments. Int Dent J 1999;49(2):90–4.

57. Wong M, Lytle WR. A comparison of anxiety levels associated with root canal therapy and oral surgery treatment. J Endod 1991;17(9):461–5.

58. Udoye CI, Oginni AO, Oginni FO. Dental anxiety among patients undergoing various dental treatments in a Nigerian teaching hospital. J Contemp Dent Pract 2005 May 15;6(2):91–8.

59. Andersson L, Emami-Kristiansen Z, Hogstrom J. Single-tooth implant treatment in the anterior region of the maxilla for treatment of tooth loss after trauma: a retrospective clinical and interview study. Dent Traumatol 2003 Jun;19(3):126–31.

60. Watkins CA, Logan HL, Kirchner HL. Anticipated and experienced pain associated with endodontic therapy. J Am Dent Assoc 2002;133(1):45–54.

61. Ekfeldt A, Carlsson GE, Borjesson G. Clinical evaluation of single-tooth restorations supported by osseointegrated implants: a retrospective study. Int J Oral Maxillofac Implants 1994;9(2):179–83.

62. Torabinejad M, Lemon RR. Procedural accidents. In: Walton R, Torabinjad M, editors. Principles and practice of endodontics. 3rd ed. Philadelphia: W.B. Saunders Company; 2002. pp. 310–30.

63. Ingle JI, Simon JH, Machtou P, Bogaerts P. Outcome of endodontic treatment and re-treatment. In: Ingle J, Bakland L, editors. Endodontics. 5th ed. London: BC Decker, Inc.; 2002. pp. 748–57.

64. Kvinnsland I, Oswald RJ, Halse A, Gronningsaeter AG. A clinical and roentgenological study of 55 cases of root perforation. Int Endod J 1989;22:75–84.

65. Farzaneh M, Abitbol S, Friedman S. Treatment outcome in endodontics: the Toronto study. Phases I and II: Orthograde retreatment. J Endod 2004;30:627–33.

66. Dugas NN, Lawrence HP, Teplitsky PE, et al. Periapical health and treatment quality assessment of root-filled teeth in two Canadian populations. Int Endod J 2003;36:181–92.

67. Ørstavik D, Kerekes K, Eriksen HM. The periapical index: a scoring system for radiographic assessment of apical periodontitis. Endod Dent Traumatol 1986;2:20–34.

68. Halse A, Molven O. A strategy for the diagnosis of periapical pathosis. J Endod 1986;12:534–8.

69. Bender IB, Seltzer S, Soltanoff W. Endodontic success—a reappraisal of criteria 1. Oral Surg Oral Med Oral Pathol Oral Radiol Endod 1966;22:780–9.

70. Goldman M, Pearson AH, Darzenta N. Endodontic success—who's reading the radiograph? Oral Surg Oral Med Oral Pathol Oral Radiol Endod 1972;33:432–7.

71. Creugers NH, Kreulen CM, Snoek PA, de Kanter RJ. A systematic review of single-tooth restorations supported by implants. J Dent 2000;28:209–17.

72. Lindh T, Gunne J, Tillberg A, Molin M. A meta-analysis of implants in partial edentulism. Clin Oral Implants Res 1998;9:80–90.

73. Iqbal MK, Kim S. For teeth requiring endodontic therapy, what are the differences in the outcomes of restored endodontically treated teeth compared to implant-supported restorations? Int J Oral Maxillofac Implants 2007;221(Suppl):96–116.

74. Paik S, Sechrist C, Torabinejad M. Levels of evidence for the outcome of endodontic retreatment. J Endod 2004;30:745.

75. Mead C, Javidan-Nejad S, Mego M, et al. Levels of evidence for the outcome of endodontic surgery. J Endod 2005;31:19.

76. Zuolo M, Ferreira M, Gutmann J. Prognosis in periradicular surgery: a clinical prospective study. Int Endod J 2000;33:91–8.

77. Rubinstein RA, Kim S. Long-term follow-up of cases considered healed one year after apical microsurgery. J Endod 2002;28:378.

78. Maddalone M, Gagliani M. Periapical endodontic surgery: a 3-year follow-up study. Int Endod J 2003;36:193.

79. Sechrist CM, Kiger R, Shabahang S, Torabinejad M. The outcome of MTA as a root end filling material: a long term clinical and radiographic evaluation. J Endod 2006;32(Abstract 58):248.

PathoBiology

CHAPTER 5

Structure and Function of the Dentin–Pulp Complex

Syngcuk Kim, Karin J. Heyeraas, Sivakami R. Haug

This chapter is dedicated to the late Dr. Yoshiaki Kishi, Department of Oral Anatomy, Kanagawa Dental College, Yokosuka, Japan, who contributed significantly toward the understanding of the microvasculature in the oral tissues.

The dental pulp is a connective tissue like other connective tissues in the body. It consists of nerves, blood vessels, ground substances, interstitial fluid, odontoblasts, fibroblasts, and other cellular components. On a radiograph, the dentist sees the pulp as a dark line running coronal to apical in the center of the root. A researcher sees the pulp as a fibrous connective tissue strip with blood (Figure 1). As the late I.B. Bender said, "The pulp is a small tissue with a big issue." The uniqueness of the pulp can be appreciated only when perturbed, since the pulp resides in a rigid capsule consisting of enamel and dentin layers.

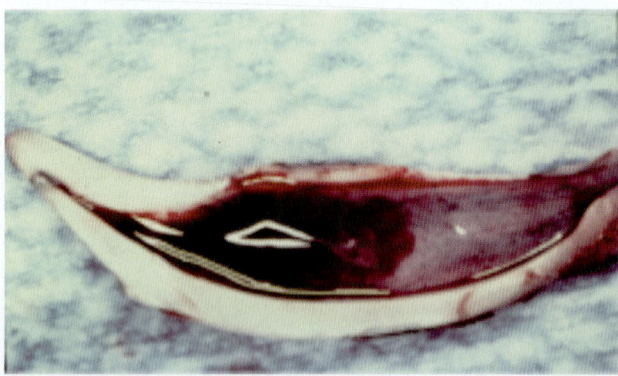

Figure 1 The young dog pulp shows highly vascularized connective tissue encased in rigid tissues that provide a unique hemodynamic environment. Pulp extirpation slide.

Unlike in other tissues this encasement creates a low-compliance environment in which a small increase in tissue volume, due to inflammation, has serious consequences. The other uniqueness of the pulp is that it consists primarily of sensory fibers. Despite its confinement by enamel and dentin, the dentin–pulp complex functions as an exquisitely responsive sensory system, using unusual mechanisms to defend it from insults. Its sensory fibers together with its microcirculatory vasculature make the pulp a unique organ to study the neurovascular interactions during various states of inflammation.

When the pulp is involved, endodontists face diagnostic dilemmas such as when presented with a tooth with thermal sensitivity, sensitivity to osmotic pressure and/or hydrostatic pressure, as well as other symptoms. The treatment option recommended to the patient must be based on sound biological/physiological knowledge. As such, one must understand the very tissue frequently eliminated by endodontic therapy.

The purpose of this chapter is to bring together the available information on the development, structure, and function of the dentin–pulp complex, with the aim that this knowledge provides a firm biological basis for clinical decision making.

EMBRYOLOGY

Human tooth development begins as early as the fifth week of gestation for primary dentition. Mineralization of primary dentition begins during the 14th week of gestation at the same time when the permanent teeth start to develop. The first primary teeth erupt around the age of 6 months and the first permanent teeth around 5 to 6 years. The third molars are the last teeth to be formed with the completion of crown development between 12 and 16 years. Thus, tooth development starts from the embryonic stage and continues into early adulthood. Recent findings have revealed multiple growth and transcription factors from several signaling families acting as critical regulators at the initiation, and subsequently throughout all stages, of tooth development. Gene-targeting experiments have demonstrated the biological function of transcription facts in regulating tooth morphogenesis. Today over 200 genes have been demonstrated to be active in the developing tooth, and a detailed list can be found in a database at http://bite-it.helsinki.fi/. This chapter will cover an overview of tooth development while referring details to excellent reviews in this field.[1-4]

Teeth derive from two principal cell types: the ectoderm and the cranial neural crest-derived ectomesenchyme. The ectodermal component gives rise to the ameloblasts that form the enamel of the tooth crown while the ectomesenchyme gives rise to the dentin, pulp, and periodontal tissue. The neural crest cells migrate from the crest of neural ectoderm. Only neural crest-derived mesenchyme has the ability to respond to the initial signals from the dental epithelium and contribute to tooth formation.[5,6] Initiation of tooth development begins with the formation of dental lamina, a thickening of the oral epithelium. Localized proliferation within the dental lamina leads to the formation of a series of epithelial outgrowths/buds at sites where the tooth should be, thus marking the time and position of tooth development. The underlying mesenchyme underneath, called the dental papilla, forms the future dentin and pulp. The dental follicle or sac surrounds the dental papilla and the enamel organ and gives rise to the supporting tissue.

There are three stages in the early tooth development: the bud, the cap, and the bell stage. During the bud stage, the mesenchyme underneath condenses and begins to appear like a cap on the dental papilla, thus leading to the stage known as the cap stage. The dental epithelium becomes to be known as the enamel organ from the cap stage. The enamel organ, the dental papilla, and the dental follicle constitute the dental organ or the tooth germ. Transition from the bud to the cap stage is a critical step in tooth morphogenesis involving multiple signaling molecules within the enamel organ epithelium. These have been implicated to regulate the expression of various transcription factors in the surrounding mesenchyme.[4,7,8]

During the cap stage, a critical signaling center, the enamel knot, is formed within the enamel organ epithelium. The enamel knot is a dense population of epithelial cells without any proliferative activity and marked by the expression of multiple signaling molecules that are critical for the proper development of the tooth organ. The enamel knot serves as a transient signaling center and is removed by programmed cell death. In molar teeth, this primary enamel knot is replaced by secondary enamel knots that are responsible for inducing cusp development. The enamel knot is critical for the patterning process such as cusp shape and size during tooth morphogenesis.[4] Determination of tooth identity depends on the expression of certain homeobox genes in the mesenchyme.[9,10] Continuous growth of the tooth germ leads to the bell stage during which the crown assumes its final shape (morphodifferentiation) and the cells that will be making the hard tissue (ameloblasts and odontoblasts) acquire their distinctive phenotype (histodifferentiation) (Figure 2). Cranial neural crest-derived

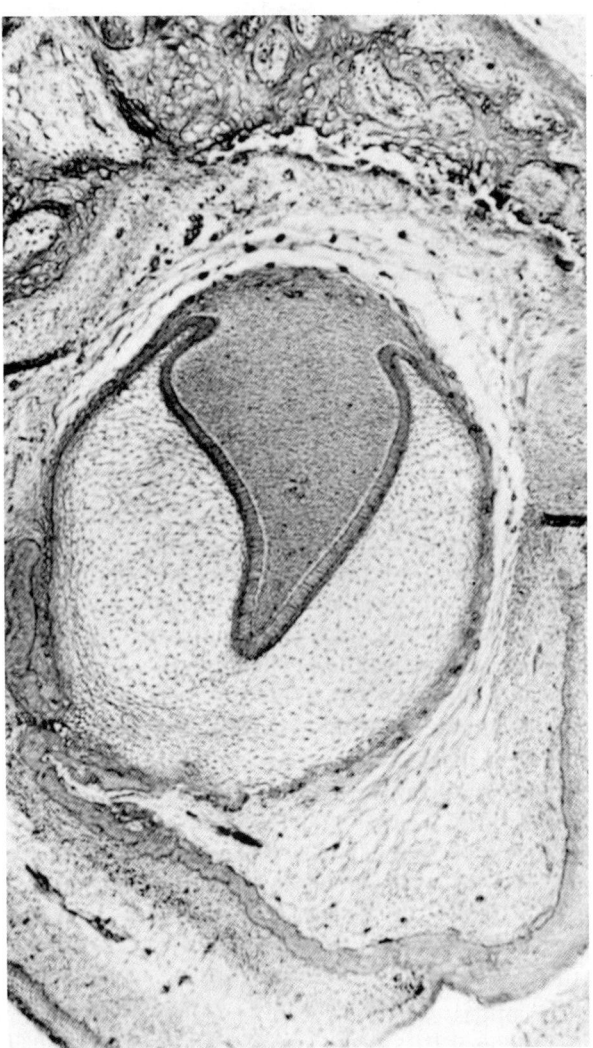

Figure 2 Early dental pulp, or dental papilla, exhibiting a cellular mass at the center of the tooth bud in the early bell stage. Nerve fiber bundles are evident in cross section as dark bodies apical to dental papilla yet are absent in the papilla itself. Human fetus, 19 weeks. Palmgren nerve stain. Reproduced with permission from Arwil T, Häggströms I. Innervation of the teeth. Transactions Royal School of Dentistry, Stockholm, 3:1958.

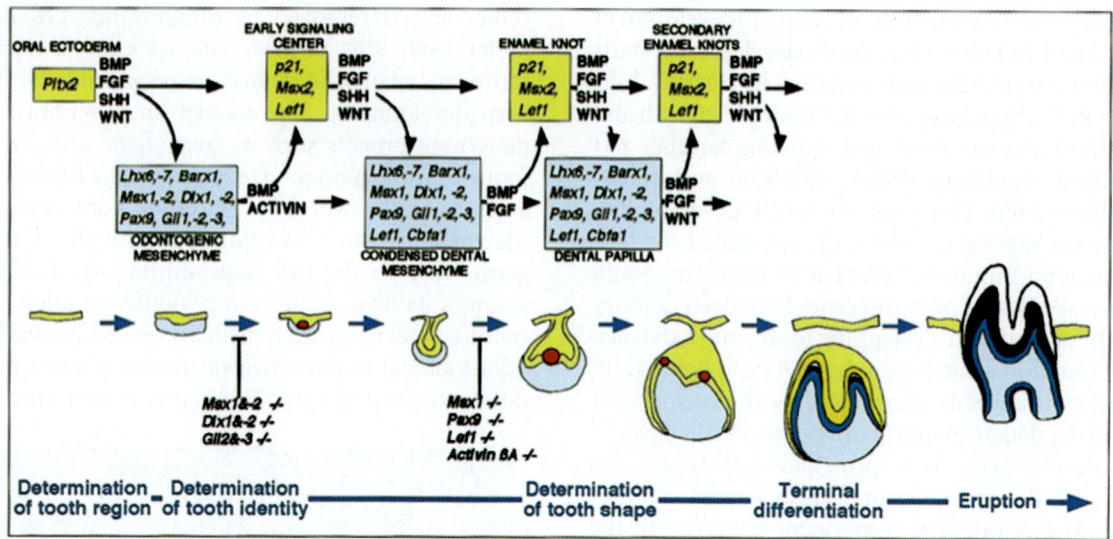

Figure 3 Schematic representation of the signals and transcription factors mediating the reciprocal signaling between epithelium and mesenchyme during advancing tooth development. The molecular cascades are shown above and the corresponding morphological stages below. The transcription factors and signals considered to be important for particular development stages are indicated in the squares and above the arrows, respectively. Note how the same signaling pathways are used reiteratively during advancing tooth development, and how tooth development arrests in the knockout mouse experiments to the early signaling center or the enamel knot stage. Yellow, tooth epithelium; red, enamel knots; blue, tooth mesenchyme. Reproduced with permission from Jernvall J and Thesleff I.[7]

odontogenic mesenchyme and its adjacent inner enamel organ epithelium differentiate into preodontoblast and preameloblast, respectively. Dentin and enamel will begin to form at the junction between odontoblasts and ameloblasts to complete the tooth-forming process (Figure 3).

Blood supply to the developing tooth is via the dental follicle during the cap stage. The enamel organ is avascular although there are numerous blood vessels in the adjacent follicle. These blood vessels ramify around the tooth germ, their number in the dental papilla increase reaching a maximum when matrix deposition begins. The vessels in the papilla are arranged in groups that coincide with the future root-forming site.

The first trigeminal nerve fibers are present in the vicinity of the tooth at the bud stage and around the tooth organ in the dental follicle during the cap and bell stages.[11–15]

In the bell stage, sensory nerve fibers containing the neuropeptides calcitonin gene-related peptide (CGRP) and substance P (SP) are present in the dental follicle but not in the dental papilla and the enamel organ.[16] In the advanced bell stage, after initiation of dentin and enamel formation, CGRP- and SP-containing nerve fibers enter the dental papilla. Sympathetic nerve-derived neuropeptide Y (NPY) appears later at the beginning of the root formation.[16] With the start of root development,

a subodontoblastic nerve plexus gradually forms with concomitant appearance of CGRP- and SP-containing nerve fibers within the dentinal tubules (Figure 4). Also

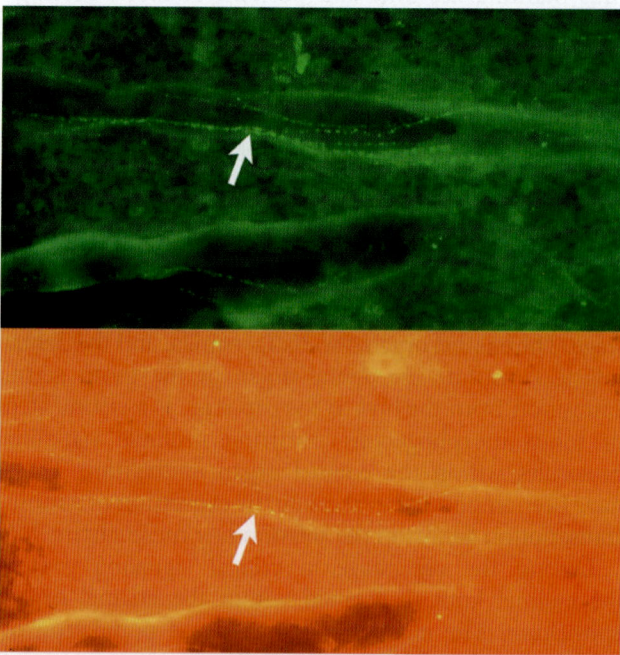

Figure 4 Expression of calcitonin gene-related peptide (CGRP) (bottom) and substance P (SP) (top) in the pulp by an immunocychemical method. CGRP and SP receptors (arrows) are colocalized and surround blood vessels.

with the start of root formation, CGRP-, SP-, and NPY-immunoreactive nerves begin to appear in the developing periodontal ligament (PDL), although a mature distribution pattern does not occur until root formation is nearly completed.[16]

The expression of nerve growth factors such as nerve growth factor, brain-derived neurotrophic factors, gondotropin neurotrophic factor, NTN, neurotrophin 3, and neurotrophin 4 (NT-4) has been shown at specific locations during various developing stages of the tooth.[17–19]

Structures and Functions

DENTAL–PULP COMPLEX

As long as dentin is covered peripherally by enamel on coronal surfaces and cementum on radicular surfaces, the dental pulp will generally remain healthy for life, unless the apical blood supply is disrupted by excessive orthodontic forces or severe impact trauma. Most pathological pulp conditions begin with the removal of one or both of these protective barriers via caries, fractures, or abrasion. The result is the communication of the pulp soft tissue with the oral cavity via dentinal tubules. A classic work done by Pashley et al.,[20] using radioactive ^{131}I in dog teeth, clearly demonstrated that once dentin tubules are opened, molecules can permeate to the pulp easily (Figure 5). This dentin permeability has a huge impact on the pathogenesis of the pulp in many clinical situations. This will be discussed later.

It is apparent that substances easily permeate dentin, permitting thermal, osmotic, and chemical insults to act on the pulpal constituents. The initial stages involve stimulation or irritation of odontoblasts and may proceed to inflammation and often to tissue destruction. First, one must examine the dentin structure.

DENTIN STRUCTURE

Dentin is a calcified connective tissue consisting of approximately 70% inorganic material and 10% water. Organic matrix accounts for 20% of dentin, of which about 91% is collagen. Most of the collagen is type I, but there is a minor component of type V. Noncollagenous matrix components include phosphoproteins, proteoglycans, g-carboxyglutamate-n-containing proteins, acidic glycoproteins, growth factors, and lipids.

Dentin is penetrated by millions of tubules; their density varies from 40,000 to 70,000 tubules per square millimeter[21,22] (Figure 6A). Tubules are from 1 μm in diameter at the dentinoenamel junction to 3 μm at their pulpal surface. These variations in the size of the tubules, in the dentin surface area, and in the surface area covered by the tubules are important in the pathogenesis of pulpal inflammation. For instance, permeation of toxic substances to the pulp created by caries or restorative procedures from the dentinoenamel junction is less likely compared to permeation from the middle of the dentin due to the degree of surface area covered by the tubules. From a purely anatomical standpoint, possible pulpal damage increases exponentially the deeper toxins reach into the dentin.

Dental tubules contain a fluid that has a composition similar to extracellular fluid.[23] If the fluid becomes contaminated with carious bacterial endotoxins and exotoxins, it becomes a reservoir of injurious agents that can permeate through dentin into the pulp to initiate inflammation.[24] It is useful to understand the important variables that control dentin permeability.

DENTIN PERMEABILITY

Dentinal tubules in the coronal dentin converge from the dentinoenamel junction to the pulp chamber.[25] This tends to concentrate permeating substances into a smaller area at their terminus in the pulp. The surface area occupied by tubules at different levels indicates the effect of tubule density and diameter. One can

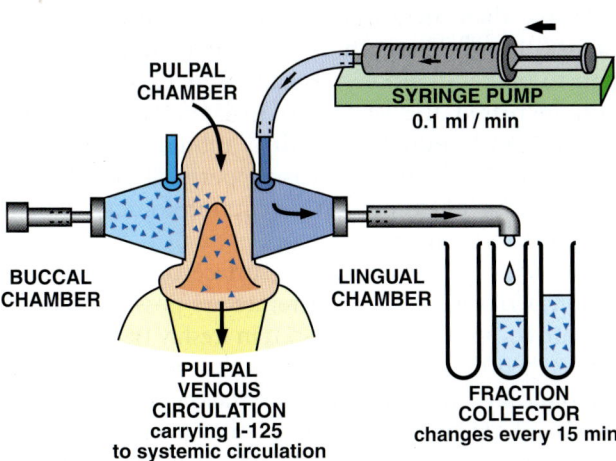

Figure 5 Pashley's experimental setup for the study of dentin permeability. ^{131}I, as the marker, was diffused through the buccal chamber attached to the naked dentin of the tooth. Blood was drawn from the venous system and checked for ^{131}I radioactivity. The appearance of ^{131}I in the blood demonstrates the degree of permeability of the dentin. Reproduced with permission from Pashley DH et al.[20]

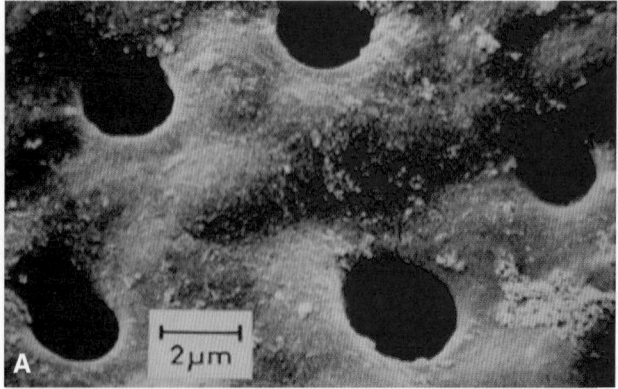

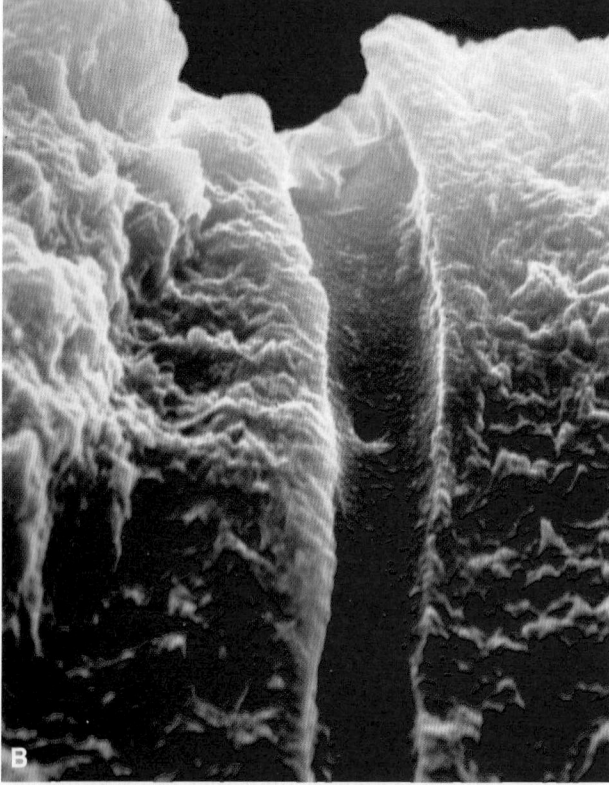

Figure 6 ***A,*** This picture shows the heterogenous nature of the dentin tubular diameters along the dentin length and dentin surface. The tubular diameter increases (up to 4 μm) and the dentin surface area occupied by the tubules increases logarithmically approaching the pulp. Courtesy of Dr. H. Trowbridge. ***B,*** Scanning electron micrograph (SEM) of a cross section of tubules. Courtesy of Dr. D. Pashley.

calculate from Garberoglio and Brännström's[22] observations that the area of dentin occupied by tubules is only 1% at the dentinoenamel junction and increases to 45% at the pulp chamber (Figure 6B).

The clinical implications of this are enormous. As dentin becomes exposed to increasing depths by restorative procedures, attrition, or disease, the remaining dentin becomes increasingly permeable.[26,27] Thus, dentin removal renders the pulp more susceptible to chemical or bacterial irritation. This functional consequence of tubule area is also responsible for the decrease in dentin microhardness closer to the pulp[28,29]; as tubule density increases, the amount of calcified matrix between the tubules decreases. This relative softness of the dentin lining the pulp chamber facilitates canal enlargement during endodontic treatment.[30]

Overall dentin permeability is directly proportional to the total surface area of exposed dentin. Obviously, a leaking restoration over a full crown preparation provides more surface for diffusion of bacterial products than would a small occlusal restoration.[31] Restorations requiring extensive and deep removal of dentin (i.e., preparation for a full crown) would open more and larger tubules and increase the rate of injurious substances diffusing from the surface to the pulp—thus the importance of "remaining dentin thickness."[32,33] The permeability of the root is 10 to 20 times less than that of a similar thickness of coronal dentin.[34] This may account for the lack of pulpal reactions to periodontal therapy that removes cementum and exposes root dentin to the oral cavity.

Recent evidence indicates that dentin permeability is not constant after cavity preparation. In dogs, dentin permeability fell over 75% in the first 6 hours following cavity preparation.[35] Although there were no histological correlates of the decreased permeability, dogs depleted of their plasma fibrinogen did not decrease their dentin permeability following cavity preparation.[36] The authors speculated that the irritation to pulpal blood vessels caused by cavity preparation increased the leakage of plasma proteins from pulpal vessels into the dentinal tubules, where they absorb to the dentin, decreasing permeability. Future study of this phenomenon is required to determine if it occurs in humans.

The character of the dentin surface can also modify dentin permeability. Two extremes are possible: tubules that are completely open, as seen in freshly fractured[37] or acid-etched dentin,[38] and tubules that are closed either anatomically[39] or with microcrystalline debris.[40] This debris creates the "smear layer" that forms on dentin surfaces whenever they are cut with either hand or rotary instruments.[41] The smear layer slows bacterial penetration,[42,43] but permits a wide range of molecules to readily permeate dentin. Small molecules permeate much faster than large molecules. Smear layers are often slowly dissolved over months to years as oral fluids percolate around microleakage channels between restorative

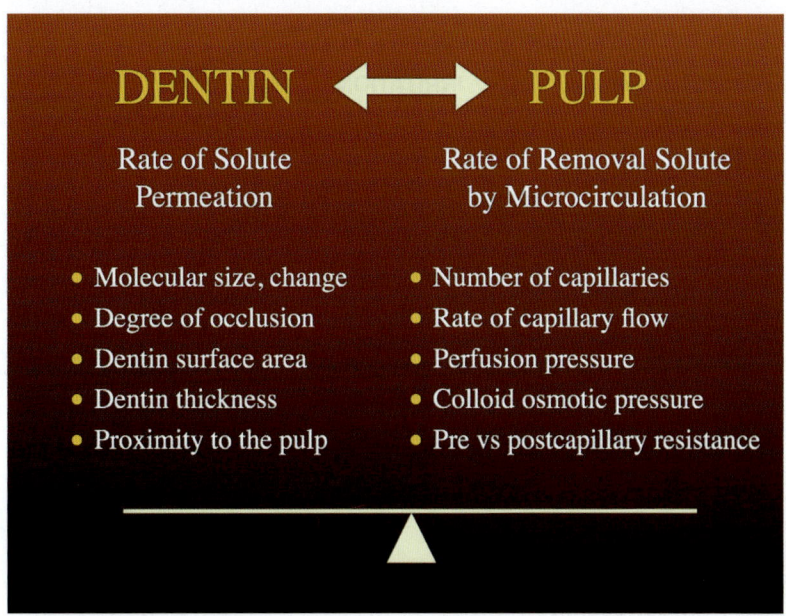

Figure 7 Diagram showing the delicate balance between the dentin and the pulp. On the left side of the balancing beam are factors governing the dentin and on the right side are factors that govern the pulp.

materials and the tooth.[44] The removal of the "smear layer" by acid etching or chelation increases dentin permeability[45] because the microcrystalline debris no longer restricts diffusion of irritants and also permits bacteria to penetrate into dentin[46] There is considerable debate as to whether smear layers created in the root canal during biomechanical preparation should be removed.[47] Its removal may increase the quality of the seal between endodontic filling materials and root dentin. It may also increase the bond strength of resin posts.[48]

PULP REACTION TO PERMEATING SUBSTANCES

What happens when permeating substances reach the pulp chamber? Although bacteria may not actually pass through dentin, their by-products[49,50] have been shown to cause severe pulp reaction.[49,51] The broad spectrum of pulp reaction, from no inflammation to abscess formation, may be related to the concentration of these injurious substances in the pulp. Although exposed dentin may permit substances to permeate, their concentrations may not reach levels high enough to trigger the cascade of events associated with inflammation. This would indicate that the interstitial fluid concentration of these substances can be maintained at low concentrations. As long as the rate of pulpal blood flow is normal, the microcirculation is very efficient at removing substances diffusing across dentin to the pulp chamber. This delicate balance between the dentin and the pulp is illustrated in Figure 7. There is enough blood flowing through the pulp each minute to completely replace between 40 and 100% of the blood volume of the pulp.[52] Since blood is confined to the vasculature, which comprises only about 7% of the total pulpal volume,[52,53] the blood volume of the pulp is replaced 5 to 14 times each minute.

If pulpal blood flow is reduced,[54–67] there will be a resultant rise in the interstitial fluid concentration of substances that permeated across dentin. The increased concentration of injurious agents may degranulate mast cells,[68–70] release histamine[70] or SP,[71–75] produce bradykinin,[76] or activate plasma proteins.[77,78] All of these effects would initiate inflammation. The endogenous mediators of inflammation produce arteriolar vasodilation, elevated capillary hydrostatic pressure, increased leakage of plasma proteins into the pulp interstitium,[79] and increased pulp tissue pressure.[80–82] These events, by causing the

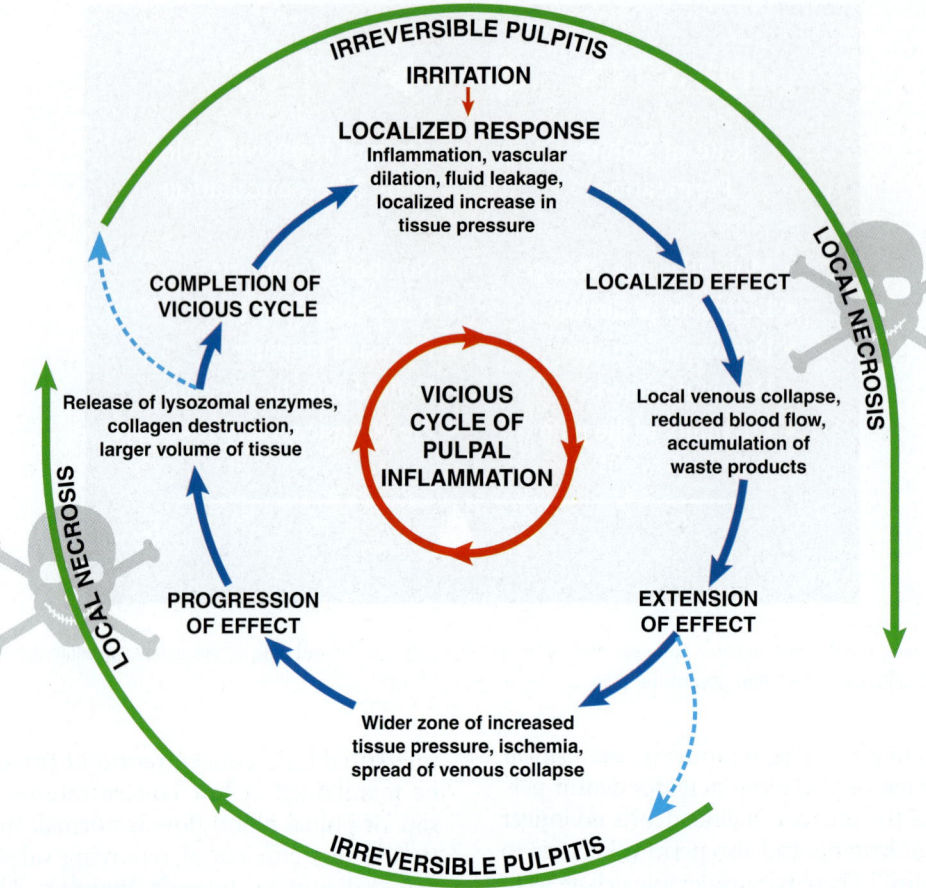

Figure 8 Vicious cycle of pulpal inflammation that begins with irritation (top), leads to a localized response, and may progress to a lesion of increasing severity and eventual irreversible pulpitis.

collapse of local venules, lead to a further reduction in pulpal blood flow.[83] With an even higher interstitial concentration of irritants, a vicious cycle[84] is created that may terminate in the pulp (Figure 8).

DENTIN SENSITIVITY

Clinicians recognize that dentin is exquisitely sensitive to certain stimuli.[85,86] It is unlikely that this sensitivity results from direct stimulation of nerves in dentin (Figure 9). As previously stated, nerves cannot be shown in peripheral dentin.[87,88] Another speculation is that the odontoblastic process may serve as excitable "nerve endings" that would, in turn, excite nerve fibers shown to exist in deeper dentin, closer to the plup.[87–89] The experiments of Anderson et al.[90] and Brännström[91] suggest that neither odontoblastic processes nor excitable nerves within dentin are responsible for dentin's sensitivity. This led Brännström et al. to propose the "hydrodynamic theory" of dentin sensitivity, which sets forth that fluid movement through dentinal tubules, moving in either direction, stimulates sensory nerves in dentin or the pulp.[91,92] Further support for the hydrodynamic theory came from electron microscopic examination of animal[93–95] and human dentin[93,96,97] demonstrating that odontoblastic processes seldom extend more than one-third the distance of the dentinal tubules. A work by LaFleche et al.[98] suggested that the process may retract from the periphery during extraction or processing. Obviously, more investigation will be required before any definitive statement can be made regarding the distribution of the process. The tubules are filled with dentinal fluid that is similar in composition to interstitial fluid.[99] The hydrodynamic theory satisfies numerous experimental observations. Although it cannot yet be regarded as fact, it has provided and will continue to provide a very useful perspective for the design of future experiments.[100–102]

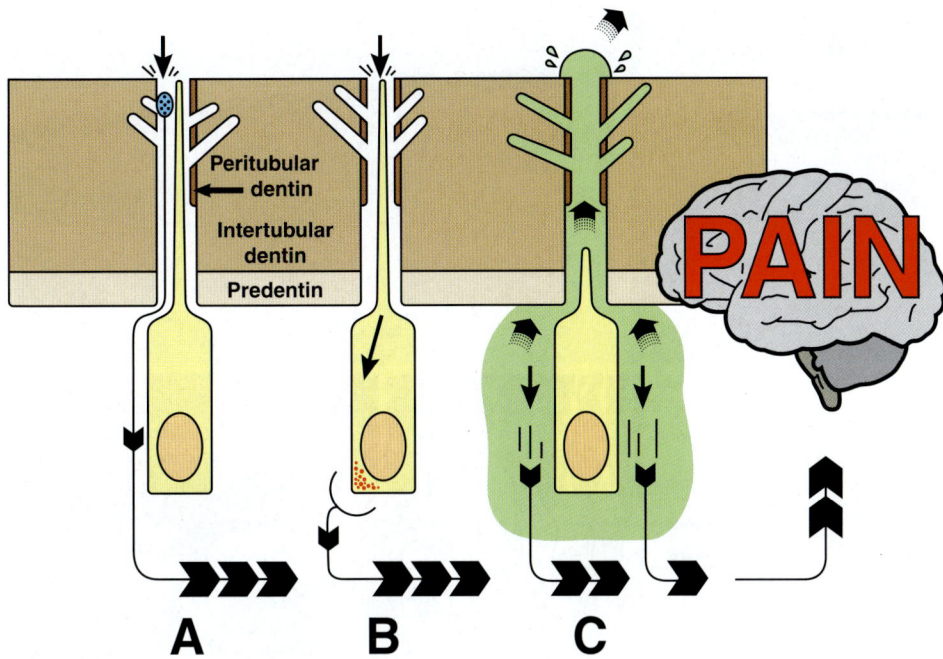

Figure 9 Schematic diagram of essentials of three theories of dentin sensitivity. *A*, Classical theory proposed that stimuli applied to dentin caused direct simulation of nerves in dentin. *B*, Modified theory proposed that stimuli applied to the odontoblastic process would be transmitted along the odontoblast and passed to the sensory nerves via some sort of synapse. *C*, Hydrodynamic theory proposed that fluid movement within tubules transmits peripheral stimuli to highly sensitive pulpal nerves. *C* more accurately represents the actual length of the odontoblastic process relative to the tubules. Nerves are seldom found more than one-third the distance from the pulp to the surface. Modified with permission Torneck.

DENTAL PULP

The dental pulp consists of a loose connective tissue. A single layer of dentin-producing cells, the odontoblasts, lines the peripheral part of the pulp separating the loose connective tissue of the pulp from the predentin. The odontoblasts represent the link between dentin and the pulp. The dental pulp connective tissue is somewhat special in regard to its encasement within rigid dentin walls (see Figure 1). The pulp receives its blood supply from arterioles and lacks a collateral blood supply. The cellular constituents of a human pulp specimen examined under the microscope are presented in Figure 10, and these are explained in subsequent sections. Also shown in Figure 11 are different layers in the pulp and its constituents.

INTERSTITIAL FLUID

The rigid encasement allows the tissue-limited possibilities to expand and keeps the extracellular fluid volume, that is, blood and interstitial fluid, relatively constant. The extracellular fluid volume in the dental pulp is normally relatively high of about 63%.[103] Due to the low compliance a small increase in the pulpal volume caused by an increase in blood or interstitial fluid will raise the hydrostatic pressure inside the tooth. This is shown to happen normally by any increase in blood flow and thus blood volume.[104] However, as long as there are no noxious stimuli that increase the vessel permeability, any change in tissue pressure caused by blood volume changes will be transitory, because interstitial fluid is absorbed back to the blood vessels, and no harm will happen to the pulp (Figure 12).

The hydrostatic pressure in this fluid is the interstitial fluid pressure, or the so-called tissue pressure. The interstitial fluid is similar to blood plasma, except for a lower concentration of plasma proteins (albumin and globulin). In health, plasma proteins do not permeate through the capillary wall and the concentration in the interstitial fluid is normally low. However, in a recent study in rat incisors, surprisingly high protein concentration in the pulp interstitial fluid during physiological conditions was reported.[103] The main function of the interstitial fluid is as a transport medium for nutrients and waste products between cells and capillary blood. Accordingly, the interstitial fluid acts as a middleman between cells and blood, or as an extension of the plasma. Every cell must have nutrition and the means to rid itself of waste products, and these metabolic requirements are taken

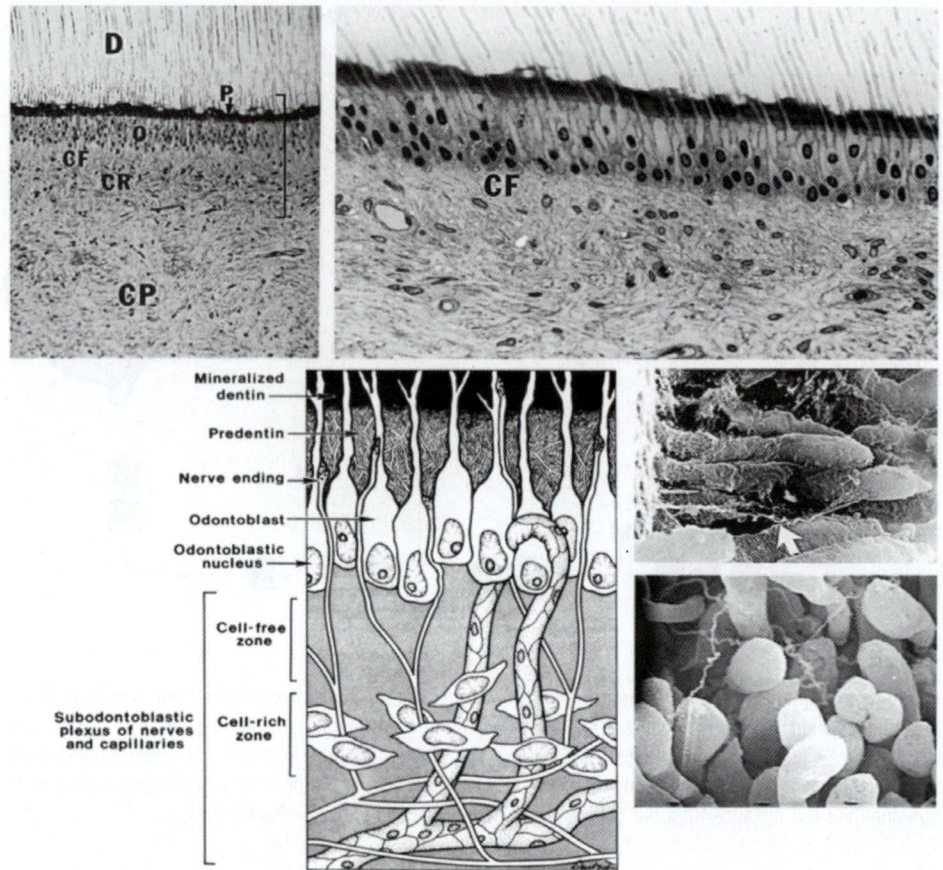

Figure 10 Top left, medium-power photomicrograph of a human pulp specimen showing dentin (D), predentin (P), odontoblast layer (O), cell-free zone (CF), cell-rich zone (CR), and central pulp (CP). **Top right,** Region similar to the area bracketed in A. CF zone contains large numbers of small nerves and capillaries not visible at this magnification. Underlying CR does not have high concentration of cells but contains more cells than the central pulp. Courtesy of Drs. Dennis Weber and Michael Gaynor. **Bottom left,** Diagram of peripheral pulp and its principal elements. **Middle right,** Scanning electron micrograph (SEM) of the dentin–pulp junction. Note corkscrew fibers between odontoblasts (arrow). Reproduced with permission from Jean A, Kerebel JB, Kerebel LM. Oral Surg Oral Med Oral Pathol Oral Radiol Endod 1986;61:592. **Bottom right,** SEM of the pulpal surface of the odontoblast layer. Thread-like structures are probably terminal raveling of nerves. Courtesy of Drs. R. White and M. Goldman.

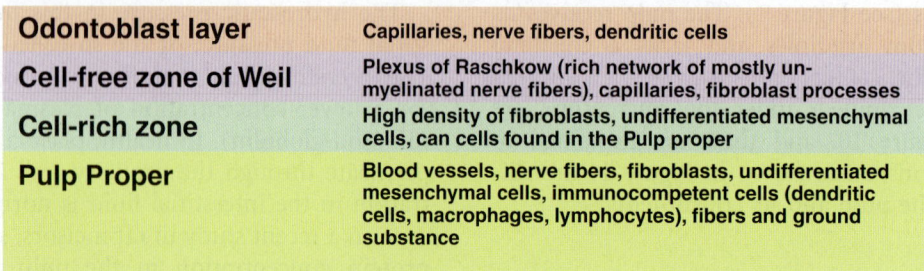

Figure 11 Illustration of different layers in the dental pulp (left) and its constituents (right).

care of by the blood and the interstitial fluid (see Figure 12). Blood is brought to the tissues by the smallest blood vessels, the capillaries. Substances are transported between the blood and the interstitial fluid mainly by diffusion through the capillary wall (see Figure 12). These capillaries are so widely distributed that no cells are more than 50 to 100 μm from the blood vessels. Due to the short distance, the exchange of substances between blood and interstitial fluid may take place rapidly by simple diffusion.

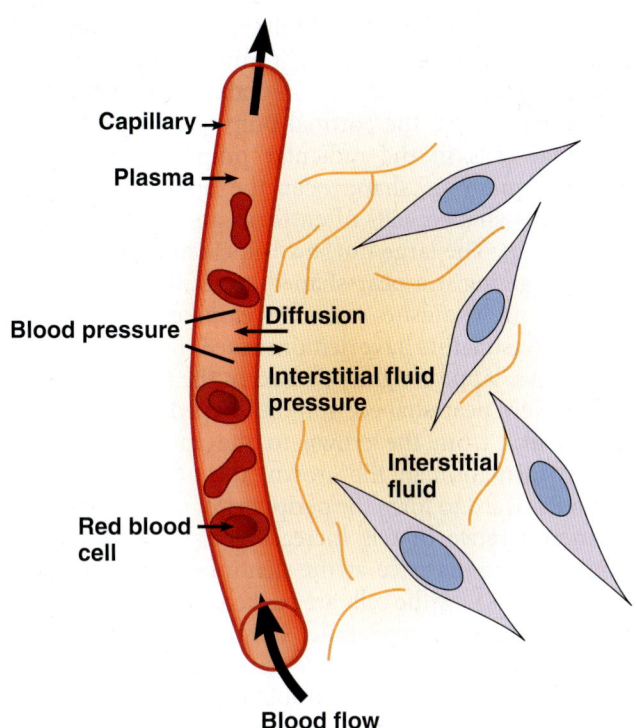

Figure 12 The interstitial fluid is the fluid that surrounds all cells in the body.

CELLULAR STRUCTURES

The odontoblasts are derived from ectomesenchymal cells and are responsible for the formation of dentin. These cells line the periphery of the pulp and consist of a cell body and a cytoplasmic/odontoblastic process. The shape of the odontoblast varies according to the functional state of the cell. The cells are tall and columnar in shape about 50 to 60 µm long in the coronal occlusal portion while they are cuboidal in the floor of the pulp chamber and the inner surface of the pulp. The odontoblast layer is separated from the mineralized dentin by a 10- to 40-µm-thick layer of unmineralized matrix, the predentin. Odontoblasts are involved in the production of predentin–dentin matrix, an extracellular framework that becomes mineralized. The matrix includes a complex mixture of proteoglycans, glycoproteins, sialoproteins, phosphoproteins, and a variety of other molecules.

FIBROBLAST

Fibroblasts originate from the ectomesenchymal tissue and are the predominant cells of the connective tissue. Fibroblasts are elongated with little cytoplasm and nucleus-containing condensed chromatin. They are responsible for the formation and maintenance of the fibrous components and ground substances of the connective tissue. Fibroblasts can synthesize and secrete a wide variety of extracellular molecules that include fibrous elements of extracellular matrix (ECM) such as collagen, elastin, proteoglycans, glycoproteins, cytokines, growth factors, and proteinases. They are also involved in the remodeling of connective tissue through the degradation of collagen and other ECM molecules and their replacement by newly synthesized molecules. Fibroblasts release proteolytic enzymes such as the matrix metalloproteinase (MMP) family. MMPs are secreted as inactive precursors and cleave to become active. Extracellular degradation often occurs in inflammatory lesions. Inhibitors to MMPs, called tissue inhibitors of metalloproteinases, are also secreted by fibroblasts to regulate extracellular degradation. Intracellular degradation is for the normal physiological turnover and remodeling of collagenous connective tissue.

ODONTOBLASTS

Odontoblast, the principal cell of the dentin-forming layer, is the first cell type encountered as the pulp is approached from the dentin (Figure 13). These cells

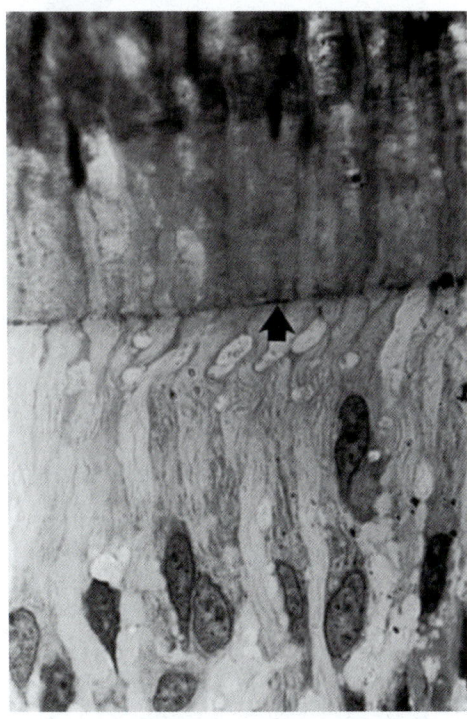

Figure 13 Pseudostratified appearance of odontoblasts. Dark horizontal line (arrow) delineates the cell body from the odontoblastic processes and predentin and was once termed "pulpodentinal membrane." Ultrastructural examination has shown this to be a terminal cell web that forms a support and attachment area between adjoining cells. Reproduced with permission from Walton R, Leonard L, Sharawy M, Gangarosa L. Oral Surg Oral Med Oral Pathol Oral Radiol Endod 1979;48:545.

arise from peripheral mesenchymal cells of the dental papilla during tooth development and differentiate by acquiring the characteristic morphology of glycoprotein synthesis and secretion[105] (Figure 14). Glycoprotein forms the predentin matrix that is rendered mineralizable by the odontoblast, a unique cell producing a unique tissue, dentin. Synthesizing and secretory activities render the odontoblast highly polarized, with synthesis occurring in the cell body and secretion from the odontoblastic process. The cell body contains organelles that represent different stages of secretion of collagen, glycoproteins, and calcium salts.[106] Matrix secretion precedes mineralization, with these two events separated in time and space by the predentin.

As happens in bones, the initial mineral seeding of predentin at the dentinoenamel junction is by the formation of "matrix vesicles."[107,108] Classic studies by Weinstock et al.,[109–111] using an autoradiographic technique, have demonstrated the functional sequence of matrix production and secretion. This material has recently been reviewed by Holland.[112] In histological sections viewed under a light microscope, odontoblasts appear to vary from tall, pseudostratified columnar cells in the coronal pulp to a single row of cuboidal cells in the radicular pulp to a flattened, almost squamous shape near the apex.[113,114] These squamous-shaped cells often form an irregular, atubular dentin. The large nucleus is located in the base of the cell, giving it a pear-shaped appearance.[115]

From an exquisite scanning electron microscopic study, investigators have demonstrated that odontoblast cell bodies "appear tightly packed in the pulp horn and successively pear-shaped, spindle-shaped, club-shaped, or globular from the crown to the apex."[116] During dentin formation in the crown, the odontoblasts are pushed inward to form the periphery of a pulp chamber, a circumference that is increasingly smaller than the original circumference at the dentinoenamel junction. This explains why the cells are packed and palisaded into a pseudostratified appearance of coronal odontoblasts. Conversely, because the space is not so compressed in the radicular pulp, the odontoblasts maintain a columnar, cuboidal, or (in the apical region) squamous shape. Also, the resulting cell and tubule density is much higher in the pulp chamber than in the root pulp.[117] This increased tubule density in the chamber may explain the greater sensitivity and permeability of the dentin of the crown. The cell body manufactures the matrix material; the material is transported to and secreted from the odontoblastic process.

Classically, the odontoblastic process has been described as extending from the cell body to the dentinoenamel junction, a distance of 2 to 3 mm. This concept was based on the observations of many light microscopists using a variety of special procedures and stains.[40] When dentin was examined by electron microscopy, the odontoblastic process was determined to be limited to the inner third of dentin, with the outer two-thirds of the tubule devoid of processes or of nerves but filled with extracellular fluid.[118–121] More recent investigations indicate that odontoblastic processes may indeed extend to the dentinoenamel junction.[122,123] However, tubular structures in dentinal tubules are not necessarily odontoblastic processes.[124,125] Unequivocal identification can be done only by identifying a trilaminar plasma membrane around the putative process using transmission electron microscopy.[126,127] The extent of the odontoblastic process remains controversial.[128] Therefore, modern interpretations of pulpal injury following conservative cavity preparation may not be attributable to amputation of odontoblastic processes but to desiccation, heat, and osmotic effects. Further, dentin sensitivity may not be related to direct stimulation of either odontoblastic processes or nerves

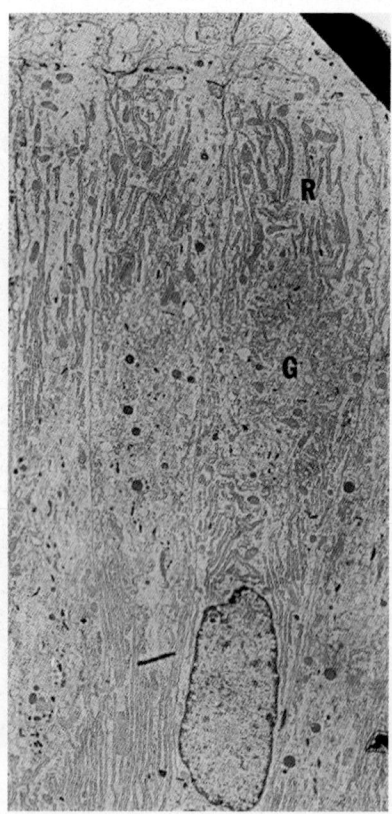

Figure 14 Odontoblasts, as viewed under the electron microscope, show organelles essential for protein synthesis: a plump nucleus filled with euchromatin, cytoplasm rich in rough endoplasmic reticulum (R), and a well-developed Golgi apparatus (G). Courtesy of Dr. Dale Eisenmann.

in the peripheral dentin since the tubules may be devoid of such structures in the periphery of dentin. After initial dentin formation, the odontoblast, via its process, can still modify the dentin structure by producing peritubular dentin. This is a hypermineralized cuff with little organic matrix within the tubule, decreasing the diameter of the tubule.[129–131] When stimulated, the odontoblast can accelerate peritubular dentin formation to the point of complete occlusion of the tubule.[132–134]

When tubule occlusions extend over a large area, it is referred to as sclerotic dentin, commonly found in teeth with cervical erosion.[135] Alternatively, irritated odontoblasts can secrete collagen, amorphous material, or large crystals into the tubule lumen; these occlusions decrease dentin permeability to irritating substances.[132–134] Although these secretions have been described as a defensive reaction by the odontoblast to protect itself and the underlying pulp, this "protection" has never been proved.

IMMUNOCOMPETENT CELLS

A normal dental pulp has a large number and a variety of indigenous immunocompetent cells that play a crucial role to maintain homeostasis.[136,137] Cells expressing Class II major histocompatibility complex (MHC) molecule are present throughout the dental pulp. Class II antigen-presenting dendritic cells are considered to participate in immunosurveillance. These cells have distinctive cytoplasmic extensions, have a high surface area for capturing antigens, while lacking intracellular lysosomes and phagocytic vacuoles, thus having phagocytic capacity of their own.[137] Dendritic cells are predominantly located in the paraodontoblastic area and along the pulp–dentin border. They are also present in the central portion of the pulp. Macrophages also express MHC molecules, and these cells are present in the central portion of the dental pulp. In the normal dental pulp, they may act as scavengers, eliminating dead odontoblasts and apoptotic bodies.[138,139] Class II MHC-expressing cells increase in number shortly after tooth eruption and continue to increase even after the completion of tooth formation.[140]

T lymphocytes are largely present in the normal dental pulp with both cytotoxic and helper subtypes present in the central pulp.[137,141] B lymphocytes have not been clearly demonstrated in the normal dental pulp. Mast cells have not been shown to exist in the uninflamed dental pulp.[136,142]

Immune cells in primary teeth are very similar to those in permanent teeth, except that the T-lymphocyte population in deciduous teeth have slightly more $CD4^+$ cells than $CD8^+$ cells, whereas in permanent teeth $CD8^+$ cells outnumber $CD4^+$ cells.[137,143,144]

EXTRACELLULAR MATRIX

ECM, or ground substance, is a structureless mass making up the bulk of the pulp tissue. It consists primarily of complexes of proteins, carbohydrates, and water. These complexes are composed of combinations of glycosaminoglycans, that is, hyaluronic acid, chondroitin sulfate, and other glycoproteins. Proteoglycans are a large group of extracellular and cell surface-associated molecules that consist of a protein core to which glycosaminoglycan chains are attached that binds them to water. Hyaluronic acid, a large glycosaminoglycan, forms a viscous hydrated gel. Proteins, glycoproteins, and proteoglycans of the ECM function in cell–matrix adhesion and signaling; regulate diffusion of nutrients, waste products, and soluble signaling molecules.

Cytokines, growth factors, and other inflammatory mediators are released by fibroblasts, endothelial cells, and immune cells in the dental pulp. Normal dental pulp contains cytokines such as interleukin-1alpha (IL-1α) and tumor necrosis factor-alpha (TNF-α),[145] however, during inflammation, orthodontic tooth movement, and other stimulation, IL-1α, IL-1β, IL-8, TNF-α, prostaglandin E2, platelet-derived growth factor, insulin-like growth factor-1, transforming growth factor-b (TGF-b1), vascular endothelial growth factor, basic fibroblast growth factor (FGF-2), hepatocyte growth factor, and keratinocyte growth factor.[146–152] These molecules mainly act locally and play important roles during development, inflammation, and wound healing.

FIBERS

Collagen is the major organic component in the dental pulp. The morphology of collagen fibers, a principal constituent in the pulp, has been described at the level of both light and electron microscopy.[153] Collagen is synthesized and secreted by both odontoblasts and fibroblasts. However, the type of collagen secreted by odontoblasts, to subsequently mineralize, differs from the collagen produced by pulpal fibroblasts that normally does not calcify. They also differ not in the basic structure but in the degree of cross-linking and in slight variation in hydroxylysine content. Tropocollagen is an immature collagen fiber that remains thin and stain black with silver nitrate, described in light microscopy as argyrophilic or reticular fibrils.

If tropocollagen molecules aggregate into larger fibers, they no longer stain with silver and are then termed "collagen fibers." If several collagen fibers aggregate (cross-link) and grow denser, they are termed "collagen bundles." Collagen generally becomes more coarse (i.e., develops more bundles) as the patient ages. Collagen fibers are inelastic but have great tensile strength, giving the tissue its consistency and strength. Collagen type I and III make up the bulk of the tissue collagen. Collagen type IV is found in basement membranes. In the pulp proper, type III collagen appears as fine-branched filaments, whose distribution is similar to reticular fibers.

Fibronectin is insoluble and the fibrils form part of the ECM. It acts as a mediator for cell–cell and cell–matrix adhesion. In the odontoblast layer, fibronectin is the fibrous structure between odontoblasts and probably corresponds to von Korff fibers, as they appear as corkscrew fibers passing from the pulp into predentin parallel to the long axis of the odontoblasts.[154] In the pulp proper, fibronectin forms a reticular network of fibrils, with an increased encasement around blood vessels. Integrins are transmembrane receptors that link intracellular actin network with ECM.

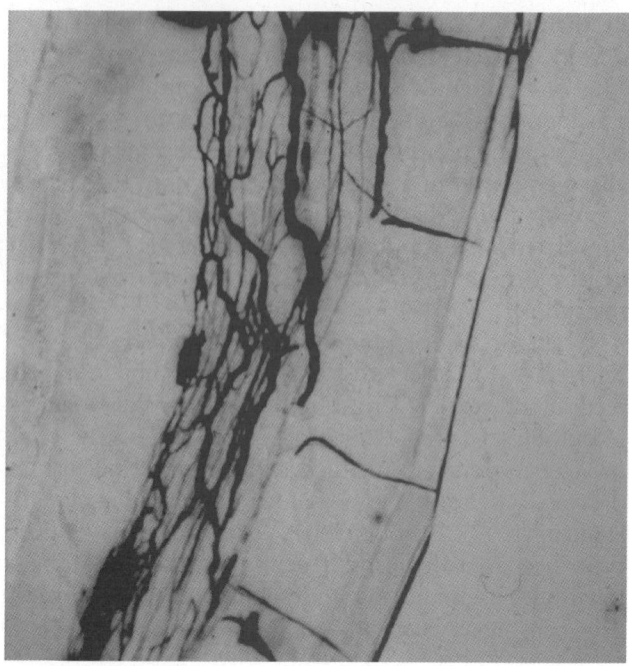

Figure 15 Vessel architecture in the pulp visualized by the India ink suction technique developed in 1950 by Dr. Kramer. This picture shows lateral canal vessels connecting the pulp and the periodontal ligament (PDL).

GROUND SUBSTANCE

This structureless mass, gel-like in consistency, makes up the bulk of the pulp organ. It occupies the space between formed elements. The ground substance resembles that of other areolar, fibrous connective tissues consisting primarily of complexes of proteins and carbohydrates and water. More specifically, these complexes are composed of combinations of glycosaminoglycans, that is, hyaluronic acid, chondroitin sulfate, and other glycoproteins. The ground substance surrounds and supports structures. It is the medium through which metabolites and waste products are transported to and from cells and vessels. Aging of the pulp alters the ground substance, although there is no substantive proof that these alterations significantly inhibit pulp functions.

PULPAL MICROVASCULATURES

The arterial supply of the pulp has its origin from the posterior superior alveolar arteries and the infraorbital and the inferior alveolar branch of the internal maxillary arteries. The main arterioles enter, and the main venules and lymphatics exit the dental pulp through the apical foramen or foraminae. Corrosion cast studies have shown that numerous arterioles and venules pass through the apex of the root.[155] Vessels also enter and leave the pulp via accessory lateral canals that may be located anywhere on the root, but most commonly in the apical region.[156,157] The tooth lacks a collateral, alternative blood supply that makes the apical region a critical point. There is evidence, however, that vessels have been identified connecting the pulp to the PDL (Figure 15). The degree to which these vessels play a role in pathogenesis remains to be investigated. Increased tooth movement in the apical area due to trauma, periodontitis, or orthodontic tooth movement may damage the pulpal blood supply.

Because the pulp itself is small, pulp blood vessels do not reach a large size. As such, the terms artery and vein cannot be used. Rather they are called arterioles (diameter in the range of 100 μm) and corresponding venules (diameter in the range of 200 to 300 μm).[158] Arterioles pass through the root pulp to supply the coronal pulp. As the arterioles travel straight to the coronal area, 90° branching patterns develop. These branching vessels have very thin smooth muscle coating at the juncture and lose the coating as they reach toward the dentin, forming a capillary network. Near the dentin, around the odontoblastic area, they form a dense terminal capillary network in the subodontoblastic region[159]

(Figure 16). Figure 17 illustrates the basic microvascular units in the pulp. Terminal capillary networks are the key vessels in the pulp and are involved in transporting nutrients and gas to the cells and removing waste products and CO_2 from the cells to maintain pulp homeostasis. Any damage or inflammation to the pulp must alter the normal function of these vessels first. And thus these vessels have been carefully investigated ultrastructurally.

ARTERIOVENOUS ANASTOMOSIS AND "U"-TURN LOOPS

Before the arterioles break up into capillary beds, arteriovenous anastomoses (AVA) often arise to connect the arteriole directly to a venule.[160] The AVAs are relatively small vessels, having a diameter approximately 10 μm.[161] Their presence is more frequent in the radicular area of the pulp. The functional role of these vascular structures is not completely known. However, one can speculate that AVAs play a role in the regulation of blood flow. Theoretically they could provide a mechanism for shunting blood away from the area of injury or inflammation, where damage to the microcirculation may result in thrombosis and hemorrhage. An interesting observation to support this view is during an intravital microscopic study, using the live rat incisor teeth. When the pulp is approached during tooth preparation, one sees a sudden appearance of AVA shunts and "U"-turn loops filled with streaming blood. "U"-turn loops are frequently found in the pulp vascular network, and it is believed that their functions are similar to the AVA's (Figure 18).

Capillary density is highest in the subodontoblastic region with loops passing between odontoblasts Y (Figure 19).[158,160,162] In the subodontoblastic region, capillaries with fenestrations occur frequently in both primary and permanent teeth.[162] However, the function of this fenestration is still disputed. Capillaries and the smallest postcapillary venules are the site of exchange between blood and the interstitial fluid. The terminal capillary network in the coronal area exhibits numerous short hairpin loops,[157] while the capillary network in the root area is similar to capillaries in the connective tissue elsewhere. Capillaries empty into small venules that connect with fewer and successively larger venules. At the apex, multiple venules exit the pulp. These venules connect with vessels that drain the PDL and adjacent alveolar bone. Vessels of the pulp have thinner muscular walls (tunica media) than vessels of comparable diameter in other parts of the body. This is probably an adaptation to the surrounding protective and unyielding walls. The vascular architecture can be divided into different vascular segments based on the morphology of periendothelial cells, such as smooth muscle cells and pericytes. These segments are muscular arterioles, terminal arterioles, precapillary arterioles, capillaries,

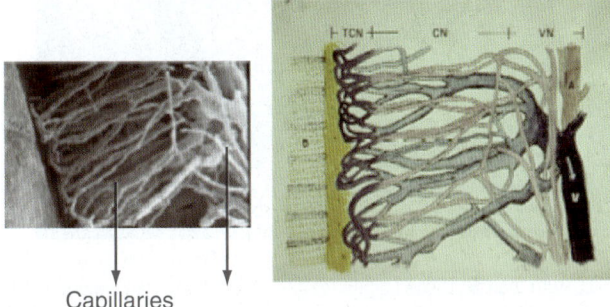

Figure 16 Pulpal microvascular units. Scanning electron micrograph (SEM) and a diagram based on the SEM are presented on the right side. The basic unit shows arterioles running parallel with venules in the center of the pulp. The small arterioles branch off almost 90° from the main arterioles. These small arterioles get smaller in diameter as they come near the dentin. These small arterioles also lose their smooth muscle coating and become capillaries forming the capillary network (CN). When they reach the odontoblastic layer, they become the terminal capillary network (TCN). They drain into the venular network (VN). Courtesy of Drs. Takahashi and Kishi.

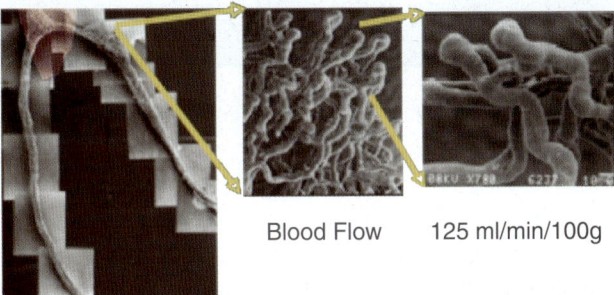

Figure 17 Corrosion resin casts of the pulp vessels of a dog premolar. These scanning electron micrographs (SEMs) clearly show heterogeneity of the pulpal microvascular architecture. *The coronal pulp*: Higher magnification of the region identified by arrows reveals many hairpin capillary loops within the pulp horn. Higher magnification of the area (left) shows an individual loop with a diameter just over 10 μm. The blood flow per unit volume per minute is 125 mL/min/100 g tissue. *The apical pulp*: Higher magnification of the root canal lesion shows a very different architecture than the coronal pulp. Here the microvessels show a net type architecture surrounding the main arteriole and venules. The blood flow in this lesion is 22 mL/min/100 g, significantly less than that in the coronal pulp. Courtesy of Drs. K. Takahashi, Y. Kishi, and S. Kim.

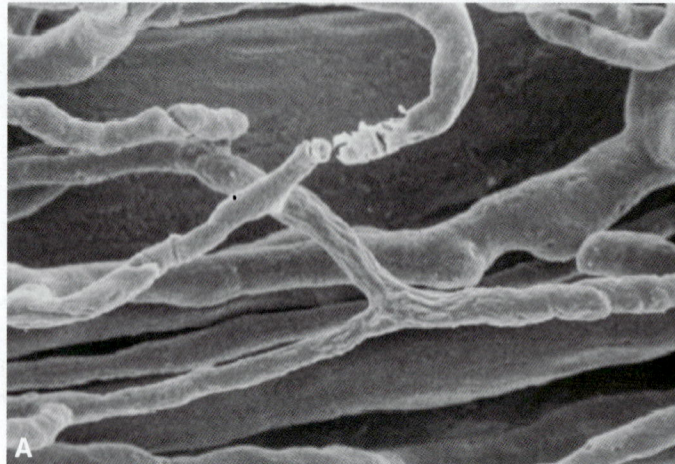
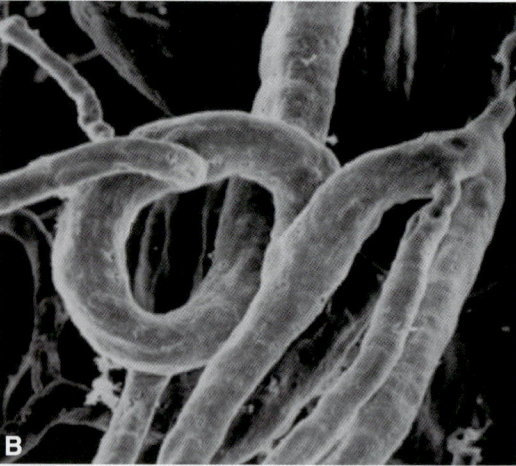

Figure 18 Corrosion resin casts of the arteriovenous anastomosis (AVA) ***A*** and a "U"-turn loop ***B***. These unique features seem to play an important role in blood flow regulation especially during the initial stages of inflammation.

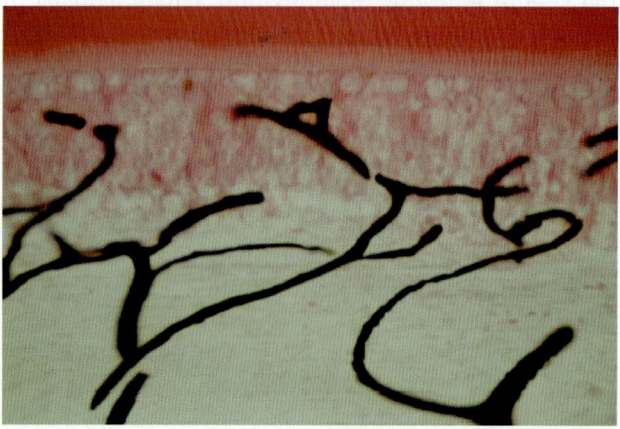

Figure 19 Capillary loops passing under or above the odontoblastic layer. Capillaries that are not in focus represent their position in relation to the cells, either under or above them. Prepared by modified H&E technique. Courtesy of Drs. Takahashi and Kishi.

Characteristics of Pulpal Vasculature

- Dense capillary network in the periphery
- Heterogenity with the pulp:
    Periphery vs. central core areas
    Coronal vs. apical areas
- Arterio-venous anastomosis
- Venous-venous anastomosis
- U-turn loop arterioles (in the apical area)
- True isolated microcirculatory network

Figure 20 Summary of characterization of the pulpal vasculature.

postcapillary venules, and collecting or muscular venules. In most arterioles and in some venules, smooth muscle cells maintain a state of partial vasoconstriction at all times, and a variety of substances such as neurotransmitters, hormones, and local factors influence this muscle tone and therefore the blood flow.[163] Nerves have intimate association with the blood vessels, with arterioles being the most densely innervated. Characteristics of pulpal vasculature are illustrated in Figure 20.

The fraction of blood in the coronal pulp of cat canines is 14.4%. Compared to other connective tissues, the dental pulp has a high resting blood flow of 40 to 50 mL/min/100 g. This is nearly as high as blood flow in the brain (Figure 21); however, the metabolic or functional requirements of this high resting blood flow in the pulp remain partly unexplained. Sometimes it is called a luxury perfusion. Figure 21 shows the comparison of blood flows among various tissues and organs, adjusted according to weight. Pulpal blood flow is intermediate between muscle and heart blood flow per unit weight.

REGULATION OF PULPAL BLOOD FLOW

Pulpal blood flow is regulated by sympathetic α-adrenergic vasoconstriction,[164] β-adrenergic vasodilation,[165] sympathetic cholinergic vasoactive system, and an antidromic vasodilation, that is, axon reflex. It has been shown

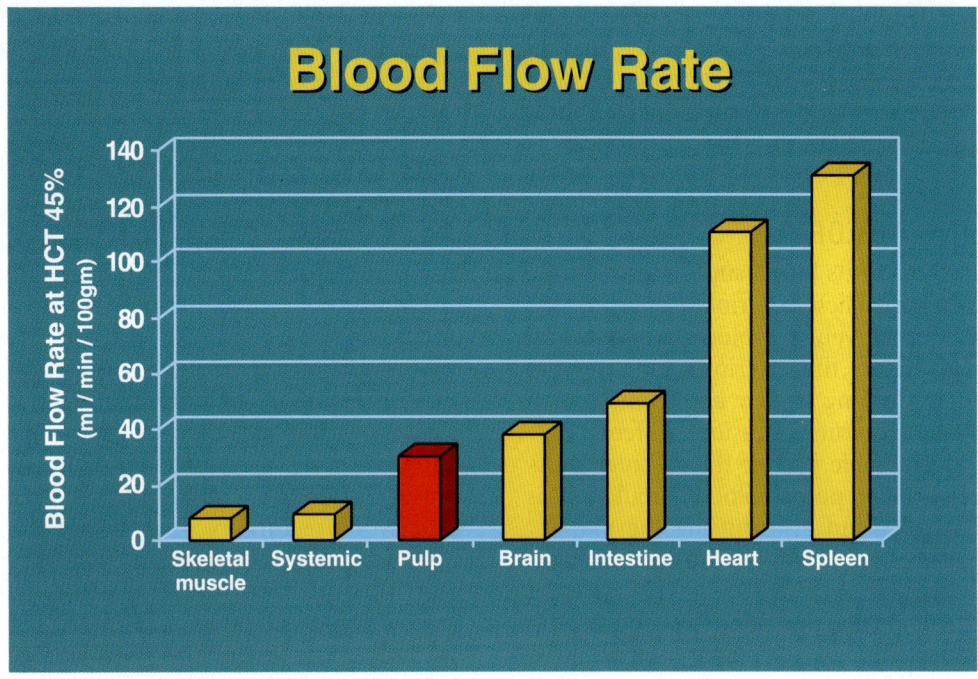

Figure 21 Blood flow rate in milliliters per minute per 100 g tissue of several important tissues and organs in a dog determined with a radioisotope-labeled microsphere technique. The pulpal blood flow is similar to that of the brain but far less than in the major organs like the heart or the spleen.

that a parasympathetic vasodilator mechanism is not present in cat dental pulp.[166]

The walls of arterioles and venules are coated with smooth muscles, innervated by unmyelinated sympathetic fibers. When stimulated, the muscle fibers contract, thus decreasing the diameter of the vessel. This phenomenon is called vasoconstriction. It has been shown experimentally that electrical stimulation of sympathetic fibers leading to the pulp results in a decrease in pulpal blood flow.[164,165] The sympathetic nerve-induced vasoconstriction of pulpal vessels is accomplished by the activation of α-adrenergic receptors in the smooth muscle of the arteriolar vessels.

Activation of α-adrenergic receptors by the administration of an α-agonist norepinephrine results in a marked decrease in pulpal blood flow. This reduction in pulpal blood flow is blocked by pretreatment of the pulpal vessels with α-antagonist. These two sets of experimental results clearly demonstrate that pulpal vessels are heavily equipped with sympathetic adrenergic receptors and their activation causes vasoconstriction.

Blood circulation in an inflamed pulp involves very complex pathophysiological reactions that have not been fully elucidated, in spite of numerous studies.[167,168] A unique feature of the pulp is that it is rigidly encased within dentin. This places it in a low-compliance environment, much like the brain, bone marrow, and nail bed. Thus pulp tissue has limited ability to expand, so vasodilation and increased vascular permeability, evoked during an inflammatory reaction, result in an increase in pulpal hydrostatic pressure.[169,170] Presumably any sudden rise in intrapulpal pressure would be distributed equally within the area of pressure increase, including the blood vessels. Theoretically if tissue pressure increases to the point that it equals the intravascular pressure, the thin-walled venules would be compressed, thereby increasing the vascular resistance and reducing the pulpal blood flow.[163] This could explain why injection of vasodilators such as bradykinin into an artery leading to the pulp results in a reduction rather than an increase in pulpal blood flow.[163,165,170] Heyeraas,[170] however, observed that an increase in intrapulpal tissue pressure promoted absorption of tissue fluid back into the blood and lymphatic vessels, thereby reducing the pressure. Thus it would appear that blood flow can increase, in spite of an elevation in tissue pressure. Obviously a combined multidisciplinary approach is needed to better understand the intricate circulatory changes occurring during the development of pulpal inflammation.

Using the laser Doppler technique to study pulpal blood flow in dogs, Sasano et al.[171] suggested that an increase or a decrease in pulpal blood flow is more dependent on systemic blood pressure than on local vasoconstriction or vasodilation.

THE STEALING THEORY

The dental pulp receives its blood supply through the so-called end arteries. These arterioles, entering the apical pulp, have a relatively low blood pressure, and the pressure drop from the arterioles entering the pulp to the venules leaving is only about one-fourth of the total arteriovenous pressure difference.[169] Accordingly a considerable part of the vascular resistance that regulates the pulpal blood circulation is located in the venules and also outside the pulp.[172] This implies that changes in circulation in the neighboring adjacent tissues, such as the gingiva, alveolar bone, and PDL, will change the blood flow to the pulp because it will affect the feeding pulpal arterial blood pressure. Any vasodilation in tissues that receive their blood supply through side branches of the end arterioles feeding the pulp will, according to the Poisseuille law, steal blood pressure from the pulp[169] (Figure 22). It should therefore be borne in mind that clinical treatment causing vasodilatation in adjacent tissues may decrease the circulation to the dental pulp. Thus the mere application of a matrix may affect the pulpal circulation and cause a fall in pulpal blood flow. The pulp may become ischemic.

LOW-COMPLIANCE SYSTEM THEORY

The dental pulp is encased in rigid structures, namely dentin, enamel, and cementum, creating a low-compliance system. In this system, any increase in blood flow or vasodilation has a limit depending on the degree of increase in tissue pressure. In normal condition, venular pressure is higher than the tissue pressure in the pulp. However, introduction of a known vasodilator, such as isoproterenol, causes an initial increase in pulpal blood flow which in turn causes a sudden increase in tissue pressure.[173] When the tissue pressure exceeds that of the venular pressure, a passive compression can cause a decrease in pulpal blood flow. Injection of various vasodilators caused a biphasic flow response, an increase followed by a decrease using the radioisotope microsphere injection technique.[174] In clinical situations, the effects of vasodilators produced by the initiation of inflammatory process on pulpal blood flow seem to be based on the low-compliance system theory. Thus, outpouring of inflammatory mediators that are mostly vasodilators has grave consequences for pulpal survival due to passive compression of the low

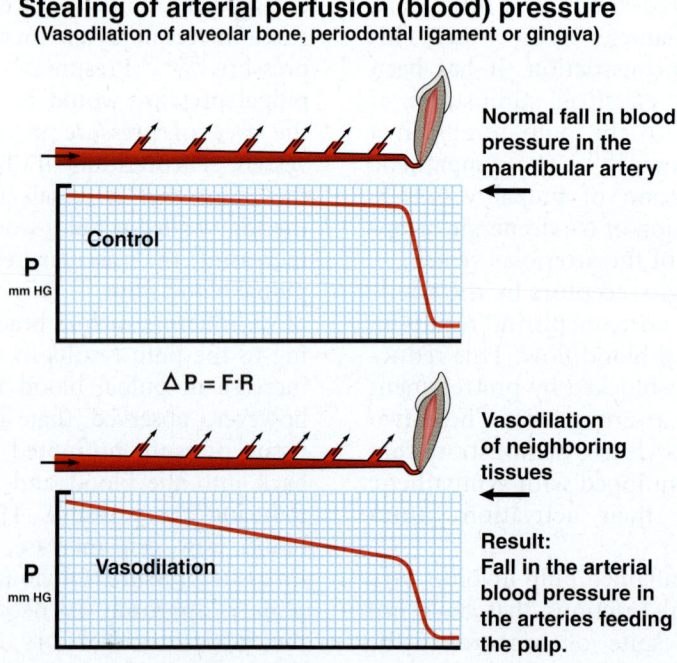

Figure 22 Stealing theory.

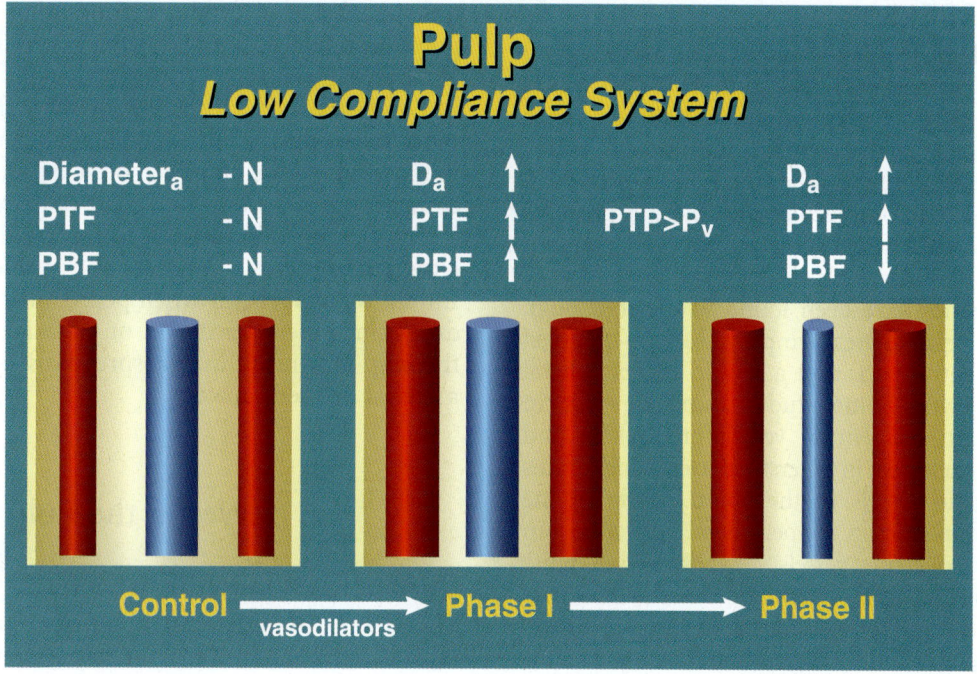

Figure 23 Schematic diagram illustrating the low-compliance system and its effects on pulpal hemodynamics.

pressure venules by a high tissue pressure. Figure 23 illustrates this theory.

TRANSCAPILLARY FLUID FLOW

At the same time the exchange of substances occurs across capillaries, another completely distinct process also takes place, that is, the bulk flow of fluid across the capillary wall. The function of this bulk flow of fluid is not the exchange of nutrients and waste products, but the distribution of the extracellular fluid. This distribution is governed by the hydrostatic pressure difference and the colloid osmotic pressure difference across the capillary wall. These pressures determine how much of the extracellular fluid will be located within the vessels as blood plasma and how much as interstitial fluid. The difference in protein concentration between plasma and interstitial fluid is important because it creates a higher colloid osmotic pressure in plasma than in the interstitial fluid, thus favoring bulk fluid movement back into the capillary. The hydrostatic pressure outside the vessels is normally considerably lower than the blood pressure inside the capillaries. Usually, this difference in hydrostatic pressure favors filtration, or bulk flow of fluid out of the vessels. However, in the dental pulp, where a small increase in volume increases the tissue pressure, absorption may take place during vasodilation. In the low-compliant pulp, a nearly simultaneous increase in blood volume and tissue pressure, as a result of vasodilation and/or venous stasis,[81] has been recorded, showing that vascular distension with an increase in blood volume compresses the pulpal tissue and raises the tissue pressure. Thus, a rapidly responding hydrostatic counterpressure develops that lowers the transmural hydrostatic pressure difference. Consequently, capillary filtration will be reduced and absorption may occur, and the tissue pressure is rapidly normalized, according to the Starling forces.[175] The interstitial fluid in the pulp reaches out in dentinal tubules and forms a continuum that extends out to the dentinoenamel and cementoenamel junctions. The mere cutting of dentin as it occurs during cavity and crown preparation may thus affect the dental pulp.[175] Furthermore, sensory nerve fibers are located in the subodontoblastic space of most tubules in the crown. Research during the last decades has shown that sensory nerves have a strong impact on the blood circulation in the dental pulp, due to liberation of vasodilating neuropeptides. In the cat pulp, most of the sensory nerve fibers contain these neuropeptides. The majority of sensory nerve fibers containing the vasodilating neuropeptides in the main pulp seem to be located in the walls of the blood vessels, a finding that implicates these neuropeptides in blood flow regulation.

LYMPH VESSELS

The only mechanism for the removal of proteins and macromolecules that may leak out from the blood vessels in any tissue is the lymphatics. The existence of lymph vessels in the dental pulp is well established.[177,178] Recovery of inflammation depends on the removal of macromolecules and plasma proteins from the tissue, thus a reversible pulpitis is dependent on functional lymph vessels.[179]

Most lymphatics have been found in the root pulp, whereas in the coronal area, lymph vessels are observed in the more central part, and a few in the peripheral odontoblastic layer. Some studies conclude that in the coronal part, real lymph vessels are lacking and that lymph is collected in interstitial clefts and drains toward lymphatic vessels in the apical region of the pulp.[180] The lymphatics in the peripheral pulp zone join to form larger collecting vessels.[181] These vessels unite with progressively larger lymphatic vessels that pass through the apex together with the blood vessels. Numerous authors, using both histological and functional methods, have described extensive anastomoses between lymph vessels of the pulp, the PDL, and the alveolar bone.[182–185] The structural identification of lymph vessels[178,185] complements the functional studies demonstrating that substances placed in the pulp chamber can be found in regional lymph nodes. The open endothelial margins and incomplete basal lamina permit the entry of large molecules and even bacteria into the lymphatics. The fact that materials placed on pulps can migrate to lymph nodes[186] indicates the possibility of the spread of bacteria or bacterial products from the pulp.[187] The anastomoses of pulpal, periodontal, and alveolar lymphatics may be important routes for the spread of pulpal inflammation into adjacent tissues during the removal of irritants and fluid from the pulp.

The architecture of the initial lymphatics, the so-called lymph capillaries, in different tissues varies considerably. Although in general they are wider than the blood capillaries, their number is much smaller. The wall of the initial lymphatics consists of a single layer of thin endothelial cells, often with overlapping margins. Open gaps between the cells, up to 2 to 5 µm, are frequent in many tissues. The initial lymphatics dilate and the number of open junctions increases during edema formation. It seems thus widely accepted that interstitial fluid pressure is the main determinant of lymph flow, and that lymph flow increases consistently when the tissue pressure is increased.[188] In the low-compliant pulp, this would imply that the increased local tissue pressure, as measured during pulpitis, induces increased lymph flow that will normalize the pressure and also drain off bacteria and bacterial products, promoting healing of the pulp. An enhanced lymph flow during inflammation has also been suggested by Feiglin and Reade.[189] They deposited radioactive microspheres in rat pulps and found more microspheres in the submandibular lymph nodes in those rats whose pulps had been exposed for 5 days in comparison with those with acute pulp exposure.[189]

The relationship of teeth to the cardiovascular and lymphatic systems is intimate and absolute. Clinicians should remember this when performing dental procedures since their placement of materials on dentin or the pulp may result in widespread distribution of that material or medicament.

Nerves in the Pulp

CLASSIFICATION OF NERVES

The dental pulp has an abundant supply of both sensory and autonomic nerves (Figure 24). This sophisticated arrangement of neural network plays an important role, although not fully understood, in managing the microenvironment of the dental pulp. The majority of these nerves are sensory. The trigeminal ganglion supplies sensory innervation to the pulp via the maxillary and mandibular nerves. Sympathetic nerves are less numerous with its source from the superior cervical ganglion. Parasympathetic fibers have been suggested to exist in the pulp, although the source of this innervation is still disputed.

Anatomical and electophysiological studies have classified nerves according to their diameter and conduction velocity (Table 1). The pulp contains two types of sensory nerve fibers: A fibers that are myelinated and C fibers that are unmyelinated. Nerve fibers enter teeth via the apical foramen, and arborize coronally to form the plexus of Rashkow in the subodontoblastic region. Some axons leave the plexus of Raschow, lose the myelin sheath to become unmyelinated, and pass between odontoblasts to reach inner dentin.[191] Nerve fibers have been found in more than 50% of tubules in inner cuspal dentin.[190–194] Coronal dentin is more densely innervated than radicular dentin. Axons do not traverse beyond 200 µm into coronal and radicular dentin but usually end less than 200 µm from the pulp.[191] A fibers include both A-β and A-δ with A-δ amounting to approximately 90% of the A fibers.[195]

Classical electrophysiological studies have shown the afferent function of sensory nerves in pain sensations. Some overlapping of functions have been

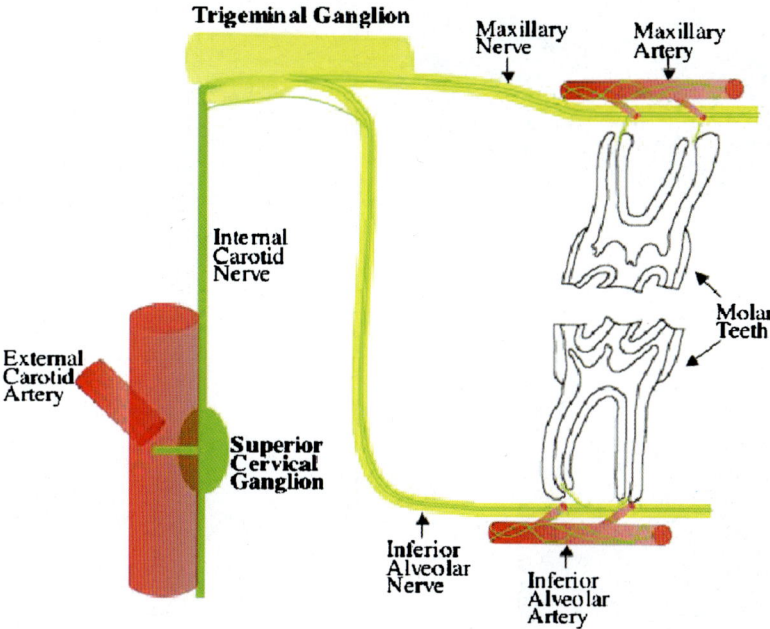

Figure 24 Schematic diagram showing the course of sensory and sympathetic nerves to the dental pulp. Sensory nerves (yellow) derive from the trigeminal ganglion while sympathetic nerves (green) are from the superior cervical ganglion. Postganglionic sympathetic nerves travel with the internal carotid nerve, reach the trigeminal ganglion, and supply teeth and supporting structures via the maxillary and the inferior alveolar nerve (yellow).

Table 1 Classification of Nerves in the Pulp			
Type of Fiber	Function	Diameter (μm)	Conduction Velocity (m/s)
Aα	Motor, proprioception	12–22	70–120
Aβ	Pressure, touch	5–12	30–70
Aγ	Motor	3–6	15–30
Aδ	Pain, temperature, touch	2–5	12–30
B	Preganglionic autonomic	<3	3–15
C	Pain	0.4–1.2	0.5–2
Sympathetic	Postganglionic sympathetic	0.3–1.3	0.7–2.3

shown between pulpal A and C fibers.[195–199] The A-δ fibers in the dental pulp have been involved in transmitting fast pain usually perceived as sharp, piercing pain, while C fibers transmit slow pain described as dull, aching pain.[200] Sympathetic nerves in general have been shown to have a vasoconstrictor effect, while parasympathetic nerves have a vasodilator effect.

NEUROPEPTIDES

In addition to their vasoactive functions, stimulated sensory and autonomic nerves release biologically active peptides, known as neuropeptides, that influence neural activity and functioning.[201–203] Neuropeptides are synthesized on ribosomes in the neuron cell body, processed through the endoplasmic reticulum and Golgi complex, transported in vesicles to the nerve terminals (Figure 25), and released from the peripheral terminals of mainly A-δ and C fibers.[204]

Neuropeptides can be classified according to the nerves from which it is derived. For example, sensory nerve-derived neuropeptides include CGRP, SP, and neurokinin A (NKA), while NPY is typically a sympathetic nerve-derived neuropeptide. Vasoactive intestinal peptide (VIP) has been shown to be in parasympathetic nerves. The introduction of immunohistochemical labeling of neuropeptides has contributed greatly to our understanding of the neural network of the dental pulp.

DISTRIBUTION

CGRP-containing or CGRP-immunoreactive (CGRP-IR) nerve fibers are the most abundant in the dental pulp (Figure 26). It is three to four times more

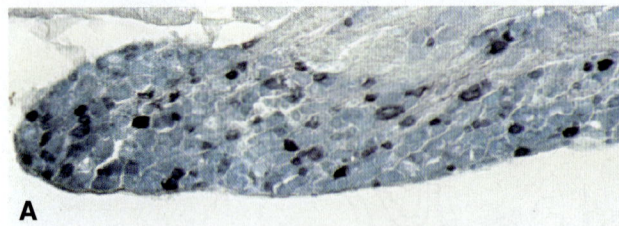
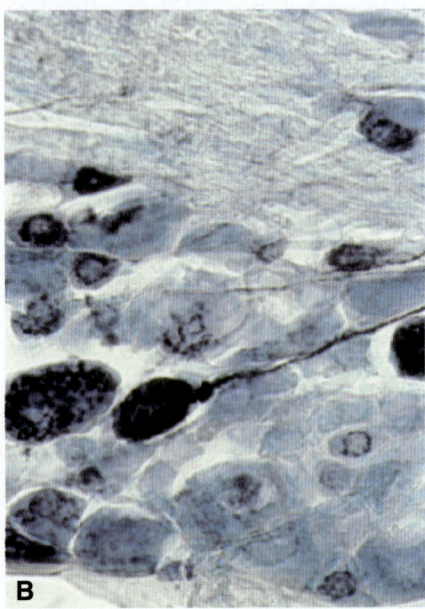

Figure 25 Calcitonin gene-related peptide-immunoreactive (CGRP-IR) neurons in the trigeminal ganglion. Low-magnification **A**, view of darkly stained neurons that contain CGRP. Higher magnification **B**, view of neurons with axons transporting CGRP to the peripheral nerve terminals. Courtesy of SR Haug and KJ Heyeraas.

abundant than SP.[205] CGRP-IR fibers enter the pulp via the apical foramen in bundles either surrounding the blood vessels or individually and ramify into a network of fine fibers in the coronal pulp.[205–207] Coronally, individual fibers penetrate the odontoblast layer and predentin to terminate in the inner 100 μm of the dental tubules. Radicular pulp fibers run parallel to the long axis of the tooth with little arborization and little penetration of the odontoblast layer.

SP is commonly found in C fibers with similar distribution to CGRP.[205,208,209] NKA fibers have similar distribution to SP-IR nerve fibers.[210] CGRP, SP, and NKA have been shown to coexist in the same nerve fibers in the dental pulp. NPY is usually found in sympathetic nerves and its distribution varies from the sensory neuropeptides. It enters the pulp mainly surrounding the blood vessels and terminates in the floor or the mid-coronal part of the pulp chamber. It is more numerous in the radicular than in the coronal pulp.[205,211–214]

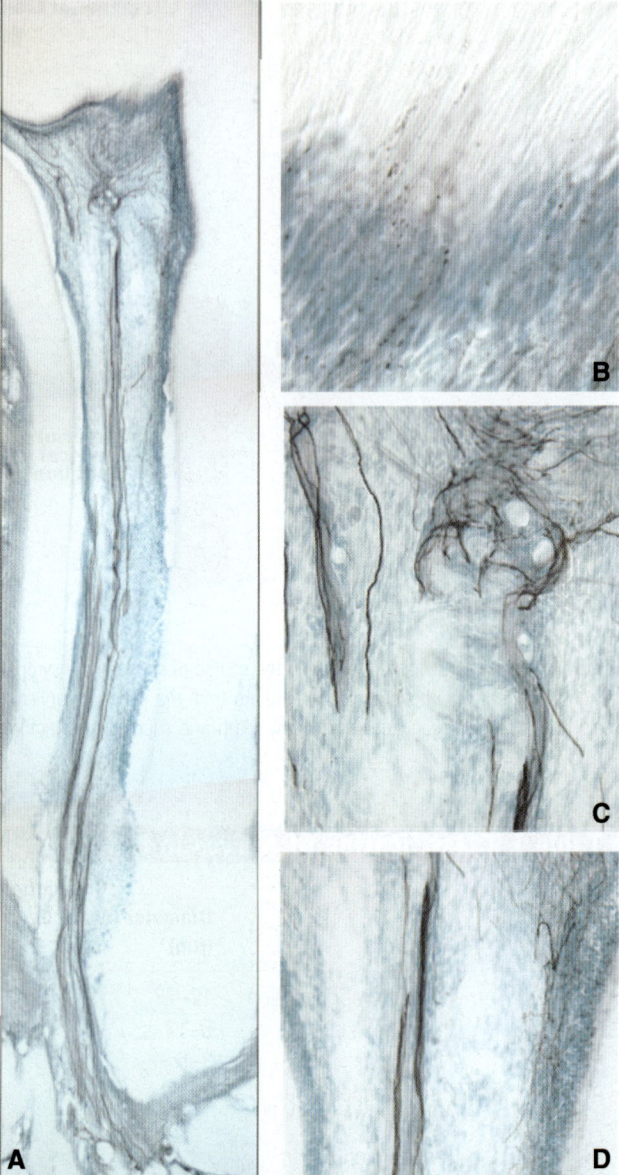

Figure 26 Immunohistochemical staining of calcitonin gene-related peptide-immunoreactive (CGRP-IR) nerve fibers in the rat dental pulp. **A,** Low-magnification view of darkly stained nerve fibers entering the apical foramen and traversing the long axis of the tooth as thick bundles. Coronally, nerve fibers branch extensively. **B,** CGRP-IR fibers penetrate the cuspal odontoblast layer and enter dentin. **C,** In the mid-coronal region, thick bundles of fibers are seen surrounding the blood vessels and in root pulp. **D,** Thick band of fibers surrounding the blood vessels are in the root pulp. Courtesy of SR Haug and KJ Heyeraas.

VIP-immunoreactive (VIP-IR) fibers in the dental pulp are associated with blood vessels[215] or occur as free and interlacing nerves in the central pulp and the subodontoblastic plexus.[215,216] Nerves containing neuro-peptides are also found in close contact with immunocompetent cells suggesting important neuroimmune interactions (Figure 27).

FUNCTION

Neuropeptides are released by various stimulations. What happens when a sensory neuropeptide is released? A classical demonstration of neuropeptide activity is the flare component of the "triple response" in the human skin: wheal (edema formation), local reddening (increased blood flow), and flare.[217] The flare is a consequence of the sensory nerve-mediated axon reflex and involves antidromic stimulation of sensory nerves to release neuropeptides such as SP and CGRP. These neuropeptides can be coreleased when an antidromic impulse depolarizes the peripheral end of the nerve. CGRP is a strong vasodilator. SP is also a vasodilator and in addition it increases vascular permeability and stimulates inflammatory and immune cells (Figure 28). NPY has many physiological effects including vasoconstriction,

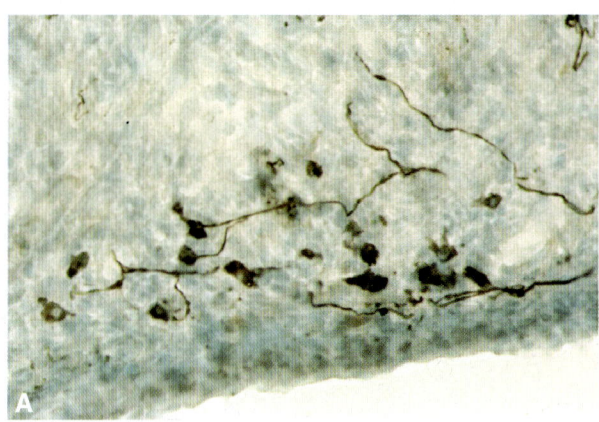
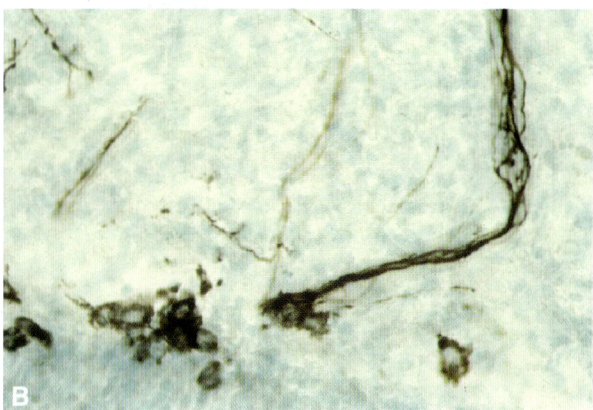

Figure 27 Calcitonin gene-related peptide-immunoreactive (CGRP-IR) nerve fibers in close proximity to immunocompetent cells in the dental pulp. Courtesy of SR Haug and KJ Heyeraas.

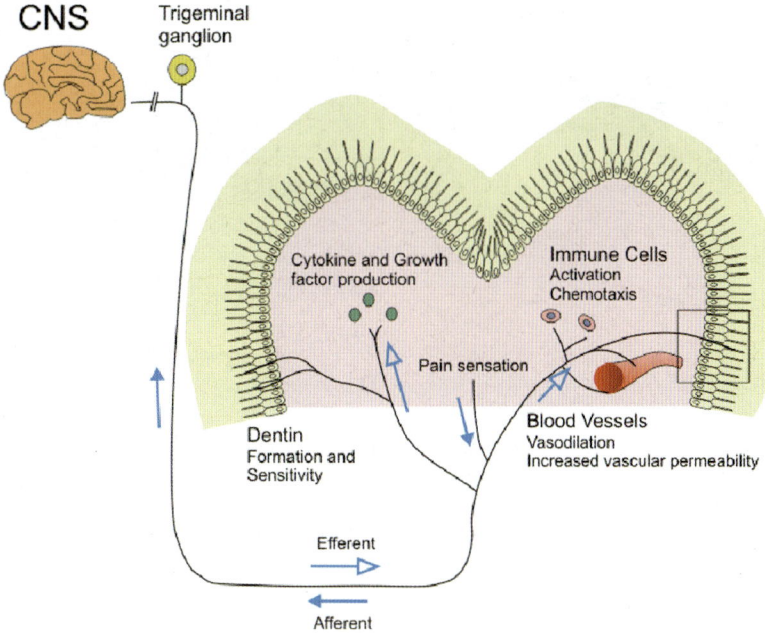

Figure 28 Schematic illustration summarizing some of the effects of neuropeptides (calcitonin gene-related protein, CGRP; substance P, SP) released from sensory nerves. Sensory nerves conduct afferent sensory information (e.g., pain sensations/dentin sensitivity) to the central nervous system and have an efferent function such as vasodilation and increased permeability of blood vessels. It affects various aspects of immune function such as activation and chemotaxis of immune cells, and release of cytokine and growth factors from various cellular structures in the dental pulp. Sensory nerves have also been shown to be involved in the formation of dentin.

immune regulation, and pain perception. In the dental pulp, CGRP and SP increases the blood flow while NPY decreases it.

Perhaps one of the most important function, although, little understood is how nerves affect the immune system, a term known as neuroimmunomodulation. SP and NKA are considered to have a proinflammatory role, while NPY and VIP are said to have an anti-inflammatory role on the immune system.[218–221] Classic work by Byers et al.[222–225] has shown that CGRP and SP-IR nerve fibers undergo sprouting during inflammation in the dental pulp. These fibers also change in quantity and architecture when inflamed (Figure 29). Recent studies have shown that NPY-IR nerve

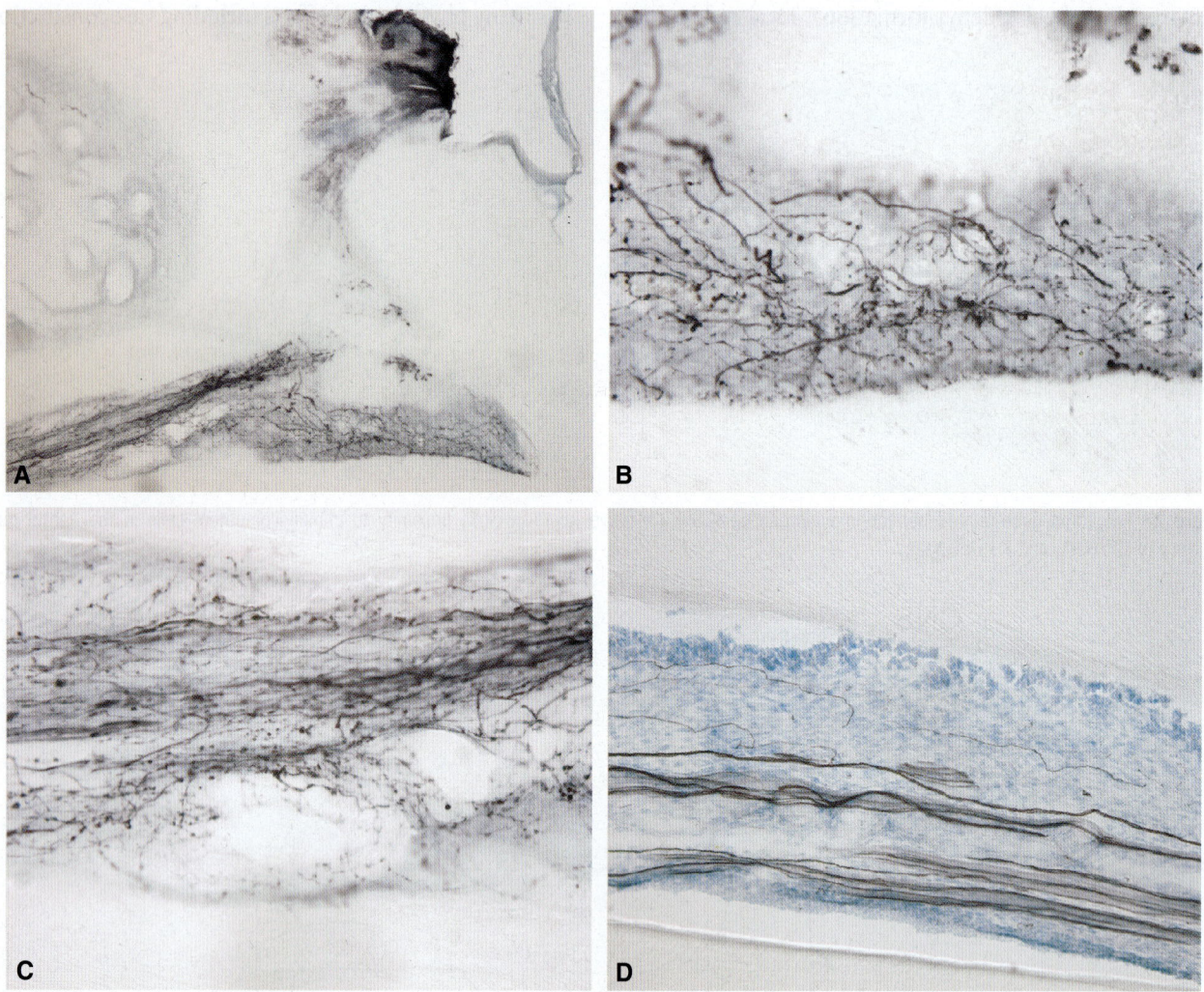

Figure 29 Calcitonin gene-related protein-immunoreactive (CGRP-IR) nerve fibers in the dental pulp. **A,** Low-magnification view of a rat molar tooth with pulp exposure (top left corner) for 20 days. Extensive formation of reparative dentin din the pulp chamber. **B,** On the right coronal pulp wall region, spouting of CGRP-IR fibers is observed. **C,** In the root pulp, sprouting of CGRP-IR nerve fibers is observed. **D,** Architecture of nerve fibers is quite different from that of a normal dental pulp from similar region. Courtesy of SR Haug and KJ Heyeraas.

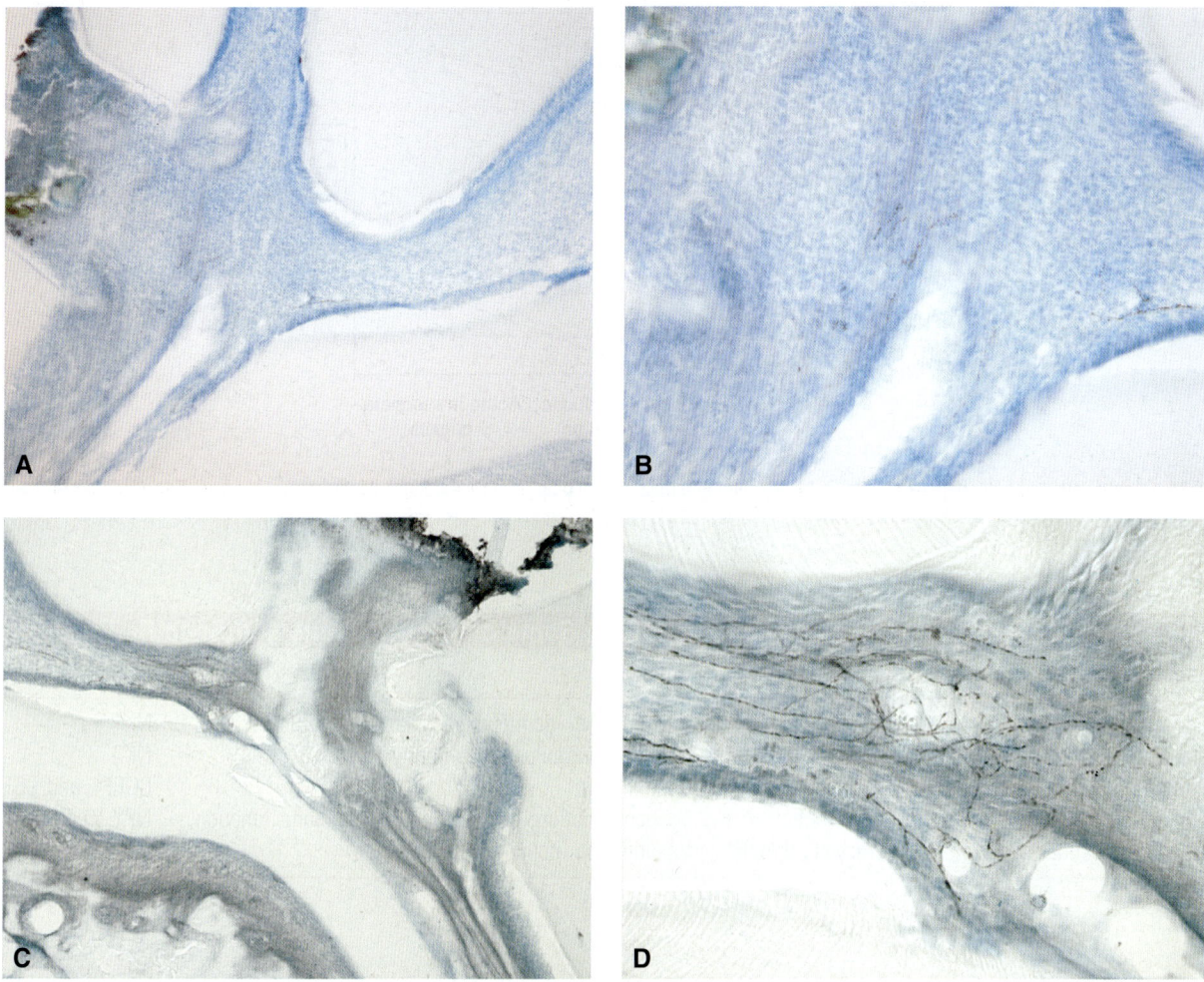

Figure 30 Neuropeptide Y-immunoreactive (NPY-IR) fibers in the inflamed dental pulp. **A,** Pulp exposure injury (top left) on a rat molar for 6 days. **B,** Higher magnification of A showing 'normal' location of NPY-IR fibers in the central pulp and on the floor of the pulp chamber. **C,** Pulp exposure injury (top right) on a rat molar tooth for 20 days. There is extensive reparative dentin formation and increased number of NPY-IR nerve fibers penetrating the region of the reparative dentin. **D,** Higher magnification. (**A** and **B**) Courtesy of SR Haug and KJ Heyeraas (**C** and **D**).[212]

fibers also sprout in long-standing inflammatory lesions (Figure 30).[212] Quantification studies have shown that SP, CGRP, NKA, NPY, and VIP are increased in pulps diagnosed clinically as irreversible pulpitis (Figure 31).[218,226]

RECEPTORS

Neuropeptides cannot cross the cell membrane and therefore their action is dependent on the existence of specific receptors (Table 2). Without the existence of a particular receptor, release of neurotransmitters or neuropeptides will have no effect. Therefore identifying the location and distribution of these receptors is important for understanding the functionality of a neuropeptide in a given location. NK1 receptors, specific for SP, are present in the blood vessels in the root pulp and smaller vessels along the odontoblast layer.[227,228] Fibroblasts express NK1 receptors during mechanical orthodontic stress.[212]

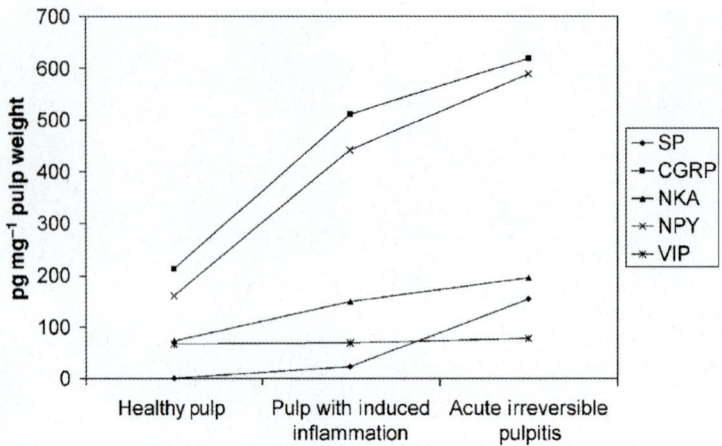

Figure 31 Quantification of neuropeptide content in healthy and inflamed human pulp tissue. Reproduced with permission from Caviedes-Bucheli J et al.[226]

Table 2	Neuropeptides and Their Origins Including Some of Their Actions and Specific Receptors		
Neuropeptides	**Released From**	**Actions**	**Receptors**
Substance P	Sensory	Vasodilation, increases vascular permeability	NK1
Neurokinin A	Sensory	Increases vascular permeability	NK2
Calcitonin gene-related peptide	Sensory	Vasodilation	CGRP1 and CGRP2
Neuropeptide Y	Sympathetic	Vasoconstriction, pain modulation, immune function	NPY Y1-6
Vasoactive intestinal peptide	Parasympathetic?	Vasodilation, immune function	VIP 1 and 2

Antagonists to these receptors are now being widely studied as therapeutic agents against inflammatory diseases or diseases involving overexpression of neuropeptides.

NEUROPHYSIOLOGY

Experimental animal model studies are widely used to investigate the role played by nerves in the dental pulp. Removing sensory nerves either by nerve transection or chemical removal has shown that sensory nerves are important for secondary dentin formation.[229] Releasing neuropeptides in the dental pulp by electrical stimulation results in transendothelial migration of inflammatory cells. This was absent when sensory nerves were previously removed from the dental pulp.[230] Recently studies have demonstrated that sympathetic nerves are involved in the modulation of the immune system (Figure 32). Sympathetic nerves inhibit the production of proinflammatory cytokines, while stimulating the production of anti-inflammatory cytokines.[220] Teeth lacking sympathetic nerves also tend to undergo necrosis more frequently.[211]

Sympathetic nerves have been shown to be important in the recruitment of granulocytes during electrical stimulation of teeth and experimental tooth movement.[231,232] Sympathetic imbalance results in the recruitment of plasma cells in an intact tooth suggesting an immune dysfunction.[233] Sympathetic nerves have also been shown to have an inhibitory effect on osteoclast resorption activity and on the cytokine IL-1α.[145,212,232] NPY that is coreleased in the sympathetic nerve terminal has recently been reported to modulate immune function in a wide range of inflammatory conditions. Therefore, the effects one sees in the dental pulp and surrounding structures could be due to the neuropeptide released from the sympathetic nerve terminal since an upregulation of NPY has been seen in the dental pulp.

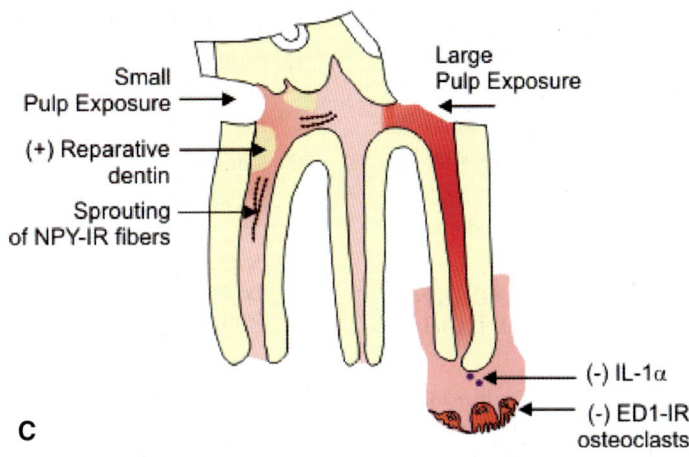

Figure 32 Schematic illustrations of rat molar teeth in three different conditions summarizing the potential effects of sympathetic nerves on teeth. Stimulating effects of sympathetic nerves are indicated by (+) and inhibitory effects by (−). **A,** Normal uninflamed pulp with sympathetic imbalance caused by unilateral sympathectomy recruits immunoglobulin-producing cells. **B,** Electrical stimulation of sympathetic nerves causes recruitment of CD43+ granulocytes in the normal dental pulp. During experimental orthodontic tooth movement (OTM), sympathetic nerves have an inhibitory effect on hard tissue resorption and a stimulating effect on CD43+ cell recruitment in the dental pulp and the periodontal ligament (PDL). **C,** The inflamed pulp shows increased reparative dentin formation and sprouting of sympathetic nerve fibers, while the periapical lesion shows decreased IL-1α production and number of osteoclasts when compared to a denervated sympathectomized tooth.[220]

References

1. Nanci A. Ten Cate's oral histology: development, structure, and function. 6th ed. St. Louis, MO: Moby; July 3, 2003.
2. Slavkin HC. Molecular determinants of tooth development: a review. Crit Rev Oral Biol Med 1990;1:1–16.
3. Slavkin HC. Molecular determinants during dental morphogenesis and cytodifferentiation: a review. J Craniofac Genet Dev Biol 1991;11:338–49.
4. Tucker AS, Sharpe PT. Molecular genetics of tooth morphogenesis and patterning: the right shape in the right place. J Dent Res 1999;78:826–34.
5. Chai Y, Bringas P Jr, Shuler C, et al. A mouse mandibular culture model permits the study of neural crest cell migration and tooth development. Int J Dev Biol 1998;42:87–94.
6. Lumsden AG. Spatial organization of the epithelium and the role of neural crest cells in the initiation of the mammalian tooth germ. Development 1988;103(Suppl):155–69.
7. Jernvall J, Thesleff I. Reiterative signaling and patterning during mammalian tooth morphogenesis. Mech Dev 2000;92:19–29.
8. Peters H, Balling R. Teeth. Where and how to make them. Trends Genet 1999;15:59–65.

9. Sharpe PT. Homeobox genes and orofacial development. Connect Tissue Res 1995;32:17–25.
10. Thomas BL, Sharpe PT. Patterning of the murine dentition by homeobox genes. Eur J Oral Sci 1998;106 (Suppl 1):48–54.
11. Løes S, Kettunen P, Kvinnsland H, Luukko K. Mouse rudimentary diastema tooth primordia are devoid of peripheral nerve fibers. Anat Embryol 2002;205:187–91.
12. Luukko K, Sainio K, Sariola H, et al. Localization of nerve cells in the developing rat tooth. J Dent Res 1997;76:1350–6.
13. Mohamed SS, Atkinson ME. A histological study of the innervation of developing mouse teeth. J Anat 1983;136:735–49.
14. Obara N, Takeda M. Expression of the neural cell adhesion molecule (NCAM) during second- and third-molar development in the mouse. Anat Embryol (Berl) 1993;188:13–20.
15. Pearson A. The early innervation of the developing deciduous teeth. J Anat 1977;123:563–77.
16. Fristad I, Heyeraas KJ, Kvinnsland I. Nerve fibres and cells immunoreactive to neurochemical markers in developing rat molars and supporting tissues. Arch Oral Biol 1994;39:633–46.
17. Fried K, Nosrat C, Lillesaar C, Hildebrand C. Molecular signaling and pulpal nerve development. Crit Rev Oral Biol Med 2000;11:318–32.
18. Luukko K. Neuronal cells and neurotrophins in odontogenesis. Eur J Oral Sci 1998;106(Suppl 1):80–93.
19. Nosrat CA, Fried K, Ebendal T, Olson L. NGF, BDNF, NT3, NT4 and GDNF in tooth development. Eur J Oral Sci 1998;106(Suppl 1):94–9.
20. Pashley DH, Kehl T, Pashley E, Palmer P. Comparison of in vitro and in vivo dog dentin permeability. J Dent Res 1981;60:763.
21. Ketterl W. Studie uber das Dentin der permanenten Zahne des Menschen. Stoma 1961;14:79.
22. Garberoglio R, Brännström M. Scanning electron microscopic investigation of human dentinal tubules. Arch Oral Biol 1976;21:355.
23. Coffey CT, Ingram MJ, Bjorndal A. Analysis of human dentinal fluid. Oral Surg 1970;30:835.
24. Bergenholtz, G. Effect of bacterial products on inflammatory reactions in the dental pulp. Scand J Dent Res 1977;85:122.
25. Walton R, Outhwaite WC, Pashley DH. Magnification—an interesting optical property of dentin. J Dent Res 1976;55:639.
26. Outhwaite W, Livingston M, Pashley DH. Effects of changes in surface area, thickness, temperature and post-extraction time on dentine permeability. Arch Oral Biol 1976;21:599.
27. Reeder OW, Walton RE, Livingston MJ, Pashley DH. Dentin permeability: determinants of hydraulic conductance. J Dent Res 1978;57:187.
28. Craig RG, Gehring PE, Peyton FA. Relation of structure to the microhardness of human dentin. J Dent Res 1959;38:624.
29. Fusayama T, Okuse K, Hosoda H. Relationship between hardness, discoloration and microbial invasion of carious dentin. J Dent Res 1966;45:1033.
30. Pashley DH, Okabe A, Parham P. The relationship between dentin microhardness and tubule density. Endod Dent Traumatol 1985;1:176.
31. Pashley DH. The influence of dentin permeability and pulpal blood flow on pulpal solute concentration. J ENDOD 1979;5:355.
32. Stanley HR. The factors of age and tooth size in human pulpal reactions. Oral Surg 1961;14:498.
33. Pashley DH. Dentin-predentin complex and its permeability: physiologic overview. J Dent Res 1985;64:613.
34. Fogel H, Marshall FJ, Pashley DH. Effect of distance from the pulp and thickness on the hydraulic conductance of human radicular dentin. J Dent Res 1988;67:1381.
35. Pashley DH, Kepler EE, Williams EC, O'Meara JA. The effect of dentine permeability of time following cavity preparation in dogs. Arch Oral Biol 1984;29:65.
36. Pashley DH, Galloway SE, Stewart FP. Effects of fibrinogen in vivo on dentine permeability in the dog. Arch Oral Biol 1984;29:725.
37. Johnson G, Brännström M. The sensitivity of dentin: changes in relation to conditions at exposed tubules apertures. Acta Odontol Scand 1974;32:29.
38. Pashley DH, Livingston MJ, Reeder OW, Horner J. Effects of the degree of tubule occlusion on the permeability of human dentin, in vitro. Arch Oral Biol 1978;23:1127.
39. Avery JK. In: Bhaskar SM, editor. Orban's oral histology and embryology. 9th ed. St. Louis, MO: CV Mosby; 1980. p. 108.
40. Pashley DH, Tao L, Boyd L, et al. Scanning electron microscopy of the substructure of smear layers in human dentine. Arch Oral Biol 1988;33:265.
41. Pashley DH. The smear layer: physiological considerations. Oper Dent 1984;Suppl 3:13.
42. Olgart L, Brännström M, Johnson G. Invasion of bacteria into dentinal tubules. Experiments in vivo and in vitro. Acta Odontol Scand 1974;32:61.
43. Michelich VJ, Schuster GS, Pashley DH. Bacterial penetration of human dentin, in vitro. J Dent Res 1980;59:1398.
44. Brännström M. Dentin and pulp in restorative dentistry. 1st ed. Nacka (Sweden): Dental Therapeutics AB; 1981.
45. Dippel HW, Broggreven JMP, Hoppenbrouwers, PMM. Morphology and permeability of the dentinal smear layer. J Prosthet Dent 1984;52:657.
46. Pashley DH, Michelich V, Kehl T. Dentin permeability: effects of smear layer removal. J Prosthet Dent 1981;46:531.
47. Goldman LB, Goldman M, Kronman JH, Lin PS. The efficacy of several irrigating solutions for endodontics: a scanning electron microscopic study. Oral Surg 1981;52:197.

48. Goldman M, DeVitre R, Pier M. Effect of the dentin smeared layer on tensile strength of cemented posts. J Prosthet Dent 1984;52:485.

49. Mjor IA, Tronstad L. Experimentally induced pulpitis. Oral Surg 1972;34:102.

50. Bergenholtz G. Inflammatory response of the dental pulp to bacterial irritation. J Endod 1981;7:100.

51. Warfringe J, Dahlen G, Bergenholtz G. Dental pulp response to bacterial cell wall material. J Dent Res 1985;64:1046.

52. Kraintz L, Conroy CW. Blood volume measurements of dog teeth. J Dent Res 1960;39:1033.

53. Kraintz L, et al. Blood volume determination of human dental pulp. J Dent Res 1980;59:544.

54. Pohto M, Scheinin A. Effects of local anesthetic solutions on the circulation of the pulp in rat incisor. Bibl Anat 1960;1:46.

55. Scheinin A. Flow characteristics of the pulpal vessels. J Dent Res 1963;438(Suppl 2):411.

56. Scott D, Scheinin A, Karjalainen S, Edwall L. Influence of sympathetic nerve stimulation on flow velocity in pulpal vessels. Acta Odontol Scand 1972;30:277.

57. Taylor AC. Microscopic observation of the living tooth pulp. Science 1950;111:40.

58. Meyer M, et al. Blood flow in the dental pulp. Proc Soc Exp Biol Med 1964;116:1038.

59. Ogilvie RW, Gillilan LA, Knapp DE. Physiologic evidence for the presence of vasoconstrictor fibers in the dental pulp. J Dent Res 1966;45:980.

60. Ogilvie RW. Direct observations of the cat dental pulp microvascular response to electrical and drug stimuli. Anat Rec 1967;157:379.

61. Edwall L, Kindlova M. The effect of sympathetic nerve stimulation on the rate of disappearance of tracers from various oral tissues. Acta Odontol Scand 1971;29:387.

62. Edwall L, Scott D. Influence of changes in microcirculation on the excitability of the sensory unit in the tooth of the cat. Acta Physiol Scand 1971;85:555.

63. Tönder KH. The effect of variations in arterial blood pressure and baroreceptor reflexes on pulpal blood flow in dogs. Arch Oral Biol 1975;20:345.

64. Ahlberg KF, Edwall L. Influence of local insults on sympathetic vasoconstrictor control in the feline dental pulp. Acta Odontol Scand 1977;35:103.

65. Olgart L, Gaelius B. Effects of adrenalin and elypressin (octapressin) on blood flow and sensory nerve activity in the tooth. Acta Odontol Scand 1977;35:69.

66. Tönder KH, Naess G. Nervous control of blood flow in the dental pulp in dogs. Acta Physiol Scand 1978;104:13.

67. Kim S. Microcirculation of the dental pulp in health and disease. J Endod 1985;11:465.

68. Jontell M, Bergenholtz G, Scheynius A, Ambrose W. Dendritic cells and macrophages expressing class II antigens in the normal rat incisor pulp. J Dent Res 1988;67:1263.

69. Kogushi M, Nakamura S, Kishi Y, et al. A study of leukocyte extravasation in early inflammatory changes in the pulp. J Endod 1988;14:475.

70. DelBalso AM, Nishimura RS, Setterstrom JA. The effects of thermal and electrical injury on pulpal histamine levels. Oral Surg 1976;41:110.

71. Olgart L, Gazelius B, Brodin E, Nilsson G. Release of substance P-like immunoreactivity from the dental pulp. Acta Physiol Scand 1977;101:510.

72. Brodin E, Gazelius B, Lundberg JM, Olgart L. Substance P in trigeminal nerve endings: occurrence and release. Acta Physiol Scand 1981;111:501.

73. Brodin E, Gazelius B, Panopoulos P, Olgart L. Morphine inhibits substance P release from peripheral sensory nerve endings. Acta Physiol Scand 1983;117:567.

74. Wakisaka S, et al. Immunohistochemical study on regeneration of substance P-like immunoreactivity in rat molar pulp and periodontal ligament following resection of the inferior alveolar nerve. Arch Oral Biol 1987;32:225.

75. Edwall L. Regulation of pulpal blood flow. J Endod 1980;6:434.

76. Inoki R, Toyoda T, Yamamoto I. Elaboration of a bradykinin-like substance in dog's canine pulp during electrical stimulation and its inhibition by narcotic and non-narcotic analgesics. Naunyn Schmiedebergs' Arch Pharmacol 1973;279:387.

77. Okamura K, Tsubakimoto K, Uobe K, et al. Serum proteins and secretory component in human carious dentin. J Dent Res 1979;58:1127.

78. Okamura K, Maeda M, Nishikawa T, Tsutsui M. Dentinal response against carious invasion: localization of antibodies in odontoblastic body and process. J Dent Res 1980;59:1368.

79. Pashley DH, Nelson R, Williams EC, Kepler EE. Use of dentine–fluid protein concentrations to measure pulp capillary reflection coefficients in dogs. Arch Oral Biol 1981;26:703.

80. Tonder KJH, Kvinsinsland I. Micropuncture measurement of interstitial fluid pressure in normal and inflamed dental pulp in cats. J Endod 1983;9:105

81. Van Hassel HJ. Physiology of the human dental pulp. Oral Surg 1971;32:126.

82. Stenvik A, Iversion J, Mjor IA. Tissue pressure and histology of normal and inflamed tooth pulps in macaque monkeys. Arch Oral Biol 1972;17:1501.

83. Kim S, Trowbridge H, Kim B, Chien S. Effects of bradykinin on pulpal blood flow in dogs. J Dent Res 1982;61:1036.

84. Heyeraas KJ. Pulpal microvascular and tissue pressure. J Dent Res 1985;64:585.

85. Rowe NH, editor. Hypersensitive dentin: origin and management. Ann Arbor, MI: University of Michigan; 1985.

86. Tronstad L, editor. Symposium on dentinal hypersensitivity. Endodont Dent Traumatol 1986;2:124.
87. Byers MR. Development of sensory innervation in dentin. J Comp Neurol 1980;191:413.
88. Byers MR. Dental sensory receptors. Int Rev Neurobiol 1984;25:39.
89. Rapp R, Avery JK, Strachan D. The distribution of nerves in human primary teeth. Anat Rec 1967;159:89.
90. Anderson DJ, Hannam AG, Matthews B. Sensory mechanisms in mammalian teeth and their supporting structures. Physiol Rev 1970;50:171.
91. Brännström M. Sensitivity of dentin. Oral Surg 1966;21:517.
92. Brännström M, Linden LA, Astrom A. The hydrodynamics of the dentinal tubule and of pulp fluid. A discussion of its significance in relation to dentinal sensitivity. Caries Res 1967;1:310.
93. Tsatsas BG, Frank RM. Ultrastructure of the dentinal tubular substances near the dentino-enamel junction. Calcif Tissue Res 1972;9:238.
94. Garant PR. The organization of microtubules within rat odontoblast processes revealed by perfusion fixation with glutaraldehyde. Arch Oral Biol 1972;17:1047.
95. Holland GR. The dentinal tubules and the odontoblast process in the cat. J Anat 1975;120:169.
96. Marion D, Jean A, Hamel H, et al. Scanning electron microscope study of odontoblasts and circum-pulpal dentin in a human tooth. Oral Surg 1991;72:473.
97. Avery JK. In: Bhaskar SM, editor. Orban's oral histology and embryology. 9th ed. St. Louis, MO: CV Mosby; 1980. p. 108.
98. LaFleche RG, Frank RM, Steuer P. The extent of the human odontoblast process as determined by transmission electron microscopy: the hypothesis of a retractable suspensor system. J Biol Buccale 1985;13:293.
99. Coffey CT, Ingram MJ, Bjorndal A. Analysis of human dentinal fluid. Oral Surg 1970;30:835.
100. Greenhill JD, Pashley DH. The effects of desensitizing agents on the hydraulic conductance of human dentin, in vitro. J Dent Res 1981;60:686.
101. Nahri MVO. Dentin sensitivity: a review. J Biol Buccale 1985;13:75.
102. Pashley DH. Dentine permeability, dentine sensitivity and treatment through tubule occlusion. J Endod 1986;12:465.
103. Bletsa A, Berggreen E, Fristad I, et al. Cytokine signalling in rat pulp interstitial fluid and transcapillary fluid exchange during lipopolysaccharide-induced acute inflammation. J Physiol 2006;573:225–36.
104. Heyeraas KJ, Kim S, Raab WH, et al. Effect of electrical tooth stimulation on blood flow, interstitial fluid pressure and substance P and CGRP-immunoreactive nerve fibers in the low compliant cat dental pulp. Microvasc Res 1994;47:329–43.
105. Gartner LP, Siebel W, Hiatt JL, Provenza DV. A fine structural analysis of mouse molar odontoblast maturation. Acta Anat 1979;103:16.
106. Garant PR. Microanatomy of the oral mineralized tissues. In: Shaw JH, Sweeney EA, Cappuccino CC, Meller SM, editors. Textbook of oral biology. Philadelphia, PA: WB Saunders; 1968. p. 181.
107. Eisenmann DR, Glick PL. Ultrastructure of initial crystal formation in dentin. J Ultrastruct Res 1972;41:18.
108. Katchburian E. Membrane-bound bodies as initiators of mineralization of dentine. J Anat 1973;116:285.
109. Weinstock M, Leblond CP. Synthesis, migration and release of precursor collagen odontoblasts as visualized by radioautography after 3H-proline administration. J Cell Biol 1974;60:92.
110. Weinstock A. Matrix development in mineralizing tissues as shown by radioautography: formation of enamel and dentin. In: Slavkin HC, Bavetta LA, editors. Developmental aspects of oral biology. New York: Academic Press; 1972.
111. Weinstock M, Leblond CP. Radioautographic visualization of a phosphoprotein at the mineralization front in the rat incisor. J Cell Biol 1973;56:838.
112. Holland GR. The odontoblast process: form and function. J Dent Res 1985;64:499.
113. Grosdenovic-Selecki S, Qvist V, Hansen HP. Histologic variations in the pulp of intact premolars from young individuals. Scand J Dent Res 1973;81:433.
114. Seltzer S, Bender IB. The dental pulp: biologic considerations in dental procedures. 2nd ed. Philadelphia, PA: JB Lippincott Co.; 1975. p. 48.
115. Jean A, Kerebel B, Kerebel L-M. Scanning electron microscope study of the predentin–pulpal border zone in human dentin. Oral Surg 1986;61:392
116. Marion D, Jean A, Hamel H, et al. Scanning electron microscope study of odontoblasts and circum-pulpal dentin in a human tooth. Oral Surg 1991;72:473.
117. Forsell-Ahlberg K, Brännström M, Edwall L. The diameter and number of dentinal tubules in rat, cat, dog and monkey. A comparative scanning electron microscopic study. Acta Odontol Scand 1975;33:243.
118. Tsatsas BG, Frank RM. Ultrastructure of the dentinal tubular substances near the dentino-enamel junction. Calcif Tissue Res 1972;9:238.
119. Holland GR. The extent of odontoblastic process in the cat. J. Anat 1976;121:133.
120. Brännström M, Garberoglio R. The dentinal tubules and the odontoblast processes. A scanning electron microscopic study. Acta Odontol Scand 1972;30:29.
121. Thomas HF. The extent of the odontoblastic process in human dentin. J Dent Res 1979;58:2207.

122. Maniatopoulos C, Smith DC. A scanning electron microscopic study of the odontoblastic process in human coronal dentine. Arch Oral Biol 1984;28:701.

123. Sigel MJ, Aubin JE, Ten Cate AR. An immunocyto-chemical study of the human odontoblast process using antibodies against tubulin, actin and vimentin. J Dent Res 1985;64:1348.

124. Thomas HF, Payne RC. The ultrastructure of dentinal tubules from erupted human premolar teeth. J Dent Res 1983;62:532.

125. Thomas HF, Carella P. Correlation of scanning and transmission electron microscopy of human dentinal tubules. Arch Oral Biol 1984;29:641

126. Thomas HF. The dentin-predentin complex and its permeability: anatomic overview. J Dent Res 1985;64:607.

127. Weber DF, Zaki AE. Scanning and transmission electron microscopy of tubular structures presumed to be human odontoblast processes. J Dent Res 1986;65:982.

128. LaFleche RG, Frank RM, Steuer P. The extent of the human odontoblast process as determined by transmission electron microscopy: the hypothesis of a retractable suspensor system. J Biol Buccale 1985;13:293.

129. Nalbandian A, Gonzales F, Sognnaes RF. Sclerotic changes in root dentin of human teeth as observed by optical, electron and X-ray microscope. J Dent Res 1960;39:598.

130. Johansen E, Parks HF. Electron-microscopic observations on sound human dentine. Arch Oral Biol 1962;7:185.

131. Mjor IA. Dentin–predentin complex and its permeability: pathology and treatment overview. J Dent Res 1985;64:621.

132. Tronstad L. Scanning electron microscopy of attrited dentinal surfaces and subjacent dentin in human teeth. Scand J Dent Res 1973;81:112.

133. Mendis BRRM, Darling AI. A scanning electron microscopic and microradiographic study of human coronal dentinal tubules related to occlusal attrition and caries. Arch Oral Biol 1979;24:725.

134. Brännström M, Garberoglio R. Occlusion of dentinal tubules under superficial attrited dentin. Swed Dent J 1980;4:87.

135. Han SS. The fine structure of cells and intercellular substance in the dental pulp. In: Finn SB, editor. Biology of the dental pulp organ. Birmingham, AL: University of Alabama Press; 1968.

136. Jontell M, Okiji T, Dahlgren U, Bergenholtz G. Immune defense mechanisms of the dental pulp. Crit Rev Oral Biol Med 1998;9:27–200.

137. Jontell M, Gunraj MN, Bergenholtz G. Immunocompetent cells in the normal dental pulp. J Dent Res 1987;66:1149–53.

138. Nishikawa S, Sasaki F. Apoptosis of dental pulp cells and their elimination by macrophages and MHC class II-expressing dendritic cells. J Histochem Cytochem 1999;47:303–12.

139. Ohshima H, Kawahara I, Maeda T, Takano Y. The relationship between odontoblasts and immunocompetent cells during dentinogenesis in rat incisors: an immunohistochemical study using OX6-monoclonal antibody. Arch Histol Cytol 1994;57:435–47.

140. Okiji T, Kosaka T, Kamal AM, et al. Age-related changes in the immunoreactivity of the monocyte/macrophage system in rat molar pulp. Arch Oral Biol 1996;41:453–60.

141. Hahn CL, Falkler WA, Siegel MA. A study of T and B cells in pulpal pathosis. J Endod 1989;15:20–6.

142. Farnoush A. Mast cells in human dental pulp. J Endod 1987;13:362–3.

143. Angelova A, Takagi Y, Okiji T, et al. Immunocompetent cells in the pulp of human deciduous teeth. Arch Oral Biol 2004;49:29–36.

144. Izumi T, Kobayashi I, Okamura K, Sakai H. Immunohistochemical study on the immunocompetent cells of the pulp in human non-carious and carious teeth. Arch Oral Biol 1995;40:609–14.

145. Bletsa A, Heyeraas KJ, Haug SR, Berggreen E. IL-1 alpha and TNF-alpha expression in rat periapical lesions and dental pulp after unilateral sympathectomy. Neuroimmunomodulation 2004;11:376–84.

146. Artese L, Rubini C, Ferrero G, et al. Vascular endothelial growth factor (VEGF) expression in healthy and inflamed human dental pulps. J Endod 2002;28:20–3.

147. Botero TM, Mantellini MG, Song W, et al. Effect of lipopolysaccharides on vascular endothelial growth factor expression in mouse pulp cells and macrophages. Eur J Oral Sci 2003;111:228–34.

148. Park SH, Hsiao GYW, Huang GTJ. Role of substance P and calcitonin gene-related peptide in the regulation of interleukin-8 and monocyte chemotactic protein-1 expression in human dental pulp. Int Endod J 2004;37:185–92.

149. Patel T, Park SH, Lin LM, et al. Substance P induces interleukin-8 secretion from human dental pulp cells. Oral Surg Oral Med Oral Pathol Oral Radiol Endod 2003;96:478–85.

150. Tran-Hung L, Mathieu S, About I. Role of human pulp fibroblasts in angiogenesis. J Dent Res 2006;85:819–23.

151. Yamaguchi M, Kojima T, Kanekawa M, et al. Neuropeptides stimulate production of interleukin-1 beta, interleukin-6, and tumor necrosis factor-alpha in human dental pulp cells. Inflamm Res 2004;53:199–204.

152. Yang LC, Tsai CH, Huang FM, et al. Induction of vascular endothelial growth factor expression in human pulp fibroblasts stimulated with black-pigmented Bacteroides. Int Endod J 2004;37:588–92.

153. Griffin CJ, Harris R. Ultrastructure of collagen fibrils and fibroblasts of the developing human dental pulp. Arch Oral Biol 1966;11:659–66.

154. Yoshiba N, Yoshiba K, Nakamura H, et al. Immunoelectron-microscopic study of the localization of fibronectin in the odontoblast layer of human teeth. Arch Oral Biol 1995;40:83–9.

155. Kishi Y, Shimozato N, Takahashi K. Vascular architecture of cat pulp using corrosive resin cast under scanning electron, microscopy. J Endod 1989;15:478–83.

156. Mjor IA, Smith MR, Ferrari M, Mannocci F. The structure of dentine in the apical region of human teeth. Int Endod J 2001;34:346–53.

157. Takahashi K, Kishi Y, Kim S. A scanning electron microscope study of the blood vessels of dog pulp using corrosion resin casts. J Endod 1982;8:131–5.

158. Kim S, Lipowsky HH, Usami S, Chien S. Arteriovenous distribution of hemodynamic parameters in the rat dental pulp. Microvasc Res 1984;27:28–38.

159. Takahashi KK. Vascular architecture of dog pulp using corrosion resin cast examined under a scanning electron microscope. J Dent Res 1985;64(Spec No):579–84.

160. Dahl E, Major IA. The fine structure of the vessels in the human dental pulp. Acta Odontol Scand 1973;31:223–30.

161. Kim S. Neurovascular interactions in the dental pulp in health and inflammation. J Endod 1990;16:48–53.

162. Sasano T, Kuriwada S, Shoji N, et al. Axon reflex vasodilatation in cat dental pulp elicited by noxious stimulation of the gingiva. J Dent Res 1994;73:277.

163. Kim S, Liu M, Simchin S, Dorscher-Kim JE. Effects of selected inflammatory mediators in blood flow and vascular permeability in the dental pulp. Proc Finn Dent Soc 1992;88(Suppl 1):387.

164. Edwall L, Kindlová M. The effect of sympathetic nerve stimulation on the rate of disappearance of tracers from various oral tissues, Acta Odontol Scand 1971;29:387.

165. Kim S, Schuessler G, Chien S. Measurement of blood flow in the dental pulp of dogs with the 133xenon washout method. Arch Oral Biol 1983;28:501.

166. Sasano T, Shoji N, Kuriwada S, et al. Absence of parasympathetic vasodilatation in cat dental pulp. J Dent Res 1995;74:1665.

167. van Hassel HJ. Physiology of the human dental pulp. Oral Surg 1971;32:126.

168. Tönder KJH, Naess G. Nervous control of blood flow in the dental pulp in dogs. Acta Physiol Scand 1978;104:13.

169. Heyerass KJ, Kvinnsland I. Tissue pressure and blood flow in pulpal inflammation. Proc Finn Dent Soc 1992;88(Suppl 1):393.

170. Heyeraas KJ. Pulpal hemodynamics and interstitial fluid pressure: balance of transmicrovascular fluid transport. J Endod 1989;15:468–72.

171. Sasano T, Kuriwada S, Sanjo D. Arterial blood pressure regulation of pulpal blood flow as determined by laser Doppler. J Dent Res 1989;68:791.

172. Tönder KJH. Effect of vasodilating drugs on external carotid and pulpal blood flow in dogs: "stealing" of dental perfusion pressure. Acta Physiol Scand 1976;97:75.

173. Kim S. Regulation of blood flow of the dental pulp: macrocirculation and microcirculation studies [PhD thesis in Physiology]. New York, N.Y.: Columbia Univ.; 1981.

174. Liu M, Kim S, et al. Comparison of the effects of intraarterial and locally applied vasoactive agents on pulpal blood flow in dog canine teeth determined by laser Doppler velocimetry. Arch Oral Biol 1990;35:405–10.

175. Starling EH. On the Absorption of Fluids from the connective tissue spaces. J Physiol 1896;19:312–26.

176. Byers MR, Narhi MV, Mecifi KB. Acute and chronic reactions of dental sensory nerve fibers to cavities and desiccation in rat molars. Anat Rec 1988;221:872–83.

177. Sawa Y, Yoshida S, Ashikaga Y, et al. Immunohistochemical demonstration of lymphatic vessels in human dental pulp. Tissue Cell 1998;30:510–16.

178. Bishop MA, Malhotra M. An investigation of lymphatic vessels in the feline dental pulp. Am J Anat 1990;187:247–53.

179. Matsumoto Y, Zhang B, Kato S. Lymphatic networks in the periodontal tissue and dental pulp as revealed by histochemical study. Microsc Res Tech 2002;56:50–9.

180. Oehmke MJ, Knolle E, Oehmke HJ. Lymph drainage in the human dental pulp. Microsc Res Tech 2003;62:187–91.

181. Bernick S. Lymphatic vessels of the human dental pulp. J Dent Res 1977;56:70–7.

182. Levy BM, Bernick S. Studies on the biology of the periodontium of marmosets: V. Lymphatic vessels of the periodontal ligament. J Dent Res 1968;47:1166–75.

183. Ruben MP, Prieto-Hernandez JR, Gott FK, et al. Visualization of lymphatic microcirculation of oral tissues. II. Vital retrograde lymphography. J Periodontol 1971;42:774–84.

184. Walton RE, Langeland K. Migration of materials in the dental pulp of monkeys. J Endod 1978;4:167–77.

185. Frank RM, Wiedemann P, Fellinger E. Ultrastructure of lymphatic capillaries in the human dental pulp. Cell Tissue Res 1977;178:229–38.

186. Kraintz L, Tyler CD, Ellis BR. Lymphatic drainage of teeth in dogs demonstrated by radioactive colloidal gold. J Dent Res 1959;38:198.

187. Barnes GW, Langeland K. Antibody formation in primates following introduction of antigens into the root canal. J Dent Res 1966;45:1111–14.

188. Aukland K, Reed RK. Interstitial-lymphatic mechanisms in the control of extracellular fluid volume. Physiol Rev 1993;73:1–78.

189. Feiglin B, Reade PC. The distribution of [^{14}C] leucine and ^{85}Sr labeled microspheres from rat incisor root canals. Oral Surg Oral Med Oral Pathol 1979;47:277–81.

190. Haug SR. Sympathetic innervation and dental inflammation: in vivo studies in rats [dissertation]. University of Bergen; 2003.

191. Byers MR. Dental sensory receptors. Int Rev Neurobiol 1984;25:39–94.
192. Byers MR, Dong WK. Autoradiographic location of sensory nerve endings in dentin of monkey teeth. Anat Rec 1983;205:441–54.
193. Byers MR, Matthews B. Autoradiographic demonstration of ipsilateral and contralateral sensory nerve endings in cat dentin, pulp, and periodontium. Anat Rec 1981;201:249–60.
194. Holland GR. The incidence of dentinal tubules containing more than one process in the cuspal dentin of cat canine teeth. Anat Rec 1981;200:437–42.
195. Matthews B. Sensory physiology: a reaction. Proc Finn Dent Soc 1992;88(Suppl 1):529–32.
196. Ikeda H, Tokita Y, Suda H. Capsaicin-sensitive A delta fibers in cat tooth pulp. J Dent Res 1997;76:1341–9.
197. Johnsen D, Johns S. Quantitation of nerve fibres in the primary and permanent canine and incisor teeth in man. Arch Oral Biol 1978;23:825–9.
198. Johnsen DC, Harshbarger J, Rymer HD. Quantitative assessment of neural development in human premolars. Anat Rec 1983;205:421–9.
199. Narhi M, Virtanen A, Kuhta J, Huopaniemi T. Electrical stimulation of teeth with a pulp tester in the cat. Scand J Dent Res 1979;87:32–8.
200. Närhi M, Jyväsjärvi E, Virtanen A, et al. Role of intradental A- and C-type nerve fibres in dental pain mechanisms. Finn Dent Soc Proc Suppl 1992;88(Suppl 1):507–16.
201. Levine JD, Clark R, Devor M, et al. Intraneuronal substance P contributes to the severity of experimental arthritis. Science 1984;226:547–9.
202. Lundberg JM, Franco-Cereceda A, Hua X, et al. Co-existence of substance P and calcitonin gene-related peptide-like immunoreactivities in sensory nerves in relation to cardiovascular and bronchoconstrictor effects of capsaicin. Eur J Pharmacol 1985;108:315–19.
203. Maggi CA. Tachykinins and calcitonin gene-related peptide (CGRP) as co-transmitters released from peripheral endings of sensory nerves. Prog Neurobiol 1995;45:1–98.
204. Brain SD. Sensory neuropeptides: their role in inflammation and wound healing. Immunopharmacology 1997;37:133–52.
205. Heyeraas KJ, Kvinnsland I, Byers MR, Jacobsen EB. Nerve fibers immunoreactive to protein gene product 9.5, calcitonin gene-related peptide, substance P, and neuropeptide Y in the dental pulp, periodontal ligament, and gingiva in cats. Acta Odontol Scand 1993;51:207–21.
206. Kimberly CL, Byers MR. Inflammation of rat molar pulp and periodontium causes increased calcitonin gene-related peptide and axonal sprouting. Anat Rec 1988;222:289–300.
207. Wakisaka S. Neuropeptides in the dental pulp: distribution, origins, and correlation. J Endod 1990;16:67–9.
208. Cuello AC, Kanazawa I. The distribution of substance P immunoreactive fibers in the rat central nervous system. J Comp Neurol 1978;178:129–56.
209. Hokfelt T, Kellerth JO, Nilsson G, Pernow B. Substance P: localization in the central nervous system and in some primary sensory neurons. Science 1975;190:889–90.
210. Wakisaka S, Ichikawa H, Nishikawa S, et al. Neurokinin A-like immunoreactivity in feline dental pulp: its distribution, origin and coexistence with substance P-like immunoreactivity. Cell Tissue Res 1988;251:565–9.
211. Haug SR, Berggreen E, Heyeraas KJ. The effect of unilateral sympathectomy and cavity preparation on peptidergic nerves and immune cells in rat dental pulp. Exp Neurol 2001;169:182–90.
212. Haug SR, Heyeraas KJ. Effects of sympathectomy on experimentally induced pulpal inflammation and periapical lesions in rats. Neuroscience 2003;120:827–36.
213. Uddman R, Grunditz T, Sundler F. Neuropeptide Y. occurrence and distribution in dental pulps. Acta Odontol Scand 1984;42:361–5.
214. Wakisaka S, Ichikawa H, Akai M. Distribution and origins of peptide- and catecholamine-containing nerve fibres in the feline dental pulp and effects of cavity preparation on these nerve fibres. J Osaka Univ Dent Sch 1986;26:17–28.
215. Wakisaka S, Ichikawa H, Nishikawa S, et al. Immunohistochemical observation on the correlation between substance P- and vasoactive intestinal polypeptide-like immunoreactivities in the feline dental pulp. Arch Oral Biol 1987;32:449–53.
216. El Karim IAM, Lamey PJM, Ardill JM, et al. Vasoactive intestinal polypeptide (VIP) and VPAC1 receptor in adult human dental pulp in relation to caries. Arch Oral Biol 2006.
217. Lewis T. The blood vessels of the human skin and their response. London: Shaw; 1927.
218. Awawdeh L, Lundy FT, Shaw C, et al. Quantitative analysis of substance P, neurokinin A and calcitonin gene-related peptide in pulp tissue from painful and healthy human teeth. Int Endod J 2002;35:30–6.
219. El Karim IA, Lamey PJ, Linden GJ, et al. Caries-induced changes in the expression of pulpal neuropeptide Y. Eur J Oral Sci 2006;114:133–7.
220. Haug SR, Heyeraas KJ. Modulation of dental inflammation by the sympathetic nervous system. J Dent Res 2006;85:488–95.
221. Rodd HD, Boissonade FM. Comparative immunohistochemical analysis of the peptidergic innervation of human primary and permanent tooth pulp. Arch Oral Biol 2002;47:375–85.
222. Byers MR, Taylor PE, Khayat BG, Kimberly CL. Effects of injury and inflammation on pulpal and periapical nerves. J Endod 1990;16:78–84.
223. Khayat BG, Byers MR, Taylor PE, et al. Responses of nerve fibers to pulpal inflammation and periapical lesions in rat molars demonstrated by calcitonin gene-related peptide immunocytochemistry. J Endod 1988;14:577–87.

224. Taylor PE, Byers MR. An immunocytochemical study of the morphological reaction of nerves containing calcitonin gene-related peptide to microabscess formation and healing in rat molars. Arch Oral Biol 1990;35:629–38.

225. Taylor PE, Byers MR, Redd PE. Sprouting of CGRP nerve fibers in response to dentin injury in rat molars. Brain Res 1988;461:371–6.

226. Caviedes-Bucheli J, Lombana N, Azuero-Holguin MM, Munoz HR. Quantification of neuropeptides (calcitonin gene-related peptide, substance P, neurokinin A, neuropeptide Y and vasoactive intestinal polypeptide) expressed in healthy and inflamed human dental pulp. Int Endod J 2006;39:394–400.

227. Fristad I, Vandevska-Radunovic V, Fjeld K, et al. NK1, NK2, NK3 and CGRP1 receptors identified in rat oral soft tissues, and in bone and dental hard tissue cells. Cell Tissue Res 2003;311:383–91.

228. Fristad I, Vandevska-Radunovic V, Kvinnsland IH. Neurokinin-1 receptor expression in the mature dental pulp of rats. Arch Oral Biol 1999;44:191–5.

229. Jacobsen EB, Heyeraas KJ. Effect of capsaicin treatment or inferior alveolar nerve resection on dentine formation and calcitonin gene-related peptide- and substance P-immunoreactive nerve fibres in rat molar pulp. Arch Oral Biol 1996;41:1121–31.

230. Fristad I, Kvinnsland IH, Jonsson R, Heyeraas KJ. Effect of intermittent long-lasting electrical tooth stimulation on pulpal blood flow and immunocompetent cells: a hemodynamic and immunohistochemical study in young rat molars. Experimental neurology 1997;146:230–9.

231. Csillag M, Berggreen E, Fristad I, et al. Effect of electrical tooth stimulation on blood flow and immunocompetent cells in rat dental pulp after sympathectomy. Acta Odontol Scand 2004;62:305–12.

232. Haug SR, Brudvik P, Fristad I, Heyeraas KJ. Sympathectomy causes increased root resorption after orthodontic tooth movement in rats: immunohistochemical study. Cell Tissue Res 2003;313:167–75.

CHAPTER 6

MORPHOLOGY OF TEETH AND THEIR ROOT CANAL SYSTEMS

BLAINE M. CLEGHORN, CHARLES J. GOODACRE, WILLIAM H. CHRISTIE

Successful root canal therapy requires a thorough knowledge of tooth anatomy and root canal morphology,[1,2] which may be quite variable within the norm. Root canal system anomalies rarely occur outside the norm. Even the incidence of the various anomalous root anatomy forms within the adult human dentition can be quite variable.

For each tooth in the permanent dentition, there is a wide range of variation reported in the literative with respect to the frequency of occurrence of the number and the shape of canals in each root, the number of roots,[2-16] and the incidence of molar root fusion.[17-23]

A number of factors contribute to the variation found in these studies (Table 1). The root canal morphology of teeth is often extremely complex and highly variable[2,3,5,12,14-16] as illustrated in the 3D models of the maxillary first molar in Figures 1–3.[5] Variations also result due to ethnic background and age and gender of the population studied. The following is a description of the normal and the many variations in human tooth anatomy and root morphology as gleaned from the available literature.

The data generated from a specialty endodontic practice may not represent the frequency of incidence in a general population, as more complex cases are

Table 1 Factors Contributing to Variations Reported Studies Assessing Number of Canals	
Factor	**Reference**
Ethnic background	10,12,24–48
Age of patient	7,49–54
Gender	10,20,53
Source of teeth (specialty endodontic practice versus general practice)	55
Study design (in vivo versus in vitro)	56–58
In vitro methods for assessing number of canals	
Clearing studies	
Decalcification	9
India ink injection	6,10,17,56,59–62
Chinese ink injection	23
Hematoxylin dye injection	13
Plastic injection	18
Metal castings	7,63
In vitro endodontic access with radiography and instruments	24,64
Instruments only	62,65
In vitro radiopaque gel infusion and radiography	22
In vitro root canal treatment	66
In vitro radiography	50,51,67
In vitro macroscopic examination	19
In vitro scanning electron microscopy of pulp floor	54

Table 1 continued on page 152

	Table 1 continued from page 151
In vitro grinding and sectioning	4,8,58,68
In vitro clinical examination with 2 loupes, 8 SOM, and histological examination of root sections	69
In vivo methods for assessing number of canals	
Clinical evaluation during endodontic treatment using magnification or surgical operating telescope (SOM)	11,53,70,71
Endodontic treatment where magnification was not specified	57–59,72–80
Retrospective evaluation of patient records of root canal-treated teeth	11,49,73,81–83
Radiography of all teeth	21
In vivo radiographic examination	20,84,85
Definition of what constitutes a canal	
Separate orifice found on floor of pulp chamber	66
Two instruments placed into two mesiobuccal canals of a maxillary first molar to a minimum of 16 mm from a cusp of an intact tooth	58
One that can be instrumented to a depth of 3–4 mm	11
A treatable canal	53
Undefined in some studies	

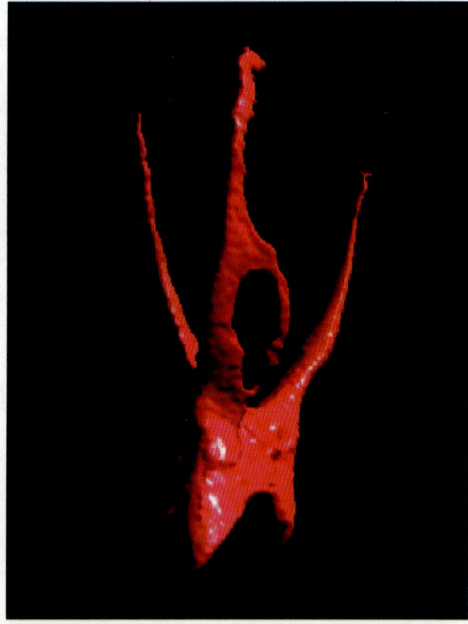

Figure 1 Mesiobuccal view of root canal system of a maxillary first molar (MB root canal system is centred); reprinted with permission from Brown P, Herbranson E. Dental Anatomy & 3D Tooth Atlas Version 3.0. Illinois: Quintessence, 2005: Maxillary First Molar- 3D Models 1. Unique Features.

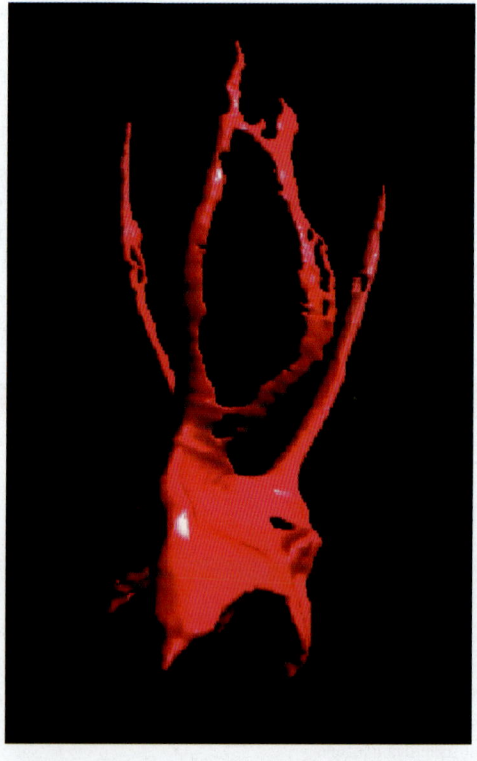

Figure 2 Mesiobuccal view of root canal system of a maxillary first molar (MB root canal system is centred); reprinted with permission from Brown P, Herbranson E. Dental Anatomy & 3D Tooth Atlas Version 3.0. Illinois: Quintessence, 2005: Maxillary First Molar- 3D Models 2. Bruce Fogel, UOP, Complex MB Root.

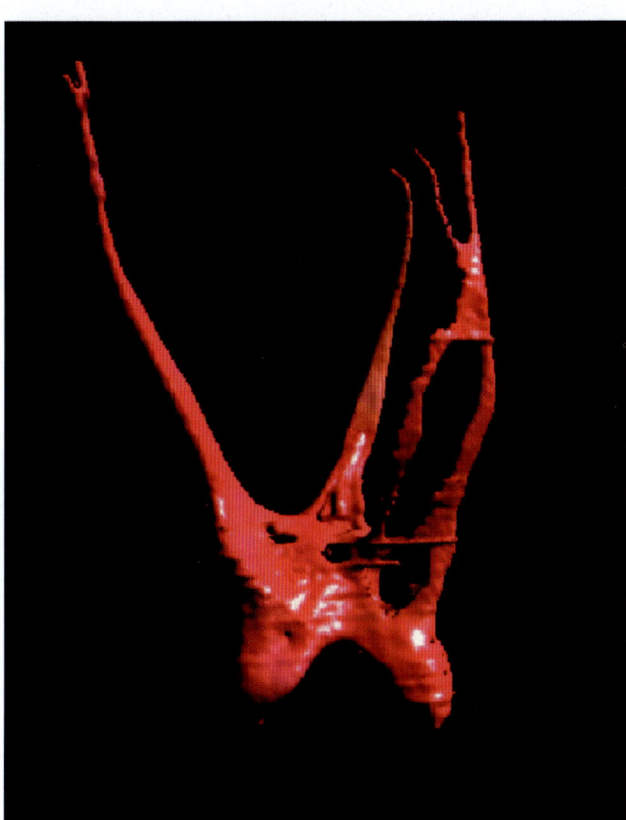

Figure 3 Mesial view of root canal system of a maxillary first molar (MB root canal system is far right). Reprinted with permission from Brown P, Herbranson E. Dental Anatomy & 3D Tooth Atlas Version 3.0. Illinois: Quintessence, 2005: Maxillary First Molar- 3D Models 3. Deep Distal Caries.

decalcification[9] injection with India ink,[6,10,17,25–29] Chinese ink,[23] hematoxylin dye,[13] plastic[18] or metal castings,[7,30] in vitro endodontic access with radiography and instruments[31,32] or instruments only,[29,33] in vitro radiopaque gel infusion and radiography,[22] in vitro root canal treatment (RCT),[34] in vitro radiography,[35–37] in vitro macroscopic examination,[19] scanning electron microscope examination of the pulp floor,[38] and grinding or sectioning.[4,8,39,40]

Clinical methods include evaluation of endodontic access openings during endodontic treatment using magnification or a surgical operating microscope (SOM),[11,41–43] or during endodontic treatment where magnification was not specified,[26,39,44–53] or retrospective evaluation of patient records of endodontically treated teeth only[11,45,54–57] or radiography of all teeth,[21] and *in vivo* radiographic examination.[20,58,59]

All of these factors contribute to variations in the reported results. There can also be variations in the number of canals reported, due to the authors' definition of what constitutes a canal. A separate canal is defined in some studies as a separate orifice found on the floor of the pulp chamber,[34] two instruments placed simultaneously into two mesiobuccal canals of a maxillary first molar to a minimum depth of 16 mm from the cusp of an intact tooth,[39] one that can be instrumented to a depth of 3–4 mm[11] or an analysis of treatable canals in retrospective clinical studies.[42] Other studies fail to provide a clear definition of what defines a canal in their reported data.

In 1969, Weine et al.[40] provided the first clinical classification of more than one canal system in a single root and used the mesiobuccal root of the maxillary first molar as the type specimen. Pineda and Kuttler[36] and Vertucci[13] further developed a system for canal anatomy classification for any tooth having a broad buccolingual diameter and more applicable for use in laboratory studies (Figure 4). All canal types reported in this chapter are based on the Vertucci classification. Additional canal types not included in Vertucci's original classification system

more likely to be referred,[24] thus skewing the sample reported in some clinical studies. Differences in reported results may also be due to the study design (clinical radiographs versus laboratory, gross morphology, or microscopic).[25] There is also a wide variety of methods used in these studies. These laboratory methods include various types of clearing studies using

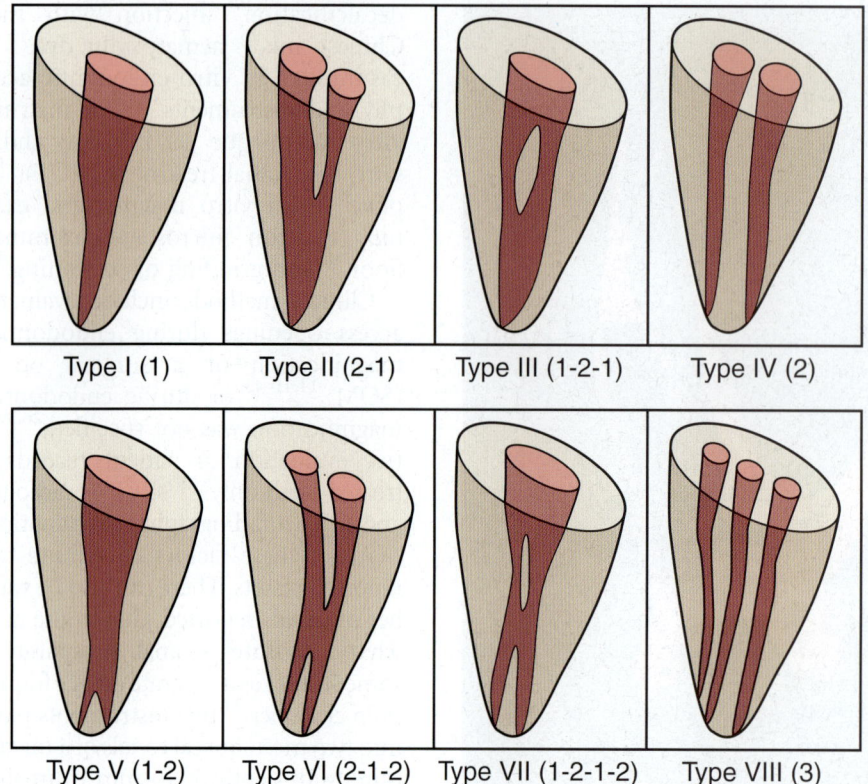

Figure 4 Vertucci's Classification of Root Canal Systems (Types I–Type VIII).

have been reported by Sert and Bayirli[10] (Figure 5) and Gulabivala et al.[60] Sert and Bayirli reported an additional 14 new canal types that have not yet been classified.[10]

Vertucci found the proximity of the canal orifices to each other as indicative of whether they joined or remained as separate canals.[13] If the separation of the orifices was greater than 3 mm, the canals tended to remain separate through their entire length. In contrast, canals usually joined together if the orifices were less than 3 mm apart. Canals were found to join more coronally as the distance between the orifices decreased.

Successful endodontic therapy is dependent on the cleaning, shaping, and obturation of the entire root canal system.[1,2] The presence of accessory canals and the ability to cleanse and seal these canals can also have an impact on prognosis.[61] Accessory canals include both lateral and furcation canals. These canals are smaller than the main canal but branch from the main canal through to the periodontium.[2,62] Pineda and Kuttler found that 30.6% of teeth had such ramifications. The majority of the ramifications or accessory canals were found in the apical third of the root.[36,61,63] Zolty and others have indicated that endodontic failure can be due to infected accessory canals.[61] Clinical studies have demonstrated that careful cleansing and sealing of the main canal and accessory canals, associated with lesions of endodontic origin, can result in healing of these defects.[61,64]

This chapter is intended to provide a review of the literature on the root and root canal morphology of each of the teeth in the permanent dentition from central incisor to second molar in both maxillary and mandibular arches. The permanent third molars have not been included in this review due to their high degree of variability of crown and root morphology. External root anatomy, canal numbers and types, and root canal system anatomy are described through a literature review of anatomical studies and case reports. The percentages reported in the tables may exceed 100% due to rounding of numbers to tenths or to incorrect tabulations from papers cited.

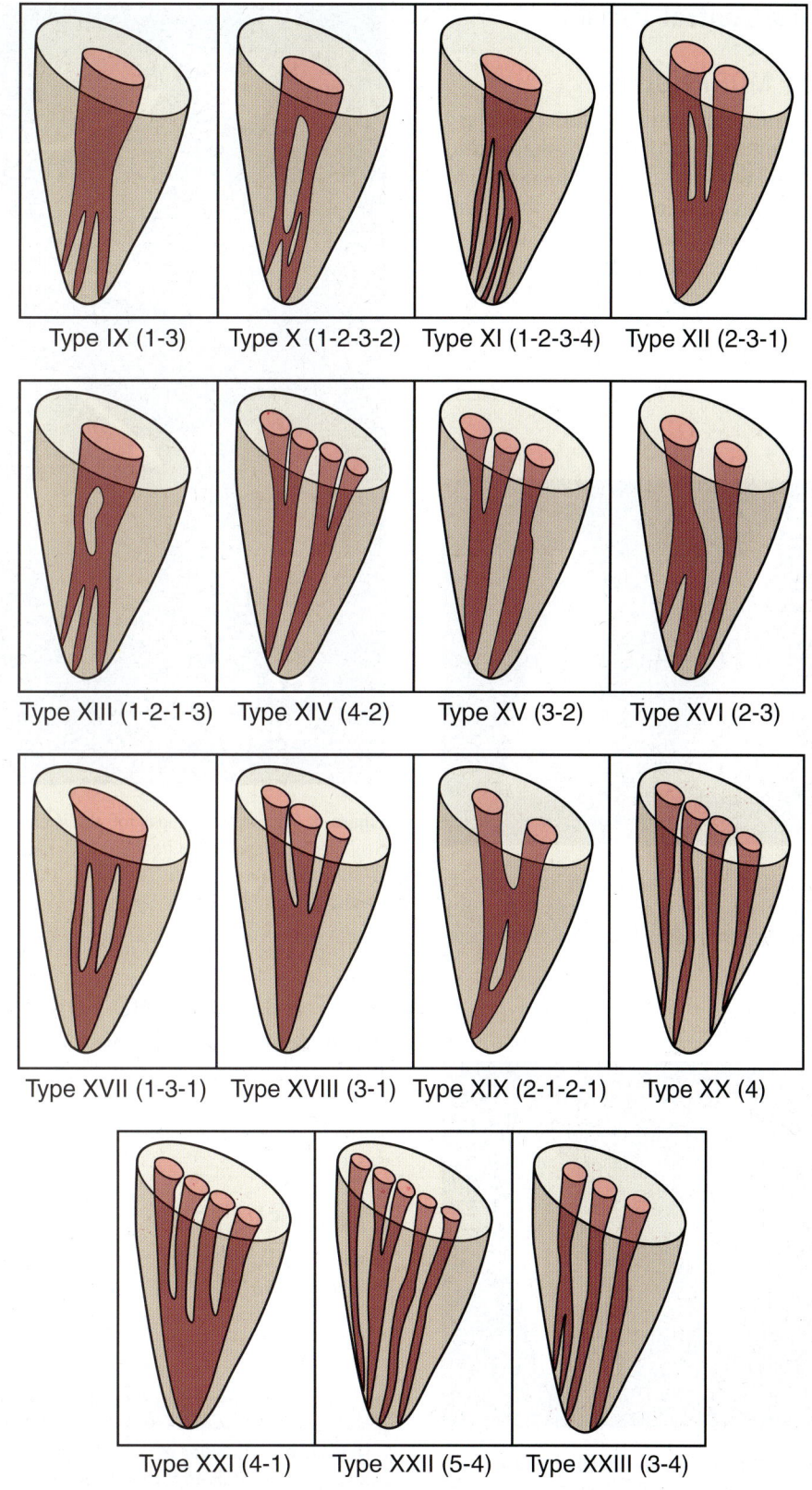

Figure 5 Sert and Bayirli's Additional Canal Types to Vertucci's Classification of Root Canal Systems (Types IX–Type XXIII).

Maxillary Central Incisor

EXTERNAL ROOT MORPHOLOGY
The cross-sectional root anatomy of the maxillary central incisor is triangular or ovoid in shape and tapers toward the lingual[3,5,12,14,16,65] as illustrated in Figures 6–8. Root concavities are normally not present in maxillary central incisors.[66] The root trunk is generally straight and tapers to a blunt apex. The overall average length of the maxillary central incisor is 23.5 mm with an average crown length of 10.5 mm and an average root length of 13 mm.[3]

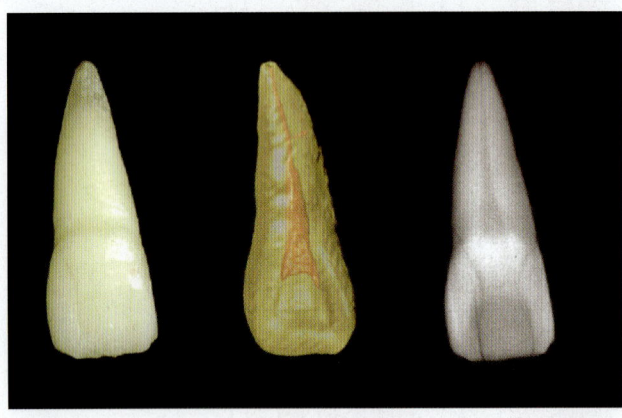

Figure 6 Labial view of maxillary right central incisor. Reprinted with permission from Brown P, Herbranson E. Dental Anatomy & 3D Tooth Atlas Version 3.0. Illinois: Quintessence, 2005: Maxillary Central Incisor-Rotations & Slices.

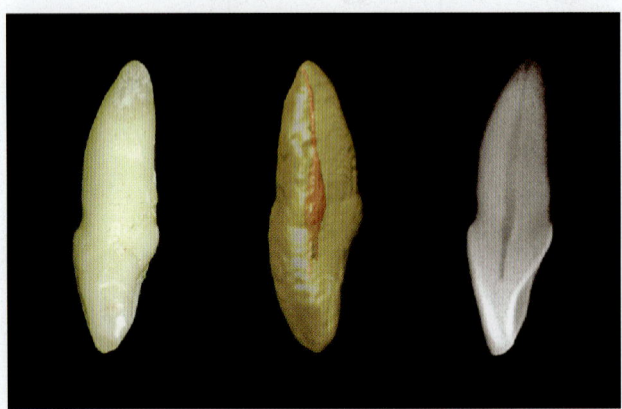

Figure 7 Mesial view of maxillary right central incisor. Reprinted with permission from Brown P, Herbranson E. Dental Anatomy & 3D Tooth Atlas Version 3.0. Illinois: Quintessence, 2005: Maxillary Central Incisor-Rotations & Slices.

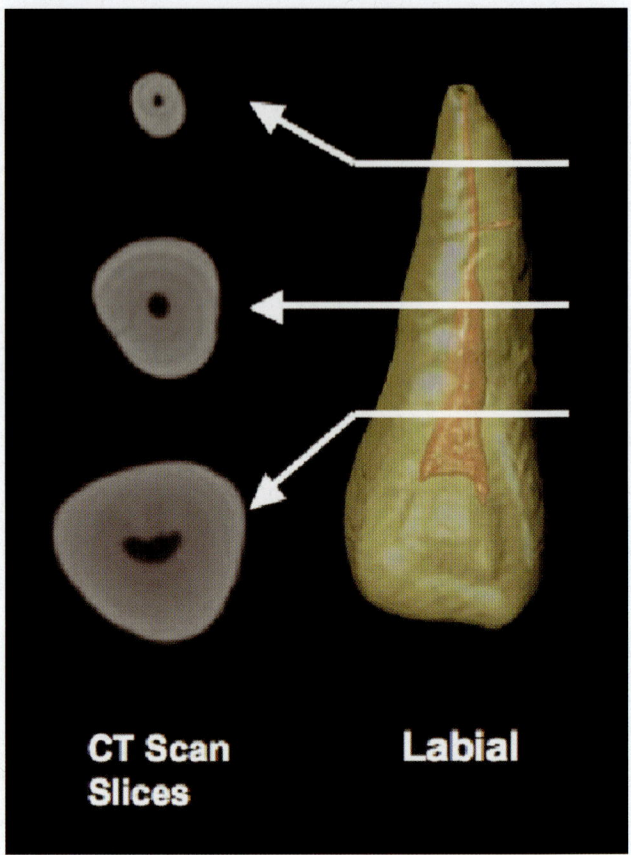

Figure 8 Root cross-sections of the maxillary right central incisor. Reprinted with permission from Brown P, Herbranson E. Dental Anatomy & 3D Tooth Atlas Version 3.0. Illinois: Quintessence, 2005: Maxillary Central Incisor- Rotations & Slices.

ROOT NUMBER AND FORM
The majority of anatomical studies found that the maxillary central incisor is a single-rooted tooth[4,6,10,13,36] (Table 2). A few case studies of anomalous root anatomy have reported more than one root or root canal system.[67–71]

CANAL SYSTEM
The maxillary central incisor is usually a single-root canal system[4,6,10,13,36] (Table 3). Mid-root and apical

Table 2 Maxillary Central Incisor			
Number of Roots	Number of Studies Cited	Number of Teeth	One Root
	5	721	100% (721)

Table 3 Maxillary Central Incisor

Number of Canals and Apices	Number of Studies Cited	Number of Teeth (Canal Studies)	One Canal	Two or More Canals	Number of Teeth (Apex Studies)	One Canal at Apex	Two or More Canals at Apex
	5	721	99.4% (717)	0.6% (4)	689	99.7% (687)	0.3% (2)

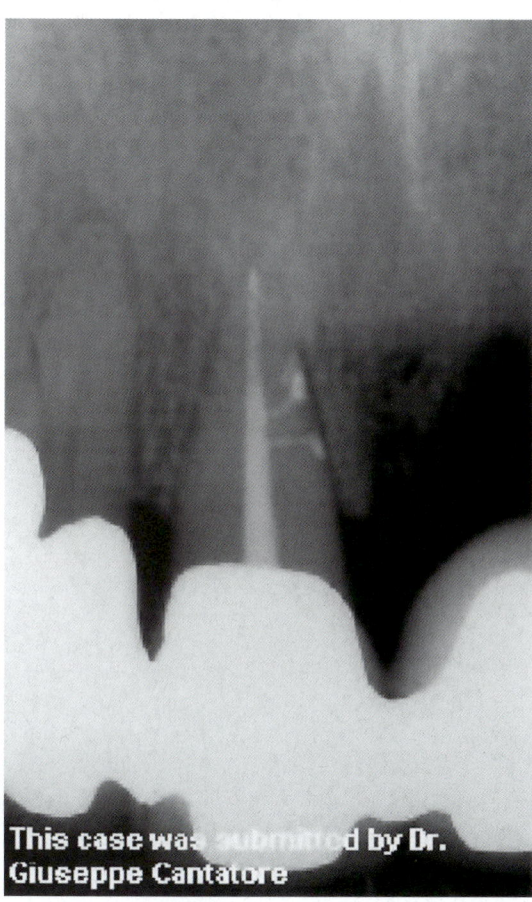

Figure 9 Maxillary right central incisor with normal anatomy; two mesial lateral canals are present. Reprinted with permission from Brown P, Herbranson E. Dental Anatomy & 3D Tooth Atlas Version 3.0. Illinois: Quintessence, 2005: Maxillary Central Incisor- X-ray Database.

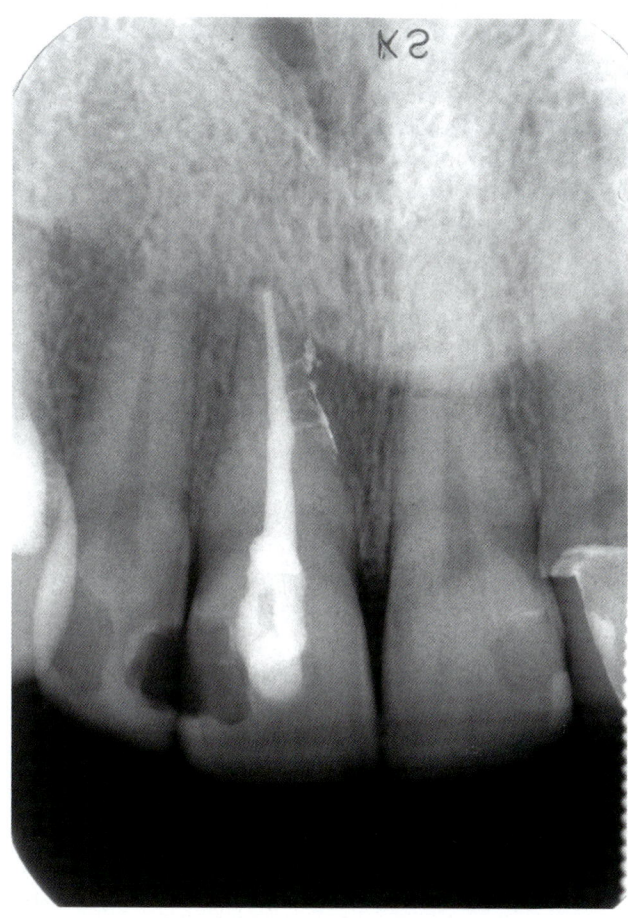

Figure 10 Maxillary right central incisor with normal anatomy; three mesial lateral canals are present. Courtesy of Dr. W.H. Christie.

lateral canals and apical delta canals are common, however (Figures 9 and 10). These lateral canals with small arterioles and venules serve as collateral circulation. When the pulp becomes diseased, Schilder referred to them as "portals of exit" into the surrounding periodontal ligament space.[64]

Relatively few studies have investigated the apical root anatomy of teeth. Altman et al.[72] investigated 20 extracted maxillary central incisors. On histological examination, accessory or lateral canals were found in three quarters of the specimens, exhibiting 1–4 accessory canals. One specimen was found to have 20 separate foramina but this anomalous canal anatomy occurred on a central incisor in a 9-year old individual. They concluded that radiographic examination was not accurate in diagnosing accessory canals and that resorptions, appositions, pulp stones, and accessory canals were commonly found in the apical 2.5 mm of the maxillary central incisors. Precise cleaning and shaping were therefore critically important.

The classic stereomicroscopic study of root apices by Green found that the average diameter of the major foramen in the 50 teeth studied was 0.4 mm while the accessory foramina were 0.2 mm in diameter. The average distance of the major apical foramen from the anatomical root apex was found to be 0.3 mm. Approximately 12% of the maxillary central incisors exhibited accessory foramina.[73]

Mizutani et al. investigated the anatomical location of the apical foramen in 30 maxillary central incisors.[74] The root apex and the apical foramen were displaced distolabially in the majority of the specimens. The coincidence of the apical foramen and the root apex was found in only one out of six specimens.

Kasahara et al.[75] assessed the apical anatomy of 510 extracted maxillary central incisors. Apical ramifications were found in 12.3% (62/510) or one-eighth of the teeth in the study. Lateral canals were present in 49.1% (247/510) or approximately half of the specimens. Only 38.6% (194/510) of the teeth had a simple main canal without lateral canals or apical ramifications. Ninety percent of the foramina in this study were located within 1.0 mm of the anatomical apex.

VARIATIONS AND ANOMALIES

Ethnic variations have been reported for some traits. Shovel-shaped incisor crowns are a common feature in Asian* populations but are relatively rare in Caucasian population.[12,76–81]

A study by Pecora and Cruz Filho[82] assessed the incidence of radicular grooves in the maxillary incisors of 642 patients (Table 4). Loss of periodontal attachment associated with these grooves can result in a deep, narrow, vertical periodontal pocket. The prognosis, even with combined periodontal–endodontic treatment in such cases, can be poor.[83] The incidence of radicular grooves was found to be 0.9% in the maxillary central incisors and 3.0% in the maxillary lateral incisors. Reports of other types of anomalies associated with the maxillary central incisor are relatively uncommon.

Table 4 Maxillary Central Incisor		
Number of Studies Cited	Number of Patients	Radicular Grooves
1	642	0.9% (6)

*Adjective of or relating to the division of Humankind including the indigenous people of East Asia, South East Asia and the Arctic regions of North America, characterestically having dark eyes, straight hair, pale ivory to dark skin, and little facial or body hair.

Table 5 Maxillary Central Incisor			
Number of Studies Cited	Number of Teeth	Fusion	Gemination
1	534	2.6% (14)	0.94% (5)

The prevalence of fusion and gemination was assessed by Hamasha and Al-Khateeb in a Jordanian population.[84] The prevalence of fusion was found to be 2.6%, while gemination was found in 0.94% of the samples for a total incidence of 3.6% of the so-called "double teeth" (Table 5). The maxillary central incisor had the highest incidence of fusion and gemination of all permanent teeth.

Al Nazhan[85] reported a case of a central incisor with enamel hypoplasia and two canals in a single root. Examples of fusion with a supernumerary tooth,[84,86–88] fusion with a maxillary lateral incisor,[89] gemination,[84,86,90,91] talon cusps,[90–94] two canals,[95,96] dens invaginatus[97] (Figures 11 and 12), and maxillary central incisors with

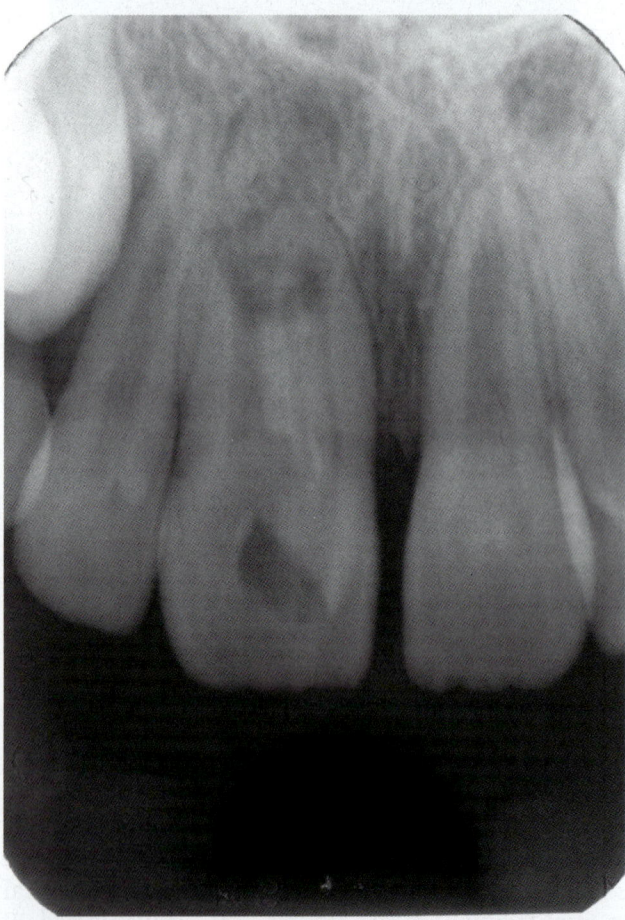

Figure 11 Dens invaginatus Type 3; three-canal maxillary right central incisor. Courtesy of Dr. W.H. Christie.

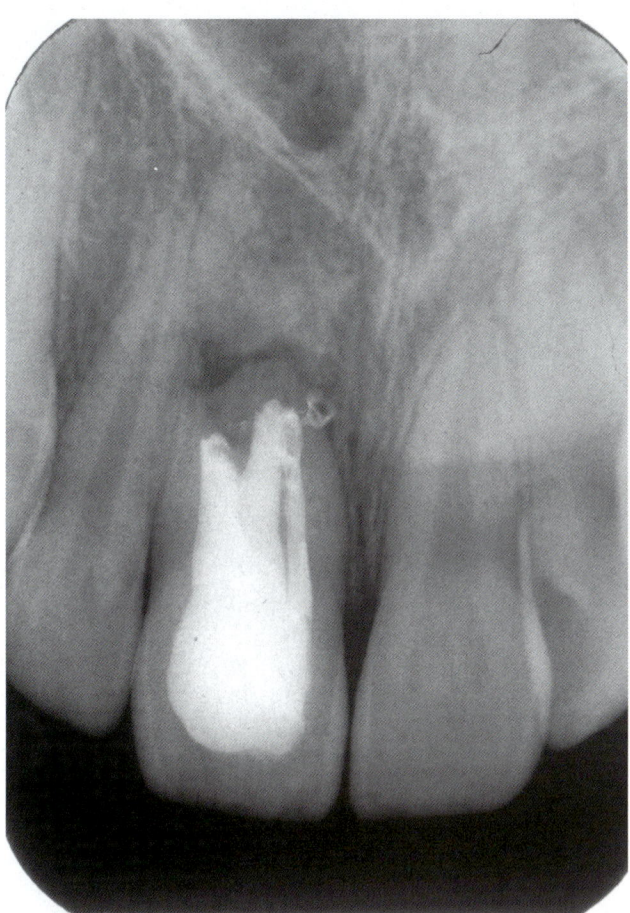

Figure 12 Dens invaginatus Type 3; three-canal maxillary right central incisor. Courtesy of Dr. W.H. Christie. (Same case as Figure 11 after completion of non-surgical root canal therapy).

Maxillary Lateral Incisor

EXTERNAL ROOT MORPHOLOGY

The cross-sectional root anatomy of the maxillary lateral incisor is described as being circular, oval, or ovoid in shape and tapers toward the lingual as illustrated in Figures 13–15.[3,5,12,14,16,65,74] Root concavities are normally not present on the root of the maxillary lateral incisors.[66] The root trunk is generally smaller than a central incisor and has a finer root tip,

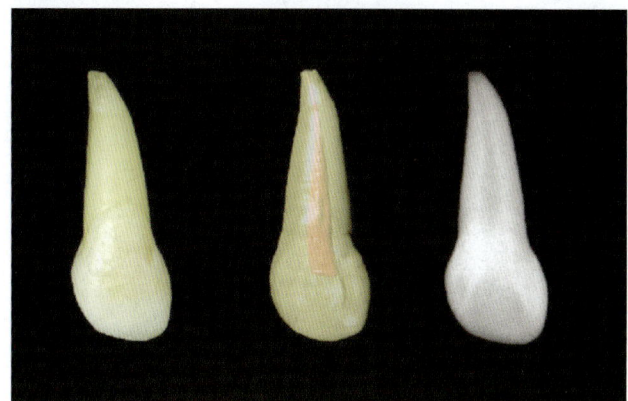

Figure 13 Labial view of maxillary right lateral incisor. Reprinted with permission from Brown P, Herbranson E. Dental Anatomy & 3D Tooth Atlas Version 3.0. Illinois: Quintessence, 2005: Maxillary Lateral Incisor-Rotations & Slices.

two roots[67–71,98] are occasionally documented in case reports. A single case of gemination and fusion with a supernumerary tooth resulting in a tooth with three canals was reported by Hosomi et al.[99]

An unusual combination of anomalies was reported by Lorena et al.[100] Anomalies in the maxillary arch included shovel-shaped incisors, dens invaginatus, peg-shaped supernumerary teeth, and Carabelli cusps on the maxillary first molars in the absence of any developmental anomaly. McNamara also reported a combination of anomalies that included maxillary central and lateral incisors that had talon cusps, short roots and dens invaginatus, premolars with short roots and Carabelli cusps on the maxillary first and second molars.[101] A rare case of a labial talon cusp on a maxillary central incisor was reported by de Sousa et al.[93]

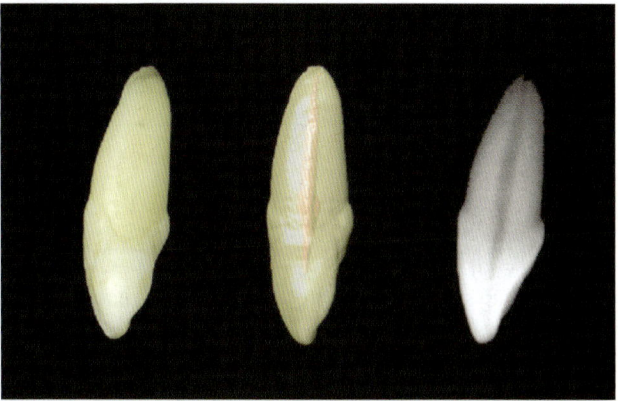

Figure 14 Mesial view of maxillary right lateral incisor. Reprinted with permission from Brown P, Herbranson E. Dental Anatomy & 3D Tooth Atlas Version 3.0. Illinois: Quintessence, 2005: Maxillary Lateral Incisor-Rotations & Slices.

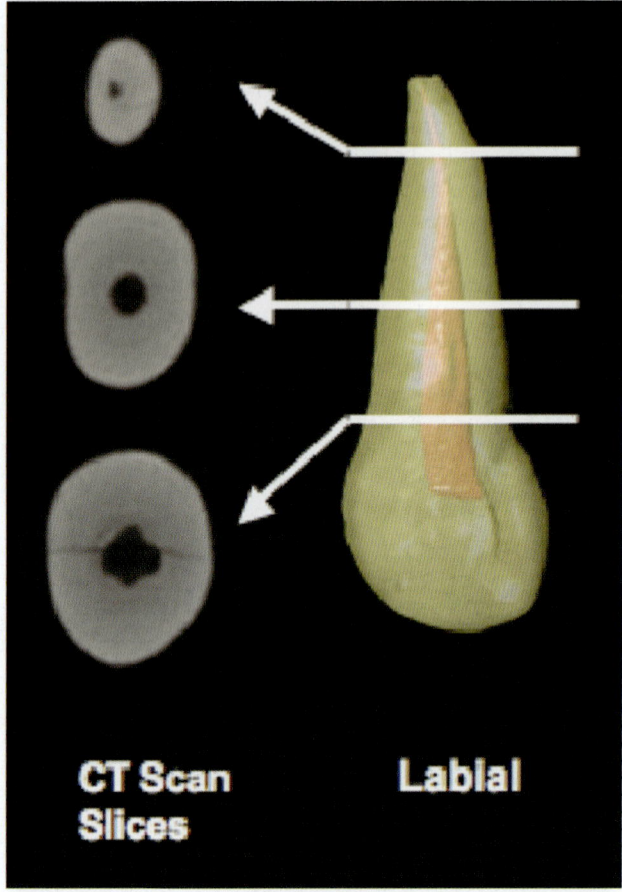

Figure 15 Root cross-sections of the maxillary right lateral incisor. Reprinted with permission from Brown P, Herbranson E. Dental Anatomy & 3D Tooth Atlas Version 3.0. Illinois: Quintessence, 2005: Maxillary Lateral Incisor- Rotations & Slices.

often terminating in a curve to the distal or the lingual, or both (Figures 13–16). The overall average length of the maxillary lateral incisor is 22 mm with an average crown length of 9 mm and an average root length of 13 mm.[3]

ROOT NUMBER AND FORM

Anatomical studies indicate that the maxillary lateral incisors are single-rooted, virtually 100% of the time,[4,6,10,13,36] as listed in Table 6. However, numerous case reports demonstrate significant variability in anatomy. Most reported cases of two-rooted maxillary lateral incisors are a result of fusion or gemination and are usually associated with a macrodont crown. There are a few reported cases of two roots associated with normal crown dimensions.[102–104] Anomalous two-rooted maxillary lateral incisors are usually associated with a developmental radicular lingual groove.

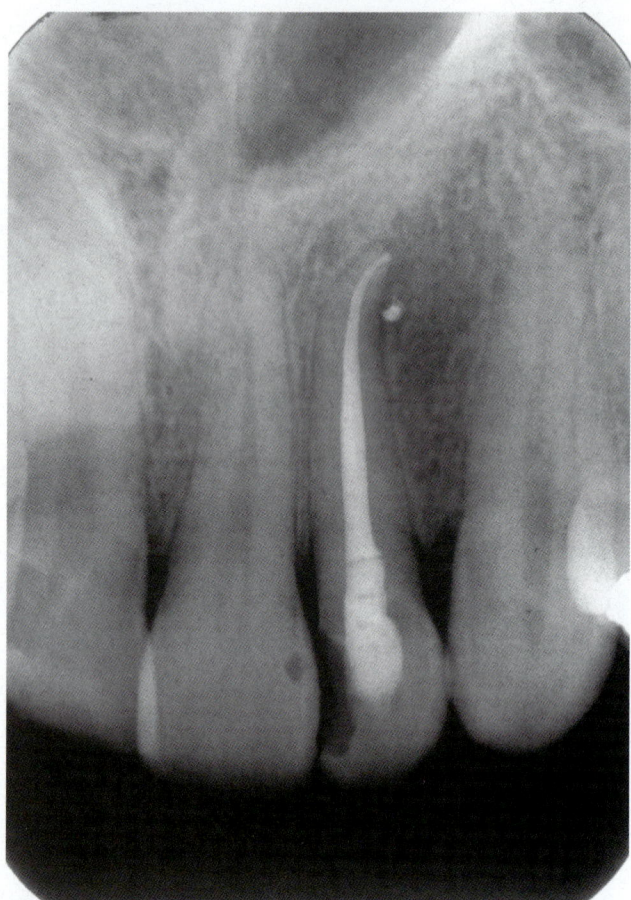

Figure 16 Maxillary left lateral incisor with moderate "J-shape" apical curvature. Courtesy of Dr. W.H. Christie.

Table 6	Maxillary Lateral Incisors		
Number of Roots	Number of Studies Cited	Number of Teeth	One Root
	6	757	100% (757)

CANAL SYSTEM

The maxillary lateral incisor usually presents with a single canal[4,6,10,13,36] as demonstrated by the anatomical studies listed in Table 7. Mizutani et al. investigated the anatomical location of the apical foramen in 30 maxillary lateral incisors.[74] The root apex and the apical foramen were displaced distolingually in a majority of the specimens. Displacements in all directions were also found in the study. The coincidence of the apical foramen and the root apex was found in only two (6.7%) of the specimens. Therefore, the exploration of the apical foramen and the constriction, with a

Table 7	Maxillary Lateral Incisors						
Number of Canals and Apices	Number of Studies Cited	Number of Teeth (Canal Studies)	One Canal	Two or More Canals	Number of Teeth (Apex Studies)	One Canal at Apex	Two or More Canals at Apex
	6	757	93.4% (707)	6.6% (50)	725	98.9% (717)	1.1% (8)

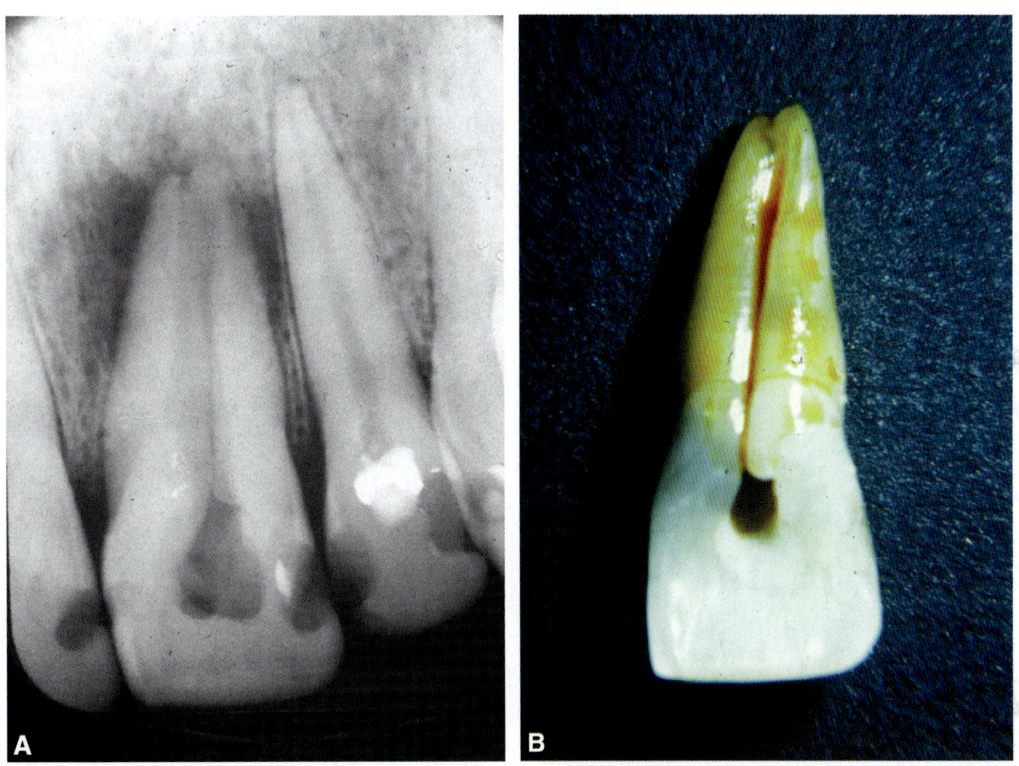

Figure 17 Radicular developmental palatogingival groove. **A,** Radiograph show lesion resulting from bacterial access along groove. **B,** Extracted tooth shows extent of groove. Courtesy, D.S. August.

fine precurved #10 size file tip and the electronic apex locator, is essential to locate the foramen.

The stereomicroscopic study of root apices by Green found that the average diameter of the major foramen in the 50 maxillary lateral incisors studied was 0.4 mm, while the accessory foramina were 0.2 mm in diameter. The average distance of the major apical foramen from the anatomical root apex was found to be 0.3 mm. Approximately 10% of the maxillary lateral incisors exhibited accessory foramina.[73]

VARIATIONS AND ANOMALIES

Maxillary lateral incisors often present anomalous anatomy resulting in diagnostic and treatment challenges. Complications resulting from radicular grooves have been well documented by Simon et al.[83] The incidence of radicular grooves is 3.0% in maxillary lateral incisors (Figure 17) in a study by Pecora and Cruz Filho,[82] as listed in Table 8, and there are several case reports in the literature

Table 8	Maxillary Lateral Incisors	
Number of Studies Cited	Number of Patients	Radicular Grooves
1	642	3.0% (19)

confirming the high probability of this finding.[105–111] Peikoff and Trott reported an endodontic failure in a maxillary lateral incisor with an accessory root and a radicular groove.[112]

An SEM investigation of 14 extracted maxillary lateral incisors with radicular grooves concluded that direct communication between the groove and the pulp was evident in these specimens and that accessory canals were the primary mechanism of communication between the periodontium and the pulp.[113] As with maxillary central incisors, the degree of shovel-shaped feature of the crown is varied and is often based on the ethnic background. Again, this feature is common in Asian populations and rare in Caucasian populations.[12,76,77,79–81] Reports of this and other coronal anomalies associated with the maxillary lateral incisor are common. Dens invaginatus or *dens in dente*[93,107,114–136] can be present in various forms.

Oehlers[137] classified dens invaginatus into three types based on the severity of the defect. Type 1 dens invaginatus is an invagination confined to the crown. Type 2 extends past the cementoenamel junction but does not involve periapical tissues. The most severe form and the most complex to treat is the Type 3 defect. The invagination extends past the cementoenamel junction and may result in a second apical foramen. A combination of nonsurgical and surgical therapy is often used to successfully treat Type 2 and Type 3 cases.[107,114,116–118,122–125,128,129,131,136,138] Nonsurgical management of the dens invaginatus, including the more severe Type 3 defects, has also been reported.[107,115,119–121,126,130,132–135] Occasionally, vitality of the pulp in the main canal has been shown to be maintained while treating (surgically, nonsurgically, or both) the accessory canal system, when there has been no communication between the two.[119,123,124,127,132]

There are reports of maxillary lateral incisors with fusion with a supernumerary tooth,[139–143] fusion with a maxillary central incisor,[89] gemination (Figure 18),[138,144–146] two roots (Figure 19),[102–104,107]

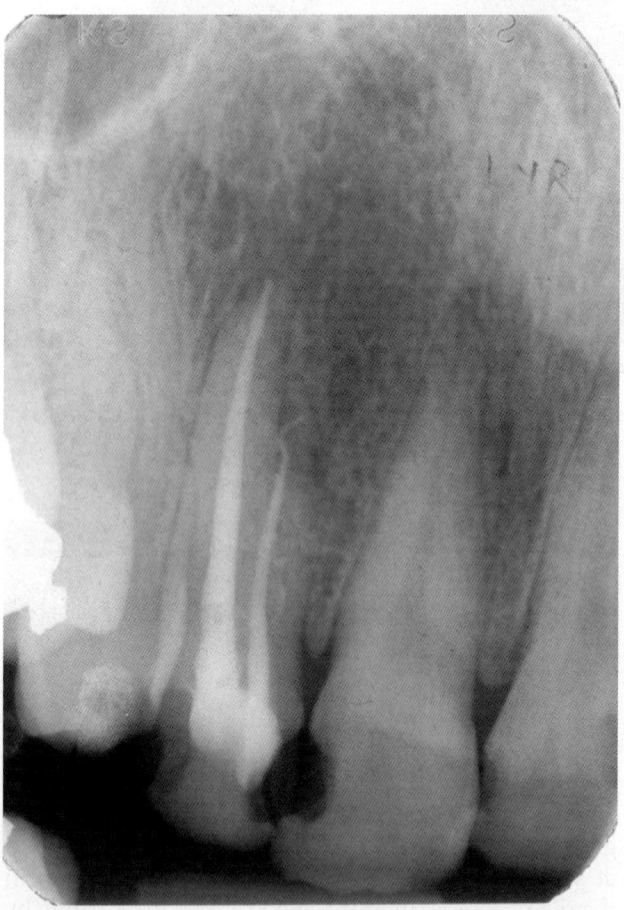

Figure 18 Gemination of a maxillary right lateral incisor. Courtesy of Dr. W.H. Christie.

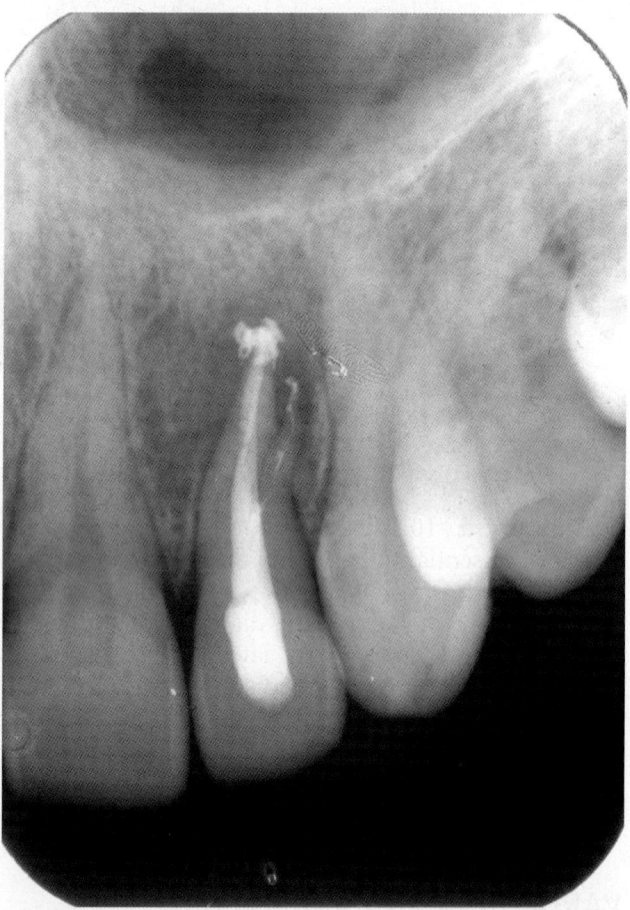

Figure 19 Accessory root with sealer filling in the canal space on the distal of a maxillary left lateral incisor. Courtesy of Dr. M.D. Peikoff.

dens evaginatus,[147,148] two canals in a single root,[96] and anomalies where gemination, fusion, or dens invaginatus could not be determined.[149,150] Mupparapu[151] reported a rare finding of both dens invaginatus and dens evaginatus associated with one maxillary lateral incisor.

Maxillary Canine

EXTERNAL ROOT MORPHOLOGY

The root of the maxillary canine is oval in shape and tapers toward the lingual as illustrated in Figures 20–22.[2,3,5,12,14,16,65] The root is wider labiolingually and is the longest root in the dentition, averaging approximately 17 mm in length.[3] Prominent developmental depressions can be present on both its mesial and distal surfaces, especially in the middle third of the root, as shown in Figures 21 and 22.[3,5] The root tip may be blunt or it may end in a fine, often curved tip (see Figures 20–22). The overall average length of the maxillary canine is 27 mm with an average crown length of 10 mm and an average root length of 17 mm.[3]

ROOT NUMBER AND FORM

Most studies have found that the maxillary canine has a single root 100% of the time,[4,6,10,13,36,152] as shown by the anatomical studies in Table 9. There are,

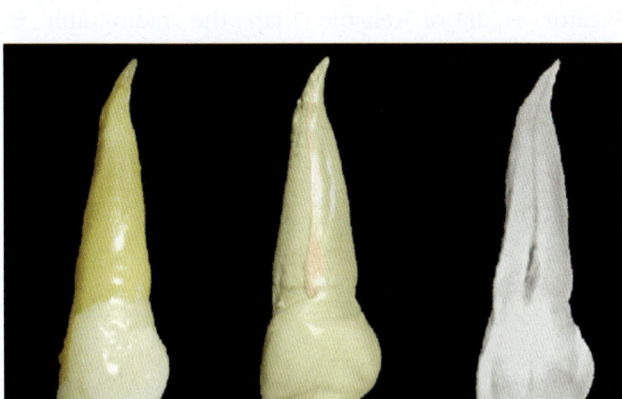

Figure 20 Labial view of maxillary left canine. Reprinted with permission from Brown P, Herbranson E. Dental Anatomy & 3D Tooth Atlas Version 3.0. Illinois: Quintessence, 2005: Maxillary Canines- Rotations & Slices.

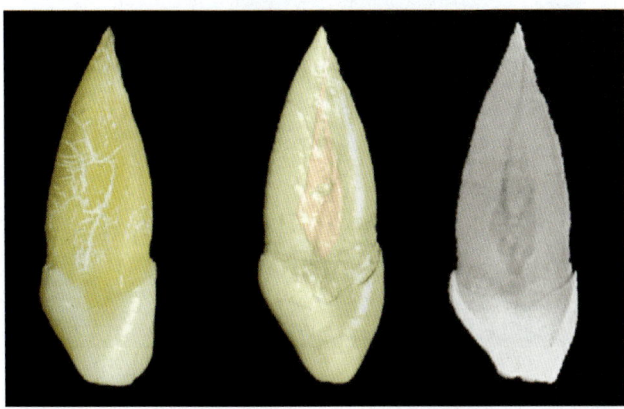

Figure 21 Mesial view of maxillary left canine. Reprinted with permission from Brown P, Herbranson E. Dental Anatomy & 3D Tooth Atlas Version 3.0. Illinois: Quintessence, 2005: Maxillary Canines- Rotations & Slices.

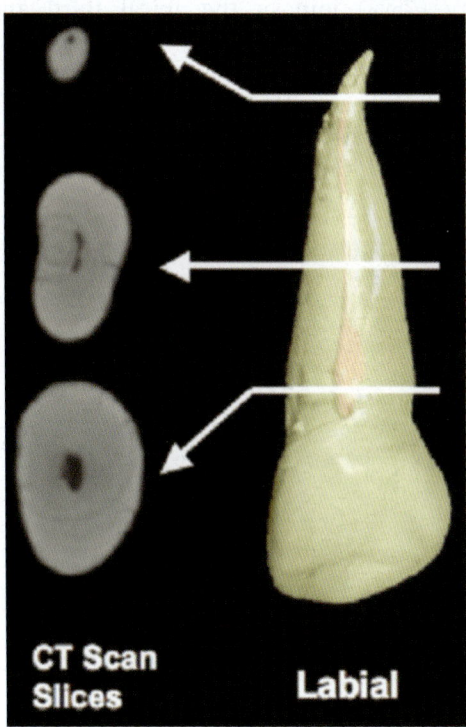

Figure 22 Root cross-sections of the maxillary left canine. Reprinted with permission from Brown P, Herbranson E. Dental Anatomy & 3D Tooth Atlas Version 3.0. Illinois: Quintessence, 2005: Maxillary Canine- Rotations & Slices.

Table 9 Maxillary Canine			
Number of Roots	Number of Studies Cited	Number of Teeth	One Root
	6	777	100% (777)

Table 10	Maxillary Canine						
Number of Canals and Apices	Number of Studies Cited	Number of Teeth (Canal Studies)	One Canal	Two or More Canals	Number of Teeth (Apex Studies)	One Canal at Apex	Two or More Canals at Apex
	5	777	96.5% (750)	3.5% (27)	745	98.8% (736)	1.2% (9)

however, rare case reports of two-rooted maxillary canines.[153,154]

CANAL SYSTEM

The maxillary canine usually has a single canal (Figures 23 and 24). A small percentage of maxillary canines have two canals (3.5%), as listed in Table 10.[4,6,10,13,36,152] Of those having two canals, the majority (75%) join in the apical third and exit through a single foramen. Accessory (lateral) canals are not uncommon and become evident radiographically after the completion of RCT (Figures 23–25). The majority of lateral canals occur in the apical third of the tooth (see Figures 23 and 24), but midroot lateral canals can also occur (see Figure 25). Mizutani et al. investigated the anatomical location of the apical foramen in 30 maxillary canines.[74] The root apex and the apical foramen were displaced distolabially in the majority of the specimens. The coincidence of the apical foramen and the root apex was found in only five (16.7%) of the specimens. The use of the electronic apex locator is more reliable than the radiograph in

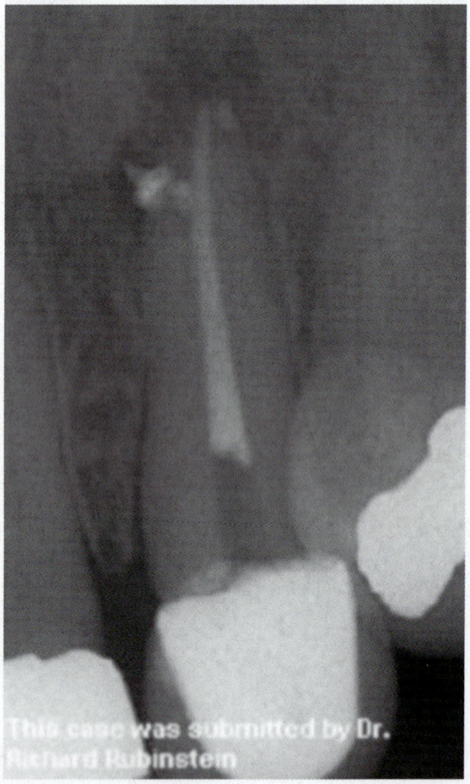

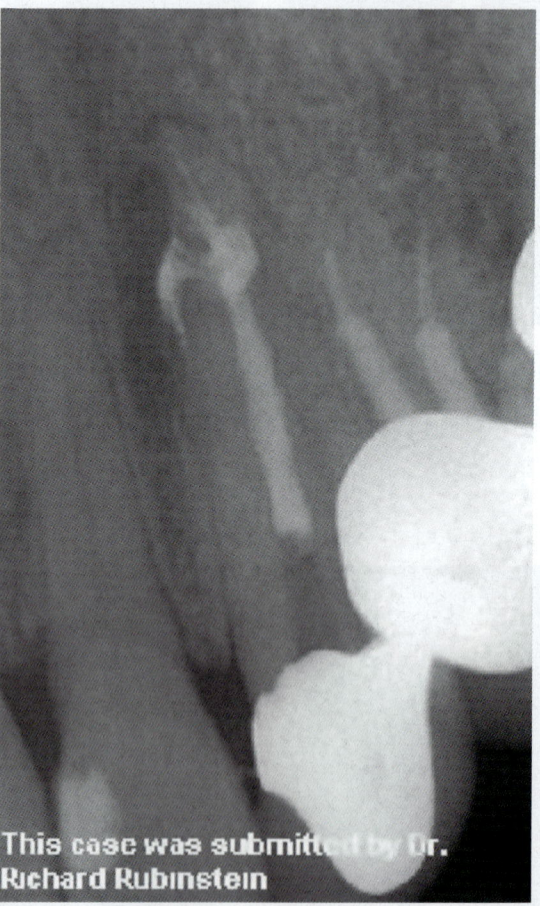

Figure 23 Maxillary left canine with normal anatomy and a mesial and apical lateral canal in the apical third. Reprinted with permission from Brown P, Herbranson E. Dental Anatomy & 3D Tooth Atlas Version 3.0. Illinois: Quintessence, 2005: Maxillary Canine- X-ray Database.

Figure 24 Maxillary left canine with normal anatomy and numerous lateral canals on the mesial aspect of the root. Reprinted with permission from Brown P, Herbranson E. Dental Anatomy & 3D Tooth Atlas Version 3.0. Illinois: Quintessence, 2005: Maxillary Canine- X-ray Database.

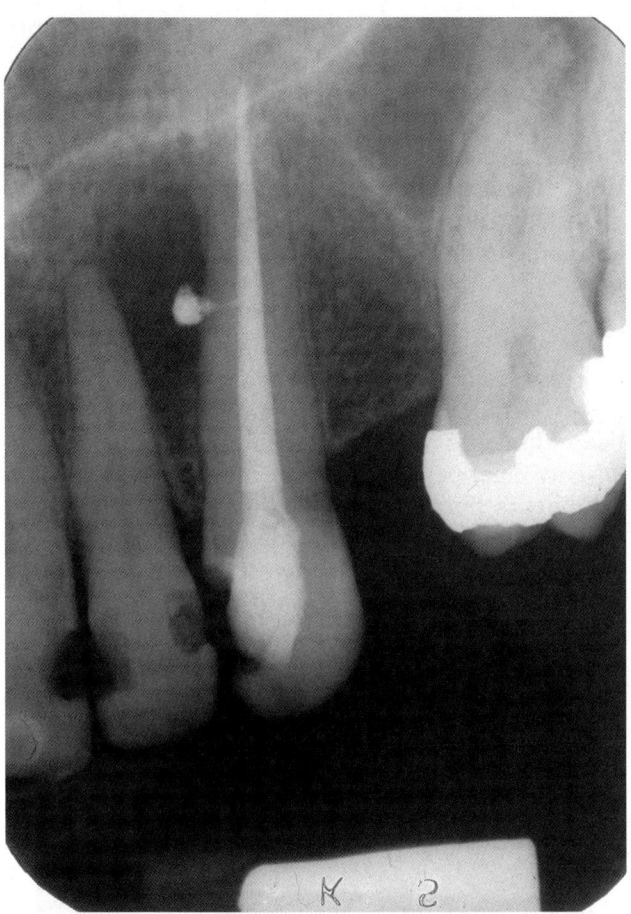

Figure 25 Maxillary left canine with large lateral canal on mesial aspect midroot. Courtesy of Dr. W.H. Christie.

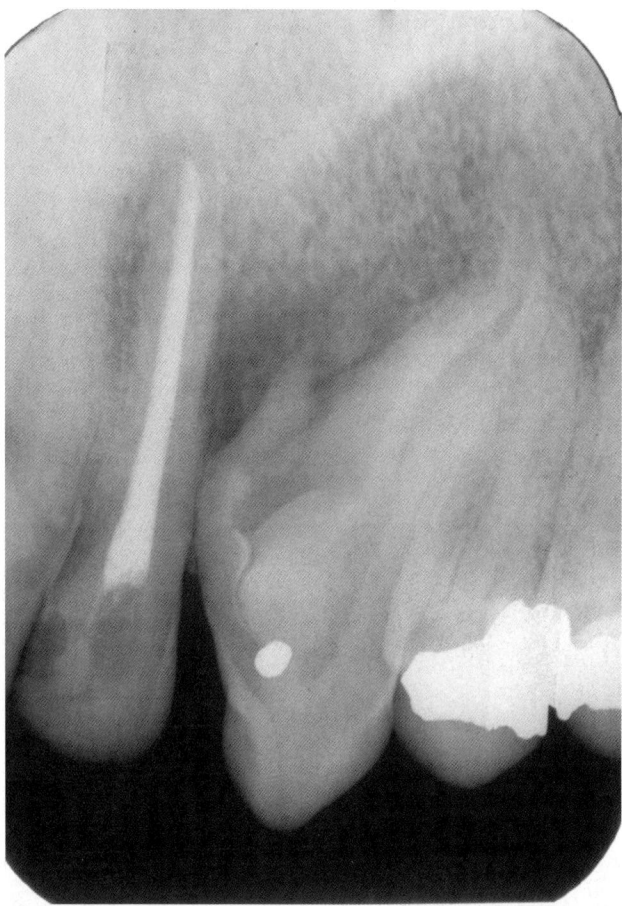

Figure 26 Maxillary left canine exhibiting radicular-form of dens invaginatus type 3. Pulp tests were vital on initial examination. Courtesy of Dr. W.H. Christie.

determining the apical foramen or the constriction in most canine teeth.

The study by Green on the root apices of permanent anterior teeth found that the average diameter of the major foramen in the 50 maxillary canines studied was 0.5 mm, while the accessory foramina were 0.2 mm in diameter. The average distance of the major apical foramen from the anatomical root apex was found to be 0.3 mm. Approximately 12% of the maxillary canines exhibited accessory foramina.[73]

VARIATIONS AND ANOMALIES

The maxillary canine usually presents few anatomical variations. When variations do occur, the root is more frequently affected than the crown. However, there are occasional reports in the literature of both coronal and radicular anomalies in the maxillary canine. The root can be dilacerated[15] or can have extreme variations in length.[2,3,5,12,15] One individual with an extremely long root length was reported by Booth in 1988 with canine teeth having an overall length of 41 mm.[155] This patient was a 5′2″, 31-year-old female of Dutch origin.

Dens evaginatus, when present, can take the form of a tubercle or a talon cusp, and is most frequently found on the lingual surface of the crown. There are also reports of labial tubercles.[156] The total incidence of dens evaginatus has been shown to be approximately 1% in an extensive literature review and a radiographic review of 15,000 anterior teeth by Dankner et al.[157] Between 1970 and 1995, there were only four case reports of dens evaginatus in the maxillary canine in their review. The radiographic survey of 15,000 anterior teeth found no occurrences of dens evaginatus in the maxillary canine.

Other variations reported in the literature include case reports with two canals in a single root,[158] two roots,[153,154] dens invaginatus[97,147,159] (Figure 26), and bilateral, supernumerary canines in a nonsyndrome case.[160]

Maxillary First Premolar

EXTERNAL ROOT MORPHOLOGY

The root anatomy of the maxillary premolar can vary depending on whether one, two, or three roots are present (Figures 27–34). The more common two-rooted form is illustrated in Figures 27–30. There are some common features to the various forms. The overall length of the maxillary first premolar is 22.5 mm with an average crown length of 8.5 mm and an average root length of 14 mm.[3]

Prominent root concavities are present on both the mesial and the distal surfaces of the root. The mesial root concavity is more prominent and extends onto the cervical third of the crown.[3,5,12,14,16,65,161] This results in a root that is broad buccolingually and narrow mesiodistally with a kidney shape when viewed in cross section at the cementoenamel junction.[3] These anatomical features have implications in restorative dentistry and in periodontal treatment, and are common areas for endodontic root perforations.

Gher and Vernino examined the external root shape as it related to the development of periodontal defects.[162] The palatal aspect of the buccal root tip of two-rooted maxillary first premolars usually has a deep longitudinal depression along its length. Seventy-eight percentage of the 45 teeth in their study exhibited a buccal furcation groove. They concluded that a buccal root furcation groove was a normal anatomical feature in these two-rooted maxillary first

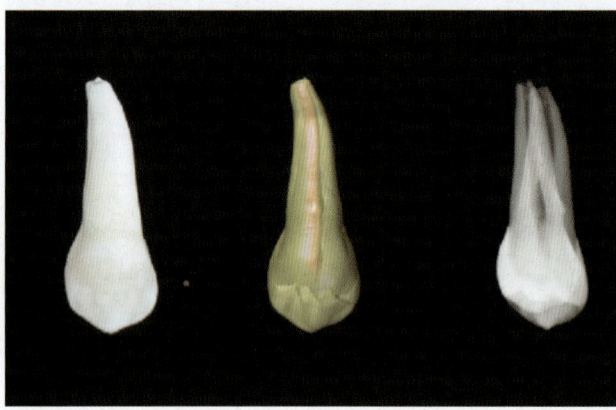

Figure 27 Buccal view of maxillary right first premolar. Reprinted with permission from Brown P, Herbranson E. Dental Anatomy & 3D Tooth Atlas Version 3.0. Illinois: Quintessence, 2005: Maxillary First Premolar- Rotations & Slices.

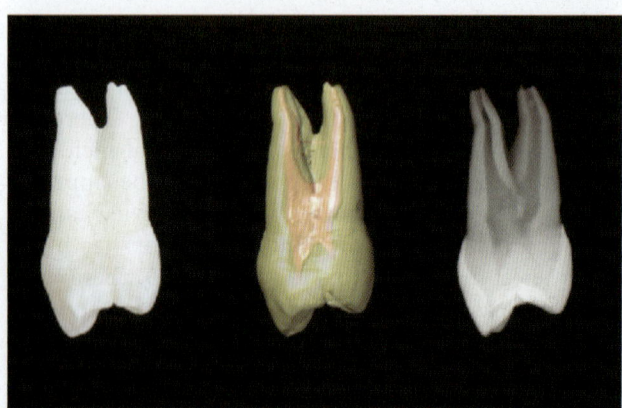

Figure 28 Mesial view of maxillary right first premolar. Reprinted with permission from Brown P, Herbranson E. Dental Anatomy & 3D Tooth Atlas Version 3.0. Illinois: Quintessence, 2005: Maxillary First Premolar- Rotations & Slices.

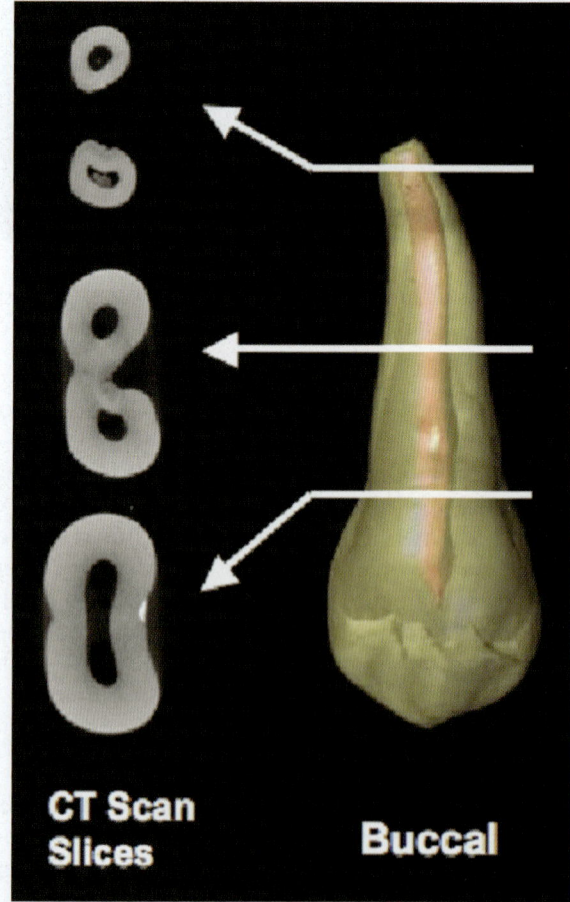

Figure 29 Root cross-sections of the maxillary right first premolar. Reprinted with permission from Brown P, Herbranson E. Dental Anatomy & 3D Tooth Atlas Version 3.0. Illinois: Quintessence, 2005: Maxillary First Premolar- Rotations & Slices.

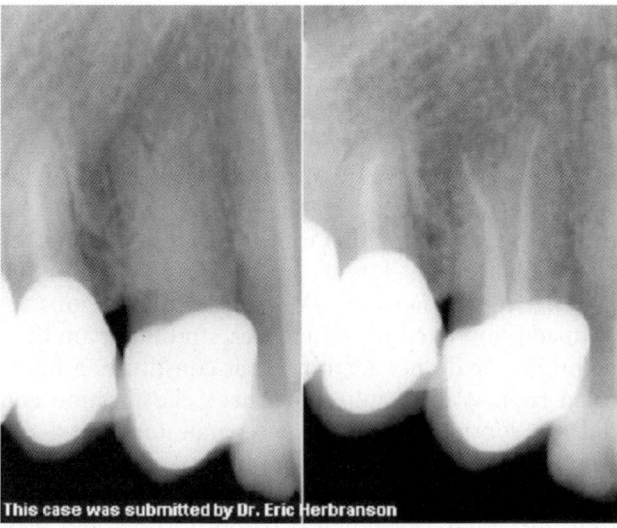

Figure 30 Maxillary right first premolar exhibiting two roots and two canals. Reprinted with permission from Brown P, Herbranson E. Dental Anatomy & 3D Tooth Atlas Version 3.0. Illinois: Quintessence, 2005: Maxillary First Premolar- X-ray Database.

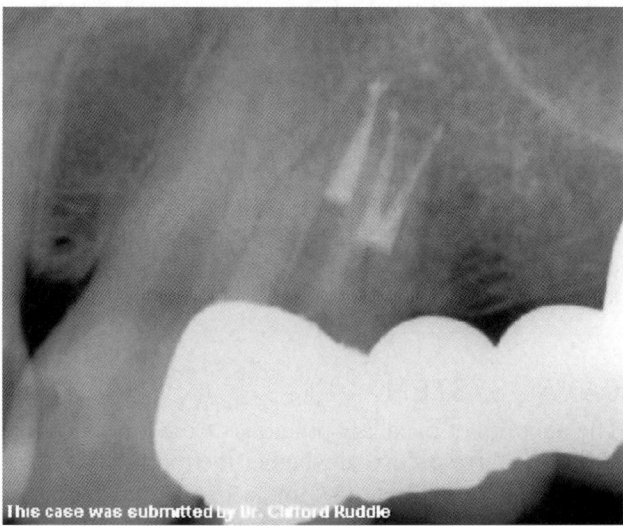

Figure 31 Maxillary left first premolar with two fused buccal roots, a lingual root and three canals (MB, DB and Palatal). Reprinted with permission from Brown P, Herbranson E. Dental Anatomy & 3D Tooth Atlas Version 3.0. Illinois: Quintessence, 2005: Maxillary First Premolar- X-ray Database.

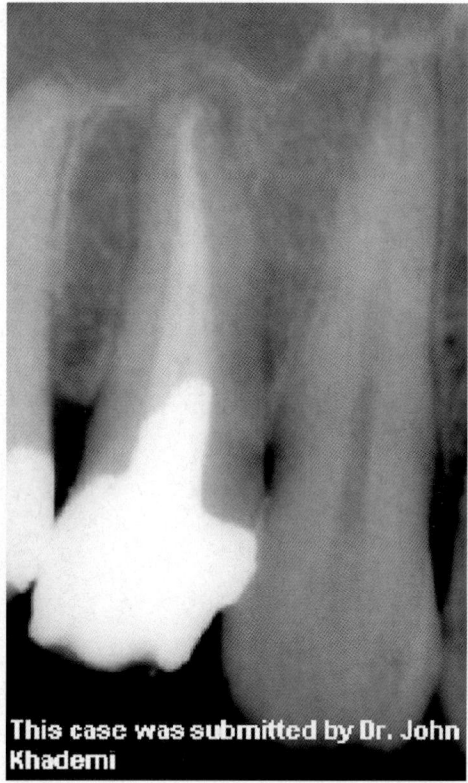

Figure 32 Maxillary right first premolar with one root and double oval canal. Reprinted with permission from Brown P, Herbranson E. Dental Anatomy & 3D Tooth Atlas Version 3.0. Illinois: Quintessence, 2005: Maxillary First Premolar- X-ray Database.

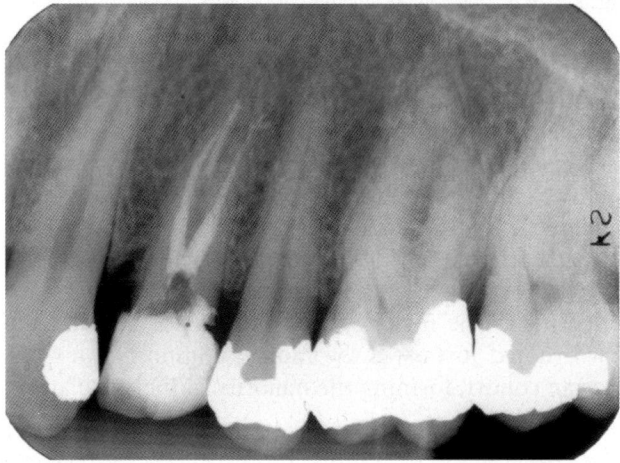

Figure 33 Maxillary left first premolar with three roots and three canals (MB, DB and Palatal). Palatal root has a coronal post-space preparation. Courtesy of Dr. W.H. Christie.

premolars that have well-formed buccal and lingual roots. The groove was not generally found in these two-rooted specimens with a furcation located in the apical third of the root. A study by Joseph et al also found an incidence of the buccal furcation groove in 62% of teeth with bifurcated roots.[163]

ROOT NUMBER AND FORM

The majority of anatomical studies found that the most common form of the maxillary first

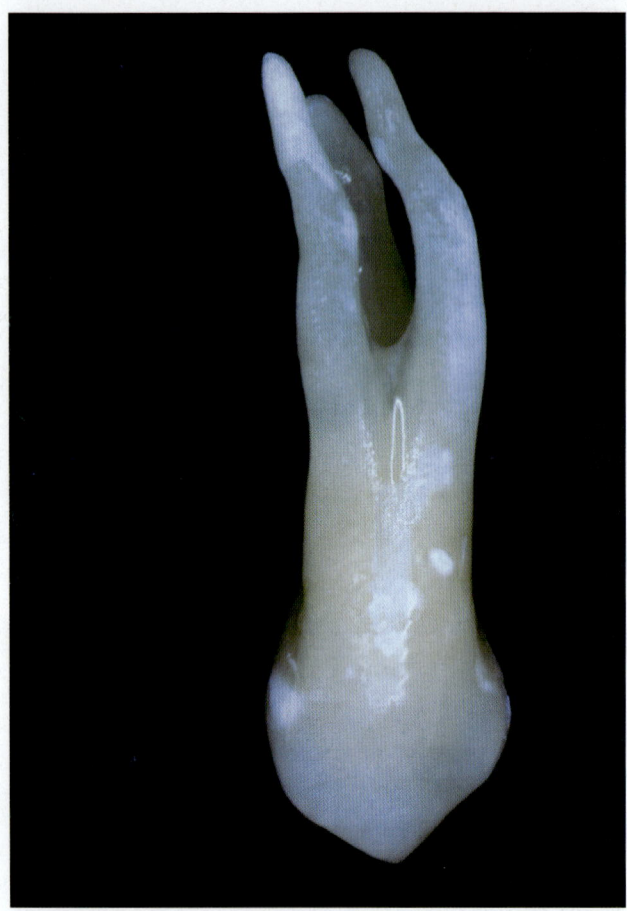

Figure 34 Extracted maxillary right first premolar with three very fine roots (MB, DB and Palatal). Courtesy of Dr. W.H. Christie.

The studies identifying ethnic background have demonstrated distinct differences between Asian and Caucasian populations. Single-rooted maxillary first premolars (see Figure 32) are the dominant form in Asian population,[164,173] and three-rooted forms are rare[164,169,173] (see Figures 33 and 34). Because of the significant influence of the ethnic background in the root number for this tooth, Table 11 reports the weighted averages for all studies and separates the data between Asian versus non-Asian populations.

In addition to ethnic differences, studies vary in their definition or do not identify what constitutes a bifurcated root. Walker utilized Turner's classification and did not consider a root to be separate unless it was a distinct and separate root for at least half of the overall root length.[173] Loh, however, grouped teeth into one root, two roots (including two-root distinct and two-root fused), and three roots. The two-root fused category was defined as teeth with roots joined almost to the apex and with two canals at their origin.[169]

The normal external three-root anatomy configuration is that of a mesiobuccal, distobuccal, and palatal root. Sabala et al. studied aberrant root and root canal morphology in 501 patient records.[21] The occurrence of the same aberration on the contralateral tooth varied according to the type of anomaly. Of the four patients, out of 501, who were found to have three-rooted maxillary first premolars, all were bilateral. Their study found that the rarer the anomaly, the greater the incidence of the anomaly occurring bilaterally. Those anomalies occurring less than 1% were found to occur bilaterally up to 90% of the time.

premolar is the two-rooted form[4,21,57,164–173] (see Figures 27–30). There was a wide variation in the incidence of the number of roots in the anatomical studies cited. Figure 31 is an example of three canals in two fused buccal roots and a lingual root. The incidence of three-rooted maxillary first premolars ranged from 0%[4,169,173] to 6%.[165] The ethnic background of the patients in many of the studies was not identified. The majority of studies reporting that the two-rooted form was the most common had a Caucasian cohort, forming the majority of the population.

CANAL SYSTEM

The majority of maxillary premolars were found to have two canals, irrespective of whether the tooth has a single or a double root (Table 12). In the 15 anatomical studies assessed, over 75% of the teeth studied had two canals.[4,6,7,10,36,57,165,167–174] Ethnicity was a factor in canal number. The incidence of a single canal was significantly higher in Asian populations compared to the mixed non-Asian population.[169,173] The Vertucci and

Table 11 Maxillary First Premolar					
Number of Roots	Number of Studies Cited	Number of Teeth	One Root	Two Roots	Three Roots
All studies	13	6241	52.2 (3256)	46.7% (2916)	1.1% (67)
Non-Asian population	10	1982	31.2% (619)	66.6% (1319)	2.1% (42)
Asian population	3	4259	61.9% (2637)	37.5% (1597)	0.6% (25)

Number of Canals and Apices	Number of Studies Cited	Number of Teeth	One Canal	Two Canals	Three Canals	Other Canal Configurations	One Canal at Apex	Two Canals at Apex
All studies	15	3721	21.3% (794)	75.8% (2821)	1.4% (51)	1.5% (55)	25.9% (386)	71.3% (1062)
	8	1488						
Non-Asian population	13	2664	11.6% (308)	84.5% (2250)	1.9% (51)	2% (55)	25.9% (386)	71.4% (1062)
	8	1488						
Asian population	2	1057	46% (486)	54% (571)	–		–	–
	0	–						

Table 12 Maxillary First Premolar

Weine classification systems are useful in exploring canal systems with double canals in single roots.[13,40]

All of the three-rooted first premolars in the anatomical studies were found to have a single canal in each root.[165,166,168] The incidence of three canal maxillary premolar teeth was reported in these and other anatomical studies, and it ranged from 0%[167,169,170,173] to 6%.[165] This finding is a rare occurrence in Asian populations.[169,173] Regardless of the number of roots, the majority of maxillary first premolars (71.3%) had two separate canals and foramina at the apex.

VARIATIONS AND ANOMALIES

Ethnic differences were demonstrated for maxillary first premolar root number in the anatomical studies reported.[81,164,169,173,175] The study by Loh reported a much lower incidence (50.6%) of the two-rooted maxillary first premolars in a Singaporean population compared to Sabala's study (98.4%) based in the United States.[169] Tratman[81] reported that the two-rooted first premolar was very uncommon in Asian stock as did Petersen[175] in his study of the East Greenland Eskimo dentition. A large anatomical study of 3,202 maxillary first premolars by Aoki (Japanese patients) found that 65.7% of the specimens were single-rooted.[164]

Three-rooted forms were reported to be a rare variation in Asian populations.[176–178] Mattuella et al. reported a variation of the maxillary first premolar with a longitudinal sulcus on the buccal surface of the buccal root.[179] This variation resulted in a two-canal system in the buccal root and three canals in teeth with two roots. Gemination of the maxillary first premolar is rarely reported in the literature.[180]

Taurodontism is another rare anomaly in premolars, as a group, and less common in the maxillary premolars compared to their mandibular counterparts. Taurodontism of roots and canal systems is explained in greater detail in section "Maxillary First Molar." Llamas found only three taurodont-like maxillary premolars in a sample of 379 extracted maxillary and mandibular premolars.[181] Of the 16 cases of taurodontism in Shifman's review of radiographs, over a 5-year period, none were maxillary first premolars.[182] Madeira's study of 4,459 premolars found a total of 11 taurodont mandibular premolars (7 mandibular first premolars and 4 mandibular second premolars) but none in the maxillary premolars.[183] The Weine type IV root canal system, with a wide buccolingual canal that branches into two apical canals and foramina in the apical third, may sometimes be confused as a taurodont-like root canal anatomy, when it occurs in single-rooted maxillary premolar teeth.

Maxillary Second Premolar

EXTERNAL ROOT MORPHOLOGY

The cross-sectional root anatomy of the maxillary second premolar in the midroot area is described as oval- or kidney-shaped.[1,3,5,12,14–16] Developmental depressions are often present on the mesial and the distal aspects of the root. The single root trunk is broad buccolingually and is narrower mesiodistally as illustrated in Figures 35–40. The root tip usually

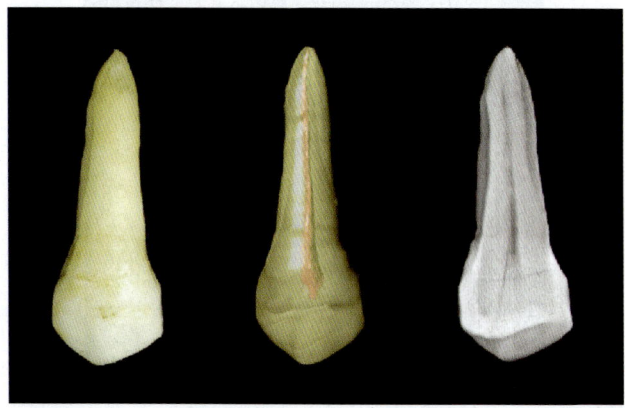

Figure 35 Buccal view of maxillary left second premolar. Reprinted with permission from Brown P, Herbranson E. Dental Anatomy & 3D Tooth Atlas Version 3.0. Illinois: Quintessence, 2005: Maxillary Second Premolar- Rotations & Slices.

ends as a single blunt apex, but it may be fine and divide into two or more, rarely three, apices. The curvature in the apical third is also not uncommon. The overall average length of the maxillary second premolar is 22.5 mm with an average crown length of 8.5 mm and an average root length of 14 mm.[3]

ROOT NUMBER AND FORM

All of the anatomical studies cited found that the most common form of the maxillary second premolar is a single root as illustrated in Figures 35–40.[4,57,153,164,184,185] The weighted averages for data from six anatomical studies of 8,513 teeth as illustrated in Table 13 result in a 90.7% incidence of single-rooted teeth. The incidence of two-rooted maxillary second premolars ranged from 5.5%[164] to 20.4%,[57] while the three-rooted form was a rare finding and ranged from 0%[4,170,184,185] to 1%.[57] The bilateral symmetry of the three-rooted form may be expected in many patients as this anomaly is quite rare.[21]

CANAL SYSTEM

The maxillary second premolar has a single canal in approximately 50% of the 2743 teeth examined in 10 anatomical studies,[6,10,13,36,57,167,168,174,184,185] as listed

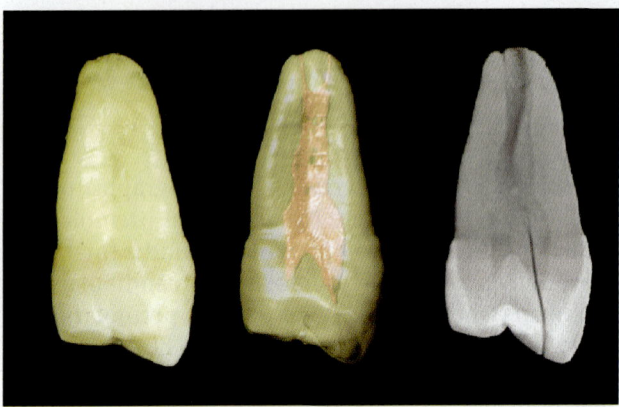

Figure 36 Mesial view of maxillary left second premolar. Reprinted with permission from Brown P, Herbranson E. Dental Anatomy & 3D Tooth Atlas Version 3.0. Illinois: Quintessence, 2005: Maxillary Second Premolar- Rotations & Slices.

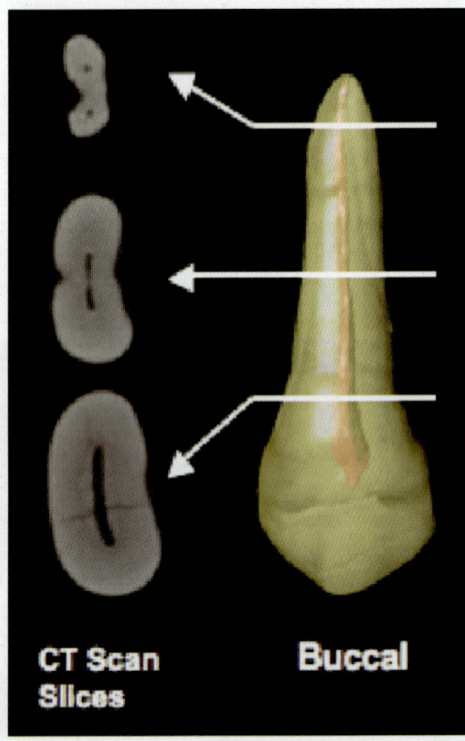

Figure 37 Root cross-sections of the maxillary left second premolar. Reprinted with permission from Brown P, Herbranson E. Dental Anatomy & 3D Tooth Atlas Version 3.0. Illinois: Quintessence, 2005: Maxillary Second Premolar- Rotations & Slices.

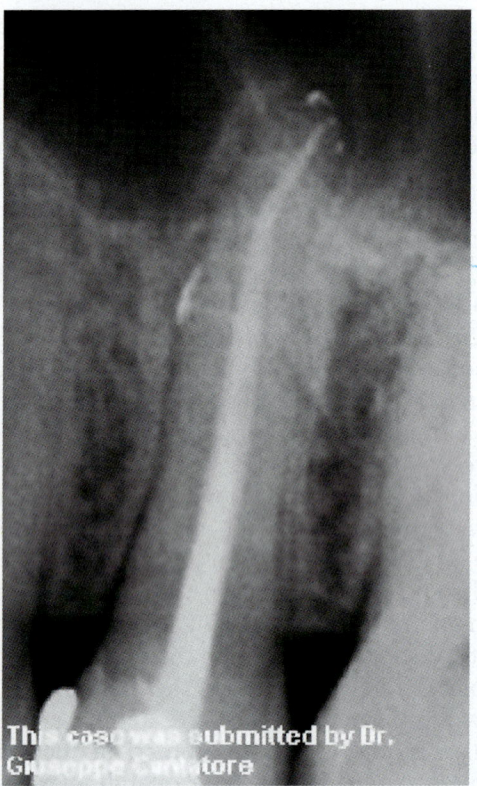

Figure 38 Maxillary left second premolar with a single root and a single canal; lateral canals are visible in the middle and apical thirds of the root. Reprinted with permission from Brown P, Herbranson E. Dental Anatomy & 3D Tooth Atlas Version 3.0. Illinois: Quintessence, 2005: Maxillary Second Premolar- X-ray Database.

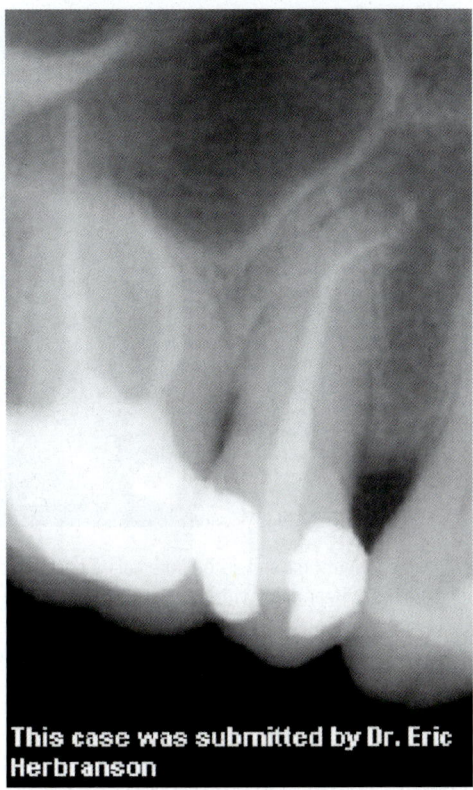

Figure 39 Maxillary right second premolar with a single root and single canal; the apical third exhibits a curvature to the mesial. Reprinted with permission from Brown P, Herbranson E. Dental Anatomy & 3D Tooth Atlas Version 3.0. Illinois: Quintessence, 2005: Maxillary Second Premolar- X-ray Database.

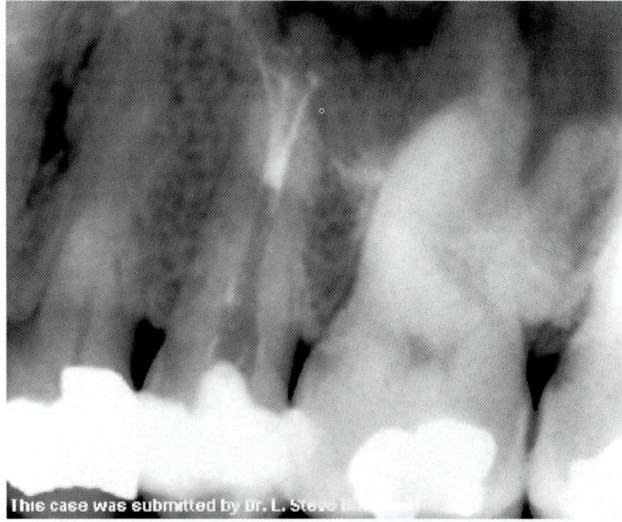

Figure 40 Maxillary left second premolar with a single root and a single main canal; two lateral (accessory) canals are visible in the apical third of the root. Reprinted with permission from Brown P, Herbranson E. Dental Anatomy & 3D Tooth Atlas Version 3.0. Illinois: Quintessence, 2005: Maxillary Second Premolar- X-ray Database.

in Table 14. Therefore, even though over 90% of these teeth have a single root, a high proportion will have two canals present. Canal exploration of maxillary second premolar teeth should be done with fine curved files, keeping in mind the Vertucci or Weine classification of two canals in one root that may not be apparent on the radiograph. The incidence of three canals in the maxillary second premolar was low in each of the anatomical studies. The majority of the teeth studied had a single canal (50.3%) and a single canal at the apex (61.4).

VARIATIONS AND ANOMALIES

Relatively few case reports of variations and anomalies in the maxillary second premolar have been published. These case reports include examples of dens

Table 13 Maxillary Second Premolar

Number of Roots	Number of Studies Cited	Number of Teeth	One Root	Two Roots	Three Roots
	6	8513	90.7% (7798)	8.2% (701)	0.2% (14)

Table 14 Maxillary Second Premolar

Number of Canals and Apices	Number of Studies Cited	Number of Teeth (Canal Studies)	One Canal	Two Canals	Three Canals	Other Canal Configurations	One Canal at Apex	Two Canals at Apex
	10	2743	50.3% (1379)	46.5% (1275)	1.2% (33)	2.0% (33)		
	8	1813					61.4% (1114)	38.1% (690)

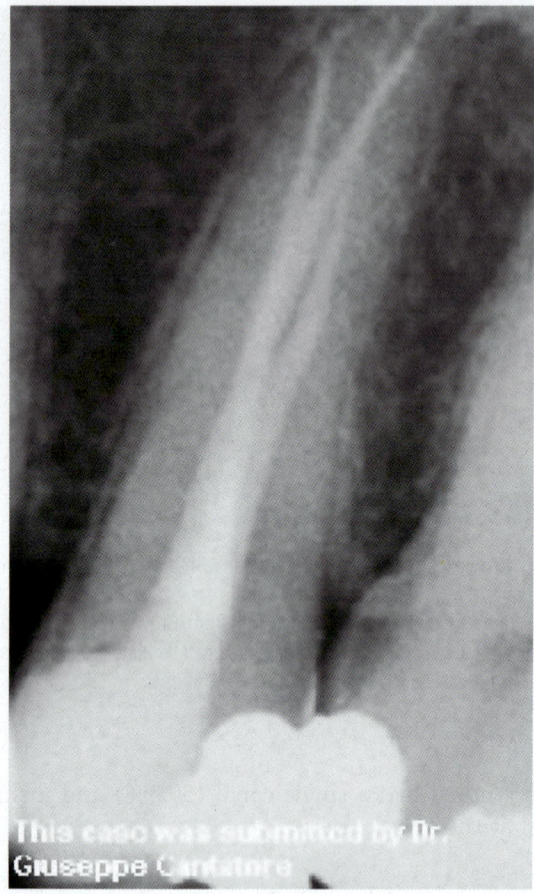

Figure 41 Maxillary left second premolar with a buccal and lingual root; the buccal root has two canals while the lingual root has one canal. Reprinted with permission from Brown P, Herbranson E. Dental Anatomy & 3D Tooth Atlas Version 3.0. Illinois: Quintessence, 2005: Maxillary Second Premolar- X-ray Database.

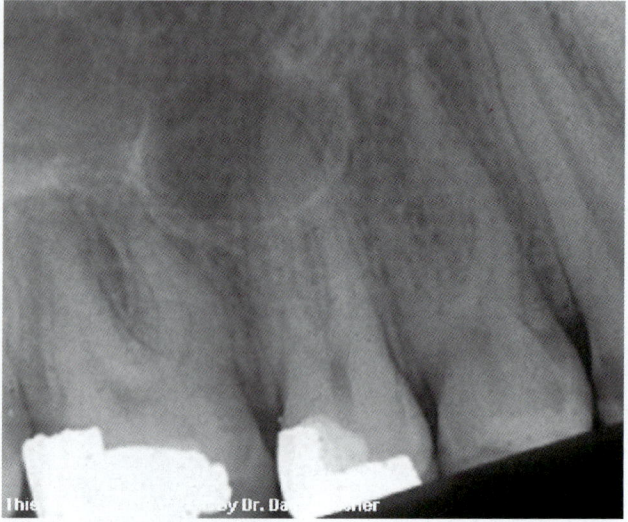

Figure 42 Maxillary right first and second premolars each have 3 roots (MB, DB and Palatal). Reprinted with permission from Brown P, Herbranson E. Dental Anatomy & 3D Tooth Atlas Version 3.0. Illinois: Quintessence, 2005: Maxillary Second Premolar- X-ray Database.

Maxillary First Molar

EXTERNAL ROOT MORPHOLOGY

The maxillary first molar normally has three roots as illustrated in Figures 43–48. The mesiobuccal root is broad buccolingually and has prominent depressions

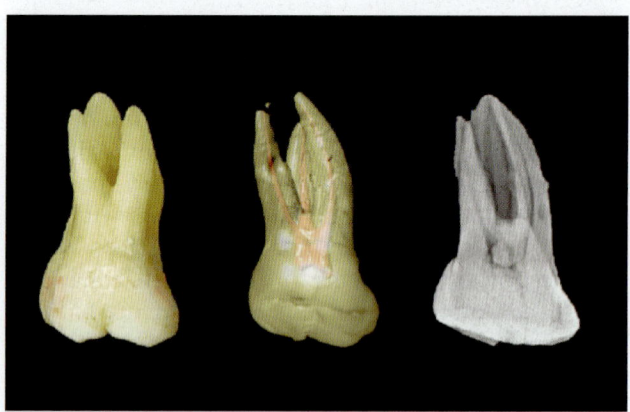

Figure 43 Buccal view of maxillary right first molar. Reprinted with permission from Brown P, Herbranson E. Dental Anatomy & 3D Tooth Atlas Version 3.0. Illinois: Quintessence, 2005: Maxillary First Molar- Rotations & Slices.

invaginatus,[186] a deep distal root concavity,[187] taurodontism,[182] two roots and three canals[5] (Figure 41), and the presence of three roots and three canals[5,178,188–191] (Figure 42). Three-rooted maxillary second premolar teeth do not seem to be as common as in first premolars. This anomaly is often bilateral and should be considered by exposing radiographs taken at different angles. Both first and second premolar triple-canal system anomalies do occur, but rarely.[178]

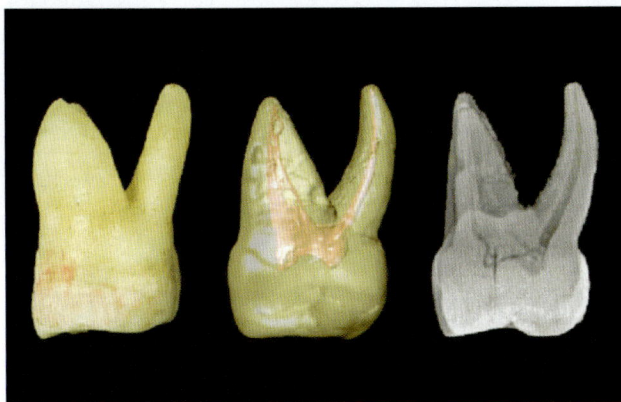

Figure 44 Mesial view of maxillary right first molar. Reprinted with permission from Brown P, Herbranson E. Dental Anatomy & 3D Tooth Atlas Version 3.0. Illinois: Quintessence, 2005: Maxillary First Molar- Rotations & Slices.

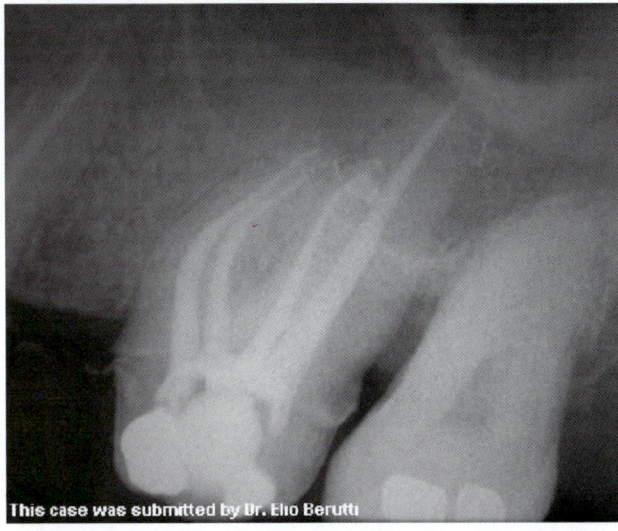

Figure 46 Maxillary left first molar with 3 roots and 4 canals (MB, ML, D and Palatal); lateral canals are visible in the apical thirds of the distobuccal and palatal roots. Reprinted with permission from Brown P, Herbranson E. Dental Anatomy & 3D Tooth Atlas Version 3.0. Illinois: Quintessence, 2005: Maxillary First Molar- X-ray Database.

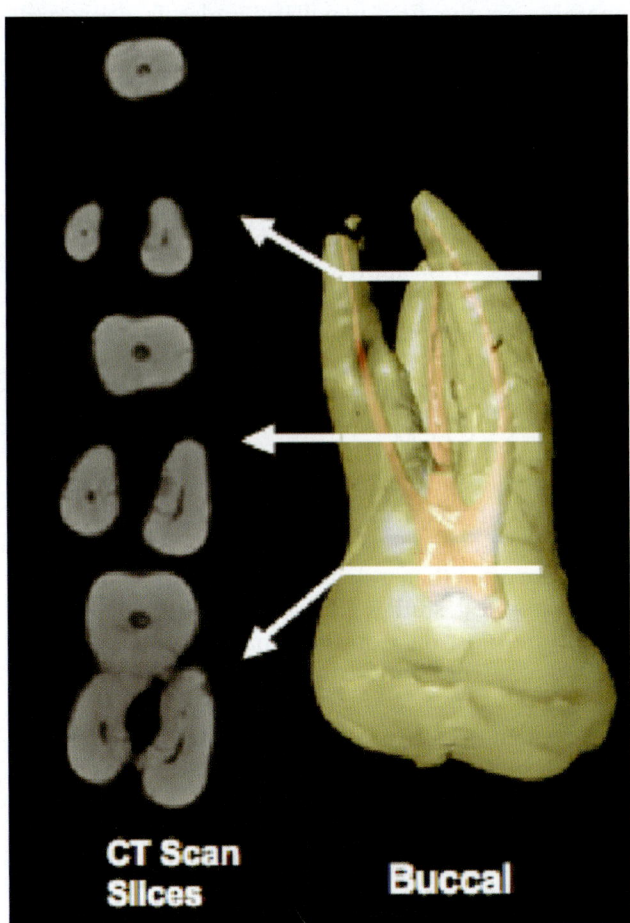

Figure 45 Root cross-sections of the maxillary right first molar. Reprinted with permission from Brown P, Herbranson E. Dental Anatomy & 3D Tooth Atlas Version 3.0. Illinois: Quintessence, 2005: Maxillary First Molar- Rotations & Slices.

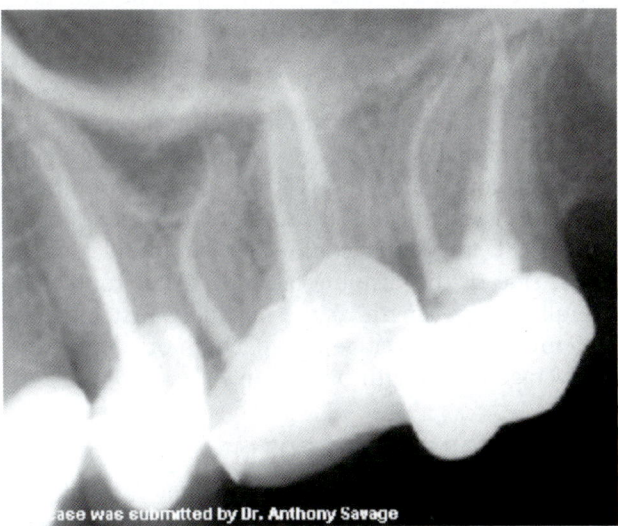

Figure 47 Maxillary left first molar with 3 roots and 3 canals (one canal in each of the MB, DB and Palatal roots); the mesiobuccal root has a distal curvature in the apical third. Reprinted with permission from Brown P, Herbranson E. Dental Anatomy & 3D Tooth Atlas Version 3.0. Illinois: Quintessence, 2005: Maxillary First Molar- X-ray Database.

or flutings on its mesial and distal surfaces.[1,3,5,14–16] The internal canal morphology is highly variable, but the majority of the mesiobuccal roots contain two canals. The distobuccal root is generally rounded or

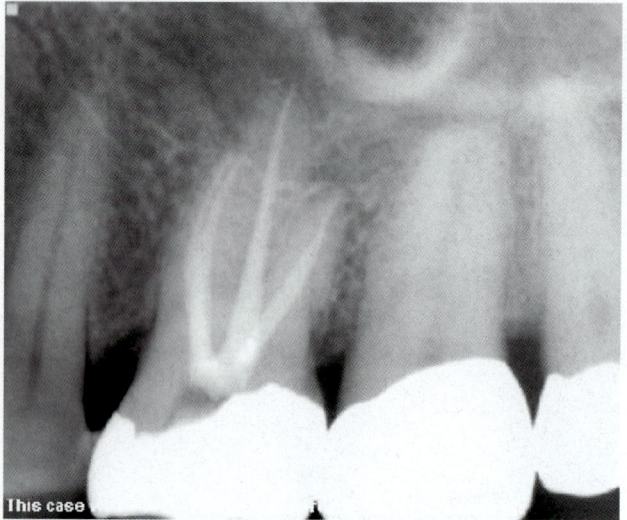

Figure 48 Maxillary left first molar with 3 roots and 4 canals (MB, ML, D and Palatal). Reprinted with permission from Brown P, Herbranson E. Dental Anatomy & 3D Tooth Atlas Version 3.0. Illinois: Quintessence, 2005: Maxillary First Molar- X-ray Database.

Table 16	Maxillary First Molar		
Fused Roots	Number of Studies Cited	Number of Teeth	Incidence of Fusion
	8	1714	6.2% (107)

Table 17	Maxillary First Molar		
C-shaped Roots	Number of Studies Cited	Number of Teeth	Incidence of Fusion
	2	2480	0.12% (3)

ovoid in cross section and usually contains a single canal. The palatal root is more broad mesiodistally than buccolingually and ovoidal in shape but normally contains only a single canal. Although the palatal root generally appears straight on radiographs, there is usually a buccal curvature in the apical third.[192] Depressions on the buccal and palatal surfaces of the palatal root can be present but are generally shallow. Gher and Vernino found prominent depressions on the distal aspect of the mesiobuccal roots.[162] Depressions could also be found on the furcal side of the distobuccal and palatal roots. The overall average length of the maxillary first molar is 20.5 mm with an average crown length of 7.5 mm and an average root length of 13 mm.[3]

ROOT NUMBER AND FORM

The maxillary first molar root anatomy is predominantly a three-rooted form, as shown in all anatomical studies[4,17,18,22] of this tooth (Table 15). The two-rooted form is rarely reported and may be due to the fusion of the distobuccal root to the palatal root or the fusion of the distobuccal root to the mesiobuccal root. The single root or the conical form of root anatomy in the first maxillary molar is very rarely reported.[4] Over 95% (95.9%) of maxillary first molars had three roots and 3.8% had two roots in four studies that included 416 teeth. The four-rooted anatomy in its various forms is also very rare in the maxillary first molar and is more likely to occur in the second or the third maxillary molar.[45,193]

The incidence of fusion (Table 16) of any two or three roots was approximately 6.2%.[17–23,194] The C-shaped root canal system morphology (Table 17) is also a rare anomaly (0.12%).[23,47]

CANAL SYSTEM

The internal root canal system morphology reflects the external root anatomy. The mesiobuccal root of the maxillary first molar contains a double root canal system more often than a single canal according to most of the anatomical studies (Table 18). This review contained the most data on the canal morphology of the mesiobuccal root with a total of 8,515 teeth from 37 studies.[6–11,13,17,18,22,25,27,28,30–34,36–43,51,52,54–57,59,195,196]

The incidence of two canals in the mesiobuccal root was 57.1% and of one canal was 42.9% in a weighted average of all reported studies. The incidence of two canals in the mesiobuccal root was higher in laboratory studies (61.1%) compared to clinical studies (54.7%). Less variation was found in the distobuccal and palatal roots, and the results were reported from 15 studies consisting of 2,606 teeth. The distobuccal root had only one canal in 98.3% of teeth studied, while the palatal root had only one canal in over 99% of the teeth studied.[24]

Table 15	Maxillary First Molar				
Number of Roots	Number of Studies Cited	Number of Teeth	One Root	Two Roots	Three Roots
	4	416	0.2% (1)	3.8% (16)	95.9% (399)

Table 18 Maxillary First Molar						
Number of Canals and Apices	Number of Studies Cited	Number of Teeth (Canal Studies)	One Canal	Two or More Canals	Two into One Canal at Apex	Two or More Canals at Apex
Mesiobuccal root (lab studies)	24	3235	38.9% (1259)	61.1% (1976)		
	18	2110			66.0% (1393)	34.0% (717)
Mesiobuccal root (clinical studies)	13	5280	45.3% (2393)	54.7% (2887)		
	6	2072			56.9% (1178)	43.1% (894)
Mesiobuccal root (all studies)	37	8515	42.9% (3652)	57.1% (4863)		
	24	4182			61.5% (2571)	38.5% (1611)
Distobuccal root (all studies)	15	2606	98.3% (2562)	1.7% (44)		
	6	1381			97.1% (1341)	2.9% (40)
Palatal root (all studies)	15	2606	99% (2581)	1% (25)		
	6	1381			98.1% (1355)	1.9% (26)

In vitro studies of the mesiobuccal root canal system are slightly more likely to report two canals in the maxillary first molar than do the vivo clinical studies, but the incidence of location of a two-canal system in clinical studies appears to be increasing with the routine use of the SOM and other aids during the modified endodontic access opening procedure.[11,59]

The two-canal system of the mesiobuccal root of the maxillary first molar has a single apical foramen roughly twice as often (66.0%) in proportion to the two-canal and two-foramen morphology, in weighted laboratory studies (see Table 18).

The single-canal system and single apical foramen in the palatal and the distobuccal root of the maxillary first molar is the most predominant form, as reported in all studies, but multiple canals and more than one apical foramen variation do exist in 1–3% of these roots in the weighted studies reported (see Table 18).

VARIATIONS AND ANOMALIES

The root and root canal morphology of teeth varies greatly in the reported literature. Many studies provided no information on ethnic background, age or gender or possible explanations for variations observed.

Walker[173,197,198] reported on the ethnic differences in the root anatomy of maxillary first premolars, mandibular first premolars, and the high incidence of three-rooted mandibular first molars in Asian patients. He did not, however, report on the incidence of a second mesiobuccal canal (MB2) in the maxillary first molar. A study by Weine et al.[32] determined that the incidence of MB2 in a Japanese population was similar to the incidence reported for other ethnic backgrounds.

Age was found to have an effect on the incidence of MB2. Fewer canals were found in the mesiobuccal root due to increasing age and calcification.[38,42,55] Sert and Bayirli[10] conducted a clearing study that identified gender, in a sample of 2800 teeth (1400 male and 1400 female) from Turkish patients. One hundred permanent teeth of each type (excluding third molars) for each gender were included in the study. Although they did not consider age in their study, they concluded that gender and race were important factors to consider in the preoperative evaluation of canal morphology for nonsurgical root canal therapy. Although only 100 of each type of tooth for each gender was included in their study, a single Vertucci Type I canal was present in the mesiobuccal root in only 3% of males compared to 10% of females. There are conflicting results with respect to gender and the number of canals.[6,10,42,55]

Some studies[39,51] compared in vivo versus in vitro techniques. Seidberg et al.[39] reported that 33.3% of the 201 teeth studied had a MB2 canal in their in vivo study. This increased to 62% in their in vitro study of 100 teeth. Similar results were reported in a study by Pomeranz and Fishelberg.[51] Only 31% of 100 teeth studied had a MB2 canal in their in vivo study compared to 69% of 100 teeth in their in vitro study. The in vitro portion of this study described the samples as extracted maxillary molars and may represent pooled data instead of maxillary first molar data alone. The definition of a canal as a treatable canal used in clinical studies[11,42] versus the more complex canal configurations visible through clearing studies[6,10,13,17,25] can also lead to different results.

The more common use of SOM or loupes in recent clinical studies has resulted in an increased prevalence of the clinical detection of the MB2 canal.[11,31,41,43] The effect of magnification on the incidence of clinical location of MB2 was assessed in a clinical study by Buhrley et al.[41] The MB2 canal was found in 41 of 58 teeth (71.1%) when using SOM. The group using loupes found MB2 in 55 of 88 teeth (62.5%). The lowest incidence of MB2 was in the group performing RCT without any magnification. MB2 was found in only 10 of 58 teeth (17.2%). A study by Sempira and Hartwell[43] found that the use of an SOM did increase the incidence of MB2. They attributed the lower incidence in their study to their characterization of a canal as one that must be negotiated and obturated to within 4 mm of the apex.

The incidence of many of the anomalies in case reports cannot be determined due to the lack of data collection. However, although rare, these anomalies can and do occur. There are reports of two palatal canals in three-rooted teeth,[54,193,199,200] three palatal canals in a reticular palatal root,[53,201] two palatal roots or four roots total,[26,44,45,193,202] five roots (two palatal, two mesiobuccal, and one distobuccal),[26] C-shaped canals,[46,47,203–205] single or multiple taurodont molar teeth,[58,182,206] root fusion,[46–48,207] two canal systems in the distobuccal root,[49,208] and a single-rooted tooth with a single canal.[209] Other rare anomalies are illustrated below in Figures 49–51.

Of all the canals in the maxillary first molar, the MB2 can be the most difficult to find and negotiate in a clinical situation. The knowledge from laboratory

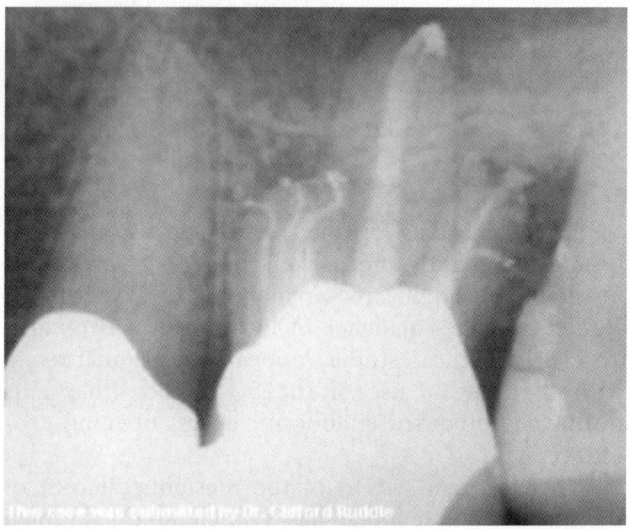

Figure 50 Maxillary left first molar 3 separate canals in the MB root. Reprinted with permission from Brown P, Herbranson E. Dental Anatomy & 3D Tooth Atlas Version 3.0. Illinois: Quintessence, 2005: Maxillary First Molar- X-ray Database.

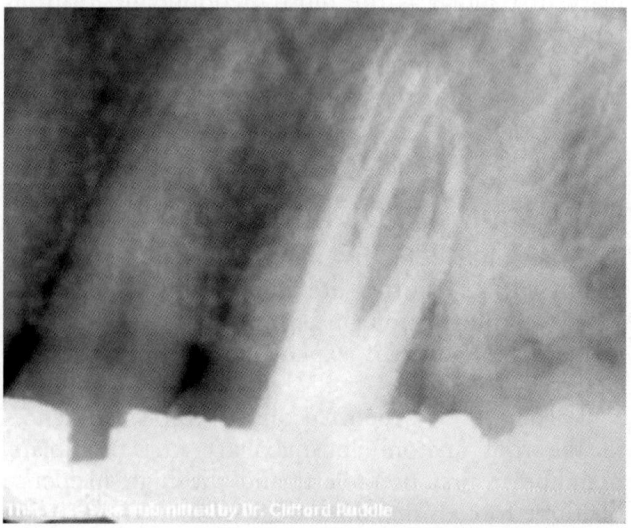

Figure 51 Maxillary left first molar with 6 canals; 2 canals were present in each of the MB, DB and Palatal roots. Reprinted with permission from Brown P, Herbranson E. Dental Anatomy & 3D Tooth Atlas Version 3.0. Illinois: Quintessence, 2005: Maxillary First Molar- X-ray Database.

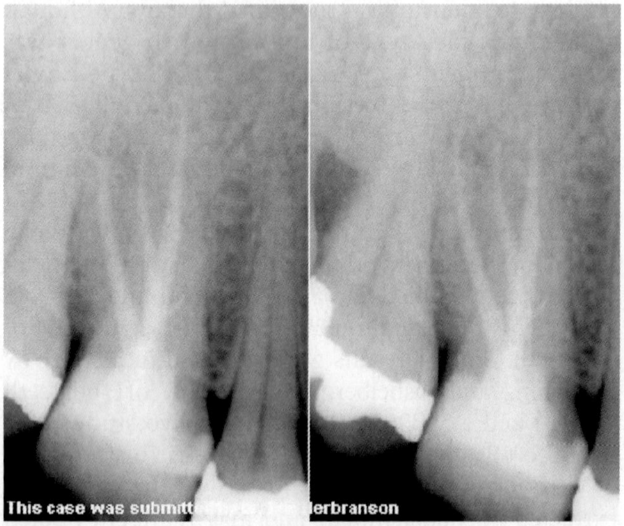

Figure 49 Maxillary right first molar exhibiting 4 roots and 4 canals; 2 MB roots, one DB and one palatal root. Reprinted with permission from Brown P, Herbranson E. Dental Anatomy & 3D Tooth Atlas Version 3.0. Illinois: Quintessence, 2005: Maxillary First Molar- X-ray Database.

studies is essential to provide insight into the complex root canal anatomy. A study by Davis et al. in 1973[210] compared the post débridement anatomy of the canals of 217 teeth. Injection of silicone impression material into the instrumented canals revealed that standard instrumentation left a significant portion of the canal walls untouched. Fins, webbing, and canals were sometimes found to be not fully instrumented. Clinical instrumentation of this tooth, especially with respect to the mesiobuccal root, can be complicated. Failure to detect and treat the second MB2 canal system will result in a decreased long-term prognosis.[52] Stropko[11] observed that by scheduling adequate clinical time, by using the recent magnification and detection instrumentation aids, and by having thorough knowledge of how and where to search for MB2, the rate of location can approach 93% in maxillary first molars.

Taurodontism or "bull-like" teeth was first described by Keith.[211] Initially, it was considered to be a primitive trait found in Neanderthal skulls from Krapina and other archaeological sites. Shaw and others[206,212,213] classified the "modern" molar form as cynodont and classified taurodontism into hypo-, meso- and hypertaurodontism. Many case reports appeared in the early dental literature with varying degrees of taurodontism. There are a few case reports to date that have described endodontic treatment on taurodont-like teeth.[214–217] Other case reports link taurodontism with inherited syndromes as well.[217,218]

Maxillary Second Molar

EXTERNAL ROOT MORPHOLOGY

The maxillary second molar normally has three roots, as shown in Figures 52–57. The relative shape of each of the roots is similar to the maxillary first molar, but the roots tend to be closer together and there is a higher tendency toward fusion of two or three roots.[15] There is also usually more of a distal inclination to the root or roots of this tooth compared to the maxillary first molar.[15]

The mesiobuccal root is broad buccolingually and has prominent depressions or flutings on its mesial and distal surfaces.[1,3,5,14–16] The internal canal morphology is variable and anatomical studies indicate that the mesiobuccal root has almost an equal incidence of one or two canals (Table 19). The distobuccal root is generally rounded or ovoid in cross section and usually contains a single canal. The palatal root is more broad mesiodistally than buccolingually and ovoidal in shape but normally contains only a single canal. Depressions on its buccal and palatal surfaces can be present but are usually shallow. Gher and Vernino found prominent depressions on the distal aspect of the mesiobuccal roots.[162] Depressions could also be found on the furcal side of the distobuccal and palatal roots. The overall average length of the maxillary second molar is 19 mm with an average crown length of 7 mm and an average root length of 12 mm.[3]

ROOT NUMBER AND FORM

The majority of maxillary second molars (88.6%) in the anatomical studies were found to be three-rooted,[4,17,219] as listed in Table 20. However, this is

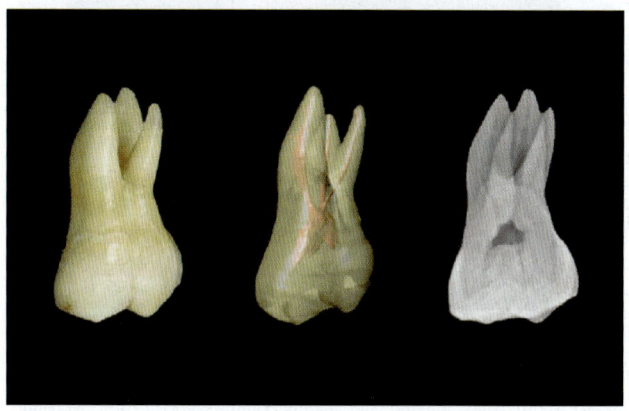

Figure 52 Buccal view of maxillary left second molar. Reprinted with permission from Brown P, Herbranson E. Dental Anatomy & 3D Tooth Atlas Version 3.0. Illinois: Quintessence, 2005: Maxillary Second Molar-Rotations & Slices.

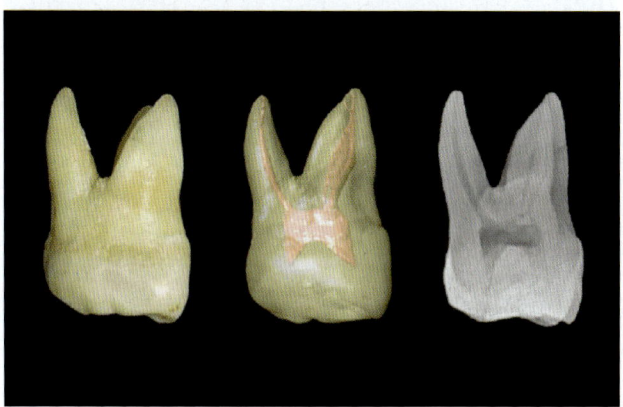

Figure 53 Mesial view of maxillary left second molar. Reprinted with permission from Brown P, Herbranson E. Dental Anatomy & 3D Tooth Atlas Version 3.0. Illinois: Quintessence, 2005: Maxillary Second Molar-Rotations & Slices.

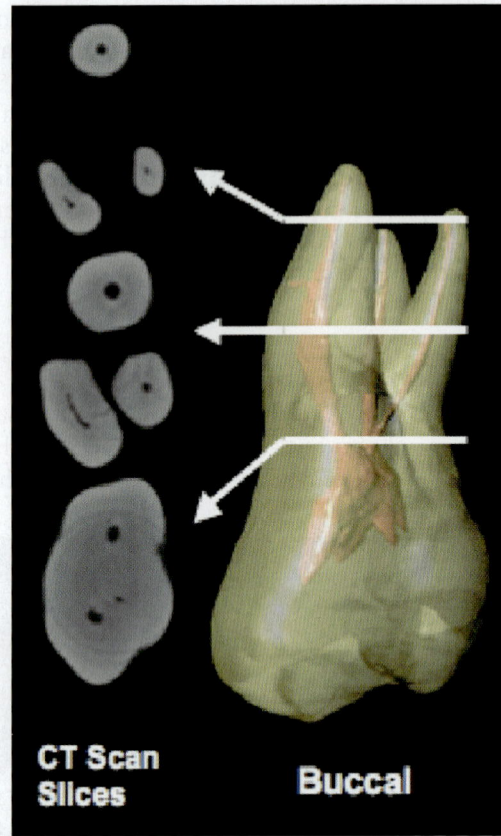

Figure 54 Root cross-sections of the maxillary left second molar. Reprinted with permission from Brown P, Herbranson E. Dental Anatomy & 3D Tooth Atlas Version 3.0. Illinois: Quintessence, 2005: Maxillary Second Molar- Rotations & Slices.

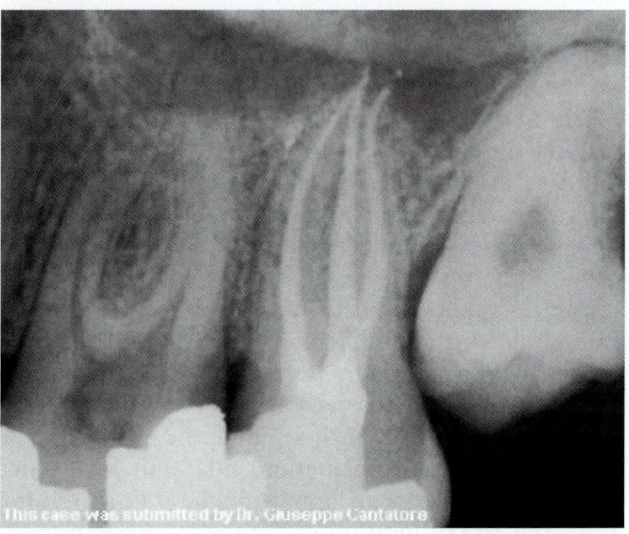

Figure 56 Maxillary left second molar with 3 roots and 3 canals; the MB and DB roots have a distal curvature. Reprinted with permission from Brown P, Herbranson E. Dental Anatomy & 3D Tooth Atlas Version 3.0. Illinois: Quintessence, 2005: Maxillary Second Molar- X-ray Database.

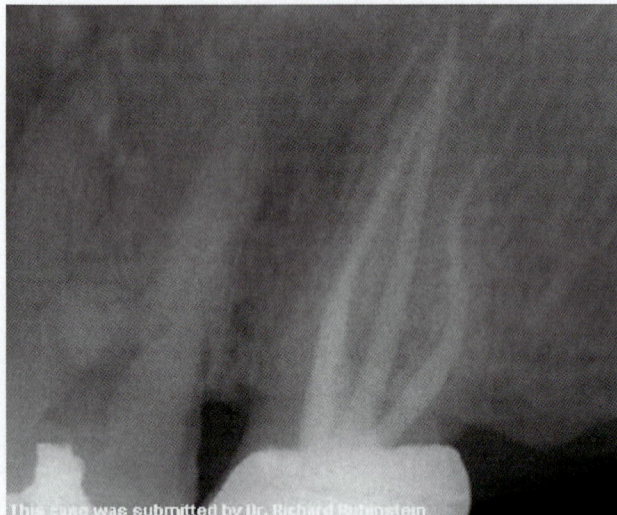

Figure 55 Maxillary left second molar 3 roots and 3 canals; the distobuccal root has an "s-shaped" curvature. Reprinted with permission from Brown P, Herbranson E. Dental Anatomy & 3D Tooth Atlas Version 3.0. Illinois: Quintessence, 2005: Maxillary Second Molar- X-ray Database.

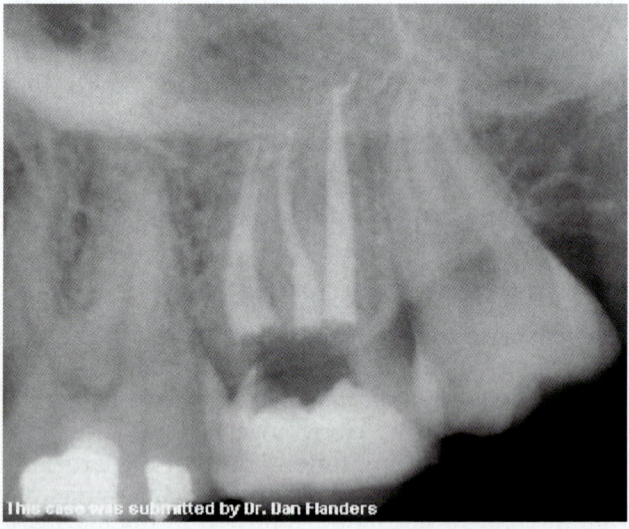

Figure 57 Maxillary left second molar with 3 roots and 4 canals (MB, ML, DB and Palatal). Reprinted with permission from Brown P, Herbranson E. Dental Anatomy & 3D Tooth Atlas Version 3.0. Illinois: Quintessence, 2005: Maxillary Second Molar- X-ray Database.

a lower incidence than that found in the maxillary first molar. The closer proximity of the roots results in a higher incidence of root fusion (25.8%),[17,19–21,23,194,220] as listed in Table 21, and C-shaped canals

Table 19	Maxillary Second Molar						
Number of Canals and Apices	Number of Studies Cited	Number of Teeth (Canal Studies)	One Canal	Two or More Canals	Number of Teeth (Apex Studies)	One Canal at Apex	Two or More Canals at Apex
Mesiobuccal root (all studies)	17	2705	52.9% (1432)	47.1% (1273)	1984	68.2% (1352)	31.8% (632)
Distobuccal root (all studies)	10	1789	99.7% (1784)	0.3% (5)	1100	100% (1100)	–
Palatal root (all studies)	10	1789	99.9% (1787)	0.1% (2)	1100	99.8% (1098)	0.2% (2)

Table 20	Maxillary Second Molar					
Number of Roots	Number of Studies Cited	Number of Teeth	One Root	Two Roots	Three Roots	Four Roots
	3	1272	2.8% (36)	7.8% (99)	88.6% (1127)	0.4% (5)

Table 21	Maxillary Second Molar		
Root Fusion	Number of Studies Cited	Number of Teeth	Incidence of Fused Roots
	7	1960	25.8% (505)

Table 22	Maxillary Second Molar		
C-shaped Canals	Number of Studies Cited	Number of Teeth	Incidence of C-shaped Canals
	1	309	4.9% (15)

(4.9%) (Table 22) when compared to the maxillary first molar.[23]

CANAL SYSTEM

The shape of the root provides an indication of the shape of the internal canal morphology.[13] The broad buccolingual and narrow mesiodistal dimension of the mesiobuccal root of the maxillary second molar may have one (see Figures 55 and 56) or two canals (Figure 57), as illustrated in Table 19. The anatomical studies found a wide range of canal incidence in the mesiobuccal root.[6,7,10,11,13,17,25,27,28,31,34,36,38,51,54,57,221] Kulild and Peters[31] reported a low incidence of a single canal of 5.3%, while Hartwell and Bellizzi[54] found a single canal in 81.8% of their specimens. It should be noted that the former was a laboratory study while the latter was clinical. The single canal is usually described as being kidney- or ribbon-shaped. Eskoz and Weine suggest that age and continued deposition of secondary dentin in the isthmus can cause narrowing and possible occlusion resulting in two canals.[221] There was a single apical foramen found in the mesiobuccal root over 68% of the time. The distobuccal and palatal roots exhibited a single canal over 99% of the time in the 10 anatomical studies reported.[6,7,10,13,17,25,28,36,54,57]

VARIATIONS AND ANOMALIES

Other variations reported in the literature include four-rooted teeth with two palatal roots and one canal in each palatal root[26,44,45,56,192,193,199,200,219,222,223]

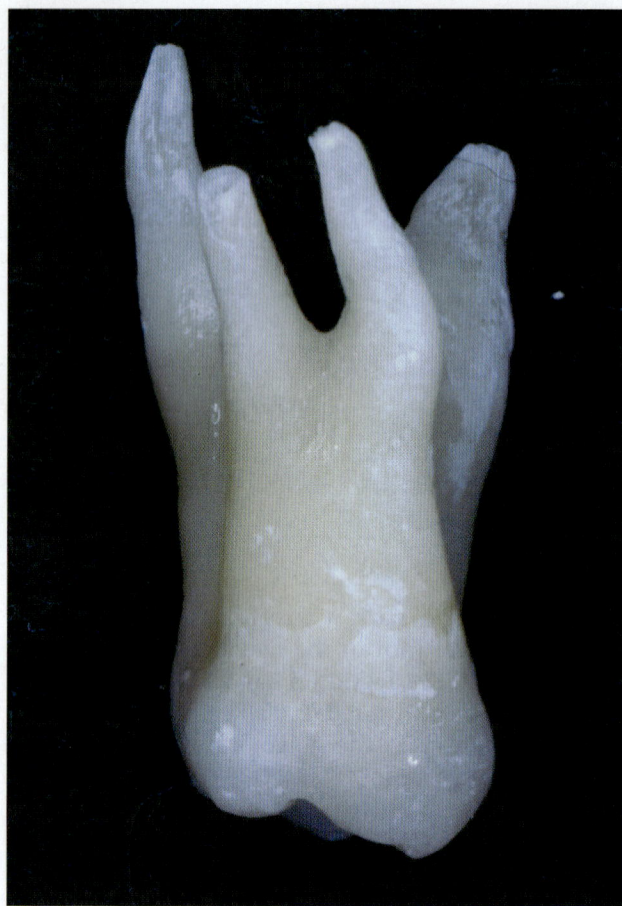

Figure 58 Maxillary right second molar (buccal view) with bifurcated double palatal root type I. (Courtesy, Dr. W. H. Christie).

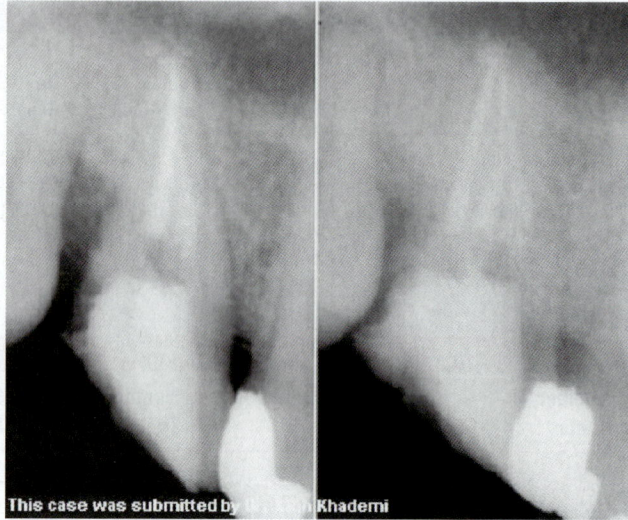

Figure 59 Maxillary right second molar with a conical C-shaped root; 3 canals join in the apical third. Reprinted with permission from Brown P, Herbranson E. Dental Anatomy & 3D Tooth Atlas Version 3.0. Illinois: Quintessence, 2005: Maxillary Second Molar- X-ray Database.

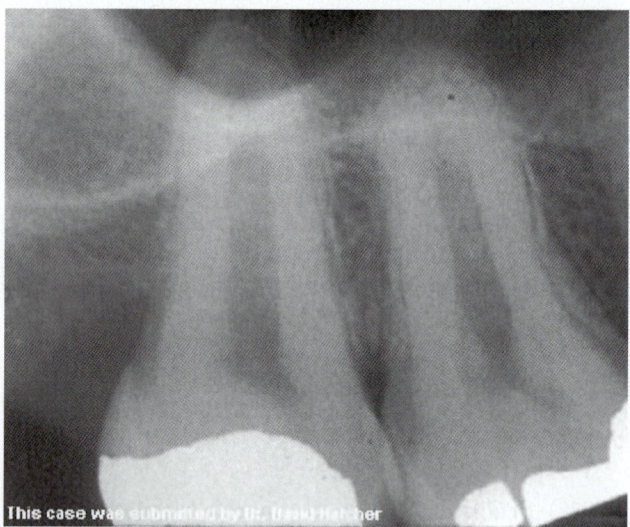

Figure 60 Maxillary right second molar (and first molar) exhibiting the large pulp chamber consistent with hypertaurodontism. Reprinted with permission from Brown P, Herbranson E. Dental Anatomy & 3D Tooth Atlas Version 3.0. Illinois: Quintessence, 2005: Maxillary Second Molar- X-ray Database.

(Figure 58), a four-rooted tooth with one palatal, one mesiobuccal, and two distobuccal roots,[224] taurodontism,[58] and a single-rooted specimen with a single canal.[225] Other rare anomalies are illustrated below in Figures 59 and 60. Darwazeh et al.[226] found the prevalence toward taurodontism in modern Jordanian patients to be highest in the maxillary second molar, while Shifman et al.[182] reported the highest incidence in the mandibular second molar.

A review article on the double palatal root by Christie, Peikoff, and Fogel[45] studied a collection of 16 clinical cases from their practice and 8 teeth from 6 case reports[56,192,193,199,219,223] from the literature to 1991. The highest occurrence of two palatal canals in double palatal roots (21/24 teeth) was found in the maxillary second molar tooth. The anomaly seemed to occur as three root anatomy types: first, the two palatal roots being long and divergent; second, the two palatal roots being shorter, nearly parallel and comparable to the two buccal roots; and third, variations of root fusion that included a two-canal system on the palatal aspect. Subsequent case reports have tended to support this observation.[44,200,227,228] Di Fiore[229] has reported on the complications that may arise in the restorative and periodontal treatment for the four-rooted maxillary molar tooth.

Mandibular Central Incisor

EXTERNAL ROOT MORPHOLOGY

The mandibular central incisor is single-rooted (Figures 61–64). The external form of the root is broad labiolingually and narrow mesiodistally. Longitudinal depressions are present on both the mesial and the distal surfaces of the root. A cross section of the root is ovoid to hourglass in shape due to the developmental depressions on each side.[3,5,12,14,16,65] The overall average length of the mandibular central incisor is 21.5 mm with an average crown length of 9 mm and an average root length of 12.5 mm.[3]

ROOT NUMBER AND FORM

All of the anatomical studies reviewed reported that 100% of the mandibular central incisors studied were single-rooted teeth, as listed in Table 23.[4,6,10,36,230,231] Variations from this form have either not been reported or not found in a review of the literature.

CANAL SYSTEM

The canal system is either ovoid or ribbon-shaped.[3,5,12,14,16,65,232] All the anatomical studies found the majority of mandibular central incisors to have a single canal. Table 24 shows that the anatomical studies found a single canal in 73.6% of the teeth

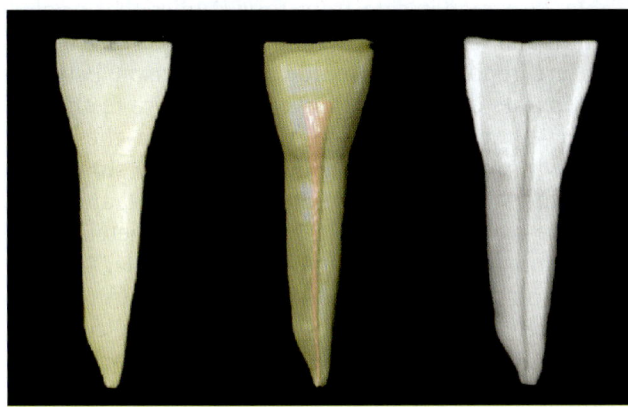

Figure 61 Labial view of mandibular right central incisor. Reprinted with permission from Brown P, Herbranson E. Dental Anatomy & 3D Tooth Atlas Version 3.0. Illinois: Quintessence, 2005: Mandibular Central Incisor- Rotations & Slices.

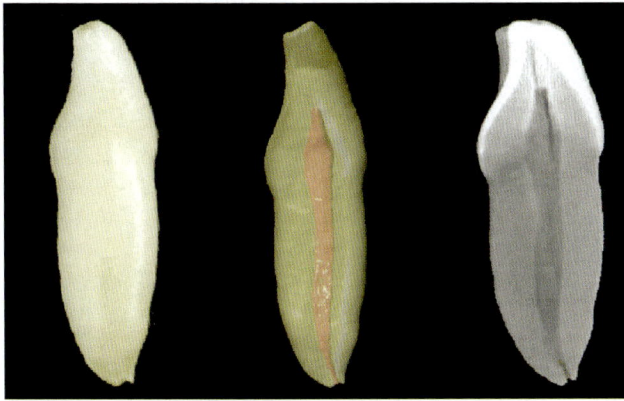

Figure 62 Mesial view of mandibular right central incisor. Reprinted with permission from Brown P, Herbranson E. Dental Anatomy & 3D Tooth Atlas Version 3.0. Illinois: Quintessence, 2005: Mandibular Central Incisor- Rotations & Slices.

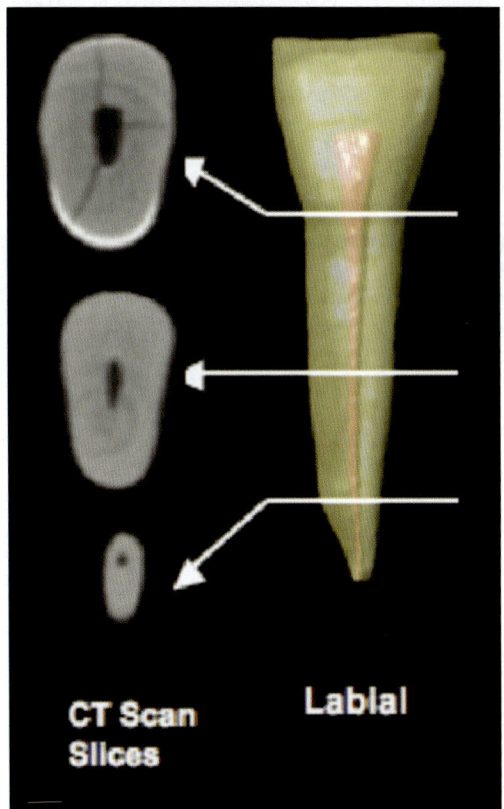

Figure 63 Root cross-sections of the mandibular right central incisor. Reprinted with permission from Brown P, Herbranson E. Dental Anatomy & 3D Tooth Atlas Version 3.0. Illinois: Quintessence, 2005: Mandibular Central Incisor- Rotations & Slices.

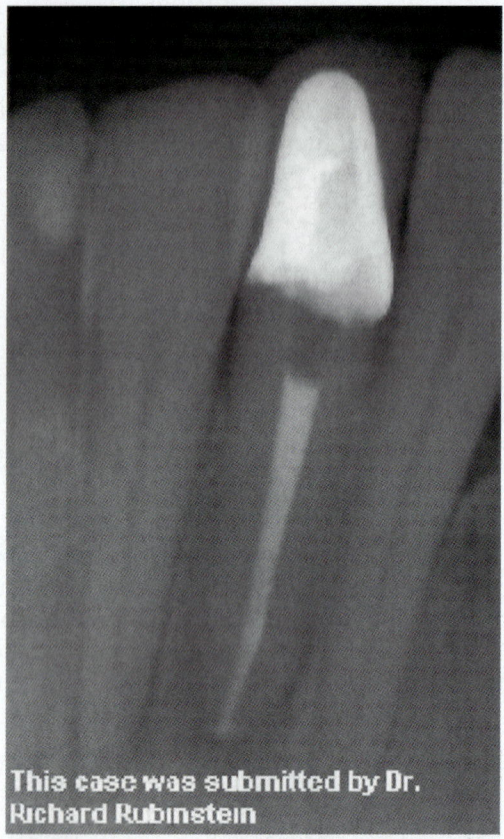

Figure 64 Mandibular right central incisor with 1 root and 1 canal.

Table 23 Mandibular Central Incisors			
Number of Roots	Number of Studies Cited	Number of Teeth	One Root
	6	1284	100% (1284)

studied. Two canals were found in 26% of the specimens.[4,6,10,36,230,231,233–240] The incidence of three or more canals was quite rare (0.4%). A single apical foramen was found in 96.4% of the teeth in the studies. Therefore, even when two separate canals have been found, the majority of these canals will join and exit in a single foramen (Figures 65 and 66). Table 25 provides data from four studies that pooled mandibular central and lateral incisors.[241–244] These data are reported to provide a comparison between the separate data reported for each of these teeth. The rationale reported for pooling data from these two teeth was that they were anatomically very similar.

A study by Green in 1956 on the root apices of anterior teeth found that the average diameter of the major foramen in the 200 pooled mandibular incisors was 0.3 mm, while the accessory foramina were 0.2 mm in diameter. Approximately 12% of the pooled mandibular incisors exhibited accessory foramina. The

Table 24 Mandibular Central Incisors							
Number of Canals and Apices	Number of Studies Cited	Number of Teeth (Canal Studies)	One Canal	Two Canals	Three or More Canals	One Canal at Apex	Two or More Canals at Apex
	14	3113	73.6% (2290)	26% (810)	0.4% (13)		
	9	1652				96.4% (1593)	2.7% (59)

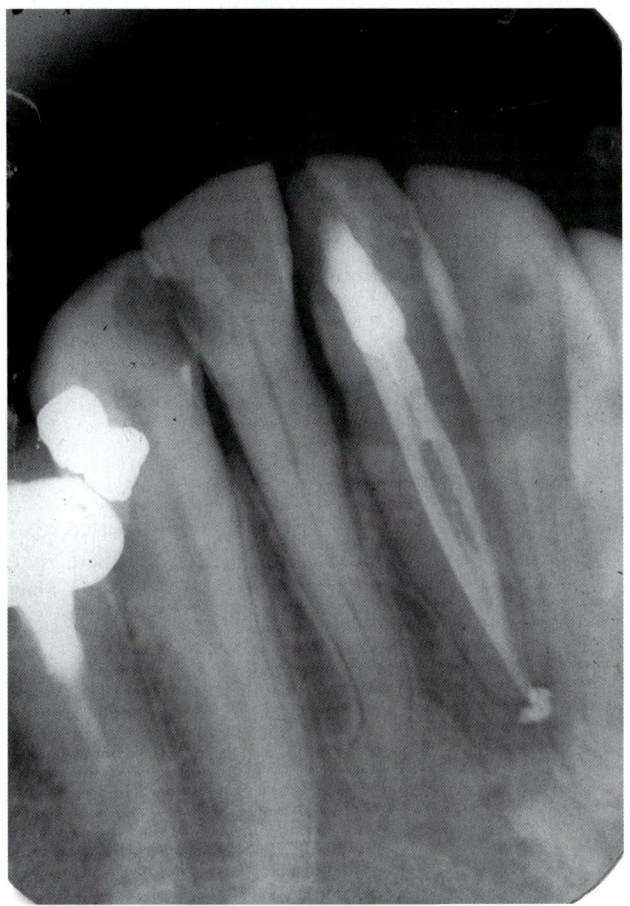

Figure 65 Mandibular left central with two canals and one apex. Courtesy of Dr. M.D. Peikoff.

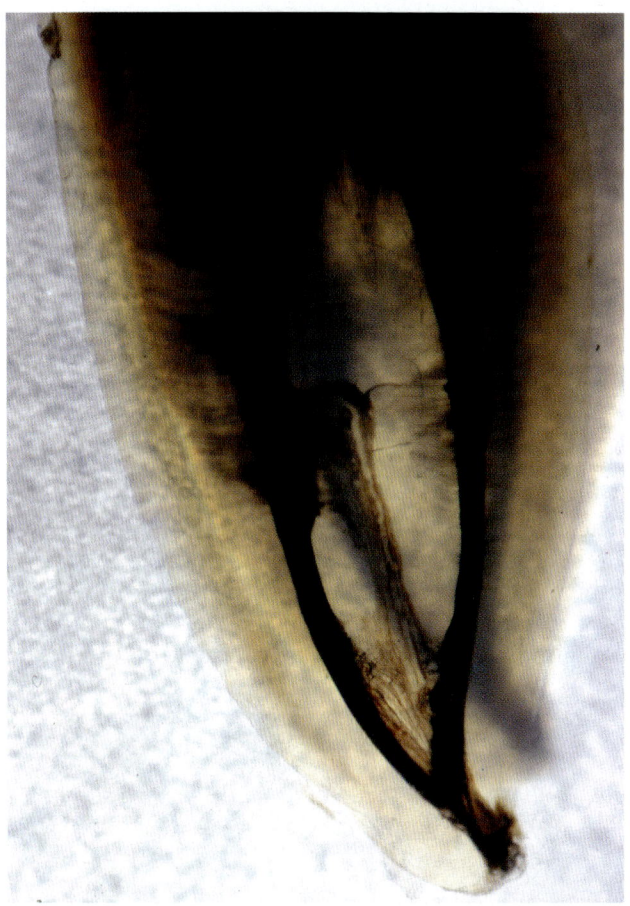

Figure 66 Mandibular central incisor with two canals, connecting apical third web-canal and one apical foramen. (India Ink infusion, 10x original magnification). Courtesy of Dr. W.H. Christie.

Table 25 Pooled Data for Mandibular Central and Lateral Incisors							
Number of Canals and Apices	Number of Studies Cited	Number of Teeth (Canal Studies)	One Canal	Two Canals	Three or More Canals	One Canal at Apex	Two or More Canals at Apex
	4	1660	77.4% (1285)	22.5% (373)	0.1% (2)	96.9% (1608)	3.1% (51)

average distance of the apical foramen from the anatomical root apex was found to be 0.2 mm.[73]

VARIATIONS AND ANOMALIES

A few anomalies are reported for this tooth in the literature. The case reports of anomalies include an example of two canals and two separate foramina (Figure 67),[245] dens invaginatus,[97,246] fusion[5] (Figure 68), gemination[5] (Figure 69), and examples of dens evaginatus that includes a lingual talon cusp[148,247] and a labial talon cusp.[156]

Mandibular Lateral Incisor

EXTERNAL ROOT MORPHOLOGY

The mandibular lateral incisor is single-rooted (Figures 70–75) and is comparable in form to the mandibular central incisor. The external form of the root is broad labiolingually and narrow mesiodistally. Longitudinal depressions are present on both the mesial and the distal midroot surfaces of the root. A cross section of the root is ovoid or hourglass in shape due to the developmental depressions on each side.[3,5,12,14,16,65] The overall length of the average mandibular lateral incisor is 23.5 mm with an average crown length of 9.5 mm and an average root length of 14 mm.[3] The major difference in tooth anatomy from the mandibular central incisor is at the incisal edge coronal anatomy. A slight angulation to the distolingual and the mesiolabial of the mandibular incisor's incisal edge should be compensated for when preparing an endodontic access opening and searching for the broader labiolingual canal system.

ROOT NUMBER AND FORM

All of the anatomical studies reviewed reported that 100% of the mandibular lateral incisors studied were single-rooted teeth, as listed in Table 26.[4,6,10,36,230,231] Variations in root number from this form have either not been reported or not found in a review of the literature.

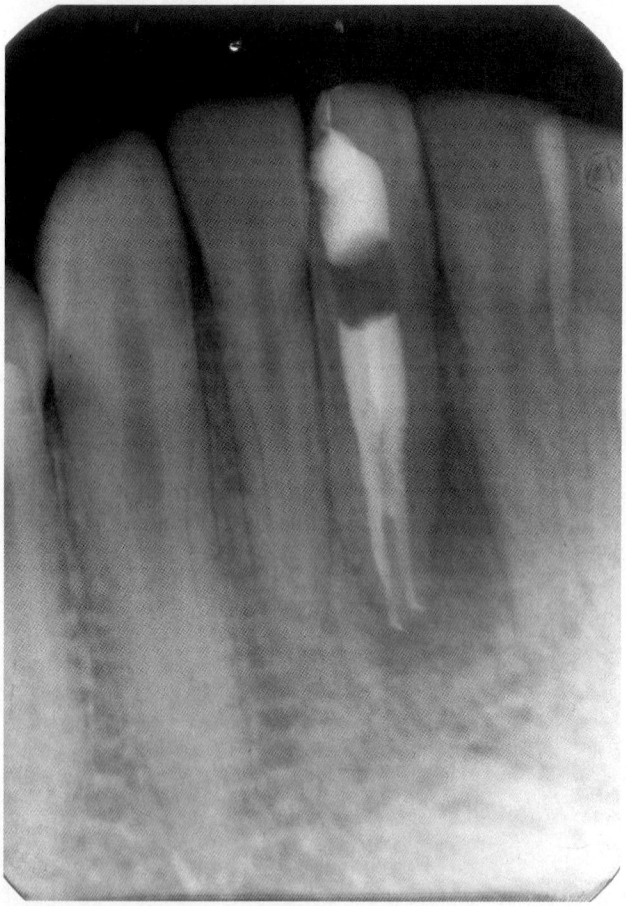

Figure 67 Mandibular left central incisor with two canals and two separate apical foramina. Courtesy of Dr. M.D. Peikoff.

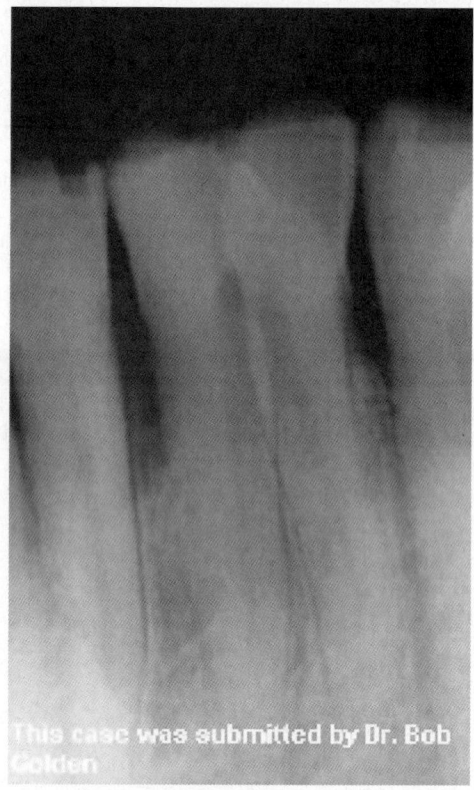

Figure 68 Mandibular left central and lateral incisors exhibiting fusion. Reprinted with permission from Brown P, Herbranson E. Dental Anatomy & 3D Tooth Atlas Version 3.0. Illinois: Quintessence, 2005: Mandibular Central Incisor- X-ray Database.

Chapter 6 / Morphology of Teeth and Their Root Canal Systems / 185

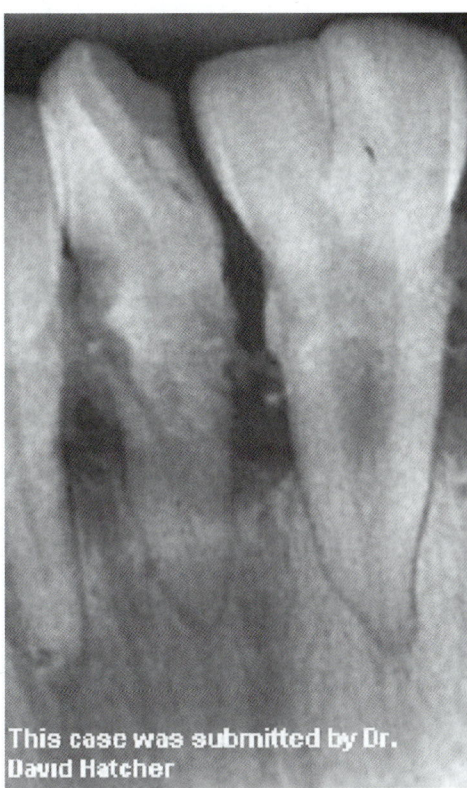

Figure 69 Mandibular left central incisor exhibiting gemination. Reprinted with permission from Brown P, Herbranson E. Dental Anatomy & 3D Tooth Atlas Version 3.0. Illinois: Quintessence, 2005: Mandibular Central Incisor- X-ray Database.

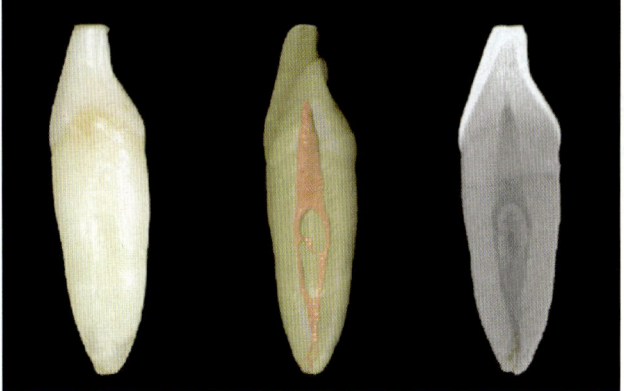

Figure 71 Mesial view of mandibular left lateral incisor. Reprinted with permission from Brown P, Herbranson E. Dental Anatomy & 3D Tooth Atlas Version 3.0. Illinois: Quintessence, 2005: Mandibular Lateral Incisor- Rotations & Slices.

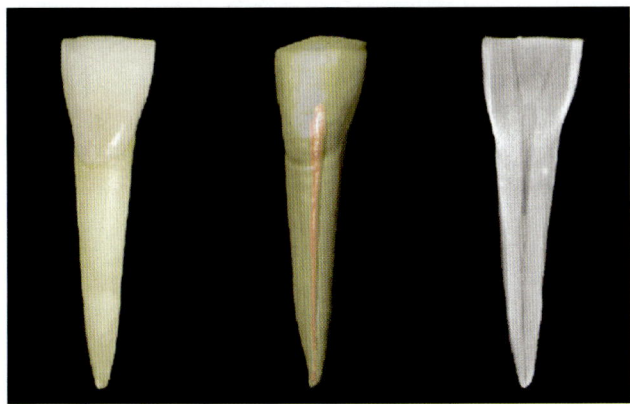

Figure 70 Labial view of mandibular left lateral incisor. Reprinted with permission from Brown P, Herbranson E. Dental Anatomy & 3D Tooth Atlas Version 3.0. Illinois: Quintessence, 2005: Mandibular Lateral Incisor- Rotations & Slices.

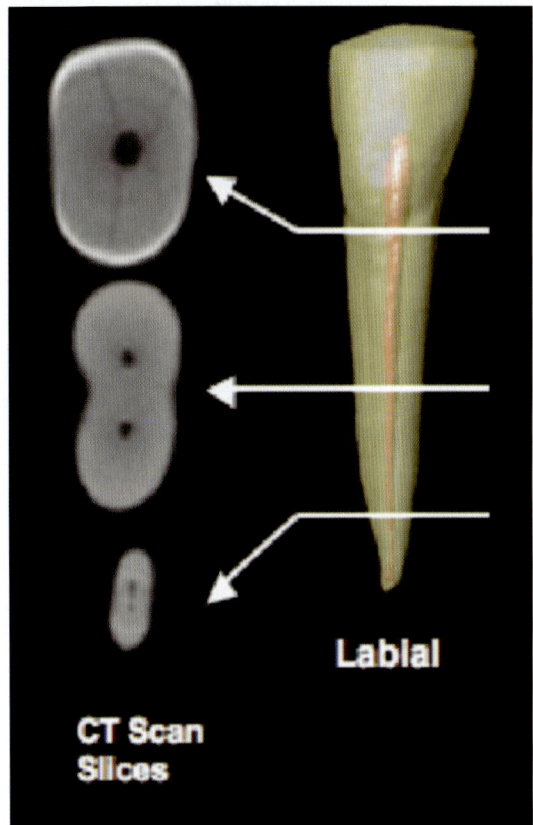

Figure 72 Root cross-sections of the mandibular left lateral incisor. Reprinted with permission from Brown P, Herbranson E. Dental Anatomy & 3D Tooth Atlas Version 3.0. Illinois: Mandibular Lateral Incisor- Rotations & Slices.

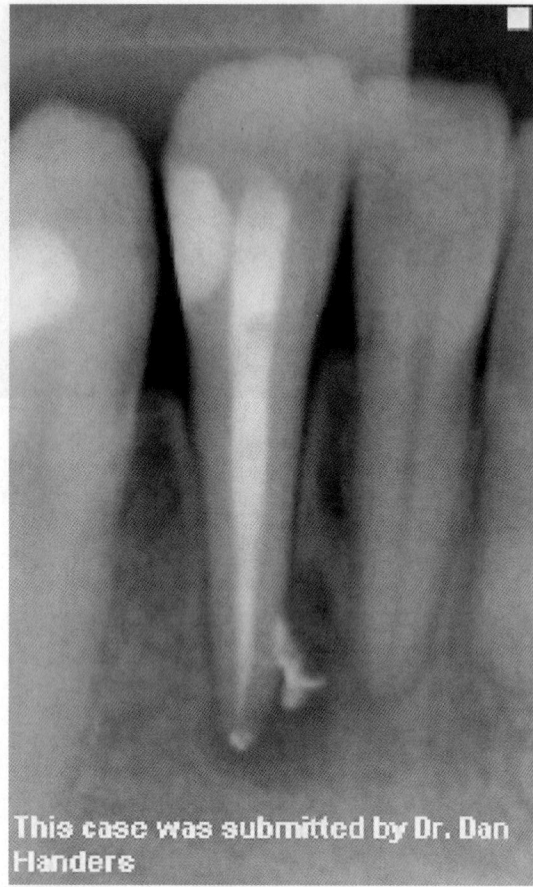

Figure 73 Mandibular right lateral incisor with 1 root and 1 canal; a lateral canal is visible on the mesial aspect of the root in the apical third. Reprinted with permission from Brown P, Herbranson E. Dental Anatomy & 3D Tooth Atlas Version 3.0. Illinois: Quintessence, 2005: Mandibular Lateral Incisor- X-ray Database.

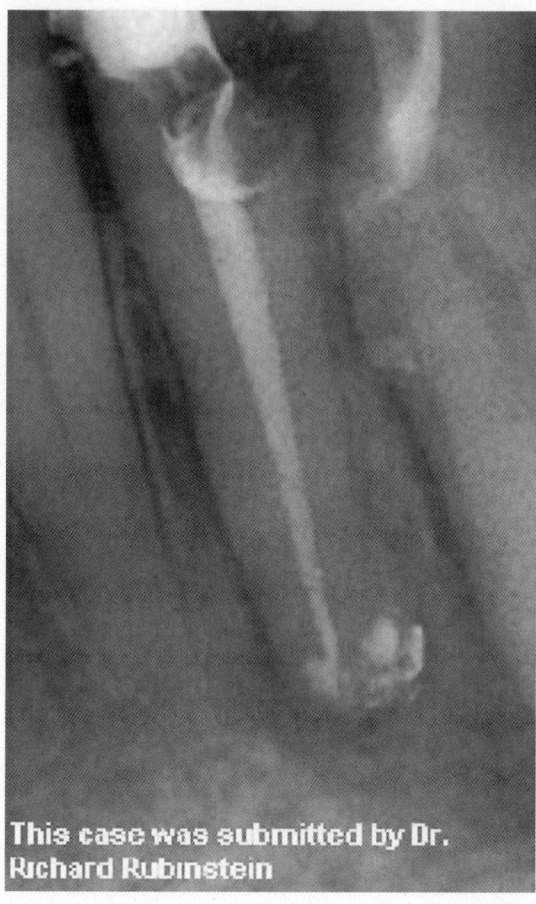

Figure 74 Mandibular lateral incisor with 1 root and 1 canal; multiple lateral canals are visible in the apical third of the root. Reprinted with permission from Brown P, Herbranson E. Dental Anatomy & 3D Tooth Atlas Version 3.0. Illinois: Quintessence, 2005: Mandibular Lateral Incisor- X-ray Database.

CANAL SYSTEM

The shape of the canal system is comparable to the mandibular central incisor and is either round or ribbon-shaped.[3,5,12,14,16,65,232] All of the anatomical studies reported found that the majority of mandibular lateral incisors have a single canal. Table 27 shows that the anatomical studies found a single canal in 71.8%

of the teeth studied. Two canals were found in 28.1% of the specimens (Figure 76).[4,6,10,36,230,231,233–240] The incidence of more than two canals was quite rare (0.1%). There was a single apical foramen found in 97.4% of the teeth included in the studies. Therefore, similar to the mandibular central incisors, even when two separate canals have been found, the majority of the canals will join and exit through a single foramen.

VARIATIONS AND ANOMALIES

Few anomalies are reported for this tooth. Case reports of anomalies include dens invaginatus,[248,249] gemination[5] (Figure 77), fusion[5,250,251] (Figure 78), and two (bifid) roots.[192]

Mandibular Canine

EXTERNAL ROOT MORPHOLOGY

The root of the mandibular canine in cross section is wider labiolingually and narrower mesiodistally, which is larger but similar to the shape of the other mandibular anterior teeth (Figures 79–83). Developmental depressions are normally present on both the mesial and the distal surfaces of the root. The depressions can be relatively deep. Normally a single-rooted tooth, one variation is a bifurcated root[3,5,12,14,16,65] (Figure 84). When this occurs, the level of furcation dividing the labial and the lingual roots can be at any level on the root and usually results in a smaller lingual rootlet at the apical region. The overall average length of the mandibular canine is 27 mm with an average crown length of 11 mm and an average root length of 16 mm.[3]

ROOT NUMBER AND FORM

As described above, the most common form of the mandibular canine is one with a single root, as listed in Table 28.[4,252,253] The three anatomical studies cited[4,252,253] that reported on the mandibular canine

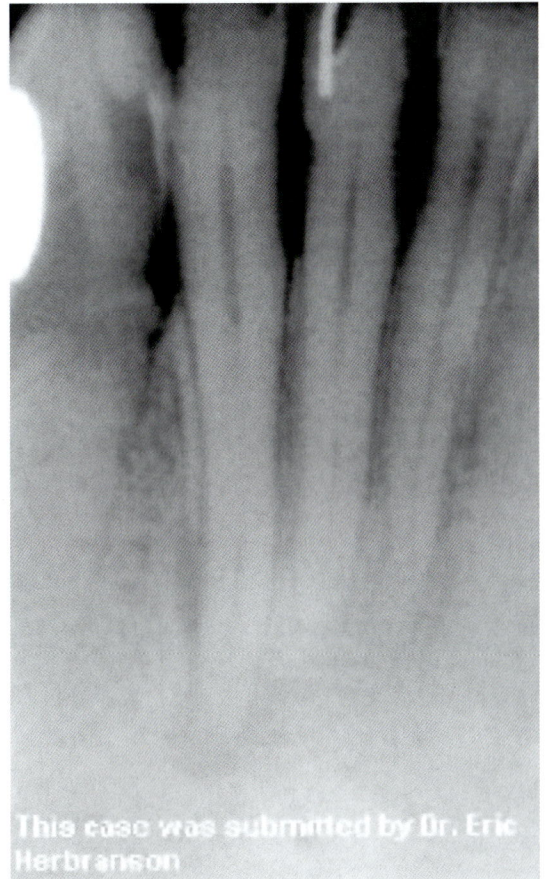

Figure 75 Mandibular right lateral incisor that exhibits a dentin island in the middle third of the root indicating a separation of the single canal into 2 canals. Reprinted with permission from Brown P, Herbranson E. Dental Anatomy & 3D Tooth Atlas Version 3.0. Illinois: Quintessence, 2005: Mandibular Lateral Incisor- X-ray Database.

Table 26 Mandibular Lateral Incisors			
Number of Roots	Number of Studies Cited	Number of Teeth	One Root
	6	1266	100% (1266)

Table 27 Mandibular Lateral Incisors							
Number of Canals and Apices	Number of Studies Cited	Number of Teeth (Canal Studies)	One Canal	Two Canals	Greater than Two Canals	One Canal at Apex	Two or More Canals at Apex
	14	2812	71.8% (2018)	28.1% (791)	0.1% (3)		
	9	1589				97.4% (1547)	2.6% (42)

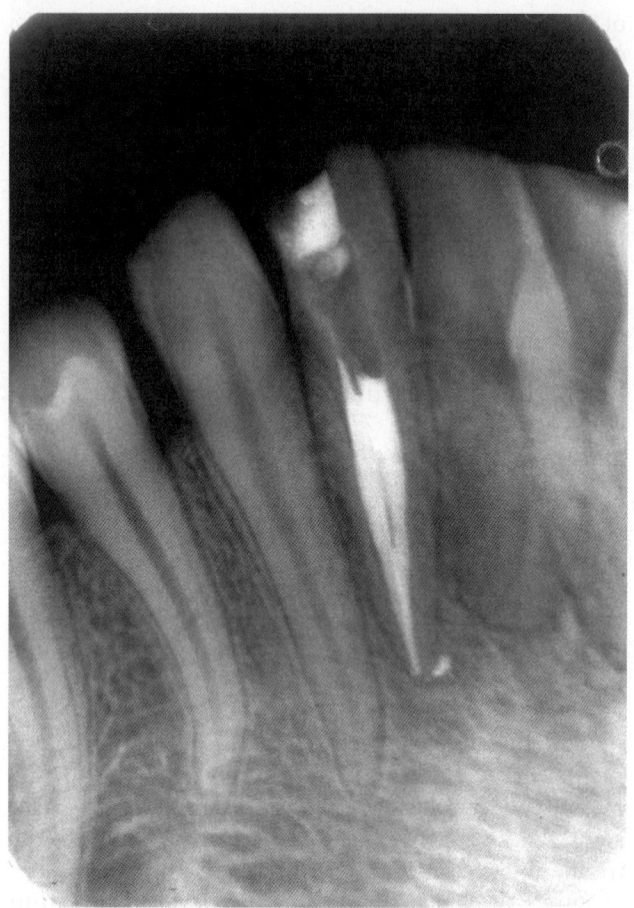

Figure 76 Mandibular right lateral incisor with two canals and one apical foramen (unpublished case report courtesy of Dr. W.H. Christie).

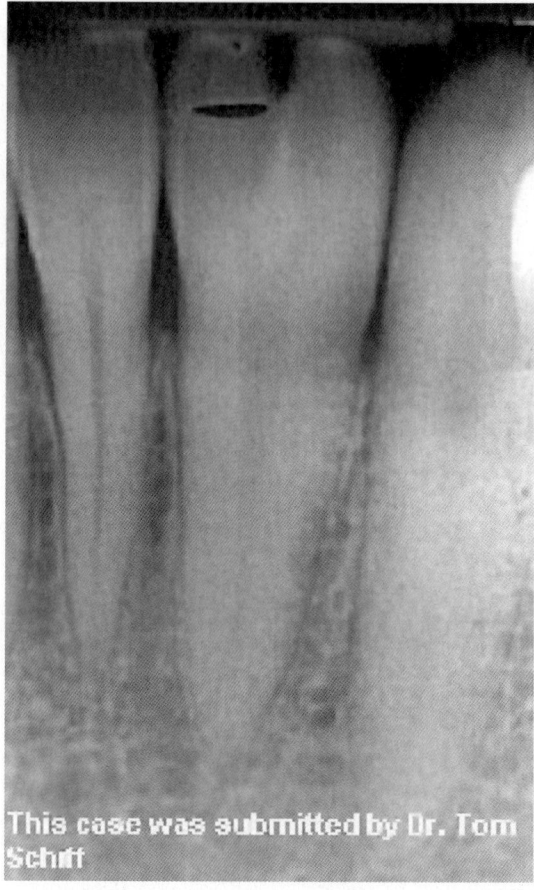

Figure 77 Mandibular left lateral incisor exhibiting gemination. Reprinted with permission from Brown P, Herbranson E. Dental Anatomy & 3D Tooth Atlas Version 3.0. Illinois: Quintessence, 2005: Mandibular Lateral Incisor- X-ray Database.

root number in certain populations found an incidence of two roots ranging from 1.7%[253] to 6.2%.[4]

CANAL SYSTEM

The mandibular canine usually presents with a single-root canal system, as cited in Table 29.[4,6,10,13,21,36,167,233,235,236,253] The incidence of a single canal is 89.4%. In the single-canal system, 96.9% have a single apical foramen.[6,13,36,253,254] Therefore, when two canals are present in a single-rooted mandibular canine, the most common configuration is the joining of the two canals before exiting at the apex (Vertucci Type II (2-1) or Vertucci Type III (1-2-1)).

A study by Green in 1956 on the root apices of the anterior teeth found that the average diameter of the major foramen, in the 50 mandibular canines studied, was 0.3 mm, while the accessory foramina were 0.2 mm in diameter. The average distance of the major apical foramen from the anatomical root apex

Chapter 6 / Morphology of Teeth and Their Root Canal Systems / 189

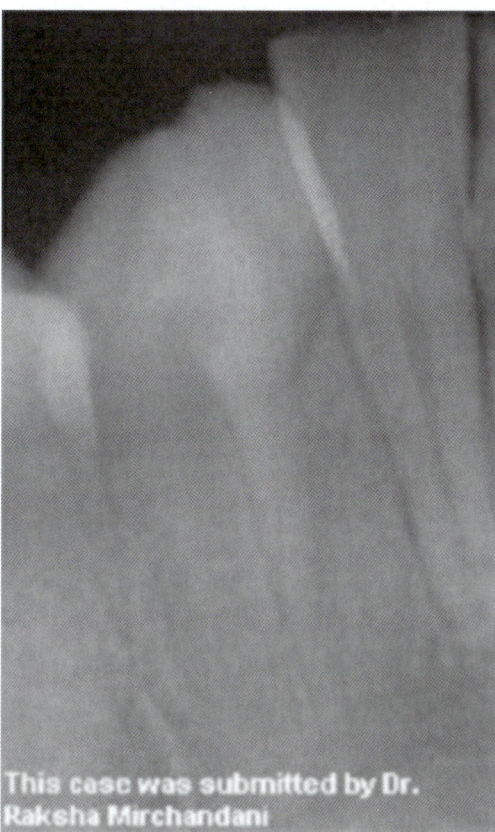

Figure 78 Mandibular right central and lateral incisor exhibiting fusion. Reprinted with permission from Brown P, Herbranson E. Dental Anatomy & 3D Tooth Atlas Version 3.0. Illinois: Quintessence, 2005: Mandibular Lateral Incisor- X-ray Database.

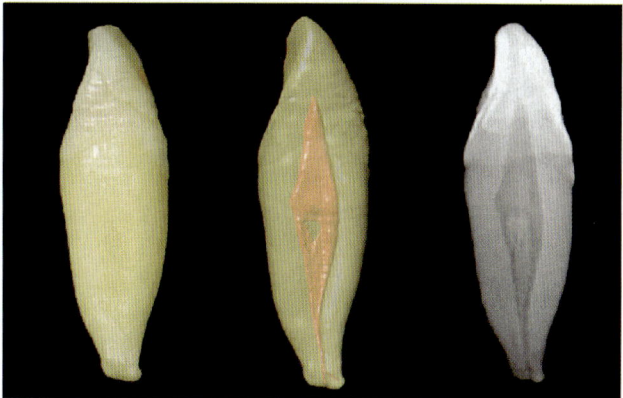

Figure 80 Mesial view of mandibular left canine. Reprinted with permission from Brown P, Herbranson E. Dental Anatomy & 3D Tooth Atlas Version 3.0. Illinois: Quintessence, 2005: Mandibular Canine- Rotations & Slices.

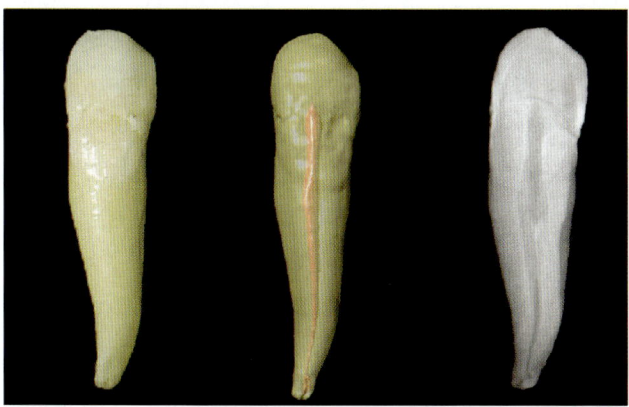

Figure 79 Labial view of mandibular left canine. Reprinted with permission from Brown P, Herbranson E. Dental Anatomy & 3D Tooth Atlas Version 3.0. Illinois: Quintessence, 2005: Mandibular Canine- Rotations & Slices.

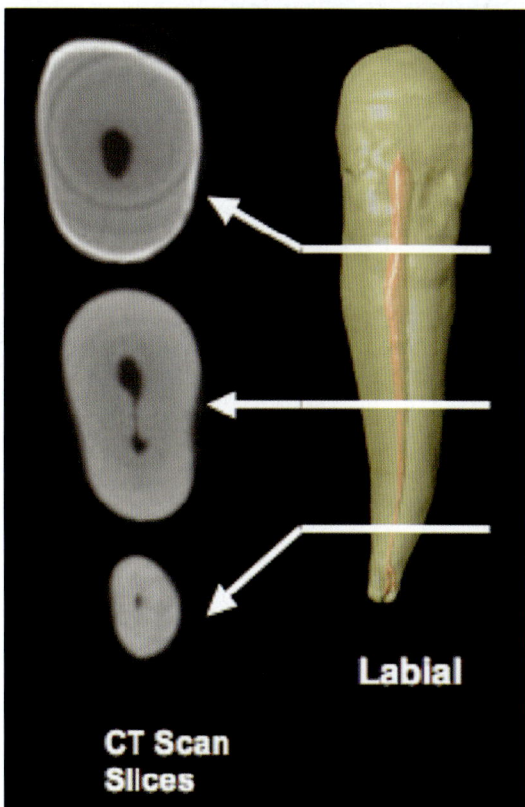

Figure 81 Root cross-sections of the mandibular left canine. Reprinted with permission from Brown P, Herbranson E. Dental Anatomy & 3D Tooth Atlas Version 3.0. Illinois: Quintessence, 2005: Mandibular Canine- Rotations & Slices.

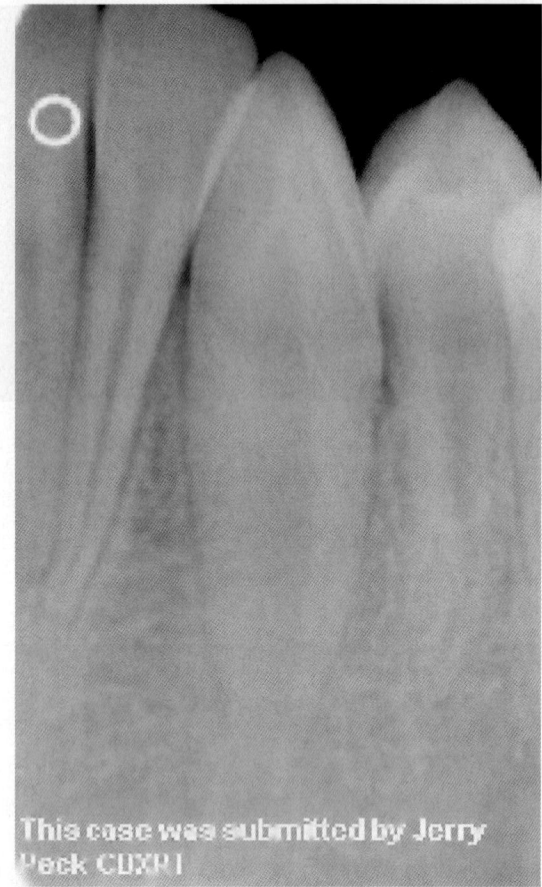

Figure 82 Rotated mandibular left canine exhibiting 1 root and 1 wide canal. Reprinted with permission from Brown P, Herbranson E. Dental Anatomy & 3D Tooth Atlas Version 3.0. Illinois: Quintessence, 2005: Mandibular Canine- X-ray Database.

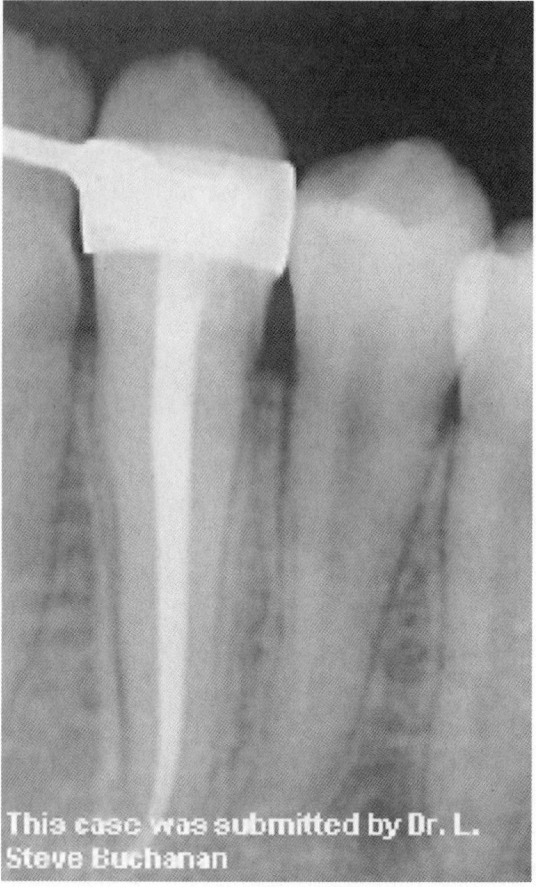

Figure 83 Mandibular left canine with 1 root and 1 canal; a mesial curvature of the root is evident in the apical third. Reprinted with permission from Brown P, Herbranson E. Dental Anatomy & 3D Tooth Atlas Version 3.0. Illinois: Quintessence, 2005: Mandibular Canine- X-ray Database.

was found to be 0.35 mm.[73] Approximately 10% of the mandibular canines exhibited accessory foramina.

VARIATIONS AND ANOMALIES

The most frequent variation found in the mandibular canine is the presence of two canals.[12] One anthropology report by Alexandersen[252] showed a high incidence of two-rooted mandibular canine teeth in an Iron-Age Danish population. Although, the data from anatomical studies vary greatly with respect to the incidence of two roots, the mandibular canine has the highest incidence of all of the anterior teeth at 5.2%. Other variations reported in the literature include two canals and two roots[255,256] (Figures 84 and 85), two canals with a single apical foramen[5,257] (Figure 86), dens evaginatus,[157] three canals in a single root,[258] fusion with a lateral incisor,[250] dens invaginatus[5] (Figure 87), and gemination[5] (Figure 88).

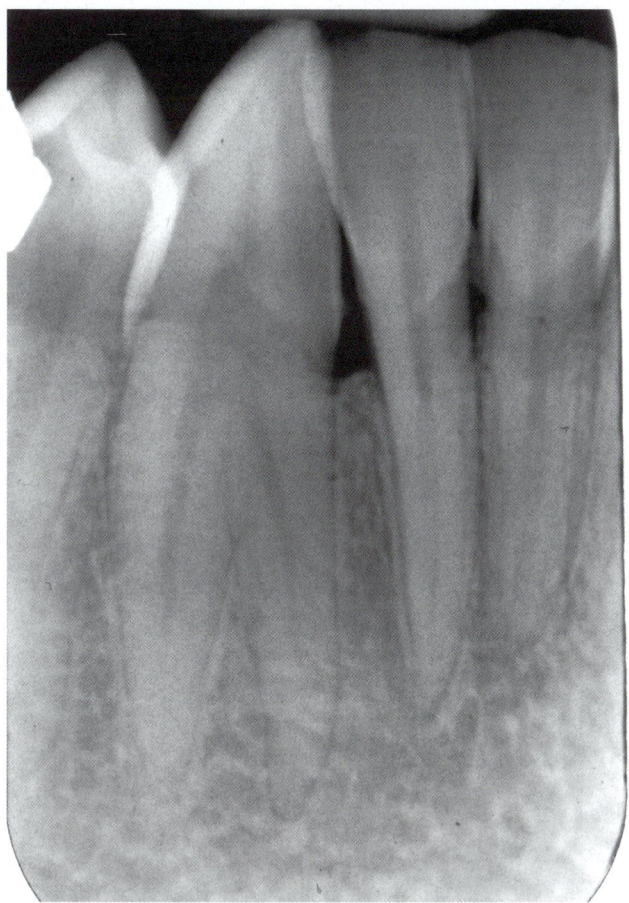

Figure 84 Rotated two-rooted mandibular right canine with radicular third root bifurcation. Courtesy of Dr. W.H. Christie.

Mandibular First Premolar

EXTERNAL ROOT MORPHOLOGY

The mandibular first premolar is typically a single-rooted tooth that is wider buccolingually and narrower mesiodistally, although two-rooted varieties do occur fairly frequently[1,3,5,14–16] (Figures 89–91). Developmental depressions or grooves are frequently found on both the mesial and the distal surfaces of the root resulting in an ovoid- or hourglass-shaped root. The depression on the distal root surface has been described as being deeper than the mesial root depression.[259] The overall average length of the mandibular first premolar is 22.5 mm with an average crown length of 8.5 mm and an average root length of 14 mm.[3]

Table 28 Mandibular Canine			
Number of Roots	Number of Studies Cited	Number of Teeth	One Root	Two Roots
	3	6259	94.8% (5935)	5.2% (324)

Table 29 Mandibular Canine						
Number of Canals and Apices	Number of Studies Cited	Number of Teeth (Canal Studies)	One Canal	Two or More Canals	One Canal at apex	Two or More Canals at apex
	11	3237	89.4% (2894)	10.6% (343)		
	5	1417			96.9% (1373)	3.1% (44)

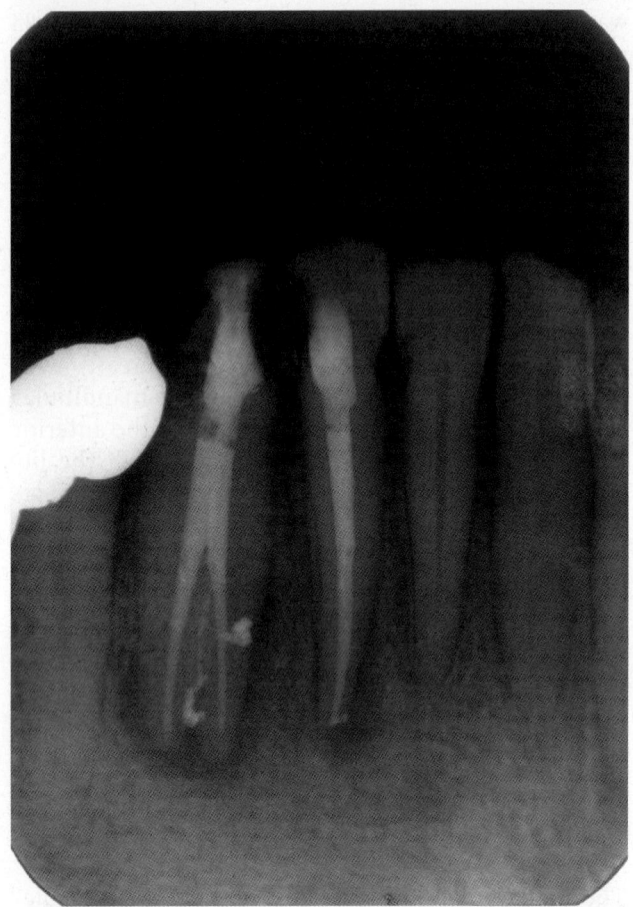

Figure 85 Rotated two-rooted mandibular right canine with two root canal systems filled and apical third separation of root tips. Courtesy of Dr. W.H. Christie.

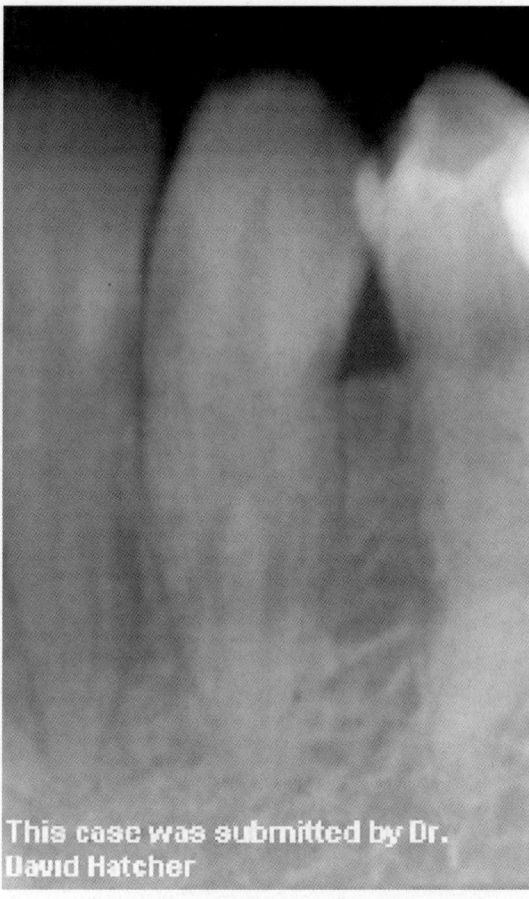

Figure 86 Mandibular right canine with two canals and two foramina in a single root. Reprinted with permission from Brown P, Herbranson E. Dental Anatomy & 3D Tooth Atlas Version 3.0. Illinois: Quintessence, 2005: Mandibular Canine- X-ray Database.

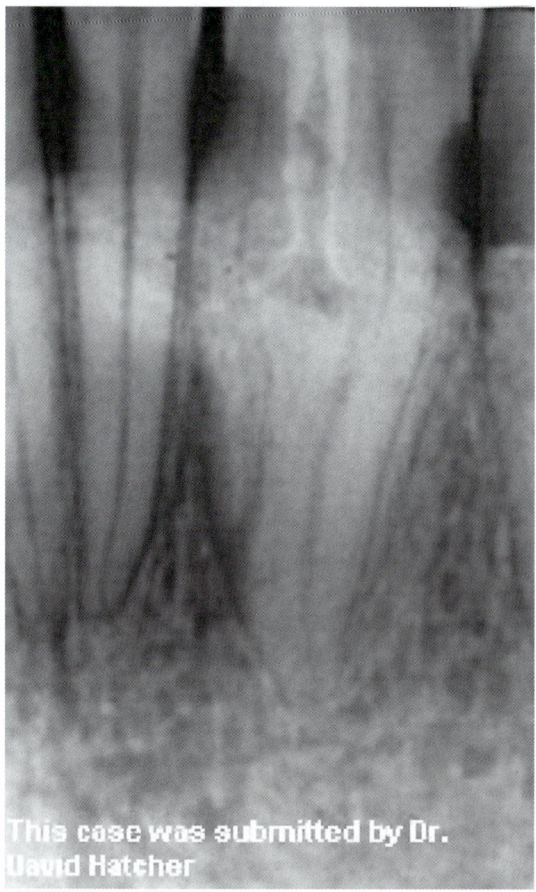

Figure 87 Mandibular left canine exhibiting dens invaginatus (dens in dente). Reprinted with permission from Brown P, Herbranson E. Dental Anatomy & 3D Tooth Atlas Version 3.0. Illinois: Quintessence, 2005: Mandibular Canine- X-ray Database.

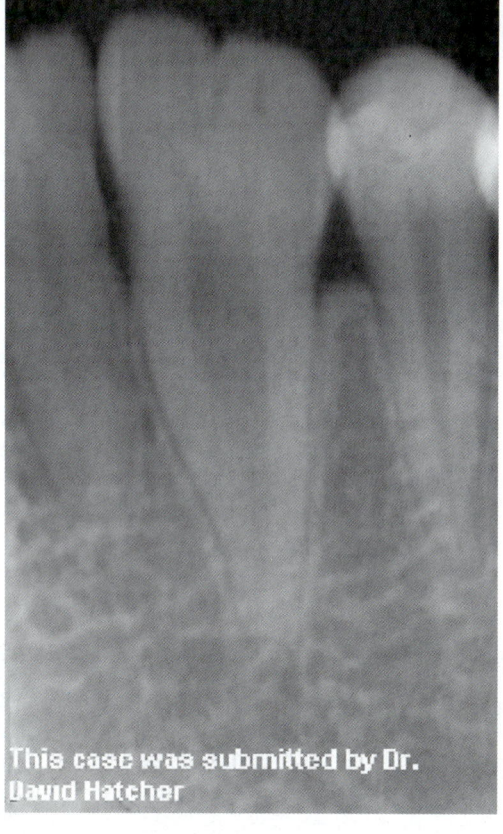

Figure 88 Mandibular left canine exhibiting gemination. Reprinted with permission from Brown P, Herbranson E. Dental Anatomy & 3D Tooth Atlas Version 3.0. Illinois: Quintessence, 2005: Mandibular Canine- X-ray Database.

ROOT NUMBER AND FORM

The mandibular first premolar is normally a single-rooted tooth, as shown in Figures 92 and 93 (Table 30); however, eight anatomical studies did reveal an incidence in approximately 1.8% of bifurcated teeth (Figure 94).[4,6,13,57,254,260–262]

Trope et al. found significant ethnic variations in the root anatomy when comparing African American and Caucasian patients.[263] Their study found an incidence of two root canals of 5.5% in the Caucasian and 16.2% in the African American group of patients. Three-rooted mandibular first premolars are rare but are occasionally found in case reports[264] (Figures 95–97). Scott and Turner[265] describe the accessory root as "Tome's root." Their anthropological review of ethnic differences indicates that aboriginal Australians and sub-Sahara African population

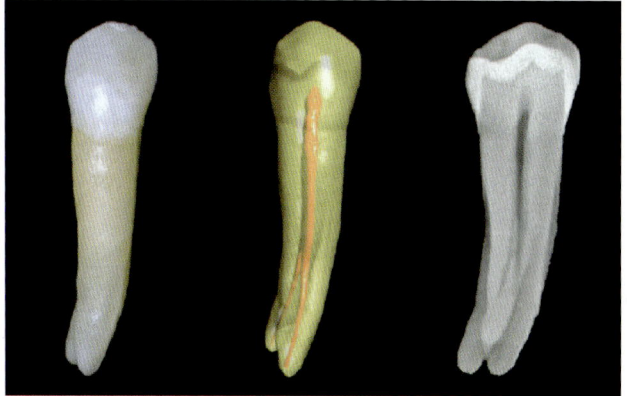

Figure 89 Buccal view of mandibular right first premolar with two canals and two roots; NOTE: the tooth pictured is a variation from normal with two roots and two canals (incidence of approximately 1.8%). Reprinted with permission from Brown P, Herbranson E. Dental Anatomy & 3D Tooth Atlas Version 3.0. Illinois: Quintessence, 2005: Mandibular First Premolar- Rotations & Slices.

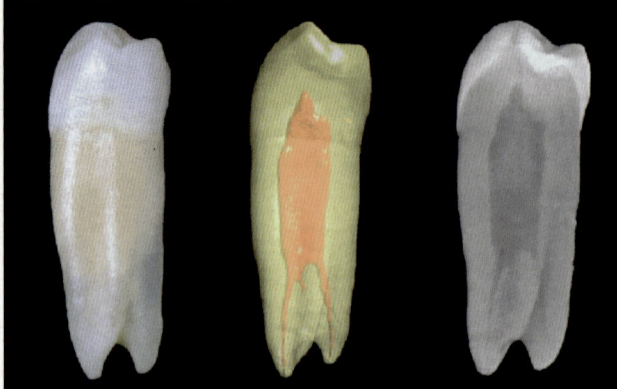

Figure 90 Mesial view of mandibular right first premolar with two canals and two roots. Reprinted with permission from Brown P, Herbranson E. Dental Anatomy & 3D Tooth Atlas Version 3.0. Illinois: Quintessence, 2005: Mandibular First Premolar- Rotations & Slices.

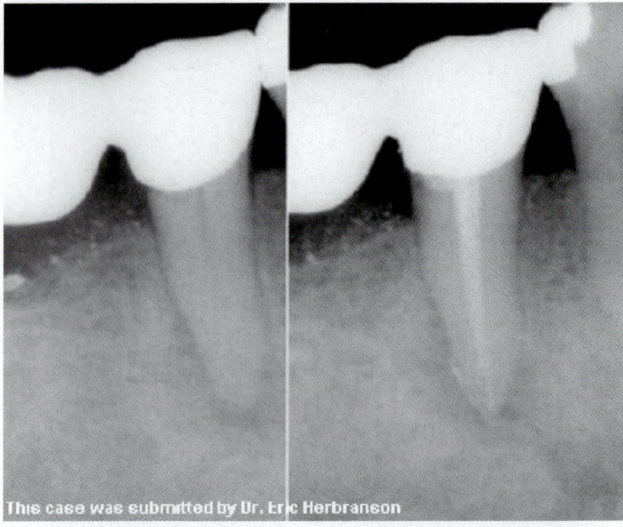

Figure 92 Mandibular right first premolar with a single root and single canal; a lateral canal is visible on the distal aspect of the apical third of the root. Reprinted with permission from Brown P, Herbranson E. Dental Anatomy & 3D Tooth Atlas Version 3.0. Illinois: Quintessence, 2005: Mandibular First Premolar- X-ray Database.

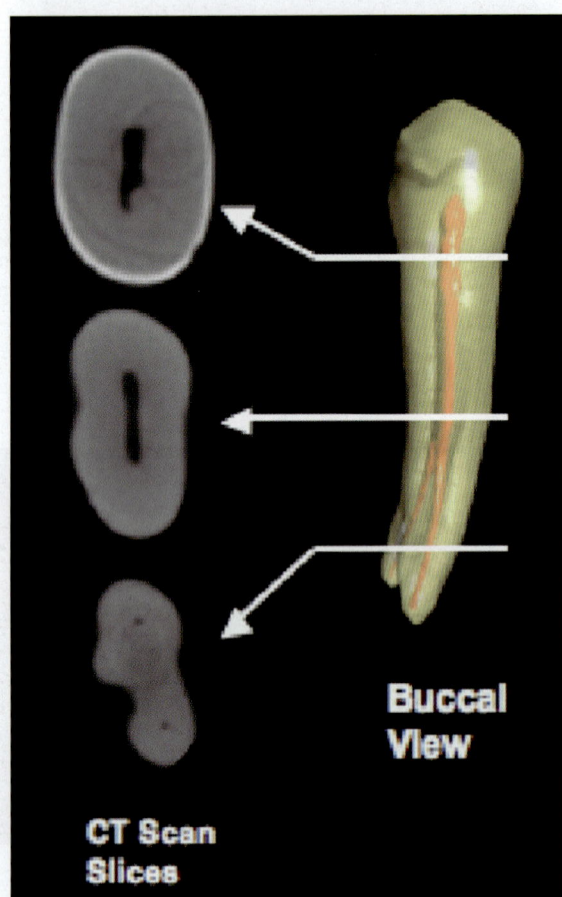

Figure 91 Root cross-sections of the mandibular right first premolar. Reprinted with permission from Brown P, Herbranson E. Dental Anatomy & 3D Tooth Atlas Version 3.0. Illinois: Quintessence, 2005: Mandibular First Premolar- Rotations & Slices.

have the highest incidence (>25%) of accessory roots. The lowest incidence (0–10%) of Tome's root occurred in American Arctic, New Guinea, Jomon, and Western Eurasian population.

CANAL SYSTEM

Slowey has suggested that the mandibular premolars may present with greatest difficulty of all teeth to treat endodontically.[192] A University of Washington study assessed the failure rate of nonsurgical RCT in all teeth. It was highest for the mandibular first premolar at 11.45%.[1] The possible reasons for a high failure rate are the numerous variations in root canal morphology and difficult access to a second canal. There is usually a straight line access to the buccal canal, while the lingual canal branches at a sharp angle, potentially resulting in a missed canal. A study by Kartal and Yanikoglu, using pooled data (Table 31) that included first and second premolars, reported a 27.8% incidence of mandibular premolars with more than one canal.[266] Serman and Hasselgren examined full mouth series of radiographs for 547 patients and found that 15.7% of patients had at least one mandibular first premolar with either a divided canal or a root.[267] The second premolars had an incidence of 7% in this study.

The data from 16 anatomical studies of the canal system that included only mandibular first premolars (Table 32) resulted in a weighted average of a single

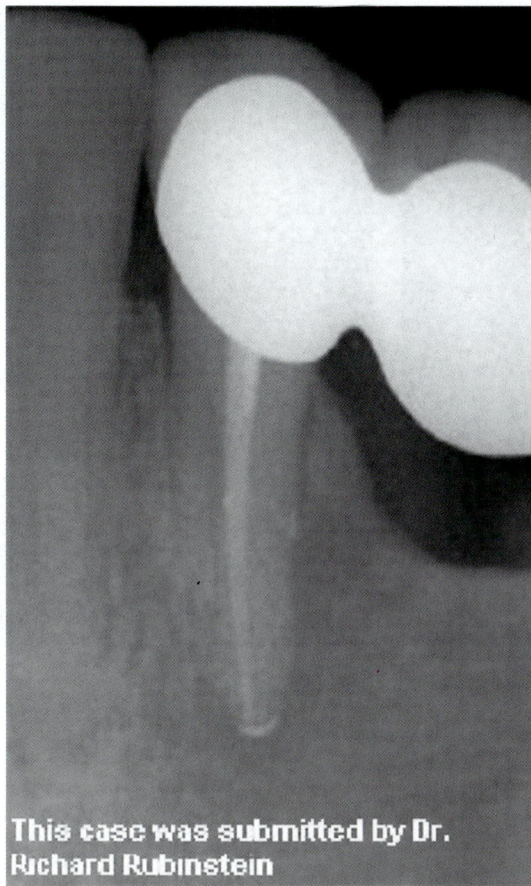

Figure 93 Mandibular left first premolar exhibiting a single root and single canal; lateral canals emanating from the main canal in the middle third of the root are present. Reprinted with permission from Brown P, Herbranson E. Dental Anatomy & 3D Tooth Atlas Version 3.0. Illinois: Quintessence, 2005: Mandibular First Premolar- X-ray Database.

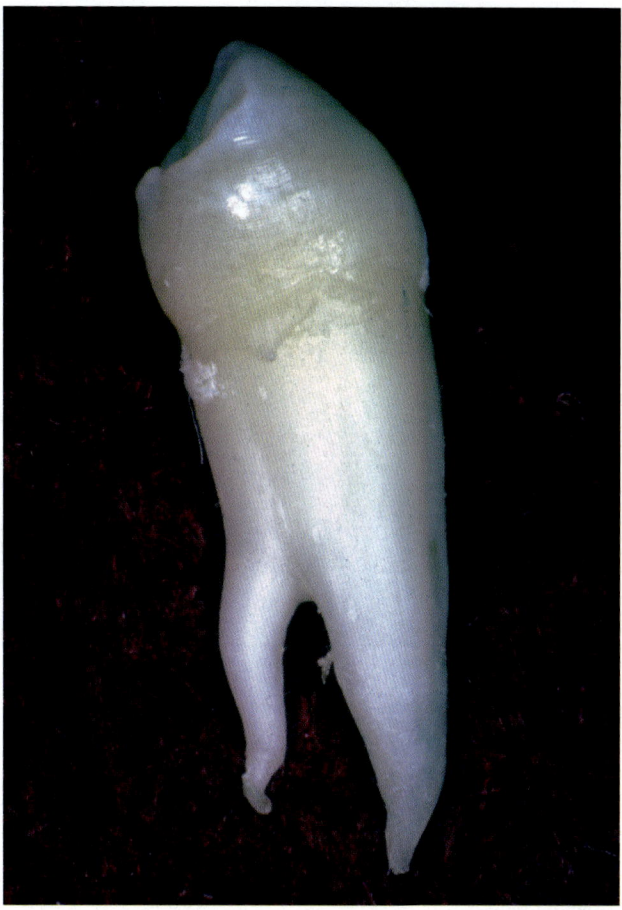

Figure 94 Extracted mandibular right first premolar with a main buccal and a vestigial mid-root lingual root. Courtesy of Dr. W.H. Christie.

Table 30 Mandibular First Premolar						
Number of Roots	Number of Studies Cited	Number of Teeth	One root	Two Roots	Three Roots	Four Roots
	8	4462	97.9% (4369)	1.8% (81)	0.2% (10)	<0.1% (2)

canal in 75.8% of the teeth studied.[4,6,21,35,57,167,170,197,236,254,260,268–272] Two or more canals were found in 24.2% of the teeth. Ten anatomical studies assessed the canal number at the apex.[6,35,57,167,197,254,268–271] These studies found a single canal at the apex 78.9% of the time.

Trope and colleague's study found significant ethnic differences between African American and Caucasian patients.[263] The incidence of two or more canals in the

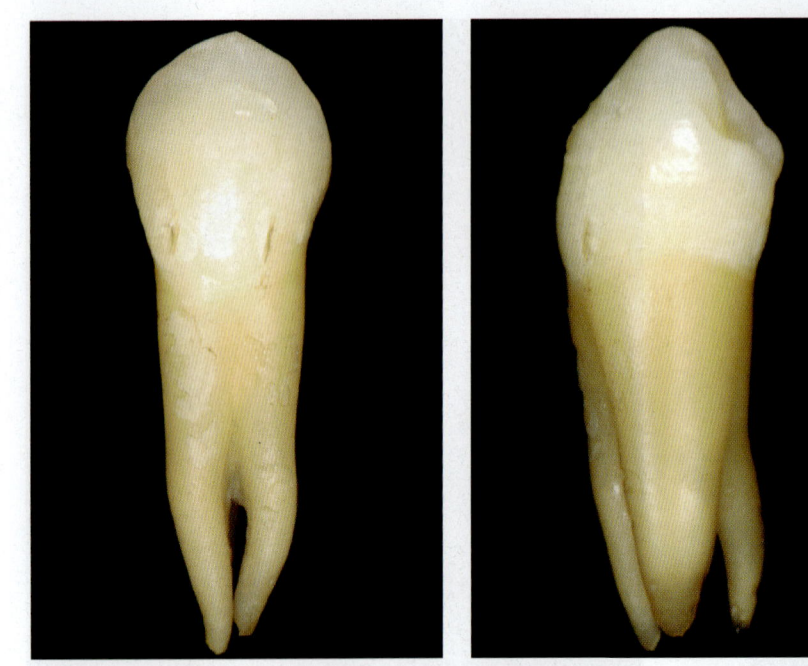
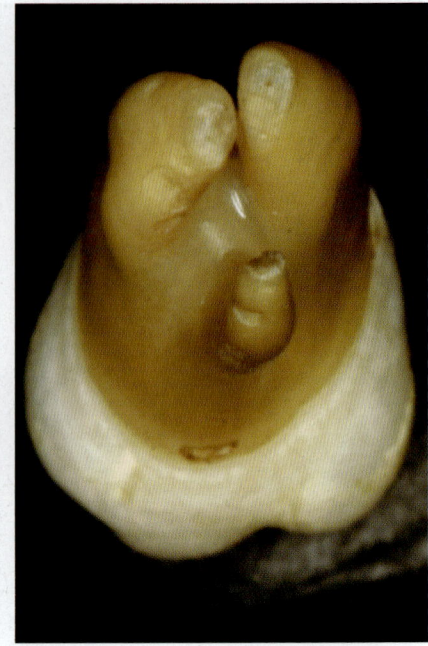

Figures 95–97 Rare three-rooted mandibular first premolar. Courtesy of Drs. BM Cleghorn and CCS Dong.

Table 31 Pooled Data for Mandibular First and Second Premolars						
Number of Canals and Apices	Number of Studies Cited	Number of Teeth (Canal Studies)	One Canal	Two or More Canals	One Canal at Apex	Two or More Canals at Apex
	1	187	72.2% (135)	27.8% (52)	76.5% (143)	23.5% (44)

Table 32 Mandibular First Premolars						
Number of Canals and Apices	Number of Studies Cited	Number of Teeth (Canal Studies)	One Canal	Two or More Canals	One Canal at Apex	Two or More Canals at Apex
	16	4733	75.8% (3586)	24.2% (1147)		
	10	2604			78.9% (2054)	21.1% (550)

African American group of 400 patients was 32.8%, while the incidence in the Caucasian group of 400 patients was 13.7%. A study of 1,000 full mouth radiographic surveys by Amos in 1955 also found ethnic differences between African American and Caucasian patients.[273] Although the number of patients in each ethnic group was not identified, Amos reported that 16% of the Caucasian patients had bifurcated canals compared to 21.6% of the African American patients. Sert and Bayirli's study of Turkish patients found an incidence of two or more canals in 35% of the males and 44% of the females, further reinforcing the importance of ethnic differences as well as gender differences.[10]

VARIATIONS AND ANOMALIES

Anomalies associated with mandibular first premolars include gemination,[274] dens evaginatus,[275] dens invaginatus,[276–278] two roots,[279] three roots (see Figures 95–97) two canals in a single root,[280–283] three canals with fused roots,[280] three canals in a single root[282,284,285] (Figure 98), three canals and two roots[286] (Figure 99), three canals and three roots,[264,287] three canals, and one case of aberrant root development and multiple roots in all mandibular premolars.[288]

A study of 45 X-chromosome females in Finland found more than one canal in one or more of the

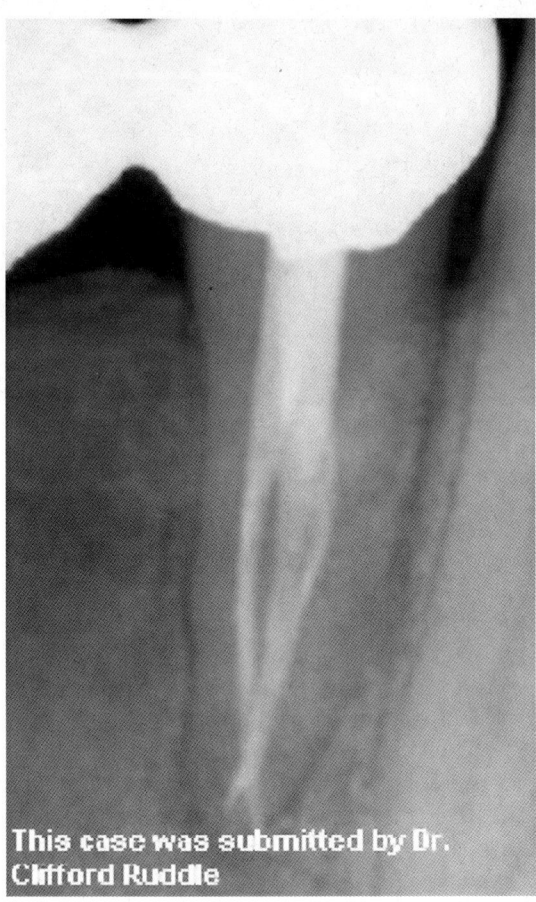

Figure 98 Mandibular right first premolar exhibiting 3 canals in a single root. Reprinted with permission from Brown P, Herbranson E. Dental Anatomy & 3D Tooth Atlas Version 3.0. Illinois: Quintessence, 2005: Mandibular First Premolar- X-ray Database.

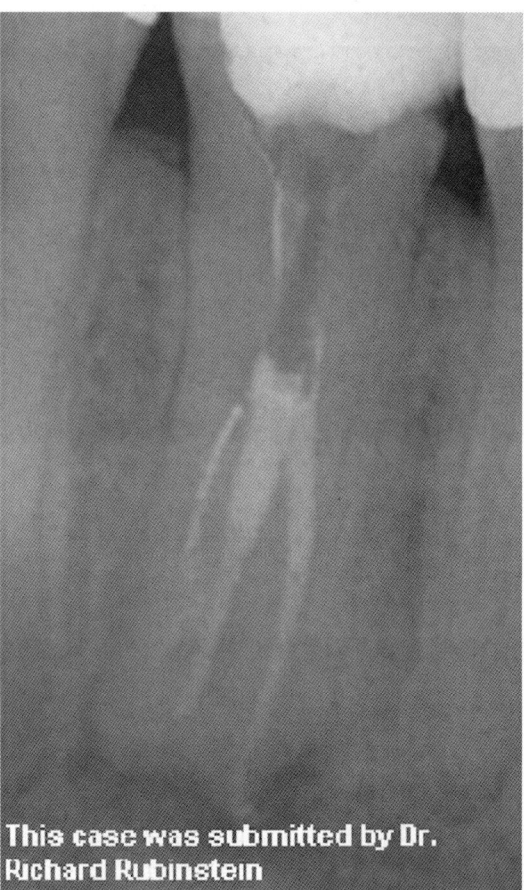

Figure 99 Mandibular left premolar with 3 canals and 2 roots. Reprinted with permission from Brown P, Herbranson E. Dental Anatomy & 3D Tooth Atlas Version 3.0. Illinois: Quintessence, 2005: Mandibular First Premolar- X-ray Database.

mandibular premolars in almost half of the 87 patients studied. Separate canals were found in 23% of the mandibular first premolars and 25% of the mandibular second premolars.[289] The study concluded that X chromosomes have a gene or genes with a regulatory function in root development.

Mandibular Second Premolar

EXTERNAL ROOT MORPHOLOGY

The mandibular second premolar is normally a single-rooted tooth (Figures 100–104) like the mandibular

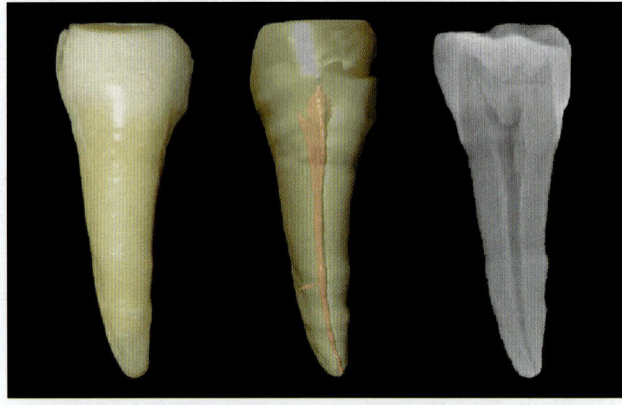

Figure 100 Buccal view of mandibular left second premolar. Reprinted with permission from Brown P, Herbranson E. Dental Anatomy & 3D Tooth Atlas Version 3.0. Illinois: Quintessence, 2005: Mandibular Second Premolar- Rotations & Slices.

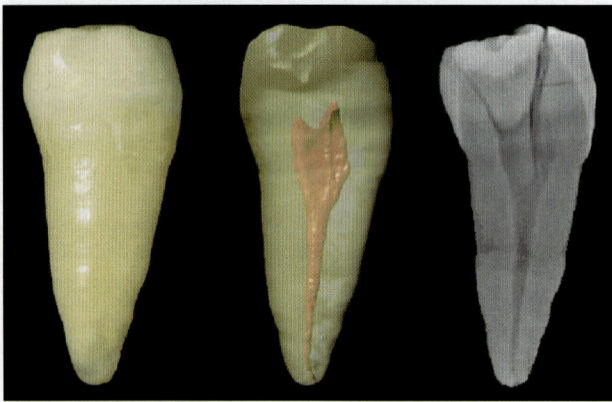

Figure 101 Mesial view of mandibular left second premolar [vertical crack in buccal cusp is an artifact]. Reprinted with permission from Brown P, Herbranson E. Dental Anatomy & 3D Tooth Atlas Version 3.0. Illinois: Quintessence, 2005: Mandibular Second Premolar- Rotations & Slices.

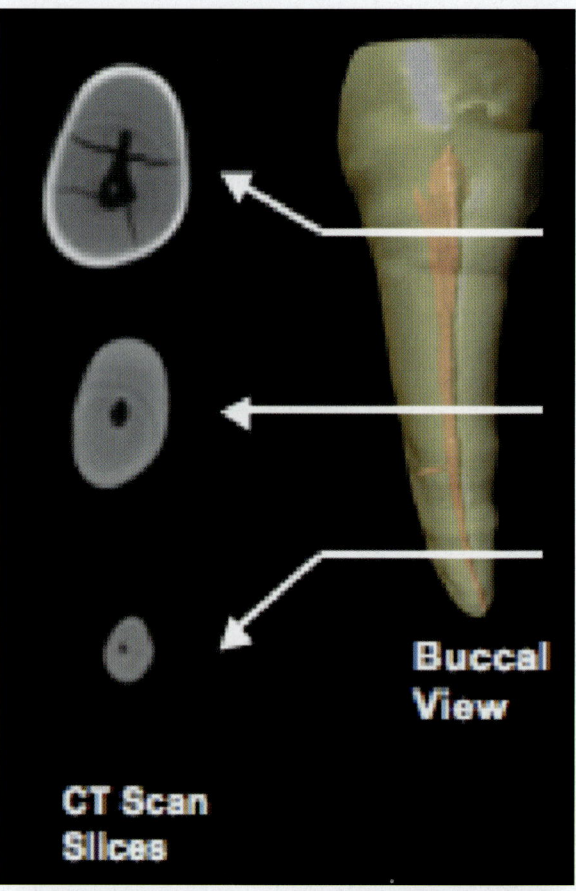

Figure 102 Root cross-sections of the mandibular left second premolar. Reprinted with permission from Brown P, Herbranson E. Dental Anatomy & 3D Tooth Atlas Version 3.0. Illinois: Quintessence, 2005: Mandibular Second Premolar- Rotations & Slices.

first premolar.[1,3,5,14–16] The root is described as flat or convex on its mesial surface, while the distal surface often (73%) has a longitudinal developmental depression.[259] A cross section of the root is usually ovoid in shape.[15] The overall average length of the mandibular second premolar is 22.5 mm with an average crown length of 8 mm and an average root length of 14.5 mm.[3]

ROOT NUMBER AND FORM

The mandibular second premolar is normally a single-rooted tooth. Trope et al. compared the root and root canal morphology in Caucasian and African American patients and found a 1.5% incidence of two roots in second premolar teeth in Caucasian and a 4.8% incidence in African American patients.[263] These differences were not statistically significant in contrast to the differences found

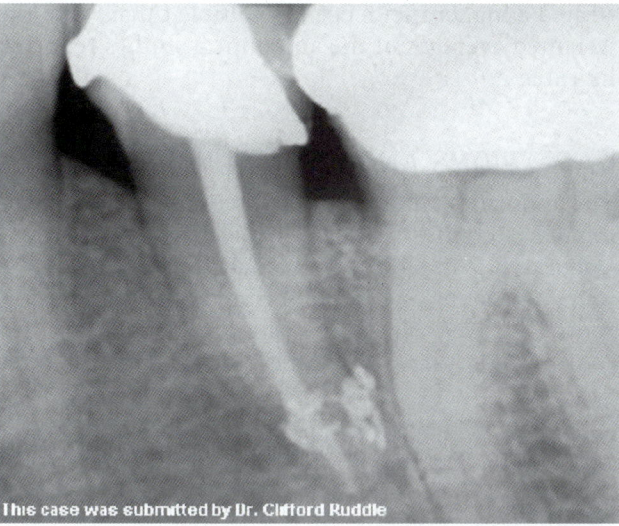

Figure 103 Mandibular left second premolar with a single root and single canal; multiple lateral canals are visible on the distal aspect of the apical third of the root. Reprinted with permission from Brown P, Herbranson E. Dental Anatomy & 3D Tooth Atlas Version 3.0. Illinois: Quintessence, 2005: Mandibular Second Premolar- X-ray Database.

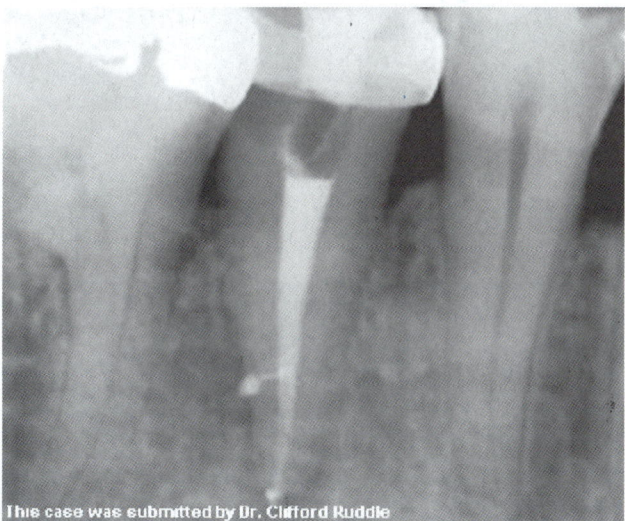

Figure 104 Mandibular right second premolar exhibiting a single root and single canal; a lateral canal emanating from the main canal in the middle third of the root is present. Reprinted with permission from Brown P, Herbranson E. Dental Anatomy & 3D Tooth Atlas Version 3.0. Illinois: Quintessence, 2005: Mandibular Second Premolar- X-ray Database.

between these two groups in the mandibular first premolars.

The eight anatomical studies cited found multi-rooted mandibular second premolars to be quite rare[4,6,10,57,260,269,271,290] (Table 33). Two-rooted varieties comprised 0.3% of the 2985 teeth in the studies. Three-rooted forms were rarely found and comprised 0.1% of these teeth.

CANAL SYSTEM

The anatomical studies found a single canal in 91.1% of the 2983 mandibular second premolars[4,6,10,36,57,167,236,260,269,271] (Table 34). When a second canal system is located, it is usually fine and branches toward the lingual surface in the middle or the apical third of the main canal. The incidence of two or more canals was 8.9%. There was a single apical foramen 91.6% of the time. Serman and Hasselgren's study of full mouth radiographic series of 547 patients found that second mandibular premolars had an incidence of a divided canal or a root of 7%.[267] Trope et al. found ethnic differences between African American and Caucasian patients.[263] The incidence of mandibular second premolars with two or more canals in

Table 33	Mandibular Second Premolars				
Number of Roots	Number of Studies Cited	Number of Teeth	One Root	Two Roots	Three Roots
	8	4019	99.6% (4001)	0.3% (12)	0.1% (6)

Table 34	Mandibular Second Premolars					
Number of Canals and Apices	Number of Studies Cited	Number of Teeth (Canal Studies)	One Canal	Two or More Canals	One Canal at Apex	Two or More Canals at Apex
	10	2983	91.1% (2717)	8.9% (266)		
	7	1970			91.6% (1804)	8.4% (166)

the African American group of 400 patients was 7.8%, while the incidence in the Caucasian group of 400 patients was 2.8%. These differences were not statistically significant in contrast to the results found with the mandibular first premolar canal systems.

Sert and Bayirli's study of Turkish patients found an incidence of two or more canals in 43% of the male patients and 15% of the female patients.[10] The gender differences in this Turkish population were significant, and this ethnic group as a whole demonstrated a higher incidence of multiple canals than the weighted averages of the anatomical studies reported in Table 2.

VARIATIONS AND ANOMALIES

The anomalies reported in the literature include mandibular second premolars with dens evaginatus[291] (Figures 105 and 106), two canals (Figures 107–109), four canals in one root,[292] four canals and three roots,[293] five canals in a single root,[294] two roots[279,287,293,295–298] (Figures 110 and 111), three

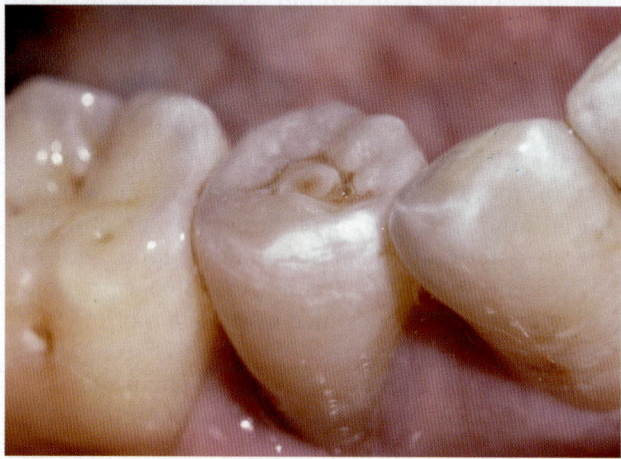

Figure 105 Non-vital mandibular right second premolar exhibiting dens evaginatus (see worn tubercle in central fossa). Courtesy of Dr. W.H. Christie.

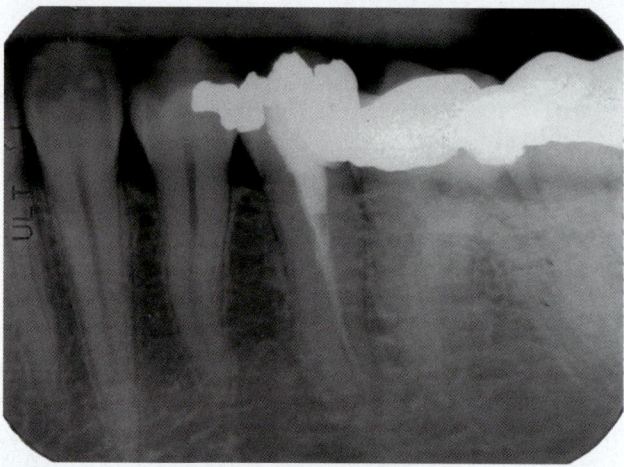

Figure 107 Failing mandibular left second premolar with incomplete root canal treatment with one canal undiscovered and left untreated. Courtesy of Dr. W.H. Christie.

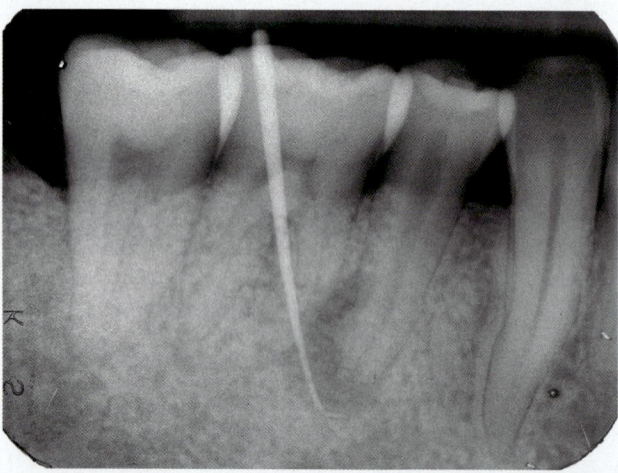

Figure 106 Radiograph of same patient seen in Figure 105 with gutta-percha point in sinus tract pointing to apex of mandibular second premolar. The mandibular first premolar was extracted for orthodontic treatment.

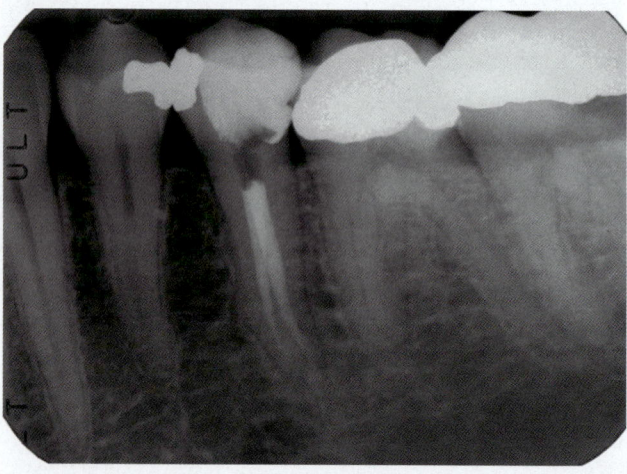

Figure 108 Same case as **Figure 6-107** after retreatment; both canal systems treated. Courtesy of Dr. W.H. Christie.

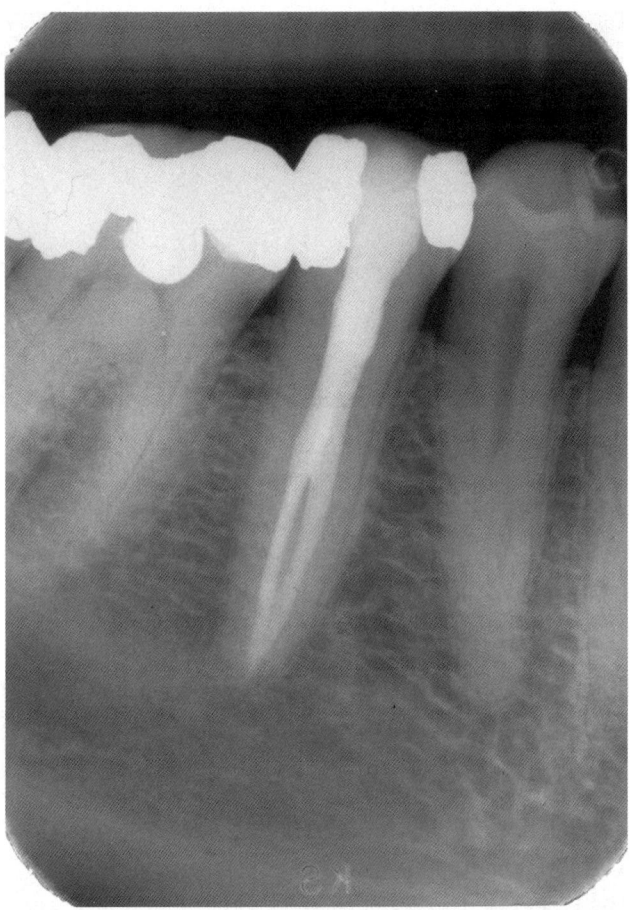

Figure 109 Mandibular right second premolar with two canals and one apical foramen. Courtesy of Dr. W.H. Christie.

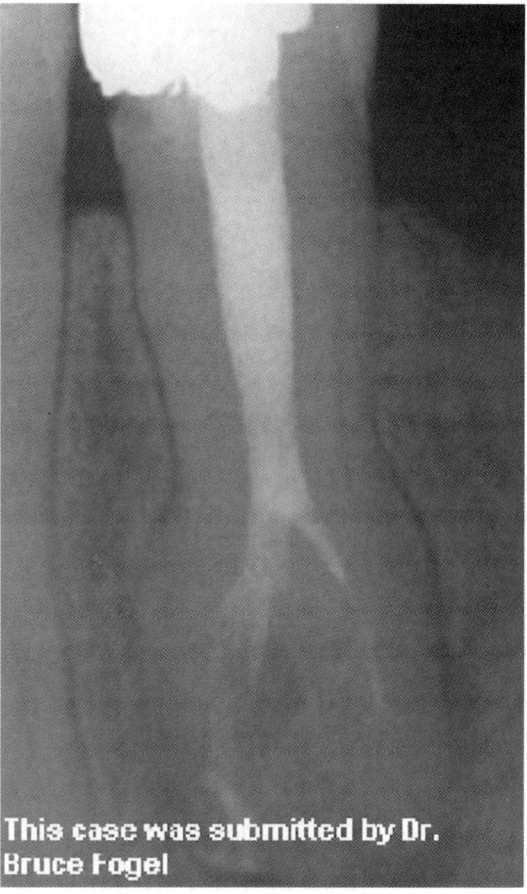

Figure 110 Mandibular left second premolar with a hypertaurodont mesial and a distal root; mesial root has multiple canals present. Reprinted with permission from Brown P, Herbranson E. Dental Anatomy & 3D Tooth Atlas Version 3.0. Illinois: Quintessence, 2005: Mandibular Second Premolar- X-ray Database.

roots and three canals,[264,287,299] three canals,[282,300–302] two canals and two roots,[280,303] two roots and four canals,[297,304] aberrant root development and multiple roots on all mandibular premolars,[288] and a four-canal system anomaly.[305] Dens evaginatus is a fairly common occurrence in Asians and is usually found in mandibular premolars. Merrill reported a high incidence (4.5%) of this anomaly in Alaskan Eskimos and

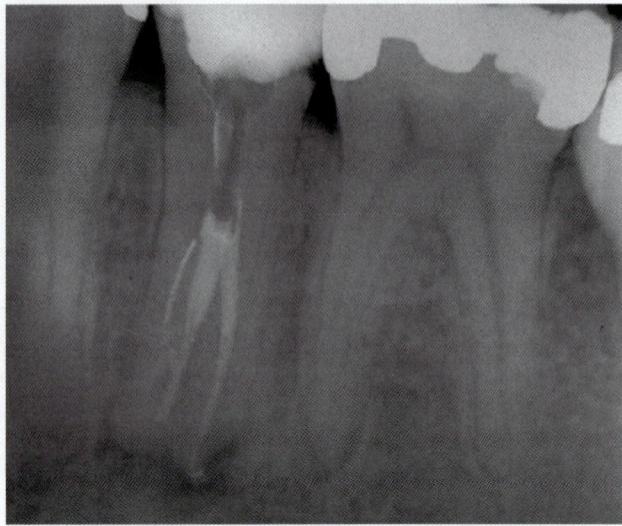

Figure 111 Mandibular left second premolar with 2 roots and 3 canals. Reprinted with permission from Brown P, Herbranson E. Dental Anatomy & 3D Tooth Atlas Version 3.0. Illinois: Quintessence, 2005: Mandibular Second Premolar- X-ray Database.

Indians, an observation serving to illustrate Alaskan natives' ties to their Asian heritage.[306]

Mandibular First Molar

EXTERNAL ROOT MORPHOLOGY

The mandibular first molar is typically a two-rooted tooth,[1,3,5,14–16] as shown in Figures 112–117. The mesial and the distal roots are normally widely separated with a furcation level buc-

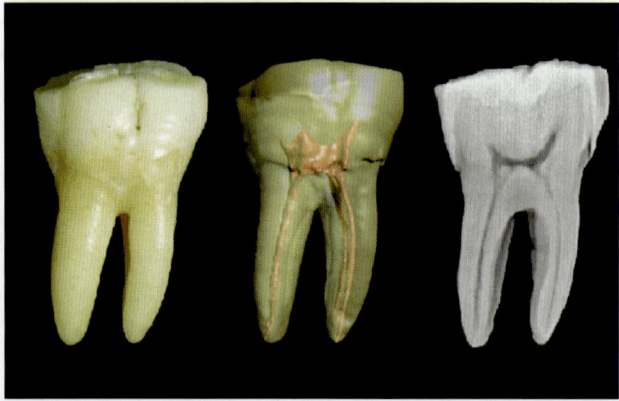

Figure 112 Buccal view of mandibular right first molar. Reprinted with permission from Brown P, Herbranson E. Dental Anatomy & 3D Tooth Atlas Version 3.0. Illinois: Quintessence, 2005: Mandibular First Molar- Rotations & Slices.

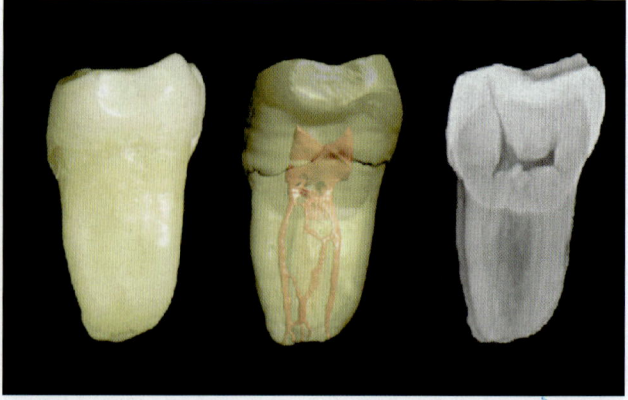

Figure 113 Mesial view of mandibular right first molar. Reprinted with permission from Brown P, Herbranson E. Dental Anatomy & 3D Tooth Atlas Version 3.0. Illinois: Quintessence, 2005: Mandibular First Molar- Rotations & Slices.

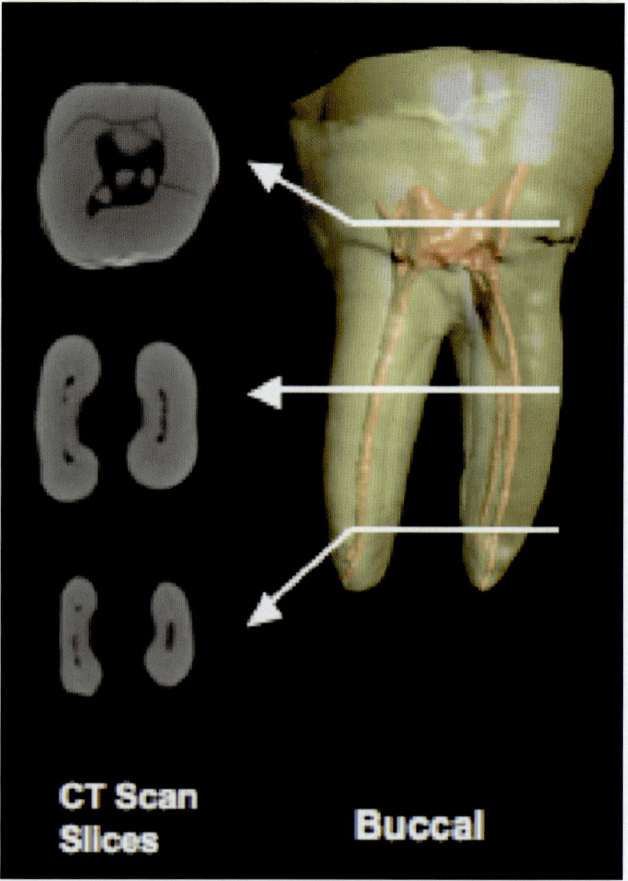

Figure 114 Root cross-sections of the mandibular right first molar. Reprinted with permission from Brown P, Herbranson E. Dental Anatomy & 3D Tooth Atlas Version 3.0. Illinois: Quintessence, 2005: Mandibular First Molar- Rotations & Slices.

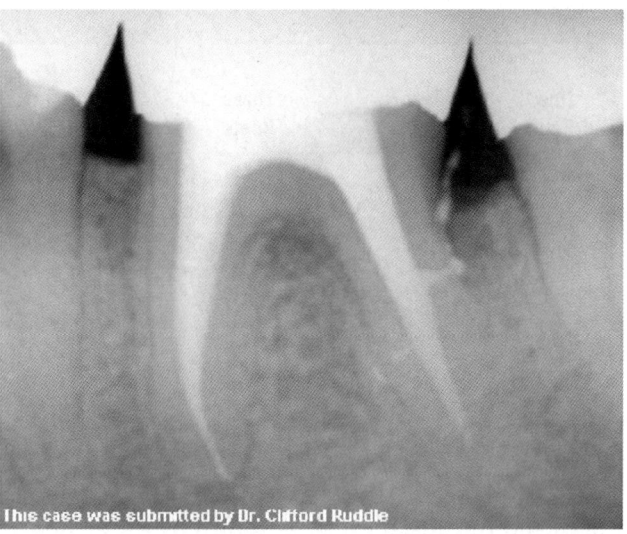

Figure 115 Mandibular left first molar has 2 roots and 3 canals. (MB, ML, and D); a lateral canal is present on the distal aspect of the distal root in the middle third. Reprinted with permission from Brown P, Herbranson E. Dental Anatomy & 3D Tooth Atlas Version 3.0. Illinois: Quintessence, 2005: Mandibular First Molar- X-ray Database.

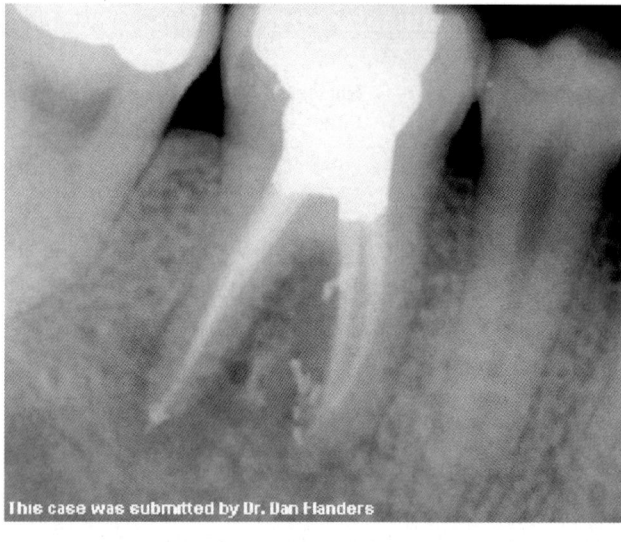

Figure 117 Mandibular right first molar with 2 roots and 3 canals (MB, ML, and D); multiple lateral canals are present on the distal aspect of the mesial root. Reprinted with permission from Brown P, Herbranson E. Dental Anatomy & 3D Tooth Atlas Version 3.0. Illinois: Quintessence, 2005: Mandibular First Molar- X-ray Database.

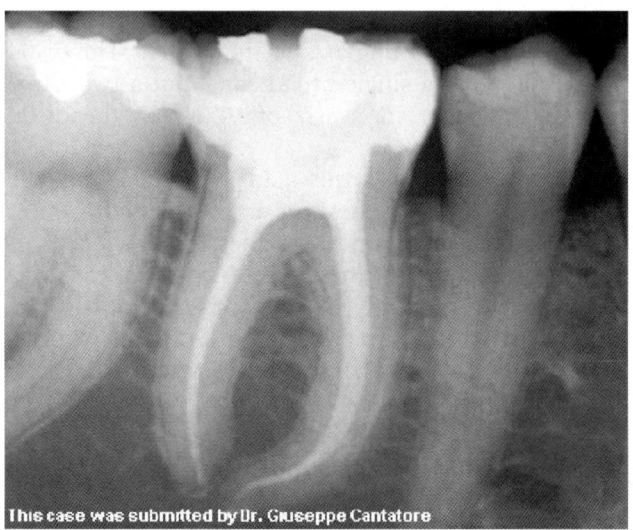

Figure 116 Mandibular right first molar with 2 roots and 3 canals (MB, ML, and D); the mesial root is curved nearly 90° distally. Reprinted with permission from Brown P, Herbranson E. Dental Anatomy & 3D Tooth Atlas Version 3.0. Illinois: Quintessence, 2005: Mandibular First Molar- X-ray Database.

cally and lingually at approximately 3 and 4 mm, respectively.[3] Both roots are broader buccolingually than mesiodistally. The mesial root has concavities on both its mesial and distal surfaces and is angled slightly mesially before curving distally approximately midroot. The mesial root is slightly rotated and tapers distally from buccal to lingual. The distal root is generally more ovoid in its cross-sectional shape.[3] The overall average length of the mandibular first molar is 21.5 mm with an average crown length of 7.5 mm and an average root length of 14 mm.[3]

ROOT NUMBER AND FORM

The mandibular first molar is typically a two-rooted form with a mesial and a distal root, as listed in Table 35.[4,57,60,198,307–320] This form has an overall incidence of 85.2%. However, there are significant differences when comparing Asian[60,198,307,309–312,

Table 35 Mandibular First Molar							
Number of Roots	Number of Studies Cited	Number of Teeth	Fused Roots (Grades I, II, and III)	One Root	Two Roots	Three Roots	Four Roots
All studies	18*	10,044	0.03% (3)	0.2% (19)	85.2% (8555)	14.6% (1465)	0.02% (2)
Non-Asian population	10	3,263	0.09% (3)	–	96.9% (3163)	2.97% (97)	–
Asian population	10	6,781	–	0.3% (19)	79.5% (5392)	20.2% (1368)	0.03% (2)

*Curzon's study[38] and de Souza-Freitas' study[46] included a Asian and a non-Asian population.

[316,318,320] with non-Asian populations.[4,57,307,308, 313–315,317,319,320] Non-Asian populations have an incidence of two roots of 96.9% while the Asian populations have an incidence of 79.5%. Therefore, three roots may occur in one of five patients from Asian populations. The 18 anatomical studies of over 10,000 teeth found that the three-rooted variety, with a bifurcated mesial or distal root or an additional supplementary root, had the next highest incidence of 14.6%. Single-rooted forms and fusion and four-rooted forms were found to be extremely rare and occurred less than 1% of the time in all population groups studied. There is a higher incidence of three roots in Asian population that includes North American Aboriginal people.[321,322] Ten of the 18 anatomical studies, which specifically included Asian populations, showed a variation in incidence even within these population groups. The incidence of three-rooted mandibular first molars in these studies ranged from 10.1% in the Burmese[309] to 26.8% in the Japanese.[312] The range of this occurrence in non-Asian groups ranged from a low of 0%[4,319] to a high of 6.0% in a Saudi Arabian population.[308]

CANAL SYSTEM

The mandibular first molar typically has two mesial canals and one distal canal, as shown by the anatomical studies of the two-rooted form in Table 36. The two-rooted forms have two canals in the mesial root 95.8% of the time.[6,13,36,54,57,60,195,196,254,308,309,313,314, 316,323,324] The mesial root canals may have a common exit foramen or can exit separately as two or more apical foramina.[192] Slowey indicated that the mesiobuccal canal usually has a distinct buccal curvature at the floor of the chamber while the mesiolingual canal is straighter in the long axis to the root.[192] The distal root usually has a single broad canal but a two-canal system can occur in nearly one-third of the distal roots.

The three-rooted forms had two canals in the mesial root 100% of the time in a weighted average of the three anatomical studies reported[60,309,316] (Table 37). However, there was a single apical foramen 93.1% of the time. The distobuccal root had one canal 97.6% of the time and the distolingual or third root had a single canal 100% of the time.

Table 36 Two-rooted Mandibular First Molars						
Number of Canals and Apices	Number of Studies Cited	Number of Teeth (Canal Studies)	One Canal	Two or More Canals	One Canal at Apex	Two or More Canals at Apex
Mesial root	16	3375	4.2% (143)	95.8% (3232)		
	13	1731			46.3% (802)	53.7% (929)
Distal root	15	3304	68.3% (2256)	31.7% (1048)		
	13	1805			82.4% (1488)	17.6% (317)

Number of Canals and Apices	Number of Studies Cited	Number of Teeth (Canal Studies)	One Canal	Two or More Canals	One Canal at Apex	Two or More Canals at Apex
Mesial root	3	208	–	100% (208)		
	2	29	–		93.1% (27)	6.9% (2)
Distobuccal root	3	208	97.6% (203)	2.4% (5)		
Distobuccal root	2	29			93.1% (27)	6.9% (2)
Distolingual root	3	208	100% (208)	–		
	2	29			100% (29)	–

VARIATIONS AND ANOMALIES

There are numerous case reports of anomalies in the literature. The most frequent anomaly relates to additional canals in one or more of the roots. There are reports of an extra canal[323,325–330] (Figure 118), supernumerary roots and canals[295,331,332] (Figures 119 and 120), taurodontism[182,206] (Figure 121), and C-shaped canals.[58,205,327,333]

Mandibular Second Molar

EXTERNAL ROOT MORPHOLOGY

The mandibular second molar normally has two roots[1,3,5,14–16] (Figures 122–127). The mesial and the distal roots are usually closer together or have a longer root trunk and are more frequently fused, compared to the mandibular first molar. The roots are broader buccolingually than mesiodistally. Root concavities are usually present on the mesial surfaces of both the mesial and the distal roots and the distal surface of the mesial root[15] (see Figure 124). The overall average length of the mandibular second molar is

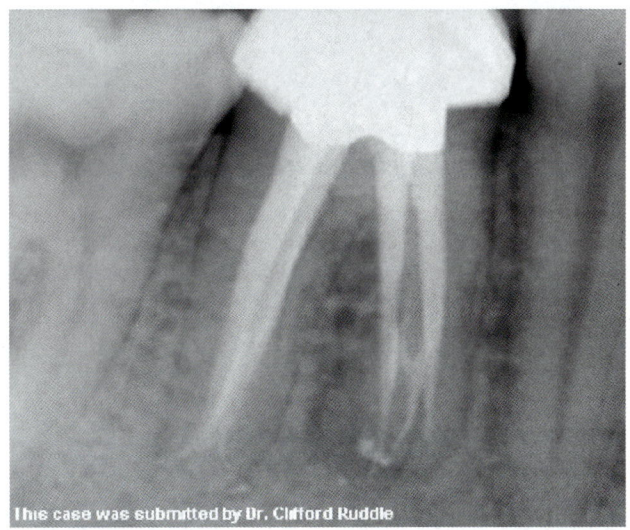

Figure 118 Mandibular right first molar with extra canal in the distal root; 2 canals are present in the mesial roots and 2 canals are present in the distal root. Reprinted with permission from Brown P, Herbranson E. Dental Anatomy & 3D Tooth Atlas Version 3.0. Illinois: Quintessence, 2005: Mandibular First Molar- X-ray Database.

206 / Endodontics

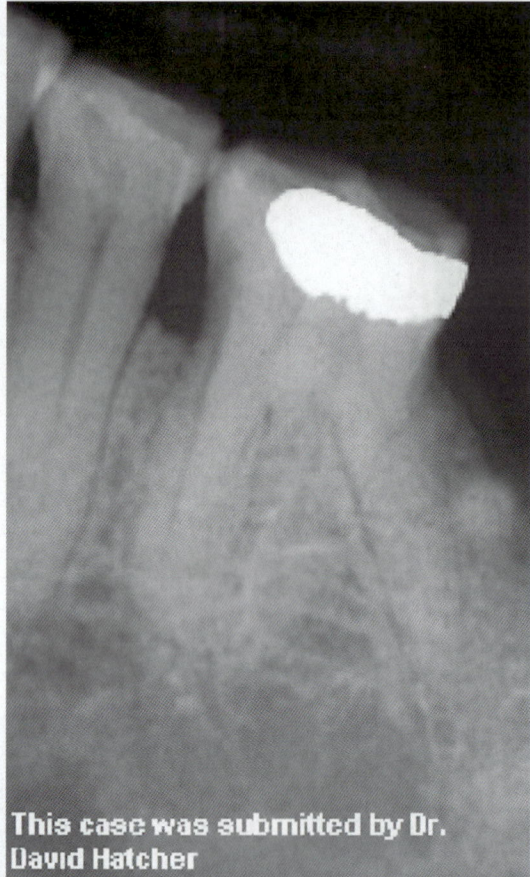

Figure 119 Mandibular left first molar with 3 roots and a 4 canal system; there is a mesial root with a double canal and 2 diverging distal roots. Reprinted with permission from Brown P, Herbranson E. Dental Anatomy & 3D Tooth Atlas Version 3.0. Illinois: Quintessence, 2005: Mandibular First Molar- X-ray Database.

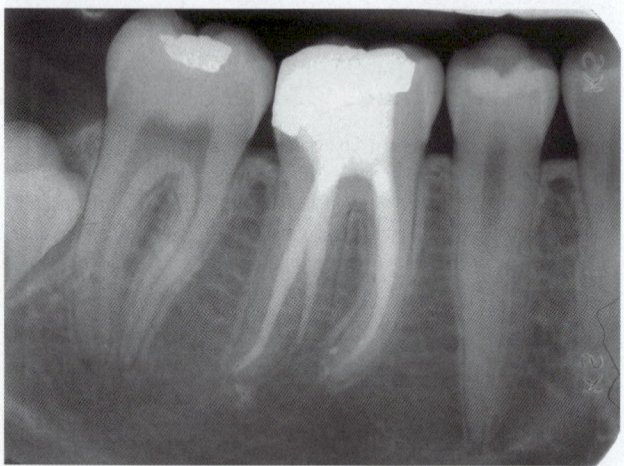

Figure 120 Mandibular right first molar with 3 roots- M, D and DL and 4 canal systems. Courtesy of Dr. W.H. Christie.

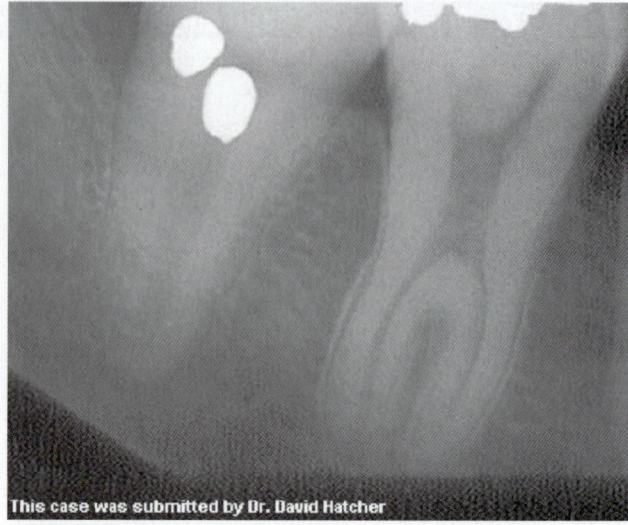

Figure 121 Mandibular right first molar exhibiting mesotaurodontism. Reprinted with permission from Brown P, Herbranson E. Dental Anatomy & 3D Tooth Atlas Version 3.0. Illinois: Quintessence, 2005: Mandibular First Molar- X-ray Database.

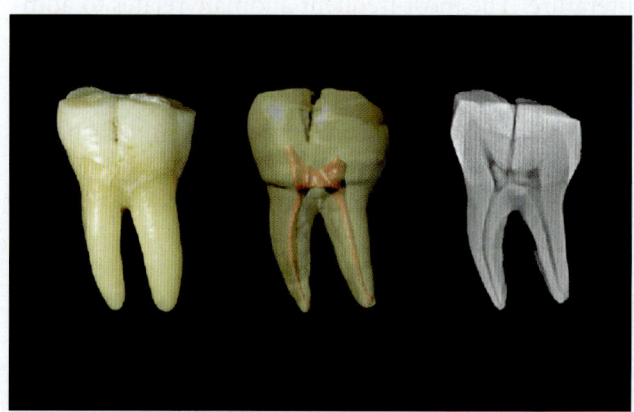

Figure 122 Buccal view of mandibular left second molar [vertical crack in crown is an artifact]. Reprinted with permission from Brown P, Herbranson E. Dental Anatomy & 3D Tooth Atlas Version 3.0. Illinois: Quintessence, 2005: Mandibular Second Molar- Rotations & Slices.

20 mm with an average crown length of 7 mm and an average root length of 13 mm.[3]

ROOT NUMBER AND FORM

The mandibular second molar is two-rooted approximately 76% of the time according to the anatomical studies reported in Table 38.[4,57,60,309,312,313,334–336] Root fusion that becomes a single-root, conical, or "C-shape" form has an incidence of approximately 21.8%.

Chapter 6 / Morphology of Teeth and Their Root Canal Systems / 207

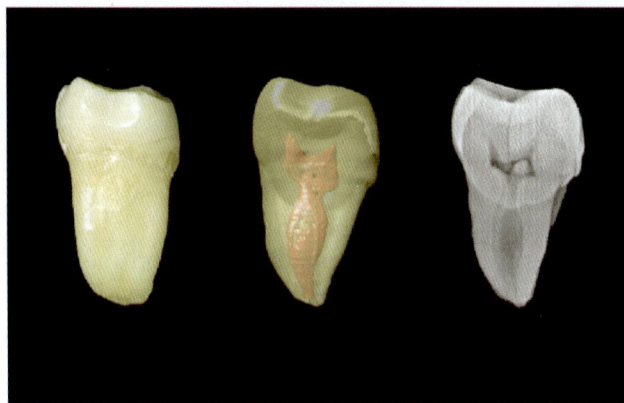

Figure 123 Mesial view of mandibular left second molar. Reprinted with permission from Brown P, Herbranson E. Dental Anatomy & 3D Tooth Atlas Version 3.0. Illinois: Quintessence, 2005: Mandibular Second Molar- Rotations & Slices.

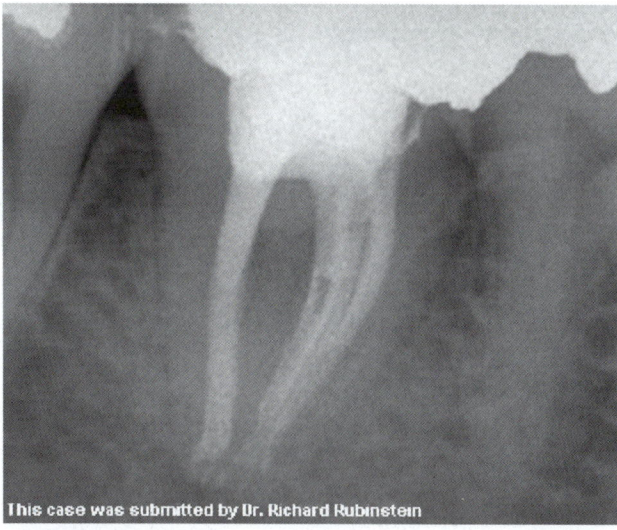

Figure 125 Mandibular right second molar with 2 roots and 3 canals; multiple apical foramina are visible radiographically after completion of RCT. Reprinted with permission from Brown P, Herbranson E. Dental Anatomy & 3D Tooth Atlas Version 3.0. Illinois: Quintessence, 2005: Mandibular Second Molar- X-ray Database.

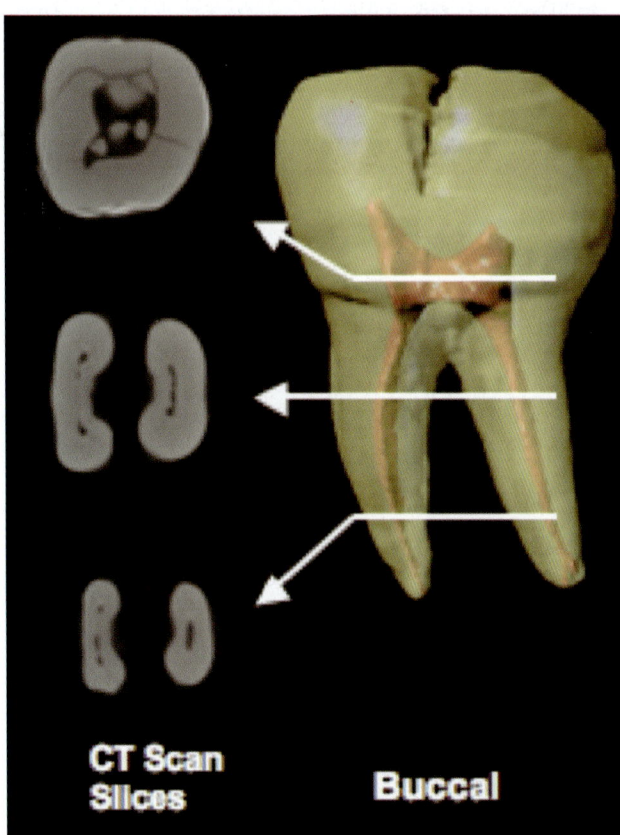

Figure 124 Root cross-sections of the mandibular left second molar. Reprinted with permission from Brown P, Herbranson E. Dental Anatomy & 3D Tooth Atlas Version 3.0. Illinois: Quintessence, 2005: Mandibular Second Molar- Rotations & Slices.

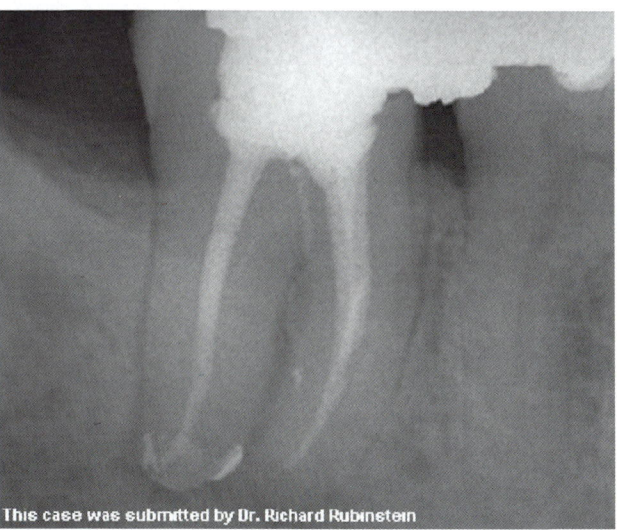

Figure 126 Mandibular right second molar with lateral canals visible in both the mesial and distal roots. Reprinted with permission from Brown P, Herbranson E. Dental Anatomy & 3D Tooth Atlas Version 3.0. Illinois: Quintessence, 2005: Mandibular Second Molar- X-ray Database.

The incidence of a third root, usually the distolingual root, in mandibular second molars (2.2%) is not as high as in first mandibular molars (14.6), as shown by the anatomical studies cited in Table 38. Asian

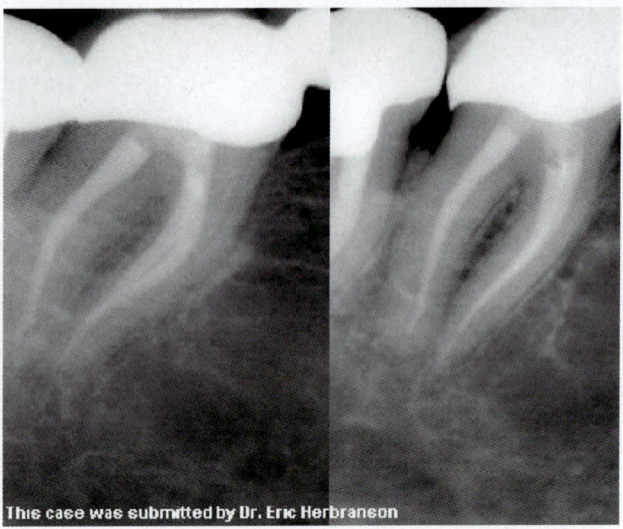

Figure 127 Two views of a mandibular right second molar with 2 roots and 3 canals; mesial canals join and exit through a common foramen. Reprinted with permission from Brown P, Herbranson E. Dental Anatomy & 3D Tooth Atlas Version 3.0. Illinois: Quintessence, 2005: Mandibular Second Molar- X-ray Database.

population reports a higher incidence of third root anatomy.[265]

CANAL SYSTEM

The mandibular second molar, like the mandibular first molar, typically has two mesial canals and one distal canal, as listed in Table 39.[6,10,13,54,57,60,309,313] The mesial root of the mandibular second molar has a higher incidence of one canal (14%) than does the mesial root of the mandibular first molar (4.2%). Mesial root canals may have a common foramen or may exit separately as two or more foramina, but the joining of the two canals is the most common form.[192]

Due to the higher incidence of root fusion in the mandibular second molar, C-shaped canals are frequent. The incidence of root fusion is generally higher in studies of Asian patients,[194,335] with Hou and Tsai reporting an incidence of 51.6% in a study of 64 patients. As would be expected, the incidence of C-shaped canals is often higher in Asian patients as well.[81] Seo and Park[337] reported an incidence of C-shaped canals of 32.7% in Korean patients and

Table 38 Mandibular Second Molar

Number of Roots	Number of Studies Cited	Number of Teeth	Total Incidence of Fused Roots (Grade I, II, and III) % (Number of Teeth)*	One Root (Conical)	One Root (C-shaped)	Two Roots	Three Roots	Four Roots
	9	997	21.8% (217)			76.2% (760)	2.2% (22)	—
	6 (studies reporting single conical root and C-shaped data)	674		8.3% (56)	8.5% (57)			

*In this table, data for fused teeth, C-shaped roots, and single conical roots are all considered to be a form of fusion; therefore, this column represents the sum of data reported in these categories.

Table 39 Mandibular Second Molars (Two-Rooted Teeth)						
Number of Canals and Apices	Number of Studies Cited	Number of Teeth (Canal Studies)	One Canal	Two or More Canals	One Canal at Apex	Two or More Canals at Apex
Mesial root	8	1194	14% (167)	86% (1027)		
	7	778			60.3% (469)	39.7% (309)
Distal root	8	1194	85.1% (1016)	14.9% (178)		
	7	778			95% (739)	5% (39)

Gulibivala et al.[309] reported an incidence of 22.4% in the Burmese. Manning[334] reported an incidence of C-shaped canals of 12.7%, and Caucasians formed the majority of the patients in his study. The studies in the United States by Weine et al.[336,338] and Sabala, Benenati, and Neas[21] reported incidences of single root or C-shape of less than 10%. Ethnicity was not identified in either of these studies, but it is likely that non-Asian patients formed the majority of the patients in both studies. The data from the six anatomical studies that differentiated single conical and C-shaped roots indicate that the incidence of these two canal systems is approximately equal (8.3% and 8.5%, respectively).[57,60,309,312,334,336]

VARIATIONS AND ANOMALIES

A variation in canal and root morphology was first termed the "C-shaped canal" by Cooke and Cox in 1979.[339] This canal shape results from the fusion of the mesial and distal roots on either the buccal or the lingual root surface. Melton et al.[340] described three categories of C-shaped canals and Haddad's group[341] added to the initial description. Category I is described as a continuous C-shaped canal from the pulp chamber to the apex. Category II is described as a "semi-colon" where one canal was separated by dentin from the C-shaped canal. Category III C-shaped anatomy is described as having a C-shaped orifice with two or more distinct and separate canals. Although there have been reported cases of C-shaped canals in other teeth such as the maxillary lateral incisor, maxillary first molar,[46,47,203–205] maxillary second molar,[342,343] maxillary third molar,[344] mandibular first premolar,[268,345] mandibular first molar,[205,327,333] and the mandibular third molar,[339,344,346] the most numerous reports are of C-shaped mandibular second molars.[60,309,334,337–341,346–358] The incidence of C-shaped canals is reported to be highest in the mandibular second molar.[339,359]

Other reported anomalies of mandibular second molars include supernumerary roots,[295,360] taurodontism,[58,182,206] fused or single roots (Figures 128 and 129),[4,5,20,194,225,309,334,335,358,361] additional canals in one or more of the roots (Figure 130),[5,326,362,363] and two canals (Figure 131).[5]

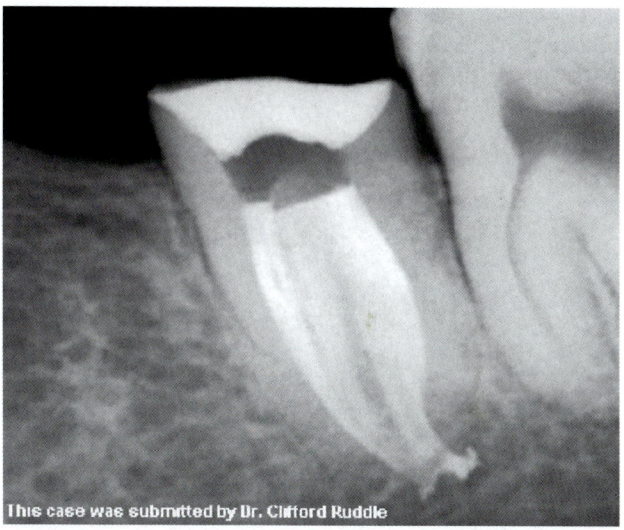

Figure 128 Mandibular left second molar exhibiting fused roots; 3 canals are present; distal canal divides into two canals with separate apical foramina. Reprinted with permission from Brown P, Herbranson E. Dental Anatomy & 3D Tooth Atlas Version 3.0. Illinois: Quintessence, 2005: Mandibular Second Molar- X-ray Database.

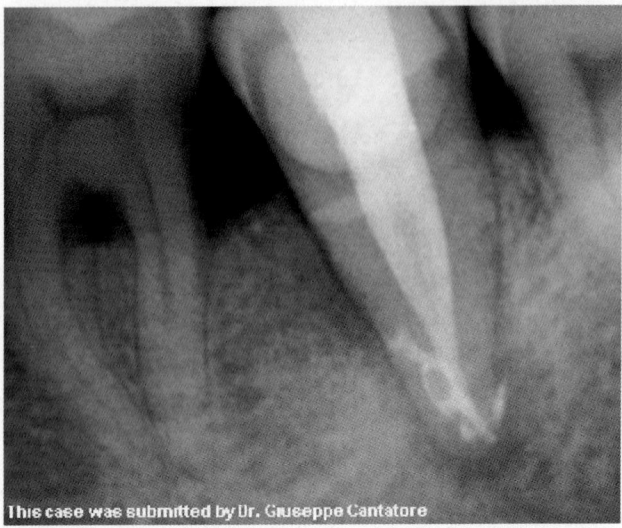

Figure 129 Mandibular left second molar with 1 root and 1 canal; multiple lateral canals are visible in the apical third. Reprinted with permission from Brown P, Herbranson E. Dental Anatomy & 3D Tooth Atlas Version 3.0. Illinois: Quintessence, 2005: Mandibular Second Molar- X-ray Database.

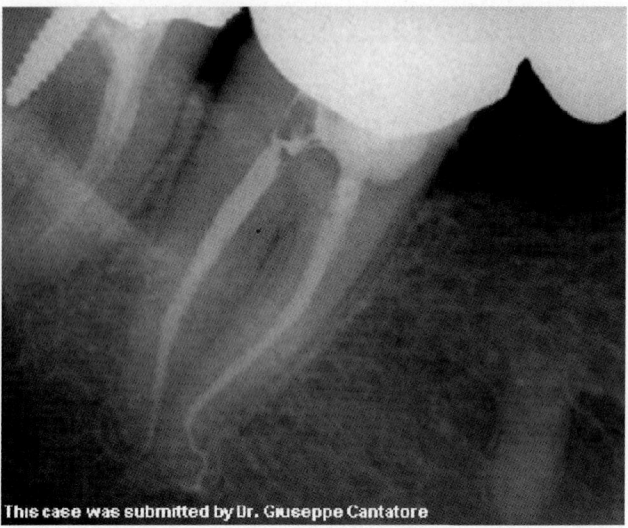

Figure 131 Mandibular right second molar with 2 roots and 2 canals; apical third of the mesial root has a significant mesial curvature on exit of the apical foramen. Reprinted with permission from Brown P, Herbranson E. Dental Anatomy & 3D Tooth Atlas Version 3.0. Illinois: Quintessence, 2005: Mandibular Second Molar- X-ray Database.

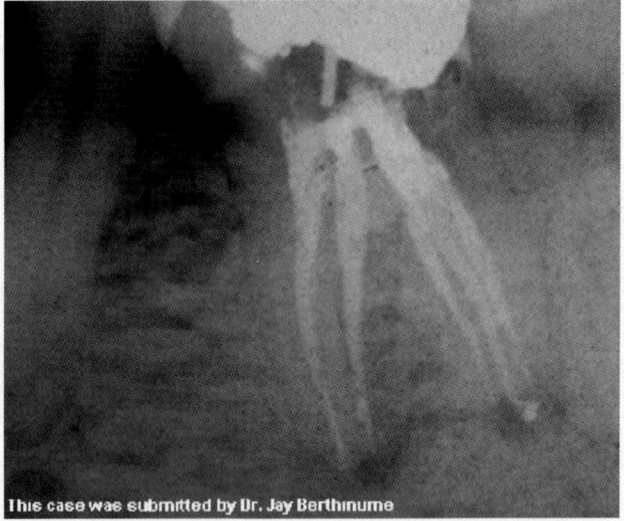

Figure 130 Mandibular left second molar with 2 mesial roots and 1 broad distal root; each mesial root contains 1 canal; the distal root contains a 3-canal system. Reprinted with permission from Brown P, Herbranson E. Dental Anatomy & 3D Tooth Atlas Version 3.0. Illinois: Quintessence, 2005: Mandibular Second Molar- X-ray Database.

References

1. Ingle J, Bakland L. Endodontics. 5th ed. Hamilton: BC Decker; 2002.
2. Walton R, Torabinejad M. Principles and Practice of Endodontics. 2nd edition ed. Philadelphia W.B. Saunders Co.; 1996.
3. Ash M, Nelson S. Wheeler's Dental Anatomy, Physiology and Occlusion. 8th ed. Philadelphia: Saunders; 2003.
4. Barrett M. The internal anatomy of the teeth with special reference to the pulp and its branches. Dent Cosmos 1925;67:581–592.
5. Brown P, Herbranson E. Dental Anatomy & 3D Tooth Atlas Version 3.0. 2nd ed. Illinois: Quintessence; 2005.
6. Çalikan M, Pehlivan Y, Sepetçiolu F, Türkün M, Tüncer SS. Root canal morphology of human permanent teeth in a Turkish population. J Endod 1995;21:200–204.
7. Hess W. The Anatomy of the Root-Canals of the Teeth of the Permanent Dentition, Part 1. New York: William Wood and Co; 1925.
8. Moral H. Ueber Pulpaausgüsse. Deutsche Monatsschrift für Zahnheilkunde 1914.

9. Okamura T. Anatomy of the root canals. J Am Dent Assoc 1927; 14:632–636.
10. Sert S, Bayirli GS. Evaluation of the root canal configurations of the mandibular and maxillary permanent teeth by gender in the Turkish population. J Endod 2004; 30:391–398.
11. Stropko JJ. Canal morphology of maxillary molars: clinical observations of canal configurations. J Endod 1999; 25:446–450.
12. Taylor R. Variations in Morphology of Teeth. Springfield, IL.: Charles C. Thomas Pub.; 1978.
13. Vertucci FJ. Root canal anatomy of the human permanent teeth. Oral Surg Oral Med Oral Pathol 1984;58:589–599.
14. Black G. Descriptive Anatomy of the Teeth. 4th ed. Philadelphia: SS White Dental Manufacturing Company; 1902.
15. Fuller J, Denehy G. Concise Dental Anatomy and Morphology. 2nd ed. Chicago: Year Book Medical Publishers, Inc; 1984.
16. Jordan R, Abrams L, Kraus B. Kraus' Dental Anatomy and Occlusion. 2nd ed. St. Louis: Mosby Year Book, Inc; 1992.
17. al Shalabi RM, Omer OE, Glennon J, Jennings M, Claffey NM. Root canal anatomy of maxillary first and second permanent molars. Int Endod J 2000;33:405–414.
18. Gray R. The Maxillary First Molar. In Bjorndal, AM, Skidmore, AE, Editors. Anatomy and Morphology of Permanent Teeth. Iowa City: University of Iowa College of Dentistry; 1983.
19. Pecora JD, Woelfel JB, Sousa Neto MD. Morphologic study of the maxillary molars. 1. External anatomy. Braz Dent J 1991;2:45–50.
20. Ross IF, Evanchik PA. Root fusion in molars: incidence and sex linkage. J Periodontol 1981;52:663–667.
21. Sabala CL, Benenati FW, Neas BR. Bilateral root or root canal aberrations in a dental school patient population. J Endod 1994;20:38–42.
22. Thomas RP, Moule AJ, Bryant R. Root canal morphology of maxillary permanent first molar teeth at various ages. Int Endod J 1993;26:257–267.
23. Yang ZP, Yang SF, Lee G. The root and root canal anatomy of maxillary molars in a Chinese population. Endod Dent Traumatol 1988;4:215–218.
24. Cleghorn B, Christie W, Dong C. Root and Root Canal Morphology of the Human Permanent Maxillary First Molar: A Literature Review. J Endod 2006;32:813–821.
25. Alavi AM, Opasanon A, Ng YL, Gulabivala K. Root and canal morphology of Thai maxillary molars. Int Endod J 2002;35:478–485.
26. Barbizam JV, Ribeiro RG, Tanomaru Filho M. Unusual anatomy of permanent maxillary molars. J Endod 2004; 30:668–671.
27. Imura N, Hata GI, Toda T, Otani SM, Fagundes MI. Two canals in mesiobuccal roots of maxillary molars. Int Endod J 1998;31:410–414.
28. Pecora JD, Woelfel JB, Sousa Neto MD, Issa EP. Morphologic study of the maxillary molars. Part II: Internal anatomy. Braz Dent J 1992;3:53–57.
29. Yoshioka T, Kikuchi I, Fukumoto Y, Kobayashi C, Suda H. Detection of the second mesiobuccal canal in mesiobuccal roots of maxillary molar teeth ex vivo. Int Endod J 2005;38:124–128.
30. Zürcher E. The Anatomy of the Root-Canals of the Teeth of the Deciduous Dentition and of the First Permanent Molars, Part 2. New York: William Wood and Co.; 1925.
31. Kulild JC, Peters DD. Incidence and configuration of canal systems in the mesiobuccal root of maxillary first and second molars. J Endod 1990;16:311–317.
32. Weine FS, Hayami S, Hata G, Toda T. Canal configuration of the mesiobuccal root of the maxillary first molar of a Japanese sub-population. Int Endod J 1999;32:79–87.
33. Acosta Vigouroux SA, Trugeda Bosaans SA. Anatomy of the pulp chamber floor of the permanent maxillary first molar. J Endod 1978;4:214–219.
34. Nosonowitz DM, Brenner MR. The major canals of the mesiobuccal root of the maxillary 1st and 2nd molars. N Y J Dent 1973;43:12–15.
35. Pineda F. Roentgenographic investigation of the mesiobuccal root of the maxillary first molar. Oral Surg Oral Med Oral Pathol 1973;36:253–260.
36. Pineda F, Kuttler Y. Mesiodistal and buccolingual roentgenographic investigation of 7,275 root canals. Oral Surg Oral Med Oral Pathol 1972;33:101–110.
37. Sykaras S, Economou P. Root canal morphology of the mesiobuccal root of the maxillary first molar. Oral Res Abstr 1971;No. 2025.
38. Gilles J, Reader A. An SEM investigation of the mesiolingual canal in human maxillary first and second molars. Oral Surg Oral Med Oral Pathol 1990;70:638–643.
39. Seidberg BH, Altman M, Guttuso J, Suson M. Frequency of two mesiobuccal root canals in maxillary permanent first molars. J Am Dent Assoc 1973;87:852–856.
40. Weine FS, Healey HJ, Gerstein H, Evanson L. Canal configuration in the mesiobuccal root of the maxillary first molar and its endodontic significance. Oral Surg Oral Med Oral Pathol 1969;28:419–425.
41. Buhrley LJ, Barrows MJ, BeGole EA, Wenckus CS. Effect of magnification on locating the MB2 canal in maxillary molars. J Endod 2002;28:324–327.
42. Fogel HM, Peikoff MD, Christie WH. Canal configuration in the mesiobuccal root of the maxillary first molar: a clinical study. J Endod 1994;20:135–137.
43. Sempira HN, Hartwell GR. Frequency of second mesiobuccal canals in maxillary molars as determined by use of an

operating microscope: a clinical study. J Endod 2000; 26:673–674.

44. Baratto-Filho F, Fariniuk LF, Ferreira EL, Pecora JD, Cruz-Filho AM, Sousa-Neto MD. Clinical and macroscopic study of maxillary molars with two palatal roots. Int Endod J 2002;35:796–801.

45. Christie WH, Peikoff MD, Fogel HM. Maxillary molars with two palatal roots: a retrospective clinical study. J Endod 1991;17:80–84.

46. Dankner E, Friedman S, Stabholz A. Bilateral C shape configuration in maxillary first molars. J Endod 1990; 16:601–603.

47. De Moor RJ. C-shaped root canal configuration in maxillary first molars. Int Endod J 2002;35:200–208.

48. Fava LR. Root canal treatment in an unusual maxillary first molar: a case report. Int Endod J 2001;34:649–653.

49. Hülsmann M. A maxillary first molar with two disto-buccal root canals. J Endod 1997;23:707–708.

50. Johal S. Unusual maxillary first molar with 2 palatal canals within a single root: a case report. J Can Dent Assoc 2001; 67:211–214.

51. Pomeranz HH, Fishelberg G. The secondary mesiobuccal canal of maxillary molars. J Am Dent Assoc 1974;88:119–124.

52. Wolcott J, Ishley D, Kennedy W, Johnson S, Minnich S. Clinical investigation of second mesiobuccal canals in endodontically treated and retreated maxillary molars. J Endod 2002;28:477–479.

53. Wong M. Maxillary first molar with three palatal canals. J Endod 1991;17:298–299.

54. Hartwell G, Bellizzi R. Clinical investigation of in vivo endodontically treated mandibular and maxillary molars. J Endod 1982;8:555–557.

55. Neaverth EJ, Kotler LM, Kaltenbach RF. Clinical investigation (in vivo) of endodontically treated maxillary first molars. J Endod 1987;13:506–512.

56. Slowey RR. Radiographic aids in the detection of extra root canals. Oral Surg Oral Med Oral Pathol 1974;37:762–772.

57. Zaatar EI, al-Kandari AM, Alhomaidah S, al-Yasin IM. Frequency of endodontic treatment in Kuwait: radiographic evaluation of 846 endodontically treated teeth. J Endod 1997;23:453–456.

58. Sert S, Bayirli G. Taurodontism in six molars: a case report. J Endod 2004;30:601–602.

59. Weller RN, Hartwell GR. The impact of improved access and searching techniques on detection of the mesiolingual canal in maxillary molars. J Endod 1989;15:82–83.

60. Gulabivala K, Opasanon A, Ng YL, Alavi A. Root and canal morphology of Thai mandibular molars. Int Endod J 2002;35:56–62.

61. Zolty G. The prevalence and significance of sealing accessory and lateral canals: a literature review. Sadj 2001;56:417–424.

62. Vertucci F. Root canal morphology and its relationship to endodontic procedures. Endo Topics 2005;10:3–29.

63. de Deus Q, Horizonte B. Frequency, location, and direction of the lateral, secondary, and accessory canals. J Endod 1975;1:361–366.

64. Schilder H. Cleaning and shaping the root canal. Dent Clin North Am 1974;18:269–296.

65. Ingle J, Beveridge E. Endodontics. 2nd ed. Philadelphia: Lea & Febiger; 1976.

66. Ong G, Neo J. A survey of approximal root concavities in an ethnic Chinese population. Arch Oral Biol 1990;35:925–928.

67. Gonzalez-Plata RR, Gonzalez-Plata EW. Conventional and surgical treatment of a two-rooted maxillary central incisor. J Endod 2003;29:422–424.

68. Heling B. A two-rooted maxillary central incisor. Oral Surg Oral Med Oral Pathol 1977;43:649.

69. Patterson JM. Bifurcated root of upper central incisor. Oral Surg Oral Med Oral Pathol 1970;29:222.

70. Lambruschini GM, Camps J. A two-rooted maxillary central incisor with a normal clinical crown. J Endod 1993;19:95–96.

71. Genovese FR, Marsico EM. Maxillary central incisor with two roots: a case report. J Endod 2003;29:220–221.

72. Altman M, Guttuso J, Seidberg BH, Langeland K. Apical root canal anatomy of human maxillary central incisors. Oral Surg Oral Med Oral Pathol 1970;30:694–699.

73. Green D. A stereomicroscopic study of the root apices of 400 maxillary and mandibular anterior teeth. Oral Surg Oral Med Oral Pathol 1956;9:1224–1232.

74. Mizutani T, Ohno N, Nakamura H. Anatomical study of the root apex in the maxillary anterior teeth. J Endod 1992;18:344–347.

75. Kasahara E, Yasuda E, Yamamoto A, Anzai M. Root canal system of the maxillary central incisor. J Endod 1990; 16:158–161.

76. Hsu JW, Tsai PL, Hsiao TH, Chang HP, Lin LM, Liu KM, et al. Ethnic dental analysis of shovel and Carabelli's traits in a Chinese population. Aust Dent J 1999;44:40–45.

77. Carbonell V. Variations in the frequency of shovel-shaped incisors in different populations. In: Brothwell D, editor. Dental Anthropology. Oxford: Pergamon Press; 1963. pp. 211–234.

78. Dahlberg A. The changing dentition of man. J Am Dent Assoc 1945;32:676–690.

79. Dahlberg A. Analysis of the American Indian dentition. In: Brothwell D, editor. Dental Anthropology. Oxford: Pergamon Press; 1963. pp. 149–177.

80. Nelson C. The teeth of the Indians of Pecos Pueblo. Am J Phys Anthrop 1938;23:261–293.

81. Tratman E. A comparison of the teeth of people (Indo-European racial stock with the Asian race stock). Dent Record 1950;70:43–44.

82. Pecora JD, da Cruz Filho AM. Study of the incidence of radicular grooves in maxillary incisors. Braz Dent J 1992; 3:11–16.

83. Simon JH, Glick DH, Frank AL. Predictable endodontic and periodontic failures as a result of radicular anomalies. Oral Surg Oral Med Oral Pathol 1971;31:823–826.

84. Hamasha AA, Al-Khateeb T. Prevalence of fused and geminated teeth in Jordanian adults. Quintessence Int 2004;35:556–559.

85. al-Nazhan S. Two root canals in a maxillary central incisor with enamel hypoplasia. J Endod 1991;17:469–471.

86. Cimilli H, Kartal N. Endodontic treatment of unusual central incisors. J Endod 2002;28:480–481.

87. Kim E, Jou YT. A supernumerary tooth fused to the facial surface of a maxillary permanent central incisor: case report. J Endod 2000;26:45–48.

88. Michanowicz AE, Michanowicz JP, Ardila J, Posada A. Apical surgery on a two-rooted maxillary central incisor. J Endod 1990;16:454–455.

89. Mehlman ES. Management of a totally fused central and lateral incisor with internal resorption perforating the lateral aspect of the root. J Endod 1978;4:189–191.

90. Cullen CL, Pangrazio-Kulbersh V. Bilateral gemination with talon cusp: report of case. J Am Dent Assoc 1985;111:58–59.

91. Hattab FN, Hazza'a AM. An unusual case of talon cusp on geminated tooth. J Can Dent Assoc 2001;67:263–266.

92. Ferraz JA, de Carvalho Junior JR, Saquy PC, Pecora JD, Sousa-Neto MD. Dental anomaly: dens evaginatus (talon cusp). Braz Dent J 2001;12:132–134.

93. de Sousa SM, Tavano SM, Bramante CM. Unusual case of bilateral talon cusp associated with dens invaginatus. Int Endod J 1999;32:494–498.

94. Bolan M, Nunes A, de Carvalho Rocha M, de Luca Canto G. Talon cusp: Report of a case. Quintessence Int 2006; 37:509–514.

95. Todd H. Maxillary right central incisor with two root canals. J Endod 1976;2:227.

96. Reid JS, Saunders WP, MacDonald DG. Maxillary permanent incisors with two root canals: a report of two cases. Int Endod J 1993;26:246–250.

97. Beltes P. Endodontic treatment in three cases of dens invaginatus. J Endod 1997;23:399–402.

98. Lin WC, Yang SF, Pai SF. Nonsurgical endodontic treatment of a two-rooted maxillary central incisor. J Endod 2006; 32:478–481.

99. Hosomi T, Yoshikawa M, Yaoi M, Sakiyama Y, Toda T. A maxillary central incisor having two root canals geminated with a supernumerary tooth. J Endod 1989;15:161–163.

100. Lorena SC, Oliveira DT, Odellt EW. Multiple dental anomalies in the maxillary incisor region. J Oral Sci 2003; 45:47–50.

101. McNamara CM, Garvey MT, Winter GB. Root abnormalities, talon cusps, dentes invaginati with reduced alveolar bone levels: case report. Int J Paediatr Dent 1998;8:41–45.

102. Hatton JF, Ferrillo PJ, Jr. Successful treatment of a two-canaled maxillary lateral incisor. J Endod 1989; 15:216–218.

103. Sykaras SN. A two-rooted maxillary lateral incisor. Oral Surg Oral Med Oral Pathol 1972;34:349.

104. Wei PC, Geivelis M, Chan CP, Ju YR. Successful treatment of pulpal-periodontal combined lesion in a birooted maxillary lateral incisor with concomitant palato-radicular groove. A case report. J Periodontol 1999;70:1540–1546.

105. Al-Hezaimi K, Naghshbandi J, Simon JH, Oglesby S, Rotstein I. Successful treatment of a radicular groove by intentional replantation and Emdogain therapy. Dent Traumatol 2004;20:226–228.

106. Estrela C, Pereira HL, Pecora JD. Radicular grooves in maxillary lateral incisor: case report. Braz Dent J 1995;6:143–146.

107. Greenfeld RS, Cambruzzi JV. Complexities of endodontic treatment of maxillary lateral incisors with anomalous root formation. Oral Surg Oral Med Oral Pathol 1986;62:82–88.

108. Mayne JR, Martin IG. The palatal radicular groove. Two case reports. Aust Dent J 1990;35:277–281.

109. Schafer E, Cankay R, Ott K. Malformations in maxillary incisors: case report of radicular palatal groove. Endod Dent Traumatol 2000;16:132–137.

110. Schwartz S, Koch M, Deas D, Powell C. Combined endodontic-periodontic treatment of a palatal groove: A case report. J Endod 2006;32:573–578.

111. Peikoff MD, Perry JB, Chapnick LA. Endodontic failure attributable to a complex radicular lingual groove. J Endod 1985;11:573–577.

112. Peikoff MD, Trott JR. An endodontic failure caused by an unusual anatomical anomaly. J Endod 1977;3:356–359.

113. Gao ZR, Shi JN, Wang Y, Gu FY. Scanning electron microscopic investigation of maxillary lateral incisors with a radicular lingual groove. Oral Surg Oral Med Oral Pathol 1989;68:462–466.

114. Benenati FW. Complex treatment of a maxillary lateral incisor with dens invaginatus and associated aberrant morphology. J Endod 1994;20:180–182.

115. Boveda C, Fajardo M, Millan B. Root canal treatment of an invaginated maxillary lateral incisor with a C-shaped canal. Quintessence Int 1999;30:707–711.

116. Creaven J. Dens invaginatus-type malformation without pulpal involvement. J Endod 1975;1:79–80.

117. da Silva Neto UX, Hirai VH, Papalexiou V, Goncalves SB, Westphalen VP, Bramante CM, et al. Combined endodontic therapy and surgery in the treatment of dens invaginatus Type 3: case report. J Can Dent Assoc 2005;71:855–858.

118. Froner IC, Rocha LF, da Costa WF, Barros VM, Morello D. Complex treatment of dens invaginatus type III in maxillary lateral incisor. Endod Dent Traumatol 1999;15:88–90.

119. Gound TG, Maixner D. Nonsurgical management of a dilacerated maxillary lateral incisor with type III dens invaginatus: a case report. J Endod 2004;30:448–451.

120. Ikeda H, Yoshioka T, Suda H. Importance of clinical examination and diagnosis. A case of dens invaginatus. Oral Surg Oral Med Oral Pathol Oral Radiol Endod 1995;79:88–91.

121. Jung M. Endodontic treatment of dens invaginatus type III with three root canals and open apical foramen. Int Endod J 2004;37:205–213.

122. Kulild JC, Weller RN. Treatment considerations in dens invaginatus. J Endod 1989;15:381–384.

123. Nallapati S. Clinical management of a maxillary lateral incisor with vital pulp and type 3 dens invaginatus: a case report. J Endod 2004;30:726–731.

124. Nik-Hussein NN. Dens invaginatus: complications and treatment of non-vital infected tooth. J Clin Pediatr Dent 1994;18:303–306.

125. Ortiz P, Weisleder R, Villareal de Justus Y. Combined therapy in the treatment of dens invaginatus: case report. J Endod 2004;30:672–674.

126. Peix-Sanchez M, Minana-Laliga R. A case of unusual anatomy: a maxillary lateral incisor with three canals. Int Endod J 1999;32:236–240.

127. Pitt Ford HE. Peri-radicular inflammation related to dens invaginatus treated without damaging the dental pulp: a case report. Int J Paediatr Dent 1998;8:283–286.

128. Sauveur G, Roth F, Sobel M, Boucher Y. Surgical treatment of a periradicular lesion on an invaginated maxillary lateral incisor (dens in dente). Int Endod J 1997;30:145–149.

129. Skoner JR, Wallace JA. Dens invaginatus: another use for the ultrasonic. J Endod 1994;20:138–140.

130. Steffen H, Splieth C. Conventional treatment of dens invaginatus in maxillary lateral incisor with sinus tract: one year follow-up. J Endod 2005;31:130–133.

131. Suchina JA, Ludington JR, Jr., Madden RM. Dens invaginatus of a maxillary lateral incisor: endodontic treatment. Oral Surg Oral Med Oral Pathol 1989;68:467–471.

132. Tsurumachi T. Endodontic treatment of an invaginated maxillary lateral incisor with a periradicular lesion and a healthy pulp. Int Endod J 2004;37:717–723.

133. Walvekar SV, Behbehani JM. Three root canals and dens formation in a maxillary lateral incisor: a case report. J Endod 1997;23:185–186.

134. Yeh SC, Lin YT, Lu SY. Dens invaginatus in the maxillary lateral incisor: treatment of 3 cases. Oral Surg Oral Med Oral Pathol Oral Radiol Endod 1999;87:628–631.

135. Zillich RM, Ash JL, Corcoran JF. Maxillary lateral incisor with two roots and dens formation: a case report. J Endod 1983;9:143–144.

136. Chen YH, Tseng CC, Harn WM. Dens invaginatus. Review of formation and morphology with 2 case reports. Oral Surg Oral Med Oral Pathol Oral Radiol Endod 1998;86:347–352.

137. Oehlers FAC. Dens invaginatus (dilated composite odontome). I. Variations of the invagination process and associated anterior crown forms. Oral Surg Oral Med Oral Pathol 1957;10:1204–1218 contd.

138. Christie WH, Peikoff MD, Acheson DW. Endodontic treatment of two maxillary lateral incisors with anomalous root formation. J Endod 1981;7:528–534.

139. Blaney TD, Hartwell GR, Bellizzi R. Endodontic management of a fused tooth: a case report. J Endod 1982;8:227–230.

140. Friedman S, Mor H, Stabholz A. Endodontic therapy of a fused permanent maxillary lateral incisor. J Endod 1984;10:449–451.

141. Itkin AB, Barr GS. Comprehensive management of the double tooth: report of case. J Am Dent Assoc 1975;90:1269–1272.

142. Tsurumachi T, Kuno T. Endodontic and orthodontic treatment of a cross-bite fused maxillary lateral incisor. Int Endod J 2003;36:135–142.

143. Wolfe RE, Stieglitz HT. A fused permanent maxillary lateral incisor: endodontic treatment and restoration. N Y State Dent J 1980;46:654–657.

144. Tagger M. Tooth germination treated by endodontic therapy. J Endod 1975;1:181–184.

145. Wong M. Treatment considerations in a geminated maxillary lateral incisor. J Endod 1991;17:179–181.

146. Yücel A, Güler E. Nonsurgical endodontic retreatment of geminated teeth: A case report. J Endod 2006;in press.

147. Hattab FN, Yassin OM, al-Nimri KS. Talon cusp in permanent dentition associated with other dental anomalies: review of literature and reports of seven cases. ASDC J Dent Child 1996;63:368–376.

148. Dash JK, Sahoo PK, Das SN. Talon cusp associated with other dental anomalies: a case report. Int J Paediatr Dent 2004;14:295–300.

149. Pereira AJ, Fidel RA, Fidel SR. Maxillary lateral incisor with two root canals: fusion, gemination or dens invaginatus? Braz Dent J 2000;11:141–146.

150. Thompson BH, Portell FR, Hartwell GR. Two root canals in a maxillary lateral incisor. J Endod 1985;11:353–355.

151. Mupparapu M, Singer SR, Goodchild JH. Dens evaginatus and dens invaginatus in a maxillary lateral incisor: report of a rare occurrence and review of literature. Aust Dent J 2004;49:201–203.

152. Bjorndal L, Carlsen O, Thuesen G, Darvann T, Kreiborg S. External and internal macromorphology in 3D-reconstructed maxillary molars using computerized X-ray microtomography. Int Endod J 1999;32:3–9.

153. Gorlin R, Goldman H. Thoma's Oral Pathology. 6th ed. St. Louis: CV Mosby; 1970.

154. Weisman MI. A rare occurrence: a bi-rooted upper canine. Aust Endod J 2000;26:119–120.

155. Booth J. The longest tooth? . Aust Endod News 1988;13:17.

156. McNamara T, Haeussler AM, Keane J. Facial talon cusps. Int J Paediatr Dent 1997;7:259–262.

157. Dankner E, Harari D, Rotstein I. Dens evaginatus of anterior teeth. Literature review and radiographic survey of 15,000 teeth. Oral Surg Oral Med Oral Pathol Oral Radiol Endod 1996;81:472–475.

158. Alapati S, Zaatar EI, Shyama M, Al-Zuhair N. Maxillary canine with two root canals. Med Princ Pract 2006;15:74–76.

159. Holtzman L, Lezion R. Endodontic treatment of maxillary canine with dens invaginatus and immature root. Oral Surg Oral Med Oral Pathol Oral Radiol Endod 1996;82:452–455.

160. Turkkahraman H, Yilmaz HH, Cetin E. A non-syndrome case with bilateral supernumerary canines: report of a rare case. Dentomaxillofac Radiol 2005;34:319–321.

161. Booker BW, 3rd, Loughlin DM. A morphologic study of the mesial root surface of the adolescent maxillary first bicuspid. J Periodontol 1985;56:666–670.

162. Gher ME, Vernino AR. Root morphology–clinical significance in pathogenesis and treatment of periodontal disease. J Am Dent Assoc 1980;101:627–633.

163. Joseph I, Varma BR, Bhat KM. Clinical significance of furcation anatomy of the maxillary first premolar: a biometric study on extracted teeth. J Periodontol 1996;67:386–389.

164. Aoki K. [Morphological studies on the roots of maxillary premolars in Japanese]. Shikwa Gakuho 1990;90:181–199.

165. Carns EJ, Skidmore AE. Configurations and deviations of root canals of maxillary first premolars. Oral Surg Oral Med Oral Pathol 1973;36:880–886.

166. Chaparro AJ, Segura JJ, Guerrero E, Jimenez-Rubio A, Murillo C, Feito JJ. Number of roots and canals in maxillary first premolars: study of an Andalusian population. Endod Dent Traumatol 1999;15:65–67.

167. Green D. Double canals in single roots. Oral Surg 1973;35:689–696.

168. Kartal N, Ozcelik B, Cimilli H. Root canal morphology of maxillary premolars. J Endod 1998;24:417–419.

169. Loh HS. Root morphology of the maxillary first premolar in Singaporeans. Aust Dent J 1998;43:399–402.

170. Mueller A. Anatomy of the root canals of the incisors, cuspids and bicuspids of the permanent teeth. J Am Dent Assoc 1933;20:1361–1386.

171. Pecora J, Saquy P, Sousa Neto M, Woelfel J. Root form and canal anatomy of maxillary first premolars. Braz Dent J 1991;2:87–94.

172. Vertucci FJ, Gegauff A. Root canal morphology of the maxillary first premolar. J Am Dent Assoc 1979;99:194–198.

173. Walker RT. Root form and canal anatomy of maxillary first premolars in a southern Chinese population. Endod Dent Traumatol 1987;3:130–134.

174. Bellizzi R, Hartwell G. Radiographic evaluation of root canal anatomy of in vivo endodontically treated maxillary premolars. J Endod 1985;11:37–39.

175. Petersen P. The East Greenland Eskimo dentition. Copenhagen: CA Reitzels Forlag; 1949.

176. Barry GN, Heyman RA, Fried IL. Endodontic treatment of a three-rooted maxillary first premolar. Case report. N Y State Dent J 1975;41:75–77.

177. Evans M. Combined endodontic and surgical treatment of a three-rooted maxillary first premolar. Aust Endod J 2004;30:53–55.

178. Soares JA, Leonardo RT. Root canal treatment of three-rooted maxillary first and second premolars–a case report. Int Endod J 2003;36:705–710.

179. Mattuella LG, Mazzoccato G, Vier FV, So MV. Root canals and apical foramina of the buccal root of maxillary first premolars with longitudinal sulcus. Braz Dent J 2005;16:23–29.

180. Nahmias Y, Rampado ME. Root-canal treatment of a trifid crown premolar. Int Endod J 2002;35:390–394.

181. Llamas R, Jimenez-Planas A. Taurodontism in premolars. Oral Surg Oral Med Oral Pathol 1993;75:501–505.

182. Shifman A, Buchner A. Taurodontism. Report of sixteen cases in Israel. Oral Surg Oral Med Oral Pathol 1976;41:400–405.

183. Madeira MC, Leite HF, Niccoli Filho WD, Simoes S. Prevalence of taurodontism in premolars. Oral Surg Oral Med Oral Pathol 1986;61:158–162.

184. Pecora J, Sousa Neto M, Saquy P, Woelfel J. In vitro study of root canal anatomy of maxillary second premolars. Braz Dent J 1992;3:81–85.

185. Sikri VK, Sikri P. Maxillary second pre-molar: configuration and deviations of root canals. J Indian Dent Assoc 1991;62:46–49.

186. Rotstein I, Stabholz A, Friedman S. Endodontic therapy for dens invaginatus in a maxillary second premolar. Oral Surg Oral Med Oral Pathol 1987;63:237–240.

187. Sussman HI. Caveat preparator: maxillary second bicuspid root invaginations. N Y State Dent J 1992;58:36–37.

188. Barkhordar RA, Sapone J. Surgical treatment of a three-rooted maxillary second premolar. Report of a case. Oral Surg Oral Med Oral Pathol 1987;63:614–616.

189. Ferreira CM, de Moraes IG, Bernardineli N. Three-rooted maxillary second premolar. J Endod 2000;26:105–106.

190. Low D. Unusual maxillary second premolar morphology: a case report. Quintessence Int 2001;32:626–628.

191. Velmurugan N, Parameswaran A, Kandaswamy D, Smitha A, Vijayalakshmi D, Sowmya N. Maxillary second premolar with three roots and three separate root canals–case reports. Aust Endod J 2005;31:73–75.

192. Slowey RR. Root canal anatomy. Road map to successful endodontics. Dent Clin North Am 1979;23:555–573.

193. Thews ME, Kemp WB, Jones CR. Aberrations in palatal root and root canal morphology of two maxillary first molars. J Endod 1979;5:94–96.

194. Hou GL, Tsai CC. The morphology of root fusion in Chinese adults (I). Grades, types, location and distribution. J Clin Periodontol 1994;21:260–264.

195. Wasti F, Shearer AC, Wilson NH. Root canal systems of the mandibular and maxillary first permanent molar teeth of south Asian Pakistanis. Int Endod J 2001;34:263–266.

196. Jung IY, Seo MA, Fouad AF, Spangberg LS, Lee SJ, Kim HJ, et al. Apical anatomy in mesial and mesiobuccal roots of permanent first molars. J Endod 2005;31:364–368.

197. Walker RT. Root canal anatomy of mandibular first premolars in a southern Chinese population. Endod Dent Traumatol 1988;4:226–228.

198. Walker RT. Root form and canal anatomy of mandibular first molars in a southern Chinese population. Endod Dent Traumatol 1988;4:19–22.

199. Stone LH, Stroner WF. Maxillary molars demonstrating more than one palatal root canal. Oral Surg Oral Med Oral Pathol 1981;51:649–652.

200. Jacobsen EL, Nii C. Unusual palatal root canal morphology in maxillary molars. Endod Dent Traumatol 1994;10:19–22.

201. Maggiore F, Jou YT, Kim S. A six-canal maxillary first molar: case report. Int Endod J 2002;35:486–491.

202. Carlsen O, Alexandersen V. Radix mesiolingualis and radix distolingualis in a collection of permanent maxillary molars. Acta Odontol Scand 2000;58:229–236.

203. Yilmaz Z, Tuncel B, Serper A, Calt S. C-shaped root canal in a maxillary first molar: a case report. Int Endod J 2006;39:162–166.

204. Newton CW, McDonald S. A C-shaped canal configuration in a maxillary first molar. J Endod 1984;10:397–399.

205. Simon J. C-shaped canals: diagnosis and treatment. Gen Dent 1993;41:482–485.

206. Bernick SM. Taurodontia. Oral Surg Oral Med Oral Pathol 1970;29:549.

207. Stabholz A, Friedman S. Endodontic therapy of an unusual maxillary first molar. J Endod 1983;9:293–295.

208. Chen IP, Karabucak B. Conventional and surgical endodontic retreatment of a maxillary first molar: unusual anatomy. J Endod 2006;32:228–230.

209. Gopikrishna V, Bhargavi N, Kandaswamy D. Endodontic management of a maxillary first molar with a single root and a single canal diagnosed with the aid of spiral CT: A case report. J Endod 2006;32:687–691.

210. Davis SR, Brayton SM, Goldman M. The morphology of the prepared root canal: a study utilizing injectable silicone. Oral Surg Oral Med Oral Pathol 1972;34:642–648.

211. Keith A. Problems relating to the teeth of the earlier forms of prehistoric man. Proc Roy Sco Med (Odontol Section) 1913;6:103–119.

212. Mena. Taurodontism. Oral Surg Oral Med Oral Pathol 1971;29:812–823.

213. Shaw J. Taurodont teeth in South African races. J Anat 1928;62:476–498.

214. Hayashi Y. Endodontic treatment in taurodontism. J Endod 1994;20:357–358.

215. Tsesis I, Steinbock N, Rosenberg E, Kaufman AY. Endodontic treatment of developmental anomalies in posterior teeth: treatment of geminated/fused teeth–report of two cases. Int Endod J 2003;36:372–379.

216. Widerman F, Serene T. Endodontic therapy involving a taurodontic tooth. Oral Surg Oral Med Oral Pathol 1971;32:618–620.

217. Yeh S, Hsu T. Endodontic treatment in taurodontism with Klinefelter's syndrome: a case report. Oral Surg Oral Med Oral Pathol 1999;88:612–615.

218. Gardner D, Girgis S. Taurodontism, shovel-shaped incisors and Klinefelter syndrome. J Can Dent Assoc 1978;44:372–373.

219. Libfeld H, Rotstein I. Incidence of four-rooted maxillary second molars: literature review and radiographic survey of 1,200 teeth. J Endod 1989;15:129–131.

220. Peikoff MD, Christie WH, Fogel HM. The maxillary second molar: variations in the number of roots and canals. Int Endod J 1996;29:365–369.

221. Eskoz N, Weine FS. Canal configuration of the mesiobuccal root of the maxillary second molar. J Endod 1995;21:38–42.

222. Alani AH. Endodontic treatment of bilaterally occurring 4-rooted maxillary second molars: case report. J Can Dent Assoc 2003;69:733–735.

223. Weiland M, Wendt A. [Acute retrograde pulpitis in molar with four roots. An interesting case]. Stomatologie der DDR 1988;38:784–786.

224. Fahid A, Taintor JF. Maxillary second molar with three buccal roots. J Endod 1988;14:181–183.

225. Fava LR, Weinfeld I, Fabri FP, Pais CR. Four second molars with single roots and single canals in the same patient. Int Endod J 2000;33:138–142.

226. Darwazeh AM, Hamasha AA, Pillai K. Prevalence of taurodontism in Jordanian dental patients. Dentomaxillofac Radiol 1998;27:163–165.

227. Deveaux E. Maxillary second molar with two palatal roots. J Endod 1999;25:571–573.

228. Di Fiore PM. A four-rooted quadrangular maxillary molar. J Endod 1999;25:695–697.

229. Di Fiore PM. Complications of surgical crown lengthening for a maxillary molar with four roots: A clinical report. J Prosthet Dent 1999;82:266–269.

230. Madeira MC, Hetem S. Incidence of bifurcations in mandibular incisors. Oral Surg Oral Med Oral Pathol 1973; 36:589–591.

231. Vertucci FJ. Root canal anatomy of the mandibular anterior teeth. J Am Dent Assoc 1974;89:369–371.

232. Mauger MJ, Waite RM, Alexander JB, Schindler WG. Ideal endodontic access in mandibular incisors. J Endod 1999; 25:206–207.

233. Bellizzi R, Hartwell G. Clinical investigation of in vivo endodontically treated mandibular anterior teeth. J Endod 1983; 9:246–248.

234. Walker RT. The root canal anatomy of mandibular incisors in a southern Chinese population. Int Endod J 1988; 21:218–223.

235. Kaffe I, Kaufman A, Littner MM, Lazarson A. Radiographic study of the root canal system of mandibular anterior teeth. Int Endod J 1985;18:253–259.

236. Miyoshi S, Fujiwara J, Tsuji YT, Yamamoto K. Bifurcated root canals and crown diameter. J Dent Res 1977;56:1425.

237. Laws AJ. Prevalence of canal irregularities in mandibular incisors: a radiographic study. N Z Dent J 1971;67:181–186.

238. Gomes BP, Rodrigues HH, Tancredo N. The use of a modelling technique to investigate the root canal morphology of mandibular incisors. Int Endod J 1996;29:29–36.

239. Karagoz-Kucukay I. Root canal ramifications in mandibular incisors and efficacy of low-temperature injection thermoplasticized gutta-percha filling. J Endod 1994;20:236–240.

240. Warren EM, Laws AJ. The relationship between crown size and the incidence of bifid root canals in mandibular incisor teeth. Oral Surg Oral Med Oral Pathol 1981;52:425–429.

241. Kartal N, Yanikoglu FC. Root canal morphology of mandibular incisors. J Endod 1992;18:562–564.

242. Miyashita M, Kasahara E, Yasuda E, Yamamoto A, Sekizawa T. Root canal system of the mandibular incisor. J Endod 1997;23:479–484.

243. Rankine-Wilson RW, Henry P. The Bifurcated Root Canal in Lower Anterior Teeth. J Am Dent Assoc 1965;70:1162–1165.

244. Benjamin KA, Dowson J. Incidence of two root canals in human mandibular incisor teeth. Oral Surg Oral Med Oral Pathol 1974;38:122–126.

245. Funato A, Funato H, Matsumoto K. Mandibular central incisor with two root canals. Endod Dent Traumatol 1998; 14:285–286.

246. Goncalves A, Goncalves M, Oliveira DP, Goncalves N. Dens invaginatus type III: report of a case and 10-year radiographic follow-up. Int Endod J 2002;35:873–879.

247. Dankner E, Harari D, Rotstein I. Conservative treatment of dens evaginatus of anterior teeth. Endod Dent Traumatol 1996;12:206–208.

248. Wells DW, Meyer RD. Vital root canal treatment of a dens in dente. J Endod 1993;19:616–617.

249. Khabbaz MG, Konstantaki MN, Sykaras SN. Dens invaginatus in a mandibular lateral incisor. Int Endod J 1995;28:303–305.

250. Reeh ES, ElDeeb M. Root canal morphology of fused mandibular canine and lateral incisor. J Endod 1989;15:33–35.

251. Peyrano A, Zmener O. Endodontic management of mandibular lateral incisor fused with supernumerary tooth. Endod Dent Traumatol 1995;11:196–198.

252. Alexandersen V. Double-rooted human lower canine teeth In: Brothwell D, editor. Dental Anthropology. Oxford: Pergamon Press; 1963. pp. 235–244.

253. Pecora JD, Sousa Neto MD, Saquy PC. Internal anatomy, direction and number of roots and size of human mandibular canines. Braz Dent J 1993;4:53–57.

254. Sert S, Aslanalp V, Tanalp J. Investigation of the root canal configurations of mandibular permanent teeth in the Turkish population. Int Endod J 2004;37:494–499.

255. D'Arcangelo C, Varvara G, De Fazio P. Root canal treatment in mandibular canines with two roots: a report of two cases. Int Endod J 2001;34:331–334.

256. Berger A. Lower canine with two roots. Dent Cosmos 1925;67:209.

257. Nandini S, Velmurugan N, Kandaswamy D. Bilateral mandibular canines with type two canals. Indian J Dent Res 2005;16:68–70.

258. Orguneser A, Kartal N. Three canals and two foramina in a mandibular canine. J Endod 1998;24:444–445.

259. Woelfel J, Scheid R. Dental Anatomy Its Relevance to Dentistry. Philadelphia: Lippincott Williams & Wilkins; 2002.

260. Geider P, Perrin C, Fontaine M. [Endodontic anatomy of lower premolars- apropos of 669 cases]. J Odontol Conserv 1989:11–15.

261. Schulze C. Developmental Abnormalities of Teeth and Jaws. In: Gorlin R, Goldman H, editors. Thoma's Oral Pathology. 6th ed. St. Louis CV Mosby Co; 1970. pp. 106–107.

262. Iyer VH, Indira R, Ramachandran S, Srinivasan MR. Anatomical variations of mandibular premolars in Chennai population. Indian J Dent Res 2006;17:7–10.

263. Trope M, Elfenbein L, Tronstad L. Mandibular premolars with more than one root canal in different race groups. J Endod 1986;12:343–345.

264. Fischer GM, Evans CE. A three-rooted mandibular second premolar. Gen Dent 1992;40:139–140.

265. Scott R, Turner II C. The Anthropology of Modern Human Teeth. Cambridge: Cambridge University Press; 2000.

266. Kartal N, Yanikoglu F. The incidence of mandibular premolars with more than one root canal in a Turkish population. J Marmara Univ Dent Fac 1992;1:203–210.

267. Serman NJ, Hasselgren G. The radiographic incidence of multiple roots and canals in human mandibular premolars. Int Endod J 1992;25:234–237.

268. Baisden MK, Kulild JC, Weller RN. Root canal configuration of the mandibular first premolar. J Endod 1992;18:505–508.

269. Vertucci FJ. Root canal morphology of mandibular premolars. J Am Dent Assoc 1978;97:47–50.

270. Yoshioka T, Villegas JC, Kobayashi C, Suda H. Radiographic evaluation of root canal multiplicity in mandibular first premolars. J Endod 2004;30:73–74.

271. Zillich R, Dowson J. Root canal morphology of mandibular first and second premolars. Oral Surg Oral Med Oral Pathol 1973;36:738–744.

272. Lu TY, Yang SF, Pai SF. Complicated root canal morphology of mandibular first premolar in a Chinese population using the cross section method. J Endod 2006;32:932–936.

273. Amos ER. Incidence of bifurcated root canals in mandibular bicuspids. J Am Dent Assoc 1955;50:70–71.

274. Aryanpour S, Bercy P, Van Niewenhuysen JP. Endodontic and periodontal treatments of a geminated mandibular first premolar. Int Endod J 2002;35:209–214.

275. Stecker S, DiAngelis AJ. Dens evaginatus: a diagnostic and treatment challenge. J Am Dent Assoc 2002;133:190–193.

276. Hartup GR. Dens invaginatus type III in a mandibular premolar. Gen Dent 1997;45:584–587.

277. Bramante CM, de Sousa SM, Tavano SM. Dens invaginatus in mandibular first premolar. Oral Surg Oral Med Oral Pathol 1993;76:389.

278. Tavano SM, de Sousa SM, Bramante CM. Dens invaginatus in first mandibular premolar. Endod Dent Traumatol 1994;10:27–29.

279. Milano M, Chavarria C, Hoppe J. Multi-rooted mandibular premolars: report of case. ASDC J Dent Child 2002;69:63–65, 12.

280. England MC, Jr., Hartwell GR, Lance JR. Detection and treatment of multiple canals in mandibular premolars. J Endod 1991;17:174–178.

281. de Almeida-Gomes F, de Sousa BC, dos Santos RA. Unusual anatomy of mandibular premolars. Aust Endod J 2006;32:43–45.

282. Nallapati S. Three canal mandibular first and second premolars: a treatment approach. J Endod 2005;31:474–476.

283. Doolittle TP, Rubel RL, Fried I. Bifid canal in a mandibular first pre-molar. A case report. N Y State Dent J 1973;39:361–362.

284. Yang ZP. Multiple canals in a mandibular first premolar. Case report. Aust Dent J 1994;39:18–19.

285. Hülsmann M. Mandibular first premolar with three root canals. Endod Dent Traumatol 1990;6:189–191.

286. Moayedi S, Lata D. Mandibular first premolar with three canals. Endodontology 2004;16:26–29.

287. Chan K, Yew SC, Chao SY. Mandibular premolar with three root canals–two case reports. Int Endod J 1992;25:261–264.

288. Prabhu NT, John R, Munshi AK. Aberrant root development of the mandibular premolars: a case report. Int J Paediatr Dent 1999;9:49–51.

289. Varrela J. Root morphology of mandibular premolars in human 45,X females. Arch Oral Biol 1990;35:109–112.

290. Visser J. Beitrag zur Kenntnis der menschlichen Zahnwurzelformen. Zürich; 1948.

291. Koh ET, Ford TR, Kariyawasam SP, Chen NN, Torabinejad M. Prophylactic treatment of dens evaginatus using mineral trioxide aggregate. J Endod 2001;27:540–542.

292. Wong M. Four root canals in a mandibular second premolar. J Endod 1991;17:125–126.

293. Shapira Y, Delivanis P. Multiple-rooted mandibular second premolars. J Endod 1982;8:231–232.

294. Macri E, Zmener O. Five canals in a mandibular second premolar. J Endod 2000;26:304–305.

295. Kannan SK, Suganya, Santharam H. Supernumerary roots. Indian J Dent Res 2002;13:116–119.

296. Oginni AO, Olusile AO, Bamise CT. Root malformation in mandibular premolars: an endodontic difficulty-report of two cases. The Nigerian postgraduate medical journal 2002;9:163–166.

297. Al-Fouzan KS. The microscopic diagnosis and treatment of a mandibular second premolar with four canals. Int Endod J 2001;34:406–410.

298. Bram SM, Fleisher R. Endodontic therapy in a mandibular second bicuspid with four canals. J Endod 1991;17:513–515.

299. Rödig T, Hülsmann M. Diagnosis and root canal treatment of a mandibular second premolar with three root canals. Int Endod J 2003;36:912–919.

300. ElDeeb ME. Three root canals in mandibular second premolars: literature review and a case report. J Endod 1982;8:376–377.

301. De Moor RJ, Calberson FL. Root canal treatment in a mandibular second premolar with three root canals. J Endod 2005;31:310–313.

302. Singh RP, Stamps HF, Tatum RC. Endodontic considerations of a tricanaled mandibular second premolar: case report and literature review. Journal of the Maryland State Dental Association 1987;30:13–16.

303. Goswami M, Chandra S, Chandra S, Singh S. Mandibular premolar with two roots. J Endod 1997;23:187.

304. Rhodes JS. A case of unusual anatomy: a mandibular second premolar with four canals. Int Endod J 2001;34:645–648.

305. Holtzman L. Root canal treatment of mandibular second premolar with four root canals: a case report. Int Endod J 1998;31:364–366.

306. Merrill RG. Occlusal Anomalous Tubercles on Premolars of Alaskan Eskimos and Indians. Oral Surg Oral Med Oral Pathol 1964;17:484–496.

307. Curzon ME. Miscegenation and the prevalence of three-rooted mandibular first molars in the Baffin Eskimo. Community Dent Oral Epidemiol 1974;2:130–131.

308. al-Nazhan S. Incidence of four canals in root-canal-treated mandibular first molars in a Saudi Arabian sub-population. Int Endod J 1999;32:49–52.

309. Gulabivala K, Aung TH, Alavi A, Ng YL. Root and canal morphology of Burmese mandibular molars. Int Endod J 2001;34:359–370.

310. Harada Y, Tomino S, Ogawa K, Wada T, Mori S, Kobayashi S, et al. [Frequency of three-rooted mandibular first molars. Survey by x-ray photographs]. Shika Kiso Igakkai Zasshi 1989;31:13–18.

311. Morita M. [Morphological studies on the roots of lower first molars in Japanese]. Shikwa Gakuho 1990;90:837–854.

312. Onda S, Minemura R, Masaki T, Funatsu S. Shape and number of the roots of the permanent molar teeth. Bull Tokyo Dent Coll 1989;30:221–231.

313. Rocha LF, Sousa Neto MD, Fidel SR, da Costa WF, Pecora JD. External and internal anatomy of mandibular molars. Braz Dent J 1996;7:33–40.

314. Skidmore AE, Bjorndal AM. Root canal morphology of the human mandibular first molar. Oral Surg Oral Med Oral Pathol 1971;32:778–784.

315. Sperber GH, Moreau JL. Study of the number of roots and canals in Senegalese first permanent mandibular molars. Int Endod J 1998;31:117–122.

316. Yew SC, Chan K. A retrospective study of endodontically treated mandibular first molars in a Chinese population. J Endod 1993;19:471–473.

317. Younes SA, al-Shammery AR, el-Angbawi MF. Three-rooted permanent mandibular first molars of Asian and black groups in the Middle East. Oral Surg Oral Med Oral Pathol 1990;69:102–105.

318. Reichart PA, Metah D. Three-rooted permanent mandibular first molars in the Thai. Community Dent Oral Epidemiol 1981;9:191–192.

319. Curzon ME. Three-rooted mandibular permanent molars in English Caucasians. J Dent Res 1973;52:181.

320. de Souza-Freitas JA, Lopes ES, Casati-Alvares L. Anatomic variations of lower first permanent molar roots in two ethnic groups. Oral Surg Oral Med Oral Pathol 1971;31:274–278.

321. Curzon ME, Curzon JA. Three-rooted mandibular molars in the Keewatin Eskimo. J Can Dent Assoc (Tor) 1971;37:71–72.

322. Somogyi-Csizmazia W, Simons AJ. Three-rooted mandibular first permanent molars in Alberta Indian children. J Can Dent Assoc (Tor) 1971;37:105–106.

323. Fabra-Campos H. Unusual root anatomy of mandibular first molars. J Endod 1985;11:568–572.

324. Goel NK, Gill KS, Taneja JR. Study of root canals configuration in mandibular first permanent molar. J Indian Soc Pedod Prev Dent 1991;8:12–14.

325. Ricucci D. Three independent canals in the mesial root of a mandibular first molar. Endod Dent Traumatol 1997;13:47–49.

326. Bond JL, Hartwell GR, Donnelly JC, Portell FR. Clinical management of middle mesial root canals in mandibular molars. J Endod 1988;14:312–314.

327. Bolger WL, Schindler WG. A mandibular first molar with a C-shaped root configuration. J Endod 1988;14:515–519.

328. Baugh D, Wallace J. Middle mesial canal of the mandibular first molar: a case report and literature review. J Endod 2004;30:185–186.

329. Mortman RE, Ahn S. Mandibular first molars with three mesial canals. Gen Dent 2003;51:549–551.

330. Martinez-Berna A, Badanelli P. Mandibular first molars with six root canals. J Endod 1985;11:348–352.

331. Kimura Y, Matsumoto K. Mandibular first molar with three distal root canals. Int Endod J 2000;33:468–470.

332. Stroner WF, Remeikis NA, Carr GB. Mandibular first molar with three distal canals. Oral Surg Oral Med Oral Pathol 1984;57:554–557.

333. Barnett F. Mandibular molar with C-shaped canal. Endod Dent Traumatol 1986;2:79–81.

334. Manning SA. Root canal anatomy of mandibular second molars. Part I. Int Endod J 1990;23:34–39.

335. Walker RT. Root form and canal anatomy of mandibular second molars in a southern Chinese population. J Endod 1988;14:325–329.

336. Weine FS, Pasiewicz RA, Rice RT. Canal configuration of the mandibular second molar using a clinically oriented in vitro method. J Endod 1988;14:207–213.

337. Seo MS, Park DS. C-shaped root canals of mandibular second molars in a Korean population: clinical observation and in vitro analysis. Int Endod J 2004;37:139–144.

338. Weine FS. The C-shaped mandibular second molar: incidence and other considerations. Members of the Arizona Endodontic Association. J Endod 1998;24:372–375.

339. Cooke HG, 3rd, Cox FL. C-shaped canal configurations in mandibular molars. J Am Dent Assoc 1979;99:836–839.

340. Melton DC, Krell KV, Fuller MW. Anatomical and histological features of C-shaped canals in mandibular second molars. J Endod 1991;17:384–388.

341. Haddad GY, Nehme WB, Ounsi HF. Diagnosis, classification, and frequency of C-shaped canals in mandibular second molars in the Lebanese population. J Endod 1999;25:268–271.

342. Carlsen O, Alexandersen V. Root canals in two-rooted maxillary second molars. Acta Odontol Scand 1997;55:330–338.

343. Carlsen O, Alexandersen V, Heitmann T, Jakobsen P. Root canals in one-rooted maxillary second molars. Scand J Dent Res 1992;100:249–256.

344. Sidow SJ, West LA, Liewehr FR, Loushine RJ. Root canal morphology of human maxillary and mandibular third molars. J Endod 2000;26:675–678.

345. Sikri VK, Sikri P. Mandibular premolars: aberrations in pulp space morphology. Indian J Dent Res 1994;5:9–14.

346. Chai WL, Thong YL. Cross-sectional morphology and minimum canal wall widths in C-shaped roots of mandibular molars. J Endod 2004;30:509–512.

347. Al-Fouzan KS. C-shaped root canals in mandibular second molars in a Saudi Arabian population. Int Endod J 2002; 35:499–504.

348. Benenati FW. Mandibular second molar with C-shaped canal morphology and five canals: report of a case. Gen Dent 2004;52:253–254.

349. Carlsen O. Root complex and root canal system: a correlation analysis using one-rooted mandibular second molars. Scand J Dent Res 1990;98:273–285.

350. Fan B, Cheung GS, Fan M, Gutmann JL, Bian Z. C-shaped canal system in mandibular second molars: Part I–Anatomical features. J Endod 2004;30:899–903.

351. Fan B, Cheung GS, Fan M, Gutmann JL, Fan W. C-shaped canal system in mandibular second molars: Part II–Radiographic features. J Endod 2004;30:904–908.

352. Jin GC, Lee SJ, Roh BD. Anatomical study of C-shaped canals in mandibular second molars by analysis of computed tomography. J Endod 2006;32:10–13.

353. Lambrianidis T, Lyroudia K, Pandelidou O, Nicolaou A. Evaluation of periapical radiographs in the recognition of C-shaped mandibular second molars. Int Endod J 2001;34:458–462.

354. Liewehr FR, Kulild JC, Primack PD. Obturation of a C-shaped canal using an improved method of warm lateral condensation. J Endod 1993;19:474–477.

355. Lyroudia K, Samakovitis G, Pitas I, Lambrianidis T, Molyvdas I, Mikrogeorgis G. 3D reconstruction of two C-shape mandibular molars. J Endod 1997;23:101–104.

356. Manning SA. Root canal anatomy of mandibular second molars. Part II. C-shaped canals. Int Endod J 1990; 23:40–45.

357. Walid N. The use of two pluggers for the obturation of an uncommon C-shaped canal. J Endod 2000;26:422–424.

358. Yang ZP, Yang SF, Lin YC, Shay JC, Chi CY. C-shaped root canals in mandibular second molars in a Chinese population. Endod Dent Traumatol 1988;4:160–163.

359. Oehlers FAC. The radicular variety of dens invaginatus. Oral Surg Oral Med Oral Pathol 1958;11:1251–1260.

360. Segura-Egea JJ, Jimenez-Pinzon A, Rios-Santos JV. Endodontic therapy in a 3-rooted mandibular first molar: importance of a thorough radiographic examination. J Can Dent Assoc 2002;68:541–544.

361. Tamse A, Kaffe I. Radiographic survey of the prevalence of conical lower second molar. Int Endod J 1981; 14:188–190.

362. Goldberg JM, Gross M, Rankow H. Endodontic therapy involving fused mandibular second and third molars. J Endod 1985;11:346–347.

363. Wells DW, Bernier WE. A single mesial canal and two distal canals in a mandibular second molar. J Endod 1984; 10:400–403.

CHAPTER 7

MICROBIOLOGY OF ENDODONTIC DISEASE

J. CRAIG BAUMGARTNER, JOSÉ F. SIQUEIRA JR., CHRISTINE M. SEDGLEY, ANIL KISHEN

Microorganisms cause virtually all pathoses of the pulp and periapical tissues. To effectively treat endodontic infections, clinicians must recognize the cause and effect of microbial invasion of the dental pulp space and the surrounding periapical tissues. Once bacterial invasion of pulp tissues has taken place, both non-specific inflammation and specific immunologic response of the host have a profound effect on the progress of the disease. Knowledge of the microorganisms associated with endodontic disease is necessary to develop a basic understanding of the disease process and a sound rationale for effective management of patients with endodontic infections. Although the vast majority of our knowledge deals with bacteria, we are now aware of the potential for endodontic disease to be associated with fungi and viruses.[1-9] The topics of this chapter are directed toward the role of microorganisms in the pathogenesis of endodontic disease. Owing to a recently resurrected controversy over the "theory of focal infection," an update on this issue will be presented.

Theory of Focal Infection (Revisited)

A focus of infection contains pathogenic microbes and can occur anywhere in the body. Foci of infection have been associated with tonsils, adenoids, sinuses, the oral cavity, the prostate, appendix, gallbladder, and the kidney.[10] In 1890, W. D. Miller associated the presence of bacteria with pulpal and periapical disease. He described "focal infection" and recommended treating and filling root canals. The first reported claim of a cure for a disease associated with focal infection was by Hippocrates[11] who believed he cured a case of arthritis by tooth extraction. In 1904, F. Billings reported a series of cures of afflictions by tonsillectomies and dental extractions. He described that cultured bacteria from septic arthritis patient could produce arthritis in rabbits.[12,13] One of his students was E. C. Rosenow, who in 1909 described the "Theory of Focal Infection" as a localized or generalized infection caused by bacteria traveling through the bloodstream from a distant focus of infection. He also introduced the concepts of "elective localization" whereby bacteria would have affinity for specific body organs. He also described "transmutation" as the process of one species of bacteria spontaneously changing into another species.[14,15] Transmutation was used to explain why other researchers could not reproduce his results. Numerous prominent physicians began advocating the removal of tonsils, adenoids, and teeth as a remedy for diseases caused by microbes and virulence factors from a distant focal infection.[16]

In 1910, a British physician, William Hunter, presented a lecture on the role of sepsis and antisepsis in medicine to the faculty of McGill University. He condemned the practice of dentistry in the United States, which emphasized restorations instead of tooth extraction. Hunter stated that the restorations were "a veritable mausoleum of gold over a mass of sepsis." He believed that this was the cause of Americans' many illnesses, including pale complexion, chronic dyspepsias, intestinal disorders, anemias, and nervous complaints.[17] This lead to an "orgy of extractions" and the recommendation of extraction for all endodontically treated teeth by the "100 percenters."[18] Many of the studies were "reverse investigation" which start with a conclusion and gather information to support it.

Weston Price began a 25-year study of pulpless and endodontically treated teeth and their association with focal infection. He published a series of rabbit experiments and case reports purporting remarkable improvement after dental extraction of non-vital teeth (teeth with non-vital pulps).[19,20] During that time frame, the dental literature contained numerous testimonials reporting cures of illnesses following tooth extraction. These reports were empirical and without adequate follow-up. However, they wrongfully supported the continued extraction of teeth without scientific reason. In many cases, diseases reoccurred, and the patients had to face the additional difficulty of living with mutilated dentitions. In the 1920s, the theory of focal infection was widely accepted and endodontic education was virtually eliminated from dental education. In the 1930s, reports began to be published critical of the theory of focal infection. Cecil and Angevine[21] reported on 200 cases of rheumatoid arthritis, which showed no benefit from tonsillectomy or dental extractions. In 1940, a critical publication by Reimann[22] raised several issues related to the theory of focal infection. They included (1) the theory of focal infection was not proved; (2) the infectious agents were unknown; (3) large groups of people with tonsils were no worse than those that had their tonsils removed; (4) patients having their teeth or tonsils removed were no better off after surgery; (5) beneficial effects could seldom be associated with the surgery; (6) harmful effects of the surgery often outweighed and benefit of surgery; (7) foci of infection often heal after recovery from a systemic disease or improved hygiene and dietary measures.

In the 1930s and 1940s, editorials and research refuted the theory of focal infection and called for a return to constructive rather than destructive dental treatment.[18,23] The studies by Rosenow and Price were flawed by inadequate controls, the use of massive doses of bacteria, and bacterial contamination of endodontically treated teeth during tooth extraction. In 1939, Fish[24] recognized four zones of reaction formed in response to bacteria implanted in the jaws of guinea pigs. He described the bacteria as being confined by polymorphonuclear neutrophil leukocytes to a zone of infection. Outside the zone of infection is the zone of contamination containing inflammatory cells, but no bacteria. Next, the zone of irritation contained histocytes and osteoclasts. On the outside was a zone of stimulation with mostly fibroblasts, capillary buds, and osteoblasts. Fish[24] theorized that removal of the nidus of infection would lead to resolution of the infection. This theory became the basis for successful root canal treatment.

Today, the medical and dental professions agree that there is no relationship between endodontically treated teeth and the degenerative diseases implicated in the theory of focal infection. However, recent publications have resurrected the focal infection theory based on the poorly designed and outdated studies by Rosenow and Price.[25,26] This body of research has been evaluated and disproved. Unfortunately, uninformed patients may receive this outdated information and believe it to be credible new findings.

Endodontic infections may be associated with metastatic infections by direct extension of the infection, via microbes carried through the blood (bacteremia), and by the release of bacterial products and inflammatory mediators. The direct extension of a periapical abscess may reach the maxillary sinuses, cavernous sinus, orbit, brain, or via parapharyngeal pathways produce Ludwig's angina.

Both non-surgical root canal instrumentation and endodontic surgery may produce bacteremia.[27-32] One study found that if the endodontic instrument was confined to inside the root canal 1 mm short of the apical foramen, the incidence of bacteremia was 4 in 13 (31%). If the instruments (sizes 15, 20, and 25) were deliberately used to a level 2 mm beyond the apical foramen, the incidence of bacteremia was 7 in 13 (54%). Ribotyping with restriction enzymes showed identical characteristics for the clinical isolates from the root canals and for the bacteria isolated from the blood. This typing method shows that the microorganisms recovered from the bloodstream during and after endodontic treatment had the root canal as their source.

Another study using both cultivation and the polymerase chain reaction (PCR) detected bacteremia in 9/30 (30%) patients undergoing non-surgical endodontic treatment.[32] Anaerobic bacteria were the predominant microbe detected in blood samples taken during endodontic treatment. In clinical practice, it is impossible to know that endodontic instruments are always confined to the canal system. In addition, infected canal debris may be extruded beyond the apical foramen. However, non-surgical endodontics is less likely to produce bacteremia than tooth extraction or surgical endodontics.[28,29] Simple tooth extraction produces an extensive bacteremia 100% of the time.[27,28] Endodontic therapy should be the treatment of choice instead of tooth extraction for patients believed to be susceptible to infective endocarditis following a bacteremia.

In a study of 20,747 positive blood cultures, 2.8% were viridens group streptococci and 4.4% were obligate anaerobes.[33] These data suggest that oral microbes are only a small percentage of the bacteria detected in blood cultures. It is also known that bacteremias from tooth brushing, flossing, and mastication produce daily bacteremias approaching that of various dental treatments.[34] There is no data on the necessary inoculum size to initiate a metastatic (focal) infection and little on the magnitude [colony-forming units (CFUs)] of a bacteremia produced by various dental procedures.[34] Currently, the most documented examples of focal infection are bacterial endocarditis, brain abscess, and prosthetic joint infections.[10] The actual risk to patients from dental treatment induced bacteremia appears to be very less.[35] The approximate risk for acquiring bacterial endocarditis from a single dental treatment ranges from 1/95,058 for a patient with previous endocarditis to 1/1,096,824 for a patient with mitral valve prolapse with regurgitation.[34] Considering a 16/1,000,000 mortality rate from penicillin anaphylaxis, penicillin prophylaxis might result in a net loss of life.[34] In addition, there is no clear mechanism of how antibiotic prophylaxis reduces bacteremias.[36] Penicillin and cephalosporin require actively dividing bacteria to be effective, and bacteriostatic antibiotics take hours to produce their effects by affecting protein synthesis. In fact, it has been shown that prophylactic antibiotics do not significantly reduce the incidence of bacteremias.[37,38] It has been proposed that antibiotic prophylaxis may prevent adherence of bacteria to valvular vegetation or eliminate the bacteria once they have attached.[39,40] Guidelines for the use of prophylactic antibiotics are found in Chapter 24.

It is believed that cardiovascular disease begins with the formation of an atheroma in response to an injury. Microorganisms may be deposited in the area and produce proinflammatory cytokines.[41] However, cardiovascular disease has many risk factors that control the progress of the atheromas and thrombogenesis.[41] Risk factors include coronary lipid profile, hypertension, diabetes mellitus, obesity, sex, age, socioeconomic factors, lifestyle stress, homocysteine levels, smoking, and genetics. Epidemiologic studies have found relationships between periodontal disease and coronary heart disease, strokes, and preterm low birth rate.[42,43] More recent studies have shown only a very limited association between periodontal disease and cardiovascular disease.[44-49] It must be kept in mind that epidemiologic research can identify relationships, but not causation.

In a health professionals' follow-up study using root canal therapy as a surrogate for pulpal inflammation, an association was found between dentists with root canal therapy and coronary heart disease.[49] Interestingly, there was no association among non-dentists in the study. Another longitudinal study evaluated whether patients with radiographic lesions of endodontic origin were more likely to develop coronary heart disease.[50] Among those patients less than 40 years old, periapical lesions of endodontic origin were associated with future diagnosis of coronary heart disease.

Further research may show that endodontic or periodontal disease constitutes an oral component of a systemic disorder or has etiologic features in common with medical diseases. They may occur without necessarily indicating a cause-effect relationship. To demonstrate cause and effect, interventional studies must be undertaken that show that elimination of a variable alters the incidence or course of the disease. More research is needed to determine the impact that endodontic disease may have on overall health of our patients.

Endodontic infections can spread to other tissues. An abscess or cellulitis may develop if bacteria invade periapical tissues, and the patient's immune system is not able to stop the spread of bacteria and bacterial by-products. This type of infection/inflammation spreads directly from one anatomic space to an adjacent space. This is not an example of the theory of focal infection, whereby bacteria travel through the circulatory system and establish an infection at a distant site.

Successfully completed root canal therapy should not be confused with an untreated infected root canal system or a tooth with a periapical abscess that may be a source of a bacteremia. Bacteremias occur every day as a result of a patient's normal daily activities. To show a causal relationship between an oral infection and systemic disease, it is not adequate to show only a potential relationship via a bacteremia. Hard evidence is needed to show that the organism in the no-oral site of infection actually came from the oral cavity. If possible, Koch's postulates should be fulfilled to establish a causal role of the microorganism from the oral cavity. Endodontics has survived the theory of focal infection because of recognition by the scientific community that successful root canal treatment is possible without endangering systemic health.

Endodontic Infections

Colonization is the establishment of microbes in a host if appropriate biochemical and physical conditions are available for growth. Normal oral microbiata is the result of a permanent microbial colonization in a symbiotic relationship with the host. Although the microbes in the normal oral microbiata participate in many beneficial relationships, they are opportunistic pathogens if they gain access to a normally sterile area of the body such as the dental pulp or periapical tissues and produce disease. An infectious disease (infection) is the result of invasion of the tissues by microbes and the reaction of the tissues to their presence which produces clinical signs and symptoms. Pulpal and periapical pathoses (diseases) result from opportunistic pathogens infecting the pulp and periapical tissues. The steps in the development of an endodontic infection include microbial invasion, multiplication, and pathogenic activity. Much of the pathogenic activity is associated with host response.

Pathogenicity is a term used to describe the capacity of a microbe to produce disease, whereas virulence describes the degree of pathogenicity. Bacteria have a number of virulence factors that may be associated with disease. They include pili (fimbriae), capsules, extracellular vesicles, lipopolysaccharides (LPS), enzymes, short-chain fatty acids, polyamines, and low molecular weight products such as ammonia and hydrogen sulfide. Pili may be important for attachment to surfaces and interaction with other bacteria in a polymicrobial infection. Bacteria including gram-negative dark-pigmented bacteria may have capsules that enable them to avoid or survive phagocytosis.[51]

Association of Microbes with Endodontic Disease

Antony van Leewenhoek,[52] the inventor of single-lens microscopes, was the first to observe oral microbiota. His description of the "animalcules" observed with his microscopes included those from dental plaque and from an exposed pulp cavity. W. D. Miller is considered to be the father of oral microbiology. In 1890, he authored a book, *Microorganisms of the Human Mouth*, which became the basis for dental microbiology in this country. In 1894, Miller[53] became the first researcher to associate the presence of bacteria with pulpal disease.

The true significance of bacteria in endodontic disease was shown in the classic study by Kakehashi et al.[54] in 1965. They found that no pathologic changes occurred in the exposed pulps or periapical tissues in germ-free rats (Figure 1A). In conventional animals, however, pulp exposures led to pulpal necrosis and periapical lesion formation (see Figure 1B). In contrast, the germ-free rats were healed with dentinal

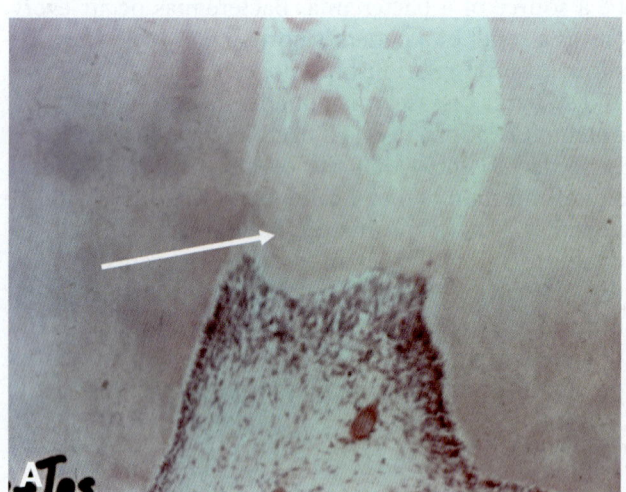 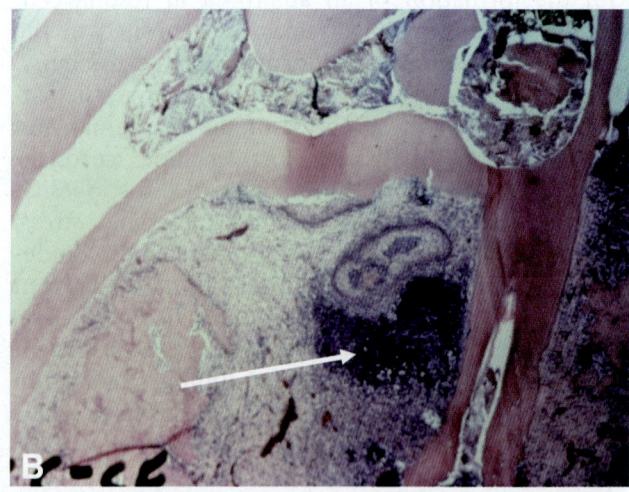

Figure 1 Role of bacteria in dentin repair following pulp exposure. *A,* Germ-free specimen obtained 100 days after pulp exposure. Normal pulp tissue can be observed beneath the dentin bridge (arrow). *B,* Exposure of pulp in control rat with normal oral flora produced pulp necrosis and Abscess formation (arrow). *A,* Reproduced with permission from Kakehashi S, Stanley HR, Fitzgerald RJ. Oral surg 1965; **20**: 340. *B,* reproduced with permission from clark JW, Stanley HR, Fitzgerald RJ. Clinical Dentistry. Hagerstown (MD): Harper & Row; 1976; **4**: 10

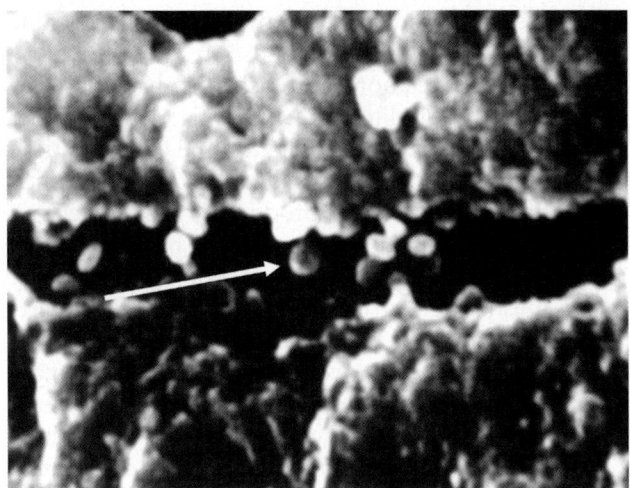

Figure 2 Coccal forms of bacteria (arrow) seen in cross-section of a fractured dentinal tubule (×5000 original magnification). Courtesy C. Baumgartner.

bridging regardless of the severity of the pulpal exposure.[54] Thus, the presence or absence of a microbiota was the major determinant for the destruction or healing of exposed rodent pulps.

Invasion of the pulp cavity by bacteria is most often associated with dental caries. Bacteria invade and multiply within the dentinal tubules (Figure 2). Dentinal tubules range in size from 1 to 4 μm in diameter, whereas the majority of bacteria are less than 1 μm in diameter. If enamel or cementum is missing, microbes may invade the pulp through the exposed tubules. A tooth with a vital pulp is resistant to microbial invasion. Movement of bacteria in dentinal tubules is restricted by viable odontoblastic processes, mineralized crystals, and various macromolecules within the tubules. Caries remains the most common portal of entry for bacteria and bacterial by-products into the pulpal space. However, bacteria and their by-products have been shown to have a direct effect on the dental pulp even without direct exposure.[55,56] These studies demonstrated inflammatory reactions adjacent to the exposed dentinal tubules. Although the inflammatory reactions could result in pulpal necrosis, the majority of pulps were able to undergo healing and repair.[55–58]

Following trauma and direct exposure of the pulp, inflammation, necrosis, and bacterial penetration are no more than 2 mm into the pulp after 2 weeks.[57] In contrast, a necrotic pulp is rapidly invaded and colonized. Peritubular dentin and reparative dentin may impede the progress of the microorganisms. However, the "dead tracts" of empty dentinal tubules following dissolution of the odontoblastic processes may leave virtual highways for the microbes' passage to the pulp cavity. Microbes may reach the pulp via direct exposure of the pulp from restorative procedures or trauma injury and from pathways associated with anomalous tooth development. It is believed that the egress of irritants from an infected root canal system through tubules, lateral or accessory canals, furcation canals, and the apical foramina may directly affect the surrounding attachment apparatus. However, it is debatable whether periodontal disease directly causes pulpal disease.[59–62] The presence of pulpitis and bacterial penetration into exposed dentinal tubules following root planing in humans has been demonstrated.[63] Langeland et al.[60] found that changes in the pulp did occur when periodontal disease was present, but pulpal necrosis occurred only if the apical foramen was involved. Kobayashi et al.[64] compared the bacteria in root canals to those in periodontal pockets. The authors believe that bacteria concurrent in both areas suggest that the sulcus or periodontal pocket is the source of the bacteria in root canal infections. To differentiate an abscess of periodontal origin from that of endodontic origin, the enumeration of spirochetes has been recommended.[65] Abscesses of periodontal origin contained 30% to 58% spirochetes, whereas those of endodontic origin were 0% to 10% spirochetes.

Anachoresis is a process by which microbes may be transported in the blood or lymph to an area of inflammation such as a tooth with pulpitis, where they may establish an infection. The phenomenon of anachoresis has been demonstrated in animal models, both non-dental inflamed tissues and inflamed dental pulps.[66–68] However, the localization of blood-borne bacteria in instrumented but unfilled canals could not be demonstrated in an animal model.[69,70] Infection of unfilled canals was possible only with overinstrumentation when bacteremia occurs to allow bleeding into the canals.[70] Anachoresis may be the mechanism through which traumatized teeth with intact crowns become infected.[71] The process of anachoresis has been especially associated with bacteremias and infective endocarditis.

Once the dental pulp becomes necrotic, the root canal system becomes a "privileged sanctuary" for clusters of bacteria, bacterial by-products, and degradation products of both the microorganisms and the pulpal tissue.[72–74]

Polymicrobial interactions and nutritional requirements make the cultivation and identification of all organisms from endodontic infections very difficult.

Prior to 1970, very few strains of strict anaerobes were isolated and identified because of inadequate anaerobic culturing methods. The importance of anaerobic bacteria in pulpal and periapical pathoses has been revealed with the development of anaerobic culturing methods and the use of both selective and non-selective culture media. However, even with the most sophisticated culturing methods, there are still many microorganisms that remain uncultivable. The bacteria in an infected root canal system are a restricted group compared to the oral microbiota.

Most of the bacteria in an endodontic infection are strict anaerobes. These bacteria grow only in the absence of oxygen but vary in their sensitivity to oxygen. They function at low oxidation-reduction potentials and generally lack the enzymes superoxide dismutase and catalase. Microaerophilic bacteria can grow in an environment with oxygen but predominantly derive their energy from anaerobic energy pathways. Facultative anaerobes grow in the presence or absence of oxygen and usually have the enzymes superoxide dismutase and catalase. Obligate aerobes require oxygen for growth and possess both superoxide dismutase and catalase.

Most species in endodontic infections have also been isolated from periodontal infections, but the root canal microbiota is not complex.[64] Using modern cultivation techniques, five or more species of bacteria are usually isolated from root canals with contiguous apical rarefactions. The number of CFUs in an infected root canal is usually between 10^2 and 10^8. A positive correlation exists between an increase in size of the periapical radiolucency and both the number of bacteria species and CFUs present in the root canal.[75,76]

The dynamics of bacteria in infected root canals have been studied in monkeys.[72,77,78] After infecting the monkey root canals with indigenous oral bacteria, the canals were sealed and then sampled for up to 3 years. Initially, facultative bacteria predominated; however, with increasing time, the facultative bacteria were displaced by anaerobic bacteria.[72,77,78] The results indicate that a selective process takes place that allows anaerobic bacteria an increased capability of surviving and multiplying. After almost 3 years (1,080 days), 98% of the cultivable bacteria were strict anaerobes.

The root canal system is a selective habitat that allows the growth of certain species of bacteria in preference to others. Tissue fluid and the breakdown products of necrotic pulp provide nutrients rich with polypeptides and amino acids. These nutrients, low oxygen tension, and bacterial by-products determine which bacteria will predominate.

Antagonistic relationships between bacteria may occur. Some metabolites (eg., ammonia) may be either a nutrient or a toxin, depending on the concentration. In addition, bacteria may produce bacteriocins, which are antibiotic-like proteins produced by one species of bacteria to inhibit another species of bacteria. When Sundqvist et al.[79] cultured intact root canals, 91% of the organisms were strict anaerobes. When Baumgartner et al.[80] cultured the apical 5 mm of root canals exposed by caries, 67% were found to be strict anaerobes. A polymicrobial ecosystem seems to be produced that selects for anaerobic bacteria over time. Gomes et al.[81,82] and Sundqvist[74,83] used odds ratios to show that some bacteria tend to be associated in endodontic infections. This suggests a symbiotic relationship that may lead to an increase in virulence by the organisms in that ecosystem. Clinicians may consider chemomechanical cleaning and shaping of the root canal system as total disruption of that microbial ecosystem.

Although no absolute correlation has been made between any species of bacteria and severity of endodontic infections, several species have been implicated with some clinical signs and symptoms. Those species include dark-pigmented bacteria, *Peptostreptococcus*, *Eubacterium*, *Fusobacterium*, and *Actinomyces*.[76,79,82,84–95] Table 1 summarizes the percentage of incidence of bacteria isolated from intact root canals from five combined studies.[76,79,96–98] Table 2 summarizes the taxonomic changes that have taken place with the bacteria formerly in the genus *Bacteroides*.

Dark (black)-pigmented bacteria have been associated with clinical signs and symptoms in several studies.[76,79,84,86–88,90,92,94] Unfortunately, taxonomic revision based on deoxyribonucleic acid (DNA) studies has made the interpretation of previous research results based on conventional identification of the bacteria at the very least confusing and in many cases impossible. Conventional identification of microbes based on Gram stain, colonial morphology, growth characteristics, and biochemical tests is often inconclusive and yield presumptive identifications. Dark-pigmented bacteria range from being tan to black colonies depending on the media and environment of incubation in the laboratory. Previously, *Prevotella intermedia* was the species of dark-pigmented bacteria most commonly isolated from endodontic infections. In 1992, isolates previously thought to be *P. intermedia* were shown to be a closely related species now

Table 1 Bacteria Cultured and Identified from the Root Canals of Teeth with Apical Radiolucencies

Bacteria	Percentage of Incidence
Fusobacterium nucleatum	48
Streptococcus spp	40
Bacteroides spp*	35
Prevotella intermedia	34
Parvimonas micra	34
Pseudorami bacter	34
Peptostreptococcus anaerobius	31
Lactobacillus spp	32
Eubacterium lentum	31
Fusobacterium spp	29
Campylobacter spp	25
Peptostreptococcus spp	15
Actinomyces spp	15
Mogibacterium timidum	11
Capnocytophaga ochracea	11
Eubacterium brachy	9
Selenomonas sputigena	9
Veillonella parvula	9
Porphyromonas endodontalis	9
Prevotella buccae	9
Prevotella oralis	8
Propionibacterium propionicum	8
Prevotella denticola	6
Prevotella loescheii	6
Eubacterium nodatum	6

Adapted from Sundqvist. Oral Surg;199478:522–30.
Other species isolated in low incidence included Porphyromonas gingivalis, Bacteroides ureolyticus, Campylobactor gracilis, Atopobium minutum Lactobacillus catenaforme, Enterococcus faecalis, Anaerococcus prevotii, Eikenella corrodens, and Pantoea agglomerans.

Table 2 Recent Taxonomic Changes for Previous "Bacteroides" Species

Porphyromonas: dark-pigmented (asaccharolytic *Bacteroides* species)
  Porphyromonas asaccharolytica (usually non-oral)
  Porphyromonas gingivalis*
  Porphyromonas endodontalis*

Prevotella: black-pigmented (saccharolytic *Bacteroides* species)
  Prevotella melaninogenica
  Prevotella denticola
  Prevotella loescheii
  Prevotella intermedia*
  Prevotella nigrescens†
  Prevotella corporis
  Prevotella tannerae

Prevotella: non-pigmented (saccharolytic *Bacteroides* species)
  Prevotella buccae*
  Prevotella bivia
  Prevotella oralis
  Prevotella oris
  Prevotella oulorum
  Prevotella ruminicola

*Studies have associated species with clinical signs and symptoms.
†Most commonly isolated species of dark-pigmented bacteria.

known as *Prevotella nigrescens*.[99] Studies have demonstrated that *P. nigrescens* is actually the dark-pigmented bacteria most commonly identified after isolation from both root canals and periapical abscesses of endodontic origin.[100,101] Another study associating dark-pigmented bacteria with endodontic infections found them in 55% of 40 intact teeth having necrotic pulps and apical periodontitis. Sixteen of the twenty-two teeth in the sample were associated with purulent drainage or an associated sinus tract.[102] Future studies will likely use molecular methods to detect and more precisely identify the microbes using extracted DNA. Strains of dark-pigmented bacteria previously identified using conventional techniques were determined to be *Prevotella tannerae* using the PCR.[103]

Several studies of endodontically treated teeth requiring re-treatment have shown a prevalence of facultative bacteria, especially *Enterococcus faecalis*, instead of strict anaerobes.[104–108] Studies using molecular methods have detected numerous other species in root canals that have failed to heal.[109–111] In addition, fungi have been shown to be associated with failed root canal treatment.[7,112] Infection at the time of refilling and the size of the periapical lesion were factors that had a negative influence on the prognosis for re-treatment.[108]

Microbiological Diagnostic Techniques

Interest in endodontic microbiology has boomed after the recognition that apical periodontitis lesions are inflammatory diseases caused by microorganisms. The growing interest in this area has become even more pronounced after the recent introduction of and further fast paced advances in methods based on detection and analysis of microbial nucleic acids. Traditionally, microorganisms involved with endodontic infections have been studied by means of culture-dependent techniques, which have been demonstrated to have several limitations when it comes to microbiological diagnosis.[113] Findings from culture-dependent methods with regard to the microbiota living in diverse ecosystems have been supplemented and significantly expanded with molecular biology techniques, and the impact of these methods on the knowledge of the endodontic microbiota in diverse clinical conditions has been astonishing.[111]

Several methodologies have been used or have the potential to be used for the study of endodontic infections. No single method can provide all the information, and the choice for a given method is indeed based on the answers the researcher or clinician is looking for. As a matter of fact, data obtained from different methods should be compiled, interpreted, and collated so that evidence can be mounted. In this regard, it is important for students, clinicians, and researchers to understand the principles behind the methodologies currently in use as well as their advantages and limitations, so that the impact of the information brought about by different methods can be properly weighed. To shed some light on these aspects, the following discussion highlights the main methods currently in use for endodontic microbiology research.

Culture

Traditionally, microbial culture has been the preferred means for examination of the endodontic microbiota. Culture is the process of propagating microorganisms in the laboratory by providing them with proper environmental conditions. Ingredients necessary for microbial pathogens can be supplied by living systems (eg., growth in an animal host or in cell culture) or artificial systems (by gathering the required conditions for growth). Artificial systems have been widely used for microbiological diagnosis of most bacterial and fungal infections that afflict humans. In order for microorganisms to multiply on/in artificial media, they must have available the required nutrients and proper physicochemical conditions, including temperature, moisture, atmosphere, salt concentration, ionic strength of the medium, and pH.[114]

In microbial culture, samples are collected and transported to the laboratory in a viability preserving, non-supportive, and anaerobic medium. They are then dispersed by sonication or by vortex mixing, distributed onto various types of agar media, and cultured under aerobic or anaerobic conditions. After a suitable period of incubation, individual colonies are subcultured and identified on the basis of multiple aspects including colony and cellular morphology, Gram-staining pattern, oxygen tolerance, comprehensive biochemical characterization, and metabolic end-product analysis by gas-liquid chromatography. The outer cellular membrane protein profile as examined by gel electrophoresis, fluorescence under ultraviolet light, and susceptibility tests to selected antibiotics can also be of great value for the identification of some species. Marketed packaged kits that test for preformed enzymes have been used for rapid identification of some species, but they can show a relatively low accuracy for identification of many anaerobes, requiring further testing.[115]

Advantages and limitations of culture-dependent methods are summarized in Table 3. The difficulties in

Table 3 Advantages and Limitations of Culture Methods

Culture Techniques	
Advantages	**Limitations**
1. Broad-range nature, identification of unexpected species	1. Impossibility of culturing a large number of extant bacterial species
2. Allow quantification of all major viable microorganisms in the samples	2. Not all viable bacteria can be recovered
3. Allow determination of antimicrobial susceptibilities of the isolates	3. Once isolated, bacteria require identification using a number of techniques
4. Physiological studies are possible	4. Misidentification of strains with ambiguous phenotypic behavior
5. Pathogenicity studies are possible	5. Low sensitivity
6. Widely available	6. Strict dependence on the mode of sample transport
	7. Samples require immediate processing
	8. Costly, time-consuming, and laborious
	9. Specificity is dependent on the experience of the microbiologist
	10. Extensive expertise and specialized equipment needed to isolate strict anaerobes
	11. Take several days to weeks to identify most anaerobic bacteria

culturing or in identification are of great importance and deserve additional discussion.

DIFFICULTIES IN CULTURING: THE HUGE AS-YET-UNCULTIVATED MAJORITY

Not all microorganisms can grow and be maintained under artificial conditions in the laboratory. In fact, there are several instances of microbial ecosystems that were thought to be well characterized by culture-dependent approaches, but which proved to be far different when assessed by culture-independent molecular biology techniques.[116] Investigations of many aquatic and terrestrial environments using culture-independent methods have revealed that the cultivable members of these systems represent less than 1% of the total extant population.[117,118] Novel culture-independent methods for microbial identification that involve amplification of the 16S rRNA gene followed by cloning and sequencing (discussed in "PCR and Its Derivatives") have recently been used to determine the bacterial diversity within different environments, including human diseased and healthy sites.[119–129] Perhaps not surprisingly, the number of recognized bacterial phyla has expanded from the original estimate of 11 in 1987 to 36 in 1998.[130] The latest tally of bacterial phyla is now probably near 53, of which one-half are as-yet-uncultivated representatives.[131,132] Taking into consideration that known bacterial pathogens fall within 7 out of the 53 candidate bacterial phyla and that culture-independent approaches have shown that 50% to 80% of the human microbiota in different sites are composed of as-yet-uncultivated bacteria,[120,121,124,128,133] it is fair to realize that there can be many human pathogens which remain to be identified.

There are many possible reasons for bacterial "unculturability." They include (1) lack of essential nutrients or growth factors in the artificial culture medium; (2) overfeeding conditions; (3) toxicity of the culture medium itself, which can inhibit bacterial growth; (4) production of substances inhibitory to the target microorganism by other species present in a mixed consortium; (5) metabolic dependence on other species for growth; and (6) disruption of bacterial intercommunication systems induced by separation of bacteria on solid culture media.[134,135] In addition, under certain stressful environmental conditions, such as starvation, some bacterial cells can be in a state of low metabolic activity and be unable to divide or form colonies onto agar plates without a preceding resuscitation phase. This state is referred to as bacterial dormancy or "viable but non-cultivable" state.[136]

Obviously, if microorganisms cannot be cultured, they cannot be identified by phenotype-based methods. While we stay relatively ignorant on the requirements of many bacteria to grow, identification methods that are not based on bacterial culturability are required. This would avoid that many pathogens pass unnoticed when one is microbiologically surveying clinical samples.

It is worth pointing out the fact that a given species is hitherto uncultivated does not necessarily imply that this species is impossible to cultivate. A myriad of strict anaerobic bacteria were uncultivated a hundred years ago, but further developments in culturing techniques have to a large extent helped solve this problem. For instance, the huge majority of anaerobic bacteria isolated from infected root canals were unnoticed in microbiologic analysis of endodontic infections before the 1970s. There is a growing trend to develop approaches and culture media that allow cultivation of as-yet-uncultivated bacteria,[137,138] allowing a better understanding of their role in nature.

DIFFICULTIES IN IDENTIFICATION: KNOWN SPECIES WITH UNCOMMON PHENOTYPES

Culture-dependent identification is based on phenotypic traits. The fact that the phenotype is inherently mutable and subject to biases of interpretation can lead culturing procedures to misidentification.[139] Interpretation of results from culturing methods is based on characteristics observed in reference strains, with predictable biochemical and physical properties under optimal growth conditions. Phenotypic characteristics are not static and can change under some conditions, including stress.[140] Thus, when common microorganisms with uncommon phenotypes are present, reliance on phenotypic traits can compromise accurate identification. Technologist bias or inexperience with an unusual phenotype or isolate may also compromise identification when results of biochemical tests are interpreted to fit expectations. Thus, one should be mindful that in some circumstances even the successful culturing of a given microorganism does not necessarily mean that this microorganism can be successfully identified.

Molecular biology technology has emerged as a more effective, accurate, and reliable means for the identification of bacteria that are difficult to identify by conventional techniques.[139,141,142] The 16S rRNA gene sequencing approach was first proposed to identify uncultivated bacteria without the need for cultivation, but it has also been widely used for identification of cultivable bacteria that shows uncommon phenotypic behavior and cannot be accurately identified by culture-dependent approaches.[142–144]

In the light of the discussion above, it may appear that the reputation of culture-dependent methods is somewhat tarnished. In addition to its historic importance and undeniable contribution to the knowledge of endodontic infections and not withstanding its numerous shortcomings, culture still has a place in studies of endodontic microbiology, particularly for the identification of microorganisms in unusual clinical conditions, after antimicrobial treatment and in situations where pure cultures are needed for additional analysis, including antibiotic susceptibility and pathogenicity tests.

Microscopy

Direct microscopic examination represents a quick, easy, and inexpensive means of screening microbial samples for major morphotypes and staining patterns. Nevertheless, microscopic findings regarding bacterial morphology may be misleading, because many species can be pleomorphic and conclusions can be influenced by subjective interpretation of the investigator. In addition, microscopy has limited sensitivity and specificity to detect microorganisms in clinical samples. Limited sensitivity is because a relatively large number of microbial cells are required before they are seen under microscopy (eg., 10^4 bacterial cells/mL of fluid).[145] Some microorganisms can even require appropriate stains and/or approaches to become visible. Limited specificity is because species cannot be distinguished.

Immunological Methods

Immunological methods employ antibodies that recognize specific microbial antigens to directly detect target species. Antibodies targeting host immunoglobulins specific to a target species can also be used for indirect detection assays. The reaction can be visualized using a variety of techniques and reactions, including direct and indirect immunofluorescence, flow cytometry, and enzyme-linked immunosorbent assay.[146] These methods may require the use of monoclonal antibodies to assure high specificity. Sensitivity is not significantly higher when compared to culture-dependent approaches.

Table 4 Advantages and Limitations of Immunological Methods

Immunological Techniques	
Advantages	Limitations
1. Rapid—no more than a few hours to identify a microbial species	1. Detect only the target species
2. Easily standardized	2. Low sensitivity
3. Low cost	3. Specificity is variable and depends on the type of antibodies used
4. Detect dead microorganisms	4. Detect dead microorganisms

Advantages and limitations of immunological methods are summarized in Table 4.

Molecular Biology Methods

The development of molecular biology techniques to investigate ecological microbial communities has provided a vast array of new techniques for study of the human microbiota in health and disease. In this regard, a significant contribution of molecular biology methods relates to the identification of previously unknown and uncharacterized human pathogens.[147–151] Moreover, molecular studies have revealed a previously unanticipated diversity of the human microbiota, with as-yet-uncultivated bacteria corresponding to more than 50% of the taxa found in the microbiota associated with diverse oral sites,[123,124,152] stomach,[133] skin,[153] and vaginosis.[154] About 80% of the taxa present in the intestinal microbiota remain to be cultivated and characterized.[120,128] As a consequence, it is fair to assume that there can exist a number of as-yet-unknown pathogens in the uncultivated segment of the human microbiota.

Several genes have been chosen as targets for bacterial identification. Some of these genes are shared by a vast majority, if not all, of bacterial species. Genes proposed for bacterial identification include the *16S rRNA* and *23S rRNA* genes, the *16S-23S rRNA* gene internal transcribed sequences, the *rpoB* gene encoding the β-subunit of RNA polymerase, the *groEL* gene encoding the heat-shock protein, the *gyrB* gene encoding the β-subunit of DNA gyrase, and homologous recombination-encoding *recA*.[155] Of these, the *16S rRNA* gene (or *16S rDNA*) has been the most widely used target because it is universally distributed among bacteria, is long enough to be highly informative and short enough to be easily sequenced, possesses conserved and variable regions, and affords reliability for inferring phylogenetic relationships.[156] Similarly, the *18S rRNA* gene of fungi and other eukaryotes have also been extensively used for identification of these organisms.

There are a plethora of molecular methods for the study of microorganisms, and the choice of a particular approach depends on the questions being addressed. Broad-range PCR followed by cloning and sequencing can be used to unravel the breadth of microbial diversity in a given environment. Microbial community structures can be analyzed via fingerprinting techniques, such as denaturing gradient gel electrophoresis (DGGE) and terminal restriction fragment length polymorphism (T-RFLP). Fluorescence in situ hybridization (FISH) can measure abundance of target species and provide information on their spatial distribution in tissues. Among other applications, DNA-DNA hybridization arrays, species-specific PCR, nested PCR, multiplex PCR, and quantitative real-time PCR can be used to survey large numbers of clinical samples for the presence of target species. Variations in PCR technology can also be used to type microbial strains. The following section will focus on the most commonly used approaches applied in the research of the endodontic microbiota.

PCR AND ITS DERIVATIVES

The PCR method is based on the in vitro replication of DNA through repetitive cycles of denaturation, primer annealing, and extension steps carried out in automated devices called thermocyclers. The target DNA serving as template denatures at high temperatures generating single strands of DNA. The temperature then decreases so that two short oligonucleotide primers can anneal to their complementary sequences on opposite strands of the target DNA. Primers are selected to encompass the desired genetic material, flanking the ends of the stretch of DNA to be copied. In sequence, a complementary second strand of new DNA is synthesized through the extension of each annealed primer by a thermostable DNA polymerase in the presence of excess deoxyribonucleoside triphosphates. All previously synthesized products act as templates for new primer-extension reactions in each ensuing cycle. The result is an exponential amplification of the DNA fragment flanked by the primers, which confers extraordinary sensitivity in detecting the target DNA.

PCR has unrivaled sensitivity (the lowest number of cells detected in a sample). While PCR can detect as few as 10 bacterial cells in a sample (with potential sensitivity to the one-cell level), other methods of identification show too higher detection limits. Culture using non-selective media can detect 10^4 to 10^5 cells in a sample, and when selective media are used, the sensitivity of culture method increases to 10^3 cells.[157] Immunological methods have a detection limit ranging from 10^3 to 10^4 cells. DNA-DNA hybridization assays can detect 10^2 to 10^4 cells in a sample. Thus, PCR methodology is at least 10 to 100 times more sensitive than the other more sensitive identification method.[158]

Numerous derivatives of the conventional PCR technology have been developed since its inception. The most used PCR-derived assays are described below.

Touchdown PCR

Touchdown PCR is a strategy to increase the specificity of the assay. The annealing temperature in the initial PCR cycle is set several degrees above the T_m of the primers. In subsequent cycles, the annealing temperature is decreased in steps of 0.5 to 2 °C per cycle until a temperature is reached that is equal to, or 2 to 5 °C below, the T_m of the primers. Touchdown techniques have been considered useful to avoid the amplification of spurious DNA fragments (non-target gene fragments and/or fragments with improper sizes).[159]

Nested PCR

Nested PCR consists of two rounds of amplification using different sets of primers in each round. A target region of DNA is amplified with an outer primer pair in an initial reaction, followed by a second amplification using an internal primer pair. This approach has been devised mainly to have increased sensitivity,[160] but can also exhibit increased specificity.[158]

Multiplex PCR

In multiplex PCR, two or more sets of primers specific for different targets are concomitantly used in the same reaction.[161] Thus, contrary to conventional PCR approaches, which can detect only one target at a time, multiplex PCR assays permit the simultaneous detection of different species in a sample.

Reverse Transcriptase PCR

Reverse transcriptase PCR (RT-PCR) was developed to amplify RNA targets and to exploit the use of the enzyme reverse transcriptase, which can synthesize a strand of complementary DNA (cDNA) from an RNA template. Most RT-PCR assays employ a two-step approach. In the first step, reverse transcriptase converts RNA into single-stranded cDNA. In the second step, PCR primers, DNA polymerase, and nucleotides are added to create the second strand of cDNA. Once the double-stranded DNA template is formed, it can be used as template for amplification as in conventional PCR.[162] The RT-PCR process may be modified into a one-step approach by using it directly with RNA as the template. In this approach, an enzyme with both reverse transcriptase and DNA polymerase activities is used, such as that from the bacteria *Thermus thermophilus* (*Tth*).

PCR-Based Microbial Typing

PCR technology can be used for clonal analysis and comparison of microbial isolates through PCR-generated fingerprinting profiles. Examples of PCR techniques used for this purpose include the arbitrarily primed PCR (AP-PCR, also referred to as random amplified polymorphic DNA, or RAPD),[163,164] which uses a single random-sequence primer at low stringency, and other assays using primers that target known genetic elements, such as enterobacterial repetitive intergenic consensus sequences (ERIC-PCR)[165,166] and repetitive extragenic palindromic sequences (REP-PCR).[167]

Real-Time PCR

PCR assays are usually qualitative or can be adjusted to be semi-quantitative. One exception is the real-time PCR, which allows the quantification of the amount of DNA in the sample by monitoring the release of fluorescence with each amplification cycle. Accumulation of PCR products is measured automatically during each cycle in a closed tube format using a thermocycler combined with a fluorimeter. Real-time PCR assays allow the quantification of individual target species as well as total bacteria in clinical samples. The advantages of real-time PCR are the rapidity of the assay (30 to 40 minutes), the ability to quantify and identify PCR products directly without the use of agarose gels, and the fact that contamination can be limited due to avoidance of postamplification manipulation.[168] There are several different real-time PCR approaches, but the most commonly used chemistries include SYBR-Green,[169] *Taq*Man,[170] and molecular beacons.[171]

Broad-Range PCR

PCR technology can be used to investigate the breadth of microbial diversity in a given environment. In broad-range PCR, primers are designed that are complementary to conserved regions of a particular gene shared by a group of microorganisms. For instance, primers that are complementary to conserved regions of the *16S rRNA* gene have been used with the intention of exploiting the variable internal regions of the amplified sequence for sequencing and further identification.[172] Initially, bacterial DNA is extracted directly from samples, and the *16S rRNA* gene is isolated via PCR amplification with oligonucleotide primers specific for conserved regions of the gene (universal or broad-range primers). Amplification with universal primers results in a mixture of the *16S rRNA* genes amplified from virtually all bacteria present in the sample. In mixed infections, direct sequencing of the PCR products cannot be performed because there are mixed products from the different species composing the consortium. PCR products are then cloned into a plasmid vector, which is used to transform *Escherichia coli* cells, establishing a clone library of *16S rRNA* gene from the sample. Cloned genes are then sequenced individually, and preliminary identification can be done by using similarity searches in public databases. Phylogenetic analysis should also be accomplished for accurate identification.[173,174] Broad-range PCR can detect the unexpected bacterial diversity in a sample, and in this regard, it is far more effective and accurate than culture. Broad-range PCR has allowed the identification of several novel fastidious or as-yet-uncultivated bacterial pathogens directly from diverse human sites.[113,134,175]

Broad-range PCR products from samples can be alternatively analyzed by fingerprinting techniques, such as DGGE and T-RFLP. Genetic fingerprinting techniques can be used to determine the structure and diversity of microbial communities living in a given environment and to monitor changes in the community over time.

DGGE The analysis of broad-range PCR products by DGGE is a useful strategy to fingerprint bacterial communities. In DGGE, DNA fragments of the same length but with different nucleotide sequences can be separated in polyacrylamide gels containing a linearly increasing gradient of DNA denaturants.[176,177] As the PCR product migrates in the gel, it encounters increasing concentrations of denaturants and becomes partially or fully denatured. DNA fragments with different sequences may have a different melting behavior and will stop migrating at different positions in the gel. Therefore, when PCR products from mixed microbial communities are subjected to DGGE, the result is a fingerprint with several different bands where, at least theoretically, each band corresponds to a single species. In DGGE, multiple samples can be analyzed concurrently, making it possible to compare the structure of the microbial community of different samples and to follow changes in microbial populations over time, including after antimicrobial treatment.[178] Specific bands can also be excised from the gels, re-amplified, and sequenced to allow species identification.

T-RFLP T-RFLP can also provide insight into the structure and function of bacterial communities.[179] In T-RFLP, the *16S rRNA* gene from different bacterial species in a community is PCR amplified using one of the universal PCR primers labeled with a fluorescent dye.[180] The mixture of PCR products is then digested with one or more restriction enzymes that have four-basepair recognition sites, generating different fluorescently labeled terminal fragment lengths, whose sizes and relative abundances are determined using an automated DNA sequencer.[181,182] The use of a fluorescently labeled primer limits the analysis to only the terminal fragments of the enzymatic digestion. All terminal fragment sizes generated from digestion of PCR products can be compared with the terminal fragments derived from sequence databases in order to infer species identification. Through application of automated DNA sequencer technology, T-RFLP has considerably greater resolution than DGGE.[179,180]

DNA-DNA HYBRIDIZATION

DNA-DNA hybridization methodology is the process of annealing the complementary bases of two single-stranded DNA molecules. It employs labeled DNA probes that can locate and bind to a target sequence, forming a new duplex molecule. The labeled duplex can then be detected.[183] Probes are segments of single-stranded DNA labeled with detection molecules that can be constructed from either whole genomic DNA or oligonucleotides. Whole genomic probes are more likely to cross-react with non-target microorganisms due to the presence of homologous sequences between different species. Oligonucleotide probes based on signature sequences of specific genes (such as the *16S rRNA* gene) may display limited or no cross-reactivity with non-target microorganisms when under optimized conditions. In addition, oligonucleotide probes can differentiate between closely related species or even subspecies and can be designed to detect as-yet-uncultivated bacteria.

Hybridization methods developed for large-scale studies include the checkerboard DNA-DNA hybridization and DNA microarray techniques. The Checkerboard DNA-DNA hybridization technique was introduced by Socransky et al.[184] for hybridizing large numbers of DNA samples against large numbers of digoxigenin-labeled whole genomic DNA or *16S rRNA* gene-based oligonucleotide probes on a single support membrane. Briefly, denatured DNA from clinical samples is placed in lanes on a nylon membrane using a Minislot apparatus. After fixation of the samples to the membrane, the membrane is placed in a Miniblotter 45 apparatus with the lanes of samples at 90° to the lanes of the device. Digoxigenin-labeled whole genomic DNA probes are then loaded in individual lanes of the Miniblotter. After hybridization, the membranes are washed at high stringency and the DNA probes detected using antibody to digoxigenin conjugated with alkaline phosphatase and chemifluorescence or chemiluminescence detection. The checkerboard method permits the simultaneous determination of the presence of a multitude of bacterial species in single or multiple clinical samples. A modification of the checkerboard method was proposed by Paster et al.[185] and consists of a PCR-based, reverse-capture checkerboard hybridization methodology. The procedure circumvents the need for in vitro bacterial culture, necessary for preparation of whole genomic probes. Up to 30 reverse-capture oligonucleotide probes that target regions of the *16S rRNA* gene are deposited on a nylon membrane in separate horizontal lanes using a Minislot apparatus. Probes are synthesized with a poly-thymidine tail, which are cross-linked to the membrane via ultraviolet irradiation or heat, leaving the probes available for hybridization. The *16S rRNA* gene from clinical samples is PCR amplified using a digoxigenin-labeled primer. Hybridizations are performed in vertical channels in a Miniblotter apparatus with digoxigenin-labeled PCR amplicons from up to 45 samples. Hybridization signals are detected using chemifluorescence or chemiluminescence procedures.

DNA microarrays were first described in 1995[186] and consist of a high-density matrix of DNA probes which are printed or synthesized on a glass or silicon slide (chip).[187] Targets incorporate either a fluorescent label or some other moiety, such as biotin, that permits subsequent detection with a secondary label. Targets are applied to the array, and those that hybridize to complementary probes are detected using some type of reporter molecule. Following hybridization, arrays are imaged using a high-resolution scanner and analyzed by sophisticated computer software programs. DNA microarrays can be used to enhance PCR product detection and identification. When PCR is used to amplify microbial DNA from clinical specimens, microarrays can then be used to identify the PCR products by hybridization to an array that is composed of species-specific probes.[188] Using broad-range primers, such as those that amplify the *16S rRNA* gene, a single PCR can be used to detect hundreds to thousands of bacterial species simultaneously.[189] When coupled to PCR, microarrays have detection sensitivity equal to conventional methods with the added ability to discriminate several species at a time.

FISH

This method uses fluorescently labeled rRNA probes and fluorescence microscopy to detect intact microbial cells directly in clinical specimens.[189] In addition to provide identification, FISH gives information about presence, morphology, number, organization, and spatial distribution of microorganisms.[190] Because oligonucleotide probes can be designed for use, FISH not only allows the detection of cultivated microbial species, but also of as-yet-uncultivated microorganisms.[191,192] A typical FISH protocol includes four steps: fixation and permeabilization of the sample; hybridization with the respective probes for detecting the respective target sequences; washing steps to remove unbound probe; and detection of labeled cells by microscopy or flow cytometry.[193]

DRAWBACKS OF MOLECULAR BIOLOGY METHODS

As with any other method, molecular methods have also limitations. The methods are summarized in Table 5. However, the issues related to the ability of PCR to detect either an extremely low number of cells or dead cells are of special interest when one interprets the results of PCR identification procedures in endodontic microbiology research. Therefore, these issues are worth a separate discussion.

THE "TOO-HIGH SENSITIVITY" ISSUE

The high detection rate of PCR may be a reason of concern, specifically when non-quantitative assays are employed. It has been claimed that because PCR can detect a very low number of cells of a given microbial species, the results obtained by this method may have no significance with regard to disease causation. However, the method's high sensitivity can represent a great advantage for microbiological diagnosis in endodontics.

When taking samples from endodontic infections, difficulties posed by the physical constraints of the root canal system and by the limitations of the sampling techniques can make it hard for the attainment of a representative sample from the main canal.[135] If cells of a given species are sampled in a number below the detection rate of the diagnostic test, species prevalence will be underestimated.

Table 5 Advantages and Limitations of Molecular Biology Methods

Molecular Biology Techniques

Advantages	Limitations
1. Detect both cultivable and as-yet-uncultivated species or strains.	1. Most assays are qualitative or semi-quantitative (exceptions: real-time PCR, microarray)
2. High specificity and accurate identification of strains with ambiguous phenotypic behavior	2. Most assays only detect one species or a few different species at a time (exceptions: broad-range PCR, checkerboard, microarray)
3. Detect species directly in clinical samples	3. Most assays detect only the target species and fail to detect unexpected species (exception: broad-range PCR)
4. High sensitivity	4. Some assays can be laborious and costly (eg., broad-range PCR)
5. Rapid—most assays take no more than minutes to a few hours to identify a microbial species	5. Biases in broad-range PCR introduced by homogenization procedures, preferential DNA amplification, and differential DNA extraction
6. Do not require carefully controlled anaerobic conditions during sampling and transportation	6. Hybridization assays using whole genome probes detect only cultivable species
7. Can be used during antimicrobial treatment	7. Can be very expensive
8. Anaerobic handling and expertise not required	8. Detect dead microorganisms
9. Samples can be stored frozen for later analysis	
10. DNA can be transported easily between laboratories	
11. Detect dead microorganisms	

PCR, polymerase chain reaction.

It is also important to take into consideration the analytical sensitivity needed for the specific clinical sample. For example, a sensitivity of no more than 10^4 microbial cells per mL is required for urine, while a sensitivity of one cell may be of extreme relevance for blood samples or cerebrospinal fluid.[194] There is no clear evidence as to the microbial load necessary for apical periodontitis to be induced. Endodontic infections are characterized by a mixed community, and individual species can play different roles in the consortium or dominate various stages of the infection. At least theoretically, all bacterial species established in the infected root canal have the potential to be considered endodontic pathogens.[195] Based on this, it would be glaringly prudent to use the method with the highest sensitivity to detect all species colonizing the root canal.

PCR detection of very low numbers of cells in clinical samples may not be as common as anticipated. There are numerous factors that can influence PCRs, sometimes dramatically reducing sensitivity for direct microbial detection in clinical samples. Thus, the analytical sensitivity of the method does not always correspond to its "clinical" sensitivity. It is well known that the effects of inhibitors are magnified in samples with low number of target DNA and therefore can significantly decrease the sensitivity of the method.[196] Another impediment refers to the aliquots of the whole sample used in PCRs. Most of the PCR assays that have been used so far in endodontic research have an analytical sensitivity of about 10 to 100 cells. If one takes into account the dilution factor dictated by the use of small aliquots (5% to 10%) of the whole sample in each amplification reaction, the actual sensitivity of the assay is 100 to 200 to 1,000 to 2,000 cells in the whole sample, without discounting the effects of inhibitors.[158] These numbers are still lower than the detection limits of other methods, but can represent more significance with regard to pathogenicity.

Therefore, the use of highly sensitive techniques is welcomed in the study of endodontic infections, decreasing the risks for potentially important species to pass unnoticed during sample analysis. Although qualitative results do not lack significance, the use of quantitative molecular assays, like the real-time PCR, can allow inference of the role of a given species in the infectious process while maintaining high sensitivity and the ability to detect fastidious or as-yet-uncultivated microbial species.

THE "DEAD-CELL" ISSUE

Detection of dead cells by a given identification method can be at the same time an advantage and a limitation. On the one hand, this ability can allow detection of hitherto uncultivated or fastidious bacteria that can die during sampling, transportation, or isolation procedures.[135,197,198] On the other hand, if the bacteria were already dead in the infected site, they may also be detected, and this might give rise to a false assumption of their role in the infectious process.[199,200]

Several studies show that bacterial DNA is rapidly cleared from the host sites after bacterial death and that DNA from different species may differ as to the elimination kinetics at different body sites.[201–204] It remains to be clarified how long bacterial DNA from dead cells can remain detectable in the infected root canal system.

It is true that detection of microbial DNA sequences in clinical specimens does not indicate viability of the microorganism. However, this issue should be addressed with common sense and without any sort of biases. The fact that some microorganisms die during the course of an infectious process does not necessarily imply that in a determined moment these microorganisms did not participate in the pathogenesis of the disease. In addition, the fate of DNA from microorganisms that have entered and not survived in root canals is unknown. DNA from dead cells might be adsorbed by dentine due to affinity of hydroxyapatite (HAP) to this molecule.[205] However, it remains to be shown if DNA from microbial dead cells can really be adsorbed in dentinal walls, and, if even, it can be retrieved during sampling with paper points. In fact, it is highly unlikely that free microbial DNA can remain intact in an environment colonized by living microorganisms. The half-life of the DNA released in the environment is considered to be very short owing to the presence of DNases in a complex background like the infected root canal. DNases released by some living species as well as at cell death can degrade free DNA in the environment. It has been reported that the presence of DNase activity on whole bacterial cells and vesicles thereof can degrade DNA.[206] These bacteria include common putative endodontic pathogens, such as *Porphyromonas endodontalis*, *Porphyromonas gingivalis*, *Tannerella forsythia*, *Fusobacterium* spp, *P. intermedia*, and *P. nigrescens*.

Thus, the DNA molecule faces an onslaught of microorganisms that can degrade macromolecules.[207] Indeed, DNases are of concern during sample storage, as they can be carried along with the sample and cause DNA degradation, with consequent false negative results after PCR amplification.

Under rare circumstances, such as when the tissue becomes rapidly desiccated after host death or the DNA becomes adsorbed to a mineral matrix, like bone or teeth, DNA may escape enzymatic and microbial degradation. Even so, slower but still relentless chemical processes start affecting the DNA. Many of these processes are similar to those that affect the DNA in the living cell, with the difference that, after cell death, these processes are not counterbalanced by cellular repair processes. Thus, damage accumulates progressively until the DNA loses its integrity and decomposes, with an irreversible loss of nucleotide sequence information.[207]

DNA is not a stable molecule, and chemical processes, like oxidation and hydrolysis, damage DNA over time. As a result, the DNA becomes fragmented and difficult or even impossible to be detected and/or analyzed. In palaeomicrobiology, certain strategies have to be developed for successful detection of ancient DNA. One of the most important strategies consists of using primers that will amplify a small DNA target size, preferably below 200 bp. Even so, the sample has to be well preserved, usually frozen or mummified. It has been stated that it is not the age of the DNA but the environmental conditions that are critical in preservation.[208] Thus, any comparisons between the use of molecular methods in palaeomicrobiology and endodontics can be considered inappropriate at best.

Based on the discussion above, although there is a possibility of detecting DNA from dead cells in endodontic infections, this possibility is conceivably low. In the event, DNA from dead cells is detected, the results by no means lack significance with regard to participation in disease causation. Nonetheless, the ability to detect DNA from dead cells poses a major problem when one is investigating the immediate effectiveness of antimicrobial intracanal treatment, as DNA released from cells that have recently died can be detected. To circumvent or at least minimize this problem, one can use some adjustments in the PCR assay or take advantage of PCR technology derivatives, such as RT-PCR. Because smaller fragments of DNA may persist for a longer time after cell death than larger sequences, designing primers to generate large amplicons may reduce the risks of positive results due to DNA from dead cells.[209] Moreover, assays directed toward the detection of RNA through RT-PCR can be more reliable for detection of living cells. RNAs are more labile and have a shorter half-life when compared to DNA, and they can be rapidly degraded after cell death.[200]

Primary Intraradicular Infections

Over 700 bacterial species can be found in the oral cavity, with any particular individual harboring 100 to 200 of these species.[210] However, only a limited assortment of species is consistently selected out of the oral microbiota for growth and survival in root canals with necrotic pulp tissue. Taken together, data from studies using culture-dependent or culture-independent identification approaches have suggested that a selected group of bacterial species can be considered as candidate endodontic pathogens based on both frequency of detection and potential pathogenicity.

Culture-dependent studies have consistently demonstrated the essential role of microorganisms in causation of the different forms of apical periodontitis.[76,211,212] Also, several putative endodontic pathogens have been recognized. More recently, with the advent of culture-independent molecular biology tools, significant technical hurdles of culture methods have been deftly overcome.[135] Not only have molecular methods corroborated findings from most culture studies, but a great deal of new information has been added to the knowledge of candidate endodontic pathogens. Molecular biology technology has enabled the recognition of new putative pathogens, which had never been previously found in endodontic infections.[111] Moreover, many species that had already been considered as putative pathogens due to their frequencies as reported by culture-dependent methods have been found in even higher prevalence values by molecular biology approaches, strengthening their association with causation of apical periodontitis.

Endodontic infections have a polymicrobial nature, and obligate anaerobic bacteria conspicuously dominate the microbiota in primary infections. Furthermore, the endodontic microbiota presents a high inter-individual variation, that is, it can significantly vary in species diversity and abundance from individual to individual,[110,213] indicating that apical periodontitis has a heterogeneous etiology and multiple bacterial combinations can play a role in disease causation.

The following is an overview of the major bacterial groups and species regarded as candidate endodontic pathogens.

Black-pigmented Gram-negative anaerobic rods include species formerly known as *Bacteroides melaninogenicus*. These bacteria have been reclassified into two genera: the saccharolytic species were transferred to the genus *Prevotella* and the asaccharolytic species to the genus *Porphyromonas*.[214,215] Some bile-sensitive non-pigmented *Bacteroides* species were also transferred to the genus *Prevotella*.[216] *Prevotella* species frequently detected in primary endodontic infections include *P. intermedia*, *P. nigrescens*, *P. tannerae*, *Prevotella multissacharivorax*, *Prevotella baroniae*, and *Prevotella denticola*.[79,89,101–103,217–225] Of the *Porphyromonas* spp, only *P. endodontalis* and *P. gingivalis* have been consistently found in endodontic infections, and they seem to play an important role in the etiology of different forms of apical periodontitis lesions, including acute apical abscesses.[79,89,94,223,226–228]

Tannerella forsythia (previously called *Bacteroides forsythus* or *Tannerella forsythensis*) is a recognized periodontal pathogen that was first detected in endodontic infections by species-specific single PCR.[229] Several studies using different culture-independent molecular biology techniques, such as species-specific single or nested PCR,[230–233] checkerboard hybridization,[227,234] and microarray,[235] have confirmed that *T. forsythia* is a common member of the microbiota associated with different types of endodontic infections, including abscesses.

Dialister species are asaccharolytic obligately anaerobic Gram-negative coccobacilli that represent another example of bacteria that have been consistently detected in endodontic infections only after the advent of molecular biology techniques. *Dialister pneumosintes* and the recently described *Dialister invisus* are amongst the most frequently detected species in asymptomatic and symptomatic primary endodontic infections in several molecular studies.[224,236–242]

Fusobacterium species are also common members of the endodontic microbiota in primary infections including abscesses, with *Fusobacterium nucleatum* being the most frequent representative of the genus.[31,83,221,230,232,243,244] PCR-based microbial typing approaches have revealed that different clonal types of *F. nucleatum* can be isolated from the same infected canal.[245] *Fusobacterium periodonticum* has been detected in acute abscesses of endodontic origin by checkerboard hybridization.[234]

Spirochetes are highly motile spiral-shaped Gram-negative bacteria with periplasmic flagella that originate at opposite poles of the cell and usually are long enough to overlap near the middle of the cell body. All oral spirochetes fall into the genus *Treponema*, which have been linked to several oral diseases.[246–248] For many years, spirochetes have been observed in samples from endodontic infections by microscopy, but they have never been reliably identified to the species level.[249–251] Culture-independent molecular biology methods allowed speciation of spirochetes in endodontic infections and revealed that all of the hitherto named oral treponemes can be found in primary endodontic infections.[235,252–262] The most prevalent treponemes in infections of endodontic origin are *Treponema denticola* and *Treponema socranskii*.[252,253,257,260] The species *Treponema parvum*, *Treponema maltophilum*, and *Treponema lecithinolyticum* have been moderately prevalent.[253,254,259,260]

Gram-positive anaerobic rods have also been found as common members of the microbiota associated with primary endodontic infections. Of these, *Pseudoramibacter alactolyticus* has been detected by culture-dependent and culture-independent studies in frequencies as high as the most prevalent Gram-negative species.[83,263,264] *Filifactor alocis* is an obligately anaerobic rod that had been only occasionally isolated from root canal infections by culture,[83] but a recent species-specific nested PCR study detected this species in about one-half of the cases of primary endodontic infections.[265] *Actinomyces* spp, *Propionibacterium propionicum*, *Olsenella* spp, *Slackia exigua*, *Mogibacterium timidum*, and *Eubacterium* spp have also been reported to occur in infected root canals in relatively high prevalence.[83,232,236,266–272]

Some Gram-positive cocci are frequently present in primary endodontic infections. *Parvimonas micra* (previously called *Peptostreptococcus micros* or *Micromonas micros*) have been isolated from about one-third of the primarily infected canals, and their prevalence in symptomatic infections has also been relatively high.[83,87,220,222,243,273] Members of the *Streptococcus anginosus* group have been reported to be the most prevalent streptococci, but *Streptococcus gordonii*, *Streptococcus mitisi*, and *Streptococcus sanguinis* can also be often recovered/detected.[83,268] *E. faecalis*, which has been closely found in association with root-filled teeth, has not been so frequent in primary infections.[268,274]

Campylobacter spp, including *Campylobacter rectus* and *Campylobacter gracilis*, are Gram-negative anaerobic rods that have been detected in primary endodontic infections, but in low to moderate prevalence values.[83,227,275–277] *Catonella morbi*, a saccharolytic obligately anaerobic Gram-negative rod associated with marginal periodontitis, has been found in about one-fourth of the cases of primary endodontic infections by a nested PCR approach.[278] Other bacteria detected more sporadically in primary infections include *Veillonella parvula*, *Eikenella corrodens*, *Granulicatella adiacens, Neisseria mucosa, Centipeda periodontii, Gemella morbillorum, Capnocytophaga gingivalis, Corynebacterium matruchotii, Bifidobacterium dentium*, and anaerobic lactobacilli.[83,227,234,278–280]

Studies using broad-range PCR associated with clone library analysis[224,236] or T-RFLP[224] have indicated that as-yet-uncultivated bacteria can participate in endodontic infections—more than 40 to 55% of the endodontic microbiota is composed of bacterial phylotypes, that is, species that are known only by a 16S rRNA gene sequence and that have yet to be cultivated and fully characterized. Several uncultivated phylotypes can be very prevalent, and there is no reason to believe that they are not important to disease causation. For instance, oral *Synergistes* clones BA121, E3_33, BH017, and W090 are hitherto uncultivated bacteria that can be commonly detected in samples from both asymptomatic and symptomatic endodontic infections.[237,239,281] Moreover, several as-yet-uncultivated phylotypes related to the genera *Dialister, Megasphaera, Solobacterium, Olsenella, Eubacterium*, and *Cytophaga*, as well as phylotypes related to the family *Lachnospiraceae* have been identified in primary endodontic infections.[224,236,242,282] A study using both 16S rRNA gene clone library and T-RFLP analyses[224] found some uncultivated phylotypes among the most prevalent bacteria in primary intraradicular infections, including *Lachnospiraceae* oral clone 55A-34, *Megasphaera* oral clone CS025, and *Veillonella* oral clone BP1-85. Two phylotypes, *Bacteroidetes* oral clone X083 and *Dialister* oral clone BS016, were detected only in asymptomatic teeth, while *Prevotella* oral clone PUS9.180, *Eubacterium* oral clone BP1-89, and *Lachnospiraceae* oral clone MCE7_60 were exclusively detected in symptomatic samples.[224] Detection of as-yet-uncultivated phylotypes in endodontic infections suggests that they can be previously unrecognized bacteria that play a role in the pathogenesis of different forms of apical periodontitis.

Figure 3 displays several cultivable and as-yet-uncultivated bacterial species found in endodontic infections by culture-dependent and culture-independent analyses. As the breadth of bacterial diversity in endodontic infections has been unraveled by molecular biology methods, the list of candidate endodontic pathogens has expanded to include several cultivable and as-yet-uncultivated species that had been underrated by culture-dependent methods. Endodontic bacteria are now recognized to belong to 8 of the 12 phyla that have oral representatives, namely *Firmicutes, Bacteroidetes, Spirochaetes, Fusobacteria, Actinobacteria, Proteobacteria, Synergistes*, and TM7. Members of the two latter phyla and several representatives of the other phyla still remain to be cultivated.

Other Microorganisms in Endodontic Infections

FUNGI

Although fungi are members of the oral microbiota, particularly *Candida* spp, they have been only occasionally found in primary root canal infections,[212,244,283,284] even though a recent molecular study[1] has reported the occurrence of *Candida albicans* in 21% of the samples from primary root canal infections.

ARCHAEA

Archaea comprise a highly diverse group of prokaryotes, distinct from bacteria. Members of this domain have been traditionally recognized as extremophiles, but recently some of these microorganisms have also been found to thrive in non-extreme environments, including the human body. To date, no member of the *Archaea* domain has been described as a human pathogen. However, methanogenic archaea have been detected in samples from subgingival plaque associated with periodontal disease.[285] Only two molecular studies surveyed endodontic samples for the presence of archaea, with conflicting results.[286,287] While one study failed to detect these microorganisms in necrotic root canals,[286] another study detected methanogenic archaea in 25% of the canals of teeth with chronic apical periodontitis.[287] Archaeal diversity was limited to a *Methanobrevibacter oralis*-like phylotype.

VIRUS

Viruses are particles structurally composed of a nucleic acid molecule (DNA or RNA) and a protein coat. Because viruses require viable host cells to infect and use the cell's machinery to replicate the viral genome, they cannot survive in a root canal containing necrotic pulp tissue. The presence of viruses in the root canal has been reported only for non-inflamed vital pulps of patients infected with the human immunodeficiency virus.[288] On the other hand, herpes viruses have been detected in apical periodontitis lesions, where living cells are found in abundance. Of the eight human herpes viruses currently identified, the human cytomegalovirus (HCMV) and the Epstein–Barr virus (EBV) have been linked to the pathogenesis of diverse forms of periodontal diseases.[289–293] More recently, molecular biology studies using single PCR or RT-PCR have

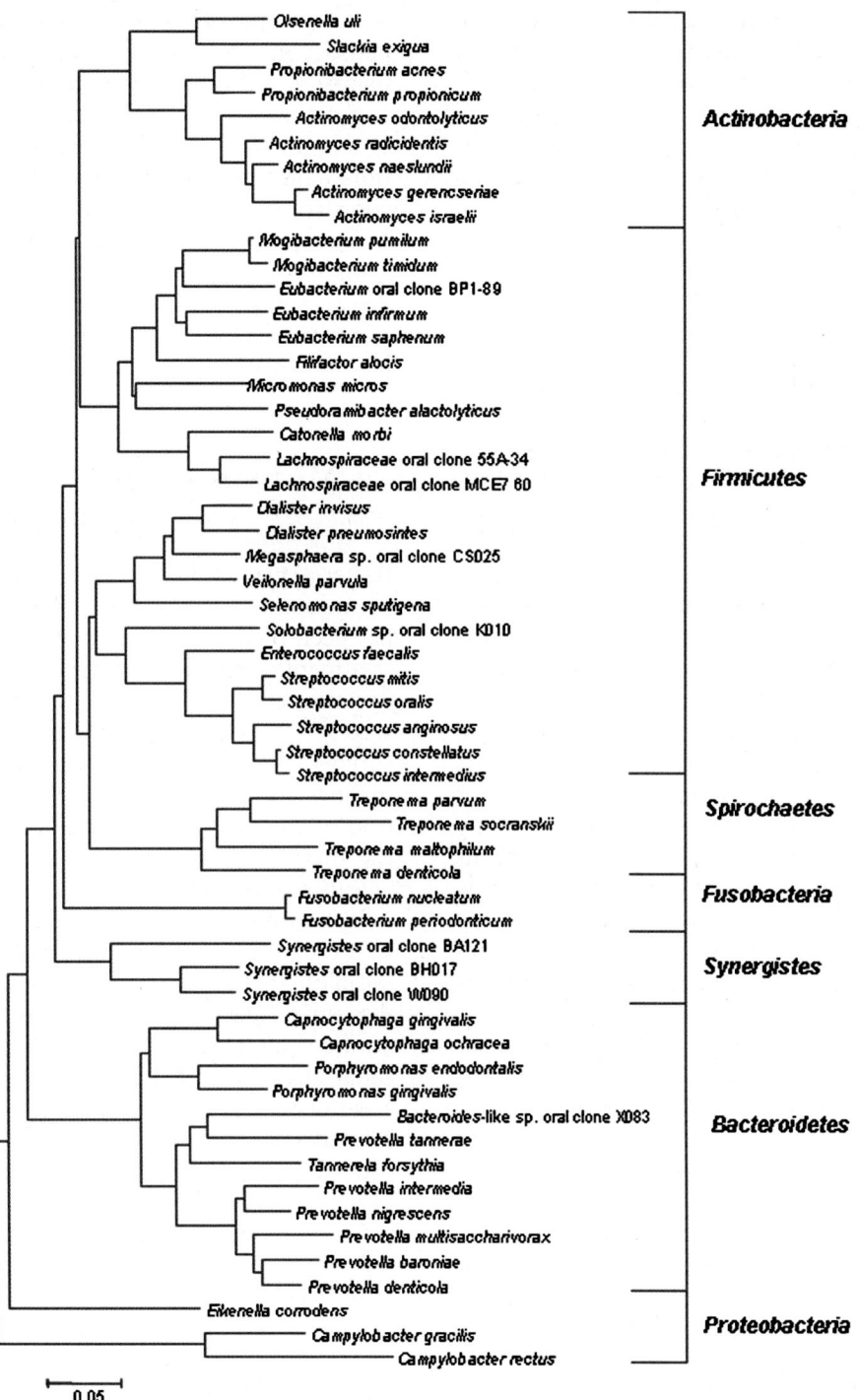

Figure 3 Phylogenetic tree of the most prevalent cultivable and as-yet-uncultivated bacterial species found in endodontic infections. Note that endodontic pathogens fall into seven major phyla. Another phylum, TM7, have been identified, but it does not contain species that are frequently detected. Courtesy J. Siqueira.

detected herpes viruses in samples from apical periodontitis lesions, and a pathogenetic role has been suggested.[5,6,294–296] HCMV and EBV transcripts have been found in high frequencies in the presence of symptoms,[5,295] in lesions exhibiting elevated occurrence of anaerobic bacteria,[6] and in cases of large periapical bone destruction.[5,6] It has been hypothesized that HCMV and EBV may be implicated in the pathogenesis of apical periodontitis as a direct result of virus infection and replication or as a result of virally induced impairment of local host defenses, which might give rise to overgrowth of pathogenic bacteria in the very apical part of the root canal.[296]

Symptomatic Infections

Whereas microbial causation of apical periodontitis is well established, there is no strong evidence disclosing specific involvement of a single species with any particular form of endodontic disease. Some Gram-negative anaerobic bacteria have been suggested to be involved with symptomatic lesions,[76,87,88,94,95,224,297] but it has been revealed that the same species can also be present in somewhat similar frequencies in asymptomatic cases.[89,102,227,230,232,234] Therefore, factors other than the mere presence of a given putative pathogenic species may play a role in the etiology of symptomatic endodontic infections. Other factors that may be involved with symptomatic infections include differences in virulence ability among strains of the same species, bacterial interactions resulting in synergism or additive effects among species, number of bacterial cells (load), environmental cues regulating expression of virulence factors, host resistance, and concomitant herpesvirus infection.[296,298,299]

Cross-sectional studies suggest that bacterial succession occurs before symptoms arise.[110] The possibility exists that, at a given moment during the endodontic infectious process, the microbiota reaches a certain degree of pathogenicity that elicits acute inflammation at the periapical tissues, with consequent development of pain and sometimes swelling. Molecular studies using DGGE or T-RFLP analysis revealed that the structure of the endodontic bacterial communities in symptomatic teeth is significantly different from that of asymptomatic teeth.[110] Differences are represented by different dominant species in the communities and larger number of species in symptomatic cases. Therefore, a shift in the structure of the microbial community is likely to occur before appearance of symptoms. Such a shift is probably a result of the arrival of new pathogenic species or of variations and rearrangements in the number of members of the bacterial consortium. Differences in the type and load of dominant species and the resulting bacterial interactions may affect virulence of the whole bacterial consortium. These findings confirmed that there is no key pathogen involved with symptomatic infections but, along with the factors mentioned above, the occurrence of certain specific bacterial combinations in infected root canals may be a decisive factor in causing symptoms.

Microorganisms: One Visit versus Two Visits

Bacteria play a major role in persistence of apical periodontitis lesions after treatment.[108,109,300–302] It has been revealed that the outcome of the endodontic treatment is significantly influenced by the presence of bacteria in the canals at the root canal-filling stage.[303–307] This suggests that persisting bacteria can survive in treated canals and sustain periapical tissue inflammation, underpinning the concept that eradication of bacteria from the root canal system should be the main goal of the endodontic treatment of teeth with apical periodontitis.

It is important to understand some aspects related to the significance of bacteria found in post-treatment samples. In this discussion, one should be aware of the time "persisters" are found in treated canals. Studies of the bacteria occurring in the root canal after treatment approaches involve three basic conditions: post-instrumentation samples (collected immediately after completion of chemomechanical procedures), post-medication samples (collected immediately after removal of interappointment dressings), and post-obturation samples (collected from root canal-treated teeth with associated apical periodontitis lesion at a given time—months to years—following treatment). Studies investigating bacteria remaining in the canals after chemomechanical procedures or intracanal medication provide a prospective view, that is, bacteria found in these samples have the potential to influence the treatment outcome. On the other hand, studies dealing with the microbiota of root canal-treated teeth evincing apical periodontitis offer a cross-sectional view, in which the bacteria found are arguably participating in the etiology of persistent disease.

Even when the endodontic treatment does not succeed in completely eradicating the infection, the huge majority of bacteria are eliminated and the environment is markedly disturbed. To survive and therefore be detected in post-treatment samples, bacteria have to resist or escape intracanal disinfection procedures and rapidly adapt to the drastically altered environment caused by treatment procedures. Bacteria detected in post-instrumentation samples are remainders of the initial infection that resisted the effects of instruments and irrigants or were introduced in the canal as a result of a breach in the aseptic chain. Whatever the source, these bacteria are temporary "persisters" but have not yet had enough time to adapt to the new environment, drastically changed by chemomechanical procedures. Their survival and involvement with the treatment outcome will be reliant on this adaptation ability. Bacteria detected in post-medication samples can be real persisters that survived both chemomechanical procedures and intracanal medication or gained entry into the canal via leakage through the temporary restoration. These bacteria have had more time for adaptation to the modified environment. Bacteria found in filled root canals in cases indicated for retreatment are conceivably adapted to the new environment and are remainders of a primary infection that resisted treatment procedures or penetrated in the canal after filling via coronal leakage (re-infection). In these cases, treatment failure is already established and the bacteria found in the canals are arguably the major culprits.

BACTERIA PERSISTING INTRACANAL DISINFECTION PROCEDURES

Diligent antimicrobial treatment can occasionally fail to promote total eradication of bacteria from root canals, with consequent selection of the most resistant segment of the microbiota. Gram-negative bacteria, which are common members of primary intraradicular infections, are usually eliminated following endodontic treatment procedures, though studies have reported that some Gram-negative anaerobic rods, such as *F. nucleatum*, *Prevotella* spp, and *C. rectus*, are amongst the most common species isolated from post-instrumentation samples.[304,308–311] However, most studies on this subject have revealed an overall higher occurrence of Gram-positive bacteria in both post-instrumentation and post-medication samples.[312] This gives support to the notion that Gram-positive bacteria can be more resistant to antimicrobial treatment measures and have the ability to adapt to the harsh environmental conditions in instrumented and medicated canals. Root canal samples positive for bacterial growth after chemomechanical procedures followed or not by intracanal medication have been shown to harbor one to six bacterial species per case. Gram-positive bacteria predominating in these samples include streptococci (*S. mitis*, *S. gordonii*, *S. anginosus*, and *Streptococcus oralis*), lactobacilli (*Lactobacillus paracasei* and *Lactobacillus acidophilus*), staphylococci, *E. faecalis*, *Olsenella uli*, *P. micra*, *P. alactolyticus* and *Propionibacterium* spp.[304,308–311,107,313–316] Other Gram-positive bacteria, including *Actinomyces* spp, *Bifidobacterium* spp, and *Eubacterium* spp, can also be found, but in lower frequencies[304,315,317] (Table 6).

With the recent findings showing as-yet-uncultivated bacteria as constituents of a significant proportion of the endodontic microbiota,[224,236] studies on the effects of intracanal antimicrobial procedures should also rely on the detection of these bacteria. A study using 16S rRNA gene clone library analysis of bacteria persisting after endodontic procedures revealed that 42% of the taxa found in post-treatment samples were as-yet-uncultivated bacteria.[311] In some cases, they even constituted the most dominant taxa in the sample. These findings suggest that previously uncharacterized bacteria may also participate in persistent endodontic infections.

PERSISTING BACTERIA INFLUENCING THE OUTCOME

Overwhelming scientific evidence demonstrates that apical periodontitis lesions are diseases of infectious origin.[72,76,318] Given the essential role played by microorganisms in causation of apical periodontitis, endodontic treatment should focus on both elimination of microbial cells colonizing the root canal system (through antiseptic means) and prevention of introduction of new microorganisms in the canal (through aseptic means). The success rate of the endodontic treatment will depend on how effective the clinician is in accomplishing these goals.[75,319] Root canal treatment of teeth containing irreversibly inflamed pulps is essentially a prophylactic treatment, as the radicular vital pulp is usually free of infection and the rationale is to prevent further infection of the root canal system.[320] On the other hand, in cases of infected necrotic pulps or in root-filled teeth associated with apical periodontitis, an intraradicular infection is established and, as a consequence, endodontic procedures should focus not only on prevention of the introduction of new microorganisms into

Table 6 Studies Showing Bacterial Persistence After Intracanal Disinfection Procedures

Study	Species Per Canal (Mean)	Irrigant	Intracanal Medication	Sample Taken After	Most Prevalent Species	Gram-Positive Bacteria
Byström and Sundqvist (1981)[96]	4.3	Saline	No	Chemomechanical preparation	Peptostreptococcus anaerobius Peptostreptococcus micros Lactobacillus species Prevotella species	70%
Byström and Sundqvist (1985)[310]	2.8	0.5% NaOCl	No	Chemomechanical preparation	Fusobacterium species Streptococcus species Eubacterium brachy Lactobacillus species Porphyromonas gingivalis Prevotella intermedia	45%
Byström and Sundqvist (1985)[310]	2.3	5% NaOCl	No	Chemomechanical preparation	Streptococcus intermedius Fusobacterium nucleatum	50%
Byström and Sundqvist (1985)[310]	2.7	5% NaOCl and EDTA	No	Chemomechanical preparation	Streptococcus species	75%
Gomes, et al. (1996)[309]	3.7	2.5% NaOCl	No	Chemomechanical preparation	Streptococcus anginosus group Peptostreptococcus micros Lactobacillus acidophilus	80%
Sjögren, et al. (1997)[304]	2.3	0.5% NaOCl	No	Chemomechanical preparation	Pseudoramibacter alactolyticus Fusobacterium nucleatum Campylobacter rectus Peptostreptococcus micros	62%
Peters, et al. (2002)[308]	3.6	2% NaOCl	No	Chemomechanical preparation	Actinomyces odontolyticus Prevotella intermedia Peptostreptococcus micros Eggerthella lenta Prevotella oralis	58%
Peters, et al. (2002)[308]	1.5	2% NaOCl	Ca(OH)$_2$	Intracanal medication	Propionibacterium acnes Peptostreptococcus micros Veillonella species Bifidobacterium species Capnocytophaga species	61%
Chavez de Paz, et al. (2003)[316]	2.4	0.5% NaOCl	Ca(OH)$_2$	Intracanal medication	Lactobacillus species Non-mutans streptococci Enterococcus species Propionibacterium species	88%
Chu, et al. (2006)[313]	2.3	0.5% NaOCl	Ca(OH)$_2$	Intracanal medication	Neisseria species Staphylococcus species Capnocytophaga species Actinomyces species	60%

the root canal system, but also on the elimination of those located therein.[321,322]

The major factor influencing the outcome of the endodontic treatment is the presence of microorganisms in the canal at the time of filling.[303–307] Better put, there is an increased risk of adverse outcome of the endodontic treatment if bacteria are left behind in the canals after intracanal procedures. It has been demonstrated that the permanent root canal filling per se has limited effect on the outcome of the endodontic treatment, even when it has been technically well performed.[303] When no bacteria are recovered from the canal at the filling stage, healing of apical periodontitis occurs uneventfully and independently of the quality of the root canal filling.

Thus, no matter whether bacteria were thoroughly eliminated after chemomechanical procedures (instrumentation and irrigation) or only after one or more sessions of intracanal medication, the success of the endodontic therapy depends on how effective the procedures are in rendering the canal bacteria-free. Therefore, the discussion on the topic "One × Two × Multiple visits" should focus on how many visits are required for the canal to be predictably disinfected. Total eradication of bacteria (or at least of culturing-detectable bacteria) can be achieved in some cases after chemomechanical procedures, and the outcome of these cases has been shown to be excellent.[304] However, microorganisms can survive the effects of chemomechanical preparation using antimicrobial irrigants in approximately 40% to 60% of the cases.[304,310,323] Studies have demonstrated that predictable disinfection of the root canal system is only achieved after proper antimicrobial medications are placed in the canals and left therein between appointments.[98,324,325]

Extraradicular Infections

Apical periodontitis lesions are formed in response to intraradicular infection and by and large comprise an effective barrier against spread of the infection to the alveolar bone and other body sites. In most situations, apical periodontitis inflammatory lesions succeed in preventing microorganisms from gaining access to the periapical tissues. Nevertheless, in some specific circumstances, microorganisms can overcome this defense barrier and establish an extraradicular infection. The most common form of extraradicular infection is the acute apical abscess, characterized by purulent inflammation in the periapical tissues in response to a massive egress of virulent bacteria from the root canal. There is, however, another form of extraradicular infection which, unlike the acute abscess, is usually characterized by absence of overt symptoms. This condition encompasses the establishment of microorganisms in the periapical tissues, either by adherence to the apical external root surface in the form of biofilm structures[326,327] or by formation of cohesive actinomycotic colonies within the body of the inflammatory lesion.[328] These extraradicular microorganisms have been discussed as one of the etiologies of persistence of apical periodontitis lesions in spite of diligent root canal treatment.[329]

Conceivably, the extraradicular infection can be dependent on or independent of the intraradicular infection.[330] For instance, the acute apical abscess is for the most part clearly dependent on the intraradicular infection—once the intraradicular infection is properly controlled by root canal treatment or tooth extraction and drainage of pus is achieved, the extraradicular infection is handled by the host defenses and usually subsides. Nonetheless, it should be appreciated that in some rare cases, bacteria that have participated in acute apical abscesses may persist in the periapical tissues following resolution of the acute response and establish a persistent extraradicular infection associated with a chronic periapical inflammation. This would then characterize an example of extraradicular infection independent of the intraradicular infection.

Except for apical actinomycosis and cases evincing sinus tracts, it is still controversial whether chronic apical periodontitis lesions can harbor bacteria for very long beyond initial tissue invasion.[331] Studies using culture-dependent[332–334] or culture-independent molecular methods, such as the checkerboard hybridization[335,336] and FISH,[337] have reported the extraradicular occurrence of a complex microbiota associated with apical periodontitis lesions that do not respond favorably to the root canal treatment. Anaerobic bacteria have been reported to be the dominant microorganisms in several of those lesions.[333,335] Because these studies did not evaluate the bacteriological conditions of the apical part of the root canal, it is difficult to ascertain whether those extraradicular infections were dependent on or independent of an intraradicular infection.

Most oral microorganisms are opportunistic pathogens and only a few species have the ability to challenge and overcome host defense mechanisms, acquire nutrients and thrive in the inflamed periapical tissues, and, then, establish an extraradicular infection. Of the several species of putative oral pathogens that have been detected in recalcitrant apical periodontitis lesions, some may have an apparatus of virulence that theoretically can allow them to invade and to survive in a hostile environment, such as the inflamed periapical tissues. For instance, it is currently recognized that some *Actinomyces* species and *P. propionicum* have the ability to participate in extraradicular infections and cause a pathological entity called apical actinomycosis, which is successfully treated only by periapical surgery.[91,330,338] Some other putative oral pathogens, such as *Treponema* spp, *P. endodontalis*, *P. gingivalis*, *T. forsythia*, *Prevotella* spp, and *F. nucleatum*, have also been detected in persistent chronic apical periodontitis lesions by culture, immunological, or molecular studies.[332,335,336,339,340] Most of these species possess an array of virulence traits that may allow them to avoid or overcome the host defenses in the periapical tissues.[341–344]

The incidence of independent extraradicular infections in untreated teeth is conceivably low,[251,345] which is congruent with the high success rate of nonsurgical root canal treatment.[319] Even in root canal-treated teeth with recalcitrant lesions, in which a higher incidence of extraradicular bacteria has been reported, a high rate of healing following retreatment[319] indicates that the major cause of post-treatment disease is located within the root canal system, characterizing a persistent or secondary intraradicular infection. This has been confirmed by studies investigating the microbiological conditions of root canals associated with persistent apical periodontitis.[109,108,300–302] Based on this, it is reasonable to assume that most of the extraradicular infections observed in root-filled teeth could have been fostered by an intraradicular infection.

There are some situations that permit intraradicular bacteria to reach the periapical tissues and establish an extraradicular infection.[346] This may be (1) a result of direct advance of some bacterial species that overcome host defenses concentrated near the apical foramen or that manage to penetrate into the lumen of pocket (bay) cysts, which is in direct communication with the apical foramen; (2) due to bacterial persistence in the apical periodontitis lesion after remission of acute apical abscesses; (3) a sequel to apical extrusion of debris during root canal instrumentation (particularly after over-instrumentation). Bacteria embedded in dentinal chips can be physically protected from the host defense cells and therefore can persist in the periapical tissues and sustain periapical inflammation. The virulence and the quantity of the involved bacteria as well as the host ability to deal with infection will be decisive factors dictating whether an extraradicular infection will develop or not.

Interactions between Microorganisms and the Host

The human commensal microbiota populates the mucosal surfaces of the oral cavity, gastrointestinal tract, urogenital tract, and the surface of the skin. A balance exists between the commensal bacteria and epithelia that allow both bacterial survival and prevention of the induction of inflammation that can damage the host.[347] The commensal microbiota, which has co-evolved with its host, has acquired the means of surviving and tolerating host defense mechanisms.[348] However, when the host is compromised, or if invading microorganisms are sufficiently pathogenic, disease can develop. Pathogenicity refers to the ability of an organism to cause disease in another organism. When microorganisms break through host barriers and multiply within host tissues, infection is initiated. The host mounts an immune response by mobilizing defense systems in an effort to ward off the invading microorganisms,[348] generally referred to as pathogens. Pathogens are capable of interfering with innate and adaptive immune responses, thereby escaping eradication by the host. They include bacteria, fungi, viruses, protozoa, and higher parasites.

Some pathogens can benefit from the inflammatory response while others are able to avoid recognition by the host,[349] or dampen host immune responses via sophisticated pathogen–host interactions.[348,349] In bacterial infections, the release of a range of bacterial components can give rise to the synthesis of local hormone-like molecules known as proinflammatory cytokines that can induce pathology.

Successful pathogens must be able to adhere, colonize, survive, propagate, and invade, while at the same time evading host defense mechanisms such as neutrophils, complement, and antibodies. In addition, pathogens can initiate tissue destruction either directly or indirectly.[350] Direct tissue damage can be induced by enzymes (eg., collagenase, hyaluronidase, and acid phosphatase), exotoxins (eg., cytolysins), and metabolites (eg., polyamines, and short chain fatty acids). Indirect damage results from a host immune reaction capable of causing tissue destruction that is stimulated by various bacterial components that include LPS, peptidoglycan (PG), lipoteichoic acid (LTA), fimbriae, outer membrane proteins, capsular components, and extracellular vesicles.

Virulence is generally understood to refer to the degree of pathogenicity or disease-producing ability of a microorganism. However, some microorganisms commonly described as "pathogens" do not necessarily cause disease in all hosts.[351] In addition, infections can be initiated by otherwise commensal organisms in immunocompromised hosts, a concept that is at odds with previously held pathogen-centered views of microbial pathogenesis. Thus, virulence is now seen as multifactorial with the susceptibility of the host playing a critical role.[348,351,352] Pathogens have generally been distinguished from nonpathogens by their expression of virulence factors, a diverse collection of proteins or molecules produced by microorganisms that facilitate adhesion, colonization, invasion, and tissue damage. Virulence factors enable a microorganism to establish itself on or within a host and enhance its potential to cause disease. For many bacterial species, cytokine induction is a major virulence mechanism related to stimulation by certain components associated with the bacterial cell wall, including LPS, proteins, lipoproteins, glycoproteins, carbohydrates, and lipids. In general, toxins that are potential virulence factors become available either directly via secretion from viable cells (exotoxins) or as a result of cell lysis (endotoxins). Toxins produced by bacteria include enterotoxins, neurotoxins, cytotoxins, and lysins.

HOST–MICROBE INTERACTIONS IN THE INFECTED ROOT CANAL SYSTEM

At the outset of carious activity, inflammatory lesions can develop in the pulp in response to dentin permeability to bacterial products and the activation of signals released from the dentinal fluids.[353] The pulp has an inherent capacity to process foreign antigens released from bacteria. Pulpal antigen presenting cells provide the necessary signals to activate T lymphocytes to mount a local immune defense.[354] Human dental pulps have immunocompetent cells in the form of helper/inducer T cells, cytotoxic/suppressor T cells, macrophages, and Class II antigen-expressing cells essential for the initiation of immunological responses.[355,356] In shallow carious lesions, the induction of type 1 cytokines in pulp tissue and the preferential activation of CD8 (+) T cells suggest that *Streptococcus mutans* may have a major influence on both the initial pulpal lesion and subsequent pulpal pathology.[357] Furthermore, in mononuclear cell cultures, *S. mutans* was the most potent and persistent interferon-gamma inducer; whereas *Lactobacillus casei* was the dominant species giving rise to interleukin-10 (IL-10).[358] The destructive aspect of inflammation may be particularly significant in the pulp due to its unique hard-tissue encasement that may be responsible for further tissue damage.[359] The repair of damaged pulp tissue may be compromised because of the limited access to appropriate repair-competent cells because of these anatomic constraints. Thus, carious pulpitis has been described as an infection where the host reaction has the capacity to produce more damage than that caused simply by the effects of the microorganisms.[359] Regardless, the interplay between pulpal injury, defense and repair can result in tissue regeneration following caries.[360]

The relationship between the microbiota in advancing caries and the histopathology of pulpitis involves irreversible tissue damage, healing, and repair in association with both specific and non-specific inflammatory reactions.[357–359,361,362] Quantitative real-time PCR has shown that the microbiota of carious dentin has significant numbers of Gram-negative bacteria that have been strongly implicated in endodontic infections subsequent to pulpitis.[363] Studies on induction of cytokines by bacteria associated with caries have provided a clearer understanding of the processes involved. Inflammatory reactions in the dental pulp of monkeys were initiated when dentin was exposed to products of certain bacteria such as *Streptococcus sanguinis*, *V. parvula*, *Rothia dentocariosa*, *Propionibacterium acnes*, and *Dialister pneumosintes*.[364] Within the pulp itself, an advancing carious lesion induced both specific and non-specific inflammatory reactions, with resultant healing and repair but also with some irreversible tissue damage.[362]

The relationship between the microbiota and the histopathology of chronic pulpitis in symptomatic teeth is less well understood. Although lactobacilli dominate in deep caries,[365] the numbers of lactobacilli and total Gram-positive rods in the carious lesions were negatively associated with the length of pain triggered by cold and heat stimulants.[366] In contrast, the less numerous Gram-positive cocci and non-black-pigmented *Prevotella* (BPB) were positively associated with thermal sensitivities. In particular, the presence of BPB, *S. mutans*, and total anaerobic counts were positively related to heat sensitivity, while *F. nucleatum*, *Actinomyces viscosus*, and enteric bacteria were associated with cold sensitivity. Furthermore, the duration of pain with thermal test was longer in teeth with low, compared to high, numbers of lactobacilli recovered from the carious lesions.[366]

As well, several physicochemical factors in the root canal have the potential to influence the pathogenicity of bacteria and in themselves modulate the host defense mechanisms. These factors include the degree of anaerobiosis, pH level, the availability of exogenous and endogenous nutrients, as well as the surfaces available for adherence and their characteristics (i.e., dentin vs cells). In infected root-filled teeth, additional factors to be considered include any medicament remnants and root filling materials.

VIRULENCE FACTORS

Many of the microorganisms found in endodontic infections have also been identified as commensals in the oral cavity that have gained entry into the pulp tissue of the root canal typically via the caries process. The transition from oral "commensal" to root canal "pathogen" may reflect an innate ability to switch on genes that encode "virulence" factors enabling survival and propagation in a different environment. Table 7 lists some virulence factors that pathogens utilize to facilitate this process. At this time, the identification and characteristics of specific virulence factors that might play a role in endodontic infections has not been widely studied. Those with known, or potential, relevance to endodontic infections will be discussed below.

Lipopolysaccharide (LPS)

One of the first virulence factors to be identified in endodontic infections is LPS, also known as endotoxin.[367] Historically, the term "endotoxin" was used

Table 7 Some Virulence Factors Utilized by Pathogens and Their Effects

Factor	Effect
Lipopolysaccharides/endotoxin	Proinflammatory
Peptidoglycans	Proinflammatory
Lipoteichoic acids	Proinflammatory
Fimbriae	Adherence
Capsules	Protection against phagocytosis and desiccation
Extracellular vesicles	Secretory products
Exotoxins	Diverse
Extracellular proteins	Diverse
Short-chain fatty acids	Proinflammatory
Polyamines	Growth factors
Superoxide anions	Denatures proteins
Chondroitin sulfatase	Digests ground substance
Hyaluronidase	Digests ground substance
Fibrinolysin	Damages fibrin
Gelatinase	Proteolytic, digests gelatin
Protease	Proteolytic
Hemolysins	Destroys erythrocytes
Leukocidin	Destroys leukocytes
Coagulases	Activates fibrin clotting
Elastase	Destroys elastin
Acids	Denatures proteins
Alcohols	Denatures proteins

based on the understanding that portions of Gram-negative bacteria caused toxicity, as opposed to "exotoxins" that were produced by bacteria and secreted into their environment. In Gram-negative bacteria, the outer membrane is constructed of a lipid bilayer, separated from the inner cytoplasmic membrane by PG with the LPS molecule embedded in the outer membrane. The lipid A portion of the molecule serves to anchor LPS in the bacterial cell wall. LPS is an integral part of the cell wall of Gram-negative bacteria regardless of their pathogenicity. When released, LPS has numerous biologic effects, including the mobilization of immunosurveillance mechanisms in the pulp. In vitro studies showed that LPS from *P. endodontalis* strains isolated from root canals and radicular cyst fluids stimulated IL-1β release from human dental pulp cells in a time- and dose-dependent manner.[368] LPS rapidly induced the expression of IL-8 in post-natal human dental pulp stem cells.[369] Both *E. coli* and *P. intermedia* LPS upregulated the expression of the pro-angiogenic vascular endothelial growth factor (VEGF) in odontoblast-like cells and macrophages[370] that was mediated, in part, by Toll-like receptor 4 (TLR4) signaling.[371]

In human clinical and animal studies, the presence of endotoxin has been associated with pulpal pain and periapical inflammation,[367,372–377] activation of complement,[372,373] and periapical bone destruction in monkeys[378] and cats.[373] Symptomatic teeth with apical rarefactions and the presence of exudate have a higher endotoxin content in root canals than do asymptomatic teeth.[375] A positive correlation was reported between the presence of endodontic signs and symptoms and the concentration of endotoxin in the root canal.[377]

Peptidoglycan (PG)

PG is the major component of Gram-positive cell walls where it forms a layer which is considerably thicker than in Gram-negative bacteria. PG functions to counteract osmotic pressure of the cytoplasm and provides cell wall strength and shape. It is a cross-linked complex consisting of polysaccharides and peptides that form a homogeneous layer outside the plasma membrane. Specifically, it is composed of interlocking chains of identical PG monomers. Each monomer consists of two joined amino sugars, *N*-acetylglucosamine and *N*-acetylmuramic acid (NAM), with a pentapeptide attached to the NAM.[379] Upon cell lysis, PG is released and can react with the innate immune system as well as induce upregulation of both proinflammatory and anti-inflammatory cytokines in T cells.[380] In T cells and monocytes, PG from *Staphylococcus aureus* induced IL-6 and IL-10 mRNA accumulation, and in *L. casei* stimulated IL-6 production in human dental pulp cells in a time- and dose-dependent manner.[381] PG may also facilitate an adaptive immune response via macrophages.[379] The potency of PG is strongly boosted in the presence of LPS.[379,382] The latter may be of particular significance to endodontic infections which are known to be typically polymicrobial, involving both Gram-positive and Gram-negative species.

Lipoteichoic Acid (LTA)

LTA is a cell wall component of Gram-positive bacteria, composed of echoic acid and lipid.[383] LTA shares with LPS many of its pathogenic properties but is reported to be much less active, on a weight-for-weight basis.[379,384] The lipid component of LTA may be involved in the binding of Gram-positive bacteria to fibronectin in cell membranes[385] and to eukaryotic cells that include neutrophils[385,386] and lymphocytes.[385] LTA is released as a result of cell lysis and can bind to target cells either non-specifically to membrane phospholipids, or specifically to TLRs and to CD14.[380] Once bound to the target cell, LTA is able to interact with circulating antibodies and activate the complement cascade. LTA can trigger the release from neutrophils and macrophages of many molecules that may act alone or together to amplify damage—

reactive oxygen and nitrogen species, acid hydrolases, highly cationic proteinases, bactericidal cationic peptides, growth factors, and cytotoxic cytokines.[387] In animals, LTA has been shown to induce a diverse range of inflammatory diseases ranging from a localized inflammatory tissue response[388] to arthritis, nephritis, meningeal inflammation, septic shock, and multiorgan failure.[387] In cell culture studies, LTA can induce expression of the pro-angiogenic VEGF in macrophages and pulp cells.[389]

Fimbriae

Fimbriae are long, filamentous macromolecules found on the surface of many Gram-negative bacteria. The thin hair-like projections are made of protein subunits. They are distinct from flagella, which are longer and involved in cell motility. Fimbriae are involved in attachment to surfaces and interactions with other bacteria.[390] Enteric pathogens, for example, E. coli and Salmonella spp, have a diverse array of fimbriae that are involved in bacterial adherence and invasion.[391] For example, type IV fimbriae, which can aggregate into bundles, have been detected on E. corrodens,[392] a periopathogen that has also been detected in root canal samples from teeth with acute periapical abscesses.[243,291] Hemagglutination activity was shown to be induced by fimbriae associated with P. intermedia.[393,394] Fimbriae have been identified on Actinomyces israelii, a species associated with failed endodontic treatment[394] and Actinomyces naeslundii.[391]

Capsules

An important element in the virulence of pathogenic microorganisms is their ability to evade or counteract host immune defenses. One strategy used by bacteria and fungi utilizes capsule formation to inhibit complement activation and resist ingestion by phagocytes. A capsule is a well-organized layer outside the cell wall of the bacteria generally composed of polysaccharides and other materials. Capsules serve to facilitate protection of the bacterial cell against desiccation, phagocytosis, bacterial viruses, and hydrophobic toxic materials such as detergents. The presence of capsules, for example, in Gram-negative black-pigmented bacteria, contributes to the persistence of the bacteria by facilitating the avoidance of, or survival after, phagocytosis.[51] In addition, capsules were identified as crucial for maturation of Streptococcus pyogenes biofilm formation on abiotic surfaces.[395]

Extracellular Vesicles

Extracellular vesicles are produced by Gram-negative bacteria and allow the release of their products into the

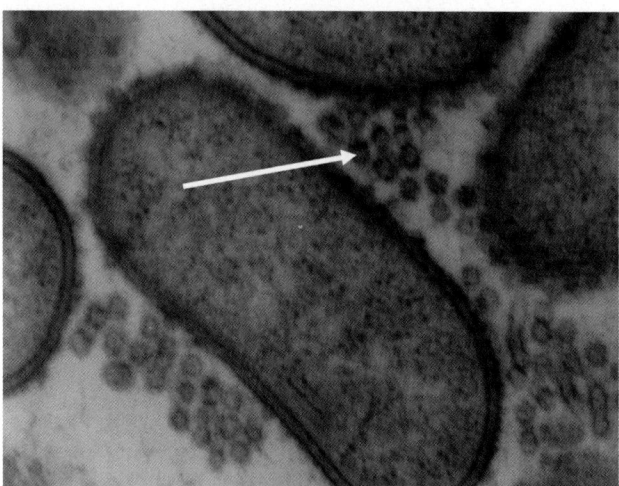

Figure 4 Extracellular vesicles (arrow) are shown between *Prevotella intermedia* cells ($\times$20,000 original magnification). Courtesy C. Baumgartner.

extracellular environment. They develop from evagination of the outer membrane and have a similar trilaminar structure as their parent cell (Figure 4). The contents of extracellular vesicles derive from the periplasm and include proteins and lipids that are involved in a diverse array of activities, including hemagglutination, hemolysis, bacterial adhesion, and proteolytic activities.[396] With an average diameter of 50 to 250 nanometers,[397] adhesive properties, toxic contents, and an ability to carry contents into host cells, extracellular vesicles are a means by which bacteria interact with both prokaryotic and eukaryotic cells.[397,398] As well, extracellular vesicles can modulate interactions between neighboring bacteria. For example, vesicles from the outer membrane of P. gingivalis can induce aggregation of a wide range of species that include Streptococcus spp, F. nucleatum, A. naeslundii, and A. viscosus.[399] In addition, specific coaggregation interactions between different species can be modulated in the presence of P. gingivalis vesicles—as was demonstrated by the coaggregation of S. aureus with the mycelium type, but not the yeast type, of C. albicans.[399] P. gingivalis releases vesicles that may also bind chlorhexidine, thereby providing its own protection.[400] Specific virulence factors associated with oral bacterial vesicles include leukotoxin produced by Aggregatibacter (formerly Actinobacillus) actinomycetemcomitans[401] and the proteases Arg- and Lys-gingipain produced by P. gingivalis.[402] Transmission electron microscopy of lesions associated with teeth with refractory apical periodontitis showed the presence of extracellular material and outer membrane vesicles, with outer membrane vesicles in close contact with the bacterial cell wall and between cells.[333]

Exotoxins

Exotoxins are toxins released by a living cell that can trigger, among other responses, excessive and aberrant activation of T cells.[403] Some exotoxins are extremely potent, for example, the toxic shock syndrome toxin-1 produced by certain strains of *S. aureus* and the pyogenic exotoxins produced by some *S. pyogenes* strains producing toxic shock-like syndrome.[403,404] Bacteria produce an array of toxins that differ in terms of structure, mode of action, and eukaryotic targets. Bacterial toxins can also target other microorganisms as bacteriocins, proteinaceous toxins produced by bacteria which are bacteriostatic or bacteriocidal to other bacteria.[405] Bacterial cytotoxins act on eukaryotic cells by targeting the cell cytostructure, either directly by modifying actin or indirectly by targeting regulators, in particular Rho GTPase regulators.[406] The Rho GTPases are essential for the functional integrity of the immune system, including transcriptional regulation of the expression of inflammatory mediators including cytokines and chemokines. A specific role for exotoxin-producing bacteria in endodontic infections has not been established.

Extracellular Proteins

Diverse arrays of extracellular proteins, many of them enzymes, are produced by bacteria. Some are enzymes released during bacterial cell lysis that can contribute to the spread of infection, including proteases that neutralize immunoglobulins and complement components.[407–410] In the "eight-strain collection" of bacteria with known pathogenicity isolated from an infected monkey root canal,[77] the enzymes hyaluronate lyase, chondroitin-sulphatase, beta-glucuronidase, DNase, and acid phosphatase contributed to tissue disintegration. Variations were observed in the ability of different strains to produce different histolytic enzymes.[411] Species demonstrating evidence of enzymes that could play a role in the pathogenesis of endodontic infections include *S. gordonii*, *S. anginosus*, *S. oralis*,[314] *P. gingivalis*,[412] and *E. faecalis*.[413,414] Extracellular proteins produced by root canal isolates of *S. gordonii*, *S. anginosus*, and *S. oralis* may be of pathogenic significance in post-treatment apical periodontitis.[314] The presence of the collagenase gene was detected in endodontic isolates of *P. gingivalis*,[412] and increased collagenase was shown to be associated with larger periapical lesions.[415] While *E. faecalis* cytolysins can enhance pathogenicity in animal models,[416] *E. faecalis*, as well as *P. acnes* showed evidence of proteolytic activity but were weak pathogens when tested in root canals or in tissue cages in both mixed and single-strain infections.[411] Serine protease, an enzyme that cleaves peptide bonds, was shown to contribute to the binding of *E. faecalis* to dentin,[414] while gelatinase production was observed in more than 70% of *E. faecalis* strains recovered from infected root canals.[413]

Short-Chain Fatty Acids

Short-chain fatty acids are major by-products of a fermentation process performed by obligate anaerobes and include butyric acid and propionic acid. These can act as virulence factors by stimulating the inflammatory response and inflammatory cytokine release via upregulation of neutrophil gene transcription, translation, and protein expression.[417] Leakage of butyric acid from coronal to apical reservoirs occurred in canals of human root sections obturated with gutta-percha and AH26.[418] Leakage of these very small molecules from root canals into the apical area could contribute to the infection process. For example, in cell culture studies, butyric acid stimulated monocyte IL-1β production, a cytokine associated with bone resorption.[419] The inhibition of cell growth induced by high levels of butyric acid resulted in inhibition of T-lymphocyte cell growth and an increase in apoptosis.[420] Other in vitro investigations showed that butyric acid increased the expression of the intercellular adhesion molecule-1 and E-selectin in endothelial cells.[421] Salts of butyric and propionic acids inhibited proliferation of mouse L929 cells and human gingival fibroblasts.[422] Clinically, the presence of the obligate anaerobe *F. nucleatum* has been associated with the most severe forms of interappointment endodontic flare-ups.[423] It is feasible that the butyric acid produced by these microorganisms might be a contributory virulence factor to endodontic flare-ups.

Polyamines

Polyamines are small, polycationic molecules that have two or more primary amino groups. They include putrescine, cadaverine, spermidine, and spermine. These molecules are essential growth factors for both eukaryotic and prokaryotic cells and act by modulating a variety of ion channels.[424] Leakage of polyamines from the infected root canal into the apical area might contribute to clinical symptoms. This hypothesis is based on an analysis of the amounts of polyamines in root canals of teeth with various clinical symptoms compared to symptom-free teeth.[425] In infected root canals of teeth with spontaneous pain and percussion pain, the levels of putrescine were significantly higher than in pain-free teeth. In the presence of a sinus tract, the levels of cadaverine from teeth with sinus tract were greater.[425]

Superoxide Anions

Superoxide anions are biologically toxic and highly reactive free radicals. Production is widespread among cells of the immune system. A few bacterial species can also produce extracellular superoxide. Blood isolates of *E. faecalis* were shown to produce large amounts of extracellular superoxide,[426] with production by an enterococcal blood isolate causing lysis of erythrocytes.[427] Superoxide production may also be involved in interspecies interactions. In a mouse model, it was shown that extracellular superoxide production by *E. faecalis* enhanced its in vivo survival in a mixed infection with *Bacteroides fragilis*.[428]

From the above, it is apparent that diverse arrays of virulence factors are potentially available in the root canal microbiota to modulate the participation of microorganisms in host–microbe interactions. However, the role of these virulence factors at this time is still mostly speculative. An absolute cause and effect relationship has not been proven between the presence of identified virulence factors and clinical signs and symptoms in root canal infections. There are additional mechanisms presently under investigation by which microorganisms might modulate the infection process. These include the ability of some intracellular bacteria to inactivate the killing mechanisms of phagocytic cells and therefore avoid being killed by macrophages and neutrophils.[429] Of potential relevance concerning commensal microorganisms is the development of host cell tolerance as a result of previous exposure that may influence the ability to counteract subsequent bacterial challenge.[352] In addition, some bacteria can genetically vary their surface antigens, making it difficult for the immune system to target these organisms.[349] Future research in these areas may clarify the role of virulence factors in endodontic infections and ultimately help identify therapeutic targets.

Interactions between Microorganisms

GENE TRANSFER SYSTEMS

The bacterial virulence factors previously described are encoded by genes usually located on chromosomal DNA, but also on extra-chromosomal DNA, for example, plasmids. The predominant means by which chromosomal genes are inherited is via replication, segregation, and cell division, also sometimes termed vertical inheritance.[430] Mechanisms of genetic variability between generations can include point mutations and genetic rearrangements.

The dissemination of genes can also occur via horizontal gene transfer (HGT, also called lateral gene transfer), whereby genetic material moves between bacterial cells. There is growing recognition of the importance of HGT for pathogenicity because genes transferred horizontally have the potential to propagate extremely rapidly across species barriers.[430] HGT provides pathogens with the means to adapt rapidly, for example, by the acquisition of genes for antibiotic resistance. Overall, these processes benefit pathogens by enabling their continual adaptation to their hosts.[350]

Virulence genes can also be transferred via pathogenicity islands, or horizontally transferable genomic islands that are located on the bacterial chromosome or may be a part of a plasmid. Pathogenicity islands have been identified in both Gram-negative and Gram-positive species including *P. gingivalis*,[431] *E. faecalis*,[432] *S. mutans*,[433] and *S. aureus*.[434] They can be associated with a particular microbial adaptation, such as antibiotic and metal resistance. For example, in *S. aureus*, a mobile pathogenicity island carries the gene for toxic shock toxin.[434]

EXTRA-CHROMOSOMAL DNA: THE HORIZONTAL GENE POOL

The accessory genetic elements, collectively described as the horizontal gene pool include plasmids (Figure 5), bacteriophages, transposons, and insertion sequences. These elements can profoundly influence genome plasticity and evolution by allowing movement of genetic information both within and between species. HGT of DNA in bacteria occurs by three basic methods: transformation, transduction, and conjugation. "Recipient" cells receive the DNA, while "donor" cells are the source of the DNA.

Transformation of bacteria involves the active uptake by a cell of free (extracellular) DNA and its subsequent incorporation into the recipient genome, giving rise to "transformants" (i.e., the recipient cell becomes "transformed"). Lysed donor cells release genomic DNA. Usually only fragments of donor genomic DNA are taken up by the recipient. This process depends on the function of specific genes located on the recipient's chromosome.[435] The DNA

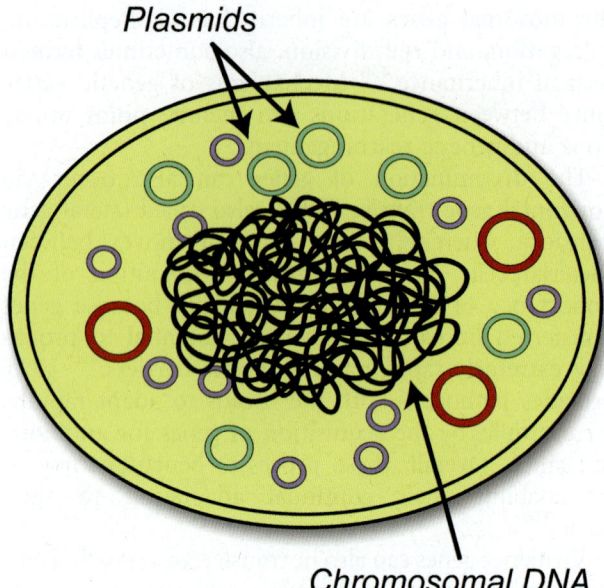

Figure 5 DNA in bacterial cells. Bacterial virulence factors are encoded by genes located usually on chromosomal DNA, but also on extra-chromosomal DNA, for example, plasmids. The dissemination of such genes can occur via vertical or inherited means and by horizontal gene transfer of extra-chromosomal DNA. Reproduced with permission from Sedgley CM and Clewell DB.[447]

acquired can include fragments of DNA that recombine with homologous regions of the recipient genome, or intact plasmids that can replicate autonomously in the recipient. Not all bacteria are capable of natural transformation. Natural transformation has been observed in the oral Gram-positive bacteria *S. mutans* in biofilms,[436] *S. gordonii*,[437] and *Streptococcus pneumoniae*.[438]

Transduction involves gene transfer whereby bacterial viruses (also termed phages or bacteriophages) carry genetic material to recipient cells that become "transductants."[439] Bacteriophages have been isolated from *A. actinomycetemcomitans*[440] and *Actinomyces* spp[441] in dental plaque and from *E. faecalis* in saliva samples.[442]

Conjugation is the most efficient gene transfer phenomenon in bacteria. The requirement for cell–cell contact distinguishes conjugation from transduction and transformation. DNA is transferred between cells that are in physical contact allowing unidirectional transfer of genetic information from donor to recipient (which then becomes a "transconjugant"). Conjugation can involve the crossing of species barriers and can also occur between bacteria and eukaryotic cells.[443] Chromosomal DNA segments, plasmids, and conjugative transposons can be transferred by conjugation.

Plasmids are extrachromosomal, autonomously replicating elements important for bacterial adaptability and survival by the provision of functions that might not be encoded by the chromosome. Bacterial plasmids are ubiquitous and can encode a variety of different traits including, in many cases, genes that specifically enable them to transfer copies of themselves to recipient bacteria. Plasmids are found in Gram-negative and Gram-positive bacteria as well as in archaea[444] and yeasts.[445] In addition, the double-stranded circular plasmids encoding the EBV, Kaposi's sarcoma-associated herpesvirus, and papillomavirus have been shown to exist "naturally" in mammalian cells.[446] From a clinical perspective, plasmids are particularly important because they are involved in the dissemination of antibiotic resistance.

In terms of structure, plasmids are typically covalently closed circular, double-stranded, supercoiled DNA molecules that replicate independently of chromosomal DNA, and range in size from approximately 1 to greater than 200 kilo base pairs (kb).[447] In contrast, the size of chromosomal DNA is much larger, for example, 3,218 kb, as reported for the clinical isolate *E. faecalis* V583.[448] The copy number of plasmids in the bacterial cell is typically characteristic for the particular plasmid and can range from greater than 30 copies per chromosome for a small plasmid (eg., <10 kb) to one to two copies for a larger plasmids (eg., >25 kb).[447] Plasmids rely on their host cell to provide essential ingredients for DNA replication. More than one type of plasmid can occur stably in a given cell provided they are compatible. Incompatibility relates to a close relationship between plasmids whereby there is competition for replication machinery, the necessary consequence being the need for a plasmid to maintain a certain copy number in the cell. Whichever plasmid is able to replicate faster, or has some other advantage, will eventually remain at the expense of its competitor. Some plasmids exhibit a broad host range and are able to propagate in many different species of bacteria. It is not always clear what genes are encoded on wild-type (or "naturally occurring") plasmids. If no known function or gene expression is associated with a plasmid, it is referred to as "cryptic." In contrast, some plasmids have had their DNA sequenced and specific genes have been identified. Figure 6 shows a simplified "map" of pAD1, a conjugative plasmid originally isolated from a clinical isolate of *E. faecalis*. Clinical strains of *E. faecalis* can carry as many as five or more coresident plasmids with different sizes and copy numbers. While not necessarily essential to the

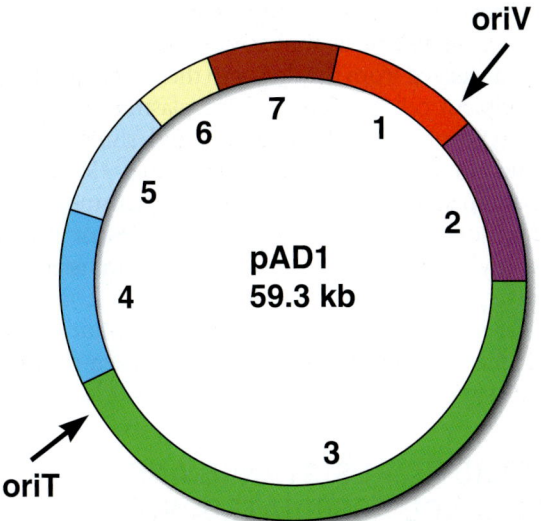

Figure 6 Simplified map of the conjugative plasmid pAD1 originally isolated from *Enterococcus faecalis* ds16. Segments are described according to the functions coded by genes contained within (1) replication and maintenance; (2) regulation of pheromone response; (3) structural genes relating to conjugation; (4) unknown; (5) cytolysin biosynthesis; (6) unknown; (7) resistance to UV light; oriV, origin of replication; oriT, origin of transfer. Reproduced with permission from Sedgley CM and Clewell DB.[447]

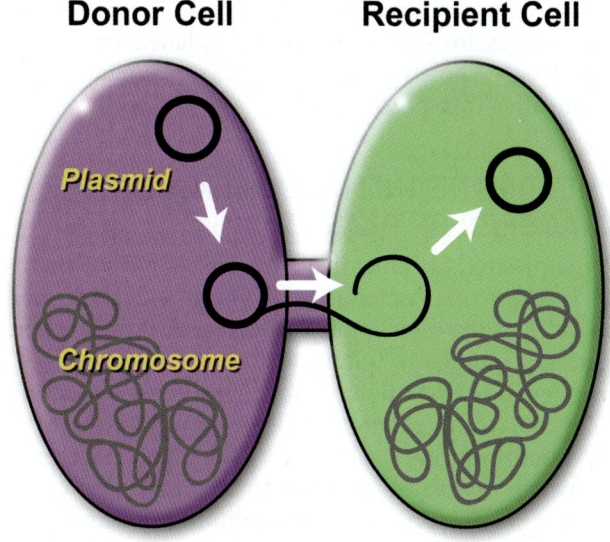

Figure 7 Conjugative transfer of plasmids in Gram-negative bacteria. Cell–cell contact is facilitated by a plasmid-encoded pilus. A single strand of DNA is then transferred from the donor to the recipient. A complementary strand is synthesized in the recipient and the resulting double-stranded DNA is circularized. Reproduced with permission from Sedgley CM and Clewell DB.[447]

bacterial host, plasmids can confer traits facilitating survival under atypical conditions such as in the presence of antibiotics and heavy metals. For example, hospital-acquired bacterial infections are often associated with the rapid spread of antibiotic resistance, traits that are often encoded on plasmids.

Transposons, sometimes also called "jumping genes," are segments of DNA that can move ("jump") from one DNA molecule to another—for example, from the chromosome to a resident plasmid. Transposons frequently accumulate on plasmids and encode functions necessary for their own transposition as well as other functions such as antibiotic resistance.[449] Insertion sequences are short DNA sequences that usually encode the ability to transpose but do not carry accessory genes like transposons do. Insertion sequences sometimes represent components of a transposon.[450]

Conjugative plasmids and conjugative transposons are transferred between cells that are in physical contact. They are ubiquitous in Gram-negative bacteria as well as in the Gram-positive *Enterococcus*, *Streptococcus*, *Staphylococcus*, *Lactococcus*, *Listeria*, *Bacillus*, *Clostridium*, *Streptomyces*, and *Rhodococcus*.[451] The conjugative transfer process in Gram-negative bacteria typically involves a single strand of DNA being transferred from the donor cell to the recipient cell after which a complementary strand is synthesized in the recipient, and the resulting double-stranded DNA is circularized (Figure 7). The size of conjugative plasmids can range from as small as 10 kb to well over 100 kb.[451,452] Perhaps due in part to the inherent differences in structures of the cell envelope, conjugative systems differ somewhat between Gram-negative and Gram-positive bacteria. For example, Gram-positive hosts generally do not make use of a pilus structure to achieve a close cell–cell contact.[453] The transfer of conjugative plasmids can also occur from the prokaryote *E. coli* to the eukaryote yeast, *Saccharomyces cerevisiae*,[454] as well as to higher eukaryotes such as Chinese hamster ovary cells (CHO K1).[443] A broad range of genes can be transported as a result of conjugation. Furthermore, otherwise non-transferable elements such as non-conjugative co-resident plasmids and even chromosomal genes can be mobilized by conjugative plasmids. Conjugative transposons are also widespread, being found for example in enteric *Bacteroides* spp.[455,456] Sometimes referred to as integrative conjugative elements, they cannot replicate autonomously, but can excise from the chromosome generating a circular intermediate that can then conjugate in a manner similar to a plasmid. Once taken up by a recipient, the transposon is believed to circularize prior to inserting itself into the chromosomal DNA. Conjugative transposons are important in the dissemination of antibiotic resistance.[451,457] Four of fifteen tetracycline-resistant bacteria isolated from root canals were shown to possess elements similar to the conjugative transposon Tn916.[458]

PHEROMONE-INITIATED CONJUGATIVE TRANSFER OF PLASMIDS

Some plasmids conjugatively transfer copies of themselves from one bacterial cell to another using small peptides called pheromones as essential signals in the process. Conjugative plasmids that make use of pheromones were first observed in an oral E. faecalis strain recovered from a patient with acute periodontitis.[459,460] The pheromones are secreted by a potential "recipient" cell which "activates" the transfer system of a potential "donor" cell. Pheromone-responding plasmids in E. faecalis can carry genes relating to antibiotic resistance as well as virulence traits. A single E. faecalis strain may secrete multiple pheromones, each one being specific for inducing transfer of different "families" of plasmids. The pheromones provide the signals essential to the conjugation process that results in transfer of the plasmid DNA to a plasmid-free cell (Figure 8). Specifically, conjugation functions are activated, including a dramatic "clumping response" mediated by the appearance of a surface adhesin ("aggregation substance" or "AS") that facilitates the attachment of the donor cells

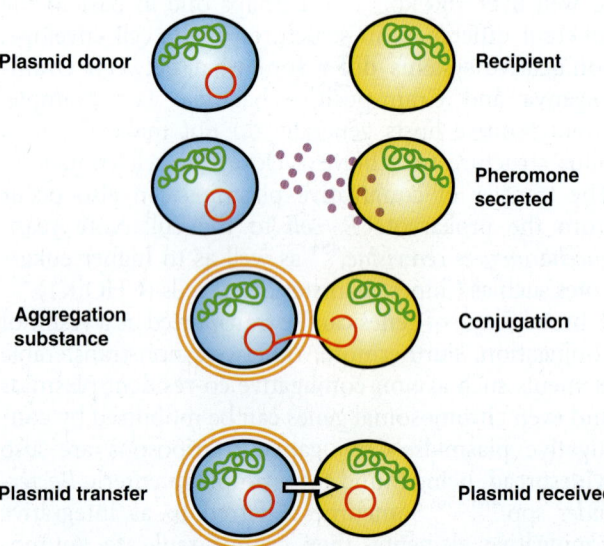

Figure 8 Pheromone-initiated conjugative plasmid transfer. The pheromone induces the appearance of a surface adhesin (aggregation substance) that facilitates the attachment of the donor and recipient cells. Aggregates give rise to conjugal channels through which the plasmid is transferred from the donor to the recipient cell. Reproduced with permission from Sedgley CM and Clewell DB.[477]

to enterococcal binding substance which is present on the surface of recipients as well as donors.[460] The plasmid is then transferred from the donor to the recipient cell. Once the recipient cell has acquired the plasmid, it assumes a phenotype of the original donor and shuts down the production of endogenous pheromone. However, the transconjugants continue to produce pheromones specific for donors harboring different classes of plasmids. Presently, the use of pheromone initiated transfer of conjugative plasmids within species other than E. faecalis has thus far not been observed. However, a peptide similar to the E. faecalis pheromone cAM373 has been detected in culture supernatants of S. aureus and S. gordonii.[461]

ANTIBIOTIC RESISTANCE AND VIRULENCE ASSOCIATED WITH PLASMIDS

In return for "lodging," plasmids can provide important survival properties to their host, in particular by conferring resistance to an antibiotic. In hospitals where patients are frequently being administered antibiotics, the selective pressure on bacteria containing plasmids bearing resistance genes has been responsible for once useful antibiotics losing their effectiveness. In addition to antibiotic resistance, a diverse range of products that may potentially contribute towards "virulence" such as cytotoxins, adhesions, and certain metabolic enzymes are also often encoded by plasmids.[462] Genes for protecting a cell against deleterious substances like mercury, copper, or silver have been found on plasmids.[463,464] Plasmids can therefore carry genes that enhance the bacterial host cell's ability to cause a disease, for example, the 92 kb plasmid (pO157) encoding a toxin that is associated with the strain E. coli O157:H7 resulting in febrile hemorrhagic colitis with potentially life-threatening complications.[465] Virulence plasmids in S. aureus can encode extracellular toxins that have been linked to systemic shock, for example, toxic shock syndrome,[466] and enterotoxins associated with food poisoning.[467] Genes on plasmids that encode cytolysins are found in E. faecalis, often in association with clinical isolates.[468,469] Cytolysins can lyse erythrocytes and other eukaryotic cells as well as kill certain Gram-positive bacteria.[59]

PLASMIDS IN THE ORAL AND ENDODONTIC MICROBIOTA

Data on plasmids associated with the oral and endodontic microbiota are limited.[447] In the oral microbiota, studies have focused on the identification[470–472] and epidemiology of plasmids in streptococci,[473–475] black-pigmented anaerobic bacteria,[476] *P. nigrescens*,[477] *F. nucleatum*,[478] oral spirochetes,[479] and *E. faecalis*.[480–482] Plasmids were found in 26.7% of *F. nucleatum* strains from periodontal patients but not in any strains from healthy subjects.[478] In contrast, no association was found between the disease status of periodontal sampling sites and the presence of a plasmid in *P. nigrescens* strains.[477] Plasmids were isolated from 7 of 11 oral *E. faecalis* strains recovered from endodontic patients.[481] The ability of plasmids in oral streptococci to transfer between species has been demonstrated.[472,483,484] Recently, it was shown that gene transfer can occur from *T. denticola* to *S. gordonii* in experimental biofilms.[437]

Information relating to plasmids associated with endodontic microbiology appears to be limited to those associated with *Enterococcus* sp. Plasmid DNA was isolated from 25 of 33 endodontic enterococcal isolates (31 *E. faecalis* and 2 *E. faecium* strains) recovered from patients in Sweden, with up to four plasmids per strain.[413] Several strains which appeared to be clones based on pulsed field gel electrophoresis analyses of total DNA were shown to have distinct plasmid types. (Figure 9). Phenotypic studies showed that 16 of the plasmid-positive strains exhibited a "clumping response" (characteristic of a response to pheromone) when exposed to a culture filtrate of a plasmid-free strain, suggesting the potential for conjugative transfer of genetic elements in these endodontic isolates. It is conceivable that if endodontic strains contain conjugative plasmids with genes that could enhance survival during or after endodontic treatment, such properties might be transferred to other strains.

COOPERATIVE AND ANTAGONISTIC INTERACTIONS BETWEEN MICROORGANISMS

Bacteria can communicate, cooperate, and alter their behavior according to changes in their communal environment. Interactions between different species, or even between different strains of the same species, can modulate the infectious process by communication processes. Some bacteria communicate and coordinate behavior via signaling molecules using a process called quorum sensing.[485] Here, cells express particular characteristics only when present as a population whose density is above a certain minimum ("quorum"). When a high density population reaches a certain threshold, the concentration of normally low levels of certain "signal molecules" becomes high enough to act as an autoinducer (AI) resulting in the increased expression of specific operons that enhance survival or are important in bringing about the next stage

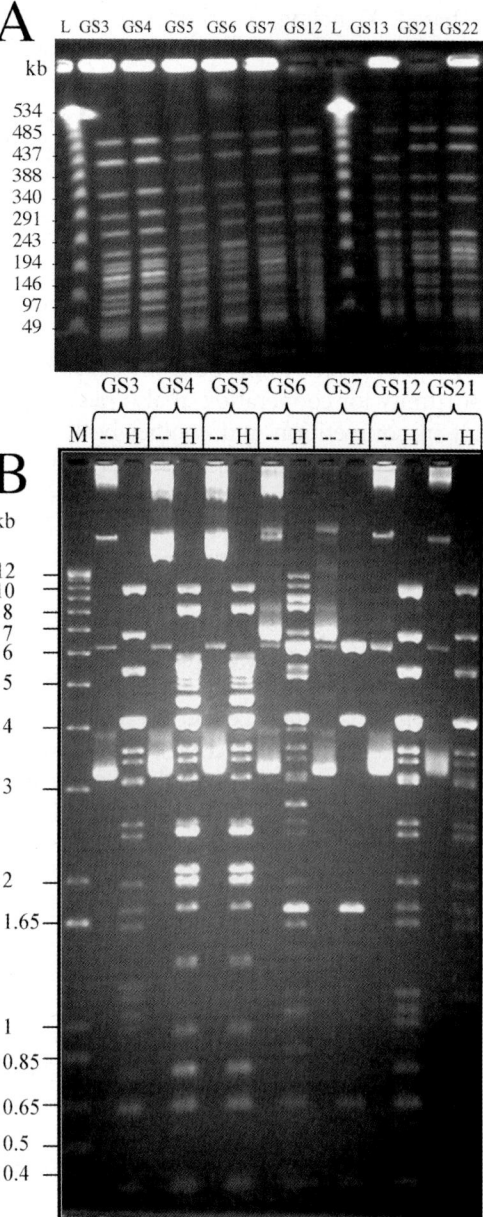

Figure 9 Total DNA and plasmid DNA analysis of endodontic *Enterococcus faecalis*. A, Pulsed field gel electrophoresis (PFGE) of SmaI-digested genomic DNA from endodontic *E. faecalis* strains GS3–GS7, GS12, GS13, GS21, GS22. Note similarities between GS3–GS7, GS12, and GS21. Reference standard: lambda phage DNA. B, Plasmid analysis of the same *E. faecalis* isolates. Lane M, molecular size marker (1 Kb plus DNA Ladder, Invitrogen); –, undigested; H, digested with *HindIII*. Strain designations are shown above the lane designations. Isolates classified based on PFGE pattern as clonal, GS3, GS12, and GS21 are similar in plasmid content. GS4 and GS5 appear to be alike in plasmid content. GS6 and GS7 each contain two similar small plasmids, however GS6 has two additional plasmids. Reproduced with permission from Sedgley CM and Clewell DB.[447]

of a colonization or virulence process. N-acyl homoserine lactone-based signaling is used by Gram-negative bacteria, while small peptides are often involved in Gram-positive bacteria. AI-2 signal is used by both Gram-negative and Gram-positive bacteria and can play a role in communication between different bacterial species. As a result of quorum sensing, the expression of key proteins can be regulated. This coordinated regulation of behavior is of particular relevance in biofilms.[486] For example, AI-2 produced by the oropharyngeal microbiota in cystic fibrosis patients modulates gene expression of *Pseudomonas aeruginosa* which enhances its pathogenicity.[487] However, while quorum sensing provides an opportunity for cooperation, it also has the potential to result in competition and conflict both within and between species, although this is not well understood.[485]

Certain microbial interactions can have beneficial or antagonistic outcomes. Examples of beneficial interactions include enzyme complementation and food chains. For example, in early dental plaque, *Veillonella atypica* requires *S. gordonii* to be present to colonize dental surfaces because *S. gordonii* ferments sugars and releases lactic acid, which is the preferred carbon source for *V. atypica*.[488] Other beneficial relationships may involve coaggregation interactions, or the recognition and adhesion between genetically distinct bacteria,[489] as distinct from "autoaggregation", or the adherence of bacteria belonging to the same strain.[490] In plaque, coaggregation commonly occurs between "early" and "late" colonizers and involves specific adhesins and complementary receptor molecules. Cell–cell adhesion occurs when cells of one microbial species adhere more or less specifically to those of a different species.[491] Coaggregation interactions have been shown to be involved in the establishment and maintenance of biofilms,[491] which may play an important role in endodontic infections.[492,493] Interactions between pairs of bacteria are highly specific. For example, recognition of the antigen I/II polypeptide facilitates coinvasion of dentinal tubules by *P. gingivalis* with *S. gordonii*, but not with *S. mutans*.[494,495] A protein adhesin and a carbohydrate receptor, often a polysaccharide,[496] mediates coaggregation. Coaggregation interactions provide an ideal environment for HGT,[497] perhaps by facilitating plasmid transfer.[447] Individual bacteria might gain a survival advantage by coaggregating with other bacteria within biofilms. By forming ordered assemblies of bacteria with species-specific molecular interactions, the bacteria are better able to adapt to fluctuating environmental conditions.[498] Recent observations suggest a potential role for specific combinations of species in endodontic infections. Using confocal microscopy, both autoaggregation and coaggregation interactions were observed, particularly in association with *Prevotella*, *Streptococcus*, and *Fusobacterium* species isolated from acute endodontic infections.[499] Coaggregation interactions were also observed between oral and endodontic isolates of *E. faecalis* and *F. nucleatum* and between *F. nucleatum* and *S. anginosus*, *Peptostreptococcus anaerobius* and *Prevotella oralis*.[500] *F. nucleatum* may provide a specific link or connection for other coaggregating microorganisms. Fusobacteria have been shown to have a wide array of coaggregation partners[501–503] and their interactions with Gram-positive and Gram-negative bacteria being distinct.[501] *F. nucleatum* and many streptococci form "corn cob" coaggregation arrangements[504] and in doing so may act as a "bridge" between early and late colonizers.[501]

Antagonistic interactions between microorganisms can occur as a consequence of pH changes and nutrient competition and subsequent to the release of hydrogen peroxide, organic acids (eg., lactic), and bacteriocins. Bacteriocins are protein or peptide "antibiotics" produced by some strains of Gram-positive and Gram-negative bacteria. Genes for bacteriocins are commonly carried on plasmids. They are bacteriostatic or bactericidal to other, often closely related, bacterial strains. The production of bacteriocins may provide the producer strain with a selective advantage over other strains, especially those closely related to the bacteriocin-producing strain.[405] Bacteriocins are diverse in terms of size and structure, ranging from short peptides to multi-component systems with induction and regulation factors. Their mechanism of action is usually characteristic for each bacteriocin. There are few data available about bacteriocins in association with endodontic infections. Fourteen of thirty-three *Enterococcus* species recovered from infected root canals, and six of 12 oral rinse strains,[481] produced bacteriocin activity, using indicator strains *E. faecalis* FA2-2, *E. faecalis* DS16, and *E. faecium* 409, but not *S. aureus* ATCC 6538, *E. coli* DH5α, and *E. coli* ATCC 29417.[413] The use of a bacteriocin as an antimicrobial agent for use in endodontics has been explored. Nisin was as effective as calcium hydroxide in the eradication of *E. faecalis* and *S. gordonii* from root canals of extracted teeth.[505]

SPECIES-SPECIFIC INTERACTIONS BETWEEN MICROORGANISMS IN ROOT CANAL INFECTIONS

Several papers have been published reporting observations of positive and negative associations of bacteria or pairs of bacteria with various clinical signs and symptoms (Table 8). For example, positive associations were found between *F. nucleatum* and *P. micra*, *P. endodontalis*, *Selenomonas sputigena*, and *Campylobacter rectus* in teeth with apical periodontitis.[83] In contradistinction, species of streptococci, *P. propionicum*, *Capnocytophaga ochracea*, and *V. parvula* showed no or negative associations with the other

Table 8 Interactions between Microorganisms

Species A	Species B	Source	Model	Observation	Reference
Animal studies					
Parvimonas micra	Black-pigmented anaerobic rods	Root canals of human necrotic teeth and periapical bone loss	Guinea pigs	Induced abscess formation and transmissible infections	Sundqvist et al. (1979)[506]
Fusobacterium nucleatum	*Porphyromonas gingivalis*, *Prevotella intermedia*	Infected human root canals	Mouse	Induced more pathogenic subcutaneous lesions in mixed compared to pure culture	Baumgartner et al. (1992)[653]
Porphyromonas endodontalis	*Prevotella intermedia*, *Prevotella nigrescens*	Infected human root canals	Mouse	No difference in induction of subcutaneous lesions in mixed compared to pure culture	Siqueira et al. (1998)
Treponema denticola	*P. gingivalis*	Non-endodontic	Mouse	*T. denticola* enhanced the virulence of *P. gingivalis*	Kesavalu et al. (1998)
Tannerella forsythia	*P. gingivalis*	Non-endodontic	Mouse	Abscess formation enhanced with combination	Kesavalu et al. (1998); Yoneda et al. (2001)
Clinical studies					
Fusobacterium nucleatum	*Streptococcus mitis*	Aspirates of periapical abscesses	Culture, Observational	Observed frequent pairing	Oguntebi et al. (1982)
Fusobacterium nucleatum	*P. micra*, *P. endodontalis*, *Selenomonas sputigena*, *Campylobacter rectus*	Infected human root canals	Culture, Odds ratio	Strong positive associations	Sundqvist (1992)[74,83]
Prevotella intermedia	*P. micra*, *P. anaerobius*, eubacteria	Infected human root canals	Culture, Odds ratio	Positive associations	Sundqvist (1992)[74,83]
Propionibacterium propionicum, *Capnocytophaga ochracea*, *Veillonella parvula*, *Streptococcus* species				No associations	Sundqvist (1992)[74,83]
Treponema maltophilum	*P. gingivalis*, *T. forsythia*	Infected human root canals	16S rDNA PCR, Odds ratio	Positive associations	Jung et al. (2001)[259]
Dialister pneumosintes	*T. denticola*, *P. endodontalis*, *F. nucleatum*, *P. micra*, *C. rectus*, *P. intermedia*, *Treponema pectinovorum*, *Treponema vincentii*	Infected human root canals	16S rDNA nested PCR, Odds ratio	Positive associations	Siqueira and Rocas (2003)

Table 8 continued on page 256

Table 8 continued from page 255

Dialister pneumosintes	T. forsythia, P. gingivalis, Actinomyces israelii			Negative associations	Siqueira and Rocas (2003)
Porphyromonas endodontalis	P. gingivalis	Infected human root canals of teeth with acute periapical abscesses	Observational, 16S rDNA PCR	P. gingivalis always found with P. endodontalis	Siqueira et al. (2001)
Prevotella intermedia	P. micra, Prevotella oralis	Infected human root canals of teeth with periapical bone loss and without signs and symptoms	Culture, Odds ratio	Positive associations	Peters et al. (2002)[308]
Actinomyces odontolyticus	Peptostreptococcus micros				Peters et al. (2002b)
Bifidobacterium species	Veillonella species				Peters et al. (2002)[308]
Peptostreptococcus species	Prevotella species	Infected human root canals of teeth without symptoms	Culture, Odds ratio	Positive associations between combination and pain and swelling	Gomes et al. (1996b)
Eubacterium species	Prevotella species, Peptostreptococcus species			Positive associations between combination and wet canal	Gomes et al. (1996b)
Bacteroides vulgatus	Fusobacterium necrophorum	Infected human root canals	Culture, Odds ratio	Negative associations	Gomes et al. (1994)[81,82,659]
Finegoldia magna	Bifidobacterium species				Gomes et al. (1994)[81,82,659]
Campylobacter gracilis	Fusobacterium nucleatum, Fusobacterium species				Gomes et al. (1994)[81,82,659]
Treponema maltophilum	Treponema socranskii, Treponema denticola	Asymptomatic infected human root canals and aspirates of periapical abscesses	16S rDNA PCR, Odds ratio	Higher incidence of spirochetes in symptomatic cases. Positive intergeneric associations	Baumgartner et al. (2003)[260]
Lactobacillus species	Gram-positive cocci	Infected human root canals of teeth with apical periodontitis	Culture, Odds ratio	Positive associations	Chavez de Paz et al. (2004)[315]
In vitro studies					
Prevotella, Streptococcus, Fusobacterium		Samples from human endodontic abscesses or cellulites	Strong intergeneric coaggregation interactions	Positive associations	Khemaleelakul et al. (2006)[499]
Enterococcus faecalis	F. nucleatum	E. faecalis from oral and human root canals	Coaggregation interactions	Positive associations	Johnson et al. (2006)[500]

PCR, polymerase chain reaction.

bacteria.[83] In monkeys, indigenous oral bacteria were able to induce apical periodontitis, with certain combinations of bacteria more potent than were single strains.[78] Combinations of bacteria obtained from teeth with purulent apical inflammation that induced transmissible infections in guinea pigs always contained strains of black-pigmented anaerobic bacteria.[506]

Microbes and Unsuccessful Endodontic Treatment

The presence of microorganisms in the dental pulp is directly associated with the development of periapical disease.[72,77,78,318] Following biomechanical preparation of the infected root canal using antimicrobial agents, followed by optimal obturation and coronal restoration procedures, a favorable long-term outcome can be expected. However, failure of root canal treatment can sometimes occur, particularly in the presence of persistent or secondary intraradicular infection.[507,508,322] A statistically significant association between the presence of microorganisms in the root canal and persistence of infection at five years recall was shown in a clinical study of 55 root canals by Sjogren et al.[322] Complete periapical healing occurred in 94% of 33 cases that had yielded a negative culture prior to root canal obturation compared to 68% of 22 cases when samples were positive prior to root filling.

It is generally understood that the microbiota associated with failed endodontic treatment differs from that associated with primary root canal infections. Culture studies have shown that primary root canal infections are polymicrobial and dominated by anaerobes,[509,510] while secondary root canal infections are composed of fewer species which are dominated by facultatively anaerobic Gram-positive bacteria, principally *Enterococcus* sp.[301,302,508] More recently, PCR-based analyses of 16S rDNA sequences in root canal samples have indicated that the microbiota associated with failed root canal infections is more diverse than previously considered, although *E. faecalis* still is frequently present.[109,111] These findings are not unexpected, considering that less than 1% of environmental microbial species are considered culturable.[118,511] In fact, numerous studies have shown that culture methods used to analyze samples from previously treated root canals are significantly far less sensitive than molecular methods in the detection of microorganisms in root canal samples.[482,512–515] However, research evaluating the contribution of unculturable organisms to the pathogenesis of endodontic infections, and their interactions, if any, with other species is still at an early stage. In the future, studies examining gene expression may be able to provide information on the viability and virulence of these putative pathogens[513] and their role in unsuccessful endodontic treatment.

Microorganisms found in failed endodontically treated teeth have either remained in the root canal from previous treatment or have entered since treatment via leakage. Regardless of methodology used for processing clinical samples, it is not possible to differentiate between viable cells or DNA remaining from primary infections and new microorganisms contributing to the secondary infection. Those remaining from the original microbiota would need to have maintained viability throughout treatment procedures, including exposure to disinfectants, and thereafter adapted to a root canal environment in which the availability of a variety of nutrients is more limited because of lack of pulp tissue. This might occur as a result of an inability of chemomechanical instrumentation procedures to completely debride the root canal system in a single visit and because of the inaccessible locations of bacteria in isthmuses, accessory canals, and apical regions of canals.[493] While it is considered that many such remaining bacteria will be unable to cause harm once entombed by the obturation material, there is little evidence for this.[516]

It is clear that studies of endodontic treatment outcomes in humans are limited by the heterogeneity of patients and the difficulty in maintaining sufficiently standardized clinical and observational conditions. Furthermore, ethical considerations prevent systematic studies of cause and effect using histopathological analyses on human material concurrent with microbiological sampling, as was possible in classic monkey studies.[72,78] Obtaining representative root canal samples from previously root-filled teeth can present considerable practical difficulties, particularly if the previous restoration and root filling are difficult to remove. For this reason, strict criteria need to be applied for inclusion and exclusion of teeth in clinical studies. For example, inclusion of previously root-filled teeth with coronal leakage introduces the potential for inclusion of oral microbiota contaminants that may have played no role in the presenting symptoms. In a recent study, the predominant cultivable species recovered from root-filled teeth with persistent periapical lesions and coronal leakage was *Staphylococcus*,[517] which differs from the findings of those studies which have sampled intact teeth.[108,301,509] Sampling guidelines using strictly aseptic conditions and appropriate controls were developed by Möller.[214] Even when these are observed, the recovery of microorganisms from root canals is usually performed using absorbent paper points. Although paper point sampling is clinically convenient, it is limited in that the paper points will only hold what is displaced from the canal into the paper and do not provide information on what remains in the root canal. Whether the microorganisms that are absorbed into the paper point are representative of those involved in the infectious process is not always, if ever, clear.

Despite the above limitations, several independent studies have shown that certain microorganisms have been repeatedly recovered from infected previously root-filled teeth. In addition to enterococci, these are chiefly *Actinomyces*, propionibacteria, yeasts, and streptococci, with occasional reports of other types. These will be discussed below.

ENTEROCOCCUS

Description

Enterococcus is a genus of Gram-positive facultatively anaerobic coccoid bacteria that until 1984 were classified as Group D streptococci.[518] Enterococcal cells are ovoid and occur singly or in pairs or short chains and can grow at temperatures ranging from 10 to 45 °C. *E. faecalis* and *E. faecium* are the most common enterococcal species found in humans. After coagulase-negative staphylococci, *E. faecalis* is the most common bloodstream nosocomial pathogen in the United States and can also cause urinary tract infections, abdominal-pelvic infections, infective endocarditis, and prosthetic joint infections, among other infections.[519,520] Multiple antibiotic resistance by *E. faecalis* is a major factor in its prominence in nosocomial infections. *E. faecalis* exhibits an intrinsic resistance to many antibiotics, for example, β-lactams antibiotics, most aminoglycosides, and clindamycin,[521] and can commonly harbor multiple antibiotic resistance determinants carried on transferable plasmids.[447]

The oral cavity is a potential reservoir of *E. faecalis* for entry to root canals. Enterococci were detected in samples from multiple oral sites in 75% of eight endodontic patients,[522] but subgingival enterococci were recovered from only 1% of 100 early-onset periodontitis patients and 5.1% of 545 adult periodontitis patients.[523] *E. faecalis* was cultured from oral rinse samples in 11% of 100 patients receiving endodontic treatment and 1% of 100 dental students with no history of endodontic treatment ($p = 0.0027$).[481] Real-time quantitative PCR reported a higher incidence of *E. faecalis* in 30 oral rinse samples (17%) than did culture techniques (5%) and showed that *E. faecalis* accounted for up to 0.005% of the total bacterial load in oral rinse samples.[515] Oral prevalence of *E. faecalis* may vary according to the sampling site and periodontal condition; *E. faecalis* was detected more in tongue than in gingival sulcus, oral rinse, and root canal samples (43, 14, 10, and 10% of patients, respectively; $p = 0.0148$) and in proportionally greater numbers from patients with gingivitis/periodontitis compared to those with healthy periodontium (73% vs 20%; $p = 0.03$).[482]

Prevalence of *Enterococci* in Previously Root-Filled Teeth

Both culture and molecular-based studies have demonstrated that *E. faecalis* could also be recovered from root canals with primary infections.[98,279,514] *E. faecalis* has been repeatedly identified as the species most commonly recovered from root canals of teeth with failed root canal treatment and persistent root canal infections.[98,108,109,285,524–526] Strains have been recovered from approximately one-third of root canals of failed endodontically treated teeth in culture studies[108,214,527] and over 70% using PCR-based methods of detection.[109,514] However, the prevalence rates of *E. faecalis* in root canal infections reported in different studies varies widely (Table 9), and in one study, enterococci were never recovered from endodontically treated teeth with asymptomatic periapical lesions.[528]

The different prevalence rates of enterococci in infected root canals might be a consequence of geographical location.[229] They could also be due to differences in methods of clinical sampling and sample analysis, particularly since the introduction of molecular methods to analyze root canal samples. For example, using sampling and culture techniques based on the "gold standard" method of Möller,[214] *E. faecalis* was recovered from root canal samples in 30% of culture-positive cases in Sweden[108] and the United States.[104] In contrast, investigations using 16S rDNA-based endpoint PCR reported that *E. faecalis* was detected in 77% of samples from 22 failed endodontically treated teeth undergoing retreatment[109] and in 67% of 30 cases of persistent endodontic infections associated with root-filled teeth[285] in Brazil. In an analysis of the same root canal samples using parallel culture and molecular techniques performed by investigators blinded to the analysis results of the other sample, *E. faecalis* was detected in 10.2% and 79.5% of 88 samples by culture and qPCR, respectively ($p < 0.0001$), and in more failed root filled teeth than primary infection samples (89.6% vs 67.5%; $p = 0.01$). In samples where *E. faecalis* was detected using qPCR, it accounted for up to 100% of total bacterial counts ranging from approximately 10^3 to 10^6 cells per sample.[514] *E. faecalis* was up to three times more prevalent in refractory than primary root canal infections sampled upon access,

Table 9 Prevalence of Enterococcus species in Endodontic Infections

Clinical Presentation	Prevalence n*	Percent	Method	Country of Sampling	Reference
Primary infections					
PI, AAP	1/22	5	PCR	Italy	Foschi et al. (2005)[272]
PI	4/53	8	DNA-DNA hybridization	Brazil	Siqueira et al. (2002)[268]
PI, AAP	1/10	10	Nested PCR	Brazil	Rocas et al. (2004b)
PI	11/91	12	Culture	Sweden	Engstrom (1964)[525]
PI	5/40	13	Culture	Sweden	Sedgley et al. (2006)[482,515]
PI, NV	28/150	19	Culture	Sweden	Möller (1966)[214]
PI, PARL, AS	7/21	33	Nested PCR	Brazil	Rocas et al. (2004b)
PI, PARL	6/15	40	Real-time qPCR	USA	Williams et al. (2006)[513]
PI	27/40	68	Real-time qPCR	Sweden	Sedgley et al. (2006)[482,515]
Secondary infections					
RF, PARL	2/36	6	PCR	USA	Kaufman et al. (2005)[529]
RF	4/48	8	Culture	Sweden	Sedgley et al. (2006)[482,515]
RF, no PARL	1/9	11	Culture	Sweden	Molander et al. (1998)[301]
RF	9/43	21	Culture	Sweden	Engstrom (1964)[525]
RF, PARL	8/37	22	PCR	USA	Fouad et al. (2005)
RF, no PARL	5/22	23	PCR	USA	Kaufman et al. (2005)[529]
RF	34/120	28	Culture	Sweden	Möller (1966)[214]
RF, PARL	10/34	30	Culture	USA	Hancock et al. (2001)[104]
RF, PARL	9/24	38	Culture	Sweden	Sundqvist et al. (1998)[108]
RF, PARL	30/68	44	Culture	Sweden	Molander et al. (1998)[301]
RF, PARL	9/14	64	PCR	Korea	Rocas et al. (2004a)
RF, PARL	21/33	64	Culture	Lithuania	Peciuliene et al. (2001)[107]
RF, PARL	20/30	67	Nested PCR	Brazil	Rocas et al. (2004b)
RF, PARL	14/20	70	Culture	Lithuania	Peciuliene et al. (2000)[106]
RF, PARL	10/14	71	Real-time qPCR	USA	Williams et al. (2006)[513]
RF, PARL	13/18	72	PCR	Italy	Foschi et al. (2005)[261]
RF, PARL	17/22	77	PCR	Brazil	Siqueira and Rocas (2004)[109,253]
RF, PARL	18/23	78	PCR	Brazil	Zoletti et al. (2006)[512]
RF, no PARL	22/27	81	PCR	Brazil	Zoletti et al. (2006)[512]
RF	43/48	90	Real-time qPCR	Sweden	Sedgley et al. (2006)[482,514]
Aspirates					
AE aspirates	1/19	5	Nested PCR	Brazil	Rocas et al. (2004b)
AE aspirates	7/43	16	PCR	USA	Baumgartner et al. (2004)[221]
AE aspirates	4/24	17	PCR	Brazil	Baumgartner et al. (2004)[221]

AAp= acute apical periodontitis; AE= abscess of endodonticsa origin; AS= asymptomatic; NV= non-vital; PARL= periapical radiolucency; PCR= polymerase chain reaction; PI= primary infection; RF= root-filled.
*In culture studies refers to prevalence in culture positive sample.

post-instrumentation/irrigation and post-calcium hydroxide treatment.[513]

Information about the prevalence of enterococci in root-filled teeth without signs of apical periodontitis but receiving endodontic retreatment for technical purposes may help elucidate its importance in persistent infection. Molander et al.[301] cultured enterococci from only 1 of 20 teeth without signs of apical periodontitis undergoing root canal retreatment. Growth was described as sparse. Recent 16S rDNA-based studies comparing the prevalence of E. faecalis in teeth with and without periapical lesions have suggested that E. faecalis, although present, does not play a significant role in post-obturation infections.[512,529] In one study, E. faecalis 16S rDNA was detected in 81.5% of 27 root-filled teeth without periapical lesions and 78% of 23 root-filled teeth with periapical lesions.[512] In a study where the overall prevalence of Enterococcus spp was low (12.1%), Kaufman et al.[529] observed a trend that the presence of enterococcal 16S rDNA was not associated with a periapical lesion.

POTENTIAL ROLE OF *ENTEROCOCCI* IN UNSUCCESSFUL ROOT CANAL TREATMENT

The pathogenicity of enterococci in endocarditis and peritonitis has long been established in animal models.[530–532] In contrast, despite their frequent recovery, whether *E. faecalis* plays a significant role in the pathogenesis of human root canal infections remains unclear. In studies concerning the survival of selected bacterial strains inoculated into monkey root canals, after 8–12 months *E. faecalis* was the only species to be re-isolated from all 24 root canals as well as produce radiographic evidence of apical periodontitis in all cases.[533] However, *E. faecalis* as a single species in the monkey model caused only low-grade periapical reactions. Only in the presence of other species within an "eight-strain collection" was lesion size larger.[78] It has been hypothesized that in periapical infections that involve *E. faecalis*, tissue damage may be predominantly caused by the host response to the bacteria rather than direct damage from bacterial products.[534] Thus, the repeated recovery of enterococci from root canal samples may instead represent an ability to survive in the root canal.

The mechanisms by which *E. faecalis* enters and survives in the root canal system for extended periods despite endodontic treatment are not well understood. However, it is well established that *E. faecalis* has the capacity to survive under various stressful environmental conditions, including intracellular survival in macrophages.[535] *E. faecalis* was capable of surviving more than 90 days on commonly used hospital fabrics and plastics[536] and for up to 4 months in water.[537] In an ex vivo model, *E. faecalis* survived in human root-filled teeth for 12 months (Figure 10). In addition, *E. faecalis* is capable of entering and recovering from the viable but nonculturable (VBNC) state, a survival strategy adopted by bacteria when exposed to environmental stress.[538,539] VBNC *E. faecalis* was detected by RT-PCR in four root canal samples that were negative by cultivation.[513] VBNC *E. faecalis* displayed cell wall alterations that might

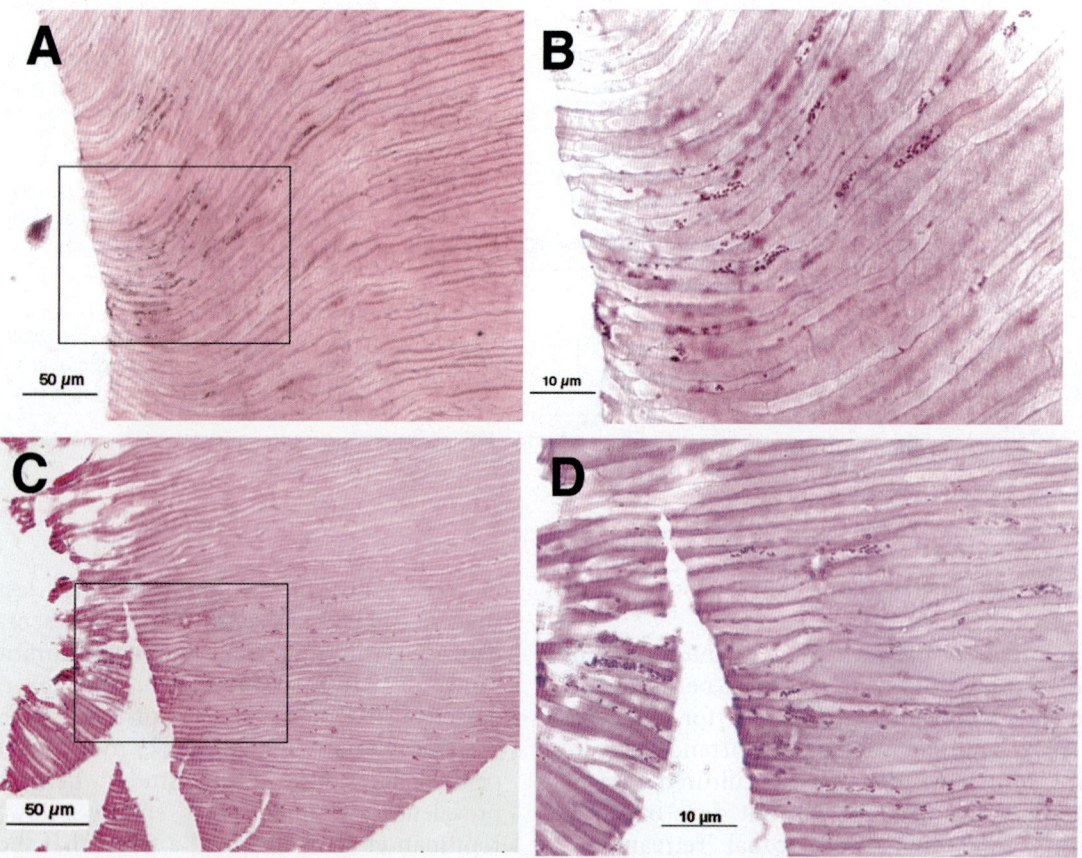

Figure 10 Infection of dentinal tubules by *Enterococcus faecalis* OG1-S after 48-hour incubation (**A** and inset in **B**), and after root canal filling and 12-month incubation (**C** and inset in **D**). Brown and Brenn stain. Reproduced with permission from Sedgley et al. Int Endod J 2005;38:735–42.

provide protection under unfavorable environmental conditions[540] and maintained adhesive properties to cultured human cells.[541] *E. faecalis* produce a variety of stress proteins when exposed to adverse environmental factors such as sodium hypochlorite,[542] salt, bile salts, acid and heat,[543] alkaline stress[544] glucose starvation,[545–547] elevated temperatures,[548] and starvation in tap water.[548]

It has been suggested that enterococci may be selected in root canals undergoing standard endodontic treatment because of low sensitivity to antimicrobial agents,[549,550] including the ability to resist the high pH of antimicrobial agents commonly used, such as calcium hydroxide paste [Ca(OH)$_2$] (pH > 11.5).[323,551,552] For example, *E. faecalis* transcripts of *ftsZ*, a gene involved in cell division, was observed to increase by 37-fold after 5 days incubation at pH 10 at 37°C.[552] Love[553] postulated that the proficiency with which *E. faecalis* can invade dentinal tubules facilitates protection from chemomechanical root canal preparation and intracanal dressing techniques. In the presence of human serum, *E. faecalis* bound better to collagen than did *S. gordonii* or *S. mutans*.[554] Another mechanism by which *E. faecalis* colonization of treated root canals with *E. faecalis* might occur is by the formation of coaggregates with other species, for example, *F. nucleatum*.[500] Coaggregation interactions occurring in biofilms may provide an effective means by which *E. faecalis* remain in the root canal. Using pure cultures of *E. faecalis* in root canals of extracted teeth, experimental biofilms have been grown[414] that appear to vary in terms of ultrastructure and physicochemical properties under different growth conditions.[555] Furthermore, as *E. faecalis* biofilms on root dentin mature, they exhibit the ability to calcify[556] which may facilitate their stability.

Virulence factors with the potential to promote adaptation and survival in different environments have been identified in enterococci recovered from infected root canals[413] as well as other sources.[414,557–559] These include enterococcus surface protein (Esp), collagen-binding protein (Ace), and AS, as well as factors that enable secretion of proteases (eg gelatinase) and toxins (eg., cytolysin).[413] Production of serine protease and Ace by *E. faecalis* have been shown to contribute to the ability to bind to dentin,[414,557] and AS can promote resistance to killing by human neutrophils.[558] Of 31 *E. faecalis* strains from infected root canals, potential virulence traits expressed included production of gelatinase by 23 strains and production of AS by 16 strains in response to pheromones in *E. faecalis* culture filtrate.[413] The latter has potential clinical significance as genes relating to antibiotic resistance, as well as virulence traits, can be found on plasmids that respond to pheromones.[447] Pheromones from *E. faecalis* were chemotactic for human neutrophils and triggered superoxide production,[559] as well as being potent chemotactic agents for rat neutrophils and inducing lysosomal granule enzyme secretion.[560] Overall, possession of the above "virulence traits" might provide a selective advantage over other species in the infected root canal that enables survival in teeth.

STREPTOCOCCUS

Description

Streptococcus is a genus of Gram-positive, asporogenous, facultatively anaerobic, catalase-negative cocci or coccoid bacteria. 16S rDNA gene sequencing has shown at least 50 species within the *Streptococcus* genus.[561] They are non-motile and typically approximately 1 μm in diameter, occurring in pairs or chains. Several species can form capsules. *Streptococcus* forms part of the normal commensal microbiota of the mouth, skin, intestine, and upper respiratory tract of humans.

Traditional classification of *Streptococcus* species relied on their phenotypic properties, with four species groups designated A, B, C, and D. Many group D streptococci have been reclassified as *Enterococcus*. Individual species of streptococci were further classified in terms of their hemolytic properties, or ability to lyse red blood cells, as one measure of potential virulence. "Alpha" hemolysis reduces iron in hemoglobin, resulting in a greenish color on blood agar. Alpha hemolytic streptococci are commonly referred to as "viridans" streptococci and are among the major causative microorganisms of infective endocarditis.[562] *S. mutans*, an important species in dental caries, is an example of alpha hemolytic oral streptococci. "Beta" hemolysis results in complete rupture of red blood cells and gives distinct, clear areas around bacterial colonies on blood agar. Beta hemolytic streptococci, for example, *S. pyogenes*, have been implicated in bacteremia and a range of streptococcal infections, including pharyngitis, rheumatic fever, and acute glomerulonephritis. Another important oral streptococcal species is *S. gordonii* (formerly *S. sanguis*), a normal inhabitant of the oral cavity and an early colonizer in the formation of dental plaque. *S. gordonii* is a causative agent for infective endocarditis, potentially due in part to its ability to avoid polymorphonuclear leukocyte (PMN) killing,[563] the presence of a sialic acid-binding adhesion,[564] and an ability of some strains to aggregate platelets.[565]

Prevalence of Streptococci in Previously Root-Filled Teeth

Streptococci were recovered from root canal samples in 6 of 24 culture-positive asymptomatic previously root-filled cases with radiographic evidence of apical periodontitis in Sweden.[108] Culture studies have shown that in teeth with clinical and radiographical signs of apical periodontitis, streptococci (and lactobacilli) appear to survive following root canal treatment although less frequently than enterococci.[108,301,316,528] In teeth with apical periodontitis receiving endodontic treatment, the most frequently isolated streptococci were S. gordonii, S. anginosus, and S. oralis.[314] In more than half of the culture positive samples, S. gordonii and S. oralis still predominated in subsequent samples. Streptococcus intermedius, S. anginosus, S. oralis, and S. gordonii recovered from root canals were strong producers of extracellular proteins suggesting that these species may play a significant role in post-treatment apical periodontitis.[314] Typically, streptococci recovered from periapical lesions are only rarely resistant to antibiotics commonly used for the treatment of endodontic infections.[566,567]

Potential Role of Streptococci in Unsuccessful Root Canal Treatment

In root-filled teeth with persisting periapical lesions, significant positive associations were observed between the presence of a sinus tract and Streptococcus spp and between coronally unsealed teeth and Streptococcus spp.[302] In endodontically treated teeth associated with asymptomatic periapical lesions in patients in Hong Kong, streptococci, as well as coagulase-negative staphylococci and P. aeruginosa were most frequently isolated.[528] The effect of streptococci on periapical tissue in humans is not well understood. Using FISH colonies with Streptococcus spp were seen in some periapical lesions of asymptomatic root-filled teeth,[337] suggesting a positive association. However, in monkeys, 8–12 months after being introduced into root canals, 85% of teeth from which Streptococcus milleri was recovered had radiographic evidence of apical periodontitis, although the contribution of anaerobic bacteria to the infection could not be eliminated.[533]

Genetic recombination and transfer of genes encoding adhesins, antibiotic resistance determinants, and virulence factors are known to occur in oral streptococci.[568] Of the oral streptococci, S. mutans has been the most widely studied. Horizontal transfer has led to widespread distribution of properties such as adhesion, acid tolerance, and acidogenicity properties.[433] The virulence factors of S. mutans are diverse and are often proteins associated with the cell wall.[569] More specifically, glucan-binding proteins participate in plaque cohesion and can play a role in the modulation of virulence.[570]

The cell walls of Gram-positive bacteria contain PG and LTA that are released upon lysis of the cell. PG and LTA can bind to cell surface receptors and induce the release of proinflammatory cytokines.[75] LTAs are present on the cell surface of most oral streptococci[383] and are important virulence factors, sharing many pathogenic properties with the LPS of Gram-negative bacteria.[387] Lysis of the bacterial cell induced by lysozyme, cationic peptides from leukocytes, or beta-lactam antibiotics results in release of LTA.

Streptococci also have a large range of cell surface adhesins that facilitate binding to various substrates including other bacterial cells, epithelial cells, and dentin.[571] S. gordonii amylase-binding protein A functions as an adhesin to amylase-coated HAP and in human saliva-supported biofilm formation.[572] Furthermore, streptococci may recognize components present within dentinal tubules, such as collagen type I. This stimulates bacterial adhesion and intra-tubular growth. S. gordonii has been shown to invade cervical and midroot dentin up to 200 microns into dentinal tubules, compared to 60 microns at apical dentin.[573] In addition, specific interactions between other bacteria and streptococci may facilitate the invasion of dentin by selected bacterial groupings. For example, recognition of the streptococcal antigen I/II polypeptide facilitates coinvasion of dentinal tubules by P. gingivalis and S. gordonii but not with S. mutans.[494,495] It has been suggested that the potential exists for infective endocarditis to result from bacteria originating in root canals under certain circumstances. For example, if the bacteria possess genes encoding functional binding regions of streptococcal fibronectin-binding protein and staphylococcal fibrinogen-binding protein, bacterial colonization of the endocardium is feasible.[574]

ACTINOMYCES

Description

Actinomyces species are non-spore-forming Gram-positive bacteria occurring as rods, branched rods or filaments, or as rudimentary mycelia. All species can grow anaerobically. Many *Actinomyces* species are commensals in the oral cavity but can become opportunistic pathogens in humans and other mammals.[575,576] Occasionally, they cause actinomycosis, a disease characterized by the formation of abscesses in the mouth, lungs, or the gastrointestinal tract. Happonen et al.[577] reported that *A. israelii* was involved in osteoradionecrosis of the jaws in 1983. Recently, *Actinomyces* has been described as an important pathogen in infected osteoradionecrosis following radiation therapy for head and neck cancer.[578]

Actinomyces species have been implicated in root caries.[579] Species recovered from active root caries include *A. israelii*, *A. naeslundii*, *Actinomyces gerencseriae*, *Actinomyces odontolyticus*, and *Actinomyces georgiae* with more than one species isolated from individual lesions.[579] In germ-free rats, *A. israelii* was shown to cause root surface caries and invasion of pulp tissue.[580] In patients with periodontally affected non-vital teeth, the periodontal pocket may provide a source of *Actinomyces*.[64]

Prevalence of *Actinomyces* in Previously Root-Filled Teeth

In primary root canal infections, reports of recovery of *Actinomyces* are not uncommon.[279,581] *Actinomyces* was predominant in the apical 5 mm of root canals of extracted teeth with carious pulpal exposures and periapical lesions contiguous with the root apex in culture studies.[80] *Actinomyces* species also have been implicated in secondary root canal infections non-responsive to conventional treatment.[315,581] However, most information is limited to that based on case reports following recovery of *Actinomyces* species from persistent lesions following root canal filling,[582,583] sometimes several years after completion of treatment.[104,322] The presence of *Actinomyces* in a periapical cyst has also been reported.[584] Strains of the species *Actinomyces radicidentis* were first found in the root canal and periapical abscesses from two patients with persisting infections following endodontic treatment.[585] Since then, there have been reports of recovery of *A. radicidentis* from previously filled root canals in endodontic patients who had persistent signs and symptoms after conventional root canal treatment[586,282] and also in two primary infection cases.[282]

Potential Role of *Actinomyces* in Unsuccessful Root Canal Treatment

Actinomyces species can be fimbriated or non-fimbriated. Fimbriae on the surface of the *A. israelii* cell wall can be detected using electron microscopy.[394] These structures may be involved in coaggregation interactions with other bacteria,[587,588] and it has been speculated that they contribute to the pathogenicity of *A. israelii*.[394] The higher cell surface interactive forces associated with fimbriated compared to non-fimbriated *Actinomyces* may contribute to modulation of their adhesion and coaggregation properties.[390] In mice, intraperitoneal injections of *A. israelii* and *A. naeslundii* produced suppurative lesions.[589] In other studies using guinea pigs, it was concluded that the pathogenicity of *A. israelii* was due to the ability of the branching filamentous organisms to evade elimination by host phagocytic cells.[590]

PROPIONIBACTERIUM

Description

Propionibacterium species are slow-growing, non-sporulating, Gram-positive anaerobic rods with propionic acid, an end product of fermentation. While *Propionibacterium* species are normal inhabitants of the skin and usually nonpathogenic,[591] they are also common contaminants of blood and body fluid cultures. The human cutaneous propionibacteria include *P. acnes*, *Propionibacterium avidum*, *Propionibacterium granulosum*, *Propionibacterium innocuum*, and *P. propionicum* (also called *Propionibacterium propionicus*, and formerly *Arachnia propionica*). They can be opportunistic pathogens, causing a diverse collection of infections that includes acnes vulgaris,[592] brain abscesses,[593] central nervous system infections,[594] and infective endocarditis.[595] *P. propionicum* is frequently associated with infections of the lacrimal apparatus[596] and has been implicated as a less common causative agent of a disease process similar to actinomycosis.[597] *P. propionicum* has been cultured from shallow and deep coronal caries[598] and deep layers of infected root canal dentin.[599]

Prevalence of *Propionibacteria* in Previously Root-Filled Teeth

P. propionicum was detected in 52% of failed endodontic cases using PCR[109]; using a nested PCR method, the same group reported that *P. propionicum* 16S rDNA was detected in samples from 7/12 (58%) root-filled teeth with chronic periapical lesions compared to 6/21 (29%) previously untreated teeth with chronic periapical lesions.[282] In teeth with apical periodontitis undergoing root canal treatment, the most frequent Gram-positive rod species cultured was *P. propionicum*, in addition to *O. uli* and *L. paracasei*.[315] *Propionibacterium* species were detected in refractory endodontic cases[282] and survived in the periapical tissues of a tooth that did not respond to conventional endodontic therapy.[600] *P. acnes* was identified in the root canal and blood of the same patient using molecular methods.[601]

Potential Role of *Propionibacteria* in Unsuccessful Root Canal Treatment

Although a *P. propionicum* isolate from a failed root-filled tooth did not survive in connective tissue in guinea pigs,[590] there is some evidence that the species possesses characteristics that might facilitate its survival in conditions found in the treated root canal, including an ability to penetrate into dentinal tubules.[602] The surface fibrillar layer that forms part of a complex cell wall structure contributes toward resistance to phagocytosis. In addition, *Propionibacterium* can survive and persist intracellularly in macrophages.[603] *P. acnes* was shown to survive for 8 months under anaerobic conditions without subculture in vitro, suggesting that it could also survive in human tissues at low oxidation potentials.[604]

Propionibacterium species produce proinflammatory mediators, including lipases, neuraminidases, phosphatases, and proteases.[605] Their virulence is thought to be associated with an ability to cause direct damage to the host by means of bioactive extracellular products and metabolites.[605] In particular, *P. acnes* can induce the production of cytokines IL-1α, IL-1β, IL-8, and tumor necrosis factor (TNF)-α by monocytes[592] and is a potent adjuvant in terms of the ability of its products to modulate the immune response to unrelated antigens.[606] Thus far, there appear to be no reports of multiply-antibiotic-resistant root canal isolates. *P. acnes* isolates from necrotic pulps were sensitive to amoxicillin, amoxicillin combined with clavulanate, and tetracycline.[287]

YEASTS

Description

Yeasts are unicellular fungi. The most clinically relevant yeasts belong to the large heterogeneous genus *Candida*, with members forming part of the commensal microbiota in many parts of the human body. *Candida* species can also be opportunistic pathogens as they have the ability to colonize and infect nearly all human tissues.[607] They make up 12% of bacteremias in intensive care units,[519] and are a leading cause of infections in immunocompromised hosts, causing systemic candidiasis in severely immunocompromised patients. *C. albicans* is the most common oral yeast, with other relevant species being *Candida glabrata*, *Candida krusei*, and *Candida tropicalis*.[607] Non-*C. albicans* yeast infections may occur in patients who have received azole-based antifungal therapy.[608] *C. albicans* cells are significantly larger than bacteria and can switch between several different phenotypes in a manner that is heritable and reversible.[609] *Candida* spp reproduce by means of multilateral budding and can form biofilms and tolerate a range of pH conditions. The cell walls are rigid and contain mannan, glucan, and chitin. Cell surface hydrophobicity and pH influence the adherence of *Candida* to host cells.[607]

Prevalence of Yeasts in Previously Root-Filled Teeth

While yeasts are occasionally recovered from primary root canal infections,[283] they may be more frequently recovered from root canals of obturated teeth in which treatment has failed.[610] Yeasts may gain access to the root canal during treatment via contamination.[527] The presence of yeasts in root canals was significantly associated with their presence in saliva[283] and with coronally unsealed teeth.[302] On the other hand, it has been suggested that the incidence of yeasts in root canals may be under-detected in some studies because selective media was not used.[611]

While there appears to be sufficient data to consider yeasts as potential non-bacterial causes of endodontic failures,[612] it is not clear if the prevalence of *Candida* is different in teeth with primary compared to secondary root canal infections. Culture studies showed that 10% of primary cases involved the presence of *Candida* spp,[283] compared to 15% and 3% of root-filled teeth with chronic periodontitis in Lithuania[107] and Sweden,[301] respectively, and 7% of culture positive samples in 967 samples from persistent endodontic infections in Finland.[613] Using PCR, *C. albicans* was detected in 21% of infected root canals[1] and 9% of cases of failed endodontic therapy.[109] Along with other species, yeasts were cultured from samples taken from periapical tissues of teeth with refractory apical periodontitis,[333] but were not detected in aspirates from cellulitis/abscesses of endodontic origin using PCR.[1] Yeasts were recovered from 2 of 18 endodontically treated teeth with asymptomatic periapical lesions.[528] Evidence for the presence of *Candida* species in refractory periapical lesions was not found using PCR methods,[614] but was found in two of 36 cases (6%) using culture methods.[316]

Potential Role of Yeasts in Unsuccessful Root Canal Treatment

In 4 of 10 extracted teeth with necrotic pulps and periapical lesions, heavy infection with yeasts was observed under scanning electron microscopy (SEM),[7] and subsequent SEM studies showed hyphae and budding yeast cells (blastospores) penetrating into dentinal tubules suggesting that *C. albicans* had an affinity to dentinal structures.[8] Penetration into dentinal tubules by *C. albicans* was less than *E. faecalis* in vitro.[615] Thick biofilm formation was associated with the presence of the smear layer, suggesting it provided a suitable substrate for attachment and growth of *C. albicans*.[8] This was supported by the observation that, following dentin treatment with ethylene diamine tetraacetic acid (EDTA) and NaOCl to remove smear layer, biofilm formation by *C. albicans* was hindered.[616]

Clinical strains of *C. albicans* recovered from infected root canals in samples in Finland revealed genotypic and phenotypic diversity,[617] but were similar to strains from other oral and non-oral sites, suggesting that *C. albicans* strains from infected root canals do not require unique characteristics to exist in the root canal environment.[618] Yeasts may play an important role in cases of persisting apical periodontitis, although the mechanisms are not clear. Nair et al.[112] studied therapy-resistant root canal infections and found yeast-like organisms in two of six specimens with microorganisms.

Streptococcus species were the most frequent facultative bacteria accompanying yeasts in root canal samples associated with persistent endodontic infections.[613] *C. albicans* has been observed to coaggregate with some oral streptococci,[503,619] a phenomenon that is enhanced when the yeast is in a starvation stage.[620] Coaggregates also form between *C. albicans* and oral *Fusobacterium*,[621] and *Actinomyces*[622] species Characteristics of *C. albicans* that might contribute to apical periodontitis were reviewed by Waltimo et al..[618] Possible factors include the ability to adhere to dental tissues, the utilization of hyphae to penetrate into dentinal tubules, and a form of contact sensing that allows hyphae to identify breaks on surfaces or between cells through which hyphae can penetrate ("thigmotropism"). Secretion of proteases that allow degradation of human proteins may also be a contributory factor. Secreted aspartyl proteinases (Sap proteins) at tissue lesion sites have been shown to directly contribute to *C. albicans* pathogenicity.[623] The Sap proteins digest molecules for nutritional purposes, disrupt host cell membranes for adhesion and invasion, and also target immune cells for digestion or to avoid killing, for example, by acting as cytolysins in macrophages after *Candida* has been phagocytosed.[624] The ability to switch between phenotypes to allow adaptation to different ecological conditions and between the yeast form and hyphae form may also contribute to pathogenicity although the mechanisms are not clear.[618]

OTHER SPECIES

Species from the family *Enterobacteriaceae* and the genera *Lactobacillus*, *Peptostreptococcus*, and *Fusobacterium* have also been occasionally cultured from previously root-filled teeth in studies from Sweden, Hong Kong, and the United States.[104,108,301,302,528] Positive associations were observed between lactobacilli and Gram-positive cocci in teeth with apical periodontitis undergoing root canal treatment.[315] *Lactobacillus* is a genus of Gram-positive asporogenous bacteria that are anaerobic, microaerophilic, or facultatively aerobic and are generally considered non-pathogens,[625] apart from their association with dental caries.[626] In culture-based studies, the obligate anaerobes, peptostreptococci, have been occasionally recovered.[104,108,301,302,528] The recovery of peptostreptococci from root-filled teeth with persisting periapical lesions was significantly associated with the presence of clinical symptoms[302] and when root canal therapy had been completed more than 3 years earlier.[104]

Using PCR- based methods, several other species have been identified as putative pathogens in samples from root-filled teeth requiring endodontic retreatment.[111] These include *P. alactolyticus* (52%), *D. pneumosintes* (48%), and *F. alocis* (48%) in 22 root-filled teeth with persistent periapical lesions selected for re-treatment.[109] In PCR assays, *T. forsythia* (previously called *B. forsythus*) was detected in 14% of samples from 14 previously root-filled teeth from a South Korean population.[627] *D. invisus*, *Synergistes* oral clone BA121, and *O. uli* were detected in canals of previously treated teeth with persistent infections.[248] The viability, pathogenicity, and relative proportion of these species in root canal infections has not been established.

In contrast, in 50 teeth with unsuccessful endodontic treatment, 16S rDNA sequences from the black-pigmented bacteria *P. gingivalis*, *P. endodontalis*, *P. intermedia*, and *P. nigrescens* were identified less frequently in teeth with failing endodontic treatment (36%) compared to teeth with necrotic pulp (64%),[223] suggesting that these species may not play an important role in infections associated with unsuccessful endodontic treatment.

From the above, it is apparent that the pathogenicity of specific bacterial species, or combinations of species identified in secondary root canal infections in humans, has yet to be unequivocally established in controlled studies. In addition, a better understanding of the role of specific virulence traits associated with microorganisms in root canal infections may help understand the process and ultimately identify therapeutic targets.

Microorganisms and Endodontic Flare-Ups

ENDODONTIC FLARE-UPS

An endodontic flare-up is defined by the American Association of Endodontists (AAE) as "an acute exacerbation of an asymptomatic pulpal and/or periapical pathosis after the initiation or continuation of root canal treatment."[628] Flare-ups are unpredictable events with reported prevalence rates varying from 1.4% to 19% (see Chapter 21). Presenting symptoms include pain with or without swelling[629–631] that is of sufficient severity for the patient to seek emergency treatment.[632]

Flare-ups can be distressing and disruptive events for both patients and clinicians. Consequently, several investigations have focused on associations between the flare-up event and corresponding pre-treatment clinical factors. The definition of a flare-up has varied among studies. However, in accordance with the current AAE definition,[628] the most likely predisposing clinical condition for its occurrence appears to be asymptomatic necrotic pulp with periapical lesion.[629,631,633] Where symptomatic pre-treatment patients have been included in the study cohort, predisposing conditions include acute apical abscess, acute apical periodontitis,[629,631,634] preoperative pain,[635] and swelling.[630]

It is well established that the presence of microorganisms in the dental pulp is directly associated with the development of periapical disease.[72,77,78,318,509] In contrast, the specific means by which microbes contribute to endodontic flare-ups is less clear. The flare-up etiology is likely multifactorial, and dependent on the interactions between the host immunological response, infection, and physical damage,[630] with the major causative factor described as microbial in origin.[632,636,637] While there is sound circumstantial evidence for the latter assumption, direct proof is lacking. Indirect support is found in studies showing that the lowest incidence of flare-ups occurred in patients without periapical pathosis[629,631,638] and when a sinus tract is present[629,634,639] the latter presumable permitting some form of drainage.

Interestingly, other factors that might be expected to contribute to a predominantly microbiological etiology have been reported to have no association with the occurrence of flare-ups. These include incomplete root canal debridement,[629,640,641] underfilled canals,[642] over-instrumentation beyond the apex[634] where extrusion of infected debris might be expected to occur, and the use of antimicrobial intracanal medicaments.[634,643] Perhaps most unexpectedly if residual viable bacteria are the major cause of flare-ups, prophylactic antibiotics are ineffective in their prevention. This has been established in a series of prospective, randomized, double-blind, placebo-controlled clinical trials that found prophylactic antibiotics (penicillin or amoxicillin) to be ineffective in preventing post-treatment flare-ups in cases of pulpal necrosis and periapical lesions in asymptomatic[644,645] and symptomatic[646] teeth as well as in untreated teeth with irreversible pulpitis.[647] Other reports indicate that the prevention of flare-ups was better managed with intracanal medicaments containing steroids[648,649] and anti-inflammatory agents.[650]

The above suggests that viable microorganisms remaining after treatment procedures may not be as critical to the development of a flare-up like the interactions between immunological factors, microbial breakdown products, and the collateral damage resulting from treatment procedures. Occasionally, environmental changes in the infected root canal and associated periodontium of a clinically asymptomatic tooth following root canal treatment procedures can trigger a severe host response. It has been hypothesized that the "immunological status of the periapical tissue may predispose patients to develop a post endodontic flare-up."[630] Fortunately, the occurrence of an endodontic flare-up does not appear to influence the long-term prognosis of the tooth. Sjögren et al.[340] reported that the occurrence of flare-ups had no significant influence on the outcome of endodontic treatment when reviewed 8 to 10 years later.

ASSOCIATIONS BETWEEN SPECIFIC BACTERIA AND ENDODONTIC FLARE-UPS

Very few studies have investigated the microbiological aspects of flare-ups, and there are no case controlled studies. The low incidence of flare-ups makes conducting prospective clinical studies with appropriate controls for microbiological analyses particularly difficult, in part because of the need for sufficiently large numbers of samples to allow statistical analyses. In addition, baseline data about the preoperative flare-up microbiota, including yeasts and viruses, should ideally be available. Future studies utilizing microarray technology that will allow rapid detection of multiple bacterial species in a single sample have the potential to make this task less arduous. In view of the importance of the role of the host, such studies could apply multiple qualifiers to account for the status of the host as well as the potential pathogens.[651]

An early study found no difference between the microbiota of asymptomatic teeth and those presenting with flare-ups; however, strict anaerobic methods were not used.[652] More recently, Chavez de Paz[423] examined the root canal microbiota of 28 patients who had originally received treatment for non-painful teeth with necrotic pulp and periapical lesions and subsequently developed symptoms necessitating emergency treatment. Correlations were made between the severity of pain and the culturable root canal microbiota. The recovery of *F. nucleatum* was associated with the most severe flare-up pain and swelling. Similarly, Peciuliene et al.[107] reported that *F. nucleatum* was isolated (along with *E. faecalis* and *A. israelii*) from an asymptomatic root-filled tooth with chronic apical periodontitis undergoing retreatment that had a flare-up after the first appointment.

Other isolates identified in the root canal microbiota of teeth with flare-ups were Gram-negative obligate anaerobic rods belonging to the genera *Prevotella* and *Porphyromonas*.[423] Chavez de Paz suggested that the combination of *F. nucleatum*, *Prevotella* species, and *Porphyromonas* species may provide a risk factor for endodontic flare-ups by acting in synergy to increase the intensity of the periapical inflammatory reaction.[423] This hypothesis is supported by an animal study demonstrating that root canal isolates of *F. nucleatum* combined with either *P. gingivalis* or *P. intermedia* induced more severe pathologic subcutaneous lesions in mice in mixed compared to pure cultures.[653]

Fusobacterium, *Prevotella*, and *Porphyromonas* are non-motile Gram-negative anaerobic rods belonging to the *Bacteroidaceae* family that are found in the human mouth and intestine. Because of their frequent recovery from asymptomatic cases[111] in addition to flare-up cases, further information is required to understand their role, if any, in endodontic flare-ups. However, it is possible that alterations in the root canal environment and surrounding periodontium as a result of treatment procedures might modulate interspecies interactions and in doing so facilitate virulence. For example, the pathogenic potential of *F. nucleatum* might be enhanced as a result of synergistic associations with *P. micra*,[366] another species frequently recovered from root canal infections.[111]

Virulence factors released by fusobacteria can engender numerous biologic effects. For example, *F. nucleatum* LPS applied to pulp tissue in rats induced a rapid immune response[654] and produced a large array of biological effects in macrophage-like cells (U937 cells) by directly upregulating several proinflammatory cytokines (IL-1, IL-6, TNF-α, and IL-8).[655] In addition, production of butyric acid by *F. nucleatum* can stimulate inflammatory cytokine release in neutrophils.[417]

Prevotella and *Porphyromonas* species have been isolated from numerous anatomic sites,[656] and are frequently detected in root canal samples from asymptomatic and symptomatic root canal infections, and aspirates from acute periapical abscesses.[89,111] They are sometimes generically identified as "BPB" based on the fact that some species form brown or black pigments when cultured on blood-containing media. Various virulence factors have been associated with these species. In vitro studies using human dental pulp cells have shown that LPS from *P. endodontalis* stimulated IL-1β release[368] and IL-8 expression.[369] The expression of the pro-angiogenic VEGF in odontoblast-like cells and macrophages was upregulated by *P. intermedia* LPS.[370] Fimbriae associated with *P. intermedia* induced hemagglutination activity.[393,394]

ASSOCIATIONS BETWEEN SPECIFIC BACTERIA AND ENDODONTIC SYMPTOMS IN GENERAL

In contrast to the paucity of data on microbiological aspects of flare-ups, there are several cohort studies that have looked for associations between specific species, or groups of species, and various clinical symptoms. Direct extrapolation of these data to the etiology of flare-ups has yet to be proven. However, it is reasonable to expect that similar virulence mechanisms are involved. In general, the release of various bacterial components (eg., LPS, LTAs, and PGs) can give rise to the synthesis of proinflammatory cytokines. For example, LPS enhances bone resorption,[367,374] inflammation,[657] and pain.[375,377,658]

Several studies have obtained microbiological samples from cohorts of patients with and without symptoms. For example, BPB species in 35 symptomatic and 27 asymptomatic root canal infections, *P. gingivalis* and *P. endodontalis*, were present only in symptomatic infections, while *P. intermedia nigrescens* was found both in symptomatic and in asymptomatic infections, and *P. denticola* occurred mostly in asymptomatic infections.[89] At 1-week review, BPB species were isolated in 9 of the 11 teeth that remained symptomatic compared to less than half of the 51 teeth that were symptom-free. This suggests that the presence of BPB at the start of treatment could be associated with the continuation of symptoms.

In single-cohort studies, the occurrence of symptoms has been associated with BPB[88,92,102,415,659,660] and *Streptococcus* species[232] in root canals. A positive correlation was noted between BPB and purulent drainage, but no other clinical signs, in samples from root canals of intact teeth with necrotic pulps and apical periodontitis.[102] Specifically, the presence of black-pigmented anaerobic bacteria and other *Bacteroides* species in infected root canals was associated with foul odor, pain, and sinus tracts in cariously and traumatically exposed non-vital teeth.[88] Gomes et al.[659] reported that both *Prevotella* and *Peptostreptococcus* species were isolated from significantly more painful than painless teeth. *P. micra* previously *Peptostreptococcus micros* has been associated with endodontic abscesses in children.[661]

Environmental changes in the infected root canal favor the development of an increasingly anaerobic environment over time.[77] The root canals of symptomatic teeth harbor more obligate anaerobes than do asymptomatic teeth.[660] Certain combinations of obligate anaerobes might be associated with certain symptoms.[662] For example, there were significant associations between (1) pain and the combination of *Peptostreptococcus* species and *Prevotella* species; (2) swelling and the combination of *P. micra* and *Prevotella* species; and (3) wet canals and the combinations of *Eubacterium* species with either *Prevotella* species or *Peptostreptococcus* species.[662] Synergistic interactions between species might enhance virulence. For example, *P. micra* from necrotic infected root canals enhanced the pathogenicity of other bacteria black-pigmented anaerobic bacteria in mixed experimental infections in guinea pigs.[506]

Significant relationships were reported concerning percussion pain and the bacteria, *Peptostreptococcus*, *Eubacterium*, and *Porphyromonas* and concerning odor and *Porphyromonas* and *Prevotella* in the infected root canals of a cohort of 25 patients.[92] Phenotypic analyses of the recovered strains showed that subacute clinical symptoms with percussion pain were associated with bacteria producing collagenase or chondroitinase and hyaluronidase. Recovery of collagenase-producing bacteria in root canal samples was associated with periapical radiolucencies larger than 5 mm in diameter.[415]

In contrast to the above, other studies have reported no association between specific clinical symptoms and BPB,[232] *P. micra*,[284] and the combination of *T. denticola*, *P. gingivalis*, and *T. Forsythia*.[240] The recovery of *Fusobacterium* species, *P. micra*, and *P. gingivalis* did not differ in cohorts of symptomatic and asymptomatic patients.[230] Associations have been made between apical periodontitis and the cytomegalovirus and EBV in the pathogenesis of symptomatic periapical lesions associated with permanent[5,6,294,296,663] and deciduous[664] teeth. Obtaining adequate controls from the same patient to control for the virus existing in latent form presents unique challenges in these studies.

Information on specific virulence factors associated with specific strains recovered from root canal infections is limited. Because different strains of a species recovered from infected root canals can express different virulence factors,[413] this suggests a capacity to modulate virulence under varying environmental conditions.[632] This may help explain the apparent disparity of the same species being recovered from both symptomatic and asymptomatic cases.[89,102,111] In addition, the importance of the host cannot be overstated and can help explain why only small numbers of virulent microorganisms may be sufficient to cause disease in an immunocompromised host.[351]

Overview of Bacterial Biofilms

Biofilm is a mode of microbial growth where dynamic communities of interacting sessile cells are irreversibly attached to a solid substratum, as well as each other, and are embedded in a self-made matrix of extracellular polymeric substances (EPS).[665] A microbial biofilm is considered a community that meets the following four basic criteria: The microorganisms living in the community (1) must possess the abilities to self-organize (*autopoiesis*); (2) resist environmental perturbations (*homeostasis*); (3) must be more effective in association than in isolation (*synergy*); and (4) respond to environmental changes as a unit rather than single individuals (*communality*).[666] Dental plaque is the typical example of a biofilm.

In the past, bacteriological studies were conducted on free-floating bacterial cells (*planktonic state*), ignoring the importance of the sessile bacterial cells (*biofilm state*).[667] Ironically, in nature, pure cultures of free-floating bacteria rarely exist. Biofilms can be formed wherever there is a flow of fluid, microorganisms, and a solid surface. It is one of the basic survival strategies employed by bacteria in all natural and industrial ecosystems in response to starvation. The sessile bacterial cells in a biofilm state differ greatly from their planktonic counterparts. Inside a biofilm, the bacterial cells exhibit altered phenotypic properties and are protected from antimicrobials, environmental stresses, bacteriophages, and phagocytic amoebae. Biofilms are responsible for most of the chronic infections and almost all recalcitrant infections in human beings, as bacteria in a biofilm are resistant to both antibiotic therapy and host defense mechanisms.[668] However, common biofilms found in the oral cavity and gastrointestinal tract are protective in nature. These biofilms featuring a large number and diverse array of commensal bacteria hinders the adherence of pathogenic microorganisms.[669]

ULTRASTRUCTURE OF BIOFILM

A fully developed biofilm is described as a heterogeneous arrangement of microbial cells on a solid surface. The basic structural unit of a biofilm is the microcolonies or cell clusters formed by the surface adherent bacterial cells. Microcolonies are discrete units of densely packed bacterial cell (single or multispecies) aggregates. There is a spatial distribution of bacterial cells (microcolony) of different physiological and metabolic states within a biofilm. A glycocalyx matrix made up of EPS surrounds the microcolonies and anchors the bacterial cell to the substrate.[670] Eighty-five percent by volume of the biofilm structure is made up of matrix material, while 15% is made up of cells. A fresh biofilm matrix is made of biopolymers such as polysaccharides, proteins, nucleic acids, and salts.[671,672] The structure and composition of a matured biofilm is known to modify according to the environmental conditions (growth conditions, nutritional availability, nature of fluid movements, physicochemical properties of the substrate, etc). Figure 11 represents the structure of a mature biofilm. Typically, a viable, fully hydrated biofilm appears as "tower-" or "mushroom"-shaped structures adherent to a substrate. The overall shape of a biofilm structure is determined by the shear forces generated by the flushing of fluid media. Biofilms formed in high-shear environments have shown that the microcolonies are deformed by these forces to produce tadpole-shaped oscillation in the bulk fluid. Advanced microscopy of living biofilms have revealed that single-species biofilms growing in the laboratories to complex multispecies biofilms growing in the natural ecosystems have similar basic community structure, with some subtle variations.[673]

The water channels, which are regarded as a primitive circulatory system in a biofilm, intersect the structure of biofilm to establish connections between the microcolonies. Presence of water channels facilitates efficient exchange of materials between bacterial cells and bulk fluid, which in turn helps to coordinate functions in a biofilm community.[665] The structural feature of a biofilm that has the highest impact in chronic bacterial infection is the tendency of microcolonies to detach from the biofilm community. During the process of detachment, the biofilm transfer particulate constituents (cells, polymers, and precipitates) from the biofilm to the fluid bathing the biofilm.[674] There are two main types of detachment process: erosion (the continual detachment of single cells and small portions of the biofilm) and sloughing (the rapid, massive loss of biofilm). Detachment has been understood to play an important role in shaping the morphological characteristics and structure of mature biofilm. It is also considered as an active dispersive mechanism (*seeding dispersal*). These detached cells, which have acquired the resistance traits from the

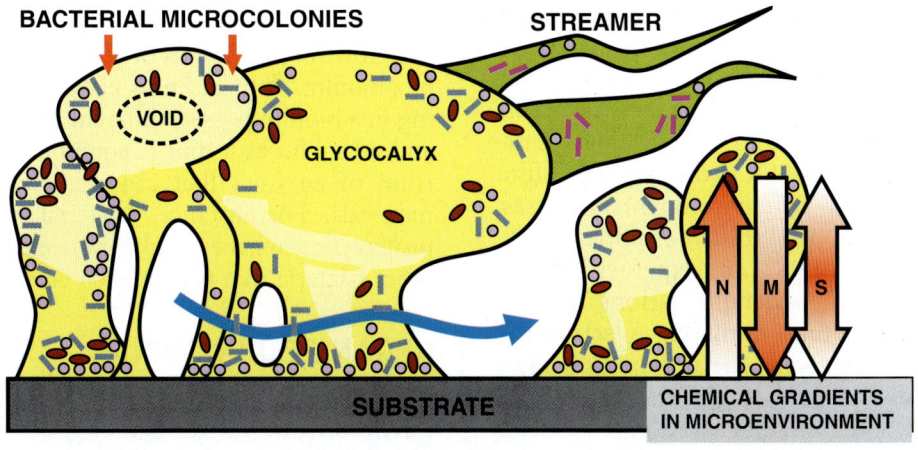

Figure 11 Schematic representation of the structure of a mature biofilm. Courtesy A. Kishen.

parent biofilm community, can be source for persistent infection.[675]

Bacterial colonization and biofilm formation can alter the physicochemical properties of many substrates. The EPS and the metabolic activities of bacteria within a biofilm determine the physicochemical characteristics of the substrate. Bacterial cell surfaces are typically anionic due to the presence of carboxylate or phosphate moieties in capsular or cell wall polymers. Therefore, a colonized substrate will acquire an anionic character, regardless of its original physicochemical properties. Under a favorable environment, metal ions including Ca^{2+}, Mg^{2+}, and Fe^{3+} will readily bind to and precipitate within anionic biofilms, inducing biofilm-mediated mineralization.[676]

CHARACTERISTICS OF BIOFILM

Bacteria in a biofilm state show distinct capacity to survive tough growth and environmental conditions. This unique capacity of bacteria in a biofilm state is due to the following features: (1) biofilm structure protects the residing bacteria from environmental threats; (2) structure of biofilm permits trapping of nutrients and metabolic cooperativity between resident cells of same species and/or different species; (3) biofilm structures display organized internal compartmentalization, which allows bacterial species with different growth requirements to survive in each compartment; (4) bacterial cells in a biofilm community may communicate and exchange genetic materials to acquire new traits.

PROTECTION OF BIOFILM BACTERIA FROM ENVIRONMENTAL THREATS

Bacteria residing in a biofilm community experience certain degree of protection and homeostasis. Many bacteria are capable of producing polysaccharides, either as cell surface structures (eg., capsule) or as extracellular excretions (eg., EPS). EPS covers biofilm communities and creates a microniche favorable for the long-term survival and functioning of the bacterial communities.[677] EPS protects the biofilm bacteria from a variety of environmental stresses, such as UV radiation, pH shifts, osmotic shock, and desiccation.[678-680] EPS can sequester metals, cations, and toxins.[681,682] Metallic cations such as magnesium and calcium minimize electrostatic repulsion between negatively charged biopolymers, increasing the cohesiveness of the EPS matrix.[683] Diffusion is the predominant transport process within cell aggregates. The diffusion distance in a planktonic cell is on the order of magnitude of the dimension of an individual cell, while the diffusion distance in a biofilm is on the order of the dimension of the multicellular aggregate. A biofilm that is 10 cells thick will exhibit a diffusion time 100 times longer than that of a single cell.[684] Furthermore, diffusion of compounds into the biofilm depends upon the nature of both the compound and the EPS matrix. EPS can physically prevent the permeability of certain compounds into the biofilm by acting as an ion exchanger.[677,678,680]

NUTRIENT TRAPPING AND ESTABLISHMENT OF METABOLIC COOPERATIVITY IN A BIOFILM

An important characteristic of biofilms growing in a nutrient-deprived ecosystem is its ability to concentrate trace elements and nutrients by physical trapping or by electrostatic interaction.[677] Besides, the highly permeable and interconnected water channels in the biofilm provide an excellent means for material exchange. The water channel connects the outer fluid medium with the interior of the biofilm, ensuring nutrient availability to microbial communities deep inside the biofilm structure.

The complex architecture of a biofilm provides the opportunity for metabolic cooperation, and niches are formed within these spatially well-organized systems. Bacterial microcolonies in a biofilm structure are exposed to distinct environmental signals. For example, cells located near the center of a microcolony are more likely to experience low oxygen tensions compared to cells located near the surface. Moreover, due to the juxtapositioning of different microorganisms, cross-feeding and metabolic cooperativity between different species of microorganisms are seen in a biofilm.[685,686] Studies have reported the production of essential growth factors such as hemin by *W. recta* to support the growth of fastidious organisms such as *P. gingivalis* in a biofilm.[686] In addition, each bacterial species residing in a biofilm possess different array of lytic enzymes, and a biofilm as a unit is equipped with a wide spectrum of enzymes that can degrade complex organic materials. For instance, bacterial species possessing proteolytic enzymes make nutrients available to all other bacteria in a protein-rich environment.[687]

ORGANIZED INTERNAL COMPARTMENTALIZATION IN BIOFILM

Environmental niches that support the physiological requirements of different bacterial species are available in a biofilm. A mature biofilm structure displays gradients in the distribution of nutrients, pH, oxygen,

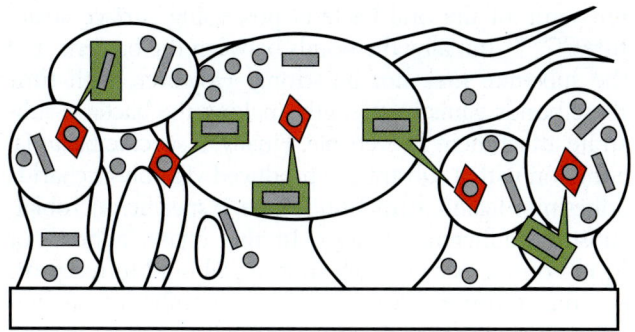

Figure 12 Schematic diagram representing cell–cell communication in a biofilm. Some bacteria can produce chemical signals (green) and other bacteria from the same species or from different species or strain can respond to them (red). Reproduced with permission from Al Cunningham et al.[684]

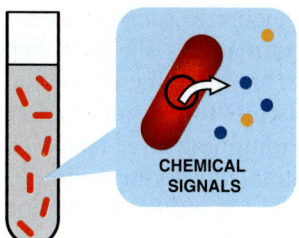

(A) Planktonic bacteria

The concentration of chemical signals secreted by the planktonic cells is low. The low concentration of signal molecules does not change genetic expression

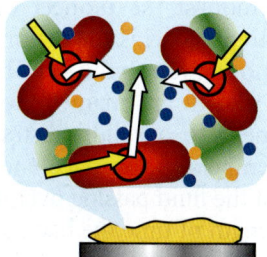

(B) Biofilm bacteria

Biofilm cells are held together in dense populations, so the secreted chemical signals higher concentrations. Signal molecules then re-cross the cell membranes and trigger changes in genetic activity.

Figure 13 Schematic diagram showing quorum sensing in biofilm bacteria. Reproduced with permission from Al Cunningham et al.[684]

metabolic products, and signaling molecules within the biofilm (Figure 12). This would create different microniche that can accommodate diverse bacterial species within a biofilm. The gradients in nutrients, chemicals, and gases, observed in a biofilm structure, are influenced by the type of nutrients and the physiological requirements of the residing microorganisms.[688] In a multispecies biofilm involving aerobic and anaerobic bacteria, oxygen is consumed by the aerobic and facultative anaerobic species, making the environment rich in carbon dioxide and other gases. When the aerobic bacteria residing on the surface of the biofilm consumes all available oxygen, the interior of the biofilm can be absolutely anaerobic that it can even support the growth of obligatory anaerobes. Despite the fact that oral cavity is abundant in oxygen, anaerobic microbes are found to dominate oral biofilms because of the possible redox gradient formed within the biofilm structure.[519]

BACTERIAL CELLS RESIDING IN A BIOFILM COMMUNICATE, EXCHANGE GENETIC MATERIALS, AND ACQUIRE NEW TRAITS

Bacterial biofilm provides a setting for the residing bacterial cells to communicate with each other. Some of these signals, produced by cells, may be interpreted not just by members of the same species, but by other microbial species too. Communications between bacterial cells residing in a biofilm is attained through signaling molecules, by a process called *quorum sensing*. Quorum sensing is mediated by low molecular weight molecules, which in sufficient concentration can alter the metabolic activity of neighboring cells, and coordinate the functions of resident bacterial cells within a biofilm.[689,690] The process of cell–cell communication and quorum sensing is illustrated in Figures 12 and 13, respectively. Exchange of genetic materials between bacterial species residing in a biofilm will result in the evolution of microbial communities with different traits. Close proximity of microbial cells in a biofilm facilitates genetic exchange between bacteria of genetically distant genera.[691] Even the possibility of gene transfer between a commensal organism (*Bacillus subtilis*) and oral biofilm bacteria (*Streptococcus* species) has been demonstrated.[692] The horizontal gene transfer is of importance in human diseases caused by bacterial biofilm as it can result in the generation of antibiotic-resistant bacterial population. Gene transfer between bacteria residing in a biofilm is thought to be mediated by bacterial conjugation. The presence of diverse bacterial species in a biofilm presents a pool of genetic codes for nutrient breakdown, antibiotic resistance, and xenobiotic metabolism. Cell–cell communication can result in the coordinated behavior of microbial population residing in a biofilm.

DEVELOPMENT OF BIOFILM

Bacteria can form biofilms on any surface that is bathed in a nutrient-containing fluid. The three major components involved in biofilm formation are bacterial cells, a solid surface, and a fluid medium. Development of biofilm is influenced by the physicochemical properties of the components involved in the biofilm and is shown in Figure 14.[689,693–695] Figure 15 shows the step-by-step manner of biofilm formation. The first step involved in the development of biofilm is the adsorption of inorganic and organic molecules to the solid surface creating what is termed a conditioning layer (stage 1). During dental plaque formation, the tooth surface is conditioned by the saliva pellicle. Once the conditioning layer is formed, the next step in biofilm formation is the adhesion of microbial cells to this layer (stage 2). Amongst the pioneer organisms, the oralis group of streptococci is the major population to form a bacterial monolayer on the salivary pellicle coated tooth surface.

There are many factors that affect bacterial attachment to a solid substrate. These factors include pH, temperature, surface energy of the substrate, flow rate of the fluid passing over the surface, nutrient availability, length of time the bacteria is in contact with the surface, bacterial growth stage, bacterial cell surface charge, and surface hydrophobicity. Physicochemical properties such as surface energy and charge density determine the nature of initial bacteria-substrate interaction (Phase 1: transport of microbe to substrate surface). In addition, the microbial adherence to a substrate is also mediated by bacterial surface structures such as fimbriae, pili, flagella, and EPS (glycocalyx). The bacterial surface structures form bridges between the bacteria and the conditioning film.[687] Molecular-specific interactions between bacterial surface structures and substrate become active in this phase (Phase 2: initial non-specific microbial-substrate adherence phase). These bridges are a combination of electrostatic attraction, covalent and hydrogen bonding, dipole interaction, and hydrophobic interaction. *P. gingivalis*, *S. mitis*, *Streptococcus salivarius*, *P. intermedia*, *P. nigrescens*, *S. mutans*, and *A. naeslundii* are some of the oral bacteria possessing surface structures.[696,697] Initially, the bonds between the bacteria and the substrate may not be strong. However, with time these bonds gains in strength, making the bacteria-substrate attachment irreversible. Finally, a specific bacterial adhesion with a substrate is produced via polysaccharide adhesin or ligand formation (Phase 3: specific microbial-substrate adherence phase). In this phase, adhesin or ligand on the bacterial cell surface will bind to receptors on the substrate. Specific bacterial adhesion is less affected by many environmental factors such as electrolyte, pH, or temperature.[698,699] The adhesive potential of microorganisms is considered to be a vital ecologic and pathogenic determinant in the development of biofilms.

Next step in the development of biofilm is the bacterial growth and biofilm expansion (stage 3). During this stage, the monolayer of microbes attracts secondary colonizers forming microcolony, and the collection of microcolonies gives rise to the final structure of biofilm.[668,700] The lateral and vertical growth of indwellers gives rise to microcolonies similar to towers. A mature biofilm will be a metabolically active community of microorganisms where individuals share duties and benefits.[701] For instance, some microorganisms help in adhering to the solid support, while some others create bridges between different species, which otherwise would not have happened. The bacterial cells in a matured biofilm will exhibit considerable variation in its genetic and biochemical constitutions compared to its planktonic counterparts. Two types of microbial interactions occur at the cellular level during the formation of biofilm. One is the process of recognition between a suspended cell and a cell already attached to substratum. This type of interaction is termed

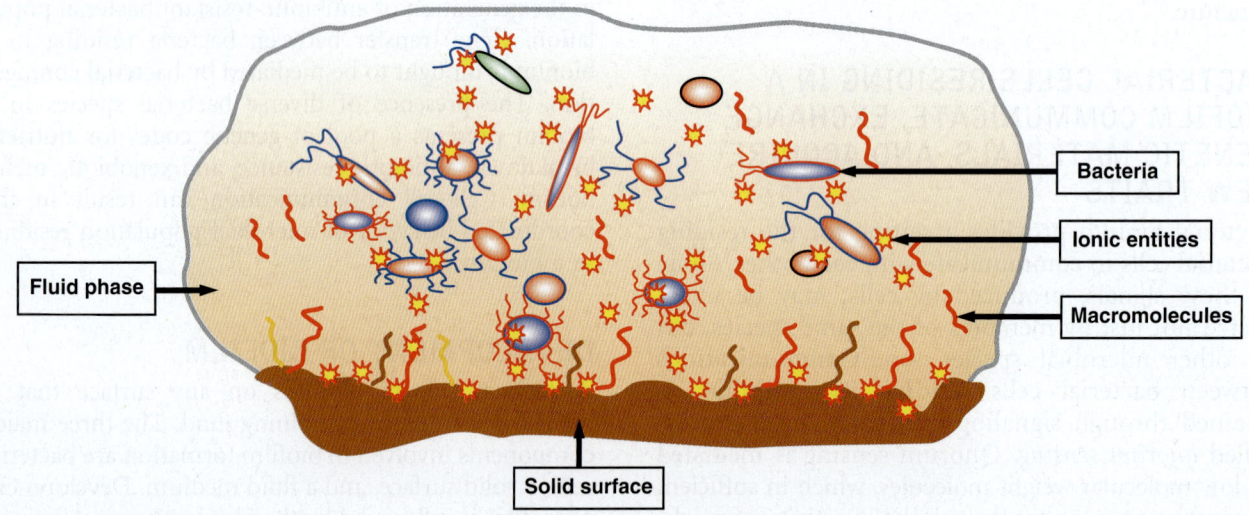

Figure 14 Schematic diagram showing different factors influencing initial bacteria–substrate interaction. Courtesy A. Kishen.

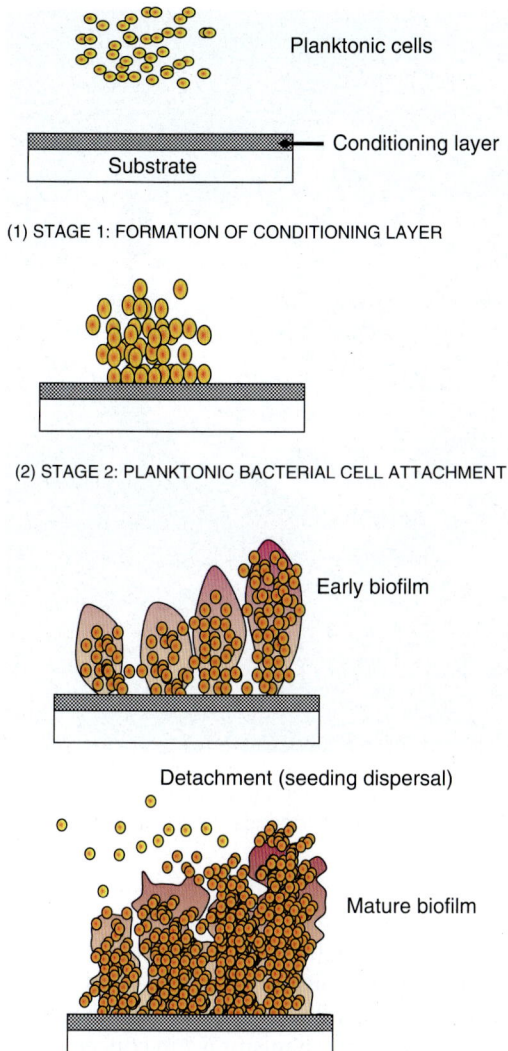

Figure 15 Stages in the development of biofilm. Courtesy A. Kishen.

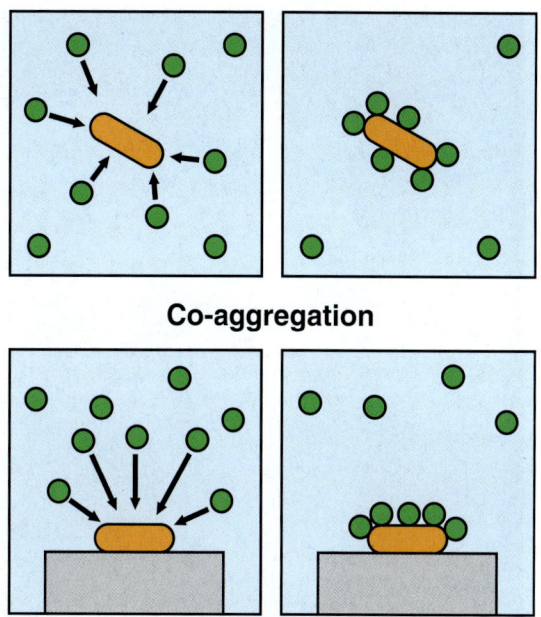

Figure 16 Schematic diagram showing co-aggregation and co-adhesion between different bacterial cells forming biofilm. Reproduced with permission from Busscher HJ and van der Mei HC.[702]

co-adhesion. In the second type of interaction, genetically distinct cells in suspension recognize each other and clump together. This type of interaction is called coaggregation.[702,703] Schematic representation of the co-adhesion and coaggregation process between bacterial cells is shown in Figure 16. These associations are highly specific and occur between co-aggregating partners only. Interestingly, most of the oral bacteria recognize each other as co-aggregating partners. *F. nucleatum*, a Gram-negative filamentous anaerobe can coaggregate with all oral bacteria tested and can act as a bridging bacterium that bind together even non-aggregating bacteria.[704,705] The association of long-filamentous bacteria and surface-adsorbed spherical-shaped cocci produce the characteristic corncob structure of oral biofilms.[706] The attachment of cocci to filamentous bacteria is said to be mediated via fimbriae of the oral streptococci.[707] Although genetic makeup of bacteria is the main determinant of coaggregation, the physicochemical characteristics of the environment also play a crucial role.[708]

Resistance of Microbes in Biofilm to Antimicrobials

The nature of biofilm structure and physiological characteristics of the resident microorganisms offer an inherent resistance to antimicrobial agents, such as antibiotics, disinfectants, or germicides. The resistance to antimicrobial agents has been found to amplify more than thousand times for microbes in biofilm, when compared to planktonic cells.[709] Figure 17 shows the scanning electron micrographs of (see Figure 17A) an untreated biofilm of *Staphylococcus epidermidis* and (see Figure 17B) an identical biofilm exposed to vancomycin and rifampin for 72 hours at concentrations exceeding the minimum inhibitory concentration (MIC) and minimum bactericidal concentration (MBC) for the microorganism. In spite of the obvious changes in the treated biofilm, viable organisms were recovered for which the MIC and MBC of both antimicrobial agents

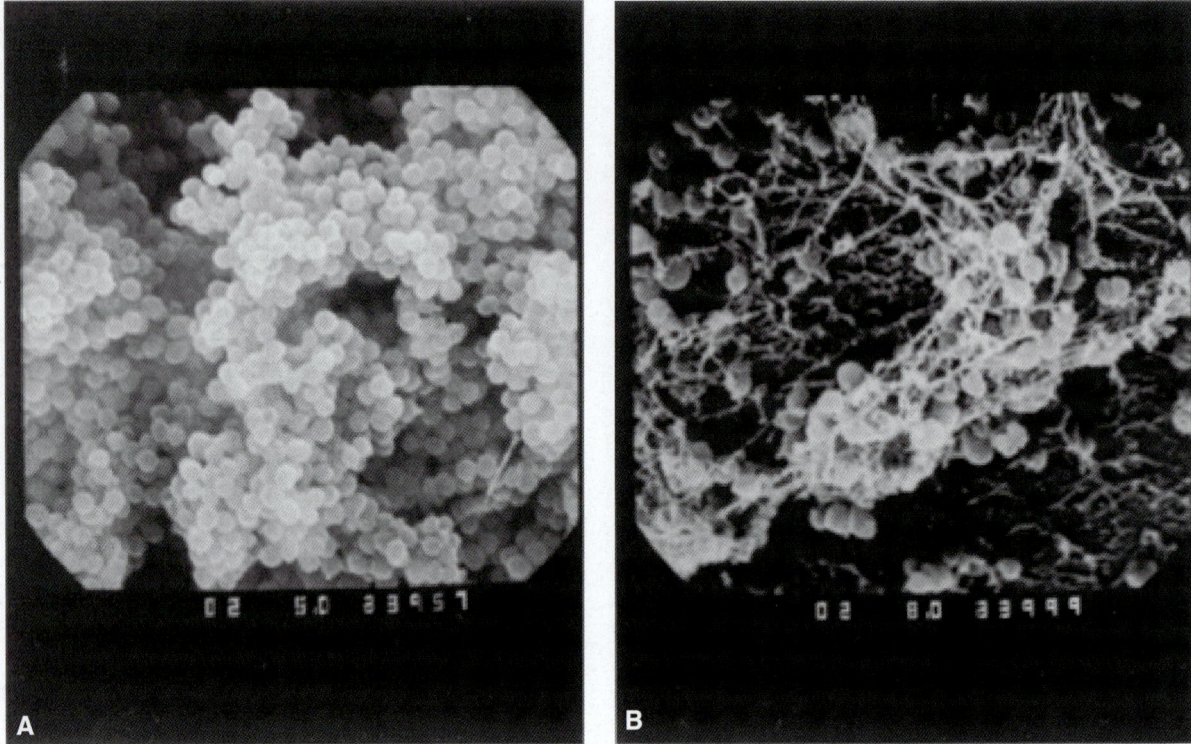

Figure 17 Scanning electron microscopy of **A**, an untreated biofilm of *Staphylococcus epidermidis* and **B**, an identical biofilm exposed to vancomycin and rifampin for 72 hours at concentrations exceeding the minimum inhibitory concentration and minimum bactericidal concentration for the organism. Reproduced with permission from Dunne WM et al.[710]

were unaltered. The observed resistance to vancomycin and rifampin was attributed to the biofilm microenvironment, altered bacterial metabolism, and EPS barrier protection.[710] The mechanisms responsible for the resistance to antimicrobial agents may include the following: (1) resistance associated with the extracellular polymeric matrix; (2) resistance associated with growth rate and nutrient availability; and (3) resistance associated with the adoption of resistance phenotype. Factors responsible for antimicrobial resistance in biofilm bacteria are shown in Figure 18. Although there are evidences to support each of these mechanisms, no single mechanism may account for the general resistance to antimicrobials. It is apparent that these mechanisms act in concert within the biofilm and amplify the effect of small variations in susceptible phenotypes.[710] Schematic diagrams of the hypothesized mechanisms of antimicrobial resistance in biofilm bacteria are shown in Figure 19.

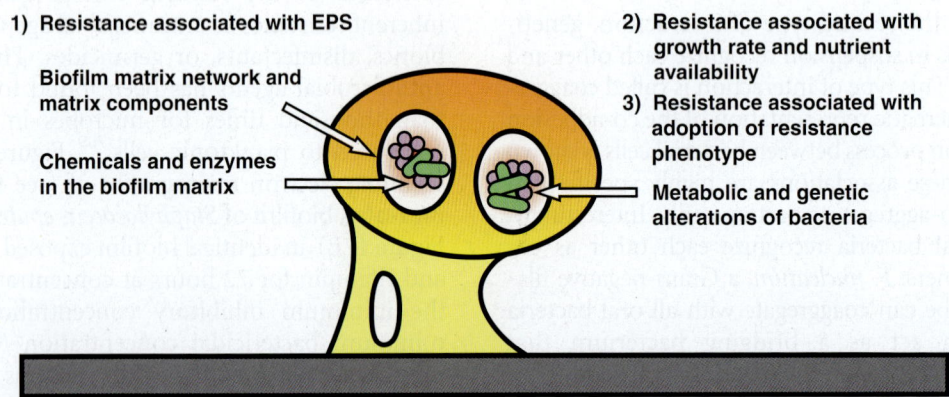

Figure 18 Schematic diagram showing factors contributing to resistance against antimicrobial agents. Courtesy A. Kishen.

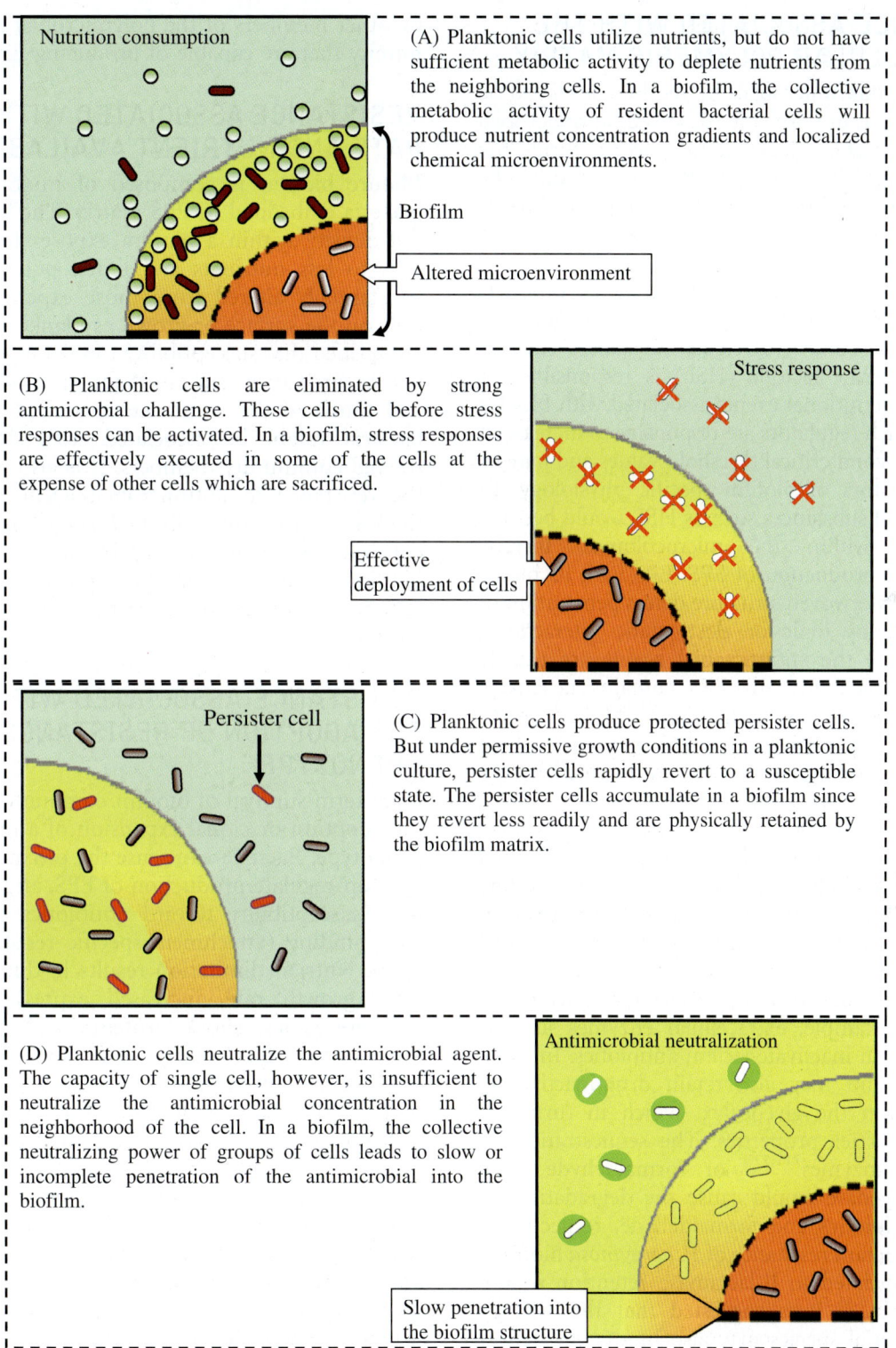

Figure 19 Schematic diagrams of some hypothesized mechanisms of antimicrobial resistance in biofilm bacteria. These schematics show how **A,** Altered microenvironment **B,** effective deployment of cells **C,** production of persister cells and **D,** slow penetration of antimicrobial agents into the biofilm leads to antimicrobial resistance in biofilm bacteria. Reproduced with permission from Cunningham AI et al.[684]

RESISTANCE ASSOCIATED WITH THE EXTRACELLULAR POLYMERIC MATRIX

Inactivation of antimicrobials by the EPS is said to be an important cause for the observed antimicrobial resistance in biofilm bacteria. EPS, which forms the biofilm matrix, has the potential to modify the response of the biofilm bacteria to antimicrobial treatments through its action as a diffusion barrier and reaction sink (neutralizer). The latter function is enhanced by the retention of extracellular products and enzymes. It has been suggested that regulation of EPS under the control of signal substances such as N-acyl hemoserine lactone (HSL) is responsible for the early transcriptional events associated with biofilm formation. Such regulators are responsive to increase in cell density beyond critical threshold values and may be general regulators of biofilm specific physiology. In biofilms, signal substances such as HSL would become concentrated within the microcolonies, thereby increasing the production of EPS. EPS with its highly charged and interwoven structure deters penetration of antimicrobials by ionic or electrostatic interactions. This is because the antimicrobial agents are usually positively charged and the EPS contains negatively charged or neutral polysaccharides.[680,684,711,712] Antibiotics such as aminoglycosides, which are hydrophilic and positively charged molecules, are retarded by the biofilm matrix for the above reason.[713]

The constituents of biofilm matrix polymer may react chemically and directly neutralize antimicrobial agents such as iodine, iodine–polyvinylpyrrolidone complexes, chlorine, and peroxygens.[714] Inactivation of antibiotics by the modified enzymes produced by the bacteria in a biofilm state has also been reported. High concentration of enzymes released by bacteria, for example, extracellular enzymes such as β-lactamase, can inactivate lactam antibiotics. In addition, the biofilm may also retain drug-inactivating enzymes within the glycocalyx, which in turn will amplify its barrier properties. The sequestration of β-lactamase enzymes[711,715] or formaldehyde lyase and dehydrogenase would cause the degradation of β-lactam antibiotics and formaldehyde, respectively. Thus, the β-lactam resistance of P. aeruginosa biofilms has been associated to β-lactamase retention in the biofilm matrix.[716] It is suggested that the synergy between bacterial species may also hinder the action of antimicrobials. For instance, E. faecalis can inactivate metronidazole, thereby protecting B. fragilis found in a multispecies biofilm.[717] In another example, Klebsiella aerogenes, which produce only limited EPS matrix, are protected from antimicrobial agents by other members of the polymicrobial biofilm community that are capable of producing EPS.[678]

RESISTANCE ASSOCIATED WITH GROWTH RATE AND NUTRIENT AVAILABILITY

Mature biofilm is composed of multiple layers of bacteria embedded in EPS matrix. The localized high cell density within a biofilm exposes the deep-lying cells to less nutrients and redox potential that are substantially altered from those experienced by the cells on the surface or grown as planktonic cells. It is established that susceptibility toward most antimicrobial agents varies as a direct function of growth rate, and much of the resistance associated with biofilm bacteria might be associated with slow growing, starved community members. It is also observed that the resistance to antimicrobial agents increases in thicker biofilms due to limited oxygen. Because nutrient and gaseous gradients will increase in extent as biofilm thickens and matures, growth rate effect on antimicrobial resistance is particularly marked in aged biofilm.[684]

RESISTANCE ASSOCIATED WITH THE ADOPTION OF RESISTANCE PHENOTYPE

Long-term survival of biofilm communities results in the adoption or clonal expansion of a more resistant phenotype. Bacteria can sense the proximity of a surface, up-regulate production of EPS, and rapidly alter their susceptibility toward antibiotics and biocides after binding (attachment-specific resistance phenotype). Nutrient limitation results in diminished bacterial growth rate, increased expression of stress response genes, shock proteins, and activation of multi-drug efflux pump. The above factors can enhance the antibiotic resistance of bacteria in a biofilm.[712] Also, sub-lethal concentration of antibiotics and biocides may act as inducers/transcriptional activators of more tolerant phenotypes such as those expressing multi-drug resistance operon and efflux pumps. It has been suggested that certain bacterial cells living in a biofilm community, when exposed to unfavorable stress or low-level antimicrobials formed specialized survivor cells called persistent cells or persistors.[679] The persistors are phenotypic variants that can regenerate the original population. Following removal of unfavorable stresses, the persistor cells would grow rapidly in the presence of nutrients released from the lysed community partners. Biofilm population are enriched in persistor cells; these cells would survive treatment procedures and proliferate in the post-treatment phase. Figure 19 shows how different regions in the structure of a matured biofilm contributed differently to its antimicrobial resistance.[684]

Biofilms in Dentistry

Oral bacteria have the capacity to form biofilms on distinct surfaces ranging from hard to soft tissues. The characteristics of the biofilm formed depend upon the residing bacterial species, the surface or substratum composition, and the conditioning layer coating the surfaces on which they are formed. Oral biofilms are formed in three basic steps, namely, pellicle formation, bacterial colonization, and biofilm maturation. These stages do not occur randomly but involves series of complex interactions.[519,718] Water constitutes 80% of the oral biofilm, while the organic and inorganic (solid) fractions form approximately 20% of the biofilm structure. Microorganisms, which makeup at least 70% to 80% of the solid fraction of the biofilm, are higher in the subgingival biofilm than in the supragingival biofilm. The chemical composition of biofilm differs among individuals, between tooth surfaces, in an individual and with age. The organic substance surrounds the microorganisms of the biofilm and contains primarily carbohydrates, proteins, and lipids. Carbohydrates are produced by many bacteria, and they include glucans, fructans, or levans. They contribute to the adherence of microorganisms to each other and are the stored form of energy in biofilm bacteria. The proteins found in the supragingival biofilm are derived from saliva, while the proteins in the subgingival biofilm are derived from gingival sulcular fluid. The lipid content may include endotoxins (LPS) from Gram-negative bacteria. The inorganic elements found in a biofilm are calcium, phosphorus, magnesium, and fluoride. The concentrations of these inorganic elements are higher in biofilm than in saliva.[719] The typical structure and development of biofilms have been discussed earlier in this chapter.

Human saliva contains proline-rich proteins that aggregate together to form micelle like globules called salivary micelle-like globules (SMGs). SMGs from saliva get adsorbed to the clean tooth surface to form acquired enamel pellicle, which acts as a "foundation" for the future multilayered biofilm.[718,720] The globular micelles of acquired enamel pellicles are characterized by a negatively charged (calcium binding) surface and hydrophobic interior.[720] Presence of calcium facilitates the formation of larger globules by bridging the negative charges on the subunits.[721] The initial attachment of bacteria to the pellicle is by selective adherence of specific bacteria from oral environment. Innate characteristics of the bacteria and the pellicle determine the adhesive interactions that cause a specific organism to adhere to the pellicle. Dental biofilm consists of a complex mixture of microorganisms that occur primarily as microcolonies. The population density is very high and increases as biofilm ages. The prospect of developing dental caries or gingivitis increases as the number of microorganisms increases.

The acquired pellicle attracts Gram-positive cocci such as S. mutans and S. sanguis, which are the pioneer organisms in the plaque formation. Subsequently, filamentous bacterium such as F. nucleatum and slender rods adheres to primary colonizers. Gradually, the filamentous form grows into the cocci layer and replaces many of the cocci. Vibrios and spirochetes appear as the biofilm thickens. More and more Gram-negative and anaerobic organisms emerge as the biofilm matures. Interestingly, it is not only the surface of tooth that can be attached by bacterial cells.[519] The surface of some bacteria (bacilli and spirochetes) also can serve as attachment sites for certain smaller coccoids. This coaggregation of F. nucleatum with coccoid bacteria gives rise to "corncob" structure, which is unique in plaque biofilms.[722] The presence of these bacteria makes it possible for other non-aggregating bacteria to coexist in the biofilm, by acting as coaggregating bridges. The existence of anaerobic bacteria in an aerobic environment is made possible by the coexistence of aerobic and anaerobic bacteria.[723]

Calcified dental biofilm is termed as calculus. It is formed by the precipitation of calcium phosphates within the organic plaque matrix. Factors that regulate the deposition of minerals on dental biofilms are physicochemical factors such as plaque pH, local saturation of Ca, P, and availability of fluoride ions and biological factors such as presence of crystallization nucleators/inhibitors from either bacteria or oral fluids.[724,725] The localized supersaturation of calcium and phosphate ions provides the driving force for mineralization. The inorganic or mineral fraction consists of calcium phosphates, magnesium, fluoride, and carbonate,[726] and they make up 70% to 80% weight of dental calculus. Various mineral phases namely, HAP, whitlockite, octacalcium phosphate, and brushite have been reported in calculus.[727]

While much emphasis is placed on the adverse effects of biofilms and the difficulty in treating biofilm-mediated diseases, it must be understood that the biofilm formed by commensals are protective in nature. The commensal bacterial biofilms inhibits

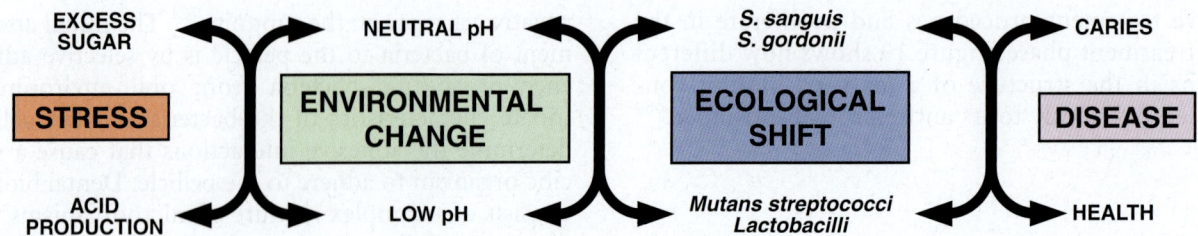

Figure 20 The ecological plaque hypothesis showing the postulated dynamic relationship between environmental factors and ecological shifts with dental caries. Reproduced with permission from Marsh PD, et al.[728]

colonization by exogenous pathogenic microorganisms by a phenomenon termed colonization resistance. For instance, dental biofilm (plaque) formed on the tooth surface is harmless under normal conditions. Nevertheless, a shift in microenvironment due to repeated use of "habit forming" substances, diet, and host immune response can lead to biofilm-mediated infections or diseases in the oral cavity. According to the "ecological plaque hypothesis," any environmental change that favors increasing colonization by potential pathogenic bacteria would cause disease.[519,718,725,728,729]

A decline in the host defense mechanisms caused by disease or immuno-suppressive medicaments may also render generally "harmless commensals" to become "opportunistic pathogens." Type of nutrients, availability of nutrients, and oxygen tension could determine the nature of bacteria associated with a biofilm at any particular location in the oral cavity. Subsequently, the nature and activity of bacteria associated with site-specific biofilms manifest as various dental infections. Some studies have emphasized the importance of an individual's threshold value of tolerance to these bacteria as the crucial factor in the shift from health to disease.[730,731] Dental caries, gingivitis, periodontitis, peri-implantitis, and periapical (apical) periodontitis are examples of diseases caused by biofilm community (biofilm-mediated disease) rather than any single organism (Koch's postulate).[728,729] Figure 20 illustrates the ecological plaque hypothesis showing the postulated dynamic relationship between environmental factors and ecological shifts in a dental biofilm with dental caries.

ENDODONTIC BIOFILMS

Endodontic microbiota is established to be less diverse compared to the oral microbiota. This transition in the microbial population is more conspicuous with the progression of infection.[520] Progression of infection alters the nutritional and environmental status within the root canal. The root canal environment apparently becomes more anaerobic and the nutritional level will be depleted. These changes will offer a tough ecological niche for the surviving microorganisms.[112,732] Furthermore, clinical investigations have shown that the complete disinfection of root canal is very difficult to achieve. Microbes are found to persist in the anatomical complexities such as isthmuses and deltas and in the apical portion of root canal system. Often, bacterial activities may not be confined to intracanal spaces, but also access regions beyond the apical foramen.[732,594] These anatomical and geometrical complexities in the root canal systems shelter the adhering bacteria from cleaning and shaping procedures.[594] Because biofilm is the manner of bacterial growth to survive unfavorable environmental and nutritional conditions, the root canal environment in both primary and post-treatment infections will favor biofilm formation. Additionally, biofilm mode of bacterial growth offers other advantages such as (1) resistance to antimicrobial agents, (2) increase in the local concentration of nutrients, (3) opportunity for genetic material exchange, (4) ability to communicate between bacterial populations of same and/or different species, and (5) produce growth factors across species boundaries. Endodontic bacterial biofilms can be categorized as (1) intracanal biofilms, (2) extra radicular biofilms, (3) periapical biofilms, and (4) biomaterial centered infections.

INTRACANAL MICROBIAL BIOFILMS

Intracanal microbial biofilms are microbial biofilms formed on the root canal dentine of an endodontically infected tooth. A detailed description on the intracanal bacterial biofilm was documented by Nair in 1987.[733] Ultra-microscopic structure of the intracanal biofilm formed on uninstrumented portion of the root canal are shown in Figure 21. It was suggested that the intracanal microbiota in an endodontically infected teeth existed as both loose collection and biofilm structures, made up of cocci, rods, and filamentous bacteria. Monolayer and/or multi-layered bacterial biofilms were found to adhere to the dentinal wall of the root canal. The extracellular matrix material of bacterial origin was also found interspersed with the cell aggregates in the biofilm.

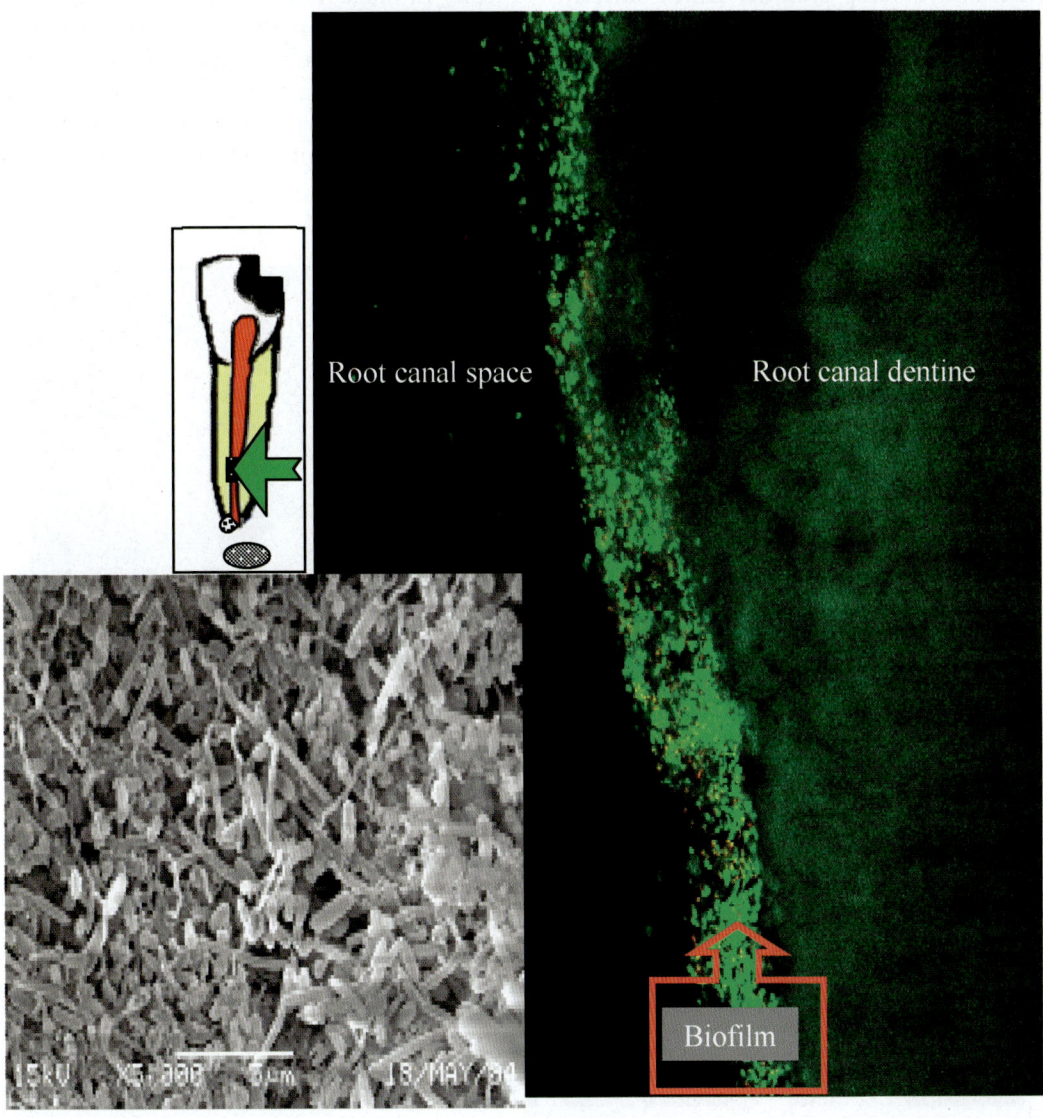

Figure 21 Endodontic intracanal microbial biofilm in a tooth with periradicular (apical) periodontitis. **A,** SEM image showing the multi-species nature of the intracanal biofilm. **B,** Laser scanning confocal microscopic image of the intracanal biofilm. Green cells on the root canal wall indicate viable cells in the biofilm. Courtesy A. Kishen unpublished.

Different morphologically distinct types of bacteria were observed in these biofilms. Bacterial microcolonies formed by the coaggregation of single morphological type and/or several morphological types of bacteria were noticed. In a multispecies biofilm, the proportion and number of different bacterial species varied according to the stage of maturation. Intracanal biofilms displayed characteristic bacteria–dentine wall relationship and distinct patterns in the organization of microbes in the biofilm. The characteristic features in cell–cell and microbe–substrate interactions were explained based on the phenomena of microbial adherence.[262,733]

Studies have established the ability of E. faecalis to resist starvation and develop biofilms under different environmental and nutrient conditions (aerobic, anaerobic, nutrient-rich, and nutrient-deprived conditions). However, the physicochemical properties of E. faecalis biofilms were noted to modify according to the prevailing environmental and nutrient conditions.

E. faecalis under nutrient-rich environment (aerobic and anaerobic) produced typical biofilm structures with characteristic surface aggregates of bacterial cells and water channels. Viable bacterial cells were present on the surface of the biofilm. Under nutrient-deprived environment (aerobic and anaerobic), irregular growth of adherent cell clumps were observed. The ultrastructure of E. faecalis biofilms formed on root dentine under different environmental and nutritional conditions is shown in Figure 22.[593] Laser scanning confocal microscopy displayed many dead bacterial cells and pockets of viable bacterial cells in this biofilm structure. In vitro experiments have revealed distinct stages in the development of E. faecalis biofilm on root canal dentine. In stage 1, E. faecalis cells adhered and formed microcolonies on the root canal dentine surface. In stage 2, they induced bacterial-mediated dissolution of the mineral fraction from the dentine substrate. This localized increase in the calcium and phosphate ions will promote mineralization (or calcification) of the

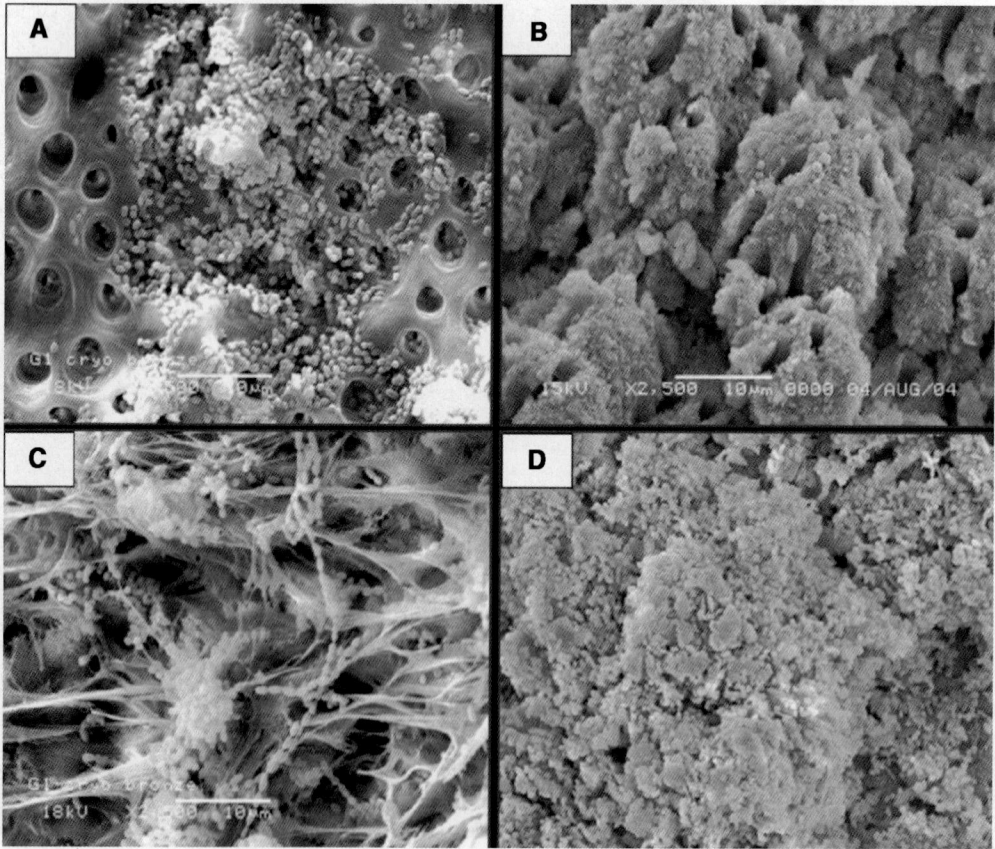

Figure 22 Scanning electron microscopy images showing the morphology of Enterococcus faecalis biofilms formed on root canal dentine under **A**, nutrient-deprived condition after 1 week, **B**, nutrient-deprived condition after 4 weeks, **C**, nutrient-rich condition after 1 week, and **D**, nutrient-rich condition after 4 weeks. Reproduced with permission from Kishen A, et al.[556]

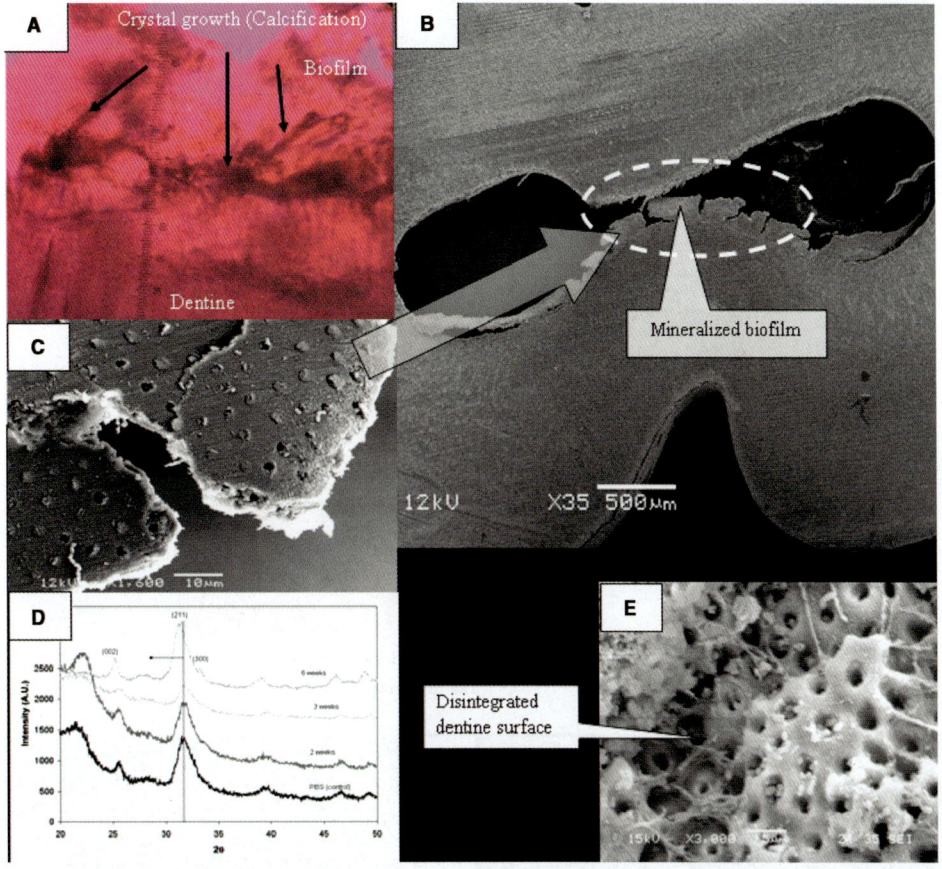

Figure 23 Cross-section of a tooth specimen incubated with *Enterococcus faecalis* for 6 weeks in vitro **A,** The ultrastructure of a typical mature *E. faecalis* biofilm on root canal dentine under light microscopy **B,** and **C,** scanning electron microscopy (SEM). X-ray diffraction spectra of *E. faecalis* biofilm at different time intervals **D,** SEM image showing *E. faecalis*-mediated dentine disintegration (E). Reproduced with permission from Kishen A, et al.[725]

E. faecalis biofilm in stage 3. The mature biofilm structure formed after 6 weeks of incubation showed signs of mineralization and subtle but distinct compositional difference (Figure 23A–D). The mineralized *E. faecalis* biofilm showed carbonated-apatite structure as compared to natural dentine which had carbonated-flor-apatite structure.[594] There were obvious signs of dentine surface degradation under nutrient-deprived environment (see Figure 23(A–C)). This degradation of dentine substrate was understood to be a consequence of the interaction of bacteria and their metabolic products on dentine.[594] A recent investigation has highlighted the ability of *E. faecalis* clinical isolate to coaggregate with *F. nucleatum*. The coaggregation interactions between *E. faecalis* and *F. nucleatum* suggested the ability of these microorganisms to coexist in a microbial community and contribute to endodontic infection.[527] The inherent capacity of *E. faecalis* to resist the bactericidal action of many antimicrobial agents,[734] along with its ability to form distinct biofilm under tough environmental and nutrient conditions, may contribute to its persistence in endodontically treated teeth.

Interestingly, the calcification of bacterial biofilms and bacterial-mediated dentine degradation observed

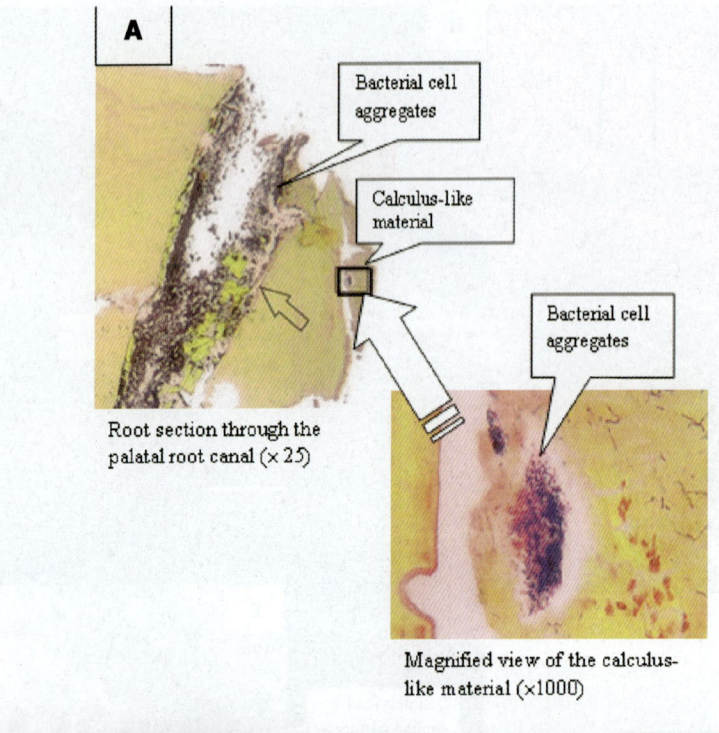

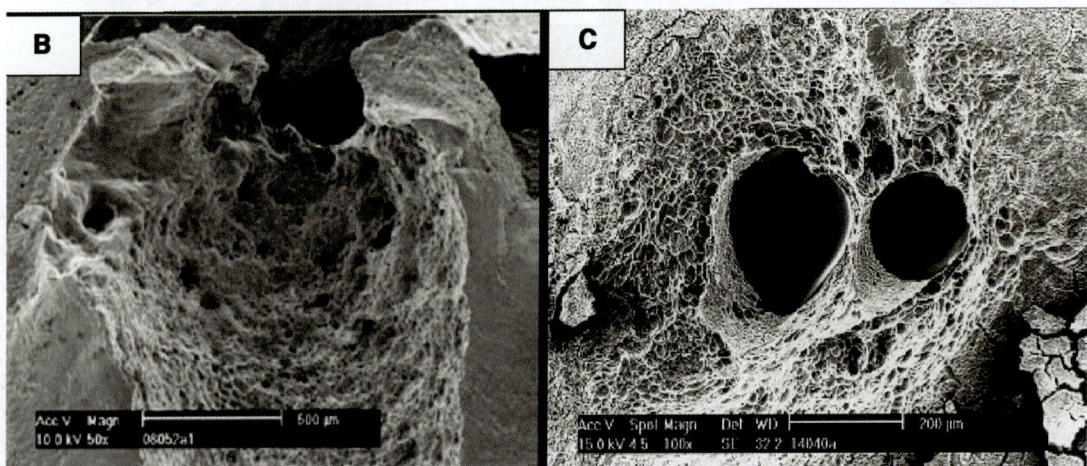

Figure 24 A calculus-like material on the external root surface in a clinical sample **A,** Magnified view showed bacterial aggregates in the deeper aspect of the amorphous material, Ricucci D, et al.[735] Scanning electron microscopy images showing apical portion of root canal with extensive internal apical resorption of the root canal, Vier FV and Figueiredo JA,[735] **B,** and root apex with extensive periforaminal and foraminal resorption exposing dentinal tubules **C,** Reproduced with permission from Vier FV and Figueiredo JA.[737]

in vitro were supported by clinical evidences. Two clinical cases were reported with mineralized calculus-like deposit on the root surface of teeth with post-treatment periapical periodontitis[735] (Figure 24A). While internal resorption of root canal dentine was reported in 74.7% of teeth associated with periapical lesions.[736] These resorptive lesions were mostly observed in the apical portion of the root canal (see Figure 24B). In another study, periforaminal resorption was reported in 87.3% and foraminal resorption in 83.2% of roots from 104 root apices extracted from teeth with periapical lesions[737] (see Figure 24C). Bearing in mind the complexities in the apical root canal anatomy, and the length and lateral limits of cleaning and shaping apical root canal, incomplete elimination of bacteria from the apical region of the root canal is very likely.[736] Investigations have also demonstrated biting force-induced retrograde fluid movement into the apical portion of the root canal (apical retrograde fluid movement).[738] Cyclic influx of ion-rich tissue fluid into the apical portion of the root canal can promote persistence of bacteria as biofilms and their mineralization, while the observed internal resorption can be a consequence of bacterial-mediated substrate dissolution.

EXTRARADICULAR MICROBIAL BIOFILMS

Extraradicular microbial biofilms also termed root surface biofilms are microbial biofilms formed on the root (cementum) surface adjacent to the root apex of endodontically infected teeth.[349] Extraradicular biofilms were reported in teeth with asymptomatic periapical periodontitis and teeth with chronic apical abscesses associated with sinus tracts. In this study, Tronstad et al. examined 10 root tips removed during surgical treatment of root-filled teeth with post-treatment disease (five teeth with the diagnosis of asymptomatic apical periodontitis and five teeth with the diagnosis of apical periodontitis with fistula). Mature bacterial biofilms were found in many areas of the apical root surfaces in all clinical specimens examined in this study. They observed bacterial biofilms in the areas of the root surfaces between fibers and cells and in crypts and holes. The biofilm contained varying degrees of extracellular matrix materials (glycocalyx). The root surface biofilms were mostly multispecies in nature.[348]

The extraradicular biofilm structures were dominated by cocci and short rods, with cocci attached to the tooth substrate. Filamentous and fibrillar forms were also observed in the biofilm. Ultrastructure of extraradicular biofilms formed on the root surface adjacent to the apical foramen is shown in Figure 25. A smooth, structureless biofilm structure consisting of extracellular matrix material with embedded bacterial cells was noticed to coat the apex of the root tip adjacent to the apical foramen. There was no obvious difference in the biofilm structures formed on the apical root surface of teeth with and without sinus tracts.[348] Clinical evidence of calcified biofilms on the extraradicular region was also reported. Ricucci et al.[735] has reported the presence of calculus-like deposit on the root apex of teeth extracted due to post-treatment periapical periodontitis. While Harn et al. noticed calculus-like deposits on apical root surface of tooth presented with lesion refractory to conventional root canal treatment. These calcified biofilms were

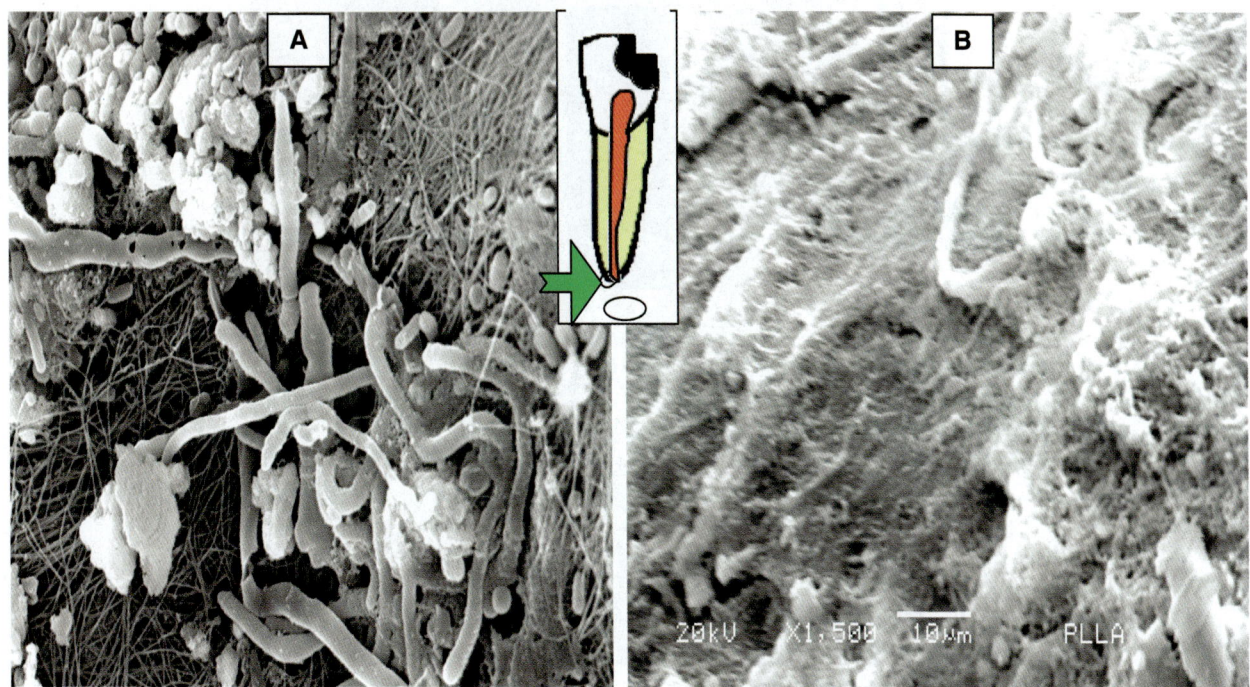

Figure 25 Extraradicular microbial biofilm formed on the root surface. It is **A,** multispecies or **B,** smooth and structureless in nature Courtesy A. Kishen unpublished.

associated with periapical inflammation and delayed periapical healing in spite of adequate orthograde root canal treatment.[739]

PERIAPICAL MICROBIAL BIOFILMS

Periapical microbial biofilms are isolated biofilms found in the periapical region of an endodontically infected teeth. Periapical biofilms may or may not be dependent on the root canal. The microbiota in the majority of teeth associated with apical periodontitis is restricted to the root canal, as most of the microbial species that infect the root canal are opportunistic pathogens that do not have the ability to survive host defense mechanism in the periapical tissues.[315] Rarely microbial species or even strains within a species may possess strategies to survive and thus infect periapical tissues.[352] Members of the genus *Actinomyces* and the species *P. propionicum* have been demonstrated in asymptomatic periapical lesions refractory to endodontic treatment. These microorganisms have the ability to overcome host defense mechanisms, thrive in the inflamed periapical tissue, and subsequently induce a periapical infection.[641,740,741] A clinical investigation detected *Actinomyces* in 72 of 129 (55.8%) clinical samples. Of those, 41 of 51 (80.4%) were from infected root canals, 22 of 48 (45.8%) were from abscesses, and 9 of 30 (30%) were associated with cellulites.[1]

Actinomyces species in tissues grow in microscopic or macroscopic aggregates, which may reach diameter of up to 3 to 4mm.[742] They are commonly referred to as "sulfur granules," because of the yellow granular appearance.[355] Microscopically, the granules give the appearance of rays projecting out from a central mass of filaments, which gave origin to the name "ray fungus" or *Actinomyces*. This granular biofilm structure consists of a central mass of intertwined branching bacterial filaments, held together by an extracellular matrix with the peripheral radiating clubs. The aggregation of *Actinomyces* cells were influenced by pH, ionic strength, and cell concentration.[743] Aggregation of cells might facilitate accumulation of cells to form a biofilm structure that differentiate, communicate, cooperate, and deploy collective defense against biological antimicrobials. It is important to note that the periapical region is "patrolled" by PMNs and macrophages, which phagocytose incoming planktonic bacteria easily.

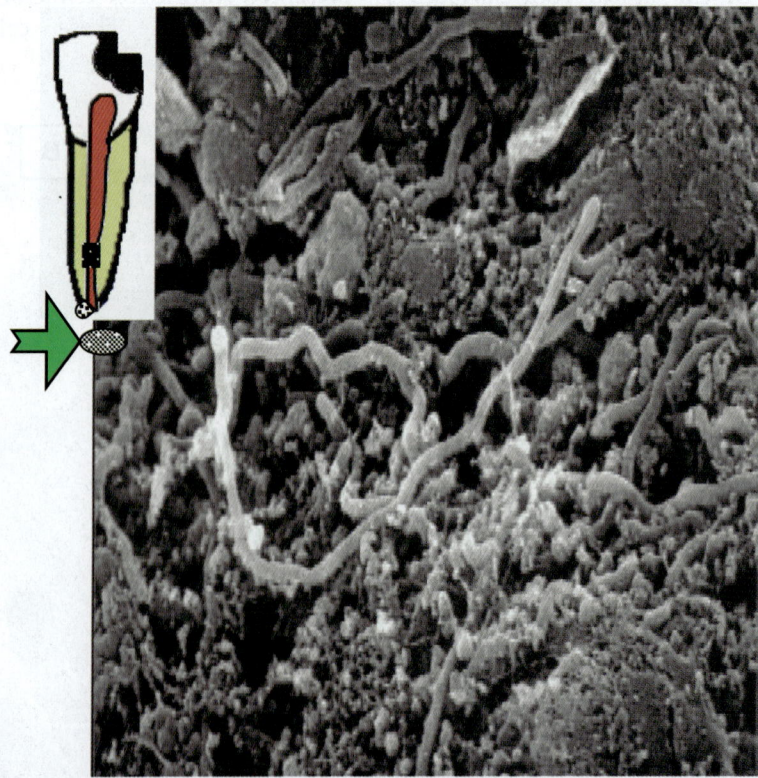

Figure 26 Endodontic periapical microbial biofilm. SEM image of the sectioned surfaces of sulfur granules showing rod-like bacteria, spiral-form bacteria, and an amorphous material between the cells. Large amounts of partly calcified extracellular material are present. Reproduced with permission from Sunde PT et al.[333]

However, the phagocytes are unable to engulf bacteria in matrix-enclosed biofilm structure.

Sunde et al. reported the incidence of "sulfur granules" in nine refractory periapical lesions and found bacteria in seven. *A. israelii*, *A. viscosus*, *A. naeslundii*, and *Actinomyces meyeri* were identified in five granules. Other bacterial species, both Gram-positive and Gram-negative, were detected in the granules as well. Two sulfur granules did not contain *Actinomyces*. SEM demonstrated rod- and spirochete-like cells in the granules, and transmission electron microscopy revealed organisms with abundant extracellular material. Many of the "sulfur granules" were calcified and the source for mineralization may have been the inflammatory exudate and/or the activity of the periapical bacteria. Although "sulfur granules" have been considered as suggestive of actinomycosis, it was confirmed that other species can form aggregates that are similar to those formed by *Actinomyces* species and *P. propionicum* (see Figure 26).[740,743] Granular biofilm structures, resembling sulfur granules, were also observed in vitro by the clumping and calcification of *E. faecalis* cells on the dentine surface. It has been shown that the lysis of adherent bacterial cells in a biofilm would induce cell calcification.[744] The calcium–phospholipid–phosphate complexes and calcifiable proteolipid, which are membrane constituents of calcified bacteria, can support biomineralization.[745]

BIOMATERIAL-CENTERED INFECTION

Biomaterial-centred infection (BCI) is caused when bacteria adheres to an artificial biomaterial surface and forms biofilm structures.[746] Presence of biomaterials in close proximity to the host immune system can increase the susceptibility to BCI. BCI is one of the major complications associated with prosthesis and/or implant-related infections. Chronic bacterial infections occur when the pathogenic bacterial population reaches a critical size and overcomes the host defense mechanisms. Both specific and non-specific interactions play important roles in the ability of the bacteria to adhere to the biomaterial surface. The comparative contribution of specific and non-specific mechanisms depends on the surface properties of the biomaterial as well as the fluid flow conditions and the nature of liquid conditioning layer. Because biofilms are extremely resistant to host defense mechanisms and antibiotic treatments, BCI are rarely resolved, and often the only solution to an infected biomaterial such as implant is its surgical removal.[747]

BCI usually reveals opportunistic invasion by nosocomial organisms. Coagulase-negative *Staphylococcus*, *S. aureus*, enterococci, streptococci, *P. aeruginosa*, and fungi are commonly isolated from infected biomaterial surfaces. Bacterial adherence to a biomaterial surface is also described in three phases—(1) phase 1: transport of bacteria to biomaterial surface, (2) phase 2: initial, non-specific adhesion phase, and (3) phase 3: specific adhesion phase. Details about bacteria–substrate interaction have been discussed in "Development of Biofilm." Concentration of electrolytes and pH value of the environment influence bacterial adherence to biomaterial surface by changing the surface characteristics of both bacteria and biomaterial.[748] Bacterial strains that do not produce EPS are less adherent and less pathogenic. Bacteria that do not adhere quickly to the surfaces are rapidly destroyed by the immune system. These features highlight the need to prevent bacterial adherence and biofilm formation to prevent BCI.

In endodontics, biomaterial-centered biofilms would form on root canal obturating materials. These biofilms can be intraradicular or extraradicular depending upon whether the obturating material is within the root canal space or has it extruded beyond the root apex. A study investigated the initial biofilm-forming ability of root canal isolates such as *E. faecalis*, *S. sanguinis*, *S. intermedius*, *S. pyogenes*, *S. aureus*, *F. nucleatum*, *P. acnes*, *P. gingivalis*, and *P. intermedia* on gutta-percha points in vitro. It was shown that *E. faecalis*, *S. sanguinis*, *S. intermedius*, *S. pyogenes*, and *S. aureus* developed biofilms on the surfaces of gutta-percha incubated in culture medium supplemented with 45% or 90% (vol/vol) serum. The *E. faecalis* and *S. sanguinis* biofilms were significantly thicker than those of *S. intermedius*, *S. pyogenes*, and *S. aureus*. *F. nucleatum*, *P. acnes*, *P. gingivalis*, and *P. intermedia* did not form biofilms on gutta-percha. The findings from this study suggested that Gram-positive facultative anaerobes have the ability to colonize and form extracellular matrices on gutta-percha points, while serum plays a crucial role in biofilm formation.[749] In a clinical investigation, six teeth and five extruded gutta-percha points associated with refractory periapical disease were investigated. Nine out of eleven samples examined showed bacterial biofilms in the extraradicular region. The gutta-percha surface was covered with glycocalyx-like structures. Filaments, long rods, and spirochete-shaped bacteria were predominant in the biofilm formed on gutta-percha.[349] Figure 27 shows the ultrastructure of (see Figure 27A) a microbial biofilm formed on extruded gutta-percha point in vivo and (see Figure 27B) *E. faecalis* biofilm formed on gutta-percha point in vitro. This study suggested that the extraradicular microbial biofilms formed on tissue or biomaterial surface were related to refractory periapical disease.[348]

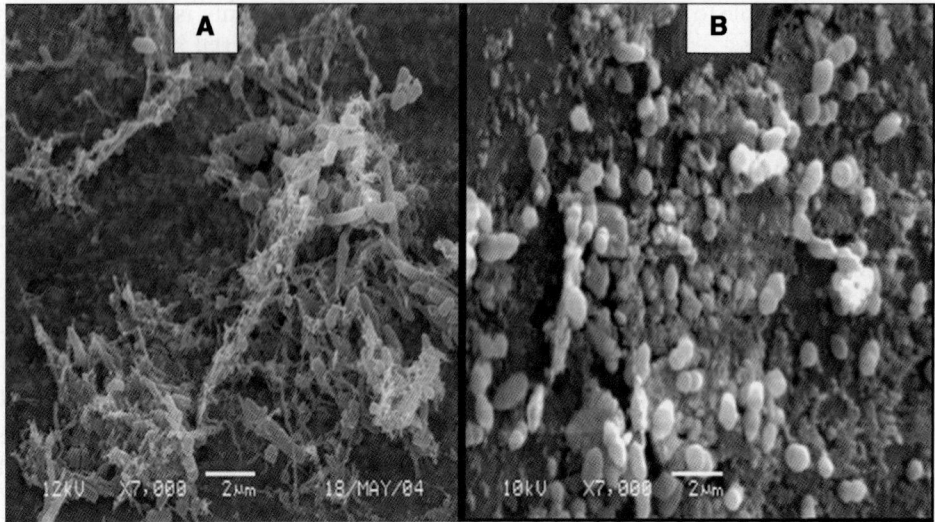

Figure 27 Scanning electron microscopy image of **A**, microbial biofilm formed on extruded gutta-percha point from a clinical sample and **B**, *E. faecalis* biofilm formed on gutta-percha in vitro. Courtesy A. Kishen.

References

1. Baumgartner JC, Watts CM, Xia T. Occurrence of *Candida albicans* in infections of endodontic origin. J Endod 2000;26(12):695–8.
2. Glick M, Trope M, Pliskin M. Detection of HIV in the dental pulp of a patient with AIDS. J Am Dent Assoc 1989;119:649–50.
3. Glick M, Trope M, Pliskin E. Human immunodeficiency virus infection of fibroblasts of dental pulp in seropositive patients. Oral Surg Oral Med Oral Pathol Oral Radiol Endod 1991;71:733–5.
4. Nair PNR, Sjögren U, Krey G, Sundqvist G. Therapy-resistant foreign body giant cell granuloma at the periapex of a root-filled human tooth. J Endod 1990;16:589–95.
5. Sabeti M, Valles Y, Nowzari H, et al. Cytomegalovirus and Epstein-Barr virus DNA transcription in endodontic symptomatic lesions. Oral Microbiol Immunol 2003;18:104–8.
6. Sabeti M, Slots J. Herpesviral-bacterial coinfection in periapical pathosis. J Endod 2004;30(2):69–72.
7. Sen BH, Piskin B, Demirci T. Observation of bacteria and fungi in infected root canals and dentinal tubules by SEM. Dent Traumatol 1995;11(1):6–9.
8. Sen BH, Safavi KE, Spangberg LSW. Growth patterns of *Candida albicans* in relation to radicular dentin. Oral Surg Oral Med Oral Pathol Oral Radiol Endod 1997;84(1):68–73.
9. Slots J, Nowzari H, Sabeti M. Cytomegalovirus infection in symptomatic periapical pathosis. Int Endod J 2004;37:519–24.
10. Pallasch TJ, Wahl MJ. Focal infection: new age or ancient history? Endod Top 2003;4:32–45.
11. Francke OC. William Hunter's "oral sepsis" and American odontology. Bull Hist Dent 1973;21:73–9.
12. Billings F. Chronic focal infection as a causative factor in chronic authritis. J Am Med Assoc 1913;61:819–23.
13. Billings F. Focal infection: the lane medical lectures. New York: Appleton and Company; 1916.
14. Rosenow EC. Immunological and experimental studies on pneumococcus and *Staphylococcus* endocarditis. J Infect Dis 1909;6:245.
15. Rosenow EC. The relation of dental infection to systemic disease. Dental Cosmos 1917;59:485.
16. Pallasch T, Wahl M. The focal infection theory: appraisal and reappraisal. J Calif Dent Assoc 2000;28(3):194–200.
17. Hunter W. The role of sepsis and antisepsis in medicine and the importance of oral sepsis as its chief cause. Dent Register 1911;44:579–611.
18. Grossman LI. Focal infection: are oral foci of infection related to systemic disease? Dent Clin North Am 1960;4:749.
19. Price WA. Fundamentals suggested by recent researches for diagnosis, prognosis, and treatment of dental focal infections. J Am Dent Assoc 1925;12:641–65.
20. Price WA, Buckley JP. Buckley-Price debate: subject: resolved, that practically all infected pulpless teeth should be removed. J Am Dent Assoc 1925;12:1468–524.
21. Cecil RL, Angevine DM. Clinical and experimental observations on focal infection with an analysis of 200 cases of rheumatoid arthritis. Ann Intern Med 1938;12:577–84.
22. Reimann HA. Focal infection and systemic disease: a critical appraisal. J Am Med Assoc 1940;114:1–6.
23. Easlick K. An evaluation of the effect of dental foci of infection on health. J Am Dent Assoc 1951;42:694–7.
24. Fish EW. Bone infection. J Am Dent Assoc 1939;26(5):691–712.

25. Meinig GE. Root canal cover-up. 2nd ed. Ojai, CA: Bion Publishing; 1994.

26. Kulacz R, Levy TE. The roots of disease. Xlibris Corporation: Philadelphia;2002.

27. Heimdahl A, Hall G, Hedberg M, Sandberg H. Detection and quantitation by lysis-filtration of bacteremia after different oral surgical procedures. J Clin Microbiol 1990;28(10):2205–9.

28. Baumgartner JC, Heggers J, Harrison J. The incidence of bacteremias related to endodontic procedures. I. Nonsurgical endodontics. J Endod 1976;2:135–40.

29. Baumgartner JC, Heggers JP, Harrison JW. The incidence of bacteremia related to endodontic procedures. I. Nonsurgical endodontics. J Endod 1976;2:135.

30. Bender IB, Seltzer S, Yermish M. The incidence of bacteremia in endodontic manipulation. Oral Surg Oral Med Oral Pathol Oral Radiol Endod 1960;13(3):353–60.

31. Debelian GJ, Olsen I, Tronstad L. Bacteremia in conjunction with endodontic therapy. Endod Dent Traumatol 1995;11(3):142–9.

32. Savarrio L, Mackenzie D, Riggio M, et al. Detection of bacteraemias during non-surgical root canal treatment. J Dent 2005;33:293–303.

33. Cockerill FR III, Hughes JG, Vetter EA, et al. Analysis of 281,797 consecutive blood cultures performed over an eight-year period: trends in microorganisms isolated and the value of anaerobic culture of blood. Clin Infect Dis 1997;24:403–18.

34. Pallasch TJ. Antibiotic prophylaxis. Endod Topics 2003;4:46–59.

35. Pallasch TJ. Antibiotic myths and reality. J Calif Dent Assoc 1986(May):40–5.

36. Pallasch TJ, Slots J. Antibiotic prophylaxis for the medically compromised patient. Periodontol 2000 1996;10:107–38.

37. Hall G, Hedstrom SA, Heindahl A, Nord CE. Prophylactic administration of penicillins for endocarditis does not reduce the incidence of postextraction bacteremia. Clin Infect Dis 1993;17(2):188–94.

38. Hall G, Nord CE, Heimdahl A. Elimination of bacteremia after dental extraction: comparison of erythromycin and clindamycin for prophylaxis of infective endocarditis. J Antimicrob Chemother 1996;37(4):783–95.

39. Durack DT. Prevention of infective endocarditis. N Engl J Med 1995;332(1):38–44.

40. Morellion P, Francioli P, Overholser D, et al. Mechanisms of successful amoxicillin prophylaxis of experimental endocarditis due to Streptococcus intermedius. J Infect Dis 1986;154(5):801–7.

41. Pallasch T, Slots J. Oral microorganisms and cardiovascular disease. J Calif Dent Assoc 2000;28(3):204–14.

42. DeStefano F, Anda R, Kahn H, et al. Dental disease and risk of coronary heart disease and mortality. Br Dent J 1993;306:688–691.

43. Offenbacher S, Katz V, Fertik G, et al. Periodontal infection as a possible risk factor for preterm low birth weight. J Periodontol 1996;67:1103–13.

44. Hujoel PP, Drangsholt M, Spiekerman C, DeRouen TA. Periodontal disease and coronary heart disease risk. J Am Med Assoc 2000;284(11):1406–10.

45. Hujoel PP, Drangsholt M, Spiekerman C, DeRouen TA. Examining the link between coronary heart disease and the elimination of chronic dental infections. J Am Dent Assoc 2001;132:883–9.

46. Hujoel PP, Drangsholt M, Spiekerman C, DeRouen TA. Pre-existing cardiovascular disease and periodontitis: a follow-up. J Dent Res 2002;81:186–91.

47. Hujoel PP, Drangsholt M, Spiekerman C, DeRouen TA. Periodontal-systemic disease associations in the presence of smoking - causal or coincidental. Periodontol 2000 2005;30:51–60.

48. Joshipura KJ, Douglas CW. Oral and cardiovascular disease associations do not call for extraction of teeth. J Evid Based Dent Pract 2002;2:261–6.

49. Joshipura KJ, Pitiphat W, Hung H-C, et al. Pulpal inflammation and incidence of coronary heart disease. J Endod 2006;32(2):99–103.

50. Caplan DJ, Chasen JB, Krall EA, et al. Lesions of endodontic origin and risk of coronary heart disease. J Dent Res 2006;85(11):996–1000.

51. Sundqvist G, Bloom GD, Enberg K, Johansson E. Phagocytosis of *Bacteroides melaninogenicus* and *Bacteroides gingivalis in vitro* by human neutrophils. J Periodont Res 1982;17:113–21.

52. Bibel DJ. The discovery of the oral flora - a 300-year retrospective. J Am Dent Assoc 1983;107:569–70.

53. Miller WD. An introduction in the study of the bacteriopathology of the dental pulp. Dent Cosmos 1894;36:505.

54. Kakehashi S, Stanley HR, Fitzgerald R. The exposed germ-free pulp: effects of topical corticosteroid medication and restoration. Oral Surg Oral Med Oral Pathol 1969;27(1):60–7.

55. Bergenholtz G, Lindhe J. Effect of soluble plaque factors on inflammatory reactions in the dental pulp. Scand J Dent Res 1975;83:153.

56. Warfvinge J, Bergenholtz G. Healing capacity of human and monkey dental pulps following experimentally-induced pulpitis. Endo Dent Traumatol 1986;2(6):256–62.

57. Cvek M, Granath L, Lundberg M. Failures and healing in endodontically treated non-vital anterior teeth with post-traumatically reduced pulpal lumen. Acta Odontol Scand 1982;40:223–8.

58. Langeland K. Tissue changes in the dental pulp. Odontol Tidskr 1957;65(239–47).

59. Czarnecki RT, Schilder H. A histological evaluation of the human pulp in teeth with varying degrees of periodontal disease. J Endod 1979;5(8):242–53.

60. Langeland K, Rodrigues H, Dowden W. Periodontal disease, bacteria, and pulpal histopathology. Oral Surg Oral Med Oral Pathol 1974;37(2):257–70.
61. Mazur B, Massler M. Influence of periodontal disease on the dental pulp. Oral Surg Oral Med Oral Pathol Oral Radiol Endod 1964;17(5):592–603.
62. Torabinejad M, Kiger RD. A histologic evaluation of dental pulp tissue of a patient with periodontal disease. Oral Surg Oral Med Oral Pathol Oral Radiol Endod 1985;59(2):198–200.
63. Wong R, Hirsch RS, Clarke NG. Endodontic effects of root planing in humans. Endod Dent Traumatol 1989;5(4):193–6.
64. Kobayashi T, Hayashi A, Yoshikawa R, et al. The microbial flora from root canals and periodontal pockets of non-vital teeth associated with advanced periodontitis. Int Endod J 1990;23:100–6.
65. Trope M, Rosenberg E, Tronstad L. Darkfield microscopic spirochete count in the differentiation of endodontic and periodontal abscesses. J Endod 1992;18(2):82–6.
66. Allard U, Nord CE, Sjoberg L, Stromberg T. Experimental infections with *Staphylococcus aureus, Streptococcus sanguis, Pseudomonas aeruginosa,* and *Bacteroides fragilis* in the jaws of dogs. Oral Surg Oral Med Oral Pathol Oral Radiol Endod 1979;48(5):454–63.
67. Gier RE, Mitchell DF. Anachoretic effect of pulpitis. J Dent Res 1968;47:564.
68. Robinson HBG, Boling LR. The anachoretic effect in pulpitis I. Bacteriologic studies. J Am Dent Assoc 1941;28:268–70.
69. Delivanis PD, Snowden RB, Doyle RJ. Localization of blood-borne bacteria in instrumented unfilled root canals. Oral Surg Oral Med Oral Pathol Oral Radiol Endod 1981;52(4):430–2.
70. Delivanis PD, Fan VSC. The localization of blood-borne bacteria in instrumented unfilled and overinstrumented canals. J Endod 1984;10(11):521–4.
71. Grossman LI. Origin of microorganisms in traumatized pulpless sound teeth. J Dent Res 1967;46:551–3.
72. Möller AJR, Fabricius L, Dahlén G, et al. Influence on periapical tissues of indigenous oral bacteria and necrotic pulp tissue in monkeys. Scand J Dent Res 1981;89:475–84.
73. Naidorf IJ. Inflammation and infection of pulp and periapical tissues. Oral Surg Oral Med Oral Pathol Oral Radiol Endod 1972;34:486–96.
74. Sundqvist G. Ecology of the root canal flora. J Endod 1992;18(9):427–30.
75. Byström A, Happonen RP, Sjögren U, Sundqvist G. Healing of periapical lesions of pulpless teeth after endodontic treatment with controlled asepsis. Endod Dent Traumatol 1987;3:58–63.
76. Sundqvist GK. Bacteriological studies of necrotic dental pulps [Odontological dissertation no. 7]. Umea, Sweden: University of Umea; 1976.
77. Fabricius L, Dahlén G, Öhman AE, Möller ÅJR. Predominant indigenous oral bacteria isolated from infected root canals after varied times of closure. Scand J Dent Res 1982;90:134–44.
78. Fabricius L, Dahlén G, Holm SE, Möller ÅJR. Influence of combinations of oral bacteria on periapical tissues of monkeys. Scand J Dent Res 1982;90:200–6.
79. Sundqvist G, Johansson E, Sjögren U. Prevalence of black-pigmented *Bacteroides* species in root canal infections. J Endod 1989;15:13–19.
80. Baumgartner JC, Falkler WA Jr. Bacteria in the apical 5 mm of infected root canals. J Endod 1991;17(8):380–3.
81. Gomes BPFA, Drucker DB, Lilley JD. Association of specific bacteria with some endodontic signs and symptoms. Int Endod J 1994;27(6):291–8.
82. Gomes BP, Drucker DB, Lilley JD. Positive and negative associations between bacterial species in dental root canals. Microbios 1994;80(325):231–43.
83. Sundqvist GK. Associations between microbial species in dental root canal infections. Oral Microbiol Immunol 1992;7:257–62.
84. Brook I, Frazier E. Clinical features and aerobic and anaerobic microbiological characteristics of cellulitis. Arch Surg 1995;130:786–92.
85. Brook I, Frazier E, Gher MJ. Microbiology of periapical abscesses and associated maxillary sinusitis. J Periodontal 1996;67(6):608–10.
86. Drucker DB, Lilley JD, Tucker D, Gibbs CC. The endodontic microflora revisited. Microbios 1992;71:225–34.
87. Gomes BP, Lilley JD, Drucker DB. Clinical significance of dental root canal microflora. J Dent 1996;24(1–2):47–55.
88. Griffee MB, Patterson SS, Miller CH, et al. The relationship of *Bacteroides melaninogenicus* to symptoms associated with pulpal necrosis. Oral Surg Oral Med Oral Pathol Oral Radiol Endod 1980;50:457–61.
89. Haapasalo M, Ranta H, Rantah K, Shah H. Black-pigmented *Bacteroides* spp. in human apical periodontitis. Infect Immun 1986;53:149–53.
90. Haapasalo M. *Bacteroides* spp. in dental root canal infections. Endod Dent Traumatol 1989;5(1):1–10.
91. Happonen RP. Periapical actinomycosis: a follow-up study of 16 surgically treated cases. Endod Dent Traumatol 1986;2:205–9.
92. Hashioka K, Yamasaki M, Nakane A, et al. The relationship between clinical symptoms and anaerobic bacteria from infected root canals. J Endod 1992;18(11):558–61.
93. Heimdahl A, Von Konow L, Satoh T, Nord CE. Clinical appearance of orofacial infections of odontogenic origin in relation to microbiological findings. J Clin Microbiol 1985;22:299–302.

94. van Winkelhoff A, Carlee A, de Graaff J. Bacteroides endodontalis and other black-pigmented Bacteroides species in odontogenic abscesses. Infect Immun 1985;49:494–7.

95. Yoshida M, Fukushima H, Yamamoto K, et al. Correlation between clinical symptoms and microorganisms isolated from root canals of teeth with periapical pathosis. J Endod 1987;13(1):24–8.

96. Byström A, Sundqvist G. Bacteriologic evaluation of the efficacy of mechanical root canal instrumentation in endodontic therapy. Scand J Dent Res 1981;89:321–8.

97. Byström A, Sundqvist G. Bacteriologic evaluation of the effect of 0.5 percent sodium hypochlorite in endodontic therapy. Oral Surg Oral Med Oral Pathol Oral Radiol Endod 1983;55(3):307–12.

98. Byström A, Claesson R, Sandqvist G. The antibacterial effect of camphorated paramonochlorophenol, camphorted phenol and calcium hydroxide in the treatment of infected root canals. Endo Dent Traumatol 1985;5(1):170–5.

99. Shah HN, Gharbia SE. Biochemical and chemical studies on strains designated *Prevotella intermedia* and proposal of a new pigmented species, *Prevotella nigrescens* sp. nov. Int J Syst Bacteriol 1992;42(4):542–6.

100. Bae KS, Baumgartner JC, Xia T, et al. SDS-PAGE and PCR for differentation of *Prevotella intermedia* and *P. nigrescens*. J Endod 1997;25(5):324–8.

101. Bae KS, Baumgartner JC, Shearer TR, David LL. Occurrence of *Prevotella nigrescens* and *Prevotella intermedia* in infections of endodontic origin. J Endod 1997;23(10):620–3.

102. Baumgartner JC, Watkins JB, Bae KS, Xia T. Association of black-pigmented bacteria with endodontic infections. J Endod 1999;25(6):413–15.

103. Xia T, Baumgartner JC, David LL. Isolation and identification of *Prevotella tannerae* from endodontic infections. Oral Microbiol Immunol 2000;15:273–5.

104. Hancock HH 3rd, Sigurdsson A, Trope M, Moiseiwitsch J. Bacteria isolated after unsuccessful endodontic treatment in a North American population. Oral Surg Oral Med Oral Pathol Oral Radiol Endod 2001;91(5):579–86.

105. Möller ÅJR. Microbiological examination of root canals and periapical tissues of human teeth. Odontol Tidskr 1966;74:1–380.

106. Peciuliene V, Balciuniene I, Eriksen H, Haapasalo M. Isolation of *Enterococcus faecalis* in previously root-filled canals in a lithuanian. J Endod 2000;26(10):593–5.

107. Peciuliene V, Reynaud AH, Balciuniene I, Haapasalo M. Isolation of yeasts and enteric bacteria in root-filled teeth with chronic apical periodontitis. Int Endod J 2001;34:429–34.

108. Sundqvist G, Figdor D, Persson S, Sjögren U. Microbiologic analysis of teeth with failed endodontic treatment and the outcome of conservative re-treatment. Oral Surg Oral Med Oral Pathol Oral Radiol Endod 1998;85(1):86–93.

109. Siqueira JF Jr, Rocas IN. Polymerase chain reaction-based analysis of microorganisms associated with failed endodontic treatment. Oral Surg Oral Med Oral Pathol Oral Radiol Endod 2004;97(1):85–94.

110. Siqueira JF Jr, Rôças IN, Rosado AS. Investigation of bacterial communities associated with asymptomatic and symptomatic endodontic infections by denaturing gradient gel electrophoresis fingerprinting approach. Oral Microbiol Immunol 2004;19:363–70.

111. Siqueira JF Jr, Rôças IN. Exploiting molecular methods to explore endodontic infections: Part 2–redefining the endodontic microbiota. J Endod 2005;31(7):488–98.

112. Nair PNR, Sjogren U, Krey G, et al. Intraradicular bacteria and fungi in root-filled, asymptomatic human teeth with therapy-resistant periapical lesions: a long-term light and electron microscopic follow-up study. J Endod 1990;16(12):580–8.

113. Relman DA. Emerging infections and newly-recognised pathogens. Neth J Med 1997;50(5):216–20.

114. Slots J. Rapid identification of important periodontal microorganisms by cultivation. Oral Microbiol Immunol 1986;1(1):48–57.

115. Engelkirk PG, Duben-Engelkirk J, Dowell VR Jr. Principles and practice of clinical anaerobic bacteriology. Belmont, CA: Star Publishing Company; 1992.

116. Hugenholtz P, Pace NR. Identifying microbial diversity in the natural environment: a molecular phylogenetic approach. Trends Biotechnol 1996;14(6):190–7.

117. Ward DM, Weller R, Bateson MM. 16S rRNA sequences reveal numerous uncultured microorganisms in a natural community. Nature 1990;345(6270):63–5.

118. Amann RI, Ludwig W, Schleifer KH. Phylogenetic identification and in situ detection of individual microbial cells without cultivation. Microbiol Rev 1995;59(1):143–69.

119. Wilson KH, Blitchington RB. Human colonic biota studied by ribosomal DNA sequence analysis. Appl Environ Microbiol 1996;62(7):2273–8.

120. Suau A, Bonnet R, Sutren M, et al. Direct analysis of genes encoding 16S rRNA from complex communities reveals many novel molecular species within the human gut. Appl Environ Microbiol 1999;65(11):4799–807.

121. Hayashi H, Sakamoto M, Benno Y. Phylogenetic analysis of the human gut microbiota using 16S rDNA clone libraries and strictly anaerobic culture-based methods. Microbiol Immunol 2002;46(8):535–48.

122. Sakamoto M, Umeda M, Ishikawa I, Benno Y. Comparison of the oral bacterial flora in saliva from a healthy subject and two periodontitis patients by sequence analysis of 16S rDNA libraries. Microbiol Immunol 2000;44(8):643–52.

123. Aas JA, Paster BJ, Stokes LN, et al. Defining the normal bacterial flora of the oral cavity. J Clin Microbiol 2005;43(11):5721–32.

124. Paster BJ, Boches SK, Galvin JL, et al. Bacterial diversity in human subgingival plaque. J Bacteriol 2001;183(12):3770–83.

125. Wang X, Heazlewood SP, Krause DO, Florin TH. Molecular characterization of the microbial species that colonize human ileal and colonic mucosa by using 16S rDNA sequence analysis. J Appl Microbiol 2003;95(3):508–20.

126. Wang M, Ahrné S, Jeppsson B, Molin G. Comparison of bacterial diversity along the human intestinal tract by direct cloning and sequencing of 16S rRNA genes. FEMS Microbiol Ecol 2005;54(2):219–31.

127. Kroes I, Lepp PW, Relman DA. Bacterial diversity within the human subgingival crevice. Proc Natl Acad Sci USA 1999;96(25):14547–52.

128. Eckburg PB, Bik EM, Bernstein CN, et al. Diversity of the human intestinal microbial flora. Science 2005;308(5728):1635–8.

129. Pei Z, Bini EJ, Yang L, et al. Bacterial biota in the human distal esophagus. Proc Natl Acad Sci USA 2004;101(12):4250–5.

130. Hugenholtz P, Goebel BM, Pace NR. Impact of culture-independent studies on the emerging phylogenetic view of bacterial diversity. J Bacteriol 1998;180(18):4765–74.

131. Rappe MS, Giovannoni SJ. The uncultured microbial majority. Annu Rev Microbiol 2003;57:369–94.

132. Keller M, Zengler K. Tapping into microbial diversity. Nat Rev Microbiol 2004;2:141–50.

133. Bik EM, Eckburg PB, Gill SR, et al. Molecular analysis of the bacterial microbiota in the human stomach. Proc Natl Acad Sci USA 2006;103(3):732–7.

134. Wade W. Unculturable bacteria–the uncharacterized organisms that cause oral infections. J R Soc Med 2002;95(2):81–3.

135. Siqueira JF Jr, Rôças IN. Exploiting molecular methods to explore endodontic infections: Part 1–current molecular technologies for microbiological diagnosis. J Endod 2005;31(6):411–23.

136. Kell DB, Young M. Bacterial dormancy and culturability: the role of autocrine growth factors. Curr Opin Microbiol 2000;3(3):238–43.

137. Breznak JA. A need to retrieve the not-yet-cultured majority. Environ Microbiol 2002;4(1):4–5.

138. Stevenson BS, Eichorst SA, Wertz JT, et al. New strategies for cultivation and detection of previously uncultured microbes. Appl Environ Microbiol 2004;70(8):4748–55.

139. Petti CA, Polage CR, Schreckenberger P. The role of 16S rRNA gene sequencing in identification of microorganisms misidentified by conventional methods. J Clin Microbiol 2005;43:6123–5.

140. Ochman H, Lerat E, Daubin V. Examining bacterial species under the specter of gene transfer and exchange. Proc Natl Acad Sci USA 2005;102:6595–9.

141. Tang YW, Ellis NM, Hopkins MK, et al. Comparison of phenotypic and genotypic techniques for identification of unusual aerobic pathogenic gram-negative bacilli. J Clin Microbiol 1998;36:3674–9.

142. Bosshard PP, Abels S, Zbinden R, et al. Ribosomal DNA sequencing for identification of aerobic gram-positive rods in the clinical laboratory (an 18-month evaluation). J Clin Microbiol 2003;41(9):4134–40.

143. Drancourt M, Bollet C, Carlioz A, et al. 16S ribosomal DNA sequence analysis of a large collection of environmental and clinical unidentifiable bacterial isolates. J Clin Microbiol 2000;38(10):3623–30.

144. Song Y, Liu C, McTeague M, Finegold SM. 16S ribosomal DNA sequence-based analysis of clinically significant gram-positive anaerobic cocci. J Clin Microbiol 2003;41:1363–9.

145. Fredricks DN, Relman DA. Application of polymerase chain reaction to the diagnosis of infectious diseases. Clin Infect Dis 1999;29(3):475–86; quiz 487–8.

146. Sanz M, Lau L, Herrera D, et al. Methods of detection of *Actinobacillus actinomycetemcomitans*, *Porphyromonas gingivalis* and *Tannerella forsythensis* in periodontal microbiology, with special emphasis on advanced molecular techniques: a review. J Clin Periodontol 2004;31(12):1034–47.

147. Anderson BE, Dawson JE, Jones DC, Wilson KH. *Ehrlichia chaffeensis*, a new species associated with human ehrlichiosis. J Clin Microbiol 1991;29(12):2838–42.

148. Relman DA, Schmidt TM, MacDermott RP, Falkow S. Identification of the uncultured bacillus of Whipple's disease. N Engl J Med 1992;327(5):293–301.

149. Relman DA. The identification of uncultured microbial pathogens. J Infect Dis 1993;168(1):1–8.

150. Relman DA. The 'emergence' of *Bartonella* and the development of molecular discovery methods for microbial pathogens. Neth J Med 1998;52(6):249–55.

151. Relman DA. Detection and identification of previously unrecognized microbial pathogens. Emerg Infect Dis 1998;4(3):382–9.

152. Kumar PS, Griffen AL, Moeschberger ML, Leys EJ. Identification of candidate periodontal pathogens and beneficial species by quantitative 16S clonal analysis. J Clin Microbiol 2005;43(8):3944–55.

153. Dekio I, Hayashi H, Sakamoto M, et al. Detection of potentially novel bacterial components of the human skin microbiota using culture-independent molecular profiling. J Med Microbiol 2005;54:1231–8.

154. Fredricks DN, Fiedler TL, Marrazzo JM. Molecular identification of bacteria associated with bacterial vaginosis. N Engl J Med 2005;353(18):1899–911.

155. Drancourt M, Raoult D. Sequence-based identification of new bacteria: a proposition for creation of an orphan bacterium repository. J Clin Microbiol 2005;43:4311–15.

156. Woese CR. Bacterial evolution. Microbiol Rev 1987;51(2):221–71.

157. Zambon JJ, Haraszthy VI. The laboratory diagnosis of periodontal infections. Periodontol 2000 1995;7:69–82.

158. Siqueira JF Jr, Rôças IN. PCR methodology as a valuable tool for identification of endodontic pathogens. J Dent 2003;31(5):333–9.

159. Don RH, Cox PT, Wainwright BJ, et al. "Touchdown" PCR to circumvent spurious priming during gene amplification. Nucleic Acids Res 1991;19:4008.

160. Haqqi TM, Sarkar G, David CS, Sommer SS. Specific amplification with PCR of a refractory segment of genomic DNA. Nucleic Acids Res 1988;16(24):11844.

161. Chamberlain JS, Gibbs RA, Ranier JE, et al. Deletion screening of the Duchenne muscular dystrophy locus via multiplex DNA amplification. Nucleic Acids Res 1988;16(23):11141–56.

162. Sambrook J, Russell DW. Molecular cloning: a laboratory manual. 3rd ed. Cold Spring Harbor, NY: Cold Spring Harbor Laboratory Press; 2001.

163. Welsh J, McClelland M. Fingerprinting genomes using PCR with arbitrary primers. Nucleic Acids Res 1990;18(24):7213–18.

164. Power EG. RAPD typing in microbiology–a technical review. J Hosp Infect 1996;34(4):247–65.

165. de Bruijn FJ. Use of repetitive (repetitive extragenic palindromic and enterobacterial repetitive intergeneric consensus) sequences and the polymerase chain reaction to fingerprint the genomes of Rhizobium meliloti isolates and other soil bacteria. Appl Environ Microbiol 1992;58(7):2180–7.

166. Arora DK, Hirsch PR, Kerry BR. PCR-based molecular discrimination of *Verticillium chlamydosporium* isolates. Mycol Res 1996;7:801–9.

167. Higgins CF, Ames GF, Barnes WM, et al. A novel intercistronic regulatory element of prokaryotic operons. Nature 1982;298(5876):760–2.

168. Raoult D, Fournier PE, Drancourt M. What does the future hold for clinical microbiology? Nat Rev Microbiol 2004;2(2):151–9.

169. Higuchi R, Dollinger G, Walsh PS, Griffith R. Simultaneous amplification and detection of specific DNA sequences. Biotechnology (N Y) 1992;10(4):413–17.

170. Heid CA, Stevens J, Livak KJ, Williams PM. Real time quantitative PCR. Genome Res 1996;6(10):986–94.

171. Tyagi S, Kramer FR. Molecular beacons: probes that fluoresce upon hybridization. Nat Biotechnol 1996;14(3):303–8.

172. Göbel UB. Phylogenetic amplification for the detection of uncultured bacteria and the analysis of complex microbiota. J Microbiol Methods 1995;23:117–28.

173. Lepp PW, Relman DA. Molecular phylogenetic analysis. In: Persing DH, Tenover FC, Versalovic J, Tang Y-W, Unger ER, Relman D, et al., editors. Molecular microbiology. Diagnostic principles and practice. Washington: ASM Press; 2004. pp. 161–80.

174. Maiwald M. Broad-range PCR for detection and identification of bacteria. In: Persing DH, Tenover FC, Versalovic J, Tang Y-W, Relman D, White TJ, editors. Molecular microbiology. Diagnostic principles and practice. Washington, DC:ASM Press;2004. pp. 379–90.

175. Pitt TL, Saunders NA. Molecular bacteriology: a diagnostic tool for the millennium. J Clin Pathol 2000;53(1):71–5.

176. Myers RM, Fischer SG, Lerman LS, Maniatis T. Nearly all single base substitutions in DNA fragments joined to a GC-clamp can be detected by denaturing gradient gel electrophoresis. Nucleic Acids Res 1985;13(9):3131–45.

177. Muyzer G, de Waal EC, Uitterlinden AG. Profiling of complex microbial populations by denaturing gradient gel electrophoresis analysis of polymerase chain reaction-amplified genes coding for 16S rRNA. Appl Environ Microbiol 1993;59(3):695–700.

178. Siqueira JF Jr, Rôças IN, Rosado AS. Application of denaturing gradient gel electrophoresis (DGGE) to the analysis of endodontic infections. J Endod 2005;31(11):775–82.

179. Marsh TL. Terminal restriction fragment length polymorphism (T-RFLP): an emerging method for characterizing diversity among homologous populations of amplification products. Curr Opin Microbiol 1999;2(3):323–7.

180. Clement BG, Kehl LE, De Bord KL, Kitts CL. Terminal restriction fragment patterns (TRFPs), a rapid, PCR-based method for the comparison of complex bacterial communities. J Microbiol Methods 1998;31:135–42.

181. Liu WT, Marsh TL, Cheng H, Forney LJ. Characterization of microbial diversity by determining terminal restriction fragment length polymorphisms of genes encoding 16S rRNA. Appl Environ Microbiol 1997;63(11):4516–22.

182. Coolen MJ, Post E, Davis CC, Forney LJ. Characterization of microbial communities found in the human vagina by analysis of terminal restriction fragment length polymorphisms of 16S rRNA genes. Appl Environ Microbiol 2005;71(12):8729–37.

183. Li J, Hanna BA. DNA probes for culture confirmation and direct detection of bacterial infections: a review of technology. In: Persing DH, Tenover FC, Versalovic J, Tang Y-W, Unger ER, Relman DA, et al., editors. Molecular microbiology. Diagnostic principles and practice. Washington, DC: ASM Press; 2004. pp. 19–26.

184. Socransky SS, Smith C, Martin L, et al. "Checkerboard" DNA-DNA hybridization. Biotechniques 1994;17(4):788–92.

185. Paster BJ, Bartoszyk IM, Dewhirst FE. Identification of oral streptococci using PCR-based, reverse-capture, checkerboard hybridization. Methods Cell Sci 1998;20:223–31.

186. Schena M, Shalon D, Davis RW, Brown PO. Quantitative monitoring of gene expression patterns with a complementary DNA microarray. Science 1995;270(5235):467–70.

187. Mothershed EA, Whitney AM. Nucleic acid-based methods for the detection of bacterial pathogens: present and future considerations for the clinical laboratory. Clin Chem Acta 2006;363(1–2):206–20.

188. Palmer C, Bik EM, Eisen MB, et al. Rapid quantitative profiling of complex microbial populations. Nucleic Acids Res 2006;34(1):e5.

189. Moter A, Gobel UB. Fluorescence in situ hybridization (FISH) for direct visualization of microorganisms. J Microbiol Methods 2000;41(2):85–112.

190. Amann R, Fuchs BM, Behrens S. The identification of microorganisms by fluorescence in situ hybridisation. Curr Opin Biotechnol 2001;12(3):231–6.

191. Moter A, Leist G, Rudolph R, et al. Fluorescence in situ hybridization shows spatial distribution of as yet uncultured treponemes in biopsies from digital dermatitis lesions. Microbiology 1998;144(Pt 9):2459–67.

192. Moter A, Hoenig C, Choi BK, et al. Molecular epidemiology of oral treponemes associated with periodontal disease. J Clin Microbiol 1998;36(5):1399–403.

193. Wagner M, Horn M, Daims H. Fluorescence in situ hybridization for the identification and characterisation of prokaryotes. Curr Opin Microbiol 2003;6(3):302–9.

194. Boissinot M, Bergeron MG. Toward rapid real-time molecular diagnostic to guide smart use of antimicrobials. Curr Opin Microbiol 2002;5(5):478–82.

195. Sundqvist G, Figdor D. Life as an endodontic pathogen. Ecological differences between the untreated and root-filled root canals. Endod Topics 2003;6(1):3–28.

196. Hayden RT. In vitro nucleic acid amplification techniques. In: Persing DH, Tenover FC, Versalovic J, Tang Y-W, Unger ER, Relman DA, et al., editors. Molecular microbiology. Diagnostic principles and practice. Washington, DC: ASM Press; 2004. pp. 43–69.

197. Wang RF, Cao WW, Cerniglia CE. PCR detection and quantitation of predominant anaerobic bacteria in human and animal fecal samples. Appl Environ Microbiol 1996;62(4):1242–7.

198. Rantakokko-Jalava K, Nikkari S, Jalava J, et al. Direct amplification of rRNA genes in diagnosis of bacterial infections. J Clin Microbiol 2000;38(1):32–9.

199. Josephson KL, Gerba CP, Pepper IL. Polymerase chain reaction detection of nonviable bacterial pathogens. Appl Environ Microbiol 1993;59(10):3513–15.

200. Keer JT, Birch L. Molecular methods for the assessment of bacterial viability. J Microbiol Methods 2003;53(2):175–83.

201. Malawista SE, Barthold SW, Persing DH. Fate of *Borrelia burgdorferi* DNA in tissues of infected mice after antibiotic treatment. J Infect Dis 1994;170:1312–16.

202. Post JC, Aul JJ, White GJ, et al. PCR-based detection of bacterial DNA after antimicrobial treatment is indicative of persistent, viable bacteria in the chinchilla model of otitis media. Am J Otolaryngol 1996;17(2):106–11.

203. Aul JJ, Anderson KW, Wadowsky RM, et al. Comparative evaluation of culture and PCR for the detection and determination of persistence of bacterial strains and DNAs in the Chinchilla laniger model of otitis media. Ann Otol Rhinol Laryngol 1998;107(6):508–13.

204. Wicher K, Abbruscato F, Wicher V, et al. Identification of persistent infection in experimental syphilis by PCR. Infect Immun 1998;66(6):2509–13.

205. Bernardi G. Chromatography of nucleic acids on hydroxyapatite. Nature 1965;206(986):779–83.

206. Leduc A, Grenier D, Mayrand D. Outer membrane-associated deoxyribonuclease activity of *Porphyromonas gingivalis*. Anaerobe 1995;1:129–34.

207. Paabo S, Poinar H, Serre D, et al. Genetic analyses from ancient DNA. Annu Rev Genet 2004;38:645–79.

208. Donoghue HD, Spigelman M, Greenblatt CL, et al. Tuberculosis: from prehistory to Robert Koch, as revealed by ancient DNA. Lancet Infect Dis 2004;4:584–92.

209. McCarty SC, Atlas RM. Effect of amplicon size on PCR detection of bacteria exposed to chlorine. PCR Methods Appl 1993;3(3):181–5.

210. Paster BJ, Olsen I, Aas JA, Dewhirst FE. The breadth of bacterial diversity in the human periodontal pocket and other oral sites. Periodontol 2000 2006;42(1):80–7.

211. Bergenholtz G. Micro-organisms from necrotic pulp of traumatized teeth. Odontol Revy 1974;25(4):347–58.

212. Möller AJR. Microbial examination of root canals and periapical tissues of human teeth. Odontologisk Tidskrift 1966;74 Suppl:1–380.

213. Machado de Oliveira JC, Siqueira JF Jr, Rôças IN, et al. Bacterial community profiles of endodontic abscesses from Brazilian and US subjects as compared by denaturing gradient gel electrophoresis analysis. Oral Microbiol Immunol 2007;22(1):14–18.

214. Shah HN, Collins DM. *Prevotella*, a new genus to include *Bacteroides melaninogenicus* and related species formerly classified in the genus *Bacteroides*. Int J Syst Bacteriol 1990;40:205–8.

215. Shah HN, Collins DM. Proposal for reclassification of *Bacteroides asaccharolyticus*, *Bacteroides gingivalis*, and *Bacteroides endodontalis* in a new genus, *Porphyromonas*. Int J Syst Bacteriol 1988;38:128–31.

216. Jousimies-Somer H, Summanen P. Recent taxonomic changes and terminology update of clinically significant anaerobic gram-negative bacteria (excluding spirochetes). Clin Infect Dis 2002;35 Suppl 1:S17–21.

217. Wasfy MO, McMahon KT, Minah GE, Falkler WA Jr. Microbiological evaluation of periapical infections in Egypt. Oral Microbiol Immunol 1992;7(2):100–5.

218. Gharbia SE, Haapasalo M, Shah HN, et al. Characterization of *Prevotella intermedia and Prevotella nigrescens* isolates from periodontic and endodontic infections. J Periodontol 1994;65(1):56–61.

219. Dougherty WJ, Bae KS, Watkins BJ, Baumgartner JC. Black-pigmented bacteria in coronal and apical segments of infected root canals. J Endod 1998;24(5):356–8.

220. Khemaleelakul S, Baumgartner JC, Pruksakorn S. Identification of bacteria in acute endodontic infections and their antimicrobial susceptibility. Oral Surg Oral Med Oral Pathol Oral Radiol Endod 2002;94(6):746–55.

221. Baumgartner JC, Siqueira JF Jr, Xia T, Rôças IN. Geographical differences in bacteria detected in endodontic infections using polymerase chain reaction. J Endod 2004;30(3):141–4.

222. Chu FC, Tsang CS, Chow TW, Samaranayake LP. Identification of cultivable microorganisms from primary endodontic infections with exposed and unexposed pulp space. J Endod 2005;31(6):424–9.

223. Gomes BP, Jacinto RC, Pinheiro ET, et al. *Porphyromonas gingivalis, Porphyromonas endodontalis, Prevotella intermedia* and *Prevotella nigrescens* in endodontic lesions detected by culture and by PCR. Oral Microbiol Immunol 2005;20(4):211–15.

224. Sakamoto M, Rôças IN, Siqueira JF Jr, Benno Y. Molecular analysis of bacteria in asymptomatic and symptomatic endodontic infections. Oral Microbiol Immunol 2006;21(2):112–22.

225. Seol JH, Cho BH, Chung CP, Bae KS. Multiplex polymerase chain reaction detection of black-pigmented bacteria in infections of endodontic origin. J Endod 2006;32(2):110–14.

226. Machado de Oliveira JC, Siqueira JF Jr, Alves GB, et al. Detection of *Porphyromonas endodontalis* in infected root canals by 16S rRNA gene-directed polymerase chain reaction. J Endod 2000;26(12):729–32.

227. Siqueira JF Jr, Rôças IN, Souto R, et al. Checkerboard DNA-DNA hybridization analysis of endodontic infections. Oral Surg Oral Med Oral Pathol Oral Radiol Endod 2000;89(6):744–8.

228. Siqueira JF, Jr, Rôças IN, Oliveira JC, Santos KR. Molecular detection of black-pigmented bacteria in infections of endodontic origin. J Endod 2001;27(9):563–6.

229. Conrads G, Gharbia SE, Gulabivala K, et al. The use of a 16s rDNA directed PCR for the detection of endodontopathogenic bacteria. J Endod 1997;23(7):433–8.

230. Jung IY, Choi BK, Kum KY, et al. Molecular epidemiology and association of putative pathogens in root canal infection. J Endod 2000;26(10):599–604.

231. Rôças IN, Siqueira JF Jr, Santos KR, Coelho AM. "Red complex" (*Bacteroides forsythus, Porphyromonas gingivalis,* and *Treponema denticola*) in endodontic infections: a molecular approach. Oral Surg Oral Med Oral Pathol Oral Radiol Endod 2001;91(4):468–71.

232. Fouad AF, Barry J, Caimano M, et al. PCR-based identification of bacteria associated with endodontic infections. J Clin Microbiol 2002;40(9):3223–31.

233. Siqueira JF Jr, Rôças IN. *Bacteroides forsythus* in primary endodontic infections as detected by nested PCR. J Endod 2003;29(6):390–3.

234. Siqueira JF Jr, Rôças IN, Souto R, et al. Microbiological evaluation of acute periradicular abscesses by DNA-DNA hybridization. Oral Surg Oral Med Oral Pathol Oral Radiol Endod 2001;92(4):451–7.

235. Vianna ME, Horz HP, Gomes BP, Conrads G. Microarrays complement culture methods for identification of bacteria in endodontic infections. Oral Microbiol Immunol 2005;20(4):253–8.

236. Munson MA, Pitt-Ford T, Chong B, et al. Molecular and cultural analysis of the microflora associated with endodontic infections. J Dent Res 2002;81(11):761–6.

237. Rôças IN, Siqueira JF Jr. Detection of novel oral species and phylotypes in symptomatic endodontic infections including abscesses. FEMS Microbiol Lett 2005;250(2):279–85.

238. Rôças IN, Siqueira JF Jr. Identification of *Dialister pneumosintes* in acute periradicular abscesses of humans by nested PCR. Anaerobe 2002;8:75–8.

239. Siqueira JF Jr, Rôças IN. Uncultivated phylotypes and newly named species associated with primary and persistent endodontic infections. J Clin Microbiol 2005;43(7):3314–19.

240. Siqueira JF Jr, Rôças IN. Positive and negative bacterial associations involving *Dialister pneumosintes* in primary endodontic infections. J Endod 2003;29(7):438–41.

241. Siqueira JF Jr, Rôças IN. *Dialister pneumosintes* can be a suspected endodontic pathogen. Oral Surg Oral Med Oral Pathol Oral Radiol Endod 2002;94(4):494–8.

242. Saito D, de Toledo Leonardo R, Rodrigues JLM, et al. Identification of bacteria in endodontic infections by sequence analysis of 16S rDNA clone libraries. J Med Microbiol 2006;55(1):101–7.

243. Weiger R, Manncke B, Werner H, Lost C. Microbial flora of sinus tracts and root canals of non-vital teeth. Endod Dent Traumatol 1995;11(1):15–19.

244. Lana MA, Ribeiro-Sobrinho AP, Stehling R, et al. Microorganisms isolated from root canals presenting necrotic pulp and their drug susceptibility in vitro. Oral Microbiol Immunol 2001;16(2):100–5.

245. Moraes SR, Siqueira JF Jr, Rôças IN, et al. Clonality of *Fusobacterium nucleatum* in root canal infections. Oral Microbiol Immunol 2002;17(6):394–6.

246. Dahle UR, Titterud Sunde P, Tronstad L. Treponemes and endodontic infections. Endod Topics 2003;6(1):160–70.

247. Edwards AM, Dymock D, Jenkinson HF. From tooth to hoof: treponemes in tissue-destructive diseases. J Appl Microbiol 2003;94:767–80.

248. Ellen RP, Galimanas VB. Spirochetes at the forefront of periodontal infections. Periodontol 2000 2005;38:13–32.

249. Miller WD. An introduction to the study of the bacteriopathology of the dental pulp. Dent Cosmos 1894;36:505–28.

250. Trope M, Tronstad L, Rosenberg ES, Listgarten M. Darkfield microscopy as a diagnostic aid in differentiating exudates

250. from endodontic and periodontal abscesses. J Endod 1988;14(1):35–8.
251. Nair PNR. Light and electron microscopic studies of root canal flora and periapical lesions. J Endod 1987;13(1):29–39.
252. Rôças IN, Siqueira JF Jr, Andrade AF, Uzeda M. Oral treponemes in primary root canal infections as detected by nested PCR. Int Endod J 2003;36(1):20–6.
253. Siqueira JF Jr, Rôças IN. *Treponema* species associated with abscesses of endodontic origin. Oral Microbiol Immunol 2004;19(5):336–9.
254. Siqueira JF Jr, Rôças IN. PCR-based identification of *Treponema maltophilum, T amylovorum, T medium*, and *T lecithinolyticum* in primary root canal infections. Arch Oral Biol 2003;48(7):495–502.
255. Siqueira JF Jr, Rôças IN. *Treponema socranskii* in primary endodontic infections as detected by nested PCR. J Endod 2003;29(4):244–7.
256. Siqueira JF Jr, Rôças IN, Favieri A, et al. Polymerase chain reaction detection of *Treponema denticola* in endodontic infections within root canals. Int Endod J 2001;34(4):280–4.
257. Siqueira JF Jr, Rôças IN, Favieri A, Santos KR. Detection of *Treponema denticola* in endodontic infections by 16S rRNA gene-directed polymerase chain reaction. Oral Microbiol Immunol 2000;15(5):335–7.
258. Siqueira JF Jr, Rôças IN, Oliveira JC, Santos KR. Detection of putative oral pathogens in acute periradicular abscesses by 16S rDNA-directed polymerase chain reaction. J Endod 2001;27(3):164–7.
259. Jung IY, Choi B, Kum KY, et al. Identification of oral spirochetes at the species level and their association with other bacteria in endodontic infections. Oral Surg Oral Med Oral Pathol Oral Radiol Endod 2001;92(3):329–34.
260. Baumgartner JC, Khemaleelakul SU, Xia T. Identification of spirochetes (treponemes) in endodontic infections. J Endod 2003;29(12):794–7.
261. Foschi F, Cavrini F, Montebugnoli L, et al. Detection of bacteria in endodontic samples by polymerase chain reaction assays and association with defined clinical signs in Italian patients. Oral Microbiol Immunol 2005;20(5):289–95.
262. Rôças IN, Siqueira JF Jr. Occurrence of two newly named oral treponemes – *Treponema parvum* and *Treponema putidum* – in primary endodontic infections. Oral Microbiol Immunol 2005;20:372–5.
263. Siqueira JF Jr, Rôças IN. *Pseudoramibacter alactolyticus* in primary endodontic infections. J Endod 2003;29(11):735–8.
264. Siqueira JF Jr, Rôças IN, Alves FR, Santos KR. Selected endodontic pathogens in the apical third of infected root canals: a molecular investigation. J Endod 2004;30(9):638–43.
265. Siqueira JF Jr, Rôças IN. Detection of *Filifactor alocis* in endodontic infections associated with different forms of periradicular diseases. Oral Microbiol Immunol 2003;18(4):263–5.
266. Hashimura T, Sato M, Hoshino E. Detection of *Slackia exigua, Mogibacterium timidum* and *Eubacterium saphenum* from pulpal and periradicular samples using the polymerase chain reaction (PCR) method. Int Endod J 2001;34(6):463–70.
267. Fouad AF, Kum KY, Clawson ML, et al. Molecular characterization of the presence of *Eubacterium* spp and *Streptococcus* spp in endodontic infections. Oral Microbiol Immunol 2003;18(4):249–55.
268. Siqueira JF Jr, Rôças IN, Souto R, et al. *Actinomyces* species, streptococci, and *Enterococcus faecalis* in primary root canal infections. J Endod 2002;28(3):168–72.
269. Tang G, Samaranayake LP, Yip HK, et al. Direct detection of *Actinomyces* spp. from infected root canals in a Chinese population: a study using PCR-based, oligonucleotide-DNA hybridization technique. J Dent 2003;31(8):559–68.
270. Xia T, Baumgartner JC. Occurrence of *Actinomyces* in infections of endodontic origin. J Endod 2003;29(9):549–52.
271. Siqueira JF Jr, Rôças IN. Polymerase chain reaction detection of *Propionibacterium propionicus* and *Actinomyces radicidentis* in primary and persistent endodontic infections. Oral Surg Oral Med Oral Pathol Oral Radiol Endod 2003;96(2):215–22.
272. Rôças IN, Siqueira JF Jr. Species-directed 16S rRNA gene nested PCR detection of *Olsenella* species in association with endodontic diseases. Lett Appl Microbiol 2005;41(1):12–16.
273. Siqueira JF Jr, Rôças IN, Andrade AF, de Uzeda M. *Peptostreptococcus micros* in primary endodontic infections as detected by 16S rDNA-based polymerase chain reaction. J Endod 2003;29(2):111–13.
274. Rôças IN, Siqueira JF Jr, Santos KR. Association of *Enterococcus faecalis* with different forms of periradicular diseases. J Endod 2004;30(5):315–20.
275. Ranta H, Haapasalo M, Ranta K, et al. Bacteriology of odontogenic apical periodontitis and effect of penicillin treatment. Scand J Infect Dis 1988;20(2):187–92.
276. Le Goff A, Bunetel L, Mouton C, Bonnaure-Mallet M. Evaluation of root canal bacteria and their antimicrobial susceptibility in teeth with necrotic pulp. Oral Microbiol Immunol 1997;12(5):318–22.
277. Siqueira JF Jr, Rôças IN. *Campylobacter gracilis* and *Campylobacter rectus* in primary endodontic infections. Int Endod J 2003;36(3):174–80.
278. Siqueira JF Jr, Rôças IN. *Catonella morbi* and *Granulicatella adiacens*: new species in endodontic infections. Oral Surg Oral Med Oral Pathol Oral Radiol Endod 2006;102:259–64.
279. Siqueira JF Jr, Rôças IN. Nested PCR detection of *Centipeda periodontii* in primary endodontic infections. J Endod 2004;30(3):135–7.
280. Rôças IN, Siqueira JF Jr. Culture-independent detection of *Eikenella corrodens* and *Veillonella parvula* in primary endodontic infections. J Endod 2006;32(6):509–12.

281. Siqueira JF Jr, Rôças IN, Cunha CD, Rosado AS. Novel bacterial phylotypes in endodontic infections. J Dent Res 2005;84(6):565–9.

282. Rolph HJ, Lennon A, Riggio MP, et al. Molecular identification of microorganisms from endodontic infections. J Clin Microbiol 2001;39(9):3282–9.

283. Egan MW, Spratt DA, Ng YL, et al. Prevalence of yeasts in saliva and root canals of teeth associated with apical periodontitis. Int Endod J 2002;35(4):321–9.

284. Siqueira JF Jr, Rôças IN, Moraes SR, Santos KR. Direct amplification of rRNA gene sequences for identification of selected oral pathogens in root canal infections. Int Endod J 2002;35(4):345–51.

285. Lepp PW, Brinig MM, Ouverney CC, et al. Methanogenic Archaea and human periodontal disease. Proc Natl Acad Sci USA 2004;101(16):6176–81.

286. Siqueira JF Jr, Rôças IN, Baumgartner JC, Xia T. Searching for Archaea in infections of endodontic origin. J Endod 2005;31(10):719–22.

287. Vianna ME, Conrads G, Gomes BPFA, Horz HP. Identification and quantification of archaea involved in primary endodontic infections. J Clin Microbiol 2006;44:1274–82.

288. Glick M, Trope M, Bagasra O, Pliskin ME. Human immunodeficiency virus infection of fibroblasts of dental pulp in seropositive patients. Oral Surg Oral Med Oral Pathol Oral Radiol Endod 1991;71(6):733–6.

289. Slots J. Herpesviruses in periodontal diseases. Periodontol 2000 2005;38:33–62.

290. Kubar A, Saygun I, Ozdemir A, et al. Real-time polymerase chain reaction quantification of human cytomegalovirus and Epstein-Barr virus in periodontal pockets and the adjacent gingiva of periodontitis lesions. J Periodontal Res 2005;40(2):97–104.

291. Parra B, Slots J. Detection of human viruses in periodontal pockets using polymerase chain reaction. Oral Microbiol Immunol 1996;11(5):289–93.

292. Contreras A, Mardirossian A, Slots J. Herpesviruses in HIV-periodontitis. J Clin Periodontol 2001;28(1):96–102.

293. Kamma JJ, Slots J. Herpesviral-bacterial interactions in aggressive periodontitis. J Clin Periodontol 2003;30(5):420–6.

294. Sabeti M, Simon JH, Nowzari H, Slots J. Cytomegalovirus and Epstein-Barr virus active infection in periapical lesions of teeth with intact crowns. J Endod 2003;29(5):321–3.

295. Sabeti M, Simon JH, Slots J. Cytomegalovirus and Epstein-Barr virus are associated with symptomatic periapical pathosis. Oral Microbiol Immunol 2003;18(5):327–8.

296. Slots J, Sabeti M, Simon JH. Herpesviruses in periapical pathosis: an etiopathogenic relationship? Oral Surg Oral Med Oral Pathol Oral Radiol Endod 2003;96(3):327–31.

297. Rôças IN, Siqueira JF Jr, Andrade AFB, Uzeda M. Identification of selected putative oral pathogens in primary root canal infections associated with symptoms. Anaerobe 2002;8:200–8.

298. Siqueira JF Jr, Barnett F. Interappointment pain: mechanisms, diagnosis, and treatment. Endod Topics 2004;7(1):93–109.

299. Siqueira JF Jr. Endodontic infections: concepts, paradigms, and perspectives. Oral Surg Oral Med Oral Pathol Oral Radiol Endod 2002;94(3):281–93.

300. Rôças IN, Siqueira JF Jr, Aboim MC, Rosado AS. Denaturing gradient gel electrophoresis analysis of bacterial communities associated with failed endodontic treatment. Oral Surg Oral Med Oral Pathol Oral Radiol Endod 2004;98(6):741–9.

301. Molander A, Reit C, Dahlen G, Kvist T. Microbiological status of root-filled teeth with apical periodontitis. Int Endod J 1998;31(1):1–7.

302. Pinheiro ET, Gomes BP, Ferraz CC, et al. Microorganisms from canals of root-filled teeth with periapical lesions. Int Endod J 2003;36(1):1–11.

303. Fabricius L, Dahlén G, Sundqvist G, et al. Influence of residual bacteria on periapical tissue healing after chemomechanical treatment and root filling of experimentally infected monkey teeth. Eur J Oral Sci 2006;114:278–85.

304. Sjögren U, Figdor D, Persson S, Sundqvist G. Influence of infection at the time of root filling on the outcome of endodontic treatment of teeth with apical periodontitis. Int Endod J 1997;30(5):297–306.

305. Waltimo T, Trope M, Haapasalo M, Orstavik D. Clinical efficacy of treatment procedures in endodontic infection control and one year follow-up of periapical healing. J Endod 2005;31(12):863–6.

306. Heling B, Shapira J. Roentgenologic and clinical evaluation of endodontically treated teeth with or without negative culture. Quintessence Int 1978;11:79–84.

307. Engström B, Hard AF, Segerstad L, et al. Correlation of positive cultures with the prognosis for root canal treatment. Odontol Revy 1964;15:257–70.

308. Peters LB, van Winkelhoff AJ, Buijs JF, Wesselink PR. Effects of instrumentation, irrigation and dressing with calcium hydroxide on infection in pulpless teeth with periapical bone lesions. Int Endod J 2002;35(1):13–21.

309. Gomes BP, Lilley JD, Drucker DB. Variations in the susceptibilities of components of the endodontic microflora to biomechanical procedures. Int Endod J 1996;29(4):235–41.

310. Byström A, Sundqvist G. The antibacterial action of sodium hypochlorite and EDTA in 60 cases of endodontic therapy. Int Endod J 1985;18(1):35–40.

311. Sakamoto M, Siqueira JF Jr, Rôças IN, Benno Y. Bacterial reduction and persistence after endodontic disinfection procedures. Oral Microbiol Immunol 2007;22(1):19–23.

312. Chavez de Paz L. Gram-positive organisms in endodontic infections. Endod Topics 2004;9(1):79–96.

313. Chu FC, Leung WK, Tsang PC, et al. Identification of cultivable microorganisms from root canals with apical periodontitis following two-visit endodontic treatment with antibiotics/steroid or calcium hydroxide dressings. J Endod 2006;32(1):17–23.

314. Chavez de Paz L, Svensater G, Dahlen G, Bergenholtz G. Streptococci from root canals in teeth with apical periodontitis receiving endodontic treatment. Oral Surg Oral Med Oral Pathol Oral Radiol Endod 2005;100(2):232–41.

315. Chavez de Paz LE, Molander A, Dahlen G. Gram-positive rods prevailing in teeth with apical periodontitis undergoing root canal treatment. Int Endod J 2004;37(9):579–87.

316. Chavez De Paz LE, Dahlen G, Molander A, et al. Bacteria recovered from teeth with apical periodontitis after antimicrobial endodontic treatment. Int Endod J 2003;36(7):500–8.

317. Tang G, Samaranayake LP, Yip HK. Molecular evaluation of residual endodontic microorganisms after instrumentation, irrigation and medication with either calcium hydroxide or Septomixine. Oral Dis 2004;10(6):389–97.

318. Kakehashi S, Stanley HR, Fitzgerald RJ. The effects of surgical exposures of dental pulps in germ-free and conventional laboratory rats. Oral Surg Oral Med Oral Pathol Endod 1965;20:340–9.

319. Sjögren U, Hagglund B, Sundqvist G, Wing K. Factors affecting the long-term results of endodontic treatment. J Endod 1990;16(10):498–504.

320. Spangberg LSW. Endodontic treatment of teeth without apical periodontitis. In: Ørstavik D, Pitt Ford T, editors. Essential endodontology. Oxford: Blackwell Science Ltd; 1998. pp. 211–41.

321. Orstavik D. Root canal disinfection: a review of concepts and recent developments. Aust Endod J 2003;29(2):70–4.

322. Siqueira JF Jr. Strategies to treat infected root canals. J Calif Dent Assoc 2001;29(12):825–37.

323. Shuping GB, Orstavik D, Sigurdsson A, Trope M. Reduction of intracanal bacteria using nickel-titanium rotary instrumentation and various medications. J Endod 2000;26(12):751–5.

324. Sjögren U, Figdor D, Spangberg L, Sundqvist G. The antimicrobial effect of calcium hydroxide as a short-term intracanal dressing. Int Endod J 1991;24(3):119–25.

325. McGurkin-Smith R, Trope M, Caplan D, Sigurdsson A. Reduction of intracanal bacteria using GT rotary instrumentation, 5.25% NaOCl, EDTA, and Ca(OH)2. J Endod 2005;31(5):359–63.

326. Tronstad L, Barnett F, Cervone F. Periapical bacterial plaque in teeth refractory to endodontic treatment. Endod Dent Traumatol 1990;6(2):73–7.

327. Noiri Y, Ehara A, Kawahara T, et al. Participation of bacterial biofilms in refractory and chronic periapical periodontitis. J Endod 2002;28(10):679–83.

328. Nair PNR, Schroeder HE. Periapical actinomycosis. J Endod 1984;10(12):567–70.

329. Tronstad L, Sunde PT. The evolving new understanding of endodontic infections. Endod Topics 2003;6(1):57–77.

330. Siqueira JF Jr. Periapical actinomycosis and infection with *Propionibacterium propionicum*. Endod Topics 2003;6(1):78–95.

331. Baumgartner JC. Microbiologic aspects of endodontic infections. J Calif Dent Assoc 2004;32(6):459–68.

332. Tronstad L, Barnett F, Riso K, Slots J. Extraradicular endodontic infections. Endod Dent Traumatol 1987;3(2):86–90.

333. Sunde PT, Olsen I, Debelian GJ, Tronstad L. Microbiota of periapical lesions refractory to endodontic therapy. J Endod 2002;28(4):304–10.

334. Wayman BE, Murata SM, Almeida RJ, Fowler CB. A bacteriological and histological evaluation of 58 periapical lesions. J Endod 1992;18(4):152–5.

335. Sunde PT, Tronstad L, Eribe ER, et al. Assessment of periradicular microbiota by DNA-DNA hybridization. Endod Dent Traumatol 2000;16(5):191–6.

336. Gatti JJ, Dobeck JM, Smith C, et al. Bacteria of asymptomatic periradicular endodontic lesions identified by DNA-DNA hybridization. Endod Dent Traumatol 2000;16(5):197–204.

337. Sunde PT, Olsen I, Gobel UB, et al. Fluorescence in situ hybridization (FISH) for direct visualization of bacteria in periapical lesions of asymptomatic root-filled teeth. Microbiology 2003;149(Pt 5):1095–102.

338. Sjögren U, Happonen RP, Kahnberg KE, Sundqvist G. Survival of *Arachnia propionica* in periapical tissue. Int Endod J 1988;21(4):277–82.

339. Barnett F, Stevens R, Tronstad L. Demonstration of Bacteroides intermedius in periapical tissue using indirect immunofluorescence microscopy. Endod Dent Traumatol 1990;6(4):153–6.

340. Sjögren U, Hanstrom L, Happonen RP, Sundqvist G. Extensive bone loss associated with periapical infection with *Bacteroides gingivalis*: a case report. Int Endod J 1990;23(5):254–62.

341. van Winkelhoff AJ, van Steenbergen TJ, de Graaff J. *Porphyromonas (Bacteroides) endodontalis*: its role in endodontal infections. J Endod 1992;18(9):431–4.

342. Fenno JC, McBride BC. Virulence factors of oral treponemes. Anaerobe 1998;4:1–17.

343. Bolstad AI, Jensen HB, Bakken V. Taxonomy, biology, and periodontal aspects of Fusobacterium nucleatum. Clin Microbiol Rev 1996;9:55–71.

344. Holt SC, Ebersole JL. *Porphyromonas gingivalis, Treponema denticola* and *Tannerella forsythia*: the "red complex", a prototype polybacterial pathogenic consortium in periodontitis. Periodontol 2000 2005;38:72–122.

345. Siqueira JF Jr, Lopes HP. Bacteria on the apical root surfaces of untreated teeth with periradicular lesions: a scanning electron microscopy study. Int Endod J 2001;34(3):216–20.

346. Siqueira JF Jr. Reaction of periradicular tissues to root canal treatment: benefits and drawbacks. Endod Topics 2005;10(1):123–47.

347. Henderson B, Wilson M. Commensal communism and the oral cavity. J Dent Res 1998;77(9):1674–83.

348. Moine P, Abraham E. Immunomodulation and sepsis: impact of the pathogen. Shock 2004;22(4):297–308.

349. Frank SA, Barbour AG. Within-host dynamics of antigenic variation. Infect Genet Evol 2006;6(2):141–6.

350. Lawrence JG. Common themes in the genome strategies of pathogens. Curr Opin Genet Dev 2005;15(6):584–8.

351. Casadevall A, Pirofski L. Host-pathogen interactions: the attributes of virulence. J Infect Dis 2001;184(3):337–44.

352. Medvedev AE, Sabroe I, Hasday JD, Vogel SN. Tolerance to microbial TLR ligands: molecular mechanisms and relevance to disease. J Endotoxin Res 2006;12(3):133–50.

353. Bergenholtz G. Pathogenic mechanisms in pulpal disease. J Endod 1990;16(2):98–101.

354. Jontell M, Okiji T, Dahlgren U, Bergenholtz G. Immune defense mechanisms of the dental pulp. Crit Rev Oral Biol Med 1998;9(2):179–200.

355. Jontell M, Gunraj MN, Bergenholtz G. Immunocompetent cells in the normal dental pulp. J Dent Res 1987;66(6):1149–53.

356. Jontell M, Bergenholtz G, Scheynius A, Ambrose W. Dendritic cells and macrophages expressing class II antigens in the normal rat incisor pulp. J Dent Res 1988;67(10):1263–6.

357. Hahn CL, Best AM, Tew JG. Cytokine induction by Streptococcus mutans and pulpal pathogenesis. Infect Immun 2000;68(12):6785–9.

358. Hahn CL, Best AM, Tew JG. Comparison of type 1 and type 2 cytokine production by mononuclear cells cultured with streptococcus mutans and selected other caries bacteria. J Endod 2004;30(5):333–8.

359. Martin FE. Carious pulpitis: microbiological and histopathological considerations. Aust Endod J 2003;29(3):134–7.

360. Smith AJ. Pulpal responses to caries and dental repair. Caries Res 2002;36(4):223–32.

361. Hahn CL, Best AM. The pulpal origin of immunoglobulins in dentin beneath caries: an immunohistochemical study. J Endod 2006;32(3):178–82.

362. Bergenholtz G. Inflammatory response of the dental pulp to bacterial irritation. J Endod 1981;7(3):100–4.

363. Martin FE, Nadkarni MA, Jacques NA, Hunter N. Quantitative microbiological study of human carious dentine by culture and real-time PCR: association of anaerobes with histopathological changes in chronic pulpitis. J Clin Microbiol 2002;40(5):1698–704.

364. Bergenholtz G. Effect of bacterial products on inflammatory reactions in the dental pulp. Scand J Dent Res 1977;85(2):122–9.

365. Hahn CL, Falkler WA Jr, Minah GE. Microbiological studies of carious dentine from human teeth with irreversible pulpitis. Arch Oral Biol 1991;36(2):147–53.

366. Hahn CL, Falkler WA Jr, Minah GE. Correlation between thermal sensitivity and microorganisms isolated from deep carious dentin. J Endod 1993;19(1):26–30.

367. Schein B, Schilder H. Endotoxin content in endodontically involved teeth. J Endod 1975;1(1):19–21.

368. Hosoya S, Matsushima K. Stimulation of interleukin-1 beta production of human dental pulp cells by Porphyromonas endodontalis lipopolysaccharide. J Endod 1997;23(1):39–42.

369. Chang J, Zhang C, Tani-Ishii N, et al. NF-kappa B activation in human dental pulp stem cells by TNF and LPS. J Dent Res 2005;84(11):994–8.

370. Botero TM, Mantellini MG, Song W, et al. Effect of lipopolysaccharides on vascular endothelial growth factor expression in mouse pulp cells and macrophages. Eur J Oral Sci 2003;111(3):228–34.

371. Botero TM, Shelburne CE, Holland GR, et al. TLR4 mediates LPS-induced VEGF expression in odontoblasts. J Endod 2006;32(10)951–5.

372. Horiba N, Maekawa Y, Yamauchi Y, et al. Complement activation by lipopolysaccharides purified from gram-negative bacteria isolated from infected root canals. Oral Surg Oral Med Oral Pathol Endod 1992;74(5):648–51.

373. Dwyer TG, Torabinejad M. Radiographic and histologic evaluation of the effect of endotoxin on the periapical tissues of the cat. J Endod 1980;7(1):31–5.

374. Schonfeld SE, Greening AB, Glick DH, et al. Endotoxic activity in periapical lesions. Oral Surg Oral Med Oral Pathol Endod 1982;53(1):82–7.

375. Horiba N, Maekawa Y, Abe Y, et al. Correlations between endotoxin and clinical symptoms or radiolucent areas in infected root canals. Oral Surg Oral Med Oral Pathol Endod 1991;71(4):492–5.

376. Khabbaz MG, Anastasiadis PL, Sykaras SN. Determination of endotoxins in the vital pulp of human carious teeth: association with pulpal pain. Oral Surg Oral Med Oral Pathol Oral Radiol Endod 2001;91(5):587–93.

377. Jacinto RC, Gomes BP, Shah HN, et al. Quantification of endotoxins in necrotic root canals from symptomatic and asymptomatic teeth. J Med Microbiol 2005;54(Pt 8):777–83.

378. Dahlen G, Magnusson BC, Möller A. Histological and histochemical study of the influence of lipopolysaccharide extracted from Fusobacterium nucleatum on the periapical tissues in the monkey Macaca fascicularis. Arch Oral Biol 1981;26(7):591–8.

379. Myhre AE, Aasen AO, Thiemermann C, Wang JE. Peptidoglycan–an endotoxin in its own right? Shock 2006;25(3):227–35.

380. Wang JE, Jorgensen PF, Almlof M, et al. Peptidoglycan and lipoteichoic acid from Staphylococcus aureus induce tumor necrosis factor alpha, interleukin 6 (IL-6), and IL-10

380. production in both T cells and monocytes in a human whole blood model. Infect Immun 2000;68(7):3965–70.

381. Matsushima K, Ohbayashi E, Takeuchi H, et al. Stimulation of interleukin-6 production in human dental pulp cells by peptidoglycans from *Lactobacillus casei*. J Endod 1998;24(4):252–5.

382. Wang JE, Jorgensen PF, Ellingsen EA, et al. Peptidoglycan primes for LPS-induced release of proinflammatory cytokines in whole human blood. Shock 2001;16(3):178–82.

383. Hogg SD, Whiley RA, De Soet JJ. Occurrence of lipoteichoic acid in oral streptococci. Int J Syst Bacteriol 1997;47(1):62–6.

384. Cohen J. Mechanisms of tissue injury in sepsis: contrasts between gram positive and gram negative infection. J Chemother 2001;13 Spec No 1(1):153–8.

385. Courtney HS, Stanislawski L, Ofek I, et al. Localization of a lipoteichoic acid binding site to a 24-kilodalton NH2-terminal fragment of fibronectin. Rev Infect Dis 1988;10 Suppl 2:S360–2.

386. Courtney H, Ofek I, Simpson WA, Beachey EH. Characterization of lipoteichoic acid binding to polymorphonuclear leukocytes of human blood. Infect Immun 1981;32(2):625–31.

387. Ginsburg I. Role of lipoteichoic acid in infection and inflammation. Lancet Infect Dis 2002;2(3):171–9.

388. Costa ED, de Souza-Filho FJ, Barbosa SV. Tissue reactions to a component of root canal system bacteria: lipoteichoic acid. Braz Dent J 2003;14(2):95–8.

389. Telles PD, Hanks CT, Machado MA, Nor JE. Lipoteichoic acid up-regulates VEGF expression in macrophages and pulp cells. J Dent Res 2003;82(6):466–70.

390. Tang G, Yip HK, Samaranayake LP, et al. Direct detection of cell surface interactive forces of sessile, fimbriated and non-fimbriated *Actinomyces* spp. using atomic force microscopy. Arch Oral Biol 2004;49(9):727–38.

391. Wu H, Fives-Taylor PM. Molecular strategies for fimbrial expression and assembly. Crit Rev Oral Biol Med 2001;12(2):101–15.

392. Hood BL, Hirschberg R. Purification and characterization of *Eikenella corrodens* type IV pilin. Infect Immun 1995; 63(9):3693–6.

393. Leung KP, Fukushima H, Nesbitt WE, Clark WB. *Prevotella intermedia* fimbriae mediate hemagglutination. Oral Microbiol Immunol 1996;11(1):42–50.

394. Figdor D, Davies J. Cell surface structures of Actinomyces israelii. Aust Dent J 1997;42(2):125–8.

395. Cho KH, Caparon MG. Patterns of virulence gene expression differ between biofilm and tissue communities of Streptococcus pyogenes. Mol Microbiol 2005;57(6):1545–56.

396. Kinder SA, Holt SC. Characterization of coaggregation between Bacteroides gingivalis T22 and Fusobacterium nucleatum T18. Infect Immun 1989;57(11):3425–33.

397. Beveridge TJ. Structures of gram-negative cell walls and their derived membrane vesicles. J Bacteriol 1999;181(16):4725–33.

398. Kuehn MJ, Kesty NC. Bacterial outer membrane vesicles and the host-pathogen interaction. Genes Dev 2005;19(22):2645–55.

399. Kamaguchi A, Nakayama K, Ichiyama S, et al. Effect of *Porphyromonas gingivalis* vesicles on coaggregation of *Staphylococcus aureus* to oral microorganisms. Curr Microbiol 2003;47(6):485–91.

400. Grenier D, Bertrand J, Mayrand D. *Porphyromonas gingivalis* outer membrane vesicles promote bacterial resistance to chlorhexidine. Oral Microbiol Immunol 1995;10(5):319–20.

401. Kato S, Kowashi Y, Demuth DR. Outer membrane-like vesicles secreted by *Actinobacillus actinomycetemcomitans* are enriched in leukotoxin. Microb Pathog 2002;32(1):1–13.

402. Duncan L, Yoshioka M, Chandad F, Grenier D. Loss of lipopolysaccharide receptor CD14 from the surface of human macrophage-like cells mediated by *Porphyromonas gingivalis* outer membrane vesicles. Microb Pathog 2004;36(6):319–25.

403. Llewelyn M, Cohen J. Superantigens: microbial agents that corrupt immunity. Lancet Infect Dis 2002;2(3):156–62.

404. Cohen J. The immunopathogenesis of sepsis. Nature 2002;420(6917):885–91.

405. Tomita H, Fujimoto S, Tanimoto K, Ike Y. Cloning and genetic and sequence analyses of the bacteriocin 21 determinant encoded on the *Enterococcus faecalis* pheromone-responsive conjugative plasmid pPD1. J Bacteriol 1997;179(24):7843–55.

406. Aktories K, Barbieri JT. Bacterial cytotoxins: targeting eukaryotic switches. Nat Rev Microbiol 2005;3(5):397–410.

407. Sundqvist GK, Carlsson J, Herrmann BF, et al. Degradation in vivo of the C3 protein of guinea-pig complement by a pathogenic strain of *Bacteroides gingivalis*. Scand J Dent Res 1984;92(1):14–24.

408. Sundqvist G, Carlsson J, Herrmann B, Tarnvik A. Degradation of human immunoglobulins G and M and complement factors C3 and C5 by black-pigmented *Bacteroides*. J Med Microbiol 1985;19(1):85–94.

409. Odell E, Pertl C. Zinc as a growth factor for *Aspergillus* sp. and the antifungal effects of root canal sealants. Oral Surg Oral Med Oral Pathol Oral Radiol Endod 1995;79(1):82–7.

410. Sundqvist G, Carlsson J, Hanstrom L. Collagenolytic activity of black-pigmented *Bacteroides* species. J Periodontal Res 1987;22(4):300–6.

411. Dahlen G, Wikstrom M, Möller A. Production of histolytic enzymes by a combination of oral bacteria with known pathogenicity. J Dent Res 1983;62(10):1041–4.

412. Odell LJ, Baumgartner JC, Xia T, David LL. Survey for collagenase gene prtC in Porphyromonas gingivalis and *Porphyromonas endodontalis* isolated from endodontic infections. J Endod 1999;25(8):555–8.

413. Sedgley CM, Molander A, Flannagan SE, et al. Virulence, phenotype and genotype characteristics of endodontic *Enterococcus* spp. Oral Microbiol Immunol 2005;20(1):10–19.

414. Hubble TS, Hatton JF, Nallapareddy SR, et al. Influence of *Enterococcus faecalis* proteases and the collagen-binding

protein, Ace, on adhesion to dentin. Oral Microbiol Immunol 2003;18(2):121–6.

415. Hashioka K, Suzuki K, Yoshida T, et al. Relationship between clinical symptoms and enzyme-producing bacteria isolated from infected root canals. J Endod 1994;20(2):75–7.

416. Jett BD, Jensen HG, Nordquist RE, Gilmore MS. Contribution of the pAD1-encoded cytolysin to the severity of experimental *Enterococcus faecalis* endophthalmitis. Infect Immun 1992;60(6):2445–52.

417. Niederman R, Zhang J, Kashket S. Short-chain carboxylic-acid-stimulated, PMN-mediated gingival inflammation. Crit Rev Oral Biol Med 1997;8(3):269–90.

418. Kersten HW, Moorer WR. Particles and molecules in endodontic leakage. Int Endod J 1989;22(3):118–24.

419. Eftimiadi C, Stashenko P, Tonetti M, et al. Divergent effect of the anaerobic bacteria by-product butyric acid on the immune response: suppression of T-lymphocyte proliferation and stimulation of interleukin-1 beta production. Oral Microbiol Immunol 1991;6(1):17–23.

420. Kurita-Ochiai T, Hashizume T, Yonezawa H, et al. Characterization of the effects of butyric acid on cell proliferation, cell cycle distribution and apoptosis. FEMS Immunol Med Microbiol 2006;47(1):67–74.

421. Miller SJ, Zaloga GP, Hoggatt AM, et al. Short-chain fatty acids modulate gene expression for vascular endothelial cell adhesion molecules. Nutrition 2005;21(6):740–8.

422. Singer RE, Buckner BA. Butyrate and propionate: important components of toxic dental plaque extracts. Infect Immun 1981;32(2):458–63.

423. Chavez de Paz Villanueva LE. *Fusobacterium nucleatum* in endodontic flare-ups. Oral Surg Oral Med Oral Pathol Oral Radiol Endod 2002;93(2):179–83.

424. Thomas T, Thomas TJ. Polyamines in cell growth and cell death: molecular mechanisms and therapeutic applications. Cell Mol Life Sci 2001;58(2):244–58.

425. Maita E, Horiuchi H. Polyamine analysis of infected root canal contents related to clinical symptoms. Endod Dent Traumatol 1990;6(5):213–17.

426. Huycke MM, Joyce W, Wack MF. Augmented production of extracellular superoxide by blood isolates of *Enterococcus faecalis*. J Infect Dis 1996;173(3):743–6.

427. Falcioni GC, Coderoni S, Tedeschi GG, et al. Red cell lysis induced by microorganisms as a case of superoxide- and hydrogen peroxide-dependent hemolysis mediated by oxyhemoglobin. Biochim Biophys Acta 1981;678(3):437–41.

428. Huycke MM, Gilmore MS. In vivo survival of *Enterococcus faecalis* is enhanced by extracellular superoxide production. Adv Exp Med Biol 1997;418:781–4.

429. Jansen A, Yu J. Differential gene expression of pathogens inside infected hosts. Curr Opin Microbiol 2006;9(2):138–42.

430. Kunin V, Goldovsky L, Darzentas N, Ouzounis CA. The net of life: reconstructing the microbial phylogenetic network. Genome Res 2005;15(7):954–9.

431. Chen T, Hosogi Y, Nishikawa K, et al. Comparative whole-genome analysis of virulent and avirulent strains of *Porphyromonas gingivalis*. J Bacteriol 2004;186(16):5473–9.

432. Nallapareddy SR, Wenxiang H, Weinstock GM, Murray BE. Molecular characterization of a widespread, pathogenic, and antibiotic resistance-receptive *Enterococcus faecalis* lineage and dissemination of its putative pathogenicity island. J Bacteriol 2005;187(16):5709–18.

433. Waterhouse JC, Russell RR. Dispensable genes and foreign DNA in *Streptococcus mutans*. Microbiology 2006;152(Pt 6):1777–88.

434. Lindsay JA, Ruzin A, Ross HF, et al. The gene for toxic shock toxin is carried by a family of mobile pathogenicity islands in *Staphylococcus aureus*. Mol Microbiol 1998;29(2):527–43.

435. Lorenz MG, Wackernagel W. Bacterial gene transfer by natural genetic transformation in the environment. Microbiol Rev 1994;58(3):563–602.

436. Li YH, Lau PC, Lee JH, et al. Natural genetic transformation of *Streptococcus mutans* growing in biofilms. J Bacteriol 2001;183(3):897–908.

437. Wang BY, Chi B, Kuramitsu HK. Genetic exchange between *Treponema denticola* and *Streptococcus gordonii* in biofilms. Oral Microbiol Immunol 2002;17(2):108–12.

438. Morrison DA, Lee MS. Regulation of competence for genetic transformation in Streptococcus pneumoniae: a link between quorum sensing and DNA processing genes. Res Microbiol 2000;151(6):445–51.

439. Canchaya C, Fournous G, Chibani-Chennoufi S, et al. Phage as agents of lateral gene transfer. Curr Opin Microbiol 2003;6(4):417–24.

440. Haubek D, Willi K, Poulsen K, et al. Presence of bacteriophage Aa phi 23 correlates with the population genetic structure of *Actinobacillus actinomycetemcomitans*. Eur J Oral Sci 1997;105(1):2–8.

441. Yeung MK, Kozelsky CS. Transfection of Actinomyces spp. by genomic DNA of bacteriophages from human dental plaque. Plasmid 1997;37(2):141–53.

442. Bachrach G, Leizerovici-Zigmond M, Zlotkin A, et al. Bacteriophage isolation from human saliva. Lett Appl Microbiol 2003;36(1):50–3.

443. Waters VL. Conjugation between bacterial and mammalian cells. Nat Genet 2001;29(4):375–6.

444. Brugger K, Redder P, She Q, et al. Mobile elements in archaeal genomes. FEMS Microbiol Lett 2002;206(2):131–41.

445. Jayaram M, Mehta S, Uzri D, Velmurugan S. Segregation of the yeast plasmid: similarities and contrasts with bacterial plasmid partitioning. Plasmid 2004;51(3):162–78.

446. Frappier L. Viral plasmids in mammalian cells. In: Plasmid biology. Washington, DC: American Society of Microbiology; 2004.

447. Sedgley CM, Molander A, Flannagan SE, Nagel AC, Appelbe OK, Clewell DB, Dahlén G. Virulence, phenotype and genotype charactteeristics of endodontic Enterococcus spp. Oral Microbiol Immunol 2005;20(1):10–19.

448. Paulsen IT, Banerjei L, Myers GS, et al. Role of mobile DNA in the evolution of vancomycin-resistant Enterococcus faecalis. Science 2003;299(5615):2071–4.

449. Hayes F. Transposon-based strategies for microbial functional genomics and proteomics. Annu Rev Genet 2003;37:3–29.

450. Mahillon J, Chandler M. Insertion sequences. Microbiol Mol Biol Rev 1998;62(3):725–74.

451. Clewell DB, Francia MV. Conjugation in Gram-positive bacteria. In: Plasmid biology. Washington, DC: American Society of Microbiology; 2004.

452. Lawley T, Wilkins BM, Frost LS. Bacterial conjugation in gram-negative bacteria. In: Plasmid biology. Washington, DC: American Society of Microbiology; 2004.

453. Grohmann E, Muth G, Espinosa M. Conjugative plasmid transfer in gram-positive bacteria. Microbiol Mol Biol Rev 2003;67(2):277–301.

454. Heinemann JA, Sprague GF Jr. Bacterial conjugative plasmids mobilize DNA transfer between bacteria and yeast. Nature 1989;340(6230):205–9.

455. Shoemaker NB, Guthrie EP, Salyers AA, Gardner JF. Evidence that the clindamycin-erythromycin resistance gene of Bacteroides plasmid pBF4 is on a transposable element. J Bacteriol 1985;162(2):626–32.

456. Gupta A, Vlamakis H, Shoemaker N, Salyers AA. A new Bacteroides conjugative transposon that carries an ermB gene. Appl Environ Microbiol 2003;69(11):6455–63.

457. Salyers AA, Shoemaker NB, Stevens AM, Li LY. Conjugative transposons: an unusual and diverse set of integrated gene transfer elements. Microbiol Rev 1995;59(4):579–90.

458. Rossi-Fedele G, Scott W, Spratt D, et al. Incidence and behaviour of Tn916-like elements within tetracycline-resistant bacteria isolated from root canals. Oral Microbiol Immunol 2006;21(4):218–22.

459. Dunny GM, Brown BL, Clewell DB. Induced cell aggregation and mating in Streptococcus faecalis: evidence for a bacterial sex pheromone. Proc Natl Acad Sci USA 1978;75(7):3479–83.

460. Dunny GM, Craig RA, Carron RL, Clewell DB. Plasmid transfer in Streptococcus faecalis: production of multiple sex pheromones by recipients. Plasmid 1979;2(3):454–65.

461. Showsh SA, De Boever EH, Clewell DB. Vancomycin resistance plasmid in Enterococcus faecalis that encodes sensitivity to a sex pheromone also produced by Staphylococcus aureus. Antimicrob Agents Chemother 2001;45(7):2177–8.

462. Martinez JL, Baquero F. Interactions among strategies associated with bacterial infection: pathogenicity, epidemicity, and antibiotic resistance. Clin Microbiol Rev 2002;15(4):647–79.

463. Silver S. Bacterial silver resistance: molecular biology and uses and misuses of silver compounds. FEMS Microbiol Rev 2003;27(2–3):341–53.

464. Silver S, Phung LT. Bacterial heavy metal resistance: new surprises. Annu Rev Microbiol 1996;50:753–89.

465. Ochoa TJ, Cleary TG. Epidemiology and spectrum of disease of Escherichia coli O157. Curr Opin Infect Dis 2003;16(3):259–63.

466. Dinges MM, Orwin PM, Schlievert PM. Exotoxins of Staphylococcus aureus. Clin Microbiol Rev 2000;13(1):16–34.

467. Balaban N, Rasooly A. Staphylococcal enterotoxins. Int J Food Microbiol 2000;61(1):1–10.

468. Ike Y, Hashimoto H, Clewell DB. High incidence of hemolysin production by Enterococcus (Streptococcus) faecalis strains associated with human parenteral infections. J Clin Microbiol 1987;25(8):1524–8.

469. Huycke MM, Gilmore MS. Frequency of aggregation substance and cytolysin genes among enterococcal endocarditis isolates. Plasmid 1995;34(2):152–6.

470. Dunny GM, Birch N, Hascall G, Clewell DB. Isolation and characterization of plasmid deoxyribonucleic acid from Streptococcus mutans. J Bacteriol 1973;114(3):1362–4.

471. Clewell DB, Franke AE. Characterization of a plasmid determining resistance to erythromycin, lincomycin, and vernamycin Balpha in a strain Streptococcus pyogenes. Antimicrob Agents Chemother 1974;5(5):534–7.

472. Yagi Y, McLellan TS, Frez WA, Clewell DB. Characterization of a small plasmid determining resistance to erythromycin, lincomycin, and vernamycin Balpha in a strain of Streptococcus sanguis isolated from dental plaque. Antimicrob Agents Chemother 1978;13(5):884–7.

473. Caufield PW, Wannemuehler YM, Hansen JB. Familial clustering of the Streptococcus mutans cryptic plasmid strain in a dental clinic population. Infect Immun 1982;38(2):785–7.

474. Caufield PW, Ratanapridakul K, Allen DN, Cutter GR. Plasmid-containing strains of Streptococcus mutans cluster within family and racial cohorts: implications for natural transmission. Infect Immun 1988;56(12):3216–20.

475. Bergmann JE, Johanna E, Oloff S, Gulzow HJ. Characterization of a Streptococcus mutans serotype e plasmid pJEB110. Arch Oral Biol 1990;35 Suppl:169S–172S.

476. Vandenbergh PA, Syed SA, Gonzalez CF, et al. Plasmid content of some oral microorganisms isolated from subgingival plaque. J Dent Res 1982;61(3):497–501.

477. Teanpaisan R, Douglas CW, Eley AR, Walsh TF. Clonality of Porphyromonas gingivalis, Prevotella intermedia and Prevotella nigrescens isolated from periodontally diseased and healthy sites. J Periodontal Res 1996;31(6):423–32.

478. Paula MO, Gaetti-Jardim Junior E, Avila-Campos MJ. Plasmid profile in oral Fusobacterium nucleatum from humans

and Cebus apella monkeys. Rev Inst Med Trop Sao Paulo 2003;45(1):5–9.
479. Chan EC, Klitorinos A, Gharbia S, et al. Characterization of a 4.2-kb plasmid isolated from periodontopathic spirochetes. Oral Microbiol Immunol 1996;11(5):365–8.
480. Oliver DR, Brown BL, Clewell DB. Characterization of plasmids determining hemolysin and bacteriocin production in *Streptococcus faecalis* 5952. J Bacteriol 1977;130(2):948–50.
481. Sedgley CM, Lennan SL, Clewell DB. Prevalence, phenotype and genotype of oral enterococci. Oral Microbiol Immunol 2004;19(2):95–101.
482. Sedgley C, Buck G, Appelbe O. Prevalence of *Enterococcus faecalis* at multiple oral sites in endodontic patients using culture and PCR. J Endod 2006;32(2):104–9.
483. Kuramitsu HK, Trapa V. Genetic exchange between oral streptococci during mixed growth. J Gen Microbiol 1984;130(10):2497–500.
484. Fitzgerald GF, Clewell DB. A conjugative transposon (Tn919) in *Streptococcus sanguis*. Infect Immun 1985;47(2):415–20.
485. Keller L, Surette MG. Communication in bacteria: an ecological and evolutionary perspective. Nat Rev Microbiol 2006;4(4):249–58.
486. Kolenbrander PE, Egland PG, Diaz PI, Palmer RJ Jr. Genome-genome interactions: bacterial communities in initial dental plaque. Trends Microbiol 2005;13(1):11–15.
487. Duan K, Dammel C, Stein J, et al. Modulation of *Pseudomonas aeruginosa* gene expression by host microflora through interspecies communication. Mol Microbiol 2003;50(5):1477–91.
488. Egland PG, Palmer RJ Jr, Kolenbrander PE. Interspecies communication in *Streptococcus gordonii-Veillonella* atypica biofilms: signaling in flow conditions requires juxtaposition. Proc Natl Acad Sci USA 2004;101(48):16917–22.
489. Gibbons RJ, Nygaard M. Interbacterial aggregation of plaque bacteria. Arch Oral Biol 1970;15(12):1397–400.
490. Kinder SA, Holt SC. Coaggregation between bacterial species. Methods Enzymol 1994;236:254–70.
491. Kolenbrander PE. Oral microbial communities: biofilms, interactions, and genetic systems. Annu Rev Microbiol 2000;54:413–37.
492. Svensäter G, Bergenholtz G. Biofilms in endodontic infections. Endod Topics 2004;9:27–36.
493. Nair PN, Henry S, Cano V, Vera J. Microbial status of apical root canal system of human mandibular first molars with primary apical periodontitis after "one-visit" endodontic treatment. Oral Surg Oral Med Oral Pathol Oral Radiol Endod 2005;99(2):231–52.
494. Love RM, Jenkinson HF. Invasion of dentinal tubules by oral bacteria. Crit Rev Oral Biol Med 2002;13(2):171–83.
495. Love RM, McMillan MD, Park Y, Jenkinson HF. Coinvasion of dentinal tubules by Porphyromonas gingivalis and Streptococcus gordonii depends upon binding specificity of streptococcal antigen I/II adhesin. Infect Immun 2000;68(3):1359–65.
496. Palmer RJ Jr, Gordon SM, Cisar JO, Kolenbrander PE. Coaggregation-mediated interactions of streptococci and *actinomyces* detected in initial human dental plaque. J Bacteriol 2003;185(11):3400–9.
497. Sorensen SJ, Bailey M, Hansen LH, et al. Studying plasmid horizontal transfer in situ: a critical review. Nat Rev Microbiol 2005;3(9):700–10.
498. Fux CA, Costerton JW, Stewart PS, Stoodley P. Survival strategies of infectious biofilms. Trends Microbiol 2005;13(1):34–40.
499. Khemaleelakul S, Baumgartner JC, Pruksakom S. Autoaggregation and coaggregation of bacteria associated with acute endodontic infections. J Endod 2006;32(4):312–18.
500. Johnson EM, Flannagan SE, Sedgley CM. Coaggregation interactions between oral and endodontic *Enterococcus faecalis* and bacterial species isolated from persistent apical periodontitis. J Endod 2006;10(32):946–50.
501. Kolenbrander PE, Andersen RN, Moore LV. Coaggregation of *Fusobacterium nucleatum*, *Selenomonas flueggei*, *Selenomonas infelix*, *Selenomonas noxia*, and *Selenomonas sputigena* with strains from 11 genera of oral bacteria. Infect Immun 1989;57(10):3194–203.
502. Coque TM, Patterson JE, Steckelberg JM, Murray BE. Incidence of hemolysin, gelatinase, and aggregation substance among enterococci isolated from patients with endocarditis and other infections and from feces of hospitalized and community-based persons. J Infect Dis 1995;171(5):1223–9.
503. Shen S, Samaranayake LP, Yip HK. Coaggregation profiles of the microflora from root surface caries lesions. Arch Oral Biol 2005;50(1):23–32.
504. Lancy P Jr, Dirienzo JM, Appelbaum B, et al. Corncob formation between *Fusobacterium nucleatum* and *Streptococcus sanguis*. Infect Immun 1983;40(1):303–9.
505. Turner SR, Love RM, Lyons KM. An in-vitro investigation of the antibacterial effect of nisin in root canals and canal wall radicular dentine. Int Endod J 2004;37(10):664–71.
506. Sundqvist GK, Eckerbom MI, Larsson AP, Sjogren UT. Capacity of anaerobic bacteria from necrotic dental pulps to induce purulent infections. Infect Immun 1979;25(2):685–93.
507. Nair PN. On the causes of persistent apical periodontitis: a review. Int Endod J 2006;39(4):249–81.
508. Siqueira JF Jr. Aetiology of root canal treatment failure: why well-treated teeth can fail. Int Endod J 2001;34(1):1–10.
509. Sundqvist G. Bacteriological studies of necrotic dental pulps [dissertation]. Umea, Sweden: University of Umea 1976.
510. Kantz WE, Henry CA. Isolation and classification of anaerobic bacteria from intact pulp chambers of non-vital teeth in man. Arch Oral Biol 1974;19(1):91–6.
511. Pace NR. A molecular view of microbial diversity and the biosphere. Science 1997;276(5313):734–40.
512. Zoletti GO, Siqueira JF Jr, Santos KR. Identification of Enterococcus faecalis in root-filled teeth with or without periradicular lesions by culture-dependent and -independent approaches. J Endod 2006;32(8):722–6.

513. Williams JM, Trope M, Caplan DJ, Shugars DC. Detection and quantitation of E. faecalis by real-time PCR (qPCR), reverse transcription-PCR (RT-PCR), and cultivation during endodontic treatment. J Endod 2006;32(8):715–21.

514. Sedgley C, Nagel A, Dahlen G, et al. Real-time quantitative polymerase chain reaction and culture analyses of Enterococcus faecalis in root canals. J Endod 2006;32(3):173–7.

515. Sedgley CM, Nagel AC, Shelburne CE, et al. Quantitative real-time PCR detection of oral Enterococcus faecalis in humans. Arch Oral Biol 2005;50(6):575–83.

516. Haapasalo M, Udnaes T, Endal U. Persistent, recurrent, and acquired infection of the root canal system post-treatment. Endod Topics 2003;6:29–56.

517. Adib V, Spratt D, Ng YL, Gulabivala K. Cultivable microbial flora associated with persistent periapical disease and coronal leakage after root canal treatment: a preliminary study. Int Endod J 2004;37(8):542–51.

518. Schleifer KH, Kilpper-Balz R. Transfer of Streptococcus faecalis and *Streptococcus faecium* to the genus *Enterococcus nom. rev Enterococcus faecalis* comb. nov. and *Enterococcus faecium* comb. nov. Int J Syst Bacteriol 1983;34:31–34.

519. Richards MJ, Edwards JR, Culver DH, Gaynes RP. Nosocomial infections in medical intensive care units in the United States. National Nosocomial Infections Surveillance System. Crit Care Med 1999;27(5):887–92.

520. Pavoni GL, Giannella M, Falcone M, et al. Conservative medical therapy of prosthetic joint infections: retrospective analysis of an 8-year experience. Clin Microbiol Infect 2004;10(9):831–7.

521. Singh KV, Weinstock GM, Murray BE. An *Enterococcus faecalis* ABC homologue (Lsa) is required for the resistance of this species to clindamycin and quinupristin-dalfopristin. Antimicrob Agents Chemother 2002;46(6):1845–50.

522. Gold OG, Jordan HV, van Houte J. The prevalence of enterococci in the human mouth and their pathogenicity in animal models. Arch Oral Biol 1975;20(7):473–7.

523. Rams TE, Feik D, Young V, et al. Enterococci in human periodontitis. Oral Microbiol Immunol 1992;7(4):249–52.

524. Bender IB, Seltzer S. Combination of antibiotics and fungicides used in treatment of the infected pulpless tooth. J Am Dent Assoc 1952;45(3):293–300.

525. Engstrom B. The significance of enterococci in root canal treatment. Odontol Revy 1964;15:87–106.

526. Haapasalo M, Ranta H, Ranta KT. Facultative gram-negative enteric rods in persistent periapical infections. Acta Odontol Scand 1983;41(1):19–22.

527. Siren EK, Haapasalo MP, Ranta K, et al. Microbiological findings and clinical treatment procedures in endodontic cases selected for microbiological investigation. Int Endod J 1997;30(2):91–5.

528. Cheung GS, Ho MW. Microbial flora of root canal-treated teeth associated with asymptomatic periapical radiolucent lesions. Oral Microbiol Immunol 2001;16(6):332–7.

529. Kaufman B, Spangberg L, Barry J, Fouad AF. *Enterococcus spp.* in endodontically treated teeth with and without periradicular lesions. J Endod 2005;31(12):851–6.

530. MacCallum WG, Hastings TW. A case of acute endocarditis caused by Micrococcus zymogenes (nov. spec.), with a description of the microorganism. J Exp Med 1899;4:521–34.

531. Dupont H, Montravers P, Mohler J, Carbon C. Disparate findings on the role of virulence factors of *Enterococcus faecalis* in mouse and rat models of peritonitis. Infect Immun 1998;66(6):2570–5.

532. Schlievert PM, Gahr PJ, Assimacopoulos AP, et al. Aggregation and binding substances enhance pathogenicity in rabbit models of *Enterococcus faecalis* endocarditis. Infect Immun 1998;66(1):218–23.

533. Möller AJ, Fabricius L, Dahlen G, et al. Apical periodontitis development and bacterial response to endodontic treatment. Experimental root canal infections in monkeys with selected bacterial strains. Eur J Oral Sci 2004;112(3):207–15.

534. Kayaoglu G, Orstavik D. Virulence factors of *Enterococcus faecalis*: relationship to endodontic disease. Crit Rev Oral Biol Med 2004;15(5):308–20.

535. Gentry-Weeks CR, Karkhoff-Schweizer R, Pikis A, et al. Survival of *Enterococcus faecalis* in mouse peritoneal macrophages. Infect Immun 1999;67(5):2160–5.

536. Neely AN, Maley MP. Survival of enterococci and staphylococci on hospital fabrics and plastic. J Clin Microbiol 2000;38(2):724–6.

537. Figdor D, Davies JK, Sundqvist G. Starvation survival, growth and recovery of *Enterococcus faecalis* in human serum. Oral Microbiol Immunol 2003;18(4):234–9.

538. Lleo MM, Pierobon S, Tafi MC, et al. mRNA detection by reverse transcription-PCR for monitoring viability over time in an Enterococcus faecalis viable but nonculturable population maintained in a laboratory microcosm. Appl Environ Microbiol 2000;66(10):4564–7.

539. Lleo MM, Bonato B, Tafi MC, et al. Resuscitation rate in different enterococcal species in the viable but nonculturable state. J Appl Microbiol 2001;91(6):1095–102.

540. Signoretto C, Lleo MM, Tafi MC, Canepari P. Cell wall chemical composition of Enterococcus faecalis in the viable but nonculturable state. Appl Environ Microbiol 2000;66(5):1953–9.

541. Pruzzo C, Tarsi R, Lleo MM, et al. In vitro adhesion to human cells by viable but nonculturable *Enterococcus faecalis*. Curr Microbiol 2002;45(2):105–10.

542. Laplace JM, Thuault M, Hartke A, et al. Sodium hypochlorite stress in *Enterococcus faecalis*: influence of antecedent growth conditions and induced proteins. Curr Microbiol 1997;34(5):284–9.

543. Flahaut S, Benachour A, Giard JC, et al. Defense against lethal treatments and de novo protein synthesis induced by NaCl in *Enterococcus faecalis* ATCC 19433. Arch Microbiol 1996;165(5):317–24.

544. Flahaut S, Hartke A, Giard JC, Auffray Y. Alkaline stress response in *Enterococcus faecalis*: adaptation, cross-protection, and changes in protein synthesis. Appl Environ Microbiol 1997;63(2):812–14.

545. Giard JC, Laplace JM, Rince A, et al. The stress proteome of *Enterococcus faecalis*. Electrophoresis 2001;22(14):2947–54.

546. Giard JC, Hartke A, Flahaut S, et al. Glucose starvation response in *Enterococcus faecalis* JH2-2: survival and protein analysis. Res Microbiol 1997;148(1):27–35.

547. Capiaux H, Giard JC, Lemarinier S, Auffray Y. Characterization and analysis of a new gene involved in glucose starvation response in *Enterococcus faecalis*. Int J Food Microbiol 2000;55(1–3):99–102.

548. Boutibonnes P, Giard JC, Hartke A, et al. Characterization of the heat shock response in *Enterococcus faecalis*. Antonie Van Leeuwenhoek 1993;64(1):47–55.

549. Molander A, Reit C, Dahlen G. Microbiological evaluation of clindamycin as a root canal dressing in teeth with apical periodontitis. Int Endod J 1990;23(2):113–18.

550. Dahlen G, Samuelsson W, Molander A, Reit C. Identification and antimicrobial susceptibility of enterococci isolated from the root canal. Oral Microbiol Immunol 2000;15(5):309–12.

551. Portenier I, Waltimo TMT, Haapasalo M. Enterococcus faecalis - the root canal survivor and 'star' in post-treatment disease. Endod Topics 2003;6:135–59.

552. Appelbe OK, Sedgley CM. Effects of prolonged exposure to alkaline pH on *Enterococcus faecalis* survival and specific gene transcripts. Oral Microbiol Immunol, 2007;22(3): 169–74.

553. Love RM. Intraradicular space: what happens within roots of infected teeth? Ann R Australas Coll Dent Surg 2000; 15:235–9.

554. Love RM. Enterococcus faecalis–a mechanism for its role in endodontic failure. Int Endod J 2001;34(5):399–405.

555. George S, Kishen A, Song KP. The role of environmental changes on monospecies biofilm formation on root canal wall by *Enterococcus faecalis*. J Endod 2005;31(12):867–72.

556. Kishen A, George S, Kumar R. Enterococcus faecalis-mediated biomineralized biofilm formation on root canal dentine in vitro. J Biomed Mater Res A 2006;77(2):406–15.

557. Kowalski WJ, Kasper EL, Hatton JF, et al. Enterococcus faecalis adhesin, Ace, mediates attachment to particulate dentin. J Endod 2006;32(7):634–7.

558. Rakita RM, Vanek NN, Jacques-Palaz K, et al. *Enterococcus faecalis* bearing aggregation substance is resistant to killing by human neutrophils despite phagocytosis and neutrophil activation. Infect Immun 1999;67(11):6067–75.

559. Ember JA, Hugli TE. Characterization of the human neutrophil response to sex pheromones from *Streptococcus faecalis*. Am J Pathol 1989;134(4):797–805.

560. Sannomiya P, Craig RA, Clewell DB, et al. Characterization of a class of nonformylated *Enterococcus faecalis*-derived neutrophil chemotactic peptides: the sex pheromones. Proc Natl Acad Sci USA 1990;87(1):66–70.

561. Facklam R. What happened to the streptococci: overview of taxonomic and nomenclature changes. Clin Microbiol Rev 2002;15(4):613–30.

562. Tak T, Dhawan S, Reynolds C, Shukla SK. Current diagnosis and treatment of infective endocarditis. Expert Rev Anti Infect Ther 2003;1(4):639–54.

563. Young Lee S, Cisar JO, Bryant JL, et al. Resistance of Streptococcus gordonii to polymorphonuclear leukocyte killing is a potential virulence determinant of infective endocarditis. Infect Immun 2006;74(6):3148–55.

564. Takahashi Y, Takashima E, Shimazu K, et al. Contribution of sialic acid-binding adhesin to pathogenesis of experimental endocarditis caused by *Streptococcus gordonii* DL1. Infect Immun 2006;74(1):740–3.

565. Douglas CW, Brown PR, Preston FE. Platelet aggregation by oral streptococci. FEMS Microbiol Lett 1990;60(1–2):63–7.

566. Vigil GV, Wayman BE, Dazey SE, et al. Identification and antibiotic sensitivity of bacteria isolated from periapical lesions. J Endod 1997;23(2):110–14.

567. Pinheiro ET, Gomes BP, Ferraz CC, et al. Evaluation of root canal microorganisms isolated from teeth with endodontic failure and their antimicrobial susceptibility. Oral Microbiol Immunol 2003;18(2):100–3.

568. Cvitkovitch DG. Genetic competence and transformation in oral streptococci. Crit Rev Oral Biol Med 2001;12(3):217–43.

569. Jenkinson HF, Lamont RJ. Streptococcal adhesion and colonization. Crit Rev Oral Biol Med 1997;8(2):175–200.

570. Banas JA, Vickerman MM. Glucan-binding proteins of the oral streptococci. Crit Rev Oral Biol Med 2003;14(2):89–99.

571. Jenkinson HF. Cell surface protein receptors in oral streptococci. FEMS Microbiol Lett 1994;121(2):133–40.

572. Rogers JD, Palmer RJ Jr, Kolenbrander PE, Scannapieco FA. Role of Streptococcus gordonii amylase-binding protein A in adhesion to hydroxyapatite, starch metabolism, and biofilm formation. Infect Immun 2001;69(11):7046–56.

573. Love RM. Regional variation in root dentinal tubule infection by *Streptococcus gordonii*. J Endod 1996;22(6):290–3.

574. Bate AL, Ma JK, Pitt Ford TR. Detection of bacterial virulence genes associated with infective endocarditis in infected root canals. Int Endod J 2000;33(3):194–203.

575. Yeung MK. Molecular and genetic analyses of *Actinomyces* spp. Crit Rev Oral Biol Med 1999;10(2):120–38.

576. Mardis JS, Many WJ Jr. Endocarditis due to *Actinomyces viscosus*. South Med J 2001;94(2):240–3.

577. Happonen RP, Viander M, Pelliniemi L, Aitasalo K. *Actinomyces israelii* in osteoradionecrosis of the jaws. Histopathologic and immunocytochemical study of five cases. Oral Surg Oral Med Oral Pathol 1983;55(6):580–8.

578. Hansen T, Kunkel M, Kirkpatrick CJ, Weber A. *Actinomyces* in infected osteoradionecrosis–underestimated? Hum Pathol 2006;37(1):61–7.

579. Brailsford SR, Tregaskis RB, Leftwich HS, Beighton D. The predominant *Actinomyces* spp. isolated from infected dentin of active root caries lesions. J Dent Res 1999;78(9):1525–34.

580. Behbehani MJ, Jordan HV, Heeley JD. Oral colonization and pathogenicity of *Actinomyces israelii* in gnotobiotic rats. J Dent Res 1983;62(1):69–74.

581. Borssen E, Sundqvist G. Actinomyces of infected dental root canals. Oral Surg Oral Med Oral Pathol 1981;51(6):643–8.

582. Figures KH, Douglas CW. Actinomycosis associated with a root-treated tooth: report of a case. Int Endod J 1991;24(6):326–9.

583. Sakellariou PL. Periapical actinomycosis: report of a case and review of the literature. Endod Dent Traumatol 1996;12(3):151–4.

584. Nair PN, Pajarola G, Luder HU. Ciliated epithelium-lined radicular cysts. Oral Surg Oral Med Oral Pathol Oral Radiol Endod 2002;94(4):485–93.

585. Collins MD, Hoyles L, Kalfas S, et al. Characterization of *Actinomyces* isolates from infected root canals of teeth: description of Actinomyces radicidentis sp. nov. J Clin Microbiol 2000;38(9):3399–403.

586. Kalfas S, Figdor D, Sundqvist G. A new bacterial species associated with failed endodontic treatment: identification and description of *Actinomyces radicidentis*. Oral Surg Oral Med Oral Pathol Oral Radiol Endod 2001;92(2):208–14.

587. Cisar JO, Curl SH, Kolenbrander PE, Vatter AE. Specific absence of type 2 fimbriae on a coaggregation-defective mutant of *Actinomyces viscosus* T14V. Infect Immun 1983;40(2):759–65.

588. Kolenbrander PE, Celesk RA. Coaggregation of human oral *Cytophaga* species and *Actinomyces israelii*. Infect Immun 1983;40(3):1178–85.

589. Coleman RM, Georg LK. Comparative pathogenicity of *Actinomyces naeslundii* and *Actinomyces israelii*. Appl Microbiol 1969;18(3):427–32.

590. Figdor D, Sjogren U, Sorlin S, et al. Pathogenicity of *Actinomyces israelii* and *Arachnia propionica*: experimental infection in guinea pigs and phagocytosis and intracellular killing by human polymorphonuclear leukocytes in vitro. Oral Microbiol Immunol 1992;7(3):129–36.

591. Roth RR, James WD. Microbial ecology of the skin. Annu Rev Microbiol 1988;42:441–64.

592. Vowels BR, Yang S, Leyden JJ. Induction of proinflammatory cytokines by a soluble factor of *Propionibacterium acnes*: implications for chronic inflammatory acne. Infect Immun 1995;63(8):3158–65.

593. Berenson CS, Bia FJ. *Propionibacterium acnes* causes postoperative brain abscesses unassociated with foreign bodies: case reports. Neurosurgery 1989;25(1):130–4.

594. Mory F, Fougnot S, Rabaud C, et al. In vitro activities of cefotaxime, vancomycin, quinupristin/dalfopristin, linezolid and other antibiotics alone and in combination against *Propionibacterium acnes* isolates from central nervous system infections. J Antimicrob Chemother 2005;55(2):265–8.

595. Delahaye F, Fol S, Celard M, et al. [*Propionibacterium acnes* infective endocarditis. Study of 11 cases and review of literature]. Arch Mal Coeur Vaiss 2005;98(12):1212–18.

596. Brazier JS, Hall V. *Propionibacterium propionicum* and infections of the lacrimal apparatus. Clin Infect Dis 1993;17(5):892–3.

597. Happonen RP, Soderling E, Viander M, et al. Immunocytochemical demonstration of *Actinomyces* species and *Arachnia propionica* in periapical infections. J Oral Pathol 1985;14(5):405–13.

598. Hoshino E. Predominant obligate anaerobes in human carious dentin. J Dent Res 1985;64(10):1195–8.

599. Ando N, Hoshino E. Predominant obligate anaerobes invading the deep layers of root canal dentin. Int Endod J 1990;23(1):20–7.

600. Sjogren U, Happonen RP, Kahnberg KE, Sundqvist G. Survival of *Arachnia propionica* in periapical tissue. Int Endod J 1988;21(4):277–82.

601. Debelian GJ, Olsen I, Tronstad L. Electrophoresis of whole-cell soluble proteins of microorganisms isolated from bacteremias in endodontic therapy. Eur J Oral Sci 1996;104(5–6):540–6.

602. Siqueira JF Jr, De Uzeda M, Fonseca ME. A scanning electron microscopic evaluation of in vitro dentinal tubules penetration by selected anaerobic bacteria. J Endod 1996;22(6):308–10.

603. Webster GF, Leyden JJ, Musson RA, Douglas SD. Susceptibility of *Propionibacterium acnes* to killing and degradation by human neutrophils and monocytes in vitro. Infect Immun 1985;49(1):116–21.

604. Csukas Z, Banizs B, Rozgonyi F. Studies on the cytotoxic effects of *Propionibacterium acnes* strains isolated from cornea. Microb Pathog 2004;36(3):171–4.

605. Perry AL, Lambert PA. *Propionibacterium acnes*. Lett Appl Microbiol 2006;42(3):185–8.

606. Roszkowski W, Roszkowski K, Ko HL, et al. Immunomodulation by propionibacteria. Zentralbl Bakteriol 1990;274(3):289–98.

607. Odds FC. Candida and candidosis—a review and bibliography. 2nd ed. London: Baillière Tindall-W.B. Saunders; 1988.

608. Ruhnke M. Epidemiology of Candida albicans infections and role of non-Candida-albicans yeasts. Curr Drug Targets 2006;7(4):495–504.

609. Slutsky B, Buffo J, Soll DR. High-frequency switching of colony morphology in Candida albicans. Science 1985;230(4726):666–9.

610. Siqueira JF Jr, Sen BH. Fungi in endodontic infections. Oral Surg Oral Med Oral Pathol Oral Radiol Endod 2004;97(5):632–41.

611. Waltimo TMT, Haapasalo H, Zehnder M, Meyer JR. Clinical aspects related to endodontic yeast infections. Endod Topics 2004;9:66–78.

612. Nair PN. Pathogenesis of apical periodontitis and the causes of endodontic failures. Crit Rev Oral Biol Med 2004;15(6):348–81.

613. Waltimo TM, Siren EK, Torkko HL, et al. Fungi in therapy-resistant apical periodontitis. Int Endod J 1997;30(2):96–101.

614. Waltimo T, Kuusinen M, Jarvensivu A, et al. Examination on Candida spp. in refractory periapical granulomas. Int Endod J 2003;36(9):643–7.

615. Waltimo TM, Orstavik D, Siren EK, Haapasalo MP. In vitro yeast infection of human dentin. J Endod 2000;26(4):207–9.

616. Sen BH, Safavi KE, Spangberg LS. Antifungal effects of sodium hypochlorite and chlorhexidine in root canals. J Endod 1999;25(4):235–8.

617. Waltimo TM, Dassanayake RS, Orstavik D, et al. Phenotypes and randomly amplified polymorphic DNA profiles of *Candida albicans* isolates from root canal infections in a Finnish population. Oral Microbiol Immunol 2001;16(2):106–12.

618. Waltimo TM, Sen BH, Meurman JH, et al. Yeasts in apical periodontitis. Crit Rev Oral Biol Med 2003;14(2):128–37.

619. Holmes AR, Gopal PK, Jenkinson HF. Adherence of *Candida albicans* to a cell surface polysaccharide receptor on *Streptococcus gordonii*. Infect Immun 1995;63(5):1827–34.

620. Jenkinson HF, Lala HC, Shepherd MG. Coaggregation of *Streptococcus sanguis* and other streptococci with *Candida albicans*. Infect Immun 1990;58(5):1429–36.

621. Grimaudo NJ, Nesbitt WE. Coaggregation of *Candida albicans* with oral *Fusobacterium* species. Oral Microbiol Immunol 1997;12(3):168–73.

622. Grimaudo NJ, Nesbitt WE, Clark WB. Coaggregation of *Candida albicans* with oral *Actinomyces* species. Oral Microbiol Immunol 1996;11(1):59–61.

623. Naglik J, Albrecht A, Bader O, Hube B. *Candida albicans* proteinases and host/pathogen interactions. Cell Microbiol 2004;6(10):915–26.

624. Monod M, Borg-von ZM. Secreted aspartic proteases as virulence factors of *Candida* species. Biol Chem 2002;383(7-8):1087–93.

625. Brouqui P, Raoult D. Endocarditis due to rare and fastidious bacteria. Clin Microbiol Rev 2001;14(1):177–207.

626. Brook I. Microbiology and management of endodontic infections in children. J Clin Pediatr Dent 2003;28(1):13–17.

627. Rocas IN, Jung IY, Lee CY, Siqueira JF Jr. Polymerase chain reaction identification of microorganisms in previously root-filled teeth in a South Korean population. J Endod 2004;30(7):504–8.

628. American Association of Endodontists. Contemporary terms of emdodontics. 7th ed; 2003.

629. Walton R, Fouad A. Endodontic interappointment flare-ups: a prospective study of incidence and related factors. J Endod 1992;18(4):172–7.

630. Walton RE. Interappointment flare-ups: incidence, related factors, prevention, and management. Endod Topics 2002;3:67–76.

631. Imura N, Zuolo ML. Factors associated with endodontic flare-ups: a prospective study. Int Endod J 1995;28(5):261–5.

632. Siqueira JF Jr. Microbial causes of endodontic flare-ups. Int Endod J 2003;36(7):453–63.

633. Genet JM, Hart AA, Wesselink PR, Thoden van Velzen SK. Preoperative and operative factors associated with pain after the first endodontic visit. Int Endod J 1987;20(2):53–64.

634. Torabinejad M, Kettering JD, McGraw JC, et al. Factors associated with endodontic interappointment emergencies of teeth with necrotic pulps. J Endod 1988;14(5):261–6.

635. O'Keefe EM. Pain in endodontic therapy: preliminary study. J Endod 1976;2(10):315–19.

636. Seltzer S, Naidorf IJ. Flare-ups in endodontics: I. Etiological factors. J Endod 1985;11(11):472–8.

637. Matusow RJ. The flare-up phenomenon in endodontics: a clinical perspective and review. Oral Surg Oral Med Oral Pathol Endod 1988;65(6):750–3.

638. Trope M. Flare-up rate of single-visit endodontics. Int Endod J 1991;24(1):24–6.

639. Clem WH. Posttreatment endodontic pain. J Am Dent Assoc 1970;81(5):1166–70.

640. Eleazer PD, Eleazer KR. Flare-up rate in pulpally necrotic molars in one-visit versus two-visit endodontic treatment. J Endod 1998;24(9):614–16.

641. Balaban FS, Skidmore AE, Griffin JA. Acute exacerbations following initial treatment of necrotic pulps. J Endod 1984;10(2):78–81.

642. Gound TG, Marx D, Schwandt NA. Incidence of flare-ups and evaluation of quality after retreatment of resorcinol-formaldehyde resin ("Russian Red Cement") endodontic therapy. J Endod 2003;29(10):624–6.

643. Walton RE, Holton IF Jr, Michelich R. Calcium hydroxide as an intracanal medication: effect on posttreatment pain. J Endod 2003;29(10):627–9.

644. Walton RE, Chiappinelli J. Prophylactic penicillin: effect on posttreatment symptoms following root canal treatment of asymptomatic periapical pathosis. J Endod 1993;19(9):466–70.

645. Pickenpaugh L, Reader A, Beck M, et al. Effect of prophylactic amoxicillin on endodontic flare-up in asymptomatic, necrotic teeth. J Endod 2001;27(1):53–6.

646. Henry M, Reader A, Beck M. Effect of penicillin on postoperative endodontic pain and swelling in symptomatic necrotic teeth. J Endod 2001;27(2):117–23.

647. Nagle D, Reader A, Beck M, Weaver J. Effect of systemic penicillin on pain in untreated irreversible pulpitis. Oral Surg Oral Med Oral Pathol Oral Radiol Endod 2000;90(5):636–40.

648. Ehrmann EH, Messer HH, Adams GG. The relationship of intracanal medicaments to postoperative pain in endodontics. Int Endod J 2003;36(12):868–75.

649. Moskow A, Morse DR, Krasner P, Furst ML. Intracanal use of a corticosteroid solution as an endodontic anodyne. Oral Surg Oral Med Oral Pathol Endod 1984;58(5):600–4.

650. Rogers MJ, Johnson BR, Remeikis NA, BeGole EA. Comparison of effect of intracanal use of ketorolac tromethamine and dexamethasone with oral ibuprofen on post treatment endodontic pain. J Endod 1999;25(5):381–4.

651. Casadevall A, Pirofski LA. Host-pathogen interactions: redefining the basic concepts of virulence and pathogenicity. Infect Immun 1999;67(8):3703–13.

652. Bartels HA, Naidorf IJ, Blechman H. A study of some factors associated with endodontic "flare-ups." Oral Surg Oral Med Oral Pathol Endod 1968;25(2):255–61.

653. Baumgartner JC, Falkler WA Jr, Beckerman T. Experimentally induced infection by oral anaerobic microorganisms in a mouse model. Oral Microbiol Immunol 1992;7(4):253–6.

654. Dahlen G. Immune response in rats against lipopolysaccharides of Fusobacterium nucleatum and *Bacteroides oralis* administered in the root canal. Scand J Dent Res 1980;88(2):122–9.

655. Grenier D, Grignon L. Response of human macrophage-like cells to stimulation by *Fusobacterium nucleatum* ssp. nucleatum lipopolysaccharide. Oral Microbiol Immunol 2006;21(3):190–6.

656. Falagas ME, Siakavellas E. *Bacteroides, Prevotella, and Porphyromonas* species: a review of antibiotic resistance and therapeutic options. Int J Antimicrob Agents 2000;15(1):1–9.

657. Pitts DL, Williams BL, Morton TH Jr. Investigation of the role of endotoxin in periapical inflammation. J Endod 1982;8(1):10–18.

658. Khabbaz MG, Anastasiadis PL, Sykaras SN. Determination of endotoxins in caries: association with pulpal pain. Int Endod J 2000;33(2):132–7.

659. Gomes BP, Drucker DB, Lilley JD. Associations of specific bacteria with some endodontic signs and symptoms. Int Endod J 1994;27(6):291–8.

660. Jacinto RC, Gomes BP, Ferraz CC, et al. Microbiological analysis of infected root canals from symptomatic and asymptomatic teeth with periapical periodontitis and the antimicrobial susceptibility of some isolated anaerobic bacteria. Oral Microbiol Immunol 2003;18(5):285–92.

661. Brook I, Grimm S, Kielich RB. Bacteriology of acute periapical abscess in children. J Endod 1981;7(8):378–80.

662. Gomes BP, Lilley JD, Drucker DB. Associations of endodontic symptoms and signs with particular combinations of specific bacteria. Int Endod J 1996;29(2):69–75.

663. Slots J, Nowzari H, Sabeti M. *Cytomegalovirus* infection in symptomatic periapical pathosis. Int Endod J 2004;37(8):519–24.

664. Yildirim S, Yapar M, Kubar A, Slots J. Human *cytomegalovirus, Epstein-Barr* virus and bone resorption-inducing cytokines in periapical lesions of deciduous teeth. Oral Microbiol Immunol 2006;21(2):107–11.

665. Costerton J, Lewandowski Z, DeBeer D, et al. Biofilms, the customized microniche. J Bacteriol 1994;176:2137–42.

666. Caldwell DE, Atuku E, Wilkie DC, et al. Germ theory vs. community theory in understanding and controlling the proliferation of biofilms. Adv Dent Res 1997;11(1):4–13.

667. Karthikeyan S, Wolfaardt GM, Korber DR, Caldwell DE. Identification of synergistic interactions among microorganisms in biofilms by digital image analysis. Int Microbiol 1999;(2):241–50.

668. Costerton J, Stewart PS, Greenberg EP. Bacterial biofilm: a common cause of persistent infections. Science 1999;(284):1318–22.

669. Gibbons R. Bacterial adhesion to oral tissues: a model for infectious diseases. J Dent Res 1989;5(68):750–60.

670. Wingender J, Neu TR, Flemming, H-C. What are bacterial extracellular polymeric substances? In: Microbial extracellular polymeric substances: characterization, structure and function. Springer Verlag; 1999.

671. Nivens D, Ohman DE, Williams J, Franklin MJ. Role of alginate and its O acetylation in formation of *Pseudomonas aeruginosa* microcolonies and biofilms. J Bacteriol 2001;3(183):1047–57.

672. Whitchurch C, Tolker-Nielsen T, Ragas PC, Mattick JS. Extracellular DNA required for bacterial biofilm formation. Science 2002;295(5559):1487.

673. Donlan R, Costerton, JW. Biofilms: survival mechanisms of clinically relevant microorganisms. Clin Microbiol Rev 2002;2(15):167–93.

674. Stewart P, Peyton BM, Drury WJ, Murga R. Quantitative observations of heterogeneities in *Pseudomonas aeruginosa* biofilms. Appl Environ Microbiol 1993;1(59):327–9.

675. Debeer D, Stoodley P, Roe F, Lewandowski Z. Effects of biofilm structures on oxygen distribution and masstransport. Biotechnol Bioeng 1994;11(43):1131–8.

676. McLean R, Fuqua C, Siegele DA, et al. Biofilm growth and an illustration of its role in mineral formation. In: Microbial biosystems: new frontiers. Proceedings of the 8th International Symposium on Microbial Ecology; 2000; Atlantic Canada Society for Microbial Ecology; pp. 255–61.

677. Stoodley P, Lewandowski Z, Boyle JD, Lappin-Scott HM. Oscillation characteristics of biofilm streamers in turbulent flowing water as related to drag and pressure drop. Biotechnol Bioeng 1998;(57):536–44.

678. Davey M, OToole, GA. Microbial biofilms: from ecology to molecular genetics. Microbiol Mol Biol Rev 2000;4(64):847–67.

679. Lewis K. Persister cells and the riddle of biofilm survival. Biochemistry (Mosc) 2005;2(70):267–74.

680. Allison D, Matthew MJ. Effect of polysaccharide interaction on antibiotic susceptibility of *Pseudomonas aeroginosa*. J Appl Bacteriol 1992;(73):484–8.

681. Gilbert P, Das J, Foley I. Biofilm susceptibility to antimicrobials. Adv Dent Res 1997;1(11):160–7.

682. Reid R, Visscher PT, Decho AW, et al. The role of microbes in accretion, lamination and early lithification of modern marine stromatolites. Nature 2000;6799(406):989–92.

683. Dewanti R, Wong AC. Influence of culture conditions on biofilm formation by Escherichia coli O157:H7. Int J Food Microbiol 1995;2(26):147–64.

684. Al Cunningham, Ross R, Stewart P, et al. Biofilms: Hypertext book. http://www.erc.montana.edu/bioflimbook/PREFACE_MATL/Contents.htm.

685. Maye RC, Moritz R, Kirschner C, et al. The role of intermolecular interactions: studies on model systems for bacterial biofilms. Int J Biol Macromol 1999;(26):3–16.

686. Costerton J, Lewandowaski Z, Caldwell DE, et al. Microbial biofilms. Annu Rev Microbiol 1995;(49):711–45.

687. Grenier D, Mayrand D. Nutritional relationships between oral bacteria. Infect Immun 1986;(53):616–20.

688. Socransky S, Haffajee AD. Dental biofilms: difficult therapeutic targets. Periodontol 2000 2000;(28):12–55.

689. Spratt D, Pratten J. Biofilms and the oral cavity. Rev Environ Sci Bio/Technology 2003;(2):109–20.

690. Stoodley P, Sauer K, Davies DG, Costerton JW. Biofilms as complex differentiated communities. Annu Rev of Microbiol 2002;(56):187–209.

691. Wtnic P, Kolter R. Biofilm, city of microbes. J Bacteriol 2000;182;(10):2675–9.

692. Drenkard E. Antimicrobial resistance of *Pseudomonas aeruginosa* biofilms. Microbes Infect 2003;13(5):1213–19.

693. Roberts AP, Pratten J, Wilson M, Mullan P. Transfer of a conjugative transposon, Tn5397 in a model oral biofilm. FEMS Microbiol Lett 1999;(177):63–66.

694. Hall-Stoodley L, Stoodley P. Developmental regulation of microbial biofilms. Curr Opin Biotechnol 2002;3(13):228–33.

695. Stoodley P, Dodds I, Boyle JD, Lappin-Scott HM. Influence of hydrodynamics and nutrients on biofilm structure. J Appl Microbiol 1999;(85):S19–28.

696. Al-Hashimi I, Levine MJ. Characterization of in vivo saliva-derived enamel pellicle. Arch Oral Biol 1989;(34):289–95.

697. Handley P, Carter PL, Fielding J. *Streptococcus salivarius* strains carry either fibrils or fimbriae on the cell surface. J Bacteriol 1984;(157):64–72.

698. Handley P, Carter PL, Wyett JE, Hesketh L. Surface structures (peritrichous fibrils and tufts of fibrils) found on *Streptococcus sanguis* strains may be related to their ability to coaggregate with other oral genera. Infect Immun 1985;(47):217–27.

699. Miron J, Ben-Ghedalia D, Morrison M. Invited review: adhesion mechanisms of rumen cellulolytic bacteria. J Dairy Sci 2001;6(84):1294–309.

700. Cowan M, Taylor KG, Doyle RJ. Energetics of the initial phase of adhesion of *Streptococcus sanguis* to hydroxyapatite. J Bacteriol 1987;(169):2995–3000.

701. Costerton J, Lewandowski Z. The biofilm lifestyle. Adv Dent Res 1997;2(11):192–5.

702. Busscher H, van der Mei HC. Physico-chemical interactions in initial microbial adhesion and relevance for biofilm formation. Adv Dent Res 1997;11(1):24–32.

703. Rickard A, Gilbert P, High NJ, Kolenbrander PE, Handley PS. Bacterial coaggregation: an integral process in the development of multi-species biofilms. Trends Microbiol 2003;2(11):94–100.

704. Busscher H, Bos R, van der Mei HC. Initial microbial adhesion is a determinant for the strength of biofilm adhesion. FEMS Microbiol. Lett 1995;(128):229–34.

705. Kolenbrander P, Andersen RN, Moore LV. Coaggregation of *Fusobacterium nucleatium, Selenomonas flueggei, Selenomonas infelix, Selenomonas noxia*, and *Selenomonas sputigena* with strains from 11 genera of oral bacteria. Infect Immun 1989;(57):3194–203.

706. Kolenbrander P, Parrish KD, Andersen RN, Greenberg EP. Intergeneric coaggregation of oral *Treponema* spp. with *Fusobacterium* spp. and intrageneric coaggregation among *Fusobacterium* spp. Infect Immun 1995;(63):4584–8.

707. Jones S. A special relationship between spherical and filamentous microorganisms in mature human dental plaque. Arch Oral Biol 1972;(17):613–16.

708. Lancy P, Appelbaum B, Holt SC, Rosan B. Quantitative invitro assay for "corncob" formation. Infect Immun 1980;(29):663–70.

709. Rosan B, Correeia FF, DiRienzo JM. Corncobs: a model for oral microbial biofilms. Harwood Academic; 1999.

710. Dunne WJ, Mason EO Jr, Kaplan SL. Diffusion of rifampin and vancomycin through a *Staphylococcus epidermidis* biofilm. Antimicrob Agents Chemother 1993;12(37):2522–6.

711. Gilbert P, Allison DG, McBain AJ. Biofilms in vitro and in vivo: do singular mechanisms imply cross-resistance? J Appl Microbiol 2002;(92):Suppl:98S–110S.

712. Davies D, Parsek MR, Pearson JP, et al. The involvement of cell-to-cell signals in the development of a bacterial biofilm. Science 1998;280:295–8.

713. Gilbert P, Allison DG. Biofilms and their resistance towards antimicobial agents. Bioline; 1999.

714. Nichols W, Evans MJ, Slack MPE, Walmsley HL. The penetration of antibiotics into aggregates of mucoid and non-mucoid *Pseudomonas aeruginosa*. J Gen Microbiol 1989;(135):1291–303.

715. Gilbert P, Allison, DG., McBain, AJ. Biofilms in vitro and in vivo: do singular mechanisms imply cross-resistance? Symposium Series (Society for Applied Microbiology) 2002(31):98S–110S.

716. Giwercman B, Jensen ET, Hoiby N, et al. Induction of beta-lactamase production in *Pseudomonas aeruginosa* biofilm. Antimicrob Agents Chemother 1991;5(35):1008–10.

717. Lambert P. Mechanisms of antibiotic resistance in *Pseudomonas aeruginosa*. J R Soc Med 2002;(95):Suppl 41:22–6.

718. Katsikogianni M, Missirlis YF. Concise review of mechanisms of bacterial adhesion to biomaterials and of techniques used in estimating bacteria-material interactions. Eur Cell Mater 2004;7(8):37–57.

719. Marsh P. Dental plaque as a microbial biofilm. Caries Res 2004;(38):204–11.

720. Esther M. Clinical practice of the dental hygienist. 2004:289–303.

721. Rolla G, Rykke M. Evidence for presence of micelle like protein globules in human saliva. Colloids Surf B Biointerfaces 1994;(3):177–82.

722. Rolla G, Waaler SM, Kjoerheim V. In oral biofilms and plaque control: concepts in dental plaque formation: Taylor & Francis, London, UK; 1999.

723. Listgarten M. Formation of dental plaque and other biofilms. 1999.

724. Li Y-H, Tang N, Aspiras MB, et al. A quorum-sensing signaling system essential for genetic competence in *Streptococcus mutans* is involved in biofilm formation. J Bacteriol 2002;(184):2699–708.

725. Jin Y, Yip HK. Supragingival calculus: formation and control. Crit Rev Oral Biol Med 2002;5(13):426–41.

726. Barone J, Nancollas GH. The seeded growth of calcium phosphates, the kinetics of growth of dicalcium dihydrate on enamel, dentin, and calculus. J Dent Res 1978;(57):153–61.

727. Gron P, Van Campen GJ, Lindstrom I. Human dental calculus. Inorganic chemical and crystallographic composition. Arch Oral Biol 1967;7(12):829–37.

728. Marsh D. Microbial ecology of dental plaque and its significance in health and disease. Adv Dent Res 1994;(8):263–71.

729. Sbordone L, Bortolaia C. Oral microbial biofilms and plaque-related diseases: microbial communities and their role in the shift from oral health to disease. Clin Oral Investig 2003;7:181–8.

730. Page R, Schroeder HE. Pathogenesis of inflammatory periodontal disease. A summary of current work. Lab Invest 1976;3(34):235–49.

731. Lamont R, Jenkinson HF. Life below the gum line: pathogenic mechanisms of *Porphyromonas gingivalis*. MicroBiol Mol Biol Rev 1998;(62):1244–63.

732. Figdor D. Apical periodontitis: a very prevalent problem. Oral Surg Oral Med Oral Pathol 2002;6(94):651–2.

733. Nair P. Apical periodontitis: a dynamic encounter between root canal infection and host response. Periodontol 2000;1997;(13):121–48.

734. Tatsuta C, Morgan LA, Baumgartner JC, Adey JD. Effect of calcium hydroxide and four irrigation regimens on instrumented and uninstrumented canal wall topography. J Endod 1999;(25):93–8.

735. Ricucci D, Martorano M, Bate AL, Pascon EA. Calculus-like deposit on the apical external root surface of teeth with posttreatment apical periodontitis: report of two cases. Int Endod J 2005;(38):262–71.

736. Vier F, Figueiredo JA. Internal apical resorption and its correlation with the type of apical lesion. Int Endod J 2004;(37):730–7.

737. Vier F, Figueiredo JA. Prevalence of different periapical lesions associated with human teeth and their correlation with the presence and extension of apical external root resorption. Int Endod J 2002;35(8):710–19.

738. Kishen A. Periapical biomechanics and the role of cyclic biting force in apical retrograde fluid movement. Int Endod J 2005;(38):597–603.

739. Harn W, Chen YH, Yuan K, et al. Calculus-like deposit at apex of tooth with refractory apical periodontitis. Endod Dent Traumatol 1998;(14):237–40.

740. Hornef M, Wick MJ, Rhen M, Normark S. Bacterial strategies for overcoming host innate and adaptive immune responses. Nat Immunol 2002;11(3):1033–40.

741. O'Grady J, Reade PC. Periapical actinomycosis involving *Actinomyces israelii*. J Endod 1988;3(14):147–9.

742. Gerencser M, Slack JM. Serological identification of *Actinomyces* using fluorescent antibody techniques. J Dent Res 1976;55:A184–91.

743. Miller C, Palenik CJ, Stamper KE. Factors affecting the aggregation of *Actinomyces naeslundii* during growth and in washed cell suspensions. Infect Immun 1978;21(3):1003–9.

744. Rosanova I, Mischenko BP, Zaitsev VV, et al. The effect of cells on biomaterial calcification: experiments with in vivo diffusion chambers. J Biomed Mater Res 1991;25:277–80.

745. Boyan B, Boskey AL. Co-isolation of proteolipids and calcium-phospholipid-phosphate complexes. Calcif Tissue Int 1984;36:214–18.

746. Wilson M. Susceptibility of oral bacterial biofilm to antimicrobial agents. J Med Microbiol 1996;44(2):79–87.

747. Gristina A, Costerton JW. Bacterial adherence to biomaterials and tissue. The significance of its role in clinical sepsis. J Bone Joint Surg Am 1985;67(2):264–73.

748. An Y, Friedman RJ. Concise review of mechanisms of bacterial adhesion to biomaterial surfaces. J Biomed Mater Res 1998;43(3):338–48.

749. Takemura N, Noiri Y, Ehara A, et al. Single species biofilm-forming ability of root canal isolates on gutta-percha points. Eur J Oral Sci 2004;112:523–9.

Chapter 8

Non-microbial Endodontic Disease

P.N.R. Nair

"In microscopy, as in nature, one recognizes only what one already knows."[1]

Apical periodontitis is an inflammatory disorder of periradicular tissues caused by irritants of endodontic origin, mostly of persistent microbes living in the root canal system of the affected tooth.[2,3] It is primarily a disease of infection. But unlike classical infectious diseases of single, specific etiologic agents, apical periodontitis is caused by a consortium of microbial species living in the root canal in an ecologically balanced community form of living[4] referred to as biofilms.[5] The microbial etiology of the disease has been discussed in Chapter 7, "Microbiology of Endodontic Disease." The purpose of this chapter is to provide a comprehensive overview of the nonmicrobial aspects of the disease, which are generally associated with asymptomatic persistent periapical radiolucencies, also referred to as endodontic failures.

Cystic Apical Periodontitis

By definition, a cyst is a closed pathologic cavity, lined by epithelium that contains a liquid or semisolid material.[6] The term *cyst* is derived from the Greek word *Kystis* meaning sac or bladder. There are several varieties of cystic lesions in the body that are commonly referred to as congenital, neoplastic, parasitic, retention, implantation, and inflammatory types. *A periapical cyst is an inflammatory jaw cyst of the periodontium of a tooth with infected and necrotic pulp and has been extensively reviewed.*[1,7,8]

INCIDENCE OF PERIAPICAL CYSTS

The epidemiology and global distribution of the disease are not yet known. Anatomically, periapical cysts are the most common of all jaw cysts and comprise about 52%[7] to 68%[9] of all the cysts affecting the human jaws. The prevalence of periapical cysts is highest among patients in their third decade of life[7,10,11] and higher among males than females.[7,10] Periapical cysts occur in all tooth-bearing sites of the jaws but are more frequent in maxillary than mandibular teeth. In the maxilla, the anterior region appears to be more affected with cysts whereas in the mandible the radicular cysts occur more frequently in the premolar region.[12]

DIAGNOSIS OF PERIAPICAL CYSTS

The clinical diagnosis of periapical cysts from other forms of apical periodontitis has been extensively debated.[13] Several radiographic features have been proposed to support a diagnosis, including size of the lesion and the presence of a radioopaque rim[14] demarcating the lesion. Although the statistical probability of cyst occurrence may be higher among larger lesions,[15] a conclusive relationship between the size of the lesion and cystic condition has not yet been substantiated by histologic data. Albeit the claim,[16] periapical lesions cannot be differentially diagnosed into cystic and noncystic lesions based on radiographic features.[10,17–21] In a recent histologic investigation, it has been conclusively shown that no correlation existed between the presence of a radioopaque rim and the histologic diagnosis of the cysts.[22] Assuming that cystic cavities may have a lower density than other apical periodontitis lesions, computer tomography[23] and densitometry[16] have been used to differentiate these conditions, but without success. Echography, ultrasonic imaging technique, has been recently introduced as a periapical diagnostic method.[24,25] The technique can detect fluid, soft tissue, and the real-time blood flow. In spite of the safety of ultrasound and the relative ease of use, the sonic waves do not pass through bone but are reflected back to the sensor, thereby enabling only detection of lesions that are not enclosed in bone. Currently, therefore, histologic serial sectioning of the lesions in toto remains to be the only reliable diagnostic method of periapical cysts.[1,8,26] This has been conclusively shown in a recent histologic investigation.[22] Histologic diagnosis, however, can only be applied after surgical removal of the root tip with the attached periapical lesion, thus making it a post hoc diagnosis.

ORIGIN OF THE CYST EPITHELIUM

The lesions of apical periodontitis often contain epithelial cells[27–38] that are generally believed to be derived from the cell rests of Malassez.[27] The cells proliferate in some lesions and serve as the *major source* of the stratified squamous epithelium[7,8] that lines the lumen of lesions that develop into cysts. In rare instances, apical cysts have also been found to be lined by ciliated columnar or muco-secretory cells of respiratory origin.[38–46] In one investigation,[46] 3 of the 256 apical periodontitis lesions examined were cysts lined with ciliated columnar epithelium (Figures 1 and 2). However, the origin of ciliated epithelium in radicular cysts has not yet been satisfactorily clarified. Currently, there are three explanations[43] for the presence of ciliated cells in radicular cysts: (1) migration of epithelial cells from the maxillary sinus or the nasal cavity; (2) metaplasia of the stratified squamous epithelium; and (3) differentiation of pluripotent cells within the jaw. Most of the reported ciliated cell-lined cysts were affecting maxillary teeth. The anatomic proximity of the periapical inflammatory lesion to the maxillary sinus may result in rarefaction of the sinus floor, perforation into the sinus cavity,[38,40] and maxillary sinusitis.[47–49] The lumen of such a periapical cyst can communicate with the sinus cavity, as has been convincingly demonstrated in photomicrographs by Kronfeld.[40] Once direct communication is established, a developing apical cyst can be lined with ciliary epithelium of sinus origin.

PREVALENCE OF CYSTS AMONG PERIAPICAL LESIONS

There have been many studies on the prevalence of periapical cysts among apical periodontitis lesions (Table 1). In this literature, the prevalence of cysts varies from 6% to 55%. However, accurate histopathologic diagnosis of radicular cysts is possible only through serial sectioning or step-serial sectioning of the lesions removed in toto.[50] There are only three studies[31,50,51] in which either one of those essential techniques was used, whereas most of the others (Table 1) analyzed specimens obtained from wide sources for routine histopathologic reports. The statistically impressive 2,308 lesions in Bhaskar's study[10] had been obtained from 314 contributors and the 800 biopsies of Lalonde and Luebke[21] originated from 134 sources. Such histopathologic diagnostic specimens, often derived through apical curettage, do not represent lesions in toto. In random sections from fragmented and epithelialized lesions, part of the specimens can give the appearance of epithelium-lined cavities that do not exist in reality. Indeed, another author[52] defined a typical radicular cyst as one in which "a real or imagined lumen was lined with stratified squamous epithelium."

It should be pointed out that the photomicrographic illustrations (Figure 3) in several studies[10,21] represent only magnified views of selected small segments of epithelialized lesions. They are not supported by overview pictures of lesser magnifications of sequential sections derived from different axial planes of the lesions in question. The wide variation in the reported incidence of periapical cysts is most probably due to the difference in the histopathologic interpretation of the sections. When the histopathologic diagnosis is based on random or limited number of serial sections, most of epithelialized periapical

Chapter 8 / Non-microbial Endodontic Disease / **311**

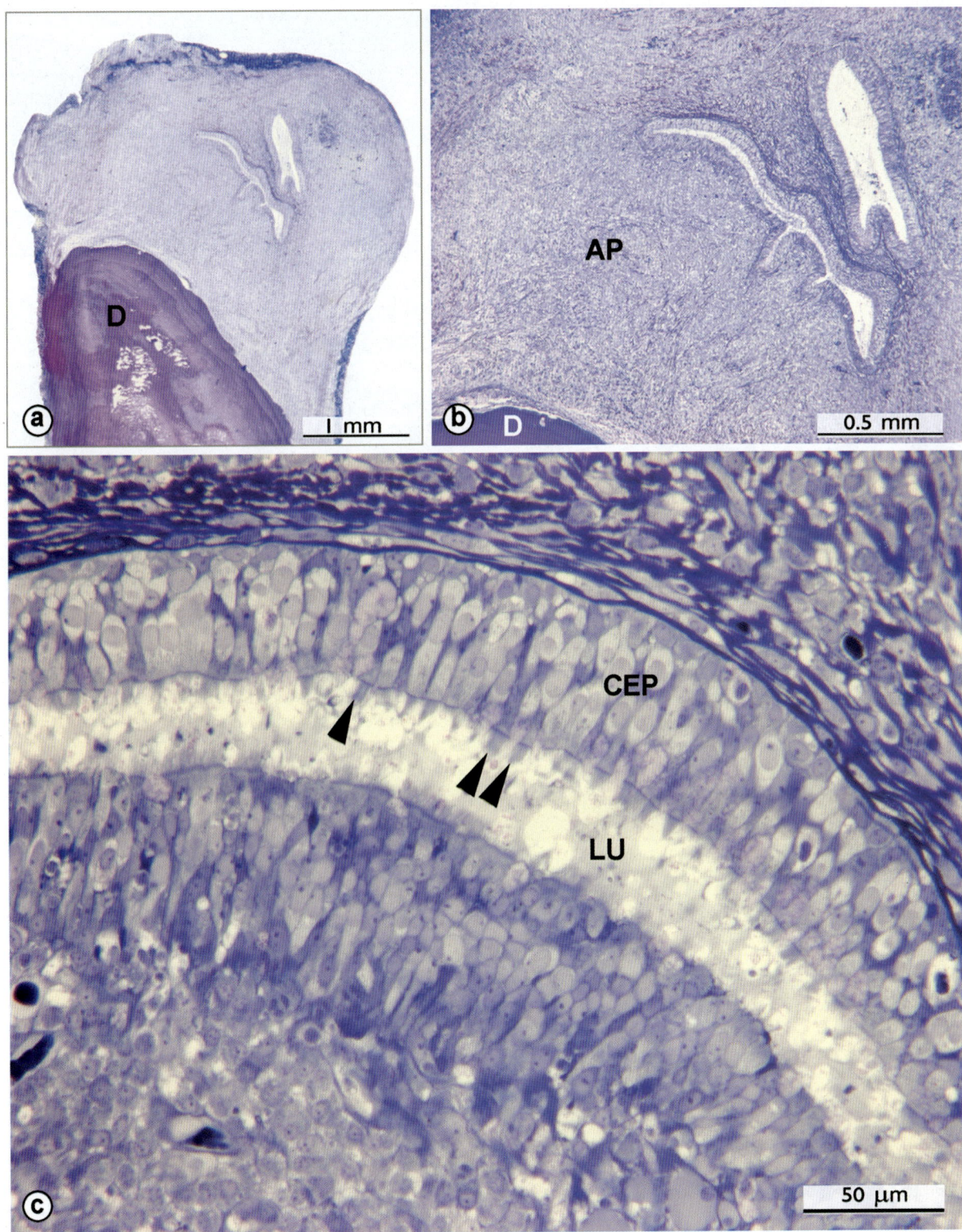

Figure 1 A photomicrograph **A,** of a cystic apical periodontitis (AP) of the left maxillary second premolar of a 34-year-old male patient. Note the two diverticula of a small cystic lumen magnified in **B,** and part of the epithelial lining enlarged in **C.** The lumen (LU) is lined with columnar epithelial cells (CEP) with distinct cilia (arrow heads). D = dentine. Original magnifications: **A** ×19, **B** ×44, **C** ×500. Reproduced with permission from Nair.[46]

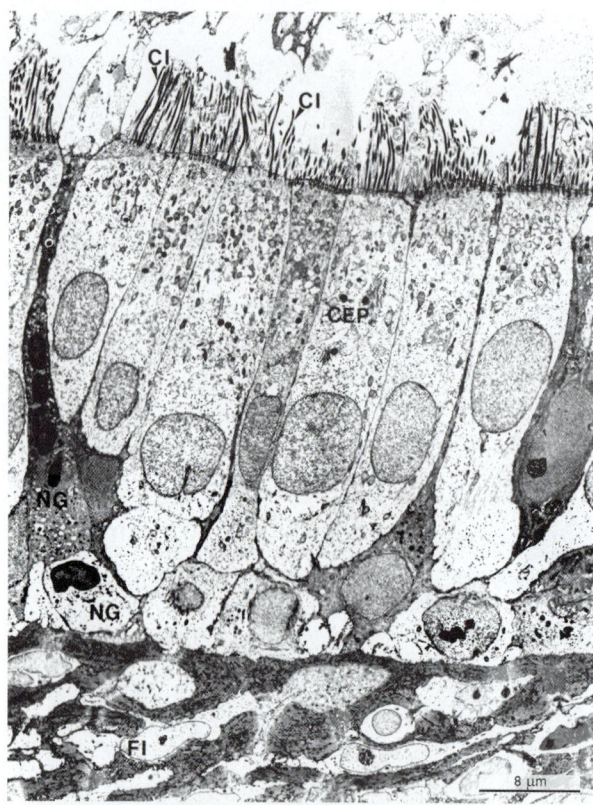

Figure 2 A transmission electron micrograph of ciliated columnar epithelial cells (CEP) lining of the cystic lumen of the lesion presented in Figure 8-1. Note the distinct cilia (CI) and the neutrophilic gametocytes (NG). FI = fibroblasts. Original magnification ×3,690. Reproduced with permission from Nair.[46]

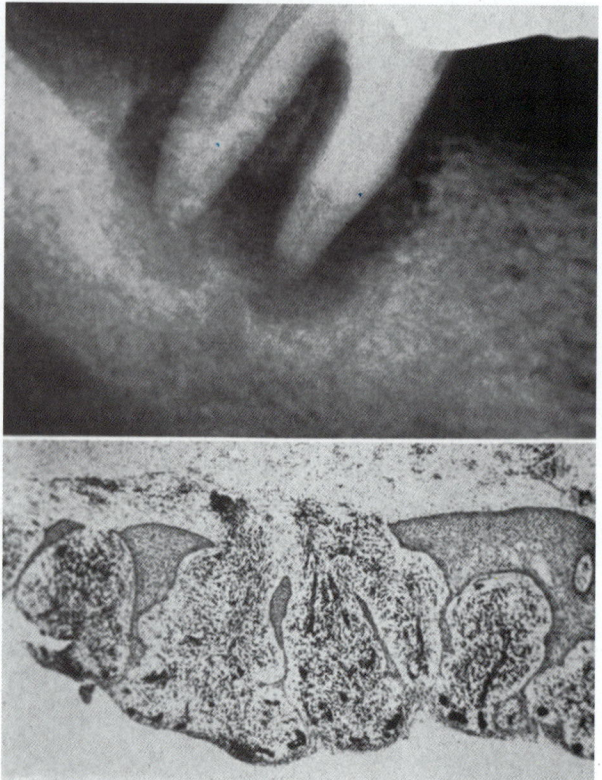

Figure 3 Roentgenogram (top) and photomicrograph (bottom) of a "radicular cyst." Original illustrations reprinted from Bhaskar.[10] Note the small selected segment of an epithelialized lesion. It is not supported by overview pictures of lesser magnification of sequential sections derived from different axial planes of the lesion. Reproduced with permission from Elsevier©.

Table 1 The Prevalence of Radicular Cysts Among Apical Periodontitis Lesions

Reference	Cysts (%)	Granuloma (%)	Others (%)	Total (n)
Sommer et al 1966[164]	6	84	10	170
Block et al 1976[165]	6	94	–	230
Sonnabend and Oh 1966[31]	7	93	–	237
Winstock 1980[166]	8	83	9	9804
Linenberg 1964[20]	9	80	11	110
Wais 1958[19]	14	84	2	50
Patterson 1964[167]	14	84	2	501
Nair 1996[50]	15	50	35	256
Simon 1980[51]	17	77	6	35
Stockdale and Chandler 1988[168]	17	77	6	1108
Lin 1991[169]	19	–	81	150
Nobuhara 1993[170]	22	59	19	150
Baumann 1956[18]	26	74	–	121
Mortensen et al 1970[11]	41	59	–	396
Bhaskar 1966[10]	42	48	10	2308
Spatafore et al 1990[171]	42	52	6	1659
Lalonde and Luebke 1968[21]	44	45	11	800
Seltzer et al 1967[52]	51	45	4	87
Priebe et al 1954[17]	55	45	–	101

Table adapted from Nair et al. 1998.[80]

lesions would be wrongly categorized as radicular cysts. This view is substantiated by the results of a study[50] in which an overall 52% of the lesions ($n = 256$) were found to be epithelialized but only 15% were actually periapical cysts.

HISTOPATHOLOGY OF PERIAPICAL CYSTS

The structure of a periapical cyst in relation to the root canal of the affected teeth has not been taken into account in routine histopathologic diagnosis. The major reason for this has been the nature of the biopsy itself. Apical specimens removed by curettage do not contain the root tips of the diseased teeth making structural reference to the root canals of the affected teeth impossible. In 1980 Simon[51] has pointed out that there are two distinct categories of radicular cysts namely, those containing cavities *completely enclosed in epithelial lining* and those containing epithelium-lined *cavities that are open to the root*

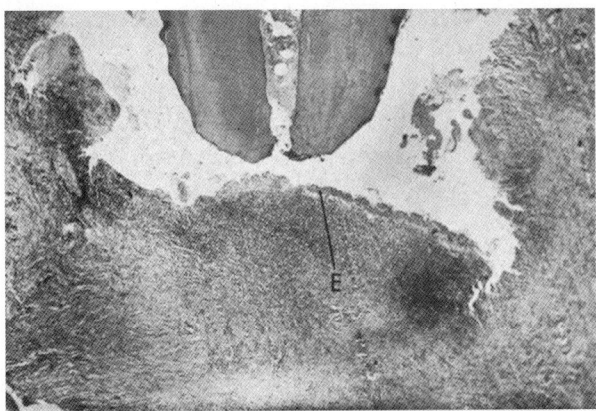
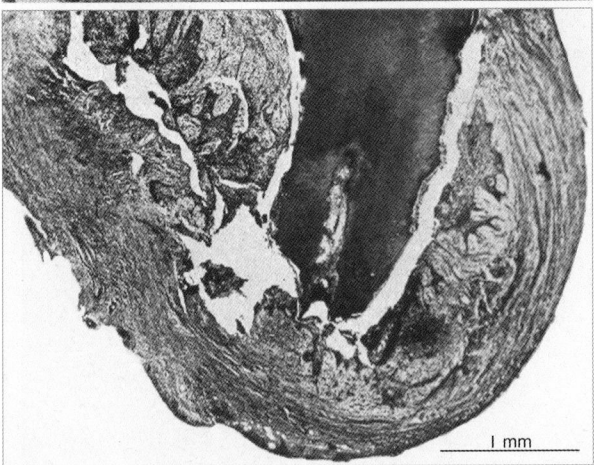

Figure 4 Root apices in cavities lined by epithelium (E in top). Original illustrations reprinted from Simon.[51] Note the severe damage of the microanatomic relationship between the root apices and the cyst epithelia that might have influenced critics to wonder whether the "bay cysts"[51] are histologic artifacts. Original magnification ×25. Reproduced with permission from Williams & Wilkins©.

canals. The latter was designated as "bay cysts"[51] and later renamed as "pocket cysts."[50] It seems that Simon[51] has observed only the large type of such lesions with voluminous cavities, into which the root apices of the affected teeth appeared to protrude. The photomicrographs in the publication reveal severe damage of the microanatomic relationship between the root apices and the cyst epithelia (Figure 4). This might have influenced critics to wonder whether the "bay cysts"[51] are histologic artifacts. We[50] analyzed 256 periapical lesions obtained in toto with extracted teeth. The specimens were processed by a modern plastic-embedding technique, and meticulous serial or step-serial sections were prepared and evaluated based on predefined histopathologic criteria. Of the 256 specimens, 35% were found to be periapical abscesses, 50% were periapical granulomas, and only 15% were periapical cysts. Equally significant was the finding that two distinct classes of radicular cysts—the *apical true cysts*, with cavities completely enclosed in epithelial linings (Figure 5), and the *apical pocket cysts*, with cyst lumina open to the root canals (Figure 6)—could be observed at the periapex when the lesions were analyzed in relation to the root canals. An overall 9% of the 256 lesions were apical true cysts and 6% were periapical pocket cysts.

GENESIS OF TRUE CYSTS

The periapical true cyst may be defined as a chronic inflammatory lesion at the periapex that contains an epithelium lined, *closed pathological cavity* (Figure 5). The pathogenesis of true cysts has been described by various authors.[8,28,50,53–59] An apical cyst is a direct sequel to apical granuloma, although a granuloma need not always develop into a cyst. Owing to still unknown reasons, only a small fraction (<10%) of the periapical lesions change into true radicular cysts.[10,21] The pathogenesis of the true cyst has been described in three phases.[7] During the *first phase*, the dormant cell-rests of Malassez begin to proliferate as a direct effect of inflammation,[57,60] probably under the influence of bacterial antigens,[61] epidermal growth factors,[62–64] cell mediators, and metabolites that are released by various cells residing in the periapical lesion. During the *second phase*, an epithelium lined cavity comes into existence. There are two main theories regarding the formation of the cyst cavity: (1) the "nutritional deficiency theory" and (2) the "abscess theory." The "nutritional deficiency theory" is based on the assumption that the central cells of the epithelial strands become removed from their source of nutrition and undergo necrosis and liquefactive degeneration.[57,65–67] The accumulating products in turn attract neutrophilic granulocytes into the necrotic area. Such microcavities containing degenerating epithelial cells, infiltrating mobile cells, and tissue fluid coalesce to form the cyst cavity lined by stratified epithelium. The "abscess theory" postulates that the

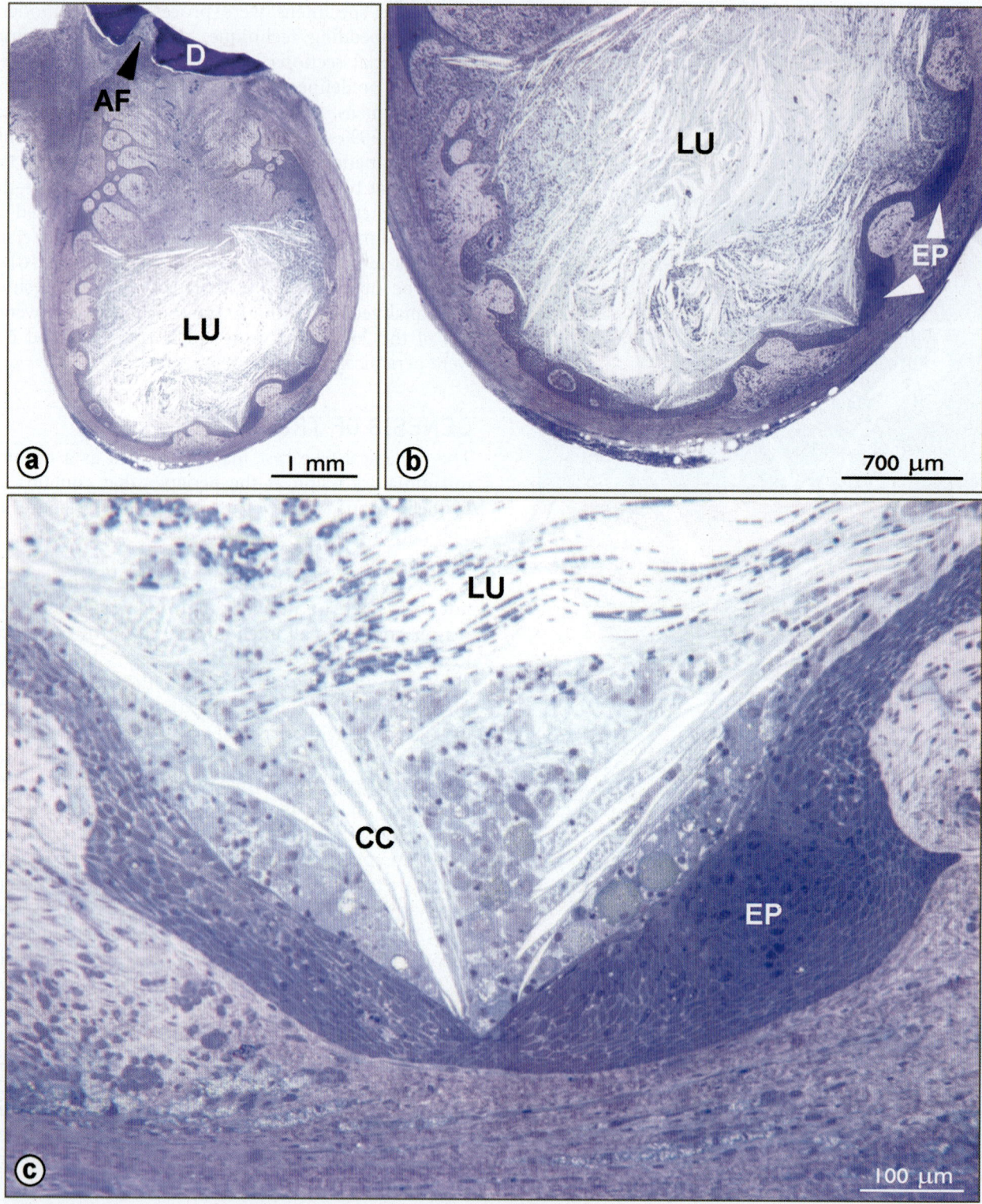

Figure 5 Periapical true cyst. Photomicrograph **A,** of an axial section passing through the apical foramen (AF). The lower half of the lesion and the epithelium (EP in *B*) are magnified in **B,** and **C,** respectively. Note the cystic lumen (LU) with cholesterol clefts (CC) completely enclosed in EP having no communication to the root canal. Original magnifications: **A** ×15, **B** ×30, **C** ×180. Reproduced with permission from Nair.[1]

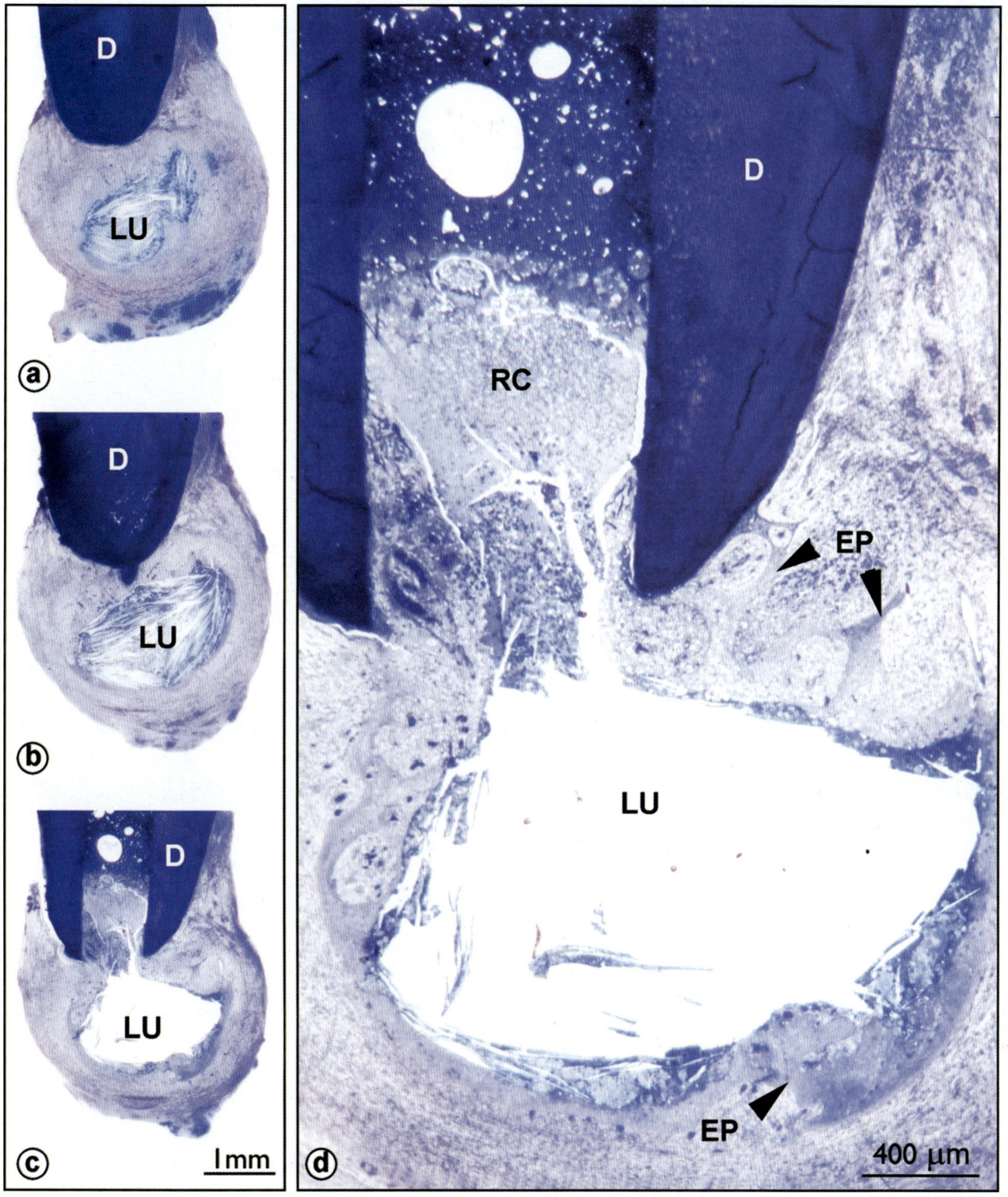

Figure 6 Periapical pocket cyst. Axial sections passing peripheral to the root canal **A, B,** give the false impression of the presence of a cyst lumen (LU) completely enclosed in epithelium. Sequential section **C,** passing through axial plane of the root canal clearly reveals the continuity of the LU with the root canal (RC in **D**. The apical foramen with the LU of the section **C,** are magnified in **D**. Note the pouch-like LU of the pocket cyst with the epithelium (EP) forming a collar at the root apex. Original magnifications: **A, B, C** ×15; **D** ×50. D = dentine. Reproduced with permission from Nair.[1]

proliferating epithelium lines an abscess cavity formed by tissue necrosis and lysis because of the innate nature of the epithelial cells to cover exposed connective tissue surfaces.[29,33] During the *third phase* the cyst grows, by which exact mechanism is still unknown. It is generally believed to be by osmosis. The presence of necrotic tissue in the cyst lumen attracts neutrophilic granulocytes, which extravasate and transmigrate through the epithelial lining (Figures 7 and 8) into the cyst cavity where they perish. The lytic products of the dying cells in the cyst lumen release a greater number of molecules. As a result, the osmotic pressure of the cyst fluid rises to a level higher than that of the tissue fluid.[68] The latter diffuses into the cyst cavity so as to raise the intraluminal hydrostatic pressure well above the capillary pressure. The increased intracyst pressure may lead to bone resorption and expansion of the cyst. However, *the fact that an apical pocket cyst with lumen open to the necrotic root canal can become larger*[50,59] suggests against osmotic pressure as a potential factor in the development of radicular cysts. Furthermore, there is increasing evidence in support of a molecular mechanism for cyst expansion.[59] The T-lymphocytes[69] and macrophages in the cyst wall may provide a continuous source of bone resorptive metabolites[70] and cytokines. The presence of effector molecules such as matrix metalloproteinases 1 and 2 have also been reported in the cyst walls.[71]

GENESIS OF POCKET CYSTS

The periapical pocket cyst contains an epithelium-lined pathologic cavity that is open to the root canal of the affected tooth (Figure 6). As mentioned previously, such lesions were originally described as "bay cysts."[51] It has been postulated that biologically, a pocket cyst constitutes an extension of the infected root canal space into the periapex. The microluminal space becomes enclosed in a stratified squamous epithelium that grows and forms an epithelial collar (Figure 9) around the root tip. The epithelial collar forms an "epithelial attachment"[37] to the root surface that seals off the infected root canal and the micro-cystic lumen from the periapical milieu and the rest of the body (Figure 9C and D). The presence of microorganisms at the apical foramen (Figure 10) attracts neutrophilic granulocytes by chemotaxis into the microlumen. However, the pouch-like lumen—biologically outside the body milieu—acts as a "death trap" to the externalized neutrophils. As the necrotic tissue and microbial products accumulate, the sac-like lumen enlarges to accommodate the debris, forming a voluminous diverticulum of the root canal

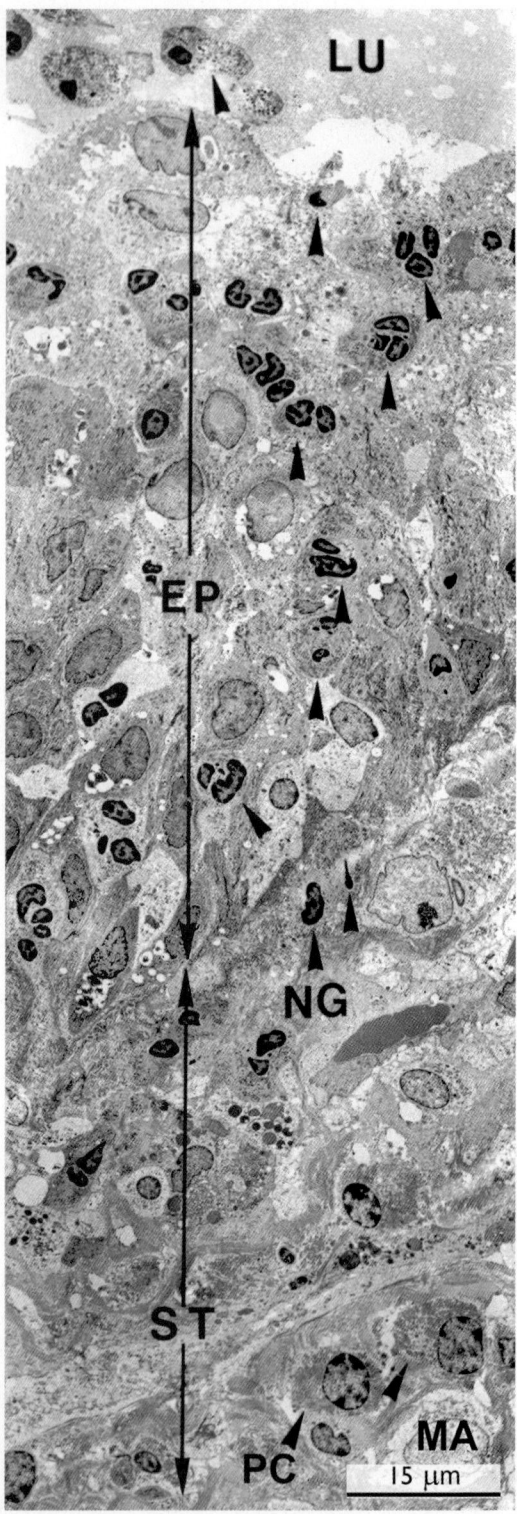

Figure 7 Composite transmission electron micrograph showing neutrophils (NG, arrowheads) apparently in the process of transmigration through the epithelial wall of a cyst (EP) into the cyst lumen (LU). ST = subepithelial tissue; PC = plasma cells; MA = macrophages. Original magnification ×1,600. Modified from Nair.[59]

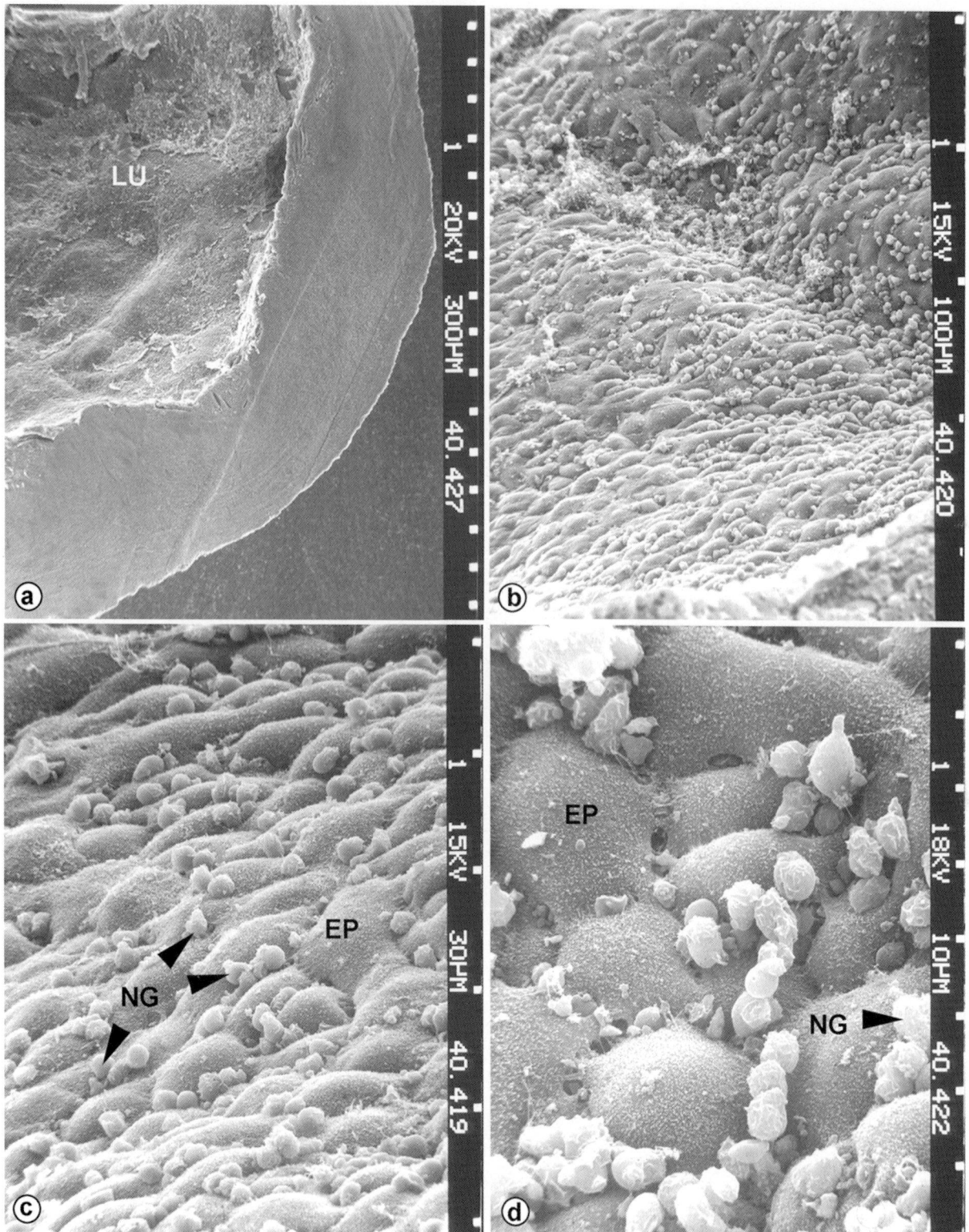

Figure 8 An intramural scanning electron microscopic view of a cyst luminal wall (LU, in ***A***) enlarged in stages (***B, C, D***). Note the flat epithelial cells (EP) and the globular neutrophilic granulocytes (NG). The latter emerge through the interepithelial cell spaces into the cyst lumen. Original magnifications: ***A*** ×20, ***B*** ×230, ***C*** ×670, ***D*** ×1,300. Reproduced with permission from Nair.[1]

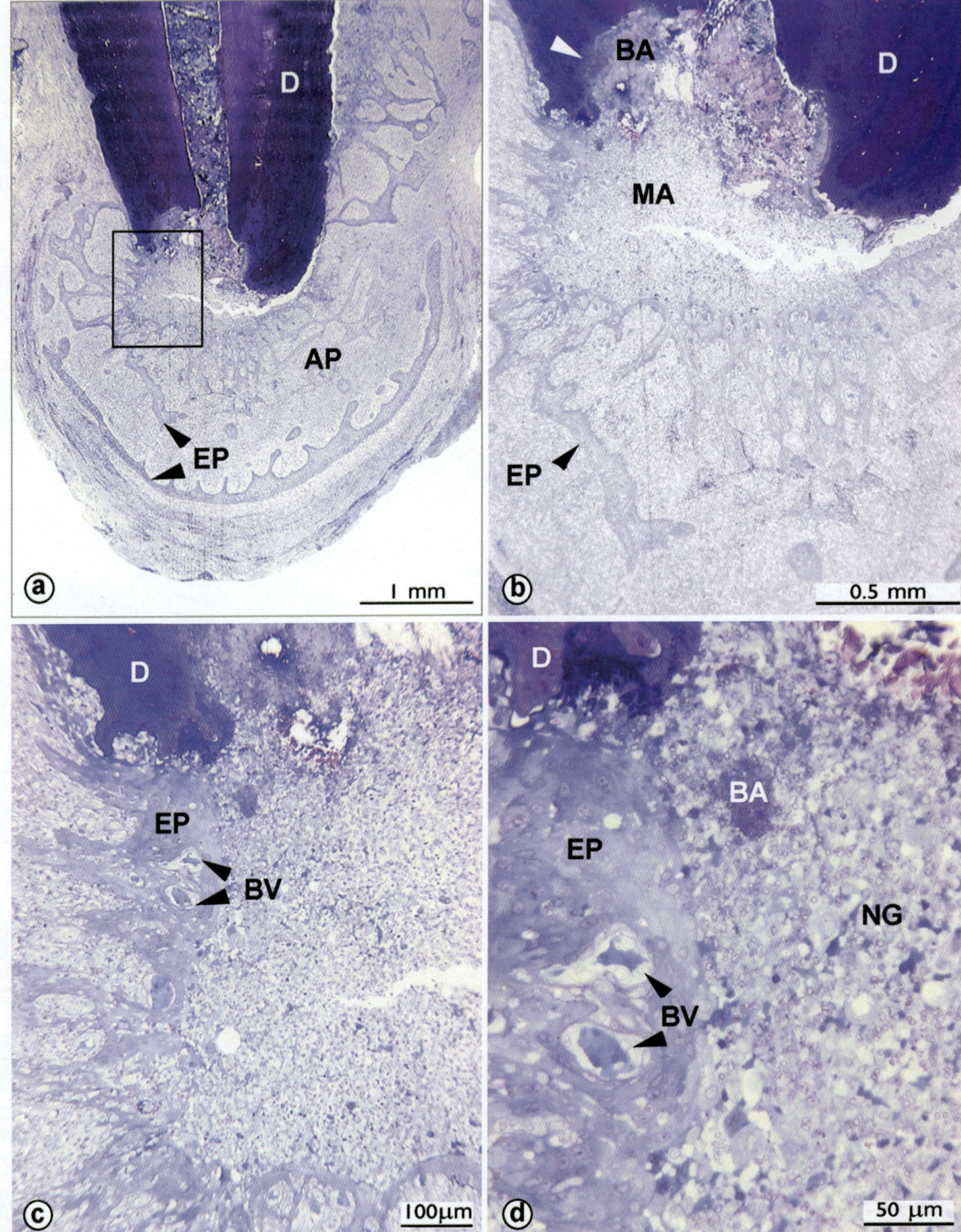

Figure 9 Overview photomicrograph **A,** of an apical periodontitis lesion (AP). The resorbed root tip with widened apical foramen is magnified in **B**. Note the bacterial plaque (white arrow head, BA) at the apical foramen and the micro-abscess (MA) externalized by an epithelial (EP) ring attached to the root tip. The rectangular demarcated area in **A,** is magnified in **C**. Note the numerous subepithelial blood vessels (BV) that are further magnified in **D**. The bacteria (BA) attract neutrophils (NG) to form the micro-abscess in front of the apical foramen which probably is the initiation of a periapical pocket cyst. D = dentine. Original magnifications: **A** ×20, **B** ×40, **C** ×130, **D** ×310. Reproduced with permission from Nair.[1]

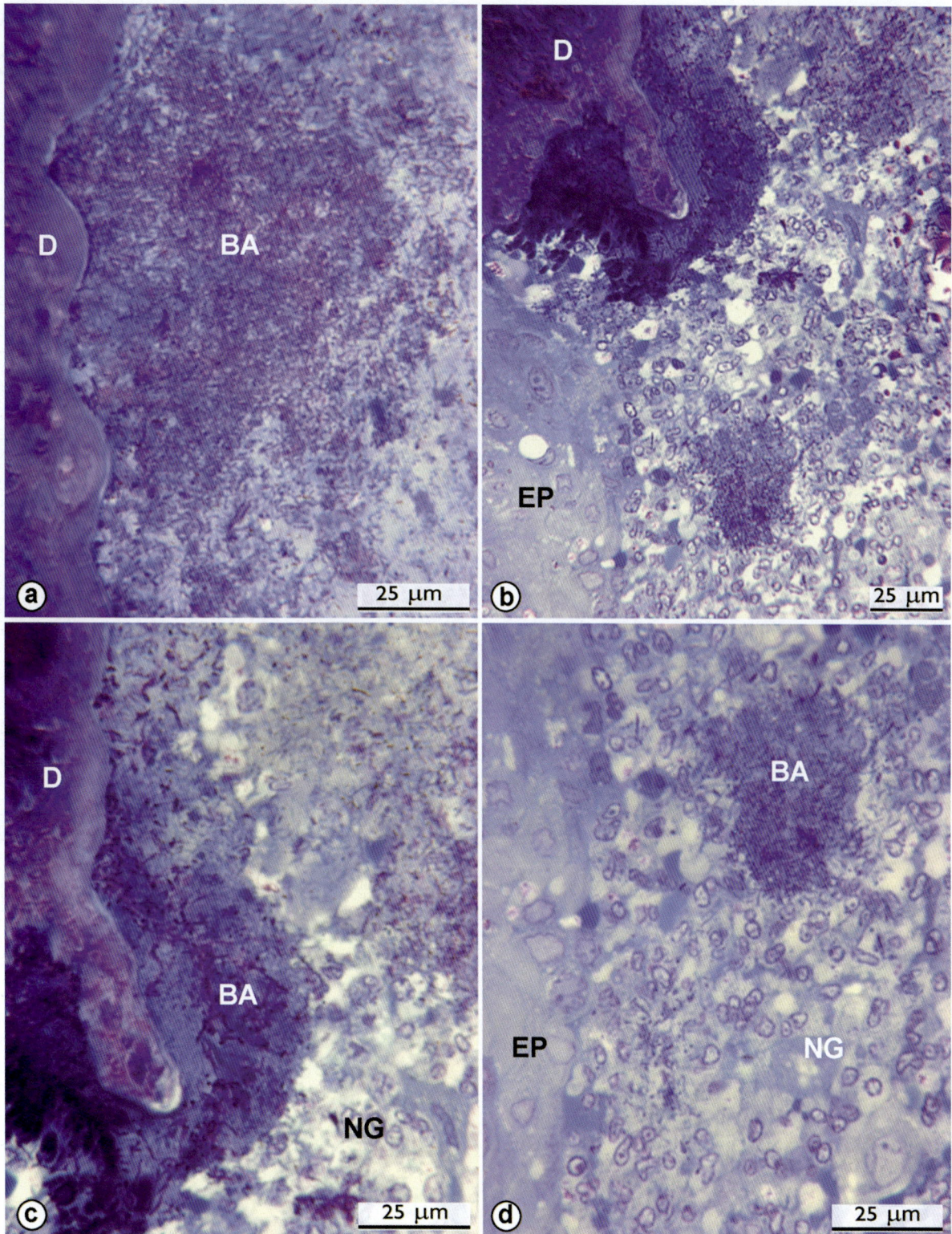

Figure 10 High-magnification photomicrographs (***A–D***) of the bacterial plaque (BA) shown in Figure 8-9 and the micro-abscess containing clusters of bacterial colonies (BA) apparently held back by a wall of neutrophils (NG). D = dentine; EP = epithelium. Original magnifications: ***A, C, D*** ×800; ***B*** ×520. Reproduced with permission from Nair.[1]

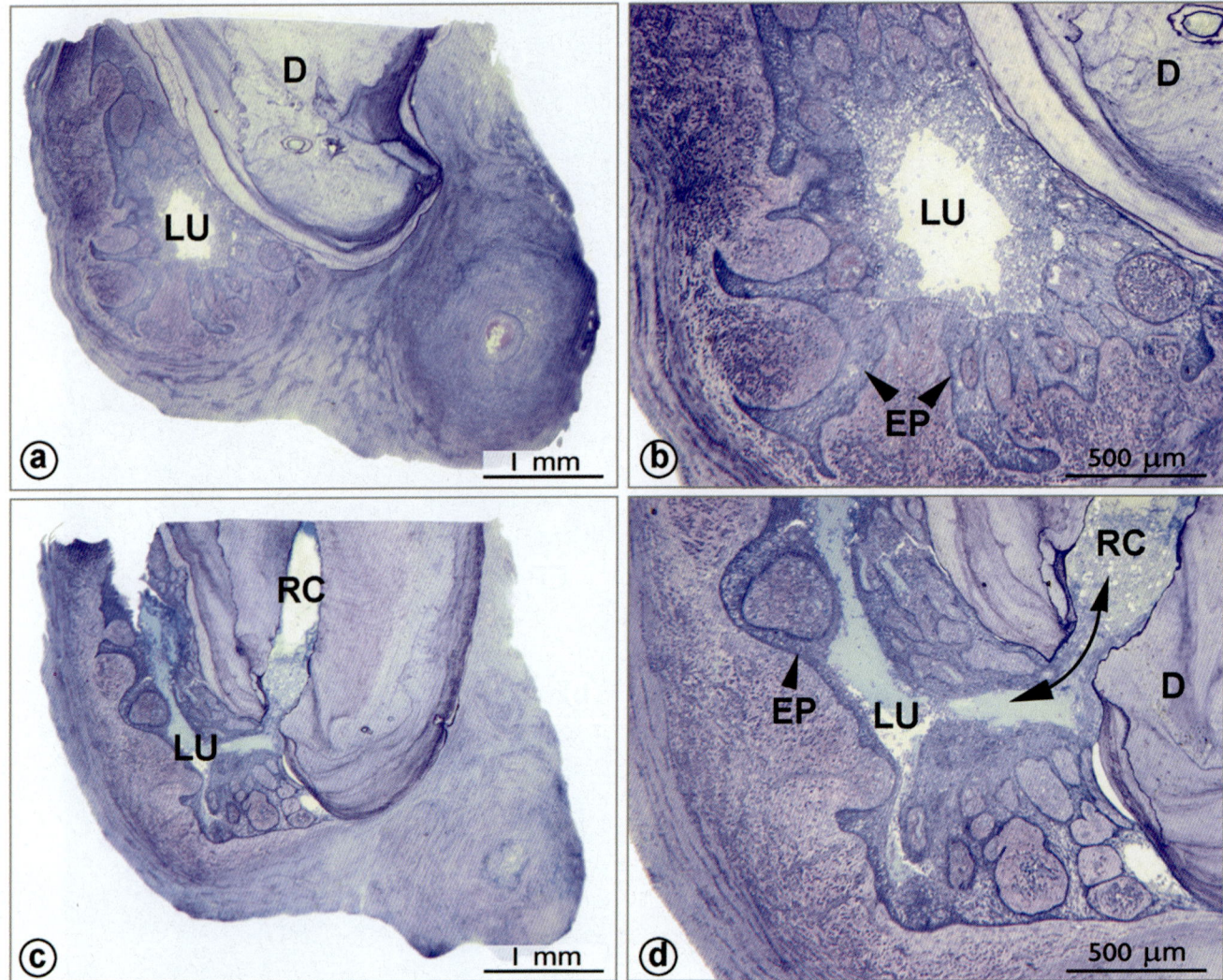

Figure 11 Photomicrograph of a well-developed pocket cyst **A**. Note the sac-like epithelial lumen (LU), enlarged in **B**. A sequential, axial serial section **C**, passing through the apical foramen in the root canal plane (RC) shows the continuity of the lumen to the root canal. D = dentine. Original magnification: **A, C** ×16; **B, D** ×40. Reproduced with permission from Nair.[1]

space into the periapical area (Figures 11 and 12). It has been pointed out[50] that from the pathogenic, structural, tissue dynamic, host-benefit, and protection stand points, the epithelium-lined pouch-like extension of the root canal space of such lesions has much in common with a marginal periodontal pocket. This appears to justify the terminology of "periapical pocket cyst" as opposed to the biologically meaningless term "bay cyst."[51] In this context, it is interesting to note that cystic lesions with morphologic features identical to those of pocket cysts have been histologically illustrated by Seltzer in a text book[72]

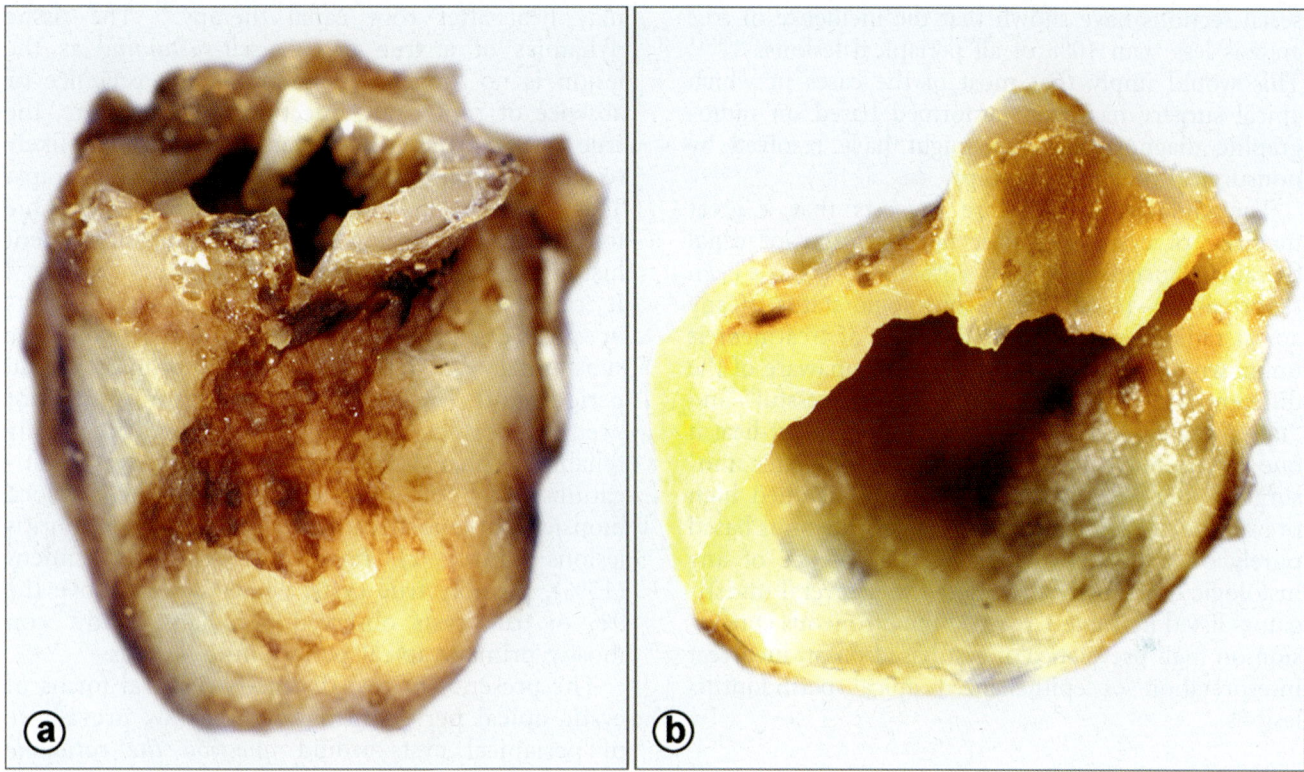

Figure 12 Macrophotographs **A, B,** of a large apical periodontitis lesion removed in toto by apical surgery **A**. The specimen after decalcification and axial subdivision **B,** shows a voluminous lumen into which the root canal opens. Reproduced with permission from Nair.[1]

and also experimentally induced in monkeys by Valderhaug.[60,73] However, these authors neither differentiated nor interpreted the lesions in relation to the root canals of the involved teeth—a reminder that in microscopy, as in nature, one recognizes only what one already knows.

CYSTS AND PERIAPICAL HEALING

The occurrence of two distinct classes of radicular cysts and the low prevalence of true cysts (<10%) are both significant considerations in clinical management of primary and particularly posttreatment apical periodontitis. Many clinicians hold the view that cysts do not heal and thus must be removed by surgery. It should be pointed out with emphasis that apical periodontitis lesions cannot be differentially diagnosed into cystic and noncystic lesions based on radiographs.[10,11,17–20,74] However, routine histopathologic diagnostic reports and publications based on retrospective reviewing of such have perpetuated the notion that nearly half of all periapical lesions are radicular cysts. As a result, a disproportionately large number of apical surgeries are performed at the tooth apex to "enucleate" lesions that are clinically diagnosed as "cysts." In fact, studies based on meticulous serial sections have shown that the incidence of *true cysts* is less than 10% of all periapical lesions.[31,50,51] This would imply that most of the cases in which apical surgery has been performed based on radiographic diagnosis of cysts might have resolved by nonsurgical root canal therapy.

The endodontic literature suggests that a great majority of cysts heal after nonsurgical root canal therapy. "Success rates" of 85% to 90% have been reported.[75–77] However, the histologic status of any apical radiolucent lesion at the time of treatment is unknown to the clinician, who is also unaware of the differential diagnostic status of the "successful" and "failed" cases. Most of the cystic lesions must heal if one should reconcile the high healing rate after nonsurgical root canal treatment and the claimed high prevalence of radicular cysts. This conclusion is based purely on a deductive logic in the absence of any histologic basis. It must be noted that several investigators listed in Table 1 reached the erroneous conclusion on high prevalence of cyst based on an incorrect interpretation of epithelialized apical periodontitis lesions.

CLINICAL RELEVANCE OF CYSTS IN PRIMARY AND POSTTREATMENT APICAL PERIODONTITIS

The aim of nonsurgical root canal therapy is the elimination of infection from the root canal and the prevention of re-infection by root filling. Periapical pocket cysts, particularly the smaller ones, may heal after root canal therapy.[51] The tissue dynamics of a true cyst is *self-sustaining* as the lesion is no longer dependent on the presence or absence of root canal infection.[50,51] Therefore, the true cysts, particularly the large ones, are less likely to be resolved by nonsurgical root canal therapy. This has been shown in a long-term radiographic follow-up (Figure 13) of a case and subsequent histologic analysis of the surgical block biopsy.[26] It can be argued that the prevalence of cysts in posttreatment apical periodontitis should be substantially higher than that in primary apical periodontitis. However, this suggestion has not been supported by data based on a statistically reliable number of specimens. Nevertheless, investigations[26,78,79] of 16 histologically reliable block biopsies of posttreatment apical periodontitis lesions (Table 2) revealed 2 cystic specimens (13%), possibly true cysts, which is well above the 9% of true cysts observed in a large study[50] on mostly primary apical periodontitis lesions.

The presence of two distinct structural forms of cystic apical periodontitis and the low prevalence of periapical cysts would *question the rationale* behind some of the current diagnostic and therapeutic concepts such as (1) disproportionate application of apical surgery based on unfounded radiographic diagnosis of apical lesions as cysts, and (2) the widely held opinion that majority of cysts heal after nonsurgical root canal therapy. Nevertheless, it should be recognized that periapical cysts could sustain persistent apical

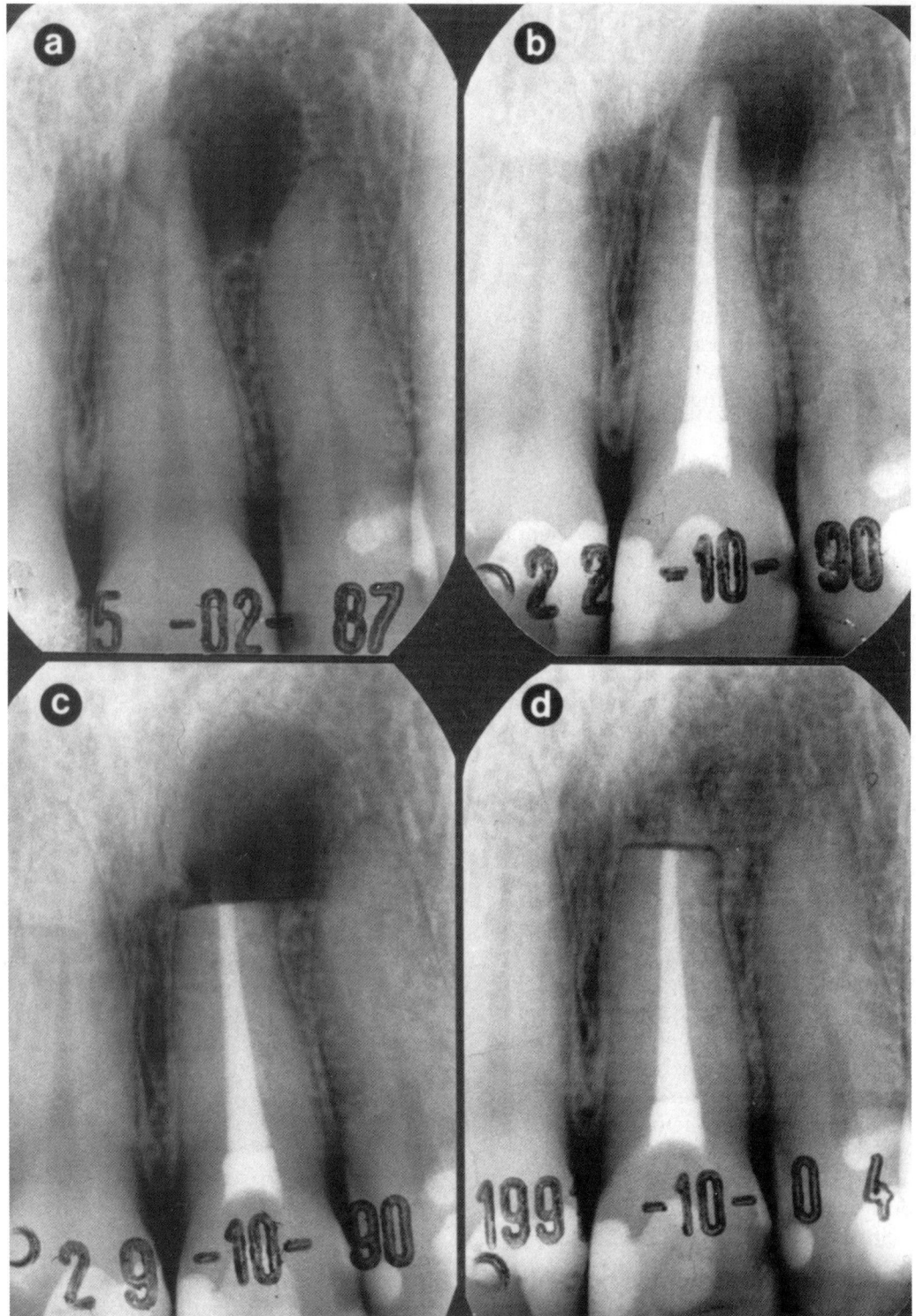

Figure 13 Longitudinal radiographs **A–D**, of a periapically affected central maxillary incisor of a 37-year-old woman for a period of 4 years and 9 months. Note the large radiolucent asymptomatic lesion before **A**, 44 months after root filling **B**, and immediately after periapical surgery **C**. The periapical area shows distinct bone healing **D**, after 1 year postoperatively. Histopathologic examination of the surgical specimen by modern tissue processing and step-serial sectioning technique confirmed that the lesion was a true radicular cyst that also contained cholesterol clefts. Selected radiographs from Nair et al.[26]

Table 2 The Prevalence of Cysts Among Posttreatment Apical Periodontitis Lesions

Reference	Cysts (n)	Granuloma (n)	Scar (n)	Total lesions (n)
Nair et al 1990[78]	0	9	0	9
Nair et al 1993[26]	1	0	–	1
Nair et al 1999[79]	1	3	2	6
Total	2	12	2	16

radiolucencies. Therefore, clinicians should consider the option of apical surgery, particularly when previous orthograde re-treatment has not resulted in radiographic healing.

CHOLESTEROL AND APICAL PERIODONTITIS

The presence of cholesterol clefts in apical periodontitis has been a common histopathologic observation. Yet, its etiologic significance to posttreatment apical periodontitis has been appreciated only recently.[26,80,81] Endogenous substances of crystalline fine particulate nature can be tissue irritating. The crystals induce cytokine-network-mediated inflammation, hard tissue resorption, and soft tissue damage. Endogenous crystalline substances that have been shown to cause pathogenic tissue reaction include monosodium urate (gout), calcium phosphate dihydrate (pseudogout), basic calcium phosphate (hydroxyapatite), and cholesterol.

Cholesterol[6] is a steroid lipid present in all animal tissues. The term is derived from *Chole-stereos* meaning "bile-solid" because of its occurrence in gall stones. Cholesterol has the characteristic core of the "cyclopentanoperhydrophenanthrene" ring (Figure 14). It is abundant in "membrane-rich" tissues (myelin) and secretory cells and is the precursor of bile acids, provitamin D3, and several hormones.[82] Cholesterol is essential to life and most of the body cholesterol is produced in the liver. The entire body requirement of cholesterol can be met by endogenous production. Nevertheless, dietary cholesterol is absorbed from the intestine and metabolized. Cholesterol, being insoluble in aqueous solution, is transported by the circulation as conjugates of lipoproteins.

CHOLESTEROL IN DISEASE

High blood level of cholesterol is suspected to play a role in atherosclerosis as a result of its deposition in the vascular walls.[82,83] Atherosclerosis is a chronic, progressive, multifactorial disease that begins as an intracellular deposition of cholesterol in previously damaged sites on the inner arterial walls. The lesions

Figure 14 The parent compound of all steroids is *Cyclopentanoperhydrophenanthrine* with four saturated rings that are designated alphabetically as shown **A**. The structural formula of cholesterol **B**. Note the four cyclohexane rings and the standard numbering system of all the carbon atoms. Reproduced with permission from Nair.[81]

eventually become fibrous calcified plaques. The consequent hardening and narrowing of the arteries promote the formation of intravascular blood clots and infarction of the dependent tissue. Although atheromas can develop in many different blood vessels, they are most common in the coronary arteries. The resultant myocardial infarction is usually fatal and is the most common cause of death in western industrialized nations.[84] Deposition of crystalline cholesterol also occurs in other tissues and organs, as in the case of otitis media and the "pearly tumor" of the cranium.[85] In the oral region, accumulation of cholesterol crystals occurs in apical periodontitis lesions[10,26,55,86–89] with clinical significance in endodontics and oral surgery.[26,90]

CHOLESTEROL IN APICAL PERIODONTITIS

Apical periodontitis lesions often contain deposits of cholesterol crystals appearing as narrow, elongated tissue clefts in histopathologic sections. The crystals dissolve in fat solvents used for the tissue processing and leave behind the spaces they occupied as clefts. The reported prevalence of cholesterol clefts in apical periodontitis varies from 18% to 44%.[55,86,88,89] The crystals are believed to be formed from cholesterol released by: (1) disintegrating erythrocytes of stagnant blood vessels within the lesion,[88] (2) lymphocytes, plasma cells, and macrophages that die in great numbers and disintegrate in chronic periapical lesions,[89] and (3) the circulating plasma lipids.[55] All these sources may contribute to the concentration and crystallization of cholesterol in the periapical area. Nevertheless, inflammatory cells that die and disintegrate within the lesion may be the major source of cholesterol, as a result of its release from membranes of such cells in long-standing lesions.[26,72] The crystals are initially formed in the inflamed periapical connective tissue, where they act as foreign bodies and provoke a giant cell reaction.

In histologic sections, numerous multinucleated giant cells can be observed around the cholesterol clefts (Figure 15). When a large number of crystals accumulate in the inflamed connective tissue, they passively move in the direction of least resistance. If the lesion happens to be a radicular cyst, the crystals move in the direction of the epithelium-lined cyst cavity, as the outer collagenous capsule of the lesion is much tougher for the crystals to move through. The slow "glacier-like" movement of the crystal mass erodes the epithelial lining and empties the crystals into the cyst lumen (Figure 15).

Radicular cysts[91] and apical granulomas[10] in which cholesterol clefts form a major component are referred to as "cholesteatoma." The term originates from general pathology where it refers to a local accumulation of cholesterol crystals that cause discomfort and dysfunction of the affected organs.[85] Therefore, the term should be used more specifically as "apical cholesteatoma" so as to distinguish the condition from cholesteatoma affecting other tissues and organs.

TISSUE REACTION TO CHOLESTEROL

Cholesterol crystals are intensely sclerogenic.[92,93] They induce granulomatous lesions in dogs,[94] mice,[92,93,95–97] and rabbits.[95,98,99] The cholesterol was applied in those studies by direct injection of its suspension into arterial walls,[94] by subcutaneous deposition of cholesterol crystals,[92,93,96,97] or by subcutaneous implantation of absorbable gelatin sponge that had been saturated with cholesterol in ether, and the solvent was allowed to evaporate before the implantation.[95,99] These studies consistently showed that the cholesterol crystals were densely surrounded by macrophages and giant cells.

There appears to be only one experimental study reported in the literature that specifically addressed the potential association of cholesterol crystals and non-resolving apical periodontitis lesions.[80] In this study in guinea pigs, the tissue reaction to cholesterol crystals was investigated by using a Teflon cage model[100] that facilitated the intact surgical retrieval of the cholesterol crystals with the surrounding host tissue after the experimentation. The study was to answer the question as to whether aggregates of cholesterol crystals would induce and sustain a granulomatous tissue reaction in guinea pigs. Pure cholesterol crystals, prepared to a mushy form, were placed in Teflon cages that were implanted subcutaneously in guinea pigs. The cage contents were retrieved after 2, 4, and 32 weeks of implantation and processed for light and correlative transmission electron microscopy. The cages revealed delicate soft connective tissue that grew in through perforations on the cage wall. The crystals were densely surrounded by numerous macrophages and multinucleated giant cells (Figures 16 and 17), forming a well circumscribed area of tissue reaction. The cells,

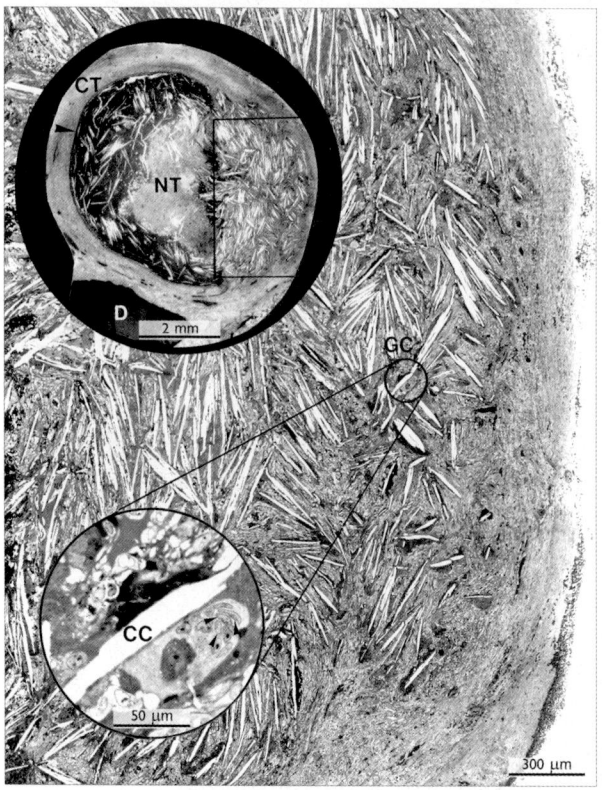

Figure 15 Cholesterol crystals and cystic condition of apical periodontitis as potential causes for endodontic failures. Overview of a histologic section (upper inset) of an asymptomatic apical periodontitis that persisted after conventional root canal treatment. Note the vast number of cholesterol clefts (CC) surrounded by giant cells (GC) of which a selected one with several nuclei (arrowheads) is magnified in the lower inset. D = dentine; CT = connective tissue; NT = necrotic tissue. Original magnifications: ×68; upper inset ×11; lower inset ×412. Reproduced with permission from Nair.[81]

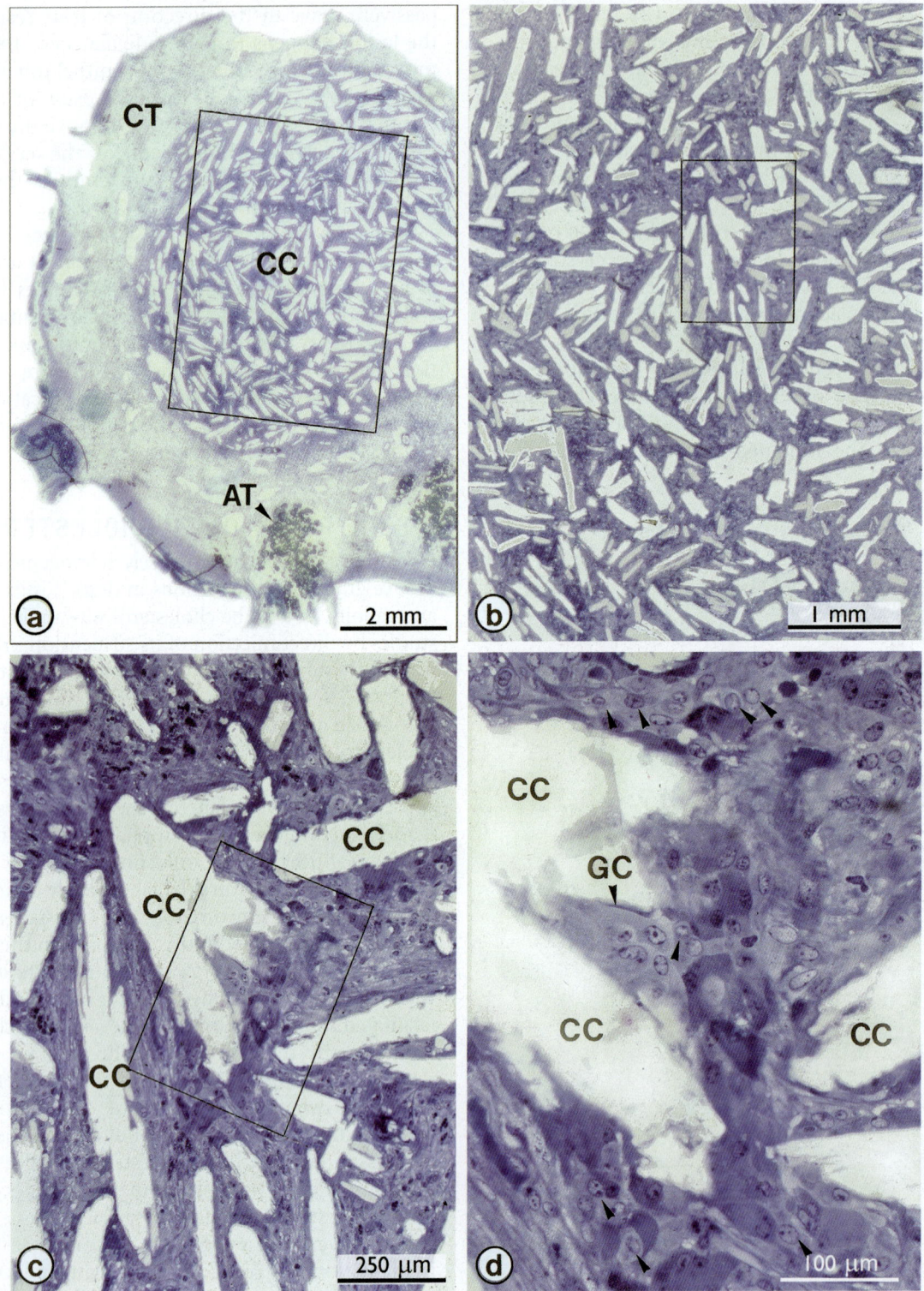

Figure 16 Photomicrograph **A,** of guinea pig tissue reaction to aggregates of cholesterol crystals after an observation period of 32 weeks. The rectangular demarcated areas in **A, B,** and **C,** are magnified in **B, C,** and **D,** respectively. Note that rhomboid clefts left by cholesterol crystals (CC) surrounded by giant cells (GC) and numerous mononuclear cells (arrowheads in *D*). AT = adipose tissue; CT = connective tissue. Original magnifications: **A** ×10, **B** ×21, **C** ×82, and **D** ×220. Reproduced with permission from Nair.[81]

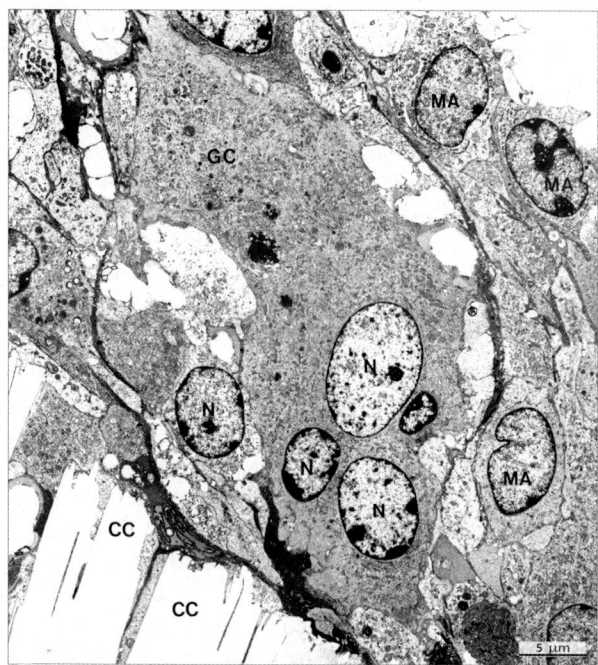

Figure 17 Ultrastructure of guinea pig tissue reaction to cholesterol crystals (CC) in cages that were removed 32 weeks after implantation. Note a large multinucleated (N) giant cell (GC) and numerous macrophages (MA) around the crystals. Original magnification: ×4,600. Reproduced with permission from Nair.[81]

however, were unable to eliminate the crystals during an observation period of 8 months.

The congregation of macrophages and giant cells around cholesterol crystals in the absence of other inflammatory cells such as neutrophils, lymphocytes, and plasma cells suggests that the crystals induced a typical foreign body reaction.[101–103] Whereas most of the macrophages may be freshly recruited blood monocyte population,[104,105] the giant cells are of local origin. Radioactive labeling studies[106,107] have conclusively shown that giant cells are monocyte derivatives formed by fusion of macrophages. Investigations on the cytogenesis of multinucleate giant cells around cholesterol crystals in subcutaneous implants suggest that they are formed by a process of "circumfusion"[93] of macrophages around individual crystals. Once formed, the giant cells can also enlarge in size by synchronous division of their nuclei.[108]

BODY CELLS CANNOT ELIMINATE CHOLESTEROL CRYSTALS

Tissue degradation of cholesterol crystals, if any, should happen via the phagocytic and/or biochemical pathways. Macrophages are efficient phagocytes[109] capable of ingesting and killing microorganisms, scavenging dead cells and necrotic tissue, and removing small foreign particles.[110] Cells belonging to the mononuclear phagocytic system[111] are involved in lipid uptake.[112] Macrophages have been shown to internalize cholesterol crystals in vitro.[93,112] Fine suspensions of cholesterol crystals administered intraperitoneally in rats were found in sternal lymph node macrophages.[113,114] In this apparently-phagocytic intake of particulate cholesterol, the size of the crystals must have been appropriately small for the macrophages to ingest them. However, when macrophages encounter larger foreign particles,[101,103] or cholesterol crystals,[92–96,99] they form multinucleate giant cells. The presence of giant cells in cholesterol granuloma is a clear sign of the large size of the crystals in relation to macrophages. However, the giant cells are poor phagocytes,[107,115] their phagocytic efficiency declining with increasing size of the cells.[116,117] The degradative power of multinucleate giant cells is mainly vested in their ability to resorb intrinsic and extrinsic substrates. Resorption is a highly specialized cellular activity in which the destruction of suitable substrates occurs extracellularly at the specialized cell/substrate interface by biochemical means.

In order to degrade tissue deposits of cholesterol crystals, the surrounding cells should have the ability to attack the crystals chemically so as to disperse them into the surrounding tissue fluid or to make them accessible to the cells themselves. Cholesterol crystals are highly hydrophobic, and their dispersal would necessitate making them hydrophilic and "soluble" in an aqueous medium.[92] The granulomatous and sclerogenic effects of cholesterol crystals can be prevented by the incorporation of phospholipids into subcutaneous implants of cholesterol.[96] This beneficial effect of phospholipids has been attributed to their "detergent" property and their role as donors of polyunsaturated fatty acids during esterification of the cholesterol.[92,97] The giant cells and macrophages are known to esterify and mobilize cholesterol in a lipid droplet form.[93] Macrophages can convert particulate cholesterol into a soluble form by incorporating it into a lipoprotein vehicle,[112,118] so that the cholesterol can be readily esterified or added into the lipoprotein pool in circulation.

These cell biologic findings obviously support the possible ability of macrophages and giant cells to degrade particulate cholesterol. But they are not consistent with the histopathologic observation of spontaneous[10,26,28] and experimentally-induced[92–96,99] cholesterol granulomas. The characteristic feature of such lesions is the accumulation of macrophages and giant cells around the cholesterol clefts and their persistence for long periods of time. *Therefore, it is to be assumed that the macrophages and the multinucleate giant cells that congregate around cholesterol crystals are unable to destroy the crystals in a way beneficial to the host.*[80] Therefore, massive accumulation of cholesterol crystals in apical periodontitis is clinically significant. The macrophages and giant cells that surround cholesterol crystals are not only unable to degrade the crystalline cholesterol but are major sources of apical inflammatory and bone resorptive mediators. Bone-resorbing activity of cholesterol-exposed macrophages due to enhanced expression of interleukin-1 has been experimentally shown.[119] Based on these considerations, it was concluded in a long-term longitudinal follow-up of a case that "the presence of vast numbers of cholesterol crystals... would be sufficient to sustain the lesion indefinitely."[26] The experimental results and other evidence presented from the literature substantiate that assumption.

FOREIGN BODIES

Foreign materials trapped in periapical tissues can cause pathologic tissue reaction. Particles of root-filling materials, other endodontic materials,[101,120] and portions of foods[121] can reach the periapical tissues and initiate a foreign body reaction that may be associated with periapical radiolucency.[101]

The most widely used solid root canal filling material is prepared from (*trans*-polyisoprene), the coagulated exudate from *Plaquium gutta* tree of Asia or from similar latex derived from the *Mimisops globsa* tree of South America.[122] Cones are composed of about 20% gutta-percha, 60% to 75% zinc oxide, and varying amounts of metal sulfates for radioopacity, waxes, and coloring agents. Based on implantation experiments in animals, cones are considered to be biocompatible and well tolerated by human tissues.[123–125] This view has not been consistent with the observation that the presence of extruded gutta-percha is associated with delayed healing of the periapex.[76,77,101,126,127] *In general, bulk form of sterile materials with smooth surfaces placed within bone or soft tissue evoke a fibrous tissue encapsulation, while particulate materials induce a foreign body and chronic inflammatory reaction.*[128–132] Apart from the particle size, the chemical composition of gutta-percha is also of significance. Leaching zinc oxide from gutta-percha cones has been shown to be cytotoxic in vitro,[133,134] tissue irritating in vivo, and associated with adjacent inflammatory reaction.[103,135] Tissue response to gutta-percha was studied[103] using subcutaneously implanted Teflon cages in which the gutta-percha evoked two distinct types of tissue reaction. Large pieces of gutta-percha were encapsulated by collagen and the surrounding tissue was free of inflammation (Figure 18). But, fine particles of gutta-percha induced an intense, localized tissue response (Figure 19), characterized by the presence of macrophages and giant cells. The

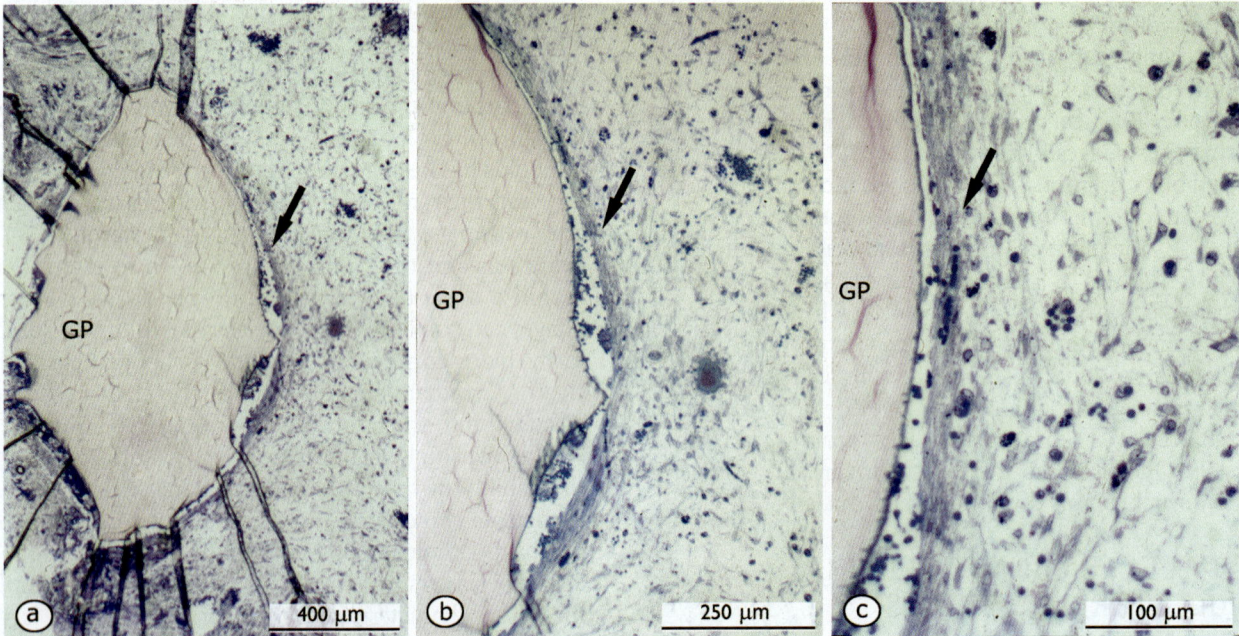

Figure 18 Guinea pig tissue reaction to gutta-percha (GP) by 1 month after subcutaneous implantation *A*. Large pieces of gutta-percha are well encapsulated by collagen fibers that run parallel to the surface of the gutta-percha particle. The interface of the gutta-percha particle and the host tissue (arrow) is magnified in stages in *B*, and *C*. The gap between the implant and the collagen capsule is artifactual. Note the noninflamed, healthy soft delicate connective tissue. Original magnifications: *A* ×17, *B* ×80, *C* ×200. Reproduced with permission from Nair.[163]

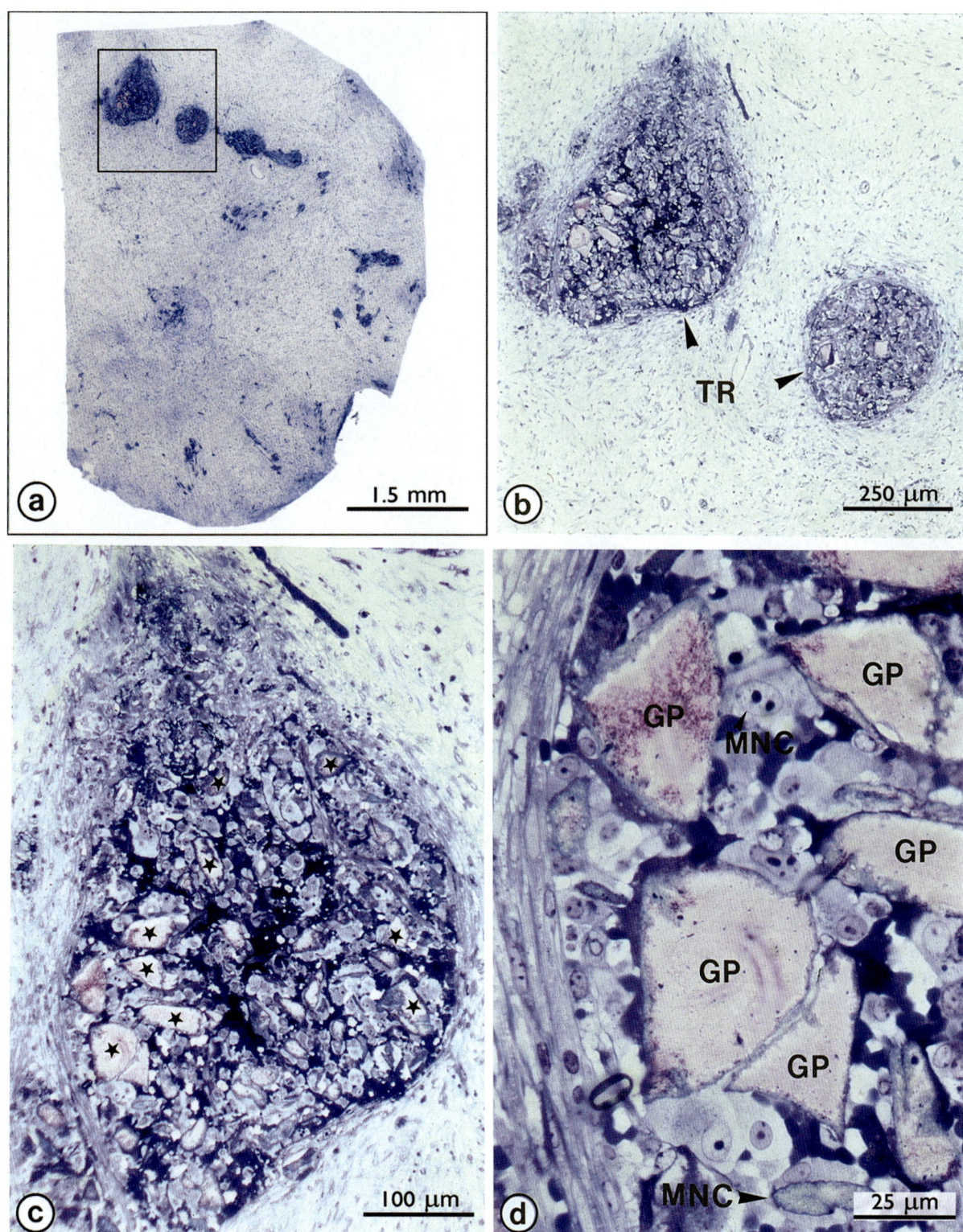

Figure 19 Disintegrated gutta-percha as potential for maintaining posttreatment apical periodontitis. As clusters of fine particles (**A, B,**) they induce intense circumscribed tissue reaction (TR) around. Note that the fine particles of gutta-percha (* in **C,** GP in **D**) are surrounded by numerous mononuclear cells (MNC). Original magnifications: **A** ×30, **B** ×80, **C** ×200, **D** ×750. From P.N.R. Nair, Pathobiology of the periapex. In: S. Cohen and R.C. Burns, editors, *Pathways of the pulp*, 8th ed., St Louis, 2002 Mosby©.

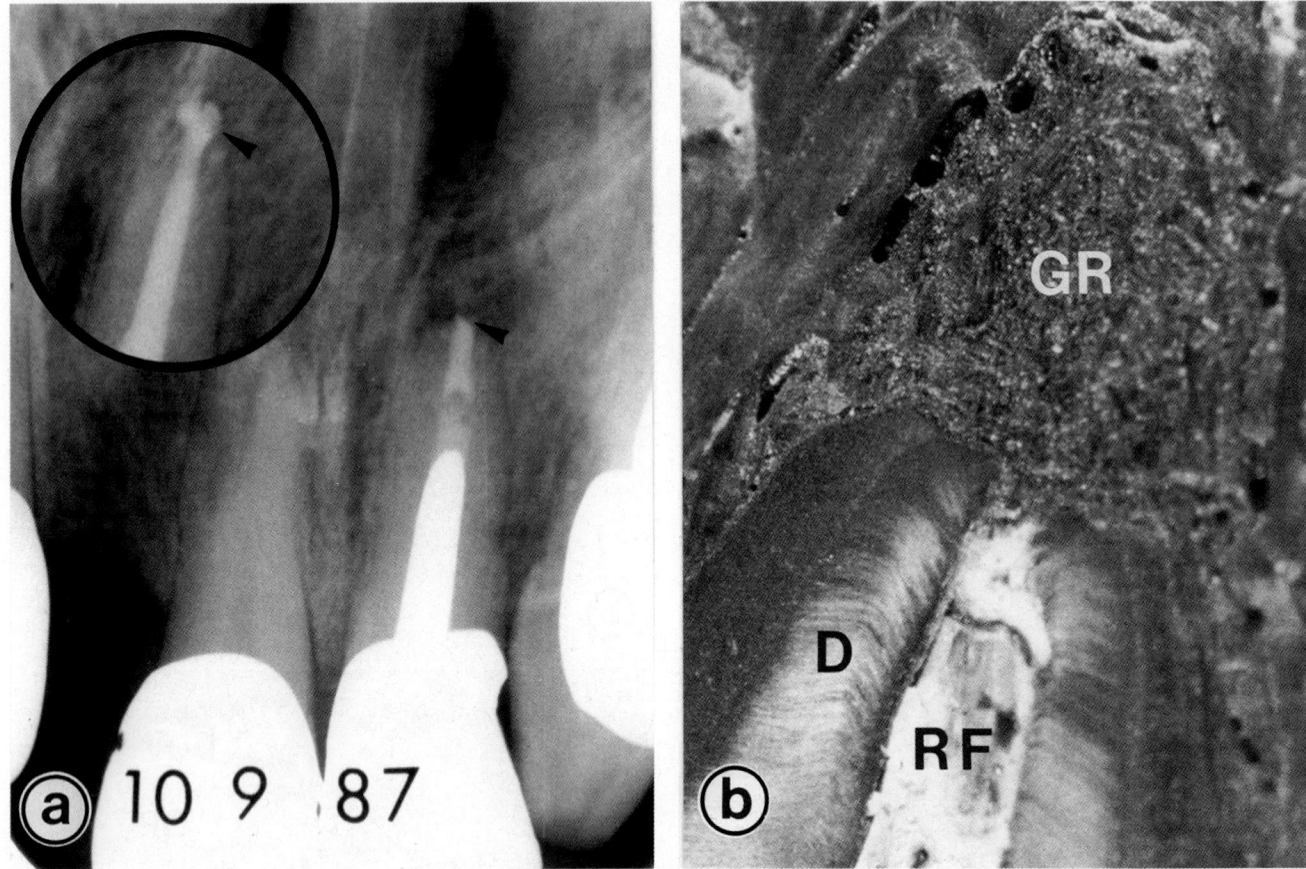

Figure 20 Two longitudinal radiographs (inset and **A**) of a root-filled and periapically affected left central maxillary incisor of a 54-year-old man. The first radiograph (inset) taken immediately after root filling in 1977 shows a small excess filling that protrudes into the periapex (arrowhead in inset). Note the excess filling has disappeared in the radiograph taken 10 years later (arrowhead in **A**) and shortly before surgery was performed. The apical block biopsy removed by surgery does not show any excess filling, as is evident from the macrophotograph of the decalcified and axially subdivided piece of the biopsy, **B**. RF = root filling; D = dentine; GR = granuloma. Original magnification: **B** ×10. Reproduced with permission from Nair.[101]

accumulation of macrophages in conjunction with the fine particles of gutta-percha is significant for the clinically observed impairment in the healing of apical periodontitis, when teeth are root filled with excess of gutta-percha. Pieces of gutta-percha cones in periapical tissue can gradually fragment into fine particles that in turn can induce a typical foreign body reaction[101–103] and activate macrophages.[136] The latter release a battery of intercellular mediators that include proinflammatory cytokines and modulators that are involved in bone resorption.[137–140]

In addition, commercial gutta-percha cones may become contaminated with tissue-irritating substances that can initiate a foreign body reaction at the periapex. In a follow-up study of nine asymptomatic persistent apical periodontitis lesions that were removed as surgical block biopsies and analyzed by correlative light and transmission electron microscopy, one biopsy (Figure 20) revealed the involvement of talc contaminated gutta-percha.[101] The radiographic lesion persisted asymptomatically and grew in size during a decade of posttreatment follow-up. The lesion was characterized by the presence of vast numbers of multinucleate giant cells with birefringent inclusion bodies (Figure 21). In transmission electron microscope, the birefringent bodies were found to be highly electron dense (Figure 22). Energy dispersive X-ray microanalysis of the

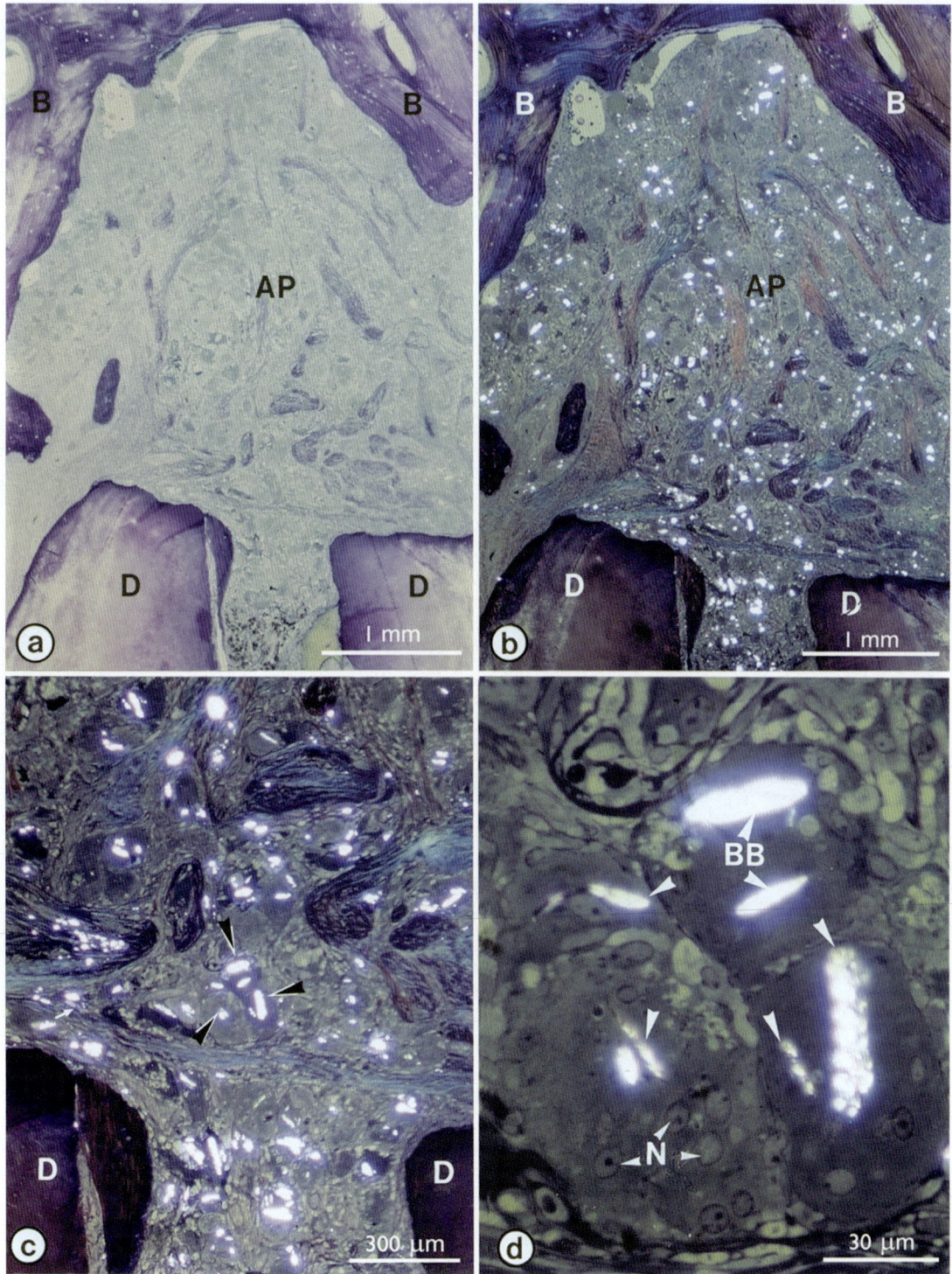

Figure 21 A bright-field photomicrograph of a plastic-embedded semithin (2 μm thick) section of the apical area shown in Figure 20B. Note the large apical periodontitis lesion (AP) ***A***. The same field when viewed in polarized lights ***B***. Note the birefringent bodies distributed throughout the lesion ***B***. The apical foramen is magnified in ***C***, and the dark arrow-headed cells in ***C***, are further enlarged in ***D***. Note the birefringence (BB) emerging from slit-like inclusion bodies in multinucleated (N) giant cells. B = bone; D = dentine. Original magnifications: ***A***, ***B*** ×23; ***C*** ×66; ***D*** ×300. From Nair, Pathology of apical periodontitis. In: D. Ørstavik and T.R. PittFord, editors, *Essential Endodontology*, Oxford, 1998, Blackwell©.

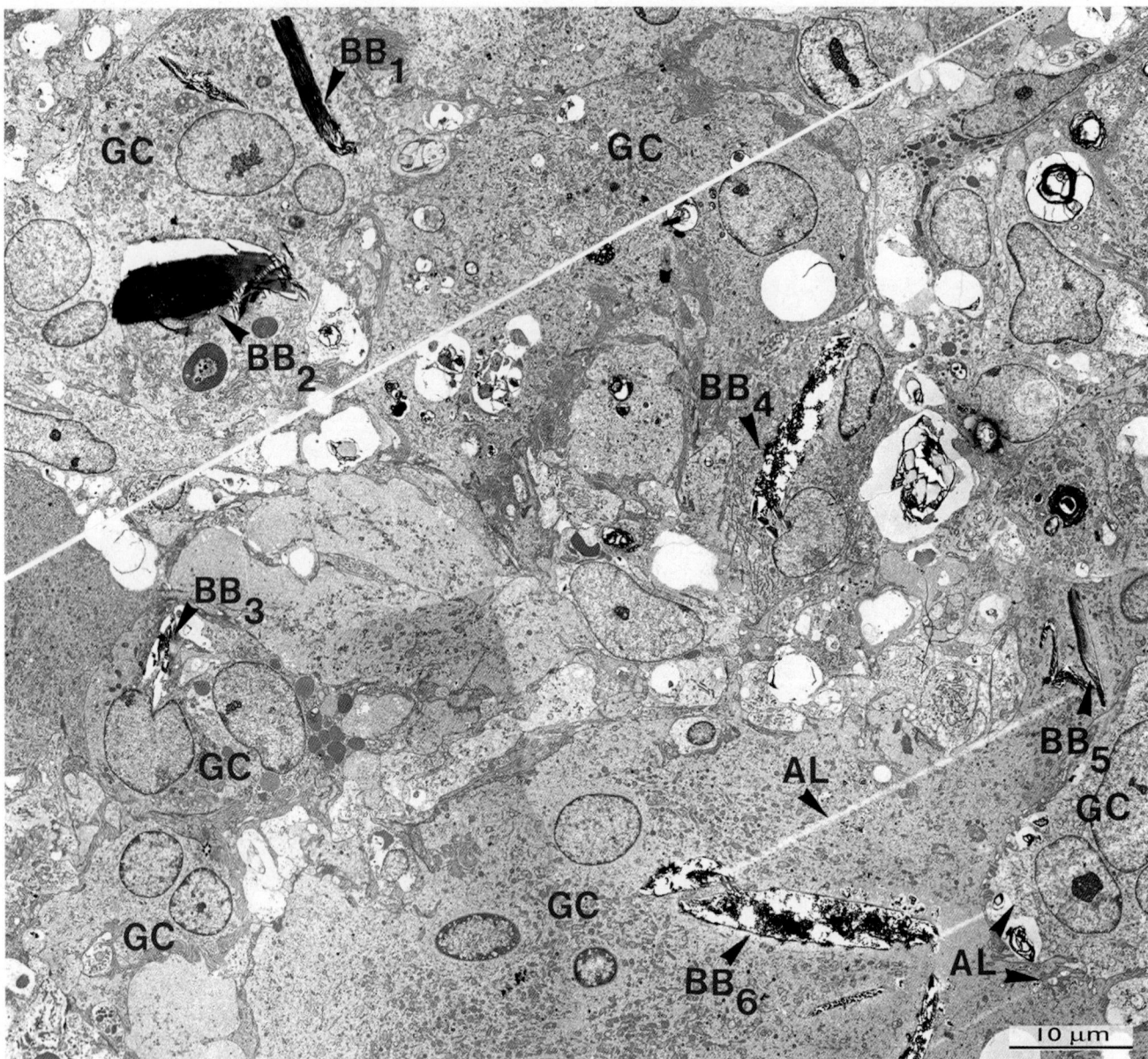

Figure 22 Low-magnification transmission electron micrograph showing the profiles of several giant cells within the apical periodontitis shown in Figures 20 and 21. Note the presence of many slit-like inclusion bodies (BB_1 to BB_6), which contain a highly electron-dense material. This material may remain intact within the inclusion body or may be pushed away from its original site (BB_2) or may appear disintegrated (BB_3 and BB_4) by the tissue processing. Note the lines of artifacts AL, which are created by portions of the electron-dense material having been carried away by the knife edge, leaving tracts behind. Original magnification: ×1,880. From P.N.R. Nair et al.[27] Reproduced with permission from Nair.[101]

inclusion bodies using scanning transmission electron microscopy (STEM) revealed the presence of magnesium and silicon (Figure 23). These elements are presumably the remnants of talc-contaminated gutta-percha that protruded into the periapex and had been resorbed during the follow-up period.

ORAL PULSE GRANULOMA

It denotes a foreign body reaction to particles of vegetable foods, particularly leguminous seeds such as peas, beans, and lentils (pulses) that get lodged in the oral tissues. The lesions are also referred to as the giant cell hyaline angiopathy,[141,142] vegetable granuloma,[143] and

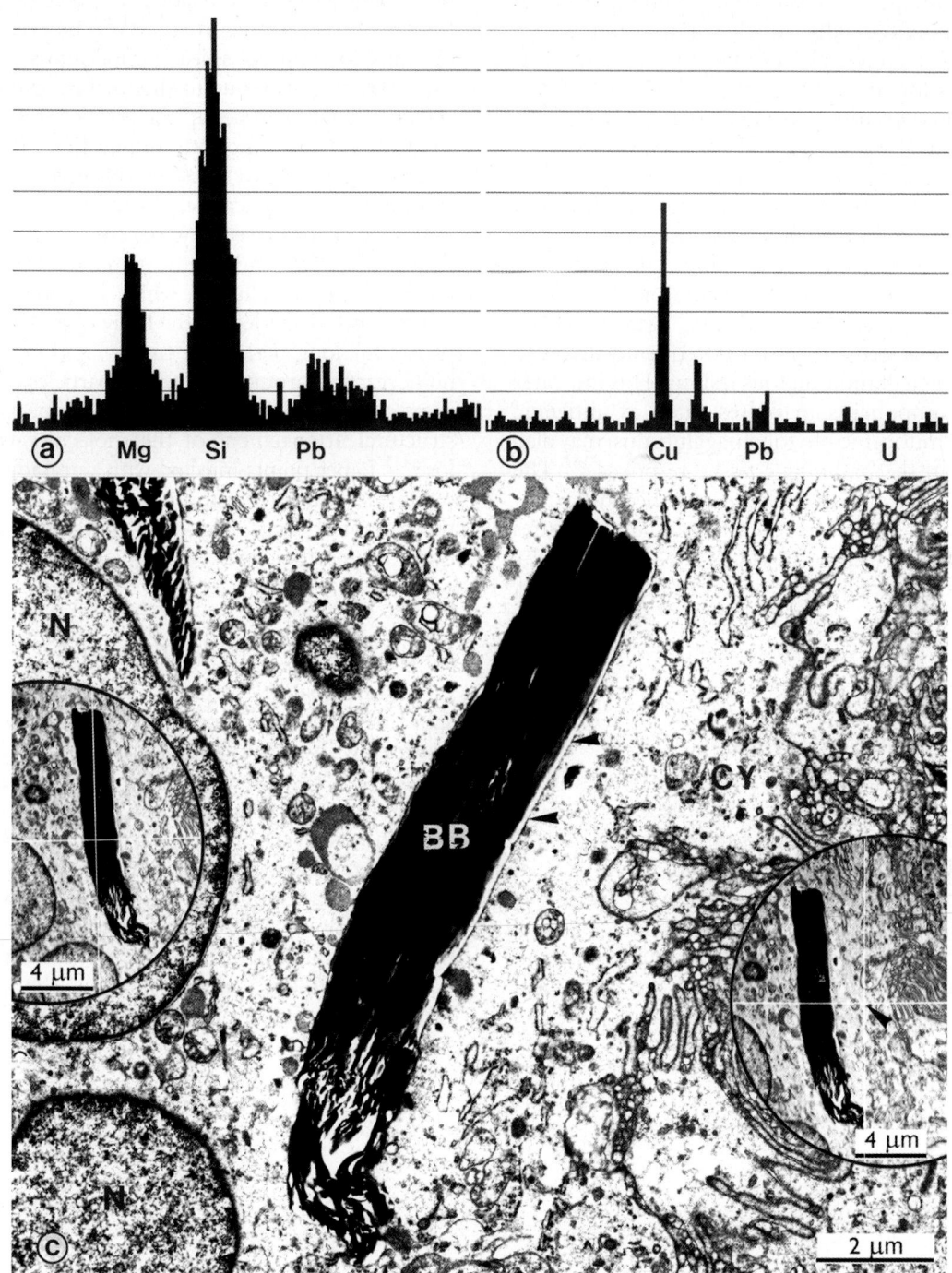

Figure 23 High-magnification transmission electron micrograph **C,** of the intact birefringent body labeled BB1 in Figure 22. Note the distinct delimiting membrane around the birefringent body (BB). Energy-dispersive X-ray microanalysis of the electron-dense material done in scanning transmission electron microscope (STEM: done at the point where the two hairlines perpendicular to each other cross in the left inset) revealed the presence of silicon (Si), magnesium (Mg), and lead (Pb) in **A,** whereas another site in the neighboring cytoplasm of the same giant cell (arrowhead in right inset) does not show the presence of Si and Mg **B**. Lead and uranium (U) are used for section contrasting, and emission in copper (Cu) is from the section-supporting grid made of copper. Original magnification ×11,000; insets ×3,300. Reproduced with permission from Nair.[101]

food-induced granuloma.[144] Pulse granuloma has been reported in lungs,[145] stomach walls, and peritoneal cavities.[146] Experimental lesions have been induced in animals by intratracheal, intraperitoneal, and submucous introduction of leguminous seeds.[147,148] Periapical pulse granulomas are associated with teeth grossly damaged by caries and with the history of endodontic therapy.[121,149] Pulse granuloma is characterized by the presence of intensely iodine and periodic acid—Schiff-positive hyaline rings/bodies surrounded by giant cells and inflammatory cells.[121,148–150] The cellulose in plants has been suggested to be the granuloma-inducing agent.[147] However, leguminous seeds are the most frequently involved vegetable in such granulomatous lesions. This indicates that other components in pulses, such as antigenic proteins and mitogenic phytohemagglutinins, may also be involved in the pathologic tissue response.[147] The pulse granulomas are clinically relevant because particles of vegetable foods can reach the periapical tissues via root canals of teeth exposed to the oral cavity by trauma, caries, or endodontic procedures.[121] However, the incidence of pulse-induced apical periodontitis may be low, as only two such cases have been reported in the literature.[121,150]

CELLULOSE GRANULOMA

Cellulose granuloma is pathologic tissue reaction to particles of predominantly cellulose-containing materials that are used in endodontic practice.[151–154] Endodontic *paper points* are utilized for microbial sampling and drying of root canals. Medicated *cotton wool* has been used in root canals as well. Particles of these thermo-sterilized materials can easily dislodge or get pushed into the periapical tissue[154] so as to induce a foreign body reaction at the periapex. Presence of cellulose fibers in periapical biopsies with a history of previous endodontic treatment has been reported.[151–153] The overall incidence of cellulose-induced apical periodontitis is unknown. This may be partly due to the inconspicuous nature of cellulose material in periapical biopsies and the difficulty to identify them without the application of special stains or techniques. In two investigations in which 13 biopsies of posttreatment apical periodontitis were histologically examined, all displayed material consistent with cellulose fibers.[151,152] The endodontic paper points and cotton wool consists of cellulose, which is neither digested by humans nor degraded by the body cells. They remain in tissues for long periods of time[153] and evoke a foreign body reaction around them. The particles, when viewed in polarized light, reveal birefringence due to the regular structural arrangement of the molecules within cellulose.[151] Paper points infected with intraradicular microorganisms can project through the apical foramen into the periapical tissue (Figure 24) and allow a biofilm to grow around the paper point (Figure 24).

OTHER FOREIGN MATERIALS

Endodontic sealer cements, amalgam, and calcium salts derived from periapically extruded calcium hydroxide also occur in periapical tissues. In a histologic and X-ray microanalytic investigation of 29 apical biopsies, 31% of the specimens were found to contain materials compatible with amalgam and endodontic sealer components.[120] However, an etiologic significance of these materials has not been conclusively shown by experiments. It is possible that these materials might have been coexisting with unidentified etiologic agents such as the presence of intraradicular infection in those cases.

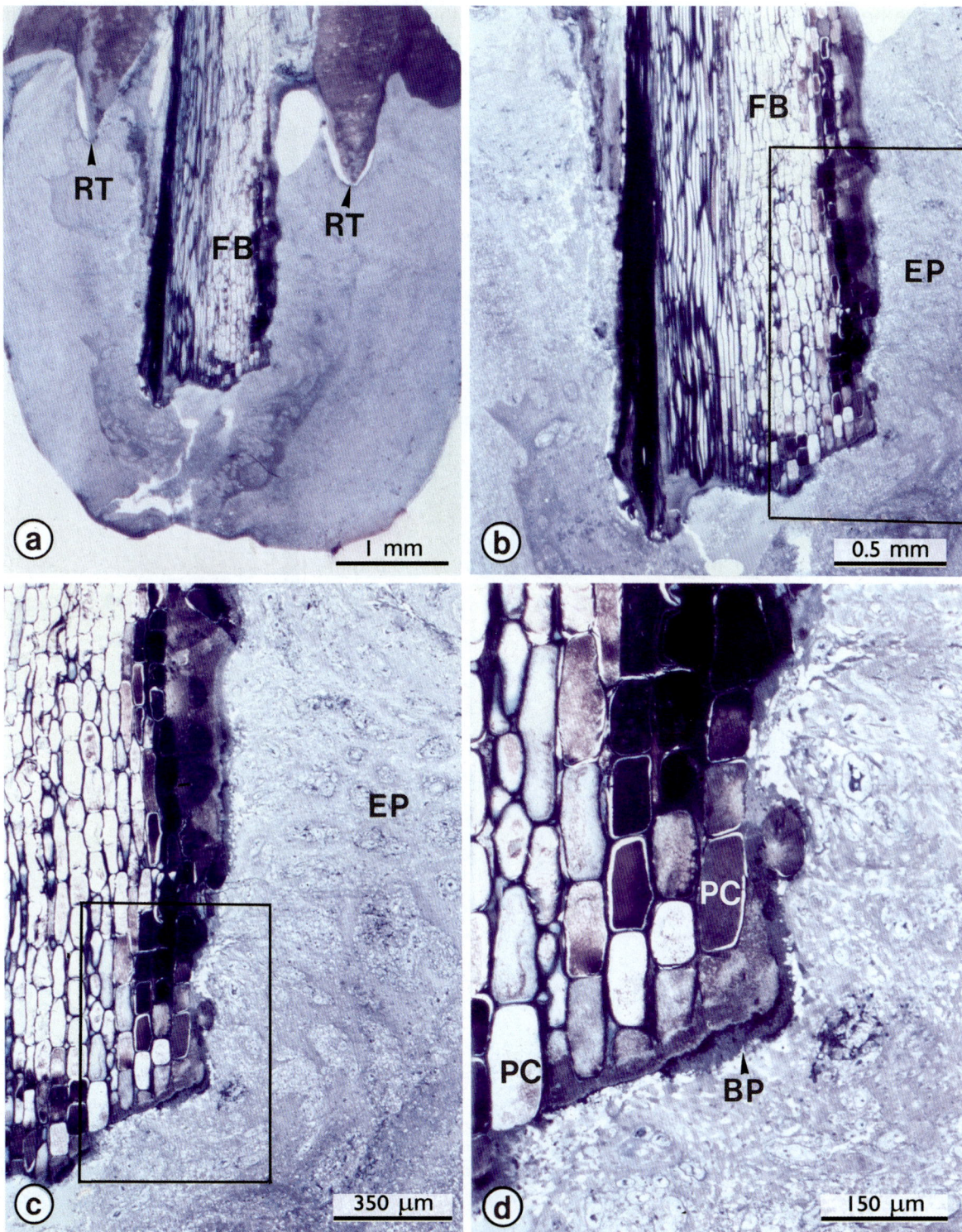

Figure 24 A massive paper-point granuloma affecting a root-canal-treated human tooth **A**. The demarcated area in **B,** is magnified in **C,** and that in the same is further magnified in **D**. Note the tip of the paper point (FB) projecting into the apical periodontitis lesion and the bacterial plaque (BP) adhering to the surface of the paper point. RT = root tip; EP = epithelium; PC = plant cell. Original magnifications: **A** ×20, **B** ×40, **C** ×60, **D** ×150. From P.N.R. Nair, Pathobiology of the periapex. In: S. Cohen and R.C. Burns, editors, *Pathways of the pulp*, 8th edition, St Louis, 2002 Mosby©.

Scar Tissue healing

There is evidence[10,52,79,155] that unresolved periapical radiolucencies may occasionally be due to healing of the lesion by scar tissue (Figure 25) that may be misdiagnosed as a radiographic sign of failed endodontic treatment. Certain deductions can be made from the

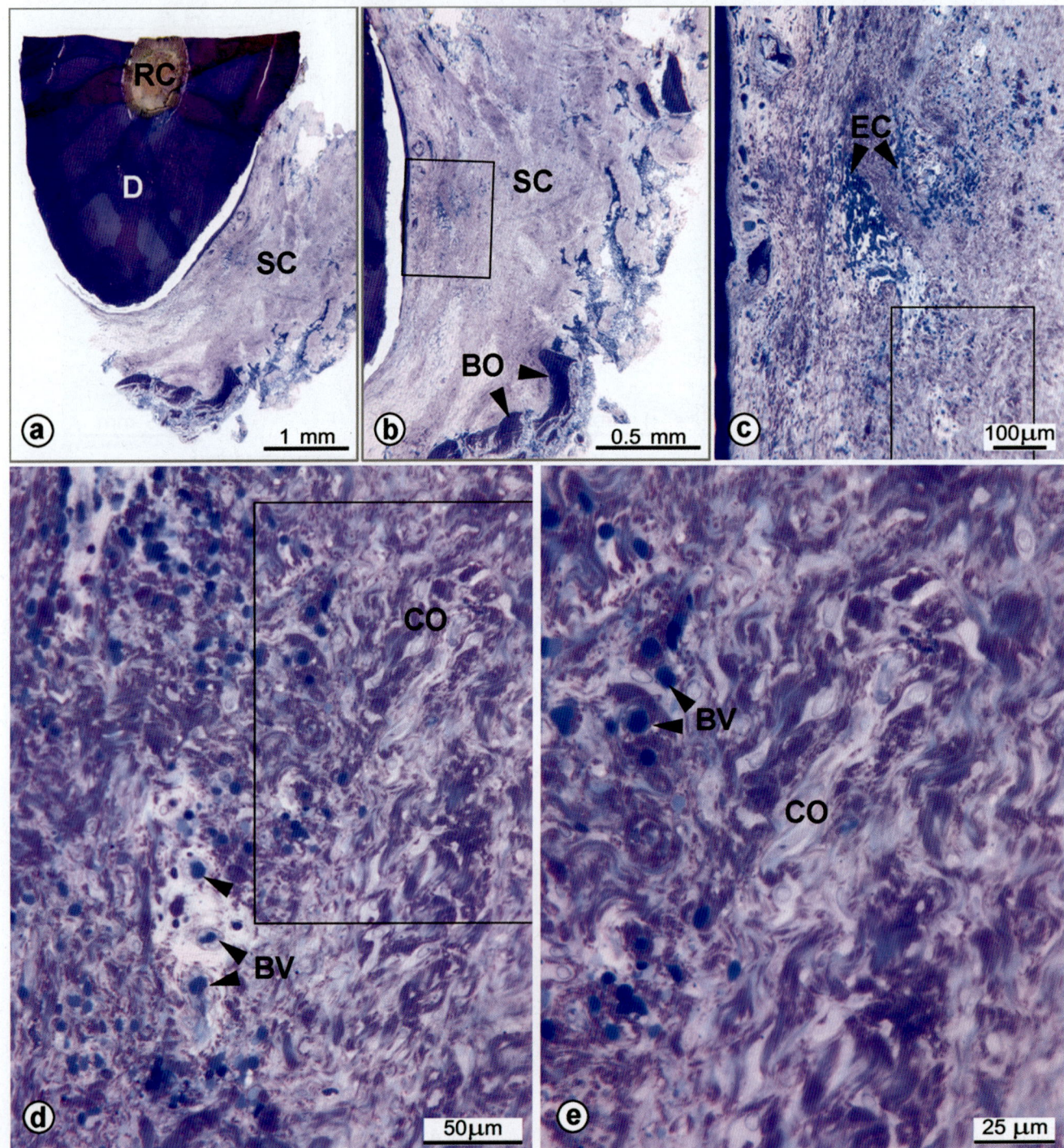

Figure 25 Periapical scar (SC) of a root canal (RC)-treated tooth after 5-year follow-up and surgery. The rectangular demarcated areas in **B–D**, are magnified in **C–E**, respectively. The scar tissue reveals bundles of collagen fibers (CO), blood vessels (BV), and erythrocytes due to hemorrhage. Infiltrating inflammatory cells are notably absent. Original magnifications: **A** ×14, **B** ×35, C ×90, **D** ×340, **E** ×560. Modified from Nair et al.[79]

data available on normal healing and guided regeneration of the marginal periodontium. Several cell populations participate in the periodontal healing process. The pattern of healing depends on several factors, two of which are decisive. They are the regeneration potential and the speed with which the tissue cells bordering the defect react.[156–159] A periapical scar probably develops because precursors of soft connective tissue colonize both the root tip and periapical tissue; this may occur before the appropriate cells, which have the potential to restore various structural components of the apical periodontium, are able to do so.[79]

Concluding Remarks

The presence of an intraradicular infection is the *essential cause* of primary apical periodontitis and the *major cause* of persistent apical radiolucencies.[160,161] This means that microbial infection is not the only etiologic agent of apical radiolucencies persisting posttreatment. The nonmicrobial factors, discussed in this chapter, include (1) true cystic lesions, (2) extruded root canal filling or other exogenous materials that cause a foreign body reaction; (3) accumulation of endogenous cholesterol crystals that irritate periapical tissues; and (4) scar tissue healing of the lesion. Although true cysts, foreign body reaction, and scar tissue healing are of rare occurrence, they are of clinical significance.

Most of the cysts, particularly larger cysts, may not be amenable to root canal treatment alone. Whereas smaller pocket cysts are likely to heal after root canal treatment, very large pocket cysts and most of the true cysts may not heal. But there are no individual statistics on them. Cysts, nevertheless, represent only a small fraction of persistent apical radiolucencies.

The fact that persistent apical radiolucencies cannot be differentially diagnosed based on etiology is of no clinical significance but of academic interest only. This is because it is not guaranteed that root canal re-treatment of an otherwise well-treated tooth will result in the removal of intraradicular microbes located in the apical canal system, which is the single most important cause of persisting radiolucencies. Furthermore, apical radiolucencies persisting because of extraradicular factors discussed in this chapter, such as foreign body reaction, including those due to cholesterol crystals, cystic condition, and scar tissue are beyond root canal system and cannot be managed by root canal re-treatment.

Therefore, with cases of asymptomatic, persistent radiolucencies, clinicians should consider the necessity of removing the extraradicular factors by an apical surgery,[162] in order to improve the long-term result of treatment. An apical surgery enables to remove the extraradicular agents that sustain the radiolucency posttreatment and also allows a retrograde access to any infection in the apical portion of the root canal system that can also be removed or sealed within the canal by a retrograde root-end filling.[163]

References

1. Nair PNR. Non-microbial etiology: periapical cysts sustain post-treatment apical periodontitis. Endod Topics 2003;6:114–34.
2. Kakehashi S, Stanley HR, Fitzgerald RJ. The effects of surgical exposures of dental pulps in germ-free and conventional laboratory rats. Oral Surg Oral Med Oral Pathol Oral Radiol Endod 1965;20:340–9.
3. Sundqvist G. Bacteriological studies of necrotic dental pulps [Dr. Odont. Thesis]. Umeå, Sweden: University of Umeå; 1976.
4. Nair PNR. Light and electron microscopic studies of root canal flora and periapical lesions. J Endod 1987;13:29–39.
5. Costerton W, Veeh R, Shirtliff M, et al. The application of biofilm science to the study and control of chronic bacterial infections. J Clin Invest 2003;112:1466–77.
6. Taylor E. Dorland's illustrated medical dictionary. 27th ed. Philadelphia: W.B. Saunders Co.; 1988. p. 324.
7. Shear M. Cysts of the oral regions. 3rd ed. Oxford: Wright; 1992. pp. 136–70.
8. Nair PNR. New perspectives on radicular cysts: do they heal? Int Endod J 1998;31:155–60.
9. Killey HC, Kay LW, Seward GR. Benign cystic lesions of the jaws, their diagnosis and treatment. 3rd ed. Edinburgh and London: Churchill Livingston; 1977.
10. Bhaskar SN. Periapical lesion—types, incidence and clinical features. Oral Surg Oral Med Oral Pathol Oral Radiol Endod 1966;21:657–71.
11. Mortensen H, Winther JE, Birn H. Periapical granulomas and cysts. Scand J Dent Res 1970;78:241–50.
12. Borg G, Persson G, Thilander H. A study of odontogenic cysts with special reference to comparisons between keratinizing and nonkeratinizing cysts. Swed Dent J 1974;67:311–25.
13. Huumonen S, Ørstavik D. Radiological aspects of apical periodontitis. Endod Topics 2002;1:3–25.
14. Sewerin IP. Radiographic examination. In: Bergenholtz G, Horsted-Bindslav P, and Reit C, editors. Textbook of endodontology. Oxford: Blackwell Munksgaard; 2003. pp. 215–35.
15. White SC, Sapp JP, Seto BG, et al. Absence of radiometric differentiation between periapical cyst and granulomas. Oral Surg Oral Med Oral Pathol Oral Radiol Endod 1994;78:650–4.

16. Shrout M, Hall J, Hildeblot C. Differentiation of periapical granulomas and radicular cysts by digital radiometric analysis. Oral Surg Oral Med Oral Pathol Oral Radiol Endod 1993;76:356–61.

17. Priebe WA, Lazansky JP, Wuehrmann AH. The value of the roentgenographic film in the differential diagnosis of periapical lesions. Oral Surg Oral Med Oral Pathol Oral Radiol Endod 1954;7:979–83.

18. Baumann L, Rossman SR. Clinical, roentgenologic and histologic findings in teeth with apical radiolucent areas. Oral Surg Oral Med Oral Pathol Oral Radiol Endod 1956;9:1330–6.

19. Wais FT. Significance of findings following biopsy and histologic study of 100 periapical lesions. Oral Surg Ora Med Oral Pathol Oral Radiol Endod 1958;11:650–3.

20. Linenberg WB, Waldron CA, DeLaune GF. A clinical roentgenographic and histopathologic evaluation of periapical lesions. Oral Surg Oral Med Oral Pathol Oral Radiol Endod 1964;17:467–72.

21. Lalonde ER, Luebke RG. The frequency and distribution of periapical cysts and granulomas. Oral Surg Oral Med Oral Pathol Oral Radiol Endod 1968;25:861–8.

22. Ricucci D, Mannocci F, Pitt Ford TR. A study of periapical lesions correlating the presence of a radioopaque lamina with histological findings. Oral Surg Oral Med Oral Pathol Oral Radiol Endod 2006;101:389–94.

23. Trope M, Pettigrew J, Petras J, et al. Differentiation of radicular cysts and granulomas using computerized tomography. Endod Dent Traumatol 1989;5:69–72.

24. Cotti E, Campisi G, Garau V, et al. A new technique for the study of periapical bone lesions: ultrasound real time imaging. Int Endod J 2002;35:148–52.

25. Cotti E, Campisi G, Garau V, et al. Ultrasound real-time imaging in the differential diagnosis of periapical lesions. Int Endod J 2003;36:556–63.

26. Nair PNR, Sjögren U, Schumacher E, et al. Radicular cyst affecting a root-filled human tooth: a long-term post-treatment follow-up. Int Endod J 1993;26:225–33.

27. Malassez ML. Sur l'existence de masses épithéliales dans le ligament alvéolodentaire chez l'homme adulte et à l'état normal. Comp Rend Soc Biol 1884;36:241–4.

28. Thoma KH. A histo-pathological study of the dental granuloma and diseased root apex. J Natl Dent Assoc 1917;4:1075–90.

29. McConnell G. The histo-pathology of dental granulomas. J Natl Dent Assoc 1921;8:390–8.

30. Freeman N. Histopathological investigation of dental granuloma. J Dent Res 1931;11:176–200.

31. Sonnabend E, Oh C-S. Zur Frage des Epithels im apikalen Granulationsgewebe (Granulom) menschlicher Zähne. Dtsch Zahnärztl Z 1966;21:627–43.

32. Seltzer S, Soltanoff W, Bender IB. Epithelial proliferation in periapical lesions. Oral Surg Oral Med Oral Pathol Oral Radiol Endod 1969;27:111–21.

33. Summers L. The incidence of epithelium in periapical granulomas and the mechanism of cavitation in apical dental cysts in man. Arch Oral Biol 1974;19:1177–80.

34. Summers L, Papadimitriou J. The nature of epithelial proliferation in apical granulomas. J Oral Pathol 1975;4:324–9.

35. Langeland MA, Block RM, Grossman LI. A histopathologic and histobacteriologic study of 35 periapical endodontic surgical specimens. J Endod 1977;3:8–23.

36. Yanagisawa W. Pathologic study of periapical lesions. I. Periapical granulomas: clinical, histologic and immuno-histopathologic studies. J Oral Pathol 1980;9:288–300.

37. Nair PNR, Schroeder HE. Epithelial attachment at diseased human tooth-apex. J Periodont Res 1985;20:293–300.

38. Nair PNR, Schmid-Meier E. An apical granuloma with epithelial integument. Oral Surg Oral Med Oral Pathol Oral Radiol Endod 1986;62:698–703.

39. Turner J. Dental cysts. Brit Dent J 1898;19:711–34.

40. Kronfeld R. Histopathology of the teeth and their surrounding structures. Philadelphia: Lea & Febiger; 1939. pp. 210–11.

41. Stafne E, Millhon J. Periodontal cysts. J Oral Surg 1945;3:102–11.

42. Gorlin R. Potentialities of oral epithelium manifest by mandibular dentigerous cysts. Oral Surg Oral Med Oral Pathol Oral Radiol Endod 1957;10:271–84.

43. Shear M. Secretory epithelium in the lining of dental cysts. J Dent Assoc South Africa 1960;15:117–22.

44. Marsland E, Browne R. Two odontogenic cysts, partially lined with ciliated epithelium. Oral Surg Oral Med Oral Pathol Oral Radiol Endod 1965;19:502–7.

45. Fujiwara K, Watanabe T. Mucous producing cells and ciliated epithelial cells in mandibular radicular cysts: an electron microscopic study. J Oral Maxillofac Surg 1988;46:149–51.

46. Nair PNR, Pajarola G, Luder HU. Ciliated epithelium lined radicular cysts. Oral Surg Oral Med Oral Pathol Oral Radiol Endod 2002;94:485–93.

47. Berry G. Dental caries in paranasal sinus infections. Arch Otolaryngol 1929;8:698–706.

48. Stevensson W. Chronic maxillary sinusitis. Arch Otolaryngol 1931;13:505–31.

49. Martensson G. Dental Sinusitiden. Dtsch Zahnärztl Z 1952;7:1417–27.

50. Nair PNR, Pajarola G, Schroeder HE. Types and incidence of human periapical lesions obtained with extracted teeth. Oral Surg Oral Med Oral Pathol Oral Radiol Endod 1996;81:93–102.

51. Simon JHS. Incidence of periapical cysts in relation to the root canal. J Endod 1980;6:845–8.

52. Seltzer S, Bender IB, Smith J, et al. Endodontic failures—an analysis based on clinical, roentgenographic, and histologic

findings. Parts I and II. Oral Surg Oral Med Oral Pathol Oral Radiol Endod 1967;23:500–30.

53. Rohrer A. Die Aetiologie der Zahnwurzelzysten. Dtsch Mschr Zahnheik 1927;45:282–94.

54. Gardner AF. A survey of periapical pathology: Part one. Dent Dig 1962;68:162–7.

55. Shear M. The histogenesis of dental cysts. Dent Practit 1963;13:238–43.

56. Main DMG. The enlargement of epithelial jaw cysts. Odont Revy 1970;21:29–49.

57. Ten Cate AR. Epithelial cell rests of Malassez and the genesis of the dental cyst. Oral Surg Oral Med Oral Pathol Oral Radiol Endod 1972;34:956–64.

58. Torabinejad M. The role of immunological reactions in apical cyst formation and the fate of the epithelial cells after root canal therapy: a theory. Int J Oral Surg 1983;12:14–22.

59. Nair PNR. Apical periodontitis: a dynamic encounter between root canal infection and host response. Periodontology 2000 1997;13:121–48.

60. Valderhaug J. A histologic study of experimentally induced periapical inflammation in primary teeth in monkeys. Int J Oral Surg 1974;3:111–23.

61. Meghji S, Qureshi W, Henderson B, et al. The role of endotoxin and cytokines in the pathogenesis of odontogenic cysts. Arch Oral Biol 1996;41:523–31.

62. Thesleff I. Epithelial rests of Malassez bind epidermal growth factor intensely. J Periodont Res 1987;22:419–21.

63. Lin LM, Wang S-L, Wu-Wang C, et al. Detection of epidermal growth factor in inflammatory periapical lesions. Int Endod J 1996;29:179–84.

64. Li T, Browne RM, Mathews JB. Immunocytochemical expression of growth factors in inflammatory periapical lesions. Mol Pathol 1997;50:21–7.

65. James WW. Do epithelial odontomes increase in size by their own tension? Proc R Soc Med 1926;19:73–7.

66. Hill TJ. The epithelium in dental granuloma. J Dent Res 1930;10:323–32.

67. Tratman EK. Diffusion as a factor in the increase in size of dental and dentigerous cysts. Br Dent J 1939;66:515–20.

68. Toller PA. The osmolarity of fluids from cysts of the jaws. Br Dent J 1970;129:275–8.

69. Torabinejad M, Kettering J. Identification and relative concentration of B and T lymphocytes in human chronic periapical lesions. J Endod 1985;11:122–5.

70. Formigli L, Orlandini SZ, Tonelli P, et al. Osteolytic processes in human radicular cysts: morphological and biochemical results. J Oral Pathol Med 1995;24:216–20.

71. Teronen O, Salo T, Laitinen J, et al. Characterization of interstitial collagenases in jaw cyst wall. Eur J Oral Sci 1995;103:141–7.

72. Seltzer S. Endodontology. 2nd ed. Philadelphia: Lea & Febiger; 1988. pp. 223–4.

73. Valderhaug J. Epithelial cells in the periodontal membrane of the teeth with and without periapical inflammation. Int J Oral Surg 1974;3:7–16.

74. Lalonde ER. A new rationale for the management of periapical granulomas and cysts. an evaluation of histopathological and radiographic findings. J Am Dent Assoc 1970;80:1056–9.

75. Staub HP. Röntgenologische Erfolgstatistik von Wurzelbehandlungen [Dr. med. dent. Thesis]. Switzerland: University of Zurich; 1963.

76. Kerekes K, Tronstad L. Long-term results of endodontic treatment performed with standardized technique. J Endod 1979;5:83–90.

77. Sjögren U, Hägglund B, Sundqvist G, et al. Factors affecting the long-term results of endodontic treatment. J Endod 1990;16:498–504.

78. Nair PNR, Sjögren U, Kahnberg KE, et al. Intraradicular bacteria and fungi in root-filled, asymptomatic human teeth with therapy-resistant periapical lesions: a long-term light and electron microscopic follow-up study. J Endod 1990;16:580–8.

79. Nair PNR, Sjögren U, Figdor D, et al. Persistent periapical radiolucencies of root filled human teeth, failed endodontic treatments and periapical scars. Oral Surg Oral Med Oral Pathol Oral Radiol Endod 1999;87:617–27.

80. Nair PNR, Sjögren U, Sundqvist G. Cholesterol crystals as an etiological factor in non-resolving chronic inflammation: an experimental study in guinea pigs. Eur J Oral Sci 1998;106:644–50.

81. Nair PNR. Cholesterol as an aetiological agent in endodontic failures—a review. Aust Endod J 1999;25:19–26.

82. Yeagle PL. The biology of cholesterol. Boca Raton: CRC Press; 1988.

83. Yeagle PL. Understanding your cholesterol. San Diego: Academic Press; 1991. pp. 35–51.

84. Voet D, Voet JD. Biochemistry. 2nd ed. New York: John Wiley & Sons; 1995. p. 323.

85. Anderson WAD. Pathology. 5th ed. St. Louis: CV Mosby; 1996. pp. 777, 1404.

86. Darlington CG. "So called" tumors of special interest to the dentists. Dental Cosmos 1933;75:310–14.

87. Nadal-Valldaura A. Fatty degeneration and the formation of fat-lipid needles in chronic granulomatous periodontitis. Rev Esp Estomat 1968;15:105.

88. Browne RM. The origin of cholesterol in odontogenic cysts in man. Arch Oral Biol 1971;16:107–13.

89. Trott JR, Chebib F, Galindo Y. Factors related to cholesterol formation in cysts and granulomas. J Can Dent Assoc 1973;38:76–8.

90. Nair PNR. Eine neue Sicht der radikulären Zysten: Sind sie heilbar? Endodontie 1995;4:169–79.

91. Thoma KH, Goldman HM. Oral pathology. 5th ed. St. Louis: CV Mosby; 1960. p. 490.

92. Abdulla YH, Adams CWM, Morgan RS. Connective tissue reactions to implantation of purified sterol, sterol esters, phosphoglycerides, glycerides and free fatty acids. J Pathol Bacteriol 1967;94:63–71.

93. Bayliss OB. The giant cell in cholesterol resorption. Br J Exp Pathol 1976;57:610–18.

94. Christianson OO. Observations on lesions produced in arteries of dogs by injection of lipids. Archs Pathol 1939;27:1011–20.

95. Spain DM, Aristizabal N, Ores R. Effect of estrogen on resolution of local cholesterol implants. Arch Pathol 1959;68:30–3.

96. Adams CWM, Bayliss OB, Ibrahim MZM, et al. Phospholipids in atherosclerosis: the modification of the cholesterol granuloma by phospholipid. J Pathol Bacteriol 1963;86:431–6.

97. Adams CWM, Morgan RS. The effect of saturated and polyunsaturated lecithins on the resorption of 4-14C-cholesterol from subcutaneous implants. J Pathol Bacteriol 1967;94:73–6.

98. Hirsch EF. Experimental tissue lesions with mixtures of human fat, soaps and cholesterol. Arch Pathol 1938;25:35–9.

99. Spain D, Aristizabal N. Rabbit local tissue response to triglycerides, cholesterol and its ester. Arch Pathol 1962;73:94–7.

100. Lundgren D, Lindhe J. Exudation inflammatory cell migration and granulation tissue formation in preformed cavities. Scand J Plast Reconstr Surg 1973;7:1–9.

101. Nair PNR, Sjögren U, Krey G, et al. Therapy-resistant foreign-body giant cell granuloma at the periapex of a root-filled human tooth. J Endod 1990;16:589–95.

102. Coleman DL, King RN, Andrade JD. The foreign body reaction: a chronic inflammatory response. J Biomed Mater Res 1974;8:199–211.

103. Sjögren U, Sundqvist G, Nair PNR. Tissue reaction to of various sizes of gutta-percha when implanted subcutaneously in guinea pigs. Eur J Oral Sci 1995;103:313–21.

104. Mariano M, Spector WG. The formation and properties of macrophage polykaryons (inflammatory giant cells). J Pathol 1974;113:1–19.

105. Ryan GP, Spector WG. Macrophage turnover in inflamed connective tissue. Proc Roy Soc Lond (Biol) 1970;175:269–92.

106. Gillman T, Wright LJ. Probable in vivo origin of multinucleate giant cells from circulating mononuclears. Nature, Lond 1966;209:263–5.

107. Spector WG, Lykke AW. The cellular evolution of inflammatory granuloma. J Pathol Bacteriol 1966;92:163–77.

108. Spector WG, Mariano M. Macrophage behaviour in experimental granulomas. In: Van Furth R, editor. Mononuclear phagocytes in immunity, infection and pathology. Oxford: Blackwell; 1975. p. 927.

109. Metchinkoff E. Lectures on the comparative pathology of inflammation. New York: Dover Publications; 1968. pp. 1–224.

110. Papadimitriou JM, Ashman RB. Macrophages: current views on their differentiation, structure and function. Ultrastruct Pathol 1989;13:343–72.

111. Van Furth R, Cohn ZA, Hirsch JG, et al. The mononuclear phagocyte system: a new classification of macrophages, monocytes and their precursors. Bull World Health Organ 1972;46:845–52.

112. Day AJ. The macrophage system, lipid metabolism and atherosclerosis. J Atheroscler Res 1964;4:117–30.

113. French JE, Morris B. The uptake and storage of lipid particles in lymph gland in the rat. J Pathol Bacteriol 1960;79:11–19.

114. Day AJ, French JE. Further observations on the storage of cholesterol and cholesterol esters in lymph gland in the rat. J Pathol Bacteriol 1961;81:247–54.

115. Carr I. Macrophages in connective tissues. The granuloma macrophage. In: Carr I and Daems WT, editors. The reticuloendothelial system. A comprehensive treatise. New York: Plenum Press; 1980. pp. 671–703.

116. Chambers TJ. Studies on the phagocytic capacity of macrophage polykaryons. J Pathol 1977;123:65–77.

117. Papadimitriou JM, Robertson TA, Walters MN. An analysis of the phagocytic potential of multinucleate foreign body giant cells. Am J Pathol 1975;78:343–58.

118. Tompkins DH. Reaction of the reticuloendothelial cells to subcutaneous injections of cholesterol. Arch Pathol 1946;42:299–319.

119. Sjögren U, Mukohyama H, Roth C, et al. Bone-resorbing activity from cholesterol-exposed macrophages due to enhanced expression of interleukin-1α. J Dent Res 2002;81:11–16.

120. Koppang HS, Koppang R, Stølen SØ. Identification of common foreign material in postendodontic granulomas and cysts. J Dent Assoc S Afr 1992;47:210–16.

121. Simon JHS, Chimenti Z, Mintz G. Clinical significance of the pulse granuloma. J Endod 1982;8:116–19.

122. American Association of Endodontists. Glossary of endodontic terms. Chicago: American Association of Endodontists; 2003. pp. 1–26.

123. Boulger EP. The foreign body reaction of rat tissue and human tissue to gutta-percha. J Am Dent Assoc 1933;20:1473–81.

124. Spångberg L. Biological effects of root canal filing materials. Experimental investigation of the toxicity of root canal filling materials in vitro and in vivo. Odontol Revy 1969;20:1–32.

125. Wolfson EM, Seltzer S. Reaction of rat connective tissue to some formulations. J Endod 1975;1:395–402.

126. Seltzer S, Bender IB, Turkenkopf S. Factors affecting successful repair after root canal treatment. J Am Dent Assoc 1963;67:651–62.

127. Strindberg LZ. The dependence of the results of pulp therapy on certain factors. An analytic study based on radiographic and clinical follow-up examinations. Acta Odontol Scand 1956;14:1–175.

128. Eley BM. Tissue reactions to implanted dental amalgam, including assessment by energy dispersive X-ray microanalysis. J Pathol 1982;138:251–72.

129. Goodmann SB, Vornasier VL, Kei J. The effects of bulk versus particulate polymethylmethacrylate on bone. Clin Orthop 1988;232:255–62.

130. Goodmann SB, Vornasier VL, Lee J, et al. The histological effects of implantation of different sizes of polyethylene particles in the rabbit tibia. J Biomed Mater Res 1990;24:517–24.

131. Stinson NE. Tissue reaction induced in guinea-pigs by particulate polymthylmethacrylate, polythene and nylon of the same size range. Br J Exp Pathol 1964;46:135–47.

132. Van Blitterswijk CA, Bakker D, Hessling SC, et al. Reactions of cells at implant surfaces. Biomaterials 1991;12:187–93.

133. Pascon EA, Spångberg LSW. In vitro cytotoxicity of root canal filling materials: 1. J Endod 1990;16:429–33.

134. Meryon SD, Jakeman KJ. The effects of in vitro of zinc released from dental restorative materials. Int Endod J 1985;18:191–8.

135. Browne RM, Friend LA. An investigation into the irritant properties of some root filling materials. Arch oral Biol 1968;13:1355–69.

136. Leonardo MR, Utrilla LS, Rothier A, et al. A comparison of subcutaneous connective tissue responses among three different formulations of used in thermatic techniques. Int Endod J 1990;23:211–17.

137. Johnston RB. Monocytes and macrophages. New Engl J Med 1988;318:747–52.

138. Murray DW, Rushton N. Macrophages stimulate bone resorption when they phagocyte particles. J Bone Joint Surg 1990;72-B:988–92.

139. Vaes G. Cellular biology and biochemical mechanisms of bone resorption: a review of recent developments on the formation, activation, and mode of action of osteoclasts. Clin Orthop 1988;231:239–71.

140. Williams JD, Czop JK, Austen KF. Release of leukotrienes by human monocytes on stimulation of their phagocytic receptor for particulate activators. J Immunol 1984;132:3034–40.

141. Dunlap CL, Barker BF. Giant cell hyalin angiopathy. Oral Surg Oral Med Oral Pathol Oral Radiol Endod 1977;44:587–91.

142. King OH. "Giant cell hyaline angiopathy": Pulse granuloma by another name? Presented at the 32nd Annual Meeting of the American Academy of Oral Pathologists, Fort Lauderdale; 1978.

143. Harrison JD, Martin IC. Oral vegetable granuloma: ultrastructural and histological study. J Oral Pathol 1986;23:346–50.

144. Brown AMS, Theaker JM. Food induced granuloma—an unusual cause of a submandibular mass with observations on the pathogenesis of hyalin bodies. Br J Maxillofac Surg 1987;25:433–6.

145. Head MA. Foreign body reaction to inhalation of lentil soup: giant cell pneumonia. J Clin Pathol 1956;9:295–9.

146. Sherman FE, Moran TJ. Granulomas of stomach. Response to injury of muscle and fibrous tissue of wall of human stomach. Am J Clin Pathol 1954;24:415–21.

147. Knoblich R. Pulmonary granulomatosis caused by vegetable particles. So-called lentil pulse granuloma. Am Rev Respir Dis 1969;99:380–9.

148. Talacko AA, Radden BG. The pathogenesis of oral pulse granuloma: an animal model. J Oral Pathol 1988;17:99–105.

149. Talacko AA, Radden BG. Oral pulse granuloma: clinical and histopathological features. Int J Oral Maxillofac Surg 1988;17:343–6.

150. Mincer HH, McCoy JM, Turner JE. Pulse granuloma of the alveolar ridge. Oral Surg Oral Med Oral Pathol Oral Radiol Endod 1979;48:126–30.

151. Koppang HS, Koppang R, Solheim T, et al. Cellulose fibers from endodontic paper points as an etiologic factor in post-endodontic periapical granulomas and cysts. J Endod 1989;15:369–72.

152. Koppang HS, Koppang R, Solheim T, et al. Identification of cellulose fibers in oral biopsies. Scand J Dent Res 1987;95:165–73.

153. Sedgley CM, Messer H. Long-term retention of a paper-point in the periapical tissues: a case report. Endod Dent Traumatol 1993;9:120–3.

154. White EW. Paper point in mental foramen. Oral Surg Oral Med Oral Pathol Oral Radiol Endod 1968;25:630–2.

155. Penick EC. Periapical repair by dense fibrous connective tissue following conservative endodontic therapy. Oral Surg Oral Med Oral Pathol Oral Radiol Endod 1961;14:239–42.

156. Karring T, Nyman S, Lindhe J. Healing following implantation of periodontitis affected roots into bone tissue. J Clin Periodontol 1980;7:96–105.

157. Karring T, Nyman S, Gottlow J, et al. Development of the biological concept of guided tissue regeneration—animal and human studies. Periodontology 2000 1993;1:26–35.

158. Nyman S, Lindhe J, Karring T, et al. New attachment following surgical treatment of human periodontal disease. J Clin Periodontol 1982;9:290–6.

159. Schroeder HE. The periodontium, Vol. V/5, handbook of micrscopic anatomy. Berlin: Springer-Verlag; 1986.

160. Nair PNR. Pathogenesis of apical periodontitis and the causes of endodontic failures. Crit Rev Oral Biol Med 2004;15:348–81.

161. Nair PNR. On the causes of persistent apical periodontitis: a review. Int Endod J 2006;39:249–81.

162. Kim S. Endodontic microsurgery. In: Cohen S and Burns RC, editors. Pathways of the pulp. Philadelphia: Mosby; 2002. pp. 683–725.

163. Nair PNR. Non-microbial etiology: foreign body reaction maintaining post-treatment apical periodontitis. Endod Topics 2003;6:96–113.

164. Sommer RF, Ostrander F, Crowley M. Clinical endodontics. 3rd ed. Philadelphia: W.B. Saunders Co.; 1966. pp. 409–11.

165. Block RM, Bushell A, Rodrigues H, et al. A histopathologic, histobacteriologic, and radiographic study of periapical endodontic surgical specimens. Oral Surg Oral Med Oral Pathol Oral Radiol Endod 1976;42:656–78.

166. Winstock D. Apical disease: an analysis of diagnosis and management with special reference to root lesion resection and pathology. Ann R Coll Surg Engl 1980;62:171–9.

167. Patterson SS, Shafer WG, Healey HJ. Periapical lesions associated with endodontically treated teeth. J Am Dent Assoc 1964;68:191–4.

168. Stockdale CR, Chandler NP. The nature of the periapical lesion—a review of 1108 cases. J Dent 1988;16:123–9.

169. Lin LM, Pascon EA, Skribner J, et al. Clinical, radiographic, and histologic study of endodontic treatment failures. Oral Surg Oral Med Oral Pathol Oral Radiol Endod 1991;71:603–11.

170. Nobuhara WK, Del Rio CE. Incidence of periradicular pathoses in endodontic treatment failures. J Endod 1993;19:315–18.

171. Spatafore CM, Griffin JA, Keyes GG, et al. Periapical biopsy report: an analysis over a 10-year period. J Endod 1990;16:239–41.

CHAPTER 9

INFLAMMATION AND IMMUNOLOGICAL RESPONSES

ASHRAF F. FOUAD, GEORGE T.-J. HUANG

Endodontic pathosis is primarily caused by infectious agents that mediate a series of inflammatory and immunological responses in the dental pulp and periradicular tissues. This chapter will describe some of the fundamental immune reactions that take place in these tissues, as well as other tissues, and will outline the basic mechanisms involved in disease initiation and progression.

The science of immunology is constantly changing and remarkable discoveries are being made about the unique molecules, cells, tissues, and pathways of reactions that take place in response to an external and autogenic stimulation. While an attempt has been made to address most of the critical and well-understood immunological data, it is impossible to address all aspects in this chapter. Immunological reactions that are either not well described in, or not relevant to the dental pulp and periradicular tissues, or simply exceed the scope of this textbook include neoplastic changes, autoimmune reactions, and some congenital and postnatal abnormalities in gene expression. Indeed, the reason why neoplastic changes are not common in the dental pulp may be of fundamental importance in understanding the pathogenesis of neoplasia in general and may have relevance in the growing field of regenerative endodontics, particularly in gene therapy. Therefore, these topics will not be addressed in this chapter, and the reader is referred to specialized textbooks or journals for more information on these topics.

The reactions and mechanisms that will be covered here are those that primarily deal with the inflammatory response and that have been described to some degree in pulpal and periradicular tissues or are widely recognized in other tissues and presumed to be in operation in endodontic tissues. In fact, wherever relevant, specific literature that addresses these questions will be cited in the text. The reader is also referred to Chapters 12 and 13 for more specific information on pulpal and periradicular inflammation and infection.

The material described in this chapter will be presented under discrete topics, for example, the individual cells and molecular mediators encountered in immunological reactions. However, the reader should always be cognizant of two fundamental concepts in immunology. The first is that there are many interrelationships between the pathways and mechanisms that will be presented, and many overlap among the functions of the cells to be described. This creates a large amount of redundancy that assures a competent and robust response. Indeed, it is commonly stated that the main purpose of treatment of various disease processes is to remove the source of irritation and provide a suitable environment for the body to heal itself, through its effective healing mechanisms. The second concept is that there is a substantial degree of variability among individuals in their response to a particular irritant. While some of this difference in response is quite extreme, and is explained by various hypersensitivity reactions, most of the variation is more subtle and is mediated by systemic conditions and diseases, or individual genetic polymorphism of different patients.

The concept of genetic polymorphism commonly refers to differences in the expression of certain inflammatory mediators or cellular activation or other immunological reactions. This variation may indeed render certain individuals more prone to a more dramatic expression of the disease process or delay in healing mechanisms. Genetic polymorphism may be explained by minor, perhaps a single nucleotide variation in the genetic make up of particular genes. Thus it is commonly referred to as single nucleotide polymorphism or SNP. SNPs have been described with respect to the expression of a number of proteins, such as interleukin-1 (IL-1), and may explain why some inflammatory reactions to seemingly similar irritants have different clinical presentations and responses to treatment in different patients.

The immune system represents a complex system of cells, tissues, organs as well as molecular mediators that act in synchrony to assure the maintenance of health and defense against disease. Cells interact with microbial irritants as well as with each other via a large number of molecular mediators and cell surface receptors that together result in various phenotypic reactions. Various host reactions will be discussed in the context of a description of the main cells of the immune response, as these cells play a critical role in mobilizing the immune response. It is appropriate initially to present the ontogeny of immune cells from hematopoietic stem cells (Figure 1).[1] A description of the mature inflammatory cells and their activities will follow, starting with the innate immune system.

Innate and Adaptive Immune Systems

The innate immune system is composed of a number of natural barriers, as well as cellular and molecular elements that represent the initial nonspecific reactions of the immune response. The barriers are epithelial, ectodermal, or ectomesenchymal in origin. Examples include the skin, oral mucosa, junctional and sulcular epithelium, as well as intact enamel and dentin. These barriers prevent the dissemination of bacteria and bacterial products into the subjacent connective tissue, which would result in a disease. Dental caries, fractures of teeth, or congenital anomalies that expose the dental pulp create a break in this barrier, resulting in the inflammation of the pulp and ultimate necrosis. Once the pulp is necrotic and the pulp space is occupied by microorganisms, there is no natural barrier to the dissemination of these irritants into the periradicular region and/or systemically through the apical, lateral, or accessory foramina. In fact, junctional complexes between odontoblasts in the vital pulp have been shown to play a role in preventing the leakage of bacterial irritants into the pulp.[2,3]

Phagocytosis is another important component of innate immunity. Likewise, the presence of certain nonspecific proteins such as lysozyme or complement—or pattern recognition receptors (PRR) such as Toll-like receptors (TLRs) (see later)—on the surface of immune cells are also constituents of the innate immune system. Inflammation is associated with a number of vascular changes such as vasodilatation, increased capillary permeability and extravasation of blood cells and inflammatory mediators, together with reduced pain threshold. Many of these nonspecific changes are caused by neurogenic elements, such as neuropeptides. These concepts will be addressed later in the chapter. Therefore, innate immunity does not involve sensitization or priming, has uniform response to all irritants that are detected, lacks memory and aims at rapidly eliminating irritants.

CELLS OF INNATE IMMUNITY

Neutrophils, also known as polymorphonuclear leukocytes or PMNs, are the most numerous white blood cells, representing about 54% to 63% of peripheral blood leukocytes. They have a short half-life, generally circulating for about 6 hours, and if not recruited to a site of inflammation, they undergo apoptosis.

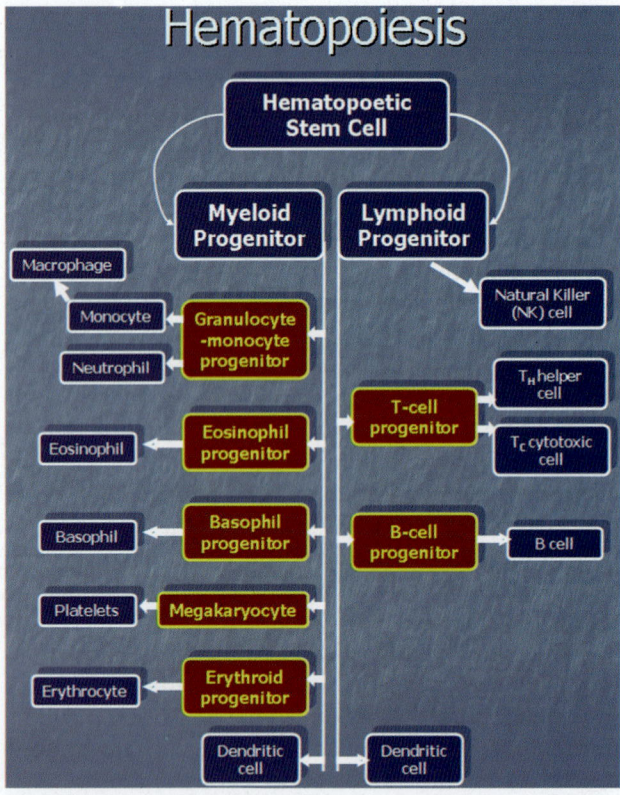

Figure 1 Hematopoiesis of immune cells. Note that dendritic cells may develop from both myeloid and lymphoid progenitor cells. Courtesy of Dr. Fouad.

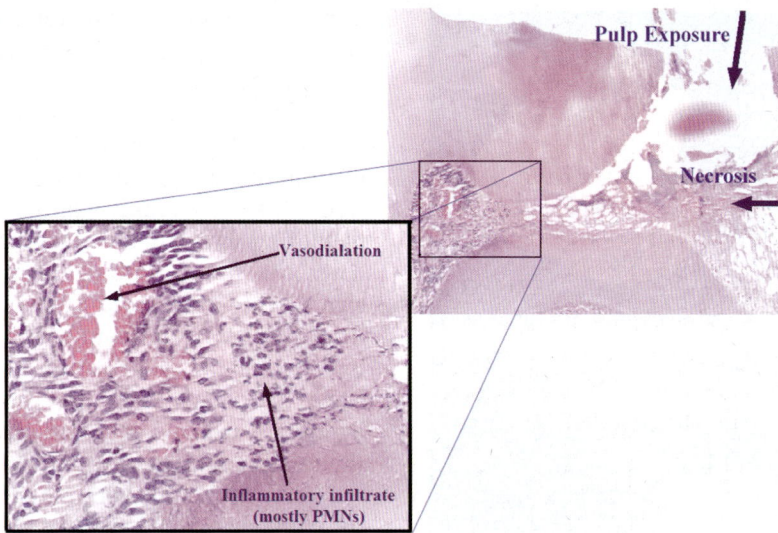

Figure 2 Experimental pulp exposure in a rodent molar, showing pulp necrosis, acute and chronic inflammation, and vasodilatation. Courtesy of Dr. Fouad.

PMNs represent the first defense line against microbial irritants, being mobilized in what is traditionally known as acute inflammation (Figure 2). PMNs utilize a large number of defense mechanisms to eliminate the invading pathogens and to inactivate their toxins. These include the production of lysosomal enzymes, cytokines, oxygen-derived free radicals, as well as phagocytosis.

Within PMNs, defense proteins are contained within two different types of granules: The first type is azurophil (large) granules (about 0.5 µm in diameter) that contain lysozyme, myeloperoxidase, defensins, acid hydrolases, and neutral hydrolases such as collagenases, elastase, cathepsin G, and other proteinases. The second type is specific (small) granules (about 0.2 µm in diameter) that contain lactoferrin, lysozyme, collagenases, plasminogen activator, histaminase, alkaline phosphatase, and membrane-bound cytochrome b_{558}. The cell also has abundant glycogen stores that enable the cell to utilize glycolysis to produce energy in anaerobic conditions,[4] such as during an abscess formation.

Monocytes are circulating leukocytes that represent 4% to 8% of blood leukocytes. *Macrophages* reside within connective tissues. Certain macrophages become especially adapted for immunological functions in certain tissues. These cells are collectively referred to as members of the mononuclear phagocyte system. Examples of these cells are Kupfer cells in the liver, microglia in the central nervous system, or alveolar macrophages in the lungs. It is generally accepted now that both macrophages and osteoclasts have a common lineage. Likewise a number of other cells commonly seen in inflammatory reaction or granulomatous disease, such as foam cells, epitheloid cells, or giant cells, may have a common lineage.

Macrophages have a relatively long half-life in tissues, commonly measured in months. They are considered among the principal inflammatory cells, commonly mobilized in areas of chronic inflammation. They possess major histocompatibility complex (MHC)-II receptor, have antigen-presenting capabilities, and are involved in phagocytosis. They are also among the principal producers of proinflammatory cytokines such as IL-1, IL-6, tumor necrosis factor-α (TNF-α), and IL-12.

Macrophages may be activated by activated Th1 cells of the specific arm of the immune response, or nonspecifically, such as by natural killer (NK) cells (Figure 3). They express surface receptors to a variety of pathogen-associated molecular patterns such as lipopolysaccharide (LPS) of gram-negative bacteria or peptidoglycan (PG) and lipoteichoic acid (LTA) of gram-positive bacteria. These receptors have intracytoplasmic component (homologous with the IL-1 receptor molecule) that transmits the signal through adapter molecules such as MyD88 and Trif to transcription factors such as NF-κB, IRF3, IRF5, and others. Eventually, these transcription factors are translocated into the nucleus to activate gene transcription followed by mRNA translation to produce certain proinflammatory proteins, such as cytokines IL-1, IL-6, and TNF-α. Molecules such as LPS are very potent biological toxins, capable of causing septic shock and killing the host. Therefore, in addition

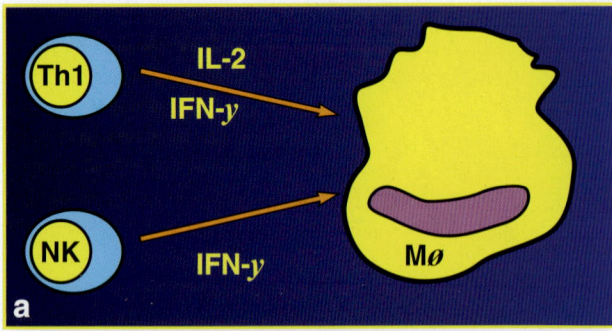
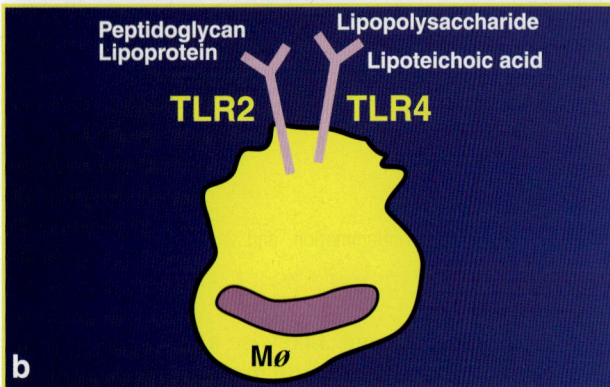
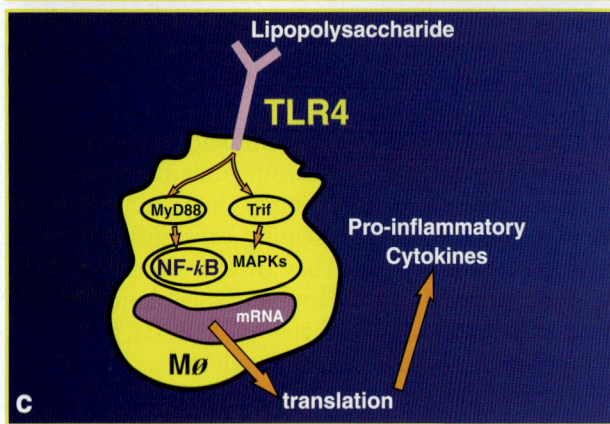

Figure 3 Macrophage activation and function. *A*, Cell is activated by cytokines from specific and nonspecific immune cells. *B*, Cell expresses various pattern recognition receptors to microbial molecules. *C*, Signal transduction through MyD88, Trif, or other intermediaries, transcription through nuclear factor kappa B, and mitogen-activated protein kinases that result in the translation of mRNA and the production of proinflammatory cytokines. Courtesy of Dr. Fouad.

component, and thus is not capable of initiating the signal transduction pathway to initiate the production of cytokines.

The PMNs and macrophages are the main cells involved in phagocytosis. The surface of phagocytes can bind to the pathogen surface pattern molecules by lectin, through complement C3b or C5b, or by binding to the Fc portion of an opsonizing antibody (Figure 4). After the initial binding of the pathogen, which is significantly enhanced by opsonins, pseudopodia develop to surround and engulf the pathogenic organism, leading to the formation of a phagosome. The final stage of phagocytosis involves lysosomal enzymes, which are released into the phagosome for degrading the microorganism or other foreign particles.

Microbial killing within the phagosome is effected through a series of oxidative reactions that require glycolysis, glycogenolysis, and the generation of reactive oxidative free radicals[5] (Figure 5). The fusion of the membranes of a phagosome and the cell's lysosomal granules (such as the azurophilic granules of PMNs) results in an oxidative burst mediated by cytoplasmic- and membrane-bound oxidases. Through the action of nicotinamide adenine dinucleotide phosphate (NADPH) oxidase, superoxide ions and hydroxyl radicals are generated (see Figure 5). While these are sufficiently antimicrobial, lysosomes of PMNs contain myeloperoxidase, which through a halide intermediate can result in the generation of hypochlorous radicals (HOCl•). As is the case with exposure to sodium hypochlorite (NaOCl), HOCl• is a powerful oxidant and antimicrobial agent that kills bacteria by halogenation, or by protein or lipid

to the membrane-bound TLRs, a number of circulating molecules such as CD14 are available that can bind to LPS in the blood rendering it less biologically active. This reaction is mediated by a plasma protein called LPS-binding protein (LBP). CD14 is also available in a membrane-bound form to the surface of macrophages and can bind LBP in this location; however, unlike TLRs, CD14 has no intracytoplasmic

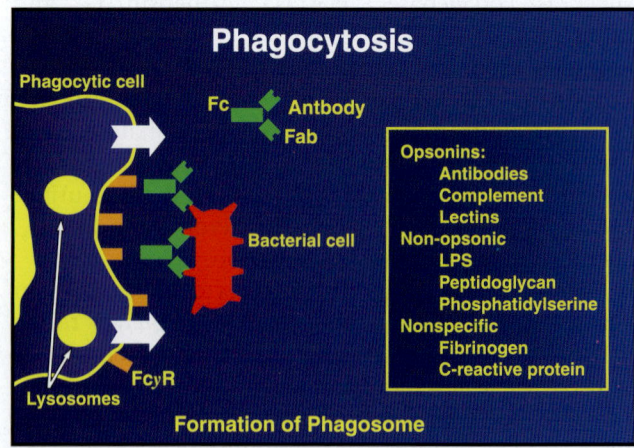

Figure 4 Phagocytic cell recognizes an opsonized bacterial cell and starts to form a phagosome (white arrows) to engulf it. Eventually, lysosomal enzymes open into the phagosome to digest the material. Courtesy of Dr. Fouad.

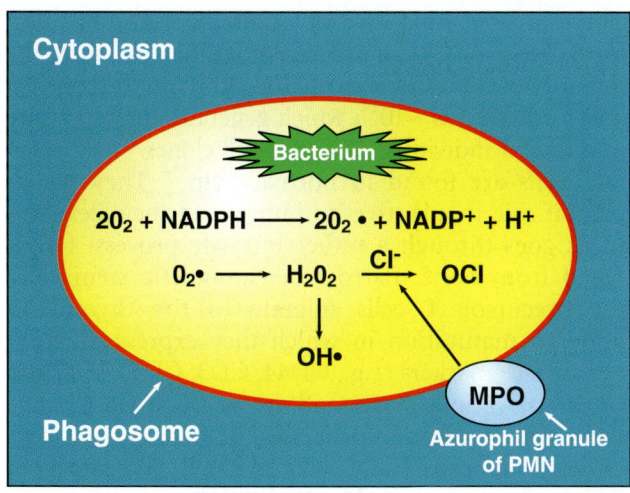

Figure 5 Oxidative burst reactions within a phagosome that result in the destruction of a pathogen. MPO, myeloperoxidase; NADPH, reduced nicotinamide adenine dinucleotide phosphate; $O_2\bullet^-$, superoxide radical; $OH\bullet$, hydroxyl radical; $OCl\bullet$, hypochlorous radical. Courtesy of Dr. Fouad.

peroxidation. Within the phagosome, other mechanisms of bacterial killing include lysozyme, which causes the degradation of bacterial coat oligosaccharides, and defensins, which are peptides that kill bacteria by forming holes through their membranes.[5]

While phagocytosis is quite effective in eliminating microbial irritants, when they are isolated or individualized, it frequently cannot deal with a microbial biofilm. A microbial biofilm has a large number of microorganisms embedded in a polysaccharide matrix. An example of this that is relevant to endodontics is a periapical infection with *Actinomyces* spp, which is generally thought to occur in the form of microbial colonies within the lesions. Inflammatory cells usually surround these colonies and attempt to eliminate them by forming phagosomes, but instead result in the release of oxygen radicals and lysosomal enzymes into the periradicular tissues, causing tissue degradation. This is referred to sometimes as "frustrated phagocytosis."

Like neutrophils, *eosinophils* are segmented leukocytes; however, they stain red with hematoxylin and eosin stains (thus the name). They are much less prevalent than PMNs, constituting only about 1 to 3% of circulating leukocytes. They are involved in allergic and some parasitic reactions. Their actions are primarily mediated by a low-affinity surface receptor for the Fc portion of the IgE molecule called FcεRII. Eosinophils express a number of inflammatory and healing mediators, most notably transforming growth factors (TGFs)-α and -β1.[6–8] Eosinophils in human periapical cysts were shown to express

Table 1 Comparison of Mast Cells and Basophils

	Mast Cells	Basophils
Size: (μm)	10–15	5–7
Location	Connective tissue	Blood
Life span	Weeks or months	Days
Terminally differentiated	No	Yes
Granule content	Histamine, heparin, PAF	Histamine, heparin, PAF
High-affinity FcεRII	Yes	Yes

PAF, Platelet-activating factor.

TGF-α, and those in both cysts and granulomas also had TGF-β1, at the mRNA and protein levels.[9]

Basophils share some similarities in shape, size, and life span with neutrophils and eosinophils; however, they are more intimately involved in the mediation of allergic reactions. In this regard, they share some features with connective tissue mast cells (Table 1).

As noted in Table 1, *mast cells* reside in connective tissues for weeks to months. They are generally dormant with little activity until they are stimulated by IgE activity in type 1 hypersensitivity reactions (see below). Complement activation also results in the production of C3a and C5a, which are both described as anaphylatoxins as they initiate the acute responses effected by mast cell degranulation. Mast cell degranulation results in local (atopic) or systemic (anaphylactic) reactions. The primary outcomes of these reactions are vasodilation and bronchoconstriction. Anaphylactic reactions can be life threatening because of the resulting apnea and reduction in peripheral circulatory tone that dramatically reduces the blood pressure. These reactions are mediated by the release of granule contents, namely histamine, arachidonic acid metabolites (especially prostaglandins: PGE2 and PGI1, and leukotrienes: LTB4 and LTD4), platelet-activating factor (PAF), eosinophil chemotactic factor A, and a number of other enzymes that cause tissue damage.

Dendritic cells (DCs) are stellate-shaped and reside in a variety of tissues including blood, lymph, epidermis, dermis, and secondary lymphoid organs.[10] They are also present in the dental pulp, where they are prevalent among the odontoblastic cell layer and around blood vessels,[11,12] and in periodontal ligament[13] and periradicular lesions.[13,14] DCs lack an Fc receptor, lack long-term adherence to immune cells or molecules, and are not involved in phagocytosis. Like other antigen-presenting cells (APCs), namely macrophages, Langerhans cells (a subset of DCs present in the epidermis),

B cells, and endothelial cells, they express MHC-II. They have a variety of phenotypes, as determined by their morphology, surface markers, and the tissue where they reside. Circulating blood DCs have two different origins: myeloid (DC1) and plasmacytoid/lymphoid (DC2). The former is characterized by the CD11c+ marker, while the latter has the $CD123^+$ marker that may have several subsets.[10] Myeloid $CD11C^+$ DCs, like macrophages, express a large number of TLRs to both bacterial and viral molecules. In contrast, $CD123^+$ plasmacytoid DCs do not express TLR-2 and -4 and thus do not respond to bacterial molecules.[15]

NK cells are lymphocytes that do not require activation like CD4 or CD8 lymphocytes. Therefore, they are members of the innate immune response. They represent about 4% to 20% of circulating mononuclear cells. They produce interferon-γ (IFN-γ) and are thus capable of activating macrophages to produce proinflammatory cytokines, without the need for activated T-lymphocytes. NK cells are particularly effective in killing host cells infected with viruses or other intracellular microorganisms.

Odontoblasts are traditionally considered as merely dentin-producing cells originated from ectomesenchymal cells. However, due to their unique anatomic location, they are the first line of cells encountering foreign antigens after enamel and dentin breakdown, in which situation they are similar to epithelial cells. Epithelial cells have been considered as an integrate part of innate immunity for being capable of producing proinflammatory cytokines and expressing antimicrobial peptides β-defensins.[16,17] Similarly, human odontoblasts have also been observed to express chemokines such as IL-8 and the antimicrobial peptides, defensins.[18–20] Furthermore, odontoblasts express TLRs[21,22] suggesting that odontoblasts play a significant role in the pulp innate immunity.

Cells of Adaptive Immunity

The adaptive immunity involves the development of specific receptor molecules made by lymphocytes that recognize and bind to foreign or self antigens. These specific receptor molecules on T cells are called T-cell antigen receptors (TCRs) and on B cells are B-cell antigen receptor (BCRs) or immunoglobulins. TCRs on T cells interact with antigens presented by MHC molecules along with other accessory molecules, whereas BCRs on B cells or as secreted form, generally known as antibodies, interact with antigens directly. The variable region of both TCR and BCR is rearranged at the genomic level via V(D)J segment recombination. The estimated total diversity after this recombination for TCR is $\sim 10^{18}$ (for αβ receptors that make up the majority of the TCR; the other minority is γδ receptor) and for BCR it is $\sim 10^{14}$, which generates the repertoire of different individual T- and B-cell clones.[23]

T cells are found in normal pulp.[24] They play a pivotal role in adaptive immunity and their development goes through a rather intricate process. Originated from bone marrow hematopoietic stem cells, the precursor T cells migrate to the thymus to undergo maturation in which they express different cell surface markers (e.g., CD44, CD3, CD4, CD8, and CD25) at various stages and are screened via positive and negative selection processes. About 97% of T cells undergo apoptosis and only a small percentage of these cells are exported to the periphery as mature T cells. During the positive selection, double-positive $CD4^+CD8^+$ T cells bearing TCRs that can interact with self peptide:self MHC complex on thymic epithelial cells are rescued from apoptosis. In the negative selection, these $CD4^+CD8^+$ T cells recognizing self peptide:self MHC complex too well are deleted via apoptosis. The positive selection ensures that mature T cells can recognize foreign antigen in the context of self MHC molecules that present the antigen, whereas the negative selection eliminates potentially self-reactive T-cell clones. Before exiting the thymus, these cells become single-positive either $CD4^+$ or $CD8^+$ along with other surface markers such as CD25. These naïve T cells then circulate back and forth between the lymphatic system and blood until they encounter foreign antigens presented by APCs.[23]

The interactions between TCR and antigen peptide:MHC and between costimulators CD28 and B7 activate signal transduction pathways in T cells leading to the synthesis of T-cell growth factor IL-2 and its receptor and T-cell clonal expansion/proliferation. Subsequently, T cells differentiate into armed effector T cells and some become memory cells. There are a number of T cell subpopulations categorized by their functions and some can be distinguished by their cell surface markers, cytokine profiles, or transcriptional factors. To date, there are four main subpopulations of T cells: T helper cells, T regulatory cells (Treg), T suppressor and T cytotoxic (cytolytic) cells.

Naïve CD4 T cells upon antigen stimulation proliferate and differentiate into Th0, which subsequently commit into Th1 or Th2 cells. Monocytoid DC (DC1) induces T helper (Th) 1-type responses and plasmacytoid DC (DC2) selectively induces Th2 responses. Each subset has distinct functions and cytokine profiles as shown in Table 2. A Th1-specific T box transcription factor, T-bet, suppresses early Th2 cytokine production

Table 2 Subpopulations of T cells

Subtype	Main CD	Key Cytokine Profile	Transcriptional Factors*	Main Function
Th0	CD4	–		Challenged Naive T cells
Th1	CD4	IFN-γ, IL-2	T-bet	Pro-inflammatory
Th2	CD4	IL-4, -5, -10, -13	GATA-3	Anti-inflammatory
Th17	CD4	IL-17	–	Pro-inflammatory
Tr	CD4, CD25	IL-10	Foxp3	Anti-inflammatory
Tr-1	CD4, CD25	TGF, IL-10	–	Anti-inflammatory
Th3	CD4, CD25	TGF	–	Anti-inflammatory
Ts	CD8		–	Anti-inflammatory
Tc	CD8		–	Kill virus-infected cells

*Transcriptional factors identified as important markers for the respective T cell subsets.

and induces Th1 T-cell development via upregulation of *IFN-γ* gene transcription and IL-12Rb2 chain expression. The differentiation of Th2 is dependent on the induction of transcription factors STAT6, c-maf, and GATA-3.[25] Th1 cells mainly produce IL-2 and IFN-γ, activate macrophages, and induce B cells to produce opsonizing antibody. Th2 cells produce IL-4, -5, -10 and -13; activate B cells to make neutralizing antibody; and have various effects on macrophages. Overall, Th1 and Th2 have mutually modulatory effect.[25]

Th17 cells are recently recognized Th cells that are closely associated with Th1 in diseased tissues and may be directly derived from naïve CD4+ T cells.[26–28] Th17 produces IL-17 and its development can be induced by IL-23, which also stimulates Th1 production of IL-17—a cytokine that is linked to autoimmune and inflammatory diseases including rheumatoid arthritis and lupus.

Treg have the cell surface markers CD4 and CD25 and therefore are generally named CD4+CD25+ Treg. They play an essential role in mediating immunosuppression and maintenance of tolerance. Those T-cell clones that may react to self antigens but are not deleted via negative selection in the thymus are considered to be suppressed by Treg cells in the periphery. Therefore, dysregulation of Treg function may illicit autoimmune diseases. There are subtypes of Treg cells based on their origin and the mechanisms of action and function.

Treg cells or naturally occurring Tr arise either in the thymus and reside in the blood and peripheral lymphoid tissues or in the periphery induced by antigen. Human Tr potently suppress the proliferation and effector functions in a cell contact-dependent manner or by acting on APCs.[29,30] The transcriptional factor FoxP3 is important to their development and a marker. Human Tr can be further divided into two subsets with distinct functions based on differential expression of integrins. α4β7 integrin-expressing Tr cells induce de novo differentiation of IL-10-producing Tr1 cells. α4β1-expressing Tr cells induce the differentiation of TGF-β-producing Th3 cells.

Tr1 cells (CD4+ type-1 Treg) arise in the periphery upon encountering an antigen presented by tolerogenic DCs which process requires IL-10. Tr1 cells produce high levels of IL-10 themselves and mediate IL-10-dependent suppression of T-cell response. In contrast, Tr cells do not produce IL-10. Defining Tr1 phenotype currently is solely based on cytokine production—IL-10, but not IL-4 and they express variable CD25. Tr1 cells regulate the response of naïve and memory T cells in vitro and in vivo and can suppress both Th1 and Th2 cell-mediated pathologies. Tr1-cell clones suppress the production of immunoglobulin by B cells. The major function of Tr1 cells is to control homeostasis of the response to foreign antigens in the periphery.[30]

Although *Th3 cells* are named under T helper cells, they are grouped with Tr cells due to their close functionality to Tr-1 cells. They are CD4+ T cells that produce TGF-β. Similar to Tr1 cells, these T cells are generated in the periphery induced by oral antigen in the mesenteric lymph nodes. They express variable CD25 and produce TGF-β and varying amounts of IL-4 and IL-10. They also inhibit Th1- and Th2-mediated adaptive immune responses. It is speculated that Tr1 and Th3 cells derive from the same population and perhaps represent adaptive Tregs, as they have a similar phenotype and usually mediate their suppressive activities via the release of IL-10 and/or TGF-β[31,32] (Figure 6).

There is a controversy regarding the recognition of *T suppressor (CD8+ T suppressor cells or Ts)* as a distinct subset of CD8+ T cells. There is also a disputable hypothesis that CD8+ Ts cells are merely cytotoxic T lymphocytes (CD8+ CTLs) based on the finding that

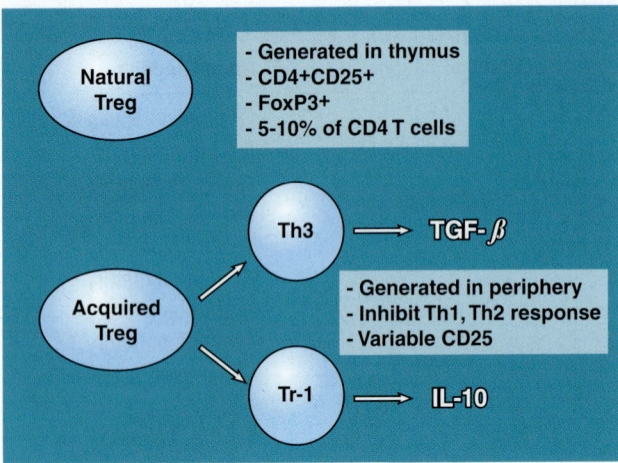

Figure 6 Regulatory T lymphocytes. Redrawn from van Oosterhout and Bloksma, Eur Respir J 2005;26:918–32. Courtesy of Dr. Huang.

both CD8$^+$ Ts and CTL play roles in immunosuppressive activities and maintenance of tolerance. Evidence has suggested that CD8$^+$ Ts and CD8$^+$ CTLs represent distinct subpopulations of CD8$^+$ T cells. Human CD8$^+$CD28$^-$ T cells have also considered another subtype of Ts cells. These cells are MHC class I-restricted CD8$^+$CD28$^-$ Ts cells that act on APCs by a contact-dependent manner, rendering them tolerogenic to Th cells. They inhibit the proliferation of Th by blocking the activation of APC and preventing the upregulation of costimulatory molecules required for efficient help. CD8$^+$CD28$^-$ Tregs can block the upregulation of costimulatory molecules on APCs such as CD80, CD86, CD54, and CD58. Suppressor function could not be abrogated using neutralizing antibodies against IL-4, IL-10, TGF-β, and CTLA-4. In contrast to the suppression of costimulatory molecules, CD8$^+$CD28$^+$ Treg have been demonstrated to upregulate the inhibitory immunoglobulin-like transcript 3 (ILT3) and ILT4 receptors on DCs. Taken together, these results suggest that CD8$^+$CD28$^-$ Tregs suppress immune responses by directly interacting with DCs and rendering these cells tolerogenic.[33]

T cytotoxic cells (CD8$^+$ T cytotoxic cells or Tc), also known as cytolytic T lymphocytes (CTLs), are a subset of T cells that kill target cells expressing MHC-associated peptide antigens, such as virus infected cells. The majority of Tc express CD8 and recognize antigens degraded in the cytosol and expressed on the class I MHC molecules of the target cells. Tc develop from "pre-Tc" that lack cytolytic functions. Two separate kinds of signals are needed for pre-Tc to differentiate to functional Tc. One is specific recognition of antigen on a target cell and the other may be provided either by costimulators expressed on professional APCs or by cytokines produced by Th cells. Functional Tc acquire specific membrane-bound cytoplasmic granules including a membrane pore-forming protein called perforin or cytolysin and enzymes called granzymes. Tc also express FasL that can deliver apoptosis-inducing signals to target cells expressing Fas protein. The killing of target cells require cell contact and is antigen-specific, that is, killing of the target cells bearing the same class I MHC-associated antigen that triggered the pre-Tc differentiation.[23]

B cells are rarely found in normal pulps.[24] Their role in adaptive immunity mainly lies in the production of antibodies that constitute the host humoral immune response. The rise and the development of B cells take place in bone marrow where the progenitor B cells rearrange their immunoglobulin (Ig) genes and turn into immature B cells with assembled antigen receptors (BCRs) in the form of cell surface IgM. The commitment to B-cell lineage occurs prior to Ig gene rearrangement. This commitment is controlled by the expression of Pax5 transcriptional factor. The bone marrow stromal cells interact with progenitor B cells and provide signals and growth factors (e.g., IL-7) important for B-cell development.

The productive and sequential rearrangement of heavy- and light-chain gene dictates the survival of B cells—positive selection. Those cells that failed to rearrange their Ig gene segments to form functional heavy- and light-chain pairs will be lost. The V(D)J gene recombination occurs in both heavy and light (κ and λ) chains. A recombinase system, which is an enzymatic complex consisting of several enzymes including recombination-activating genes 1 and 2 (RAG-1, RAG-2), terminal deoxynucleotidyl transferase (TdT), DNA ligase IV, Ku proteins, and XRCC4, is essential to the recombination process. This recombinase system is also used for TCR recombination.[23]

Similar to T-cell selection, B cells also undergo negative selection. Developing B cells expressing BCRs that recognize self cell-surface molecules are deleted via apoptosis. Immature B cells that bind soluble self antigens are rendered unresponsive to the antigen—anergic. Only those B cells that do not interact with self antigens mature normally and enter the peripheral lymphoid tissues bearing both IgM and IgD on their surface. Mature IgM/IgD coexpressing B cells undergo isotype switching via a process called switch recombination after encountering antigen. The rearranged V(D)J gene segment recombines with a downstream C region gene (γ, ε, or α) and the intervening

DNA sequence is deleted. This gives rise to other classes of Ig, that is, IgG, IgE, and IgA besides IgM. In addition to isotype switching, activated B cells undergo somatic mutation in V region gene leading to affinity maturation of antibodies and alternative splicing of VDJ RNA to membrane or secreted Ig mRNA. A large quantity of antibody is secreted when B cells terminally differentiate into plasma cells.[23]

MHC AND ANTIGEN PRESENTATION

Multistep antigen-processing pathways within the APC are involved in the generation of cell-surface antigen:MHC complex. Distinct subcellular pathways take place to generate complexes of peptides with class I versus class II.

Class I MHC molecule consists of α (heavy) chain and β chain (β2 microglobulin that is located only extracellularly). Almost all cells express class I MHC that display peptide antigens presented to $CD8^+$ TCRs. Endogenously synthesized foreign proteins (e.g., viral proteins) or products of mutated genes in tumor cells are degraded into peptides by proteosomes in the cytosol and transported via transporter associated with antigen processing (TAP) peptide transporter into ER in which the peptides are bound onto assembled class I MHC. Subsequently, this peptide:MHC complex is transported onto the cell surface. $CD8^+$ T cells (mostly CTLs) recognize the peptide antigen associated with class I MHC.

The molecules involved in the interactions between peptide antigen:class I MHC complex and TCR include CD8, CD3/ζ, CD2, CD28 and LFA-1 (on T cells) and ICAM-1, LFA-3, and B7-1/B7–2 on APC (Figure 7).

Class II MHC molecules are composed of two noncovalently associated polypeptide chains—α and β chains, both of which have peptide-binding, immunoglobulin-like, transmembrane, and cytoplasmic domains. Unlike MHC class I, only restricted group of cells normally express class II MHC. They are APCs: (1) DCs, (2) macrophages, (3) B cells, (4) vascular endothelial cells, and (5) epithelial cells. The former three are considered professional APCs. The latter two nonprofessional APCs are induced by IFN-γ to express class II MHC.

DCs and macrophages phagocytose antigens while B cells utilize the membrane immunoglobulin to bind and internalize antigens. Other nonprofessional APCs endocytose antigens into cytoplasm for antigen processing. These internalized antigens are localized in endosomes in which the antigens are

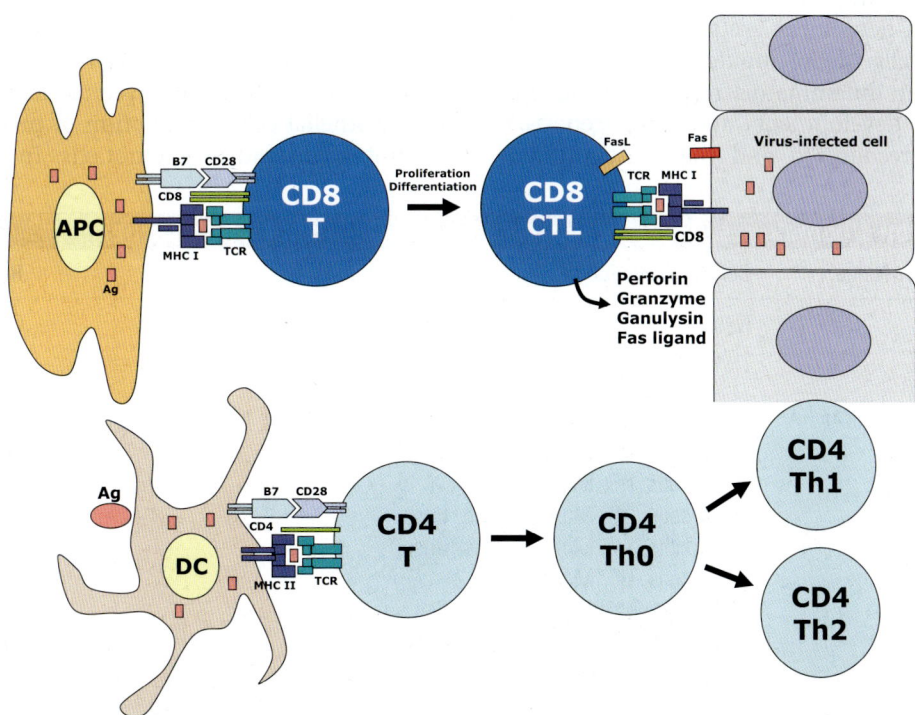

Figure 7 Cells and molecules involved in the interaction of antigen-presenting cells (APCs) and CD4/CD8 T lymphocytes. Courtesy of Dr. Huang.

degraded and then further processed in lysosomes. The processed antigens turn into small peptides, and many of them are 10–30 amino acid long and are capable of binding onto the newly synthesized class II MHC molecules within intracellular vesicles before this antigen:class II MHC complex is transported to the surface of cells and presented to TCRs of $CD4^+$ T cells (see Figure 7).

Molecular Mediators of the Proinflammatory Response

CHEMOKINES

Chemokines are a group of about 45 to 47 chemoattractant cytokines. There are two main types of chemokines:

1. *CC Chemokines.* Macrophage/monocyte chemoattractant proteins (MCP-1–4); macrophage inflammatory protein (MIP)-1α, MIP-1β, eotaxin, RANTES.
2. *CXC Chemokines.* IFN-inducible protein 10 (IP-10); monokine-inducible IFN-γ (MIG); interleukin-8 (IL-8/CXCL8). These chemokines have currently been renamed to include CXCL1–16; XCL1, 2; CX3CL1; and CCL1–28.

Table 3 lists different names of the commonly studied chemokines. Chemokines are primarily involved in trafficking of cells of the innate immune system toward the site of an inflammatory response or during lymphoid organ development and angiogenesis.[4] Among the first recognized and the most studied chemokines is IL-8 (CXCL8), which has also been most studied in endodontic pathosis.[18,19,34–37] There is some redundancy with respect to the cells that express chemokine receptors and receptor specificity for various chemokines (see Table 3).

ADHESION MOLECULES

There are a variety of adhesion molecule classes that are expressed at the site of an inflammatory process (Table 4). Adhesion molecules that serve a critical role with respect to halting the inflammatory cells that are circulating in the capillaries at high speed and that are then through the function of chemokines are directed to the site of inflammation. This process is achieved in steps: the cells initially slow down, they roll on the endothelial wall, and then start to bind to the endothelial cells. Eventually, they become extravasated through diapedesis and migrate to the area of inflammation. The slowing down of circulating leukocytes is mediated by selectins, then integrins, and Ig superfamily proteins mediate the binding of the cells to endothelial cells. The expression of these adhesion molecules is mediated by a number of inflammatory mediators, most notable IL-1 and TNF-α.

PLATELET-ACTIVATING FACTOR

PAF is a ubiquitous factor that is secreted by many different cells and plays a role in a number of immune mechanisms. It is secreted by platelets, basophils, monocytes/macrophages, PMNs, and endothelial cells. It is primarily involved in leukocyte adhesion to endothelial cells, production of prostaglandins and thromboxane and in chemotaxis. In low doses, PAF

Table 3 Common Chemokines, Their Receptors and the Cells that They Target[4,38,39]

Chemokine	Other Name	Cell for Chemotaxis	Receptor
CXCL8	IL-8	Neutro	CXCR1, CXCR2
CXCL9	Mig	T cells (T), NK cells (NK)	CXCR3-A, CXCR3-B
CXCL10	IP-10	T, NK cells	CXCR3-A, CXCR3-B
CCL2	MCP-1/MCAF	T, NK cells, dendritic cells (DC), monocytes (Mono), basophils (Baso)	CCR2
CCL3	MIP-1α	T, NK cells, DC, Mono, eosinophils (Eosino)	CCR1, CCR5
CCL4	MIP-1β	T, NK cells, DC, Mono	CCR5
CCL5	RANTES	T, NK cells, DC, Mono, Eosino, Baso	CCR1, CCR3, CCR5
CCL7	MCP-3	T, NK cells, DC, Mono, Eosino, Baso	CCR1, CCR2, CCR3
CCL8	MCP-2	T, NK cells, DC, Mono, Baso	CCR3
CCL11	Eotaxin-1	T, DC, Eosino, Baso	CCR3
CCL13	MCP-4	T, NK cells, DC, Mono, Eosino, Baso	CCR2, CCR3
CCL24	Eotaxin-2	T, DC, Eosino, Baso	CCR3
CCL26	Eotaxin-3	T	CCR3

DC, Dendritic cells; NK, natural killer.

Table 4	Important Adhesion Molecules, Their Tissue Distribution and Ligands[23]		
	Name	**Tissue Distribution**	**Ligand**
Selectins	P-selectin (PADGEM)	Activated endothelium and platelets,	PSGL-1, Sialyl-Lewis
Bind carbohydrates. Initiate leukocyte-endothelial interaction	E-selectin (PADGEM)	Activated endothelium	Sialyl-Lewis
Integrins	$\alpha_L : \beta_2$ (LFA-1, CD11a/CD18)	Monocytes, T cells, macrophages, neutrophils, dendritic cells	ICAMs
Bind to cell-adhesion molecules and extracellular matrix.	$\alpha_M : \beta_2$ (CR3, Mac-1, CD11b/CD18)	Neutrophils, monocytes, macrophages,	ICAM-1, iC3b, fibrinogen
Strong adhesion	$\alpha_X : \beta_2$ (CR4, p150.95, CD11c/CD18)	Dendritic cells, macrophages, neutrophils	iC3b
	$\alpha_5 : \beta_1$ (VLA-1, CD49d/CD29)	Monocytes, macrophages	Fibronectin
Immunoglobulin superfamily	ICAM-1 (CD54)	Activated endothelium	LFA-1, Mac-1
Various roles in cell adhesion. Ligand for integrins	ICAM-2 (CD102)	Resting endothelium, dendritic cells	LFA-1
	VCAM-1 (CD106)	Activated endothelium	VLA-4
	PECAM (CD31)	Activated leukocytes, endothelial cell–cell junctions	CD31

may cause vasodilatation; however, in regular doses, it is involved in vasoconstriction.

PLASMA PROTEASES

There are a large number of enzymatic changes that take place during an immune response and that aim to remove antigenic or foreign material, kill microbial cells, control hemorrhage, as well as initiate and promote the healing process that takes place following the elimination of irritants. These enzymatic processes are closely regulated so that the response is proportionate to the irritation; however, they frequently result in side effects causing break down of host tissues, which frequently accompanies an inflammatory response. The main pathways that are involved in these reactions will be described here. The principal mediators and interactions of these pathways are summarized in Figure 8.

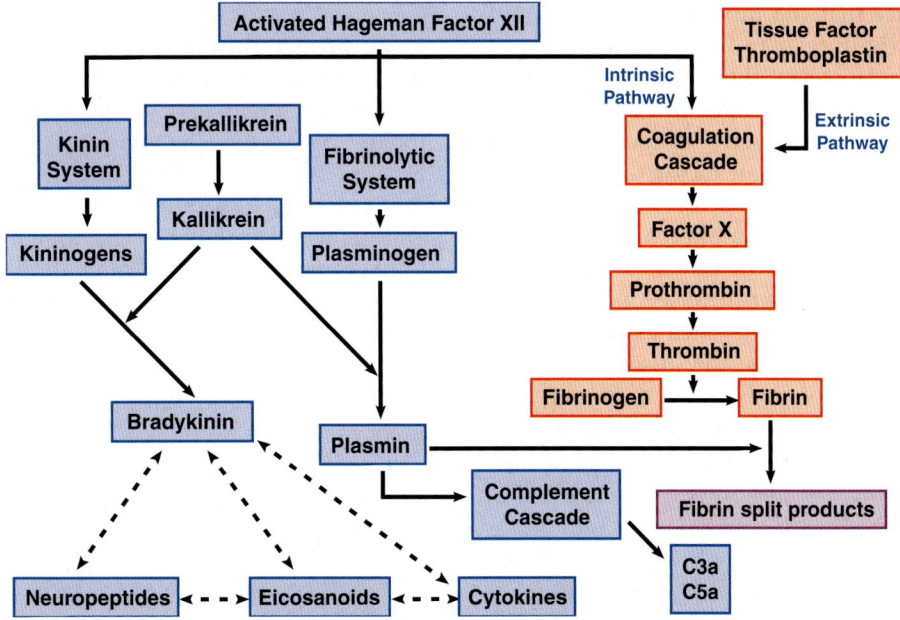

Figure 8 Diagram showing various pathways that are activated during an inflammatory response. Dotted lines indicate a synergistic or costimulatory function. Courtesy of Dr. Fouad.

Kinin System: Bradykinin

As can be seen in Figure 8, the activated Hageman factor causes the formation of kinins from kininogen, a reaction that is mediated by kallikrein. The most important of the kinins is bradykinin. This protein causes vasodilatation, extravasation of plasma proteins, and reduction of pain threshold.[40] Bradykinin performs its actions through the binding with two receptors, B1 and B2. B1 is primarily associated with chronic pain syndromes, while B2 is constitutively present in tissues and is over expressed in acute pain situations,[41] including pulpal pain.[42] It has been shown that bradykinin can act synergistically with neuropeptides, thrombin, and other factors to enhance the production of a number of eicosanoids, such as PGE2, and cytokines, such as IL-1 and TNF-α.[43-46] Once released, bradykinin levels are controlled by a number of kininases, and their effects on pain are controlled by endogenous opiates and steroids. Nonsteroidal anti-inflammatory drugs (NSAIDs) have also been shown to reduce bradykinin levels.[47]

The Coagulation Cascade and Fibrinolytic Systems

Tissue injury and severe inflammation frequently result in hemorrhage, at macroscopic or microscopic levels. Therefore, one of the principal initial mechanisms of healing is the coagulation cascade. Traditionally, the coagulation cascade has been divided into intrinsic and extrinsic pathways (see Figure 8). This was due to the fact that the intrinsic pathway could occur in vitro by the Hageman factor, in the absence of thromboplastin. However, there are many interactions between both pathways, and the distinction is now less critical.[5] Through a series of localized enzymatic activations, the Hageman factor/thromboplastin result in the formation of Factor X; this in turn results in the formation of thrombin from prothrombin. Thrombin (activated Factor II) has a number of critical functions, including positive feedback activation of a number of other factors such as Factors VIII and V, but essentially forms the insoluble fibrin clot from the soluble protein fibrinogen. In order to limit the size of the clot and prevent disseminated coagulation, the fibrinolytic system is activated and results in the formation of plasmin.

Complement System

The complement system consists of a series of about 20 proteins that play a number of critical roles in the immune system (Figure 9). Complement is activated through one of the two main pathways. The classical pathway involves antigen–antibody reaction and results in the activation of C1 to form a molecule commonly referred to as C3 convertase. Certain microbial cell wall molecules such as LPS can activate the alternate pathway in which C3 through coenzymatic interaction from Factors B and D and a protein called properdin result in the formation of another C3 convertase of a different structure. The enzyme C3 convertase, in whichever formulation, mediates the formation of C3b from C3, with C3a as a by product. Together with C5 convertases, C3b activates C5 to C5b, with C5a as a by-product. C5b combines with C6, C7, C8, and C9 to form a complex that forms holes through the bacterial cell membrane resulting in death of the cell. Complement molecules may also act as opsonins for phagocytosis, as discussed previously. Finally, C3a and C5a are known as anaphylatoxins because they cause degranulation of mast cells with the release of histamine, which causes vasodilatation and increased vascular permeability. C5a activates the lipoxygenase pathway of arachidonic acid in neutrophils and monocytes and is itself a potent chemotactic agent for these cells.

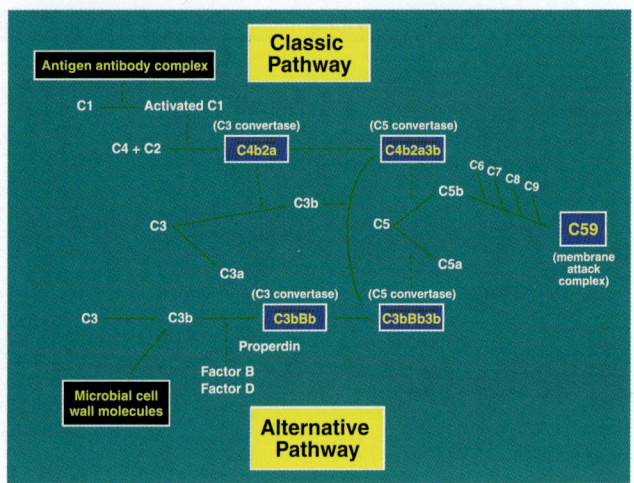

Figure 9 Complement cascade. Courtesy of Dr. Fouad.

Matrix Metalloproteinases

Matrix metalloproteinases (MMPs) are a number of endopeptidases (Table 5) that are responsible for tissue remodeling during structural development and for tissue break down during pathological states such as the inflammatory and neoplastic changes and caries. Occasionally, some of these enzymes, such as collagenase, may be of microbial origin. Host MMPs are typically modulated by levels of cytokines and growth factors in various tissues. They are

Table 5 Commonly Identified Matrix Metalloproteinases that are Zinc-dependant Endopeptidases	
Common Name	MMP
Collagenases	1, 8, 13, 18
Gelatinases	2, 9
Stromelysins	3, 10, 11
Membrane Ttype MMPs (MT MMPs)	14, 15, 16, 17, 24, 25
Minimal domain MMPs	7, 26
Others MMPs	12, 19, 20, 21, 22, 23, 27, 28

MMP, Matrix metalloproteinases.

upregulated by IL-1β and TNF-α and by growth factors such as platelet-derived growth factor (PDGF), epidermal growth factor (EGF), and nerve growth factor (NGF). They are abrogated by IFN-γ and TGF-β.[40] They are also inactivated by a group of molecules collectively known as tissue inhibitors of metalloproteinases (TIMPs) and by α$_2$-macroglobulin (which also inhibits neutrophil elastase—see below). MMPs and tissue inhibitors of metalloproteinases have been identified in the dental tissues during health and disease.[48–52] It is noteworthy, though, that in the oral cavity, MMPs can be released in saliva, and so the sources of MMPs that degrade dentin matrix in caries may be salivary rather than pulpal.

It has been documented through a significant body of evidence that tetracyclines and some tetracycline analogues and chemically modified tetracyclines may degrade MMPs at subantibiotic levels.[53,54] This is thought to be one of a number of anti-inflammatory properties that are exhibited by some antibiotics.[55]

Neutrophil Elastase

During pulpal and periradicular tissue inflammation, a number of other proteases may contribute to the tissue destruction frequently encountered. Among these proteolytic enzymes is neutrophil elastase, a neutral serine protease that is released from azurophilic granules in the PMNs during the activation of these cells. Neutrophil elastase can cleave a wide variety of structurally important proteins and glycoproteins, such as elastin, type III and IV collagen, fibronectin, and core proteins of proteoglycan molecules. It was recently reported that neutrophil elastase was increased in periradicular lesions that were symptomatic,[56] and that its levels although correlated with prostaglandin E2 did not change following root canal instrumentation.[57]

NITRIC OXIDE

Nitric oxide (NO) is a gaseous free radical that has been described to have several proinflammatory and modulatory effects in tissues. It is produced through a reaction that involves the enzyme NO synthase (NOS) and several cofactors including NADPH. Several NOS isoforms are present, including inducible (iNOS), neuronal (nNOS), and endothelial (eNOS). The nNOS and eNOS are constitutively expressed in the respective tissues and are calcium-dependent, whereas the iNOS is induced in macrophages and a number of other cells, primarily by cytokines such as IL-1 and TNF-α or microbial products such as LPS, and are calcium-independent.[40] Because it is relatively volatile and short-lived, the detection of NO is frequently assessed through the presence of NOS, particularly iNOS.

Under normal conditions, NO is primarily involved in vasodilatation through the relaxation of smooth muscles and prevention of adhesion of leukocytes to endothelial wall, which is considered as an anti-inflammatory function. However, during inflammation, including that of the pulp and periradicular tissues, and due to the action of cytokines, large amounts of NO are released.[58–63] NO contributes to the killing of microbial cells and tumor cells by macrophages through its interaction with superoxide free radical as follows[5]:

$$NO + O_2^{\bullet -} \rightarrow OH^{\bullet} + NO_2$$

NO is also an antagonist for platelet activation, adhesion, and degranulation. Moreover, it was recently shown that NO can regulate the proliferation, growth and apoptosis of pulp cells in vitro.[64]

OXYGEN-DERIVED FREE RADICALS

These are highly reactive, short-lived molecules produced by macrophages and neutrophils in normal and pathological states. The most important molecules are the superoxide anion ($O_2^{\bullet -}$), which eventually is converted to hydrogen peroxide (H_2O_2), and the hydroxyl radical (OH•) and toxic NO derivatives.[5] The main role that these molecules play is to increase the inflammatory response by increasing cytokines, chemokines, and adhesion molecules. However, in large amounts they cause thrombosis and tissue damage. The antioxidant activity is mediated through enzymes such as catalase, glutathione peroxidases, and superoxide dismutase (SOD). There are two main forms of SODs: copper–zinc (Cu, Zn-SOD) found primarily in cytoplasm and manganese (Mn-SOD) found primarily in mitochondria. While the presence of SOD in normal pulp has been described a long time ago,[65] the effect of inflammation on the levels of both isoforms of this enzyme has been controversial. Several studies have shown an increase of SOD,[65,66] or both Cu, Zn-SOD and Mn-SOD,[67] in pulpal inflammation. In fact, one study showed an anti-inflammatory effect that Cu, Zn-SOD has on pulpal inflammation in an animal model.[68] However, a more recent study showed that there is a reduction of Cu, Zn-SOD in human pulpitis, possibly due to depletion.[69] Using quantitative real-time RT-PCR, which is more sensitive than traditional protein assays, it has just been reported that the expression of mRNA for both enzymes does increase in pulpitis in patients and that the elevation of Mn-SOD is significantly higher than that of Cu, Zn-SOD.[70]

CYTOKINES

Cytokines are low molecular weight proteins that stimulate or inhibit proliferation, differentiation, or function of immune cells.[4] Approximately 40 cytokines have been described with various functions that mediate or modulate the immune system and bone resorption. Cytokines may exert their actions through autocrine (acting on receptors of the same cell that produced them), paracrine (acting on other cells in the local vicinity), and endocrine (acting systemically) modes. Because of the involvement of cytokines in several areas of interest in endodontics, their various roles and functions have been and will be described in various sections of this chapter and in other chapters dealing with pulpal and periradicular pathosis. In order to avoid redundancy, a brief description of the main features of some cytokines will be described here, with other information provided elsewhere in the chapter. Table 6 presents a summary of the role, sources, and main actions of cytokines.

Proinflammatory Cytokines

TNF-α is the principal mediator of the response to gram-negative bacteria. LPS stimulates the functions of mononuclear phagocytes and acts as a polyclonal activator of B cells, thus contributing to the elimination of the invading bacteria. The major cellular source of TNF is the LPS-activated mononuclear phagocyte and the minor source is antigen-stimulated T cells, activated NK cells, and activated mast cells. IL-1 derived from mononuclear phagocytes has a principal function, similar to TNF, as a mediator of the host inflammatory response in innate immunity. LPS can trigger monocytes to secrete IL-1 or TNF. T cells are more effective

Table 6 Summary of the Origin and Actions of the Commonly Investigated Cytokines [1,4,23]

Cytokine	Special Function*	Secreted by	Effector Function
Interleukins			
IL-1α, IL-1β	Pro-inflammatory; bone-resorptive	Mono, MΦ, DC, NK, B, Endo	Co-stimulates T activation by enhancing the production of cytokines including IL-2 and its receptor; enhances B proliferation and maturation; NK cytotoxicity; induces IL-1, -6, -8, TNF, GM-CSF, and PGE$_2$ by MΦ; proinflammatory by inducing chemokines and ICAM-1 and VCAM-1 on endothelium; induces fever, APP, bone resorption by osteoclasts
IL-2	Pro-inflammatory	Th1	Induces proliferation of activated T- and B-cells; enhances NK cytotoxicity and killing of tumor cells and bacteria by monocytes and MΦ
IL-3		T, NK, MC	Growth and differentiation of hematopoietic precursors; MC growth
IL-4	Anti-inflammatory; bone modulatory	Th2, Tc2, NK, NKT, γδ T, MC	Induces Th2 cells; stimulates proliferation of activated B, T, MC; upregulates MHC class II on B and MΦ, and CD23 on B; downregulates IL-12 production and thereby inhibits Th1 differentiation, increases MΦ phagocytosis; induces switch to IgG1 and IgE
IL-5	Anti-inflammatory	Th2, MC	Induces proliferation of eosino and activated B; induces switch to IgA
IL-6	Pro-/Anti-inflammatory; bone modulatory	Th2, Mono, MΦ, DC, BM stroma	Differentiation of myeloid stem cells and of B into plasma cells; induces APP; enhances T proliferation
IL-7		BM and thymic stroma	Induces differentiation of lymphoid stem cells into progenitor T and B; activates mature T
IL-8		Neutro; Mono, MΦ, Endo	Chemokine; mediates chemotaxis and activation of neutrophils

Table 6 Continued on Page 357

Table 6 Continued from Page 356

IL-9		Th	Induces proliferation of thymocytes; enhances MC growth; synergizes with IL-4 in switch to IgG1 and IgE
IL-10	Anti-inflammatory; bone modulatory	Th (Th2 in mouse), Tc, B, Mono, MΦ	Inhibits IFN-γ secretion by mouse, and IL-2 by human, Th1 cells; downregulates MHC class II and cytokine (including IL-12) production by Mono, MΦ and DC, thereby inhibiting Th1; differentiation; inhibits T proliferation; enhances B differentiation
IL-11	Bone resorptive	BM stroma	Promotes differentiation of pro-B and megakaryocytes; induces APP
IL-12	Pro-inflammatory	Mono, MΦ, DC, B	Critical cytokine for Th1 differentiation; induces proliferation and IFN-γ production by Th1, $CD8^+$ and γδ T and NK; enhances NK and $CD8^+$ T cytotoxicity; but may inhibit osteoclast formation in vitro
IL-13	Anti-inflammatory	Th2, MC	Inhibits activation and cytokine secretion by MΦ; co-activates B proliferation; upregulates MHC class II and CD23 on B and Mono; induces switch to IgG1 and IgE; induces VCAM-1 on endo
IL-14			
IL-15		T, NK, Mono, MΦ, DC, B	Induces proliferation of T-, NK an d activated B and cytokine production and cytotoxicity in NK and $CD8^+$ T; chemotactic for T; stimulates growth of intestinal epithelium
IL-16		Th, Tc	Chemoattractant for CD4 T, Mono and eosino; induces MHC class II
IL-17		T	Proinflammatory; stimulates production of cytokines including TNF, IL-1β, -6, -8, G-CSF
IL-18	Bone resorptive	MΦ, DC	Induces IFN-γ production by T; enhances NK cytotoxicity; but may inhibit osteoclast formation in vitro
IL-19		Mono	Modulation of Th1 activity
IL-20		Mono, keratinocytes	Regulation of inflammatory responses to skin
IL-21–33			(Sources and actions of these cytokines are overlapping and not well characterized. The reader is referred to reference [4] for a complete list)
Tumor Necrosis Factors			
TNF-α	Pro-inflammatory; bone resorptive	Th, Mono, MΦ, DC, MC, NK, B	Tumor cytotoxicity; cachexia (weight loss); induces cytokine secretion; induces E-selectin on endo; activates MΦ; antiviral
Lymphotoxin (LT), TNF-β	Pro-inflammatory	Th1, Tc	Tumor cytotoxicity; enhances phagocytosis by neutro and MΦ; involved in lymphoid organ development, antiviral
Interferons			
IFN-α		Leukocytes	Inhibits viral replication; enhances MHC class I
IFN-β		Fibroblasts	Inhibits viral replication; enhances MHC class I
IFN-γ	Pro-inflammatory	Th1, Tc1, NK	Inhibits viral replication; enhances MHC class I and II; activates MΦ; induces switch to IgG2a; antagonizes several IL-4 actions; inhibits proliferation of Th2
Colony-Stimulating Factors			
GM-CSF	Pro-inflammatory	Th, MΦ, Fibro, MC, Endo	Stimulates growth of progenitors of mMono, neutro, eosino and baso; activates MΦ
G-CSF	Pro-inflammatory	Fibro, Endo	Stimulates growth of neutro progenitors
M-CSF	Pro-inflammatory	Fibro, Endo, Epith	Stimulates growth of mMono progenitors
SLF		BM stroma	Stimulates stem cell division (c-kit ligand)
Others			
TGFβ		Th3, B, MΦ, MC	Not only proinflammatory by, for example, chemoattraction of Mono and MΦ but also anti-inflammatory by, for example, inhibiting lymphocyte proliferation; induces switch to IgA; promotes tissue repair
LIF		Thymic epith, BM stroma	Induces APP
Eta-1		T	Stimulates IL-12 production and inhibits IL-10 production by MΦ
Oncostatin M		T, MΦ	Induces APP

APP, acute phase proteins; B, B cell; baso, basophile; BM, bone marrow; Endo, endothelium; eosino, eosinophil; Epith, epithelium; Fibro, fibroblast; GM-CSF, granulocyte–macrophage colony-stimulating factor; IL, interleukin; LIF, leukemia inhibitory factor; MΦ, macrophage; MC, mast cell; Mono, monocyte; neutro, neutrophil; NK, natural killer; SLF, steel locus factor; T, T cell; TGF-β, transforming growth factor-β. Note that there is no interleukin-14. This designation was given to an activity that, upon further investigation, could not be unambiguously assigned to a single cytokine. IL-30 also awaits assignment. IL-8 is a member of the chemokine family. These cytokines are listed separately in Table 9.5.
*Recognized actions in pulpal and periradicular lesions.

than LPS at eliciting IL-1 synthesis by monocytes. IL-1 is made by diverse cell types, epithelium and endothelium providing local sources of IL-1 in the absence of macrophage-rich infiltrate.

The effect of IL-1 is similar to that of TNF. At low quantity, it acts on endothelium to increase the expression of adhesion molecules and on monocytes to secrete chemokines. It shares many features of TNF but is also different; for example, it enhances rather than suppresses the actions of colony-stimulating factors (CSFs) (see Table 6) on bone marrow cells. IL-6 serves as a growth factor for activated B cells.[71,72]

Systemic Effects of Cytokines

As noted before, during an acute infection or after tissue injury, there is an increase in the concentration of proinflammatory cytokines in the blood, primarily IL-1, TNF, and IL-6. IL-1 and TNF cause fever through their action on the thermoregulatory center in the hypothalamus due to the release of local eicosanoids.[5] IL-1 causes an increase in IL-6 that acts on hepatocytes to synthesize a number of plasma proteins called acute phase proteins, and the reaction is known as acute phase reaction. Among the most intensely secreted proteins are C-reactive protein (CRP), mannose-binding lectin (MBL), serum amyloid P component (SAP) and α_1-acid glycoprotein. CRP and MBL are important in fixing complement and deposit C3b, which is an opsonins, on the microbial cell.[4] SAP can, together with chondroitin sulfate, bind to lysosomal enzymes such as cathepsin B released in inflammation. This complex becomes a component of the amyloid fibrillar deposits that accompany chronic infections.[4] Other proteins that are released in moderate amounts in an acute phase reaction include fibrinogen, fibronectin, haptoglobin, angiotensin, ceruloplasmin, complement proteins C3, C9, and factor B, α_1-proteinase inhibitors and α_1-antichymotrypsin. Finally, cytokines may also act on bone marrow to cause the increased production of white cells causing leukocytosis, where white cells may reach 15,000 to 20,000/µL rather than the 4,000 to 10,000/µL normal count.[5]

The discussion of bone-resorptive cytokines and bone resorption modulatory actions of cytokines will be provided under the role of cytokines in bone resorption (see page 42). The discussion of anti-inflammatory cytokines is under molecular mediators of anti-inflammatory reactions (see page 42).

NEUROPEPTIDES

Neuropeptides are proteins produced by neural tissues and are released at the sites of nerve endings. Under normal conditions they function to maintain the vascular tone of blood vessels, thus modulating the vascularity and regulating the innervation of the tissue. During an inflammatory response, there is vasodilatation, extravasation of plasma proteins, and sprouting of nerve endings within the inflamed tissue. These changes result in an increase in the levels of certain neuropeptides. It is now recognized that certain neuropeptides such as Substance P (SP) have decidedly proinflammatory actions, whereas a number of other neuropeptides such as vasoactive intestinal peptide (VIP), α-melanocyte-stimulating hormone, neuropeptide Y (NPY), and somatostatin are members of an anti-inflammatory repertoire of immune modulators.[73,74] The newly discovered neuropeptides, such as urocortin, adrenomedullin, and cortistatin, also appear to have anti-inflammatory actions in that they inhibit T-cell proliferation, Th1 response, and IL-2 production.[74] Calcitonin gene-related peptide (CGRP) may have proinflammatory as well as anti-inflammatory actions.[74] SP was the first neuropeptide described around 1931; it is localized in sensory nerves, is related to neurokinins A and B, and its receptors are NK1, NK2, and NK3.[75] CGRP was described in 1983 and it binds to CGRP1, CGRP2, and AM2, whereas NPY was discovered in 1982, is localized in sympathetic, cholinergic, sensory, enteric, and central neurons and binds to Y1, Y2, Y4, and Y5 receptors.[75]

With respect to pulpal and periradicular region, denervation experiments have shown that, in the pulp, SP-, neurokinin A-, and CGRP-containing nerve fibers originate from the trigeminal ganglion and that NPY-containing nerve fibers come from the superior cervical ganglion. The origin of VIP-containing fibers may be parasympathetic nerve fibers since it has been associated with acetylcholine in other tissues.[40,76]

Since the dental pulp is highly innervated, neuropeptides play a significant role in mediating and modulating the inflammatory response in it. The neuropeptides that have been studied the most in endodontic pathosis are SP and CGRP and to a lesser degree VIP and NPY. In the normal rat molar pulp, SP and CGRP were shown to be present in close proximity to macrophages, an association that was more prevalent in the odontoblastic layer than in the central pulp.[77] During inflammation, sprouting of pulpal nerve fibers was shown to be associated with an increased expression of SP and CGRP closely surrounding the areas of irritation.[78,79] However, severe irritation by experimental pulp exposures caused a drop in the overall pulpal levels of SP and CGRP, possibly due to the depletion of neuropeptide stores in the nerve endings.[80] In vitro experiments showed that below a certain threshold, the addition of SP increased, and CGRP

(EMDs), PDGF, and insulin-like growth factor (IGF). These proteins have been extensively investigated with respect to their ability to induce, potentiate, and accelerate bone regeneration, whether as purified proteins or as components of demineralized freeze-dried bones.[9,105–110]

There have been considerable interests in whether BMPs,[112–115] TGF-β,[116–120] EMD,[121] or other growth factors may enhance the formation of reparative dentin following pulp exposure. In vivo trials in animal models have initially been conducted via protein deposition directly on experimentally exposed pulp.[114,122,123] However, more recently gene transfer strategies have been employed to assure prolonged effect of the induced protein[112,118] or transplantation of cells in which the growth factor genes have been induced in vitro to a polyglycolic acid scaffold in the pulp.[124] However, it was later realized that in the presence of inflammation, as induced by applying LPS to the model, these strategies fail to produce the desired outcome.[112,113]

Within a pathological pulpal or periapical tissue, or even during an orthodontic movement, growth factors are frequently expressed and are thought to modulate the inflammatory process and aid in the healing that ensues after the removal of irritants.[9,125–131] For example, it has been shown that TGF-β1 downregulates the expression of matrix metaprotein-8 (MMP-8) in human odontoblasts and dental pulp cells in vitro.[49]

Molecular Mediators of Anti-Inflammatory Reactions

MEMBRANE PHOSPHOLIPIDS/ ARACHIDONIC ACID METABOLIC PATHWAYS

An inflammatory process is fine tuned by proinflammatory and anti-inflammatory mediators. There is more information known about proinflammatory mediators, whereas less is known regarding anti-inflammatory factors. In fact, in the pathways leading to the production of proinflammatory mediators such as prostaglandins and leukotrienes, there is also the production of anti-inflammatory mediators such as lipoxins (Figure 10). In the host defense mechanism, acute inflammation executed by neutrophils is resolved by proceeding to chronic inflammation in which proinflammatory mediators are produced or to resolution in which protective mediators are released.[132–136]

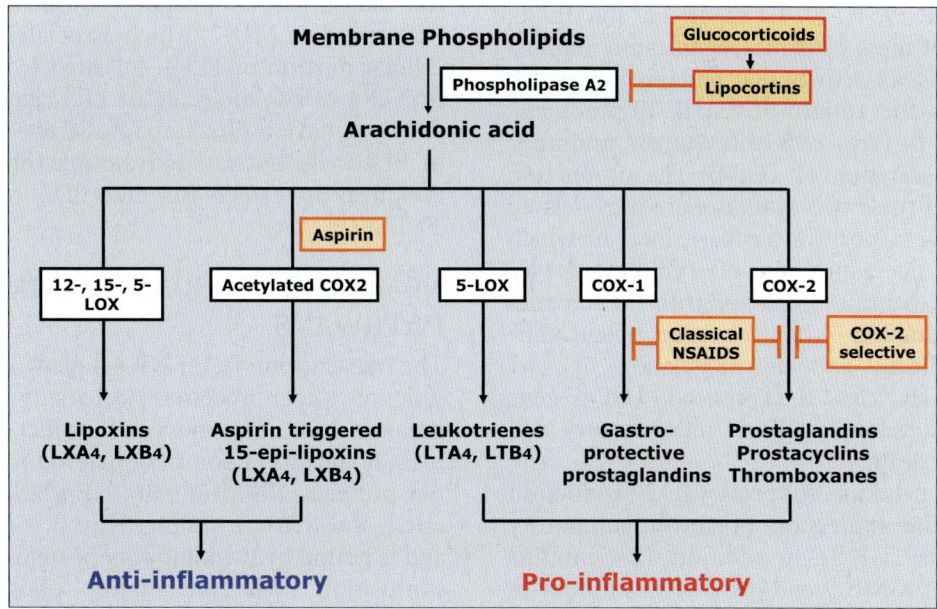

Figure 10 Pathways of lipid mediator production from membrane phospholipids. LOX, lipoxygenase; COX, cyclooxygenase; NSAIDs, nonsteroidal anti-inflammatory drugs; LX, lipoxin. Courtesy of Dr. Huang.

This proresolution against acute inflammation is an active process that involves the activation of specific biochemical and cellular programs of resolution. Lipoxins are potent counter-regulatory signals for endogenous proinflammatory mediators, including lipids (e.g., leukotrienes) and cytokines (TNF-α and IL-6), resulting in the inhibition of leukocyte-dependent inflammation. Lipoxins are rapidly biosynthesized in response to stimuli, act locally, and then are rapidly enzymatically inactivated.[133,137–139]

ANTI-INFLAMMATORY CYTOKINES: IL-10, TGF-β, IL-4, AND IL-6

Several cytokines have predominantly anti-inflammatory effects including IL-1 receptor antagonist (IL-1Ra), TGF-β, and IL-10. Monocytes and B cells are the major sources of IL-10 in human subjects. The primary T-cell source for IL-10 is regulatory T lymphocytes (Tr), as mentioned above. IL-10 inhibits the production of many proinflammatory cytokines such as IL-1β, IL-6, IL-8, IL-12, IFN-γ, and TNF-α. In addition, IL-10 inhibits MHC class II, CD23, intercellular adhesion molecule 1 (ICAM-1), and CD80/CD86 expression by DCs and other APCs. IL-10 plays an important role in human allergic diseases. Asthma and allergic rhinitis are associated with diminished IL-10 expression in the allergic airway by both alveolar macrophages and DCs. Newer members of the IL-10 family include IL-19, IL-20, IL-22, IL-24, and IL-26; however, none of these cytokines significantly inhibits cytokine synthesis, an activity that remains unique for IL-10.[140] Besides the antigen-driven IL-10-producing Treg, Th3 (TGF-β–Treg) cells also regulate immunosuppression via secretion of TGF-β. The production and the action of these two cytokines are inter-related and likely involve a positive feedback loop in which IL-10 enhances the expression of TGF-β and vice versa.[140–143] TGF-β has a broad spectrum of activities including the induction of oral tolerance, potent anti-inflammatory effects, and downregulation of Th1 activities and MHC class II expression. TGF-β gene knockout mice develop multifocal inflammatory disease resulting in death.[144]

IL-4, as a Th2 cytokine, suppresses IL-2 production and promotes the expression of anti-inflammatory cytokines such as TGF-β$_1$. In addition, IL-4 inhibits the expression of MMP-9 and MMP-1 in monocytes and macrophages.[145] IL-6 is a highly pleiotropic cytokine that mediates the host response to injury and infection and is considered both a proinflammatory and an anti-inflammatory cytokine; it is secreted during inflammation and after TNF-α and IL-1 secretion. IL-6 subsequently inhibits the secretion of TNF-α and IL-1.[146]

Intracellular Signaling Pathways of Inflammatory Mediators

TLR SIGNAL TRANSDUCTION PATHWAYS

Upon binding the ligands, TLRs activate the same signaling molecules that are used for IL-1R signaling,[147] triggering downstream signaling cascades that leads to the activation of proinflammatory cytokine and chemokine genes. The stimulation of most TLRs leads to Th1 rather than Th2 differentiation. Thus, innate immunity is a key element in the inflammatory response as well as the immune response against pathogens. Microbial cell-wall components stimulate immune cells and serve as pathogen associated molecular patterns (PAMPs), recognized by individual TLRs. LPS, also known as an endotoxin, is generally the most potent immunostimulant among these cell-wall components. Earlier studies have shown that endotoxin plays an important role in the initiating and perpetuating of periradicular inflammation and bone resorption.[148–151] LPS liberated from gram-negative bacteria binds LBPs that are present in the bloodstream, and then binds to CD14 expressed on the cell surface of phagocytes. Subsequently, LPS is transferred to MD-2, which associates with the extracellular portion of TLR4, followed by oligomerization of TLR4, a key molecule of LPS signaling.[152,153] LPS does not have a direct apoptotic effect on osteoblasts or PDL cells, but can activate macrophages to induce apoptosis in osteoblasts and PDL cells via released TNF-α.[154]

NF-κB AND NF-κB-ACTIVATING PATHWAYS

The transcription factor NF-κB plays a pivotal role in a series of cellular processes, particularly those involved in inflammation, immunity, cell proliferation, and apoptosis. It consists of homo- or heterodimers of a group of five proteins, NF-κB1 (p50), NF-κB2 (p52), p65/RelA, c-Rel, and RelB. In resting, NF-κB is in the cytoplasm and is bound by the inhibitory proteins IκBs. Upon cell stimulation, IκBs are rapidly phosphorylated and degraded, freeing the NF-κB to translocate into the nucleus and bind onto the transcriptional regulatory sequence motifs of multiple target genes. NF-κB activation is divided into two main pathways—the classical and the alternative pathways of NF-κB activation. The classical pathway is induced by a variety of innate and adaptive immunity mediators including proinflammatory cytokines (TNF-α and IL-1β), TLRs, and antigen receptors (TCR and BCR) ligation. While these NF-κB inducers signal through different receptors and adaptor proteins, all converge to the activation of IκB–kinase (IKK) complex, which phosphorylates IκB leading to its degradation. The freed NF-κB then translocates into the nucleus where it activates the transcription of target genes such as cytokines, chemokines, adhesion molecules, and inhibitors of apoptosis (see Figure 3). The alternative pathway of NF-κB activation is important for secondary lymphoid organ development, homeostasis, and adaptive immunity. It is induced by B cell-activating factor, lymphotoxin b, CD40 ligand, and human T-cell leukemia and Epstein-Barr virus. It enhances NF-κB inducing kinase- and IKKα-dependent processing of p100 into p52, which binds DNA in association with its partners, like RelB. These stimuli also activate the classical pathway. NF-κB inducers trigger the formation of reactive oxygen species (ROS), which may be the reason why that such a diversity of inducers activates NF-κB via the same IKK-dependent pathway. Both IL-β and TNF-α activation of NF-κB involve ROS.[155]

Inflammation-Induced Bone Resorption

The formation of periradicular lesion as the result of pulpal infection involves features that are somewhat different from a typical microbial infection of other tissues. Pulp tissue ends and transits into the periodontal ligament tissue at the apical cementodentinal junction. Apical periodontal ligament begins to be affected as the pulpal inflammation spread toward it. Inflamed apical portion of the pulp and the periodontal ligament releases factors that induce bone resorption to build and maintain a defense line against the incoming microbial invasion. The resorbed bone space is replaced with abscesses and/or granulomatous tissue rife with inflammatory cells and fibroblasts. The proliferation of epithelial cell rest of Malassez leads to scattered epithelial cell clusters within the inflamed periradicular lesion. With time, these epithelial cell clusters may form a cyst that occurs in 7% to 54% of the periradicular lesions examined.[156–162] Nair found that 52% (133/256) of the periradicular lesions examined histologically demonstrated epithelial proliferation, but only 15% were actually determined to be periapical cysts.[163]

The epithelial cells in the PDL are involved not only in the formation of cysts but may also be in the regulation of cementum and bone metabolism as they express osteopontin and osteoprotegerin (OPG) that are not expressed in gingival epithelial cells.[164] Based on animal studies, periradicular lesions expand in the early phase of the lesion formation and become self-limited at later stage.

MICROBIAL ROLE IN THE PATHOGENESIS OF PERIRADICULAR LESION

Although inflammation is generally associated with infection, inflammation can be the mere result of an aseptic trauma or a dysregulated immune reaction. The classic study by Kakehashi et al. (1965)[165] verified this notion that without the presence of microbes, exposed pulp tissue will heal after a transient inflammatory response without the development of periradicular lesions. Endodontic infection is characterized as a polymicrobial infection with predominately anaerobes, many of which are gram-negative. The damage of host tissues from infection is the result of (1) direct infliction from microbial products such as collagenase, trypsin-like enzymes, and fibronectin-degrading enzymes and (2) host immune response that leads to the destruction of tissue such as periradicular bone.

As mentioned above, host innate immunity exerts certain extent of specificity to the microbial components via PRRs such as TLRs. TLR4-mutated C3H/HeJ mice (LPS hyporesponsive) have reduced response to gram-negative bacteria and are highly susceptible to infection by *Salmonella typhimurium* or *Neisseria meningitis*.[166] There is a reduced expression of IL-1 and IL-12 and a decreased periradicular bone destruction in TLR-4-deficient mice when subjected to pulpal exposure and infection with a mixture of four anaerobic pathogens, *Prevotella intermedia*, *F. nucleatum*, *Streptococcus intermedius* (gram-negative), and *Peptostreptococcus micros* (gram-positive). Also, no dissemination of infection occurs in the TLR-4-deficient mice.[167]

If the pulp is exposed to the microorganisms in the oral environment, these LPS hyporesponsive mice do not show significant difference in the level of cytokine production or periradicular bone destruction from the normal controls.[168] Studies have indicated that the variations of microflora obtained from molar surfaces of mouse within a same experimental group are as great as the variation between mice in different groups,[169] which could contribute to the discrepancies of findings by different investigators.

Components such as LTA of gram-positive bacterial cell walls can also stimulate innate immunity in a similar manner as LPS. TLR2 plays a major role in detecting gram-positive bacteria and is involved in the recognition of a variety of microbial components, including LTA, lipoproteins, and PG. The importance of TLR2 in the host defense against gram-positive bacteria has been demonstrated using TLR2-deficient (TLR2-/-) mice that were found to be highly susceptible to challenge with *Staphylococcus aureus* or *Streptococcus pneumoniae*.[170,171]

LTA can cause apoptotic cell damage including that of *Enterococcus faecalis*, which induces apoptosis in osteoblasts, osteoclasts, periodontal ligament fibroblasts, macrophages, and neutrophils. It also stimulates leukocytes to release mediators that are known to play a role in various phases of the inflammatory response including TNF-α, IL-1β, IL-6, IL-8, and PGE2. These factors have all been detected in periapical samples, and each has a well-known tissue-damaging property.[172]

ROLE OF IMMUNE CELLS IN PERIAPICAL LESION FORMATION

Immune cells present in human periradicular lesion consist of lymphocytes, macrophages, plasma cells, neutrophils, and NK cells with the former two types as the majority.[173,174] Within lymphocytes, T cells are in greater number or equal to B cells.[175] APCs and T suppressor/cytotoxic cells are associated with both pre-existing and newly formed epithelium.[174]

By using rodents as study models, the dynamics of periradicular lesion development in rodents is characterized by having an active bone resorption phase within 15 days after pulp exposure followed by a chronic phase with little lesion expansion.[176–179] Th cells are predominant during the active phase, whereas increased numbers of Ts cells are associated with chronicity. The subpopulations of specific Th cells involved in the periradicular lesion development remain unclear.

The role of lymphocyte subpopulations in the formation of periradicular lesions was studied using lymphocyte-deficient rodents. T cell-deficient rodents develop periradicular lesion in a similar manner compared to the normal counter animals except some minor differences. Wallstrom et al.[180] used athymic rat model (T cell-deficient) and found no significant difference between periapical tissue responses of the conventional and athymic groups. Tani et al. (1995) used nude mice (T cell-deficient) and immunostaining to study the involvement of lymphocytes in the kinetics of periradicular lesion development. They found that at 2 weeks after pulp exposure, nude mice develop larger periradicular lesion than normal mice, but the lesion sizes are similar between the two experimental groups at 4 and 6 weeks after pulp exposure. At 8 weeks, however, normal mice have slightly larger lesion size. No T cells and reduced number of B cells are present in the lesions of nude mice. T cells (more Th than Ts) begin to emerge in lesions after 4 weeks in normal mice.[181] Fouad[182] employed severe combined immunodeficiency (SCID, T-, and B cell-deficient) mice as a study model and found that the SCID mice lesions are significantly smaller than the controls at only the 3-week period. In these studies, the pulp was exposed to oral microbes.

By using RAG-2 SCID mice (both T and B cell-deficient) and an infection protocol—equalized bacterial challenge of the exposed pulp with mixed microbes *P. intermedia*, *F. nucleatum*, *P. micros*, and *S. intermedius* and the access sealed—Teles et al.[183] found that approximately one-third of the RAG-2 mice develop endodontic abscesses, while no immunocompetent controls have abscesses. In another study, specific knockout (k/o) mice RAG 2, Igh-6 (B cell-deficient, Ig heavy chain k/o), Tcrb Tcrd (T cell-deficient, β and δ chain TCR k/o), and Hc⁰ (C5-deficient) were used to determine which immune element is important for the defense mechanism in endodontic infection. Their results demonstrate that B cells, not T cells or C5, play a pivotal role in preventing the dissemination of endodontic infection.[184]

MECHANISMS OF BONE RESORPTION: REGULATION OF OSTEOCLAST FORMATION AND ACTIVATION

Under normal conditions, osteoclastogenesis mainly occurs within the bone marrow as a continuing process of bone modeling and remodeling. Compared to the generalized bone loss seen in osteoporosis, localized bone loss in jaw bones resulting from endodontic infection is a combination of a focal inflammatory immune reaction and a localized osteoclastogenesis. Inflammatory cells, including lymphocytes and macrophages, produce cytokines, such as TNF and IL-1, and chemokines to recruit and activate more inflammatory cells (Table 9). Lymphocytes, monocytes and DCs found in

Table 9 Mediators Promote or Inhibit Bone Resorption

Action	Mediator
Promote bone resorption	IL-1, TNF-α, PGE2, IL-6, IL-11, RANK/RANKL, M-CSF, IGF-I
Inhibit bone resorption	IL12, IL-18, IL-4, OPG
Dual functions	PGs, TGF-β, IFN-γ, glucocorticoids

periapical granulomas synthesize receptor activator of nuclear factor-κB ligand (RANKL). There is a significantly higher RANKL gene expression in the granulomas compared with the control tissues in both humans and rats.[185–187] Macrophage colony-stimulating factor (M-CSF) and RANKL are two cytokines essential for promoting the differentiation of osteoclast precursors (OCPs) into mature osteoclasts. OCPs, generated in the bone marrow from hematopoietic stem cells, mobilize to diseased sites through the bloodstream and differentiate into osteoclasts to resorb bones. OCPs migrate along chemokine gradients.

The RANKL/RANK system is essential for mature osteoclast formation, a critical player in T-lymphocyte-mediated osteoclastogenesis, and induces OCPs to produce proinflammatory cytokines and chemokines.[188–190] RANKL not only delivers a final differentiation signal, but also activates osteoclasts and promotes their survival. Mature B and T cells do not form osteoclasts but affect osteoclastogenesis indirectly by producing RANKL or OPG, a soluble decoy RANKL receptor (Figure 11). OPG binds RANKL thereby preventing RANKL activity. OPG is expressed in the human pulp of healthy and inflamed tissues[191]; however its role in pulp tissue is unclear. The expression of OPG in periradicular lesion has not been reported. The influence of immune cells on osteoclastogenesis becomes significant when they accelerate osteoclast formation, and then both cell types contribute to the pathogenesis of the disease, as seen in inflammatory arthritis or periodontal disease.

RANKL is expressed by almost all cell types in the body. In the immune system, RANKL is expressed by activated T cells, B cells, and DCs (see Figure 11). OPG is produced by cells of mesenchymal origin. RANKL and OPG expression is regulated by many factors, and the ratio of RANKL/OPG controls osteoclastogenesis in vivo and in vitro. Periodontal ligament cells produce both RANKL and OPG.[192,193] In contrast to the broad expression of RANKL, RANK, the receptor for RANKL, is identified only on mature osteoclasts, DCs, and OCPs, which are therefore the major target cells for RANKL and OPG. TNF is overproduced by many cell types at inflammatory foci, including macrophages, T cells, DCs, osteoclasts, and OCPs.[194,195]

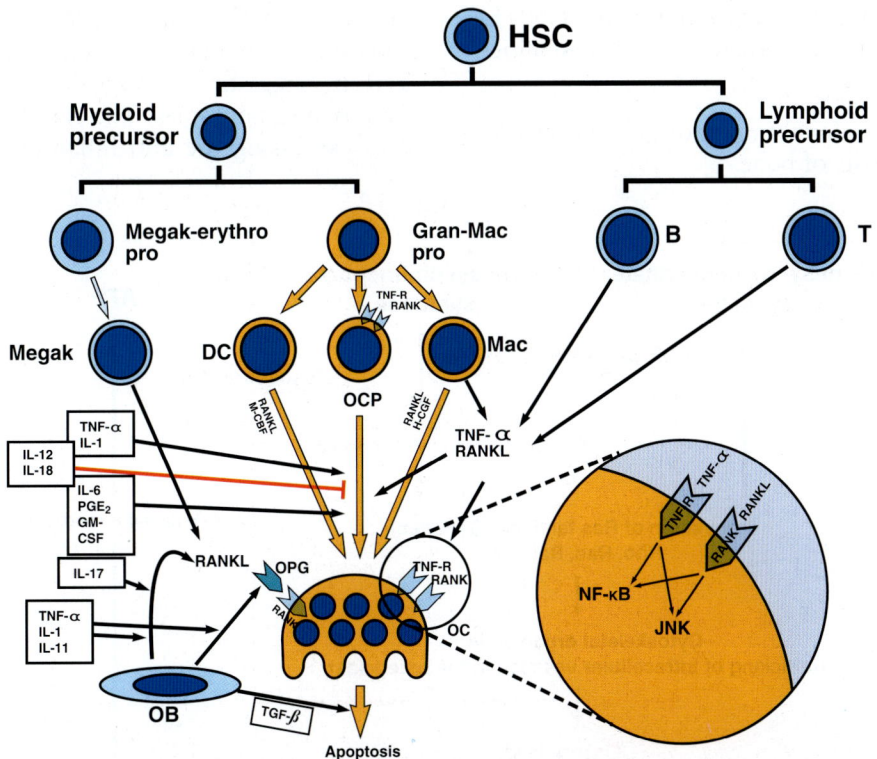

Figure 11 Regulations of osteoclast differentiation and the involved key cytokines. HSC, hematopoietic stem cells; OCP, osteoclast precursor; OC, osteoclast; OB, osteoblast; DC, dendritic cells; GC, granulocyte; Mac, macrophage; E, erythrocyte; OPG, osteoprotegerin. Courtesy of Dr. Huang.

INHIBITION OF BONE RESORPTION BY BISPHOSPHONATES

Bisphosphonates (BPs) have a unique high-affinity binding property to hydroxyapatite mineral, generating high local concentrations of drug on bone surfaces where these agents can preferentially interfere with osteoclast-mediated bone resorption. BPs comprise amino- and nonamino-containing compounds. Aminobisphosphonates such as pamidronate, alendronate, risedronate, and zoledronate exert their inhibitory effects on osteoclast function by inhibiting farnesyl pyrophosphate synthase, an enzyme in the mevalonate pathway necessary for lipid modification (prenylation) of small guanosine triphosphate (GTP)-binding proteins. Interference with the activity of the binding proteins alters cytoskeletal organization and intracellular trafficking in osteoclasts, resulting in the inhibition of osteoclast function. Ruffled border formation is a process that is highly dependent on cytoskeletal function, strongly regulated by geranylgeranylated GTP-binding proteins, such as Rac, Rho. Nonaminobisphosphonates such as etidronate and clodronate are metabolized to nonhydrolysable analogues of adenosine triphosphate (ATP) and act as inhibitors of ATP-dependent enzymes, leading to enhanced osteoclast apoptosis (Figure 12).[196]

The mechanism of osteonecrosis of the jaw (ONJ) by BPs is not completely clear. There are two possibilities:

(1) BPs are antiangiogenic.
(2) Osteoclast functional inhibition may affect normal homeostasis of bone.

Precipitating factors of ONJ include severe periodontitis, spontaneous exposure, periodontal surgery, dental implants, and root canal surgery.[197–199]

ROLES OF CYTOKINES IN PERIRADICULAR BONE RESORPTION

Many cytokines are involved in the initiation and maintenance of inflammation, some of which are also responsible directly or indirectly for the induction of bone resorption. Periradicular bone resorption induced by cytokines is a destructive and an undesirable process indicative of the magnitude of endodontic infection. On the other hand, cytokines are also important for the establishment of local immune defense mechanism. The role of specific cytokines in a variety of immune and inflammatory diseases, including endodontic pathoses, is difficult to elucidate due to the intricate and overlapping functions of these inflammatory cytokines and mediators.

Cytokines, TNF-α, IL-1, IL-6, and IL-11 are involved in promoting bone resorption and mediating inflammation both systemically and locally. In human dental granulomas, there is a correlation between the intensity of inflammatory infiltrate and the percentage of mononuclear cells positive for IL-4, suggesting a predominant Th2 response. There is also a correlation between the frequency of cells expressing IL-6 and TNF-α, suggesting synergistic activities of IL-6 and TNF-α in granulomas. The number of inflammatory cells expressing the anti-inflammatory molecules far

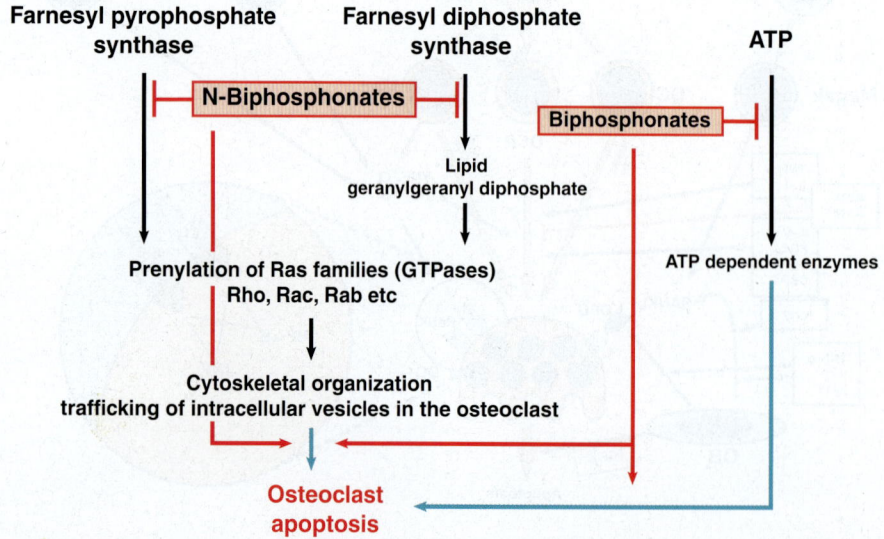

Figure 12 Mechanism of bisphosphonate (BP)-induced, osteoclast apoptosis. Courtesy of Dr. Huang.

outnumbered the cells that expressed proinflammatory cytokines.[200,201]

In mice, TNF-α and IL-1α are highly expressed in areas that contain a mixed inflammatory infiltrate or fibroblasts in periradicular lesions. The number of cells expressing these two cytokines is proportional to the lesion size.[182] The expression of IL-11 is not modulated by pulp exposure. Most of the Th1-type cytokines, including IL-2, IL-12, and IFN-γ, increase in mRNA and/or protein expression in periapical lesions after pulpal exposure; the expression of Th2-type cytokines (IL-4, IL-6, IL-10, and IL-13) is similarly increased, but declines after 28 days. Th1-modulated pro-inflammatory pathways appears to predominate during periapical bone destruction in mice.[202–206]

The role of specific cytokines in the development of periradicular lesions has been studied using mice with gene knockouts of different cytokines or their receptors, such as IL-1, IL-6, and TNF.[169,207,208] Mice with functional deletions of receptors to IL-1 (IL-1RI(-/-)), TNF (TNFRp55(-/-)-p75(-/-)), or both (TNFRp55(-/-)–IL-1RI(-/-)) infected with multiple anaerobic pathogens after pulp exposure lead to increased polymorphonuclear and mononuclear phagocyte recruitment in the periradicular lesions and bacterial penetration into the host tissue. Osteolytic lesion formation is also greater in animals lacking TNF and/or IL-1 receptors than in control mice, indicating that IL-1 or TNF receptor signaling is not required for bacteria-induced osteoclastogenesis and bone loss, but does play a critical role in protecting the host against mixed anaerobic infections. Although TNF-α enhances osteoclastogenesis and mediates LPS-induced bone loss, deletions of TNFRp55(-/-) do not reduce bacteria-induced bone resorption.[207] Between IL-1 and TNF-α, IL-1 receptor signaling is more important than TNF receptor signaling in preventing the spread of infection into the surrounding fascial planes.[209]

IL-6 production in mouse periapical lesions reaches its peak (~two-fold higher than the baseline) on day 14 after pulpal exposure and then decreases to the basal level after 28 days.[204] Depleting IL-6 negatively affects the host defense mechanism against local infection in the periradicular area.[169,208] In IL-6-/- mice, periradicular lesions rapidly develop in week 2, whereas in the IL-6+/+ mice the development of the lesion is 1 week slower.[169] The increased bone resorption in IL-6-deficient animals correlated with increases in osteoclast numbers, as well as with elevated expression of bone-resorptive cytokines IL-1α and IL-1β, in periapical lesions and with decreased expression of the anti-inflammatory cytokine IL-10. These data demonstrate that endogenous IL-6 expression has significant anti-inflammatory effects in modulating infection-stimulated bone destruction in vivo.[208]

The functional role of the Th2-type cytokines IL-4 and IL-10 in infection-stimulated bone resorption in vivo has also been assessed using gene knock-out mice. IL-10(-/-) mice have significantly greater infection-stimulated bone resorption compared with wild-type mice, while IL-4(-/-) have no increased resorption. IL-10(-/-) mice show markedly elevated IL-1α production within periapical inflammatory tissues (>10-fold), whereas IL-4(-/-) exhibit decreased IL-1α production. These findings suggest that IL-10, but not IL-4, is an important endogenous suppressor of infection-stimulated bone resorption in vivo, likely acting via inhibition of IL-1α expression.[210]

The functional roles of the Th1 cytokine IFN-γ and IFN-γ-inducing cytokines IL-12 and IL-18 has also been determined with a similar approach using IL-12-/-, IL-18-/- and IFN-gamma-/- mice.[211] Although in vitro evidence has demonstrated that IL-12 and IL-18 have inhibitory effects on osteoclast formation,[212] no difference was found in the infection-stimulated periapical bone resorption between knock-out and wild-type control mice.[211] Therefore, it appears that there is a functional redundancy in proinflammatory pathways.

Hypersensitivity Reactions

Hypersensitivity reactions represent a group of immunological responses where the reaction observed by the host far exceeds that normally triggered in the immune response described before. This results in excessive tissue damage and even death in certain cases. There are four types of immunological hypersensitivity reactions recognized. They vary in their severity and extent from a mild subclinical response to a life-threatening reaction. It is important for the clinician to understand the underlying mechanisms of these conditions in order to recognize and manage these reactions in their patients effectively.

Type I: IgE-mediated degranulation of mast cells and basophils, with release of histamine. This may be either systemic (anaphylaxis) or local (atopy). Type 1 hypersensitivity is fundamentally caused by the initial sensitization of the patient to a particular allergen. Some of the common allergens here include penicillin, certain foods, pollen, and insect bite. Upon exposure to a second challenge to this allergen, cross-linking of IgE on the surface of mast cells occurs, and release of C3a and C5a complement molecules cause degranulation of mast cells and release of inflammatory mediators. The most important of these mediators is histamine; however, other mediators including eicosanoids, Th2 cytokines, and chemokines are released. The patient experiences vasodilatation, which may be local or systemic, as well as bronchoconstriction, which causes wheezing and may cause asphyxia. The patient is considered to have a medical emergency that should be immediately managed with subcutaneous injection of epinephrine. A proportion of patients with chronic exposure to allergens develop asthma.

Type II: Antibody-dependent cytotoxic hypersensitivity. Antigens on the cell surface can cause cell damage through the interaction with inflammatory cells that have Fcγ or C3b receptors. Recall from the discussion of phagocytosis that this reaction primes the microbial surface by opsonins that aid in phagocytosis. In this case, however, phagocytosis does not occur, occasionally because the target is too large for phagocytosis such as for large target cells or in parasitic infections. Examples of type II reactions include blood factor (ABO) or rhesus (Rh) factor incompatibility and autoimmune hemolytic anemia.

Type III: Immune complex-mediated hypersensitivity. Excessive accumulation of antigen–antibody complexes in tissues, such as when there is excessive chronic accumulation of antigen, can stimulate an immune response through phagocyte-, complement-, and/or cytokine-mediated reactions. Frequently, neutrophils and macrophages attempt to perform phagocytosis, but due to the large amount of antigen, such as a microbial colony, they spill their proteases and oxygen- and nitrogen-reactive intermediates in the tissue causing tissue damage. Examples of this reaction include arthus reactions, serum sickness, systemic lupus erythematosus, and immune complex glomerulonephritis.

Type IV: Cell-mediated (delayed-type) hypersensitivity. This reaction is mediated by T_H1, $CD4^+$, or $CD8^+$ cells, causing cytokine-mediated tissue damage. Examples of this reaction include allergic reactions to bacteria, viruses and fungi, contact dermatitis reactions, chronic granulomas such as tuberculosis and leprosy, and the skin tuberculin test (Mantoux reaction) in which subcutaneous administration of antigen causes accumulation of mononuclear inflammatory cells within 24 to 48 hours.

Type V: Stimulatory hypersensitivity. The prime example of this reaction is Graves disease, in which plasma cells continue to produce a self antibody against the thyroid-stimulating hormone (TSH) receptor in the thyroid gland, which itself stimulates the gland to keep producing thyroxine, and does not respond to negative feedback mechanisms.

Innate hypersensitivity reactions. The severe disseminated reaction to LPS in gram-negative bacteria is known as septic shock syndrome. In this reaction, LPS causes the release of systemic cytokines IL-1, TNF-α, and IL-6, which in excessive amounts activate compliment, cause respiratory distress by excess circulating neutrophils, and disseminated intravascular coagulation. More recently, gram-positive septic shock has also been recognized due to enterotoxins of streptococci or staphylococci.

References

1. Goldsby RA, Kindt TJ, Osborne BA. Cells and organs of the immune system. Kuby immunology. 5th ed. New York: W. H. Freeman; 2003.

2. Izumi T, Inoue H, Matsuura H, et al. Changes in the pattern of horseradish peroxidase diffusion into predentin and dentin after cavity preparation in rat molars. Oral Surg Oral Med Oral Pathol Oral Radiol Endod 2001;92(6):675–81.

3. Turner DF, Marfurt CF, Sattelberg C. Demonstration of physiological barrier between pulpal odontoblasts and its perturbation following routine restorative procedures: a horseradish peroxidase tracing study in the rat. J Dent Res 1989;68(8):1262–8.

4. Delves PJ, Martin SJ, Burton DR, Roitt IM. Roitt's essential immunology. 11th ed. Malden, MA: Blackwell Publishing; 2006.

5. Kumar V, Cotran RS, Robbins SL. Robbins basic pathology. 7th ed. Philadelphia, PA: Saunders; Elsevier Science; 2003.

6. Elovic AE, Ohyama H, Sauty A, et al. IL-4-dependent regulation of TGF-alpha and TGF-beta1 expression in human eosinophils. J Immunol 1998;160(12):6121–7.

7. Levi-Schaffer F, Garbuzenko E, Rubin A, et al. Human eosinophils regulate human lung- and skin-derived fibroblast properties in vitro: a role for transforming growth factor beta (TGF-beta). Proc Natl Acad Sci USA 1999;96(17):9660–5.

8. Ohno I, Lea RG, Flanders KC, et al. Eosinophils in chronically inflamed human upper airway tissues express transforming growth factor beta 1 gene (TGF beta 1). J Clin Invest 1992;89(5):1662–8.

9. Tyler LW, Mastossian K, Todd R, et al. Eosinophil-derived transforming growth factors (TGF-alpha and TGF-beta 1) in human periradicular lesions. J Endod 1999;25(9):619–24.

10. Cutler CW, Jotwani R. Dendritic cells at the oral mucosal interface. J Dent Res 2006;85(8):678–89.

11. Jontell M, Gunraj MN, Bergenholtz G. Immunocompetent cells in the normal dental pulp. J Dent Res 1987;66(6):1149–53.

12. Okiji T, Jontell M, Belichenko P, et al. Perivascular dendritic cells of the human dental pulp. Acta Physiol Scand 1997;159(2):163–9.

13. Zhao L, Kaneko T, Okiji T, et al. Immunoelectron microscopic analysis of CD11c-positive dendritic cells in the

periapical region of the periodontal ligament of rat molars. J Endod 2006;32(12):1164–7.

14. Kaneko T, Okiji T, et al. Heterogeneity of dendritic cells in rat apical periodontitis. Cell Tissue Res 2006 (online publication: http://www.springerlink.com/content/01812247gp331163).

15. Kadowaki N, Ho S, Antonenko S, et al. Subsets of human dendritic cell precursors express different toll-like receptors and respond to different microbial antigens. J Exp Med 2001;194(6):863–9.

16. Kusumoto Y, Hirano H, Saitoh K, et al. Human gingival epithelial cells produce chemotactic factors interleukin-8 and monocyte chemoattractant protein-1 after stimulation with *Porphyromonas gingivalis* via toll-like receptor 2. J Periodontol 2004;75(3):370–9.

17. Pazgier M, Hoover DM, Yang D, et al. Human beta-defensins. Cell Mol Life Sci 2006;63(11):1294–313.

18. Huang GT, Chugal N, Potente AP, Zhang X. Constitutive expression of interleukin-8 and intercellular adhesion molecule-1 in human dental pulps. Int J Oral Biol 1999;24(4):163–8.

19. Huang GT, Potente AP, Kim JW, et al. Increased interleukin-8 expression in inflamed human dental pulps. Oral Surg Oral Med Oral Pathol Oral Radiol Endod 1999;88(2):214–20.

20. Dommisch H, Winter J, Acil Y, et al. Human beta-defensin (hBD-1, -2) expression in dental pulp. Oral Microbiol Immunol 2005;20(3):163–6.

21. Durand SH, Flacher V, Romeas A, et al. Lipoteichoic acid increases TLR and functional chemokine expression while reducing dentin formation in in vitro differentiated human odontoblasts. J Immunol 2006;176(5):2880–7.

22. Jiang H-W, Zhang W, Ren B-P, et al. Expression of toll like receptor 4 in normal human odontoblasts and dental pulp tissue. J Endod 2006;32(8):747–51.

23. Janeway CA, Travers P, Walport M, Shlomchik MJ. Immunobiology: the immune system in health and disease. 6th ed. New York: Garland Science; 2005.

24. Hahn CL, Falkler WA Jr, Siegel MA. A study of T and B cells in pulpal pathosis. J Endod 1989;15(1):20–6.

25. Davide A, Carla SRL, Jay B, et al. Cytokines and transcription factors that regulate T helper cell differentiation: new players and new insights. J Clin Immunol 2003;V23(3):147–61.

26. Wynn TA. T(H)-17: a giant step from T(H)1 and T(H)2. Nat Immunol 2005;6(11):1069–70.

27. McKenzie BS, Kastelein RA, Cua DJ. Understanding the IL-23–IL-17 immune pathway. Trends Immunol 2006;27(1):17–23.

28. Dong C. Diversification of T-helper-cell lineages: finding the family root of IL-17-producing cells. Nat Rev 2006;6(4):329–33.

29. O'Garra A, Vieira P. Regulatory T cells and mechanisms of immune system control. Nat Med 2004;10(8):801–5.

30. Damoiseaux J. Regulatory T cells: back to the future. Neth J Med 2006;64(1):4–9.

31. van Oosterhout AJ, Bloksma N. Regulatory T-lymphocytes in asthma. Eur Respir J 2005;26(5):918–32.

32. Izcue A, Coombes JL, Powrie F. Regulatory T cells suppress systemic and mucosal immune activation to control intestinal inflammation. Immunol Rev 2006;212:256–71.

33. Beissert S, Schwarz A, Schwarz T. Regulatory T cells. J Invest Dermatol 2006;126(1):15–24.

34. Bando Y, Henderson B, Meghji S, et al. Immunocytochemical localization of inflammatory cytokines and vascular adhesion receptors in radicular cysts. J Oral Pathol 1993;22(5):221–7.

35. Honma M, Hayakawa Y, Kosugi H, Koizumi F. Localization of mRNA for inflammatory cytokines in radicular cyst tissue by in situ hybridization, and induction of inflammatory cytokines by human gingival fibroblasts in response to radicular cyst contents. J Oral Pathol 1998;27(8):399–404.

36. Lukic A, Vojvodic D, Majstorovic I, Colic M. Production of interleukin-8 in vitro by mononuclear cells isolated from human periapical lesions. Oral Microbiol Immunol 2006;21(5):296–300.

37. Marton IJ, Rot A, Schwarzinger E, et al. Differential in situ distribution of interleukin-8, monocyte chemoattractant protein-1 and Rantes in human chronic periapical granuloma. Oral Microbiol Immunol 2000;15(1):63–5.

38. Kabashima H, Yoneda M, Nagata K, et al. The presence of chemokine receptor (CCR5, CXCR3, CCR3)-positive cells and chemokine (MCP1, MIP-1alpha, MIP-1beta, IP-10)-positive cells in human periapical granulomas. Cytokine 2001;16(2):62–6.

39. Yoshie O, Imai T, Nomiyama H. Chemokines in immunity. Adv Immunol 2001;78:57–110.

40. Fouad A. Molecular mediators of pulpal inflammation. In: Hargreaves KM, Goodis HE, editors. Seltzer and Bender's dental pulp. Surrey, UK: Quintessence Publishing Co., Inc.; 2002. Pp. 247–79.

41. Hall JM. Bradykinin receptors: pharmacological properties and biological roles. Pharmacol Ther 1992;56(2):131–90.

42. Lepinski AM, Haegreaves KM, Goodis HE, Bowles WR. Bradykinin levels in dental pulp by microdialysis. J Endod 2000;26(12):744–7.

43. Goodis H, Saeki K. Identification of bradykinin, substance P, and neurokinin A in human dental pulp. J Endod 1997;23(4):201–4.

44. Lerner UH. Effects of kinins, thrombin, and neuropeptides on bone. In: Gowen M, editor. Cytokines and bone metabolism. Chapter 10. Ann Arbor, MI: CRC Press; 1992.

45. Sundqvist G, Lerner UH. Bradykinin and thrombin synergistically potentiate interleukin 1 and tumour necrosis factor induced prostanoid biosynthesis in human dental pulp fibroblasts. Cytokine 1996;8(2):168–77.

46. Sundqvist G, Rosenquist JB, Lerner UH. Effects of bradykinin and thrombin on prostaglandin formation, cell

proliferation and collagen biosynthesis in human dental-pulp fibroblasts. Arch Oral Biol 1995;40(3):247–56.

47. Swift JQ, Garry MG, Roszkowski MT, Hargreaves KM. Effect of flurbiprofen on tissue levels of immunoreactive bradykinin and acute postoperative pain. J Oral Maxillofac Surg 1993;51(2):112–6; discussion 6–7.

48. Palosaari H, Pennington CJ, Larmas M, et al. Expression profile of matrix metalloproteinases (MMPs) and tissue inhibitors of MMPs in mature human odontoblasts and pulp tissue. Eur J Oral Sci 2003;111(2):117–27.

49. Palosaari H, Wahlgren J, Larmas M, et al. The expression of MMP-8 in human odontoblasts and dental pulp cells is down-regulated by TGF-beta1. J Dent Res 2000;79(1):77–84.

50. Tjaderhane L, Larjava H, Sorsa T, et al. The activation and function of host matrix metalloproteinases in dentin matrix breakdown in caries lesions. J Dent Res 1998;77(8):1622–9.

51. Paakkonen V, Ohlmeier S, Bergmann U, et al. Analysis of gene and protein expression in healthy and carious tooth pulp with cDNA microarray and two-dimensional gel electrophoresis. Eur J Oral Sci 2005;113(5):369–79.

52. Shin SJ, Lee JI, Baek SH, Lim SS. Tissue levels of matrix metalloproteinases in pulps and periapical lesions. J Endod 2002;28(4):313–5.

53. Golub LM, McNamara TF, Ryan ME, et al. Adjunctive treatment with subantimicrobial doses of doxycycline: effects on gingival fluid collagenase activity and attachment loss in adult periodontitis. J Clin Periodontol 2001;28(2):146–56.

54. Ramamurthy NS, Rifkin BR, Greenwald RA, et al. Inhibition of matrix metalloproteinase-mediated periodontal bone loss in rats: a comparison of 6 chemically modified tetracyclines. J Clin Periodontol 2002;73(7):726–34.

55. Fouad AF. Are antibiotics effective for endodontic use? An evidence-based review. Endod Topics 2002;3:52–66.

56. Alptekin NO, Ari H, Ataoglu T, et al. Neutrophil elastase levels in periapical exudates of symptomatic and asymptomatic teeth. J Endod 2005;31(5):350–3.

57. Alptekin NO, Ari H, Haliloglu S, et al. The effect of endodontic therapy on periapical exudate neutrophil elastase and prostaglandin-E2 levels. J Endod 2005;31(11):791–5.

58. Law AS, Baumgardner KR, Meller ST, Gebhart GF. Localization and changes in NADPH-diaphorase reactivity and nitric oxide synthase immunoreactivity in rat pulp following tooth preparation. J Dent Res 1999;78(10):1585–95.

59. Hama S, Takeichi O, Hayashi M, et al. Co-production of vascular endothelial cadherin and inducible nitric oxide synthase by endothelial cells in periapical granuloma. Int Endod J 2006;39(3):179–84.

60. Shimauchi H, Takayama S, Narikawa-Kiji M, et al. Production of interleukin-8 and nitric oxide in human periapical lesions. J Endod 2001;27(12):749–52.

61. Takeichi O, Saito I, Hayashi M, et al. Production of human-inducible nitric oxide synthase in radicular cysts. J Endod 1998;24(3):157–60.

62. Kerezoudis NP, Olgart L, Edwall L. Involvement of substance P but not nitric oxide or calcitonin gene-related peptide in neurogenic plasma extravasation in rat incisor pulp and lip. Arch Oral Biol 1994;39(9):769–74.

63. Di Nardo Di Maio F, Lohinai Z, D'Arcangelo C, et al. Nitric oxide synthase in healthy and inflamed human dental pulp. J Dent Res 2004;83(4):312–16.

64. Yasuhara R, Suzawa T, Miyamoto Y, et al. Nitric oxide in pulp cell growth, differentiation, and mineralization. J Dent Res 2007;86(2):163–8.

65. Davis WL, Jacoby BH, Craig KR, et al. Copper–zinc superoxide dismutase activity in normal and inflamed human dental pulp tissue. J Endod 1991;17(7):316–18.

66. Tulunoglu O, Alacam A, Bastug M, Yavuzer S. Superoxide dismutase activity in healthy and inflamed pulp tissues of permanent teeth in children. J Clin Ped Dent 1998;22(4):341–5.

67. Baumgardner KR, Law AS, Gebhart GF. Localization and changes in superoxide dismutase immunoreactivity in rat pulp after tooth preparation. Oral Surg Oral Med Oral Pathol Oral Radiol Endod 1999;88(4):488–95.

68. Baumgardner KR, Sulfaro MA. The anti-inflammatory effects of human recombinant copper–zinc superoxide dismutase on pulp inflammation. J Endod 2001;27(3):190–5.

69. Varvara G, Traini T, Esposito P, et al. Copper–zinc superoxide dismutase activity in healthy and inflamed human dental pulp. Int Endod J 2005;38(3):195–9.

70. Bodor C, Matolcsy A, Bernath M. Elevated expression of Cu, Zn-SOD and Mn-SOD mRNA in inflamed dental pulp tissue. Int Endod J 2007;40(2):128–32.

71. Riggs BL. The mechanisms of estrogen regulation of bone resorption. J Clin Invest 2000;106(10):1203–4.

72. Hofbauer LC, Khosla S, Dunstan CR, et al. The roles of osteoprotegerin and osteoprotegerin ligand in the paracrine regulation of bone resorption. J Bone Miner Res 2000;15(1):2–12.

73. Reinke E, Fabry Z. Breaking or making immunological privilege in the central nervous system: the regulation of immunity by neuropeptides. Immunol Lett 2006;104(1–2):102–9.

74. Gonzalez-Rey E, Chorny A, Delgado M. Regulation of immune tolerance by anti-inflammatory neuropeptides. Nat Rev 2007;7(1):52–63.

75. Brain SD, Cox HM. Neuropeptides and their receptors: innovative science providing novel therapeutic targets. Br J Pharmacol 2006;147 (Suppl 1):S202–11.

76. Wakisaka S, Akai M. Immunohistochemical observation on neuropeptides around the blood vessel in feline dental pulp. J Endod 1989;15(9):413–16.

77. Okiji T, Jontell M, Belichenko P, et al. Structural and functional association between substance P- and calcitonin gene-

related peptide-immunoreactive nerves and accessory cells in the rat dental pulp. J Dent Res 1997;76(12):1818–24.

78. Kimberly CL, Byers MR. Inflammation of rat molar pulp and periodontium causes increased calcitonin gene-related peptide and axonal sprouting. Anat Rec 1988;222(3):289–300.

79. Byers MR. Effects of inflammation on dental sensory nerves and vice versa. Proc Finn Dent Soc 1992;88(Suppl 1): 499–506.

80. Grutzner EH, Garry MG, Hargreaves KM. Effect of injury on pulpal levels of immunoreactive substance P and immunoreactive calcitonin gene-related peptide. J Endod 1992; 18(11):553–7.

81. Calland JW, Harris SE, Carnes DL Jr. Human pulp cells respond to calcitonin gene-related peptide in vitro. J Endod 1997;23(8):485–9.

82. Gazelius B, Edwall B, Olgart L, et al. Vasodilatory effects and coexistence of calcitonin gene-related peptide (CGRP) and substance P in sensory nerves of cat dental pulp. Acta Physiol Scand 1987;130(1):33–40.

83. Hargreaves KM, Swift JQ, Roszkowski MT, et al. Pharmacology of peripheral neuropeptide and inflammatory mediator release. Oral Surg Oral Med Oral Pathol Oral Radiol Endod 1994;78(4):503–10.

84. Rodd HD, Boissonade FM. Substance P expression in human tooth pulp in relation to caries and pain experience [In Process Citation]. Eur J Oral Sci 2000;108(6):467–74.

85. Todd WM, Kafrawy AH, Newton CW, Brown CE Jr. Immunohistochemical study of gamma-aminobutyric acid and bombesin/gastrin releasing peptide in human dental pulp. J Endod 1997;23(3):152–7.

86. Gibbs J, Flores CM, Hargreaves KM. Neuropeptide Y inhibits capsaicin-sensitive nociceptors via a Y1-receptor-mediated mechanism. Neuroscience 2004;125(3):703–9.

87. Jaber L, Swaim WD, Dionne RA. Immunohistochemical localization of mu-opioid receptors in human dental pulp. J Endod 2003;29(2):108–10.

88. Wadachi R, Hargreaves KM. Trigeminal nociceptors express TLR-4 and CD14: a mechanism for pain due to infection. J Dent Res 2006;85(1):49–53.

89. Payan DG. Neuropeptides and inflammation: the role of substance P. Ann Rev Med 1989;40:341–52.

90. Brain SD. Sensory neuropeptides: their role in inflammation and wound healing. Immunopharmacology 1997;37 (2–3):133–52.

91. Goodis HE, Bowles WR, Hargreaves KM. Prostaglandin E2 enhances bradykinin-evoked iCGRP release in bovine dental pulp. J Dent Res 2000;79(8):1604–7.

92. Gibbs JL, Diogenes A, Hargreaves KM. Neuropeptide Y modulates effects of bradykinin and prostaglandin E(2) on trigeminal nociceptors via activation of the Y(1) and Y(2) receptors. Br J Pharm 2007;150(1):72–9.

93. Fried K. Changes in pulpal nerves with aging. Proc Finn Dent Soc 1992;88(Suppl 1):517–28.

94. Akira S, Uematsu S, Takeuchi O. Pathogen recognition and innate immunity. Cell 2006;124(4):783–801.

95. Uematsu S, Akira S. The role of Toll-like receptors in immune disorders. Expert Opin Biol Ther 2006;6(3):203–14.

96. Huang GT, Zhang HB, Yin C, Park SH. Human beta-defensin-2 gene transduction of dental pulp cells: a model for pulp antimicrobial gene therapy. Int J Oral Biol 2004; 29(1):7–12.

97. Joly S, Maze C, McCray PB Jr, Guthmiller JM. Human beta-defensins 2 and 3 demonstrate strain-selective activity against oral microorganisms. J Clin Microbiol 2004;42(3):1024–9.

98. Yin C, Dang HN, Gazor F, Huang GT. Mouse salivary glands and human beta-defensin-2 as a study model for antimicrobial gene therapy: technical considerations. Int J Antimicrob Agents 2006;28(4):352–60.

99. Yin C, Dang HN, Zhang HB, et al. Capacity of human beta-defensin expression in gene-transduced and cytokine-induced cells. Biochem Biophys Res Commun 2006;339(1):344–54.

100. Harder J, Meyer-Hoffert U, Wehkamp K, et al. Differential gene induction of human beta-defensins (hBD-1, -2, -3, and -4) in keratinocytes is inhibited by retinoic acid. J Invest Dermatol 2004;123(3):522–9.

101. Harder J, Schroder JM. Psoriatic scales: a promising source for the isolation of human skin-derived antimicrobial proteins. J Leukoc Biol 2005;77(4):476–86.

102. Jia HP, Schutte BC, Schudy A, et al. Discovery of new human beta-defensins using a genomics-based approach. Gene 2001;263(1–2):211–18.

103. Premratanachai P, Joly S, Johnson GK, et al. Expression and regulation of novel human beta-defensins in gingival keratinocytes. Oral Microbiol Immunol 2004;19(2):111–17.

104. Feucht EC, DeSanti CL, Weinberg A. Selective induction of human beta-defensin mRNAs by *Actinobacillus actinomycetemcomitans* in primary and immortalized oral epithelial cells. Oral Microbiol Immunol 2003;18(6):359–63.

105. Bergenholtz G, Wikesjo UM, Sorensen RG, et al. Observations on healing following endodontic surgery in nonhuman primates (*Macaca fascicularis*): effects of rhBMP-2. Oral Surg Oral Med Oral Pathol Oral Radiol Endod 2006;101(1):116–25.

106. Chen D, Zhao M, Mundy GR. Bone morphogenetic proteins. Growth Factors 2004;22(4):233–41.

107. He J, Jiang J, Safavi KE, et al. Emdogain promotes osteoblast proliferation and differentiation and stimulates osteoprotegerin expression. Oral Surg Oral Med Oral Pathol Oral Radiol Endod 2004;97(2):239–45.

108. Hughes FJ, Turner W, Belibasakis G, Martuscelli G. Effects of growth factors and cytokines on osteoblast differentiation. Periodontology 2000 2006;41:48–72.

109. Jiang J, Fouad AF, Safavi KE, et al. Effects of enamel matrix derivative on gene expression of primary osteoblasts. Oral

Surg Oral Med Oral Pathol Oral Radiol Endod 2001;91(1):95–100.

110. Werner H, Katz J. The emerging role of the insulin-like growth factors in oral biology. J Dent Res 2004;83(11):832–6.

111. Smith AJ. Vitality of the dentin-pulp complex in health and disease: growth factors as key mediators. J Dent Educ 2003;67(6):678–89.

112. Rutherford RB. BMP-7 gene transfer to inflamed ferret dental pulps. Eur J Oral Sci 2001;109(6):422–4.

113. Rutherford RB, Gu K. Treatment of inflamed ferret dental pulps with recombinant bone morphogenetic protein-7. Eur J Oral Sci 2000;108(3):202–6.

114. Rutherford RB, Spangberg L, Tucker M, Rueger D, Charette M. The time-course of the induction of reparative dentine formation in monkeys by recombinant human osteogenic protein-1. Arch Oral Biol 1994;39(10):833–8.

115. Sloan AJ, Rutherford RB, Smith AJ. Stimulation of the rat dentin–pulp complex by bone morphogenetic protein-7 in vitro. Arch Oral Biol 2000;45(2):173–7.

116. D'Souza RN, Cavender A, Dickinson D, et al. TGF-beta1 is essential for the homeostasis of the dentin–pulp complex. Eur J Oral Sci 1998;106(Suppl 1):185–91.

117. Farges JC, Romeas A, Melin M, et al. TGF-beta1 induces accumulation of dendritic cells in the odontoblast layer. J Dent Res 2003;82(8):652–6.

118. Nakashima M, Akamine A. The application of tissue engineering to regeneration of pulp and dentin in endodontics. J Endod 2005;31(10):711–18.

119. Sloan AJ, Smith AJ. Stimulation of the dentine-pulp complex of rat incisor teeth by transforming growth factor-beta isoforms 1-3 in vitro. Arch Oral Biol 1999;44(2):149–56.

120. Tziafas D. The future role of a molecular approach to pulp-dentinal regeneration. Caries Res 2004;38(3):314–20.

121. Jiang J, Goodarzi G, He J, et al. Emdogain-gel stimulates proliferation of odontoblasts and osteoblasts. Oral Surg Oral Med Oral Pathol Oral Radiol Endod 2006;102(5):698–702.

122. Nakashima M. Induction of dentin formation on canine amputated pulp by recombinant human bone morphogenetic proteins (BMP)-2 and -4. J Dent Res 1994;73(9):1515–22.

123. Rutherford RB, Wahle J, Tucker M, et al. Induction of reparative dentine formation in monkeys by recombinant human osteogenic protein-1. Arch Oral Biol 1993;38(7):571–6.

124. Buurma B, Gu K, Rutherford RB. Transplantation of human pulpal and gingival fibroblasts attached to synthetic scaffolds. Eur J Oral Sci 1999;107(4):282–9.

125. Derringer KA, Linden RW. Vascular endothelial growth factor, fibroblast growth factor 2, platelet derived growth factor and transforming growth factor beta released in human dental pulp following orthodontic force. Arch Oral Biol 2004;49(8):631–41.

126. Caviedes-Bucheli J, Munoz HR, Rodriguez CE, et al. Expression of insulin-like growth factor-1 receptor in human pulp tissue. J Endod 2004;30(11):767–9.

127. Ohnishi T, Suwa M, Oyama T, et al. Prostaglandin E2 predominantly induces production of hepatocyte growth factor/scatter factor in human dental pulp in acute inflammation. J Dent Res 2000;79(2):748–55.

128. Matsushita K, Motani R, Sakuta T, et al. The role of vascular endothelial growth factor in human dental pulp cells: induction of chemotaxis, proliferation, and differentiation and activation of the AP-1-dependent signaling pathway. J Dent Res 2000;79(8):1596–603.

129. Lin SK, Hong CY, Chang HH, et al. Immunolocalization of macrophages and transforming growth factor-beta 1 in induced rat periapical lesions. J Endod 2000;26(6):335–40.

130. Lin LM, Wang SL, Wu-Wang C, et al. Detection of epidermal growth factor receptor in inflammatory periapical lesions. Int Endod J 1996;29(3):179–84.

131. Derringer KA, Jaggers DC, Linden RW. Angiogenesis in human dental pulp following orthodontic tooth movement. J Dent Res 1996;75(10):1761–6.

132. Serhan CN. Mediator lipidomics. Prostaglandins Other Lipid Mediat 2005;77(1–4):4–14.

133. Serhan CN. Lipoxins and aspirin-triggered 15-epi-lipoxins are the first lipid mediators of endogenous anti-inflammation and resolution. Prostaglandins Leukot Essent Fatty Acids 2005;73(3–4):141–62.

134. Serhan CN. Novel eicosanoid and docosanoid mediators: resolvins, docosatrienes, and neuroprotectins. Curr Opin Clin Nutr Metab Care 2005;8(2):115–21.

135. Serhan CN. Novel omega-3-derived local mediators in anti-inflammation and resolution. Pharmacol Ther 2005;105(1):7–21.

136. Serhan CN, Savill J. Resolution of inflammation: the beginning programs the end. Nat Immunol 2005;6(12):1191–7.

137. Cook JA. Eicosanoids. Crit Care Med 2005;33(12 Suppl):S488–91.

138. Fierro IM, Serhan CN. Mechanisms in anti-inflammation and resolution: the role of lipoxins and aspirin-triggered lipoxins. Braz J Med Biol Res 2001;34(5):555–66.

139. Pelletier JP, Boileau C, Boily M, et al. The protective effect of licofelone on experimental osteoarthritis is correlated with the down regulation of gene expression and protein synthesis of several major cartilage catabolic factors: MMP-13, cathepsin K and aggrecanases. Arthritis Res Ther 2005;7(5):R1091–102.

140. Steinke JW, Borish L. 3. Cytokines and chemokines. J Allergy Clin Immunol 2006 Feb;117(2 Suppl Mini-Primer):S441–5.

141. Mocellin S, Marincola FM. The challenge of implementing high-throughput technologies in clinical trials. Pharmacogenomics 2005;6(4):435–8.

142. Mocellin S, Marincola FM, Young HA. Interleukin-10 and the immune response against cancer: a counterpoint. J Leukoc Biol 2005;78(5):1043–51.

143. Steinke JW, Borish L. Genetics of allergic disease. Med Clin North Am 2006;90(1):1–15.

144. Ohtsuka Y, Sanderson IR. Transforming growth factor-beta: an important cytokine in the mucosal immune response. Curr Opin Gastroenterol 2000;16(6):541–5.

145. Li J, Leschka S, Rutschow S, et al. Immunomodulation by interleukin-4 suppresses matrix metalloproteinases and improves cardiac function in murine myocarditis. Euro J Pharma. [In Press, Corrected Proof]

146. Schindler R, Mancilla J, Endres S, et al. Correlations and interactions in the production of interleukin-6 (IL-6), IL-1, and tumor necrosis factor (TNF) in human blood mononuclear cells: IL-6 suppresses IL-1 and TNF. Blood 1990;75(1):40–7.

147. Akira S, Takeda K. Toll-like receptor signalling. Nat Rev 2004;4(7):499–511.

148. Schein B, Schilder H. Endotoxin content in endodontically involved teeth. J Endod 1975;1(1):19–21.

149. Schonfeld SE, Greening AB, Glick DH, et al. Endotoxic activity in periapical lesions. Oral Surg Oral Med Oral Pathol Oral Radiol Endod 1982;53:82–7.

150. Moller AJ, Fabricius L, Dahlen G, et al. Influence on periapical tissues of indigenous oral bacteria and necrotic pulp tissue in monkeys. Scand J Dent Res 1981;89(6):475–84.

151. Dwyer TG, Torabinejad M. Radiographic and histologic evaluation of the effect of endotoxin on the periapical tissues of the cat. J Endod 1980;7(1):31–5.

152. Poltorak A, He X, Smirnova I, et al. Defective LPS signaling in C3H/HeJ and C57BL/10ScCr mice: mutations in Tlr4 gene. Science 1998;282(5396):2085–8.

153. Shimazu R, Akashi S, Ogata H, et al. MD-2, a molecule that confers lipopolysaccharide responsiveness on Toll-like receptor 4. J Exp Med 1999;189(11):1777–82.

154. Thammasitboon K, Goldring SR, Boch JA. Role of macrophages in LPS-induced osteoblast and PDL cell apoptosis. Bone 2006 Jun; 38(6):845–52.

155. Gloire G, Legrand-Poels S, Piette J. NF-κB activation by reactive oxygen species: Fifteen years later. Biochem Pharmacol 2006; 72(11):1493–505.

156. Bhaskar SN. Oral surgery—oral pathology conference No. 17, Walter Reed Army Medical Center. Periapical lesions—types, incidence, and clinical features. Oral Surg Oral Med Oral Pathol Oral Radiol Endod 1966;21(5):657–71.

157. Lalonde ER, Luebke RG. The frequency and distribution of periapical cysts and granulomas. An evaluation of 800 specimens. Oral Surg Oral Med Oral Pathol Oral Radiol Endod 1968;25(6):861–8.

158. Priebe WA, Lazansky JP, Wuehrmann AH. The value of the roentgenographic film in the differential diagnosis of periapical lesions. Oral Surg Oral Med Oral Pathol Oral Radiol Endod 1954;7(9):979–83.

159. Block RM, Bushell A, Rodrigues H, Langeland K. A histopathologic, histobacteriologic, and radiographic study of periapical endodontic surgical specimens. Oral Surg Oral Med Oral Pathol Oral Radiol Endod 1976;42(5):656–78.

160. Patterson SS, Shafer WG, Healey HJ. Periapical lesions associated with endodontically treated teeth. J Am Dent Assoc 1964;68:191–4.

161. Stockdale CR, Chandler NP. The nature of the periapical lesion—a review of 1108 cases. J Dent 1988;16(3):123–9.

162. Ramachandran Nair PN, Pajarola G, Schroeder HE. Types and incidence of human periapical lesions obtained with extracted teeth. Oral Surg Oral Med Oral Pathol Oral Radiol Endod 1996;81(1):93–102.

163. Nair PN. On the causes of persistent apical periodontitis: a review. Int Endod J 2006;39(4):249–81.

164. Mizuno N, Shiba H, Mouri Y, et al. Characterization of epithelial cells derived from periodontal ligament by gene expression patterns of bone-related and enamel proteins. Cell Biol Int 2005;29(2):111–17.

165. Kakehashi S, Stanley HR, Fitzgerald RJ. The effects of surgical exposures of dental pulps in germfree and conventional laboratory rats. Oral Surg Oral Med Oral Pathol Oral Radiol Endod 1965;20:340–8.

166. Cook DN, Pisetsky DS, Schwartz DA. Toll-like receptors in the pathogenesis of human disease. Nat Immunol 2004;5(10):975–9.

167. Hou L, Sasaki H, Stashenko P. Toll-like receptor 4-deficient mice have reduced bone destruction following mixed anaerobic infection. Infect Immun 2000;68(8):4681–7.

168. Fouad AF, Acosta AW. Periapical lesion progression and cytokine expression in an LPS hyporesponsive model. Int Endod J 2001;34(7):506–13.

169. Huang GT, Do M, Wingard M, et al. Effect of interleukin-6 deficiency on the formation of periapical lesions after pulp exposure in mice. Oral Surg Oral Med Oral Pathol Oral Radiol Endod 2001;92(1):83–8.

170. Echchannaoui H, Frei K, Schnell C, et al. Toll-like receptor 2-deficient mice are highly susceptible to *Streptococcus pneumoniae meningitis* because of reduced bacterial clearing and enhanced inflammation. J Infect Dis 2002;186(6):798–806.

171. Takeuchi O, Hoshino K, Akira S. Cutting edge: TLR2-deficient and MyD88-deficient mice are highly susceptible to *Staphylococcus aureus* infection. J Immunol 2000;165(10):5392–6.

172. Kayaoglu G, Orstavik D. Virulence factors of *Enterococcus faecalis*: relationship to endodontic disease. Crit Rev Oral Biol Med 2004;15(5):308–20.

173. Niederman R, Westernoff T, Lee C, et al. Infection-mediated early-onset periodontal disease in P/E-selectin-deficient mice. J Clin Periodontol 2001;28(6):569–75.

174. Liapatas S, Nakou M, Rontogianni D. Inflammatory infiltrate of chronic periradicular lesions: an immunohistochemical study. Int Endod J 2003;36(7):464–71.

175. Torabinejad M, Kettering JD. Identification and relative concentration of B and T lymphocytes in human chronic periapical lesions. J Endod 1985;11(3):122–5.

176. Wang CY, Stashenko P. Kinetics of bone-resorbing activity in developing periapical lesions. J Dent Res 1991;70(10):1362–6.

177. Stashenko P, Yu SM, Wang CY. Kinetics of immune cell and bone resorptive responses to endodontic infections. J Endod 1992;18(9):422–6.

178. Stashenko P, Wang CY. Characterization of bone resorptive mediators in active periapical lesions. Proc Finn Dent Soc 1992;88 (Suppl 1):427–32.

179. Stashenko P, Yu SM. T helper and T suppressor cell reversal during the development of induced rat periapical lesions. J Dent Res 1989;68(5):830–4.

180. Wallstrom JB, Torabinejad M, Kettering J, McMillan P. Role of T cells in the pathogenesis of periapical lesions. A preliminary report. Oral Surg Oral Med Oral Pathol Oral Radiol Endod 1993;76(2):213–18.

181. Tani N, Kuchiba K, Osada T, et al. Effect of T-cell deficiency on the formation of periapical lesions in mice: histological comparison between periapical lesion formation in BALB/c and BALB/c nu/nu mice. J Endod 1995;21(4):195–9.

182. Fouad AF. IL-1 alpha and TNF-alpha expression in early periapical lesions of normal and immunodeficient mice. J Dent Res 1997;76(9):1548–54.

183. Teles R, Wang CY, Stashenko P. Increased susceptibility of RAG-2 SCID mice to dissemination of endodontic infections. Infect Immun 1997;65(9):3781–7.

184. Hou L, Sasakj H, Stashenko P. B-Cell deficiency predisposes mice to disseminating anaerobic infections: protection by passive antibody transfer. Infect Immun 2000;68(10):5645–51.

185. Sabeti M, Simon J, Kermani V, et al. Detection of receptor activator of NF-kappa beta ligand in apical periodontitis J Endod 2005;31(1):17–18.

186. Vernal R, Chaparro A, Graumann R, et al. Levels of cytokine receptor activator of nuclear factor kappaB ligand in gingival crevicular fluid in untreated chronic periodontitis patients. J Periodontol 2004;75(12):1586–91.

187. Zhang X, Peng B. Immunolocalization of receptor activator of NF kappa B ligand in rat periapical lesions. J Endod 2005;31(8):574–7.

188. Xing L, Schwarz EM, Boyce BF. Osteoclast precursors, RANKL/RANK, and immunology. Immunol Rev 2005;208:19–29.

189. Boyce BF, Li P, Yao Z, et al. TNF-alpha and pathologic bone resorption. Keio J Med 2005;54(3):127–31.

190. Yao Z, Li P, Zhang Q, et al. Tumor necrosis factor-alpha increases circulating osteoclast precursor numbers by promoting their proliferation and differentiation in the bone marrow through up-regulation of c-Fms expression. J Biol Chem 2006;281(17):11846–55.

191. Kuntz KA, Brown CE Jr, Legan JJ, Kafrawy AH. An immunohistochemical study of osteoprotegerin in the human dental pulp. J Endod 2001;27(11):666–9.

192. Hasegawa T, Yoshimura Y, Kikuiri T, et al. Expression of receptor activator of NF-kappa B ligand and osteoprotegerin in culture of human periodontal ligament cells. J Periodont Res 2002;37(6):405–11.

193. Kanzaki H, Chiba M, Shimizu Y, Mitani H. Dual regulation of osteoclast differentiation by periodontal ligament cells through RANKL stimulation and OPG inhibition. J Dent Res 2001;80(3):887–91.

194. Bezerra MC, Carvalho JF, Prokopowitsch AS, Pereira RM. RANK, RANKL and osteoprotegerin in arthritic bone loss. Braz J Med Biol Res 2005;38(2):161–70.

195. Gyurko R, Shoji H, Battaglino RA, et al. Inducible nitric oxide synthase mediates bone development and P. gingivalis-induced alveolar bone loss. Bone 2005;36(3):472–9.

196. Romas E. Bone loss in inflammatory arthritis: mechanisms and therapeutic approaches with bisphosphonates. Best Pract Res Clin Rheumatol 2005;19(6):1065–79.

197. Marx RE. Pamidronate (Aredia) and zoledronate (Zometa) induced avascular necrosis of the jaws: a growing epidemic. J Oral Maxillofac Surg 2003;61(9):1115–17.

198. Melo MD, Obeid G. Osteonecrosis of the jaws in patients with a history of receiving bisphosphonate therapy: strategies for prevention and early recognition. J Am Dent Assoc 2005;136(12):1675–81.

199. Sarathy AP, Bourgeois SL Jr, Goodell GG. Bisphosphonate-associated osteonecrosis of the jaws and endodontic treatment: two case reports. J Endod 2005;31(10):759–63.

200. Walker KF, Lappin DF, Takahashi K, et al. Cytokine expression in periapical granulation tissue as assessed by immunohistochemistry. Eur J Oral Sci 2000;108(3):195–201.

201. de Sa AR, Pimenta FJ, Dutra WO, Gomez RS. Immunolocalization of sinterleukin 4, interleukin 6, and lymphotoxin alpha in dental granulomas. Oral Surg Oral Med Oral Pathol Oral Radiol Endod 2003;96(3):356–60.

202. Bsarkhordar RA, Hayashi C, Hussain MZ. Detection of interleukin-6 in human dental pulp and periapical lesions. Endod Dent Traumatol 1999;15(1):26–7.

203. Ishimi Y, Miyaura C, Jin CH, et al. IL-6 is produced by osteoblasts and induces bone resorption. J Immunol 1990;145(10):3297–303.

204. Kawashima N, Stashenko P. Expression of bone-resorptive and regulatory cytokines in murine periapical inflammation. Arch Oral Biol 1999;44(1):55–66.

205. Stashenko P, Teles R, D'Souza R. Periapical inflammatory responses and their modulation. Crit Rev Oral Biol Med 1998;9(4):498–521.

206. Takahashi K. Microbiological, pathological, inflammatory, immunological and molecular biological aspects of periradicular disease. Int Endod J 1998;31(5):311–25.

207. Chen CP, Hertzberg M, Jiang Y, Graves DT. Interleukin-1 and tumor necrosis factor receptor signaling is not required for bacteria-induced osteoclastogenesis and bone loss but is essential for protecting the host from a mixed anaerobic infection. Am J Pathol 1999;155(6):2145–52.

208. Balto K, Sasaki H, Stashenko P. Interleukin-6 deficiency increases inflammatory bone destruction. Infect Immun 2001;69(2):744–50.

209. Graves DT, Chen CP, Douville C, Jiang Y. Interleukin-1 receptor signaling rather than that of tumor necrosis factor is critical in protecting the host from the severe consequences of a polymicrobe anaerobic infection. Infect Immun 2000;68(8):4746–51.

210. Sasaki H, Hou L, Belani A, et al. IL-10, but not IL-4, suppresses infection-stimulated bone resorption in vivo. J Immunol 2000;165(7):3626–30.

211. Sasaki H, Balto K, Kawashima N, et al. Gamma interferon (IFN-gamma) and IFN-gamma-inducing cytokines interleukin-12 (IL-12) and IL-18 do not augment infection-stimulated bone resorption in vivo. Clin Diagn Lab Immunol 2004;11(1):106–10.

212. Horwood NJ, Elliott J, Martin TJ, Gillespie MT. IL-12 alone and in synergy with IL-18 inhibits osteoclast formation in vitro. J Immunol 2001;166(8):4915–21.

Chapter 10

Mechanisms of Odontogenic and Non-odontogenic Pain

Jennifer L. Gibbs, Kenneth M. Hargreaves

Overview of the Trigeminal Pain System

Perceived association of pain with endodontic therapy represents a source of fear for many of our patients and equally represents a meaningful challenge to many practitioners. However, considerable and ongoing research now provides a solid framework for understanding the biological basis of odontogenic and non-odontogenic pain. Moreover, it is our belief that effective diagnosis and treatment flows from this conceptual framework. Accordingly, this chapter provides a comprehensive review of pain mechanisms that forms the basis for clinical recommendations of the diagnosis and management of orofacial pain detailed in other chapters (see Chapters 11 and 21).

Organization and Function of the Peripheral Trigeminal Pain System

A fundamental function of the peripheral nervous system is detecting the magnitude, quality, location, and temporal characteristics of innocuous (light touch, vibration, warm, and cool) and noxious (thermal, mechanical, and chemical) sensory input. This detection is mediated by receptors expressed on subclasses of primary afferent neurons that are activated by various stimuli,[1] leading to intracellular changes. As detailed below, these intracellular changes may activate neurons, inhibit neurons, or alter their responsiveness to subsequent stimuli. The cell bodies of nearly all nociceptive neurons innervating the oral and craniofacial region are found in the trigeminal ganglia. The cell body is classically viewed where protein synthesis of receptors as well as peptidergic neurotransmitters takes place (Figure 1), although emerging evidence now points to protein synthesis occurring at terminal endings as well.[2] The synthesis of receptors and peptidergic neurotransmitters by the trigeminal ganglia is a dynamic process that is very sensitive to injury and inflammation detected in the peripheral terminals. For example, animal studies have demonstrated the amount of certain neurotransmitters such as neuropeptide Y, substance P (SP), and galanin detected in the trigeminal ganglia will change dramatically after a peripheral injury such as a tooth extraction or pulpitis.[3,4] Moreover, nerve injury induces a rapid trafficking of sodium channels from the cell body out to the terminal endings.[5] Collectively, these studies demonstrate the potential for striking plasticity of the sensory neurons in response to tissue injury or inflammation.

As illustrated in Figure 1, the pain system can be conceptualized as having three main organizational elements: *detection*, *processing*, and *perception*. Although the anatomical basis is considerably more complex than illustrated, and still incompletely understood, this model provides a framework for interpretation of experimental findings and for developing a biological basis for pain diagnoses and pain management strategies.

Upon detection of an appropriate stimulus, primary afferent neurons encode this information by the frequency and temporal characteristics (e.g., duration) of action potential discharge, and this digitized information is conveyed to second-order neurons by the release of neurotransmitters such as glutamate, SP and calcitonin gene-related peptide (CGRP) from the central terminal of the primary afferent neuron. In addition to the central release of neurotransmitters, primary afferent neurons also release these substances from the peripheral terminals located in dental pulp and periradicular tissue.[6–14] Several dental pulp

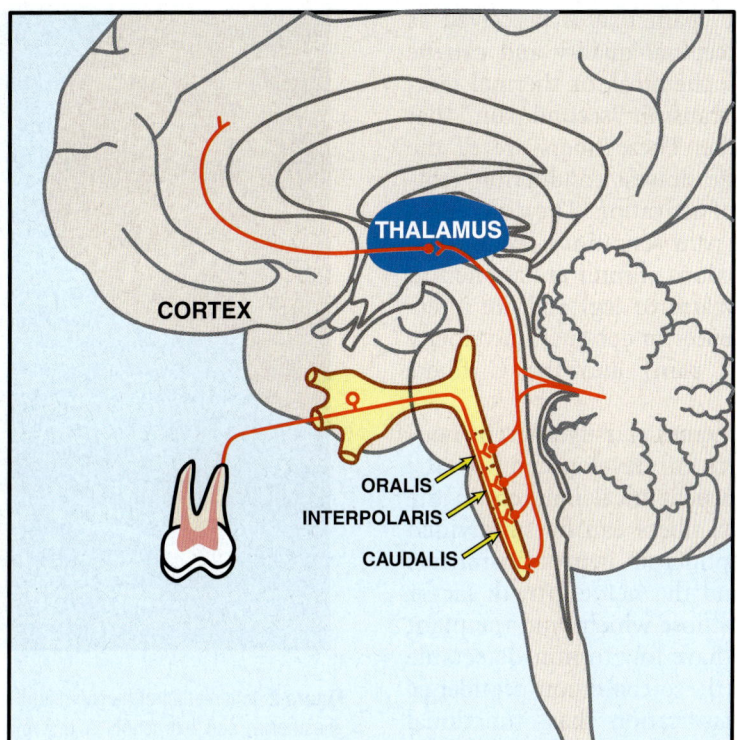

Figure 1 A conceptual model for the trigeminal pain system. Acute dental pain is due to detection of peripheral stimuli by sensory nociceptive neurons that innervate teeth and the periodontal ligament and convey information on stimulus intensity, location, and duration to the nuclei oralis, interpolaris, and caudalis of the trigeminal brainstem complex. Considerable processing occurs in these central sites leading to either an amplification of the nociceptive signal (e.g., central sensitization) or an inhibition of the signal (due to activity of endogenous analgesic systems). Finally, nociceptive information is integrated in cortical structures with affective, psychosocial, and other cognitive elements resulting in the perception of pain.

studies have demonstrated the presence, as well as the stimulated release, of SP and CGRP.[15–18] The release of theses peptides is important for causing vasodilation and plasma extravasation and is critical for the recruitment of immune cells to the site of injury.

With advancements in neuroscience research, the classification of peripheral sensory neurons has become increasingly complex. The classic scheme for categorizing neurons was based historically on the diameter and the amount of myelination of the neurons as well as their conduction velocity, which is a function of both of these factors. Based on this classification system, we can identify three broad categories of primary afferents (Table 1). The Aβ class of sensory neurons is heavily myelinated and has a large diameter that allows for rapid transmission of information to the central nervous system. This fiber class detects stimuli such as touch, vibration, and pressure. Although the Aβ class of afferent fibers is classically described as conveying innocuous mechanical stimuli, it should be recognized that they innervate dentinal tubules and are capable of encoding stimuli that induce dentinal pain in humans and, in addition, may be important in certain chronic pain conditions.[19–22] The two classic neuronal categories of nociceptors are the Aδ and the C fibers. The Aδ class of primary afferents has a smaller diameter than the Aβ class, is lightly myelinated, and has a higher threshold of activation. These neurons function in

Table 1 Classification Scheme of Peripheral Neurons

Fiber	Function	Size (μm)	Conduction Velocity (m/s)
Aα	Motor, proprioceptor	12–20	60–120
Aβ	Touch, pressure	5–10	35–70
Aγ	Muscle spindles	3–6	15–30
Aδ	Pain, temperature, touch	2–5	12–30
B	Pre-ganglionic autonomic nervous system (ANS)	<3	3–15
C	Pain, sympathetic	0.5–1	0.5–2

the transmission of "first" pain that is perceived as sharp or "bright" in perceptual quality and can be stimulated by mechanical, chemical, or thermal noxious stimuli. The C fibers transmit "second pain" that is perceived as a dull ache. These fibers are of the smallest diameter, have the slowest conduction velocity, and a high threshold of activation. The differences between first and second pain sensations are derived from studies in which noxious stimuli are applied to peripheral tissues (usually arm or leg) and are interpreted to be due to differences in conduction velocity between the Aδ ("first" pain) and the C fibers ("second" pain).

More contemporary schemes classify afferent neurons based upon genetics of development or the expression of certain neurochemical markers in the adult.[23,24] For example, C fibers can be subdivided into those expressing peptidergic neurotransmitters such as CGRP and SP and the nerve growth factor (NGF) receptor trkA and those which bind the plant lectin, IB4, and generally have low to non-detectable amounts of CGRP and SP (the so-called non-peptidergic nociceptors).[25] This classification has functional significance as the trkA subpopulation is thought to primarily encode inflammatory pain while the IB4 subpopulation is thought to be more responsible for neuropathic pain.[26] This finding is of clear endodontic significance as the development of pulpal necrosis represents a unique tissue condition that has some similarity to both inflammatory and neuropathic pain conditions.[27] In addition, this neurochemical classification has a correlation with the anatomic organization of the central terminals of these neurons in the spinal and medullary dorsal horns.[23,28,29] However, the relative contribution of the trkA and IB4 subpopulations of nociceptors in mediating odontogenic pain over the course of pulpitis to pulpal necrosis still remains unclear. Interestingly, the dental pulp is apparently unique in which the IB4 population of C fibers represents a much lower proportion of the neurons compared to other peripheral tissues such as skin.[30]

Innervation of the Pulp–Dentin Complex

Given that pain is the dominant, although not exclusive,[31] sensory modality elicited by stimulation of the pulpodentin complex, it is not surprising that the dental pulp is densely innervated by nociceptive sensory neurons.[20,32–35] Sensory neurons in the dental pulp travel in nerve bundles through the apical and midroot portions of the pulp and then branch exten-

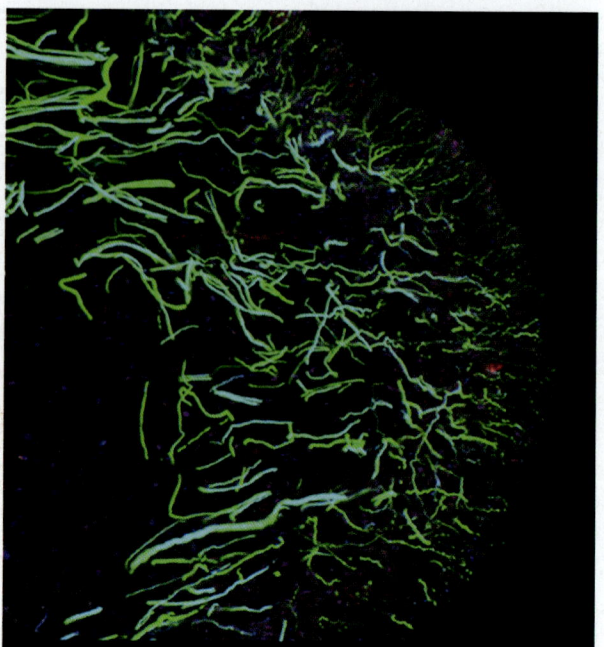

Figure 2 Innervation of human dental pulp. Following informed consent, anesthesia, and extraction, a first molar was split and processed for immunohistochemistry using antibodies directed to nerve filament proteins (N52 and PGP9.5), and the image of the coronal pulp was collected by confocal microscopy. For orientation, the fibers traverse through the odontoblastic layer to the dentinal tubules (on the right). Reproduced with permission from Henry MA and Hargreaves KM.[1]

sively in the coronal pulp (Figure 2). The nerve terminals are either found in the pulp proper (generally the unmyelinated C fibers) or they can travel through the odontoblast layer and terminate a short distance (150–200 μm) within the dentinal tubule (generally the Aδ or A-β fibers). An intricate layer of neuronal branching is found below the odontoblast layer and is termed the plexus of Rashkow. This branching is especially dense and complex within the pulp horns. The dense innervation of the pulpo–dentin border found in the coronal region is reduced in cervical regions. Studies have demonstrated that approximately 50% of the tubules present in the area of the cusp tips contain nerve fibers while dentinal tubules in the cervical region are much less innervated.[36]

Anatomic and electrophysiologic studies have demonstrated the presence of Aδ, C, and Aβ fibers in the dental pulp,[30,37,38] although the myelin sheaths are lost as the axons traverse the apical foramen and are thus not apparent in pulpal histological images. These fibers appear to be organized anatomically in a manner consistent with their observed functionality. For example, small myelinated fibers (likely Aδ) generally terminate in the dentin, pre-dentin, and odontoblast regions of the pulp. Electrophysiologic recordings of the dental pulp demonstrate that Aδ fibers are activated by hydrodynamic stimuli such as the application of a burst of air onto exposed dentin, drilling, and rapid temperature change.[21,39,40] The hydrodynamic theory and its relation to dental pain will be discussed in more detail later in this chapter. Application of hydrodynamic-type stimuli in human volunteers elicits a quick, sharp, or bright type pain consistent with perceptual qualities from activation of Aδ fibers.[41] In contrast to the superficial localization of the Aδ fibers, the pulpal C fibers are found deeper within the pulp and often adjacent to blood vessels. Electrophysiologic studies demonstrate that C fibers are more likely to become activated by inflammatory mediators such as bradykinin, prostaglandins, and histamine.[42,43] They also can respond to intense heat or cold and it is surmised that the delayed response likely corresponds to the time it takes for detection of the temperature change in the well-insulated mass of the pulp tissue.[42–44] Studies in human volunteers have demonstrated that the same stimuli which activate pulpal C fibers in vitro produce a dull, throbbing, or burning pain which is often difficult to localize when applied in vivo.[45]

It is somewhat surprising that Aβ fibers are found within the pulp, as these fibers are classically not associated with detection of painful stimuli. However, anatomic and electrophysiologic studies have demonstrated their presence in dental pulp and their responsiveness to noxious stimuli. In dental pulp, these fibers are functionally indistinct from Aδ fibers and as such primarily respond to hydrodynamic stimuli.[35] They generally terminate at the dentin–pulp border and innervate dentinal tubules particularly at the pulp horn tip.[37,46] Other neuronal structures innervating the dental pulp include postganglionic sympathetic fibers that cause vasoconstriction in the pulp when activated,[47–49] and the resulting reduced pulpal blood flow may be due to both direct vasoconstriction and indirect mechanisms via inhibition of CGRP release from afferent neurons.[10,11] Comparatively less is known about parasympathetic innervation in dental pulp.[50–53]

It has long been debated whether odontoblasts, that are obviously non-neuronal cells, are involved in the sensory function of the dental pulp. Ultrastructure studies have demonstrated that although odontoblasts come in close contact with pulpal neurons they do not form a classical synaptic-like connection and therefore likely are not responsible for directly activating pulpal neurons.[54,55] However, recent studies demonstrating that odontoblasts are capable of generating action potentials[56] and express the transient receptor potential V1 also known as the capsaicin receptor (TRPV1)[57] and sodium channels (discussed in the Peripheral Pain Mechanisms Section) suggest that this debate is likely to continue.

Organization and Function of the Central Trigeminal Pain System

The second major functional element of the pain system is processing and this is thought to occur, at least in part, in the trigeminal nuclei. Peripheral trigeminal neurons enter the medulla forming the trigeminal spinal tract and terminate in the trigeminal brainstem nuclear complex (VBSNC). The VBSNC consists of the principle sensory nucleus of V, which receives non-nociceptive sensory input, and the spinal tract nucleus of V. The spinal tract nucleus of V is further divided in a rostro-caudal direction into the nucleus caudalis (most caudal section), the nucleus interpolaris, and the nucleus oralis (most rostral section) (see Figure 1). The nucleus caudalis is a primary site for integration and processing of orofacial nociceptive input. The nucleus caudalis is a laminated structure similar to the spinal dorsal horn, and in fact, the most caudal extent of this nucleus is continuous with the cervical spinal dorsal horn. For this reason, this region is often referred to as the medullary dorsal horn. However, despite these similarities, numerous studies have demonstrated that there are several unique features of the nucleus caudalis that distinguish it from the spinal dorsal horn.[58–61] For example, the neuronal inputs from peripheral tissues often terminate over a broader region in the VBSNC, whereas the spinal dorsal horn is organized in more of a segmental manner (e.g., C1-C2-C3). Specifically, anatomic and electrophysiologic studies have demonstrated that pulpal neurons terminate in the nucleus caudalis, nucleus interpolaris, and nucleus oralis.[62–65] This may partially account for the clinical observation of patients experiencing symptomatic pulpitis and having difficulty localizing the painful tooth. Furthermore, the observation that all three nuclei as well as other regions (e.g., cervical dorsal spinal cord) receive orofacial nociceptive input indicates nociceptive processing in the trigeminal system is multifocal.[59]

The processing of a nociceptive signal that takes place in the VBSNC is highly complex involving numerous neurons and supportive structures and

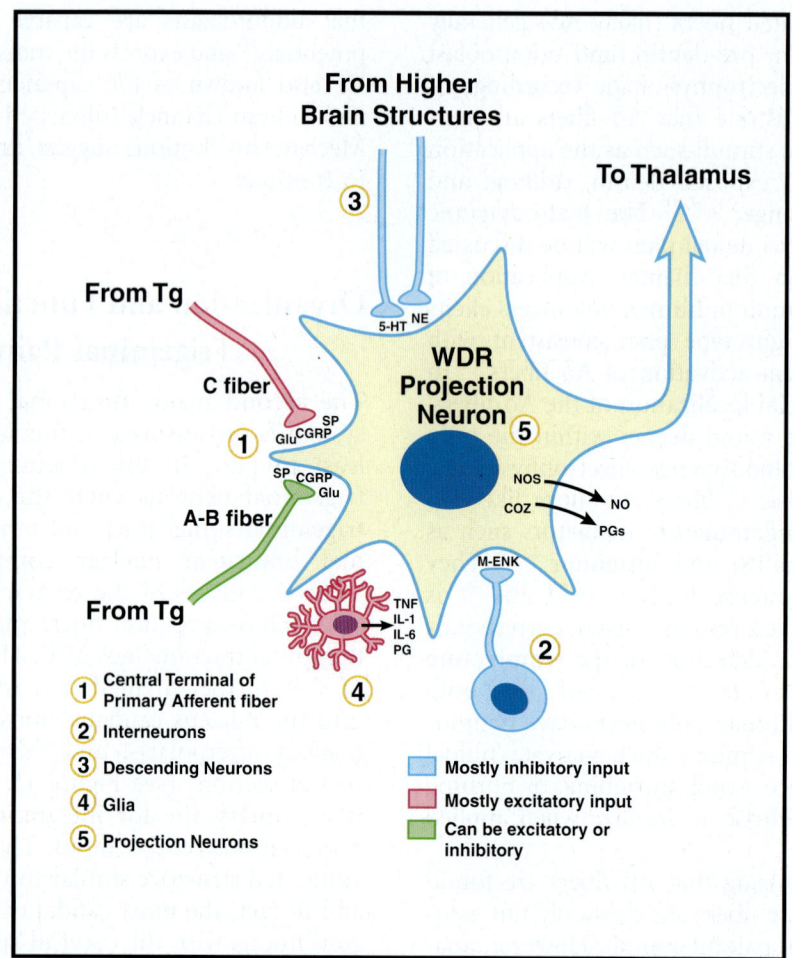

Figure 3 Illustration of a wide dynamic range (WDR) projection neuron in the medullary dorsal horn and the major components that alter the processing of nociceptive input from a C nociceptor. 5HT = serotonin; CGRP = calcitonin gene-related peptide; COX = cyclooxygenase; Glu = glutamate; NE = norepinephrine; NO = nitric oxide; NOS = nitric oxide synthase; PG = prostaglandin; SP = substance P; Tg = trigeminal ganglia.

can result in either the amplification or the diminution of a peripheral nociceptive signal (Figure 3). The key components mediating this process include (1) the central terminal of the primary afferent fiber; (2) the interneurons; (3) the descending neurons; (4) the glia; and finally (5) the projection neurons.

When a noxious stimulus activates a peripheral trigeminal nociceptor, an action potential is generated that propagates the length of the neuron and ultimately results in the release of neurotransmitters from the central terminals, including the excitatory amino acid glutamate, as well as neuropeptides such as CGRP and SP. Although activation of many of the cognate receptors for these neurotransmitters plays a role in the generation of pain, the glutamate receptors are particularly relevant. Glutamate activates the NMDA and AMPA receptors, and numerous studies have demonstrated that these receptors are critical for the generation of hyperalgesia and mediate certain phenomena such as central sensitization, described in the Central Mechanisms section.[66]

Local interneurons make connections between different neurons within the medullary dorsal horn, and depending upon the neurotransmitters they express and can either inhibit or facilitate nociceptive transmission.

The third component of the medullary dorsal horn is the terminals of the descending neurons. These neurons arise from higher level structures in the brain such as the periaquiductal gray and the rostral ventromedial medulla and descend to modulate the nociceptive signal at the level of the projection neuron. Both inhibitory function and excitatory modulation of the descending neurons has been demonstrated.[67] The endogenous opioid system is an important component of this descending modulation. We know from clinical studies that the endogenous opioid system is important in modulating dental pain. Prior to a dental procedure, administration of the opioid receptor antagonist naloxone significantly increases the perception of pain.[68–70]

The fourth component of nociceptive processing in the medullary dorsal horn is the glia. These are the microglia and astrocytes that until recently were only believed to function as supportive structure for neurons. Glia are now known to express receptors for many neurotransmitters involved in pain and activated glia-release cytokines and prostaglandins that can subsequently activate or sensitize neighboring neurons.[71,72] Accordingly, the central mechanism of action for the non-steroidal anti-inflammatory drugs (NSAID) is thought to be mediated by inhibition of central cyclooxygenase.

The final component of the medullary dorsal horn is the projection neuron whose activity is modulated by all of the previously described components. After processing peripheral neuronal input, these neurons project to the thalamus via the trigeminothalamic tract. The thalamocortical tract relays sensory information from the thalamus to the cerebral cortex, where perception occurs. The three major classes of projection neurons are the low-threshold mechanoreceptor (LTM) neurons, the wide dynamic range (WDR) neurons, and the nociceptive-specific (NS) neurons. The LTM projection neurons receive input from non-nociceptive fibers (i.e., Aβ fibers). The WDR neurons receive input from both nociceptive and non-nociceptive fibers while the NS projection neurons only receive input from nociceptors.[58]

An important concept in understanding the implications of central processing at the level of the projection neurons is that of convergence. One projection neuron can often receive afferent input from numerous distinct afferent inputs, such as cutaneous tissues, dental pulp, dura, and/or cornea.[58,73] This represents the physiologic basis for referred pain. Referred pain is frequently encountered by endodontists. For example, a patient with irreversible pulpitis in a mandibular first molar may also complain of pain in the right pre-auricular region. Referred pain can also work in the other direction where a fibromyalgia patient with a trigger point in the lower belly of the masseter muscle might present with a chief complaint of throbbing pain in the mandibular first premolar on the same side. Both of these scenarios can be explained by the concept of central convergence.

The Inflamed Dental Pulp

Under normal conditions, the nociceptors of dental pulp are thought to be quiescent. In the absence of any pathology, pulpal nociceptors are usually not activated by the modest temperature changes they are exposed to when eating or drinking a hot or cold substance, and they are protected from chemical or mechanical activation by dentin and enamel. However, in the presence of tissue injury, such as caries, trauma, or enamel abrasion, the nociceptors are readily activated by various stimuli. The development of pulpitis and apical periodontitis and the experience of pain that often (but not always) accompanies them involve complex neuro-immune interactions. Both the peripheral primary afferent neuron and the central projection neurons are critical for the initiation and maintenance of pain, and important features of these mechanisms are described below.

The three characteristics of an acute inflammatory process are (1) allodynia or a decreased threshold for detecting painful stimuli, whereby an innocuous stimulus is able to produce a sensation of pain; (2) hyperalgesia or an enhanced response to a frankly noxious stimulus; and (3) spontaneous pain. These characteristics are present in patients experiencing symptomatic pulpitis and/or symptomatic apical periodontitis. For example, a patient with acute apical periodontitis might report pain on chewing (i.e., mechanical allodynia). Moreover, an exaggerated painful response to the cold test and percussion test are signs of thermal and mechanical hyperalgesia, respectively.

Peripheral Pain Mechanisms

The activity of nociceptors in an inflamed environment is markedly altered from those in a native or uninjured state. When present in sufficient concentration, inflammatory mediators can either activate (e.g., bradykinin) or sensitize (e.g., prostaglandins such as prostaglandin E2) nociceptors via interactions with their receptors. Sensitization is characterized as a decrease in threshold (i.e., contributing to allodynia), an increased response to suprathreshold stimuli (i.e., contributing to hyperalgesia), and spontaneous activity (i.e., contributing to spontaneous pain). Although some inflammatory mediators are capable of immediately activating peripheral nociceptors, many other inflammatory mediators primarily function to change the transduction sensitivity of the peripheral neuron. Peripheral sensitization refers to the altered activity and excitability of peripheral neurons in the presence

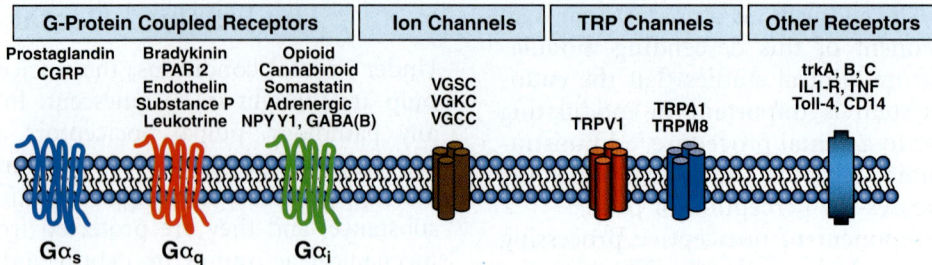

Figure 4 A schematic illustration of the primary families of receptor or ion channels expressed on peripheral terminals dental nociceptors that serve to detect physical stimuli and chemical substances, leading to altered nerve activity. Not all receptors/ion channels are present on all neurons, and several have been shown to be altered during inflammation or nerve injury. PAR-2 = protease-activated receptor subtype 2; PG = prostaglandin; TRPA1= transient receptor potential A1; TRPM8 = transient receptor potential M8; TRPV1 = transient receptor potential V1 aka the capsaicin receptor; VGCC = voltage-gated calcium channel; VGKC = voltage-gated potassium channel; VGSC = voltage-gated sodium channel. Reproduced with permission from Henry MA and Hargreaves KM.[1]

of inflammatory mediators and is one peripheral mechanism mediating inflammatory pain.

A key concept in understanding the function of peripheral nociceptors is their expression of receptors and ion channels. Peripheral terminals of nociceptors express receptors that detect chemical or physical stimuli resulting in activation of ion channels leading to generation of action potentials sent back to the brain (Figure 4). Although considerable research has focused on receptors that increase nociceptor activity (e.g., receptors for bradykinin, prostaglandins), it should be appreciated that receptors are present that inhibit nociceptor activity (e.g., receptors for opioid or adrenergic drugs) and thus overall activity is due to an integration of these receptor signaling pathways. The activation of certain G protein-coupled receptors (GPCR) can lead to activation of intracellular signaling pathways leading to Gs stimulation of protein kinase A (e.g., Prostagland E2 (PGE2) or to Gq activation of protein kinase C (e.g., bradykinin). Both of these pathways phosphorylate key receptors, altering their kinetics, and increasing the overall excitability of the neuron. Conversely, many peripheral analgesic drugs bind to GPCRs coupled to the Gi protein that inhibits Protein kinase A(PKA) activity contributing to reduced nociceptor function. An example of this interaction is presented in (Figure 5). Capsaicin is the active ingredient in hot chili peppers and activates nociceptors by binding to the TRPV1 channel (see Figure 4), resulting in chemical activation of pulpal nociceptors. When applied to isolated superfused dental pulp, capsaicin evokes a significant activation of pulpal nociceptors as indicated by release of CGRP (see Figure 5). However, if the pulpal neurons are first pretreated with epinephrine, a drug that binds to adrenergic receptors coupled to Gi, there is an inhibition of nociceptor activity. Thus, an understanding of receptors and signaling pathways allows one to predict whether a drug might increase or inhibit pain perception. Moreover, these data suggest that the epinephrine contained in local anesthetic cartridges might have direct peripheral analgesic properties independent of the "vasoconstrictor" effect of the drug.[10]

Numerous inflammatory mediators and their corresponding receptors are present in dental pulp including bradykinin, arachidonic acid metabolites

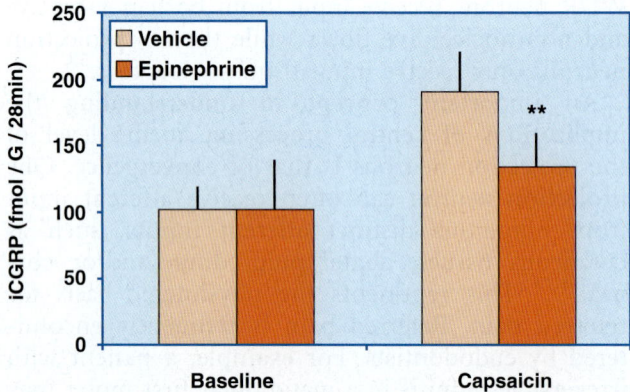

Figure 5 Effect of pretreatment with epinephrine or vehicle on the release of immunoreactive calcitonin gene-related peptide (iCGRP) evoked by capsaicin. Bovine dental pulp was sliced into 200 μm^2 slices, superfused with oxygenated Kreb's buffer, and the iCGRP released over a 28-minute period was measured by radioimmunoassay. Epinephrine (10 nM) or vehicle was administered before and concurrently with capsaicin (10 µM). Error bars are SEM **$p < 0.01$ versus vehicle. N = 7 to 8 per group. Reproduced with permission from Hargreaves KM, et al.[10]

(e.g., prostaglandins and leukotrienes), histamine, serotonin, cytokines, protons, and adenosine and adenosine phosphates (e.g., AMP, ADP, and ATP). Because inflammatory mediators evoke their effects by binding to protein receptors, their tissue concentration must be sufficient to occupy an appreciable fraction of the receptors on the cell's membrane. Thus, interventions that reduce tissue levels of inflammatory mediators (e.g., NSAID reduction of PGE2 levels) lead to reduced activation of these receptors. Other pharmacological interventions work by blocking the receptor to prevent endogenous mediators from activating it (e.g., antihistamine blockade of the histamine receptor). Also, the combination of inflammatory mediators present is important as many inflammatory mediators activate receptors leading to a rich potential for interactions that could substantially increase nociceptor activities. For example, the pain evoked in human volunteers by infusion of a mixture of inflammatory mediators into the skin was 10-fold greater when the skin was previously exposed to a low pH (i.e., higher proton concentration).[74] Studies in the dental pulp have also demonstrated that a positive interaction exists between bradykinin and prostaglandin E2 signaling in nociceptors.[13]

Trophic factors such as NGF, that play an important role in neural development, are also important in inflammation. Cytokines increase NGF production in inflamed tissues, including dental pulp, and NGF can sensitize nociceptors as well as mediate some of the transcriptional changes which occur after inflammatory injury.[75,76] Specifically, NGF has been demonstrated to increase expression of TRPV1, transient receptor potential A1 (TRPA1), as well as the sodium channels Na_v 1.8.[77–79] For example, the local infusion of NGF evokes a three-fold increase in the expression of TRPA1 transcripts (Figure 6A) and significantly increased the neuronal depolarization induced by a chemical stimulus of the TRPA1 channel (see Figure 6B). The importance of these receptors to inflammatory pain is described below. It is important to note that these changes contribute to the phenomenon of peripheral sensitization, but because they are transcription dependent (i.e., requiring synthesis of new proteins), they manifest over a time from hours to days.

The use of local anesthetics is essential to the practice of endodontics. Therefore, the target of local anesthetics, voltage-gated sodium channels (VGSC), is clearly an important molecular target when discussing pain management (see Figure 4). These sodium channels are termed "voltage gated" as the channels undergo a conformation change in response to application of a voltage, leading to sodium influx and membrane depolarization. Dentists take advantage of this property by using electrical pulp tests that apply

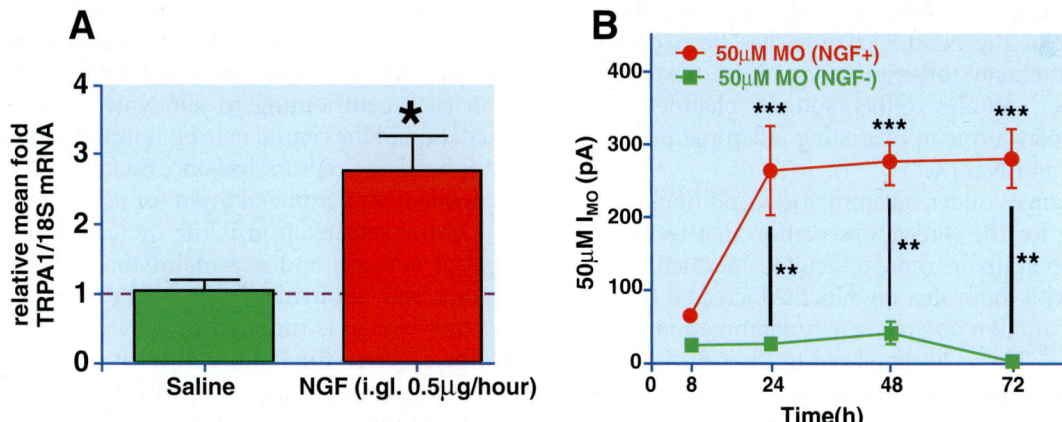

Figure 6 *A*, Local administration of nerve growth factor (NGF) significantly upregulated the expression of transient receptor potential A1 (TRPA1) mRNA in the trigeminal (TG) neurons in vivo. Rats received intraganglionic (i.gl.) infusion of NGF at a constant rate of 0.5 μg/h/7 d or vehicle via a cannula attached to a osmotic mini pump. Real time reverse transcriptase-polymerase chain reaction was performed with specific primers against the TRPA1 sequence, and the data were normalized to the mRNA levels found in the contralateral ganglion for each rat per group. *B*, The exposure of TG neurons to NGF (100 ng/ml) time dependently increased mustard oil-evoked currents (iMO) (red line) as compared to vehicle-treated neurons (green line). TG neurons were grown in culture for a total of 72 hours in the presence of NGF (100 ng/ml) or vehicle. Whole-cell patch voltage clamp was performed at 8, 24, 48, and 72 hours of culture. Data are presented as mean ± SEM (N = 8–16, ***p < 0.001 for time 0 hours versus 8, 24, 48, 72 hours within each treatment group, and **p < 0.01 NGF⁻ versus NGF⁺ for each time point; two-way analysis of variance with Boferroni's post hoc test). Reproduced with permission from Diogenes A et al.[77]

an ascending ramp of voltage across pulpal tissue leading to activation of the channels and the brief sensation of pain. There are several subtypes of sodium channels, and although most are involved in the transmission of non-noxious sensory information via action potential initiation and propagation, a few of these channels may be nociceptor specific and therefore are more favorable therapeutic targets for drug development (for reviews see refs 80–82). The first evidence in support of the hypothesis of nociceptor-specific (or "nociceptor enriched") expression of certain VGSCs was a result of the observation that sodium currents in nociceptors have the distinct physical property of resistance to tetrototoxin (TTX) and that sodium currents in Aβ sized neurons were TTX-sensitive; importantly, the TTX-resistant currents were increased following exposure to inflammatory mediators.[83-85]

Molecular cloning led to the identification of the Nav1.8 and Nav1.9 sodium channels subtypes as mediating the TTX-resistant current.[86,87] Further studies demonstrate that the Nav1.8 channel mediates the majority of the TTX-resistant current and that this channel plays a key role in the generation and maintenance of inflammatory pain. It was demonstrated that inflammatory mediators, including prostaglandins, alter the kinetics of the channels activity resulting in increased neural depolarization or firing.[84,88] Also, the channel itself is expressed at higher levels under conditions of inflammation.[89-91] Finally, using animal studies evaluating pain behaviors, the knock-down or elimination of the Nav1.8 channel has been demonstrated to attenuate inflammatory pain in most,[79,92-95] but not all,[79] studies. Other sodium channels, that potentially play a role in mediating inflammatory pain, are Nav1.7 and Nav1.9.[81,96,97]

These changes under inflammatory conditions possibly account for the clinical observation that teeth with irreversible pulpitis are more difficult to anesthetize. Pretreatment with ibuprofen inhibits the increased sodium channel production observed after inflammation in animal studies.[89] This is likely related to clinical trials indicating that local anesthesia in irreversible pulpitis patients may be improved by premedication with ibuprofen.[98,99] Therefore, for patients who can tolerate NSAIDs, it is possible that the preoperative administration of fast-acting NSAIDs to patients experiencing acute symptoms will provide improved local anesthetic efficacy.

Recently, several lines of evidence have led to the observation that some members of the transient receptor potential (TRP) family of ion channels are able to respond to temperature changes and are important for the development of inflammatory pain.[100] The most well-studied channel to date is the TRPV1 channel that is activated by noxious heat (>43°C) as well as capsaicin, the pungent ingredient of chili peppers that produces a burning sensation when administered to human volunteers.[101] Inflammatory mediators such as PGE2 and bradykinin (BK) can sensitize the TRPV1 channel, and mice that have been genetically altered so as to not express the TRPV1 channel exhibit less thermal hyperalgesia/allodynia after inflammatory injury.[25,102,103] Other TRP receptors such as TRPV2, TRPM8, and TRPA1 have been identified which have different temperature activation thresholds and chemical activators.[104] Given the exquisite temperature sensitivity present in many irreversible pulpitis patients, it is likely that certain TRP receptors at least partially mediate pain of pulpal origin. Several studies have demonstrated the presence of TRP receptors in the dental pulp, but the role of these receptors has yet to be clearly defined and is an important area for future research.[105,106] Several TRP antagonists have been developed and are now being evaluated as a potential novel class of analgesic drugs.[107]

Central Mechanisms

In addition to the neuronal changes that occur in peripheral nociceptors during inflammation, changes can occur in the central projection neurons that can cause expansion of the receptive field, an increased spontaneous firing (i.e., contributing to spontaneous pain), increased response to noxious stimuli (i.e., contributing to hyperalgesia), and a lowered threshold for nociceptor activation (i.e., contributing to allodynia). This increase in excitation of the central neuron is initiated by input from peripheral nociceptors, but once established becomes less dependent on peripheral input for its maintenance.

Central sensitization is the increased excitability of central neurons and is a major mechanism of hyperalgesia and allodynia.[19,108,109] The sensitization of a central neuron is initiated by a barrage of input from C fibers. When the C-fiber input is of sufficient intensity and duration (e.g., that which occurs in symptomatic pulpitis), neuronal changes occur in the central projection neurons whereby they exist in an excited state. The C fibers release neurotransmitters including glutamate and SP that act on post-synaptic NMDA and AMPA receptors or NK1 receptors, respectively. A signal transduction cascade is initiated in the central neuron involving numerous cellular signals of which nitric oxide and protein kinase C are particularly important.[110-112] Central sensitization can also affect low-threshold Aβ fibers. These changes cause an

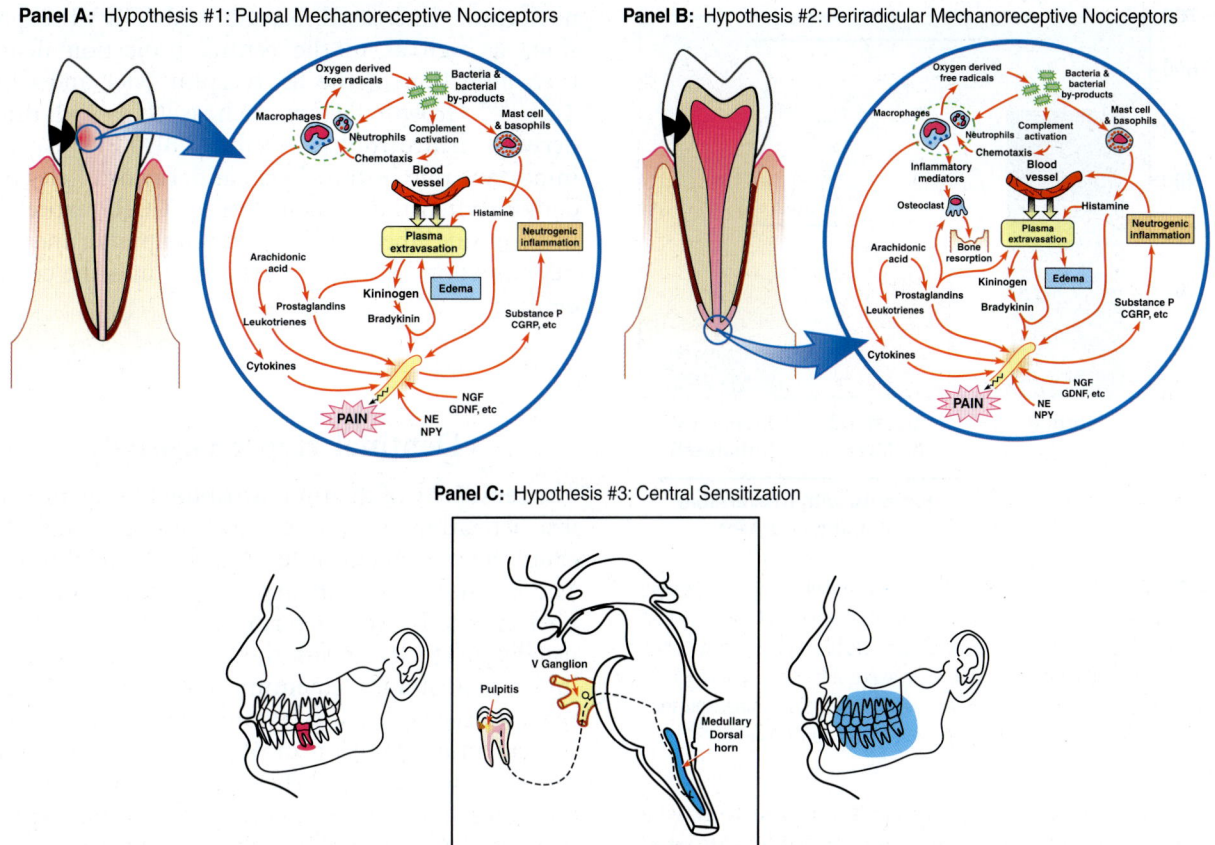

Figure 7 Three alternative hypotheses to explain the presence of mechanical allodynia in patients with irreversible pulpitis. *A,* Pulpal mechanoreceptive nociceptors. Diagrammatic representation of mechanical allodynia due to activation of pulpal mechanoreceptive neurons. Carious lesion allows bacteria and bacterial byproducts access to pulp tissue. Inflammation develops causing activation of pulpal mechanoreceptors by bacterial byproducts and inflammatory mediators and subsequent mechanical allodynia. *B,* Periradicular mechanoreceptive nociceptors. Diagrammatic representation of mechanical allodynia due to activation of periradicular mechanoreceptive neurons. Inflammatory mediators and bacterial byproducts from dental pulp diffuse apically into periradicular tissues causing inflammation, activation of periradicular mechanoreceptors, and subsequent mechanical allodynia. *C,* Central sensitization. Diagrammatic representation of mechanical allodynia due to central sensitization. Bacterial byproducts and inflammatory mediators activate nociceptors on pulpal nociceptive neurons. This afferent barrage causes central sensitization in the medullary dorsal horn leading to rapid expansion of the receptive fields leading to the development of mechanical allodynia at distant sites. Reproduced with permission from Owatz C et al.[128]

amplification of noxious and non-noxious input to the central neuron.

The process of central sensitization plays a significant role in the pain experienced by patients who are experiencing symptomatic irreversible pulpitis. We know from animal studies that central sensitization occurs in the nucleus caudalis after induction of inflammation in the dental pulp.[66,113] Clinically, central sensitization plays a role in the maintenance of pain after seemingly successful endodontic treatment. Central sensitization is also an important mechanism of referred pain and certain chronic pain conditions.

A recent series of studies has evaluated mechanical allodynia in odontogenic pain patients. Mechanical allodynia is defined as a reduction in pain thresholds where innocuous mechanical stimuli are now capable of causing pain. In the first study, approximately 1,000 patients were surveyed for pain reports prior to dental procedures, and 57% of patients diagnosed with irreversible pulpitis reported mechanical allodynia in response to a percussion test.[114] As shown in Figure 7, mechanical allodynia that is due to irreversible pulpitis might be due to activation of pulpal mechanonociceptive neurons and application of periapical mechanonociceptive neurons or due to central sensitization. In follow-up studies, a digital bite force device was constructed that permitted quantitative measurement of mechanical pain thresholds.[115] Using this device,

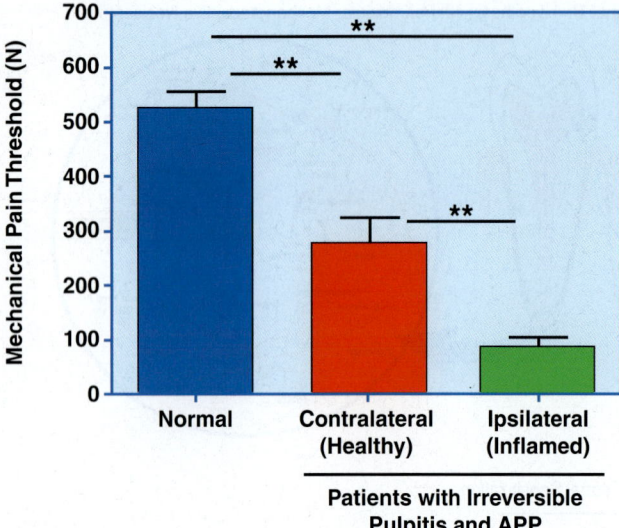

Figure 8 Mechanical pain thresholds of the first molars of subjects with no odontogenic or orofacial pain ($n = 40$) as compared with that of subjects with a clinical diagnosis of irreversible pulpitis and acute periradicular periodontitis ($n = 30$). Data were analyzed by using one-way analysis of variance and Newman–Keuls multiple comparison test. $**p \_ 0.001$. Reproduced with permission from Khan AA, et al.[116]

patients with irreversible pulpitis were found to have a 77% reduction in mechanical pain thresholds compared to their contralateral teeth (Figure 8).[116] These findings are consistent with the hypothesis that central sensitization occurs in patients with irreversible pulpitis as the contralateral teeth, which had no detectable pathosis, exhibited mechanical pain thresholds that were reduced by 50% as compared to healthy control patients without any intraoral pathosis.

Transcription-Dependent Changes

When peripheral neurons are exposed to inflammatory mediators, they become sensitized which leads to an increase in peripheral input to the central projection neuron. This input initiates and sustains central sensitization. These processes also cause transcription-dependent changes, in other words a change in the expression pattern of proteins (such as peptidergic neurotransmitters and receptors) in the affected neurons, fundamentally altering their function for extended periods. An example of transcription-dependent changes is the increased expression of the sodium channel Nav1.8 and peptidergic neurotransmitters such as CGRP and SP under conditions of inflammation. Transcription-dependent changes can occur in the peripheral nociceptor (increased Nav1.8 and TRPV1 expression) as well as in the central projection neuron (i.e., induction of the SP receptor NK1 and COX-2).[117,118] Growth factors such as NGF and Brain-derived neurotrophic factor (BDNF) play an important role in this. Byers and Taylor[119] elegantly demonstrated the upregulation of CGRP expression in sprouting fibers in the dental pulp after inducing inflammation by preparing a cavity into the cervical dentin.

Dentinal Hypersensitivity

The sensitivity of dentin is attributed to the mechanical activation of A fibers by various stimuli that cause the movement of fluid in the dentinal tubules. The hydrodynamic theory of activation of pulpal nociceptors is well described.[20,35,120] The pulp is usually protected from these types of stimuli by intact enamel and cementum. However, in the presence of caries, leaking restorations, or enamel and/or cementum abrasion or absence, dentinal tubules can become exposed. When patent dentinal tubules are exposed, the A fibers either innervating the dentinal tubules or located in the pulp adjacent to the tubules can be activated by stimuli such as air blast from an air/water syringe, scratching the dentin with an explorer tip, rapid cooling, or the presence of a hypertonic solution (usually sweets). Numerous studies have demonstrated that these stimuli cause a transient, sharp pain in human subjects and that similar stimuli applied to the teeth in animal studies causes activation of A fibers.[20,35,43] It is also clear that the patency of the dentinal tubules is critical to activate A fibers by hydrodynamic stimuli, as removal of the smear layer is critical for eliciting the response, and occlusion of the dentinal tubules with resin can prevent the activation of A fibers by hydrodynamic stimuli.[121,122]

Although dentin sensitivity is usually not an issue in intact teeth, it is possible to activate neurons with a high intensity stimulus such as that occurs during vital pulp testing with ethyl chloride spray to evaluate a response to cold. This scenario represents normal dentinal sensitivity. On the other hand, dentinal hypersensitivity describes the clinical situation where the dentin is more sensitive than normal. Pain is commonly evoked in these patients by cold stimuli as well as mechanical (i.e., probing with explorer tip) and hypertonic stimuli (i.e., sweets).[123–125] There is evidence that A fibers can be sensitized to hydrodynamic stimuli in the presence of inflammatory mediators.[20] This indicates first that pulpal inflammation can contribute to the symptoms of dentinal hypersensitivity and second that there is some evidence for the blurring of diagnostic categories of reversible and irreversible pulpitis and dentinal hypersensitivity. It is up to the astute clinician to consider all of the contributing factors and come up with an appropriate diagnosis. Typically, the symptoms of dentinal hypersensitivity are reversible, even when presenting with concomitant symptoms of pulpal inflammation. There is evidence supporting the use of toothpaste, gels, or mouthwash containing potassium salts for the treatment dentinal hypersensitivity.[126] There is also evidence that the application of resins to exposed dentinal tubules[121,127] can effectively treat dentinal hypersensitivity.

To date, the majority of studies support the hypothesis that hydrodynamic stimuli activate neurons located in or near dentinal tubules. However, it has also been hypothesized that odontoblasts, in addition to their function in dentinogenesis, could function as a sensory receptor cell. Histological studies have failed to demonstrate anatomic evidence of synapse or gap-junction type connections forming between odontoblasts and neurons.[128,129] However, electrophysiological evidence has demonstrated that odontoblasts have membrane potentials similar to those found in excitable cells.[130] A recent study demonstrated that odontoblasts contain the same subtypes of sodium channels as found in neural tissues and that under in vitro conditions these cells can be depolarized and generate action potentials.[56] This study also demonstrated a clustering of these receptors in regions of apparent odontoblast to neuron contact. In addition, another recent study suggests the presence of the TRPV1 receptor in odontoblasts, giving further evidence that this cell is potentially functioning in a sensory capacity.[57]

In summary, there is a good deal of evidence in support of the theory that dentinal sensitivity and hypersensitivity is due to the detection of movement of fluid in dentinal tubules. The question remains whether the detection occurs by direct activation of pulpal nociceptors or whether the nociceptors are indirectly activated by odontoblasts that may be functioning as the primary or secondary sensory cell in the dentin. Also, if pulpal nociceptors are directly activated by movement of fluid in the dentinal tubules, what is the molecular receptor mediating the mechanical activation of these neurons?

Conclusions

Research conducted in the last two decades has led to a dramatically increased understanding of orofacial pain mechanisms. Our knowledge of the biological basis of pain offers, for the first time, new opportunities to develop and evaluate analgesics designed to improve our ability to care for our patients. This conceptual framework, when combined with subsequent chapters on clinical pharmacology, provides a strong basis for improved diagnosis and treatment of odontogenic pain conditions.

References

1. Henry MA, Hargreaves KM. Peripheral mechanisms of odontogenic pain. Dent Clin North Am 2007;51(1):19–44.
2. Price TJ, Flores CM, Hargreaves KM. RNA binding and transport proteins are expressed by rat and human primary afferent neurons and localize to rat sensory axons: Implications for RNA transport in the PNS. Neuroscience 2006;141(4):2107–16.
3. Hokfelt T, Zhang X, Wiesenfeld-Hallin Z. Messenger plasticity in primary sensory neurons following axotomy and its functional implications. Trends Neurosci 1994; 17(1):22–30.
4. Wakisaka S, Kajander KC, Bennett GJ. Increased neuropeptide Y (NPY)-like immunoreactivity in rat sensory neurons following peripheral axotomy. Neurosci Lett 1991;124(2):200–3.
5. Novakovic SD, et al. Distribution of the tetrodotoxin-resistant sodium channel PN3 in rat sensory neurons in normal and neuropathic conditions. J Neurosci 1998;18(6):2174–87.
6. Bowles WR, et al. Beta 2-adrenoceptor regulation of CGRP release from capsaicin-sensitive neurons. J Dent Res 2003;82(4):308–11.
7. Lynn B. Efferent function of nociceptors. In: Neurobiology of nociceptors. C.Belmonte and F. Cervero, editors. Oxford: Oxford University Press; 1996. p. 419–38.
8. Goodis, HE, Poon A, Hargreaves KM. Tissue pH and temperature regulate pulpal nociceptors. J Dent Res 2006;85(11):1046–9.
9. Bowles WR, et al. Chronic nerve growth factor administration increases the peripheral exocytotic activity of capsaicin-sensitive cutaneous neurons. Neurosci Lett 2006;403(3):305–8.
10. Hargreaves KM, Jackson DL, Bowles WR. Adrenergic regulation of capsaicin-sensitive neurons in dental pulp. J Endod 2003;29(6):397–9.
11. Hargreaves KM, Bowles WR, Jackson DL. Intrinsic regulation of CGRP release by dental pulp sympathetic fibers. J Dent Res 2003;82(5):398–401.

12. Bowles WR, et al. Tissue levels of immunoreactive substance P are increased in patients with irreversible pulpitis. J Endod 2003;29(4):265–7.
13. Goodis HE, Bowles WR, Hargreaves KM. Prostaglandin E2 enhances bradykinin-evoked iCGRP release in bovine dental pulp. J Dent Res 2000;79(8):604–7.
14. Jackson DL, Hargreaves KM. Activation of excitatory amino acid receptors in bovine dental pulp evokes the release of iCGRP. J Dent Res 1999;78(1):54–60.
15. Olgart L, et al. Release of substance P-like immunoreactivity from the dental pulp. Acta Physiol Scand 1977;101(4):510–12.
16. Heyeraas KJ, et al. Effect of electrical tooth stimulation on blood flow, interstitial fluid pressure and substance P and CGRP-immunoreactive nerve fibers in the low compliant cat dental pulp. Microvasc Res 1994;47(3):329–43.
17. Hargreaves KM, et al. Pharmacology of peripheral neuropeptide and inflammatory mediator release. Oral Surg Oral Med Oral Pathol Oral Radiol Endod 1994;78(4):503–10.
18. Hargreaves KM, Bowles WR, Garry MG. An in vitro method to evaluate regulation of neuropeptide release from dental pulp. J Endod 1992;18(12):597–600.
19. Woolf CJ, Doubell TP. The pathophysiology of chronic pain–increased sensitivity to low threshold A beta-fibre inputs. Curr Opin Neurobiol 1994;4(4):525–34.
20. Närhi M, et al. Role of intradental A- and C-type nerve fibres in dental pain mechanisms. Proc Finn Dent Soc 1992;88(Suppl 1):507–16.
21. Närhi MV, Hirvonen TJ, Hakumaki MO. Responses of intradental nerve fibres to stimulation of dentine and pulp. Acta Physiol Scand 1982;115(2):173–8.
22. Närhi MV, Hirvonen T. The response of dog intradental nerves to hypertonic solutions of CaCl2 and NaCl, and other stimuli, applied to exposed dentine. Arch Oral Biol 1987;32(11):781–6.
23. Chen CL, et al. Runx1 determines nociceptive sensory neuron phenotype and is required for thermal and neuropathic pain. Neuron 2006;49(3):365–77.
24. Hjerling-Leffler J, et al. Emergence of functional sensory subtypes as defined by transient receptor potential channel expression. J Neurosci 2007;27(10):2435–43.
25. Julius D, Basbaum AI. Molecular mechanisms of nociception. Nature 2001;413(6852):203–10.
26. Snider WD. McMahon SB.Tackling pain at the source: new ideas about nociceptors. Neuron 1998;20(4):629–32.
27. Wakisaka S, et al. Neuropeptide Y-like immunoreactive primary afferents in the periodontal tissues following dental injury in the rat. Regul Pept 1996;63(2–3): 163–9.
28. Stucky CL, Lewin GR. Isolectin B(4)-positive and -negative nociceptors are functionally distinct. J Neurosci 1999; 19(15):6497–505.
29. Hunt SP, Rossi J. Peptide- and non-peptide-containing unmyelinated primary afferents: the parallel processing of nociceptive information. Philos Trans R Soc Lond B Biol Sci 1985;308(1136):283–9.
30. Fried K, et al. Combined retrograde tracing and enzyme/immunohistochemistry of trigeminal ganglion cell bodies innervating tooth pulps in the rat. Neuroscience 1989;33(1):101–9.
31. Virtanen AS, et al. The effect of temporal parameters on subjective sensations evoked by electrical tooth stimulation. Pain 1987;30(3):361–71.
32. McGrath PA, et al. Non-pain and pain sensations evoked by tooth pulp stimulation. Pain 1983;15(4):377–88.
33. Mumford JM, Newton AV. Spatial summation of pre-pain and pain in human teeth. Pain 1985;22(3):320–1.
34. Nair PN. Neural elements in dental pulp and dentin. Oral Surg Oral Med Oral Pathol Oral Radiol Endod 1995;80(6):710–19.
35. Närhi MV. The characteristics of intradental sensory units and their responses to stimulation. J Dent Res 1985;64(Spec. No):564–71.
36. Fearnhead RW. Histological evidence for the innervation of human dentine. J Anat 1957;91(2):267–77.
37. Byers MR, Närhi MV. Dental injury models: experimental tools for understanding neuroinflammatory interactions and polymodal nociceptor functions. Crit Rev Oral Biol Med 1999;10(1):4–39.
38. Sugimoto T, Takemura M, Wakisaka S. Cell size analysis of primary neurons innervating the cornea and tooth pulp of the rat. Pain 1988;32(3):375–81.
39. Närhi MV. Dentin sensitivity: a review. J Biol Buccale 1985;13(2):75–96.
40. Brännström M, Linden LA, Åström A. The hydrodynamics of the dental tubule and of pulp fluid. A discussion of its significance in relation to dentinal sensitivity. Caries Res 1967;1(4):310–17.
41. Brännström M, Johnson G. The sensory mechanism in human dentin as revealed by evaporation and mechanical removal of dentin. J Dent Res 1978;57(1):49–53.
42. Ikeda H, Sunakawa M, Suda H. Three groups of afferent pulpal feline nerve fibres show different electrophysiological response properties. Arch Oral Biol 1995;40(10):895–904.
43. Jyvasjarvi E, Kniffki KD. Studies on the presence and functional properties of afferent C-fibers in the cat's dental pulp. Proc Finn Dent Soc 1992;88(Suppl 1):533–42.
44. Närhi M, et al. Activation of heat-sensitive nerve fibres in the dental pulp of the cat. Pain 1982;14(4):317–26.
45. Mengel MK, et al. Pain sensation during cold stimulation of the teeth: differential reflection of A delta and C fibre activity? Pain 1993;55(2):159–69.

46. Maeda T, et al. Immunohistochemical demonstration of nerves in the predentin and dentin of human third molars with the use of an antiserum against neurofilament protein (NFP). Cell Tissue Res 1986;243(3):469–75.

47. Arwill T, et al. Ultrastructure of nerves in the dentinal-pulp border zone after sensory and autonomic nerve transection in the cat. Acta Odontol Scand 1973;31(5):273–81.

48. Aars H, et al. Effects of autonomic reflexes on tooth pulp blood flow in man. Acta Physiol Scand 1992;146(4):423–9.

49. Vongsavan N, Matthews B. Changes in pulpal blood flow and in fluid flow through dentine produced by autonomic and sensory nerve stimulation in the cat. Proc Finn Dent Soc 1992;88(Suppl 1):491–7.

50. Sasano T, et al. Absence of parasympathetic vasodilatation in cat dental pulp. J Dent Res 1995;74(10):1665–70.

51. Borda E, et al. Nitric oxide synthase and PGE2 reciprocal interactions in rat dental pulp: cholinoceptor modulation. J Endod 2007;33(2):142–7.

52. Caviedes-Bucheli J, et al. The effect of cavity preparation on substance P expression in human dental pulp. J Endod 2005;31(12):857–9.

53. Olgart L. Neural control of pulpal blood flow. Crit Rev Oral Biol Med 1996;7(2):159–71.

54. Byers MR. Dental sensory receptors. Int Rev Neurobiol 1984;25:39–94.

55. Holland GR. Odontoblasts and nerves; just friends. Proc Finn Dent Soc 1986;82(4):179–89.

56. Allard B, et al. Voltage-gated sodium channels confer excitability to human odontoblasts: Possible role in tooth pain transmission. J Biol Chem 2006;281(39):29002–10.

57. Okumura R, et al. The odontoblast as a sensory receptor cell? The expression of TRPV1 (VR-1) channels. Arch Histol Cytol 2005;68(4):251–7.

58. Sessle BJ. Acute and chronic craniofacial pain: brainstem mechanisms of nociceptive transmission and neuroplasticity, and their clinical correlates. Crit Rev Oral Biol Med 2000;11(1):57–91.

59. Bereiter DA, Hirata H, Hu JW. Trigeminal subnucleus caudalis: beyond homologies with the spinal dorsal horn. Pain 2000;88(3):221–4.

60. Sugimoto T, et al. Central projection of calcitonin gene-related peptide (CGRP)- and substance P (SP)-immunoreactive trigeminal primary neurons in the rat. J Comp Neurol 1997;378(3):425–42.

61. Ambalavanar R, Morris R. The distribution of binding by isolectin I-B4 from Griffonia simplicifolia in the trigeminal ganglion and brainstem trigeminal nuclei in the rat. Neuroscience 1992;47(2):421–9.

62. Hu JW, Shohara E, Sessle BJ. Patterns and plasticity of dental afferent inputs to trigeminal (V) brainstem neurons in kittens. Proc Finn Dent Soc 1992;88(Suppl 1):563–9.

63. Takemura M, et al. The central projections of the monkey tooth pulp afferent neurons. Somatosens Mot Res 1993;10(2):217–27.

64. Barnett EM, et al. Anterograde tracing of trigeminal afferent pathways from the murine tooth pulp to cortex using herpes simplex virus type 1. J Neurosci 1995;15(4):2972–84.

65. Shigenaga Y, et al. Topographic representation of lower and upper teeth within the trigeminal sensory nuclei of adult cat as demonstrated by the transganglionic transport of horse-radish peroxidase. J Comp Neurol 1986;251(3):299–316.

66. Chiang CY, et al. NMDA receptor mechanisms contribute to neuroplasticity induced in caudalis nociceptive neurons by tooth pulp stimulation. J Neurophysiol 1998;80(5):2621–31.

67. Ren K, Dubner R. Descending modulation in persistent pain: an update. Pain 2002;100(1–2):1–6.

68. Hargreaves KM, et al. Naloxone, fentanyl, and diazepam modify plasma beta-endorphin levels during surgery. Clin Pharmacol Ther 1986;40(2):165–71.

69. Gracely RH, et al. Placebo and naloxone can alter post-surgical pain by separate mechanisms. Nature 1983;306(5940):264–5.

70. Levine JD, Gordon NC, Fields HL. The mechanism of placebo analgesia. Lancet 1978;2(8091):654–7.

71. Watkins LR, Maier SF. The pain of being sick: implications of immune-to-brain communication for understanding pain. Annu Rev Psychol 2000;51:29–57.

72. Watkins LR, Milligan ED, Maier SF. Spinal cord glia: new players in pain. Pain 2001;93(3):201–5.

73. Sessle BJ, et al. Convergence of cutaneous, tooth pulp, visceral, neck and muscle afferents onto nociceptive and non-nociceptive neurones in trigeminal subnucleus caudalis (medullary dorsal horn) and its implications for referred pain. Pain 1986;27(2):219–35.

74. Steen KH, et al. Inflammatory mediators potentiate pain induced by experimental tissue acidosis. Pain 1996;66(2–3):163–70.

75. Woodnutt DA, et al. Neurotrophin receptors and nerve growth factor are differentially expressed in adjacent non-neuronal cells of normal and injured tooth pulp. Cell Tissue Res 2000;299(2):225–36.

76. Pezet S, McMahon SB. Neurotrophins: Mediators and Modulators of Pain. Annu Rev Neurosci 2006;29:507–38.

77. Diogenes A, Akopian AN, Hargreaves KM. NGF Upregulates TRPA1: Implications for Orofacial Pain. J Dent Res 2007;86:550–5.

78. Fjell J, et al. Sodium channel expression in NGF-overexpressing transgenic mice. J Neurosci Res 1999;57(1):39–47.

79. Kerr BJ, et al. A role for the TTX-resistant sodium channel Nav 1.8 in NGF-induced hyperalgesia, but not neuropathic pain. Neuroreport 2001;12(14):3077–80.

80. Waxman SG, et al. Sodium channels and pain. Proc Natl Acad Sci USA 1999;96(14):7635–9.

81. Wood JN, et al. Voltage-gated sodium channels and pain pathways. J Neurobiol 2004;61(1):55–71.

82. Lai J, et al. Voltage-gated sodium channels and hyperalgesia. Annu Rev Pharmacol Toxicol 2004;44:371–97.

83. Arbuckle JB, Docherty RJ. Expression of tetrodotoxin-resistant sodium channels in capsaicin-sensitive dorsal root ganglion neurons of adult rats. Neurosci Lett 1995;185(1):70–3.

84. Gold MS, et al. Hyperalgesic agents increase a tetrodotoxin-resistant Na+ current in nociceptors. Proc Natl Acad Sci USA 1996;93(3):1108–12.

85. Brock JA, McLachlan EM, Belmonte C. Tetrodotoxin-resistant impulses in single nociceptor nerve terminals in guinea-pig cornea. J Physiol 1998;512(Pt. 1):211–17.

86. Akopian AN, Sivilotti L, Wood JN. A tetrodotoxin-resistant voltage-gated sodium channel expressed by sensory neurons. Nature 1996;379(6562):257–62.

87. Dib-Hajj SD, et al. NaN, a novel voltage-gated Na channel, is expressed preferentially in peripheral sensory neurons and down-regulated after axotomy. Proc Natl Acad Sci USA 1998;95(15):8963–8.

88. Gold MS, Levine JD, Correa AM. Modulation of TTX-R INa by PKC and PKA and their role in PGE2-induced sensitization of rat sensory neurons in vitro. J Neurosci 1998; 18(24):10345–55.

89. Gould HJ, III, et al. Ibuprofen blocks changes in Na v 1.7 and 1.8 sodium channels associated with complete Freund's adjuvant-induced inflammation in rat. J Pain 2004; 5(5):270–80.

90. Villarreal CF, et al. The role of Na(V)1.8 sodium channel in the maintenance of chronic inflammatory hypernociception. Neurosci Lett 2005;386(2):72–7.

91. Coggeshall RE, Tate S, Carlton SM. Differential expression of tetrodotoxin-resistant sodium channels Nav1.8 and Nav1.9 in normal and inflamed rats. Neurosci Lett 2004;355(1–2):45–8.

92. Porreca F, et al. A comparison of the potential role of the tetrodotoxin-insensitive sodium channels, PN3/SNS and NaN/SNS2, in rat models of chronic pain. Proc Natl Acad Sci USA 1999;96(14):7640–4.

93. Ekberg J, et al. muO-conotoxin MrVIB selectively blocks Nav1.8 sensory neuron specific sodium channels and chronic pain behavior without motor deficits. Proc Natl Acad Sci USA 2006;103(45):17030–5.

94. Akopian AN, et al. The tetrodotoxin-resistant sodium channel SNS has a specialized function in pain pathways. Nat Neurosci 1999;2(6):541–8.

95. Khasar SG, Gold MS., Levine JD. A tetrodotoxin-resistant sodium current mediates inflammatory pain in the rat. Neurosci Lett 1998;256(1):17–20.

96. Dib-Hajj S, et al. NaN/Nav1.9: a sodium channel with unique properties. Trends Neurosci 2002;25(5):253–9.

97. Waxman SG, Dib-Hajj S. Erythermalgia: molecular basis for an inherited pain syndrome. Trends Mol Med 2005;11(12):555–62.

98. Modaresi J, Dianat O, Mozayeni MA. The efficacy comparison of ibuprofen, acetaminophen-codeine, and placebo premedication therapy on the depth of anesthesia during treatment of inflamed teeth. Oral Surg Oral Med Oral Pathol Oral Radiol Endod 2006;102(3):399–403.

99. Ianiro SR, et al. The effect of preoperative acetaminophen or a combination of acetaminophen and Ibuprofen on the success of inferior alveolar nerve block for teeth with irreversible pulpitis. J Endod 2007;33(1):11–14.

100. Tominaga M, Caterina MJ. Thermosensation and pain. J Neurobiol 2004;61(1):3–12.

101. Caterina MJ, et al. The capsaicin receptor: a heat-activated ion channel in the pain pathway. Nature 1997;389(6653):816–24.

102. Caterina MJ, et al. Impaired nociception and pain sensation in mice lacking the capsaicin receptor. Science 2000; 288(5464):306–13.

103. Premkumar LS, Ahern GP. Induction of vanilloid receptor channel activity by protein kinase C. Nature 2000; 408(6815):985–90.

104. Wang H, Woolf CJ. Pain TRPs. Neuron 2005;46(1):9–12.

105. Renton T, et al. Capsaicin receptor VR1 and ATP purinoceptor P2X3 in painful and nonpainful human tooth pulp. J Orofac Pain 2003;17(3):245–50.

106. Park CK, et al. Functional expression of thermo-transient receptor potential channels in dental primary afferent neurons: implication for tooth pain. J Biol Chem 2006; 281(25):17304–11.

107. Zheng X, et al. From arylureas to biarylamides to aminoquinazolines: discovery of a novel, potent TRPV1 antagonist. Bioorg Med Chem Lett 2006;16(19):5217–21.

108. Woolf CJ, Costigan M. Transcriptional and posttranslational plasticity and the generation of inflammatory pain. Proc Natl Acad Sci USA 1999;96(14):7723–30.

109. Basbaum AI. Spinal mechanisms of acute and persistent pain. Reg Anesth Pain Med 1999;24(1):59–67.

110. Wu J, et al. Nitric oxide contributes to central sensitization following intradermal injection of capsaicin. Neuroreport 1998;9(4):589–92.

111. Lin Q, Peng YB, Willis WD. Possible role of protein kinase C in the sensitization of primate spinothalamic tract neurons. J Neurosci 1996;16(9):3026–34.

112. Brenner GJ, et al. Peripheral noxious stimulation induces phosphorylation of the NMDA receptor NR1 subunit at the PKC-dependent site, serine-896, in spinal cord dorsal horn neurons. Eur J Neurosci 2004;20(2):375–84.

113. Sessle BJ. Peripheral and central mechanisms of orofacial pain and their clinical correlates. Minerva Anestesiol 2005; 71(4):117–36.

114. Owatz C, Khan AA, Schindler WG, et al. The incidence of mechanical allodynia in patients with irreversible pulpitis. J Endod 2007;33:552–6.

115. Khan AA, McCreary B, Owatz CB, et al. The development of a diagnostic instrument for the measurement of mechanical allodynia. J Endod 2007;33:663–6.

116. Khan AA, Owatz CB, Schindler WG, et al. Measurement of mechanical allodynia and local anesthetic efficacy in patients with irreversible pulpitis and acute periradicular periodontitis. J Endod 2007;33(7):796–9.

117. Noguchi K, Ruda MA. Gene regulation in an ascending nociceptive pathway: inflammation-induced increase in preprotachykinin mRNA in rat lamina I spinal projection neurons. J Neurosci 1992;12(7):2563–72.

118. Hay CH, et al. The potential role of spinal cord cyclooxygenase-2 in the development of Freund's complete adjuvant-induced changes in hyperalgesia and allodynia. Neuroscience 1997;78(3):843–50.

119. Taylor PE, Byers MR. An immunocytochemical study of the morphological reaction of nerves containing calcitonin gene-related peptide to microabscess formation and healing in rat molars. Arch Oral Biol 1990;35(8):629–38.

120. Brännström M, Åström A. A study on the mechanism of pain elicited from the dentin. J Dent Res 1964;43:619–25.

121. Brännström M, Johnson G, Nordenvall KJ. Transmission and control of dentinal pain: resin impregnation for the desensitization of dentin. J Am Dent Assoc 1979;99(4):612–18.

122. Matthews B, Vongsavan N. Interactions between neural and hydrodynamic mechanisms in dentine and pulp. Arch Oral Biol 1994;39(Suppl):87S–95S.

123. Irwin CR, McCusker P. Prevalence of dentine hypersensitivity in a general dental population. J Ir Dent Assoc 1997;43(1):7–9.

124. Gillam DG, et al. Perceptions of dentine hypersensitivity in a general practice population. J Oral Rehabil 1999;26(9):710–14.

125. Holland GR. Morphological features of dentine and pulp related to dentine sensitivity. Arch Oral Biol 1994;39(Suppl):3S–11S.

126. Orchardson R, Gillam DG. The efficacy of potassium salts as agents for treating dentin hypersensitivity. J Orofac Pain 2000;14(1):9–19.

127. Nordenvall KJ, Malmgren B, Brännström M. Desensitization of dentin by resin impregnation: a clinical and light-microscopic investigation. ASDC J Dent Child 1984;51(4):274–6.

128. Ibuki T, et al. An ultrastructural study of the relationship between sensory trigeminal nerves and odontoblasts in rat dentin/pulp as demonstrated by the anterograde transport of wheat germ agglutinin-horseradish peroxidase (WGA-HRP). J Dent Res 1996;75(12):1963–70.

129. Tsukada K. Ultrastructure of the relationship between odontoblast processes and nerve fibres in dentinal tubules of rat molar teeth. Arch Oral Biol 1987;32(2):87–92.

130. Magloire H, Vinard H, Joffre A. Electrophysiological properties of human dental pulp cells. J Biol Buccale 1979;7:251–62.

CHAPTER 11

NON-ODONTOGENIC TOOTHACHE AND CHRONIC HEAD AND NECK PAIN

BERNADETTE JAEGER, MARCELA ROMERO REYES

Pain is perfect misery, the worst of evils; and excessive, overturns all patience.

–John Milton, Paradise Lost

Patients with chronic oral or facial pain, or headache, present a true diagnostic and therapeutic challenge to the practitioner. For many in the dental profession, the only solution to problems of pain lies with a scalpel, forceps, or ever-increasing doses of analgesics, narcotics, or sedatives. Many patients with chronic pain have suffered this mistreatment and stand as an indictment of a poorly trained, insecure, and disinterested segment of dentistry. Attending to patients who have been unable to obtain resolution of their pain complaint, despite extensive evaluation and treatment, requires a compassionate reappraisal and fresh approach. Fortunately, accurate diagnosis and successful management of these patients can be among the most rewarding experiences in dental or medical practice.

What Is Pain?

Pain is not a simple sensation but rather a complex neurobehavioral event involving at least two components. First is an individual's discernment or perception of the stimulation of specialized nerve endings designed to transmit information concerning potential or actual tissue damage (nociception). Second is the individual's reaction to this perceived sensation (pain behavior). This is any behavior, physical or emotional, that follows pain perception. Culture or environment often influences these behaviors. Beyond this is the suffering or emotional toll the pain has on any given individual. Suffering is so personal that it is difficult to quantify, evaluate, and treat.

The fact that pain is difficult to define, quantify, and understand is reflected in the numerous ways in which it has been described. *Dorland's Medical Dictionary* defines pain as "a more or less localized sensation of discomfort, distress, or agony resulting from the stimulation of specialized nerve endings."[1] In this definition, the behavioral reaction to nociception is already assumed to be distress or agony, which is not always the case. Take, for example, the observations made by Beecher in 1956 that only 25% of soldiers wounded in battle requested narcotic medications for pain relief, compared to more than 80% of civilian patients with surgical wounds of a similar magnitude.[2] Clearly, the behavioral reaction to similar nociceptive stimuli varies from person to person and depends on a number of factors, including the significance of the injury to that individual. The wounded soldier may be relieved to be out of a life-threatening situation; the surgical patient may be concerned about recurrence of a tumor just removed. *Dorland's* definition also implies that stimulation of nociceptors is required for perception of pain, yet the dental patient who has been anxious for weeks in anticipation of the "needle" at the dentist's office may jump in agony at the slightest touch of his cheek.

Fields[3] defined pain as "an unpleasant sensation that is perceived as arising from a specific region of the body and is commonly produced by processes that damage or are capable of damaging bodily tissue." He emphasized the need to be able to localize the painful source in order to distinguish it from psychological pain and suffering, for example, the "pain" of a broken heart.

A more complete definition is cast by the *International Association for the Study of Pain* (*IASP*) in its taxonomy of painful disorders.[4] That definition of pain is as follows: "An unpleasant sensory and emotional experience associated with actual or potential tissue damage, or described in terms of such damage." Added to this definition, however, is the following, emphasizing the subjective nature of pain that distinguishes and separates it from the simple stimulation of nociceptors:

Pain is always subjective. Each individual learns the application of the word through experiences related to injury in early life. It is unquestionably a sensation in a part of the body, but it is also always unpleasant and therefore also an emotional experience. Many people report pain in the absence of tissue damage or any likely pathophysiological cause, usually this happens for psychological reasons. There is no way to distinguish their experience from that due to tissue damage, if we take the subjective report. If they regard their experience as pain and if they report it in the same ways as pain caused by tissue damage, it should be accepted as pain. This definition avoids tying pain to a stimulus. The activity induced in the nociceptor and nociceptive pathways by a noxious stimulus is not pain, which is always a psychological state, even though we may well appreciate that pain most often has a proximate physical cause.[4]

The IASP definition of pain makes the point that *pain is pain even if a nociceptive source is not readily identified*. Pain owing to psychological causes is as real as any pain associated with actual nociception and should be treated as such.

To understand pain better, this chapter first looks at what is currently known about the anatomy and physiology of the nociceptive pathways and some of the modulating influences that modify the nociceptive input into the central nervous system (CNS). Following this, various psychological and behavioral factors that influence the perception of, and the reaction to pain, are reviewed.

Neurophysiology of Pain

The following summarizes what is known about the basic anatomy and physiology of pain under normal physiological conditions.[5]

ACUTE PAIN PATHWAYS

The body has specialized neurons that respond only to noxious or potentially noxious stimulation. These neurons are called primary afferent nociceptors and are very complex in structure. They express several types of receptors such as ion channels and G protein-coupled receptors that are implicated in inflammation and pain activation signaling[6,7] and are made up of

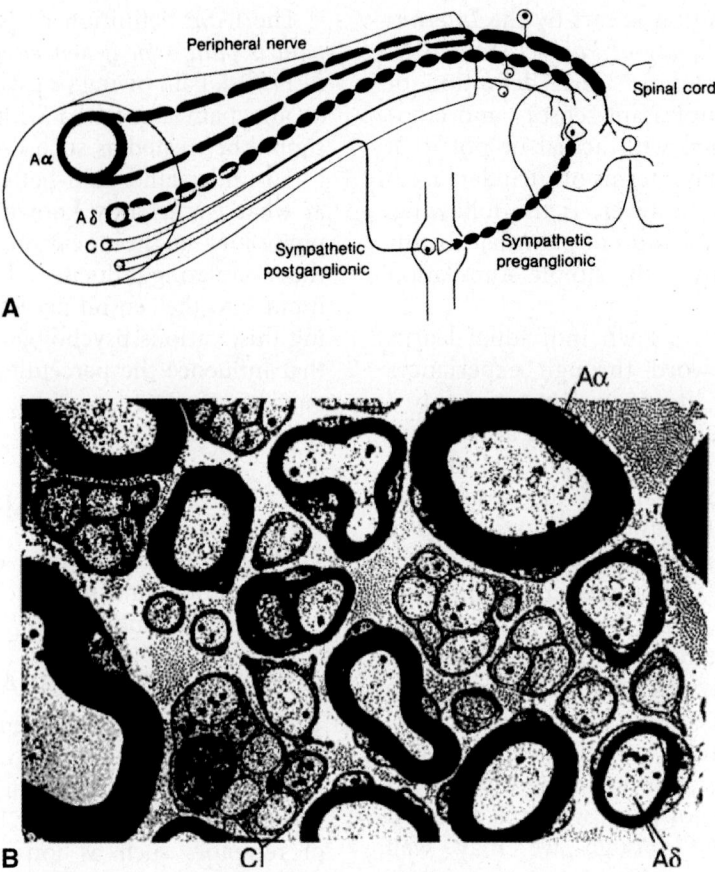

Figure 1 Components of a typical cutaneous nerve. **A,** It illustrates that there are two distinct functional categories of axon: primary afferents with cell bodies in the dorsal root ganglion and sympathetic postganglionic fibers with cell bodies in the sympathetic ganglion. Primary afferents include those with large-diameter myelinated (Aα), small-diameter myelinated (Aδ), and unmyelinated (C) axons. All sympathetic postganglionic fibers are unmyelinated. **B,** Electron micrograph of cross section of a cutaneous nerve illustrating the relative size and degree of myelination of its complement of axons. The myelin appears as black rings of varying thickness. The unmyelinated axons (C) occur singly or in clusters. Reproduced with permission from Ochoa JL [and Dyck PJ et al. (eds)] First edn. WB Saunders: 1975.

small-diameter thinly myelinated Aδ and unmyelinated C fibers (Figure 1). Other types of nociceptors are known as "silent" and respond only to tissue injury.[8] These primary sensory neurons synapse in the substantia gelatinosa of the dorsal horn of the spinal cord with neurons known as second-order pain transmission neurons. From here the signals are transmitted along specialized pathways (spinothalamic and reticulothalamic tracts) to the medial and lateral regions of the thalamus and then to the brain (Figure 2).

Fields[3] divided the processing of pain from the stimulation of primary afferent nociceptors to the subjective experience of pain into four steps: transduction, transmission, modulation, and perception. *Transduction* is the activation of the primary *afferent* nociceptor. Primary afferent nociceptors can be activated by intense thermal, mechanical stimuli, noxious chemicals, and immunological stimuli.[9] Stimulation from endogenous inflammatory mediators is produced in response to tissue injury, immune effectors,

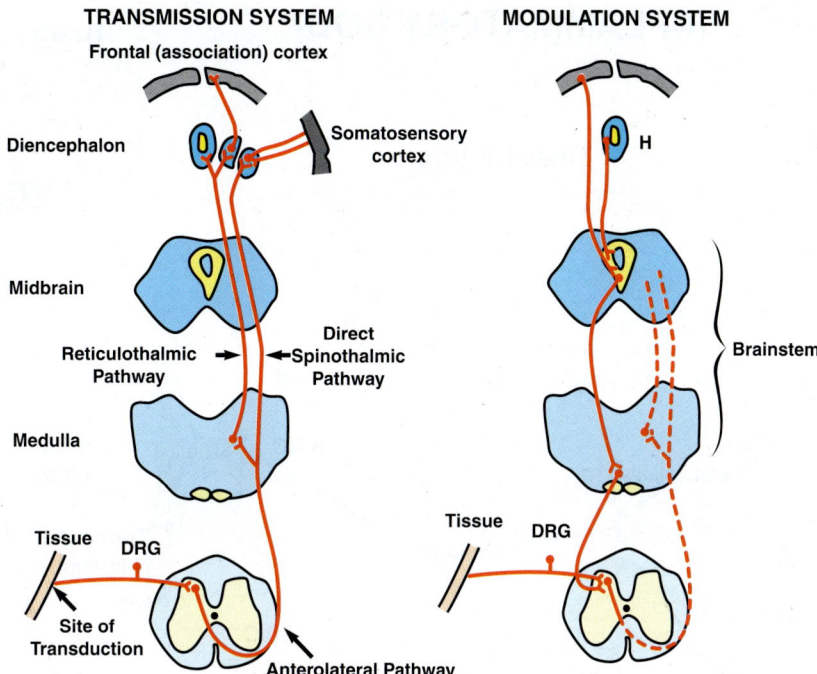

Figure 2 A diagrammatic outline of major neural structures relevant to pain. Sequence of events leading to pain perception begins in the transmission system with transduction (lower left), in which a noxious stimulus produces nerve impulses in the primary afferent nociceptor. These impulses are conducted to the spinal cord, where primary afferent nociceptors contact central pain transmission cells that relay the message to the thalamus either directly via the spinothalamic tract or indirectly via the reticular formation and the reticulothalamic pathway. From the thalamus, the message is relayed to the cerebral cortex and the hypothalamus (H). The outflow is through the midbrain and the medulla to the dorsal horn of the spinal cord, where it inhibits pain transmission cells, thereby reducing the intensity of perceived pain. Reproduced with permission from National Academy of Sciences; 1987.

and glia,[10,11] producing an "inflammatory soup" and plasma extravasation (Figure 3). These mediators are bradykinin, neuropeptides such as the potent vasodilator calcitonin gene-related peptide (CGRP), and substance P, growth factors, cytokines, chemokines, amines, purines, protons, ions, and arachidonic acid.[12,13] These inflammatory mediators interact with the multiple receptors expressed in the nociceptive afferences inducing their excitation.

Arachidonic acid is processed by two different enzyme systems to produce *prostaglandins* and *leukotrienes*, which, along with bradykinin, act as inflammatory mediators (see Figure 3). Whereas prostaglandins stimulate the primary afferent nociceptor directly, the leukotrienes contribute indirectly by causing *polymorphonuclear neutrophil leukocytes* to release another chemical that, in turn, stimulates the nociceptor. Bradykinin further contributes by causing the *sympathetic* nerve terminal to release a prostaglandin that also stimulates the nociceptor.[14] Additionally, in an area of injury or inflammation, the *sympathetic nerve terminal* will release yet another prostaglandin in response to its own neurotransmitter, *norepinephrine*. The presence of such an ongoing inflammatory state causes physiological sensitization of the primary afferent nociceptors.[14] Sensitized nociceptors display ongoing discharge, a lowered activation threshold to *normally nonpainful stimuli* (*allodynia*), and an *exaggerated response* to noxious stimuli (*primary hyperalgesia*).[15]

In addition to sending nociceptive impulses to synapse in the dorsal horn of the spinal cord or, in the case of trigeminal input, to synapse in the trigeminal nucleus, activation of cutaneous C fibers causes their cell bodies to synthesize the neuropeptides, *substance P* and *CGRP*. These neuropeptides are then antidromically transported along axon branches to the periphery by an axon transport system where they induce further plasma extravasation and increase inflammation. The release of these algogenic substances at the peripheral axon injury site produces the flare commonly seen around an injury site and is referred to as *neurogenic inflammation*,[7,16–18] or the *axon reflex*[15,19,20] (Figure 4). *Transmission* refers to the process by which peripheral nociceptive information is relayed to the CNS. The primary afferent nociceptor synapses with a second-order pain transmission

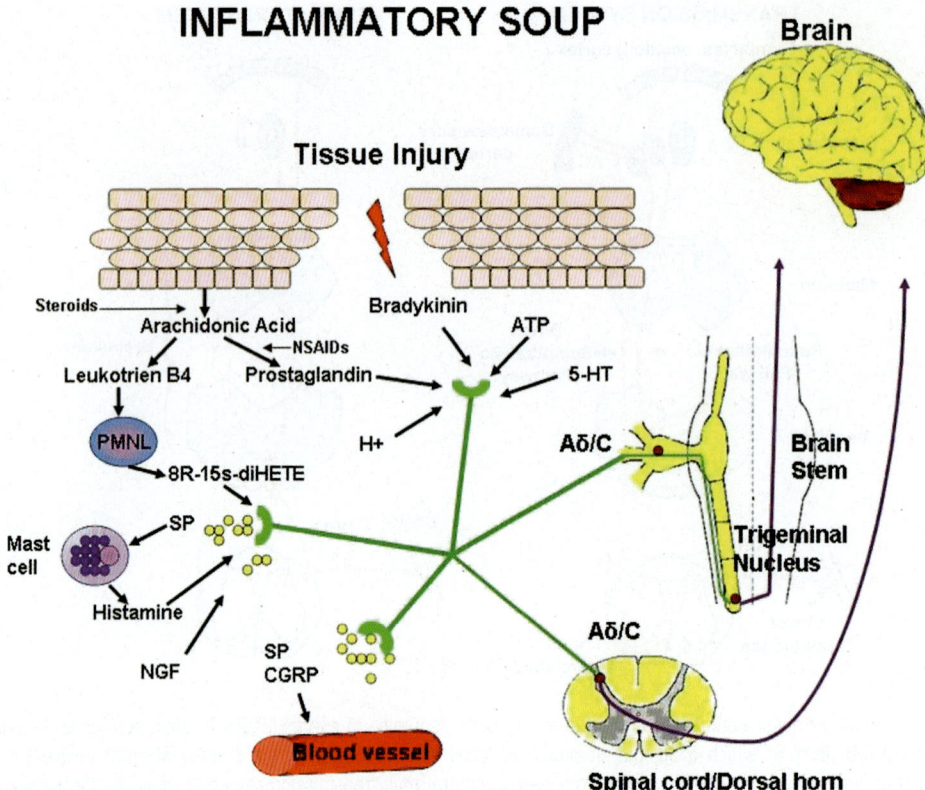

Figure 3 Membrane lipids produce arachidonic acid, which is converted to prostaglandins by the cyclooxygenase enzyme and to leukotriene B4 by the lipoxygenase enzyme. Prostaglandins act directly on the primary afferent nociceptor to lower the firing threshold and therefore cause "sensitization." Leukotriene B4 causes polymorphonuclear neutrophil leukocytes to produce another leukotriene that, in turn, acts on the primary afferent nociceptor to cause sensitization. Steroids prevent the synthesis of arachidonic acid altogether, thus inhibiting both pathways of prostaglandin production. Nonsteroidal anti-inflammatory drugs (NSAIDs), on the other hand, inhibit only the cyclooxygenase pathway.

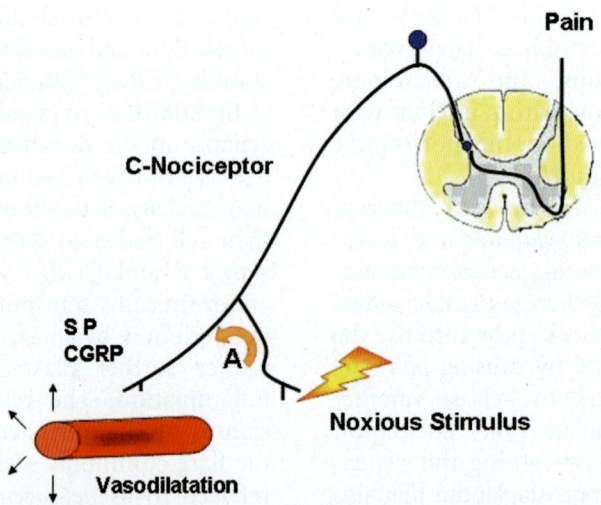

Figure 4 The axon reflex. Activation of cutaneous nociceptive C fibers elicits impulses that are conveyed centrally to induce pain and antidromically via axon branches (A). The antidromically excited peripheral C-fiber terminals release vasoactive substances, for example, calcitonin gene-related peptide (CGRP) and substance P (SP), causing cutaneous vasodilation, which produces the flare that develops around the site of noxious stimulation. Reproduced with permission from Field HL et al. *Neurobiol Dis;* 1998.

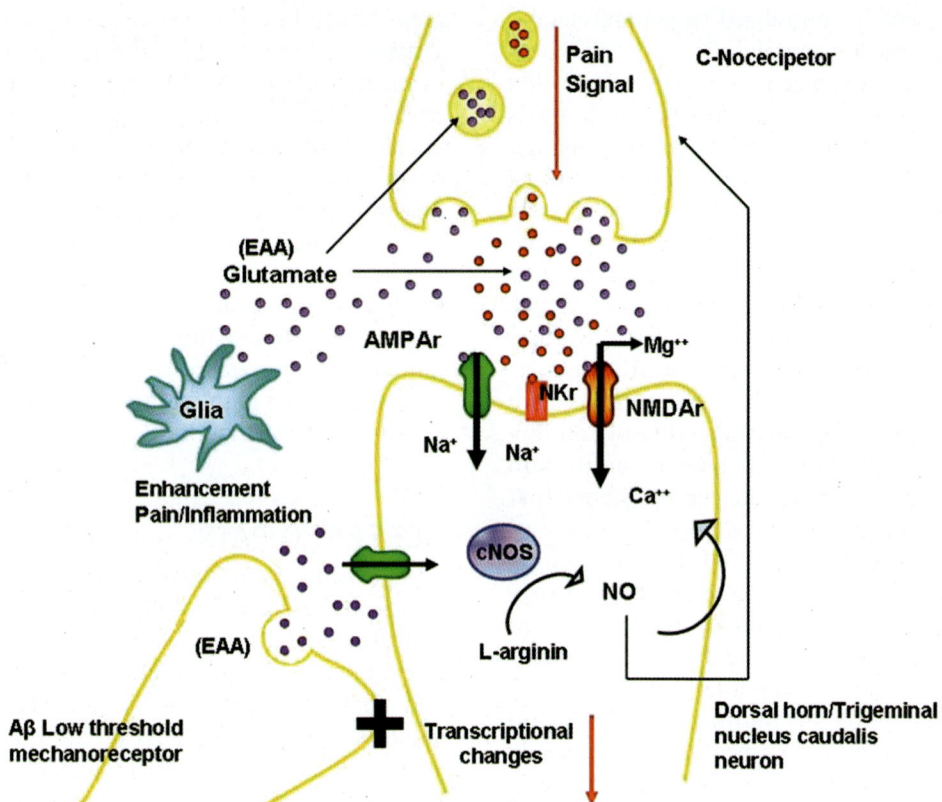

Figure 5 Central sensitization and allodynia. Input from C-nociceptors enhances the response of dorsal horn pain-signaling neurons to subsequent afferent inputs (central sensitization). This involves neuropeptides such as substance P (SP) acting at neurokinin receptors (NKR) and excitatory amino acids (EAA) acting at both the AMPA/KA and N-methyl-D-aspartate (NMDA) receptors, triggering secondary nitric oxide (NO) mechanisms. Large-diameter low-threshold mechanoreceptive primary afferents (A fibers) respond maximally to innocuous tactile stimuli and normally produce tactile sensation. When central sensitization is present, A fibers become capable of activating central nervous system (CNS) pain-signaling neurons (+), leading to touch-evoked pain (allodynia). Modified from Fields HL et al. Neurobiol Dis, 1998.

neuron in the dorsal horn of the spinal cord where a new action potential heads toward higher brain structures (see Figures 2 and 3). It is at this point that repeated or intense C fiber activation facilitates and increases responsiveness in the second-order pain transmission neuron, enhancing synaptic transmission and depressing inhibition in the dorsal horn.[21] This process further induces physiological, neurochemical, anatomical, and genetic changes.[22,17] Excitatory amino acids such as glutamate stimulate the activation of the N-methyl-D-aspartate receptor (NMDAr), which is a major component of inflammatory and chronic neuropathic pain[21,23,24] resulting in *central sensitization*.[15] Long-term changes in the response of second-order pain transmission neurons to nonpainful and painful input are induced with intense or prolonged nociceptive stimuli.[15] The response of these spinal cord dorsal horn neurons increases progressively and is enhanced with repeated identical noxious cutaneous input from the periphery, a process called "wind-up."[25–27] In addition, the size of the receptive field of the second-order pain transmission neuron increases.[28] The subjective correlate of wind-up is "temporal summation," for which a slowly repeated noxious stimulus is associated with a progressive increase in the intensity of perceived pain.[15,29] In addition, with central sensitization, stimulation of Aβ fibers (large-diameter low-threshold mechanoreceptors that normally respond only to painless tactile stimuli) will also establish connections with second-order nociceptive dorsal horn neurons, producing what is called a "secondary mechanical hyperalgesia"[15,30,31] (Figure 5). These plastic changes result in nonpainful stimuli causing pain. This can be observed in the hypersensitivity and allodynea present during a migraine headache or in the diffuse referred and aching pain in myofascial pain (MFP) disorders,[22,32] as well as in the ongoing persistent aching burning pain present in centralized trigeminal neuropathies such as atypical odontalgia.[33]

Modulation refers to mechanisms by which the transmission of noxious information to the brain is reduced. Numerous *descending inhibitory* systems that originate supraspinally and strongly influence spinal nociceptive transmission exist.[34] In the past, only midline structures such as the periaqueductal gray, rostroventral medulla, and nucleus raphe magnus were known to be involved in descending nociceptive modulation (see Figure 2). Now many sites previously thought to be primarily involved in cardiovascular function and autonomic regulation (e.g., nucleus tractus solitarius; locus ceruleus/subceruleus, among others) have also been shown to play a role in pain modulation.[34] The ascending nociceptive signal that synapses in the midbrain area activates the release of norepinephrine and *serotonin*, two of the main neurotransmitters involved in the descending inhibitory pathways.[34,35] Activity in the pain modulation system means that there is less activity in the pain transmission pathway in response to noxious stimulation.

An endogenous opioid system for pain modulation also exists.[36] *Endogenous opioid peptides* are naturally occurring pain-dampening neurotransmitters and neuromodulators that are *implicated in pain suppression* and modulation because they are present in large quantities in the areas of the brain associated with these activities (subnucleus caudalis and the substantia gelatinosa of the spinal cord).[36–38] They reduce nociceptive transmission by preventing the release of the excitatory neurotransmitter substance P from the primary afferent nerve terminal. The presence of these natural opioid receptors for endogenous opiates permits morphine-like drugs to exert their analgesic effect. However, evidence suggests that exogenous opioids, when used extensively, can paradoxically induce hyperalgesia.[39]

The final step in the subjective experience of pain is *perception*. How and where the brain perceives pain is still under investigation. Part of the difficulty lies in the fact that the pain experience has at least two components: the sensory-discriminatory dimension and the affective (emotional) dimension. The affective dimension of pain is made up of feelings of expectations, unpleasantness, and emotions associated with future implications related to the pain.[40,41]

Neuroimaging studies have demonstrated the involvement of the thalamus and multiple cortical areas (including the primary and secondary somatosensory cortices (S1,S2), the insular cortex (IC), the prefrontal cortex (PFC), and the anterior cingulated cortex (ACC)[42] in the perception of pain. However, it is clear from intersubject variability in the activation of any one of these areas that affective reactions and possibly motor responses are also involved.[43]

Of significance is the fact that, with high levels of modulation or with damage in the pain transmission system, it is possible to have nociception without pain perception. Conversely, with certain types of damage to the nervous system, there may be an overreaction to pain stimuli or pain perception without nociception.[3]

REFERRED PAIN

Pain arising from deep tissues, muscles, ligaments, joints, and viscera is often perceived at a site distant from the actual nociceptive source. Thus, the pain of angina pectoris is often felt in the left arm or the jaw, and diaphragmatic pain is often perceived in the shoulder or the neck. Whereas cutaneous pain is sharp, burning, and clearly localized, referred pain from musculoskeletal and visceral sources is usually deep, dull, aching, and more diffuse.

Referred pain presents a diagnostic dilemma. If left unrecognized, it may result in a clinician telling a patient that his pain is psychogenic in origin. Treatments directed at the site of the pain are ineffective and, if invasive, subject the patient to unnecessary risks, expense, and complications. However, referred pain is dependent on a primary pain source and will cease if this source is eliminated.

The mechanism of referred pain is still somewhat enigmatic. The two most popular theories are convergence-projection and convergence-facilitation.

1. *Convergence-projection theory*. This is the most popular theory. Primary afferent nociceptors from both visceral and cutaneous neurons often converge onto the same second-order pain transmission neuron in the spinal cord,[44] and convergence has been well documented in the trigeminal brainstem nuclear complex.[23,45–47] The trigeminal spinal tract nucleus also receives converging input from cranial nerves VII, IX, and X, as well as the upper cervical nerves.[48,49] The brain, having more awareness of cutaneous than of visceral structures through past experience, interprets

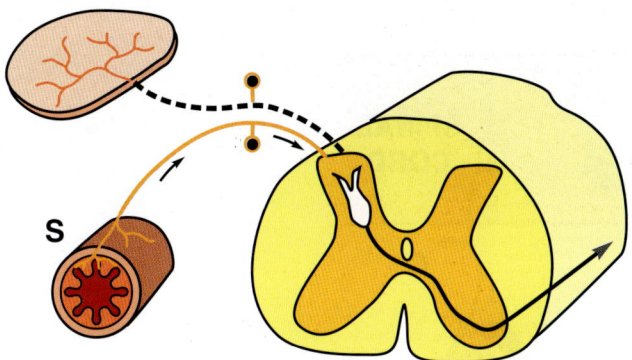

Figure 6 The convergence-projection hypothesis of referred pain. According to this hypothesis, visceral afferent nociceptors (S) converge on the same pain-projection neurons as the afferents from the somatic structures in which the pain is perceived. The brain has no way of knowing the actual source and mistakenly "projects" the sensation to the somatic structure. Reproduced with permission from Fields HL, McGraw-Hill; 1987.

the pain as coming from the regions subserved by the cutaneous afferent fibers (Figure 6).

2. *Convergence-facilitation theory.* This theory is similar to the convergence-projection theory, except that the nociceptive input from the deeper structures causes the resting activity of the second-order pain transmission neuron in the spinal cord to increase or be "facilitated." The resting activity is normally created by impulses from the cutaneous afferents. "Facilitation" from the deeper nociceptive impulses causes the pain to be perceived in the area that creates the normal, resting background activity. This theory tries to incorporate the clinical observation that blocking sensory input from the reference area, with either a local anesthetic or cold, can sometimes reduce the perceived pain. This is particularly true with referred pain from *myofascial trigger points (TrPs)*, for which application of a vapocoolant spray is actually a popular and effective modality used for pain control.

The mechanism of referred pain from myofascial TrPs is also under speculation. According to Mense,[50] the convergence-projection and convergence-facilitation models of referred pain do not directly apply to muscle pain because there is little convergence of neurons from *deep* tissues in the dorsal horn. Based on experimentally induced changes in the receptive field properties of dorsal horn neurons in the cat in response to a deep noxious stimulus,[51] Mense proposed that convergent connections from other spinal cord segments are "unmasked" or opened by the nociceptive input from skeletal muscles and that referral to other myotomes is owing to the release and spread of substance P and CGRP to adjacent spinal segments.[50] Simons has expanded on this theory to specifically explain the referred pain from TrPs[52] (Figure 7). MFP is discussed in more detail later in the chapter.

TRIGEMINAL SYSTEM

An appreciation of the arrangement of the trigeminal nociceptive system provides some insight into the interesting pain and referral patterns that are encountered in the head and neck region. The primary afferent nociceptors of the fifth cranial nerve synapse is the nucleus caudalis of the brainstem.[53] The nucleus caudalis is the caudal portion of the trigeminal spinal tract nucleus and corresponds to

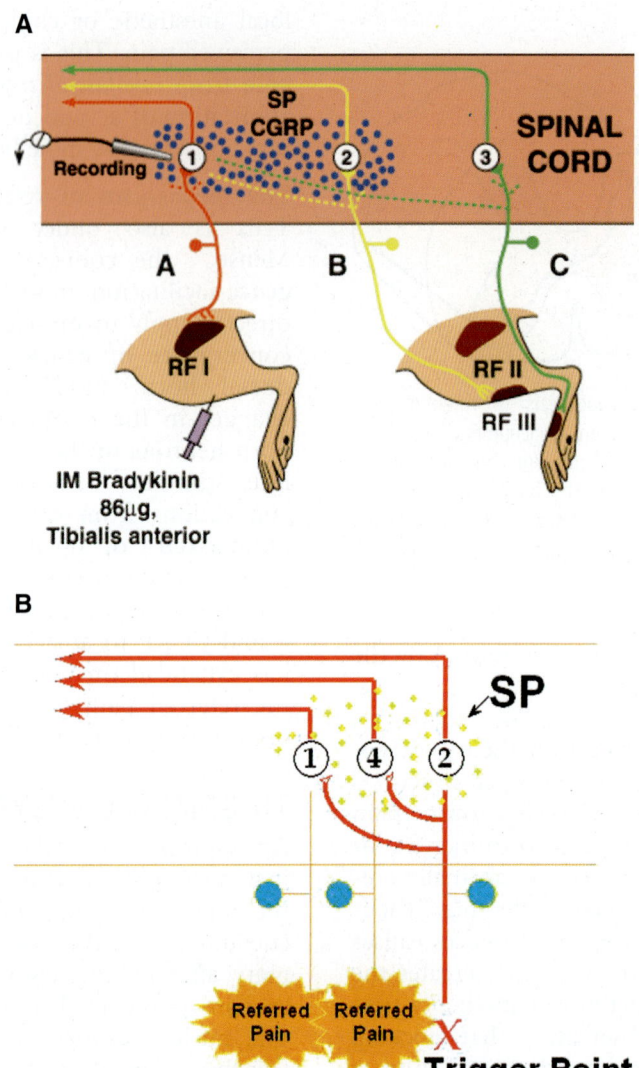

Figure 7 ***A,*** Neuroanatomic model explaining the apperance of new receptive fields (RF's) (see Figure 7A) by unmasking latent connections in the dorsal horn. The activity of neuron 1 was recorded with a microelectrode introduced into the spinal cord. The neuron is connected by pathway A to its original RF in the biceps femoris muscle (RF I). Synaptically effective connections are drawn as solid lines, ineffective (latent) connections as dashed lines. The injection of bradykinin was made outside RF I into the tibialis anterior (TA) muscle, which contains the RF of neuron 2 (RF II). The Bradykinin-induced excitation of nociceptive fibers of pathway B is assumed to release substance P (SP) and calcitonin gene-related peptide (CGRP) in the dorsal horn, which diffuse (stippling) to neuron 1 and increase the efficacy of latent connections from pathways B and C to this cell. Now neuron 1 can be activated also from RF II and RF III. ***B,*** Extension of the neuroanatomic model presented of Mense's model of deep referred pain. Although no direct experimental evidence substantiates this modification, it is compatible with the mechanisms described by Mense and helps to explain some trigger point characteristics not accounted for by his model. Neurons 1 and 2 correspond to neurons 1 and 2 in the Mense model. Neurons 1 and 4 are connected by solid lines to their respective receptive fields. These fields are the areas that would be identified as the source of nociception when neurons 1 and 4 are activated. Nociceptive input from the trigger point would activate neuron 2 and could account for the initial localized pain in response to pressure applied to the trigger point. This activity is assumed to release substance P (SP) and calcitonin gene-related peptide (CGRP) in the dorsal horn that diffuses (stippling) to neurons 1 and 4. This increases the efficacy of latent connections (dashed lines) to these cells. Now neurons 1 and 4 can be activated by nociceptive activity originating in the trigger point and would be perceived as referred pain. ***A,*** reproduced with permission from Menses S, *Am Pain Soc J;* 1994; ***B,*** reproduced with permission from Simons DG, *Am Pain Soc J;* 1994.

the substantia gelatinosa of the rest of the spinal dorsal horn (Figure 8). From here the nociceptive input is transmitted to the higher centers via the trigeminal lemniscus. Of significance is the arrangement of the trigeminal nerve fibers within this nucleus and the fact that the nucleus descends as

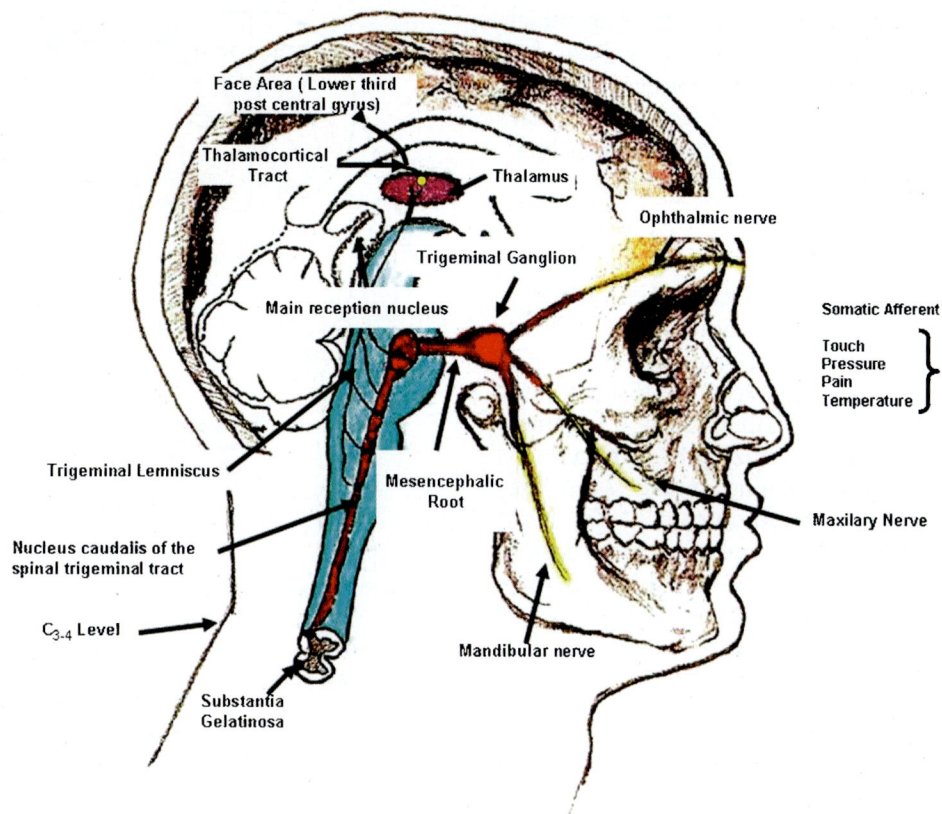

Figure 8 Primary afferent nociceptive fibers of the trigeminal nerve (cranial nerve V) synapse in the nucleus caudalis of the spinal trigeminal tract. The nucleus caudalis descends as low as C3–4 in the spinal cord. Many nociceptors from deep cervical structures synapse on the same second-order pain transmission neurons as the trigeminal nerve. This may explain why cervical pain disorders are often perceived as facial pain or headache.

low as the third and fourth cervical vertebrae (C3–4) in the spinal cord. Fibers from all three trigeminal branches are found at all levels of the nucleus, arranged with the mandibular division highest and the ophthalmic division lowest.[54] In addition, they are arranged in such a manner that fibers closest to the midline of the face synapse in the most cephalad portion of the tract. The more lateral the origin of the fibers on the face, the more caudal the synapse in the nucleus (Figure 9). Understanding this "laminated" arrangement helps to explain why a maxillary molar toothache may be perceived as pain in a mandibular molar on the same side (referred pain) but not in an incisor. Similarly, pain perceived in the ear may actually be owing to (or referred from) an infected third molar.

Because the trigeminal nucleus descends to the C3–4 level in the spinal cord, primary afferent nociceptors from deep cervical structures synapse on the same second-order pain transmission neurons that subserve the fifth cranial nerve.[55] This convergence

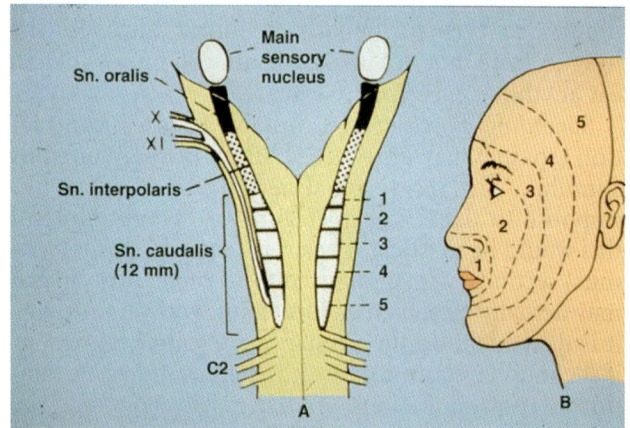

Figure 9 The arrangement of the trigeminal nociceptive fibers of the spinal trigeminal tract is significant. Fibers from all three trigeminal branches are found at all levels of the nucleus, arranged with the mandibular division highest and the ophthalmic division lowest. Fibers closest to the midline of the face synapse in the most cephalad portion of the tract. The more lateral the origin of the fibers on the face, the more caudal the synapse in the nucleus. Modified from Kunc Z, Georg Thieme Verlag, 1970.

of primary afferent nociceptors from the trigeminal region and the cervical region provides a basis for understanding why *cervical pain* disorders may be perceived as pain in the head and face, particularly in the *forehead and temple*—the lateral ophthalmic trigeminal fibers synapse the lowest (see Figure 9).

CHRONIC PAIN

Pain becomes complicated and difficult to manage when it is prolonged. Often the clinician is frustrated by the apparent discrepancy between the identifiable nociceptive source, which may seem very small, and the amount of suffering and disability seen. It becomes easy to label these patients as "crazy" or "malingering" (deliberately, fraudulently feigning an illness for the purpose of a consciously desired outcome).[1] Yet there are both physiological and psychological mechanisms that may increase pain perception—mechanisms that help to explain why there may be a discrepancy between actual nociception, perceived pain, and the apparent resultant suffering and disability.

PHYSIOLOGICAL MECHANISMS MODIFYING PAIN

Sensitization. As previously discussed, primary afferent nociceptors become sensitized through the release of endogenous substances caused by tissue injury. As a result, normally innocuous stimuli become painful[14] For example, acute arthritis of the temporomandibular joint (TMJ) results in pain on joint movement or with increased pressure from chewing, normally innocuous events. Similarly, a minor burn on the tongue from hot tea makes it almost impossible to eat anything, even mildly spicy.

Spreading muscle spasm. Sustained muscle contraction (spasm) may arise as a result of primary noxious stimulus. This is a spinal reflex and a protective response to tissue injury (Figure 10). An example of this would be masticatory elevator muscle spasm (trismus) secondary to an infected third molar. The spasm may actually be the chief complaint, and yet, initially, it is dependent on the primary pain source. However, if the muscle spasm results in ischemia and accumulation of potassium ions, muscle nociceptors may be activated, resulting in the development of an independent, self-perpetuating primary pain source in the muscle (see Figure 10). Successful treatment of the infection or removal of the painful third molar will no longer correct the muscle pain problem since use of the muscle produces pain, causing more spasm, causing more pain. In addition, studies have shown that this type of deep musculoskeletal pain causes spasm

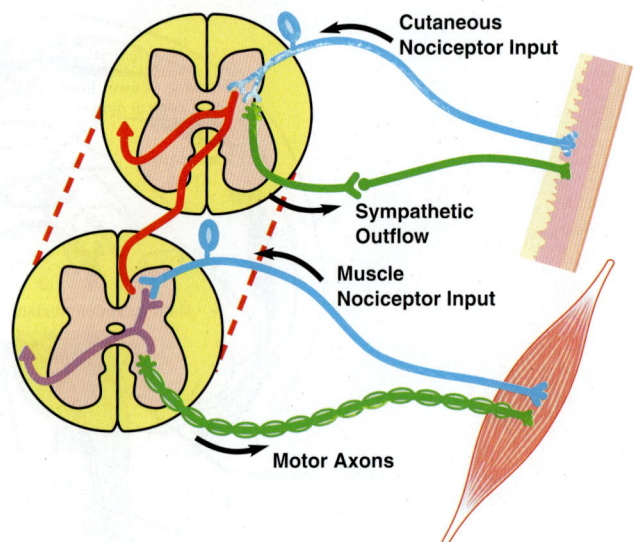

Figure 10 Reflex activation of nociceptors in self-sustaining pain. There are two important reflex pathways for pain. The top loop illustrates the sympathetic component. Nociceptor input activates sympathetic reflexes, which activate or sensitize nociceptor terminals. The bottom loop illustrates the muscle contraction loop. Nociceptors induce muscle contraction, which, in some patients, activates muscle nociceptors that feed back into the same reflex to sustain muscle contraction and pain. Modified from National Acad Sciences, 1987.

and pain in other muscles innervated by the same spinal segment.[56,57] Long-standing conditions of this sort may result in the recruitment of more muscles and more pain, with the ultimate establishment of a vicious spreading pain cycle. This may partly explain the development and some of the characteristics of myofascial TrPs, to be discussed in detail later in the chapter.

Autonomic factors. Just as primary afferent nociceptive input may activate motoneurons, so may it also activate the sympathetic nervous system (see Figure 10). Efferent discharge from the sympathetic nervous system has been shown, in animals at least, to activate primary afferent nociceptors, especially when injured.[58] Thus, a peripheral injury may set up a positive feedback loop through activation of the sympathetic nervous system that will perpetuate the activation of the primary afferent nociceptors. The extreme result of this type of sympathetic hyperactivity is a condition known as "reflex sympathetic dystrophy" (RSD) included in the complex regional pain syndromes[59] (discussed in more detail later in this chapter). In this syndrome, the pain, even from a minor injury, does not subside and, in fact, develops into a progressive, excruciating burning pain with cutaneous hypersensitivity. The pain may occur in a site larger than and different from that of the original injury; autonomic signs such as vasoconstriction or sweating of the painful area are usually present. The sympathetic nervous system is strongly implicated because sympathetic blockade abolishes the pain. Mild forms of this self-perpetuating loop of sympathetic activity and primary nociceptive response may explain why pain sometimes worsens, even when the injury has healed.

PSYCHOLOGICAL FACTORS MODIFYING PAIN

Psychological and social factors are inextricably linked with the perception of pain and illness.[60] The traditional dualistic view of mind and body as separate, independently functioning entities is wholly inadequate. As a result of the need for a new approach to illness and pain, the biopsychosocial model for disease and illness was developed. In this model, disease is defined as "definite pathologic process with a characteristic set of signs and symptoms."[1] Illness refers to the subjective experience of that disease or the belief that disease is present.[61] An explosion of research in chronic pain over the last 10 years has documented the complex interrelationship between genetics, neurophysiology, pain, and emotion.[60] For example, emotional distress may predispose a person to experience pain, amplify or inhibit the intensity of the pain, perpetuate the pain, or be a result of the pain.[60] Anxiety and depression have long been studied with respect to their complexly intertwined relationship with chronic pain, but anger also plays an interesting role. These emotional concomitants to chronic pain are important to appreciate because they affect treatment motivation and compliance to treatment recommendations. For successful treatment, clinicians treating patients with pain, acute or chronic, must pay attention to their emotional/psychological states, as well as the somatically identified nociceptive cause.

Cognitive and affective factors. Sensory factors refer to the detection, localization, quantification, and identification of the quality of a particular stimulus. However, the reaction to the stimulus and the intensity of desire to terminate the stimulus are determined by cognitive and affective variables. *Cognitive variables* include such things as an individual's *past experience* with similar stimuli, their *psychological makeup*, and *societal* and *cultural* factors. *Affective variables* relate to emotions and feelings and determine how unpleasant the stimulus is to the individual. *Affective descriptors* of a sensory experience might include words such as "nagging," "uncomfortable," "intense," or "killing," in contrast to sensory features such as "mild burning," "localized to the palate," or "aching over the TMJ."

Affective variables may be accompanied by *anxiety or depression* and are influenced by expectation and suggestion. Interestingly, the meaning that a person ascribes to their pain, threatening, benign or irrelevant, and their perception of the control they have over their pain, affects that individual's affective and behavioral response to the pain. For example, most people are not particularly distressed about having a headache since the vast majority of headaches are not pathological. Yet someone whose sibling recently died of a brain tumor might be much more worried and anxious about this same symptom, even if it is very mild. Similarly, recurrence of pain owing to cancer carries with it the knowledge that the disease may be progressing and may remind the individual of his mortality. This type of pain will have many more emotional components and may be perceived as much more severe.[62]

Another good example is the anxious dental patient who jumps in agony at the first touch of the cheek. Even though the sensation of touch is well below his experimental pain threshold, the patient perceives it and reacts to it as painful. Conversely, a person experiencing analgesia through hypnosis may perceive no sensations or only nonpainful sensations while undergoing normally painful procedures such as tooth extraction or pulp extirpation.[63,64]

BEHAVIORAL FACTORS

Suffering and pain are communicated through actions such as moaning, limping, grimacing, guarding, pill taking, or visiting the doctor. These actions are termed *pain behaviors*. Pain behaviors follow basic learning principles and tend to increase unconsciously if they are rewarded by positive consequences. Positive consequences may include attention from loved ones and/or the medical/dental system and avoidance of various aversive tasks and responsibilities. Since chronic pain conditions, by definition, last a long time, they provide an opportunity for unconscious learning to occur. The pain behaviors observed in a patient with chronic pain may be the cumulative result of intermittent *positive reinforcement* over months or years. In addition, *well behaviors* are often totally ignored and nonreinforced, causing them to decrease. Just as positive reinforcement causes an increase in particular behaviors, so will nonreinforcement cause a decrease. Thus, even when the nociceptive source has diminished or healed, pain perception and attendant disability may be maintained through *learned pain behaviors* along with physical, cognitive, and affective factors.[65]

Pain Assessment Tools

Pain is a subjective experience that is communicated to us only through words and behaviors. Unlike measuring blood pressure, temperature, or erythrocyte sedimentation rate, measuring pain intensity is extremely difficult. As discussed above, there are several physiological and psychological factors that will influence the intensity of pain perceived. Other cognitive, affective, behavioral, and learning factors affect how this pain is communicated.

Nonetheless, measuring pain is important, not just for studying pain mechanisms in a laboratory but also to *assess treatment outcome*. To this end, a number of instruments have been developed and tested for their reliability and validity in measuring different aspects of the pain experience.

Quantifying the Pain Experience

VISUAL ANALOG SCALES

A visual analog scale is a line that represents a continuum of a particular experience, such as pain. The most common form used for pain is a 10-cm line, whether horizontal or vertical, with perpendicular stops at the ends. The ends are anchored by "no pain" and "worst pain imaginable" (Figure 11). Numbers should not be used along the line to ensure a better, less biased distribution of pain ratings. Otherwise, a disproportionately high frequency of 5 and 10 cm will be chosen.[65] Patients are asked to place a slash mark somewhere along the line to indicate the intensity of their current pain complaint. For scoring purposes, a millimeter ruler is used to measure along the line and obtain a numeric score for the pain ratings. Most people understand this scale quickly and can easily rate their pain. Children as young as 5 years are able to use this scale.[66] Its reliability and validity for measuring pain relief have been demonstrated[67,68] Caution is advised with photocopying because this process usually lengthens the line and introduces error.

The use of the scale should be clearly explained to the patient. For measuring treatment outcome, relief scales (a line anchored with "no pain relief" and "complete pain relief") may be superior to asking absolute pain intensities.[69] Similarly, if a pain intensity visual analog scale was used, patients may be more accurate if they are allowed to see their previous scores.[70]

Numeric rating scales, where "0" is no pain and "10" is the worst pain imaginable, are also very useful and preferred by adults without cognitive impairment.[71] Children and older adults, either minority or cognitively impaired, may do better with colored analog scales or faces pain scales.[72–74] Colored analog scales use a 0 to 10 scale and verbal markers on a scale that is colored from green to yellow to red depicting increasing levels of pain. Faces pain scales use faces depicting various expressions from smiling to crying along a continuum with verbal descriptors underneath. Studies have shown that pain ratings are lower if the scale starts with a nonsmiling face.[75]

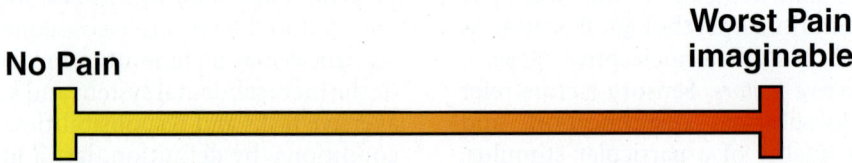

Figure 11 Visual analog pain scale used to indicate patient's level of daily pain. The patient places a mark at the perceived level of discomfort. The scale is 10 cm, so direct measurement can subsequently be made.

MCGILL PAIN QUESTIONNAIRE

The McGill Pain Questionnaire (Table 1) is a verbal pain scale that uses a vast array of words commonly used to describe a pain experience. Different types of pain and different diseases and disorders have different qualities of pain. These qualitative sensory descriptors are invaluable in providing key clues to possible diagnoses. Similarly, patients use different words to describe the affective component of their pain.

To facilitate the use of these words in a systematic way, Melzack and Torgerson set about categorizing many of these verbal descriptors into classes and subclasses designed to describe these different aspects of the pain experience. In addition to words describing the sensory qualities of pain, affective descriptors including such things as fear and anxiety and evaluative words describing the overall intensity of the pain experience were included.[76]

The words are listed in 20 different categories (see Table 1). They are arranged in order of magnitude from least intense to most intense and are grouped according to distinctly different qualities of pain. The patients are asked to circle only one word in each category that applies to them. Patients are usually happy to select from this list of pain-describing adjectives, often saying, "Now I can tell exactly how it feels. Before I couldn't think of just the right words."

The first 10 categories represent different sensory descriptors covering various temporal, spatial, pressure, and thermal qualities of pain. The next five categories are affective or emotional descriptors, category 16 is evaluative (i.e., how intense is the pain experience), and the last four categories are grouped as miscellaneous.

To score the questionnaire, the words in each category are given a numeric value. The first word in each category ranks as 1, the second as 2, and so on. The scores for each category are added up separately for the sensory, affective, evaluative, and miscellaneous groupings. Then the total number of words chosen is also noted. Using this questionnaire, it is possible to obtain a sense of the quality of a patient's pain complaint (categories 1 through 10), its intensity (category 16), and the amount of emotional or psychological overlay accompanying the pain (categories 11 through

Table 1 Sample of Classic McGill Pain Questionnaire

Terms Describing Pain

Sensory

1	2	3	4	5
Flickering	Jumping	Pricking	Sharp	Pinching
Quivering	Flashing	Boring	Cutting	Pressing
Pulsing	Shooting	Drilling	Lacerating	Gnawing
Throbbing		Stabbing		Cramping
Beating		Lancinating		Crushing
Pounding				

6	7	8	9	10
Tugging	Hot	Tingling	Dull	Tender
Pulling	Burning	Itchy	Sore	Taut
Wrenching	Scalding	Smarting	Hurting	Rasping
	Searing	Stinging	Aching heavy	Splitting

Affective

11	12	13	14	15
Tiring	Sickening	Fearful	Punishing	Wretched
Exhausting	Suffocating	Frightful	Gruelling	Blinding
		Terrifying	Cruel vicious	
			Killing	

Evaluative | **Miscellaneous**

16	17	18	19	20
Annoying	Spreading	Tight	Cool	Nagging
Troublesome	Radiating	Numb	Cold	Nauseating
Miserable	Penetrating	Drawing	Freezing	Agonizing
Intense	Piercing	Squeezing		Dreadful
Unbearable		Tearing		Torturing

15). Changes in a patient's pain experience can be monitored by administering the questionnaire at various time points during treatment and follow-up.

Melzack used this master list of words to derive quantitative measures of clinical pain that can be treated statistically; if used correctly, it can also detect changes in pain with different treatment modalities.[72]

PSYCHOLOGICAL ASSESSMENT

Chronic pain is the most complicated pain experience and the most perplexing and frustrating problem in medicine and dentistry today. Because chronic pain syndromes have such a complex network of psychological and somatic interrelationships, it is critical to view the patient as an integrated whole and not as a sum of individual parts. Determining the emotional, behavioral, and environmental factors that perpetuate chronic pain is as essential as establishing the correct physical diagnosis or, in many chronic cases, multiple diagnoses.

Almost all patients with chronic head and neck pain have physical findings contributing to their complaint. Similarly, almost all patients with chronic head and neck pain have psychological components to their pain as well. Contributing to the complex neurobehavioral aspects of pain is the fact that chronic pain is not self-limiting, seems as though it will never resolve, and has little apparent cause or purpose. As such, multiple psychological problems arise that confuse the patient and perpetuate the pain. Patients feel helpless, hopeless, and desperate in their inability to receive relief. They may become hypochondriacal and obsessed about any symptom or sensation they perceive. Vegetative symptoms and overt depression may set in, with sleep and appetite disturbances. Irritability and great mood fluctuations are common. Loss of self-esteem, libido, and interest in life activities add to the patient's misery. All of this may erode personal relationships with family, friends, and health professionals. Patients focus all of their energy on analyzing their pain and believe it to be the cause of all of their problems. They shop from doctor to doctor, desperately searching for an organic cure. They can become belligerent, hostile, and manipulative in seeking care. Many clinicians make gallant attempts with multiple drug regimens or multiple surgeries, but failure frustrates the clinician and adds to the patient's ongoing depression.

Near the end of this progression, in addition to their continuing pain, many of these patients have multiple drug dependencies and addictions or high stress levels; they may have lost their jobs, be on permanent disability, or be involved in litigation.

Herein lies the importance of proper *psychological diagnosis* as well as accurate physical diagnosis. An appropriate evaluation should include consideration of all factors that reinforce and perpetuate the pain complaints. Examining factors contributing to pain aggravation can include a look at stress (current and cumulative), interpersonal relationships, any secondary gain the patient may be receiving for having the pain, perceptual distortion of the pain, and poor lifestyle habits such as inadequate diet, poor posture, and lack of exercise. This information may well point to the reasons why patients have been unsuccessfully treated in the past. Obtaining baseline measures of pain levels, drug intake, functional impairment, and emotional state is important and will help monitor a patient's progress through rehabilitation. Additionally, systematic assessment of psychosocial difficulties that interfere with work and interpersonal activities is important but often neglected. The dentist should include questions to elicit information about oral habits, depression, anxiety, stressful life events, lifestyle changes, and secondary gain (operant pain) in the clinical interview.

To decide whether a patient should be referred for a full psychological assessment, the clinician evaluating the patient with chronic pain may choose to use simple questionnaires that are easy to administer, do not take long to fill out, and are reliable and adequate psychological screening tools. The Brief Battery for Health Improvement (BBHI-2) is a basic screening device that has been normed with a range of pain/orofacial pain/TMD patients.[77,78] It is short and gives three main dimensions of pain that practitioners should screen for: (1) mood (with suicide ideation); (2) functional limitations; and (3) somatization. A brief tutorial on the use and interpretation of the BBHI-2 can be found on the web at http://www.pearsonassessments.com/medical/bbhi2-tutorial.htm.

Another extremely useful screening tool is the Beck Depression Inventory (BDI/BDI-II),*[79,80] Patients who score high on any of these inventories should be sent to a psychologist or a psychiatrist familiar with chronic pain for a more complete workup. Psychologists or psychiatrists may use the Minnesota Multiphasic Personality Inventory (*MMPI/MMPI-II*),[81] in addition to the BDI-II and other psychological instruments, as part of their comprehensive assessment.

---

*The BDI and BDI-II can be obtained by contacting the Psychological Corporation, 555 Academic court, San Antonio, TX 78204.

Making a Diagnosis

Diagnosing orofacial disease and headaches follows the same principles as any medical diagnosis. Of primary importance is a careful and exhaustive history. This alone will often point directly to a specific diagnosis or at least reveal a diagnostic category. The history is followed by a physical examination that should help to confirm or rule out the initial diagnostic impression. If necessary, further diagnostic studies such as pulp testing, nerve blocks, radiographs, or blood tests may be carried out or ordered at this time. These may help rule out serious disorders and provide information complementing the history and physical examination. Finally, if doubt concerning the diagnosis persists, or pathosis out of one's area of expertise exists, other medical specialists and health care providers may provide valuable consultation.

Begin by pondering the scenario of the following case:

Case history. A 33-year-old woman presents herself for evaluation of intense left-sided facial pain. The pain is described as a constant burning sensation that radiates from the left preauricular area to the orbit, zygoma, mandible, and, occasionally, shoulder. Her pain is exacerbated by cold air, cold liquids, chewing, smiling, and light touch over certain areas of her face. She also reports a constant "pinching" sensation over her left eyebrow and mandible and photophobia in the left eye. She is currently taking high doses of narcotics with little relief. The pain began 1 year previously, after the extraction of a left maxillary molar. The extraction site apparently developed a "dry socket" (localized osteomyelitis of the alveolar crypt). This was treated appropriately but without relief of the patient's symptoms. Subsequently, two mandibular molars on the same side were extracted in an attempt to relieve the pain. These extraction sites likewise developed "dry sockets" and were treated, again without pain relief. Local anesthetic injections twice daily for many months and a 4-week course of cephalosporin, given empirically for possible periodontal infection or osteomyelitis of the mandible were also unsuccessful in releiving the pain.

To properly evaluate these rather confusing signs and symptoms, additional information is necessary.

CLASSIFICATION

In evaluating orofacial pains and headaches, an easy-to-use, practical, and clinical classification of these pains will facilitate diagnosis (Table 2). In developing such a classification, it is important to remember that local pathosis of the extracranial or intracranial structures and referred pain from pathema of more distant organs such as the heart must be ruled out first. This covers a wide variety of infectious, inflammatory, degenerative, neoplastic, or obstructive processes that can affect any organ in the head, neck, and thorax, including the brain (see Tables 7–9). Most dentists and physicians are well trained to evaluate a patient for such pathosis.

There are other disorders, however, causing pain in the head and neck region that cannot be attributed to any obvious diseases of the craniofacial, craniocervical, thoracic, or intracranial organs. These disorders are less well appreciated and, for ease of clinical use, are best classified according to the apparent tissue origin of the pain (see Table 2). For an exhaustive classification of headaches and facial pain that includes very specific diagnostic criteria, the reader is referred to the International Headache Society's publication.[82]

The primary distinguishing feature of these diagnostic categories is the quality of the pain. For example, *vascular* pain, such as migraine, generally has a throbbing, pulsing, or pounding quality; *neuropathic* pain, for example, trigeminal neuralgia, is usually described as sharp, shooting, or burning and is restricted to the peripheral distribution of the affected nerve branch; *muscle* pain is usually deep, steady, and aching or produces a sensation of tightness or pressure.

Table 2 Practical Clinical Classification of Craniofacial Pain

General Classification	Origin of Pain	Basic Quality of Pain
Local pathosis of extracranial structures	Craniofacial organs	Any
Referred pain from remote pathologic sites	Distant organs and structures	Aching, pressing
Intracranial pathosis	Brain and related structures	Any
Neurovascular	Blood vessels	Throbbing
Neuropathic	Sensory nervous system	Shooting, sharp, burning
Causalgic	Sympathetic nervous system	Burning
Muscular	Muscles	Deep aching, tight
Unclassifiable	Etiology as yet unknown	Any

In contrast, *extracranial* or *intracranial* pathema may present with any quality of pain. An inflamed tooth pulp may throb with each heartbeat. A tumor pressing on a nerve may cause sharp, lancinating, neuralgic-like pain. A sinus infection may be dull and aching. *Referred pain* tends to be deep and poorly localized and has an aching or pressing quality.

Once organic pathosis has been ruled out, a preliminary diagnostic category can be chosen based on the location and the quality of the pain. Therefore, when taking a pain history, the first questions to ask are "*Where*, exactly, do you feel your pain?" "*How*, exactly, does your pain feel to you?" "Please mark on this line how severe you consider your pain to be at its worst, usual, and lowest." This will help guide further questioning to confirm or rule out a specific diagnosis within that group. For example, a patient may complain of a constant dull ache in front of the ear and a paroxysmal lancinating pain that shoots from the ear to the chin and tongue. In this situation, two patterns of pain are described. One points to a possibly myofascial or rheumatic diagnosis for the ear pain and the other to a paroxysmal neuralgia for the shooting pain. Further history, examination, and diagnostic tests will help establish more definitive physical diagnoses. This systematic approach is particularly helpful in chronic pain, in which there are often multiple diagnoses, and psychological distress and pain behavior may confuse the diagnostic process.

If the patient in the case outlined above does not have any ongoing pathological lesions of the extracranial or intracranial structures, which categories of pain would fit her description best? Based on the limited information given, namely, a *constant burning quality*, the most likely preliminary diagnostic categories are neuropathic and sympathetic. To make a specific diagnosis within a category, more specific information regarding the pain, its temporal pattern (timing of occurrence), associated symptoms, and aggravating and alleviating factors is needed.

HISTORY

The key elements of taking a history for a pain complaint are delineated in Table 3. Establishing the patient's chief complaint requires listening carefully as the patient describes each type of pain or complaint present, including the *location, quality, and severity* of each symptom. Chronic pain patients often have multiple pain complaints with different descriptions that may indicate that multiple diagnoses are involved. When this is the case, obtaining complete information on each pain complaint separately simplifies the diagnostic process.

Table 3 History of Pain

Chief complaint
Characteristics of pain
Location
Quality
Temporal patterns
Constant or intermittent
Duration of each attack if intermittent
Diurnal or nocturnal variation in intensity if constant
Seasonal variation of symptoms if any
Associated symptoms
Precipitating factors if intermittent
Aggravating factors
Alleviating factors
Symptoms severity range (lowest, usual, and highest pain intensities)
Onset and history
Past and present medications or other treatments for pain
Past medical and dental history
Family history
Social history
Review of systems

The patient in this case scenario complains of only one pain. The location is over the left side of the face, radiating from the preauricular area. The quality of the pain is described primarily as burning. Her usual pain intensity on a 0 to 10 scale is 8, 5 being the lowest, and 9 being the highest.

Different pains also have different *temporal patterns* or patterns of occurrence. For example, a patient may complain of an intermittent, unilateral throbbing head pain. This would be the hallmark of a diagnosis in the vascular category. The exact pattern of the pain will help determine which vascular headache the patient is suffering. For example, *migraines* last from 4 to 48 hours and occur once or twice a year up to several times per month. *Cluster headaches* last less than 90 minutes each but occur several times a day, for several months, before going into remission. Similar distinctions can be made with neuropathic pains. The pain of trigeminal neuralgia is seconds in duration and may be triggered frequently throughout the day. The pain of a posttraumatic neuropathy or postherpetic neuralgia (PHN) is constant.

The temporal pattern for this patient's burning pain is constant, with little daily variation.

Often there are associated symptoms such as nausea, vomiting, ptosis, nasal congestion, tingling, numbness, blurred vision, or visual changes that may precede or accompany the pain. These symptoms may point to a specific diagnosis. For example, visual changes may precede a migraine with aura. Nausea and vomiting often accompany severe headaches, especially migraine. Generalized malaise may accompany a temporal arteritis. Autonomic changes, such as ptosis, nasal congestion, or conjunctival injection, almost always accompany cluster headaches or chronic paroxysmal hemicrania (CPH). Tingling and numbness may occur with deafferentation (nerve damage) pains such as postherpetic or posttraumatic neuralgias.

Unexplained neurological symptoms, however, such as cognitive or memory changes, transient sensory or motor loss of the face or extremities, tinnitus, vertigo, loss of consciousness, or any of the above symptoms not fitting an appropriate pain picture, must alert the health professional to the possibility of an intracranial lesion, requiring further workup. Some of these symptoms may be normal bodily sensations enhanced through distorted perceptions. Similarly, others, such as tinnitus, vertigo, or sensory tingling, may be associated with the referred symptoms of *myofascial TrP pain*.[83] Further diagnostic tests or consultations may be needed to rule out more serious pathosis.

Associated symptoms of this patient include a constant "pinching" sensation over her left eyebrow and mandible and photophobia of the left eye. She also describes occasional "electric" attacks that radiate out from the left TMJ. The "electric" attacks she describes last anywhere from 30 minutes to 24 hours.

Precipitating, aggravating, and *alleviating factors* also add clues to the origin of pain. Withdrawal from alcohol or caffeine may trigger a migraine attack.[84,85] Light touch, shaving, or brushing teeth may precipitate an attack of trigeminal neuralgia. Cold weather, maintaining any one body position for a prolonged period of time, or overexercise will aggravate MFP. A dark room and rest will alleviate migraine but aggravate cluster headache. Heat and massage will alleviate muscular pain and MFP but may aggravate an inflamed joint.

The burning pain is constant, without precipitating factors. Aggravating factors include cold air, cold liquids, chewing, smiling, and light touch. The "electric" attacks are precipitated by light touch over the preauricular area. At this stage, nothing alleviates the pain. High doses of narcotics barely serve to "take the edge off."

Gathering information about the *onset* and *history* of the problem will provide further clues as to the etiology of the complaint. Of interest are the events surrounding the initiation of the pain, how the pain has changed since onset, and what evaluations and treatments have been tried in the past. For example, a history of skin lesions and malaise (herpes zoster) typically precedes PHN. Acute trauma may precede a myofascial TrP pain complaint. In contrast, psychological stress can trigger almost any type of pain complaint.

Knowing which specialists the patient has seen, which tests and radiographs have already been completed, what the previous diagnostic impressions have been, and which treatments have been tried, helps the practitioner in several ways. First, which workups are still needed? Did the past workups adequately rule out organic or life-threatening pathema? How long ago were these workups completed? Have the symptoms changed since then? Do any of these workups need to be repeated? Second, what diagnoses were considered in the past? Were appropriate medications or treatments tried, in adequate doses and for long enough periods of time? With acute pain, the history is usually quite short, but with chronic pain, the history may take hours to obtain, the patient having seen many different health care providers in the past. With chronic pain, the effect of past medications, surgeries, and other treatments may provide insight not only into the etiology of the pain but also into the psychological or behavioral status of the patient.

The pain began 1 year previously, after the extraction of a left maxillary molar. The extraction site apparently developed a "dry socket." This was treated appropriately but without relief of the patient's symptoms. Subsequently, two left mandibular molars were extracted in an attempt to relieve the pain. These extraction sites likewise developed "dry sockets" and were treated, again without pain relief. Local anesthetic injections twice daily for many months and a 4-week course of cephalosporin given empirically for a possible periodontal infection or osteomyelitis of the mandible were also unsuccessful.

This history tells us that, initially, local tooth pathosis was suspected as the etiology of the pain. However, extraction of teeth provided no relief. Osteomyelitis and possibly periodontal disease had also been suspected, but high-dose antibiotic treatment for osteomyelitis also failed to provide pain relief. Are there other extracranial or intracranial pathemas that may need to be ruled out?

A *family history* should include information regarding the patient's parents and siblings. Are they alive and well? If not, why not? Does anyone in the immediate family suffer from a similar pain problem? For example, 70% of migraine patients have a relative who also has or had migraine. Does anyone in the family have a chronic illness? This person may provide a model for pain behavior and coping.

The patient's parents and siblings are alive and well. There is no history of similar illness or chronic illness in her family.

A *social history* should not only cover demographic information, marital status, household situation, and occupation but also seek to uncover any potential perpetuating factors to the pain. Look for potential stressors at work and at home and ask about postural habits, body mechanics, dietary habits, environmental factors, and drug and alcohol use.

This patient lives in a rural farm area, has been married to the same man for 15 years, and has three children. She used to work on the farm but has been unable to do so for the last 6 months because of the pain. The patient has smoked one pack a day for 18 years. She does not drink alcohol. Currently she spends most of her day in bed because of the pain.

Since the patient lives in a rural area, the possibility of a coccal infection must be considered and ruled out.

The *past medical history* may reveal some underlying illnesses such as lupus erythematosus or hypothyroidism that may predispose the patient to developing pain. Past surgeries and medications for other purposes, any psychiatric history, allergies, hospitalizations, and other illnesses must be included and may reveal health care abuse.

The patient states that she is otherwise in good health. She had the usual childhood diseases, has no known allergies, and had been hospitalized only for the birth of her children. There is no history of trauma other than the tooth extractions previously mentioned.

A *review of systems* screens the person's present state of health. It includes asking about any recent symptoms related to the head and neck; the skin; and the cardiovascular, respiratory, gastrointestinal, genitourinary, endocrine, neurological, obstetric–gynecologic, and musculoskeletal systems.

The patient complains of decreased energy and sleep disturbance secondary to the pain. She has no other complaints.

In acute pain problems, a firm diagnosis may be established almost immediately from the history. In contrast, diagnosis of a chronic pain complaint may take months of tests or trials despite an exhaustive history. The next step in diagnosis is a thorough physical examination.

PHYSICAL EXAMINATION

The physical examination for craniofacial pain may vary slightly, depending on its location and the apparent cause. Pathosis of extracranial structures, particularly the oral cavity, must be sought and ruled out first. This usually involves inspection, palpation, percussion, transillumination, and auscultation of the tissues and structures suspected of causing pain. Intraoral examination that must include inspection of all intraoral tissues, teeth, and periodontium is discussed in detail in Chapters 14 and 15. Once acute pathema has been ruled out, the physical examination must be augmented to include evaluation of the cranial nerves, TMJ, cervical spine, and head and neck muscles. In specific cases, a more comprehensive neurological examination may be indicated. The basic components of a physical examination are listed in Table 4.

General inspection can reveal a great deal about a patient to the alert clinician. A slouching posture can point to *depression*. Rigidity in posture or clenching is an indication of excess *muscle tension* in the neck, shoulders, or jaws. Asymmetry, swelling, redness, and other signs may indicate a neoplastic or infectious process. Closer inspection of the head and neck may reveal scars of past surgeries, trophic skin changes associated with RSD, or color changes from local infection, systemic anemia, or jaundice.

The examination of the TMJs involves testing the range and quality of motion of the mandible, palpating and listening to joint noises, and palpating the lateral and dorsal joint capsules for tenderness. The normal range of jaw opening is 40 to 60 mm. Laterotrusive and protrusive movements should be 8 to 10 mm. The path of opening and laterotrusive and protrusive movements should be straight, without deflections or deviations. Joint capsule palpation anterior to the tragus of the ear for the lateral capsule and from the external auditory meatus for the dorsal capsule may be "uncomfortable" but should not be painful.

As discussed later in the chapter, the cervical spine is often the source of persistent referred pain to the orofacial and TMJ regions. Similarly, poor posture is one of the most important contributing factors to TMJ dysfunction and *myofascial TrP* pain. For these reasons, the cervical spine and the posture must be evaluated in any chronic head and neck or facial pain

Table 4 Physical Examination

General inspection
Head and neck inspection
Stomatognathic examination
Cervical spine examination
Myofascial examination
Cranial nerve examination

problem. The examination of the cervical spine includes testing its range and quality of motion as a whole, as well as testing the range and quality of motion of the first two cervical joints individually.[86–88] Posture, especially anterior head positioning, must also be systematically evaluated. For details on how and why this is important, the reader is referred to Travell and Simons' *Trigger Point Manual*.[83]

Myofascial TrP examination requires a thorough, systematic palpation of all of the masticatory and cervical muscles, looking for tight muscle bands and the focal tenderness associated with myofascial TrPs. Myofascial TrP is the most prevalent cause of chronic pain, both in the head and neck region and in general.[89–93] Also, it is frequently an accompanying diagnosis to other chronic pain conditions.

A *cranial nerve examination* (Table 5) is indicated when the history points to a neuropathic type of pain; if disturbances in touch, taste, smell, sight, hearing, motor function, balance, or coordination are suspected; or if there are any subjective complaints or objective signs of cranial nerve involvement. Lesions of the cranial nerve nuclei or their efferent or afferent pathways will result in an abnormal examination. For example, meningitis may cause double vision; an acoustic neuroma may cause hearing loss. Symptoms of numbness or tingling may accompany nasopharyngeal carcinoma or other intracranial pathema. Sensory deficits can be verified using accurate two-point discrimination testing, pinprick tests, and light touch tests. Complaints of transient or persistent paralysis, weakness, or spasticity of any of the head and neck muscles dictate the need for evaluation of the nerves that control their motor function.

The motor function of the head and neck is mediated through several cranial nerves. The *trigeminal nerve, cranial nerve V*, controls the masticatory muscles. The *facial nerve, cranial nerve VII*, controls the muscles of facial expression. The *hypoglossal nerve, cranial nerve XII*, controls the tongue. The *spinal accessory nerve, cranial nerve XI*, controls the trapezius and sternocleidomastoid muscles. Detailed information on how to perform a cranial nerve examination is available in Bates's textbook on physical examination and history taking.[94] If intracranial pathosis is suspected, a complete *neurological examination*, including mental status; cerebellar, motor, and sensory function; and reflexes, is indicated. This requires referral to a competent neurologist.

General inspection of the patient reveals an obese female in moderate distress. Closer inspection of the head and neck reveals slight swelling of the left cheek with a distinct increase in skin temperature over this site. On intraoral examination, the intraoral tissues are firm, pink,

Table 5 Cranial Nerve Examination

I	Olfactory test: sense of smell of each nostril separately by using soap, tobacco, or coffee with patient's eyes closed
II	Optic test visual acuity
	Examining fundi ophthalmoscopically
	Test visual fields
III, IV, VI	Oculomotor, trochlear, abducens
	Test pupillary reactions to light and accommodation
	Test extraocular movements
	Check for ptosis or nystagmus
V	Trigeminal
	Motor—palpate masseter and temporalis during contraction
	Sensory—Test discrimination of pinprick, V1, V2, V3 temperature, V1, V2, V3, and light touch, V1, V2, V3
	Test corneal reflex
VII	Facial
	Observe patient's face during rest and conversation
	Check for symmetry, tics
	Examine for symmetric smile, ability to wrinkle forehead, hold air in cheeks, and tense the platysma muscle
VIII	Acoustic
	Whisper, rub fingers, or hold watch next to ear, use tuning fork for Rinne and Weber tests
IX, X	Glossopharyngeal, vagus
	Check for symmetric movement of the soft palate and the uvula when patient says "Ah"
	Check gag reflex by touching back of throat. Note any hoarseness
XI	Spinal accessory
	Have patient shrug shoulders against resistance (trapezius) (partially innervated by C4)
	Have patient turn head against resistance (SCM)
XII	Hypoglossal. Observe tongue in mouth: check for atrophy or asymmetry
	Check for deviation by having patient stick tongue out

and stippled without lesions. The patient is missing the maxillary left third molar and all three mandibular left molars. TMJ examination *reveals an active oral opening of only 33 mm with little translation of the left condyle (the jaw deflects to the left with opening). Definitive intraoral or extraoral palpation is impossible because the patient complains of pain at the slightest touch.*

The patient has *full range of motion of the cervical spine. The first two cervical joints similarly show good range and quality of motion. Her posture is slightly abnormal, with elevation of the left shoulder and a forward head position.*

Myofascial TrP examination *is restricted to the cervical muscles and unaffected side owing to the extreme sensitivity of the left side of the face. Even so, active myofascial TrPs are found in the left upper trapezius that intensifies the patient's pain over the left temple and angle of the jaw.*

Cranial nerve examination *is normal except for the extreme cutaneous sensitivity on the left side of the face.* Neurological examination *is similarly unremarkable.*

At this stage, one must still rule out acute pathological changes. Pathosis of the various organs and structures of the head and neck should always be suspected first in any orofacial pain. The teeth, pulp and periodontium, TMJs, eyes, ears, nose, throat, sinuses, and salivary glands should be thoroughly evaluated (see Table 6). As mentioned previously, the quality of pain from this group varies depending on the etiology. Equally important are many referred pain problems (see Table 7). These are very often difficult to diagnose and include pathological conditions such as the tight, pressing pain of coronary artery disease that may be felt in the sternum and the jaws.

This patient demonstrates swelling and temperature change as well as cutaneous hyperesthesia over the painful area. She could still have a chronic osteomyelitis despite the previous course of antibiotics. She could have a retropharyngeal abscess or a neoplastic disease affecting or surrounding the fifth cranial nerve, either intracranially or extracranially. She could also have a localized coccal infection since she lives in a rural area. The limited range of motion of the left TMJ and the fact that much of her pain seems to emanate from there bring up the possibility of severe degenerative joint disease or neoplastic disease involving the joint. The myofascial TrPs in the left trapezius have probably developed in response to the chronic pain problem. It is unlikely that myofascial TrP pain is the primary cause of this patient's pain.

The next step involves choosing appropriate diagnostic studies to help rule out the pathema suspected.

DIAGNOSTIC STUDIES

Table 8 is a list of some of the more common diagnostic studies available to help facilitate diagnosis.

Panoramic and periradicular radiographs reveal an area of bony sclerosis in the mandibular extraction sites, consistent with the history of curettage of dry sockets and not at all typical of osteomyelitis. TMJ *tomograms reveal flattening of the left condyle consistent with mild to moderate degenerative joint disease. Computed tomographic (CT) scans of the brain, mandible, and retropharyngeal area are normal. A gallium scan, which is used to identify soft tissue inflammation, is also normal. Skin tests for coccal infection are negative.* Complete

Table 6 Local Pathosis of Extracranial Structures

Structures	Diseases
Tooth pulp, periradicular structures	Inflammation
Periodontium, gingival, mucosa	Infection
Salivary glands	Degeneration
Tongue	Neoplasm
Ears, nose, throat, sinuses	Obstruction
Eyes	
Temporomandibular joints	

Table 7 Referred Pain from Remote Pathological Sites

Structures	Diseases
Heart	Angina pectoris, myocardial infarction
Thyroid	Inflammation
Carotid artery	Inflammation, other obscure causation
Cervical spine	Inflammation, trauma, dysfunction
Muscles	Myofascial trigger points

Table 8 Common Diagnostic Studies

Pulp testing
Radiography
Tomography
Laboratory studies (blood, urine)
CT or MRI scan
Bone scan
Gallium scan
Arthrography
Thermography
Nerve conduction studies
EEG
Lumbar puncture
Differential diagnostic analgesic blocking

blood count and erythrocyte sedimentation rate also fail to show any signs of infection or inflammation. No pathosis of the extracranial and intracranial structures can be identified.

What, then, could be causing this patient's pain? At this point in the workup of a pain patient, practitioners are often tempted to ascribe the pain to some "psychogenic" problem. Clearly, if there is no obvious pathological process, and the patient is in severe distress or does not respond well to treatments, then she must be suffering from a "psychogenic" pain. Do not be too sure!

PSYCHOGENIC PAIN

Many clinicians use the term "psychogenic" to refer to patients with a chronic pain problem that has a strong emotional component or to patients who do not respond well to somatic treatment. It must be re-emphasized, however, that psychological factors are intimately involved in the expression of all pain, regardless of etiology or time course.

By definition, chronic pain has been present for a protracted period (at least 6 months), and the patient has usually received multiple treatments with little or no results. This creates an emotional strain for the patient and frustration for the clinician, sometimes resulting in the inappropriate label of "psychogenic pain." Patients with chronic pain invariably have a somatic diagnosis. What frustrates the clinician is often the discrepancy between the identifiable somatic cause and the disproportionate amount of perceived pain and disability that accompanies this cause.

"Psychogenic pain" or "somatoform disorders" are described in the DSM-IV, the Diagnostic and Statistical Manual of Mental Disorders,[95] and include physical complaints that, after appropriate medical workup and testing, either cannot be explained by a medical condition or substance (ab)use or, if due to an identifiable medical condition, cause physical, social or occupational impairment greater than what would be expected given the objective findings. In addition, they have been present for over 6 months and cannot be explained by other psychological disorders such as depression or anxiety. Despite their inclusion in the Diagnostic and Statistical Manual of Mental Disorders, somatoform disorders have been the subject of continuing criticism by both professionals and patients[96] mostly because no empirical evidence exists to support these psychodynamic diagnoses and to date no psychodynamic treatment has been shown to be effective in treating these disorders. Thus the validity of these diagnoses is under debate.[97]

Myofascial TrP pain is frequently overlooked as an organic finding and is thus often mislabeled as psychogenic pain.[98] Occasionally, there are patients in whom no etiology for their pain can be identified and who have no psychological findings consistent with a psychological disorder. This situation simply speaks to the limitations of our current medical knowledge and the complexity of the human nervous system and is not an indication of the mental state of the patient.

OPERANT PAIN (PAIN BEHAVIOR)

Although pain behaviors (the behavioral manifestations of pain, distress, and suffering) likely result from a complex interaction of various psychological and physical factors,[65] understanding the basic concepts of learning and "operant" conditioning is essential to understanding the chronic pain patient.

In combination with cognitive and affective factors, learned behavior and "operant conditioning" are powerful psychological or "psychogenic" factors that play an important role in any patient with a chronic or persistent pain problem. Fordyce and Steger[99,100] described operant pain and conditioning as follows:

> ...in chronic pain, the normal responses to a noxious stimulus, such as moaning, complaining, grimacing, limping, asking for medication, or staying in bed, are present for a long enough period of time to allow learning to occur. By using the above set of actions, termed operants, the patient either purposely or unintentionally communicates to those around him that he has pain. The significance of these operants is that they can be influenced by certain consequences. For example, if a certain behavior or action is consistently followed by a favorable consequence (a positive reinforcer), then the probability that the behavior or action will be repeated again in response to a similar stimulus is increased (as in Pavlov's dog). If, however, a certain behavior or action is not consistently followed by a favorable consequence, the behavior will diminish in frequency and disappear. This is known as "extinction."

It is generally accepted that all chronic pain begins at some point with a true pathological or nociceptive stimulus. This stimulus elicits a pain response or "pain behavior." Most people live in an environment that systematically and positively reinforces pain behaviors while ignoring or punishing healthy behaviors.[92] In acute pain, these behaviors and their rewards subside quickly, but in chronic or persistent pain, pain behaviors become more prominent and may persist even after the noxious stimulus is gone: "The degree of pain behavior has little or no direct relationship to pathogenic [or nociceptive] factors."[90]

It is easy to label the behavioral manifestations of pain, distress, and suffering as pain of psychogenic origin. Unfortunately, this term usually implies some kind of personality disorder such as *hypochondriasis* (excessive concern with one's health and bodily functions) or *hysteria* (also known as conversion reaction), and often this is not present, or, if it is, it generally has little or nothing to do with the pain. As Fordyce said,[100] "It is not necessary to have personality problems to learn a pain habit, because learning occurs automatically if the conditions are favorable." Therefore, other psychological labels, such as *somatization* (conversion of mental states into bodily symptoms similar to hysteria but with more elaborate complaints), *malingering* (conscious exhibition of pain or illness for secondary gain), and *Munchausen syndrome* (a type of malingering characterized by habitual presentation for hospital treatment of an apparent acute illness with a plausible and dramatic but fictitious history),[1] are also usually inappropriate. The astute clinician will try to ascertain which environmental factors are acting to maintain and reinforce a particular behavior instead of assuming that the patient has a character disorder.

It is important to realize that, whether or not the pain has an ongoing identifiable organic basis, it is still very real to the patient and can be as intense as any somatic pain. Management typically requires a multidisciplinary approach that includes identification and elimination of any positive reinforcers to the pain behaviors. All treatment and follow-up visits, medications, exercises, rest, and so on must be scheduled on a time-contingent and not on a pain-contingent basis, regardless of the somatic diagnosis. The family must also be educated to reinforce well behaviors and ignore sick behaviors. Then activity levels must be increased and medications gradually decreased and eliminated. The help of a behaviorally oriented psychologist or psychiatrist familiar with chronic pain patients is highly recommended.

Occasionally, situational insight, supportive therapy, guidance, or counseling is sufficient to resolve the problem. Other cases may require more long-term outpatient psychotherapy. Sometimes medications such as antidepressants, antipsychotics, hypnotics, or tranquilizers will help alleviate the pain. Inpatient psychiatric care is indicated for anyone at risk of committing suicide or inflicting bodily injury on themselves or others.

An interview with a psychologist and the MMPI did not reveal a psychopathological state in this particular patient. So, clearly, there must be other factors that have not been considered that are causing this patient's pain.

Instead of falling into the trap of calling unidentified pain "psychogenic," one should go back to the classification of pain (see Table 2) to answer this question. Based on the burning quality of pain, it is clear that neuropathic or sympathetic pains would be the categories most likely to carry a diagnosis that accounts for this patient's pain. These pains and specific diagnoses within each category are described in more detail later in the chapter.

Specifics for Each Broad Category of Pain Origin

The remainder of the chapter will be devoted to discussing many of the specific diagnoses that fall into each broad diagnostic category. This classification is by no means exhaustive. The disorders discussed are those with which dentists should be familiar. An exhaustive treatise of orofacial pains has been published by Bell[101] and an official classification with diagnostic criteria by the International Headache Society.[82]

Extracranial Pathosis

LOCAL PATHOSIS OF EXTRACRANIAL STRUCTURES

Local pathosis of extracranial structures and referred pain from remote pathologic *sites* are listed in Tables 7 and 8. Acute pain arising from pathosis of the extracranial structures is commonly seen in dental practice. Some extracranial acute pain is well localized, easily identifiable, and straightforward to treat. However, some pains from local pathema are more elusive because they are referred to other head and neck structures. Similarly, pathosis of some distant structures such as the heart and thyroid may refer pain into the head, neck, or jaws. These more unusual pains will be discussed.

Tooth Pulp, Periodontium, Periradicular Structures, Gingiva, and Mucosa

Diseases of the intraoral structures, including referred pain from pulpalgia, are fully discussed in Chapter 10,

"Mechanisms of Odontogenic and Non-Odontogenic Pain" and will not be covered here.

Salivary Gland Disorders

The salivary glands can be affected by many diseases, including ductal obstruction, infection, inflammation, cystic degeneration, and tumor growth. Pain and tenderness are typically found in association with ductal obstruction, inflammation, or infection.

The salivary glands are also affected by various medications, especially those with anticholinergic activity against the M3 muscarinic receptor including some sympathomimetic drugs, antidepressants, amphetamines, protease inhibitors, and cytokines.[102] Medication use is the most common cause of reduced salivary flow and, while not painful, may result in subjective complaints of dry mouth and occasionally true xerostomia.

Etiology. The most common causes of salivary gland pain are mumps and acute parotitis in children and blockage of salivary flow by a mucus plug or a sialolith in adults. The latter results in pressure from salivary retention and may cause ascending infection. Sjögren's syndrome, a disease of unknown etiology typically seen in older women, is characterized by dry eyes, dry oropharyngeal mucosa, and enlargement of the parotid glands.[103] This disorder may also cause salivary gland pain if the glands become inflamed. The use of various medications may contribute to or aggravate symptoms or signs of dry mouth or xerostomia in susceptible individuals.

Symptoms. Salivary gland pain is typically localized to the gland itself, and the gland is tender to palpation. Precipitating and aggravating factors to the pain are salivary production prior to meals, eating, and swallowing. Mouth opening may aggravate the pain because of pressure on the gland from the posterior border of the mandible during this movement. This, and increased pain with chewing, may lead the clinician to mistake the pain as being from the masticatory system. Associated symptoms include salivary gland swelling and, occasionally, fever and malaise. Salivary flow from the affected gland may be minimal or nonexistent. Cancer of the parotid gland should not be ruled out. It may be characterized by persistent Bell's palsy.

Symptoms of dry mouth may include symptoms such as a painful tongue, the tongue sticks to the palate, lipstick sticks to the teeth, dentures are painful, hoarseness, difficulty in swallowing food, needing to sip water a lot, and taste changes.[104]

Examination. The pain can be localized fairly well by palpation. Other signs of inflammation may be present. With parotid gland disorders, to determine diminished or absent flow, the gland can be manually milked while observing salivary flow from the parotid duct.

Screening tests for dry mouth include visual inspection of the lips, gingiva, and mucosa looking for evidence of dryness, visual inspection for the presence or the absence of salivary pooling, and placing a tongue blade against the buccal mucosa to see if it sticks (sticking indicates dryness).[104]

Diagnostic tests. Radiographs of the gland and ducts may reveal a calcific mass in the region of the gland. Sialography (radiographic examination of a gland using a radiopaque dye injected into the ductal system) may also show obstruction or abnormal ductal patterns.

Salivary flow testing is useful to verify salivary gland hypofunction, and the saliva can also be tested for pH and buffering capacity.[105] The standard procedure for evaluating dry mouth is to have the patient expectorate into a graduated measuring cup for 5 minutes (the unstimulated test) and the volume of the saliva is recorded. The patient is then given a piece of paraffin (the stimulated test) to chew while expectorating into the graduated cup for another 5 minutes, and the unstimulated and stimulated volumes are compared. If the volume of the unstimulated test is within the range of normal, the patient does not have dry mouth or xerostomia. If the volume of the unstimulated test is below normal but the volume of the stimulated test comes up to the normal range, the patient has dry mouth, not xerostomia. If, however, the volume of the stimulated test continues to be in the low range, the patient has xerostomia.

Treatment. The mucus plug or sialolith should be removed in the case of obstruction. Antibiotics may be needed if infection accompanies the pain.

Management of dry mouth or xerostomia can range from simple home care including frequent brushing and flossing, using fluoridated toothpaste, rinsing and wiping the oral cavity immediately after meals, drinking more water, avoiding liquids and foods with high sugar content, overly salty foods, citrus juices and mouthwash containing alcohol, and using lip balm regularly, use of prescription mouthwash, toothpaste, and fluoride as well as sialogogues. Depending on the severity of the salivary gland hypofunction, increased frequency of regular dental cleanings and periodontal maintenance may be required.[105]

Patients with otitis externa (inflammation of the external auditory canal) may present themselves to the dentist first because this pain is aggravated by swallowing. Otitis externa may be misdiagnosed as arthralgia of the TMJ if the condyle is palpated through the external auditory canal without first evaluating the ear. Glossopharyngeal neuralgia, also aggravated by swallowing, may need to be considered if ear and dental pathosis are absent.

Examination. The dentist must carefully examine the dentition for pulpal disease and the oropharyngeal mucosa for inflammation to rule out referred ear pain from oral or dental sources. Myofascial TrPs in the lateral and medial pterygoid muscles frequently refer pain to the ear as well. Deep masseter and SCM TrPs may cause tinnitus.[54]

If primary ear pain is suspected, referral to a competent ENT specialist should be made. However, screening examination should include visual inspection of the ear and ear canal. The use of an otoscope facilitates this examination. Wiggling the auricle itself or tugging on the earlobe will aggravate otitis externa and will help distinguish an ear lesion from a TMJ problem. Pumping on the ear with the palm of the hand will exacerbate pain from otitis media. Hearing can be grossly evaluated by rubbing the fingers together in front of each ear or using a watch tick or coin click. The practitioner can use his own hearing as a control.

Treatment. Primary ear pain should be diagnosed and managed by an ENT specialist. Dental sources of ear pain are treated by treating the oral pathema. Of importance is the fact that primary ear pain may also induce *secondary myospasm*, and development of *myofascial TrPs* may persist beyond the course of primary ear disease. These TrPs and the resulting masticatory dysfunction are self-perpetuating, even after the acute ear problem resolves. Appropriate treatment of this secondary masticatory dysfunction will be required for resolution of the complaint.

Case history. A good example of this phenomenon is a 27-year-old woman who presented with an 18-month history of right-sided facial pain that started after a middle ear infection. During the initial illness, she experienced dizziness, and a spinal tap was performed to rule out viral meningitis. This was negative, and a diagnosis of a viral syndrome was made. Several months later, persistent pain led the patient to seek a further ENT consultation. A cyst discovered in the right maxillary sinus was removed through a Caldwell-Luc procedure, with only transient relief of symptoms.

On evaluation, the patient complained of intermittent, deep, dull, aching pain in the right side of her face, including her eye, ear, and neck. The pain was associated with blurred vision, ptosis, and redness of both eyes. She also complained of unilateral hearing loss and nasal congestion on the symptomatic side. The pain occurred one or two times per week and lasted 24 to 48 hours.

Examination revealed multiple active myofascial TrPs in the right masseter, temporalis, medial pterygoid, sternocleidomastoid, and suboccipital muscles that reproduced all of her symptoms, including blurred vision. In contrast, there were essentially no TrPs in any of the muscles on the asymptomatic side. Treatment directed at rehabilitation of the involved muscles provided significant reduction in the intensity and frequency of her pain.

Ear Pain

Most patients who have a primary complaint of ear pain will seek the help of their primary care physician or an ear, nose, and throat (ENT) specialist. Ear pain is typically seen with disorders such as otitis media, otitis externa, and mastoiditis and may be associated with headache. When a medical workup is negative, patients may be referred to the dentist for evaluation of ear pain. Astute physicians will want to know whether the TMJ or pulpalgia is referring the symptoms. Patients may also present themselves to the dentist with another primary pain complaint such as toothache or headache, whereupon when taking a careful history, ear pain is found to be an associated symptom. The dentist needs to rule out dental disease or temporomandibular disorders (TMDs) as a cause of ear pain. Additionally, the dentist must decide when a referral for a medical workup of ear pain is indicated.

Etiology. The ear is innervated by cranial nerves V, VII, VIII, IX, X, and XI and also branches of the upper cervical roots that supply the immediate adjacent scalp and muscles. Therefore, pain can be referred to the ear from inflammatory or neoplastic disease of the *teeth*, tonsils, larynx, nasopharynx, thyroid, *TMJ*, and cervical spine, as well as from inflammation or tumors in the posterior fossa of the brain.[106] Ear pains are also associated with neuralgias such as herpes zoster of the cranial nerve V or VII, glossopharyngeal neuralgia, and nervus intermedius neuralgia. These will be discussed later.

Symptoms. Primary ear pains are usually described as a constant aching pressure. Their onset is usually recent. Inflammatory or infectious disorders may be associated with fever and malaise. These complaints should be diagnosed and managed by an ENT specialist.

Sinus and Paranasal Pain

The most common extraoral source of dental pain arises from the maxillary sinus and associated pain-sensitive nasal mucosa. Many teeth have been mistakenly extracted because of an incorrect diagnosis of this syndrome.

Etiology. The sinuses themselves are relatively pain-insensitive structures. Reynolds and Hutchins[108] demonstrated that most so-called "sinus" pain actually arises from the nasal mucosa or from the stimulation of the nasal ostia. Minor disease in critical locations within the nasal ostia and meata may give rise to greater symptomatology than diffuse disease in the sinuses.[109] Conversely, various intranasal and sinus abnormalities, anatomic variations or subclinical inflammation, may present as primary headache disorders.[110]

Allergies may also cause boggy, edematous nasal mucosa. This may cause swelling of the turbinates, that may, in turn, block off the ostia of the maxillary sinuses. This has been implicated in causing referred symptoms to the teeth (Figure 12) Sicher[111] pointed out that the superior alveolar nerves, supplying the maxillary molar and premolar teeth, pass along the thin wall of the sinuses. The canaliculi of the teeth often open toward the sinus, and pulpal nerves may be in direct contact with the inflamed mucoperiosteum of the sinus lining. Their direct irritation may cause dental symptoms. The reverse is also true. Inflammation or infection from the root of a tooth in contact with the sinus floor may cause sinusitis. This, in turn, will not resolve until the dental problem is corrected.

Symptoms. Contrary to popular belief, infection and inflammation of the sinuses rarely cause facial pain or headache. Many headache patients with autonomic features will probably have tension-type headaches or migraines. Most authors feel that acute or chronic headache processes are not a result of overt paranasal sinus disease.[107]

Chronic sinusitis may cause symptoms of fullness or pressure but rarely pain. The location of these symptoms may vary from the maxilla and maxillary teeth in maxillary sinusitis to the upper orbit and frontal process in frontal sinusitis, between and behind the eyes in ethmoid sinusitis, and at the junction of the hard and soft palate, occiput, and mastoid process in sphenoid sinusitis.

The sinusitis patient who reports to the dentist does so with a chief complaint of "toothache." In this case, constant but rather mild pain in a number of posterior maxillary teeth on one side is almost pathognomonic. All of the teeth on this side, the roots of which are related to the floor of the sinus, may be aching mildly.

The teeth feel elongated, as if they "touch first" when the patient closes. The teeth are also tender, and the patient clenches against them, saying it "hurts good" to do so. These same maxillary teeth are hypersensitive to cold fluids. Occasionally, all of the maxillary teeth on the involved side, to the midline, feel uncomfortable and elongated. The pain, mild but deep and nonpulsating, radiates out of this area onto the face, upward toward the temple and forward toward the nose. A referred frontal headache and cutaneous hyperalgesia along the side of the face and the scalp may also be present. The patient frequently reports that the pain begins in the early afternoon or may give a history of increased pain at altitude when crossing a high mountain pass or when making a plane flight. Patients may also complain of a "stuffy nose," blood- or pus-tinged mucus, postnasal drip, fever, and malaise.

Examination. The dentist's contribution will be to rule out dental disease as the cause of the pain and

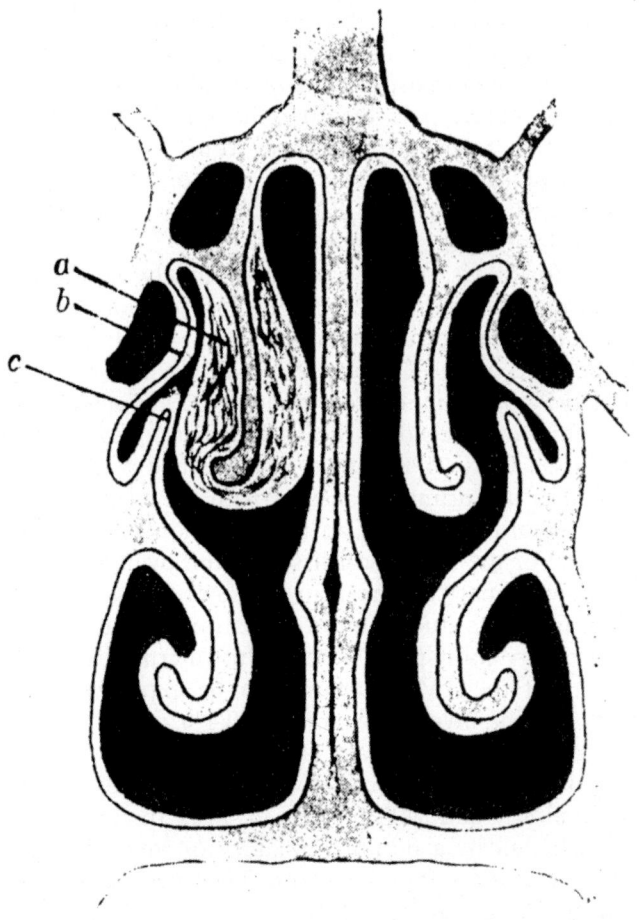

Figure 12 Inflammation of nasal mucosa causes swelling of the turbinate and blocks off the ostium of the maxillary sinus. Pain referred to maxillary teeth may then develop. Reproduced with permission from Ballenger JJ, Lea & Febiger; 1969.

correctly refer the patient for complete diagnosis and treatment.

The extraoral examination should include palpation of the maxillary sinuses under the zygomatic process bilaterally. If maxillary sinusitis is present and unilateral, the cheek on the involved side, from the canine fossa back to the base of the zygomatic process, will be tender to heavy palpation. The patient may say it feels as if he has been hit in the area, or "frostbitten" is another term used in northern climes. It may also hurt to smile.

If the patient complains of frontal headache, the dentist should check the frontal sinuses for tenderness by pressing up against the inferior surface of the supraorbital ridge on each side of the nose. All of the anterior sinuses, maxillary, frontal, and anterior ethmoidal, may be involved at one time. Such pansinusitis may follow an upper respiratory infection.

The intraoral examination should include mobility, percussion, thermal and electric pulp tests, and radiographs. The teeth adjacent to the affected maxillary sinus often are mobile when moved between the two index fingers. Furthermore, the teeth are painful and sound "mushy" when percussed and may be hypersensitive to cold or when pulp tested electrically compared to the uninvolved side. Illuminating the sinuses with a fiber optic in a darkened room may reveal changes in the affected sinus. Direct inspection of the nasal passages with a speculum may reveal engorged nasal mucosa and turbinates.

Radiographically, the involved teeth are likely to be normal, reconfirming that nothing is wrong orally. The roots of the teeth, however, may be found extending well up into or against the sinus floor, which would account for their involvement. On the other hand, the radiograph and the pulp test may show a pulpless tooth with a periapical lesion. Periapical infections may extend into the sinus.[112] As stated previously, this could be the cause of a unilateral sinus inflammation. Nenzen and Welander[113] found "local hyperplasia of the maxillary sinus mucosa" in 58% (14 of 24) of the patients who had pulpless teeth with periradicular lesions associated with the floor of the sinus.

Persistent pain in this area may be caused by a cyst or neoplasm of the maxillary sinus. In these cases, the pain syndrome is the same as for sinusitis but more long-standing. A radiographic study of the area may reveal the lesion.

The diagnosis of maxillary sinusitis may be confirmed by spraying 4% lidocaine anesthetic from a spray bottle into the nostril on the affected side. This will anesthetize the sensitive area around the ostium. The pain from the congested nasal mucosa and accompanying maxillary sinusitis should be substantially reduced within a minute or two.

Treatment. Complete diagnosis and treatment of maxillary sinusitis are left to the ENT specialist. Treatment usually consists of the use of decongestants and analgesics. If there is persistent purulent discharge, cultures should be taken and appropriate antibiotics prescribed. For a more complete discussion of "Rhinosinusitis and Endodontic Disease" refer to Chapter 17, "Rhinosinusitis and Endodontic Disease."

Temporomandibular Joint Articular Disorders

Before discussing TMJ disorders, a distinction must be made between pain and dysfunction arising from the TMJ itself, TMD, and MFP owing to TrPs. TMD is an umbrella term that refers to various painful and nonpainful conditions involving the TMJ and the associated masticatory musculature. MFP is a distinct muscle pain disorder that produces various local and referred symptoms from TrPs in taut bands of skeletal muscle, and may or may not be associated with a TMJ disorder. MFP is reviewed in detail later in this chapter.

Historically, there has been much confusion around TMD and the differential contribution of pain from the joint versus the muscles and MFP. In a study conducted at the University of Minnesota TMJ and Facial Pain Clinic, doctors evaluated 296 consecutive patients with chronic head and neck pain complaints.[89] Only 21% of these patients had a TMJ disorder as the primary cause of pain. In all 21%, the joint disorder included an inflammation of the TMJ capsule or the retrodiscal tissues. MFP owing to TrPs was the primary diagnosis in 55.4% of the patients in the Minnesota study, almost three times the incidence of primary joint pain. Nonpainful internal derangements of the TMJs were felt to be a perpetuating factor to the myofascial TrPs in 30.4%.[89]

Considering these data, it is important to make a distinction between true TMJ pain, MFP owing to TrPs alone, and MFP owing to TrPs that is being perpetuated by a noninflammatory or intermittently inflammatory joint condition. Treatment priorities will be affected accordingly.

Table 9 Temporomandibular Joint Articular Disorders
Inflammatory disorders
Capsulitis/synovitis
Polyarthritides
Disk derangement disorders
Disk displacement with reduction
Disk displacement without reduction
Osteoarthritis (noninflammatory disorders)
Primary
Secondary
Congenital or developmental disorders
Aplasia
Hypoplasia
Hyperplasia
Neoplasia
Temporomandibular joint dislocation
Ankylosis
Fracture (condylar process)

Adapted from Okeson.[90]

Table 9 provides a simple breakdown of TMJ disorders, the vast majority of which are nonpainful. Included in this category are inflammatory disorders, disk derangement disorders, and osteoarthritis. It is possible to have several of these diagnoses affecting one joint. It is also very common to find myofascial TrP pain associated with TMJ pathosis.

The term *internal derangement* applies to all joints and encompasses those disorders causing mechanical interference to normal joint functions. In the TMJs, this primarily involves displacement and distortion of the articular disk, as well as remodeling of the articular surfaces, and joint hypermobility.[114] Many of the articular disorders affecting the TMJs involve an abnormal or restricted range of motion and noise but are relatively painless. These include the congenital or developmental disorders, disk derangement disorders, osteoarthritis, and ankylosis listed in Table 9. Any pain associated with these disorders is usually momentary and associated with pulling or stretching of ligaments. In the case of *ankylosis*, pain ensues if the mandible is forcibly opened beyond adhesive restrictions. Forcible opening can cause acute inflammation. Primary or secondary *osteoarthritis*, unless accompanied by synovitis, is also associated with minimal pain or dysfunction,[90] although crepitus and limited range of motion may be present.

As far as the incidence of TMJ pain in the general population is concerned, the National Institute of Dental Research, reporting on the National Center for Health Statistics' 1989 survey of 45,711 US households over 6 months, has estimated that 9,945,000 Americans were suffering from what they termed "jaw joint pain." They further estimated that 5.3% of the US population was experiencing this condition at any one time. Twice as many women as men complained of jaw pain.[104]

Inflammatory Disorders Of The Joint. It is the inflammatory joint disorders that cause pain. Included in this group are *capsulitis and synovitis* and *polyarthritides* (see Table 9).[115–117]

Symptoms. Capsulitis and synovitis present with similar signs and symptoms and are difficult to differentiate. The chief symptom is continuous pain over the joint, aggravated by function. Swelling may be evident, and the patient may complain of an acute malocclusion ("back teeth on the same side don't touch"), restricted jaw opening, and ear pain. There is usually a history of trauma, infection, polyarthralgia, or chronic, nonpainful degenerative arthritis that is now in an acute stage.[90,116] Because the pain is fairly constant, the clinical picture is often complicated by referred pain, masticatory muscle spasm, or myofascial TrP pain.[116] The pain tends to wax and wane with the course of the inflammation. Inflammatory disorders of the joint may occur alone or in combination with an internal derangement.

Polyarthritides are relatively uncommon and occur with other rheumatological diseases, such as rheumatoid arthritis. Symptoms may include pain at rest and with mandibular function, crepitus, and a limited range of motion.

Etiology. Inflammation of the capsule or synovium may occur secondary to localized trauma or infection, through overuse of the joint, or secondary to other joint disorders. Synovitis may also occur secondary to primary osteoarthritis. The inflammatory conditions occur most commonly in young people with a history of trauma, clenching, bruxism, or internal derangement.[118]

Inflammation and degenerative changes in the TMJ caused by systemic rheumatological illnesses that affect multiple joints are called polyarthritides. They most commonly include rheumatoid arthritis, juvenile rheumatoid arthritis (Figure 13A,B), psoriatic arthritis, and gout. The autoimmune disorders and mixed connective tissue diseases such as scleroderma, Sjögren's syndrome, and lupus erythematosus may also affect the TMJ.[90]

Examination. For capsulitis and synovitis, palpation over the joint itself is painful. Posterior or superior joint loading and any movement that stretches the capsule may also increase the pain. Range of motion is not usually restricted except owing to pain. Initiation of mandibular movement after a period of rest may be slow and "sticky." Inflammatory effusion in the joint may cause acute malocclusion with slight disclusion of the homolateral posterior teeth. Although clenching may be painful, biting on a tongue depressor may reduce the pain by preventing intercuspation and full closure.

In the polyarthritides, palpation of the joint is also painful. Range of motion is not affected except owing to

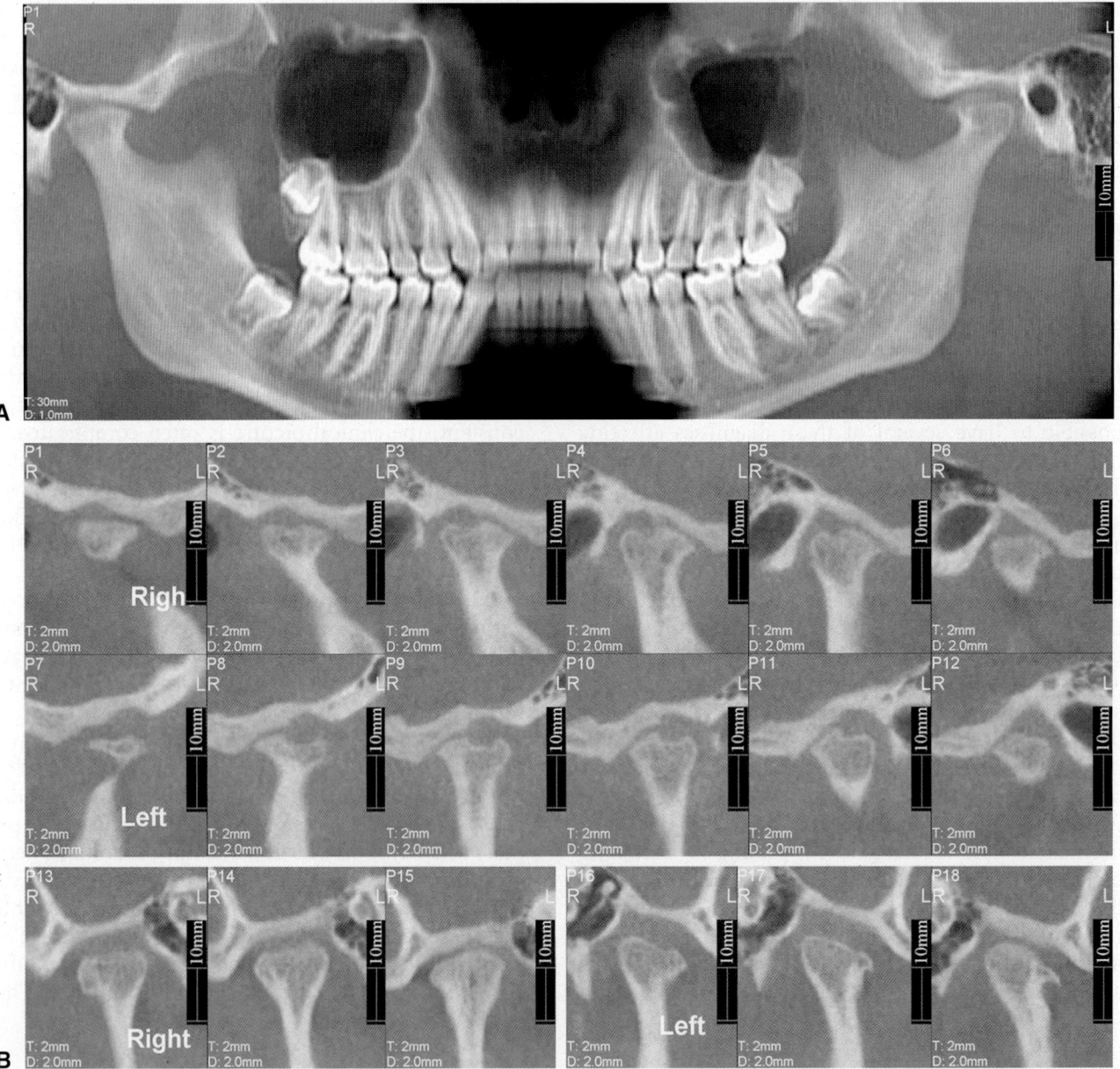

Figure 13 Tomography of a juvenile rheumatoid arthritic temporomandibular joint (TMJ). ***A,*** Observe the flattened surface of both TMJ condyles. ***B,*** Note the resorption of both articular surfaces of the TMJ and in particular, the important resorption of the left condyle. Courtesy, Dr. Marcela Romero.

pain and may be accompanied by crepitus; malocclusion is related to inflammatory effusion or lateral pterygoid muscle spasm secondary to the primary pain.[87] In severe cases of rheumatoid arthritis, rapid resorption of the condyles causes an acute anterior open bite.[90] Ankylosis may also occur.

Diagnostic tests. Plain radiographs and tomography will show a few, if any, bony changes in the joint with capsulitis or synovitis unless these are secondary to osteoarthritis. Magnetic resonance imaging, on the other hand, will show a bright T_2-weighted signal secondary to the presence of fluid.

The polyarthritides will show extensive TMJ changes on radiographic examination. Radiographic changes include more gross deformities than are seen in osteoarthritis, including erosions, marginal proliferations, and flattening. Of particular diagnostic value in the polyarthritides are various serologic tests screening for evidence of rheumatoid disease such as antinuclear antibodies, elevated erythrocyte sedimentation rate, rheumatoid factor, or anemia, although not all rheumatologic diseases are seropositive. Definitive diagnosis and management of the polyarthritides are left to the rheumatologist. The dentist's role is to manage concomitant TMJ symptoms should they occur.

Treatment. In treating inflammatory TMJ disorders, palliative care is an appropriate first step. This includes jaw rest, a soft diet, and *nonsteroidal anti-inflammatory drugs* (NSAIDs). Intermittent application of ice or moist heat may also be helpful. Office physical therapy, including ultrasonography, may be indicated in some patients. Single supracapsular or intra-articular injections of steroids may be effective in reducing inflammation and pain if simpler methods prove ineffective. Pain relief from steroid injection can be expected to last 1 1/2 to 2 years provided that the patient limits joint use appropriately. It is generally accepted that steroid injections into the TMJ should be limited: no more than two in 12 months, and two or three in a lifetime. This is because of concern about inducing joint deterioration owing to the steroid.[119] More recent data suggest that these injections may be better tolerated than previously thought.[120]

Definitive therapy is aimed at reducing the causative or contributing factors. This must involve the patient who alone controls the functional demands placed on the joint. The dentist must enlist his help and compliance. This is best achieved through reassurance and education. The patient must be motivated to reduce joint use and eliminate abusive habits. Home exercises, application of heat and ice, and massage are also important. In addition to the self-help program, construction of a *stabilization splint may help reduce bruxism* and decrease intra-articular pressure on the joint. If necessary, a psychological approach to decrease bruxism or clenching may also be instituted. Surgery is seldom, if ever, indicated.

If the condition is owing to polyarthritis, management is similar to treating the systemic disease itself. It includes analgesics and anti-inflammatory agents such as aspirin, indomethacin, and ibuprofen, corticosteroids such as prednisone, gold salts, and penicillamine. Physical therapy, home exercises, appropriate jaw use, reduction of abusive habits, occlusal stabilization, and periodic intra-articular steroid injections are other supportive measures. Surgical intervention is limited to severe cases with marked dysfunction.

Disk Derangement Disorders. The disk derangement disorders include disk displacement with and without reduction.

Symptoms. Both of these disorders are typically painless. With *disk displacement with reduction*, pain, when present, is intermittent and related to interference or "jamming" of the disk and function of the condyle against ligaments. Patients may complain of difficulty in opening the jaws, particularly in the morning. Sometimes they have to manipulate their jaws, with a resultant loud crack, before they can function normally for the rest of the day.

Patients who present with *disk displacement without reduction* usually relate a history of TMJ clicking that stopped when the joint "locked." In addition to the limited range of motion, they may also complain of mild hyperocclusion on the affected side. Acutely, there may be pain that is usually secondary to attempts to open the mouth. Over time, the mandibular range of motion gradually improves and the pain subsides, often being replaced with a feeling of stiffness.

Etiology. The development of a disk displacement disorder is often attributed to external trauma, such as a blow, or to chronic microtrauma, such as *habitual parafunction (especially bruxism)* in the TMJ in which structural or functional incompatibilities exist. Occlusal disharmony, such as loss of posterior teeth or occlusal interferences in retruded and lateral movements, may contribute to the problem but is rarely causative.

Discrete clicks and pops are the result of the rapid reduction of an anteriorly displaced disk on opening

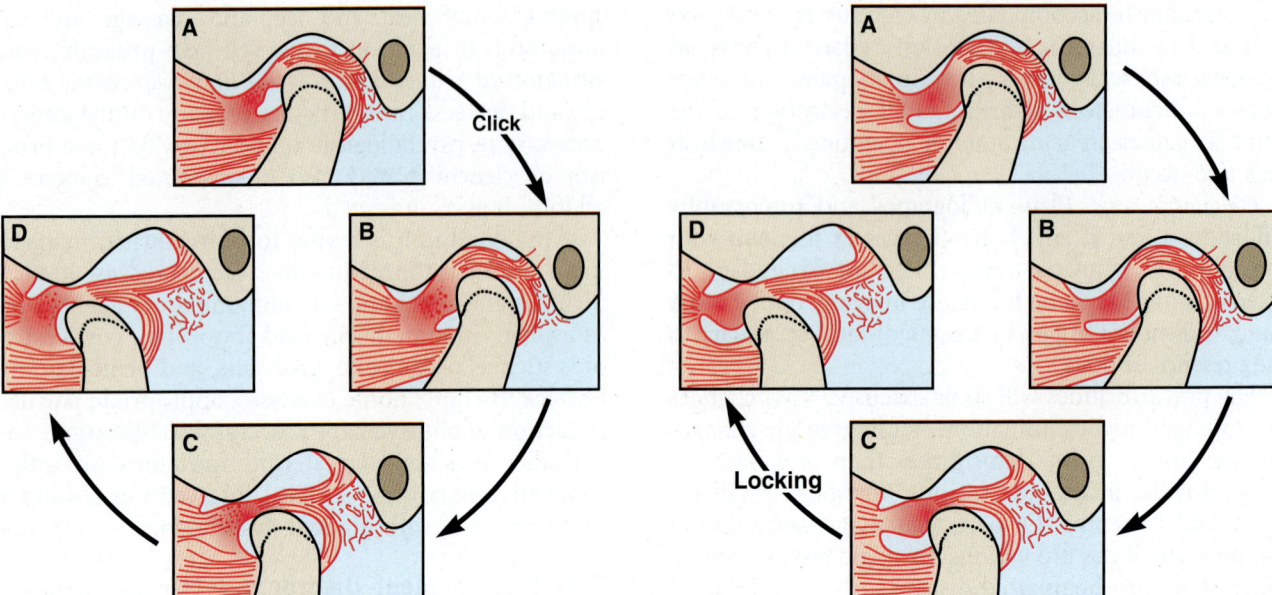

Figure 14 Internal temporomandibular joint (TMJ) derangement—the early click. Notice in the closed position **A,** that the disk (stippled) is situated completely anterior to the articulating surface of the condyle. As the condyle begins to translate anteriorly, it passes beneath the thickened rim of the disk at the same time the patient notices a "click" within the joint. At one fingerbreadth opening **B,** and throughout the remaining opening sequence **C,** and **D,** the relationship between the disk and the bony structure is normal and not painful. Reproduced with permission from Wilkes CH, *Minn Med;* 1978.

Figure 15 Severe disk derangement—the closed lock situation. In the closed projection **A,** notice that the stippled disk has been deformed from a normal biconcave wafer to an amorphous mass. The disk is situated entirely anterior to the condylar articulating surface. During jaw opening **B,** and **C,** the condyle progressively forces the disk mass anteriorly, causing greater deformation. At no point in the sequence does the condyle negotiate its way past the thickened posterior aspect of the disk to acquire a normal relationship. Locking **D,** and discomfort ensue. Reproduced with permission from Wilkes CH, *Minn Med;* 1978.

(Figure 14). Locking results when the disk is so severely displaced or deformed that it can no longer relocate itself on top of the condyle during normal opening movements (Figure 15).

Examination. With disk displacement with reduction, there is a normal mandibular range of movement. Palpation of the joint on opening and closing will reveal a fairly distinct click or pop that is often accompanied by a slight deviation of mandibular movement. These clicks and pops are usually found at approximately 25 to 30 mm of opening, the point at which the condyle shifts from rotation to translation in the opening cycle. Often these joint noises are reciprocal. That is, there is another, very soft click just at the end of the closing path. It is at this time that the disk once again slips off the condyle and into its anterior position.

With disk displacement without reduction, there is clear restriction of jaw range of motion to approximately 25 to 30 mm. If only one joint is locking, the midline will deviate toward the affected joint. Forced opening results in pain. Laterotrusive movement is restricted to the unaffected side; bilateral restriction exists if the disorder affects both joints.

Diagnostic tests. For both disk displacement with and without reduction, tomograms of the joints may reveal a mild posterior displacement of the condyle in the glenoid fossa, although this is not a consistent finding and should not be used alone to make a diagnosis. Bony contour of the condyle will usually show only mild degenerative changes. Arthrography or magnetic resonance imaging (MRI) reveals anterior displacement of the articular disk in both conditions. In disk displacement with reduction, the anterior displacement typically normalizes during jaw function.

Treatment. Because most disk displacement disorders are nonpainful, many patients only require an explanation for their symptoms and reassurance. There is no clear evidence that all disk displacement disorders are progressive[121] or that intervention prevents progression. In fact, most TMDs are self-limiting.[122–124]

Specific treatment, when indicated, will depend on the specific nature of the derangement. Conservative, reversible treatments such as patient education and self-care, physical therapy, behavior modification, orthopedic appliances, and medications are appropriate. Since most TMDs are self-limiting and resolve without serious long-term effects,[125,124] extensive occlusal rehabilitation or surgery should be avoided except in carefully selected cases.[126]

Osteoarthritis (noninflammatory).

Osteoarthritis (noninflammatory) is found in many of the joints of the body and is classified according to the perceived etiology. *Primary osteoarthritis* is so-called because its etiology is unrelated to any other currently identifiable local or systemic disorders.[127] It may affect the TMJ alone or may include other joints of the body.[124,128,129] When other joints are involved, any of the weight-bearing joints in the body may be affected. Heberden's nodes of the terminal phalangeal joints are a clinical feature.

Secondary osteoarthritis, on the other hand, is considered to be the result of a specific precipitating event (such as trauma or infection) or other disease or disorder (such as rheumatoid arthritis, endocrine disturbance or gout, or a TMJ disk derangement disorder).

Symptoms. Despite their classification as noninflammatory disorders, *primary and secondary osteoarthritis* may be associated with a secondary synovitis. As a result, the patient may complain of pain with function and tenderness over the joint. In the absence of synovitis, crepitus and limited range of motion are the most likely complaints.

Etiology. Osteoarthritis is a degenerative joint condition characterized by joint breakdown involving erosion and attrition of the articular tissue along with remodeling of the underlying subchondral bone[130] (Figure 16). Degenerative change is thought to be induced when the joint's natural physiological remodeling capabilities are exceeded owing to factors that overload and stress the joint.[130,131]

Examination. The distinguishing clinical feature of osteoarthritis is crepitus: grating or multiple cracking noises within the joint during opening and closing. There may also be limitation of the movement of the condyle and deviation to the affected side with opening. When accompanied by synovitis, there is pain with function and point tenderness over the joint on palpation.

Diagnostic tests. Radiographic examination of the condyle may reveal decreased joint space, subchondral sclerosis, cystic formation, surface erosions, osteophytes, or marginal lipping. The articular eminence may be flattened or eroded or may contain osteophytes (see Figure 16). All clinical laboratory findings are usually within normal limits.

Treatment. Since most osteoarthritis is nonpainful and dysfunction is minimal, patients often do well with appropriate explanation of their symptoms and reassurance without specific treatment. When accompanied by synovitis and pain, treatment strategies for the acute inflammatory disorders are appropriate. In *secondary osteoarthritis*, identification of a precipitating disease or event may simplify treatment since correction of the underlying cause may facilitate the resolution of any symptoms associated with the osteoarthritis.

Congenital or developmental disorders.

Congenital or developmental disorders such as *aplasia*, *hypoplasia*, and *hyperplasia* tend to cause esthetic and functional problems and are rarely accompanied by pain.

Temporomandibular joint dislocation.

TMJ dislocation refers to that situation when a patient is unable to close his mouth because the condyle is trapped either anterior to the articular eminence or anterior to a posteriorly dislocated disk.[132] Elevator muscle spasm usually aggravates the situation by forcing the condyle superiorly and opposing attempts to relocate the condyle in the glenoid fossa or on the articular disk. There is usually a history of nonpainful hypermobility and sometimes of previous dislocations that the patient was able to reduce himself.

Symptoms. The patient is distressed because of the inability to close the mouth and sometimes associated pain. There is acute malocclusion.

Examination. This reveals an anterior open bite with only the posterior teeth in contact. Visual inspection or palpation of the articular fossa may reveal a depression where the condyle would normally be.[133]

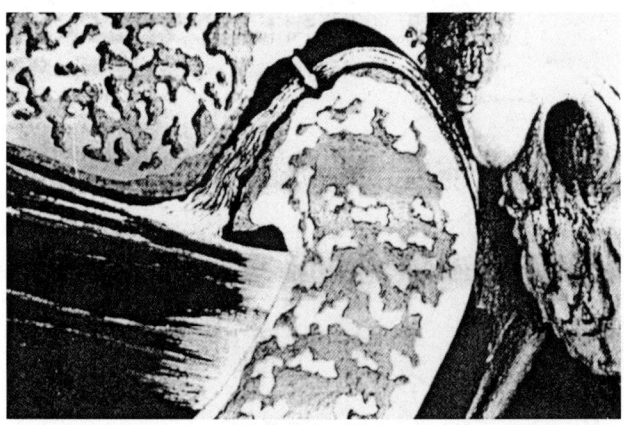

Figure 16 Degenerative joint changes that occur to the disk and condylar surfaces. Disk perforation (arrow), allowing bone-to-bone contact, may cause crepitus and pain on opening and closing. Reproduced with permission from Dr. Samuel Higdon.

Diagnostic tests. Radiographic examination shows the condyles anterior to the articular eminence or anteriorly displaced within the fossa.

Treatment. Reduction of the mandibular displacement is the goal and usually requires some kind of manual manipulation of the mandible. Initial steps include reassurance followed by gentle jaw opening against resistance to relax the elevator muscles. Manipulation procedures to reduce the mandible range from simple downward and posterior pressure on the chin during voluntary yawning, to downward and backward pressure on the mandibular molar teeth during yawning, to the administration of muscle relaxants or local anesthetics or even intravenous sedation followed by manual manipulation. Patients can expect some mild residual pain for one to several days following reduction.

Ankylosis in the TMJ refers to a fibrous or bony union between the condyle, disk, and fossa causing restricted mandibular range of motion with deflection of the mandible to the affected side but no pain. Ankylosis may follow joint inflammation caused by direct trauma, mandibular fracture, surgery, or a systemic disease such as arthritis. Treatment depends on the degree of dysfunction: arthroscopy and physical therapy may improve function for fibrous ankylosis (most common); open joint surgery is needed to create a new articulating surface in bony ankylosis (relatively rare). Elevator muscle shortening must be addressed as part of the management protocol for both conditions.

REFERRED PAIN FROM REMOTE PATHOLOGICAL SITES

Angina Pectoris

Severe pain of cardiac origin can be referred to the mandible and the maxillary region. The opposite pain reference has also been reported—pain from pulpalgia referring down the homolateral neck, shoulder, and arms.[134] That cardiac pain can be referred as far away as the jaws is fascinating. Yet remembering that dorsal root ganglion cells have been shown to branch in the periphery[135,136] and that, in the rat at least, the dorsal root ganglion cell supplying the heart also supplies the arm[135] helps to provide a probable explanation to this referred pain phenomenon (Figure 17). Potential convergence of nerve fibers from different sensory dermatomes in the dorsal horn of the spinal cord provides a basis for a "convergence-projection" phenomenon for the pain referral (see Figure 6). The thoracic dermatomes, innervating the chest and arms, overlap with the cervical dermatomes, some of which innervate the arm and shoulder, as well as part of the lower face. The second cervical dermatome, in turn, slightly overlaps with the fifth cranial nerve that innervates the entire oral complex.

Symptoms. Angina pectoris is typically characterized by heaviness, tightness, or aching pain in the mid or the upper sternum. These symptoms may radiate upward from the epigastrium to the mandible—the left more frequently than the right. In addition, the inner aspects of the arms may ache, again the left

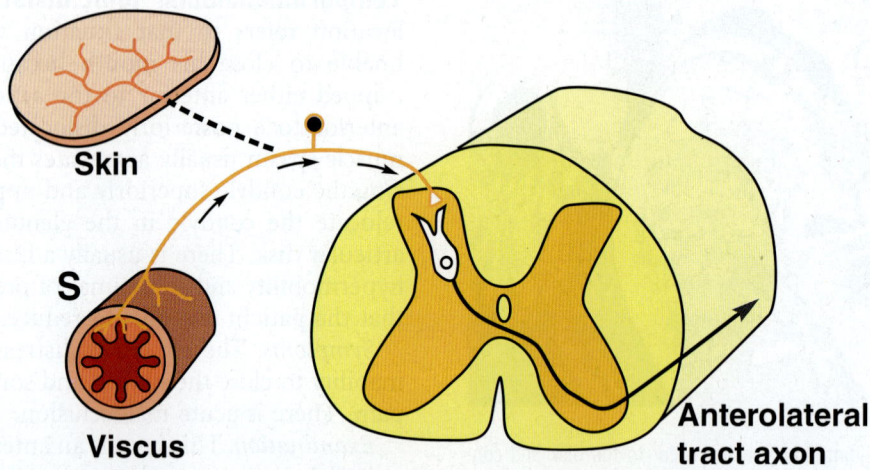

Figure 17 Branched primary afferent hypothesis of referred pain. According to this theory, a single primary afferent branches to supply both the deep structure stimulated and the structure(s) in which the pain is perceived. Reproduced with permission from Fields HL, McGraw-Hill; 1987.

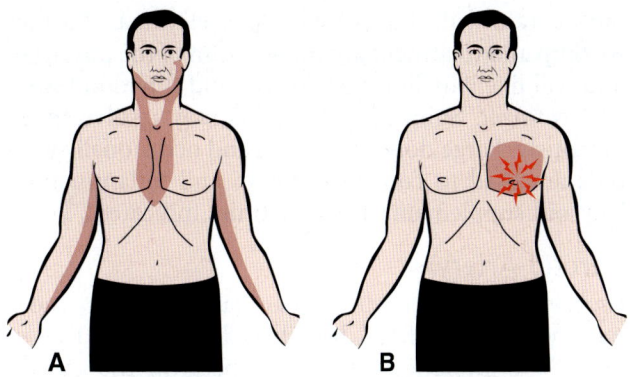

Figure 18 ***A,*** Pattern of pain and referred pain emanating from myocardial infarction. Central necktie pattern and greater left jaw and arm pain than on the right side are typical. ***B,*** Harmless noncardiac pain in the left chest. Reproduced with permission from Turner GO, Med World News; 1973.

more frequently and extensively than the right. This pattern is similar to that seen with myocardial infarction (Figure 18A). Precipitating factors include exertion and emotional excitement or ingestion of food.[137] Angina attacks are usually short-lasting, rarely longer than 15 minutes. A number of patients with recurrent angina pectoris, who know they have the disease and who use nitroglycerine to control the attacks, have reported left mandibular pain with each spasm. Anginal pain referred to the teeth may be experienced with or without concomitant chest pain.[138]

Myocardial Infarction

Myocardial infarction is characterized by a symptom complex that includes a sudden, gradually increasing precordial pain, with an overwhelming feeling of suffocation. The squeezing pain radiates in a pattern similar to that described for angina pectoris (see Figure 18A). Accompanying these symptoms may be a sense of impending doom, nausea, and the attendant signs of shock: sweating, cold clammy skin, and a gray complexion. In advanced stages, the patient becomes unconscious and cyanotic. If conscious, the patient generally complains of severe pain and rubs the chest, jaw, and arms. Thus myocardial infarct pain is similar to angina but is more pronounced, long-lasting, and does not resolve with rest. Severe pain in the left maxilla and mandible related to angina pectoris or myocardial infarction may occur without any other symptoms. Bonica reported an incidence as high as 18% for the presentation of cardiac pain as jaw or tooth pain alone.[139] The distribution of this cardiac pain may vary. One patient had the unusual symptoms of referred pain in the left maxilla and right arm but no chest pain. Matson reported a case of coronary thrombosis during which the patient experienced "pain in both sides of the mandible and neck that radiated to the lateral aspects of the zygoma and temporal areas. She specifically denied having chest, shoulder, or arm pains…."[140] Norman[141] discussed four unusual cases of myocardial infarction with pain referred to the right and left jaws. The left maxilla is also a common site. Batchelder and her colleagues[137] also reported a case in which mandibular pain was the sole clinical manifestation of coronary insufficiency. Krant[139] reported referred pain in the left mandibular molars that proved to be a manifestation of a malignant mediastinal lymphoma.[142] It is these patients with jaw pain in the absence of other symptoms of heart disease who report to the dental office for diagnosis.[138]

Etiology. Angina pectoris refers to pain in the thoracic region and surrounding areas owing to transient and reversible myocardial ischemia.[143] Coronary atherosclerosis with or without coronary artery spasm is the most common cause of myocardial ischemia. Any other cause of reduced myocardial blood flow may also cause angina, such as in aortic stenosis or isolated coronary artery spasm

Myocardial infarction refers to necrosis of the cardiac muscle secondary to a severe reduction in coronary blood supply.[143] Coronary artery occlusion is usually an abrupt event related to unstable atherosclerotic plaques. Predisposing factors include heredity, obesity, tobacco use, lack of physical exercise, diets high in saturated fats, emotional stress, and hostility and anger.

Examination. A careful history is important in diagnosing the referred oral pain of cardiac origin. Usually, the patient has a rather unusual story to tell, with a fairly severe pain that began rather suddenly in the left jaw and grew in intensity. The symptoms may sound very much like a pulpitis. The pain might even have moved from the mandible to the maxilla. The dentist must rule out dental pathosis quickly and efficiently.

Diagnostic tests. Radiographs and pulp testing of all of the teeth in the site of pain or rinsing with ice water will be equivocal. Analgesic block of the involved tooth or teeth will fail to relieve the pain.

After localized dental or TMJ origins have been ruled out, referred pain from the chest must be considered.

Treatment. If previously undiagnosed cardiac pain is suspected, the patient must be referred to an emergency room immediately. The patient should be transported by paramedic or emergency services personnel and not allowed to drive. It is wise to call the hospital and have them ready to receive the patient.

If the patient loses consciousness, basic cardiopulmonary resuscitation should be applied until help arrives. This may be lifesaving. Every dental office should be equipped with a defibrillator.

Thyroid

The thyroid is a butterfly-shaped gland situated in the neck superficial to the trachea at or below the cricoid cartilage. Thyroid hormone regulates the metabolic state of the body. Disorders of the thyroid gland are prevalent in medical practice, second only to diabetes as an endocrine disorder.[144] *Subacute thyroiditis* (viral inflammation of the thyroid gland) is of interest to the dentist because it may refer *pain to the jaws and ears*.

Symptoms. The typical symptom picture includes a sore throat with pain over at least one lobe of the thyroid gland or pain radiating up the sides of the neck and into the lower jaws, ears, or occiput. Swallowing may aggravate the symptoms. This is usually associated with a feeling of pressure or fullness in the throat. There may be mild fever, asthenia, and malaise.[144] Symptoms may wax and wane over a period of months and then finally resolve with return of normal thyroid function.

Etiology. Subacute thyroiditis is reported to occur 2 to 3 weeks after an upper respiratory infection and is viral in origin.[144]

Examination. The thyroid gland may be visibly enlarged and will be exquisitely tender to palpation with nodularity (Figure 19). If thyroiditis or other thyroid disease is suspected, referral to the patient's physician should be made for a complete medical workup.

Diagnostic tests. A complete blood count may show an elevated leukocyte count. The erythrocyte sedimentation rate will be substantially elevated. Further workup and treatment are in the realm of the physician and will likely include various thyroid function tests.

Treatment. Subacute thyroiditis may resolve spontaneously. Large doses of aspirin and occasionally steroids are used to control the pain and inflammation. Thyroid supplements are sometimes indicated.[144]

Carotid Artery

Carotidynia is a symptom of unilateral vascular neck pain which was first described by Temple Fay in 1927.[145] Stimulation of various parts of the carotid artery in the region of the bifurcation was shown to cause pain in the *ipsilateral jaw, maxilla, teeth, gums*, scalp, eyes, or nose.[146] Long thought to be a benign complaint, frequently associated with migraine, and often responding to migraine therapy,[147] carotidynia was removed from International Headache Society (IHS) classification in 2004 due to an apparent lack of radiological or pathological findings.[148] More recently, various systematic MRI and ultrasonic studies have found evidence of abnormal soft tissue infiltration surrounding the symptomatic carotid arteries, renewing the interest in carotidynia as a distinct disease entity.[50]

Symptoms. The patient with *carotidynia* will most likely complain of constant or intermittent dull aching, rarely pulsing jaw and neck pain, with intermittent sore throat or swollen glands. The pain may also involve the *temple and TMJ region* and radiate forward into the *masseter muscle* with occasional concomitant tenderness and fullness. Aggravating factors may include *chewing, swallowing*, bending over, or straining. Females outnumber males in the ratio of approximately 4:1.[147] A history of migraine may be present. Precipitating factors may include an inflammatory response secondary to physical trauma or bacterial or viral infection, drugs, or alcohol.

Etiology. The nerves innervating the adventitial and intimal walls of the carotid artery are considered part of the visceral nervous system. The convergence-projection theory of referred visceral pain discussed earlier in this chapter may explain why pain is referred from the carotid artery to the skin and muscles of the head and neck region.

Recent studies support the idea that there is inflammation and abnormal soft tissue infiltration surrounding the symptomatic tender carotid bulb.[149]

Examination. The examination may reveal tenderness and swelling over the ipsilateral carotid artery along with pronounced throbbing of the carotid pulse. Palpation may aggravate the pain. The thyroid is nontender. All other tests and examinations are

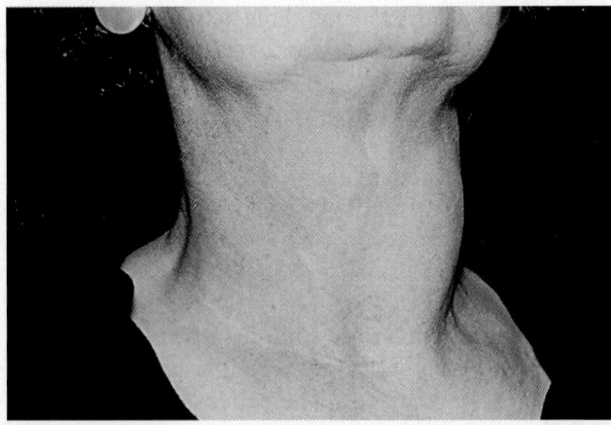

Figure 19 Benign thyroid tumor that recurred following thyroidectomy is referring pain into the mandibular first molar on the homolateral side.

normal. Carotidynia has an extensive *differential diagnosis*, including such conditions as pharyngitis, otitis, bruxism, TMJ syndrome, neuralgia, myalgia, and temporal arteritis,[150] and these should be ruled out with appropriate history and examination prior to making a diagnosis of carotidynia.

Treatment. Medications used in the treatment and prevention of migraine headaches have been shown to be effective in controlling the symptoms of carotidynia.[151] Some authors advocate the use of steroids and NSAIDs.[151] Concomitant treatment of any myofascial TrPs will ameliorate the symptoms to some extent as well.

Cervical Spine

Disorders of the cervical spine and neck area may refer pain into the *facial region* owing to the convergence of cervical and trigeminal primary afferent nociceptors in the nucleus caudalis of the spinal trigeminal tract. The normal cervical spine has 37 individual joints, making it the most complicated articular system in the body.[152] Most of the structures in the neck have been shown to produce pain when stimulated.[153] Pain may be elicited through several different pathological processes including trauma; inflammation or misalignment of the vertebral bodies; inflammation or herniation of the intervertebral disks; trauma or strain in the spinal ligaments; and strains, spasms, or tears of the cervical muscles.

Nonmusculoskeletal pain-producing structures of the neck include the cervical nerve roots and nerves and the vertebral arteries.[153] Trauma, inflammation, and compression are implicated in the etiology of pain from these structures as well.

Acute trauma and primary pathological processes of the neck are obviously not in the realm of the dentist to diagnose and treat; therefore, these will not be discussed. However, the cervical spine must be recognized as a potential source of dermatomal and referred pain into the head and the *orofacial* region. Chronic subclinical dysfunction of the cervical spine may produce complaints that first appear in the dental office. This dysfunction may serve as a powerful perpetuating factor in temporomandibular and facial pain disorders and must be screened for and appropriately managed for successful treatment outcome.

Cervical Joint Dysfunction. Cervical joint dysfunction refers to a lack of normal anatomical relationship and/or restricted functional movement of individual cervical vertebral joint segments.

Etiology. In the craniocervical region, cervical joint dysfunction may occur as the result of trauma (e.g., a *whiplash injury*), degenerative osteoarthritis, or chronic poor postural habits that result in sustained muscular contraction and immobility. As the cervical spine loses mobility and adapts to abnormal positions, nerve compression, nerve root irritation, neurovascular compression, posterior vertebral joint irritation, and peripheral entrapment neuropathies may result.[88,151,152] Entrapment or chronic irritation of the nerve roots in the C4 to C7 area generally produces pain in the respective dermatomes in the shoulder and arm regions (see Figure 10). Although C1, C2, and C3 nerve roots are not thought to be involved in compression or peripheral entrapment-type problems,[156] they do become inflamed through mechanical irritation by other neighboring structures such as the vertebral processes, muscles, or connective tissue capsules. When this occurs, pain may be experienced in the craniofacial, orofacial, mandibular, and temporomandibular regions (the C2–C3 dermatomes) (see Figures 10 and 20). Pain impulses from the first four upper cervical roots are thought to be referred to the trigeminal region (mainly V1 and V2) as a result of the proximity of the nucleus caudalis in the spinal trigeminal tract.[55] The nucleus caudalis descends into the spinal cord as far as C3–C4. These dermatomal and referred pain syndromes are particularly important to the dentist.

Symptoms. Local symptoms of cervical dysfunction may include stiffness, pain, and a limited range of motion of the head and neck.[153] The patient may also complain of throat tightness and difficulty in swallowing.[154]

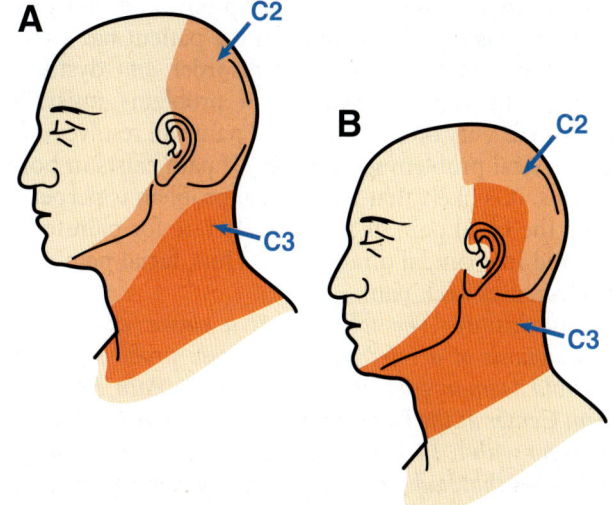

Figure 20 A study by Poletti revealed a slightly different distribution of C2–C3 dermatomes for pain than those previously defined by using tactile criteria. The upper figure **A**, depicts the C2 and C3 tactile dermatomes previously defined by Foerster. **B**, depicts C2 and C3 pain dermatomes as defined by Poletti. Reproduced with permission from Poletti CE, Cephalgia; 1991.

Dermatomal pains may have an aching or neuritic quality and typically follow the distribution of the cervical nerve root involved. *Referred pains* are usually deep and aching and may present as a unilateral headache, as in a headache syndrome known as "cervicogenic headache."[55,157,158] This headache has a clinical picture similar to migraine except the pain is strictly or predominantly unilateral and always on the same side. The patient may note that cervical movement or pressure on certain spots in the neck will precipitate a headache.

Examination. Postural evaluation is essential for all facial pain patients. Of particular importance is anterior head position. The examination of the cervical spine should include range of motion in flexion, extension, lateral flexion, and rotation. Additionally, the movement of the individual upper cervical segments (occiput—C1 and C1–C2) should be evaluated.[86,88] Range of motion is often restricted with cervical dysfunction. Upper cervical dysfunction may be unilateral or bilateral.

Radiographic evaluation may reveal osteoarthritis or show a decreased cervical lordosis, evidence of soft tissue spasm, or muscular shortening. Most commonly, however, no pathological radiographic findings are present. More sophisticated radiographic techniques can pick up decreased cervical mobility.[159]

Treatment. Physical therapy, including cervical joint mobilization along with a comprehensive home exercise program and postural retraining, is required to treat pain of cervical origin.

Local treatment of referred symptoms does not provide long-lasting, if any, relief. If the patient has a true dental or temporomandibular disorder *and* dysfunction of the cervical spine, both problems must be addressed. Very often craniofacial pain will resolve once the cervical problem is corrected. If pain exists in both regions, it is likely that the cervical problem is perpetuating the facial pain. It is extremely rare for pain to be referred in a caudal direction.[101] Thus, facial pain only rarely causes neck pain.

Case history. The following is a classic example of misdiagnosis of a referred cervical pain problem. A 38-year-old woman presented herself to the Pain Management Center at the University of California at Los Angeles (UCLA) with a 14-year history of severe left hemicranial headaches that had forced her to give up working. Because of the unilateral distribution, they had previously been misdiagnosed and unsuccessfully treated as migraine. However, the pain was strictly unilateral and was present on a continuous daily basis (unlike migraine), with intermittent exacerbations. The quality of the pain was described as dull and aching, progressing to throbbing only when severe. The patient also had an endodontic history involving the upper left second premolar, reportedly still sensitive. The dental examination revealed slight hyperocclusion of the involved premolar that was corrected. Thorough musculoskeletal range of motion examination of the TMJ and cervical spine revealed a very prominent Cervical spine dysfunction of atlas on axis on the left. There was no evidence of any internal derangement of the TMJ. Myofascial examination revealed several active TrPs that reproduced her pain complaint.

Physical therapy, including cervical joint mobilization along with a comprehensive home exercise program and postural retraining, was instituted. As treatment progressed, the painful area began to decrease in size until all that remained was the left TMJ and left lower-border mandible pain—the precise distribution of the C2 tactile dermatome (see Figure 20A) and C3 pain dermatome (see Figure 20B).

Myofascial TrP injections into the left splenius capitis muscle in conjunction with further physical therapy and a continued home program completely resolved the C1–C2 dysfunction and the associated dermatomal pain. The patient has now been pain free for 18 years.

The case of this patient illustrates how easy it would be to search in the TMJ and dental area for a cause for the pain when the true culprit is actually the neck. The role of cervical dysfunction and myofascial TrPs in this type of pain presentation has been thoroughly discussed.[134]

A TMJ disorder is unlikely to be causing all of our initial patient's pain. However, on examination, a restricted mandibular range of motion was found, as well as radiographic evidence of degenerative joint disease. Perhaps these are incidental findings. Alternatively, if the internal derangement is painful or the joint is inflamed, it may also be a contributing factor.

Muscles

Myofascial TrP pain is discussed under section "Muscular pains" in this chapter.

Intracranial Pathosis

Although rare, intracranial lesions can cause pain referral to all areas of the head, face, and neck, including the oral cavity. Neurological or neurosurgical evaluation is critical to rule out space-occupying lesions, intracranial infections, or neurological syndromes.

Intracranial causes of head and neck pain can be classified into two groups: those caused by *traction on pain-sensitive structures* (which include the venous sinuses, dural and cerebral arteries, pia and dura mater, and cranial nerves) and those caused by *specific*

Table 10 Intracranial Causes of Pain	
Neoplasm	Neurofibromatosis
Aneurysm	Meningitis
Hematoma/hemorrhage	Thalamic pain
Edema	
Abscess	Cerebrovascular accidents
Angioma	Venous thrombosis

CNS syndromes, such as neurofibromatosis, meningitis, or thalamic pain[159] (Table 10). Different types of cerebrovascular accidents and venous thrombosis may also cause painful CNS lesions. Most of these problems will, however, not be seen in the dental office and therefore will not be discussed in detail.

Intracranial lesions are rarely painful, but when they are, the pain is severe and difficult to treat.[161] The quality of pain may vary from a generalized throbbing or aching to a more specific paroxysmal sharp pain. *Neurofibromatosis*, a condition in which there are numerous pedunculated tumors of the neurolemmal tissue all over the body, is not painful unless the tumors press on nerves. Intracranial lesions are usually associated with different focal neurological signs or deficits such as weakness, dizziness, difficulty in speaking or swallowing, ptosis, areas of numbness, memory loss, or mental confusion. If such neurological signs or deficits appear with a pain complaint, pain from intracranial sources must be ruled out. This will require referral to a competent neurologist or neurosurgeon. Treatment will depend on the diagnosis and may range from antibiotic or antiviral therapy for infective processes to surgical intervention for aneurysms and tumors to palliative pain management for inoperable cases.

In our patient, presented earlier, extensive examinations and sophisticated imaging techniques have already ruled out extracranial and intracranial pathosis as causes for her pain, although she does have active myofascial TrPs in the trapezius muscle referring pain into the angle of the jaw. This, however, does not account for her entire pain presentation. The other sources of pain must still be sought.

Neurovascular Pains

This category of pain encompasses several of the primary headache disorders (headaches not of pathological origin) such as migraines, trigeminal autonomic cephalalgias (Iwata, Imai et al.), and simple intracranial vasodilation, as well as some headaches associated with pathological vascular disorders, such as temporal arteritis (Table 11). The list includes only those headaches that have a higher likelihood of presenting in the dental office.

In general, these headache types share the following features. They all have primarily a deep, throbbing, pulsing, or pounding quality, occasionally sharp, and occasionally with an aching or burning background. The pain is exclusively or *predominantly unilateral* with pain-free or almost pain-free periods between attacks. The main difference between the different headache types lies

Table 11 Neurovascular Pains
Migraines
Migraine with aura (classic)
Migraine without aura (common)
Migraine with prolonged aura (complicated)
Cluster headaches and chronic paroxysmal hemicrania
Cluster headache
Episodic
Chronic
Chronic paroxysmal hemicrania
Miscellaneous headaches unassociated with structural lesion
External compression headache
Cold stimulus headache
Benign cough headache
Benign exertional headache
Headache associated with sexual activity
Headaches associated with vascular disorders
Arteritis
Carotid or vertebral artery pain
Hypertension
Headaches associated with substances or their withdrawal
Acute substance use/exposure (nitrates, monosodium glutamate, carbon monoxide, alcohol)
Chronic substance use/exposure (ergotamine, analgesics)
Acute use withdrawal (alcohol)
Chronic use withdrawal (ergotamine, caffine, narcotics)
Headaches associated with metabolic disorder
Hypoxia
Hypoglycemia
Dialysis

Adapted from Headache Classification Committee of the International Headache Society, 2004.[82]

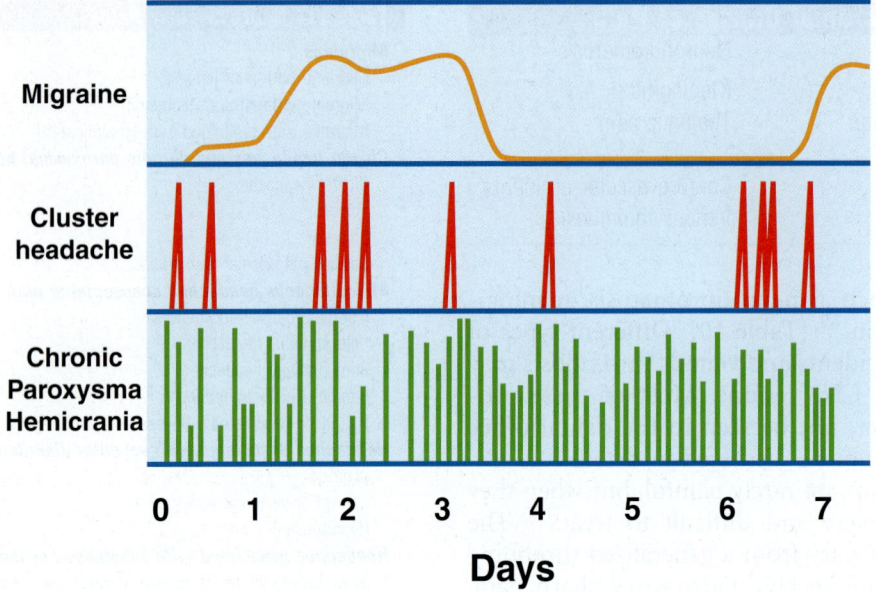

Figure 21 Comparison of temporal pattern of three main "vascular" head ache types.

in their temporal patterns (Figure 21) and their associated symptoms.

MIGRAINE

Migraine is a debilitating, inherited, episodic disorder and a form of sensory processing disturbance in the CNS.[162]

Symptoms. Migraine with aura, commonly known as "classic" migraine, is distinguished by the occurrence of transient focal neurological symptoms (the aura), 10 to 30 minutes prior to the onset of headache pain.

Visual auras are most common and may present as flashing lights, halos, or loss of part of the visual field. Somatosensory auras are also common and consist of dysesthesias that start in one hand and spread up to involve the ipsilateral side of the face, nose, and mouth.[163] The headache itself is predominantly unilateral in the frontal, temporal, or retrobulbar areas, although it may occur in the face or in a single tooth. The pain may begin as an ache but usually develops into a pain of throbbing, pulsating, or beating nature. Associated symptoms may include nausea, vomiting, photo- and phonophobia, cold extremities, water retention, and sweating. The headaches are episodic and can last anywhere from several hours to 3 days, with variable pain-free periods (days to years).

Migraine without aura or "common" migraine is similar to migraine with aura except that the headache occurs without a preceding aura. Migraine headaches are more common in females and may begin in early childhood. The usual onset is between the ages of 20 and 40 years, with 70% of these patients reporting *a family history* of migraine. Some factors that may precipitate the headache include stress and fatigue, foods rich in tyramine (ripe cheese) or nitrates, red wines and alcohol, histamines, and vasodilators. Often patients with migraine, especially migraine without aura, have *overlying MFP*, causing additional dull, aching headache pain. The prevalence of TMDs and various orofacial pain (OF) disorders in relation to headaches has been reported.[164–167]

Case history. The following is an example of an unusual presentation of a migraine headache of particular interest to the dentist. The patient was a 52-year-old woman who had a 7-year history of pain in the upper right quadrant, second premolar area, radiating to the right temple. The quality of pain was described as pulsing, sharp, and penetrating. The temporal pattern was intermittent, with 2 to 3 days of pain followed by 1 to 2 weeks without pain. The symptoms occurred without any identifiable precipitating factor, although loud noise seemed to make the pain worse. Associated autonomic symptoms were absent. Previous unsuccessful treatments included endodontic treatment of the right maxillary second premolar and an exploratory open flap in the same area, looking for fractures or external resorption. Topical anesthetics over the gingiva surrounding tooth #4 were similarly ineffective in relieving the symptoms. A diagnosis of migraine without aura was made based on the quality

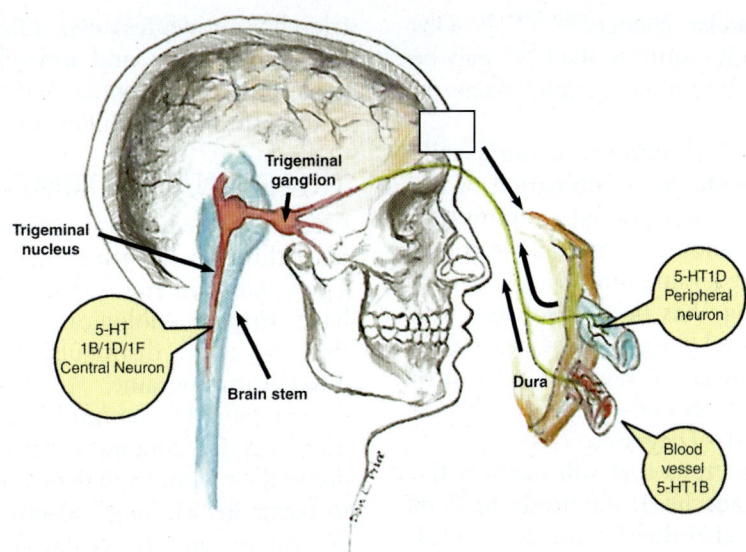

Figure 22 Potential binding sites of the action of triptans in the trigeminovascular complex. Modified from Burstein et al.[174]

and temporal pattern of the pain and the absence of dental pathema to explain the symptoms. Treatment with abortive migraine medications proved quite successful.

Etiology. The exact etiology and pathogenesis of *migraine with aura* headaches remain controversial. Evidence suggests that migraine is a disorder of cortical brain excitability,[168] which may be due to an increase or a disturbance of excitatory neurotransmitters and as a result enhancing the probability of cortical spreading depression (CSD). CSD is the experimental correlate of the aura.[169] The pain is thought to be *referred* to the more superficial cranial structures through convergence of vascular and somatic nerve fibers on single second-order pain transmission neurons in the trigeminal nucleus caudalis.[170] In addition, a sterile neurogenic inflammation caused by the release of vasoactive neuropeptides from nerves surrounding the affected intracranial vasculature is thought to be the nociceptive source. While the mechanism of pain generation in migraine is still controversial, evidence suggests that central sensitization in the trigeminocervical complex (the trigeminal nucleus caudalis and the dorsal horns of C1 and C2), together with the reflex connections of the trigeminal system with the cranial parasympathetic neuronal flow mediated through the pterigopalatine, otic and carotid ganglia, results in headache and cutaneous allodynia.[168,171–174] It has been proposed that vasodilatation of the dural blood vessels activates the trigeminal sensory afferents that surround them. They then transmit the input to the trigeminocervical complex, cervicomedullary junction, and C1–C2 levels of the dorsal horn. From there the signals are transmitted to the higher centers.[168,175] The activation of the trigeminal sensory afferents around the dural blood vessels induces the release of SP, CGRP, glutamate, serotonin (5-HT), and nitric oxide (NO) from the trigeminal afferents exacerbating the vasodilation and neurogenic inflammation.[169,173,174] The efficacy of the *ergot* alkaloids and a family of tryptamine-based drugs called "triptans" appears to be due to the ability of these drugs to cause a vasoconstriction in the cranial blood vessels.[169,175] They do this through their binding action to serotonin 5-HT1B and 5-HT1D receptors (Figure 22). Furthermore, experimental pharmacological evidence suggests that triptans also act on the second-order neurons of the trigeminocervical complex reducing cell activity[178] and repressing the CGRP promoter,[180,181] thereby inhibiting the transcription of this neuropeptide.

Many headache researchers and clinicians feel that *migraine without aura* is the same as migraine with aura, except that the aura is absent or not dramatic enough to be noted. Thus, the mechanism is thought to be similar. The cortical blood flow changes resemble closely those observed in migraine with aura.[182] In addition, data indicate the possibility of a clinically silent CSD in migraine without aura not only in the cortex but also in the cerebellum.[182,183]

There is, however, fairly good evidence that the *pain* of migraine without aura may actually be due to muscle tenderness and referred pain from myofascial TrPs rather than cerebral vascular changes.[167,184–187] This indicates that the nociceptive input to the CNS may be increased as a result of sensitization of peripheral sensory afferents.[188]

Examination. The diagnosis of migraine can usually be made by history. Nonetheless, examination of the patient complaining of undiagnosed intermittent toothache or facial pain should include a thorough dental, TMJ, and muscle evaluation. Once obvious dental and joint pathology has been ruled out, and the qualitative and temporal pattern of the pain raises the possibility of dental or facial migraine, referral to an orofacial pain dentist should be made. Dental heroics should be avoided—*Diagnostic Tests.*

There are no diagnostic tests that will confirm the diagnosis of migraine headache. If the headache is of recent onset, a neurological evaluation including a CT scan or an MRI may be indicated. Thermography during an acute attack of migraine does show areas of increased blood flow on the side of the headache.[189,190]

Treatment. Long-term management of migraine headache typically requires identification and control of any obvious precipitating factors. Restriction of alcohol intake and elimination of tyramine-containing foods[191] are simple yet sometimes effective means of decreasing the frequency of migraine attacks. Regular meals and good sleep hygiene also help prevent the onset of migraine. If myofascial TrPs or musculoskeletal dysfunction is present, competent treatment of these will significantly reduce the frequency of vascular headache symptoms and reduce the need for migraine medications. For those patients in whom stress, depression, or anxiety play a role, psychological interventions such as stress management and relaxation training, biofeedback, or cognitive behavioral therapy may be indicated.

Medications used in the treatment of migraine include abortive and prophylactic drugs, the choice of which depends on the frequency of migraine attacks. Individuals who suffer less than three or four migraines per month may do well with abortive drugs that are taken during the onset of the headache or migrainous facial pain. Abortive drugs are particularly useful in migraine with aura for which the aura warns the patient that a headache is pending. The serotonin 5-HT(1B/1D) agonists or "triptans" are highly effective. They improve headache as well as nausea, photo- and phonophobia. Prophylactic medications are used when headache frequency exceeds three or four per month since the triptans may cause coronary vasospasm or ischemia. Prophylactic medications include β-blockers, tricyclic antidepressants, calcium channel blockers, 5-HT antagonists, and antiepileptic drugs such as valproic acid, Gabapentin, and topiramate. The use of botulinum toxin is under investigation.[192]

TRIGEMINAL AUTONOMIC CEPHALAGIAS

Cluster headaches and chronic paroxysmal hemicrania belong to the trigeminal autonomic cephalagias. They share several clinical characteristics and may have similar etiological mechanisms. Nonetheless, they are easily distinguishable clinically and clearly differ from migraine.

Symptoms. Cluster headaches are probably one of the most painful conditions known by humankind and derive their name from their temporal pattern. They tend to occur in "clusters," a series of one to eight 20- to 180-minute attacks per day lasting for several weeks or months, followed by remissions of months or years[82,193,194] (see Figure 21). These headaches are found five to eight times more frequently in men than in women, particularly in *men aged 20 to 50 years who smoke*. The pain is a severe, unilateral, continuous, intense ache or burning that often occurs at night. Movements that increase the blood flow to the head may result in throbbing. The most common sites are either around or behind the eye radiating to the forehead and temple or around and behind the eye radiating infraorbitally *into the maxilla and occasionally into the teeth*, rarely to the lower jaw and neck. Because of the oral symptoms, serious diagnostic errors are committed by dentists. Researchers from UCLA reported that 42% of 33 patients suffering cluster headache had been seen by dentists and that 50% of these patients *received inappropriate dental treatment.*[195]

Prodromal auras are absent with cluster headaches, but nasal stuffiness, lacrimation, rhinorrhea, conjunctival injection, perspiration of the forehead and face, and Horner's syndrome (ptosis of upper lid and miosis) are characteristics. Precipitating factors may include alcohol or other vasodilating substances, such as nitroglycerine. Cluster headache patients typically pace the floor during their headaches owing to the intensity of pain. This is in contrast to the migraine patient who retreats to a dark room to sleep.

Cluster headaches may progress from the more classic episodic form, occurring in periods lasting 1 week to 1 year, with at least 2-week pain-free periods between, to a chronic form in which remissions are absent or last less than 2 weeks.[82] Rarely is the chronic form present from the onset.

Case History. The following history was obtained from a 42-year-old man who had suffered from cluster headaches for 27 years. The pain, located retro-orbitally on the right side, was described as intermittent, sharp, excruciating, and knife-like. Associated symptoms included tearing of the right eye, stuffiness of the right nostril, numbness on the right side of the face, and right conjunctival injection. The pain occurred one or two times per year in "cluster periods" of 1 to 5 weeks duration. The headaches typically lasted 60 to 75 minutes and could occur multiple times per day. During an attack, the patient would pace the floor and hit his head against doors and walls. He noted that red wine could precipitate an attack and avoided alcohol during headache periods. Past trials of various migraine medications were all without benefit. Oxygen inhalation at the onset of a headache attack, however, immediately relieved the pain. Of importance was a past medical history of myocardial infarction at age 35 and poorly controlled hypertension. These factors impacted treatment and will be discussed.

Chronic Paroxysmal Hemicrania (CPH)

As the name implies, it is typically an unremitting, unilateral headache disorder, although episodic versions have been identified.[196] CPH is characterized by short-lasting (2 to 30 to 45 minutes), frequently occurring attacks of pain (five per day for more than half of the time).[82,197,198] The quality of pain is throbbing or pounding, with an intensity that parallels that of cluster headaches, the patient often choosing to pace the floor during an attack. Pain location is predominantly oculotemporal and frontal, always on the same side, and can spread to involve the entire side of the head and the neck, shoulder, and arm.[198] Cases involving CPH presenting as *intermittent toothache* have been reported.[199] Turning or bending the head forward may precipitate an attack in some cases.[200] Associated symptoms include unilateral lacrimation, nasal stuffiness, and conjunctival injection. Nausea and vomiting are usually absent, as are visual or somatosensory auras. In contrast to cluster headache, CPH is seen *predominantly in women*.[201] Age at onset appears to be 20 years, although a variable pre-CPH period may exist.[201]

Case history. A 21-year-old woman presented with a 3-year history of right-sided supraorbital headaches. These headaches had a full, tight, aching quality with shooting, stabbing exacerbations brought on by rapid head movement, sneezing, or running. Associated symptoms included ptosis and tearing of the right eye. The pain lasted approximately 1 hour and occurred three to four times per day. The longest the patient had ever been without pain since the onset of the headaches was less than 5 days. The headache was completely responsive to indomethacin (NSAID), which is typical of CPH. Of interest was a family history of cluster headaches in her father and a cousin of her mother.

Etiology of trigeminal autonomic cephalalgias. The exact etiology or pathophysiology of *cluster headaches*, and *CPH* for that matter, is as yet unknown; however, involvement of the posterior hypothalamus is suspected.[202,203] Over the years, many theories have been advanced to try to explain the pronounced sympathetic and parasympathetic symptomatology, the trigeminal distribution of the pain, and the periodicity. To date, no consensus has been reached. Vasodilation, once considered an important element in the pathogenesis of cluster, is now thought to be secondary to trigeminal activation.[194] This is because the pain of cluster headache typically precedes any extracranial blood flow changes, and intracranial blood flow studies have shown inconsistent results.[194] The unusual temporal pattern of cluster headaches implicates the hypothalamus that regulates autonomic functions and also largely controls circadian rhythms, as possibly triggering the primary neuronal discharge resulting in cluster headache pain.[190,201] Studies of circadian changes in various hormone levels in cluster patients versus controls do support activation of the hypothalamic gray matter region during cluster headache.[191,205,206] Others propose a complex neuroimmunological mechanism.[207]

The pathophysiology of Chronic Paroxysmal Hemicranic (CPH) is also unknown. Because of the autonomic and temporal similarities of CPH with cluster headache, similar mechanisms are implicated, yet studies of the cardiovascular and sweat responses as well as cognitive processing in the two headaches suggest that they are different.[208,209]

Examination: Cluster headaches. The diagnosis is based on signs and symptoms. There are no diagnostic tests to confirm a diagnosis of cluster headache. Either the patient presents with a typical history and no abnormalities on physical and neurological examination or the examination may cause suspicion of organic lesions with an ultimately normal neuroimaging scan.[82] Mild ptosis and miosis with or without periorbital swelling and conjunctival congestion may be present on the side of the headache if the patient is seen during or shortly after an attack.[189]

As with cluster headaches, a careful history is the primary basis for diagnosis. Organic lesions should always be ruled out with any new headache disorder.

Treatment. Definitive treatment of cluster headaches and CPH is best left to the orofacial pain dentist or other health care providers with a specific interest in headache management.

Cluster Headaches

Many of the treatments used for migraine therapy are also useful in cluster headaches, including symptomatic use of subcutaneous or intranasal triptans.[210–212] In general, however, prophylactic medications are more appropriate in cluster headache because of the frequency of attacks and because prodromal warning symptoms are rare. Cluster headache patients are often wakened from sleep, and the pain reaches its high intensity very quickly. Once the cluster period subsides, patients are weaned from their prophylactic medications until the headaches recur.

Oxygen inhalation (100% 7 to 8 L/min with a non-rebreathing mask), given at the very beginning of an attack for 15 minutes, may be successful in aborting an attack. Oxygen and subcutaneous sumatriptan or intranasal zolmatriptan are also useful as abortive options for the patient taking prophylactic medications who is experiencing breakthrough headaches. In rare cases of resistant chronic cluster headache, trigeminal ganglion lysis or gamma knife treatment may be considered.[213–216]

Chronic Paroxysmal Hemicrania

Indomethacin is the medication of choice for CPH. If the pain does not resolve with this medication, it is unlikely to be CPH. Aspirin and naproxen have a partial effect, but the relief is not as dramatic as with indomethacin.[198]

MISCELLANEOUS HEADACHES UNASSOCIATED WITH STRUCTURAL LESION

Symptoms. These headaches that include external compression headache, cold stimulus headache, benign cough headache, benign exertional headache, and headache associated with sexual activity[82] are usually bilateral, short-lasting, and clearly related to a well-defined precipitating factor. For example, cold stimulus headache may result from exposure of the head to cold or from ingestion of cold substances.

The latter headache, also known as "ice cream headache," typically occurs in the middle of the forehead after cold food or drink passes over the teeth and the palate and lasts less than 5 minutes. *Benign cough headache* is a bilateral headache of extremely short duration (1 minute) that is precipitated by coughing. Physical exertion may also result in bilateral throbbing headaches that may last anywhere from 5 minutes to 24 hours. In some individuals, *sexual excitement* precipitates bilateral headache. This headache intensifies with increasing sexual arousal and may become "explosive" at orgasm.

Etiology. External compression headache is precipitated by prolonged stimulation of the cutaneous nerves through pressure from a tight band, hat, swim goggles, or sunglasses. *Cold stimulus headaches* are caused by exposure of the head to cold or from sudden stimulation of the nasopalatine or posterior palatine nerves with cold foods such as ice cream.[82] *Benign cough* and *exertional headaches*, as well as headaches associated with sexual activity, seem to occur more commonly in people with a history of migraine. The exact mechanism underlying these headaches is unknown but may be related to increased venous pressure in the head, transient hypertension, muscle contraction, increased sympathetic tone, or possibly the release of vasoactive substances.[217]

Treatment. Most of these headaches can be prevented by avoiding the precipitating cause (e.g., pressure from swim goggles, exposure of the head to cold, rapid ingestion of cold substances, exertion). If necessary, frequent exertional headaches can be treated with prophylactic medications such as propranolol or NSAIDs.[207]

HEADACHES ASSOCIATED WITH VASCULAR DISORDERS

This category includes headaches that are attributable to demonstrable pathosis, such as *giant cell arteritis* or *acute hypertension*. Other pathological vascular causes of headache include vertebral or carotid artery dissection and intracranial ischemia owing to intracranial hematoma, subarachnoid hemorrhage, arteriovenous malformations, or venous thrombosis (see Table 11). Headaches owing to such intracranial pathosis are unlikely to appear in the dental office and are therefore not further described. Giant cell arteritis, however, which does, on occasion, present with dental symptoms, may produce serious, irreversible consequences if left unrecognized and untreated.

Giant Cell Arteritis (Temporal Arteritis)

Headache or facial pain from giant cell arteritis is relatively rare, but the dentist must know about this disorder and be able to recognize it because blindness is a serious potential complication.

Symptoms. The patient with giant cell arteritis is usually over 50 years old and may have other rheumatic symptoms, such as polymyalgia rheumatica. Involvement of the temporal artery may bring the patient in to see the dentist first because pain with mastication ("jaw claudication") may be the first or only symptom. Friedlander and Runyon[218] reported patients with *a burning tongue and claudication of the muscles of mastication*. Guttenberg et al.[216] reported a case mimicking dental pain that led to *inappropriate, ineffective endodontic surgery*.[219]

The pain is usually unilateral and in the anatomic area of the artery and may also radiate down to the ear, *teeth*, and occiput with generalized scalp tenderness. Temporal arteritis may resemble a migraine attack because it, too, has a persistent throbbing quality that may last hours to days and the location is unilateral, over the temple area.[210] *Temporal arteritis*, however, has an *additional burning, ache-like quality*. The pain increases with lowering of the head, *mastication*, and movements that create increased blood flow to that artery. The patient may present with complaints of malaise, fatigue, anorexia, and weight loss if the arteritis occurs as a febrile illness. In advanced cases, patients may complain of transient visual loss on the side of the headache. This is a particularly severe symptom and requires immediate, aggressive treatment since thrombosis of the ophthalmic artery may result in partial or complete blindness.

Etiology. Arterial inflammation, which may often be associated with immunological disorders, is the causative factor in this headache. Arterial biopsy often reveals frayed elastic tissues and giant cells in the vessel walls on histological examination.[220]

Examination. Dental examination is negative. The temporal artery may be tender to palpation, thickened, and enlarged and may lack a normal pulse. Digital pressure with occlusion of the common carotid artery on the same side will frequently alleviate the symptoms. Ophthalmological examination or evaluation of optic ischemia is mandatory. Occasionally patients will have signs and symptoms that mimic other disorders.[221]

Diagnostic tests. In giant cell arteritis, erythrocyte sedimentation rate, although a nonspecific test, will be significantly elevated above 60 mm/h Westergren. Definitive diagnosis is based on arterial biopsy. The entire temporal artery is typically removed to ensure sampling of diseased sections; skip lesions are common. Biopsy of the artery is essential because treatment involves high doses of steroids, but treatment is never delayed if visual disturbance is present.

Treatment. The dentist who suspects temporal arteritis should immediately refer the patient to a rheumatologist or an internist for complete workup. If optic symptoms are present, emergency ophthalmological examination is essential without delay.

Treatment of the condition consists of emergency dosages of steroids. When the elevated sedimentation rate has been reduced, maintenance doses of *prednisone* are administered as clinically determined.

Carotid Or Vertebral Artery Pain. The dissection of the carotid or vertebral arteries causes headache and cervical pain on the same side as the dissection. This serious, life-threatening condition is typically acute and accompanied by symptoms of transient ischemic attack or stroke. Since patients with this problem are unlikely to appear in the dental office, there need be no further discussion of this type of syndrome. *Idiopathic carotidynia* is discussed under the category of "Referred Pain From Remote Pathosis."

Hypertension

Symptoms. Generalized throbbing headache may be a symptom of acute hypertension, especially if the diastolic pressure rises 25%.[82]

Etiology. Usually, abrupt increases in blood pressure are associated with ingestion of a substance that causes vasoconstriction or a systemic disorder such as pheochromocytoma, preeclampsia, or eclampsia in pregnancy, or malignant hypertension. Chronic arterial hypertension is not reported to cause headache.[221]

Examination. A routine blood pressure check is useful to rule out hypertension as a medical problem requiring treatment.

Treatment. Patients with acute or chronic hypertension should be referred to their family practitioner for management. Associated headaches resolve within 24 hours to 7 days after the resolution of the hypertension.

HEADACHE ASSOCIATED WITH ABUSE SUBSTANCES OR THEIR WITHDRAWAL AND HEADACHE ASSOCIATED WITH METABOLIC DISORDERS

These headache types are unlikely to present as a primary complaint in the dental office and thus will not be discussed further here.

Our patient's pain had none of the characteristics described in this category of pain. Therefore, vascular headaches can be excluded in the differential diagnosis.

Neuropathic Pains

Neuropathic pains are caused by some form of structural abnormality or pathosis affecting the peripheral nerves themselves. This is in contrast to the normal transmission of noxious stimulation along these nerves from organic disease or trauma. The structural abnormality or pathosis affecting the nerve(s) may have many different etiologies, including genetic disorders such as porphyria; mechanical damage from compression, trauma, entrapment,

Table 12 Neuropathic Pains
Paroxysmal
Trigeminal neuralgia
Glossopharyngeal neuralgia
Nervus intermedius neuralgia
Occipital neuralgia
Neuroma
Continuous
Postherpetic neuralgia
Posttraumatic neuralgia
Anesthesia dolorosa

traction, or scarring; metabolic disorders such as diabetes, alcoholism, nutritional deficiencies, or multiple myeloma; toxic reactions to drugs, metals, or certain organic substances; or infectious or inflammatory processes such as herpes, hepatitis, leprosy, or multiple sclerosis.

Not all neuropathies are painful. When they are, they may be dramatically so. The distinguishing feature of peripheral neuropathic pains in the head and neck region is the quality of pain, which is burning, sharp, shooting, lancinating, or electric-like. The distribution of the pain is limited to the anatomical pathways of the nerve involved and is almost always unilateral. Sensory abnormalities may include diminished pain sensation in the presence of hypersensitivity to typically nonpainful stimuli.

In general, *neuropathic pains* in the head and neck can be divided into two main groups, *paroxysmal* or *continuous*, based on their temporal pattern (Table 12).

PAROXYSMAL NEURALGIAS

Symptoms. Paroxysmal, lancinating, sharp, unilateral pain that follows a distinct dermatomal pattern is common to all paroxysmal neuralgias. The pain is often described as electric-like, shooting, cutting, or stabbing. The attacks may last only a few seconds to minutes, with virtually no discomfort between attacks. Sometimes patients notice vague prodromata of tingling and occasionally ache or burn after an attack. The attacks may occur intermittently, with days to months between a series of attacks. Usually, patients complain of "trigger areas" that, when stimulated, precipitate an attack. These are frequently located within the distribution of the nerve affected, usually on the skin or the oral mucosa. Neural blockade of the trigger area almost always relieves the pain for the duration of action of the local anesthetic. Should neural blockade fail to relieve the symptoms, either the diagnosis or the nerve block technique must be questioned. Each type of paroxysmal neuralgia has its own distinct characteristics.

Trigeminal Neuralgia and Pretrigeminal Neuralgia

Trigeminal neuralgia or tic douloureux usually affects one or at most two divisions of the fifth cranial nerve.[82] The *mandibular and maxillary* divisions are most commonly involved together, causing pain to shoot down the mandible and across the cheek into the teeth or the tongue. The maxillary or mandibular divisions alone are the next most frequently affected, with ophthalmic division neuralgias being the least common. The pain is unilateral 96% of the time. Touching and washing the face, tooth brushing, shaving, chewing, talking, or even cold wind against the face may set off the trigger and result in pain. Deep pressure or painful stimuli are usually tolerated without a painful episode. Patients go to extraordinary lengths, such as not shaving, washing, or brushing their teeth, to avoid stimulating the trigger area. Between attacks, patients are completely pain-free. Long remissions for months or years are not uncommon but tend to decrease with increasing age.

Trigeminal neuralgia is almost twice as common in women as in men and usually starts after the age of 50.[223] Anyone under the age of 40 with this disorder should be referred to a neurologist to be worked up for a structural lesion or multiple sclerosis.

A syndrome of pain preceding the onset of true paroxysmal trigeminal neuralgia, known as *pretrigeminal neuralgia*, has been described.[224–226] Patients may present themselves up to 2 years before developing trigeminal neuralgia, with pain usually *localized to one alveolar quadrant* and sometimes a sinus. They may describe this pain as dull, aching, and/or burning, or as a sharp (burning) toothache, not unlike pain arising from the dental pulp. Some patients may also report a "pins and needles" sensation. The duration of PTN pain may be 2 hours to several months, with variable periods of remission. Movement, usually opening of the mouth, may trigger the pain.

Dental pathosis may be minimal or absent. Retained root tips are the most common finding, and their removal has been associated with remission of pain. Obvious dental pathosis should be treated, but dental heroics in the absence of clinical or radiographic findings should be avoided. A UCLA group reported that 61% of the cases with PTN or trigeminal neuralgia were incorrectly diagnosed and treated for dental conditions.[226] Onset of classic trigeminal neuralgia may be quite sudden and occurs in the same division affected by the PTN symptoms. The onset may follow remission produced by previous dental treatment.

Case history. A 67-year-old man underwent extensive dental treatment, including endodontic therapy and hemisection of tooth #30, followed by the placement of two different intraoral stabilization appliances, for a pain complaint that turned out to be trigeminal neuralgia. He had also seen a general medical practitioner and a neurologist, who were unable to identify a cause for his pain. A diagnosis of psychogenic pain was made. The reason the true diagnosis was not obvious was because the patient described the pain as constant and related to tooth #30, worsened by eating and talking. Careful questioning, however, revealed that the pain was not constant. Indeed, if he sat very still without talking or moving his mouth, he was pain-free. Movement of the tongue, touching the lower lip, and biting anywhere in the mouth seemed to be precipitating factors. Observation of an attack during the history and physical examination confirmed the diagnosis: the patient became very quiet, his lips began to tremble, and tears came to his eyes because the pain was so intense. The whole episode lasted less than a minute, after which the patient resumed normal conversation.

Glossopharyngeal neuralgia

Glossopharyngeal neuralgia is 70 to 100 times less common than trigeminal neuralgia.[227] The symptoms include unilateral and rarely nonconcurrent bilateral stabbing pain in the lateral posterior pharyngeal and tonsillar areas, the base of the tongue, down into the throat, the eustachian tube or ear, and down the neck.[228] Sometimes pain radiates into the vagal region and *may be associated with salivation*, flushing, sweating, tinnitus, cardiac arrhythmias, hypertension, vertigo, or syncope. *Throat movements*, pressure on the tragus of the ear, *yawning*, or *swallowing* may trigger the pain. Again, local anesthesia of the trigger area temporarily prevents precipitation of attacks. This can be accomplished by spraying the posterior pharynx with a topical anesthetic.

Eagle's syndrome may be the cause of symptoms similar to those of glossopharyngeal neuralgia,[229–231] although some believe that this syndrome is not sufficiently validated.[82] The symptoms that include a "sore throat" and *posterior tongue and pharyngeal pain* are thought to be related to the compression of the area of the glossopharyngeal nerve by a calcified elongation of the *stylohyoid process* of the temporal bone. Precipitating factors include fast rotation of the head, swallowing, and pharyngeal motion from talking and chewing. Blurring of vision and vertigo are rarely seen.

Nervus intermedius neuralgia

Nervus intermedius neuralgia is extremely rare.[232] The pain is described as a lancinating "hot poker" in the ear.[228] It can occur anterior to, posterior to, or on the pinna; in the auditory canal; or, occasionally, in the soft palate. A duller background pain may persist between attacks. Attacks may be accompanied by *salivation, tinnitus*, vertigo, or *dysgeusia*.[233] The trigger area is usually in the external auditory canal. This neuralgia has also been termed *Ramsay Hunt syndrome*, geniculate neuralgia, or Wrisberg's neuralgia and is often associated with *herpes zoster* (or shingles).

Superior laryngeal neuralgia

Superior laryngeal neuralgia is also a rare neuralgia with paroxysmal neuralgic pains of varying duration, minutes to hours, located in the throat, in the submandibular region, or under the ear. Triggering factors include swallowing, turning the head, loud vocalizations, or stimulating the site overlying the hypothyroid membrane where the nerve enters the laryngeal structures.

Occipital neuralgia

Occipital neuralgia occurs in the distribution of the greater or lesser occipital nerves to the back of the head and mastoid process. The *ear and the underside of the mandible* may be involved because of the dermatomal patterns of C2 and C3 (see Figure 20). The pain often radiates into the *frontal and temporal regions*, occasionally with the same sharp, electric-like character of the other neuralgias, but may last hours instead of seconds. Sometimes the pain takes on a more continuous burning, aching nature. A case of maxillary right posterior quadrant dental pain owing to occipital neuralgia has been reported.[234] Trauma, especially rotational injuries to the neck, may precede the onset. Trigger zones, such as those seen with trigeminal neuralgia, are rare. The pain may be associated with neck and back pain, and emotional stress is a common aggravating factor.

Etiology. The paroxysmal neuralgias are considered *symptomatic* if a specific pathological process affecting the involved nerve can be identified and *idiopathic* if not. Paroxysmal neuralgias rarely occur in young people unless there is a distinct compression of the nerve by a tumor or other structural lesion. Compression of the nerve either peripherally or centrally by bone, scar tissue, tumors, aberrant arteries, or arteriovenous malformations causes *focal demyelination*, which is postulated to result in ectopic firing and reduced segmental inhibition of the low-threshold mechanoreceptors and wide-dynamic-range relay neurons.[235] The net effect is a *lowered threshold* of neuronal firing for which ordinary orofacial maneuvers such as chewing, swallowing, talking, or smiling may precipitate a neuralgic attack.

Trigeminal neuralgia, along with other paroxysmal cranial neuralgias, is typically considered idiopathic, although nerve compression by intracranial arteries that have become slack and tortuous with age is thought to be the likely culprit.[236] The *demyelinating* lesions associated with *multiple sclerosis* may also precipitate trigeminal neuralgia in younger individuals. The symptoms of trigeminal neuralgia associated with diabetic polyradiculopathy have also been reported.[237]

Glossopharyngeal neuralgia is more commonly, secondary to another pathologic disorder. For example tumors are found in 25% of cases. Local infection, neck trauma, elongation of the styloid process (Eagle's syndrome), and compression of the nerve root by a tortuous vertebral or posterior inferior cerebellar artery[238] are other symptomatic causes of this ninth-nerve neuralgia. Unlike trigeminal neuralgia, glossopharyngeal neuralgia is almost never associated with multiple sclerosis,[224] and has been reported to be associated with an anomaly of the nerve itself.[239]

Occipital neuralgia may be secondary to hypertrophic fibrosis of subcutaneous tissue around the occipital nerve following trauma, irritation of the nerve by the atlantoaxial ligament, spondylosis of the upper cervical spine, spinal cord tumors, or tubercular granulomas.[240] Myofascial TrPs in the semispinalis capitis and splenius cervicus muscles may mimic this type of pain or may cause neuralgia-like symptoms owing to the entrapment of the greater occipital nerve as it passes through the tense semispinalis muscle fibers.[83] Since treatment of myofascial TrPs is noninvasive, with very low morbidity and no mortality, they must be carefully ruled out before neurectomy or other neuroablative techniques are considered.[241]

Examination. A patient presenting with symptoms of *trigeminal neuralgia* must be worked up for dental disorders, sinus disease, and head and neck infections or neoplasms.[90,242,243] Since nerve compressions from intracranial tumors, aneurysms or vascular malformations, or central lesions from multiple sclerosis may also cause symptomatic trigeminal neuralgia,[244,245] all patients with trigeminal neuralgia-like symptoms should be worked up with an *imaging study* of the head, either contrast-*enhanced CT or MRI*, in addition to routine films.

Diagnosis of *pretrigeminal neuralgia* is based on the clinical presentation of constant *dull toothache pain* in the absence of dental or neurological findings and normal radiographic, CT, or MRI examinations.

Since *glossopharyngeal neuralgia* is more often associated with nasopharyngeal, tonsillar, or posterior fossa tumors or other pathosis than is trigeminal neuralgia, imaging studies including skull films, panoramic films, and MRI are essential.

In *Eagle's syndrome*, the diagnosis is usually established on the basis of radiographs, as well as intraoral finger palpation of the posterior pharyngeal area. Panoramic films should reveal a *stylohyoid process that is so long* that its image projects beyond the ramus of the mandible. Anything shorter is not significant, and other causes for the patient's pain should be sought. Pain is alleviated temporarily by neural block of the suspected compressive area. Treatment is primarily surgical shortening of the styloid process either through an intraoral or an extraoral approach.[229]

Occipital neuralgia requires a thorough musculoskeletal evaluation in addition to a cervical spine radiographic series to rule out neoplasms or other local destructive lesions. Digital palpation of the greater occipital nerve along the nuchal line may be painful. Caudal pressure to the vertex of the head while it is flexed and rotated toward the side of the pain may reproduce cervical compression symptoms.[246] Sensory loss is rare. Because myofascial TrPs may mimic or accompany this disorder, careful palpation of the posterior cervical muscles for the tight bands and focal tenderness with referred pain, characteristic of myofascial TrPs, is essential.[242]

Treatment. Obviously, if a neuralgia is "symptomatic" or the result of identifiable pathema or structural lesion, treatment is directed at correction of the cause. For example, stylohyoid resection may be indicated if this is the cause of glossopharyngeal neuralgia. However, for idiopathic paroxysmal neuralgias, the first treatment of choice is the drug *carbamazepine (Tegretol)*. Carbamazepine is most efficacious in trigeminal neuralgia but has some success in glossopharyngeal or nervus intermedius neuralgias as well. Baclofen (Lioresal), gabapentin (Neurontin), pregabalin (Lyrica) and diphenylhydantoin (Dilantin) are also used, alone or in combination. All of these medications may cause varying degrees of dizziness, drowsiness, and mental confusion. In addition, carbamazepine may cause hematopoietic changes and baclofen may affect liver enzymes. Although such side effects are not as common as once thought and are less common with gabapentin and diphenylhydantoin; patients taking any of these medications must be monitored very closely initially. Patients on Dilantin must be very careful to not develop gingivitis that can lead to gingival hypertrophy.

In those infrequent instances for which these medications or combinations thereof are ineffective, or the patient becomes refractory to the medications or cannot tolerate them, either owing to severe drowsiness or frank allergy, neurosurgical intervention remains an option. In *trigeminal neuralgia*, gamma knife radiosurgery is the newest alternative for treatment. *Gamma knife radiosurgery* is a neurosurgical technique using a single-fraction high-dose ionizing radiation focused on a small (4 mm), stereotactically defined intracranial target.[247] The targeted cells necrotize without apparent harm to adjacent tissues. In *trigeminal neuralgia*, the beam is focused on the trigeminal sensory root adjacent to the pons. The results have been so good[248,249] that some authors advocate gamma knife radiosurgery as the "safest and most effective form of treatment currently available for trigeminal neuralgia."[248] The procedure carries with it low morbidity (infrequent reports of delayed onset of facial tactile hypesthesia or paresthesias) and no mortality.[247] Nonetheless, the long-term effects of this form of treatment have yet to be evaluated, and more traditional approaches to the surgical treatment of trigeminal neuralgia are still used, especially in younger patients.

Younger, healthier patients may choose to undergo *suboccipital craniotomy with microvascular decompression*.[250] In this major neurosurgical procedure, which in some centers is now performed endoscopically, an attempt is made to relieve any pressure on the trigeminal sensory root from blood vessels or other proximal structures. The superior cerebellar artery is the most common offender because it tends to kink under the ganglion itself. Muscle or sponge may be used to hold the vessel away from the nerve root. In this way, pain relief may be obtained with no or minimal loss of sensation or damage to the fifth cranial nerve.[250–253]

For older or medically infirm patients, alternatives to gamma knife radiosurgery include injection of glycerol into the arachnoid cistern of the gasserian ganglion or radiofrequency neuroablation of the trigeminal sensory root to destroy Aδ and C pain fibers.[253,254] Both of these procedures involve the percutaneous insertion of a needle through the cheek into Meckel's cave. They are usually carried out by a neurosurgeon under local anesthesia with fluoroscopic control and take less than 45 minutes. The patient is conscious for both of these percutaneous procedures. Because they are relatively simple procedures, with low morbidity and mortality, they can be easily repeated should the symptoms return. Rare complications include corneal anesthesia, anesthesia dolorosa, injury to the carotid artery, and sixth cranial nerve palsy.[255]

Therapies, especially medications, used to treat true trigeminal neuralgia have been reported to work for *pretrigeminal neuralgia* as well.[256]

Idiopathic *glossopharyngeal neuralgia* can be managed with the same medications used for trigeminal neuralgia. If these fail, microvascular decompression has been reported effective.[257,258] Nerve section or radiofrequency rhizotomies have mixed results.[258,259]

Because of its predominantly musculoskeletal etiology, *occipital neuralgia* lends itself best to nonpharmacological and nonsurgical treatments. Consequently, physical therapy, postural re-education, corrected ergonomics, home neck-stretching exercises, TrP injections, and even C2 nerve blocks, with or without corticosteroids, are the first line of approach.[240] Surgical interventions, such as neurectomy,[260] rarely provide long-term relief.[261]

Surgical section of the nervus intermedius or the chorda tympani has been reported to relieve the pain of *nervus intermedius neuralgia*, as has neurectomy in the case of recalcitrant *superior laryngeal neuralgia*.[262–264]

Neuromas

Neuromas are non-neoplastic, nonencapsulated, tangled masses of axons, Schwann cells, endoneurial cells, and perineurial cells in a dense collagenous matrix (Figure 23).

Etiology. Neuromas tend to develop when a nerve axon is transected, as might occur with a dental extraction, surgery, or trauma. The proximal stump of a transected nerve is still connected to its cell body and, in a few days postinjury, it will start to

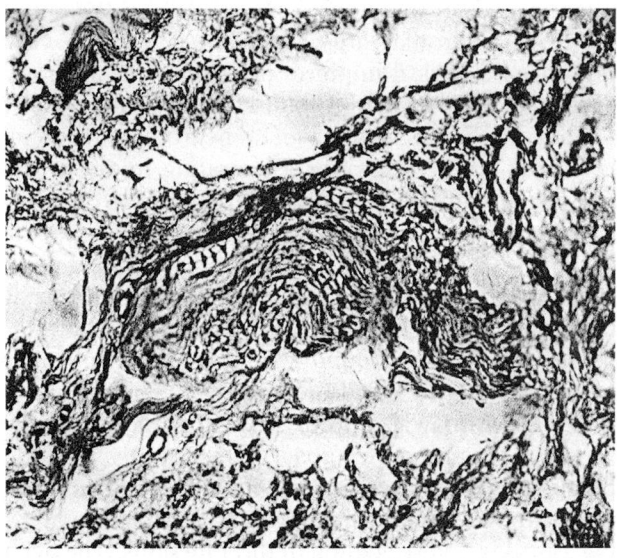

Figure 23 Amputation neuroma revealed by biopsy. Strikingly clear-cut, tangled, and well-myelinated fibers, cut at various angles, are massed with irregular sheath and perineural connective tissues into an abnormal aggregate of varying size and surrounded by well-vascularized fibrous tissue. Biopsy was occasioned by sharp, intermittent pricking "nerve pain," 6 months in duration, becoming more diffuse and steady. Courtesy, Dr. Gordon Agnew.

sprout axons, in an attempt to re-establish continuity with its distal segment. Usually, this process is unsuccessful, especially in soft tissue; therefore, a tangled mass of tissue results.[265,266] In the orofacial region, neuromas most commonly develop in the area of the mental foramen, followed by the lower lip, tongue, and buccal mucosa, all easily traumatized sites. Neuromas are least likely to occur in the inferior alveolar canal because the bone guides the tissue growth.

In a seminal research effort, Hansen[264] found neuromas forming quite routinely in the extraction sockets of the rat alveolus. Four months after extraction, he noted axon and myelin sheath degeneration at the bottom of the alveolus. At 10 months, the appearance was that of a small traumatic neuroma. If this same phenomenon occurs as frequently in humans as in experimental animals, it might well account for persistent postextraction pain, for which the patient is finally classified as neurotic and the pain as psychogenic. Of 45 oral traumatic neuromas reviewed for clinicopathological features, 15 were painful, and 53% of these demonstrated inflammatory infiltrate under light microscopy.[265] This was in contrast to only 17% of asymptomatic neuromas. Only 4 (9%) in this series were associated with extractions. Anoxia and local scar formation are thought to contribute to the production of pain.[267]

Symptoms. A neuroma may be completely asymptomatic, and, in fact, approximately 25% of them are. However, neuromas are capable of generating very prolonged electrical impulses in response to a variety of stimuli.[265] They may even discharge spontaneously.

The diagnostic features of a neuroma include a history of prior surgery or a lacerating injury at the site of the pain, along with precipitation of the pain with local pressure or traction. The pain is short-lasting, with a burning, tingling, radiating quality. A drop of local anesthetic will abolish the response. If the neuroma has developed on the inferior alveolar nerve, it may be visible radiographically as a widening of the mandibular canal.

Neuromas may also occur in the *TMJ postsurgically* or post-lacerating trauma.[101] Symptoms include restricted joint movement owing to adhesions and pain with neuropathic qualities (sharp, shooting, itching, burning) on stretching of the adhesions. The deep aching pain of musculoskeletal disorders is lacking.

Examination. In the oral cavity, neuromas may appear as nodules of normal surface color but usually are not visible or palpable. Of greater interest is the presence of a scar, indicating previous injury or surgery. In the TMJ, movement against adhesive restrictions, as with jaw opening, should elicit short-lasting neuropathic pain.

Treatment. A one-time excision of a sensitive neuroma located in the accessible scar tissue is worth trying provided that the pain is localized and can be relieved by infiltration with a local anesthetic.[69] Unfortunately, neuroma excision and other peripheral neuroablative procedures provide significant relief in very few patients.[268] *Neuromas often re-form*, and the pain may return. Medications such as carbamazepine (Tegretol) or amitriptyline (Elavil) may be helpful but should be used only if the patient feels that the pain is severe enough to warrant tolerating the side effects that may accompany these medications.

CONTINUOUS NEURALGIAS

Continuous neuralgias typically occur after some kind of peripheral nerve damage or "deafferentation." This category includes postherpetic, post-traumatic, and postsurgical neuralgias, as well as anesthesia dolorosa. As with paroxysmal neuralgias, the continuous neuralgias follow the distribution of the damaged nerve but differ in that the pain is more or less continuous, with some fluctuation over time. Patients report altered sensations, dysesthesias, or pain in the distribution of the nerve that varies from tingling, numbness, and twitching to prickling or burning. They may also report "formication," which is a sensation of worms under the skin or ants crawling over the skin. The dysesthesias are generally discomforting to the patient because they are continuous and exacerbated by movement or touching of the area. As with paroxysmal neuralgias, local anesthetic blocks of the nerve eliminate all paresthesias except numbness.

Postherpetic Neuralgia

Etiology. PHN follows an acute attack of *herpes zoster* ("shingles"). Herpes zoster is an acute viral infection produced by the deoxyribonucleic acid[269] virus varicella zoster. Varicella zoster causes chickenpox in the young and afterward remains in the ganglia of sensory nerve endings in a dormant "provirus" form. Periodically, the virus reverts to its infectious state and is held in check by circulating antibodies. If an individual is immunocompromised or is older and has a low antibody titer, the infectious virus is able to retrace its path down the sensory nerve and escape into the skin, where it causes the typical skin eruptions and vesicles of zoster. Acute hemorrhagic inflammation with demyelination and axonal degeneration of dorsal root ganglion cells has been demonstrated in early and more recent pathological studies.[270–274]

Acute herpes zoster affects individuals over 70 years of age 12 times more frequently than persons under 10 presumably because their antibody titer decreases as their exposure to children with chickenpox diminishes. One or two of every 100 elderly people suffer an attack of shingles in a single year. They may have repeated attacks, often in the same distribution; 3.4 per 1,000 individuals develop PHN annually.[275]

Symptoms. Continuous pain in the distribution of the affected nerve and malaise commonly precedes the eruption of *acute herpes zoster*, sometimes along with paresthesia and shooting pains. Vesicles form, become infected, scab over, and heal. Small and sometimes severe scars are left behind. The scars are usually anesthetic, the skin between being hyperesthetic.

Ten to 15% of patients with herpes zoster develop lesions in the head and neck region, and 80% of these are in the ophthalmic division of the trigeminal nerve[82,101] (Figure 24). C1–3 are also sometimes affected. When cranial nerve V1 is affected, vesicles may appear on the cornea, and the risk of impaired vision is high. If the infection affects the *maxillary division of the trigeminal nerve*, intraoral eruptions may develop concomitantly with those on the skin. Involvement of the oral mucosa without cutaneous involvement may occur and must be differentiated from aphthous stomatitis.[101] Multiple devitalized teeth, isolated in a single quadrant, have been reported as a rare complication of herpes zoster infection.[276] If the *facial nerve (cranial nerve VII)* is involved, facial palsy may occur owing to pressure on the nerve from inflammatory swelling in the bony canal. The pupil may become permanently paralyzed, and the upper eyelid may droop. Involvement of the geniculate ganglion causes lesions to erupt in the external auditory canal, may cause acoustic symptoms, and is known as Ramsey Hunt syndrome.[101]

PHN results when the pain of acute zoster does not subside as the acute eruption clears. The pain of PHN often has several distinct components.[15] Patients complain of a steady, deep, aching pain along with superimposed sharp, stabbing pains similar to trigeminal neuralgia. In addition, many complain of *allodynia*, pain in response to light brushing of the skin, an innocuous event under normal circumstances. The pain is limited to the distribution of the affected nerve, and there is usually cutaneous scarring and sensory loss also.[276,277] Complaints of *formication* are not infrequent. Since this pain is severe and unrelenting, it places a large emotional burden on the elderly patients who suffer from it. Interruption of sleep, drug reliance, depression, and even contemplation of suicide are common.

Examination. The history of acute zoster infection and the obvious scars it leaves behind make diagnosis relatively simple in most cases. PHN, on the other hand, may occur up to a month or two after the vesicular stage of herpes zoster has healed. If the patient knows he has had severe herpes zoster infection, the diagnosis may well be self-evident. The dentist, however, should carefully check the mouth to ascertain that a concomitant severe pulpitis is not superimposed on the condition.

Difficulty in diagnosis arises when the severe vesicular herpetic attack is not manifested but rather one or two small aphthous ulcers appear in the oral cavity or on the lips or face. This mild attack is often forgotten by the patient, and a careful history is essential.[278]

Treatment. In the future, new vaccines may reduce the overall incidence of chickenpox in the population or boost immunity to varicella-zoster virus in middle-

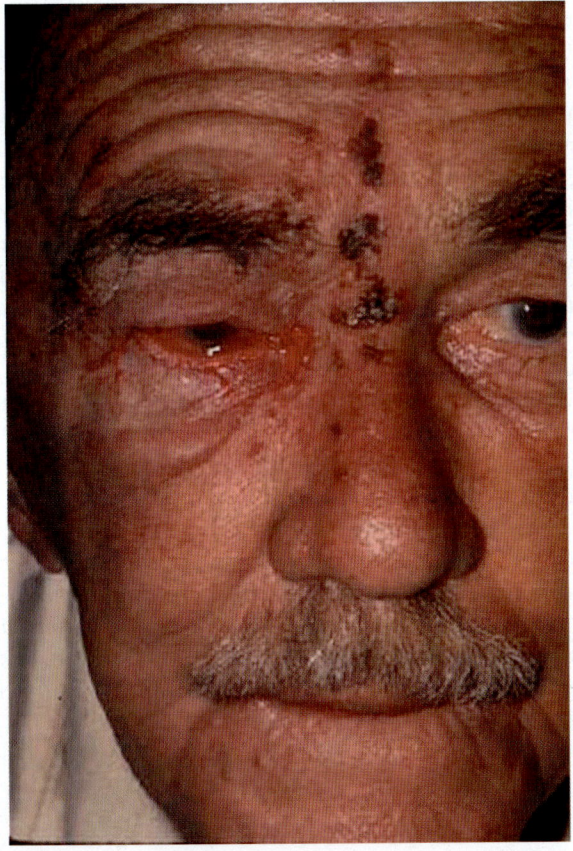

Figure 24 Herpes zoster infection of the first division of the trigeminal cranial nerve. Courtesy of Faculty of Medicine, University of Toronto, Canada.

aged persons, thus preventing the emergence of the virus from its latent phase.[279] Although age is the most important risk factor for the development of this painful chronic disorder, early treatment during the *acute phase of herpes zoster* with antiviral agents or certain tricyclics such as amitriptyline (antidepressants),[280] combined with psychosocial support, may be effective in preventing the development of PHN.[281] Although sympathetic nerve blocks do tend to reduce acute herpetic pain, they have not been proven to be effective in preventing PHN.[276,282,283] The treatment of PHN is often difficult and unrewarding. The longer the infection continues and the longer the patient has PHN, the more difficult pain management becomes. Tricyclic antidepressants, gabapentin, and opioids are the only medications that have shown efficacy in randomized clinical trials.[280] Topical agents also work[284] but are rarely effective alone.[280] *Amelioration of the depression* that invariably accompanies this condition is as significant in therapy as reduction of the primary pain.

Posttraumatic Neuralgias

Traumatic injury to the peripheral nerves often results in persistent discomfort that is qualitatively different from PHN.

Symptoms. The pain is described as a continuous tingling, numb, twitching, or prickly sensation but without the intense, burning hyperesthesia usually seen with PHN or painful neuromas. The onset is following damage to the nerve by trauma or surgery. The discomfort can be self-limited, but total nerve regeneration is a slow, inaccurate process and can result in permanent dysesthesias or the formation of a neuroma.

Etiology. Peripheral degeneration or scarring of the nerve may be found on histopathological examination. Substance P has been implicated as a mediator of the pain, and depletion of this neurotransmitter has been shown to reduce the pain.

Treatment. Treatment of traumatic trigeminal dysesthesias may be met with varying success and can include any of the pharmacological therapies used for the other neuralgias as well as acupuncture, transcutaneous electrical nerve stimulation, and hypnosis. Capsaicin, a substance P depleter with significant long-term effects, has been used topically in the treatment of posttraumatic neuralgia with some success.[285] All of the available therapies may be used individually or in combination with other interventions. In some cases of trigeminal neuropathy, in which peripheral nerve damage has resulted in continuous severe pain, electrical stimulation of the gasserian ganglion via an implanted electrode has been shown to provide good pain relief.[286]

Anesthesia Dolorosa

This literally means "painful anesthesia" or pain in a numb area.

Etiology. Anesthesia dolorosa is considered a complication of deafferentation procedures such as trigeminal rhizotomy or thermocoagulation used to treat trigeminal neuralgia. It may also follow trauma or damage to the trigeminal nuclear complex or after vascular lesions of the central trigeminal pathways.[82]

Symptoms. Patients complain of pain in an area that is otherwise numb or has decreased ability to detect tactile or thermal stimuli. Onset follows deafferentation of part or all of the trigeminal nerve, and the pain typically follows the distribution of the deafferented branches.

Examination. The painful area is numb or has diminished sensation to pinprick.

Treatment. Anesthesia dolorosa is a chronic intractable pain syndrome[101] that is very difficult to treat. Centrally acting medications such as tricyclics or anticonvulsants may provide some relief.

Case history. Our patient, described initially, has complaints that have characteristics of both the continuous and paroxysmal neuralgias. The constant burning pain could be a continuous neuralgia. Since there is no history of viral infection or herpes zoster outbreak, it is unlikely to be PHN. Since there is no history of deafferentation procedures, anesthesia dolorosa is also unlikely. However, multiple extractions and repeated dry sockets may have resulted in the development of deafferentation pain in V2 and V3. It does not explain the pain in V1, however.

What about the sharp, shooting, electric-like pains the patient complained about? These are reminiscent of trigeminal neuralgia. However, the temporal pattern is inconsistent. Trigeminal neuralgia attacks are over in seconds to minutes; this patient complains of pains lasting 30 minutes to 24 hours. Also, the patient is too young for an idiopathic trigeminal neuralgia, and CT scans have failed to show any structural lesion that could account for such a pain. Thus, at this point, there is one possible diagnosis on our differential list, namely, post-traumatic deafferentation pain.

Causalgic Pains

Causalgia is a word derived from the Greek words *kausos,* meaning "heat," and *algia,* meaning "pain." Causalgia was first described by Mitchell in 1864 as a pain that appears following damage to a major peripheral nerve by a high-velocity missile injury.[287] Consequently, it is typically seen in the extremities. In 1947, Evans[288] used the term RSD to describe the same burning pain. He noted that the pain had many features of sympathetic stimulation such as redness, swelling, sweating, and atrophic changes in the skin, muscles, and bones. He also found that minor injuries, such as fractures or sprains, could precipitate this pain, not just major nerve trauma. That same year, Bingham published the first report of RSD of the face.[289]

Today, RSD and in particular causalgia are considered the most dramatic forms of a class of pains called *sympathetically maintained pains* (SMPs), RSD occurring without and causalgia with a definable nerve lesion. Because the exact contribution of the sympathetic nervous system to RSD and causalgia is still under investigation, an effort was made in the mid-1990s to rename these types of pain disorders as "complex regional pain syndromes," *type I and type II*, respectively.[290,291] These terms eliminate the implied causal association of the sympathetic nervous system to these pain disorders. This terminology, along with clinical criteria, was included in the second edition of the IASP Classification of Chronic Pain Syndromes but has shown marginal reliability when tested clinically,[291,292] and the terms SMP, RSD, and causalgia continue to be used.

Symptoms. The characteristic pain is a constant, hot, burning sensation with painful cutaneous hypersensitivity (hyperalgesia) and muscle tenderness.[3] The pain is worse with light touch, heat, cold, or emotional stress.

Typically, *RSD* begins a few days to several weeks after an injury to or an inflammation of sensory afferent pathways.[293] In the head and neck region, RSD has been reported to develop after maxillofacial surgery for cancer, head injury, *molar extraction*, and sinus surgery.[294] If allowed to progress undiagnosed or untreated, RSD passes through an initial or "traumatic" stage characterized by a burning ache, edema, and hyperthermia to a second or "dystrophic" stage, with cool, cyanotic skin, spreading pain, and edema. The third or "atrophic" stage is evidenced by muscle atrophy; osteoporosis; smooth, glossy, mottled-appearing skin; and intractable pain. However, because of the abundant collateral blood circulation in the head and neck region, the bony, vascular, and trophic changes so typical in the extremities are less common in the face.[294]

Etiology. The exact pathophysiological mechanisms of RSD are unknown. What is known is that after experimental nerve injury, surviving primary afferent nociceptors develop noradrenergic receptors and become sensitive to noradrenalin,[279,294,295] as do primary afferents that are experimentally cut and surgically repaired.[296] Other experimental studies suggest that some regenerating primary afferents may anastomose with the regenerating postganglionic sympathetic axons that run with them.[297,298] Posttraumatic sympathetic-afferent coupling also appears to occur in the dorsal root ganglion where sympathetic fibers that innervate the vasculature subserving the dorsal root ganglion begin to sprout around the primary afferent fibers[299,300] (Figure 25).

Clinically, the sympathetic nervous system is implicated in these pains because sympathetic blockade provides profound relief, and electrical stimulation of

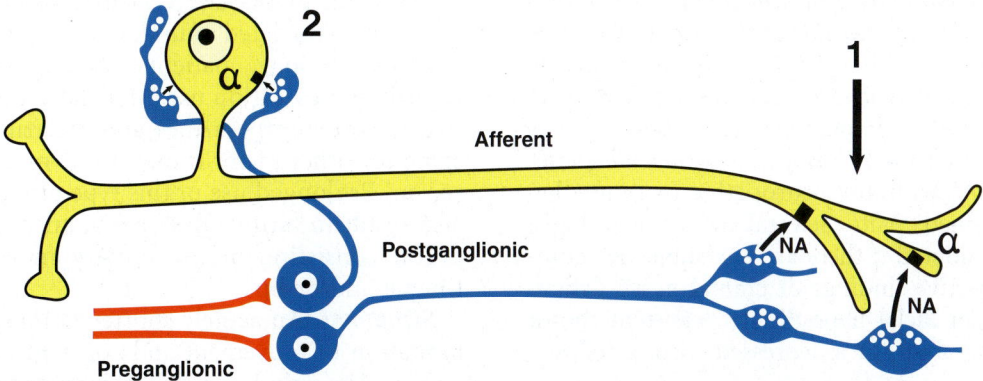

Figure 25 The influence of sympathetic activity and catecholamines on sensitized and damaged primary afferents. Normally, primary afferent neurons do not have catecholamine sensitivity, and their activity is unaffected by sympathetic outflow. After nerve lesion (1) or in the presence of inflammation, afferent terminals in the periphery or afferent somata in the dorsal root ganglion acquire sensitivity to noradrenaline (NA) by expressing a-receptors at their membrane. Activity in postganglionic sympathetic neurons is now capable of activating afferent neurons by the release of NA. In addition, sympathetic postganglionic neurons sprout around dorsal root ganglion cells (2). Reproduced with permission from Fields HL et al., *Neurobiol Dis*; 1998.

sympathetic outflow makes the pain worse.[301] Neither of these conditions exists in a normal individual. Changes in central pain pathways are also implicated in the RSD picture.[3]

Examination. The patient with causalgia/RSD complains of pain at the slightest touch and is difficult to examine. The skin may be flushed and dry or cold and sweaty, and a temperature difference may be discernible.

Diagnostic tests. Definitive diagnosis of the condition in the head and neck can be accomplished through immediate reduction of pain and hyperesthesia with a successful local anesthetic block of the stellate ganglion. This procedure requires a trained anesthesiologist since the stellate ganglion is located in close proximity to several vital structures, including the vertebral artery and the apex of the lung.

Treatment. Repeated sympathetic blocks are the treatment of choice for sympathetically maintained pains. Early intervention is best. For the upper extremities and the head and neck region, this involves repeated blocks of the stellate ganglion.[294] Oral medications such as calcium channel blockers or low-dose tricyclic antidepressants with or without an anticonvulsant or systemic local anesthetic may be a useful adjunct.[302] Biofeedback and relaxation techniques may help reduce generalized sympathetic activity. Transcutaneous electrical nerve stimulation or acupuncture in combination with physical therapy may be helpful in providing relief and increasing function. Surgical removal of the upper sympathetic chain is the last resort procedure when all else has failed. If an inadequate sympathectomy is performed, the pain may return.

Case history. Our patient complains of pain with many of the characteristics described for RSD and causalgic pain. The pain has a burning quality. The skin is hypersensitive. The affected side of the face is warmer to touch and slightly swollen. The pain is made worse with any type of stimulation. She has a history of tooth extraction with alveolar osteitis (dry socket). RSD of the face is definitely worth listing as a possible diagnosis.

When dealing with any neuropathic or sympathetically maintained pain, referral to a neurologist should be considered if there are any subjective complaints or objective findings of cranial nerve deficits such as areas of facial hypesthesia, persistent motor weakness or paralysis, or a depressed corneal reflex.

Muscular Pains

Pain of muscular origin is generally described as a continuous, deep, dull ache or as tightness or pressure.

Table 13 Muscular Pains

Myospasm pain
Myositis pain
Local myalgia—unclassified
Myofascial pain
    Tension-type headaches
    Coexisting migraine and tension-type headaches

Adapted from Okeson.[90]

It is undoubtedly the most prevalent cause of pain in the head and neck region.[91,92,303] According to Bell,[101] "a good rule to follow in diagnosing pains about the face and mouth is initially to assume that the pain is dental until proved otherwise, then muscular until proved otherwise." Myospasm, myositis, and myofascial TrP pain will be discussed as part of this group (Table 13). "Local myalgia—unclassified" includes muscle splinting, which is grouped with other muscle disorders such as delayed-onset muscle soreness or pain owing to ischemia, bruxism, or fatigue. This is because there are a few clinical characteristics that differentiate these muscle disorders from each other.[90]

Myospasm

Etiology. Myospasm, involuntary continuous contraction of a muscle or group of muscles, may occur owing to acute overuse, strain, or overstretching of muscle previously weakened through protective reflex contraction (see Figure 9). Commonly termed a "charley horse," muscle spasm may occur, for example, after sustained opening of the patient's mouth for dental treatment. Deep pain input from other sources such as joint inflammation, dental infection, or myofascial TrPs may also result in reflex spasm of associated muscles. In the absence of an obvious etiology, patients should be questioned regarding medication use. Medications such as Compazine (prochlorperazine) and Stelazine (trifluoperazine) or other major tranquilizers may cause muscle spasm. Prolonged use of this type of medication may also result in tardive dyskinesia, an irreversible condition consisting of involuntary movement of the tongue and/or lips.

Symptoms. An acutely shortened muscle with gross limitation of movement and constant pain is characteristic. The pain has a dull, aching quality with occasional sharp, lancinating pains in the ear, temple, or face. Depending on which muscles are involved, acute malocclusion may result. Patients may complain of increased pain on chewing or functioning of the spastic muscle. Headache may also result.

Examination. A normal jaw opening of 40 to 60 mm may be reduced to 10 to 20 mm with spasm. Malocclusion and abnormal jaw opening may be evident.

Diagnostic tests. Electromyography (EMG), surface, needle, or fine wire, will show substantially increased muscle activity even at rest.[90,304] Injection of suspected muscles with plain 0.5% or 1% procaine or lidocaine should provide relief and confirm the diagnosis.

Treatment. If left untreated, the pain will subside. However, as a result of decreased function, there is a risk of developing contracture. Many episodes of "lock jaw" and torticollis (wry neck) are attributable to contracture. Therefore, patients should continue to use the jaw within pain-free limits. Heat may provide symptomatic relief. As the pain decreases, gradual active stretching of the muscle over a period of 3 to 7 days, with simultaneous application of counterstimulation or injection of the muscle with a weak solution of plain procaine or lidocaine, may facilitate restoration of normal function.

Myositis

Myositis is *inflammation* of muscles that, in the head and neck region, most frequently involves the masseter and medial pterygoid muscles. According to Bell,[101] "*the familiar trismus associated with dental sepsis, injury, surgery, or needle abscess typifies this condition.*"

Etiology. Myositis is usually the result of external trauma (e.g., contact sports), excessive muscle overuse, or spreading infection (e.g., dental abscess).[101] In fact, many of the same things that cause myospasm may cause myositis if prolonged or severe enough. The associated mandibular dysfunction is related to pain and to the presence of inflammatory exudate in the muscles. Myositis may progress to fibrous scarring or contracture.[101]

Symptoms. Characteristically, the patient complains of continuous pain over the muscle aggravated by jaw opening, limited jaw opening, and swelling over the involved muscle. There is usually a history of trauma or infection. If the cause is attributable to infection, the patient may also complain of malaise and fever.

Examination. Myositis can be distinguished from myospasm owing to the presence of swelling. The muscle is diffusely tender. Mandibular range of motion is severely restricted. *Regional lymphadenitis* is present if there is infection.

Treatment. Treatment of both myositis and contracture is similar to that used for myospasm, except that NSAIDs are also recommended. Exercises, massage, and injections are contraindicated until acute symptoms have subsided.

Local Myalgia: Unclassified

Myospasm and myositis present with specific characteristics that allow a definite clinical distinction to be made. Other kinds of myalgias owing to ischemia, muscle overuse (fatigue and postexercise muscle soreness), or protective "splinting" or co-contraction also exist. However, currently, there is little scientific information to allow clear distinction between these disorders, and for this reason they are grouped together as unclassified myalgias.[90]

Myofascial Pain

MFP, a regional referred pain syndrome associated with focally tender Trigger Points (TrPs) in muscle, is a prevalent cause of pain in all parts of the body and has been reported as a common source of pain in numerous medical specialties.[91,93] For example, almost 30% of patients presenting themselves with a complaint of pain in an internal medicine practice[61] and over 80% of patients in a chronic pain center[93] had MFP as a primary diagnosis. It is also the most prevalent cause of painful symptoms in TMDs.[93,302]

In a study conducted at the University of Minnesota TMJ and Facial Pain Clinic, doctors evaluated 296 consecutive patients with chronic head and neck pain complaints.[165] MFP was the primary diagnosis in 55.4% of these patients. Nonpainful internal derangements of the TMJs were felt to be a perpetuating factor to the MFP in 30.4%. In contrast, only 21% of these patients had a true TMD disorder as the primary cause of pain. In this 21%, the joint disorder included inflammation of the TMJ joint capsule or the retrodiscal tissues.

Despite its prevalence and the recent surge in scientific documentation, *MFP* remains poorly understood and frequently unrecognized by most health care providers. Many physicians and dentists alike insist on calling it MFP and think of it as a myalgia of the facial muscles and masticatory muscles. Others feel that it is a syndrome that involves some internal derangement of the TMJ plus associated local muscle soreness.

Symptoms. In *MFP*, the presenting pain complaint is usually a *referred symptom* with a *deep, dull aching quality* located in or about normal muscular or, importantly, nonmuscular structures. In the head and neck region, the patient may complain of such things as toothache, sinus pain, TMJ pain, or headache, yet evaluation of these areas does not yield any pathological change. In fact, *any undiagnosed deep, dull, aching pain may be myofascial in origin.* The intensity of MFP should not be underestimated: the pain intensity has been documented to be equal or slightly greater than that of pain from other causes.[91]

Associated symptoms, thought to be owing to the physiological sensory, motor, and autonomic effects seen with prolonged pain, are common and may confuse the clinical picture.[305,306] These effects were discussed earlier in the section under "Neurophysiology of pain." Associated sensory complaints may include tenderness in the referred pain site, such as scalp pain on brushing the hair, or abnormal sensitivity of the teeth.[307] Motor effects include increased EMG activity in the pain reference zone[308,306,309] although patients rarely complain about this specifically. Autonomic changes such as localized vasoconstriction (pallor),[308] sweating, lacrimation, coryza, increased salivation, and nausea and vomiting have also been reported.[83]

Patients note worsening of symptoms with increased psychological stress, cold weather, immobility, and overuse of involved muscles. Hot baths, rest, warm weather, and massage are typical alleviating factors.

Etiology. Myofascial TrPs can be primary or secondary. When primary, injury to the muscle owing to *macrotrauma* or *cumulative microtrauma* is typically involved. Macrotrauma is easily identified and includes injuries such as those caused by falls, blows, sports injuries, motor vehicle accidents, or even *prolonged jaw opening* at the dental office. Microtrauma is more insidious and includes muscle overuse owing to poor posture and body mechanics, abnormal strain, and repetitive motion-type injuries.

Secondary myofascial TrPs develop in response to prolonged underlying disease, especially if painful, for which any process that activates nociceptors may induce secondary muscle contraction and TrP development (described under section "Physiological mechanisms modifying pain" at the beginning of this chapter). Secondary MFP may prolong and complicate pain owing to other causes.[305] Examples include migraine, inflammatory disorders of the TMJ, chronic ear infections, persistent pulpalgia, PHN, cancer, or any other chronic painful condition[305] including *bursitis of the tensor villi palatini muscle* as it passes over the hamulus.[310] MFP needs to be identified and treated to reduce pain and improve response to other therapies. Patients with what appears to be primary MFP, in whom TrPs and pain recur despite appropriate initial response to TrP therapies and compliance to home exercise, must be reevaluated for occult underlying disease or other perpetuating factors.

In MFP, the presenting pain complaint is always associated with a TrP located in a taut band of skeletal muscle that is often distant from the site of pain. TrPs are focally tender, firm, nodular areas in muscle that, with the application of 2 to 4 kg of pressure for 6 to 10 seconds, produce spontaneous referred pain or intensify existing pain in local or distant locations.[311] Patients are typically unaware of the existence of these TrPs. TrPs are considered active when the referred pain pattern and associated symptoms are clinically present and latent when they are not. TrPs will vacillate between active and latent states depending on the amount of psychological stress the individual is under and the amount of muscle overload placed on the affected muscle.

The location of TrPs and their associated referred pain patterns are predictable and reproducible from patient to patient[83,312,313] (Figures 26–29). A meticulous discussion

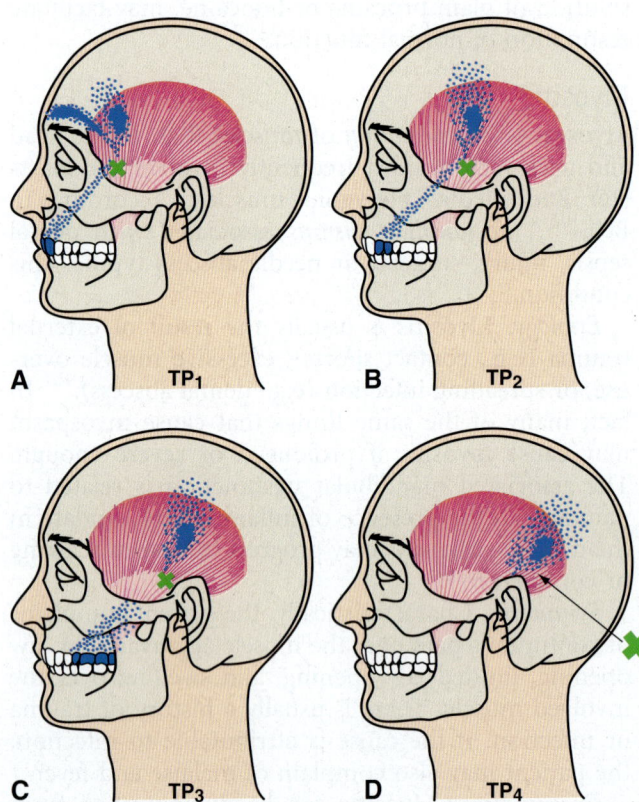

Figure 26 Referred pain patterns from trigger points (TrPs) (crosses) in the temporalis muscle (essential zone, blue, spillover zone, green). *A,* Anterior "spokes" of pain arising from anterior fibers (trigger point, TP1). Note reference to anterior teeth. *B* and *C,* Middle "spokes" of TP2 and TP3 referring to maxillary posterior teeth, sinus, and zygomatic area. *D,* Posterior, TP4, supra-auricular "spoke" referral. Reproduced with permission from Travell JG & Simons DG, Vol I, 2nd Edn; 1999.

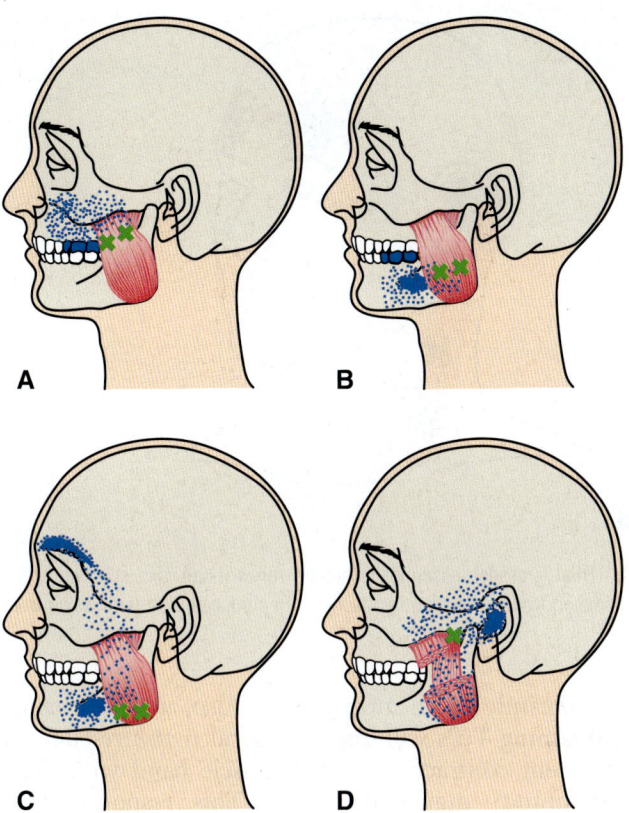

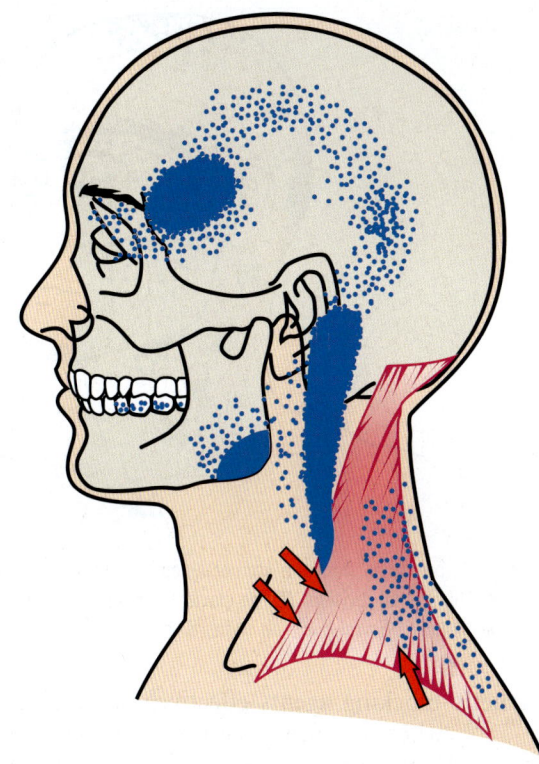

Figure 27 Central and referred pain from the masseter muscle. The green crosses locate trigger points (TrPs) in various parts of the masseter; the blue areas show essential referred pain zones and stippled areas are spillover pain zones. **A,** Superficial layer, upper portion. Note reference to maxillary posterior teeth. **B,** Superficial layer, midbelly. Note spillover reference to the mandible and posterior teeth. **C,** Superficial layer; lower portion refers to the mandible and frontal "headache." **D,** Deep layer; upper part refers to the temporomandibular joint area and ear. Reproduced with permission from Travell JG & Simons DG, Vol I, 2nd ed. Wms & Wilkins; 1999.

Figure 28 Composite pain reference patterns of the trapezius muscle, suprascapular region. Trigger points (TrPs) are indicated by arrows, essential pain reference zones by blue on posterior teeth. Spillover pain zones are stippled. Note temporal "tension headache" and reference to the angle of the mandible with spillover to posterior teeth. Reproduced with permission from Travell JG, J. Prosthet Dent; 1960.

of MFP, as well as a complete compendium of the pain referral patterns for most muscles of the body, has been brilliantly detailed by Travell and Simons.[83,313]

Pathophysiology. With some training, myofascial TrPs are relatively easy to palpate. Despite the comparative ease of clinical identification of TrPs, controversy still exists about their structure and exact pathophysiology, but progress has been made. Muscle biopsy studies using light and electron microscopy, as well as histochemical analyses, have not shown consistent abnormalities, and there is no evidence for inflammation.[314,315] However, careful monopolar needle EMG evaluation revealed *spontaneous electrical activity* or "SEA" at the TrP sites, while evaluation of the muscle surrounding the TrP was normal.[316] This objective laboratory finding opened the door for establishing MFP as a clinical entity with an electromyographical marker. The SEA is significantly higher in subjects with clinical pain due to active TrPs than in subjects without clinical pain who have latent or no TrPs.[316,317] SEA can be recorded only if the needle is precisely placed in the nidus of the TrP; movement of the needle tip as little as 1 mm is enough to lose the signal.[316]

In addition, Shah et al.,[95] using a unique in vivo microanalytical technique, have demonstrated that concentrations of protons, bradykinin, CGRP, substance P, tumor necrosis factor-α, interleukin-1β, serotonin, and norepinephrine are significantly higher in active TrP sites than in latent TrP sites or in normal muscle. In addition, pH was significantly lower in the active TrP sites than in the other two groups.

Psychological stress, that causes increased sympathetic output, has been shown to increase the SEA recorded from TrPs, whereas the EMG activity of adjacent non-TrP sites remains unchanged.[318] These data parallel the clinical observation that emotional stress activates or aggravates pain from TrPs. Similarly, intramuscular or intravenous administration of

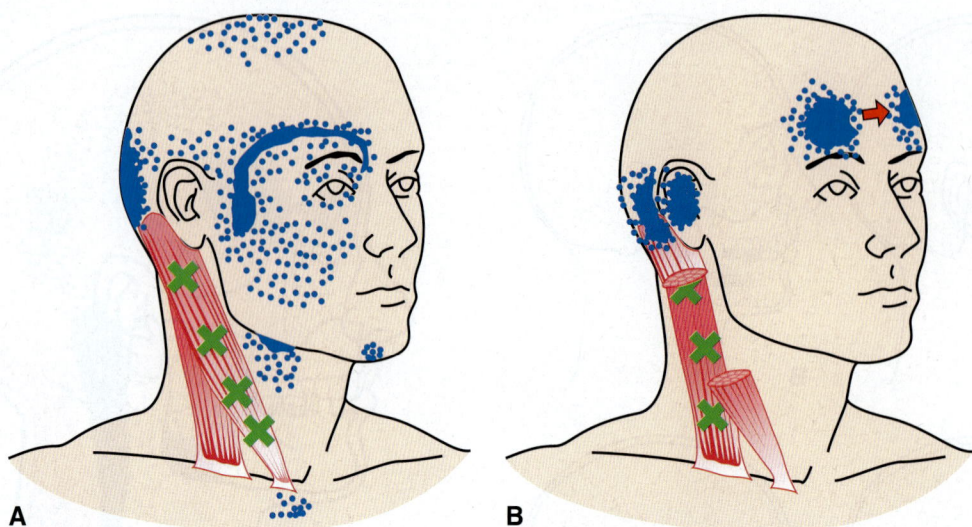

Figure 29 Pain reference from the sternocleidomastoid muscle. Trigger points (TrPs) (crosses), essential reference zones (blue), and spillover areas (stippled). ***A,*** The sternal division. ***B,*** The clavicular (deep) division refers most common frontal "tension headaches." Reproduced with permission from Travell JG & Simons DG, Vol I, 2nd ed. Wms & Wilkins; 1999.

sympathetic blocking agents effectively abolishes the SEA,[319–321] whereas curare and botulinum toxin, postsynaptic and presynaptic cholinergic blockers, respectively, have no effect on SEA in randomized, controlled studies.[316,319]

Based on the psychophysical evidence available to date and the observation that myofascial TrPs are frequently located in and around the motor end-plate area of muscles,[323,324] Simons and Reeves et al.[325] hypothesized that the myofascial TrP represents an area of isolated sustained muscle contraction due to excess acetylcholine release. This would result in uncontrolled metabolism, and localized ischemia that is initiated by acute muscle injury or strain.[309,325] This theory does provide a credible explanation for the palpable nodules and taut muscle bands associated with TrPs. The TrP nodule is described as a group of "contraction knots" in which a number of individual muscle fibers are maximally contracted at the end-plate zone, making them shorter and wider at that point than the noncontracted neighboring fibers. If enough fibers are so activated, a *palpable nodule* could result. As for the taut band, both ends of these affected muscle fibers would be maximally stretched out and "taut," producing the palpable taut band (Figure 30).

Clinically, data exist documenting that TrPs are truly focally tender areas in muscles; pain with palpation is not owing to generalized muscle tenderness.[325,326] Indeed, tenderness to palpation over non-TrP sites in subjects with MFP does not differ significantly from normals.[325] Also, muscle bands containing TrPs will display a local *twitch response*, a transient contraction of the muscle band with deep "snapping" digital palpation. This response, best appreciated in more superficial muscle fibers, has also been substantiated experimentally.[327] A rabbit model of the twitch response has documented that, at least in rabbits, the twitch response is a spinally mediated reflex.[328,329]

The mechanism of referred pain from myofascial TrPs is also under speculation. According to Mense[50] and Vecchiet et al.,[330] the convergence-projection and convergence-facilitation models of referred pain (described earlier under section "Referred pain") do not directly apply to muscle pain because there is little convergence of neurons from deep tissues in the dorsal horn.[50] These authors propose that convergent connections from other spinal cord segments are "unmasked" or opened by nociceptive input from skeletal muscle and that referral to other myotomes is owing to the release and spread of substance P to adjacent spinal segments[50,331] (see Figure 6). Simons[52] has expanded on this theory to specifically explain the referred pain from TrPs (see Figure 7).

The following is an excellent example of myofascial TrP pain developing in response to an acutely inflamed TMJ.

Case history. A 47-year-old man with a long-standing history of painless osteoarthrosis of both TMJs presented himself with an acute left TMJ inflammation.

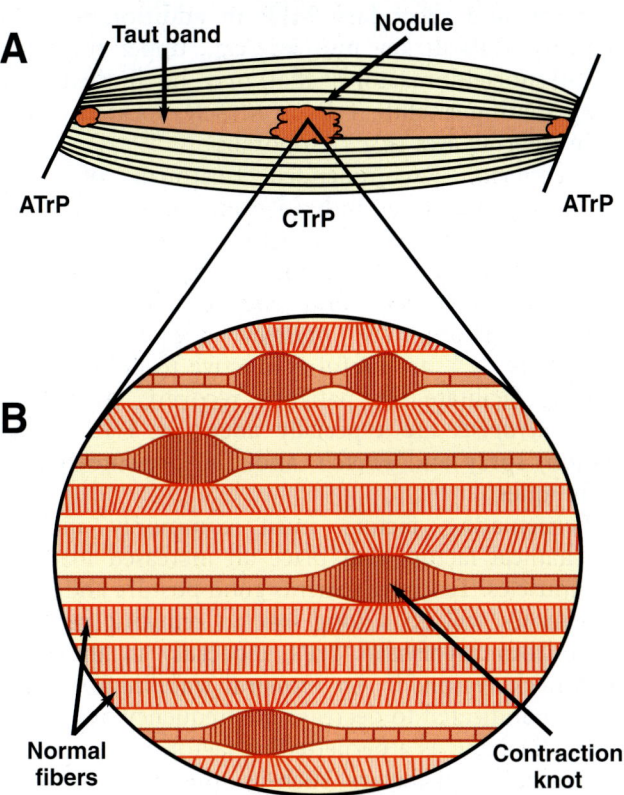

Figure 30 Schematic of a trigger point (TrP) complex of a muscle in the longitudinal section. **A,** The central TrP, which is drawn in the muscle end-plate zone, contains numerous "contraction knots," maximally contracted individual muscle fibers that are shorter and wider at the end plate than the noncontracted neighboring fibers. **B,** is an enlarged view of part of the central TrP showing the distribution of five contraction knots. The vertical lines in each muscle fiber identify the relative spacing of its striations. The space between two striations corresponds to the length of one sarcomere. Each contraction knot identifies a segment of the muscle fiber experiencing maximal contracture of its sarcomeres. The sarcomeres within these contraction knots are markedly shorter and wider than the sarcomeres of the neighboring normal muscle fibers. In fibers with these contraction knots (note the lower three individual knots), the sarcomeres on the part of the muscle fiber that extends beyond both ends of the contraction knot are elongated and narrow compared with normal sarcomeres. At the top of this enlarged view is a pair of contraction knots separated by an interval of empty sarcolemma between them that is devoid of contractile elements. This configuration suggests that the sustained maximal tension of the contractile elements in an individual contraction knot could have caused mechanical failure of the contractile elements in the middle of the knot. If that happened, the two halves would retract, leaving an interval of empty sarcolemma between them. In patients, the central TrP would feel nodular as compared to the adjacent muscle tissue because it contains numerous "swollen" contraction knots that take up additional space and are much more firm and tense than uninvolved muscle fibers. If enough fibers are so activated, a palpable nodule could result. As for the taut band, both ends of these affected muscle fibers would be maximally stretched out and "taut," producing the palpable taut band. Reproduced with permission from Travell JG & Simons DG, Vol I, 2nd edn. Wms & Wilkins; 1999.

This was conservatively treated with rest, soft diet, and anti-inflammatory medications. Severe symptoms subsided, but the patient continued to complain of persistent "aching of the left jaw." Clenching the teeth together produced a high-pitched ringing in his left ear. Careful history revealed that the pain was no longer specifically over the joint but was actually inferior and anterior to the left TMJ over the masseter muscle. Active range of motion of the mandible had increased from 41 to 47 mm, and the joint was nontender to palpation. Despite the negative joint examination, the less astute clinician may still direct his or her energies toward treating the TMJs, especially since there is documented osteoarthrosis bilaterally, worse on the left. However, the source of pain is now from myofascial TrPs and not the joint. Palpation of the masseter muscle, particularly the deep fibers, reproduced the patient's current symptoms, including the ringing in his left ear (Figure 31). TrPs in this part of the masseter muscle have also been reported to cause unilateral tinnitus[52] and accounted for the high-pitched sound that the patient complained of with clenching. Treatment must be directed at rehabilitating the masseter muscle and not at the asymptomatic joint.

Examination. Because the patient's pain complaint is typically a referred symptom, it is usually distant from the muscle containing the guilty TrP,[83,331] although some TrPs also cause more localized pain symptoms. Multiple TrPs can produce overlapping

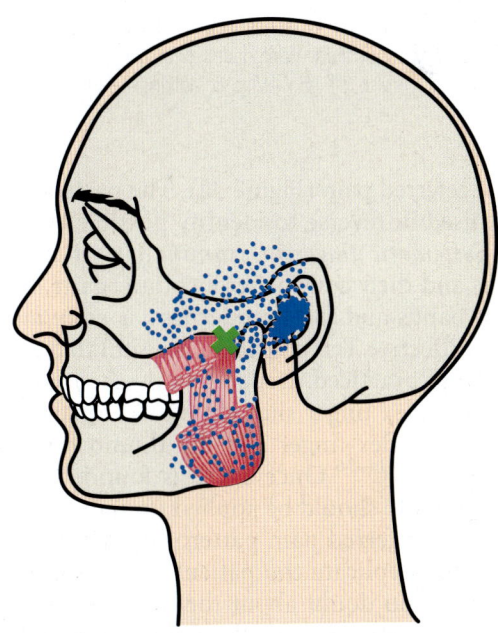

Figure 31 Deep layer, upper part of the masseter muscle refers pain to the temporomandibular joint (TMJ) area and the ear. Reproduced with permission from Travell JG & Simons DG, Vol I, 2nd edn. Wms & Wilkins; 1999.

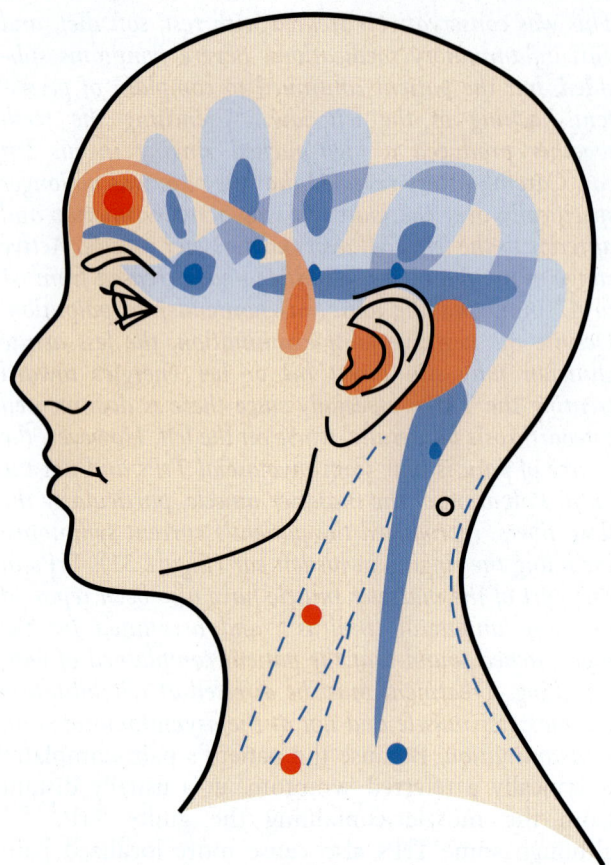

Figure 32 Overlapping pain referral patterns from the temporalis, sternocleidomastoid, upper trapezius, and suboccipital muscles produce a clinical picture of "tension-type headache." Unilateral symptoms may mimic migraine without aura. Reproduced with permission from Travell JG & Simons DG, Vol I, 2nd edn. Wms & Wilkins; 1999.

areas of referred pain (Figure 32). The pattern of pain can be used in reverse to identify possible etiological TrPs. *Systematic fingertip examination* of suspected muscles and their contralateral counterparts, looking for taut bands and focal tenderness, is *essential* (Figure 33). Effective TrP palpation is a skill that must be learned and practiced. Depending on the muscle, the tip of the index finger should be used for flat palpation or the index finger and the thumb for pincer-type palpation.[11–36] Once a TrP is found, 2 to 4 kg/cm^2 of pressure should be applied for 6 to 10 seconds to elicit the referred pain pattern, if any. The examination may replicate the patient's pain so precisely that there is no doubt about the diagnosis. If uncertainty exists, specific TrP therapies, such as "spray and stretch" or TrP injections, described below, may be used diagnostically. *All head and neck muscles should be routinely examined* in patients with a persistent pain complaint. This will help identify both primary and secondary MFP in addition to help identify TrPs in key muscles (e.g., upper trapezius or sternocleidomastoid) that may be inducing or perpetuating satellite TrPs in muscles located in the pain referral sites (e.g., temporalis).[83,306]

Treatment. Recommended treatment of MFP involves most importantly identification and control of causal and perpetuating factors, patient education, and specific home stretching exercises. Therapeutic techniques such as "spray and stretch," voluntary contract release, TrP pressure release, and TrP injections[332,333] are useful adjunctive techniques that usually facilitate the patient's recovery. *Myofascial TrP therapists* are especially adept at TrP examination, spray and stretch, and TrP pressure release techniques.

Perpetuating factors most commonly include mechanical factors that place an increased load on the muscles. Teaching patients good posture and body mechanics will go a long way in reducing referred pain from myofascial TrPs, especially in the head and neck region.[334] An *intraoral stabilization splint* may be indicated to decrease the frequency of clenching or bruxing as a perpetuating factor.

Psychological factors, such as *stress* that has been shown to cause TrP, activation, or *depression* that lowers pain thresholds, will contribute to MFP. Sleep disturbance and inactivity are also common perpetuating factors. Simple stress management and relaxation skills are invaluable in controlling involuntary muscle tension if this is a problem. Mild depression and sleep disturbance can be treated with low doses of *tricyclic antidepressant drugs* and a structured exercise/activation program.

Other perpetuating factors include metabolic, endocrine, or nutritional inadequacies that affect muscle metabolism.[83] Patients should be screened for general good health and referred to their physician for management of any systemic abnormalities. In secondary MFP, the primary concomitant painful disorder, such as TMJ capsulitis, pulpitis, or PHN, must also be treated or managed.

Spray and stretch is a highly successful technique for the treatment of myofascial TrPs that uses a vapocoolant spray (Gebbauer, Co., Cleveland, OH) to facilitate muscle stretching. Muscle stretching has been shown to reduce the intensity of referred pain and TrP sensitivity in patients with MFP.[335] The vapocoolant is applied slowly in a systematic pattern over the muscle being stretched and into the pain reference

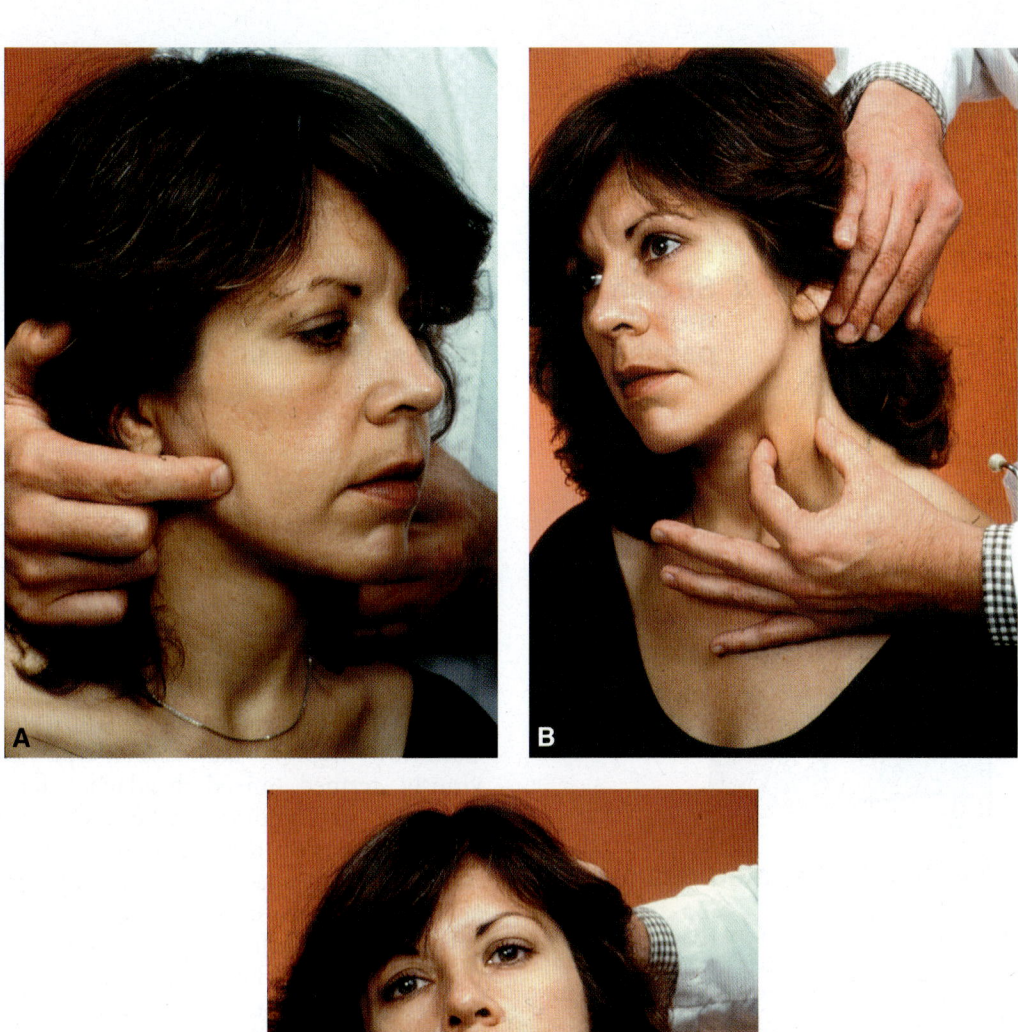

Figure 33 Muscle palpation for myofascial trigger points (TrPs). ***A,*** "Flat" fingertip palpation of the masseter muscle looking for taut bands and focal tenderness characteristic of myofascial TrPs. The flat palpation technique is also useful for temporalis, suboccipital, medial pterygoid, and upper back muscles. ***B,*** "Pincer" palpation of the deep clavicular head of the sternocleidomastoid muscle. ***C,*** "Pincer" palpation of the superficial sternal head. Heads should be palpated separately. The upper border of the trapezius also lends itself to pincer palpation. Reproduced with permission from and courtesy of Dr. Bernadette Jaeger.

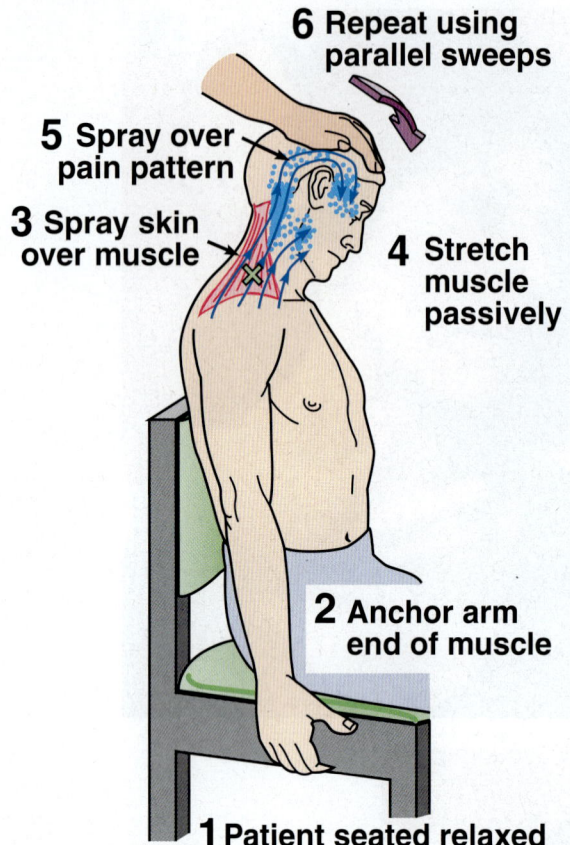

Figure 34 Sequence of steps when stretching and spraying any muscle for myofascial trigger points (TrPs), here applied to the upper trapezius. **1**, Patient supported in a comfortable relaxed position. **2**, One end of the muscle is anchored. **3**, Skin sprayed with three to four parallel sweeps of vapocoolant over the length of the muscle in the direction of the pain pattern (arrows). **4**, Immediately after the first sweep of spray, pressure is applied to stretch the muscle and continues as the spray is applied. **5**, Sweeps of spray cover the referred pain pattern of the muscle. **6**, Steps 3, 4, and 5 repeated only two or three times or less. Hot packs and several cycles of full active range of motion follow. Reproduced with permission from Travell JG & Simons DG, Vol I, 2nd edn. Wms & Wilkins; 1999.

zone (Figure 34). This technique and alternatives not using a vapocoolant are described in detail in the Travell & Simons text.[83]

Needling of TrPs with or without injection of solution has also been shown to be helpful in reducing the TrP activity to allow stretching.[333,335–339] Dry needling or injection of "key" myofascial TrPs has been shown to reduce the activity and tenderness in related satellite TrPs.[340] Although dry needling is effective, the use of a local anesthetic reduces postinjection soreness.[335] If a local anesthetic is to be injected, 0.5% procaine or 0.5% lidocaine is recommended. Longer-acting amide local anesthetics or local anesthetics containing epinephrine cause permanent muscle damage.[341] Injection must always be followed by stretch.[83] Trigger point injection in the absence of a home program that addresses relevant perpetuating factors will provide only temporary relief. Randomized controlled studies looking at the efficacy of botulinum toxin in comparison to dry needling, saline or other placebo solutions in trigger point injections have shown that overall Botox is no more effective than dry needling or other solutions.[342,343]

Tension-type headaches. *Tension-type headaches are usually bilateral, with a pressing, nonpulsating quality. They last 20 minutes to 7 days when episodic and may be daily without remission when chronic.*[82] Overlapping referred pain patterns from myofascial TrPs can produce a typical tension-type headache (see Figure 31). Studies have documented the presence of focally tender points and referred pain in this type of headache.[184,344] Thus, the same treatment strategies used for MFP also work well for the reduction of tension-type headache.[332,344]

Coexisting migraine and tension-type headache. *Coexisting migraine and tension-type headache* (previously termed mixed headache, tension-vascular headache, or combination headache and now often described under the term transformed migraine, chronic daily headache, or new daily persistent headache) combine features of both tension-type and neurovascular headaches. These patients have varying degrees of each of these two headache types. Typically, they complain of dull, aching, pressing head pain that progresses into a throbbing headache. This type of headache has an even higher incidence of pericranial muscle tenderness and referred pain than tension-type headache.[184] Treatment requires management of the MFP as well as judicious use of abortive or prophylactic migraine medications.

Although our patient did not complain specifically of deep, aching pains, secondary MFP does occur with most types of chronic pain input into the CNS system. Therefore, it is likely that secondary myofascial TrPs have developed. In fact, when the patient was initially examined, TrPs were found in the upper trapezius muscle that referred pain to the side of the temple and the face (see Figure 26). Even if this is not the primary cause of the pain, it is likely to be a contributing factor.

Unclassifiable Pains/Atypical Facial Pains

Mock et al.[345] have stated, "The diagnoses of atypical facial pain and atypical facial neuralgia are often applied interchangeably to the patient with poorly localized, vaguely described facial pain, nonanatomic in distribution with no evidence of a defined organic cause." Technically, these are not "atypical" pains but idiopathic pains, pains for which we do not yet have a diagnosis or sufficient understanding. Yet if we look at the retrospective analysis of data collected on 493 consecutive patients who presented to a university orofacial pain clinic, a different picture emerges.[346] A diagnosis of atypical facial pain was made if patients had persistent orofacial pain for more than 6 months for which previous treatments had been unsuccessful and the diagnosis was unknown on referral to the clinic. Of the 493 patient charts reviewed, 35 (7%) met these criteria. Using the American Academy of Orofacial Pain diagnostic criteria,[90] all but 1 (97%) had diagnosable physical problems and sometimes multiple overlapping physical diagnoses causing the pain. Over half (19 of 35 or 54%) were found to have MFP owing to TrPs as a primary cause or a significant contributing factor to the pain. Eleven (31%) had periodontal ligament sensitivity, eight had referred pain from dental pulpitis, three had neuropathic pain, and one each had burning mouth from oral candidiasis, sinus pathology, burning tongue from an oral habit, pericoronitis, or an incomplete tooth fracture.

There is currently significant controversy in the field about the diagnosis and classification of atypical facial pain. Myofascial TrP pain is clearly under-recognized[296,296] and trigeminal neuropathies or "dysesthesias," which many believe to be at fault for various "atypical" facial pains, are still inadequately understood.[347] Although proposals for nomenclature and classification changes abound,[347–349] this "atypical" nomenclature is likely to haunt the dental/orofacial pain profession for several years to come.

Two types of atypical pain that commonly appear in the dental office are *atypical odontalgia* (idiopathic toothache, phantom odontalgia,[349] or trigeminal dysesthesia) and *burning mouth syndrome* (BMS) (Table 14). Although deafferentation (neuropathic pain) is believed to play a role in both of these pain syndromes, the mechanism and the etiology are still largely speculative. Therefore, it is as yet difficult to reliably classify them under any of the diagnostic categories already discussed.

Table 14 Unclassifiable Pains
Atypical odontalgia
Burning mouth syndrome

Atypical Odontalgia

In 1979, Rees and Harris[350] described a disorder they called atypical odontalgia. Synonymous or almost synonymous terms include phantom tooth pain,[349] idiopathic orofacial pain,[351] vascular toothache,[101] and, more recently, trigeminal dysesthesia. Patients present with chronic toothache or tooth site pain with no obvious cause.[352,353] It is extremely important for dentists to be aware of the existence of this syndrome to avoid performing unnecessary dental procedures and extractions. It has been postulated that as many as 3% to 6% of endodontic patients may suffer from this type of tooth pain, especially if they had pain prior to pulp extirpation.[349]

Symptoms. The chief complaint is a deep, dull, aching pain in a tooth or tooth site that is unchanging over weeks or months. The pain is fairly constant, with some diurnal fluctuation, and usually worsens as the day progresses. The molars are most commonly involved, followed by premolars. Anterior teeth and canines are less frequently affected.[354] The vast majority of patients present themselves with unilateral pain, although other quadrants may become involved and other oral and facial sites may hurt.

Most patients are *female* and *over 40 years* of age. Table 15 lists the clinical characteristics of patients with atypical odontalgia as reported by several different authors. The onset of the pain may coincide with or develop within a month or so after dental treatment (especially endodontic therapy or extraction) or trauma or medical procedures related to the face.[349] Patients may have a history of repeated dental therapies that have failed to resolve the problem. Chewing or clenching on painful teeth, heat, cold, and stress are typical but inconsistent aggravating factors.

Etiology. The true etiology of atypical odontalgia remains elusive. Bell[101] classified it as a vascular disorder, as did Rees and Harris, who postulated a "painful migraine-like disturbance" in the teeth and periodontal tissues, possibly triggered by depression.[350] There are no data to support this idea, although a study using subcutaneous sumatriptan in 19 atypical facial pain patients did show some small temporary positive effects,

Table 15 Clinical Characteristics of Patients with Atypical Odontalgia*
N = 30
Age 58.4 years
Duration 4.4 years
90% female

*Seen at the University of Florida College of Dentistry.[356]

possibly supporting a vascular contribution to the pain.[355,356] Others have suggested depression or some other psychological disorder as the cause[357,357] since many patients with atypical odontalgia report depressive symptoms on clinical interview.[349,359,360] However, these results must be questioned owing to poor, uncontrolled study methodology and because there is a generally higher incidence of depression in patients with chronic pain. Of interest is the fact that standard *MMPI scores* for patients with *atypical odontalgia* compared with standard scores for a chronic headache group (matched for age, sex, and chronicity) were similar, and scales for both groups were within normal ranges,[354,361] making a psychological cause unlikely.

A more probable cause of atypical odontalgia is *deafferentation* (partial or total *loss of the afferent nerve supply* or sensory input) with or without sympathetic involvement. Atypical odontalgia usually follows a dental procedure, and most dental procedures, including cavity preparation, cause varying degrees of deafferentation. Studies supporting this theory are also lacking, yet the symptoms and clinical presentations are consistent with *posttraumatic neuropathic pain*. Many cases respond to sympathetic blocks[354] or phentolamine infusion,[362] implying that at least some may be sympathetically mediated or maintained. This theory would also explain why the pain remains even after the painful tooth is extracted. In addition, the preponderance of females suffering from this disorder raises the question of the role of estrogen and other female hormones as a risk factor in atypical odontalgia and related idiopathic orofacial pains.[363]

Examination. Intraoral and radiographic examinations are typically unrevealing. If the pain is in a tooth as opposed to an extraction site, responses to percussion, thermal testing, and electric pulp stimulation are variable. Clinically, there is no observable cause, yet thermographic evaluation is always abnormal.[364] The majority of patients report little or no relief with diagnostic local anesthetic blocks,[354,365] although sympathetic blocks seem to be helpful.[354]

Treatment. Invasive, irreversible treatments, such as endodontic therapy, exploratory surgery, extraction, or even occlusal adjustments, are contraindicated.[349,365] This is because, despite possible transient relief, the pain is likely to recur with equal or greater intensity.

The current treatment of choice is the use of *tricyclic antidepressant agents* such as *amitriptyline* or *imipramine*.[349,353,354] Pregabalin has also shown some promise.[365] If the pain has a *burning quality*, the addition of a *phenothiazine*, such as *trifluoperazine*, may be helpful.[349,365] Tricyclic antidepressants have analgesic properties independent of their antidepressant effects and often provide good pain relief at a fraction of the dose typically used to treat depression.[360,367,368] Pain relief normally occurs at doses from 50 to 100 mg. Dry mouth is an expected and usually unavoidable side effect. A history of significant cardiac arrhythmias or recent myocardial infarction, urinary retention, and glaucoma are contraindications for the use of tricyclic medications because of their atropine-like action. Patients may need reassurance that the pain is *real and not psychogenic* but that invasive procedures will not help.

If a patient complains of associated gingival hyperesthesia, the use of topical agents such as local anesthetic or capsaicin has been shown to be beneficial.[362] Unwanted stimulation of the area can be reduced by construction of an acrylic stent that can also be used to help apply any topical medication.

Burning Mouth Syndrome

BMS is an intraoral pain disorder that most commonly affects postmenopausal women. The National Institutes of Dental and Craniofacial Research report on the national Centers for Disease Control household health survey stated that 1,270,000 Americans (0.7% of the US population) suffered from this disorder.[124] When it primarily affects the tongue, it is referred to as burning tongue or glossodynia. Grushka and her colleagues[369–372] have conducted several studies to systematically characterize the features of this syndrome.

Symptoms. Patients complain of intraoral burning, the tip and sides of the tongue being the most common sites, followed by the palate. Dry mouth, thirst, taste and sleep disturbances, headaches, and other pain complaints are frequently associated symptoms. Onset is often related to a dental procedure. The intensity of pain is quantitatively similar to that of toothache, although the quality is burning rather than pulsing, aching, or throbbing. The pain increases as the day progresses and tends to peak in the early evening. Patients with BMS may complain of spontaneous tastes or "taste phantoms" (dysgeusia).[373]

Etiology. There are many obvious oral and systemic conditions that are associated with mucogingival and glossal pains. These include candidiasis, geographic tongue, allergies to dental materials, denture dysfunction, xerostomia, various anemias and vitamin deficiencies (iron, vitamin B_{12}, or folic acid), diabetes mellitus, several dermatological disorders (lupus, lichen planus, erythema multiforme), human immunodeficiency virus, or systemic medications (either directly or indirectly through resultant xerostomia).[124,374,375] However, in BMS, controlled studies have documented that the oral mucosa appears normal, and no obvious organic cause can be identified.[372,375] There is evidence for a higher incidence of immunological abnormalities in BMS patients than would be expected in a normal population, and several BMS patients have been shown to have Sjögren's syndrome.[369]

Recent research supports a theory that damage to or dysfunction of the chorda tympani branch of CN VII contributes to the dysguesia and pain of burning mouth.[376] The special sense of taste from the tongue is mediated by the chorda tympani (anterior two-thirds) and CN IX (posterior one-third). The chorda tympani innervates the fungiform papillae of the tongue, which, in turn, are surrounded by pain fibers from cranial nerve V. The chorda tympani normally inhibits both cranial nerve V (pain fibers) and cranial nerve IX (taste). Damage or partial deafferentation of the chorda tympani appears to release inhibition of both cranial nerves V and IX, producing both pain and taste phantoms, respectively.[374,377]

BMS is not to be confused with postmenopausal oral discomfort that has a burning component. In the latter condition, estrogen replacement therapy is effective about half of the time.[378] Psychological factors, although present in some of this population, do not appear to be etiological.[379]

Examination. The patient with BMS generally has a negative intraoral examination.[375] Obvious tissue-irritating causes such as denture soreness, rough crowns or teeth, and other causes of tissue irritation such as candidiasis or true vitamin deficiencies must, of course, be ruled out.

Tests. Candidiasis should be tested for, even if the mucosa looks normal. *Local anesthetic rinse* will decrease the pain of other conditions such as geographical tongue or candidiasis but increase the pain of burning mouth. This increase in pain is thought to be owing to further loss of Aβ fiber inhibition. Sedimentation rate may be mildly elevated, and, in view of the higher incidence of immunological abnormalities, rheumatological evaluation should be considered.

Treatment. The management of BMS is still not satisfactory. Studies assessing therapeutic outcome are lacking and BMS does not appear to remit spontaneously. Few studies report relief without intervention. Emerging evidence supports the effectiveness of the antioxidant, alpha lipoic acid,[380,381] but because BMS is thought to be neuropathic in origin, treatment is typically with medications that may suppress neurological transduction, transmission, and even pain signal facilitation more centrally.[382]

Recapitulation

The pain our patient complains of has none of the characteristics of either atypical odontalgia or BMS except for the burning quality. It is therefore unlikely that these diagnoses are causing her pain.

Thus we have the following differential:

1. Rule out RSD (sympathetically maintained pain) of the left side of the face.
2. Rule out posttraumatic neuralgia of cranial nerve V1–V3 on the left.
3. Myofascial TrP pain is likely to be contributing to the pain complaint.
4. There is internal derangement of the left TMJ with questionable contribution to the total pain complaint.

How can one differentiate between 1 and 2? Sensory blocks of the trigeminal nerve in the past have provided temporary but not long-lasting relief. In fact, the pain returned with the return of sensation. To differentiate between a purely sensory neuralgia and RSD (sympathetically maintained pain), the definitive test is a stellate ganglion block. This will provide dramatic relief if the pain is sympathetically mediated and no relief if it is owing to a neuralgia.

Left sympathetic stellate ganglion block does indeed relieve this patient's pain, and the pain relief outlasts the duration of the local anesthetic. Now that the patient is pain-free, it is possible to complete a thorough musculoskeletal examination. Range of motion is restricted in the left TMJ, with deviation of the jaw to that side on opening. At 30 mm of the mandibular depression, a loud "crack" is audible, and the patient is able to open wider. Active myofascial TrPs that refer pain into the forehead and along the side of the face are found in the upper trapezius, masseter, and lateral pterygoid muscles.

Management of this patient's pain will require repeated sympathetic blockade to control the sympathetically maintained pain. In addition, postural and stretching exercises, along with an intraoral stabilization splint, are indicated to reduce the MFP and stabilize the left TMJ. Spray and stretch, TrP pressure release, and/or TrP injections may facilitate the resolution of the MFP even further. Ultimately, dental treatment to restore left posterior dental support is indicated. Stress management and relaxation training may further help this patient control her pain. This is true because somatic and psychological factors are never separate in maintaining pain. Stress and anxiety will increase the sympathetic activity, which will activate RSD and myofascial TrPs, which are intimately involved in the patient's pain.

This case illustrates the complexity of dealing with patients with persistent orofacial head and neck pain complaints. Multiple diagnoses and contributing factors are common. The biopsychosocial model of chronic pain and illness emphasizes the need for an interdisciplinary pain management approach, including cognitive behavioral therapy, in order to be effective.[382,383] As mentioned previously, in addition to changes in their neurophysiology resulting in increased pain perception and nociceptive dysregulation, patients with chronic pain may develop anxiety, depression, and anger, and may have poor coping skills.[60] Interdisciplinary or multidisciplinary treatments are often required for successful rehabilitation. Rehabilitation includes treatment of the pathema causing the pain, as well as altering lifestyle habits and psychological concomitants that perpetuate the problem. A good liaison with a competent psychologist and a physical therapist is invaluable when evaluating and treating these patients. Even a brief intervention with cognitive behavioral therapy, either in a group setting or individually, has been shown to drastically improve overall coping, pain and activity levels.[384]

Conclusion

In conclusion, it is a time-consuming and difficult task to understand and manage people suffering chronic pain. Many interdisciplinary pain clinics employ orofacial pain dentists; physicians; psychologists; nurses; physical, occupational, and myotherapists; and other health professionals to coordinate patient care and to provide a comprehensive healthy environment for rehabilitation. Chronic pain management, including orofacial pain, has become a growing specialty in health care. It takes years of training and experience to gain adequate insight into these complex cases. Several dental schools across the United States now offer 2-year postgraduate orofacial pain programs to train interested dentists in the field of orofacial pain. Dentists with competence in this field can be identified by contacting the American Board of Orofacial Pain. This organization awards diplomate status to qualified dentists who pass their certification examination. Orofacial pain dentists, armed with knowledge, interest, curiosity, and patience, and, finally, the instruments of diagnosis, enjoy the most rewarding experience—identifying the source of pain and relieving the suffering of a fellow human being. The orofacial pain dentist, oriented toward looking at the patient as a whole person, can gain much satisfaction from arriving at a correct diagnosis and saving teeth or preventing unnecessary surgery.

The complex and personal nature of good diagnosis cannot be overemphasized. This is the area in which the dentist is most likely, on a professional basis, to earn the respect and friendship of colleagues, both dental and medical, as well as patients.

References

1. Dorland's illustrated medical dictionary. 31st ed. Philadelphia, PA: WB Saunders; 2007.
2. Beecher HK. Relationship of significance of wound to the pain experienced. JAMA 1956;161:1609.
3. Fields H. Pain. New York: McGraw-Hill Information Services Company, Health Professions Division; 1987.
4. Merskey H, Bogduk N, editors. Classification of chronic pain. Descriptions of chronic pain syndromes and definitions of pain terms. IASP Task Force on Taxonomy. Seattle, WA: IASP Press; 1994.
5. Committee on Pain, Disability and Chronic Illness Behaviar The anatomy and physiology of pain. In: Osterweis M, Kleinman A, Mechanic D, editors. Pain and disability. Clinical, behavioral, and public policy perspectives, Institute of Medicine, Committee on Pain Disability, and Chronic Illness Behavior. Washington, DC: National Academy Press; 1987.
6. Basbaum AI, Woolf CJ. Pain. Curr Biol 1999;9(12):R429–31.
7. Julius D, Basbaum AI. Molecular mechanisms of nociception. Nature 2001;413(6852):203–10.
8. Schmidt R, Schmelz M, Forster C, et al. Novel classes of responsive and unresponsive C nociceptors in human skin. J Neurosci 1995;15(1 Pt 1):333–41.
9. Watkins LR, Maier SF. Immune regulation of central nervous system functions: from sickness responses to pathological pain. J Intern Med 2005;257(Davis, Reeves et al.):139–55.
10. Watkins LR. Immune and glial regulation of pain. Brain Behav Immun 2007.
11. Watkins LR, Hutchinson MR, Johnston IN, Maier SF. Glia: novel counter-regulators of opioid analgesia. Trends Neurosci 2005;28(12):661–9.
12. Boddeke EW. Involvement of chemokines in pain. Eur J Pharmacol 2001;429(1–3):115–19.
13. Wang H, Ehnert C, Brenner GJ, Woolf CJ. Bradykinin and peripheral sensitization. Biol Chem 2006;387(1):11–14.
14. Basbaum AI, Levine JD. The contribution of the nervous system to inflammation and inflammatory disease. Can J Physiol Pharmacol 1991;69:647.
15. Fields HL, Rowbotham M, Baron R. Neuralgia: irritable nociceptors and deafferentation. Neurobiol Dis 1998;5:209.

16. Fields HL, Levine JD. Pain—mechanics and management. West J Med 1984;141(McClelland, Barnett et al.):347–57.

17. Merrill RL. Central mechanisms of orofacial pain. Dent Clin North Am 2007;51(1):45–59.

18. Basbaum, AI, Jessell TM. In principles of Neuroscience. Kandel ER, Schwartz JH, Jessell TM.472–491 New York:-MacGraw-Hill;2000.

19. Chapman LF. Mechanisms of the flare reaction in human skin. J Invest Dermatol 1977;69:88.

20. Pernow B. Substance P. Pharmacol Rev 1983;35:85.

21. Woolf CJ, Salter MW. Neuronal plasticity: increasing the gain in pain. Science 2000;288(5472):1765–9.

22. Merrill RL. Orofacial pain mechanisms and their clinical application. Dent Clin North Am 1997;41(Davis, Reeves et al.):167–88.

23. Petrenko AB, Yamakura T, Baba H, Shimoji K. The role of N-methyl-D-aspartate (NMDA) receptors in pain: a review. Anesth Analg 2003;97(4):1108–16.

24. Thompson SW, Urban L, Dray A. Contribution of NK1 and NK2 receptor activation to high threshold afferent fibre evoked ventral root responses in the rat spinal cord in vitro. Brain Res 1993;625(1):100–8.

25. Mendell LM, Wall PD. Responses of single dorsal cord cells to peripheral cutaneous unmyelinated fibers. Nature 1965;206:97.

26. Price DD, Hayes RL, Ruda M, Dubner R. Spatial and temporal transformations of input to spinothalamic tract neurons and their relation to somatic sensations. J Neurophysiol 1978;41:933–47.

27. Dickenson AH. Central acute pain mechanisms. Ann Med 1995;27:223.

28. Cervero F, Laird JM, Pozo MA. Selective changes of receptive field properties of spinal nociceptive neurones induced by noxious visceral stimulation in the cat. Pain 1992;51:513.

29. Price DD, Hu JW, Dubner R, Gracely RH. Peripheral suppression of first pain and central summation of second pain evoked by noxious heat pulses. Pain 1977;3:57.

30. Simone DA, Sorkin LS, Oh U, et al. Neurogenic hyperalgesia: central neural correlates in responses of spinothalamic tract neurons. J Neurophysiol 1991Jul;66:(1)228–46.

31. Scholz J, Woolf CJ. Can we conquer pain? Nat Neurosci 2002;5 (Suppl):1062–7.

32. Graff-Radford SB. Regional myofascial pain syndrome and headache: principles of diagnosis and management. Curr Pain Headache Rep 2001;5(4):376–81.

33. Clark GT. Persistent orodental pain, atypical odontalgia, and phantom tooth pain: when are they neuropathic disorders? J Calif Dent Assoc 2006;34(8):599–609.

34. Jones SL. Descending noradrenergic influences on pain. Prog Brain Res 1991;88:381.

35. Lu Y, Perl ER. Selective action of noradrenaline and serotonin on neurones of the spinal superficial dorsal horn in the rat. J Physiol 2007;582(1):127–136.

36. Basbaum AI, Fields HL. Endogenous pain control systems: brainstem spinal pathways and endorphin circuitry. Annu Rev Neurosci 1984;7:309.

37. Kanjhan R. Opioids and pain. Clin Exp Pharmacol Physiol 1995;22:397.

38. Urban MO, Smith DJ. Nuclei within the rostral ventromedial medulla mediating morphine antinociception from the periaqueductal gray. Brain Res 1994;652(1):9.

39. Juni A, Klein G, Pintar JE, Kest B. Nociception increases during opioid infusion in opioid receptor triple knock-out mice. Neuroscience 2007;147(Davis, Reeves et al.):439.

40. Price DD. Psychological and neural mechanisms of the affective dimension of pain. Science 2000;288:1769.

41. Goffaux P, Redmond WJ, Rainville P, Marchand S. Descending analgesia—when the spine echoes what the brain expects. Pain 2007;130(1–2):137–43.

42. Moisset X, Bouhassira D. Brain imaging of neuropathic pain. Neuroimage 2007; 37 (Suppl 1): S80-8. Epub Apr 10, 2007.

43. Davis KD. The neural circuitry of pain as explored with functional MRI. Neurol Res 2000;22:313.

44. Milne RJ, Foreman RD, Giesler GJ Jr, Willis WD. Convergence of cutaneous and pelvic visceral nociceptive inputs onto primate spinothalamic neurons. Pain 1981;11:163–83.

45. Sessle BJ, Greenwood LF. Inputs to trigeminal brain stem neurons from facial, oral, tooth pulp and pharyngolaryngeal tissues: I. Responses to innocuous and noxious stimuli. Brain Res 1976;117:211.

46. Broton JG, Hu JW, Sessle BJ. Effects of temporomandibular joint stimulation on nociceptive and nonnociceptive neurons of the cat's trigeminal subnucleus caudalis (medullary dorsal horn). J Neurophysiol 1988;59:1575.

47. Kojima Y. Convergence patterns of afferent information from the temporomandibular joint and masseter muscle in the trigeminal subnucleus caudalis. Brain Res Bull 1990;24:609.

48. Sessle BJ. The neurobiology of facial and dental pain: present knowledge, future directions. J Dent Res 1987;66:962.

49. Kerr FWL. Facial, vagal and glossopharyngeal nerves in the cat: afferent connections. Arch Neurol 1962;6:624.

50. Mense S. Referral of muscle pain. New aspects. Am Pain Soc J 1994;3:1.

51. Hoheisel U, Mense S, Simons DG, Yu X-M. Appearance of new receptive fields in rat dorsal horn neurons following noxious stimulation of skeletal muscle: a model for referral of muscle pain? Neurosci Lett 1993;153:9–12.

52. Simons DG. Neurophysiological basis of pain caused by trigger points. APS J 1994;3:17–19.

53. Bereiter DA, Hirata H, Hu JW. Trigeminal subnucleus caudalis: beyond homologies with the spinal dorsal horn. Pain 2000;88(McClelland, Barnett et al.):221–4.

54. Kunc Z. Significant factors pertaining to the results of trigeminal tractotomy. In: Hassler R, Walker AE, editors. Trigeminal neuralgia: pathogenesis and pathophysiology. Stuttgart: Georg Thieme Verlag; 1970. pp. 90–100.

55. Pfaffenrath V, Dandekar R, Pöllmann W. Cervicogenic headache—the clinical picture, radiological findings and hypotheses on its pathophysiology. Headache 1987;27:495–9.

56. Head H. On disturbance of sensation with special reference to the pain of visceral disease. Brain 1893;16:1.

57. Kellgren JH. Observations on referred pain arising from muscle. Clin Sci 1938;3:175.

58. Devor M. The pathophysiology and anatomy of damaged nerve. In: Wall PD, Melzack R, editors. Textbook of pain. Edinburgh: Churchill Livingstone; 1984.

59. Schott GD. Complex? Regional? Pain? Syndrome? Pract Neurol 2007;7(McClelland, Barnett et al.):145–57.

60. Gatchel, RJ, Peng, YB, Peteres, ML, et al. The biopsychosocial approach to chronic pain: scientific advances and future directions. Psychol Bull 2007:133 (4)581–624.

61. Gatchel, RJ. Comorbitiy of chronic pain and mental health: The biopsychosocial perspective. Am Psychol 2004;59:792–4.

62. Smith, WB, Gracely, RH, Safer, MA. The meaning of pain. Cancer patients' rating and recall of cancer pain and affect. Pain 1998:78;123–9.

63. Barber J. Rapid induction analgesia: a clinical report. Am J Clin Hypn 1977;19:138.

64. Barber TS. Toward a theory of pain: relief of chronic pain by prefrontal leukotomy, opiates, placebos, and hypnosis. Psychol Bull 1959;56:430.

65. Turk DC, Okifuji A. Evaluating the role of physical, operant, cognitive, and affective factors in the pain behaviors of chronic pain patients. Behav Modif 1997;21:259.

66. Scott PJ, Ansell BM, Huskisson EC. The measurement of pain in juvenile chronic polyarthritis. Ann Rheum Dis 1977 Apr;36(2):186–7.

67. Huskisson EC. Visual analog scales. In: Melzack R, editor. Pain measurement and assessment. New York: Raven Press; 1973. pp. 33–7.

68. Price DD, McGrath PA, Rafii A, Buckingham B. The validation of visual analogue scale measures for chronic and experimental pain. Pain 1983;17:45–56.

69. Huskisson EC. Measurement of pain. Lancet 1974;ii:127.

70. Scott J, Huskisson EC. Accuracy of subjective measurements made with or without previous scores: an important source of error in serial measurements of subjective states. Ann Rheum Dis 1979;38:558.

71. Scott J, Huskisson EC. Accuracy of subjective measurements made with or without previous scores: an important source of error in serial measurements of subjective states. Ann Rheum Dis 1979;38:558.

72. Kim EJ, Buschmann MT. Reliability and validity of the Faces Pain Scale with older adults. Int J Nurs Stud 2006 May;43(4):447–56. Epub Feb 28, 2006.

73. Ware LJ, Epps CD, Herr K, Packard A. Evaluation of the Revised Faces Pain Scale, Verbal Descriptor Scale, Numeric Rating Scale, and Iowa Pain Thermometer in older minority adults. Pain Manage Nurs 2006 Sep;7(3):117–25.

74. Chambers CT, Giesbrecht K, Craig KD, et al. A comparison of faces scales for the measurement of pediatric pain: children's and parents' ratings. Pain 1999 Oct;83(1):25–35

75. Miro J, Huguet A. Evaluation of reliability, validity, and preference for a pediatric pain intensity scale: the Catalan version of the faces pain scale—revised. Pain 2004 Sep;111(1–2):59–64.

76. Melzack R, Torgeson WS. On the language of pain. Anesthesiology 1971;34:50.

77. Bruns D, Disorbio JM. Chronic pain and biopsychosocial disorders. The BHI-2 approach to assessment and management. Pract Pain Manage 2005;5(7):52–61.

78. Disorbio JM, Bruns D, Barolat G. Assessment and treatment of chronic pain. A physician's guide to a biopsychosocial approach. Pract Pain Manage 2006;6(2):11–27.

79. Steer RA, Rissmiller DJ, Beck AT. Use of the Beck Depression Inventory-II with depressed geriatric patients. Behav Res Ther 2000;38:311.

80. Beck AT, Steer RA, Shaw BF, Emery G Psychometric properties of the Beck Depression Inventory: twenty-five years of evaluation. Clin Psychol Rev 1988;8:77.

81. Melzack R. The McGill Pain Questionnaire: major properties and scoring methods. Pain 1975;1.

82. International Classification of Headache Disorders, 2nd ed. International Headache Society. Cephalalgia 2004;24(Suppl 1):1–160.

83. Simons DG, Travell JG, Simons LS. Travell and Simons' myofascial pain and dysfunction. The trigger point manual. Vol. 1. Upper half of body. 2nd ed. Baltimore, MD: Williams and Wilkins; 1999.

84. Holzhammer J, Wöber C. Alimentary trigger factors that provoke migraine and tension-type headache [Article in German] Schmerz. 2006 Apr;20(2):151–9.

85. Zivadinov R, Willheim K, Sepic-Grahovac D, Jurjevic A, Bucuk M, Bunabic-Razmilic O, Relja G, Zorzon M. Migraine and tension-type headache in Croatia: a population-based survey of precipitating factors. Cephalalgia 2003 Jun;23(5):336–43.

86. Clark GT. Examining temporomandibular disorder patients for cranio-cervical dysfunction. J Craniomandib Pract 1984;2:55.

87. Hoppenfield S. Physical examination of the spine and extremities. New York: Appleton-Century Crofts; 1976.
88. Stiesch-Scholz M, Fink M, Tschernitschek H. Comorbidity of internal derangement of the temporomandibular joint and silent dysfunction of the cervical spine. J Oral Rehabili 2003;30 (4):386–91.
89. Fricton JR, Kroening R, Haley D, Siegert R. Myofascial pain syndrome of the head and neck: a review of clinical characteristics of 164 patients. Oral Surg 1985;160:615.
90. Okeson JP, editor. Orofacial pain. Guidelines for assessment, diagnosis, and management. American Academy of Orofacial Pain. Chicago, IL: Quintessence; 1996.
91. Skootsky SA, Jaeger B, Oye RK. Prevalence of myofascial pain in general internal medicine practice. West J Med 1989;151:157.
92. Solberg WK. Myofascial pain and dysfunction. In: Clar JW, editor. Clinical dentistry. Hagerstown, MD: Harper and Row; 1976.
93. Couppe C, Torelli P, Fuglsang-Frederiksen A, et al. Myofascial trigger points are very prevalent in patients with chronic tension-type headache: a double-blinded controlled study. Clin J Pain 2007 Jan;23(1):23–7.
94. Bates' guide to physical examination and history taking. by Lynn S. Bickley, M.D. , Barbara Bates, Peter G. Szilagyi; Lippincott Williams & Wilkins, December 2005.
95. American Psychiatric Association Diagnostic and Statistical Manual of Mental Disorders, 4th ed. Text Revision, Washington, D.C., American Psychiatric Association, 2000.
96. Giovanni A, Fava MD, Thomas N, Wise MD. Issues for DSM-V: Psychological Factors Affecting Either Identified or Feared Medical Conditions: A Solution for Somatoform Disorders Am J Psychiatry 164:1002–3, July 2007
97. Mayou R, Kirmayer LJ, Simon G, et al. Somatoform disorders: time for a new approach in DSM-V. Am J Psychiatry. 2005 May;162(5):847–55
98. Jaeger B, Skootsky SA. Male and female chronic pain patients categorized by DSM-III psychiatric diagnostic criteria [letter]. Pain 1987;29:263.
99. Fordyce WE, Steger JC. Chronic pain. In: Pomerleau OF, Brady JP. Behavioral medicine: theory and practice. Baltimore: Williams & Wilkins; 1978. pp. 125–54.
100. Fordyce WE. An operant conditioning method for managing chronic pain. Postgrad Med 1973;53:123.
101. Bell's Orofacial Pains by Jeffrey P. Okeson and Welden E. Bell; Quintessence Publishing, 5th ed. 1995.
102. Scully C. Drug effects on salivary glands: dry mouth. Oral Dis. 2003 Jul;9(4):165–76.
103. Arthritis Foundation. Primer on the rheumatic diseases. 12th ed. Arthritis Foundation, 2001.
104. Navazesh M. ADA Council on Scientific Affairs and Division of Science: How can oral health care providers determine if patients have dry mouth? J Am Dent Assoc. 2003 May;134(5):613–20.
105. Bardow A, Nyvad B, Nauntofte B. Relationships between medication intake, complaints of dry mouth, salivary flow rate and composition, and the rate of tooth demineralization in situ. Arch Oral Biol. 2001 May;46(5):413–23.
106. Shah RK, Blevins NH. Otalgia. Otolaryngol Clin North Am 2003;36(6):1137–51.
107. Schor DI. Headache and facial pain-the role of the paranasal sinuses: a literature review. Cranio. 1993 Jan;11(1):36–47. Review.
108. Reynolds OE, Hutchins HC, et al. Aerodontalgia occurring during oxygen indoctrination in low pressure chamber. US Naval Med Bull 1946;46:845.
109. Kennedy DW, Loury MC. Nasal and sinus pain: current diagnosis and treatment. Neurol 1988;8:303.
110. Clerico DM. Sinus headaches reconsidered: referred cephalgia of rhinologic origin masquerading as refractory primary headaches. Headache. 1995 Apr;35(4):185–92.
111. Sicher H. Problems of pain in dentistry. Oral Surg Oral Med Oral Pathol Oral Radiol Endod 1954;7:149.
112. Hauman CH, Chandler NP, Tong DC. Endodontic implications of the maxillary sinus: a review.Int Endod J. 2002 Feb;35(2):127–41. Review.
113. Nenzen B, Welander U. The effect of conservative root canal therapy on local mucosal hyperplasia of the maxillary sinus. Odontol Rev 1967;18:295.
114. Solberg WK. Temporomandibular disorders. Br Dent J 1986.
115. American Academy of Orofacial Pain. McNeill C, editor. Temporomandibular disorders: guidelines for classification, assessment, and management. Chicago: Quintessence; 1993.
116. Bell W. Clinical management of temporomandibular disorders. Chicago: Yearbook Medical Publishers; 1982.
117. de Leeuw R, Albuquerque R, Okeson J, Carlson C. The contribution of neuroimaging techniques to the understanding of supraspinal pain circuits: Implications for orofacial pain. Oral Surg Oral Med Oral Pathol Oral Radiol Endod 2005;100:308–14.
118. Guralnick W, Raban LB, Merrill RG. Temporomandibular joint afflictions. N Engl J Med 1978;123:299.
119. Gangarosa LP, Mahan PE. Pharmacologic management of TMD-MPDS. Ear Nose Throat J 1982;61:670.
120. Wenneberg B, Kopp S, Grondahl HG. Long-term effect of intra-articular injections of a glucocorticosteroid into the TMJ: a clinical and radiographic 8-year follow-up. J Craniomandib Disord 1991;5(1)11.
121. Rasmussen OC. Description of population and progress of symptoms in longitudinal study of temporomandibular arthropathy. Scand J Dent Res 1981;89:196.
122. Fricton JR. Recent advances in temporomandibular disorders and orofacial pain. J Am Dent Assoc 1991;122:25.

123. Greene CS, Laskin DM. Long term evaluation of treatment of myofascial pain-dysfunction syndrome: a comparative analysis. J Am Dent Assoc 1983;107:235.

124. Magnusson T, Carlsson GE, Egermark I. Changes in subjective symptoms of craniomandibular disorders in children and adolescents during a 10 year period. J Orofac Pain 1993;7:76.

125. Lipton JH, Ship JA, Larach-Robinson D. Estimated prevalence and distribution of reported orofacial pain in the United States. J Am Dent Assoc 1993;124:115.

126. Greene CS, Laskin DM. Long-term status of TMJ clicking in patients with myofascial pain and dysfunction. J Am Dent Assoc 1988;117:461.

127. Brandt KD, Slemenda CW. Osteoarthritis: epidemiology, pathology, and pathogenesis. In: Schumacher HR, editor. Primer on the rheumatic diseases. 10th ed. Atlanta: Arthritis Foundation; 1993. pp.184–8.

128. Kreutziger KL, Mahan PE. Temporomandibular degenerative joint disease. Part I. Anatomy, pathophysiology, and clinical description. Oral Surg 1975;40:165.

129. Christian CL. Diseases of the joints. Part VII. In: Wyngaarden JB, Smith LH Jr. Cecil textbook of medicine. 15th ed. Philadelphia: WB Saunders; 1979. pp. 185–93.

130. De Bont LGM, Boering G, Liem RSB, et al. Osteoarthritis of the temporomandibular joint: a light microscopic and scanning electron microscopic study of the articular cartilage of the mandibular condyle. J Oral Maxillofac Surg 1985;43:481.

131. Stegenga B, de Bont LGM, Boering G, et al. Tissue responses to degenerative changes in the temporomandibular joint: a review. J Oral Maxillofac Surg 1991;49:1079.

132. Katzberg RW, Westesson PL. Diagnosis of the temporomandibular joint. Philadelphia: WB Saunders; 1993.

133. Bell WE. Temporomandibular disorders: classification, diagnosis and management. 3rd ed. Chicago: Year Book; 1990.

134. Senia ES, Klarich JD. Arm pain of dental origin. Abbreviated case report. Oral Surg Oral Med Oral Pathol. 1974 Dec;38(6):960–1.

135. Alles A, Dom RM. Peripheral sensory nerve fibers that dichotomize to supply the brachium and the pericardium in the rat: a possible morphological explanation for referred cardiac pain? Brain Res 1985;342:382.

136. Laurberg S, Sorensen KE. Cervical dorsal root ganglion cells with collaterals to both shoulder skin and the diaphragm. A fluorescent double labeling study in the rat. A model for referred pain? Brain Res 1985;331:160.

137. Batchelder BJ, Krutchkoff DJ, Amara J. Mandibular pain as the initial and sole clinical manifestation of coronary insufficiency: report of case. J Am Dent Assoc 1987;115:710–12.

138. Kreiner M, Okeson JP, Michelis V, et al. Craniofacial pain as the sole symptom of cardiac ischemia: a prospective multicenter study. J Am Dent Assoc. 2007 Jan;138(1):74–9.

139. Bonica JJ. The management of pain. Vol. II. Philadelphia, PA: Lea & Febiger; 1990.

140. Matson MS. Pain in orofacial region associated with coronary insufficiency. Oral Surg 1963;16:284.

141. Norman JE de B. Facial pain and vascular disease: some clinical observations. Br J Oral Surg 1970;8:138.

142. Krant KS. Pain referred to teeth as the sole discomfort in undiagnosed mediastinal lymphoma. J Am Dent Assoc 1989;118:587.

143. Lee, Thomas H. Chest discomfort. In: Harrsion's principles of internal medicine. 16th ed. New York: Mc Graw-Hill; 2007.

144. Larry Jameson J, Anthony P Weetman. Diseases of the thyroid gland. In: Harrison's Principles of Internal Medicine. 16th ed. Boston, MA: McGraw-Hill; 2007

145. Fay T. Atypical facial neuralgia. Arch Neurol Psychiat.1927;18:309–15.

146. Fay T. Atypical facial neuralgia, a syndrome of vascular pain. Ann Otol Rhinol Laryngol 1932;41:1030.

147. Chambers BR, Donnan GA, Riddell RJ, Bladin PF. Carotidynia: aetiology, diagnosis and treatment. Clin Exp Neurol. 1981;17:113–23.

148. Burton BS, Syms MJ, Petermann GW, Burgess LP. MR imaging of patients with carotidynia. AJNR Am J Neuroradiol. 2000 Apr;21(4):766–9.

149. Kosaka N, Sagoh T, Uematsu H, et al. Imaging by multiple modalities of patients with a carotidynia syndrome. Eur Radiol. 2007 Sep;17(9):2430–3. Epub 2007 Jan 13.

150. Cannon CR. Carotidynia: an unusual pain in the neck. Otolaryngol Head Neck Surg 1994;110:387.

151. Clark HV, King DE, Yow RN. Carotidynia. Am Fam Physician 1994 Oct;50(5):987–90. Review.

152. Bland JH editor. Disorders of the cervical spine. 2nd ed. Philadelphia: WB Saunders; 1994.

153. Edmeads V. Headaches and head pains associated with diseases of the cervical spine. Med Clin North Am 1978;62:533.

154. Rocabado M. Diagnosis and treatment of abnormal craniocervical and craniomandibular mechanics. In: Head, neck and temporomandibular joint dysfunction manual. Tacoma (WA): Rocabado Institute; 1981. pp. 1–21.

155. Jacques P Meloche MD, Yves Bergeron MD, F.R.C.P.(C) F.A.C.P, Andre Bellavance M.D.,Ph.D, Marcel Morand M.D., F.R.C.P.(C), Jean Huot M.D, Gabriel Belzile M.D (1993)Painful Intervertebral Dysfunction: Robert Maigne's Original Contribution to Headache of Cervical OriginHeadache: The Journal of Head and Face Pain 33 (6), 328–34.

156. Bogduc N. The anatomy of occipital neuralgia. J Clin Exp Neuropsychol 1981;17:167.

157. Sjaastad O, Saunte C, Hovdahl H, Breivik H, Gronbaek E. "Cervicogenic" headache. A hypothesis. Cephalalgia 1983;3:249.

158. Jaeger B. Are "cervicogenic" headaches due to myofascial pain and cervical spine dysfunction? Cephalalgia 1989;9:157.

159. Pfaffenrath V, Dandekar R, Mayer ET, Hermann G, Pollmann W. Cervicogenic headache: results of computer-based measurements of cervical spine mobility in 15 patients. Cephalalgia 1988;8:45.

160. Jannetta PJ. Pain problems of significance in head and face, some of which often are misdiagnosed. Curr Prob Surg 1973;47:53.

161. Nurmikko TJ. Mechanisms of central pain. Clin J Pain 2000;16 (Suppl 2):S21.

162. Goadsby PJ. Headache: a good year for research. Lancet Neurol 2006;5(1):5–6.

163. Spierings ELH. Recent advances in the understanding of migraine. Headache 1988;28:655.

164. Kemper JT, Jr., Okeson JP. Craniomandibular disorders and headaches. J Prosthet Dent 1983;49(5):702–5.

165. Molina OF, dos Santos J, Jr., Nelson SJ, Grossman E. Prevalence of modalities of headaches and bruxism among patients with craniomandibular disorders. Cranio 1997;15(4):314–25.

166. Lipton RB, Stewart WF. The epidemiology of migraine. Eur Neurol 1994;34 (Suppl 2):6–11.

167. Mitrirattanakul S, Merrill RL. Headache impact in patients with orofacial pain. J Am Dent Assoc 2006;137(9):1267–74.

168. Goadsby PJ, Lipton RB, Ferrari MD. Migraine–current understanding and treatment. N Engl J Med 2002;346(4):257–70.

169. Silberstein SD. Migraine pathophysiology and its clinical implications. Cephalalgia 2004;24 (Suppl 2):2–7.

170. Moskowitz MA. Basic mechanisms in vascular headache. Neurol Clin 1990;8:801.

171. Burstein R, Yarnitsky D, Goor-Aryeh I, et al. An association between migraine and cutaneous allodynia. Ann Neurol 2000;47(5):614–24.

172. Yarnitsky D, Goor-Aryeh I, Bajwa ZH, et al. 2003 Wolff Award: Possible Parasympathetic Contributions to Peripheral and Central Sensitization During Migraine. Headache: The Journal of Head and Face Pain 2003;43(7):704–14.

173. Shibata K, Yamane K, Iwata M. Change of Excitability in Brainstem and Cortical Visual Processing in Migraine Exhibiting Allodynia. Headache: The Journal of Head and Face Pain 2006;46(10):1535–44.

174. Burstein R, Collins B, Jakubowski M. Defeating migraine pain with triptans: a race against the development of cutaneous allodynia. Ann Neurol 2004;55(1):19–26.

175. Malick A, Burstein R. Peripheral and central sensitization during migraine. Funct Neurol 2000;15 (Suppl 3):28–35.

176. Durham PL. CGRP receptor antagonists: a new choice for acute treatment of migraine? Curr Opin Investig Drugs 2004;5(7):731–5.

177. Durham PL. Calcitonin gene-related peptide (CGRP) and migraine. Headache 2006;46 (Suppl 1):S3–8.

178. Rapoport AM. Acute treatment of headache. J Headache Pain 2006;7(5):355–9.

179. Goadsby PJ. Migraine: emerging treatment options for preventive and acute attack therapy. Expert Opinion on Emerging Drugs 2006;11(McClelland, Barnett et al.):419–27.

180. Durham PL, Sharma RV, Russo AF. Repression of the calcitonin gene-related peptide promoter by 5-HT1 receptor activation. J Neurosci 1997;17(24):9545–53.

181. Storer RJ, Akerman S, Goadsby PJ. Calcitonin gene-related peptide (CGRP) modulates nociceptive trigeminovascular transmission in the cat. Br J Pharmacol 2004;142(7):1171.

182. Geraud G, Denuelle M, Fabre N, et al. [Positron emission tomographic studies of migraine]. Rev Neurol (Paris) 2005;161(6–7):666–70.

183. Sanchez-Del-Rio M, Reuter U, Moskowitz MA. New insights into migraine pathophysiology. Curr Opin Neurol 2006;19(McClelland, Barnett et al.):294–8.

184. Tfelt-Hansen P, Lous I, Olesen J. Prevalence and significance of muscle tenderness during common migraine attacks. Headache 1981;2:45.

185. Lous I, Olesen J. Evaluation of pericranial tenderness and oral function in patients with common migraine, muscle contraction headache and combination headache. Pain 1982;12:385.

186. Jensen R, Rasmussen BK, Pedersen B, et al. Prevalence of oromandibular dysfunction in a general population. J Orofac Pain 1993;7(Davis, Reeves et al.):175–82.

187. Jensen R. Pathophysiological mechanisms of tension-type headache: a review of epidemiological and experimental studies. Cephalalgia 1999;19(6):602–621.

188. Bendtsen L. Sensitization: its role in primary headache. Curr Opin Investig Drugs 2002;3(McClelland, Barnett et al.):449–53.

189. Rapoport AM, et al. Correlations of facial thermographic patterns and headache diagnosis. In: Abernathy M, Uematsu S, editors. Medical thermology. Washington (DC): American Academy of Thermology; 1986. p. 56.

190. Volta GD, Anzola GP. Are there objective criteria to follow up migrainous patients? A prospective study with thermography and evoked potentials. Headache 1988;28:423.

191. Diamond S, Dalessio DJ. Migraine headache. In: Diamond S, Dalessio DJ, editors. The practicing physician's approach to headache. 4th ed. Baltimore: Williams and Wilkins; 1986. pp. 50–6.

192. Freitag FG. Botulinum toxin type A in chronic migraine. Expert Rev Neurother 2007;7(5):463–70. Review.

193. Diamond S, Dalessio DJ. Cluster headache. In: Diamond S, Dalessio DJ, editors. The practicing physician's approach to headache. 4th ed. Baltimore: Williams and Wilkins; 1986. pp. 66–75.

194. Goadsby PJ. Cluster headache: new perspectives. Cephalalgia 1999;19 (Suppl 25):39–41.
195. Bittar G, Graff-Radford SB. A retrospective study of patients with cluster headache. Oral Surg 1992;73:519.
196. Benoliel R, Sharav Y. Paroxysmal hemicrania. Case studies and review of the literature. Oral Surg Oral Med Oral Pathol Oral Radiol Endod 1998;85:285–92.
197. Sjaastad O, Dale I. A new(?) clinical headache entity, "chronic paroxysmal hemicrania." Acta Neurol Scand 1976;54:140.
198. Goadsby PJ, Cohen AS, Matharu MS. Trigeminal autonomic cephalalgias: diagnosis and treatment. Curr Neurol Neurosci Rep 2007;7(Davis, Reeves et al.):117–25.
199. Delcanho RE, Graff-Radford SB. Chronic paroxysmal hemicrania presenting as toothache. J Orofac Pain 1993;7:300–6.
200. Sjaastad O, Eggl K, Horven I, et al. Chronic paroxysmal hemicrania: mechanical precipitation of attacks. Headache 1979;19:31
201. Sjaastad O, Apfelbaum R, Caskey W, et al. Chronic paroxysmal hemicrania (CPH). The clinical manifestations. A review. Ups J Med Sci Suppl1980;31.
202. Goadsby PJ, May A. PET demonstration of hypothalamic activation in cluster headache. Neurology 1999;52(7):1522.
203. May A, Bahra A, Buchel C, et al. Hypothalamic activation in cluster headache attacks. Lancet 1998;352(9124):275–8.
204. Dodick DW, Rozen TD, Goadsby PJ, Silberstein SD. Cluster headache. Cephalalgia 2000;9:787–803.
205. Waldenlind E, Ekborn K, Wetterberg L, et al. Decreased nocturnal serum melatonin levels during active cluster headache periods. Opus Med 1984;29:109.
206. May A, Bahra A, Buchel C, et al. Hypothalamic activation in cluster headache attacks. Lancet 1998;352:275–8.
207. Martelletti P, Giacovazzo M. Putative neuroimmunological mechanisms in cluster headache. An integrated hypothesis. Headache 1996;36:312.
208. Russel D. Clinical characterization of the cluster headache syndrome. In: Olesen J, Edvinnson L, editors. Basic mechanisms of headache. Amsterdam: Elsevier Science; 1988. p. 21.
209. Evers S, Bauer B, Suhr B, et al. Cognitive processing is involved in cluster headache but not in chronic paroxysmal hemicrania. Neurology 1999;53:357–63.
210. Ekbom K. Treatment of cluster headache: clinical trials, design and results. Cephalalgia 1995;15 (Suppl 15):33–6.
211. Gobel H, Lindner V, Heinze A, et al. Acute therapy for cluster headache with sumatriptan: findings of a one-year long-term study. Neurology 1998;51:908–11.
212. Cittadini E, May A, Straube A, et al. Effectiveness of intranasal zolmitriptan in acute cluster headache: a randomized, placebo-controlled, double-blind crossover study. Arch Neurol 2006;63(11):1537–42.
213. Cirkpatrick PJ, O'Brien MD, MacCabe JJ. Trigeminal nerve section for chronic migrainous neuralgia. Br J Neurosurg. 1993;7(5):483–90.
214. Delassio DJ. Surgical therapy of cluster headache. In: Mathew N, editor. Cluster headache. New York:Spectrum;1984. p. 119.
215. Salvesen R. Cluster headache. Curr Treat Option Neurol 1999;1:441.
216. Ford RG, Ford KT, Swaid S, et al. Gamma knife treatment of refractory cluster headache. Headache 1998;38:3–9.
217. Kunkel RS. Complications and rare forms of migraine. In: Olesen J, Edvinnson L, editors. Basic mechanisms of headache. Amsterdam: Elsevier Science; 1988. p. 82.
218. Friedlander AH, Runyon C. Polymyalgia rheumatic and temporal arteritis. Oral Surg 1990;69:317.
219. Guttenberg SA, Emery RW, Milobsky SA, Geballa M. Cranial arteritis odontogenic pain: report of a case. J Am Dent Assoc 1989;119:621.
220. Diamond S, Dalessio DJ. The practicing physician's approach to headache. 5th ed. Baltimore: Williams & Wilkins; 1992.
221. Kleinegger CL, Lilly GE. Cranial arteritis: a medical emergency with orofacial manifestations. J Am Dent Assoc 1999
222. Waters WE. Headache and blood pressure in the community. BMJ 1971;1:142.
223. Penman J. Trigeminal neuralgia. In: Vinken PJ, Bruyn GW, editors. Handbook of clinical neurology. Vol 5. Amsterdam: Elsevier; 1968. pp. 296–322.
224. Evans RW, Graff-Radford SB, Bassiur JP. Pretrigeminal Neuralgia. Headache: The Journal of Head and Face Pain 2005;45(McClelland, Barnett et al.):242–4.
225. Mitchell RG. Pre-trigeminal neuralgia. Br Dent J 1980;149:167.
226. Merrill RL, Graff-Radford SB. Trigeminal neuralgia: how to rule out the wrong treatment. J Am Dent Assoc 1992;123:63.
227. Rushton JG, Stevens JC, Miller RH. Glossopharyngeal (vagoglossopharyngeal) neuralgia: A Study of 217 Cases. Arch Neurol 1981;38:201.
228. Walker AE. Neuralgias of the glossopharyngeal, vagus and nervus intermedius nerves. In: Knighton PR, Dumke PR, editors. Pain. Boston, MA: Little, Brown; 1966. pp. 421–9.
229. Balbuena L Jr, Hayes D, Ramirez SG, Johnson R. Eagle's syndrome. South Med J 1997;90:331.
230. Massey EW, Massey J. Elongated styloid process (Eagle's syndrome) causing hemicrania. Headache 1979;19:339.
231. Sivers JE, Johnson GK. Diagnosis of Eagle's syndrome. Oral Surg 1985;59:575.
232. Dubuisson D. Nerve root damage and arachnoiditis. In: Wall PD, Melzack R, editors. Textbook of pain. New York: Churchill Livingstone; 1984. p. 436.

233. White UC, Sweet WH. Pain and the neurosurgeon. Springfield (IL): Charles C. Thomas; 1969.
234. Sulfaro MA, Gobetti JP. Occipital neuralgia manifesting as orofacial pain. Oral Surg Oral Med Oral Pathol Oral Radiol Endod 1995;80:751.
235. Fromm GH, Terrence CF, Maroon JC. Trigeminal neuralgia. Current concepts regarding etiology and pathogenesis. Arch Neurol 1984;41:1204.
236. Janetta PJ. Surgical treatment: microvascular decompression. In: Fromm GH, Sessle BJ, editors. Trigeminal neuralgia: current concepts regarding pathogenesis and treatment. Boston, MA: Butterworth-Heinemann; 1991. pp. 145–57.
237. Casamassimo PS, Tucker-Lammert JE. Diabetic polyradiculopathy with trigeminal nerve involvement. Oral Surg Oral Med Oral Pathol Oral Radiol Endod 1988;66:315.
238. Laha RK, Jannetta PJ. Glossopharyngeal neuralgia. J Neurosurg 1977;47:316.
239. Khan NU, Iyer A. Glossopharyngeal neuralgia associated with anomalous glossopharyngeal nerve. Otolaryngology - Head and Neck Surgery 2007;136(McClelland, Barnett et al.):502.
240. Andrychowski J, Nauman P, Czernicki Z. Occipital nerve neuralgia as postoperative complication. Views on etiology and treatment. Neurol Neurochir Pol 1998;32:871.
241. Graff-Radford SB, Jaeger B, Reeves JL. Myofascial pain may present clinically as occipital neuralgia. Neurosurgery 1986;19:610.
242. Pinsaesdi P, Seltzer S. The induction of trigeminal neuralgia-like pain and endodontically treated teeth. JOE 1988;14:360.
243. Francica F, Brickman J, Lo Monaco CJ, Lin LM. Trigeminal neuralgia and endodontically treated teeth. JOE 1988;14:360.
244. Fromm GH. Etiology and pathogenesis of trigeminal neuralgia. In: Fromm GH, editor. The medical and surgical management of trigeminal neuralgia. Mount Kisco (NY): Futura; 1987. pp. 31–41.
245. Cheng TMW, Cascino TL, Onofrio BM. Comprehensive study of diagnosis and treatment of trigeminal neuralgia secondary to tumors. Neurology 1993;43:2298.
246. Druigan MC, et al. Occipital neuralgia in adolescents and young adults. N Engl J Med 1962;267:1166.
247. Varady P, Dheerendra P, Nyary I, et al. Neurosurgery using the gamma knife. Orv Hetil 1999;14;140:331.
248. Young RF, Vermulen S, Posewitz A. Gamma knife radiosurgery for the treatment of trigeminal neuralgia. Stereotact Funct Neurosurg 1998;70 (Suppl 1):192.
249. Pollock BE, Gorman DA, Schomberg PJ, Kline RW. The Mayo Clinic gamma knife experience: indications and initial results. Mayo Clin Proc 1999;74:5.
250. Brisman R. Microvascular decompression vs. gamma knife radiosurgery for typical trigeminal neuralgia: preliminary findings. Stereotact Funct Neurosurg 2007;85(2–3):94–8.
251. Lee KH, Chang JW, Park YG Chung SS. Microvascular decompression and percutaneous rhizotomy in trigeminal neuralgia. Stereotact Funct Neurosurg 1997;68(1–4 Pt 1):196.
252. Broggi G, Ferroli P, Franzini A, et al. Microvascular decompression for trigeminal neuralgia: comments on a series of 250 cases, including 10 patients with multiple sclerosis. J Neurol Neurosurg Psychiatry 2000;68:59.
253. Henson CF, Goldman HW, Rosenwasser RH, et al. Glycerol rhizotomy versus gamma knife radiosurgery for the treatment of trigeminal neuralgia: an analysis of patients treated at one institution. Int J Radiat Oncol Biol Phys 2005;63(1):82–90
254. Cappabianca P, Spaziante R, Graziussi G, et al. Percutaneous retrogasserian glycerol rhizolysis for treatment of trigeminal neuralgia. Technique and results in 191 patients. J Neurosurg Sci 1995;39:37.
255. Pollock BE. Percutaneous retrogasserian glycerol rhizotomy for patients with idiopathic trigeminal neuralgia: a prospective analysis of factors related to pain relief. J Neurosurg 2005;102(2):223–8.
256. Fromm GH, Graff-Radford SB, Terrence CF, Sweet WH. Pretrigeminal neuralgia. Neurology 1990;40:1493.
257. Kondo A. Follow-up results of using microvascular decompression for treatment of glossopharyngeal neuralgia. J Neurosurg 1998;88:221.
258. Tronnier VM, Rasche D, Hamer J, Kunze S. [Neurosurgical therapy of facial neuralgias] Schmerz. 2002;16(5):404–11.
259. Laha JM, Tew JM Jr. Long-term results of surgical treatment of idiopathic neuralgias of the glossopharyngeal and vagal nerves. Neurosurgery 1995;36:926.
260. Hunter CR, Mayfield SH. Role of the upper cervical roots in the production of pain in the head. Am J Surg 1949;78:743.
261. Campbell JK, Cassel RD. Headache and other craniofacial pain. In: Bradley, W. G. Neurology in Clinical Practice. 3rd ed. Boston, MA: Butterworth-Heinemann, 2000.
262. Lovely TJ, Jannetta PJ. Surgical management of geniculate neuralgia. Am J Otol 1997;18:512.
263. Bruyn GW. Nervus intermedius neuralgia (Hunt). Superior laryngeal neuralgia. In: Rose FC, editor. Headache. Handbook of clinical neurology. Vol 4. Amsterdam: Elsevier; 1986. pp. 487–500.
264. Hansen HJ. Neuro-histological reactions following tooth extractions. Int J Oral Surg 1980;9:411.
265. Neurobiology of Pain. In: Stephen McMahon, Martin Koltzenburg, editors. Wall and Melzack's. Textbook of pain. 5th ed. Churchill-Livingstone;2005.
266. Peszkowski MJ, Larsson A. Extraosseous and intraosseous oral traumatic neuromas and their association with tooth extraction. J Oral Maxillofac Surg 1990;48:963.
267. Robinson M, Slavkin H. Dental amputation neuromas. J Am Dent Assoc 1965;70:662.

268. Burchiel KJ, Johans TJ, Ochoa J. The surgical treatment of painful traumatic neuromas. J Neurosurg 1993;78:714.
269. Liverton NJ, Bednar RA, Bednar B, et al. Identification and characterization of 4-methylbenzyl 4-[(pyrimidin-2-ylamino)methyl]piperidine-1-carboxylate, an orally bioavailable, brain penetrant NR2B selective N-methyl-D-aspartate receptor antagonist. J Med Chem 2007;50(4):807–19.
270. Head H, Campbell AW. The pathology of herpes zoster and its bearing on sensory location. Brain 1900;23:353.
271. Lhermitte J, Nicholas M. Les lésions spinales du zona. La myelte zosterienne. Rev Neurol 1924;1:361.
272. Denny-Brown D, et al. Pathologic features of herpes zoster: a note on "geniculate herpes." Arch Neurol Psychiatry 1944;77:337.
273. Watson CP, Evans RJ, Watt VR. Post-herpetic neuralgia and topical capsaicin. Pain 1988;33:333.
274. Watson CP, Deck JH, Morshead C, et al. Post-herpetic neuralgia: further post-mortem studies of cases with and without pain. Pain 1991;44:105.
275. Tyring SK. Advances in the treatment of herpes virus infection: the role of famciclovir. Clin Ther 1998;20:661.
276. Goon WWY, Jacobsen PL. Prodromal odontalgia and multiple devitalized teeth caused by a herpes zoster infection of the trigeminal nerve: report of case. J Am Dent Assoc 1988;116:500.
277. Nurmikko T, Bowsher D. Somatosensory findings in postherpetic neuralgia. J Neurol Neurosurg Psychiatry 1990;53:135.
278. Barrett AP, Katelaris CH, Morri JG, Schift M. Zoster sine herpete of the trigeminal nerve. Oral Surg Oral M Oral Pathol 1993;75:173.
279. Johnson RW. Herpes zoster and postherpetic neuralgia. Optimal treatment. Drugs Aging 1997;10:80.
280. Graff-Radford SB, Shaw LR, Naliboff BN. Amitriptyline and fluphenazine in the treatment of postherpetic neuralgia. Clin J Pain 2000;16(McClelland, Barnett et al.):188–92.
281. Beydoun A. Postherpetic neuralgia: role of gabapentin and other treatment modalities. Epilepsia 1999;40 (Suppl 6):S51–6.
282. Diamond S. Postherpetic neuralgia. Prevention and treatment. Postgrad Med 1987;81:321.
283. Boas RA. Sympathetic nerve blocks: in search of a role. Reg Anesth Pain Med 1998;23:292.
284. Juel-Jenson BE, MacCallum FO, Mackenzie SM, Pike Mc. Treatment of zoster with idoxuridine in dimethyl sulphoxide. Results of two double blind controlled trials. Br Med J. 1970 Dec26;4(5738);776–80.
285. Canavan D, Graff-Radford SB, Gratt B. Traumatic dysesthesia of the trigeminal nerve. J Orofac Pain 1994;4:391.
286. Meyerson BA, Hakanson S. Suppression of pain in trigeminal neuropathy by electrical stimulation of the gasserian ganglion. Neurosurgery 1986;18:59.
287. Mitchell SW, Morehouse GR, Keen WW. Gunshot wounds and other injuries of nerves. Philadelphia: JB Lippincott; 1864.
288. Evans JA. Reflex sympathetic dystrophy: report on 57 cases. Ann Intern Med 1947;26:417.
289. Bingham JAE. Causalgia of the face. Two cases successfully treated by sympathectomy. BMJ 1947;1:804.
290. Schott, GD. Complex regional pain syndrome. Pract Neurol 2007;7(3):145–57.
291. Galer BS, Bruehl S, Harden RN. IASP diagnostic criteria for complex regional pain syndrome: a preliminary empirical validation study. International Association for the Study of Pain. Clin J Pain 1998;14(1):48.
292. Bruehl S, Harden RN, Galer BS, et al. External validation of IASP diagnostic criteria for complex regional pain syndrome and proposed research diagnostic criteria. International Association for the Study of Pain. Pain 1999;81:147.
293. Detakats G. Sympathetic reflex dystrophy. Med Clin North Am 1963;49:117.
294. Jaeger B, Singer E, Kroening R. Reflex sympathetic dystrophy of the face: report of two cases and a review of the literature. Arch Neurol 1986;43:693.
295. Sato J, Perl ER. Adrenergic excitation of cutaneous pain receptors induced by peripheral nerve injury. Science 1991;251:1608.
296. Habler HJ, Janig W, Koltzenburg M. Activation of unmyelinated afferents in chronically lesioned nerves by adrenaline and excitation of sympathetic efferents in the cat. Neurosci Lett 1987;82:35.
297. Aguayo AJ, Bray GM. Pathology and pathophysiology of unmyelinated nerve fibers. In: Dyck PJ, Thomas PK, Lambert EH, editors. Peripheral neuropathy. Philadelphia: WB Saunders;1975. pp. 363–78.
298. Belenky M, Devor M. Association of postganglionic sympathetic neurons with primary afferents in sympathetic-sensory co-cultures. J Neurocytol 1997;26:715.
299. Chung K, Yoon YW, Chung JM. Sprouting sympathetic fibers form synaptic varicosities in the dorsal root ganglion of the rat with neuropathic injury. Brain Res 1997;751:275.
300. McLachlan EM, Jang W, Devor M, Michaelis M. Peripheral nerve injury triggers noradrenergic sprouting within dorsal root ganglia. Nature 1993;363:543.
301. Walker AE, Nulson F. Electrical stimulation of the upper thoracic portion of the sympathetic chain in man. Arch Neurol Psychiatry 1948;59:559.
302. Lipman AG. Analgesic drugs for neuropathic and sympathetically maintained pain. Clin Geriatr Med 1996;12:501.
303. Fricton JR, Kroening R, Hakey D, Sieger R. Myofascial pain and dysfunction of the head and neck: a review of the clinical characteristics of 164 patients. Oral Surg Oral Med Oral Pathol Oral Radiol Endod 1985;60:615.

304. Layzer RB. Diagnostic implications of clinical fasciculations and cramps. In: Rowland LP, editor. Human motor neuron diseases. New York: Raven; 1982. pp. 23–7.

305. Jaeger B. Myofascial referred pain patterns: the role of trigger points. Can Dent Assoc J 1985;13:27.

306. Carlson CR, Okeson JP, Falace DA, et al. Reduction of pain and EMG activity in the masseter region by trapezius trigger point injection. Pain 1993;55:397.

307. Travell J. Temporomandibular joint dysfunction: temporomandibular joint pain referred from muscles of the head and neck. J Prosthet Dent 1960;10:745.

308. Travell J, et al. Effects of referred somatic pain on structures in the reference zone. Fed Proc 1944;3:49.

309. Simons DG. Referred phenomena of myofascial trigger points. In: Vecchiet L, Albe-Fessard D, Lindblom U, Giamberardino MA, editors. New trends in referred pain and hyperalgesia. Pain research and clinical management. No 27. Amsterdam: Elsevier Science; 1993. pp. 341–57.

310. Salins PC, Bloxham GP. Bursitis: a factor in the differential diagnosis of orofacial neuralgias and myofascial pain dysfunction syndrome. Oral Surg Oral Med Oral Pathol. 1989 Aug;68(2):154–7.

311. Hong C-Z, Chen Y-N, Twehous D, Hong DH. Pressure threshold for referred pain by compression on the trigger point and adjacent areas. J Musculoskel Pain 1996;4:61.

312. Simons DG. Myofascial pain syndrome of head, neck, and low back. In: Dubner R, Gebhart GF, Bond MR, editors. Pain research and clinical management. Vol 3: proceedings of the Fifth World Congress on Pain. Amsterdam: Elsevier Science; 1988.

313. Travell JG, Simons DG. Myofascial pain and dysfunction. The trigger point manual. Vol 2. The lower extremities. Baltimore: Williams and Wilkins; 1992.

314. Miehlke K, Schulze G, Eger W. Clinical and experimental studies on the fibrositis syndrome. Z Rheumaforsch 1960;19:310–30.

315. Yunus M, Kalyan-Raman UP. Muscle biopsy findings in primary fibromyalgia and other forms of non-articular rheumatism. Rheum Dis Clin North Am 1989;15:115.

316. Hubbard DR, Berkoff GM. Myofascial trigger points show spontaneous needle EMG activity. Spine 1993;18:1803.

317. Kuan TS, Hsieh YL, Chen SM, et al. The myofascial trigger point region: correlation between the degree of irritability and the prevalence of endplate noise. Am J Phys Med Rehabil 2007;86(3):183–9.

318. McNulty WH, Gevirtz RN, Hubbard DR, Berkoff GM. Needle electromyographic evaluation of trigger point response to a psychological stressor. Psychophysiology 1994;31:313.

319. Hong C-Z, Simons DG. Pathophysiologic and electrophysiologic mechanisms of myofascial trigger points. Arch Phys Med Rehabil 1998;79:863.

320. Hubbard DR. Chronic and recurrent muscle pain: pathophysiology and treatment, and review of pharmacologic studies. J Musculoskel Pain 1996;4:123–4.

321. Chen JT, Chen SM, Kuan TS, et al. Phentolamine effect on the spontaneous electrical activity of active loci in a myofascial trigger spot of rabbit skeletal muscle. Arch Phys Med Rehabil 1998;79:790.

322. Wheeler AH, Goolkasian P, Gretz SS. A randomized double-blind prospective pilot study of botulinum toxin. Injection for refractory unilateral cervical-thoracic paraspinal myofascial pain syndrome. Spine 1998;23:1662.

323. Simons D. Clinical and etiological update of myofascial pain from trigger points. J Musculoskel Pain 1996;4:93.

324. Simons DG, Hong C-Z, Simons LS. Nature of myofascial trigger points, active loci [abstract]. J Musculoskel Pain 1995;3 (Suppl 1):62.

325. Reeves JL, Jaeger B, Graff-Radford SB. Reliability of the pressure algometer as a measure of trigger point sensitivity. Pain 1986;24:313.

326. Vecchiet L, Giambardino MA, de Bigontina P, Dragani L. Comparative sensory evaluation of parietal tissues in painful and non-painful areas in fibromyalgia and myofascial pain syndrome. In: Gebhart GF, Hammond DL, Jensen TS, editors. Proceedings of the 7th World Congress on Pain. Progress in pain research and management. Vol 2. Seattle, WA: IASP Press; 1994. pp. 177–249.

327. Fricton JR, et al. Myofascial pain syndrome: electromyographic changes associated with local twitch response. Arch Phys Med Rehabil 1986;66:314.

328. Hong C-Z, Torigoe Y, Yu J. The localized twitch responses in responsive taut bands of rabbit skeletal muscle fibers are related to the reflexes at spinal cord level. J Musculoskel Pain 1995;3:15.

329. Hong C-Z, Torigoe Y. Electrophysiological characteristics of localized twitch responses in responsive taut bands of rabbit skeletal muscle. J Musculoskel Pain 1994;2:17.

330. Vecchiet L, Vecchiet J, Giamerardino MA. Referred muscle pain: clinical and pathophysiologic aspects. Curr Rev Pain 1999;3;489.

331. Travell JG, Rinzler, SH. The myofascial genesis of pain. Postgrad Med 1952;11:425.

332. Graff-Radford SB, Reeves JL, Jaeger B. Management of head and neck pain: the effectiveness of altering perpetuating factors in myofascial pain. Headache 1987;27:186.

333. Sola A. Trigger point therapy. In: Roberts JR, Hedges JR, editors. Clinical proceedings in emergency medicine. 2nd ed. Philadelphia, PA:WB Saunders; 1991. p. 828.

334. Komiyama O, Kawara M, Arai M, et al. Posture correction as part of behavioural therapy in treatment of myofacial pain with limited opening. J Oral Rehabil 1999;26:428.

335. Jaeger B, Reeves JL. Quantification of changes in myofascial trigger point sensitivity with the pressure algometer. Pain 1986;27:203.

336. Hong C-Z. Lidocaine injection versus dry needling to myofascial trigger point. The importance of the local twitch response. Am J Phys Med Rehabil 1994;73:256.

337. Frost FA, Jessen B, Siggaard-Anderson J. A control, double-blind comparison of mepivacaine injection versus saline injection for myofascial pain. Lancet 1980;1:499.

338. Hameroff SR, Crago BR, Blitt CD, Womble J, Kanel J. Comparison of bupivacaine, etidocaine, and saline for trigger-point therapy. Anesth Analg 1981;60:752.

339. Lewit K. The needle effect in the relief of myofascial pain. Pain 1979;6:83.

340. Hsieh YL, Kao MJ, Kuan TS, et al. Dry needling to a key myofascial trigger point may reduce the irritability of satellite MTrPs. Am J Phys Med Rehabil. 2007 May;86(5):397–403.

341. Benoit PW. Microscarring in skeletal muscle after repeated exposures to lidocaine with epinephrine. J Oral Surg 1978;36:530.

342. Qerama E, Fuglsang-Frederiksen A, Kasch H, et al. A double-blind, controlled study of botulinum toxin A in chronic myofascial pain. Neurology. 2006 Jul 25;67(2):241–5.

343. Ho KY, Tan KH. Botulinum toxin A for myofascial trigger point injection: a qualitative systematic review. Eur J Pain. 2007 Jul;11(5):519–27. Epub 2006 Oct 27. Review.

344. Jaeger B. Tension-type headache and myofascial pain. In: Fricton JR, Dubner R, editors. Advances in pain research and therapy. Vol 21. New York:Raven Press; 1995.

345. Mock D, Frydman W, Gordon AS. Atypical facial pain: a retrospective study. Oral Surg Oral Med Oral Pathol 1985;59:472.

346. Fricton JR. Atypical orofacial pain disorders: a study of diagnostic subtypes. Curr Rev Pain 2000;4:142–7.

347. Graff-Radford SB. Facial pain. Curr Opin Neurol 2000;13:291–6.

348. Pfaffenrath V, Rath M, Pollmann W, Keeser W. Atypical facial pain—application of the IHS criteria in a clinical sample. Cephalalgia 1993;13 (Suppl 12):84–8.

349. Marbach JJ, Raphael KG. Phantom tooth pain: a new look at an old dilemma. Pain Med 2000;1(1):68.

350. Rees RT, Harris M. Atypical odontalgia. Br J Oral Surg 1978–9;16:212.

351. Woda A, Pionchon P. A unified concept of idiopathic orofacial pain: clinical features. J Orofac Pain 1999;13:172.

352. Clark GT, Minakuchi H, Lotaif AC. Orofacial pain and sensory disorders in the elderly. Dent Clin North Am 2005;49(Davis, Reeves et al.):343–62.

353. Graff-Radford SB, Solberg WK. Atypical odontalgia. J Craniomandib Disord 1992;6(4):260–5.

354. Solberg WK, Graff-Radford SB. Orodental considerations in facial pain. Semin Neurol 1988;8:318.

355. al Balawi S, Tariq M, Feinmann C. A double-blind, placebo-controlled, crossover, study to evaluate the efficacy of subcutaneous sumatriptan in the treatment of atypical facial pain. Int J Neurosci 1996;86:301.

356. Harrison SD, Balawi SA, Feinmann C, Harris M. Atypical facial pain: a double-blind placebo-controlled crossover pilot study of subcutaneous sumatriptan. Eur Neuropsychopharmacol 1997;7:83.

357. Marbach JJ. Is phantom tooth pain a deafferentation (neuropathic syndrome)? Part I. Oral Surg Oral Med Oral Pathol Oral Radiol Endod 1993;75:95.

358. Marbach JJ. Is phantom tooth pain a deafferentation (neuropathic syndrome)? Part II. Oral Surg Oral Med Oral Pathol Oral Radiol Endod 1993;75:225.

359. Reik L. Atypical facial pain. Headache 1985;25:30.

360. Feinman C. Pain relief by antidepressants: possible modes of action. Pain 1985;23:1.

361. Graff-Radford SB, Solberg WK. Is atypical odontalgia a psychological problem? Oral Surg Oral Med Oral Pathol Oral Radiol Endod 1993;75:579.

362. Vickers ER, Cousins MJ, Walker S, Chisholm K. Analysis of 50 patients with atypical odontalgia. A preliminary report on pharmacological procedures for diagnosis and treatment. Oral Surg 1998;85:24.

363. Woda A, Pioncho P. A unified concept of idiopathic orofacial pain: pathophysiologic features. J Orofac Pain 2000;14:196.

364. Graff-Radford SB, Ketelaer MC, Gratt BM, Solberg WK. Thermographic assessment of neuropathic facial pain. J Orofac Pain 1995;9:138.

365. Bates RE Jr, Stewart CM. Atypical odontalgia: phantom tooth pain. Oral Surg 1991;72:479.

366. Backonja MM, Serra J. Pharmacologic management part 1: better-studied neuropathic pain diseases. Pain Med. 2004 Mar;5 (Suppl 1):S28–47

367. McQuay HJ, Tramer M, Nye BA, et al. A systematic review of antidepressants in neuropathic pain. Pain 1996;68:217.

368. Grushka M. Clinical features of burning mouth syndrome. Oral Med 1987;63:30.

369. Grushka M, et al. Psychophysical evidence of taste dysfunction in burning mouth syndrome. Chem Senses 1986;11:485.

370. Grushka M, et al. Pain and personality profiles in burning mouth syndrome. Pain 1987;28:155.

371. Grushka M, Sesse BJ. Demographic data and pain profile of burning mouth syndrome (BMS). J Dent Res 1985;64:1648.

372. Bartoshuk LM, Grushka M, Duffy VB, et al. Burning mouth syndrome: a pain phantom in supertasters who suffer taste damage? [abstract]. San Diego (CA): American Pain Society; 1998.

373. Mott AE, Grushka M, Sessle BJ. Diagnosis and management of taste disorders and burning mouth syndrome. Dent Clin North Am 1993;37:33.

374. Grushka M, Bartoshuk LM. Burning mouth syndrome and oral dysesthesia. Can J Diagn 2000;17:99.

375. Danhauer SC, Miller CS, Rhodus NL, Carlson CR. Impact of criteria-based diagnosis of burning mouth syndrome on treatment outcome. J Orofac Pain 2002 Fall;16(4):305–11.

376. Eliav E, Kamran B, Schaham R, et al. Evidence of chorda tympani dysfunction in patients with burning mouth syndrome. J Am Dent Assoc. 2007 May;138(5):628–33.

377. Forabosco A, Criscuolc M, Coukos G, Uccell E, Weinstein R, Spinat S, Bottice A, Volpe A. Efficacy of hormone replacement therapy in postmenopausal women with oral discomfort. Oral Surg Oral Med Oral Pathol 1992;73:570.

378. Grushka M, Sessle BJ. Burning mouth syndrome. Dent Clin North Am 1991;35:171.

379. Bogetto F, Maina G, Ferro G, et al. Psychiatric comorbidity in patients with burning mouth syndrome. Psychosom Med 1998;60:378.

380. Patton LL, Siegel MA, Benoliel R, De Laat A. Management of burning mouth syndrome: systematic review and management recommendations. Oral Surg Oral Med Oral Pathol Oral Radiol Endod. 2007 Mar;103 (Suppl):S39.e1–13.

381. Zakrzewska JM, Forssell H, Glenny AM. Interventions for the treatment of burning mouth syndrome. Cochrane Database Syst Rev. 2005 Jan 25;(1):CD002779.

382. Suarez P, Clark GT. Burning mouth syndrome: an update on diagnosis and treatment methods. J Calif Dent Assoc. 2006 Aug;34(8):611–22.

383. Reeves JL, Merrill RL: The Complex Orofacial Pain Patient: A Case for Collaboration. In Roger Kessler, Dale Stafford (editors). Collaborative Medicine Case Studies. Springer Publications, in press.

384. Turner JA, Mancl L, Aaron LA. Short- and long-term efficacy of brief cognitive-behavioral therapy for patients with chronic temporomandibular disorder pain: a randomized, controlled trial. Pain. 2006 Apr;121(3):181–94.

385. Turner-Stokes L, Erkeller-Yuksel F, Miles A, et al. Outpatient cognitive behavioral pain management programs: a randomized comparison of a group-based multidisciplinary versus an individual therapy model. Arch Phys Med Rehabil. 2003 Jun;84(6):781–8.

386. Scott J, Huskisson EC. Graphic representation of pain. Pain 1976;2:175.

387. Hathaway SR, McKinley JC. The Minnesota Multiphasic Personality Inventory manual. New York: Psychological Corporation; 1967.

388. Lewit K. Manipulative therapy in rehabilitation of the locomotor system. 2nd ed. Oxford: Butterworth Heinemann; 1991.

389. Shah JP, Phillips TM, Danoff JV, Gerber LH. An in vivo microanalytical technique for measuring the local biochemical milieu of human skeletal muscle. J Appl Physiol 2005 Nov;99(5):1977–84. Epub 2005 Jul 21.

CHAPTER 12

PULPAL PATHOSIS

G. R. HOLLAND, STEPHEN B. DAVIS

"The pulp lives for the dentin and the dentin lives by the grace of the pulp. Few marriages in nature are marked by a greater affinity." Alfred L. Ogilvie

Response of the Pulp to Dental Caries

BACTERIA ARE RESPONSIBLE FOR MOST PULPAL DISEASE

Bacteria are responsible for most pulpal disease. The classic study by Kakehashi et al.[1] proved that exposed pulps in gnotobiotic (germ free) rats did not become inflamed while similarly exposed pulps in rats with a full oral flora did. Dental caries and the pulpal inflammation beneath it are clearly microbial in origin. The pulpal injury beneath restorations is also microbial and not due to cytotoxicity of the materials. Bacteria and their products occur between the restoration and the dentin as a result of microleakage.[2–4]

DENTAL CARIES IS THE MOST COMMON SOURCE OF BACTERIA AND THEIR BY-PRODUCTS AFFECTING THE PULP

Dental caries begins beneath a biofilm of dental plaque when environmental factors favor the growth and metabolism of acidogenic bacteria. The population of bacteria that are present in carious lesions is mixed and variable. Chhour et al.[5] demonstrated the presence of 75 species in 10 samples of carious dentin. Up to 31 taxa were represented in each sample. A diverse collection of lactobacilli were found to comprise 50% of the species, with prevotellae also abundant, comprising 15% of the species. In another study significant positive associations were found between *Micromonas micros* and *Porphyromonas endodontalis* detection and inflammatory changes in the pulp.[6] These anaerobes have been strongly implicated in endodontic infections that occur as sequelae to carious pulpitis. Accordingly, the data suggest that the presence of high levels of these bacteria in carious lesions may be indicative of irreversible pulpal pathosis.

A variety of products are released or formed on the death of the bacteria. These include acids and proteinases that dissolve and digest the enamel and dentin, and toxins including lipopolysaccharide (LPS) and lipotechoic acid (LTA). Although bacteria can readily travel within dentinal tubules (Figure 1), toxins pass through dentin and enamel well ahead of the bacteria themselves. Thus, the pulp's inflammatory response is to the toxins rather than the bacteria themselves. Bacteria only invade the pulp at a late stage of the caries process that clinically would present as a carious exposure. More detail of the microbial basis of caries will be found in Chapter 7. Diverse groups and different proportions of species are found in carious lesions. Thus, it has not been possible to produce an antibiotic to inhibit the progress of caries or a vaccine to prevent

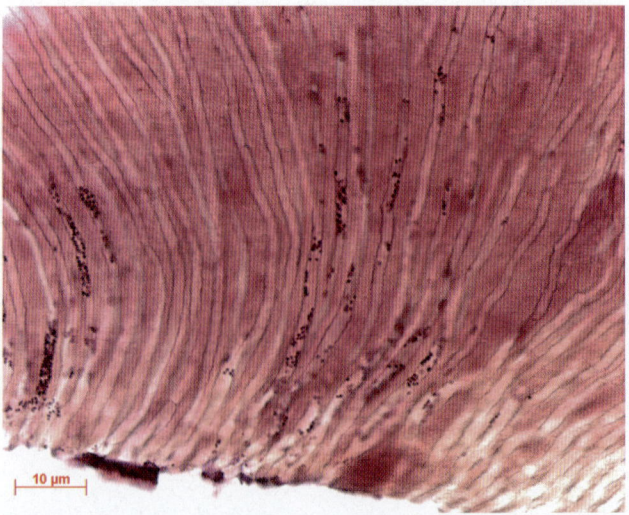

Figure 1 Bacteria in dentinal tubules in vitro. Brown and Brenn.[197] Photo courtesy of Dr. C. Sedgley.

it. The bacteria inhabiting the margins between restorations and dentin are similarly highly variable.

A variety of by-products are produced by cariogenic bacteria. The investigation of these is incomplete and our knowledge about them limited. The toxins that have thus far been recognized include LPS and LTA. LPS results from the breakdown of the walls of gram-negative bacteria and LTA from the breakdown of gram-positive bacteria. As gram-negative bacteria predominate in the plaque over carious lesions, we may assume that LPS is the primary toxin. LPS is a generic term and there are many variations of its molecular structure, and differing virulence, depending on the species of bacteria producing it. The speed of progress of both dental caries and pulpal inflammation is variable, perhaps as a result of variations in the quantity, nature, and combination of toxins.

BACTERIA AND THEIR BY-PRODUCTS CAN REACH THE PULP FROM OTHER SOURCES

Anomalous Crown Morphology, Fractures, and Cracks

Any feature that allows the accumulation of bacteria will increase the likelihood of pulpal inflammation. In most cases, the inflammation will be secondary to caries. In cracked teeth, if they are symptomatic, the cracks will be lined with bacteria that have easy direct access to the pulp (Figure 2).[7]

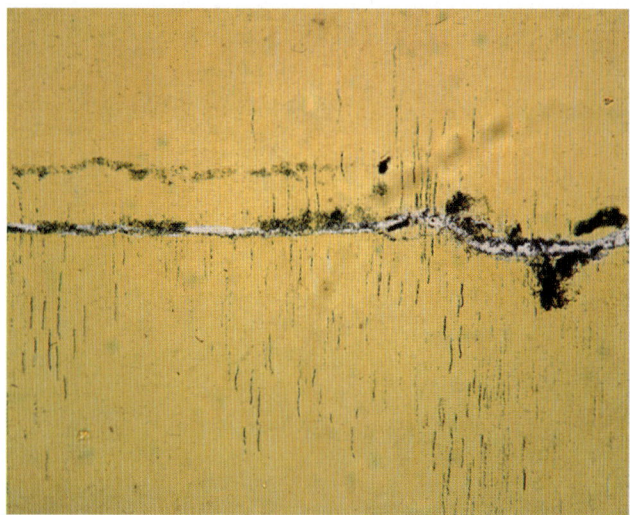

Figure 2 Bacteria within a crack in dentine extending from the crack into dentinal tubules. Brown and Brenn.[197] Photo courtesy of Dr. H. Trowbridge.

Periodontal Disease

Biofilms form on the root surface of periodontal pockets. Their flora is similar to dental caries and would, presumably, release similar toxins. Caries itself is not commonly found in this situation, but toxins may enter the pulp via lateral canals or by diffusing along dentinal tubules. The outward flow of dentinal fluid would oppose this and the relative impermeability of radicular dentin would prevent or reduce it. It has been demonstrated by the examination of extracted teeth with periodontal disease, but no caries, that pathologic changes do occur in the pulp when periodontal disease is present.[8] By removing the cementum layer, periodontal scaling might be thought to allow greater ingress of bacteria and toxins. This has not been supported experimentally.[9] That the pulp has considerable powers to oppose invasion via the dentinal tubules has been clearly demonstrated by observations showing bacteria invading dentinal tubules of devitalized teeth much more readily than the tubules of vital control teeth.[10] Teeth with periodontal disease reaching the apex often remain vital. The consensus seems to be that periodontal diseases may lead to some pulpal changes but they rarely, if ever, lead to necrosis unless there is apical involvement.

Blood Stream (Anachoresis)

Bacteria in circulating blood may be deposited in the pulp. An experimental study on dogs in which some pulps were exposed and capped and then bacteria released in to the blood stream showed accumulations of bacteria in the capped pulps but not in normal pulps.[11] Whether this phenomenon is of clinical significance is unknown.

THE IMMUNE RESPONSE IN THE DENTAL PULP IS THE SAME BASIC PROCESS THAT OCCURS ELSEWHERE BUT IN A UNIQUE ENVIRONMENT

All connective tissues are capable of mounting an immune response that will follow the same basic pattern but is affected by local factors. The pulp's response differs from that in some other tissues. Because bacteria enter the tissue only at a very late stage, the pulp's blood supply is limited and the tissue is within a low-compliance chamber. If the tissue is presented with a new antigen, the innate immune response is initiated and is followed a few days later by the specific response. If the tissue is presented with an antigen it has met before, the specific response will be initiated immediately.

The tissue response to foreign antigens is described in molecular terms in Chapter 9, "Inflammation and

Immunological Response." This present chapter will relate these processes to histologic and physiologic changes in the pulp and to the tissue's attempts at repair.

ANTIGEN RECOGNITION IN THE DENTAL PULP

All three antigen-presenting cell types expressing the type II major histocompatibility complex (MHC) surface proteins, macrophages, dendritic cells, and B lymphocytes, are present and active in the pulp's response to bacteria and toxins. In addition, it is now becoming clear that odontoblasts, being in the ideal position to detect antigens via Toll-like receptors (TLRs), produce a variety of cytokines and chemokines.[12]

In a normal healthy pulp, *macrophages* (Figure 3)[13] are present in a resting form, as monocytes. Macrophages require stimulation by bacteria or cytokines before they express type II MHC molecules.[14] At rest they are found predominantly around blood vessels[15] though a few are distributed throughout the tissue.

Dendritic cells (Figure 4) are characterized by the shape that provides their name. They form a network throughout the pulp concentrating around blood vessels (Figure 5)[15,16] and the odontoblast layer. Some of the dendritic cells in the odontoblast layer extend their processes into the dentinal tubules (Figure 6).[17] They constantly express the MHC

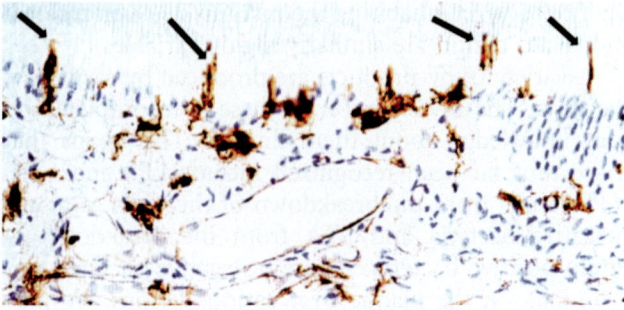

Figure 4 Dendritic cells (brown) in and around the odontoblast layer. Some dendritic cells have processes extending into dentinal tubules (arrows). Immunohistochemistry with blue counterstain. Reproduced with permission from Yoshiba K et al.[17]

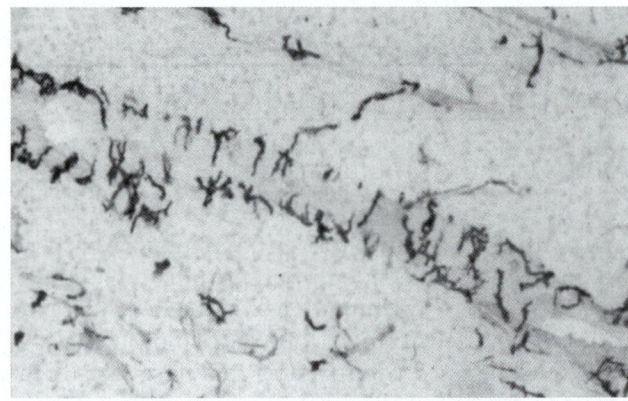

Figure 5 Dendritic cells surrounding and adjacent to blood vessels. Immunohistochemistry. Reproduced with permission from Jontell et al.[13]

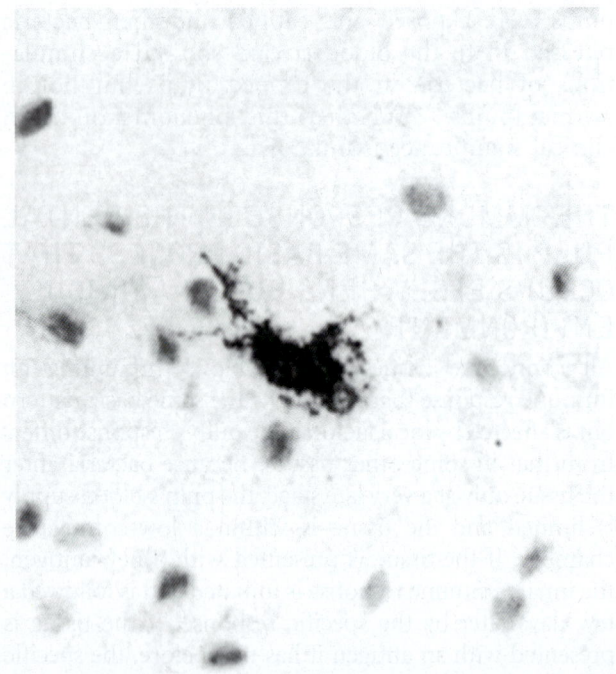

Figure 3 Macrophage from the central pulp. Immunohistochemistry. Reproduced with permission from Jontell et al.[13]

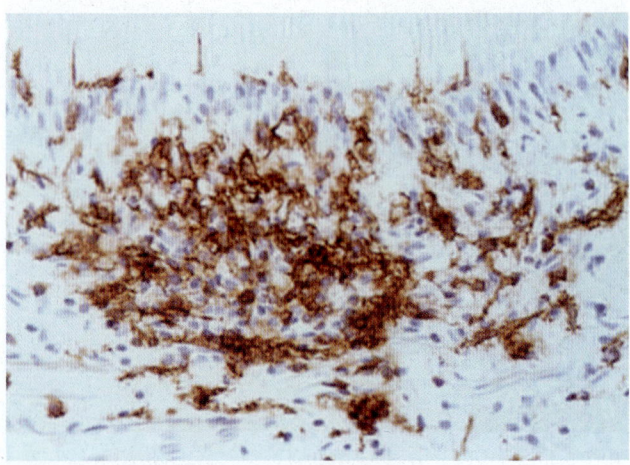

Figure 6 Dendritic cells (brown) congregating in an area of inflammation. Reproduced with permission from Yoshiba K et al.[17]

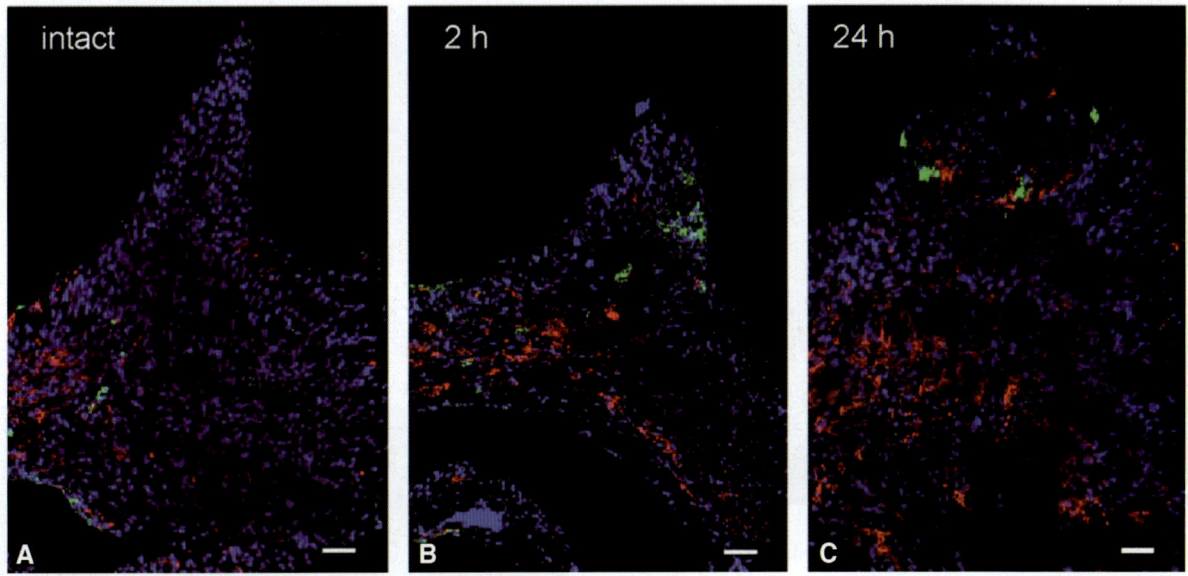

Figure 7 Two different types of dendritic cells (here stained red or green) differentiated by immunohistochemistry. The nuclei of odontoblasts and fibroblasts are stained blue. In this experiment, the pulp was injured and the three images were taken at different time points after the injury. Reproduced with permission from Zhang J et al.[18]

molecules on their surface without provocation. Recent studies[18] indicate that there are two populations of dendritic cell in the dental pulp, one beneath the odontoblast layer and the other around the blood vessels (Figure 7). The number of dendritic cells increases in the pulp when it becomes inflamed and they accumulate beneath the carious lesion (see Figure 6).[17]

B cells are specialized lymphocytes that will become plasma cells. They secrete antibodies during the specific immune response and express the MHC molecules. They have also been reported in the normal pulp but are rather rare.[19,20] Their role in the initial stages of antigen recognition and presentation in the pulp is unclear. Occasional T cells are found in normal pulp (Figure 8) and may be activated by antigen-presenting cells locally.

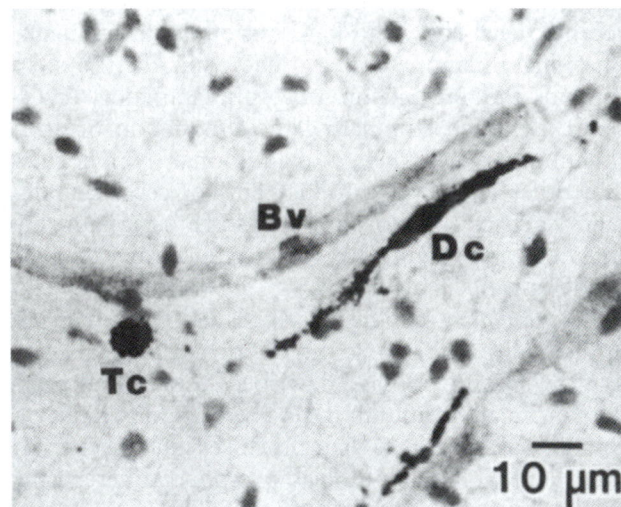

Figure 8 Dendritic cell (Dc) and a T-helper cell (Tc) adjacent to a blood vessel in the pulp. Immunohistochemistry. Reproduced with permission from Jontell et al.[13]

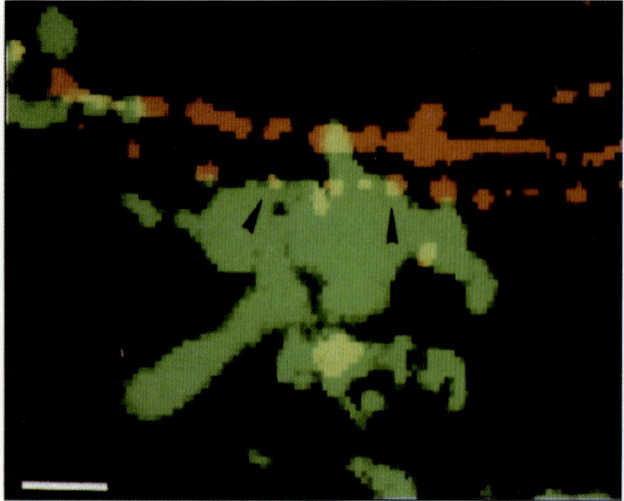

Figure 9 Confocal miscroscope image of a dendritic cell (red) and a nerve fiber (green). Where they are close together is yellow. Reproduced with permission from Okiji et al.[15]

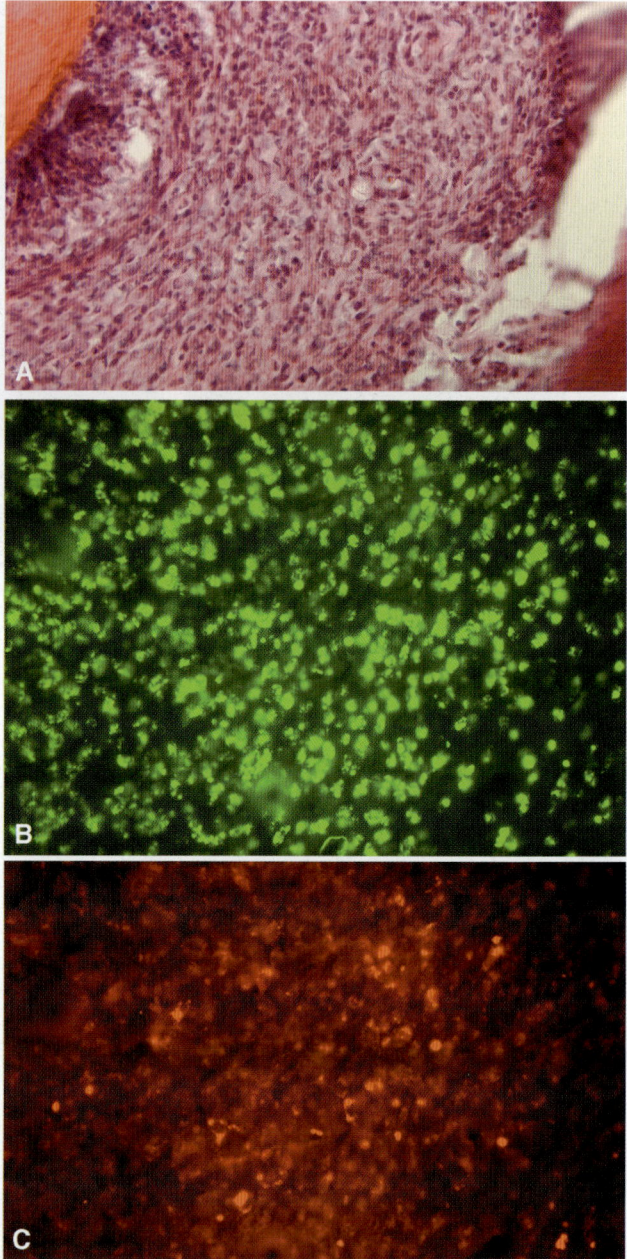

Figure 10 **A,** Area of inflammation in a pulp exposed 1 week earlier and left untreated (hematoxylin and eosin). **B,** and **C,** Same section of the pulp photographed through different color filters after immunofluorescent staining. In **B,** the staining for β-endorphin is seen and in **C,** the staining for T lymphocytes. Some cells are labeled by both stains indicating that T lymphocytes produce β-endorphin. Reproduced with permission from Mudie and Holland.[25]

In the pulp, there is a close anatomic relationship between nerve fibers and dendritic cells (Figure 9), and both increase in parallel when the pulp is inflamed.[17,21] The sympathetic nervous system has recently been shown to have a modulating influence on pulpal inflammation.[22-24] The sympathetic system inhibits the production of proinflammatory cytokines, although stimulating the production of anti-inflammatory cytokines.[22] In addition, T lymphocytes and other leukocytes produce antinociceptive molecules such as β-endorphin and somatostatin during inflammation (Figure 10) which reduce the excitability of pain fibers.[25]

Odontoblasts are the first cells to encounter an antigen diffusing along the dentinal tubules. Veerayutthwilai et al.[12] have described how several markers of innate immunity have been demonstrated on odontoblasts and that their processes include chemokines and TLRs. Odontoblasts respond differentially to the toxins produced by gram-positive and gram-negative bacteria. A gram-negative toxin activating TLR-4 up-regulates mRNAs for interleukin-1β, interleukin-8, tumor necrosis factor-α, and chemokines and TLRs. A synthetic peptide mimicking a toxin from gram-positive bacteria activating TLR-2 down-regulates these mRNAs. Interleukin-1β, tumor necrosis factor-α, and chemokine (C-C motif) ligand 20 were also up-regulated from 6-fold to 30-fold in odontoblast preparations from decayed teeth. These data show that odontoblasts express microbial pattern recognition receptors in situ, allowing differential responses to gram-positive and gram-negative bacteria. They also suggest that pro-inflammatory cytokines and innate immune responses in decayed teeth may result from TLR signaling[12] (Figure 11).

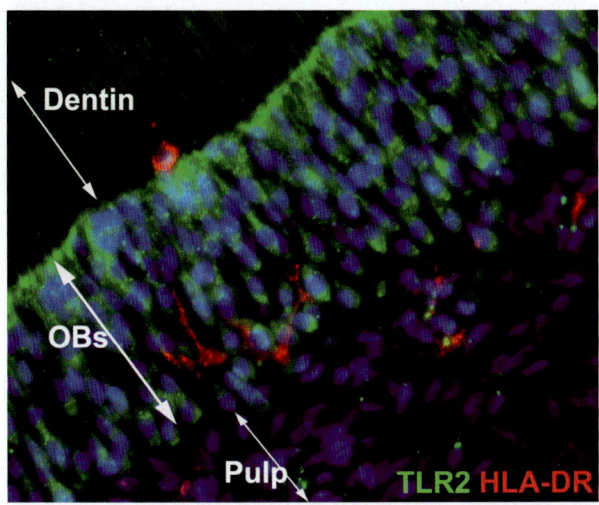

Figure 11 Immunohistochemistry showing Toll-like receptors (green) for bacterial components on odontoblasts (blue nuclei). Some dendritic cells are also stained (red). Toll-like receptors when activated by bacterial components lead to the release of chemokines that participate in the immune response. Reproduced with permission from Zhang et al.[12]

Other studies on odontoblasts in vitro suggest that in response to a bacterial toxin they produce chemokines that attract dendritic cells.[26]

The Process of Antigen Recognition

Dendritic cells and macrophages bind to and phagocytize antigen that is then processed intracellularly, bound to MHC molecules, and moved to the cell membrane for recognition by T cells. B cells bind antigen to specific cell surface receptors. All the antigen-presenting cell types enter the blood stream and carry the surface molecules to the lymph nodes where T cell activation takes place, though some may occur locally (see Figure 8).[16] Each type of antigen-presenting cell carries different types of antigen. The T cells respond not to the antigen itself but to the modified complex in the cell membrane of the antigen-presenting cells. Being stationary, the odontoblast does not participate directly in the activation of T cells but, presumably, activates dendritic cells.

HISTOLOGIC CHANGES IN THE EARLY STAGES OF CARIOUS ATTACK DURING THE NONSPECIFIC IMMUNE RESPONSE ("ACUTE INFLAMMATION")

The classic description of the histology of the inflamed dental pulp beneath caries was published by Seltzer et al. in 1963.[27] They attempted, with limited success, to find a relationship between the clinical presentation of the patient and the histology of the pulp. In so doing, they looked at many examples of pulpitis at many different stages. This and other studies[19,20] have made it possible to piece together a hypothetical description of pulpal changes during the progression of dental caries.

The description is very much hypothetical as dental caries is a highly variable disease and its progress has never been followed continuously in a single tooth. This description was obtained largely by examining paraffin-embedded sections stained with hematoxylin and eosin under the light microscope. Other approaches have been used more recently, particularly immunohistochemistry, electron microscopy, and molecular techniques, but the original microscopic description provides a framework on which newer data may be hung.

Cariogenic bacteria in the dental plaque produce a mixture of acids and enzymes that dissolve the mineral elements of enamel and dentin and then digest the organic matrix. The initial removal of mineral makes the enamel more permeable and the bacterial toxins will diffuse well ahead of cavitation. Once the dentin is reached, the toxins and, much later, the bacteria themselves will travel along the dentinal tubules (see Figure 1). Clearly, variations in the composition and thickness of enamel and dentin, and particularly the patency of the dentinal tubules, will determine the rate at which these toxins reach the pulp. In vital teeth, this movement will be opposed by the outward flow of dentinal fluid. Toxins, however, reach the pulp at a very early stage relative to surface changes. Brannstrom and Lind[28] looked at a large number of extracted teeth and found that in approximately 50% of teeth with white spot lesions and no cavitation, there was histologic evidence of inflammation in the underlying pulp (Figure 12).

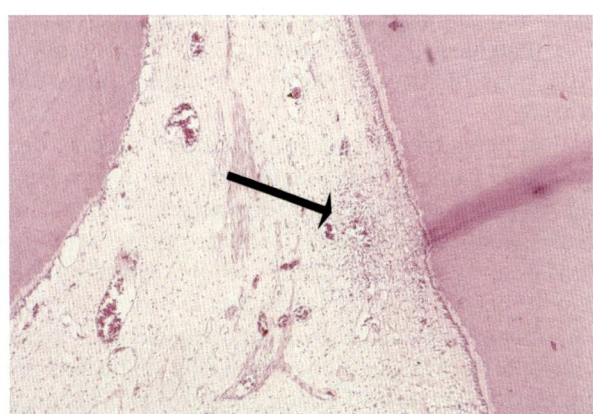

Figure 12 Early inflammatory response (arrow) beneath a non-cavitated carious lesion (hematoxylin and eosin).

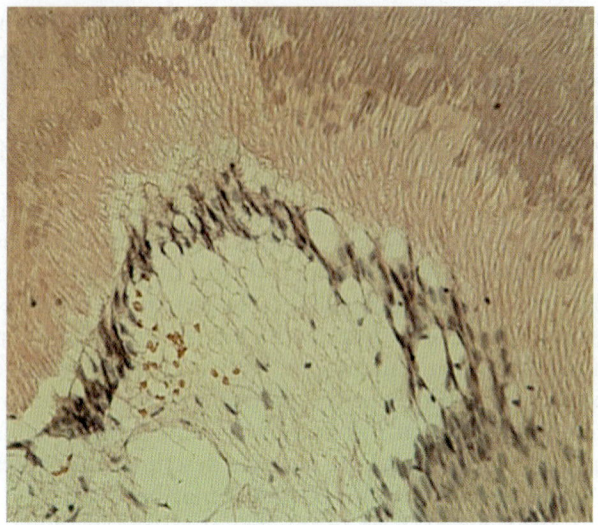

Figure 13 Poorly fixed section of pulp and dentin. The vacuoles and disruption of the odontoblast layer are artifacts (hematoxylin and eosin).

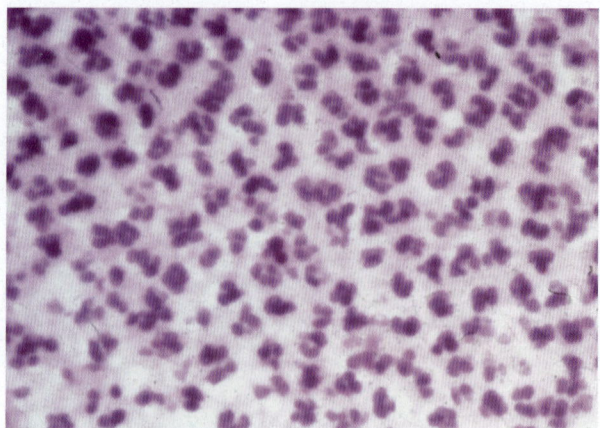

Figure 14 Polymorphonuclear leukocytes in early inflammation (hematoxylin and eosin). Photo courtesy of Dr. H. Trowbridge.

The first cells contacted by the toxic bacterial broth, diffusing down the dentinal tubules, will be the odontoblasts. Some studies describe structural changes in the odontoblast layer even at an early stage. This may not be truly happening when seen in hematoxylin and eosin stained sections. All histologic procedures are subject to artifacts; man-made changes which are not linked to any biologic change. Teeth that have been examined in this way have probably been extracted with forceps and compressed in the process, causing aspiration and damage to the odontoblast layer. The teeth are then fixed usually in formaldehyde, which often causes the pulp to shrink away from the dentin. The later stages of preparation, demineralization, embedding in wax, and sectioning may also cause damage (Figure 13). From studies using other techniques, we now know that odontoblasts respond to toxins and can create a reactionary dentin barrier. It is more than likely that the morphologic changes reported in the odontoblast layer early in the carious process are artifactual.

With hematoxylin and eosin stained sections, dendritic cells cannot be distinguished, but macrophages and neutrophils can be distinguished. The macrophages (and dendritic cells) will recognize a foreign antigen and carry its details to the lymph nodes, though this is a histologically invisible process. Resting macrophages (monocytes) enlarge and become active. Neutrophils leave the blood stream by diapedesis and migrate to the scene of action (Figure 14). This accumulation of phagocytic cells is dominated numerically by neutrophils, recognizable by their lobed nuclei, and is the key morphologic feature in the early response to caries. Mast cells may also be present,[29,30] but they are difficult to detect in routine preparations due to their extreme fragility. They are most common in surface tissues in response to inhaled or ingested antigens. At the same time, vascular and then neural changes (described elsewhere in this chapter) occur. Nerves are not well visualized in hematoxylin and eosin stained sections, and observations of changes in them during inflammation require other techniques. Sometimes an apparent dilation of local blood vessels may be seen.

HISTOLOGIC CHANGES IN THE LATER STAGES OF CARIOUS ATTACK DURING THE SPECIFIC IMMUNE RESPONSE ("CHRONIC INFLAMMATION")

The immediate "inflammatory" phase of the immune response begins very shortly after the antigen arrives in the tissue. If the body has been exposed to the antigen on a previous occasion, then the record of that exposure will have been maintained by the memory T cells. The production of lymphocytes synthesizing specific antibodies will begin very quickly (within a few hours). If the antigen has not been encountered before, new clonal lines of lymphocytes will be developed, which takes several days. In either case, the production of specific lymphocytes will take place in the lymph nodes. With a known antigen, however, there may also be a second challenge, a local interaction between antigen-presenting cells and resident T lymphocytes.[16]

Whether the antigen is new or returning, the histologic appearance of the tissue will be the same, only the time scale will be different. At this stage, the appearance of the pulpal response is characterized by the

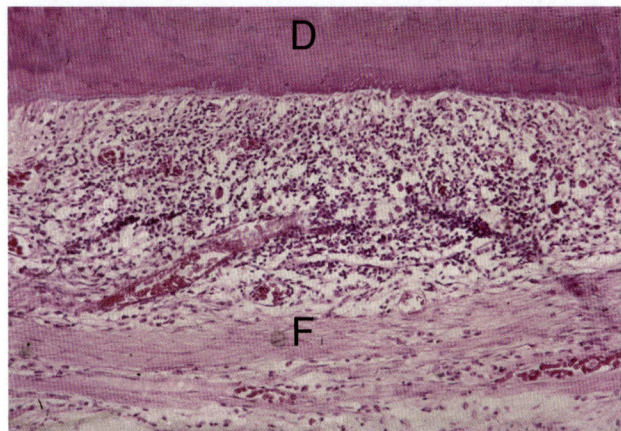

Figure 15 Chronic inflammation. D = dentin. An attempt at fibrous repair (F) is going on at the same time as inflammation. The inflammatory cells are predominantly lymphocytes (hemotoxylin as eosin). Photo courtesy of Dr. H. Trowbridge.

dominating presence of lymphocytes (Figure 15). The numbers of lymphocytes present increases with the severity of clinical symptoms.[21]

A commonly used definition of chronic inflammation, often called a granuloma, is "inflammation of slow progress marked chiefly by the presence of lymphocytes and the formation of reparative tissue" (see Figure 15). This is commonly seen in the dental pulp of extracted carious teeth, some of which may be asymptomatic.

The pulp is a remarkably robust tissue and can, by the production of tertiary dentin, protect itself from persistent carious attacks. If the carious lesion is not treated, however, the increasing quantity of irritants will eventually cause irreversible changes. These are at first limited in size and may even form a "pulpal abscess." The bulk of the tissue around it appears healthy (Figure 16). This local necrosis, unless checked, will progress gradually throughout the tissue and into the periradicular tissues. The progress of tissue damage in the pulp is determined by the presence and spread of bacterial toxins and is not due to the "strangulation" of blood vessels.

HEMODYNAMIC CHANGES IN THE PULP DURING CARIES

An understanding of the vascular component of the immune response in the dental pulp is critical to planning or executing vital pulp therapy. Unfortunately, there are relatively few studies on pulpal vascular changes under carious lesions in humans.[31–36] Several investigators have looked at the effect of experimentally induced inflammation in animal models.[37–41] There are some excellent recent reviews of the vascular physiol-

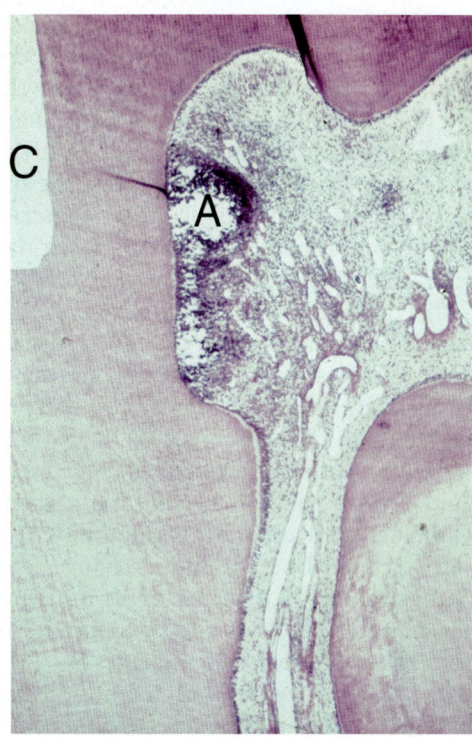

Figure 16 Pulpal abscess (A) beneath a deep cavity preparation (C). Away from the diseased area, the appearance of the pulp is normal (hematoxylin and eosin). Photos courtesy of Dr. H. Trowbridge.

ogy of the dental pulp[40] as well as well the description contained in Chapter 5.

Blood Flow

Measuring blood flow in the dental pulp, even in experimental animals, is a difficult procedure, and data generated are a challenge to interpret. Using plaque extract to initiate inflammation in a rat incisor model, Kim et al.[42] reported a 40% increase in blood flow in a "moderately inflamed" pulp but a 35% reduction in a "partially necrotic" pulp. A more recent study by Bletsa et al.,[41] in a similar model, showed that the application of LPS to the pulp resulted, after 10 minutes, in a reduction in blood flow that continued for the 3-hour duration of the experiments. This was interpreted as a limited ability of the pulp to respond.

Interstitial Fluid Pressure

The healthy dental pulp has an interstitial pressure of 5 to 10 mm Hg.[37,43] One of the key changes during inflammation is the movement of fluid from within the capillaries into the interstitial space. By the laws of physics, increasing the amount of fluid in a rigid chamber leads to an increase in pressure. It was assumed, for a long time, that such a pressure rise in the pulp would cause compression of the blood vessels leading to vascular stasis and necrosis. It was even suggested that this pressure change could lead to strangulation of the vessels at the apex causing necrosis in areas of the pulp not directly affected by the bacterial toxins. Experimental work by Tonder[37] (later Heyeraas) and by Van Hassel[43] measured interstitial fluid pressure in the pulps of experimental animals and showed that although the pressure rose in the area immediately beneath an injury a short distance (2 mm) away, the pressure stayed within normal limits. Even within areas of raised interstitial fluid pressure, capillaries remain patent because of a balancing increase in intra-luminal pressure. The increased interstitial fluid pressure may be beneficial as, when combined with increased capillary permeability, it would lead to an accelerated rate of fluid exchange across the capillary membrane.[40] Any net increase in tissue fluid, especially macromolecules, will be removed by the lymphatics. The presence of lymphatics in the dental pulp has been controversial, but recent studies using ultrastructural and histochemical techniques have established their existence.[44–46] Necrosis occurs beneath persisting carious lesions only when bacterial toxins, spreading throughout the pulp, poison cells directly.

NEURAL CHANGES DURING PULPAL INFLAMMATION

Sympathetic nerves control blood flow by constricting precapillary sphincters[47–49] and by interaction with other elements of inflammation. Sympathetic activity inhibits the production of proinflammatory cytokines although stimulating the production of anti-inflammatory cytokines[50] and is involved in the recruitment of inflammatory cells to the area.[23,51,52] Sympathetic nerves have an inhibitory effect on odontoclasts and stimulate reparative dentin production. In the dental pulp, sympathectomy has no apparent effect on the degree of inflammation induced by mustard oil,[53] whereas Haug et al.[51] found less abscess formation 4 days after deep cavity preparation in normal teeth when compared with sympathectomized teeth. Nor is it possible to detect any differences in the extent or severity of inflammation after pulp exposure injury in sympathectomized rat molars after a waiting period of more than 20 days.[51]

Afferent sensory fibers from the trigeminal system also play an important role in the response to toxins and injury. The afferent fibers release two important neuropeptides, substance P and calcitonin gene-related peptide (CGRP). Both cause vasodilatation and increased capillary permeability. Sympathetic activity causes vasoconstriction and also reduces the release of peptides from afferents. Thus, the sympathetics and the afferents seem to act in opposing directions.

In injured pulps, there is an increased expression of nerve growth factor (NGF) and its receptors.[54,55] A concomitant sprouting of the afferent terminals and increased presence of substance P and CGRP[55–60] also takes place. Sprouting of sensory nerve fibers occurs as early as 1 day after dental injury[61] and decreases 3 to 4 weeks after pulp exposure injury, a time when sympathetic nerve sprouting occurs.[62–65]

Pulpal injury and inflammation are also associated with neural changes outside the pulp itself. In the trigeminal ganglion after pulpal injury, the expression of various neuropeptides increases,[66,67] Trk-B receptors (associated with pain) increase,[68] and nitric oxide synthesis is enhanced.[69] There are also detectable changes in the supporting cells of the ganglion.[70] In the trigeminal nucleus (pars caudalis has been the most studied), pulpal injury and inflammation lead to degenerative changes[71] and to cFos expression, an indication of possible changes in the pain system.[72] Perhaps, most significantly from a clinical point of view are changes in the nucleus related to central sensitization.[73–77] This may help explain the variable presentation of pulpitis in terms of pain.

ANTI-INFLAMMATORY AND ANTINOCICEPTIVE MECHANISMS IN THE DENTAL PULP

During inflammation, there are important interactions between the nervous and immune systems.[78] Neuroimmune interactions control pain through the activation of opioid receptors on sensory nerves by immune-derived opioid peptides.[79] Opioid-containing leukocytes migrate to peripheral sites of inflammation. On exposure to stress, opioid peptides are released, bind to opioid receptors on peripheral sensory neurons, and induce endogenous antinociception. Although much of the research in this area has been done on skin and joints (in relation to arthritis), the efficacy of adding as little as 1 mg of morphine to the local anesthetic used in oral surgery has been demonstrated.[80] Although no published studies focus directly on the effect of local opioids on pulpalgia, the underlying elements have been demonstrated. Opioid receptors are present on pulpal nerves[22,81] and β-endorphin has been shown to be present in, at least, lymphocytes in the inflamed pulp[25] (see Figure 10). Pulpal pain and its modulation and management are discussed in depth in Chapter 10, "Mechanisms of Odontogenic and Nonodontogenic Pain." It is important to see this as a part of the pulpal response to injury. The extent of this antinociceptive mechanism may be variable depending on, for one possibility, the exact nature of the antigen presented. This may, in part, explain the wide variation in the pain experienced as a result of pulpal inflammation.

LESS COMMON PULPAL RESPONSES: CALCIFICATION AND RESORPTION

Calcification of the pulp takes a variety of forms. Discrete pulp stones occur in a large proportion of the population. In one Australian study of young adults (dental students), 46% of the group had radiographic evidence of pulp stones in at least one tooth. Ten percent of all the teeth included in the study contained a pulp stone.[82] The vast majority of pulp stones are found in molars (Figure 17). Although the etiology of pulp stone formation is unknown, there is evidence that pulp stones are more common in patients with atheromatous cardiovascular disease (74%) than in those without (39%).[83] A higher incidence of pulpal mineralization is associated with some genetic disorders such as Ehlers–Danlos syndrome[84] and amelogenesis imperfecta.[85] A generalized, more diffuse mineralization of the pulp may occur after trauma[86,87] and is one of

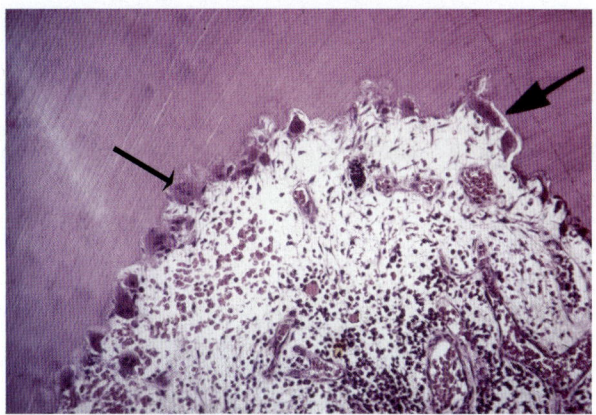

Figure 18 Internal resorption. Multinuclear odontoclasts can be seen within lacunae in thee dentin (arrows) (hematoxylin and eosin). Photo courtesy of Dr. H. Trowbridge.

several good reasons for follow-up radiographs. In this case, there is a clear indication for root canal therapy. Discrete pulp stones are not considered pathologic. Their only clinical significance is that they can add to the adventure of locating and instrumenting root canals.

Internal resorption has been considered an alternative sequela to trauma though most of the literature on this condition consists of case reports (Figure 18). An alternative is to suggest that internal resorption is "idiopathic." The difficulty in establishing a correlation with trauma is probably related to the length of time between the traumatic incident and the diagnosis.

WHEN THE PULPAL RESPONSE SUCCEEDS: REPAIR AND REGENERATION

The immune response, including inflammation, is only one part of the pulp's total response to toxins or injury. When effective, it neutralizes and removes any foreign material and allows and probably initiates the second part, recovery, repair, and regeneration. The repair process can take several forms. The most obvious distinctions relate to the severity of the injury. When no cells are killed, the original odontoblasts can form reactionary (tertiary) dentin (Figure 19). When the odontoblasts are killed, new dentin-forming

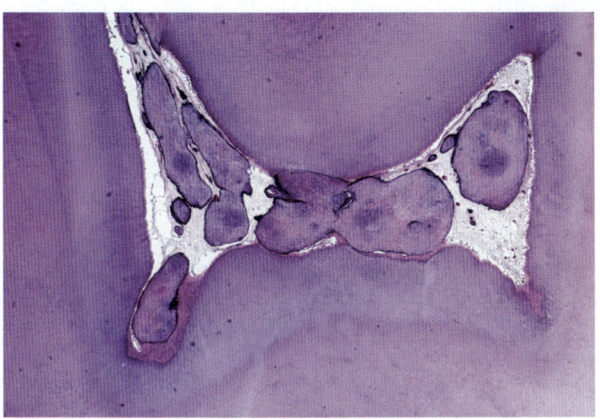

Figure 17 Multiple pulp stones in the pulp chamber of a molar (hematoxylin and eosin). Photo courtesy of Dr. H. Trowbridge.

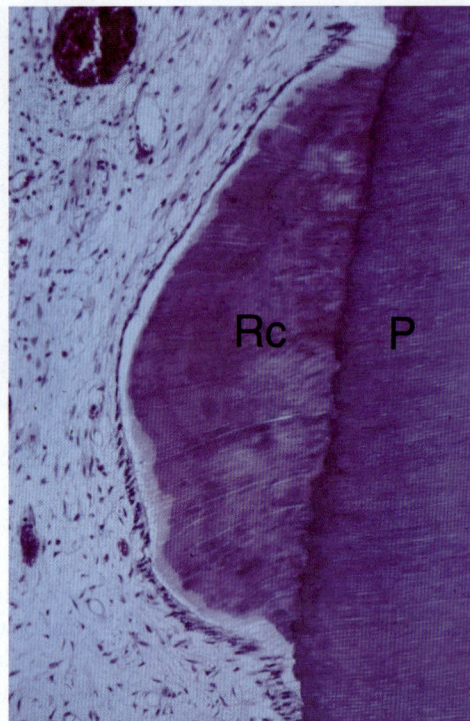

Figure 19 Reactionary (tertiary) dentin (Rc) that has developed beneath a deep cavity preparation. The tubules in the reactionary dentin are continuous with those of the primary dentin (P) (hematoxylin and eosin). Photo courtesy of Dr. H. Trowbridge.

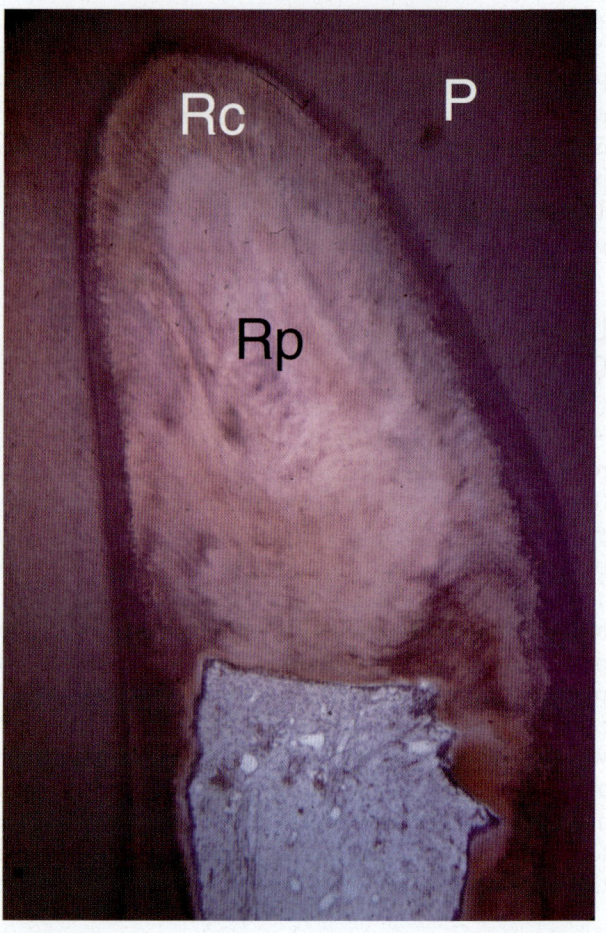

Figure 20 A layer of reactionary (tertiary) dentin (Rc) has formed beneath an injury which has then become severe enough to kill the original odontoblasts resulting in the formation of reparative (tertiary) dentin (Rp), which having been formed by new odontoblasts is atubular (hematoxylin and eosin). P = primary dentin. Photo courtesy of Dr. H. Trowbridge.

cells develop from stem cells (undifferentiated mesenchymal cells) and form reparative (tertiary) dentin (Figure 20).[88,89] The repair of larger areas of damage is more variable and depends on the nature of any clinical intervention. It seems that normally organized pulp tissue does not re-form. An example of extensive tissue damage from which the pulp recovers is the pulp polyp (Figure 21). Rapidly advancing caries in young molars can result in collapse of the crown with a large but self-cleansing pulp exposure. Epithelial cells from the oral mucosa settle on the exposed pulp and form an epidermis (Figure 22). This attests to the pulps ability to respond to injury, but in this case it is futile as the molars involved are often not restorable.

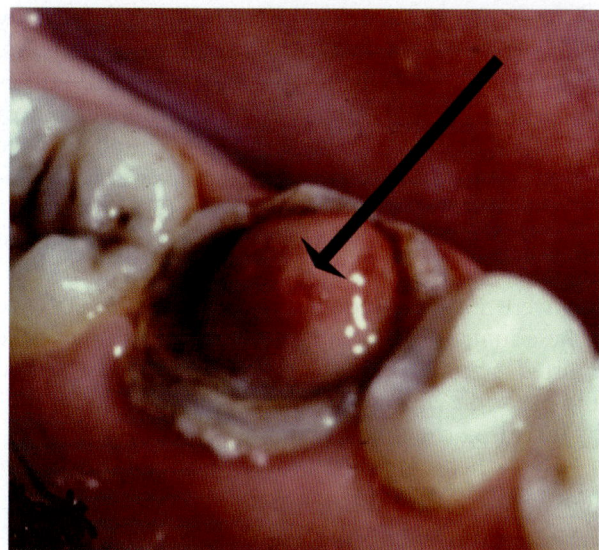

Figure 21 Pulp polyp, also known as hyperplastic pulpitis (arrows). Caries of the lower first permanent molars in a young patient has proceeded so quickly that the walls of the cavity collapsed, leaving a largely self-cleansing area. The pulp survives and its surface has been colonized by epithelial cells shed from the buccal mucosa. Photo courtesy of Dr. H. Trowbridge.

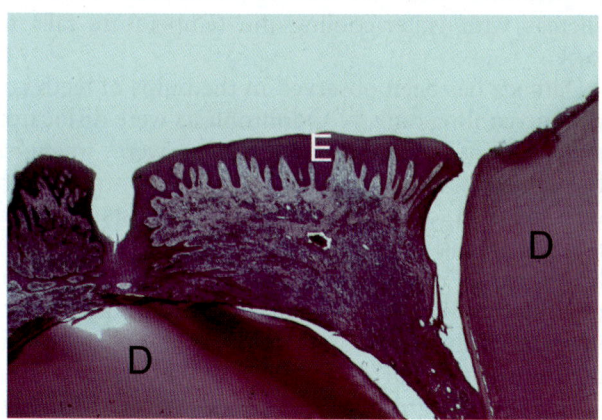

Figure 22 Structure of a pulp polyp. The epithelial cells shed from the buccal mucosa form an epithelium (E) that is normal in appearance. Dentin (D) is present on each side of the polyp that has a dense infiltrate of inflammatory leukocytes (hematoxylin and eosin). Photo courtesy of Dr. H. Trowbridge.

Sometimes the progress of caries and the defensive response can reach a stalemate. The irritant continues but is contained. This, by one definition, is chronic inflammation with injury and repair going on at the same time. Many inflammatory cells, largely lymphocytes, are present as well as areas of fibrous tissue representing an attempt to "wall off" the diseased tissue.

ENCOURAGING A SUCCESSFUL RESPONSE

From a clinical standpoint, it is important to recognize that the pulp has a strong innate ability to respond and repair. Most of our strategies for encouraging pulpal repair involve removal of the irritant and diseased tissue and the prevention of further injury. Calcium hydroxide, for example, probably does nothing directly to stimulate reparative dentin formation but is permissive of the pulp's inherent activity. Mineral trioxide aggregate may have some stimulatory activity, but its main property may be its high level of biocompatibility and its success in preventing recontamination. With the discovery of biologically active molecules such as growth factors and matrix proteins, there is the possibility of stimulating repair.[90,91] The development of cultures of pulpal cells and supporting scaffolds may allow tissue regeneration. Neither of these approaches is, at present, ready for clinical adoption.[92]

FACTORS LIMITING THE PULP'S RESPONSE

The only significant factor that limits the pulp's ability to respond to injury is age. The older pulp has a reduced number of cells,[93] innervation,[94] and vascularity,[95,96] but the immune response remains active.[88,89]

Iatrogenic Effects on the Dental Pulp

LOCAL ANESTHETICS

Local anesthetics reduce pulpal blood flow by approximately half when they contain vasoconstrictors.[97,98] This effect is due almost entirely to the vasoconstrictor. It is important to remember that when preparing a cavity in an anesthetized tooth the pulp is in a suboptimal condition to respond. Much of what we know about the pulp's response to cavity preparation and materials has been from animal experiments in which general rather than local anesthetics were used.

CAVITY/CROWN PREPARATION

Heat: Experimental Observations

The basic effect of heat on mineralized tissue has been best documented on bone.[99-102] From this work, a value of 10°C above body temperature is frequently cited as the threshold to cause irreversible damage to vital tissues.[99] Higher temperatures and increased application times lead to greater damage. An increase of surface temperature to 47°C held for only 1 minute resulted in minor reversible injury. Increasing the duration to 5 minutes caused irreversible damage to calcified bone and marrow that healed by repair. Raising the temperature to 50°C but reducing the duration back to 1 minute produced injury similar to the injury caused by raising the temperature to 47°C at 5 minutes. Temperatures of 60°C and higher will result in bone necrosis.[99] Severe cold will, of course, also damage tissue. The formation of water crystals within cytoplasm will kill a cell. This occurs at a temperature of approximately 2°C below zero,[103] a temperature never likely to be experienced in the mouth.

Moderate elevation of temperature on the external surface of a tooth can raise the internal temperature of the pulp to the point that injury occurs. A temperature increase of 5.5°C above body temperature as observed by Zach and Cohen[104] is frequently cited as the threshold for damage to the pulp. This observation was made after applying a soldering iron preheated to 275°C to the teeth of monkeys for a limited time. When the same temperature was applied for a longer period of time, generating an 11.1°C increase in pulp temperature, 60% of pulps became necrotic. However, this very abrupt application of high heat may not translate directly to clinical situations.

A more recent study applied a gradually increasing heat stimulus until the patient indicated sensitivity then sustained it for 30 seconds. The temperature change across the dentin was measured after extraction. The maximum temperature increase was 14.7°C reaching a measured temperature of 50.9°C. Histologic examination of the heated pulp revealed neither necrosis nor even alteration of the odontoblast layer. All the patients remained symptom free through the duration of the study, and all teeth responded to cold testing just before extraction.[105] These in vivo experimental observations were made on un-restored, noncarious human teeth scheduled for extraction for orthodontic treatment. These are young patients and their pulps will have a good blood supply and will not have been affected by previous injury. This model may not be fully revealing of the effects of heat on the mature pulp.

The more moderate pulp responses observed by Baldissara et al.[105] are borne out by earlier studies. Pulps from human subjects that were examined immediately and 1 month after a 30-second application of 150°C to dentin 0.5 mm thick were found to have localized areas of injury though no pulps were completely necrotic.[106] The most common histologic observation was a breakdown of the odontoblast layer. Some of the pulps had localized areas of necrosis. The affected areas were not surrounded by inflammatory cells. None of these injuries was symptomatic. Other studies have reported similar results.[107,108] It appears the dental pulp has some capacity to adapt to a moderate, gradually increased rise in temperature.

Heat: Cutting Dentin

The amount of heat produced during cutting is determined by the sharpness of the bur, the amount of pressure exerted on the bur, and the length of time the cutting instrument contacts tooth structure. The temperature on the surface of a rotating dental bur in contact with dentin has been reported to be as high as 417°C.[107] High-speed air-driven handpieces require some method of cooling the tooth in order to safely use these handpieces. The two cooling methods most frequently applied have been air-cooling and water-cooling. Pulp temperatures with air-cooling alone rise to 60°C whereas with water-cooling the temperature falls to 26°C.[109]

Damage has been observed in the pulps of teeth cut with air-cooling only.[110] Odontoblasts were dislocated into dentinal tubules and there were vacuoles throughout the odontoblast layer. By contrast, with water-cooling, displacement of odontoblasts occurred in less than half the teeth and was less marked when it did occur. Fifteen days after cavity preparation, inflammation was noted in all the pulps under cavities prepared with air-cooling only. On the other hand, inflammation occurred in only 25% of water-cooled group. In both groups, recovery occurred within 200 days with the formation of tertiary reparative dentin.

Dentin is a good insulator and thus careful cutting is not likely to damage the pulp unless the thickness of dentin between preparation and pulp is less than 1.0 mm.[111] Even then, the response should be mild.

The "blushing" of dentin during crown preparation is thought to be due to frictional heat resulting in vascular injury (hemorrhage) in the pulp.[106] The dentin takes on an underlying pinkish hue soon after the operative procedure. The most intense level of frictional heat is generated with a large diamond stone when teeth are prepared for a full crown. Crown preparation performed without the use of a coolant leads to a marked reduction in pulpal blood flow, presumably because of vascular stasis and thrombosis.

The safest way to prepare tooth structure is to use ultrahigh speeds of rotation (100,000–250,000 rpm), with an efficient water-cooling system, light pressure, and intermittent cutting. During cutting at high speeds, the revolving bur creates an area of turbulence that tends to deflect a stream of water. Therefore, an air–water spray with sufficient volume and pressure must be used if the coolant is to overcome the rotary turbulence. The bur–dentin interface should be constantly wet. Cavity preparation with a low-speed handpiece, sharp bur, and light, intermittent pressure is only slightly more injurious than cutting at high speeds. Hand instruments and low-speed cutting are relatively safe ways to finish a cavity preparation, rather than using a high-speed handpiece with the water coolant shut off.

Heat: Laser Beams

The use of laser beams to fuse enamel and reduce the likelihood of carious invasion has been suggested.[108] Different lasers with different energy levels may also be used to remove caries. Laser irradiation can generate a large increase in temperature within dentin and pulp tissue.[112] Proper power setting, time of application, and use of water spray will mitigate the temperature increase to levels below the heat threshold of pulp damage.[113,114] The use and effects of laser irradiation in endodontic treatment is thoroughly reviewed in Chapter 26E, "Lasers in Endodontics."

PINS

Pulp damage may result from pinhole preparation or pin placement. Coolants do not reach the depth of the pin preparation. During pinhole preparation, there is always the risk of pulp exposure. Furthermore, friction-locked pins often produce micro-fractures that may extend to the pulp, subjecting the pulp to irritation and the effects of microleakage. The use of pins should be discouraged.[115,116]

CAVITY CLEANSING

A prolonged blast of compressed air aimed onto freshly exposed vital dentin will cause a rapid outward movement of fluid in patent dentinal tubules.[117] Tubule diameter midway between the pulp and the dentin-enamel junction (DEJ) is only 1.5 μm. Therefore, the removal of fluid from the tubules by a blast of air activates strong capillary forces. These in turn lead to a rapid outward flow of dentinal fluid.[118] Fluid removed from the tubules at the dentin surface is replaced by fluid from the pulp.

The rapid outward flow of fluid in the dentinal tubules stimulates nociceptors in the dental pulp producing pain. Rapid outward fluid movement may also result in odontoblast displacement.[118] Odontoblasts are dislodged from the odontoblast layer and drawn outward into the tubules. Within a short time, the displaced cells undergo autolysis and disappear. Providing the pulp has not been severely injured either by caries or by other factors, displaced odontoblasts are replaced by new cells derived from stem cells deeper in the pulp. In this way, the odontoblast layer is reconstituted by "replacement" odontoblasts capable of producing tertiary dentin. Even vigorous drying of dentin alone does not result in severe injury to the underlying pulp. Drying agents containing lipid solvents such as acetone and ether have been used to clean cavity floors. Because of their rapid rate of evaporation, application of these agents to exposed dentin produces strong hydrodynamic forces in the tubules causing odontoblast displacement. Cavities should be dried with cotton pellets and short blasts of air rather than harsh chemicals. Disinfectants have, in the past, been used in cavity cleansing. There seems to be no particular benefit to this, and they are now rarely used as they are potentially toxic to the pulp.

Etching Dentin/Smear Layer

Cutting dentin results in a smear layer on the cut surface consisting of fragments of microscopic mineral crystals and organic matrix.[119–125] This layer may interfere with the adherence of adhesive restorative materials although some newer bonding agents reportedly bond well to the smear layer. Acidic cavity-cleansing products and chelating agents have been used to remove the smear layer, but the use of these depends on the nature of the restorative material. The smear layer does have one desirable property. By blocking the orifices of dentinal tubules, the smear plugs greatly decrease the permeability of dentin. While the smear layer is a semipermeable membrane, it is not a barrier to bacteria or bacterial products.

Complete dissolution of the smear layer opens the dentinal tubules, significantly increasing the permeability of dentin. If the dentin is left unsealed, the diffusion of irritants to the pulp may intensify and prolong the severity of pulpal reactions. Available experimental evidence is contradictory. Some evidence indicates that etching as a step in restoration may reduce microleakage.[126] Other evidence suggests that etching, when there is less then 300 μm of remaining dentin thickness (RDT), causes pulpal damage.[127]

In the absence of microleakage, acid etching of dentin does not appear to produce injury to the pulp, because calcium and phosphate ions are released producing a buffering action. Even when placed in deep cavities, acid etchants produce only a small increase in hydrogen ion concentration in the pulp.[128]

IMPRESSIONS AND TEMPORARY CROWNS

Temperatures of up to 52°C have been recorded in the pulp during impression taking with modeling compound. Modeling compound may be damaging because of the combination of heat and pressure.[129–132] Fortunately, this technique is no longer used. Rubber base and hydrocolloid materials do not injure the pulp.

The heat generated during the exothermic polymerization of autopolymerizing resins may also injure the pulp. Cooling is strongly recommended when provisional crowns are fabricated directly. Before cementing provisional crowns, the crown preparation should be carefully lined with temporary cement to minimize microleakage. The temporary crown/cement should be in place for a short period of time; temporary cements are not stable and will eventually wash out. Microleakage around temporary crowns is a common cause of postoperative sensitivity.

CROWN CEMENTATION

During the cementation of crowns, inlays, and bridges, strong hydraulic forces may be exerted on the pulp as cement compresses the fluid in the dentinal tubules.[133] In deep preparations, this can result in a separation of the odontoblast layer from the predentin. Vents in the casting will allow cement to escape and facilitate seating.

DENTAL MATERIALS

Microleakage

The most important characteristic of any restorative material, in determining its effect on the pulp, is its ability to form a seal that prevents the leakage of bacteria and their products onto dentin and then into the pulp.[2,127,134]

Cytotoxicity

Certain restorative materials are composed of chemicals having the potential to irritate the pulp. However, when placed in a cavity, the intervening dentin usually neutralizes or prevents leachable ingredients from reaching the pulp in a high enough concentration to cause injury. For example, eugenol in zinc oxide–eugenol (ZnOE) is potentially irritating, but very little can reach the pulp. Phosphoric acid is a component of silicate and zinc orthophosphate (ZnOP) cements and was thought to be highly injurious to the pulp. However, the buffering capacity of dentin greatly limits the ability of hydrogen ions to reach the pulp. It is now clear that the problems following use of these materials were due to their high degree of shrinkage and subsequent microleakage.[4]

Clearly, the thickness and permeability of dentin between a material and the pulp affect the response to the material. In addition, the penetration of some materials through dentin may be limited by the outward flow of fluid through the tubules that will be increased if the pulp is inflamed.[135] This is a factor that has been overlooked in many in vitro studies focusing on the passage of materials through dentin.

Many cytotoxicity studies focus on isolated cell types in culture and do not take into account the immunocompetent cells present in the intact pulp. Materials may have a differential effect on these cells by either stimulating or inhibiting their activity.[136]

Materials are more toxic when they are placed directly on an exposed pulp. Cytotoxicity tests carried out on materials in vitro or in soft tissues may not predict the effect these materials have on the dental pulp. The toxicity of the individual components of a material may vary.[137,138] A set material may differ in toxicity from an unset material. The immediate pulpal response to a material is much less significant than the long-term response. Upon examination a few days after placement, there may be a strong inflammatory response. After a few months, the inflammatory response may have receded and repair has taken over. The best measure of long-term response is the thickness of tertiary dentin laid down by the affected pulp.

Heat upon Setting

Many restorative materials have exothermic setting reactions. Temperature increases during setting procedures may be over 10°C[139] but can be limited to 2 to 3°C with care.[132,140] Cooling techniques include the use of air-/water-cooling and removing the temporary upon initial polymerization.[141]

Some luting cements generate heat during setting; it has been suggested that this might cause pulpal injury. The most exothermic luting material is ZnOP cement. However, during setting, an intrapulpal temperature increase of only 2°C was recorded. Heat of this magnitude is not sufficient to injure the pulp.

Desiccation by Hygroscopy

Some hygroscopic materials may potentially cause injury by withdrawing fluid from dentin. However, little relationship exists between the hydrophilic properties of materials and their effect on the pulp. Moisture absorbed by materials is probably much less than that removed from dentin during cavity drying, a procedure that produces an insignificant amount of pulpal inflammation.[140]

Specific Materials

ZINC OXIDE–EUGENOL

ZnOE has many uses in dentistry, having had a long history as a temporary filling material, cavity liner, cement base, and luting agent for provisional cementation of castings. Before the introduction of calcium hydroxide, ZnOE was the material of choice for direct pulp capping.[127,142–144]

Eugenol, biologically the most active ingredient in ZnOE, is a phenol derivative and is toxic when placed in direct contact with tissue.[145] It also possesses antibacterial properties.[146] Eugenol's usefulness in pain control is attributed to its ability to block the transmission of nerve impulses.[147] A thin mix of ZnOE significantly reduces intradental nerve activity when placed in a deep cavity preparation in cat's teeth; a dry mix of ZnOE has no effect.[148]

When included in cements to temporize crown preparation, some eugenol does reach the pulp, but the amounts are small and unrelated to RDT. In in vitro studies "desensitizing" agents do not seem to reduce the penetration of eugenol, though time does.[149] The release of eugenol is by a hydrolytic mechanism that is dependent on the presence of fluid. With little fluid available, release is low.[142,143]

The most important property of ZnOE is that it provides a tight marginal seal preventing microleakage. Its superiority as a temporary restorative material is enhanced by its antimicrobial properties.

ZINC PHOSPHATE CEMENT

ZnOP is a popular luting and basing agent. It has a high modulus of elasticity and therefore is commonly used as a base beneath amalgam restorations. The phosphoric acid liquid phase was formerly thought to injure the pulp. However, recent studies have shown that this is not the case. Cementation of castings with ZnOP is well tolerated by the pulp. Researchers reported that ZnOP is more likely to produce pulpal sensitivity at the time of cementation and 2 weeks after cementation than glass ionomer. However, 3 months after cementation, there is no difference in sensitivity.[150–153]

POLYCARBOXYLATE CEMENT

When placed in cavities or used as a luting cement, zinc polycarboxylate does not irritate the pulp. In cementing well-fitting crowns and inlays, neither polycarboxylate nor ZnOP cements contract enough to permit the ingress of bacteria. Consequently, it is unnecessary to apply a varnish or liner to cavity walls; doing so only reduces cement adhesion.[153–155]

RESTORATIVE RESINS

The first adhesive bonding and resin composite systems that were developed contracted during polymerization, resulting in gross microleakage and bacterial contamination of the cavity. Bacteria on cavity walls and within axial dentin are associated with moderate pulpal inflammation. Over a period of time, some composites absorb water and expand; this tends to compensate for initial contraction. To limit microleakage and improve retention, enamel margins are beveled and acid etched to facilitate mechanical bonding. When compared with unfilled resins, the newer resin composites present a coefficient of thermal expansion similar to that of tooth structure. With recently developed hydrophilic adhesive bonding composite systems, the problem of marginal leakage appears to have been diminished.[156–158]

GLASS IONOMER CEMENTS

Glass ionomer cement's original use was as an esthetic restorative material but now has also found use as liners, luting agents, and pulp-capping agents (sometimes in conjunction with calcium hydroxide). When placed on exposed pulps in noncarious teeth, glass ionomer cement shows a degree of bacterial microleakage similar to that of composite resins but less than half that of calcium hydroxide cement.[159,160] The incidence of severe pulpal inflammation or necrosis caused by glass ionomer cement on exposed healthy pulps is similar to that for calcium hydroxide but greater than that for composite resins.[160] When placed in cavities in which the pulp is not exposed and where there is a narrow RDT (0.5–0.25 μm), both calcium hydroxide and composite resin show faster deposition of tertiary dentin than glass ionomer cements.[161]

When used as a luting agent, the pulpal response to glass ionomer cements is similar to that of polycarboxylate and ZnOP cements.[151] For some time after their introduction as luting agents, glass ionomer cements were associated with post-cementation sensitivity. A more recent clinical trial has shown that, using appropriate technique, the incidence of sensitivity using these agents is no greater than that with other commonly used luting agents.[152]

AMALGAM

Amalgam alloy is widely used material for restoring posterior teeth. There is shrinkage during setting, which results in microleakage.[162] This decreases as corrosion products accumulate between restoration and cavity walls and can be reduced by the use of liners.[163] Amalgam is the only restorative material in which the marginal seal improves with time. Esthetics and public concern with the mercury content of amalgams have lead to an accelerated use of composite resins as posterior restorative materials. Their use, however, is more technique sensitive than amalgams. In deep cavities in posterior teeth, composites are associated with more pulpal injury than amalgams because of microleakage.[158]

Polishing Restorations

Polishing glass ionomer and composite restorations does not cause an increased temperature at the pulp–dentin interface.[164] Polishing amalgam restorations, however, can produce temperatures that may be damaging. With high contact pressure, high speed, and no coolant, in vitro temperature increases of greater than 20 °C have been recorded within 30 seconds.[127] However, a handpiece rotating at 2,500 rpm that was held for 60 seconds with a relatively light (55 gm) force generated a maximum temperature increase of only 6.2 °C.[121] This occurred when a Burlew disk without coolant was used as the polishing agent. With air-cooling, the increase was 2.0 °C. When polishing an amalgam restoration with continuous pressure and no water coolant, it is recommended to not exceed 4,000 rpm.[165] With use of coolant, light pressure, and intermittent contact during polishing, there is a low likelihood of heat-generated pulp damage.

Post-restorative Hypersensitivity

Many patients complain of hypersensitivity after a restorative procedure.[139,152] This may be due to any one or an accumulation of the factors listed above. Discomfort is usually of short duration. If pain is prolonged, a preexisting pulpitis may have been exacerbated. If delayed in onset by days, the cause may be microleakage of bacterial toxins under a poorly sealed temporary restoration. The absence of postoperative sensitivity after restoration with modern composites of both class I and II preparations has been demonstrated in clinical studies suggesting that variations in technique may be responsible for the anecdotal reports of sensitivity.[164,166] The use of hydroxymethacrylate and glutaraldehyde "desensitizer" does not reduce the incidence of sensitivity.[165] Self-etching, self-priming dentin-bonding systems reduce the incidence of sensitivity following the restoration of deep carious cavities.[121]

If pain evoked is by biting on a recently restored tooth, an intracoronal restoration may be exerting a strong shearing force on the dentin walls of the preparation. It is more likely to be due to injury to the periodontal ligament resulting from hyperocclusion. Hyperocclusion from an extra-coronal restoration is not injurious to the pulp but may cause a transient hypersensitivity.

Vital Tooth Bleaching

Overnight external bleaching of anterior teeth with 10% carbamide peroxide causes mild pulpitis that is reversed within 2 weeks.[167] In vitro studies show that the principle bleaching agent, hydrogen peroxide, can reach the pulp[168] after application to the enamel. Whether this occurs in vivo is unknown. Outward fluid flow in dentinal tubules and other factors would reduce the effect. Both short-term and long-term (9–12 years) clinical observations on bleached teeth report no significant pulpal changes.[169] Heat-activated bleaching agents can cause intrapulpal temperatures to rise by 5 to 8 °C when measured in vitro.[170]

Vitality Testing

Thermal "vitality" testing utilizes media at temperatures that certainly have the potential to damage tissues. Heated gutta-percha reaches a temperature of around 200 °C just before the smoke point, and a cold-test substance like carbon dioxide snow has an inherent temperature of –78 °C. A heat-testing device like the System B with the appropriate tip is recommended to be set at a temperature of 200 °C. The question must be asked whether these extreme temperatures are transmitted to dental pulp during clinical testing and whether there is any likelihood that the tissue may be damaged. Rickoff et al.[171] reported combined in vivo and in vitro findings with no damage to pulp tissue following use of flame-heated gutta-percha and carbon dioxide snow. Gutta-percha was heated to the smoke point and then applied to a tooth surface in vivo. The gutta-percha remained in contact for 1 to 10 seconds. For cold testing, a carbon dioxide pencil of 3.5 mm diameter was held to the tooth for 5 seconds to 5 minutes. The teeth were extracted and examined histologically. To measure the temperatures generated at the pulpal–dentin junction (PDJ), a thermistor was placed onto the dentin surface of an extracted tooth. Internal temperature was recorded as the external surface was heated to different temperatures. The maximum PDJ temperature reached with heat testing was 39.9°C (10-second application) and for cold was 9.5°C (5-minute application). These temperatures do not reach the thresholds at which tissue damage will occur. Additionally, the time of application falls within the range of likely clinical application.

Augsburger et al.[172] observed similar temperature decreases with their in vitro and in vivo measurements. The greatest temperature drop in their in vitro evaluation was 6.3°C. This fall in temperature occurred in a tooth with a full gold crown, which received a 5-second application of carbon dioxide snow. The greatest temperature drop in noncarious teeth was 2.5°C (also with carbon dioxide). They also tested water and skin refrigerant that had maximum temperature drops at the PDJ of 2.8 and 1.8°C, respectively. The greatest temperature transference between adjacent teeth was a decrease of 1.7°C between a tooth with a gold crown and one with an amalgam. Rickoff et al.[171] experienced a similar, very small temperature drop of 0.9°C, after applying carbon dioxide to four premolar teeth in vitro. In vivo histologic analysis revealed no alteration from normal tissue appearance after a 2-minute[173] or a 5-minute[174] application of carbon dioxide. When carbon dioxide was held to a tooth for 20 minutes, the pulp suffered with necrosis of odontoblasts.[175] It is safe to conclude that heat and cold testing within normal clinical parameters will not damage the dental pulp.

Orthodontics

TOOTH MOVEMENT

Orthodontic tooth movement of a routine nature does not cause clinically significant changes in the dental pulp. Responses to pulp testing, especially electrical, may be unreliable.[175] The heavy forces used to reposition impacted canines frequently lead to pulp necrosis or calcific metamorphosis.[176] Intrusion but not extrusion reduces pulpal blood flow for a few minutes as the pressure is applied.[177] Capillaries proliferate in the pulps of moving teeth.[177] A variety of growth factors are produced including vascular endothelial growth factor (VEGF) that may explain this increase in vascularity.[178–180]

REMOVAL OF ORTHODONTIC BRACKETS

Some of the methods of removing brackets at completion of orthodontic treatment have the potential to cause injury to the pulp.[181–186] Brackets may be simply ground off, or pincher-type pliers may be used to mechanically remove an orthodontic bracket. A third method of bracket removal is use of an electrothermal device (ETD) that heat-softens the bonding composite expediting removal of the bracket. Heat transferred from the ETD has been measured as high as 45.6°C[187] on the pulpal side of dentin in vitro experiments, though most reports have been in a lower range.[181,188,189] When residual composite is cleaned up by grinding it away, pulp-side temperature actually decreased below ambient temperature when water coolant was used.[181] Metal brackets seem to have a greater capacity to transmit heat to inner dentinal surfaces than ceramic brackets.[183]

In vivo evaluation has recorded much lower temperatures and has reported limited pulpal damage. Jost-Brinkman et al.[182] observed no pulpal inflammation 4 weeks after electrothermally debonding brackets from human teeth. The maximum temperature recorded was 6.9°C over a period of 43 seconds. There has been consensus that electrothermal debonding does not cause gross damage or necrosis of dental pulp. However, there may be limited peripheral disruption of odontoblasts with slight inflammation.[181,185,186,190]

Ultrasonic Scaling

Activation of ultrasonic instruments generates large amounts of heat. Although dentin is not a particularly good thermal conductor, this heat can still transfer through dentin to affect pulp tissue. Ultrasonic scaling of roots requires prolonged contact of an ultrasonic device, and the potential for pulp damage exists. As with other heat-generating dental procedures, proper cooling with water prevents gross pulpal damage. In live dogs, ultrasonic scaling did not create heat-induced pulpal damage when water coolant was used.[191] Interestingly, histologic examination did reveal acute pulpitis, but it was attributed to the vibratory effects of the ultrasonic device rather than the temperature, because the measured temperature did not reach a level sufficient to cause damage. An interesting phenomenon of ultrasonic dental scalers is that the load of force with which the ultrasonic tip is held against the tooth has a much greater effect (4×) on the heat generated in the dentin substrate than the power setting.[192] One investigation found greater heat generation with diamond sonic tips versus smooth surface tips and greater heat production with heavy versus light force (1 N and 0.3 N).[193] A diamond tip with heavy pressure resulted with in vitro measurement of 36°C increase. When water coolant was used, all measurements were below 4.2°C increase. Proper water-cooling of both ultrasonic and sonic scalers will prevent excessive heat production in the pulp.

Systemic Factor

HEREDITARY HYPOPHOSPHATEMIA

An unusual and rare cause of pulpal dystrophy and necrosis is found in individuals afflicted with hereditary

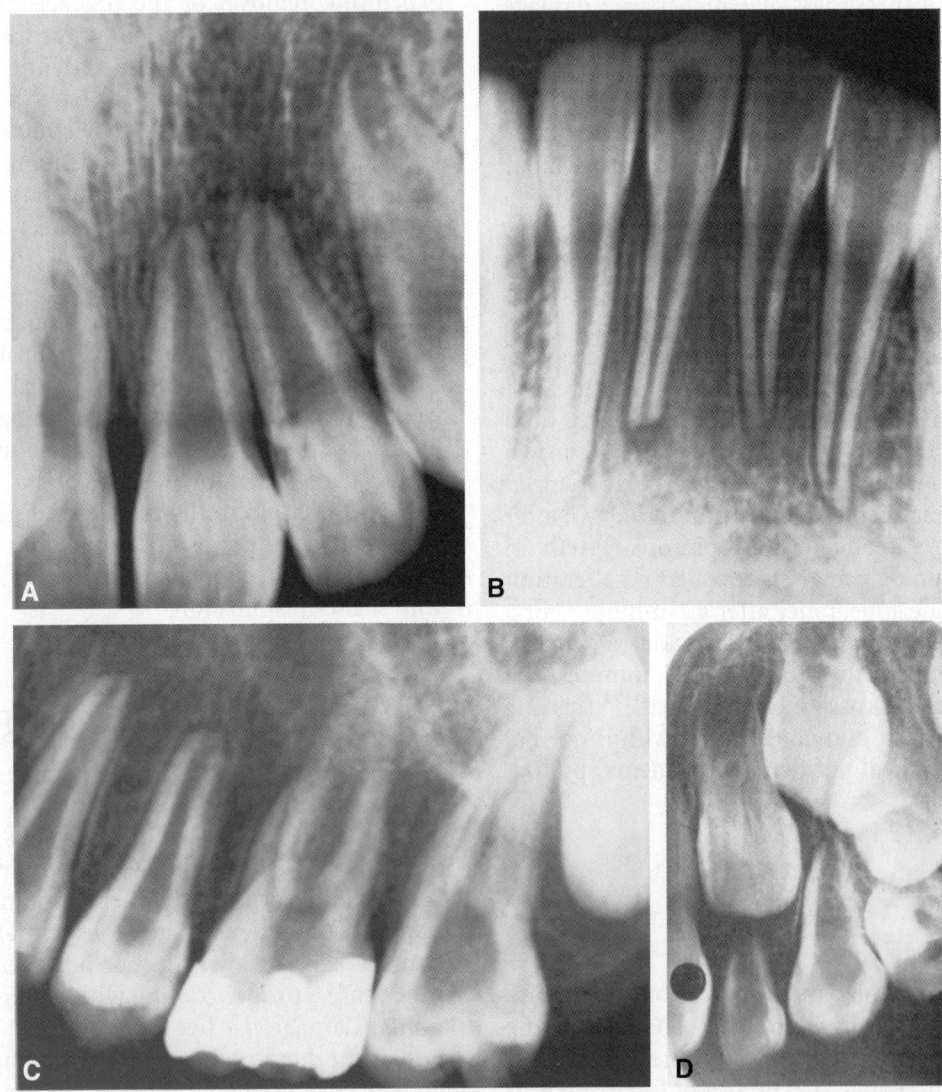

Figure 23 Unusual pulp dystrophy in *hereditary hypophosphatemia*. Incomplete calcification of dentin and large pulps leave these teeth vulnerable to infection and necrosis. *A,* Maxillary incisors at the age of 13. Note large pulp spaces. *B,* Mandibular incisors have been traumatized and pulp necrosis has developed. *C,* Large pulps can be seen in molar and premolar teeth. The pulp in the first molar later became necrotic. *D,* Large pulp size and shape are also apparent in the deciduous dentition. On the basis of these childhood radiographs, diagnosis can be made early about the patient's condition. Timely vitamin D therapy may prevent dwarfing. From Ingle JI. Endodontics, 1st ed. 1965. Ingle JI. Etilology of pulpal inflammation, necrosis or dystrophy.

hypophosphatemia. This disease, which results in dwarfism and "tackle deformity" of the legs, was formerly called refractory rickets, renal rickets, or vitamin D-resistant rickets. Its involvement in dentistry was first reported by Everett and Ingle.[194] It is characterized dentally by the abnormally large pulps and incomplete calcification of the dentin (Figure 23). The pulps in these teeth appear to be fragile and succumb to minor irritating stimuli. In one report, the patient had 11 pulpless teeth requiring endodontic treatment.

The diagnosis of this condition can be made through viewing oral radiographs, even of the deciduous teeth. It allows differentiation of this condition from achondroplastic dwarfism, which does not affect tooth pulps.

A report from Montreal pointed out that two different diseases are operative in this syndrome, namely autosomal dominant hypophosphatemic bone disease (HBD) and X-linked hypophosphatemia (XLH).[195] Although victims of HBD and XLH share similar dental abnormalities (large pulp spaces and pulp necrosis), patients with XLH have severe malocclusions as well. Unfortunately, the dental abnormalities are not prevented by early systemic treatment.[195]

The classic oral features of hypophosphatasia, namely, premature tooth loss and large pulp spaces, were found in a young adult woman with bone and joint pains. A study of 22 family members revealed several with dental abnormalities such as abnormal enamel, dentin, or cementum formation, decreased mandibular bone density, and abnormally large pulp spaces. Only a sister fulfilled the biochemical criteria for hypophosphatasia.[196] Biochemical examination of an extracted tooth from this sister showed phosphate and alkaline phosphate values 7 to 10 times lower than normal.

References

1. Kakehashi S, Stanley H, Fitzgerald R. The effects of surgical exposures of dental pulps in germ-free and conventional laboratory rats. Oral Surg Oral Med Oral Pathol Oral Radiol Endod 1965;20:340–9.
2. Bergenholtz G. Effect of bacterial products on inflammatory reactions in the dental pulp. Scand J Dent Res 1977;85:122–9.
3. Bergenholtz G. Evidence for bacterial causation of adverse pulpal responses in resin-based dental restorations. Crit Rev Oral Biol Med 2000;11:467–80.
4. Bergenholtz G, Cox CF, Loesche WJ, Syed SA. Bacterial leakage around dental restorations: its effect on the dental pulp. J Oral Pathol 1982;11:439–50.
5. Chhour K-L, Nadkarni MA, Byun R, et al. Molecular analysis of microbial diversity in advanced caries. J Clin Microbiol 2005;43:843–49.
6. Martin FE, Nadkarni MA, Jacques NA, Hunter N. Quantitative microbiological study of human carious dentine by culture and real-time PCR: association of anaerobes with histopathological changes in chronic pulpitis. J Clin Microbiol 2002;40:1698–704.
7. Kahler B, Moule A, Stenzel D. Bacterial contamination of cracks in symptomatic vital teeth. Aust Endodontic J 2000;26:115–18.
8. Langeland K, Rodrigues H, Dowden W. Periodontal disease, bacteria, and pulpal histopathology. Oral Surg Oral Med Oral Pathol Oral Radiol Endod 1974;37:257–70.
9. Bergenholtz G, Lindhe J. Effect of experimentally induced marginal periodontitis and periodontal scaling on the dental pulp. J Clin Periodontol 1978;5:59–73.
10. Nagaoka S, Miyazaki Y, Liu HJ, et al. Bacterial invasion into dentinal tubules of human vital and nonvital teeth. J Endod 1995;21:70–3.
11. Tziafas D. Experimental bacterial anachoresis in dog dental pulps capped with calcium hydroxide. J Endod 1989;15:591–5.
12. Veerayutthwilai O, Byers MR, Pham TTT, et al. Differential regulation of immune responses by odontoblasts. Oral Microbiol Immunol 2007;22:5–13.
13. Jontell M, Gunraj MN, Bergenholtz G. Immunocompetent cells in the normal dental pulp. J Dent Res 1987;66:1149–53.
14. Nakanishi T, Takahashi K, Hosokawa Y, et al. Expression of macrophage inflammatory protein 3alpha in human inflamed dental pulp tissue. J Endod 2005;31:84–7.
15. Okiji T, Jontell M, Belichenko P, et al. Structural and functional association between substance P- and calcitonin gene-related peptide-immunoreactive nerves and accessory cells in the rat dental pulp. J Dent Res 1997;76:1818–24.
16. Jontell M, Okiji T, Dahlgren U, Bergenholtz G. Immune defense mechanisms of the dental pulp. Crit Rev Oral Biol Med 1998;9:179–200.
17. Yoshiba K, Yoshiba N, Iwaku M. Class II antigen-presenting dendritic cell and nerve fiber responses to cavities, caries, or caries treatment in human teeth. J Dent Res 2003;82:422–7.
18. Zhang J, Kawashima N, Suda H, et al. The existence of CD11c+ sentinel and F4/80+ interstitial dendritic cells in dental pulp and their dynamics and functional properties. Int Immunol 2006;18:1375–84.
19. Hahn CL, Falkler WA, Jr., Siegel MA. A study of T and B cells in pulpal pathosis. J Endod 1989;15:20–6.
20. Izumi T, Kobayashi I, Okamura K, Sakai H. Immunohistochemical study on the immunocompetent cells of the pulp in

20. human non-carious and carious teeth. Arch Oral Biol 1995;40:609–14.
21. Sakurai K, Okiji T, Suda H. Co-increase of nerve fibers and HLA-DR- and/or factor-XIIIa-expressing dendritic cells in dentinal caries-affected regions of the human dental pulp: an immunohistochemical study. J Dent Res 1999;78:1596–608.
22. Fristad I, Berggreen E, Haug SR. Delta (delta) opioid receptors in small and medium-sized trigeminal neurons supporting the dental pulp of rats. Arch Oral Biol 2006;51:273–81.
23. Haug SR, Heyeraas KJ. Immunoglobulin producing cells in the rat dental pulp after unilateral sympathectomy. Neuroscience 2005;136:571–7.
24. Haug SR, Heyeraas KJ. Effects of sympathectomy on experimentally induced pulpal inflammation and periapical lesions in rats. Neuroscience 2003;120:827–36.
25. Mudie AS, Holland GR. Local opioids in the inflamed dental pulp. J Endod 2006;32:319–23.
26. Durand SH, Flacher V, Romeas A, et al. Lipoteichoic acid increases TLR and functional chemokine expression while reducing dentin formation in in vitro differentiated human odontoblasts. J Immunol 2006;176:2880–7.
27. Seltzer S, Bender IB, Ziontz M. The dynamics of pulp inflammation: correlations between diagnostic data and actual histologic findings in the pulp. Oral Surg Oral Med Oral Pathol Oral Radiol Endod 1963;16:969–77.
28. Brannstrom M, Lind PO. Pulpal response to early dental caries. J Dent Res 1965;44:1045–50.
29. Miller GS, Sternberg RN, Piliero SJ, Rosenberg PA. Histologic identification of mast cells in human dental pulp. Oral Surg Oral Med Oral Pathol Oral Radiol Endod 1978;46: 559–66.
30. Zachrisson BU. Mast cells in human dental pulp. Arch Oral Biol 1971;16:555–6.
31. Baume LJ. Diagnosis of diseases of the pulp. Oral Surg Oral Med Oral Pathol Oral Radiol Endod 1970;29:102–16.
32. Bernick S. Morphological changes in lymphatic vessels in pulpal inflammation. J Dent Res 1977;56:841–9.
33. Marchetti C, Poggi P, Calligaro A, Casasco A. Lymphatic vessels of the human dental pulp in different conditions. Anat Rec 1992;234:27–33.
34. Rodd HD, Boissonade FM. Vascular status in human primary and permanent teeth in health and disease. Eur J Oral Sci 2005;113:128–34.
35. Di Nardo Di Maio F, Lohinai Z, D'Arcangelo C, et al. Nitric oxide synthase in healthy and inflamed human dental pulp. J Dent Res 2004;83:312–16.
36. Trowbridge HO. Pathogenesis of pulpitis resulting from dental caries. J Endod 1981;7:52–60.
37. Tonder KJ, Kvinnsland I. Micropuncture measurements of interstitial fluid pressure in normal and inflamed dental pulp in cats. J Endod 1983;9:105–9.
38. Tonder KJ. Vascular reactions in the dental pulp during inflammation. Acta Odontol Scand 1983;41:247–56.
39. Takahashi K. Changes in the pulpal vasculature during inflammation. J Endod 1990;16:92–7.
40. Heyeraas KJ, Berggreen E. Interstitial fluid pressure in normal and inflamed pulp. Crit Rev Oral Biol Med 1999;10:328–36.
41. Bletsa A, Berggreen E, Fristad I, et al. Cytokine signalling in rat pulp interstitial fluid and transcapillary fluid exchange during lipopolysaccharide-induced acute inflammation. J Physiol 2006;573:225–36.
42. Kim S, Liu M, Simchon S, Dorscher-Kim JE. Effects of selected inflammatory mediators on blood flow and vascular permeability in the dental pulp. Proc Finn Dent Soc 1992;88 (Suppl 1):387–92.
43. Van Hassel HJ. Physiology of the human dental pulp. Oral Surg Oral Med Oral Pathol Oral Radiol Endod 1971;32:126–34.
44. Matsumoto Y, Zhang B, Kato S. Lymphatic networks in the periodontal tissue and dental pulp as revealed by histochemical study. Microscopy Res Tech 2002;56:50–9.
45. Marchetti C, Poggi P. Lymphatic vessels in the oral cavity: different structures for the same function. Microscopy Res Tech 2002;56:42–9.
46. Bishop MA, Malhotra M. An investigation of lymphatic vessels in the feline dental pulp. Am J Anat 1990;187:247–53.
47. Anneroth G, Norberg KA. Adrenergic vasoconstrictor innervation in the human dental pulp. Acta Odontol Scand 1968;26:89–93.
48. Christensen K. Sympathetic nerve fibres in the alveolar nerves and nerves of the dental pulp. J Dent Res 1940;19:227–42.
49. Tonder KH, Naess G. Nervous control of blood flow in the dental pulp in dogs. Acta Physiol Scand 1978;104:13–23.
50. Bletsa A, Heyeraas KJ, Haug SR, Berggreen E. IL-1 alpha and TNF-alpha expression in rat periapical lesions and dental pulp after unilateral sympathectomy. Neuroimmunomodulation 2004;11:376–84.
51. Haug SR, Berggreen E, Heyeraas KJ. The effect of unilateral sympathectomy and cavity preparation on peptidergic nerves and immune cells in rat dental pulp. Exp Neurol 2001;169:182–90.
52. Fristad I, Heyeraas KJ, Kvinnsland IH, Jonsson R. Recruitment of immunocompetent cells after dentinal injuries in innervated and denervated young rat molars: an immunohistochemical study. J Histochem Cytochem 1995;43:871–9.
53. Komorowski RC, Torneck CD, Hu JW. Neurogenic inflammation and tooth pulp innervation pattern in sympathectomized rats. J Endod 1996;22:414–17.
54. Woodnutt DA, Wager-Miller J, O'Neill PC, et al. Neurotrophin receptors and nerve growth factor are differentially expressed in adjacent nonneuronal cells of normal and injured tooth pulp. Cell Tissue Res 2000;299:225–36.

55. Byers MR, Wheeler EF, Bothwell M. Altered expression of NGF and P75 NGF-receptor by fibroblasts of injured teeth precedes sensory nerve sprouting. Growth Factors 1992; 6:41–52.

56. Byers MR, Taylor PE. Effect of sensory denervation on the response of rat molar pulp to exposure injury. J Dent Res 1993;72:613–18.

57. Byers MR, Suzuki H, Maeda T. Dental neuroplasticity, neuro-pulpal interactions, and nerve regeneration. Microsc Res Tech 2003;60:503–15.

58. Byers MR. Dynamic plasticity of dental sensory nerve structure and cytochemistry. Arch Oral Biol 1994;39 (Suppl): 13S–21S.

59. Byers MR, Narhi MV, Mecifi KB. Acute and chronic reactions of dental sensory nerve fibers to cavities and desiccation in rat molars. Anat Rec 1988;221:872–83.

60. Byers MR. Effects of inflammation on dental sensory nerves and vice versa. Proc Finn Dent Soc 1992;88 (Suppl 1):499–506.

61. Byers MR, Taylor PE, Khayat BG, Kimberly CL. Effects of injury and inflammation on pulpal and periapical nerves. J Endod 1990;16:78–84.

62. Rodd HD, Boissonade FM. Comparative immunohistochemical analysis of the peptidergic innervation of human primary and permanent tooth pulp. Arch Oral Biol 2002; 47:375–85.

63. Oswald RJ, Byers MR. The injury response of pulpal NPY-IR sympathetic fibers differs from that of sensory afferent fibers. Neurosci Lett 1993;164:190–4.

64. El Karim IA, Lamey P-J, Linden GJ, et al. Caries-induced changes in the expression of pulpal neuropeptide Y. Eur J Oral Sci 2006;114:133–7.

65. El Karim IA, Lamey PJ, Ardill J, et al. Vasoactive intestinal polypeptide (VIP) and VPAC1 receptor in adult human dental pulp in relation to caries. Arch Oral Biol 2006; 51:849–55.

66. Buck S, Reese K, Hargreaves KM. Pulpal exposure alters neuropeptide levels in inflamed dental pulp and trigeminal ganglia: evaluation of axonal transport. J Endod 1999;25:718–21.

67. Itotagawa T, Yamanaka H, Wakisaka S, et al. Appearance of neuropeptide Y-like immunoreactive cells in the rat trigeminal ganglion following dental injuries. Arch Oral Biol 1993;38:725–8.

68. Behnia A, Zhang L, Charles M, Gold MS. Changes in TrkB-like immunoreactivity in rat trigeminal ganglion after tooth injury. J Endod 2003;29:135–40.

69. Cao Y, Deng Y. Histochemical observation of nitric oxide synthase in trigeminal ganglion of rats with experimental pulpitis. J Tongji Med Univ 1999;19:77–80.

70. Stephenson JL, Byers MR. GFAP immunoreactivity in trigeminal ganglion satellite cells after tooth injury in rats. Exp Neurol 1995;131:11–22.

71. Henry MA, Westrum LE, Johnson LR, Canfield RC. Ultrastructure of degenerative changes following ricin application to feline dental pulps. J Neurocytol 1987; 16:601–11.

72. Chattipakorn SC, Sigurdsson A, Light AR, et al. Trigeminal c-Fos expression and behavioral responses to pulpal inflammation in ferrets. Pain 2002;99:61–9.

73. Kwan CL, Hu JW, Sessle BJ. Effects of tooth pulp deafferentation on brainstem neurons of the rat trigeminal subnucleus oralis. Somatosens Mot Res 1993;10:115–31.

74. Zhang S, Chiang CY, Xie YF, et al. Central sensitization in thalamic nociceptive neurons induced by mustard oil application to rat molar tooth pulp. Neuroscience 2006;142: 833–42.

75. Chiang CY, Park SJ, Kwan CL, et al. NMDA receptor mechanisms contribute to neuroplasticity induced in caudalis nociceptive neurons by tooth pulp stimulation. J Neurophysiol 1998;80:2621–31.

76. Torneck CD, Kwan CL, Hu JW. Inflammatory lesions of the tooth pulp induce changes in brainstem neurons of the rat trigeminal subnucleus oralis. J Dent Res 1996;75:553–61.

77. Hu JW, Dostrovsky JO, Lenz YE, et al. Tooth pulp deafferentation is associated with functional alterations in the properties of neurons in the trigeminal spinal tract nucleus. J Neurophysiol 1986;56:1650–68.

78. Labuz D, Berger S, Mousa SA, et al. Peripheral antinociceptive effects of exogenous and immune cell-derived endomorphins in prolonged inflammatory pain. J Neurosci 2006;26: 4350–8.

79. Machelska H, Schopohl JK, Mousa SA, et al. Different mechanisms of intrinsic pain inhibition in early and late inflammation. J Neuroimmunol 2003;141:30–9.

80. Likar R, Koppert W, Blatnig H, et al. Efficacy of peripheral morphine analgesia in inflamed, non-inflamed and perineural tissue of dental surgery patients. J Pain Symptom Manage 2001;21:330–7.

81. Jaber L, Swaim WD, Dionne RA. Immunohistochemical localization of mu-opioid receptors in human dental pulp. J Endod 2003;29:108–10.

82. Ranjitkar S, Taylor JA, Townsend GC. A radiographic assessment of the prevalence of pulp stones in Australians. Aust Dent J 2002;47:36–40.

83. Edds AC, Walden JE, Scheetz JP, et al. Pilot study of correlation of pulp stones with cardiovascular disease. J Endod 2005;31:504–6.

84. De Coster PJ, Martens LC, De Paepe A. Oral health in prevalent types of Ehlers-Danlos syndromes. J Oral Pathol Med 2005;34:298–307.

85. Collins MA, Mauriello SM, Tyndall DA, Wright JT. Dental anomalies associated with amelogenesis imperfecta: a radiographic assessment. Oral Surg Oral Med Oral Pathol Oral Radiol Endod 1999;88:358–64.

86. Robertson A, Andreasen FM, Bergenholtz G, et al. Incidence of pulp necrosis subsequent to pulp canal obliteration from trauma of permanent incisors. J Endod 1996;22:557–60.

87. Fried I, Erickson P, Schwartz S, Keenan K. Subluxation injuries of maxillary primary anterior teeth: epidemiology and prognosis of 207 traumatized teeth. Pediatr Dent 1996; 18:145–51.

88. Kawagishi E, Nakakura-Ohshima K, Nomura S, Ohshima H. Pulpal responses to cavity preparation in aged rat molars. Cell Tissue Res 2006;326:111–22.

89. Izumi T, Inoue H, Matsuura H, et al. Age-related changes in the immunoreactivity of the monocyte/macrophage system in rat molar pulp after cavity preparation. Oral Surg Oral Med Oral Pathol Oral Radiol Endod 2002;94:103–10.

90. Smith AJ. Vitality of the dentin-pulp complex in health and disease: growth factors as key mediators. J Dent Educ 2003; 67:678–89.

91. Goldberg M, Six N, Decup F, et al. Bioactive molecules and the future of pulp therapy. Am J Dent 2003;16:66–76.

92. Murray PE, Garcia-Godoy F, KM. H. Regenerative endodontics: a review of current status and a call for action. J Endod 2007;33:377–90.

93. Murray PE, Matthews JB, Sloan AJ, Smith AJ. Analysis of incisor pulp cell populations in Wistar rats of different ages. Arch Oral Biol 2002;47:709–15.

94. Fried K, Erdelyi G. Changes with age in canine tooth pulp-nerve fibres of the cat. Arch Oral Biol 1984;29:581–5.

95. Bernick S. Age changes in the blood supply to human teeth. J Dent Res 1967;46:544–50.

96. Bennett CG, Kelln EE, Biddington WR. Age changes of the vascular pattern of the human dental pulp. Arch Oral Biol 1965;10:995–8.

97. Ahn J, Pogrel MA. The effects of 2% lidocaine with 1:100,000 epinephrine on pulpal and gingival blood flow. Oral Surg Oral Med Oral Pathol Oral Radiol Endod 1998;85: 197–202.

98. Kim S, Edwall L, Trowbridge H, Chien S. Effects of local anesthetics on pulpal blood flow in dogs. J Dent Res 1984; 63:650–2.

99. Eriksson AR, Albrektsson T. Temperature threshold levels for heat-induced bone tissue injury: a vital-microscopic study in the rabbit. J Prosthet Dent 1983;50:101–7.

100. Eriksson A, Albrektsson T, Grane B, McQueen D. Thermal injury to bone. Int J Oral Surg 1982;11:115–21.

101. Eriksson AR, Albrektsson T, Albrektsson B. Heat caused by drilling cortical bone. Acta Orthop Scand 1984;55:629–31.

102. Eriksson RA, Adell R. Temperatures during drilling for the placement of implants using the osseointrgration technique. J Oral Maxillofac Surg 1986;44:4–7.

103. Frank U, Freundlich J, Tansy MR, et al. Vascular and cellular responses of teeth after localized controlled cooling. Cryobiology 1972;9:526–33.

104. Zach L, Cohen G. Pulp response to externally applied heat. Oral Surg Oral Med Oral Pathol Oral Radiol Endod 1966; 19:515–30.

105. Baldissara P, Catapano S, Scotti R. Clinical and histological evaluation of thermal injury thresholds in human teeth: a preliminary study. J Oral Rehabil 1997;24:791–801.

106. Nyborg H, Brannstrom M. Pulp reaction to heat. J Prosthet Dent 1968;19:605–12.

107. Lisanti V, Zander H. Thermal injury to normal dog teeth: in vivo measurements of pulp temperature increases and their effect on the pulp tissue. J Dent Res 1952;31:548–58.

108. Dachi SF, Stigers RW. Pulpal effects of water and air coolants used in high-speed cavity preparations. J Am Dent Assoc 1968;76:95–8.

109. Carlton ML, Jr., Dorman HL. Comparison of dentin and pulp temperatures during cavity preparation. Tex Dent J 1969; 87:7–9.

110. Marsland EA, Shovelton D. Repair in the human dental pulp following cavity preparation. Arch Oral Biol 1970; 15:411–23.

111. Fernandez-Seara MA, Wehrli SL, Wehrli FW. Diffusion of exchangeable water in cortical bone studied by nuclear magnetic resonance. Biophysics J 2002;82:522–29.

112. Attrill DC, Davies RM, King TA, et al. Thermal effects of the Er: YAG laser on a simulated dental pulp: a quantitative evaluation of the effects of a water spray. J Dent Res 2004; 32:35–40.

113. Louw NP, Pameijer CH, Ackermann WD, et al. Pulp histology after Er:YAG laser cavity preparation in subhuman primates - a pilot study. S Afr Dent J 2002;57:31.

114. Rizoiu I, Kohanghadosh F, Kimmel AI, Eversole LR. Pulpal thermal responses to an erbium, chromium:YSGG pulsed laser hydrokinetic system. Oral Surg Oral Med Oral Pathol Oral Radiol Endod 1998;86:220–3.

115. Felton DA, Webb EL, Kanoy BE, Cox CF. Pulpal response to threaded pin and retentive slot techniques: a pilot investigation. J Prosthet Dent 1991;66:597–602.

116. Knight JS, Smith HB. The heat sink and its relationship to reducing heat during pin-reduction procedures. Oper Dent 1998;23:299–302.

117. Murray PE, About I, Lumley PJ, et al. Cavity remaining dentin thickness and pulpal activity. Am J Dent 2002;15:41–6.

118. Stevenson TS. Odontoblast aspiration and fluid movement in human dentine. Arch Oral Biol 1967;12:1149–58.

119. Tziafas D, Koliniotou-Koumpia E, Tziafa C, Papadimitriou S. Effects of a new antibacterial adhesive on the repair capacity of the pulp-dentine complex in infected teeth. Int Endod J 2007;40:58–66.

120. Shimada Y, Seki Y, Uzzaman MA, et al. Monkey pulpal response to an MMA-based resin cement as adhesive luting for indirect restorations. J Adhes Dent 2005;7:247–51.

121. Unemori M, Matsuya Y, Akashi A, et al. Self-etching adhesives and postoperative sensitivity. Am J Dent 2004; 17:191–5.
122. Costa CAD, Giro EMA, do Nascimento ABL, et al. Short-term evaluation of the pulpo-dentin complex response to a resin-modified glass-ionomer cement and a bonding agent applied in deep cavities. Dent Mater J 2003;19:739–46.
123. Pashley DH. The effects of acid etching on the pulpodentin complex. Oper Dent 1992;17:229–42.
124. Stanley HR. Pulpal consideration of adhesive materials. Oper Dent 1992;5 (Suppl 5):151–64.
125. Medina VO, 3rd, Shinkai K, Shirono M, et al. Histopathologic study on pulp response to single-bottle and self-etching adhesive systems. Oper Dent 2002;27:330–42.
126. Murray PE, Smyth TW, About I, et al. The effect of etching on bacterial microleakage of an adhesive composite restoration. J Dent 2002;30:29–36.
127. Camps J, Dejou J, Remusat M, About I. Factors influencing pulpal response to cavity restorations. Dent Mater J 2000; 16:432–40.
128. Hiraishi N, Kitasako Y, Nikaido T, et al. Detection of acid diffusion through bovine dentine after adhesive application. Int Endod J 2004;37:455–62.
129. Castelnuovo J, Tjan AH. Temperature rise in pulpal chamber during fabrication of provisional resinous crowns. J Prosthet Dent 1997;78:441–6.
130. Grajower R, Kaufman E, Stern N. Temperature of the pulp chamber during impression taking of full crown preparations with modelling compound. J Dent Res 1975;54:212–17.
131. Kim S, Dorscher-Kim JE, Liu M, Grayson A. Functional alterations in pulpal microcirculation in response to various dental procedures and materials. Proc Finn Dent Soc 1992; 88 (Suppl 1):65–71.
132. Moulding MB, Teplitsky PE. Intrapulpal temperature during direct fabrication of provisional restorations. Int J Prosthodont 1990;3:299–304.
133. Jackson CR, Skidmore AE, Rice RT. Pulpal evaluation of teeth restored with fixed prostheses. J Prosthet Dent 1992; 67:323–5.
134. Bergenholtz G. Evidence for bacterial causation of adverse pulpal responses in resin-based dental restorations. Crit Rev Oral Biol Med 2000;11:467–80.
135. Vongsavan N, Matthews RW, Matthews B. The permeability of human dentine in vitro and in vivo. Arch Oral Biol 2000;45:931–5.
136. Jontell M, Hanks CT, Bratel J, Bergenholtz G. Effects of unpolymerized resin components on the function of accessory cells derived from the rat incisor pulp. J Dent Res 1995; 74:1162–7.
137. Al-Hiyasat AS, Darmani H, Milhem MM. Cytotoxicity evaluation of dental resin composites and their flowable derivatives. Clin Oral Investig 2005;9:21–5.
138. Lonnroth EC, Dahl JE. Cytotoxicity of liquids and powders of chemically different Dent Mater J evaluated using dimethylthiazol diphenyltetrazolium and neutral red tests. Acta Odontol Scand 2003;61:52–6.
139. Silvestri AR, Jr., Cohen SH, Wetz JH. Character and frequency of discomfort immediately following restorative procedures. J Am Dent Assoc 1977;95:85–9.
140. Brannstrom M. The effect of dentin desiccation and aspirated odontoblasts on the pulp. J Prosthet Dent 1968;20: 165–71.
141. Plant CG, Jones DW, Darvell BW. The heat evolved and temperatures attained during setting of restorative materials. Br Dent J 1974;137:233–8.
142. Hume WR. An analysis of the release and the diffusion through dentin of eugenol from zinc oxide-eugenol mixtures. J Dent Res 1984;63:881–4.
143. Hume WR. Influence of dentine on the pulpward release of eugenol or acids from restorative materials. J Oral Rehabil 1994;21:469–73.
144. Murray PE, Lumley PJ, Smith AJ. Preserving the vital pulp in Oper Dent: 3. Thickness of remaining cavity dentine as a key mediator of pulpal injury and repair responses. Dent Update 2002;29:172–8.
145. Al-Nazhan S, Spangberg L. Morphological cell changes due to chemical toxicity of a dental material: an electron microscopic study on human periodontal ligament fibroblasts and L929 cells. J Endod 1990;16:129–34.
146. Olasupo NA, Fitzgerald DJ, Gasson MJ, Narbad A. Activity of natural antimicrobial compounds against Escherichia coli and Salmonella enterica serovar Typhimurium. Lett Appl Microbiol 2003;37:448–51.
147. Brodin P. Neurotoxic and analgesic effects of root canal cements and pulp-protecting dental materials. Endod Dent Traumatol 1988;4:1–11.
148. Trowbridge H, Edwall L, Panopoulos P. Effect of zinc oxide-eugenol and calcium hydroxide on intradental nerve activity. J Endod 1982;8:403–6.
149. Camps J, About I, Gouirand S, Franquin JC. Dentin permeability and eugenol diffusion after full crown preparation. Am J Dent 2003;16:112–16.
150. Fitzgerald M, Heys RJ, Heys DR, Charbeneau GT. An evaluation of a glass ionomer luting agent: bacterial leakage. J Am Dent Assoc 1987;114:783–6.
151. Heys RJ, Fitzgerald M, Heys DR, Charbeneau GT. An evaluation of a glass ionomer luting agent: pulpal histological response. J Am Dent Assoc 1987;114:607–11.
152. Johnson GH, Powell LV, DeRouen TA. Evaluation and control of post-cementation pulpal sensitivity: zinc phosphate and glass ionomer luting cements. J Am Dent Assoc 1993; 124:38–46.
153. Watts A. Bacterial contamination and the toxicity of silicate and zinc phosphate cements. Br Dent J 1979;146:7–13.

154. About I, Murray PE, Franquin JC, et al. Pulpal inflammatory responses following non-carious class V restorations. Oper Dent 2001;26:336–42.

155. Jendresen MD, Trowbridge HO. Biologic and physical properties of a zinc polycarboxylate cement. J Prosthet Dent 1972;28:264–71.

156. Heys RJ, Heys DR, Fitzgerald M. Histological evaluation of microfilled and conventional composite resins on monkey dental pulps. Int Endod J 1985;18:260–6.

157. Kitasako Y, Murray PE, Tagami J, Smith AJ. Histomorphometric analysis of dentinal bridge formation and pulpal inflammation. Quintessence Int 2002;33:600–8.

158. Whitworth JM, Myers PM, Smith J, et al. Endodontic complications after plastic restorations in general practice. Int Endod J 2005;38:409–16.

159. Graver H, Trowbridge H, Alperstein K. Microleakage of castings cemented with glass-ionomer cements. Oper Dent 1990;15:2–9.

160. Murray PE, Kitasako Y, Tagami J, et al. Hierarchy of variables correlated to odontoblast-like cell numbers following pulp capping. J Dent 2002;30:297–304.

161. Murray PE, Windsor LJ, Smyth TW, et al. Analysis of pulpal reactions to restorative procedures, materials, pulp capping, and future therapies. Crit Rev Oral Biol Med 2002;13:509–20.

162. Shimada Y, Seki Y, Sasafuchi Y, et al. Biocompatibility of a flowable composite bonded with a self-etching adhesive compared with a glass Ionomer cement and a high copper amalgam. Oper Dent 2004;29:23–8.

163. Morrow LA, Wilson NH. The effectiveness of four-cavity treatment systems in sealing amalgam restorations. Oper Dent 2002;27:549–56.

164. Sarrett DC, Brooks CN, Rose JT. Clinical performance evaluation of a packable posterior composite in bulk-cured restorations. J Am Dent Assoc 2006;137:71–80.

165. Sobral MA, Garone-Netto N, Luz MA, Santos AP. Prevention of postoperative tooth sensitivity: a preliminary clinical trial. J Oral Rehabil 2005;32:661–8.

166. Casselli DS, Martins LR. Postoperative sensitivity in Class I composite resin restorations in vivo. J Adhes Dent 2006;8:53–8.

167. Fugaro JO, Nordahl I, Fugaro OJ, et al. Pulp reaction to vital bleaching. Oper Dent 2004;29:363–8.

168. Gokay O, Tuncbilek M, Ertan R. Penetration of the pulp chamber by carbamide peroxide bleaching agents on teeth restored with a composite resin. J Oral Rehabil 2000;27:428–31.

169. Ritter AV, Leonard RH, Jr., St Georges AJ, et al. Safety and stability of nightguard vital bleaching: 9 to 12 years post-treatment. J Esthet Restor Dent 2002;14:275–85.

170. Baik JW, Rueggeberg FA, Liewehr FR. Effect of light-enhanced bleaching on in vitro surface and intrapulpal temperature rise. J Esthet Restor Dent 2001;13:370–8.

171. Rickoff B, Trowbridge H, Baker J, et al. Effects of thermal vitality tests on human dental pulp. J Endod 1988;14:482–5.

172. Augsburger RA, Peters DD. In vitro effects of ice, skin refrigerant, and CO2 snow on intrapulpal temperature. J Endod 1981;7:110–16.

173. Peters DD, Lorton L, Mader CL, et al. Evaluation of the effects of carbon dioxide used as a pulpal test. 1. In vitro effect on human enamel. J Endod 1983;9:219–27.

174. Ingram TA, Peters DD. Evaluation of the effects of carbon dioxide used as a pulpal test. Part 2. In vivo effect on canine enamel and pulpal tissues. J Endod 1983;9:296–303.

175. Hall CJ, Freer TJ. The effects of early orthodontic force application on pulp test responses. Aust Dent J 1998;43:359–61.

176. Woloshyn H, Artun J, Kennedy DB, Joondeph DR. Pulpal and periodontal reactions to orthodontic alignment of palatally impacted canines [see comment] [erratum appears in Angle Orthod 1994;64(5):324]. Angle Orthod 1994;64:257–64.

177. Nixon CE, Saviano JA, King GJ, Keeling SD. Histomorphometric study of dental pulp during orthodontic tooth movement. J Endod 1993;19:13–16.

178. Derringer KA, Jaggers DC, Linden RW. Angiogenesis in human dental pulp following orthodontic tooth movement. J Dent Res 1996;75:1761–6.

179. Derringer KA, Linden RW. Angiogenic growth factors released in human dental pulp following orthodontic force. Arch Oral Biol 2003;48:285–91.

180. Derringer KA, Linden RW. Vascular endothelial growth factor, fibroblast growth factor 2, platelet derived growth factor and transforming growth factor beta released in human dental pulp following orthodontic force. Arch Oral Biol 2004;49:631–41.

181. Uysal T, Eldeniz AU, Usumez S, Usumez A. Thermal changes in the pulp chamber during different adhesive clean-up procedures. Angle Orthod 2005;75:220–5.

182. Jost-Brinkmann PG, Radlanski RJ, Artun J, Loidl H. Risk of pulp damage due to temperature increase during thermodebonding of ceramic brackets. Eur J Orthod 1997;19:623–8.

183. Lee-Knight CT, Wylie SG, Major PW, et al. Mechanical and electrothermal debonding: effect on ceramic veneers and dental pulp. Am J Orthod Dentofacial Orthop 1997;112:263–70.

184. Takla PM, Shivapuja PK. Pulpal response in electrothermal debonding. Am J Orthod Dentofacial Orthop 1995;108:623–9.

185. Dovgan JS, Walton RE, Bishara SE. Electrothermal debracketing: patient acceptance and effects on the dental pulp. Am J Orthod Dentofacial Orthop 1995;108:249–55.

186. Jost-Brinkmann PG, Stein H, Miethke RR, Nakata M. Histologic investigation of the human pulp after

diffusible factors, C3a and C5a, while the third is a larger molecule, C3b, that remains attached to the bacterium and serves as a signal that marks the targets for PMNs to engage and phagocytize.

Effective phagocytosis requires marking the bacteria with a dual signal, the other signal being a specific IgG molecules attached to the bacterium. PMNs have two distinct receptors, C3b receptor and Fc receptor, on their membrane that engage the relevant molecules allowing for effective phagocytosis. The latter attaches to the Fc portion of an IgG molecule that has been attached to the bacterial surface antigen via its binding sites (located at its Fab region). This mechanism is termed "opsonization" and is essential for the effective elimination of bacteria by the PMNs.[7] Antibodies may come from the bloodstream, but evidence for their local production will be discussed below.

It is also clear that an effective and continuous local supply of complement constituent is essential for the above-mentioned process to take place. This is achieved by an increased permeability of the capillaries in the area, induced by C3a and C5a via activation and degranulation of local mast cells. When vascular permeability is normal, large molecules are kept within the blood vessels. They serve to maintain the essential osmotic pressure that will draw water back into the venous part of the capillaries and maintain the blood and tissue volumes at equilibrium.

From the above sequence of events, it becomes apparent that even though the PMNs are responsible for phagocytizing and killing bacteria, an elaborate infrastructure of cells is required to locally provide at least two main types of molecules, without which the PMN response will be handicapped: IgG *specific* to the involved bacteria and the cytokines IL-1 and TNF.

CELLS, IMMUNOGLOBULINS AND CYTOKINES IN PERIAPICAL LESIONS

Qualitative and quantitative studies of the cellular composition of periapical granulomas have been profoundly influenced by the methodology available. Initial attempts to characterize the cells participating in these lesions were based on the classical morphology of the cells, followed by the use of electron microscopy. With the introduction of immunohistological methods, the first attempts to specifically identify plasma cells in periapical lesions by their immunoglobulin content were reported.[8] In recent decades, the intensive use of monoclonal antibodies against subsets of T lymphocytes, B lymphocytes, macrophages, dendritic cells, plasma cells, and PMNs resulted in a major breakthrough in the understanding of the immunobiology of the periapical host response, in both naturally occurring human periapical lesions and those experimentally induced in the rat. The most recent approach involves molecular biology methods, such as in situ hybridization or the polymerase chain reaction.

Cells with distinct morphology, such as PMNs, mast cells, lymphocytes, plasma cells, and osteoclasts, have been easily identifiable. However, in earlier studies only cells with "classical" macrophage morphology could be identified as such. Monoclonal antibodies make it possible to identify macrophages and dendritic cells of diverse morphology as well as to recognize subsets of these and other cells.

EVOLUTION OF THE IMMUNOBIOLOGICAL CONCEPT OF PERIAPICAL LESIONS

The availability of new methodologies has influenced the type of studies performed and eventually affected the evolution of the immunobiological understanding of the complex nature of the periapical host response.[9-11] Initially, the commercial availability of specific antibodies directed against human IgG, IgM, IgA, and IgE allowed for the immunofluorescent or immunohistochemical detection of these molecules in periapical lesions, either in a free form or as markers of subsets of B lymphocytes and plasma cells.[12] Later, the combination of these antibodies with those directed against human complement allowed the demonstration of *activity* rather the *simple presence* of immunoglobulins in periapical lesions. Johannessen et al. demonstrated intracellular colocalization of IgG and C3b in macrophages in periapical inflammatory lesions, suggesting phagocytosis of bacteria via dual opsonization by both opsonins.[13]

The availability of monoclonal antibodies against various T lymphocyte subsets made it possible to explore the presence of these cells in both human periapical lesions as well as in those experimentally induced in rats. T-cells in human periapical granulomas were studied by Cymerman and others.[14-16] It became apparent that both T helper (CD4$^+$) and T suppressor (CD8$^+$) lymphocytes were present in these lesions.[14] In delayed hypersensitivity in humans, a typical T helper/T suppressor relation is about 2:1.[17] It was therefore of interest to define whether T lymphocytes in periapical lesions follow this trend. Babal et al. found a T helper/T suppressor ratio of <1.0 in periapical granulomas, while Barkhordar and Desouza reported a ratio of ~1.0.[15] It seemed that the predominance of T helper lymphocytes, which is typical of delayed hypersensitivity, does not exist in a chronic periapical granuloma. Nevertheless, this is not a uniform finding, as Kopp and Schwarting found a T helper/T suppressor ratio of 3:2 in periapical granulomas, which diminished to ~1.0 in periapical scars.[18]

In a rat model, Stashenko and Yu demonstrated that during the early, active, phase of lesion development, helper (CD4$^+$) T cells predominated, while at the later chronic stage, suppressor (CD8$^+$) T cells outnumbered the helper T-cell population.[19] The initial Th/Ts ratio of 1.7 lessened to <1.0 at the later stage, as compared to a Th/Ts ratio of 2.0 in peripheral blood. These findings were interpreted as the initial active function of T lymphocytes, which is later downregulated and controlled by suppressor T cells. The balance of their activities is expressed in chronic periapical lesions, such as those encountered in humans.

THE PROTECTIVE FUNCTION OF T LYMPHOCYTES IN THE PERIAPICAL GRANULOMA

A protective role of helper T lymphocyte function should eventually be expressed as a better ability of the host to prevent bacteria from spreading from the infected root canal. This may be accomplished by (1) the local production of antibodies and (2) increasing the local availability and enhancing the function of phagocytes (Figure 1). Local activation of antigen-specific T helper lymphocytes is a prerequisite for the local production of antibodies that are specific to the bacteria that periodically emerge from the root canal.[20,21] This in turn will enable effective opsonization of the bacteria, followed by phagocytosis and killing.

Local macrophage activation is accomplished mainly by interferon-γ (INF-γ) produced by the activated T helper cells (see Figure 1). Even though activation of the lymphocytes is antigen-specific, once macrophages are activated, the result is nonspecific, and their phagocytic and killing abilities, as well as cytokine production, will be greatly enhanced. IL-1 and TNF production by activated macrophages will locally elevate ICAM-1 molecule expression by endothelial cells in the capillaries, thus enhancing the local attachment of PMNs and monocytes and enhancing their migration into the periapical area.[3,6] IL-8 produced by these macrophages will chemotactically attract the PMNs and activate them, making them more available and more competent to engage and kill the bacteria[22–24] (see Figure 1). Thus, macrophage activation has a major role in maintaining the two lines of phagocytic cell defense that are typically

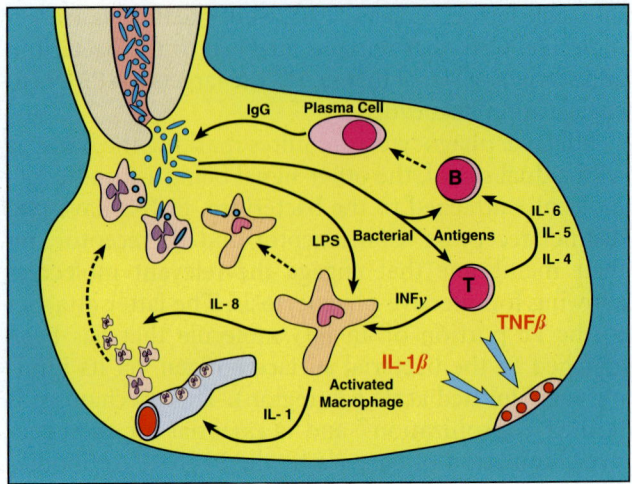

Figure 1 Protective functions of T lymphocytes and macrophages in the periapical granuloma. Specifically activated T lymphocytes produce a plethora of cytokines, some of which promote activation, proliferation, and maturation of B lymphocytes to become plasma cells producing immunoglobulins specific to the root canal bacteria. Macrophage activation is mediated by interferon-γ (INF-γ) produced also by these cells. Activated macrophages produce IL-1 and IL-8 that are essential for effective local recruitment and activation of PMNs. Bacterial endotoxin (LPS) can bypass the T lymphocytes and directly activate macrophages. Bone resorption in apical granuloma is mediated by IL-1β (an activated macrophage product) and by TNF-β (an activated T lymphocyte product). It may be considered a negative side effect of the ongoing protective process in the apical granuloma.

described in the periapical lesion: an inner area, closer to the apex, in which PMNs predominate and the area around it in which the phagocytic macrophages are observed.[25] The defensive function of helper T lymphocytes is achieved *indirectly* by allowing (1) activated specific B lymphocytes to proliferate and mature into plasma cells that will produce antibodies and (2) the activation of nonspecific effector cells, the macrophages. In order to avoid an endless loop of mutual activation of macrophages and T lymphocytes, the process is actively controlled and downregulated by suppressor T lymphocytes.[26–28]

The essential role of the T lymphocytes in this process was well established and accepted by the late 1980s of the last century.[28,29] A turning point occurred with the first studies that utilized athymic mice and rats to study the formation of periapical inflammatory lesions to determine the critical role of T lymphocytes in the formation of these lesions.[30,31] Unexpectedly, both groups demonstrated that periapical lesions could also develop independent of T-lymphocyte activity, thus leaving the center stage to another key actor: the macrophage (as will be detailed below).

B CELLS, PLASMA CELLS, AND IMMUNOGLOBULIN PRODUCTION

The presence of *plasma cells*, the cells that produce immunoglobulins, in apical granulomas has been well documented by many investigators.[16,32–35] In addition, the presence of *B lymphocytes*, the precursors of plasma cells, has also been documented in apical granulomas.[12,36,37] Immunoglobulin-containing cells (B Ly + plasma cells) may constitute 11–50% of the mononuclear cells in apical granulomas.[12,36] Among these cells, a majority of them produce IgG (70–85%) while small fractions of them produce IgA, IgE, and IgM.[12,36] It must be kept in mind that the presence of IgG and IgG-producing cells in the periapical tissue does not necessarily mean that the immunoglobulins will be specific to the bacteria that reside in necrotic infected root canals. Baumgartner and Falkler[20] and Kettering et al.[21] demonstrated that antibodies specific to root canal bacteria are indeed present in the periapical tissue. Both groups independently demonstrated that specific immunoglobulins that bind to bacteria typically found in infected root canals are present in human periapical granulomas.[20,38] IgG concentrations reported in periapical exudates are four times higher than those found in the serum of the same patients.[37] This may indicate but not prove the local production of these immunoglobulins in periapical lesions. Baumgartner and Falkler[39,40] convincingly demonstrated that the local production of immunoglobulins does indeed take place in the human apical granuloma.

Immunoglobulin production by plasma cells is the end result of a complex and well-controlled process that starts with the exposure of antigen-presenting cells (APCs) to the relevant antigen. In turn, they present the antigen, in conjunction with their major histocompatibility complex class II (MHC II) surface molecule, to specific T lymphocytes. This specific signal, together with a nonspecific signal in the form of the cytokine IL-1, results in the activation of the antigen-specific set of T cells.[41] Once activated, the T cells proliferate and produce several cytokines, two of which are essential for immunoglobulin production, IL-4 and IL-5, which induce the proliferation of B lymphocytes and their maturation into plasma cells. Both serve as nonspecific signals that allow a clone of antigen-specific B cells that were exposed to the same specific antigen to respond by proliferation and maturation into specific plasma cells. These cells will eventually produce immunoglobulin that is specific to that antigen.

MHC II molecules expressing macrophages and dendritic cells were found by Kaneko et al. in experimentally induced periapical lesions in rats.[42,43] The presence of HLA-DR+ cells, which are the human equivalent of the MHC II-positive cells, was studied in human granulomas in a dispersed cell cytometric flow immunochemistry study.[44] Activated macrophages (HLA-DR+, CD14$^+$) and mature dendritic cells (HLA-DR+, CD83$^+$) were found in great numbers. Thus, antigen presentation is possible and likely in the confinement of the apical granuloma.

T LYMPHOCYTES IN THE PERIAPICAL GRANULOMA

T lymphocytes are a major constituents of the chronic inflammatory response at the periapical region.[16,18,19,25,34–36,45] They may constitute up to 40% of the mononuclear inflammatory cells.[35,36] During the active phase of development of an induced apical periodontitis in rats, T helper cells outnumbered T suppressor lymphocytes with a Th/Ts ratio of 1.7.[19] When active lesion expansion subsided, by day 20, this ratio reversed to 0.9 and remained at 0.7 for the remaining 70 days of the experiment. In an established human apical granuloma, T helper (CD4$^+$) cells outnumber T suppressor cells (CD8$^+$) by a ratio of 1.5–2.0.[19] Even though large numbers of T cells are present, it is most likely that only the *activated T cells* play a role in the protective response, and these may constitute as few as 6% of the total T-cell population.[35] When activated, these cells produce a plethora of cytokines that regulate the immune response. T helper (CD4$^+$) lymphocytes may be divided according to their cytokine expression pattern and classified as either T helper 1 (Th1) cells that produce and secrete IL-2 and INF-γ or Th2 cells that produce and secrete IL-4, IL-5, IL-6, IL-10, and IL-13. Th1 type cytokines augment cytotoxic T-cell functions and stimulate proinflammatory cytokine production in other cells, such as macrophages, while Th2 type cytokines participate in B-cell stimulation to mount a humoral immune response and in downregulation of inflammatory reactions.[46,47] Among the cytokines produced by activated T cells, IL-2 is involved in T-lymphocyte proliferation while IL-4, IL-5, and IL-6 are involved in B-cell proliferation, differentiation, and maturation into plasma cells, thus leading to immunoglobulin production (see Figure 1). INF-γ is the key proinflammatory cytokine produced by activated T lymphocytes. Its major function is to activate macrophages that have several key roles, as will be discussed below. Activated macrophages, in turn, are the major source of IL-1 in the periapical lesion and, thus, may contribute to several protective processes including immunoglobulin production, at its initiation stage. TNF-β is another important cytokine produced by activated T cells, which has been implicated as a major factor in the activation of osteoclastic bone resorption in humans, as will be discussed below.[48]

MACROPHAGES IN THE PERIAPICAL GRANULOMA

Macrophages have a major role in several processes that take place in these lesions.[49] Macrophages make up to 46% of the periapical inflammatory cells found in tissue sections of human periapical granulomas.[45] When Stern et al.[50] dispersed periapical granulomas to cell suspensions, 30% of the resulting cells were macrophages. Macrophages were also found as the predominant inflammatory cell when Kopp and Schwarting[18] used monoclonal antibodies to identify them in human periapical lesions. Piatelli et al.[35] similarly reported that macrophages outnumbered T lymphocytes in human periapical granulomas. In the rat model, Kawashima et al.[25] recently demonstrated that macrophages were the predominant immunocompetent cell type throughout the development of the lesion. The kinetics of their presence in these experimental periapical lesions was studied by Akamine et al.,[32] who followed the periapical lesions for as long as 150 days. Macrophages increased in number during the first 10 days and maintained their numbers through day 60, followed by a gradual decline thereafter (Figure 2A,B).

POTENTIAL ROLE OF MACROPHAGES IN THE PERIAPICAL GRANULOMA

Macrophages have a central role in (1) innate, nonspecific immunity; (2) the onset, regulation, and outcome of antigen-specific, acquired immunity; and (3) the regulation of connective tissue destruction and repair. Macrophages are "professional" phagocytic cells that can internalize and kill bacteria by several mechanisms, some of which are part of innate immunity, while others require the presence of specific antibodies against the bacterium and should be considered to be part of the effector arm of specific, acquired immunity. Bacteria, new to the host, may activate the complement system by the alternative pathway, resulting in their opsonization by the C3b component. This, in turn, will result in their phagocytosis by the macrophages via a C3b receptor–mediated process. Other bacteria may attach to the macrophages through lectin-mediated mechanisms, leading to lectinophagocytosis that is independent of the common C3b receptor–ligand binding.[51] Once specific antibodies to a strain of bacteria are present, either

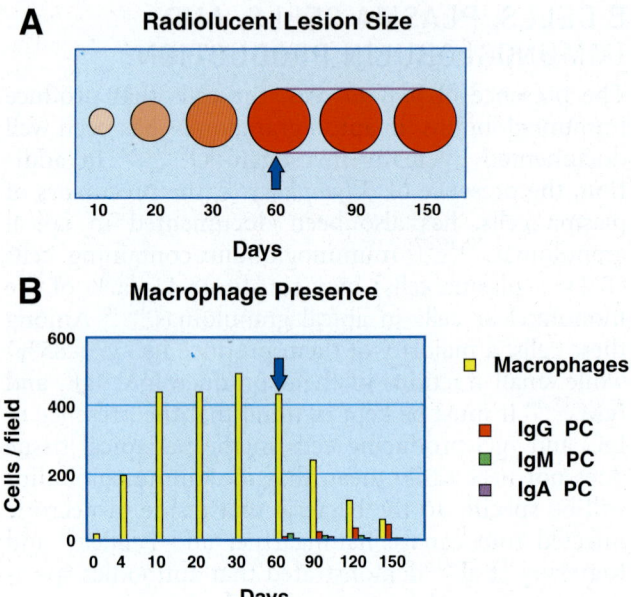

Figure 2 Macrophages and bone resorption in developing periapical lesions in rats. **A,** The periapical lesion gradually enlarges up to 60 days, and then its size remains stable. **B,** Macrophage domination in the lesion coincides with the period in which the lesion grows and diminishes afterwards, with the appearance of plasma cells. Adapted from Akamine A et al.[32]

by developing through the course of the current infection or as a result of a former encounter with these bacteria, a more efficient form of phagocytosis will occur, involving *dual* opsonization by IgG and C3b and engagement of both the Fc and C3b macrophage receptors.

It is the innate immunity that enables the host to survive the initial steps of infection, while the acquired, specific immunity allows the host to efficiently eliminate the invading microorganisms. Macrophages present in the periapical granuloma may contribute, by their function as phagocytes, to the effective prevention of the dissemination of bacteria from the infected root canal. Macrophages may also serve as "APCs" in the essential initial steps of the induction of acquired immunity. They process the antigen and present it to the antigen-specific clones of helper T lymphocytes by a process involving recognition of an MHC II molecule on macrophages by lymphocytes. Additionally, they produce the cytokine IL-1, which is an essential complementary signal for the activation of these lymphocytes. Macrophages that carry MHC II molecules, and thus may serve as APCs, have been identified in periapical granulomas in both humans and the rat model (also termed HLA-DR or Ia antigen-positive cells).[18,52]

Macrophages are considered to be a main source of the cytokines IL-1α, IL-1β, and TNF-α that contribute to the initiation and regulation of the inflammatory process. Additionally, they produce a plethora of other active molecules, including metalloproteases (collagenase and elastase) and prostaglandins that may also contribute to the destructive outcome of the periapical inflammatory process. Some of these products directly damage connective tissue constituents, while others, including the cytokines produced by the macrophages, activate other cells to exhibit either (1) destructive activities such as osteoclast activation and bone resorption or (2) constructive repair processes by activation of fibroblast proliferation and collagen production by these cells.

Though it is commonly assumed that *all* of the above-listed potential activities of the macrophage take place in the periapical granuloma, this is not entirely true. Subsets of macrophages that may exist in relatively small numbers are responsible for a specific activity. Emerging evidence indicates that some of these functions, such as active production of IL-1, involve only a small number of activated macrophages. In chronic human periapical granulomas, these cells do not exceed 2% to 3% of the macrophages present in these lesions, and only these cells have been shown to express mRNA for IL-1β.[9,53]

KINETICS OF MACROPHAGE PRESENCE IN PERIAPICAL LESIONS

The unique study by Akamine et al.[32] followed rat periapical lesions for as long as 150 days. An analysis of their data reveals that the active growing stage of periapical lesions in the rat, which lasted for the first 60 days, coincides with a peak of macrophage presence in this lesion. When the active growth stops and a stationary stage is reached, the presence of macrophages in the lesion gradually declines (Figure 2). This may be a coincidence, but nevertheless, it may indicate a significant correlation. Further support may be found in a recent study by Kawashima et al. that showed that macrophage infiltration in the periapical lesions was associated with bone resorption in the area.[25] In their study, macrophage infiltration preceded that of lymphocytes and gradually increased throughout the 56 days of the experiment.

IL-1 AND MACROPHAGES IN THE PERIAPICAL GRANULOMA

The presence of IL-1β in association with a subpopulation of the macrophages in periapical lesions has been reported by several investigators.[9,53,54] Artese et al.[53] reported that there were very few cells (2% to 3%) in established human periapical granulomas with immunoreactivity of IL-1β and TNF-α and that these cells had a macrophage morphology. Tani-Ishii et al.[54] used a rat model to demonstrate that IL-1α and TNF-α were associated with macrophages in the periapical lesion as soon as two days after the exposure of the pulp and persisted through the 30 days of the experiment. In contrast, TNF-β and IL-1β could not be detected in their sections.

It should be kept in mind that the presence of cytokines, in association with these cells, does not necessarily prove that they are the source of these molecules. A cytokine may potentially have been attached to or may have been taken up by the macrophages, rather than produced by them. Recently, direct proof has been provided that clearly demonstrates that the activated macrophages actually produce IL-1β in periapical lesions. In an in situ hybridization study, Hamachi et al.[9] demonstrated the presence of IL-1β mRNA in macrophages in human periapical lesions. This proves not only that these cells are capable of producing cytokines in general and that cytokines are associated with them in the periapical lesion, but also that subpopulations of macrophages are actively engaged in the production of this cytokine in periapical granulomas.

BACTERIA IN PERIAPICAL LESIONS

For many years, periapical lesions were considered "not an area in which bacteria *live*, but in which they are *destroyed*."[55] This concept had its origin in experiments that failed to produce viable bacteria from closed apical granulomas,[56] and it gained support from the common clinical experience that once bacteria are eliminated from the root canal, most lesions will heal. With the development of adequate anaerobic cultivation methods,[57] it became apparent that this concept may be true "in most cases" but clearly not in all of them. Initially, the concept that viable bacteria may be present outside of the root canal in the periapical tissue was accepted for few specific bacteria.[58–61] The concept that *extraradicular infection* may survive independent of what occurs in the root canal has recently become more widely accepted.[62–68] It is widely accepted that viable bacteria may be cultured from chronic periapical abscesses with a sinus tract and that some closed periapical lesions may contain viable bacteria outside of the root canal: an extraradicular infection. The latter point was initially considered to be a unique condition related only to specific bacteria, such as strains of Actinomyces and

Arachnia.[58–61] However, evidence has accumulated that other bacteria may also survive outside of the root canal in certain lesions.[62–68] Even though this concept is not yet uniformly accepted,[69,70] the original concept that the periapical granuloma is *always* a sterile lesion should be reconsidered in favor of the more moderate statement that it is sterile in *most* cases. This inevitably leads to an understanding that the equilibrium between bacteria and the host, in the periapical environment, is more complicated than believed in the past.

THE EQUILIBRIUM BETWEEN BACTERIA AND THE HOST

An apical granuloma and a chronic periapical abscess with a sinus tract represent two distinct types of equilibriums established between bacteria in the root canal and the host response. The front between bacteria and the host response is established at or near the apical foramen where bacteria or bacterial products/antigens are immediately engaged by the immune system. PMNs will attempt to kill any bacteria within their reach. PMNs are relatively short-lived cells and once they migrate into the tissues they have up to a 3-day life span. Those arriving into the area adjacent to the bacteria will remain there and spontaneously die within a short period, followed by cellular disintegration. The remaining dead bacteria and remnants of the PMNs are taken up by abundant local tissue macrophages. When enzyme-containing PMNs disintegrate, they also release lytic enzymes, such as collagenase, elastase, and hyaluronidase, in the area that damage the host tissue.[71] In histological sections taken under such conditions, only the long-living cells, such as lymphocytes, plasma cells, and macrophages, will be found. The short-lived PMNs will be found only in small numbers, either on their way from adjacent blood vessels or where they accumulate, adjacent to the apical foramen. It is important to realize that macrophages, lymphocytes, and fibroblasts, seen in the histological sections, were there a few days ago and would have been there many days after the section was taken. On the other hand, any PMN seen in the section is a new comer: it left the bloodstream a few hours beforehand and would have died, disintegrated, and disappeared within a few hours or a couple of days. They are not residents of the tissue, but rather are temporary visitors.

An apical granuloma may develop into an acute apical abscess or into a chronic periapical abscess with a sinus tract.[72] A shift in the balance between bacteria and the host may be the likely cause. Such a change may be quantitative, qualitative, or both. If the amount of bacteria introduced into the lesion suddenly increases, the amount of complement-derived chemotactic factor will increase, followed by an increased number of PMNs reaching the area per given time period. More PMNs will die and more damage will be caused by the released enzymes. This rate of destruction may exceed the cleaning capacity of local macrophages and the local tissue may become solubilized by proteolytic and hydrolytic enzymes, resulting in a liquefied area surrounded by migrating PMNs in a background of chronically inflamed tissue. This results in the formation of an abscess.

If the change in the amount of bacteria is transient in nature, macrophages will clean the area, repair will take over, and the tissue will return to its previous state with connective tissue heavily infiltrated with lymphocytes, plasma cells, and macrophages.

A shift in the equilibrium could also be qualitative in nature: a shift in the bacterial population. Some bacterial strains developed a variety of phagocytosis-evading mechanisms that allow them to survive a massive host PMN attack. Some *Porphyromonas gingivalis* strains isolated from suppurating periapical lesions have the capacity to evade phagocytosis due to an antiphagocytic capsule they possess.[73] Other strains have a potent protease that attacks and destroys the C3 and/or C5 complement molecules, thus disrupting this essential antibacterial mechanism.[74–76] Some strains developed a unique evasion strategy and have proteases that clip off the Fc portion of IgG molecules that attach to their surface, thus creating host-derived shields made of Fab fractions that protect them from phagocytes.[77] Strains of *Actinomyces israelii* have yet another strategy: they form aggregates and biofilms that cannot be penetrated by the PMNs and are too large to be phagocytized.[59,61,78–80] A frustrated host response will continuously pour large amounts of PMNs into the battle field only to result in local tissue destruction and pus formation but without any real effect on the bacteria. A draining sinus tract is the clinical expression of the resulting chronic apical abscess.

FLARE-UPS IN PERIAPICAL LESIONS: AN IMMUNOBIOLOGICAL VIEW

A flare-up represents a shift from the equilibrium previously established between bacteria in the root canal and the host response[81] (Chapters 7 and 20). The immune response to extruded bacteria and bacterial by-products results in two main events that occur concomitantly and result in the above symptoms: a vascular and a chemotactic response. Antibodies bind to their specific bacterial antigens, thus activating the complement system via C1q and the "classical pathway." Large amounts of C3a and C5a are generated that drive these two main events. C5a and C3 bind to receptors on local mast cells, causing them to degranulate and release vasoactive amines, such as histamine, in the area.[12,35] The resulting vasodilatation and increased vascular permeability provide additional complement and systemic, plasma-derived, specific antibodies to the ongoing response. Other large proteins also leave the blood vessels. This, in turn, results in a disturbance of the osmotic system that is responsible for the water balance between blood and adjacent tissues. Normally, fluid that leaves the blood vessels in the arterial part of the capillary bed, under the driving force of hydrostatic blood pressure, should be drawn back into the bloodstream in the venous part. This occurs due to the osmotic pressure generated by the large molecules that stay in the blood vessels. When this gradient is disrupted by the large molecules that leave the blood vessels, due to the increased permeability, water stays in the tissue, which results in edema. Since the bony crypt, in which the periapical lesion is contained, cannot expand, this process will result in increased pressure. The one direction in which this pressure may be partially relieved is moving the tooth occlusally, as far as the periodontal ligament fibers will allow. This tooth may now occlude prior to the adjacent teeth, causing an additional mechanical trauma, and the patient experiences more pain.

The other process caused by local complement activation will be a massive chemotactic signal that will attract large amounts of PMNs into the area that may result in abscess formation by the mechanisms discussed above.

PAIN IN APICAL PERIODONTITIS

Pain associated with symptomatic apical periodontitis is sometimes of moderate or severe nature, whereas most periapical lesions are not associated with pain at all.[82,83] It may be a spontaneous pain or a painful response to mechanical stimuli such as percussion, occlusal loading, or sensitivity to palpation of the periapical tissues.[84] Pain is defined as "an unpleasant sensory and emotional experience associated with actual or potential tissue damage."[85] Accordingly, it has peripheral, as well as central, components and is subjected to modulation at each of these levels.

The key peripheral event is the stimulation of nociceptors, neurons that are preferentially sensitive to noxious stimuli or to stimuli that would become noxious in a prolonged exposure.[85] Peripheral nociceptors may respond to mechanical, chemical, or thermal stimuli, the first two being of significance in apical periodontitis. Local sensitization of nociceptors may be induced by numerous mediators that are present in the inflamed periapical tissue (Figure 3). Some of these mediators, such as IL-1α, IL-1β, TNF-α, IL6, or nerve growth factor (NGF), are locally produced by cells of the immune system.[86–89] Others such as CGRP and Substance P derive from stimulated nerve fibers that may become abundant in the area by a sprouting process associated with chronic inflammation.[90] Blood-derived bradykinin may also be locally present.[91] Some local, peripheral mediators, such as bradykinin and serotonin, may directly induce action potential in the nociceptors.[91] The effect of others, such as prostaglandins, NGF, cytokines, serotonin, nitric oxide and adenosine, is indirect, as they lower the stimulatory threshold of these nerve fibers.[86] Pressure building up in the bony crypt, due to edema, is unable to release by swelling, as would be the case in soft tissues. Triggering of pressure nociceptors that have a lowered threshold will result in pain that is often described as an "excruciating pain" and may be relieved only by either natural or artificial drainage.[92]

The proalgesic effect of some cytokines such as IL-1β, IL6 and TNF-α may be partially explained by

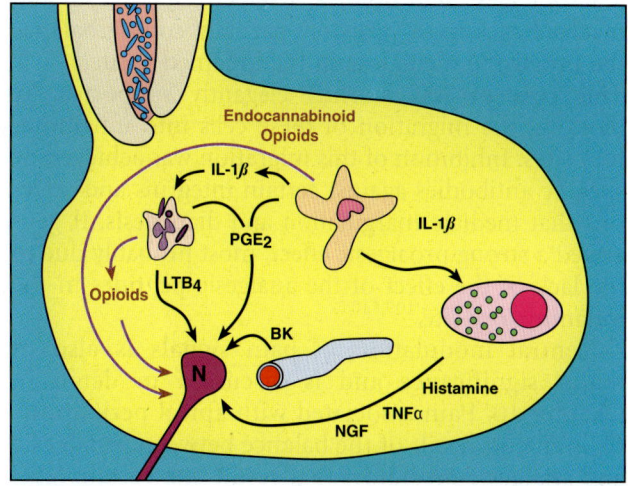

Figure 3 Local activation of nociceptors in an apical granuloma. Nociceptors (N) respond to mechanical and chemical stimuli. Bradykinin (BK) may directly induce action potential in a nociceptor. Others such as prostaglandins, nerve growth factor (NGF), and cytokines may act indirectly by lowering the stimulatory threshold of the nociceptors or by increasing their expression of BK receptors. All the mediators above have a proalgesic effect (black arrows). Opioids, endocannabinoids, and somatostatin (SRIF) generated by macrophages and PMNs have an analgesic effect (purple arrows).

enhancement of local prostaglandin production.[88] Nevertheless, some will have additional indirect effects. IL-1β enhances the production of NGF by mast cells and T lymphocytes.[93,94] NGF, in turn, binds to its receptors on the primary afferent neuron, resulting in the release of neurotransmitters.[95] It will also increase the expression of bradykinin receptors and increase the neuron's sensitivity to acidic pH that is often encountered in inflamed tissues.[96] IL-1β also enhances the local formation of another pain-inducing arachidonic acid metabolite: LTB_4.[88] In addition, bradykinin itself may initiate a cascade of cytokine release that mediates hyperalgesic state by contributing to the above-mentioned mechanisms.[97]

The presence of the above-mentioned mediators in symptomatic periapical tissues is well documented.[22,98,99,100] Nevertheless, pain is not a typical symptom of asymptomatic apical periodontitis. This may be a simple quantitative issue: it could be that only when local proalgesic mediators reach a certain threshold, pain does appear.[98,101,102] Nevertheless, it seems to be more complicated.

Local proalgesic effects of the mediators mentioned above are partially balanced by analgesic mediators derived from inflammatory cells (see Figure 3). Macrophages release somatostatin (SRIF) that has a local analgesic effect.[103] Endocannabinoids secreted by macrophages and opioids released by PMNs and macrophages most probably partially counterbalance the proalgesic mediators in the inflamed tissue.[104–108] This concept was recently elegantly supported by blocking the migration of these cells into inflammatory sites. Inhibition of this migration was achieved by specific antibodies against certain integrins and selectins that mediate margination and diapedesis. It generated a strong proalgesic effect, most probably due to the lack of the effect of the analgesic peptides in the inflammatory site.[109,110]

Central modulation of pain signals is also of major significance and is discussed in detail in Chapter 10. Pain associated with apical periodontitis is an end result of the balance between proalgesic and analgesic mediators that result in a certain level of stimulation of local peripheral nociceptors that is then transmitted centrally, where it is further modulated, resulting in a sensation of "pain."

BONE RESORPTION IN PERIAPICAL LESIONS

Bone resorption is one of the clinical hallmarks of periapical pathosis. The resorption may be viewed either as an undesirable destructive by-product of the host response, as is the case with periodontal disease, or alternatively, as is traditionally presented, as a process by which a bone is removed from a risky area, thus allowing a "buffer zone" to be formed in which host response constituents engage the bacteria. In any case, it is bone resorption in the periapical area that serves the clinician as a major indicator of the presence of a periapical pathological process and the progression of its healing. As such, it has been thoroughly studied in both humans and animal models.

POTENTIAL VERSUS ACTUAL BONE-RESORBING AGENTS

Bone resorption occurs through the activation of the bone-resorbing cells: the osteoclasts. A wide range of biologically active molecules have been demonstrated to have the capacity to activate osteoclastic bone resorption in in vitro models. These include prostaglandins,[111] bacterial endotoxin,[112] complement activation products, as well as the inflammatory cytokines IL-1α, IL-1β, TNF-α, TNF-β, IL-6, and IL-11 that, as a group, were previously referred to as "osteoclast-activating factor."[113] Among these, IL-1β is the most active cytokine and its bone-resorbing capacity is 13-fold of that of IL-1α and 1000-fold of that of TNF-α or TNF-β.[114] When considering the periapical bone resorption associated with infected root canals, all of these have been mentioned and most of them were demonstrated in periapical lesions.[6,12,33,48,53,98,100–102,115,116] The question was which of these *potential* bone-resorbing stimuli is actually involved in the activation of osteoclasts in these lesions?

Two studies by Wang and Stashenko[48] have provided convincing evidence that among the long list of *potential* mediators that may activate osteoclasts and cause periapical bone resorption, the main factors and those that are most important in human chronic periapical lesions are IL-1β and TNF-β. In the rat model of induced active periapical bone resorption, IL-1α and, to a lesser extent, IL-1β and TNF-β are the major bone-resorbing cytokines.[117] Both studies suggest that osteoclast activation by these cytokines may be mediated in part by de novo formation of cyclooxygenase pathway products such as prostaglandins, as the effect could be significantly blocked by nonsteroid anti-inflammatory drugs (NSAIDs).[48,117]

The formation of periapical lesions was studied in the rat model by Kakehashi, Stashenko, and others.[9,19,25,31,118,119] Following exposure and bacterial contamination of the pulp chamber and the root canal, an inflammatory response is activated in the periapical region that is associated with rapid growth of a periapical lesion, the size of which can be monitored using either radiographs or histological sections. This rapid growth persists for 15 days and is associated with "bone-resorbing activity" that can be detected in homogenates of the lesions and measured using an in vitro bone resorption assay.[119] Following the active resorptive phase, the lesions remain at a stable size for as long as 30 days.[120] During this stationary phase, the bone-resorbing activity declined to 10% to 30% of that in the active growing stage. This last stationary phase is considered to be equivalent to an existing chronic, periapical granuloma in humans that also contains bone-resorptive activity.[48] The cytokines defined in the above studies are found in human periapical lesions in measurable amounts. Lim et al.[102] found significant amounts of IL-1β in homogenates of human periapical lesions, even though none of the patients had detectable serum levels of this cytokine. Noninflamed pulp tissue, which served as a control, was also free of the cytokine. Periapical exudates were studied by Matsuo et al.[121] for their IL-1α and IL-1β contents. Exudates, obtained through the root canal, contained an average level of 6.57 (±0.73) ng/mL of IL-1β and 3.23 (±0.66) ng/mL of IL-1α. The cytokine profile change following root canal treatment with a tendency of IL-1α to increase and of IL-1β to decrease.[122,123]

CELLULAR SOURCES OF BONE-RESORBING CYTOKINES

Even though IL-1 and TNF may be produced by many cell types, the activated macrophage is considered to be the main source of IL-1α, IL-1β, and TNF-α.[124] On the other hand, TNF-β is commonly considered to be an activated T-lymphocyte product.[125] In view of the above, two cell types should be considered as being responsible for bone-resorbing activity in human periapical lesions: activated T cells and activated macrophages. Not all T lymphocytes or macrophages in the periapical lesion are in a state of activation. Kopp and Schwaring[18] have found that only 6% of the T lymphocytes in human periapical granulomas were activated. Artese et al.,[53] who also used human periapical granulomas, demonstrated that while 41% of the mononuclear inflammatory cells were macrophages, only 2% to 3% of these cells were activated and produced IL-1β and TNF-α. The activation states of these cells are closely related to each other: T helper lymphocytes may be activated in an antigen-specific manner by antigen-presenting macrophages that also produce the IL-1 required to accomplish this process. Macrophage activation, as part of the acquired, specific immune response, may be achieved by cytokines such as IFN-γ that are produced by the activated T lymphocytes (see Figure 1). Macrophages may also be activated by other routes, such as by exposure to bacterial endotoxin (LPS), as part of innate, nonspecific immunity.[126]

STUDIES IN ATHYMIC ANIMALS

Athymic rats and mice are powerful tools used to study and demonstrate the essential role of T lymphocytes in other immunobiological processes.[127,128] These animals lack T cells, and consequently T-cell function is missing, rendering a variety of immune responses inactive. Such animals were used in two studies that assumed that periapical bone resorption and the development of periapical lesions would be defective in athymic animals. The results of these studies should be viewed as a turning point in the understanding of the immunobiology of the host response and bone resorption in periapical lesions. Wallstrom et al.[129] demonstrated that no significant difference existed between the periapical bone resorption of conventional and athymic rats. Similar results were reported in a study by Tani-Ishii et al.[31] using athymic mice. They also found that periapical lesions developed in the T-cell-lacking animals at a rate that precluded the possibility that T lymphocytes are essential prerequisites in the development of these lesions. Even though T lymphocytes may, and most probably do, contribute to the process, alternative routes likely exist, enabling the formation of lesions in their absence.

Activated macrophages may serve in such a route in the formation of periapical lesions. Macrophage activation may occur by a variety of pathways. Cytokines such as IFN-γ, produced by antigen-specific activated T lymphocytes, are the main immune response-related activators of the macrophage.[124,130] In their absence, bacterial endotoxin (LPS) may successfully accomplish this task.[126,131,132] This activation of the macrophage may be viewed as part of innate immunity, independent of a specific response to antigens. This may have been the mechanism by which the lesions developed in the athymic animals. The bacterial content of the infected root canals in these animals gradually developed to 46% gram-negative flora.[133] LPS, derived from these gram-negative bacteria, could activate macrophages in the periapical area, independent of T lymphocytes. These macrophages, in turn, produce their cytokines IL-1α, IL-1β and TNF-α that activate osteoclastic bone resorption. This does not preclude the participation of T cells in the process in normal animals, but rather turns the spotlight to *the main effector cell*: the macrophage. This result is in agreement with the finding that in the rat model, IL-1α is the major bone-resorbing cytokine while TNF-β, the T-cell product, could not be detected in these lesions by antibody-blocking or immunohistochemical studies.[54,117]

OSTEOCLAST ACTIVATION: UPDATED CONCEPT

The concept of osteoclast activation had a missing link for many years. It was well known that both systemic factors such as parathyroid hormone (PTH) and local factors such as IL-1β activate osteoclastic bone resorption. Nevertheless, osteoclasts do not have receptors for either of these agents. The presence of other cells such as osteoblasts or stromal bone marrow cells that do have the proper receptors is required.[134] An intermediate factor, produced by other bone cells and affecting the osteoclasts, had been hypothesized in an attempt to solve this enigma.[113] It was also recognized that bone cells and osteoclasts have to be *in proximity* to each other to allow the activation to take place.[134,135]

The missing link has recently been discovered.[134,136–139] (Figure 4A,B). A group of cell surface receptors and ligands as well as soluble ligands is responsible for up-and-down regulation of osteoclastic bone resorption. When bone cells are activated by either PTH or IL-1β, they express a ligand named osteoprotegerin ligand (OPGL, RANK-Ligand) on their surface that has the following two main functions:

(1) Binding to a surface receptor RANK (receptor activator of nuclear factor κB) on mononuclear preosteoclasts, thus inducing their maturation to multinucleated mature osteoclasts
(2) Binding to RANK, also expressed on the surface of mature but inactive osteoclasts, thus activating them to become active bone-resorbing cells with a fully expressed ruffled border.[134]

This process results in increased numbers of active osteoclasts and bone resorption. Such a mechanism also explains the well-established need for cell proximity during osteoclast activation: both receptors and ligands are *surface molecules* that require proximity for binding. Inflammatory bone resorption may have yet another avenue of osteoclast activation, as activated T cells may also express OPGL on their surface, allowing them to directly activate the osteoclasts.[140–142] Down-regulation of bone resorption is carried out by a soluble inhibitor, osteoprotegerin ("bone protector," OPG), that binds to OPGL and serves as a competitive inhibitor of RANK, preventing its binding to OPGL. This soluble inhibitor was among the first to be discovered. It has been clinically tested as an osteoporosis preventing agent with promising results.[143]

OPGL was recently demonstrated to be present in human periapical granulomas where it was found on macrophages and dendritic cells.[144,145] This, taken together with the recent demonstration of OPG production by periodontal ligament fibroblasts, may have important future implications and applications.[146]

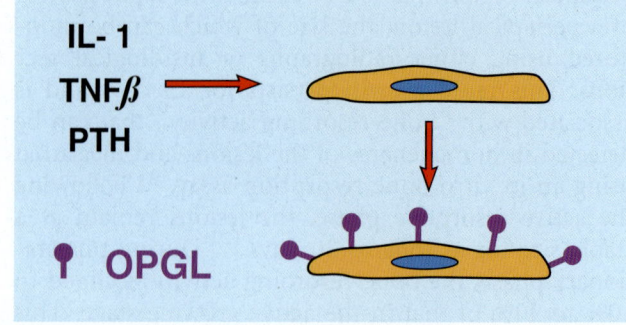

Figure 4 Osteoclast activation via osteoprotegerin ligand (OPGL) (RANK-ligand). ***A***, Osteoblasts and bone marrow stromal cells express OPGL (RANK-ligand) when stimulated by either PTH (parathyroid hormone) or the cytokines IL-1 and tumor necrosis factor-β (TNF-β). ***B***, Osteoclast precursors that carry the receptor RANK on their surface are activated to develop into multinucleated osteoclasts, thus increasing the number of osteoclasts in the area. Osteoclasts that are present are activated through their receptor RANK to become active in bone resorption, expressing a ruffled border. Osteoclast activation is downregulated by the soluble competitive inhibitor osteoprotegerin (OPG) that inhibits the binding of RANK to its ligand OPGL.

Histopathology of Periapical Lesions of Endodontic Origin

The discussion of the histopathology of periapical lesions includes the *apical granuloma*, as well as two entities that may develop within it or from it: *apical abscess* and *apical cyst*.

The *apical granuloma* is an inflammatory lesion dominated by macrophages, lymphocytes, and plasma cells (Figure 5A,B). Abundant capillaries may be found with numerous fibroblasts and connective tissue fibers. It is often encapsulated in collagenous connective tissue. Epithelial cell proliferation is a common finding in apical granuloma. Serial sectioning reveals that epithelial proliferation occurs in 6% to 55% of these lesions.[81,147] They are believed to originate from the epithelial cell rests of Mallasez that proliferate under the influence of cytokines and growth factors generated in the periapical granuloma (Figure 6). Thus, the presence of epithelial cells in a granuloma is a common finding, and its development into a cyst may be considered to be an event that occurs with time within an existing apical granuloma.

PMNs are found in varying numbers in an apical granuloma and may reach a local dominancy within a given area of the granulomatous tissue when an abscess is formed. Thus, an apical abscess may be considered to be a transient or persistent event (in the case of a chronic apical abscess) that occurs within an existing apical granuloma. In general, the histological picture of granulomas varies considerably.[81,148] The simple, well-organized morphological description of apical periodontitis, based on a zonal pattern, hardly represents the common reality. It was originally an extrapolation from observations by Fish in an experimental model.[149] The experimental lesions were produced in guinea pigs by drilling holes in bones and packing them with wool fibers saturated with microorganisms and were not associated with infected root canals. This zonal pattern has been a conceptually useful teaching aid and, as such, has survived through the generations.[150–152] Nevertheless, one should not expect to find it in random biopsies of periapical granulomas, as it does not seem to represent the actual structural variation

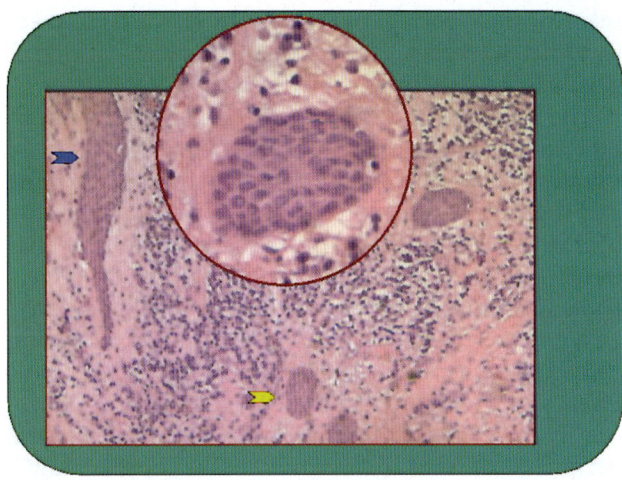

Figure 6 Epithelial strands in an apical granuloma. Epithelial strands form a network in an apical granuloma. They may be observed in a longitudinal section (blue arrow) or at cross section (yellow arrow and enlargement). This epithelium originated from the rest cells of Malassez that proliferate under the influence of cytokines and growth factors in the apical granuloma. They are the source of the epithelial lining of cysts that may develop in apical granulomas.

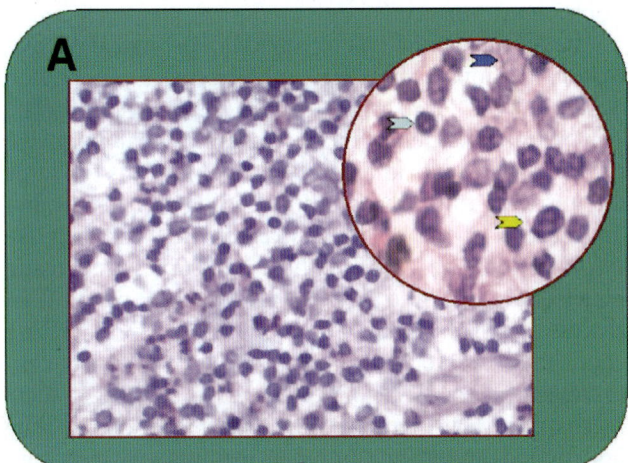

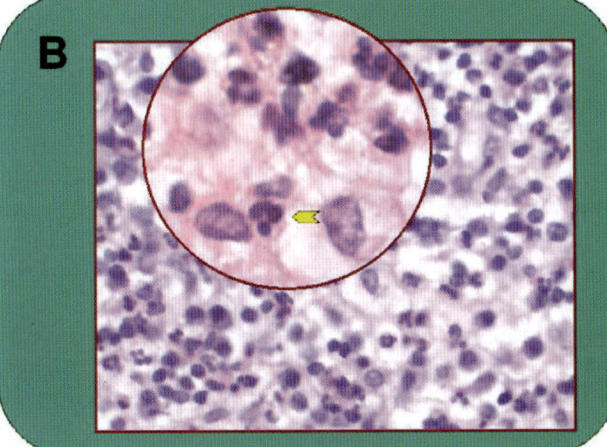

Figure 5 Apical granuloma: histopathology. ***A***, The lesion is dominated by lymphocytes (green arrow) and macrophages (yellow arrow), with abundant fibroblasts (blue arrow). ***B***, A chronic periapical lesion with a polymorphonuclear leukocyte (PMN) infiltrate (yellow arrow).

seen in most periapical lesions. In fact, great structural heterogeneity is the *norm* for apical periodontitis, particularly in chronic lesions.[81,148]

The hallmark of an *apical abscess* is the presence of pus: an area containing liquefied tissue. Abscesses are usually found within a pre-existing apical granuloma and represent a shift in cellular dynamics. The influx of PMNs is dramatically increased to the extent that tissue macrophages are no longer able to effectively cope with the tissue damage caused by hydrolytic enzymes released from a vast number of dying PMNs. Connective tissue constituents such as collagen and hyaluronic acid are degraded and the tissue in the center of the abscess is liquefied. On the periphery of the abscess, the tissue of the apical granuloma persists and its adjacent layer is infiltrated with a large number of PMNs that are migrating from the nearest blood vessel to end their life in the pus-containing center of the abscess.

A histological continuum may be found between an apical granuloma that contains a small number of infiltrating PMNs, through a granuloma with a large number of infiltrating PMNs, and an established apical abscess. The former may be histologically termed a granuloma with acute inflammation, but only the latter warrants the term apical abscess.

An *apical cyst* is an epithelium-lined cavity that contains fluid or semisolid material and is commonly surrounded by dense connective tissue (Figure 7). Apical cysts are associated with teeth that have necrotic pulps and an infected root canal system and develop within the periapical inflammatory lesion, the granuloma. The cyst cavity is most commonly lined with stratified squamous epithelium of varying thickness that originates from the epithelial rest cells of Malassez. Nevertheless, lining with ciliary epithelium that originates from an adjacent maxillary sinus may also be found.[153] The epithelial lining may be continuous, but it is often disrupted or even completely missing, most probably due to a secondary infection. Periapical cysts are divided into *pocket cysts* (bay cyst) and *true cysts*.[154–156]

A periapical pocket cyst (bay cyst) is an apical inflammatory cyst that contains a sac-like, epithelium-lined cavity that is open to and continuous with the root canal space.[154–156] True apical cysts are located within the periapical granuloma with no connection between their cavity and that of the root canal space. More than half of the apical cysts are true apical cysts while the remainder are of the pocket cyst variety.[81,154–156]

The mechanism of cyst formation in periapical inflammatory lesions has been the subject of much debate.[81,157–159] Two main theories were proposed. The "nutritional deficiency theory" assumes that epithelial proliferation results in an epithelial mass that is too large for nutrients to reach its core, resulting in necrosis and liquefaction of the cells in its center, thus forming the cystic cavity. The "abscess theory" assumes that tissue liquefaction occurred first, at the central part of an abscess, that was later lined by locally proliferating epithelium, due to the inherent nature of epithelial cells to cover the exposed connective tissue surfaces.[159] The mechanism by which cysts grow and expand is not fully understood and most probably involves inflammatory mediators that are present in the lesion.[81]

CLINICAL MANIFESTATION AND DIAGNOSTIC TERMINOLOGY

Periapical lesions of endodontic origin vary greatly in their clinical manifestation. Their classification is based on the clinical presentation at a given time point; it may shift from one diagnosis to another, with time. Such shifts may be understood and explained on the basis of the biological events discussed above.

The diagnostic terminology used here will include *normal periapical tissues, symptomatic apical periodontitis* (acute apical/periradicular periodontitis), *asymptomatic apical periodontitis* (chronic apical/periradicular periodontitis), *acute apical abscess* (acute periradicular abscess), *chronic apical abscess* (chronic periradicular abscess and suppurative apical/periradicular abscess), *cellulitis, condensing osteitis* (focal sclerosing osteomyelitis, periradicular

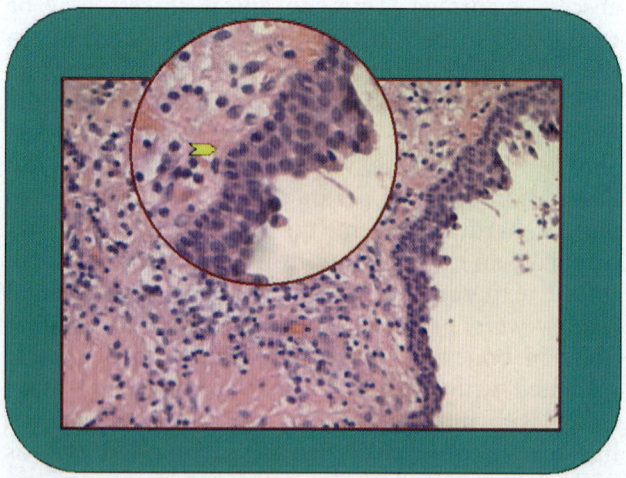

Figure 7 Apical cyst. A partial view of the wall of a space that was filled with liquid and lined with stratified cuboidal epithelium (yellow arrow and enlargement), originating from the epithelial rests of Malassez.

osteosclerosis, sclerosing osteitis, and sclerotic bone), and *apical scar*.

Clinical manifestations that are used to make a periapical diagnosis derive from (1) subjective information derived from a patient's anamnesis and objective data derived from (2) radiographic examination, as well as (3) results of direct observation and physical examination of the patient, the subjected tooth, and surrounding tissues.

A correlation between the clinical diagnosis and that derived from histopathological examination of the tissue is limited. An apical abscess may be clinically recognized by the presence of pus; however, clinical findings and conventional radiographs cannot predict if another lesion is a granuloma or a cyst.[160,161] Accordingly, clinical manifestations and diagnostic terminologies were discussed in this chapter separately from histopathological features of periapical lesions. A discussion of the latter was in terms of form and function in order to allow the reader to understand the processes that lead to the clinical manifestations.

Inflammatory lesions of endodontic origin appear in response to stimuli originating from a root canal. As such, they are located around any of the root canal system portals of exit. Pathogenesis and pathology of the inflammatory lesions will be similar at any of those portals of exit; nevertheless, the clinical and radiographic manifestation may vary greatly with the location of the involved portal. The term *periradicular* rather than periapical has often been used to express this diversity.[66,102,162–165] The terms *apical* or *periapical* were used throughout this text for the sake of simplicity, as well as to express the fact that this is the most common manifestation of inflammatory lesions of endodontic origin.

NORMAL PERIAPICAL TISSUES

In normal periapical tissues, the tooth is not tender to percussion or pressure and there is not any tenderness to palpation of the mucosa overlying the periapical region. There is no swelling and there are no symptoms noted by the patient.[166] Radiographically, the lamina dura is intact and the periodontal ligament space has a normal and consistent width along the entire root, which is similar to that of the adjacent teeth.[166] Recognition of "normal" is essential to estimate changes that may occur with disease, as well as their gradual disappearance with healing.

SYMPTOMATIC APICAL PERIODONTITIS

Symptomatic apical periodontitis occurs within a previously healthy periapical region in response to either microbiological or physical irritation.[166] The former may result from an initial emergence of bacteria or their products from an infected root canal into the apical periodontium. The latter may result from endodontic treatment when there is mechanical or chemical injury to the apical tissues. They may occur together when the physical insult carry bacteria with it, from the infected root canal into the apical periodontium.

If the insult was short in nature, such as with trauma induced by a file passing through a sterile, noninfected pulp tissue, the symptoms will usually soon subside and healing will take place. On the other hand, if the insult is continuous and persistent, such as the permanent communication between bacteria growing in the root canal and the host response in the apical periodontium, events may take one of two other routes. It may either become more and more symptomatic, a process that may develop into an acute apical abscess and facial cellulitis. Alternatively, it may take a quieter route and gradually become asymptomatic apical periodontitis, with slight or no symptoms and with typical periapical bone resorption. Factors that dictate which route will be taken are not completely clear, but they most probably involve the nature of the bacteria. Their susceptibility or ability to survive the host response may shift the balance one way or the other. Symptomatic apical periodontitis may also represent a shift of the balance established between the bacteria and the host, in an asymptomatic apical periodontitis lesion (see below). Such shifts may occur due to a variety of reasons, starting with naturally occurring events and ending with iatrogenically induced exacerbation.

ASYMPTOMATIC APICAL PERIODONTITIS

Asymptomatic apical periodontitis is a long-standing periapical inflammatory lesion with radiographically visible periapical bone resorption but with minimal or no clinical symptoms. Its development may be uneventful and often goes unnoticed by the patient until it is discovered on a radiograph or until it develops into a symptomatic lesion. Histologically, the radiolucent area associated with asymptomatic apical periodontitis will be either a granuloma or a cyst. The radiological appearance of the lesion may take a wide range of shapes and sizes that has tempted clinicians to search for a correlation between size and morphology of the lesion and its histological nature. The appearance of the radiolucent area in conventional radiographs cannot predict its histological diagnosis.[160,161,167,168] Recent innovative technologies may be more predictive (see Chapter 15).

ACUTE APICAL ABSCESS

An acute apical abscess is characterized by rapid onset, spontaneous pain, tenderness of the tooth to pressure, pus formation, and eventual swelling of the associated tissues. At the initial stages of its formation, the process may be extremely painful, as pressure builds up in the restricted periapical space. The establishment of drainage through the root canal may, in some cases, end the agonizing process. Left to natural events, an acute apical abscess will sometimes subside. In most cases, the overlying cortical plate will eventually perforate and purulence will accumulate under the periosteum producing a painful condition. Only with the perforation of the periosteum will the pus be able to drain into over lying tissues and allow the major pain to subside. At this stage, a local swelling will appear and an incision for drainage should be made in the overlying tissues to allow final drainage. In some cases, natural drainage will be established within a few days by perforation of the covering tissue. In other cases, the swelling will remain for some time before it gradually subsides.

CHRONIC APICAL ABSCESS

A sinus tract is the hallmark of the *chronic apical abscess*. The inflammatory process perforates one of the cortical plates and a draining sinus tract is established that allows for continuous discharge of pus forming in the periapical lesion through the oral mucosa or, in rare cases, through the skin. Typically, a stoma of a parulis can be detected that, from time to time, will discard the pus. Sometimes a sinus tract will lead to the maxillary sinus and will go unobserved. A sinus tract may also exit in the gingival sulcus a furcation area and must be differentiated from periodontal disease. A chronic apical abscess is most commonly, but not always, associated with an apical radiolucency. It is asymptomatic or only slightly symptomatic, and the patient may often be unaware of its presence. This may last as long as the sinus tract is not obstructed. Even when such an obstruction occurs, it is most likely that any swelling will be of limited duration and will be limited to the local area of the sinus tract, as both the bone and the periosteum are already perforated.

CELLULITIS

Cellulitis is a symptomatic edematous inflammation associated with diffuse spreading of invasive microorganisms throughout connective tissue and facial planes. Diffuse swelling of facial or cervical tissues is its main clinical feature. Cellulitis is usually a sequel of an apical abscess that penetrated the bone, allowing the spread of pus along the paths of least resistance, between facial structures. This usually implies the facial planes between the muscles of the face or the neck (see Chapter 20). Spreading of an infection may or may not be associated with systemic symptoms such as fever and malaise. Since cellulitis is usually a sequel of an uncontrolled apical abscess, other clinical features typical of an apical abscess are also expected. Spreading of an infection into adjacent and more remote connective tissue compartments may result in serious or even life-threatening complications. Cases of Ludwig's angina,[169] orbital cellulites,[170] cavernous sinus thrombosis,[171] and even death from a brain abscess[172] originating from a spreading dental infection have been reported.

CONDENSING OSTEITIS

Condensing osteitis (focal sclerosing osteomyelitis) is a diffuse radiopaque lesion believed to represent a localized bony reaction to a low-grade inflammatory stimulus, usually seen at the apex of a tooth (or its extraction site) in which there has been a long-standing pulp pathosis. It is characterized by overproduction of bone in the periapical area, mostly around the apices of mandibular molars and premolars that had long-standing pulp pathosis. The pulp of the involved tooth may be chronically inflamed, but since such inflammation may lead to pulp necrosis, it may be expected that, at some stage, the involved pulp is nonvital. The radiopacity may or may not respond to endodontic treatment.

APICAL SCAR

Apical scar is not an inflammatory lesion, but rather an uncommon pattern of healing of an apical inflammatory lesion. It consists of a dense collagenous connective tissue in the bone at or near the apex of a root with a distinctive radiolucent presentation.[173,174] It represents a form of healing that is usually associated with a root that has been treated surgically. Perforation of both facial and lingual osseous cortices is believed to result in collagenous rather than osseous healing.[173,175] Maxillary lateral incisors are the most frequently affected teeth. Definitive clinical diagnosis is very difficult without histopathological examination. A case history may be helpful, especially when a detailed surgical report is included. Periapical inflammation that, with time, resorbed and perforated both cortices may also result in an apical scar. Since such cases are quite rare,[160,174,176] the probability that a given nonresponsive periapical lesion, with no surgical involvement, is actually an apical scar is extremely low when compared to that of a rather common posttreatment disease.

Traditional Concepts Versus a Futuristic View

The current concept and rational of endodontic treatment of periapical lesions has not changed significantly for many years. It is centered on one issue: stopping the bacterial stimulation of the host response at the apical foramen/foramina that would allow healing of the lesion. Methods used to achieve this goal include the following:

(1) Cleaning, shaping, and disinfection, aimed at thorough elimination of bacteria from the root canal system, followed by obturation
(2) In case the above procedure fails, surgical removal of residual infected tissue in apical ramifications of the root canal system inaccessible to the above-mentioned procedure and thus may still harbor bacteria
(3) Root-end sealing of the root canal system to prevent continuous bacterial stimulus that may still exist after the completion of stages "1" and/ or "2" described above.

This comprises a simple and rather mechanistic rational that has worked well for several generations. Nevertheless, by limiting itself to this concept alone, the profession may ignore, or at least make no use of the vast information and potential tools generated over the last two decades in bone biology research and in studies aimed to pharmacologically modulate destructive immune responses.

The ideas, information, and concepts that follow should not be taken as proven or approved clinical therapeutic protocols. They should rather provide a conceptual framework for understanding possibilities and new avenues of thought that will most probably become possible in the coming years. They are aimed to prepare the minds and hearts of future leaders of the profession and inspire them to look into additional therapeutic avenues. Endodontics should not limit itself only to better ways of cleaning, shaping, and obturation. Biological research may provide, in the not so far future, new concepts and methods to supplement traditional ones.

Endodontic treatment is aimed to eliminate bacteria from infected root canals that will later be sealed to prevent recontamination. With the elimination of the bacterial stimuli that evoked the periapical inflammation, the periapical lesion should resolve and repair should take place. Healing of the lesions may take many months.[177–180] It may be argued that if a given lesion eventually heals in 12, 24, or even 36 months, there is no benefit in rushing the process. Nevertheless, shortening the healing time may have clinical importance, as it may (1) allow earlier decisions in regard to the restorative treatment plan related to the treated teeth and (2) limit the period for which temporary crowns and bridges are used; temporary restorations that may leak and allow recontamination of the treated root canal.

The prolonged healing process of many periapical lesions raises the possibility that the activated cells in the lesion may maintain their state of activation long after the initial cause of their activation has been eliminated. Namely, the activation state may outlive its useful purpose and become a burden. Macrophages are known to persist in tissues for many months and if their state of activation persists, they may inhibit the fibroblasts, maintain osteoclastic activity, and inhibit osteogenesis, thus preventing both soft connective tissue and bone repair from taking place.[126,181] Indirect support for this notion may be found in a study carried out, for a totally different purpose, by Kvist and Reit.[178] Healing of periapical lesions was compared following surgical and nonsurgical retreatment. At 12 months, a significant difference was found in favor of surgical treatment that faded by 48 months to almost no difference between the groups (Figure 8). If

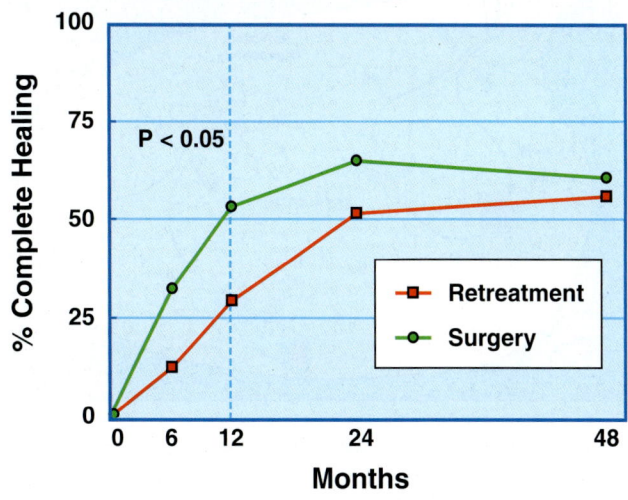

Figure 8 Healing of periapical lesions following surgical removal of the chronically inflamed tissue, compared to healing after retreatment. By 48 months, no difference was found between the groups. Nevertheless, healing was much faster when the tissue was surgically removed, with a significant difference at 12 months. Adapted from Kvist T and Reit C.[178]

the idea presented above is true, these results may support the concept that early surgical removal of the tissue containing activated macrophages, allowed its replacement with fresh granulation tissue that contains a fresh set of cells that will not delay repair.

If this concept is valid, it may be important and possible to monitor the state of activation of periapical macrophages by sampling the interstitial fluid of the lesion through the root canal.[121,123,182] Recently Kuo et al.[122] were successful in performing such measurements and were able to quantify the IL-1β concentration in apical exudates and correlate it with clinical and radiological features of the lesions. A longitudinal study that evaluates the correlation between the diminishing IL-1β content of the lesions and their gradual radiographic repair will be required to prove this point.

Assuming that such inhibitory mechanisms are involved in the prolonged and delayed repair of periapical lesions, pharmacological modulation of the process may be considered (Figure 9). Stashenko et al.[113] demonstrated that an IL-1 receptor antagonist may be used in animals to reduce the bone-resorbing activity and the formation of periapical lesions. Similarly, NSAIDs were successfully used for a similar purpose in both experimental and human periodontal diseases, as well as in the cat model for periapical lesions.[183,184]

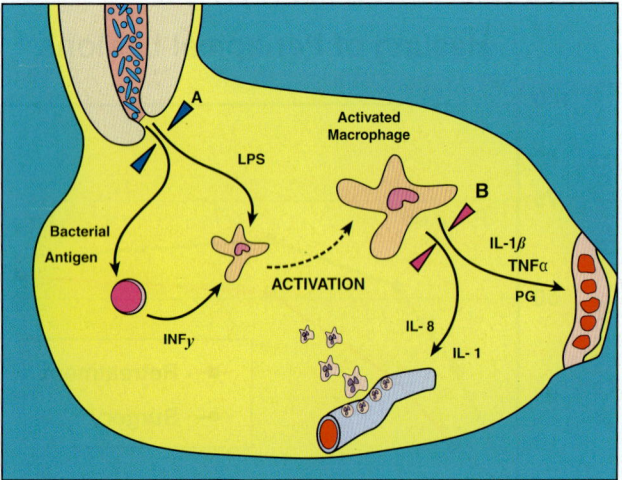

Figure 9 Potential pharmacological modulation of the healing of apical granuloma. *A,* Traditional endodontic approach: elimination of the bacteria from the root canal, followed by obturation of the root canal to prevent recontamination. *B,* Potential additional sites for pharmacological modulation. Either the local production and release of bone-resorbing cytokines or their effect on bone cells is a potential target for "turning off" the lesion, once its activity had outlived its useful, protective purpose.

These two approaches were directed at either blocking the *binding* of the already produced cytokine to its target cells or *interfering with its action* on osteoclasts and osteoblasts that may involve prostaglandin production.[48,117]

Tetracyclines may be used to inhibit cytokine *secretion* by activated macrophages.[185,186] Shapira et al.[186] studied tetracycline inhibition of TNF and IL-1 production by LPS-activated macrophages and found its effect to be at a post-transcriptional level: both mRNA and the cytokines themselves were produced but they were not secreted into the cells' surroundings. Tetracyclines may also inhibit bone resorption by other mechanisms that are unrelated to their antimicrobial capacity. This is mediated by inhibition of connective tissue metalloproteases.[187] Accordingly, it has recently been demonstrated that systemic low-dose tetracycline inhibits the formation of periapical lesions in rats by a mechanism(s) that is (are) unrelated to their antimicrobial effects.[188]

An alternative strategy may be to try to locally "turn off" the activated macrophages, thus lowering the local *production* of IL-1 in the lesion. Modulation of macrophage activation has been attempted both in vivo and in vitro using glucocorticoid steroids.[126,130,189,190] Macrophages, activated to become tumoricidal, were "turned off" in vivo by a process involving cortico steroids.[189] Recently, Metzger et al.[126] reported that suppression of fibroblast proliferation by LPS-activated macrophages was reversed using hydrocortisone. Dexamethasone also inhibited periapical lesion formation in the rat model, most probably by a similar mechanism.[191] Such effects on macrophage activation and production of its mediators have also been reported by others and were attributed to inhibitory effects of the steroids at the gene transcription level.[130,192,193]

If and when bacteria are no longer present in the root canal, the state of activation of the macrophages may outlive its useful and beneficial purpose. Attempts to "turn off" the host response and its effects in the lesion may represent a *new biological treatment modality* that may alleviate suppression and enhance repair in these lesions (see Figure 9). Local delivery of desired pharmacological agents should be simpler in the closed environment of the periapical lesion, as compared to similar attempts in periodontal pockets. *Local sustained delivery* of drugs aimed at this goal may easily be achieved. By using biodegradable slow release devices in the form of a point that may be inserted through the root canal into periapical tissues, it may locally deliver the drug or drug combination for a predetermined period of time.

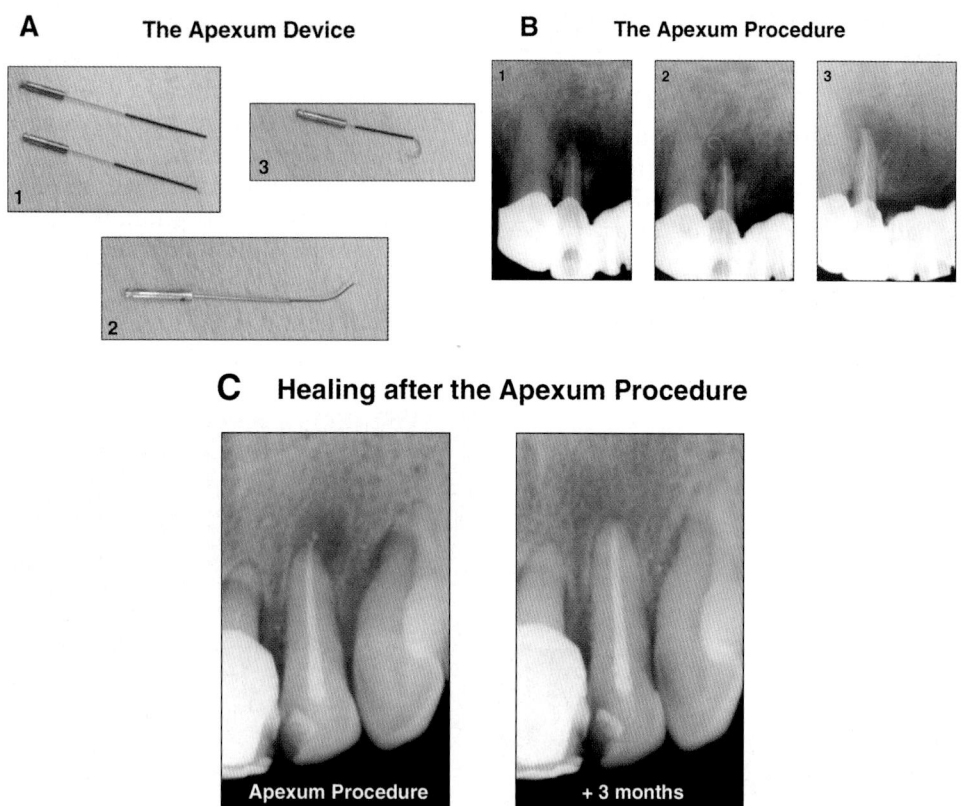

Figure 10 Apexum©: A method for minimally invasive removal of periapical tissues through the root canal. **A,** The Apexum NiTi Ablator© (1, 2). The black tube contains a nickel–titanium wire that is protruded when pushed through the apical foramen. Upon entering the periapical area, it takes a specially designed form (2) and is rotated at 300 rpm, mincing the soft tissue, while being deflected from the surrounding bone. The Apexum PGA Ablator© (3) has a fiber made of biodegradable material that is rotated in the periapical area at 5000 rpm, grinding the tissue to a thin suspension that is then washed out with saline. **B,** (1) The nickel–titanium tube is inserted to the working length. (2) The Apexum NiTi Ablator is pushed and inserted into the periapical area. (3) Once the Apexum procedure is completed, the root canal is obturated with a root canal filling. **C,** A maxillary incisor immediately after the completion of the procedure and 3 months later. Note the rapid bone healing in the periapical area.

A better understanding of the immunobiology of periapical lesions may eventually result in a different endodontic practice than is encountered today. Chairside diagnostic kits that will allow definition of a periapical lesion as "active" or "healing," by sampling via the root canal prior to obturation, seem logical and possible. Similarly, pharmacological modulation of the healing process may also be near.

An alternative, simpler, approach has recently emerged with the development of a device that allows enucleation of the periapical tissue, through the root canal and the apical foramen. The Apexum™ protocol is applied just before root canal obturation. Once cleaning, shaping, and disinfection of the root canal is completed, the apical foramen is enlarged by passing a No. 35 rotary file to 1 to 2 mm beyond the apex. This passage is used to insert a specially designed nickel–titanium wire into the periapical tissue that rotates and minces the tissue (Figure 10A,B). This is followed by a biodegradable fiber rotated at a higher speed that turns the tissue into a thin suspension that is then washed out with saline using a 30-G needle. A fresh blood clot forms in the periapical bony crypt. Ongoing clinical trials indicate that much faster periapical healing occurs, similar to that encountered with apical surgery (see Figure 10C).

ALVEOLAR OSTEOPOROSIS ASSOCIATED WITH BRUXISM

Ingle[194] and then Natkin and Ingle[195] have described a syndrome ("Ingle's Syndrome") affecting adolescent females related to protrusive bruxism. By the age of 13 or 14, over one-third of the mandibular incisors had been "ground away" (see Figure 11A–D). Most of the lingual enamel of the maxillary incisors were also destroyed. In one case, a pulpal horn had already been exposed. In all the cases, osteoporotic bone destruction in the mental area of the mandible is apparent radiographically. Also seen radiographically, from left to right, is a graceful curve formed by the worn incisal edges of the lower anterior teeth.

When one realizes that this amount of destruction had occurred since eruption, within 6 or 7 years, one recognizes the intensity of the habit. The first girl seen was also a serious nail biter; "down to the quick" as she stated.

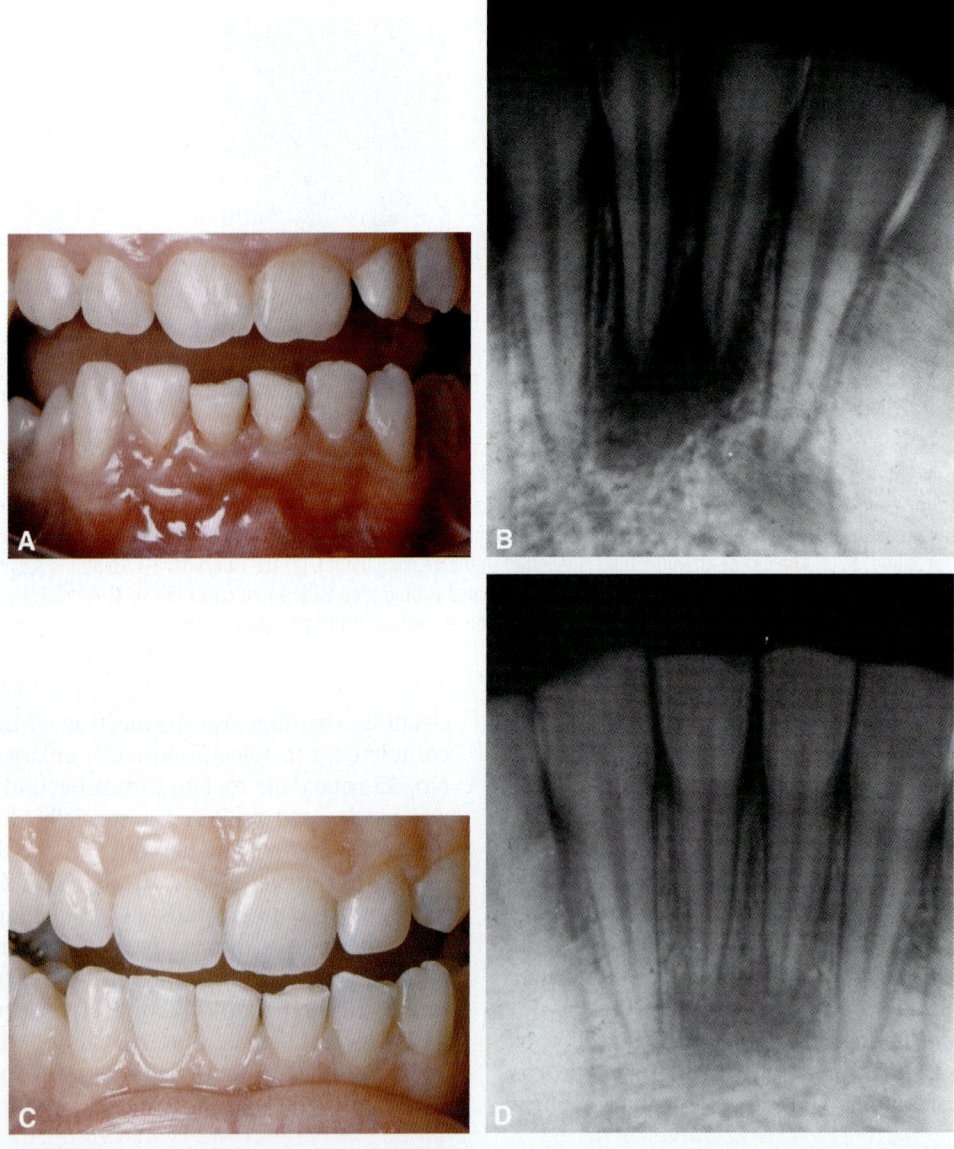

Figure 11 *A–D,* Osteoporosis and pulp death in 14-year-old identical twin sisters with the same syndrome—Adolescent Female Protrusive Bruxism. In both cases, incisal wear involving mandibular anterior teeth from compulsive protrusive bruxism. Nearly one-third of the teeth have been destroyed in 7 or 8 years. Radiographs demonstrate the osteoporotic bone loss, the periapical lesions, and the graceful curve, left to right, of the worn incisal edges common to this condition.

Not only the involved teeth were mobile, even though normal periodontal attachments were present, but also some of the pulps were necrotic. Consulting pathologists termed the bony destruction "traumatic osteoporosis" comparable to leg bone destruction seen in industry wherein a worker constantly presses a treadle downward, day after day.

Why do these girls grind their teeth in a protrusive motion rather than the usual lateral grinding chewing motion seen in most bruxers? The answer might be that they derive pleasure from this habit. One consulting psychiatrist suggested that this protrusive motion is the same suckling motion used by infants in nursing. Babies do not nurse by sucking (as adults do through a straw), but by moving the mandible forth and back, "milking" the nipple. This is a pleasurable and satisfying period of time in a baby's life. And these girls might well have some psychological need to continue the habit. Following endodontic therapy, "night guards" were constructed for these patients. They either threw them away after 2 or 3 months or chewed through them.

References

1. Genco CA, Cutler CW, Kapcynski D, et al. A novel mouse model to study the virulence of and host response to *Porphyromonas (Bacteroides) gingivalis*. Infect Immun 1991;59:1255–63.
2. Baumgartner JC, Falkler WA Jr, Beckerman T. Experimentally induced infection by oral anaerobic microorganisms in a mouse model. Oral Microbiol Immunol 1992;7:253–6.
3. Luscinskas FW, Cybulsky MI, Kiely JM, et al. Cytokine-activated human endothelial monolayers support enhanced neutrophil transmigration via a mechanism involving both endothelial-leukocyte adhesion molecule-1 and intercellular adhesion molecule-1. J Immunol 1991;146:1617–25.
4. Lane TA, Lamkin GE, Wancewicz EV. Protein kinase C inhibitors block the enhanced expression of intercellular adhesion molecule-1 on endothelial cells activated by interleukin-1, lipopolysaccharide and tumor necrosis factor. Biochem Biophys Res Commun 1990;172:1273–81.
5. Issekutz AC, Rowter D, Springer TA. Role of ICAM-1 and ICAM-2 and alternate CD11/CD18 ligands in neutrophil transendothelial migration. J Leukoc Biol 1999;65:117–26.
6. Kabashima H, Nagata K, Maeda K, Iijima T. Involvement of substance P, mast cells, TNF-alpha and ICAM-1 in the infiltration of inflammatory cells in human periapical granulomas. J Oral Pathol Med 2002;31:175–80.
7. Cutler CW, Kalmar JR, Arnold RR. Phagocytosis of virulent *Porphyromonas gingivalis* by human polymorphonuclear leukocytes requires specific immunoglobulin G. Infect Immun 1991;59:2097–104.
8. Naidorf IJ. Immunoglobulins in periapical granulomas: a preliminary report. J Endod 1975;1:15–18.
9. Hamachi T, Anan H, Akamine A, et al. Detection of interleukin-1 beta mRNA in rat periapical lesions. J Endod 1995;21:118–21.
10. Siqueira JF, Rocas IN, De Uzeda M, et al. Comparison of 16S rDNA-based PCR and checkerboard DNA–DNA hybridization for detection of selected endodontic pathogens. J Med Microbiol 2002;51:1090–6.
11. Sunde P, Tronstad L, Eribe R, et al. Assessment of periradicular microbiota by DNA–DNA hybridization. Endod Dent Traumatol 2000;16:191–6.
12. Pulver WH, Taubman MA, Smith DJ. Immune components in human dental periapical lesions. Arch Oral Biol 1978;23:435–43.
13. Johannessen AC, Nilsen R, Skaug N. Deposits of immunoglobulins and complement factor C3 in human dental periapical inflammatory lesions. Scand J Dent Res 1983;91:191–9.
14. Cymerman JJ, Cymerman DH, Walters J, et al. Human T lymphocyte subpopulations in chronic periapical lesions. J Endod 1984;10:9–11.
15. Barkhordar RA, Desouza YG. Human T-lymphocyte subpopulations in periapical lesions. Oral Surg Oral Med Oral Pathol Oral Radiol Endod 1988;65:763–6.
16. Babal P, Soler P, Brozman M, et al. In situ characterization of cells in periapical granuloma by monoclonal antibodies. Oral Surg Oral Med Oral Pathol Oral Radiol Endod 1987;64:348–52.
17. Poulter LW, Seymour GJ, Duke O, et al. Immunohistological analysis of delayed-type hypersensitivity in man. Cell Immunol 1982;74:358–69.
18. Kopp W, Schwarting R. Differentiation of T lymphocyte subpopulations, macrophages, and HLA-DR-restricted cells of apical granulation tissue. J Endod 1989;15:72–75.
19. Stashenko P, Yu SM. T helper and T suppressor cell reversal during the development of induced rat periapical lesions. J Dent Res 1989;68:830–4.
20. Baumgartner JC, Falkler WA Jr. Reactivity of IgG from explant cultures of periapical lesions with implicated microorganisms. J Endod 1991;17:207–12.
21. Kettering JD, Torabinejad M, Jones SL. Specificity of antibodies present in human periapical lesions. J Endod 1991;17:213–16.
22. Shimauchi H, Takayama S, Narikawa-Kiji M, et al. Production of interleukin-8 and nitric oxide in human periapical lesions. J Endod 2001;27:749–52.
23. Wuyts A, Proost P, Put W, et al. Leukocyte recruitment by monocyte chemotactic proteins (MCPs) secreted by human phagocytes. J Immunol Meth 1994;174:237–47.
24. Lukic A, Vojvodic D, Majstorovic I, Colic M. Production of interleukin-8 in vitro by mononuclear cells isolated from human periapical lesions. Oral Microbiol Immunol 2006;21:296–300.

25. Kawashima N, Okiji T, Kosaka T, Suda H. Kinetics of macrophages and lymphoid cells during the development of experimentally induced periapical lesions in rat molars: a quantitative immunohistochemical study. J Endod 1996;22:311–16.

26. Stashenko P, Wang CY, Tani IN, Yu SM. Pathogenesis of induced rat periapical lesions. Oral Surg Oral Med Oral Pathol Oral Radiol Endod 1994;78:494–502.

27. Stashenko P, Teles R, D'Souza R. Periapical inflammatory responses and their modulation. Critic Rev Oral Biol Med 1998;9:498–521.

28. Stashenko P, Yu SM. T helper and T suppressor cell reversal during the development of induced rat periapical lesions. J Dent Res 1989;68:830–4.

29. Stashenko P, Wang CY, Tani-Ishii N, Yu SM. Pathogenesis of induced rat periapical lesions. Oral Surg Oral Med Oral Pathol Oral Radiol Endod 1994;78:494–502.

30. Wallstrom JB, Torabinejad M, Kettering J, McMillan P. Role of T cells in the pathogenesis of periapical lesions. A preliminary report. Oral Surg Oral Med Oral Pathol Oral Radiol Endod 1993;76:213–18.

31. Tani-Ishii N, Kuchiba K, Osada T, et al. Effect of T-cell deficiency on the formation of periapical lesions in mice: histological comparison between periapical lesion formation in BALB/c and BALB/c nu/nu mice. J Endod 1995;21:195–9.

32. Akamine A, Hashiguchi I, Toriya Y, Maeda K. Immunohistochemical examination on the localization of macrophages and plasma cells in induced rat periapical lesions. Endod Dent Traumatol 1994;10:121–8.

33. Babal P, Brozman M, Jakubovsky J, et al. Cellular composition of periapical granulomas and its function. Histological, immunohistochemical and electron microscopic study. Czech Med 1989;12:193–215.

34. Marton IJ, Kiss C. Characterization of inflammatory cell infiltrate in dental periapical lesions. Int Endod J 1993 26:131–6.

35. Piattelli A, Artese L, Rosini S, et al. Immune cells in periapical granuloma: morphological and immunohistochemical characterization. J Endod 1991;17:26–9.

36. Matsuo T, Ebisu S, Shimabukuro Y, et al. Quantitative analysis of immunocompetent cells in human periapical lesions: correlations with clinical findings of the involved teeth. J Endod 1992;18:497–500.

37. Matsuo T, Nakanishi T, Ebisu S. Immunoglobulins in periapical exudates of infected root canals: correlations with the clinical findings of the involved teeth. Endod Dent Traumatol 1995;11:95–9.

38. Kettering JD, Torabinejad M, Jones SL. Specificity of antibodies present in human periapical lesions. J Endod 1991;17:213–16.

39. Baumgartner JC, Falkler WA Jr. Biosynthesis of IgG in periapical lesion explant cultures. J Endod 1991;17:143–6.

40. Baumgartner JC, Falkler WA Jr. Detection of immunoglobulins from explant cultures of periapical lesions. J Endod 1991;17:105–10.

41. Mustelin T, Coggeshall KM, Isakov N, Altman A. T cell antigen receptor-mediated activation of phospholipase C requires tyrosine phosphorylation. Science 1990;247:1584–7.

42. Kaneko T, Okiji T, Kan L, et al. Ultrastructural analysis of MHC class II molecule-expressing cells in experimentally induced periapical lesions in the rat. J Endod 2001;27:337–42.

43. Kaneko T, Okiji T, Kan L, et al. An immunoelectron-microscopic study of class II major histocompatibility complex molecule-expressing macrophages and dendritic cells in experimental rat periapical lesions. Arch Oral Biol 2001;46:713–20.

44. Lukic A, Vasilijic S, Majstorovic I, et al. Characterization of antigen-presenting cells in human apical periodontitis lesions by flow cytometry and immunocytochemistry. Int Endod J 2006;39:626–36.

45. Stern MH, Dreizen S, Mackler BF, et al. Quantitative analysis of cellular composition of human periapical granuloma. J Endod 1981;7:117–22.

46. Harris DP, Goodrich S, Mohrs K, et al. Cutting edge: the development of IL-4-producing B cells (B effector 2 cells) is controlled by IL-4, IL-4 receptor alpha, and Th2 cells. J Immunol 2005;175:7103–7.

47. Naldini A, Morena E, Filippi I, et al. Thrombin inhibits IFN-gamma production in human peripheral blood mononuclear cells by promoting a Th2 profile. J Interferon Cytokine Res 2006;26:793–9.

48. Wang CY, Stashenko P. Characterization of bone-resorbing activity in human periapical lesions. J Endod 1993;19:107–11.

49. Metzger Z. Macrophages in periapical lesions. Endod Dent Traumatol 2000;16:1–8.

50. Stern MH, Dreizen S, Mackler BF, Levy BM. Isolation and characterization of inflammatory cells from the human periapical granuloma. J Dent Res 1982;61:1408–12.

51. Ofek I, Goldhar J, Keisari Y, Sharon N. Nonopsonic phagocytosis of microorganisms. Annu Rev Microbiol 1995;49:239–76.

52. Okiji T, Kawashima N, Kosaka T, et al. Distribution of Ia antigen-expressing nonlymphoid cells in various stages of induced periapical lesions in rat molars. J Endod 1994;20:27–31.

53. Artese L, Piattelli A, Quaranta M, et al. Immunoreactivity for interleukin 1-beta and tumor necrosis factor-alpha and ultrastructural features of monocytes/ macrophages in periapical granulomas. J Endod 1991;17:483–7.

54. Tani-Ishii N, Wang CY, Stashenko P. Immunolocalization of bone-resorptive cytokines in rat pulp and periapical lesions following surgical pulp exposure. Oral Microbiol Immunol 1995;10:213–19.

55. Grossman LI. Endodontic practice. 6th ed. Philadelphia, PA: Lea & Febiger; 1965.

56. Shindell E. A study of some periapical radiolucencies and their significance. Oral Surg Oral Med Oral Pathol Oral Radiol Endod 1961;14:1057–65.

57. Moller AJ. Microbiological examination of root canals and periapical tissues of human teeth. Methodological studies. Odontol Tidskr 1966;74:Suppl-380.

58. Happonen RP, Arstila P, Viander M, et al. Comparison of polyclonal and monoclonal antibodies to *Actinomyces* and *Arachnia* species. Scand J Dent Res 1987;95:136–43.

59. Happonen RP, Soderling E, Viander M, et al. Immunocytochemical demonstration of *Actinomyces* species and *Arachnia propionica* in periapical infections. J Oral Pathol 1985;14:405–13.

60. Sjogren U, Happonen RP, Kahnberg KE, Sundqvist G. Survival of *Arachnia propionica* in periapical tissue. Int Endod J 1988;21:277–82.

61. Figdor D, Sjogren U, Sorlin S, et al. Pathogenicity of *Actinomyces israelii* and *Arachnia propionica*: experimental infection in guinea pigs and phagocytosis and intracellular killing by human polymorphonuclear leukocytes in vitro. Oral Microbiol Immunol 1992;7:129–36.

62. Abou-Rass M, Bogen G. Microorganisms in closed periapical lesions. Int Endod J 1998;31:39–47.

63. Iwu C, MacFarlane TW, MacKenzie D, Stenhouse D. The microbiology of periapical granulomas. Oral Surg Oral Med Oral Pathol Oral Radiol Endod1990;69:502–5.

64. Tronstad L, Barnett F, Riso K, Slots J. Extraradicular endodontic infections. Endod Dent Traumatol 1987;3:86–90.

65. Wayman BE, Murata SM, Almeida RJ, Fowler CB. A bacteriological and histological evaluation of 58 periapical lesions. J Endod 1992;18:152–5.

66. Siqueira JF Jr, Lopes HP. Bacteria on the apical root surfaces of untreated teeth with periradicular lesions: a scanning electron microscopy study. Int Endod J 2001;34:216–20.

67. Sunde PT, Olsen I, Lind PO, Tronstad L. Extraradicular infection: a methodological study. Endod Dent Traumatol 2000;16:84–90.

68. Noguchi N, Noiri Y, Narimatsu M, Ebisu S. Identification and localization of extraradicular biofilm-forming bacteria associated with refractory endodontic pathogens. Appl Environ Microbiol 2005;71:8738–43.

69. Nair PN. Pathogenesis of apical periodontitis and the causes of endodontic failures. Crit Rev Oral Biol Med 2004;15:348–81.

70. Nair PN. On the causes of persistent apical periodontitis: a review. Int Endod J 2006;39:249–81.

71. Ding Y, Haapasalo M, Kerosuo E, et al. Release and activation of human neutrophil matrix metallo- and serine proteinases during phagocytosis of *Fusobacterium nucleatum*, *Porphyromonas gingivalis* and *Treponema denticola*. J Clin Periodontol 1997;24:237–48.

72. AAE. Glossary of endodontic terms. Chicago, IL: American Association of Endodontists; 2003.

73. Sundqvist G, Figdor D, Hanstrom L, et al. Phagocytosis and virulence of different strains of *Porphyromonas gingivalis*. Scand J Dent Res 1991;99:117–29.

74. Sundqvist GK, Carlsson J, Herrmann BF, et al. Degradation in vivo of the C3 protein of guinea-pig complement by a pathogenic strain of *Bacteroides gingivalis*. Scand J Dent Res 1984;92:14–24.

75. Cutler CW, Arnold RR, Schenkein HA. Inhibition of C3 and IgG proteolysis enhances phagocytosis of *Porphyromonas gingivalis*. J Immunol 1993;151:7016–29.

76. Sundqvist G, Carlsson J, Herrmann B, Tarnvik A. Degradation of human immunoglobulins G and M and complement factors C3 and C5 by black-pigmented *Bacteroides*. J Med Microbiol 1985;19:85–94.

77. Jansen HJ, van-der HJ, van-den KC, et al. Degradation of immunoglobulin G by periodontal bacteria. Oral Microbiol Immunol 1994;9:345–51.

78. Hirshberg A, Tsesis I, Metzger Z, Kaplan I. Periapical actinomycosis: a clinicopathologic study [see comment]. Oral Surg Oral Med Oral Pathol Oral Radiol Endod Oral Radiol Endod 2003;95:614–20.

79. Weiss EI, Shaniztki B, Dotan M, et al. Attachment of *Fusobacterium nucleatum* PK1594 to mammalian cells and its coaggregation with periopathogenic bacteria are mediated by the same galactose-binding adhesin. Oral Microbiol Immunol 2000;15:371–7.

80. Shaniztki B, Hurwitz D, Smorodinsky N, et al. Identification of a *Fusobacterium nucleatum* PK1594 galactose-binding adhesin which mediates coaggregation with periopathogenic bacteria and hemagglutination. Infect Immun 1997;65:5231–7.

81. Nair PNR. Pathobiology of primary apical periodontitis, In: Cohen S, Hargreaves KM, editors. Pathways of the pulp. 9th ed. Amsterdam: Elseiver; 2006. pp. 541–79.

82. Fouad AF, Burleson J. The effect of diabetes mellitus on endodontic treatment outcome: data from an electronic patient record. J Am Dent Assoc 2003;134:43–51.

83. Mattscheck DJ, Law AS, Noblett WC. Retreatment versus initial root canal treatment: factors affecting posttreatment pain. Oral Surg Oral Med Oral Pathol Oral Radiol Endod Oral Radiol Endod 2001;92:321–4.

84. Yu CY. Role of occlusion in endodontic management: report of two cases. Aus Endod J 2004;30:110–15.

85. IASP Task Force on Taxonomy. Classification of chronic pain. In: Mersky H, Bogduk N, editors. 2nd ed. Seattle, WA: IASP Press; 1994. pp. 209–14.

86. Rittner HL, Brack A, Stein C. Pro-algesic versus analgesic actions of immune cells. Curr Opin Anaesthesiol 2003;16:527–33.

87. Cunha JM, Cunha FQ, Poole S, Ferreira SH. Cytokine-mediated inflammatory hyperalgesia limited by interleukin-1 receptor antagonist. Brit J Pharmacol 2000;130:1418–24.

88. Cunha FQ, Poole S, Lorenzetti BB, Ferreira SH. The pivotal role of tumour necrosis factor alpha in the development of inflammatory hyperalgesia. Brit J Pharmacol 1992;107:660–4.

89. Aloe L, Simone MD, Properzi F. Nerve growth factor: a neurotrophin with activity on cells of the immune system. Micros Res Tech 1999;45:285–91.

90. Byers MR, Taylor PE, Khayat BG, Kimberly CL. Effects of injury and inflammation on pulpal and periapical nerves. J Endod 1990;16:78–84.

91. Wang H, Ehnert C, Brenner GJ, Woolf CJ. Bradykinin and peripheral sensitization. Biol Chem 2006;387:11–14.

92. Sorkin LS, Wallace MS. Acute pain mechanisms. Surg Clin North Am 1999;79:213–29.

93. Safieh-Garabedian B, Kanaan SA, Jalakhian RH, et al. Involvement of interleukin-1 beta, nerve growth factor, and prostaglandin-E2 in the hyperalgesia induced by intraplantar injections of low doses of thymulin. Brain Behav Immun 1997;11:185–200.

94. Kawamoto K, Aoki J, Tanaka A, et al. Nerve growth factor activates mast cells through the collaborative interaction with lysophosphatidylserine expressed on the membrane surface of activated platelets. J Immunol 2002;168:6412–19.

95. Price TJ, Louria MD, Candelario-Soto D, et al. Treatment of trigeminal ganglion neurons in vitro with NGF, GDNF or BDNF: effects on neuronal survival, neurochemical properties and TRPV1-mediated neuropeptide secretion. BMC Neurosci 2005;6:4.

96. Petersen M, Segond B, Heppelmann B, Koltzenburg M. Nerve growth factor regulates the expression of bradykinin binding sites on adult sensory neurons via the neurotrophin receptor p75. Neuroscience 1998;83:161–8.

97. Ferreira SH, Lorenzetti BB, Poole S. Bradykinin initiates cytokine-mediated inflammatory hyperalgesia. Br J Pharmacol 1993;110:1227–31.

98. McNicholas S, Torabinejad M, Blankenship J, Bakland L. The concentration of prostaglandin E2 in human periradicular lesions. J Endod 1991;17:97–100.

99. Radics T, Kiss C, Tar I, Marton IJ. Interleukin-6 and granulocyte-macrophage colony-stimulating factor in apical periodontitis: correlation with clinical and histologic findings of the involved teeth. Oral Microbiol Immunol 2003;18:9–13.

100. Shimauchi H, Takayama S, Miki Y, Okada H. The change of periapical exudate prostaglandin E2 levels during root canal treatment. J Endod 1997;23:755–8.

101. Torabinejad M, Cotti E, Jung T. Concentrations of leukotriene B4 in symptomatic and asymptomatic periapical lesions. J Endod 1992;18:205–8.

102. Lim GC, Torabinejad M, Kettering J, et al. Interleukin 1-beta in symptomatic and asymptomatic human periradicular lesions. J Endod 1994;20:225–7.

103. Elliott DE, Blum AM, Li J, et al. Preprosomatostatin messenger RNA is expressed by inflammatory cells and induced by inflammatory mediators and cytokines. J Immunol 1998;160:3997–4003.

104. Matias I, Pochard P, Orlando P, et al. Presence and regulation of the endocannabinoid system in human dendritic cells. Eur J Biochem 2002;269:3771–8.

105. Labuz D, Berger S, Mousa SA, et al. Peripheral antinociceptive effects of exogenous and immune cell-derived endomorphins in prolonged inflammatory pain. J Neurosci 2006;26:4350–8.

106. Brack A, Labuz D, Schiltz A, et al. Tissue monocytes/macrophages in inflammation: hyperalgesia versus opioid-mediated peripheral antinociception. Anesthesiology 2004;101:204–11.

107. Rittner HL, Machelska H, Stein C. Leukocytes in the regulation of pain and analgesia. J Leukoc Biol 2005;78:1215–22.

108. Fiset ME, Gilbert C, Poubelle PE, Pouliot M. Human neutrophils as a source of nociceptin: a novel link between pain and inflammation. Biochemistry 2003;42:10498–505.

109. Machelska H, Brack A, Mousa SA, et al. Selectins and integrins but not platelet-endothelial cell adhesion molecule-1 regulate opioid inhibition of inflammatory pain. Br J Pharmacol 2004;142:772–80.

110. Machelska H, Mousa SA, Brack A, et al. Opioid control of inflammatory pain regulated by intercellular adhesion molecule-1. J Neurosci 2002;22:5588–96.

111. Klein DC, Raisz LG. Prostaglandins: stimulation of bone resorption in tissue culture. Endocrinology 1970;86:1436–40.

112. Hausmann E, Raisz LG, Miller WA. Endotoxin: stimulation of bone resorption in tissue culture. Science 1970;168:862–4.

113. Stashenko P, Teles R, D'Souza R. Periapical inflammatory responses and their modulation. Crit Rev Oral Biol Med 1998;9:498–521.

114. Stashenko P, Dewhirst FE, Peros WJ, et al. Synergistic interactions between interleukin 1, tumor necrosis factor, and lymphotoxin in bone resorption. J Immunol 1987;138:1464–8.

115. Kawashima N, Stashenko P. Expression of bone-resorptive and regulatory cytokines in murine periapical inflammation. Arch Oral Biol 1999;44:55–66.

116. Shimauchi H, Takayama S, Imai TT, Okada H. Balance of interleukin-1 beta and interleukin-1 receptor antagonist in human periapical lesions. J Endod 1998;24:116–19.

117. Wang CY, Stashenko P. The role of interleukin-1 alpha in the pathogenesis of periapical bone destruction in a rat model system. Oral Microbiol Immunol 1993;8:50–6.

118. Kakehashi S, Stanley HR, Fitzgerald RJ. The effect of surgical exposures of dental pulps in germ-free and conventional laboratory rats. Oral Surg Oral Med Oral Pathol Oral Radiol Endod 1965;20:340–9.

119. Wang CY, Stashenko P. Kinetics of bone-resorbing activity in developing periapical lesions. J Dent Res 1991;70:1362–6.
120. Wang CY, Stashenko P. Kinetics of bone-resorbing activity in developing periapical lesions. J Dent Res 1991;70:1362–6.
121. Matsuo T, Ebisu S, Nakanishi T, et al. Interleukin-1 alpha and interleukin-1 beta periapical exudates of infected root canals: correlations with the clinical findings of the involved teeth. J Endod 1994;20:432–5.
122. Kuo ML, Lamster IB, Hasselgren G. Host mediators in endodontic exudates. II. Changes in concentration with sequential sampling. J Endod 1998;24:636–40.
123. Kuo ML, Lamster IB, Hasselgren G. Host mediators in endodontic exudates. I. Indicators of inflammation and humoral immunity. J Endod 1998;24:598–603.
124. Dinarello CA. Interleukin-1. Ann NY Acad Sci 1988;546:122–32.
125. Pennica D, Nedwin GE, Hayflick JS, et al. Human tumour necrosis factor: precursor structure, expression and homology to lymphotoxin. Nature 1984;312:724–9.
126. Metzger Z, Berg D, Dotan M. Fibroblast growth in vitro suppressed by LPS-activated macrophages. Reversal of suppression by hydrocortisone. J Endod 1997;23:517–21.
127. Vos JG, Kreeftenberg JG, Kruijt BC, et al. The athymic nude rat. II. Immunological characteristics. Clin Immunol Immunopathol 1980;15:229–37.
128. Pritchard H, Riddaway J, Micklem HS. Immune responses in congenitally thymus-less mice. II. Quantitative studies of serum immunoglobulins, the antibody response to sheep erythrocytes, and the effect of thymus allografting. Clin Exp Immunol 1973;13:125–38.
129. Wallstrom JB, Torabinejad M, Kettering J, McMillan P. Role of T cells in the pathogenesis of periapical lesions. A preliminary report. Oral Surg Oral Med Oral Pathol Oral Radiol Endod 1993;76:213–18.
130. Politis AD, Sivo J, Driggers PH, et al. Modulation of interferon consensus sequence binding protein mRNA in murine peritoneal macrophages. Induction by IFN-gamma and down-regulation by IFN-alpha, dexamethasone, and protein kinase inhibitors. J Immunol 1992;148:801–7.
131. Metzger Z, Hoffeld JT, Oppenheim JJ. Suppression of fibroblast proliferation by activated macrophages: involvement of H2O2 and a non-prostaglandin E product of the cyclooxygenase pathway. Cell Immunol 1986;100:501–14.
132. Metzger Z, Hoffeld JT, Oppenheim JJ. Macrophage-mediated suppression. I. Evidence for participation of both hydrogen peroxide and prostaglandins in suppression of murine lymphocyte proliferation. J Immunol 1980;124:983–8.
133. Tani-Ishii N, Wang CY, Tanner A, Stashenko P. Changes in root canal microbiota during the development of rat periapical lesions. Oral Microbiol Immunol 1994;9:129–35.
134. Hofbauer LC, Heufelder AE. Role of receptor activator of nuclear factor-kappaB ligand and osteoprotegerin in bone cell biology. J Mol Med 2001;79:243–53.
135. Lacey DL, Timms E, Tan HL, et al. Osteoprotegerin ligand is a cytokine that regulates osteoclast differentiation and activation. Cell 1998;93:165–76.
136. Hofbauer LC, Kuhne CA, Viereck V. The OPG/RANKL/RANK system in metabolic bone diseases. J Musc Neur Interact 2004;4:268–75.
137. Lacey DL, Timms E, Tan HL, et al. Osteoprotegerin ligand is a cytokine that regulates osteoclast differentiation and activation. Cell 1998;93:165–76.
138. Suda T, Takahashi N, Udagawa N, et al. Modulation of osteoclast differentiation and function by the new members of the tumor necrosis factor receptor and ligand families. Endocr Rev 1999;20:345–57.
139. Teitelbaum SL. Bone resorption by osteoclasts. Science 2000;289:1504–8.
140. Kong YY, Feige U, Sarosi I, et al. Activated T cells regulate bone loss and joint destruction in adjuvant arthritis through osteoprotegerin ligand. Nature 1999;402:304–9.
141. Taubman MA, Kawai T. Involvement of T-lymphocytes in periodontal disease and in direct and indirect induction of bone resorption. Crit Rev Oral Biol Med 2001;12:125–35.
142. Kawai T, Matsuyama T, Hosokawa Y, et al. B and T lymphocytes are the primary sources of RANKL in the bone resorptive lesion of periodontal disease. Am J Pathol 2006;169:987–98.
143. Bekker PJ, Holloway D, Nakanishi A, et al. The effect of a single dose of osteoprotegerin in postmenopausal women. J Bone Miner Res 2001;16:348–60.
144. Vernal R, Dezerega A, Dutzan N, et al. RANKL in human periapical granuloma: possible involvement in periapical bone destruction. Oral Dis 2006;12:283–9.
145. Sabeti M, Simon J, Kermani V, et al. Detection of receptor activator of NF-kappa beta ligand in apical periodontitis. J Endod 2005;31:17–18.
146. Wada N, Maeda H, Tanabe K, et al. Periodontal ligament cells secrete the factor that inhibits osteoclastic differentiation and function: the factor is osteoprotegerin/osteoclastogenesis inhibitory factor. J Periodont Res 2001;36:56–63.
147. Nair PN. On the causes of persistent apical periodontitis: a review. Int Endod J 2006;39:249–81.
148. Nair PN. Apical periodontitis: a dynamic encounter between root canal infection and host response. Periodontology 2000 1997;13:121–48.
149. Fish EW. Bone infection. J Am Dent Assoc 1939;26:691.
150. Happonen RP, Bergengoltz G. Apical periodontitis, In: Bergenholtz G, Horsted-Bindslev, Reit C, editors. Textbook of endodontology. 1st ed. Oxford: Blackwell; 2003. pp. 130–44.

151. Kiss C. Cell to cell interactions. Endod Top 2004;8:88–103.
152. Marton IJ, Kiss C. Protective and destructive immune reactions in apical periodontitis. [Review] [169 refs]. Oral Microbiol Immunol 2000;15:139–50.
153. Nair PN, Pajarola G, Luder HU. Ciliated epithelium-lined radicular cysts. Oral Surg Oral Med Oral Pathol Oral Radiol Endod 2002;94:485–93.
154. Nair PN, Sjogren U, Schumacher E, Sundqvist G. Radicular cyst affecting a root-filled human tooth: a long-term posttreatment follow-up. Int Endod J 1993;26:225–33.
155. Nair PN, Pajarola G, Schroeder HE. Types and incidence of human periapical lesions obtained with extracted teeth. Oral Surg Oral Med Oral Pathol Oral Radiol Endod 1996;81:93–102.
156. Simon JH. Incidence of periapical cysts in relation to the root canal. J Endod 1980;6:845–8.
157. Ten Cate AR. The epithelial cell rests of Malassez and the genesis of the dental cyst. Oral Surg Oral Med Oral Pathol Oral Radiol Endod1972;34:956–64.
158. Shafer W, Hine M, Levy B. A textbook of oral pathology. 3rd ed. Philadelphia, PA: W.B. Saunders; 1974.
159. Summers L. The incidence of epithelium in periapical granulomas and the mechanism of cavitation in apical dental cysts in man. Arch Oral Biol 1974;19:1177–80.
160. Bhaskar SN. Periapical lesions—types, incidence, and clinical features. Oral Surg Oral Med Oral Pathol Oral Radiol Endod1966;21:657–71.
161. Natkin E, Oswald RJ, Carnes LI. The relationship of lesion size to diagnosis, incidence, and treatment of periapical cysts and granulomas. Oral Surg Oral Med Oral Pathol 1984;57:82–94.
162. Cotti E, Torabinejad M. Detection of leukotriene C4 in human periradicular lesions. Int Endod J 1994;27:82–6.
163. Cummings GR, Torabinejad M. Effect of systemic doxycycline on alveolar bone loss after periradicular surgery. J Endod 2000;26:325–7.
164. Kaufman B, Spangberg L, Barry J, Fouad AF. *Enterococcus* spp. in endodontically treated teeth with and without periradicular lesions. J Endod 2005;31:851–6.
165. Torabinejad M. Mediators of acute and chronic periradicular lesions. Oral Surg Oral Med Oral Pathol Oral Radiol Endod1994;78:511–21.
166. Abbott PV. Classification, diagnosis and clinical manifestation of apical periodontitis. Endod Top 2004;8:36–54.
167. Ricucci D, Mannocci F, Ford TR. A study of periapical lesions correlating the presence of a radiopaque lamina with histological findings. Oral Surg Oral Med Oral Pathol Oral Radiol Endod Oral Radiol Endod 2006;101:389–94.
168. Gundappa M, Ng SY, Whaites EJ. Comparison of ultrasound, digital and conventional radiography in differentiating periapical lesions. Dento-Maxillo-Facial Radiol 2006;35:326–33.
169. Hought RT, Fitzgerald BE, Latta JE, Zallen RD. Ludwig's angina: report of two cases and review of the literature from 1945 to January 1979. J Oral Surg 1980;38:849–55.
170. Bullock JD, Fleishman JA. The spread of odontogenic infections to the orbit: diagnosis and management. J Oral Maxill Surg 1985;43:749–55.
171. Fielding AF, Cross S, Matise JL, Mohnac AM. Cavernous sinus thrombosis: report of case. J Am Dent Assoc 1983;106:342–5.
172. Henig EF, Derschowitz T, Shalit M, et al. Brain abscess following dental infection. Oral Surg Oral Med Oral Pathol Oral Radiol Endod1978;45:955–8.
173. Molven O, Halse A, Grung B. Incomplete healing (scar tissue) after periapical surgery—radiographic findings 8 to 12 years after treatment. J Endod 1996;22:264–8.
174. Nair PN, Sjogren U, Figdor D, Sundqvist G. Persistent periapical radiolucencies of root-filled human teeth, failed endodontic treatments, and periapical scars. Oral Surg Oral Med Oral Pathol Oral Radiol EndodOral Radiol Endod 1999;87:617–27.
175. Pecora G, De Leonardis D, Ibrahim N, et al. The use of calcium sulphate in the surgical treatment of a 'through and through' periradicular lesion. Int Endod J 2001;34:189–97.
176. Seltzer S, Bender IB, Smith J, et al. Endodontic failures—an analysis based on clinical, roentgenographic, and histologic findings. II. Oral Surg Oral Med Oral Pathol Oral Radiol Endod 1967;23:517–30.
177. Orstavik D. Time-course and risk analyses of the development and healing of chronic apical periodontitis in man. Int Endod J 1996;29:150–5.
178. Kvist T, Reit C. Results of endodontic retreatment: a randomized clinical study comparing surgical and nonsurgical procedures. J Endod 1999;25:814–17.
179. Friedman S. Prognosis of initial endodontic therapy. Endod Top 2002;2:59–88.
180. Fristad I, Molven O, Halse A. Nonsurgically retreated root filled teeth—radiographic findings after 20–27 years. Int Endod J 2004;37:12–18.
181. Stashenko P, Dewhirst FE, Rooney ML, et al. Interleukin-1 beta is a potent inhibitor of bone formation in vitro. J Bone Miner Res 1987;2:559–65.
182. Shimauchi H, Miki Y, Takayama S, et al. Development of a quantitative sampling method for periapical exudates from human root canals. J Endod 1996;22:612–15.
183. Williams RC, Jeffcoat MK, Howell TH, et al. Altering the progression of human alveolar bone loss with the nonsteroidal anti-inflammatory drug flurbiprofen. J Periodontol 1989;60:485–90.
184. Torabinejad M, Clagett J, Engel D. A cat model for the evaluation of mechanisms of bone resorption: induction of

bone loss by simulated immune complexes and inhibition by indomethacin. Calcif Tissue Int 1979;29:207–14.

185. Shapira L, Barak V, Soskolne WA, et al. Effects of tetracyclines on the pathologic activity of endotoxin: in vitro and in vivo studies. Adv Dent Res 1998;12:119–22.

186. Shapira L, Soskolne WA, Houri Y, et al. Protection against endotoxic shock and lipopolysaccharide-induced local inflammation by tetracycline: correlation with inhibition of cytokine secretion. Infect Immun 1996;64:825–8.

187. Golub LM, Lee HM, Ryan ME, et al. Tetracyclines inhibit connective tissue breakdown by multiple non-antimicrobial mechanisms. Adv Dent Res 1998;12:12–26.

188. Metzger Z, Belkin D, Kariv N, et al. Low-dose doxycycline inhibits development of periapical lesions in rats. Int Endod J [In press].

189. Schultz RM, Chirigos MA, Stoychkov JN, Pavilidis RJ. Factors affecting macrophage cytotoxic activity with particular emphasis on corticosteroids and acute stress. J Reticuloendothel Soc 1979;26:83–91.

190. Nakamura Y, Murai T, Ogawa Y. Effect of in vitro and in vivo administration of dexamethasone on rat macrophage functions: comparison between alveolar and peritoneal macrophages. Eur Respir J 1996;9:301–6.

191. Metzger Z, Klein H, Klein A, Tagger M. Periapical lesion development in rats inhibited by dexamethasone. J Endod 2002;28:643–5.

192. Knudsen PJ, Dinarello CA, Strom TB. Glucocorticoids inhibit transcriptional and post-transcriptional expression of interleukin 1 in U937 cells. J Immunol 1987;139:4129–34.

193. Waage A, Slupphaug G, Shalaby R. Glucocorticoids inhibit the production of IL6 from monocytes, endothelial cells and fibroblasts. Eur J Immunol 1990;20:2439–43.

194. Ingle JI. Alveolar osteoporosis and pulpal death associated with compulsive bruxism. Oral Surg Oral Med Oral Pathol Oral Radiol Endod 1960;13 Nov:1371–81.

195. Natkin, E, Ingle JI. A further report on alveolar osteoporosis and pulpal death associated with compulsive bruxism. Periodont J Am Soc Periodont 1963; 1 Nov/Dec:260–3.

EXAMINATION, EVALUATION, DIAGNOSIS AND TREATMENT PLANNING

CHAPTER 14

DIAGNOSIS OF ENDODONTIC DISEASE

A. ENDODONTIC EXAMINATION

ROBERT A. HANDYSIDES, DAVID E. JARAMILLO, JOHN I. INGLE

"For I seek the truth by which no man has ever been harmed."

—Marcus Aurelius, *Meditations VI. 21*, 173 AD

Diagnosis is arguably the most critical component of all dental treatment, and endodontics is no exception. *Stedman's Medical Dictionary* describes clinical diagnosis as "the determination of the nature of a disease made from a study of the signs and symptoms of a disease."[1] The diagnostic process therefore is an essential part of treatment and treatment planning. Collection of information, history, signs and symptoms, a thorough clinical examination, and objective testing are mandatory prior to recommending and initiating treatment. Only after collecting this information can one come up with a diagnosis that benefits the patient. "Providing the wrong treatment for a patient could not only intensify a patient's symptom but make it even more difficult to arrive at the correct diagnosis."[2] The Hippocratic Oath counsels "First, do no harm."

To achieve this goal, one must dedicate oneself to becoming an astute diagnostician.

To become this type of diagnostician, one must develop numerous personal attributes that will complement and enhance one's ability and efficiency for arriving at the correct diagnosis. The art of listening has often been a neglected diagnostic tool. Most clinicians have tried to develop a thorough knowledge of examination procedures: percussion, palpation, probing, and pulp testing. Knowledge of endodontic disease, radiographic interpretation, and clinical manifestations is an integral and important part to achieving the correct diagnosis. But the most basic skill of all is **listening** to the patient. Through careful and attentive listening one develops a strong patient-clinician rapport. Such relationships enhance the patient's reliability as a historian.[3]

Requirements of a Diagnostician

Diagnosis is often derived from personal and cognitive experiences. Good diagnosticians use past experience, based on knowledge and diagnostic tools. Diagnosing any orofacial disease, odontogenic or non-odontogenic, is similar to other medical diagnoses. Radiographs and other testing procedures can facilitate the diagnosing of dental or facial disease, just as a host of various other radiographs and testing can facilitate medical diagnosis.

To become a successful diagnostician, one must develop a number of assets. The most important of these are **knowledge, interest, intuition, curiosity, and patience.** The successful diagnostician must also have acute senses and the necessary examining equipment for diagnosis.

KNOWLEDGE

Knowledge must be listed as the most important attribute a clinician possesses. Typically clinicians, practicing dentistry by themselves, are in relative isolation from outside help. They must be prepared to assess various types of orofacial pain, and the sources vary from odontogenic to numerous systemic, neurologic, and psychological causes. They must intimately understand the changes that pain can bring in patients. These changes range from physical and perceptual to emotional and behavioral. Every clinician has a different level of experience and knowledge that is ever evolving. One of the most important aspects of knowledge is recognizing when one needs help. The astute clinician will recognize that the problem is outside the scope of his or her field of training. Rather than pursue what is hoped is the best, consultation from an appropriate source is advisable. Even if the problem appears to be within the scope of one's training, yet the diagnosis or treatment is beyond the comfort level of the practitioner, referral is often appropriate. Recognition of one's limitations and fallibility is a major asset not only for the clinician but also for the patient.

INTEREST

Interest is an attitude. If one is interested in a subject, usually one excels in that area. It is human nature to develop one's interests, but it is difficult to do so if one is uninterested. The uninterested clinician often makes a guess, prescribes inappropriate treatments, and shows a lack of concern for the patient's condition. The interested clinician will be supportive and understanding of the patient seeking the source of a problem.

INTUITION

Intuition is a very helpful tool in diagnosis. A good diagnostician will sense something out of the ordinary. This sense allows the clinician to delve deeper and look more closely into atypical situations. Intuition allows one to suspect the unusual, and then curiosity takes over. Intuition needs to be used with common sense. It is not good to get sidetracked to the obscure when the obvious is right in front of you. Unless one is on a safari in Africa, one must recall the saying, "When you hear hoof beats, think horses, not zebras."

CURIOSITY

As stated in the 5th edition of **Endodontics**, "the clinician must pursue or develop a natural curiosity about the patient and his condition if perseverance is to be maintained in arriving at a diagnosis."[4] Dr. Harry Sicher often likened dental diagnosis to "the actions of a good detective, and curiosity is a detective's greatest asset" (H. Sicher, personal communication with Dr. John Ingle, 1954). Medawar described diagnosis as the "use of the hypothetico-deductive system."[5]

PATIENCE

Patience is something that is often in short supply for both the clinician and the patient when it comes to pain. A definitive diagnosis of unusual pain may take anywhere from hours to months to develop. Some patients may have suffered this pain for years, so it is unreasonable for the clinician to expect to always make a diagnosis in a matter of minutes. This is one reason why a difficult diagnosis may be unrewarding financially but very rewarding emotionally.

History

The first step in arriving at a diagnosis is the recollection of the patient's signs and symptoms, the past as well as the present. The importance of this "history" goes beyond medicolegal protection. A complete history (Table 1) will often modify endodontic treatment and may even determine the total treatment. It may also deny treatment, although it seldom does. The "history" should be broken down into a medical and a dental history.

A complete medical history is very important as the overall picture of a patient's health. A thorough history may help define risks to the clinician and staff, as well as identify risks to the patient. The medical history must be regularly updated to monitor any changes in the patient's health status. Recording the patients' vital signs, at the onset of the examination, is strongly encouraged. Vital signs may give early warning of unsuspected systemic disease. If indicated, the patient should be encouraged to visit his or her physician for an examination and appropriate treatment. The American Society of Anesthesiologists has developed a system for organizing and assigning risk (see Figure 1 in Chapter 23, "Management of Medically Complex Patients").

As stated in the 5th edition of **Endodontics**, once the status of the patient's general health has been established, a dental history follows.[4] This is best developed by following the time-honored formula of determining the **chief complaint,** enlarging on this complaint with questions about the **present dental illness,** relating the history of past dental illness to the chief complaint, and combining this with information about the patient's general health (**medical history**) and the examination results.

Table 1 Medical History Form*

MEDICAL HISTORY

Name _____ Sex _____ Date of Birth _____
Address _____
Telephone _____ Height _____ Weight _____
Date _____ Occupation _____ Marital Status _____

MEDICAL HISTORY   CIRCLE

1. Are you having pain or discomfort at this time? .... YES   NO
2. Do you feel very nervous about having dentistry treatment? .... YES   NO
3. Have you ever had a bad experience in the dentistry office? .... YES   NO
4. Have you been a patient in the hospital during the past 2 years? .... YES   NO
5. Have you been under the care of a medical doctor during the past 2 years? ... YES   NO
6. Have you taken any medicine or drugs during the past 2 years? .... YES   NO
7. Are you allergic to (ie, itching, rash, swelling of hands, feet, or eyes)
   or made sick by penicillin, aspirin, codeine, or any drugs or medications? ... YES   NO
8. Have you ever had any excessive bleeding requiring special treatment? .... YES   NO
9. Circle any of the following which you have had or have at present:

Heart Failure	Emphysema	AIDS or HIV
Heart Disease or Attack	Cough	Hepatitis A (infectious)
Angina Pectoris	Tuberculosis (TB)	Hepatitis B (serum)
High Blood Pressure	Asthma	Liver Disease
Heart Murmur	Hay Fever	Yellow Jaundice
Rheumatic Fever	Sinus Trouble	Blood Transfusion
Congenital Heart Lesions	Allergies or Hives	Drug Addiction
Scarlet Fever	Diabetes	Hemophilia
Artificial Heart Valve	Thyroid Disease	Venereal Disease (Syphilis, Gonorrhea)
Heart Pacemaker	X-ray or Cobalt Treatment	Cold Sores
Heart Surgery	Chemotherapy (Cancer, Leukemia)	Genital Herpes
Artificial Joint	Arthritis	Epilepsy or Seizures
Anemia	Rheumatism	Fainting or Dizzy Spells
Stroke	Cortisone Medicine	Nervousness
Kidney Trouble	Glaucoma	Psychiatric Treatment
Ulcers	Pain in Jaw Joints	Sickle Cell Disease
		Bruise Easily

10. When you walk up stairs or take a walk, do you ever have to stop because
    of pain in your chest, or shortness of breath, or because you are very tired? ... YES   NO
11. Do your ankles swell during the day? .... YES   NO
12. Do you use more than two pillows to sleep? .... YES   NO
13. Have you lost or gained more than 10 pounds in the past year? .... YES   NO
14. Do you ever wake up from sleep short of breath? .... YES   NO
15. Are you on a special diet? .... YES   NO
16. Has your medical doctor ever said you have a cancer or tumor? .... YES   NO
17. Do you have any disease, condition, or problem not listed? .... YES   NO
18. WOMEN: Are you pregnant now? .... YES   NO
              Are you practicing birth control? .... YES   NO
              Do you anticipate becoming pregnant? .... YES   NO

To the best of my knowledge, all of the preceding answers are true and correct. If I ever have any change in my health, or if my medicines change, I will inform the doctor of dentistry at the next appointment without fail.

_____   _____   _____
Date   *Dentist Signature*   *Signature of Patient, Parent, or Guardian*

MEDICAL HISTORY/PHYSICAL EVALUATION UPDATE

Date   Addition   Signatures
_____   _____   _____   _____
_____   _____   _____   _____
_____   _____   _____   _____

This comprehensive medical history responds to contemporary advances in physical evaluation and to increasing malpractice claims.

*Reproduced with permission from McCarthy FM. A new patient administered history developed for dentistry. J Am Dent Assoc 1985;111:595.

CHIEF COMPLAINT

The chief complaint is the reason the patient is seeking care. It is usually documented in the patient's words, or in the case of a young minor, the parent's or guardian's words. This verbal description of the problem is often aided by hand gestures and the patient pointing to a general area of discomfort. After obtaining the **chief complaint,** the examination process is continued by obtaining a dental history of the **present illness.** This helps establish the correct diagnosis. Treatment should not be rendered unless the clinician is certain of the diagnosis. Patients suffering excruciating pain often have difficulty in cooperating with the diagnostic procedures, but until a diagnosis has been made, treatment must not be started. Nonodontogenic pains need to be managed appropriately, which usually does not involve endodontic treatment (see Chapter 11, "Nonodontogenic Toothache and Chronic Head and Neck Pains").

PRESENT DENTAL ILLNESS

A history of the present illness should help determine the severity and the urgency of the problem. When questioning the patient regarding the problem, questions should be put forth in a manner that leaves them open for patient discussion. Closed questions that allow the patient to respond with "yes" or "no" are of less help than open-ended questions. Start asking questions with words such as "how," "when," "where," or "what." Questions of this type encourage even the poor historian to verbalize more specifically problems that persist.

In obtaining information regarding the present illness, certain areas should be covered, such as whether there has been any recent dental treatment. This information may help localize a particular problem or give an impression of how frequently the patient seeks dental care. A history of trauma is important in determining the course of examination as well as treatment. Discomfort, and what triggers it, is also very important in determining severity and urgency. Questions should be posed in regard to the character of pain, its location, what initiates or relieves the symptoms, the duration of the symptoms, and what medications the patient is taking to alleviate the symptoms. Not only will this help determine the pain intensity level, but analgesic ingestion can interfere with testing results.[6–8]

MEDICAL HISTORY

Patients need to share their medical problems with their clinicians so the data can be used in planning treatment.[9] Today, with patients on so many medications, it is essential to communicate properly with patients. Health history is one of the most important steps in diagnosis and treatment planning What are the patient's medical conditions, concerns, and contraindications? Technology facilitates communicating with the patient's physician by telephone, fax, and/or the Internet. An almost instantaneous access to concerns by the physician is an improvement over past methods.

To begin the medical history, one needs to provide patients with a standard medical history form for them to fill out (such as the one in Table 1). This can be done in the reception room and with the help of office staff.

In the past, patients often felt uncomfortable revealing their medical history to staff, let alone the clinician. Fortunately, today patients are much more open to completing a detailed medical history form or discussing a "condition" with the clinician in the presence of staff. However, in those instances in which a patient does feel uncomfortable, it is the clinician's duty to thoroughly review with the patient the health treatment as certain aspects can result in adverse reactions with treatment.

In reviewing the medical history, particular emphasis must be placed on **illnesses, history of bleeding, and medications. Illness** often means hospitalization to patients; consequently, they may not list weight changes, accidents, or problems related to stress and tension. Patients of African American heritage should be questioned about sickle cell anemia; there is a report of pulp necrosis occurring in patients with this distressing condition.[10] The term **bleeding** is usually interpreted by the patient to mean frank blood and seldom elicits answers related to bruising or healing time. Chronic use of aspirin[11] (not considered a drug by many people) or a history of liver disease should be of concern to the clinician. These should all be specifically mentioned in the medical history form. **Medication** means to many people only those items obtained by written prescription. Clinicians must also ask about "pills" and "drugs." Many people are self-medicating with diet pills, sleep inducers, and vitamins, as well as "recreational drugs," to mention only a few.

Investigating self-administered medication is also important to find out what "over-the-counter" medications the patient is actually taking. Women should be asked if they are pregnant or nursing, or if they have menstrual or menopausal problems.

Positive answers to these questions must be weighed and evaluated along with the other responses to determine the risk of treatment against the risk of nontreatment. When the history uncovers a serious problem, and a review of the systems involved (e.g., cardiac, respiratory) does not explain the problem, the patient's physician must be consulted. Then it is important to obtain the patient's physician's written permission to perform any dental treatment.

During these interviews, the clinician-patient relationship tends to crystallize. Patients feel more confident in the relationship. This is the time when high-strung patients may be calmed and reassured, although they may not be completely at ease until the first treatment is completed. Kindness and attention to their concerns or problems (chief complaint) during the history taking will greatly reduce most patients' emotional trauma and stress.

Clinical Examination

In general, the clinical examination should follow a logical sequence, from the general to the specific, from the more obvious to the less obvious, from the external to the internal. The results of the examination, along with information from the patient's history, will be combined with the clinical testing to establish the diagnosis, formulate a treatment plan, and determine the prognosis.

VITAL SIGNS

The first step in an examination is to obtain and record the patient's vital signs. These include blood pressure, pulse, respiratory rate, and temperature. Establishing a baseline or a **"norm"** for each patient is considered standard of care. Patients with test values well outside the range of acceptable norms are at risk, as is the clinician who treats them.[9] Common sense suggests that this risk should be shared with the patient's physician. Communication with the physician and the information received should be recorded in the chart and dated.

The vital signs may be recorded by any trained member of the office team. However, abnormal values must be evaluated and signed by the doctor. Any additional observations of abnormalities such as breathlessness, color change, altered gait, or unusual body movements observed during the initial meeting must be recorded.

Blood Pressure (normal: 120/80 mm Hg for persons under age 60 years; 130/90mm Hg for persons over age 60 years)

The Joint National Committee on Prevention, Detection, Evaluation, of High Blood Pressure recently added a new category, prehypertension, for patients with blood pressure of 120 to 139/80 to 89 mm Hg (see Chapter 23). Routine use of the sphygmomanometer not only establishes a baseline blood pressure but also occasionally brings to light unsuspected cases of hypertension in patients who are not regularly seeing a physician or are not maintaining prescribed regimens of therapy. Some ethnic groups are predisposed to hypertension. Halpern reported that only 18% of the dental clinic patients attending Temple University Dental School "were seeing their physicians."[9] At times, however, elevated blood pressure is caused only by the stress and anxiety of the moment and can be dealt with by reassurance or, if necessary, pretreatment sedation.

The emphasis of this procedure stresses the importance of the examination. Both the patient and the doctor are inclined to be more serious in their questions and answers when the examination begins with blood pressure records. It must be stressed that no patient, with or without a dental emergency, should be treated when the **diastolic** blood pressure is over 100 mm Hg.[12]

Blood Pressure, Pulse Rate and Respiration (normal: pulse 60 to 100 beats per minute; respiration 16 to 18 breaths per minute)

Blood Pressure When these examinations are added to the recording of blood pressure, the clinician increases the opportunity to know the patient better. These examinations also show the patient, by physical contact, how further examination will proceed—deliberately, gently, and completely. Pulse and respiration rates may also be elevated owing to stress and anxiety; in fact, these elevated signs may be even better indicators of stress than is blood pressure. Tests with markedly positive findings should be repeated later in the appointment or at a subsequent appointment.

Temperature (normal body temperature, 98.6°F [37°C])

The taking and recording of body temperature is a simple, significant procedure. An elevated temperature (fever) is one indication of a total body reaction to inflammatory disease. If the body temperature is not elevated, one can assume that the body is "managing" its defenses well, whatever the local signs (pain, swelling of an abscess formation). Systemic treatment with antibiotics, with its attendant risks, will likely not be required. A temperature above 98.6°F but less than 100°F indicates localized disease.[13] Localized disease can usually be treated by removing the cause (e.g., cleaning and disinfecting the root canal) and/or incision and drainage.

Cancer Screen (soft tissue examination: lumps, bumps, white spots)

Every new patient must be routinely screened for cancer and other soft tissue non-odontogenic conditions as part of the examination and informed of the results.

Table 2 Oral Cancer Warning Signals*
Swelling, lump, or growth anywhere in or about the mouth
White, scaly patches inside the mouth
Any sore that does not heal
Numbness or pain anywhere in the mouth area
Repeated bleeding in the mouth without cause

*"Open Wide." Reproduced with permission from the American Cancer Society, New York.

This examination should include a survey of the face, lips, neck, and intraoral soft tissues. When such examinations are made routinely, without secrecy, they will usually dispel the unstated fears of the cancerphobe and add to the confidence and rapport of all patients with their clinicians. The sooner this examination is completed the better. It is sometimes argued that clinicians are liable if they inform patients that they are performing an examination and then miss finding disease when it is present. In fact, clinicians are more liable if they miss reporting the disease because they have not made an examination. Extraorally, a cancer survey includes palpation of the floor of the mouth for masses, and examination for asymmetry and color changes. Intraorally, this examination is repeated with the additional care of directed lighting and of moving the tongue in such a manner so that all areas can be clearly seen (Table 2).

EXTRAORAL EXAMINATION

Inflammatory changes originating intraorally and observable extraorally may indicate a serious, spreading problem.[14] The patient must be examined for asymmetries, localized swelling, changes in color or bruises, abrasions, cuts or scars, and similar signs of disease, trauma, or previous treatment. Positive findings, combined with the chief complaint and information about past injuries or previous treatment to teeth or jaws, will begin to clarify the extent of the patient's problem. The extraoral examination includes the face, lips, and neck, which may need to be palpated if the patient reports soreness or if there are apparent areas of inflammation. Painful and/or enlarged lymph nodes are of particular importance. They denote the spread of inflammation and possible malignant disease. The extent and manner of jaw opening can provide information about possible myofascial pain, neuralgia, and dysfunction.[15] The temporomandibular joint should be examined during function for sensitivity to palpation, joint noise, and irregular movement.[16] (See Chapter 11 for more details on this topic.)

INTRAORAL EXAMINATION

The intraoral examination begins with a general evaluation of the oral structures. The lips and cheeks are retracted while the teeth are in occlusal contact, and the oral vestibules and buccal mucosa are examined for localized swelling, sinus tract, or color changes. With the patient's jaws apart, the clinician should evaluate in a similar manner the lingual and palatal soft tissues. Also, the presence of tori should be noted. Finally, as part of the general inspection, carious lesions, enamel fractures, discolorations, and other obvious abnormalities associated with the teeth, including loss of teeth and the presence of supernumerary or retained deciduous teeth, should be noted. Often the particular tooth causing the complaint is readily noted during this visual examination if it has not already been pointed out by the patient. Complaints associated with discolored or fractured teeth or with enamel crack lines could involve not only enamel but dentin as well. Teeth with extensive caries or large restorations, or teeth restored by full coverage, are, for the most part, readily located. Sinus tracts should be traced to the origin of lesions. True "puzzlement" begins when the complaint centers on teeth fully crowned and/or are part of extensive bridges or splints, or when only a few teeth are restored, and then only with minimal restorations.

Transillumination with a fiber-optic light, directed through the crowns of teeth, can add further information.[17] By this method, a previously treated tooth, not noticeably discolored, may show a gross difference in translucency when the shadow produced on a mirror is compared with that of adjacent teeth. Transillumination may also locate teeth with vertical cracks or fractures (see Chapter 19, "Infractions and Vertical Root Fractures," for more information).

CORONAL EVALUATION

The most obvious tooth is examined first, particularly when the patient, the history, or the general examination calls attention to a certain tooth. Using a mouth mirror and an explorer, and possibly a fiber-optic light, the clinician carefully and thoroughly examines the suspected tooth or teeth for caries, defective restorations, discoloration, enamel loss, periodontal problems, or defects that allow direct passage of stimuli to the pulp. Sometimes sealing off such leakage with temporary cements or periodontal dressings can be diagnostic. Vertical and horizontal fractures, located by transillumination, should be further investigated by having the patient bite on a firm object such as the Tooth Slooth (Professional Results Inc., Laguna Nigel, CA) or a wet cotton roll.[18] Occlusal wear facets and parafunctional patterns are also sought out, as is tooth mobility. Since the use of the operating microscope, diagnosis of crack lines has improved since many of these lines are not visible to the naked eye.

Pulpal Diagnosis

For convenience, diagnosis has been divided into two areas, pulpal and apical. The diagnostic terminology for both the pulp and the periapex is consistent with the terms recommended by the American Board of Endodontics. Pulpal diagnosis is addressed first (Table 3).

PULPALGIA

In the first edition of *Endodontics*, Ingle introduced the term *pulpalgia*.[19] Pulpalgia (pulpal pain) had numerous classifications that described its degree of severity and pathologic process. Today this term is not often used, and the terms *reversible* and *irreversible pulpitis* are the generally accepted clinical diagnostic terms. Clinicians, however, must deal with patients suffering from pulpalgia and have an understanding of the role of pulpal pain. Pulpal pain (toothache) is the symptom that brings patients into the clinician's office. It comes in many forms, rising from mild discomfort to raging pain, and then disappears, but the pulp is left in a worsening condition. Histologically, the pulp ranges from normal, to severely inflamed, to becoming totally necrotic. Prior

Table 3 Endodontic Diagnostic Terminology*

PULPAL

Normal pulp: a clinical diagnostic category in which the pulp is symptom free and normally responsive to vitality testing

Reversible pulpitis: a clinical diagnosis based on subjective and objective findings indicating that the inflammation should resolve and the pulp return to normal

Irreversible pulpitis: a clinical diagnosis based on subjective and objective findings indicating that the vital inflamed pulp is incapable of healing

Additional descriptions:
  Symptomatic: lingering thermal pain, spontaneous pain, referred pain

  Asymptomatic: no clinical symptoms but inflammation produced by caries, caries excavation, trauma, etc.

  Hyperplastic pulpitis (pulp polyp): growth of an exposed pulp into occlusal surfaces

  Internal resorption: the pulp has dentinoclastic activity

Pulp necrosis: a clinical diagnostic category indicating death of the dental pulp

Previously treated: a clinical diagnostic category indicating that the tooth has been endodontically treated and the canals are obturated with various filling materials, other than intracanal medicaments

Previously initiated therapy: a clinical diagnostic category indicating that the tooth has been previously treated by partial endodontic therapy (e.g., pulpotomy, pulpectomy)

Additional pulpal terms:
  Calcific metamorphosis: a pulpal response to trauma characterized by rapid deposition of hard tissue within the canal space

  Dystrophic calcification: diffuse foci of calcification frequently found in the aging pulp; usually described as being perivascular or perineural

APICAL (PERIAPICAL)

Normal apical (periapical) tissues: Teeth with normal periradicular tissues that will not be abnormally sensitive to percussion or palpation testing. The lamina dura surrounding the root is intact and the periodontal ligament space is uniform.

Symptomatic apical periodontitis (acute apical periodontitis): inflammation, usually of the apical periodontium, producing clinical symptoms including a painful response to biting and percussion. It may or may not be associated with an apical radiolucent area.

Additional descriptions:
  Lateral or **furcal** for additional spatial clarification

Asymptomatic apical periodontitis (chronic apical periodontitis): inflammation and destruction of apical periodontium that is of pulpal origin, appears as an apical radiolucent area, and does not produce clinical symptoms

Additional descriptions:
  Lateral or **furcal** for additional spatial clarification

Table 3 Continued on Page 527

Table 3 Continued from Page 526
Acute apical (periapical) abscess: an inflammatory reaction to pulpal infection and necrosis characterized by rapid onset, spontaneous pain, tenderness of the tooth to pressure, pus formation, and eventual swelling of associated tissues *Additional descriptions:* **Lateral** or **furcal** for additional spatial clarification
Chronic apical (periapical) abscess (suppurative periapical abscess): an inflammatory reaction to pulpal infection and necrosis characterized by gradual onset, little or no discomfort, and the intermittent discharge of pus through an associated sinus tract *Additional descriptions:* **Lateral** or **furcal** for additional spatial clarification *Additional periradicular terms:* **Apical scar:** dense collagenous connective tissue in the bone at or near the apex of a tooth with a distinctive radiolucent presentation; a form of repair usually associated with a root that has been treated surgically and usually associated with a perforation of both the facial and lingual osseous cortices **Cellulitis:** a symptomatic edematous inflammatory process associated with invasive microorganisms that spread diffusely through connective tissue and fascial planes. **Condensing osteitis (focal sclerosing osteomyelitis, periradicular osteosclerosis, sclerosing osteitis, sclerotic bone):** a diffuse radiopaque lesion believed to represent a localized bony reaction to a low-grade inflammatory stimulus, usually seen at the apex of a tooth (or its extraction site) in which there has been a long-standing pulp pathosis
*The diagnostic terminology for both the pulp and the periapex is consistent with the terms recommended by the American Board of Endodontics, 2007.

to opening into the pulp, one must make a diagnosis based on the signs and symptoms with which the patient presents. In some cases, no treatment will be needed, only advice and reassurance.

Pulpal pain can be classified as hyperreactive, acute, or chronic. *Acute* and *chronic* refer to the timing of the pain, not to its intensity. Hyperreactive pulpalgia, also known as dentinal sensitivity, is non-inflammatory, yet a remarkable number of patients present with this condition, brought on by heat or cold, sweet or sour foods, or touch to the tooth. They consider it toothache, not realizing that the pain from eating ice cream is not pathologic. Today it can be quite easily controlled with desensitization or sealant application by the clinician or with special toothpastes.

Acute pulpalgia ranges from incipient, to moderate, to advanced and reflects the degree of inflammation the pulp is suffering. Incipient pulpalgia is rarely irreversible. Some moderate pulpalgias are reversible and some are irreversible. This is where many diagnostic mistakes are made.

Incipient pulpalgia is the mild discomfort experienced following cavity or crown preparation or, in some patients, incipient caries. It could be gone in a day or two. Histologically, one would find a marginal increase in leukocytes and some edema causing pressure. When the edema subsides, the discomfort disappears. But it still causes patients to return for assurance, and, of course, incipient caries should be removed if that is the cause.

Moderate acute pulpalgia is a true but tolerable toothache; however, now there is true inflammation of the pulp. The pulp may not yet be infected by bacteria but is reacting to their acidic output. The symptoms may be "nagging" but mild and of short duration. Pulpalgia may be spontaneous but more likely is precipitated by an irritant such as hot or cold fluid. Mild analgesics may control the pain, and the pulpal condition is still reversible.

If bacteria have invaded and infected the pulp, the patient may initially have symptoms that he or she can "live with" and does live with, even though the pain is more intense and longer lasting once it begins. Temperature tests result in lingering pain, pointing to irreversible pulpitis. "Watchful waiting" may lead to the next level of pulpalgia, excruciating pain. That pain comes from advanced acute pulpalgia, the **ultimate toothache.** It is deemed irreversible. The patient may be in exquisite agony, at the point of hysteria. Relief can often be achieved temporarily with cold water or an ice cube. The patient may report to the office with a jar of ice water. Histologically, the coronal pulp is necrotic and gas has formed, causing the pressure that can be relieved by the cold. Testing with heat gives an immediate explosive response, so one must be prepared to immediately bathe the tooth with ice water. Immediate pulp extirpation is required.

Chronic pulpalgia is associated with irreversible pulpitis. The pain is not severe, and some patients have lived with it for months or even years, suppressing the pain with analgesics. They may not even have had any overt symptoms. Eventually, the tooth starts to ache at night. Radiographically, there may be resorption of the roots and condensing osteitis of the surrounding bone. Pulp testing results may be inconclusive. There is usually no pulpalgia with a totally necrotic pulp because the pulp tissue, including its sensory nerves, is destroyed.

Today these terms are not often used, and the terms *reversible* and *irreversible pulpitis* are the generally accepted clinical diagnostic terms. Clinicians, however, must deal with patients suffering from pulpalgia, and an understanding of the role pulpal pain—pulpalgia—plays can assist in developing a correct diagnosis necessary for proper treatment.

NORMAL PULP

This is a clinical diagnostic category in which the pulp is symptom free and normally responsive to vitality testing. Temperature sensitivity will disappear once the stimulus, such as ice cream, has been removed. The normal pulp may exhibit a strong response but is not painful. (see Table 3)

REVERSIBLE PULPITIS

Reversible pulpitis is a clinical diagnosis based on subjective and objective findings, indicating that the inflammation should resolve and the pulp return to normal. Signs of reversible pulpitis often include a normal periapical diagnosis but an increased response to cold that is nonlingering in nature (disappearing within seconds). The term *lingering* is often a confusing term to some, but it is used on an individual basis. If the patient response is equal in duration on all teeth, it would be nonlingering. If one tooth (or more) stands out above the rest of the teeth in terms of a variation or duration of symptoms, that is classified as lingering. Reversible pulpitis is commonly related to recent restorations, root scaling, traumatic brushing techniques, incipient caries, and small infractions in the tooth crown. Patients who complain of symptoms related to sweets also are typically exhibiting a reversible pulpitis. The patient who is undergoing vital bleaching may develop reversible pulpitis.[20] Pohjola et al. mentioned this sensitivity as the most frequently reported side effect.[21] Whatever the reason for the reversible pulpitis, stopping the irritation typically allows the pulp to return to normal. However, if the stimulus is not stopped, resolved, or treated, and the pulp is sufficiently irritated, pulpitis will progress into an irreversible state.

IRREVERSIBLE PULPITIS

Irreversible pulpitis, like reversible pulpitis, is a clinical diagnosis based on subjective and objective findings. It is defined as the point where an inflamed pulp is no longer capable of healing and returning to normal. This type of pulpitis exhibits many forms and symptoms. Lingering painful thermal responses, particularly to cold, are the classic form of irreversible pulpitis. This pain is intensified by a stimulus but can be spontaneous. It is typically episodic in nature initially but may progress into a constant intense pain or toothache.

Because the pulp is considered a deep tissue, it can be very difficult to isolate and pinpoint the exact tooth. Referred pain is common. Pulp testing needs to be thorough and methodical. Irreversible pulpitis, although commonly associated with its symptomatic form, also presents in numerous other ways. Many times, an asymptomatic tooth may have an irreversible pulpitis. Lin and Langeland showed that when caries invaded the pulp space, bacteria were present, and a root canal filling is the appropriate treatment.[22] The exception to this will be the young patient who still exhibits open apices or incomplete root development. For further discussion of this, see Chapter 34 on vital pulp therapy.

Another form of irreversible pulpitis is hyperplastic pulpitis.[23] Also referred to as a pulp polyp, this is a growth of pulp tissue from the pulp chamber that is usually covered with epithelium. This is typically seen again in a younger population and can be found in both primary and permanent dentition.

Aerodontalgia or barodontalgia has often been referred to as an irreversible pulpitis. This was first documented in World War II pilots when they were flying at elevations of 5,000 to 38,000 feet. In 1945, Orban and Ritchey published a research article in which they placed pilots into a decompression chamber and simulated different altitudes and flights.[24] They found that the healthy pulps were asymptomatic, but irreversible pulpitis that was "sealed" in the tooth elicited intense pain when barometric pressure decreased with altitude. This phenomenon also occurs when traveling in high mountainous countries.

PULP NECROSIS

This is a clinical diagnostic category, indicating partial or complete death of the dental pulp. This could be due to persisting inflammation of pulp tissue. The pulp is nonresponsive to vitality testing and is often pain free, although it can often be very painful to heat stimulation. Apical inflammatory response is primarily caused by a bacterial invasion from the infected pulp but may also be due to trauma or continual chemical irritation.

PREVIOUSLY TREATED

A clinical diagnostic category indicating that the tooth has been endodontically treated and the canals are obturated. Obturation may occur with various filling materials, including hard and soft pastes and resins, gutta-percha, and many other materials. Intracanal medicaments, such as calcium hydroxide, are not considered completely treated. They would fall into the category of previously initiated treatment.

PREVIOUSLY INITIATED THERAPY

This is a relatively new term that is being introduced to clarify the clinical scenarios encountered. This clinical diagnostic category indicates that the tooth has been previously treated by partial endodontic therapy (e.g., pulpotomy, pulpectomy), but no definitive treatment has been done.

Apical Diagnosis

The second part in determining a comprehensive diagnosis is apical diagnosis. In the past, various other terminologies have been used and sometimes referred to as periapical or periradicular diagnosis. For a description of a tooth's signs and symptoms, the diagnostic terminology is divided into five main categories. As these topics have already been extensively described in Chapter 13, they are mentioned here briefly for the purpose of completeness in the diagnosis.

NORMAL PERIAPICAL TISSUES

Teeth with normal apical tissues are asymptomatic. They will not be abnormally sensitive to percussion, or palpation, or thermal or electric testing. Radiographically, the lamina dura surrounding the root is intact and the periodontal ligament space is uniform. There is no sign or symptom of a pathologic change evident from either a clinical or a radiographic examination.

SYMPTOMATIC APICAL PERIODONTITIS

When the term *symptomatic* is used, it is done so to describe a clinical scenario representing some form of altered sensation for the patient. Inflammation, usually in the apical periodontium, produces clinical symptoms ranging from mild discomfort to an exquisitely painful response to biting and/or percussion. It may or may not be associated with an apical radiolucent area. These symptoms usually are of shorter onset but may exhibit mild discomfort. If a radiographic image reveals a radiolucency, the terms *lateral* or *furcal* may be used for additional spatial clarification of the lesion.

ASYMPTOMATIC APICAL PERIODONTITIS

Asymptomatic is a term used to describe a clinical scenario in which there is noted radiographically, inflammation and destruction of the apical periodontium with possible root and bone resorption but not necessarily producing clinical symptoms. Again, the terms *lateral* and *furcal* may be used to give additional clarification as to the position of the lesion.

ACUTE APICAL ABSCESS

The term *abscess* is used when signs of swelling or exudate are present or believed to be occurring. The term *acute* is used when an inflammatory reaction to pulpal infection and necrosis is characterized by rapid onset, spontaneous pain, and exquisite tenderness of the tooth to pressure. These patients are typically in moderate to severe discomfort owing to the sudden onset. Often few, if any, changes to the apical periodontium will be noted radiographically. The most commonly noted change is a widened periodontal ligament (PDL). As with all apical diagnoses, the terms *lateral* and *furcal* may be used to give additional clarification as to the position of the lesion or widened PDL.

CHRONIC APICAL ABSCESS

Chronic apical abscess is usually characterized by a gradual onset, with little or no discomfort to the patient. An intermittent discharge of pus through an associated sinus tract is commonly found. Radiographically, a large periapical lesion may be present. As with all endodontic abscess formations, it is an inflammatory reaction to pulpal infection and necrosis.

CELLULITIS

This is another form of abscess characterized by a symptomatic edematous inflammatory process. Invasive microorganisms spread diffusely through the connective tissue and fascial planes, to create various degrees of swelling and discomfort. It can be very rapid in its spread and requires close observation in its treatment.

APICAL SCAR

The apical scar is a dense collagenous connective tissue "scar" in the bone with a distinctive presentation. It is a dark radiolucency found at or near the apex of a tooth that has been surgically treated. It is a form of repair but is commonly associated with lesions that have been involved with the destruction of both the facial and lingual osseous cortical plates.

CONDENSING OSTEITIS

Condensing osteitis is a diffuse radiopaque lesion noted usually at the apex of a tooth or extraction site. It is believed to be associated with a low-grade inflammatory stimulus. It is a localized bony reaction commonly found in cases of long-standing pulpal pathosis.

PROGNOSIS AND INFORMED CONSENT

Today patients are demanding to be more informed and to actively participate in the choices available to them when it comes to treatment. This area must be divided into two parts: prognosis and informed consent.

Prognosis, as described by *Stedman's Medical Dictionary*, "is a forecast of the probable course and/or outcome of a disease."[25] The ability to accurately prognosticate is a major factor and a key to obtaining positive outcomes. One clinician's view of success or a positive outcome may differ from another's depending on the factors used to define success. Chapter 31, "Outcomes of Endodontic Treatment," explores in detail many aspects of treatment outcomes. It is important to remember when discussing treatment options with a patient that one does not omit the prognosis. Some patients may choose to "gamble" more than others when it comes to saving their teeth, but it is ultimately their choice after having received a detailed informed consent.

Informed consent consists of the risks, benefits, alternatives, and consequences associated with these choices. (See Chapter 3, "Ethics and the Law," for more details.) These areas need to be explored completely. Patients do not understand dental terminology for the most part, and it is important to relate these items in lay terms so as to reduce confusion for the patient. It is not necessary to explain every miniscule detail of the procedure or risk, but it is important to relay a general overview and the most likely complications that might ensue. Patients should feel comfortable and participatory in their treatment.[3] It is also of the utmost importance to have a written informed consent that patients sign at the end of this explanation, acknowledging that they were informed of the risks, benefits, and alternatives to treatment and that they had the option to have any questions they had, answered prior to treatment. From a medico-legal perspective, this will not stop litigation, but it will show due diligence to the attorneys that the patient was involved in the treatment choices. In today's litigious society, one cannot be too careful in protecting oneself.

References

1. Stedman's medical dictionary. 26th ed. Baltimore: Williams and Wilkins; 1995. Diagnosis.
2. Jaeger B. Pain Diagnosis Presented at Loma Linda University School of Dentistry; 2000; Loma Linda, CA.
3. Krasny RM. Seven steps to better doctor-patient communications. Dent Econ 1982;60:26.
4. Ingle JI, et al. Endodontic diagnostic procedures. In Ingle JI, Bakland LK. Endodontics. 5th ed. Hamilton (ON): BC Decker; 2002 pp. 203–58.
5. Medawar PD. The art of the soluble. London: Methuen, 1967.
6. Cecic PA, Hartwell GR, Bellizzi R. Cold as a diagnostic aid in cases of irreversible pulpitis. Oral Surg Oral Med Oral Pathol Oral Radiol Endod 1983;56:647.
7. Abou-Raas M. The stressed pulp condition: an endodontic restorative diagnostic concept. J Prosthet Dent 1982; 48:264.
8. Bolden TE, et al. Effect of prolonged use of analgesics on pulpal responses: a preliminary investigation. J Dent Res 1975;54:198.
9. Halpern IL. Patient's medical status—a factor in dental treatment. Oral Surg Oral Med Oral Pathol Oral Radiol Endod 1975;39:216.
10. Andrews CH, et al. Sickle cell anemia: an etiological factor in pulpal necrosis. J Endod 1983;9:249.
11. Biesterfeld RC, et al. Aspirin: an update. J Endod 1978;4:198.
12. Abbey LM, Hargrove B. Guidelines for a dental office high blood pressure screening program. Va Dent J 1974;51:52.
13. Summers GW. The diagnosis and management of dental infections. Otolaryngol Clin North Am 1976;8:717.
14. Tarsitano JJ. The use of antibiotics in dental practice. Dent Clin North Am 1970;14:697.
15. Cohen SR. Follow-up evaluation of 15 patients with myofascial pain-dysfunction syndrome. J Am Dent Assoc 1978;97:825.
16. Guralnick W, Kaban LB, Merrill RB. Temporomandibular joint affliction. N Engl J Med 1978;299:123.
17. Hill CM. The efficacy of transillumination in vitality tests. Int Endod J 1986;19:198.

18. Cameron CE. The cracked tooth syndrome. J Am Dent Assoc 1976;93:971.
19. Ingle JI, et al. Differential diagnosis and treatment of oral and perioral pain. In Ingle JI. Endodontics. 1st ed. Philadelphia: Lea & Febiger; 1965, pp. 420–71.
20. Leonard RH Jr. Efficacy, longevity, side effects, and patient perception of night guard vital bleaching. Compend Contin Educ Dent 1998;19:766.
21. Pohjola RM, et al. Sensitivity and tooth whitening agents. J Esthet Restor Dent 2002;14:85.
22. Lin LM, Langeland K. Light and electron microscopic study of teeth with carious pulp exposures. Oral Surg Oral Med Oral Pathol Oral Radiol Endod 1981;51:292.
23. Caliskan MK, Oztop F, Caliskan G. Histological evaluation of teeth with hyperplastic pulpitis caused by trauma or caries: case reports. Int Endod J 2003;36:64.
24. Orban B, Ritchey BT. Toothache under conditions simulating high altitude flight. J Am Dent Assoc 1945;32:145.
25. Stedman's medical dictionary. 26th ed. Baltimore: Williams and Wilkins; 1995. Prognosis.

B. Diagnostic Testing

James C. Kulild

An accurate diagnosis is the cornerstone of any subsequent endodontic therapy. To achieve the critical goal of this accurate diagnosis, a clinician must follow a systematic diagnostic evaluation process. This process must assess all possible orofacial areas that could have an influence on decision making and subsequent possible endodontic treatment, or referral, if the chief complaint is not of endodontic origin.

The overall goal of diagnostic testing is two-fold. The first is to gain objective data from the patient's signs and symptoms as well as from the results of diagnostic testing. The second is to reproduce the patient's chief complaint, if the patient has had past painful episodes. If the chief complaint cannot be reproduced during the evaluation, the practitioner should be wary of providing any treatment that might be well-intentioned but might result in a poor outcome, as that treatment may not be related to the chief complaint and may not, in fact, have been necessary.

At the present time, the capabilities of diagnostic testing are well short of the objective science needed to definitively determine the health or disease status of the pulp. This is because pulp tissue is contained in the noncompliant environment of the root canal system that does not allow direct visual inspection, histological, or other direct evaluation techniques. Van Hassel[1] stated that the unique encasement of the pulp in a low-compliance environment directly affects its ability to respond to injury and/or disease. However, within these limitations, the clinician must still attempt to determine the health or disease status of the pulp so that appropriate treatment decisions can be made.

The clinician must clearly understand that any, and all, diagnostic tests are merely adjuncts in the decision-making process that leads to both pulpal and periapical diagnoses. Treatment decisions should not be made on the basis of one piece of diagnostic data. There must be corroborating data from at least one other test before treatment is recommended. In 1937, Stephen[2] reported a poor correlation between diagnostic data, clinical signs and symptoms and actual histological findings. Mitchell and Tarplee[3] attempted a similar in vivo experiment in 1960 and also could not identify consistent findings in teeth with painful pulpitis. Seltzer et al.[4,5] reported a poor correlation between diagnostic data and actual histological findings in their exhaustive studies. They stated that a history of previous pain was an important diagnostic sign of pulp inflammation. They also found that the presence of large deposits of tertiary dentin did not result in delayed responses to pulp testing, but surprisingly generated responses more quickly. They also stated that inflammation was not necessarily irreversible and that the pulp may have the capability to repair itself. Conversely, the pulp may become necrotic without ever manifesting pain. Johnson et al.[6] stated that false-positive pulp testing results were obtained in half of the teeth that were histologically necrotic. Conversely, negative pulp testing results had a much greater chance of indicating histological pulp necrosis. In 1973, Garfunkel et al.[7] reported the correlation between a clinical diagnosis and the histological status of the pulp that was about 50%. Bhaskar and Rappaport[8] reported on 25 anterior teeth, that had been previously traumatized and reacted negatively to conventional pulp testing, all contained vital pulps when examined histologically. Hyman and Cohen[9] concluded that it was possible to erroneously reason that a tooth contained a pulp with irreversible pulpitis when, in fact, it contained either a normal or irreversibly involved pulp. They also stated that a diagnosis of irreversible pulpitis should be substantiated by multiple tests to prevent unnecessary endodontic treatment. In 1945, Herbert[10] attempted to correlate clinical signs and symptoms with the histological condition of the pulp in an in vivo experiment and determined that the results were not always consistent.

However, if a clinician has performed the correct diagnostic procedures and performed them correctly with clear results, he should put his faith in them in spite of apparent conflicting data or signs. For example, a tooth that has been treated previously with nonsurgical root canal treatment (NS RCT) can still illicit a positive response to pulp vitality tests.[11,12] Adjacent teeth that seem to manifest two separate and distinct

Table 1 Example of Diagnostic Grid for Recording Pulp Testing Results						
Tooth	Cold*	Hot	Percussion	Palpation	Mobility	Periodontal Probing†
13	WNL	N/A	–	–	WNL	F: 2 2 3
						L: 2 3 3
14	WNL	N/A	–	–	WNL	F: 2 2 3
						L: 3 2 2
15	L	N/A	–	–	WNL	F: 2 2 2
						L: 2 2 2
2	NR	N/A	+	+	Class I	F: 2 3 4
						L: 3 3 4
3	WNL	N/A	–	–	WNL	F: 3 3 3
						L: 2 2 2

N/A = not applicable; NR = no response; WNL = within normal limits.
–, not sensitive to percussion/palpation; +, sensitive to percussion/palpation.
*L = lingering.
†L = lingual, measurements go from mesial to distal.

periapical radiolucencies may, in fact, reflect pathology of only one of those teeth if pulp vitality tests indicate a normal pulp in one of the teeth.[11,12]

Practically speaking, a diagnostic table for recording diagnostic testing results can be easily created for each clinically tested tooth. It can include responses for a variety of tests (Table 1). The information should be recorded and placed in the patient's dental record. The information can also be recorded in an electronic record with the help of a dental assistant as the tests are being performed. Both pulpal and periapical diagnoses should be recorded based on the documented clinical findings (see Table 1 in section 14A in this chapter).

Caring, competent, and capable clinicians must be confident enough to tell the patient that the diagnosis is based on the best available evidence. There are many physiological and psychological processes occurring that could cloud any diagnostic testing results that might be performed.[13–25] Patients must understand that diagnostic testing is not pure science and that ultimate treatment recommendations may be based on not only the tests themselves but on the clinical judgment of the clinician formed by a variety of factors: education and training, updating current information by reading appropriate literature, attending related continuing education courses, and always giving each and every patient full attention and expertise. A variety of various pulp testing methodologies and techniques have been used in the past with and without consistent success.[14,23,25]

Visual Oral Examination and Review of Systems

A clinician should perform a thorough general visual examination that evaluates the entire orofacial region. This soft and hard tissue exam avoids "tunnel vision" that can occur by examining only the single tooth or the specific area in question. A cancer screening exam should always be conducted particularly in the danger areas on the ventral and/or lateral surfaces of the tongue and the floor of the mouth. A visual exam is also helpful in determining any facial asymmetries that may or may not be helpful in subsequent determination of the patient's chief complaint.

Croll et al.[26] published a guide for a rapid neurological assessment and initial management for the patient with traumatic dental injuries that could require immediate referral, as well as prevent significant second- and third-order effects from neurological damage. It is important to point out that pain appearing to be of endodontic origin may in fact be referred from another source, particularly when evaluating teeth in the mandibular left quadrant. A patient may be experiencing either a coronary insufficiency or a myocardial infarct.[27,28] If the pain does not resolve, vital signs should be repeated and the patient should be questioned on any other possible symptoms, for example, chest pain, pain radiating down the left arm, nausea, or sweating. When in doubt, it is always prudent to activate the emergency response system, prepare to administer cardiopulmonary resuscitation if needed, and have a staff member ready the office automated external defibrillator for any possible eventuality. Never assume "everything is OK" until the facts provide substance for that assumption.

Thermal Tests

Thermal tests are commonly employed diagnostic pulpal tests. If properly done, they have proven to be reasonably effective and generally cause no irreversible negative effects on either soft or hard tissues. Any thermal test, at best, merely identifies the presence of pulp nerve tissue that is capable of responding to a change in temperature. Reiss and Furedi[29] stated, back in 1933, that dentists should not be interested in just the condition of the nerves in the pulp but in the condition of the pulp itself.

Mullaney et al.[30] reported that only 2 of 48 pulps that had not responded to either the electric pulp tester (EPT) or cold thermal tests exhibited a normal histological appearance. However, every patient in the study had a painful response when the pulpal tissue in the canal was broached, indicating remaining neural innervation. The authors attributed the response to the movement of the necrotic tissue putting pressure on the periapical tissues.

England et al.[31] histologically examined 30 human pulps, in which clinical diagnostic testing indicated the pulps had either irreversible pulpitis or were necrotic. The nerve fibers of both types of pulps were compared with those of normal pulps. Functioning nerve tissue was reported in the pulps with irreversible pulpitis. In the necrotic pulps, only the connective tissue sheaths remained. They were incapable of transmitting any neural impulses. The nerve fibers in pulps with irreversible pulpitis resisted degeneration longer than the surrounding tissue.[31] A thermal test may provide information that suggests whether the pulp is reversibly or irreversibly inflamed or necrotic.

Ice has been used for cold thermal tests as it is readily available and inexpensive. However, ice is not as cold as some other available materials and has many shortcomings that limit its effectiveness. The primary shortcoming is that melted ice water can spread to either soft tissue or another tooth and cause a false-positive result. A false positive is defined as the patient responding to a pulp test, when in fact the pulp tissue in the tooth being examined is necrotic, or another tooth is responding, not the tooth being examined. A false negative is defined as the patient not responding to a pulp test when in fact the pulp tissue in the tooth being examined is vital. Cold tests are most likely to give a positive response in the cervical area compared to the occlusal surface.[32] Cold response seems to be related to the thickness and type of tooth structure between the source of the cold and the pulp. It is important to emphasize that just because the pulp tissue in the tooth being tested responds "positive," it does not necessarily indicate that the pulp is either healthy or diseased. The pulp could be either normal or suffering from reversible or irreversible pulpitis. A normal pulp is a clinical diagnostic category in that the pulp is symptom free and normally responsive to vitality testing.[33] Reversible pulpitis is a clinical diagnosis based on subjective and objective findings indicating that the inflammation should resolve and the pulp return to normal.[33] Irreversible pulpitis is a clinical diagnosis based on subjective and objective findings indicating that the vital inflamed pulp is incapable of healing.[33] Seltzer et al.[34] tried to simplify the previously complicated pulpal diagnostic terminology by coining earlier similar terms, treatable or non-treatable. The fact that a tooth responds quickly and dramatically does not, in and of itself, indicate that endodontic treatment is indicated. If the sensation remits relatively "quickly," the pulp can reasonably be presumed to be either normal or suffering from reversible pulpitis. However, if the sensation "lingers," it may indicate that the pulp is irreversibly involved and NS RCT is indicated. The time periods represented by the words "quickly" and "lingers" are relative and can vary from patient to patient. Generally, "quickly" implies that the sensation returns to normal within a few seconds. The term "lingers" implies that the sensation lasts much longer extending perhaps 30 seconds or more. Materials with temperatures colder than ice include skin refrigerant, Endo Ice, carbon dioxide snow (CO_2) and Spray and Stretch (Gebauer Co., Cleveland, OH).

White and Cooley[35] compared in vitro the temperature changes in a human tooth when skin refrigerant (ethyl chloride), an ice water bath, and an ice stick were applied to the crown of an extracted canine tooth. They reported that skin refrigerant produced a greater thermal change (58.4°F) than ice water (69.2°F) or an ice stick (75.4°F).

Tetrafluoroethane (Endo-Ice, Hygenic Corp., Akron, OH) is approximately –50°F.[36] It is available in a convenient spray that can be used to apply the liquid material to a medium- or large-sized cotton pellet held

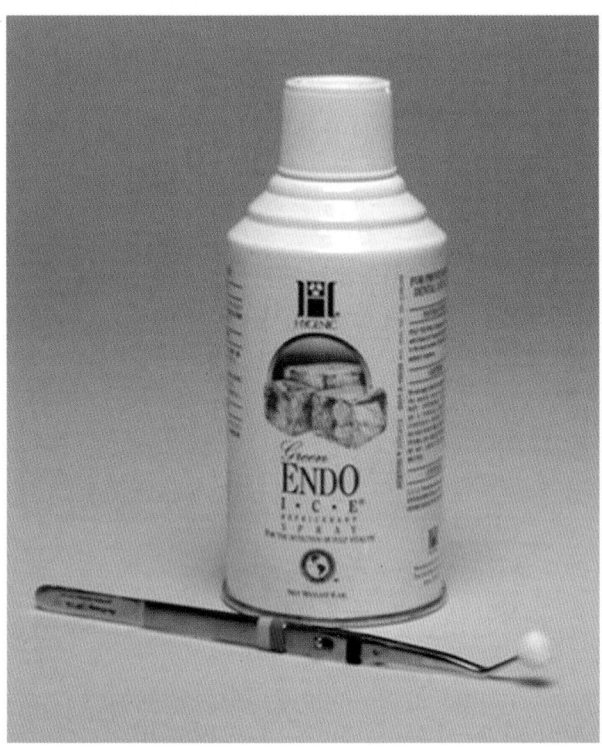

Figure 1 Endo-Ice (Hygenic Corp., Akron, OH) is tetrafluoroethane, can be applied to teeth with cotton forceps and large cotton pellets.

in a pair of cotton forceps (Figure 1). During the testing procedure, the patient is shown the cold test materials to help alleviate any anxiety they may have about the procedure. The patient is told to raise their hand when they feel any cold, burning, or tingling sensation and at that time the pellet will be immediately removed from the tooth being tested. They are told to warm the tooth with their tongue and cheek and keep their hand up until the sensation returns to normal. After testing control teeth, the clinician can then move the testing process to the tooth (teeth) in question and determine their response.

Jones[37] reported that a large cotton pellet produced the largest temperature change in the pulp chamber compared to a small cotton pellet, a cotton-tipped applicator, and/or cotton roll. Jones et al.[38] reported that Endo-Ice and CO_2 produced similar results in determining pulpal response, but the Endo-Ice elicited faster response. Miller et al.[39] conducted an in vitro experiment to determine whether ice, 1,1,1,2,-tetrafluoroethane (the new formulation for Endo-Ice), or CO_2 produced the greatest temperature change in teeth restored with full coverage. They reported that Endo Ice produced the greatest temperature reduction in intact teeth and those restored with gold, porcelain fused to metal, and porcelain crowns, when tested for less than 15 seconds.

Fuss et al.[36] evaluated the in vivo effectiveness of the EPT, CO_2, dichlorodifluoromethane, (Spray and Stretch), ethyl chloride, and ice in producing a response in patients during pulp testing. They reported that the EPT, CO_2, and dichlorodifluoromethane were more dependable in producing a response than ethyl chloride or ice. However, in young patients, they reported that CO_2 and dichlorodifluoromethane were the most dependable. They also reported in the same study that CO_2 and dichlorodifluoromethane were more effective in lowering the internal temperature of the tooth than ethyl chloride or ice.

Carbon dioxide snow, more commonly known as dry ice, became popular because it was predictable as a cold thermal material in diagnostic testing. Ehrmann[40] popularized the use of the CO_2 pencil ($-78°C$) that had been previously introduced by Obwegeser and Steinhauser in 1963. A small amount of the CO_2 is expressed through the end of the syringe that is then placed on the crowns of the teeth being evaluated. Figure 2A shows the solid CO_2 being extruded from the syringe in the form of a pencil, that can then be applied to the tooth (Figure 2B). In order to avoid the danger involved if a tank of this type falls to the floor breaking the regulator in the top of the tank and turning it into a potential lethal missile, the tank should be secured with a chain or in a box (Figure 3) Despite the very cold temperature, numerous investigations have demonstrated the safety of CO_2 on both the enamel and the pulp. Augsburger and Peters[41] reported that a 5-second application of CO_2 resulted in a statistically significantly greater temperature decrease on the crowns of extracted teeth compared to ice or skin refrigerant. Peters et al.[42] reported that CO_2 produced no cracks or fissures in the enamel of human teeth in vitro after being subjected to it for 15, 45, and 60 seconds on the same spot on the enamel, a time that is significantly longer than that used clinically. A follow-up in vivo scanning electron microscope and histological investigation using canine teeth as the experimental model resulted in no damage to either the enamel or the pulp.[43] Using the scanning electron microscopy, Peters et al.[44] evaluated the effects of 2 minutes of exposure of CO_2 on human teeth scheduled for extraction and reported that there was no subsequent damage to the enamel surface. An in vivo investigation showed

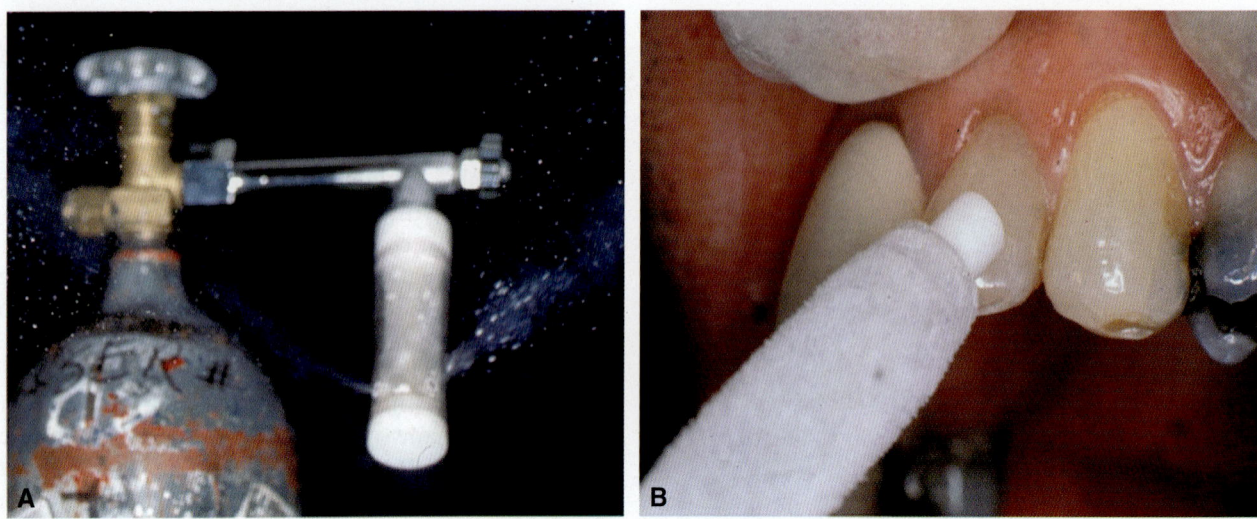

Figure 2 ***A***, Solid CO_2 being extruded from the syringe in the form of a pencil. ***B***, The pencil is held with a gauze pad and applied to the tooth.

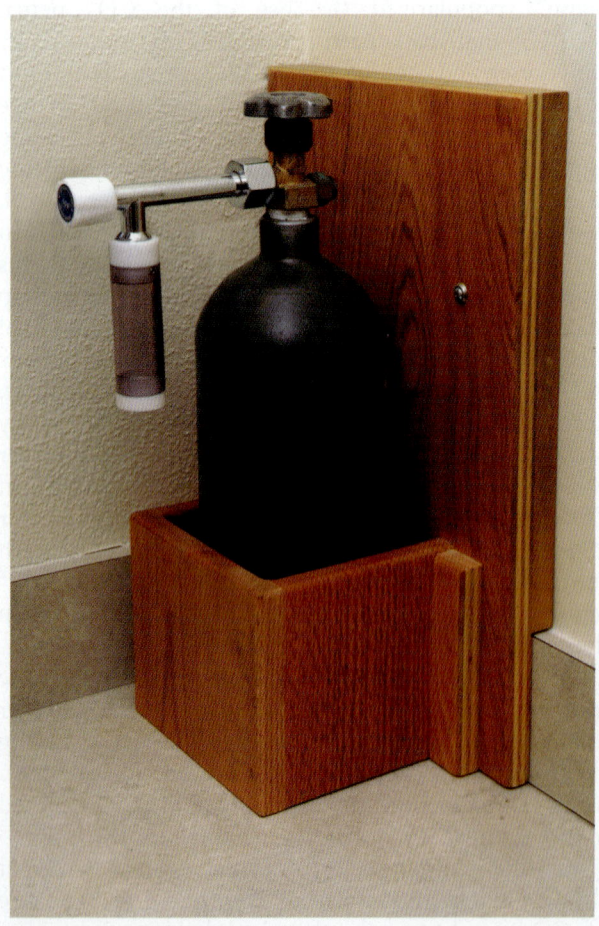

Figure 3 The CO_2 tank is stored securely in a box.

that a 5-minute application of CO_2 to the surface of a tooth had no effect on intact human pulps.[45]

Warm thermal testing is not employed as frequently as cold testing as most patients are more sensitive to cold stimuli and the fact that warm thermal tests have been traditionally more difficult to perform. Some traditional ways to apply warm thermal testing include the following: a heated ball burnisher, a rotating Burlew rubber wheel, heated base plate gutta-percha (GP), or warm water. White and Cooley[35] evaluated the temperature changes in a human tooth when hot water from the tap, hot GP stopping material, a hot burnisher, or a Burlew wheel were applied to the crown of an extracted canine tooth. The hot GP stopping material, hot burnisher, and Burlew wheel produced temperature rises within 2°F of each other after an 8-second application. However, flooding the tooth with water at 136°F produced a temperature rise approximately 7°F higher. The authors preferred the Burlew wheel because of its convenience and because of the inherent difficulties involved in isolating each individual tooth with a rubber dam before the warm water is applied.[35] The warm thermal test can be accomplished by isolating an individual tooth, filling a syringe with very warm water from the tap, applying the water to the tooth, and then quickly suctioning the water from the site if the patient demonstrates a severe response. The practitioner must be prudent when using a heated ball burnisher or a Burlew wheel as there is no way to gauge the temperatures being

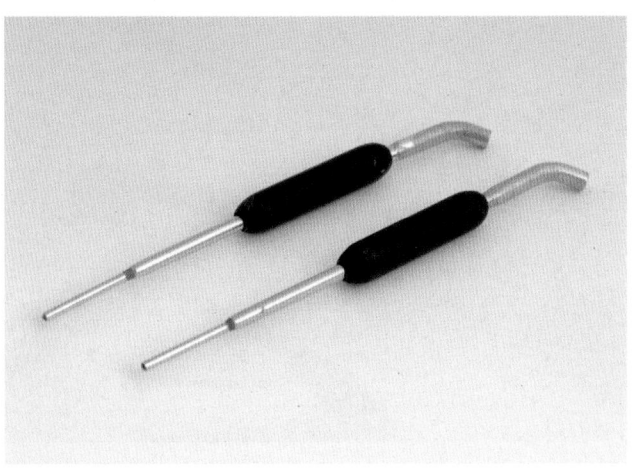

Figure 4 System B Hot Pulp Test Tip (Sybron Endo, Orange, CA).

produced on the surface of a tooth or within the pulp chamber, and possible irreversible damage to either the enamel or the pulp can occur.

Selden[46] reported a warm thermal technique whereby the patient rinses their mouth with extremely warm water, and then ice is applied to the most likely tooth to determine if the pain is diminished by the application of ice. Using heated GP is an adequate testing procedure if a suitable lubricant is placed on the buccal surface of the tooth to prevent the GP from sticking to it. One investigation showed that after 10 seconds of exposure to heated GP on the enamel of a tooth that there was no evidence of injury.[45]

The System B (Sybron Endo, Orange, CA) allows the dentist to set specific temperatures for warm thermal testing. After the surface of the tooth has been lubricated, a hot pulp test tip can be attached to the handle of the System B and the temperature set at 150°F. The tip is placed on the surface(s) of the tooth, and the patient's response is evaluated (Figure 4). This temperature is used as it represents the temperature of very warm tap water. This can be done without fear of damage to either the hard or soft tissues of the tooth.

Electric Pulp Testing

The EPT gauges the ability of nerves in the pulp to respond to electrical stimulation. The patient generally does not feel a true "electrical" stimulation but feels a warm, "tingly," burning, or pain sensation. This is because the nerves in the pulp responding to EPT are A-delta nociceptors and do not transmit electric, thermal, touch, or proprioceptive sensations to the central nervous system, but only pain. The EPT also causes the patient some anxiety knowing the instrument passes an electrical current through their teeth. False-positive responses can also occur just as in thermal tests in adjacent teeth.[47] The EPT gives the clinician no information on the status of inflammation in the pulp or the health or disease of the vasculature system. Reynolds[48] accurately stated this fact when he reported after getting accurate EPT readings that those results still could not distinguish between various states of vitality. The clinician should evaluate contralateral teeth as control teeth. Chilton and Fertig[49] reported that there was no significant difference in the pulp test results of contralateral vital teeth.

Jacobson[50] reported that the optimal placement of the probe tip in vitro was the occlusal two-thirds on the labial or buccal surfaces of teeth. Other investigators have reported that the incisal edge was the optimal placement site to achieve the lowest possible threshold for an EPT response.[32,51] The threshold increased as the probe tip was moved toward the gingival margin.

Van Hassel and Harrington[52] reported that precautions needed to be taken during pulp testing procedures to prevent electrical current from spreading to adjacent teeth, especially those with contacting metal fillings, and that multirooted teeth had the greatest chance of giving false readings.

Historically, EPT relied on direct or indirect current applied directly to the tooth. In 1909, Tousey[53] described the faradic current that was suitable for pulp testing through enamel and dentin. Early EPT instruments were not well calibrated, and the design sometimes allowed a tooth to receive full power on the first application causing the patient needless discomfort. In 1953, Taylor[54] reported on the capabilities of the Burton Vitalometer that used frequencies between 2 and 3,000 cycles. The instrument had a manual sliding device that would increase the current on a scale from 1 to 14.

Mumford[55] reported that the shape of the area produced by the current emitted during use of the EPT was triangular in shape, with the base of the triangle at the interface between the pulp tester tip and the enamel. The apex was oriented toward the pulp. He further stated that teeth with incompletely formed root apices require a stronger current to illicit a response, because the pulp has a greater cross-sectional area and requires greater current density.

Fulling and Andreasen[56] reported a higher EPT threshold value for teeth with immature root apices. They also reported that the CO_2 pencil provided

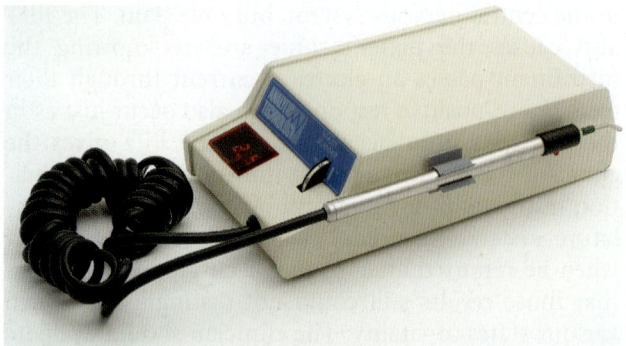

Figure 5 The Analytic Technology pulp tester (Sybron Endo, Orange, CA) was the first digital pulp tester marketed in the 1980s.

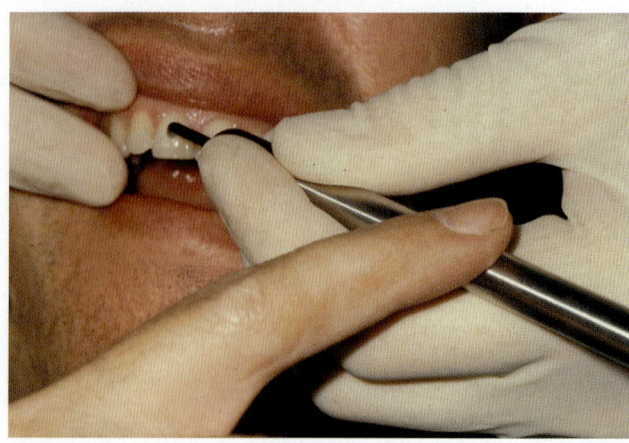

Figure 6 Patient placing finger lightly on the metal part of the probe handle.

similar pulp test reactions regardless of status of root formation.

Newer instruments introduced since the 1980s use either battery or AC power that is applied logarithmically and automatically to the tooth being tested (Figure 5). This design precludes the chance of a patient receiving a full charge on the first application. The clinician can adjust the speed of delivery of the small amount of electric current based on personal preference. Cooley et al.[57] reported that the Analytic Technology pulp tester (Sybron Endo) included some technological advances that improved both performance, comfort to the patient, and ease of operation for the dentist. These enhancements included the following: the ability to turn on automatically when the probe made contact with the tooth, the ability to turn off automatically when the probe tip was removed from the tooth surface, a numerical digital display, a red light on the probe handle indicating to the clinician that a good contact with the tooth was made, and voltage was electronically stabilized. Kitamura et al.[58] reported similar positive results when evaluating the Analytic Technology pulp tester both in vitro and in vivo. Wahab and Kennedy[59] reported in an investigation that more accurate results were obtained with the EPT if there was a slower rate of current increase.

Martin et al.[60] investigated various conductive media to transmit current used during use of the EPT. They reported that a water-based jelly was the most conductive of the materials evaluated including toothpaste, saline pads, prophylaxis paste, and direct contact with no media. The type of media was not significant except for direct contact with no media. Michaelson et al.[61] reported no difference between toothpastes, water, or Electrocardiogram (EKG) paste. Dry contact did not evoke a response. Before the routine use of gloves in the dental clinic, the circuit between the EPT instrument was closed by contact of the clinicians' ungloved hands or a lip clip in contact with the patients lips, cheek, or gingival. Anderson and Pantera[62] reported on a modified EPT technique that not only allows the use of gloves and predictably accurate measurements, but also puts the patient "in charge" of the procedure alleviating much of the anxiety many patients feel when told a small amount of electric current will be used on their tooth. The technique consists of placing the probe tip of the EPT on the tooth, asking the patient to place their finger lightly on the metal part of the probe handle and informing them to remove their finger from the probe handle when they feel a warm, tingling sensation (Figure 6). Cailleteau and Ludington[63] reported a similar technique, but also stated that the lip clip may still be necessary if a patient has limited or restricted ability to control their hand movements, for example, physically debilitated or handicapped patients.

A clinician may need to use EPT on a tooth with full coverage. This may preclude using a pulp tester probe tip because its relatively large size would contact either the gingival tisssue or the metal of the restoration. Pantera et al.[64] reported that small metal endodontic instruments such as files, explorers, or the like could be used in a bridging procedure. The tip of a small bridging instrument is coated with a contact medium and placed on the enamel or dentin of the tooth being evaluated. The probe tip is then placed on the metal of the bridging instrument.

Some have questioned the use of dental electrical diagnostic or treatment equipment applying current to a patient with an embedded cardiac pacemaker that could potentially interfere with its function.[65] This includes the EPT, electric desensitizing equipment, ultrasonics, electrosurgical instruments, and related equipment. Using an animal model, the authors reported that the magnitude of currents used in those type of instruments could modify pacemaker function and cautioned against their use in patients with artificial pacemakers. However, Simon et al.[66] in an exhaustive in vitro and in vivo investigation reported that three dogs with implanted artificial pacemakers were unaffected by short or sustained stimulation with pulp vitality testers. Wilson et al.[67] recently demonstrated no effect on implanted cardiac pacemakers or cardioverters/defibrillators with either the EPT or electronic apex locators. Investigators do recommend contacting the patient's physician or cardiologist for specific guidance regarding the use of electrical devices.

Percussion

Percussion is one of the oldest pulp vitality tests used because it requires no armamentarium. Generally, patients who have a tooth sensitive to mastication have already percussed the tooth in question with their own finger tip(s) and informed the dentist which teeth are sensitive. Percussion is an indirect means of testing pulp vitality because teeth that are sensitive to percussion often have existing periapical lesions associated with a necrotic pulp. However, this is not always the case, and false positives can result if the clinician is evaluating a cracked tooth or a "high" restoration. If a crack has developed in the crown of a tooth with a vital pulp, the tooth can still be exquisitely sensitive, because of the crown segments, moving microscopically causes pain due to the movement of fluid in the odontoblastic tubules. The tooth is sensitive to thermal stimuli as the pulp is vital. These mutually exclusive diagnostic findings, pain to percussion/mastication and thermal sensitivity, are pathognomonic for a cracked tooth.

Sometimes, the solution to percussion sensitivity might be as simple as performing an occlusal adjustment. Periapical lesions cause discomfort to the patient because when the tooth is compressed in the socket during percussion, pressure is added to the bone and periodontal ligament (PDL) causing discomfort. Clinicians should move cautiously when percussing a tooth known to be sensitive to mastication. Although the standard instrument used to percuss teeth by many clinicians has been the end of the mirror handle, there is another way to employ this test that causes minimal discomfort but still achieves

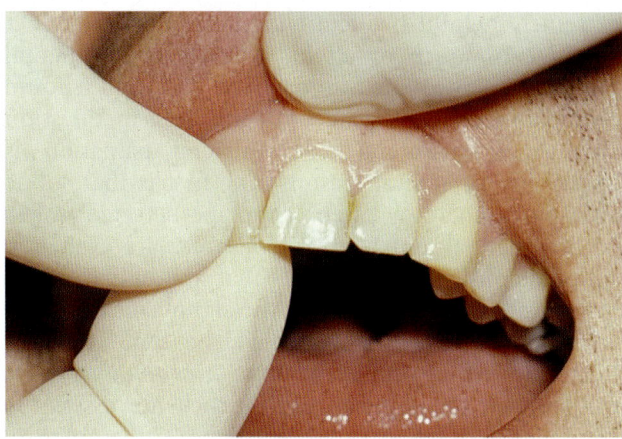

Figure 7 Clinician grasping a tooth between his thumb and forefinger at the level of the middle third of the crown.

the desired results. To begin with, control teeth and then the tooth to be tested are compressed into the socket with increasing force until the clinician is assured the tooth is not sensitive to percussion (Figure 7). If the clinician is not confident with the pressure findings, one can gently tap with the end of the mirror handle to determine percussion sensitivity. One of the advantages of using digital pressure to assess percussion sensitivity is that the mobility of the tooth can be assessed simultaneously as discussed in "Mobility." A calibrated percussion instrument has been suggested that can more objectively identify the percussion test.[68]

Mobility

The advantage of performing both mobility and percussion testing simultaneously makes the testing process more tolerable for the patient while decreasing the number of separate diagnostic tests. The following Miller Index[69] is an objective system to use, and the results can be easily communicated:
- Class I: First distinguishable sign of movement greater than normal.
- Class II: Movement of the tooth as much as 1 mm in any direction.
- Class III: Movement of the tooth more than 1 mm in any direction and/or depression or rotation of the tooth.

Palpation

Manual digital palpation of the soft and hard tissues around or adjacent to the tooth in question can be extremely helpful in identifying areas that are either sensitive to touch or altered due to developmental reasons, disease, or trauma. The clinician should always bilaterally palpate both the area in question and the contralateral side. Bilateral palpation is important for several reasons. The first is that subtle changes in anatomy often cannot be detected unless both ipsilateral and contralateral areas are evaluated simultaneously. The second is that a swelling on the ipsilateral side may appear to be significant until the contralateral side is palpated at the same time. A bilateral swelling could be *toris mandibularis*. The third is that the clinician can much better assess the consistency of either a neoplastic or inflammatory swelling by palpating bilaterally, for example, fluctuant or indurated. Absence of discomfort during palpation does not mean that disease is not present or that the tissues are healthy. For example, the swelling might be a painless ameloblastoma. Conversely, the presence of discomfort does not mean that disease is present, for example, palpating over the mental foramen.

Transillumination

Diagnostic use of transillumination was reported in 1927 when Cameron[70] reported its use for diagnostic procedures. Friedman and Marcus[71] reported that it was a useful test for detection of caries, calculus, and soft tissue lesions. It is a vital and extremely effective tool in the evaluation process and one that is frequently overlooked. It is primarily used to help determine the presence of a crown or root fracture. It can also be used to aid in the determination of pulp vitality. When a bright light is projected through the tooth being tested, the transmitted light can be interrupted by cracks present as well as changes in the color of the pulp. There are many devices available for transillumination. These include specifically designed fiberoptic lights, a high speed handpiece with the fiberoptic-activated or other bright point light sources. Inexpensive alternatives are also available.[72]

To evaluate a tooth for a crown fracture, the dental unit light should be turned off and only the fiberoptic light used. The fiberoptic light is placed sequentially on all sides of the tooth. If a crack is present in the dentin, the light will be interrupted at that crack and the clinician will see a dark line marking its location. The dentin on the opposite side of the crack from the light source will be darker in color (Figure 8). If a crack of this type is observed in a tooth, the tooth may also exhibit symptoms such as sensitivity to thermal stimulation and mastication and/or percussion.[73] Ritchey et al.[74] previously described these defects as incomplete tooth fractures and discussed the diagnostic frustrations

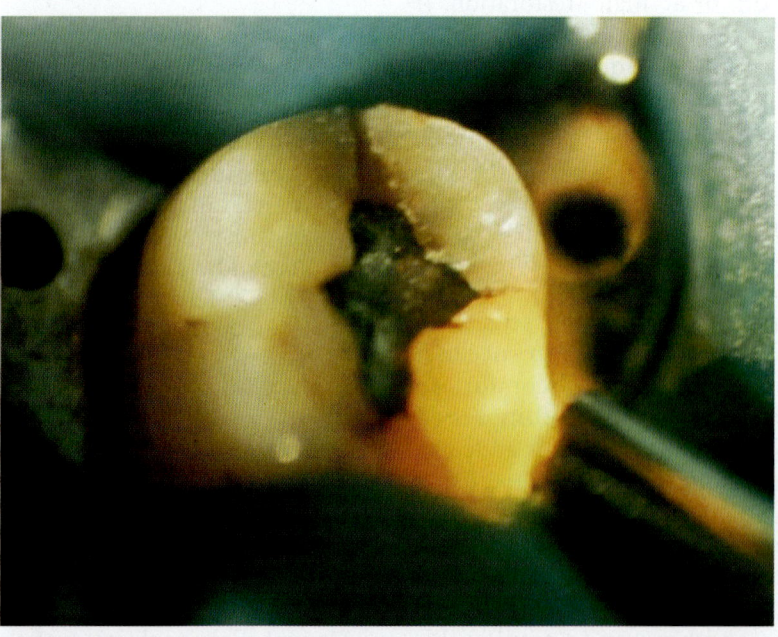

Figure 8 Photo of crown of tooth with crack located using a transilluminator.

they presented to the clinician. If multiple signs and symptoms are observed, endodontic treatment is indicated followed by a full coverage restoration. Frequently, the sensitivity to mastication occurs when the pressure is released after it is applied.[75] These fractures have been referred to as greenstick fractures.[76,77]

Fiberoptic illumination is also a helpful adjunct to evaluate pulp vitality in anterior teeth after trauma. Loss of tooth translucency is reported to be an accurate indication of pulpal health or disease.[78] The dental unit light should be turned off, and the fiberoptic light is placed on the lingual surfaces of the anterior teeth. The color of a tooth with normal uninflamed pulp has yellow, white, and pink hues indicating a combination of the yellow dentin, the white enamel, and the pink healthy pulp. The color of a tooth with a necrotic pulp often exhibits a darker brown or black color indicating the change in color of the necrotic pulp. These color changes are often subtle and not observable when using only the dental unit light.

Periodontal Probing

Periodontal probing is an essential part of the diagnostic process, but it is also one that is frequently omitted by practitioners, particularly if the patient does not have generalized periodontal disease. A periodontal probe should always be readily available. Double-ended instruments are available with an explorer on one end and a periodontal probe on the other (Figure 9). The tooth should be evaluated interproximately as well as in at least three locations on both the buccal and the lingual surfaces. In addition, each furcation should also be explored with a periodontal probe. Periodontal defects could be a sign of either an endodontic or a periodontal problem. Simon et al.[79] described a classification of endodontic/periodontal presentations that can aid in not only diagnosis but also determination of an acceptable treatment plan and prognosis. Harrington et al.[80] reported diagnostic criteria to aid the practitioner in

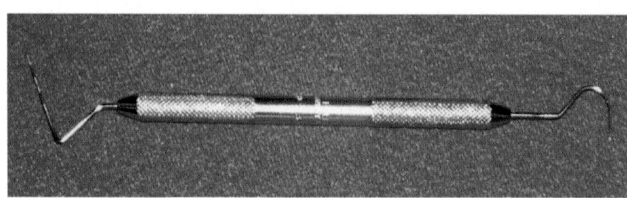

Figure 9 Instrument with periodontal probe on one end and number 23 explorer on the other end.

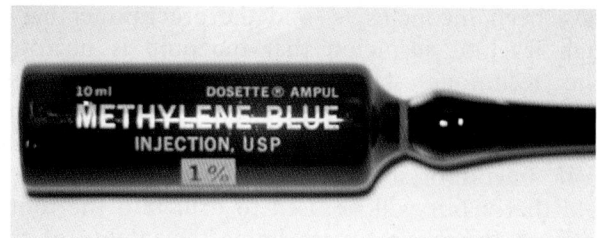

Figure 10 Methylene blue dye (Sullivan-Schein, Melville, NY).

determining whether a periodontal defect is of periodontal or endodontic origin. If the periodontal probe sinks abruptly into an isolated periodontal defect, the level of suspicion for a vertical root fracture (VRF) increases (see Chapter 19). Conversely, if the periodontal probe steps down into a periodontal defect, the level of suspicion of a generalized periodontal condition increases. This is particularly true if a similar situation exists on the contralateral side of the arch. If a VRF is suspected but cannot be visualized, with or without magnification, a dye can be used to help in identifying a crack. Methylene blue has also been used to stain cracks (Figures 10).

Although the presence of a furcation defect does not directly imply pulp necrosis, it is extremely important in the health or disease status of the tooth. Furcation canals have been reported to be a portal of exit for necrotic pulp tissue by-products and/or bacteria from a necrotic pulp into the adjacent periodontal ligament.[81] The following Glickman Classification System is commonly used[82]:

- Grade I: Incipient lesion when the pocket is suprabony involving soft tissue and there is slight bone loss.
- Grade II: Bone is destroyed on one or more aspects of the furcation but a probe can only penetrate partially into the furcation.
- Grade III: Intraradicular bone is completely absent but tissue covers the furcation.
- Grade IV: A through-and-through furcation defect.

The practitioner, using furcation probing as well as other endodontic diagnostic results, must also make a reasonable determination whether any furcation lesion is the result of periodontal disease, endodontic disease, or a true combined endodontic/periodontal lesion.

Test Cavity

A test cavity has been advocated for pulp vitality testing after all other diagnostic evaluation tests have been inconclusive, and the practitioner has a high level of suspicion that the pulp is necrotic. The technique starts with fully informing the patient of the exact procedure so there are no surprises because this procedure has the potential to be uncomfortable for the patient. The patient is told that a bur will be used to drill into the tooth without anesthesia to determine the vitality of the pulp tissue. Air water coolant should be used to avoid injury to a vital pulp. If the patient does not respond to the bur, once the dentin is exposed, the tooth can be tested with an EPT or a cold thermal test. A tooth with calcification producing pulpal obliteration may still not give clear test results. If the pulp is vital, the test cavity should be restored with a bonded restoration.

Anesthetic Test

When other appropriate diagnostic tests have been inconclusive, the anesthetic test may be performed by injection of local anesthetic into a painful area with an end toward making a diagnosis. Administration of the local anesthetic could be by block, infiltration, or intraosseous injection. A diagnostic block anesthetic test can be used effectively if the practitioner desires to evaluate the effects of anesthetizing large areas when a patient reports a vague location(s) for the pain. For example, a patient explains that the discomfort covers the entire left cheek and associated hard and soft structures. If a left inferior alveolar (IA) nerve block is successful and the pain remits, the practitioner can feel confident that the chief complaint is associated with pathosis within the distribution of the IA nerve (V3) and its branches. A second example is a patient who reports vague and intense pain in the mandibular left arch that contains teeth that are carious or have faulty restorations. After a successful IA nerve block, the intense pain does not remit but remains constant. This block anesthetic test may have identified the chief complaint as being a myocardial infarct, as there was no decrease in the pain after the nerve block. Cardiac pain may be referred to the left mandible and occasionally to the maxilla or the right mandible and can easily mimic pain of dental or orofacial origin.[27,28]

The infiltration anesthetic test may be used in an area suspected of being the source of the patient's chief complaint, and then waiting to see if the pain remits. It can be a useful test, particularly in the maxillary arch, in differentiating pain between the maxillary and mandibular arches. An example would be a patient who reports sharp and lingering pain to hot coffee on the left side of the face, but cannot narrow it down to either an individual tooth or even which arch. Thermal pulp tests are inconclusive, but the patient is now experiencing the same pain once again and cannot narrow the location to either arch. If the clinician believes the pain emanates from the posterior maxillary arch, he can inject local anesthetic in that area to see if the pain remits. If the pain remits, the practitioner can be reasonably sure the pain is due to pulpitis in the maxilla. If the pain does not remit, the practitioner may conclude that the pain source is in the mandibular arch and now administer a mandibular block with a reasonable assurance that the pain should abate. If after all the above have been accomplished and the pain does not abate, the practitioner may draw the conclusion that the pain is not of endodontic origin and refer the patient to the appropriate healthcare practitioner for further evaluation. The pain could be referred from the heart or the thyroid.

The PDL injection may be helpful in identifying a source of pulpally related pain. However, a common misperception is that the anesthetic remains in the PDL and does not diffuse into the surrounding bone and to adjacent teeth. Studies have shown that the PDL injection is an intraosseous injection with the local anesthetic passing into the surrounding cancellous bone and anesthetizing adjacent teeth.[83] Thus, PDL anesthetic provides the same type diagnostic information as the infiltration of anesthetic but on a more localized basis.

Magnification

Magnification allows the clinician to visualize what cannot be observed using only the unaided eye. Chapter 25F provides an extensive description of the use of aids in magnification in endodontics.

Dyes

Dyes can aid greatly in the diagnosis of either caries or fractures. Caries detector dyes have been used effectively to identify caries not otherwise evident with either visual inspection methods or traditional

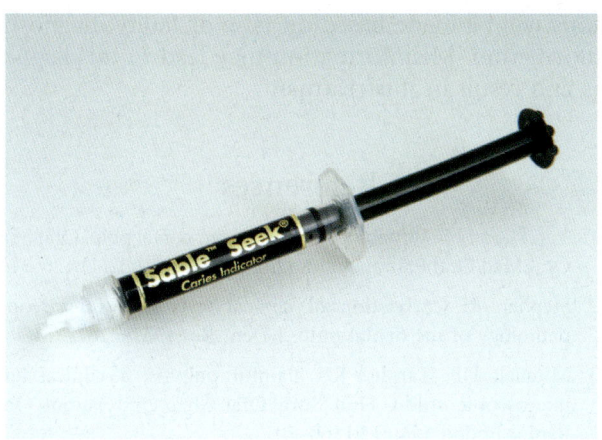

Figure 11 Caries indicator solutions can highlight tooth cracks; shown here is Sable-Seek (Ultradent, South Jordan, UT).

hand instruments (Figure 11).... Caries can contribute to the patient's chief complaint and perhaps require conservative pulp therapy. Methylene blue dye and India ink have been very effective dyes used to diagnose the presence of crown or root fractures (see Figure 10). A very small amount of the dye is placed on a small cotton pellet and the crown/root is coated with it. Any dye remaining on the surface is washed away and, if a fracture is present, the dye remains within the crack and can be observed through loupes or a dental operating microscope.

Measurement of Tooth Surface Temperatures

Even though not widely used, measurement of tooth surface temperatures could represent another testing technique. Fanibunda[84] reported that the pulp circulation was much more efficient than supporting tissue circulation in maintaining the temperature of the crown in vitro. His results indicate that measurement of crown surface temperatures may be a step in the right direction in determining whether vital tissue or necrotic tissue fills the pulp chamber. However, even the most sensitive temperature measurement device may not be able to distinguish whether a vital pulp is reversibly or irreversibly involved.

Cholesteric liquid crystals are a possible vehicle for measuring the surface temperature of a tooth. Howell et al.[85] experimented with various liquid crystals until they arrived at a combination that would indicate temperatures in 30° to 40°C range. They used cholesteric compounds that were in a 10% solution in a chlorinated hydrocarbon solvent. When applied to the tooth surface, the crystals went through color changes that were compared with adjacent or contralateral teeth. Although their reported results were equivocal, this diagnostic test might be helpful when taken into consideration with other diagnostic information.

Banes and Hammond[86] evaluated the ability of a thermistor to accurately measure the surface temperatures of teeth with vital pulps and contralateral teeth that had previously received NS RCT both with and without full gold crowns. They reported that the surface temperatures of the endodontically treated teeth without full gold crowns were statistically significantly lower than those of the contralateral teeth with vital pulps. There was no temperature difference, however, between those two groups when restored with full gold crowns. Stoops and Scott[87] used thermistors in vivo to determine the surface temperature of contralateral teeth and reported thermisters to be extremely consistent in recording the temperatures of teeth with both necrotic and vital pulps. They stated that there was a statistically significant difference between the surface temperatures recorded for teeth with vital pulps and those that were pulpless. They also reported that the thermistors, like any other sensitive temperature measuring devices, were affected by a small amount of saliva on the tooth or a current of air in the room.

Electronic thermography produces color images of the body that indicate relative differences in temperature in both superficial and deep areas. Components include an infrared sensor, control unit, thermal image computer, software, a color monitor, and printer. A review of the literature reports that current technology is not sensitive enough to identify periapical lesions deep within the bone that would indicate a necrotic pulp or irreversible pulpitis.[88]

The use of the Hughes Probeye 4300 thermal video system (Hughes Aircraft Co., Carlsbad, CA) was reported to be sensitive enough to measure temperature differences of as little as 0.1°C.[89] The authors conducted their investigation on 20 human subjects and measured the surface temperatures on maxillary incisor teeth after they had been isolated with a rubber dam. The teeth had a variety of restorations with some containing normal pulps and others containing necrotic pulps or prior root canal-filling materials. They reported no difference in the surface temperatures between those categories of teeth. However, when the teeth were cooled by air spray to approximately 22°C and then allowed to re-warm to their original resting temperature of approximately 29°C, the teeth containing normal pulps took about 5 seconds to re-warm whereas the others containing necrotic pulps or prior root canal-filling materials took about 15 seconds to re-warm. The investigators suggested that electronic thermography could be a useful adjunct to other pulp diagnostic tests if the prohibitive expense of the current system could be reduced and if an alternative could be found to the requirement for routine isolation of the effected teeth with a rubber dam.

Measurement of Pulpal Blood Flow

It is recognized that measuring pulpal blood flow can aid in determining pulpal healthy; to that end efforts using laser Doppler flowmetry and pulse oximetry are currently investigated (see Chapter 14C).

Ultraviolet Light

Some objects possess the unusual feature of being able to emit light of a higher wavelength when illuminated with ultraviolet (UV) light. That principle is called fluorescence. Foreman[90] reported that teeth with necrotic pulps and teeth with endodontic treatment did not fluoresce when exposed to UV light while teeth with vital pulps fluoresced normally. He cautioned that lighting in the operatory needed to be suppressed to fully observe any changes in the tooth color. Moreover, the patient and staff need to wear suitable goggles to protect them from the harmful effects of UV light on their eyes.

Patient Temperature

The importance of obtaining a baseline temperature as well as follow-on readings at subsequent appointments cannot be underestimated. Patients frequently state they do not have a fever when, in fact, they have not taken their temperature before they came in for the evaluation appointment. A temperature over 100°F indicates a systemic response to an infection. Having a baseline temperature gives the clinician one more diagnostic tool that can be used to determine whether the patient's condition is either improving or worsening.

Communication with other practitioners must employ an objective and understandable language so the facts can be conveyed clearly about a patient's current condition. Otherwise, poor treatment decisions will be made based on false or faulty diagnostic information. Misinformation may lead to misdiagnosis and result in mistreatment.

References

1. Van Hassel HJ. Physiology of the human dental pulp. Oral Surg Oral Med Oral Pathol Oral Radiol Endod 1971;32(1):126–34.
2. Stephen R. Correlation of clinical tests with microscopic pathology of the dental pulp. J Dent Res 1937;6:267–78.
3. Mitchell DF, Tarplee RE. Painful pulpitis; a clinical and microscopic study. Oral Surg Oral Med Oral Pathol Oral Radiol Endod 1960;13:1360–70.
4. Seltzer S, Bender IB, Ziontz M. The dynamics of pulp inflammation: correlations between diagnostic data and actual histologic findings in the pulp. Part I. Oral Surg Oral Med Oral Pathol Oral Radiol Endod 1963;16:846–71.
5. Seltzer S, Bender IB, Ziontz M. The dynamics of pulp inflammation: correlations between diagnostic data and actual histologic findings in the pulp. Part II. Oral Surg Oral Med Oral Pathol Oral Radiol Endod 1963;16:969–77.
6. Johnson RH, Dachi SF, Haley JV. Pulpal hyperemia–a correlation of clinical and histologic data from 706 teeth. J Am Dent Assoc 1970;81(1):108–17.
7. Garfunkel A, Sela J, Ulmansky M. Dental pulp pathosis. Clinicopathologic correlations based on 109 cases. Oral Surg Oral Med Oral Pathol Oral Radiol Endod 1973;35(1):110–17.
8. Bhaskar SN, Rappaport HM. Dental vitality tests and pulp status. J Am Dent Assoc 1973;86(2):409–11.
9. Hyman JJ, Cohen ME. The predictive value of endodontic diagnostic tests. Oral Surg Oral Med Oral Pathol Oral Radiol Endod 1984;58(3):343–6.
10. Herbert W. A correlation between nervous accommodation, symptomatology and histological condition of the pulps of 52 teeth. Brit Dent J 1945;78:161–73.
11. Kulild JC, Weller RN. Endodontic diagnostic dilemmas. Med Bulletin 1988;PB-8–88:50–3.
12. Keir DM, Walker WA III Schindler WG, Dazey SE. Thermally induced pulpalgia in endodontically treated teeth. J Endod 1991;17(1):38–40.
13. Ardekian L, Peleg M, Samet N, et al. Burkitt's lymphoma mimicking an acute dentoalveolar abscess. J Endod 1996;22(12):697–8.
14. Bellizzi R, Drobotij E, Keller D, Kenevan R. Sinusitis secondary to pregnancy rhinitis, mimicking pain of endodontic origin: a case report. J Endod 1983;9(2):60–4.
15. Chelm-Berger D, Gutmann JL. Focal myositis mimicking posttreatment pain of periradicular origin. J Endod 1986;12(3):119–23.
16. Glickman GN. Central giant cell granuloma associated with a non-vital tooth: a case report. Int Endod J 1988;21(3):224–30.

17. Guttenberg SA, Emery RW, Milobsky SA, Geballa M. Cranial arteritis mimicking odontogenic pain: report of case. J Am Dent Assoc 1989;119(5):621–3.
18. Harris WE. Endodontic pain referred across the midline: report of case. J Am Dent Assoc 1973;87(6):1240–3.
19. Keller EE, Gunderson LL. Bone disease metastatic to the jaws. J Am Dent Assoc 1987;115(5):697–701.
20. Merrill RL, Graff-Radford SB. Trigeminal neuralgia: how to rule out the wrong treatment. J Am Dent Assoc 1992;123(2):63–8.
21. Orsini G, Fioroni M, Rubini C, Piattelli A. Hemangioma of the mandible presenting as a periapical radiolucency. J Endod 2000;26(10):621–2.
22. Roz TM, Schiffman LE, Schlossberg S. Spontaneous dissection of the internal carotid artery manifesting as pain in an endodontically treated molar. J Am Dent Assoc 2005;136(11):1556–9.
23. Selden HS. The interrelationship between the maxillary sinus and endodontics. Oral Surg 1974;38:623–9.
24. Selden HS, Manhoff DT, Hatges NA, Michel RC. Metastatic carcinoma to the mandible that mimicked pulpal/periodontal disease. J Endod 1998;24(4):267–70.
25. Senia ES, Cunningham KW, Marx RE. The diagnostic dilemma of barodontalgia. Report of two cases. Oral Surg Oral Med Oral Pathol Oral Radiol Endod 1985;60(2):212–17.
26. Croll TP, Brooks EB, Schut L, Laurent JP. Rapid neurologic assessment and initial management for the patient with traumatic dental injuries. J Am Dent Assoc 1980;100(4):530–4.
27. Natkin E, Harrington GW, Mandel MA. Anginal pain referred to the teeth. Report of a case. Oral Surg Oral Med Oral Pathol Oral Radiol Endod 1975;40(5):678–80.
28. Batchelder BJ, Krutchkoff DJ, Amara J. Mandibular pain as the initial and sole clinical manifestation of coronary insufficiency: report of case. J Am Dent Assoc 1987;115(5):710–12.
29. Reiss H, Furedi A. Significance of the pulp test as revealed in a microscopic study of the pulp of 130 teeth. Dental Cosmos 1933;75:272–81.
30. Mullaney TP, Howell RM, Petrich JD. Resistance of nerve fibers to pulpal necrosis. Oral Surg Oral Med Oral Pathol Oral Radiol Endod 1970;30(5):690–3.
31. England MC, Pellis EG, Michanowicz AE. Histopathologic study of the effect of pulpal disease upon nerve fibers of the human dental pulp. Oral Surg Oral Med Oral Pathol Oral Radiol Endod 1974;38(5):783–90.
32. Peters DD, Baumgartner JC, Lorton L. Adult pulpal diagnosis I. evaluation of the positive and negative responses to cold and electrical pulp tests. J Endod 1994;20(10):506–11.
33. Hargreaves, KM. Glossary contemporary terminology for endodontics. Chicago, Il: American Association of Endodontists; 2003.
34. Seltzer S, Bender IB, Nazimov H. Differential diagnosis of pulp conditions. Oral Surg Oral Med Oral Pathol Oral Radiol Endod 1965;19:383–91.
35. White JH, Cooley RL. A quantitative evaluation of thermal pulp testing. J Endod 1977;3:453–7.
36. Fuss Z, Trowbridge H, Bender IB, et al. Assessment of reliability of electrical and thermal pulp testing agents. J Endod 1986;12(7):301–5.
37. Jones DM. Effect of the type carrier used on the results of dichlorodifluoromethane application to teeth. J Endod 1999;25(10):692–4.
38. Jones VR, Rivera EM, Walton RE. Comparison of carbon dioxide versus refrigerant spray to determine pulpal responsiveness. J Endod 2002;28(7):531–3.
39. Miller SO, Johnson JD, Allemang JD, Strother JM. Cold testing through full-coverage restorations. J Endod 2004;30(10):695–700.
40. Ehrmann EH. Pulp testers and pulp testing with particular reference to the use of dry ice. Aust Dent J 1977;22(4):272–9.
41. Augsburger RA, Peters DD. In vitro effects of ice, skin refrigerant, and CO2 snow on intrapulpal temperature. J Endod 1981;7(3):110–16.
42. Peters DD, Lorton L, Mader CL, et al. Evaluation of the effects of carbon dioxide used as a pulpal test. 1. In vitro effect on human enamel. J Endod 1983;9(6):219–27.
43. Ingram TA, Peters DD. Evaluation of the effects of carbon dioxide used as a pulpal test. Part 2. In vivo effect on canine enamel and pulpal tissues. J Endod 1983;9(7):296–303.
44. Peters DD, Mader CL, Donnelly JC. Evaluation of the effects of carbon dioxide used as a pulpal test. 3. In vivo effect on human enamel. J Endod 1986;12(1):13–20.
45. Rickoff B, Trowbridge H, Baker J, et al. Effects of thermal vitality tests on human dental pulp. J Endod 1988;14(10):482–5.
46. Selden HS. Diagnostic thermal pulp testing: a technique. J Endod 2000;26(10):623–4.
47. Myers JW. Demonstration of a possible source of error with an electric pulp tester. J Endod 1998;24(3):199–200.
48. Reynolds R. The determination of pulp vitality by means of thermal and electrical stimuli. Oral Surg 1966;22:231–40.
49. Chilton NW, Fertig JW. Pulpal responses of bilateral intact teeth. Oral Surg Oral Med Oral Pathol Oral Radiol Endod 1972;33(5):797–800.
50. Jacobson JJ. Probe placement during electric pulp-testing procedures. Oral Surg Oral Med Oral Pathol Oral Radiol Endod 1984;58(2):242–7.
51. Bender IB, Landau MA, Fonsecca S, Trowbridge HO. The optimum placement-site of the electrode in electric pulp testing of the 12 anterior teeth. J Am Dent Assoc 1989;118(3):305–10.
52. Van Hassel HJ, Harrington GW. Localization of pulpal sensation. Oral Surg Oral Med Oral Pathol Oral Radiol Endod 1969;28(5):753–60.
53. Tousey C. The faradic current in dental diagnosis. Dent Cosmos 1909;LI:513–22.

54. Taylor PP. The evaluation and use of the high frequency vitalometer. Oral Surg Oral Med Oral Pathol Oral Radiol Endod 1953;6(8):1020–4.

55. Mumford J. Path of direct current in electric pulp-testing. Brit Dent J 1959:23–6.

56. Fulling HJ, Andreasen JO. Influence of maturation status and tooth type of permanent teeth upon electrometric and thermal pulp testing. Scand J Dent Res 1976;84(5):286–90.

57. Cooley RL, Stilley J, Lubow RM. Evaluation of a digital pulp tester. Oral Surg Oral Med Oral Pathol Oral Radiol Endod 1984;58(4):437–42.

58. Kitamura T, Takahashi T, Horiuchi H. Electrical characteristics and clinical application of a new automatic pulp tester. Quint Int 1983;1:45–53.

59. Abdel Wahab MH, Kennedy JG. The effect of rate of increase of electrical current on the sensation thresholds of teeth. J Dent Res 1987;66(3):799–801.

60. Martin H, Ferris C, Mazzella W. An evaluaion of media used in electric pulp testing. Oral Surg Oral Med Oral Pathol Oral Radiol Endod 1969;27(3):374–8.

61. Michaelson RE, Seidberg BH, Guttuso J. An in vivo evaluation of interface media used with the electric pulp tester. J Am Dent Assoc 1975;91(1):118–21.

62. Anderson RW, Pantera EA Jr. Influence of a barrier technique on electric pulp testing. J Endod 1988;14(4):179–80.

63. Cailleteau JG, Ludington JR. Using the electric pulp tester with gloves: a simplified approach. J Endod 1989;15(2):80–1.

64. Pantera EA Jr, Anderson RW, Pantera CT. Use of dental instruments for bridging during electric pulp testing. J Endod 1992;18(1):37–8.

65. Woolley LH, Woodworth J, Dobbs JL. A preliminary evaluation of the effects of electrical pulp testers on dogs with artificial pacemakers. J Am Dent Assoc 1974;89(5):1099–101.

66. Simon AB, Linde B, Bonnette GH, Schlentz RJ. The individual with a pacemaker in the dental environment. J Am Dent Assoc 1975;91(6):1224–9.

67. Wilson BL, Broberg C, Baumgartner JC, et al. Safety of electronic apex locators and pulp testers in patients with implanted cardiac pacemakers or cardioverter/defibrillators. J Endod 2006;32(9):847–52.

68. Weisman MI. The use of a calibrated percussion instrument in pulpal and periapical diagnosis. Oral Surg Oral Med Oral Pathol Oral Radiol Endod 1984;57(3):320–2.

69. Miller S. Textbook of peridontics. 3rd. ed. Blackstone; 1950:125.

70. Cameron W. Diagnosis by transillumination. Cameron's Publishing Co.; 1927.

71. Friedman J, Marcus MI. Transillumination of the oral cavity with use of fiber optics. J Am Dent Assoc 1970;80(4):801–9.

72. Liewehr FR. An inexpensive device for transillumination. J Endod 2001;27(2):130–1.

73. Cameron CE. Cracked-tooth syndrome. J Am Dent Assoc 1964;68:405–11.

74. Ritchey B, Mendenhall R, Orban B. Pulpitis resulting from incomplete tooth fracture. Oral Surg Oral Med Oral Pathol Oral Radiol Endod 1957;10(6):665–70.

75. Ehrmann EH, Tyas MJ. Cracked tooth syndrome: diagnosis, treatment and correlation between symptoms and post-extraction findings. Aust Dent J 1990;35(2):105–12.

76. Sutton P. Greenstick fracture of the toothe crown. Brit Dent J 1962;112:362–3.

77. Turp JC, Gobetti JP. The cracked tooth syndrome: an elusive diagnosis. J Am Dent Assoc 1996;127(10):1502–7.

78. Hill CM. The efficacy of transillumination in vitality tests. Int Endod J 1986;19(4):198–201.

79. Simon JH, Glick DH, Frank AL. The relationship of endodontic-periodontic lesions. J Periodontol 1972;43(4):202–8.

80. Harrington GW. The perio-endo question: differential diagnosis. Dent Clin North Am 1979;23(4):673–90.

81. Gutmann JL. Prevalence, location, and patency of accessory canals in the furcation region of permanent molars. J Periodontol 1978;49(1):21–6.

82. Carranza F. Glickman's clinical periodontology. 7th ed. Philadelphia: W. B. Saunders; 1990. p. 860.

83. Walton RE. Distribution of solutions with the periodontal ligament injection: clinical, anatomical, and histological evidence. J Endod 1986;12(10):492–500.

84. Fanibunda KB. A laboratory study to investigate the differentiation of pulp vitality in human teeth by temperature measurement. J Dent 1985;13(4):295–303.

85. Howell RM, Duell RC, Mullaney TP. The determination of pulp vitality by thermographic means using cholesteric liquid crystals. A preliminary study. Oral Surg Oral Med Oral Pathol Oral Radiol Endod 1970;29(5):763–8.

86. Banes JD, Hammond HL. Surface temperatures of vital and nonvital teeth in humans. J Endod 1978;4(4):106–9.

87. Stoops LC, Scott D Jr. Measurement of tooth temperature as a means of determing pulp vitality. J Endod 1976;2(5):141–5.

88. Gratt BM, Sickles EA. Future applications of electronic thermography. J Am Dent Assoc 1991;122(5):28–36.

89. Pogrel MA, Yen CK, Taylor RC. Studies in tooth crown temperature gradients with the use of infrared thermography. Oral Surg Oral Med Oral Pathol Oral Radiol Endod 1989;67(5):583–7.

90. Foreman PC. Ultraviolet light as an aid to endodontic diagnosis. Int Endod J 1983;16(3):121–6.

C. Laser Doppler Flowmetry

Asgeir Sigurdsson

Having information about the blood flow, or re-establishment of circulation, in the pulp can be of great value, particularly in situations in which teeth have been traumatized. All traumas to developing teeth have the potential to cause irreversible damage that ultimately may lead to pulpal necrosis. In many situations, there is the possibility of revascularization of the injured pulp, a development that is most desirable for the continued development of the tooth. The risk in waiting for revascularization is that bacteria may enter the damaged pulp leading to inflammatory root resorption.[1] However, if the endodontic treatment is initiated while blood vessels are attempting to re-grow through the apical opening, healing of the pulp is arrested and there is no further growth or development of the root structure. It is therefore very desirable to have a reliable method for assessing blood flow in the pulp.

The usual diagnostic instruments like the electric pulp tester (EPT) and various temperature tests have been shown to be not at all reliable in diagnosing the pulpal status of teeth following a traumatic injury, especially for teeth with immature root formation and open apex.[2-5] Compounding the problem with these testing methods is that they all are very subjective, dependent on cooperation and understanding of the situation by the patient, something which can lead to further difficulty in cases involving young children. It is important to note that the usual pulp tests provide information only about the presence or absence of nerve receptors in the pulp and not about pulpal blood supply.

Current efforts to assess pulpal circulation involve the use of laser Doppler flowmetry (LDF) and pulse oximetry. Both methods are in their infancy and are not ready for general clinical application yet, but hopefully before long, these technologies can become part of dentists' diagnostic armamentaria.

Technology

DEVELOPMENT AND PRINCIPLE OF THE LDF TECHNOLOGY

Laser Doppler Flowmetry (LDF) was first introduced in the early 1970s. Initially, it was suggested for use in measuring blood flow in the retina.[6] Soon, other applications for this technology were suggested, such as measuring blood flow in skin and in renal cortex.[6] The technology employs a beam of infrared (780 to 820 nm) or near infrared (632.8 nm) light, directed into the tissue by optical fibers. As light enters tissue, it is scattered by stationary tissue cells and moving blood cells (Figure 1).

Photons that hit stationary tissue cells are scattered, but their frequency is not shifted. Photons that hit moving blood cells are scattered, and the light frequency is shifted according to the Doppler principle. A small proportion of the light, containing both Doppler-shifted and transmitted light, is backscattered to a photodetector (or more commonly, in newer instruments, to two or more photodetectors) built into the probe from which the laser light is beamed. A signal is then calculated with a preset algorithm in the LDF machine (Figure 2A,B).

Because red blood cells represent the vast majority of objects moving within a tooth, measurement of the Doppler-shifted backscattered light from them could give an indication of pulpal blood flow. The outcome signal depends on the number and velocity of the illuminated red blood cells, most commonly termed flux; that is the number of moving red cells per second times their mean velocities. Most current laser Doppler instruments give a readout, in addition to the flux, in perfusion units (PUs). It is important to remember that these PUs are arbitrary and calculated by the software that accompanies each instrument. No current Laser

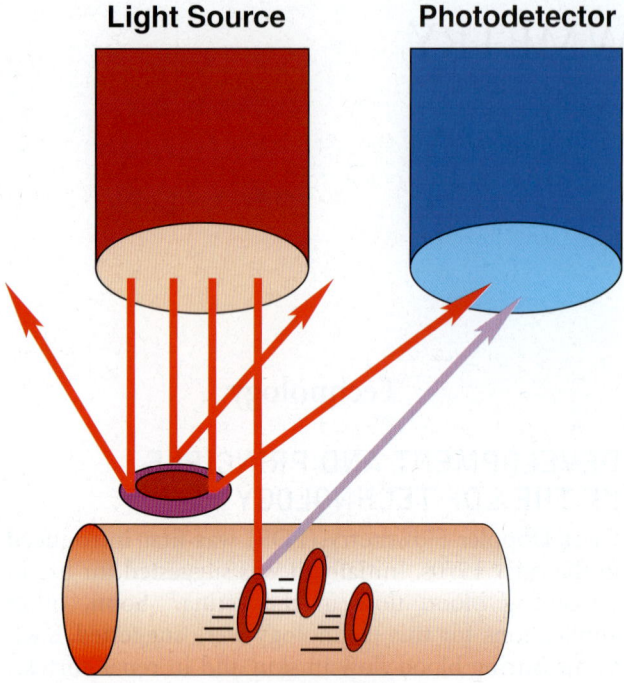

Figure 1 Red light is emitted from a light source; if the light beam is scattered off stationary tissue or cells, there is no shift in the light spectrum. If, however, the light hits a moving cell in a blood vessel, there is a shift in the light spectrum of the scattered light according to the Doppler principle.

Doppler instrument can present absolute perfusion values of blood flow (e.g., mL/min/100 gram tissue). Because of this, the PUs are never comparable between various types of instruments, and even for the same instrument they could vary at different times unless the instrument is calibrated frequently using special suspensions of particles in liquid that have a known inherent vibration.

Initially, there was some concern that the power of the laser light would be hazardous to living tissues and could possibly burn or cause other permanent damage. That fear has been shown to be unfounded as the laser light in all currently used medial instruments is far below the maximum limit permitted for clinical applications and temperature changes in the illuminated tissue.[7]

For many LDF instruments, it can be difficult to objectively analyze the output of the instrument. Therefore, earlier, it was suggested to use the so-called Fast Fourier Transform (FFT) analysis associated with the LDF measurements.[8] Subsequently, numerous studies have confirmed its usefulness in evaluating blood flow in soft tissues. This analysis identifies the presence of consistency of time between peaks in pulses. For example, a peak at or around 1.3 Hz, which is equivalent to approximately 78 heartbeats per minute, would give an indication of vitality in a tooth pulp (Figure 3A–C).

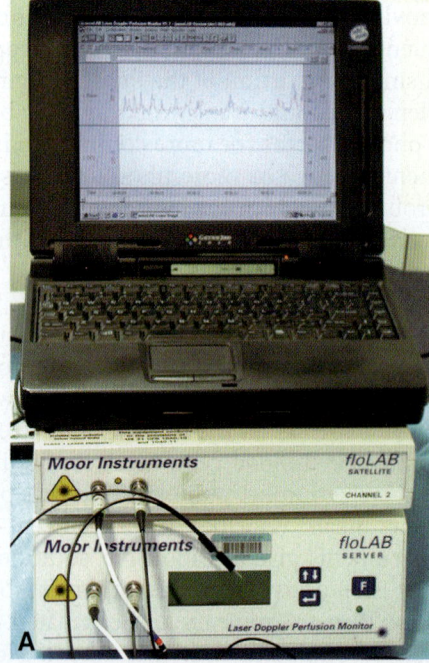
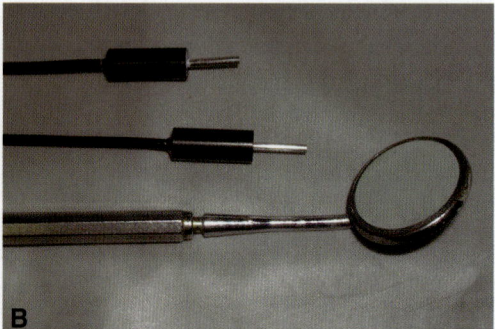

Figure 2 ***A***, Example of a laser Doppler setup. The machine is from Moor Instruments Ltd, Devon, UK and has two sets of probes, so it is possible to record two different sites or two teeth simultaneously. ***B***, The two probes from the Moor laser Doppler flow meter. Note that for practical purposes a one-probe machine is sufficient for most clinical applications.

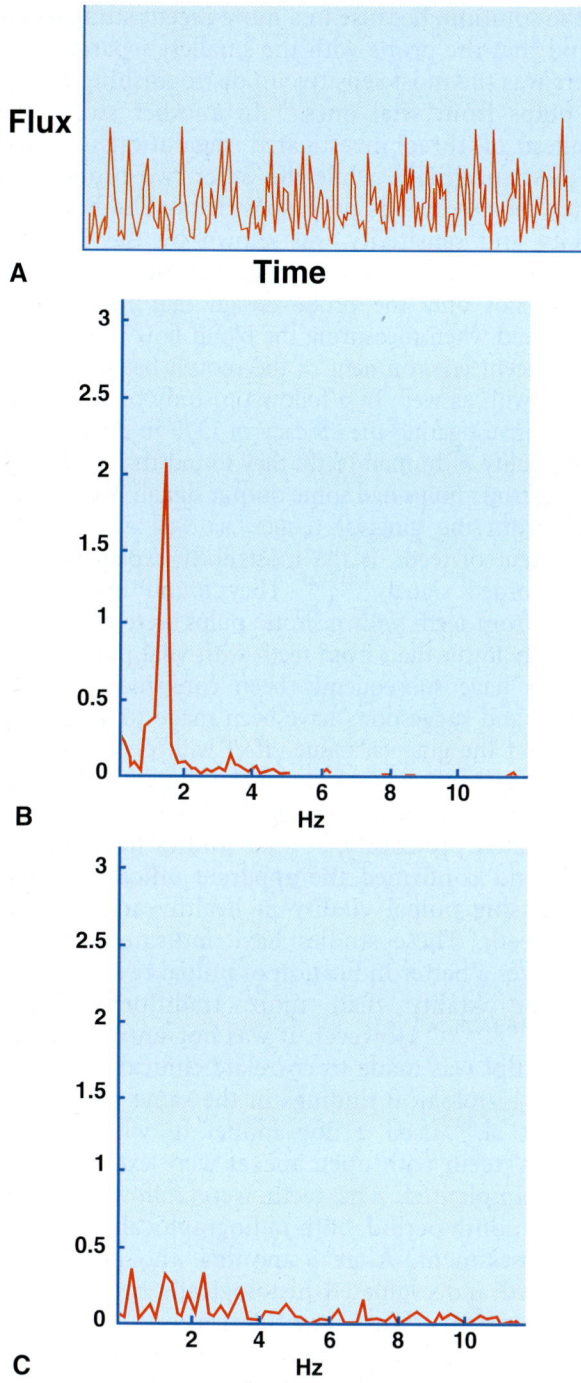

Figure 3 ***A***, A typical readout of a laser Doppler machine. Even though there are several spikes, it is hard to determine if those represent heartbeats or just movement artifacts. ***B***, When the readout in panel A is analyzed by Fast Fourier Transform analysis, it is clear that there is a constant amplitude spike of about 1.3 Hz or about 78 beats per minute indicating blood circulation in the pulp. ***C***, A readout from a different tooth and analyzed by Fast Fourier Transform analysis indicates no vitality. There is no consistent amplitude spike and therefore the pulp is deemed to be necrotic.

To date, only few investigations of pulpal vitality have been done with the FFT analytical approach.[9,10] A recent study investigating revascularization of tooth pulp in a dog model applied this analysis to readings from teeth with vital pups. A peak appeared at or around 2 Hz, that is, at around 120 beats per minute of the dog's heart rate. When readings from teeth with non-vital pulps were analyzed, this dominant peak was absent. This method of analysis thereby established that the pulsatile reading is of similar frequency to the heart rate and is due to blood flow rather than of movement artifacts.[10] It was of interest to note that the investigators found that two teeth had been classified as having non-vital pulps based on a net flux value of only 18% of the pre-extraction flux, a reading that indicated a very low if not absent blood flow. But the FFT analysis indicated that both teeth had the typical peak of 2 Hz, indicating vitality of the pulps. Based on the FFT analysis, the teeth were correctly categorized as having vital pulps. Histological evaluation later confirmed that revascularization had occurred in both teeth. Based on their experience, the authors suggested that FFT analysis might prove a more feasible method than net flux calculation if this method is to be used in dentistry.[10] However, further research is warranted because only a few studies have used this analytical method in dental application of the LDF.

Initial Suggestions for Dentistry

The first study showing that LDF could differentiate between vital and non-vital pulps in humans was published in 1986 by Gazelius et al.[11] They confirmed in five human subjects that there was a correlation between their heart rates as measured by electrocardiograms and peaks of flow measured in healthy and responsive maxillary central incisors. In addition, they showed that local injection of lidocaine (20 mg/mL) with adrenaline (12.5 mg/mL) caused a pronounced and long-lasting reduction of the flowmetric values in the same pulps. In this initial report on use of LDF in dentistry, the authors also mentioned, but did not investigate any further, the fact that a tooth with history of trauma and that did not respond to traditional vitality tests also did not show typical flow characteristics of a healthy pulp.

Two years later, Gazelius et al.[12] reported a case history on four luxated mandibular incisors in an 11-year-old boy in which the LDF showed no flux 1 week after the traumatic injury. After 6 weeks, however, the LDF indicated partial restoration of the blood flow in the pulps, and 9 months later the blood flow appeared normal. The same teeth were not responsive to EPT until 9 months to a year after the trauma.

Subsequently, there have been several studies investigating the accuracy and, more importantly, the usefulness of the LDF technology in dentistry. One of the first studies to confirm that it was actually blood flow that was being measured in the pulp with the LDF was by Kim et al. in 1990.[13] In a dog model study, they compared blood flow measurements, gathered by LDF, to data from a 133Xe washout method that enables the researcher to accurately calculate blood flow in real time. However, this requires injection of 133Xe into the blood stream close to the tissue of interest. All measurements were done on the same teeth and conducted at the same time. During the experiment, they used an intra-arterial injection of norepinephrine to affect the blood flow to the pulps. They found a significant correlation between the two measurement approaches, and both followed the expected effect of the norepinephrine on the blood flow.

All these findings are promising; however, it was pointed out, earlier, that the position of the probe on the tooth crown had a significant effect on pulpal blood flow estimates. For example, measurements recorded have not been consistent across all the testing sessions.[14] It has been suggested, therefore, that to achieve reliable and comparable readings at different times, an accurate repositioning of the light probe each time is mandatory. Custom-made stents have been found to ensure accurate and reproducible positioning of the measurement probe at each session.[14]

Another question that surfaced is with regard to the applicability of LDF technology for dental situations. As mentioned above, the initial use of LDF was exclusively for direct soft tissue blood flow measurements, without any interference of hard tissue like dentin and enamel. All the engineering of light sources and photodetectors was designed with that in mind. It first had to be confirmed that the commercially available machines could be used in clinical settings in dentistry. A study published in 1993 by Ingolfsson et al.[15] reported an investigation on the influence of probe design on the LDF signal output from the dental pulp. Recordings were made from anterior teeth in humans with different probe designs. All tested instruments had in common one light source and two photodetectors, the variable was the distance between the photodetectors. They found that the probe with the largest separation of the fibers produced significantly higher output than the other probes.[15] This observation may not, however, be the solution, because in a more recent study it was found that the probe with the smallest separation of fibers was the most sensitive in distinguishing necrotic pulps from vital ones.[16] In another study, the smallest of three investigated separations showed the best specificity, while the other two probes had better sensitivity but poor specificity. The best specificity and sensitivity was shown by the 0.5 mm probe/3.1 KHz bandwidth combination.[9]

It is not only the probe design that needs to be considered when measuring the blood flow in the pulp; the adjacent environment of the mouth has to be contended with as well. In a follow-up study by Ingolfsson et al.[17] investigating the efficacy of LDF in determining pulp vitality of human teeth, they found that even teeth with necrotic pulps had some output signal. Background noise from the gingival tissues, as well as from the movement of teeth, is the most likely explanation for the recorded signals.[14,17–21] They found that output signals from teeth with necrotic pulps were always significantly lower than from teeth with vital pulps. These findings have subsequently been confirmed in other studies, and suggestions have been made to attempt to block out the gingival tissue effect with dental dam or aluminum foil covering the gingival tissues prior to placement of the custom-made stent (Figure 4A).[18,20,22]

As stated previously, several studies have investigated and confirmed the apparent efficacy of LDF in assessing pulpal vitality in healthy and traumatized teeth. These studies have indicated that the LDF gives a better indication of pulpal revascularization or vitality than more traditional vitality tests.[11,16,18,23,24] However, it was not until 2001 that an attempt was made to correlate clinical LDF findings to histological findings in the same teeth. Yanpiset et al.[10] used a dog model in which young puppies' teeth with open apexes were extracted and then reimplanted. The teeth were followed weekly over 3-month period, both radiographically and with LDF assessment. After 3 months, the pulps were harvested and evaluated histologically by "blinded" evaluators for signs revascularization. This study confirmed previous findings that the LDF technology was very effective in determining revascularization or lack thereof. LDF readings correctly predicted the pulpal status (vital vs non-vital) in 83.7% of the teeth; 73.9% (17 of 23) were correct for the vital pulps and 95% (19 of 20) were correct for the non-vital pulps. It was of interest that in this dog model the flux value increased significantly from week 2 to week 4 in the revascularizing pulps indicating that the LDF could provide information about healing progress in the pulps earlier.

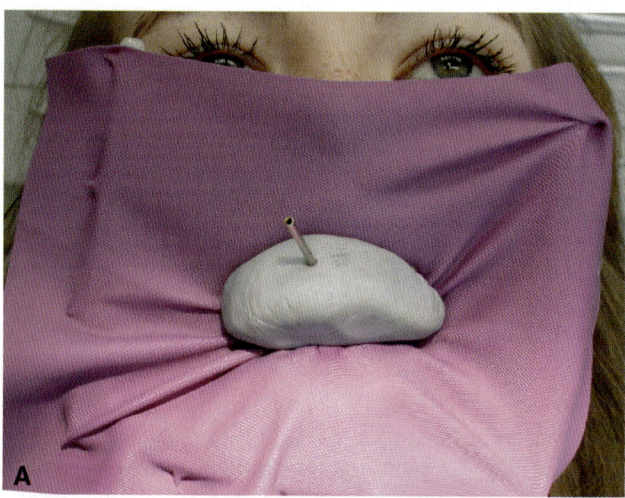 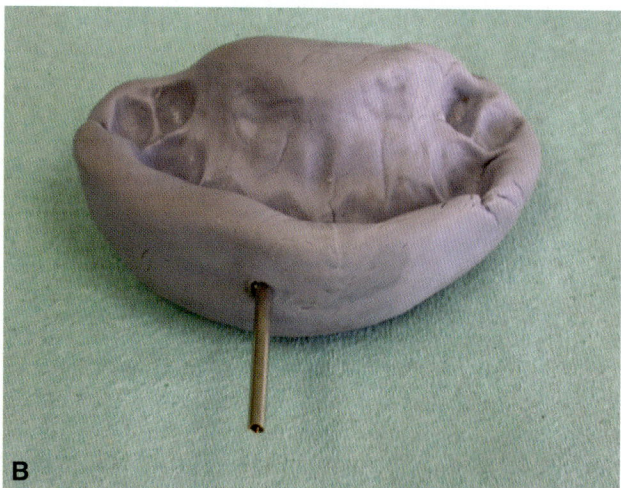

Figure 4 ***A***, When recording a traumatized tooth pulp, effort must be taken to block out as much as possible of the gingiva and other soft tissues immediately surrounding the tooth. It is recommended to use a dental dam as opaque as possible. In this figure, a vinyl (non latex) dental dam is used. ***B***, An individual bite stent is made for every patient. By using heavy dental impression putty the stent can be made quickly and inexpensively. To ensure consistency in measurements, a hollow cylinder is placed into the putty through which the laser Doppler probe is placed. That way, the same area of the tooth can be measured each time, and it is easier to control for needed spacing from the gingiva.

Current Applications of LDF in Dentistry

CLINICAL DENTISTRY

It appears that the LDF technology has a future in clinical dentistry. It is, if properly conducted, an objective way to assess pulpal blood flow. Tests like EPT and temperature stimulation rely on subjective responses by the patient and only measure the neurological status of the pulp, not the vitality. Additionally, the LDF technology has also been shown to work in primary incisors. In a clinical study, it was shown that the LDF readings were different for primary incisor teeth prior to pulpotomy or extraction compared to the same teeth at an earlier time.[25]

There are some recognized drawbacks with the current application of the LDF technology in dentistry. Apart from the initial high setup cost, the other drawbacks can be fairly easily overcome. The main issue is ensuring consistent and accurate reading of the LDF assessment over time. To be able to obtain accuracy and consistency, certain critical steps needs to be taken. First, because of the sensitivity to movement, it is not possible to hold the probe manually against a crown surface. A stabilizing stent, most easily made out of rubber impression material, needs to be fabricated individually for each patient (see Figure 4A,B). This will not only reduce the artificial movements that might be picked up by the photodetectors but also ensure that the tooth is always tested on the same part of the crown. Prior to placing the stent, the gingiva should be covered with a dark dental dam or aluminum foil. Additionally, the patient should be in a similar, if not identical, position in the dental chair each time while the recording is done, as body position might affect the reading.[26] With commercially available equipment and computer technology storing and comparing the recorded data should not be any obstacle for using this technology.

DENTAL TRAUMA

The use of LDF in dental trauma has proven to be even more valuable than in assessing vitality in healthy pulps.[27–29] The LDF test can, for example, be a useful diagnostic adjunct for luxated teeth showing signs of adverse outcomes. In a series of studies, it was suggested that a predictive modeling may provide opportunity to identify "at-risk" teeth early after the trauma. Treatment, therefore, could be initiated with confidence prior to the tooth being lost from pulpal necrosis and infection.[30–32] There is also a good indication, in case of avulsion, the LDF can detect revascularization after a few weeks, and well in advance of other more traditional clinical tests.[10,27]

Other Potential Modalities

Pulse oximetry is routinely used in medicine to assess blood oxygen saturation. This technology uses a noninvasive and objective way to record the oxygen saturation, and, as with the laser Doppler technology, it requires no subjective response from the patient. This technology is based on the principles of spectrophotometry and optical plethysmography[33] rather than the law of light frequency shift in LDF technology. The machinery consists of a light source probe that emits simultaneously two light beams; one transmits red light (640 nm) and the other transmits infrared light (940 nm). The light has to pass through the tissue of interest and a photodetector on the opposite side to the light source captures whatever light gets through. Oxygenated hemoglobin and deoxygenated hemoglobin absorb different amounts of red and infrared light. After the light from the probe has passed through living tissue with circulating blood, the machine calculates how much light has been absorbed and then calculates the ratio of the two lights. The output is in percentages of oxygenated arterial blood.

Over the years, pulse oximetry has been suggested and tested for use in dentistry with reasonable good results.[34] However, all that work has been done using testing machines designed to be used on earlobes or fingers but not teeth. Some authors have concluded that the accuracy of these commercial instruments, adapted for dental use, has been disappointing and they did not have predictable diagnostic value.[35] Recently, a study was published that used a custom-made probe specifically made for dental application.[33] In that study, the accuracy rate of detecting vital and non-vital pulp was found to be 86% for the cold test, 81% for the electrical test, and 97.5% for the pulse oximetry test, indicating that this approach is more accurate than more traditional methods. The custom-made probe is, as of yet, not commercially available, but when it is, it should be considered as an important adjunct to pulpal evaluation.

Future Suggestions for Use and Development

Early research has indicated that there are no differences between various LDF machines.[24,27] However, no recent work has been published on this matter. With the fast developments in computer technology and equipment, vigilance must be kept and new and supposedly improved machines need to be tested and compared. There are still some questions about the probe design, the effect of different wavelength, frequency, and intensity of the laser light not fully answered for dental application of this technology. And algorithms like FFT analysis should be investigated further and confirmed for use in dentistry.

References

1. Tronstad L. Root resorption-etiology, terminology, and clinical manifestations. Endod Dent Traumatol 1988;4:241.
2. Pileggi R, Dumsha TC, Myslinski NR. The reliability of the electric pulp test after concussion injury. Endod Dent Traumatol 1996;12:16–19.
3. Andreasen JO, Ravn, JJ. Epidemiology of traumatic dental injuries to primary and permanent teeth in a Danish population sample. Int J Oral Surg 1972;1:235.
4. Fuss Z, Trowbridge H, Bender IB, et al. Assessment of reliability of electrical and thermal pulp testing agents. J Endod 1986;12:301–5.
5. Fulling HJ, Andreasen JO. Influence of maturation status and tooth type of permanent teeth upon electrometric and thermal pulp testing procedures. Scand J Dent Res 1976;84:286–90.
6. Holloway GA, Watkins DW. Laser Doppler measurement of cutaneous blood flow. J Invest Dermatol 1977;69:306–12.
7. Tozer BA. The calculation of maximum permissible exposure levels for laser radiation. J Pliys E Sci Instium 1979;12:922–6.
8. Histand MB, Daigle R, Miller CW, McLeod F. Proceedings: Evaluation of the pulsed Doppler with a Fast Fourier Transform. Biomed Sci Instrum 1974;10:61–6.
9. Odor TM, Ford TR, McDonald F. Effect of probe design and bandwidth on laser Doppler readings from vital and root-filled teeth. Med Eng Phys 1996;18:359–64.
10. Yanpiset K, Vongsavan N, Sigurdsson A, Trope M. Efficacy of laser Doppler flowmetry for the diagnosis of revascularization of reimplanted immature dog teeth Dental Traumatol 2001;17:63–70.
11. Gazelius B, Olgart L, Edwall B, Edwall L. Non-invasive recording of blood flow in human dental pulp. Endod Dent Traumatol 1986;2:219–21.
12. Gazelius B, Olgart L, Edwall B. Restored vitality in luxated teeth assessed by laser Doppler flowmeter. Endod Dent Traumatol 1988;4:265–8.
13. Kim S, Liu M, Markowitz K, et al. Comparison of pulpal blood flow in dog canine teeth determined by the laser Doppler and the 133xenon washout methods. Arch Oral Biol 1990;35:411–43.
14. Ramsay DS, Artun J, Martinen SS. Reliability of pulpal blood-flow measurements utilizing laser Doppler flowmetry. J Dent Res 1991;70:1427–30.
15. Ingolfsson AR, Tronstad L, Hersh EV, Riva CE. Effect of probe design on the suitability of laser Doppler flowmetry in vitality testing of human teeth. Endod Dent Traumatol 1993;9:65–70.
16. Ingólfsson AR, Tronstad L, Hersh EV, Riva CE. Efficacy of laser Doppler flowmetry in determining pulp vitality of human teeth. Endod Dent Traumatol 1994;10:83–7.
17. Ingolfsson, AE, Tronstad, L, Riva, CE. Reliability of laser Doppler flowmetry in testing vitality of human teeth. Endod Dent Traumatol 1994;10:185–7.

18. Vongsavan N, Matthews B. Experiments in pigs on the sources of laser Doppler blood-flow signals recorded from teeth. Arch Oral Biol 1996;41:97–103.
19. Ikawa M, Vongsavan N, Horiuchi H. Scattering of laser light directed onto the labial surface of extracted human upper central incisors. J Endod 1999;25:483–5.
20. Soo–ampon S, Vongsavan N, Soo-ampon M, et al. The sources of laser Doppler blood-flow signals recorded from human teeth. Arch Oral Biol 2003;48:353–60.
21. Polat S, Er K, Akpinar KE, Polat NT. The sources of laser Doppler blood-flow signals recorded from vital and root canal treated teeth. Arch Oral Biolm 2004;49:53–7.
22. Hartmann A, Azerad J, Boucher Y. Environmental effects on laser Doppler pulpal blood-flow measurements in man. Arch Oral Biol 1996;41:333–9.
23. Vongsavan N, Matthews B. Some aspects of the use of laser Doppler flow meters for recording tissue blood flow. Exp Physiol 1993;78:1–14.
24. Mesaros S, Trope M, Maixner W, Burkes EJ. Comparison of two laser Doppler systems on the measurement of blood flow of premolar teeth under different pulpal conditions. Int Endod J 1997;30:167–74.
25. Fratkin RD, Kenny DJ, Johnston DH. Evaluation of a laser Doppler flowmeter to assess blood flow in human primary incisor teeth. Pediatr Dent 1999;21:53–6.
26. Firestone AR, Wheatley AM, Thuer UW. Measurement of blood perfusion in the dental pulp with laser Doppler flowmetry. Int J Microcirc Clin Exp 1997;17:298–304.
27. Mesaros SV, Trope M. Revascularization of traumatized teeth assessed by laser Doppler flowmetry: a case report. Endod Dent Traumatol 1997;13:24–30.
28. Lee JY, Yanpiset K, Sigurdsson A, Vann WF. Laser Doppler flowmetry for monitoring traumatized teeth. Dent Traumatol 2001;17:231–5.
29. Ritter AL, Ritter AV, Murrah V, et al. Pulp revascularization of replanted immature dog teeth after treatment with minocycline and doxycycline assessed by laser Doppler flowmetry, radiography, and histology. Dent Traumatol 2004;20:75–8.
30. Emshoff R, Moschen I, Strobl H. Use of laser Doppler flowmetry to predict vitality of luxated or avulsed permanent teeth. Oral Surg Oral Med Oral Pathol Oral Radiol Endod 2004;98:750–5.
31. Emshoff R, Emshoff I, Moschen I, Strobl H. Laser Doppler flowmetry of luxated permanent incisors: a receiver operator characteristic analysis. J Oral Rehabil 2004; 31:866–72.
32. Emshoff R, Emshoff I, Moschen I, Strobl H. Laser Doppler flow measurements of pulpal blood flow and severity of dental injury. Int Endod J 2004;37:463–7.
33. Gopikrishna V, Tinagupta K, Kandaswamy D. Evaluation of efficacy of a new custom-made pulse oximeter dental probe in comparison with the electrical and thermal tests for assessing pulp vitality. J Endod 2007;33:411–14.
34. Schnettler JM, Wallace JA. Pulse oximetry as a diagnostic tool of pulpal vitality. J Endod 1991;17:488–90.
35. Kahan RS, Gulabivala K, Snook M, Setchell DJ. Evaluation of a pulse oximeter and customized probe for pulp vitality testing. J Endod 1996;22:105–9.

CHAPTER 15

Diagnostic Imaging
A. Endodontic Radiography

Richard E. Walton

Radiographs are the "eyes" of the dentist when performing many procedures. They are essential for diagnosis and treatment planning, determining anatomy, managing treatments, and assessing outcome. Now considered essential, the use of the X-ray was not available to the dental profession until early in the last century.

No single scientific development has contributed as greatly to improved dental health as the discovery of the amazing properties of cathode rays by Professor Wilhelm Konrad Roentgen in 1895. The significant possibilities of their application to dentistry were seized upon 14 days after Roentgen's announcement. Dr. Otto Walkoff took the first dental radiograph in his own mouth.[1] In the United States, within 5 months, Dr. William James described Roentgen's apparatus and displayed several radiographs. Three months later, Dr. C. Edmund Kells gave the first clinic in this country on the use of the X-ray for dental purposes. Three years later (1899), Kells was using the X-ray to determine tooth length during root canal therapy. "I was attempting to fill the root canal of an upper central incisor," Kells later said. "It occurred to me to place a lead wire in this root canal and then take a radiogram to see whether it extended to the end of the root or not. The lead wire was shown very plainly in the root canal."

One year later (1900), Dr. Weston A. Price "called attention to incomplete root canal fillings as evidenced in radiographs." By 1901, Price was suggesting that radiographs be used to check the adequacy of root canal fillings.[2] Price is also credited with developing the bisecting angle technique, whereas Kells described what today is called the paralleling technique, made popular some 40 years later by Dr. Gordon Fitzgerald.

Although these early attempts were rarely of diagnostic quality, they were the beginning of a new era. For the first time, dentists could see the accumulation of past dental treatment—therapy done without knowledge of what lay beneath the gingiva. Yet even today, with all of the technical refinements, the sleekness of operation, and the reduction of hazards, a discouraging segment of our profession continues to deprive their patients by failing to use radiography to its full potential. Dentists often under use or over use, under interpret or over interpret radiographs or fail to use careful and appropriate techniques.

Application of Radiography to Endodontics

In endodontics, radiographs have several essential functions:

1. Aid in diagnosis of hard tissue alterations of the teeth and periradicular structures.
2. Determine the number, location, shape, size, and direction of roots and root canals.[3]
3. Estimate and confirm the length of canals.
4. Localize hard-to-find, or disclose unsuspected, pulp canals by examining the position of an instrument within the root (Figure 1).
5. Aid in locating a pulp space markedly calcified and/or receded (Figure 2).
6. Determine the relative position of structures in the facial–lingual dimension.
7. Confirm the position and adaptation of master cones.
8. Aid in the evaluation of obturation.

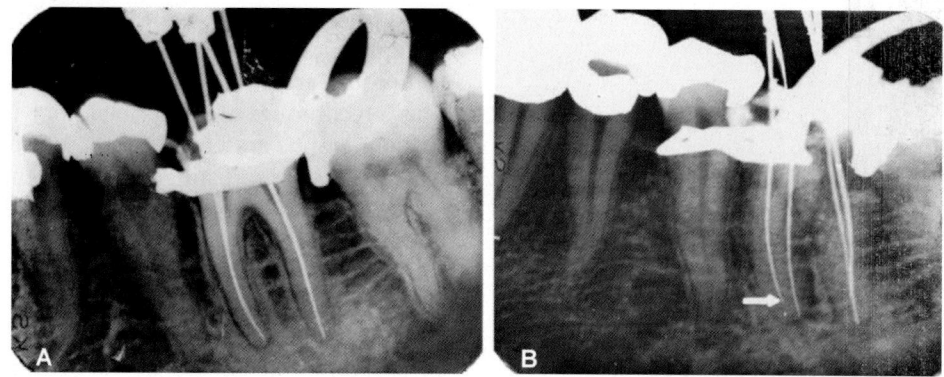

Figure 1 Disclosing canals by radiography. **A,** Right angle horizontal projection reveals four files in separate canals superimposed. **B,** Horizontal angulation varied 30° mesially reveals all four canals and file short of working length in mesiolingual canal (arrow).

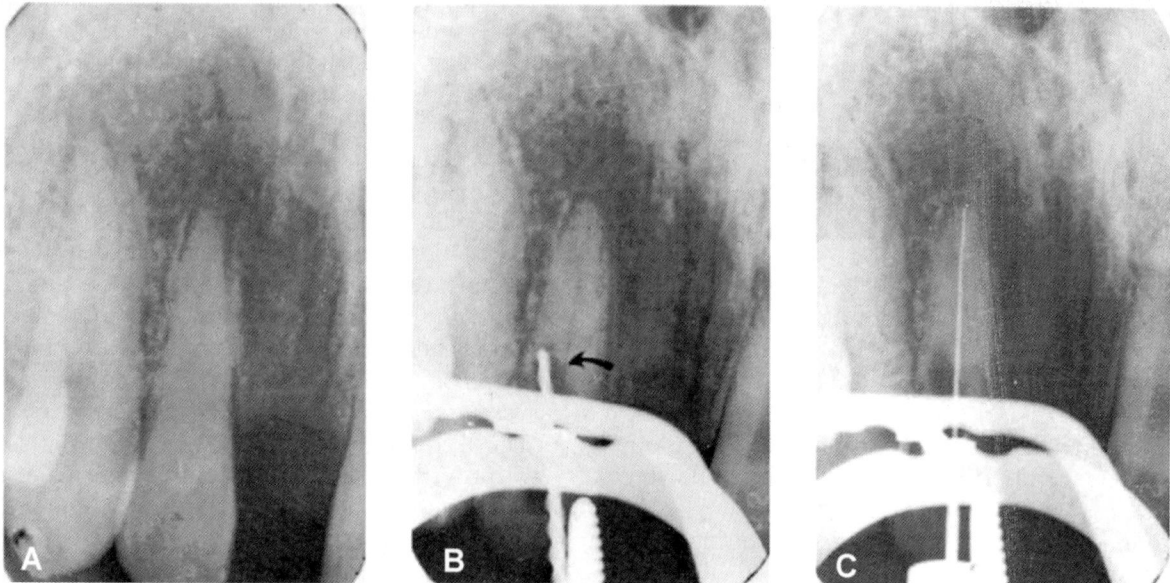

Figure 2 Locating canal. **A,** Advanced calcification and receded pulp. **B,** Radiograph reveals angulation of preparation and canal (arrow) at mesial of cut. **C,** Canal, seen in radiograph, is discovered with a fine file.

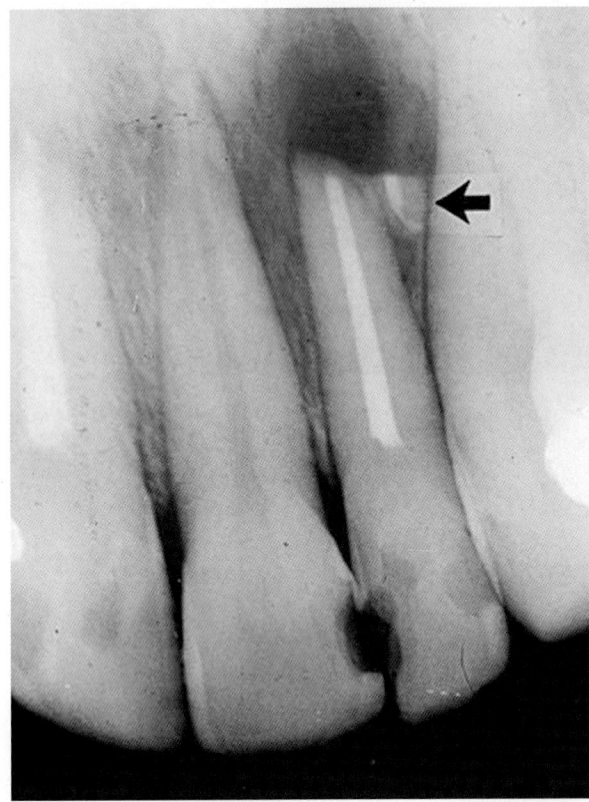

Figure 3 Radiograph taken *after* suturing and developed after patient left the office. The patient had to return to the office for removal of the root tip.

9. Facilitate the examination of soft tissues for tooth fragments and other foreign bodies following trauma.
10. Aid in localizing a hard-to-find apex during root-end surgery.
11. Confirm, following root-end surgery and before suturing, that all tooth fragments and excess filling material have been removed from the apical region and the surgical flap (Figure 3).
12. Evaluate, in follow-up films, the outcome of treatment.

LIMITATIONS OF RADIOGRAPHS

Radiographs are two-dimensional shadows on a single film. They are suggestive only and are not the singular final evidence in judging a clinical problem. There must be correlation with other subjective and objective findings. The greatest fault with the radiograph relates to its physical state. As with any shadow, these dimensions are easily distorted through improper technique, anatomic limitations, or processing errors. In addition, the buccal–lingual dimension is absent on a single film and is frequently overlooked, although techniques are available to define the third dimension. These techniques are described later in detail.

Radiographs are not infallible. Various states of pulpal pathosis are indistinguishable in the X-ray shadow. Neither healthy nor necrotic pulps cast an unusual image. Correspondingly, the bacterial status of hard or soft tissue is not detectable other than by inference. Only bacteriologic evidence can determine this. Furthermore, periradicular soft tissue lesions cannot be accurately diagnosed by radiographs; they require histologic verification.[4] Chronic inflammatory tissue cannot, for example, be differentiated from healed, fibrous, "scar" tissue, nor can a differential diagnosis of periradicular radiolucencies usually be made on the basis of size, shape, and density of the adjacent bone.[3–7] A common misconception is that an inflammatory lesion is present only when there is at least a perceptible "thickening" of the periodontal ligament space. In fact, investigators have demonstrated that lesions of the *medullary bone* often go undetected unless there is marked resorption or until the resorption has eroded a portion of the *cortical plate*.[8–11]

The fallibilities and inherent errors in radiographic interpretation were clearly demonstrated by Goldman et al.,[12] who submitted recall radiographs of endodontic treatments, for clinical evaluation, to a group of radiologists and endodontists. They assessed success and failure by observation of radiodensities. There was *more disagreement than agreement* among the examiners.

The techniques outlined in the following sections have proved to be successful and predictable. If followed, they will greatly simplify difficulties in root canal treatment.

Technology Systems

There are basically two radiographic approaches. The traditional is the X-ray exposure of film, that is chemically processed to produce an image. The newer digital systems rely on an electronic detection of an X-ray-generated image that is then electronically processed and reproduced on a computer screen. Overall, the resulting image is similar in interpretative quality to the traditional radiograph.[13–16] Advantages of digital radiography include reduced radiation, speed of obtaining the image, enhancement of the image, computer storage, transmissibility, and a system that does not require chemical processing.[17] Disadvantages are cost and more difficulty in placing the sensor. Many endodontists are finding that the advantages outweigh the disadvantages to their practice. As costs decrease and technology improves, use of the digital system will undoubtedly increase. Digital radiography is discussed in full later in the chapter.

TRADITIONAL MACHINES

Two basic types of X-ray machines are commonly used in dental offices. One type has a range of kilovoltage and two milliamperage settings with which the long (16-inch) cone is frequently used. The other type offers only one kilovoltage and milliamperage setting and only the short (8-inch) cone. Either type provides adequate radiographs. However, each has advantages that, under different circumstances, will yield a more satisfactory result. The long-cone system is superior for diagnostic radiographs, whereas the flexible short-cone machine is more appropriate for treatment or "working" films. However, either the "long cone" or the "short cone" is satisfactory if used properly.

LONG CONE

Because of the clarity of detail and minimum distortion inherent in the long-cone parallel technique,[18–21] the long-cone machine is preferred for exposing diagnostic, final, and follow-up radiographs.

SHORT CONE

Because of the number of working radiographs taken in the course of endodontic therapy, the practitioner treating more than the occasional tooth will find that a short-cone machine, with a small, easily manipulated head, saves time, energy, and frustration.

FILM

Industrial technological advances have allowed film exposure time to be reduced to fractions of a second. Recent improvements in emulsion thickness allow rapid processing of the new films, which are used for diagnostic and "working films" alike. A study of Kodak Ektaspeed film ("E" film), that is coated with larger silver bromide crystals and has one-half the exposure time of standard Kodak Ultraspeed film, concluded that the "Ektaspeed film had comparable accuracy with the Ultraspeed film in measuring root length," even though the new Ektaspeed is somewhat grainier.[22] A double-blind study found the slower Ultraspeed film superior "in terms of contrast, image, quality, and rater satisfaction."[23] However, another study found both films "adequate for routine endodontic use."[24]

An even faster film (F speed) has been introduced. This film requires 20% less radiation but is grainier. There are no conclusive studies to date on the suitability of this new film for endodontic use.

For endodontists, duplicate film packets are recommended for the diagnostic, final treatment, and recall radiographs—one set for the permanent office record, the other for the referring dentist. The front film in the double pack, the one closest to the X-ray machine, "had significantly superior image quality compared to back films."[25]

The standard periradicular size film is used for most situations. In addition, every office should have 3 by 2 1/4-inch *occlusal* film available for use when

1. periradicular lesions are so extensive that they cannot be demonstrated in their entirety on one periradicular film;
2. there is interest in or involvement of the nasal cavity, sinuses, or roof or floor of the mouth;
3. trauma or inflammation prohibits normal jaw opening required to place and hold a periradicular film;
4. a disabled person is unable to hold a periradicular film by the usual means;
5. detection of fractures of the anterior portion of the maxilla or mandible is needed; and
6. very young children are being examined.

INTRAORAL FILM PLACEMENT

Film placed parallel to the long axis of the teeth and exposed by cathode rays at a right angle to the surface of the film yields accurate images, with no

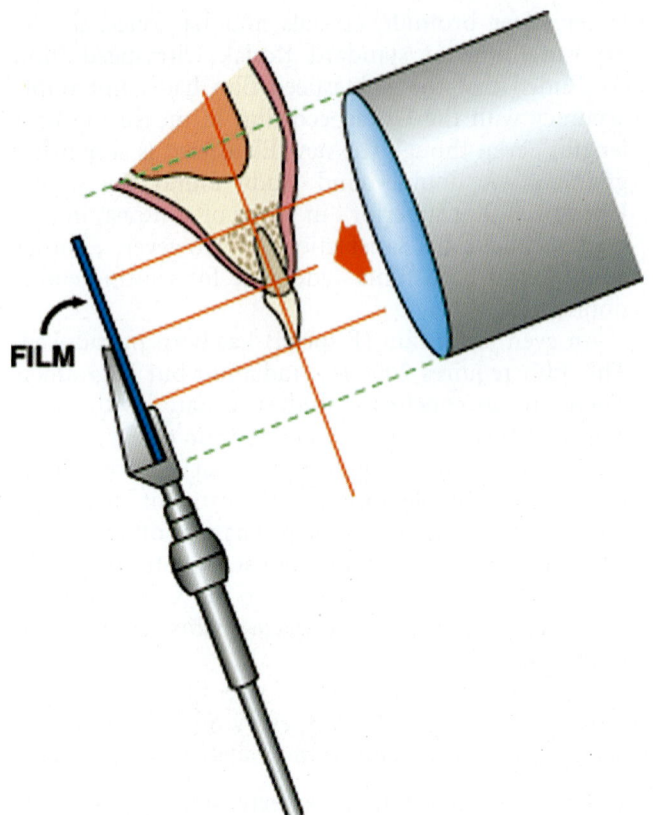

Figure 4 Radiographic parallelism. The long axis of the film, the long axis of the tooth, and the leading edge of the cone are parallel and perpendicular to the X-ray central beam. Reproduced with permission from Goerig AC. In: Besner E, et al., editors. Practical endodontics. St Louis (MO): Mosby; 1993, p. 56.

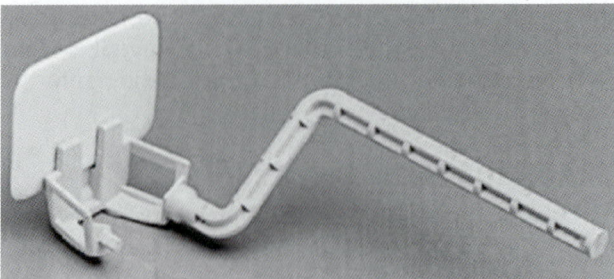

Figure 5 The Universal Rinn Endo Ray plastic film holder is designed for horizontal posterior films or anterior vertical films, maxilla or mandible, right or left. Here it is set for a maxillary posterior view. The "cupped-out" area accommodates the tooth, clamp, and extruding endodontic files. Photo courtesy of Rinn Corp. USA.

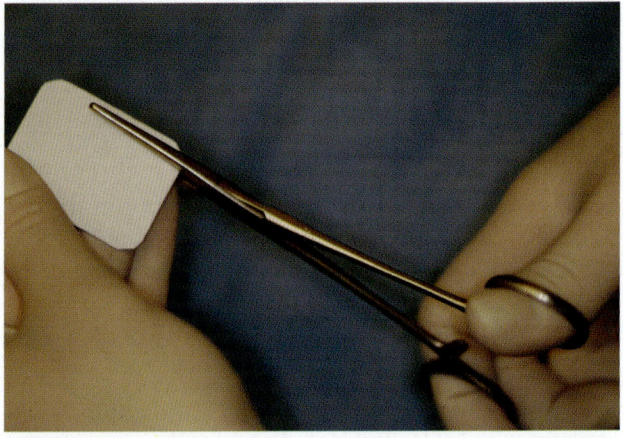

Figure 6 A hemostat is used for grasping the film and as a cone positioning and orientation device.

foreshortening or elongation[26] (Figure 4). If this principle is applied, it is unnecessary to memorize fixed cone angulations. Also, a patient need not be returned to an upright position for each exposure.

Because of the complicating presence of the rubber dam, the methods for placement of *working* films differ somewhat from the methods for placement of diagnostic, final, and follow-up films.

DIAGNOSTIC RADIOGRAPHS

These must be the *best radiographs possible*. There are advantages to parallelism, that permits more accurate visualization of structures as well as reproducibility. This facilitates comparison of follow-up radiographs.

There are a number of devices on the market that ensure film placement and parallelism. The *Rinn XCP* (Dentsply/Rinn, Elgin, IL) virtually guarantees distortion-free films but cannot be used with the rubber dam in place. The *Rinn Endoray II endodontic film holder* is designed specifically to ensure parallelism yet avoid rubber dam clamps while allowing space for files protruding from the tooth (Figure 5). A disadvantage to this system is that the paralleling bar interferes with the cone when varying the horizontal cone angulations. Finger retention of the film should never be used. A *straight hemostat* is a good film holder and additionally serves as a cone-positioning device (Figure 6).

WORKING RADIOGRAPHS

One great difficulty in root canal therapy is the clumsy, aggravating method of making treatment radiographs with the rubber dam in place. The rubber dam frame should not be removed for access in film placement because doing so allows saliva entry to contaminate the operating field. A film-placement technique is used so that the *rubber dam frame need not be removed*. Use of a radiolucent N-Ø

(Nygaard–Østby) frame (Coltene/Whaledent/Hygenic, Mahwah, NJ), Lexicon hinge dam frame (Dentsply-Tulsa-Dental) or the *Star VisiFrame* (Dentaleze/Star, USA) will ensure that apices are not obscured.

With the rubber dam in place, a *hemostat-held* film has significant advantages:

1. The film placement is easier when the opening is restricted by the rubber dam and frame.
2. The patient may close somewhat with the film in place, a particular advantage in *mandibular posterior areas* where closing relaxes the mylohyoid muscle, permitting the film to be positioned farther apically.
3. The handle of the hemostat is a guide to align the cone in the proper vertical and horizontal angulation (see Figure 6).
4. There is less risk of distortion of the radiograph caused by too much finger pressure bending the film.
5. Patients can hold a hemostat handle more securely with less possibility of film displacement.
6. Any movement can be detected by the shift of the handles and corrected before exposure.

The *identifying dimple* should be placed at the incisal or occlusal edge to prevent its obscuring an important apical structure.

CONE POSITIONING

It is often a mistake to rely on only one film. Additional exposures taken from varied horizontal or vertical projections give visualization of the third dimension (Figure 7).

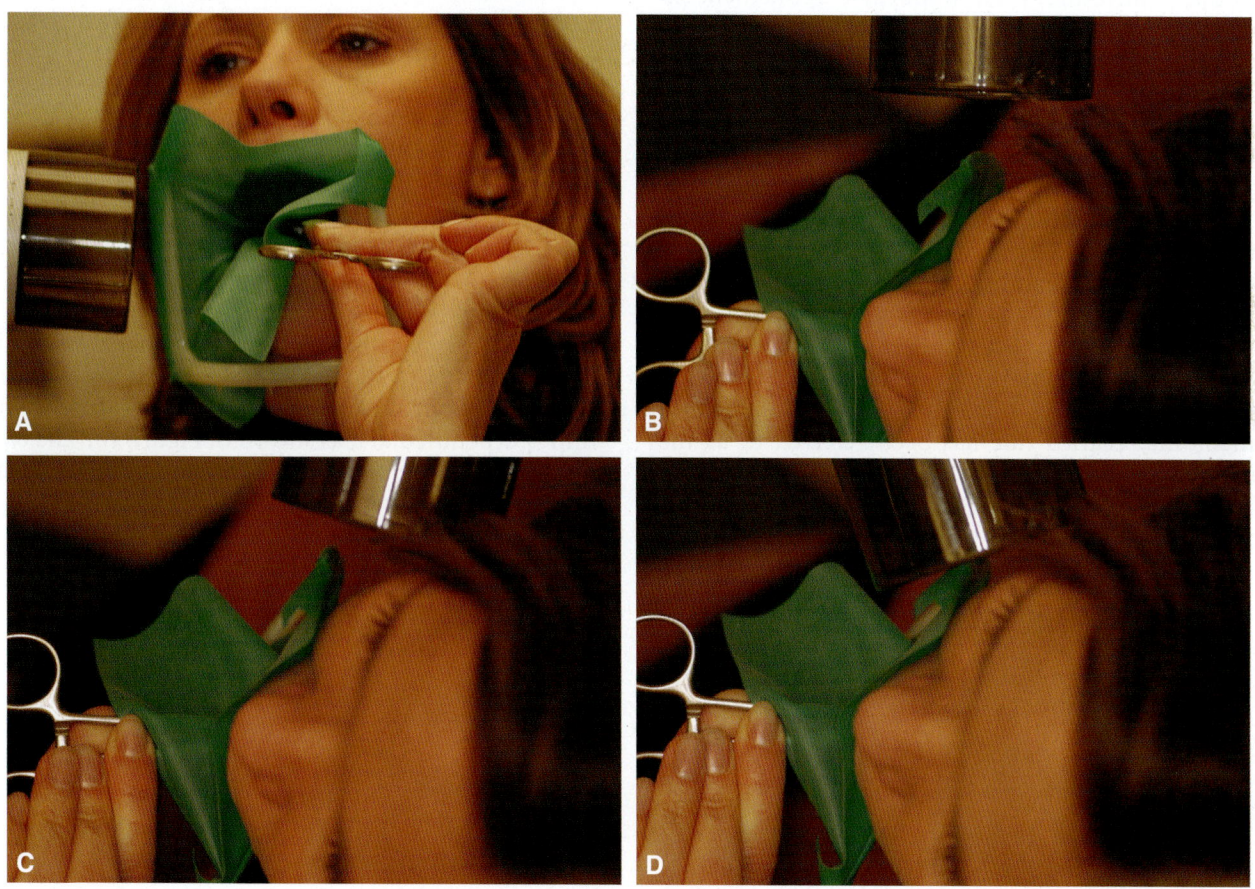

Figure 7 "Working" film properly placed and held under rubber dam with hemostat. ***A***, Vertical angle. Cone is aligned so that central beam is parallel with the handle. ***B***, Cone is aligned at right angle to handle and film. ***C***, Varying horizontal angle. Vertical angle is maintained. ***D***, Cone is shifted 20–25° to the mesial.

VERTICAL ANGULATION

Ordinarily, it is preferable to align the cone so the beam strikes the film at a right angle. This alignment ensures a fairly accurate vertical image. Elongation of an image, however, *may be corrected by increasing the vertical angle* of the central ray. Conversely, *foreshortening is corrected by decreasing* the vertical angle of the central ray.

Frequently, an impinging palatal vault prevents parallel alignment of the film and the teeth. However, if the film angle is no greater than 20° in relation to the long axis of the teeth, and the beam is directed at a right angle to the film, no distortion occurs, although there is a less effective orientation of structures.[26] The resulting radiograph is still adequate.

HORIZONTAL ANGULATION

Walton[27] introduced an important refinement in dental radiography that has materially improved the endodontic interpretive film. He demonstrated a simple technique whereby the *third dimension* may be readily visualized. Specifically, the anatomy of superimposed structures, the roots and pulp canals, may be better defined. The basic technique is to vary the *horizontal angulation* of the central ray of the X-ray beam. By this method, overlying canals may be separated, and by applying Clark's rule,[28] the separate canals may then be identified. Clark's rule states that "the most distant object from the cone (lingual) moves toward the direction of the cone." Stated in another way, using a helpful mnemonic, Clark's rule has been referred to as the SLOB rule (*S*ame *L*ingual, *O*pposite *B*uccal): the object that moves in the *S*ame direction as the cone is located toward the *L*ingual. The object that moves in the *O*pposite direction from the cone is located toward the *B*uccal. The SLOB rule, simply stated, is "The lingual object follows the tube head." Goerig and Neaverth[29] cleverly applied the SLOB rule to determine, from a single film, from which direction a radiograph was taken: mesial, straight on, or distal. Knowing the direction, one is then able to determine lingual from buccal (Figure 8). Stated more simply, Ingle's rule is *MBD*: Always "shoot" from the *M*esial and the *B*uccal root will be to the *D*istal.

HORIZONTAL CONE ANGULATIONS

For working and/or interpretive diagnostic radiographs, the following cone angles are preferred:

1. Maxillary anterior teeth (straight facial)
2. Maxillary premolars and molars (mesial angle)
3. Mandibular incisor teeth (distal angle)
4. Mandibular canines (mesial angle)
5. Mandibular premolars (mesial)
6. Mandibular molars (distal).

All teeth require specific film placement and cone positioning for working films (Figure 9).

Mandibular Molars

As previously emphasized, the film must be positioned parallel to the lower arch. The *standard* horizontal X-ray projection then is at a right angle to the film (perpendicular), as shown in Figure 10. The two mesial canals are superimposed one upon the other and appear as a single line.

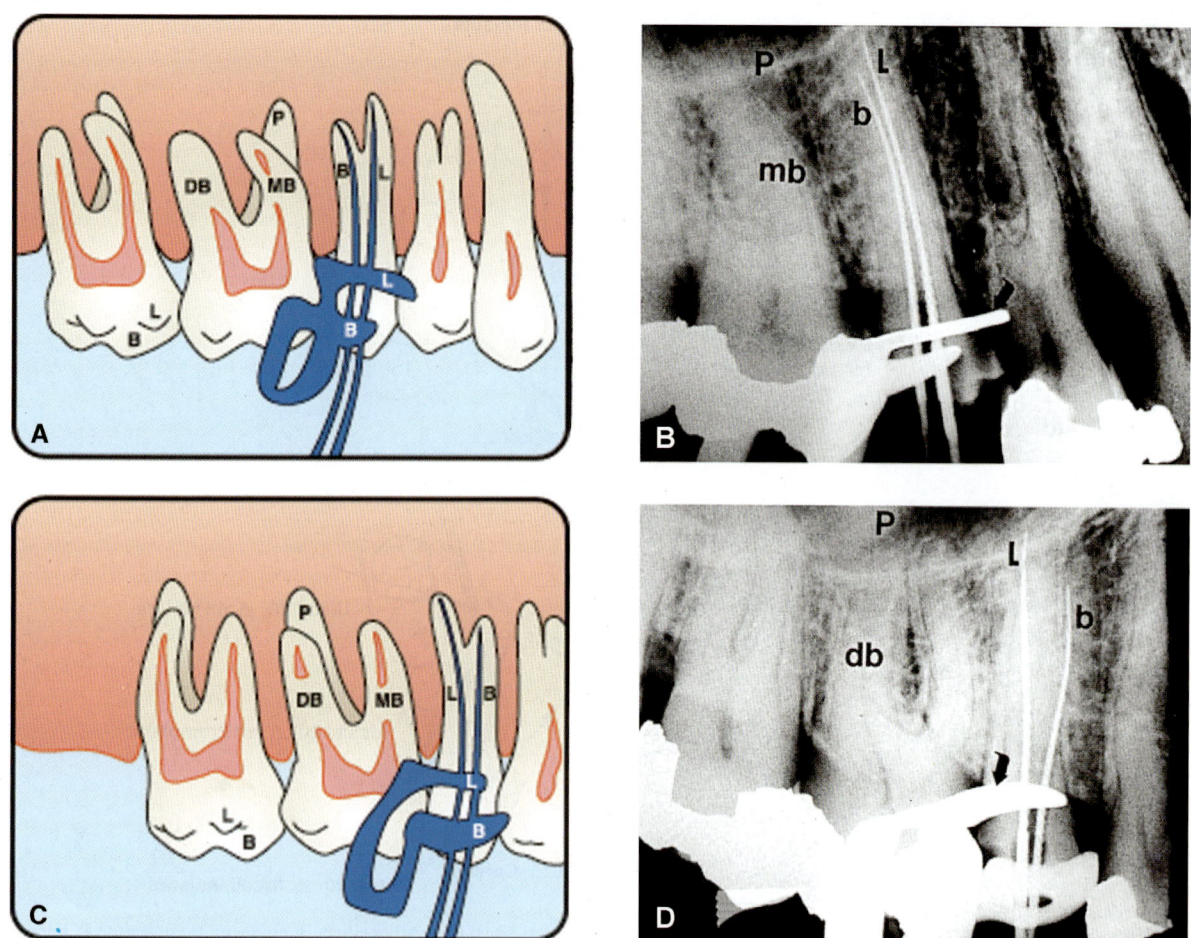

Figure 8 Applying the SLOB (*s*ame *l*ingual, *o*pposite *b*uccal) rule to determine the cone angle. Clues that the cone is oriented from the mesial: **A,** and **B,** The mesial–buccal (MB) root lies over the palatal (P) root, that is, the lingual (palatal) root has moved mesially; the lingual arm of the rubber dam clamp (arrow) has moved mesially. The canine is visible. Once it has been determined that the radiograph was taken from the mesial, the lingual root (toward the mesial) of the premolar is defined. **C,** and **D,** Radiograph of the same teeth taken from the distal. Clues are reversed. The canine is not visible. The lingual premolar canal is now toward the distal. Reproduced with permission from Goerig AC. In: Besner E, et al., editors. Practical endodontics. St Louis (MO): Mosby; 1993, p. 54.

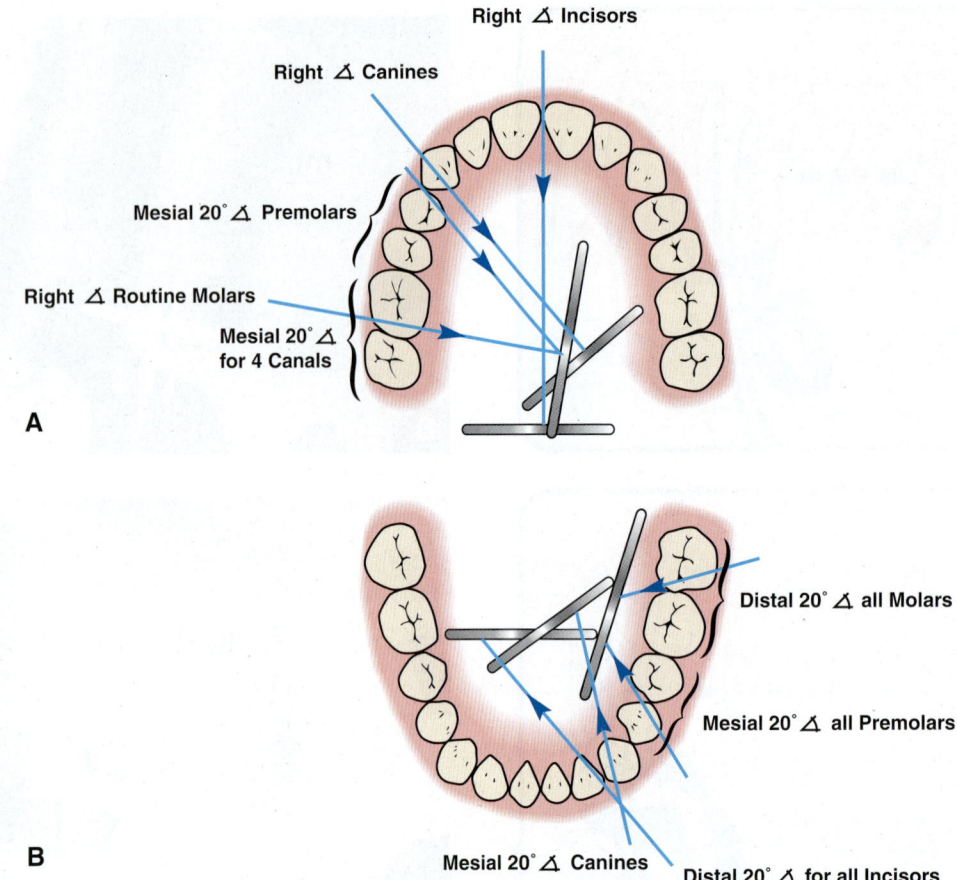

Figure 9 ***A,*** maxillary film/central beam (arrows) position. ***B,*** mandibular film/central beam (arrows) position. Reproduced from Walton R. Principles and practice of endodontics, 3rd ed. Philadelphia: Saunders and Co.; 2002 p.147.

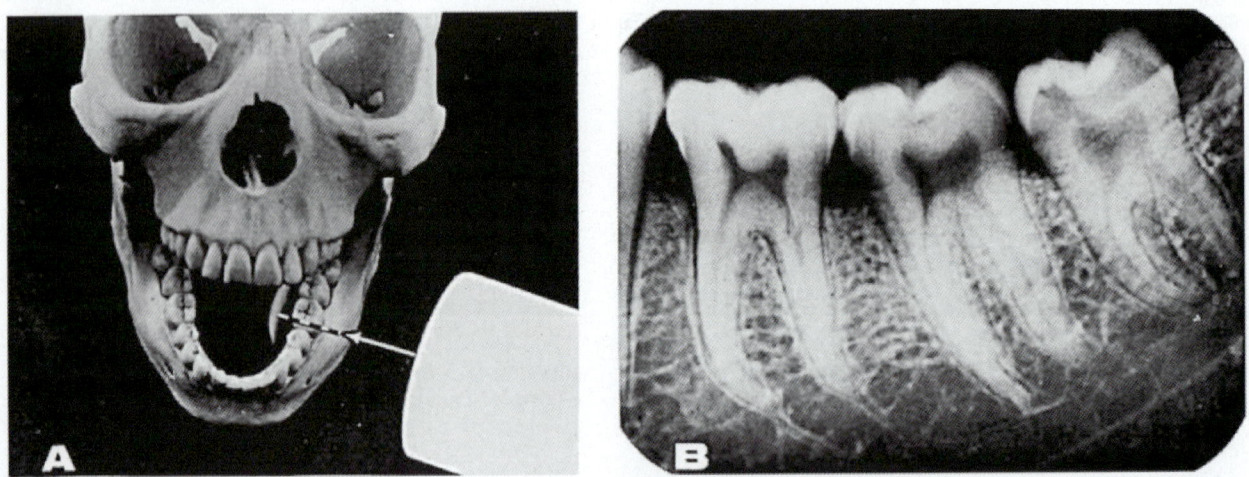

Figure 10 Mandibular molars. ***A,*** Central ray directed at right angle to film positioned parallel to arch. ***B,*** Limited information is gleaned from the radiograph because of superimposition of structures and canals. Reproduced with permission from Walton RE.[27]

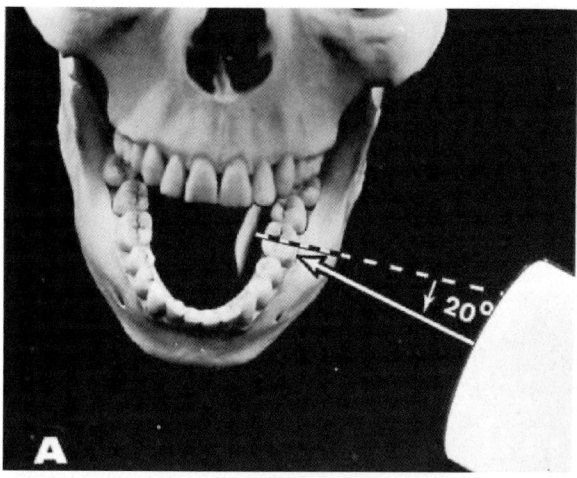 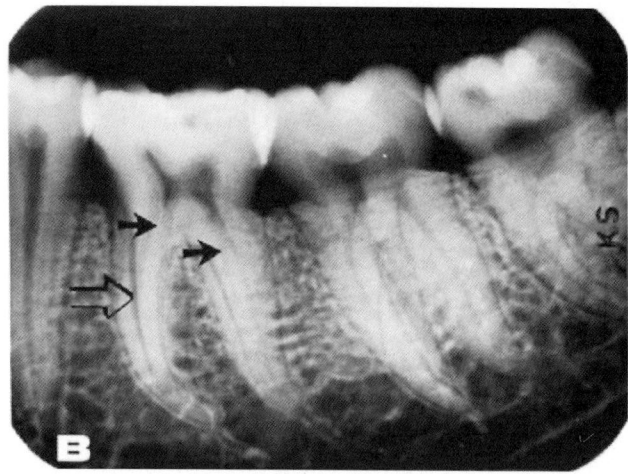

Figure 11 Mandibular molars. ***A,*** Central ray directed at 20° mesially to film positioned parallel to arch. ***B,*** Two canals are now visible in both roots of the first molar (black arrows). Open arrow indicates confusing root outlines. Reproduced with permission from Walton RE.[27]

Through the *Walton projection*, however, the roots can be made to "open up." This is done by directing the central beam 20 to 30° from the mesial (Figure 11A). In Figure 11B (black arrows), the two canals in each root can now be readily discerned. The contrast gained by varying the horizontal projection is seen in a clinical case with four canals. Figure 12A taken at a right angle, clearly shows the four instruments superimposed on one another. Figure 12B, on the other hand, taken from a 30° variance in horizontal projection, emphasizes the third dimension: the separation of the instruments in the canals. By applying Ingle's rule (MBD: project the central beam from the *mesial*), the *buccal* canals are toward the *distal*, the *lingual* canals toward the *mesial*.

Another point concerns a frequent mistake in "reading" periradicular radiographs. It can best be

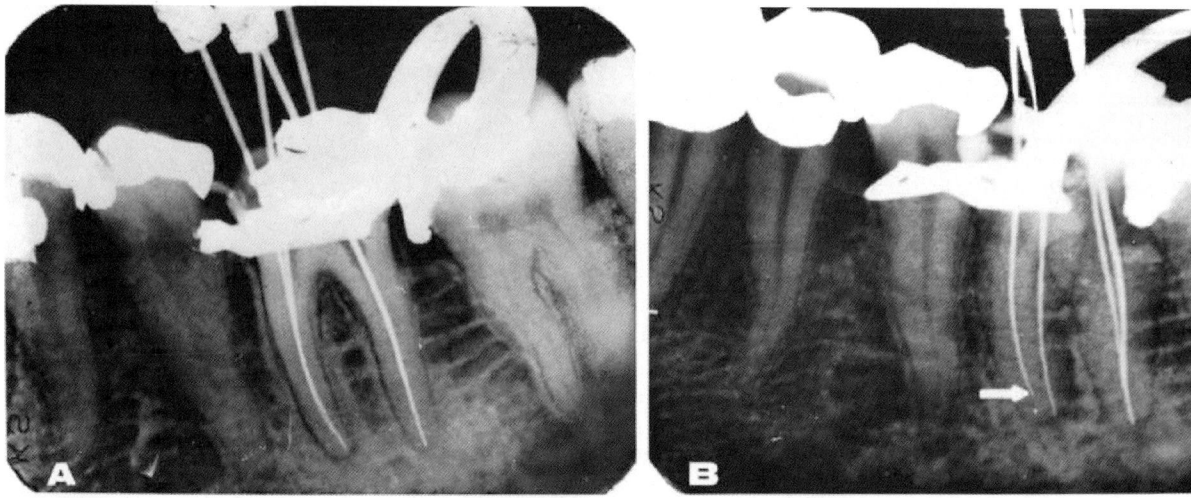

Figure 12 Mandibular molars. ***A,*** Right-angle horizontal projection superimposes four files, one on the other. ***B,*** Horizontal variance of 30° separates four canals. SLOB (*s*ame *l*ingual, *o*pposite *b*uccal) rule proves lingual canals are to the mesial. Reproduced with permission from Walton RE.[27]

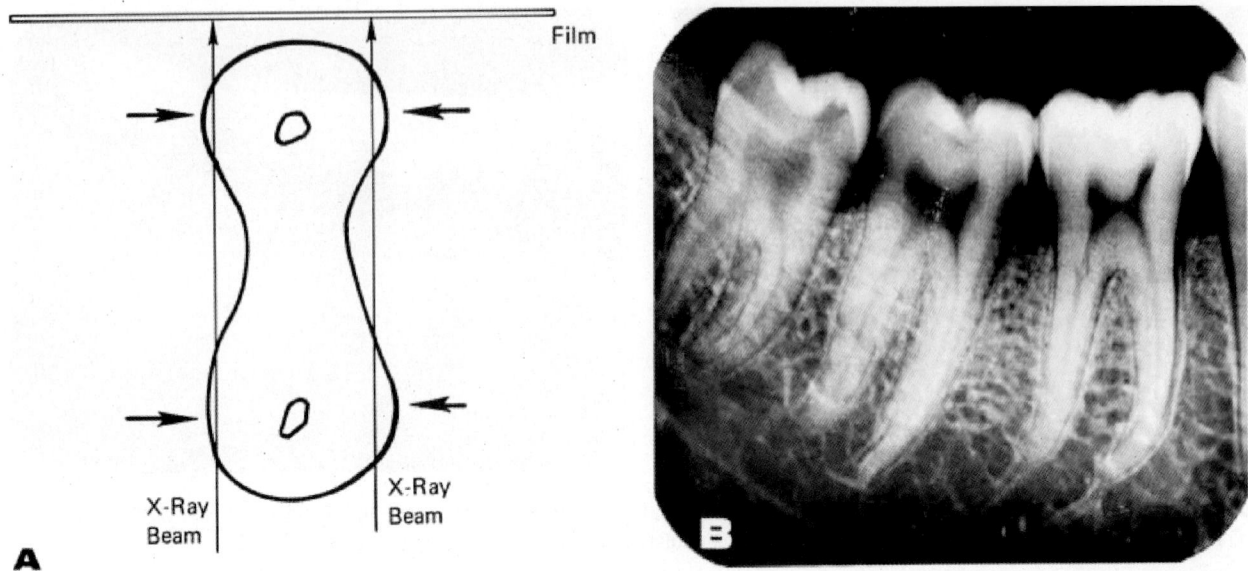

Figure 13 ***A***, X-ray beam passing directly through two thicknesses of root structure presents intensified image on film. ***B***, Note radiopaque root outline inside lamina dura. B reproduced with permission from Walton RE.[27]

illustrated by a cross-sectional drawing of molar root structure. Roots containing two canals are often hourglass-shaped (Figure 13A). When an X-ray beam passes directly through this structure, the buccal and lingual portions of the root are in the same path (arrows). Because a double thickness of tooth structure is penetrated by the X-rays, it is seen in the film as a radiopaque root outline in close contact with the *lamina dura*. This is readily apparent on the radiograph (Figure 13B).

By aiming the cone 20° from the mesial, however, the central beam passes through the hourglass-shaped root at an angle (Figure 14A). In this case, the two thicknesses of the root are projected separately onto the film. Because less tooth structure is penetrated by the X-ray, the image on the film is less dense. A

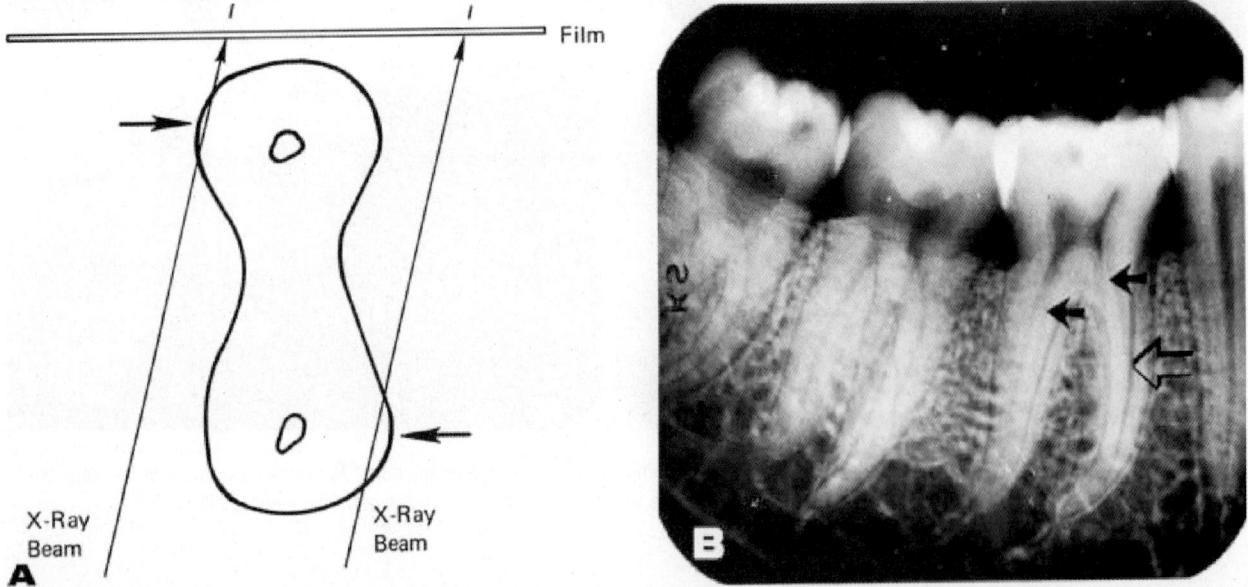

Figure 14 ***A***, X-ray beam aimed 20° passes through single thicknesses of hourglass root, leaving less dense impression on film. ***B***, Radiolucent line is apparent (open arrow) and may be confused with root canal. Note that it emerges at gingival, not into pulp chamber. Black arrows indicate regular canals. B reproduced with permission of Walton RE.[27]

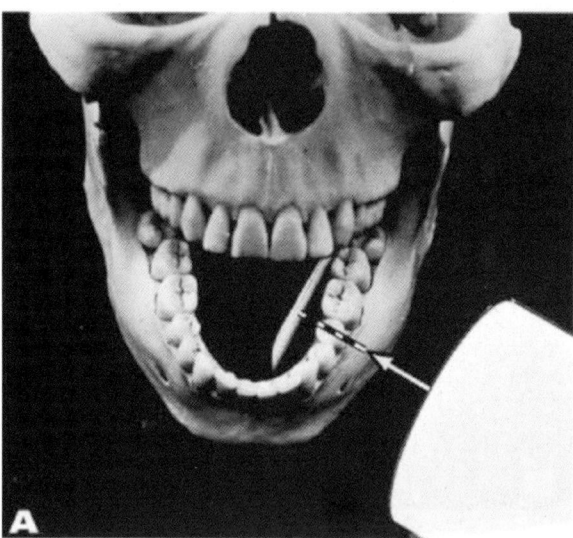
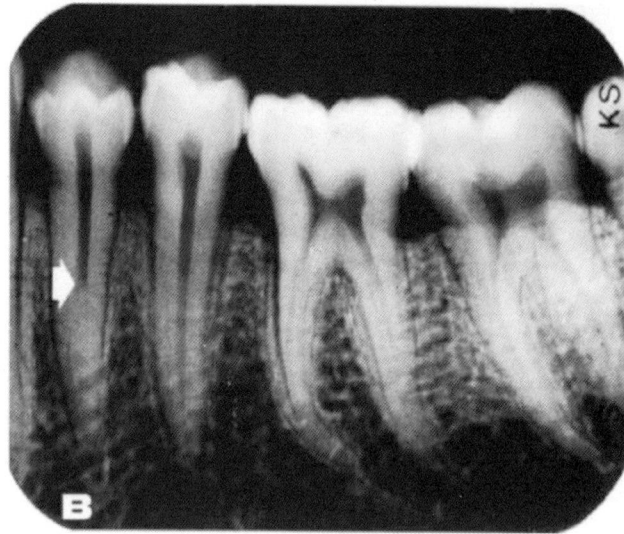

Figure 15 Mandibular premolars. ***A***, Central ray directed at right angle to film positioned parallel to arch. ***B***, Radiograph reveals one canal in each premolar, although abrupt change in density (arrow) may indicate bifurcation. Reproduced with permission from Walton RE.[27]

radiolucent line is clearly seen in Figure 14B (open arrow). This radiolucent line can be erroneously interpreted as a root canal. By following up the length of the line, instead of entering the pulp chamber, the line can be traced to the gingival surface of the root; this is the lamina dura. This simple interpretive error can easily lead to gross mistakes.

Mandibular Premolars

The importance of varying the horizontal angulation when radiographing mandibular premolars is demonstrated in Figure 15A. The central beam is directed at a right angle to the film. What appears to be a single straight canal is discernible in each premolar (Figure 15B). There is an indication, however, in the image of the first premolar that the canal might bifurcate at the point of the abrupt change ("fast-break") in density (arrow).

Directing the central ray 20° from the mesial in the *first premolar* (Figure 16A) causes the bifurcation to separate into two canals (Figure 16B). The tapering outline of the tooth, seen in both projections, would

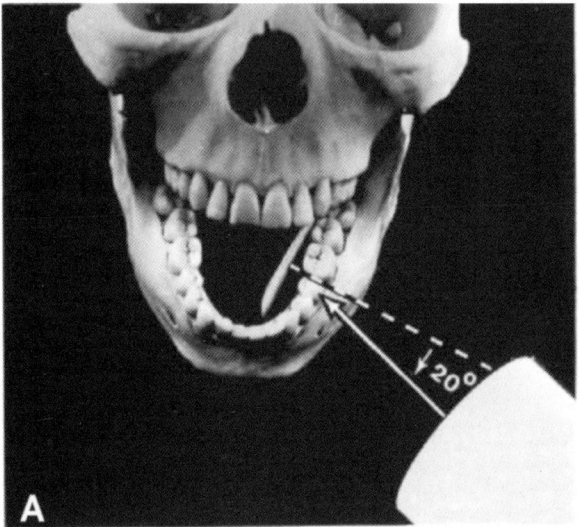
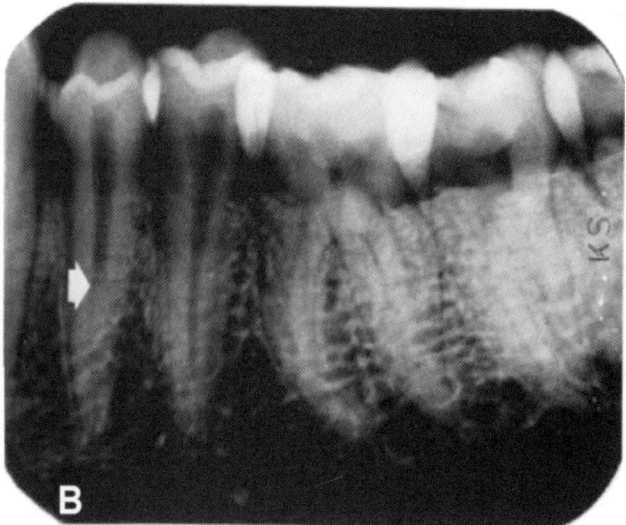

Figure 16 Mandibular premolars. ***A***, Central ray directed at 20° mesially to film, parallel to arch. ***B***, In first premolar, two canals that are clearly visible (arrow) probably reunite, as indicated by sharply tapered root. Reproduced with permission from Walton RE.[27]

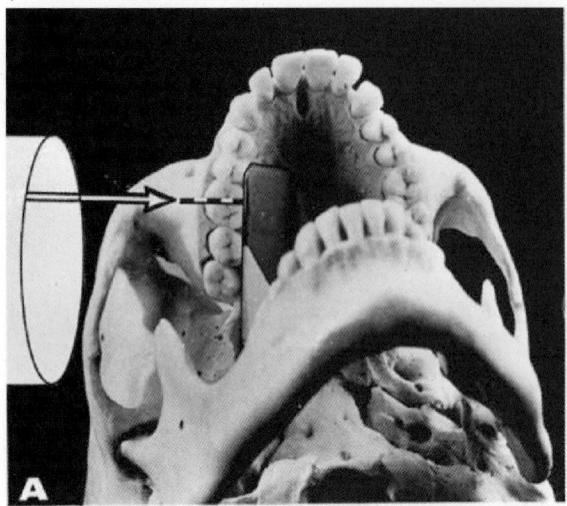 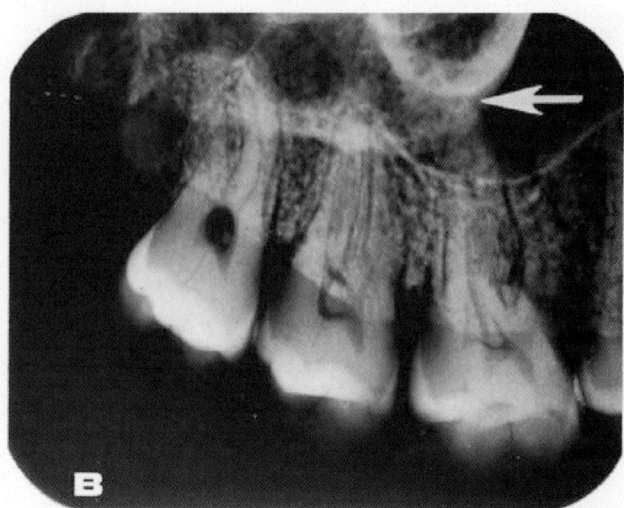

Figure 17 Maxillary molars. **A,** Central ray is directed through maxillary molar at right angle to inferior border of film. Arrow and dotted line passing through malar process indicate it will superimpose over first molar. **B,** Superimposition of first molar roots, sinus floor, and malar process (white arrow) confuse the diagnosis. Reproduced with permission from Walton RE.[27]

indicate, on the other hand, that the two canals undoubtedly rejoin to form a common canal at the apex. In both the right-angle and 20° variance projections, the *second premolar* appears as a single canal.

Maxillary Molars

Maxillary molars are consistently the most difficult to radiograph because of their more complicated root and pulp anatomy, the frequent superimposition of portions of the roots on each other, the superimposition of bony structures (sinus floor, zygomatic process) on root structures, and the shape and depth of the palate. Each of these, singly or in combination can be a major impediment.

As is true of the mandible, the complex root anatomy and superimpositions may be dealt with *by varying the horizontal* angulations. Film placement must again be parallel to the posterior maxillary arch, not to the palate.

The standard right-angle projection for a maxillary first molar, illustrated in Figure 17A, produces the image seen in Figure 17B, wherein the zygomatic process is superimposed on the apex of the palatal root (arrow) and the distobuccal root appears to

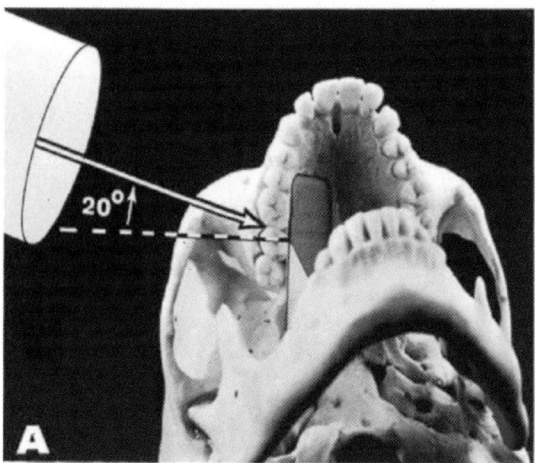
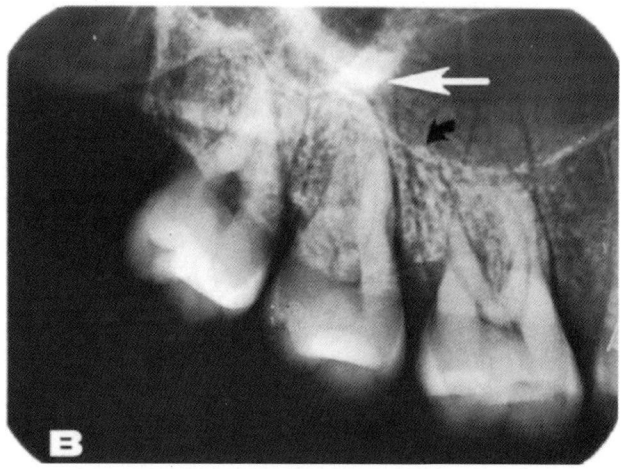

Figure 18 Maxillary molars. **A,** Central ray directed at 20° mesially skirts malar process, projecting it distally. **B,** Distobuccal root is cleared of palatal root and malar process is projected far distal (white arrow). Between right-angle and 20° projection, all three roots are clearly seen. Reproduced with permission from Walton RE.[27]

overlie the palatal root. The sinus floor is also superimposed on the apices of both the first and second molars. When the horizontal angulation is varied by 20° to the mesial (Figure 18A), the zygomatic process is "moved" to the distal of the first molar and the distobuccal root is cleared of the palatal root (Figure 18B, arrows).

The *opposite projection* also can be used to isolate the mesiobuccal root of the first molar, that is, the central ray may be projected from *20° distal* to the right angle (Figure 19A). Although this projection distorts the shape of the mesiobuccal root, it also isolates it (Figure 19B), so that the canal is readily discernible (arrow). Also the zygomatic process is moved completely away from any root structure, including the second molar. The same technique illustrated here for the maxillary first molar can be applied to the second or third molars by directing the central beam at a horizontal variance through those teeth.

Maxillary Premolars

Variance in the horizontal projection has great value in maxillary premolar radiography, particularly for the *first* premolar, which generally has two roots and canals, but sometimes three. The clinical efficacy of the Walton

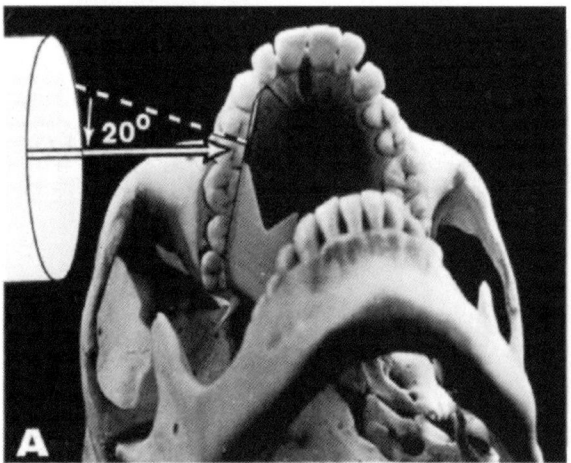
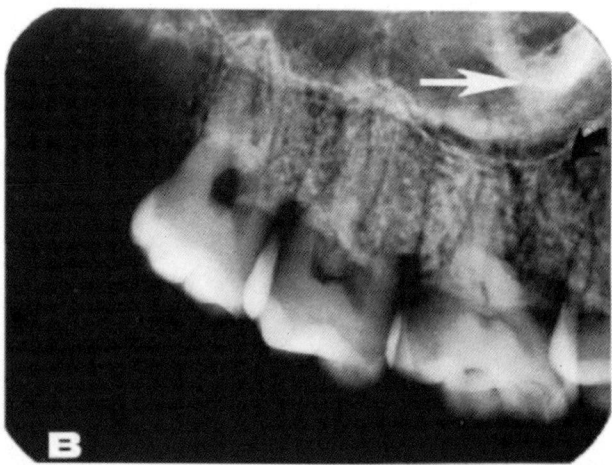

Figure 19 Maxillary molars. **A,** Central beam projected 20° from the distal. **B,** Mesiobuccal root of the first molar is isolated (black arrow) and second and third molars are cleared of malar process, which is projected forward (white arrow). Sinus floor may be "lowered" or "raised" by changing vertical angulation. Reproduced with permission from Walton RE.[27]

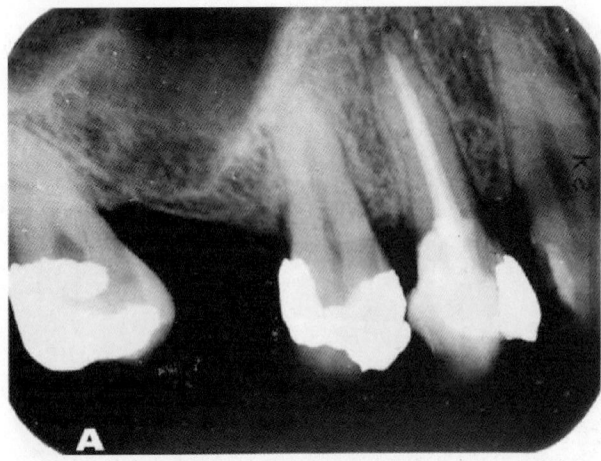
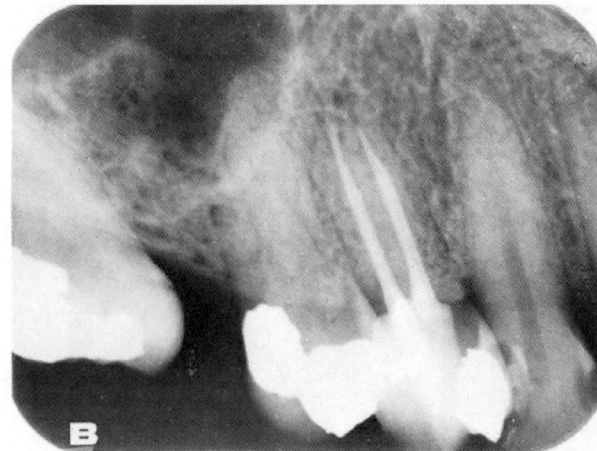

Figure 20 Maxillary premolars. ***A,*** Horizontal right-angle projection produces illusion that maxillary first premolar has only one canal. ***B,*** Varying horizontal projection by 20° from the mesial separates two canals. Buccal canal is distal (MBD). Reproduced with permission from Walton RE.[27]

technique is well illustrated in Figure 20. The right-angle horizontal projection produces the single canal image seen in Figure 20A. By varying the angulation by 20°, however, the two canals are separated (Figure 20B), giving an unobstructed view of the obturation quality in both canals.

Mandibular Anterior Teeth

Aberrations in canal anatomy in the *mandibular* anterior teeth are infamous. Variance of the horizontal X-ray projections in this region will bring out the differences. Figure 21A illustrates the standard X-ray projection bisecting the film held parallel to the arch. The incisor

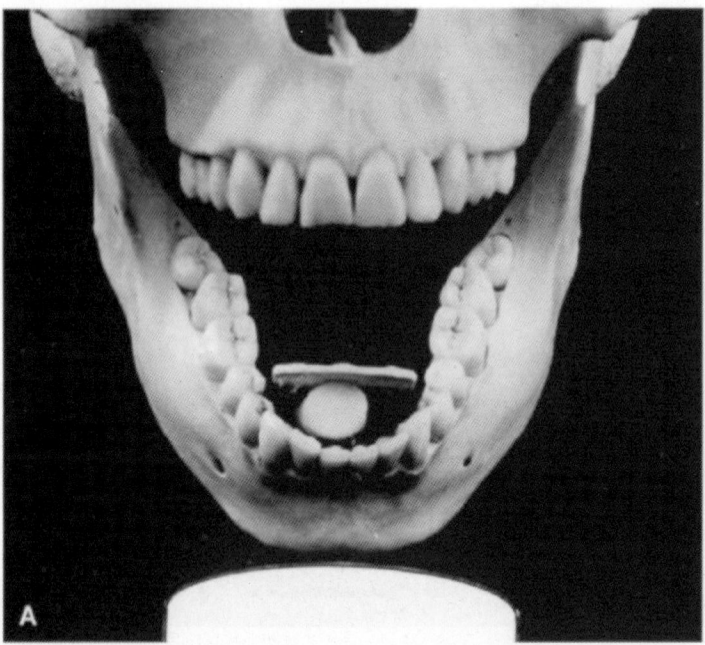
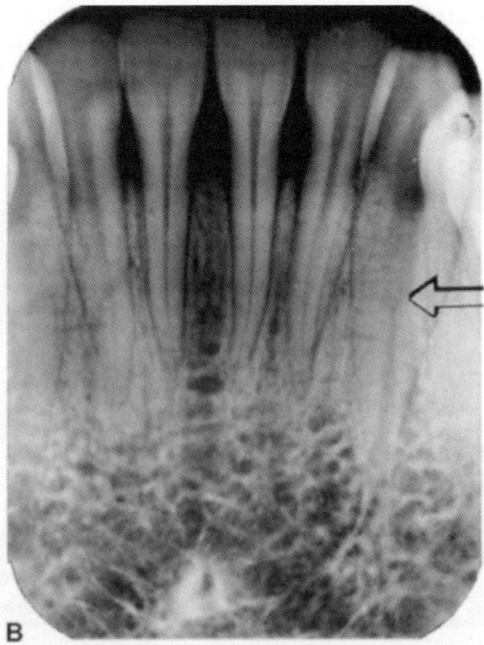

Figure 21 Mandibular anterior teeth. ***A,*** Film placement for modified parallel technique. Horizontal central beam projection at right angle to film. ***B,*** Single canals seen in central incisors with only suggestion of two canals in lateral incisor. In distorted image of canine, note broad labiolingual canal dimension (arrow). Reproduced with permission from Walton RE.[27]

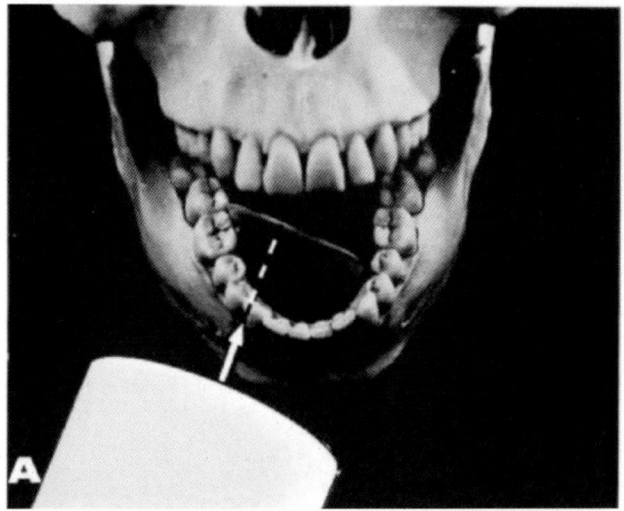 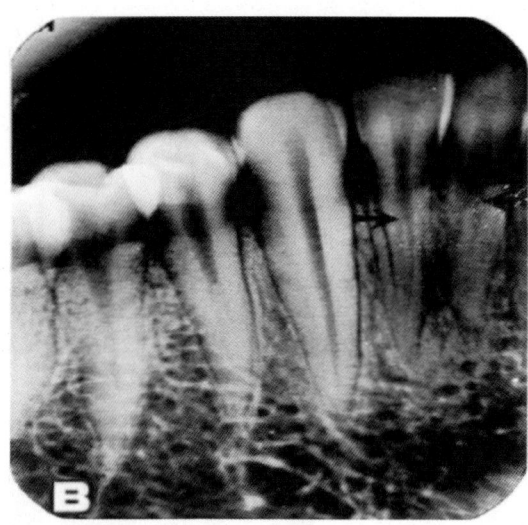

Figure 22 Mandibular canine. **A,** Film is positioned for canine radiograph. Horizontally, central beam is projected at right angle to film. **B,** Canine image is single straight canal, but incisor image reveals bifurcated canals that reunite in narrow tapered root (arrows). Note "bonus" image of bifurcated canals. First premolar. Reproduced with permission from Walton RE.[27]

teeth appear to have single canals. But a broad single canal is seen in the distorted canine image (Figure 21B).

By varying the film placement and projecting directly through the canine, as seen in Figure 22A (which is about 30° variance for the incisors), separate canals appear in the incisors (Figure 22B, arrow); the canals join at the apex. This would be expected, however, when viewing the tapered incisor roots seen in both horizontal projections; the roots are far too narrow to support two separate canals and foramina. Once again, the abrupt change in canal radiodensity in the premolars (arrow) indicates a canal bifurcation.

Maxillary Anterior Teeth

Although canal or root aberrations appear less frequently in the maxillary anterior teeth, root curvature in the maxillary lateral incisors is a particularly vexing problem. Grady and Clausen[30] have shown, for example, how difficult it is to determine when foramina exit

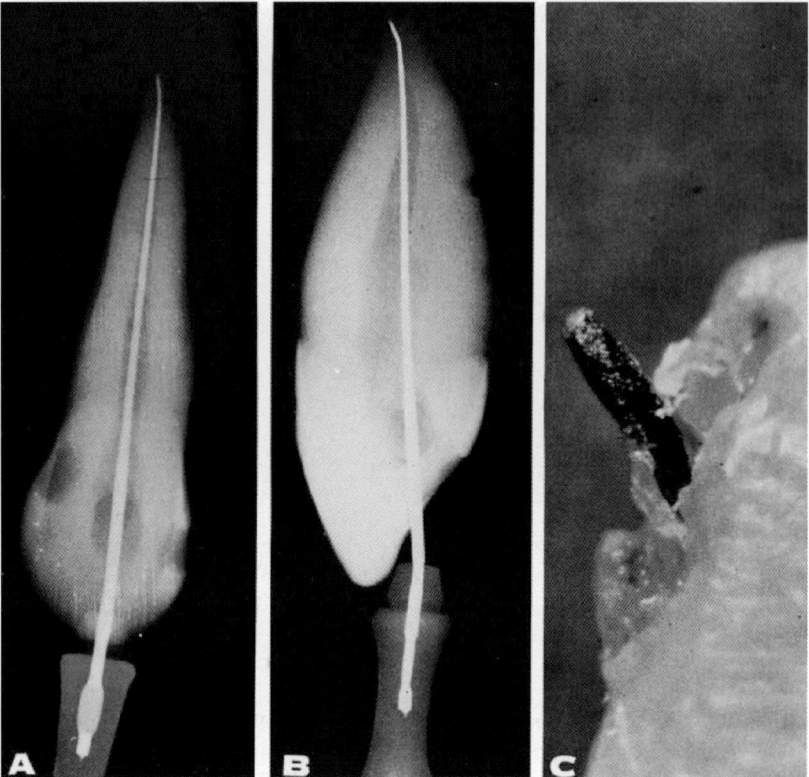

Figure 23 ***A***, Labiolingual projection through canine shows instrument apparently at apex with slight distal curvature. ***B***, Mesiodistal projection reveals instrument actually emerging from labial short of apex. ***C***, Instrument perforating foramen to labial well short of radiographic root end. Photos courtesy of Dr. John R. Grady and Dr. Howard Clausen.

to the labial or lingual. Their radiographs of extracted teeth matched with photographs of instrument perforation short of the apex are a warning to all (Figure 23).

EXTRAORAL FILM PLACEMENT

This is useful for patients who cannot accommodate or tolerate intraoral film placement, usually because of gagging or trismus. Acceptable diagnostic and working films are possible.[31] This requires special positioning of cone and film (Figure 24).

PROCESSING

Another deterrent has been the length of time required to process films. Old, weakened solutions greatly increase the time required for processing. Moreover, adherence to the manufacturer's recommended temperature and time (68°F for 5 to 7 minutes) for developing and clearing has hampered "on-the-spot" processing and viewing.

Ingle et al.[32] demonstrated, in a well-controlled blind study, the effects of varied processing temperatures. A processing temperature of 92°F yielded, in less than 1 minute, the most acceptable radiographs. At 92°F, using Kodak developer and fixer mixed to company specifications, *development required only 30 seconds* and fixation required 25 to 35 seconds, with no loss of quality. By comparison, at 70°F temperature, it required 5 minutes' developing time and 10 minutes' fixing time for Ultraspeed film. Ektaspeed is slightly better: 72 to 80°F for 2 1/2 to 4 minutes' developing and 2 to 4 minutes' fixing time. All films need to be *final washed* for at least 30 minutes.

For rapid processing, small quart-size tanks are adequate and economical. Frequent change of solutions is recommended.

RAPID-PROCESSING SOLUTIONS

Concentrated chemicals, such as *Kodak's Rapid Access* solution, have become very popular in endodontic practice. Although more expensive, they save measurable time, requiring only 15 seconds' developing and 15 seconds' clearing time in the fixer at room temperature.

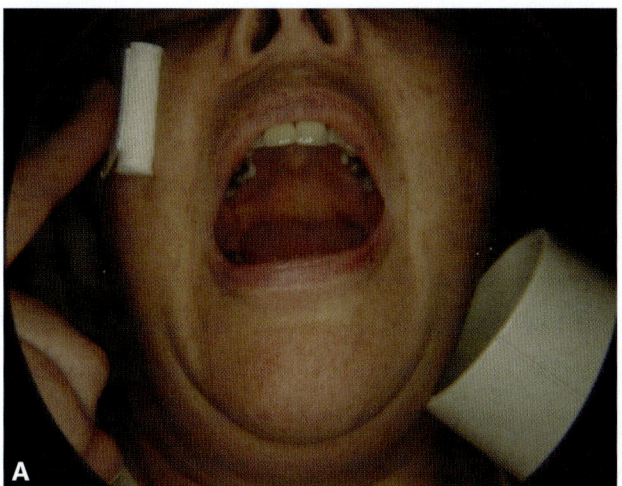 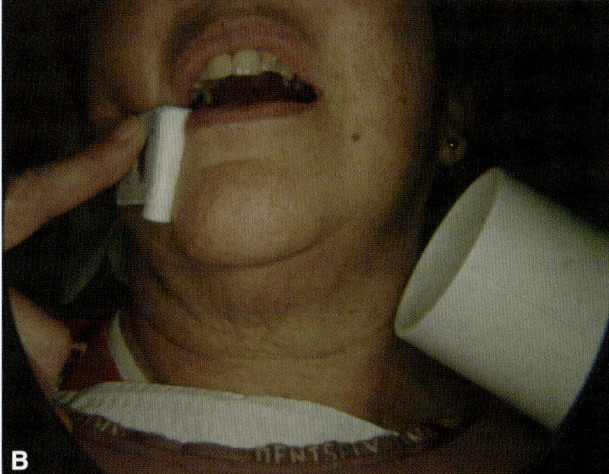

Figure 24 Extraoral film placement. Useful for patients who cannot accommodate or tolerate an intraoral film. The film or sensor is placed on the cheek. Increasing the exposure time is necessary—approximately double. **A,** Maxillary posterior: The cone is positioned a negative 45° to the occlusal plane. **B,** Mandibular posterior: The cone is positioned a negative 35°.

Four rapid-developing solutions were compared, processing both Ultraspeed and Ektaspeed films. Film fog became a problem as the solutions deteriorated with time. Kodak Rapid Access had to be changed every day, whereas the other solutions, Colitts (Buffalo Dental, Syosset, NY), IFP, and Instaneg (Neo-Flo, Inc., Chicago, IL, USA), deteriorated over 60 days. Developing time and 3 to 5 seconds' rinse time between developing and fixing are essential.[33] These rapidly processed films will fade or discolor with time.[34] This change can be prevented, after viewing, by returning the wet film for a few minutes of fixation, followed by washing for 30 minutes, and then drying. The films will then retain their quality indefinitely.

TABLE-TOP DEVELOPING

For quick turnaround and ease of processing, combining rapid-speed solutions with a *table-top processing hood* greatly improves radiographic reporting, particularly working films. These hoods are often used right in the operatory. The film is passed through light-proof cuffs; hand movement is seen through the red Plexiglas cover. The rapid solutions and rinse water can be in small cups.

References

1. Ennis LM, Berry HM. Dental roentgenology. 5th ed. Philadelphia: Lea & Febiger; 1959. p. 13.
2. Glenner RA. Eighty years of dental radiography. J Am Dent Assoc 1975;90:549.
3. Lambrianidis T, Lyroudia K, Pandelidou O, Nicolaou A. Evaluation of periapical radiographs in the recognition of C-shaped mandibular second molars. Int Endod J 2001;34:458.
4. Ricucci D, Mannocci F, Ford T. A study of periapical lesions correlating the presence of a radiopaque lamina with histological findings. Oral Surg Oral Med Oral Pathol Oral Radiol Endod 2006;101:389.
5. Baumann L, Rossman SR. Clinical roentgenologic and histopathologic findings in teeth with apical radiolucent areas. Oral Surg Oral Med Oral Pathol Oral Radiol Endod 1956;9:1330.
6. Linenberg WB, Waldron CA, DeLaune GF. A clinical, roentgenographic and histologic evaluation of periradicular areas. Oral Surg Oral Med Oral Pathol Oral Radiol Endod 1964;17:467.
7. LaLonde ER. A new rationale for the management of periradicular granulomas and cysts: an evaluation of histopathological and radiographic findings. J Am Dent Assoc 1970;80:1056.
8. Ardran GM. Bone destruction not demonstrable by roentgenography. Br J Radiol 1951;24:107.
9. Bender IB, Seltzer S. Roentgenographic and direct observation of experimental lesions of bone. J Am Dent Assoc 1961;62:153.
10. Lee S, Messer H. Radiographic appearance of artificially prepared periapical lesions confined to cancellous bone. Int Endod J 1986;19:64.
11. Schwartz SF, Foster JK. Roentgenographic interpretation of experimentally produced bony lesions. Oral Surg Oral Med Oral Pathol Oral Radiol Endod 1971;32(Pt I):606.
12. Goldman M, Pearson A, Darzenta N. Endodontic success—who's reading the radiograph? Oral Surg Oral Med Oral Pathol Oral Radiol Endod 1972;23:432.

13. Holtzman D, Johnson W, Southard T, et al. Storage-phosphor computed radiography versus film radiography in the detection of pathological periradicular bone loss in cadavers. Oral Surg Oral Med Oral Pathol Oral Radiol Endod 1998;86:90.
14. Akdeniz B, Sogur B. An ex vivo comparison of conventional and digital radiography for perceived image quality of root fillings. Int Endod J 2005;38:397.
15. Burger C, Mork T, Hutter J, et al. Direct digital radiography versus conventional radiography for estimation of canal length in curved canals. J Endod 1999;25:260.
16. Scarfe W, Czerniejewski W, Farman A, et al. *In vivo* accuracy and reliability in color-coded image enhancements for the assessment of periradicular lesion dimensions. Oral Surg Oral Med Oral Pathol Oral Radiol Endod 1999;88:603.
17. Baker W, Loushine R, West L. Interpretation of artificial and *in vivo* periapical bone lesions comparing conventional viewing versus a video conferencing system. J Endod 2000;26:39.
18. Fitzgerald GM. Dental roentgenography I: an investigation in adumbration, or the factors that control geometric unsharpness. J Am Dent Assoc 1947;34:1.
19. Fitzgerald GM. Dental roentgenography II: vertical angulation, film placement and increased object-film distance. J Am Dent Assoc 1947;34:160.
20. Waggener DT. The right-angle technique using the extension cone. Dent Clin North Am 1968;783.
21. Forsberg J. A comparison of the paralleling and bisecting-angle radiographic techniques in endodontics. Int Endod J 1987;20:177.
22. Girsch WJ, Matteson SR, McKee MN. An evaluation of Kodak Ektaspeed periradicular film for use in endodontics. J Endod 1983;9:282.
23. Kleier DJ, Benner SJ, Averbach RE. Two dental X-ray films compared for rater preference using endodontic views. Oral Surg Oral Med Oral Pathol Oral Radiol Endod 1985;59:201.
24. Donnelly JC, Hartwell GR, Johnson WB. Clinical evaluation of Ektaspeed X-ray film for use in endodontics. J Endod 1985;11:90.
25. Jarvis WD, Pifer R, Griffen J, Skidmore A, et al. Evaluation of image quality in individual films of double film packs. Oral Surg Oral Med Oral Pathol Oral Radiol Endod 1990;69:764.
26. Barr JH, Gron P. Palate contour as a limiting factor in intraoral X-ray technique. Oral Surg Oral Med Oral Pathol Oral Radiol Endod 1959;12:459.
27. Walton RE. Endodontic radiographic techniques. Dent Radiogr Photogr 1973;46:51.
28. Clark CA. A method of ascertaining the relative position of unerupted teeth by means of film radiographs. Odont Sec R Soc Med Trans 1909–1910;3:87.
29. Goerig AC, Neaverth EJ. A simplified look at the buccal object rule in endodontics. J Endod 1987;13:570.
30. Grady JR, Clausen H. Establishing your point. Clinic Am Assoc Endod New Orleans, LA 1975.
31. Newman M, Friedman S. Extraoral radiographic technique: an alternative approach. J Endod 2003:29:419.
32. Ingle JI, Beveridge EE, Olson C. Rapid processing of endodontic "working" films. Oral Surg Oral Med Oral Pathol Oral Radiol Endod 1965;19:101.
33. Kaffe I, Gratt BM. E-speed dental films processed with rapid chemistry: a comparison with D-speed film. Oral Surg Oral Med Oral Pathol Oral Radiol Endod 1987;64:367.
34. Maddalozzo D, Knoeppel RO, Schoenfeld CM. Performance of seven rapid radiographic processing solutions. Oral Surg Oral Med Oral Pathol Oral Radiol Endod 1990;69:382.

Chapter 15B

B. Digital Imaging for Endodontics

Allan G. Farman, Ramya Ramamurthy, Lars G. Hollender

Many acronyms have come about as a result of the development of technology in radiography and the need for terms to describe concepts. The following glossary of the acronyms used in this chapter will assist the reader in understanding these new concepts.

Glossary of Acronyms

AEC: Automatic Exposure Compensation is an enhancement feature that compensates for image variations due to exposure.

ALARA: Acronym for "As Low As Reasonably Achievable," an important principle in radiation protection.

CBCT: Cone-Beam Computed Tomography is a 3D imaging device that integrates a series of transmission images taken over an arc of 180° or greater.

CBVCT: Cone-Beam Volumetric Computed Tomography (synonym of CBCT).

CCD: A Charge-Coupled Device is an image sensor consisting of an integrated circuit containing an array of linked or coupled, energy-sensitive capacitors.

CDR: Computed Dental Radiography. Digital intraoral sensor manufactured by Schick Technologies (A Division of Sirona AG).

CMOS: Complementary Metal Oxide Semiconductor. This represents a major class of integrated circuits including image sensors.

CMOS-APS: CMOS Active Pixel System.

DICOM: Digital Imaging and Communication in Medicine. The internationally referenced standard for improving the likelihood of interoperability of diagnostic images by setting file format standards and transmission protocols.

dpi: Dots per inch.

H&D: Hurter and Driffield. Descriptor applied to a curve relating optical density to exposure for film photography and radiography.

IP: Imaging Plate. The sensor plate used for photostimulable phosphor (PSP) imaging.

ISO: International Standards Organization.

MB2: For maxillary molar, mesiobuccal root second canal.

PSP: Photostimulable phosphor. An imaging system using IPs that store energy from transmitted X-rays. The PSP IP is processed using laser scanning.

RVG: RadioVisioGraphy. Radiographic system proprietary to Kodak Dental Imaging: Term applied to the first commercial dental digital detector.

SNR: Signal-to-Noise Ratio.

TACT: Tuned Aperture Computed Tomography. A system developed by Richard Webber that integrates a series of transmission images taken from varying beam geometry to tomosynthesize a limited 3D perception.

The success of endodontic treatment is dependent on the identification of teeth requiring such treatment, and then the recognition of the root canal system, so it can be cleaned, shaped, and obturated.[1] Endodontic therapy relies on a series of radiographic images made at different stages of the treatment: preoperatively, periodically during instrumentation, and postoperatively. Radiographs provide important clues about hard and soft tissues of the teeth, including the pulp chamber and root canals. They also facilitate the estimation of root canal length. Furthermore, they aid in detecting tooth fractures and foreign bodies following trauma, provide useful information of the periradicular region, and assist in evaluating post-treatment healing. Hence, radiography is an important adjunct to endodontic diagnosis and image-guided treatment. The use of digital technologies can facilitate the process by speeding image acquisition and display.

The first dental radiograph is attributed to Walkhoff of Braunschweig, Germany, who on January 14, 1896 made images of the crowns of teeth on both sides of his own jaw using silver halide emulsion on glass plates.[2] The exposure time was 25 minutes. The thickness and rigidity of the glass plate were akin to those of present-day solid-state digital X-ray detectors; today, however, acquisition can be as fast as one-tenth of a second.

Edison invented the fluoroscope as film imaging was obviously too slow in the 1890s; Eastman, founder of the Eastman Kodak Corporation, was quick to point out, though, that the fluoroscope could not fit inside the mouth. He tasked Stuber, a future President of Eastman Kodak, with the development of a silver halide X-ray film specifically for dentistry.[3] Eastman Kodak produces this product to this day.[3-8]

Kells, in 1899, was among the first to use a radiograph to determine tooth length during root canal therapy.[9] One year later, Price drew attention to incomplete root canal therapies resulting in failure as evidenced by radiographs.[9] The discovery of the X-ray laid a foundation for a new era in the field of endodontics. It took more than eight decades for the next major advance in dental X-ray sensor technology to occur; a patent was issued in Europe to Mouyen in 1983 and in the United States in 1986.[10] Solid-state imaging, using indirect exposure of a charge-coupled device (CCD), became commercially available around 1989 in Europe, with FDA approval for use of the technology in the United States being granted later that same year.

The invention of digital intraoral radiography has "endodontic roots." In the 1970s Mouyen, then a dental student at the University of Toulouse, France, tells the story that because the distance between the endodontic clinic and the film processors several floors below spurred the idea of finding a way to create instant X-ray images for "operative" purposes. Mouyen realized that the chip in his video camera could detect light and that X-rays could be converted to light by scintillators such as the screens used in extraoral radiography cassettes. In other words, almost 90 years after the discovery of the X-ray, available technology could indeed permit the placement of a "fluoroscope" in the patient's mouth.

A few years following graduation as a dentist, Mouyen[10] completed the DERSO—a French equivalent to the PhD in engineering—and went on to develop a prototype digital radiographic system that he named RadioVisioGraphy (RVG). The RVG patent was licensed by a French Company, Trophy Radiologie, and digital imaging for operative radiology in dentistry was born (Figure 1). In 1989, in a special issue of the "National Geographic," celebrating the bicentennial of the French Revolution, the RVG was included among 10 major French inventions, alongside such inventions as the Train Grand Vitesse (TVG), the Concorde, and the Arienne space rocket. Trophy Radiologie has since been acquired by Kodak Dental Imaging.

Since 1989, there have been seven new generations of RVG, and there are now many alternate solid-state systems (e.g., Figure 2) that can produce almost instant images electronically. Although these images are essentially "instant," most are not "direct" as the solid-state systems, for the most part, employ a scintillator to convert X-rays to light, and it is the analog light signal that is then converted to a digital image.

Furthermore, it is possible to replace silver halide film by photostimulable phosphor (PSP) plates that interact directly with X-rays but require the added step of subsequent processing by laser scanning to convert the latent image to one that can be viewed on a computer monitor screen.

Digital Intraoral X-Ray Imaging Options

DIGITIZATION USING SECONDARY CAPTURE OF ANALOG FILM IMAGES

Conventional X-ray films consist of a polyester sheet covered on both sides by a thin layer of silver halide emulsion that absorbs X-ray photons resulting in a latent image. When the latent image is developed using developing chemicals, the silver halide crystals are converted into metallic silver (silver is not black but gives such an impression in granular from within the processed radiograph). The unexposed crystals are later removed from the emulsion during the fixing process. This procedure, including the unpacking of the film in a light safe environment, usually takes several minutes and can produce a visible image of high diagnostic quality even when automatic processing is utilized, as long as optimal procedures are employed. Unfortunately, optimal procedures are not always employed in dental practices. To digitize the analog film image adds another time-consuming step, and the extra step also leads to the possibility of impaired image quality.

Once a visible film-based image has been produced, it is possible to use a flat bed scanner with a

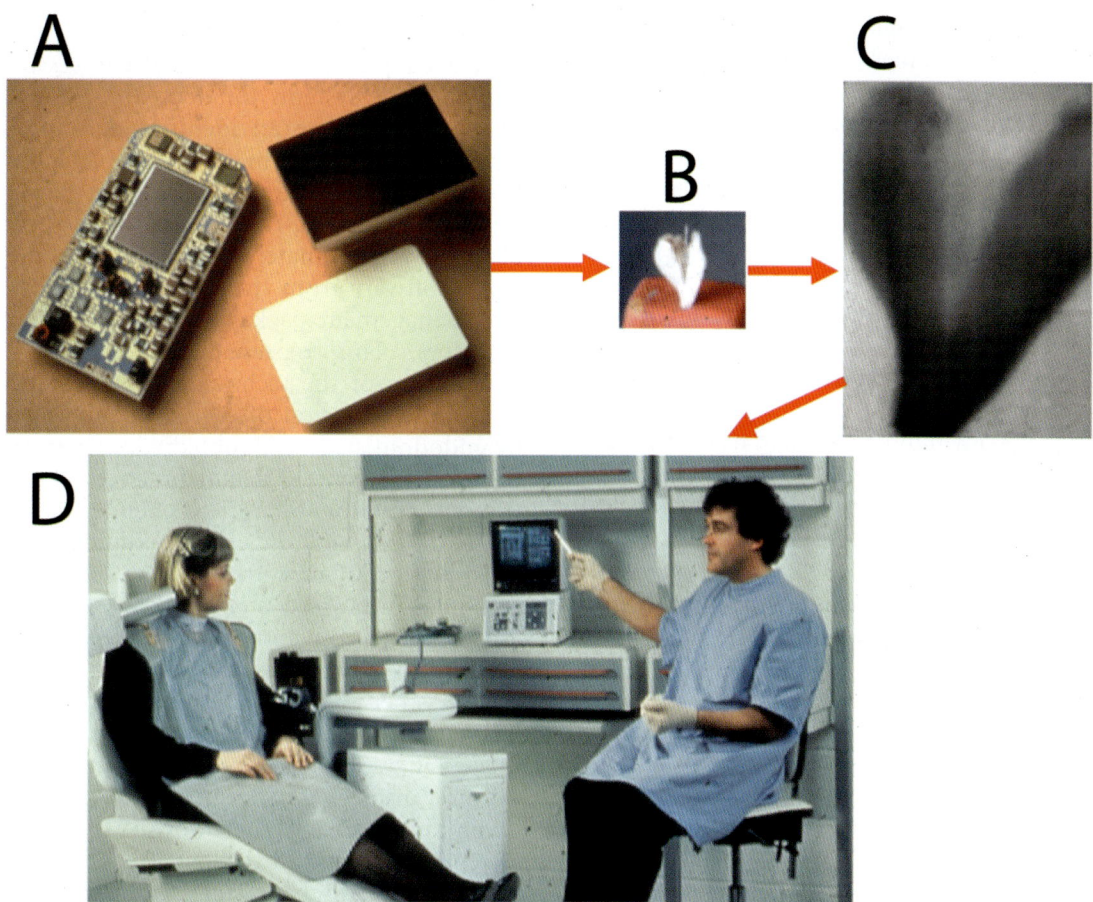

Figure 1 *A,* Components of the RadioVisioGraphy (RVG)-32000 showing the solid-state electronics board with charge-coupled device (CCD) chip, the scintillator, and the fiber optic plate used to reduce the size of the image to the size of the CCD. The fiber optic was made of tungsten glass that protected the CCD from direct exposure to X-rays. *B,* Primary tooth of Mouyen's daughter. *C,* The first "clinical" RVG image achieved in Dr. Mouyen's living room of this tooth. *D,* Commercial version of the RVG with Mouyen himself in the blue gown.

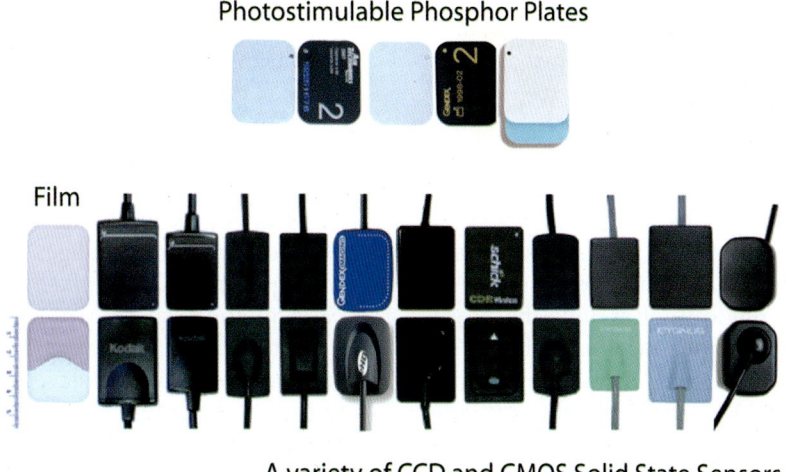

Figure 2 Demonstration of the diversity of available intraoral X-ray sensors.

transparency adaptor to digitize the image by secondary capture. Flat bed scanners are preferred over cameras as the latter is more prone to optical distortion and added noise from light reflected from the surface of the radiograph film. For scanning, the parameters should be set at high-definition grayscale images and scanned at a minimum of 300 dots per inch (dpi) using a transparency adaptor and acquisition software parameters set to "transparency." Secondary capture images are dependent on the person making the input and associate such information as right versus left, patient name, procedure date, and so forth. This can be subject to "human error."

Conventional X-ray film has survived more than 110 years in dental radiography. It obviously is capable of providing useful diagnostic information. However, disadvantages of analog X-ray film include the following:

1. Inefficiency as photon detectors, therefore requiring a relatively high radiation exposure.
2. Film packet is thin and can be felt by the patient to "cut into the tissues."
3. Film is not rigid and hence can bend resulting in a distorted radiographic image.
4. Produce static images with no availability of post-image treatments other than varying the brightness of the viewbox illumination.
5. Exposure errors and suboptimal processing conditions can result in poor image quality that is not immediately obvious.
6. Film processing is relatively time-consuming.
7. Costs for maintaining a darkroom.
8. Silver in spent processing chemicals has the potential to cause environmental pollution.
9. Duplicate radiograph in a double film packet is of very slightly lower density compared with the top film. Physicochemical duplication of film radiographs results in copies of higher contrast and less detail.
10. Archiving radiographic film radiographs in physical patient files requires extra storage space in the office. Retrieving radiographs can take time.
11. Intraoral film radiographs not appropriately mounted and labeled cannot in themselves be associated for certainty with a given patient or time of exposure. Although one cannot exclude the possibility that digital radiographs may be attributed to the wrong patient, the use of a Digital Imaging and Communications in Medicine (DICOM) file format that is appropriately populated makes this less likely to occur.

DIGITAL RADIOGRAPHY

Figure 2 represents some recent choices in intraoral digital X-ray systems for dentistry. Several of these systems may share an identical detector; however, they generally differ in electronics and the application software supplied. There is increasing acceptance of filmless X-ray alternatives in dentistry. As of 2006, approximately 28% to 40% of US dentists using software from the three top vendors of practice management packages were using digital X-ray detectors. This represented a fivefold increased penetration of the technology over the past 2 to 3 years. The adoption of digital imaging technologies by endodontists is undoubtedly much greater than is the case for general dental practice. With the continuous addition of improvements and sophistications in the already existing digital systems and introduction of new systems, the diagnostic quality of digital intraoral systems is now generally considered equal to conventional X-ray film even for tasks where film is known to do well such as in endodontic assessment and detection of proximal dental caries.[11]

Digital systems utilize computer technology in the capture, display, enhancement, and storage of radiographic images. Computers work on the binary number system consisting of two digits (0 and 1) to represent data. These two characters are called bits (binary digits), and they form "words" of eight or more bits in length called bytes. The total number of possible bytes for 8-bit language is $2^8 = 256$. The analog-to-digital converter (ADC) transforms analog data to digital data based on binary number system. The strength of the output signal is measured and assigned a number from 0 (black or white depending on designation) to 255 (white or black—opposite of "0") according to the intensity of the electric signal. These numeric assignments translate into 256 shades of gray in an 8-bit system. A digital image consists of a number of pixels (picture elements), and each pixel is represented by a number corresponding to its gray level. The pixel is the smallest picture element of the image, and the resolution of an image is directly related to the pixel size among other factors. Images of 12, 14, or 16 bits will have a greater range of pixel values and also consume greater memory space of the computer. For instance, a 12-bit image can have a range up to 4,096 gray values, and window and level adjustments can permit selection of the gray levels to be displayed on the monitor as the latter is usually restricted to 256 gray levels at one time.

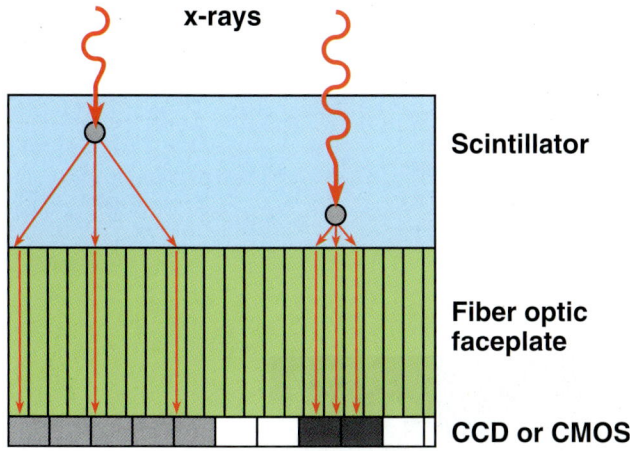

Figure 3 Indirect solid-state X-ray sensor using a scintillator to convert X-rays to light photons. The image represents a small section of such a sensor.

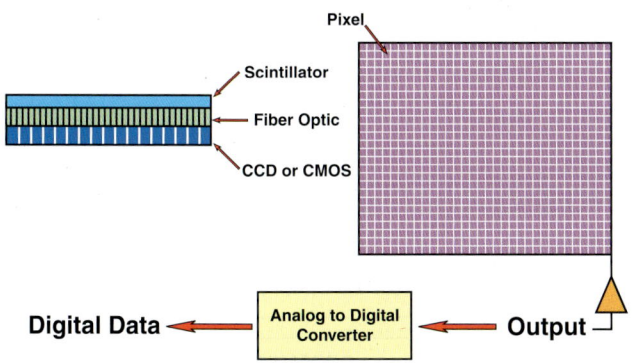

Figure 4 Solid-state sensor process. With the charge-coupled device (CCD), the pixel wells are read out in sequence, whereas with the complimentary metal oxide semiconductor (CMOS), each pixel can be read independently.

The two major technologies presently used in intraoral digital X-ray systems are as follows:

1. Solid-state detectors (Figures 3 and 4)
    a. Charge-coupled device (CCD)
    b. Complimentary metal oxide semiconductor (CMOS)

Solid-state detectors (CCD and CMOS) can be indirect detectors using a scintillating screen such as cesium iodide or gadolinium oxysulfide, or (less commonly) can use direct conversion of X-ray photons to electrons (e.g., Cadmium-Telluride technology).

2. Storage phosphor detectors (Figures 5 and 6)
    a. Photostimulable phosphor (PSP)

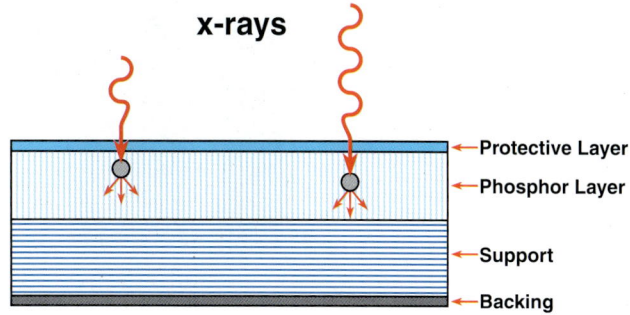

Figure 5 The intraoral photostimulable phosphor (PSP) is composed of a phosphor layer, a thin protective layer, support, and backing. X-ray energy is stored during exposure and subsequently released as photoluminescence on application of energy from a scanning laser. The emitted light is photomultiplied and then converted to an electronic signal that is digitized. (Note that this figure is of the PSP during exposure only and represents only a small section of a PSP.)

Working Principles of Digital Systems[12]

SOLID-STATE SYSTEMS

Charge-Coupled Device

The CCD is composed of an electronic circuit embedded in several thin layers of silicon. The silicon chip usually is composed of an array of light sensitive pixels (picture elements), and each pixel consists of a small electron well into which the X-ray or light energy is deposited upon exposure. Each silicon atom in the detector chip is covalent with another silicon atom. When light photons strike the silicon and the energy exceeds the strength of the covalent bond, an electron hole pair is formed. Alternatively, electrons can be produced by a coating layer when direct technology is used instead of a scintillator layer. Either way, an electric charge is established by release of electrons. The electric charge in each "pixel" well is proportional to the incident X-ray or photon energy. Charge-coupling is a process by which the electrons from one well are transferred to another in a sequential manner, and this transfer concept has been compared to a "bucket brigade." The charge of each pixel is converted from an analog electric signal representing the energy absorbed by the solid-state chip to a digital signal representing the discrete numeric pixel values for image display on a computer monitor.

Complimentary Metal Oxide Semiconductor Active Pixel Technology (CMOS-APS)

CMOS chips are commonly used in digital cameras, video cameras, and computers. Externally, CMOS

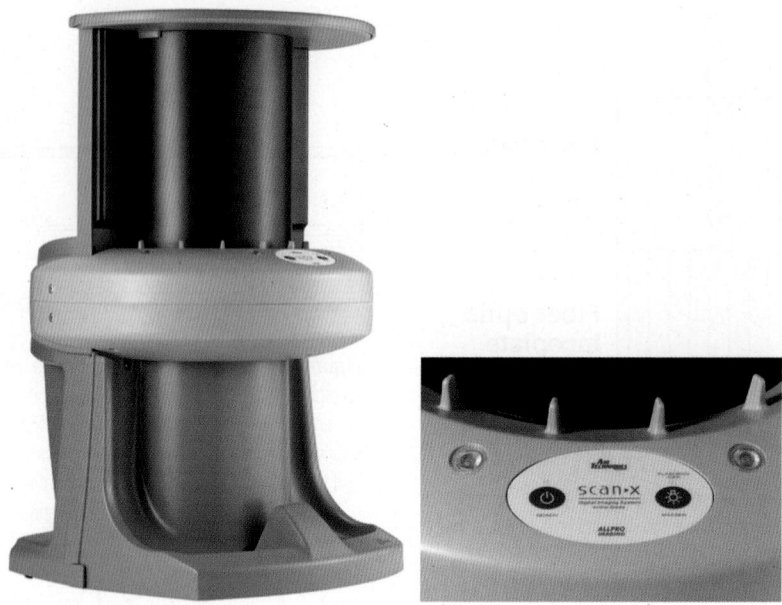

Figure 6 Example of a photostimulable phosphor (PSP) laser scanner (Scan-X; Air Techniques, NY). Detail shows loading area for the individual PSPs. Scanners come in a variety of sizes and configurations from the various vendors of this technology.

detectors appear similar to CCDs, but the former use an active pixel technology, that is, each CMOS-APS has an active transistor built into each pixel and provides a reduction by a factor of up to 100 in the system power (translating into electric voltage) required when compared with CCDs. This has permitted the introduction of wireless radio frequency (RF) transmission of the acquired image. Other advantages of the CMOS-APS include design integration and a potential for relatively low cost manufacture that, however, has not so far translated into cost savings for the consumer. In addition, the APS system eliminates the need for charge transfer between adjacent pixel wells extending the exposure latitude by suppressing "pixel blooming."

STORAGE PHOSPHOR DETECTORS

Photostimulable Phosphor

The PSP imaging plate (Figure 7) works on the principle of radiation-induced emission of photostimulated luminance. PSPs generally contain barium fluorohalide crystals with small amounts of bivalent europium atoms as an activator. When a storage phosphor imaging plate is exposed to X-radiation, the europium atoms in the phosphor crystalline lattice are ionized liberating a valence electron. This results in the formation of electron vacancy. The valence electrons are exited to the level of conduction band where they travel

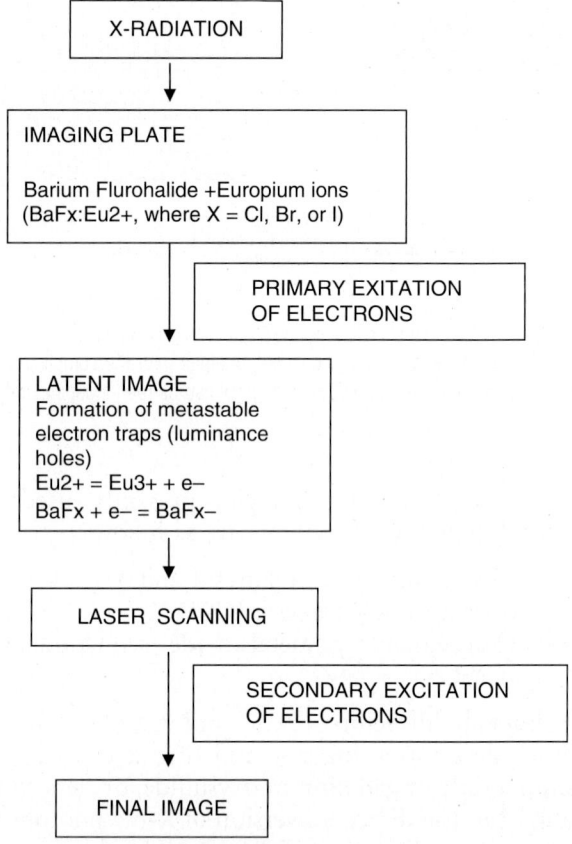

Figure 7 Flow diagram to demonstrate the sequence involved in the formation of a photostimulable phosphor (PSP) image.

freely until trapped by so-called Farbzentren centers present in halide crystals to form metastable electrons with an energy level slightly lower than the conduction band but greater than that of the valence bond. These trapped metastable electrons constitute the latent image and their number is proportional to the number of incident X-rays. When the latent image is exposed to the red light of solid state laser, the metastable electrons are again exited to reach high-energy conduction band where they recombine with Eu^{3+} atoms and return to low-energy valence bond ($Eu^{3+} + e^- = Eu^{2+}$). This results in the liberation of energy, emitted as blue light. The light is registered by a photo multiplier tube and converted into an analog electric output signal that is digitized, resulting in a digital image. Each pixel has a numeric value that is proportional to the amount to light emitted from the corresponding area of the PSP imaging plate.

Advantages of Digital X-Ray Imaging

Potential advantages of digital X-ray over analog film imaging include the following:

1. Reduced time between exposure and image formation when using solid-state detectors.
2. Reduced radiation dose per image sometimes possible.
3. Multiple exposures, from various angles, both vertical and horizontal, may be made without moving the sensor once positioned.
4. Elimination of chemical processing and disposal of spent chemicals.
5. Images can be duplicated any number of time without any loss of image quality (each is a perfect clone of the original).
6. Images can be stored and retrieved electronically.
7. Images can be transmitted electronically for referrals and other purposes.
8. Dynamic nature of the image with the ready option of post-imaging enhancements.
9. Digital systems also have measurement tools that given a suitably positioned fiducial reference (e.g., an endodontic instrument of known length placed in a root canal) can accurately measure, for example, the root canal working length.
10. Reusable detector reduces expenditure on consumables.
11. With DICOM image file usage, digital images can provide greater security regarding radiographic image integrity and tags include such information as patient name, date of exposure, and laterality.
12. Wired detectors have an advantage when working on special needs patients as the wire makes swallowing or ingesting the detector unlikely.

Potential Disadvantages of Digital Imaging over Films

There are also some potentially negative issues that should be considered:

1. Relatively high initial investment cost if the practice has previously sunk costs in film-processing facilities.
2. Issues related to infection control as the detectors cannot be autoclaved.
3. Solid-state detectors are somewhat thicker and more rigid (however, this can also be an advantage in preventing disproportionate distortion from film bending).
4. Packaged PSP imaging plates (IPs) are thinner than prepackaged analog intraoral X-ray films and may not be held firmly in position in film holders.
5. As most current versions of CCD and CMOS detectors are wired, this could create patient psychological discomfort. It might also be a drawback for the inexperienced operator, requiring adjustments in technique and patience through the learning curve of a new methodology.
6. Competency using software may take time to master. The learning curve may be longer or shorter depending on the computer literacy of the operator.
7. With PSPs, the intraoral imaging plates have been prone to mechanical degradation necessitating replacement of plates to sustain image quality.
8. Although unlikely to occur given reasonable diligence, mishandling can cause mechanical damage with high replacement costs for CCD and CMOS detectors.

Examples of Digital Images Used in Endodontics

It is now appropriate to illustrate some examples of digital radiographic images used in the practice of endodontics so one might get a better appreciation of attainable image quality (Figures 8–10). It should, however, be remembered that the printed page is static and does not permit the modifications to image

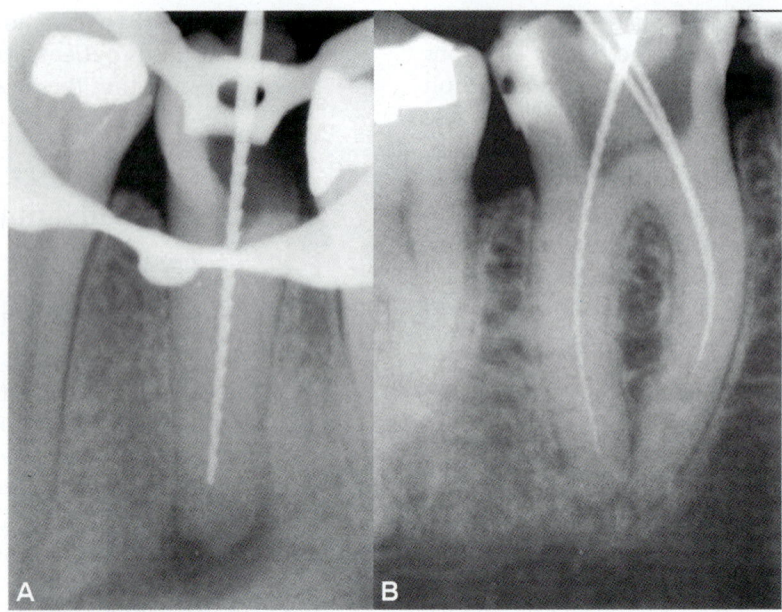

Figure 8 ***A,*** Endodontic instruments in a mandibular second premolar tooth with a radiolucent periapical pathosis. ***B,*** Mandibular molar with slight widening of the apical periodontal ligament space of the distal root. These images were made using the DentX Eva (CMOS) system from AFP/DentX (New York).

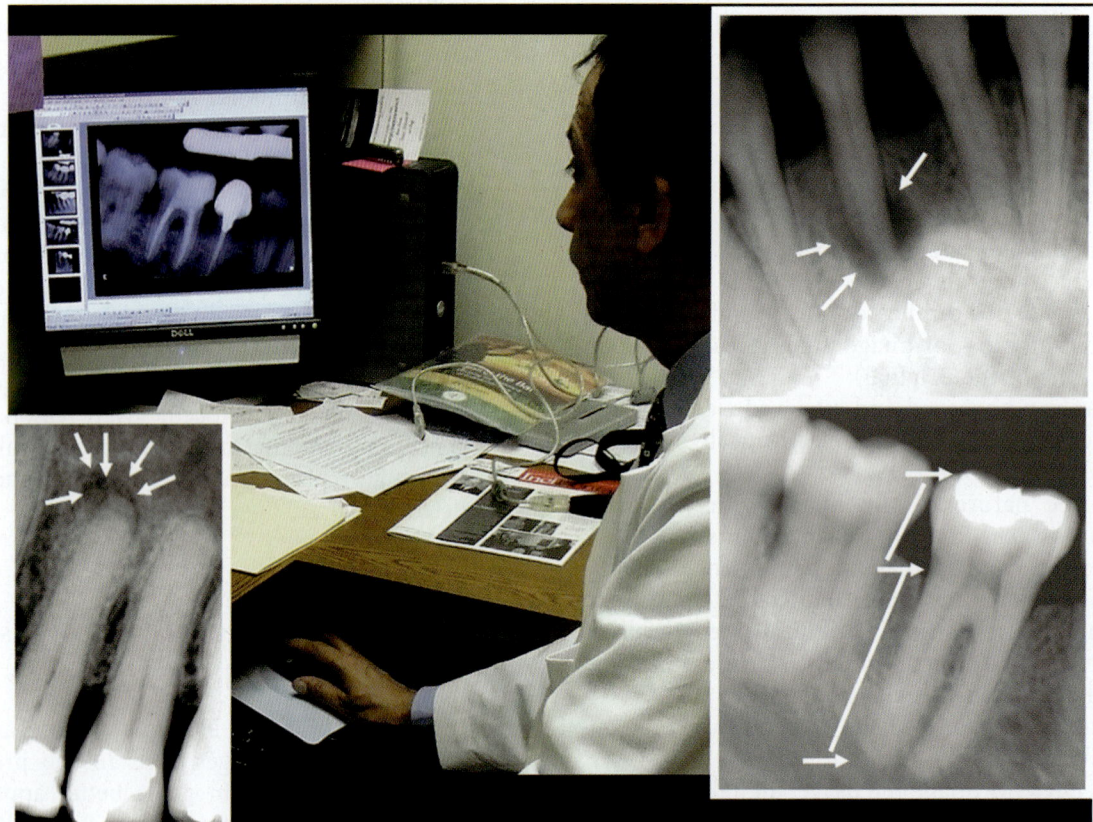

Figure 9 Endodontic evaluations using the Kodak RVG-6000 (Kodak Dental Imaging, Marne-la-Vallée, France) CMOS system. These details clearly demonstrate the ability of solid-state sensors to demonstrate periapical lesions and tooth length (even with long root length in rhizodontia).

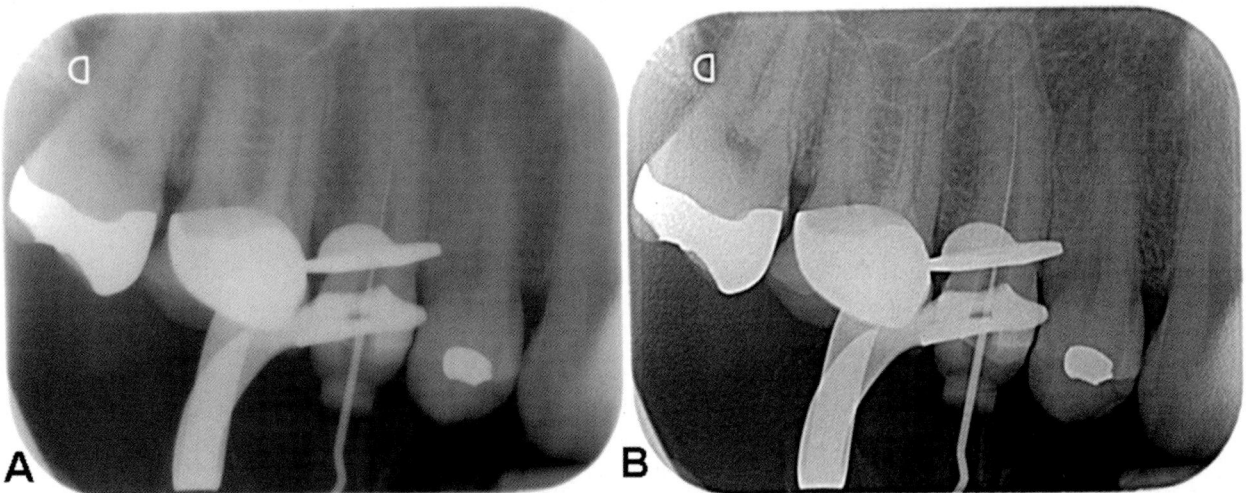

Figure 10 Dürr Vista-Scan photostimulable phosphor image of endodontic instrument in place in tooth: **A,** Without enhancement. **B,** With high pass sharpness filter applied.

density and contrast that are available when the digital images are viewed on the computer monitor.

CONVENTIONAL VERSUS DIGITAL: WHICH IS BETTER?

With the introduction of digital imaging systems in dentistry, a question arises: "How effective are these systems when compared with film for specific diagnostic tasks in endodontic practice?" The reported studies are rather consistent and have shown that the diagnostic ability of the digital image is equivalent to film-based radiographs as referenced in the subsequent sections of this chapter. The following discussion concentrates on investigations concerning diagnostic tasks in endodontology.

DETECTION OF PERIAPICAL LESIONS

Accurate assessment of the periradicular status is crucial in diagnosis, treatment, and evaluation of healing in endodontic therapy. However, from some reported studies, it is believed that periapical lesion cannot be detected until a comparatively advanced bone destruction, that is, not until the lesion erodes the junction between cortical and cancellous bone.[13,14] Alternatively, it has been postulated that changes in the lamina dura are key to the detection of periapical lesions.[15,16] Several studies have evaluated the efficacy of digital images in detecting periradicular bone changes. Most of the studies, concluded that digital imaging did not increase the rate of detection of lesions.[15,17–20] Paurazas et al.,[19] for instance, found no difference in diagnostic accuracy between film radiographs, CCD, and CMOS-APS systems in detecting periradicular lesions. However, the use of CMOS-APS system has been supported because of perceived functional advantages over CCD systems such as "low cost," reduced electric power requirement, and suggested increased life time of the product. Digital imaging was preferred over film-based imaging as the former, according to one report, requires 50% less radiation than the latter.

In 1994, Yokota et al.[17] studied mechanically created lesions in human cadaver specimens using film radiographs and an early vintage RVG CCD X-ray detector. It was concluded that (1) when no lesion exists, conventional radiograph were more accurate than the vintage RVG; (2) when the lesion is enlarged to involve lamina dura and medullary bone, the vintage RVG was superior; and (3) when the lesion involved the cortical bone, there was no difference between a conventional radiograph and vintage RVG. This study was in agreement with a similar study conducted by Tirrell et al.[21]

It has been reported that digital images have been found to be more accurate than conventional radiographs when image enhancements are performed.[22] In another study, image processing was found to be of limited value on diagnostic quality, but altering the basic functions such as contrast and brightness were preferred for the detection of periapical lesions.[23] However, Wallace et al.[24] concluded that enhanced digital images perform inferior to film-based images in periapical lesion detection. This was attributed to the observers' lack of familiarity with digital images and lack of experience with the image enhancement procedures.

Other image-processing functions such as color enhancement and reverse imaging have been found to be of limited diagnostic value in the detection of periapical lesions.[25] In this context, it should be noted that many times the enhancement leads to worse performance, although the subjective impression is that of improvement. It should be remembered that when enhancements are applied, they generally hide information, thereby making certain features stand out. Also many studies have used rather underexposed films or digital detectors, before the enhancement of the digital images leading to improved performance of the digital system. One has to caution the readers about these inherent fallacies and also point out the great variation sometimes reported among observers in periapical radiographic diagnosis. When high variability between observers is present, one can predict that the studies concerned will result in no proven differences between the modalities compared. Woolhiser et al.[26] even reported great variation in the seemingly straightforward task of estimation of root length, with variations for the same observation being as great as 1.5 to 8 mm. Nevertheless, they did conclude that observers using enhanced digital images outperformed the same observers using conventional radiographs.

EVALUATION OF ASSESSMENT OF ROOT CANAL LENGTH

A too short working length can result in infected tissue being left in the root canal, and this can then continue to damage the periapical tissue. Hence, a correct estimation of working length is crucial for endodontic success. The radiographic apex does not always coincide with true apex. Even though, the ISO recommended smallest file size for a working length radiograph is #15, files smaller than #15 are required for initial instrumentation in fine, curved, and calcified canals to prevent root perforation or ledge formation within the canal. The problem encountered with small-sized files is that the instrument tip will not always be clearly visible on a radiograph. Comparative studies have been conducted between film radiographs and digital detectors to evaluate their accuracy in estimating endodontic length and perceived clarity in visualizing fine endodontic files. It has been reported that digital systems closely approximate film radiographs in the accuracy they provide for practitioners in estimating root length.[27,28] However, digital images were found to be inferior to film images when #10 rather than #15 files are used.[29,30]

Cederberg et al.[31] compared the difference in interpretation of the position of endodontic file tips between PSP imaging (Digora; Soredex, Helsinki, Finland) and intraoral radiographic film (Ektaspeed Plus; Kodak, Rochester, NY) for a limited number of patients ($n = 13$). Film radiographs were viewed using a 7× measuring magnifier. PSP was reported to outperform film radiographs in that a smaller difference was found between the file tip and root apex with digital imaging.

Eikenberg and Vandre[28] sectioned human skulls into 15 sextants. Teeth were then removed and 45 canals were instrumented to their apical foramina. Endodontic files were glued in place at random distances from the apical foramina. Image geometry was maintained by a custom mounting jig. Images were captured with two types of analog film and a solid-state digital radiographic system (Dexis). Digital images were read on a conventional color monitor (cathode ray tube) and a laptop screen (active-matrix liquid crystal display). Fifteen dentists measured the distance from the file tip to the apical foramen of the tooth. Results showed that the measurement error was significantly less for the digital images than for the film radiographs.

Martinez-Lozano et al.[32] evaluated the diagnostic efficacy of an electronic system for the determination of working length, in comparison with two radiologic methods (conventional film and digital radiography). The study sample consisted of 28 root canals in 20 human mandibular teeth. A comparison was made between the working length measurements obtained by the radiologic methods and an apex locator, using as "gold standard" the observation of the actual file position within the root following selective grinding of the root tissue. It was concluded that none of the techniques was totally satisfactory in establishing the true working length. No statistical differences were proven comparing the techniques investigated.

DETECTION OF ROOT CANAL ANATOMY

Success of endodontic treatment depends mainly on the identification of all the canals in the tooth that can then be cleaned, shaped, and obturated. The ability to locate all the canals is crucial in determining the eventual success of the therapy, and radiographs are considered one of the important tools apart from clinical examination. Reported studies are contradictory to one another. Naoum et al.[33] compared conventional with PSP images to visualize the root canal system contrasted with radiographic contrast medium. The image clarity on conventional radiographs was found to be better than with Digora PSP images.

Nance et al.[34] studied maxillary and mandibular molars using conventional D-speed film radiographs versus tuned aperture computed tomography (TACT) in the identification of root canals. TACT, using arrays of several digital images to tomosynthesize the third dimension, was reported to be superior to conventional film radiographs in the detection of root canal in molars. There was a reported 36% detection rate of the (elusive) second mesiobuccal canal (MB2) in maxillary molars and 80% detection rate of the mesiolingual canal in the mandibular molar using the TACT system. By contrast, with the film-based images, there was a somewhat unbelievable 0% detection of MB2 canals. This highly skewed result might be caused by using a standard paralleling technique for making conventional images, leading to overlap of canals.

In a similar study by Barton et al.,[35] parallax analog and parallax digital images were compared with TACT in the ability to detect MB2 canals in maxillary first molars. With TACT, there was 37.9% chance of locating the MB2 canal, which is consistent with the results of Nance's study. However, in this study, the success rate of detecting MB2 canals using film-based images was approximately equal to that using TACT, and TACT did not significantly affect the rate of detection of MB2 canals. It was also observed that the distance between first mesiobuccal and the MB2 canal is quite small and perhaps too minute for current TACT applications.

Stereoscopic radiographs might be helpful and would probably be superior to parallax radiographs viewed one by one. High-resolution cone-beam volumetric computed tomography (CBVCT) might provide a solution to this problem in the near future. The CBVCT characterization in three-dimensions of an apical dental cyst affecting the palatal root of a right maxillary first permanent molar tooth is demonstrated in Figure 11.

Recent studies using high-resolution CBVCT have shown that this technology might well have a role in defining the number of canals present in a tooth and the positions of the apical foramen.[36]

Digital Subtraction Radiography

Given radiographs taken in precisely the same position and with the same beam geometry and exposure parameters, images can be subtracted to show changes over time. This technique has been largely conducted for research purposes in view of the difficulties experienced in practice in achieving images with reproducible projection geometry over time.

Digital subtraction has been performed for endodontic tasks, and digital detectors have been used for this purpose (Figure 12).[37–39] Yoshioka et al.[37] evaluated the efficacy of digital subtraction radiography using an old version of the RVG system (RVG-S) in a follow-up study of endodontically treated teeth. The intra-image variation of the original RVG-S image caused by dark current and sensitivity variations among pixels in this vintage digital system was corrected pixel-to-pixel. The inter-image variation was further corrected using a copper step-wedge attached to the detector. Standardized images were obtained using the same beam geometry at patient follow-up. Pixel values at the regions of interest, positioned on the periapical lesion, increased after endodontic treatment, and this change continued during an observation period of up to 545 days. It was concluded that subtraction radiology is possible for the purpose of endodontic follow-up.

Nicopoulou-Karayianni et al.[38] also evaluated the effect of root canal treatment on periapical lesions by conventional and subtracted digital radiographic images of patients. Better observer agreement was achieved by digital subtraction radiography during the evaluation than without digital subtraction at follow-ups 3 to 12 months after treatment.

Mikrogeorgis et al.[39] evaluated the suitability of digital radiograph registration and subtraction in the assessment of the progress of chronic apical periodontitis. Ninety cases of teeth with chronic apical periodontitis were studied. In each case, a preoperative radiograph was made, root canals were prepared, and a calcium hydroxide paste was placed in the root canals. Radiographic control and replacement of calcium hydroxide paste took place at 15-day intervals before final obturation. The root canals were obturated 1.5 months after the first appointment, and recall radiographs were made 2 weeks, 6 weeks, 3, 6, and 12 months after the obturation. Digital radiography using a solid-state detector was employed. Changes to the periapical tissue structure were detectable using digital subtraction, even during short time intervals.

Radiation Dose

The ALARA (As Low As Reasonably Achievable) principle advocates the use of the smallest possible radiation dose that can still produce an image without compromising diagnostic quality. Conventional direct exposure emulsion X-ray films are relatively poor detectors of radiation and can require relatively high radiation dosages to produce images of optimal diagnostic value.

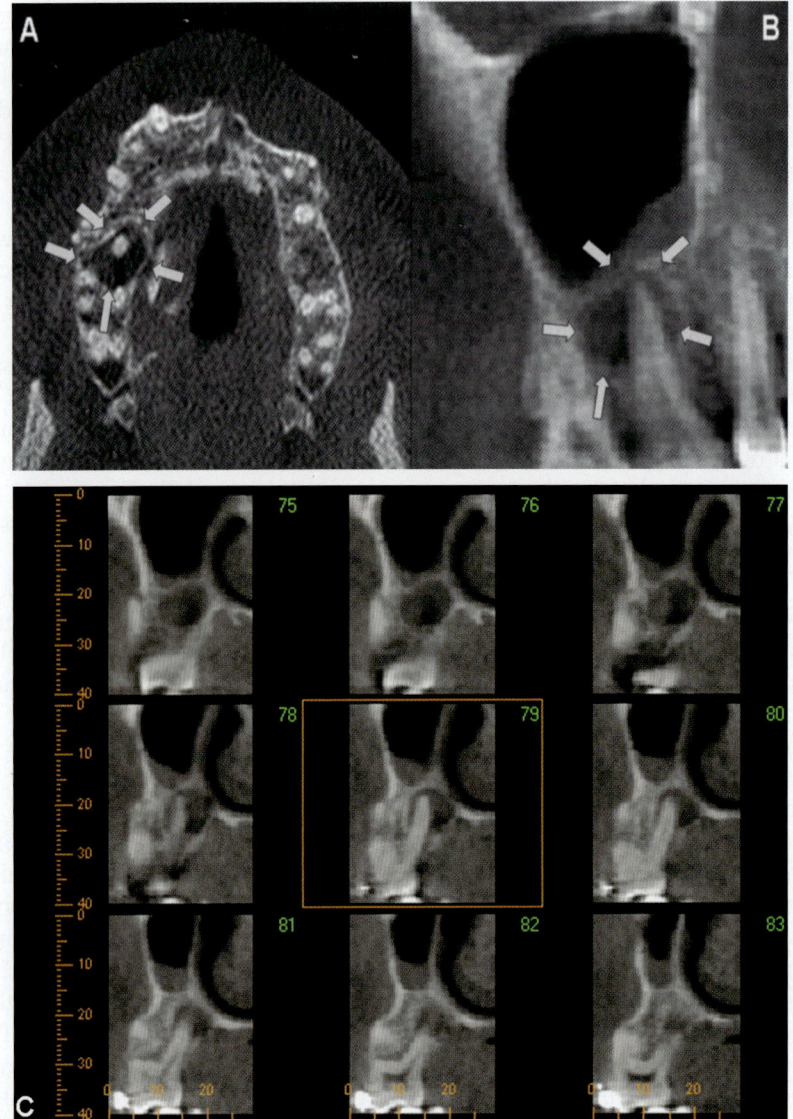

Figure 11 i-CAT cone-beam volumetric computed tomography (CBVCT) demonstrating an apical dental cyst (green arrows). ***A,*** Axial section through the lesion. ***B,*** Constructed panoramic detail (magnified) of the same lesion. ***C,*** Buccolingual cross-sections of the lesion at 1 mm intervals. The lesion is clearly demonstrated for clinical diagnosis despite the relatively low-resolution 0.4 mm scan that was used in this case where the cyst was an incidental finding. High-resolution images with isotrophic voxel dimensions of less than 0.1 mm can be performed with some CBVCT systems if needed to help in diagnosis.

By contrast, digital detectors can be more quantum efficient and, therefore, require lower radiation exposure. On the other hand, intraoral X-ray films are now available in higher speed than heretofore and this has greatly increased film's quantum efficiency to radiation. Hence, with the use of high-speed films, it is possible to obtain high-contrast images at relatively low exposure. Underexposing X-ray film still tends to increase radiographic "mottle" and graininess of the images, giving an impression of a lack of sharpness in the image.[40] This finding was supported by Sheaffer et al.,[41] who found that underexposed radiographs, in an attempt to minimize radiation dosage, result in inferior images irrespective of film speed.

With the invention of increasingly more efficient digital X-ray detector technologies, with an added advantage of contrast enhancement as well as reported reduction in radiation dose, it might be possible to achieve diagnostically efficient images at lower

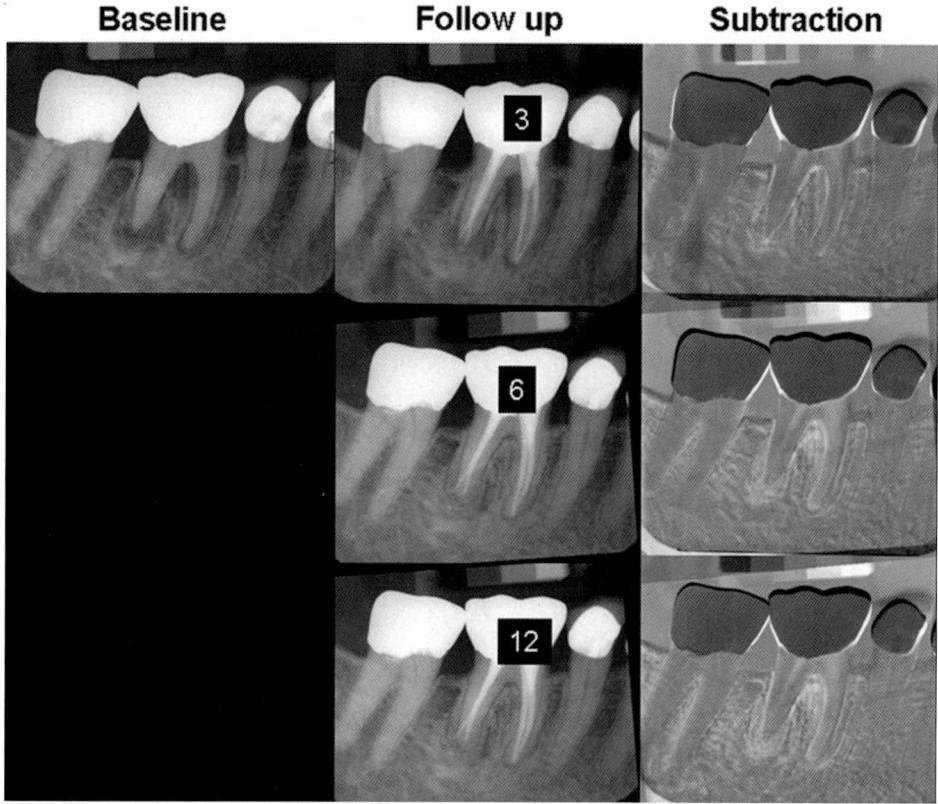

Figure 12 Digital subtraction comparing baseline (column 1) to follow-up images made at 3, 6, and 12 months following endodontic therapy (column 2). Column 3 indicates subtraction of respective follow-up images from the baseline radiograph. Progressive remineralization of the radiolucency at the apex of the distal root of the first molar is evident.

exposures than with conventional film. Velders et al.[42] found that it was possible to achieve a dose reduction of approximately 95% compared with Ektaspeed film when digital systems were used for dental radiographic imaging. One should remember, however, that the use of such low dosages can impair image quality because of a reduced signal-to-noise ratio (SNR).

Although the possible dose reduction for thinner objects has, however, been questioned for a PSP detector, in a study by Huda et al.,[43] the low-contrast discrimination of PSPs was found to be superior to that of X-ray films when using the same exposure time. By way of contrast, in a study by Berkhout et al.,[44] it was found that the PSPs required 10 times more radiation than the minimally acceptable dose to produce images of preferred quality. Further these authors state that PSPs require more radiation than E-speed films and that dose reduction with digital technology can be achieved only when using solid-state systems. PSP systems have a wide dynamic range, much larger than CCD systems and films. PSPs are said theoretically to have an exposure latitude ratio of approximately 10,000:1.[43] Hence, they should be capable of producing usable images over a wide range of exposures.[43–48] The actual exposure latitude for PSP systems is dependent on the acquisition software and scanning electronics. It does not exceed 25:1 for PSP intraoral radiography when the relative exposure latitude is determined using clear discrimination of the enamel–dentin junction as the lower limit and pixel blooming or unacceptable levels of cervical burnout as the upper limit.[49]

The effective latitude range for solid-state detectors can exceed 20:1 for some CMOS systems. However, intraoral X-ray systems using a CCD generally have narrower recording latitudes (<10:1), because high exposure results in pixel blooming.[49]

Dynamic range, also known as latitude, corresponds to the range of exposures that will produce images within the useful density range. Radiographic modalities, that produce diagnostic images over a wide range of exposures, are said to have a wide dynamic range and vise versa. The Hurter and

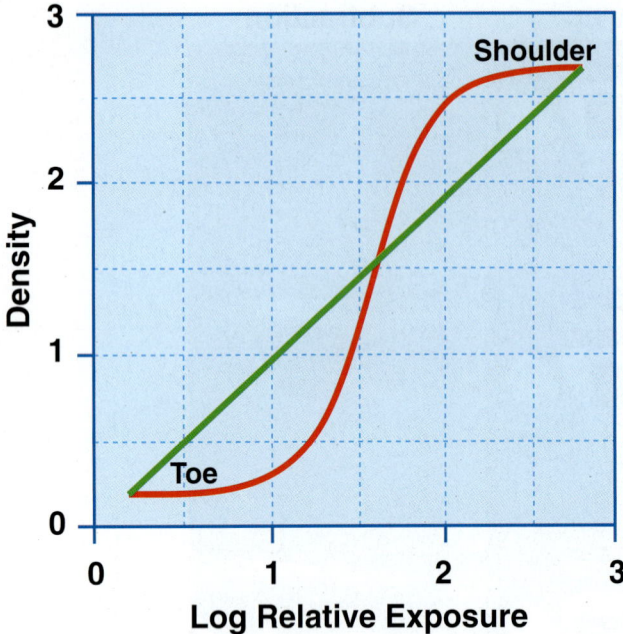

Figure 13 Hurter and Driffield curve relating radiograph density to exposure.

Driffield (H&D) curve was invented to characterize photographic emulsion some 5 years before the discovery of the X-ray but was extended to include X-ray film radiographs (Figure 13). Using pixel values rather than film density, the H&D curve concept can also be applied to digital imaging. The straight-line portion of the curve for film corresponds to the dynamic range. This curve demonstrates for conventional film the relationship between exposure (log number of X-rays) and the optical density (darkness) of an image detector. The scale of useful densities for film radiographs ranges approximately from 0.5, which produces low density or light images, to 3.0, which results in darker images of high density. However, outside this range, images tend to lose diagnostic detail. For films, this curve takes a form of stretched letter S appearance, with the top horizontal portion of the curve called "shoulder" that corresponds to higher exposure and the lower portion called "toe" that corresponds to lower exposure. Exposure changes in these portions of the curve have little effect on density. Even little changes in the straight-line and vertical portion of the curve significantly affect image density. Thus, the more vertical the straight-line portion of the curve, the smaller is the latitude. This explains the relatively wider dynamic range of digital receptors, especially storage phosphors. The curve can be linear and wider with no shoulder or toe when compared with film images (Figure 14).

Many digital systems have an option of using an "image equalize" function, and this is commonly the automated default setting. Equalization is a method of enhancing the contrast in a nonlinear fashion by stretching the pixel values disproportionately to obtain images of optimum image quality. In a study by Hayakawa et al.,[50] equalization exposure compensation for computed dental radiography (CDR) was found to be useful only for underexposed images but not for overexposed images. They also found that this compensation for underexposure did not significantly change the SNR. Furthermore, other studies have found that lower exposures, when severe, can in fact result in increased background noise and thus negatively affect the detection of small and low-contrast details within an object or tissue.[51]

Similar to equalize function in PSP images, the fourth generation RVG (RVG-4) had an option of automatic exposure compensation (AEC), which compensated for exposure errors by stretching the pixel value range to increase the contrast of structures within the images. It was found that both under- and overexposed images can be compensated using this algorithm. Because it can compensate for overexposure, it might lead to the risk of practitioners overexposing their patients. Moreover, it was also found that AEC reduces the SNR and produces disproportionate pixel values relative to exposure.[50] Newer versions, such as the RVG-6000, have dose indicator that warns the dentist in cases of exposure errors.

There is evidence that dentists, particularly endodontists, routinely prefer and view high-contrast and relatively dense images when performing endodontic tasks.[41] Likewise, detection of occlusal caries was found to be more accurate when using darker radiographs.[52] This is probably because higher exposure allows easier discrimination between small and low-contrast objects. Moving the exposure difference up on the H&D curve increased contrast results. The smaller the change in structure, the greater the contrast required to differentiate between adjacent structures. One of the methods employed to achieve required contrast is increasing the exposure. Furthermore, if there is superimposition of structure by the images of other objects, the signal of the latter has to be handled as additional noise. Thus, the dose has to be increased in order to notice the structure in the image. This is proposed by Thoms,[53] who believes that attempting a dose reduction will result in images having a low SNR and thereby reducing the visibility of small structures. However, higher exposures also negatively affect the diagnostic accuracy. Whereas images with lower exposures resulted in more false negatives, overexposed images resulted in higher false-positive responses.[54] With these rather contrasting studies in the literature and unanswered questions, there is confusion regarding the exposure time that is actually required to produce images of diagnostic quality and more so in the detection of low-contrast objects. Questions that still need to be addressed are as follows: (1) What is the optimal exposure time or range of exposures required by each of the intraoral radiographic systems that are presently used? (2) Is high radiation exposure really necessary for endodontic tasks? (3) What are the effects of radiation dose on the detection of low-contrast objects such as fine root canals? Many of these questions have not yet been fully answered even for analog film radiography.

Summary

Digital imaging systems, using solid-state detectors, have definite advantages over analog film in terms of immediacy of image display and seem to be equal to film imaging for most tested diagnostic purposes. There is still a need, however, for further scientific validation of the best exposure strategies for imaging optimizing specific diagnostic tasks including those used for endodontics.

References

1. Vertucci FJ. Root canal anatomy of human permanent teeth. Oral Surg Oral Med Oral Pathol Oral Radiol Endod 1984;58:589–99.
2. Langland OE, Sippy FH, Langlais RP. Textbook of dental radiology, 2nd ed. Springfield, Illinois: Charles C. Thomas, Publisher;1984. p. 13.
3. Brayer E. George Eastman: a biography. Baltimore amp; London: The Johns Hopkins University Press; 1996. pp. 111–12.
4. Morton WJ. The X-ray: or photography of the invisible and its value in surgery. American Technical Book Co.; 1896. Reported in http://books.google.com/books?q=Morton++%2B+Dental+Cosmos+1896&btnG=Search+Books (accessed Sep 1, 2006).
5. Raper HR. Elementary and dental radiography. London: Claudius Ash, Son amp; Co., Ltd.; 1913.
6. Satterlee F, Le Roy Jr. Dental radiology. New York: Swenarton Stationery Company; 1913.
7. Thoma KH. Oral roentgenology. Boston, Mass.: Ritter amp; Company; 1917.
8. Ivy RH. Dental and maxillary roentgenograms. St Louis: C.V. Mosby, Company; 1918.
9. Burns RC, Herbranson EJ. Tooth morphology and cavity preparation. In: Cohen S, Burns RC, editors. Pathways of the pulp. 8th ed. Mosby: St. Louis; 2002. pp. 173–229.
10. Mouyen F. Apparatus for providing a dental radiological image and intra-oral sensor used therewith. US patent 4593400. 1986 Jun 3.
11. van der Stelt PF. Filmless imaging: the uses of digital radiography in dental practice. J Am Dent Assoc 2005;136:1379–87.
12. Farman AG. Fundamentals of image acquisition and processing in the digital era. Orthod Craniofac Res 2003;6(Suppl 1):17–22.
13. Bender IB, Seltzer S. Roentgenographic and direct observation of experimental lesions in bone: I. J Am Dent Assoc 1961;62:152–6.
14. Bender IB, Seltzer S. Roentgenographic and direct observation of experimental lesions in bone: II. J Am Dent Assoc 1961;62:707–12.
15. Barbat J, Messer HH. Detectability of artificial periapical lesions using direct digital and conventional radiography. J Endod 1998;24:837–42.
16. Barkhordar RA, Meyer JR. Histologic evaluation of a human periapical defect after implantation with tricalcium phosphate. Oral Surg Oral Med Oral Pathol Oral Radiol Endod 1986;61:201–6.
17. Yokota ET, Miles DA, Newton CW, Brown CE Jr. Interpretation of periapical lesions using RadioVisioGraphy. J Endod 1994;20:490–4.
18. Holtzmann DJ, Johnson WT, Southard TE, et al. Storage-phosphor computed radiology versus film radiography in detection of pathologic periradicular bone loss in cadavers. Oral Surg Oral Med Oral Pathol Oral Radiol Endod 2000;86:90–7.
19. Paurazas SB, Geist JR, Pink FE, et al. Comparison of diagnostic accuracy of digital imaging by using CCD and CMOS-APS sensors with E-speed film in the detection of periapical bony lesions. Oral Surg Oral Med Oral Pathol Oral Radiol Endod 2000;89:356–62.
20. Mistak EJ, Loushine RJ, Primack PD, et al. Interpretation of periapical lesions comparing conventional, direct digital and telephonically transmitted radiographic images. J Endod 1998;24:262–6.
21. Tirrell BC, Miles DA, Brown CE Jr, Legan JJ. Interpretation of chemically created lesions using direct digital imaging. J Endod 1996;22:74–8.
22. Farman AG, Avant SL, Scarfe WC, et al. In vivo comparison of Visualix-2 and Ektaspeed Plus in the assessment of periradicular lesion dimensions. Oral Surg Oral Med Oral Pathol Oral Radiol Endod 1998;85:203–9.
23. Kullendorff B, Nilsson M. Diagnostic accuracy of direct digital dental radiography for the detection of periradicular bone lesions. II. Effects on diagnostic accuracy after application of image processing. Oral Surg Oral Med Oral Pathol Oral Radiol Endod 1996;82:585–9.
24. Wallace JA, Nair MK, Colaco MF, Kapa SF. A comparative evaluation of the diagnostic efficacy of film and digital sensors for detection of simulated periapical lesions. Oral Surg Oral Med Oral Pathol Oral Radiol Endod 2001;92:93–7.

25. Scarfe WC, Czerniejewski VJ, Farman AG, et al. In vivo accuracy and reliability of color-coded image enhancements for the assessment of periradicular lesion dimensions. Oral Surg Oral Med Oral Pathol Oral Radiol Endod 1999;88:603–11.

26. Woolhiser GA, Brand JW, Hoen MM, et al. Accuracy of film-based, digital, and enhanced digital images for endodontic length determination. Oral Surg Oral Med Oral Pathol Oral Radiol Endod 2005;99:499–504.

27. Vandre RH, Pajak JC, Abdel-Nabi H, et al. Comparison of observer performance in determining the position of endodontic files with physical measures in the evaluation of dental X-ray imaging systems. Dentomaxillofac Radiol 2000;29:216–22.

28. Eikenberg S, Vandre R. Comparison of digital dental X-ray systems with self-developing film and manual processing for endodontic file length determination. J Endod 2000;26:65–7.

29. Sanderink GC, Huiskens R, van der Stelt PF, et al. Image quality of direct digital intraoral x-ray sensors in assessing root canal length. The RadioVisioGraphy, Visualix/VIXA, Sens-A-Ray, and Flash Dent systems compared with Ektaspeed films. Oral Surg Oral Med Oral Pathol Oral Surg Endod 1994;78:25–32.

30. Li G, Sanderink GC, Welander U, et al. Evaluation of endodontic files in digital radiographs before and after employing three image processing algorithms. Dentomaxillofac Radiol 2004;33:6–11.

31. Cederberg RA, Tidwell E, Frederiksen NL, Benson BW. Endodontic working length assessment. Comparison of storage phosphor digital imaging and radiographic film. Oral Surg Oral Med Oral Pathol Oral Radiol Endod 1998;85:325–8.

32. Martinez-Lozano MA, Forner-Navarro L, Sanchez-Cortes JL, Llena-Puy C. Methodological considerations in the determination of working length. Int Endod J 2001;34:371–6.

33. Naoum HJ, Chandler NP, Love RM. Conventional versus storage phosphor-plate digital images to visualize the root canal system contrasted with radiopaque medium. J Endod 2003;29:349–52.

34. Nance R, Tyndall D, Levin LG, Trope M. Identification of root canals in molars by tuned-aperture computed tomography. Int Endod J 2000;33:392–6.

35. Barton DJ, Clark SJ, Eleazer PD, et al. Tuned-aperture computed tomography versus parallax analog and digital radiographic images in detecting second mesiobuccal canals in maxillary first molars. Oral Surg Oral Med Oral Pathol Oral Radiol Endod 2003;96:223–8.

36. Gröndahl H-G. CBCT in implantology with special reference to small volume unit. Invited presentation, 17th International Congress on Head and Neck Radiology; 2006; Budapest.

37. Yoshioka T, Kobayashi C, Suda H, Sasaki T. An observation of the healing process of periapical lesions by digital subtraction radiography. J Endod 2002;28:589–91.

38. Nicopoulou-Karayianni K, Bragger U, Patrikiou A, et al. Image processing for enhanced observer agreement in the evaluation of periapical bone changes. Int Endod J 2002;35:615–22.

39. Mikrogeorgis G, Lyroudia K, Molyvdas I, et al. Digital radiograph registration and subtraction: a useful tool for the evaluation of the progress of chronic apical periodontitis. J Endod 2004 Jul;30:513–17.

40. Sanderink GC. Imaging: new versus traditional technological aids. Int Dent J 1993;43:335–42.

41. Sheaffer JC, Eleazer PD, Scheetz JP, et al. Endodontic measurement accuracy and perceived radiograph quality: effects of film speed and density. Oral Surg Oral Med Oral Pathol Oral Radiol Endod 2003;96:441–8.

42. Velders XL, Sanderink GC, van der Stelt PF. Dose reduction of two digital sensor systems measuring file lengths. Oral Surg Oral Med Oral Pathol Oral Radiol Endod 1996;81:607–12.

43. Huda W, Rill LN, Benn DK, Pettigrew JC. Comparison of a photostimulable phosphor system with film for dental radiology. Oral Surg Oral Med Oral Pathol Oral Radiol Endod 1997;83:725–31.

44. Berkhout WE, Beuger DA, Sanderink GC, van der Stelt PF. The dynamic range of digital radiographic systems: dose reduction or risk of overexposure? Dentomaxillofac Radiol 2004;33:1–5.

45. Matsuda Y, Okana T, Igeta A, Seki K. Effects of exposure reduction on the accuracy of an intraoral photostimulable phosphor imaging system in detecting incipient proximal caries. Oral Radiology (Japan) 1995;11:11–16.

46. Borg E, Gröndahl H-G. On the dynamic range of different X-ray photon detectors in intra-oral radiography: a comparison of image quality in film, charge-coupled device and storage phosphor systems. Dentomaxillofac Radiol 1996;25:82–8.

47. Borg E, Attaelmanan A, Gröndahl HG. Subjective image quality of solid-state and photostimulable phosphor systems for digital intra-oral radiography. Dentomaxillofac Radiol 2000;29:70–5.

48. Borg E. Some characteristics of solid-state and photo-stimulable phosphor detectors for intra-oral radiography. Swed Dent J Suppl 1999;139:i–viii, 1–67.

49. Farman AG, Farman TT. A comparison of 18 different x-ray detectors currently used in dentistry. Oral Surg Oral Med Oral Pathol Oral Radiol Endod 2005;99:485–9.

50. Hayakawa Y, Farman AG, Scarfe WC, Kuroyanagi K. Pixel value modification using RVG-4 automatic exposure compensation for instant high-contrast images. Oral Radiol (Japan) 1996;12:11–17.

51. Ramamurthy R, Canning CF, Scheetz JP, Farman AG. Impact of ambient lighting intensity and duration on the signal-to-noise ratio of images from photostimulable phosphor plates processed using DenOptix and ScanX systems. Dentomaxillofac Radiol 2004;33:307–11.

52. Skodje F, Espelid I, Kvile K, Tveit AB. The influence of radiographic exposure factors on the diagnosis of occlusal caries. Dentomaxillofac Radiol 1998;27:75–9.
53. Thoms M. The effect of dose reduction on the diagnoses on the small structural sizes in two-dimensional imaging. In: Lemke HU, Vannier MW, Inamura K, et al., editors. Computer assisted radiology and surgery. International Congress Series 1256. Amsterdam: Elsevier; 2003. pp. 1206–11.
54. Svenson B, Welander U, Anneroth G, Soderfeldt B. Exposure parameters and their effects on diagnostic accuracy. Oral Surg Oral Med Oral Pathol Oral Radiol Endod 1994;78:544–50.

Chapter 15C

C. Ultrasonic Imaging

Elisabetta Cotti

Given the importance of imaging systems in the diagnosis, description, follow-up, and study of endodontic lesions in the mandible and maxilla, as well as the development of advanced diagnostic systems in traditional radiology, alternative imaging techniques are constantly being investigated.[1,2]

Osteolytic endodontic lesions in the jaws are a consequence of pulpal and periapical inflammation.[3–5] The clinical diagnosis of a tooth with a root-end radiolucency of endodontic origin is apical periodontitis. However, following biopsy and depending on the microscopic features of an apical lesion, it may receive a histopathologic diagnosis of either granuloma or cyst. The possibility of making a clinical differential diagnosis between a granuloma and a cyst may be important in the management of such lesions, especially in predicting the outcome of endodontic treatment or explaining lack of healing.[4,6–9] Unfortunately, radiographs allow visualization of hard tissues only and not soft tissues. Therefore, radiographs are not good guides for differentiating these types of lesions.[1]

Basic Principles of Ultrasound Real-Time Imaging

Ultrasound real-time imaging, also called real-time echotomography or echography, has been a widely used diagnostic technique in many fields of medicine since 1942.[10,11] The production of ultrasonic images is based on the generation and reflection of ultrasound waves. Ultrasound waves are generated as a result of the so-called *piezoelectric effect* by quartz or a synthetic ceramic crystal, when it is exposed to an alternating electric current of 3 to 10 MHz. Ultrasound waves, oscillating at the same frequency, are bundled by means of an acoustic lens and directed toward the area of interest in the body via an ultrasonic probe (transducer) (Figure 1A).

Various biologic tissues of the body possess different mechanical and acoustic properties. When the ultrasound waves encounter the interface between two biologic tissues with different acoustic impedance, they undergo the phenomena of reflection and refraction. The echo is the part of the ultrasound wave that is reflected back from the tissue interface toward the crystal (Figure 1B). The crystal is capable of transforming an incoming ultrasound wave (echo) of the same frequency back to an electromagnetic wave. The echo is then transformed into electric energy, which in turn is transformed into a light spot,

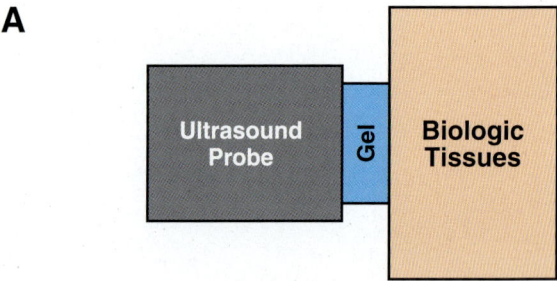

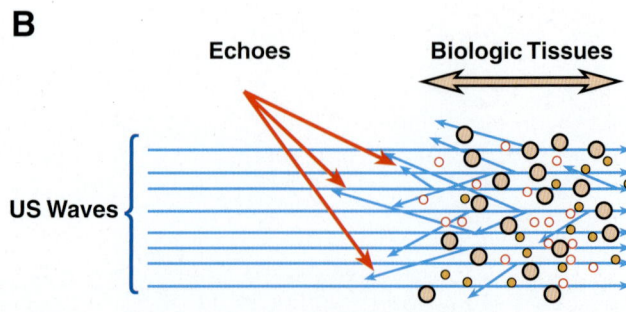

Figure 1 *A*, Schematic representation of sending ultrasounds into biologic tissue with a probe. *B*, Production of echoes from ultrasound waves sent into biologic tissues and reflected back.

thermodebonding of metal and ceramic brackets. Am J Orthod Dentofacial Orthop 1992;102:410–17.

187. Cummings M, Biagioni P, Lamey PJ, Burden DJ. Thermal image analysis of electrothermal debonding of ceramic brackets: an in vitro study. Eur J Orthod 1999;21:111–18.

188. Crooks M, Hood J, Harkness M. Thermal debonding of ceramic brackets: an in vitro study. Am J Orthod Dentofacial Orthop 1997;111:163–72.

189. Ma T, Marangoni RD, Flint W. In vitro comparison of debonding force and intrapulpal temperature changes during ceramic orthodontic bracket removal using a carbon dioxide laser. Am J Orthod Dentofacial Orthop 1997; 111:203–10.

190. Sheridan JJ, Brawley G, Hastings J. Electrothermal debracketing. Part I. An in vitro study. Am J Orthod 1986; 89:21–7.

191. Verez-Fraguela JL, Vives Valles MA, Ezquerra Calvo LJ. Effects of ultrasonic dental scaling on pulp vitality in dogs: an experimental study. J Vet Dent 2000; 17:75–9.

192. Lea SC, Landini G, Walmsley AD. Thermal imaging of ultrasonic scaler tips during tooth instrumentation. J Clin Periodontol 2004;31:370–5.

193. Kocher T, Ruhling A, Herweg M, Plagman HC. Proof of efficacy of different modified sonic scaler inserts used for debridement in furcations—a dummy head trial. J Clin Periodontol 1996;23:662–9.

194. Ingle JI. Hereditary hypophosphatemia. In: Ingle JI, editor. Endodontics. 1st ed. Philadelphia, PA: Lea & Febiger; 1965. pp. 289–91.

195. Schwartz S, et al. Oral finding in patients with autosomal dominant hypophosphatemic bone disease and X-linked hypophatemia: further evidence that they are different diseases. Oral Surg Oral Med Oral Pathol Oral Radiol Endod 1988;66:310.

196. Macfarlane JD, Swart JGN. Dental aspects of hypophosphatasia: a case report, family study and literature review. Oral Surg Oral Med Oral Pathol Oral Radiol Endod 1989; 67:521.

197. Brown JH, Brenn L. Bull. Johns Hopkins Hosp., 48:69 (1931). AFIP Manual of Histologic Staining Techniques: 3rd. ed., G. Luna (ed.); New York: McGraw-Hill Publications, c.1968. p. 222.

CHAPTER 13

PERIAPICAL LESIONS OF ENDODONTIC ORIGIN

ZVI METZGER, ITZHAK ABRAMOVITZ

Periapical lesions of endodontic origin will be discussed in this chapter in terms of function and form. An emphasis is placed on the understanding of the biological function of the lesion, with special attention to processes leading to its formation and to changes it may go through, as observed by either the clinician or the histopathologist. The content of this chapter requires some knowledge of microbiology and immunology. The reader is referred to Chapters 7 and 9 dedicated to these subjects, which provide the essential background in detail. Periapical lesions, *not inflammatory in nature,* will be discussed in Chapter 8.

Periapical lesions of endodontic origin are produced by an inflammatory response at the root apices of teeth with nonvital pulps. Because the necrotic pulp cavity is relatively inaccessible to the immune response, it becomes a reservoir of infection. The establishment of an inflammatory response is believed to be an attempt to prevent the spread of infection to periapical tissues. Periapical lesions of endodontic origin are generated by the immune system. The response may occur at any portal of exit from the root canal system. Since most such portals are found in the apical area, and for the sake of convenience for the reader, the terms "periapical" or "apical" will be used as a uniform term, for inflammatory lesions of endodontic origin.

Bacterial Elimination in Periapical Lesions

The elimination of bacteria emerging from the apical foramen and the prevention of their spread to other tissues are important functions of apical periodontitis.[1,2] Even though bacteria are present in infected root canals, most periapical lesions successfully contain them. Thus, periapical inflammatory lesions may be considered to be a successful host response to bacteria and bacterial by-products in an infected root canal system. The elimination of the invading bacteria is one of the main functions of the immune response. The key role in this process is played by the polymorphonuclear leukocytes (PMNs) that eventually phagocytize and kill the bacteria. PMNs originate from progenitor cells in the bone marrow and enter the bloodstream where they circulate for 7–10 hours, ready to be called to duty. To reach the bacteria emerging from the apical foramen, PMNs must first leave the bloodstream and find their way to that site. This process is initiated by a stage termed "margination," which is mediated by a locally elevated expression of attachment molecules such as intercellular attachment molecule-1 (ICAM-1) on the surface of the endothelial cells in the area.[3–5] The "right area" for margination is defined for the PMNs by local production of IL-1 and tumor necrosis factor (TNF) that results in an elevated expression of the attachment molecules.[3,6] Once attached, the PMNs can leave the blood vessels by passing between endothelial cells in a process termed "diapedesis." PMNs follow the gradient of the chemotactic factor C5a that is generated by the activation of the complement system at the site where bacteria are present. This gradient serves as a chemotactic signal; the random motion of the PMNs becomes directional and they follow this gradient from low to high concentration. Complement may be activated directly by bacterial constituents such as bacterial endotoxin (lipopolysaccharide, LPS), using the "alternative" or "properidin" pathway. This represents the basic, innate immune response of the host. The "classical pathway" of complement activation is dependent on specific IgG or IgM that binds to antigens present on the bacterial surface. This, in turn, triggers complement activation by C1q molecules of the complement cascade. Complement activation is a "chain reaction" type of response that generates large amounts of three types of molecules that may be considered as major life-sustaining factors. Two of them are small and readily

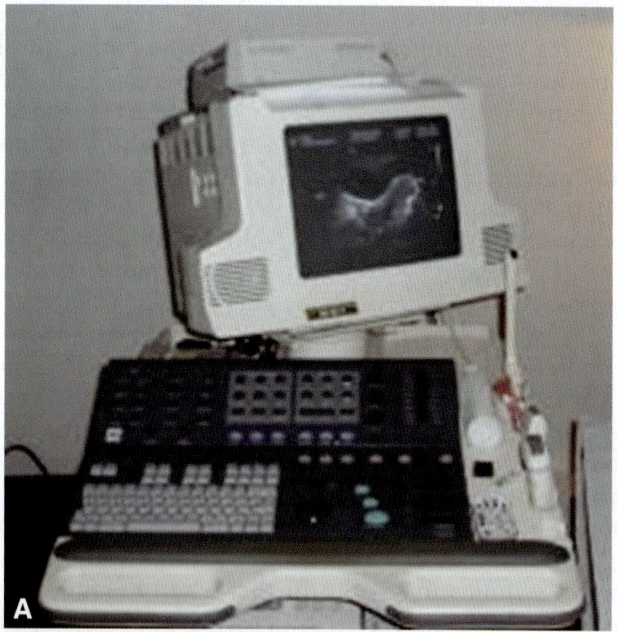
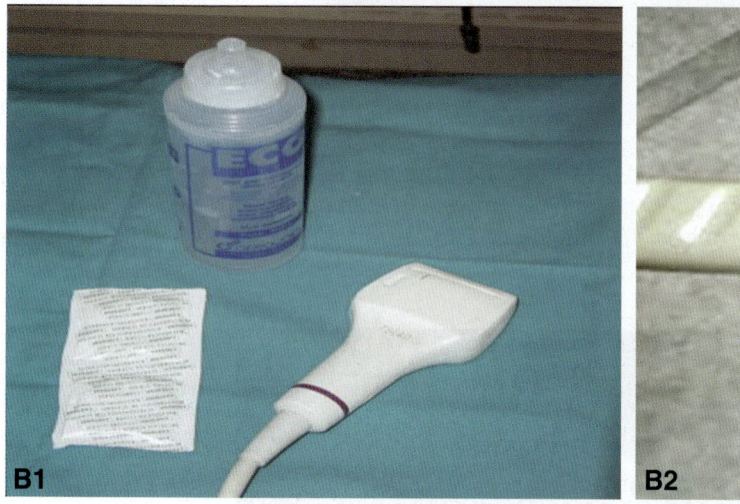
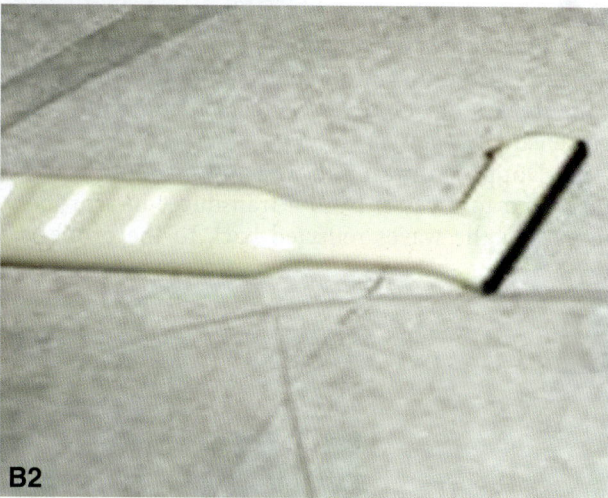

Figure 2 Ultrasound technical equipment. **A,** Ultrasound imaging apparatus. **B,** Echographic probes and gel.

using a gray scale, into a computer monitor built into the ultrasound apparatus (Figure 2A and B).[11]

The intensity of the echoes depends on the difference in acoustic properties between two adjacent tissue compartments: the greater the difference, the greater the amount of reflected ultrasound energy, the higher the echo intensity. Low echo signals appear as dark spots whereas high echo signals appear as bright/white spots. The point in the tissue where the echo originates is calculated by the computer from the time delay between the beginning of the wave signal and the return of the echo. The ultrasound images seen on the monitor are produced by the automatic movement of the crystal over the tissue of interest. Because each movement of the crystal gives one image of the tissue (depending on its plane), and an average of 30 images per second are produced, the tissue being examined will appear on the monitor as a sequence of moving images. The movement by the operator of the probe, on the area of examination, creates a change on the sector plane, thus allowing the creation of a "real-time three-dimensional image of that space."[10,11]

The interpretation of the gray values on the images is based on a comparison with those of normal tissues. When an area in a given tissue has *high echo intensity*, it is called "hyperechoic." When it displays *low echo intensity*, it is termed "hypoechoic"; if characterized by *absence of echo intensity*, it is called "anechoic." Any fluid-filled area where no reflection occurs is anechoic, whereas bone, from which total reflection occurs, is hyperechoic. Areas that contain different types of tissues show a "dishomogeneous echo."[11]

The ultrasound examination can be supplemented by the use of color power Doppler (CPD) ultrasound to determine the perfusion of the tissue of interest. When applied to the ultrasound, examination with the CPD offers the opportunity to observe the presence and direction of the blood flow and the intensity of the Doppler signal with its changes in real time (*Doppler*), in the format of color spots superimposed on the images of blood vessels (*color*), and with very high sensitivity (*power*).[11]

The Doppler ultrasound test uses sound waves transmitted to a vessel from a transducer in a probe. The part of the waves reflected back to the probe is processed by a computer that creates graphs or pictures representing the blood flow within the vessel. The movement of blood cells causes a change in pitch in the reflected sound waves (*Doppler effect*). The Doppler shift of the moving blood is monitored continuously to form the Doppler signal. Because the transmit frequency is about 2 to 4 MHz, the Doppler shift of moving blood is in the audible range. The CPD technique combines ultrasound real-time imaging with the color encoding of the Doppler frequency shift and is used to visualize the presence and velocity of blood flow within an image plane. The frequency shift is color-encoded depending on the velocity and the direction of the blood flow relative to the transducer and is superimposed on the grayscale image. The way in which the frequency shifts are encoded is defined by the color bar located to the left of the image (Figure 3). Blood flow is assigned different hues that reflect the flow velocity and the insonation angle. Fast flow is assigned lighter hues whereas slow flows appear with deeper hues (Figure 3).[12–14]

Positive Doppler shifts are caused by the blood moving toward the transducer and are encoded as red; negative Doppler shifts are caused by blood moving opposite to the transducer and are encoded as blue. Because CD (Color Doppler) presents some shortcomings such as dependency on the insonation angle and the "aliasing," PD (Power Doppler) is best

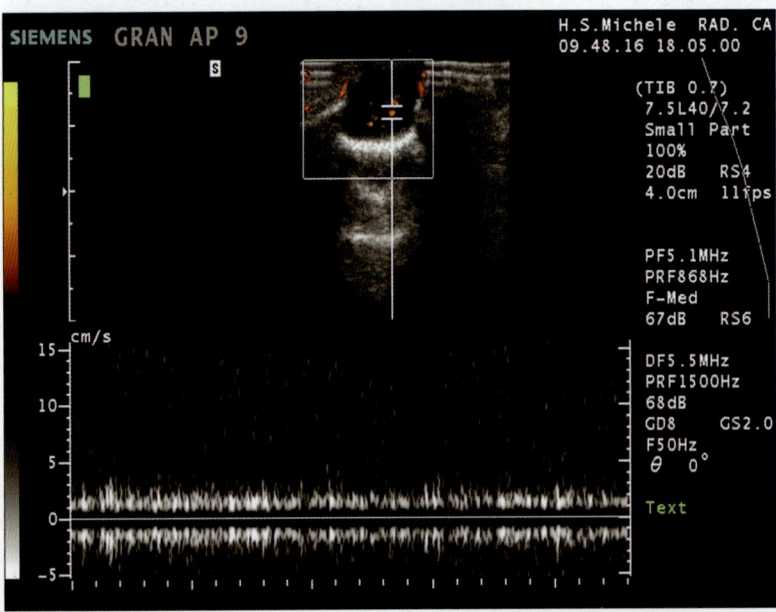

Figure 3 Picture representing the echo color power Doppler applied to the echographic examination of a periapical lesion. On the upper right the ultrasound image of the lesion is showed (framed), the colored spots represent the presence and direction of the blood flow (color Doppler). The intensity of the Doppler signal with its modification in time is represented in the lower part of the figure.

associated with it to improve its sensitivity to low flow rates. CPD is based on the integrated power spectrum, is angle independent, and is up to five times more sensitive in detecting blood flow than color Doppler.[12–14]

Intravenous injections of contrast media increase the echogenicity of the blood by enhancing the difference in acoustic impedance in the area of interest, thus rendering the CPD examination more sensitive.[11,13]

Ultrasound imaging is considered to be a relatively safe technique. Ultrasound waves targeted into biologic tissues are absorbed in the form of heat energy. This could be hazardous because it causes cavitation and vibration.[11] On the other hand, it is important to note that the crystal emits energy only during 0.1% of its activity, whereas the remainder of the time it receives echoes: it is "listening." Any potential adverse effects of the system depend on the length of application time of the sound energy; safety, therefore, is achieved by limiting the number and the repetitions of the examinations. No adverse effects of ultrasound waves have been reported in experimental and clinical studies.[15–17] In any case, the risk entailed is much lower than that associated with radiographic investigations.[17]

Ultrasound Imaging in the Study of Periapical Lesions

In 2001, a pilot project was conducted at the University of Cagliari, Italy, to try ultrasound real-time examination in the study of periapical lesions of endodontic origin. Several patients diagnosed with apical periodontitis, based on clinical signs and symptoms and intraoral and panoramic radiographs, were asked to participate. They signed an informed consent and had echographic examinations of the areas affected by the apical lesions. An endodontist, an oral surgeon, and a radiologist expert in echography were involved in the project.

After a few trials, it was possible to consistently trace the lesions within the mandible and maxilla and describe them by means of echography. A protocol was subsequently developed and used in the first published investigation.[18] Twelve patients diagnosed with endodontic periapical lesions were chosen to participate. In each patient, the area of interest was selected for the echographic examination. Intraoral and/or panoramic radiographs were used as a guide. Patients were placed in the echographic "bed" and an Elegra Siemens apparatus (Siemens, Erlangen, Germany) with a standard, high-definition multi-frequency ultrasound probe of 7 to 9 MHz was used for the examinations (Figure 4).

The echographic probe, covered with a latex protection and topped with echographic gel, was then moved into the buccal area of the mandible or maxilla, corresponding to the radicular area of the tooth of interest. When the bony defect was identified, the probe was moved slightly around the area to obtain an adequate number of transversal scans to define the lesion.

The images were evaluated, based on the echographic principles used to describe the appearance of bone pathosis, and compared with the radiographic appearances of the lesions. The data were accurately reported in a descriptive chart. It was noted that the examinations were relatively easy to perform and that the patients reported no discomfort. In all the cases examined, it was possible to obtain an echographic three-dimensional image of a given lesion, to measure its dimensions, and to evaluate its content (fluids, solid, or a combination of both).

Following the application of CPD to echography, it was possible to see the presence of blood vessels within a lesion. One drawback was that it was not easy to distinguish specific anatomic reference points within the echographic image (i.e., roots of teeth).

Based on these first data, it was possible to confirm the following information:

1. Alveolar bone, if healthy, is hyperechoic because it exhibits a total reflecting surface that appears white in the image.
2. The roots of the teeth are also hyperechoic and appear as an even whiter shade than bone and can be seen in three dimensions.
3. Solid lesions in the bone are echogenic or hypoechoic presenting various intensities of echoes and appear as different shades of gray (Figure 4A).
4. A bone cavity filled with clear fluids (i.e., serous) is anechoic (or transonic) because it has no reflection and it appears dark (Figure 4B).
5. A bone cavity filled with fluids containing inclusions is hypoechoic and exhibits various degrees of darkness, depending on the contents of the fluid.
6. The irregular bone (resorbed) around a lesion shows a dishomogeneous echo (Figure 4A).
7. The reinforced bony contour of a lesion is usually very bright (hyperechoic) (Figure 4B).

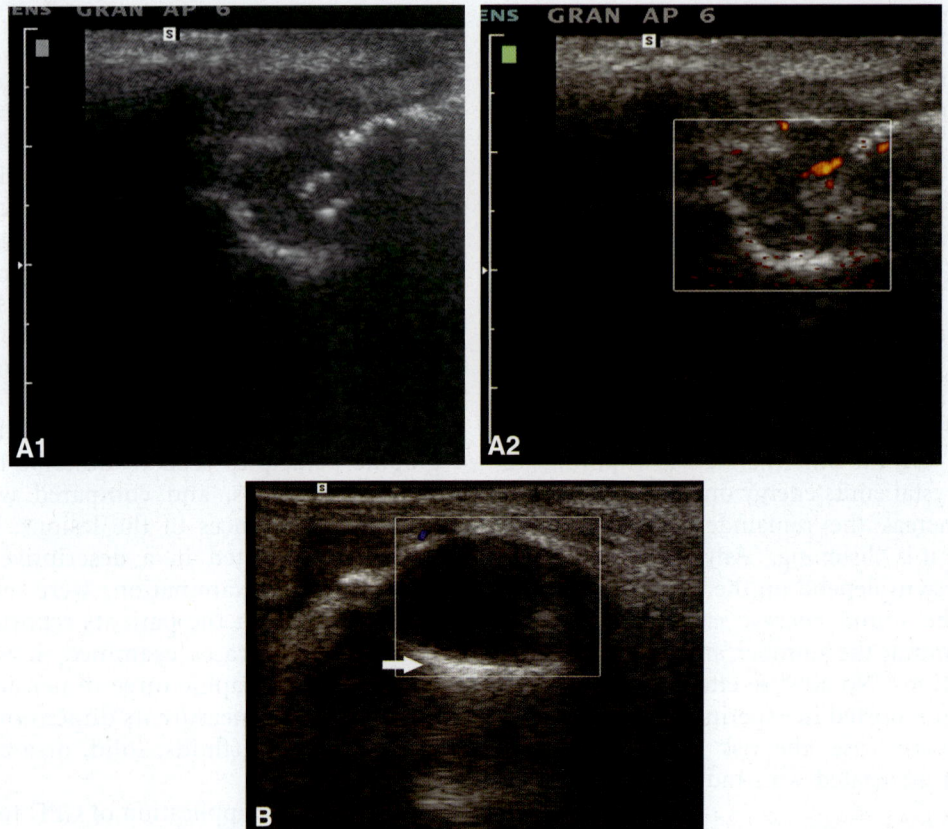

Figure 4 Ultrasound real-time imaging of two different lesions in the jaws. ***A1,*** Periapical lesion (granuloma) as seen in the ultrasound image (framed); it is an "echogenic" area where echoes are reflected at different intensities. ***A2,*** The same lesion after the application of color power Doppler. The colored spots represent the vascularization within the lesion. ***B,*** Ultrasound image of a cystic lesion (framed): it shows an "anechoic"/"transonic" cavity; the reinforced lower bone contour of this lesion is hyperechoic" (arrow).

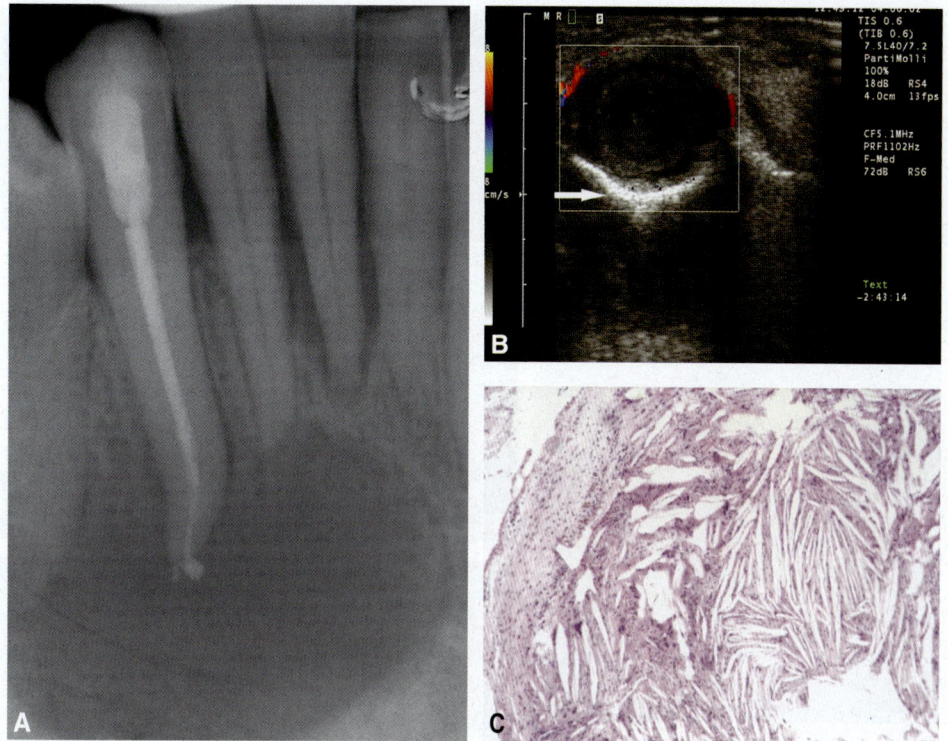

Figure 5 Ultrasound real-time imaging of a lesion of endodontic origin in the mandible. **A,** Periapical lesion as seen in the intraoral radiograph; the lesion involves the periapical area of the lower right lateral incisor, canine, and first premolar. **B,** The same lesion as seen in the ultrasound image (framed): it is a "transonic" cavity with reinforced, hyperechoic bony contour (arrow). The vascular supply appearing at the CPD (red spots) is external to the lesion. **C,** Histopathologic features of the previous lesion that has confirmed the echographic diagnosis of "cystic lesion."

8. By applying the CPD to the examination procedure, the presence and direction of blood vessels around and within the lesion can be detected (Figure 4A).
9. The mandibular canal, the mental foramen, and the maxillary sinus can often be distinguished and appear mostly transonic.

Given all this information, a second study was done to differentiate between cystic lesions and granulomas based on the ultrasound examination complemented with the CPD procedure.[19] Eleven patients, with clinical diagnoses of apical periodontitis and whose treatment plan included endodontic surgery with apicoectomy, retrograde filling, and biopsy, were chosen for this study. The ultrasound examination with CPD was performed in each area of diagnostic interest in the maxilla. A representative echographic image was selected for each lesion, analyzed, and recorded. An attempt was made to make a differential diagnosis between cystic lesions and granulomas based on the following principles:

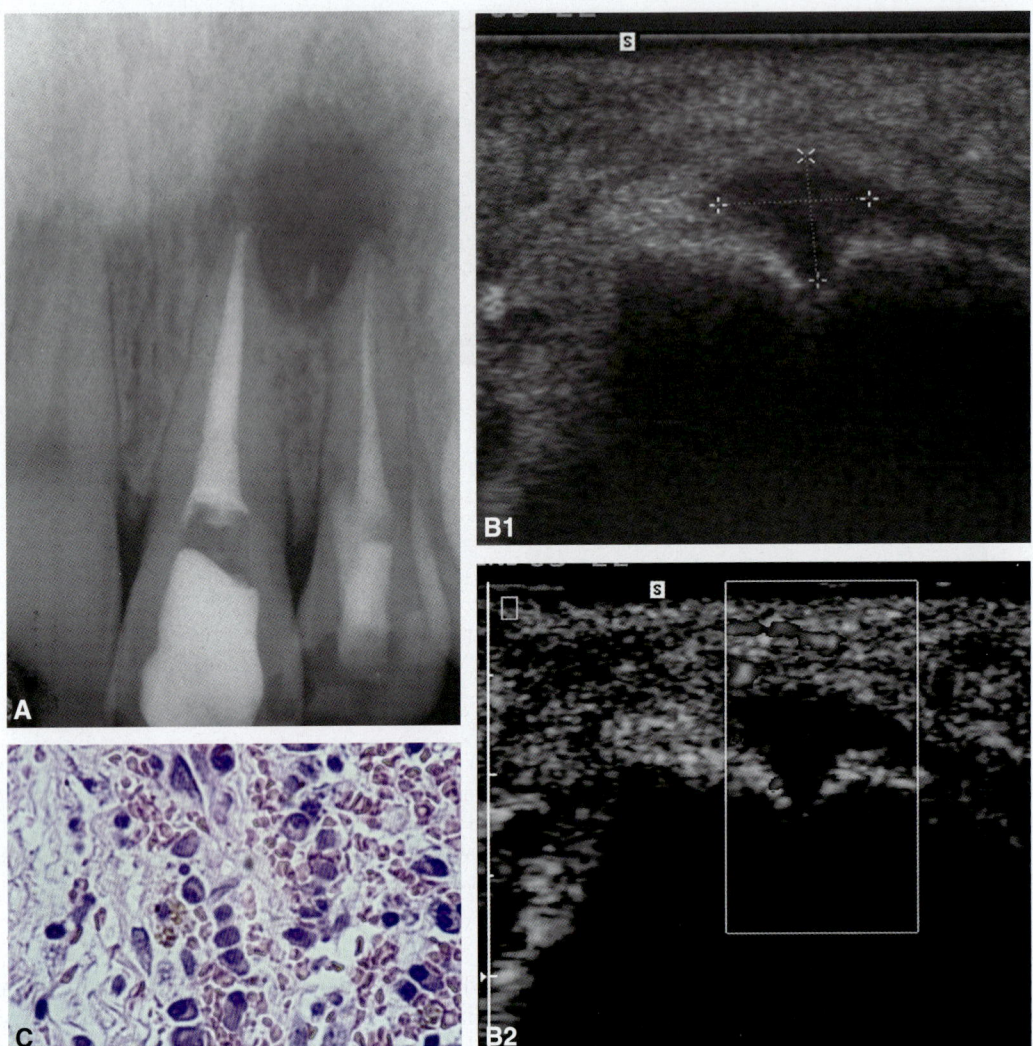

Figure 6 Ultrasound real-time imaging of a lesion of endodontic origin in the maxilla. **A,** Intraoral radiograph showing a periapical lesion involving the upper left central and lateral incisors. **B1,** Periapical lesion as seen in the ultrasound images. It is possible to distinguish an "echogenic" area with irregular contours; the dotted areas correspond to the diameters of the lesion. **B2,** The same lesion with the CPD which shows the presence of blood vessels within the lesion. The lesion was diagnosed as periapical granuloma. **C,** Histopathologic features of the previous lesion confirming the echographic diagnosis.

Cystic lesion: a transonic, well-contoured cavity filled with fluid, surrounded by reinforced bony walls with no evidence of internal vascularization based on CPD (Figure 5A–C).

Granulomas: a distinct lesion that could be echogenic or mixed in content, with non-precisely defined contours and exhibiting the presence of blood vessels based on CPD (Figure 6A–C).

The results from the histopathologic examination confirmed the tentative echographic diagnosis. Six of eleven lesions that were described as transonic cavities, well contoured, and without blood vessels corresponded to the histopathologic feature of a cyst: a cavity lined with stratified squamous epithelium with necrotic debris and impressions from cholesterol crystals within its lumen. One lesion, whose transonic content showed also scattered echogenic particles, revealed a cystic lumen with areas of secretory epithelium. This case supports the specific sensitivity of this technique with respect to the content of the studied bone pathosis.

Four of the remaining lesions were echographically diagnosed as granulomas because of their echogenic appearance and the presence of internal blood vessels. Their histopathologic reports described the typical appearance of granulomas: connective tissue with peripheral mononuclear (PMN) cells, lymphocytes, monocytes, and newly formed blood vessels. The only case that presented with both an echogenic appearance in the lower portion and a hypoechoic aspect toward the upper end showed the histopathologic feature of a large granuloma containing a cyst. Based on these findings, ultrasound imaging showed enough potential sensitivity to allow the distinction between a cyst and a granuloma, to define a mixed type of lesion, and to evaluate the various degrees of turbidity of the fluid content in the bony lesion.[19,20]

Furthermore, these findings were recently confirmed by researchers[21] who replicated our study and evaluated the efficacy of ultrasound as opposed to digital radiographs and conventional radiographs, in the differential diagnosis of 15 periapical lesions. Their results were consistent with our findings even if they used the ultrasonic probe to conduct the examination only from outside the mouth; the echographic apparatus and the probe were different from the ones we used, and the clinical situation of the selected patients might not have been the same.

The possibility of monitoring inflammatory changes in diseased bone using the ultrasound real-time examination associated with CPD has been the subject of a recently concluded pilot project. The rationale was that the various degrees of inflammation of a given lesion can be assumed by evaluating the diffusion of blood vessels within or/and around the lesion, and that the application of CPD has the sensitivity to detect the presence of newly formed vessels. Six clinical cases diagnosed with clinical diagnoses of apical periodontitis, whose treatment plan included endodontic orthograde treatment, were included in this experiment. A clinical protocol was established and it was decided to complete the treatment in two appointments using calcium hydroxide as an intermediate medication. Besides routine radiographs, echographic examinations of each case were carried out as follows: (1) before treatment; (2) 1 week after root canal cleaning, disinfection, and application of intermediate medication; and (3) 1 month after completion of root canal treatment.

The results from this investigation have shown an active response to endodontic treatment in all phases of all examined cases. A reduction in the vascularization within the lesions, both after application of the intermediate medication and after filling the root canals with gutta-percha and cement, was observed in all cases (Figure 7A–E). The degree of reduction of vascular supply was not the same in each case, but it was not possible to quantify it in this experiment.

These data are very preliminary and cannot yet lead to general conclusions, but they open new horizons on the follow-up of endodontic treatment with special regard to tissue reactions at different stages and protocols for endodontic treatment.

Recently, real-time ultrasound examination with CPD was used to monitor five apical lesions in the mandible and maxilla 6 months after orthograde treatment was completed. The rationale was that when the healing process starts within a lesion in bone, the Doppler signal will show the formation of new vessels. As the bone is remodeled, the flow signal will progressively decrease to the point of disappearing when the lesion is completely healed.[22] In conclusion, ultrasound imaging appears to be clinically useful in the dimensional assessment of lesions, the evaluation of their content (fluid versus mixed or solid), and obtaining information on the patterns of expansion, vascularization, evolution in time, and response to treatment. In terms of its potential in differential diagnosis, cysts may be distinguished from granulomas, and cystic content may be defined as "clear" or "turbid."[19,20]

Trope et al.[8] reported that a granuloma could be differentiated from a cyst by density using CT scan. Ultrasound imaging is more convenient than CT because it is less expensive and entails lower biologic adverse effects.[23,24] Other investigators have used digital radiographs to measure grayscale values to differentiate cysts from granulomas.[25] Recently, cone-beam CT has been applied to the differential diagnosis of large apical radiolucencies, based on the negative and positive gray values with promising results.[9]

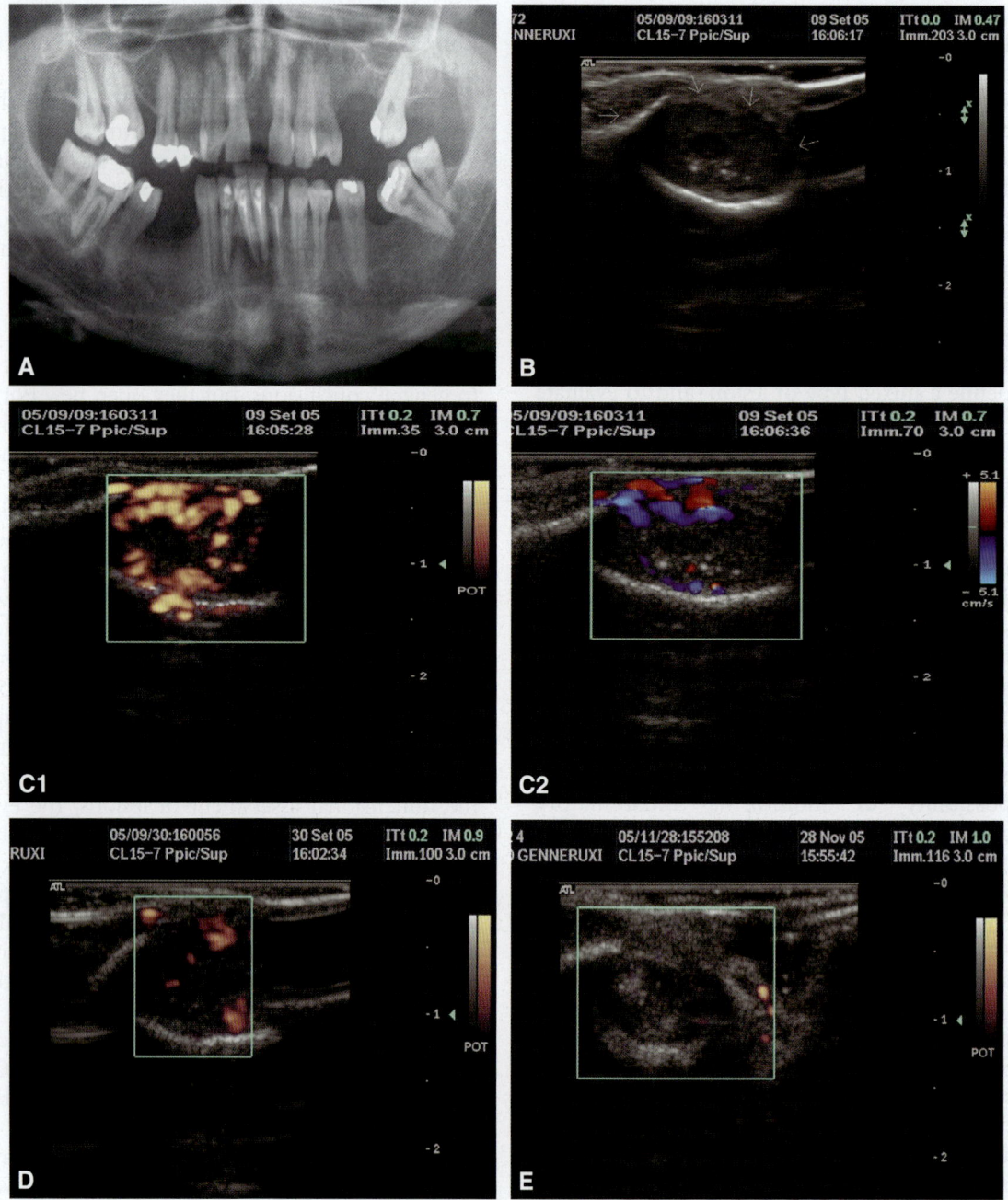

Figure 7 Ultrasound real-time imaging follow-up of an endodontic treatment with application of CPD. **A,** Panoramic radiograph showing periapical lesion involving all four mandibular incisors, before endodontic re-treatment. **B,** The same lesion seen in the ultrasound image (framed and arrowed): it is an "echogenic" image with solid content and well-defined contours. **C,** The two echographic images of the same lesion after the application of the power Doppler (1) and Color Doppler (2) show the presence of vascular supply. The diagnosis was periapical granuloma. **D,** Echography of the lesion (framed) 1 week after endodontic re-treatment was initiated and an intracanal medication was placed. The CPD shows reduced vascularization. **E,** Ultrasound image of the same lesion (framed) 1 month after completion of re-treatment on all four teeth. The CPD indicated that the vascular supply was greatly reduced.

Ultrasonic imaging may find a place in research of apical radiolucencies and may also become a part of clinical procedures for dental diagnosis. But as with many other technological improvements, it will take some time for equipment and training to catch up with the possibilities of using these new modalities.

References

1. Huumonen S, Orstavik D. Radiological aspects of apical periodontitis. Endod Topics 2002;1:3–25.
2. Cotti E, Campisi G. Advanced radiographic techniques for the detection of lesions in bone. Endod Topics 2004;7:52–72.
3. Torabinejad M, Eby WC, Naidorf IJ. Inflammatory and immunological aspects of the pathogenesis of human periapical lesions. J Endod 1985;11:479–84.
4. Nair PNR. Pathology of apical periodontitis. In: Orstavik D, Pitt Ford TR, editors. Essential endodontology. Prevention and treatment of apical periodontitis. 1st ed. Oxford: Blackwell Science Ltd; 1998:68–95.
5. Stashenko P, Teles R, D'Souza R. Periradicular inflammatory responses and their modulation. Crit Rev Oral Biol Med 1998;9:498–521.
6. Simon JH. Incidence of periapical cysts in relation to the root canal. J Endod 1980;6:845–8.
7. Nair R. New perspective on radicular cysts: do they heal? Int Endod J 1998;31:155–60.
8. Trope M, Pettigrew J, Petras J, et al. Differentiation of periapical granulomas and radicular cysts by digital radiometric analysis. Endod Dent Traumatol 1989;5:69–72.
9. Simon JH, Enciso R, Malfaz J, et al. Differential diagnosis of large periapical lesions using cone-beam computed tomography measurements and biopsy. J Endod 2006;32:833–7.
10. French LA, Wild JJ, Neal D. Detection of cerebral tumors by ultrasonic pulses. Pilot studies on post-mortem material. Cancer 1950;3:705–8.
11. Auer LM, Van Velthoven V. Intraoperative ultrasound imaging in neurosurgery. Berlin: Springer Verlag; 1990.
12. Fleischer A, Emerson DS. Color Doppler sonography in obstetrics and gynecology. New York: Churchill Livingstone Inc.; 1993.
13. Nanda NC, Schlief R, Goldberg BB. Advances in echo imaging using contrast enhancement. 2nd ed. Dordrecht: Kluwer; 1997.
14. Wolf KJ, Fobbe F. Color duplex sonography. Principles and clinical applications. New York: Thieme; 1995.
15. Martin AO. Can ultrasound cause genetic damage? J Clin Ultrasound 1984;12:1–20.
16. Barnett SB, Rott HD, Ter Haar GR, et al. The sensitivity of biological tissue to ultrasound. Ultrasound Med Biol 1997;23:805–12.
17. Barnett SB, Ter Haar GR, Ziskin MC, et al. International recommendations and guidelines for the safe use of diagnostic ultrasound in medicine. Ultrasound Med Biol 2000;20:355–66.
18. Cotti E, Campisi G, Garau V, Puddu G. A new technique for the study of periapical bone lesions: ultrasound real time imaging. Int Endod J 2002;35:148–52.
19. Cotti E, Campisi G, Ambu R, Dettori C. Ultrasound real-time imaging in the differential diagnosis of periapical lesions. Int Endod J 2003;36:556–64.
20. Cotti E, Simbola V, Dettori C, Campisi G. Echographic evaluation of bone lesions of endodontic origin: report of two cases in the same patient. J Endod 2006;32:901–5.
21. Gundappa M, Ng SY, Whaites EJ. Comparison of ultrasound, digital and conventional radiography in differentiating periapical lesions. Dentomaxillofac Radiol 2006;35:326–33.
22. Rajendran N, Sundaresan B. Efficacy of Ultrasound and Color Power Doppler as a monitoring tool in the healing of endodontic periapical lesions. J Endod 2007;33:181–6.
23. Dula K, Mini R, van der Stelt PF, et al. Hypothetical mortality risk associated with spiral computed tomography of the maxilla and mandible. Eur J Oral Sci 1996;104:503–10.
24. Berrington de Gonzalez A, Darby S. Risk of cancer from diagnostic X-rays: estimates for the UK and 14 other countries. Lancet 2004;363(9406):345–51.
25. Shrout MK, Hall JM, Hidebolt CE. Differentiation of periapical granuloma and cysts by digital radiometric analysis. Oral Surg Oral Med Oral Pathol Oral Radiol Endod 1993;76:356–61.

Chapter 16

Radiographic Interpretation

Dag Ørstavik, Tore Arne Larheim

Radiographs are indispensable in most aspects of endodontic practice. They are important for diagnosis, treatment planning, monitoring details during treatment, control of details at conclusion of treatment, and for follow-up control of treatment outcome. The main focus in this chapter will be on interpretation of periapical radiographic images as intraoral films or digital counterparts, sensors, and image plates are the most frequently used means of radiographic examinations for endodontic diagnosis.

More sophisticated methods for radiographic diagnosis have become available, providing better details of normal and pathological structures with multiplanar imaging. Examples of such advanced imaging interpretation are also given, mainly in the section dealing with differential diagnosis.

Biological Processes Related to Radiographic Diagnosis

It is basic knowledge that radiographic details portray variations in mineral density in tissues and that conventional film- or sensor-detected exposures are two-dimensional reflections of a three-dimensional reality. Normal anatomical structures are recognized by density variations in tooth and bone tissues. The interpretation is done by relating the radiographic signs to our mental image of what the three-dimensional image normally should look like, and how we perceive this to be projected to the film. With time and experience, we rely increasingly on how a given radiograph relates to other radiographs we have seen and learned to accept as normal or pathological structures.

Obviously, interpretation of even simple radiographic exposures is subject to a great deal of bias: the knowledge base of basic, three-dimensional anatomy will vary among observers, there is bias and variation in the learning process from peers et al., and we develop individual preferences in attaching importance to specific elements of the radiograph. As clinical and radiographic signs of endodontic disease often are small and rather unspecific, there is always pressure on the diagnostician to read as much as possible into small variations in radiographic appearance of tooth and periapical structures. This bias and individual variation in diagnosis of periapical disease by radiography was elegantly demonstrated by Goldman et al.[1] and more scientifically by Reit and Gröndahl.[2]

CARIES

In caries diagnosis, the endodontic dilemma is to determine the spatial relationship of the carious lesion to the pulp. On the one hand, we are conditioned to think that proximal caries goes deeper than what can be seen in the radiograph; on the other, caries located on the buccal or lingual aspect may project over the pulp and give the false impression of pulpal involvement. Interpretation of radiographic findings in crowned teeth represents special challenges.[3]

PULPAL CHANGES: CALCIFICATION, OBLITERATION, AND RESORPTION

Abnormal pulp calcification may be reactionary (tertiary) dentin to caries or trauma (operative procedures); degenerative localized or diffuse calcifications in the coronal and, characteristically, the radicular pulp; and pulp obliteration following traumas such as tooth concussion or luxation or intentional or necessary replantation.[4–7]

Internal resorptions are usually associated with the replacement of dentin by a soft tissue with resorbing cells causing a balloon-shaped lesion starting from the radicular pulp.[8–12] The radiographic end result is a round or ovoid radiolucent area observed on the

PATHOLOGICAL REACTIONS OF TOOTH STRUCTURE: FRACTURE, RESORPTIVE PROCESSES

Fracture of a root can be difficult to diagnose but may result in reparative processes that become recognizable in later radiographs.[13–16] Diagnosis of root fractures may be made easier by using multiple projections (Figure 2) or advanced radiographic techniques, particularly computed tomography (CT).[14,16] There may be a hard tissue union of the two fragments if they are in close apposition to each other, the pulp is vital, and the fracture line is in its entirety within the periodontal ligament (PDL). Remodeling may then lead to a near normalization of the radiographic appearance of the root (Figure 3). In the case of fibrous repair, the fragments remain separated by a structure resembling periodontal membrane, and remodeling processes in the form of blunting of the fragment edges may become visible in the radiograph.

Resorptive processes of the tooth structure induce changes in radiographic structures that may be challenging both from a diagnostic and therapeutic point of view.[17–20] Surface resorption and repair may be seen as the body's way of coping with damage to the cementum, and these processes are sometimes extensive enough to be detectable radiographically. In cases of trauma with pulp damage, it then becomes a diagnostic challenge to differentiate resorption and repair from progressive inflammatory resorption, which, when uncontrolled, will lead to rapid loss of tooth substance.

Cervical root resorption[21] attacks dentin from pinpoint openings in cementum at the bottom of the gingival pocket and progresses either in irregular pathways in all directions into dentin or as semilunar, distinct caries- or erosion-like lesions (Figure 4), sometimes in multiple locations. As the process tends to halt when the inner dentin and predentin

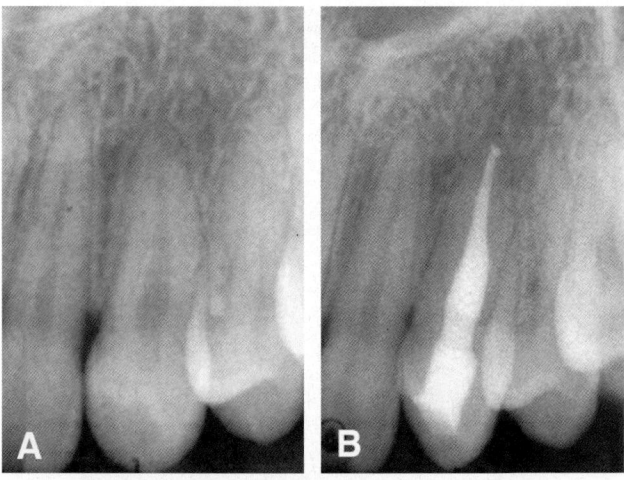
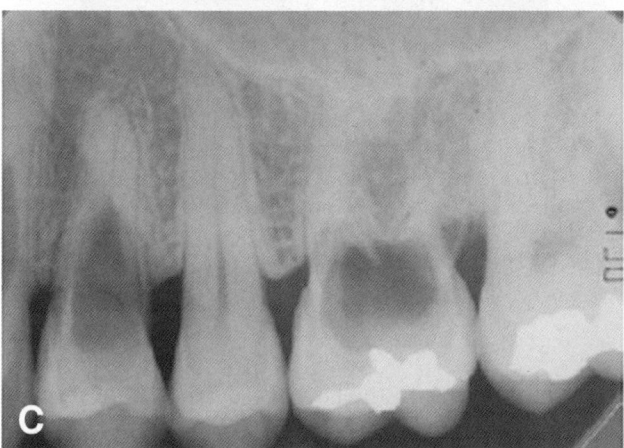

Figure 1 *A, B,* Internal resorption of left upper canine before and after endodontic treatment (Courtesy, Dr. Harald Prestegaard); *C,* Rare case of multiple resorptions (Courtesy, Dr. Elisabeth Samuelsen).

radiograph (Figure 1). It is a characteristic radiographic sign that the internal pulpal wall is destroyed, whereas cementum and periodontium are not affected, at least not initially.

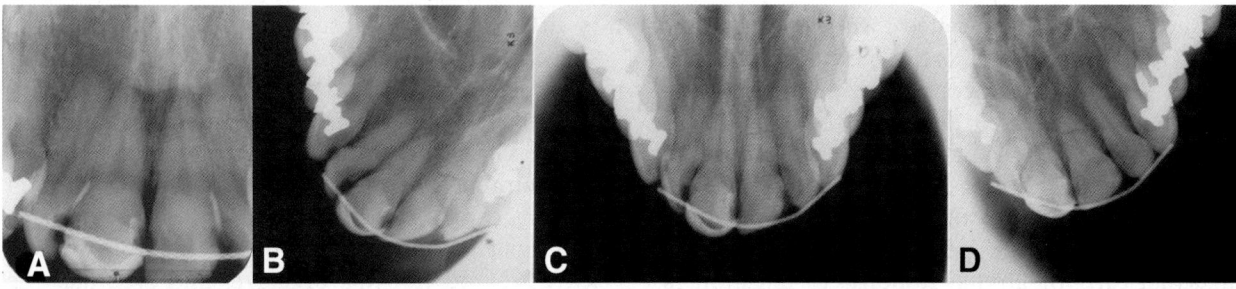

Figure 2 Root fracture examined two days after trauma. *A,* Uncertain diagnosis on the periapical radiograph. *B, C, D,* Fracture is evident when multiple projections are obtained.

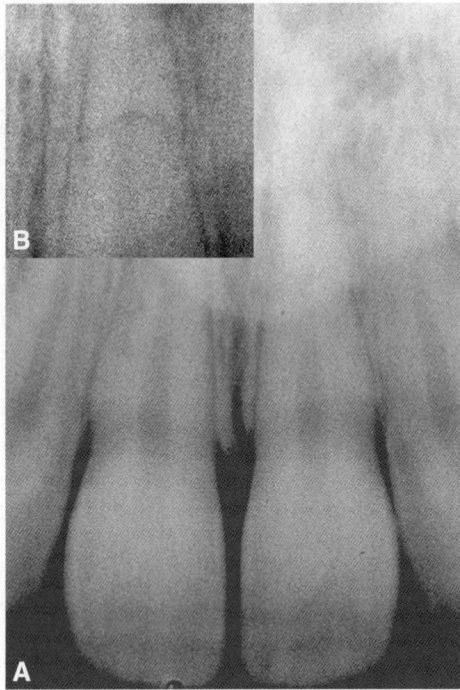
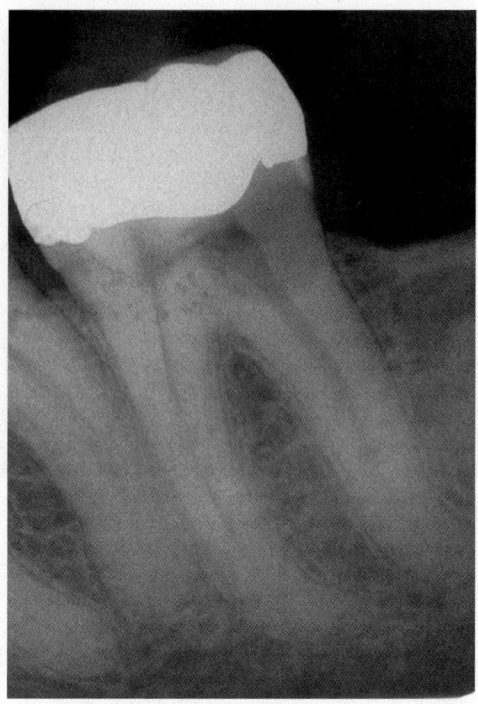

Figure 3 **A,** Tooth remodeling of fragments after healing of horizontal root fracture. **B,** Blunting of edges shown in insert with artificially increased contrast.

Figure 4 Cervical root resorption; erosive type.

are reached, radiographically the lesions are often characterized by an outline of the pulp space appearing through the radiolucent area caused by the resorption (Figure 5).

PERIAPICAL CHANGES: WIDTH OF PERIODONTAL LIGAMENT, BONE TEXTURE CHANGES, DEMINERALIZATION, BONE FORMATION, APICAL SURGERY

Apical root resorption, bone resorption, cementum formation, and bone deposition are the biological processes primarily associated with radiographic changes in the periapical area. Furthermore, there are often structural changes in the periapical bone reflecting either increased density of bone (condensing apical osteitis)[22,23] or altered organization of trabeculae (incipient apical osteitis) (Figure 6).

Resorption/remodeling of the apical lamina dura and a widening of the periodontal ligament may occur as an early or limited response to infection in the root canal system, but is also common as a consequence of increased tooth mobility, as in marginal periodontal inflammation or during orthodontic tooth movement. In the latter case, apical root resorption and remodeling of the root apex may be very extensive (Figure 7).

Apical periodontitis leads to demineralization of periapical bone with subsequent lesion development. Preceded by structural changes in the bone, this lesion may be evident in radiographs before overt demineralization has begun in the area.

Apical periodontitis (granuloma, radicular cyst) develops with variable speed, and the effects on the surrounding bone will also vary. Bone deposition with the formation of a distinct bony rim may occur, which has been associated with stable lesions more likely to have cyst formation; however, there is little evidence to support this concept.[24,25] On the other hand, cyst formation is more likely to be found in large lesions compared to small.[26] Histological studies have indicated that in lesions with acute characteristics there are changes in bone structure peripherally to the outer margin of the lesion proper.[27]

Surgical endodontic or other periapical procedures leave a blood clot that organizes and eventually heals by formation of cortical and medullary bone. This healing process is faster than healing of apical lesions after conservative endodontic therapy,[28] and leads to

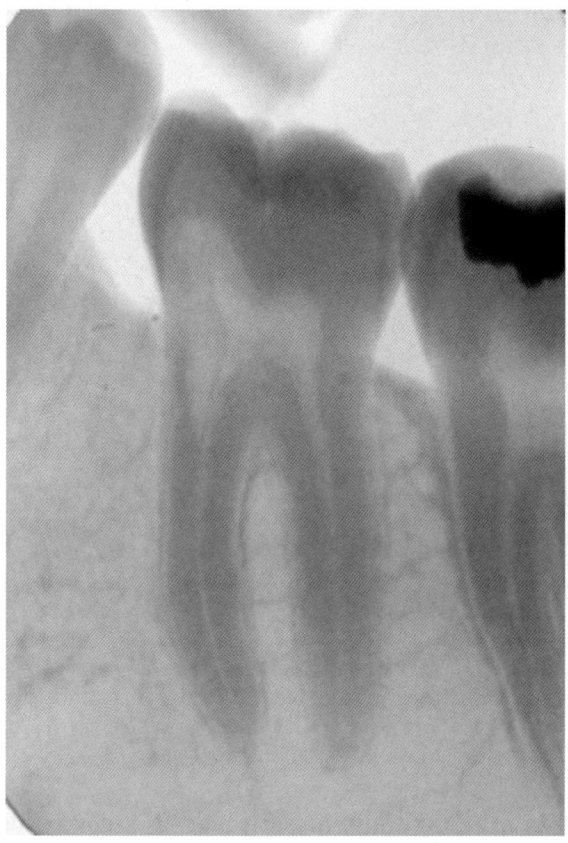

Figure 5 Cervical root resorption progressing apically with characteristic outline of pulp chamber clearly visible (Courtesy, Dr. Nabeel Mekhlif).

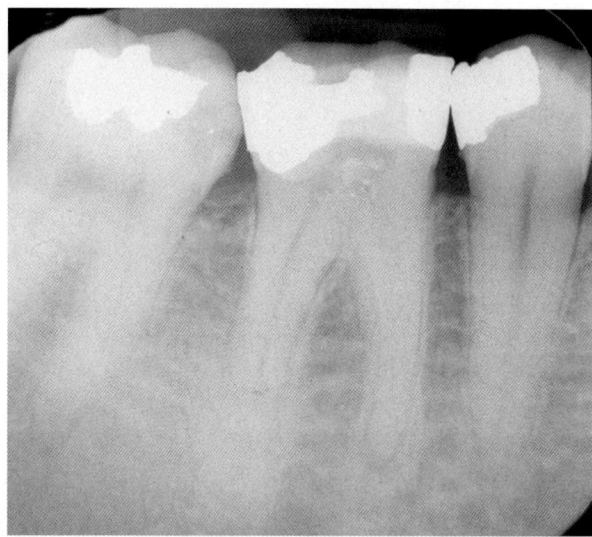

Figure 6 Condensing apical periodontitis at distal root, incipient apical periodontitis at mesial root of mandibular first right molar. Note foreign material in pulp chamber, a likely cause of chronic pulpitis or pulp necrosis.

radiographic signs that may differ from normal periapical structures, particularly if scar tissue with reduced mineral content is formed.[29,30]

OTHER ENDODONTIC APPLICATIONS OF PERIAPICAL RADIOLOGY

There are several situations and cases where other aspects of endodontic treatment are detected and monitored by radiographs. Examples are iatrogenic mishaps such as root perforations and overfillings, root fractures and special procedures such as root resection and hemisection.

Periapical Diagnosis

Apical periodontitis is typically a droplet-shaped radiolucent area associated with the root apex surrounded by bone in continuity with the lamina dura at some distance from the pulpal exit.[31] Being dependent on the egress of infectious material through the apical pulp orifice, lesions of apical periodontitis may be situated in lateral or furcal locations in association with lateral or furcal accessory canals, respectively.

Apical periodontitis is a defense mechanism against infection. When apical cementum and dentin are invaded by microbes, the structures are attacked by resorbing cells, and root resorption, albeit limited, is integral to lesion development.[32,33] The development of a granuloma and/or a cyst may be seen as the mobilization of an area where host defense mechanisms are concentrated, and the resorption of bone is a process necessary to provide space for the defending tissues.[34] The granuloma/cyst is also protecting from direct infection of the bone marrow (osteomyelitis). While the granuloma/cyst is defined to a degree by the relative resistance of the bone, it occupies a place that is effective for the mobilization of a host defense, and cortical bone may be eroded for this purpose even if the path of least resistance would have pointed in another direction.

As the cortex makes up a very large percentage of the bone mass in the radiograph of a normal periapical area,[35] the proposition has been made that involvement of cortical bone loss is necessary for detection of a lesion in a radiograph. While it is a matter of course that any lesion involving the cortex is more easily detectable,[36,37] research has documented that the changes induced by resorptions and changes in the medullary and subcortical, trabecular bone can also be seen.[37,38]

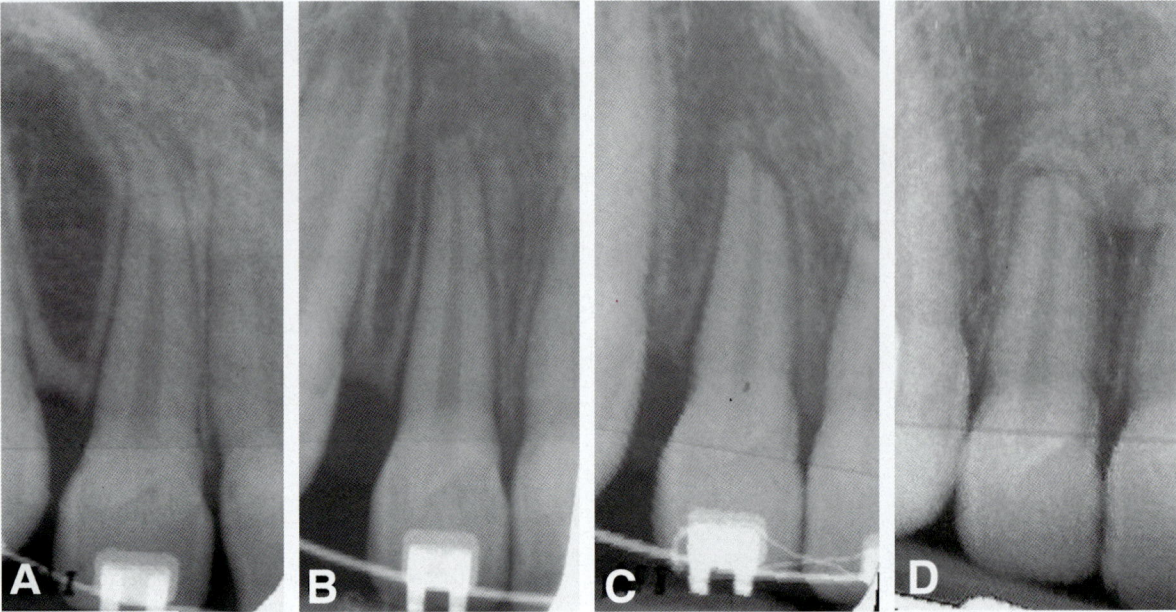

Figure 7 ***A,*** Periapical radiographs of maxillary premolar made before orthodontic treatment, ***B,*** at 5.2 months and ***C,*** 11.9 months after bracket placement, and ***D,*** at end of 22.1 months of orthodontic treatment. Projections ***A, C*** and ***D*** are reconstructed according to projection ***B.*** Note apical root resorption of 2.6mm at 5.2 months ***B,*** of 5.1mm at 11.9 months ***C,*** and of 7.0mm at end of treatment ***D.*** (Modified with permission from Årtun J, Van 't Hullenar R., Doppel D., Kuijpers-Jagtman A.M. Identification of orthodontic patients at risk of severe apical root resorption. Am J Orthod Dentofacial Orthop 2007; 132:in press.)

Radiographic signs must be correlated with macroscopic or microscopic anatomical and pathological features. Several studies have compared the radiographic and histological appearance of apical periodontitis, of which Brynolf's[27] is by far the most extensive and detailed. Table 1 lists some of her findings that relate radiographic signs to histological characteristics of periapical inflammation.

There are few things easier than the radiographic diagnosis of a well-established, chronic apical periodontitis. Two particular radiographic aspects of apical periodontitis, however, may be difficult and frustrating: the detection of incipient changes and the monitoring of healing or post-treatment development of disease.

Advanced Multiplanar Imaging

Advanced imaging of the periapical area usually means section imaging. With computer technology it is possible to obtain an image of virtually any plane through a structure, greatly improving the diagnostic information of its three-dimensional morphology. However, the interpretation of multiple sections versus one projectional radiographic image is challenging and may require collaboration between specialists in endodontics and oral and maxillofacial radiology as given in the following paragraphs.

Advanced imaging, in particular CT, may be used supplementary to conventional periapical radiography for demonstration of complex anatomy of the root and surrounding structures, including associated lesions (Figure 8). With the development of cone beam CT, the root and periapical bone can be examined in axial, coronal, and sagittal sections with less patient exposure than with conventional CT to evaluate, for instance, the integrity of the cortical bone (Figure 9).

Table 1 Histological and Radiographic Correlates

Histological Appearance	Radiographic Features
Incipient apical periodontitis	Bone structural changes
Initial inflammation with acute features	Bone structural changes
Chronic inflammation	Bone demineralization; lesion area defined
Granuloma or cyst formation	Radiolucent area; peripheral bony rim
Lesion with features of exacerbation	Bone structural changes peripheral to lesion

Adapted from Brynolf[27]

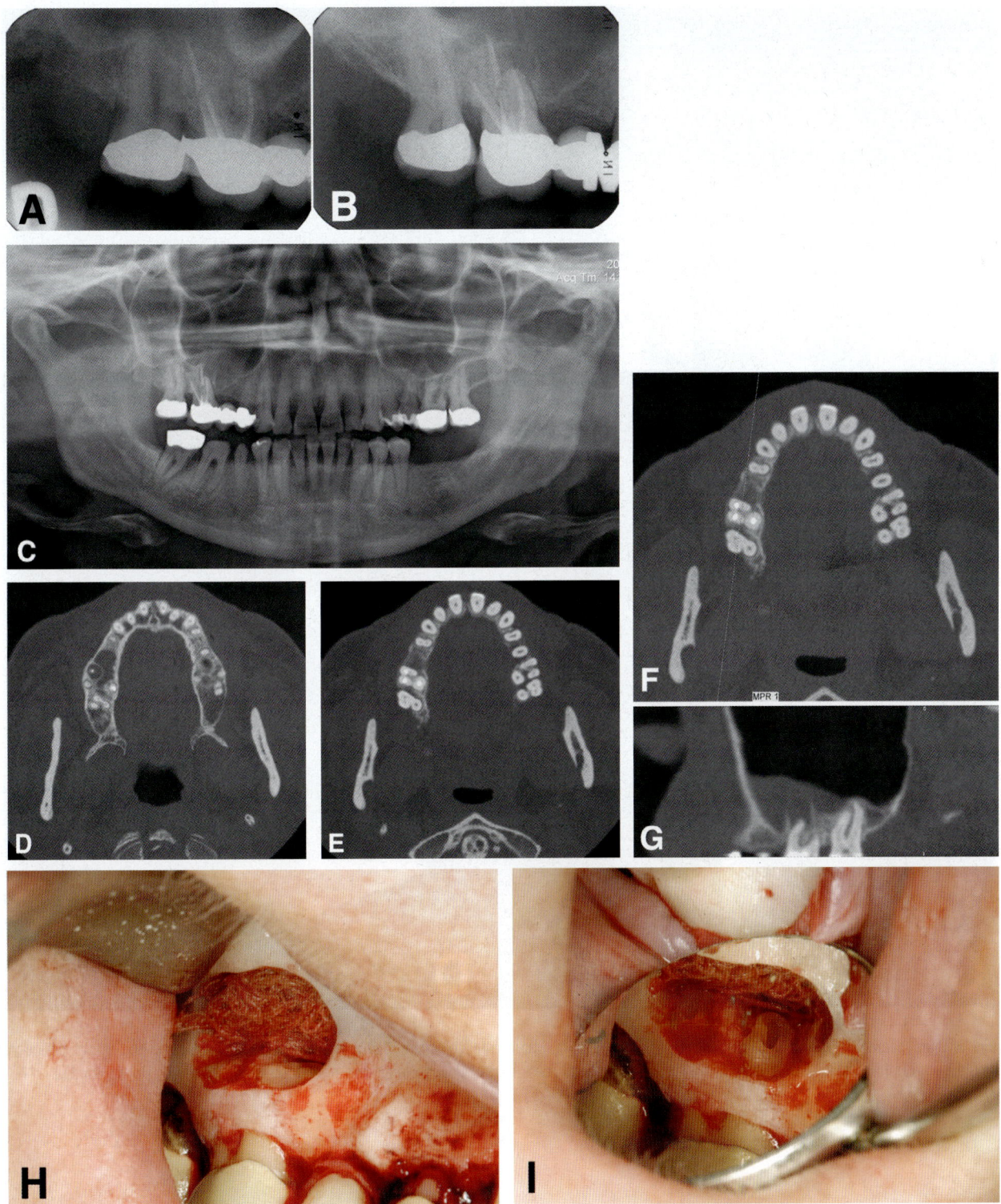

Figure 8 Molar with one canal in the mesiobuccal root unfilled and with apical periodontitis. *A, B, C,* Unfilled root canal is not seen on periapical or panoramic radiographs. *D, E, F, G,* Unfilled root canal and apical periodontitis seen on CT scans. *H, I,* Clinical photos confirm two root canals in the mesiobuccal root (of which only the most buccal was found to be root filled). (*H, I,* Courtesy, Dr. Homan Zandi)

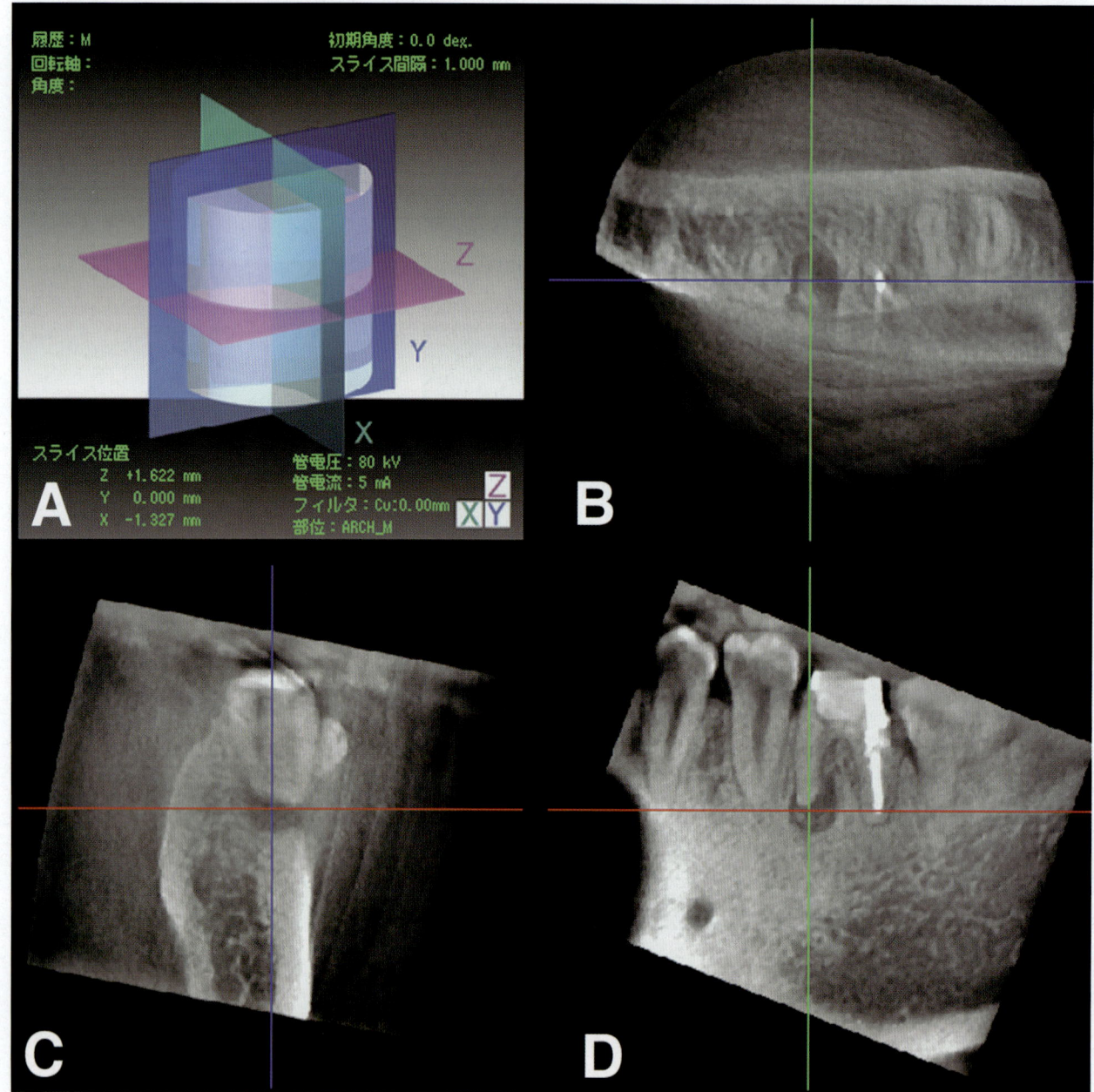

Figure 9 Cone beam CT. **B,** axial, **C,** coronal, **D,** sagital sections. Root filled distal root with normal periapical structure and apical periodontitis associated with unfilled mesial root with destroyed buccal cortex. The different image planes are illustrated in **A.** (Courtesy, Dr. K. Honda.)

Problems and Potentials of Periapical Radiographic Diagnosis and Follow-up of Apical Periodontitis

INCIPIENT CHANGES

Based on a concept of apical periodontitis (granuloma, cyst) formation as an expanding balloon starting at the apical orifice of the pulp, it has been held that the first sign of disease can be recognized as a widened periodontal ligament. Brynolf's[27] and later studies[39,40] have documented that this is a poor indicator of disease development. Rather, it may reflect increased tooth mobility or a limited tissue reaction to root filling surplus, or traumatic occlusion. Initial or limited inflammatory processes in relation to root canal infection can be detected by changes in the bone structure periapically rather than by overt demineralization.[27] While it may be possible through extensive training to obtain proficiency in observing these changes,[41] it should probably be accepted that such initial changes cannot reliably be diagnosed by conventional radiographic methods. In keeping with standard procedures for diagnosing disease in clinical practice and epidemiological studies, a high threshold should be set to exclude weak radiographic signs.

HEALING OF APICAL PERIODONTITIS

The biological dynamics of healing apical periodontitis are rarely studied and therefore not well known. It is a slow process,[28] probably because of the resistance to resorption/replacement of the tissue components of cysts and, particularly, granulomas. By quantitative analyses of radiographs, healing may be seen as early as 3 months after therapy,[42,43] and by 1 year, almost all cases that will eventually heal completely, show unequivocal, radiographic signs of healing[44] (Figure 10). But healing processes that were not in evidence for as long as 10 to 17 years after treatment can be activated later to re-establish normal radiographic structures.[45]

ANATOMICAL LIMITATIONS

Normal anatomical structures and their variable location, size, and characteristics in different individuals, interfere with the interpretation of the periapical tissue responses in endodontic diagnosis. It is not simple in individual cases to account for variations of this kind; for example, while the alveolar bone surrounding roots of mandibular second and third molars is often free of confounding anatomical structures and thus should lead to an unquestionable diagnosis of periapical changes, the variations in trabecular pattern in this area is a frequent source of misdiagnosis of apical lesions that do not actually exist.

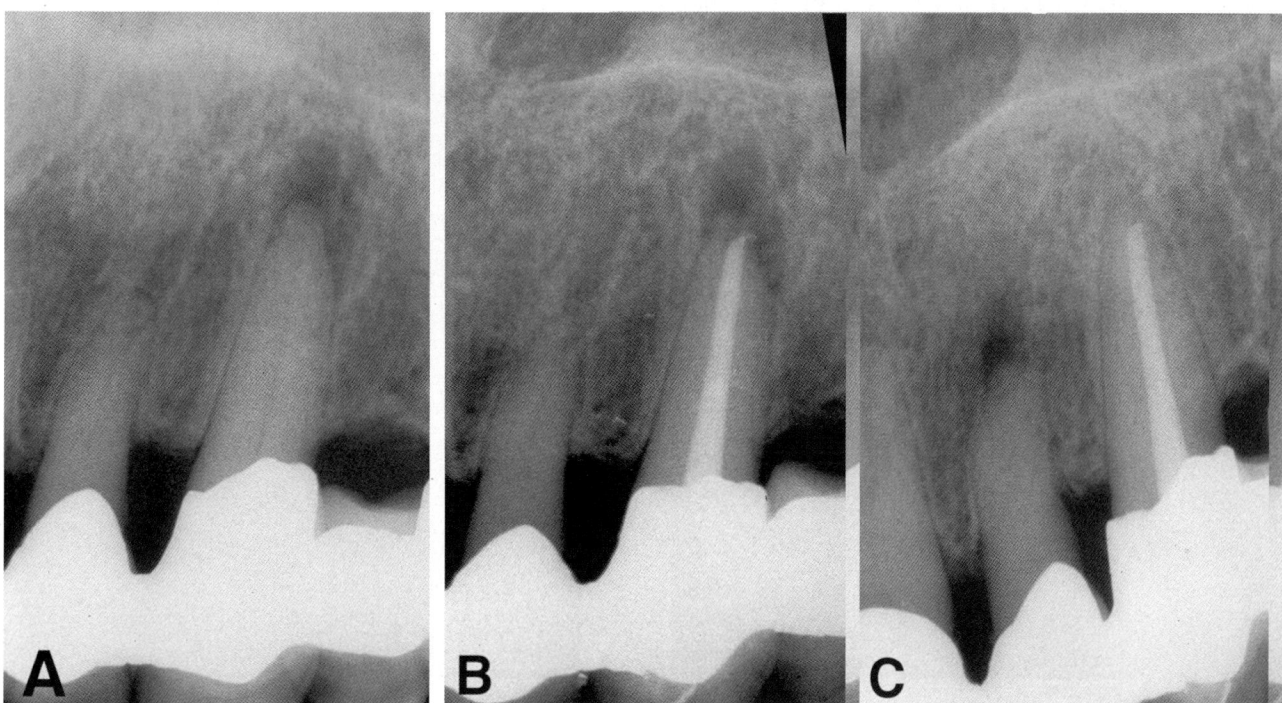

Figure 10 *A, B, C,* Complete healing of apical periodontitis within 17 months of treatment.

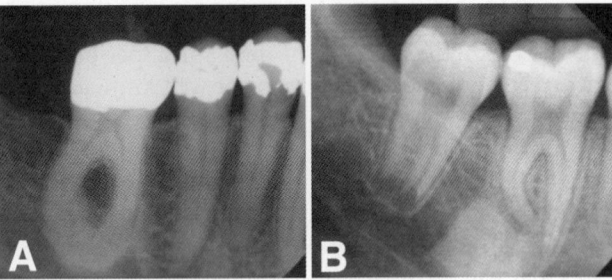

Figure 11 Idiopathic osteosclerosis. ***A***, Closely located to the apex of a vital tooth. ***B***, Separated from the apex of a tooth with vital pulp.

DIFFERENTIAL DIAGNOSIS

Although conventional periapical radiography will be sufficient for differential diagnostic radiographic evaluation in most cases, the usefulness of advanced imaging is evident in the examination of a number of conditions, particularly when more serious disease is suspected.[46]

Hypercementosis may occur in response to pulpal inflammation without infection in the apical part of the canal. While the pulpitis usually requires endodontic treatment, the cementum deposited is not remodeled and will persist after endodontic treatment. Condensing apical osteitis is also associated with chronic pulpitis and will resolve following adequate therapy. It is the bone structure that is altered, and remodeling is possible and likely, although areas of persistent condensed bone may be seen in apposition to apparently adequately treated teeth. Idiopathic osteosclerosis may be a differential diagnostic problem if located close to the apices (Figure 11). Marginal periodontitis may show radiographic features similar to apical periodontitis, and when presenting with a necrotic and infected pulp may need combined treatment (Figure 12). Root fractures may indeed be seen as a variant of apical periodontitis; if the pulp canal space and the fracture slit are infected, this will result in a periodontitis where the fracture communicates with the periodontal space (Figure 13). The radiographic signs are somewhat characteristic in the case of vertical fractures, in that the whole length of the root may be affected, producing a diffuse halo of radiolucent bone around the root (Figure 14). Similarly,

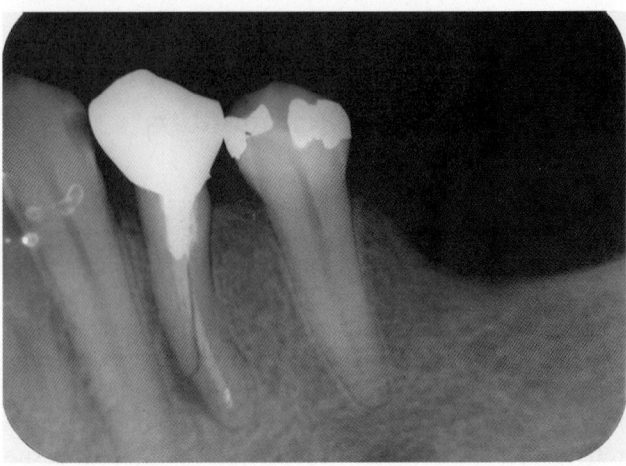

Figure 13 Oblique-vertical root fracture with laterally widened periodontal ligament due to infection.

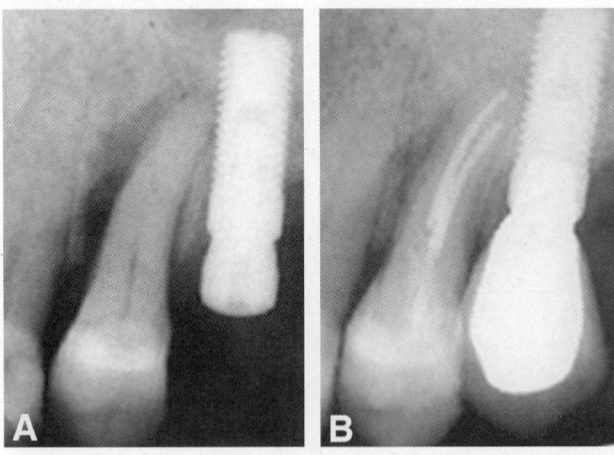

Figure 12 ***A***, Typical endodontic-periodontal lesion. ***B***, Healing 10 months after endodontic treatment. (Courtesy, Dr. Birte N. Myrvang)

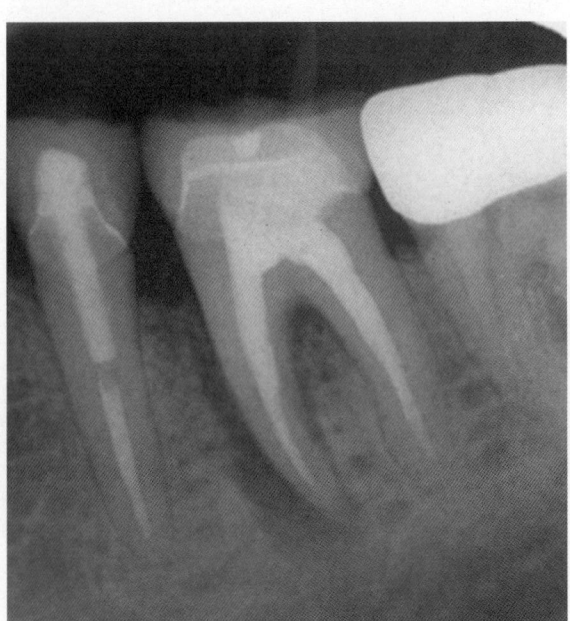

Figure 14 Vertical root fracture with bone resorption along the entire length of the mesial root.

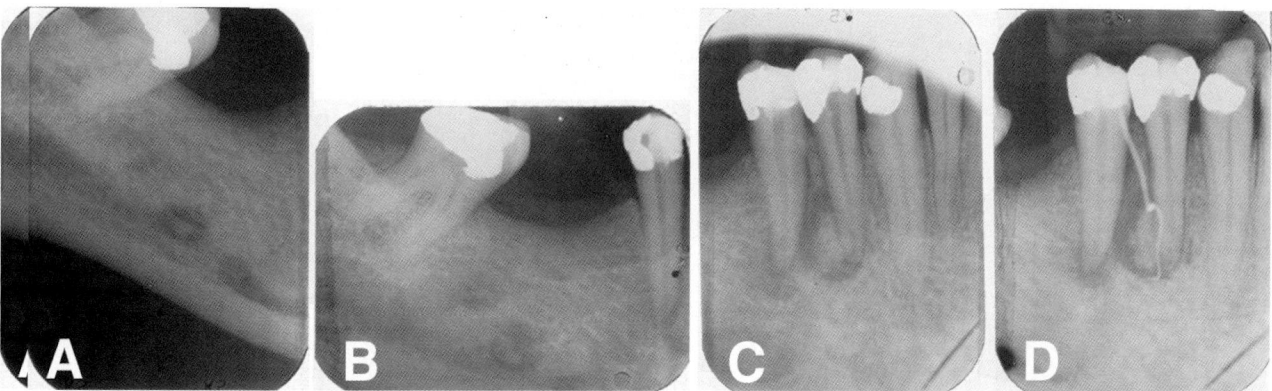

Figure 15 Osteomyelitis with fistula formation and sequestration. **A, B,** Destructive foci, apparently with normal bone structures in between. **C, D,** Apical periodontitis with sequestrum and gutta-percha point in sinus tract.

osteomyelitis may follow an initial root canal infection that for some reason has escaped the protective functions of the cyst or granuloma and invaded the bone marrow spaces (Figures 15, 16). Osteomyelitis characteristically may show sequestration and apparently normal bone structures between areas of bone destruction (see Figure 15). Another characteristic feature is periosteal bone formation that in young patients may become extensive (Figures 16, 17). In patients with irradiated mandibles, osteoradionecrosis may develop

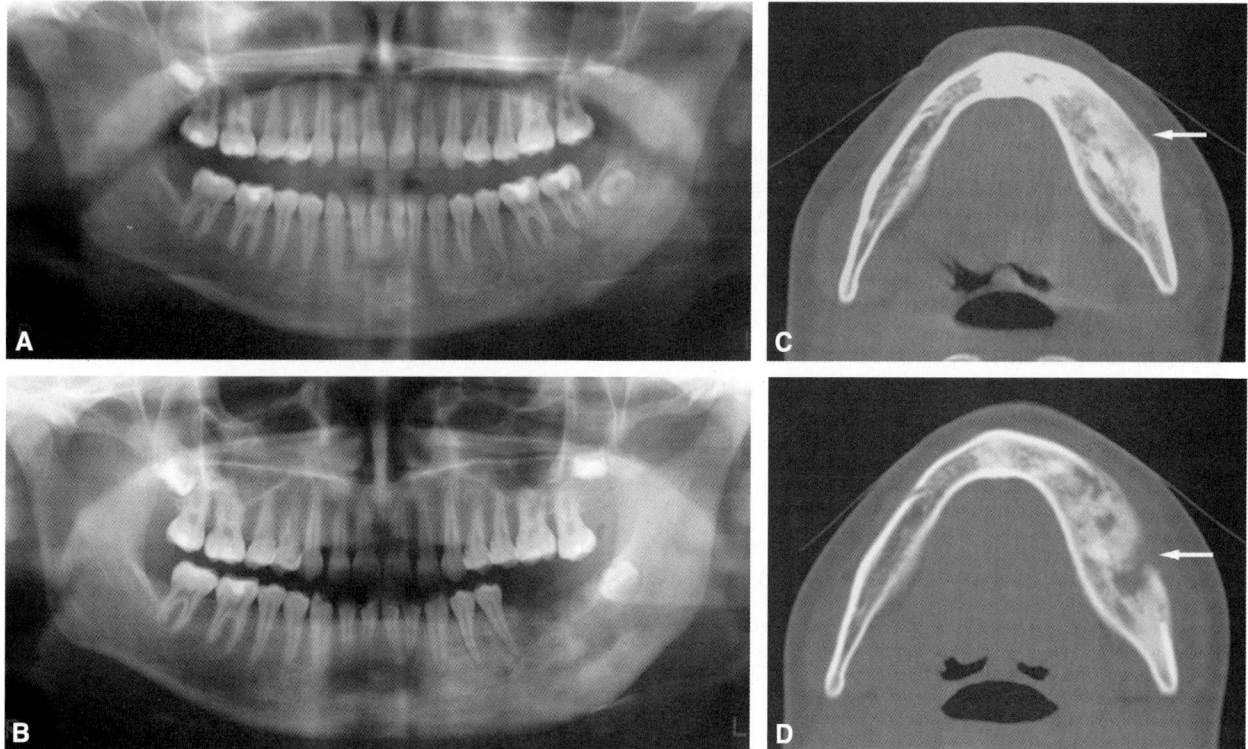

Figure 16 Osteomyelitis in 12-year old patient with extensive periosteal reaction. **A,** Apical periodontitis associated with both molars with necrotic pulps in left mandible and onion-peel bone formation of the lower mandibular border. **B, C,** One year later extensive bone formation is evident (arrow). **D,** Two years after baseline new bone destruction because of increased disease activity is clearly seen (arrow). (Reproduced with permission from Larheim, T.A., Westesson, P.-L. Maxillofacial Imaging, Springer 2006.)

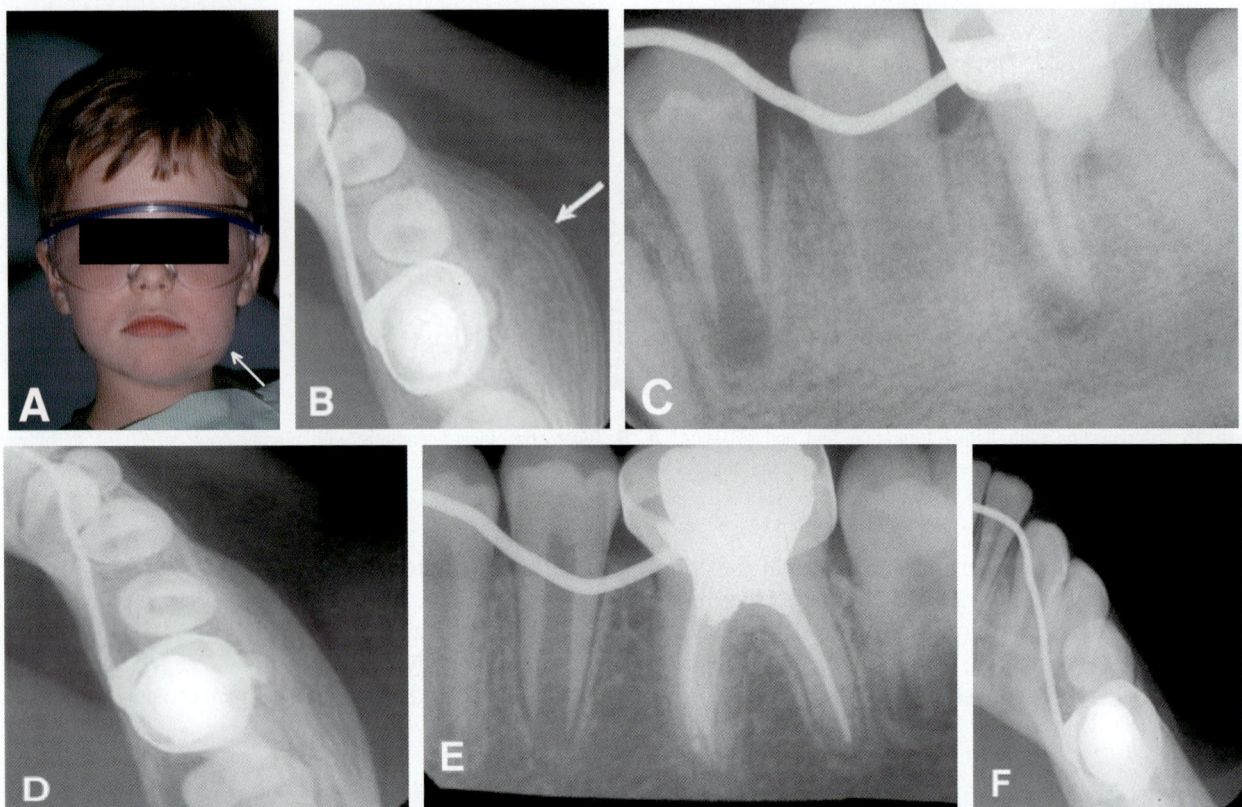

Figure 17 Proliferative periostitis of Garré. *A,* Clinical photo of 8-year-old boy with swelling associated with the left mandible (arrow). *B,* Occlusal radiograph shows classic onion skin osseous expansion around the mesial root of the first molar. *C,* Periapical radiograph shows a large lesion associated with the mesial root of the molar. *D,* Occlusal view 5 months after endodontic treatment; note significant reduction in swelling. *E,* Periapical radiograph taken 1 year after treatment; note resolution of apical lesion. *F,* Occlusal view 1 year later; note resolution of osseous expansion. (Reproduced with permission from Jacobson H.L.J., Baumgartner J.C., Marshall J.G., Beeler W.J. Proliferative periostitis of Garré: Report of a case. Oral Surg Oral Med Oral Pathol Oral Radiol Endod 2002;94:111-14.)

that is indistinguishable from osteomyelitis, although usually with less prominent periosteal reaction (Figure 18). This may occur even many years after the radiation therapy of the malignancy. Bisphosphonate-related osteonecrosis of the jaws with a similar radiographic picture has been reported to occur with increasing frequency.[47]

The inflammatory paradental cyst is a rare entity, occurring exclusively in the mandibular molar area, and should not cause major difficulties in differentiation from apical periodontitis.[48] However, the cyst may be projected over the apex on a conventional radiograph, making advanced imaging a valuable supplement for diagnosis (Figure 19). The lateral periodontal cyst is a developmental cyst occurring primarily in the premolar area of the mandible and may be difficult to distinguish radiographically from apical periodontitis.[49] It can also occur in the maxilla, and when

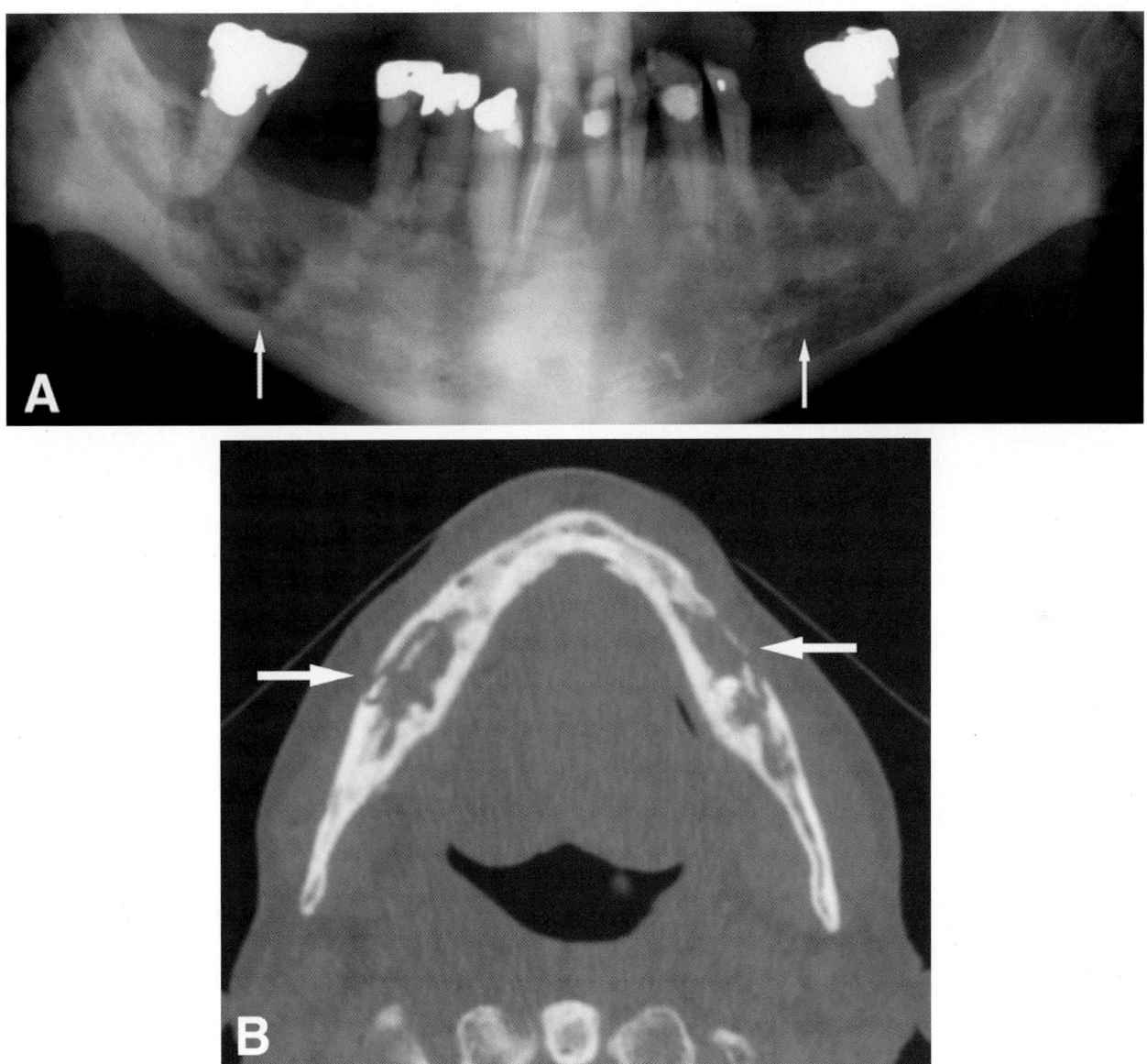

Figure 18 Osteoradionecrosis two years after radiation therapy and surgery of malignancy in maxilla. ***A, B,*** Extensive bilateral bone destruction with sequestration (arrows). (Reproduced with permission from Larheim, T.A., Westesson, P.-L. Maxillofacial Imaging, Springer 2006.)

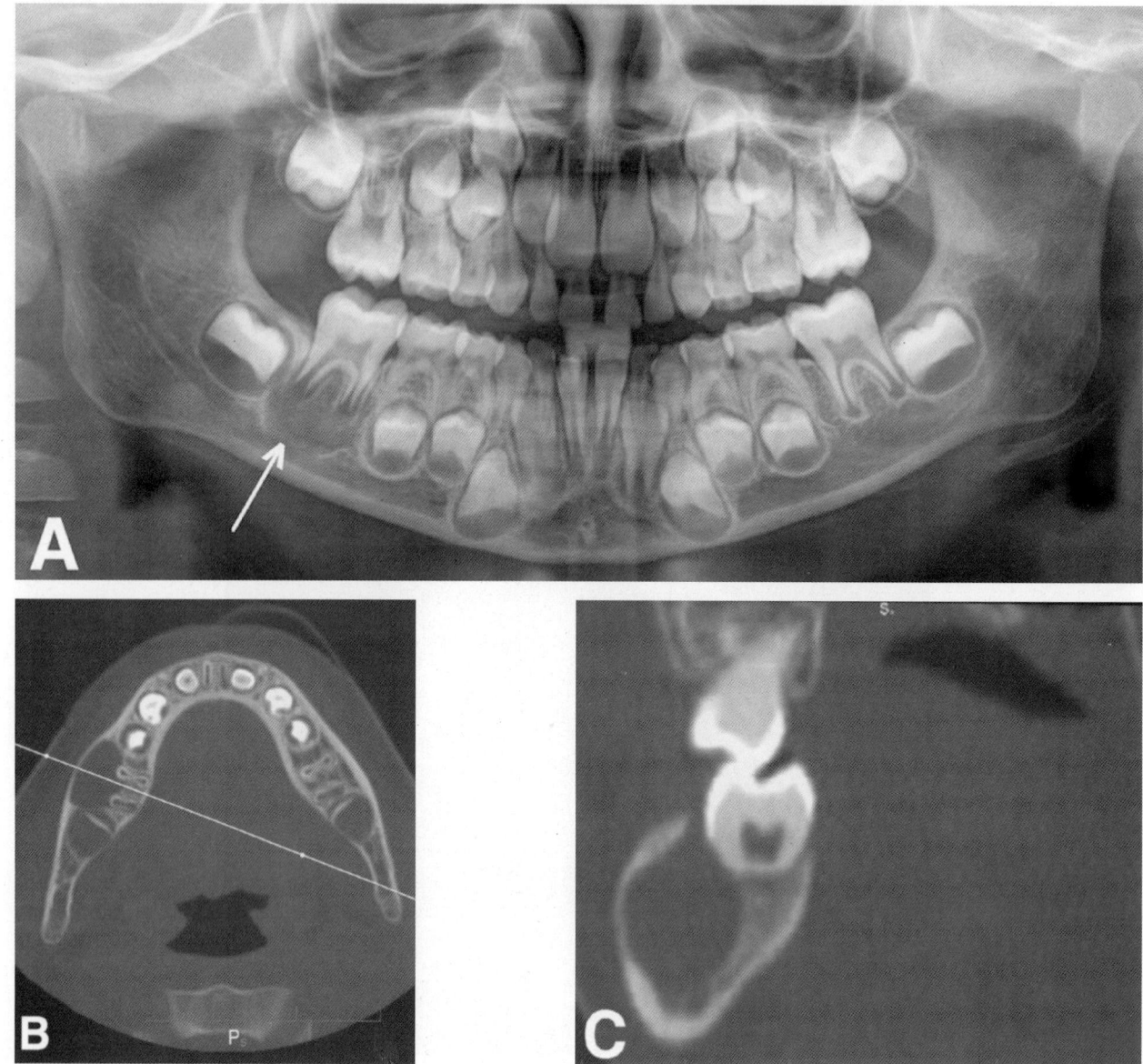

Figure 19 Paradental cyst. ***A,*** Apical radiolucency of first mandibular molar (Arrow). ***B, C,*** Buccal radiolucency with marginal communication, typically of a buccally infected paradental cyst.

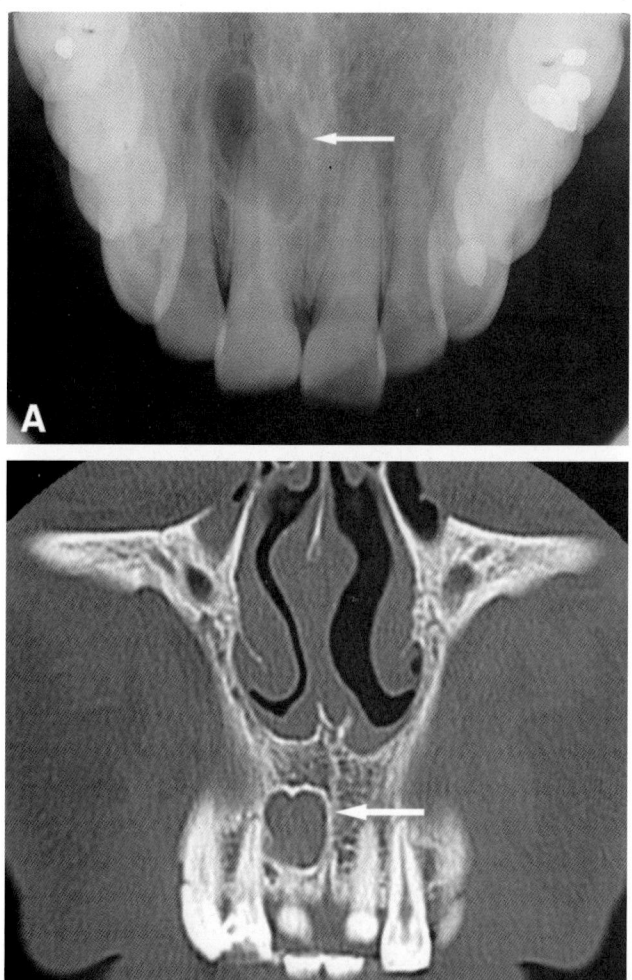

Figure 20 Lateral periodontal cyst. ***A,*** Occlusal view shows apical radiolucency (arrow). ***B,*** CT scan shows cyst not connected to the tooth (arrow). (Reproduced with permission from Larheim, T.A., Westesson, P.-L. Maxillofacial Imaging, Springer 2006.)

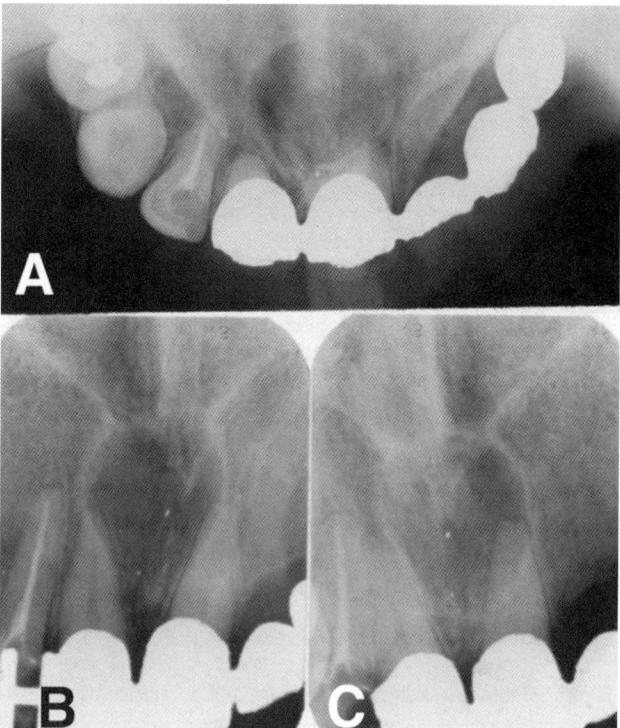

Figure 21 Incisive canal cyst. ***A, B, C,*** Occlusal view and conventional periapical radiographs show the cyst palatally located to the incisors.

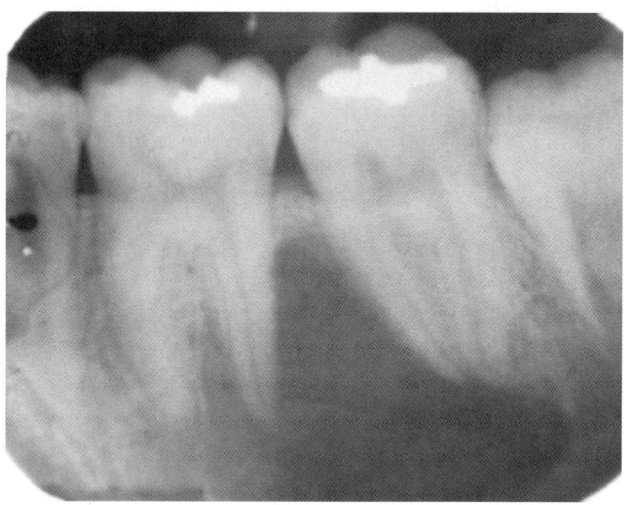

Figure 22 Simple bone cyst. Periapical radiograph showing radiolucency between first and second molars. There was no expansion of the mandible.

projected over the apex on a conventional radiograph, supplementary advanced imaging may add decisive diagnostic information (Figure 20). The non-odontogenic incisive canal developmental cyst is located centrally between the maxillary incisors and may be easily mistaken for apical periodontitis if projected over the apex. An axial view may be helpful to identify the cyst in a palatal position in the jaw (Figure 21). A normal apical periodontium and pulp sensitivity will rule out apical periodontitis in such cases. The simple bone cyst (traumatic bone cyst) is not a true cyst but an empty hole in the jaw bone without epithelial coverage and of unknown origin, usually found in young individuals (Figure 22). Osseous (cemental) dysplasia may completely mimic almost any phase, productive or resorptive, of chronic apical periodontitis. The condition may be

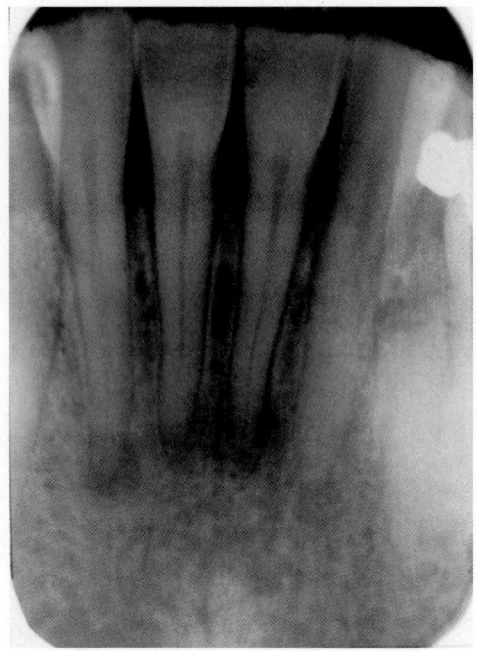

Figure 23 Osseous (cemental) dysplasia. Apical radiolucencies (early stage dysplasia) around apices of three incisors.

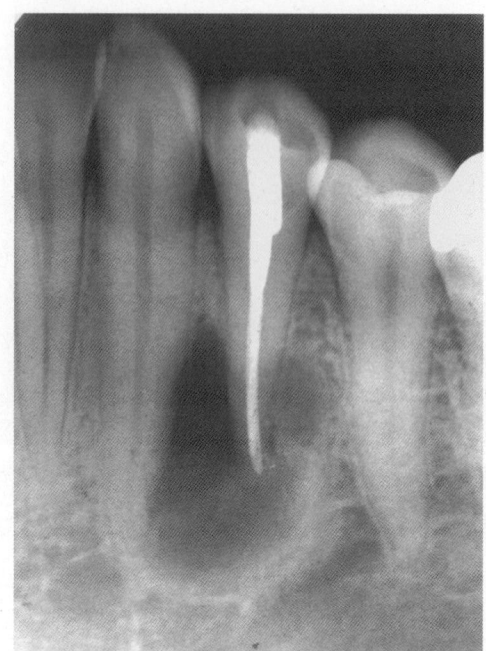

Figure 24 Giant cell granuloma mimicking apical periodontitis.

multiple and is predominantly found in the incisal region of the lower jaw (Figure 23). It is characteristic of most of the conditions mentioned in this paragraph that the pulps are vital and there are no clinical symptoms The giant cell granuloma is another lesion that usually presents as a large, sometimes multilocular, radiolucent area. It may also be more unilocular (Figures 24, 25), like eosinophilic granuloma, and sometimes give radiographic signs not unlike apical periodontitis. The value of advanced imaging is clearly demonstrated with the case of giant cell granuloma; it could be determined

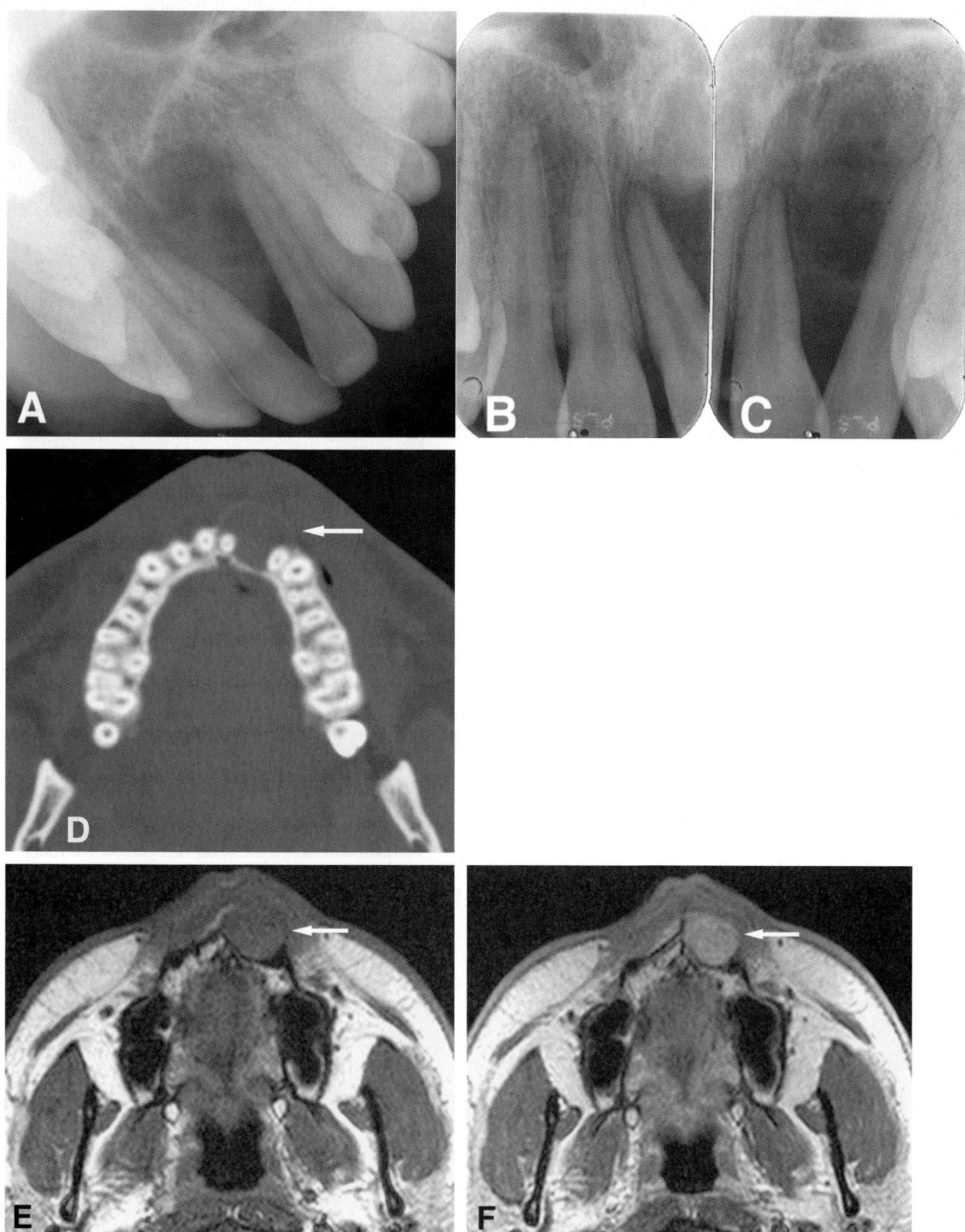

Figure 25 Giant cell granuloma. *A, B, C,* Unilocular radiolucency with displacement of two incisors; *D,* CT scan shows severe expansion buccally without corticated outline (arrow); *E, F,* MR imaging scans before *E* and after *F* intravenous contrast injection show contrast enhancement of entire lesion, consistent with solid tumor (arrow). (Reproduced with permission from Larheim, T.A., Westesson, P.-L. Maxilofacial Imaging, Springer 2006.)

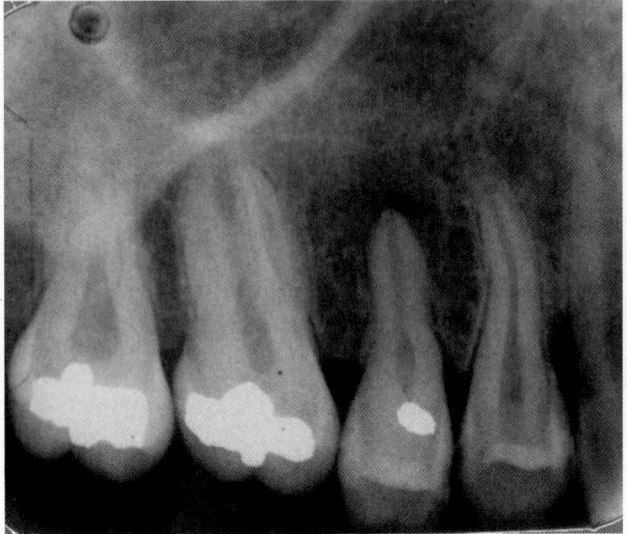

Figure 26 Primary hyperparathyreoidism. Defects in dentin structure and wide pulp chambers and root canals make the pulp tissue highly susceptible to damage and infection.

before surgery and histology that the lesion was solid and not cystic when supplementary magnetic resonance imaging was performed (see Figure 25).

Hyperparathyroidism (Figure 26) is a systemic condition predisposing for pulpal and periapical infections.

Tumors of the jaw present radiolucencies that sometimes may mimic apical periodontitis. Pulp sensitivity will normally rule out apical periodontitis. The odontogenic keratocyst (keratocystic odontogenic tumor) and the ameloblastoma may appear close to root apices in singlelobular or multilobular forms, the latter tumor frequently demonstrates evident root resorption (Figure 27). A case of ameloblastoma, seen as a unilocular radiolucency on a conventional radiograph, proved to be multicystic with advanced imaging (Figure 28). Ossifying fibroma may also simulate apical periodontitis

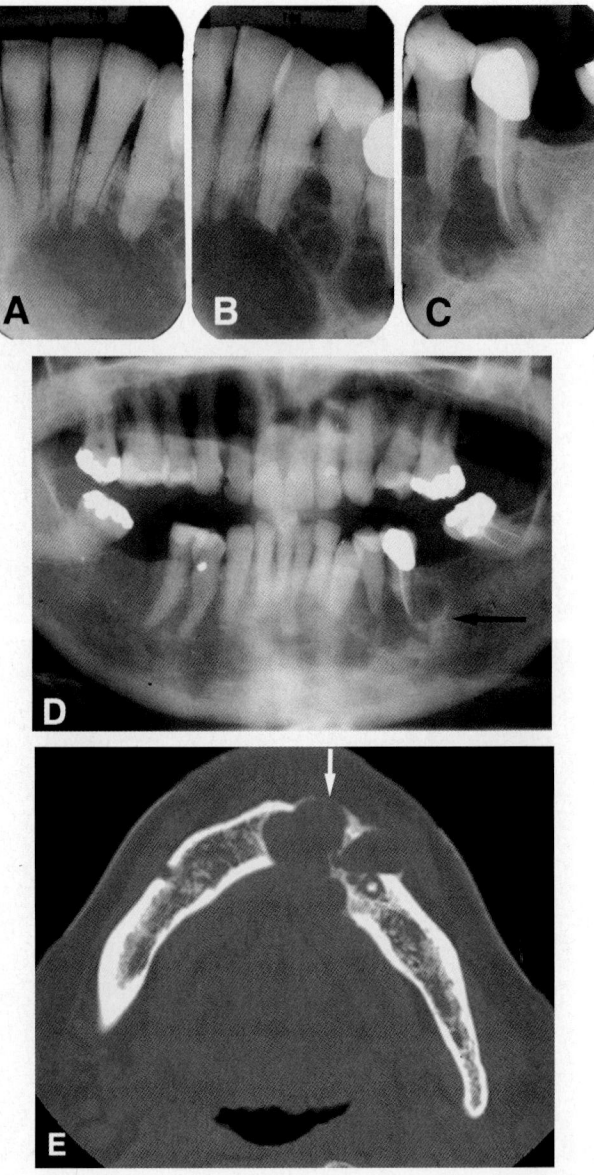

Figure 27 Ameloblastoma, multicystic/solid type. ***A, B,*** Multilocular radiolucencies with evident root resorptions (arrow). ***C,*** CT scan shows severe bone destruction and evident buccal expansion with destroyed lingual cortical bone (arrow). (Reproduced with permission from Larheim, T.A., Westesson, P.-L. Maxillofacial Imaging, Springer 2006.)

(Figure 29), but unlike the other conditions mentioned (except cemental dysplasia), it also produces bone giving a mixed radiographic appearance.[50]

Malignant tumors in the jaws are rare but may cause severe bone destruction, and displace, but rarely resorb, adjoining teeth; floating teeth are more typical.[46] A case of metastatic breast carcinoma in the mandible is shown in Figure 30, detected when the patient had a postoperative follow-up after apicoectomy.

Periapical Radiographs in Clinical and Epidemiological Endodontic Research

Clinical radiographic research in endodontics is primarily concerned with apical periodontitis: its emergence following pulp extirpation or its healing after root canal treatment of infected teeth.

SPECIFICITY AND SENSITIVITY, REPRODUCIBILITY

Any system for registering disease must address the issue of specificity and sensitivity: how specific is a given criterion for the disease in question (i.e., how often will the diagnosis be wrong) and how quickly/early the criterion can be detected (i.e., how sensitive is the sign). From the discussions above, it is apparent that initial signs of apical periodontitis in radiographs may be of low specificity (widened periodontal ligament (PDL) reflecting increased mobility rather than disease), and increasing the sensitivity may come at the expense of specificity in registering initial disease. Also with reference to the discussion above, the personal bias in interpreting radiographs makes it imperative that for research purposes, harmonization and calibration of observers, while difficult, is carried out.

SUCCESS AND FAILURE

Endodontic treatment is performed under conditions with a theoretical potential for complete asepsis or effective antisepsis. This leads to a concept of a potential also for absolute "success" (complete elimination of infection) or "failure" (residual, recurrent or de novo infection). Complete radiographic maintenance or reestablishment of normal periapical structures have thus been defined as "success," whereas persistence or emergence of radiographic signs of disease is termed "failure."[51] The concept is simple

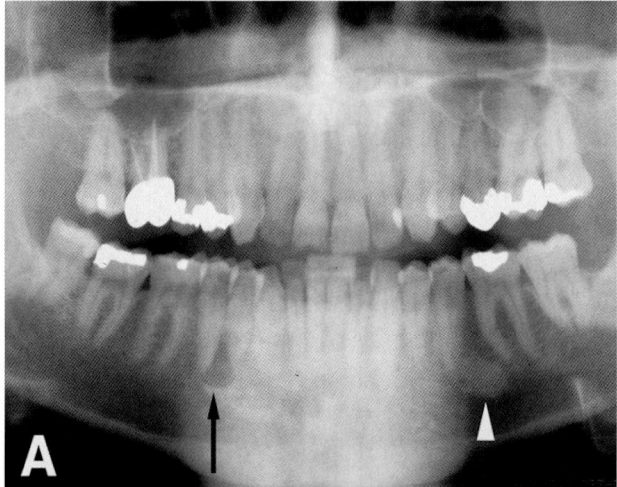
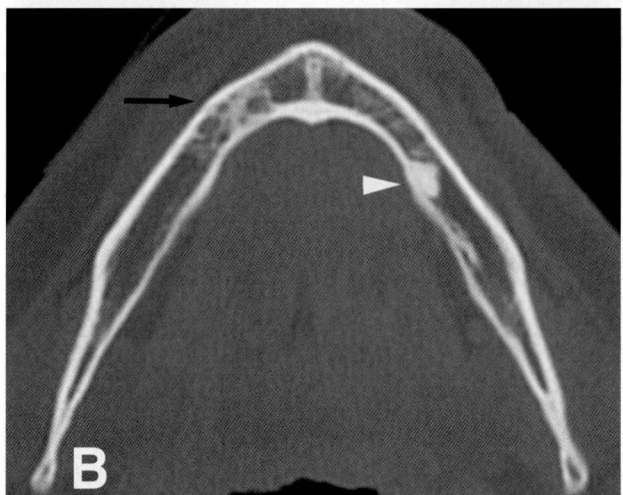
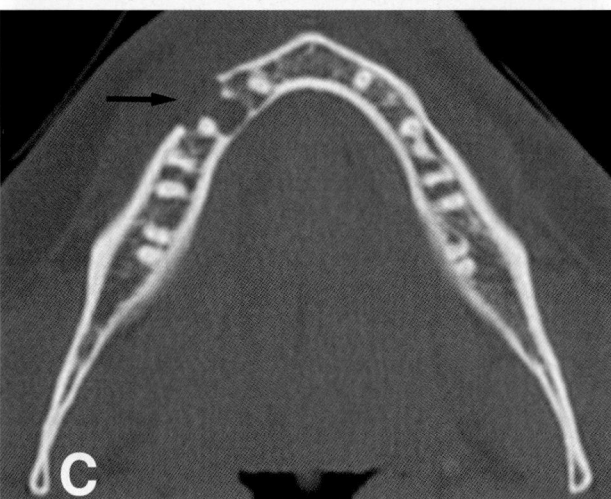

Figure 28 Ameloblastoma, desmoplastic type. ***A, B, C, D,*** Apical unilocular radiolucency in the premolar region (arrow). Note also idiopathic osteosclerosis (arrow head). ***E,*** CT scan shows multilocular radiolucences (arrow) and sclerosis (arrow head). ***C,*** CT scan shows evident destruction including buccal cortex (arrow). (Reproduced with permission from Larheim, T.A., Westesson, P.-L. Maxillofacial Imaging, Springer 2006.)

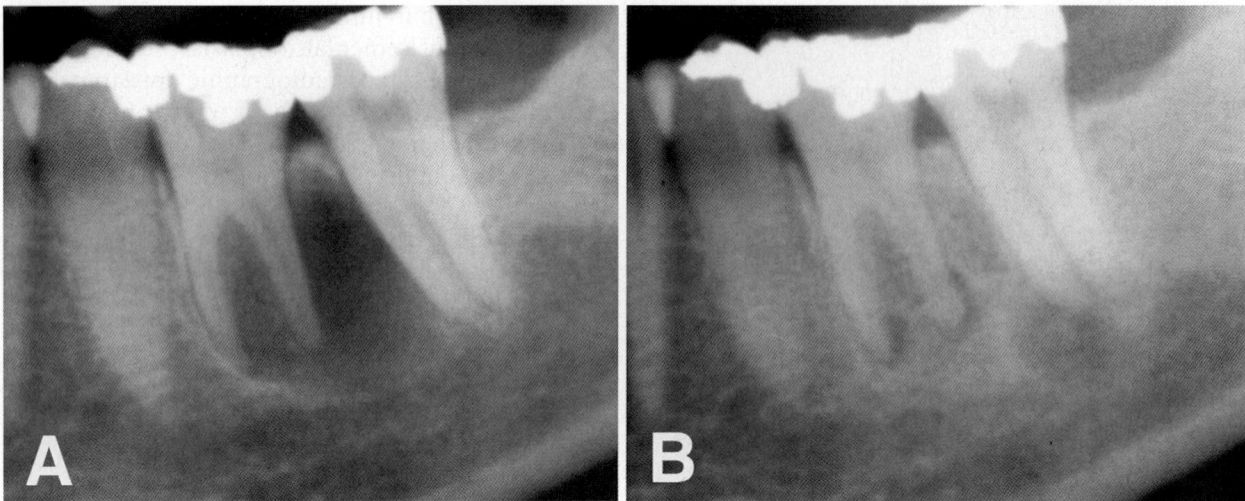

Figure 29 Ossifying fibroma. ***A,*** Apical radiolucency (and pulp sensitivity). ***B,*** 2.5 years later a mixed lesion was found including second molar. (Reproduced with permission from Mork Knutsen B., Larheim T.A., Johannessen S., Hillestad J., Solheim T., Strømme Koppang H. Recurrent conventional cemento-ossifying fibroma of the mandible. Dentomaxillofac Radiol 2002; 31:65-8.)

and easily understandable to patient, clinician, and researcher and has been widely used for assessments of treatment outcome (for review see refs 52, 53). However, the bias and variation in observers' perceptions of what constitutes success or failure has made comparisons among studies with different observers problematic.

PROBABILITY ASSESSMENTS

Acknowledging the bias and difficulties in calibration, Reit and Gröndahl[54] and Zakariasen et al.[55] applied a probability scoring system for monitoring apical disease: the observers were assigned to assess the probability that disease be present on a 5- or 6-point scale. The system provides numerical data amenable to more sophisticated analyses than the dichotomous scoring, but it does in no way address the problem of harmonization of observers.

THE PERIAPICAL INDEX SCORING SYSTEM

This was developed[56] for two reasons: to integrate radiographic score with histological characteristics of the disease and to make possible harmonization of observers across studies and geographical distance. The histological reference was to the studies by Brynolf,[27] by adoption of her findings with a degree of simplification deemed necessary for calibration of scorers (Figure 31). Bias was reduced by making scoring a visual exercise rather than relying on verbal descriptors in characterization of radiographic findings and controlled by providing a

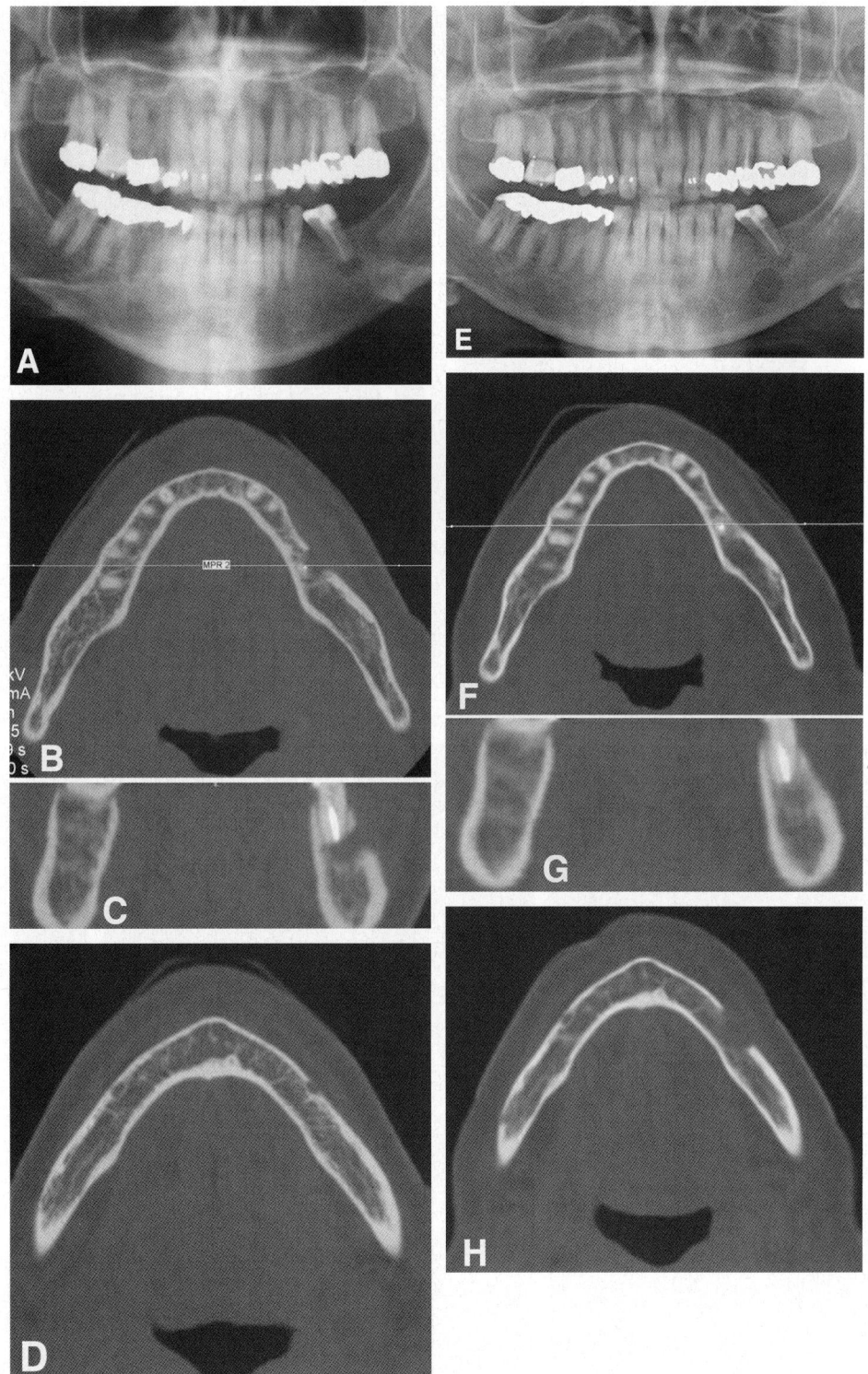

Figure 30 Metastasis to the mandible from breast cancer. ***A,*** Periapical radiolucency after apicectomy of premolar in left mandible. ***B, C, D,*** CT scans show the postoperative defect and otherwise normal bone. ***E,*** Healed surgical defect, but new radiolucency had developed one year and 4 months later. ***F, G, H,*** CT scans confirm healed area and bone destruction including buccal cortex.

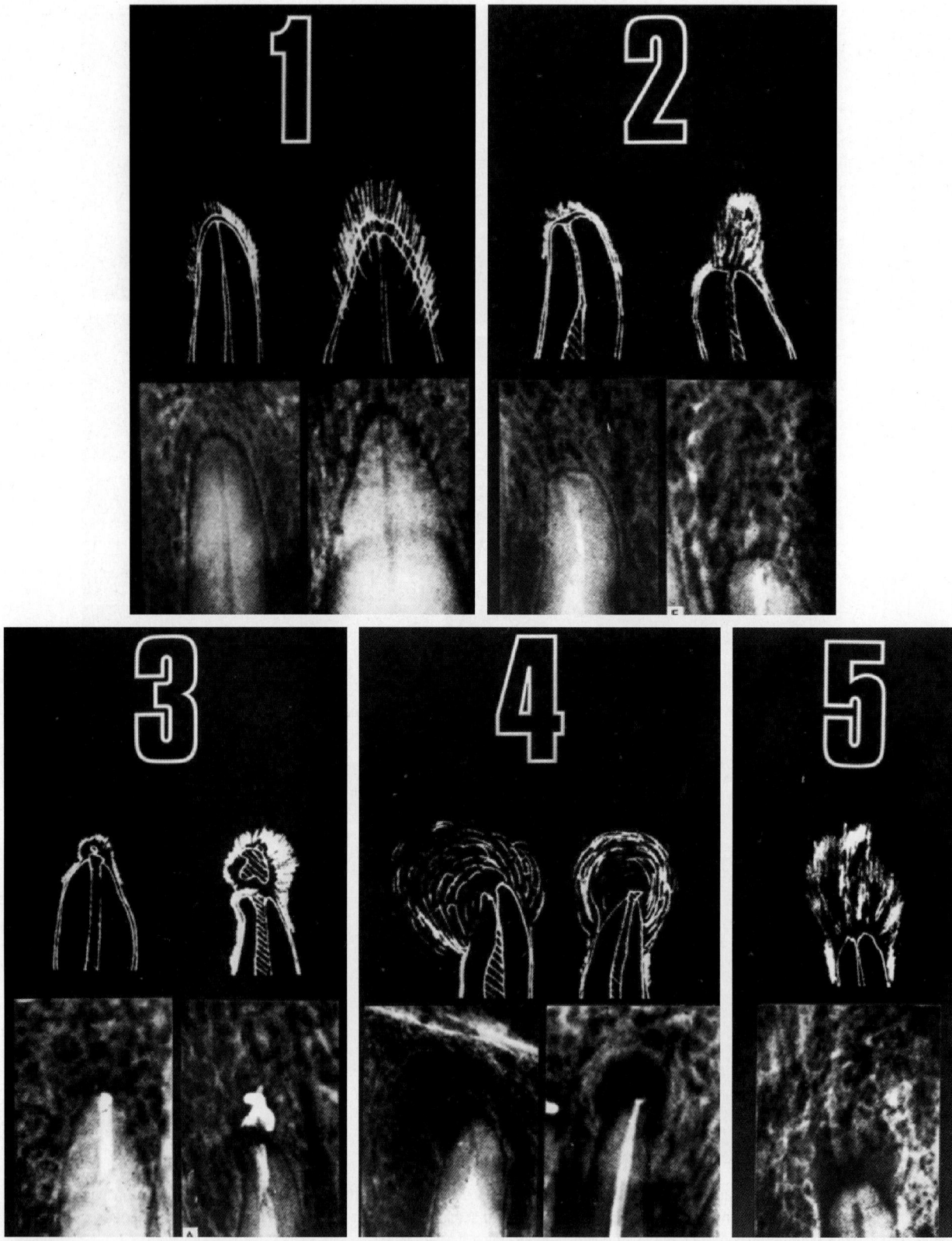

Figure 31 The periapical index scoring system. (Reproduced with permission from Ørstavik D., Kerekes K., Eriksen H.M. The periapical index: a scoring system for radiographic assessment of apical periodontitis. Endod Dent Traumatol 1986;2:20-34.)

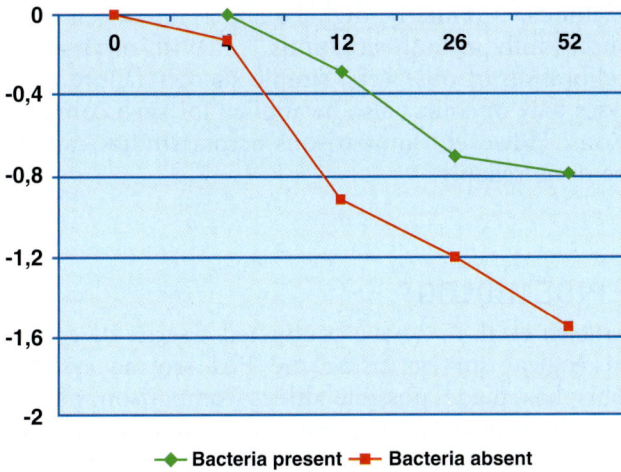

Figure 32 Periapical index scores used to monitor and compare healing of teeth with apical periodontitis with and without cultivable bacteria at the filling session. Average change in PAI score from baseline at 4, 12, 26 and 52 weeks used as indicator of healing (Data from Waltimo T., Trope M., Haapasalo M., Ørstavik D. Clinical efficacy of treatment procedures in endodontic infection control and one year follow-up of periapical healing. J Endod 2005;31:863-6.)

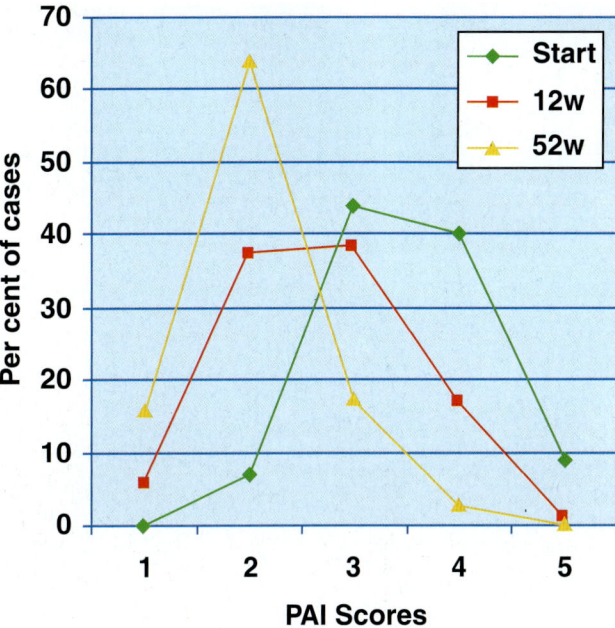

Figure 33 Periapical index scores used to monitor healing in a group of teeth treated for apical periodontitis (Data from Sathorn C., Parashos P., Messer H.H. Effectiveness of single- versus multiple-visit endodontic treatment of teeth with apical periodontitis: a systematic review and meta-analysis. Int Endod J 2005;38:347-55.)

calibration kit with precise measurement of a given observer's performance in relation to a set of "true" scores. The system has been applied to more than 30 peer-reviewed publications since 2001, from Canada to China, with applications typically in endodontic epidemiology[57] and clinical, follow-up studies[58] (Figures 32, 33).

DIGITAL QUANTIFICATION OF RADIOGRAPHIC DATA

Using direct digital or digitized, conventional radiographs, the numerical information in the acquired image may be used for quantitative assessment of grey level/mineral content changes. Digital subtraction is one attractive option for this purpose, but despite several attempts to apply this procedure to endodontic, periapical radiographs,[42,59] this has not been successful. A method whereby lesion grey levels are related to a peripheral area in the same jaw, unaffected by pathological or healing processes in the bone, has proven more robust and found application in quantitative studies[42,60–63] (Table 2) (Figure 34).

Table 2 Application of the Ratio Method in Evaluation of Healing After Treatment of Apical Periodontitis with Three Modalities

Treatment	n	Ratio Gray Value at 52 Weeks
Ca(OH)$_2$	23	0.9897
Empty canal	21	0.9279
Immediate fill	41	0.9555

Adapted from Delano et al.[60]

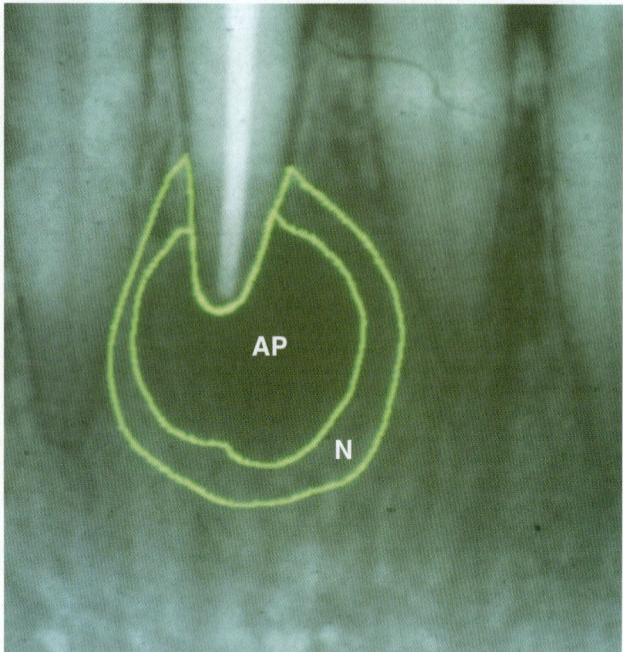

Figure 34 Delineation of areas to be monitored during healing. AP, lesion as outlined at start, N, peripheral, stable normal bone (Modified from Ørstavik D., Farrants G., Wahl T., Kerekes K. Image analysis of endodontic radiographs: digital subtraction and quantitative densitometry. Endod Dent Traumatol 1990;6:6-11.)

APPLICATIONS TO CLINICAL RESEARCH

New procedures, materials, and medicaments keep emerging for use in endodontics with claims of superior performance. While many such products and methods may be evaluated for their feasibility by in vitro technological and biological tests, true progress in treatment outcome can only be measured in controlled, follow-up studies with randomized design and in comparison with conventional methods of reference. Very few such studies have been performed and that is reflected in the scarcity of solid data at the higher levels of evidence found when endodontic treatment is studied in systematic reviews and meta-analyses.[52,64–67] Extensive, at times costly, randomized clinical trials are necessary for documentation of performance, and it is unfortunate that many new techniques and products do not have such data available.

The Periapical Index (PAI) scoring system has been used in several studies with randomization of techniques and has proven useful for strict comparisons of, particularly, root filling materials[68,69] (see Figure 34), but also for comparison of treatment methods.[70] Similarly, digital analyses have been used successfully in both situations.[42,61] With intra-study calibration of observers, simple success–failure analyses may of course also be applied for such comparisons. However, comparisons across studies cannot be done reliably.

EPIDEMIOLOGY

Eriksen et al.[71–77] have conducted a series of epidemiological surveys using the PAI scoring system. This has made possible direct comparison of the distribution of apical periodontitis and endodontic treatment results in several different regions and countries. Other investigators[78,79] have also produced epidemiological data with the index, adding to our knowledge base with the same methodology. Based on these surveys, with a standardized interpretation of radiographic information, the realization is growing that chronic apical periodontitis is quite prevalent in most societies all over the world and that periapical disease is an important dental health issue and a major cause of tooth extraction in many populations[80] (Figure 35).

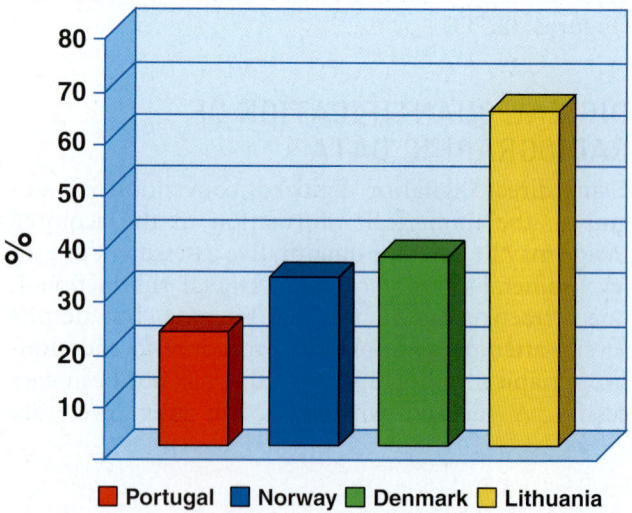

Figure 35 Periapical index scores used to record the prevalence of apical periodontitis in 35–45 year-olds in selected countries (Data from Skudutyte-Rysstad R., Eriksen H.M. Endodontic status amongst 35-year-old Oslo citizens and changes over a 30-year period. Int Endod J 2006;39:637-42.)

Radiography in the Future of Endodontics

The periapical radiograph has successfully maintained a position of ubiquity and remains indispensable in endodontic practice. The ease and precision with which relatively detailed knowledge can be obtained with this diagnostic tool makes it superior for routine applications today and in the foreseeable future. Critical and evidence-based knowledge of how endodontically relevant changes in teeth and bone are reflected in radiographs remains crucial, and it is an ever challenging task to reduce personal and institutional bias in radiographic interpretation. The dose and cost of scans and the difficulty to use other, sophisticated methods in real time at chairside make it unlikely that these techniques will affect the basic procedures in endodontic diagnosis and treatment. The continued reinforcement of clinicians' proficiency in reading and interpreting the information in periapical radiographs is therefore a key for maintaining and improving the quality in endodontic practice.

On the other hand, tremendous advances are being made with the development of, particularly, the computer-assisted scanning techniques. The technology producing localized scans of areas in the jaw with much reduced dosage holds a promise for future improvements in diagnostic and treatment procedures. New insights and concepts may have to be developed of how the three-dimensional appearance and localizations of apical periodontitis lesions appear in areas of the jaw, where conventional radiography offers limited if any help.

References

1. Goldman M, Pearson AH, Darzenta N. Endodontic success – who's reading the radiograph? Oral Surg Oral Med Oral Pathol Oral Radiol Endod 1972;33:432–7.
2. Reit C, Gröndahl HG. Endodontic decision-making under uncertainty: a decision analytic approach to management of periapical lesions in endodontically treated teeth. Endod Dent Traumatol 1987;3:15–20.
3. Zoellner A, Diemer B, Weber HP, et al. Histologic and radiographic assessment of caries-like lesions localized at the crown margin. J Prosthet Dent 2002;88:54–9.
4. Torneck CD. The clinical significance and management of calcific pulp obliteration. Alpha Omegan 1990;83:50–4.
5. Piattelli A. Generalized "complete" calcific degeneration or pulp obliteration. Endod Dent Traumatol 1992;8:259–63.
6. Piattelli A, Trisi P. Pulp obliteration: a histological study. J Endod 1993;19:252–4.
7. Cavalleri G, Zerman N. Traumatic crown fractures in permanent incisors with immature roots: a follow-up study. Endod Dent Traumatol 1995;11:294–6.
8. Cabrini RL, Manfredi EE. Internal resorption of dentine; histopathologic control of eight cases after pulp amputation and capping with calcium hydroxide. Oral Surg Oral Med Oral Pathol Oral Radiol Endod 1957;10:90–6.
9. Caliskan MK, Turkun M. Prognosis of permanent teeth with internal resorption: a clinical review. Endod Dent Traumatol 1997;13:75–81.
10. Rabinowitch BZ. Internal resorption. Oral Surg Oral Med Oral Pathol Oral Radiol Endod 1972;33:263–82.
11. Magnusson BO. Therapeutic pulpotomies in primary molars with the formocresol technique. A clinical and histological follow-up. Acta Odontol Scand 1978;36:157–65.
12. Holmes JP, Gulabivala K, van der Stelt PF. Detection of simulated internal tooth resorption using conventional radiography and subtraction imaging. Dentomaxillofac Radiol 2001;30:249–54.
13. Zachrisson BU, Jacobsen I. Long-term prognosis of 66 permanent anterior teeth with root fracture. Scand J Dent Res. 1975;83:345–54.
14. Youssefzadeh S, Gahleitner A, Dorffner R, et al. Dental vertical root fractures: value of CT in detection. Radiology 1999;210:545–9.
15. Cvek M, Andreasen JO, Borum MK. Healing of 208 intra-alveolar root fractures in patients aged 7–17 years. Dent Traumatol 2001;17:53–62.
16. Mora MA, Mol A, Tyndall DA, Rivera EM. In vitro assessment of local computed tomography for the detection of longitudinal tooth fractures. Oral Surg Oral Med Oral Pathol Oral Radiol Endod. 2007;103:825–9. Epub 2006 Dec 22.
17. Andreasen FM. Transient root resorption after dental trauma: the clinician's dilemma. J Esthet Restor Dent 2003;15:80–92.
18. Cohen S, Blanco L, Berman LH. Early radiographic diagnosis of inflammatory root resorption. Gen Dent 2003;51:235–40.
19. Holan G. Development of clinical and radiographic signs associated with dark discolored primary incisors following traumatic injuries: a prospective controlled study. Dent Traumatol 2004;20:276–87.
20. Smale I, Årtun J, B ehbehani F, et al. Apical root resorption 6 months after initiation of fixed orthodontic appliance therapy. Am J Orthod Dentofacial Orthop 2005;128:57–67.
21. Heithersay GS. Invasive cervical resorption following trauma. Aust Endod J 1999;25:79–85.
22. Eliasson S, Halvarsson C, Ljungheimer C. Periapical condensing osteitis and endodontic treatment. Oral Surg Oral Med Oral Pathol Oral Radiol Endod 1984;57:195–9.

23. Marmary Y, Kutiner G. A radiographic survey of periapical jawbone lesions. Oral Surg Oral Med Oral Pathol Oral Radiol Endod 1986;61:405–8.

24. Zain RB, Roswati N, Ismail K. Radiographic features of periapical cysts and granulomas. Singapore Dent J 1989;14:29–32.

25. Ricucci D, Mannocci F, Ford TR. A study of periapical lesions correlating the presence of a radiopaque lamina with histological findings. Oral Surg Oral Med Oral Pathol Oral Radiol Endod 2006;101:389–94.

26. Zain RB, Roswati N, Ismail K. Radiographic evaluation of lesion sizes of histologically diagnosed periapical cysts and granulomas. Ann Dent 1989;48:3–5, 46.

27. Brynolf I. Histological and roentgenological study of periapical region of human upper incisors. Odontol Revy 1967;18 Suppl 11.

28. Kvist T, Reit C. Results of endodontic retreatment: a randomized clinical study comparing surgical and nonsurgical procedures. J Endod 1999;25:814–17.

29. Nair PN, Sjögren U, Figdor D, Sundqvist G. Persistent periapical radiolucencies of root-filled human teeth, failed endodontic treatments, and periapical scars. Oral Surg Oral Med Oral Pathol Oral Radiol Endod 1999;87:617–27.

30. Maddalone M, Gagliani M. Periapical endodontic surgery: a 3-year follow-up study. Int Endod J 2003;36:193–8.

31. Ørstavik D, Larheim TA. Radiology of apical periodontitis. In: Ørstavik D, Pitt Ford TR, editors. Essential Endodontology. Blackwell, Oxford, UK, 2008, pp. 197–234.

32. Vier FV, Figueiredo JA. Prevalence of different periapical lesions associated with human teeth and their correlation with the presence and extension of apical external root resorption. Int Endod J 2002;35:710–19.

33. Vier FV, Figueiredo JA. Internal apical resorption and its correlation with the type of apical lesion. Int Endod J 2004;37:730–7.

34. Ørstavik D, Pitt Ford TR. Apical periodontitis: microbial infection and host responses. In: Ørstavik D, Pitt Ford TR, editors. Essential Endodontology. Blackwell, Oxford, UK, 2008, pp. 1–9.

35. Christgau M, Hiller KA, Schmalz G, et al. Accuracy of quantitative digital subtraction radiography for determining changes in calcium mass in mandibular bone: an in vitro study. J Periodontal Res 1998;33:138–49.

36. Bender IB, Seltzer S. Roentgenographic and direct observation of experimental lesions of bone. J Am Dent Assoc 1961;62:157–62.

37. Colosi D, Potluri A, Islam S, Geha H, Lurie A. Bone trabeculae are visible on periapical images. Oral Surg Oral Med Oral Pathol Oral Radiol Endod 2003;96:772–3.

38. Cavalcanti MG, Ruprecht A, Johnson WT, et al. The contribution of trabecular bone to the visibility of the lamina dura: an in vitro radiographic study. Oral Surg Oral Med Oral Pathol Oral Radiol Endod 2002;93:118–22.

39. Molven O, Halse A, Fristad I, MacDonald-Jankowski D. Periapical changes following root-canal treatment observed 20–27 years postoperatively. Int Endod J 2002;35:784–90.

40. Halse A, Molven O. Increased width of the apical periodontal membrane space in endodontically treated teeth may represent favourable healing. Int Endod J 2004;37:552–60.

41. Brynolf I. Roentgenologic periapical diagnosis. I. Reproducibility of interpretation. Sven Tandläk Tidskr 1970;63:339–44.

42. Ørstavik D, Farrants G, Wahl T, Kerekes K. Image analysis of endodontic radiographs: digital subtraction and quantitative densitometry. Endod Dent Traumatol 1990;6:6–11.

43. Kerosuo E, Ørstavik D. Application of computerised image analysis to monitoring endodontic therapy: reproducibility and comparison with visual assessment. Dentomaxillofac Radiol 1997;26:79–84.

44. Ørstavik D. Time-course and risk analyses of the development and healing of chronic apical periodontitis in man. Int Endod J 1996;29:150–5.

45. Fristad I, Molven O, Halse A. Nonsurgically retreated root filled teeth – radiographic findings after 20–27 years. Int Endod J 2004;37:12–18.

46. Larheim TA, Westesson P-L. Maxillofacial Imaging. Springer Berlin, Germany; 2006.

47. Hewitt C, Farah CS. Bisphosphonate-related osteonecrosis of the jaws: a comprehensive review. J Oral Pathol Med 2007;36:319–28.

48. Philipsen HP, Reichart PA, Ogawa I, et al. The inflammatory paradental cyst: a critical review of 342 cases from a literature survey, including 17 new cases from the author's files. J Oral Pathol Med 2004;33:147–55.

49. Carter LC, Carney YL, Perez-Pudlewski D. Lateral periodontal cyst. Multifactorial analysis of a previously unreported series. Oral Surg Oral Med Oral Pathol Oral Radiol Endod 1996;81:210–16.

50. Mork Knutsen B, Larheim TA, Johannessen S, et al. Recurrent conventional cemento-ossifying fibroma of the mandible. Dentomaxillofac Radiol 2002;31:65–8.

51. Strindberg LZ. The dependence of the results of pulp therapy on certain factors. An analytical study based on radiographic and clinical follow-up examinations. Dissertation. Acta Odontol Scand 1956;14(Suppl 21):1–174.

52. Torabinejad M, Kutsenko D, Machnick TK, et al. Levels of evidence for the outcome of nonsurgical endodontic treatment. J Endod 2005;31:637–46.

53. Friedman S. Endodontic treatment outcome: the potential for healing and retained function. In: Ingle JI, editor. Endodontics. 6th ed. London, Canada: BC Decker; 2007a in press.

54. Reit C, Gröndahl HG. Application of statistical decision theory to radiographic diagnosis of endodontically treated teeth. Scand J Dent Res 1983;91:213–18.

55. Zakariasen KL, Scott DA, Jensen JR. Endodontic recall radiographs: how reliable is our interpretation of endodontic success or failure and what factors affect our reliability? Oral Surg Oral Med Oral Pathol Oral Radiol Endod 1984;57:343–47.

56. Ørstavik D, Kerekes K, Eriksen HM. The periapical index: a scoring system for radiographic assessment of apical periodontitis. Endod Dent Traumatol 1986;2:20–34.

57. Kirkevang LL, Vaeth M, Horsted-Bindslev P, et al. Risk factors for developing apical periodontitis in a general population. Int Endod J 2007;40:290–9.

58. Waltimo T, Trope M, Haapasalo M, Ørstavik D. Clinical efficacy of treatment procedures in endodontic infection control and one year follow-up of periapical healing. J Endod 2005;31:863–6.

59. Tyndall DA, Kapa SF, Bagnell CP. Digital subtraction radiography for detecting cortical and cancellous bone changes in the periapical region. J Endod 1990;16:173–8.

60. Delano EO, Ludlow JB, Ørstavik D, et al. Comparison between PAI and quantitative digital radiographic assessment of apical healing after endodontic treatment. Oral Surg Oral Med Oral Pathol Oral Radiol Endod 2001;92:108–15.

61. Pettiette MT, Delano EO, Trope M. Evaluation of success rate of endodontic treatment performed by students with stainless-steel K-files and nickel–titanium hand files. J Endod 2001;27:124–7.

62. Yoshioka T, Kobayashi C, Suda H, Sasaki T. An observation of the healing process of periapical lesions by digital subtraction radiography. J Endod 2002;28:589–91.

63. Vakalis SV, Whitworth JM, Ellwood RP, Preshaw PM. A pilot study of treatment of periodontal–endodontic lesions. Int Dent J 2005;55:313–18.

64. Messer HH. Review of one-visit endodontic treatment. Aust Endod J 2000;26:81.

65. Law A, Messer H. An evidence-based analysis of the antibacterial effectiveness of intracanal medicaments. J Endod 2004;30:689–94.

66. Paik S, Sechrist C, Torabinejad M. Levels of evidence for the outcome of endodontic retreatment. J Endod 2004;30:745–50.

67. Sathorn C, Parashos P, Messer HH. Effectiveness of single- versus multiple-visit endodontic treatment of teeth with apical periodontitis: a systematic review and meta-analysis. Int Endod J 2005;38:347–55.

68. Waltimo TM, Boiesen J, Eriksen HM, Ørstavik D. Clinical performance of 3 endodontic sealers. Oral Surg Oral Med Oral Pathol Oral Radiol Endod 2001;92:89–92.

69. Huumonen S, Lenander-Lumikari M, Sigurdsson A, Ørstavik D. Healing of apical periodontitis after endodontic treatment: a comparison between a silicone-based and a zinc oxide-eugenol-based sealer. Int Endod J 2003;36:296–301.

70. Trope M, Delano EO, Ørstavik D. Endodontic treatment of teeth with apical periodontitis: single vs. multivisit treatment. J Endod 1999;25:345–50.

71. Eriksen HM, Bjertness E. Prevalence of apical periodontitis and results of endodontic treatment in middle-aged adults in Norway. Endod Dent Traumatol 1991;7:1–4.

72. Eriksen HM, Berset GP, Hansen BF, Bjertness E. Changes in endodontic status 1973–1993 among 35-year-olds in Oslo, Norway. Int Endod J 1995;28:129–32.

73. Marques MD, Moreira B, Eriksen HM. Prevalence of apical periodontitis and results of endodontic treatment in an adult, Portuguese population. Int Endod J 1998;31:161–5.

74. Sidaravicius B, Aleksejuniene J, Eriksen HM. Endodontic treatment and prevalence of apical periodontitis in an adult population of Vilnius, Lithuania. Endod Dent Traumatol 1999;15:210–15.

75. Aleksejuniene J, Eriksen HM, Sidaravicius B, Haapasalo M. Apical periodontitis and related factors in an adult Lithuanian population. Oral Surg Oral Med Oral Pathol Oral Radiol Endod 2000;90:95–101.

76. Peciuliene V, Balciuniene I, Eriksen HM, Haapasalo M. Isolation of Enterococcus faecalis in previously root-filled canals in a Lithuanian population. J Endod 2000;26:593–5.

77. Skudutyte-Rysstad R, Eriksen HM. Endodontic status amongst 35-year-old Oslo citizens and changes over a 30-year period. Int Endod J 2006;39:637–42.

78. Kirkevang LL, Vaeth M, Hørsted-Bindslev P, Wenzel A. Longitudinal study of periapical and endodontic status in a Danish population. Int Endod J 2006;39:100–7.

79. Ridell K, Petersson A, Matsson L, Mejare I. Periapical status and technical quality of root-filled teeth in Swedish adolescents and young adults. A retrospective study. Acta Odontol Scand 2006;64:104–10.

80. Eriksen HM, Kirkevang LL , Petersson K. Endodontic epidemiology and treatment outcome: general considerations Endod Top 2002, 2:1–9.

81. Årtun J, Van 't Hullenar R, Doppel D, Kuijpers-Jagtman AM. Identification of orthodontic patients at risk of severe apical root resorption. Am J Orthod Dentofacial Orthop 2007; 132, in press.

CHAPTER 17

RHINOSINUSITIS AND ENDODONTIC DISEASE

RODERICK W. TATARYN

Maxillary Rhinosinusitis as a Source of Dental Pain

The most common nonodontogenic cause of dental pain arises from the maxillary sinus and associated pain-sensitive ostial mucosa.[1] Maxillary rhinosinusitis therefore deserves important consideration when developing a differential diagnosis for maxillary discomfort. Despite its prevalence, differentiating pain caused by rhinosinusitis from that of pulpal etiology can be one of the more difficult diagnostic challenges faced by the clinician. The result of a misdiagnosis in this area has lead to unnecessary endodontic therapy, periapical surgery, and even multiple tooth extractions, with no effective pain relief for the patient.

In order to effectively distinguish rhinosinusitis from odontalgia, it is imperative that clinicians understand the anatomy and functions of the paranasal sinuses both in healthy and diseased states, and recognize the signs and symptoms associated with sinus inflammation. It should be made clear that it is not expected of the endodontist, and is in fact outside the scope of dentistry, to definitively diagnose or provide treatment for a sinus condition. This diagnosis and treatment is best left to an otorhinolaryngologist, or ear, nose, and throat physician (ENT). Nevertheless, it is essential that the endodontist have a thorough understanding of this system and its potential disease processes to effectively diagnose and treat or rule out pain of odontogenic origin and to make an appropriate ENT referral if rhinosinusitis is suspected. A knowledge of these structures is also crucial to understanding the effects of periapical infection on the adjacent sinus tissues and the role of endodontic disease in acute and chronic rhinosinusitis.

Paranasal Sinuses: Anatomy and Function

Sinuses are hollow air spaces or cavities located within the skull surrounding the nasal cavity. There are four pairs of paranasal sinuses: the maxillary, the frontal, the ethmoid, and the sphenoid (Figure 1). The sinuses are lined with a membrane of ciliated and nonciliated pseudostratified columnar epithelium that is continuous with the nasal cavities. The columnar cells are interspersed with mucous-producing goblet cells that constantly produce a thin layer of mucinous fluid. The mucous is rich with immune cells, antibodies, and antibacterial proteins that serve in immune defense and air filtration by trapping and filtering particles such as dust, spores, and bacteria. The cilia beat in a coordinated, rhythmic wavelike pattern moving the mucous toward a small opening or ostium into the nasal cavity and then on to the throat where it is swallowed and finally dissolved by digestive acids. In addition to air filtration, the paranasal sinuses serve to humidify and warm inspired air and are also important in giving the voice resonance, defining tonal quality and voice amplification as well as reducing the weight of the skull.[2]

The largest of the paranasal sinuses and most prone to infection are the maxillary sinuses. The maxillary sinus, also known as the antrum, is somewhat pyramidal in shape with the lateral wall of the nasal cavity forming the base and the apex extending into the zygoma. The floor of the maxillary sinus is the maxillary alveolar and palatine process, the roof is the floor of the orbit, and the posterior wall is adjacent to the infratemporal fossa. The ostium of the maxillary sinus is located approximately two-thirds up the medial sinus wall and is a small (1 to 3 mm diameter) passageway into the nasal cavity.

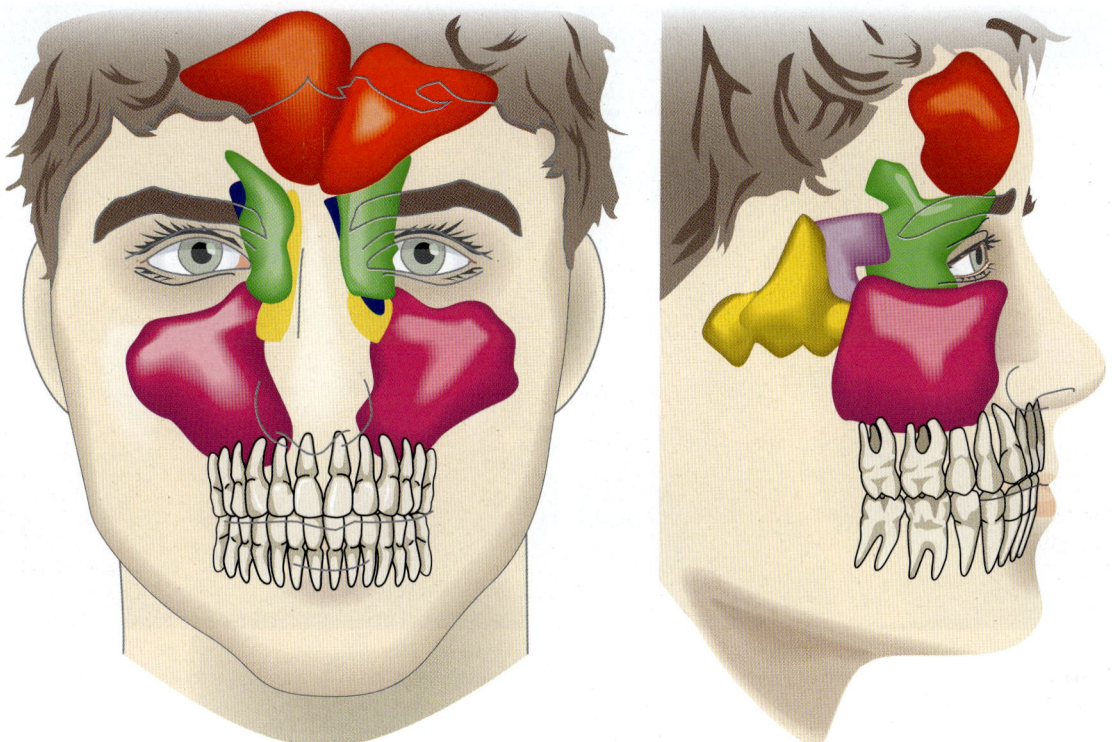

Figure 1 The paranasal sinuses. Maxillary sinuses (red), frontal sinuses (orange), anterior ethmoid sinuses (green), posterior ethmoid sinuses (purple), and sphenoid sinus (yellow).

This ostium opens into the semilunar hiatus of the middle meatus of the nasal cavity and is a highly innervated structure and is extremely sensitive when inflamed or stimulated during sinus-related pain episodes.[3] Although the mucosa of the sinuses is rather insensitive to pain, the region of the ostia of the sinuses is the most sensitive of any of the nasal structures.[4]

Rhinosinusitis: Etiology, Epidemiology, Symptoms, and Treatment

The sinus openings or ostia are the focal point for sinus disease with blockage of the sinus ostia initiating the cycle of events leading to rhinosinusitis. Obstruction is commonly caused by inflammatory edema of the nasal lining mucosa usually in response to a virus, an allergen, or bacteria. This blockage can also occur from an anatomic obstruction such as a septal deviation or polyp, or a foreign body obstruction such as dried mucous. When a blockage occurs, mucous secretions, normally expelled through the ostium, accumulate within the sinus cavity where they begin to stagnate and thicken. The lack of sinus ventilation and stagnation of the secretions results in a lowered oxygen tension and a decrease in pH, providing an excellent environment for bacterial pathogens to colonize.[5] As the condition progresses, the cilia and the epithelium become damaged, preventing fluid movement, and there is further mucosal thickening creating a more severe obstruction. The condition of sinusitis has recently been redefined as *rhinosinusitis* due to the contiguous lining membrane of the paranasal and nasal cavities and its similar responses to therapy; however, both terms are presently used in the current literature.[6,7]

Rhinosinusitis is the single most common chronic medical condition in the United States affecting approximately 16% of the population and accounting for up to 5% of all visits to primary care physicians.[8] Rhinosinusitis is more prevalent in patients with congenital or acquired immunodeficiency, asthma, or allergic rhinitis. Symptoms may include nasal congestion, facial pain and pressure, purulent rhinorrhea, cough, headache, fever and fatigue, and pain in the maxillary posterior teeth.[9] In a prospective study of 247 men, Williams et al.[10] found that the symptom with the highest specificity for maxillary rhinosinusitis was a maxillary toothache at 93%.

A diagnosis of rhinosinusitis is generally made through clinical examination and is based on the

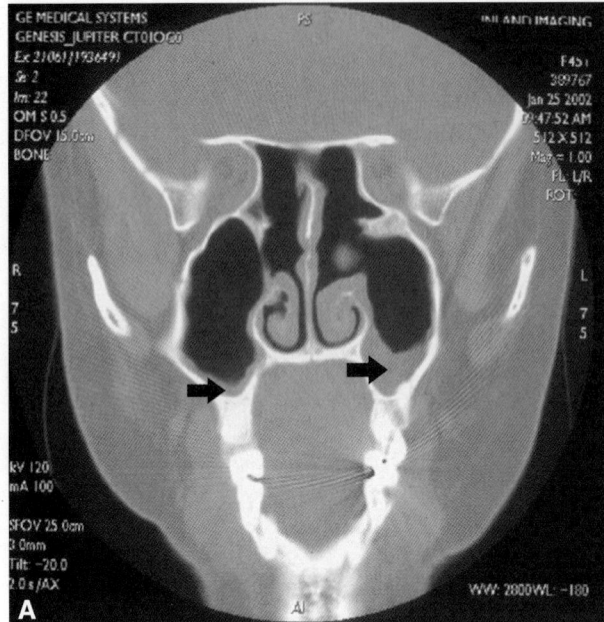 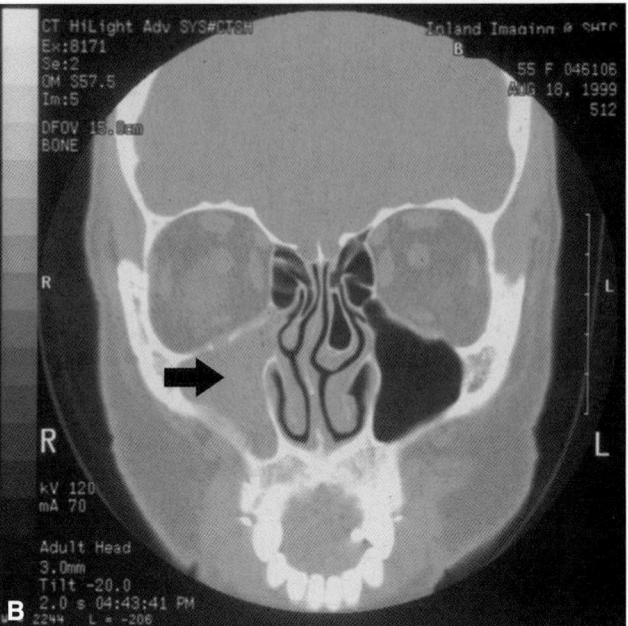

Figure 2 Maxillary rhinosinusitis. ***A***, Coronal CT image of mucosal thickening and fluid accumulation in the maxillary sinuses (arrows). ***B***, Coronal CT image of a completely obstructed right maxillary sinus (arrow).

patient's history and physical signs and symptoms, with no single clinical finding being conclusively predictive of the condition.[10] In recurrent acute or chronic cases, endoscopy and CT scanning may be helpful in the diagnosis.[6] Coronally viewed sections of a CT scan can reveal ostial patency or blockage, soft tissue changes, or any retained fluids that may be indicative of sinus disease (Figure 2). Although CT scanning has a high sensitivity, it has a low specificity for demonstrating rhinosinusitis. More than 40% of asymptomatic patients and 87% of patients with common colds show sinus abnormalities on sinus CT.[11,12] It is also important to note that sinus inflammation and symptoms can occur in the absence of CT findings, thus the physician's overall clinical impression is superior to any single physical or radiological finding.[13] Treatment of sinus disease is centered on re-establishing and then maintaining adequate drainage.

Rhinosinusitis is classified as acute, subacute, and recurrent acute or chronic according to the temporal course of the disease.[6,9] Acute rhinosinusitis by definition lasts less than 4 weeks. Four or more episodes of acute rhinosinusitis within a 1-year period are defined as a recurrent acute rhinosinusitis. Subacute rhinosinusitis is a continuation of an acute form lasting between 4 and 12 weeks. Persistent signs and symptoms that continue unresolved for more than 12 weeks are classified as a chronic rhinosinusitis.

Acute rhinosinusitis usually has a sudden onset, usually with severe symptoms, but 40 to 50% of patients will recover spontaneously and the remainder will respond fairly well to antibiotic and/or adjunctive treatments. The predominant bacterial flora isolated in acute rhinosinusitis includes *Streptococcus pneumoniae*, *Haemophilus influenzae*, and *Moraxella catarrhalis*. Amoxicillin or trimethoprim–sulfamethoxazole is the preferred antibiotic as a first-line treatment although the role of antibiotics in uncomplicated rhinosinusitis has been questioned because of concern regarding its overuse.[5,14,15] The bacterial species isolated from acute rhinosinusitis has not changed in the last 50 years; however, antibiotic resistance in these organisms is a growing problem due to a significant increase in the production of β-lactamase. It has been estimated that up to 40% of *H. influenza* strains and more than 90% of *M. catarrhalis* isolates are now resistant to amoxicillin.[16]

Chronic rhinosinusitis usually has less severe symptoms, yet is more difficult to resolve. Because symptoms are poorly localized and mild, this condition may be extremely difficult to recognize. The bacterial flora of chronic rhinosinusitis tends to be a more mixed infection with *Staphlococcus aureus* and anaerobes being the more frequent isolates.[17] Narrow spectrum antibiotic regimens are typically ineffective against chronic rhinosinusitis. Current treatment includes the use of broader spectrum antibiotics such as amoxycillin–clavulanate, clindamycin, or the combination of metronidazole and penicillin.[18] Other adjunctive treatments include the use of steroid nasal sprays, decongestants, or saline irrigation. If antibiotic therapy and adjunctive treatments prove ineffective, then endoscopic sinus surgery is currently the recommended procedure to surgically remove any diseased tissue or blockage and open the natural ostium in an attempt to re-establish drainage.[18]

Referral of Maxillary Sinus Pain to the Teeth

The referral of pain from the maxillary sinus to the maxillary dentition is primarily due to the close anatomic relationship between the floor of the maxillary sinus and the roots of the posterior maxillary teeth. In a highly pneumatized antrum, the sinus floor will extend between adjacent teeth and between individual roots of the maxillary molars (Figure 3). In a study of adults, Eberhardt[19] found the average thickness of the bony partition between the apices of the maxillary second molar teeth and the antral mucosa to be only 0.83 mm. Occasionally, no bony partition exists at all with the roots apices and the sinus separated only by the mucosal lining.[3] With such an intimate relationship, increased sinus pressure during sinusitis can produce the sensation of pain and pressure in the maxillary alveolar process and the corresponding teeth. Percussion of these proximate teeth produces acute tenderness due to the direct transfer of shock pressure to the inflamed sinus and the sensitive ostium. Often, for some patients, the most sensitive trigger for their sinus pain is by manipulation of the maxillary posterior teeth, leading them to believe with near certainty that teeth are the source of their pain.

Heterotropic or neurologically referred pain can also be responsible for a patient mistaking rhinosinusitis for odontalgia.[20] It has been demonstrated that stimulation of the maxillary sinus ostium can induce dental pain in the maxillary posterior teeth.[21-23] It has also been demonstrated that the local topical anesthetic applied to the maxillary sinus ostium can relieve perceived dental pain in the case of referred sinus pain.[24] Anesthetic nerve blocks, however, may not be reliable in differentiating maxillary rhinosinusitis from odontalgia due to mutual dental and antral innervations. Sensory innervation of the maxillary sinus is via the maxillary division of the trigeminal nerve with branches coming from the anterior, middle, and posterior superior alveolar nerves, the infraorbital nerve, and the anterior palatine nerve.[4] These nerves travel along the floor of the maxillary sinus innervating the related teeth.[25]

Distinguishing Differences between Symptoms of Odontalgia and Sinus Pain

Proper diagnosis always starts with a complete medical and dental history. An important question to ask the patient during the endodontic exam as well as on the medical history form is, "Do you have chronic allergies, a current cold, congestion, or nasal drainage, or a history of sinus infections or problems?" Although many patients suffering with maxillary rhinosinusitis may perceive dental pain, they usually complain of a dull aching pain that is difficult to pinpoint or localize to a single tooth. In addition, the patients often feel pressure in their cheeks and below their eyes, which usually can be reproduced by external palpation of the cheeks. Positional changes can cause increased pain due to the movement of mucosal fluid over the sensitive sinus ostium as well as from increased intracranial pressure from blood flow.[26] The pain usually increases when patients are lying down, usually on one side more than the other, or if they bend over and place their heads below their knees. In addition, patients with acute rhinosinusitis can have potentially severe symptoms, but then experience sudden and total relief if the sinus pressure is temporarily alleviated.

In contrast, pain of pulpal origin is more easily localized, unchanged with variations in position and rarely intermittent in intensity. In cases of maxillary rhinosinusitis, often all teeth that are proximate to the sinus floor test positive to percussion, whereas with

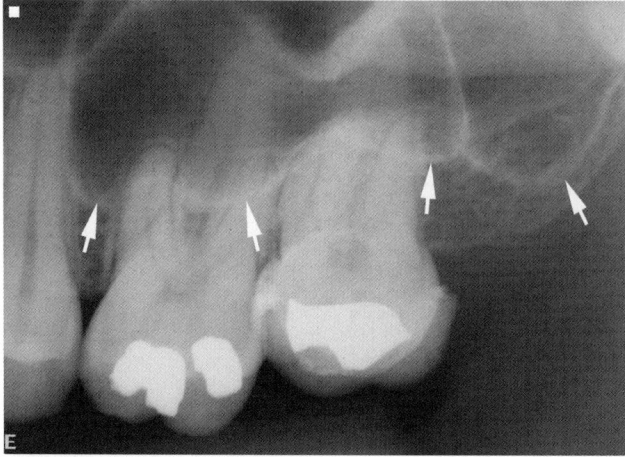

Figure 3 Radiograph of a highly pneumatized left maxillary sinus in close approximation to the roots of the maxillary posterior teeth. The dense cortical bone defines the inferior border of the antrum (arrows).

odontalgia usually only the offending teeth are percussion-sensitive. The key diagnostic test in differentiating maxillary sinus etiology from pain of pulpal origin is the pulp vitality test. If the tooth in question responds within normal limits to a pulpal stimulus such as Electric pulp test (EPT) or ice, when compared with other healthy teeth, then pulpal etiology is effectively ruled out. Regardless of percussion sensitivity or the patient's complaint of spontaneous dental pain, endodontic therapy is not indicated, as removal of a healthy pulp will surely not provide pain relief.

Although periapical radiographs are crucial to a thorough endodontic examination, the clinician must be careful not to establish the entire diagnosis on radiographic interpretation alone, particularly when evaluating the posterior maxillary area. A variation in bone density, the presence of the maxillary sinus and its bony septa as well as the zygomatic and palatal processes can impede important periradicular details necessary for accurate interpretation. Ambiguous radiographic conclusions are often the result, and multiple radiographic angles are highly recommended in combination with a thorough clinical examination.

Periapical Mucositis

A maxillary posterior tooth with apical periodontitis can produce a localized mucosal thickening in the adjacent sinus mucosa. This localized mucosal response to periapical odontogenic inflammation has been termed *periapical mucositis*.[27] Periapical mucositis is the inflammation or the swelling of the sinus membrane secondary to periapical inflammation, and will present as a radiopaque soft-tissue dome directly above the offending tooth[28] (Figures 4 and 5).

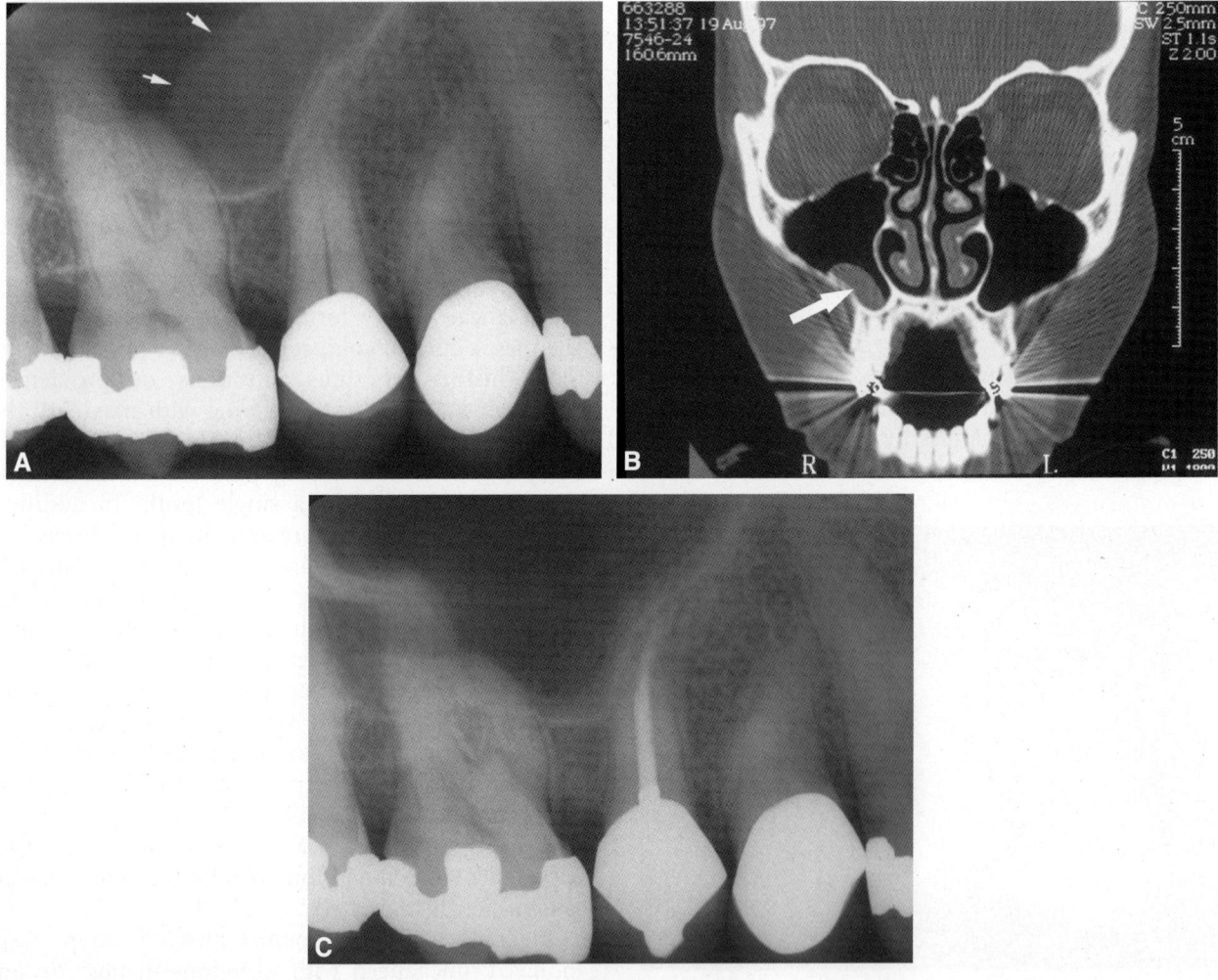

Figure 4 Periapical mucositis. **A,** Radiograph of a mucositis lesion (white arrows) in the right maxillary sinus apical to tooth #4 with necrotic pulp. **B,** Corresponding coronal CT image of the mucositis lesion (arrow). **C,** Follow-up radiograph taken 4 weeks after Root Canal Theraphy (RCT) demonstrating full resolution of the mucositis.

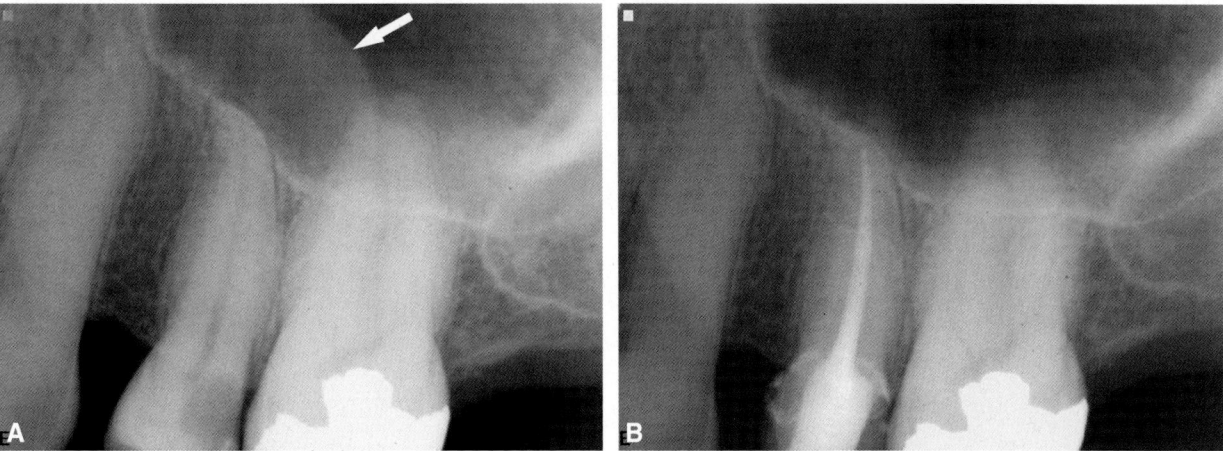

Figure 5 Periapical mucositis. **A,** Radiograph of a mucositis lesion in the left maxillary sinus apical to tooth #13 (arrow). **B,** Follow-up radiograph taken 6 weeks after RCT showing full resolution of the mucositis.

Mucositis is usually asymptomatic and can be expected to resolve following endodontic treatment. It is important not to confuse a periapical mucositis with a mucous retention cyst or a mucocele on the floor of the maxillary sinus. Mucous retention cysts are seen in approximately 10% of the routine sinus CTs and are considered incidental findings. They can develop in all areas of the sinus and normally do not require surgical intervention by the physician unless they are blocking the ostium.[9] Careful pulp testing is imperative in distinguishing a routine mucosal abnormality on the floor of the sinus from a mucositis secondary to periapical inflammation. Occasionally, apical periodontitis will not penetrate the antral floor, but rather will displace the periosteum, which in turn will deposit a thin layer of new bone on the periphery of the disease process. This has been termed periapical osteoperiostitis or "halo" shadow and will resolve following endodontic treatment of the offending tooth[27] (Figure 6).

Maxillary Sinusitis of Dental Origin

The link between dental and sinus pathosis is widely recognized in both the dental and the medical literature.[28-39] This condition was first referred to by Bauer in 1943 as maxillary sinusitis of dental origin (MSDO) and occurs when a dental infection extends directly through the mucosal floor of the antrum causing a secondary maxillary sinus infection.[29] Bauer's classic study on cadavers showed histological evidence of the extension of endodontic disease into the maxillary sinus, destruction of the cortical bone normally separating the teeth from the sinus floor, and causing pathological damage to the sinus tissues.

The pathological extension of dental disease into the maxillary sinus has since been well documented. Abrahams et al.[36] have reported that infections of the maxillary posterior teeth show maxillary sinus pathology in 60% of the cases, while Matilla[37] found sinus mucosal hyperplasia present in approximately 80% of teeth with periapical osteitis. Sinus inflammation in response to dental infection is usually localized to the floor of the sinus; however, if ostial obstruction occurs, this can lead to bacterial colonization and a sinus infection. The reported frequency of MSDO varies considerably, between 4.6 and 47% of all sinus infections.[40] This wide variation may be due to the difference in criteria and definitions as well as the inherent difficulty in establishing an exact causal relationship in maxillary sinusitis.[41]

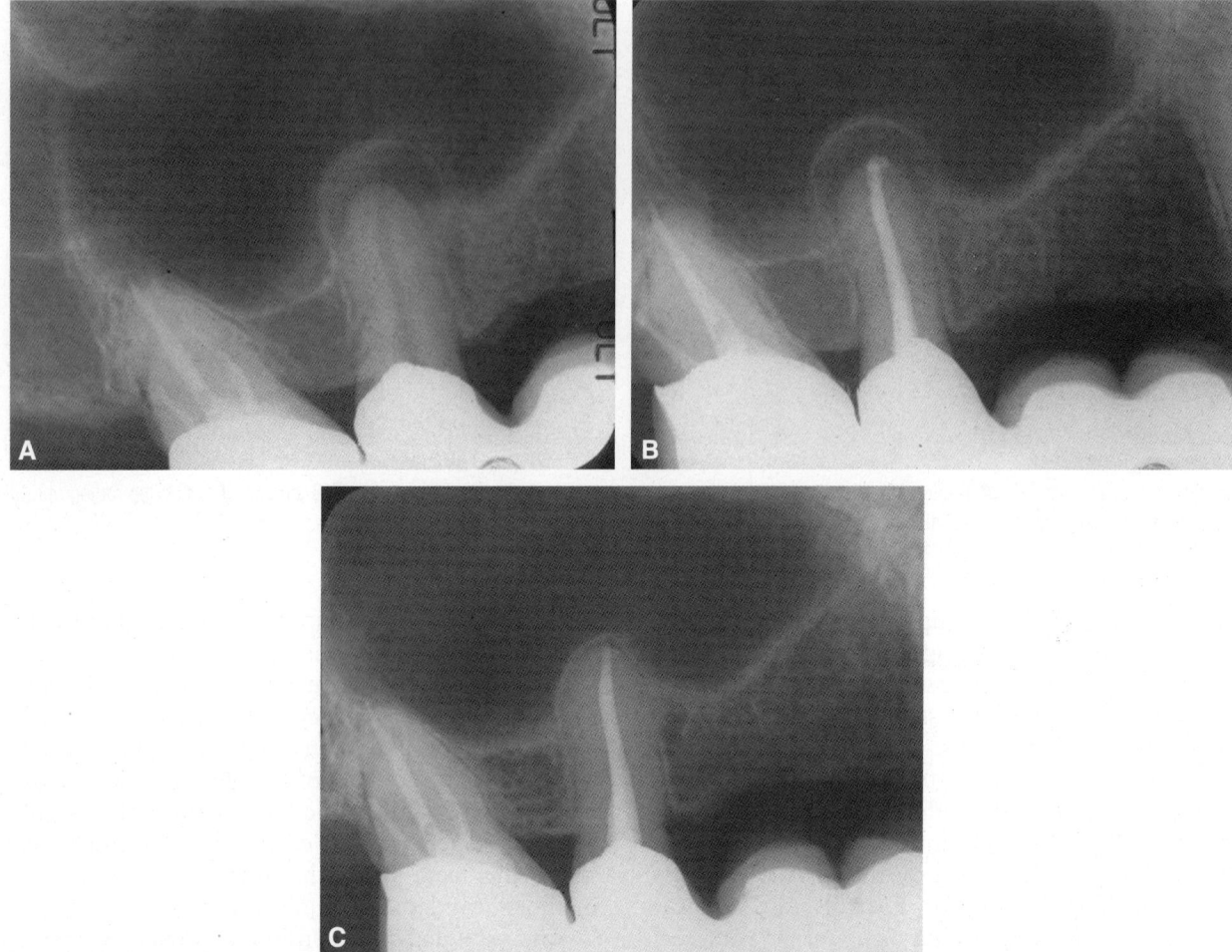

Figure 6 Periapical osteoperiositis ("halo" lesion). **A,** Radiograph showing expansive bone formation resulting from a displaced periostium by the periapical infection from pulp necrosis in tooth #4. **B,** Post-operative radiograph of RCT in tooth #4. **C,** Follow-up radiograph taken 1 year after RCT demonstrating full resolution of the halo lesion.

It is generally accepted that dental infections account for approximately 10 to 15% of the cases of acute maxillary sinusitis.[9,40] This phenomenon however, may be much higher in chronic cases. Melen et al.[38] in a study of 198 patients with 244 cases of chronic bacterial maxillary sinusitis, found dental etiology in 40.6% of the cases. It is also well documented that the predominant anaerobic bacterial isolates frequently found in chronic sinusitis are *Prevotella* sp., *Porphyromonas* sp., *Fusobacterium nucleatum*, and *Peptostreptococcus* sp., the same bacterial species that are found in endodontic infections.[17,42–44] It is unclear if the presence of these species is an indication of dental etiology or simply develops due to environmental changes within the sinus as the condition becomes more chronic.

If a sinus infection is secondary to a dental infection, sinus healing cannot occur unless the offending tooth is endodontically treated or removed. The dental literature provides numerous case reports of the resolution of maxillary sinusitis following endodontic treatment or extraction.[45–47] The challenge for patients with MSDO is that they often have primary symptoms of maxillary sinusitis yet are rarely able to localize pain to a specific tooth or sense any dental pain. These patients typically first seek care from their physicians or ENTs who may diagnose and treat the condition as a primary sinus infection, as dental infections are easily overlooked during routine ENT examinations.[48] Regrettably, some patients have undergone multiple antibiotic regimens and even sinus surgery before a dental condition is finally diagnosed as the primary etiology[49] (Figure 7).

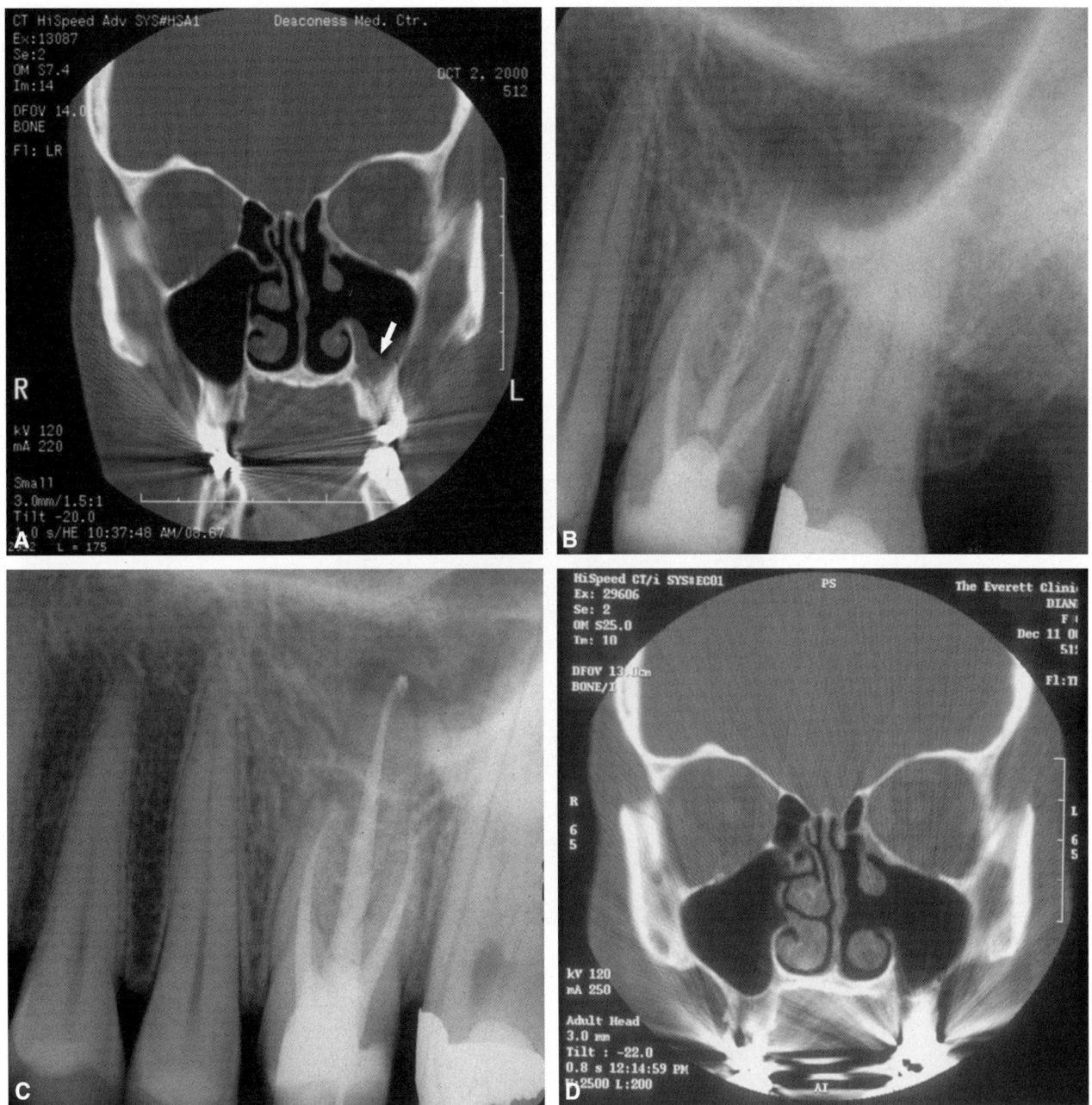

Figure 7 Maxillary sinusitis of dental origin (MSDO). **A,** Coronal CT image of chronic unresolved rhinosinusitis despite extensive sinus surgery and more than 2 years of multiple antibiotic regimens (arrow). **B,** Periapical radiograph shows evidence of a failing RCT in tooth #14 adjacent to the antral floor. **C,** Post-operative radiograph following retreatment of RCT in tooth #14. **D,** Follow-up coronal CT image taken 6 weeks after endodontic retreatment showing full resolution of sinus infection.

This unfortunately occurs despite strong suggestions in the medical literature for careful oral examination including dental radiographs in all patients with recurrent acute or chronic maxillary sinusitis.[38,44,48,50]

The importance of properly diagnosing and treating MSDO is heightened with reports in the literature of dental infections spreading rapidly through the maxillary sinus causing orbital cellulitis, blindness, meningitis, subdural empyema, brain abscess, and life-threatening cavernous sinus thrombosis.[50–52] More recent medical literatures on sinus management have emphasized the need to rule out and treat any possible dental etiology for both acute and chronic rhinosinusitis.[16,41] However, to date none of the current medical guidelines for management of acute or chronic rhinosinusitis include the recommendation for referral to a dentist or an endodontist to rule out a possible dental etiology.[18,53–55] An improved communication between the endodontic and ENT communities is essential in providing improved patient care and resolving a greater number of cases of MSDO.

When diagnosing a possible dental etiology for a patient with maxillary rhinosinusitis, the endodontist must seek out any pulpal necrosis and periapical disease and must carefully evaluate all previous endodontic treatments for failure in the suspected quadrant. In order for a periapical infection to occur, bacteria must be present within the root canal system.[56] A vital pulp, whether healthy or inflamed, will not contribute significantly to any periapical or secondary sinus infection. Thus, in order for MSDO to occur, the causative tooth must either have necrotic pulp tissue or have a failing endodontic treatment.

Properly angled periapical radiographs can offer helpful information regarding sinus pathosis. A generalized inflammatory reaction of the sinus mucosa will result in mucosal hyperplasia, which may be seen as a radiopaque band of tissue following the contours of the sinus floor.[57] Periapical and panoramic radiographs may also reveal the presence of significant mucosal fluid buildup in the sinus floor or complete opacification, which can be confirmed with a corresponding CT scan and through communication with the ENT physician (Figure 8). If the sinus infection is

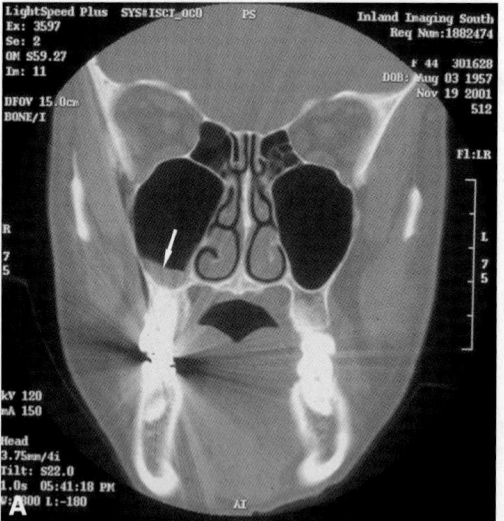

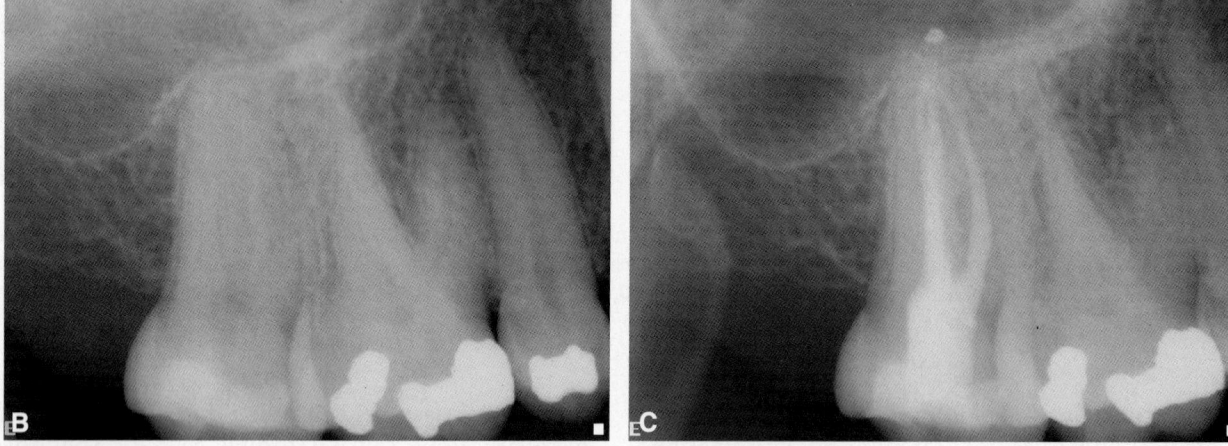

Figure 8 Maxillary sinusitis of dental origin (MSDO). **A,** Coronal CT image of a patient diagnosed with right maxillary sinusitis (arrow). **B,** Periapical radiograph shows no evidence of periapical radiolucency; however, the right maxillary sinus appears clouded. Clinical tests reveal the pulp in tooth #2 to be necrotic. **C,** Follow-up radiograph taken 4 weeks after RCT in tooth #2 with patient reporting resolution of sinusitis symptoms. The sinus appears less clouded than preoperatively on the periapical radiograph.

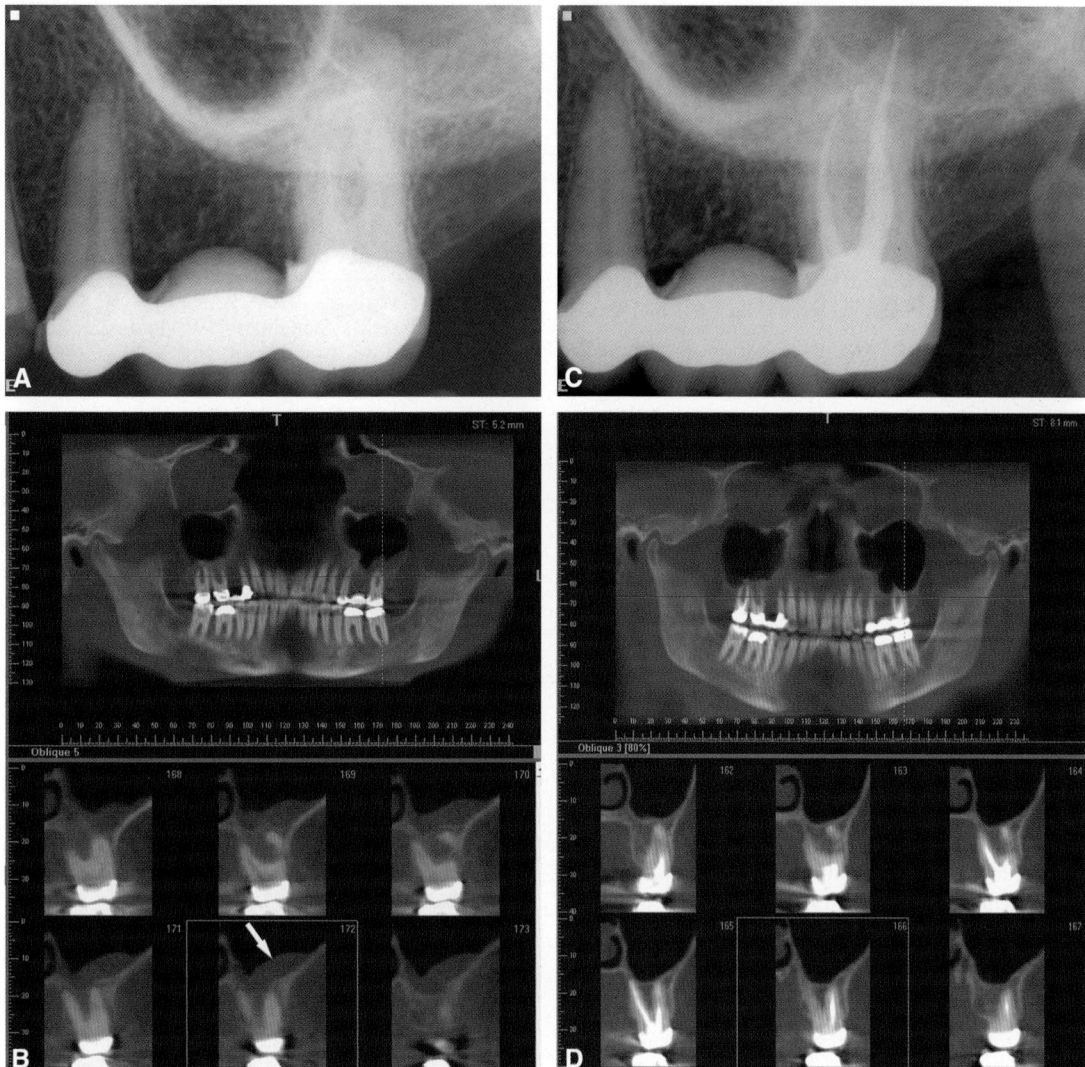

Figure 9 Maxillary sinusitis of dental origin (MSDO). *A,* Patient presented with radiating spontaneous pain in the upper left quadrant. Tooth #15 tested necrotic; however, radiographic evidence was inconclusive for periradicular or sinus pathosis. *B,* Digital CT imaging reveals significant left maxillary sinus pathosis apical to tooth #15 (arrow) and evidence of periapical radiolucency associated with the palatal root of tooth #15. *C,* Postoperative radiograph following RCT of tooth #15. *D,* One-year follow-up digital CT images show complete resolution of left maxillary sinus pathosis and endodontic disease.

determined to be secondary to periapical infection, endodontic therapy or extraction should resolve the problem. However, concomitant management of the associated rhinosinusitis may be necessary to ensure complete resolution of the infection and to prevent any complications.[43] The resolution should be confirmed with a follow-up radiograph or a CT scan and a positive patient report. The increased availability and resolution of digital CT imaging should be of great future benefit in the diagnosis of MSDO as well as for the post-treatment follow-up confirming the resolution of the mucosal inflammation (Figure 9).

References

1. Ingle JI, Bakland LK. Endodontics. 5th ed. Hamilton, Ont.: BC Decker; 2002.

2. AAOMS Surgical Update. Maxillary sinuses, guidelines for diagnosis and treatment. Am Assoc Oral Maxillofac Surg 1986;2:4–6.

3. Alberti PW. Applied surgical anatomy of the maxillary sinus. Otolaryngol Clin North Am 1976;9:3–20.

4. Stammberger H, Wolf G. Headaches and sinus disease: the endoscopic approach. Ann Otol Rhinol Laryngol 1988; (Suppl)134:3–23.

5. Fagnan LJ. Acute sinusitis: a cost-effective approach to diagnosis and treatment. Am Fam Physician 1998;58: 1795–806.
6. Osguthorpe JD, Hadley JA. Rhinosinusitis. Current concepts in evaluation and management. Med Clin North Am 1999;83:27–41.
7. Hamilos DL, Lanza DC, Kennedy DW. Rhinosinusitis and the revised "sinusitis practice parameters". J Allergy Clin Immunol 2005;116:1267–8.
8. Benson V, Marano MA. Current estimates from the National Health Interview Survey 1992. Vital Health Stat 1994;189:1–269.
9. Lanza DC, Kennedy DW. Adult rhinosinusitis defined. Otolaryngol Head Neck Surg 1997;117:1–7.
10. Williams JW, Simel DL, Roberts L, Samsa GP. Clinical evaluation for sinusitis: making the diagnosis by history and physical evaluation. Ann Intern Med 1992;117:705–10.
11. Havas TE, Motbey JA, Gullane PJ. Prevalence of incidental abnormalities on computed tomographic scans of the paranasal sinuses. Arch Otolarngol Head Neck Surg 1988;114:856–9.
12. Gwaltney JM, Phillips CD, Miller RD, Riker DK. Computed tomography study of the common cold. N Engl J Med 1994;330:25–30.
13. Benninger MS, Ferguson BJ, Hadley JA, et al. Adult chronic rhinosinusitis: definitions, diagnosis, epidemiology, and pathophysiology. Otolaryngol Head Neck Surg 2003;129(3 Suppl):S1–32.
14. Poole MD. A focus on acute sinusitis in adults: changes in disease management. Am J Med 1999;106:38S–47S.
15. Snow V, Mottur-Pilson C, Hickner JM. Principles of appropriate antibiotic use for acute sinusitis in adults. Ann Intern Med 2001;134:495–7.
16. Brook I. Microbiology and antimicrobial management of sinusitis. J Laryngol Otol 2005;119:251–8.
17. Brook I. Bacteriology of chronic maxillary sinusitis in adults. Ann Otol Rhinol Laryngol 1989;98:426–8.
18. Slavin RG, Spector SL, Bernstein IL, et al. The diagnosis and management of sinusitis: a practice parameter update. J Allergy Clin Immunol 2005;116:S13–47.
19. Eberhardt JA, Torabinejad M, Christiansen EL. A computed tomographic study of the distances between the maxillary sinus floor and the apices of the maxillary posterior teeth. Oral Surg Oral Med Oral Pathol Oral Radiol Endod 1992;73:345–6.
20. Okeson JP, Falace DA. Nonodontogenic toothache. Dent Clin North Am 1997;41:367–83.
21. Reynolds OE, Hutchins HC, Werner AY, Philbrook FR. Aerodontalgia occurring during oxygen indoctrination in low pressure chamber. US Naval Med Bull June 1946;46:845.
22. Dalessio DJ. Wolff's headache and other head pain. 3rd ed. New York: Oxford University Press; 1972.
23. Ballenger JJ. Diseases of the nose, throat and ear. 11th ed. Philadelphia, PA: Lea amp; Febiger; 1969.
24. Radman WP. The maxillary sinus: revisited by an endodontist. J Endod 1983;9:382–3.
25. Wallace JA. Transantral endodontic surgery. Oral Surg Oral Med Oral Pathol Oral Radiol Endod 1996;82:80–4.
26. Hauman CHJ, Chandler NP, Tong DC. Endodontic implications of the maxillary sinus: a review. Int Endod J 2002;35:127–41.
27. Worth HM, Stoneman DW. Radiographic interpretation of antral mucosal changes due to localized dental infection. J Can Dent Assoc 1972;38:111–16.
28. Berry G. Further observations on dental caries as a contributing factor in maxillary sinusitis. Arch Otol 1930;11:55.
29. Bauer WH. Maxillary sinusitis of dental origin. Am J Orthod Oral Surg 1943;29:133–51.
30. Nenzen B, Welander U. The effect of conservative root canal therapy on local mucosal hyperplasia in the maxillary sinus. Odontol Revy 1967;18:295–302.
31. Maloney PL, Doku HC. Maxillary sinusitis of odontogenic origin. J Can Dent Assoc 1968;34:591–603.
32. Seldon HS. The interrelationship between the maxillary sinus and endodontics. Oral Surg Oral Med Oral Pathol Oral Radiol Endod 1974;38:623–9.
33. Yoshiura K, Ban S, Hijiya T, et al. Analysis of maxillary sinusitis using computed tomography. Dentomaxillofac Radiol 1993;22:86–92.
34. Bertrand B, Rombaux P, Eloy P, Reychler H. Sinusitis of dental origin. Acta Otorhinolaryngol Belg 1997; 51;315–22.
35. Connor SEJ, Chavda SV, Pahor AL. Computed tomography evidence of dental restoration as aetiological factor for maxillary sinusitis. J Laryngol Otol 2000; 114:510–13.
36. Abrahams JJ, Glassberg RM. Dental disease: a frequently unrecognized cause of maxillary sinus abnormalities? Am J Roentenol 1996;166:1219–23.
37. Matilla K. Roentgenological investigations of the relationship between periapical lesions and conditions of the mucous membrane of the maxillary sinuses. Acta Odontolog Scand 1965;23:42–6.
38. Melen I, Lindahl L, Andreasson L, Rundcrantz H. Chronic maxillary sinusitis. Definition, diagnosis and relation to dental infections and nasal polyposis. Acta Otolaryngol 1986;101:320–7.
39. Mehra P, Murad H. Maxillary sinus disease of odontogenic origin. Otolarngol Clin North Am 2004; 37:347–64.
40. Kretzschmar DP, Kretzschmar JL. Rhinosinusitis: review from a dental perspective. Oral Surg Oral Med Oral Pathol 2003;96:128–35.

41. Legert KG, Zimmerman M, Stierna P. Sinusitis of odontogenic origin: pathophysiological implications of early treatment. Acta Otolaryngol 2004;124:655–63.

42. Brook I, Frazier EH, Foote PA. Microbiology of the transition from acute to chronic maxillary sinusitis. J Med Microbiol 1996;45:372–5.

43. Brook I. Microbiology of acute and chronic maxillary sinusitis associated with an odontogenic origin. Laryngoscope 2005;115:823–5.

44. Brook I, Frazier EH, Gher ME Jr. Microbiology of periapical abscesses and associated maxillary sinusitis. J Periodontol 1996;67:608–10.

45. Seldon HS, August DS. Maxillary sinus involvement – an endodontic complication. Oral Surg Oral Med Oral Pathol Oral Radiol Endod 1970;30:117–22.

46. Seldon HS. The endo-antral syndrome. J Endod 1977;3:462–4.

47. Dodd RB, Dodds RN, Hocomb JB. An endodontically induced maxillary sinusitis. J Endod 1984;10:504–6.

48. Lindahl L, Melen I, Ekedahl C, Holm SE. Chronic maxillary sinusitis. Differential diagnosis and genesis. Acta Otolaryngol 1982;93:147–50.

49. Kulacz R., Fishman G, Levine H. An unsuccessful sinus surgery caused by dental involvement within the floor of the maxillary sinus. Opt Tech Otolaryngol Head Neck Surg 2004;15:2–3.

50. Ngeow WC. Orbital cellulitis as a sole symptom of odontogenic infection. Singap. Med J 1999;40:101–3.

51. Wagenmann M, Naclerio RM. Complications of sinusitis. J Allergy Clin Immunol 1992;90:552–4.

52. Gold RS, Sager E. Pansinusitis, orbital cellulitis, and blindness as sequelae of delayed treatment of dental abscess. J Oral Surg 1974;32:40–3.

53. Gwaltney JM Jr, Jones JG, Kennedy DW. Medical management of sinusitis: educational goals and management guidelines. The International Conference on Sinus Disease. Ann Otol Rhinol Laryngol Suppl 1995;167:22–30.

54. Benninger MS, Anon J, Mabry RL. The medical management of rhinosinusitis. Otolaryngol Head Neck Surg 1997;117:41–9.

55. Brook I, Gooch WM III, Jenkins SG. Medical management of acute bacterial sinusitis – recommendations of a clinical advisory committee on pediatric and adult sinusitis. Ann Otol Rhinol Laryngol 2000;109:1–20.

56. Kakehashi S, Stanley HR, Fitzgerald RJ. The effects of surgical exposures of dental pulps in germ-free and conventional laboratory rats. Oral Surg Oral Med Oral Pathol Oral Radiol Endod 1965;20:340–9.

57. Van Dis ML, Miles DA. Disorders of the maxillary sinus. Dent Clin North Am 1994;38:155–66.

CHAPTER 18

ENDODONTIC–PERIODONTAL INTERRELATIONSHIPS

ILAN ROTSTEIN, JAMES H.S. SIMON

Endodontic–Periodontal Communication

Understanding the interrelationship between endodontic and periodontal diseases is crucial for correct diagnosis, prognosis, and treatment decision making. The dental pulp and the periodontium are closely related, and pathways of communications between these structures often determine the progress of disease in these tissues. The main pathways for communication between the dental pulp and the periodontium are (1) dentinal tubules, (2) lateral and accessory canals, and (3) the apical foramen.

DENTINAL TUBULES

Direct communication between the pulp and the periodontium may occur via patent dentinal tubules if the cementum layer is interrupted. This is usually attributed to developmental defects, disease processes, or surgical procedures involving root surfaces. Exposed dentinal tubules, in areas devoid of cementum, may serve as communication pathways between the pulp and the periodontal ligament (Figure 1).

Radicular dentin tubules extending from the pulp to the cemento-dentinal junction run a relatively straight course.[1] Their diameter ranges from 1 μm at the periphery to 3 μm near the pulp.[2] The tubular lumen decreases with age or as a response to chronic low grade stimuli causing apposition of highly mineralized peritubular dentin. The density of dentin tubules varies from approximately 15,000/mm^2 in the cervical portion of the root down to 8,000/mm^2 near the apex. At the pulpal end, however, tubular numbers increase to 57,000/mm^2.[2] When the cementum and enamel do not meet at the cemento-enamel junction (CEJ), these tubules remain exposed, thus creating pathways of communication between the pulp and the periodontal ligament. Cervical dentin hypersensitivity is a classic example of such tubular exposure.

Scanning electron microscopic studies have demonstrated that dentin exposure at the CEJ occurs in about 18% of teeth.[3] This incidence is even higher in anterior teeth reaching up to 25%.[3] The same tooth may also have several different CEJ characteristics, presenting dentin covered with cementum on one side while the other sides have dentin exposure.[4] Dentin exposure plays an important role in the progression of endodontic or periodontal pathogens, as well as cementum root scaling and planing, trauma, and chemically induced pathosis.[5–8]

LATERAL AND ACCESSORY CANALS

Lateral and accessory canals may be found anywhere along the root[9–15] (Figure 2). It is estimated that 30 to 40% of all teeth have lateral or accessory canals, mostly found in the apical third of the root.[1] De Deus[12] found that 17% of the teeth examined presented lateral canals in the apical third of the root, about 9% in the middle third, and less than 2% in the coronal third. Kirkham,[13] however, reported that only 2% of lateral canals were associated with periodontal pockets.

Accessory canals in the furcation of molars may also be pathways of communication between the pulp and periodontium.[10,14] The reported incidence of furcal accessory canals varies from 23 to 76%.[11,12,16] In vital pulps, these accessory canals contain connective tissue and blood vessels that connect the circulatory system of the pulp with the periodontium. However, not all these canals extend the full length from the

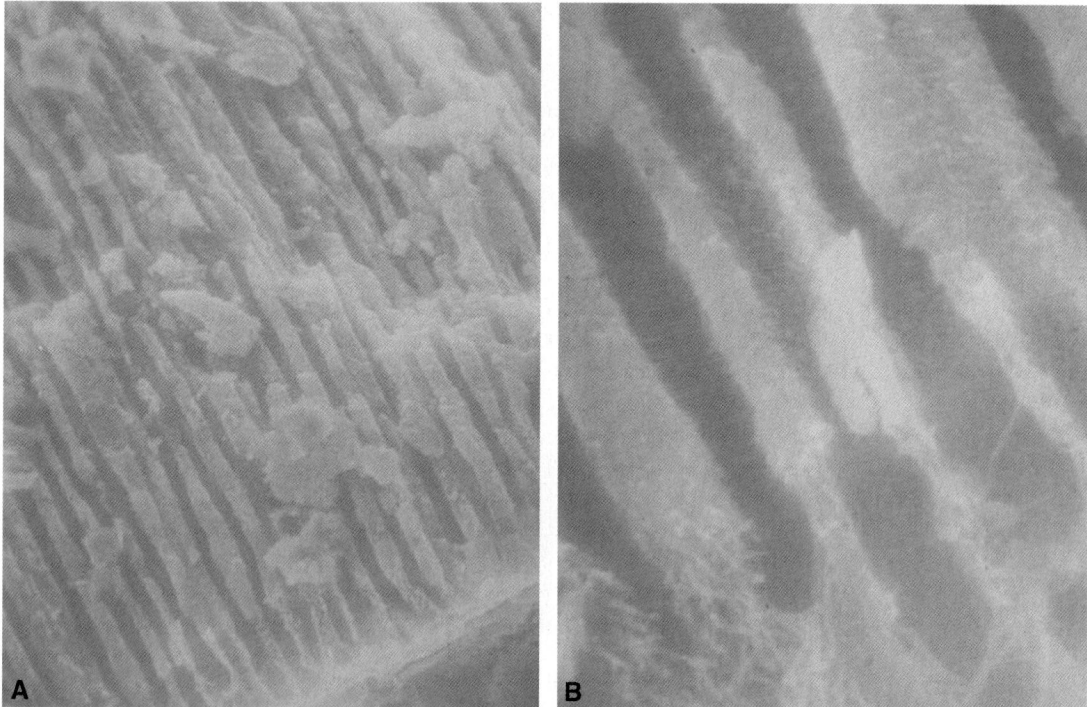

Figure 1 ***A,*** Scanning electron micrograph of open dentinal tubules. ***B,*** Higher magnification demonstrates absence of odontoblastic processes.

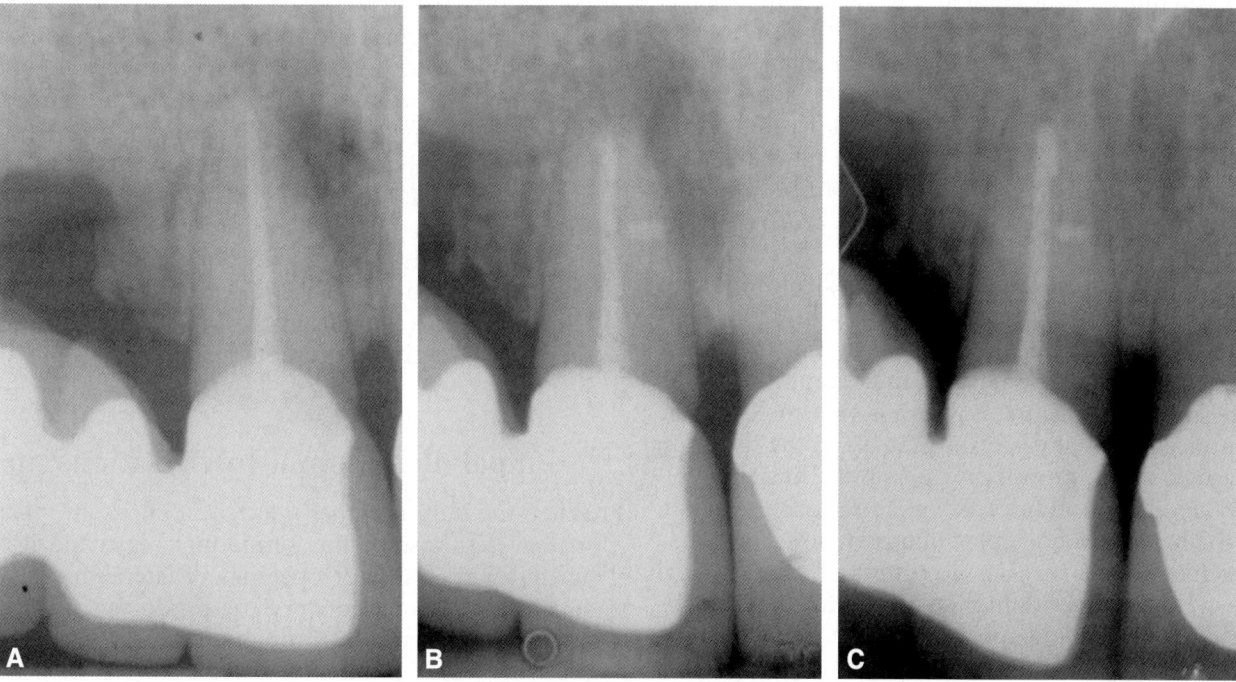

Figure 2 Non-surgical endodontic treatment of a maxillary central incisor with a lateral radiolucency. ***A,*** Pre-operative radiograph showing previously treated canal with mesial lateral lesion. ***B,*** Tooth was re-treated and the root canal filled with thermoplasticized gutta-percha. Note, lateral canal extending toward the lesion. ***C,*** One-year recall shows evidence of active healing.

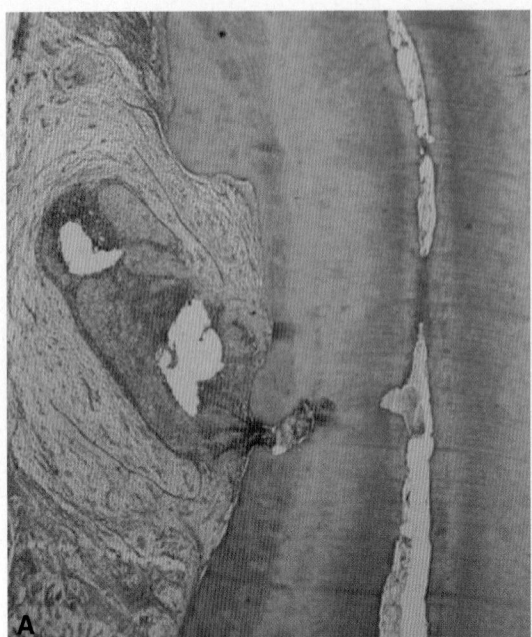 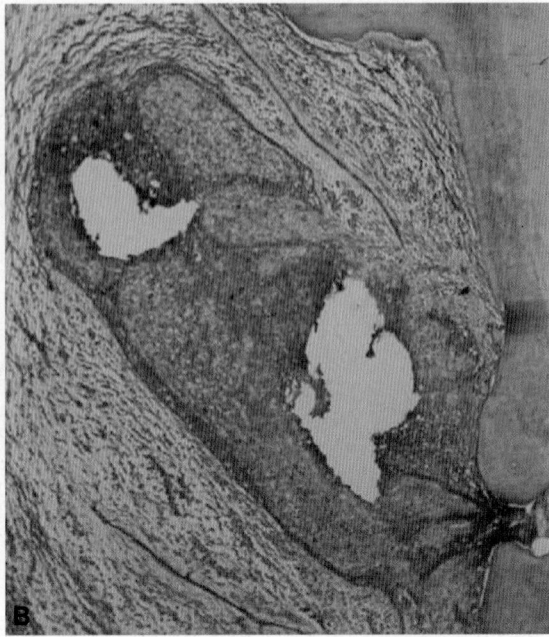

Figure 3 Micrograph stained with Masson's trichrome of a maxillary lateral incisor with a necrotic pulp associated with a lateral inflammatory process in the periodontal ligament. **A,** Main canal, accessory canal, and the resultant inflammatory response in the periodontal ligament are evident. **B,** Higher magnification of the area shows chronic inflammation with proliferating epithelium.

pulp chamber to the floor of the furcation.[16] Seltzer et al.[17] suggested that pulpal inflammation or necrosis may cause inflammatory reaction in the inter-radicular periodontal tissues. Patent accessory canals are a potential pathway for the spread of microorganisms and their toxic byproducts, as well as other irritants, from the pulp to the periodontal ligament and vice versa, resulting in an inflammatory process in the involved tissues (Figure 3).

Clinically, lateral canals are very difficult to detect. Pineda and Kuttler[18] reported that about 30% of lateral canals could be identified through use of two-view radiographs, whereas standard radiographs identified only about 8%. Moreover, using this method, the identification of any accessory canals in the furcation area of molar teeth was also possible. Clinically, predictable identification of lateral and accessory canals, on the basis of radiographic interpretation alone, may be achieved in a very small number of cases. Several clinical aids, however, may be helpful for their identification: (1) a radiographic image of a discrete lateral lesion associated with a necrotic pulp; (2) radiographic identification of a "notch" on the lateral root surface suggesting the presence of an orifice; and (3) demonstration of root canal filling material, or sealer, extruding through the patent orifices.

APICAL FORAMEN

The apical foramen is the main pathway of communication between the pulp and periodontium. Irritants from a diseased pulp may permeate readily through the apical foramen resulting in periapical pathosis. The apical foramen may also be a portal of entry of irritants from deep periodontal pockets into the pulp. Often, such irritants cause a local inflammatory response associated with bone and root resorption. Elimination of the etiologic irritants from the root canal, as well as from the periodontal tissues, is therefore essential to promote healing.

Pulpal–Periodontal Interrelationship

When the pulp becomes infected, it elicits an inflammatory response of the periodontal ligament at the apical foramen and/or openings of lateral and accessory canals. Inflammatory by-products of pulpal origin may permeate through the apex, lateral and accessory canals, and dentinal tubules to trigger an inflammatory vascular response in the periodontium. Among those products are living pathogens such as certain bacterial strains, fungi, and viruses[19–27] as well as several non-living pathogens.[28–31] In certain cases, pulpal disease may stimulate epithelial growth that will affect the integrity of the periradicular tissues.[32,33]

The result of pulp inflammation can range in extent from minimal inflammation, confined to the periodontal ligament to extensive destruction of the periodontal ligament, tooth socket, and surrounding bone. Such a lesion may result in a localized or diffuse swelling that occasionally involves the gingival attachment. A lesion related to pulpal necrosis may result in a sinus tract that drains through the alveolar mucosa or attached gingival. Occasionally, it may also drain through the gingival sulcus of the involved tooth or the gingival sulcus of an adjacent tooth. In most instances, after adequate root canal treatment, lesions resulting from pulpal necrosis resolve uneventfully, and the integrity of the periodontal tissues are re-established.[34]

Certain procedures involved in root canal treatment as well as irrigants, intra-canal medicaments, sealers, and filling materials have the potential to cause an inflammatory response in the periodontium. These inflammatory responses, however, are usually transient in nature and quickly resolved if the materials are confined within the canal space. Periodontal defects, resulting from attachment breakdown, may occur after procedural mishaps, such as perforations of the floor of a pulp chamber or the root surface apical to the gingival attachment, strip perforations, or root perforations from cleaning and shaping procedures. Periodontal defects may also be caused by vertical root fractures associated with excessive force used during canal obturation or restorative procedures.

Periodontal–Pulpal Interrelationship

The effect of periodontal inflammation on the pulp is more controversial.[17,35–49] It appears that, clinically, the pulp is usually not affected by periodontal disease until the defect has exposed an accessory canal to the oral environment.[9] At this stage, pathogens that pass from the oral cavity through the accessory canal into the pulp may cause a localized inflammatory reaction that could be followed by pulp necrosis. On the other hand, if the microvasculature of the apical foramen remains intact, the pulp may test positive to pulp vitality tests. The effect on the pulp of periodontal treatment is similar during scaling, curettage, or periodontal surgery if accessory canals are severed and/or opened to the oral environment. In such cases, pathogenic invasion and secondary inflammation and necrosis of the pulp may result.[44] It has been suggested that endodontic infection in molars, involved with periodontal disease, might enhance progression of periodontitis by spreading pathogens through accessory canals and dentinal tubules.[47,48]

Etiological Factors

Among the pathogens from a diseased pulp, that can cause lesions in the apical tissues and periodontium, are bacteria (Figure 4), fungi (Figure 5), and viruses (Figure 6). These pathogens and their by-products must be eliminated during endodontic treatment. Pathogens and other irritants associated with apical periodontitis other than microbes are discussed in Chapter 8, "Non-microbial Endodontic Disease."

BACTERIA

Bacteria play a critical role in both endodontic and periodontal diseases.[25,50–57] Periapical tissues become involved following bacterial invasion of the pulp, leading to partial or total pulp necrosis. Kakehashi et al[50] demonstrated the relationship between the presence of bacteria in the pulp and periapical disease. Pulps of normal rats were exposed and left open to the oral environment. Pulp necrosis ensued followed by periapical inflammation, lesion formation, and furcal inflammation. On the other hand, when the same procedure was performed in germ-free rats, the pulps remained vital and relatively non-inflamed and the exposure sites were repaired by dentin. The study demonstrated that without bacteria and their products, periapical lesions would not occur from exposed pulps. Möller et al.[52] confirmed these findings in monkeys.

Proteolytic bacteria predominate in the root canal flora, which changes over time to a more anaerobic microbiota.[58,59] Specific profiles of periodontal pathogens in pulpal and periodontal diseases associated with the same tooth were also studied.[60] It appears that periodontal pathogens and endodontic pathogens are similar and that endodontic–periodontal interrelationships are a critical pathway for both diseases.

Spirochetes are associated with both endodontic and periodontal diseases. Spirochetes are found more frequently in subgingival plaque than in root canals. As several studies have shown a large diversity of oral treponemes present in subgingival biofilms of periodontal pockets,[61–63] it has been assumed that the presence or absence of oral spirochetes can be used to differentiate between endodontic and periodontal abscesses.[20] However, today, the presence of spirochetes in the root canal system is well documented and has been demonstrated by different identification

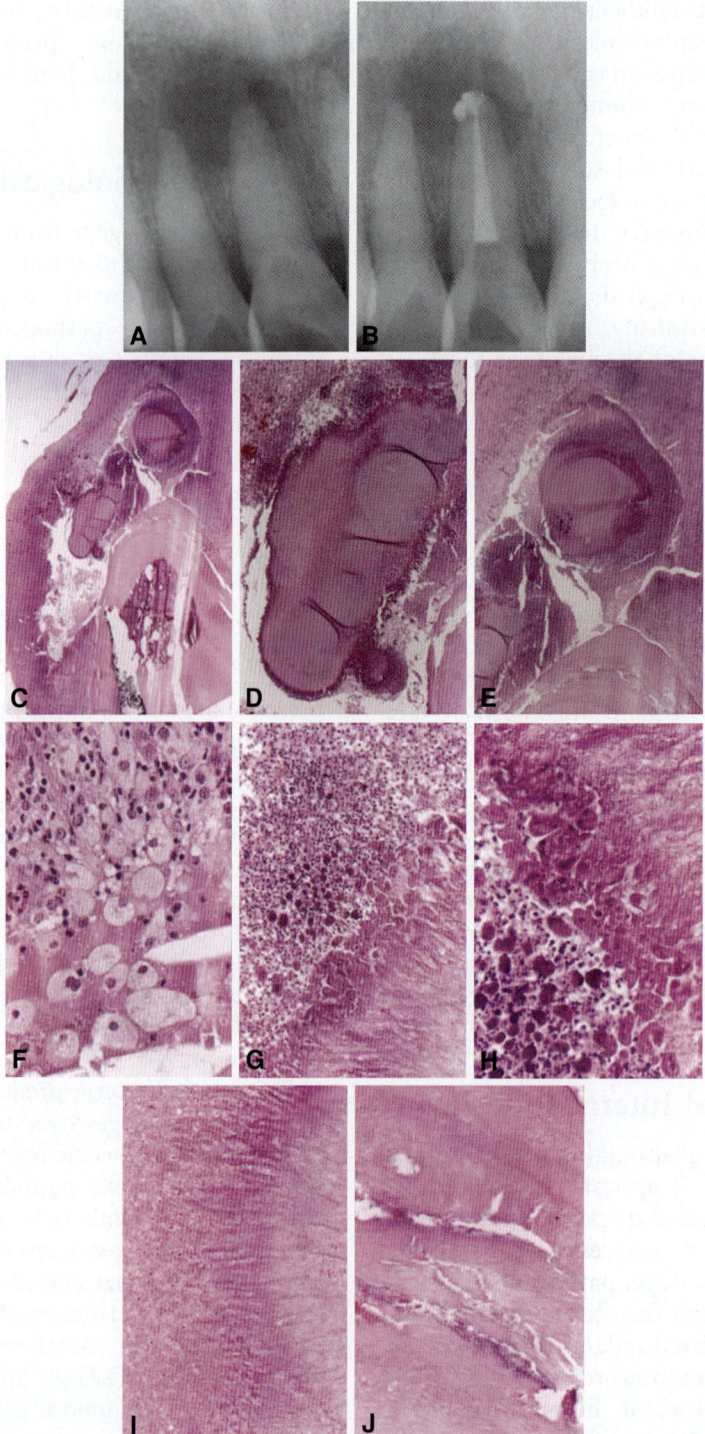

Figure 4 Periapical *Actinomyces* infection. This case demonstrates the growth of bacteria past the apical foramen and their invasion of apical cementum and periapical tissues. ***A,*** Radiograph of a maxillary central incisor with a necrotic pulp showing a large periapical lesion. ***B,*** Non-surgical endodontic therapy was done but symptoms persisted. ***C,*** Apical surgery was then performed. Photomicrograph shows part of the root with the attached lesion. ***D,*** Colonies of *Actinomyces* in the lumen of the lesion are evident. ***E,*** Higher magnification shows large colony of *Actinomyces*. ***F,*** Foamy macrophages attacking the bacteria. ***G,*** Edge of the bacterial mega-colony showing the absence of inflammatory cells unable to penetrate the colony. ***H,*** Higher magnification of the bacterial colony. ***I,*** Center of the colony devoid of inflammatory cells. ***J,*** Viable bacteria within the apical cementum.

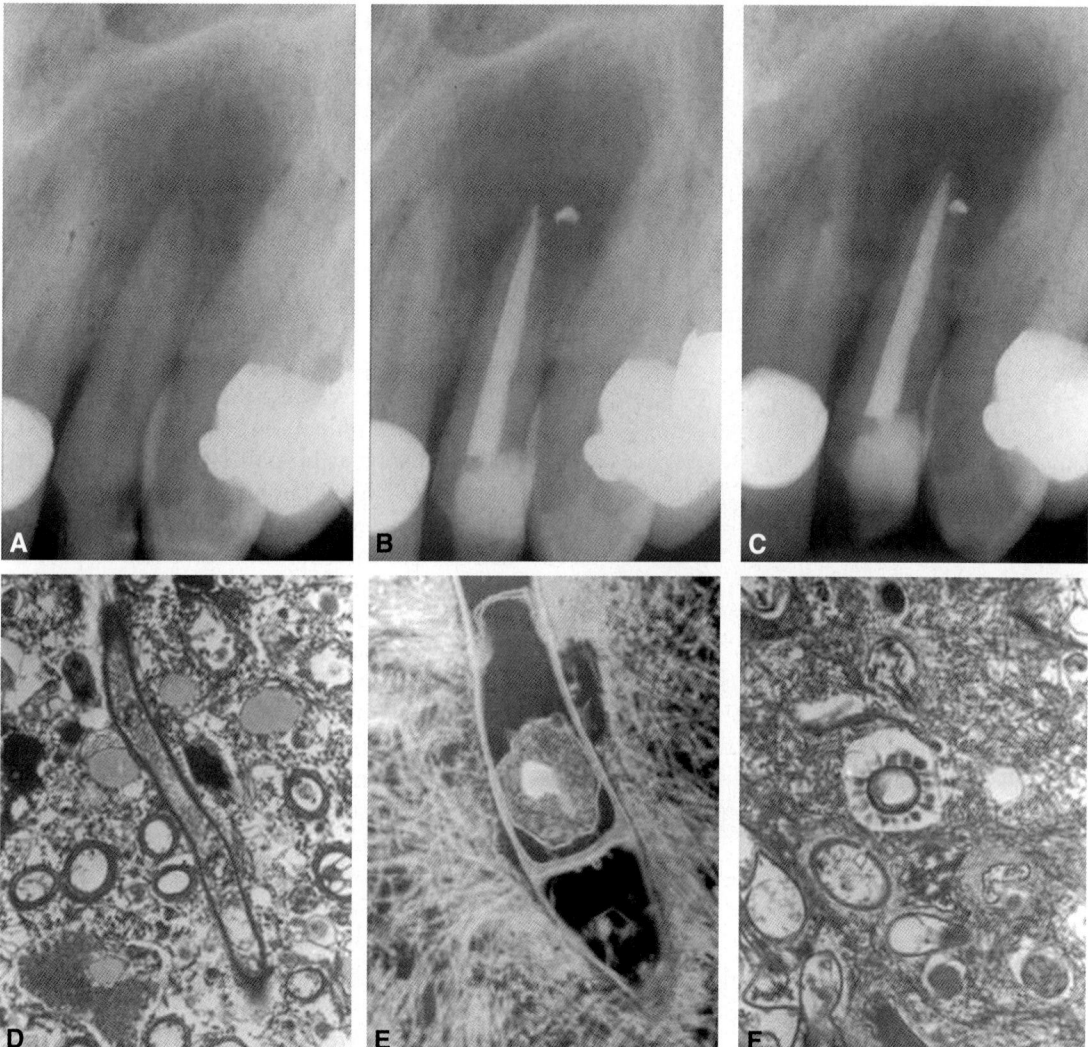

Figure 5 Fungi in a persistent periapical lesion. ***A***, Radiograph of maxillary lateral incisor with necrotic pulp and periapical radiolucency. ***B***, Immediate postoperative radiograph of non-surgical treatment ***C***, At 3-month recall, the patient is still symptomatic and the periapical radiolucency is larger. ***D***, Transmission electron micrograph shows growing hyphae of a fungus. ***E***, Higher magnification of the hyphae showing the cell wall. ***F***, Reproductive fungi spores.

techniques.[22,23,64,65] The spirochete species most frequently found in root canals are *Treponema denticola*[66,67] and *Treponema maltophilium*.[68]

L-form bacteria may also have a role in endodontic disease.[69] Some bacteria strains can undergo morphological transition to their L-form after exposure to certain agents, particularly penicillin. L-form bacteria may transform with several intermediate L-form transitional stages. This may occur either spontaneously or by induction in a cyclic manner. Under certain conditions, depending on host resistance factors and bacterial virulence, the L-forms revert to their original pathogenic bacterial form and may then be responsible for acute exacerbation of chronic apical lesions.[69]

FUNGI

The presence and prevalence of fungi associated with endodontic infections is well documented.[26,70–78] The majority of these fungi are *Candida albicans*.[79,80] Fungi may also colonize canal walls and invade dentinal tubules.[81] Other species such as *Candida glabrata*, *Candida guillermondii*, *Candida incospicia*,[79] and *Rodotorula mucilaginosa*[24] have also been detected.

Factors affecting the colonization of the root canal by fungi are not fully understood. It has been suggested that the reduction of specific strains of bacteria in the root canal during endodontic treatment may allow fungal overgrowth in the remaining low nutrient environment.[75,82] Another possibility is that fungi

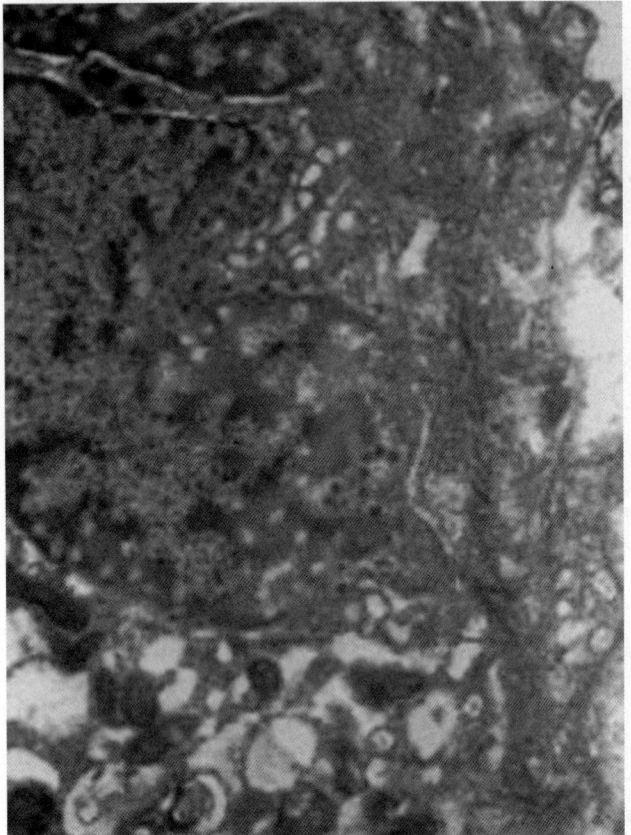

Figure 6 Trasmission electron micrograph of the nucleus of a macrophage in a periapical lesion suggesting a possible viral infection.

may gain access to the root canal from the oral cavity as a result of poor asepsis during endodontic treatment or post-preparation procedures. It has been found that approximately 20% of adult periodontitis patients also harbor subgingival yeasts.[83,84] As in endodontic infections, *C. albicans* was the most common species isolated.[85]

It has also been demonstrated that the presence of fungi in root canals is directly associated with their presence in saliva.[24] These findings further stress the importance of using aseptic endodontic and periodontal techniques, maintaining the integrity of dental hard tissues, and covering the tooth crown as soon as practical with a well-sealed permanent restoration in order to prevent re-infection.

VIRUSES

Viruses may also play a role in the pathogenesis of both endodontic and periodontal diseases. In patients with periodontal disease, herpes simplex virus was frequently detected in gingival crevicular fluid and in gingival biopsies of periodontal lesions.[86] Human cytomegalovirus was observed in about 65% of periodontal pocket samples and in about 85% of gingival tissue samples. Epstein–Barr virus type I was observed in more than 40% of pocket samples and in about 80% of the gingival tissue samples.[86] Gingival herpesviruses were found to be associated with increased occurrence of subgingival *Porphyromonas gingivalis*, *Bacteroides forsythus*, *Prevotella intermedia*, *Prevotella nigrescens*, *T. denticola*, and *Actinobacillus actinomycetemcomitans*, thus suggesting a role in overgrowth of periodontal pathogenic bacteria.[87]

Recent data suggest that certain viruses may also be involved in pulpal disease and associated periapical pathoses such as human cytomegalovirus and Epstein–Barr virus.[88] Thus far, however, herpes simplex virus has not been detected in periapical lesions. It appears that active virus infection may give rise to production of an array of cytokines and chemokines with the potential to induce immunosuppression and tissue destruction.[89] Herpesvirus activation in periapical inflammatory cells may impair the host defense mechanisms and give rise to overgrowth of bacteria, as seen in periodontal lesions. Herpesvirus-mediated immune suppression may also be detrimental in periapical infections due to already compromised host resistant factors and affected connective tissues in situ.[90] Alterations between prolonged periods of herpesvirus latency interrupted by periods of activation may explain some burst-like symptomatic episodes of periapical disease. Absence of herpesvirus infection or viral reactivation may be the reason that some periapical lesions remain clinically stable and asymptomatic for extended periods of time.[88] However, more research is needed to further clarify the relationship between viral infections and pulpal and/or periodontal diseases.

Contributing Factors

Periapical disease of non-endodontic origin is reviewed in Chapter 8, "Non-microbial Endodontic Disease".[91–98]

INADEQUATE ENDODONTIC TREATMENT

It is essential to clean, shape, and obturate the canal system well in order to enhance successful outcomes.[99–101] Poor endodontic treatment often results in treatment failure. Endodontic failures can be treated either by orthograde retreatment or by endodontic surgery with good success rates. In recent years, retreatment techniques have improved dramatically due to use of the operating microscope and development of new armamentarium.

CORONAL LEAKAGE

The term coronal leakage refers to leakage of microbes and other irritants to the root canal filling. Coronal leakage is a major cause of endodontic treatment failure.[102–104] Root canals may also become contaminated by microorganisms due to delay in placement of a coronal restoration and fracture of the coronal restoration and/or the tooth.[102] Defective restorations and adequate root canal fillings will have a higher incidence of failures than teeth with inadequate root canal fillings and adequate restorations.[103] In an in vitro study, it was found that packing excess gutta-percha and sealer over the floor of the pulp chamber, after completion of root canal filling, did not provide a better seal of the root canals.[104] It is therefore recommended that excess of gutta-percha filling should be removed to the level of the canal orifices and the floor of the pulp chamber be protected with a well-sealed restorative material. An adequate coronal restoration is the primary barrier against coronal leakage and bacterial contamination of the root canal treatment.[100] It is essential that the root canal system be protected by good endodontic obturation and a well-sealed coronal restoration.

TRAUMATIC INJURIES

Traumatic injuries to teeth may involve the pulp and the surrounding periodontal attachment apparatus. Dental injuries may vary but generally can be classified as enamel fractures, crown fractures without pulp involvement, crown fractures with pulp involvement, crown-root fracture, root fracture, luxation, and avulsion.[105] Treatment and prognosis will depend on the type of injury.[105–113] Surgical exposure of the remaining tooth structure is one option (Figure 7). Treatment of traumatic injuries is

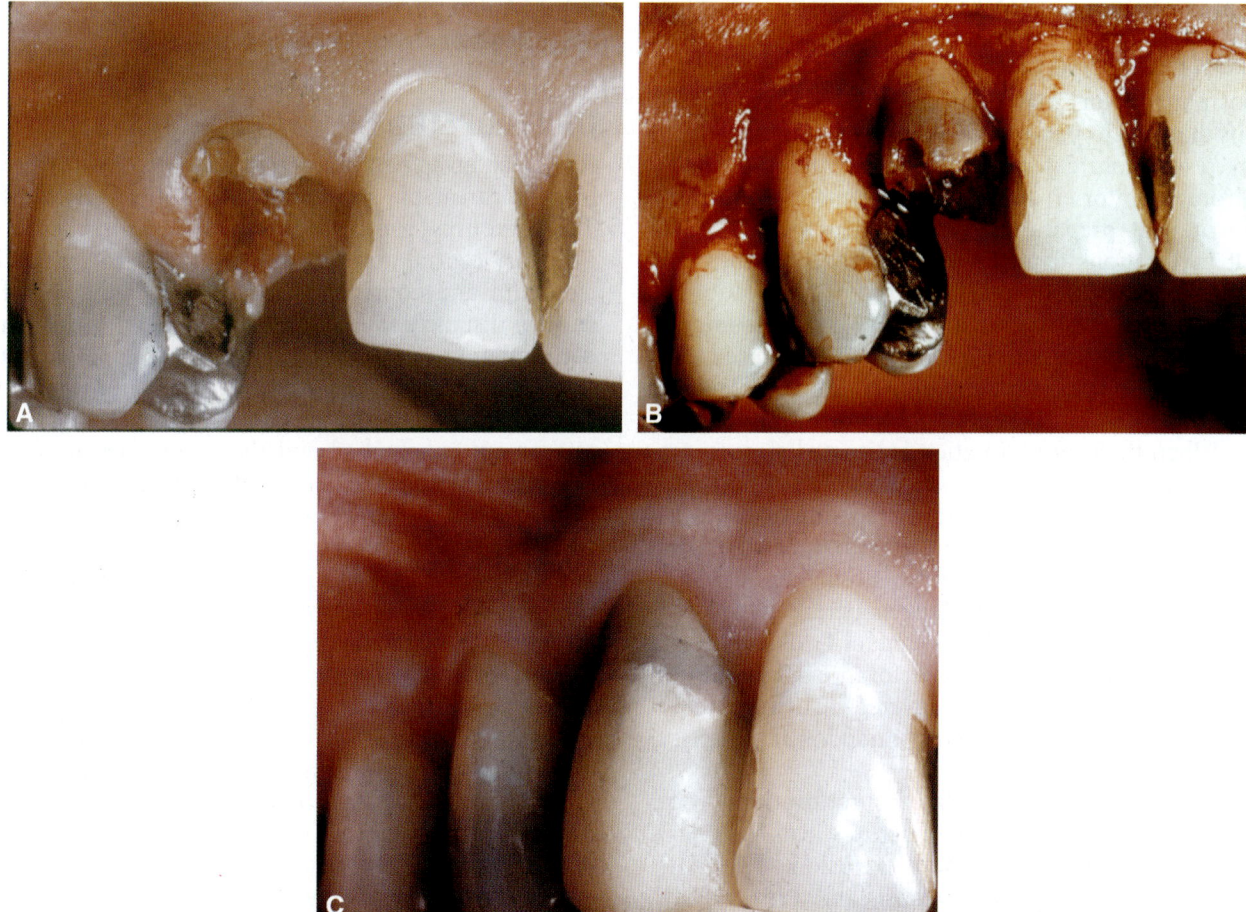

Figure 7 *A*, Canine fractured below the gingival level, compromising root canal treatment. *B*, Gingivoplasty and osteoplasty to remove gingival tissue and bone uncovering the root while maintaining normal gingival architecture. Strip of attached gingiva must be retained. Root canal filling is completed. *C*, Temporary crown has been placed and attached gingiva has regrown at new level. (Courtesy, Dr. Edward E. Beveridge)

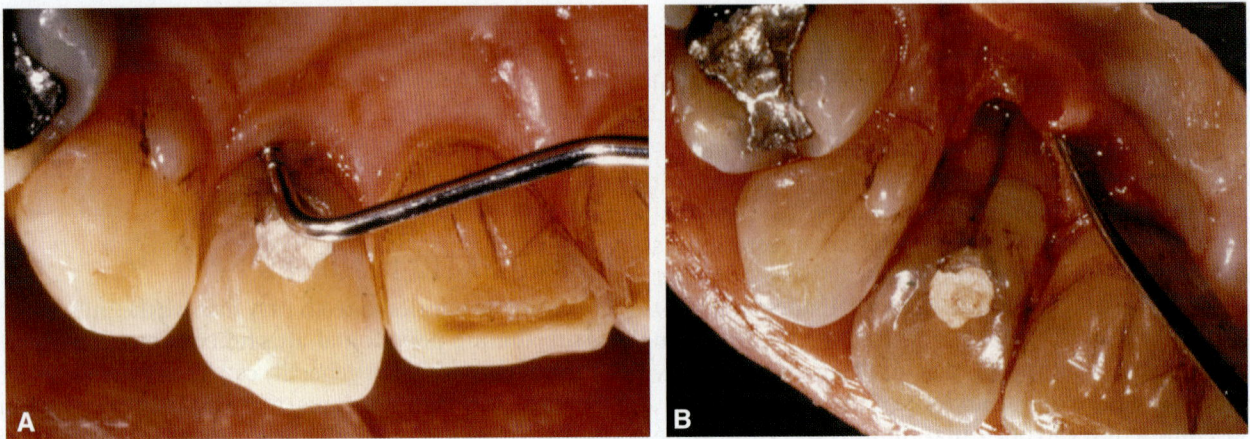

Figure 8 ***A***, Probing deep lingual pocket associated with radicular invagination. ***B***, Raised flap reveals the depth and length of deep lingual groove.

covered in Chapter 35 "Endodontic Considerations in Dental Trauma."

ROOT PERFORATIONS

Root perforations may often cause clinical complications that lead to periodontal lesions. Root perforations may result from extensive carious lesions, resorption, or from operator error during root canal instrumentation or post preparation.[114] Treatment prognosis of root perforations depends on the size, location, time of diagnosis and treatment, degree of periodontal damage as well as the sealing ability and biocompatibility of the repair material. It has been recognized that treatment success depends mainly on immediate sealing of the perforation and appropriate infection control. When the root perforation is situated close to the alveolar crest, it may be possible to raise a flap and repair the defect with an appropriate filling material. In deeper perforations, or in a furcation, immediate repair of the perforation has a better prognosis than management of an infected one. Many materials have been used to seal root perforations. Mineral Trioxide Aggregate is widely used to seal root perforations. Techniques for perforation repair are covered in Chapter 30 "Retreatment of Non-Healing Endodontic Therapy and Management of Mishaps."

Another treatment modality for perforations, root resorptions, and certain root fractures in the cervical third region is orthodontic root extrusion.[115–118] The procedure has very good prognosis and a low risk of relapse. It can be performed either immediately or over a few weeks period depending on each individual case. The goal of controlled root extrusion is to modify the soft tissues and bone and is therefore used to correct gingival discrepancies and osseous defects of periodontally involved teeth.[116] It is also used in the management of non-restorable teeth and as a non-surgical alternative to crown lengthening.[117]

DEVELOPMENTAL MALFORMATIONS

Radicular invaginations or radicular grooves can lead to an untreatable periodontal condition (Figure 8). These grooves usually begin in the central fossa of maxillary central and lateral incisors crossing over the cingulum and continuing apically down the root for varying distances. Such a groove is probably the result of an attempt of the tooth germ to form another root. As long as the epithelial attachment remains intact, the periodontium remains healthy. However, once this attachment is breached and the groove becomes contaminated, a self-sustaining infrabony pocket can be formed along its entire length. This fissure-like defect provides a nidus for accumulation of microorganisms and an avenue for the progression of periodontal disease that can also affect the pulp. Radiographically, the area of bone destruction follows the course of the groove.

Clinically, the patient may present symptoms of a periodontal abscess or a variety of asymptomatic endodontic conditions. If the condition is purely periodontal, it can be diagnosed by visually following the groove to the gingival margin and by probing the depth of the pocket, which is usually tubular in form and localized to this one area, as opposed to a more generalized periodontal problem. The tooth will also respond to pulp testing procedures. If this condition is also associated with an endodontic disease, the patient may present clinically with any of the spectrum of endodontic symptoms. While performing clinical examination, the clinician must look for the groove as it may have been altered by a previous access opening or restoration placed in the access cavity. The appearance of a teardrop-shaped area on the radiograph should immediately arouse suspicion. The developmental groove may be visible on the radiograph as a dark vertical line. This condition must be differentiated from a vertical fracture, which may give a similar radiographic appearance.

The prognosis of root canal treatment in such cases is guarded, depending on the apical extent of the groove. Radicular grooves are self-sustaining infra-bony pockets and therefore scaling and root planing will not suffice. Although the acute nature of the problem may be alleviated initially, the source of the chronic or acute inflammation must be eradicated by a surgical approach. Treatment consists of burring out the groove, placing bone substitutes, and surgical management of the soft tissues and underlying bone. A clinical case using Emdogain as a treatment adjunct was recently described.[119] If unsuccessful, the tooth needs to be extracted due to poor prognosis.

Differential Diagnosis

Differential diagnosis for treatment and prognosis of endodontic-periodontal diseases can be achieved by using the following classification: (1) primary endodontic diseases, (2) primary periodontal diseases, and (3) combined diseases.[120] The combined diseases include (1) primary endodontic disease with secondary periodontal involvement, (2) primary periodontal disease with secondary endodontic involvement, and (3) true combined diseases. This classification is based on how these lesions are formed. By understanding the pathogenesis, the clinician can then offer an appropriate course of treatment and better assess the prognosis.

PRIMARY ENDODONTIC DISEASE

A chronic apical abscess may drain coronally through the periodontal ligament into the gingival sulcus. This condition may clinically mimic the presence of a periodontal abscess draining through a pseudo-pocket. In reality, the pocket is a sinus tract from pulpal origin that opens through the periodontal ligament area. A deep solitary pocket in the absence of periodontal disease may indicate the presence of a lesion of endodontic origin. For diagnosis purposes, a gutta-percha cone, or another tracking instrument, should be inserted into the sinus tract and radiographs taken. This will determine the origin of the lesion. A sulcular pocket of endodontic origin is typically very narrow compared to a pocket of periodontal origin. A similar condition occurs where drainage from the apex of a molar extends coronally into the furcation area. This may also occur in the presence of lateral canals extending from a necrotic pulp into the furcation area. A vertical root fracture or a radicular crack should always be ruled out as they may give initially similar periodontal clinical findings. Primary endodontic lesions usually heal following root canal treatment. The sinus tract extending into the gingival sulcus or furcation area quickly heals once the affected pulp has been removed and the root canals cleaned, shaped, and obturated (Figures 9, 10).

PRIMARY PERIODONTAL DISEASE

These types of conditions are caused primarily by periodontal pathogens. In this process, chronic marginal periodontitis progresses apically along the root surface. In most cases, pulp tests indicate a clinically normal pulpal reaction (Figure 11). There is frequently an accumulation of plaque and calculus and the pockets are wider. The prognosis depends upon the stage of periodontal disease and the efficacy of periodontal treatment. The clinician must also be aware of the radiographic appearance of periodontal disease associated with developmental radicular anomalies (Figures 12, 13).

PRIMARY ENDODONTIC DISEASE WITH SECONDARY PERIODONTAL INVOLVEMENT

Untreated suppurating primary endodontic disease may sometimes become secondarily involved with marginal periodontal breakdown. In such cases, marginal periodontitis is developed as a result of plaque formation at the gingival margin of the sinus tract. When plaque or calculus is present, the treatment and prognosis of the tooth are different than those of teeth involved with only primary endodontic

648 / Endodontics

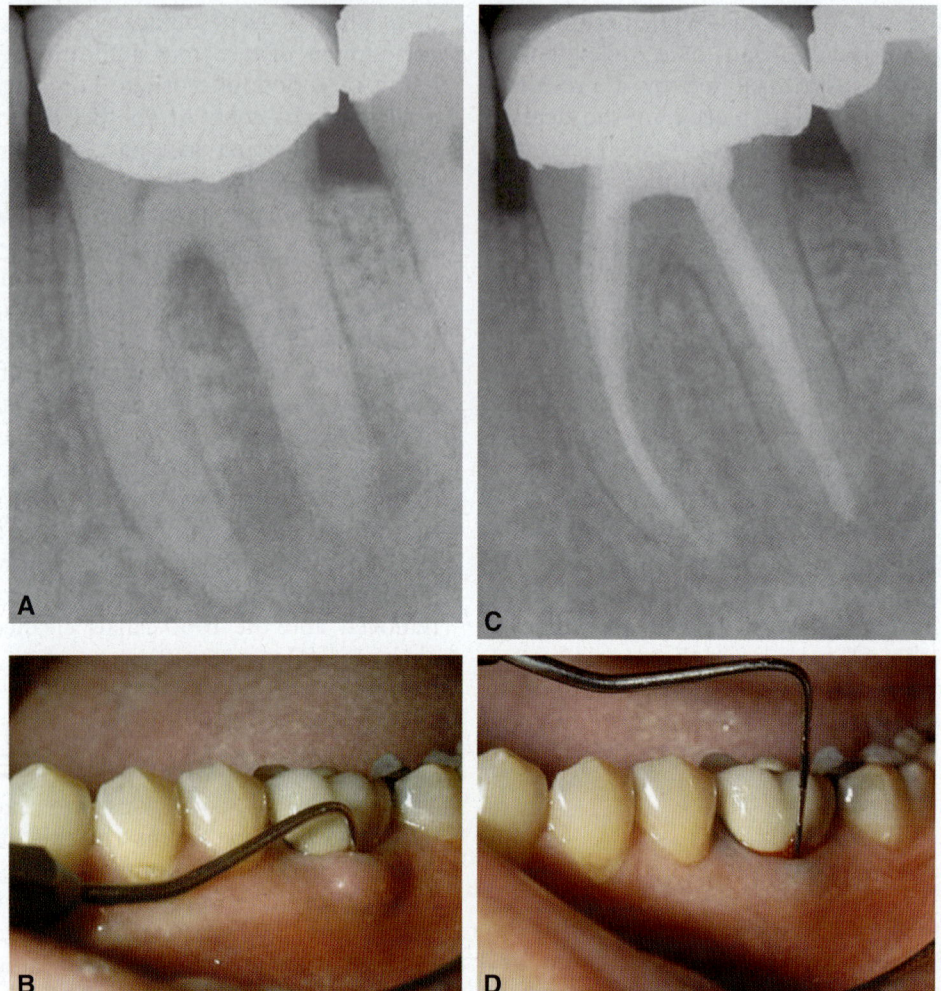

Figure 9 Primary endodontic disease in a mandibular first molar with necrotic pulp. ***A,*** Preoperative radiograph showing periradicular radiolucency associated with the distal root. ***B,*** Clinically, a deep narrow buccal periodontal defect can be probed. ***C,*** One-year after root canal therapy, resolution of the periradicular bony radiolucency is evident. ***D,*** Clinically, the buccal defect healed and probing is normal.

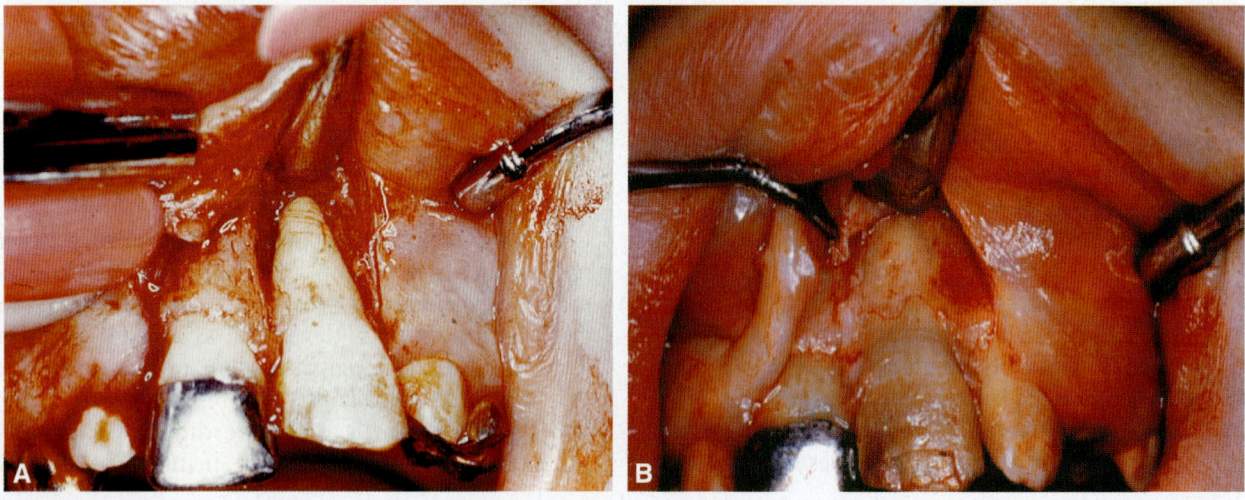

Figure 10 Osseous repair of primary endodontic lesion following trauma. ***A,*** Following root canal treatment, surgical approach removed inflammatory tissue to initiate repair. There was no periodontal disease. ***B,*** "Reentry" 2 years later reveals excellent repair with regrowth of alveolar bone, cementum, and periodontal ligament. (With permission, Hiatt W. J Am Soc Periodont; 1963;1:152.)

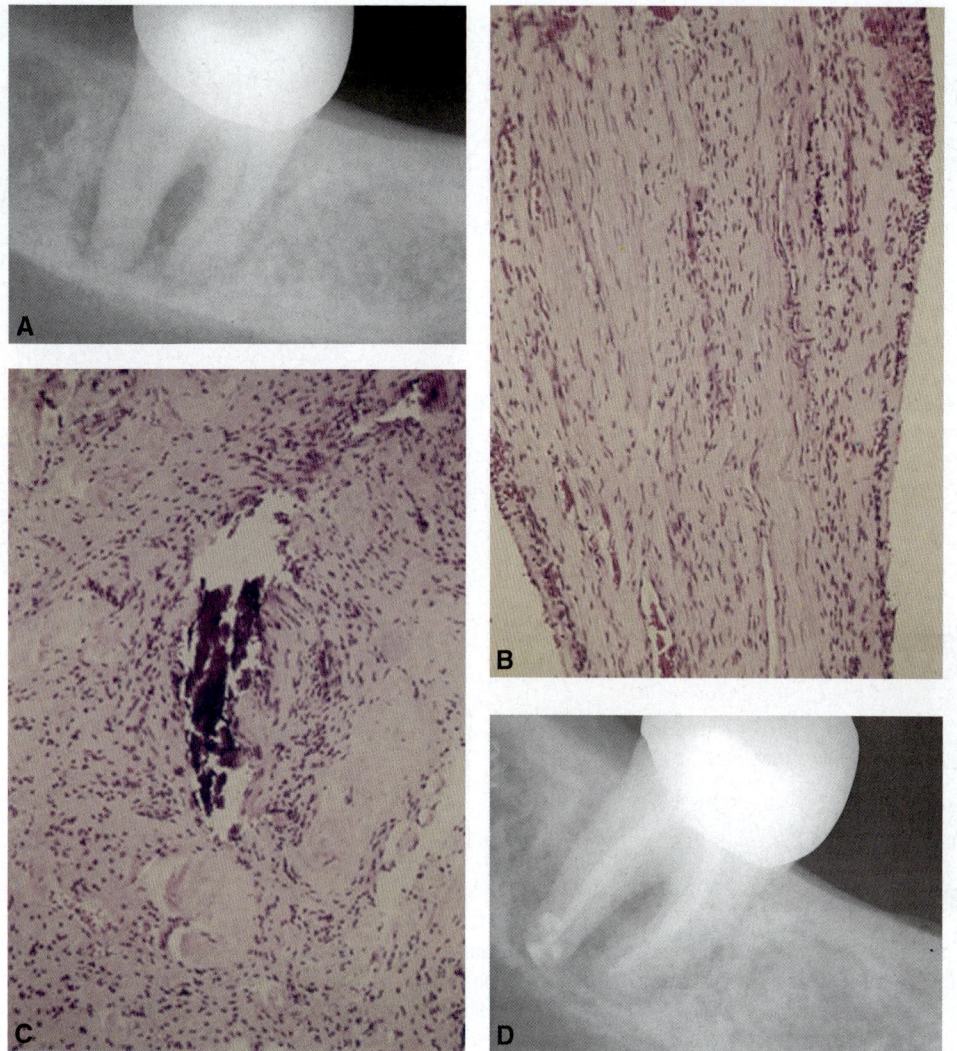

Figure 11 Primary periodontal disease in a mandibular second molar. Patient was referred for endodontic therapy. ***A,*** Preoperative radiograph showing periradicular radiolucency; however, the tooth responded to pulp sensitivity tests. The referring dentist insisted that endodontic therapy should be done. ***B,*** Photomicrograph of the pulp tissue removed during treatment. Note normal appearance of the pulp. ***C,*** Higher magnification shows normal cellular components as well as blood microvasculature. ***D,*** Post-operative radiograph. The tooth was subsequently lost due to the periodontal disease.

disease. The tooth now requires both endodontic and periodontal treatments. If the endodontic treatment is adequate, the prognosis depends on the severity of the marginal periodontal damage and the efficacy of periodontal treatment. With endodontic treatment alone, only part of the lesion will heal to the level of the secondary periodontal lesion (Figure 14).

A similar clinical picture may also occur as a result of root perforation during root canal treatment, or where pins or posts have been misplaced during coronal restoration. Sometimes, symptoms may be acute, with periodontal abscess formation associated with pain, swelling, purulent exudate, and pocket formation and tooth mobility. A more chronic response may also occur without pain and involves the sudden

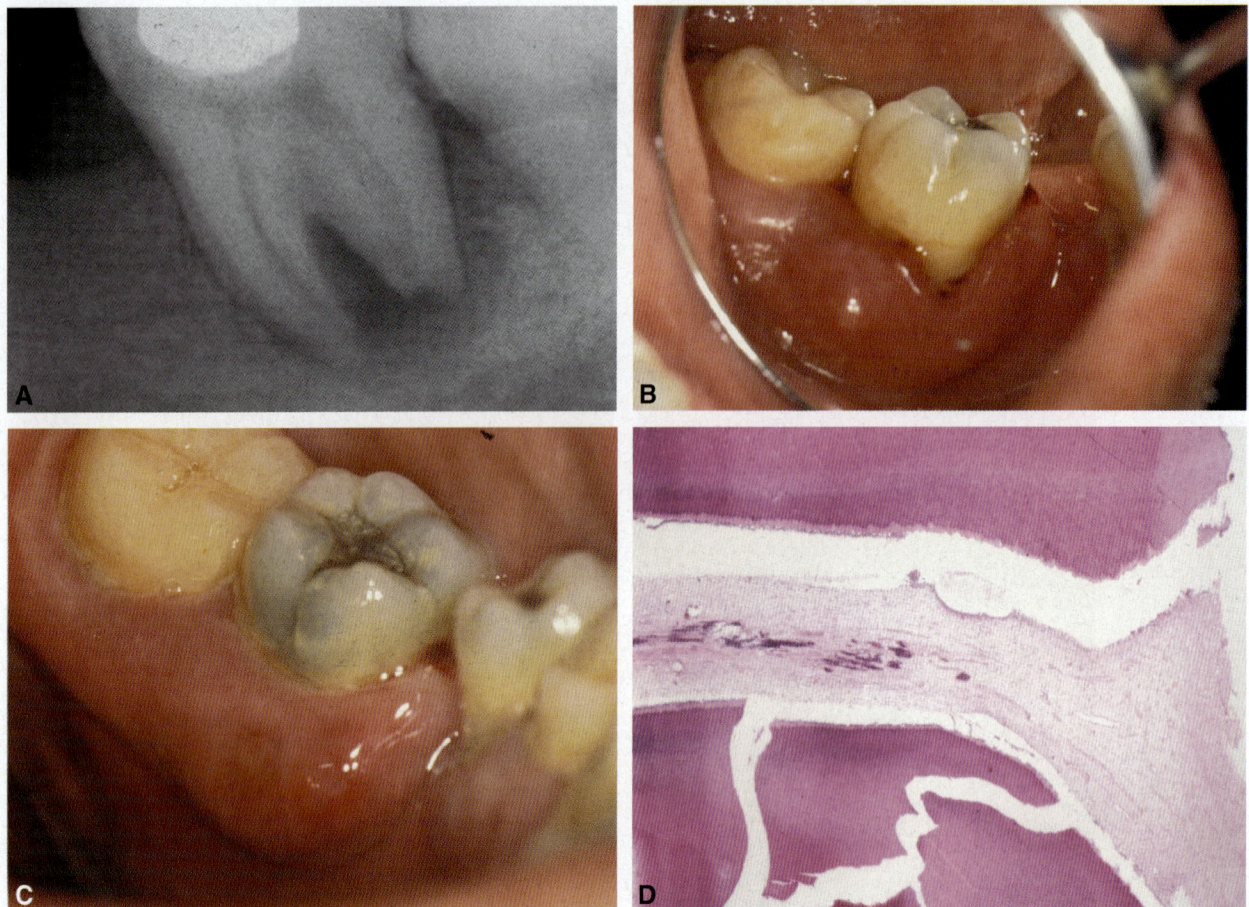

Figure 12 Primary periodontal lesion simulating endodontic lesion. **A,** Radiograph of mandibular first molar showing periradicular radiolucency and periapical resorption. **B,** and **C,** Buccal and lingual views of the affected tooth. Note, gingival swelling and evidence of periodontal disease. In addition, an occulsal filling is present close to the pulp chamber. Inspite of the clinical and radiographic picture, the pulp responded normal to vitality testing procedures indicating the radiolucency, resorption and gingival swelling are of periodontal origin. **D,** Microphotograph stained with H&E showing floor of the pulp chamber and entrance to the mesial canal containing normal pulp tissue.

appearance of a pocket with bleeding on probing or exudation of pus.

Root fractures may also mimic the appearance of primary endodontic lesions with secondary periodontal involvement. These typically occur on endodontically treated teeth often with a large post. In such cases, a local deepening of a periodontal pocket and more acute periodontal abscess symptoms can be found.

PRIMARY PERIODONTAL DISEASE WITH SECONDARY ENDODONTIC INVOLVEMENT

A periodontal pocket may continue and progress until the apical tissues are involved. In this case, the pulp may become infected due to irritants entering via lateral canals or the apical foramen and subsequently become necrotic. In single-rooted teeth, the prognosis is usually poor. In molar teeth, the prognosis may be better because not all the roots may suffer the same loss of supporting tissues. In some of these cases, root resection can be considered as a treatment alternative.

Bacteria originating from the periodontal pocket can be a source of root canal infection. A strong correlation between the presence of microorganisms in root canals and their presence in periodontal pockets of advanced periodontitis has been demonstrated indicating that similar pathogens may be involved in both diseases.[121,122] As long as the neurovascular supply of the pulp remains intact, prospects for survival are good. If the neurovascular suppy is lost to periodontal disease, pulpal necrosis will ensue.[42]

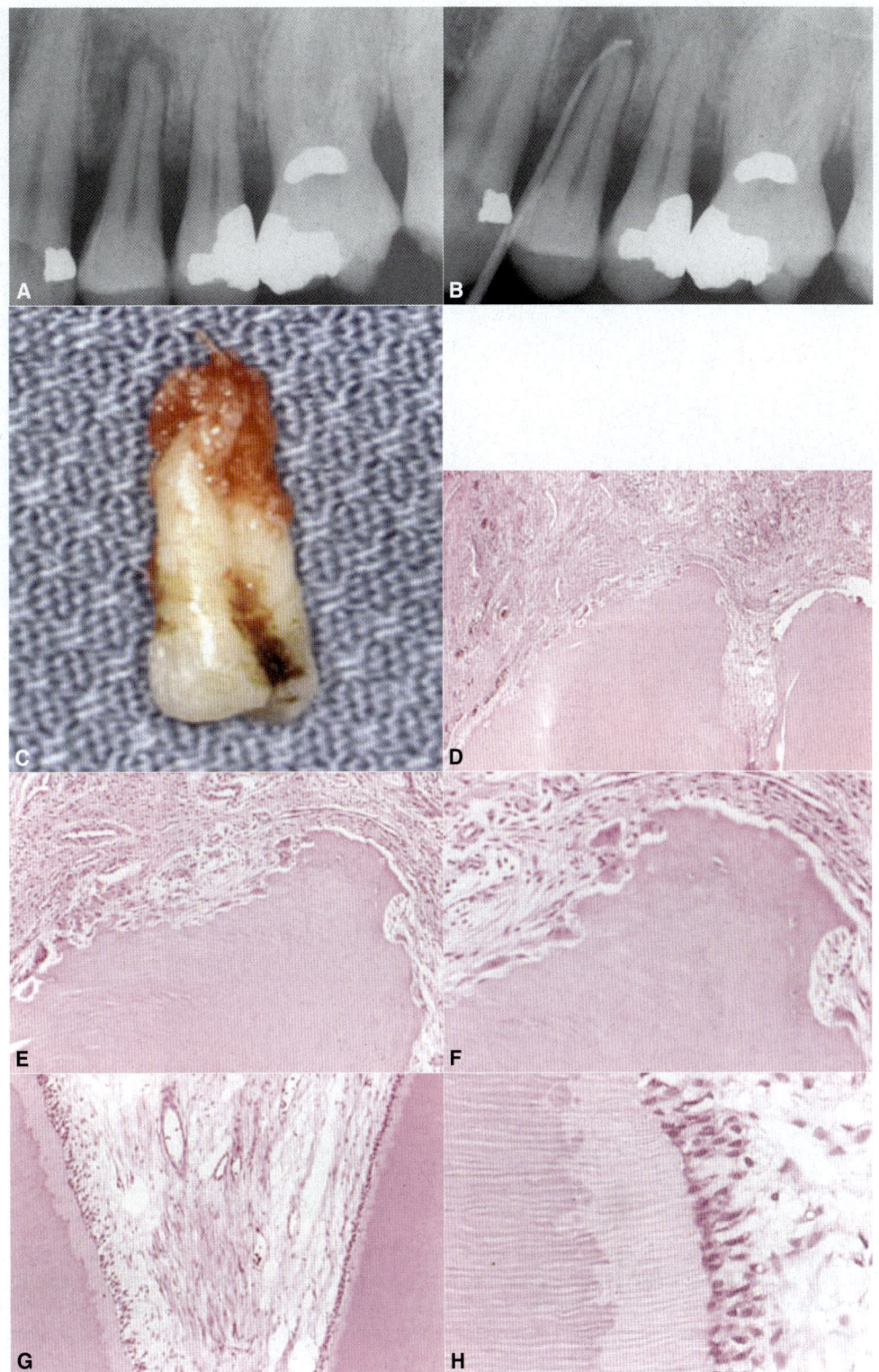

Figure 13 Primary periodontal disease in a maxillary first premolar. **A,** Radiograph showing alveolar bone loss and a periapical lesion. Clinically, a deep narrow pocket was found on the mesial aspect of the root. There was no evidence of caries, and the tooth responded normally to pulp sensitivity tests. **B,** Radiograph showing pocket tracking with gutta-percha cone to the apical area. It was decided to extract the tooth. **C,** Clinical view of the extracted tooth with the attached lesion. Note a deep mesial radicular development groove. **D,** Photomicrograph of the apex of the tooth with the attached lesion. **E,** and **F,** Higher magnification shows the inflammatory lesion, cementum and dentin resorption, and osteoclasts. **G,** and **H,** Histologic sections of the pulp chamber shows uninflamed pulp, odontoblastic layer, and intact predentin.

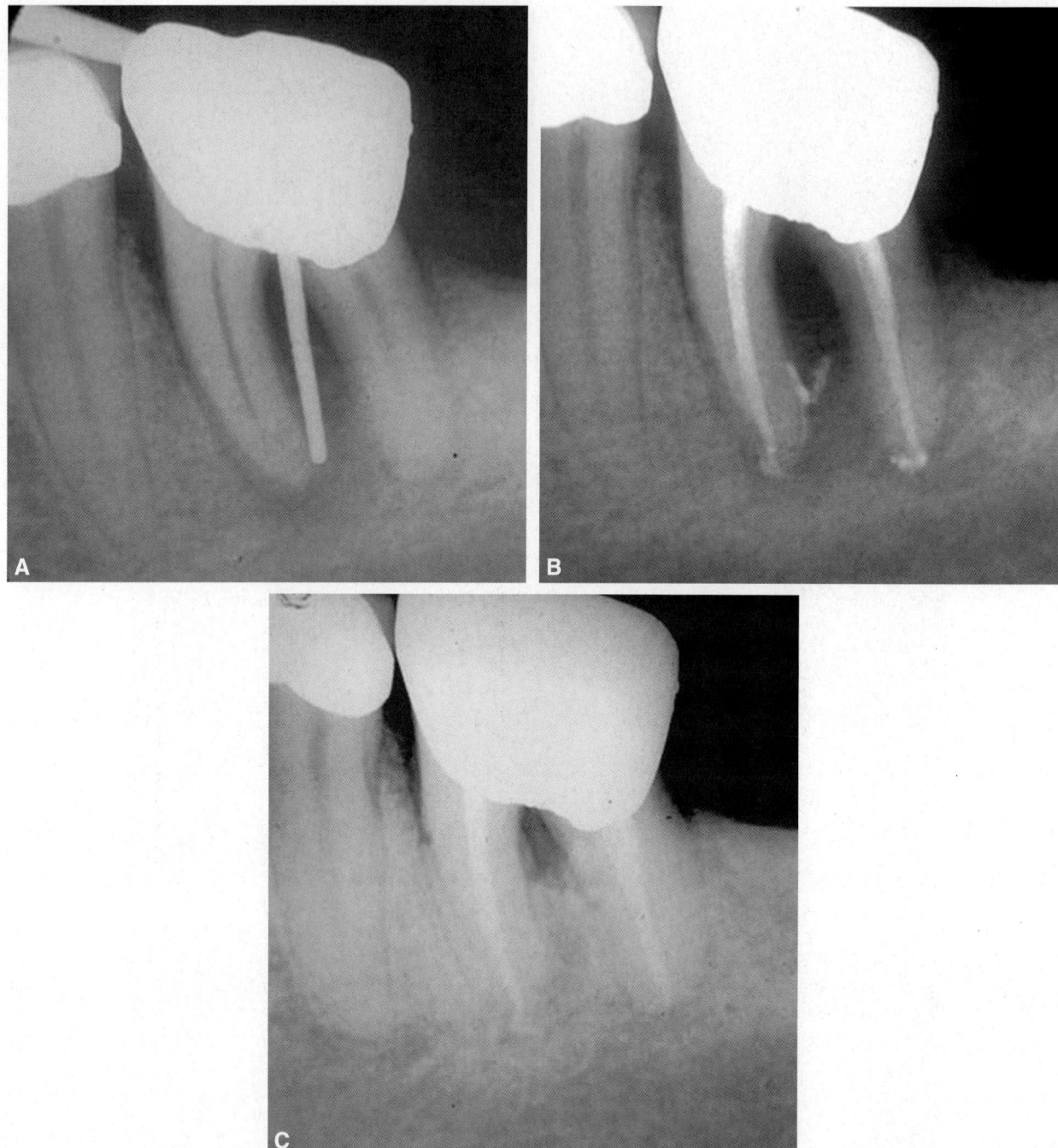

Figure 14 Primary endodontic disease with secondary periodontal involvement in a mandibular first molar. **A**, Preoperative radiograph demonstrating interradicular defect extending to the apical region of the mesial root. **B**, Radiograph taken at completion of root canal therapy. **C**, One-year follow-up radiograph showing resolution of most of the periradicular lesion; however, a bony defect at the furcal area remained. Note that endodontic treatment alone did not yield complete healing of the defect. Periodontal treatment is necessary for further healing of the furcal area and inflamed gingival tissues.

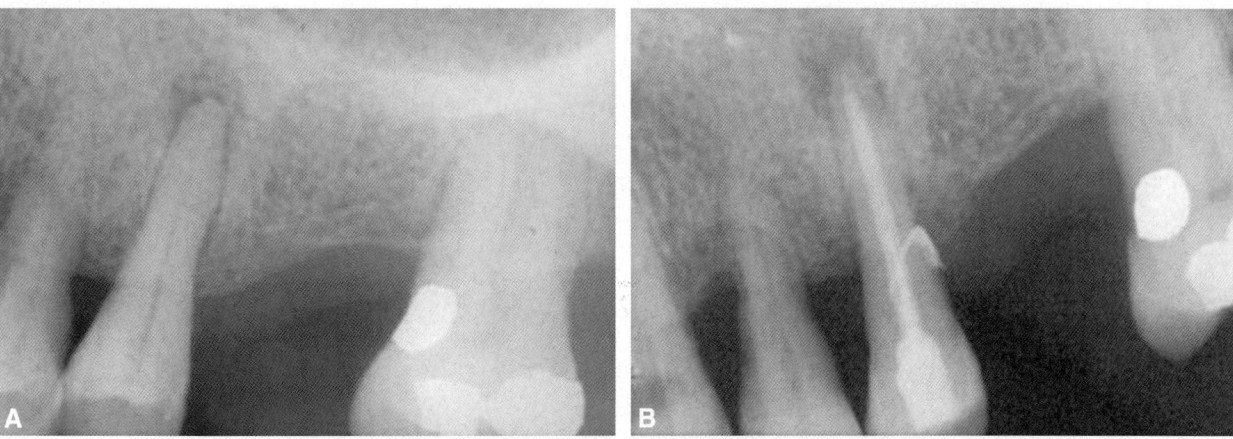

Figure 15 Primary periodontal disease with secondary endodontic involvement in a maxillary premolar. ***A,*** Radiograph showing bone loss in one-third of the root and separate periapical radiolucency. The crown was intact, but pulp sensitivity tests were negative. ***B,*** Radiograph taken immediately after root canal therapy showing sealer in lateral canal that was exposed due to bone loss.

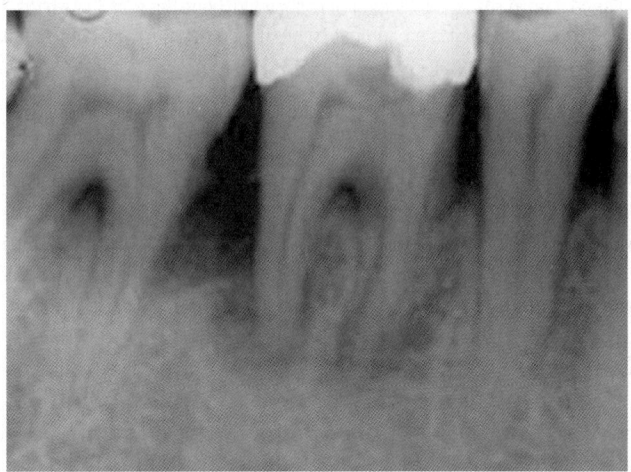

Figure 16 True combined endodontic–periodontal disease in a mandibular first molar. Radiograph showing separate progression of endodontic disease and periodontal disease. The tooth remained untreated and consequently the two lesions joined together.

Treatment complications of periodontal disease can also lead to secondary endodontic involvement. Lateral canals and dentinal tubules may be opened to the oral environment by curettage, scaling, or surgical flap procedures. In such cases, blood vessels within a lateral canal can be severed by a curette and microorganisms introduced into the area during treatment. This may often result in pulp inflammation and necrosis (Figure 15).

TRUE COMBINED DISEASES

True combined diseases occur less often. They are usually formed when an endodontic disease progressing coronally joins with an infected periodontal pocket progressing apically.[17,123] The degree of attachment loss in this type of lesions is large and the prognosis guarded in single-rooted teeth (Figures 16, 17, 18). In most cases, periapical healing may be anticipated

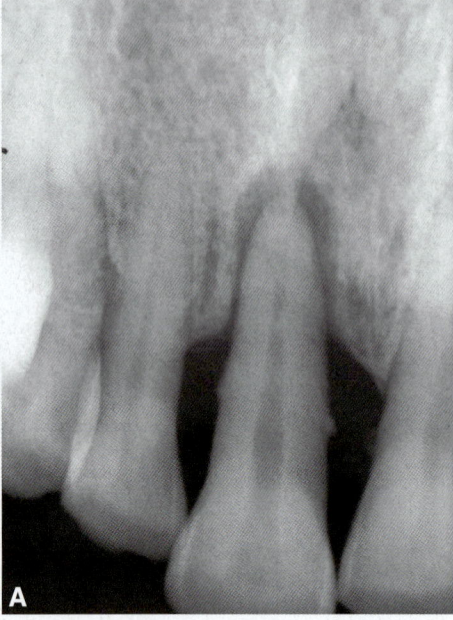
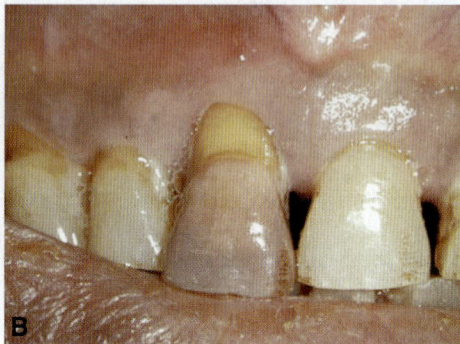

Figure 17 True combined endodontic–periodontal disease. **A,** Radiograph showing bone loss in two-thirds of the root with calculus present and separate periapical radiolucency. **B,** Clinical examination revealed coronal color change of the tooth involved and pus exuding from the gingival crevis. Pulp sensitivity tests were negative.

following successful endodontic treatment. However, the periodontal tissues may not respond well to treatment, and healing will depend on the severity of the condition.

The radiographic appearance of combined endodontic-periodontal disease may be similar to that of a vertically fractured tooth. A fracture that has invaded the pulp space causing pulp necrosis may also be considered a true combined lesion and yet not be amenable to successful treatment. Often, it is necessary to perform surgical exploration of the affected site to confirm the diagnosis.

Prognosis

Correct diagnosis of the etiology of the disease process, whether endodontic, periodontal, or combined, will determine the treatment and long-term prognosis. The main factors to consider are pulp vitality and type and extent of the periodontal condition. For example, the prognosis for a tooth with a necrotic pulp, with or without a sinus track, is excellent following adequate root canal therapy. However, the prognosis of root canal treatment in a tooth with severe periodontal disease is dependent on the success of the periodontal therapy.

Primary endodontic disease need only be treated by endodontic therapy. Good prognosis is to be expected if appropriate endodontic treatment is carried out. Primary periodontal disease should only be treated by periodontal therapy. In this case, the prognosis depends on severity of the periodontal disease and the patient's tissues response.

Primary endodontic disease with secondary periodontal involvement should first be treated with endodontic therapy. Treatment results should be evaluated in 2 to 3 months and only then periodontal treatment should be considered. This sequence of treatment allows sufficient time for initial tissue healing and better assessment of the periodontal condition.[15,124] It also reduces the potential risk of introducing bacteria and their byproducts during the initial phase of healing. Aggressive removal of the periodontal ligament and underlying cementum during interim endodontic therapy might adversely affect periodontal healing.[125] What is of endodontic etiology will heal, in most cases, following adequate endodontic therapy, leaving periodontal disease to be treated.

Primary periodontal disease with secondary endodontic involvement and true combined endodontic-periodontal diseases require both endodontic and periodontal considerations. The prognosis of primary periodontal disease with secondary endodontic

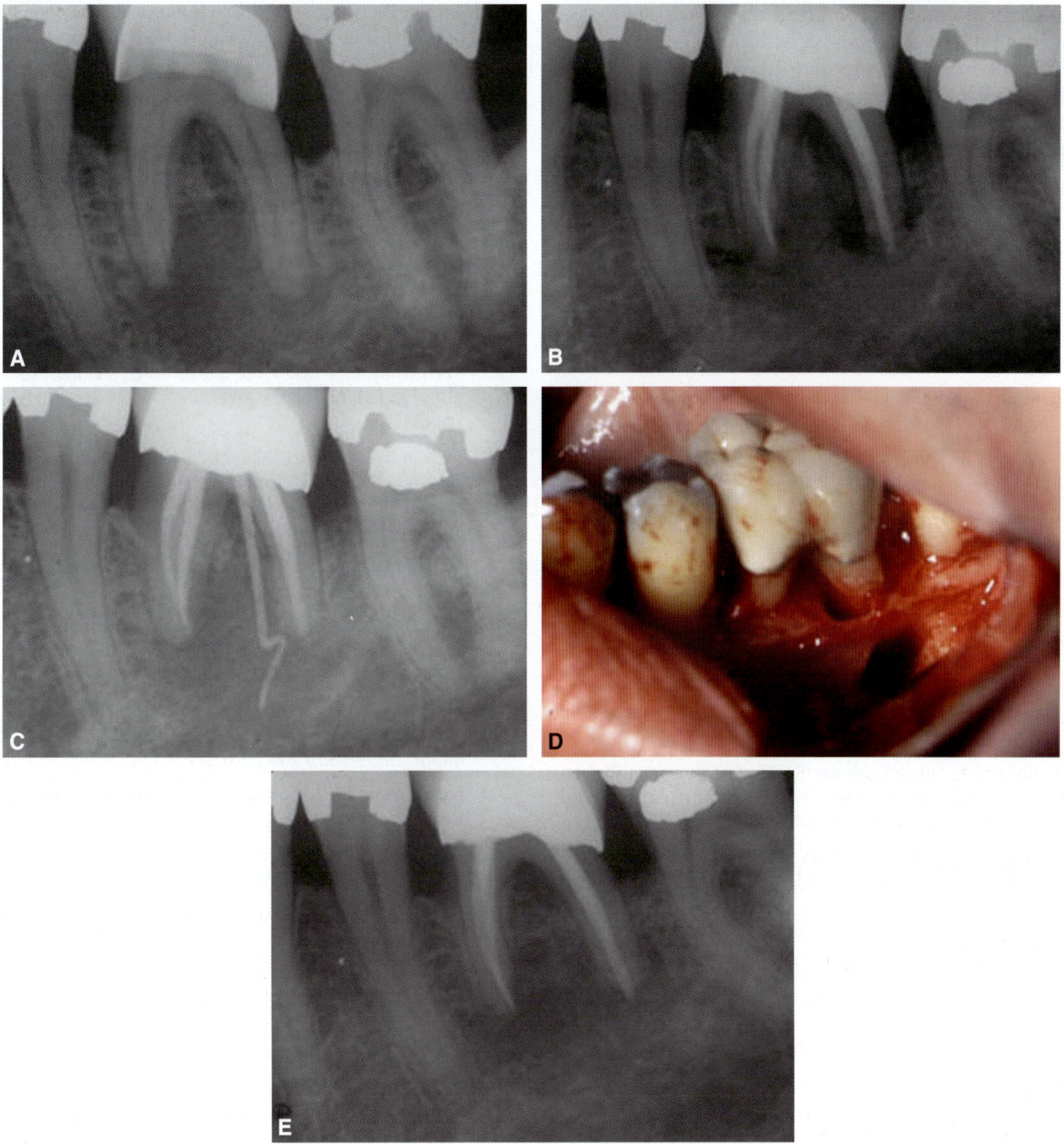

Figure 18 True combined endodontic–periodontal diseases in a mandibular first molar. **A,** Preoperative radiograph showing periradicular radiolucencies. Pulp sensitivity tests were negative. **B,** Immediate post-operative radiograph of non-surgical endodontic treatment. **C,** Six-month follow-up radiograph showing no evidence of healing. Gutta-percha cone is inserted in the buccal gingival sulcus. **D,** Clinical photograph showing treatment of the root surfaces and removal of the periradicular lesion. **E,** One-year follow-up radiograph demonstrates evidence of active healing.

involvement and true combined diseases depends primarily upon severity of the periodontal disease and periodontal tissues response to treatment. True combined diseases usually have a more guarded prognosis. The prognosis of combined diseases depends mainly on the success of periodontal therapy.

References

1. Harrington GW, Steiner DR. Periodontal-endodontic considerations. In: Walton RE and Torabinejad M, Principles and Practice of Endodontics, 3rd ed., Philadelphia: W.B. Saunders 2002; p. 466.
2. Mjør IA, Nordahl I. The density and branching of dentinal tubules in human teeth. Arch Oral Biol 1996;41:401.
3. Muller CJ, Van Wyk CW. The amelo-cemental junction. J Dent Assoc S Africa 1984;39:799.
4. Schroeder HE, Scherle WF. Cemento-enamel junction-revisited. J Periodont Res 1988;23:53.
5. Ehnevid H, Jansson L, Lindskog S, et al. Endodontic pathogens: propagation of infection through patent dentinal tubules in traumatized monkey teeth. Endod Dent Traumatol 1995;11:229.
6. Rotstein I, Friedman S, Mor C, et al. Histological characterization of bleaching-induced external root resorption in dogs. J Endod 1991;17:436.
7. Rotstein I, Torek Y, Misgav R. Effect of cementum defects on radicular penetration of 30% H_2O_2 during intracoronal bleaching. J Endod 1991;17:230.
8. Simon JHS, Dogan H, Ceresa LM, Silver GK. The radicular groove: it's potential clinical significance. J Endod 2000;26:295.
9. Rubach WC, Mitchell DF. Periodontal disease, accessory canals and pulp pathosis. J Periodontol 1965;36:34.
10. Lowman JV, Burke RS, Pellea GB. Patent accessory canals: incidence in molar furcation region. Oral Surg Oral Med Oral Pathol Oral Radiol Endod 1973;36:580.
11. Burch JG, Hulen S. A study of the presence of accessory foramina and the topography of molar furcations. Oral Surg, Oral Med, Oral Pathol Oral Radiol Endod 1974;38:451.
12. De Deus QD. Frequency, location and direction of the lateral, secondary and accessory canals. J Endod 1975;1:361.
13. Kirkham DB. The location and incidence of accessory pulpal canals in periodontal pockets. J Am Dent Assoc 1975;91:353.
14. Gutmann JL. Prevalence, location, and patency of accessory canals in the furcation region of permanent molars. J Periodont 1978;49:21.
15. Paul BF, Hutter JW. The Enodontic-periodontal continuum revisited: new insights into etiology, diagnosis and treatment. J Am Dent Assoc 1997;128:1541.
16. Goldberg F, Massone EJ, Soares I, Bittencourt AZ. Accessory orifices: anatomical relationship between the pulp chamber floor and the furcation. J Endod 1987;13:176.
17. Seltzer S, Bender IB, Ziontz M. The interrelationship of pulp and periodontal disease. Oral Surg Oral Med Oral Pathol Oral Radiol Endod 1963;16:1474.
18. Pineda F, Kuttler Y. Mesiodistal and buccolingual roentgenographic investigation of 7,275 root canals. Oral Surg Oral Med Oral Pathol Oral Radiol Endod 1972;33:101.
19. Haapasalo M, Ranta H, Ranta K, Shah H. Black-pigmented Bacteroides spp. in human apical periodontitis. Infec Immunol 1986;53:149.
20. Trope M. Tronstad L. Rosenberg ES, Listgarten M. Darkfield microscopy as a diagnostic aid in differentiating exudates from endodontic and periodontal abscesses. J Endod 1988;14:35.
21. Jansson L, Ehnevid H, Blomlof L, et al. Endodontic pathogens in periodontal disease augmentation. J Clin Periodontol 1995;22:598.
22. Dahle UR, Tronstad L, Olsen I. Characterization of new periodontal and endodontic isolates of spirochetes. Eur J Oral Sci 1996;104:41.
23. Jung IY, Choi BK, Kum KY, et al. Molecular epidemiology and association of putative pathogens in root canal infection. J Endod 2000;26:599–604.
24. Egan MW, Spratt DA, Ng YL, et al. Prevalence of yeasts in saliva and root canals of teeth associated with apical periodontitis. Int Endod J 2002;35:321.
25. Baumgartner JC. Microbiologic aspects of endodontic infections. J Calif Dent Assoc 2004;32:459.
26. Siqueira JF, Sen BH. Fungi in endodontic infections, Oral Surg Oral Med Oral Pathol Oral Radiol Endod 2004;97:632.
27. Nair PNR. Pathogenesis of apical periodontitis and the causes of endodontic failures. Crit Rev Oral Biol Med 2004;15:348.
28. El-Labban NG. Electron microscopic investigation of hyaline bodies in odontogenic cysts. J Oral Pathol 1979;8:81.
29. Nair PNR. Cholesterol as an aetiological agent in endodontic failures- a review. Aust Endod J 1999;25:19.
30. Tagger E, Tagger M, Sarnat H. Russell bodies in the pulp of a primary tooth. Oral Surg Oral Med Oral Pathol Oral Radiol Endod 2000;90:365.
31. Silver GK, Simon JHS. Charcot-Leyden crystals within a periapical lesion. J Endod 2000;26:679.
32. Nair PNR, Pajarola G, Schroeder HE. Types and incidence of human periapical lesions obtained with extracted teeth. Oral Surg Oral Med Oral Pathol Oral Radiol Endod 1996;8:93.
33. Simon JHS. Incidence of periapical cysts in relation to the root canal. J Endod 1980;6:845.
34. Sjögren U, Hägglund B, Sundqvist G, Wing K. Factors affecting the long-term results of endodontic treatment. J Endod 1990;16:498.

35. Bender IB, Seltzer S. The effect of periodontal disease on the pulp. Oral Surg Oral Med Oral Pathol Oral Radiol Endod 1972;33:458.
36. Czarnecki RT, Schilder H. A histologic evaluation of the human pulp in teeth with varying degrees of periodontal disease. J Endod 1979;5:242.
37. Torabinejad M, Kiger RD. Histologic evaluation of dental pulp tissue of a patient with periodontal disease. Oral Surg Oral Med Oral Pathol Oral Radiol Endod 1985;59:198.
38. Gold SI, Moskow BS. Periodontal repair of periapical lesions: the borderland between pulpal and periodontal disease. J Clin Periodontol 1987;14:251.
39. Adriaens PA, De Boever JA, Loesche WJ. Bacterial invasion in root cementum and radicular dentin of periodontally diseased teeth in humans. A reservoir of periodontopathic bacteria. J Periodontol 1988;59:222.
40. Adriaens PA, Edwards CA, De Boever JA, Loesche WJ. Ultrastructual observations on bacterial invasion in cementum and radicular dentin of periodontally diseased human teeth. J Periodontol 1988;59:493.
41. Wong R, Hirch RS, Clarke NG. Endodontic effects of root planning in humans. Endod Dent Traumatol 1989;5:193.
42. Langeland K, Rodrigues H, Dowden W. Periodontal disease, bacteria, and pulpal histopathology. Oral Surg Oral Med Oral Pathol Oral Radiol Endod 1974;37:257.
43. Mandi FA. Histological study of the pulp changes caused by periodontal disease. J Br Endod Soc 1972;6:80.
44. Bergenholtz G, Lindhe J. Effect of experimentally induced marginal periodontitis and periodontal scaling on the dental pulp. J Clin Periodontol 1978;5:59.
45. Blomlöf L, Lengheden A, Lindskog S. Endodontic infection and calcium hydroxide treatment. Effects on periodontal healing in mature and immature replanted monkey teeth. J Clin Periodontol 1992;19:652.
46. Jansson L, Ehnevid J, Lindskog SF, Blomlöf LB. Radiographic attachment in periodontitis-prone teeth with endodontic infection. J Periodontol 1993;64:947.
47. Jansson L, Ehnevid H, Lindskog S, Blomlöf L. The influence of endodontic infection on progression of marginal bone loss in periodontitis. J Clin Periodontol 1995;22:729.
48. Jansson L, Ehnevid H. The influence of endodontic infection on periodontal status in mandibular molars. J Periodontol 1998;69:1392.
49. Miyashita H, Bergenholtz G, Gröndahl K. Impact of endodontic conditions on marginal bone loss. J Periodontol 1998;69:158.
50. Kakehashi S, Stanley HR, Fitzgerald RJ. The effects of surgical exposures of dental pulps in germ-free and conventional laboratory rats. Oral Surg Oral Med Oral Pathol Oral Radiol Endod 1965;18:340.
51. Korzen BH, Krakow AA, Green DB. Pulpal and periapical tissue responses in conventional and monoinfected gnotobiotic rats. Oral Surg Oral Med Oral Pathol Oral Radiol Endod 1974;37:783.
52. Möller AJ, Fabricius L, Dahlén G, et al. Influence on periapical tissues of indigenous oral bacteria and necrotic pulp tissue in monkeys. Scand J Dent Res 1981;89:475.
53. Ranta K, Haapasalo M, Ranta H. Monoinfection of root canals with Pseudomonas aeruginosa. Endod Dent Traumatol 1988;4:269.
54. Fouad AF, Walton RE, Rittman BR. Induced periapical lesions in ferret canines: histologic and radiographic evaluation. Endod Dent Traumatol 1992;8:56.
55. Van Winkelhoff AJ, Boutaga K. Transmission of periodontal bacteria and models of infection. J Clin Periodontol 2005l;32(Suppl 6):16.
56. Curtis MA, Slaney JM, Aduse-Opoku J. Critical pathways in microbial virulence. J Clin Periodont 2005;32 (Suppl 6):28.
57. Vitkov L, Krautgartner WD, Hannig M. Bacterial internalization in periodontitis. Oral Microbiol Immunol 2005;20:317.
58. Fabricius L, Dahlen G, Ohman A, Möller A. Predominant indigenous oral bacteria isolated from infected root canals after varied times of closure. Scand J Dent Res 1982;90:134.
59. Sundqvist G. Ecology of the root canal flora. J Endod 1992;18:427.
60. Rupf S, Kannengiesser S, Merte K, et al. Comparison of profiles of key periodontal pathogens in the periodontium and endodontium. Endod Dent Traumatol 2000;16:269.
61. Choi BK, Paster BJ, Dewhirst FE, Gobel UB. Diversity of cultivable and uncultivable oral spirochetes from a patient with severe destructive periodontitis. Infect Immun 1889, 1994;62.
62. Dewhirst FE, Tamer MA, Ericson RE, et al. The diversity of periodontal spirochetes by 16S rRNA analysis. Oral Microbiol Immunol 2000;15:196.
63. Kasuga Y, Ishihara K, Okuda K. Significance of detection of *Porphyromonas gingivalis*, *Bacteroides forsythus* and *Treponema denticola* in periodontal pockets. Bull Tokyo Dent Coll 2000;41:109.
64. Molven O, Olsen I, Kerekes K. Scanning electron microscopy of bacteria in the apical part of root canals in permanent teeth with periapical lesions. Endod Dent Traumatol 1991;7:226.
65. Dahle UR, Tronstad L, Olsen I. Observation of an unusually large spirochete in endodontic infection. Oral Microbiol Immunol 1993;8:251.
66. Siqueira JF Jr, Rocas IN, Souto R, et al. Checkboard DNA-DNA hybridization analysis of endodontic infections. Oral Surg Oral Med Oral Pathol Oral Radiol Endod 2000;89:744.
67. Rocas IN, Siqueira JF Jr, Santos KR, Coelho AM. "Red complex" *Bacteroides forsythus*, *Porphyromonas gingivalis*, and *Treponema denticola* in endodontic infections: a

68. Jung IY, Choi BK, Kum KY, et al. Identification of oral spirochetes at the species level and their association with other bacteria in endodontic infections. Oral Surg Oral Med Oral Pathol Oral Radiol Endod 2001;92:329.
69. Simon JHS, Hemple PL, Rotstein I, Salter PK. The possible role of L-form bacteria in periapical disease. Endodontology 1999;11:40.
70. Waltimo T, Haapasalo M, Zehnder M, Meyer J. Clinical aspects related to endodontic yeast infections. Endod Topics 2005;8:1.
71. Wilson MI, Hall J. Incidence of yeasts in root canals. J Brit Endod Soc 1968;2:56.
72. Sen BH, Piskin B, Demirci T. Observations of bacteria and fungi in infected root canals and dentinal tubules by SEM. Endod Dent Traumatol 1995;11:6.
73. Nair PNR, Sjogren U, Krey G, et al. Intraradicular bacteria and fungi in root-filled, asymptomatic human teeth with therapy resistant periapical lesions: a long term light and electron microscopic follow-up study. J Endod 1990;16:580.
74. Molander A, Reit C, Dahlen G, Kvist T. Microbiological status of root filled teeth with apical periodontitis. Int Endod J 1998;31:1.
75. Sundqvist G, Figdor D, Persson S, Sjogren U. Microbiologic analysis of teeth with failed endodontic treatment and the outcome of conservative re-treatment. Oral Surg Oral Med Oral Pathol Oral Radiol Endod 1998;85:86.
76. Peciuliene V, Reynaud AH, Balciuniene I, Haapasalo M. Isolation of yeasts and enteric bacteria in root-filled teeth with chronic apical periodontitis. Int Endod J 2001;34:429.
77. Lomicali G, Sen BH, Camkaya H. Scanning electron microscopic observations of apical root surfaces of teeth with apical periodontitis. Endod Dent Traumatol 1996;12:70.
78. Tronstad L, Barnett F, Riso K, Slots J. Extraradicular endodontic infections. Endod Dent Traumatol 1987;3:86.
79. Waltimo TM, Siren EK, Torkko HL, et al. Fungi in therapy-resistant apical periodontitis. Int Endod J 1997;30:96.
80. Baumgartner JC, Watts CM, Xia T. Occurrence of *Candida albicans* in infections of endodontic origin. J Endod 2000;26:695.
81. Peterson K, Soderstrom C, Kiani-Anaraki M, Levy G. Evaluation of the ability of thermal and electrical tests to register pulp vitality. Endod Dent Traumatol 1999;15:127.
82. Siren EK, Haapasalo MPP, Ranta K, et al. Microbiological findings and clinical treatment procedures in endodontic cases selected for microbiological investigation. Int Endod J 1997;30:91.
83. Slots J, Rams TE, Listgarten MA. Yeasts, enteric rods and pseudomonas in the subgingival flora of severe adult periodontitis. Oral Microbiol Immunol 1988;3:47.
84. Dahlen G, Wikstrom M. Occurrence of enteric rods, staphylococci and Candida in subgingival samples. Oral Microbiol Immunol 1995;10:42.
85. Hannula J, Saarela M, Alaluusua S, et al. Phenotypic and genotypic characterization of oral yeasts from Finland and the United States. Oral Microbiol Immunnol 1997;12:358.
86. Contreras A, Nowzari H, Slots J. Herpesviruses in periodontal pocket and gingival tissue specimens. Oral Microbiol Immunol 2000;15:15.
87. Contreras A, Umeda M, Chen C, et al. Relationship between herpesviruses and adult periodontitis and perioodontopathic bacteria. J Periodontol 1999;70:478.
88. Sabeti M, Simon JH, Nowzari H, Slots J. Cytomegalovirus and Epstein-Barr virus active infection in periapical lesions of teeth with intact crowns. J Endod 2003;29:321.
89. Contreras A, Slots J. Herpesvirus in human periodontal disease. J Periodontol Res 2000;35:3.
90. Marton LJ, Kiss C. Protective and destructive immune reactions in apical periodontitis. Oral Microbiol Immunol 2000;15:139.
91. Nair PNR. New perspectives on radicular cysts: do they heal? Int Endod J 1998;31:155.
92. Browne RM. The origin of cholesterol in odontogenic cysts in man. Arch Oral Biol 1971;16:107.
93. Nair PNR, Sjogren U, Schumacher E, Sundqvist G. Radicular cyst affecting a root filled human tooth: a long-term post treatment follow-up. Int Endod J 1993;26:225.
94. Cotran SR, Kumar V, Collins T. In. Robbins pathologic basis of disease. 6th ed. Philadelphia:WB Saunders;1999, pp. 40–1.
95. Allison RT. Electron microscopic study of "Rushton" hyaline bodies in cyst linings. Br Dent J 1974;137:102.
96. Ackerman SJ, Corrette SE, Rosenberg HF, et al. Molecular cloning and characterization of human eosinophils Charcot-Leyden crystal protein (lysophospholipase). J Immunol 1993;150:456.
97. Lao LM, Kumakiri M, Nakagawa K, et al. The ultrastructural findings of Charcot-Leyden crystals in stroma of mastocytoma. J Dermatol Sci 1998;17:198.
98. Dvorak AM, Weller PF, Monahan-Earley RA, et al. Ultrastructural localization of Charcot-Leyden crystal protein (lysophospholipase) and peroxidase in macrophages, eosinophils, and extracellular matrix of the skin in the hypereosinophilic syndrome. Lab Invest 1990;62:590.
99. Lazarski MP, Walker WA, Flores CM, et al. Epidemiological evaluation of the outcomes of nonsurgical root canal treatment in a large cohort of insured dental patients. J Endod 2001;27:791.
100. Salehrabi R, Rotstein I. Endodontic treatment outcomes in a large patient population in the USA: an epidemiologic study. J Endod 2004;30:846.

101. Rotstein I, Salehrabi R, Forrest JL. Endodontic treatment outcome: survey of oral health care professionals. J Endod 2006;32:399.
102. Saunders WP, Saunders EM. Coronal leakage as a cause of failure in root canal therapy: a review. Endod Dent Traumatol 1994;10:105.
103. Ray HA, Trope M. Periapical status of endodontically treated teeth in relation to the technical quality of the root filling and the coronal restoration. Int Endod J 1995;28:12.
104. Saunders WP, Saunders EM. Assessment of leakage in the restored pulp chamber of endodontically treated multi-rooted teeth. Int Endod J 1990;23:28.
105. Bakland LK, Andreasen FM, Andreasen JO. Management of traumatized teeth. In: Walton RE, Torabinejad T, Principles and practice of endodontics. 3rd ed. Philadelphia:WB Saunders, 2002; p. 445.
106. Tronstad L. Root resorption: etiology, terminology and clinical manifestations. Endod Dent Traumatol 1988;4:241.
107. Magnusson I, Claffey N, Bogle G, et al. Root resertption following periodontal flap procedures in monkeys. J Periodont Res 1985;20:79.
108. Karring T, Nyman S, Lindhe J, Sirirat M. Potentials for root resorption during periodontal wound healing. J Clin Periodont 1984;11:41.
109. Andreasen JO. Periodontal healing after replantation of traumatically avulsed human teeth. Assessment by mobility testing and radiography. Acta Odont Scand 1975;33:325.
110. Heithersay GS. Clinical, radiographic, and histopathologic features of invasive cervical resorption. Quint Int 1999;30:27.
111. Heithersay GS. Invasive cervical root resorption: An analysis of potential predisposing factors. Quint Int 1999;30:83.
112. Delzangles B. Apical periodontitis and resorption of the root canal wall. Endod Dent Traumatol 1988;4:273.
113. Wedenberg C, Lindskog S. Experimental internal resorption in monkey teeth. Endod Dent Traumatol 1985;1:221.
114. Torabinejad M, Lemon RL. Procedural accidents. In: Walton RE, Torabinejad M: Principles and practice of endodontics. 2nd Ed. Philadelphia:W.B. Saunders;1996, p. 306.
115. Simon JHS. Root extrusion- rationale and techniques. Dent Clin North Am 1984;28:909.
116. Stevens BH, Levine RA. Forced eruption: a multidisciplinary approach for form, function, and biologic predictability. Compendium 1998;19:994.
117. Emerich-Poplatek K, Sawicki L, Bodal M, Adamowitz-Klepalska B. Forced eruption after crown/root fracture with a simple and aesthetic method using the fractured crown. Dent Traumatol 2005;21:165.
118. Simon JHS, Lythgoe JB, Torabinejad M. Clinical and histological evaluation of extruded endodonticall treated teeth in dogs. Oral Surg Oral Med Oral Pathol Oral Radiol Endod 1980;50:361.
119. Al-Hezaimi K, Naghshbandi J, Simon JHS, et al. Successful treatment of a radicular groove by intentional replantation and Emdogain therapy. Dent Traumatol 2004;20:226.
120. Rotstein I, Simon JHS. Diagnosis, prognosis and decision-making in the treatment of combined periodontal-endodontic lesions. Periodontol 2000–2004;34:165.
121. Kipioti A. Nakou M, Legakis N, Mitsis F. Microbiological finding of infected root canals and adjacent periodontal pockets in teeth with advanced periodontitis. Oral Surg Oral Med Oral Pathol Oral Radiol Endod 1984;58:213.
122. Kobayashi T, Hayashi A, Yoshikawa R, et al. The microbial flora from root canals and periodontal pockets of nonvital teeth associated with advanced periodontitis. Int Endod J 1990;23:100.
123. Simon JHS, Glick DH, Frank AL. The relationship of endodontic-periodontic lesions. J Periodontol 1972;43:202.
124. Chapple I, Lumley P. The periodontal–endodontic interface. Dent Update 1999;26:331.
125. Blomlöf LB, Lindskog S, Hammarstrom L.Influence of pulpal treatments on cell and tissue reactions in the marginal periodontium. J Periodontol 1988;59:577.

CHAPTER 19

TOOTH INFRACTIONS

LEIF K. BAKLAND

Tooth fractures include trauma-related crown, crown–root, and root fractures (see Chapter 36) and a broad group of cracked teeth. The latter is divided into five categories by the American Association of Endodontists (AAE)[1]: *Craze lines*—confined to enamel (Figure 1A,B); *cuspal fracture*—usually diagonal fractures that do not involve the pulp directly (Figure 2A,B); *cracked teeth*—incomplete vertical fractures, often involving the pulp (Figure 3A,B); *split tooth*—complete vertical fractures (Figure 4); and vertical root fractures (VRFs)—longitudinal complete fractures, usually of endodontically treated teeth (Figure 5). This is a fairly representative classification of cracked teeth and will be used in the descriptions to follow.

The term "cracked tooth" is one of many used for this condition. Others include *cuspal fracture odontalgia*,[2] *incomplete tooth fracture*,[3] *cracked tooth syndrome*,[4] *green stick fracture*,[5] *split root syndrome*,[6] *hairline fracture*,[7] and *tooth infraction*.[8]

The number of terms used to show the confusion about this complex situation of tooth fractures is estimated to be responsible for about one-third of the loss of molars and premolars.[9] A review of the rather extensive available literature points to the presence of two main categories: (1) *tooth infraction* and (2) *vertical root fracture* (VRF).

Tooth infraction can be defined as an incomplete tooth fracture extending partially through a tooth. It

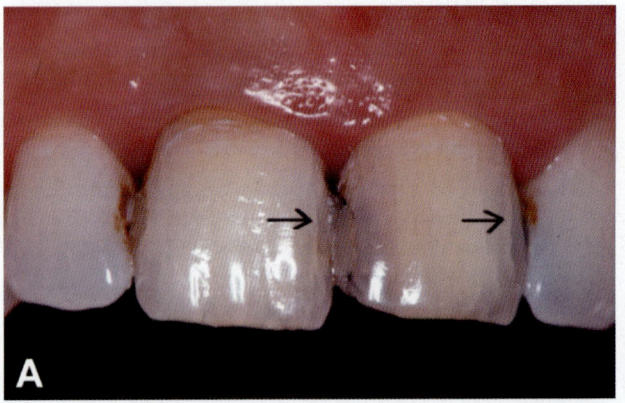
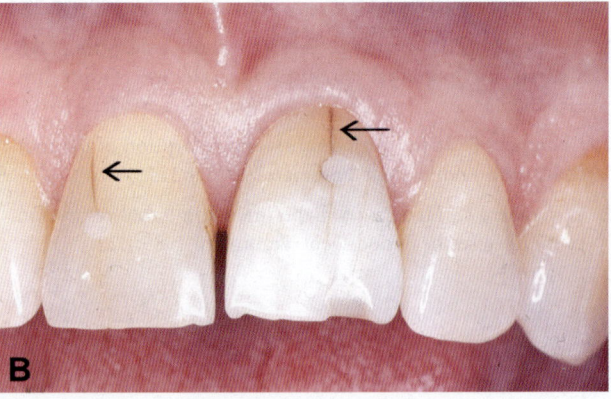

Figure 1 *A,* Multiple craze lines are common in teeth (arrows). *B,* When an enamel fracture line becomes larger, organic debris will fill the crack and discolor (arrow).

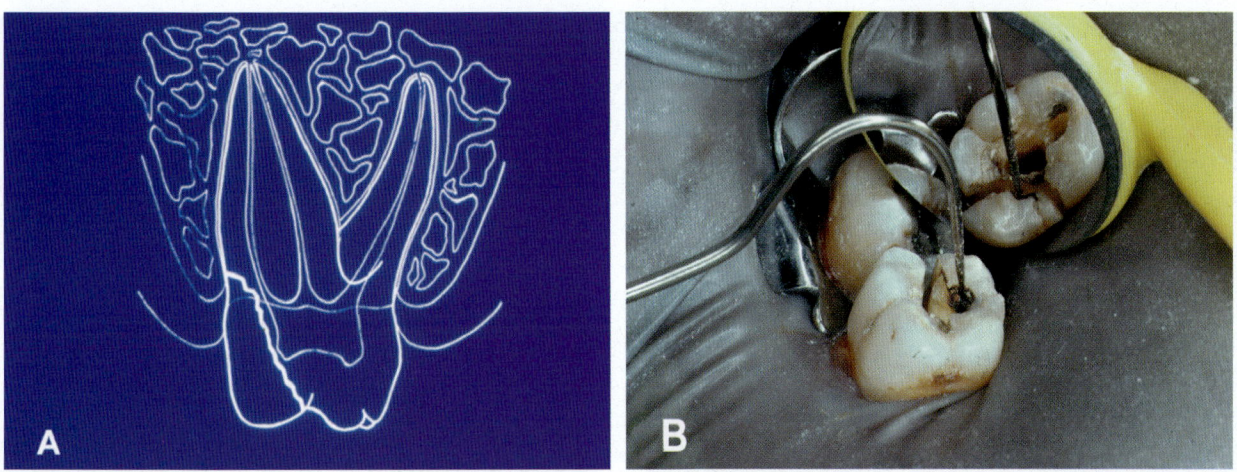

Figure 2 ***A,*** Graphical illustration of cuspal fracture. ***B,*** Clinical example of cuspal fracture; these often do not communicate directly with the pulp.

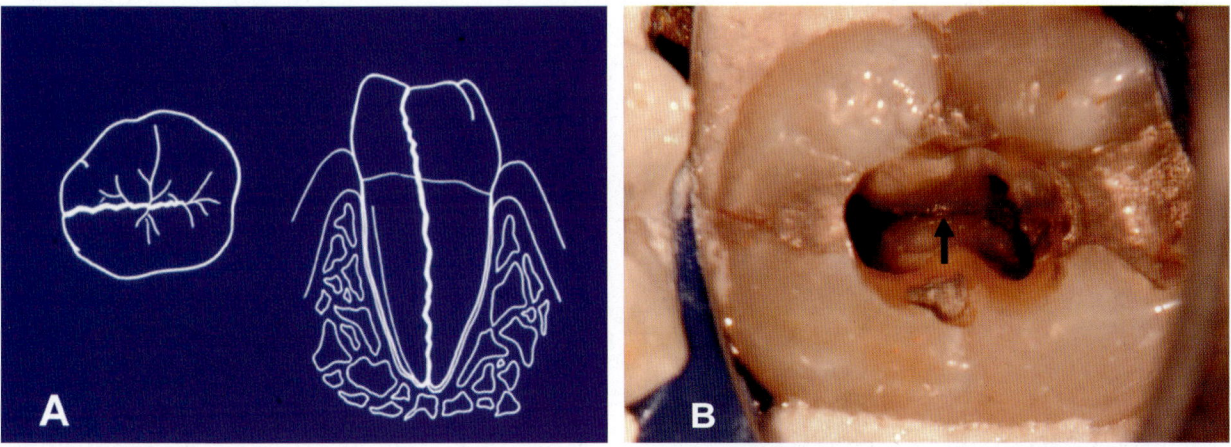

Figure 3 ***A,*** Graphical illustration of an infraction located centrally and which is likely to communicate with the pulp; it also typically runs in a mesiodistal direction and involves one or both marginal ridges. ***B,*** Clinical example of fracture line that extends to the floor of the chamber (arrow). Note mesiodistal direction of the fracture.

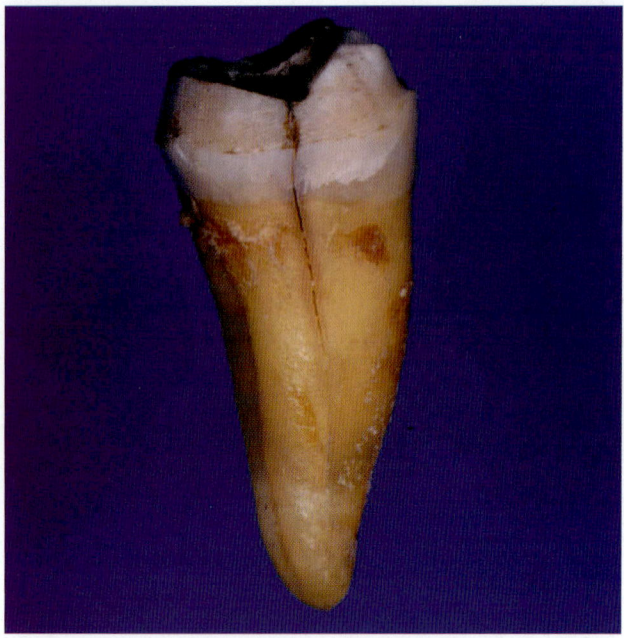

Figure 4 Example of a split tooth, a vertical fracture not involving an endodontically treated tooth.

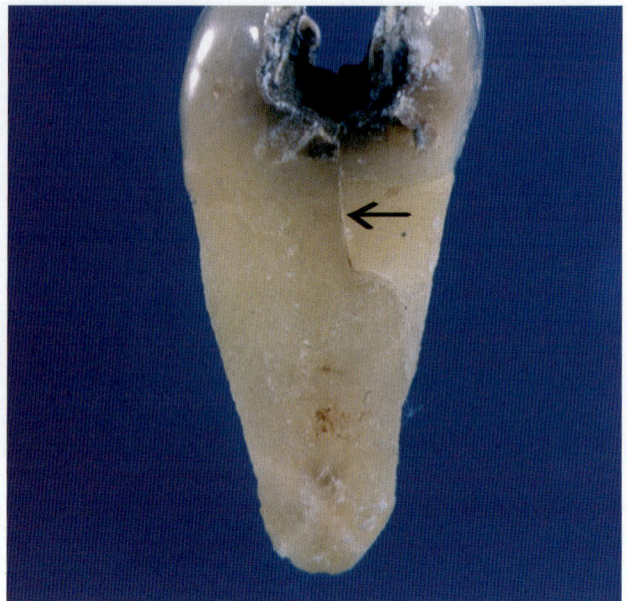

Figure 6 Extracted tooth shows tooth infraction (arrow), having started in the crown and propagating apically.

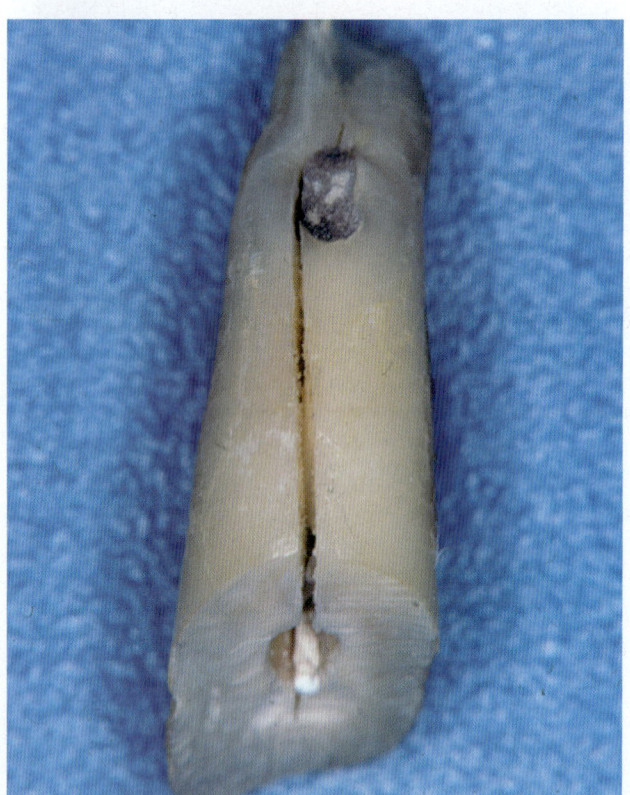

Figure 5 Vertical root fracture (VRF) of an endodontically treated tooth.

is an accurate description that matches the use of the term 'infraction' in other medical situations.[10] Tooth infraction can be further described as originating in the tooth crown, originating from the pulp toward the dentinoenamel junction, and propagating apically in the root[11–13] (Figure 6).

Tooth infractions can be identified as three fairly distinct types: (1) those confined to enamel ("craze lines") and usually do not require treatment, (2) those related to cuspal fracture that typically do not involve the pulp, and (3) those more centrally located that do involve the pulp. Diagnosis, treatment, and prognosis are different for the latter two types and will be described.

Vertical root fractures are longitudinal fractures that originate in the roots of teeth, in contrast to tooth infractions that originate in the crowns.[14,15] With few exceptions,[14,15] these fractures occur almost exclusively in endodontically treated teeth.

In summary, there are two main groups of cracked teeth: (1) tooth infractions, including craze lines, cuspal fractures, and cracked teeth; and (2) VRFs that occur in endodontically treated teeth. The latter will be discussed in Chapter 20 "Vertical Root Fractures of Endodontically Treated Teeth".

Characteristics of Tooth Infractions

PROBLEMS IN DIAGNOSIS

Gibbs[2] was one of the first to describe the problem of pain during mastication that was unrelated to caries or infected teeth. He noted cracks associated with cusps in posterior teeth and termed the condition "cuspal fracture odontalgia." He pointed out the problem in identifying the involved tooth, a situation also described by Ritchey et al.[3] as a vague discomfort during mastication and often associated with elevated sensitivity to cold. They suspected the likelihood of incomplete tooth fractures.

Clinically, symptomatic tooth infractions are confusing because they often mimic symptoms from other conditions such as earache, sinusitis, temporomandibular joint dysfunction, and even trigeminal neuralgia and other neurological pain conditions.[4,7,8,16] When the problem is difficult to identify, it can lead to a long-standing pain condition that becomes more diffuse and makes localization of the offending tooth very difficult.[8,13] Many reported cases of problematic infraction diagnosis are usually long-standing, from months to many years.[8,17]

Because infractions typically originate internally and extend peripherally,[13] a tooth with infraction is not likely to be identified by percussion until the fracture extends to involve the periodontal ligament (PDL).[18] Further, since most infractions are situated in a mesiodistal direction, radiographs are not very diagnostic.[13] Also, it can be challenging to differentiate between masticatory pain from infractions and similar pain from microleakage associated with restorations.[12] Finally, without magnification, infractions are not readily visualized, unless they are at least 20 μm.[7] Fortunately, most instances of tooth infractions can readily be diagnosed using various diagnostic aids, to be described later.

DISTRIBUTION

The incidence of tooth infractions is not extensively reported. Two studies[16,19] indicate that 2% to 3% of dental patients have infractions in their molars and premolars; most are asymptomatic, so the incidence of symptomatic teeth may be less than 1%. The low incidence may contribute to the difficulty many dentists seem to have in identifying this condition.

Molars and premolars appear to be the teeth almost exclusively involved.[4,8,17,19–21] The location of fractures occurs overwhelmingly in the mesiodistal direction, with only a few in the buccolingual direction, and some in a combination of both.[4,8,12,17,20] Brynjulfsen et al.[8] noted that 10% of the infractions were centrally located, meaning pulpal involvement. It is interesting that in their study, in maxillary teeth, the majority (70%) of fracture lines were toward the buccal tooth surface, while in the mandibular teeth they were toward the lingual, also at 70%.

Many reports appear to point to mandibular teeth, in particular the second molar as being most frequently involved,[4,14,17] but other studies identify maxillary molars more frequently.[8,21] Both of the latter studies involved specific groups of patients: the first, a group of patients that had long histories of undiagnosed infractions and the second group, exclusively Korean. How much such factors influence incidence is not entirely clear.

In the rare case, when an infracted anterior tooth is involved, it is probably the result of a sudden traumatic blow to the tooth. Makkes and Folmer[22] described a situation in which a central incisor suffered a luxation injury when the patient was very young. The immature root fractured vertically, but the fracture was not detected until years later because the split was not visible on radiographs.

The question has been raised about which tooth is more likely to fracture—one with or without a restoration? As with other aspects of tooth infraction, the available evidence is not conclusive. Most investigators agree that teeth with restorations are more likely to develop infractions,[12,13,16,19,23–26] but there are also reports about non-restored teeth with infractions.[20,21] Hiatt,[20] however, selectively chose teeth with no proximal restorations, and Roh and Lee[21] studied a group of elderly Korean patients in which the majority of teeth were non-restored. They speculated that diet and racial anatomical characteristics as well as restorative procedures contribute to the development of infractions.

When looking at the total picture of cracked teeth—infractions and VRFs—it appears that clinicians encounter VRFs more often than infractions.[15,27] But because of the rather minimal epidemiological evidence, one cannot be certain about which type of fracture is more common.

PAIN CHARACTERISTICS

Pain is generally a complaint that draws patients' attention to problem teeth. This is also true with respect to tooth infractions.[2–5,8,9,12,13,20,28–31] All of the authors cited pointed out that pain to chewing is the most common finding in symptomatic tooth infractions.

Brännström[30] has proposed that the masticatory pain is due to sudden movement of dentinal fluid when the fractured tooth portions move independently, activating myelinated A-δ fibers in the pulp and creating a rapid, acute pain response. Stimulation of the A-δ fibers does not require inflammation of pulp tissue, which explains why chewing discomfort occurs in the very early stages of infraction and appears to be a symptom common to all infractions, both cuspal infractions and those involving the pulp. Sutton[5] also suggested that the occasional sharp, momentary lancinating masticatory pain was due to bending and rubbing of dentin along fracture lines.

A unique pain response to chewing experienced by many patients is the pain that occurs when they release the pressure of biting, variously referred to as "rebound" or "relief" pain.[9,12,13] This response can be duplicated diagnostically by having the patient bite on a moist cotton roll and if "rebound" pain occurs on release, it is very likely that one of the two teeth, maxillary or mandibular, has an infraction[12] (Figure 7).

Pain that is stimulated by temperature changes, particularly with application of cold stimuli, is also a common feature of teeth with infractions, but less common than chewing discomfort.[3,4,12,13,17,18,20,29,30]

Ritchey et al.[3] noted an elevated response to cold, a condition attributed to pulpal inflammation caused by the infractions communicating with the pulp and likely containing bacteria[13,18,29,30] (Figure 8). Brännström[30] proposed that the inflammation sensitizes the pulpal C-fiber receptors that respond to temperature changes. While hot stimuli are not often mentioned as producing symptoms, they no doubt can cause pain, particularly as pulpal inflammation increases, making C-fiber receptors more sensitive and lowering threshold levels to both cold and hot stimuli.

One would think that teeth, painful due to masticatory forces, would be uniformly hypersensitive to percussion stimuli. This does not appear to be the case in tooth infarctions.[21] Swepston and Miller[31] have suggested that sensitivity to percussion occurs when the pulp becomes involved, which is not always the case in tooth infractions, at least not initially. Rosen[18] pointed out that until the infraction has propagated all the way from the pulp to the PDL, localization of an infracted tooth by percussion is very difficult. Thus, in cases of cuspal infractions in which the pulp is not directly involved, percussion may not produce a painful response.

It is well known that teeth with infarctions are associated with unusual pain conditions.[3,4,7,8,13,18] Ritchey et al.[3] described the patients' chief complaint as vague discomfort to mastication, and Cameron[4]

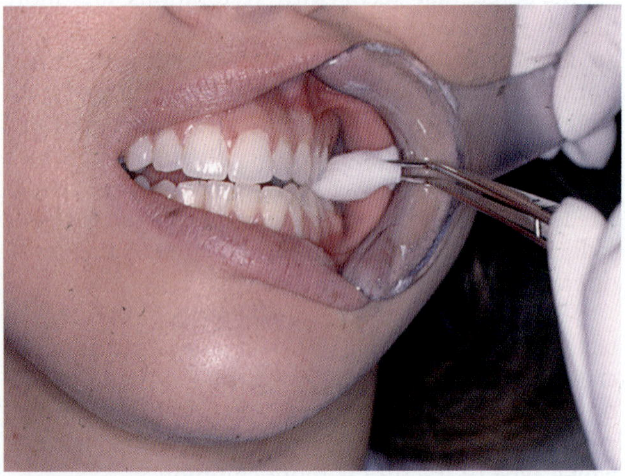

Figure 7 Clinical test for detecting tooth infraction. The patient bites on a moist cotton roll and on release, pain will often be quite noticeable ("rebound" or "relief" pain).

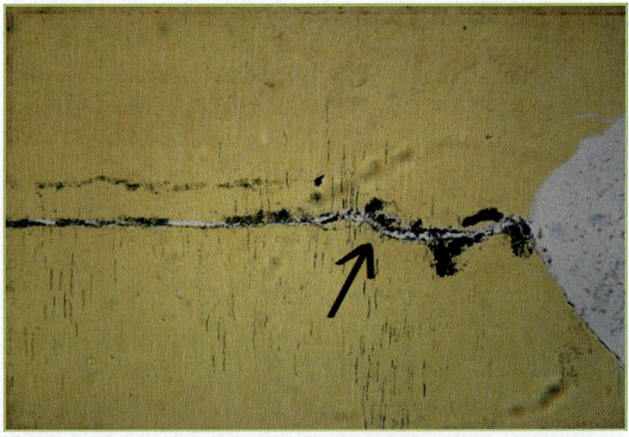

Figure 8 Infraction (arrow) in tooth extending from the pulp and filled with bacteria. Courtesy of Dr. H. Trowbridge.

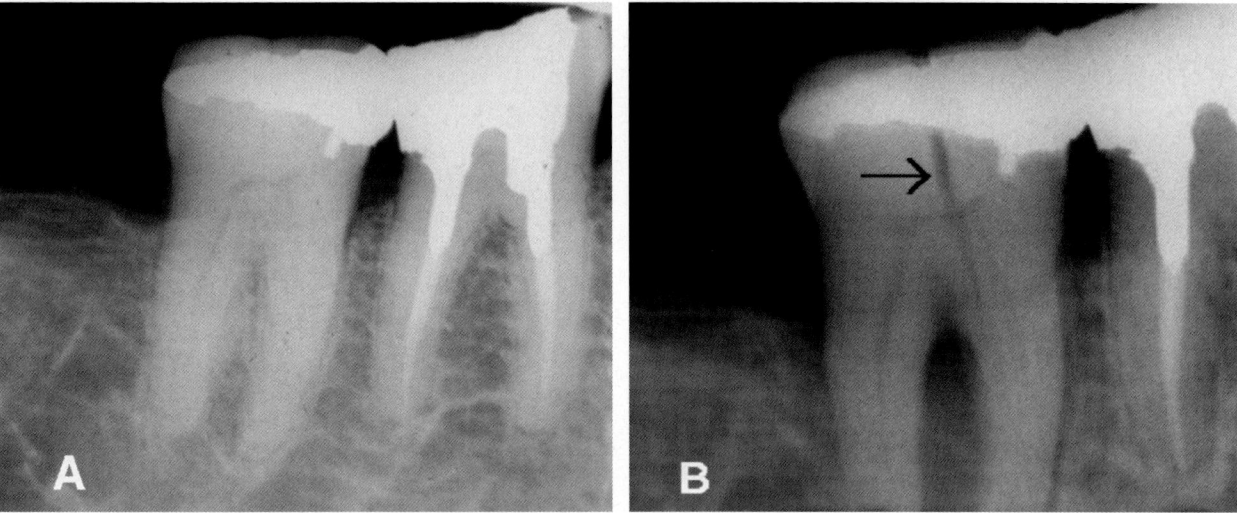

Figure 9 A 78-year-old patient mistakenly diagnosed with trigeminal neuralgia. *A,* Patient was referred from neurology service for dental evaluation for complaint related to typical symptoms of neuralgia: excruciating, lancinating pain to touch (mandibular right side). Initial dental examination revealed no dental pathosis. *B,* Four months later, the patient returned with a "sore tooth." The initial symptoms had subsided within a few days and he had taken only one carbamazepine (Tegretol) tablet. In retrospect, it was most likely that the initial symptoms he had were related to tooth infraction (arrow) that was not evident on the first examination.

observed that in addition to being vague, the pain complaint could mimic other conditions, such as trigeminal neuralgia (Figure 9A,B). This was also reported by Caufield.[7] Further confounding pain description in tooth infraction is that the resultant pulpal inflammation tends to refer pain responses to other areas served by the fifth cranial nerve[18] with the result that pain can be experienced in other noninvolved teeth, and adjacent anatomical locations. Both Kahler et al.[13] and Brynjulfsen et al.[8] have made a point of the fact that tooth infraction pain is associated with protracted histories of pain. The latter reported a range of 3 months to 11 years in a group of 32 patients with undiagnosed long-standing orofacial pain from tooth infraction. They indicated that such protracted histories could lead to development of chronic orofacial pain with hyperalgesia. Another observation by Brynjulfsen et al.[8] was that in some cases the symptoms of pain were not provoked by chewing or application of cold stimuli, but rather were spontaneous pain experiences involving diffuse orofacial areas. Often, the pain would be felt anterior to the tooth responsible for the symptom when not referred to an anatomical area apart from teeth. The pattern of pain referral noted by Brynjulfsen et al.[8] was that pain from mandibular teeth was frequently distributed to maxillary teeth, the neck, ear, muscles of mastication, and temporomandibular joint (TMJ). Pain from maxillary teeth seldom projected to the mandible. An important observation was that the longer the duration of pain, the more diffuse it became and often led to headaches.

Pain response to sweets has been reported;[13,20,26,28] likely the response is from pulps that have become inflamed due to exposure to infractions with bacteria present. While pain responses in teeth with infractions can mimic many other conditions, such as cariously affected teeth, it is prudent to maintain a high degree of suspicion when symptoms and examination findings do not match.

ETIOLOGY

Considering that restored teeth are more often associated with infractions than non-restored teeth,[12,13,16,19,23–26] it would not be surprising that investigators have looked at a number of restorative factors for clues to the etiology of tooth infractions. In fact several aspects of restorative dentistry have been identified as potential culprits. Most often mentioned are excessively large and incorrectly designed restorations.[12,16,18,23–25,32] Another contributing factor has been the use of pins for supporting large restorations, especially self-threading and friction-lock pins[18,23,32–34] (Figure 10).

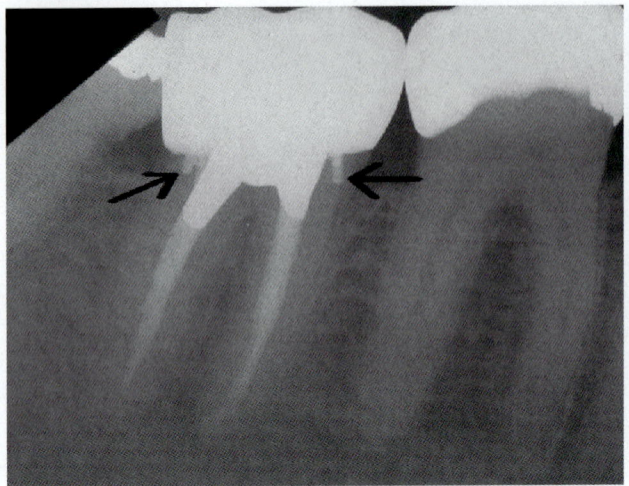

Figure 10 The use of pins for coronal buildup can be detrimental if the friction-grip or self-locking types are used (arrows). This tooth had developed infractions, but it was difficult to determine if they were connected with the pin placements.

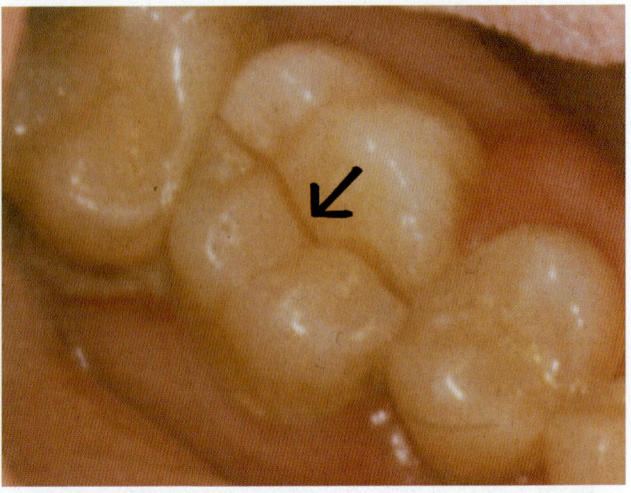

Figure 11 Vertical fracture (arrow) of the crown, running mesiodistally and resulting from traumatic injury.

Abrasion, erosion, and caries may also contribute to the development of infractions,[25] along with age changes in dentin,[12] oral habits,[12,18] and thermal cycling.[35,36] The latter is suspected of initiating infractions near the dentin–enamel junction and leading to breakdown of the dentin–enamel bond. Resisting these damaging forces is the dentin's collagenous structure that prevents fractures from forming and propagating. As the dentin loses the ability for plastic deformation, it becomes more inclined to develop infractions, evidenced by the increase in infractions with age.[13]

In addition to cavity designs and size, the act of preparing a tooth for restoration can also be hazardous. It is suspected that the use of both high-speed handpieces[34] and course diamond burs[37] can lead to infractions. When course diamond burs are used, subsurface cracks develop from enamel into dentin. It is not clear if such infractions are more likely to progress further than the frequently observed enamel infractions. These craze lines can range from 1 to 20 μm in size and are usually filled with an organic material that appears to stain quite readily[36] (see Figure 1B).

The act of chewing is also implicated in the development of infractions.[9,13–15,18,20,21,26,32] Masticatory forces from repeated occlusal loads and perhaps certain types of foods can contribute to this problem.[9,13–15,21,26,32] Certainly, accidental biting on hard objects, such as bird shots and hard candy, has resulted in tooth infraction and VRFs[9,18] (Figure 11), and bruxism and clenching often combined with a wedging effect of cusps in opposing fossae can be stressful on teeth.[14,15,20,21] Considering a biting force of up to 90 kg on first molars,[26] it is obvious that these teeth are subjected to extensive stress. Yeh[14] coined the term "fatigue root fracture" to describe the stress on teeth that can be very damaging when combined with a course diet.

Acute trauma to teeth is also responsible for tooth infractions,[18] and Makkes and Folmer[22] described a situation in which an injury to a central incisor in a child resulted in a VRF that was not discovered until years later. Because anterior teeth are subjected to acute trauma more than posterior teeth, trauma is likely to be the etiology of vertical fractures in anterior teeth (Figure 12A,B).

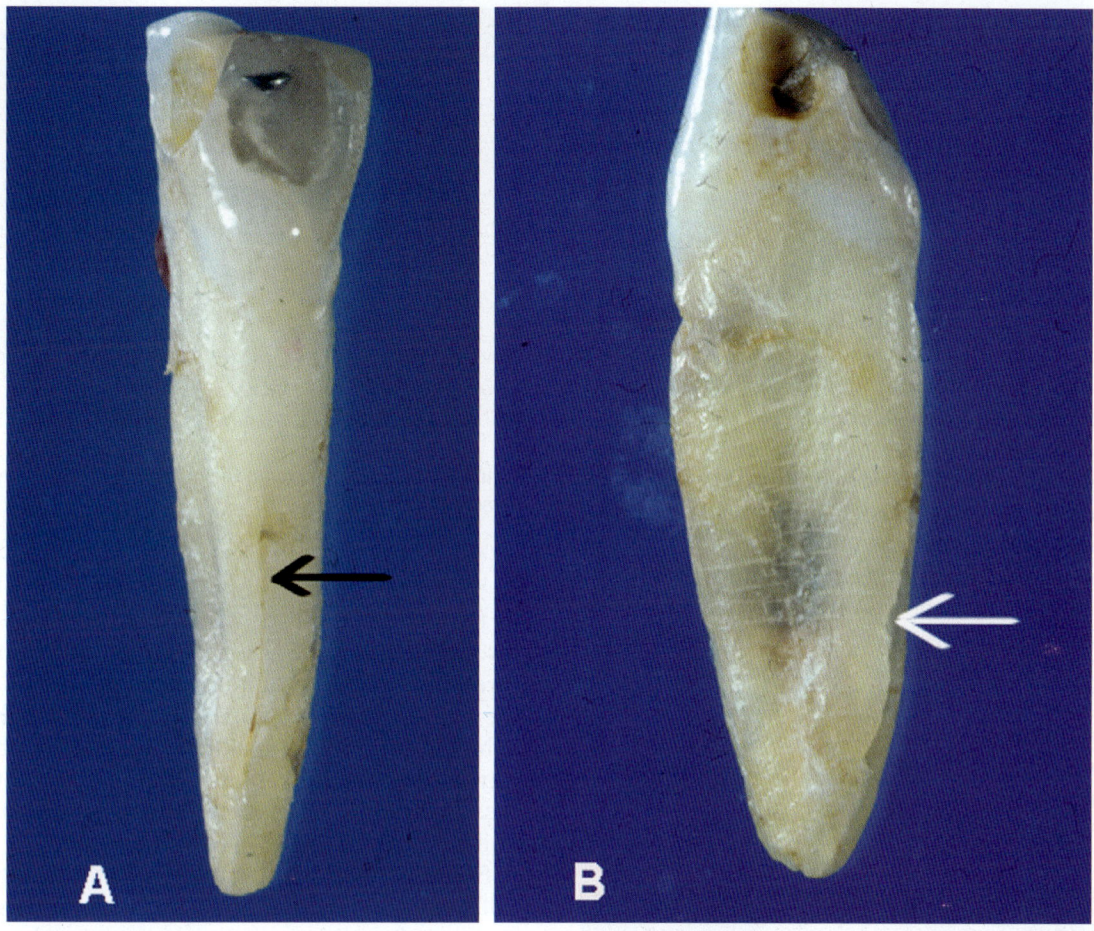

Figure 12 *A*, Traumatic injury to the mandibular incisors resulted in a vertical fracture (arrow). *B*, Another view of small fracture (arrow).

Teeth are subjected to a variety of traumatic and stressful events, many resulting in damage such as infractions and fractures. In contrast to bones where repair of such injuries can readily take place, in dentin and enamel, similar repair following development of fracture lines does not occur.

Diagnosis of Tooth Infractions

Diagnosis of symptomatic tooth infractions is usually quite easily made based on symptoms, clinical and radiographic findings, and history. A suspicion of infraction is raised when symptoms of toothache are not readily connected to evidence of caries, periodontal disease, or recent trauma. If the initial examination fails to provide a definitive diagnosis, it can be difficult to proceed and also becomes more likely that an incorrect diagnosis will be made. Many patients with infracted teeth may suffer symptoms for long periods of time before a correct diagnosis is made.[8,13,17,22] Brynjulfsen et al.[8] pointed out that the longer it takes to make a diagnosis, the more diffuse the pain becomes.

SYMPTOMS

The most common symptoms associated with symptomatic tooth infractions are pain to chewing,[2,4,5,12,13,17,21,26] followed by pain to exposure to cold food,[3,4,12,13,21,26,29] and in some cases to sweets.[13,26,28]

It should be noted that not all teeth with infractions are symptomatic.[19] Symptoms probably develop when infractions involve the pulp, especially when the infractions become populated with bacteria,[13,29,31] and localization may also be possible when infractions reach the PDL, usually starting in the area of the crestal ligament.[18]

The history of a patient's symptoms can be helpful in forming a diagnosis. Diffuse, protracted pain, not associated with more easily diagnosed conditions of caries-induced pulpitis, should at least attract a suspicion of tooth infraction.[8,13,16–18] Considering that symptomatic infractions are in fact not a common dental condition, it is prudent for the careful diagnostician to keep this option as a possibility, when other definitive diagnoses are not applicable.

CLINICAL EXAMINATION

As with other dental diagnoses, making a definitive diagnosis of symptomatic tooth infractions requires obtaining adequate information, both from the patient's history and from clinical examination. It usually begins with a chief complaint of pain to chewing, possibly elevated sensitivity to cold food and sweets. The absence of an obvious carious etiology should trigger a suspicion of a possible infraction and in most cases the following clinical examination procedures should identify teeth with infractions.

Visual examination should reveal many instances of infractions, especially when aided by the use of transillumination[8,12] (Figure 13) and a dye such as methylene blue[8,12,17,38] (Figure 14). The use of transillumination is dependent on the part of the tooth to be examined to be without restoration to allow the light beam to pass through the tooth; when it encounters a fracture line in the dentin, the light beam will bend and not pass through the fracture line and the opposite tooth structure will be dark.[12] Additionally, to aid in visualization, the use of a microscope can be very valuable,[8,12] although magnification alone may not be a predictable way of detecting infractions.[39] But in combination with the application of a dye, infractions become quite visible.[8]

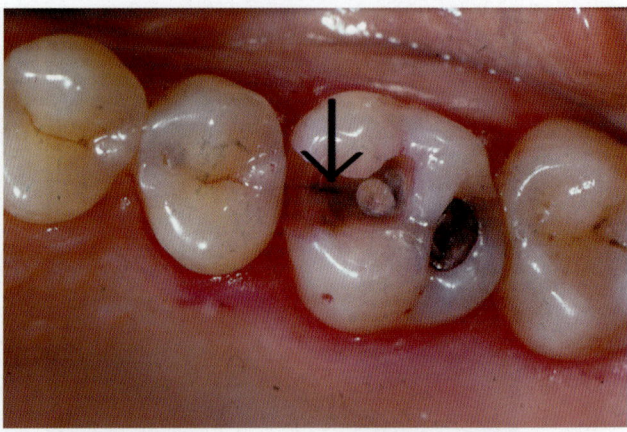

Figure 14 Removal of restoration and highlighting with a dye to detect infraction (arrow).

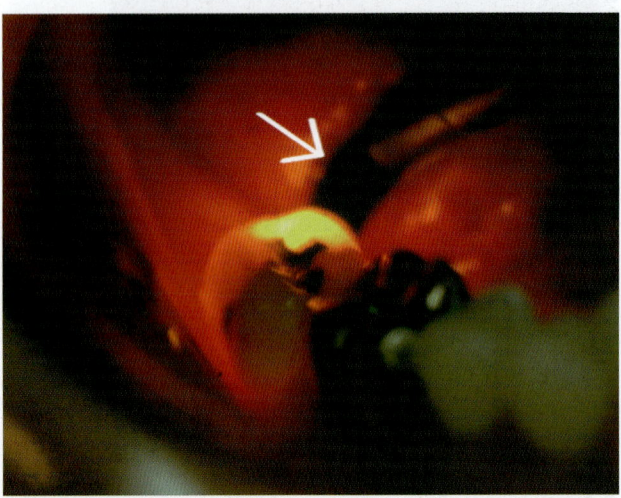

Figure 13 Clinical illustration of the use of fiber optic light source (arrow) to identify an infraction. Note that the light beam does not cross the infraction.

Because existing restorations in a tooth with infractions may hide infractions, it is often necessary to remove the filling materials to reveal infraction lines[8,12] (see Figure 14). This becomes an important step in the clinical examination when the symptoms are vague and the location of pain is diffuse and not localized. Brynjulfsen et al.[8] methodically removed restorations, one tooth at a time, to locate teeth with infractions in patients with long-standing, undiagnosed orofacial pain.

An important step in clinical examinations is the application of a *biting test*. Various techniques have been recommended, such as biting on burlew wheels,[17] rubber wheels,[11] cotton tip applicators,[11] moist cotton rolls[12] (see Figure 7), and commercial biting applicators such as Tooth Slooth (Professional Results Inc., Laguna Nigel, CA) and Fracfinder (Svenoka Dental Instruments, Vasby, Sweden). To differentiate between biting pain from restorations with microleakage and pain from tooth infraction, a Tooth Slooth can be

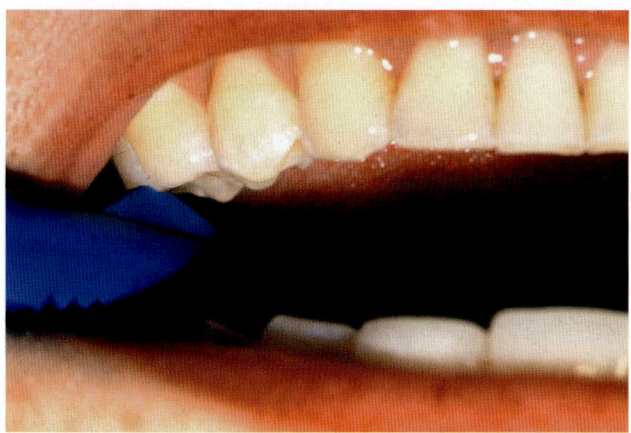

Figure 15 The use of Tooth Slooth to test biting sensitivity to differentiate between pain from infraction and pain from microleakage related to a restoration.

positioned so that pressure is first placed on the filling and then on the tooth cusps[12] (Figure 15).

A very significant response to biting is when pain is experienced on release of biting pressure[9,12,13] and is referred to as either "rebound pain"[13] or "relief pain."[9] Kahler et al.[13] explain the pain associated with the release of pressure as resulting from fluid movement as the crack rapidly closes. For the author, the moist cotton roll has been very effective in stimulating rebound pain, providing a good clue to the tooth in question.

Cold stimulus application and electric pulp testing (EPT) will provide information about the status of the pulp, and there is evidence that teeth with infractions respond at lower threshold levels to cold and EPT stimulation compared to noncracked teeth.[3,29] Since any tooth with pulpal inflammation is likely to have a lowered pain threshold, it is not particularly significant that teeth with infractions also do. But it can add to the total information about the tooth.

Percussion sensitivity in teeth with infractions is not as frequent as biting sensitivity[21] and appears to require pulpal involvement.[31] One could speculate that if the infraction is a cuspal infraction and not directly involving the pulp, percussion may not be as likely to produce a symptomatic response as percussion of teeth with infractions in direct contact with the pulp.

Cameron[17] has suggested the use of a thin sharp *explorer* to probe around the cervical circumference of teeth suspected of having infractions, particularly in interproximal areas not readily visible if the tooth crown has a large or full coverage restoration. Both the "click" of the explorer tip encountering the crack and perhaps the patient's response can provide a clue.

Periodontal probing has been recognized as an indispensable part of clinical dental examinations in general and also when examining teeth with potential infractions.[12,20] Hiatt[20] described the result of probing to be narrow pockets adjacent to fracture lines, and Ailor[12] has suggested that if the probing extends below the alveolar crest, the tooth is not suitable for restoration (Figure 16A,B). Since the pockets adjacent to infractions are extremely narrow—in contrast to those adjacent to

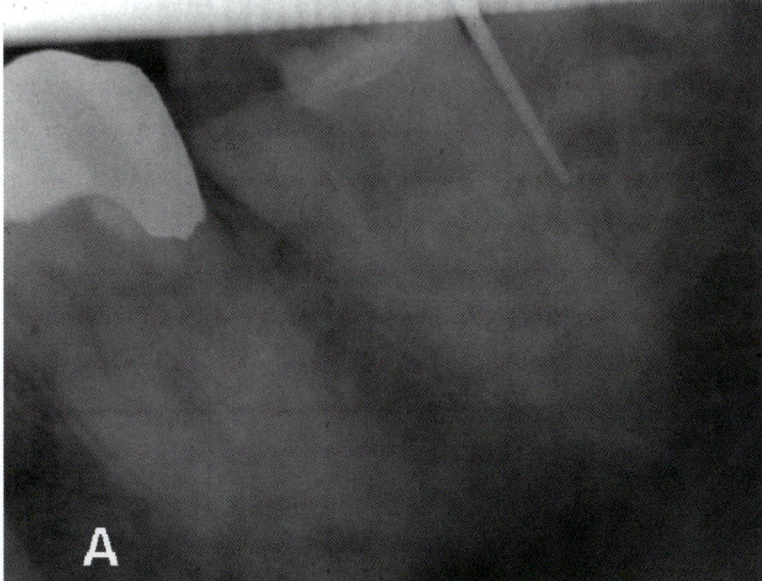
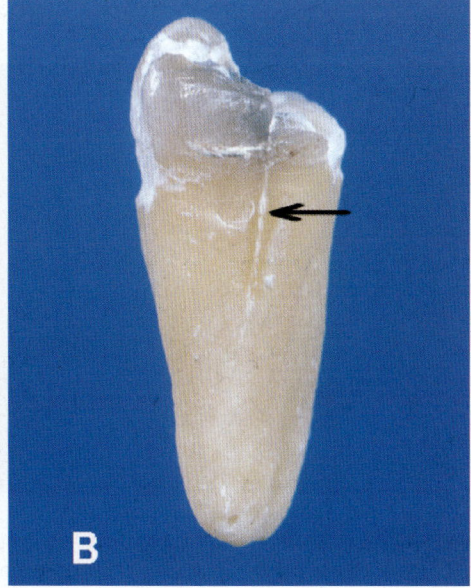

Figure 16 Periodontal probing of a tooth with infraction. Anesthesia is necessary because the pocket is very narrow. *A,* Radiograph shows periodontal probe extending well below the alveolar crest. *B,* Extracted tooth shows infraction (arrow).

VRFs in endodontically treated teeth—it is usually necessary to anesthetize the tissues surrounding the tooth prior to probing.

RADIOGRAPHIC EXAMINATION

It is generally recognized that radiographic examination, while obviously necessary for a number of reasons, does not provide much information with respect to tooth infractions.[8,12,13,40] This is because the infraction lines usually run mesiodistally in the majority of cases[17] and the X-ray beam travels perpendicular to the fracture lines. If, however, the tooth infraction is located in a buccolingual direction, the X-ray beam may produce a clear image of the fracture line on the film or the sensor (Figure 17). If computed tomography technology continues to improve with respect to imaging smaller and smaller entities, one may expect that in the future, infractions in the size of 5 μm may be detectable.[40–42]

One aspect of tooth infractions that can be detected radiographically is the rare instance in which bacteria in the infraction has stimulated clastic activity in the pulp, resulting in internal resorptive lesions.[43] This type of internal resorption is unique in many respects in that it appears to occur adjacent to the pulp space and may be mistaken for invasive external resorption. The presence of an infraction in connection with the resorption defect, and no communication of the resorptive defect with the periodontal tissues, confirms the diagnosis (Figure 18).

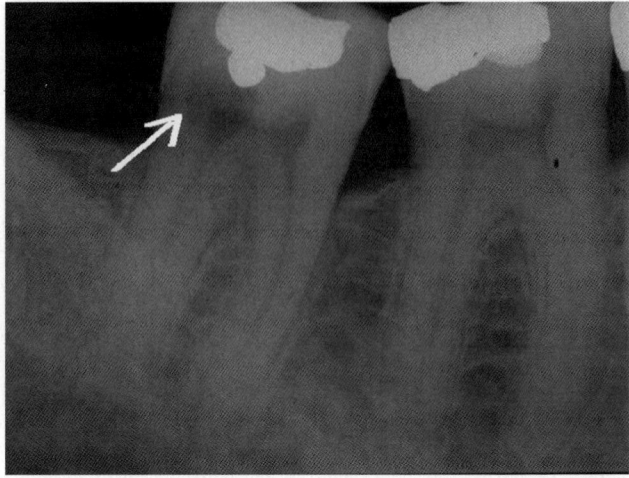

Figure 18 Radiograph of a tooth with internal resorption (arrow) as a consequence of an infraction. The pulp was vital and the infraction was in the mesiodistal direction, communication with the pulp in the distal aspect of the crown.

FUTURE DIRECTION

Some tooth infractions can be diagnosed quite readily with just a few examination steps, while other cases are very difficult to solve and require extensive efforts.[8] There is a need for additional means of detecting infractions and fractures in teeth; various avenues are being explored including the application of *ultrasound* to this problem. Ultrasound may have the potential to complement radiography as an imaging technique by identifying physical discontinuances (cracks) in hard tissues such as enamel and dentin. The application of ultrasound is used in industry for a similar purpose and would, if developed in dentistry, be of great help in the detection of tooth infractions.[44]

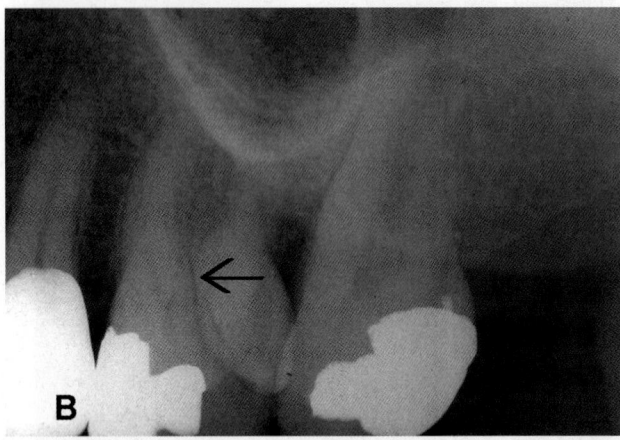

Figure 17 Radiograph of a maxillary molar with a buccopalatal infraction. Because of the fracture direction, it is readily identified radiographically (arrow).

Treatment

Any discussion of the treatment of tooth infractions must include an acknowledgement that neither dentin nor enamel can be permanently reunited once a fracture line develops. All treatment efforts therefore are attempts—some better than others—at preventing separation of the hard tissue entities, and perhaps keeping bacteria from colonizing the space caused by infractions. Further, root canal therapy, while contributing to reductions or elimination of symptoms, also will not change the fact that a tooth with infraction is a weakened tooth that likely will not last as long as a non-infracted tooth.

Endodontists appear to be in agreement that teeth with infractions can be treated,[45] but it is not clear if all teeth with infractions need root canal therapy. The lack of clear understanding in this regard is probably related to the difficulty in determining if an infraction communicates directly with the pulp (in which case endodontic treatment would reasonably be a part of the overall treatment for the tooth), or the infraction is a cuspal infraction that may not communicate with the pulp.

One approach to the question of treating endodontically or not is that used by the author and also recommended by Ailor[12] and Brynjulfsen et al.[8]: Stabilize the tooth with an orthodontic band before beginning root canal therapy. If the initial pulpal diagnosis is less than irreversible pulpitis (no lingering pain to cold or spontaneous, severe pain), wait for about 2 weeks before scheduling root canal therapy. If all the symptoms have subsided after the placement of the orthodontic band, the patient may be offered the option of only placing a restoration that binds the tooth crown together, with the understanding that the tooth may later need root canal therapy (Figure 19A–C). If a full coverage crown is the recommended restorative procedure, it may be wise to include the root canal treatment prior to crown placement to avoid having to make an access through a prosthetic crown later. The reason for waiting a while after placement of the

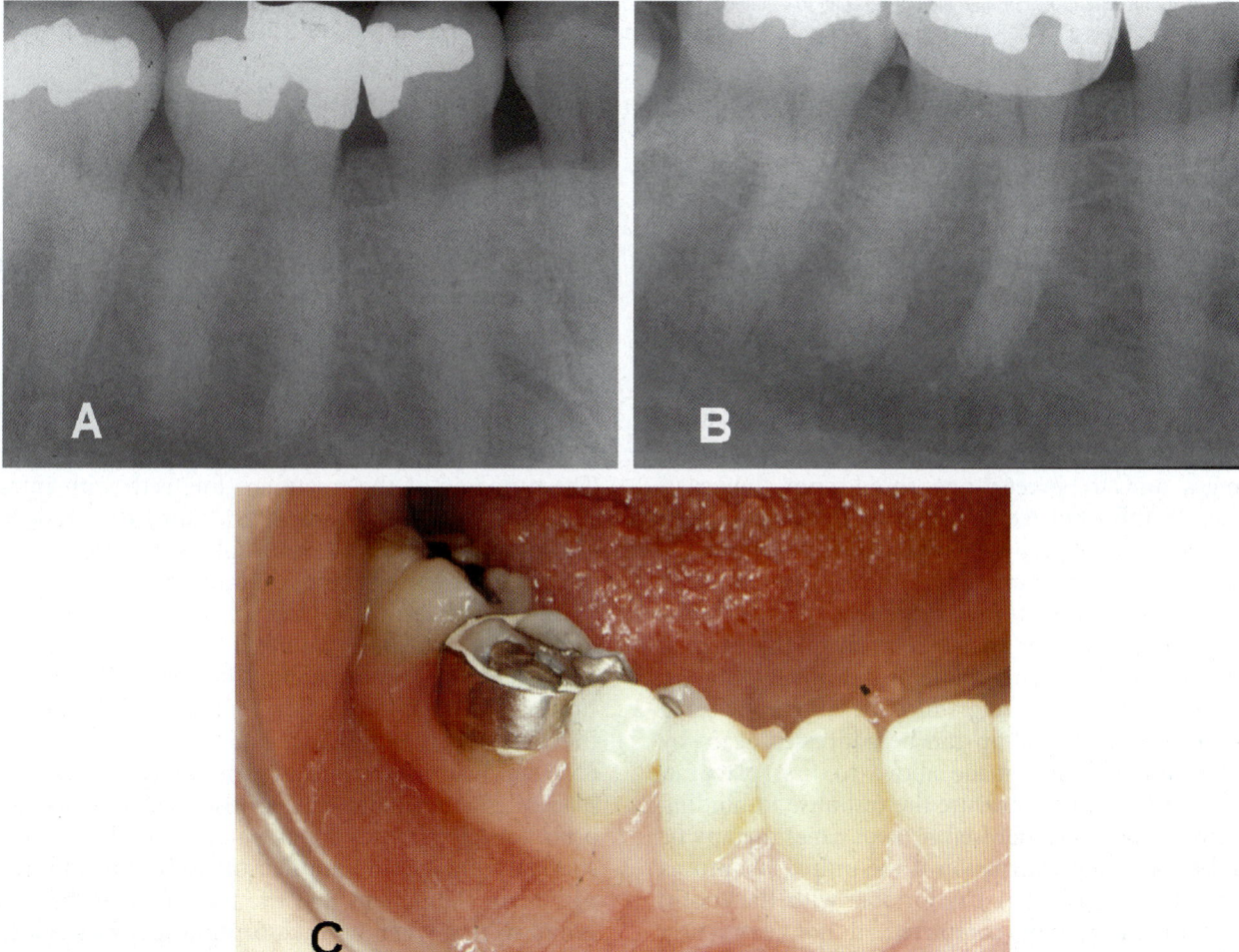

Figure 19 Initial treatment of a tooth with infraction to determine pulpal involvement **A,** Radiograph of a tooth that was painful to chewing and slightly sensitive to cold. **B, C,** Orthodontic band placed to bind the crown together. After 3 weeks the tooth was completely asymptomatic and the patient chose to have it restored with a crown.

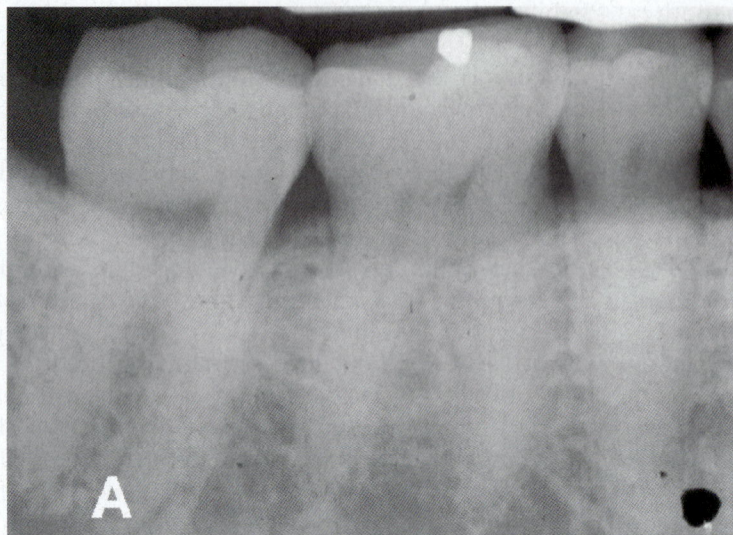
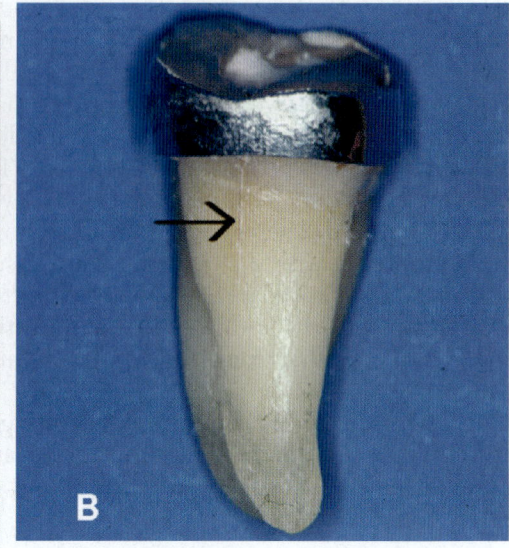

Figure 20 Tooth with infraction that did not respond to treatment. **A,** Radiograph of a tooth that was painful to chewing and had lingering pain to ice. Orthodontic band was placed and the pulp was extirpated. The tooth continued to be painful to chewing and the patient chose extraction. **B,** Photo of the extracted tooth shows infraction (arrow).

orthodontic band is that it takes some time before cold sensitivity subsides. Davis and Overton[11] found that it took 2 weeks for cold sensitivity to subside after binding infracted teeth with bonded amalgam restorations.

When teeth with infractions also have pulps that are irreversibly involved or necrotic, the need for root canal treatment is self-evident if the tooth is to be retained. Root canal treatment will obviously eliminate pulpal pain and sensitivity to temperature changes and to sweets; one should not, however, expect all infracted teeth to be free of chewing pain after root canal therapy. Pain to mastication forces is associated with inflammation in the PDL and one can expect such inflammation to be generated by bacteria-containing infractions that extend from the coronal area apically.[13,18,20] The problem of not being able to predict if pain to chewing will cease after root canal treatment and restoration can be addressed again by the recommendation made above to first place an orthodontic band to measure the response to binding the crown together, followed by root canal therapy or possibly just pulp extirpation if the pulpal symptoms persist. If the patient is comfortable with the tooth, the treatment can be completed; if not, extraction becomes the alternative treatment (Figure 20A,B).

Treatments designed to bind infracted teeth together include the use of adhesives,[46–49] amalgam with retention on both sides of the infractions,[11] and full coverage crowns.[8,11,12,50,51] Experimental approaches using lasers (CO_2, Nd:YAG) have not yet produced any promising results.[52]

PROGNOSIS

The outcome of the treatment for teeth with infractions is not extensively reported. Cameron[17] reported a 75% success after 10 years following placement of crowns, and Guthrie and DiFiore[50] found that 24 of 25 teeth restored with acrylic crowns were asymptomatic after 1 year. Brynjulfsen et al.[8] achieved pain relief in 90% of their patients after protective restorations of teeth with infraction (endodontic therapy was included when indicated), and Tan et al.[51] had an 85% survival rate 2 years after protective crowns were placed. The available data is insufficient to use as a basis for giving individual patient's odds on tooth survival for a specific number of years. It is important to inform the patient that the teeth need to be monitored so that when bone resorption becomes evident, the tooth should be extracted to prevent alveolar bone

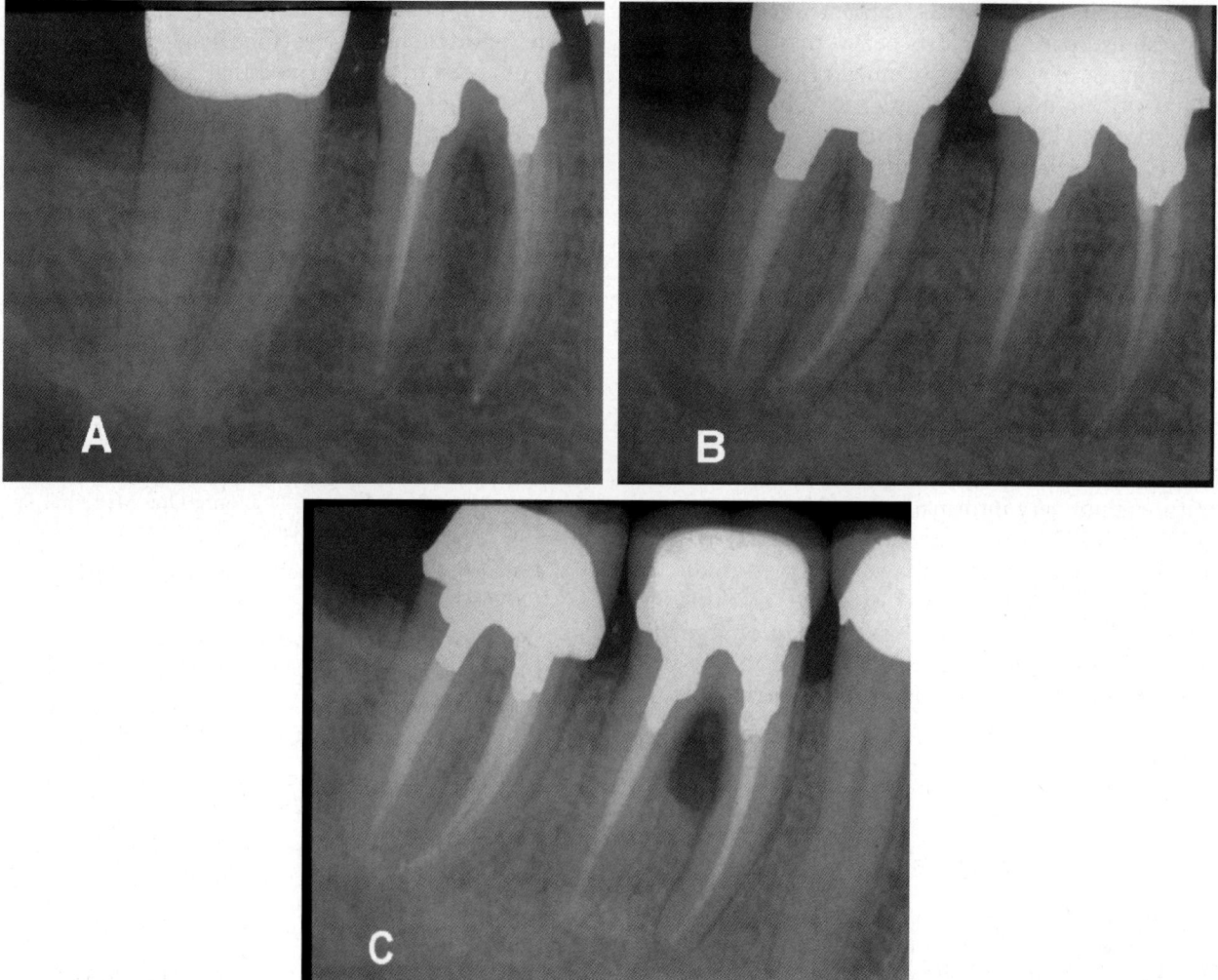

Figure 21 Long-term follow-up of an endodontically treated tooth with infraction. **A,** The diagnosis and endodontic treatment was done in 1987 for the mandibular first molar. **B,** The tooth was monitored yearly and this radiograph shows the tooth in 1992 (at the time of treatment of the second molar that did not have infraction but pulpitis due to recurrent decay). The first molar continued to be asymptomatic, and the patient missed the following year recall. **C,** Radiograph in 1994 (17 years after original treatment) shows bone loss associated with the development of vertical root fracture (VRF) as a result of the initial infraction. The tooth was extracted and the patient chose to replace it with an implant.

loss (Figure 21A–C). In the author's clinical experience, a 5-year survival prediction appears reasonable in most cases. Patients must be fully informed of the uncertainty based on the lack of data. What one can recognize is that in some situations the prognosis is poor: terminal teeth, teeth with periodontal involvement related to infractions, and teeth with multiple infractions.[51] As with other dental treatment recommendations, clinicians can provide advice based on what is available in the literature and the clinician's own experience, and the patient can contribute his/her preferences.

Prevention

A number of factors have been recognized as steps that can be taken to reduce the incidence of tooth infraction. They include cavity design and size,[11,12,18,23,24,32] proper design of intracoronal cast restorations,[24,32] avoiding the use of self-threading and friction-lock pins,[18,23,32,33] avoiding extensive use of course diamond burs and vibrating high-speed handpieces,[12,37] and restoring teeth with attention to occlusion to avoid interference from working premature contacts.[12,18] It may also be beneficial to advise patients about potential damage from oral habits (pipes, pencils, carpenter nails)[12,18] and the stress excessive repetitive heavy mastication can produce in teeth.[14,15,26] Yeh[14] coined the term "fatigue root fracture" to describe the result of a coarse Chinese diet in patients who usually used heavy mastication over the years of their lives. Many often developed VRFs in non-restored teeth with no endodontic treatment history. The biting force on first molars is up to 90 kg[26] and if there is sudden external trauma, such as biting unexpectedly on something hard in the food, an infraction may result. Kahler et al.[13] described how infraction can occur from "cyclic fatigue"—repeated occlusal loads. As with all body parts, teeth are not indestructible and care in the use of one's teeth is advised.

With respect to care of teeth, a question sometimes raised is, is it damaging to chew on ice? The dental literature is not very informative on this topic; Brown et al.[35] in 1972 used thermal cycling—alternating exposure to very cold and very hot stimuli to extracted teeth—and reported extensive cracking in the teeth. It is not clear if this information can be applied to the question of ice chewing, but until more information becomes available, it seems reasonable to advise against chewing on ice.

Summary

Tooth infraction in dentistry is not a major problem in terms of incidence,[16,19] but it is a problem in diagnosis when the symptoms and clinical findings are not definitive.[3,4,7,8,12,13,17,20] Current information supports the notion that tooth infraction is an incomplete fracture of the tooth, most often starting in the crown, but sometimes in the root.[4,6,11–13,15,18,21] Tooth infractions may be cuspal infractions that usually do not communicate directly with the pulp. They may, however, propagate from the pulp toward the dentin–enamel and dentin–cementum junctions. In the former situation, treatment may not need to include endodontic therapy, while in the latter situation, the pulp is likely to be at least irreversibly involved and root canal treatment is included with the restorative procedure.[1,11,21,51] Restorative treatment involves procedures that provide a binding effect on the tooth infraction; this can be accomplished by using amalgam restorations that incorporate retention on both sides of the infractions,[11] amalgam in combination with bonding agents or full coverage crowns.[8,11,12,51,53]

Adequate data is not available to determine prognosis for teeth with infractions; symptomatic teeth that have received treatment—either restorative alone or in combination with root canal therapy—have been reported to survive for many years,[17,50,51] but patients need to be informed that long-term retention is questionable. In spite of probable unfavorable long-term outcome, retaining a tooth with infraction may still be an excellent option in many instances.

References

1. American Association of Endodontists. Endodontists. Colleagues for Excellence Cracking the cracked tooth code American Association of Endodontists; Fall/Winter 1997.
2. Gibbs JW. Cuspal fracture odontalgia. Dent Dig 1954;60:158.
3. Ritchey B, Mendenhall R, Orban B. Pulpitis resulting from incomplete tooth fracture. Oral Surg Oral Med Oral Pathol Oral Radiol Endod 1957;10:665.
4. Cameron CE. Cracked-tooth syndrome. J Am Dent Assoc 1964;68:405–11.
5. Sutton PRN. Greenstick fracture of the tooth crown. Br Dent J 1962;112:362–6.
6. Luebke RG. Vertical crown–root-fractures in posterior teeth. Dent Clin North Am 1984;28:883–95.
7. Caufield JB. Hairline tooth fracture: a clinical case report. J Am Dent Assoc 1981;102:501–2.
8. Brynjulfsen A, Fristad I, Grevstad T, Hals-Kvinsland I. Incompletely fractured teeth associated with diffuse longstanding orofacial pain: diagnosis and treatment outcome. Int Endod J 2002;35:461–6.
9. Geurtsen W, Schwarze T, Günay H. Diagnosis, therapy, and prevention of the cracked tooth syndrome. Quintessence Int 2003;34:409–17.
10. Stedman's Medical Dictionary. 26th ed., Baltimore, MD: Williams and Wilkins; 1995.
11. Davis R, Overton JD. Efficacy of bonded and nonbonded amalgam in the treatment of teeth with incomplete fractures. J Am Dent Assoc 2000;131:469–78.
12. Ailor JE. Managing incomplete tooth fractures. J Am Dent Assoc 2000;131:1168–74.
13. Kahler B, Moule A, Stenzel D. Bacterial contamination of cracks in symptomatic vital teeth. Aust Endod J 2000;26:115–18.
14. Yeh C-J. Fatigue root fracture: a spontaneous root fracture in non-endodontically treated teeth. Br Dent J 1997;182:261–6.
15. Chan C-P, Lin C-P, Tseng S-C, Jeng J-H. Vertical root fractures in endodontically versus nonendodontically treated teeth. Oral Surg Oral Med Oral Path Oral Radiol Endod 1999;87:504–7.
16. Snyder DE. The cracked tooth syndrome and fractured posterior cusp. Oral Surg Oral Med Oral Pathol Oral Radiol Endod 1976;41:698–704.

17. Cameron CE. The cracked tooth syndrome: additional findings. J Am Dent Assoc 1976;93:971–5.
18. Rosen H. Cracked tooth syndrome. J Prosthet Dent 1982;47:36–43.
19. Motsch A. Pulpitische Symptome als Problem in der Praxis. Deutsche Zahnarz Zeit 1992;47:78–83.
20. Hiatt WH. Incomplete crown–root fracture. J Periodontol 1973;44:369–79.
21. Roh BD, Lee YE. Analysis of 154 cases of teeth with cracks. Dent Traumatol 2006;22:118–23.
22. Makkes PC, Folmer T. An unusual vertical fracture of the root. J Endod 1979;5:315–16.
23. Silvestri AR. The undiagnosed split-root syndrome. J Am Dent Assoc 1976;92:930–5.
24. Cavel WT, Kelsey WP, Blankenau RJ. An in vitro study of cuspal fracture. J Prosthet Dent 1985;53:38–42.
25. Eakle WS, Maxwell EH, Braly BV. Fractures of posterior teeth in adults. J Am Dent Assoc 1986;112:215–18.
26. Homewood CI. Cracked tooth syndrome-incidence, clinical findings and treatment. Aust Dent J 1998;43:217–22.
27. Gher ME, Dunlap RM, Anderson MH, et al. Clinical survey of fractured teeth. J Am Dent Assoc 1987;174–7.
28. Stanley HR. The cracked tooth. J Am Acad Gold Foil Operators 1968;X1:36–47.
29. Wahab MHA, Kennedy JG. Response of cracked teeth to cold and electrical stimulation. Br Dent J 1985;158:250–60.
30. Brännström M. The hydrodynamic theory of dentinal pain: sensation in preparations, caries, and the dentinal crack syndrome. J Endod 1986;12:453–7.
31. Swepston JH, Miller AW. The incompletely fractured tooth. J Prosthet Dent 1986;55:413–16.
32. Rosen H. The cracked tooth syndrome. Additional findings. J Am Dent Assoc 1976;93:971–5.
33. Standlee JP, Collard EW, Caputo AA. Dentinal defects caused by some twist drills and retentive pins. J Prosthet Dent 1970;24:185–92.
34. Schweitzer JL, Gutmann JL, Bliss RQ. Odontiatrogenic tooth fracture. Int Endod J 1989;22:64–74.
35. Brown WS, Jacobs HR, Thompson RE. Thermal fatigue in teeth. J Dent Res 1972;51:461–7.
36. Despain RR, Lloyd BA, Brown WS. Scanning electron microscope investigation of cracks in teeth through replication. J Am Dent Assoc 1974;88:580–4.
37. National Institute of Standards and Technology. Tech Beat; January 1998.
38. Ibsen RL. A rapid method for diagnosis of cracked teeth. Quintessence Int 1978;10:21–3.
39. Slaton CC, Loushine RJ, Weller RN, et al. Identification of resected root-end dentinal cracks: a comparative study of visual magnification. J Endod 2003;29:519–22.
40. Youssefzadeh S, Gahleitner A, Dorffner R, et al. Dental vertical root fractures: value of CT in detection. Radiology 1999;210:545–9.
41. Hannig C, Dullin C, Hülsmann M, Heidrich G. Three-dimensional, non-destructive visualization of vertical root fractures using flat panel volume detector computer tomography: an ex vivo in vitro case report. Int Endod J 2005;38:904–13.
42. Cotton TP, Geisler TM, Holden DT, et al. Endodontic applications of cone-beam volumetric tomography. J Endod 2007;33:1121–32.
43. Walton RE, Leonard LA. Cracked tooth: an etiology for "idiopathic" internal resorption. J Endod 1986;12:167–9.
44. Culjat MO, Singh RS, Brown ER, et al. Ultrasound crack detection in a simulated human tooth. Dentomax Radiol 2005;34:80–5.
45. Maxwell EH, Braly BV, Eakle WS. Incompletely fractured teeth – a survey of endodontists. Oral Surg Oral Med Oral Pathol Oral Radiol Endod 1986;61:113–17.
46. Oliet S. Treating vertical root fractures. J Endod 1984;10:391–6.
47. Friedman S, Moshonov M, Trope M. Resistance to vertical fracture of roots, previously fractured and bonded with glass ionomer cement, composite resin and cyanoacrylate cement. Endod Dent Traumatol 1993;9:101–5.
48. Gutmann JL, Rakusin H. Endodontic and restorative management of incompletely fractured molar teeth. Int Endod J 1994;27:343–8.
49. Belli S, Erdemir A, Ozcopur M. Fracture resistance of endodontically treated molar teeth: various restoration techniques. IADR Abstracts #1748; 2004.
50. Guthrie RC, DiFiore PM. Treating the cracked tooth with a full crown. J Am Dent Assoc 1991;122:71–3.
51. Tan L, Chen NN, Poon CY, Wong HB. Survival of root filled cracked teeth in a tertiary institution. Int Endod J 2006;39:886–9.
52. Arakawa S, Cobb CM, Rapley JW, et al. Treatment of root fracture by CO_2 and ND:Yag lasers: an in vitro study. J Endod 1996;22:662–7.
53. Pilo R, Brosh T, Chweidan H. Cusp reinforcement by bonding of amalgam restorations. J Dent 1998;26:467–72.

CHAPTER 20

VERTICAL ROOT FRACTURES OF ENDODONTICALLY TREATED TEETH

AVIAD TAMSE

Vertical root fractures (VRFs) occur mainly in endodontically treated and restored teeth, but have been found in mesial roots of mandibular molars in nonendodontically treated teeth in a Chinese population.[1] According to the American Association of Endodontists,[2] "a vertical root fracture is a longitudinally oriented fracture of the root that originates from the apex and propagates to the coronal part." From a horizontal aspect, the fracture initiates in the root canal wall and extends to the root surface,[3] involving either one side (incomplete) or both sides (complete fracture)[3,4] (Figure 1A,B).

VRFs present numerous problems for both patients and clinicians. VRFs can be difficult to differentiate from failing endodontically treated teeth or teeth associated with periodontal disease.[5–8] Often the definitive diagnosis is made years after extensive treatment.[9,10] The etiology tends to be multifactorial[6,10,11] and the need to extract the tooth or the root when the definitive diagnosis is made is disappointing.[3,12]

Endodontically treated teeth may need to be extracted if they cannot be restored or have become periodontally involved; both causes are unrelated to the endodontic treatment itself. Survival rate studies have shown VRF to be one reason to extract endodontically treated teeth,[13–15] but only a few studies show the prevalence of VRF teeth. Gher et al.[16] suggest a low incidence (2.3%), similar to the 2 to 5% prevalence found in retrospective "success and failure" studies on prosthetic reconstructions.[17,18] However, the percentage of extracted teeth with VRF can be much higher, between 10 and 20%.[19,20]

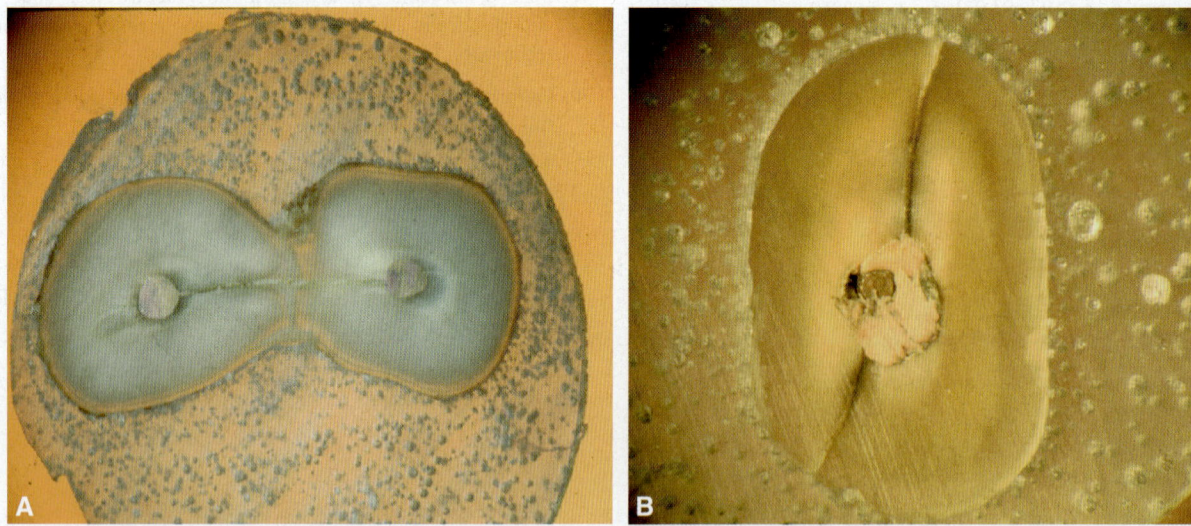

Figure 1 *A,* Incomplete fracture in a maxillary premolar. *B,* Complete fracture in a mandibular premolar.

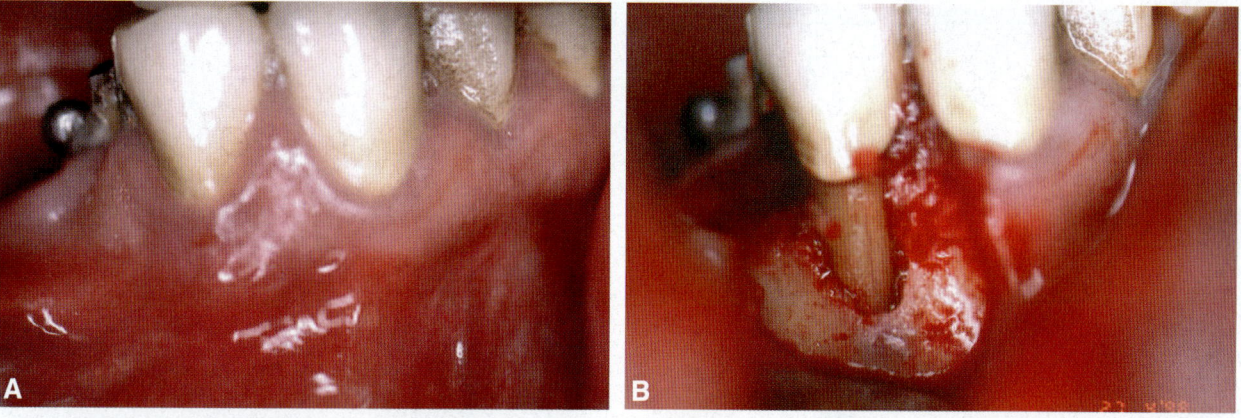

Figure 2 **A,** Mandibular premolar suspected of vertical root fracture (VRF). **B,** Buccal exploratory flap procedure reveals the nearly complete loss of buccal bone—dehiscence type.

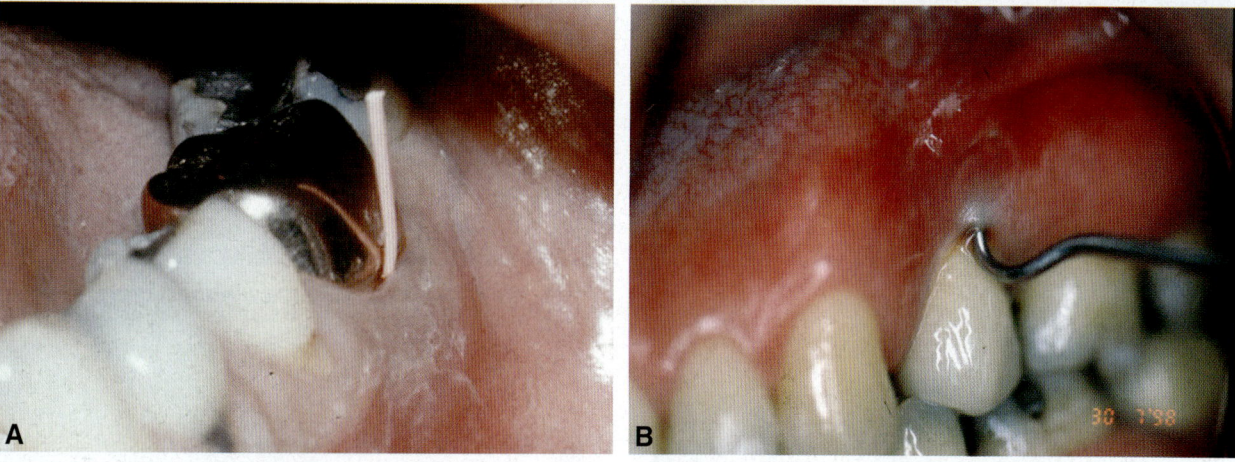

Figure 3 **A,** Gutta-percha cone demonstrating a deep osseous defect on the buccal aspect of the mesial root in a mandibular molar. **B,** Periodontal probe in a buccal osseous defect of a maxillary premolar.

Clinical Diagnosis

Arriving at the correct diagnosis for VRF of endodontically treated teeth based on clinical and radiographic findings can be challenging for any clinician. There are several reasons for this diagnostic difficulty.

1. It is often difficult radiographically to make an early detection of a crack.
2. Signs and symptoms, such as spontaneous dull pain, mastication pain, tooth mobility, presence of sinus tracts, osseous defects, periodontal-type abscesses, and bony radiolucencies, are often similar to those found in failed root canal treatment or in periodontal disease.[5,6,21–23]
3. Often an existing crack or an incomplete fracture is not visually detected when intraradicular procedures are performed (instrumentation, obturation, or dowel preparation), and tooth restoration is completed over the existing crack or fracture. A definitive diagnosis may not be made for years after treatment has been completed.[10,21]

To complicate matters even more, early diagnosis needs to be made because of the direct correlation between bone resorption around a root with VRF and time.[24] That is, the longer the inflammatory process continues, the more bone resorption occurs.

The typical bone loss associated with VRF is loss of the alveolar bone buccal to the affected root (Figure 2A,B), a process that continues until the tooth or the root is removed.[24] Common clinical signs that can help clinicians make the correct diagnosis are a deep osseous defect (Figure 3A,B) and a sinus tract located near the cervical area (Figure 4A,B). In four retrospective clinical surveys of teeth with VRFs, deep osseous defects were found between 64 and 93% of the time, and cervically located sinus tracts between 13 and 35% of the cases.[5,6,8,22]

When a root fracture line propagates coronally and laterally to the periodontal ligament (PDL), local

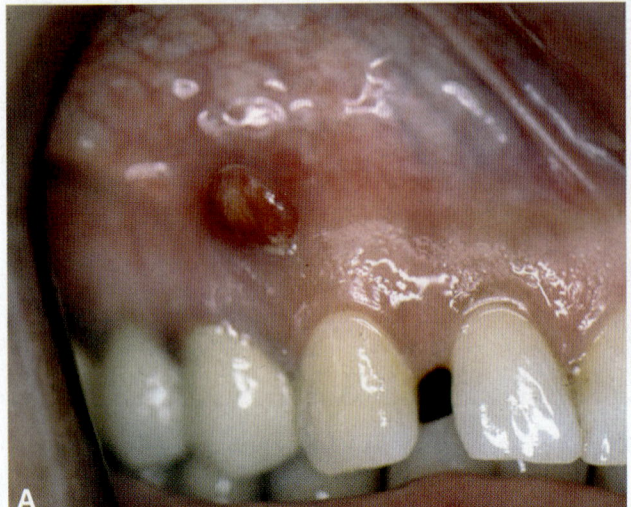
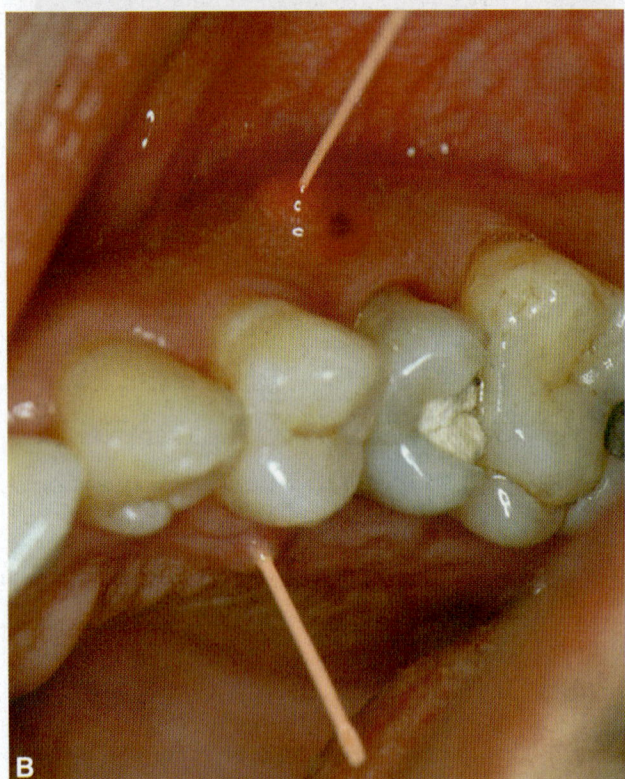

Figure 4 *A*, Coronally located sinus tract near a maxillary premolar. *B*, Buccal and lingual sinus tracts from a complete vertical root fracture (VRF) of a second maxillary premolar. The lingual sinus tract is located mesially to the fractured tooth.

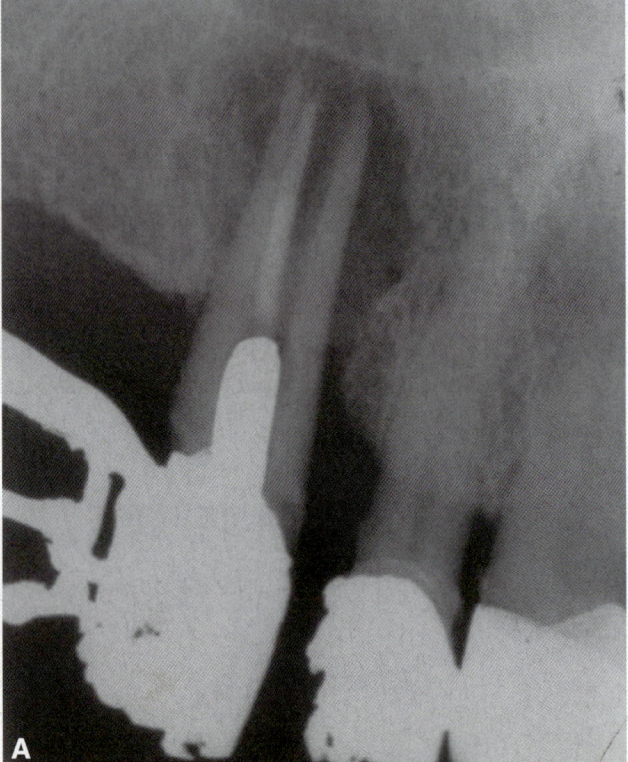
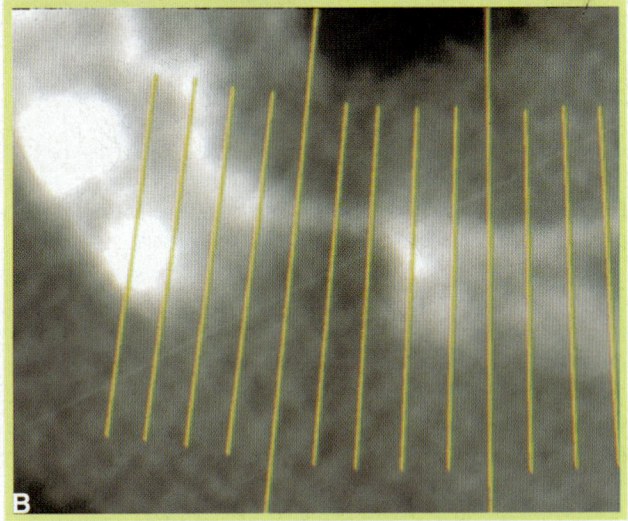

Figure 5 *A*, Late diagnosis of a vertical root fracture (VRF) showing separated root segments and inflammatory process around them. *B*, Axial computed tomography (CT) scan showing complete bone loss on the buccal aspect.

inflammation develops in the PDL associated with the crack. It is caused by bacteria from the oral cavity and the root canal space penetrating into the crack.[3] The local inflammatory process leads to periodontal breakdown followed by development of a deep osseous defect. An abscess forms when this chronic situation exacerbates over time and is similar to periodontal disease abscesses.[5,6,8,22,25] An exploratory surgical procedure to visualize the VRF allows definitive diagnosis.[24–27]

Lustig et al.[24] have described the typical bone resorption patterns in teeth with VRF. In 90% of teeth with VRF extracted during exploratory surgery, buccal bone dehiscence along the entire root length was noted. There is a direct correlation between the amount of bone resorbed facing the fracture line and time (Figure 5A,B). A fenestration type of bone loss (Figure 6A-D) was found in only 10% of maxillary premolars and mesial roots of mandibular molars. Walton and Torabinejad[28] described the fracture initiation as apicocoronal propagation of initial bone resorption. In a later stage, when the fracture extends to the gingival margin, resorption is more oblong, with resorption rapidly progressing apically and laterally to the interproximal areas. Radiographically, even if the buccal plate is completely resorbed, with no interproximal involvement, a single

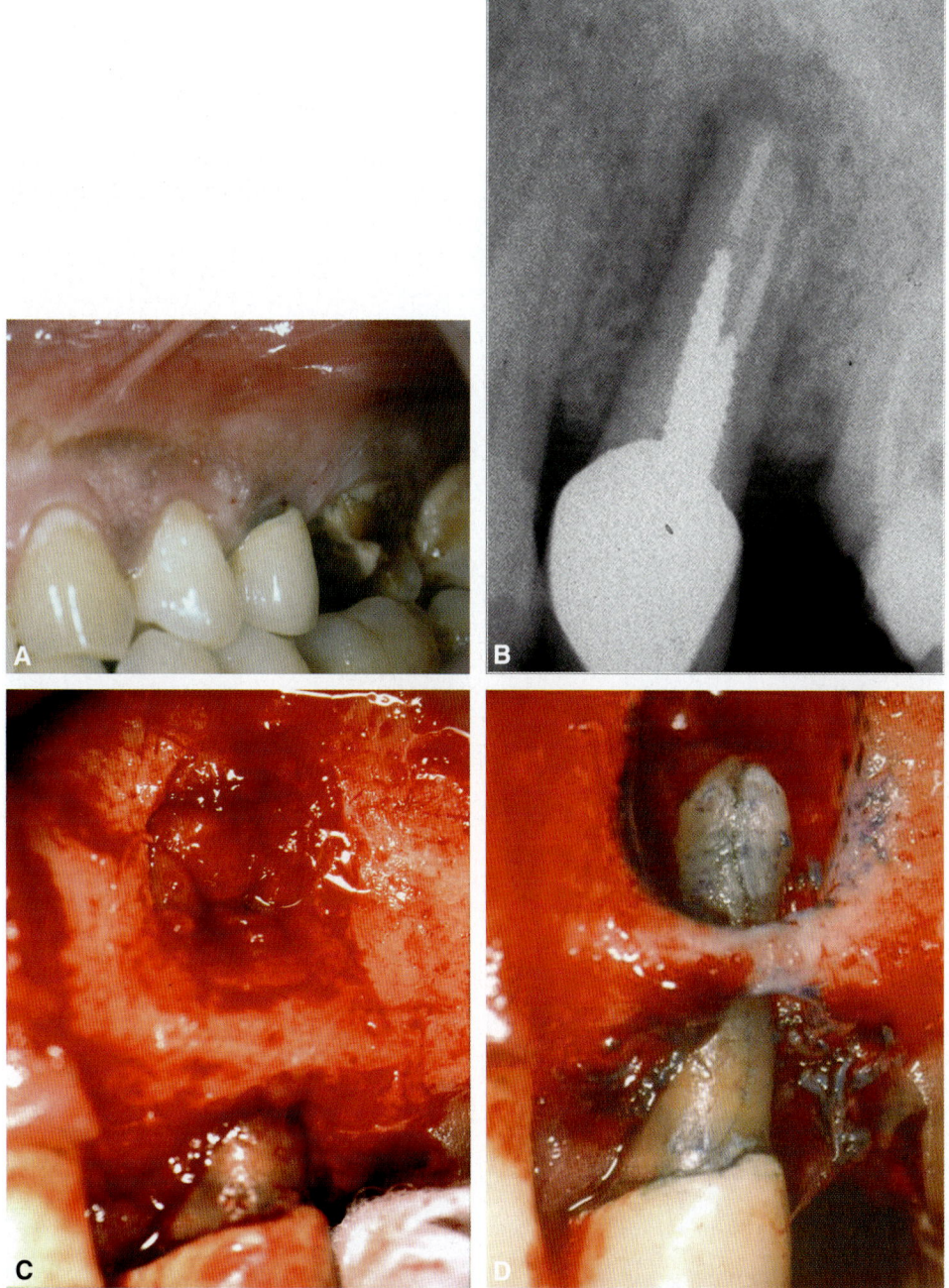

Figure 6 *A*, Vertical root fracture (VRF) in a maxillary premolar. New restorative treatment was needed for the posterior segment. *B*, Periapical radiograph shows the "halo" radiolucency around the root. *C*, Exploratory flap procedure reveals buccal fenestration filled with granulation tissue *D*, Removal of the soft tissue reveals fracture line from apical to cervical root area. Methylene blue dye helped to demonstrate the fracture.

periapical view would, most likely, not reveal the bone loss (Figure 7A, B).

On the lingual aspect of a tooth with VRF, the bone resorbs into a shallow, rounded U-shaped defect because spongeous bone is much thicker and resorbs away from the root, and only later extends laterally. It is interesting to note that in 10% of the fenestrations, an abscess similar to a chronic apical abscess of endodontic origin, with no probable osseous defect on the buccal side, was the only clinical sign.[24]

During exploratory surgery, when the typical dehiscence appearance combined with a visible fractured root is seen, the root or the tooth can be extracted to prevent further bone loss.[24] Sinus tracts associated with VRF, unlike those from a chronic apical abscess, are usually not located in the apical area. They tend to be within several millimeters of the gingival margin.[8,21] This type of sinus tract has been found in 14 to 42% of the VRF cases.[5,6,8,10,22] A deep osseous defect, a cervically located sinus tract, and typical bone loss upon exploratory surgery are very helpful in making a diagnosis.

Radiographic Diagnosis

It is possible to detect a VRF in an endodontically treated tooth radiographically in only two instances.

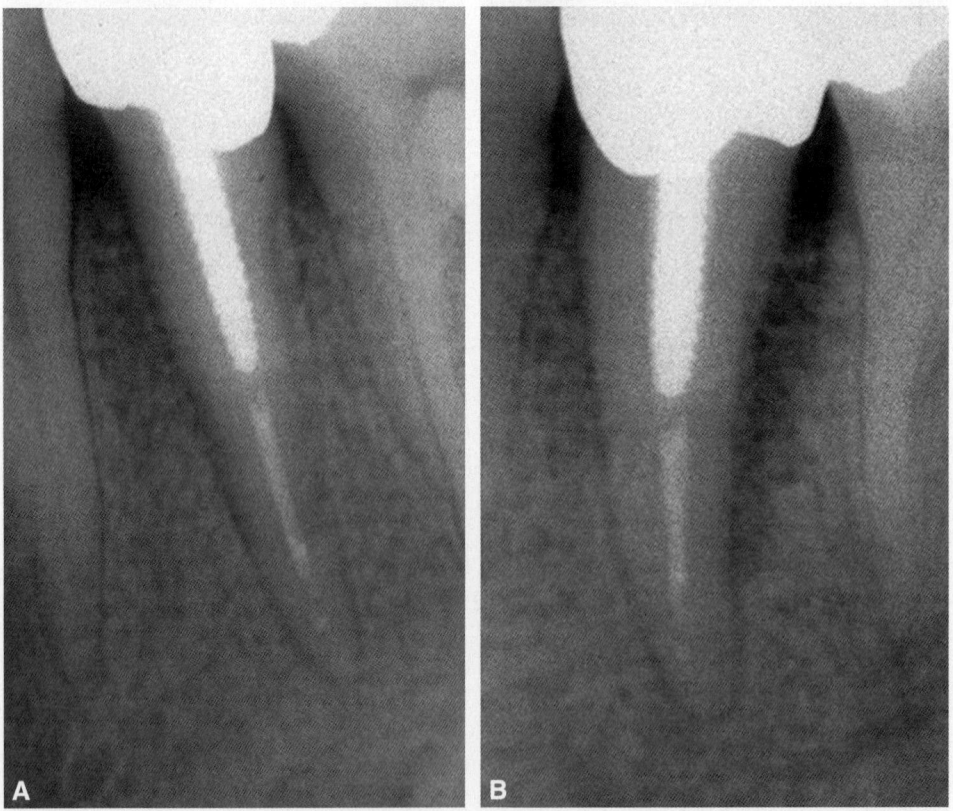

Figure 7 *A*, Periapical radiograph of a mandibular premolar reveals widening of the periodontal ligament (PDL) on the mesial tooth aspect. *B*, Change of horizontal angulation reveals radiolucency along most of the distal aspect from the coronal aspect, not involving the periapical area—periodontal radiolucency.

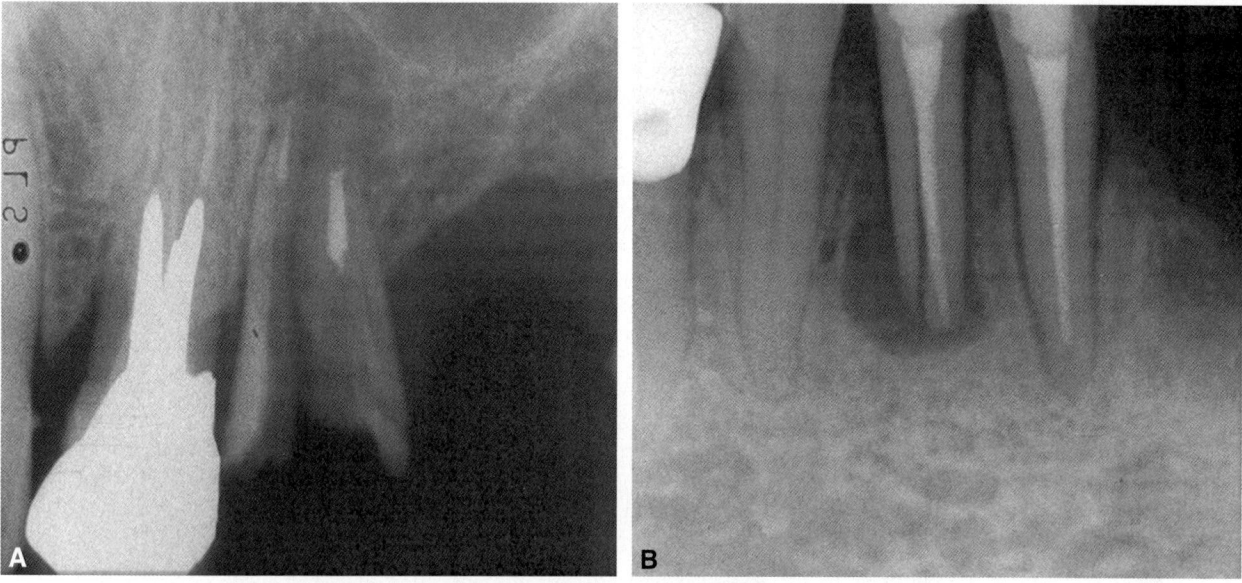

Figure 8 ***A***, Separation of root segments of a maxillary premolar and a mandibular incisor ***B***,.

The first is when there is evidence of separation of the root segments (Figure 8A,B), usually accompanied by a large radiolucency surrounding the bone between the roots that is actually inflammatory tissue separating the segments.[7,21,29] The second is when a "hair-like" fracture line radiolucency can be detected in a periapical radiograph (Figure 9). Rud and

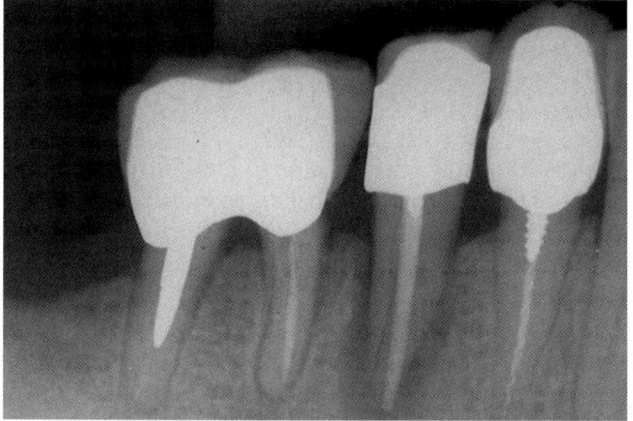

Figure 9 "Hair-like" radiolucent line can be seen at the distal aspect of a fractured mandibular premolar.

Omnell[21] claimed that it was possible to see fracture lines in 35.7% of the cases in their study. However, many of their cases were not true VRF cases. In clinical practice, it is still rare, when only a single periapical radiograph is taken, to have the X-ray beam lined up with the fracture line. Two or three periapical radiographs should be taken from different angulations when a fracture is suspected. Often the clinician can speculate, from bony radiolucencies surrounding or between the roots, whether or not there is a root fracture. Since some of these radiolucencies are similar to those in "endodontic"- or "periodontal"-type lesions,[8,21,23,30,31] the correct diagnosis based on radiographs is often difficult and can delay the definitive diagnosis.

The appearance of a radiolucency associated with a VRF is influenced by the extent of bone destruction, direction and location of the fracture, and time elapsed since the initiation of the fracture.[5,21] A possible helpful diagnostic factor is the observation that some radiolucencies have been found to be more often associated with VRFs than with cases of failed root canal treatment or periodontal disease.[23,31–33]

The most frequent feature in VRFs, both in maxillary premolars and in mesial roots of mandibular

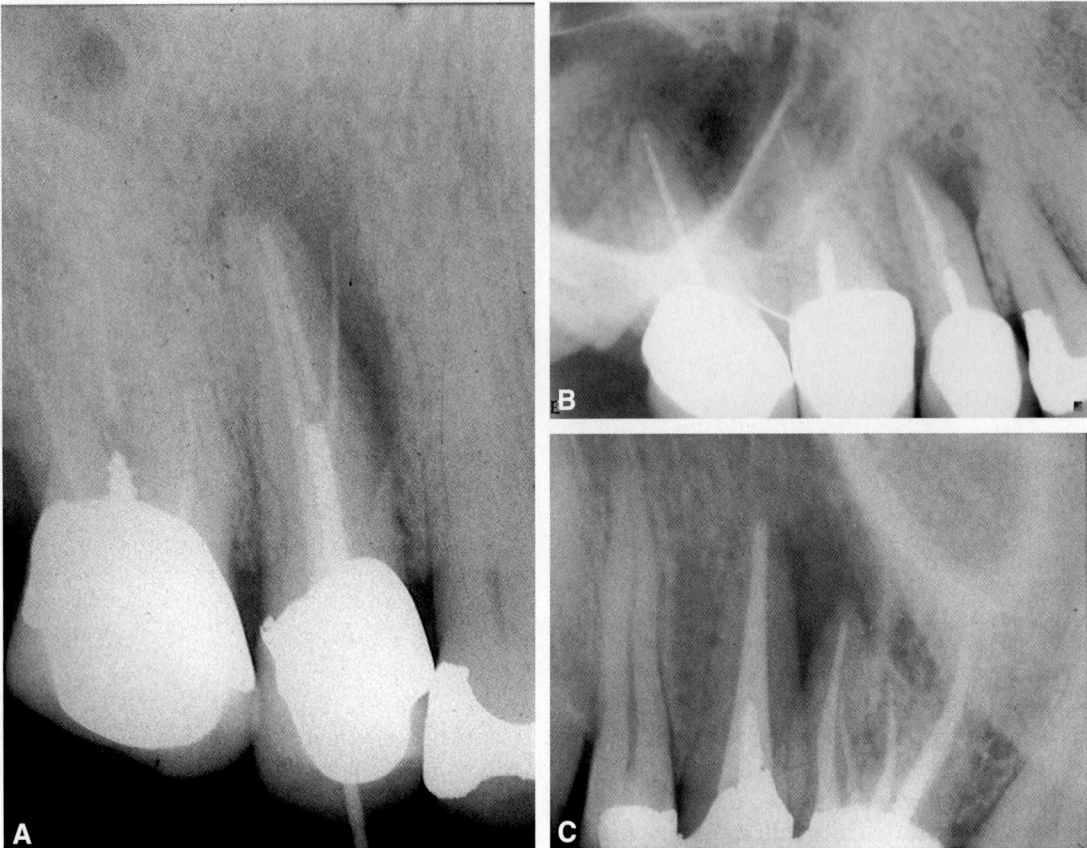

Figure 10 *A,* "Halo" appearance radiolucency around the apical and mesial aspects of a maxillary premolar. *B,* "Halo" type radiolucency including the mesial and distal aspects of the apical third of the root. *C,* Isolated lateral radiolucency in a maxillary premolar. The apical and coronal areas are not involved.

molars, is the "halo" appearance, a combined periapical and periradicular radiolucency on one or both sides of the involved root[23,33] (Figure 10A-C). In mandibular molars, in addition to the "halo" appearance of the lesion, typical in these roots, a bifurcation radiolucency is also found in 63.3% of the cases[23] (Figure 11A-D). Observing such radiolucencies can help clinicians make the correct diagnosis of VRF teeth, especially when combined with the other signs and symptoms.

With digital radiography, it is possible to acquire, enhance, store, retrieve, and transfer radiographic information with reduced radiation dosage compared to conventional radiography. When digital radiography was compared with analog radiography in detecting VRF, neither had any advantage over the other.[34,35]

The use of tomography to detect root fractures is not new,[36] and recently additional imaging techniques to detect and visualize root fractures have been introduced.[37–40] These new techniques could be in clinical use in the near future, providing opportunities for early detection of VRFs.

Etiology

Since VRFs occur mostly in endodontically treated and restored teeth, some root canal procedures, such as excessive removal of dentin during canal preparation[19,22] and post space preparation and post placement,[41] have been identified as causes of VRF.

These VRF etiologies are iatrogenic.[10] There are also several predisposing factors to fractures, making VRF etiology more complex and multifactorial. Understanding the etiological factors may help clinicians better understand how to prevent and manage VRFs.

PREDISPOSING ETIOLOGIC FACTORS

Predisposing factors for VRF are root anatomy, amount of remaining sound tooth structure, loss of moisture in the dentin, amount of bony support,

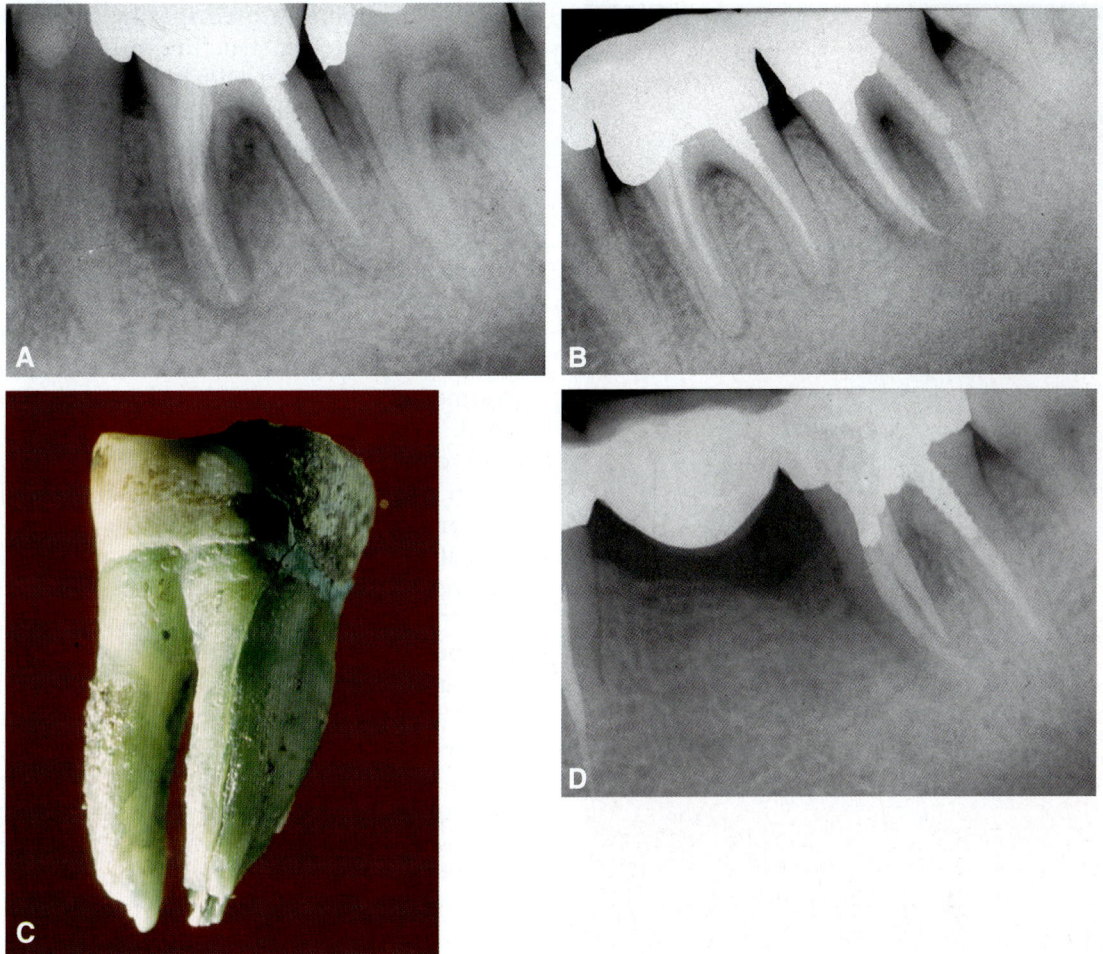

Figure 11 Typical bony periradicular radiolucencies around mesial roots of mandibular molars. **A,** Lateral radiolucency on the mesial aspect and at the bifurcation area of a mandibular first molar. **B,** Periapical and bifurcation radiolucency around a second mandibular molar. **C,** Extracted tooth from **D,** shows the fracture line on the buccal aspect of the mesial root. **D,** Angular and bifurcation radiolucency.

pre-existing cracks, and biochemical properties of root dentin.

The most susceptible roots to fracture are those in which the mesiodistal diameter is narrow compared to the buccolingual dimension (oval, triangular, kidney-shaped, ribbon-shaped).[42] Examples of such teeth would be maxillary and mandibular premolars, mesial roots of mandibular molars, and mandibular incisors.[43] In a retrospective study of fractured roots, Tamse et al.[8] found that these were the most frequently fractured roots and teeth (79%). To minimize the risk of VRF, familiarity with the root anatomy and morphology is essential for appropriate root canal treatment and restoration of endodontically treated teeth.[42]

Root curvature[44] and root depressions in the mesial root of mandibular molars and the buccal root of bifurcated maxillary premolars are anatomical entities that can predispose the roots to fracture and perforation[42,44–46] (Figure 12).

The canal and root shape, combined with dentin thickness, affect tensile stress distribution during intracanal procedures.[47] Canal shape is the most important factor of the two since the area of reduced curvature radius (the buccal and lingual areas) is strongly influenced by stress concentrations. More than likely, this is the reason these roots fracture in a buccolingual direction and not mesiodistally, although more tooth structure is removed from the mesial and distal aspects at the stage of canal instrumentation and post space preparation.[48,49]

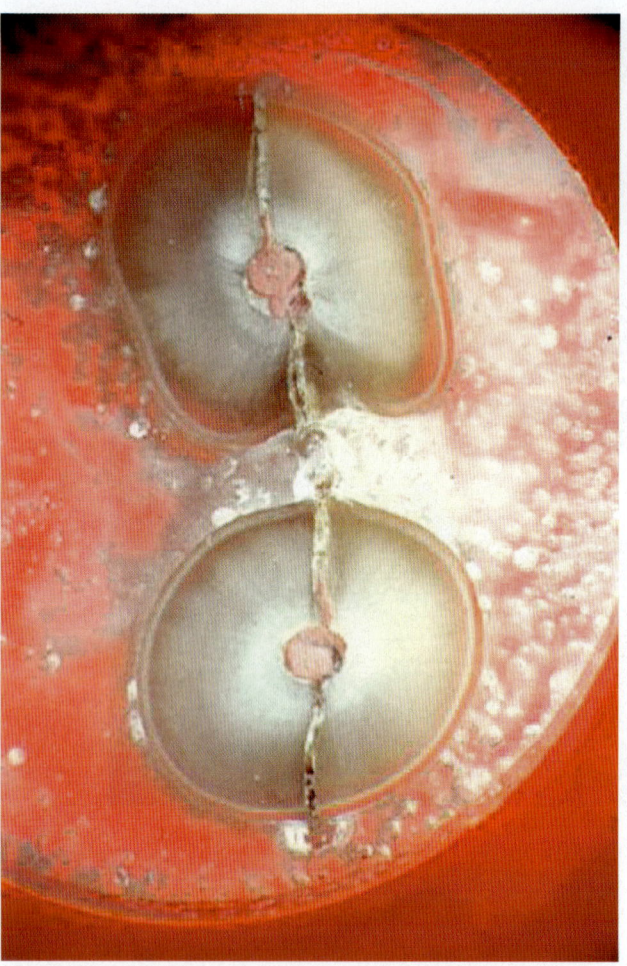

Figure 12 Complete vertical root fracture (VRF) in buccal and lingual roots of a maxillary bifurcated premolar. Note the depression on the bifurcation aspects of the buccal root.

Another important predisposing factor for VRF is the amount of tooth structure missing due to caries or trauma. Combined with the reduced amount of radicular dentin, the result of various intracanal procedures (initial root canal therapy, retreatment, post space preparation), the remaining tooth structure is directly related to the ability of endodontically treated teeth to resist fracture[42,48–53] (Figure 13A,B). A common clinical speculation is that an endodontically treated tooth is more brittle compared to one with a vital pulp, and that the dentin undergoes changes in collagen cross-linking after root canal treatment.[54] However, this has not been validated.[55–57] Moisture loss in endodontically treated teeth, compared with teeth with vital pulps, is not a major etiological factor but rather a predisposing one for fracture.[58]

Small cracks are often present in dentin, parallel or perpendicular to the root canal space in intact teeth.[3,59–61] During intracanal procedures when dentin is removed, especially in the mesiodistal areas, such cracks may be exposed (incomplete fractures or infractions), and then later may propagate in buccal and/or lingual directions (complete fracture).[61]

The specific biochemical properties of dentin are also predisposing factors in VRFs. In a study on the stress–strain response in human dentin, Kishen et al.[62] found that the dentin adaptation to functional strain–stress distribution results in greater mineralization in the buccolingual areas. This may increase the likelihood for a fracture to propagate in this direction, compared with the less mineralization and more collagen in the mesiodistal areas.

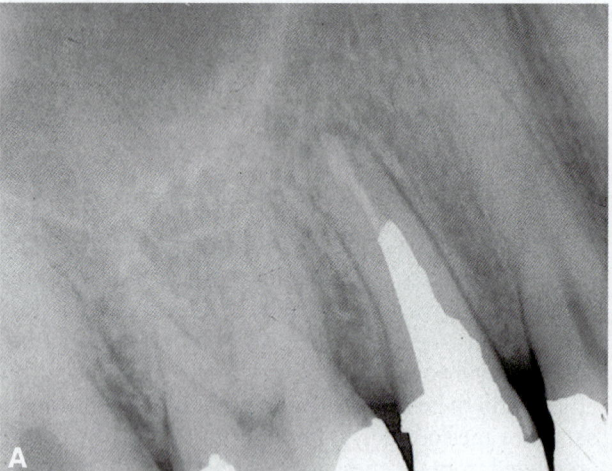
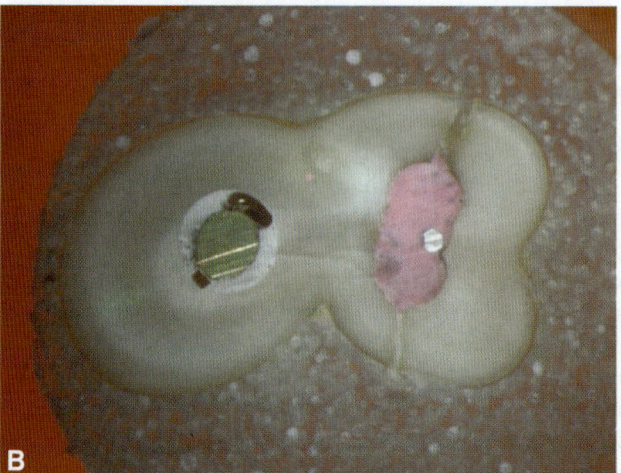

Figure 13 *A*, Thin dentin walls after excessive preparation of a post in a maxillary premolar. *B*, Complete vertical root fracture (VRF) in the buccal part of a single-rooted maxillary premolar. Excessive preparation of the root canal space is evident.

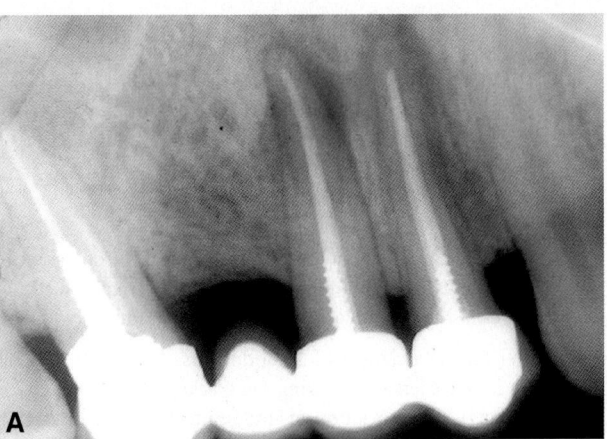 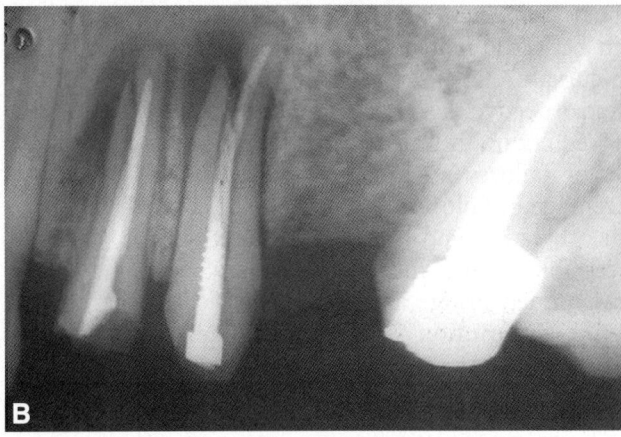

Figure 14 Endodontically treated maxillary premolars as abutments. **A**, Typical periradicular radiolucencies around two premolars serving as abutments. **B**, Six months after the diagnosis of vertical root fracture (VRF).

Reinhardt et al.[63] found, by evaluating radiographs, a correlation between the height of the alveolar crest and the stress in the apical part of a post. One may assume that loss of bone support due to periodontal disease, pre-endodontic and prosthetic treatment, can result in reduced ability of the tooth to withstand functional stresses.

IATROGENIC ETIOLOGICAL FACTORS

Iatrogenic factors contribute to the susceptibility of a root to fracture. These factors are a combination of the residual tooth structure after dentin removal from the coronal area[64] and residual dentin thickness after completion of all intracanal procedures combined, along with the stress generated during these procedures, such as lateral condensation of gutta-percha, followed by post placement.[5,10,65–67] A common procedure is the enlargement of the coronal third of the root canal as an early step in root canal preparation. The result is loss of tooth structure that may weaken the root. Obviously, enlargement of the coronal third of the root canal enables better access to the apical part of the canal, but excessive removal of dentin during root canal and post space preparation can leave thin dentin walls[48,49] (see Figure 13A).

The risk of root fracture may increase as well with the use of spreaders during gutta-percha obturation. The stress generated during lateral condensation of gutta-percha may be from the wedging effect of the spreader, either on the canal walls or through the gutta-percha.[66] The spreader design or the metal used can also be a contributing factor for a VRF.[68] Since the introduction of NiTi instruments for canal preparation, a NiTi spreader has been designed that is more elastic than stainless steel spreaders; it exerts less strain in the root canal during lateral condensation.[69] The exact contribution of stress to the inception of a fracture in clinical situations is not known. What is known is that the vertical load during obturation is only between 1 and 3 kg.[65,66,70]

An important correlation has been shown by Sathorn et al.[71,72] between the anatomy of the root canals, as a major predisposing factor, and major operative factors, such as stress distribution, residual dentin thickness, and types of canal preparation. Canal diameter, along with shape and proximal concavity, even plays a more major role in fracture susceptibility. On the other hand, residual dentin thickness, although an important factor in itself, does not appear to increase the susceptibility for fracture.

Another factor playing a major role in fracture susceptibility is canal irregularities. Their removal will decrease VRF susceptibility. Recently, Zandbiglari et al.[73] addressed the correlation of canal preparation to fracture susceptibility and stated that roots may be weakened significantly by preparation with greater taper instruments. Rundquist and Versluis[53] have shown that although more dentin may be removed, increased taper of the root canal causes less stress during obturation. However, this stress increases during masticatory loading.

Restorative procedures after root canal therapy, such as post space preparation, selection of tapered posts, traumatic seating of the post creating hydrostatic pressure, and expansion of posts due to corrosion, are additional iatrogenic causes for VRF.[5,29,74–76] Post space preparation and post selection are of utmost importance, especially in VRF-susceptible teeth because of their specific cross-section contours and curvatures.[42,43,77]

Retrospective surveys of success and failure of restored endodontically treated teeth have shown that 10% of failures are due to root fractures.[78,79] The percentage of failures by root fracture is much higher with threaded posts.[80] The selection of VRF-susceptible teeth, such as maxillary premolars as post-retained bridge abutments, should also be considered with caution[9,81,82] (Figure 14A,B).

Treatment

The constant ingress of bacteria into VRFs provides an open pathway from the oral cavity to the supporting periodontal and alveolar tissues. Various treatment modalities have been suggested to save vertically fractured roots, but all of them have proved to be ineffective in the long run.[7,83–88] In posterior teeth, a fractured root can sometimes be amputated and the other roots retained with a new coronal restoration, or partially resected to provide some additional use of the tooth. In recent in vitro studies, some epoxy resin sealers have shown a positive effect in increasing the resistance of roots against fracture.[52,89]

Prevention

As described above, a fractured root cannot be repaired despite some anecdotal sporadic attempts. Prevention, knowledge, and appreciation of the multifactorial etiology of fractures in endodontically treated teeth are the best solutions that the clinician can accomplish by

1. recognizing the roots and teeth susceptible to fracture;
2. preserving as much tooth structure as possible, thus finding the necessary "golden path" between the need to achieve canal cleanliness and removing only the amount of dentin necessary for the specific intracanal procedure;
3. judicious use of force during obturation of the root canal space;
4. placing a post only when necessary for additional core support;
5. using dowels with a parallel wall with passive fit and round edges, or fiber-reinforced resin-based composite posts when indicated[90,91]; and
6. preparing coronal restoration ferrules with a vertical length of 1.5 to 2 mm on sound dentin.

Acknowledgments

The author thanks Ms. R. Lazar for editorial assistance and Dr. I. Tsesis for technical assistance.

References

1. Chan CP, Lin CP, Tseng SC, Jeng JH. Vertical root fracture in endodontically versus non-endodontically treated teeth. Oral Surg Oral Med Oral Pathol Oral Radiol Endod 1999;87:504–7.
2. American Association of Endodontists. Endodontics: Colleagues for excellence– Cracking the cracked tooth code. Chicago, IL: American Association of Endodontists; Fall/Winter 1997.
3. Walton RE, Michelich RJ, Smith GN. The histopathogenesis of vertical root fractures. J Endod 1984;10:48–56.
4. Bergenholtz G, Hasselgren G. Endodontics and periodontics. In: Lindhe J, editor. Clinical periodontology and implant dentistry. 4th ed. Copenhagen: Munksgaard 2003.
5. Meister F, Lommel TJ, Gerstein H. Diagnosis and possible causes of vertical root fractures. Oral Surg Oral Med Oral Pathol Oral Radiol Endod 1980;49:243–53.
6. Tamse A. Iatrogenic vertical root fractures in endodontically treated teeth. Endod Dent Traumatol 1988;4:190–6.
7. Moule AJ, Kahler B. Diagnosis and management of teeth with vertical fractures. Aust Dent J 1999;44:75–87.
8. Tamse A, Fuss Z, Lustig J, Kaplavi J. An evaluation of endodontically treated vertically fractured teeth. J Endod 1999;25:506–8.
9. Tamse A, Zilburg I, Halpern J. Vertical fractures in adjacent maxillary premolars. An endodontic–prosthetic perplexity. Int Endod J 1998;31:127–32.
10. Fuss Z, Lustig J, Katz A, Tamse A. An evaluation of endodontically treated vertically fractured roots: impact of operative procedures. J Endod 2001;1:46–8.
11. Sedgley CM, Messer HH. Are endodontically treated teeth more brittle? J Endod 1992;18:332–5.
12. Morfis AS. Vertical root fractures. Oral Surg Oral Med Oral Pathol Oral Radiol Endod 1990;68:631–5.
13. Sjögren U, Högglund B, Sundqvist G, Wing K. Factors affecting long term results of endodontic treatment. J Endod 1990;16:498–504.
14. Vire DE. Failure of endodontically treated teeth: classification and evaluation. J Endod 1991;17:338–42.
15. Caplan DJ, Weintraub JA. Factors related to loss of root canal filled teeth. J Public Health Dent 1997;57:31–9.
16. Gher ME, Dunlap RM, Anderson MH, Huhl LV. Clinical survey of fractured teeth. J Am Dent Assoc 1987;117:174–7.
17. Bergman B, Lundquist P, Sjögren U, Sundquist G. Restorative and endodontic results after treatment with cast posts and cores. J Prosthet Dent 1989;61:10–5.

86. Aesert G. Management of vertical root fractures. Endod Pract 2001;4:32–8.

87. Kawai K, Masaka N. Vertical root fracture treated by bonding fragments and rotational replantation. Dent Traumatol 2002;18:42–5.

88. Kudou Y, Kubota M. Replantation with intentional rotation of complete vertically fractured root using adhesive resin. Dent Traumatol 2003;18:115–17.

89. Lertchirakarn V, Timyan A, Messer HH. Effects of root canal sealers on vertical root fracture resistance of endodontically treated teeth. J Endod 2002;28:217–19.

90. Christensen GJ. Post concepts are changing. J Am Dent Assoc 2004;135:1308–10.

91. Schwartz RS, Robbins JW. Post placement and restoration of endodontically treated teeth: A literature review. J Endod 2004;30:289–301.

MANAGEMENT

CHAPTER 21

TREATMENT OF ENDODONTIC INFECTIONS, CYSTS, AND FLARE-UPS

J. CRAIG BAUMGARTNER, PAUL A. ROSENBERG, MICHAEL M. HOEN, LOUIS M. LIN

Periapical abscesses and cellulitis occur when microbes invade these tissues. The severity of the periapical infections is related to the virulence of the organisms and host resistance. An abscess is a localized collection of pus within a tissue or confined space.[1] Cellulitis is a symptomatic edematous inflammatory process that spreads diffusely through connective tissue and fascial planes.[1] Clinically, cellulitis and the associated abscess should be considered a continuum of the infectious inflammatory process.

After bacteria have invaded periapical tissues, an otherwise healthy patient will eventually exhibit clinical signs and symptoms of infection. The patient may experience swelling and mild to severe pain. As the infection and inflammatory response spreads further, the patient may experience systemic signs and symptoms such as chills, fever, lymphadenopathy, nausea, and headache. The tooth that is the reservoir of the endodontic infection will usually be sensitive to biting and percussion (touch), and eventually the overlying tissues will be sensitive to palpation. There may or may not be radiographic evidence of periapical disease. The pulp cavity of an infected tooth is the source of the infection spreading to periapical tissues and for secondary (metastatic) infection that may spread to fascial spaces of the head and neck. Appropriate treatment includes removing the reservoir of infection either by debridement of the infected root canal system or removal of the tooth, along with drainage from swollen tissues. Adjunctive pharmacotherapeutics may also be indicated with cellulitis, progressive swellings, and systemic signs and symptoms of infection.

The spread of infection into fascial spaces may be life-threatening. There are potential spaces between anatomic structures of the head and neck which may be involved in infection and inflammation. These fascial spaces are recognized by their anatomic boundaries.[2] An anatomic space that may be involved in mandibular infections is the mandibular buccal vestibule. The swelling occurs between the cortical plate and the buccinator muscle in the posterior of the mandible and the mentalis muscle in the anterior. Mandibular anterior teeth may produce swelling of the mental or submental spaces (Figure 1). The mental space is located between the mentalis muscle and the

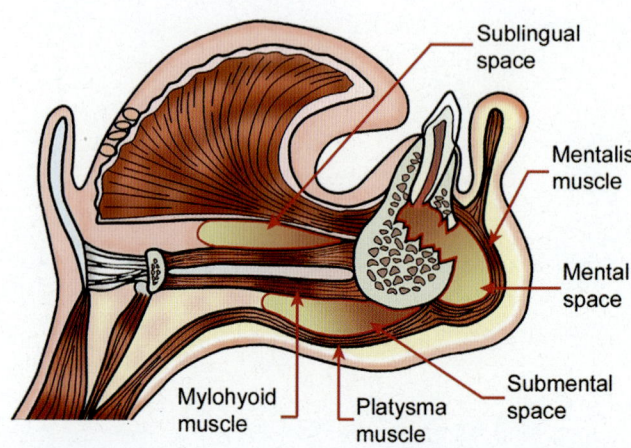

Figure 1 Mental, submental, and sublingual spaces. Courtesy Dr. Wm. Girsch.

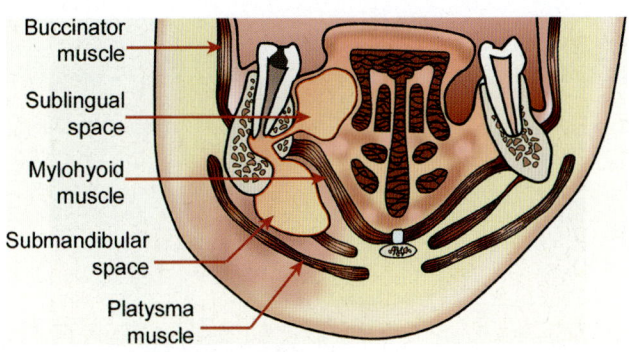

Figure 2 Submandibular and sublingual spaces. Courtesy Dr. Wm. Girsch.

platysma muscle. The submental space is between the mylohyoid muscle and the platysma muscle. Mandibular anterior teeth may also lead to swelling in the sublingual space (see Figure 1) located between the floor of the mouth and the inferiorly located mylohyoid muscle. The submandibular space (Figure 2) is between the mylohyoid and the platysma muscles. The source of infection in this space is usually a mandibular posterior tooth. Ludwig's angina is an infection that includes the submental, sublingual, and submandibular spaces. Cellulitis may extend to the pharyngeal and cervical spaces and produce airway obstruction.

Anatomic spaces involved in lateral face swelling include the maxillary buccal vestibule. This space is located between the cortical plate of the maxilla and the superior attachment of the buccinator muscle and associated with infections of maxillary posterior teeth. The buccal space (Figure 3) is between the lateral surface of the buccinator muscle and the overlying skin of the cheek. The source of the infection may be either a maxillary or a mandibular posterior tooth. The submasseteric space (see Figure 3) lies between the lateral surface of the ramus of the mandible and the masseter muscle. The source of the infection is usually the mandibular third molar. The deep temporal space is between the lateral surface of the skull and the medial surface of the temporal muscle while the superficial temporal space lies between the temporal muscle and the overlying fascia.

Anatomic spaces involved in the pharyngeal and cervical areas include the pterygomandibular space (see Figure 3). That space is usually associated with infection of the mandibular second or third molars. The pterygomandibular space is bounded by the lateral surface of the medial pterygoid muscle and the medial surface of the mandible. The bilateral parapharyngeal space is between the medial surface of the medial pterygoid muscle and the superior constrictor muscle. The superior border is the base of the skull and the inferior border is the hyoid bone. The carotid space contains the carotid artery, internal jugular vein, and the vagus nerve. The retropharyngeal space (Figure 4) is posterior to the superior constrictor muscle and extends to the mediastinum. The pretracheal space surrounds the trachea and extends from the thyroid cartilage to the level of the aortic arch. The retrovisceral space extends from the base of the skull into the posterior mediastinum. The danger space (see Figure 4) extends from the base of the skull into the posterior mediastinum. The prevertebral space surrounds the vertebral column.

The anatomic spaces involved in midface swellings are the palate, the base of the upper lip, the

Figure 3 Buccal, submasseteric, pterygomandibular, and parapharyngeal spaces. Courtesy Dr. Wm. Girsch.

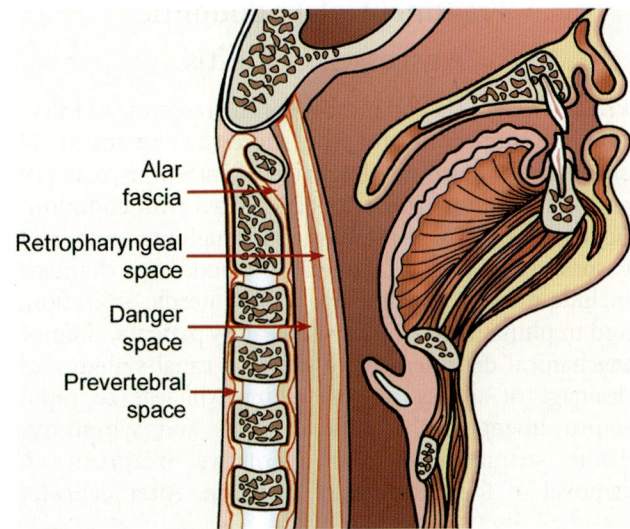

Figure 4 Pretracheal, prevertebral, and danger spaces. Courtesy Dr. Wm. Girsch.

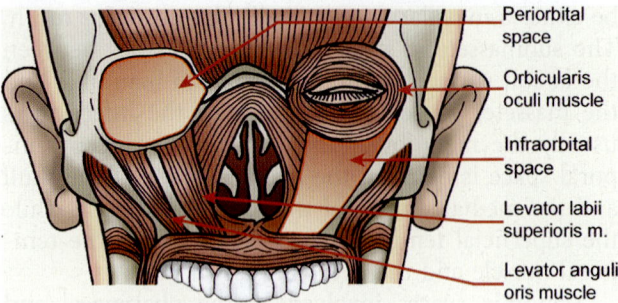

Figure 5 Periorbital and canine spaces. Courtesy Dr. Wm. Girsch.

infraorbital (canine) space, and the periorbital spaces. The source of infection for the palate is the maxillary teeth. Swelling of the base of the nose is typically caused by a maxillary central incisor with its root apex above the attachment of the orbicularis oris muscle. The infraorbital space (Figure 5) is between the levator anguli oris muscle and the levator labii superioris muscle. The source of the infection is usually the maxillary cuspid or first premolar. The periorbital space lies deep to the orbicularis oculi muscle and becomes involved as a result of the spread of infection from the buccal or infraorbital space. Infections of the midface are of special concern because of the possibility that they may result in cavernous sinus thrombosis. If the inflammation and resulting edema cause blood to back up into the cavernous sinus, the infected thrombi may escape into circulation and produce a life-threatening event.

Treatment of Endodontic Abscesses/Cellulitis

Prompt diagnosis and removal of the reservoir of infection are important for the successful treatment of endodontic infections. Drainage of infectious material and inflammatory mediators associated with endodontic infections may be established through the tooth, soft tissues, or alveolus. Surgical methods for drainage include incision for drainage (I&D), needle aspiration, and trephination. In otherwise healthy patients, chemomechanical debridement of the root canal system and drainage of an associated swelling will lead to rapid improvement of the patient's signs and symptoms. Tooth extraction is the alternative treatment to removal of the reservoir of infection. After debride-

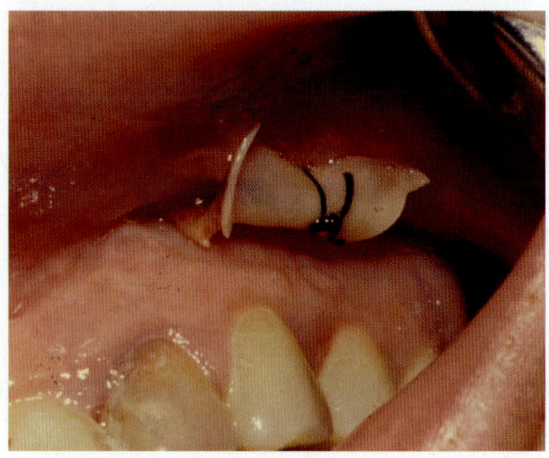

Figure 6 Drain sutured in place. Courtesy Dr. Craig Baumgartner.

ment of the root canal system, I&D is indicated for periapical swellings. A recent study found that even with drainage through the access opening into the pulp cavity, there was not a significant reduction in pain, percussion pain, swelling, or number of analgesics taken.[3]

INCISION FOR DRAINAGE

Successful resolution of an infection requires removal of the source of infection and drainage of the accumulated exudate. Drainage from a swelling caused by an abscess/cellulitis decreases the number of bacteria, bacterial by-products, and inflammatory mediators associated with the swelling. The removal of pockets of purulence and edematous fluid also improves circulation and allows delivery of prescribed antibiotics in a minimum inhibitory concentration. An I&D or needle aspiration of a swelling associated with cellulitis will often reveal accumulations of purulence consistent with an abscess. An incision provides a pathway for additional drainage to prevent the further spread of the abscess/cellulitis. Nerve block anesthesia should be used and if necessary supplemented with local infiltration (see Chapter 22).

To achieve drainage from a swelling, a stab incision through the periosteum is made at the most dependent site of the swelling. A periosteal elevator or hemostat is then used for blunt dissection to allow drainage of any accumulated exudate and inflammatory mediators. Except for very small localized swellings, a drain should be sutured into place (Figure 6).

Chapter 21 / Treatment of Endodontic Infections, Cysts, and Flare-ups / **693**

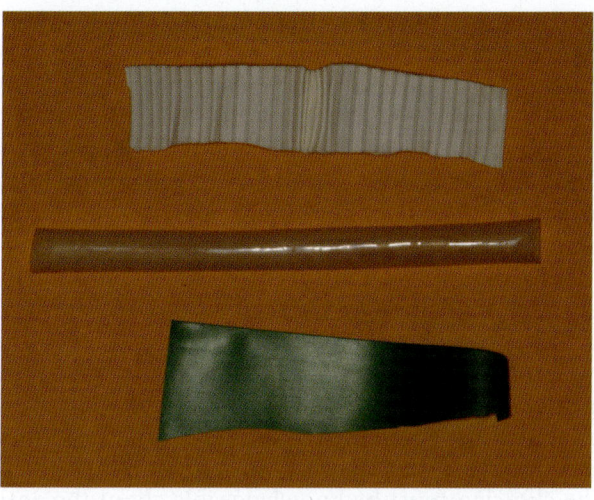

Figure 7 Top drain is a capillary drain, middle is a penrose drain, bottom is a rubber dam drain. Courtesy Dr. Craig Baumgartner.

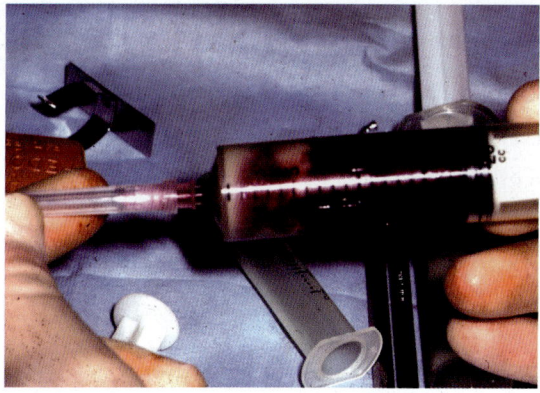

Figure 8 Aspirate from abscess/cellulitis. Courtesy Dr. Mike Hoen.

Drains may be a piece of rubber dam, a Penrose drain, or a capillary drain (Figure 7). The latter is ribbed and seems to stay under the tissues better than the non-ribbed drains. Non-latex drains should be used for those allergic or sensitive to latex. A sutured drain keeps the incision open for continued drainage and encourages compliance by the patient to return for follow-up evaluations. The use of warm intraoral rinses may help promote drainage. The drain can usually be removed in 1 or 2 days when there is improvement in the patient's clinical signs and symptoms. Consultation with, and referral to other specialists in the management of facial infections, is indicated for severe or persistent infections.

NEEDLE ASPIRATION

Needle aspiration may be described as the use of suction to remove fluids from a cavity or space. It is a surgical procedure that may provide information as to the presence and volume of exudate, cystic fluid, or blood. Aspirated samples may be used for microbial isolation and identification, using either culturing or molecular methods[4–6] (Figure 8). In addition, the sample may be used for immunohistochemical analysis (Figure 9). In 1995, Simon et al.[7] described the clinical use of needle aspiration for intraoral swelling as an alternative technique to I&D. Following regional and local anesthesia, the technique involved the use of a syringe with an 18-gauge needle to aspirate the contents of a swelling. Clinical advantages of needle aspiration over I&D include reduced scarring, evaluation of volume and character of the aspirate, use of the aspirate for culture and sensitivity testing, and the lack of postoperative drain removal.

ANTIBIOTICS IN ENDODONTICS

The vast majority of infections of endodontic origin can be effectively managed without the use of antibiotics. Systemically administered antibiotics are not a substitute for timely endodontic treatment. Chemomechanical debridement of the infected root canal system with drainage through the root canal and by incision and drainage of swollen tissues will decrease the bioburden so that a normal healthy patient can

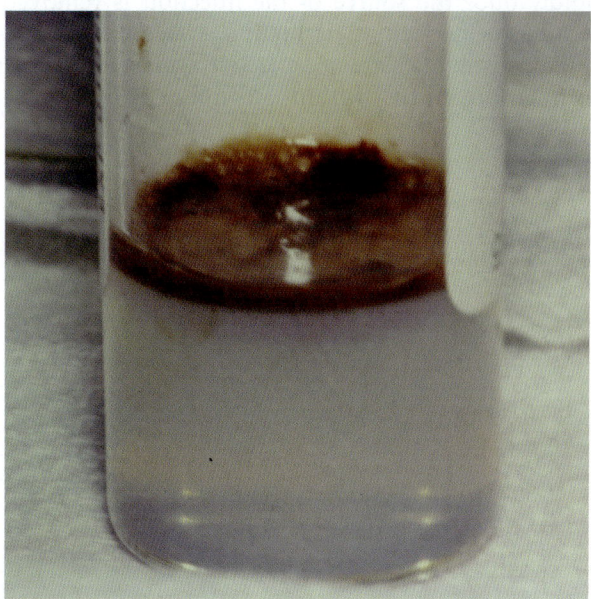

Figure 9 The aspirated sample is injected through the stopper into an anaerobic transport vial. Courtesy Dr. Craig Baumgartner.

Table 1 Conditions not Requiring Adjunctive Antibiotics
1. Pain without signs and symptoms of infection
a. Symptomatic irreversible pulpitis
b. Symptomatic apical periodontitis
2. Teeth with necrotic pulps and a radiolucency
3. Teeth with a sinus tract (chronic apical abscess)
4. Localized fluctuant swellings

begin the healing process. Antibiotics are not recommended for healthy patients with symptomatic pulpitis, symptomatic apical periodontitis, a draining sinus tract, a localized swelling of endodontic origin, or following endodontic surgery[8–13] (Table 1). An antibiotic regimen should be prescribed in conjunction with endodontic treatment when there are systemic signs and symptoms of infection or a progressive/persistent spread of infection. The presence of a fever (>100°F), malaise, cellulitis, unexplained trismus, and progressive swelling are all signs and symptoms of systemic involvement and spread of infection (Table 2). Under these circumstances, an antibiotic is indicated in addition to debridement of the root canal harboring the infecting microbes and drainage of any accumulated purulence. Patients with serious endodontic infections should be closely followed on a daily basis. Their conditions will usually improve rapidly once the source of the infection is removed. Because of the lack of circulation, systemically administered antibiotics are not effective against a reservoir of microorganisms within an infected root canal system. Furthermore, a minimum inhibitory concentration of an antibiotic may not reach an anatomic space filled with purulence and edematous fluid because of poor circulation and the diffusion gradient that it must traverse. Pus consists mainly of neutrophils, cellular debris, bacteria, bacterial by-products, enzymes, and edematous fluid. An I&D will allow drainage of the purulent material and improve circulation to the area. Drainage provides a pathway for removal of inflammatory mediators and helps prevent further spread of cellulitis.

Empirical selection of an antibiotic (antimicrobial agent) should be based on knowledge of which bacteria are most commonly associated with endodontic infections and their antibiotic susceptibility.[4,5,14–18] The clinician must be knowledgeable about the antibiotic and inform the patient of its benefits, possible side effects, and possible sequelae of failing to take the recommended dosage. A loading dose is important to provide an initial adequate therapeutic blood level of antibiotic. It should generally be continued for 2 to 3 days following resolution of the major clinical signs and symptoms of the infection. Following removal of the source of the infection and adjunctive antibiotic therapy, significant improvement in the patient's status should be seen in 24 to 48 hours. A prescription written for a 7-day regimen of antibiotic therapy is usually adequate.

Penicillin VK is the antibiotic of choice because of its effectiveness against both facultative and anaerobic microorganisms commonly found in polymicrobial endodontic infections.[4,5,14,17–19] However, up to 10% of the population may be allergic to this medication, so a careful history of drug hypersensitivity is important. A loading dose of 1,000 mg of penicillin VK should be orally administered followed by 500 mg every 4 to 6 hours.

Amoxicillin has an expanded spectrum of activity that includes bacteria not routinely associated with infections of endodontic origin.[4,5,15,16] It is rapidly absorbed and provides sustained serum levels which make it ideal for use with medically compromised patients who require antibiotic prophylaxis. The usual oral dosage for amoxicillin to treat infections is 1,000-mg loading dose followed by 500 mg every 8 hours. An alternate dosage for amoxicillin is 875 mg every 12 hours.

Clavulanate is a competitive inhibitor of beta-lactamase. Antibiotic susceptibility tests have shown excellent results against bacteria isolated from endodontic infections when clavulanate is used in combination with amoxicillin (Augmentin).[4,5,15,16] This combination should be considered for patients who

Table 2 Indications for Adjunctive Antibiotics (Antimicrobial Therapy)
1. Systemic involvement
Fever >100°F.
Malaise
Lymphadenopathy
Trismus
2. Progressive infections
Increased swelling
Cellulitis
Osteomyelitis
3. Persistent infections

are immunocompromised. The usual oral dosage for amoxicillin with clavulanate is 1,000-mg loading dose followed by 500 mg every 8 hours. An alternate dosage is 875 mg every 12 hours.

Erythromycin has traditionally been the alternative choice for patients allergic to penicillin, but it is not effective against anaerobes associated with endodontic infections. Clarithromycin and azithromycin are macrolides like erythromycin, with some advantages over the latter. They have a spectrum of antimicrobial activity that includes facultative bacteria and some anaerobic bacteria associated with infections of endodontic origin. They also have less gastrointestinal upset than erythromycin. The oral dosage for clarithromycin is a 500-mg loading dose followed by 250 mg every 12 hours. The oral dosage for azithromycin is a 500-mg loading dose followed by 250 mg once a day.

Clindamycin is effective against both facultative and strict anaerobic bacteria associated with endodontic infections. It is well distributed throughout the body, especially to bone, where its concentration approaches that of plasma. Both penicillin and clindamycin have been shown to produce good results in treating odontogenic infections.[4,5,20] Clindamycin is rapidly absorbed even in the presence of food in the stomach.[21] The oral adult dosage for serious endodontic infections is a 600-mg loading dose followed by 300 mg every 6 hours.

Metronidazole is a nitroimidazole that is active against parasites and anaerobic bacteria. However, it is ineffective against facultative bacteria.[4,5,22] It is a valuable antimicrobial agent in combination with penicillin when penicillin alone has been ineffective.[22] The usual oral dosage for metronidazole is a 1,000-mg loading dose followed by 500 mg every 6 hours. Consultation with, and referral to other specialists in the management of facial infections, is indicated for severe or persistent infections.

Cephalosporins are usually not indicated for the treatment of endodontic infections. First-generation cephalosporins do not have activity against the anaerobes usually involved in endodontic infections. Second-generation cephalosporins have some efficacy for anaerobes, however, there is a possibility of cross-allergenicity of cephalosporins with penicillin.

Doxycycline occasionally may be indicated when the above antibiotics are contraindicated. However, many strains of bacteria have become resistant to the tetracyclines.

Ciprofloxacin is a quinilone antibiotic that is not effective against anaerobic bacteria usually found in endodontic infections. With a persistent infection, it may be indicated if culture and sensitivity tests demonstrated the presence of susceptible organisms.

PROPHYLACTIC ANTIBIOTICS FOR MEDICALLY COMPROMISED PATIENTS

Prophylactic antibiotic coverage may be indicated for medically compromised patients requiring endodontic treatment. The American Heart Association (AHA) and the American Academy of Orthopaedic Surgeons have made guidelines for prophylactic antibiotic coverage.[23,24] The guidelines are meant to aid practitioners but are not intended as the standard of care or as a substitute for clinical judgment. The incidence of endocarditis following most procedures on patients with underlying cardiac disease is low (see Chapter 7 "Microbiology of Endodontic Disease").

A reasonable approach for prescribing prophylactic antibiotics considers the degree to which the underlying disease creates a risk for endocarditis, the apparent risk for producing a bacteremia, adverse reactions to the prophylactic antibiotic, and the cost-benefit aspect of the regimen.[23] Antibiotic prophylaxis is employed to prevent surgical infections or their postoperative sequelae, to prevent metastatic bacteremias, and to prevent accusation that "all was not done for the patient."[25] It is suspected that antibiotic prophylaxis is often prescribed to prevent malpractice claims.[25]

How antibiotics quickly kill bacteria in the blood is difficult to answer when many antibiotics are only effective with actively dividing bacteria. It is speculated that antibiotics may reduce metastatic infections by preventing adhesion of bacteria to tissues or inhibiting growth after attachment.[26] The principles of antibiotic prophylaxis state that the antibiotic must be in the system prior to an invasive procedure. If a patient has not taken the prescribed antibiotic, he or she should be rescheduled or wait an hour after administration of the antibiotic for treatment. However, there is data to support the use of an antibiotic up to 2 hours after the onset of bacteremia.[25]

The incidence of bacteremia has been shown to be low during root canal therapy. A transient bacteremia can result from the extrusion of microorganisms from the root canal to the periapical tissues of the tooth.[27–31] In addition, positioning rubber dam clamps and accomplishing other dental procedures may produce bleeding and can lead to a bacteremia. Medically compromised dental patients who are at risk of infection should receive a regimen of antibiotics that either follows the recommendations of the AHA or an alternate regimen determined in consultation with the patients' physicians.[23] Chapter 24 gives the antibiotic regimens recommended for dental procedures. It is believed that amoxicillin, ampicillin, and penicillin V are equally effective against alpha-hemolytic streptococci; however, amoxicillin is recommended because it is better absorbed from the gastrointestinal tract and provides higher and more sustained serum levels.[23]

For cardiac conditions associated with endocarditis, prophylaxis is recommended for both non-surgical and surgical endodontic procedures.[23] Antibiotic prophylaxis is recommended for cardiac conditions associated with endocarditis at a high or risk category (see Chapter 24). Dental procedures for which antibiotic prophylaxis is recommended (see Chapter 24) include endodontic instrumentation beyond the apex or surgery, but not intracanal endodontic treatment, post-placement and buildup.[23] From a practical standpoint, it is difficult to determine with certainty that endodontic instruments do not pass beyond the apical foramen. Also included for prophylaxis antibiotics is intraligamentary period-ontal ligament (PDL) local anesthetic injections, but not non-intraligamentary ones.[23]

In 2003, a joint committee of the American Dental Association and American Academy of Orthopaedic Surgeons published their first advisory statement on antibiotic prophylaxis for patients with prosthetic joints. The dental procedures of concern and the antibiotic regimens are the same as for endocarditis Chapter 24. Patients of potential increased risk of having a hematogenous total joint infection include all patients during the first 2 years following joint replacement, immunocompromised/immunosuppressed patients, and patients with comorbidities as shown in Chapter 24.[32]

COLLECTION OF A MICROBIAL SAMPLE

Adjunctive antibiotic therapy for endodontic infections is most often prescribed empirically based on knowledge of the bacteria most often associated with endodontic infections. At times, culturing may provide valuable information to better select the appropriate antibiotic regimen. For example, an immunocompromised/immunosuppressed patient (not immunocompetent) or patients at high risk of developing infections (e.g., history of infective endocarditis) following a bacteremia require close monitoring. These patients may have an infection caused by bacteria usually not associated with the oral cavity. Other examples include a seemingly healthy patient who has persistent or progressive symptoms following surgical or non-surgical endodontic treatment. An aseptic microbial sample from a root canal is collected by first isolating the tooth with a rubber dam and disinfecting the tooth surface and rubber dam with sodium hypochlorite or other disinfectant. Sterile burs and instruments must be used to gain access to the root canal system. Intracanal irrigation should not be used until after the microbial sample has been taken. If there is drainage from the canal, it may be sampled with a sterile paper point or aspirated into a sterile syringe with a sterile 18- to 25-gauge needle, depending on the viscosity of the exudate. The aspirate should either be taken immediately to a microbiology laboratory in the syringe or injected into pre-reduced transport media. To sample a dry root canal, a sterile syringe should be used to place some pre-reduced transport medium into the canal. A sterile endodontic instrument is then used to scrape the walls of the canal to suspend microorganisms into the medium.

To prevent contamination by the normal oral flora, a microbial sample from a soft tissue swelling should be obtained before making an I&D. Once profound anesthesia is achieved, the surface of the mucosa should be dried and disinfected with an iodophor swab. A sterile 16- to 20-gauge needle and syringe is used to aspirate the exudate. The aspirate should be handled as described above. A sample can be collected on a swab after the I&D has been made, but great care must be taken to prevent microbial contamination with normal oral flora. After collecting the specimen on a swab, it should be quickly placed in pre-reduced medium for transport to the laboratory.

Good communication with the laboratory personnel is important. The sample should be Gram-stained to demonstrate which types of microorganisms predominate. The culture results should show the prominent isolated microorganisms and not just be identified as "normal oral flora." Antibiotics can usually be chosen to treat endodontic infections based on the identification of the prominent microorganisms in the culture. With persistent infections, susceptibility testing can be undertaken to establish which antibiotics are the most effective against resistant microbial isolates. At present, it may take 1 to 2 weeks to identify anaerobes using conventional methods. Some laboratories may have molecular methods available to rapidly detect and identify known opportunistic bacteria.

CORTICAL TREPHINATION

Cortical trephination is defined as the surgical perforation of the alveolar cortical plate to release accumulated tissue exudates.[1] Its use is indicated for patients with severe pain of endodontic origin without intraoral or extraoral swelling and when drainage cannot be accomplished through the root canal, for example, in the presence of posts, filling material, or ledging. Cortical trephination involves exposing the cortical bone, making an opening in the bone, and making a pathway through the cancellous bone to the root end.[33–40] Occasionally, an instrument may be used to penetrate the mucosa and cortical plate without an incision (Figure 10A,B). Several studies have demonstrated that a patient with severe periapical pain without swelling will have significant relief following trephination.[34,41–43] A technique for trephination recommended by Henry and Fraser[41] involves a submarginal horizontal full thickness flap to access the alveolar bone, the use of a surgical high speed round bur to access the involved root apex and abscessed area, and the placement of a sutured drain.

Some studies have shown cortical trephination may not be predictable in relieving periapical pain.[36–38] A prospective randomized blinded clinical trial raised concern about the assumed clinical effectiveness of trephination.[38] In that study, pain logs were evaluated after non-surgical endodontic treatment and either real or simulated trephination. It was found that the routine use of trephination for the reduction of pain or swelling in symptomatic necrotic pulps in teeth with periapical radiolucencies was not predictable. A systematic review of the literature concerning the emergency management of acute apical periodontitis in the permanent dentition also concluded that routine cortical trephination did not show significant benefit.[44] While there is no higher level of evidence justifying the routine use of surgical trephination, there are limited instances in which it is a reasonable treatment alternative. Patients with severe periapical pain of endodontic origin without swelling may benefit from the procedure.

DECOMPRESSION: ASPIRATION AND IRRIGATION

The terms decompression and marsupialization are often used interchangeably. Decompression is the surgical exposure of a cyst wall and insertion of a tube or other type of drain to decompress the lesion during healing.[1] It is not uncommon for chronic periapical pathosis to remain clinically asymptomatic and develop a bony defect of significant size. If left undiagnosed and untreated, periapical pathosis may develop into self-perpetuating entities that erode osseous supporting structures and encroach on adjacent teeth, sinus cavities, neurovascular bundles, and even the nasal cavity. Bony lesions radiographically exceeding 200 mm^2 have a higher statistical chance of being cystic.[45] There are radicular cysts that may have progressed to the extent that they are truly independent, and non-surgical endodontic treatment may no longer be enough to result in bony healing.[46,47] When non-surgical endodontics does not resolve apical pathosis, surgical intervention is an alternative treatment recommendation.

Surgical treatment, including the enucleation of extensive bony lesions, may involve unintentional interruption of periapical vascular and neural structures, development of soft tissue defects, and damage to adjacent anatomic structures. Decompression is a more conservative treatment option that allows the progressive reduction in lesion size and may eliminate

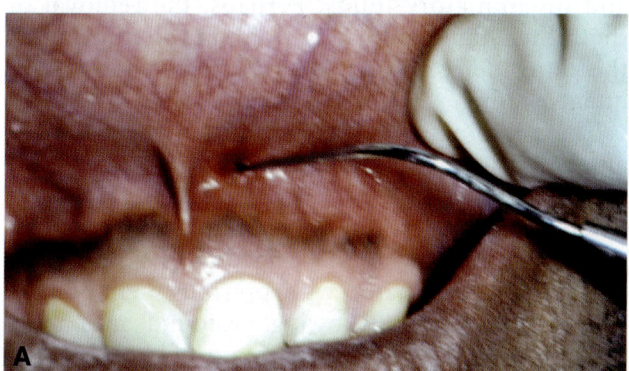
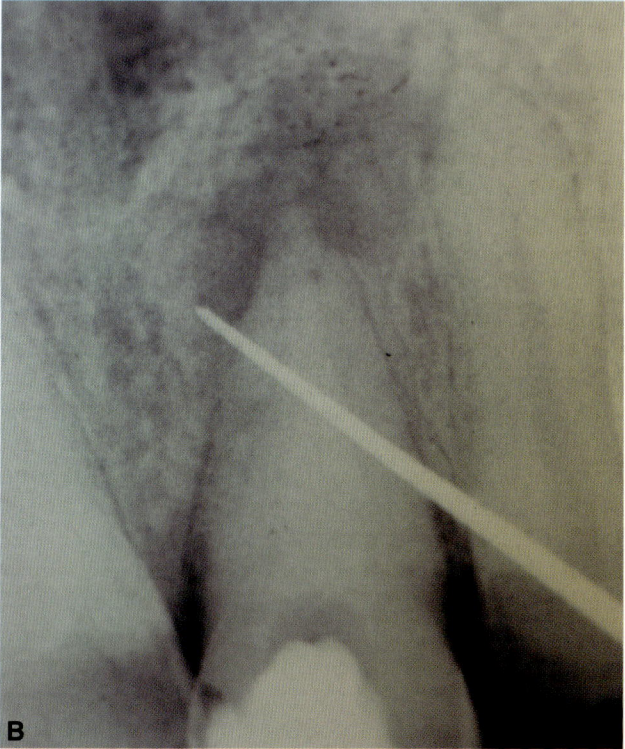

Figure 10 *A*, Trephination using a #3 spreader. *B*, Radiograph showing tip of a #3 spreader near root end. Courtesy Dr. Craig Baumgartner.

the necessity for surgical enucleation. Decompression is intended to disrupt the integrity of the lesion wall, reduce the internal osmotic pressure, and permit osseous regeneration (Figure 11).

In 1982, Suzuki[48] suggested treating jaw cysts using an irrigational technique. In that study, the contents of 36 cysts were irrigated weekly for months and even years. This irrigation method involved the use of Ringer's solution, glucose, and antibiotics. The fluids aspirated from the cysts were quantitatively analyzed for electrolytes, inorganic substances, proteins, and lipids. Irrigation of the lesions eventually resulted in the reduction in the volume and size of the cysts. The irrigation method is effective for the treatment of cysts in jaws.[48] Large cysts have been decompressed using acrylic stents, obturators, and tubing that extends into the lesion.[49–53] Acrylic stents or tubing was often left in for months with irrigation of the lesion. Neaverth and Berg[52] described several cases of large lesion decompression that lasted from several weeks to more than a year. The method used radiopaque tubing in conjunction with water irrigation by the patient. The tube was removed once there was evidence of elimination of the cystic lesion.

A surgical technique was described in case series format by Wong[54] in 1991. After flap reflection, a surgical fenestration was used to obtain some tissue for biopsy, but the majority of bony defect was left intact. Copious drainage was accomplished and the defect irrigated with saline prior to suturing. This surgical treatment was effective in producing healing while avoiding potential complications.[54] Rees[55] in 1997 reviewed and highlighted the treatment of large maxillary cysts by root canal treatment and subsequent decompression. The described technique used a drain made from surgical suction tubing. This seems to be the consensus treatment sequence currently in the dental literature. Figure 12 shows the radiographic and clinical appearance of decompression tube that was left in position for 1 week and the 6-month follow-up radiograph after non-surgical root canal filling.

A 20-patient cohort study of decompression results by Enislidis et al.[56] is perhaps the best evidence of the technique's effectiveness. The authors described the advantages as ease of treatment, confirmed diagnosis with biopsy, low morbidity, and low incidence of complications. The quickest evidence of successful decompression was related by Loushine et al.[57] in 1991. This case report related the removal of the decompression tube after only 2 days with follow-up examinations showing progressive osseous repair at 3, 6, and 12 months. The use of decompression to treat odontogenic keratocyst (OKC) has been reported by August et al.[58] A pediatric nasal airway was modified and placed in 14 OKCs for an average of 8.4 months. They were irrigated twice a day with chlorhexidine. At the time of cystectomy, 9 of 14 no longer showed histological features of OKCs. The epithelium had dedifferentiated and lost cytokeratin 10 production in 64% of the patients.

Mejia et al.[59] reported, in a case series format, the use of a vacuum system within the root canal system. The technique produced a vacuum effect capable of removing copious amounts of exudate and inflammatory fluids. Perhaps, the removal of the rather high osmolarity fluid and disruption of the bony defect lining is the impetus for subsequent healing.

The combination of aspiration and irrigation as an alternative to surgical endodontic treatment was reported by Hoen et al.[60] in 1990. This case series demonstrated successful outcomes using a single-visit aspiration and saline irrigation of non-healing bony lesions associated with previously endodontically treated teeth. Following profound anesthesia, mucosa disinfection and aspiration of the cyst contents was accomplished using a 16- or 18-gauge needle attached to a syringe. Several milliliters of viscous aspirate was routinely obtained. The aspirates were submitted for aerobic and anaerobic culturing, Gram-staining, and immunoglobulin quantification. The level of immunoglobulin (Ig) G was significantly elevated in each specimen. Above normal levels of IgG have been shown to be consistent with cyst fluid.[61] It has also been shown there is a high level of albumin and globulin in cysts compared to "granulomas".[62] No bacteria were seen or cultured from any of the aspirates. At the 1-year follow-up appointments, the patients were asymptomatic and significant bony healing was seen on radiographs. It is important to develop a clear differential diagnosis and to have timely re-evaluations of the patient's signs and symptoms to determine if further treatment is needed.[60]

An additional use of aspiration is to obtain a biopsy sample. August et al.[58] concluded that the use of needle aspiration for biopsy is a useful technique to distinguish between malignant and benign intraosseous jaw lesions. The described technique involved the use of a 10-mL syringe containing 1 or 2 mL of air attached to 23- or 25-gauge needles. Once within the lesion, suction was applied and several quick passes were performed to obtain cellular

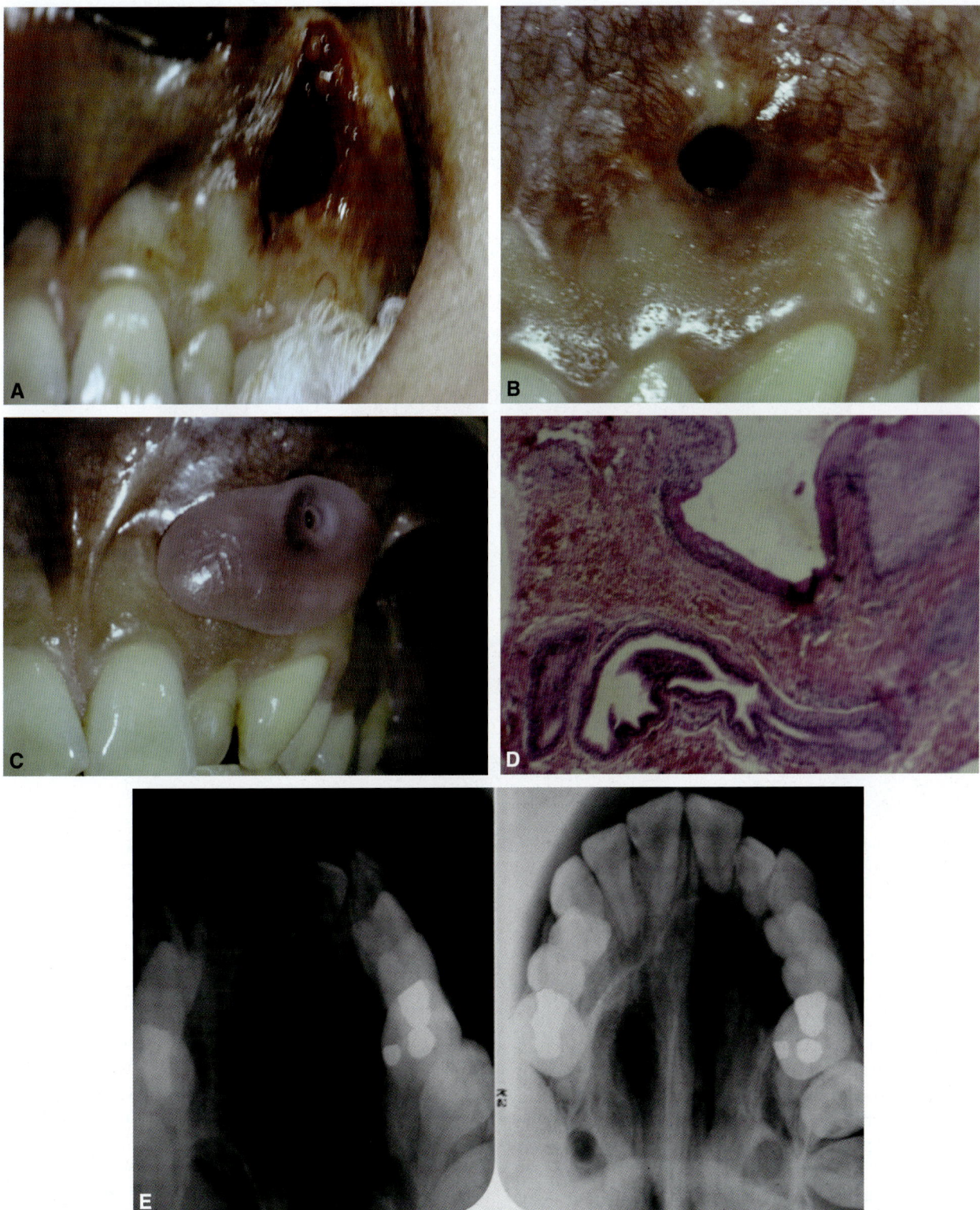

Figure 11 *A,* Surgical window into cyst. *B,* Healed surgical window. *C,* Acrylic stint in place for decompression. *D,* Biopsy from window consistent with radicular cyst. *E,* Palatal radiographs showing loss of bone on left and bone fill after 3 months of decompression. Courtesy Dr. Craig Baumgartner.

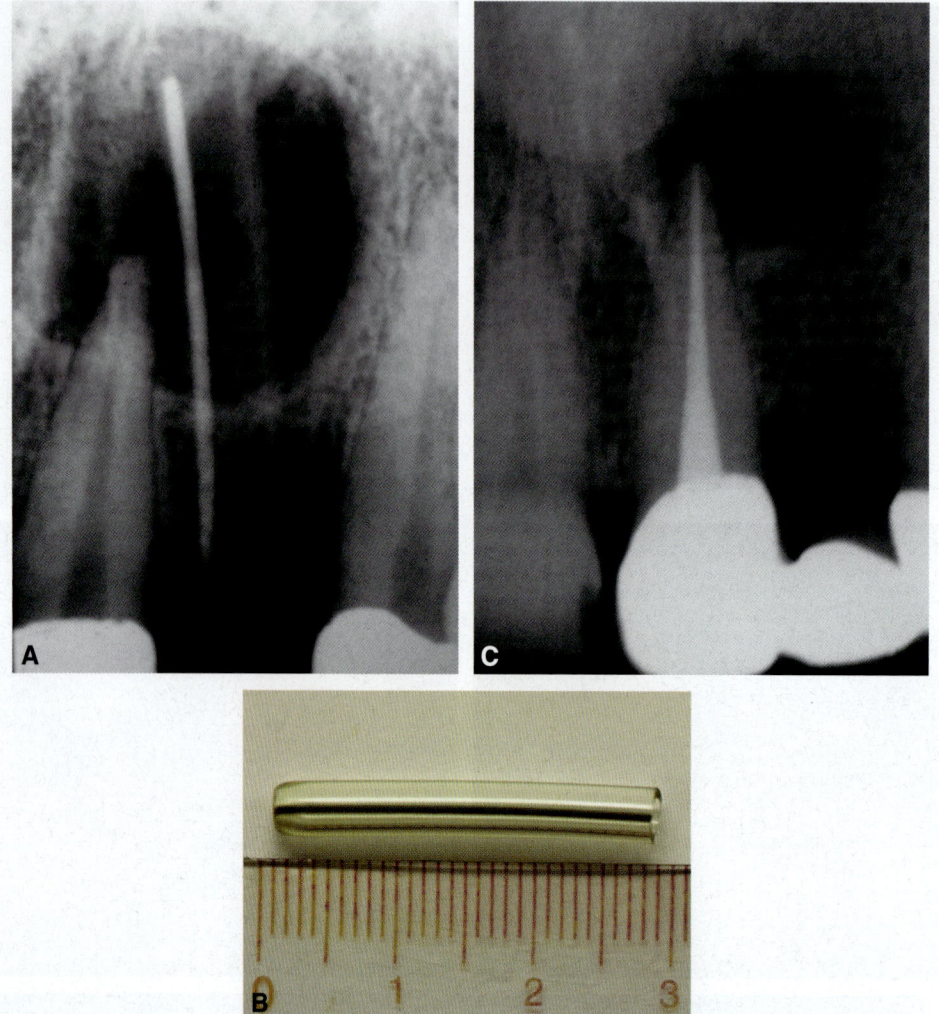

Figure 12 ***A***, A 20-mm piece of nasogastric tubing in cyst for decompression. ***B***, Tubing used next to ruler was in place for 1 week. ***C***, Six-month follow-up after non-surgical root canal filling. Courtesy Dr. Craig Baumgartner.

material. The specimens were then placed on glass slides for smear preparation. The authors suggested that aspiration may be the diagnostic tool of choice in a hospital setting due to its simplicity, suitability as an outpatient procedure, rapidity of interpretation, and minimal morbidity.[63] The accuracy of fine-needle aspiration biopsy of head and neck tumors has been reviewed in 218 patients.[64] The technique was determined to be a useful modality for the diagnosis of head and neck tumors. The use of such a technique requires coordination with a pathologist familiar with needle biopsy specimens.

Endodontic Flare-ups

The American Association of Endodontics' *Glossary of Endodontic Terms* offers the following definition: "A flare-up is an acute exacerbation of an asymptomatic pulp/or periapical pathosis after the initiation or continuation of root canal treatment."[1] Treating similar teeth in patients with comparable medical and dental histories is no assurance of a common outcome. While one patient remains asymptomatic, another may have a flare-up. The contrasting clinical outcomes may seem to occur in a random manner or lead to erroneous conclusions about the cause–effect relationship of endodontic procedures to the flare-up. The development of moderate to severe inter-appointment pain, with or without swelling, is an infrequent but challenging problem. The severe pain and swelling associated with flare-ups represent the clinical manifestation of complex pathologic changes occurring at a cellular level. There is increasing evidence pointing to multiple complex factors involved in producing a flare-up. These factors include mechanical, microbial, chemical, immunological, gender, and psychological components. The regulation of periapical inflammation is highly complex and is another factor in patients' response to endodontic procedures.[22,65–70]

The reported incidence of inter-appointment emergencies ranges from 1.4 to 19%.[66,69–74] While one study found pain and swelling occurred in as many as 20 to 40% of patients,[75] the incidence of severe pain conditions is most frequently reported at less than 5%.[65,70,76,77] Variations in the findings are the result of a number of factors. For example, differences exist in the definition of a flare-up. Some investigators have used swelling as the sole criteria for a flare-up after treating asymptomatic teeth with pulp necrosis and chronic apical periodontitis.[71] Others have used broader definitions of a flare-up which do not require swelling.[65,66,69,70] Some investigators used a retrospective approach in their research,[69,73] while others used prospective methodologies.[65,66,70] There have also been variations in sample size, treatment procedures, number of visits, endodontic medications, and other variables that are neither well-defined nor controlled.

AGE OF PATIENT

There is a lack of agreement concerning the influence of age on the incidence of flare-ups. Prospective studies assessing the incidence of flare-ups in endodontic patients found no correlation between flare-ups and the age of the patient.[70] However, a large retrospective study reached a different conclusion. Records of 2,000 patients were examined, and it was determined that when age was evaluated (20–39, 40–59, over age 60), a significant difference was found among age groups ($p = 0.0001$). Patients in the 40- to 59-year range had the most flare-ups and those under the age of 20 had the least.[69] Conflicting conclusions regarding the influence of age on the incidence of flare-ups can be attributed to variations in research methodologies, definitions, sample size, and clinical procedures.

GENDER AND FLARE-UPS

An extensive review concerning gender variation in clinical pain experience reported that women are more likely than men to experience a variety of recurrent pain.[78] In most studies, women have reported more severe levels of pain, more frequent pain, and pain of longer duration than men.[79] While a number of studies found a significantly higher percentage of females than males had postoperative pain,[69,70,75,80] others have not found gender to be a significant factor.[66,81] It should be noted that there are considerable variations between different types of clinical pain.[82] Experimental pain, produced under controlled conditions by brief, noxious stimuli, differs from procedural and post-surgical pain. These differences make the study of pain more complex.[79]

SYSTEMIC CONDITIONS

It seems reasonable to assume that host resistance, for example, medical status of the patient, is an important variable in the occurrence of flare-ups. Unfortunately, there is little conclusive evidence concerning the relationship between host resistance and flare-ups. One study found a highly significant association between flare-ups and the presence of allergies to various substances (sulfa medication, pollen, dust, and foodstuffs) and the frequency of inter-appointment pain.[69] It was suggested that this could have been due to an immediate hypersensitivity reaction occurring in the periapical tissues in response to the egress of antigens from the root canal. Although the components of the immediate hypersensitivity reactions (IgE, mast cells, and mast cell-derived mediators) have been found in periapical lesions, evidence is lacking as to whether these reactions actually occur in the periapical tissues and are responsible for inter-appointment pain.[68] An association between allergy and inter-appointment pain has not been confirmed.[70]

ANATOMIC LOCATION

Examining the incidence of flare-ups by tooth groups or between arches (maxillary versus mandibular) has usually shown no significant difference.[66,70,80] An exception was a retrospective study of 2,000 patients who had received root canal treatment for necrotic pulps. Mandibular teeth were associated with more inter-appointment emergencies than their maxillary counterparts ($p = 0.0247$). Mandibular premolars followed by mandibular incisors were the most problematic teeth after cleaning and shaping of their root canals.[69]

ANXIETY

A high incidence of fear and anxiety among patients concerning an endodontic procedure may have a marked effect on the patient's intra-operative and postoperative response to treatment. It has been shown that if a patient expects pain to occur during dental treatment, this increases the likelihood of pain being perceived.[83] An anxious patient with a previous memory of dental pain is more likely to expect pain during subsequent treatment. The slightest pressure on the tooth can be interpreted as pain and initiate a pain reaction. Anxiety may also lead to increased sympathetic activity and muscle tension that may cause more pain.[79] Patients' descriptions of their pain can be influenced by their level of anxiety and complicate the diagnostic process.[79]

A multivariate analysis of the effectiveness of local anesthesia in pediatric patients indicated anxiety as the strongest predictor of poor pain control.[84] A large retrospective study noted an association between apprehension and postoperative pain.[72] The dental procedures causing the highest levels of stress and anxiety are oral surgery and endodontics. There is a high probability that endodontic patients are anxious and expect to experience pain during treatment[79] (see Chapter 22).

PREOPERATIVE HISTORY OF THE TOOTH

Most studies have found a highly significant relationship between the presence of preoperative pain and/or swelling and the incidence of inter-appointment emergencies.[65,66,69,70] Studies have also shown a statistically significant higher incidence of flare-ups in patients taking analgesics and anti-inflammatory drugs.[66,70] It is reasonable to assume that patients taking those drugs were having preoperative pain.

PULP/PERIAPICAL STATUS

There is no universal agreement concerning the influence of pulp status and/or the presence of a periapical lesion on the incidence of inter-appointment emergencies. A prospective study found that teeth with vital pulps resulted in relatively few flare-ups, with an overall percentage of 1.3%.[66,70] In contrast, pulp necrosis correlated to an incidence of flare-ups of 6.5%, a statistically significant increase when compared to vital pulps. A low number of flare-ups following root canal treatment of teeth with vital pulps is consistent with findings in other studies.[73,74]

The periapical diagnosis of acute apical abscess was also related to significantly greater incidence of flare-ups when compared with less symptomatic or less severe apical pathosis.[70] As one might expect, the presence of a sinus tract did not correlate with flare-ups.[69,70] Investigators found the presence of a periapical radiolucency was significantly related to inter-appointment flare-ups.[65,66,71,74] These findings are in contrast to others who found a higher incidence of inter-appointment emergencies in teeth without apical radiolucencies.[69,81,85,86] The differences in findings may be attributable to variations in research methodologies, sample size, clinical procedures, patients studied, and definition of flare-ups.

NUMBER OF TREATMENT VISITS

A number of studies have determined that less postoperative pain results from a single-visit approach to endodontics than a multi-visit course of treatment.[66,87,88] Other investigators concluded that little or no difference occurred between single- and multiple-visit endodontic therapy.[70,89–91] Significant variables exist among the studies that may account for the different conclusions.

CAUSES OF INTER-APPOINTMENT PAIN

Inter-appointment pain is caused by mechanical, chemical, and/or microbial injury to the pulp or periapical tissues that are induced or exacerbated during endodontic treatment.[68,69,92] The cause of injury may vary, but the intensity of the inflammatory response is usually directly proportional to the intensity of tissue injury.[93] Mechanical and chemical injuries are often associated with iatric factors, but microbial-induced injury is a major cause of inter-appointment pain.[68,92,94] Microbial factors may be combined with iatric factors to cause inter-appointment pain. Even when endodontic procedures are performed within accepted guidelines, microbes can cause a flare-up.[68] Development of pain precipitated by microbial factors can depend on the interrelationship of several factors that are discussed in Chapter 7.

TREATMENT OF TEETH WITH VITAL AND NON-VITAL PULPS

Treatment of teeth with vital (pulpitis) and non-vital (necrotic) pulps represent pathological conditions that require different approaches to therapy.[95] It has been suggested that if the pulp is free of infection, the endodontic treatment should be completed in one visit if other factors permit. Temporization after removal of a vital pulp entails the risk of micro-leakage and contamination of the canal.[95] A high level of asepsis during pulpectomy and subsequent obturation is an essential part of treatment. Although asepsis is also an important part of treating a tooth with a non-vital pulp, the principle concern is the presence of bacteria in the root canal system. Infected canals may contain 10 to 100 million bacterial cells.[95–97] Clinicians are faced with the challenge of disinfecting the canal system through instrumentation, irrigation, and medication without pushing debris into the periapical tissues.

RE-TREATMENT CASES

Re-treatment cases, in most studies, have had a significantly higher incidence of flare-ups than conventional cases[69,70] (Figure 13). One study found an extremely high incidence of flare-ups (13.6%) in re-treatment teeth with apical periodontitis.[77] It can be hypothesized that re-treatment cases are often technically difficult to treat, and there is a tendency to push remnants of gutta-percha, solvents, and other debris into the periapical tissues. Microbes may also be pushed apically during the re-treatment process. Extrusion of infected debris or solvents into the periapical tissues during preparation of the canals is allegedly one of the principal causes of postoperative pain.[92,96,98] Re-treatment cases are usually associated with a persistent or secondary root canal infection by therapy-resistant microorganisms that may be more difficult to eradicate when compared to primary infections.[67,98,99] In contrast, others have found no statistical significance in the relation of re-treatment to flare-ups.[70]

WORKING LENGTH

The apical portion of the root canal system has been considered the most critical anatomic area with regard to the need for cleaning, disinfection, and sealing.[67,100]

Overextension should be avoided as it can result in postoperative pain.[67] Teeth with non-vital (necrotic) pulps associated with a periapical lesion, as well as root-filled teeth with recalcitrant lesions, represents a different biological challenge.[67] In these cases, microorganisms may be at or near the apical foramen and accessory foramina that are in close contact with the periapical tissues.[67,101–104] Thus, correct working length in infected teeth is essential.[67,105] Inaccurate working length or inadvertent over- or under-instrumentation can result in negative outcomes for the patient. Over-instrumentation may force infected debris into the periapical tissues eliciting a severe inflammatory response and pain. Under-instrumentation will leave microorganisms in close proximity to the apical foramina where they or their virulence factors can gain access to the periapical tissues[67,106] (see Chapter 7). Incomplete instrumentation can disrupt the balance within the microbial flora and allow previously inhibited species to overgrow.[107] If those strains of bacteria are virulent and/or reach sufficient numbers, damage to the periapical tissues may be intensified and result in an exacerbation of the lesion. Furthermore, environmental changes, induced by incomplete debridement, have the potential to activate virulence genes.[68]

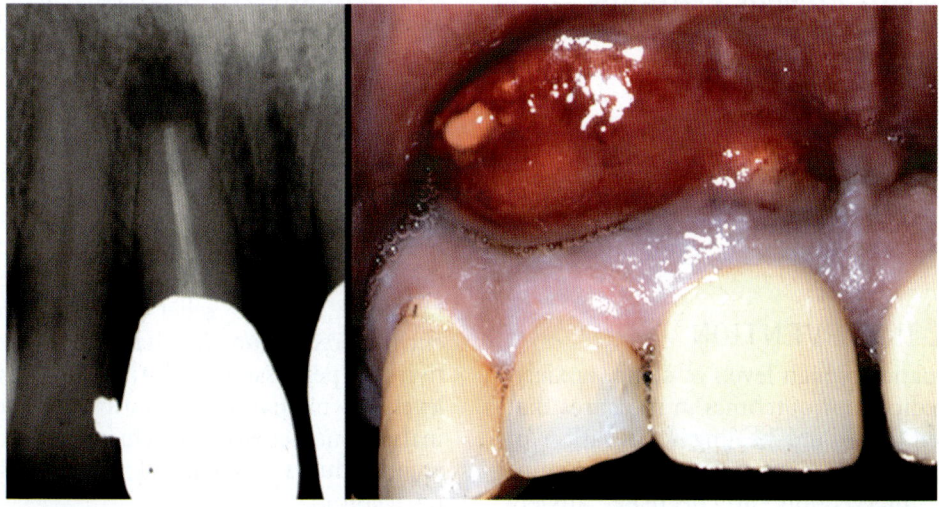

Figure 13 Swelling associated with flare-up following revision of previous endodontic treatment. Courtesy Dr. Paul Rosenberg.

A change in host resistance or microbial virulence may allow a previously asymptomatic situation to become symptomatic.[68] Clinical studies, however, have not linked incomplete canal preparation to flare-ups.[70,91,108,109]

OBTURATION

Overfilling can cause postoperative pain particularly when a substantial amount of filling material extrudes through the apical foramen. Gross overfilling involves the introduction of excess sealer (and its cytotoxic components) into the periapical tissues causing tissue damage and inflammation.[67] A recent study found that overfilling was significantly associated with increased rate of pain and percussion sensitivity in 1-week follow-up examinations in comparison with teeth not overfilled.[110] Scheduling of the obturation visit in relation to instrumentation may be another important factor. Obturation in the presence of acute apical periodontitis can be considered to be a predictor of postoperative pain. In order to avoid increased postoperative pain, patients who present for obturation but have significant acute apical periodontitis should have the procedure postponed until the tooth is more comfortable. Relief of pain can be achieved by treatment directed at reducing tissue levels of factors that stimulate peripheral terminals of nociceptors or by reducing mechanical stimulation of sensitized nociceptors (e.g., occlusal adjustment). Thus by deferring obturation of a tooth with pericementitis, further stimulation of sensitized nociceptors is avoided.[111,112]

Strategies to Prevent Flare-ups

ANXIETY REDUCTION

The causes of endodontic flare-ups are varied, and an effective preventive strategy must be multifaceted (see Chapter 23). There is a well-documented relationship between anxiety, pain threshold, and postoperative pain.[72,79,83,84]

BEHAVIORAL INTERVENTION

In preoperative patients, high levels of stress, anxiety, or pessimism predict poor outcomes in measures that range from speed of wound healing to duration of hospital stay. Over 200 studies indicate that preemptive behavioral intervention, to decrease anxiety before and after surgery, reduces postoperative pain intensity and intake of analgesics improves treatment compliance, cardiovascular and respiratory indices, and accelerates recovery.[113] In a landmark study, it was found that preoperative discussion of likely postsurgical treatments and associated discomfort halved the requirement for postoperative morphine and reduced time to discharge. Patients in that study also received instructions in a relaxation technique.[114]

Providing information about the procedure is an important step in preparing patients for endodontic treatment. Information about profound dental anesthesia and preventive pain strategies is an important anxiety reduction technique. Perhaps most importantly, the dentist should assure the patient that pain prevention is a primary concern. It was determined that patients given a running commentary concerning procedures and associated sensations rated themselves as less anxious and experiencing less pain than a normal control group.[115] Information about sensations experienced during treatment as well as a description of procedures appears to have a significant impact in reducing patient anxiety.[115] Patients should not be allowed to watch surgical procedures in a mirror.

OCCLUSAL REDUCTION

Occlusal reduction is a valuable pain preventive strategy in appropriate cases.[116,117] Some earlier studies raised questions concerning the value of prophylactic occlusal reduction as a pain preventive measure.[118,119] The results of a more recent study indicated that occlusal reduction should result in less post-treatment pain in patients whose teeth exhibit pulp vitality, preoperative pain, percussion pain, or absence of a periapical radiolucency.[120] While the presence of all four conditions is the strongest predictor, the presence of any one or more of the conditions is enough to indicate the need for occlusal reduction (Figure 14).

Occlusal reduction when performed in appropriate cases is a highly predictable, simple strategy for the prevention of postoperative pain and relief of pain due to acute apical periodontitis. There is a biologic rationale for the relief of pain provided by the occlusal reduction. Mechanical allodynia (i.e., sensitivity to percussion or biting forces) is due to tissue levels of mediators that stimulate peripheral terminals of nociceptors. Occlusal adjustment, in either arch, reduces mechanical stimulation of sensitized nociceptors.[120,121]

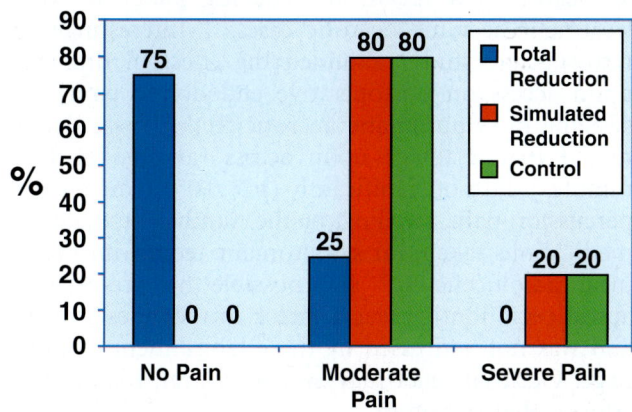

Figure 14 Effect of occlusal reduction on pain. Courtesy Dr. Paul Rosenberg.

Pharmacologic Strategies for Flare-ups

ANTIBIOTICS

Antibiotics are frequently prescribed to endodontic patients without a rational biologic basis.[122,123] An evidence-based review determined that the use of systemic antibiotics for the prevention of post-treatment endodontic pain should be discouraged.[124] Antibiotic treatment is generally not recommended for healthy patients with localized endodontic infections. Systemic antibiotics should be considered if there is a spreading infection that indicates failure of local host responses to control bacterial irritants or the patient has a medical condition that compromises defense mechanisms and could expose the patient to higher systemic risks.[124]

NSAIDS AND ACETOMINOPHEN

Nonsteroidal anti-inflammatory drugs (NSAIDs) have been shown to be effective for managing pulpal and periapical pain.[111,125] However, due to the renal effects of NSAIDs as well as interactions with many anti-hypertensive drugs, acetaminophen should be considered for post-treatment pain in patients with known sensitivity to NSAIDs or aspirin. Acetaminophen should also be considered for those with the following disorders: ulcers, ulcerative colitis, asthma, or hypertension. Pretreatment with NSAIDs or acetaminophen has also been shown to be effective for reducing postoperative pain.[68,121] Pretreatment with NSAIDs for irreversible pulpitis should have the effect of reducing pulpal levels of the inflammatory mediator prostaglandin E2 (PGE2).[68,71]

It is advisable to have endodontic patients take their analgesics "by the clock" rather than on an "as needed basis".[121] Patients should take an NSAID or acetaminophen just prior to, or immediately after, treatment. If they wait to take medication until after the onset of pain, there is usually a delay of up to 1 hour before they experience pain relief. It has been suggested that instructing patients to take their analgesics by the clock for the first few days provides a more consistent blood level of the drug and may contribute to more consistent pain relief.[121] The combination of ibuprofen and acetaminophen taken together has been shown to produce additive analgesia when treating dental pain.[111,121,126–128] Opioids may be added when indicated (see Chapter 22).

LONG-ACTING LOCAL ANESTHETICS

Long-acting local anesthetics (e.g., bupivicaine) can provide an increased period of post-treatment analgesia beyond the usual duration of anesthesia.[129,130] By blocking the activation of unmyelinated C-fiber nociceptors, the anesthetic decreases the potential for central sensitization.[121] Long-acting local anesthetics can provide a period of analgesia for up to 8 to 10 hours following block injections and may reduce pain even 48 hours later.[121,129] Use of long-acting local anesthetics is a valuable biologically based strategy that provides analgesia during the immediate postoperative period.[121] Endodontic treatment by itself can be expected to provide significant pain relief (see Chapter 22).

Treatment of Endodontic Flare-ups

Selecting the appropriate treatment after an endodontic flare-up is dependent upon understanding its biological cause. For example, the clinician must determine if a flare-up is primarily iatrogenic in nature, as in the case of inaccurate measurement control, or microbiologically based, as in an infected necrotic situation.

DIAGNOSIS AND DEFINITIVE TREATMENT

History of the onset of pain is important in determining if the pain is spontaneous or provoked by a specific stimulus. For example, if a tooth had a history of acute apical periodontitis and its occlusion had not been reduced, that could be identified as a probable cause of postoperative pain, appropriate treatment should be provided.[120] In contrast, a complaint of swelling, pressure, and throbbing in the interproximal area might suggest a periodontal component of the problem that should be explored. If inaccurate measurement control was used or proper measurement not maintained, the clinician must determine if the canal was under- or over-instrumented. Working length should be reconfirmed, patency to the apical foramen obtained, and thorough debridement with copious irrigation completed. Remaining tissue, microorganisms and their products, and extrusion beyond the apex are major factors responsible for post-treatment symptoms.[94] Pain relief in the over-instrumented case is often dependent on an analgesic strategy. The under-instrumented case may require further instrumentation to the correct measurement, as well as the use of analgesics.

Drainage Through the Coronal Access Opening

A cardinal principle in the treatment of suppurative lesions is the establishment of drainage (Figure 15). Drainage, upon access to the pulp cavity, releases purulent or hemorrhagic exudate from the periapical tissues and may reduce periapical pressure in symptomatic teeth with radiolucent areas.[131] Obtaining drainage through the coronal access opening has been advocated as a means of reducing pain following treatment in some necrotic cases.[132] Interestingly, a retrospective study examined the effect of drainage upon access on postoperative endodontic pain and swelling in symptomatic necrotic teeth. It was determined that drainage upon access (average of 1.85 minutes) did not significantly ($p > 0.05$) reduce pain, percussion pain, swelling, or the number of analgesic medications taken, for symptomatic teeth with periapical radiolucencies.[131] It is possible that pre-existent apical periodontitis was a factor in the cases studied and was not addressed by the establishment of drainage. Occlusal relief may also have been required to address that symptom.

I&D

The goal of emergency treatment for an endodontic flare-up with a swelling is to achieve drainage.[132] The object of drainage is to evacuate exudate from the periapical spaces (Figure 16). Drainage is best achieved through a combination of canal instrumentation and I&D. Even in cases where an I&D is to be implemented, the canal should be accessed, instrumented, irrigated, medicated, and closed as soon as active drainage stops. Systemic antibiotics can be expected to be more effective once the canal has been debrided, medicated, and closed.[133,134]

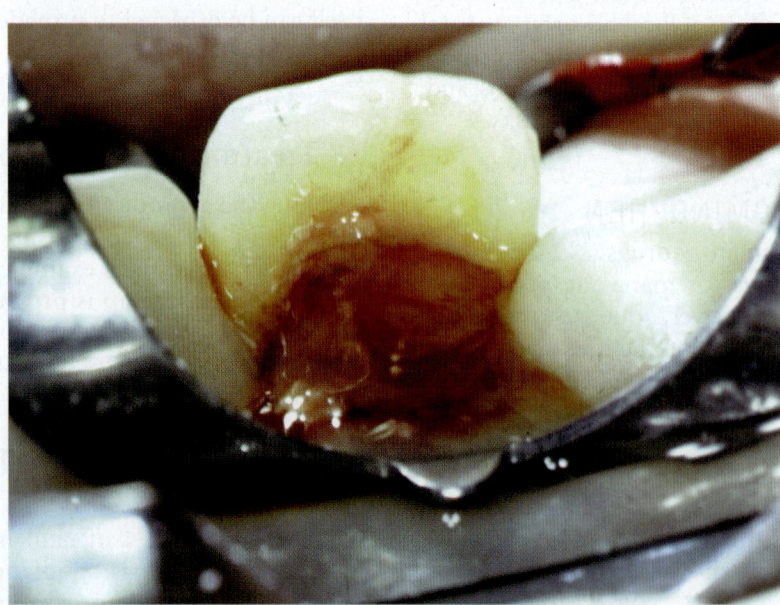

Figure 15 Purulent drainage upon access to the pulp cavity. Courtesy Dr. Craig Baumgartner.

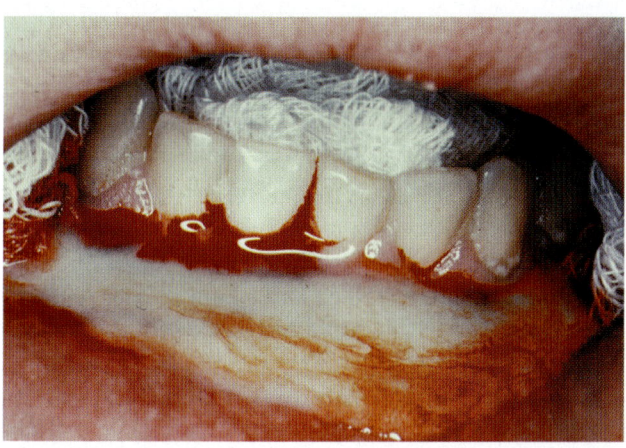

Figure 16 Purulent drainage following incision of a fluctuant abscess involving a mandibular anterior tooth (Courtesy Dr. John Ingle).

INSTRUMENTATION

After considering the biological cause of the flare-up, the clinician may decide to re-enter the symptomatic tooth. Profound local anesthesia is necessary before re-entry. Enhanced magnification and illumination are helpful in reassessing the chamber morphology for canals that might have been missed at the prior visit.[135–137] Working lengths should be reconfirmed, patency to the apical foramen obtained, and a thorough debridement with copious irrigation performed.[68] Remaining necrotic tissue, microorganisms, and toxic products are important factors responsible for flare-ups.[94] Enlarging the apical constriction has been advocated to encourage drainage.[138] Others have found that instrumenting through the apical foramen does not ensure drainage of periapical exudation.[68,138]

In some cases, however, drainage may be established through the root canal system upon instrumentation. Drainage allows for exudate to be released from the periapical tissues thus reducing localized tissue pressure and pain.[131] Leaving a tooth open after drainage is complete will result in re-infection from oral microbes.[73,94]

TREPHINATION

As discussed earlier in the chapter, trephination is the surgical perforation of the alveolar cortical plate over the root end, to release accumulated tissue exudate that is causing pain.[1] It may be indicated for patients with a flare-up when there is exquisite pain, no swelling, and drainage cannot be accomplished through the tooth.

COMPLEX DIAGNOSES

The clinician must be sensitive to the potential of non-odontogenic pain being confused with a flare-up. For example, the words "tingling" or "burning" when used as descriptors of pain are signals of non-odontogenic pain rather than a flare-up. Similarly, although rare, it is possible for a tooth, other than one undergoing endodontic treatment, to suddenly become painful and confuse the diagnosis. A previously undetected periodontal component may also pose a diagnostic problem.

Bacterial Factors Associated with Flare-ups

Bacteria are capable of acting as irritants and induce non-specific innate or specific adaptive immune responses in the host.[139,140] The host's responses to a bacterial challenge depend largely on virulence factors and the numbers of pathogens, as well as the host's innate and adaptive immunity. If the host's defense mechanisms are capable of overcoming a bacterial challenge, bacteria will be eliminated. In contrast, if the bacterial challenge overwhelms the host's defense mechanisms, an inflammatory response, as a result of innate or adaptive immunity, will occur. Microorganisms have been suggested as the major causative agents of flare-ups.[68,92,94] Unlike elsewhere in the body, bacteria in the root canal system are well protected from the host's immune defenses and antimicrobial agents. The microbes and virulence factors associated with pulpal and periapical infections are discussed in Chapter 7 "Microbiology of Endodontic Disease."

The bacterial community in an infected root canal is closely related to the nutrient supply, bacterial interaction, and oxidation–reduction potential.[107] Endodontic procedures cause changes in the root canal environment, favoring growth of some pathogens remaining in the incompletely instrumented canals, thus predisposing the patient to a flare-up.[94] Some bacterial species may, under certain conditions such as changes in oxidation-reduction potential, bacterial interaction, or environmental stresses, become more virulent and induce higher concentrations of inflammatory molecules and/or cytokines from damaged periapical tissues, thus intensifying the inflammatory response.[68,94] This is exemplified in some asymptomatic infected teeth with pulpal and/or periapical pathosis, as well as some asymptomatic re-treatment cases with periapical pathosis. After initiation or continuation of root canal treatment, those cases suddenly develop a flare-up. Preoperative symptomatic teeth have been shown to produce a higher incidence of flare-ups than asymptomatic teeth,[69,70] although the mechanism is not clear. It is possible, in teeth that are symptomatic, the canals are dominated by pathogens often found associated with pain or an acute periapical abscess. Therefore, these cases are predisposed to flare-up if the canals are not completely debrided or critical numbers of pathogens are forced into the apical tissues to overwhelm the host's defenses. A shift in the microbial community in the root canal may occur before the appearance of a flare-up.[94]

Therapeutically, it is easier to reduce the intracanal bacterial count than to control specific pathogens in the infected root canals. Mechanical instrumentation and antiseptic irrigation have been shown to greatly reduce bacterial count in infected root canals.[141] Intracanal medication between visits with calcium hydroxide may further reduce the bacterial count.[97,142] However, studies have not demonstrated an ability to eliminate all bacteria in infected root canals using contemporary endodontic procedures. Usually, the pathogenicity of microorganisms is related to their virulence factors and numbers. Although complete chemo-mechanical preparation, in combination with intracanal medication, may not eliminate specific pathogens and their virulence factors, the procedures will significantly reduce the intracanal bacterial count and the nutrient supply, thus possibly preventing critical numbers of pathogens from causing a flare-up. Many species of bacteria have been demonstrated in teeth with clinical signs and symptoms; however, the cause of a flare-up by a specific species of bacteria or combinations of bacteria requires further clarification. The presence of specific species of bacteria in teeth with clinical symptoms does not necessarily imply they are the cause of a flare-up.

References

1. American Association of Endodontists. Glossary of endodontic terms. Chicago, IL. 7th edition; 2003.
2. Hohl TH, Whitacre RJ, Hooley JR, Williams B. A self instructional guide: diagnosis and treatment of odontogenic infections. Seattle: Stoma Press, Inc; 1983.
3. Nusstein JM, Reader A, Beck M. Effect of drainage upon access on postoperative endodontic pain and swelling in symptomatic necrotic teeth. J Endod 2002;28(8):584–8.
4. Baumgartner JC, Xia T. Antibiotic susceptibility of bacteria associated with endodontic abscesses. J Endod 2003;29(1):44–7.
5. Khemaleelakul S, Baumgartner JC, Pruksakorn S. Identification of bacteria in acute endodontic infections and their antimicrobial susceptibility. Oral Surg Oral Med Oral Pathol Oral Radiol Endod 2002;94(6):746–55.
6. Siqueira JF Jr, Rôças IN, Favieri A, et al. Polymerase chain reaction detection of *Treponema denticola* in endodontic infections within root canals. Int Endod J 2001;34:280–4.
7. Simon JHS, Warden JC, Bascom LK. Needle aspiration: an alternative to incision and drainage. Gen Dent 1995;1:42–5.
8. Fouad AF, Rivera EM, Walton RE. Penicillin as a supplement in resolving the localized acute apical abscess. Oral Surg Oral Med Oral Pathol Oral Radiol Endod 1996;81(5):590–5.
9. Henry M, Reader A, Beck M. Effect of penicillin on postoperative endodontic pain and swelling in symptomatic necrotic teeth. J Endod 2001;27(2):117–23.
10. Lindeboom JAH, Frenken JWH, Valkenburg P, van den Akker HP. The role of preoperative prophylactic antibiotic administration in periapical endodontic surgery: a randomized, prospective double-blind placebo-controlled study. Int Endod J 2005;38:877–81.
11. Nagle D, Reader A, Beck M, Weaver J. Effect of systemic penicillin on pain in untreated irreversible pulpitis. Oral Surg Oral Med Oral Pathol Oral Radiol Endod 2000;90:636–40.
12. Pickenpaugh L, Reader A, Beck M, et al. Effect of Prophylactic amoxicillin on endodontic flare-up in asymptomatic, necrotic teeth. J Endod 2001;27(1):53–6.
13. Walton RE, Chiappinelli J. Prophylactic penicillin: effect on post-treatment symptoms following root canal treatment of asymptomatic periapical pathosis. J Endod 1993;19(9):466–70.
14. Baker PT, Evans RT, Slots J, Genco RJ. Antibiotic susceptibility of anaerobic bacteria from the human oral cavity. J Dent Res 1985;64:1233–44.
15. Jacinto RC, Gomes BP, Ferraz CC, et al. Microbiological analysis of infected root canals. Oral Microbiol Immunol 2003;18(5):285–92.
16. Jacinto RC, Gomes BPFA, Shah HN, et al. Incidence and antimicrobial susceptibility of *Porphyromonas gingivalis* isolated from mixed endodontic infections. Int Endod J 2006;39:62–70.
17. Ranta H, Haapasalo M, Kontiainen S, et al. Bacteriology of odontogenic apical periodontitis and effect of penicillin treatment. Scand J Infect Dis 1988;20:187–92.
18. Vigil GV, Wayman BE, Dazey SE, et al. Identification and antibiotic sensitivity of bacteria isolated from periapical lesions. J Endod 1997;23(2):110–14.
19. Yamamoto Y, Fukushima H, Tsuchiya H, Sagawa H. Antimicrobial susceptibilities of *Eubacterium, Peptostreptococcus,* and *Bacteroides* isolated from root canals of teeth with periapical pathosis. J Endod 1989;15(3):112–16.
20. Gilmore WC, Jacobus NV, Gorbach SL, Doku HC. A prospective double-blind evaluation of penicillin versus clindamycin in the treatment of odontogenic infections. J Oral Maxillofac Surg 1988;46:1065–70.

21. Babe KS, Serafin WE. Histamine, Bradykinin, and their antagonists. In: Hardman JG, Limbird LE, editors. Goodman and Gilman's The pharmacological basis of therapeutics. New York: McGraw-Hill; 1996.
22. Hardman JG, Limbird LE, Molinoff PB, et al, editors. Goodman & Gilman's the pharmacological basis of therapeutics. 10th ed. New York: McGraw-Hill; 2005.
23. Lockhart PB, Loven B, Brennan MT, Fox PC. The evidence base for the efficacy of antibiotic prophylaxis in dental practice. J Am Dent Assoc 2007;138:458–74.
24. Wilson W, Taubert KA, Gewitz M, Lockhart PB, Baddour LM, Levison M, et al. Prevention of infective endocarditis: guidelines from the American Heart Association. J Am Dent Assoc 2007;138:739–60.
25. Pallasch TJ. Antibiotic prophylaxis. Endod Topics 2003;4:46–59.
26. Morellion P, Francioli P, Overholser D et al. Mechanisms of successful amoxicillin prophylaxis of experimental endocarditis due to *Streptococcus intermedius*. J Infect Dis 1986;154(5):801–7.
27. Baumgartner JC, Heggers JP, Harrison JW. The incidence of bacteremia related to endodontic procedures. I. Non-surgical endodontics. J Endod 1976;2:135.
28. Baumgartner JC, Heggers JP, Harrison JW. Incidence of bacteremias related to endodontic procedures. II. Surgical endodontics. J Endod 1977;3(10):399–404.
29. Bender IB, Seltzer S, Yermish M. The incidence of bacteremia in endodontic manipulation. Oral Surg Oral Med Oral Pathol Oral Radiol Endod 1960;13(3):353–60.
30. Debelian GF, Olsen I, Tronstad L. Bacteremia in conjunction with endodontic therapy. Endod Dent Traumatol 1995;11(3):142–9.
31. Savarrio L, Mackenzie D, Riggio M, et al. Detection of bacteraemias during non-surgical root canal treatment. J Dent 2005;33:293–303.
32. American Dental Association. Antibiotic prophylaxis for dental patients with total joint replacements. J Am Dent Assoc 2003;134(July):895–9.
33. Bence R. Trephination technique. J Am Dent Assoc 1980;6(7):657–8.
34. Elliott JA, Holcomb JB. Evaluation of a minimally traumatic alveolar trephination procedure to avoid pain. J Endod 1988;14:405–7.
35. Henry B, Fraser J. Trephination for acute pain management. J Endod 2003;29(2):144–6.
36. Houck V, Reader A, Beck M, et al. Effect of trephination on postoperative pain and swelling in symptomatic necrotic teeth. Oral Surg Oral Med Oral Pathol Oral Radiol Endod 2000;90(4):507–13.
37. Moos HL, Bramwell JD, Roahen JO. A comparison of pulpectomy alone versus pulpectomy with trephination for the relief of pain. J Endod 1996;22(8):422–5.
38. Nist E, Reader A, Beck M. Effect of apical trephination on postoperative pain and swelling in symptomatic necrotic teeth. J Endod 2001;27(6):415–20.
39. Serene TP, McKelvy BD, Scaramella JM. Endodontic problems resulting from surgical fistulation: report of two cases. J Am Dent Assoc 1978;96:101–4.
40. Werts R. Apical aeration technic: Artificial fistulation. Dent Surv 1971;47:17–18.
41. Henry BM, Fraser JG. Trephination for acute pain management. J Endod 2003;29(2):144–6.
42. Peters DD. Evaluation of prophylactic alveolar trephination to avoid pain. J Endod 1980;6:518–26.
43. Chestner SB, Selman AJ, Friedman J, Heyman RA. Apical fenestration: solution to recalcitrant pain in root canal therapy. J Am Dent Assoc 1968;77:846–8.
44. Sutherland S, Matthews DC. Emergency management of acute apical periodontitis in the permanent dentition: a systematic review of the literature. J Can Dent Assoc 2003;69(3):160.
45. Natkin E, Oswald RJ, Carnes LI. The relationship of lesion size to diagnosis, incidence, and treatment of periapical cysts and granulomas. Oral Surg Oral Med Oral Pathol Oral Radiol Endod 1984;51(1):82–94.
46. Nair PNR. New perspectives on radicular cysts: do they heal? Int Endod J 1998;31(3):155–60.
47. Simon JHS. Incidence of periapical cysts in relation to the root canal. J Endod 1980;6:845–8.
48. Suzuki M. Treatment of jaw cysts with an irrigational method. On the significance of the method and the progress of cysts. Int J Oral Surg 1982;11(4):217–25.
49. Freedland JB. Conservative reduction of large periapical lesions. Oral Surg Oral Med Oral Pathol Oral Radiol Endod 1970;29:455–64.
50. Gunraj MN. Decompression of a large periapical lesion utilizing an improved drainage device. J Endod 1990;16:140–3.
51. Harris WE. Conservative treatment of a large radicular cyst: report of case. J Am Dent Assoc 1971;82:1390–4.
52. Neaverth EJ, Burg HA. Decompression of large periapical cystic lesions. J Endod 1982;8(4):175–82.
53. Samuels HS. Marsupialization: effective management of large maxillary cysts. Oral Surg Oral Med Oral Pathol Oral Radiol Endod 1965;20:676–83.
54. Wong M. Surgical fenestration of large periapical lesions. J Endod 1991;17(10):516–21.
55. Rees JS. Conservative management of a large maxillary cyst. Int Endod J 1997;30(1):64–7.
56. Enislidis G, Fock N, Sulzbacher I, Evers R. Conservative treatment of large cystic lesions of the mandible: a prospective study of the effect of decompression. Br J Oral Maxillofac Surg 2004;42(6):546–50.

57. Loushine RJ, Weller RN, Bellizzi R, Kulild JC. A 2-day decompression: a case report of a maxillary first molar. J Endod 1991;17(2):85–7.

58. August M, Gaquin W, Ferraro N, Kaban L. Fine-needle aspiration biopsy of intraosseous jaw lesions. J Oral Maxillofac Surg 1999;57:1282–6.

59. Mejia JL, Donado JE, Basrani B. Active non-surgical decompression of large periapical lesions-3 case reports. J Can Dent Assoc 2004;70(10):691–4.

60. Hoen MM, LaBounty GL, Strittmatter EJ. Conservative treatment of persistent periradicular lesions using aspiration and irrigation. J Endod 1990;16(4):182–7.

61. Toller PA, Holborow EJ. Immunoglobulins and immunoglobulin-containing cells in cysts of the jaws. Lancet 1969;2:178–81.

62. Morse DR, Patnik JW, Schacterle GR. Electrophoretic differentiation of radicular cysts and granulomas. Oral Surg Oral Med Oral Pathol Oral Radiol Endod 1973;35(2):249–64.

63. August M, Faquin WC, Troulis MJ, Kaban LB. Dedifferentiation of odontogenic deratocyst epithelium after cyst decompression. J Oral Maxillofac Surg 2003;61(6):678–83.

64. Fulciniti F, Califano L, Zupe A, Vetrani A. Accuracy of fine needle aspiration biopsy in head and neck tumors. J Oral Maxillofac Surg 1997;55:1094–7.

65. Genet J, Hart A, Wesselink P, Thoden van Velzen S. Preoperative and postoperative factors associated with pain after the first endodontic visit. Int Endod J 1987;20:53–64.

66. Imura N, Auolo M. Factors associated with endodontic flare-ups: A prospective study. Int Endod J 1995;28:261–5.

67. Siqueira J. Reaction of periradicular tissues to root canal treatment: Benefits and drawbacks. Endod Topics 2005;10:123–47.

68. Siqueira J, Barnett F. Interappointment pain: mechanisms, diagnosis and treatment. Endod Topics 2004;79:93–109.

69. Torabinejad M, Kettering J, McGraw J, et al. Factors associated with endodontic interappointment emergencies of teeth with necrotic pulps. J Endod 1988;14:261–6.

70. Walton R, Fouad A. Endodontic interappointment flare-ups: a prospective study of incidence and related factors. J Endod 1992;18:172–7.

71. Morse D, Korzen L, Esposito J, et al. Asymptomatic teeth with necrotic pulps and associated periapical radiolucencies: relationship of flare-ups to endodontic instrumentation, antibiotic usage and stress in three separate practices at three different periods Parts 1–5. Int J Psychol 1986;33:5–87.

72. Torabinejad M, Cymerman J, Frankson M, et al. Effectiveness of various medications on postoperative pain following complete instrumentation J Endod 1994;20:345–54.

73. Barnett F. The incidence of flare-ups following endodontic treatment. [Special Issue] J Dent Res 1989;68:1253.

74. Trope M. Relationship of intracanal medicaments to endodontic flare-ups. Endod Dent Traumatol 1990;6:226–9.

75. Genet J, Wesselink P, Thoden van Velzen S. The incidence of preoperative and postoperative pain in endodontic therapy. Int Endod J 1986;19:221–9.

76. Harrison J, Baumgartner J, Zielke D. Analysis of interappointment pain associated with the combined use of endodontic irrigants and medicaments. J Endod 1981;7:272–6.

77. Trope M. Flare-up rate of single-visit endodontics. Int Endod J 1991;24:24–6.

78. Unruh A. Gender variations in clinical pain experience. Pain 1996;65:123–67.

79. Eli I. The multidisciplinary nature of pain: textbook of endodontology. Munksgaard Blackwell, Copenhagen, Denmark;2003.

80. Oguntebi B, DeSchepper E, Taylor T, et al. Postoperative pain incidence related to the type of emergency treatment of symptomatic pulpitis. Oral Surg Oral Med Oral Pathol Oral Radiol Endod 1992;73:479–83.

81. Marshall J, Liesinger A. Factors associated with endodontic post treatment pain. J Endod 1993;19:573–5.

82. Erskine A, Morley S, Pearce S. Memory of pain: a review. Pain 1990;41:255–65.

83. Anderson D, Pennebaker J. Pain and pleasure: alternative interpretations for identical stimulation. Eur J Soc Psychol 1980;10:207–12.

84. Nakai Y, Milgram P, Mancl L, et al. Effectiveness of local anesthesia in a pediatric dental practice. J Am Dent Assoc 2000;1221:1699–705.

85. Frank A, Glick D, Weichman J, Harvey H. The intracanal use of sulfathiazole in endodontics to reduce pain. J Am Dent Assoc 1968;77:102–6.

86. Fox J, Atkinson J, Dinin A et al. Incidence of pain following one-visit endodontic treatment. Oral Surg Oral Med Oral Pathol Oral Radiol Endod 1970;30:123–30.

87. Pekruhn B. Single-visit endodontic therapy: a preliminary clinical study. J Am Dent Assoc 1981;103:875–7.

88. Roane J, Dryden J, Grimes E. Incidence of post operative pain after single and multiple visit endodontic precedures. Oral Surg Oral Med Oral Pathol Oral Radiol Endod 1983;55:68–72.

89. Mulhern J, Patterson S, Newton C, Ringel A. Incidence of postoperative pain after one-appointment endodontic treatment of asymptomatic pulpal necrosis single rooted teeth. J Endod 1992;8:370–5.

90. Fava L. A comparison of one versus two appointment endodontic therapy in teeth with non-vital pulps. I Endod J 1989;22:179–83.

91. Eleazer P, Eleazer K. Flare-up rate in pulpally necrotic molars in one visit versus two-visit endodontic treatment. J Endod 1998;24:614–16.

92. Seltzer S, Naidorf I. Flare-ups in endodontics I. Etiology factors. J Endod 1985;11:472–278.
93. Trowbridge H, Emling R. Inflammation. A review of the process. 5th ed. Quintessence, Pub. Co., Chicago;1997.
94. Siqueira J. Microbial causes of endodontic flare-ups. Int Endod J 2003;36:453–63.
95. Spangberg L, Haapasalo M. Rationale and efficacy of root canal medicaments and root filling materials with emphasis on treatment outcome. Endod Topics 2002;2:35–58.
96. Bystrom A, Sunquist G. Bacteriological evaluation of the effect of 0.5% sodium hypochlorite in endodontic therapy. Oral Surg Oral Med Oral Pathol Oral Radiol Endod 1983;55:307–12.
97. Sjogren U, Figdor D, Spangberg L, Sunqvist G. The antimicrobial effect of calcium hydroxide as a short-term intracanal dressing. Int Endod J 1991;24:119–25.
98. Siqueira J. Aetiology of the endodontic failure: why well treated teeth can fail. Int Endod J 2001;34:1–10.
99. Sundqvist G, Figdor D. Life as an endodontic pathogen. Ecological differences between the untreated and root-filled canals. Endod Topics 2003;6:3–28.
100. Simon J. The apex: how critical is it? Gen Dent 1994;42:330–4.
101. Nair P, Sjogren U, Krey G, et al. Intraradicular bacteria and fungi in root-filled asymptomatic human teeth with therapy-resistant periapical lesions: a long term light and electron microscope follow-up study. J Endod 1990;16:580–8.
102. Nair P. Light and electron microscopic studies of root canal flora and periapical lesions. J Endod 1987;13:29–39.
103. Fukushima H, Yamamoto K, Hirohata K, et al. Localization and identification of root canal bacteria in clinically asymptomatic periapical pathosis. J Endod 1990;16:534–8.
104. Siqueira J, Lopes H. Bacteria on the apical root surfaces of untreated teeth with periradicular lesions: a scanning electron microscopy study. Int Endod J 2001;34:216–20.
105. Molven O. The apical level of root fillings. Acta Odontol Scand 1976;34:89–116.
106. Siqueira J. Endodontic infections: concepts, paradigms and perspectives. Oral Surg Oral Med Oral Pathol Oral Radiol Endod 2002;94:281–93.
107. Sundqvist G. Ecology of the root canal flora. J Endod 1992;18:427–30.
108. Balaban F, Skidmore A, Griffen J. Acute exacerbations following initial treatment of necrotic pulps. J Endod 1984;10:78–80.
109. Walton R. Interappointment flare-ups: incidence, related factors, prevention and management. Endod Topics 2002;3:67–76.
110. Gesi A, Hakeberg M, Warfinge J, Bergenholtz G. Incidence of periapical lesions and clinical symptoms after pulpectomy: a clinical and radiographic evaluation of one- versus two-session treatment. Oral Surg Oral Med Oral Pathol Oral Radiol Endod 2006;101:379–88.
111. Hargreaves K, Seltzer S. Pharmacological control of dental pain. In: Hargreaves KM, Goodis HE, editors. Seltzer and Bender's Dental Pulp. Chicago: Quintessence; 2002.
112. Hargreaves K. Pain mechanisms of the pulpodentin complex. In: Hargreaves KM, Goodis HE, editors Chicago: Quintessence; 2002.
113. Carr D, Goudas L. Acute pain. Lancet 1999;353:2051–8.
114. Egbert A, Bettit G, Welch C, Barttett M. Reducation of postoperative pain by encouragement and instruction of patients. N Engl J Med 1964;270:825–7.
115. Wardle J. Psychological management of anxiety and pain during dental treatment. J Psychosom Res 1983;27:399–402.
116. Natkin E. Treatment of endodontic emergencies. Dent Clin North Am 1974;18:243–55.
117. Antrim D, Bakland L, Parker M. Treatment of endodontic urgent care cases. Dent Clin North Am 1986;30:549–72.
118. Creech J, Walton R, Kaltenbach R. Effect of occlusion relief on endodontic pain. J Am Dent Assoc 1984;109:64–7.
119. Jostes J, Holland G. The effect of occlusal reduction after canal preparation on patient comfort. J Endod 1984;10:34–7.
120. Rosenberg P, Babick P, Schertzer L, Leung A. The effect of occlusal reduction on pain after endodontic instrumentation. J Endod 1998;24:492–6.
121. Keiser K, Hargreaves K. Building effective strategies for the management of endodontic pain. Endod Topics 2002;3:93–105.
122. Whitten B, Gardiner D, Jeansonne B, Lemon R. Current trends in endodontic treatment: report of a national survey. J Am Dent Assoc 1996;127:1333–14.
123. Yingling N, Byrne B, Hartwell G. Antibiotic use by members of the American Association of Endodontists in the year 2000: report of a national survey. J Endod 2002;28:396–404.
124. Fouad A. Are antibiotics effective for endodontic pain? Endod Topics 2002;3:52–6.
125. Holstein A, Hargreaves K, Niederman R. Evaluation of NSAIDs for treating post-endodontic pain: a systemic review. Endod Topics 2002;3:3–13.
126. Wright CI, Antal E, Gillespie W, Albert K. Ibuprofen and acetaminophen kinetics when taken concurrently. Clin Pharmacol Ther 1983;34:707–10.
127. Cooper S. The relative efficacy of ibuprofen in dental pain. Compend Contin Educ Dent 1986;7–11.
128. Breivik E, Barkvoll P, Skovlund E. Combining diclofinac with acetaminophen-codeine after oral surgery: a randomized, double blind single dose study. Clin Pharmacol Ther 1999;66:625–35.

129. Cout R, Koraido G, Moore P. A clinical trial of long-acting abesthetics for periodontal surgery. Anesth Prog 1990;37:194–9.

130. Gordon S, Dionne R, Brahim J, et al. Blockage of periapical neuronal barrage reduced post-operative pain. Pain 1997;709:209–15.

131. Nusstein J, Reader A, Beck M. Effect of drainage upon access on postoperative endodontic pain and swelling in symptomatic necrosis teeth. J Endod 2002;28:584–8.

132. Harrington G, Natkin E. Midtreatment flare-ups. Dent Clin North Am 1992;36:409–23.

133. Baumgartner J, Hutter J. Endodontic microbiology and treatment of infection. In: Pathways of the pulp. Cohen, S. and Hargreaves, K. 8th ed. St. Louis: Mosby; 2002.

134. Hutter J. Facial space infections of odontogenic origin. J Endod 1991;17:422.

135. Schwarze T, Baethge C, Stecher T, Guertsen W. Identification of second canals in the mesiobuccal root of maxillary first and second molars using magnifying loupes or an operating microscope. Aust Endod J 2002;28:57–60.

136. Wolcott J, Ishley D, Kennedy W, et al. Clinical investigation of second mesiobuccal canals in endodontically treated and retreated maxillary molars. J Endod 2002;28:477–9.

137. Buhrley L, Barrows M, BeGole E, Wenckus C. Effect of magnification on location the MB2 canal in maxillary molars. J Endod 2002;28:324–7.

138. Weine F. Endodontic therapy. 2nd ed. St. Louis: Mosby; 1976.

139. Mims C, Playfair J, Roitt I, et al. Medical microbiology. 2nd ed. Philadelphia: Mosby; 1999.

140. Abbas A, Lichtman A, Pober J. Cellular and molecular immunology. 4th ed. Philadelphia: WB Saunders; 2000.

141. Bystrom A, Sundqvist G. Bacteriologic evaluation of the efficacy of mechanical root canal instrumentation in endodontic therapy. Scand J Dent Res 1981;89:321–8.

142. Bystrom A, Claesson R, Sundqvist G. The antibacterial effect of camphorated paramonochlorophenol, camphorated phenol and calcium hydroxide in the treatment of infected root canals. Endod Dent Traumatol 1985;1:170–5.

CHAPTER 22

PHARMACOLOGIC MANAGEMENT OF ENDODONTIC PAIN

KENNETH M. HARGREAVES, AL READER, JOHN M. NUSSTEIN, J. GORDON MARSHALL, JENNIFER L. GIBBS

The management of pain represents both a challenge and an opportunity for the endodontist. It is a challenge due to pharmacological (e.g., reduced anesthetic success), behavioral (e.g., patient apprehension), and practice management (e.g., relationship with referring practitioner) issues. Many of these factors can increase the stress of providing high-quality clinical care to our patients. However, effective pain management also represents a unique opportunity to integrate pharmacological, procedural, and behavioral skills in providing outstanding pain control to grateful patients. A tremendous increase in our knowledge of the pain system and its dynamic plasticity in response to tissue inflammation occurred over the last decade (Chapter 10, "Mechanisms of Odontogenic and Non-Odontogenic Pain" and Chapter 11, "Non-Odontogenic Toothache and Chronic Head and Neck Pains"). Equally important, a commensurate increase in analgesic clinical trials provides the clinician with a unique opportunity to develop biologically and evidence-based strategies for effectively treating endodontic pain patients. This chapter contributes to that skillset by comprehensively reviewing this clinical literature and formulating strategies based on the latest results from clinical research. To accomplish this goal, the chapter will sequentially review major drug classes available to the practitioner and then use this information to summarize evidence-based approaches for pain control.

Local Anesthesia

Profound pain control starts with effective local anesthesia. In addition to the obvious ethical and moral obligation of providing appropriate high-quality care, the technical challenges of endodontic procedures are greatly increased without effective anesthesia. Background reviews on local anesthetic techniques and pharmacology should be reviewed as needed by the reader. This section provides an evidence-based rationale of various local anesthetic agents and primary and supplemental routes of administration, with an emphasis on clinical implications.

Before reviewing the clinical trial literature, several preliminary factors should be considered. First, subjective approaches for assessing the depth of anesthesia ("are you numb?") are fraught with a lack of sensitivity and specificity.[1–4] Instead, testing for pulpal responses in vital teeth, by an application of a cold refrigerant or by using an electric pulp tester (EPT), are effective methods for evaluating anesthesia in pain-free[5–9] or symptomatic vital teeth[5,9–11] in nearly[5,9,10] all patients. Simply put, the lack of profound anesthesia after an initial injection becomes a major indication for supplemental injection of local anesthetic solutions. Second, a prior history of incomplete anesthesia often predicts subsequent problems with obtaining complete anesthesia.[12] This issue should be considered when reviewing the patient's dental history. Third, preoperative pain is a risk factor for incomplete local anesthesia, with up to an eight-fold increase in the prevalence of incomplete anesthesia observed in patients with irreversible pulpitis.[13] Although the mechanism(s) mediating this clinical problem is incompletely understood, several hypotheses have been advanced including (1) ion trapping of local anesthetic molecules due to lower pH (only possible for infiltration injections; block injections are not likely to involve acidotic tissue); (2) altered membrane excitability of peripheral nociceptors[14,15]; (3) increased activity of the tetrodotoxin-resistant (TTXr) class of sodium channels that may also be resistant to the action of local anesthetics[16]; (4) increased overall expression of sodium channels in pulps diagnosed with irreversible pulpitis[17]; and/or (5) central sensitization that amplifies peripheral input from afferent neurons. Importantly, supplemental techniques such as intraosseous[9,10,18,19] or periodontal ligament (PDL)[11] injections have been demonstrated to increase anesthetic efficacy when an inferior alveolar nerve (IAN) block fails to provide effective anesthesia. Fourth, preoperative apprehension, possibly due to previous dental procedures including injections,[20–22] may contribute to patient management issues. Topical anesthetics have been reported to be effective in reducing injection discomfort in some,[23–26] but not all,[27–29] studies, and both pharmacological and psychological components may contribute to the effectiveness of topical anesthetics.[29] Fifth, a slow rate of injection (60 versus 15 seconds) reduces patient discomfort[30] and can be accomplished either manually or by a computer-controlled anesthetic delivery system. Automated anesthetic delivery systems have been shown to produce less pain in some studies,[31–36] or either no difference or greater pain in other studies[37,38]; at least some discomfort has been noted in most studies.[32–38] Sixth, epinephrine-containing local anesthetics, with their associated lowered pH, are thought to be associated with more injection discomfort in some[39,40] but not all[41] studies. As noted in Chapter 10, "Mechanisms of Odontogenic and Non-Odontogenic Pain," the TRPV1 "capsaicin receptor" is expressed on pain neurons and is profoundly activated by pH solutions of <6.0, which might provide a biological basis for this observation. Seventh, permanent damage to the lingual nerve and IANs are very rare, with a calculated incidence of about 0.0006 to 0.3%.[42] Of these reported injuries, the lingual nerve is affected ~70 to 79%, while the IAN is affected ~21 to 30% of these cases.[42,43] In one case series, the lingual nerve was affected in 18 out of 12,104 patients (~0.1%), with 17 of these 18 cases resolved within 6 months.[44] Collectively, these general principles of local anesthesia provide foundation knowledge when using this important class of drugs.

Mandibular Anesthesia

Numerous studies have evaluated pulpal anesthesia using a standardized testing protocol involving repeated application of an EPT using a 0–80 scale of current.[1–4,45–49] This method permits controlled clinical trials in which either normal healthy control subjects or odontogenic pain patients using the same dependent measure for study outcome. In these studies, anesthetic success is defined as the percentage of subjects who achieve two consecutive 80 readings

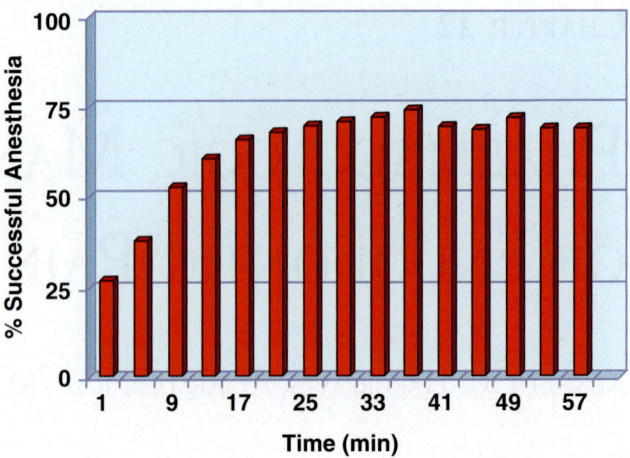

Figure 1 Time–response curve for the development of pulpal anesthesia (defined as no response on Analytical Technologies EPT at setting = 80) of mandibular first molars following inferior alveolar nerve (IAN) block injection of 1.8 mL of 2% lidocaine with 1:100,000 epinephrine. Data courtesy of Dr. A. Reader et al.

(EPT) within 15 minutes and continuously demonstrate a lack of responsiveness for 60 minutes. Conversely, anesthetic failure is defined as the percentage of subjects who never achieved two consecutive 80 EPT readings at any observation time. In general, studies performing IAN block injections with one cartridge of 2% lidocaine with 1:100,000 epinephrine report different proportions of anesthetic success/failure for the mandibular first molar (53% success/17% failure), first premolar (61%/11%), and the lateral incisor (35%/32%)[1–4,45–49] (Figure 1). It is important to note, however, that 100% of the subjects[1–4,45–49] reported profound lip numbness. Therefore, this outcome has no predictable value for determining the depth of pulpal anesthesia. Although the presence of lip sign does not indicate effective pulpal anesthesia, the absence of a lip sign indicates a failed IAN block injection and should prompt a second injection of local anesthetic before treatment begins.

Several local anesthetics have been compared in clinical trials using designs similar to that described above. As summarized in Table 1, these studies have demonstrated that many local anesthetics produce similar levels of anesthesia for IAN block injections. In particular, the equivalency of 3% mepivacaine and 2% lidocaine with 1:100,000 epinephrine, in patients with irreversible pulpitis, is an important finding. It provides a vasoconstrictor-free alternative when medical conditions or drug therapies suggest caution in administering epinephrine-containing solutions.

Mepivacaine is available in a formulation containing levonordefrin, an adrenergic agonist with 75% α

Table 1 Comparison of Local Anesthetics for Inferior Alveolar Nerve Anesthesia

Local Anesthetic I	Local Anesthetic II	Patient Population	Finding	Reference
3% Mepivacaine plain	2% Lidocaine with 1:100,000 epinephrine	Healthy volunteer subjects	I = II	2
3% Mepivacaine plain	2% Lidocaine with 1:100,000 epinephrine	Irreversible pulpitis	I = II	11
2% Mepivacaine with 1:20,000 levonordefrin	2% Lidocaine with 1:100,000 epinephrine	Healthy volunteer subjects	I = II	4
4% Prilocaine plain	2% Lidocaine with 1:100,000 epinephrine	Healthy volunteer subjects	I = II	2
4% Prilocaine with 1:200,000 epinephrine	2% Lidocaine with 1:100,000 epinephrine	Healthy volunteer subjects	I = II	4
4% Articaine with 1:100,000 epinephrine	2% Lidocaine with 1:100,000 epinephrine	Healthy volunteer subjects	I = II	71
4% Articaine with 1:100,000 epinephrine	2% Lidocaine with 1:100,000 epinephrine	Irreversible pulpitis	I = II	72
4% Articaine with 1:100,000 epinephrine	4% Articaine with 1:200,000 epinephrine	Healthy volunteer subjects	I = II	73

activity and only 25% β activity, making it seem more attractive than epinephrine (50% α activity and 50% β activity).[50] However, levonordefrin is marketed as a 1:20,000 concentration in dental cartridges.[50] Clinically, the higher concentration of levonordefrin makes it equipotent to epinephrine in clinical and systemic effects.[4,51] Therefore, 1:20,000 levonordefrin offers no clinical advantage over 1:100,000 epinephrine.

Articaine is available in the United States as a 4% solution containing 1:100,000 and 1:200,000 epinephrine.[52] Articaine is an amide anesthetic that contains a thiophene ring and an ester linkage unlike other amide local anesthetics.[52] The extra ester linkage is susceptible to hydrolysis by plasma esterases.[52] Several studies have reported that articaine is safe when used in appropriate doses.[52–60] Although lidocaine and articaine have the same maximum 500 mg dose for the adult patient,[50] the manufacturer's recommended maximum dose for a healthy 70 kg adult would be 7 cartridges of 4% articaine solution compared to 13 cartridges of 2% lidocaine solution.[50] Articaine, like prilocaine, has the potential to cause methemoglobinemia and neuropathies.[52] While the incidence of methemoglobinemia is rare, dentists should be aware of this complication in patients who are at an increased risk of developing this condition.[61] The incidence of neuropathies (involving the lip and/or the tongue), associated with articaine and prilocaine, is approximately five times more than that found with either lidocaine or mepivacaine.[62,63] In one retrospective study, the incidence of paresthesia was approximately one in 785,000 injections.[62] Therefore, while the paresthesia incidence is statistically higher for articaine and prilocaine, it is a clinically rare event that nevertheless imposes some medicolegal implications. Available literature indicates that articaine is equally effective when statistically compared to other local anesthetics,[60,64–71] with relatively few studies demonstrating a statistical superiority of articaine over lidocaine for nerve blocks. Recent studies have reported that articaine was significantly better than lidocaine for anesthesia after buccal infiltration of the mandibular first molar, with articaine producing a success rate of about 64 to 87%.[72,73]

Long-acting local anesthetics, including bupivacaine and etidocaine, have been advocated for *prolonged* pain control, with support from several clinical trials.[74–79] Recently, etidocaine has been withdrawn from the market by Dentsply Pharmaceuticals. Although bupivacaine exhibits sustained anesthesia and pain control, patients should be informed of prolonged soft tissue anesthesia (lip sign) since this may preclude their willingness to use this drug.[75] Bupivacaine has a somewhat slower onset than 2% lidocaine but almost twice the duration of pulpal anesthesia (approximately 4 hours) in the mandible[48] (Figure 2).

Ropivacaine is a structural homologue of bupivacaine that appears to have a lower potential for central

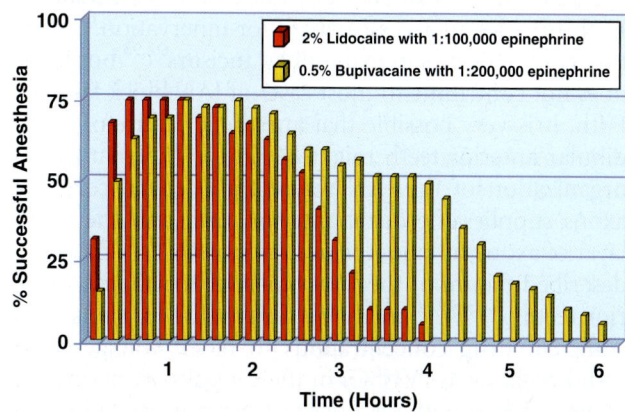

Figure 2 Time–response curve for the development of pulpal anesthesia (defined as no response on Analytical Technologies EPT at setting = 80) of mandibular first molars following inferior alveolar nerve (IAN) block injection of either 1.8 mL of 2% lidocaine with 1:100,000 epinephrine or 1.0 mL of 0.5% bupivacaine with 1:200,000 epinephrine. Data courtesy of Dr. A. Reader et al.

nervous system (CNS) and cardiovascular toxic effects.[80] Anesthesia from injection of 0.5% ropivacaine with 1:200,000 epinephrine was equivalent to 0.5% bupivacaine with 1:200,000 epinephrine. One study found that 0.5 and 0.75% concentrations of ropivacaine without epinephrine were effective for IAN blocks.[81]

IAN block injections are not always successful. As noted above, patients with preoperative pain are at risk for reduced rates of successful anesthesia. However, even in patients without pain, the IAN block injection is not always successful. Several hypotheses have been advanced for this lack of complete success.[69] First, the mylohyoid nerve has been suggested to provide accessory innervation that might contribute to the clinical failure of IAN block injections.[82,83] However, clinical studies in which IAN block injections were compared to an IAN block as well as with mylohyoid nerve block failed to demonstrate any increase in anesthetic success. This led to the conclusion that the mylohyoid nerve is not a major contributor to failed IAN block injections.[84] Second, it is possible that inaccurate positioning of the needle might contribute to IAN block failures; however, confirming the needle position with either a medical ultrasound device[45] or radiographs[85,86] failed to increase success rates of IAN injections. Third, it is possible that needle deflection might be a cause for IAN block failures.[87–89] However, neither a bidirectional rotation method, using the Wand (CompuDent, Milestone Scientific Inc., Deerfield, IL),[89] nor insertion with the needle bevel oriented away from the mandibular ramus (so the needle would deflect toward the mandibular foramen)[90,91] substantially improved anesthetic success. Fourth, it is possible that the contralateral IAN provides an accessory path for innervation. Cross-innervation occurs in mandibular incisors[92,93] but likely does not contribute to most cases of IAN block failures. Fifth, it is very possible that anesthetic failure of mandibular anterior teeth might be due to the anatomical organization of the IAN where the "central core" of axons supplies the distal anterior teeth and the outer layer of axons supplies the posterior teeth.[94,95] The well-described failure of the IAN block to anesthetize anterior teeth[1–4,45–49,96] might be simply due to the lack of sufficient drug concentrations to block voltage-gated sodium channels (VGSC) in the central core axons. Of course, this hypothesis does not explain the failure to block posterior mandibular teeth. Collectively, these findings have prompted much research to increase the success of IAN nerve block injections.

Several procedures have been evaluated for increasing the rate of successful anesthesia of the IAN block. First, increasing the volume of 2% lidocaine with epinephrine (from 1.8 to 3.6 mL) does not increase anesthetic success.[1,49,84,97,98] Second, increasing epinephrine concentration (from 1:100,000 to 1:50,000) does not appear to increase anesthetic success in normal teeth.[46,99] Third, hyaluronidase, an enzyme that reduces tissue viscosity[100] with favorable anesthetic enhancement properties,[101,102] was not found to improve the success of lidocaine anesthesia in a recent double-blind, randomized clinical study.[103] Fourth, *carbonated* solutions are thought to trap the anesthetic within the nerve as well as impose a direct depressant action on nerves.[3] Lidocaine hydrocarbonate, however, was no more effective for anesthetic success.[3] Fifth, diphenhydramine, an antihistamine with reported local anesthetic properties,[104,105] did not improve lidocaine anesthesia when injected as a combined solution.[106] Sixth, meperidine, an opioid analgesic with demonstrated anesthetic properties,[107] did not improve the success of lidocaine anesthesia after coinjection.[107,108] Although these experimental approaches using pharmacological methods were not successful in improving IAN block anesthesia, other studies evaluating alternative methods of drug delivery proved more successful in addressing this problem.

Alternative or supplemental injections are indicated when IAN block is not successful. One alternative approach is to reduce the speed of injection for an IAN block. A slow IAN block injection (60 seconds) significantly increases anesthesia success rates (electric pulp testing), compared to a rapid injection (15 seconds).[30] There are three supplemental routes of injection that will be discussed in the following sections, "The intraligamentary injection," "The intraosseous injection," and "The intrapulpal injection." They are included in the section under "Mandibular anesthesia" because this is the major, though not exclusive, area for their clinical application.

THE SUPPLEMENTAL INTRALIGAMENTARY INJECTION

The technique of intraligamentary anesthesia can be reviewed in other published papers or textbooks. Studies have reported that about 0.2 mL of solution is delivered with each mesial and distal injection using a traditional or pressure syringe, that different needle gauges (25, 27, or 30 gauge) are equally effective,[109,110] and that standard syringes are as effective as special ligamental syringes.[110–112] Several studies have shown that the intraligamentary injection produces initial success rates of about 63 to 74% and that, if needed, reinjections produce an overall success rate of about 92 to

96%.[11,110–113] The intraligamentary injection will not be successful in mandibular anterior teeth.[114,115] This route of injection should be considered a type of intraosseous injection since the solutions are forced through the cribriform plate into the marrow spaces around the tooth[116–120] and *not* via the PDL. Although backpressure upon injection is the most important factor for anesthetic success,[116,118] this simply reflects forces necessary to penetrate the cribriform plate and does not produce pressure anesthesia[121,122] like the intrapulpal injection.[123,124] The presence of a vasoconstrictor significantly increases the efficacy of intraligamentary injection,[122,125–128] and anesthetic solutions with reduced vasoconstrictor concentrations (e.g., bupivacaine with 1:200,000 epinephrine) are not very effective with this technique.[128,129] The onset of anesthesia is immediate[110–112,114,121,122] and if anesthesia is still not adequate, reinjection is indicated. Since the duration of pulpal anesthesia in asymptomatic cases following the IAN nerve block plus supplemental intraligamentary injections is only about 23 minutes,[113] the operator must work fairly quickly and be prepared to reinject if profound anesthesia is lost. Although it has been reported that the intraligamentary injection can be used in the differential diagnosis of pulpally involved teeth,[130,131] experimental studies have demonstrated that adjacent teeth also become anesthetized with the intraligamentary injection of a single tooth.[114,121,122] Therefore, the intraligamentary PDL injection should *not* be used for differential diagnosis.

Several studies have evaluated potential adverse effects that may occur with the intraligamentary route of injection. First, intraligamentary injections are more painful when anesthetizing teeth with irreversible pulpitis, as compared to normal teeth,[5,111,114,122] and this may be due to the mechanical allodynia that often occurs in cases of irreversible pulpitis.[132] The patient should be made aware of this possibility. Second, intraligamentary injections typically produce mild postinjection pain in the majority of patients for 14 to 72 hours after injection,[111,114,122] and this would be additive to any postendodontic pain. Third, about 40% of the patients will report that their tooth feels high in occlusion.[114,122] Fourth, although a letter to the editor reported avulsion of a tooth following intraligamentary injections,[133] no clinical or experimental study has reported avulsion or loosening of teeth with this technique,[114,121,122] and therefore, avulsion should not be a concern when using the intraligamentary injection technique. Fifth, initial studies in dogs reported cardiovascular responses to intraligamentary injection of epinephrine-containing solutions[134]; however, this has not been confirmed in clinical studies evaluating tachycardia.[135,136] Sixth, minor damage to the periodontium does occur, but only at the site of needle penetration and this subsequently undergoes repair in nearly all cases. In very rare instances, periodontal abscesses and deep pocket formation[113,114] or root resorption[137,138] have occurred after intraligamentary injections. Seventh, clinical and animal studies have shown no effect on the pulp following intraligamentary injections[114,121,122,138–140] other than a rapid and prolonged decrease in pulpal blood flow caused by epinephrine.[127] No histological induction of pulpal inflammation has been observed in studies comparing restorative procedures to restorative procedures combined with intraligamentary injections.[141] Therefore, intraligamentary injections are unlikely to cause pulpal necrosis. Eighth, the intraligamentary injection of primary teeth may cause enamel hypoplasia of the developing permanent teeth.[142] However, the effect was not due to the injection itself but due to the anesthetic agents used. The same effect would seemingly be produced by an infiltration injection next to the developing tooth. Ninth, intraligamentary injection has been reported to be safe in the presence of mild to moderate gingival inflammation or incipient periodontitis.[143] Taken together, the intraligamentary route of injection provides a useful supplemental route for increasing anesthesia success with minimal adverse events reported in the great majority of studies.

A recent modification of the intraligamentary supplemental injection is the computer-assisted local anesthetic delivery system such as the Wand or CompuDent (CompuDent, Milestone Scientific Inc.) that accommodates a standard local anesthetic cartridge that is linked by sterile microtubing to a disposable, pen-like handpiece with a Luer-Lok needle attached to the end. The device is activated by a foot control that automates the infusion of local anesthetic solution at a controlled rate. A slow or fast flow rate may be initiated and maintained by a foot pedal control. A 1.4-mL aliquot of solution is delivered in 1 minute in the fast mode and in about 4 minutes and 45 seconds in the slow mode. The slow rate is used for the intraligamentary injection.

A recent study,[144] using experimental subjects, demonstrated that the Wand method of primary intraligamentary injection of 1.4 mL of 4% articaine with 1:100,000 epinephrine, versus injection of 1.4 mL of 2% lidocaine with 1:100,000 epinephrine, produced similar rates of successful anesthesia of the mandibular first molar (86 versus 74%, respectively, using EPT). The duration of anesthesia (31–34 minutes) was much longer than that reported previously using a pressure syringe and 0.4 mL of a lidocaine solution

(10 minutes).[114] Another study evaluated patients with irreversible pulpitis and a failed IAN block. Success of the intraligamentary injection (none or mild pain upon endodontic access or initial instrumentation) was obtained in only 56% of the patients.[145] The results were somewhat disappointing because the computer-controlled anesthetic delivery system should have been capable of delivering approximately 1.4 mL of anesthetic solution via intraligamentary injection by consistently maintaining a precise flow rate. Thus, other supplemental injection procedures may be indicated in patients with irreversible pulpitis.

INTRAOSSEOUS ANESTHESIA

A second route for supplemental injection is the intraosseous injection. There are three intraosseous systems in the commercial market, including the Stabident system (Fairfax Dental Inc., Miami, FL), the X-tip system (Dentsply, Tulsa, OK), the IntraFlow (IntraVantage, Plymouth, MN). However, to date, most published clinical trials have used either the Stabident or X-tip systems. The Stabident system is comprised of a slow-speed handpiece-driven perforator, a solid 27-gauge wire with a beveled end that, when activated, drills a small hole through the cortical plate. The anesthetic solution is delivered to the cancellous bone through the 27-gauge ultra-short injector needle placed into the hole made by the perforator; the modified nonbevel needle is recommended for ease of negotiation. The X-tip anesthesia delivery system consists of a special hollow needle that serves as the drill penetrating the cortical plate, whereupon it is separated and withdrawn. The guide sleeve is designed to accept a 27-gauge needle to inject the anesthetic solution and is removed after injection (Figure 3).

Several characteristics are similar among the studied intraosseous delivery systems. First, anesthetic success is improved following injection into a site distal rather than mesial to the selected tooth.[19,51,146–152] The exception to this rule is the maxillary and mandibular second molars where the mesial site should be selected.[19,51,146–152] Second, the onset of anesthesia is essentially immediate.[19,51,146–153] Third, manufacturer's instructions locate the perforation site in attached gingival, where the cortical bone is often thinner and one can inject at a site equidistant between adjacent root structures. However, two studies have successfully used the X-tip system, with its guide sleeve design, in alveolar mucosa at a more apical location,[19,148] providing a potential clinical advantage over the Stabident system when apical injections are considered.

As described above, a regular IAN block often provides poor anesthetic success in patients with irreversible pulpitis (i.e., only 19 to 56% of patients report no/mild pain upon access).[9–11,19,71,153] Thus, several studies have evaluated whether supplemental intraosseous injections improve anesthetic success after IAN nerve block in odontogenic pain patients.

Several studies have evaluated the Stabident system in patients with irreversible pulpitis in mandibular posterior molars after failed conventional IAN nerve block injections. In general, these trials have demonstrated that a Stabident injection of 2% lidocaine with 1:100,000 epinephrine produced 79% anesthetic success at a volume of 0.45 to 0.9 mL[18] and 91% success rate at an intraosseous injection volume of 1.8 mL.[9] The intraosseous injection was more successful than the PDL injection,[113] probably due to the greater amount of anesthetic solution delivered with the intraosseous injection. Other studies using a similar patient population and experimental design have demonstrated that supplemental intraosseous injection of 3% mepivacaine produced 80% success after one cartridge and 98% success following a second intraosseous injection.[10] Another study demonstrated that a supplemental intraosseous injection of 1.8 mL of 4% articaine with 1:100,000 epinephrine was 87% successful after the failure of IAN blocks for posterior teeth diagnosed with irreversible pulpitis.[153] Two conclusions are evident from this analysis. First, a supplemental intraosseous injection after a failed IAN nerve block significantly improves anesthetic success. Second, it appears that an intraosseous injection of one cartridge of 3% mepivacaine plain may not be as efficacious as one cartridge of 2% lidocaine with 1:100,000 epinephrine. However, as noted below, an advantage of mepivacaine is that 3% mepivacaine not does evoke the tachycardia typically observed with epinephrine-containing anesthetic solutions.

Parallel studies have evaluated the X-Tip system in patients with irreversible pulpitis in mandibular posterior molars after failed conventional IAN nerve block injections. In one study evaluating apical positioning of the perforator, the X-tip injection site was 3 to 7 mm apical to the mucogingival junction of the mandibular molar or premolar tooth, and 1.8 mL of 2% lidocaine with 1:100,000 epinephrine was administered.[19] The authors reported that in the absence of the backflow of anesthetic solution into the oral cavity, the success rate was 82%, but that in the presence of a backflow, the success rate dropped to 18%.[19]

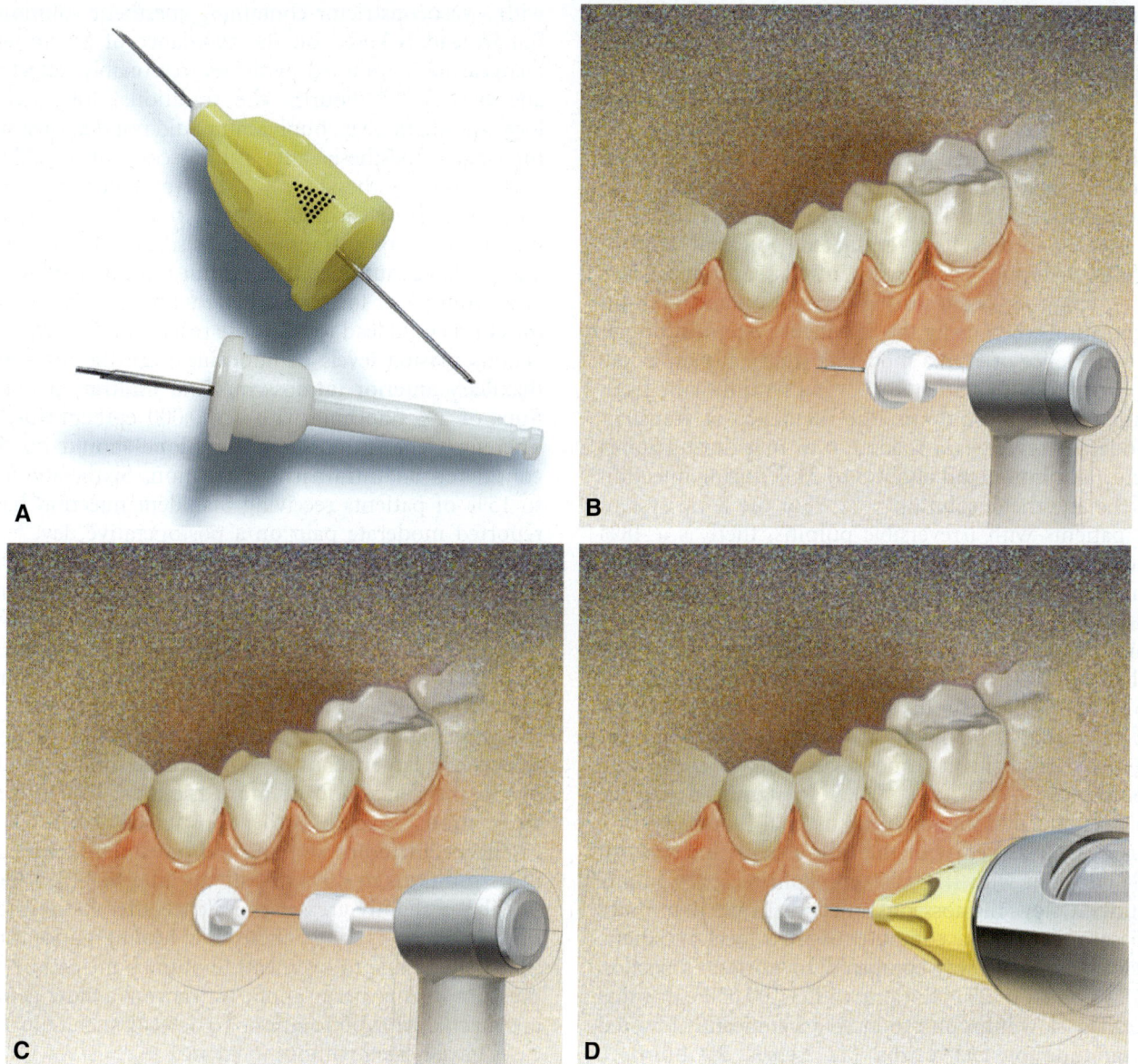

Figure 3 Intraosseous anesthesia delivery system X-tip. ***A,*** The X-tip system comes in two parts: the drill and the guide sleeve and special injection needle. First, anesthetize the mucobuccal fold and select a site 2 to 4 mm apical to the alveoli crest and between the roots. ***B,*** Place the X-tip drill in a slow-speed handpiece (15,000 to 20,000 rpm) and drill at maximum speed at 90° to the bone. In 2 to 4 seconds the drill will perforate the cortical bone into the cancellous bone. ***C,*** Hold the guide sleeve in place and withdraw the drill. ***D,*** Insert the special short needle into the hole in the guide sleeve and slowly inject a few drops of anesthetic solution. In the event, additional anesthesia is needed later; the guide sleeve can be left in place until the end of treatment.

Several clinical implications can be derived from these studies. First, given the relatively high failure rate of IAN blocks in patients with irreversible pulpitis, it would be prudent to consider using these combined methods in all patients with irreversible pulpitis. Second, anesthetic success requires deposition of the solution into the cancellous bone. If backflow occurs, the clinician should consider reperforation at the same or another site. A second intraosseous injection of 1.4 mL of 2% lidocaine with 1:100,000 epinephrine 30 minutes after the initial intraosseous injection provided an additional 15 to 20 minutes of pulpal anesthesia.[154] Third, in studies using either the Stabident or the X-tip system, the duration of anesthesia was sufficient for the entire debridement appointment.[9,19,153] Fourth, no clinical study has reported the anesthetic success rate or adverse events of supplemental intraosseous injection in painful teeth with necrotic pulps and periradicular radiolucencies. Therefore, no evidence-based clinical recommendations for necrotic cases can be made due to this lack of data. This is an area for future research.

Several studies have evaluated potential adverse effects that may occur with intraosseous injections. First, pain may occur during perforation and solution deposition when using the Stabident system, although the incidence of even a moderate transient pain is low in asymptomatic patients.[146–151] In symptomatic teeth with irreversible pulpitis, the incidence of transient moderate–severe pain is about 0 to 16% during Stabident perforation and about 5 to 31% during injection of the anesthetic solution.[9,10,153] For the X-tip system in patients with irreversible pulpitis, there is a 48% incidence of moderate to severe pain with perforation and a 27% incidence with injection of anesthetic.[19] Second, it has been estimated that about 1% of perforators "separate" during use, requiring removal with a hemostat.[19,146–151] Third, a transient tachycardia (12 to 32 bpm) can occur for about 4 minutes in 46 to 93% of patients after Stabident or X-tip intraosseous injection of epinephrine- and levonordefrin-containing solutions.[9,19,51,146–150,152,153,155] No significant change in diastolic, systolic, or mean arterial blood pressure has been observed with the intraosseous injection of 2% lidocaine with 1:100,000 epinephrine.[155,156] In one study, a slow intraosseous injection (over 4 minutes 45 seconds using a computer-assisted local anesthetic delivery system) was compared to a "fast" injection (45 seconds) of 2% lidocaine with 1:100,000 epinephrine. The slow infusion produced a significantly lowered magnitude of tachycardia (12 versus 25 bpm).[157] Although transient tachycardia is noticeable to the patient, it is thought to be not clinically significant in otherwise healthy patients.[155] Importantly, there is no significant increased tachycardia when 3% mepivacaine is used for intraosseous anesthesia.[155,158] This represents an alternative approach for patients whose medical condition (moderate-to-severe cardiovascular disease) or drug therapies (patients taking tricyclic antidepressants or nonselective β-adrenergic blocking agents) suggest caution in administering epinephrine- or levonordefrin-containing solutions. Based upon these considerations, the intraosseous injection of 1.8 mL of 3% mepivacaine without a vasoconstrictor (e.g., 3% Carbocaine) could be recommended as a local anesthetic of first choice. This is not based on the potential cardiovascular risks associated with a vasoconstrictor-containing anesthetic solutions, but instead is based on the avoidance of a transient tachycardia combined with its reasonably effective anesthesia.[155,158] Fourth, the traditional long-acting local anesthetic (e.g., bupivacaine) did not demonstrate prolonged anesthesia after intraosseous or maxillary infiltration anesthesia.[152,159–161] Given concerns about its potential for cardiotoxicity,[162] bupivacaine should not be used for intraosseous anesthesia. Fifth, some authors have cautioned that administration of an overly large volume of local anesthetic with an intraosseous injection could lead to overdose reactions.[163] However, venous plasma levels of lidocaine were the same for maxillary anterior intraosseous and infiltration injections of 2% lidocaine with 1:100,000 epinephrine.[164] Therefore, the intraosseous technique should not be considered an intravascular injection. Sixth, about 2 to 15% of patients receiving Stabident injection have reported moderate pain on a postoperative day,[51,146,149,150,155] although this is less than that reported after intraligamentary injection.[122] Gallatin et al.[165] found that significantly more males experienced postoperative pain with the X-tip system than with the Stabident system. They felt that this was related to a denser and more mineralized bone in the posterior mandible in males and the fact that the X-tip perforating system diameter is larger than the Stabident perforator resulting in the generation of more frictional heat during perforation. Seventh, other postinjection problems can occur, including swelling and/or exudate at the site of perforations in <5% of patients after Stabident and possibly a slightly greater prevalence after X-tip injections.[51,146,149,150,155,165] These slow-healing perforation sites may be due to overheating of the bone caused by pressure during perforation, warranting a slow gentle approach during perforation. To date, all such reported cases have healed without incidence.

THE INTRAPULPAL INJECTION

In about 5 to 10% of mandibular posterior teeth with irreversible pulpitis, supplemental intraosseous injections, even when repeated, do not produce profound anesthesia; pain persists when the pulp is entered. This is an indication for an intrapulpal injection. The advantage of the intrapulpal injection is that it works well for profound anesthesia if given under backpressure.[123,124] Onset will be immediate and no special syringes or needles are required. The major drawback of the technique is that needle placement and injection are directly into a vital and very sensitive pulp; the injection may be moderately to severely painful and the patient should be warned of this potentiality.[9]

Maxillary Anesthesia

Descriptions of conventional techniques for maxillary anesthesia are available for review in numerous articles and textbooks. Clinically, maxillary anesthesia is more successful than mandibular anesthesia and the infiltration route is by far the dominant approach.[12] Numerous studies have demonstrated that infiltration injection of anesthetics such as 2% lidocaine with 1:100,000 epinephrine results in 90 to 95% successful pulpal anesthesia (obtaining an 80 reading) in anterior and posterior maxillary teeth.[67,68,160,166–169] Although the onset of infiltration anesthesia usually occurs within 5 to 7 minutes, the duration is fairly short in both anterior (20 to 30 minutes) and posterior (30 to 45 minutes) maxillary teeth.[160,166–169] This may require additional anesthetic injections depending on the length of the procedure. For maxillary infiltration injections, increasing the volume of 2% lidocaine with 1:100,000 epinephrine to 3.6 mL will increase the duration of pulpal anesthesia.[167] As with mandibular anesthesia, pulpal anesthesia does not last as long as soft tissue anesthesia.[160,166–169] The infiltration injection of 4% prilocaine (1:200,000 epinephrine) is similar in action to an infiltration injection using 2% lidocaine (1:100,000 epinephrine).[169] In most,[65–68] but not all,[170] studies, maxillary infiltration injections of articaine with 1:100,000 epinephrine were equivalent to both prilocaine and lidocaine with epinephrine. Although bupivacaine provides long-acting anesthesia in the mandible, it does not provide prolonged pulpal anesthesia in maxillary infiltration injections.[80,159,160] The infiltration injection of anesthetics without vasoconstrictors, 3% mepivacaine plain and 4% prilocaine plain, produce a brief duration (15 to 20 minutes) of pulpal anesthesia and accordingly are generally used only for brief procedures.[168,169]

Since many endodontic procedures are done on one tooth at a time, the infiltration route is most commonly employed. However, for the sake of completeness, major maxillary block injections that are effective for anesthetizing multiple teeth will be briefly reviewed. The posterior superior alveolar (PSA) nerve block anesthetizes some first molars, and all second and third molars.[7] Generally, to ensure patient comfort for the first molar, an *additional buccal infiltration* injection after the PSA block may be needed. The *infraorbital nerve block* injection will anesthetize the first and second premolars and the lip, but not the central or lateral incisors.[171,172] The *second division nerve block* will successfully anesthetize the pulps of molar teeth and about 50% of the second premolars.[173,174] The high tuberosity approach is preferred over the greater palatine approach because the success rate is similar and it is less painful.[173] The *palatal-anterior superior alveolar* (P-ASA) injection deposits the anesthetic solution into the incisive canal and derives its name from the injection's ability to supposedly anesthetize both the right and the left anterior superior alveolar nerves leading to bilateral anesthesia of maxillary incisors and canines.[175] However, needle insertion results in 54 to 58% of the subjects reporting moderate/severe pain following needle placement.[34,176] The *anterior middle superior alveolar* (AMSA) injection is a new route for anesthetizing the maxillary central and lateral incisors, canines, and first and second premolars.[177–179] The AMSA injection site is located palatally at a point that bisects the premolars and is approximately halfway between the midpalatine raphe and the crest of the free gingival margin. However, studies evaluating the AMSA route have reported rather modest to low success rates,[180,181] and 32% to 38% incidence of moderate injection pain.[35]

Non-Narcotic Analgesics: Nonsteroidal Anti-Inflammatory Analgesics and Acetaminophen

The major analgesic drug class for treating endodontic pain is the non-narcotic drugs, consisting of the nonsteroidal anti-inflammatory analgesics (NSAIDs) and acetaminophen. The reader is referred to basic pharmacology texts for an overview of these drugs. The present review will instead focus on newer evidences and clinical implications from controlled clinical trials. The NSAID class of drugs are thought to produce their analgesic and anti-inflammatory effects by the inhibition of cyclooxygenase (COX).[182] Other mechanisms such as inhibition of cell signaling molecules (e.g., NFκB) have also been proposed.[183] Two major isotypes of COX have been described,[184,185] and NSAID drugs can be classified based upon their preference for blocking COX1 or COX2. NSAIDs such as ibuprofen should be considered "mixed COX" inhibitors since they can inhibit both enzymes at clinical dosages. Moreover, a recent study has reported that the analgesic efficacy of ibuprofen depends upon the genetic mutation of COX1, with patients having certain polymorphisms of COX1 displaying significantly better analgesic responses than patients having other polymorphisms.[186] If confirmed, then variations in patient responses to NSAIDs might be due to variations in the mutations on the gene encoding the COX1 enzyme. Blockade of COX1 is associated with increased risk for gastrointestinal side effects such as ulcers, whereas blockade of COX2 is associated with increased

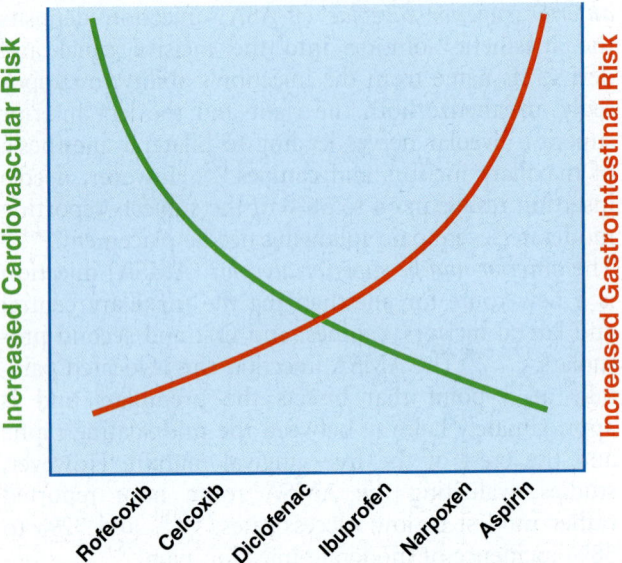

Figure 4 Schematic illustration of the relationship between risk for adverse side effect profile of non-narcotic analgesics based on the relative inhibition of COX1 versus COX2. Adapted from FitzGerald GA.[187]

Table 2 Meta-Analysis of Non-Narcotic Analgesics for Relief of Postoperative Pain

Drug	Percentage of Patients with ≥50% pain relief	N (No. of patients)
Ibuprofen 200 mg	46	1,194
Ibuprofen 400 mg	56	3,402
Ibuprofen 600 mg	79	203
Diclofenac 50 mg	50	367
Diclofenac 100 mg	70	204
Acetaminophen 600–650 mg	36	1,265
Acetaminophen 600–650 mg plus codeine 60 mg	48	911
Placebo	~13	6,497

Data adapted from Barden J et al.[192]

cardiovascular risk such as thrombotic events.[187] Instead of a bimodal classification, the NSAIDs should be viewed as having an inhibitory continuum,[187] where drugs can have varying efficacy for inhibiting COX1 versus COX2, and accordingly would be expected to vary in their clinical side effect profile (Figure 4). Based upon findings demonstrating rapid upregulation of prothrombic enzymes[188] and cardiac events,[189,190] it has been suggested that most patients would be best managed with the non-COX2-selective NSAIDs such as ibuprofen.[191]

Several systematic reviews have been published describing the efficacy and adverse effect profile of NSAIDs for treating both postsurgical pain[192–194] and postendodontic pain.[195] In general, these studies have demonstrated that NSAIDs produce excellent analgesic responses in patients who can tolerate this class of drugs. For example, in a meta-analysis of >14,000 third molar patients,[192] several NSAIDs were shown to produce a dose-related analgesic effect (defined as >50% pain relief). These data are summarized in Table 2. Since many clinicians were originally taught that acetaminophen/codeine combinations provide superior pain control, it is worth carefully reviewing these data. The lowest studied dose of ibuprofen (200 mg) actually has about the same analgesic response as acetaminophen 600 to 650 mg/codeine 60 mg. Moreover, the 400 mg and 600 mg doses of ibuprofen produce substantially greater levels of analgesia. Equally important, only the acetaminophen/codeine combination was associated with any significant increase in adverse effects.[192] Fortunately, these findings mirror the responses of endodontists published in a recent survey[196] where non-narcotics, especially ibuprofen 600 mg, were dominantly selected for pain control over the acetaminophen/opiate combination drugs.

Other studies have evaluated the analgesic benefit of NSAIDs for treating pain after nonsurgical endodontic procedures.[197–215] In general, the randomized placebo-controlled endodontic studies have demonstrated significant analgesic benefits for patients treated with flurbiprofen,[202] flurbiprofen/tramadol,[197] intracanal ketorolac,[198] IM ketorolac,[208] intraoral ketorolac (in some,[201,207] but not all[216] studies), piroxicam,[210] mefanamic acid,[211] aspirin,[211] diclofenac,[209] ketoprofen (in some,[199,209] but not all[200] studies), ibuprofen,[199,204] and ibuprofen/acetaminophen.[204]

Interestingly, ibuprofen 600 mg produced only a modest/moderate analgesic effect in several postendodontic studies.[217–220] It is not clear if this modest analgesic effect reflects a non-COX pain mechanism in endodontic pain patients reflective of chronic inflammatory conditions (e.g., cytokines), or whether it represents a "floor effect" where nonsurgical root canal treatment by itself reduces pain to the extent that it is difficult to detect further reduction by the addition of an analgesic. This latter point has been observed in many endodontic trials where non-surgical root canal treatment (NS-RCT) plus a placebo pill resulted in a 50 to 80% pain reduction, 24 to 48 hours after treatment.[197,199] However, the overall interpretation of these data provide strong support for the use of NSAIDs as a primary class of analgesics for treating acute inflammatory pain due to either surgical or nonsurgical procedures.

As noted in Chapter 10, "Mechanisms of Odontogenic and Non-Odontogenic Pain," the VGSC play the dominant role in the signaling of nociceptor activity from the periphery to the CNS. In particular, the TTX-resistant class of VGSCs expressed on nociceptors is relatively resistant to lidocaine and is sensitized by prostaglandins.[16,221,222] One interpretation of these basic science findings is that NSAIDs would be expected to increase the effectiveness of local anesthetics by virtue of their ability to reduce prostaglandin levels in inflamed tissue. A preemptive approach to improve anesthesia in patients with irreversible pulpitis is to give ibuprofen 1 hour before anesthetic administration. A recent study[223] evaluated ibuprofen given before local anesthetic injection in patients with irreversible pulpitis. It concluded that *it significantly improved the depth of anesthesia* using an EPT testing paradigm. Another study pretreated patients with either a placebo or with acetaminophen 650 mg or the combination of ibuprofen 600 mg with acetaminophen 650 mg. They concluded that the odds ratio for the *combination group* tended to favor successful anesthesia in the active groups as compared to the placebo.[224] However, both of the studies have fairly small sample sizes, and further research is needed on this potentially important clinical finding.

Acetaminophen represents the second major member of the non-narcotic class of analgesics. Its utility is largely based on the finding that its side effect profile is less adverse than the NSAIDs, and that the drug can be used in patients for whom NSAIDs are contraindicated.[225] Although acetaminophen has been used for nearly 100 years, its mechanism of action remains mostly unknown. Acetaminophen does inhibit peripheral COX activity in inflamed tissues but only at doses of about 1,000 mg.[226] Recent studies have suggested additional mechanisms by which acetaminophen may act by metabolic conversion to a compound previously called AM404, which is a cannabinoid-like analgesic.[227] Indeed, acetaminophen antinociception is reversed in mice by pretreatment with a cannabinoid receptor antagonist.[228] However, other potential mechanisms have been proposed including modulation of the serotonin receptor 5HT1A.[229]

In humans, acetaminophen inhibits central sensitization under conditions that exclude a potential peripheral site of action,[230] suggesting that this drug also has a CNS site of action. Interestingly, animal studies demonstrate that acetaminophen produces synergistic effects with a variety of NSAIDs (i.e., ibuprofen, diclofenac, ketoprofen, meloxicam, metamizol, naproxen, nimesulide, parecoxib, and piroxicam) using a mouse model of tissue hyperalgesia.[231] This finding appears to have clinical implications since acetaminophen/NSAID combinations appear to be very effective for pain control following surgical[232,233] or endodontic[204] procedures.

Steroids

Various classes of drugs have been studied for the management of endodontic posttreatment pain.[197] These include non-narcotic analgesics comprising NSAIDs and acetaminophen, opioids and glucocorticoids (steroids). This section will consider the use of glucocorticoids for the management of endodontic pain. For an in-depth description of the pharmacology, pharmacodynamics, mechanisms and sites of action, as well as their anti-inflammatory actions, the reader is directed to review articles.[198,199,234–238]

The potent anti-inflammatory properties of glucocorticoids were first appreciated and utilized as an adjunct to endodontic therapy more than 50 years ago.[239–241] Steroids have been used as a pulp-capping agent,[242] as an intracanal medicament either alone or in combination with antibiotics/antihistamines,[198,240,241,243–247] and systemically[199,248,234–236,239,249–253] as a means to decrease pain and inflammation in endodontic patients.

In critically evaluating the literature, it must be kept in mind that the most powerful conclusions are generated from studies that are prospective, randomized, double-blind, and placebo-controlled. However, none of the endodontic reports on the use of corticosteroids published prior to 1984 meets these criteria, and the results therefore should be considered as lower levels of evidence. Results from studies that used corticosteroids in combination with other agents (antibiotics and/or antihistamines) are also difficult to interpret, as results ascribed to one of the agents may reflect the activity of the combination.[199,200] Equally difficult to interpret are results from studies using intracanal steroid delivery.[198,240,241,243–247] The methodology in these studies cannot account for either the dosage or the delivery period of the intracanal medicament to reach the site of action (periapical tissues). In these studies, very small dosages of the steroid are placed into the canal(s). Even assuming apical patency of unknown size, the steroid must pass through the apical foramen via passive diffusion along a concentration gradient, and this may be opposed by a potential backpressure from periapical transudate or exudate. For a critical assessment of these studies, the reader is directed to review an article by Marshall.[238] Studies evaluating the systemic administration of corticosteroid as the sole agent, in a known dose, are the critical ones in evaluating the efficacy of the steroid's ability to decrease endodontic posttreatment pain.

In a randomized, prospective, double-blind, placebo-controlled study, Marshall and Walton[235] evaluated the effect of the intramuscular injection of dexamethasone on posttreatment endodontic pain when compared to a placebo. After endodontic instrumentation and/or obturation, patients received an IM injection of 1.0 mL of either dexamethasone (4 mg/mL) or sterile saline. Pain levels of none, mild, moderate, or severe were recorded preoperatively at 4, 24, and 48 hours posttreatment. Teeth with vital and necrotic pulps as well as retreatment cases were included. No antibiotics were taken by the patients and no postoperative infections were reported. The amount of additional postoperative pain medication required was not recorded. Results indicated that dexamethasone significantly reduced both pain incidence and severity at 4 hours posttreatment. At 24 hours posttreatment, patients in the corticosteroid group showed a trend toward less pain.

Another double-blind study evaluated the effect of oral dexamethasone on posttreatment pain.[252] Fifty patients presenting for endodontic treatment were studied. Retreatment cases and patients presenting with purulent drainage or cellulitis were excluded. Teeth were instrumented and closed with no intracanal medication. Pretreatment, 8, and 24 hours posttreatment pain levels were recorded on a visual analog scale (0–100). Patients randomly received dexamethasone (0.75-mg tablet) or a placebo, with instructions to take three tablets immediately and then one tablet every 3 hours until bedtime for a total of seven tablets. Results showed that patients receiving dexamethasone had significantly less pain at 8 and 24 hours when compared to those receiving the placebo ($p<0.01$)

A third study[250] evaluated the effect of oral dexamethasone on endodontic interappointment pain, but at a much higher dosage than the preceding study.[252] Forty patients with "asymptomatic vital inflamed" pulps were evaluated. After endodontic instrumentation and temporization, alternate patients were given either dexamethasone (4 mg per tablet) or a placebo. Instructions were to take one tablet immediately and then one tablet at 4 and 8 hours posttreatment for a total dose of 12 mg in the dexamethasone group. Pain was recorded on a visual analog scale at 8, 24, and 48 hours posttreatment. Patients receiving dexamethasone had a statistically significant reduction in pain at all post treatment periods.

Liesinger et al.[234] in a double-blind, randomized, prospective, placebo-controlled study evaluated the effect of four different dosages of dexamethasone on posttreatment endodontic pain. All patients ($N=106$) presented with pretreatment pain. Pulp status was recorded (vital and necrotic cases were included). Endodontic instrumentation and/or obturation was performed after which patients randomly received a 1.0-mL intraoral injection of either a placebo (sterile saline) or dexamethasone (2, 4, 6, 8 mg/mL). The injection was given into the masseter, internal ptyergoid, or buccinator muscle; preference was given to introoral muscles anesthetized for treatment. Patients recorded their pain levels on a 0 to 9 scale. Pretreatment and posttreatment (4, 8, 24, 48, and 72 hours) pain levels were recorded. The type and the amount of posttreatment analgesics taken were also recorded. No antibiotics were given at any time. Results showed patients receiving dexamethasone had significantly less severe pain at 4 and 8 hours postoperatively ($p<0.05$) and took significantly less pain medication compared to the placebo (dexamethasone mean, 1.98 tablets; placebo mean, 4.64 tablets). When evaluated on a milligram per kilogram dosage basis, patients who received 0.07 to 0.09 mg/kg of IM dexamethasone had significantly less pain at 8 hours and required significantly less postoperative pain medication when compared to the IM placebo.

Kaufman et al.[254] were the first to evaluate the effect of the *intraligamentary delivery* of dexamethasone on endodontic posttreatment pain. Forty-five patients were randomly assigned to one of three experimental groups. Endodontic treatment was completed in one appointment on both vital and necrotic pulps, with and without periapical radiolucencies. After the administration of local anesthesia, but prior to endodontic treatment, patients in Group 1 received 4 to 8 mg of slow-release methylprednisolone (Depo-Medrol) via an intraligamentary syringe. Single-rooted teeth received 4 mg, and multirooted teeth received 8 mg. Group 2 received a PDL injection of 3% mepivacaine in a similar fashion to Group 1. Patients in Group 3 received no PDL injection. Pretreatment pain levels were not recorded. Patients were telephoned at 24 hours posttreatment and reported their pain intensity on a 1–10 scale. The results showed a significant decrease in postoperative pain in the methylprednisolone group compared to the active and passive placebo groups ($p<0.05$).

Gallatin et al.[248] evaluated pain reduction in patients with untreated irreversible pulpitis using an intraosseous injection of methylprednisolone. Forty patients with a clinical diagnosis of irreversible pulpitis actively associated with moderate–severe pain participated in this prospective double-blind study. The involved tooth was anesthetized followed by an intraosseous injection of 1 mL of either methylprednisolone (Depo-Medrol 40 mg/mL) or saline. The blinded solutions were administered using the Stabident system (Fairfax Dental Inc.). No endodontic treatment was performed at this time. Patients were given a 7-day pain diary as well as analgesic medication. Over the 7-day observation period, patients who received Depo-Medrol reported significantly less pain ($p<0.05$) compared to a placebo while taking significantly fewer analgesics ($p<0.05$).

Bramy et al.[236] evaluated the intraosseous administration of corticosteroid for pain reduction in symptomatic necrotic teeth. Thirty-eight patients with a clinical diagnosis of pulpal necrosis with associated periapical radiolucency participated in the study. All patients experienced moderate–severe pain at the time of presentation with mild or no clinical swelling. After complete canal debridement, patients in a double-blind fashion randomly received an intraosseous injection of 1 mL of either methylprednisolone (Depo-Medrol 40 mg/mL) or sterile saline. All subjects received ibuprofen and Tylenol #3 (with codeine) and were instructed to take the medication as needed for pain. Patients recorded their pain levels and the type and amount of pain medications taken for 7 days postoperatively. The results showed that the steroid group had significantly less postoperative pain and took significantly less pain medication over the 7 days when compared to the placebo group ($p<0.05$). No antibiotics were taken by patients at any time.

In a follow-up study, Claffey et al.[249] evaluated pain reduction in symptomatic teeth with necrotic pulps using an oral dose regimen of methylprednisolone. The materials and methods were nearly identical to Bramy et al.[236] except that no patient had clinical swelling, and after canal debridement, patients randomly received either oral methylprednisolone (48 mg/day for 3 days) or an oral placebo (lactose 48 mg/day for 3 days) in a double-blind fashion. All patients received ibuprofen and Tylenol #3 and a diary to record pain, percussion pain, swelling, and number and type of pain medication taken. Clinical success was defined as any patient who experienced only none–mild pain, none–mild percussion pain, none–mild swelling, and did not take any Tylenol #3. No antibiotics were prescribed or taken. The results showed that patients who received methylprednisolone had a significantly higher level of clinical success when compared to the placebo ($p<0.05$).

Ouyang et al.[253] evaluated the effect of submucosally injected dexamethasone on both the incidence and the severity of endodontic interappointment pain. Teeth with a diagnosis of asymptomatic pulpal necrosis were endodontically treated in one appointment. Eighty patients received a submucosal injection of 5 mg dexamethasone; the control group of 80 patients had endodontic treatment performed but no submucosal injection. Pain incidence and severity was evaluated for 3 days postoperatively. Results indicated that the patients in the dexamethasone group had a statistically significant decreased incidence and severity of endodontic interappointment pain.

Prior to interpreting these studies,[248,234–236,249–251,253] it is critical to remember that endodontic treatment has a major effect in reducing posttreatment pain regardless of pharmacologic intervention. As stated by Hargreaves,[255] "This reduction in posttreatment pain, combined with variable levels of preoperative pain, reduces the statistical power of endodontic clinical trials for detecting active analgesics over time in all patient groups (the so-called floor effect). This limitation is a problem in interpreting clinical studies in general and may explain why some endodontic clinical trials fail to detect analgesic treatment or only detect it in those patients with moderate/severe pain." This has been shown by Torabinejad et al.[199] and Rogers et al.[198] where various agents including corticosteroid significantly reduced posttreatment pain but only in those patients who presented for treatment with at least moderate/severe pretreatment pain. It would seem that the systemic administration of a corticosteroid to ameliorate endodontic posttreatment pain would be appropriate only for those patients who present with at least moderate levels of preoperative pain. Three independent studies[234,236,249] meet the criteria of being prospective, randomized, double-blind, placebo-controlled with no drug combinations, and including patients who presented with the required level of pretreatment pain. Importantly, these studies showed that the systemic administration of corticosteroid not only significantly reduces posttreatment pain at various times but also significantly reduces the amount of additional pain medication required.

Interestingly, the reports by Bramy et al.[236] and Claffey et al.[249] show significant pain relief with the administration of a steroid for up to 7 days posttreatment, in contrast to Liesinger et al.[234] who found significant differences in pain reduction only in the first 8 hours. It is possible that these findings are due to differences in dosages of different corticosteroids or due to the routes of administration. This is probably not the case, as dexamethasone is approximately five times as potent as methylprednisolone. The 6 to 8 mg intramuscular dosage used by Liesinger et al.[234] would be equivalent to 30 to 40 mg of methylprednisolone. Intraosseous 40 mg of methylprednisolone was the dosage used by Bramy et al.[236] It may be speculated that these differences in the duration of action might be related to differences in the preoperative pulpal and periapical status of the patient populations of these studies. All of the patients in the studies by Bramy et al.[236] and Claffey et al.[249] presented for treatment with necrotic pulps, associated periapical radiolucencies, and either mild or no swelling. The majority of patients in the study by Liesinger et al.[234] had a preoperative diagnosis of irreversible pulpitis and acute apical periodontitis. Those patients with necrotic pulps had no associated periapical radiolucencies. It is plausible that corticosteroids may be more efficacious in attenuating the pain associated with pulpal necrosis and an associated radiolucency compared to pain associated with irreversible pulpitis. Necrosis/radiolucency is associated with a more complex chronic inflammatory process. Thus the efficacy of corticosteroids, in endodontic pain patients, may be related to variations in the periapical immunological/inflammatory dynamics of teeth with irreversibly inflamed pulps compared to necrotic pulps.

On the basis of the work of Bramy et al.[236] and Claffey et al.,[249] it is plausible that corticosteroids would have efficacy in cases of endodontic flare-up that result after treatment of previously asymptomatic teeth with necrotic pulps with or without associated periapical radiolucencies. This premise has not been investigated. The low incidence of this type of flare-up[256] would require a multicenter study over a period of years to achieve an adequate sample size.

It appears that the route of systemic administration of a steroid is not a determinant in the efficacy of action.[234,236,249] When given in equivalent dosages, agents such as dexamethasone and methylprednisolone appear to be interchangeable. If a systemic steroid is to be administered, an intraoral IM injection or an intraosseous injection would seem to be preferable over an extraoral IM injection. Clinicians are familiar with intraoral and intraosseous injections, and the site of injection is already anesthetized. Intraoral injection of steroid would be preferable to a written prescription for glucocorticoid as no assumption to patient compliance is required. An injection dosage of 6 to 8 mg of dexamethasone or 40 mg of methylprednisolone appears to be appropriate for the adult patient. If an oral route is chosen, 48 mg of methylprednisolone per day for 3 days and by extrapolation 10 to 12 mg of dexamethasone per day for 3 days should provide significant posttreatment pain relief.

It has been stated that antibiotics must be given in conjunction with steroids to prevent an infection secondary to a decrease in the inflammatory response.[239,257–259] The implication is that suppression of inflammation also means a decrease in local defenses permitting unchecked proliferation of pathogenic microorganisms. None of the studies published since 1984 supports this premise, including those cases with a diagnosis of pulpal necrosis with periapical radiolucency where the potential for dissemination of an infectious process might be expected.[236,249] Antibiotics were not given or needed at any time during these studies nor were the steroids associated with any increase in infection rate compared to the control groups. It can be concluded that antibiotics are not routinely required or recommended in conjunction with corticosteroids for the management of endodontic posttreatment pain in the otherwise healthy patient.

Opioid Analgesics

Because opioids are not anti-inflammatory, nonopioids with anti-inflammatory efficacy (e.g., aspirin, ibuprofen) are the analgesics of first choice for endodontic pain.[260] It has been shown that codeine in a 30 mg dose provides no more analgesia than a placebo.[261,262] However, a 60 mg dose of codeine produces significantly more analgesia than a placebo. Thus, opioids in the appropriate dosage may be of benefit when additional pain control in needed. For example, if an NSAID is not controlling a patient's discomfort, an opioid combination such as acetaminophen/hydrocodone may be prescribed in addition to the NSAID. Opioids in combination with an NSAID produce additional analgesia beyond the ceiling effect of the NSAID. Opioid analgesics activate mu receptors that inhibit the transmission of nociceptive signals from the trigeminal nucleus to the higher brain centers and activate peripheral receptors to reduce pain.[263,264] Although opioid analgesics may be effective for the relief of moderate to severe pain, their use is limited by adverse side effects that include nausea, vomiting, drowsiness, dizziness, constipation, and respiratory depression. In addition, chronic use is associated with tolerance and dependence. Because of the numerous side effects, opioids are usually used in combination with other analgesics to manage endodontic pain. Table 3 has a list of opioids

Table 3 Opioid Analgesic Combinations

Opioid Combination	Usual Dose
Acetaminophen (300 mg) and codeine (30 mg)	2 tablets q4h
Aspirin (325 mg) and codeine (30 mg)	2 tablets q4h
Acetaminophen (500 mg) and hydrocodone (5 mg)	1-2 tablets q6h
Acetaminophen (325/500 mg) and oxycodone (5 mg)	1 tablet q6h
Aspirin (325 mg) and oxycodone (5 mg)	1 tablet q6h
Ibuprofen (200 mg) and hydrocodone (7.5 mg)	1 tablet q6h

in combination with aspirin, acetaminophen, and ibuprofen that may be used to alleviate pain of endodontic origin. Clinicians must be aware of drug-seeking patients who request a specific opioid.

Conclusions

A thorough knowledge of the biological (Chapter 10, "Mechanisms of Odontogenic and Non-Odontogenic Pain") and pharmacological aspects of odontogenic pain reveals several important conclusions that are summarized as follows:

- There is no single magic bullet for treating pain. Clinicians need to develop skills for differential diagnoses of pain disorders, delivering positive behavioral management strategies, identifying risk factors for postprocedural pain, effective intraosseous injection of local anesthetics (particularly in cases of painful mandibular teeth, especially irreversible pulpitis), using combinations of an NSAID with acetaminophen (in patients who can tolerate these drugs), delivering effective and appropriate dental treatment, and following up all patients to ensure their appropriate response.
- The intensity of preoperative pain is a useful predictor of post-endodontic pain,[199,202,265] and this risk factor should be considered when developing the pain treatment plan before treatment commences.
- Preoperative pain in a mandibular tooth is a risk factor for anesthetic failure of IAN block injections. The best evidence to date, which balances efficacy with minimal adverse effects, would support treating patients with an irreversible pulpitis of a mandibular tooth first with an IAN block injection, followed immediately by an intraosseous injection of 3% mepivacaine. Little is known about benefits/risks of an intraosseous injection of symptomatic mandibular teeth with pulpal necrosis and periapical radiolucencies.
- Emerging clinical evidence provides qualitative support that a preoperative NSAID would be expected to enhance the magnitude of anesthesia, although additional research is needed.
- In patients who can tolerate the drug classes, there is strong preclinical and clinical trial data demonstrating that the combination of an NSAID with acetaminophen provides effective pain control in both postsurgical and postendodontic patients. One possible strategy to treat patients in moderate-to-severe pain would be to consider combinations of up to ibuprofen 600 mg and acetaminophen 1,000 mg, four times a day for no more than 2 to 3 days after the procedure. This combination of analgesics provides a useful alternative to the classical use of narcotic-containing analgesic drugs.
- It is our belief that the integration of high-quality clinical research findings together with the clinician's own skills, the patient's desires and the particulars of each case, represents the highest level of clinical care. From this perspective, this chapter represents an important contribution, but is only one source of information on the pharmacology of pain control. Clinicians must supplement this information and evaluate its application to any particular clinical case.

References

1. Vreeland DL, Reader A, Beck M, et al. An evaluation of volumes and concentrations of lidocaine in human inferior alveolar nerve block. J Endod 1989;15(1):6–12.
2. McLean C, Reader A, Beck M, et al. An evaluation of 4% prilocaine and 3% mepivacaine compared with 2% lidocaine (1:100,000 epinephrine) for inferior alveolar nerve block. J Endod 1993;19(3):146–50.
3. Chaney MA, Kerby R, Reader A, et al. An evaluation of lidocaine hydrocarbonate compared with lidocaine hydrochloride for inferior alveolar nerve block. Anesth Prog 1991;38(6):212–16.
4. Hinkley SA, Reader A, Beck M, Meyers WJ. An evaluation of 4% prilocaine with 1:200,000 epinephrine and 2% mepivacaine with 1:20,000 levonordefrin compared with 2% lidocaine with 1:100,000 epinephrine for inferior alveolar nerve block. Anesth Prog 1991;38(3):84–9.
5. Dreven LJ, Reader A, Beck M, et al. An evaluation of an electric pulp tester as a measure of analgesia in human vital teeth. J Endod 1987;13(5):233–8.
6. Certosimo A, Archer R. A clinical evaluation of the electric pulp tester as an indicator of local anesthesia. Oper Dent 1996;21:25–30.
7. Loetscher C, Melton D, Walton R. Injection regimen for anesthesia of the maxillary first molar. J Am Dent Assoc 1988;117:337–40.
8. Jones VR, Rivera EM, Walton RE. Comparison of carbon dioxide versus refrigerant spray to determine pulpal responsiveness. J Endod 2002;28(7):531–3.
9. Nusstein J, Reader A, Nist R, et al. Anesthetic efficacy of the supplemental intraosseous injection of 2% lidocaine with 1:100,000 epinephrine in irreversible pulpitis. J Endod 1998;24(7):487–91.
10. Reisman D, Reader A, Nist R, et al. Anesthetic efficacy of the supplemental intraosseous injection of 3% mepivacaine in

irreversible pulpitis. Oral Surg Oral Med Oral Pathol Oral Radiol Endod 1997;84(6):676–82.

11. Cohen H, Cha B, Spangberg L. Endodontic anesthesia in mandibular molars: a clinical study. J Endod 1993;19:370–3.

12. Kaufman E, Weinstein P, Milgrom P. Difficulties in achieving local anesthesia. J Am Dent Assoc 1984;108:205–8.

13. Hargreaves K, Keiser K. Local anesthetic failure in endodontics: Mechanisms and management. Endod Top 2002;1:26–39.

14. Wallace JA, Michanowicz AE, Mundell RD. A pilot study of the clinical problem of regionally anesthetizing the pulp of an acutely inflamed mandibular molar. Oral Surg Oral Med Oral Pathol Oral Radiol Endod 1985;59(5):517–21.

15. Byers MR, Taylor PE, Khayat BG, et al. Effects of injury and inflammation on pulpal and periapical nerves. J Endod 1990;16(2):78–84.

16. Roy M, Nakanishi T. Differential properties of tetrodotoxin-sensitive and tetrodotoxin-resistant sodium channels in rat dorsal root ganglion neurons. J Neurosci 1992;12:2104–11.

17. Sorensen H, Skidmore L, Rzasa R, et al. Comparison of pulpal sodium channel density in normal teeth to diseased teeth with severe spontaneous pain [abstract]. J Endod 2004;30:287.

18. Parente SA, Anderson RW, Herman WW, et al. Anesthetic efficacy of the supplemental intraosseous injection for teeth with irreversible pulpitis. J Endod 1998;24(12):826–8.

19. Nusstein J, Kennedy S, Reader A, et al. Anesthetic efficacy of the supplemental X-tip intraosseous injection in patients with irreversible pulpitis. J Endod 2003;29(11):724–8.

20. Milgrom P, Coldwell SE, Getz T, et al. Four dimensions of fear of dental injections. J Am Dent Assoc 1997;128:756–66.

21. Kleinknecht R, Klepac R, and Alexander L. Origins and characteristics of fear of dentistry. J Am Dent Assoc 1993;86:842–8.

22. Milgrom P, Fiset L, Melnick S, et al. The prevalence and practice management consequences of dental fear in a major US city. J Am Dent Assoc 1988;116:641–7.

23. Rosivack R, Koenigsberg S, Maxwell K. An analysis of the effectiveness of two topical anesthetics. Anesth Prog 1990;37:290–2.

24. Hersh E, Houpt MI, Cooper SA, et al. Analgesic efficacy and safety of an intraoral lidocaine patch. J Am Dent Assoc 1996;127:1626–34.

25. Hutchins HS Jr, Young FA, Lackland DT, Fishburne CP. The effectiveness of topical anesthesia and vibration in alleviating the pain of oral injections. Anesth Prog 1997;44:87–9.

26. Nusstein JM, Beck M. Effectiveness of 20% benzocaine as a topical anesthetic for intraoral injections. Anesth Prog 2003;50(4):159–63.

27. Gill C, and Orr D. A double-blind crossover comparison of topical anesthetics. J Am Dent Assoc 1979;98:213–14.

28. Keller B. Comparison of the effectiveness of two topical anesthetics and a placebo in reducing injection pain. Hawaii Dent J 1985;16:10–1.

29. Martin M, Ramsay DS, Whitney C, et al. Topical anesthesia: differentiating the pharmacological and psychological contributions to efficacy. Anesth Prog 1994;41:40–7.

30. Kanaa M, Meechan JG, Corbett IP, Whitworth JM. Speed of injection influences efficacy of inferior alveolar nerve blocks: a double-blind randomized controlled trial in volunteers. J Endod 2006;32:919–23.

31. Hochman M, Chiarello D, Hochman CB, Lopatkin R, Pergola S. Computerized local anesthetic delivery vs. traditional syringe technique. NY State Dent J 1997; 63:24–9.

32. Nicholson J, Berry TG, Summitt JB, et al. Pain perception and utility: a comparison of the syringe and computerized local injection techniques. Gen Dent 2001;49:167–73.

33. Primosch R. and Brooks R. Influence of anesthetic flow rate delivered by the Wand local anesthetic system on pain response to palatal injections. Am J Dent 2002; 15:15–20.

34. Nusstein, J, Burns Y, Reader A, et al. Injection pain and postinjection pain of the palatal-anterior superior alveolar injection, administered with the Wand Plus system, comparing 2% lidocaine with 1:100,000 epinephrine to 3% mepivacaine. Oral Surg Oral Med Oral Pathol Oral Radiol Endod 2004;97(2):164–72.

35. Nusstein J, Lee S, Reader A, et al. Injection pain and post-injection pain of the anterior middle superior alveolar injection administered with the Wand or conventional syringe. Oral Surg Oral Med Oral Pathol Oral Radiol Endod 2004;98:124–31.

36. Kudo M. Initial injection pressure for dental local anesthesia: effects on pain and anxiety. Anesth Prog 2005;52:95–101.

37. Saloum FS, Baumgartner JC, Marshall G, Tinkle J. A clinical comparison of pain perception to the Wand and a traditional syringe. Oral Surg Oral Med Oral Pathol Oral Radiol Endod 2000;86:691–5.

38. Goodell G, Gallagher F, Nicoll B. Comparison of a controlled injection pressure system with a conventional technique. Oral Surg Oral Med Oral Pathol Oral Radiol Endod 2000;90:88–94.

39. Meechan J, Day P. A comparison of intraoral injection discomfort produced by plain and epinephrine-containing lidocaine local anesthetic solutions: a randomized, double-blind, split-mouth, volunteer investigation. Anesth Prog 2002;49:44–8.

40. Wahl M, Schmitt MM, Overton DA, Gordon MK. Injection pain of bupivacaine with epinephrine vs. prilocaine plain. J Am Dent Assoc 2002;133:1652–6.

41. Wahl M, Overton D, Howell J, et al. Pain on injection of prilocaine plain vs. lidocaine with epinephrine; a prospective double-blind study. J Am Dent Assoc 2001;132:1396–401.

42. Pogrel M. and Thamby S. Permanent nerve involvement resulting from inferior alveolar nerve blocks. J Am Dent Assoc 2000;131:901.

43. Pogrel M, Schmidt BL, Sambajon V, Jordan RC. Lingual nerve damage due to inferior alveolar nerve blocks: a possible explanation. J Am Dent Assoc 2003;134:195–9.

44. Krafft T and Hickel R. Clinical investigation into the incidence of direct damage to the lingual nerve caused by local anesthesia. J Craniomaxillofac Surg 1994;22:294.

45. Hannan L, Reader A, Nist R, et al. The use of ultrasound for guiding needle placement for inferior alveolar nerve blocks. Oral Surg Oral Med Oral Pathol Oral Radiol Endod 1999;87(6):658–65.

46. Wali M, Reader A, Beck M, Meyers W. Anesthetic efficacy of lidocaine and epinephrine in human inferior alveolar nerve blocks [abstract]. J Endod 1988;14:193.

47. Simon F, Reader A, Meyers W, Beck M, Nist R. Evaluation of a peripheral nerve stimulator in human mandibular anesthesia [abstract]. J Dent Res 1990;69:278.

48. Fernandez C, Reader A, Beck M, Nusstein J. A prospective, randomized, double-blind comparison of bupivacaine and lidocaine for inferior alveolar nerve blocks. J Endod 2005;31:499–503.

49. Nusstein J, Reader A, Beck FM. Anesthetic efficacy of different volumes of lidocaine with epinephrine for inferior alveolar nerve blocks. Gen Dent 2002;50(4):372–5.

50. Malamed S. Handbook of local anesthesia. Vol. 5. St. Louis, MO: Mosby; 2004 pp. 41, 65, 72, 237, 242.

51. Guglielmo A, Reader A, Nist R, Beck M, Weaver J. Anesthetic efficacy and heart rate effects of the supplemental intraosseous injection of 2% mepivacaine with 1:20,000 levonordefrin. Oral Surgery, Oral Surg Oral Med Oral Pathol Oral Radiol Endod 1999;87(3):284–93.

52. Malamed SF, Gagnon S, Leblanc D. Articaine hydrochloride: a study of the safety of a new amide local anesthetic. J Am Dent Assoc 2001;132(2):177–85.

53. Wright G, Weinberger SJ, Friedman CS, Plotzke OB. The use of articaine local anesthesia in children under 4 years of age—a retrospective report. Anesth Prog 1989;36:268–71.

54. Hidding J, Khoury F. General complications in dental local anesthesia. Dtsch Zahnarztl Z 1991;46:831–6.

55. Moller R, Covino B. Cardiac electrophysiologic effects of articaine compared with bupivacaine and lidocaine. Anesth Analg 1993;76:1266–73.

56. Jakobs W, Ladwig B, Cichon P, et al. Serum levels of articaine 2% and 4% in children. Anesth Prog 1995;42:113–15.

57. Daublander M, Muller R, Lipp M. The incidence of complications associated with local anesthesia in dentistry. Anesth Prog 1997;44:132–41.

58. Simon M, Gielen MJ, Alberink N, et al. Intravenous regional anesthesia with 0.5% articaine, 0.5% lidocaine, or 0.5% prilocaine. A double-blind randomized clinical study. Reg Anesth 1997;22:29–34.

59. Oertel R, Ebert U, Rahn R, Kirch W. The effect of age on pharmacokinetics of the local anesthetic drug articaine. Reg Anesth Pain Med 1999;24:524–8.

60. Malamed S, Gagnon S, Leblanc D. A comparison between articaine HCl and lidocaine HCl in pediatric dental patients. Pediatr Dent 2000;22:307–11.

61. Wilburn-Goo D, Lloyd L. When patients become cyanotic: acquired methemoglobinemia. J Am Dent Assoc 1999;130:826–31.

62. Haas, DA, Lennon D. A 21 year retrospective study of reports of paresthesia following local anesthetic administration. J Can Dent Assoc 1995;61(4):319–20, 323–6, 329–30.

63. Miller P, Lennon D. Incidence of local anesthetic-induced neuropathies in Ontario from 1994–1998. J Dent Res 2000;Abstract (3869):627.

64. Malamed S, Gagnon S, Leblanc D. Efficacy of articaine: a new amide local anesthetic. J Am Dent Assoc 2000;131:635–42.

65. Donaldson D, James-Perdok L, Craig BJ, et al. A comparison of Ultracaine DS (articaine HCl) and Citanest forte (prilocaine HCl) in maxillary infiltration and mandibular nerve block. J Can Dent Assoc 1987;53:38–42.

66. Haas D, Harper DG, Saso MA, Young ER. Comparison of articaine and prilocaine anesthesia by infiltration in maxillary and mandibular arches. Anesth Prog 1990;37:230–7.

67. Haas D, Harper DG, Saso MA, Young ER. Lack of differential effect by Ultracaine (articaine) and Citanest (prilocaine) in infiltration anaesthesia. J Can Dent Assoc 1991;57:217–23.

68. Vahatalo K, Antila H, Lehtinen R. Articaine and lidocaine for maxillary infiltration anesthesia. Anesth Prog 1993;40:114–16.

69. Wright G, Weinberger SJ, Marti R, Plotzke O. The effectiveness of infiltration anesthesia in the mandibular primary molar region. Pediatr Dent 1991;13:278–83.

70. Mikesell P, Nusstein J, Reader A, et al. A comparison of articaine and lidocaine for inferior alveolar nerve blocks. J Endod 2005;31:265–70.

71. Claffey E, Reader A, Nusstein J, et al. Anesthetic efficacy of articaine for inferior alveolar nerve blocks in patients with irreversible pulpitis. J Endod 2004;30:568–71.

72. Robertson D, Nusstein J, Reader A, et al. The anesthetic efficacy of articaine in buccal infiltration of mandibular posterior teeth. J Am Dent Assoc 2007;138(8):1104–12.

73. Kanaa MD, Whitworth J, Corbett I, Meechan J. Articaine and lidocaine mandibular buccal infiltration anesthesia: a prospective randomized double-blind cross-over study. J Endod 2006;32:296.

74. Davis W, Oakley J, Smith E. Comparison of the effectiveness of etidocaine and lidocaine as local anesthetic agents during oral surgery. Anesth Prog 1984;31:159–64.

75. Rosenquist J, Rosenquist K, Lee P. Comparison between lidocaine and bupivacaine as local anesthetics with diflunisal for postoperative pain control after lower third molar surgery. Anesth Prog 1988;35:1–4.

76. Dunsky JL, Moore PA. Long-acting local anesthetics: a comparison of bupivacaine and etidocaine in endodontics. J Endod 1984;10(9):457–60.

77. Moore PA, Dunsky JL. Bupivacaine anesthesia—a clinical trial for endodontic therapy. Oral Surg Oral Med Oral Pathol Oral Radiol Endod 1983;55(2):176–9.

78. Linden E, Abrams H, Matheny J, et al. A comparison of postoperative pain experience following periodontal surgery using two local anesthetic agents. J Periodontol 1986;57:637–42.

79. Crout RJ, Koraido G, Moore PA. A clinical trial of long-acting local anesthetics for periodontal surgery. Anesth Prog 1990;37(4):194–8.

80. Kennedy M, Reader A, Beck M, Weaver J. Anesthetic efficacy of ropivacaine in maxillary anterior infiltration. Oral Surg Oral Med Oral Pathol Oral Radiol Endod 2001;91(4):406–12.

81. El-Sharrawy E. Anesthetic efficacy of different ropivacaine concentrations for inferior alveolar nerve block. Anesth Prog 2006;53:3.

82. Frommer J, Mele F, Monroe C. The possible role of the mylohyoid nerve in mandibular posterior tooth sensation. J Am Dent Assoc 1972;85:113–17.

83. Wilson S, Johns P, Fuller P. The inferior alveolar and mylohyoid nerves: an anatomic study and relationship to local anesthesia of the anterior mandibular teeth. J Am Dent Assoc 1984;108:350–2.

84. Clark S, Reader A, Beck M, Meyers WJ. Anesthetic efficacy of the mylohyoid nerve block and combination inferior alveolar nerve block/mylohyoid nerve block. Oral Surg Oral Med Oral Pathol Oral Radiol Endod 1999;87(5):557–63.

85. Berns J, Sadove M. Mandibular block injection: a method of study using an injected radiopaque material. J Am Dent Assoc 1962;65:736–45.

86. Galbreath J, Eklund M. Tracing the course of the mandibular block injection. Oral Surg Oral Med Oral Pathol Oral Radiol Endod 1970;30:571–82.

87. Cooley R, Robison S. Comparative evaluation of the 30-gauge dental needle. Oral Surg Oral Med Oral Pathol Oral Radiol Endod 1979;48:400–4.

88. Davidson M. Bevel-oriented mandibular injections: needle deflection can be beneficial. Gen Dent 1989;37:410–12.

89. Hochman M, Friedman M. In vitro study of needle deflection: a linear insertion technique versus a bidirectional rotation insertion technique. Quintessence Int 2000;31:33–8.

90. Kennedy S, Reader A, Nusstein J, et al. The significance of needle deflection in success of the inferior alveolar nerve block in patients with irreversible pulpitis. J Endod 2003;29(10):630–3.

91. Steinkruger G, Nusstein J, Reader A, et al. The significance of needle bevel orientation in success of the inferior alveolar nerve block. J Am Dent Assoc 2006;137(12):1685–91.

92. Yonchak T, Reader A, Beck M, Meyers WJ. Anesthetic efficacy of unilateral and bilateral inferior alveolar nerve blocks to determine cross innervation in anterior teeth. Oral Surg Oral Med Oral Pathol Oral Radiol Endod 2001;92(2):132–5.

93. Rood J. The nerve supply of the mandibular incisor region. Br Dent J 1977;143:227–30.

94. DeJong R. Neural blockade by local anesthetics. J Am Dent Assoc 1997;238:1383–5.

95. Strichartz G. Molecular mechanisms of nerve block by local anesthetics. Anesthesiology 1967;45:421–44.

96. Agren E, Danielsson K. Conduction block analgesia in the mandible. A comparative investigation of the techniques of Fischer and Gow-Gates. Swed Dent J 1981;5:91–9.

97. Yared GM, Dagher FB. Evaluation of lidocaine in human inferior alveolar nerve block. J Endod 1997;23(9):575–8.

98. Yonchak T, Reader A, Beck M, et al. Anesthetic efficacy of infiltrations in mandibular anterior teeth. Anesth Prog 2001;48(2):55–60.

99. Dagher FB, Yared GM, Machtou P. An evaluation of 2% lidocaine with different concentrations of epinephrine for inferior alveolar nerve block. J Endod 1997;23(3):178–80.

100. Anonymous. Wydase lyophilized hyaluronidase 150 units, package insert. Philadelphia, PA: Wyeth Laboratories Inc.

101. Looby J, Kirby C. Use of hyaluronidase with local anesthetic agents in dentistry. J Am Dent Assoc 1949;38:1–4.

102. Kirby C, Eckenhoff J, Looby J. The use of hyaluronidase with local anesthetic agents in nerve block and infiltration anesthesia. Surgery 1949;25:101–3.

103. Ridenour S, Reader A, Beck M, Weaver J. Anesthetic efficacy of a combination of hyaluronidase and lidocaine with epinephrine in inferior alveolar nerve blocks. Anesth Prog 2001;48(1):9–15.

104. Meyer RA. Use of tripelenamine and diphenhydramine as local anesthetics. J Am Dent Assoc 1964;69:112.

105. Welborn JF. Conduction anesthesia using diphenhydramine HCl. J Am Dent Assoc 1964;69:706.

106. Willett J, Reader A, Beck M, Meyers W, Nist R. Benadryl and combination Benadryl/lidocaine for mandibular anesthesia [abstract]. J Endod 1994;20:191.

107. Goodman A, Reader A, Nusstein J, et al. Anesthetic efficacy of lidocaine/meperidine for inferior alveolar nerve blocks. Anesth Prog 2006;53:131–9.

108. Bigby J, Reader A, Nusstein J, Beck M. Anesthetic efficacy of lidocaine/meperidine for inferior alveolar nerve blocks in patients with irreversible pulpitis. J Endod, 2006 in press.

109. Malamed S. The periodontal ligament (PDL) injection: an alternative to inferior alveolar nerve block. Oral Surg Oral Med Oral Pathol Oral Radiol Endod 1982;53:117–21.

110. Walton R, Abbott B. Periodontal ligament injection: a clinical evaluation. J Am Dent Assoc 1981;103:571–5.

111. D'Souza J, Walton R, Peterson L. Periodontal ligament injection: an evaluation of extent of anesthesia and postinjection discomfort. J Am Dent Assoc 1987;114:341–4.

112. Smith G, Walton R, Abbott B. Clinical evaluation of periodontal ligament anesthesia using a pressure syringe. J Am Dent Assoc 1983;107:953–6.

113. Childers M, Reader A, Nist R, et al. Anesthetic efficacy of the periodontal ligament injection after an inferior alveolar nerve block. J Endod 1996;22(6):317–20.

114. White JJ, Reader A, Beck M, Meyers WJ. The periodontal ligament injection: a comparison of the efficacy in human maxillary and mandibular teeth. J Endod 1988;14(10):508–14.

115. Meechan J, Ledvinka J. Pulpal anesthesia for mandibular central incisor teeth: a comparison of infiltration and intraligamentary injections. Int Endod J 2002;35:629–34.

116. Smith G, Walton R. Periodontal ligament injections: distribution of injected solutions. Oral Surg Oral Med Oral Pathol Oral Radiol Endod 1983;55:232–8.

117. Dreyer WP, van Heerden JD, de V Joubert JJ. The route of periodontal ligament injection of local anesthetic solution. J Endod 1983;9(11):471–4.

118. Walton RE. Distribution of solutions with the periodontal ligament injection: clinical, anatomical, and histological evidence. J Endod 1986;12(10):492–500.

119. Tagger M, Tagger E, Sarnat H. Periodontal ligament injection: spread of the solution in the dog. J Endod 1994;20(6):283–7.

120. Rawson R, Orr D. Vascular penetration following intraligamental injection. J Oral Maxillofac Surg 1985;43:600–4.

121. Moore KD, Reader A, Meyers WJ, et al. A comparison of the periodontal ligament injection using 2% lidocaine with 1:100,000 epinephrine and saline in human mandibular premolars. Anesth Prog 1987;34(5):181–6.

122. Schleder JR, Reader A, Beck M, Meyers WJ. The periodontal ligament injection: a comparison of 2% lidocaine, 3% mepivacaine, and 1:100,000 epinephrine to 2% lidocaine with 1:100,000 epinephrine in human mandibular premolars. J Endod 1988;14(8):397–404.

123. Birchfield J, Rosenberg PA. Role of the anesthetic solution in intrapulpal anesthesia. J Endod 1975;1(1):26–7.

124. VanGheluwe J, Walton R. Intrapulpal injection—factors related to effectiveness. Oral Surg Oral Med Oral Pathol Oral Radiol Endod 1997;19:38–40.

125. Gray R, Lomax A, Rood J. Periodontal ligament injection: with or without a vasoconstrictor? Br Dent J 1987;162:263–5.

126. Kaufman E, Solomon V, Rozen L, Peltz R. Pulpal efficacy of four lidocaine solutions injected with an intraligamentary syringe. Oral Surg Oral Med Oral Pathol Oral Radiol Endod 1994;78:17–21.

127. Kim S. Ligamental injection: a physiological explanation of its efficacy. J Endod 1986;12(10):486–91.

128. Meechan J. A comparison of ropivacaine and lidocaine with epinephrine for intraligamentary anesthesia. Oral Surg Oral Med Oral Pathol Oral Radiol Endod 2002;93:469–73.

129. Johnson G, Hlava G, Kalkwarf K. A comparison of periodontal intraligamental anesthesia using etidocaine HCl and lidocaine HCl. Anesth Prog 1985;32:202–5.

130. Littner MM, Tamse A, Kaffe I. A new technique of selective anesthesia for diagnosing acute pulpitis in the mandible. J Endod 1983;9(3):116–19.

131. Simon D, Jacobs JL, Senia E, Walker WA. Intraligamentary anesthesia as an aid in endodontic diagnosis. Oral Surg Oral Med Oral Pathol Oral Radiol Endod 1982;54:77–8.

132. Owatz CB, Khan AA, Schindler WG, et al. The incidence of mechanical allodynia in patients with irreversible pulpitis. J Endod 2007;33(5):552–6.

133. Nelson P. Letter to the editor. J Am Dent Assoc 1981;103:692.

134. Smith G, Pashley D. Periodontal ligament injection: evaluation of systemic effects. Oral Surg Oral Med Oral Pathol Oral Radiol Endod 1983;56:571–4.

135. Cannell H, Kerawala C, Webster K, Whelpton R. Are intraligamentary injections intravascular? Br Dent J 1993;175:281–4.

136. Nusstein J, Berlin J, Reader A, Beck M, Weaver J. Comparison of injection pain, heart rate increase and post-injection pain of articaine and lidocaine in a primary intraligamentary injection administered with a computer-controlled local anesthetic delivery system. Anesth Prog 2004;51:126–33.

137. Pertot W, Dejou J. Bone and root resorption. Effects of the force developed during periodontal ligament injections in dogs. Oral Surg Oral Med Oral Pathol Oral Radiol Endod 1992;74:357–65.

138. Roahen JO, Marshall FJ. The effects of periodontal ligament injection on pulpal and periodontal tissues. J Endod 1990;16(1):28–33.

139. Lin L, Lapeyrolerie M, Skribner J, Shovlin F. Periodontal ligament injection: effects on pulp tissue. J Endod 1985;11(12):529–34.

140. Peurach J. Pulpal response to intraligamentary injection in cynomologus monkey. Anesth Prog 1985;32:73–5.

141. Plamondon T, Walton R, Graham GS, Houston G, Snell G. Pulp response to the combined effects of cavity preparation and periodontal ligament injection. Oper Dent 1990;15:86–93.

142. Brannstrom M, Lindskog S, Nordenvall K. Enamel hypoplasia in permanent teeth induced by periodontal

ligament anesthesia of primary teeth. J Am Dent Assoc, 1984;109:735–6.

143. Cromley N, Adams D. The effect of intraligamentary injections on diseased periodontiums in dogs. Gen Dent 1991;39:33–7.

144. Berlin J, Nusstein J, Reader A, Beck M, Weaver J. Efficacy of articaine and lidocaine in a primary intraligamentary injection administered with a computer-controlled local anesthetic delivery system. Oral Surg Oral Med Oral Pathol Oral Radiol Endod 2005;99:361.

145. Nusstein J, Claffey E, Reader A, Reader A, Nist R, Beck M, Meyers W. Anesthetic effectiveness of the supplemental intraligamentary injection, administered with a computer-controlled local anesthetic delivery system, in patients with irreversible pulpitis. J Endod 2005;31:354–8.

146. Coggins R, Reader A, Nist R, Beck M, Meyers W. Anesthetic efficacy of the intraosseous injection in maxillary and mandibular teeth. Oral Surgery, Oral Medicine, Oral Surg Oral Med Oral Pathol Oral Radiol Endod 1996;81(6):634–41.

147. Dunbar D, Reader A, Nist R, et al. Anesthetic efficacy of the intraosseous injection after an inferior alveolar nerve block. J Endod 1996;22(9):481–6.

148. Gallatin J, Reader A, Nusstein J, et al. A comparison of two intraosseous anesthetic techniques in mandibular posterior teeth. J Am Dent Assoc 2003;134(11):1476–84.

149. Reitz J, Reader A, Nist R, Beck M, Meyers W. Anesthetic efficacy of the intraosseous injection of 0.9 mL of 2% lidocaine (1:100,000 epinephrine) to augment an inferior alveolar nerve block. Oral Surg Oral Med Oral Pathol Oral Radiol Endod 1998;86(5):516–23.

150. Reitz J, Reader A, Nist R, et al. Anesthetic efficacy of a repeated intraosseous injection given 30 min following an inferior alveolar nerve block/intraosseous injection. Anesth Prog 1998;45(4):143–9.

151. Replogle K, Reader A, Nist R, Beck M, Meyers W. Anesthetic efficacy of the intraosseous injection of 2% lidocaine (1:100,000 epinephrine) and 3% mepivacaine in mandibular first molars. Oral Surg Oral Med Oral Pathol Oral Radiol Endod 1997;83(1):30–7.

152. Stabile P, Reader A, Gallatin E, Beck M, Weaver J. Anesthetic efficacy and heart rate effects of the intraosseous injection of 1.5% etidocaine (1:200,000 epinephrine) after an inferior alveolar nerve block. Oral Surg Oral Med Oral Pathol Oral Radiol Endod 2000;89(4):407–11.

153. Bigby J, Reader A, Nusstein J, et al. Articaine for supplemental intraosseous anesthesia in patients with irreversible pulpitis. J Endod 2006;32(11):1044–7.

154. Jensen J, Nusstein J, Reader A, Beck M. Anesthetic efficacy of a repeated intraosseous injection following a primary intraosseous injection [abstract]. J Endod 2006;32(3):237.

155. Replogle K, Reader A, Nist R, et al. Cardiovascular effects of intraosseous injections of 2 percent lidocaine with 1:100,000 epinephrine and 3 percent mepivacaine. J Am Dent Assoc 1999;130(5):649–57.

156. Chamberlain T, Davis RD, Murchison DF, et al. Systemic effects of an intraosseous injection of 2% lidocaine with 1:100,000 epinephrine. Gen Dent 2000;48(3)May–June:299–302.

157. Susi L, Reader A, Nusstein J, Beck M. Heart rate changes associated with intraosseous injections using slow and fast rates [abstract]. J Endod 2006;32:238.

158. Gallatin E, Stabile P, Reader A, Nist R, Beck M. Anesthetic efficacy and heart rate effects of the intraosseous injection of 3% mepivacaine after an inferior alveolar nerve block. Oral Surg Oral Med Oral Pathol Oral Radiol Endod 2000;89(1):83–7.

159. Danielsson K, Evers H, Nordenram A. Long-acting local anesthetics in oral surgery: an experimental evaluation of bupivacaine and etidocaine for oral infiltration anesthesia. Anesth Prog 1985;32:65–8.

160. Gross R, Reader A, Beck M, Meyer W. Anesthetic efficacy of liodaine and bupivacaine in human maxillary infiltration [abstract]. J Endod 1988;14:193.

161. Hull T, Rothwell B. Intraosseous anesthesia comparing lidocaine and etidocaine [abstract]. J Dent Res 1998;77:197.

162. Bacsik C, Swift J, Hargreaves K. Toxic systemic reactions of bupivacaine and etidocaine. Oral Surg Oral Med Oral Pathol Oral Radiol Endod 1995;79:18–23.

163. Ingle J, Bakland L. Endodontics. In: Ingle J, Bakland L, editors. Vol. 5. Hamilton, ON: BC Decker; 2002, p. 391.

164. Wood M, Reader A, Nusstein J, et al. Comparison of intraosseous and infiltration injections for venous lidocaine blood concentrations and heart rate changes after injection of 2% lidocaine with 1:100,000 epinephrine. J Endod 2005;31:435.

165. Gallatin J, Nusstein J, Reader A, Beck M, Weaver J. A comparison of injection pain and postoperative pain of two intraosseous anesthetic techniques. Anesth Prog 2003;50(3):111–20.

166. Nusstein J, Wood M, Reader A, et al. Comparison of the degree of pulpal anesthesia achieved with the intraosseous injection and infiltration injection using 2% lidocaine with 1:100,000 epinephrine. Gen Dent 2005;53:50–3.

167. Mikesell P, ReaderA, Beck M, Meyers W. Analgesic efficacy of volumes of lidocaine in human maxillary infiltration [abstract]. J Endod 1987;13:128.

168. Mason R, Reader A, Beck M, Meyers W. Comparisons of epinephrine concentrations and mepivacaine in human maxillary anesthesia [abstract]. J Endod, 1989;15:173.

169. Katz S, Reader A, Beck M, Meyers W. Anesthetic comparison of prilocaine and lidocaine in human maxillary infiltrations [abstract]. J Endod 1989;15:173.

170. Costa CG, Tortamano IP, Rocha RG, Froncischone CE, Tortamano N. Onset and duration periods of articaine and

lidocaine on maxillary infiltration. Quintessence Int 2005;36:197.

171. Berberich G, Reader A, Beck M, Meyer W. Evaluation of the infraorbital nerve block in human maxillary anesthesia [abstract]. J Endod 1990;16:192.

172. Karkut B, Reader A, Nist R, Beck M, Meyer W. Evaluation of the extraoral infraorbital nerve block in maxillary anesthesia [abstract]. J Dent Res 1993;72:274.

173. Broering R, Reader A, Beck M, Meyer W. Evaluation of second division nerve blocks in human maxillary anesthesia [abstract]. J Endod 1991;17:194.

174. Martinkus A, Reader A, Nusstein J, Beck M, Weaver J. Anesthetic efficacy of lidocaine and mepivacaine in the maxillary second division nerve block [abstract]. J Endod 2004;30:263.

175. Friedman M, Hochman M. P-ASA block injection: a new palatal technique to anesthetize maxillary anterior teeth. J Esthetic Dent 1999;11:63–71.

176. Meechan JG, Howlett PC, Smith BD. Factors influencing the discomfort of intraoral needle penetration. Anesth Prog 2005;52:91–4.

177. Friedman M, Hochman M. Using AMSA and P-ASA nerve blocks for esthetic restorative dentistry. Gen Dent 2001;5:506–11.

178. Friedman M, Hochman M. The AMSA injection: a new concept for local anesthesia of maxillary teeth using a computer-controlled injection system. Quintessence Int 1998;29:297–303.

179. Friedman M, Hochman M. A 21st century computerized injection system for local pain control. Compend Cont Dent Educ 1997;18:995–1003.

180. Lee S, Reader A, Nusstein J, et al. Anesthetic efficacy of the anterior middle superior alveolar (AMSA) injection. Anesth Prog 2004;51:80–9.

181. Fukayama H, Yoshikawa F, Kohase H, et al. Efficacy of anterior and middle superior alveolar (AMSA) anesthesia using a new injection system: The Wand. Quintessence Int 2003;34:537–41.

182. Rainsford KD. Anti-inflammatory drugs in the 21st century. Subcell Biochem 2007;42:3–27.

183. Lleo A, Galea E, Sastre M. Molecular targets of non-steroidal anti-inflammatory drugs in neurodegenerative diseases. Cell Mol Life Sci 2007;64(11):1403–18.

184. Khan AA, Dionne RA. The COX-2 inhibitors: new analgesic and anti-inflammatory drugs. Dent Clin North Am 2002;46(4):679–90.

185. Cicconetti A, et al. COX-2 selective inhibitors: a literature review of analgesic efficacy and safety in oral-maxillofacial surgery. Oral Surg Oral Med Oral Pathol Oral Radiol Endod 2004;97(2):139–46.

186. Lee YS, et al. Genetically mediated interindividual variation in analgesic responses to cyclooxygenase inhibitory drugs. Clin Pharmacol Ther 2006;79(5):407–18.

187. FitzGerald GA. COX-2 in play at the AHA and the FDA. Trends Pharmacol Sci 2007;28(7):303–7.

188. Wang XM, et al. Rofecoxib regulates the expression of genes related to the matrix metalloproteinase pathway in humans: implication for the adverse effects of cyclooxygenase-2 inhibitors. Clin Pharmacol Ther 2006;79(4):303–15.

189. Graham DJ, et al. Risk of acute myocardial infarction and sudden cardiac death in patients treated with cyclooxygenase 2 selective and non-selective non-steroidal anti-inflammatory drugs: nested case–control study. Lancet 2005;365(9458):475–81.

190. Salzberg DJ, Weir MR. COX-2 inhibitors and cardiovascular risk. Subcell Biochem 2007;42:159–74.

191. Huber MA, Terezhalmy GT. The use of COX-2 inhibitors for acute dental pain: a second look. J Am Dent Assoc 2006;137(4):480–7.

192. Barden J, et al. Relative efficacy of oral analgesics after third molar extraction. Br Dent J 2004;197(7):407–11.

193. Barden J, et al. Pain and analgesic response after third molar extraction and other postsurgical pain. Pain 2004;107(1–2):86–90.

194. Bandolier; 2007 (cited 2007 September 17, 2007); Available from: http://www.jr2.ox.ac.uk/bandolier/booth/painpag/Acutrev/Analgesics/lftab.html.

195. Hohman A, Neiderman R, Hargreaves K. Evaluation of NSAIDs for treating post-endodontic pain. Endod Top 2002;3:3–13.

196. Mickel AK, et al. An analysis of current analgesic preferences for endodontic pain management. J Endod 2006;32(12):1146–54.

197. Doroschak AM, Bowles WR, Hargreaves KM. Evaluation of the combination of flurbiprofen and tramadol for management of endodontic pain. J Endod 1999;25(10):660–3.

198. Rogers MJ, et al. Comparison of effect of intracanal use of ketorolac tromethamine and dexamethasone with oral ibuprofen on post treatment endodontic pain. J Endod 1999;25(5):381–4.

199. Torabinejad M, et al. Effectiveness of various medications on postoperative pain following complete instrumentation. J Endod 1994;20(7):345–54.

200. Torabinejad M, et al., Effectiveness of various medications on postoperative pain following root canal obturation. J Endod 1994;20(9):427–31.

201. Battrum D, Gutmann J. Efficacy of ketorolac in the management of pain associated with root canal treatment. J Can Dent Assoc 1996;62(1):36–42.

202. Flath RK, et al. Pain suppression after pulpectomy with preoperative flurbiprofen. J Endod 1987;13(7):339–47.

203. Segura JJ, et al. A new therapeutic scheme of ibuprofen to treat postoperatory endodontic dental pain. Proc West Pharmacol Soc 2000;43:89–91.

204. Menhinick KA, et al. The efficacy of pain control following nonsurgical root canal treatment using ibuprofen or a

combination of ibuprofen and acetaminophen in a randomized, double-blind, placebo-controlled study. Int Endod J 2004;37(8):531–41.

205. Nekoofar MH, Sadeghipanah M, Dehpour AR. Evaluation of meloxicam (A cox-2 inhibitor) for management of postoperative endodontic pain: a double-blind placebo-controlled study. J Endod 2003;29(10):634–7.

206. Sadeghein A, Shahidi N, Dehpour AR. A comparison of ketorolac tromethamine and acetaminophen codeine in the management of acute apical periodontitis. J Endod 1999;25(4):257–9.

207. Penniston SG, Hargreaves KM. Evaluation of periapical injection of Ketorolac for management of endodontic pain. J Endod 1996;22(2):55–9.

208. Curtis P Jr, Gartman LA, Green DB. Utilization of ketorolac tromethamine for control of severe odontogenic pain. J Endod 1994;20(9):457–9.

209. Negm MM. Effect of intracanal use of nonsteroidal anti-inflammatory agents on posttreatment endodontic pain. Oral Surg Oral Med Oral Pathol Oral Radiol Endod 1994;77(5):507–13.

210. Negm MM. Management of endodontic pain with nonsteroidal anti-inflammatory agents: a double-blind, placebo-controlled study. Oral Surg Oral Med Oral Pathol Oral Radiol Endod 1989;67(1):88–95.

211. Rowe NH, et al. Control of pain resulting from endodontic therapy: a double-blind, placebo-controlled study. Oral Surg Oral Med Oral Pathol Oral Radiol Endod 1980;50(3):257–63.

212. Modaresi J, Dianat O, Mozayeni MA. The efficacy comparison of ibuprofen, acetaminophen–codeine, and placebo premedication therapy on the depth of anesthesia during treatment of inflamed teeth. Oral Surg Oral Med Oral Pathol Oral Radiol Endod 2006;102(3):399–403.

213. Menke ER, et al. The effectiveness of prophylactic etodolac on postendodontic pain. J Endod 2000;26(12):712–15.

214. Gopikrishna V, Parameswaran A. Effectiveness of prophylactic use of rofecoxib in comparison with ibuprofen on postendodontic pain. J Endod 2003;29(1):62–4.

215. Morse DR, et al. Comparison of diflunisal and an aspirin–codeine combination in the management of patients having one-visit endodontic therapy. Clin Ther 1987;9(5):500–11.

216. Mellor AC, Dorman ML, Girdler NM. The use of an intra-oral injection of ketorolac in the treatment of irreversible pulpitis. Int Endod J 2005;38(11):789–92.

217. Rogers MJ, et al. Comparison of effect of intracanal use of ketorolac tromethamine and dexamethasone with oral ibuprofen on post treatment endodontic pain. J Endod 1999;25(5):381–4.

218. Gopikrishna V, Parameswaran A. Effectiveness of prophylactic use of rofecoxib in comparison with ibuprofen on post-endodontic pain. J Endod 2003;29(1):62–4.

219. Kusner G, et al. A study comparing the effectiveness of Ibuprofen (Motrin), Empirin with Codeine #3, and Synalgos-DC for the relief of postendodontic pain. J Endod 1984;10(5):210–14.

220. Torabinejad M, et al. Effectiveness of various medications on postoperative pain following root canal obturation. J Endod 1994;20(9):427–31.

221. Gold M, et al. Hyperalgesic agents increase a tetrodotoxin-resistant Na^+-current in nociceptors. Proc Natl Acad Sci 1996;93:1108–12.

222. Black JA, et al. Changes in the expression of tetrodotoxin-sensitive sodium channels within dorsal root ganglia neurons in inflammatory pain. Pain 2004;108(3):237–47.

223. Modaresi J, Dianat O, Mozayeni MA. The efficacy comparison of ibuprofen, acetaminophen–codeine, and placebo premedication therapy on the depth of anesthesia during treatment of inflamed teeth. Oral Surg Oral Med Oral Pathol Oral Radiol Endod 2006;102:399.

224. Ianiro SR, et al, The effect of preoperative acetaminophen or a combination of acetaminophen and Ibuprofen on the success of inferior alveolar nerve block for teeth with irreversible pulpitis. J Endod 2007;33(1):11–14.

225. Whelton A. Clinical implications of nonopioid analgesia for relief of mild-to-moderate pain in patients with or at risk for cardiovascular disease. Am J Cardiol 2006;97(9A):3–9.

226. Lee YS Kim H, Brahim JS, et al. Acetaminophen selectively suppresses peripheral prostaglandin E2 release and increases COX-2 gene expression in a clinical model of acute inflammation. Pain, 2007;129(3):279–86.

227. Hogestatt ED, Jönsson BA, Ermund A, et al. Conversion of acetaminophen to the bioactive N-acylphenolamine AM404 via fatty acid amide hydrolase-dependent arachidonic acid conjugation in the nervous system. J Biol Chem 2005;280(36):31405–12.

228. Ottani A, Leone S, Sandrini M, et al. The analgesic activity of paracetamol is prevented by the blockade of cannabinoid CB1 receptors. Eur J Pharmacol 2006;531(1–3):280–1.

229. Bonnefont J, Daulhac L, Etienne M, et al. Acetaminophen recruits spinal p42/p44 MAPKs and GH/IGF-1 receptors to produce analgesia via the serotonergic system. Mol Pharmacol 2007;71(2):407–15.

230. Koppert W, Wehrfritz A, Körber N, et al. The cyclooxygenase isozyme inhibitors parecoxib and paracetamol reduce central hyperalgesia in humans. Pain 2004;108(1–2):148–53.

231. Miranda HF, Puig MM, Prieto JC, Pinardi G. Synergism between paracetamol and nonsteroidal anti-inflammatory drugs in experimental acute pain. Pain 2006;121(1–2):22–8.

232. Cooper SA. The relative efficacy of ibuprofen in dental pain. Compend Contin Educ Dent 1986;7(8):578, 580–1, 584–8.
233. Breivik EK, Barkvoll P, Skovlund E. Combining diclofenac with acetaminophen or acetaminophen–codeine after oral surgery: a randomized, double-blind single-dose study. Clin Pharmacol Ther 1999;66(6):625–35.
234. Liesinger A, Marshall FJ, Marshall JG. Effect of variable doses of dexamethasone on posttreatment endodontic pain. J Endod 1993;19(1):35–9.
235. Marshall JG, Walton RE. The effect of intramuscular injection of steroid on posttreatment endodontic pain. J Endod 1984;10(12):584–8.
236. Bramy E, Reader A, Gallatin E, et al. The intraosseous injection of Depo-Medrol on postoperative endodontic pain in symptomatic necrotic teeth [Abstract OR29]. J Endod 1999;25:289.
237. Barnes PJ. Molecular mechanisms and cellular effects of glucocorticosteroids. Immunol Allergy Clin North Am 2005;25(3):451–68.
238. Marshall JG. Contribution of steroids for endodontic pain. Endod Top 2002;3:41–51.
239. Stewart G, Chilton NW. The role of antihistamines and corticosteroids in endodontic practice. Oral Surg Oral Med Oral Pathol Oral Radiol Endod 1958;11:433.
240. Wolfson B. The role of hydrocortisone in the control of apical periodontitis. Oral Surg Oral Med Oral Pathol Oral Radiol Endod 1954;7:314–21.
241. Blitzer M. Root canal therapy. Use of a combination of antibacterial agents, hydrocortisone and hyaluronidase. NY State Dent J 1956;22:503–8.
242. Fry AE, Watkins, RF, Phatak NM. Topical use of corticosteroids for the relief of pain sensitivity of dentine and pulp. Oral Surg Oral Med Oral Pathol Oral Radiol Endod 1960;13:594–7.
243. Ehrman G. The effect of triamcinalone with tetracycline on the dental pulp and apical periodontium. J Prosthet Dent 1965;15:149–52.
244. Langeland K, Langeland LK, Anderson DM. Corticosteroids in dentistry. Int Dent J 1977;27(3):217–51.
245. Chance K, Lin L, Shovlin FE, Skribner J. Clinical trial of intracanal corticosteroid in root canal therapy. J Endod 1987;13(9):466–8.
246. Moskow A, et al. Intracanal use of a corticosteroid solution as an endodontic anodyne. Oral Surg Oral Med Oral Pathol Oral Radiol Endod 1984;58(5):600–4.
247. Negm MM. Intracanal use of a corticosteroid-antibiotic compound for the management of posttreatment endodontic pain. Oral Surg Oral Med Oral Pathol Oral Radiol Endod 2001;92(4):435–9.
248. Gallatin, E, Reader A, Nist R, Beck M. Pain reduction in untreated irreversible pulpitis using an intraosseous injection of Depo-Medrol. J Endod 2000;26(11):633–8.
249. Claffey D, et al. Pain reduction in symptomatic, necrotic teeth using an oral dose regimen of methylprednisolone [Abstract OR34]. J Endod 2001;27:233.
250. Glassman G, et al. A prospective randomized double-blind trial on efficacy of dexamethasone for endodontic interappointment pain in teeth with asymptomatic inflamed pulps. Oral Surg Oral Med Oral Pathol Oral Radiol Endod 1989;67(1):96–100.
251. Kaufman E, et al. Intraligamentary injection of slow-release methylprednisolone for the prevention of pain after endodontic treatment. Oral Surg Oral Med Oral Pathol Oral Radiol Endod 1994;77(6):651–4.
252. Krasner, P, Jackson E. Management of posttreatment endodontic pain with oral dexamethasone: a double-blind study. Oral Surg Oral Med Oral Pathol Oral Radiol Endod, 1986;62(2):187–90.
253. Ouyang Y, Tang Z, Chen S. Clinical study on preventing endodontic interappointment pain with dexamethasone. Zhonghua Kou Qiang Yi Xue Za Zhi 2001;36(3):206–8.
254. Kaufman E, Chastain DC, Gaughan AM, Gracely RH. Staircase assessment of the magnitude and time-course of 50% nitrous-oxide analgesia. J Dent Res 1992;71(9):1598–603.
255. Hargreaves K, Seltzer S. Pharmacologic control of dental pain. In: K. Hargreaves, HE. Goodis, editors. Seltzer and Bender's dental pulp.. Chicago, IL: Quintessence; 2002, pp. 205–26.
256. Walton R, Fouad A. Endodontic interappointment flare-ups: a prospective study of incidence and related factors. J Endod, 1992;18(4):172–7.
257. Klotz MD, Gerstein H, Bahn AN. Bacteremia after topical use of prednisolone in infected pulps. J Am Dent Assoc 1965;71(4):871–5.
258. Sinkford JC, Harris SC. The case against topical use of adrenocorticosteroids in dentistry. J Am Dent Assoc 1964;68:765–7.
259. Williamson LW, Lorson EL, Osbon DB. Hypothalamic–pituitary–adrenal suppression after short-term dexamethasone therapy for oral surgical procedures. J Oral Surg 1980;38(1):20–8.
260. Cooper SA, Engel J, Ladov M, et al. Analgesics efficacy of an ibuprofen–codeine combination. Pharmacotherapy 1982;2:162–7.
261. Beaver W. Mild analgesics: a review of their clinical pharmacology. Am J Med Sci 1966;251:576.
262. Troullos E, Freeman R, Dionne R. The scientific basis for analgesic use in dentistry. Anesth Prog 1986;33:123.
263. Dionne R, Lepinski AM, Gordon SM, et al. Analgesic effects of peripherally administered opioids in clinical models of acute and chronic inflammation. Clin Pharmacol Ther 2001;70:66.
264. Hargreaves K, Joris J. The peripheral analgesic effects of opioids. J Am Pain Soc 1993;2:51.
265. Glennon JP, Ng YL, Setchell DJ, Gulabivala K. Prevalence of and factors affecting postpreparation pain in patients

undergoing two-visit root canal treatment. Int Endod J 2004;37(1):29–37.

266. Oguntebi B, et al. Postoperative pain incidence related to the type of emergency treatment of symptomatic pulpitis. Oral Surg Oral Med Oral Pathol Oral Radiol Endod 1992;73:479–83.

267. Nagle, D, Reader A, Beck M, Weaver J. Effect of systemic penicillin on pain in untreated irreversible pulpitis. Oral Surg Oral Med Oral Pathol Oral Radiol Endod 2000;90(5):636–40.

268. Keenan JV, Farman AG, Fedorowicz Z, Newton JT. A Cochrane systematic review finds no evidence to support the use of antibiotics for pain relief in irreversible pulpitis. J Endod 2006;32:87–92.

269. Isett J, Reader A, Gallatin E, et al. Effect of an intraosseous injection of Depo-Medrol on pulpal concentrations of PGE2 and IL-8 in untreated irreversible pulpitis. J Endod 2003;29(4):268–71.

270. Agarwala V, Reader A, Nusstein J, Beck M. Anesthetic efficacy of a preemptive intraosseous injection of Depo-Medrol in untreated irreversible pulpitis [abstract]. J Endod 2006;32:238.

CHAPTER 23

ANXIETY AND FEAR IN THE ENDODONTIC PATIENT

STANLEY F. MALAMED

Fear and anxiety is far from being a uniquely endodontic problem; it is, however, a more significant problem within because of the commonplace nature of the patients' underlying problem: pain. Dentistry consistently appears in lists of our most common fears along with fear of heights, flying, mice, and public speaking.[1] Common dental fears include fear of the unknown, fear of pain, and, perhaps most commonly, fear of the "shot."

Studies over the years have evaluated the incidence of dental phobia (odontophobia) in the general population.[2–4] They indicate that between 10 and 30% of the adult population suffer from moderately severe to extreme odontophobia. Chanpong et al.[4] in a survey ($n = 1101$) of Canadian adults found 7.6% stating they had "missed, cancelled or avoided a dental appointment because of fear or anxiety." In response to the question "How would you assess your feelings towards having dental treatment done?", 5.5% assessed themselves as either "very afraid" (2.0%) or "terrified" (3.5%). In this "high fear" group, 49.2% had missed, cancelled, or avoided a dental appointment because of fear or anxiety compared with only 5.2% of the "low or no fear" group.

Enkling et al.[5] reported that in 67% of odontophobic patients a prior painful dental or medical experience was the primary cause of their fear, followed by fear of needles (33%).

Dental fear is real and it hurts. For the patient, it is palpable. For the doctor and office staff, it stands as a barrier to the delivery of quality dental care. Within the realm of endodontics, many patients requiring treatment do so as a result of their extreme odontophobia. The first endodontic appointment, during which access will be gained and pulpal tissues removed, provides the greatest challenge to the endodontist, confronted with a patient who is in pain and having possibly been in pain for several months, and who is fearful not just of the local anesthetic injection but of "root canal work" itself.

Other chapters have information on the management of endodontic infection (Chapter 20, "Treatment of Endodontic Infections, Cysts, and Flare-Ups") and endodontic pain (Chapter 10, "Mechanisms of Odontogenic and Nonodontogenic Pain") and pain of nonendodontic origin (Chapter 11, "Nonodontogenic Toothache and Chronic Head and Neck Pains").

Fear and pain are a potent combination capable of provoking some of the most catastrophic situations imaginable in the dental office, such as cardiac arrest. Surveying the incidence of medical emergencies in the dental environment, Malamed[6] found that 54.9% occurred during the administration of the local anesthetic with an additional 22.0% occurring during dental treatment. When a medical emergency arose during dental treatment, 65.8% occurred either during extirpation of the pulp (26.9%) or extraction of the tooth (38.9%).[7] Over three-quarters of medical emergencies seen in dentistry are stress-related. Potentially stress-related medical emergencies include syncope, angina pectoris, bronchospasm, seizures, hyperventilation, and the so-called "epinephrine reaction."

Recognition of Fear and Anxiety

Recognition of dental fear should not be left until the patient is seated in the dental chair. Quite often the receptionist is asked revealing questions by patients, such as "Is the doctor gentle?", "Does the doctor give good shots?" Patients in the reception area may converse amongst themselves, discussing their upcoming treatment, perhaps in lurid ways. This invaluable information must be relayed to chair-side personnel who can now act to prevent a "problem" from developing.

Once seated in the dental chair, the patient's fears usually become more obvious. Fearful patients simply do not "look" comfortable. Legs remain crossed and fingers clutch the armrest of the dental chair, the so-called "white-knuckle syndrome." The patient closely watches everything, not wanting to be "snuck up on" by the doctor. Responses to questions are unusually prompt; speech is rapid. Perspiration may be observed on the patient's forehead, upper lip, and perhaps underarms.

If any of the above is noted, it is important for the doctor to confront the patient, asking them "if anything about the upcoming procedure bothers them." Once the patient admits to having fears and once the fears are out in the open, the "problem" should be manageable.

Management problems occurring during the local anesthetic administration can be almost entirely prevented by taking a patient's "feelings" about receiving "shots" into consideration. Most people do not relish the thought of receiving intraoral local anesthetic injections as demonstrated by the high incidence of adverse reactions occurring at this time. Fifty-five percent of all medical emergencies reported by Malamed[6] were fainting, and over 54% of all emergencies occurred during administration of the local anesthetic. Syncope accounted for 61.1% of dental office medical emergencies reported during a 1-year period in New Zealand.[8]

Fainting during injection is preventable by following a few simple steps aimed at making all local anesthetic injections as comfortable (atraumatic) as possible: (1) placing the patient about to receive an intraoral injection into a supine position *prior* to injection, (2) slow administration of the local anesthetic solution, and (3) use of sedation, if warranted, prior to the administration of the local anesthetic.

Management of Fear and Anxiety

The concept behind the successful use of sedation is that fearful patients are overly focused on everything that happens around them, and to them, in the dental environment. Administration of a central nervous system (CNS)-depressant drug lessens the patients' awareness, moving their minds away from the dental chair. They no longer over-respond to stimulation. They no longer care about the procedure and, in effect, become more "normal" patients. Stated even more simply, sedation is about distraction.

DEFINITIONS

Sedation occurs as a result of depression of the CNS. Although various levels of CNS depression will be discussed, one is in fact dealing with a continuum, from the earliest manifestations of a drug's action, *anxiolysis*, through the controlled loss of consciousness, *general anesthesia*. As most jurisdictions require a licensed dentist to obtain a permit before being allowed to administer CNS-depressant drugs via various routes and to varying levels of CNS depression, a number of dental (and medical) organizations have published guidelines for the safe and effective use of these drugs.[9–11]

When describing, and defining, the various levels of CNS depression, the precise wording of the definition may vary slightly from state to state and organization to organization, but the essence of the definitions is the same. The reader is strongly advised to adhere to those definitions that have been established in the jurisdiction in which he/she is licensed. Until recently, the terms used to describe the levels of CNS depression were (in order of increasing levels of depression): anxiolysis → conscious sedation → deep sedation → general anesthesia. New definitions, first proposed by the American Society of Anesthesiologists, describe the degree of CNS depression ultimately achieved (Table 1).[12] The definitions that follow are taken from the American

Table 1	Continuum of Depth of Sedation: Definition of General Anesthesia and Levels of Sedation/Analgesia			
	Minimal Sedation (Anxiolysis)	Moderate Sedation/Analgesia (Conscious Sedation)	Deep Sedation/Analgesia	General Anesthesia
Responsiveness	Normal response to verbal stimulation	Purposeful* response to verbal or tactile stimulation	Purposeful* response after repeated or painful stimulation	Unarousable, even with painful stimulus
Airway	Unaffected	No intervention required	Intervention may be required	Intervention often required
Spontaneous ventilation	Unaffected	Adequate	May be inadequate	Frequently inadequate
Cardiovascular function	Unaffected	Usually maintained	Usually maintained	May be impaired

*Source: American Society of Anesthesiologists Task Force on Sedation and Analgesia by Non-Anesthesiologists.[12]

Dental Association's (ADA's) Guidelines for the Use of Sedation and General Anesthesia by Dentists.[11]

Minimal Sedation

Minimal sedation was previously associated with *anxiolysis*—a minimally depressed level of consciousness that retains the patient's ability to independently and continuously maintain an airway and respond appropriately to physical stimulation or verbal command, and that is produced by a pharmacologic or nonpharmacologic method or a combination thereof. Although cognitive function and coordination may be modestly impaired, ventilatory and cardiovascular functions are unaffected.[11–12] In accord with this particular definition, the drug(s) and/or techniques used should carry a margin of safety wide enough to render unintended loss of consciousness unlikely. Furthermore, patients whose only response is a reflexive withdrawal from repeated painful stimuli would not be considered to be in a state of minimal sedation.

When the intent is minimal sedation for adults, the appropriate dosing of enteral drugs is no more than the maximum recommended dose of a single drug that can be prescribed for unmonitored home use.

Nitrous oxide/oxygen (N_2O–O_2) when used in combination with sedative agents may produce minimal, moderate, or deep sedation or general anesthesia.

The following definitions apply to administration of *minimal sedation*:

Maximum recommended therapeutic dose (MRTD): maximum FDA-recommended dose of a drug approved for unmonitored home use. *Incremental dosing*: administration of multiple doses of a drug until a desired effect is reached, but not to exceed the MRTD. *Titration*: administration of incremental doses of a drug until a desired effect is reached. Knowledge of each drug's time of onset, peak response, and duration of action is essential. Although the concept of titration of a drug to effect is critical, when the intent is minimal sedation, one must know whether the previous dose has taken full effect before administering an additional drug dose.

Moderate Sedation

This was previously associated with *conscious sedation*—a drug-induced depression of consciousness during which patients respond purposefully to verbal commands, either alone or accompanied by light tactile stimulation. No interventions are required to maintain a patent airway, and spontaneous ventilation is adequate. Cardiovascular function is usually maintained.[11,12] In accord with this particular definition, the drugs and/or techniques used should carry a margin of safety wide enough to render unintended loss of consciousness unlikely. Repeated dosing of an agent before the effects of previous dosing can be fully appreciated may result in a greater alteration of the state of consciousness than is the intent of the dentist. Furthermore, a patient whose only response is a reflexive withdrawal from a painful stimulus is not considered to be in a state of moderate sedation.

Deep Sedation

This is a drug-induced depression of consciousness during which patients cannot be easily aroused but respond purposefully following repeated or painful stimulation. The ability to independently maintain ventilatory function may be impaired. Patients may require assistance in maintaining a patent airway, and spontaneous ventilation may be inadequate. Cardiovascular function is usually maintained.[11,12]

General Anesthesia

This is a drug-induced loss of consciousness during which patients are not arousable, even by painful stimulation. The ability to independently maintain ventilatory function is often impaired. Patients often require assistance in maintaining a patent airway, and positive pressure ventilation may be required because of depressed spontaneous ventilation or drug-induced depression of neuromuscular function. Cardiovascular function may be impaired.[11,12] Because sedation and general anesthesia are a continuum, it is not always possible to predict how an individual patient will respond. Hence, practitioners intending to produce a given level of sedation should be able to diagnose and manage the physiologic consequences (rescue) for patients whose level of sedation becomes deeper than initially intended.[12]

For all levels of sedation, the practitioner must have the training, skills, and equipment to identify and manage such an occurrence until either assistance arrives (emergency medical service) or the patient returns to the intended level of sedation without airway or cardiovascular complications.

REGULATION

Through the 1960s, upon receiving a dental degree and a license to practice dentistry, the dentists were allowed to administer any form of anesthesia (from local anesthesia to sedation to general anesthesia). No prohibitions, except for common sense, existed. As no formal training had been received in these techniques (aside from local anesthesia) in dental school, most new doctors prudently avoided their use, managing fearful patients as best they could. Some, however, felt that they could easily administer anesthesia (in the broad sense) to their patients. Although some were successful, a large enough number became involved in serious untoward events, leading to death or severe neurologic damage, that governmental agencies (state dental boards and/or legislatures) began to seriously question whether dentists should be allowed to perform these techniques.

In the early 1970s, an Alaskan dentist had several deaths occur under halothane general anesthesia. As this dentist had little or no formal training in general anesthesia, Alaska became the first state to ban the administration of general anesthesia in the dental office. In 1974, in response to four patient deaths under general anesthesia in a short span of time in the office of an untrained dentist, Ohio became the first state to limit the use of general anesthesia to dentists who could prove adequate training, either through an oral surgery program or a 1-year anesthesiology residency[13] (J. Weaver, personal communication, January 2006).

As of 21 December 2006, all 50 states have enacted regulation governing the administration of general anesthesia and deep sedation in dental offices.[14] Deep sedation, by virtue of the fact that the patient's ventilatory status and ability to maintain an airway may be impaired, requires a level of training equal to that of general anesthesia. Education and training in general anesthesia requires a minimum of a 1-year or 2-year, full-time residency in anesthesiology.

Some dentists, untrained and now unable to administer general anesthesia, began administering CNS-depressant drugs parenterally, either intramuscularly or intravenously, as these techniques had not yet been regulated. Not surprisingly, a number of deaths occurred, as well as other serious morbidities over the ensuing years. And also, not surprisingly, legislative bodies began to regulate parenteral sedation. All 50 states now regulate the administration of parenteral conscious sedation.[15] (Intranasal [IN] sedation, a relatively new approach to CNS-depressant drug administration in dentistry, is classified as a parenteral route of drug administration.)

The oral route, the least effective and least controllable common mode of drug delivery, had always enjoyed a somewhat limited use in dentistry. As other routes of drug delivery and levels of sedation encountered increased scrutiny and regulation, interest burgeoned in this, as yet, unregulated mode of drug administration.

Orally administered drugs had always been an important management technique within the specialty practice of pediatric dentistry, with chloral hydrate, hydroxyzine, and promethazine forming a triad of oft-used drugs. In 1985 the American Academy of Pediatric Dentistry developed guidelines for the use of sedation by pediatric dentists who received adequate clinical and didactic experience in this technique during their residencies. These guidelines have been reevaluated several times with the most recent version accepted and published in 2006.[16]

Unfortunately, some untrained nonpediatric dentists (e.g., general dentists), now unable to administer drugs parenterally, began using oral sedative drugs to achieve more profound levels of CNS depression, with predictable results: death and severe morbidity (e.g., brain damage). Legislation to require permits for oral conscious sedation (OCS) in children appeared in the late 1990s. Enacted in 2000, California's legislation requires a permit for OCS in patients less than 13 years of age.[17] At present, 11 states require advanced education and awarding of a permit for a licensed dentist to administer OCS to a pediatric patent.[15]

OCS for adult dental patients had an increase in popularity in the mid-1990s, which continues today. Although many oral drugs are available, one, triazolam, has proven the most popular.[18,19]

And now, for the first time, state dental boards have acted proactively rather than reactively, as in the past, enacting legislation mandating continuing dental education (CDE) and a permit to administer OCS to the adult dental patient. As of December 2006, 19 states have requirements for CDE and a permit for adult OCS.[15]

One route of drug administration has yet to be discussed: inhalation. In contrast to the oral route, the inhalation route represents *the* most controllable technique of drug administration. In dentistry in the United States, the combination of N_2O and O_2 is available and used, with varying frequency, in approximately 35% of dental offices.[20] The ADA, in concert with manufacturers of inhalation sedation units, mandated the inclusion of safety features into these machines. The goal of these safety features is to make it close to impossible the administration of levels of O_2 less than 21% (ambient air) to a patient.[21] Deaths and serious morbidity associated with N_2O–O_2 inhalation sedation in dentistry have not occurred in recent years due primarily to the addition of these safety features and the requirement of the ADA's Commission on Dental Accreditation that all graduating dental students be trained to proficiency in inhalation sedation.[22] As of December 2006, only a handful of states require a permit for the use of inhalation sedation.

SEDATION: NONDRUG TECHNIQUES (IATROSEDATION)

Management of a patient's dental fear begins as soon as the patient enters the office. The environment, the ambiance of the office, establishes a mood either of quiet relaxation or of a hurried, frenetic pace. The dental staff should be alert to any tell-tale signs of dental fear and, if noted, report it to the dentist immediately. "Forewarned is forearmed." Relaxation of a patient by the doctor's behavior has been termed *iatrosedation*, a term formulated by Dr. Nathan Friedman, for many years chairman of the Section of Human Behavior at the University of Southern California, School of Dentistry.[23] The word is derived from the Greek prefix *iatro*, "pertaining to the doctor," and *sedation*, "the relief of anxiety."

The concept on which iatrosedation is based is rather basic: that the behavior of the doctor and staff has a profound influence on the behavior of the patient. Other terms applied to this concept include suggestion, chairside/bedside manner, and the laying on of hands. The underlying premise of all these techniques is similar: that one can use nonchemical means to aid in relaxing the patient. For a more in-depth discussion of nondrug techniques of sedation, the reader is referred to *Sedation: a guide to patient management*.[24] Examples of iatrosedative techniques include hypnosis, acupuncture, audioanalgesia, and biofeedback.

Iatrosedation forms the building block for all sedation techniques requiring drug administration. Simply put, a patient who remains fearful, perhaps with distrust of the doctor, is less likely to "allow" their CNS-depressant drug to work. Although true for all routes of drug administration, it is especially relevant with the oral and inhalation routes.

Consider the patients' frame of mind in the dental office: afraid that something/everything is going to be painful. Their dentist is telling them, nonverbally, to "trust me." "Allow me, a stranger, to give you a drug that will decrease your level of consciousness so that you are less aware of what is happening around you." "I will take good care of you." The doctor who establishes a bond of trust with their patients will have them sit back in the dental chair and "let the drug work." Conversely, where the doctor–patient relationship is strained or uncomfortable, patients are much less likely to surrender to the clinical effects of the drug, not wanting to "lose control" of the situation. The level defined as minimal sedation is highly unlikely to succeed in this situation. Moderate sedation would have a somewhat greater success rate but still with a significant, perhaps unacceptably high, failure rate (Table 2).

Table 2 Efficacy of Sedation by Routes of Drug Administration

Technique Route	Titrate to Effect	Rapid Reversal	Expected Success Rate(%)
Intravenous	Yes	Yes*	90
Inhalation	Yes	Yes	80
Intramuscular Intranasal	No	No	67
Oral (adult)	No	No	50–60
Oral (child)	No	No	Older: 50–60 Younger: 35–40
General anesthesia†	Yes	Yes#	0

*Opioids, benzodiazepines.
†General anesthesia is *not* a sedation technique. It is included for comparative purposes only.
#Dependent on route of administration and drug.

SEDATION: DRUG TECHNIQUES (PHARMACOSEDATION)

In dentistry, CNS-depressant drugs are administered by four routes: commonly by oral and inhalation, and less commonly by intravenous (IV) and intramuscular (IM). IN drug administration is a relatively recent addition to this armamentarium, primarily employed to provide moderate sedation in children.[25]

The following is a brief overview of these routes of CNS-depressant drug administration in dentistry. It is not meant to substitute for a complete course in pharmacology or in the safe and effective technique of drug administration. The doctor wishing to administer drugs by any of these routes should check with their state Board of Dental Examiners for specific education and permit requirements for each technique or level of sedation.

INHALATION SEDATION (N_2O–O_2)

Inhalation sedation with N_2O–O_2 represents the most controllable technique of sedation available. Inhalation sedation possesses a number of compelling clinical properties that serve to increase its success rate and its safety, including (1) rapid onset of action (~20–30 seconds); (2) a level of CNS depression that can rapidly be increased, if necessary; (3) the level of CNS depression that can be rapidly decreased, if needed—a significant factor in increasing the safety of inhalation sedation; (4) complete recovery following the delivery of 100% O_2 at the conclusion of the procedure, permitting almost all N_2O–O_2 patients to be discharged from the dental office unescorted, and with no prohibitions on their postinhalation sedation activities. No other route of drug administration offers this significant advantage. Because of its rapid onset, inhalation sedation with N_2O–O_2 may be titrated. The ability to titrate increases both the success and safety of the technique.

In order for a drug to be titrated, it must enter into the cardiovascular system rapidly. When possible, titration allows the doctor to individualize the dosage of the drug for each patient, negating the so-called "bell-shaped" or "normal distribution" curve.

The technique of inhalation sedation with N_2O–O_2 possesses very few significant disadvantages. One factor, common to it and several other techniques, is that of patient cooperation. The patient breathes the gasses through a small mask placed on the nose, the nasal hood. Uncooperative patients, usually odontophobic younger children, or any patient who is claustrophobic, might not allow the nasal hood to be placed, condemning the inhalation route to failure. Persons unable to breathe through their nose, for whatever reason, will be unable to receive inhalation sedation in a dental office. A recommended technique of administration of N_2O–O_2 is outlined in Table 3.

Inhalation sedation with N_2O–O_2 may be employed to provide minimum to moderate sedation. It may also be used, in conjunction with drugs administered by other routes, to supplement the CNS depression they provide. N_2O–O_2 when used in combination with sedative agents may produce minimal, moderate, or deep sedation or general anesthesia.[11]

The use of N_2O–O_2 inhalation sedation in endodontics should become more common given the positive attributes of the technique. A common complaint from endodontists is that the nasal hood is in the way (Figure 1). Once experience is gained in the technique, this ceases to be a concern. Inhalation sedation with N_2O–O_2 has a success rate of approximately 80% in adult patients.

ORAL CONSCIOUS SEDATION

The oral route of drug administration is the least controllable route of drug administration. A number of factors work against an orally administered drug being effective, including a slow onset of action (~1 hour for most drugs); erratic absorption of the drug from the gastrointestinal (GI) tract; and, for some drugs, a significant hepatic first-pass effect. For these reasons, titration of the drug to clinical effect is not possible, eliminating the most important safety factor in drug administration.

Once administered, the level of CNS depression reached by oral drugs is not easily increased (providing deeper sedation) or decreased (lighter sedation).

Table 3 Technique of Administration of Inhalation Sedation with N_2O–O_2

1. Prior to placing nasal hood, start a flow of 5 to 6 LPM (liters per minute) of O_2.
2. Have patient assist in proper placement and securing of the nasal hood.
3. Determine if patient can "breathe comfortably" with 100% oxygen ("Is the flow volume adequate?"). Increase the flow, if necessary.
4. Start titration of N_2O by increasing its flow to 1 LPM, decreasing the O_2 flow by 1 LPM.
5. After 1 minute determine what, if any, signs and symptoms the patient may be experiencing.
6. If needed, increase N_2O by 0.5 LPM, decreasing O_2 0.5 LPM.
7. Repeat steps 5 and 6 until the patient reaches the desired level of sedation.
8. Administer local anesthesia as would be done if the patient were not receiving N_2O–O_2.
9. At the conclusion of the procedure, increase the O_2 flow to the level determined in step 3 and return the N_2O to 0 LPM.
10. Permit the patient to breathe 100% O_2 for not less than 3 to 5 minutes before considering removal of the nasal hood.
11. Assess recovery from sedation. If considered recovered, remove nasal hood before terminating the flow of O_2.
12. Permit the patient to leave dental chair. Have a staff person close to the patient so as to prevent any possible injury when standing, due to postural hypotension.
13. Document treatment in the patient's chart.

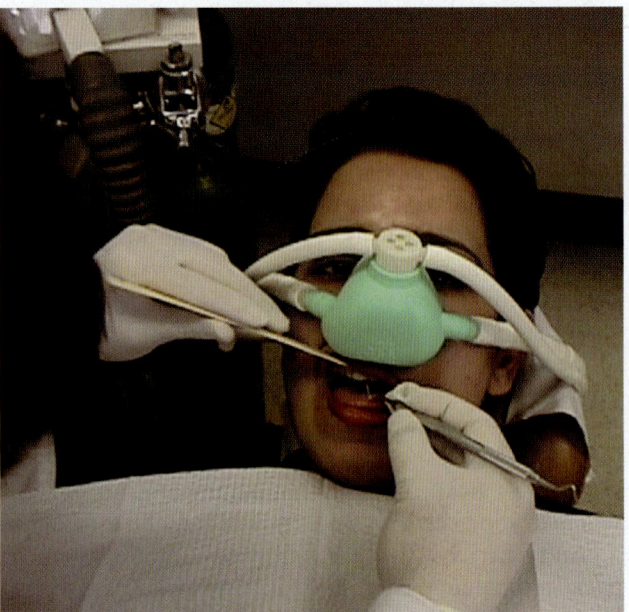

Figure 1 N_2O–O_2 nasal hood.

The duration of CNS depression from orally administered drugs greatly exceeds the typical length of the dental visit so these patients will always require an escort on being discharged from the office. This escort should be a responsible adult who has a vested interest in the health and safety of the patient.

The only advantages associated with the oral route of drug administration are that it is easier for both the doctor and the patient.

Having just described a technique that seems quite mediocre compared with other routes of administration, it must be stated that there is a legitimate place for orally administered CNS depressants in dentistry.

Odontophobic patients, especially when faced with the fear of root canal treatment, frequently require management with CNS depressants (1) the night prior to the planned appointment, in order for the patient to experience a restful night's sleep, and (2) in the morning, 1 hour prior to the scheduled dental visit, to assist them in overcoming any last minute increase in their anxiety.

In the absence of other sedation techniques in a dental office, the oral route may also be used for intraoperative sedation. However, owing to the lack of control maintained over this technique by the doctor, the goal in administering oral CNS depressants should be limited to minimal to moderate CNS depression.

Many excellent oral preparations are currently available for administration. Table 4 presents some commonly used drugs and their recommended dosages.[26,27]

When used alone, and in recommended dosages, orally administered drugs will have only an approximately 50 to 60% success rate with adult patients. This success rate is even lower in younger children.

INTRAVENOUS CONSCIOUS SEDATION

CNS-depressant drugs administered intravenously in the dorsum of the hand reach the brain in approximately 20 seconds. With this rapid onset, IV drug administration allows patients to be titrated to a desired level of CNS depression, thereby increasing control over the effect of the administered drug and, ultimately, the safety of the technique. Other advantages of IV drug administration include the ability to rapidly increase the level of sedation, if needed, and the reversibility of many intravenously administered drugs (benzodiazepines and opioids).

Disadvantages associated with intravenously administered CNS depressants include the requirement of

Table 4 Common Orally Administered CNS Depressants

Generic Name	Proprietary Name	Availability (mg)	Usual Dental Dosage
Benzodiazepines			
Alprazolam	Niravam, Xanax	Tab: 0.25, 0.5, 1.0, 2.0	0.25–0.5 (max 4 mg/day)
Diazepam	Valium	Tab: 2, 5, 10	2–10 mg bid-qid
Flurazepam	Dalmane	Cap: 15, 30	15–30 mg at bedtime
Lorazepam	Ativan	0.5, 1.0, 2.0	2–3 mg/day given bid-tid
Midazolam	Versed	Syr: 2 mg/mL	Pediatrics: 0.25–1.0 mg/kg single dose
Oxazepam	Serax	Cap: 10, 15, 30 Tab: 15	Adults (Anxiety): mild to moderate: severe: 15–30 tid-qid
Triazolam	Halcion	Tab: 0.125, 0.25	0.25 qhs, max 0.5
Miscellaneous, non-benzodiazepine anxiolytics, sedatives			
Eszopiclone	Lunesta	Tab: 1.0, 2.0, 3.0	Initial: 2mg qhs
Zaleplon	Sonata	Cap: 5, 10	Insomnia: 10 qhs
Zolpidem	Ambien	Tab: 5, 10	Adult: usual 10 mg qhs
Miscellaneous sedative-hypnotic			
Chloral hydrate	n/a	Syr: 500 mg/5ml	Adults: 500 mg – 1gr 15–30 mg hs; max 2 g/day
Hydroxyzine HCl	Atarax	Syr: 10 mg/5mL Tab: 25, 50, 100	Adults (Sedation): 50–100 mg
Hydroxyzine pamoate	Vistaril	Cap: 25, 50, 100 Sus: 25 mg/5mL	

Tab = Tablet; Syr = Syrup; Cap = Capsule; Sus = Suspension.
Sources: (1) ADA/PDR Guide to Accepted Dental Therapeutics[26].
(2) www.ePocrates.com[27]

fasting prior to the procedure (NPO status); an inability to quickly lessen the level of CNS depression; an inability to reverse the clinical actions of some drugs (e.g., barbiturates); and prolonged clinical recovery with an attendant need for an adult escort for the patient when discharged from the dental office.

Venipuncture is a learned skill and, though normally quite easy to achieve, represents the most difficult part of the entire IV sedation procedure. Once venous access is obtained, titration to the desired level of CNS depression is normally accomplished easily.

Many CNS-depressant drugs are available for IV administration, but those most often employed are the benzodiazepines, midazolam (Versed), and diazepam (Valium).

State requirements for a permit to employ IV conscious sedation (also termed "parenteral sedation" or "moderate sedation") most often mandate 60 hours of didactics and either 10 or 20 cases of IV sedation administered by the doctor in a supervised environment.[15] Variation may exist from jurisdiction to jurisdiction, so it is strongly advised that specific state dental board regulations be consulted.

Basic IV sedation techniques have evolved over the past three decades. The combination of pentobarbital (Nembutal), meperidine (Demerol), and scopolamine represented the original IV technique introduced in the 1950s by Dr. Neils Björn Jörgensen at Loma Linda University.[28] As described by Jörgensen, the drugs were injected directly into the vein via the syringe that was then removed.[29] The Jörgensen technique provided a duration of CNS depression of approximately 2 hours, a function of the barbiturate, a pentobarbital. With the introduction in the early 1960s of the benzodiazepine diazepam, a shorter duration of CNS depression became possible.[30] An additional benefit of diazepam was a brief period (approximately 10 minutes) of retrograde amnesia, permitting potentially traumatic procedures to be done with a likelihood of the patient not having any recall. For the patient this meant, in essence, that the fearful event (e.g., local anesthetic injection) never happened.

IV conscious sedation with a benzodiazepine has become the most popular technique in dentistry. IV benzodiazepine sedation meets the needs of contemporary dental practice, that is, sedation for approximately 1 hour. Introduced in the United States in 1986, midazolam (Versed) has now supplanted diazepam (Valium) as the most used IV benzodiazepine in the area of 1-hour IV conscious sedation. Midazolam, unlike diazepam, is water soluble, thus capable of being administered intramuscularly and intranasally (see following discussions of these techniques). The amnestic properties of midazolam are considerably greater than diazepam's, providing lack of recall for most, if not all, of the dental appointment. Clinical sedation, however, from the dentist's perspective, is not quite as good with midazolam compared with diazepam. Both drugs, with one titrating dose, provide the doctor with approximately 1 hour of working time.

Direct injection of a drug into a vein, followed by removal of the syringe at the start of the dental procedure, gave way to the continuous IV infusion, in which venous access is maintained for the duration of the procedure. Initially, winged needles, also known as "scalp vein" and "butterfly needles," were used (Figure 2). Easy to insert, the winged needle has the disturbing propensity to perforate the vein during the dental procedure, leading to loss of venous access and formation of a hematoma. In recent years, the indwelling catheter has become increasing popular.

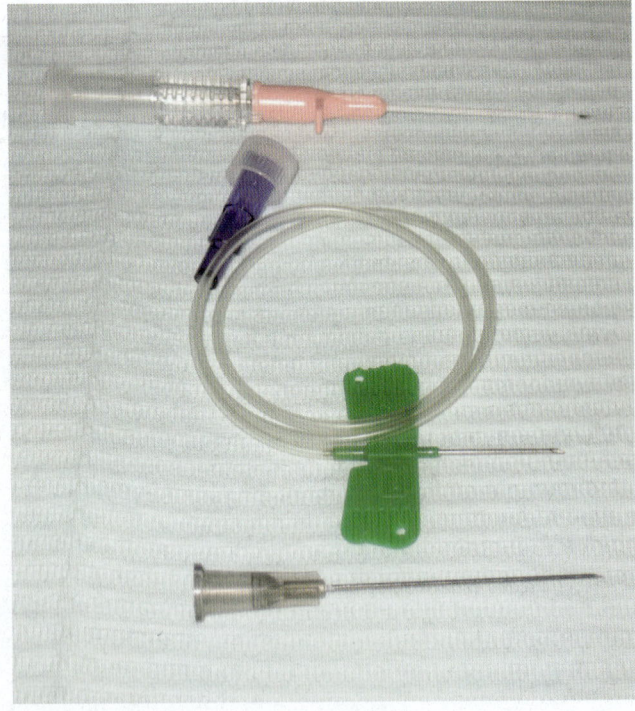

Figure 2 IV needles.

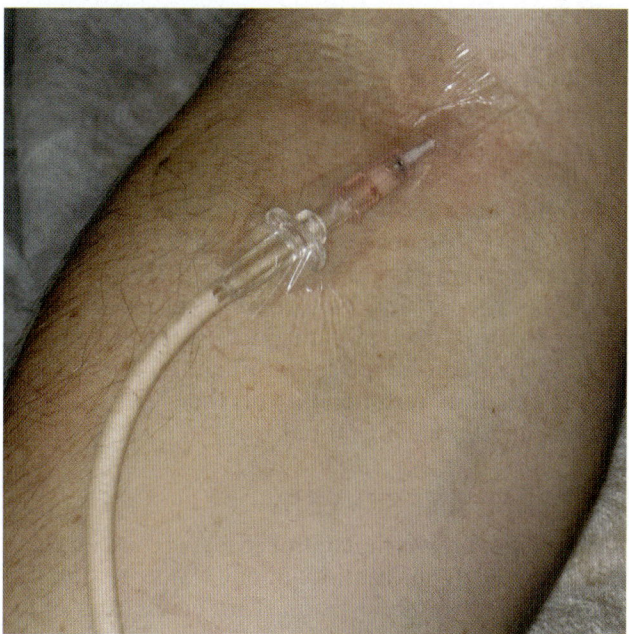

Figure 3 Indwelling catheter.

Once inserted and secured in a vein, the 3″ plastic catheter is unlikely to accidentally become dislodged (Figure 3).

Opioids, specifically the short-acting fentanyl, have also been used in IV conscious sedation with increased frequency. When the primary goal of IV drug administration is management of fear, there is usually little or no need for opioid administration. Indeed, in the vast majority of successful IV sedation cases, the only drug(s) administered are either midazolam and/or diazepam. However, in situations in which surgery or other dental procedures that may prove painful are planned, or in which successful pain control may not be easily achieved with local anesthesia alone, opioid administration may be justified.

When administered carefully via titration, success rates of 90% may be achieved with IV sedation. The IV route can be used to achieve moderate and deep sedation, as well as general anesthesia.

INTRAMUSCULAR

IM, like IV, is a parenteral route of administration, in which the drug by-passes the GI tract, being absorbed directly into the systemic (venous) circulation. The hepatic first-pass effect is negated, leading to more reliable absorption and more rapid onset of action (~10–20 minutes) than with enterally administered drugs. However, titration is not possible, as the onset is not rapid enough, thus denying the IM route a major safety benefit and thereby limiting its indications for use in sedation in dentistry.

Doses of IM drugs are primarily determined on a weight (e.g., mg/kg) basis. Given the appropriate dosage, approximately 70% of patients should be CNS depressed to the desired level of sedation. However, another 15% will likely be undersedated with that same dose, whereas the remaining 15% are CNS depressed to a level beyond that which is being sought. This latter group, hyperresponders to the drug, may be CNS depressed to a level beyond which the doctor is able to safely manage them. For example, an IM drug is administered to a patient to achieve a level of moderate sedation (formerly termed "conscious sedation"). However, the resultant level of CNS depression is deep sedation. At this level, patients are unable to adequately maintain their airway without assistance (e.g., head-tilt, chin-lift). Dental care would, of course, need to be postponed as the doctor is required to "rescue" patients from this unintended level of CNS depression. Airway management and, possibly, ventilatory assistance are continued until the level of CNS depression lightens, a process that could require several hours.

Along with the inability to titrate IM drugs, it is also not possible to rapidly lessen or deepen the level of sedation. Reversal of intramuscularly administered drugs, if possible, by intravenously administered flumazenil or naloxone, would be somewhat successful for a period of time. However, as a reservoir of the IM drug exists within the muscle into which it was injected previously, the drug will continue to be absorbed over several hours leading to the likelihood of a rebound sedation effect occurring as the action of the intravenously administered reversal agent diminishes. IM administration of the reversal agent is generally not recommended as its onset, 10 to 20 minutes, is too slow to provide any immediate relief in the event of oversedation. Additionally, the degree of the intramuscularly administered reversal agent's effectiveness would be less than that seen following its administration IV.

IM drugs are not as controllable as intravenously administered drugs. Sedation should therefore be limited to a moderate level, with the doctor trained to recognize and manage (e.g., rescue) the patients should they inadvertently enter deep sedation. Patients receiving IM drugs for sedation must also maintain NPO status prior to sedation.

Recovery from IM drugs is prolonged; thus, the patient must have an adult escort when being discharged from the office. This being said, it would seem that IM drugs have few indications in dentistry. However, used judiciously by the doctor trained in parenteral conscious sedation (IV, IM, IN), the technique can be employed with a likelihood of success of about 67%. Midazolam is the most commonly employed IM CNS-depressant drug in conscious sedation.

INTRANASAL

The IN administration of CNS-depressant drugs is relatively new within medicine and dentistry, though it has been used for many years by drug abusers (e.g., cocaine) and for the administration of nasal decongestants.

Nasal mucosa is highly vascular; therefore, absorption of drugs instilled into the nares is more rapid than for other routes of administration. Lam et al.[25] compared the efficacy, in children, of IN midazolam with that of its IM administration, finding the level of sedation to be comparable. IN midazolam has also been adopted in emergency medicine in the management of acute seizures in pediatric patients.[31] Primosch[32] compared nasal drops versus nasal spray as a technique of IN drug administration and found that although the effectiveness of conscious sedation was not influenced by the method of nasal administration, spray administration produced significantly less aversive behavior than administering drops in 2- to 3-year-old dental patients of similar behavioral characteristics.

Most studies and clinical usage of the IN route of drug administration appear in pediatrics, there being few reports of the use of this technique, and of its effectiveness, in adults, thereby limiting its utility in most endodontic cases.

The advantages of IN drug administration include its more rapid onset of action (compared with enteral routes) and the lack of need for injection and the accompanying trauma, both psychological and physical, associated with it.

Disadvantages of IN drug administration are similar to those of IM. IN drugs cannot be titrated. Dosages are based on weight (mg/kg). Along with the inability to titrate IN drugs, it is also not possible to rapidly lessen or deepen the level of the resultant CNS depression. Reversal of intranasally administered drugs, if possible, by intravenously administered flumazenil or naloxone, would be somewhat successful. IM or IN administration of a reversal agent is generally not recommended as its onset, 10 to 20 minutes, is too slow to provide any immediate relief in the event of oversedation. Additionally, the efficacy of an IM or IN reversal agent would be less than that seen with its IV administration.

IN drugs are not as controllable as intravenously administered drugs. The level of CNS depression sought should, therefore, be limited to moderate, with the doctor trained to recognize and manage (e.g., rescue) the patients should they enter into deep sedation. Patients receiving IN drugs for sedation must also maintain NPO status prior to sedation.

Recovery from IN drugs is prolonged, thus the requirement for an adult escort for the patient when discharged from the office.

Techniques of conscious sedation will enable the endodontist to manage the dental fears of the overwhelming majority of odontophobic patients. Table 6 illustrates the possible uses of the techniques of conscious sedation in endodontic practice. Unfortunately, not all fears can be successfully managed with conscious sedation techniques. For these few patients, general anesthesia is required.

GENERAL ANESTHESIA

General anesthesia is the controlled loss of consciousness, the final step in our continuum of CNS depression that started with minimal sedation. The success rates of the sedation techniques described above, along with the amnestic properties of some of the drugs employed, specifically the benzodiazepines midazolam and triazolam, has decreased the need for general anesthesia as a method of managing significant numbers of odontophobic patients.

All 50 states regulate the use of general anesthesia in dentistry.[14] A residency in anesthesiology of either 1- or 2-year duration usually represents the educational requirement. As of November 2007, seven residencies in anesthesiology for dentists were accredited by the American Dental Board of Anesthesiology.[33]

Doctors who have completed accredited residencies, dentist anesthesiologists, provide anesthesia services for other dentists either (1) by establishing a free-standing outpatient surgical center, in which the endodontist (or any other dentist) brings the odontophobic patient to the surgical center to carry out the scheduled procedures while the patient receives general anesthesia provided by the dentist anesthesiologist, or (2) by traveling to the office of the dentist who will be managing the dental needs of the fearful patient, wherein dentist anesthesiologists bring along all of their anesthesia drugs, equipment, and expertise.

Once general anesthesia has been induced by the dentist anesthesiologist, the dentist can then proceed with the endodontic procedure on a now more nearly "ideal" patient.

SUMMARY

Dental fears exist and are a fact of life, especially in the specialty of endodontics. The primary obstacles to successful endodontic treatment are the presence of dual

Table 5 Comparison of Routes of Drug Administration

Route of Drug Administration	Onset of Action	Titrate Yes–No	Advantages	Disadvantages
Inhalation	Rapid (~20 seconds)	Yes	Patient need not be NPO; rapid onset; titration; rapidly increase or decrease level of CNS depression; full recovery in most patients; no prohibitions of postoperative functions	Patient cooperation required; ineffective if unable to breathe through nose
Oral	Slow (~ 1 hour for maximal clinical effect)	No	Easy for patient; easy for doctor	Patient cooperation needed; slow onset; inability to titrate; erratic absorption from GI tract; significant hepatic 1st-pass effect for some drugs; no control over ultimate level of CNS depression; inability to quickly increase or decrease level of CNS depression; inability to reverse CNS depression; prolonged recovery; requirement for escort for patient on leaving dental office
Parenteral: Intramuscular	Intermediate (10–20 minutes)	No	More reliable absorption than oral; minimal patient cooperation required	Patient must be NPO; potential needle injury; relatively slow onset; inability to titrate; no control over ultimate level of CNS depression; inability to quickly increase or decrease level of CNS depression; inability to reverse CNS depression; prolonged recovery; requirement for escort for patient on leaving dental office
Parenteral: Intravenous	Rapid (~20 seconds)	Yes	Rapid onset; titration; rapidly increase level of CNS depression; most drugs reversible	Venipuncture is learned technique; patient must be NPO; inability to quickly decrease level of CNS depression; prolonged recovery; requirement for escort for patient on leaving dental office
Parenteral: Intranasal	Intermediate (10–20 minutes)	No	More reliable absorption than oral; minimal patient cooperation required	Unpleasant (bitter) taste if liquid enters oral cavity; may irritate nasal mucosa; inability to titrate; no control over ultimate level of CNS depression; inability to quickly increase or decrease level of CNS depression; inability to reverse CNS depression; prolonged recovery; requirement for escort for patient on leaving dental office

Table 6 Techniques of Conscious Sedation—Summary

	Preoperative		Perioperative	Ability to Titrate	CNS Depression Level When Used Alone	CNS Depression Level Used in Combination
	Night prior to treatment	Morning of treatment				
Oral sedation	Yes	Yes	Yes	No	Min, mod	Min, mod, deep, GA
Inhalation			Yes	Yes	Mod	Mod, deep, GA
IV			Yes	Yes	Mod, deep, GA	Mod, deep, GA
IM/IN			Yes	No	Mod, deep, GA	Mod, deep, GA

Min = minimal sedation; Mod = moderate sedation; Deep = deep sedation; GA = general anesthesia.

problems: pain and fear. To ignore fear, in the best of circumstances, will complicate dental treatment unnecessarily, as the patient remains an unwilling participant throughout the procedure. Fear lowers the pain reaction threshold, with odontophobic patients being unable to sit still during their treatment, adding to the frustration of the treating doctor. Fear increases catecholamine release into the cardiovascular system with a resultant rise in the incidence and severity of medical emergency situations.

The recognition of fear, and its management, removes the primary obstacle to the delivery of health care. Once fear is eliminated, clinically adequate pain control is normally accomplished quite readily. As Peter Milgrom wrote, "Deal with the fear first, then pain will be a minor problem."[5,34]

References

1. Our most common fears. Dental Health Advisor, Spring 1987.
2. Dionne DA, Gordon SM, McCullagh LM, Phero JC. Assessing the need for anesthesia and sedation in the general population. J Am Dent Assoc 1998;129(2):167–73.
3. Gatchel RJ, Ingersoll BD, Bowman L, et al. The prevalence of dental fear and avoidance: a recent survey study. J Am Dent Assoc 1983;107(4):609–10.
4. Chanpong B, Haas DA, Locker D. Need and demand for sedation or general anesthesia in dentistry: a national survey of the Canadian population. Anesth Prog 2005;52(1):3–11.
5. Enkling N, Martwinski G, Johren P. Dental anxiety in a representative sample of residents of a large German city. Clin Oral Investig 2006;10(1):84–91.
6. Malamed SF. Beyond the basics: emergency medicine in dentistry, J Am Dent Assoc 1997;128(7):843–54.
7. Matsuura H. Analysis of systemic complications and deaths during dental treatment in Japan. Anesth Prog 1990;36:219–28.
8. Broadbent JM, Thomson WM. The readiness of New Zealand general dental practitioners for medical emergencies. NZ Dent J 2001;97:82–6.
9. American Association of Oral and Maxillofacial Surgeons. Parameters of care for oral and maxillofacial surgery: a guide for practice, monitoring and evaluation, Rosemont, Ill: The Association of Oral and Maxillofacial Surgeons; 1995.
10. Academy Report: The use of conscious sedation by periodontists. J Periodontol 2003;74:933.
11. American Dental Association. Guidelines for the use of sedation and general anesthesia by dentists. Draft 11 November 2006.
12. American Society of Anesthesiologists Task Force on Sedation and Analgesia by Non-Anesthesiologists. Practice guidelines for sedation and analgesia by non-anesthesiologists. Anesthesiology 2002;96(4):1004–17.
13. Ohio State Dental Board, Ohio State Dental Board Law and Rules, Columbus, Ohio, 1974.
14. Department of State Government Affairs, 30a Statutory Requirements for general anesthesia/deep sedation, American Dental Association, December 21, 2006, Chicago, IL.
15. Department of State Government Affairs, 30b Conscious Sedation Permit Requirement, American Dental Association, December 21, 2006, Chicago, IL.
16. American Academy of Pediatrics. American Academy of Pediatric Dentistry. Cote CJ, Wilson S. Work Group on Sedation. Guidelines for monitoring and management of pediatric patients during and after sedation for diagnostic and therapeutic procedures: an update. Pediatrics 2006;118(6):2587–602.
17. Dental Board of California, Chapter 2, Article 5.5. Oral conscious sedation. Dental Board of California, Sacramento, CA. www.dentalboard@dca.ca.gov 2000 accessed 9 Febuary 2007.
18. Feck AS. Goodchild JH. The use of anxiolytic medications to supplement local anesthesia in the anxious patient. Compend Contin Educ Dent 2005;26(3):183–6, 188, 190.
19. Dionne RA, Yagiela JA, Cote CJ, et al. Balancing efficacy and safety in the use of oral sedation in dental outpatients. J Am Dent Assoc 2006;137(4):502–13.
20. Clark M, Brunick A. Handbook of nitrous oxide and oxygen sedation. 2nd ed. St. Louis: C.V. Mosby; 2003.
21. American Dental Association Seal of Acceptance Program. www.ada.org/ada/seal/index.asp accessed 9 Febuary 2007.
22. Commission on Dental Accreditation, Accreditation standard 23, American Dental Association, Chicago, IL 2006.
23. Friedman N. Iatrosedation. In: McCarthy FM, editor. Emergencies in dental practice. 3rd ed. Philadelphia: WB Saunders; 1979.
24. Malamed SF. Iatrosedation. In: Malamed SF, editor. Sedation: a guide to patient management. 4th ed. St. Louis: CV Mosby; 2002.
25. Lam C, Udin RD, Malamed SF, et al. Midazolam premedication in children: a pilot study comparing intramuscular and intranasal administration. Anesth Prog 2005;52(2):56–61.
26. Byrne BE, Tibbetts LS, editors. Conscious sedation and agents for the control of anxiety. In: ADA/PDR guide to accepted dental therapeutics, 4th ed. Chicago, IL: ADA Publishing Division; 2006, pp. 23–51.
27. www.ePocrates.com
28. Jorgensen NB, Leffingwell FE. Premedication in dentistry. J South Calif Dent Assoc 1953;21:25.
29. Jorgensen NB, Hayden J Jr. Premedication, local and general anesthesia in dentistry. Philadelphia: Lea amp; Febiger; 1967.
30. O'Neill R, Verrill PJ, Aellig WH, et al. Intravenous diazepam in minor oral surgery. Br Dent J 1970;128:15.
31. Harbord MG, Kyrkou NE, Kyrkou MR, et al. Use of intranasal midazolam to treat acute seizures in paediatric community settings. J Paediatr Child Health 2004;40(9–10):556–8.
32. Primosch RE, Guelmann M. Comparison of drops versus spray administration of intranasal midazolam in two- and three-year-old children for dental sedation. Pediatr Dent 2005;27(5):401–8.
33. www.asdahq.org/training.html accessed 23 November 2007.
34. Milgrom P, Weinstein P, Getz T. Treating fearful dental patients: a patient management handbook. 2nd ed. Seattle, WA: University of Washington Continuing Dental Education; 1995.[12]

CHAPTER 24

THE MEDICALLY COMPLEX ENDODONTIC PATIENT

BRADFORD R. JOHNSON, DENA J. FISCHER, JOEL B. EPSTEIN

One of the challenges faced by dental specialists today is in the assessment and management of patients with increasingly complex medical conditions. Not only has the average life expectancy increased dramatically over the past 50 years, but our geriatric patients are much more likely to be at least partially dentulous and have a complex medical history with multiple medical problems and the use of multiple medications.[1] Approximately 25% of patients aged 65 to 74 and 35% of patients aged 75 and older have a medical condition that would place them in the ASA (American Society of Anesthesiologists' Health Classification System) category III or IV (Figure 1).[2] An aging population with both the desire and resources to preserve their natural dentition will drive the demand for root canal therapy for patients with complex medical conditions. Even in a typical population of younger and presumably healthier patients, approximately 50% of patients referred to a dental specialty practice can be expected to report at least one positive finding on their health history questionnaire.[1,3] Since medical complexity is often an indication for referral to a dental specialist,[4,5] endodontists should be prepared to accurately evaluate medically complex patients and identify situations that require a modification of normal treatment procedures and identify oral and systemic conditions requiring diagnosis and management.

The purpose of this chapter is to serve as a brief overview of common medical conditions that require some modification of the treatment protocol to ensure safe endodontic treatment in an ambulatory dental setting. It is not intended as a substitute for case-specific clinical judgment or consultation with medical experts. For the purposes of this chapter, a medically complex patient will be defined as any patient requiring modification of the usual treatment procedure.

MEDICAL HISTORY AND PATIENT INTERVIEW

"Never Treat a Stranger" (Attributed to Sir William Osler)

The value of a thorough medical history and patient interview cannot be overemphasized. Recognition of a medical condition that requires treatment modification prior to treatment can avert significant treatment complications. Approximately 25 to 30% of patients seeking treatment in a dental office can be expected to report at least one medical condition that has potential relevance to dental treatment, although not all of these conditions will require treatment modification.[6,7] An adverse outcome, due to failure to recognize a known risk factor and modify treatment accordingly, is a major predictor of a successful liability claim.[8] Cardiovascular disease, drug allergies, diabetes, and concerns about the safety of vasoconstrictor use are some of the most common medical reasons for referral to a specialist.[1,9,10] This is consistent with an analysis of the most common medical emergencies in the dental office: angina, hypoglycemia, adverse reaction to local anesthetics, and seizures.[11]

A standard health history questionnaire should cover all common medical conditions (both treated and untreated), surgeries, hospitalizations, medications, and allergies. Although many standard forms are readily available and are usually convenient and easy to complete, most of these forms do not clearly lead to a specific determination of risk for dental treatment. More useful medical risk assessment models are under development and will be briefly discussed later in this section. The written health history questionnaire should always be supplemented with a patient interview to help decrease

ASA physical classification	Description	Therapy modifications (McCarthy and Malamed, 1979)
ASA 1	A normal healthy patient	None (stress reduction as indicated)
ASA 2	A patient with mild systemic disease	Possible stress reduction and other modifications as needed
ASA 3	A patient with a severe systemic disease that limits activity, but is not incapacitating	Possible strict modifications; stress reduction and medical consultation are priorities
ASA 4	A patient with an incapacitating systemic disease that is a constant threat to life	Minimal emergency care in office (may consist of pharmacologic management only); hospitalize for stressful elective treatment; medical consultation urged
ASA 5	A moribund patient who is not expected to survive without the operation	Treatment in the hospital is limited to life support only; for example, airway and hemorrhage management
ASA 6	A declared brain-dead patient whose organs are being removed for donor purposes	Not applicable

Figure 1 American Society of Anesthesiologists' (ASA) health classification system and suggested treatment modifications. Adapted from Tables 1 and 2, Goodchild J and Glick M.[27]

false-positive and false-negative findings and to further explore positive findings.[12] The clinician should review any positive findings with the patient and determine the patient's level of compliance with medical treatment recommendations. For example, a compliant patient with well-managed hypertension presents a relatively low risk compared to a patient who refuses to take prescribed medications or does so erratically. Unfortunately, for a variety of reasons, the reliability of self-reported information in the health history may be less than ideal. Patients may simply forget to report important medical information, but it has also been shown that some patients will intentionally omit relevant information due to concerns over privacy or failure to understand how the information could be relevant to dental practice.[13,14]

MEDICATIONS AND ALLERGIES

The list of medications and allergies should be consistent with the disclosed medical conditions and can alert the clinician to unlisted medical conditions as well as potential drug interactions. Relevant medical conditions and severity of systemic disease can often be determined by a careful analysis of the patient's list of medications.[15] Allergies to materials used in endodontic treatment are covered later in this chapter and drug interactions are covered in Chapter 25, "Drug Interactions and Laboratory Tests."

Herbs, dietary supplements, vitamins, and other over the counter medications can contribute to complications in the dental setting, although patients often fail to report the use of these substances in the initial evaluation.[16] In a recent survey of surgical patients, approximately one-third reported the use of a nonprescription medication that could potentially inhibit coagulation or interact with anesthetics.[17] In particular, *Ginkgo biloba*, ginger, garlic, ginseng, feverfew, and vitamin E all inhibit platelet aggregation and can increase the risk of bleeding.[18] Ingredients in over-the-counter (OTC) weight loss products can potentiate the effect of epinephrine and increase cardiac stress, although the most obvious example of this phenomenon, ephedra, has been removed from the US market by FDA order.

PREVIOUS DENTAL TREATMENT

A standard screening question for all patients should enquire about any problems with previous dental treatment. This line of questioning serves several important functions. First, it allows the patient to discuss any previous negative dental experiences as well as express possible anxiety related to the proposed treatment. A report of difficulty in achieving profound local anesthesia is a common finding, especially for root canal therapy. This provides an opportunity to demonstrate concern for your patient and discuss how you plan to avoid a repeat of the previous experience. Second, potential adverse reactions to dental materials or drugs may emerge in response to this question. Finally, since this question is designed at least in part to help develop rapport with your patient, it can serve as a good lead into other important but potentially more sensitive questions (e.g., use of oral contraceptives, history of human immunodeficiency virus (HIV))

PHYSICAL EXAM: VITAL SIGNS

In addition to the mandatory health history questionnaire and patient interview, vital signs (blood pressure, heart rate, respiratory rate, temperature, height, and weight) should be recorded prior to dental treatment whenever possible. In particular, blood pressure, heart rate, and respiratory rate provide the essential risk assessment baseline information for all patients. Temperature may be routinely recorded but is specifically indicated in the presence of infection or signs of generalized malaise or toxicity. Height and weight can usually be obtained from the patient or the guardian, and this information is particularly important in determining appropriate drug dosages in pediatric and geriatric patients and in assessing unexplained changes in weight.

RELATIVE STRESS OF THE PLANNED PROCEDURE AND BEHAVIORAL CONSIDERATIONS

A patient's ability to tolerate the stress of dental treatment depends on the procedure planned, time required to complete the procedure, physical health status, and psychological factors. Anticipation of a stressful dental procedure can increase the heart rate and endogenous secretion of epinephrine in otherwise healthy adults.[19,20] In fact, even anticipation of a routine dental checkup can result in increased blood pressure in some patients.[21] Most changes in heart rate and blood pressure are within the normal physiological range, although more significant changes have been observed before administration of local anesthetic, during subgingival scaling and during extractions.[22] Since there are no specific guidelines for assigning stress levels to various dental procedures, clinical judgment is essential in determining whether or not stress-reducing treatment modifications should be employed. Dental specialists, by virtue of additional training and experience, should be expected to provide treatment in a shorter time period and should be better prepared to manage perioperative complications than a general practitioner.

Endodontic treatment in general is often considered a high-stress dental visit, especially among patients with no prior endodontic treatment experience or patients who have had a previous negative experience with endodontic treatment. For many, the perception of the treatment often differs from the reality that most current endodontic treatment is minimally invasive, relatively comfortable, efficient and very well tolerated by the majority of patients when skillfully performed. In a study that measured salivary cortisol levels in patients undergoing a variety of dental procedures, root canal treatment was no different than a routine dental exam, prophylaxis, or restorative treatment, and only tooth extraction resulted in a significant increase in salivary cortisol.[23] Surgical root canal procedures, the presence of acute pain, self-reported dental anxiety, or difficulty with previous treatment, and lengthy procedures would all be expected to increase the level of stress.[22,24] If any of these conditions are present in addition to significant systemic disease, treatment modification including a stress reduction protocol should be considered (see Chapter 23, "Anxiety and Fear in Endodontics").

PHYSICAL HEALTH STATUS

The American Society of Anesthesiologists' (ASA) Health Classification System is the most widely used system for assessing physical health status and helps to determine the potential need for medical consultation and treatment modifications prior to dental and medical procedures (see Figure 1). In general, ASA I status represents a healthy patient who does not require any treatment modification. An ASA II patient presents with well-controlled systemic disease and usually will not require significant treatment modification, although stress reduction may be indicated. Patients in the ASA III category or above will almost always require medical consultation and possible treatment modifications. However, the ASA classification system has several significant limitations and should be used only as a general guide for determining peri- and postoperative risk. Even experienced anesthesiologists exhibit differences of opinion in the classification of cases.[25,26] In addition, when used alone, the ASA system is not a good predictor of operative risk.[27] Various authors have proposed a medical risk assessment process that focuses more clearly on medical conditions specifically relevant to dental practice.[2,6,27,28] Clinicians may want to consider health history questionnaires and verbal questions that focus primarily on medical conditions that would, when present, elevate the patient to ASA II status or above. That is, any positive response to one of the health history questions would automatically classify the patient as at least ASA II and further exploration would be necessary to determine the extent of systemic disease. de Jong et al.[12,28,29] have developed and validated a patient questionnaire consisting of approximately 30 questions for use in assessing the risk for dental treatment.

MEDICAL CONSULTATIONS

Approximately one-third of patients referred for a medical consultation result in recommendations for some modification of treatment procedures.[9] A request for consultation may occur by phone or letter and each approach has certain advantages and disadvantages. A phone conversation is immediate and may allow for the discovery of additional useful information. However, the lack of a written letter from the physician increases the risk for potential misunderstanding and provides a lower level of documentation from a medicolegal standpoint. The substance of all medical consultation conversations should be documented in the patient's record and, whenever possible, a letter detailing the physician's recommendations should be requested. A letter provides more formal documentation of the communication between health care providers.

When requesting a medical consultation, the clinician should be specific and concise. The medical condition in question should be identified and the nature of dental procedure planned should be described (e.g., a brief description of the procedure, the type of anesthetic planned, the potential for bleeding, the expected length of procedure). The clinician should specifically ask the physician if the patient's medical condition requires any modification in the usual treatment protocol and, if so, what modifications are recommended. Since the ultimate responsibility for providing safe treatment rests with the dentist, any concerns about recommended treatment modifications should be resolved with the physician prior to treatment.

Assessing the Need for Treatment Modifications

MULTIDIMENSIONAL RISK ASSESSMENT MODEL (MD-RAM)

Systemic disease can result in the loss of reserve capacity to handle stress.[15] A patient's ability to handle stress decreases in direct relation to the extent of systemic disease. The three primary components of risk assessment for dental treatment are physical health status (reserve capacity), emotional or psychological status, and type of dental procedure planned.[30] Lapointe et al.[15] proposed a two-dimensional risk assessment model that correlated the severity of disease and procedural stress. However, this model presented only two specific medical conditions as examples (ischemic heart disease and chronic obstructive pulmonary disease (COPD)) and did not explicitly consider patient anxiety as a variable. Dental anxiety can increase sympathetic activity and for some patients can potentially precipitate a medical emergency.[31]

We propose a new model, the Multidimensional Risk Assessment Model (MD-RAM; Figures 2 and 3), that incorporates the three primary aspects of risk assessment into a unified approach for evaluating perioperative risk related to treatment for the ambulatory dental patient. In this model, the dental patient is assigned a score ranging from 1 to 4 in each of the three domains: physical health status (using the ASA classification system); procedural stress (type of procedure, length of time to complete the procedure, and clinician expertise—Figure 4); and psychological status (self-reported dental anxiety—Figure 5). As with any model, the output is only as good as the information input.

This model may provide a general guide for patient assessment and is not intended to be all inclusive or a substitute for case-specific clinical judgment. The primary purpose of this model is to assist clinicians in determining if treatment modification, often a stress reduction protocol, may be indicated prior to dental treatment. Disease-specific recommendations will be discussed later in the chapter.

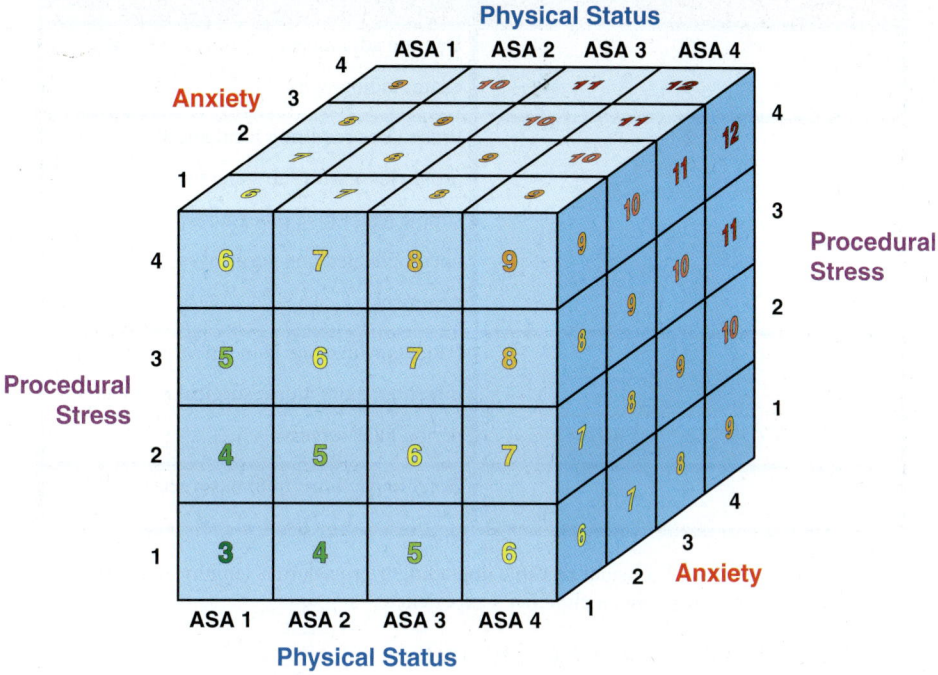

Figure 2 Multidimensional Risk Assessment Model (MD-RAM).

MD-RAM score	Interpretation
3-5	No treatment modification usually indicated
6-7	Possible medical consultation and treatment modification
8-9	Medical consultation often indicated and probable treatment modification
10-12	Medical consultation strongly advised; may require treatment in a hospital or specially equipped out-patient facility

Figure 3 Interpretation of MD-RAM score.

Procedural stress scale	Examples*
1	Denture adjustment; non-invasive oral exam; radiographs
2	Procedures requiring local anesthesia; prophylaxis with sub-gingival scaling; simple restorative procedures; uncomplicated non-surgical root canal treatment
3	Patients with acute pain and/or significant infection; extractions; surgical root canal; periodontal surgery
4	Bony impactions; trauma surgery

* = The clinician should consider possible upgrading if procedure is lengthy and move either up or down depending on clinician's experience.

Figure 4 Estimating procedural stress. Adapted in part from Lapointe HJ et al.[15]

Dental anxiety scale	Verbal descriptor
1	No anxiety
2	Mild anxiety
3	Moderate anxiety
4	Severe anxiety

Figure 5 Behavioral scale—patient's self-reported dental anxiety.

Cardiovascular Disease

HYPERTENSION

Hypertension is one of the most common medical conditions likely to be encountered in a dental office. Hypertensive patients are defined as those receiving treatment for hypertension or those with a mean systolic blood pressure (SBP) of 140 mg Hg or greater and/or a mean diastolic blood pressure (DBP) of 90 mg Hg or greater. By this definition, approximately 24% of the adult population of the United States is hypertensive with about half of this group untreated and only one-quarter receiving successful treatment for hypertension.[32] The goal for patients with diabetes or renal disease is to maintain blood pressure below SBP of 130 and DBP of 80. Since hypertension is typically asymptomatic, approximately one-third of patients with high blood pressure are unaware of their condition.[33] Even patients with normal blood pressure at the age of 55 to 65 years have an almost 90% risk of developing hypertension by the age of 80 to 85 years.[34] Patients with untreated or inadequately treated hypertension are at significantly increased risk for acute complications such as myocardial infarction (MI) and stroke and chronic complications of hypertension.

Classification	Systolic Blood Pressure (SBP) in mm Hg	Diastolic Blood Pressure (DBP) in mm Hg
Normal	< 120	and < 80
Prehypertension	120-139	or 80-89
Stage 1 Hypertension*	140-159	or 90-99
Stage 2 Hypertension	≥ 160	or ≤ 100

* For patients with diabetes or renal disease, the goal is to maintain blood pressure less than 130/80 mm Hg.

Figure 6 Blood pressure classification for adult patients. Adapted from Herman WW et al.[36]

The clinical significance to the dental practitioner is clear—since at least 15% of all adult dental patients have either untreated or inadequately treated hypertension, initial blood pressure measurement is an essential screening tool prior to dental treatment. In addition, it is appropriate to measure blood pressure at least annually during recall visits for all patients and at every visit for patients when an invasive dental procedure is planned.

Guidelines for the classification of blood pressure were recently revised in the seventh report of the Joint National Committee on Prevention, Detection, Evaluation, and Treatment of High Blood Pressure (JNC 7, 2003) (Figure 6). The JNC 7 report added a new category, prehypertension, for patients with SBP of 120 to 139 and/or DBP of 80 to 89 in recognition of the fact that this group was at greater risk for developing hypertension and should receive lifestyle modification advice and subsequent monitoring. The report also combined the previous Stage 2 and Stage 3 categories into a new Stage 2 category for patients with SBP greater than or equal to 160 and/or DBP greater than or equal to 100. From a practical standpoint, patients with well-controlled hypertension or SBP below 160 and DBP below 100 should tolerate all routine dental procedures,[35] although referral for evaluation by the patient's physician is appropriate due to the well-documented benefits of maintaining blood pressure in the normal range. Patients with SBP between 160 and 180 or DBP between 100 and 110 should also be able to tolerate most dental procedures without significantly increased risk of perioperative cardiovascular complications; however, complexity and stress of the planned treatment should be carefully considered with attention given to stress reduction strategies prior to treatment.[36] Although clear guidelines for establishing a cutoff point for dental treatment (emergency or routine) are lacking, it is generally accepted that patients with SBP greater than 180 and/or DBP greater than 110 should be referred for medical consultation and treatment prior to dental treatment and only emergency management of pain or acute infection should be considered.[36] Patients with SBP above 210 and/or DBP above 120 should be referred for emergent medical evaluation.

VASOCONSTRICTOR USE IN PATIENTS WITH CARDIOVASCULAR DISEASE

Vasoconstrictors are used routinely in endodontic therapy as a component of local anesthetics and often as a hemostatic agent during periapical surgery. Local anesthetic with a vasoconstrictor, most commonly lidocaine with 1:100,000 epinephrine, is the usual anesthetic of choice for root canal therapy, although many nonsurgical procedures can be performed using local anesthetics without vasoconstrictor.[37] When a vasoconstrictor is indicated, epinephrine is preferred over norepinephrine or levonordefrin due to a decreased potential for alpha-1 receptor stimulation. Surgical procedures typically require greater quantities of local anesthetic with a vasoconstrictor than nonsurgical root canal treatment. In particular, patients with advanced cardiovascular disease, geriatric patients, and patients taking certain medications (e.g., MAO inhibitors and nonselective beta blockers) may have a reduced tolerance for vasoconstrictor-containing local anesthetics. Since local anesthetics with vasoconstrictors are very helpful in obtaining adequate hemostasis and visibility during periapical surgery, it may be difficult to perform the procedure using anesthetics without vasoconstrictors.[38]

The use of local anesthetics with vasoconstrictors in patients with cardiovascular disease has been somewhat controversial and was addressed by the JNC 7 report. While the general goal should be to minimize the use of vasoconstrictors in patients with cardiovascular disease, the benefit of greater depth and duration of anesthesia when local anesthetics with a vasoconstrictor are used is a significant argument in favor of their use. Adequate pain control is an essential component of endodontic therapy since pain-related stress could stimulate the release of significant quantities of endogenous catecholamines. Different kinds of stress can increase the release of endogenous epinephrine by as much as 20 to 40 times over baseline values.[39] Pooled results from six studies of patients undergoing extraction or other minor oral surgery procedure demonstrated an average increase in SBP and DBP of 11.7 and 3.3 mm Hg, respectively, as well as an increase in heart rate of 4.7 beats per minute (bpm). The use of local anesthetics containing epinephrine for these procedures resulted in an additional relatively minor increase in SBP of 4 mm Hg and 6 bpm.[32] Careful aspiration and use of adequate gauge needle to facilitate aspiration during injection is required to minimize the chance of intravascular injection. Most authors feel that 0.036 to 0.054 mg of epinephrine (approximately two to three cartridges of local anesthetic with 1:100,000 epinephrine) should be safe for all patients except those with severe cardiovascular disease or other specific risk factors, and those with SBP requiring urgent medical attention.[36,40,41] Local anesthetics with vasoconstrictors should be avoided or used with extreme caution in patients with the following cardiovascular conditions: severe or poorly controlled hypertension, arrhythmias that are refractory to treatment, MI within the past month, stroke within the past 6 months, coronary artery bypass graft within the past 3 months, and uncontrolled congestive heart failure (CHF).[30]

An important exception to this general rule regarding vasoconstrictors is the choice of local anesthetic for intraosseous (IO) injections in patients with cardiovascular disease. IO injections are most commonly used as a supplemental anesthetic technique for teeth that are otherwise difficult to anesthetize. A transient increase in heart rate can be expected in about two-thirds of patients receiving an IO injection using lidocaine with 1:100,000 epinephrine, although heart rate returns to near baseline within 4 minutes after injection.[42] No increase in heart rate was found in patients receiving an IO injection with a 3% mepivacaine solution. Although in this study no significant change in blood pressure was found in either group, the authors recommended 3% mepivacaine without vasoconstrictor for patients with any medical condition that could reduce their tolerance for epinephrine.

Although most experts agree that the use of gingival retraction cord containing epinephrine should be avoided in patients with significant cardiovascular disease,[36,40] some uncertainty exists over the use of racemic epinephrine-impregnated pellets as recently advocated for improved hemostasis during periapical surgery.[38,43] In two clinical studies, no significant changes were observed in blood pressure or heart rate when epinephrine pellets (either cotton or collagen) were placed in the bony crypt to improve hemostasis during periapical surgery.[44,45] It is unlikely that a patient healthy enough to tolerate two or three cartridges of local anesthetic with 1:100,000 epinephrine would experience any untoward effects from the proper use of epinephrine-impregnated pellets during periapical surgery. Regardless, other alternative topical hemostatic agents are available and should be considered for patients with significant cardiovascular disease.

ISCHEMIC HEART DISEASE

When coronary atherosclerotic heart disease becomes sufficiently advanced to produce symptoms, it is referred to as ischemic heart disease. Ischemic heart disease is relatively common in the general population, especially with increasing age, and typically presents as angina or heart failure.[46] In most cases, diminished blood perfusion of the myocardium due to coronary artery disease (atherosclerosis) is the underlying cause with hypertension as a common contributing factor in heart failure. CHF and enlargement of the heart result from weakening of the damaged heart muscle.

Chest pain secondary to ischemic heart disease results when the oxygen demand of the myocardium exceeds the oxygen supply. Transient pain is referred to as angina pectoris and is often described as an aching, squeezing sensation or tightness in the middle of the chest. Angina is often precipitated by physical activity or stress and may radiate to the arm or jaw and may present as facial or dental pain. Fear and anxiety associated with dental treatment may be a precipitating factor for angina in some patients.[46] Sublingual or other forms of nitrates are the standard treatment for angina and should result in rapid reversal of symptoms. Patients should always be instructed to bring their usual antianginal medicine with them for dental appointments. If symptoms are not relieved with oral nitrates and suspension of stress-inducing activity, then MI should be suspected and immediate emergency treatment should be initiated. Since angina is usually a transient event, patients with progressive pain or pain at rest are considered to have unstable angina and present a significant perioperative risk for MI.[30] These patients are usually categorized as ASA IV. Chest pain that is manageable with rest or medication and relatively unchanged in duration, frequency, or severity over time is termed stable angina and represents a better prognosis and somewhat lower risk level than unstable angina. Typically, patients with stable angina would be classified as ASA II or ASA III.

Compared to other surgical procedures, most dental and oral surgery procedures are considered relatively low risk.[47,48] However, a history of significant cardiac disease can be a major predictor of perioperative risk, even for procedures with relatively low procedural stress. Recent MI (less than 1 month), unstable angina, past MI with significant residual damage, decompensated CHF, significant arrhythmias, and severe valvular disease are all considered major predictors of increased perioperative cardiovascular risk, and these patients would usually be classified as ASA IV. Patients with stable angina, past history of MI (greater than 1 month) with minimal residual myocardial damage, compensated CHF, or diabetes mellitus (DM) should be considered at intermediate risk and would usually be classified as ASA II or ASA III.[30,47] The presence of multiple risk factors creates an additive increase in the overall perioperative risk.[49] Even patients with a history of recent MI or unstable angina should be able to tolerate routine dental procedures with local anesthesia, although medical consultation is required and conscious sedation with monitoring is often recommended.[48,50]

Treatment modification considerations for patients with ischemic heart disease should include morning appointments, short appointments, oral premedication with an anxiolytic drug and/or nitrous oxide/oxygen sedation, limited use of vasocontrictors (as previously discussed), adequate pain management (during and after the dental appointment), and possible cardiac monitoring.[30] Sedation with a short acting oral benzodiazepine (e.g., triazolam or ativan) and/or nitrous oxide can reduce the stress of a dental procedure and increase the effectiveness of local anesthesia.[31] Clinicians must be aware of the medical need and legal requirements that include special training, permits, and monitoring when anxiolysis crosses over into conscious sedation. If conscious sedation is required, it is best performed by a trained provider of anesthesia/sedation and with another operator providing the dental care.

HEART MURMURS AND VALVULAR DISEASE

Patients with valvular disease present two primary considerations for dental treatment: potential risk for infective endocarditis and risk of excessive bleeding in patients on anticoagulant therapy.[46] Management considerations for patients on anticoagulant therapy are discussed later in this chapter. Most heart valve abnormalities affect either the aortic or the mitral valve and represent partial obstruction of blood flow (stenosis) or valve incompetence (regurgitation). Heart murmurs are common and may be benign or signify major underlying diseases such as degenerative valve disorders (e.g., aortic stenosis), rheumatic heart disease, congenital valve lesions, prosthetic valves, atrial fibrillation, or CHF.[51] Two other conditions that place patients at increased risk for infective endocarditis are systemic lupus erythematosus and certain medications used for weight reduction (dexfenfluramine and fenfluramine–phentermine).[51,52] Dental management requires evaluation of the type of heart condition and the risk of bacteremia from the planned dental procedure. New guidelines for the prevention of infective endocarditis were published in 2007 and represent a significant change from previous American Heart Association guidelines.[53] For example, antibiotic prophylaxis is no longer recommended for patients with a history of mitral valve prolapse (with or without regurgitation), rheumatic heart disease, bicuspid valve disease, aortic stenosis, and certain congenital heart conditions. Antibiotic prophylaxis is now recommended only for patients with valvular disease associated with the highest risk of adverse outcomes from infective endocarditis. For patients in the highest risk category, antibiotic

Antibiotic prophylaxis recommended

<u>Highest risk of adverse outcome from infective endocarditis:</u>

Prosthetic heart valve

Previous infective endocarditis

Congenital heart disease (CHD)*

- Unrepaired cyanotic CHD, including palliative shunts and conduits

- Completely repaired congenital heart defect with prosthetic material or device, whether placed by surgery or catheter, during the first six months after the procedure

- Repaired CHD with residual defects at the site or adjacent to the site of a prosthetic patch or prosthetic device

Cardiac transplantation recipients who develop cardiac valvulopathy

* antibiotic prophylaxis is not recommended for other forms of CHD

Figure 7 Recommendations for antibiotic prophylaxis based on risk stratification for infective endocarditis. Adapted from Wilson W et al.[53]

Antibiotic prophylaxis recommended *only for patients at highest risk* for adverse outcome from infective endocarditis (Figure 24-7):

All dental procedures that involve manipulation of gingival tissue or the periapical region of teeth or perforation of the oral mucosa (does not include routine local anesthetic injections through noninfected tissue)

Figure 8 Risk of dental procedures. Adapted from Wilson W et al.[53]

---

prophylaxis is recommended for dental procedures that involve manipulation of gingival tissues or the periapical region of teeth or perforation of the oral mucosa. For all other patients with valvular disease, the risks associated with routine antibiotic prophylaxis are greater than potential benefits.[53] Figures 7 and 8 list the specific heart valve abnormalities and dental procedures that are considered highest risk for infective endocarditis. In general, procedures associated with nonsurgical root canal treatment such as local anesthetic injection, placement of the rubber dam, and instrumentation when contained within the canal system do not place the patient at significant risk for infective endocarditis.[54] The incidence and magnitude of bacteremia when canal instrumentation does not extend into the periapical tissues is very low, and almost all bacteria are eliminated from the blood within 10 minutes.[55,56] Canal instrumentation beyond the apex, intraligamentary and IO injections, and periapical surgery can all be expected to result in a higher risk for transient bacteremia. In these situations, antibiotic premedication is recommended for patients in the highest risk disease categories. Infective endocarditis is only rarely directly linked to dental procedures and the efficacy of the recommended antibiotic regimen is

Standard oral regimen	Adults: 2.0g Amoxicillin
	Children: 50mg/kg
Alternative oral regimen for patients allergic to penicillin or patients who are currently taking a penicillin class antibiotic	Adults: 2.0g Cephalexin or other 1st or 2nd generation cephalosporin in equivalent dosage* OR 600mg Clindamycin OR 500mg Azithromycin or clarithromycin Children: 50mg/kg Cephalexin or other 1st or 2nd generation cephalosporin in equivalent dosage* OR 20mg/kg Clindamycin OR 15mg/kg Azithromycin or clarithromycin
Patients unable to take oral medications	Adults: 2.0g IM or IV Ampicillin OR 1.0g IM or IV Cefazolin or ceftriaxone* Children: 50mg/kg IM or IV Ampicillin OR 50mg/kg IM or IV Cefazolin or ceftriaxone*
Alternative IM/IV regimen for patients allergic to penicillin and unable to take oral medications	Adults: 1.0g IM or IV Cefazolin or ceftriaxone* OR 600mg IM or IV Clindamycin Children: 50mg/kg IM or IV Cefazolin or ceftriaxone* OR 20mg/kg IM or IV Clindamycin within 30 minutes before the procedure

* = Cephalosporins should be used with caution in patients reporting an allergy to penicillin since approximately 5%–15% of patients who are allergic to penicillin will demonstrate cross reactivity with cephalosporins, especially first and second generation cephalosporins.

Figure 9 Antibiotic prophylaxis for dental procedures—all regimens are a single dose given 30 to 60 minutes before the procedure. Adapted from Wilson W et al.[53]

questionable.[53,57–61] The current regimen and drugs of choice for antibiotic prophylaxis are presented in Figure 9.

According to Lessard et al., some patients with significant heart murmurs may have dyspnea, fatigue and difficulty in breathing when reclined in the dental chair[51] and therefore the dental procedure may need to be performed with the chair in a more upright position. They also suggest that the use of a rubber dam may be contraindicated for some of these patients due to restriction of air flow; however, this may be overcome with careful application of the rubber dam. Failure to use the rubber dam is considered below the standard of care for root canal therapy and extraction may be the only option for these patients if a rubber dam cannot be used.

ANTICOAGULANT THERAPY AND BLEEDING DISORDERS

Management of patients on anticoagulant therapy depends on the type of anticoagulant, the reason for anticoagulant therapy, and the type of procedure planned. Warfarin (Coumadin—DuPont Pharmaceuticals, Wilmington, DE) anticoagulants are commonly prescribed for the treatment or the prevention of thromboembolic events. This category of anticoagulant works by blocking the formation of prothrombin and other clotting factors. The international normalized ratio (INR) value is the accepted standard for measuring prothrombin time (PT). The desired therapeutic range for INR is usually between 2 and 3.5, depending on the underlying medical indication for anticoagulant therapy.

Limited oral surgery procedures, defined as simple forceps extraction of one to three teeth, may be safely performed on patients with INR values within the normal therapeutic range.[62–64] Nonsurgical root canal treatment does not usually require modification of anticoagulant therapy, although it is important to ascertain that the patient's INR is within the therapeutic range, especially if a nerve block injection is required. Periapical surgery may present a greater challenge for hemostasis even for patients well maintained within the therapeutic range. The clear field visibility normally required for proper surgical management of the root end may not be possible in patients on anticoagulant therapy. Consultation with the patient's physician is required to assist in developing an appropriate treatment plan. Some patients may be able to tolerate discontinuation of warfarin therapy 2 days prior to a planned surgical procedure to allow for the INR to "drift" downward. In a prospective cohort study, Russo et al.[65] report that suspension of warfarin 2 days prior to a surgical procedure resulted in no bleeding problems and no thromboembolic events. They found that the average time spent at an INR less than 2.0 (critical value) was 28 hours and that 90% of the patients returned to the desired therapeutic INR value within 7 days. However, this strategy may place certain patients at greater risk for a thromboembolic event and in these cases discontinuation of anticoagulant therapy would not be recommended.

In general, patients on warfarin anticoagulant therapy should present minimal risk for significant bleeding during or after oral surgery and local measures to control bleeding should be adequate.[66,67] Jeske and Suchko,[68] in a review prepared for the American Dental Association Council on Scientific Affairs and Division of Science, recommend against routine discontinuation of anticoagulant therapy prior to dental procedures, including surgical procedures. Regardless of the management approach selected, consultation with the patient's physician and an INR test on the day of surgery are strongly recommended. Hospitalization and conversion to heparin therapy may be considered in special cases, but the patient, physician, and surgeon must carefully weigh the potential risks against the expected outcome and benefits. A new category of heparin anticoagulant, low molecular weight heparins (LMWHs), allows for patient self-administration and may present a viable alternative for some patients who need to remain at a high level of anticoagulation but wish to reduce the cost and time associated with traditional heparin conversion therapy.

Low-dose aspirin therapy is known to increase bleeding time by irreversibly inhibiting platelet aggregation. No treatment modifications should be necessary for nonsurgical root canal procedures. However, surgical procedures require evaluation of the reason for and the necessity of aspirin therapy. It has been a common practice to advise patients to discontinue aspirin therapy for 7 to 10 days prior to an oral surgical procedure.[69] At low-dose therapeutic levels (<100 mg/day), aspirin may increase bleeding time and potentially complicate surgical procedures. However, Ardekian et al.[69] concluded that low-dose aspirin therapy (<100 mg/day) should *not* be discontinued prior to oral surgery procedures and that bleeding could be controlled by local measures. Higher dose therapy may present a greater risk for bleeding either during or after surgery. Even though a patient on aspirin therapy may not be at high risk for significant intra- or postoperative bleeding, a concern for periapical surgery is the visibility problems created by oozing blood. Consultation with the patient's physician is advised to determine the medical reason for aspirin therapy and to weigh the risks and benefits of discontinuing aspirin prior to the proposed surgery. It should be possible to perform periapical surgery without discontinuing aspirin therapy if necessary, but the visibility during the procedure may be compromised and the prognosis may decrease accordingly.[38]

Nonsteroidal anti-inflammatory drugs (NSAIDs) also have an antiplatelet effect but, unlike aspirin, the effect is reversible when discontinued and platelet activity should be expected to return to normal within approximately three half-lives of the drug. Other commonly prescribed antiplatelet drugs include dipyridamole, ticlopidine, clopidogrel, abciximab, integrelin, tyrafiban, and lamifiban. Heavy alcohol consumption, liver disease, and certain medications can increase the risk of perioperative bleeding in patients taking antiplatelet medications. Medical consultation is advised prior to surgical procedures and lab tests to determine platelet count and function (PFA-100 and Ivy BT) may be indicated. Some herbs and dietary supplements may also affect bleeding risk.

Patients with inherited or acquired bleeding disorders are also at risk for excessive bleeding during and after periapical surgery procedures and may be at risk from local anesthetic injections particularly when using nerve block injections. Impaired liver function secondary to past or current alcohol or drug abuse may also predispose a patient to excessive bleeding during surgery. A medical consultation, usually with a hematologist, is required prior to dental treatment for patients with serious bleeding disorders such as thrombocytopenia, hemophilia, and von Willebrand's disease. Replacement of deficient coagulation factors or platelet transfusion may be required prior to dental treatment,[70] particularly if an inferior alveolar nerve block is required or a surgical treatment is planned. If non-surgical root canal treatment can be performed with only infiltration local anesthesia, replacement may not be necessary.[71] However, this decision must be reached in consultation with the patient's hematologist.

ARRHYTHMIAS AND CARDIAC PACEMAKERS

Cardiac arrhythmias are a heterogeneous group of conditions defined as any disturbance in the normal rate or rhythm of the heartbeat. Arrhythmias are the result of abnormal impulse generation, impulse conduction, or both and can range from harmless to life threatening.[46] The overall prevalence of cardiac arrhythmias in the general dental patient population is 15% to 17% with approximately 2 to 4% representing serious, potentially life-threatening arrhythmias.[30] Although arrhythmias are not uncommon in normal, healthy adults, the possibility of underlying cardiovascular disease, systemic disease, or medication-induced arrhythmia should be carefully evaluated prior to dental treatment. Anxiety associated with dental treatment may induce arrhythmias in susceptible patients. In addition, patients with cardiovascular disease are more prone to arrhythmias during oral surgery procedures with local anesthesia.[72] Patients taking digoxin for atrial fibrillation or CHF are especially at risk for arrhythmias during oral surgery procedures.[73]

Medications are usually the first line of treatment for cardiac arrhythmias, although many of these have a narrow therapeutic safety range (e.g., digoxin) and must be carefully monitored. Surgery, cardioversion, and pacemakers are also used to treat arrhythmias. It is common for patients with atrial fibrillation to be treated with an anticoagulant (typically warfarin sodium—management considerations discussed previously in this chapter). A history of cardiac arrhythmia is often disclosed in the medical history. In addition to the medical history, patients with an irregular pulse, unusually rapid or slow pulse, reports of syncope, palpitations, dizziness, angina, or dyspnea should be referred to a physician for evaluation prior to dental treatment. Once the nature of arrhythmia and the stability of the condition have been determined, most dental treatment can be safely performed using the same stress reduction treatment modifications listed in the discussion of ischemic heart disease. As always, the clinician and staff should be prepared to manage a medical emergency if necessary.

Electrical interference from certain dental devices is a potential concern for patients with implanted cardiac pacemakers or cardioverter/defibrillators. In particular, electronic apex locators (EAL) and electric pulp testers (EPT) are commonly used in root canal therapy. Manufacturers of EAL and EPT devices warn against the use of these devices in patients with cardiac pacemakers. However, current cardiac pacemakers are very well shielded from external electrical fields and the possibility for electrical interference seems to be very low. A recent clinical study supports previous *in vitro* research and a case report in concluding that EAL and EPT devices should be safe to use in patients with cardiac pacemakers and cardioverter/defibrillators.[74–76] One caveat from this study is that a mucosal lip clip was used to complete the circuit with the EPT device instead of the common clinical practice of having the patient hold the EPT wand in their hand. This lip clip technique is recommended if one elects to use an EPT device on a patient with a cardiac pacemaker, since the practice of using the patient's hand to complete the circuit may allow for electrical current to pass through an area of the body in closer proximity to the pacemaker. The safety of this variation of the EPT technique has not yet been tested.

CONGESTIVE HEART FAILURE

CHF is the fourth most common medical diagnosis in all age groups and represents the end-stage of other common cardiovascular diseases such as coronary

New York Heart Association CHF classification	Signs and symptoms	Dental management considerations
Class I	No limitations on physical activity; no dyspnea, fatigue, or palpitations with ordinary physical activity	Should be able to tolerate routine dental treatment; stress reduction protocol as needed
Class II	Slight limitation on physical activity; comfortable at rest but may experience fatigue, palpitations, and dyspnea with ordinary physical activity	Should be able to tolerate routine dental treatment; stress reduction protocol as needed; possible medical consultation
Class III	Significant limitation of activity; comfortable at rest but even minor activity results in symptoms	Medical consultation; consider treatment in hospital dental clinic or similar facility; avoid vasoconstrictors
Class IV	Symptoms present at rest; symptoms exacerbated by any physical activity	Medical consultation; conservative treatment only; treatment in hospital dental clinic; avoid vasoconstrictors

Figure 10 New York Heart Association's classification system for patients with congestive heart failure (CHF) and dental management considerations. Adapted from Little JW et al.[30]

artery disease, hypertension, cardiomyopathy, and valvular heart disease.[30] CHF results in an inability of the heart to efficiently pump blood that can involve one or both ventricles. Patients with CHF typically present with significantly diminished reserve capacity for handling stress (including dental treatment) and are often taking multiple medications with the potential for drug interactions.

Patients with well-managed CHF should tolerate routine dental treatment with possible minor treatment modifications, similar to those recommended for patients with ischemic heart disease. In addition, the underlying causes (coronary artery disease, hypertension, valve disease, etc.) and medications should be considered and managed appropriately. Patients with moderate to advanced CHF may require a more upright chair position due to the presence of pulmonary edema. The clinician should be alert for orthostatic hypotension when making adjustments in chair position. Uncompensated, advanced CHF requires medical consultation prior to dental treatment and vasoconstrictors should be avoided. These patients may require treatment in special care facilities or hospital-based clinics. The New York Heart Association (NYHA) has developed a classification system for CHF that can be adapted to assist in assessing risk for dental treatment (Figure 10).

Diabetes

Diabetes mellitus (DM) is a complex metabolic disorder characterized by abnormalities in carbohydrate, fat, and protein metabolism resulting either from a deficiency of insulin (type 1) or from target tissue resistance to its cellular metabolic effects (type 2). Hyperglycemia is the most clinically important metabolic aberration in DM and the basis for its diagnosis. Chronic hyperglycemia is associated with ophthalmic, renal, cardiovascular, cerebrovascular, and peripheral neurological complications. DM is defined as a fasting blood glucose level greater than 125 mg/dL and the normal fasting blood glucose level is considered to be less than 110 mg/dL. Patients with fasting plasma glucose levels greater than 110 mg/dL but less than 126 mg/dL represent a transitional condition between normal and DM and are considered to have impaired glucose tolerance.[77] Identification of patients at this stage can allow for earlier preventive interventions and possibly delay or prevent progression to DM. There are 20.8 million children and adults in the United States, or 7% of the population, who have DM. While an estimated 14.6 million have been diagnosed with DM, 6.2 million people (or nearly one-third) are unaware that they have the disease.[78] The epidemic of obesity in the United States is anticipated to result in an increase in the prevalence of diabetes.

When reviewing medical histories, the clinician should be aware of cardinal symptoms of DM, such as polydipsia, polyuria, polyphagia, weight loss, and weakness, and should be referred to a physician for diagnosis and treatment.[30] In diabetic patients, the clinician should ascertain how well controlled the condition may be. Dental appointment scheduling should take into account the importance of nutritional consistency and the avoidance of appointments that will overlap with or prevent scheduled meals. Symptoms of hypoglycemia may range from mild, such as anxiety, sweating, tachycardia, to severe, such as mental status changes, seizure, and coma. Severe hypoglycemic episodes are a medical emergency and should promptly be treated with 15 g of oral carbohydrate, such as 6 oz orange juice, three to four teaspoons of table sugar, five Life Savers, or three glucose or dextrose tablets. If a patient is unable to cooperate or swallow, 1 mg glucagon may be administered by subcutaneous or intramuscular injection. Side effects of glucagon include nausea, vomiting, and headache.

It has been well established that hyposalivation, gingivitis, periodontitis, and periodontal bone loss are associated with DM, especially when poorly controlled.[79,80] The well-controlled diabetic is at no greater risk of postoperative infection than is the nondiabetic.[81] Therefore, surgical procedures in well-controlled diabetics do not require prophylactic antibiotics. However, when surgery is necessary in the poorly controlled diabetic, prophylactic antibiotics should be considered due to the altered function of neutrophils in diabetics. Surgery may also increase insulin resistance such that a diabetic may become hyperglycemic in the postoperative period. Preoperative antibiotics should be administered in these instances.[82] Furthermore, delayed alveolar healing following dentoalveolar surgery should raise the suspicion of osteomyelitis, for which prompt surgical consultation should be arranged. Finally, patients with DM may present with systemic complications, each of which should be taken into account prior to dental procedures.

Pulmonary Disorders: Asthma, COPD, and Tuberculosis

Asthma is a chronic inflammatory respiratory disease with recurrent episodes of chest tightness, coughing, dyspnea, and wheezing resulting from hyperresponsiveness and inflammation of bronchiole tissue. Overt attacks may be provoked by allergens, upper respiratory tract infections, genetic and environmental factors, certain medications, and highly emotional states such as anxiety, stress, and nervousness.

The endodontist should obtain a good history to determine the severity and stability of disease. Patients should be instructed to bring their inhalers (bronchodilators) to each appointment and inform the endodontist of the earliest sign or symptom of an asthma attack. During dental treatment, the most likely times for an acute exacerbation of asthma are during and immediately after local anesthetic administration and with stimulating procedures such as pulp extirpation.[83] Because stress is implicated as a precipitating factor in asthma attacks, sedation may be beneficial. While nitrous oxide may be used in patients with mild-to-moderate asthma, its use is contraindicated in patients with severe asthma due to its potential to cause airway irritation.[84] Alternatively, oral premedication may be accomplished with small doses of a short-acting benzodiazepine. In patients taking theophylline, macrolide antibiotics should be avoided, as they have the potential to develop toxic levels of theophylline. In addition, it is important to note that aspirin and other NSAIDs may trigger asthma attacks in a proportion of patients.[85]

COPD is a term for pulmonary disorders characterized by chronic irreversible obstruction of airflow from the lungs and represents the fourth most common cause of death in the United States.[86] The three most common forms of COPD are chronic bronchitis, emphysema, and bronchial asthma. Patients with pulmonary diseases typically present with one or more of the following symptoms: cough, dyspnea, sputum, hemoptysis, wheezing, or chest pain.[87] Patients should be placed in a semisupine position. Since the use of a rubber dam may induce a feeling of airway constriction, careful application of the rubber dam and administration of humidified low-flow oxygen, generally between 2 and 3 L/min, may be considered. Nitrous oxide should not be used in patients with severe COPD.

Tuberculosis (TB) is an infectious disease that is spread by way of bacilli-containing airborne droplets, typically by coughing, sneezing, or talking. The signature lesion of TB is the tubercle, a granuloma formed by the continuing ingress of macrophages and lymphocytes to the site of infection.[88] In the lung, tuberculous granulomas are frequently associated with regions of tissue necrosis, termed *caseous necrosis* due to its gross appearance. After the infection is established, symptomatic individuals will show pulmonary manifestations of the disease, often limited to the periphery of the middle and lower regions of the lung,[88] though reactivated disease is most commonly found in the lung apices.[89] Oral tubercular infections are rare, occurring in 0.05 to 5% of patients with TB, though when lesions are present, they typically consist of ulcers, fissures, or swellings on the dorsum of the tongue.[90] Despite the declining incidence of TB in the United States, health care workers including endodontists and their staff remain at high risk for contracting the disease. It is imperative for the endodontist to educate office staff about TB prevention and recognition of symptoms and oral manifestations of the disease to protect the staff and other patients from becoming infected. A thorough medical history should be obtained, and any elective dental procedures on a patient with established or suspected active TB should be delayed until the individual can be treated and subsequently proved noninfectious. Routine dental treatment is appropriate after it has been established that the patient has been adequately treated and there are no signs or symptoms of active disease. The clinician should be aware of potential drug interactions when managing dental patients undergoing antitubercular treatment. In patients taking medications such as rifampin and isoniazid, acetaminophen should be avoided due to the potential for liver damage. The use of aspirin and muscle relaxants is discouraged in those individuals taking streptomycin due to a heightened risk of ototoxicity and respiratory paralysis, respectively.[91] Streptomycin is also known to cause facial paresthesia and pancytopenia.

Central Nervous System: Stroke, Seizure Disorders, and Hydrocephalic Shunts

Cerebrovascular accident or stroke is defined as the acute onset of neurologic deficits persisting for at least 24 hours. Strokes are subclassified into ischemic insults, occurring secondary to thrombosis or embolization, or hemorrhagic, which usually indicate an arterial process. The lack of blood flow leads to deprivation of oxygen and glucose in a localized area of the brain. The endodontist should be aware of how to identify the patient having a stroke in his/her office. Regardless of the procedure, a patient's blood pressure should be checked before treatment to identify a patient whose blood pressure is elevated and who might be at risk for a stroke if subjected to stress. Slurred speech, loss of motor control over a portion of the body, unilateral facial droop, unilateral visual changes, and unilateral severe headache are all potential signs of a stroke or a transient ischemic attack. Should any of these events occur, the patient should have his/her vital signs checked, be placed in a supine position, have vital signs monitored, and be transported to an emergency facility immediately, as treatment must be activated in a timely manner. Patients with a history of stroke may be at risk for aspiration due to swallowing abnormalities, so they should be positioned in a semisupine position, and rubber dams should be carefully applied and should always be used. Poststroke patients may be on oral anticoagulants; so if surgical intervention is planned, the endodontist should contact the physician to determine whether or not the risk of a thromboembolic event outweighs the benefits of postoperative hemostasis (please refer to section "Anticoagulant therapy and bleeding disorders"). The endodontist should also be aware that the poststroke patient may experience emotional problems, including depression and behavior inappropriate to the situation.

Seizures are one of the most commonly encountered neurological disorders and can manifest as an isolated incident with unknown etiology or as a symptom of a condition that requires long-term treatment. A seizure is a temporary involuntary disturbance of brain function that results in synchronous, excessive, abnormal electrical discharges of the neurons in the central nervous system.[92] This manifestation can take the form of motor disturbances, altered feelings, or changes in the patient's level of consciousness. The two main categories of seizure classification are partial and generalized. Most people who have seizures have good control and are capable of receiving routine dental care. The endodontist should be aware of the patient's seizure medications, since many antibiotics are contraindicated. Should a seizure occur in the dental office, the procedure should be stopped immediately and all instruments should be removed from the oral cavity. The patient should be placed in a supine position and low to the ground. Basic life support should begin immediately, including opening the airway, obtaining vital signs such as heart rate and blood pressure, and contacting emergency medical services.

The risk of shunt infection following invasive dental treatment for patients with hydrocephalic shunts (ventriculoperitoneal and ventriculoatrial) is believed to be about 3.0 to 5.0% and because of this there is a lack of consensus regarding the need for antibiotic prophylaxis.[93] The authors of this study found that pediatric dentists were more likely to be concerned about streptococcal microorganisms and neurosurgeons were more concerned about staphylococcal microorganisms in shunt infection. The majority of both groups recommended penicillin prophylaxis, although there are more appropriate antibiotics if staphylococcal microorganisms are presumed to be responsible for most shunt infections (please refer to the discussion in section "Prosthetic joints and other prosthetic devices"). Consultation with the patient's neurosurgeon is advised and close attention to any changes in prophylaxis guidelines is important.

Renal Disease and Dialysis

Chronic renal failure is a slowly progressive condition characterized by an irreversible reduction in the glomerular filtration rate. The progression of this disease begins with an asymptomatic decrease in the kidney function and eventually results in end-stage renal disease (ESRD). Throughout the decline in function, multiple systems are affected, directly related to the kidney dysfunction. ESRD is potentially fatal unless the patient undergoes dialysis or kidney transplantation (please see section "Solid Organ Transplantation" regarding kidney transplantation). Dialysis may take the form of hemodialysis, which represents 90% of dialysis treatment,[94] or peritoneal dialysis. This treatment removes fluid and wastes and equilibrates electrolytes and acid–bases via diffusion and osmosis across a semipermeable membrane.

The clinician should be aware of the ESRD patient's type and days of dialysis treatment as well as comorbid conditions such as hypertension and/or diabetes. Mechanical trauma to platelets and anticoagulants such as heparin used during hemodialysis may increase the renal patient's tendency for bleeding. While it is recommended that dental procedures be performed on nondialysis days, typically the day after dialysis,[95] the endodontist should be aware that abnormal platelet function may cause a greater risk of bleeding during surgical procedures. In addition, patients with ESRD require aggressive treatment of odontogenic infections. Antibiotic premedication has also been recommended for hemodialysis patients with shunts who undergo invasive dental procedures,[96–98] and other authors have recommended antibiotic prophylaxis for all hemodialysis patients undergoing procedures that cause mucosal bleeding to prevent vascular access infections, bacteremia, and infective endocarditis.[97] Renal osteodystrophy and secondary hyperparathyroidism may occur in late-stage disease due to disorders in calcium, phosphorous, and abnormal vitamin D metabolism. Such a manifestation may predispose renal patients to jaw fracture during surgical procedures.

Because many drugs are metabolized via the kidney, renal dosing should account for the drug's extended half-life by lengthening the interval between medication doses. In particular, antibiotic medications should be adjusted for renal dosing. NSAIDs should be avoided in patients with renal insufficiency due to their nephrotoxic effects, but no longer need to be avoided when the patient has ESRD.

Cancer Chemotherapy and Radiation Therapy

Oropharyngeal cancer encompasses a variety of malignant diseases. More than 90% of oral cancers are squamous cell cancers, 9% are salivary gland tumors, sarcomas and lymphomas, and the remaining 1% are metastatic cancers originating in other parts of the body.[99] In the year 2006, the American Cancer Society reported 31,000 people with newly diagnosed oropharyngeal cancers and 7800 deaths from this disease.[100] Numerous risk factors have been implicated in the etiology of oropharyngeal cancer, including tobacco, excessive alcohol, ultraviolet light exposure, immunosuppression, and viruses. Oral cancer has a variable appearance, including white or red patches, an exophytic mass, an ulceration, a granular raised lesion, a submucosal mass, or a combination thereof. Treatment of oropharyngeal cancer is composed of surgical intervention, radiation treatment, and chemotherapy and for systemic cancers possibly hematopoietic stem cell transplantation (HSCT). Multimodality therapy is now more commonly used for oropharyngeal cancer in order to obtain increased survival rates.

Cancers that are amenable to surgery and do not affect the oral cavity require few treatment plan modifications. However, oropharyngeal cancer treatments and complications may cause significant changes in the oral cavity. Preceding cancer treatment, all sources of inflammation and potential infection should be eliminated. Whenever possible, nonrestorable teeth and teeth with a poor long-term periodontal prognosis (i.e., not expected to be retained for the patient's lifetime) within the field of high-dose radiation should be extracted more than 2 weeks prior to radiation therapy. Symptomatic nonvital teeth can be endodontically treated at least 1 week before initiation of head and neck radiation or chemotherapy although dental treatment of asymptomatic teeth even with periapical involvement can be delayed, particularly if treatment can be limited to intracanal therapy. Many cancer patients have indwelling catheters that may be susceptible to infection and, while controversial, the American Heart Association (AHA) regimen for antibiotic prophylaxis (see Figure 9) has been recommended before invasive dental procedures.[101] If an individual is receiving chemotherapy, the endodontist should be familiar with the patient's white blood count (WBC) count and platelet status. Endodontic procedures can be performed if the neutrophil count is greater than 2000 cells per cubic millimeter and platelets are greater than 50,000 cells per cubic millimeter. Postradiation osteonecrosis (PRON) results from radiation-induced changes in the jaws, may arise in bones exposed to high-dose radiation, and is characterized by asymptomatic or painful bone exposure. Protocols to reduce the risk of osteonecrosis include selection of endodontic therapy over extraction, expert atraumatic surgical procedures, considering the use of nonlidocaine local anesthetics that contain no or low concentration of epinephrine, and prophylactic antibiotics plus antibiotics during the week of healing.[102]

BISPHOSPHONATE-ASSOCIATED OSTEONECROSIS OF THE JAWS

Bisphosphonates are bone resorption inhibitor medications that are commonly used in conjunction with cancer chemotherapy and the prevention or treatment of osteoporosis. Recent reports have suggested that bisphosphonates (e.g., pamidronate, zoledronic acid) may cause osteonecrosis of the maxillary and mandibular bones, either spontaneously or following dental surgical procedures or oral trauma.[103–107] Although the mechanism of action is unknown, it is suggested that a decrease in bone cellularity and antiangiogenic effects and decreased blood flow resulting from bisphosphonate therapy could lead to a generalized impairment in bone remodeling.[105] There appears to be a dose–response relationship in that patients taking IV formulations appear to be at greater risk for bisphosphonate-associated osteonecrosis (BON).[108] There are currently no scientific data to support any specific treatment protocol for the management of patients with BON, though minimally invasive procedures have been recommended.[106] Before initiation of bisphosphonate therapy, aggressive preventive treatment should be performed including oral hygiene, caries control, and extraction of teeth with a poor long-term prognosis. For patients who have been taking bisphosphonate medication, preventive care for high-risk patients is important to reduce the risk of developing BON. Nonsurgical endodontic treatment of teeth that would otherwise be extracted should be considered. Teeth with extensive carious lesions might be treated by nonsurgical endodontic therapy possibly followed by crown resection and restoration similar to preparing an overdenture abutment.[109] For patients at higher risk of developing BON, surgical procedures including surgical endodontic procedures should be avoided if possible. Informed consent for endodontic procedures should involve a discussion of risks, benefits, and alternative treatments with the patient.

Bone Marrow and Solid Organ Transplantation

HEMATOPOIETIC STEM CELL TRANSPLANTATION

HSCT may be indicated in patients with hematological malignancy, nonhematological malignancy, and some nonmalignant disorders. Patients may undergo an autologous (self) or an allogeneic (nonself) transplantation, each of which has its own pros and cons. The goal is to treat bone marrow disease or to intensify therapy that would destroy the bone marrow, following which the patient is "rescued" by the infusion of previously stored autologous hematopoietic stem cells or hematopoietic stem cells from a matched donor. Prior to transplantation, patients should undergo a thorough dental examination and treatment to permit adequate healing before the HSCT. Pretreatment endodontic therapy should be completed at least 10 days prior to initiation of cancer therapy. Teeth with poor prognoses should be extracted, utilizing the 10-day window as a guide. The current AHA protocol for antibiotic prophylaxis prior to invasive oral procedures may be warranted in patients who have indwelling catheters (e.g., Hickman catheter). Prophylactic antibiotics are also recommended in patients who are neutropenic (<1,000 neutrophils per cubic millimeter).

During and following high-dose chemotherapy/HSCT, aggressive oral hygiene measures should be instituted. Numerous oral complications may develop, including mucositis, graft-versus-host disease, infection, taste changes, and bleeding. Patients should not resume routine dental treatment, including dental scaling and polishing, until adequate immunological reconstitution has taken place; this typically occurs no less than 1 year posttransplant. The aerosolization of debris and bacteria during the use of high-speed rotary cutting instruments can put the patient at risk for aspiration pneumonia; additionally, bacteremias occur as a result of dental treatment and can cause serious outcomes. Should treatment be deemed necessary within 1 year posttransplant, the endodontist must consult with the oncologist to determine appropriate treatment.

SOLID ORGAN TRANSPLANTATION

It is important to reduce the risk of infection in the immunosuppressed recipient of a transplant.[110] Pretransplant patients should undergo eradication of dental disease, including endodontic procedures as warranted to remove any potential sources of infection, and deferral of any elective treatments. Of course, the endodontist should take into account the underlying condition for which the transplant is required. In the immediate posttransplant period, emergency dental procedures may be necessary. At this stage, patients are highly immunosuppressed to prevent organ rejection, so the AHA regimen of antibiotic prophylaxis with possible postoperative antibiotics may be recommended for invasive procedures. Further, patients may have indwelling catheters that may lead to a recommendation for antibiotic prophylaxis. Should a patient experiences transplant rejection, dental care provided should be limited to emergency care only until stabilization is again achieved. After the posttransplantation patient has stabilized, indicated dental procedures may be performed after consultation with the patient's transplant team. Postoperative guidelines regarding prophylactic antibiotics have not been established but, if recommended, AHA guidelines may be used.[110] Finally, the endodontist should be aware that posttransplant recipients will likely be on immunosuppressant therapy, regardless of the length of time posttransplant.

Prosthetic Joints and Other Prosthetic Devices

Patients with prosthetic joints may be at increased risk for developing a hematogenous joint infection following dental procedures. Since the necessity of prophylactic antibiotics in this group of patients is controversial, consultation with the patient's orthopedic surgeon is advised. Current recommendations include antibiotic coverage with higher risk dental procedures (see Figure 8) within 2 years following prosthetic joint surgery, for those who have had previous hematogenous prosthetic joint infections and for those with some medical conditions (Figure 11).[111]

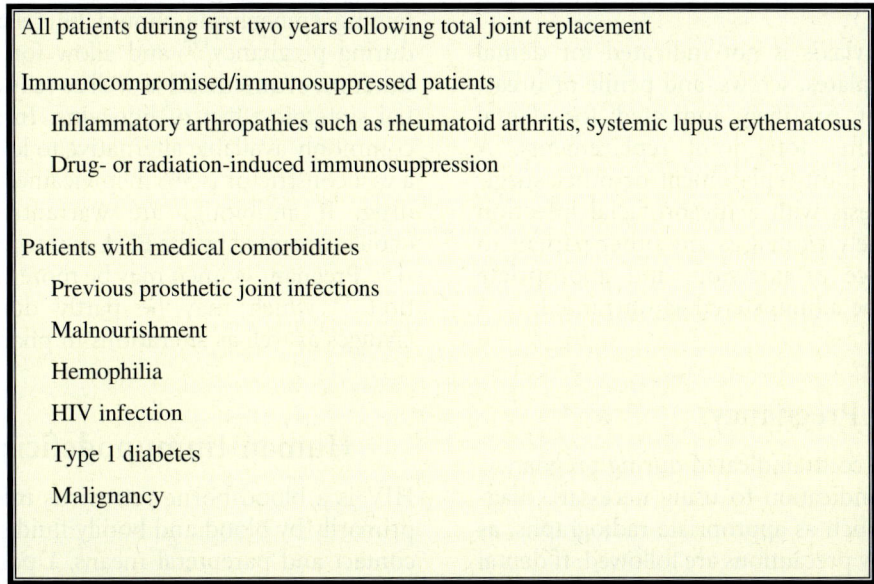

Figure 11 Patients at potential increased risk of experiencing hematogenous total joint infection. Adapted from ADA, AAOS Advisory statement.[111]

Patient Type	Suggested Drug	Regimen
Patients not allergic to penicillin	Cephalexin, cephradine or amoxicillin	2 grams orally 1 hour prior to dental procedure
Patients not allergic to penicillin and unable to take oral medications	Cefazolin or ampicillin	Cefazolin 1g or ampicillin 2g intramuscularly or intravenously 1 hour prior to the dental procedure
Patients allergic to penicillin	Clindamycin	Clindamycin 600 mg orally 1 hour prior to the dental procedure
Patients allergic to penicillin and unable to take oral medications	Clindamycin	600mg intravenously 1 hour prior to the dental procedure

Figure 12 Suggested antibiotic prophylaxis regimens for patients with total joint replacement. Adapted from ADA, AAOS Advisory statement.[111]

The selection of antibiotic and dosage regimen differs slightly from the commonly accepted regimen for prevention of bacterial endocarditis since different microorganisms are more commonly associated with late joint infections (Figure 12). These guidelines suggest prophylaxis for recently placed large joint prostheses even though there is little evidence that oral flora account for many infections in joint prostheses. These guidelines will be continually reviewed and current guidelines must be followed for medicolegal purpose.

Antibiotic prophylaxis is not indicated for dental patients with pins, plates, screws, and penile or breast implants, nor is it routinely indicated for dental patients 2 years after total joint replacements. A patient with a total joint replacement or other surgically placed prosthesis with acute orofacial infection should be aggressively treated as any other patient to eliminate the source of infection, and appropriate antibiotics should be administered as warranted.

Pregnancy

Few procedures are contraindicated during pregnancy. There is no contraindication to using necessary diagnostic procedures, such as appropriate radiographs, as long as normal safety precautions are followed. If dental caries is the source of pain or infection, invasive care such as endodontic therapy should be provided regardless of the patient's phase of pregnancy.[112] Elective dental procedures may often be performed in the second trimester, when the pregnancy is mostly devoted to maturation. While some medications may be harmful to the fetus, safe alternatives are often available. Lidocaine and prilocaine local anesthetics have an FDA category B rating and consequently should be first-line choices for use with pregnant women. A common misconception is concern over the use of local anesthetics containing epinephrine. Local anesthetics containing epinephrine should be relatively safe for use during pregnancy[113] and allow for greater depth and duration of anesthesia as well as reduction of any potential systemic effect of lidocaine. In addition, the only commonly available alternative to local anesthetics with a vasoconstrictor is 3% mepivicaine, an FDA category C drug. If antibiotics are warranted, many first-line choices are rated by the FDA as category B for pregnancy risk. Pregnant women may be more susceptible to infection,[114] which may be partly due to physiological changes as well as alterations in pharmacokinetics.

Human Immunodeficiency Virus

HIV is a blood-borne retrovirus infection transmitted primarily by blood and bodily fluids by intimate sexual contact and parenteral means. Upon infection, a viral enzyme reverse transcriptase allows the virus to integrate its own DNA into the genome of an infected cell and replicate using the infected cell's ribosomes and protein synthesis. Initially, immune seroconversion with antiviral antibody production occurs followed by a significant decrease in $CD4^+$ lymphocytes over a period of up to years. The most effective management in the progression of HIV infection and AIDS is a combination of antiviral agents known as highly active antiretroviral therapies (HAART), which has significantly increased the lifespan and the quality of life of individuals infected with HIV. Upon initial assessment of an HIV-infected individual, the patient's physician should be contacted to determine $CD4^+$ counts as well as baseline kidney and liver function. It is safe and desirable to assure that comprehensive dental care is available to HIV-positive patients. No modification of irreversible procedures or surgical treatment is recommended unless patients have reduced platelet count (<50,000 cells per microliter) or neutrophil counts <1,000 cells per mm^3, at which time a patient may require antibiotic prophylaxis. Routine antibiotic use is contraindicated. The prognosis for successful healing of necrotic teeth with chronic apical periodontitis following root canal treatment is essentially the same for HIV-positive patients as for noninfected patients.[115,116] The endodontist should examine oral tissues, as oral conditions associated with HIV may identify a person who is unknowingly infected with HIV, may be used in staging and classification, and/or may denote progression to AIDS. Surgically treated teeth do not show delayed healing. Antibiotics are used only if warranted by the clinical infection, and in a neutropenic patient.

Sickle Cell Anemia

Sickle cell anemia (SCA) affects approximately 1 in 400 African-Americans and as much as 30% of the population of some Central and West African countries. Clinical concerns in endodontic practice include the propensity for painful vasoocclusive episodes and bacterial infections.[117] Since patients with SCA may be considered immunocompromised and infections can trigger a sickle cell crisis, these patients usually require aggressive treatment of infections, including the use of systemic antibiotics.[117] The vasoocclusive aspects of the disease can result in tissue and bone necrosis and pulpal necrosis in an otherwise intact and healthy tooth.[118] Since teeth with asymptomatic necrotic pulps can become infected, patients with SCA require careful pulpal evaluation. Nonsurgical root canal treatment of asymptomatic necrotic teeth prior to the development of acute symptoms and infection is indicated. There is a lack of consensus regarding the value of prophylactic antibiotics for patients with SCA, although the majority of pediatric dentistry program directors and pediatric hematologists recommend antibiotic coverage for invasive procedures such as extraction or other surgical procedures.[119] The use of a local anesthetic with no vasoconstrictor (or minimal vasoconstrictor) may be advisable for nonsurgical procedures since the microvasculature is often already compromised by SCA. Osteomyelitis is much more common in patients with SCA[117] and the risk/benefit ratio for surgical endodontic procedures should be carefully considered for patients with SCA.

Liver Disease

End-stage chronic liver disease (cirrhosis) is the result of hepatocellular injury and necrosis that leads to fibrosis and nodular regeneration. Cirrhosis may be asymptomatic for long periods of time and may be undiagnosed until systemic signs are apparent. Ultimately, chronic liver disease affects multiple body systems. For more information on the preliver transplant patient, please see section "Solid organ transplantation" earlier in this chapter.

Performing any surgery in the preliver transplant patient involves the risk of severe hemorrhage due to thrombocytopenia or reduced hepatic synthesis of coagulation factors. Preoperative evaluation should include a complete blood count with platelet count, PT or INR, and partial thromboplastin time to ensure an intact coagulation system. Patients with cirrhosis have an increased susceptibility to infection. Odontogenic infections should be treated aggressively with appropriate antibiotic treatment. Antibiotic prophylaxis prior to dental procedures is recommended only if the patient has a history of spontaneous bacterial peritonitis (SBP), ascites (accumulation of excess fluid in the abdomen), another medical indication for antibiotic prophylaxis, or whose medical condition would drastically deteriorate should SBP develop. When antibiotic prophylaxis is indicated in the patient with end-stage liver disease, a recommended oral regimen is 2.0 g of amoxicillin plus 500 mg of metronidazole 1 hour before the dental procedure, or patients may be given 2.0 g of ampicillin plus 500 mg of metronidazole intravenously 1 hour before the procedure.[120] Finally, the pharmacokinetics of drugs commonly used in dentistry can be altered in patients with end-stage liver disease. Alteration of medication dosage based upon hepatic compromise, additional medications, and site of metabolism of the medication may require consultation with the patient's physician.

Adrenal Suppression and Long-Term Steroid Use

The adrenal cortex produces mineralocorticoids, such as aldosterone, and glucocorticoids, such as cortisol, which are important in maintaining fluid volume. Adrenocortical insufficiency may result primarily from Addison's disease, an autoimmune condition, or secondarily from hypothalamic or pituitary disease or from the administration of exogenous corticosteroids (30 mg per day or more of cortisol equivalent [about 5 mg prednisone]). Supplemental steroids are often recommended before and possibly following surgery to prevent adrenal crisis in patients who receive chronic daily steroid therapy.[121] In these patients, for minor surgical procedures such as routine endodontic surgeries, the glucocorticoid target is about 25 mg of hydrocortisone equivalent (5 mg of prednisone) on the day of surgery. If a moderate risk surgery is to be performed, the glucocorticoid target is about 50 to 75 mg per day of hydrocortisone equivalent on the day of surgery and for one postoperative day. Nonsurgical dental procedures, including nonsurgical root canal treatment, generally require no supplementation; however, this should be reviewed on a case-by-case basis and consideration given to the anticipated procedural stress and patient tolerance for dental treatment.[121] As a rule of thumb, a patient who recently discontinued the use of exogenous corticosteroids should wait 2 weeks before undergoing surgical procedures. Patients on alternate day steroids do not likely require steroid supplementation. Efforts to control pain and infection can decrease the risk of an adrenal crisis.

Allergy to Materials Used in Endodontic Therapy

The prevalence of allergies and allergy-related diseases has increased significantly in recent years.[122] Approximately 15 to 20% of dental patients report some form of allergy on their medical history questionnaire and approximately 5% report allergy to one or more drugs.[123] In fact, allergy is the single most common positive finding on the medical history questionnaire.[2] Fortunately, with the exceptions of latex and certain antibiotics, the majority of reported allergies are to substances not typically used in dental treatment. Even so, many materials used in root canal therapy have the potential for eliciting an allergic reaction. The medical history questionnaire serves as the first stage in screening for allergies but should always be supplemented with direct patient questioning about the history of allergic reactions to any drugs or substances. True allergic reactions are characterized by one or more of the following signs and symptoms: skin rash, swelling, urticaria, chest tightness, shortness of breath, rhinorrhea, and conjunctivitis.[123]

Type I (immediate or anaphylactic, IgE-mediated) and Type IV (delayed, cell-mediated) are the two types of allergic reactions most likely to be encountered as a result of exposure to a substance used in endodontic treatment. Type I hypersensitivity requires previous exposure to the antigen and can occur after a single prior exposure or multiple prior exposures to the allergen. The reaction occurs shortly after exposure and can rapidly progress to life-threatening anaphylaxis. Type IV hypersensitivity typically appears 48 to 72 hours after exposure and is mediated by T lymphocytes in contrast to the humoral immune system (antibody)-mediated Type I reaction. Contact dermatitis is a classic Type IV reaction. When materials used in endodontic treatment come in contact with the periapical tissues (either intentionally or inadvertently), there is the potential for a delayed Type IV hypersensitivity reaction. The allergic potential of various materials commonly used in endodontic treatment is summarized in Figure 13.

LOCAL ANESTHETICS

True Type I allergy to an amide local anesthetic is extremely rare. Nevertheless, patients reporting a history of allergic reaction to a local anesthetic require thorough evaluation prior to proceeding with treatment (assuming that a local anesthetic is needed for root canal treatment) since true allergic reactions have been reported.[124–133] Perhaps the most common response elicited upon exploration of the presumed allergic reaction is a report of tachycardia, syncope or general uneasiness following local anesthetic injection. Such a response almost certainly represents a psychogenic reaction rather than true allergy.[132,134] Careful aspiration during injection can help prevent an inadvertent intravascular injection and subsequent increased toxicity and potential for adverse reaction.

In a recent prospective study of 5,018 dental patients who received a local anesthetic, 25 (0.5%) adverse reactions were recorded.[124] Twenty-two of the reactions were mild, quickly reversible, and considered to be psychogenic in nature. Only two of the reactions were initially viewed as possible allergic reactions and both of these were excluded as true allergic reactions after provocative challenge tests. In another study of 236 patients who experienced an adverse reaction after injection of local anesthetic, all tested negative following

Category	Material	Allergic potential
Barriers	Natural rubber latex	+
	Vinyl (polyvinyl chloride)	–*
	Nitrile (acrylonitrile and butadiene)	–*
	Polychloroprene (Neoprene)	–*
Irrigating solutions and disinfectants	Sodium hypochlorite (0.5%–6%)	+
	Hydrogen peroxide (3%–30%)	–
	Chlorhexidine (0.2%–2%)	+
	Iodine Potassium iodide (2%–5%)	+
	Ethylenediamine tetraacetic acid (EDTA) (10%–17%)	–
	Citric acid (10%–50%)	–
	MTAD (mixture of tetracycline, citric acid and detergent)	?
Intracanal medications	Phenols	+
	Aldehydes	+
	Calcium hydroxide	–
	Iodine containing pastes	+
Sealers and filling materials	ZnOE materials (various sealers and temporary filling materials)	+
	Epoxy resins	+
	Glass ionomers	–
	Composite resins	?
	Mineral trioxide aggregate (MTA)	–
	Calcium chelate/polyvinyl resin	–
	Gutta percha (trans 1,4-isoprene polymer)	?

* = Type I allergic reactions are generally not seen with use of these synthetic materials; however, chemicals used in processing and powders in gloves may still cause Type IV reactions in sensitive individuals
? = allergic potential is uncertain or unknown but probably low; allergy to one of the components is possible.

Figure 13 Allergic potential of materials commonly used in endodontic treatment. Adapted in part from Hensten A and Jacobsen N,[158] and Zehnder M.[151]

intradermal injection of local anesthetic containing epinephrine and preservative.[135]

Both sulfite preservatives used in local anesthetics containing epinephrine and latex allergen released into the anesthetic solution from the vial stopper are potential causes of allergic reactions. Although reaction to the sulfite preservative is also believed to be rare,[135] allergic reactions to preservatives used in local anesthetics have been reported.[136–138] Since preservatives are used only in local anesthetics containing a vasoconstrictor, the risk of allergic reaction from this potential source can be eliminated by using an anesthetic without vasoconstrictor and preservative (e.g., 3% mepivicaine). Local anesthetic cartridges contain two potential sources of latex allergen that could possibly leach into the anesthetic solution—the rubber stopper and the diaphragm. A recent review of the literature found no case reports or controlled studies demonstrating that the latex present in a dental local anesthetic cartridge could cause an allergic reaction.[139] However, the same review found several case reports of allergic reactions attributed to trace amounts of latex found in other medication vial stoppers and intravenous tubing. Even though there is no strong evidence to support the avoidance of local anesthetic cartridges in patients with a known latex allergy, experts in the area have recommended using local anesthetic from glass-enclosed vials to avoid any potential risk of exposure to latex allergens.[140,141] If it can be determined that the local anesthetic cartridge contains non-latex materials for the diaphragm and stopper, then there is no need for concern.

It should also be noted that a documented allergy to one type of amide local anesthetic does not necessarily imply allergy to all amide local anesthetics and often a readily available alternative can be found after testing.[128,132] As a practical matter, patients referred for allergy testing should be given sample cartridges of at least two different local anesthetics so that the allergist can test with the same solution that will be used for dental treatment. Options for patients with a documented allergy to all commonly used local anesthetics include sedation, general anesthesia, electronic anesthesia,[132,142] and injectable diphenhydramine. A solution of 1% diphenhydramine with 1:100,000 epinephine can be compounded by a local pharmacist and used for infiltration or mandibular block injections. The dosage should be limited to a maximum of 50 mg at each appointment.[123]

LATEX

Of the many materials used in the dental office with the potential for initiating an allergic reaction, natural rubber latex (NRL) is the most common.[143] Reports of allergic reactions to NRL began in 1987 coincident with the widespread adoption of universal precautions, including the use of latex gloves for practically all medical and dental procedures.[144,145] Type IV sensitivity is the most common type and is related to the various chemicals used in processing NRL. The potentially much more serious Type I sensitivity to NRL is a reaction to proteins found in NRL. Approximately 6% of the general population is believed to have Type I sensitivity to NRL and this number increases to as much as 17% for health care workers.[146] Urticaria is the most common initial finding in Type I sensitivity reaction to NRL.[144] Patients with a history of multiple surgeries (especially spina bifida) or atopy (multiple allergies) and health care workers all have an increased risk of sensitivity to NRL. Some food allergies (e.g., avocado and banana) are associated with an increased risk of latex allergy. Considering the multiple potential sources of exposure to NRL in the dental office (e.g., rubber dam material, gloves, local anesthetic cartridges, rubber mouth props, rubber tubing, and even some blood pressure cuffs), history of allergy to NRL requires special treatment modifications. In addition, clinicians who treat patients with known or suspected sensitivity to NRL should be prepared to provide initial management of an acute allergic reaction if necessary.

Consultation with the patient's primary care physician or allergist is advised to help assess the degree of risk, previous reactions and treatment, and possible premedication with a corticosteroid. All potential sources of NRL exposure in the dental office should be considered. Non-latex gloves and rubber dam materials are now readily available from commercial sources, and these items may be easily substituted for NRL-containing products. Since latex allergens can be transferred by contact with powder from latex gloves and other sources, it may be prudent to schedule the patient as the first of the day to decrease the chance of contact with residual latex allergens on environmental surfaces, clothing, and room air.[147] The potential for cross-reaction with gutta-percha in NRL-sensitive patients has not been demonstrated although caution should be exercised to avoid extrusion of any filling material beyond the confines of the root canal space (for more on this subject, please refer to section "Intracanal medications, cements, and filling materials"). Also, as previously discussed, the potential for reaction to latex allergens present in the local anesthetic cartridge stopper or diaphragm should be considered.

ANTIBIOTICS AND ANALGESICS

Allergy to penicillin is one of the most common drug allergies and affects approximately 2.5 million people in the United States.[123] Although many reported allergic reactions cannot be confirmed unless the patient is willing to undergo testing to rule out allergy to penicillin, it is safest to assume the allergy is real and select an alternative antibiotic. In the case of allergy to penicillin, it should be presumed that the patient is also allergic to the synthetic penicillins. In addition, cephalosporins show cross-reactivity in approximately 5% to 10% of penicillin allergic patients.[123] Clindamycin is an appropriate alternative to penicillin for treatment of endodontic infections and bacterial endocarditis prophylaxis.[54,148] Clarithromycin is another medication that can be considered. More information about antibiotic selection and dosage is found in Chapter 21, "Treatment of Endodontic Infections, Cysts, and Flare-Ups."

NSAIDs are the usual drugs of first choice for management of endodontic-related pain and are tolerated well by most patients. However, caution should be used in prescribing NSAIDs in patients with asthma and/or known allergy or sensitivity to aspirin. Reports of allergy to codeine are most commonly related to gastrointestinal side effects rather than true allergy, although allergy to opioid analgesics does occur. If the patient's history suggests an adverse reaction related to gastrointestinal distress (including nausea, emesis, or constipation), an alternative synthetic narcotic or a combination pain medicine may be considered. Analgesics are discussed in more detail in Chapter 22, "Management of Endodontic Pain."

IRRIGATING SOLUTIONS

Sodium hypochlorite, in concentrations varying from 0.5% to 6%, is currently the most commonly used canal disinfectant and irrigating solution in endodontics.[149–151] Sodium hypochlorite not only possesses excellent tissue solvent and antimicrobial properties but also demonstrates concentration-related tissue toxicity. Although an allergic reaction and/or hypersensitivity to sodium hypochlorite when used as an endodontic irrigating solution is rare, several cases have been reported.[150,152,153] It has been suggested that some patients may be sensitized by exposure to household bleaching products.[150] Alternatives to sodium hypochlorite include sterile saline or water, chlorhexidine (0.2% to 2%), iodine potassium iodide (2% to 5%), hydrogen peroxide (3%), ethylenediamine tetraacetic acid (EDTA, 10% to 17%), citric acid (10%), and a recently introduced material, MTAD.[151,154–157] Of these alternatives, iodine potassium iodide and chlorhexidine possess the potential for stimulating an allergic reaction. A recent review article provides an excellent overview of the relative advantages and disadvantages of these selected irrigating solutions.[151]

INTRACANAL MEDICATIONS, CEMENTS, AND FILLING MATERIALS

Intracanal medications such as formocresol, formaldehyde, eugenol, camphorated phenols, and cresatin are all known to be potential allergens.[158,159] Fortunately, these canal medications are not frequently used in current endodontic therapy. Calcium hydroxide paste, a commonly used intra-appointment medication, is not allergenic. Temporary filling materials containing zinc oxide and eugenol (ZnOE) have the potential for allergic reactions and, unlike materials contained exclusively within the confines of the root canal space, are likely to have contact with mucosal tissues.[160]

Zinc oxide and eugenol, a potential allergen, is a common component of many root canal sealers and two common root-end filling materials (IRM and Super EBA). Sealers containing formaldehyde or paraformaldehyde (such as N2 paste and Endometazone), especially when extruded beyond the apex, have been demonstrated to stimulate often severe allergic reactions.[161–164] Resin-based sealers such as AH26 and AHPlus also have the potential to stimulate an allergic response,[158] although this is believed to be rare. Calcium hydroxide-based sealers such as Sealapex or glass ionomer sealers such as Ketac-Endo could be reasonable alternatives for patients with known allergy to any of the components of ZnOE or resin-based sealers. As always, one should carefully read the list of ingredients since at least one sealer marketed as a calcium hydroxide-based sealer contains a significant ZnOE component.

Dentin-bonded resin-type root-end filling materials have demonstrated excellent biocompatibility in long-term clinical studies with no evidence of allergic reactions in treatment failures.[165–167] However, the choice of resin filling material is important since some resins are known to release formaldehyde when setting. Mineral trioxide aggregate (MTA), a relatively new material used for root-end fillings, apexification, perforation repair, and pulp capping, has demonstrated excellent biocompatibility and no suspected allergic potential.[168–170]

Although there have been case reports of suspected allergic reactions to gutta-percha in patients who were allergic to NRL,[171,172] the possibility that the reactions were due to another material used in root canal treatment could not be ruled out. In fact, cross-reactivity between commercially available gutta-percha and NRL has not been demonstrated.[173,174] In addition, gutta-percha is normally well contained within the confines of the root canal space and therefore should not have the potential to elicit an immune response. Gutta-percha manufactured for root canal treatment contains other ingredients such as barium sulfate, zinc oxide, waxes, and coloring agents; so potential allergy to any of these materials should be considered, especially if there is a potential for extrusion of filling material. Newer non-gutta-percha filling materials (e.g., Resilon) show promise but could be expected to contain many of the same added ingredients as commercially available gutta-percha. In patients with multiple allergies (atopy) and suspected allergy to any of the components of gutta-percha, consultation with the patient's physician is advised. If safe use of the standard obturating material cannot be confirmed, one alternative is to fill the root canal space with MTA. This technique presents some technical challenges, especially in smaller canals, but should be manageable by an experienced clinician. MTA has a relatively long setting time (about 4 hours) but once final hardening has occurred, removal of the filling material through an orthograde approach is extremely difficult and is possible only in large, straight canals.

References

1. Peacock ME, Carson RE. Frequency of self-reported medical conditions in periodontal patients. J Periodontol 1995;66(11):1004–7.
2. Smeets EC, de Jong KJ, Abraham-Inpijn L. Detecting the medically compromised patient in dentistry by means of the medical risk-related history. A survey of 29,424 dental patients in The Netherlands. Prev Med 1998;27(4):530–5.
3. Kaufman DW, Kelly JP, Rosenberg L, et al. Recent patterns of medication use in the ambulatory adult population of the United States: the Slone survey. J Am Med Assoc 2002;287(3):337–44.
4. Dietz GC Sr, Dietz GC Jr. The endodontist and the general dentist. Dent Clin North Am 1992;36(2):459–71.
5. American Association of Endodontists. AAE endodontic case difficulty assessment form and guidelines. Chicago, IL: American Association of Endodontists; 2005.
6. Chandler-Gutierrez L, Martinez-Sahuquillo A, Bullon-Fernandez P. Evaluation of medical risk in dental practice through using the EMRRH questionnaire. Med Oral 2004;9(4):309–20.
7. Fenlon MR, McCartan BE. Medical status of patients attending a primary care dental practice in Ireland. J Ir Dent Assoc 1991;37(3–4):75–7.
8. Drinnan AJ. Medical conditions of importance in dental practice. Int Dent J 1990;40(4):206–10.
9. Jainkittivong A, Yeh CK, Guest GF, Cottone JA. Evaluation of medical consultations in a predoctoral dental clinic. Oral Surg Oral Med Oral Pathol Oral Radiol Endod 1995;80(4):409–13.
10. Absi EG, Satterthwaite J, Shepherd JP, Thomas DW. The appropriateness of referral of medically compromised dental patients to hospital. Br J Oral Maxillofac Surg 1997;35(2):133–6.
11. Chapman PJ. Medical emergencies in dental practice and choice of emergency drugs and equipment: a survey of Australian dentists. Aust Dent J 1997;42(2):103–8.
12. de Jong KJ, Abraham-Inpijn L, Vinckier F, Declerck D. The validity of a medical risk-related history for dental patients in Belgium. Int Dent J 1997;47(1):16–20.
13. Fenlon MR, McCartan BE. Validity of a patient self-completed health questionnaire in a primary care dental practice. Community Dent Oral Epidemiol 1992;20 (3):130–2.
14. McDaniel TF, Miller D, Jones R, Davis M. Assessing patient willingness to reveal health history information. J Am Dent Assoc 1995;126(3):375–9.
15. Lapointe HJ, Armstrong JE, Larocque B. A clinical decision making framework for the medically compromised patient: ischemic heart disease and chronic obstructive pulmonary disease. J Can Dent Assoc 1997;63(7):510–12, 515–16.
16. Norred CL, Brinker F. Potential coagulation effects of preoperative complementary and alternative medicines. Altern Ther Health Med 2001;7(6):58–67.
17. Norred CL. Complementary and alternative medicine use by surgical patients. AORN J 2002;76(6):1013–21.
18. Chang LK, Whitaker DC. The impact of herbal medicines on dermatologic surgery. Dermatol Surg 2001;27(8):759–63.
19. Beck FM, Weaver JM II. Blood pressure and heart rate responses to anticipated high-stress dental treatment. J Dent Res 1981;60(1):26–9.
20. Palmer-Bouva C, Oosting J, deVries R, Abraham-Inpijn L. Stress in elective dental treatment: epinephrine, norepinephrine, the VAS, and CDAS in four different procedures. Gen Dent 1998;46(4):356–60.
21. Brand HS, Gortzak RA, Abraham-Inpijn L. Anxiety and heart rate correlation prior to dental checkup. Int Dent J 1995;45(6):347–51.
22. Brand HS. Cardiovascular responses in patients and dentists during dental treatment. Int Dent J 1999;49(1):60–6.
23. Miller CS, Dembo JB, Falace DA, Kaplan AL. Salivary cortisol response to dental treatment of varying stress. Oral Surg Oral Med Oral Pathol Oral Radiol Endod 1995;79(4):436–41.
24. Brand HS. Anxiety and cortisol excretion correlate prior to dental treatment. Int Dent J 1999;49(6):330–6.
25. Owens WD, Felts JA, Spitznagel EL Jr. ASA physical status classifications: a study of consistency of ratings. Anesthesiology 1978;49(4):239–43.
26. Haynes SR, Lawler PG. An assessment of the consistency of ASA physical status classification allocation. Anaesthesia 1995;50(3):195–9.
27. Goodchild J, Glick M. A different approach to medical risk assessment. Endod Top 2003;4:1–8.
28. de Jong KJ, Oosting J, Abraham-Inpijn L. Medical risk classification of dental patients in The Netherlands. J Public Health Dent 1993;53(4):219–22.
29. de Jong KJ, Borgmeijer-Hoelen A, Abraham-Inpijn L. Validity of a risk-related patient-administered medical questionnaire for dental patients. Oral Surg Oral Med Oral Pathol Oral Radiol Endod 1991;72(5):527–33.

30. Little JW, Falace DA, Miller CS, Rhodus NL. Dental management of the medically compromised patient. 6th ed. St. Louis, MO: Mosby; 2002.
31. Feck AS, Goodchild JH. The use of anxiolytic medications to supplement local anesthesia in the anxious patient. Compend Contin Educ Dent 2005;26(3):183–6, 188, 190; quiz 191, 209.
32. Bader JD, Bonito AJ, Shugars DA. Cardiovascular effects of epinephrine on hypertensive dental patients. Evidence Report/Technology Assessment Number 48. Rockville, MD: Agency for Healthcare Research and Quality; 2002 July. AHRQ Publication No. 02-E006.
33. Little JW. The impact on dentistry of recent advances in the management of hypertension. Oral Surg Oral Med Oral Pathol Oral Radiol Endod 2000;90(5):591–9.
34. Glick M. The new blood pressure guidelines: a digest. J Am Dent Assoc 2004;135(5):585–6.
35. Muzyka BC, Glick M. The hypertensive dental patient. J Am Dent Assoc 1997;128(8):1109–20.
36. Herman WW, Konzelman JL Jr, Prisant LM. New national guidelines on hypertension: a summary for dentistry. J Am Dent Assoc 2004;135(5):576–84; quiz 653–4.
37. Walton RE, Torabinejad M. Principles and practice of endodontics. 2nd ed. Philadelphia, PA: W.B. Saunders Company; 1996.
38. Johnson BR, Witherspoon DE. Periradicular surgery. In: Cohen S, Hargreaves KM, Keiser K, editors. Pathways of the pulp. 9th ed. St. Louis, MO: Mosby; 2006. pp. 724–85.
39. Perusse R, Goulet JP, Turcotte JY. Contraindications to vasoconstrictors in dentistry: Part I. Cardiovascular diseases. Oral Surg Oral Med Oral Pathol Oral Radiol Endod 1992;74(5):679–86.
40. Bader JD, Bonito AJ, Shugars DA. A systematic review of cardiovascular effects of epinephrine on hypertensive dental patients. Oral Surg Oral Med Oral Pathol Oral Radiol Endod 2002;93(6):647–53.
41. Yagiela JA. Injectable and topical local anesthetics. In: Ciancio SG, editor. ADA guide to dental therapeutics. 3rd ed. Chicago, IL: American Dental Association; 2003. pp. 1–16.
42. Replogle K, Reader A, Nist R, et al. Cardiovascular effects of intraosseous injections of 2 percent lidocaine with 1:100,000 epinephrine and 3 percent mepivacaine [see comments]. J Am Dent Assoc 1999;130(5):649–57.
43. Kim S, Rethnam S. Hemostasis in endodontic microsurgery. Dent Clin North Am 1997;41(3):499–511.
44. Vickers FJ, Baumgartner JC, Marshall G. Hemostatic efficacy and cardiovascular effects of agents used during endodontic surgery. J Endod 2002;28(4):322–3.
45. Vy CH, Baumgartner JC, Marshall JG. Cardiovascular effects and efficacy of a hemostatic agent in periradicular surgery. J Endod 2004;30(6):379–83.
46. Jowett NI, Cabot LB. Patients with cardiac disease: considerations for the dental practitioner. Br Dent J 2000;189(6):297–302.
47. Eagle KA, Brundage BH, Chaitman BR, et al. Guidelines for perioperative cardiovascular evaluation for noncardiac surgery. Report of the American College of Cardiology/American Heart Association Task Force on Practice Guidelines (Committee on Perioperative Cardiovascular Evaluation for Noncardiac Surgery). J Am Coll Cardiol 1996;27(4):910–48.
48. Cintron G, Medina R, Reyes AA, Lyman G. Cardiovascular effects and safety of dental anesthesia and dental interventions in patients with recent uncomplicated myocardial infarction. Arch Intern Med 1986;146(11):2203–4.
49. Eagle KA, Froehlich JB. Reducing cardiovascular risk in patients undergoing noncardiac surgery. N Engl J Med 1996;335(23):1761–3.
50. Niwa H, Sato Y, Matsuura H. Safety of dental treatment in patients with previously diagnosed acute myocardial infarction or unstable angina pectoris. Oral Surg Oral Med Oral Pathol Oral Radiol Endod 2000;89(1):35–41.
51. Lessard E, Glick M, Ahmed S, Saric M. The patient with a heart murmur: evaluation, assessment and dental considerations. J Am Dent Assoc 2005;136(3):347–56; quiz 380–1.
52. Connolly HM, Crary JL, McGoon MD, et al. Valvular heart disease associated with fenfluramine–phentermine. N Engl J Med 1997;337(9):581–8.
53. Wilson W, Taubert KA, Gewitz M, et al. Prevention of infective endocarditis: guidelines from the American Heart Association Rheumatic Fever, Endocarditis and Kawasaki Disease Committee, Council on Cardiovascular Disease in the Young, and the Council on Clinical Cardiology, Council on Cardiovascular Surgery and Anesthesia, and the Quality of Care and Outcomes Research Interdisciplinary Working Group. J Am Dent Assoc 2007;138(6):739–45, 747–60.
54. Dajani AS, Taubert KA, Wilson W, et al. Prevention of bacterial endocarditis: recommendations by the American Heart Association. J Am Dent Assoc 1997;128(8):1142–51.
55. Heimdahl A, Hall G, Hedberg M, et al. Detection and quantitation by lysis-filtration of bacteremia after different oral surgical procedures. J Clin Microbiol 1990;28(10):2205–9.
56. Bender IB, Naidorf IJ, Garvey GJ. Bacterial endocarditis: a consideration for physician and dentist. J Am Dent Assoc 1984;109(3):415–20.
57. Strom BL, Abrutyn E, Berlin JA, et al. Dental and cardiac risk factors for infective endocarditis. A population-based, case–control study. Ann Intern Med 1998;129(10):761–9.
58. Morris AM, Webb GD. Antibiotics before dental procedures for endocarditis prophylaxis: back to the future. Heart 2001;86(1):3–4.
59. Delahaye F, De Gevigney G. Should we give antibiotic prophylaxis against infective endocarditis in all cardiac patients, whatever the type of dental treatment? Heart 2001;85(1):9–10.

60. Epstein JB. Infective endocarditis and dentistry: outcome-based research. J Can Dent Assoc 1999;65(2):95–6.

61. Pallasch TJ. Antibiotic prophylaxis. Endod Top 2003;4:46–59.

62. Scully C, Wolff A. Oral surgery in patients on anticoagulant therapy. Oral Surg Oral Med Oral Pathol Oral Radiol Endod 2002;94(1):57–64.

63. Cannon PD, Dharmar VT. Minor oral surgical procedures in patients on oral anticoagulants—a controlled study. Aust Dent J 2003;48(2):115–18.

64. Jafri SM. Periprocedural thromboprophylaxis in patients receiving chronic anticoagulation therapy. Am Heart J 2004;147(1):3–15.

65. Russo G, Corso LD, Biasiolo A, et al. Simple and safe method to prepare patients with prosthetic heart valves for surgical dental procedures. Clin Appl Thromb Hemost 2000;6(2):90–3.

66. Campbell JH, Alvarado F, Murray RA. Anticoagulation and minor oral surgery: should the anticoagulation regimen be altered? J Oral Maxillofac Surg 2000;58(2):131–5; discussion 135–6.

67. Wahl MJ. Dental surgery in anticoagulated patients. Arch Intern Med 1998;158(15):1610–16.

68. Jeske AH, Suchko GD. Lack of a scientific basis for routine discontinuation of oral anticoagulation therapy before dental treatment. J Am Dent Assoc 2003;134(11):1492–7.

69. Ardekian L, Gaspar R, Peled M, et al. Does low-dose aspirin therapy complicate oral surgical procedures? J Am Dent Assoc 2000;131(3):331–5.

70. Gomez-Moreno G, Cutando-Soriano A, Arana C, Scully C. Hereditary blood coagulation disorders: management and dental treatment. J Dent Res 2005;84(11):978–85.

71. Brewer AK, Roebuck EM, Donachie M, et al. The dental management of adult patients with haemophilia and other congenital bleeding disorders. Haemophilia 2003;9(6):673–7.

72. Campbell RL, Langston WG, Ross GA. A comparison of cardiac rate–pressure product and pressure-rate quotient with Holter monitoring in patients with hypertension and cardiovascular disease: a follow-up report. Oral Surg Oral Med Oral Pathol Oral Radiol Endod 1997;84(2):125–8.

73. Blinder D, Shemesh J, Taicher S. Electrocardiographic changes in cardiac patients undergoing dental extractions under local anesthesia. J Oral Maxillofac Surg 1996;54(2):162–5; discussion 165–6.

74. Wilson BL, Broberg C, Baumgartner JC, et al. Safety of electronic apex locators and pulp testers in patients with implanted cardiac pacemakers or cardioverter/defibrillators. J Endod 2006;32(9):847–52.

75. Garofalo RR, Ede EN, Dorn SO, Kuttler S. Effect of electronic apex locators on cardiac pacemaker function. J Endod 2002;28(12):831–3.

76. Beach CW, Bramwell JD, Hutter JW. Use of an electronic apex locator on a cardiac pacemaker patient. J Endod 1996;22(4):182–4.

77. Lalla RV, D'Ambrosio JA. Dental management considerations for the patient with diabetes mellitus. J Am Dent Assoc 2001;132(10):1425–32.

78. American Diabetes Association. www.diabetes.org; 2006; October 26, 2007.

79. Grossi SG. Treatment of periodontal disease and control of diabetes: an assessment of the evidence and need for future research. Ann Periodontol 2001;6(1):138–45.

80. Taylor GW, Burt BA, Becker MP, et al. Non-insulin dependent diabetes mellitus and alveolar bone loss progression over 2 years. J Periodontol 1998;69(1):76–83.

81. McKenna SJ. Dental management of patients with diabetes. Dent Clin North Am 2006;50(4):591–606.

82. Clark R. The hyperglycemic response to different types of surgery and anaesthesia. Br J Anaesth 1970;42:45.

83. Steinbacher DM, Glick M. The dental patient with asthma. An update and oral health considerations. J Am Dent Assoc 2001;132(9):1229–39.

84. Malamed SF. Asthma. In: Medical emergencies in the dental office. 5th ed. St. Louis, MO: Mosby; 2000. pp. 209–23.

85. Kacso G, Terezhalmy GT. Acetylsalicylic acid and acetaminophen. Dent Clin North Am 1994;38(4):633–44.

86. Centers for Disease Control and Prevention. Annual Smoking-Attributable Mortality, Years of Potential Life Lost, and Productivity Losses–United States, 1997–2001. Morb Mortal Weekly Rep 2005;54(25):625–8.

87. Bricker SL, Langlais RP, Miller CS. In: Oral diagnosis, oral medicine, and treatment planning. 2nd ed. Haminton, ON (Canada): BC Decker; 2002. pp. 165–91.

88. Milburn HJ. Primary tuberculosis. Curr Opin Pulm Med 2001;7(3):133–41.

89. Maartens G. Advances in adult pulmonary tuberculosis. Curr Opin Pulm Med 2002;8(3):173–7.

90. Mignogna MD, Muzio LL, Favia G, et al. Oral tuberculosis: a clinical evaluation of 42 cases. Oral Dis 2000;6(1):25–30.

91. Little JW, Falace DA, Miller CS, Rhodus NL. Pulmonary disease. In: Dental management of the medically compromised patient. St. Louis, MO: Mosby; 2002. pp. 125–46.

92. Brodie MJ, French JA. Management of epilepsy in adolescents and adults. Lancet 2000;356(9226):323–9.

93. Acs G, Cozzi E. Antibiotic prophylaxis for patients with hydrocephalus shunts: a survey of pediatric dentistry and neurosurgery program directors. Pediatr Dent 1992;14(4):246–50.

94. Kerr AR. Update on renal disease for the dental practitioner. Oral Surg Oral Med Oral Pathol Oral Radiol Endod 2001;92(1):9–16.

95. Proctor R, Kumar N, Stein A, et al. Oral and dental aspects of chronic renal failure. J Dent Res 2005;84(3):199–208.
96. Manton SL, Midda M. Renal failure and the dental patient: a cautionary tale. Br Dent J 1986;160(11):388–90.
97. Naylor GD, Hall EH, Terezhalmy GT. The patient with chronic renal failure who is undergoing dialysis or renal transplantation: another consideration for antimicrobial prophylaxis. Oral Surg Oral Med Oral Pathol Oral Radiol Endod 1988;65(1):116–21.
98. De Rossi SS, Glick M. Dental considerations for the patient with renal disease receiving hemodialysis. J Am Dent Assoc 1996;127(2):211–19.
99. National Cancer Institute (U.S.). Division of Cancer Control and Rehabilitation; National Institutes of Health (U.S.). Management guidelines for head and neck cancer: U.S. Department of Health, Education and Welfare, Public Health Service, National Institutes of Health (Bethesda, MD), 1979.
100. Cancer facts & figures. Atlanta, GA: American Cancer Society; 2006.
101. Dajani AS, Taubert KA, Wilson W, et al. Prevention of bacterial endocarditis. Recommendations by the American Heart Association. J Am Med Assoc 1997;277(22):1794–801.
102. Maxymiw WG, Wood RE, Liu FF. Postradiation dental extractions without hyperbaric oxygen. Oral Surg Oral Med Oral Pathol Oral Radiol Endod 1991;72(3):270–4.
103. Marx RE. Pamidronate (Aredia) and zoledronate (Zometa) induced avascular necrosis of the jaws: a growing epidemic. J Oral Maxillofac Surg 2003;61(9):1115–17.
104. Migliorati CA. Bisphosphanates and oral cavity avascular bone necrosis. J Clin Oncol 2003;21(22):4253–4.
105. Migliorati CA, Schubert MM, Peterson DE, Seneda LM. Bisphosphonate-associated osteonecrosis of mandibular and maxillary bone: an emerging oral complication of supportive cancer therapy. Cancer 2005;104(1):83–93.
106. Migliorati CA, Casiglia J, Epstein J, et al. Managing the care of patients with bisphosphonate-associated osteonecrosis: an American Academy of Oral Medicine position paper. J Am Dent Assoc 2005;136(12):1658–68.
107. Ruggiero SL, Mehrotra B, Rosenberg TJ, Engroff SL. Osteonecrosis of the jaws associated with the use of bisphosphonates: a review of 63 cases. J Oral Maxillofac Surg 2004;62(5):527–34.
108. Woo SB, Hellstein JW, Kalmar JR. Narrative [corrected] review: bisphosphonates and osteonecrosis of the jaws. Ann Intern Med 2006;144(10):753–61.
109. American Association of Endodontists. Endodontic implications of bisphosphonate associated osteonecrosis of the jaws. AAE Position Paper; 2006.
110. Guggenheimer J, Eghtesad B, Stock DJ. Dental management of the (solid) organ transplant patient. Oral Surg Oral Med Oral Pathol Oral Radiol Endod 2003;95(4):383–9.
111. American Dental Association, American Academy of Orthopaedic Surgeons. Antibiotic prophylaxis for dental patients with total joint replacements. J Am Dent Assoc 2003;134(7):895–9.
112. Livingston HM, Dellinger TM, Holder R. Considerations in the management of the pregnant patient. Spec Care Dentist 1998;18(5):183–8.
113. Little JA, Falace DA, Miller CS, Rhodus N. Pregnancy and breast-feeding. In: Dental management of the medically compromised patient. 6th ed. St. Louis, MO: Mosby; 2002.
114. Silver R, Peltier M, Branch D. The immunology of pregnancy. In: Creasy R, Resnik R, Iams J, editors. Maternal-fetal medicine: principles and practice. Philadelphia, PA: W.B. Saunders; 2004. pp. 89–110.
115. Suchina JA, Levine D, Flaitz CM, et al. Retrospective clinical and radiologic evaluation of nonsurgical endodontic treatment in human immunodeficiency virus (HIV) infection. J Contemp Dent Pract 2006;7(1):1–8.
116. Quesnell BT, Alves M, Hawkinson RW Jr, et al. The effect of human immunodeficiency virus on endodontic treatment outcome. J Endod 2005;31(9):633–6.
117. Kelleher M, Bishop K, Briggs P. Oral complications associated with sickle cell anemia: a review and case report. Oral Surg Oral Med Oral Pathol Oral Radiol Endod 1996;82(2):225–8.
118. Andrews CH, England MC, Jr., Kemp WB. Sickle cell anemia: an etiological factor in pulpal necrosis. J Endod 1983;9(6):249–52.
119. Tate AR, Norris CK, Minniti CP. Antibiotic prophylaxis for children with sickle cell disease: a survey of pediatric dentistry residency program directors and pediatric hematologists. Pediatr Dent 2006;28(4):332–5.
120. Douglas LR, Douglass JB, Sieck JO, Smith PJ. Oral management of the patient with end-stage liver disease and the liver transplant patient. Oral Surg Oral Med Oral Pathol Oral Radiol Endod 1998;86(1):55–64.
121. Miller CS, Little JW, Falace DA. Supplemental corticosteroids for dental patients with adrenal insufficiency: reconsideration of the problem. J Am Dent Assoc 2001;132(11):1570–9; quiz 1596–7.
122. Kay AB. Allergy and allergic diseases. First of two parts. N Engl J Med 2001;344(1):30–7.
123. Little JA, Falace DA, Miller CS, Rhodus NL. Dental management of the medically compromised patient. St. Louis, MO: Mosby; 2002. pp. 314–27.
124. Baluga JC, Casamayou R, Carozzi E, et al. Allergy to local anaesthetics in dentistry. Myth or reality? Allergol Immunopathol (Madr) 2002;30(1):14–19.
125. El-Qutob D, Morales C, Pelaez A. Allergic reaction caused by articaine. Allergol Immunopathol (Madr) 2005;33(2):115–16.
126. Finder RL, Moore PA. Adverse drug reactions to local anesthesia. Dent Clin North Am 2002;46(4):747–57, x.

127. Brown RS, Paluvoi S, Choksi S, et al. Evaluating a dental patient for local anesthesia allergy. Compend Contin Educ Dent 2002;23(2):125–8, 131–2, 134 passim; quiz 140.

128. Malanin K, Kalimo K. Hypersensitivity to the local anesthetic articaine hydrochloride. Anesth Prog 1995;42(3–4):144–5.

129. Bosco DA, Haas DA, Young ER, Harrop KL. An anaphylactoid reaction following local anesthesia: a case report. Anesth Pain Control Dent 1993;2(2):87–93.

130. MacColl S, Young ER. An allergic reaction following injection of local anesthetic: a case report. J Can Dent Assoc 1989;55(12):981–4.

131. Ravindranathan N. Allergic reaction to lignocaine. A case report. Br Dent J 1975;138(3):101–2.

132. Ball IA. Allergic reactions to lignocaine. Br Dent J 1999;186(5):224–6.

133. Seng GF, Kraus K, Cartwright G, et al. Confirmed allergic reactions to amide local anesthetics. Gen Dent 1996;44(1):52–4.

134. Rood JP. Adverse reaction to dental local anaesthetic injection—'allergy' is not the cause. Br Dent J 2000;189(7):380–4.

135. Berkun Y, Ben-Zvi A, Levy Y, et al. Evaluation of adverse reactions to local anesthetics: experience with 236 patients. Ann Allergy Asthma Immunol 2003;91(4):342–5.

136. Campbell JR, Maestrello CL, Campbell RL. Allergic response to metabisulfite in lidocaine anesthetic solution. Anesth Prog 2001;48(1):21–6.

137. Schwartz HJ, Sher TH. Bisulfite sensitivity manifesting as allergy to local dental anesthesia. J Allergy Clin Immunol 1985;75(4):525–7.

138. Seng GF, Gay BJ. Dangers of sulfites in dental local anesthetic solutions: warning and recommendations. J Am Dent Assoc 1986;113(5):769–70.

139. Shojaei AR, Haas DA. Local anesthetic cartridges and latex allergy: a literature review. J Can Dent Assoc 2002;68(10):622–6.

140. Malamed SF. Medical emergencies in the dental office. 5th ed. St. Louis, MO: Mosby; 2000. p. 394.

141. Roy A, Epstein J, Onno E. Latex allergies in dentistry: recognition and recommendations. J Can Dent Assoc 1997;63(4):297–300.

142. Malamed SF, Quinn CL. Electronic dental anesthesia in a patient with suspected allergy to local anesthetics: report of case. J Am Dent Assoc 1988;116(1):53–5.

143. Scully C, Ng Y-L, Gulabivala K. Systemic complications due to endodontic manipulations. Endod Top 2003;4:60–8.

144. Huber MA, Terezhalmy GT. Adverse reactions to latex products: preventive and therapeutic strategies. J Contemp Dent Pract 2006;7(1):97–106.

145. Hamann CP, DePaola LG, Rodgers PA. Occupation-related allergies in dentistry. J Am Dent Assoc 2005;136(4):500–10.

146. Clarke A. The provision of dental care for patients with natural rubber latex allergy: are patients able to obtain safe care? Br Dent J 2004;197(12):749–52; discussion 746.

147. Kosti E, Lambrianidis T. Endodontic treatment in cases of allergic reaction to rubber dam. J Endod 2002;28(11):787–9.

148. Baumgartner JC, Xia T. Antibiotic susceptibility of bacteria associated with endodontic abscesses. J Endod 2003;29(1):44–7.

149. Johnson BR, Remeikis NA. Effective shelf-life of prepared sodium hypochlorite solution. J Endod 1993;19(1):40–3.

150. Kaufman AY, Keila S. Hypersensitivity to sodium hypochlorite. J Endod 1989;15(5):224–6.

151. Zehnder M. Root canal irrigants. J Endod 2006;32 (5):389–98.

152. Caliskan MK, Turkun M, Alper S. Allergy to sodium hypochlorite during root canal therapy: a case report. Int Endod J 1994;27(3):163–7.

153. Dandakis C, Lambrianidis T, Boura P. Immunologic evaluation of dental patient with history of hypersensitivity reaction to sodium hypochlorite. Endod Dent Traumatol 2000;16(4):184–7.

154. Torabinejad M, Khademi AA, Babagoli J, et al. A new solution for the removal of the smear layer. J Endod 2003;29(3):170–5.

155. Shabahang S, Pouresmail M, Torabinejad M. In vitro antimicrobial efficacy of MTAD and sodium hypochlorite. J Endod 2003;29(7):450–2.

156. Beltz RE, Torabinejad M, Pouresmail M. Quantitative analysis of the solubilizing action of MTAD, sodium hypochlorite, and EDTA on bovine pulp and dentin. J Endod 2003;29(5):334–7.

157. Vianna ME, Gomes BP, Berber VB, et al. In vitro evaluation of the antimicrobial activity of chlorhexidine and sodium hypochlorite. Oral Oral Surg Oral Med Oral Pathol Oral Radiol Endod 2004;97(1):79–84.

158. Hensten A, Jacobsen N. Allergic reactions in endodontic practice. Endod Top 2005;12:44–51.

159. Gawkrodger DJ. Investigation of reactions to dental materials. Br J Dermatol 2005;153(3):479–85.

160. Hensten-Pettersen A, Jacobsen N. Perceived side effects of biomaterials in prosthetic dentistry. J Prosthet Dent 1991;65(1):138–44.

161. Forman GH, Ord RA. Allergic endodontic angio-oedema in response to periapical endomethasone. Br Dent J 1986;160(10):348–50.

162. Kunisada M, Adachi A, Asano H, Horikawa T. Anaphylaxis due to formaldehyde released from root-canal disinfectant. Contact Dermititis 2002;47(4):215–18.

163. Haikel Y, Braun JJ, Zana H, et al. Anaphylactic shock during endodontic treatment due to allergy to formaldehyde in a root canal sealant. J Endod 2000;26(9):529–31.

164. Braun JJ, Zana H, Purohit A, et al. Anaphylactic reactions to formaldehyde in root canal sealant after endodontic treatment: four cases of anaphylactic shock and three of generalized urticaria. Allergy 2003;58(11):1210–15.
165. Rud J, Rud V, Munksgaard EC. Long-term evaluation of retrograde root filling with dentin-bonded resin composite. J Endod 1996;22(2):90–3.
166. Rud J, Rud V, Munksgaard EC. Periapical healing of mandibular molars after root-end sealing with dentine-bonded composite. Int Endod J 2001;34(4):285–92.
167. Andreasen JO, Munksgaard EC, Fredebo L, Rud J. Periodontal tissue regeneration including cementogenesis adjacent to dentin-bonded retrograde composite fillings in humans. J Endod 1993;19(3):151–3.
168. Torabinejad M, Chivian N. Clinical applications of mineral trioxide aggregate. J Endod 1999;25(3):197–205.
169. Torabinejad M, Hong CU, Pitt Ford TR, Kaiyawasam SP. Tissue reaction to implanted super-EBA and mineral trioxide aggregate in the mandible of guinea pigs: a preliminary report. J Endod 1995;21(11):569–71.
170. Koh ET, McDonald F, Pitt Ford TR, Torabinejad M. Cellular response to mineral trioxide aggregate. J Endod 1998;24(8):543–7.
171. Gazelius B, Olgart L, Wrangsjo K. Unexpected symptoms to root filling with gutta-percha. A case report. Int Endod J 1986;19(4):202–4.
172. Boxer MB, Grammer LC, Orfan N. Gutta-percha allergy in a health care worker with latex allergy. J Allergy Clin Immunol 1994;93(5):943–4.
173. Costa GE, Johnson JD, Hamilton RG. Cross-Reactivity studies of gutta-percha, gutta-balata, and natural rubber latex (*Hevea brasiliensis*). J Endod 2001;27(9):584–7.
174. Hamann C, Rodgers PA, Alenius H, et al. Cross-reactivity between gutta-percha and natural rubber latex: assumptions vs. reality. J Am Dent Assoc 2002;133(10):1357–67.

CHAPTER 25

DRUG INTERACTIONS AND LABORATORY TESTS

PAUL D. ELEAZER

Drug Interactions

Drug interaction discussions are often exhaustive, but may not be directed to probabilities of interactions clinicians are more likely to experience. Drug–drug interactions as well as some food–drug and herbal medicine–drug interactions that are likely to occur will be considered in this chapter. While dentists are not obliged to treat every patient, they cannot deny treatment based on a patient's disability, such as a medical condition. Therefore, it is important to be prepared to treat patients taking multiple drugs by becoming aware of dangerous drug interactions.

The drug interaction information in this chapter is derived from the work of a panel of pharmacologists who factor likelihood of an interaction with severity of the possible reaction to arrive at a level of clinical significance.[1] Some less likely reactions with serious potential adverse results are also included. Certainly new reactions, some serious, will be discovered as more knowledge accumulates. On-line resources are available for updated information.[2,3]

Principles of pharmacology and history taking can help the clinician determine probable risk for individual patients. Drug interactions can be classed as pharmacokinetic or pharmacodynamic. Pharmacokinetic reactions include changes of rate or extent of absorption, distribution, metabolism, or excretion. Pharmacodynamic drug interactions involve a change in the patient's response without a change in drug plasma level.

An example of a pharmacokinetic absorption is the anti-diarrheal Kao-Pectate (kaolin and pectin) which decreases absorption of tetracycline antibiotics. An example of pharmacokinetic drug interaction of distribution is epinephrine and β-blocker drugs competing for the same binding site on albumin. Metabolism-type pharmacokinetic interactions include the macrolide family of antimicrobials competing for the breakdown liver enzyme pathway with drugs such as Tagamet (cimetidine). Elimination drug reactions include the competition of methotrexate and nonsteroidal anti-inflammatory drugs (NSAIDs) for removal by the kidney.

An example of pharmacodynamic reaction is ethanol and a benzodiazepine combining to increase central nervous system (CNS) sedation without a detectable difference in plasma levels in either of the drugs from their levels if administered alone.

Interviewing the patient may provide valuable clues about possible drug reactions or interactions. When drug action is plotted against response in a large patient population, the graph is almost always a bell-shaped curve, meaning that a few patients develop an exaggerated response and some show very little effect. Most people have the expected response. If a patient has a history of over- or under-response to a drug, the clinician should be alert to a similar response. Drug interactions for members of the same drug class are likely to be analogous, but there are exceptions. A second major consideration in history taking is the possibility of inaccurate reporting by the patient. Such may be the case with a patient who denies a medical problem based on a sense of bravado or one who vainly wants to postpone admission of the encroachment of age. Furthermore, patients may simply forget important details of their drugs or dosages. Also, many lay persons who are not well versed in medical conditions may not grasp the importance of reporting all their specific conditions or chronic medications.

Some authors have suggested that generic medications may not be as effective as brand name drugs, especially for certain categories of drugs. An example of this is illustrated by the discovery of imperfections with enteric coatings that would not protect the medication from adverse effects of acidic stomach contents.[4]

The prudent practitioner should observe drug interaction reports for newly introduced drugs and be cautions about prescribing these drugs until sufficient time has elapsed to elucidate all reactions. Often, drug interactions are discovered after a drug is introduced to the market, even though many lab tests, animal tests, and human trials were performed before release of the drug for sale. An example of such a situation is the drug ketorolac (Toradol). It was found very effective in controlling postoperative dental pain and was widely prescribed before being associated with stomach and kidney problems that eventually lead to withdrawal of the oral form from the market, except for brief follow-up to parenteral use.[5]

Dentists are fortunate in that they seldom need to prescribe drugs for chronic use. Brief exposure limits drug interactions and side effects compared to long-term use. Even so, some important drug interactions occur rapidly.

For many drug interactions, the net result is simply a change in reaction to one or both drugs. The change can be an increased response or a decreased effect. Sometimes, a combination of drugs results in an unexpected interaction. An example of a surprising increased drug effect occurs when administering benzodiazepine drugs to patients taking the calcium channel blocker diltiazem (Cardizem). The combination causes little change to diltiazem action, but results in a rapid increase in benzodiazepine sedation, apparently because the calcium channel blocker decreases metabolic breakdown of the benzodiazepine. In one study, the area under the curve of drug concentration over time for a benzodiazepine was nearly tripled.[6]

Individual variation plays an important role in much of what we know about drug interactions. Generally, those affected more are the elderly, whose metabolic systems are less robust. Often, those with chronic systemic disease, and those taking multiple medicines, are more likely to have drug interactions, perhaps because unknown reactions may be at work. Patients taking herbal medicines and those on atypical diets also may be more likely to have an unexpected drug reaction.

Some patients may not be greatly affected by a drug interaction and might not report it to their prescribing doctor. Even among observant patients, the number of dramatic drug interactions that affect every patient every time is probably very low. This inconsistency of effect may allow the practitioner to gain confidence in prescribing drugs if they see their patients having no problems. Even for a specific individual, past experience with combining drugs is no guarantee of safety.

The most serious reactions of concern to dentists are listed in Tables 1–12. With theophylline, the margin between therapeutic dose and toxic level is narrow. With international travel now commonplace, drugs removed from the market in one country may be brought in from another, making the need to know overseas trade names as well as the generic labels. Such is the case with nonsedating antihistamines astemizole (Hismanal) and terfenadine (Seldane), which can cause life-threatening *torsades de pointes* cardiac arrhythmias if combined with macrolide antibiotics.

Systemic epinephrine can adversely affect a patient without drug interaction by increasing anxiety and causing frightening tachycardia. Keeping the local anesthetic in the local area minimizes the possibility of drug interaction. However, Lipp et al.[7] experimented with labeled epinephrine and found a 22% incidence of intravascular injection without positive aspiration, meaning that the clinician should not derive a false sense of security from a lack of aspiration of blood during an anesthetic injection. Avoidance of systemic interaction can best be assured by slow injection with observation of the patient for signs of systemic injection of epinephrine, such as pallor, tachycardia, and anxiety.

The concept of decreased drug effect of oral contraceptives by orally administered antibiotics has received attention in the lay press. Careful research has led to the belief that antibacterial drugs commonly used by dentists are very unlikely to cause a failure in oral contraception. Research suggests that the antifungal drug ketoconazole and the antituberculosis drug rifampin may have an effect on oral contraceptives. It is prudent for clinicians to suggest alternative methods of contraception to female patients of childbearing age because birth control pills are not 100% effective and because of the misinformation in the lay press.

Over-the-counter drugs can cause drug interactions of concern to the dentist. Herbals can also cause drug interaction problems. One problem with herbals is that many patients consider them to be dietary supplements and fail to report that they are taking an herbal. Recent study has elucidated many drug interactions with herbals.

Dentists commonly use antimicrobial drugs, pain relievers, and local anesthetics. Antimicrobial drugs have eliminated many risks of life. The first true antibiotic, penicillin, came into common use among dentists following World War II. Because so many patients have taken antibiotics, it is a little wonder that many drug interactions have been identified.

Tetracyclines were developed after penicillin. As they were gaining in popular usage, penicillin drugs were undergoing structural changes to offer different forms to counter antimicrobial resistance. Erythromycin, the original macrolide antibiotic, was introduced after tetracyclines. For a time, erythromycin was widely popular among dentists, who chose it because there was no risk of anaphylactic reaction and because antibiotic resistance to this drug originally seemed to be a limited problem. While severe allergic problems have not arisen, bacterial resistance and serious drug interactions have limited use of erythromycin and its congeners, clarithromycin (Biaxin) and azithromycin (Zithromax). The many drugs now known to interact with macrolides do so because of shared metabolic pathways that delay metabolism. Higher levels of one or both drugs commonly result in severe cardiac rhythm problems, some life-threatening. Surprisingly, even anti-arrhythmic drugs may cause such arrhythmias when administered with macrolides. One should note that combinations do not always cause a predictable reaction, meaning that prescribing a certain dose for a particular individual without untoward reaction does not guarantee a similar result for subsequent prescriptions.

Severe muscle wasting serious reactions may occur with macrolides when combined with "statin" drugs, very commonly used for lowering cholesterol. These drugs inhibit HMG-CoA reductase, a key enzyme in the production pathway of the "bad" or low density cholesterol. Muscle aches are among the first symptoms that can occur with the drug alone, but occur much more often when the macrolide antibiotic effectively increases its concentration by impeding metabolism through their common liver pathway. The symptoms may take a few days to appear. Damaged muscle leads to increased creatine phosphokinase enzyme levels, which are typically used to confirm a clinician's suspicion of this potentially very serious drug interaction. Early reports question whether rosuvastatin (Crestor) is subject to this interaction.[8]

Ergot derivatives, which mitigate vascular headaches, may interact with macrolide antibiotics, inducing peripheral ischemia secondary to vasospasm. Not all patients respond to reversal therapy for this drug interaction, making this a very serious potential problem.

Yet another category of classic interaction with drugs slowing metabolic pathways occurs with macrolides. To reach therapeutic levels, theophylline is often administered in doses close to the toxic threshold. When paired with erythromycin, the decreased elimination may push the concentration of the bronchodilator into the danger zone. Obviously, the higher the patient's therapeutic dose, the greater the risk. Early studies indicate azithromycin probably acts similarly, while clarithromycin may not.[9,10]

Table 1 contains more serious and more probable reactions of drugs with macrolide antibiotics. Dentists who prescribe macrolides should maintain vigilance for signs of any interaction.

Table 2 ranks potential reactions to metronidazole (Flagyl), a drug many dentists prescribe. This drug's antibacterial spectrum is for obligate anaerobes, but some obligate anaerobes are resistant. Clinicians often use this DNA impeding agent with a penicillin or cephalosporin bactericidal drug. Research has shown that most endodontic infections contain multiple organisms, characteristically with many facultative microbes.[11] Outcome analysis of microbial susceptibilities of cultures from endodontic infections shows that metronidazole alone is not effective for these infections.[12]

Metronidazole shares the adverse interaction of anticoagulant drugs with all antibiotics. By killing normal gut flora, the production of vitamin K decreases, thus altering the balance between the normal clotting enhancing vitamin and the clot-preventing anticoagulant. The result is that a clinical bleeding problem is more likely. Metronidazole has an additional interaction of importance to the clotting balance. It further increases bleeding proclivity by a direct inhibition of metabolism of warfarin (Coumadin).[13]

Also of note, metronidazole shows interaction with ethanol, just like with disulfram (Antabuse),

Table 1 Potential Reactions between Macrolide* Antibiotics and All Drugs

Rapid Reactions	Delayed Reactions
Very significant	
Established reaction	Established reactions
▲ Carbamazepine (Tegretol) (→ toxicity) (76b)	▲ Cispride (Propulcid) (→ arrhythmia) (192)
	▲ Digoxin (→ toxicity) (285a)
Probable reaction	Probable reactions
Ergot derivatives (→ peripheral ischemia) (315a)	▲ Anticoagulants (→ bleed) (79)
	▲ Statins (→ myopathy) (rhabdomyolysis) (368hb)
	▲ Primozide (Orap) antipsychotic (→ cardiotoxicity) (575d)
	Suspected reactions
	▲ Antiarrhythmics (→ arrhythmia) (36a)
	▲ Eplerenone (hyperkalemia) (→ arrhythmia) (312c)
	Grapefruit = ▲ absorption (→ toxicity) (479f)
	Some quinolones = (→ arrhythmia) (479h)
	Verapamil, ▲ macrolide (→ cardiotoxicity) (759)
Somewhat less significant	Established reactions
	▲ Theophylline (→ toxicity) (714a)
	▲ Corticosteroid (→ possible toxicity) (221)
	▲ Cyclosporine = (→ nephrotoxicity amp; neurotoxicity) (236a)
	Probable reaction
	Rifampin (→ ▼ antibacterial/▲ gut effects) (479i)
Suspected reaction	Suspected reactions
▲ Benzodiazepines (→ sedation) (131a)	Tacrolimus (Prograf) (→ ▲ tacrolimus toxicity) (685d)
	Repag. (Prandin) (→ ▲ Repag = ▼ blood glucose) (613b)

Numbers indicate page number in *Facts and Comparisons, Drug Interactions*.[1]
*Macrolides share liver metabolic pathways with many other drugs, generally resulting in delayed metabolism of both drugs, which increases drug levels.
▼ Drug action is probably diminished.
▲ Drug action is probably increased.

resulting in nausea and vomiting in many patients. The clinician should caution patients to avoid ethanol while taking metronidazole and for 1 full day thereafter to ensure no untoward drug interaction. Another drug interaction of metronidazole is, when combined with Antabuse, patients taking metronidazole have experienced acute psychotic reactions.

Except for potentially fatal allergic reactions (anaphylaxis), the penicillin family of antibiotics, and the cephalosporins, have remained relatively free of serious drug interactions (Table 3). The penicillins are very effective against common endodontic pathogens.[12] Most cephalosporins are not

Table 2 Metronidazole* (Flagyl) and All Drugs

Rapid Reactions	Delayed Reactions
Very significant	▲ Anticoagulants (bleed) (82)
Somewhat less significant	Suspected reactions
Suspected reaction	Barbiturates speed metabolism of
Ethanol (→ disulfram	metronidazole (→ ▼ antibacterial)
reaction) (335)	(512), Disulfram (→ acute psychosis) (304)

Numbers in brackets indicate page number in *Facts and Comparisons, Drug Interactions*.[1]
*This antibiotic decreases metabolism of warfarin. It also may cause nausea if combined with ethanol or disulfram (Antabuse), but reaction is inconsistent.
▼ Drug action is probably diminished.
▲ Drug action is probably increased.

Table 3 Penicillins/Cephalosporins and All Drugs

Delayed Reactions

Suspected reactions
  Tetracyclines (→ cidal drug) (560)
  Methotrexate (→ toxicity) (496c)
Somewhat less significant
Suspected reactions
  Allopurinol (Zyloprim) (→ rash) (555)
  Food decreases → absorption (559)
  Beta-blockers (▼ antihypertensive + antianginal) (155)
  Warfarin, ▲ bleeding (51)
  Aminoglycosides, inactivated by parenteral Penicillin (PCN) (22)
  Aminoglycosides + cephalosporin (→ nephrotoxicity) (18)

Numbers in brackets indicate page number in *Facts and Comparisons Drug Interactions*.[1]
▼ Drug action is probably diminished.
▲ Drug action is probably increased.

effective against the strict anaerobes found in endodontic infections. There may be cross-allergenicity between penicillins and cephalosporins.

Methotrexate, a powerful anti-metabolite for some types of cancer and for refractory arthritis patients, combined with penicillin has caused severe toxicity, including renal failure, myelosuppression, neutropenia, thrombocytopenia, and skin ulcers. Cephalosporins have not been reported to cause this drug interaction.

Quinolone antibiotics have potential to cause severe interactions with several drugs (Table 4). As with macrolides, quinolones cause serious cardiac rhythm problems in the presence of many other drugs. The macrolide–quinolone combination is one of the drug interactions that can cause fatal arrhythmias. Macrolides or quinolones plus cisapride (Propulcid) may interrupt normal nerve impulse conduction within the heart that may threaten life. Yet another problem that quinolones have is the drug interaction with theophylline. The shared metabolic pathway similarly causes theophylline concentrations to increase to toxic levels. These similarities occur even though the molecular structures of the two drug classes are quite different.

Coumadin plus a quinolone may produce a cardiac rhythm problem.[14] All antibiotics can cause bleeding problems for patients taking anticoagulants because the antibiotic kills gut flora that produce vitamin K, a natural substance that enhances clotting. Lack of this balance means patient takes longer to clot. When healthy patients take an antibiotic, the reduction in vitamin K causes no clinically apparent change in clotting parameters. The well-informed dentist should be able to evaluate blood clotting tests such as bleeding time and International Normalized Ratio (INR) with the patient's physician.

Tetracyclines have seen resurgence in popularity among dentists because of their actions against collagenase and their effectiveness against periodontal pathogens, many shared with endodontic diseases. Both of these advantages carry over into endodontics. While there is a long list of drugs that interact with tetracyclines, the reactions tend to be inconsistent and are rarely life-threatening (Table 5). The digoxin–tetracycline interaction arguably has the most serious potential. In a small portion of the population, the gut flora metabolizes a significant percentage of their digoxin dose, meaning that they need a fairly high dose to achieve the proper steady-state digoxin level.

Table 4 Quinolone* Antibiotics and All Drugs

Rapid Reactions	Delayed Reactions
Very significant	Probable reaction
	Anticoagulants ▲ bleed (92)
	Suspected reactions
	Serious arrhythmias with:
	phenothiazines (573);
	Cisapride (Propulsid) (610b);
	Macrolide antibiotics (479h);
	Tricyclic antidepressants (750a);
	Ziprasidone (Geodon) (773e);
	Antiarrhythmics (36b)
Somewhat less significant	
Antacids, ▼ Quinolone absorption (610)	Suspected reactions
	Cyclosporine, nephrotoxicity (238j)
	Theophylline ▲ Theo → toxicity (716)
Probable reactions	
Sulcralfate (Carafate) = ▼ Quinolone absorption (610j)	
Heavy metal salts = ▼ Quinolone absorption (610f)	
Suspected reactions	
Sevelamer (Ranagel) = ▼ Quinolone absorption (610i)	
Tizanidine (Zanaflex) = ▼ Tizanidine metabolism → toxicity (735 ab)	
Food = ▼ Quinolone absorption (610d)	

Numbers in brackets indicate page number in *Facts and Comparisons Drug Interactions*.[1]
*Note that serious psychotic reactions can occur with these drugs. Such reactions may persist long after the drug is discontinued.
▼ Drug action is probably diminished.
▲ Drug action is probably increased.

Table 5 Tetracycline and All Drugs

Delayed Reactions

Suspected reactions
  Pens/Cephs, cidal/ static (560)
  Digoxin, ▲ dig. (295)
Somewhat less significant
Suspected reactions
  Activated charcoal, absorbs (182)
  Heavy metal salts = chelation (686) (687) (688) (693) (696)
  Retinoids (Accutane) risk of (614) benign intracranial hypertension

Numbers in brackets indicate page number in *Facts and Comparisons Drug Interactions*.[1]
▼ Drug action is probably diminished.
▲ Drug action is probably increased.

Tetracyclines can induce significant microflora changes, such that greater digoxin absorption leads to toxic levels. As noted above, macrolides interact with digoxin in a different way, inhibiting renal excretion of digoxin, also reaching potentially toxic levels, and this change can last for many days after macrolide is stopped.

While it may be nice to contemplate treating endodontic patients without antibiotics, such is an unrealistic dream. No antibiotic is without potential interaction with other drugs. The rapid discovery of new interactions mandates that those who treat infected patients keep abreast of contemporary information.

Pain control drugs fall into a similar situation. Certainly, modern endodontic techniques and better appreciation of the value of "not" harming tissues adjacent to root canals have helped reduce the need for pain-relieving drugs. Yet, postoperative pain will remain a factor in treating some endodontic maladies. Clinical experience of many dentists reinforces the experimental observations that NSAIDs are effective pain relievers. Most practitioners find NSAIDs as effective as codeine or hydrocodone for most patients. Chronic NSAID use has revealed stomach and kidney problems, especially among the elderly, but only a few problems have been associated with short-term use.

Serious drug interactions with NSAIDs are relatively rare (Table 6). The effect of Coumadin is potentiated by NSAIDs. The prescription of NSAIDs for only a few doses limits the clinical appearance of this interaction. But a very serious NSAID reaction is with methotrexate, resulting in kidney failure. This reaction is more likely with high-dose methotrexate, typically used for antineoplastic therapy, as opposed to the lower doses used for rheumatoid arthritis refractory to less powerful drugs.

Patients taking β-blockers may experience hypertension breakthrough when taking NSAIDs. Sulindac (Clinoril) apparently does not have the propensity to cause this reaction.[15]

Lithium toxicity induced by adding NSAIDs has occurred. The decrease of lithium metabolism has not resulted in clinical problems in healthy patients.[16]

NSAIDs and the very popular antidepressants that work by selective serotonin re-uptake inhibition (SSRI) drugs within brain synapses can interact adversely. Increased gastrointestinal (GI) bleeding has been reported, although the problem has also occurred when an SSRI drug was used alone.[17]

Narcotic pain relievers will continue to play a useful role for dentists, albeit less necessary because of improved understanding and better instruments and techniques. Demerol (meperidine) is the most troublesome for potential interactions. The most serious, sometimes resulting in death, is less likely now because oxidase inhibitors are rarely prescribed. Other reactions are listed in Table 7.

Control of intra-operative pain is a standard by which patients judge their endodontic caregiver. Pilots are judged by how smoothly they can land a plane even though this is a small part of a pilot's skill. Similarly, patients judge us by our skill at giving an "easy shot."

There are two separate drug interaction considerations with local anesthetics, the anesthetic itself

Table 6 Nonsteroidal Anti-inflammatory Drugs and All Drugs

Delayed Reactions

Very significant
    Probable reaction
        Anticoagulants ▲ bleed (86a, 86b)
    Suspected reaction
        Methotrexate ▲ Methotrexate (→ toxicity) (496)
Somewhat less significant
    Probable reaction
        Beta-blockers = ▼ antihypertensive (154)
    Suspected reactions
        Aminoglycosides, ▲ antibiotic (21)
        ▲ Lithium (→ Li toxicity) (464)
        SSRI, ▲ gut bleed (548)

SSRI, selective serotonin re-uptake inhibition. Numbers in brackets indicate page number in *Facts and Comparisons Drug Interactions*.[1]
▼ Drug action is probably diminished.
▲ Drug action is probably increased.

Table 7 Narcotics* and All Drugs

Rapid Reactions	Delayed Reactions
Very significant	
Demerol and Mao inhibitors (488)	
Somewhat less significant	
Probable reaction	Suspected reaction
Demerol + Phenothiazines (488a)	Demerol + Ritonavir (Norvir) (488b)
Suspected reaction	
Barbiturates (112)	

Numbers in brackets indicate page number in Facts and Comparisons Drug Interactions.[1]
Note that death has been reported from giving Demerol to Manomine oxidase (MAO) inhibitor patients.
*Most reactions are due to additive central nervous system effects.

and the vasoconstrictor. Epinephrine is very rapidly metabolized, so any drug interaction is rapidly apparent (Table 8). Tolerance of the vasoconstrictor in one dose means that an additional dose after about 5 minutes can be given with similar result, given that neither is injected systemically.

Hypertensive events have been documented in patients taking β-blockers, Furazolidone (Furoxone) tricyclic antidepressants, methyl dopa, and the anti-hypertensive drugs guanethedine (Ismelin) and Rauwolfia alkaloids. Beta-blocker interactions are potentially the most serious. It is advisable to take a preoperative blood pressure reading to establish a baseline for that patient. Furthermore, intravascular injection occurs without a positive aspiration of blood.[7]

The anesthetic itself does not cause any known very serious drug interactions (Table 9). The problem with the anesthetic is that repeated injections build to overdose levels because, unlike the very rapidly metabolized vasoconstrictor, the anesthetic agent is metabolized over hours. This is especially important for pediatric patients whose body mass cannot tolerate as much anesthetic as an adult.

Beta-blockers may interact with lidocaine, lowering the number of doses to reach the toxic range. This drug interaction is believed to be via inhibition of hepatic metabolic enzymes.[18]

Cimetidine (Tagamet) increases lidocaine levels too, probably by the same general effect on liver enzymes. Yet, the reaction does not occur every time the drugs are combined.[19] Research on other histamine H2 antagonists failed to show this interaction.

Benzodiazepine reactions are typically one of the increased drug effects and can be accounted for by beginning with a lower dose, perhaps a half pill, until the patient's own reaction is defined. The protease inhibitor reactions however have been reported to induce severe sedation and respiratory depression. As noted in Table 10, no drug interactions with benzodiazepines have been ranked in the very significant category.

Table 11 lists drugs that may be used by dentists that interact with Coumadin (warfarin). This extensive list calls for careful consideration by the

---

Table 9 Local Anesthetics and All Drugs

Rapid Reaction

Somewhat less significant
  Established reactions
    Beta blockers [→ (Lido. toxicity)] (450a)
    Histamine H2 Antagonists (Tagamet) (→ Lido. toxicity) (451)
  Suspected reaction
    Succinylcholine, ▲ succinylcholine half-life (636)

Numbers in brackets indicate page number in *Facts and Comparisons Drug Interactions*.[1]
▼ Drug action is probably diminished.
▲ Drug action is probably increased.

Table 8 Epinephrine*-Containing Local Anesthetics and All Drugs

Rapid Reactions

Very significant
  Established reaction
    Beta Blockers → hypertension then bradycardia (312)
  Suspected reaction
    Furazolidone (Furozone) antibiotic → hypertension (674a)
Somewhat less significant
  Established reaction
    Tricyclic antidepressants → hypertension (683)
  Suspected reactions
    Rauwolfia alkaloids → hypertension (682)
    Methyldopa → hypertension (680)
    Guanethidine → hypertension (354)

Numbers in brackets indicate page number in *Facts and Comparisons Drug Interactions*.[1] Epinephrine is rapidly metabolized, so delayed reactions do not occur.
*Minimize risk by injecting slowly and watching patient reaction.

Table 10 Benzodiazepine* and All Drugs

Rapid Reaction	Delayed Reaction
Somewhat less significant	
Established reactions	
Ethanol (325)	Suspected reactions
Azole antifungals (122b)	Carbamazepine (Tegretol) (123a)
	Hydantoins (Dilantin) (375)
	Modafinil (Provigil) (131b)
	Non-nucleoside reverse transcriptase (131d)
	Inhibitors
	Protease inhibitors (133)
	St. John's Wort (136a)
	Macrolide antibiotics (131a)
	Rifampin (136)
Probable reactions	
Diltiazem (Cardizem) (128)	
Food (129b)	

Numbers in brackets indicate page number in *Facts and Comparisons Drug Interactions*.[1]
*In most reactions, benzodiazepine effect is increased, but decreased with Rifampin. Generally, titration of dosage is indicated.

Table 11 Drugs Prescribed by Dentists That May Interact with Warfarin Anticoagulant

Delayed Reactions

Very significant
  Established reactions
    Sulfonamides, bleed (98)
    Metronidazole, bleed (82)
    Vitamin E, bleed *(197a)
    Aspirin (ASA), bleed (94)
  Probable reaction
    NSAIDs/(86a) CoX_2 inhibitors (86b) = bleed
    Quinolones = bleed (92)
    Macrolides = bleed (79)
Somewhat less significant
  Established reaction
    Suspected reactions
      Acetaminophen = ▲ vitamin K, thus ▼ bleed (39)
      Carbamazepine (Tegretol), ▼ bleed (50)
      Vitamin K = ▼ bleed (109)
      Most antibiotics kill vitamin K bacteria = bleed (51, 89, 92, 47, 82, 93, 98)

NSAIDs, nonsteroidal anti-inflammatory drugs. Numbers in brackets indicate page number in *Facts and Comparisons Drug Interactions*.[1] Most drug interactions result in increased bleeding. Tylenol, Tegretol, rifampin, and vitamin K increase bleeding. The Tylenol reaction is apparently not consistent and, if reported, exceeded six doses/week. Vitamin K reverses the action of warfarin. However, there is currently no antidote for Plavix.
▼ Drug action is probably diminished.
▲ Drug action is probably increased.

Table 12 Drugs Prescribed by Dentist That May Interact with Herbal Medicines

Significance levels	
1	Amoxicillin + Khat → ▼ amoxicillin (85, 86)
1	ASA or NSAIDs + Ginkgo biloba → bleed by platelet aggregation) (19, 20)
1	Benzodiazepines + Kava → ▲ benzo levels (sedation) (84)
	Benzodiazepine + St. John's Wort → ▼ Benzodiazepine (sedation)
2	Corticosteroids + Licorice → ▲ corticosteroid (87)
1	Ciprofloxacin + Calcium-supplemented orange juice → ▲ Cipro (95a) ↓ antibiotic absorption
1	Cipro + Zinc → ▲ Cipro (154ba) ↓ antibiotic absorption
1	Acetaminophen + Ethyl Alcohol → Hepatotoxic Metabolite (14e)
1	Macrolide antibiotics + Grapefruit → ▲ absorption of macrolide (toxicity) (44a)
2	Tetracycline + Zinc → ▲ tetracycline ↓ antibiotic absorption
1	Tetracycline + dairy products → ↓ Tetracycline due to chelation (12a–12d)
	Levofloxacin + orange juice (plain or with ca^{++}) → ↓ Levoflox (95f)

Numbers in brackets indicate page number in *Facts and Comparisons Drug Interactions*.[1]
Significance level 1 = herbal drug should not be combined. Significance level 2 = herbal drug may be continuously allowed.
▼ Drug action is probably diminished.
▲ Drug action is probably increased.

dentist and alerting the patient to watch for signs of bleeding. Notably, the rapid reaction category is empty, indicating that short-term use carries less harmful potential.

Drug Interactions with Food and Herbals

Many patients are now taking herbal medicines, yet consider them as harmless food supplements. Table 12 lists more serious interactions with prescription drugs that should be reviewed (the table is derived from the panel of experts described in the beginning of this chapter). Facts and comparisons herbal supplements and food publication ranks potential interactions into only three categories, of which the more serious two are included.[20] However, many new drug interactions with herbals and food are currently under study and the fact that more people are now taking herbals means that more interactions will be elucidated.

Grapefruit–drug absorption interactions account for many newly discovered drug level changes. Apparently, this citrus fruit speeds absorption far more than other similar fruits. The result can be damagingly high levels of drug, even in the absence of other drugs. This action contradicts the typical finding that food binds with drugs to decrease absorption, or at least slows drug absorption.

Khat is a stimulant plant from East Africa that is usually chewed. It has been imported into the United States and other counties as a recreational euphoric agent. It sometimes is smoked to achieve higher concentrations, which may induce hallucinations. Khat has been shown to decrease absorption of amoxicillin and its close congener, ampicillin. This may lead to persistence of an infection. A small study demonstrated the maximum decrease to occur 2 hours after chewing khat.[21] Other potential drug interactions with khat have not been investigated thoroughly.

Ginkgo biloba, which is commonly used as a memory enhancer, interacts with salicylates and NSAIDs to increase bleeding. The apparent mechanism is by lowered platelet aggregation.

Kava, an herbal drug from the South Pacific plant of the same name, is drunk as a tea or now available in pill form to relieve stress and produce a sense of well-being. A single, but serious drug interaction-induced coma has been reported. While the reaction occurred when combined with alprazolam (Xanax), experts anticipate that the danger likely extends to the entire benzodiazepam family.[22]

Another herbal anxiolytic–benzodiazepine interaction has been anticipated, but not yet reported, between a benzodiazepine and the weed-derived St. John's Wort. Experimental evidence demonstrated that the combination of the herbal and clonazepam (Klonapin) decreased the benzodiazepine levels.[23]

Licorice has been shown to alter levels of corticosteroids, either increasing or decreasing the drug.[24] The interaction would be more serious in patients on high-dose steroid. No evidence exists yet as to exact mechanism of the interaction or about any potential problems with natural steroid drugs or overall action on inflammation or healing.

Orange juice, particularly when calcium-fortified, lowers the levels of the fluoroquinones Cipro (ciprofloxacin) and Levaquin (levofloxacin). While the exact mechanism is unknown, the suspicion is that the orange juice and the drug compete for transportation across the intestinal membrane.[25]

Cipro absorption is also diminished in the presence of zinc, as are tetracycline concentrations. This essential heavy metal additive is common in multivitamin preparations. The net result of the interactions is lowering of antibiotic levels in the 25 to 40% range.[26,27]

Tetracycline absorption is also hindered by dairy products, which all contain the heavy metal ion calcium. Doxycycline is the least affected of the tetracycline family to bind with heavy metal ions, a process called chelation.[28]

Ethyl alcohol is discussed in "Drug Interactions", but there is a brief review in here.[20] Perhaps, because it is so often used or abused among patients, alcohol is sometimes considered a food. Generally, its interactions are to increase action of drugs that act on the CNS. It delays gastric emptying, so can delay absorption of almost any drug taken by mouth. It specifically interacts with metronidazole in a disulfram class reaction, inducing nausea and vomiting. All the above reactions are dose related, so the astute clinician should caution patients accordingly. The interaction with Tylenol (acetaminophen) is different and potentially lethal. Chronic use of ethyl alcohol increases the enzyme that metabolizes acetaminophen, resulting in the rapid metabolism of acetaminophen with consequent high levels of a toxic acetaminophen metabolite, known as NAPQI, N-acetyl-p-benzoquinone.

Lab Tests of Potential Importance in Endodontics

Dentists may be uncomfortable in ordering laboratory tests. Referral to a physician is always appropriate, but there is no reason for a dentist to be intimidated by the process. Dentists are often the first healthcare provider to identify systemic disease. Frequently, this is the case because oral tissues are the first to be affected. Also, many patients do not regularly visit their physician, or many receive only cursory information on subtleties of oral changes from disease. Leukemia, bacterial endocarditis-induced oral petechiae, bleeding disorders, various cancers, and many other diseases are first suspected in the dental office. Ordering a laboratory test to confirm or rule-out suspicions is perfectly appropriate for any dentist. Culture and sensitivity testing for identification of the cause of an infection and the most likely effective antimicrobial should be in every dentist's armamentarium.

Laboratory tests are commonly helpful to dentists. The list of lab tests commonly helpful to dentists is not exhaustive, and dentists should not be limited to those tests listed below. Disorders of inflammation, perhaps related to a chronic dental infection, may cause an increased erythrocyte sedimentation rate. Blood tests can be helpful in identifying blood dyscrasias from cellular imbalances to inflammatory system evaluation and to clotting factors. Most classic hemophiliacs are diagnosed early in life and can provide the dentist with important information by history. Every dentist should be aware of the risks associated with altered blood clotting profiles of their patients. Newly identified risk assessment studies have shown the mortality and morbidity of decreasing anti-clotting parameters. The dentist should be comfortable in interpreting these tests to determine if a patient is a candidate for a surgical procedure.

The prothrombin time test has been largely replaced by the INR, which uses a standardized control and expresses the result in a percent of normal clotting time. This test evaluates the extrinsic clotting mechanism. With an INR of 1 being the normal level, minor dental-alveolar surgery can be carried out to an INR level <3.5 with local methods of hemostasis sufficing. For other than minor surgery, consultation should be obtained with consideration for modification of the anticoagulation or hospitalization.

The partial thromboplastin time test remains valuable to determine the intrinsic clotting pathway, which is the clotting factors in blood plasma.

Bleeding time, the number of minutes required for a standard wound to clot, may help diagnose later onset problems of importance to the dentist such as von Willebrand's disease, where the intrinsic factor VIII is diminished by this hereditary defect. Also, bleeding time identifies disorders of the platelet system, including those induced by salicylates or NSAIDs.

Complete blood counts enumerate platelets, different white blood cells, and red blood cells and can confirm or rule out many suspicious findings. An increased number of red cells, polycythemia vera, can reveal itself as darker gingival, because of the engorgement of the vascular system. Bleeding gingival can be seen in many forms of leukemia. Petechiae due to sickle cell anemia can be diagnosed by the occasional characteristic shaped red blood cells.

While it is easier to direct patients and staff who are accidentally exposed to blood-borne pathogens to someone trained in counseling for such risks, tests for such infectious agents may be ordered by the dentist who suspects a disease.

Patients with unexplained radiolucencies of their jaws may need testing for certain disorders. For example, a multiple myeloma patient will have the abnormal Bence Jones protein in their urine. A patient with hyperparathyroidism-caused bone radiolucencies will have elevated blood calcium and decreased blood phosphorus. Urine levels of calcium may be lower, with increased urine phosphorus. Serum alkaline phosphatase is elevated in hyperparathyroidism, although not as markedly as with Paget's disease.

Diabetes mellitus has broad implications in healing. Blood or urine glucose elevations can be the impetus needed to send a patient for medical care.

Allergies can make life unpleasant for many. They may stem from food allergies which can cause nutritional imbalances which may be suggested by changes in oral tissues. They may include dental materials, such as nickel or eugenol, making the patient less likely to have a favorable treatment outcome. The dentist who suspects such a problem will probably refer the patient to an allergist for skin or other tests and then help manage the dental aspects of the patient's care.

Summary

There is a limited understanding of drug interaction incidence because of under-reporting. Also, animal studies may not transfer directly to the human. Animals cannot express mood changes effectively and there are some metabolic differences between animals and man.

The astute clinician should explain possible adverse or undesirable reactions with patients so that they may watch for an adverse outcome. This chapter emphasizes drug reactions that are potentially very serious and/or very likely to occur. Some practitioners will see interactions of drugs beyond those covered here. It is important to report suspected drug interactions to the Food and Drug Administration (FDA) for evaluation. The FDA periodically sends information about newly discovered serious drug interactions to practitioners registered by state license to practice dentistry. Furthermore, the reader should remember that information about drug interactions is constantly changing, mostly with newly discovered interaction reports.

References

1. Tatro DS, editor. Facts and comparisons, drug interactions facts. St. Louis: Wolters Klewer Health; 2006.
2. Lexi-Comp, Inc. http://www.lexi.com.
3. Epocrates, Inc. http://www.epocrates.com.
4. Agyilirah GA, Banker GS. Polymers for enteric coating applications. In: Tarcha PJ, editor. Polymers for controlled drug delivery. Cleveland, OH: CRC Press; 1990.
5. Fick DM, Cooper JW, Wade WE, et al. Updating the Beers criteria for potentially inappropriate medication use in older adults. Arch Intern Med 2003;163:2716–24.
6. Bachman JT, Olkkola KT, Aranko K, et al. Dose of midazolam should be reduced during diltiazem and verapamil treatments. Br J Clin Pharmacol 1994;37:221–5.
7. Lipp M, Dick W, Daublander M, et al. Exogenous and endogenous plasma levels of epinephrine during dental treatment under local anesthesia. Reg Anesth 1993;18(1):6–12.

8. Cooper KJ, Martin PD, Dane AL, et al. The effect of erythromycin on the pharmacokinetics of rosuvastatin. Eur J Clin Pharmacol 2003;59:51–6.

9. Gillum GJ, Israel DS, Scott RB, et al. Effect of combination therapy with ciprofloxacin and clarithromycin on theophylline pharmacokinetics in healthy volunteers. Antimicrob Agents Chemother 1996;40:1715–16.

10. Pollak TP, Slayter KL. Reduced serum theophylline concentrations after discontinuation of azithromycin: evidence for an unusual interaction. Pharmacotherapy 1997;17(4):827–9.

11. Munson MA, Pitt-Ford T, Chong B, et al. Molecular and cultural analysis of the microflora associated with endodontic infections. J Dent Res 2002;81(11):761–6.

12. Baumgartner JC, Xia T. Antibiotic susceptibility of bacteria associated with endodontic abscesses. J Endod 2002;29:44–7.

13. Yacobi A, Lai C, Levy G. Pharmacokinetic and pharmacodynamic studies of acute interaction between warfarin enantiomers and metronidazole in rats. J Pharmacol Exp Ther 1984;231:72–9.

14. Linville T, Matani D. Norfloxacin and warfarin. Ann Intern Med 1989;110:751–2.

15. Pope JE, Anderson JJ, Felson DT. A meta-analysis of the effects of nonsteroidal anti-inflammatory drugs on blood pressure. Arch Intern Med 1993;153:477–84.

16. Levin GM, Grum C, Eisele G. Effect of over-the-counter dosages of naproxen sodium and acetaminophen on plasma lithium concentrations in normal volunteers. J Clin Psychopharmacol 1998;18:237–40.

17. Dalton SO, Johansen C, Mellemkjaer L, et al. Use of selective serotonin reuptake inhibitors and risk of upper gastrointestinal tract bleeding. Arch Intern Med 2003;163:59–64.

18. Bax NDS, Al-Asady LD, Deacon CS, et al. Inhibition of drug metabolism by β-adrenoceptor antagonists. Drugs 1983;26(Suppl 2):121–6.

19. Jackson JE, Bentley JB, Glass SJ, et al. Effects of histamine-2 receptor blockade on lidocaine kinetics. Clin Pharmacol Ther 1985;37:544–8.

20. Tatro DS, editor. Facts and comparisons, drug interactions facts, Herbal supplements and food. St. Louis: Wolters Klewer Health; 2006.

21. Attef OA, Ali AA, Ali HM Effect of khat chewing on the bioavailability of ampicillin and amoxicillin. J Antimicrob Chemother 1997;39:523–5.

22. Almeida JC, Grimsley EW. Coma from the health food store: interaction between kava and alprazolam. Ann Intern Med 1996;125:940–1.

23. Wang Z, Gorski JC, Hamman MA, Huang SM, Lesko LJ, Hall SD. The effects of St. John's Wort (Hypericum perforatum) on human Cytochrome P450 activity. Clin Pharmacol Ther 2001;70:317–26.

24. Homma M, Oka K, Ikeshima K, Takahashi N, Nitsuma T, Fukudu T, Itah H. Different effects of traditional Chinese medicines containing similar herbal constituents on prednisolone pharmacokinetics. J Pharm Pharmacol 1995;47:687–92.

25. Wallace AW, Victory JM, Amsden GW. Lack of bioequivalence when levofloxacin and calcium-fortified orange juice are coadministered to healthy volunteers. J Clin Pharmacol 2003;43:539–44.

26. Polk RE, Healy DP, Sahai J, Drwal L, Racht E. Effect of ferrous sulfate and multivitamins with zinc on absorption of ciprofloxacin in normal volunteers. Antimicrob Agents Chemother 1989;33:1841–4.

27. Penttilä O, Hurme H, Neuvonen PJ. Effect of zinc sulfate on the absorption of tetracycline and doxycycline in man. Eur J Clin Pharmacol 1975;9:131–4.

28. Matilla MJ, et al. Interference of iron preparations and milk with the absorption of tetracyclines. Excerpta Medica International Congress Series No. 254. Toxicological Problems of Drug Combinations. 1927:128–33.

Chapter 26

Endodontics Instruments and Armamentarium

A. Dental Dam and its Application

William G. Schindler

It may be difficult, if not impossible, to achieve a sterile field in endodontics; however, every effort should be made to work as much as possible in a bacteria-free field. That being said, *the use of dental dam is absolutely essential during nonsurgical endodontic therapy.* For root canal treatment, rapid, simple, and effective methods of dam applications have been developed. In all but the most unusual circumstances, the dental dam can be placed on the tooth being treated in less than a minute. Its routine use will enhance every aspect of endodontic therapy.

Although the modern nonsurgical endodontic approach to the use of dental dam has changed, the importance and purposes of the dam remain the same:

1. It provides a dry, clean, and disinfected operating field removed from saliva and blood.
2. It protects the patient from possible aspiration or swallowing of tooth debris, restorative materials, bacteria, necrotic pulp tissue, and instruments[1–3] (Figure 1).
3. It protects the adjacent soft tissues (tongue, lips, cheek) by retracting them out of the way.
4. It protects the patient's soft tissues from irritating irrigating solutions and drugs that may be used during treatment.
5. Visibility and efficiency are improved.
6. Its routine use protects the clinician from litigation related to instrument aspiration or swallowing. Even swallowing diluted sodium hypochlorite can be dangerous in addition to it having an unpleasant taste.[4] *Use of dental dam for nonsurgical endodontics is the standard of care.*[5]

The clinician should be aware that there may be rare instances when coronal access to root canals might be made prior to the placement of the dental dam. Examples of this situation may include severe tipping of teeth, extreme calcification of the canal system, and orientation difficulties related to coronal restoration. However, once the chamber or canals have been located and before instruments or irrigating solutions have been used, the dental dam must be placed.

Equipment

DAM MATERIAL

Dental dam is available in a variety of thicknesses, colors, sizes, and material. The medium-weight thickness is highly recommended for general all-around use. It has the advantage of nicely adapting to the cervical area of the tooth, providing a fluid seal without the use of floss or ligature ties around each tooth. Also, it does not tear easily and provides more protection from injury to the adjacent soft tissues and increased visibility than does the thinner material. There are, however, some advantages in the use of thin-weight dam material on mandibular anterior teeth and partially erupted posterior teeth. These teeth have very little bulk of contour and the thinner material will exert less dislodging force on the clamp. The disadvantage is that it is easily torn.

Dam materials may be purchased in precut 5" × 5" (127 mm × 127 mm) or 6" × 6" (152 mm × 152 mm) sheets. The choice of light- or dark-colored material is largely up to the practitioner. Darker material provides a contrasting color as a background for the light-colored tooth.

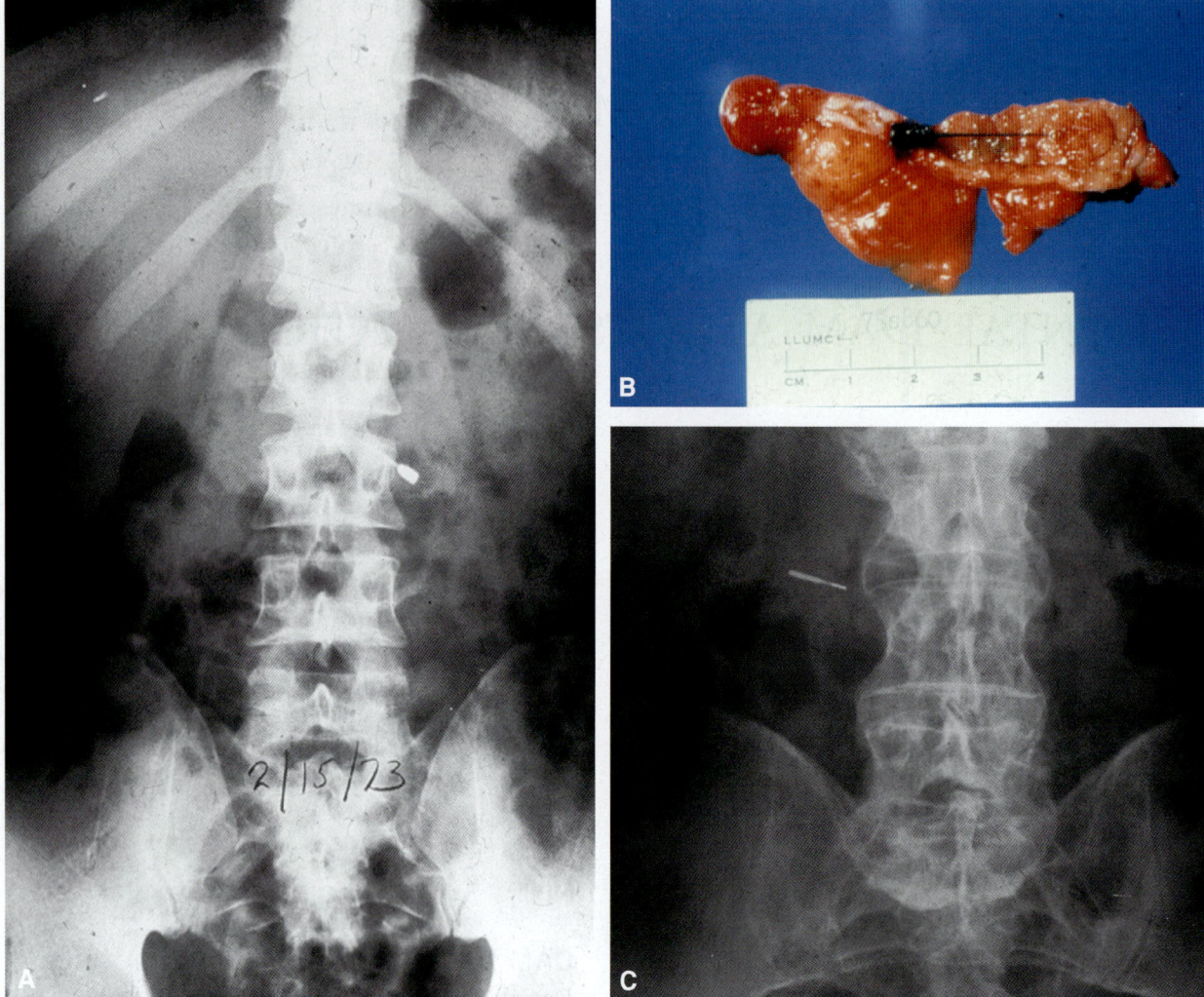

Figure 1 ***A***, Swallowed endodontic file ended up in the appendix resulting in acute appendicitis. ***B***, Specimen shows file in the appendix removed by appendectomy. Use of dental dam would have prevented this complication. ***C***, Dental burs can sometimes disengage from hand pieces and be swallowed, as shown here. This is also preventable with dental dam. (***A*** and ***B***, Reproduced with permission from Thomsen LC, Appleton SS, Engstrom HI. Appendicitis induced by an endodontic file. Gen Dent 1989;37:50.)

Dental dam is available in latex or non-latex material. With the apparent increasing incidence of patients allergic to latex, non-latex dental dam must be available in all offices.[6,7] Latex-free dams are available (Coltene Whaledent, Inc., Cuyahoga Falls, OH) and supplied in a powder-free, 6″ × 6″, medium thickness. In an emergency, non-latex glove material can also be used (Figure 2).

PUNCH

Any dental dam punch that is convenient for the operator and creates a sharp, clean hole in the dam material is satisfactory. All too often the punch has not been correctly centered over the hole, and a "nick" on the cutting margin results, producing an incomplete jagged cut in the dam material. This results in a poor seal at the time of placement and may make the dam susceptible to tearing.

FRAMES

In addition to supporting the dam, frames should be radiolucent to prevent obstruction of an important area on radiographs that are taken during treatment. There are a variety of dental dam frames that meet this requirement. The U-shaped Young's frame is made of radiolucent plastic for endodontic

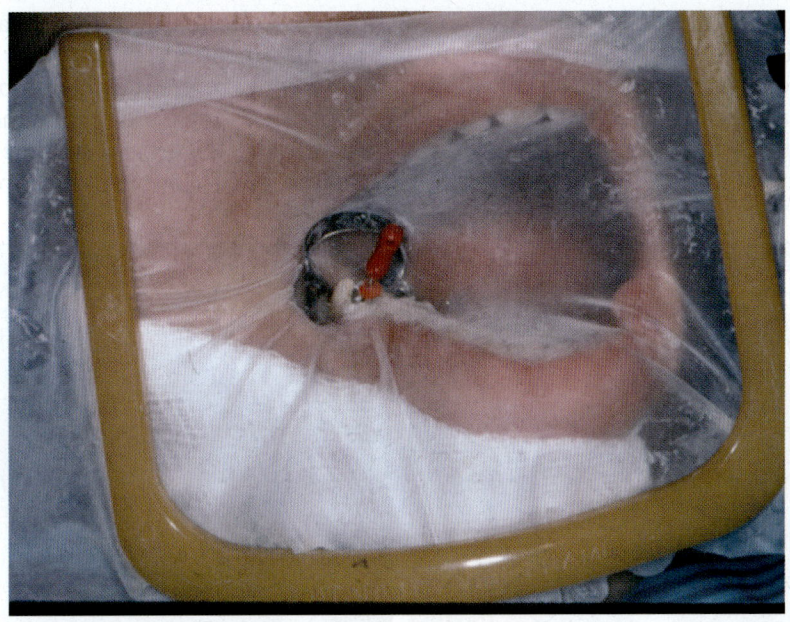

Figure 2 Latex-free barrier dams must be used for patients sensitive to latex; in this case a latex-free glove was cut up and used as a barrier.

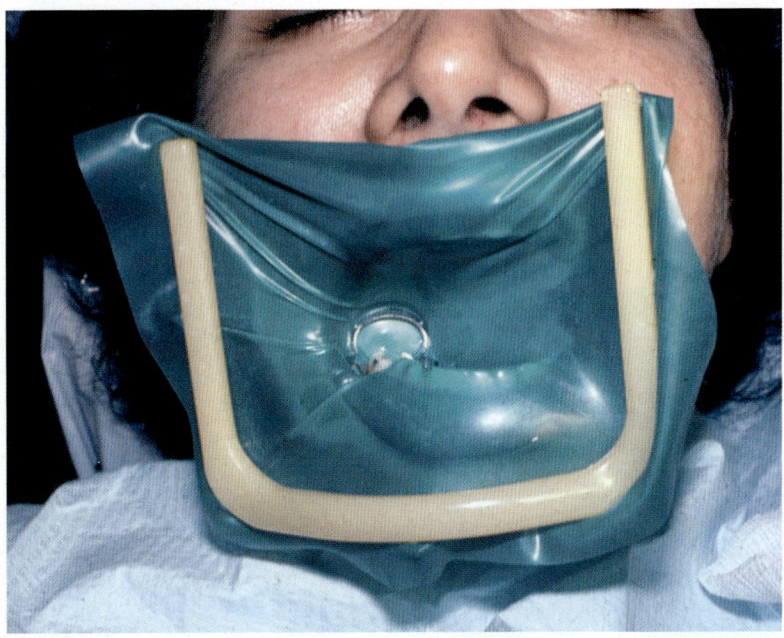

Figure 3 The U-shaped Young's dental dam frame is an example of commonly used frames.

applications. It is easily manipulated and is used widely (Figure 3). The Nygaard-Østby (N-Ø) dental dam frame (Coltene Whaledent, Inc.) is shield-shaped to fit the face, is made of radiolucent nylon, and may be in place while a tooth is subjected to X-rays without interfering with the radiographic image.

An articulated frame developed to facilitate endodontic radiography (Figure 4) is also curved to fit the face. It is hinged in the middle to fold back, allowing easier access for film and sensor placement. Derma-Frame (Ultradent Products, Inc., South Jordan, UT) is a soft metal frame that may be formed to fit the patient's face. The frame retains its configuration but may then be reshaped after use.

Recently, several dental companies have introduced disposable, single-use, pre-framed dental dams. The HandiDam (Figure 5) and the InstaDam (Zirc Co., Buffalo, NY) allow the clinician to quickly apply the

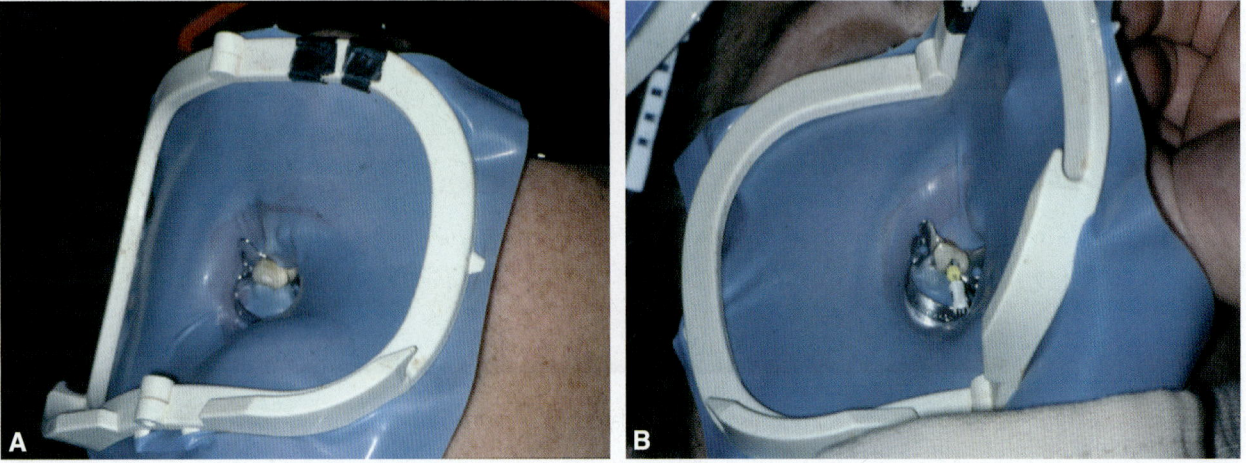

Figure 4 Hinged dental dam frame. **A,** In closed position, frame is curved to fit face. **B,** Open position, from either side, allows passage of radiographic film holder.

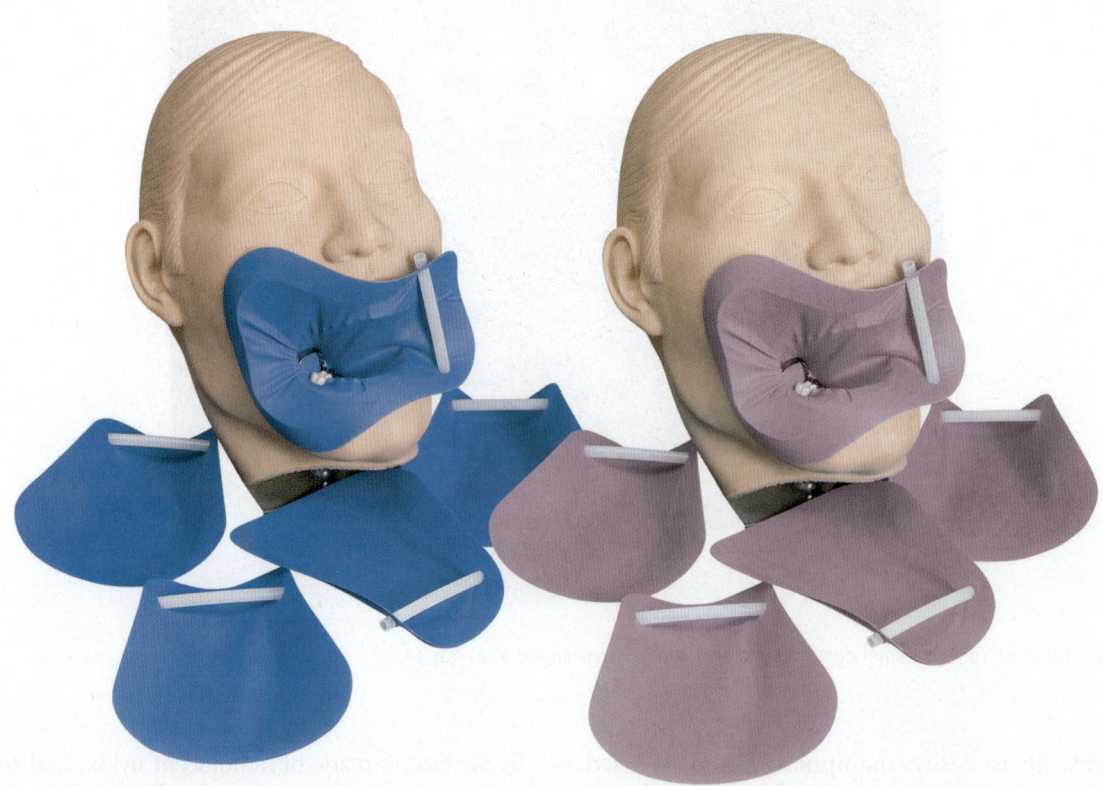

Figure 5 Frame and dam combinations such as the HandiDam (Aseptico, Inc., Woodinville, WA) allow convenient placement of a dental dam barrier for single teeth; the material is available both in latex and latex-free.

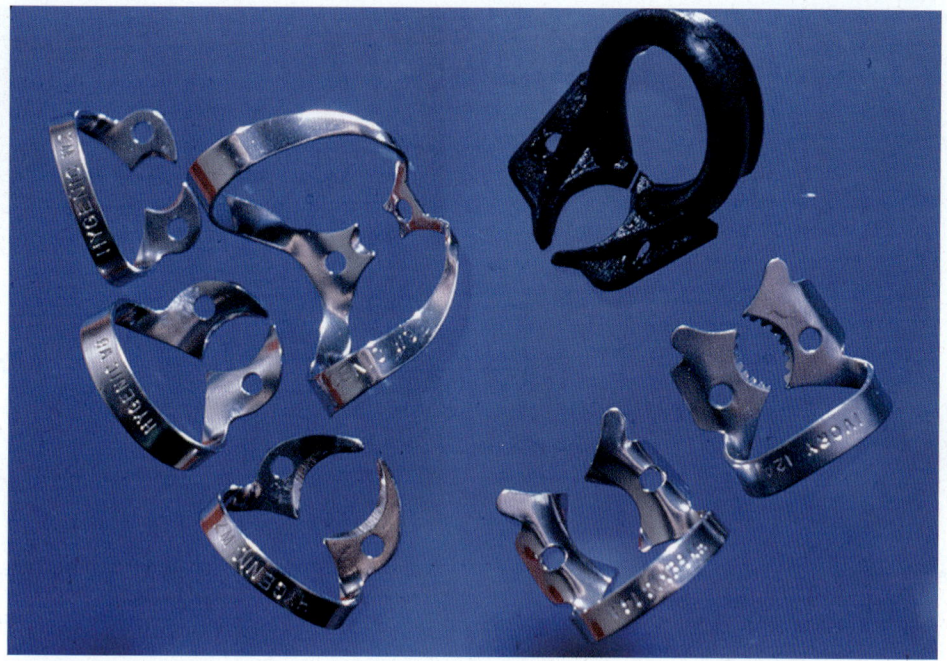

Figure 6 There are a variety of clamps available for all situations, including plastic clamps.

dam without the addition of a conventional frame. Both of these innovative devices are available in latex and latex-free versions.

CLAMPS

The dental dam clamp secures the dam to the tooth and helps in soft-tissue retraction. Although the selection of five to seven clamps will permit the clinician to isolate the majority of teeth treated, the experienced operator will expand that number. Teeth that are rotated, partially erupted, fractured, unusual in crown form, or with severe carious involvement all present problems requiring special clamps or clamping techniques. There are a variety of clamps available to meet any clinical situation that may arise (Figure 6). Table 1 lists a suggested assortment of metal clamps for various teeth.

For endodontic treatment particularly, the use of clamps with wings allows a more rapid, efficient means of applying the dental dam. The wings allow the dentist to place the clamp, dam, and frame in one operation (Figure 7). In addition, the wings cause a broader buccal–lingual deflection of the dam from the isolated tooth, thus allowing increased access. One disadvantage of the use of winged clamps is that the wings may occasionally interfere with radiographic interpretation of file or master cone positioning.

Plastic clamps (Moyco/Union Broach, York, PA) are also available in two sizes, large and small, and are used in selected cases. When metal clamp obstruction is a problem, radiolucent plastic clamps allow for an unobstructed film-view of the tooth.

FORCEPS

Either the Ash- or Ivory-style clamp forceps is acceptable. One advantage of the Ivory forceps, however, is

Table 1 Dental Dam Clamp Selection

	Clamps
Maxillary teeth	
Central incisor	6, 9, 210, 212
Lateral incisor	6, 9, 210, 00
Canine	6, 9, 210
Premolars	0, 2, 2A, W2A
Molars	3, W3, W8A, 14, 14A
Mandibular teeth	
Incisors	6, 9, 210, 212
Canine	6, 9, 210
Premolars	0, 00, 2, W2A
Molars	3, W3, W8A, 14, 14A

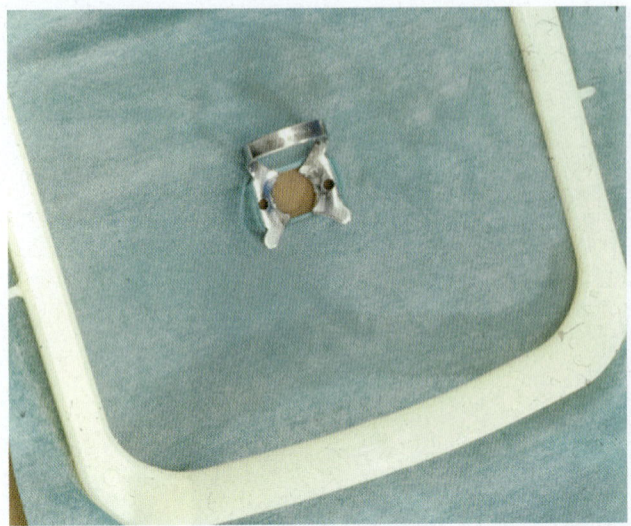

Figure 7 Winged clamp, dental dam, and frame ready for placement on tooth. Bow of clamp is oriented to the distal.

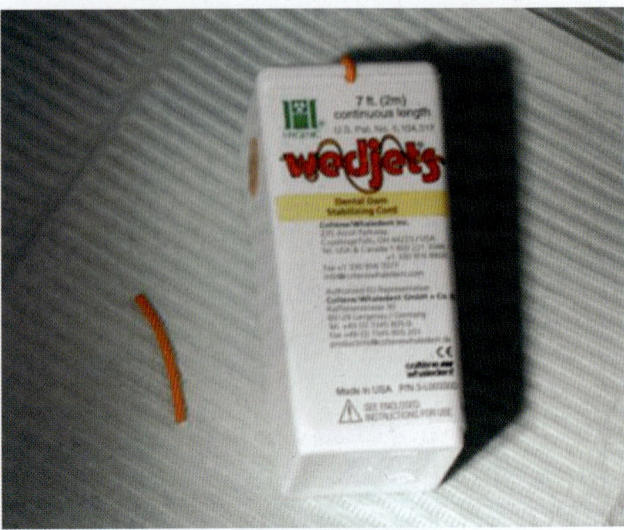

Figure 8 Wedjets cord (Coltene Whaledent, Inc.) can help stabilize the interproximal area of the dental dam.

the projections from the engaging beaks. These allow the clinician the opportunity to exert a gingivally directed force, which is often necessary to direct the clamp beyond the bulk of contour and into proximal undercuts. The Ash-style forceps beaks, however, afford a fulcrum point for posterior or anterior rotation of the clamp.

ADJUNCTS TO DENTAL DAM PLACEMENT

In addition to the previously mentioned materials, several other items will be of benefit for the efficient application of the dental dam.

A plastic or cement instrument can be used to shed the dental dam off the wings of the clamp once the clamp has been positioned. It is also used, along with a stream of air, to invert or "tuck" the edges of the dam into the gingival sulcus, thus ensuring a fluid-proof seal. This is particularly necessary in multi-tooth applications.

Dental floss is an essential adjunct to dam placement, even for endodontic therapy. Floss can be used for testing of contacts prior to dam application and for passing the dam material through the contacts after placement. It is recommended that the operator release the lingual grasp of the floss after passing it through the contact and pulling it out to the buccal, rather than back through the contact. Another product that may help with the stabilization of the interproximal dam is the Wedjets stabilizing cord (Coltene Whaledent, Inc.) (Figure 8). Small strips of the cord can be wedged into the interproximal space over the dam to fix the dam in place.

Even with proper techniques of placement of the dental dam, there will still be clinical situations in which some small amount of leakage of fluids can be anticipated. Adjustments can be made including repositioning of the clamp and closer attention to inversion of the dam material around the tooth. When those techniques are ineffective, leakage can usually be effectively controlled by the placement of a "patching" material at the interface of the tooth and the dam material. Orabase, rubber base adhesive, Cavit, a mixture of Super Poly-Grip Denture Adhesive with zinc oxide powder, and periodontal packing have been used in the past with limited success.[8] Currently, the application of OraSeal Caulking (Ultradent Products, Inc.) seems to provide a quick, easy-to-apply solution to the problem of seepage of fluids around the dental dam (Figure 9).

Techniques of Application

ROUTINE TECHNIQUES

Two techniques of dental dam application that can be used routinely are next described, followed by examples of special situations that may complicate the process.

Prior to application of the dental dam, it is suggested that the patient should rinse for 30 seconds with an effective antibacterial agent. A mouth rinse of

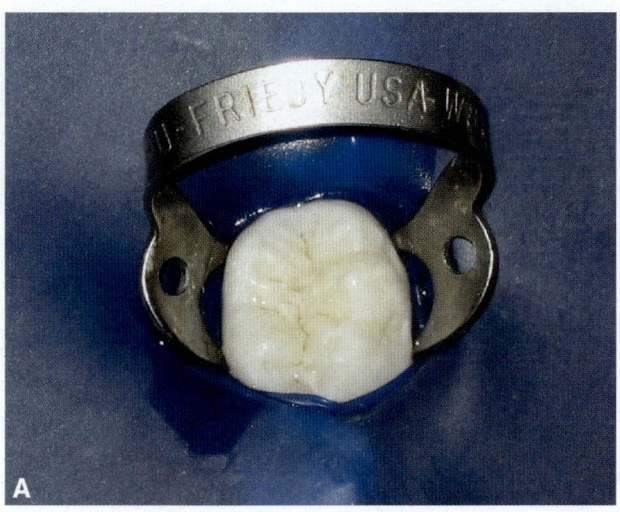 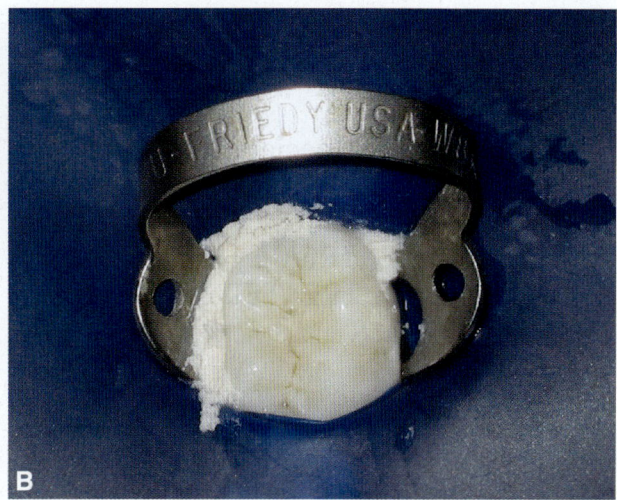

Figure 9 ***A***, Partially erupted first molar clamped with a W8A with leakage toward the lingual and distal. ***B***, Leakage controlled with Oraseal (Ultradent Products, Inc.).

0.12% chlorhexidine gluconate, such as Peridex (Proctor & Gamble, Cincinnati, OH), will reduce the number of microorganisms in the mouth prior to dam placement.[9]

SINGLE MOTION TECHNIQUE

This is the most efficient endodontic dam application technique through the use of winged clamps resulting in the dam, clamp, and frame being taken to the tooth to be isolated in a single motion (see Figure 7).

1. Select the clamp to be used.
2. Punch one appropriate-sized hole just off center of a 6″ × 6″ piece of dam material.
3. Stretch the dam over the frame and fit the clamp through the punched hole so that the wings retain the clamp.
4. Place the clamp over the tooth with the accompanying frame and dam attached so the clamp is seated over the bulk of contour of the tooth.
5. Use a plastic or cementing instrument to flick the dam off of the wings of the clamp. The dam material should be positioned on the tooth below the clamp.
6. Use floss to aid in passing the dam through contacts.

DOUBLE MOTION TECHNIQUE

This technique is still very efficient, requires the use of a winged or wingless clamp, and involves a seven-steps procedure.

1. Select the clamp to be used.
2. Punch one appropriate-sized hole just off center of a 6″ × 6″ piece of dam material.
3. Loosely attach the dam material to the four corners of the frame.
4. Place the clamp over the bulk of contour of the tooth to be isolated and ensure the clamp is secure.
5. Stretch the dam over the clamp so the dam material is seated under the clamp and hugging the cervical area of the tooth.
6. Completely stretch the dental dam onto all prongs of the frame.
7. Use floss to aid in passing the dam through contacts.

Regardless of the technique used, the surface of the tooth and dental dam should be disinfected with an appropriate disinfectant (i.e., 2.5% sodium hypochlorite, 10% iodine tincture, 2% chlorhexidine) prior to access of the root canal system.[10]

REMOVAL OF DAM

1. For single-tooth applications, simply remove the clamp with the forceps and remove the dam.
2. For multiple-tooth applications, first remove the clamp, then place a finger under the dam in the vestibule, and stretch the dam to the facial, away from the teeth. Cut the stretched interproximal dam with scissors and then remove the dam. After removal, it is essential that the dam be

inspected to ensure that no interproximal dam has been left between the teeth.

Techniques for Special Situations

MULTIPLE ADJACENT TEETH REQUIRING TREATMENT OR EXTREME MOBILITY OF THE TOOTH BEING TREATED

The posterior tooth is clamped normally whereas a second clamp is reversed (with the bow pointing mesially) on the most anterior tooth (Figure 10). Or, the most posterior tooth is clamped normally, whereas the anterior portion of the dam is retained without a clamp. A strip of dental dam, a piece of floss, or a Wedjets cord can be placed interproximally to hold the anterior portion of the dam in place.

INSUFFICIENT TOOTH STRUCTURE OR PORCELAIN CROWNS OF VENEERS WHERE AN INTACT POSTERIOR TOOTH IS IN PLACE

The split-dam technique can be effectively used utilizing a clamped tooth posterior to the tooth to be treated (Figure 11). Two holes can be punched, one for the clamped tooth and one for the tooth anterior to the tooth to be treated. The dam between the two holes can be cut with iris scissors. Once the clamp is placed on the posterior tooth, the dam can be placed on the clamped tooth and stretched mesially to anterior tooth and held in place with a Wedjets cord, floss, or a cut piece of dental dam. A cotton role can be

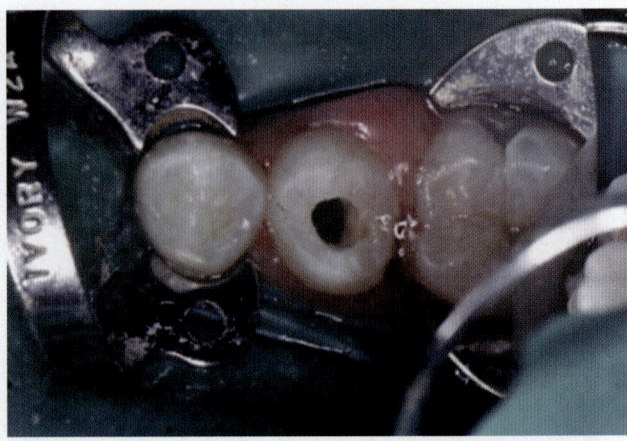

Figure 10 The posterior tooth is clamped normally whereas a second clamp is reversed (with the bow pointing mesially) on the more anterior tooth.

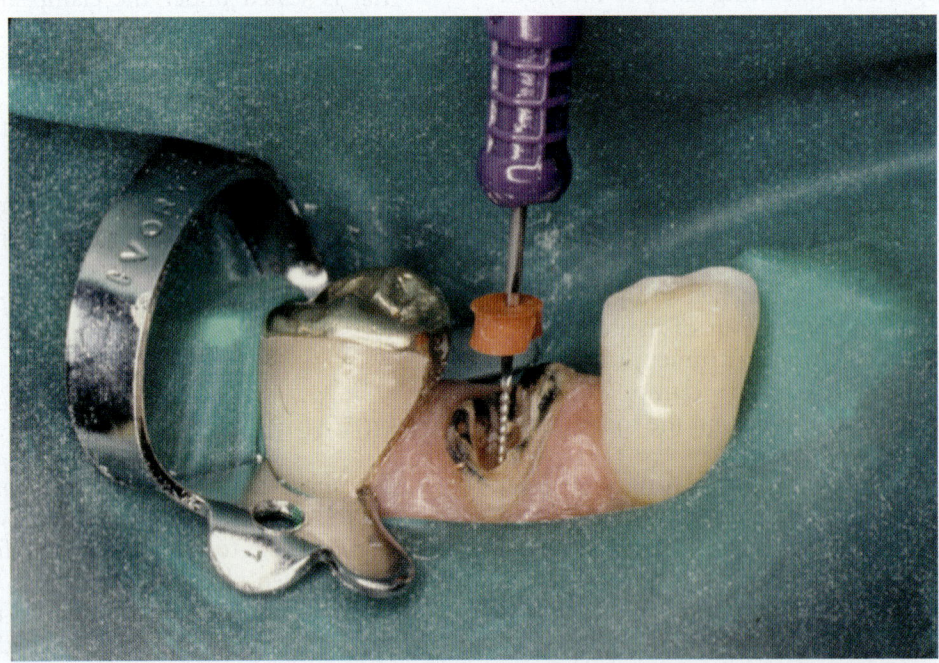

Figure 11 The split-dam technique can be effectively used by clamping a tooth posterior to the one to be treated and stretching over a tooth anteriorly.

placed under the lip or cheek in the mucobuccal fold over the tooth to be treated.

BRIDGE ABUTMENTS, SPLINTS, AND ORTHODONTICS WITH WIRES

Punch a larger-than-normal hole in the dam. Place OraSeal around the punched hole on the underside of the dam. Clamp the tooth in the normal manner. If leakage is a problem, add more Oraseal around the abutment at the site of leakage.

TOOTH WITH CALCIFIED PULP CHAMBER AND CANAL(S)

Use the three-tooth dental dam isolation technique previously described in the multiple adjacent teeth requiring treatment technique. The involved tooth is without a clamp, allowing the clinician to better visualize the Cemento Enamel Junction (CEJ) region of the tooth. A periodontal probe can be traced along the root surface to orientate oneself to the crown–root angulations during difficult access cavity preparations.

TERMINAL TOOTH WITH INSUFFICIENT TOOTH STRUCTURE

If insufficient tooth structure is present to allow a clamp from being placed on the tooth and the tooth is the terminal tooth in an arch, the clinician must first determine whether the tooth is sufficiently periodontally sound and restorable. If the tooth is determined to be retainable, perhaps a clamp with prongs extending apically can be used to effectively engage and hold on the tooth, followed by dam placement. If that is unsuccessful, the tooth may require coronal build-up restoration with pin-retained restorative materials so the retainer can be properly placed. Additionally, the terminally positioned tooth can undergo periodontal crown lengthening to expose more tooth structure to allow for clamp placement[11] (see Chapter 18, "Endodontic–Periodontic Differentiation").

Summary

Clinicians will find endodontic procedures more rewarding and less frustrating as their mastery of dental dam applications increases. The use of simplified techniques, improved materials, and organized procedures, as well as patience and practice, will hasten this mastery. Endodontists have long recognized that the use of dental dam is imperative in the practice of endodontics.

References

1. Goultschin J, Heling B. Accidental swallowing of an endodontic instrument. Oral Surg Oral Med Oral Pathol Oral Radiol Endod 1971;32:621–2.

2. Govila CP. Accidental swallowing of an endodontic instrument. A report of two cases. Oral Surg Oral Med Oral Pathol Oral Radiol Endod 1979;48:269–71.

3. Lambrianidis T, Beltes P. Accidental swallowing of endodontic instruments. Endod Dent Traumatol 1996;12:301–4.

4. The Dentist Insurance Company, California Dental Association. Rubber dam it. Liability Lifeline 2004;80:1–7.

5. Cohen S, Schwartz, S. Endodontic complications and the law. J Endod 1987;13:191–7.

6. de Andrade ED, Ranali J, Volpato MC, de Oliveira MM. Allergic reaction after rubber dam placement. J Endod 2000;26:182–3.

7. Kosti E, Lambrianidis T. Endodontic treatment in cases of allergic reaction to rubber dam. J Endod 2002;28:787–9.

8. Weisman MI. Remedy for dental dam leakage problems. J Endod 1991;17:88–9.

9. Miller CH. Infection control. Dent Clin North Am 1996;40:437–56.

10. Ng Y, Spratt D, Sriskantharajah S, Gulabivala K. Evaluation of protocols for field decontamination before bacterial sampling of root canals for contemporary microbiology techniques. J Endod 2006;29:317–20.

11. Lovdahl PE, Gutmann JL. Periodontal and restorative considerations prior to endodontic therapy. Gen Dent 1980;28:38–45.

CHAPTER 26B

B. INTRODUCTION OF NICKEL–TITANIUM ALLOY TO ENDODONTICS

WILLIAM A. BRANTLEY

Prior to the prescient review article by Civjan et al.[1] on the potential uses of nickel–titanium alloys for dentistry, pioneering feasibility studies for orthodontics were performed by George Andreasen et al.[2,3] This work led to the commercial development of the first NiTi alloy for orthodontics (Nitinol) by the Unitek Corporation (now 3M Unitek, Monrovia, CA). The mechanical properties of this alloy, along with its notable clinical applications, were presented in a classic article by Andreasen and Morrow.[4] Particularly important were the very low elastic modulus and very wide elastic working range of the NiTi alloy, compared with stainless steel, which was the major orthodontic wire alloy for clinical use at that time.

Subsequently, Harmeet Walia thought that this nickel–titanium (NiTi: see next section) alloy might have enormous potential for endodontic files, because its very low elastic modulus would permit the negotiation of curved root canals with much greater facility than stainless steel instruments available at the time. Using special large-diameter orthodontic wires contributed by the Unitek Corporation, Quality Dental Products (Johnson City, TN) fabricated the first prototype NiTi hand files by machining rather than the conventional manner of twisting the tapered stainless steel wire blanks. The properties of these first NiTi files in bending and torsion were compared with those for stainless steel hand files of the same size manufactured by a similar machining process. The highly promising initial results of these pioneering laboratory studies were first presented by Walia et al.[5] at the annual meeting of the International Association for Dental Research in 1987, and a more complete description of this work was published the next year in a seminal article in the *Journal of Endodontics*.[6] Subsequently, more information about torsional ductility, which was superior to that for machined stainless steel instruments,[5,6] and cutting ability of the NiTi hand files, was reported by Walia et al.[7] at the 1989 annual meeting of the American Association for Endodontists.

Based on these promising research results, innovative dental manufacturers began to market NiTi endodontic instruments in the 1990s. A major impetus was the merger of Quality Dental Products with Tulsa Dental Products (now Dentsply Tulsa Dental, Tulsa, OK), and this latter company introduced Pro-File NiTi rotary files in 1993. Subsequently, many other manufacturers introduced NiTi rotary instruments for endodontics, and studies of the properties and performance of these instruments became an intensive area for endodontics research. In January 2007, PubMed listed over 350 articles dealing with various aspects of the NiTi endodontic instruments since their inception.

Mechanical Behavior and NiTi Phases for Nickel–Titanium Alloys

The NiTi alloy used in orthodontics and endodontics was developed by Buehler and associates. This alloy was termed "Nitinol" from *ni*ckel, *ti*tanium, and the *N*aval *O*rdnance *L*aboratory, the site of this development work that is described in a classic review article by Buehler and Wang.[8] The alloy is based on the NiTi intermetallic compound and can exhibit superelastic behavior (termed "pseudoelastic" in materials science) and shape memory with appropriate processing conditions.[9] Because of the difference in atomic weights of nickel and titanium, the equiatomic NiTi alloy composition is 55 wt% Ni and 45 wt% Ti.

When a superelastic NiTi wire is loaded in tension, normal elastic behavior initially occurs. With further tensile loading, the elastic stress reaches a certain level at which there is an extended horizontal region of elastic strain (upper superelastic plateau). Up to about 10% elastic strain can occur in a superelastic NiTi orthodontic wire at this constant stress.[10] During subsequent tensile unloading, the alloy will exhibit a horizontal region of elastic strain at a lower stress (lower superelastic plateau) on the stress–strain plot. With further unloading, the strain reaches the end of the lower superelastic plateau, and the final portion on the stress–strain plot again corresponds to the linear elastic unloading.

Khier et al.[11] compared the bending properties of superelastic and nonsuperelastic NiTi orthodontic

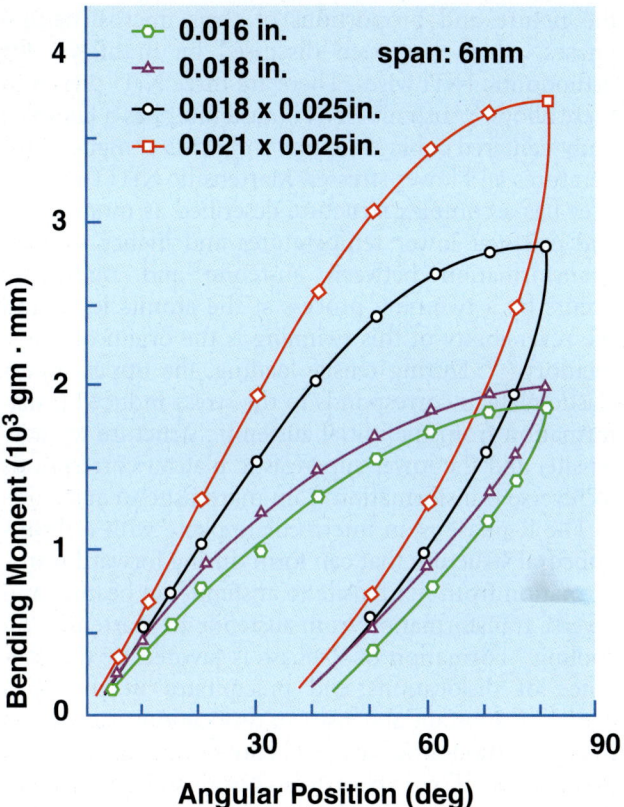

Figure 2 Cantilever bending plots for 6 mm test spans of four different sizes of the nonsuperelastic NiTi alloy Nitinol (3M Unitek). Reprinted from Khier et al.[11] with permission from the American Association of Orthodontists.

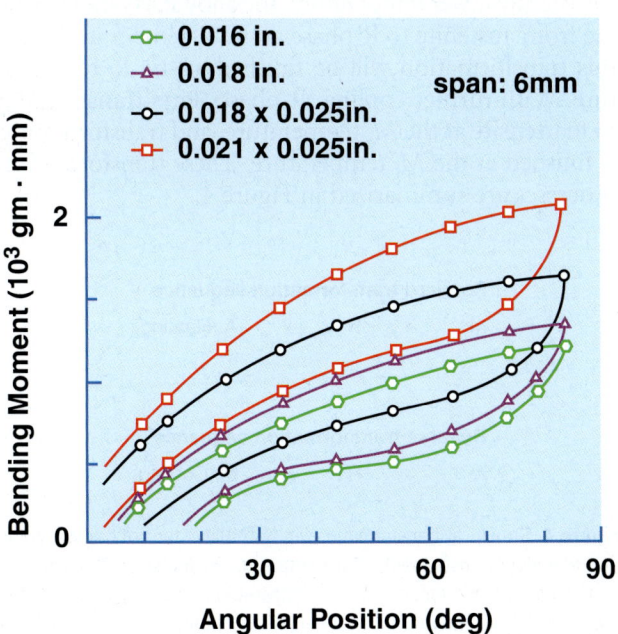

Figure 1 Cantilever bending plots for 6 mm test spans of four different sizes of the superelastic NiTi alloy Nitinol SE (3M Unitek). Reprinted from Khier et al.[11] with permission from the American Association of Orthodontists.

wires. For elastic bending of superelastic NiTi orthodontic wires having clinically relevant test spans, the upper and lower superelastic plateaus are less well defined (Figure 1), because stress varies linearly over the cross-section. The regions on the bending plots that correspond to these plateaus have greater slopes for nonsuperelastic NiTi wires, such as the original 3M Unitek Nitinol orthodontic wire (Figure 2). If the superelastic alloy is loaded in tension to a value of strain beyond the upper plateau region, there will be some permanent strain after unloading. This permanent strain will be greater for a nonsuperelastic NiTi wire having the same dimensions and loaded to the same overall strain as the superelastic wire. By contrast, a NiTi wire alloy that exhibits shape memory behavior in the oral environment will have no residual permanent strain after unloading from beyond the upper plateau region; the wire will completely return to its initial dimensions before loading.[9]

The mechanical behavior of the superelastic, nonsuperelastic, and shape memory NiTi alloys arises from the nature and proportions of their microstructural phases, which has been discussed by Brantley[12] for orthodontic NiTi wires. There are three NiTi phases in these alloys.[9] Austenitic NiTi (austenite) has a complex body-centered cubic structure, and exists at higher temperatures and lower stresses. Martensitic NiTi (martensite) has a complex structure described as monoclinic, and exists at lower temperatures and higher stresses. Transformation between austenite and martensite occurs by a twinning process at the atomic level, and the reversibility of this twinning is the origin of shape memory.[9,12] During tensile loading, the upper superelastic plateau corresponds to the stress-induced transformation from the initial austenitic structure to martensite, and the lower superelastic plateau corresponds to reverse transformation from martensite to austenite.

The R-phase is an intermediate phase with a rhombohedral structure that can form during forward transformation from martensite to austenite on heating and reverse transformation from austenite to martensite on cooling.[9] Formation of R-phase is favored by the presence of dislocations and precipitates in the NiTi alloy.[13] A substantial density of dislocations is expected in NiTi orthodontic wires and endodontic instruments, because the alloy experiences considerable permanent deformation during the manufacturing processes. Because of the relatively narrow range of the equiatomic NiTi phase field in the nickel–titanium phase diagram at low temperatures, Ti_2Ni and Ni_3Ti precipitates are expected in Ti-rich and Ni-rich alloys, respectively.[14] Oxide particles also form during processing of the NiTi alloy by manufacturers.[9] Such nickel–titanium oxide precipitates have been observed by Alapati et al.[15] on the cutting tip of a rotary instrument (Figure 3) and were presumably elongated during the manufacturing process for the starting wire blank.

Several phase transformation temperatures are important: A_s, the starting temperature for transformation to austenite; A_f, the temperature at which transformation to austenite is finished; M_s, the starting temperature for transformation to martensite; and M_f, the temperature at which transformation to martensite is finished. The R_s and R_f temperatures for transformations involving the R-phase are defined in a similar manner.

If a NiTi orthodontic wire or endodontic instrument is cooled to a sufficiently low temperature (shown in later differential scanning calorimetry [DSC] plots), it will consist entirely of martensite. Upon heating, martensite will start transforming to R-phase at the R_s temperature, and this transformation will be finished at the R_f temperature. With further heating, R-phase starts transforming to austenite at the A_s temperature, and transformation is finished at the A_f temperature. Alternatively, if the NiTi orthodontic wire or endodontic instrument is heated above the A_f temperature, it will be converted entirely to austenite. Then, upon cooling to sufficiently lower temperature, the alloy starts transforming from austenite to R-phase at the R_s temperature, and this transformation will be finished at the R_f temperature. With further cooling, R-phase starts transforming to martensite at the M_s temperature, and transformation is finished at the M_f temperature. These transformation processes are summarized in Figure 4.

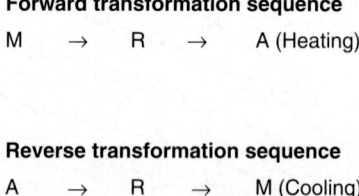

Forward transformation sequence

M → R → A (Heating)

Reverse transformation sequence

A → R → M (Cooling)

Figure 4 Structural transformations in NiTi alloys for orthodontic wires and endodontic instruments: M, martensite; R, R-phase; A, austenite. Beginning with martensite at low temperatures, starting temperatures are R_s and A_s for forward transformations on heating, which are finished at R_f and A_f temperatures. Beginning with austenite at high temperatures, starting temperatures are R_s and M_s for reverse transformations on cooling, which are finished at R_f and M_f temperatures. Starting and finishing temperatures for the same transformation can be different for heating and cooling.

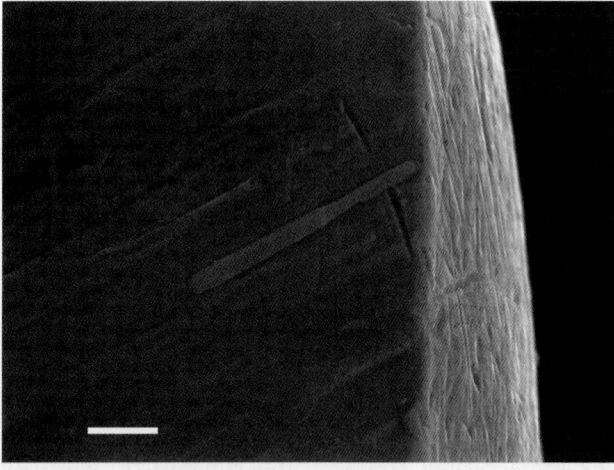

Figure 3 SEM photograph of the cutting tip for a LightSpeed instrument after one simulated clinical use, showing elongated nickel-titanium oxide precipitates and flattening of the rollover. Scale bar length is 5 μm. Reprinted from Alapati et al.[15] with permission from the American Association of Endodontists.

Use of Differential Scanning Calorimetry to Study Nickel–Titanium Alloys

DSC can be used to easily determine the transformation temperature ranges (TTRs) for NiTi phases and enthalpy changes in NiTi alloys.[16,17] A test sample is heated or cooled at the same rate (typically 10°C/min) as an inert control material. The difference in thermal energy to heat both materials at this rate is plotted as heat flow per unit sample weight (W/g) as a function of temperature. Bradley et al.[18] used DSC to compare superelastic, nonsuperelastic, and shape memory NiTi orthodontic wires.

In their first published article on the use of DSC to investigate NiTi rotary instruments, Brantley et al.[19] compared ProFile (Dentsply Tulsa Dental) and Light-Speed (LightSpeed Technology, San Antonio, TX) instruments in the as-received condition. Figure 5 presents heating and cooling DSC plots for a test sample consisting of several segments from an as-received ProFile instrument. The temperature range from –75°C to 75°C is shown. The lower curve is for the initial heating cycle and the upper curve is for the subsequent cooling cycle. Exothermic reactions are represented by peaks in the upward direction. The two endothermic peaks on the heating curve correspond to initial transformation from martensite to R-phase (M → R), followed by transformation from R-phase to austenite (R → A). This latter transformation is completed at an A_f temperature of approximately 25°C, so the as-received instrument will be in the superelastic condition at 37°C, which Thompson reported to be desired by manufacturers.[20] (Some investigators determine the A_f temperature from the intersection of a tangent line to the right side of the peak with an extension of the adjacent baseline, which gives a lower value.) A single exothermic peak is observed on the cooling curve, because the peaks associated with the reverse transformations of A → R followed by R → M could not be resolved.

Figure 6 presents DSC plots for the tip segment from another as-received ProFile instrument (Dentsply Tulsa Dental) in a subsequent study by Brantley et al.,[21] investigating instruments subjected to simulated clinical use. This test sample was also in the superelastic condition, but the A_f temperature on the heating curve was less than 0°C. The endothermic peak on the heating curve corresponds to the M → R transformation, followed by R → A, which could not be resolved as two separate peaks. The weaker broad exothermic peak over the same temperature range on the cooling curve corresponds to the reverse transformations of A → R, followed by R → M. The broad low-temperature peak has been reported by Brantley et al.[22] to arise from twinning within martensite, and similar low-temperature peaks have been observed by Brantley et al.[23,24] in NiTi orthodontic wires, using temperature-modulated DSC.

Figure 7 presents DSC plots for the tip segment of a ProFile instrument, from the same batch as the

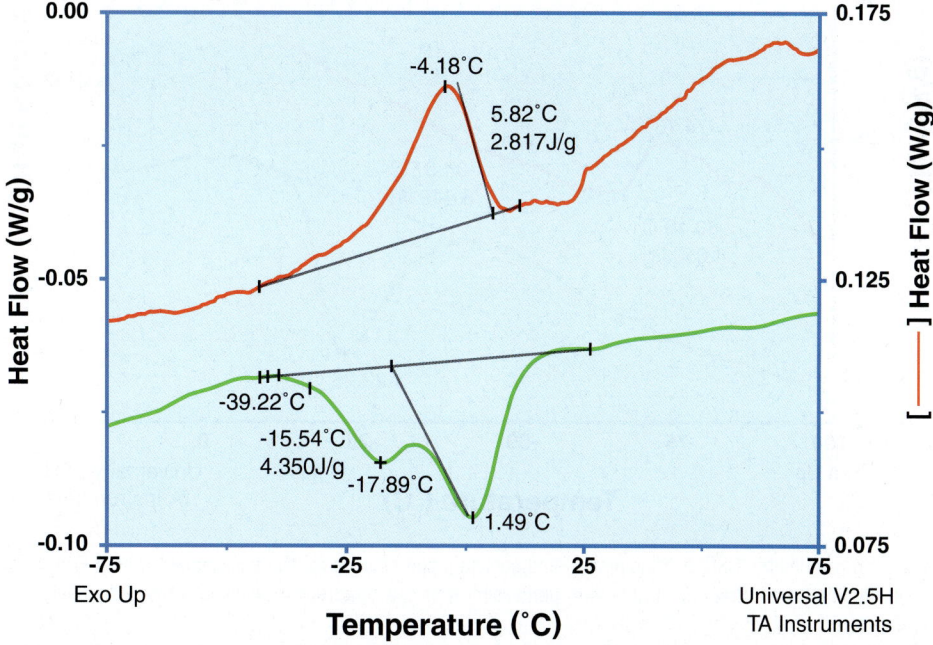

Figure 5 Differential scanning calorimetry (DSC) heating (lower) and cooling (upper) curves for a test sample of several segments from one as-received ProFile NiTi instrument. Reprinted from Brantley et al.[19] with permission from the American Association of Endodontists.

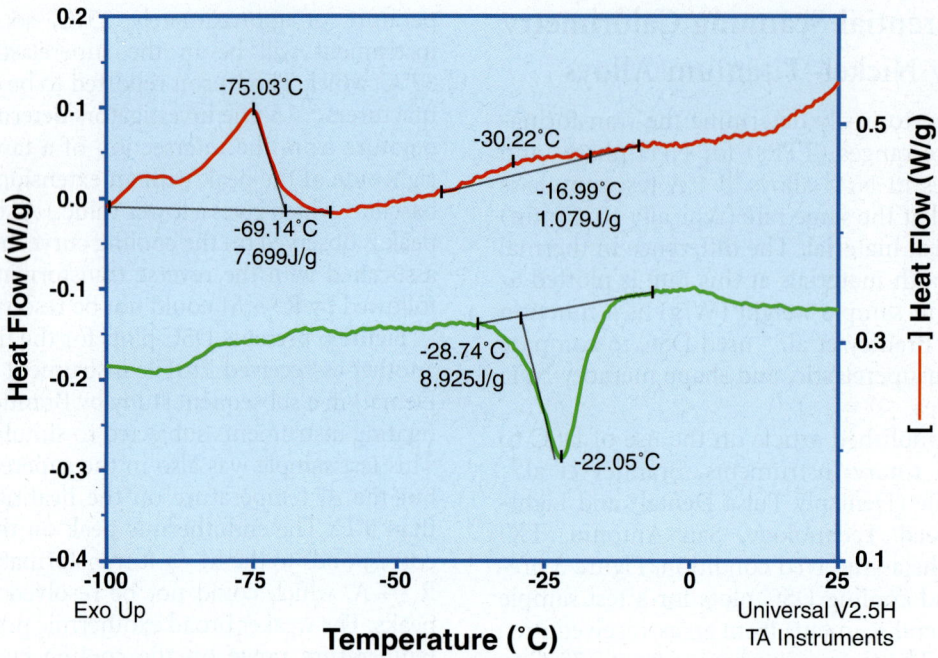

Figure 6 Differential scanning calorimetry (DSC) heating (lower) and cooling (upper) curves for the tip segment from another as-received ProFile instrument. Reprinted from Brantley et al.[21] with permission from the American Association of Endodontists.

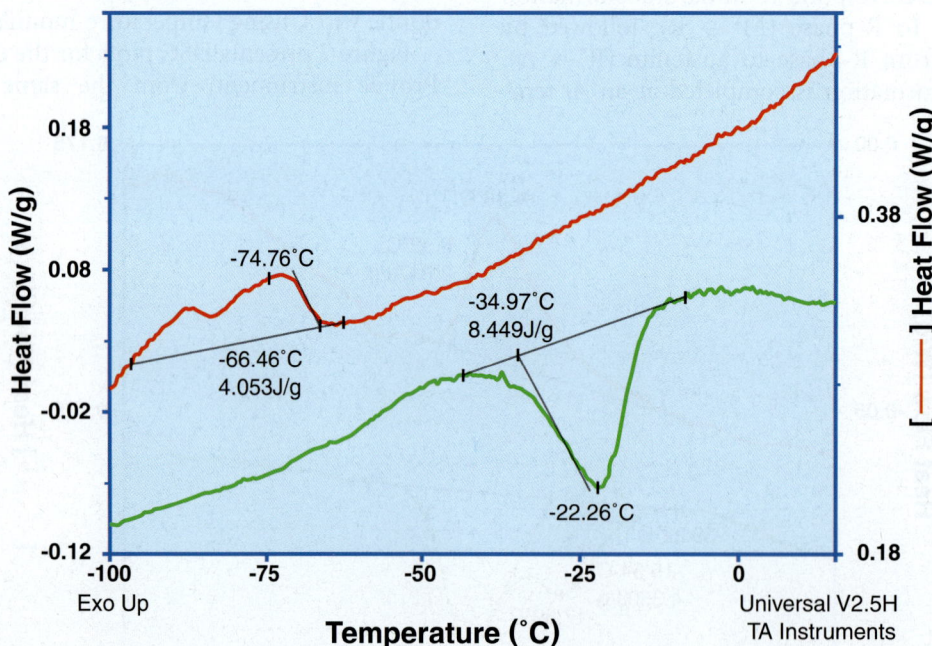

Figure 7 Differential scanning calorimetry (DSC) heating (lower) and cooling (upper) curves for the tip segment from a ProFile instrument subjected to one simulated clinical use. Reprinted from Brantley et al.[21] with permission from the American Association of Endodontists.

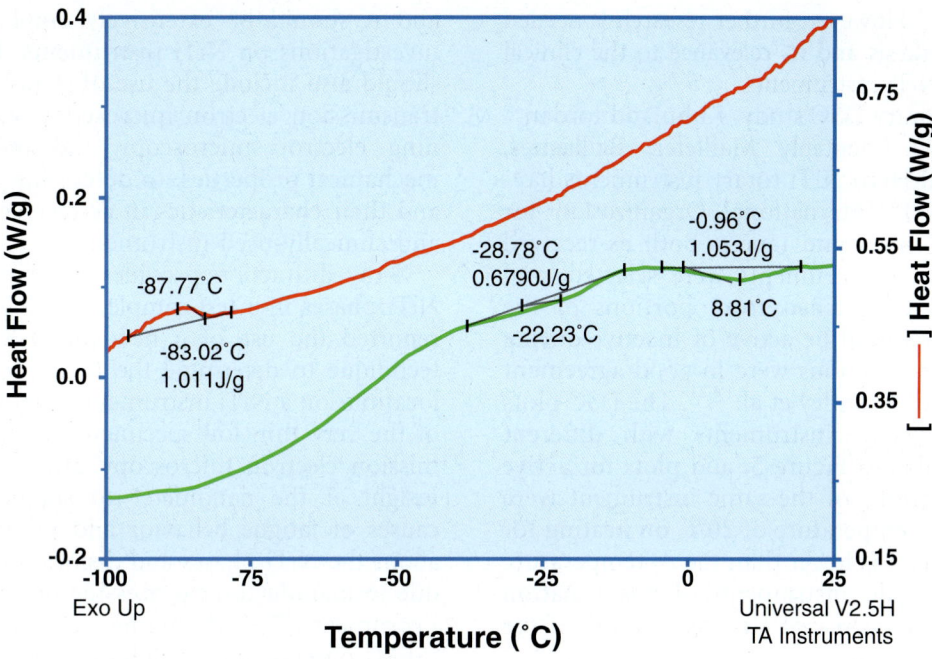

Figure 8 Differential scanning calorimetry (DSC) heating (lower) and cooling (upper) curves for the tip segment from a LightSpeed instrument subjected to one simulated clinical use. Reprinted from Brantley et al.[21] with permission from the American Association of Endodontists.

instrument for Figure 6, which had been subjected to one simulated clinical use.[21] Similar DSC plots were obtained for tip segments from other ProFile instruments in this batch, which had been subjected to three and five simulated clinical uses. After one, three, and five simulated clinical uses, the tip segments still remained in the superelastic condition, with the A_f temperature on the heating curve less than 0°C. Thus, DSC was unable to detect effects from up to five simulated clinical uses on the tip segments of these instruments.

Figure 8 shows DSC plots for the tip segment from a LightSpeed NiTi rotary instrument that had been subjected to one simulated clinical use.[21] This tip segment is also in the superelastic condition, because the A_f temperature on the heating DSC curve is less than 25°C. There were minimal differences compared with Figure 8 for the DSC plots from tip segments of other LightSpeed instruments from the same batch that were subjected to three and five simulated clinical uses, as well as with DSC plots from the tip segment of an as-received LightSpeed instrument.[21] Interestingly, the DSC plots for a test sample consisting of several segments for a LightSpeed instrument from a different batch were similar to Figure 5 for an as-received ProFile instrument.[19]

These two DSC studies by Brantley et al.[19,21] showed that there are substantial differences in the character of the NiTi phases for segments taken from different portions of the same rotary NiTi instrument. Moreover, evident batch effects were observed in the DSC plots for instruments from the same manufacturer. The DSC results also indicated that the stresses experienced by a rotary instrument during manufacturing vary with position along its axis and that there may be differences in the manufacturing procedure and starting NiTi alloy. Nevertheless, regardless of the considerably different character of the various DSC plots,[19,21] test samples from the ProFile and LightSpeed instruments, in either the as-received condition or after simulated clinical use, always displayed superelastic behavior at 37°C, although there were relatively large differences in the A_f values for test samples.

From these DSC studies,[19,21] it is tempting to assume that the optimum microstructure for superelastic NiTi rotary instruments would have the maximum amount of austenite that could reversibly transform to martensite, with a large enthalpy change (peak area). When there is substantial stable work-hardened martensite in the microstructure, the enthalpy change for reversible transformation to austenite is much smaller.[18,23] However, further research is needed to test this hypothesis and its relevance to the clinical performance of NiTi instruments.

In a contemporary DSC study, Kuhn and Jordan[25] analyzed ProFile (Dentsply Maillefer, Baillagues, Switzerland) and Hero NiTi rotary instruments having different ISO (International Organization for Standardization) sizes and tapers. Both as-received and clinically used instruments were selected, and test samples were obtained from portions of the instruments that would be active or inactive during cutting. Their observations were in good agreement with the results by Brantley et al.[19,21]. The DSC plots for as-received Hero instruments with different tapers were similar to Figure 5, and plots for active and inactive portions of the same instrument were different. The A_f temperature of 20°C on heating for Hero instruments was lower than the A_f temperature of 35°C for ProFile instruments. Transformation temperatures were decreased after clinical use of the instruments.

Kuhn and Jordan[25] also studied the effects of heat treatments at six temperatures from 350° to 700°C. Whereas only single peaks were observed on the heating and cooling DSC plots for as-received instruments (interpreted as direct transformations of M → A and A → M, respectively), the DSC plots were altered for annealed test samples. Heat treatments below 510°C resulted in two DSC peaks during heating (M → R followed by R → A) and two peaks during cooling (A → R followed by R → M). After heat treatments above 510°C, one peak was observed during heating (interpreted as M → A) and one peak during cooling (interpreted as A → M). Heat treatment shifted the martensite transformation to lower temperatures. When heat treatment was performed at 600°C, recrystallization of the NiTi microstructure occurred in the instruments, as previously found for NiTi orthodontic wires.[12] Kuhn and Jordan[25] observed that heat treatments below 600°C caused test samples to have increased bending flexibility, whereas flexibility was decreased by heat treatments above 600°C. They recommended that heat treatment at 400°C, corresponding to the recovery annealing stage before recrystallization,[12] be utilized by manufacturers prior to machining the NiTi instruments to decrease the work hardening of the alloy.

Alapati et al.[26] have recently reported the first use of temperature-modulated DSC to investigate heat-treated NiTi rotary instruments. This technique provides much greater resolution about the complex structural transformations in the NiTi orthodontic wires than is possible with conventional DSC,[23,24] and it should be extensively employed for future investigations on NiTi instruments. Future research should also include the use of X-ray diffraction and transmission electron microscopy, along with scanning electron microscopy and measurements of mechanical properties, to determine the NiTi phases and their characteristics in as-received, heat-treated, and clinically-used instruments.

X-ray diffraction provides information about the NiTi phases in a test sample, and Iijima et al.[27] have reported the use of a new micro-X-ray diffraction technique to determine the NiTi phases at different locations on a NiTi instrument. Although preparation of the very thin foil specimens is challenging, transmission electron microscopy can be used to obtain insight at the nanometer to submicron level into causes of fatigue behavior and provide information about the NiTi phases and dislocation configurations due to manufacturer processing or clinical use of the instruments.[28–30] Scanning electron microscopic (SEM) observations of polished and etched test samples can show whether the rotary instrument has a conventional wrought microstructure or provide evidence of heat treatment that caused recrystallization to yield equiaxed grains.[12] Vickers hardness measurements can be used to verify whether the NiTi instrument is in the superelastic condition and to investigate the extent of work hardening.[12,31]

As another example of combining experimental techniques, Miyai et al.[32] recently investigated torsional and bending properties of EndoWave, Hero 642, K3, ProFile .06, and ProTaper instruments and found that their functional properties (particularly flexible bending load level) were related to phase transformation behavior determined by DSC. Transformation temperatures for Hero and K3 instruments were significantly lower than for EndoWave, ProFile, and ProTaper instruments. However, the clinical significance and predictability from such DSC results for performance of the NiTi instruments remain to be established in future research.

Effects of Heat Sterilization on Properties of Nickel–Titanium Instruments

There have been numerous laboratory studies of NiTi instruments subjected to multiple heat sterilization cycles. Repeated sterilization has been found by Silvaggio and Hicks[33] and Canalda-Sahli et al.[34] to cause changes in torsion and bending properties, and by Rapisarda et al.[35] and Schäfer[36] to affect cutting efficiency. However, Hilt et al.[37] found no effects on the torsional properties, hardness, and microstructure of NiTi files from the number of sterilization cycles and the type of autoclave sterilization.

Whereas Mize et al.[38] found that repeated heat sterilization did not affect the number of cycles for fatigue failure, Chaves Craveiro de Melo et al.[39] and Viana et al.[40] reported that repeated heat sterilization caused substantial increases in the number of cycles for failure. These observations indicate the necessity of having a standard technique for evaluation of the fatigue behavior of NiTi instruments.

Recent DSC studies by Alexandrou et al.[41] have shown that after 11 sterilization cycles, ProFile and Flexmaster instruments had the completely austenitic structure needed for superelastic behavior in the oral environment. Alexandrou et al.[42] also found that after 11 sterilization cycles, the Mani NRT instruments were either austenite or a mixture of austenite and R-phase at 37°C and concluded that these instruments are also capable of superelastic behavior under clinical conditions.

In future studies, it would be worthwhile to compare etched microstructures of the NiTi alloy for instruments subjected to multiple heat sterilization cycles with etched microstructures for as-received instruments to determine whether changes occurred in the original wrought structure due to the sterilization cycles. Comparison of the X-ray diffraction patterns and Vickers hardness for sterilized and as-received instruments would reveal[12,27,31] whether sterilization caused relief of the residual stresses present in the as-received instruments from the manufacturing process. Such residual stresses may contribute to the clinical failure of the NiTi instruments.

Failure of Nickel–Titanium Instruments and Failure Mechanisms

The manufacturing process of machining the NiTi rotary instruments from starting wire blanks[20] results in rollover at the edges of the flutes[6] and a variety of surface defects.[6,43–45] Machining grooves, microcracks, and surface debris are evident when as-received instruments are examined with a scanning electron microscope, and instrument fracture generally occurs at surface defects.

Recent extensive clinical studies by Knowles et al.[46] for LightSpeed instruments and by Di Fiore et al.[47] for ProFile, ProTaper, ProFile GT, and K3 Endo instruments reported separation (fracture) rates of less than 1.5% and much less than 1%, respectively. No statistically significant difference in incidence of fracture was found for the ProFile, ProTaper, ProFile GT, and K3 Endo instruments.[47] Although these rates are very low and justify the widespread use of rotary NiTi instruments, clinical failures are sources of anguish for both the patient and endodontist. Accordingly, there have been substantial research efforts to characterize the instrument failures and determine their origins and to develop new instruments that would minimize the occurrence of failures.

One contributing mechanism for clinical failure of NiTi instruments, reported by Alapati et al.,[48] may be the widening of surface machining grooves by tenacious dentin debris deposits. The SEM photograph in Figure 9 shows an example of this phenomenon for a clinically fractured ProTaper instrument. The potential role of dentin debris for failure of rotary NiTi instruments requires further study.

Alapati et al.[49] have also performed an extensive SEM study of clinically failed NiTi rotary instruments to characterize the major aspects of their fracture processes. Instruments generally appeared to exhibit

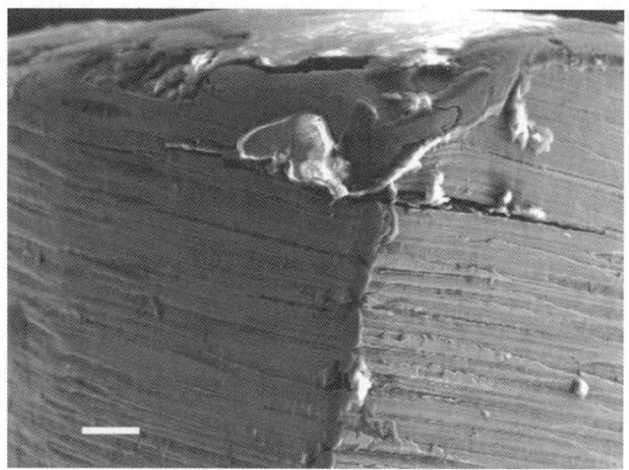

Figure 9 SEM photograph of a clinically fractured ProTaper instrument showing a widened machining groove containing dentin debris that was close to the area in which the fracture occurred. Scale bar length is 22 μm. Reprinted from Alapati et al.[48] with permission from the American Association of Endodontists.

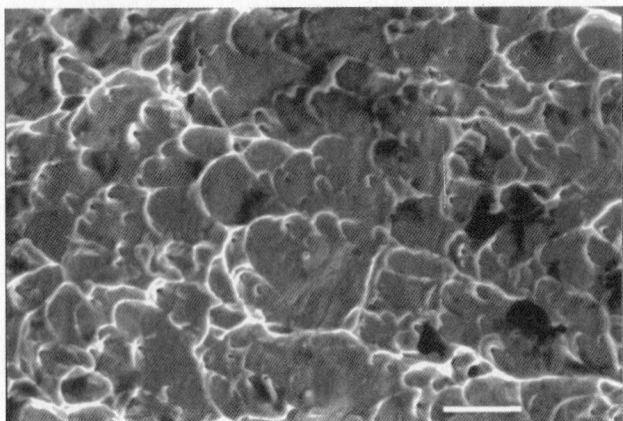

Figure 10 Secondary electron image of the fracture surface of a ProTaper rotary instrument that failed during clinical use, showing elongated dimples indicative of ductile fracture and secondary phase particles that may be nickel-titanium oxides. Scale bar length is 6 μm. Reprinted from Alapati et al.[49] with permission from the American Association of Endodontists.

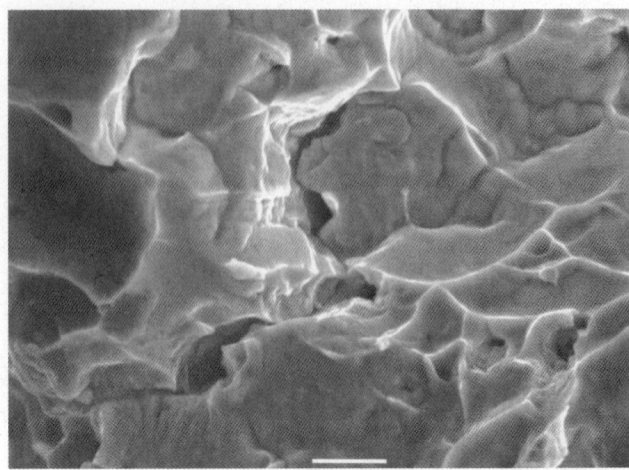

Figure 11 SEM photograph of the fracture surface of a ProFile GT instrument that failed during clinical use, showing transgranular (cleavage) fracture and intergranular fracture along grain boundaries. Scale bar length is 3 μm. Reprinted from Alapati et al.[49] with permission from the American Association of Endodontists.

ductile fracture, rather than brittle fracture, as shown in Figure 10 of a clinically fractured ProTaper instrument,[49] where the surface has the characteristic dimpled appearance for ductile fracture.[50,51] SEM observations at high magnification show that these dimples are nucleated at secondary phase particles in the microstructure, such as nickel–titanium oxides.[9] The volume fraction of such particles may indicate the quality of the starting NiTi wire alloy used for manufacturing the instruments.

An example of a more complex fracture surface is shown for a clinically failed ProFile GT instrument in Figure 11.[49] Transgranular fracture occurred across the fine grains in this microstructure, as well as intergranular fracture along some grain boundaries. Voids or regions of separation between some grains can also be seen in Figure 11 and suggest the loss of small grains, subgrains, or secondary phase particles during the fracture process.[49] Although this rotary instrument may have experienced overall ductile fracture during clinical failure, the features in Figure 11 do not resemble those for ductile fracture in Figure 10.

Two other major failure processes, excessive torsional deformation without separation and axial fracture, were observed by Alapati et al.[49] for these clinically retrieved NiTi rotary instruments. Permanent torsional deformation, giving an "unfluted appearance," and permanent bending deformation without instrument separation, as well as instruments that fractured in these modes, under clinical conditions, have been observed by other investigators.[44,52–56] The axial fracture mode for clinically retrieved instruments[49] involved crack propagation in a direction approximately parallel to the flutes that connected pitted regions on the surface. These pits may have been former sites of secondary phase particles.

Alapati et al.[49] did not observe the characteristic striations[50,51] for cyclic fatigue on the fracture surfaces of clinically failed NiTi instruments, presumably because the instrumentation time before fracture of the retrieved instruments was insufficiently long. These investigators concluded that separation of the used instruments, retrieved for their study, was generally caused by a single overload event that resulted in ductile fracture. By contrast, Cheung et al.[55] observed striations indicative of fatigue failure for numerous ProTaper instruments that had fractured during clinical use, and these authors concluded that fatigue failure is an important mode of separation during clinical instrumentation. An example of the fine-scale striations is shown in Figure 12 from a laboratory study by Luebke et al.[57] of

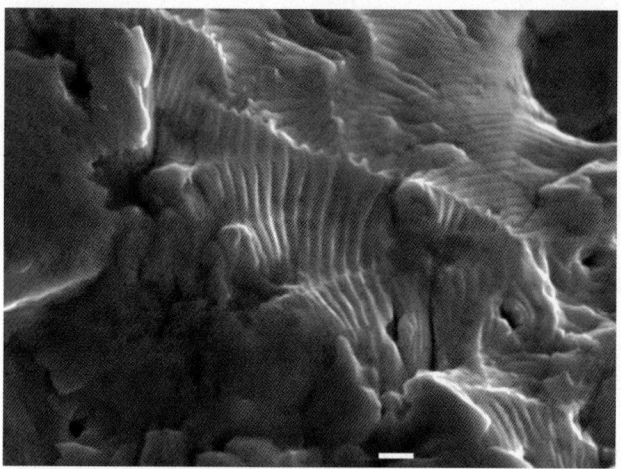

Figure 12 SEM photomicrograph of the in vitro fracture surface of a NiTi Gates Glidden drill tested to failure in bending fatigue, showing fine striations that form during fatigue crack propagation. Scale bar length is 0.7 μm. Reprinted from Luebke et al.[57] with permission from the American Association of Endodontists.

NiTi Gates Glidden drills subjected to cyclic cantilever bending.

In summary, numerous studies have shown that NiTi alloys for rotary instruments can possess significant ductility in bending and torsion, without experiencing separation in certain clinical cases, where the canals have substantial curvature or where rotation of the tip is hindered. Fracture initiation often appears to occur at machining grooves, with a possible role from retained dentin debris in these grooves. Retrieved instruments, which failed during clinical use, may fracture from cyclic fatigue after longer periods of use or from single overload events after relatively brief periods of use. Clearly, the manufacturing process for NiTi rotary instruments and the need for a starting NiTi wire alloy of high metallurgical quality are major factors for reducing the incidence of clinical failure of these instruments.

Strategies for Improved Nickel–Titanium Instruments

Several strategies have been employed to develop NiTi instruments that should have improved clinical performance. These strategies have included electropolishing the machined surfaces, ion implantation to create harder surfaces, and use of special surface coatings. Research has also suggested that heat treatment of these instruments may yield beneficial results.

Tripi et al.[58] recently compared the effects of instrument design and surface treatment on the cyclic fatigue of ProFile, RaCe, K3, Hero, and Mtwo instruments. While the best fatigue resistance was found for the ProFile instruments, the electropolishing surface treatment for RaCe instruments increased their fatigue resistance by reducing the presence of microcracks, surface debris, and other machining damage.

Lee et al.[59] first proposed the application of ion implantation to NiTi instruments. They reported that boron-ion implantation more than doubled the surface hardness of Nitinol at the nanoindentation depth of 0.05 μm, yielding a hardness value greater than that of stainless steel.

Rapisarda et al.[60] subsequently employed both a thermal nitriding technique and nitrogen-ion implantation to increase the wear resistance of NiTi instruments. The ion-implanted samples had a higher N:Ti ratio, which suggested the presence of a titanium nitride layer. Both the thermal-nitrided and nitrogen-ion-implanted instruments had higher wear resistance and increased cutting ability in acrylic blocks compared with control instruments without surface modifications. An SEM study of nitrogen-ion-implanted instruments by these investigators[61] revealed the absence of surface wear and morphology changes that occurred in control instruments after the same period of simulated clinical use.

Schäfer[36] used a physical vapor deposition (PVD) process to create a TiN surface coating on NiTi instruments. Surface-coated instruments had greater cutting efficiency (penetration into plastic samples with cylindrical canals) compared with control instruments, and their cutting efficiency was not altered by repeated autoclave or sodium hypochlorite sterilization.

Lastly, use of heat treatments for the NiTi instruments, or general modifications in proprietary thermomechanical processing procedures for the starting wire blanks, may provide other strategies.[62] It has been noted that Kuhn and Jordan[25] explored the use of heat treatments at temperatures ranging from 350° to 700°C. They concluded that annealing around 400°C yields a suitable proportion of NiTi microstructural phases and a beneficial effect (limiting brittleness) on the mechanical properties of these instruments. Previous research on NiTi orthodontic wires has shown that heat treatment at 400°C does not affect the bending properties of superelastic wires, whereas heat treatment at 600°C causes loss of superelastic behavior.[10,11] Heat treatment for 10 minutes at 500°C had minimal effect on the cantilever bending plots, but 2 hours of heat treatment at this temperature decreased the average superelastic bending moment during unloading of the wire test span.

Heat treatment can alter the phase transformation temperatures for the NiTi alloy, such as reduction of the M_s temperature to subambient levels to yield a completely austenitic structure at room temperature.[12] Heat treatment within only the recovery annealing stage for the NiTi alloy would reduce residual stresses of potential importance for fracture behavior without altering the microstructure. Presumably, heat treatment at temperatures of 600°C and higher, causing recrystallization of the wrought microstructure,[12,25] should be avoided for the rotary instruments. Given the special nature of the NiTi alloy phases and their transformations,[9] one can envision the future development of complex thermomechanical processing cycles to optimize the starting NiTi wire blanks or new heat treatments to improve the cutting efficiency and fatigue resistance of the instruments after machining from these blanks.

References

1. Civjan S, Huget EF, DeSimon LB. Potential applications of certain nickel-titanium (Nitinol) alloys. J Dent Res 1975;54:89–96.
2. Andreasen GF, Brady PR. A use hypothesis for 55 nitinol wire for orthodontics. Angle Orthod 1972;42:172–7.
3. Andreasen GF, Hilleman TB. An evaluation of 55 cobalt substituted nitinol wire for use in orthodontics. J Am Dent Assoc 1971;82:1373–5.
4. Andreasen GF, Morrow RE. Laboratory and clinical analyses of nitinol wire. Am J Orthod 1978;73:142–51.
5. Walia H, Brantley W, Gerstein H, Arpaio J. New metallurgy root canal files. J Dent Res 1987;66(Special Issue):349, Abstract No. 1943.
6. Walia H, Brantley WA, Gerstein H. An initial investigation of the bending and torsional properties of Nitinol root canal files. J Endod 1988;14:346–51.
7. Walia H, Costas J, Brantley W, Gerstein H. Torsional ductility and cutting efficiency of the Nitinol file. J Endod 1989;15:174 [Abstract 22].
8. Buehler WJ, Wang FE. A summary of recent research on the nitinol alloys and their potential application in ocean engineering. Ocean Eng 1968;1:105–20.
9. Duerig TW, Melton KN, Stöckel D, Wayman CM, editors. Engineering aspects of shape memory alloys. London: Butterworth-Heinemann; 1990. pp. 3–45, 369–93.
10. Miura F, Mogi M, Ohura Y, Hamanaka H. The super-elastic property of the Japanese NiTi alloy wire for use in orthodontics. Am J Orthod Dentofacial Orthop 1986;90:1–10.
11. Khier SE, Brantley WA, Fournelle RA. Bending properties of superelastic and nonsuperelastic nickel-titanium orthodontic wires. Am J Orthod Dentofacial Orthop 1991;99:310–128.
12. Brantley WA. Orthodontic wires. In: Brantley WA, Eliades T, editors. Orthodontic materials: scientific and clinical aspects. Stuttgart: Thieme; 2001. pp. 15–21, 84–97.
13. Miyazaki S, Otsuka K. Development of shape memory alloys. Iron Steel Inst Jpn Int 1989;29:353–77.
14. Goldstein D, Kabacoff L, Tydings J. Stress effects on nitinol phase transformations. J Metals 1987;39:19–26.
15. Alapati SB, Brantley WA, Svec TA, et al. Scanning electron microscope observations of new and used nickel-titanium rotary files. J Endod 2003;29:667–9.
16. Todoroki T, Tamura H. Effect of heat treatment after cold working on the phase transformation in TiNi alloy. Trans Jpn Inst Metals 1987;28:83–94.
17. Yoneyama T, Doi H, Hamanaka H, et al. Super-elasticity and thermal behavior of Ni-Ti alloy orthodontic arch wires. Dent Mater J 1992;11:1–10.
18. Bradley TG, Brantley WA, Culbertson BM. Differential scanning calorimetry (DSC) analyses of superelastic and nonsuperelastic nickel-titanium orthodontic wires. Am J Orthod Dentofacial Orthop 1996;109:589–97.
19. Brantley WA, Svec TA, Iijima M, et al. Differential scanning calorimetric studies of nickel titanium rotary endodontic instruments. J Endod 2002;28:567–72.
20. Thompson SA. An overview of nickel-titanium alloys used in dentistry. Int Endod J 2000;33:297–310.
21. Brantley WA, Svec TA, Iijima M, et al. Differential scanning calorimetric studies of nickel-titanium rotary endodontic instruments after simulated clinical use. J Endod 2002;28:774–8.
22. Brantley WA, Guo WH, Clark WAT, Iijima M. TEM confirmation of low-temperature martensite transformation in nickel-titanium orthodontic wire. J Dent Res 2003;82(Special Issue A): Abstract No. 1535.
23. Brantley WA, Iijima M, Grentzer TH. Temperature-modulated DSC study of phase transformations in nickel-titanium orthodontic wires. Thermochimica Acta 2002;392–3:329–37.
24. Brantley WA, Iijima M, Grentzer TH. Temperature-modulated DSC provides new insight about nickel-titanium wire transformations. Am J Orthod Dentofacial Orthop 2003;124:387–94.
25. Kuhn G, Jordan L. Fatigue and mechanical properties of nickel-titanium endodontic instruments. J Endod 2002;28:716–20.
26. Alapati SB, Brantley WA, Schricker SR, et al. Investigation of transformations in used and heat-treated nickel-titanium endodontic instruments. J Dent Res 2006;85(Special Issue A): Abstract No. 38.
27. Iijima M, Brantley WA, Alapati SB, Nusstein JM. Micro-XRD study of nickel-titanium rotary endodontic instruments after

clinical use. J Dent Res 2005;84(Special Issue A): Abstract No. 1479.

28. Guo WH, Brantley WA, Li D, et al. Fatigue studies of high-palladium dental casting alloys: Part II. Transmission electron microscopic observations. J Mater Sci: Mater Med 2002;13:369–74.

29. Guo WH, Brantley WA, Clark WAT, et al. Transmission electron microscopic investigation of a Pd-Ag-In-Sn dental alloy. Biomaterials 2003;24:1705–12.

30. Guo WH, Brantley WA, Clark WAT, et al. Transmission electron microscopic studies of deformed high-palladium dental alloys. Dent Mater 2003;19:334–40.

31. Alapati SB, Brantley WA, Nusstein JM, et al. Vickers hardness investigation of work-hardening in used NiTi rotary instruments. J Endod 2006;32:1191–3.

32. Miyai K, Ebihara A, Hayashi Y, et al. Influence of phase transformation on the torsional and bending properties of nickel-titanium rotary endodontic instruments. Int Endod J 2006;39:119–26.

33. Silvaggio J, Hicks ML. Effect of heat sterilization on the torsional properties of rotary nickel-titanium endodontic files. J Endod 1997;23:731–4.

34. Canalda-Sahli C, Brau-Aguade E, Sentis-Vilalta J. The effect of sterilization on bending and torsional properties of K-files manufactured with different metallic alloys. Int Endod J 1998;31:48–52.

35. Rapisarda E, Bonaccorso A, Tripi TR, Condorelli GG. Effect of sterilization on the cutting efficiency of rotary nickel-titanium endodontic files. Oral Surg Oral Med Oral Pathol Oral Radiol Endod 1999;88:343–7.

36. Schäfer E. Effect of sterilization on the cutting efficiency of PVD-coated nickel-titanium endodontic instruments. Int Endod J 2002;35:867–72.

37. Hilt BR, Cunningham CJ, Shen C, Richards N. Torsional properties of stainless-steel and nickel-titanium files after multiple autoclave sterilizations. J Endod 2000;26:76–80.

38. Mize SB, Clement DJ, Pruett JP, Carnes DL Jr. Effect of sterilization on cyclic fatigue of rotary nickel-titanium endodontic instruments. J Endod 1998;24:843–7.

39. Chaves Craveiro de Melo M, Guiomar de Azevedo Bahia M, Lopes Buono VT. Fatigue resistance of engine-driven rotary nickel-titanium endodontic instruments. J Endod 2002;28:765–9.

40. Viana ACD, Gonzalez BM, Buono VTL, Bahia MGA. Influence of sterilization on mechanical properties and fatigue resistance of nickel-titanium rotary endodontic instruments. Int Endod J 2006;39:709–15.

41. Alexandrou GB, Chrissafis K, Vasiliadis LP, et al. SEM observations and differential scanning calorimetric studies of new and sterilized nickel-titanium rotary endodontic instruments. J Endod 2006;32:675–9.

42. Alexandrou G, Chrissafis K, Vasiliadis L, et al. Effect of heat sterilization on surface characteristics and microstructure of Mani NRT rotary nickel-titanium instruments. Int Endod J 2006;39:770–8.

43. Eggert C, Peters O, Barbakow F. Wear of nickel-titanium Lightspeed instruments evaluated by scanning electron microscopy. J Endod 1999;25:494–7.

44. Sattapan B, Nervo GJ, Palamara JEA, Messer HH. Defects in rotary nickel-titanium files after clinical use. J Endod 2000;26:161–5.

45. Tripi TR, Bonaccorso A, Tripi V, et al. Defects in GT rotary instruments after use: an SEM study. J Endod 2001;27:782–5.

46. Knowles KI, Hammond NB, Biggs SG, Ibarrola JL. Incidence of instrument separation using LightSpeed rotary instruments. J Endod 2006;32:14–16.

47. Di Fiore PM, Genov KA, Komaroff E, et al. Nickel-titanium rotary instrument fracture: a clinical practice assessment. Int Endod J 2006;39:700–8.

48. Alapati SB, Brantley WA, Svec TA, et al. Proposed role of embedded dentin chips for the clinical failure of nickel-titanium rotary instruments. J Endod 2004;30:339–41.

49. Alapati SB, Brantley WA, Svec TA, et al. SEM observations of nickel-titanium rotary endodontic instruments that fractured during clinical use. J Endod 2005;31:40–3.

50. Dieter GE. Mechanical metallurgy. 3rd ed. New York: McGraw-Hill; 1986. pp. 254–6, 262–4, 394–8.

51. Kerlins V, Phillips A. Modes of fracture. In: Metals handbook. Vol 12. 9th ed. Fractography. Metals Park, OH: ASM International; 1987. pp. 12–71.

52. Tygesen YA, Steiman HR, Ciavarro C. Comparison of distortion and separation utilizing ProFile and Pow-R nickel-titanium rotary files. J Endod 2001;27:762–4.

53. Arens FC, Hoen MM, Steiman HR, Dietz GC Jr. Evaluation of single-use rotary nickel-titanium instruments. J Endod 2003;29:664–6.

54. Parashos P, Gordon I, Messer HH. Factors influencing defects of rotary nickel-titanium endodontic instruments after clinical use. J Endod 2004;30:722–5.

55. Cheung GSP, Peng B, Bian Z, et al. Defects in ProTaper S1 instruments after clinical use: fractographic examination. Int Endod J 2005;38:802–9.

56. Shen Y, Cheung GSP, Bian Z, Peng B. Comparison of defects in ProFile and ProTaper systems after clinical use. J Endod 2006;32:61–5.

57. Luebke NH, Brantley WA, Alapati SB, et al. Bending fatigue study of nickel-titanium Gates Glidden drills. J Endod 2005;31:523–5.

58. Tripi TR, Bonaccorso A, Condorelli GG. Cyclic fatigue of different nickel-titanium endodontic rotary instruments. Oral Surg Oral Med Oral Pathol Oral Radiol Endod 2006;102:E106–14.

59. Lee DH, Park B, Saxena A, Serene TP. Enhanced surface hardness by boron implantation in Nitinol alloy. J Endod 1996;22:543–6.

60. Rapisarda E, Bonaccorso A, Tripi TR, et al. The effect of surface treatments of nickel-titanium files on wear and cutting efficiency. Oral Surg Oral Med Oral Pathol Oral Radiol Endod 2000;89:363–8.

61. Rapisarda E, Bonaccorso A, Tripi TR, et al. Wear of nickel-titanium endodontic instruments evaluated by scanning electron microscopy: effect of ion implantation. J Endod 2001;27:588–92.

62. Alapati SB. An investigation of phase transformation mechanisms for nickel-titanium rotary endodontic instruments (PhD dissertation). Columbus, OH: The Ohio State University, 2006.

Chapter 26C

C. Instruments for Cleaning and Shaping

Timothy A. Svec

Instrumentation of the root canal system requires both hand and rotary files. No canal system can or should be instrumented with rotary files alone. The development of hand and engine-driven files will be discussed with an emphasis on nickel–titanium rotary files.

Basic Endodontic Instruments

After the introduction of standardized instruments,[1] about the only changes made were the universal use of stainless rather than carbon steel and the addition of smaller (Nos. 6 and 8) and larger (Nos. 110–150) sizes as well as color coding. It was not until 1976 that the first approved specification for root canal instruments was published (ADA Specification No. 28).

ENDODONTIC INSTRUMENT STANDARDIZATION

In 1959, a new line of standardized instruments and filling material was introduced to the profession:[2]

1. A formula for the diameter and taper in each size of instrument and filling material was agreed on.
2. A formula for a graduated increment in size from one instrument to the next was developed.
3. A new instrument numbering system based on instrument metric diameter was established.

This numbering system, last revised in 2002,[3] using numbers from 6 to 140, is based on the diameter of the instruments in hundredths of a millimeter at the beginning of the tip of the blades, a point called D0 (diameter 1 mm) (Figure 1), and extending up the blades to the most coronal part of the cutting edge at D16 (diameter 2–16 mm in length). Additional revisions are under way to cover instruments constructed with new materials, designs, and tapers greater than 0.02 mm/mm.

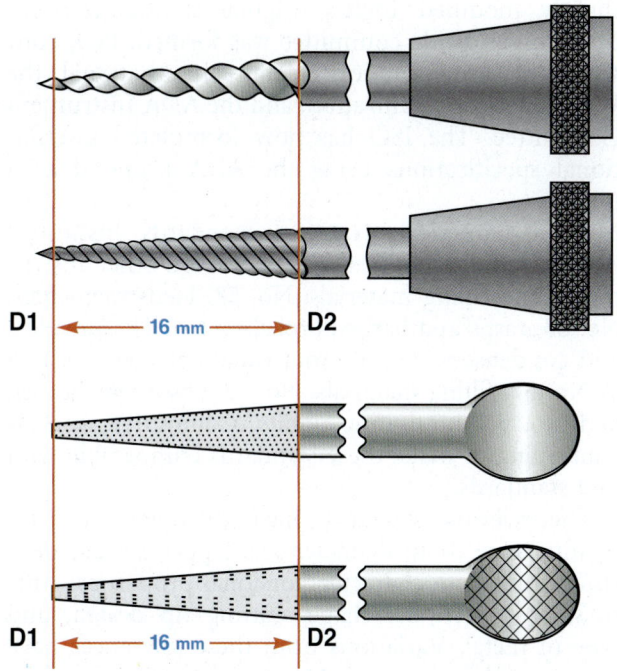

Figure 1 Original recommendation for standardized instruments. Cutting blades 16 mm in length are of the same size and numbers as standardized filling points. The number of the instrument is determined by diameter size at D1 in hundredths of millimeters. Diameter 2 (D2) is uniformly 0.32 mm greater than D1, a gain of 0.02 mm/1 mm of cutting blades. Reproduced with permission from Ingle JI. In Grossman, LI, editor. Transactions of the Second International Conference on Endodontics. Philadelphia: University of Pennsylvania; 1958. p. 123.

Instruments with a taper greater than the ISO (International Standards Organization) standard of 0.02 mm/mm have become popular: 0.04, 0.06, 0.08, 0.10, and 0.12. This means that for every millimeter gain in the length of the cutting blade, the width (taper) of the instrument increases in size by 0.04, 0.06, 0.08, 0.10, or 0.12 of a millimeter rather than the ISO standard of 0.02 mm/mm. These new instruments allow for greater coronal flaring than the 0.02 instruments.

The full extent of the shaft, up to the handle, comes in three lengths: standard, 25 mm; long, 31 mm; and short, 21 mm. The long instruments are often necessary when treating canines over 25 mm long. Shorter instruments are helpful in second and third molars or in the patient who cannot open widely. Other special lengths are available.

Ultimately, to maintain these standards, the American Association of Endodontists (AAE) urged the American Dental Association (ADA) and the United States Bureau of Standards to appoint a committee for endodontic instrument standardization. A committee was formed and produced a specification package that slightly modified Ingle's original standardization.[1] Then a worldwide committee was formed: ISO, consisting of the Fédération Dentaire International, the World Health Organization, and the ADA Instrument Committee. The ISO has now formulated international specifications using the ADA proposal as a model.

ANSI (American National Standards Institute)/ ADA standards have also been set for other instruments and filling materials: No. 58, Hedstroem files; No. 63, rasps and barbed broaches; No. 71, spreaders and condensers; No. 95, root canal enlargers; as well as No. 57, filling materials; No. 73, absorbent points; and No. 78, obturating points. Committee work is continuing to make these standards comparable with ISO standards.

The relevant standards have tolerances for size maintenance (both diameter and taper), surface debris, cutting flute character, torsional properties, stiffness, cross-sectional shape, cutting tip design, and type of metal. Variations from these tolerances have been noted[4–9] (Figure 2). More recently, Stenman and Spångberg[10] noted that few brands are within acceptable dimensional standards.

Cormier et al.[6] have warned of the importance of using only one brand of instruments because of discrepancies in instrument size among manufacturers. Seto et al.[7] noted that grinding the flutes in files rather than twisting them "does not improve the strength or ductility of the instrument... (and) may also create more undesirable fluting defects." Since then, however, grinding has improved and gained importance because most nickel–titanium instruments must be machined, not twisted. Several recent studies have indicated that this type of manufacturing does not weaken instruments. In fact, most studies indicate that both manufacturing processes produce files that meet or exceed ISO standards.[11–13]

It has also been found that autoclaving has no significant deleterious effects on stainless steel or nickel–titanium endodontic instruments.[14,15] Now made universally of nickel–titanium and stainless steel rather than carbon steel, K-type instruments are produced using one of two techniques. The more traditional is produced by grinding graduated sizes of round wire into various shapes such as square, triangular, or rhomboid. A second grinding operation properly tapers these pieces. To give the instruments the spirals that provide the cutting edges, the square or triangular stock is then grasped by a machine that twists it counterclockwise a programed number of times—tight spirals for files, loose spirals for reamers. The cutting blades that are produced are the sharp edges of either the square or the triangle. In any instrument, these edges are known as the "rake" of the blade. The more acute the angle of the rake, the sharper the blade. There is approximately twice the

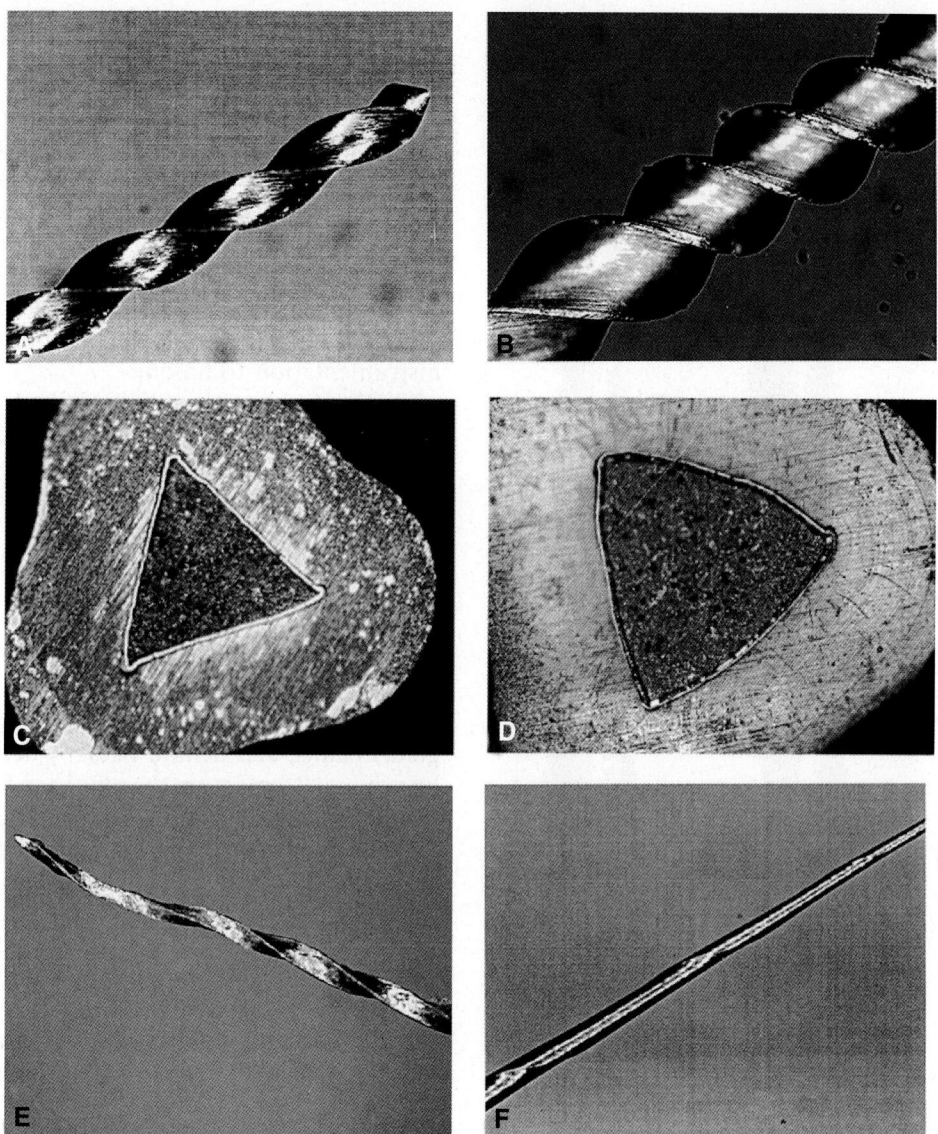

Figure 2 Comparisons of the condition of *unused* instruments from different manufacturers. ***A,*** New No. 30 K-file with consistently sharp blades and point. ***B,*** New No. 35 K-file, different brand, exhibiting dull blades. ***C,*** Cross-sectional profile of triangular No. 20 file showing consistency in angles. ***D,*** Cross-section of competing No. 20 file with dull, rounded angles of cutting blades. ***E,*** No. 15 file showing lack of consistency in the blade, reflecting poor quality control. ***F,*** New No. 08 file with no cutting blades at all.

number of spirals on a file than on a reamer of a corresponding size (Figure 3A and B).

The second and newer manufacturing method is to grind the spirals into the tapered wire rather than twist the wire to produce the cutting blades. Grinding is usually necessary for nickel–titanium instruments. Because of their superelasticity, they cannot be twisted.

Originally, the cross-section of the K-file was square and the reamer triangular. However, manufacturers have started using many configurations to achieve better cutting and/or flexibility. Cross-section is now the prerogative of individual companies.

K-Style Modification

K-style endodontic instruments came into a series of modifications beginning in the 1980s. Not wholly satisfied with the characteristics of their K-style instrument, the Kerr Manufacturing Company in

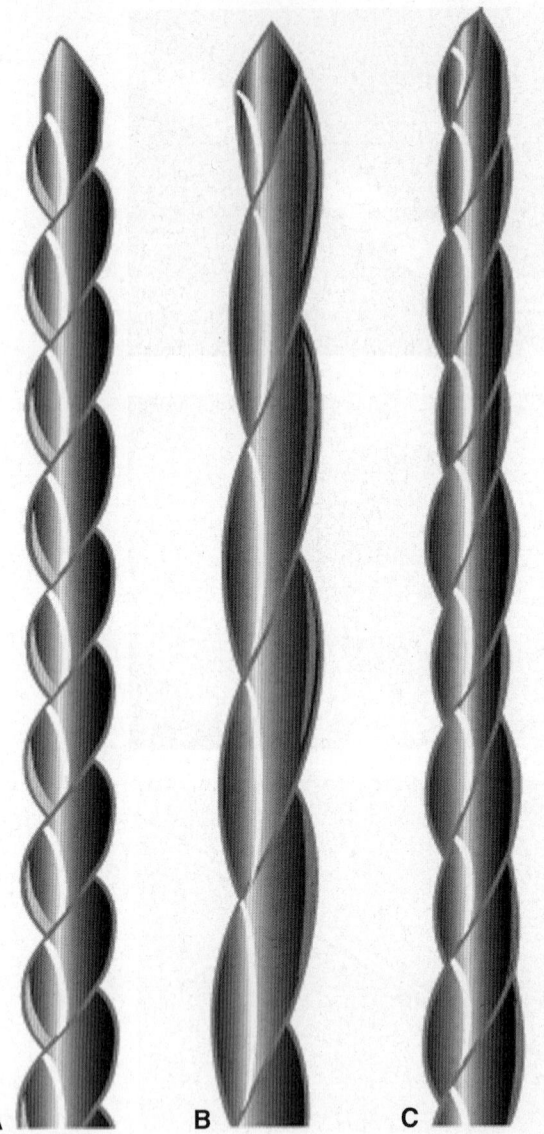

Figure 3 ISO Group I, K-style endodontic instruments. **A,** K-style file. **B,** K-style reamer. **C,** K-flex file.

acute angles of the rhombus and present increased sharpness and cutting efficiency. The alternating low flutes formed by the obtuse angles of the rhombus are meant to act as an auger, providing more area for increased debris removal. The decreased contact by the instrument with the canal walls provides a space reservoir that, with proper irrigation, further reduces the danger of compacting dentinal filings in the canal. Schafer[16] found that the cross-sectional design and the number of flutes will influence canal shape in severely curved canals when employing the same instrumentation technique.

Testing five brands of K-type files for stiffness, Roth et al.[17] found K-Flex files to be the most flexible. Moreover, not a single K-Flex fractured in torque testing, even when twisted twice the recommended level in the ADA specification.

REAMERS

The clinician should understand the importance of differentiating endodontic files and reamers from burs. Burs are used for boring holes in solid materials such as gold, enamel, and dentin. Files, by definition, are used by rasping. Reamers, on the other hand, are instruments that ream (twisting)—specifically, a sharp-edged tool for enlarging or tapering holes (see Figure 3B). Endodontic reamers cut by being tightly inserted into the canal, twisted clockwise one quarter- to one half-turn to engage their blades into the dentin, and then withdrawn—penetration, rotation, and retraction. The cut is made during retraction. The process is then repeated, penetrating deeper and deeper into the canal. When working length is reached, the next size instrument is used, and so on.

FILES

The tighter spiral of a file (see Figure 3A) establishes a cutting angle (rake) that achieves its primary action on withdrawal, although it will cut in the push motion as well. The cutting action of the file can be effected in either a filing (rasping) or a reaming (drilling) motion. In a filing motion, the instrument is placed into the canal at the desired length, pressure is exerted against the canal wall, and while this pressure is maintained, the rake of the flutes rasps the wall as the instrument is withdrawn without turning. The file need not contact all walls simultaneously. For example, the entire length and circumference of large-diameter canals can be filed by inserting the instrument to the desired working distance and filing circumferentially around all of the walls.

1982 introduced a new instrument design that they termed the K-Flex File (Sybron-Endo/Kerr, Orange, CA), a departure from the square and triangular configurations (Figure 3C).

The cross-section of the K-Flex is rhombus or diamond shaped. The spirals or flutes are produced by the same twisting procedure used to produce the cutting edge of the standard K-type files; however, this new cross-section presents significant changes in instrument flexibility and cutting characteristics. The cutting edges of the high flutes are formed by the two

To use a file in a reaming action, the motion is the same as for a reamer—penetration, rotation, and retraction. The file tends to set in the dentin more readily than the reamer and must therefore be treated more gingerly. Withdrawing the file cuts away the engaged dentin.

To summarize the basic action of files and reamers, it may be stated that either files or reamers may be used to ream out a round, tapered apical cavity but that files are also used as push-pull instruments to enlarge by rasping certain curved canals as well as the ovoid portion of large canals. In addition, copious irrigation and constant cleansing of the instrument are necessary to clear the flutes and prevent packing debris at or through the apical foramen.

Oliet and Sorin[18] evaluated endodontic reamers from four different manufacturers and found "considerable variation in the quality, sharpness of the cutting edges, cross sectional configuration, and number of flutes of the 147 different reamers tested." They further found that "triangular cross sectional reamers cut with greater efficiency than do the square cross sectional reamers," but the failure rate of the triangular instruments was considerably higher. Webber et al.[19] found that "instruments with triangular cross sections were initially more efficient but lost sharpness more rapidly than square ones of the same size."

Oliet and Sorin[18] also found that "wear does not appear to be a factor in instrument function, but rather instruments generally fail because of deformation or fracture of the blades. Once an instrument became permanently distorted, additional rotation only caused additional distortion, with minimum cutting frequently leading to fracture." A more recent in vitro study of stainless steel files demonstrated that significant wear and potential loss of efficiency occurred after only one use of 300 strokes. It was proposed that endodontic instruments should be available in sterile packaging for single-patient use.[20] Another study concluded that stainless steel instruments, in small sizes, should be used once, and the No. 30 could be used three times. The No. 30 nickel–titanium instruments, however, "even after five times, did not show appreciable abnormalities in shape."[21] Of course, this study was done with one type of hand nickel–titanium files, and there was no assessment of instrumentation time as compared with stainless steel files.[21]

Webber et al.[19] used a linear cutting motion in moist bovine bone and found that "there was a wide range of cutting efficiency between each type of root canal instrument, both initially and after successive use." Similar findings were found when comparing K-type files with five recently introduced brands in three different sizes, Nos. 20, 25, and 30.[22] Significant differences were noted in the in vitro cutting efficiency among the seven brands. Wear was exhibited by all instruments after three successive 3-minute test periods. Depth of groove is also a significant factor in improving cutting ability (Figure 4).

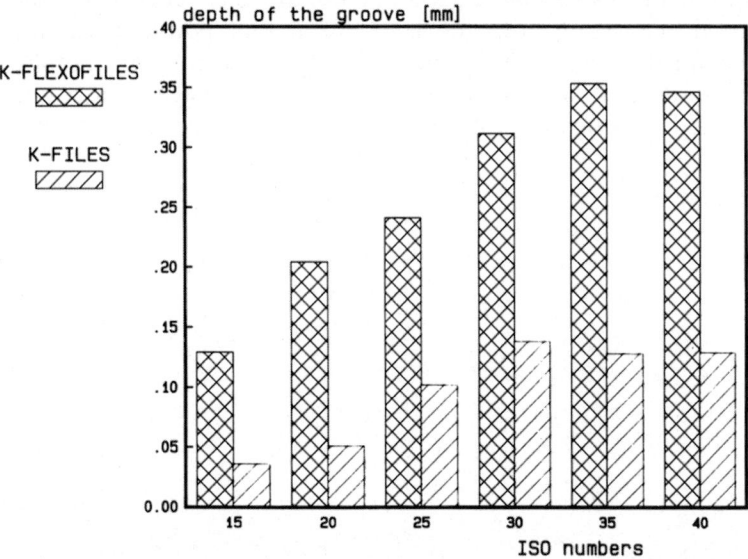

Figure 4 Comparison between two competing brands of endodontic instruments showing widely different cutting ability related to the depth of the blade groove.

Neal et al.[23] also studied the cutting ability of K-type files. A wide variance in the cutting ability of individual files was found. This study appears to confirm what dentists have long noted: the wide variance in cutting ability among individual instruments, even from the same manufacturer. Contrary to the study by Newman et al.,[22] this study reported an insignificant role played by wear in decreasing the cutting ability of regular K-type stainless steel files.[23] Current studies have shown that stainless steel hand files have better cutting efficiency than nickel–titanium hand files and are not adversely affected by sodium hypochlorite.[24,25] A study by Schafer[26] also demonstrated that the cross-sectional design of stainless steel hand files has more of an influence on cutting efficiency than the number of flutes. In two other studies that compared a recently introduced stainless steel file with one that has been in use for 20 years, it was confirmed that stainless steel files that are more flexible have less machining efficiency than a stiffer file.[27,28]

Studies by Oliet and Sorin,[18] Webber et al.,[19] and Neal et al.[23] all alluded to certain weaknesses in K-style instruments. In addition, Luks[29] has shown that the smaller reamers and files may be easily broken by twisting the blades beyond the limits of the metal until the metal separated. On the other hand, Gutierrez et al.[30] found that although the instrument did not immediately break, a progression of undesirable features occurred. Locking and twisting clockwise led to unwinding and elongation as well as the loss of blade cutting edge and blunting of the tip. With continued clockwise twisting, a reverse "roll-up" occurred. Cracks in the metal eventually developed that finally resulted in breakage. These findings were unusual in that breakage would have normally resulted long before "roll-up" occurred. It may reflect a variance in the quality of metal used by manufacturing companies. This point was borne out in a study by Lentine,[31] in which he found a wide range of values within each brand of instrument as well as between brands.

An additional study of 360° clockwise rotation (ISO revision of ADA Specification No. 28) found only 5 K-style files failing of 100 instruments tested. They were sizes 30 to 50, all from one manufacturer.[17]

Attempts to "unscrew" a locked endodontic file also present a problem. Chernick et al.[32] demonstrated that "endodontic files twisted in a counterclockwise manner were extremely brittle in comparison with those twisted in a clockwise manner." They warned that dentists "should exercise caution when 'backing-off' embedded root canal instruments." This finding was supported by Lautenschlager et al.,[33] who found that "all commercial files and reamers showed adequate clockwise torque, but were prone to brittle fracture when placed in counterclockwise torsion."

By contrast, Roane and Sabala[34] found that clockwise rotation was more likely (91.5%) to produce separation and/or distortion than counterclockwise rotation (8.5%) when they examined 493 discarded instruments. Seto et al.[7] also found greater rotational failure in clockwise rotation and greater failure as well in machined stainless steel K-files over twisted K-files.

Sotokawa[35] also studied discarded instruments and indicted metal fatigue as the culprit in breakage and distortion. "First a starting point crack develops on the file's edge and then metal fatigue fans out from that point, spreading towards the file's axial center" (Figure 5). Sotokawa[35] also classified the types of damage to instruments (Figure 6). He found the No. 10 file to be the most frequently discarded.

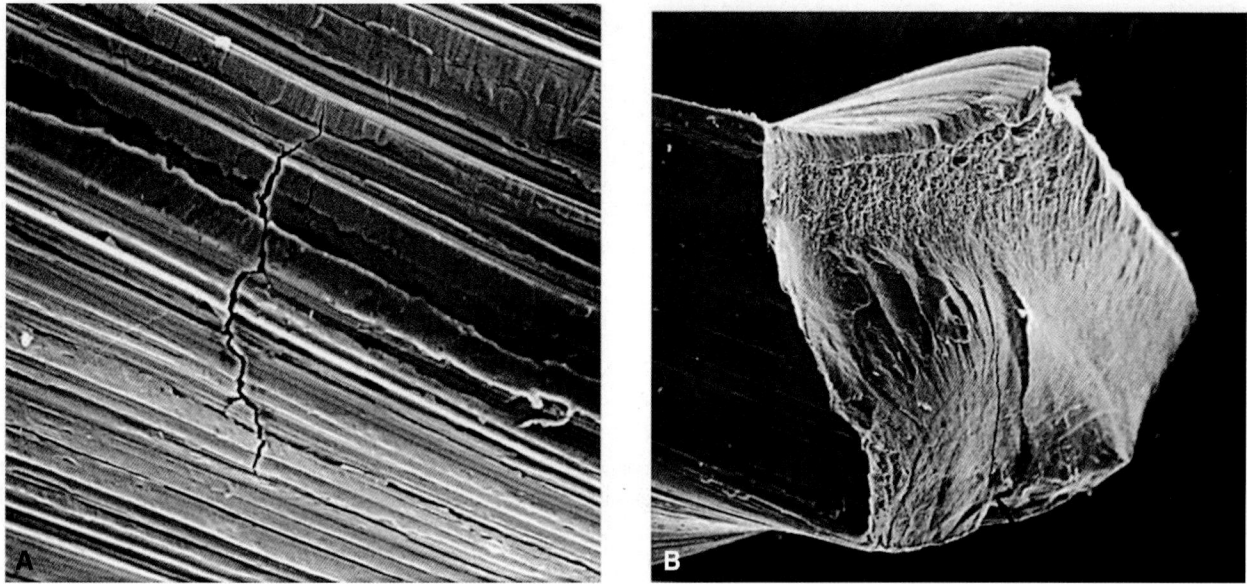

Figure 5 Instrument breakage. **A,** Initial crack across the shaft near the edge of the blade, Type V (original magnification ×1,000). **B,** Full fracture of file broken in a 30° twisting simulation, Type VI (original magnification ×230).

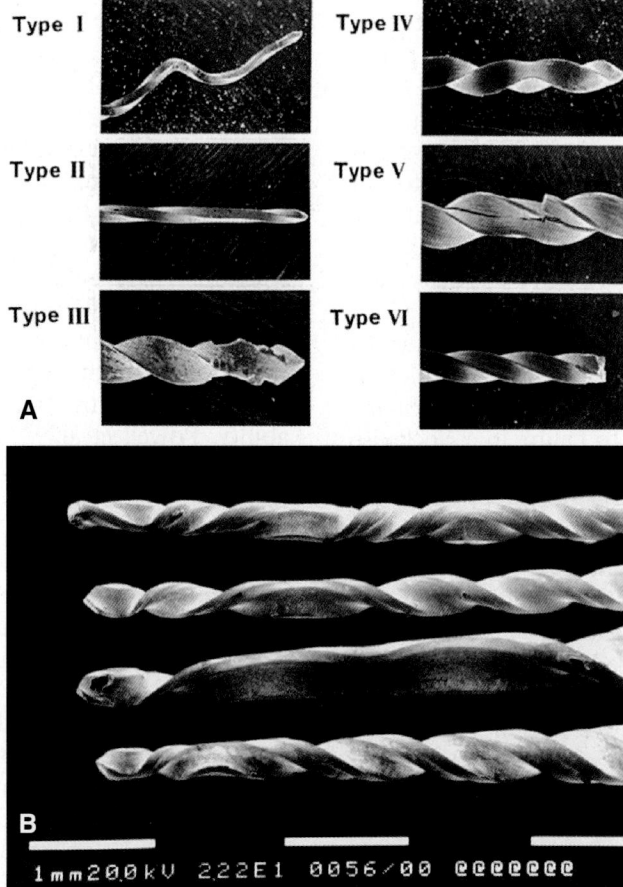

Figure 6 A, Sotokawa's classification of instrument damage. Type I, Bent instrument. Type II, Stretching or straightening of twist contour. Type III, Peeling-off metal at blade edges. Type IV, Partial clockwise twist. Type V, Cracking along axis. Type VI, Full fracture. **B,** Discarded rotary nickel–titanium files showing visible defects without fracture. All files show unwinding, indicating a torsional defect, and are very dangerous to be used further. Reproduced with permission from Sattapan B, Nervo GJ, Palamara JEA, Messer, HH. J Endod 2000;26:161.

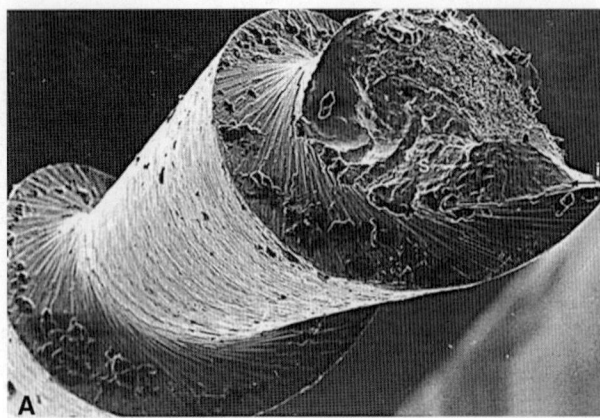 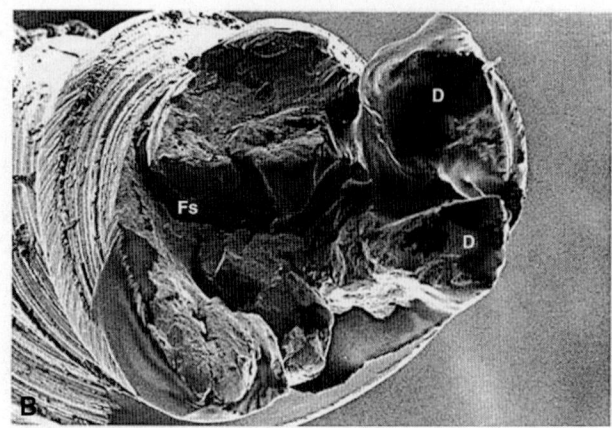

Figure 7 Instrument fracture by cracks and deformation. ***A,*** Broken Hedstrom file with starting point at (i) (far right) spreading to cracks (S) and ductile fracture (F). ***B,*** Broken K-Flex file with plastic deformations at (D) and axial fissure at (Fs). Reproduced with permission from Haikel Y, et al. J Endod 1991;17:217.

Haikel et al.[36] compared instrument fracture between traditional K and Hedström files and the newer "hybrid" instruments. They found that "the instruments with triangular cross sections, in particular the Flexofile (Dentsply/Maillefer, Tulsa, OK), were found to be the most resistant to fracture." Starting-point cracks and ductile fracture as well as plastic deformations and axial fractures were found (Figure 7). Schafer and Tepel[37] showed that the cross-sectional design had more to do with a stainless steel files flexibility and its ability to resist fracture than the number of flutes.

Rowan et al.[38] compared rotation and torque to failure of stainless steel and nickel–titanium files of various sizes. An interesting relation was noted. Stainless steel had greater rotations to failure in a clockwise direction, and the nickel–titanium was superior in a counterclockwise direction. Despite these differences, the actual force to cause failure was the same. It should be noted that the test instrument used in this study is not the one specified in ADA Specification No. 28. To overcome the problems chronicled above—distortion, fracture—Walia et al.[39] suggested that nickel–titanium, with a very low modulus of elasticity, be substituted for stainless steel in the manufacture of endodontic instruments.

TIP MODIFICATION

Early interest in the cutting ability of endodontic instruments centered around the sharpness, pitch, and rake of the blades. By 1980, interest had also developed in the sharpness of the instrument tip and the tip's effect in penetration and cutting as well as its possible deleterious potential for ledging and/or transportation—machining the preparation away from the natural canal anatomy.

Villalobos et al.[40] noted that tip design, as much as flute sharpness, led to improved cutting efficiency. Felt et al.[41] designed experiments to exclude tip design because the tip might "overshadow the cutting effects of flute design." Later, it was reported that "tips displayed better cutting efficiency than flutes" and that triangular pyramidal tips outperformed conical tips, which were least effective.[42,43]

At the same time that a pitch was being made for the importance of cutting tips, other researchers were redesigning tips that virtually eliminated their cutting ability. Powell et al.[44,45] began modifying the tips of K-files by "grinding to remove the transition angle" from tip to first blade.

By 1988, Sabala et al.[46] confirmed previous findings that the modified tip instruments exerted "less transportation and more inner curvature preparation. The modified files maintained the original canal curvature better and more frequently than did the unmodified files."

Powell et al.[45] noted that each stainless steel "file's metallic memory to return to a straight position, increases the tendency to transport or ledge and eventually to perforate curved canals." This action takes place on the outer wall, the convex curvature of the canal. They pointed out that when this tip "angle is reduced, the file stays centered within the original canal and cuts all sides (circumference) more evenly." This modified-tip file has been marketed as the

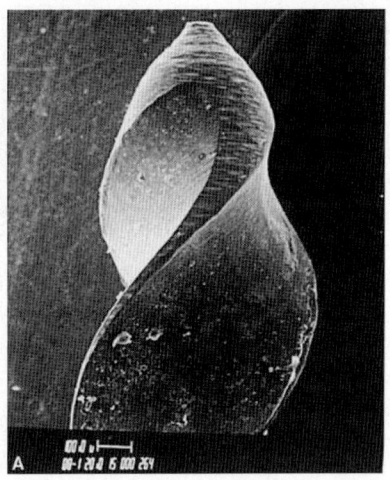 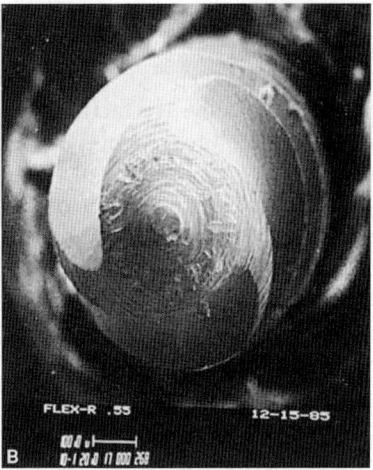

Figure 8 Flex-R-file with noncutting tip. **A,** Note rounded tip. **B,** "Nose" view of a noncutting tip ensures less gouging of the external wall and reduced cavity transport. From Ingle JI, Bakland LK. Endodontics, 5th ed. 2002, Ingle JI. et al. Endodontic Cavity Preparation. Page 483.

Flex-R-file (Moyco/Union Broach, Miller Dental, Bethpage, NY) (Figure 8).

Rounded-tipped files, developed by Roane,[34] were compared with other files with triangular cross-sections and various forms of tip modification. Although the round-tipped files were the least efficient, they prepared canals more safely and with less destruction than did the other files.[47] This study was done with stainless steel hand files in plastic blocks with balanced forces instrumentation.[47]

HEDSTROM FILES

H-type files are made by cutting the spiraling flutes into the shaft of a piece of round, tapered, stainless steel wire. Actually, the machine used is similar to a screw-cutting machine. This accounts for the resemblance between the Hedstrom configuration and a wood screw (Figure 9A).

It is impossible to ream or drill with this instrument. To do so locks the flutes into the dentin much as a screw is locked in wood. To continue the drilling action would fracture the instrument. Furthermore, the file is impossible to withdraw once it is locked in the dentin and can be withdrawn only by backing off until the flutes are free. This action also "separates" files. Zinelis and Margelos[48] stated that fatigue is the primary cause of failure of Hedstrom files, whereas Kosti et al.[49] feel that the instrumentation technique that is used with the Hedstrom files also can contribute to their failure. Kazemi et al.[50] used two different materials to fabricate identical Hedstrom type of instruments. One set was made with stainless steel

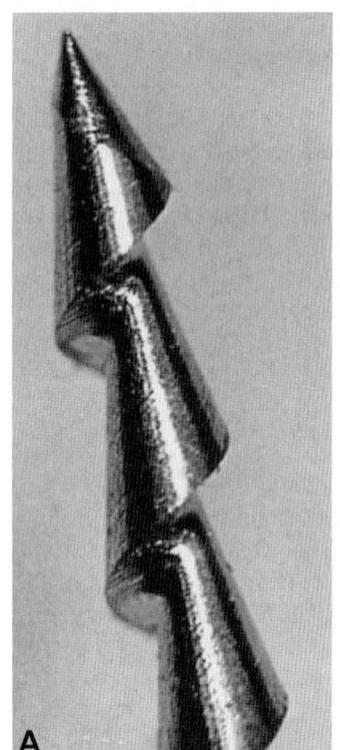 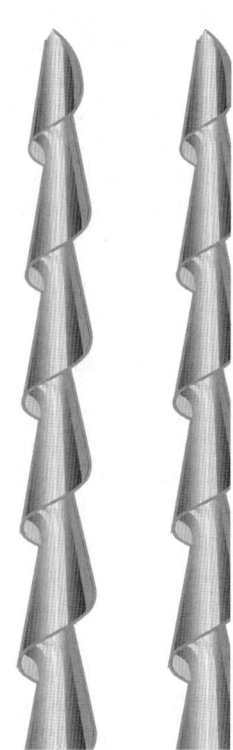

Figure 9 ISO Group I, H-style instruments. **A,** Maillefer Hedstrom file resembling a wood screw. **B,** Modified Hedstrom file (left) with noncutting tip. "Safety" Hedstrom (right) with flattened noncutting side to prevent "stripping." Reproduced with permission from Keate KC, Wong M. J Endod 1990;16:488.

and the other with nickel–titanium. These files were then tested for flexibility and resistance to fracture. The torsional moment for the stainless steel files was significantly higher than the nickel–titanium although the angular deflection for the nickel–titanium was significantly higher than the stainless steel.[50]

Hedstrom files cut in one direction only—retraction. Because of the very positive rake of the flute design, they are more efficient as files per se.[51–55] Yguel-Henry et al.[54] reported on the importance of the lubricating effect of liquids on cutting efficiency, raising this efficiency by 30% with H-style files and 200% with K-files. Mizrahi et al.,[52] however, reported the proclivity that H-files have for packing debris at the apex. On the other hand, El Deeb and Boraas[55] found that H-files tended not to pack debris at the apex and were the most efficient.

Hedstrom files are not to be used in a torquing action. For this reason, ADA Specification No. 28 could not apply, and a new specification, No. 58, was approved by the ADA and the American National Standards Committee.[56]

H-STYLE FILE MODIFICATION

The Hyflex file (Coltene/Whaledent/Hygenic, Mahwah, NJ) in cross-section presents an "S" shape rather than the single-helix teardrop cross-sectional shape of the true Hedstroem file. The "S" File (J-S Dental, Ridgefield, CT) also appears to be a variation of the H-style file in its double-helix configuration. Reports on this instrument are very favorable.[57] Buchanan has further modified the Hedstroem file, the Safety Hedstrom (Sybron-Endo/Kerr), which has a noncutting side to prevent ledging in curved canals (Figure 9, B).

U-FILE

An instrument for which there is no ISO or ANSI/ADA specification as yet is the U-File. It is marketed as ProFiles, GT Files (Dentsply/Tulsa Dental, Tulsa, OK), and LIGHTSPEED (LightSpeed Technology Inc., San Antonio, TX). The U-File's cross-sectional configuration has two 90° cutting edges at each of the three points of the blade (Figure 10). The flat cutting surfaces act as a planing instrument and are referred to as radial lands. A noncutting pilot tip ensures that the file remains in the lumen of the canal, thus avoiding transportation and "zipping" at the apex. The files are used in both a push-pull and rotary motion and

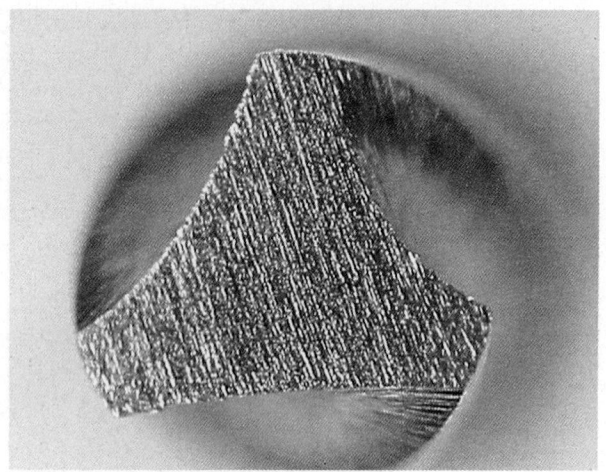

Figure 10 Cross-sectional view of a U-File reveals six corners in cutting blades compared with four corners in square stock and three corners in triangular stock K-files. Courtesy of John McSpadden.

are very adaptable to nickel–titanium rotary instruments. ProFiles are supplied in a variety of tapers and ISO tip sizes of 15 through 80.

GT ProFiles, developed by Buchanan in the U-design, are unusual in that the cutting blades extend up the shaft only 6 to 8 mm rather than 16 mm, and the tapers start at 0.06 mm/mm (instead of 0.02), as well as 0.08 and 0.10, tapered instruments. They are made of nickel–titanium and come as hand instruments and rotary files. GT instruments all start with a noncutting tip ISO size 20.

LIGHTSPEED LSX

The distinctive design of LightSpeed instruments (Discus Dental, Culver City, CA) maximizes flexibility and allows larger apical preparations without unnecessary removal of dentin. The LSX has a non-cutting shaft and very short blade. After making straight-line access to about mid-root, the coronal third is flared with the instrument of choice (not with the LSX). After flaring, at least a #15 K-file is used to obtain patency to working length (WL). A #20 LSX and sequentially larger sizes are used to prepare the apical third. The final apical instrument size (FAS) is

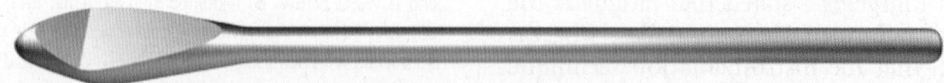

Figure 11 The newly designed LightSpeed LSX NiTi rotary instrument (Discus Dental, Culver City, CA) maximizes flexibility that allows for enlarged apical preparations. The distinctive cutting head terminates a noncutting shaft. It should be used at 2500-3000 RPM and irrigation is required throughout the enlarging procedure. The new LSX is used to prepare a tapered and circular apical preparation in an ovoid canal.

the blade size that encounters 4mm or more of cutting resistance apically. A 4mm step back with the next larger (than the FAS) instrument completes the apical preparation. The mid-root is then cleaned and tapered with the next two or three sequentially larger LSX sizes, blending mid-root instrumentation with the previously prepared coronal third. Recapitulation usually is necessary only once – with the FAS – at the end of canal preparation. The new LSX is to be used at 2500 rpm, and irrigation is required throughout the procedure.

GATES GLIDDEN MODIFICATION

Another hand instrument also designed for apical preparation was the Flexogate (Dentsply/Maillefer), but it is no longer manufactured. Briseño et al.[62] compared Flexogates and Canal Master (Brasseler, Savannah, GA) in vitro and found Flexogates less likely to cause apical transportation.

QUANTEC "FILES"

The Quantec instrument (Sybron-Endo/Kerr), although called a "file," was more like a reamer. It was not designed to be used in the file's push-pull action but rather in the reamer's rotary motion. The radial lands of the Quantec were slightly relieved to reduce frictional contact with the canal wall, and the helix angle is configured to remove debris. It is no longer manufactured.

HAND INSTRUMENT CONCLUSIONS

The literature is replete with references to the superiority of one instrument or one method of preparation over all others.[55,63–66] Quite true is Briseño's[67] statement, "Regardless of the instrument type, none was able to reproduce ideal results; however, clinically acceptable results could be obtained with all of them." All too often clinicians report success with instruments and techniques with which they are most comfortable. No ulterior motive is involved, but often a report reflects badly on an instrument when it is the clinician's inexperience with an unfamiliar technique that is unknowingly being reported. Stenman and Spångberg[68] said it "is difficult to assess, as results from published investigations often vary considerably."

BARBED BROACHES

Barbed broaches are short-handled instruments used primarily for vital pulp extirpation. They are also used to loosen debris in necrotic canals or to remove paper points or cotton pellets. ISO Specification No. 63 sets the standards for barbed broaches. Rueggenberg and Powers[69] tested all sizes of broaches from three manufacturers and found significant differences in shape, design, and size, as well as results from torsion and deflection tests. The authors warned that a "jammed broach" should be removed vertically without twisting.

Broaches are manufactured from round wire, the smooth surface of which has been notched to form barbs bent at an angle from the long axis (Figure 12A). These barbs are used to engage the pulp as the broach is rotated within the canal until it begins to meet resistance against the walls of the canal. The broach should never be forced into a canal beyond the length where it first begins to bind. Forcing it farther apically causes the barbs to be

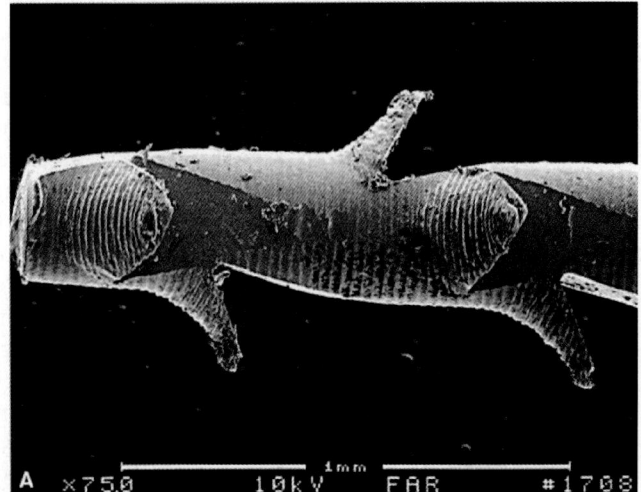
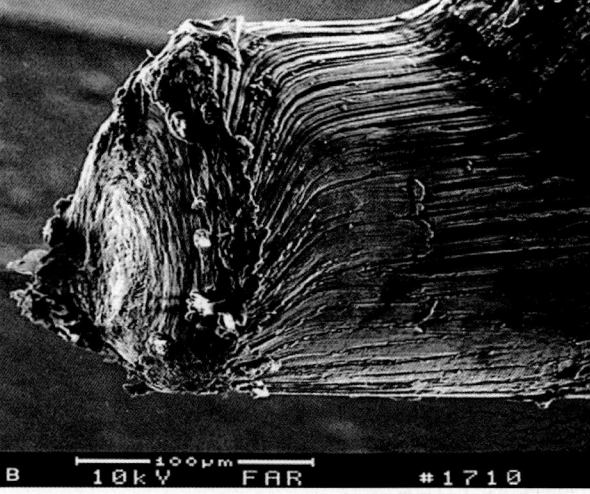

Figure 12 A, Barbed broach. As a result of a careless barbing process, the effective shaft diameter is greatly reduced. Size "coarse." **B**, Ductile failure of size "xx fine" barbed broach fractured after axial twisting greater than 130°. Reproduced with permission from Rueggenberg FA, Powers JM. J Endod 1988;14:133.

compressed by the canal walls. Subsequent efforts to withdraw the instrument will embed the barbs in the walls. Increased withdrawal pressure to retrieve the instrument results in breaking off the embedded barbs or the shaft of the instrument itself at the point of engagement (Figure 12B). A broken barbed broach embedded in the canal wall is seldom retrievable.

Nickel–Titanium Endodontic Instruments

A new generation of endodontic instruments, made from nickel–titanium, has added a new dimension to the practice of endodontics.[70,71] The superelasticity of nickel–titanium, the property that allows it to return to its original shape following significant deformation, differentiates it from other metals, such as stainless steel, that sustain deformation and retain permanent shape change. These properties make nickel–titanium endodontic files more flexible and better able to conform to canal curvature, resist fracture, and wear less than stainless steel files (see Chapter 25B, "Introduction of Nickel–Titanium Alloy to Endodontics").

SUPERELASTICITY

Alloys such as nickel–titanium, that show superelasticity, undergo a stress-induced martensitic transformation from a parent structure, which is austenite. On release of the stress, the structure reverts back to austenite, recovering its original shape in the process. Deformations involving as much as a 10% strain can be completely recovered in these materials, as compared with a maximum of 1% in conventional alloys.

In a study comparing piano wire and a nickel–titanium wire, Stoeckel and Yu[71] found that a stress of 2,500 MPa was required to stretch a piano wire to 3% strain, as compared with only 500 MPa for a nickel–titanium wire. At 3% strain, the music wire breaks. On the other hand, the nickel–titanium wire can be stretched much beyond 3% and can recover most of this deformation on the release of stress. The superelastic behavior of nickel–titanium also occurs over a limited temperature window. Minimum residual deformation occurs at approximately room temperature.[71] A composition consisting of 50 atomic percent nickel and 50 atomic percent titanium seems ideal, both for instrumentation and manufacture.

MANUFACTURE

Today, nickel–titanium instruments are precision ground into different designs (K style, Hedstrom, Flex-R, U-files, and drills) and are made in different sizes and tapers. The nickel–titanium alloy is difficult to machine as the properties of the alloy can be changed during the manufacturing process. Variables such as feed rate, lubrication, and heat treating during the fabrication process can influence the final product.[72] Just now there are new manufacturing methods that employ casting of the alloy or stamping wire blanks. In addition, spreaders and pluggers are also available. Nickel–titanium instruments are as effective as or better than comparable stainless steel instruments in machining dentin, and nickel–titanium instruments are more wear resistant.[73] U and drill designs make it possible to use mechanical (i.e., rotary handpiece) instrumentation. Moreover, rotary motors now offer the potential for improved torque control with automatic reversal that may decrease rotary instrument breakage.

Finally, nickel–titanium files are biocompatible and appear to have excellent anticorrosive properties.[74] In addition, implantation studies have verified that nickel–titanium is biocompatible and acceptable as a surgical implant.[75]

With the ability to machine flutes, many new designs such as radial lands have become available. Radial lands allow nickel–titanium files to be used as reamers in a 360° motion as opposed to the traditional reamers with more acute rake angles. Although the most common use of this new design has been as a rotary file, the identical instrument is available as a hand instrument. In addition, a converter handle is available that allows the operator to use the rotary file as a hand instrument.

TORSIONAL STRENGTH AND SEPARATION

The clinician switching from stainless to nickel–titanium hand instruments should not confuse nickel–titanium's superelastic characteristics with its torsional strength and so assume that it has super strength. This misconception has led to unnecessary file breakage when first using this new metal. Studies indicate that instruments, whether stainless steel or nickel–titanium, meet or exceed ANSI/ADA Specification No. 28. However, when reviewing the literature on this subject the results are mixed. Canalda-Sahli et al.[76] found nickel–titanium files (Nitiflex and Naviflex) (Dentsply) to be more flexible than the stainless files tested (Flexofile and Flex-R). However, the stainless steel files were found to be more resistant to fracture. Both types of metal exceeded all ANSI/ADA specifications. Canalda-Sahli et al.,[77] in another study, compared identical instruments: CanalMaster (aka LIGHTSPEED) stainless steel and CanalMaster nickel–titanium. Within these designs, the nickel–titanium values were superior in all aspects to those of stainless steel of the same design.

Tepel et al.[12] looked at bending and torsional properties of 24 different types of nickel–titanium, titanium–aluminum, and stainless steel instruments. They found the nickel–titanium K-files to be the most flexible, followed in descending order by titanium–aluminum, flexible stainless steel, and conventional stainless steel. When testing for resistance to fracture for 21 brands, however, they found that No. 25 stainless steel files had a higher resistance to fracture than their nickel–titanium counterpart.

Wolcott and Himel[13] compared the torsional properties of stainless steel K-type and nickel–titanium U-type instruments. As in previous studies, all of the stainless steel instruments showed no significant difference between maximum torque and torque at failure, whereas the nickel–titanium instruments showed a significant difference between maximum torque and torque at failure. Essentially, this means that the time between "windup" and fracture in nickel–titanium instruments is extended, which could lead to a false sense of security.

While studying cyclic fatigue using nickel–titanium LightSpeed instruments, Pruett et al.[78] determined that canal curvature and the number of rotations determined file breakage. Separation occurred at the point of maximum curvature of the shaft.

Cyclic fatigue should be considered a valid term, even for hand instrumentation, in light of the fact that many manufacturers are placing handles on files designed for rotational use. From these studies, it seems that if the clinician is changing from a high-torque instrument, such as stainless steel, to a low-torque instrument, such as nickel–titanium, it would be wise to know that nickel–titanium instruments are more efficient and safer when used passively. Although instrument breakage should be rare, any instrument, hand or rotary, can break. It is the clinician's knowledge and experience, along with the manufacturer's quality control, that will ultimately minimize breakage. If breakage occurs, the fractured piece can occasionally be removed or bypassed using ultrasonics and hand instruments in conjunction with magnification. Dentists having problems with file breakage should seek help in evaluating one's technique. One should practice on extracted teeth until a level of confidence is reached that will help ensure safe and efficient patient care.

The following is a list of situations that place nickel–titanium hand or rotary instruments at risk along with suggestions for avoiding problems.

Nickel–Titanium Precautions and Prevention

1. Often too much pressure is applied to the file. Never force a file! These instruments require a passive technique. If resistance is encountered, stop immediately, and before continuing, increase the coronal taper and negotiate additional length, using a smaller, 0.02 taper stainless steel hand file. Stainless steel files should be used in sizes smaller than a No. 15. If one is using more finger pressure than that required to break a No. 2 pencil lead, too much pressure is being used.
2. Canals that join abruptly at sharp angles are often found in roots such as the mesiobuccal root of maxillary molars, all premolars, and mandibular incisors and the mesial roots of mandibular molars. The straighter of the two canals should first be enlarged to working length and then the other canal, only to where they join. If not, a nickel–titanium file may reverse its direction at this juncture, bending back on itself and damaging the instrument.
3. Curved canals that have a high degree and small radius of curvature are dangerous.[78] Such curvatures (over 60° and found 3 to 4 mm from working length) are often seen in the distal canals of mandibular molars and the palatal roots of maxillary first molars.
4. Files should not be overused! Clinicians have experienced more fracture after files have been used a number of times. Remember that all uses of a file are not equal. A calcified canal stresses the file more than an uncalcified canal. A curved canal stresses the file more than a straight canal. One must also bear in mind operator variability and the use of lubricants, which will affect stress. Consider discarding a file after abusive use in calcified or severely curved canals even though it has been used only in one tooth. Use new files in hard cases and older files in easier cases. No one knows the maximum or ideal number of times a file can be used. Follow manufacturers' instructions. Once only is the safest number.
5. Instrument fatigue occurs more often during the initial stages of the learning curve. The clinician changing from stainless steel to nickel–titanium should take continuing education courses with experienced clinicians and educators, followed

by in vitro practice on plastic blocks and extracted teeth.
6. Ledges that develop in a canal allow space for deflection of a file. The nickel–titanium instrument can then curve back on itself. A nickel–titanium instrument should not be used to bypass ledges.
7. Teeth with "S"-type curves should be approached with caution! Adequate flaring of the coronal third to half of the canal, however, will decrease problems in these cases. It may also be necessary to go through a series of instruments an additional time or two in more difficult cases.
8. If the instrument is progressing easily in a canal and then feels as if it hits bottom, do not apply additional pressure! This will cause the instrument tip to bind. Additional pressure applied at this point may cause weakening or even breakage of the instrument. In this situation, remove the instrument and try a smaller, 0.02 taper hand instrument, either stainless steel or nickel–titanium, carefully flaring and enlarging the uninstrumented apical portion of the canal.
9. Avoid creating a canal the same size and taper of the instrument being used. On removal from the canal, the debris pattern on the file should be examined. Debris should appear on the middle portion of the file. Except for negotiating calcified canals and enlarging the apical portion of the canal, the tip and coronal section of the file should not carry debris. Avoid cutting with the entire length of the file blade. This total or frictional fit of the file in the canal will cause the instrument to lock. If this occurs, rotate the instrument in a counterclockwise direction and remove it from the canal. The greater the distance a single file is advanced into the canal, the greater will be the chance of files "locking up." When the file feels tight throughout the length of blade, it is an indication that the orifice and coronal one-third to two-thirds of the canal need increased taper. Instruments of varying design and/or taper can be used to avoid frictional fit. Nickel–titanium instruments with tapers from 0.04, 0.06, and greater, as well as Gates Glidden drills and sonic/ultrasonic instruments, serve this purpose well.
10. Sudden changes in the direction of an instrument caused by the operator (i.e., jerky or jabbing movements) must be avoided. A smooth gentle reaming or rotary motion is most efficient.
11. As with any type instrument, poor access preparation will lead to procedural errors.
12. Advancing or pushing an instrument into a canal in too large an increment causes it to act as a drill or piston and greatly increases stress on the metal. Except for the most difficult cases and the necessity of using small instruments, the tip should not be used to cut into or drill into the canal; it should act only as a guide. Regardless of the technique being used, nickel–titanium instruments should be advanced in small increments with a more passive pressure than that used with stainless steel.
13. Do not try to make nickel–titanium do more than it is designed to do.
14. Inspection of instruments, particularly used instruments, by staff and doctor is critical. Prior to insertion and on removal, look at the blade. Rotate the file, looking for deflections of light. This indicates a damaged instrument. Also remember that, unlike stainless steel, nickel–titanium has an excellent memory. The file should be straight. If any bend is present, the instrument is fatigued and should be replaced.
15. Do not assume that the length of files is always accurate; measure each file. Some files are longer from handle to tip than others. Files may also become longer or shorter if they are unraveled or twisted.

COMPARATIVE STUDIES

Nickel–titanium instruments function differently than those made of stainless steel, even when the cross-sectional design, taper, flutes, and tip are identical. Himel et al.[79] compared hand nickel–titanium filing of plastic blocks with curved canals to stainless steel filing.

Working length was maintained significantly more often ($p < .05$) in the nickel–titanium group than in the stainless steel group. There was no ledging of canals using the more flexible nickel–titanium files compared with 30.4% ledging when stainless steel files were used. Apical zipping occurred 31.7% less often with the Nitinol files.[79] Stripping of the canal walls was less with the nickel–titanium files. An observation from these studies was the creation of a smooth belly shape on the outer aspect of the apical third of the canals instrumented with nickel–titanium instruments. This seemed to replace the ledging that occurred with stainless steel.

Using computed tomography, Gambill et al.[80] reamed extracted teeth with either stainless steel or nickel–titanium files and reported that the nickel–titanium files caused less canal transportation, removed less dentin, were more efficient, and produced more centered canals. On the other hand, not all studies are in agreement concerning cutting efficiency. Tepel et al.[81] tested 24 brands of hand instruments specifically for cutting efficiency. They found that flexible stainless steel files were more efficient than nickel–titanium. However, they did not address the quality of the completed canal.

Elliot et al.[82] used resin blocks to compare stainless steel (Flexofiles) and nickel–titanium (Nitiflex) instruments used with either a balanced force or step-back technique. They concluded that it is preferable to use nickel–titanium instruments in a balanced force technique and stainless steel in a filing technique because stainless steel files can be precurved. Considering these results, nickel–titanium instruments should be used as reamers, not files.

ROTARY NICKEL–TITANIUM FILES

It needs to be emphasized that the previously stated guidelines apply to all of the rotary nickel–titanium files that are and will be available. Just as most of the preceding papers apply to hand nickel–titanium files, there now exists an extensive body of literature on rotary nickel–titanium files. This literature covers a variety of aspects from the metallurgy of the files to how well they clean and shape the canal system.

A number of studies have utilized a variety of test instruments to investigate the properties of new and used nickel–titanium rotary files. These researchers have used such things as X-ray diffraction (XRD), scanning electron microscopy (SEM), microhardness testing, differential scanning calorimetry (DSC), and temperature-modulated DSC (TMDSC). In a series of studies, Kuhn et al.[83,84] have shown that the alloy of various files (both new and used) is fully austenitic at room temperature by means of XRD and DSC. They also exposed the files to various heat treatments to determine what if any influence these treatments would have on the flexibility of the files. Kim et al.[85] performed cryogenic treatment on nickel–titanium instruments. They showed that the microhardness of the files was increased but that there was no noticeable change in cutting efficiency, nor was there any change in the crystalline phase composition of the files. Although these results did show some differences, it is doubtful that the differences are clinically relevant. Brantley et al.[86] looked at two different types of rotary files as well as the wire blanks that were used to fabricate the files. They compared new files with ones that had been used to instrument canals in extracted teeth. Their analysis with DSC showed that although there were differences between the files and the blanks, all of the instruments were still fully austenitic at room temperature. In another study that compared the wire blanks with the final product (ProFile instruments), Bahia et al.[87] found that cyclic loading did change the wire blanks as well as the instruments. However, these changes did not compromise the instruments, nor did DSC or XRD demonstrate any significant differences. Another study utilized DSC to compare five types of rotary nickel–titanium files and correlate these findings with torsional and bend testing of these instruments. It was seen that a lower transformation temperature as disclosed by DSC was correlated with an instrument that required a higher torsional load to fail and a higher load to bend to the maximum deflection of 4 mm.[88] Clinically, this would equate to an instrument that had increased stiffness. Whether this would be a noticeable increase in stiffness would depend in some degree on the operator. Some of these studies have remarked on machining defects that are revealed by SEM and speak to the possible relationship of these defects to the clinical failure of the instruments.

FATIGUE AND FLEXIBILITY OF ROTARY NICKEL–TITANIUM FILES

There have been a number of approaches to ascertaining the fatigue and flexibility of rotary nickel–titanium files. Some have looked at mathematical models and employed finite element analysis to develop theoretical values. In a comparison of a triple U (ProFile) versus triple helix (HERO 642) theoretical cross-sections, it was determined that the triple U was more flexible but had less torsional strength.[89] When these same cross-sections were used to calculate theoretical torsional and bending moments, it was determined that the triple U model had a larger and higher range for torsional stress and a higher maximum stress value.[90] The translation of these values into determining the clinical usability of the respective instruments is not easily done because there are so many other variables such as rpm, canal curvature, canal radius of curvature, and insertion rate/force that must also be considered.

In another study utilizing a computer model, the ProTaper instrument was compared with the ProFile instrument. Although the ProTaper was shown to be a stiffer instrument, it was also shown that the stress distribution during torsional loading and bending loads was more evenly distributed. The authors suggest that the ProTaper design will accumulate less stress during usage and thus would be indicated for instrumenting small curved canals.[91]

In a finite element analysis of existing nickel–titanium instruments, it was confirmed that as the cross-sectional area of the files increases, the file is more resistant to torsional forces.[92] Such an interpretation is limited by a number of factors including heat treating during manufacture, modification of the nickel–titanium alloy used, and changes in any number of parameters during fabrication such as feed rate or newness of the machining tools. A series of studies, more closely related to the clinical usage of rotary nickel–titanium files, have brought out some interesting results. One study stated that there was no significant difference in fatigue resistance between new and used ProFile instruments after clinical usage. However, the used instruments did fail sooner when rotated in a 90° curved tube.[93] Another study states there is a significant difference between the fatigue resistance of new and used files and that larger files will fail sooner after they are used.[94,95] A clinical usage study by Bahia et al.[96] confirmed these results. These results were then verified in another study by Bahia et al.[97] done under more controlled conditions. They demonstrated that a used file will fail sooner than a new file. A number of other studies have verified these results.[98–101] When other parameters are addressed such as angle and radius of curvature, it is seen that an increase in the angle of curvature or a decrease in the radius of curvature causes files to fail sooner.[99,102,103] It is also seen that a larger file is more resistant to torque.[104–106]

When Gates Glidden drills were fabricated from nickel–titanium, it was shown that the larger the size of the drill, the sooner it would fail when rotated in a device that imparted a bend to the instrument while being rotated.[107] An interesting sidelight in one report demonstrated that dry heat sterilization seemed to increase the files' ability to resist fatigue.[98] However, it required five cycles of dry heat sterilization to achieve these results. One could question the advisability of using a rotary file many times. Finally, a study looked at the cross-sectional geometry of five different types of rotary nickel–titanium files and determined that as the cross-section area increased, the file became more resistant to bending.[108] This would seem to verify the theoretical studies that were mentioned previously.

FORCES ENCOUNTERED

During canal preparation, forces are generated by the insertion of the rotating file into the canal system. In a series of studies utilizing a test instrument developed by Blum et al.,[109] they reported some interesting findings. They have shown that the crown-down technique with ProFile instruments produced less force than the step-back technique. In another study, they demonstrated that forces were lowest when there was less engagement of the file with the canal walls.[110] When the same type of study was done with the ProTaper instrument in narrow and large canals, the same conclusions were reached. The more a file was in contact with the canal wall, the higher the forces on the instrument and the canal wall.[111] These results were confirmed by others utilizing different test instruments and test methods. When Quantec rotary files were used in extracted teeth, it was seen that a file with a larger taper generated more forces particularly in a smaller canal.[112] Peters[113] confirmed these findings; when a ProTaper instrument was used in smaller canals, higher forces were generated. When a step-back technique utilizing RaCe rotary nickel–titanium instruments was compared with ProFile instrumentation, it was found that the RaCe instruments produced less force in the canal system.[114]

Another study compared the use of a sequence of 0.04 tapered instruments with a sequence using 0.04 and 0.06 instruments. The sequence using the two different tapers produced less force.[115] A study performed with photoelastic material showed that with less engagement of the canal wall, there were smaller forces generated.[116] It was also shown that when more flutes per unit length are engaged, higher forces are the result.[117] Lubrication also influences the forces that can be generated during canal instrumentation. In particular, the use of an EDTA chelation solution significantly reduced maximum torque values for ProFile instruments.[118]

SEPARATION AND DISTORTION

A separated instrument is an undesirable occurrence during endodontic therapy. Unfortunately, it is very difficult to avoid when any type of rotary instrument is used in the canal system. Two recent studies looked at file separation and distortion. In one, only one file type (ProFile Series 29) was utilized. These files were used in only one patient before being discarded. The failure rate (separation) was less than 1%. The distortion rate was 15%. It is not known how many canals were treated with any one instrument.[119] A similar study looked at the LightSpeed instrument and found that for a total of 3,543 canals treated, the separation rate was 1.3%.[120] When ProFile instruments were used by dental students in their preclinical simulation laboratory, there was a separation rate of 0.31%.[121] A clinical study that compared ProFile with ProTaper systems found a separation rate of 7% for ProFile and 14% for ProTaper.[122] In this study, each instrument was used in at least four molars or 20 premolars or 50 incisors and canines. It would seem that these instruments were over used. In the other study, over 7,000 instruments of 8 different types were examined. The overall distortion rate was 12% and the fracture rate was 5%. However, these instruments were not discarded after being used in one patient. The mean use of the distorted instruments was three times, and the mean use of the undistorted instruments was four times.[123] In both studies, the patient treatment was done by endodontists. In other studies, an attempt has been made to delineate what factors are important in the distortion or separation of these files.

A series of studies considered rpm as a primary factor. Two studies concluded that higher rpm resulted in more separation and distortion.[124,125] Another concluded that lower rpm resulted in more file distortion, but none were fractured in the study.[126] When two different file types were compared at the same rpm, there were no significant differences.[127] When canal curvature was factored in, Zelada et al.[128] stated that rpm was not a significant factor but that a canal curvature of greater than 30° was significant. However, when some of the same researchers did a similar study, they concluded that a higher rpm did result in more separated files.[129] They also stated that the angle of curvature was a significant factor in file breakage whereas the radius of curvature was not a factor. Yared et al.[130] considered other factors in a series of studies. In one study, they used sets of ProFile instruments up to 10 times. They concluded that a higher rpm resulted in more deformation and separation of the instruments. They also showed that changing the torque setting for the motors did not influence the results. In the final analysis, they determined that operator experience was a significantly important factor. In another study, they looked at the use of an air motor and compared it with a high-torque motor and a low-torque motor. There were no significant differences.[131] When a similar study was done at a higher rpm setting, there were no significant differences when comparing the air motor with a high- or low-torque electric motor.[132] Finally, they looked at operator experience as a factor with the ProTaper instrument. They concluded that operator experience was a significant factor in instrument separation and deformation. Unfortunately, the use of a low-torque motor did not prevent the inexperienced operator from separating or deforming files.[133]

A study affirming the comparison between the electric and air motors showed that there were no significant differences in file distortion when either of these types of motors was used.[134] In addition to considering separation and distortion of files, there have been those who have looked at the wear of nickel–titanium rotary files. Interestingly, they have found that in some aspects the files improve with use. That is, metal strips and pitted surfaces decreased after being used.[135] When a similar study was performed on GT rotary files, Tripi et al.[136] found that the frequency of defects such as disruption of the cutting edge, fretting, and craters increased. Both of these studies were done on human teeth. A study of ProTaper S1 instruments used clinically determined that multiple uses of these instruments resulted in microcrack formation in instruments that were not separated. It was also found that debris was seen to be trapped in crack-like structures.[137]

SURFACE TREATMENT

In an effort to decrease the effects of usage, there have been attempts to modify the surface of the nickel–titanium alloy by various means. These methods include ion implantation[138,139] and vapor deposition[140–142] by various modalities. All of these methods were successful in changing the chemical composition of the nickel–titanium alloy surface as determined by XRD and other testing methods. However, in two studies, the efficacy of the vapor deposition was not confirmed by testing the wear or cutting efficiency.[140,142] In two studies by Rapisarda et al.,[138,139] they determined that there was better cutting efficiency and less wear because of the changes in the surface of the instruments. Schafer[141] confirmed these findings by verifying that a vapor deposition of titanium nitride did increase the cutting efficiency of the instruments. However, when one considers the additional cost of modifying these instruments, there is a question as to whether the gain in wear resistance or cutting efficiency warrants the additional expense for an instrument that is already considered to be disposable after as little as one use.

IRRIGANTS AND STERILIZATION

The most common irrigant used during endodontic instrumentation is sodium hypochlorite. It is important to know whether this or any other irrigant will have a deleterious effect on canal instruments. Haikel[143] showed that even lengthy exposure to sodium hypochlorite did not cause nickel–titanium files to fail at lower torsional moment values. In another study, Haikel[25] determined that the same long-term exposure to sodium hypochlorite did not decrease the cutting efficiency of nickel–titanium files. Stokes[144] determined that nickel–titanium files have a very high corrosion resistance even when immersed in full-strength sodium hypochlorite. A more recent study by Darabara et al.[145] showed that nickel–titanium files were highly corrosion resistant when exposed to sodium hypochlorite or R-EDTA. These instruments are also sterilized and, depending on clinical circumstances, may be sterilized multiple times before being discarded. Mize et al.[15] looked at LightSpeed nickel–titanium instruments and found that multiple sterilization cycles did not influence the cyclic fatigue of these instruments. In a study that compared nickel–titanium files with stainless steel files, it was shown that even 40 sterilization cycles had no effect on the torsional moment at failure for either file type.[146]

CANAL CLEANLINESS

Cleaning the canal system is a primary goal in endodontic therapy. Many instrumentation techniques and instruments have been developed to accomplish this important task. When only the removal of smear layer was considered, it was shown that the Quantec Series 2000 instruments removed significantly more of the smear layer in the apical third of the canal system when compared with K-file hand instrumentation.[147] Smear layer production by K3 was compared with ProFile, and it was found that K3 instruments produced less of a smear layer in the apical third of the canal system. However, both instruments did produce a smear layer.[148] In a comparison of RaCe and Pro-Taper rotary files, there was no difference in canal cleanliness, but in the apical third, the RaCe system did produce significantly less smear layer.[149] When the K3 system was compared with the NiTi-TEE system, there were no significant differences in canal cleanliness or smear layer removal.[150] When the K3 system was compared with the RaCe system and the Mtwo system, the Mtwo system was significantly better at cleaning the canal, but there were no significant differences for removal of the smear layer.[151]

Another study that compared nickel–titanium instrumentation with stainless steel hand files showed that canal cleanliness was equivalent if the size of the master apical file was the same. However, with an increase in size of the apical preparation, it was found that a cleaner canal was the result regardless of the instrument type that was used.[152] A similar study was performed utilizing GT files. All parameters except the size of the apical preparation were kept the same. The results were a larger apical preparation that left a canal system significantly cleaner.[153] These results are somewhat contradicted by the following studies. When Ahlquist et al.[154] compared stainless steel instrumentation with ProFiles, they found that the stainless steel instrumentation produced a significantly cleaner canal system in the apical third of the canal. When canal shape or curvature was considered, the results were similar. Barbizam et al.[155] found that oval canals were cleaned significantly better by hand instrumentation with stainless steel K-files. Schafer[156] reported the same results with stainless steel K-Flexofiles as compared with K3 rotary nickel–titanium files. Iqbal et al.[157] demonstrated that a combination technique was the best. The use of modified stainless steel Hedstrom files in combination with Pro-File instrumentation produced the cleanest canals. In another study by Schafer,[158] hand instrumentation was compared with engine-driven stainless steel files and motor-driven ProFile instruments. None of the instruments produced a completely clean canal especially in the apical third of the canal system. Hand instrumentation with Hedstrom files produced the cleanest canals. When another engine-driven system of stainless steel files was compared with the ProFile or the HERO 642, it was shown that the HERO 642 produced the least amount of smear layer.[159] A more recent development in automated handpieces AET (Anatomic Endodontic Technology) utilizing stainless steel instruments was compared with the ProFile system and hand instrumentation with K-Flexofiles. The AET system produced significantly cleaner canal walls with significantly less smear layer.[160] These results were to be expected because the AET system specifies that the apical third of the canal is to be prepared with hand instruments.

No canal system can be properly prepared without the use of irrigants. Gambarini[161] compared three irrigation regimes and concluded that the cleanest canal system was produced by a combination of EDTA, sodium hypochlorite, and a surfactant. Light-Speed instrumentation was compared with ProFile with two different irrigation techniques. There were differing results at different levels, but essentially there were no differences, particularly when consideration is given to the larger apical instrumentation with the LightSpeed group.[162] When canal curvature was brought in as a variable, it was shown that the RaCe instrument system produced a significantly cleaner canal system than the ProTaper instrument system.[163] In a comparative study with the Mtwo system, the ProTaper system produced a canal system that was as clean as the Mtwo system.[164] It may be presumed, if the canal system is being cleaned, that there is a reduction or elimination of bacteria. A group of studies has confirmed this presumption. Dalton et al.[165] compared stainless steel K-file instrumentation of the canal system with ProFile Series 29. There were no significant differences in the reduction of bacterial counts with saline irrigation. Another study compared hand nickel–titanium filing with the GT system with the ProFile Series 29 preparation of the canal system. There was no significant difference in bacterial counts with saline as an irrigant.[166]

If sodium hypochlorite was used as an irrigant, there were no significant differences in the reduction of bacterial counts when comparing hand nickel–titanium preparation of the canal system with the GT system of canal preparation.[167] If a combination of irrigants (5.25% NaOCl, EDTA, and calcium hydroxide) was used with GT rotary instrumentation, bacterial counts were significantly reduced. It was also confirmed that larger apical instrumentation resulted in the removal of more bacteria.[168]

As in the past, an additional concern with canal instrumentation is the amount of apical extrusion of debris. Ferraz et al.[169] compared two different stainless steel hand filing techniques (step-back versus balanced forces) with three different nickel–titanium instrument systems (ProFile versus Quantec 2000 versus Pow-R). As expected, there was significantly more debris extruded through the apical foramen by the step-back filing technique. In looking at the amount of bacteria that were extruded past the apex, a comparison was made between the ProTaper system and the GT system. There were no significant differences.[170] Unfortunately, these results were not compared with hand instrumentation or any other instrumentation technique. A recent study made comparisons between three rotary systems (ProTaper versus ProFile versus HERO). All systems produced apical extrusion of debris. ProTaper caused the extrusion of significantly more debris.[171] The question remains as to how much bacteria or debris the body can tolerate. It is doubtful any instrumentation technique would be able to eliminate extruding any bacteria or debris.

A final concern in the cleanliness of the canal system is whether or not the instruments themselves may be clean before use or be able to be cleaned after being used. Linsuwanont et al.[172] showed that new rotary nickel–titanium files have metal filings and debris present on them. This will vary from manufacturer to manufacturer and from lot to lot. They also determined that most files can not be rendered completely clean after use. When a similar study utilized pre-soaking in an enzymatic cleaner and an ultrasonic bath, it was found that the enzymatic cleaner did not have a significant effect. However, the ultrasonic bath did render the instruments significantly cleaner but was not able to remove calcium hydroxide deposits on all of the files.[173]

CANAL SHAPE

Just as canal anatomy may limit one's ability to clean the canal system, it also limits one's ability to shape the canal system before placing the obturation material. A major concern with any instrumentation system or technique is whether or not the canal system will be distorted in some fashion. When Schafer[24] compared hand nickel–titanium files with stainless steel files of the same cross-sectional geometry, he found that the nickel–titanium files removed less material than the stainless steel files. Another study compared hand filing of the canal system between nickel–titanium GT files, nickel–titanium K-files, and stainless steel K-files. In this study, Song et al.[174] found significantly less transportation with the nickel–titanium files. Whenever, in a series of studies, stainless steel hand filing was compared with either nickel–titanium hand filing or nickel–titanium rotary files, there was significantly less transportation of the canal system with the nickel–titanium files. This applied to LightSpeed nickel–titanium rotary files, GT nickel–titanium rotary files, ProFile Series 29, ProFile rotary files, Pow-R, K3, RaCe, and HERO 642 files.[156,175–182] However, there were two exceptions. When Peters et al.[183] utilized high-resolution computed tomography to assess canal transportation, they found that the ProFile system transported the most when compared with stainless steel hand files or LightSpeed rotary nickel–titanium files. The other exception was the study by Imura et al.[184] that compared stainless steel Flex-R filing of the canal system with two rotary nickel–titanium systems and found that all of the instruments transported the canal system to some degree. However, when hand nickel–titanium filing was compared with rotary nickel–titanium filing, there were no significant differences in canal transportation.[185–187] The same results were usually obtained when various rotary nickel–titanium files were compared with each other. That is, there were no significant differences in canal transportation. This applied to ProFile versus Naviflex,[188] HERO 642 versus Quantec SC,[189] ProTaper versus K3,[190] Flexmaster versus HERO 642,[191] ProFile versus GT rotary versus Quantec versus ProTaper,[192] and ProTaper versus GT rotary.[193] Of course, there were exceptions. When ProTaper was compared with RaCe, the RaCe instruments had significantly less transportation.[163] However, when ProTaper was compared with ProFile Series 29, there was significantly more transportation at 4 mm from the working length with the ProFile Series 29 files.[194] But, ProFile instruments showed significantly less transportation than K3 files depending on canal curvature.[195]

In later studies, some of the previous comparisons were confirmed and some were not confirmed. A study done in simulated S-shaped canals in plastic blocks compared the ProTaper system with K3 and RaCe instruments. It was found that the ProTaper system caused significantly more widening of the canal.[196] However, the clinical relevance of the results are questionable when one considers that the differences in canal widening were on the order of tenths of a millimeter. When comparing Mtwo with K3 and RaCe, it was found that the Mtwo system was significantly better at maintaining canal curvature.[151] Again, what is the clinical relevance of the results when it was found that the differences in canal curvature were less than two degrees? When Paque et al.[149] compared ProTaper with RaCe in extracted teeth, they found no significant differences for canal straightening or canal shape.

What needs to be remembered here is that canal anatomy should dictate what instruments can be used and how they should be used. Any instrument or instrumentation system can cause irreversible damage to the canal system. Any instrument or instrumentation system can produce excellent results if they are properly employed.

Rotary nickel–titanium files are not only used to prepare the canal system, they are also used to remove gutta-percha during re-treatment procedures. One study showed that ProFile instrumentation alone leaves significantly less gutta-percha debris after re-treatment.[197] However, other studies have shown no differences when compared with other rotary systems or hand filing with chloroform.[198,199] One study did show that hand K-files left significantly less debris than the Quantec SC system.[200] Other studies have looked at a number of different methodologies to remove either gutta-percha or a polymer-based material. When K-files activated by the M4 or Endo-gripper automated handpieces were compared with K-files alone or K3 rotary files, there were no overall differences in removing gutta-percha.[201] When H-files were compared with the ProFile system, there were no significant differences.[202] In a study comparing H-files, Flexmaster, ProTaper, and RaCe, it was determined that RaCe was significantly better than Flexmaster of H-files. It was also determined that there were no significant differences between ProTaper and all the other techniques.[203]

Finally, when H-files were compared with RaCe for the removal of gutta-percha or a polymer-based material, there were no significant differences between the techniques.[204] In all of these studies, there was no technique or instrumentation system that was able to remove all of the obturation materials. One would not expect that this could occur because it is not possible to completely clean any canal system.

NITI SPREADERS

There are also nickel–titanium spreaders developed for use in canal obturation. Berry et al.[205] showed these spreaders could penetrate further than stainless steel spreaders when used in curved canals. Schmidt et al.[206] compared penetration depth and force required to insert the spreader to place with a master cone in place in a curved canal. The nickel–titanium spreaders required less force and penetrated deeper than stainless steel spreaders. Gharai et al.[207] confirmed these results and tested the adequacy of the obturation by subjecting the molar teeth to a microleakage test. The nickel–titanium finger spreaders produced significantly less force, but there were no significant differences in microleakage.

ENGINE-DRIVEN INSTRUMENTS

Engine-driven instruments can be used in three types of contra-angle handpieces: a full rotary handpiece, latch or friction grip, a reciprocating/quarter-turn handpiece, or a special handpiece that imparts a vertical stroke but with an added reciprocating quarter-turn that "cuts in" when the instrument is stressed. In addition, there are battery-powered, slow-speed handpieces that are combined with an apex locator, designed to prevent apical perforations. Because the instruments used in these handpieces are generally designed for the type of action delivered, it is best to describe the handpiece before discussing their instruments.

ROTARY CONTRA-ANGLE HANDPIECE INSTRUMENTS

Instrumentation with a full rotary handpiece is by straight-line drilling or side cutting. Mounted with round or tapered burs or diamond points, full rotary contra-angle handpieces can be used to develop coronal access to canal orifices. Special reamers may be used to funnel out orifices for easier access, to clean and shape canals with slow-turning nickel–titanium reamer-type instruments, and to prepare post channels for final restoration of the tooth.

Because some of these instruments (stainless) do not readily bend and should be used in perfectly straight canals and because they are often misdirected or forced beyond their limits, they can cause perforations or break.

One solution to these problems is to use a slower handpiece: the Medidenta/Micro Mega MM 324 reduction gear Handpieces (Medidenta/Micro Mega, Woodside, NY), the Aseptico Electric Motor Handpiece (Aseptico International, Woodinville, WA), the Quantec ETM Electric torque control motor (Sybron-Endo, Irving, CA), and the Moyco/Union Broach Sprint EDM Electronic Digital Motor handpiece (Miller Dental). These electric motors are specifically designed to power the new nickel–titanium instruments in canal preparation. The speeds vary from 300 rpm suggested for ProFiles (Tulsa Dental) to 2,000 rpm recommended for LightSpeed instruments.

Electric handpieces are available wherein not only the speed can be controlled but the torque as well, that is, the speed and torque can be set for a certain size instrument and the handpiece will "stall" and reverse if the torque limit is exceeded. Some of these motors are the Aseptico ITR Motor handpiece (Aseptico International), the Nouvag TCM ENDO motor (Nouvag, Switzerland), the Endo-Pro Electric (Medidenta/Micro Mega), and the ProTorq motor handpiece (Micro Motors Inc., Santa Ana, CA).

There is also the Morita Tri Auto-ZX (J. Morita USA Inc., Irvine, CA), a cordless, battery-powered, endodontic, slow-speed (280 rpm) handpiece with a built-in apex locator. It uses rotary nickel–titanium instruments held by a push-button chuck. The Tri Auto-ZX has three automatic functions: The handpiece automatically starts when the file enters the canal and stops when the file is removed. If too much pressure is applied, the handpiece automatically stops and reverses rotation. It also automatically stops and reverses rotation when the file tip reaches the apical stop, as determined by the built-in apex locator. The Tri Auto-ZX works in a moist canal.

RECIPROCATING HANDPIECE

A commonly used flat plane reciprocating handpiece is the Giromatic (Medidenta/Micro Mega). It accepts only latch-type instruments. In this device, the quarter-turn motion is delivered 3,000 times per minute. Kerr has the M4 Safety Handpiece (Sybron-Kerr, Orange, CA), which has a 30° reciprocating motion and a chuck that locks regular hand files in place by their handles (Figure 13). The Kerr Company recommends their Safety Hedstrom Instrument be used with the M4. Zakariasen et al.[208,209] found the M4, mounted with Safety Hedstrom files, to be somewhat superior to "step-back

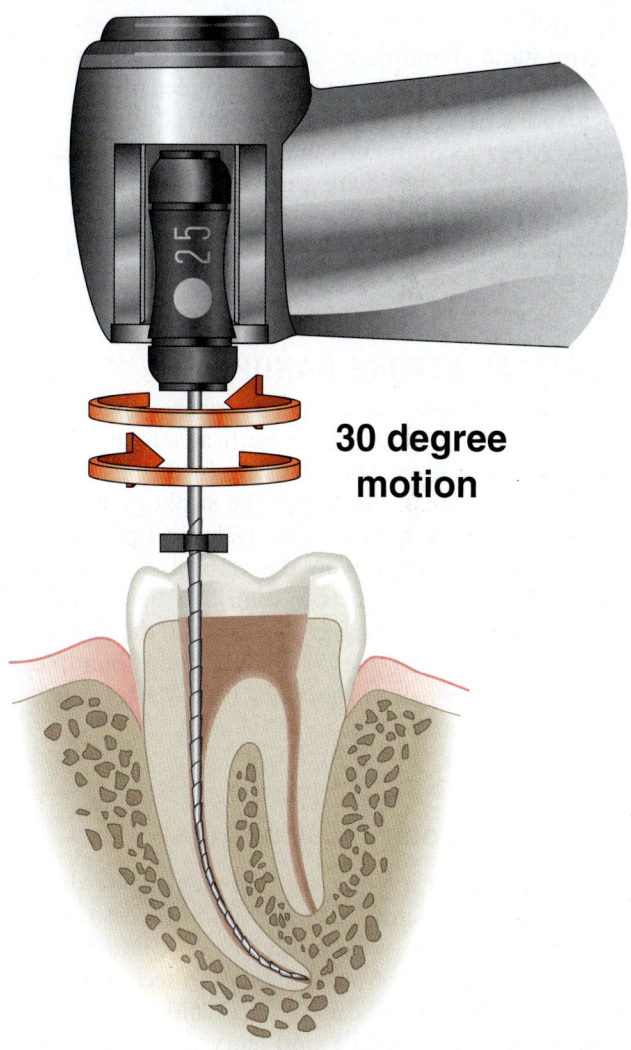

Figure 13 The M4 Safety Handpiece reciprocates in a 30° motion and locks regular hand files in place. The manufacturer recommends that Safety Hedstrom files be used. Courtesy of Sybron-Endo/Kerr.

hand preparations and a shorter time of preparation." Hulsman and Stryga[210] found much the same for both the M4 and the Giromatic.

The Endo-Gripper (Moyco/Union Broach) is a similar handpiece, with a 10:1 gear ratio and a 45° turning motion. As with the Kerr M4, the Endo-Gripper also uses regular hand, not contra-angle, instruments. Union Broach recommends their Flex-R and Onyx-R files. In a comparison of nickel–titanium rotary engine-driven instruments with the Endo-Gripper and the Kerr M4, it was found that there were no significant differences among the groups for the direction of transportation. The one nickel–titanium rotary instrument that did have significant transportation has subsequently been redesigned.[211]

Giromatic handpiece instrumentation was not effective when broaches were used. Hedstroem-type files and K-style reamers were more effective.[212–214] Micro Mega recommends that Rispi Sonic or Triocut instruments be used with the Giromatic handpiece. The reports are mixed, however, between "zipping" at the apical foramen versus round, tapered preparation.[215–218]

VERTICAL STROKE HANDPIECE

The vertical stroke handpiece is driven either by air or electrically that delivers a vertical stroke ranging from 0.3 to 1 mm. The more freely the instrument moves in the canal, the longer the stroke. The handpiece also has a quarter-turn reciprocating motion that "kicks in," along with the vertical stroke, when the canal instrument starts to bind in a tight canal. If it is too tight, the motion ceases, and the operator returns to a smaller file. The Endo Pulse handpiece (Endo Technic, San Diego, CA) uses Master Files, a variation of the H-files.

Rotary Instruments

Two of the most historic and popular engine-driven instruments are Gates Glidden drills and Peeso reamers (drills) (Figure 14, A and B). Gates Glidden drills are an integral part of instrumentation techniques for both initial opening of canal orifices and deeper penetration in both straight and curved canals. Gates Glidden drills are designed to have a weak spot in the part of the shaft closest to the handpiece so that, if the instrument separates, the separated part can be easily removed from the canal. They come in sizes 1 through 6.

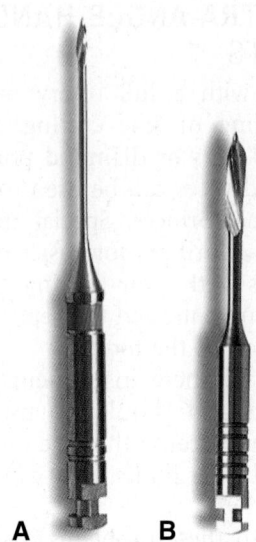

Figure 14 Engine-driven instruments used in a slow-speed handpiece. *A*, Gates Glidden drills come in sizes 1 through 6, end cutting or non–end cutting, and are used extensively in enlarging the straight part of the canal. *B*, Peeso reamer (drill) used primarily for post preparation. Photos courtesy of Dentsply/Maillefer.

In a laboratory study, Luebke and Brantley[219] tested two brands of Gates Glidden drills by clamping the head of the drill and then twisting the handles either clockwise or counterclockwise. There was no specific pattern to their fracture except that some broke at the head and some high on the shaft near the shank. Luebke and Brantley[220,221] later repeated the experiment, allowing the drill head to turn as it would in a clinical situation. This time, all of the drills fractured near the shank, "a major departure from the previous test."

The Peeso reamer (Dentsply/Maillefer) is most often used in preparing the coronal portion of the root canal for a post and core. One must be careful to use the "safe-ended" Peeso drill to prevent lateral perforation. Gutta-percha should have previously been removed to post depth with a hot plugger.

ULTRASONIC AND SONIC HANDPIECES

Instruments used in the handpieces that move near or faster than the speed of sound range from standard K-type files to special broach-like instruments. "Ultrasonic endodontics is based on a system in which sound as an energy source (at 20 to 25 kHγ) activates an endodontic file resulting in three-dimensional activation of the file in the surrounding medium."[222] "The main debriding action of ultrasonics was initially thought to be by cavitation, a process by which bubbles formed from the action of the file, become unstable, collapse, and cause a vacuum-like 'implosion.' A combined shock, shear and vacuum action results."[222] Ultrasonic handpieces use K-files as a canal instrument. Before a size 15 file can fully function, however, the canal must be enlarged with hand instruments to at least a size 20.

Although Richman[223] in 1957 must be credited with the first use of ultrasonics in endodontics, Martin and Cunningham[224–232] were the first to develop a device, test it, and see it marketed in 1976. Ultimately named the Cavitron Endodontic System (no longer manufactured), it was followed on the market by the Enac unit (Osada Electric Co., Los Angeles, CA) and the Piezon Master 400 (Electro Medical Systems, SA, Switzerland).

These instruments all deliver an irrigant/coolant, usually sodium hypochlorite, into the canal space while cleaning and shaping are carried out by a vibrating K-file. The results achieved by the ultrasonic units have ranged from outstanding[224–239] to disappointing.[240–244] What is the explanation for such a wide variance in results? The answer seems to lie in the extensive experimentation on ultrasonic instruments carried out by Ahmad et al.[245–247] They thoroughly studied the mechanisms involved and questioned the role that cavitation and implosion play in the cleansing process. It is believed that a different physical phenomenon, "acoustic streaming," is responsible for the debridement. They concluded that "transient cavitation does not play a role in canal cleaning with the CaviEndo unit; however, acoustic streaming does appear to be the main mechanism involved."[245] They pointed out that acoustic streaming "depends on free displacement amplitude of the file" and that the vibrating file is "dampened" in its action by the restraining walls of the canal.

Ahmad et al.[246] found that the smaller files generated greater acoustic streaming and hence much cleaner canals. After canals are fully prepared, by whatever means, they recommended returning with a fully oscillating No. 15 file for 5 minutes with a free flow of 1% sodium hypochlorite. In another study, Ahmad et al.[247] found that root canals had to be enlarged to the size of a No. 40 file to permit enough clearance for the free vibration of the No. 15 file at full amplitude. Others, including Martin, the developer, have recommended that the No. 15 file be used exclusively.[227,241] The efficacy of ultrasound to thoroughly debride canals following stepback preparation was demonstrated by Archer et al.[248] There was a difference in cleanliness between canals needle-irrigated during preparation and those canals prepared and followed by 3 minutes of ultrasonic instrumentation with a No. 15 file and 5.25% sodium hypochlorite.

Walmsley and Williams[249] reached similar conclusions about the oscillatory pattern of endosonic files. They pointed out that the greatest displacement amplitude occurs at the unconstrained tip and that the greatest restraint occurs when the instrument is negotiating the apical third of a curved canal. This is the damping effect noted by Ahmad et al.,[245] the lack of freedom for the tip to move freely to either cut or cause acoustic streaming to cleanse. Krell et al.[250] observed the same phenomenon that the irrigant could not advance to the apex "until the file could freely vibrate." Lumley and Walmsley[251] reported better results if K-files were precurved when used in curved canals.

Ahmad et al.[252] noted another interesting phenomenon about ultrasonic canal preparation—that, contrary to earlier reports, ultrasonics alone actually increased the viable counts of bacteria in simulated root canals. This was felt to be caused by the lack of cavitation and the dispersal effects of the bacteria by acoustic streaming. On substitution of sodium hypochlorite (2.5%) for water, however, all of the bacteria were killed, proving once again the importance of using an irrigating solution with bactericidal properties.

Ahmad and Pitt Ford[253] also compared two ultrasonic units—CaviEndo versus Enac. They evaluated canal shape and elbow formation: "There was no significant difference...in the amount of apical enlargement." They did find, however, that the Enac unit had a greater propensity for producing "elbows," as well as apical deviation and change of width. Ahmad[254] suggested that "the manufacturers of ultrasonic units consider different file designs." She found the K-Flex to be more efficient than the regular K style.

ULTRASONIC CONCLUSIONS

One can draw the conclusion that ultrasonic endodontics has added to the practice of root canal therapy. There is no question that canals are better debrided if ultrasonic oscillation with sodium hypochlorite is used at the conclusion of cavity preparation. But the files must be small and loose in the canal, particularly in curved canals, to achieve optimum cleansing.

SONIC HANDPIECES

The principal sonic endodontic handpiece available today is the Micro Mega 1500 (or 1400) Sonic Air

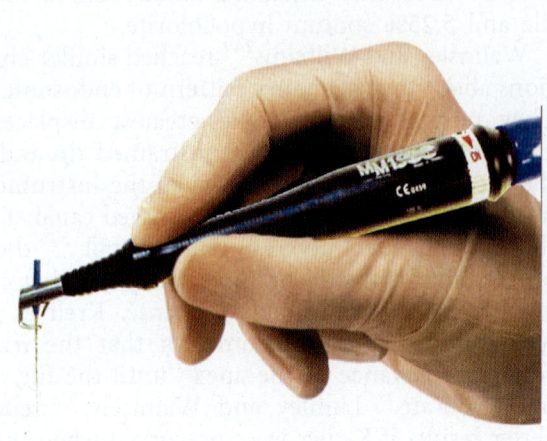

Figure 15 Micro Mega 1500 Sonic Air handpiece. Activated by pressure from the turbine air supply, the Micro Mega 1500 can be mounted with special instruments easily adjusted to the length of the tooth. Water spray serves as an irrigant. Photo courtesy of Medidenta/Micro Mega.

Endo System (Medidenta International, Inc.; Woodside, NY) (Figure 15). Like the air rotor handpiece, it attaches to the regular airline at a pressure of 0.4 MPa. The air pressure may be varied with an adjustable ring on the handpiece to give an oscillatory range of 1,500 to 3,000 cycles per second. Tap water irrigant/coolant is delivered into the preparation from the handpiece.

Walmsley et al.[255] studied the oscillatory pattern of sonically powered files. They found that out in the air, the sonic file oscillated in a large elliptical motion at the tip. When loaded, as in a canal, they found that the oscillatory motion changed to a longitudinal motion, up and down, "a particularly efficient form of vibration for the preparation of root canals."

The strength of the Micro Mega sonic handpiece lies in the special canal instruments used and the ability to control the air pressure and hence the oscillatory pattern. The three choices of file that are used with the Micro Mega 1500 are the Rispi Sonic, the Shaper Sonic, and the Trio Sonic (Medidenta International, Inc.) (Figure 16). The Rispi Sonic resembles the old rat-tail file. The Shaper Sonic resembles a barbed broach. The Trio Sonic resembles a triple-helix Hedstroem file. All of these instruments have safe-ended noncutting tips.

The Rispi Sonic has 8 cutting blades and the Shaper Sonic has 16. The ISO sizes range from 15 to 40.

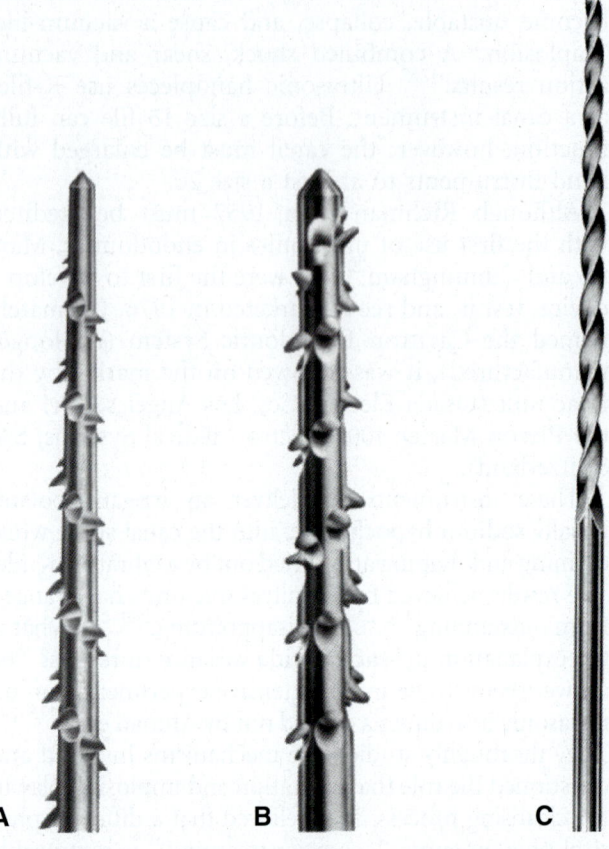

Figure 16 Three instruments used with the Micro Mega 1500 Sonic Air handpiece. **A**, Rispi Sonic. **B**, Shaper Sonic. **C**, Trio Sonic (aka Heliosonic or Triocut). Courtesy of Medidenta/Micro Mega.

Because graduated-size instruments have varying shaft sizes, the instrument must be tuned with the unit's tuning ring to optimum tip amplitude of 0.5 mm. As with the ultrasonic canal preparation, these instruments must be free to oscillate in the canal, to rasp away at the walls, and to remove necrotic debris and pulp remnants. To accommodate the smallest instrument, a size 15, the canal must be enlarged to the working length with hand instruments through size No. 20. The sonic instruments, with the 1.5 to 2.0 mm safe tips, begin their rasping action this far removed from the apical stop. This is known as the "sonic length." As the instrument becomes loose in the canal, the next-size instrument is used, and then the next size, which develops a flaring preparation. The sonic instruments are primarily for step-down enlarging, not penetration.

Three commonly held objectives of shaping the root canal are (1) developing a continuous tapering conical form, (2) making the canal narrow apically with the narrowest cross-sectional diameter at its terminus, and (3) leaving the apical foramen in its original position spatially. To satisfy these requirements, two of the sonic instruments have been quite successful. Dummer et al.[256] found the Rispi Sonic and Shaper Sonic files to be the most successful, the Trio Sonic less so. "In general, the Shaper Sonic files widened the canals more effectively than the Rispi Sonic files, whilst the Heliosonic [Trio Sonic] files were particularly ineffective...."[256]

Bolanos et al.[257] found essentially the same results. They recommended that the Shaper Sonic files be used first and that the remaining two-thirds of the canal be finished with the Rispi Sonic. Ehrlich et al.[258] compared canal apical transport using Rispi Sonic and Trio Sonic files versus hand instrumentation with K-files. They found no difference in zipping among the three instruments. Tronstad and Niemczyk[259] also tested the Rispi and Shaper files against other instruments. They reported no complications (broken instruments, perforations, etc.) with either of the Sonic instruments. Miserendino et al.[260] also found that the "Micro Mega sonic vibratory systems using Rispi Sonic and Shaper files were significantly more efficient than the other systems tested."

COMPARISONS IN EFFICACY AND SAFETY OF AUTOMATED CANAL PREPARATION DEVICES

Before making an investment in an automated endodontic device, one should know the comparative values of the different systems and their instruments. Unfortunately, the ultimate device and instrument has not been produced and tested as yet. Some are better in cutting efficiency, some in following narrow curved canals, some in producing smooth canals, and some in irrigating and removing smear layer, but apparently none in mechanically reducing bacterial content.

As stated above, Miserendino et al.[260] found that the cutting varied considerably. They ranked the Rispi Sonic file at the top, followed by the Shaper Sonic, the Enac "U" file (Osada Electric Co.), and the CaviEndo K-file.

Tronstad and Niemczyk's[259] comparative study favored the Canal Finder System in narrow, curved canals. On the other hand, the Rispi and Shaper files in the Micro Mega Sonic handpiece proved the most efficacious "in all types of root canals." The Cavitron Endo System was slow, blocked and ledged canals, and fractured three files in severely curved canals. They also found the Giromatic with Rispi files to be effective in wide straight canals, less so in curved canals, where four Rispi files fractured.

Bolanos et al.[257] also tested the Giromatic with Rispi files against the Micro Mega Sonic handpiece with Rispi and Shaper files. They found the Rispi Sonic best in straight canals, the Shaper Sonic best in curved canals, and both better than the Giromatic/Rispi and/or hand instrumentation with K-Flex files. The Shaper files left the least debris and the Giromatic/Rispi left "an extensive amount of debris."

Kielt and Montgomery[261] also tested the Micro Mega Sonic unit with Trio Sonic files against the ultrasonic Cavitron Endo and Enac units with K-files. Even though others found the Trio Sonic files less effective (than the Rispi or Shaper files), Kielt and Montgomery[261] concluded that "overall the Medidenta unit was superior to the other endosonic systems and to the hand technique (control)." Zakariasen et al.[262] reported success in combining hand instrumentation with sonic enlargements using the Micro Mega 1500.

Walker and del Rio[263] also compared the efficacy of the Cavitron Endo and Enac ultrasonic units against the Micro Mega Sonic unit and found "no statistically significant difference among the groups, however, liquid extruded from the apical foramen in 84% of their test teeth." They felt that "sodium hypochlorite may improve the debridement of the canal."

Yahya and El Deeb[264] tested ultrasonic units against sonic units. The researchers found the Micro Mega Sonic to be the fastest in preparation time and caused the "least amount of straightening of the canals." On the other hand, Reynolds et al.[265] found hand preparation with the step-back technique superior to sonic and ultrasonic preparation except in the important apical area, where they were similar. Lumley et al.[266] found that ultrasonic and sonic files best cleaned ovoid canals.

Lev et al.[267] prepared the cleanest canals using the step-back technique followed by 3-minute use of a CaviEndo ultrasonic file with sodium hypochlorite.

Stamos et al.[268] also compared cleanliness following ultrasonic debridement with sodium hypochlorite or tap water. Using water alone, the Enac system was more effective, but when sodium hypochlorite was used, the CaviEndo unit (which has a built-in tank) was superior. They also reported ultrasonic preparation to be "significantly faster" than hand instrumentation.

Goldman et al.[269] tested sonic versus ultrasonic units and concluded that they were all effective in canal preparation but judged the Micro Mega Sonic Air System, using Rispi and Shaper Sonic files, "as the best system tested."

Pugh et al.[270] compared four techniques according to the amount of debris extruded from the apex. The sonic technique extruded the least and hand instrumentation the most debris. Ultrasonic was halfway between. Whether the debris discharged into the apical tissue contains bacteria was of the utmost importance. Using sterile saline as an irrigant, Barnett et al.[271] found sodium hypochlorite to be four times more effective than sterile saline. Fairbourn et al.[272] found essentially the same thing.

COMPARATIVE CONCLUSION OF AUTOMATED DEVICES

It appears safe to say that no one automated device will answer all needs in canal cleaning and shaping. Hand instrumentation is essential to prepare and cleanse the apical canal, no matter which device, sonic or ultrasonic, is used. Recent research has confirmed the previous findings. Sonic or ultrasonic instrumentation is significantly better than hand instrumentation of the canal system as far as producing a cleaner canal system.[273–275] In one study, Lee et al.[276] confirmed that ultrasonic instruments perform better in a larger canal space. In a similar study by van der Sluis et al.,[277] it was found that there was a tendency for ultrasonic irrigation to produce a cleaner canal system in a larger canal, but the differences were not significant. Another study by Lee et al.[278] demonstrated that the volume of irrigant is also essential in ridding the canal system of dentinal debris.

References

1. Ingle JI. A standardized endodontic technique using newly designed instruments and filling materials. Oral Surg Oral Med Oral Pathol Oral Radiol Endod 1961;14:83–91.
2. Ingle JI, LeVine M. The need for uniformity of endodontic instruments, equipment and filling materials. In: Transactions of the 2nd international conference of endodontics. Philadelphia: Univ. of Pennsylvania Press; 1958. pp. 123–43.
3. American Dental Association Council on Dental Materials, Instruments and Equipment. Revised ANSI/ADA specification no. 28 for root canal files and reamers, type-K, type-K for hand use. Chicago: American Dental Association Press; 2002.
4. Kerekes K. Evaluation of standardized root canal instruments and obturating points. J Endod 1979;5:145–50.
5. Serene TP, Loadholt C. Variations in same-size endodontic files. Oral Surg Oral Med Oral Pathol Oral Radiol Endod 1984;57:200–2.
6. Cormier CJ, von Fraunhofer JA, Chamberlain JH. A comparison of endodontic file quality and file dimensions. J Endod 1988;14:138–42.
7. Seto BG, Nicholls JI, Harrington GW. Torsional properties of twisted and machined endodontic files. J Endod 1990;16:355–60.
8. Keate KC, Wong M. A comparison of endodontic file tip quality. J Endod 1990;16:486–91.
9. Stenman E, Spångberg L. Machining efficiency of endodontic K-files and Hedstroem files. J Endod 1990;16:375–82.
10. Stenman E, Spångberg L. Root canal instruments are poorly standardized. J Endod 1993;19:327–34.
11. Canalda-Sahli C, Brau-Aguade E, Berastegui-Jimeno E. A comparison of bending and torsional properties of K-files manufactured with different metallic alloys. Int Endod J 1996;29:185–9.
12. Tepel A, Schafer E, Hoppe W. Properties of endodontic hand instruments used in rotary motion. Part 3: resistance to bending and fracture. J Endod 1997;23:141–5.
13. Wolcott J, Himel VT. Torsional properties of nickel-titanium versus stainless steel endodontic files. J Endod 997;23:217–20.

Table 1 Dimensions in Millimeters (Revision of ADA Specification No. 28 Added Instrument Sizes 08 and 110–150 to the Original Specification Diameter [Tolerance ± 0.02 mm])

Handle Size	D1 mm	D2 mm	D3 mm	Color Code
08	0.08	0.40	0.14	Gray
10	0.10	0.42	0.16	Purple
15	0.15	0.47	0.21	White
20	0.20	0.52	0.26	Yellow
25	0.25	0.57	0.31	Red
30	0.30	0.62	0.36	Blue
35	0.35	0.67	0.41	Green
40	0.40	0.72	0.46	Black
45	0.45	0.77	0.51	White
50	0.50	0.82	0.56	Yellow
55	0.55	0.87	0.61	Red
60	0.60	0.92	0.66	Blue
70	0.70	1.02	0.76	Green
80	0.80	1.12	0.86	Black
90	0.90	1.22	0.96	White
100	1.00	1.32	1.06	Yellow
110	1.10	1.42	1.16	Red
120	1.20	1.52	1.26	Blue
130	1.30	1.62	1.36	Green
140	1.40	1.72	1.46	Black
150	1.50	1.82	1.56	White

New diameter measurement point (D3) was added 3 mm from the tip of the cutting end of the instrument. Handle color coding is official. From Ingle and Bakland, Endodontics, 5th ed., 2002, Table 10-1, Ingle, JI et al, Endodontic cavity preparation.

14. Mitchell BF, James GA, Nelson RC. The effect of autoclave sterilization on endodontic files. Oral Surg Oral Med Oral Pathol Oral Radiol Endod 1983;55:204–7.
15. Mize SB, Clement DJ, Pruett JP, Carnes DL. Effect of sterilization on cyclic fatigue of rotary nickel-titanium endodontic instruments. J Endod 1998;24:843–7.
16. Schafer E. Relationship between design features of endodontic instruments and their properties. Part 2. Instrumentation of curved canals. J Endod 1999;25:56–9.
17. Roth WC, Gough RW, Grandich RA, Walker WA. A study of the strength of endodontic files. J Endod 1983;9:228–32.
18. Oliet S, Sorin SM. Cutting efficiency of endodontic reamers. Oral Surg Oral Med Oral Pathol Oral Radiol Endod 1973;36:243–52.
19. Webber J, Moser JB, Heuer MA. A method to determine the cutting efficiency of root canal instruments in linear motion. J Endod 1980;6:829–34.
20. Kazemi RB, Stenman E, Spångberg LSW. The endodontic file is a disposable instrument. J Endod 1995;21:451–5.
21. Filho IB, Esberard M, Leonardo RD, del Rio CE. Microscopic evaluation of three endodontic files, pre- and post-instrumentation. J Endod 1998;24:461–4.
22. Newman JG, Brantley WA, Gerstein H. A study of the cutting efficiency of seven brands of endodontic files in linear motion. J Endod 1983;9:316–22.
23. Neal RG, Craig RG, Powers JM. Cutting ability of K-type endodontic files. J Endod 1983;9:52–7.
24. Schafer E, Lau R. Comparison of cutting efficiency and instrumentation of curved canals with nickel-titanium and stainless-steel instruments. J Endod 1999;25:427–30.
25. Haikel Y, Serfaty R, Wilson P, et al. Cutting efficiency of nickel-titanium endodontic instruments and the effect of sodium hypochlorite treatment. J Endod 1998;24:736–9.
26. Schafer E. Relationship between design features of endodontic instruments and their properties. Part 1. Cutting efficiency. J Endod 1999;25:52–5.
27. Dearing GJ, Kazemi RB, Stevens RH. An objective evaluation comparing the physical properties of two brands of stainless steel endodontic hand files. J Endod 2005;31:827–30.
28. Dearing GJ, Kazemi RB, Stevens RH. A comparison of the machining efficiency of two brands of stainless steel endodontic hand files. J Endod 2005;31:873–6.
29. Luks S. An analysis of root canal instruments. J Am Dent Assoc 1959;58:85–92.
30. Gutierrez JH, Gigoux C, Sanhueza I. Physical and chemical deterioration of endodontic reamers during mechanical preparation. Oral Surg Oral Med Oral Pathol Oral Radiol Endod 1969;28:394–403.
31. Lentine FN. A study of torsional and angular deflection of endodontic files and reamers. J Endod 1979;5:181–91.
32. Chernick LB, Jacobs JJ, Lautenschlauger EP, Heuer MA. Torsional failures of endodontic files. J Endod 1976;2:94–7.
33. Lautenschlager EP, Jacobs JJ, Marshall GW, Heuer MA. Brittle and ductile torsional failures of endodontic instruments. J Endod 1977;3:175–8.
34. Roane JB, Sabala C. Clockwise or counterclockwise. J Endod 1984;10:349–53.
35. Sotokawa T. An analysis of clinical breakage of root canal instruments. J Endod 1988;14:75–82.
36. Haikel Y, Gasser P, Allemann C. Dynamic fracture of hybrid endodontic hand instruments compared with traditional files. J Endod 1991;17:217–20.
37. Schafer E, Tepel J. Relationship between design features of endodontic instruments and their properties. Part 3. Resistance to bending and fracture. J Endod 2001;27:299–303.
38. Rowan MB, Nicholls JI, Steiner J. Torsional properties of stainless steel and nickel-titanium endodontic files. J Endod 1996;22:341–5.
39. Walia H, Brantley WA, Gerstein H. An initial investigation of the bending and torsional properties of Nitinol root canal files. J Endod 1988;14:346–51.
40. Villalobos RL, Moser JB, Heuer MA. A method to determine the cutting efficiency of root canal instruments in rotary motion. J Endod 1980;6:667–71.
41. Felt RA, Moser JB, Heuer MA. Flute design of endodontic instruments: Its influence on cutting efficiency. J Endod 1982;8:253–9.
42. Miserendino LJ, Moser JB, Heuer MA, Osetek EM. Cutting efficiency of endodontic instruments. Part 2: analysis of tip design. J Endod 1986;12:8–12.
43. Miserendino LJ, Moser JB, Heuer MA, Osetek EM. Cutting efficiency of endodontic instruments. Part 1: a quantitative comparison of the tip and fluted regions. J Endod 1985;11:435–41.
44. Powell SE, Simon JHS, Maze BB. A comparison of the effect of modified and nonmodified instrument tips on apical configuration. J Endod 1986;12:293–300.
45. Powell SE, Wong PD, Simon JHS. A comparison of the effect of modified and nonmodified tips on apical canal configuration. Part II. J Endod 1988;14:224–8.
46. Sabala CL, Roane JB, Southard LZ. Instrumentation of curved canals using a modified tipped instrument: a comparison study. J Endod 1988;14:59–64.
47. Dummer PMH, Al-Omari MAO, Bryant S. Comparison of the performance of four files with rounded tips during shaping of simulated root canals. J Endod 1998;24:364–71.
48. Zinelis S, Margelos J. Failure mechanism of hedstroem endodontic files in vivo. J Endod 2002;28:471–3.
49. Kosti E, Zinelis S, Lambrianidis T, Margelos J. A comparative study of crack development in stainless-steel Hedstrom files used with step-back or crown-down techniques. J Endod 2004;30:38–41.

50. Kazemi R, Stenman E, Spångberg L. A comparison of stainless steel and nickel-titanium H-type instruments of identical design: Torsional and bending tests. Oral Surg Oral Med Oral Pathol Oral Radiol Endod 2000;90:500–6.

51. Machian GR, Peters DD, Lorton L. The comparative efficiency of four types of endodontic instruments. J Endod 1982;8:398–402.

52. Mizrahi SJ, Tucker JW, Seltzer S. A scanning electron microscopic study of the efficacy of various endodontic instruments. J Endod 1975;1:324–33.

53. Miserendino LJ, Brantley WA, Walia HD, Gerstein H. Cutting efficiency of endodontic hand instruments. Part 4. Comparison of hybrid and traditional designs. J Endod 1988;14:451–4.

54. Yguel-Henry S, Vannesson H, von Stebut J. High precision, simulated cutting efficiency measurement of endodontic root canal instruments: influence of file configuration and lubrication. J Endod 1990;16:418–22.

55. El Deeb ME, Boraas JC. The effect of different files on the preparation shape of curved canals. Int Endod J 1985;18:1–7.

56. American National Standards Institute/ADA specification no. 58 for root canal files, Type H (Hedstroem). J Am Dent Assoc 1989;118:239–40.

57. Stenman E, Spångberg LSW. Machining efficiency of Flex-R, K-Flex, Trio-Cut and S-Files. J Endod 1990;16:575–9.

58. Wildey WL, Senia S. A new root canal instrument and instrumentation technique: a preliminary report. Oral Surg Oral Med Oral Pathol Oral Radiol Endod 1989;67:198–207.

59. Leseberg DA, Montgomery S. The effects of Canal Master, Flex-R, and K-Flex instrumentation on root canal configuration. J Endod 1991;17:59–65.

60. Wildey WL, Senia ES, Montgomery S. Another look at root canal instrumentation. Oral Surg Oral Med Oral Pathol Oral Radiol Endod 1992;74:499–507.

61. Baumgartner JC, Martin H, Sabala CC, et al. Histomorphometric comparison of canals prepared by four techniques. J Endod 1992;18:530–4.

62. Briseño BM, Kremers L, Hamm G, Nitsch C. Comparison by means of a computer-supported device of the enlarging characteristics of two different instruments. J Endod 1993;19:281–7.

63. Cirnis GJ, Boyer TJ, Pelleu GB. Effect of three file types on the apical preparations of moderately curved canals. J Endod 1988;14:441–4.

64. Sepic AO, Pantera EA, Neaverth EJ, Anderson RW. A comparison of Flex-R files and K-type files for enlargement of severely curved molar root canals. J Endod 1989;15:240–5.

65. Calhoun G, Montgomery S. The effects of four instrumentation techniques on root canal shape. J Endod 1988;14:273–7.

66. Alodeh MHA, Dummer PMH. The comparison of the ability of K-files and Hedstroem files to shape simulated root canals in resin blocks. Int Endod J 1989;22:226–35.

67. Briseño BM, Sonnabend E. The influence of different root canal instruments on root canal preparation: an *in vitro* study. Int Endod J 1991;24:15–23.

68. Stenman E, Spångberg LSW. Machining efficiency of endodontic files: a new methodology. J Endod 1990;16:151–7.

69. Rueggenberg FA, Powers JM. Mechanical properties of endodontic broaches and effects of bead sterilization. J Endod 1988;14:133–7.

70. Civjan S, Huget EF, DeSimon LB. Potential applications of certain nickel-titanium (nitinol) alloys. J Dent Res 1975;54:89–96.

71. Stoeckel D, Yu W. Superelastic Ni-Ti wire. Wire J Int 1991 March: 45–50.

72. Thompson SA. An overview of nickel-titanium alloys used in dentistry. Int Endo J 2000;33:297–310.

73. Kazemi RB, Stenman E, Spångberg LSW. Machining efficiency and wear resistance of nickel-titanium endodontic files. Oral Surg Oral Med Oral Pathol Oral Radiol Endod 1996;81:596–602.

74. Serene TP, Adams JD, Saxena A. Physical tests, in nickel-titanium instruments: application in endodontics. St. Louis: Ishiyaku EuroAmerica; 1995.

75. Hsich M, Yu F. The basic research on NiTi shape-memory alloy-anti-corrosive test and corrosive test and histological observation. Chin Med J 1982;1:105–20.

76. Canalda-Sahli C, Brau-Aguade E, Berastegui-Jimeno E. A comparison of bending and torsional properties of K files manufactured with different metallic alloys. Int Endod J 1996;29:185–9.

77. Canalda-Sahli C, Brau-Aguade E, Berastegui-Jimeno E. Torsional and bending properties of stainless steel and nickel-titanium CanalMaster U and Flexogate instruments. Endod Dent Traumatol 1996;12:141–5.

78. Pruett JP, Clement DJ, Carnes DL. Cyclic fatigue testing of nickel-titanium endodontic instruments. J Endod 1997;23:77–85.

79. Himel VT, Ahmed KM, Wood DM, Alhadainy HA. An evaluation of Nitinol and stainless steel files used by dental students in a laboratory proficiency exam. Oral Surg Oral Med Oral Pathol Oral Radiol Endod 1995;79:232–7.

80. Gambill JM, Alder M, del Rio CE. Comparison of nickel-titanium and stainless steel hand file instrumentation using computed tomography. J Endod 1996;22:369–75.

81. Tepel J, Schafer E, Hoope W. Properties of endodontic hand instrumentation used in rotary motion. Part 1. Cutting efficiency. J Endod 1995;21:418–21.

82. Elliot LM, Curtis RV, Pitt Ford TR. Cutting pattern of nickel titanium files using two preparation techniques. Endod Dent Traumatol 1998;14:10–15.

83. Kuhn G, Tavernier B, Jordan L. Influence of structure on nickel-titanium endodontic instruments failure. J Endod 2001;27:516–20.

84. Kuhn G, Jordan L. Fatigue and mechanical properties of nickel-titanium endodontic instruments. J Endod 2002;28:716–20.
85. Kim JW, Griggs JA, Regan JD, et al. Effect of cryogenic treatment on nickel-titanium endodontic instruments. Int Endo J 2005;38:364–71.
86. Brantley WA, Svec TA, Iijima M, et al. Differential Scanning Calorimetric studies of nickel-titanium rotary endodontic instruments after simulated clinical use. J Endod 2002;28:774–8.
87. Bahia MGA, Martins RC, Gonzalez BM, Buono VTL. Physical and mechanical characterization and the influence of cyclic loading on the behavior of nickel-titanium wires employed in the manufacture of rotary endodontic instruments. Int Endo J 2005;38:795–801.
88. Miyai K, Ebihara A, Hayashi Y, et al. Influence of phase transformation on the torsional and bending properties of nickel-titanium rotary endodontic instruments. Int Endo J 2006;39:119–26.
89. Turpin Y, Chagneau F, Vulcain J. Impact of two theoretical cross-sections ontorsional and bending stresses of nickel-titanium root canal instrument models. J Endod 2000;26:414–17.
90. Turpin YL, Chagneau F, Bartier O, et al. Impact of torsional and bending inertia on root canal instruments. J Endod 2001;27:333–6.
91. Berutti E, Chiandussi G, Gaviglio I, Ibba A. Comparative analysis of torsional and bending stresses in two mathematical models of nickel-titanium rotary instruments: ProTaper versus ProFile. J Endod 2003;29:15–19.
92. Xu X, Eng M, Zheng Y, Eng D. Comparative study of torsional and bending properties for six models of nickel-titanium root canal instruments with different cross-sections. J Endod 2006;32:372–5.
93. Yared GM, Bou Dagher FE, Machtou P. Cyclic fatigue of ProFile rotary instruments after clinical use. Int Endo J 2000;33:204–7.
94. Gambarini G. Cyclic fatigue of ProFile rotary instruments after prolonged clinical use. Int Endo J 2001;34:386–9.
95. Gambarini G. Cyclic fatigue of nickel-titanium rotary instruments after clinical use with low- and high-torque endodontic motors. J Endod 2001;27:772–4.
96. Bahia MGA, Buono VTL. Decrease in the fatigue resistance of nickel-titanium rotary instruments after clinical use in curved canals. Oral Surg Oral Med Oral Pathol Oral Radiol Endod 2005;100:249–55.
97. Bahia MGA, Melo MCC, Buono VTL. Influence of simulated clinical use on the torsional behavior of nickel-titanium rotary endodontic instruments. Oral Surg Oral Med Oral Pathol Oral Radiol Endod 2006;101:675–80.
98. de Melo MCC, Bahia MGA, Buono VTL. Fatigue resistance of engine-driven rotary nickel-titanium endodontic instruments. J Endod 2002;28:765–9.
99. Booth JR, Scheetz JP, Lemons JE, Eleazer PD. A comparison of torque required to fracture three different nickel-titanium rotary instruments around curves of the same angle but of different radius when bound at the tip. J Endod 2003;29:55–7.
100. Yared G, Kulkarni K. An in vitro study of the torsional properties of new and used rotary nickel-titanium files in plastic blocks. Oral Surg Oral Med Oral Pathol Oral Radiol Endod 2003;96:466–71.
101. Ullmann CJ, Peters OA. Effect of cyclic fatigue on static fracture loads in ProTaper nickel-titanium rotary instruments. J Endod 2005;31:183–6.
102. Li U-M, Lee B-S, Shih C-T, et al. Cyclic fatigue of endodontic nickel titanium rotary instruments: Static and dynamic tests. J Endod 2002;28:448–51.
103. Best S, Watson P, Pillier R, et al. Torsional fatigue and endurance limit of a size 30.06 ProFile rotary instrument. Int Endo J 2004;37:370–3.
104. Peters OA, Kappeler S, Bucher W, Barbakow F. Engine-driven preparation of curved root canals: Measuring cyclic fatigue and other physical parameters. Aust Endo J 2002;28:11–17.
105. Guilford WL, Lemons JE, Eleazer PD. A comparison of torque required to fracture rotary files with tips bound in simulated curved canal. J Endod 2005;31:468–70.
106. Yao JH, Schwartz SA, Beeson TJ. Cyclic fatigue of three types of rotary nickel-titanium files in a dynamic model. J Endod 2006;32:55–7.
107. Luebke NH, Brantley WA, Alapati SB, et al. Bending fatigue study of nickel-titanium Gates Glidden drills. J Endod 2005;31:523–5.
108. Schafer E, Dzepina A, Danesh G. Bending properties of rotary nickel-titanium instruments. Oral Surg Oral Med Oral Pathol Oral Radiol Endod 2003;96:757–63.
109. Blum JY, Cohen A, Machtou P, Micallef JP. Analysis of forces developed during mechanical preparation of extracted teeth using Profile NiTi rotary instruments. Int Endo J 1999;32:32–46.
110. Blum J, Machtou P, Micallef J. Location of contact areas on rotary profile instruments in relationship to the forces developed during mechanical preparation on extracted teeth. Int Endo J 1999;32:108–14.
111. Blum J-Y, Machtou P, Ruddle C, Micallef JP. Analysis of mechanical preparations in extracted teeth using ProTaper rotary instruments: Value of the Safety Quotient. J Endod 2003;29:567–75.
112. Sattapan B, Palamara J, Messer H. Torque during canal instrumentation using rotary nickel-titanium files. J Endod 2000;26:156–60.
113. Peters OA, Peters CI, Schonenberger K, Barbakow F. ProTaper rotary root canal preparation: assessment of torque and force in relation to canal anatomy. Int Endo J 2003;36:93–9.

114. da Silva FM, Kobayashi C, Suda H. Analysis of forces developed during mechanical preparation of extracted teeth using RaCe rotary instruments and ProFiles. Int Endo J 2005;381:17–21.

115. Schrader C, Peters OA. Analysis of torque and force with differently tapered rotary endodontic instruments in vitro. J Endod 2005;31:120–3.

116. Mayhew J, Eleazer P, Hnat W. Stress analysis of human tooth root using various root canal instruments. J Endod 2000;26:523–4.

117. Diemer F, Calas P. Effect of pitch length on the behavior of rotary triple helix root canal instruments. J Endod 2004;30:716–18.

118. Peters OA, Boessler C, Zehnder M. Effect of liquid and paste-type lubricants on torque values during simulated rotary root canal instrumentation. Int Endo J 2005;38:223–9.

119. Arens FC, Hoen MM, Steiman HR, Dietz GC. Evaluation of single-use rotary nickel-titanium instruments. J Endod 2003;29:664–6.

120. Knowles KI, Hammond NB, Biggs SG, Ibarrola JL. Incidence of instrument separation using LightSpeed rotary instruments. J Endod 2006;32:14–16.

121. Di Fiore PM, Genov KI, Komaroff E, et al. Fracture of ProFile nickel-titanium rotary instruments: a laboratory simulation assessment. Int Endo J 2006;39:502–9.

122. Shen Y, Cheung GSP, Bian Z, Peng B. Comparison of defects in ProFile and ProTaper systems after clinical use. J Endod 2006;32:61–5.

123. Parashos P, Gordon I, Messer HH. Factors influencing defects of rotary nickel-titanium endodontic instruments after clinical use. J Endod 2004;30:722–5.

124. Gabel W, Hoen M, Steiman R, et al. Effect of rotational speed on nickel-titanium file distortion. J Endod 1999;25:752–4.

125. Dietz D, Di Fiore P, Bahcall J, Lautenschlager E. Effect of rotational speed on the breakage of nickel-titanium rotary files. J Endod 2000;26:68–71.

126. Daugherty DW, Gound TG, Comer TL. Comparison of fracture rate, deformation rate, and efficiency between rotary endodontic instruments driven at 150 rpm and 350 rpm. J Endod 2001;27:93–5.

127. Tygesen YA, Steiman HR, Ciavarro C. Comparison of distortion and separation utilizing Profile and Pow-R nickel-titanium rotary files. J Endod 2001;27:762–4.

128. Zelada G, Varela P, Martin B, et al. The effect of rotational speed and the curvature of root canals on the breakage of rotary endodontic instruments. J Endod 2002;28:540–2.

129. Martin B, Zelada G, Varela P, et al. Factors influencing the fracture of nickel-titanium rotary instruments. Int Endo J 2003;36:262–6.

130. Yared GM, Bou Dagher FE, Machtou P. Influence of rotational speed, torque and operator's proficiency on ProFile failures. Int Endo J 2001;34:47–53.

131. Yared GM, Bou Dagher FE, Machtou P. Failure of ProFile instruments used with high and low torque motors. Int Endo J 2001;34:471–5.

132. Yared G, Sleiman P. Failure of ProFile instruments used with air, high torque control, and low torque control motors. Oral Surg Oral Med Oral Pathol Oral Radiol Endod 2002;93:92–6.

133. Yared G, Bou Dagher F, Kulkarni K. Influence of torque control motors and the operator's proficiency on ProTaper failures. Oral Surg Oral Med Oral Pathol Oral Radiol Endod 2003;96:229–33.

134. Bortnick KL, Steiman HR, Ruskin A. Comparison of nickel-titanium file distortion using electric and air-driven handpieces. J Endod 2001;27:57–9.

135. Eggert C, Peters O, Barbakow F. Wear of nickel-titanium Lightspeed instruments evaluated by scanning electron microscopy. J Endod 1999;25:494–7.

136. Tripi TR, Bonaccorso A, Tripi V, et al. Defects in GT rotary instruments after use: An SEM study. J Endod 2001;27:782–5.

137. Peng B, Shen Y, Cheung GSP, Xia TJ. Defects in ProTaper S1 instruments after clinical use: longitudinal examination. Int Endo J 2005;38:550–7.

138. Rapisarda E, Bonaccorso A, Tripi T, et al. The effect of surface treatments of nickel-titanium files on wear and cutting efficiency. Oral Surg Oral Med Oral Pathol Oral Radiol Endod 2000;89:363–8.

139. Rapisarda E, Bonaccorso A, Tripi TR, et al. Wear of nickel-titanium endodontic instruments evaluated by scanning electron microscopy: Effect of ion implantation. J Endod 2001;27:588–92.

140. Tripi TR, Bonaccorso A, Rapisarda E, et al. Depositions of nitrogen on NiTi instruments. J Endod 2002;28:497–500.

141. Schafer E. Effect of physical vapor deposition on cutting efficiency of nickel-titanium files. J Endod 2002;28:800–2.

142. Tripi TR, Bonaccorso A, Condorelli GG. Fabrication of hard coatings on NiTi instruments. J Endod 2003;29:132–4.

143. Haikel Y, Serfaty R, Wilson P, et al. Mechanical properties of nickel-titanium endodontic instruments and the effect of sodium hypochlorite treatment. J Endod 1998;24:731–5.

144. Stokes OW, Di Fiore PM, Barss JT, et al. Corrosion in stainless-steel and nickel-titanium files. J Endod 1999;25:17–20.

145. Darabara M, Bourithis L, Zinelis S, Papadimitriou GD. Susceptibility to localized corrosion of stainless steel and NiTi endodontic instruments in irrigating solutions. Int Endo J 2004;37:705–10.

146. Hilt B, Cunningham C, Shen C, Richards N. Torsional properties of stainless-steel and nickel-titanium files after multiple autoclave sterilizations. J Endod 2000;26:76–80.

147. Bertrand M, Pizzardini P, Muller M, et al. The removal of the smear layer using the Quantec system. A study using the scanning electron microscope. Int Endo J 1999;32:217–24.

148. Kum K-Y, Kazemi RB, Cha BY, Zhu Q. Smear layer production of K3 and ProFile Ni-Ti rotary instruments in curved root canals: A comparative SEM study. Oral Surg Oral Med Oral Pathol Oral Radiol Endod 2006;101:536–41.

149. Paque F, Musch U, Hulsmann M. Comparison of root canal preparation using RaCe and ProTaper rotary Ni-Ti instruments. Int Endo J 2005;38:8–16.

150. Jodway B, Hulsmann M. A comparative study of root canal preparation with NiTi-TEE and K3 rotary Ni-Ti instruments. Int Endo J 2006;39:71–80.

151. Schafer E, Erler M, Dammaschke T. Comparative study on the shaping ability and cleaning efficiency of rotary Mtwo instruments. Part 2. Cleaning effectiveness and shaping ability in severely curved root canals of extracted teeth. Int Endo J 2006;39:203–12.

152. Lumley PJ. Cleaning efficacy of two apical preparation regimens following shaping with hand files of greater taper. Int Endo J 2000;33:262–5.

153. Usman N, Baumgartner JC, Marshall JG. Influence of instrument size on root canal debridement. J Endod 2004;30:110–12.

154. Ahlquist M, Henningsson O, Hultenby K, Ohlin J. The effectiveness of manual and rotary techniques in the cleaning of root canals: a scanning electron microscope study. Int Endo J 2001;34:533–7.

155. Barbizam JVB, Fariniuk LF, Marchesan MA, et al. Effectiveness of manual and rotary instrumentation techniques for cleaning flattened root canals. J Endo 2002;28:365–6.

156. Schafer E, Schlingemann R. Efficiency of rotary nickel-titanium K3 instruments compared with stainless steel hand K-Flexofile. Part 2. Cleaning effectiveness and shaping ability in severely curved root canals of extracted teeth. Int Endo J 2003;36:208–17.

157. Iqbal MK, Karabucak B, Brown M, Menegazzo E. Effect of modified Hedstrom files on instrumentation area produced by ProFile instruments in oval canals. Oral Surg Oral Med Oral Pathol Oral Radiol Endod 2004;98:493–8.

158. Schafer E, Zapke K. A comparative scanning electron microscopic investigation of the efficacy of manual and automated instrumentation of root canals. J Endod 2000;26:660–4.

159. Jeon I-S, Spångberg LSW, Yoon T-C, et al. Smear layer production by 3 rotary reamers with different cutting blade designs in straight root canals: A scanning electron microscope study. Oral Surg Oral Med Oral Pathol Oral Radiol Endod 2003;96:601–7.

160. Zmener O, Pameijer CH, Banegas G. Effectiveness in cleaning oval-shaped root canals using Anatomic Endodontic Technology, ProFile and manual instrumentation: a scanning electron microscope study. Int Endo J 2005;38:356–63.

161. Gambarini G. Shaping and cleaning the root canal system: a scanning electron microscopic evaluation of a new instrumentation and irrigation technique. J Endod 1999;25:800–3.

162. Peters O, Barbakow F. Effects of irrigation on debris and smear layer on canal walls prepared by two rotary techniques: a scanning electron microscopic study. J Endod 2000;26:6–10.

163. Schafer E, Vlassis M. Comparative investigation of two rotary nickel-titanium instruments: ProTaper versus RaCe. Part 2. Cleaning effectiveness and shaping ability in severely curved root canals of extracted teeth. Int Endo J 2004;37:239–48.

164. Foschi F, Nucci C, Montebugnoli L, et al. SEM evaluation of canal wall dentine following use of Mtwo and ProTaper NiTi rotary instruments. Int Endo J 2004;37:832–9.

165. Dalton BC, Orstavik D, Phillips C, et al. Bacterial reduction with nickel-titanium rotary instrumentation. J Endod 1998;24:763–7.

166. Siqueira J, Lima K, Magalhaes F, et al. Mechanical reduction of the bacterial population in the root canal by three instrumentation techniques. J Endod 1999;25:332–5.

167. Siqueira JF, Rocas IN, Santos SRLD, et al. Efficacy of instrumentation techniques and irrigation regimens in reducing the bacterial population within root canals. J Endod 2002;28:181–4.

168. McGurkin-Smith R, Trope M, Caplan D, Sigurdsson A. Reduction of intracanal bacteria using GT rotary instrumentation, 5.25% NaOCl, EDTA, and $Ca(OH)_2$. J Endod 2005;31:359–63.

169. Ferraz CCR, Gomes NV, Gomes BPFA, et al. Apical extrusion of debris and irrigants using two hand and three engine-driven instrumentation techniques. Int Endo J 2001;34:354–8.

170. Er K, Sumer Z, Akpinar KE. Apical extrusion of intracanal bacteria following use of two engine-driven instrumentation techniques. Int Endo J 2005;38:871–6.

171. Tanalp J, Kaptan F, Sert S, et al. Quantitative evaluation of the amount of apically extruded debris using 3 different rotary instrumentation systems. Oral Surg Oral Med Oral Pathol Oral Radiol Endod 2006;101:250–7.

172. Linsuwanont P, Parashos P, Messer H. Cleaning of rotary nickel-titanium endodontic instruments. Int Endo J 2004;37:19–28.

173. Aasim SA, Mellor AC, Qualtrough AJE. The effect of presoaking and time in the ultrasonic cleaner on the cleanliness of sterilized endodontic files. Int Endo J 2006;39:143–9.

174. Song YL, Bian Z, Fan B, et al. A comparison of instrument-centering ability within the root canal for three contemporary instrumentation techniques. Int Endo J 2004;37:265–71.

175. Shadid DB, Nicholls JI, Steiner JC. A comparison of curved canal transportation with balanced force versus Lightspeed. J Endod 1998;24:651–4.

176. Pettiette M, Metzger S, Phillips C, Trope M. Endodontic complications of root canal therapy performed by dental students with stainless-steel K-files and nickel-titanium hand files. J Endod 1999;25:230–4.

177. Barthel C, Gruber S, Roulet J. A new method to assess the results of instrumentation techniques in the root canal. J Endod 1999;25:535–8.

178. Park H. A comparison of Greater Taper files, ProFiles, and stainless steel files to shape curved root canals. Oral Surg Oral Med Oral Pathol Oral Radiol Endod 2001;91:715–18.

179. Schafer E. Shaping ability of Hero 642 rotary nickel-titanium instruments and stainless steel hand K-Flexofiles in simulated curved root canals. Oral Surg Oral Med Oral Pathol Oral Radiol Endod 2001;92:215–20.

180. Tasdemir T, Aydemir H, Inan U, Unal O. Canal preparation with Hero 642 rotary Ni-Ti instruments compared with stainless steel hand K-file assessed using computed tomography. Int Endo J 2005;38:402–8.

181. Guelzow A, Stamm O, Martus P, Kielbassa AM. Comparative study of six rotary nickel-titanium systems and hand instrumentation for root canal preparation. Int Endo J 2005;38:743–52.

182. Schirrmeister JF, Strohl C, Altenburger MJ, et al. Shaping ability and safety of five different rotary nickel-titanium instruments compared with stainless steel hand instrumentation in simulated curved root canals. Oral Surg Oral Med Oral Pathol Oral Radiol Endod 2006;101:807–13.

183. Peters OA, Laib A, Gohring TN, Barbakow F. Changes in root canal geometry after preparation assessed by high-resolution computed tomography. J Endod 2001;27:1–6.

184. Imura N, Kato AS, Novo NF, et al. A comparison of mesial molar root canal preparations using two engine-driven instruments and the balanced-force technique. J Endod 2001;27:627–31.

185. Deplazes P, Peters O, Barbakow F. Comparing apical preparations of root canals shaped by nickel-titanium rotary instruments and nickel-titanium hand instruments. J Endod 2001;27:196–202.

186. Peters OA, Schonenberger K, Laib A. Effects of four Ni-Ti preparation techniques on root canal geometry assessed by micro computed tomography. Int Endo J 2001;34:221–30.

187. Kaptan F, Sert S, Kayahan B, et al. Comparative evaluation of the preparation efficacies of HERO Shaper and Nitiflex root canal instruments in curved root canals. Oral Surg Oral Med Oral Pathol Oral Radiol Endod 2005;100:636–42.

188. Ottosen S, Nicholls J, Steiner J. A comparison of instrumentation using naviflex and profile nickel-titanium engine-driven rotary instruments. J Endod 1999;25:457–60.

189. Hulsmann M, Schade M, Schafers F. A comparative study of root canal preparation with HERO 642 and Quantec SC rotary Ni-Ti instruments. Int Endo J 2001;34:538–46.

190. Bergmans L, Van Cleynenbreugel J, Beullens M, et al. Progressive versus constant tapered shaft design using NiTi rotary instruments. Int Endo J 2003;36:288–95.

191. Hulsmann M, Gressman G, Schafers F. A comparative study of root canal preparation using FlexMaster and HERO 642 rotary Ni-Ti instruments. Int Endo J 2003;36:358–66.

192. Yun H, Kim SK. A comparison of the shaping abilities of 4 nickel-titanium rotary instruments in simulated root canals. Oral Surg Oral Med Oral Pathol Oral Radiol Endod 2003;95:228–33.

193. Veltri M, Mollo A, Pini PP, et al. In vitro comparison of shaping abilities of ProTaper and GT rotary files. J Endod 2004;30:163–6.

194. Iqbal MK, Firic S, Tulcan J, et al. Comparison of apical transportation between ProFile and ProTaper NiTi rotary instruments. Int Endo J 2004;37:359–64.

195. Ayar LR, Love RM. Shaping ability of ProFile and K3 rotary Ni-Ti instruments when used in a variable tip sequence in simulated curved root canals. Int Endo J 2004;37:593–601.

196. Yoshimine Y, Ono M, Akamine A. The shaping effects of three nickel-titanium rotary instruments in simulated S-shaped canals. J Endod 2005;31:373–5.

197. Sae-Lim V, Rajamanickam I, Lim B, Lee H. Effectiveness of ProFile .04 taper rotary instruments in endodontic retreatment. J Endod 2000;26:100–4.

198. Ferreira JJ, Rhodes JS, Pitt Ford TR. The efficacy of gutta-percha removal using ProFiles. Int Endo J 2001;34:267–74.

199. Barrieshi-Nusair KM. Gutta-percha retreatment: Effectiveness of nickel-titanium rotary instruments versus stainless steel hand files. J Endod 2002;28:454–6.

200. Betti LV, Bramante CM. Quantec SC rotary instruments versus hand files for gutta-percha removal in root canal retreatment. Int Endo J 2001;34:514–19.

201. Masiero AV, Barletta FB. Effectiveness of different techniques for removing gutta-percha during retreatment. Int Endo J 2005;38:2–7.

202. Kosti E, Lambrianidis T, Economides N, Neofitou C. *Ex vivo* study of the efficacy of H-files and rotary ni-ti instruments to remove gutta-percha and four types of sealer. Int Endo J 2006;39:48–54.

203. Schirrmeister JF, Wrbas K-T, Meyer KM, et al. Efficacy of different rotary instruments for gutta-percha removal in root canal retreatment. J Endod 2006;32:469–72.

204. Schirrmeister JF, Meyer KM, Hermanns P, et al. Effectiveness of hand and rotary instrumentation for removing a new synthetic polymer-based root canal obturation material (Epiphany) during retreatment. Int Endo J 2006;39:150–6.

205. Berry KA, Loushine RJ, Primack PD, Runyan DA. Nickel-titanium versus stainless steel finger spreaders in curved canals. J Endod 1998;24:752–4.

206. Schmidt K, Walker T, Johnson J, Nicoli B. Comparison of nickel-titanium and stainless-steel spreader penetration and accessory cone fit in curved canals. J Endod 2000;26:42–4.

207. Gharai SR, Thorpe JR, Strother JM, McClanahan SB. Comparison of generated forces and apical microleakage using nickel-titanium and stainless steel finger spreaders in curved canals. J Endod 2005;31:198–200.

208. Zakariasen KA, Zakariasen KL. Comparison of hand, hand/sonic, and hand/mechanical instrumentation methods. J Dent Res 1994;73:215.

209. Zakariasen KL, Buerschen GH, Zakariasen KA. A comparison of traditional and experimental instruments for endodontic instrumentation. J Dent Res 1995;74:100.

210. Hulsman M, Stryga F. Comparison of root canal preparation using different automated devices and hand instrumentation. J Endod 1993;19:141–5.

211. Kosa D, Marshall G, Baumgartner J. An analysis of canal centering using mechanical instrumentation techniques. J Endod 1999;25:441–5.

212. Molven O. A comparison of the dentin removing ability of five root canal instruments. Scand J Dent Res 1970;78:500–11.

213. O'Connell DT, Brayton SM. Evaluation of root canal preparation with two automated endodontic handpieces. Oral Surg Oral Med Oral Pathol Oral Radiol Endod 1975;39:298–303.

214. Klayman S, Brilliant J. A comparison of the efficacy of serial preparation versus Giromatic preparation. J Endod 1975;1:334–7.

215. Weine FS, Kelly RF, Bray KE. Effect of preparation with endodontic handpieces on original canal shape. J Endod 1976;2:298–303.

216. Harty F, Stock C. The Giromatic system compared with hand instrumentation in endodontics. Br Dent J 1974;137:239–44.

217. Felt RA, Moser JB, Heuer MA. Flute design of endodontic instruments: its influence on cutting efficiency. J Endod 1982;8:253–9.

218. Spyropoulos S, El Deeb ME, Messer HH. The effect of Giromatic files on the preparation shape of severely curved canals. Int Endod J 1987;20:133–42.

219. Luebke NH, Brantley WA. Physical dimensions and torsional properties of rotary endodontic instruments. I. Gates-Glidden drills. J Endod 1990;16:438–41.

220. Luebke NH. Performance of Gates-Glidden drill with an applied deflection load. J Endod 1989;15:175.

221. Luebke NH, Brantley WA. Torsional and metallurgical properties of rotary endodontic instruments. II Stainless steel Gates-Glidden drills. J Endod 1991;17:319–23.

222. Johnson TA, Zelikow R. Ultrasonic endodontics: a clinical review. J Am Dent Assoc 1987;114:655–7.

223. Richman MJ. The use of ultrasonics in root canal therapy and root resection. J Dent Med 1957;12:12–18.

224. Cunningham WT, Martin H. A scanning electron microscope evaluation of root canal debridement with the endosonic ultrasonic synergistic system. Oral Surg Oral Med Oral Pathol Oral Radiol Endod 1982;53:527–31.

225. Martin H. Ultrasonic disinfection of the root canal. Oral Surg Oral Med Oral Pathol Oral Radiol Endod 1976;42:92–9.

226. Martin H, Cunningham WT, Norris JP, Cotton WR. Ultrasonic versus hand filing of dentin: a quantitative study. Oral Surg Oral Med Oral Pathol Oral Radiol Endod 1980;49:79–81.

227. Martin H, Cunningham WT, Norris JP. A quantitative comparison of the ability of diamond and K-type files to remove dentin. Oral Surg Oral Med Oral Pathol Oral Radiol Endod 1980;50:566–8.

228. Martin H, Cunningham WT. The effect of endosonic and hand manipulation on the amount of root canal material extruded. Oral Surg Oral Med Oral Pathol Oral Radiol Endod 1982;53:611–13.

229. Martin H, Cunningham WT. An evaluation of postoperative pain incidence following endosonic and conventional root canal therapy. Oral Surg Oral Med Oral Pathol Oral Radiol Endod 1982;54:74–6.

230. Cunningham WT, Martin H, Forrest WR. Evaluation of root canal debridement with the endosonic ultrasonic synergistic system. Oral Surg Oral Med Oral Pathol Oral Radiol Endod 1982;53:401–4.

231. Cunningham WT, Martin H. A scanning electron microscope evaluation of root canal debridement with the endosonic ultrasonic synergistic system. Oral Surg Oral Med Oral Pathol Oral Radiol Endod 1982;53:527–31.

232. Cunningham WT, Martin H, Pelleu GB, Stoops DE. A comparison of antimicrobial effectiveness of endosonic and hand root canal therapy. Oral Surg Oral Med Oral Pathol Oral Radiol Endod 1982;54:238–41.

233. Cameron JA. The use of ultrasonics in the removal of the smear layer: a scanning electron microscope study. J Endod 1983;9:289–92.

234. Scott GL, Walton RE. Ultrasonic endodontics: the wear of instruments with usage. J Endod 1986;12:279–83.

235. Krell KV, Neo J. The use of ultrasonic endodontic instrumentation in the retreatment of a paste-filled endodontic tooth. Oral Surg Oral Med Oral Pathol Oral Radiol Endod 1985;60:100–2.

236. Yamaguchi M, Matsumori M, Ishikawa H et al. The use of ultrasonic instrumentation in the cleansing and enlargement of the root canal. Oral Surg Oral Med Oral Pathol Oral Radiol Endod 1988;65:349–53.

237. Cameron JA. The effect of ultrasonic endodontics on the temperature of the root canal wall. J Endod 1988;14:554–9.

238. Haidet J, Reader A, Beck M, Meyers W. An *in vivo* comparison of the step-back technique versus a step-back/ultrasonic technique in human mandibular molars. J Endod 1989;15:195–9.

239. Briggs PFA, Gulabivala K, Stock CJR, Setchell DJ. The dentine-removing characteristics of an ultrasonically energized K-file. Int Endod J 1989;22:259–68.

240. Pedicord D, El Deeb ME, Messer HH. Hand versus ultrasonic instrumentation: its effect on canal shape and instrumentation time. J Endod 1986;12:375–81.

241. Chenail BL, Teplitsky PE. Endosonics in curved root canals. Part II. J Endod 1988;14:214–17.

242. Baker MC, Ashrafi SH, Van Cura JE, Remeikis NA. Ultrasonic compared with hand instrumentation: a scanning electron microscope study. J Endod 1988;14:435–40.

243. Krell KV, Johnson RJ. Irrigation patterns of ultrasonic files. Part II. Diamond coated files. J Endod 1988;14:535–7.

244. Walsh CL, Messer HH, El Deeb ME. The effect of varying the ultrasonic power setting on canal preparation. J Endod 1990;16:273–8.

245. Ahmad M, Pitt Ford TR, Crum LA. Ultrasonic debridement of root canals: an insight into the mechanisms involved. J Endod 1987;13:93–101.

246. Ahmad M, Pitt Ford TR, Crum LA. Ultrasonic debridement of root canals: acoustic streaming and its possible role. J Endod 1987;13:490–9.

247. Ahmad M, Pitt Ford TR, Crum LA, Walton AJ. Ultrasonic debridement of root canals: acoustic cavitation and its relevance. J Endod 1988;14:486–93.

248. Archer R, Reader A, Nist R, et al. An *in vivo* evaluation of the efficacy of ultrasound after step-back preparation in mandibular molars. J Endod 1992;18:549–52.

249. Walmsley AD, Williams AR. Effects of constraint on the oscillatory pattern of endosonic files. J Endod 1989;15:189–94.

250. Krell KV, Johnson RJ, Madison S. Irrigation patterns during ultrasonic canal instrumentation. Part I. K-type files. J Endod 1988;14:65–8.

251. Lumley PJ, Walmsley AD. Effect of precurving on the performance of endosonic K-files. J Endod 1992;18:232–6.

252. Ahmad M, Pitt Ford TR, Crum LA, Wilson RF. Effectiveness of ultrasonic files in the disruption of root canal bacteria. Oral Surg Oral Med Oral Pathol Oral Radiol Endod 1990;70:328–32.

253. Ahmad M, Pitt Ford TR. Comparison of two ultrasonic units in shaping curved canals. J Endod 1989;15:457–62.

254. Ahmad M. Shape of the root canal after ultrasonic instrumentation with K-Flex files. Endod Dent Traumatol 1990;6:104–8.

255. Walmsley AD, Lumley PJ, Laird WR. The oscillatory pattern of sonically powered endodontic files. Int Endod J 1989;22:125–32.

256. Dummer PMH, Alodeh MHA, Doller R. Shaping of simulated root canals in resin blocks using files activated by a sonic handpiece. Int Endod J 1989;22:211–25.

257. Bolanos OR, Sinai IH, Gonsky MR, Srinivasan R. A comparison of engine and air-driven instrumentation methods with hand instrumentation. J Endod 1988;14:392–6.

258. Ehrlich AD, Boyer TJ, Hicks ML, Pelleu GB. Effect of sonic instrumentation on the apical preparation of curved canals. J Endod 1989;15:200–3.

259. Tronstad L, Niemczyk SP. Efficacy and safety tests of six automated devices for root canal instrumentation. Endod Dent Traumatol 1986;2:270–6.

260. Miserendino LJ, Miserendino CA, Moser JB, et al. Cutting efficiency of endodontic instruments. Part III. Comparison of sonic and ultrasonic instrument systems. J Endod 1988;14:24–30.

261. Kielt LW, Montgomery S. The effect of Endosonic instrumentation in simulated root canals. J Endod 1987;13:215–19.

262. Zakariasen KL, Zakariasen KA, McMinn M. Today's sonics: using the combined hand/sonic endodontic technique. J Am Dent Assoc 1992;123:67–78.

263. Walker TL, del Rio CE. Histological evaluation of ultrasonic and sonic instrumentation of curved root canals. J Endod 1989;15:49–59.

264. Yahya AS, El Deeb ME. Effect of sonic versus ultrasonic instrumentation on canal preparation. J Endod 1989;15:235–9.

265. Reynolds MA, Madison S, Walton RE, et al. An *in vitro* histological comparison of the step-back, sonic and ultrasonic instrumentation techniques in small curved canals. J Endod 1987;13:307–14.

266. Lumley PJ, Walmsley AD, Walton RE, Rippin JW. Cleaning of oval canals using ultrasonic or sonic instrumentation. J Endod 1993;19:453–7.

267. Lev R, Reader A, Beck M, Meyers W. An *in vitro* comparison of the step-back technique versus a step-back/ultrasonic technique for 1 and 3 minutes. J Endod 1987;13:523–30.

268. Stamos DE, Sadeghi EM, Haasch GC, Gerstein H. An *in vitro* comparison study to quantitate the debridement ability of hand, sonic and ultrasonic instrumentation. J Endod 1987;13:434–40.

269. Goldman M, Sakurai-Fuse E, Turco J, White RR. A silicone model method to compare three methods of preparing the root canal. Oral Surg Oral Med Oral Pathol Oral Radiol Endod 1989;68:457–61.

270. Pugh RJ, Goerig AC, Glaser CG, Luciano WJ. A comparison of four endodontic vibration systems. Gen Dent 1989;37:296–301.

271. Barnett F, Trope M, Khoja M, Tronstad L. Bacteriologic status of the root canal after sonic, ultrasonic and hand instrumentation. Endod Dent Traumatol 1985;1:228–31.

272. Fairbourn DR, McWalter GM, Montgomery S. The effect of four preparation techniques on the amount of apically extruded debris. J Endod 1987;13:102–8.

273. Jensen S, Walker T, Hutter J, Nicoll B. Comparison of the cleaning efficacy of passive sonic activation and passive ultrasonic activation after hand instrumentation inmolar root canals. J Endod 1999;25:735–8.
274. Sabins RA, Johnson JD, Hellstein JW. A comparison of the cleaning efficacy of short-term sonic and ultrasonic passive irrigation after hand instrumentation in molar root canals. J Endod 2003;29:674–8.
275. Gutarts R, Nusstein J, Reader A, Beck M. In vivo debridement efficacy of ultrasonic irrigation following hand-rotary instrumentation in human mandibular molars. J Endod 2005;31:166–70.
276. Lee SJ, Wu MK, Wesselink PR. The efficacy of ultrasonic irrigation to remove artificially placed dentine debris from different-sized simulated plastic root canals. Int Endo J 2004;37:607–12.
277. van der Sluis LWM, Wu M-K, Wesselink PR. The efficacy of ultrasonic irrigation to remove artificially placed dentine debris from human root canals pre-pared using instruments of varying taper. Int Endo J 2005;38:764–8.
278. Lee SJ, Wu MK, Wesselink PR. The effectiveness of syringe irrigation and ultrasonics to remove debris from simulated irregularities within prepared root canal walls. Int Endo J 2004;37:672–8.

CHAPTER 26D

D. ELECTRONIC APEX LOCATORS

ADAM LLOYD, JOHN I. INGLE

The dentin–cementum junction has been recommended as an ideal apical termination for root canal preparation.[1-3] The position of this histologic entity varies around the internal circumference of the canal by up to 3 mm across opposing walls.[4,5] It is located approximately 1 mm away from the apical foramen.[6] An apical constriction usually occurs in the region of the dentin–cementum junction and often forms a natural apical matrix. It is the narrowest portal of entry of the pulpal vasculature from the periapical tissues and would be the smallest wound following pulp removal.[7] The topography of the apical constriction is variable[8] and undetectable radiographically. Kuttler[9] investigated the root apices of teeth and provided a dimensional analysis of the apical morphology. He noted that the distance from the apical constriction to the vertex of the root increased with age and was recorded as between 0.5 and 0.6 mm. This distance was considered as a measurement to subtract from the radiographic apex to approximate the location of the apical constriction.[10]

Working length, the apical extent of canal preparation and obturation, is often the main variable in determining success or failure.[11-16] Seltzer et al.[17] were the first to report greater success in terminating cleaning and obturating the root canal system just short of the radiographic apex, rather than overfilling or underfilling. Sjögren et al.[18] investigated endodontic outcomes over an 8- to 10-year period in over 350 patients. They reported the best outcome was when the root canal filling was between 0 to 2 mm short of the radiographic apex. Distances beyond the radiographic apex, or more than 2 mm short of this point, resulted in significantly lower success rates. These findings are in agreement with research conducted by other investigators[14-19] and most recently by meta-analysis of the literature.[20]

Chugal[21] found variations in success rate of teeth root filled at different levels. Teeth with normal preoperative pulps and periapical tissues enjoyed a higher success rate when filled over 1 mm from the radiographic apex. On the other hand, teeth with necrotic pulps and apical periodontitis showed greater success when the canal filling was closer to the level of the radiographic apex. From all the evidence cited, it is clearly prudent to be able to accurately prepare and fill root canals to a predetermined location in the canal short of the actual apical foramen—ideally the dentin–cementum junction.

The common method of determining root canal length for the past 100 years has been by radiography (see Chapter 15A, "Endodontic Radiography"). This method unfortunately often leads to inaccuracies, even though various techniques for improved radiographic length determination have been developed.[22-29] Interpretation of the file's position on the radiograph and the surrounding anatomy is also prone to errors when using the bisecting angle technique.[29] Estimation of the canal length often varies greatly from actual working length. The long-cone paralleling technique has been shown to be more accurate.[29] Furthermore, radiographs only provide a two-dimensional representation of the three-dimensional object and can also be interpreted differently between clinicians.[30,31] In fact, reports of observer agreement in determining file position found that agreement decreased as the distance from the radiographic apex increased.[32]

Many digital radiographic techniques do not easily permit obtaining endodontic working films with the long-cone paralleling technique, which necessitates using the bisecting angle method.[33] The use of digital radiography has reduced radiation exposure of patients,[34,35] increased the speed of delivery, and created the ability to "enhance" images.[36] However, studies have shown that digital radiographs have no greater resolution than conventional radiographs.[37-41]

In addition to radiography, tactile sensation has been used with questionable success, plus the drawbacks cited about radiographic length determination, along with the increasing concern about radiation exposure, the introduction and development of the electronic apex locator (EAL) has been received with enthusiasm by clinicians performing endodontic procedures.

The first reported use of electric current to measure root canal working length was in 1918 by Custer.[42] He noted a marked increase in the conductivity of a tooth at the apical foramen when the canal was dry or filled with a nonconductive medium. By placing a broach inside a tooth and applying a voltage across it and the alveolus, Custer was able to identify the apical foramen by observing a change in the value on the milliammeter of the time.[42]

Suzuki[43] found that an electrode placed on the oral mucosa, and an instrument placed in the root canal, gave consistent measurements of electrical resistance. This is the basis for the resistance-based EALs. As the advancing file, surrounded by insulating dentin and cementum, approaches the conductive periodontal ligament, the resistance decreases until the circuit is complete.

Sunada[44] used this principle to create a device, using direct current, to estimate the root canal length *in vivo*. He found that when the file reached the canal terminus, regardless of tooth shape, tooth type, or age of the patient, the resistance measured was consistent at 6.5 KΩ. Furthermore, the same resistance was recorded when the file encountered an accidental perforation.[44]

Direct current apex locators have also been associated with patients experiencing electric shocks.[45–46] Suchde and Talim[45] proposed changing to alternating current, which would result in less tissue damage and increased stability of the electrolyte's resistance in a wet canal. The disadvantage, however, in determining canal length in this manner, is the change in the capacitance of the circuit, along with many other variables that affect accuracy.[45,47] Meredith and Gulabivala[48] discovered that impedance in a tooth and periradicular tissues consists of resistive and capacitance circuits that provide a model for EALs.

The *first* generation of EALs was based on resistance, and the resistance was measured between the two electrodes to determine location within a canal. The *second* generation employed single-frequency impedance, in which impedance measurements instead of resistance was used to measure location within a canal. The improvement of the second over the first generation was essentially that it would gather more information. Impedance is a complex property comprised of resistance and capacitance. Whereas resistance has constant amplitude, impedance is sinusoidal. The frequency of an impedance-based unit can be varied to compensate for canal conditions. The *third* generation of EAL was similar to the second, but it used multiple frequencies to determine distances from the end of the canal. The *fourth* generation of EALs breaks impedance down into its primary components (resistance and capacitance) and measures them independently during use. This eliminates erroneous readings because different combinations of these properties provide the same impedance reading. This prevents EALs from being "jumpy" and erratic. Multiple frequencies are still used to compensate for canal conditions. The Elements Diagnostic Unit (SybronEndo, Glendora, CA) (Figure 1) does not make calculations internally as third-generation units do. Instead, all combinations of capacitance and resistance relating to location within the canal have been loaded into a matrix database within the unit (Figure 2). This decreases processing time, making the displayed information much more stable.

Accuracy of Electronic Apex Locators

A concern for accuracy in determining working length has generated many investigations using various EALs. Concern for accuracy also affected its acceptance for use in practices which has varied from 10% in the United States to 90% in Japan.[49–54]

RESISTANCE-BASED ELECTRONIC APEX LOCATORS

As the file approaches the periodontal ligament, the voltage change divided by the current (amperes) results in decreasing resistance, per Ohm's law, until a value of 6.5 KΩ is reached.[44] The accuracy of resistance-based apex locators can be high provided certain conditions are adhered to. Dry canals provided the most accurate readings. Strong electrolytes such as endodontic irrigants, purulence, excess hemorrhage, or pulp tissue lead to inaccurate and even unstable results.[55–59] In 1969, Bramante and Berbert[60] looked at the first commercially available apex locator, the Root Canal Meter, and found it to be consistently more accurate than radiographs in the palatal roots of maxillary molars and premolars. The original device, however, often elicited a painful response by the patient. Further refinements were made in later

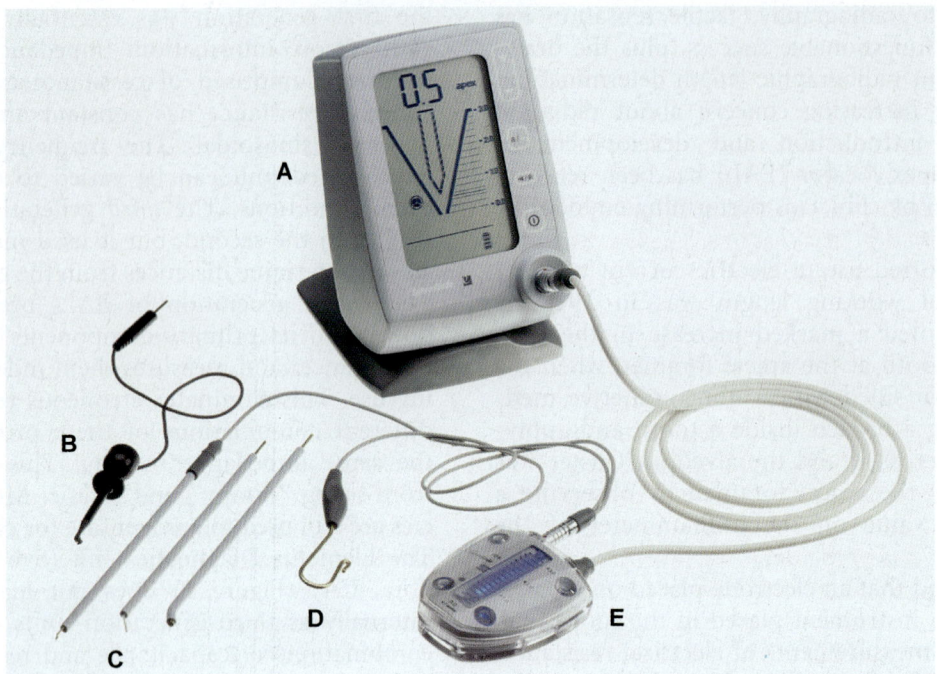

Figure 1 The Sybron Elements Diagnostic Unit is an example of a current electronic apex locator with a vitality scanner. *A,* Elements Diagnostic Unit; *B,* file clip; *C,* vitality probes; *D,* lip hook; *E,* satellite.

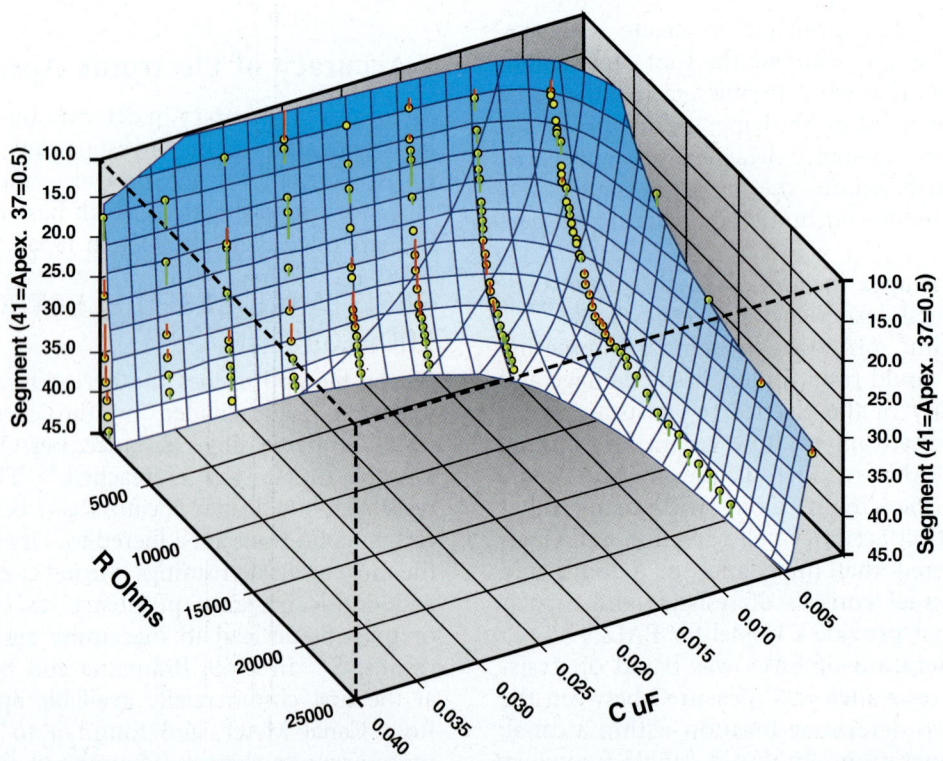

Figure 2 Matrix database for the Elements Diagnostic software: The left axis identifies the measured resistance in ohms, the right axis identifies the measured capacitance in microfarads, and the vertical axis illustrates the resultant apex location that is displayed. It is shown in segments on the unit display, "41 segments" being the "0" reading, "37 segments" being "0.5 mm," and so on.

EAL models measuring resistance such as the Endodontic Meter and the Endodontic Meter S II.[61] The more recent resistance-based apex locators provided accurate location of the apical constriction 55 to 75% of the time.[62] However, their accuracy was still diminished in the presence of fluids.[63]

LOW-FREQUENCY APEX LOCATORS

The resistance-based circuit proved insufficient to accurately and consistently measure root canal length.[48,64,65] Impedance rather than resistance became the characteristic used to mark the depth of canal penetration. In 1972, the Sono-Explorer was introduced by Inoue[64,66] on the premise that although the many parameters that determine impedance are varied in different canals under altered conditions, the impedance between the oral mucosa and depth of the gingival sulcus should be coincident with the impedance value of a circuit across the oral mucosa and the periodontal ligament. Thus, the device would indicate the canal terminus when the two impedance values approached each other. The frequency of the impedance was heard as an audible "marker tone" that signaled the endpoint of the canal, generated by low-frequency oscillation. The device had to be calibrated at the periodontal sulcus before each use. This involved placing a file, shielded along its length except for its tip, into the gingival sulcus, and listening for the "gingival crevice sound." A file was then introduced into the canal, and when the sound became identical to the "gingival crevice sound," the canal terminus had been reached. A disadvantage of the first model Sono-Explorer was the depth at which the probe could be placed into the gingival sulcus. If the reference tuner was placed deeper than 0.5 mm into the crevice when tuning the device, the gingival frequency increases resulted in the tip of the file protruding through the apical foramen.[67] The Sono-Explorer II rectified this with a coated gingival frequency me-asuring probe, but the accuracy still remained disappointing.

HIGH-FREQUENCY APEX LOCATORS

The Endocater was introduced by Hasegawa in 1979[59,62] with the premise that operating with a high-frequency wave (400 kHz) as a measuring current produces a more stable single electrode.[68,69] The device is able to perform accurate measurements in the presence of electrolytes and pulp tissue due to the file having a special coating except for the exposed tip, thereby decreasing the variable capacitive properties.[70] Accuracy with the Endocater has been reported between 67 and 93.4%.[62,65,71] A problem occurred in constricted canals when the coating of the file caused it to bind prematurely.[65] In addition, the coating did not withstand repeated autoclaving.[72] Fouad et al.[62] tested the Endocater with uncoated files and found grossly inaccurate results.

VOLTAGE GRADIENT APEX LOCATORS

Custer[42] and subsequently Sunada[44] relied on a constant resistance value of 6.5 KΩ between the canal and the periodontal membrane, and Ushiyama[73] used both monopolar and bipolar electrodes coated in lacquer with just the tip exposed, similar to the Endocater. Ushiyama found the voltage gradient was greatest at the most constricted point in the canal, where the current density is the highest. The principle of Ushiyama's device differs from Sunada's[44] resistance-based device in that separate electrodes are used to apply current to the probe and to record the voltage. Ushiyama pointed out a potential flaw in the resistance value of 6.5 KΩ quoted by Sunada[44] reporting that this more likely reflected the resistance of the metal electrode in contact with the canal contents, as a result of the polarization produced. The effect was minimized by Ushimaya's coated electrodes. Further investigation, using the monopolar and bipolar electrodes, respectively, were found to be successful in all but two cases tested.[74] Unfortunately, the thickened bipolar electrodes did not allow them to travel freely to the constriction in narrow canals.

DUAL-FREQUENCY ELECTRONIC APEX LOCATORS

In 1990, Saito and Yamashita[75] investigated the use of the Endex, developed by Yamaoka, describing the method of determining the canal terminus as the difference between two impedance values at two different frequencies. Calibration of the device in the coronal region is required to compensate for the dielectric capacity of the electrolyte in the canal. The findings from the study concluded that there were no differences in locating the apical foramen when different file sizes were used, a different apical diameter was encountered, or in the presence of saline, 5% sodium hypochlorite, 14% EDTA, or 3% hydrogen peroxide. The Endex was also marketed under the Apit brand name and further studied by Fouad et al.,[63] who also found the Endex superior to other apex locators in the presence of electrolytes, especially where the apical foramen was widened.

In 1993, Frank and Torabinejad,[76] using the Endex, took canal measurements of 99 teeth *in vivo* and were able to locate the file tip, in moist canals, to within 0.5 mm of the apical constriction in nearly 90% of the specimens. Mayeda et al.[77] studied the Endex to determine whether there were differences in accuracy in vital or necrotic cases in vivo, finding that there was no statistical difference based on pulpal status, and that generally file tips were found between +0.50 mm to 0.86 mm from the apical foramen.

Felippe and Soares[78] investigated 350 extracted teeth *in vitro* and found the Endex to locate the apical foramen within 0 to 0.5 mm in 96.5% of the specimens studied. Arora and Gulabivala[79] compared the Endex with the RCM Mark II EAL *in vivo*. They used sodium hypochlorite, pus, water, and vital and necrotic pulp tissue as possible electrolytes. They also exposed a radiograph before extracting the tooth and then examined the file position visually. What was evident from the study was an overestimation of the file's position based solely on the radiograph, with the file extending beyond the foramen. The extensions were affected by the canal's contents. The Endex was found to be within 0.5 mm of the apical foramen 71.7% of the time, whereas the RCM Mark II AEL had only a 43.5% rate of accuracy. The Endex performed better than the RCM Mark II in the presence of sodium hypochlorite.

MULTIPLE-FREQUENCY ELECTRONIC APEX LOCATORS

By the ratio method of canal length determination, these dual-frequency AELs overcame differences in the changing dielectric constant of different electrolytes left in the root canal system.[80,81] The position of the file tip is derived from the simultaneous measurement of the impedance of two different frequencies that are used to calculate the quotient of the impedances. The Root ZX (J. Morita Manufacturing Co., Kyoto, Japan) was one of these. It was initially introduced between 1991 and 1994 by Kobayashi and Suda.[82] The Root ZX simultaneously uses two waveforms, a high (8 kHz) and low (400 Hz) frequency waveform. As the content of the fluid changes within the root canal, the ratio of the impedances would be modified by the same rate as each other, yielding a ratio that would not differ. This results in the same positioning of the file tip regardless of the canal contents.[82] *In vitro* studies of the Root ZX have shown it to be accurate in the presence of electrolytes.[83] Varying concentrations of sodium hypochlorite made no significant difference in performance.[84,85] The accuracy of the Root ZX has been reported to range from 64% to 100%. If 1.0 mm difference is deemed acceptable, the accuracy is reported at 100%.[86] Lesser deviations from the apical constriction are reproducible.[87,88]

The Bingo 1020 (Forum Technologies, Rishon LeZion, Israel) compared favorably with the Root ZX regardless of canal contents or irrigants. Both were deemed more reliable than the radiographic interpretation.[89] An *in vitro* study also found the Bingo 1020 and the Root ZX performed equally well in the hands of clinicians with varying degrees of experience.[90] The Bingo 1020 is also marketed as the Raypex 4 (Roydent Dental Products, Johnson City, TN) and as the ProPex (Dentsply Maillefer, Ballaigues, Switzerland).

Welk et al.[91] tested the accuracy of the five-frequency Endo Analyzer Model 8005 (Analytic, Sybron Dental, Orange, CA) against the Root ZX and found the latter able to locate the apical foramen ±0.5 mm over 90% of the time with a mean difference less the 0.2 mm, compared with the Endo Analyzer at over 1.0 mm. Lucena-Martin et al.[92] found the Root ZX to be consistently reliable at 85%. A similar clinical comparison was conducted in Hungary in 2006, where Gyorfi et al.[93] determined the working lengths of 10 canals using radiographs and then compared these findings with four different apex locators. The Root ZX and the Foramatron D10 (Parkell Co., Edgewood, NY) agreed with the radiographic analysis in all 10 canals. The Apex Finder AFA 7005 (Analytic, Sybron Dental) agreed on seven canals and the ProPex (Dentsply Maillefer) agreed on five canals.

Tselnik et al.[94] recently tested the Elements Diagnostic EAL (Sybron Endo, Sybron Dental, Orange, CA) against the Root ZX *in vivo*. Both devices were accurate to 75% of the time to ±0.5 mm from the minor diameter. Haffner et al.[95] reported a similar finding for the latter at 78%. Plotino et al.[96] tested the Root ZX, the Elements Diagnostic Unit, and the ProPex unit and found their accuracy at 97.4, 94.3, and 100%, respectively, although the majority of the ProPex readings were beyond the apex.

In 2005, Goldberg et al.[97] compared the Root ZX, the ProPex (Dentsply Maillefer), and the NovApex (Forum Technologies) for accuracy in re-treatment cases. At 0.5 mm from the foramen, they reported an accuracy level of 95, 80, and 85%, respectively.

Foramina of unusual width can cause unreliable apex locator readings, particularly if a fine diameter file is used. However, Ebrahim et al.[98] concluded that when a tight-fitting file was used to determine working length of canals with large diameter foramina, the Foramatron D10 (Parkell Co.) and the Root ZX were significantly more accurate than the Apex NRG (Kibbutz Afikim, Israel) or the Apit 7 (Osada, Tokyo, Japan).

A number of other studies have been done assessing the qualities of these newest AELs. It was found, for instance, that stainless steel and nickel–titanium files were equally effective as canal "electrodes."[99] It was also noted that EALs are effective devices in determining resorptive defects and their location[100] and in measuring the working length in resorbing deciduous teeth.[101]

Morita has modified the Root ZX, applying the principle to the Solfy ZX, marketed only in Japan, which enables the operator to stop at any distance from the desired length,[68] as well as the Tri-Auto ZX and the Dentaport ZX that combine the apex locator with plug-in and/or cordless battery-operated handpieces that have an auto-reverse feature when the apex is reached or if the instrument binds in the canal.[102–104]

Parameters for Use of Electronic Apex Locators

The original apex locators proved to be more reliable in a dry canal than in the presence of saline or distilled water.[45] Manufacturers of newer models claim the ability of their apex locators to work in both dry and wet conditions, including in the presence of blood, pulp tissue, and the common endodontic irrigants. Although these claims have now shown the accuracy to be between 83 and 96%,[59,83,84,88,105,106] there are other factors that need to be considered in using an apex locator in practice. Contemporary root canal preparation with nickel–titanium rotary endodontic instruments typically involves crown-down preparations and some form of preflaring and removal of coronal obstructions. It has been shown that preflaring increases the accuracy of EAL.[107,108] Furthermore, the choice of file alloy, stainless steel, or nickel–titanium appears to have no bearing on apex locator accuracy.[90] Choosing a file that closely matches the canal diameter appears to no longer be a concern in locating the working length, with studies showing files of sizes much smaller than the canal, working equally well.[106,109] Contact of the file or probe to metallic restorations or fluid in contact with the metallic restorations will cause the apex locator to give a false reading.

Garofalo et al.[110] connected EALs directly to a pacemaker in an *in vitro* study and found that four of five EALs showed no effect on cardiac pacemaker function. However, the Bingo 1020 produced an irregular pace recording and oscilloscope pattern. Wilson et al.[111] recently demonstrated no effect on implanted cardiac pacemakers or cardioverters/defibrillators with either the Root ZX or the Elements Diagnostic EALs. However, manufacturers of EALs continue to warn against the use of their devices in patients with cardiac pacemakers. It is recommended to contact the patient's physician or cardiologist for specific guidance regarding the use of any electrical devices.

References

1. Grove C. Why canals should be filled to the dentinocemental junction. J Am Dent Assoc 1930;17:293–6.
2. Kettle Y. Microscopic investigation of root apexes. J Am Dent Assoc 1955;50:544–52.
3. Kuttler Y. A precision and biologic root canal filling technic. J Am Dent Assoc 1958;56:38–50.
4. Ponce EH, Vilar Fernandez JA. The cemento-dentino-canal junction, the apical foramen, and the apical constriction: evaluation by optical microscopy. J Endod 2003;29:214–19.
5. Gutierrez JH, Aguayo P. Apical foraminal openings in human teeth. Number and location. Oral Surg Oral Med Oral Pathol Oral Radiol Endod 1995;79:769–77.
6. Smulson MH, Hagen JC, Ellenz SJ. Pulpo-periapical pathology and immunologic considerations. In: Weine FS, editor. Endodontic therapy. 5th ed. St. Louis: Mosby-Yearbook Inc.; 1996. pp. 166–7.
7. Ricucci D, Langeland K. Apical limit of root canal instrumentation and obturation, part 2. A histological study. Int Endod J 1998;31:394–409.
8. Dummer PM, McGinn JH, Rees DG. The position and topography of the apical canal constriction and apical foramen. Int Endod J 1984;17:192–8.
9. Kuttler Y. Microscopic investigation of root apexes. J Am Dent Assoc 1955;50:544–52.
10. Stein TJ, Corcoran JF. Radiographic "working length" revisited. Oral Surg Oral Med Oral Pathol Oral Radiol Endod 1992;74:796–800.
11. Bender IB, Seltzer S, Soltanoff W. Endodontic success—a reappraisal of criteria. II. Oral Surg Oral Med Oral Pathol Oral Radiol Endod 1966;22:790–802.

12. Bender IB, Seltzer S, Soltanoff W. Endodontic success—a reappraisal of criteria. I. Oral Surg Oral Med Oral Pathol Oral Radiol Endod 1966;22:780–9.
13. Matsumoto T, Nagai T, Ida K, et al. Factors affecting successful prognosis of root canal treatment. J Endod 1987;13:239–42.
14. Kerekes K. Radiographic assessment of an endodontic treatment method. J Endod 1978;4:210–13.
15. Kerekes K, Tronstad L. Long-term results of endodontic treatment performed with a standardized technique. J Endod 1979;5:83–90.
16. Harty FJ, Parkins BJ, Wengraf AM. Success rate in root canal therapy. A retrospective study of conventional cases. Br Dent J 1970;128:65–70.
17. Seltzer S, Soltanoff W, Sinai I, et al. Biologic aspects of endodontics. III. Periapical tissue reactions to root canal instrumentation. Part II. Oral Surg Oral Med Oral Pathol Oral Radiol Endod 1968;26:694–705.
18. Sjögren U, Haglund B, Sundqvist G, Wing K. Factors affecting the long-term results of endodontic treatment. J Endod 1990;16:498–504.
19. Swartz DB, Skidmore AE, Griffin JA, Jr. Twenty years of endodontic success and failure. J Endod 1983;9:198–202.
20. Schaeffer MA, White RR, Walton RE. Determining the optimal obturation length: a meta-analysis of literature. J Endod 2005;31:271–4.
21. Chugal NM, Clive JM, Spångberg LS. A prognostic model for assessment of the outcome of endodontic treatment: effect of biologic and diagnostic variables. Oral Surg Oral Med Oral Pathol Oral Radiol Endod 2001;91:342–52.
22. Pineda F, Kuttler Y. Mesiodistal and buccolingual roentgenographic investigation of 7,275 root canals. Oral Surg Oral Med Oral Pathol Oral Radiol Endod 1972;33:101–10.
23. Green D. Double canals in single roots. Oral Surg Oral Med Oral Pathol Oral Radiol Endod 1973;35:689–96.
24. Vertucci FJ. Root canal anatomy of the human permanent teeth. Oral Surg Oral Med Oral Pathol Oral Radiol Endod 1984;58:589–99.
25. Burch JG, Hulen S. The relationship of the apical foramen to the anatomic apex of the tooth root. Oral Surg Oral Med Oral Pathol Oral Radiol Endod 1972;34:262–8.
26. Palmer MJ, Weine FS, Healey HJ. Position of the apical foramen in relation to endodontic therapy. J Can Dent Assoc 1971;37:305–8.
27. Ingle JI. PDQ Endodontics. Hamilton, Ont.: BC Decker; 2005. p. 125.
28. Olson AK, Goerig AC, Cavataio RE, Luciano J. The ability of the radiograph to determine the location of the apical foramen. Int Endod J 1991;24:28–35.
29. Forsberg J. A comparison of the paralleling and bisecting-angle radiographic techniques in endodontics. Int Endod J 1987;20:177–82.
30. Tidmarsh BG. Radiographic interpretation of endodontic lesions—a shadow of reality. Int Dent J 1987;37:10–15.
31. Goldman M, Pearson AH, Darzenta N. Endodontic success—who's reading the radiograph? Oral Surg Oral Med Oral Pathol Oral Radiol Endod 1972;33:432–7.
32. Cox VS, Brown CE, Jr., Bricker SL, Newton CW. Radiographic interpretation of endodontic file length. Oral Surg Oral Med Oral Pathol Oral Radiol Endod 1991;72:340–4.
33. Forsberg J. Radiographic reproduction of endodontic "working length" comparing the paralleling and the bisecting-angle techniques. Oral Surg Oral Med Oral Pathol Oral Radiol Endod 1987;64:353–60.
34. Brunton PA, Abdeen D, MacFarlane TV. The effect of an apex locator on exposure to radiation during endodontic therapy. J Endod 2002;28:524–6.
35. Saad AY, al-Nazhan S. Radiation dose reduction during endodontic therapy: a new technique combining an apex locator (Root ZX) and a digital imaging system (RadioVisioGraphy). J Endod 2000;26:144–7.
36. Shearer AC, Horner K, Wilson NH. Radiovisiography for length estimation in root canal treatment: an in-vitro comparison with conventional radiography. Int Endod J 1991;24:233–9.
37. Martinez-Lozano MA, Forner-Navarro L, Sanchez-Cortes JL, Llena-Puy C. Methodological considerations in the determination of working length. Int Endod J 2001;34:371–6.
38. Melius B, Jiang J, Zhu Q. Measurement of the distance between the minor foramen and the anatomic apex by digital and conventional radiography. J Endod 2002;28:125–6.
39. Radel RT, Goodell GG, McClanahan SB, Cohen ME. *In vitro* radiographic determination of distances from working length files to root ends comparing Kodak RVG 6000, Schick CDR, and Kodak insight film. J Endod 2006;32:566–8.
40. Velders XL, Sanderink GC, van der Stelt PF. Dose reduction of two digital sensor systems measuring file lengths. Oral Surg Oral Med Oral Pathol Oral Radiol Endod 1996;81:607–12.
41. Piepenbring ME, Potter BJ, Weller RN, Loushine RJ. Measurement of endodontic file lengths: a density profile plot analysis. J Endod 2000;26:615–18.
42. Custer LE. Exact methods of locating the apical foramen. Natl Dent Assoc J 1918;5:815–19.
43. Suzuki K. Experimental study on iontophoresis. J Jpn Stomatol 1942;16:411–29.
44. Sunada I. New method for measuring the length of the root canal. J Dent Res 1962;41:375–87.
45. Suchde RV, Talim ST. Electronic ohmmeter. An electronic device for the determination of the root canal length. Oral Surg Oral Med Oral Pathol Oral Radiol Endod 1977;43:141–50.
46. Kim E, Lee SJ. Electronic apex locator. Dent Clin North Am 2004;48:35–54.

47. O'Neill LJ. A clinical evaluation of electronic root canal measurement. Oral Surg Oral Med Oral Pathol Oral Radiol Endod 1974;38:469–73.
48. Meredith N, Gulabivala K. Electrical impedance measurements of root canal length. Endod Dent Traumatol 1997;13:126–31.
49. Whitten BH, Gardiner DL, Jeansonne BG, Lemon RR. Current trends in endodontic treatment: report of a national survey. J Am Dent Assoc 1996;127:1333–41.
50. Saunders WP, Chestnutt IG, Saunders EM. Factors influencing the diagnosis and management of teeth with pulpal and periradicular disease by general dental practitioners. Part 2. Br Dent J 1999;187:548–54.
51. Chandler NP, Koshy S. Radiographic practices of dentists undertaking endodontics in New Zealand. Dentomaxillofac Radiol 2002;31:317–21.
52. Yoshikawa G, Sawada N, Wettasinghe KA, Suda H. Survey of endodontic treatment in Japan. J Endod 2001;27:236.
53. Hommez GM, Braem M, De Moor RJ. Root canal treatment performed by Flemish dentists. Part 1. Cleaning and shaping. Int Endod J 2003;36:166–73.
54. Bjørndal L, Reit C. The adoption of new endodontic technology amongst Danish general dental practitioners. Int Endod J 2005;38:52–8.
55. Nekoofar MH, Ghandi MM, Hayes SJ, Dummer PM. The fundamental operating principles of electronic root canal length measurement devices. Int Endod J 2006;39:595–609.
56. Gordon MPJ, Chandler NP. Electronic apex locators. Int Endod J 2004;37:425–37.
57. McDonald NJ. The electronic determination of working length. Dent Clin North Am 1992;36:293–307.
58. Venturi M, Breschi L. A comparison between two electronic apex locators: an *in vivo* investigation. Int Endod J 2005;38:36–45.
59. Fouad AF, Krell KV. An *in vitro* comparison of five root canal length measuring instruments. J Endod 1989;15:573–7.
60. Bramante CM, Berbert A. A critical evaluation of some methods of determining tooth length. Oral Surg Oral Med Oral Pathol Oral Radiol Endod 1974;37:463–73.
61. Kobayashi C, Suda H. A basic study on the electronic root canal length measurement: Part 4. A comparison of 6 apex locators. Jpn J Conserv Dent 1993;36:185–92.
62. Fouad AF, Krell KV, McKendry DJ, et al. Clinical evaluation of five electronic root canal length measuring instruments. J Endod 1990;16:446–9.
63. Fouad AF, Rivera EM, Krell KV. Accuracy of the Endex with variations in canal irrigants and foramen size. J Endod 1993;19:63–7.
64. Inoue N. An audiometric method for determining the length of root canals. J Can Dent Assoc 1973;39:630–6.
65. McDonald NJ, Hovland EJ. An evaluation of the Apex Locator Endocater. J Endod 1990;16:5–8.
66. Inoue N. Dental 'stethoscope' measures root canal. Dent Surv 1972;48:38–9.
67. Inoue N, Skinner DH. A simple and accurate way to measuring root canal length. J Endod 1985;11:421–7.
68. Kobayashi C. Electronic canal length measurement. Oral Surg Oral Med Oral Pathol Oral Radiol Endod 1995;79:226–31.
69. Iizuka H, Hasegawa K, Takei M, et al. A study on electric method for measuring root canal length. J Nihon Univ Sch Dent 1987;29:278–86.
70. Hasegawa K, Iizuka H, Takei M, et al. A new method and apparatus for measuring root canal length. J Nihon Univ Sch Dent 1986;28:117–28.
71. Keller ME, Brown CE, Jr., Newton CW. A clinical evaluation of the Endocater—an electronic apex locator. J Endod 1991;17:271–4.
72. Himel VT, Schott RN. An evaluation of the durability of apex locator insulated probes after autoclaving. J Endod 1993;19:392–4.
73. Ushiyama J. New principle and method for measuring the root canal length. J Endod 1983;9:97–104.
74. Ushiyama J, Nakamura M, Nakamura Y. A clinical evaluation of the voltage gradient method of measuring the root canal length. J Endod 1988;14:283–7.
75. Saito T, Yamashita Y. Electronic determination of root canal length by newly developed measuring device. Influences of the diameter of apical foramen, the size of K-file and the root canal irrigants. Dent Jpn 1990;27:65–72.
76. Frank AL, Torabinejad M. An *in vivo* evaluation of Endex electronic apex locator. J Endod 1993;19:177–9.
77. Mayeda DL, Simon JH, Aimar DF, Finley K. *In vivo* measurement accuracy in vital and necrotic canals with the Endex apex locator. J Endod 1993;19:545–8.
78. Felippe MC, Soares IJ. *In vitro* evaluation of an audiometric device in locating the apical foramen of teeth. Endod Dent Traumatol 1994;10:220–2.
79. Arora RK, Gulabivala K. An *in vivo* evaluation of the ENDEX and RCM Mark II electronic apex locators in root canals with different contents. Oral Surg Oral Med Oral Pathol Oral Radiol Endod 1995;79:497–503.
80. Kobayashi C, Suda H, Sunada I. A basic study on the electronic root canal measurement. Part 2. Measurement using impedance analyzer. Jpn J Conserv Dent 1991;34:1208–21.
81. Kobayashi C, Okiji T, Kawashima N, et al. A basic study on the electronic root canal length measurement: Part 3. Newly designed electronic root canal length measuring device using division method. Jpn J Conserv Dent 1991;34:1442–8.
82. Kobayashi C, Suda H. New electronic canal measuring device based on the ratio method. J Endod 1994;20:111–14.

83. Jenkins JA, Walker WA, III, Schindler WG, Flores CM. An *in vitro* evaluation of the accuracy of the root ZX in the presence of various irrigants. J Endod 2001;27:209–11.
84. Weiger R, John C, Geigle H, Lost C. An *in vitro* comparison of two modern apex locators. J Endod 1999;25:765–8.
85. Tinaz AC, Sevimli LS, Gorgul G, Turkoz EG. The effects of sodium hypochlorite concentrations on the accuracy of an apex locating device. J Endod 2002;28:160–2.
86. Pagavino G, Pace R, Baccetti T. A SEM study of *in vivo* accuracy of the Root ZX electronic apex locator. J Endod 1998;24:438–41.
87. Vajrabhaya L, Tepmongkol P. Accuracy of apex locator. Endod Dent Traumatol 1997;13:180–2.
88. Shabahang S, Goon WW, Gluskin AH. An *in vivo* evaluation of Root ZX electronic apex locator. J Endod 1996;22:616–18.
89. Kaufman AY, Keila S, Yoshpe M. Accuracy of a new apex locator: an *in vitro* study. Int Endod J 2002;35:186–92.
90. Tinaz AC, Maden M, Aydin C, Turkoz E. The accuracy of three different electronic root canal measuring devices: an *in vitro* evaluation. J Oral Sci 2002;44:91–5.
91. Welk AR, Baumgartner JC, Marshall JG. An *in vivo* comparison of two frequency-based electronic apex locators. J Endod 2003;29:497–500.
92. Lucena-Martin C, Robles-Gijon V, Ferrer-Luque CM, de Mondelo JM. *In vitro* evaluation of the accuracy of three electronic apex locators. J Endod 2004;30:231–3.
93. Gyorfi A, et al. An *in vivo* comparison of different apex locators during endodontic treatment. Hungarian Society of Endodontology and Dent-Maxillo-Facial-Radiological Section of the Hungarian Dental Association. June 04, 2006.
94. Tselnik M, Baumgartner JC, Marshall JG. An evaluation of root ZX and elements diagnostic apex locators. J Endod 2005;31:507–9.
95. Haffner C, Folwaczny M, Galler K, Hickel R. Accuracy of electronic apex locators in comparison to actual length—an *in vivo* study. J Dent 2005;33:619–25.
96. Plotino G, Grande NM, Brigante L, et al. *Ex vivo* accuracy of three electronic apex locators: Root ZX, elements diagnostic unit and apex locator and propex. Int Endod J 2006;39:408–14.
97. Goldberg F, Marroquin BB, Frajlich S, Dreyer C. *In vitro* evaluation of the ability of three apex locators to determine the working length during retreatment. J Endod 2005;31:676–8.
98. Ebrahim AK, Wadachi R, Suda H. *Ex vivo* evaluation of four different apex locators to determine the working length in teeth with various foramen diameters. Aust Dent J 2006;51(3):258–62.
99. Thomas AS, Hartwell GR, Moon PC. The accuracy of the Root ZX electronic apex locator using stainless-steel and nickel-titanium files. J Endod 2003;29:662–3.
100. Goldberg F, De Silvio AC, Manfre S, Nastri N. *In vitro* measurement accuracy of an electronic apex locator in teeth with simulated apical root resorption. J Endod 2002;28:461–3.
101. Mente J, Seidel J, Buchalla W, Koch MJ. Electronic determination of root canal length in primary teeth with and without root resorption. Int Endod J 2002;35:447–52.
102. Alves AM, Felippe MC, Felippe WT, Rocha MJ. *Ex vivo* evaluation of the capacity of the Tri Auto ZX to locate the apical foramen during root canal retreatment. Int Endod J 2005;38:718–24.
103. Kobayashi C, Yoshioka T, Suda H. A new engine-driven canal preparation system with electronic canal measuring capability. J Endod 1997;23:751–4.
104. Grimberg F, Banegas G, Chiacchio L, Zmener O. *In vivo* determination of root canal length: a preliminary report using the Tri Auto ZX apex-locating handpiece. Int Endod J 2002;35:590–3.
105. Meares WA, Steiman HR. The influence of sodium hypochlorite irrigation on the accuracy of the Root ZX electronic apex locator. J Endod 2002;28:595–8.
106. Ebrahim AK, Yoshioka T, Kobayashi C, Suda H. The effects of file size, sodium hypochlorite and blood on the accuracy of Root ZX apex locator in enlarged root canals: an *in vitro* study. Aust Dent J 2006;51:153–7.
107. Ibarrola JL, Chapman BL, Howard JH, et al. Effect of preflaring on Root ZX apex locators. J Endod 1999;25:625–6.
108. Davis RD, Marshall JG, Baumgartner JC. Effect of early coronal flaring on working length change in curved canals using rotary nickel-titanium versus stainless steel instruments. J Endod 2002;28:438–42.
109. Nguyen HQ, Kaufman AY, Komorowski RC, Friedman S. Electronic length measurement using small and large files in enlarged canals. Int Endod J 1996;29:359–64.
110. Garofalo RR, Elias N, Dorn SO, Kuttler S. Effect of electronic apex locators on cardiac pacemaker function. J Endod 2002;28:831–3.
111. Wilson BL, Broberg C, Baumgartner JC, et al. Safety of electronic apex locators and pulp testers in patients with implanted cardiac pacemakers or cardioverter/defibrillators. J Endod 2006;32:847–52.

CHAPTER 26E

E. Lasers in Endodontics

ADAM STABHOLZ, JOSHUA MOSHONOV, SHARONIT SAHAR-HELFT, JEAN-PAUL ROCCA

The rapid development of laser technology, as well as a better understanding of laser interaction with biological tissues, has widened the spectrum of possible applications of lasers in endodontics. The development of new delivery systems, including thin and flexible fibers as well as new endodontic tips, has made it possible to apply this technology to various endodontic procedures, including pulpal diagnosis, pulp capping/pulpotomy, cleaning and disinfecting the root canal system, obturation of the root canal system, endodontic retreatment, and apical surgery.

Although interest in the clinical use of laser systems for endodontic procedures is increasing, there are still some concerns associated with their use, mainly, lack of sufficient well-designed clinical studies that clearly demonstrate advantages of lasers over conventional methods and techniques. Selection of suitable wavelengths from the various laser systems requires advanced training and an educated understanding of the different characteristics in each laser system. The purpose of this chapter is to describe the principles of operation and discuss possible clinical applications of lasers in endodontics.

Principles of Operation

Dental lasers used today for clinical procedures and research operate in the infrared, visible, or ultraviolet range of the electromagnetic spectrum[1] (Figure 1). The word LASER is an acronym for Light Amplification by the Stimulated Emission of Radiation. Although "L" stands for light, the actual physical process that takes place within the laser device is amplification by stimulated emission of radiation. A light beam is composed of packets of energy known as photons such as produced by a light bulb or other light sources. The natural state of an atom when all its electrons are moving around its nucleus is the ground state. When an atom is excited by an external energy source, an electron moves to a higher energy level. As the atom tendency is to revert to its ground level, the electron falls back to its basic orbit, while emitting energy in the form of photons.[2] This emission is called "spontaneous emission" because it occurs without additional interference and results in the formation of "individual" waves from each atom not in phase with one another that is, a non-coherent, broadband spectrum (polychromatic) light.

The laser beam, on the other hand, implies stimulated emission of radiation. It is a single wavelength (monochromatic), collimated (very low divergence), coherent (photons in phase), and intense.[2] The laser principle accounts for the creation of this kind of light: The construction of a light source based on stimulated emission of radiation requires an active medium, a collection of atoms or molecules. The active medium that can be a gas, liquid, or a solid material and is contained in a glass or ceramic tube has to be excited to emit the photons by stimulated emission. Energy in the form of electric current or a flash lamp is applied to the medium, and once there are more atoms in the excited state than in the ground state, a population inversion is created. By adding a mirror to each end of the laser medium, a population of photons can be directed back and forth through the medium stimulating the emission of radiation from multiple excited electrons. Some of the photons produced can be released by allowing them to pass through one of the mirrors. The light can be coupled to a delivery device and used as a "surgical" beam[3] (Figure 2).[3]

The medium producing the beam is what identifies the laser and distinguishes one from another. Different types of lasers used in dentistry, such as carbon dioxide (CO_2), erbium (Er), and neodymium (Nd), and various other substances used in the medium [e.g., yttrium, aluminum, garnet (YAG) and yttrium, scandium, gallium, garnet (YSGG)], and argon, diode, and excimer types, all produce light of a specific

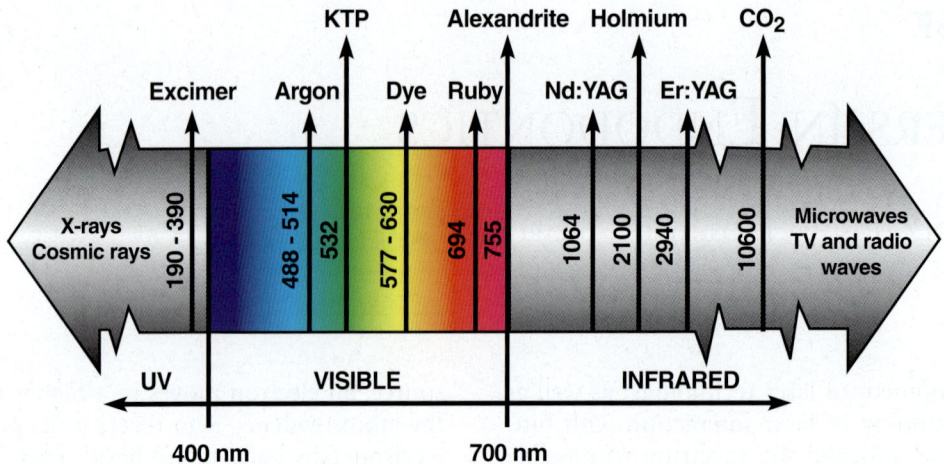

Figure 1 The wavelengths of various types of lasers according to their emission spectra.

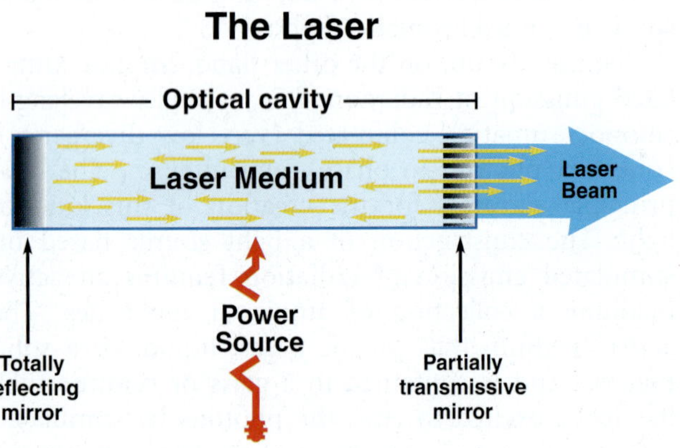

The Laser

Figure 2 Schematic diagram of a laser.

wavelength. The CO_2, the Er:YAG, the Er, Cr:YSGG, and the Nd:YAG lasers emit invisible beams in the infrared range (10.6 μm, 2.94 μm, 2.79 μm, and 1.06 μm, respectively). The Argon laser emits a visible light beam at 488 or 514 nm, while the excimer lasers emit invisible ultraviolet light beams at various predetermined wavelengths (ArF, 193 nm; KrF, 248 nm; and XeCl, -308 nm).[4]

Laser photons interact with tissue in one of four ways: they are transmitted through tissue, reflected from tissue, scattered within tissue, or absorbed by tissue.[5] Transmission of light transfers energy through the tissue without any interaction and thus does not cause any effect or injury. Reflection results in little or no absorption, so that there is no thermal effect on the tissue. When scattered, light travels in different directions and energy is absorbed over a greater surface area, producing a less intense and less precise thermal effect; when absorbed, light energy is converted into thermal energy (Figure 3).[6] A single laser device cannot perform all the required functions as the beam is absorbed or reflected according to its wavelength and the color of the object impacted.[3]

The particular properties of each type of laser and the specific target tissue render them suitable for various procedures. The CO_2 laser is highly absorbed by all biological soft and hard tissues and thus is most effective in tissues with high water content, such as the soft tissues of the oral cavity. However, its high thermal absorption makes this laser unsuitable for drilling and cutting enamel and dentin as damage to the dental pulp may occur.[7]

The Er:YAG laser is the most efficient for drilling and cutting enamel and dentin as its energy is well absorbed by water as well as by hydroxyapatite. Argon lasers are more effective on pigmented or highly vascular tissues, whereas Nd:YAG laser photons are transmitted through tissues by water and interact well with dark pigmented tissue.

The excimer lasers generate light in the ultraviolet range of the electromagnetic spectrum and function by breaking molecular bonds and reducing the tissue to its atomic constituents before their energy is dissipated as heat. Different types of lasers may have various effects on the same tissue, and the same laser can have varying effects on diverse tissue.

Unlike the CO_2 and the Er:YAG lasers, the Nd:YAG, argon, and excimer laser beams can be delivered through fiber optic, allowing greater

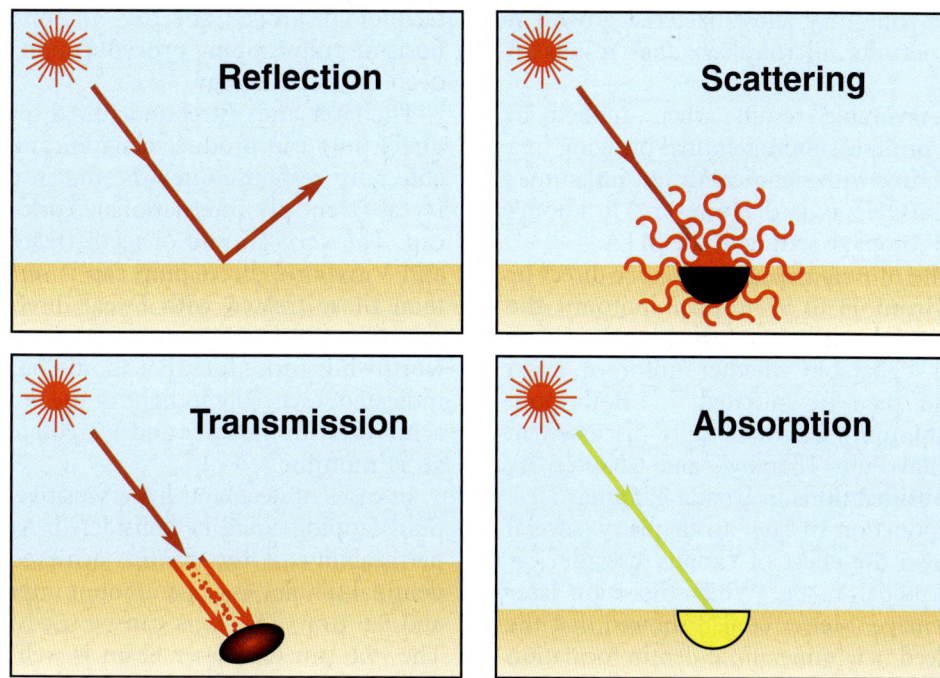

Figure 3 Four basic types of laser interactions occur when light hits the target tissue: reflection, scattering, transmission, and absorption.

accessibility to different areas and structures in the oral cavity.[7] The extent of the interaction of laser energy with a tissue is generally determined by two dependent variables: the specific wavelength of the laser emission and the optical characteristics of the particular target tissue.[5] These variables dictate absorption (i.e., the ability to effect tissue changes and generation of heat) and are important for pulp protection.[8] The clinician controls four parameters when operating the laser: (1) the level of applied power (power density), (2) the total energy delivered over a given surface area (energy density), (3) the rate and duration of the exposure (pulse repetition), and (4) the mode of energy delivery to the target tissue (i.e., continuous versus pulsed energy and direct contact or no contact with the target tissue).

Pulpal Diagnosis

A diagnosis of pulp vitality may be, at times, difficult to assess, in view of the fact that current vitality tests are poor indicators. A false diagnosis may lead to an unnecessary removal of the pulp tissue. Histological evaluation of the exact state of the pulp tissue is not feasible since an opening into the pulp chamber will result with the need to remove this tissue and subsequently perform a root canal treatment. Laser Doppler flowmetry (LDF) was developed to assess blood flow in micro vascular systems. It also can be used as a diagnostic system for measurements of blood flow in the dental pulp.[9,10] Laser Doppler flowmetry (LDF), is discussed in Chapter 14C.

Pulp Capping and Pulpotomy

Pulp capping, as defined by the American Association of Endodontists,[11] is a procedure in which a dental material such as calcium hydroxide $Ca(OH)_2$ or mineral trioxide aggregate (MTA) is placed over a pulpal wound to encourage the formation of reparative dentin. Pulpotomy entails surgical removal of the coronal portion of the pulp as a means of preserving the remaining radicular pulp tissues.

Pulp capping is recommended when the exposure is very small, 1.0 mm or less,[12,13] and the patients are young; pulpotomy is recommended when the young pulp is already exposed to caries and the roots are not yet fully formed (open apices). The traditionally used pulp capping agent is $Ca(OH)_2$.[14,15] When it is applied to pulp tissue, a necrotic layer is produced subjacent to which a dentin bridge is expected to form. The same may occur when a pulpotomy procedure is done. The disadvantage of both techniques is that the necrotic zone may allow bacterial growth if the restoration permits microleakage that results in pulpal problems.

MTA shows favorable results when applied to exposed pulp. It produces more dentinal bridging in a shorter period of time with significantly less inflammation than when Ca(OH)$_2$ is used. However, 3 to 4 hours are necessary for complete setting of the MTA.[16–18]

The success rate of pulp capping, whether direct or indirect, ranges from 44 to 97%. In pulpotomy, the same agents are used until root formation has been completed. It is debatable whether full root canal treatment should then be initiated.[19,20] Both pulp capping and pulpotomy are more fully discussed in Chapter 35, "Vital Pulp Therapy" and Chapter 36, "Endodontic Considerations in Dental Trauma."

Since the introduction of laser to dentistry, several studies have shown the effect of various laser devices on dentin and pulpal tissue. While the ruby laser caused pulpal damage, Melcer et al.[21] showed that the CO$_2$ laser produced new mineralized dentin formation without cellular modification of pulpal tissue when tooth cavities were irradiated in beagles and primates. Shoji et al.[22] applied CO$_2$ laser to the exposed pulps of dogs, using a focused and defocused laser mode and a wide range of energy levels (3, 10, 30, and 60 W). Charring, coagulation necrosis, and degeneration of the odontoblastic layer occurred, although no damage was detected in the radicular portion of the pulp. Jukic et al.[23] used CO$_2$ and Nd:YAG lasers with an energy density of 4 and 6.3 J/cm^2, respectively, on exposed pulp tissue. In both experimental groups, carbonization, necrosis, an inflammatory response, edema, and hemorrhage were observed in the pulp tissue. In some specimens, a dentinal bridge was formed.

In patients in whom direct pulp capping treatment was indicated, Moritz et al.[24] used the CO$_2$ laser. An energy level of 1 W at 0.1-second exposure time with 1-second pulse intervals was applied until the pulps exposed areas were completely irradiated. They were then dressed with Ca(OH)$_2$ (Kerr Life, Orange, CA). In the control group, the pulps were only capped with Ca(OH)$_2$. Symptoms were recorded and vitality tests were made after 1 week and monthly for 1 year: 89% of the experimental group had no symptoms and responded normally to vitality tests versus only 68% of the control.

The importance of pulp capping that considerably improves the prognosis of the tooth justifies the quest for new techniques and technologies: the most recent literature reports more predictable results (~90%) with capping performed using laser of different wavelengths, compared to traditional procedures that report a success rate of approximately 60%. Laser technology proved effective in improving the prognosis of pulp capping procedures on teeth affected by deep caries pathology.[25]

The laser and Vitrebond (3M Espe, St. Paul, MN) direct pulp cap produce a significantly more predictable pulp response after the first 6 months than the Dycal (Dentsply International, York, PA) direct pulp cap. The survival rate of teeth treated with the laser and Vitrebond direct pulp cap is significantly greater than those treated with Dycal direct pulp cap over intervals of 9 to 54 months. Direct pulp capping is a worthwhile procedure that should be performed when indicated, especially in light of the 90.3% survival rate achieved with the laser and Vitrebond direct pulp cap at 54 months.[26]

In cases of deep and hypersensitive cavities, indirect pulp capping could be considered. A reduction in the permeability of the dentin, achieved by sealing the dentinal tubules, is of paramount importance. Nd:YAG and 9.6 μm CO$_2$ lasers can be used for this purpose. The 9.6 μm CO$_2$ laser beam is well absorbed by the hydroxyapatite of enamel and dentin and causes tissue ablation, melting, and re-solidification.[27] The use of a 9.6 μm CO$_2$ laser did not cause any noticeable damage to the pulpal tissue in dogs.[28] The effect of the Nd:YAG laser on intrapulpal temperature was investigated by White et al.[29] They found that the use of pulsed a Nd:YAG laser, with an energy of below 1 W, a 10-Hz repetition rate and overall 10-second exposure time, did not significantly elevate the intrapulpal temperature. According to their results, these may be considered safe parameters, as the remaining dentinal thickness in cavity preparations cannot be measured in vivo. It is recommended, therefore, that clinicians choose laser parameters lower than these safety limits.

In a study of the effects of Nd:YAG laser pulpotomy on human primary molars, it was shown that 66 out of 68 laser-treated teeth were clinically successful with no signs or symptoms of pathosis. The clinical success rate was 97% and the radiographic success rate was 94.1%. In the formocresol control group (69 teeth), the clinical success was 85.5% and the radiological success was 78.3%.[30] More clinical studies are required to verify the advantages of the use of lasers in pulp capping and pulpotomy procedures.

Cleaning and Disinfecting the Root Canal System

Bacterial contamination of the root canal system is considered the principal etiologic factor for the development of pulpal and periapical lesions.[31–33] Obtaining a root canal system free of irritants is a major goal of root canal therapy. Biomechanical instrumentation of the root canal system has been suggested to achieve this task. However, because of the complexity of the root canal system, it has been shown that the complete elimination of debris and achievement of a sterile root canal system is very difficult[34,35] and that a smear layer containing bacteria, covering the instrumented walls of the root canal, is formed.[36–38]

The smear layer consists of a superficial layer on the surface of the root canal wall approximately 1 to 2 μm thick and a deeper layer packed into the dentinal tubules to a depth of up to 40 μm.[38] It contains inorganic and organic substances including microorganisms and necrotic debris.[39] In addition to the possibility that the smear layer may be infected, it can also protect the bacteria already present in the dentinal tubules by obstructing intra-canal disinfection agents.[40] Pashley[41] considered that a smear layer containing bacteria or bacterial products might provide a reservoir of irritants. Thus, complete removal of the smear layer would be consistent with the elimination of irritants from the root canal system.[42] Peters et al.[43] moreover demonstrated that 35% of the canals' surface area remained unchanged following instrumentation of the root canal prepared with four Ni-Ti preparation techniques.

Because most currently used intra-canal medicaments have a limited anti-bacterial spectrum and a limited ability to diffuse into the dentinal tubules, it has been suggested that newer treatment strategies designed to eliminate microorganisms from the root canal system should be considered. These must include agents that can penetrate the dentinal tubules and destroy the microorganisms, located in areas beyond the host defense mechanisms, where they cannot be reached by locally administered antibacterial agents.[44]

Numerous studies have documented that CO_2,[45] Nd:YAG,[45–47] argon,[45,48] Er,Cr:YAG,[49] and Er:YAG[50,51] laser irradiation has the ability to remove debris and smear layer from the root canal walls following biomechanical instrumentation. The task of cleaning and disinfecting a root canal system that contains microorganisms gathered in a biofilm became very difficult; certain bacterial species become more virulent when harbored in biofilm, demonstrating stronger pathogenic potential and increased resistance to antimicrobial agents as biofilm has the ability to prevent the entry and action of such agents.[52]

Bergman et al.[53] tried to define the role of laser as a disinfection tool by using Nd:YAG laser irradiation on some endodontic pathogens ex vivo. They concluded that Nd:YAG laser irradiation is not an alternative but a possible supplement to existing protocols for canal disinfections, as the properties of laser light may allow a bactericidal effect beyond 1 mm of dentin. Endodontic pathogens that grow as biofilms are difficult to eradicate even upon direct laser exposure.

However, there are several limitations that may be associated with the intra-canal use of lasers that cannot be overlooked.[54] The emission of laser energy from the tip of the optical fiber or the laser guide is directed vertically along the root canal and not necessary laterally to the root canal walls.[55] Thus, it is almost impossible to obtain uniform coverage of the canal surface using a laser.[54,55] Furthermore, thermal damage to the periapical tissues is potentially possible, so safety of the procedures must always be considered.[55] Direct emission of laser irradiation from the tip of the optical fiber in the vicinity of the apical foramen of a tooth may result in transmission of the irradiation beyond the foramen into periapical tissues. This, in turn, may also be hazardous in teeth in close proximity to the mental foramen or to the mandibular nerve.[55] In their review, *Lasers in Endodontics*, Matsumoto et al.[56] emphasized the possible limitations of the use of lasers in the root canal system. They suggested that "removal of smear layer and debris by laser is possible, however it is difficult to clean all root canal walls, because the laser beam is emitted straight ahead, making it almost impossible to irradiate the lateral canal walls." They strongly recommended improving the endodontic tip to enable irradiation of all areas of the root canal walls. The Er:YAG laser has gained increasing popularity among clinicians following its approval by the US Food and Drug Administration for use on dental hard tissues.[57]

Stabholz et al.[55] recently reported the development of a new endodontic tip to be used with an Er:YAG laser system. The beam of the Er:YAG laser is delivered through a hollow tube, with an endodontic tip that allows lateral emission of the irradiation (side-firing), rather than direct emission through a single opening at its far end. This new endodontic side-firing spiral tip was designed to fit the shape and the volume of root canals prepared by Ni-Ti rotary instrumentation. It emits the Er:YAG laser irradiation laterally to the walls of the root canal through a spiral slit located all along the tip. The tip is sealed at its far end, preventing the transmission of irradiation to and through the apical foramen of the tooth (Figures 4 and 5).

The efficacy of the endodontic1 side-firing spiral tip, in removing debris and smear layer from distal and

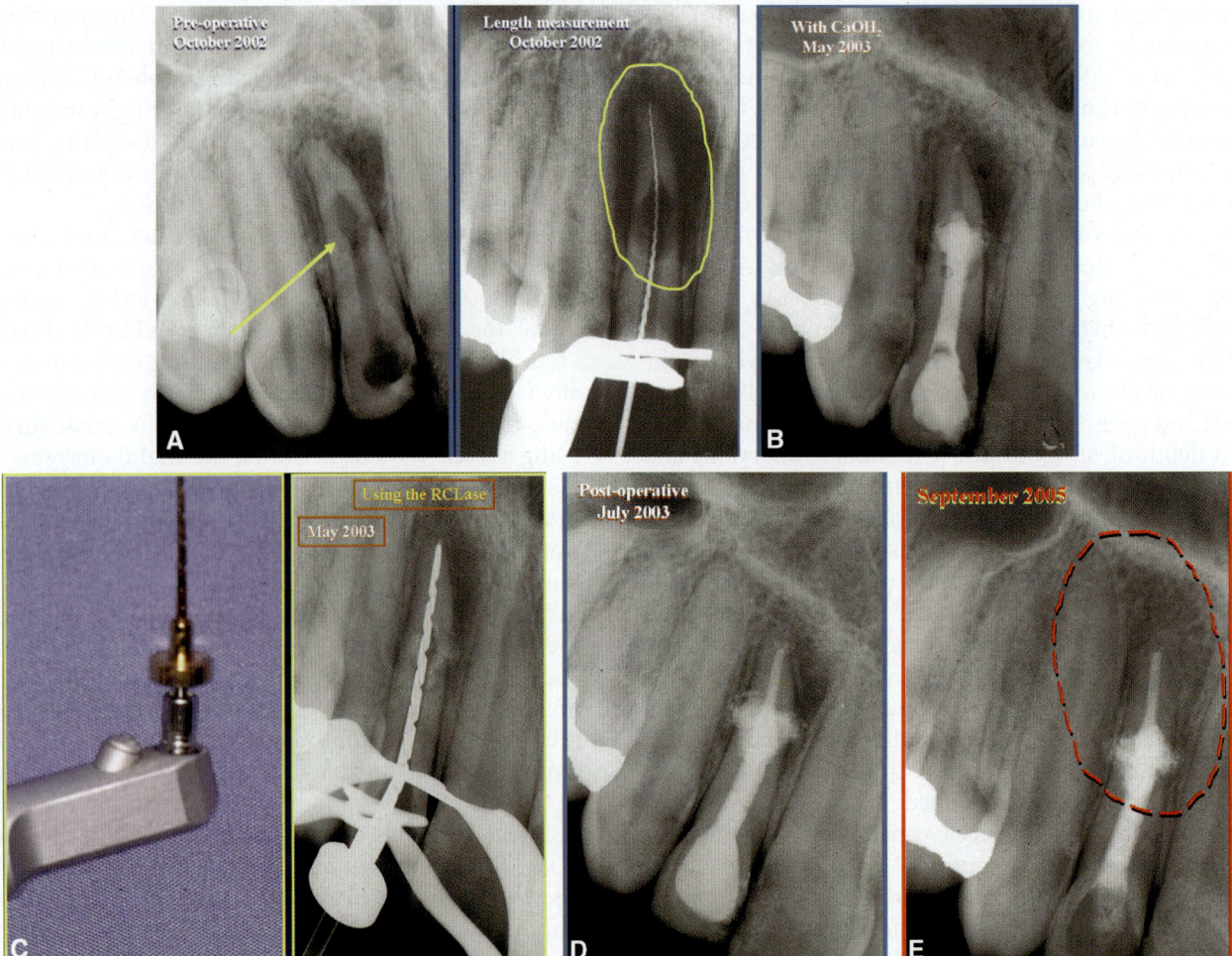

Figure 4 An 18-year-old patient came to the endodontic clinic complaining about a bad taste in her mouth and a lesion on the gums in the anterior area of the mouth. The clinical examination revealed a sinus tract opening close to the apex of the maxillary right lateral incisor. **A,** The radiograph showed an area of internal resorption and a large radiolucent area around the root apex. A diagnostic/length measurement radiograph suggested the presence of root perforation associated with the internal resorption. The patient was given the option of root canal treatment with poor prognosis, or replacing the tooth with an implant. The patient chose endodontic treatment. **B,** After cleaning and shaping the canal, Ca(OH)$_2$ was placed and replaced after 3 months. After 6 months, the sinus tract was still present with no sign of healing. **C,** The patient was offered the opportunity to have the tooth treated with the newly developed prototype of the RCLase Side Firing Spiral Tip that might provide better disinfection of the root canal system. The picture shows the RCLase tip positioned in the contra angle (left) and the radiograph shows the tip inside the root canal. **D,** Radiograph shows the lateral incisor following completion of the root canal filling using warm gutta-percha technique. **E,** A two-year follow-up radiograph shows complete healing of the periapical lesion. The sinus tract had disappeared and the patient was free of symptoms.

palatal root canals of freshly extracted human molars, was examined. Scanning electron microscopy (SEM) of the lased root canal walls revealed clean surfaces, free of smear layer and debris.[55] The dentinal tubules in the root run a relatively straight course between the pulp and the periphery, in contrast to the typical S-shaped contours of the tubules in the tooth crown.[41] Studies have shown that bacteria and their byproducts, present in infected root canals, may invade the dentinal tubules. Their presence in the tubules of infected teeth, at junction, was also reported.[58,59] These findings justify the rationale and need for developing effective means of removing the smear layer from root canal walls following biomechanical instrumentation. This would allow disinfectants and laser irradiation to reach and destroy microorganisms harbored in the dentinal tubules.

In various laser systems used in dentistry, the emitted energy can be delivered into the root canal system by a either thin optical fiber (Nd:YAG, KTP-Nd:YAG, Er;YSGG, argon, and diode) or by a hollow tube (CO_2 and Er:YAG). Thus, the potential

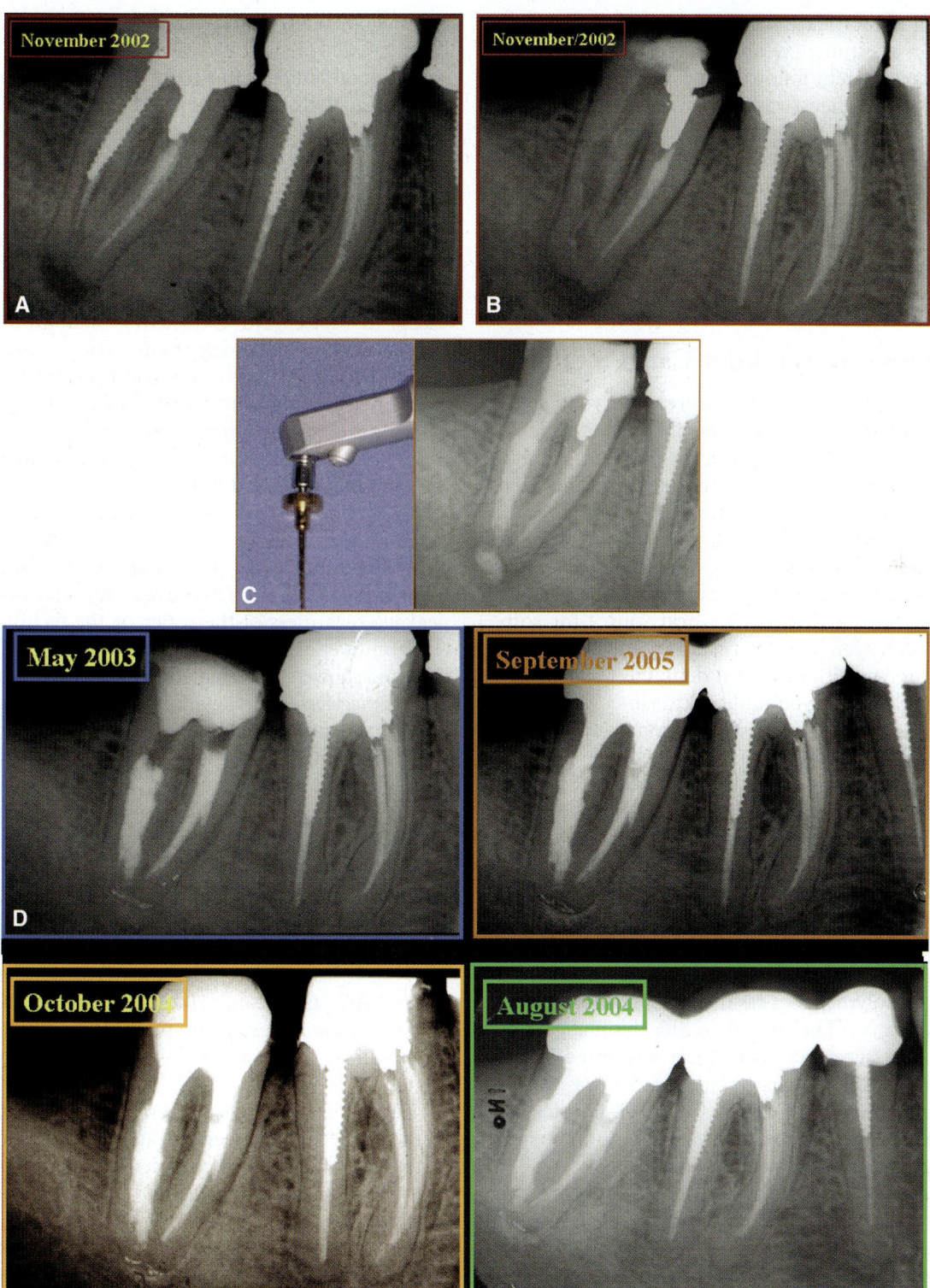

Figure 5 ***A,*** Radiograph of a 42-year-old male patient with a suspected vertical root fracture on the second mandibular right molar. The tooth had been restored 12 years earlier after root canal therapy. He reported several episodes of pain and swelling during the past several years. ***B,*** At the first appointment, the leaky restoration and the screw post were removed, the distal root canal was thoroughly cleaned and irrigated using sodium hypochlorite, and $Ca(OH)_2$ dressing was placed. ***C,*** On a later appointment, the canal was treated with the prototype of the RCLase Side Firing Spiral Tip. ***D,*** The endodontic treatment was completed 6 months later (May 2003). Follow-up radiographs that were taken 1, 2 and 4 years after the completion of the endodontic treatment show complete healing of the periapical lesion.

bactericidal effect of laser irradiation can be effectively utilized for additional cleansing and disinfecting of the root canal system following biomechanical instrumentation. This effect was extensively studied using lasers such as CO_2,[60,61] Nd:YAG,[62–65] KTP-Nd:YAG,[66] excimer,[67,68] diode,[69] and Er:YAG.[70–72]

The emerging consensus is that laser irradiation emitted from laser systems adapted to dentistry has the potential to kill microorganisms. In most cases, the effect is directly related to the amount of irradiation and to its energy level.

Obturation of the Root Canal System

The purpose of obturating the prepared root canal space is twofold: (1) to eliminate all avenues of leakage from the oral cavity or from the periapical tissues and (2) to seal within the system any irritants that cannot be fully removed during the cleaning and shaping procedures.[73] The rationale in introducing laser technology to assist in obturating the root canal system is based on two major assumptions: the ability to use the laser irradiation as a heat source for softening the gutta-percha to be used as obturating material and for conditioning the dentinal walls before placing an obturating bonding material.

The concept of thermoplasticized compaction is not new and covers any technique based entirely on heat softening gutta-percha combined primarily with vertical compaction. The pioneering technique using vertical compaction of warm gutta-percha was described 40 years ago by Schilder[74] as a way to fill canals in all dimensions and is an example of thermoplasticized compaction.

The first laser-assisted root canal filling procedure involved using the wavelength of Argon 488 nm laser. This wavelength that can be transmitted through dentin was used to polymerize a resin that was placed in the main root canal. The ability of this biomaterial to penetrate into accessory root canals was tested and it was shown that the resin in the lateral canals was readily polymerized at low energy levels (30m W). Further use of this wavelength became irrelevant due to its unsuitable properties in other dental procedures.[75]

Anic and Matsumoto[76] were the first to compare different root canal filling techniques for single-rooted teeth. Lateral condensation, vertical condensation, low-temperature gutta-percha (Ultrafil, Coltène/Whaledent, New York, NY), and laser-cured resin with different wavelengths (Argon, CO_2, and Nd-YAG) were the techniques used. The apical sealing ability achieved by the various filling techniques was compared by measuring the apical dye penetration following placement of the samples in a 1% solution of methylene blue. Gutta-percha softened with Argon laser created an apical seal similar to that obtained with lateral condensation and Ultrafil techniques.

Maden et al.[77] used the dye penetration method to measure apical leakage by comparing lateral condensation, System B technique, and Nd-YAG softened gutta-percha. No statistically significant differences were reported. In another study, Anic and Matsumoto[78] demonstrated that the temperature elevation induced on the outer root surface when Nd-YAG and Argon lasers were used ranged from $12.9°C$ (Argon laser) to $14.4°C$ (Nd-YAG laser). Such an increase in temperature may be detrimental to the tissues of the attachment apparatus of the teeth. The implication of such methodologies remains questionable.

In order to examine whether laser irradiation improves the adhesion of endodontic materials to the dentinal walls and thus reduce apical leakage, Park et al.[79] used different sealers and two root canal filling techniques. Using an Nd-YAG laser irradiation at the end of the root canal preparation (5 W, 20 Hz), they concluded that Nd-YAG irradiation reduced apical leakage regardless of the sealer or the technique used.

Kimura et al.[80] used Er-YAG laser (170 to 250 mJ, 2 Hz) and showed that irradiation of the root canal did not affect apical leakage following obturation when compared with conventional methods. They later demonstrated that the use of Nd-YAG laser was useful for the reduction of apical leakage.[81] Because Nd:YAG laser irradiation is very well absorbed by black color, an absorbent paper point soaked with black ink was introduced to working length and the apical root canal walls were painted.[81]

Significant improvement in the quality of the apical sealing of root canals was reported by Gekelman et al.[82] who used an Nd:YAG laser (100 mJ/pulse, 1 W, 10 Hz). It has also been demonstrated that application of Er-YAG laser beam (200 mJ, 4 Hz) for 60 seconds enhanced the adhesion of epoxy resin-based sealers in comparison with zinc oxide–eugenol-based root canal sealers.[83]

The clinical evidence from reported studies concerning the use of lasers to assist in obturating root canals is currently not sufficient. For example, it has not been determined whether the use of an optical fiber as a heat source to soften gutta-percha is safe for the surrounding structures of the tooth. It is also not clear if the softening of gutta-percha is homogeneous in all parts of the filling when vertical condensation techniques were described.[84] The significant role of endodontic sealers, when warm gutta-percha compaction techniques are employed, has been clearly demonstrated.[85] It is recognized that root canal sealers affect the quality of the apical seal of vertically condensed gutta-percha and that without a sealer significantly more apical leakage occurs.

Some questions remain concerning the effectiveness of lasers contributing to the obturating procedures of root canals: what is the most suitable wavelength and what are adequate parameters? These areas should be explored and assessed.

Endodontic Retreatment

Endodontic failures can be attributed to inadequacies in cleaning, shaping, and obturation, iatrogenic events, or re-infection of the root canal system. Regardless of the initial cause, the sum of causes is bacterial contamination. The objective of non-surgical retreatment is to eliminate from the root canal space sources of irritation to the attachment apparatus.[86] Some of these failures may be managed by endodontic retreatment, proven to be effective in eliminating clinical and radiographic signs of pathosis. A variety of techniques have been described to remove deficient root canal filling and/or metallic obstructions that may lead to undesirable results[87] (see Chapter 31 "Retreatment of Non-Healing Endodontic Therapy and Management of Mishaps")

The rationale for using laser irradiation in non-surgical retreatment may be ascribed to the need to remove foreign material from the root canal system that may otherwise be difficult to remove by conventional methods. Farge et al.[88] examined the efficacy of the Nd-YAP laser (1340 nm) in root canal retreatment (200 mJ and a frequency of 10 Hz). They attempted to remove gutta-percha and zinc oxide–eugenol sealer previously placed. In addition, they also reported an attempt to remove silver cones and broken instruments. They concluded that using laser radiation alone would not completely remove debris and obturating materials from the root canal.

Yu et al.[89] used an Nd-YAG laser at three output powers (1, 2, 3 W) to remove gutta-percha and broken files from root canals. They were able to remove filling material in more than 70% of the samples while broken files were removed 55% of the time.

Anjo et al.[90] reported that the time required for removal of any root canal-filling materials using laser ablation was significantly shorter than that required using conventional methods. It appeared that following laser irradiation, some orifices of dentinal tubules were blocked with melted dentin. They concluded that Nd:YAG laser irradiation is an effective technique for removal of root canal-filling materials and may offer advantages over conventional methods.

The efficacy of the Er-YAG laser in removing zinc oxide sealers and phenoplastic resins has also been studied.[91] In straight root canals, laser irradiation with 250 mJ/pulse and 10 Hz frequency was useful in eliminating zinc oxide sealers.

Hand instruments without the use of any specific solvent were also used. In curved root canals, however, the procedure had to be stopped because of the risk of lateral root perforation. Under the same experimental conditions when laser irradiation was delivered to remove phenoplastic resins, ledging of the root canal occurred and it was not possible to return to the previously established working length.

A clinical advantage that should be further explored is the possibility of eliminating the use of toxic solvents when removing semi-solid materials from root canals. Although it was shown[89–92] that root canal-filling materials can be removed from the root canal using lasers, such as the Nd:YAG and the Er:YAG, the decisive advantage in using lasers for this purpose still remains to be confirmed.

Apical Surgery

Surgical endodontic therapy is indicated when teeth have responded poorly to conventional treatment or when they cannot be treated appropriately by non-surgical means. The goal of endodontic surgery is to eliminate the disease and prevent its recurrence.[93] Surgical options should be considered only when better results cannot be achieved by non-surgical treatment.[94,95]

Egress of irritants from the root canal system into the periapical tissues is considered the main cause of failure following apicoectomy and apical filling. The irritants penetrate mainly through gaps between the filling and the dentin.[96] A second possible pathway for irritants to egress into the periapical tissues is through dentinal tubules on the cut root surface. It has been shown that the dentin of apically resected roots is more permeable to fluids than the dentin of non-resected roots.[97]

The first attempt to use a laser in endodontic surgery was performed by Dr. Weichman at the University of Southern California (at the suggestion of Dr. Ingle). He attempted to seal the apical foramina of extracted teeth from which the pulps had been extirpated.[98] The apices of those specimens were irradiated using a high power CO_2 laser. Melting of the cementum and dentin was observed with a "cap" formation that could, however, be easily removed.

Miserendino[99] used a CO_2 laser to irradiate the apex of a tooth during apicoectomy. He described the advantages associated with laser application for periapical surgery such as improved hemostasis and concurrent visualization of the operative field. He also emphasized the potential sterilizing effect of the contaminated root apex as well as the reduction in permeability of the root surface dentin. Moreover, he described re-crystallization of the apical root dentin that appeared to be smooth and suitable for placement of an apical filling material. Duclos et al.[100] used a CO_2 laser to perform apicoectomies in patients and advocated the use of a mini contra-angle head for efficient delivery of the laser irradiation at a 90° angle to the root apexes of teeth in the posterior areas.

However, unfavorable results of an in vivo study on dogs where the success rate following apicoectomies using the CO_2 laser was not improved have failed to support the rationale previously described by Miserendino.[99] A prospective study of two apical preparations with and without CO_2 laser, in which 320 cases were evaluated, did not show that CO_2 laser use improved the healing process.[102] In vitro studies[103–106] with Nd:YAG lasers have shown a reduction in penetration of dye or bacteria through resected roots. It was suggested that the reduced permeability in the lased specimens was probably the result of structural changes in the dentin following laser application.[104] Although SEM examination showed melting, solidification, and re-crystallization of the hard tissue, the structural changes were not uniform and the melted areas appeared connected by areas that looked like those in the non-lased specimens. It was postulated that this was the reason why the permeability of the dentin was reduced, but not completely eliminated. It is reasonable to assume that homogenously glazed surfaces would be less permeable than partially glazed ones.

Ebihara et al.[107] used Er:YAG laser for apical cavity preparations of extracted teeth. They found no significant difference in dye penetration between the laser-treated groups and those in which ultrasonic tips were used. These results were not surprising as the Er:YAG laser neither melts nor seals the dentinal tubules; therefore, any reduction in dentin permeability should not be expected. A different result was obtained by Gouw-Soares et al.[108] who evaluated the marginal permeability in teeth after apicoectomy and apical dentin surface treatment using two different lasers (Er:YAG and 9.6 μm TEA CO_2). Both laser systems showed a reduction of permeability to methylene blue dye.

Recently it has been reported that when using an Er:YAG laser in a low output power in apical surgery, it was possible to resect the apex of extracted teeth. Smooth and clean resected surfaces devoid of charring were observed.[109,110] It was also found that although the cutting speed of the Er:YAG laser was slightly slower than conventional high-speed burs, absence of discomfort and vibration and less chance for contamination at the surgical site, as well as reduced risk of trauma to adjacent tissues may compensate for the additional time required.[111]

In a 3-year clinical study, Gouw-Soares et al.[112] reported a new protocol for use in apical surgery. An Er-YAG laser was used for osteotomy and root resection, whereas the Nd:YAG laser irradiation served to seal the dentinal tubules to reduce possible bacterial contamination of the surgical cavity. Improvement in healing was achieved by the use of a LILT Ga-Al-As diode laser. The radiographic follow-up showed significant decrease in the radiolucent periapical areas with no adverse clinical signs and symptoms.[112]

The preparation of apical cavities by Er:YAG laser and ultrasonics was also studied by Karlovic et al.[113] They found lower values of microleakage when the root end cavities were prepared with the Er:YAG laser irrespective of the material used to seal those cavities.

It has been suggested that after the appropriate wavelength to melt the hard tissues of the tooth has been established, the main contribution of laser technology to surgical endodontics is to convert the apical dentin and cementum structure into a uniformly glazed area that does not allow egress of microorganisms through dentinal tubules and other openings in the apex of the tooth. Hemostasis and sterilization of the contaminated root apex will have an additional significant input.[114]

References

1. Coluzzi DJ. An overview of laser wavelengths used in dentistry. Den Clin N Am 2000;44:753–65.
2. Harris DM, Pick RM. Laser physics. In: Miserendino LJ and Pick RM. Lasers in dentistry. Chicago: Quintessence; 1995.
3. Nelson SJ, Berns MW. Basic laser physics and tissue interactions. Contemp Dermatol 1982;2:1–15.
4. Sulewski JG. Historical survey of laser dentistry. Dent Clin N Am 2000;44:717–52.
5. Dederich DN. Laser tissue interaction. Alpha Omegan 1991;84:33–6.
6. Miserendino LJ, Levy G, Miserendino CA. Laser interaction with biologic tissues. In: Miserendino LJ and Pick RM. Lasers in dentistry. Chicago: Quintessence, 1995.
7. Goodis HE, Pashley D, Stabholz A. Pulpal effects of thermal and mechanical irritants In: Hargreaves KM, Goodies HE. Seltzer's and Bender's Dental Pulp. Chicago: Quintessence; 2002.
8. Arcoria CJ, Miserendino LJ. Laser effects on the dental pulp. In: Miserendino LJ, Pick RM. Lasers in dentistry. Chicago: Quintessence; 1995.
9. Kimura Y, Wilder-Smith P, Matsumoto K. Lasers in endodontics: a review. Int Endod J 2000;33:173–85.
10. Cohen S, Liewehr F. Diagnostic procedures. In: Cohen S, Burns RC. Pathways of the pulp. 8th ed. St. Louis:Mosby; 2002.

11. American Asoociation of Endodontics. Glossary of endodontic terms. 7th ed. AAE, Chicago,IL 2003.
12. Isermann GT, Kaminski EJ. Pulpal response to minimal exposure in presence of bacteria and Dycal. J Endod 1979;5:322–7.
13. Cvek M, Cleaton-Jones PE, Austin JC, et al. Pulp reaction to exposure after experimental crown fractures or grinding in adult monkeys. J Endod 1982;8:391–7.
14. Cvek M: Endodontic treatment of traumatized teeth. In: Andreasen JO. Traumatic injuries of the teeth, 2nd ed. Philadelphia:WB Saunders; 1981.
15. Seltzer S, Bender IB. Pulp capping and pulpotomy. In: Seltzer S, Bender IB. The dental pulp, biologic considerations in dental procedures. 2nd ed. Philadelphia: JB Lippincott;1975.
16. Torabinejad M, Chivian N. Clinical applications of mineral trioxide aggregate. J Endod 1999;25:197–20.
17. Pitt-Ford TR, Torabinejad M, Abedi HR. Mineral trioxide aggregate as a pulp capping material. J Am Dent Assoc 1996;27:1491.
18. Myers K, Kaminski E, Lautenschlager EP. The effect of mineral trioxide aggregate on the dog pulp. J Endod 1996;22:198–202.
19. Klein H, Fuks A, Eidelman E, et al. Partial pulpotomy following complicated crown fracture in permanent incisors: a clinical and radiographical study. J Pedod 1985;9(2):142–7.
20. Fuks AB, Chosack A, Klein H, et al. Partial pulpotomy as a treatment alternative for exposed pulps in crown-fractured permanent incisors. Endod Dent Traumatol 1987;3:100–102.
21. Melcer J, Chaumate MT, Melcer F, et al. Preliminary report of the effect of CO_2 laser beam on the dental pulp of the Macaca Mulatta primate and the beagle dog. J Endod 1985;11:1–5.
22. Shoji S, Nakamura M, Horiuchi H. Histopathological changes in dental pulps irradiated by CO_2 laser: a preliminary report on laser pulpotomy. J Endod 1985;11:379–84.
23. Jukic S, Anic I, Koba K. The effect of pulpotomy using CO_2 and Nd:YAG lasers on dental pulp tissue. Int Endod J 1977;30:175–188.
24. Moritz A, Schoop U, Goharkhay K. The CO_2 laser as an aid in direct pulp capping. J Endod 1998;24:248–51.
25. Olivi G, Genovese MD, Maturo P, Docimo R. Pulp capping: advantages of using laser technology. Eur J Peadiatr Dent 2007;8:89–95.
26. Santucci PJ. Dycal versus Nd:YAG laser and Vitrebond for direct pulp capping in permanent teeth. J Clinc Laser Med Surg. 1999;17:69–75.
27. Fried D, Glena RE, Featherstone JD, et al. Permanent and transient changes in the reflectance of CO_2 laser-irradiated dental hard tissues at lambda = 9.3, 9.6, 10.3, and 10.6 microns and at fluences of 1-20 J/cm2. Lasers Surg Med 1997;20:22–31.
28. Wigdor HA, Walsh JT Jr. Histologic analysis of the effect on dental pulp of a 9.6-microm CO_2 laser. Laser Surg Med 2002;30:261–6.
29. White JM, Fagan MC, Goodis HE. Intrapulpal temperatures during pulsed Nd:YAG laser treatment, in vitro. J Periodontol 1994;65:255–9.
30. Jeng-fen Liu. Effects of Nd:YAG laser pulpotomyon human primary molars. J Endod 2006;32:404–7.
31. Kakehashi S, Stanley HR, Fitzgerald RJ. The effect of surgical exposures of dental pulps in germ-free and conventional laboratory rats. Oral Surg Oral Med Oral Pathol Oral Radiol Endod 1965;20:340–9.
32. Bergenholz G. Microorganisms from necrotic pulps of traumatized teeth. Odontol Revy 1974;25:347–58.
33. Möller AJ, Fabricius L, Dahlen G, et al. Influence on periapical tissues of indigenous oral bacteria and necrotic pulp tissue in monkeys. Scand J Dent Res 1981;89:475–84.
34. Bystrom A, Sundquist G. Bacteriologic evaluation of the efficacy of mechanical root canal instrumentation in endodontic therapy. Scand J Dent Res 1981;89:321–8.
35. Sjogren U, Hagglund B, Sundquist G, et al. Factors affecting the long-term results of endodontic treatment. J. Endod 1990;16:498–504.
36. McComb D, Smith DC. A preliminary scanning electron microscope study of root canals after endodontic procedures. J Endod 1975;1:238–42.
37. Moodnik RM, Dorn SO, Feldman MJ, et al. Efficacy of biomechanical instrumentation; a scanning electron microscopy study. J Endod 1976;2:261–6.
38. Mader CL, Baumgartner JC, Peters DD. Scanning electron microscopic investigation of the smeared layer on root canal walls. J Endod 1984;10:477–83.
39. Torabinejad M, Handysides R, Khademi AA, et al. Clinical implications of the smear layer in endodontics: A review. Oral Surg Oral Med Oral Pathol Oral Radiol Endod 2002;94:658–66.
40. Haapasalo M, Orstavik D. In vitro infection and disinfection of dentinal tubules. J Dent Res 1986;66:1375–9.
41. Pashley DH. Smear layer physiological considerations. Oper Dent (Suppl) 1984;3:13–29.
42. Drake DR, Wiemann AH, Rivera EM, et al. Bacterial retention in canal walls in vitro: effect of smear layer. J Endod 1994;20:78–82.
43. Peters OA, Schonenberger K, Laib A. Effects of four Ni-Ti preparation techniques on root canal geometry assessed by micro computed tomography. Int Endod J 2001;34:221–30.
44. Oguntebi BR. Dentin tubule infection and endodontic therapy implications. Int Endod J 1994;27:218–22.
45. Anic I, Tachibana H, Matsumoto K, et al. Permeability, morphologic and temperature changes of canal dentin walls induced by Nd:YAG, CO_2 and argon lasers. Int Endod J 1996; 29:13–22.
46. Harashima T, Takeda FH, Kimura, et al. Effect of Nd:YAG laser irradiation for removal of intracanal debris and smear

layer in extracted human teeth. J Clin Laser Med Surg 1997;15:131–5.

47. Saunders WP, Whitters CJ, Strang R, et al. The effect of an Nd:YAG pulsed laser on the cleaning of the root canal and the formation of a fused apical plug. Int Endod J 1995;28:213–20.

48. Moshonov J, Sion A, Kasirer J, et al. Efficacy of argon laser irradiation in removing intracanal debris. Oral Surg Oral Med Oral Pathol Oral Radiol Endod 79;1995:221–5.

49. Yamazaki R, Goya C, Yu DG, et al. Effect of Erbium, Chromium:YSGG laser irradiation on root canal walls: A scanning electron microscopic and thermographic study. J Endod 2001;27:9–12.

50. Takeda FH, Harashima T, Kimura Y, et al. Efficacy of Er:YAG laser irradiation in removing debris and smear layer on root canal walls. J Endod 1998;24:548–51.

51. Kimura Y, Yonaga K, Yokoyama K, et al. Root surface temperature increase during Er:YAG laser irradiation of root canals. J Endod 2002;28:76–8.

52. Svenstater G, Bergenholz G. Biofilms in endodontic infections. Endod Topics 2004; 9:27–36.

53. Bergmans L, Moisiadis P, Teughels W, et al. Bactericidal effects of Nd:YAG laser irradiation on some endodontic pathogens ex vivo. Int Endodo J 2006;39:547.

54. Goodis HE, Pashley D, Stabholz A. Pulpal effects of thermal and mechanical irritants. In: Hargreaves KM, Goodis HE. Seltzer and Bender's dental pulp. Carol Stream IL: Quintessence publishing 2002.

55. Stabholz A, Zeltzser R, Sela M, et al. The use of lasers in dentistry: principles of operation and clinical applications. Compend 2003;24:811–24.

56. Matsumoto K. Lasers in endodontics. Dent Clin of North Am 2000;44:889–906.

57. Cozean C, Arcoria CJ, Pelagalli J, et al. Dentistry for the 21st century? Erbium:YAG laser for teeth. J Am Dent Assoc 1997;128:1080–7.

58. Ando N, Hoshino E. Predominant obligate anaerobes invading the deep layers of root canal dentine. Int Endod J 1990;23:20–7.

59. Armitage GC, Ryder MI, Wilcox SE. Cemental changes in teeth with heavily infected root canals. J Endod 1983;9:127–30.

60. Zakariasen KL, Dederich DN, Tulip J, et al. Bactericidal action of carbon dioxide laser radiation in experimental root canals. Can J Microbiol 1986;32:942–6.

61. Le Goff A, Morazin-Dautel A, Guigand M, et al. An evaluation of the CO_2 laser for endodontic disinfection. J Endod 1999;25:105–8.

62. Moshonov J, Orstavik D, Yamauchi S, et al. Nd:YAG laser irradiation in root canal disinfection. Endod Dent Traumatol 1995;11:220–4.

63. Fegan SE, Steiman HR. Comparative evaluation of the antibacterial effects of intracanal Nd:YAG laser irradiation: An in vitro study. J Endod 1995;21:415–7.

64. Rooney J, Midda M, Leeming J. A laboratory investigation of the bactericidal effect of Nd:YAG laser. Br Dent J 1994;176:61–4.

65. Gutknecht N, Moritz A, Conrads G. Bactericidal effect of the Nd:YAG laser in in vitro root canals. J Clin Laser Med Surg 1996;14:77–80.

66. Nammour S, Kowaly k, Powell L, et al. External temperature during KTP-Nd:YAG laser irradiation in root canals: an invitro study. Lasers Med Science 2004;19:27–32.

67. Stabholz A, Kettering J, Neev J, et al. Effects of XeCl excimer laser on *Streptococcus mutans*. J Endod 1993;19:232–5.

68. Folwaczny M, Liesenhoff T, Lehn N, et al. Bactericidal action of 308nm excimer-laser radiation: An in vitro investigation. J Endod 1998;24:781–5.

69. Gutknecht N, Alt T, Slaus G, et al. A clinical comparison of the Bactericidal effect of the diode laser and a 5% sodium hypochlorite in necrotic root canals J Oral Laser Applications 2002;2:151–7.

70. Mehl A, Folwaczny M, Haffner C, et al. Bactericidal effects of 2.94μ Er:YAG laser irradiation in dental root canals. J Endod 1999;25:490–3.

71. Dostalova T, Jelinkova H, Housova D, et al. Endodontic treatment with application of Er:YAG laser waveguide radiation disinfection. J Clin Laser Med Surg 2002;20:135–9.

72. Schoop U, Moritz A, Kluger W, et al. The Er;YAG laser in endodontics: results of an in vitro study. Lasers Surg Med 2002;30:360–4.

73. Gutmann JL, Whitherspoon DE. Obturation of the cleaned and shaped root canal system. In: Cohen S, Burns RC. Pathways of the pulp 8th ed. St. Louis MO: Mosby;2002.

74. Schilder H. Filling root canals in three dimensions. Dent Clin North Am 1967;11:723–9.

75. Potts TV, Petrou A. Laser photopolymerization of dental materials with potential endodontic applications. J Endod 1990;16:265–8.

76. Anic I, Matsumoto K. Comparison of the sealing ability of laser softened, laterally condensed and low-temperature thermoplasticized gutta-percha. J Endod 1995;21:464–9.

77. Maden M, Gurgul G, Tinaz AC. Evaluation of apical leakage of root canals obturated with Nd:YAG laser-softened gutta-percha, System-B, and lateral condensation techniques. Contemp Dent Pract 2002;15:16–26.

78. Anic I, Matsumoto K. Dentinal heat transmission induced by a laser-softened gutta-percha obturation technique. J Endod. 1995;21:470–4.

79. Park DS, Yoo HM, Oh TS. Effect of Nd:YAG laser irradiation on the apical leakage of obturated root canals: an electrochemical study. Int Endod J 2001;4:318–21.

80. Kimura Y, Yonaga K, Yokoyama K, et al. Apical leakage of obturated canals prepared by Er:YAG laser. J Endod 2001;27:567–70.

81. Kimura Y, Yamazaki R, Goya C, et al. A comparative study on the effects of three types of laser irradiation at the apical stop and apical leakage after obturation. J Clin Laser Med Surg 1999;17:261–6.

82. Gekelman D, Prokopowitsch I, Eduardo CP. In vitro study of the effects of Nd:YAG laser irradiation on the apical sealing of endodontic fillings performed with and without dentin plugs. J Clin Laser Med Surg 2002;20:117–21.

83. Sousa-Neto MD, Marchesan MA, Pecora JD, et al. Effect of Er:YAG laser on adhesion of root canal sealers. J Endod. 2002;28:185–7.

84. Blum JY, Parahy E, Machtou P. Warm vertical compaction sequences in relation to gutta-percha temperature. J Endod 1997;23:307–11.

85. Yared GM, Bou Dagher F. Sealing ability of the vertical condensation with different root canal sealers. J Endod 1996;21:6–8.

86. Ruddle CJ. Non surgical endodontic retreatment. In: Cohen S, Burns RC. Pathways of the pulp. 8th ed. St. Louis MO: Mosby;2002.

87. Hulssman R. Methods for removing metal obstructions from the root canal. Endod Dent Traumatol 1983;9:223–23.

88. Farge P, Nahas P, Bonin P. In vitro study of a Nd-YAP laser in endodontic retreatment. J Endod 1998;42:359–3.

89. Yu DG, Kimura Y, Tomita Y, et al. Study on removal effects of filling materials and broken files from root canals using pulsed Nd:YAG laser. J Clin Laser Med Surg 2000;18:23–8.

90. Anjo T, Ebihara A, Takeda A, et al. Removal of two types of root canal filling material using pulsed Nd-YAG laser irradiation. Photomed Laser Surg 2004;22:470–6.

91. Warembourg P, Rocca JP, Bertrand MF: Efficacy of an Er:YAG laser to remove endodontic pastes. An in vitro. J Oral Laser Appl 2001;1:43–7.

92. Viducic D, Jukic S, Karlovic Z, et al. Removal of gutta-percha using an Nd-YAG laser. Int Endod J 2003;36:670–3.

93. Carr GB. Surgical endodontics. In: Cohen S, Burns RC. Pathways of the pulp. 6th ed. St. Louis MO: Mosby;1994.

94. Gutmann JL. Principles of endodontic surgery for the general practitioner. Dent Clin North Am 1984;28:895–908.

95. Leubke RG. Surgical endodontics. Dent Clin North Am 1974;18:379.

96. Stabholz A, Shani J, Friedman S, et al. Marginal adaptation of retrograde fillings and its correlation with sealability. J Endod 1985;11:218–23.

97. Ichesco E, Ellison R, Corcoran J. A spectrophotometric analysis of dentinal leakage in the resected root [Abstract]. J Endod 1986;12:129.

98. Weichman JA, Johnson FM. Laser use in endodontics. A preliminary investigation. Oral Surg Oral Med Oral Pathol Oral Radiol Endod 1971;31:416–20.

99. Miserendino LL. The laser apicoectomy: endodontic application of CO_2 laser for periapical surgery. Oral Surg Oral Med Oral Pathol Oral Radiol Endod 1988;66:615–9.

100. Duclos P, Behlert V, Lenz P. New technique of surgical treatment of periapical lesions using carbon dioxide laser. Rev. Odontostomatol 1990;19:143–50.

101. Friedman S, Rotstein I, Mahamid A. In vivo efficacy of various retrofills and of CO_2 laser in apical surgery. Endodon Dent Traumatol 1991;7:19–25.

102. Bader G, Lejeune S. Prospective study of two retrograde endodontic apical preparations with and without the use of $CO2$ laser. Endod Dent Traumatol 1998;14:75–8.

103. Stabholz A, Khayat A, Ravanshad SH, et al. Effects of Nd:YAG laser on apical seal of teeth after apicoectomy and retrofill. J Endod 1992;18:371–5.

104. Stabholz A, Khayat A, Weeks DA, et al. Scanning electron microscopic study of the apical dentine surfaces lased with Nd:YAG laser following apicectomy and retrofill. Int Endod J 1992;25:288–91.

105. Arens DL, Levy GC, Rizoiu IM. A comparison of dentin permeability after bur and laser apicoectomies. Compendium 1993;14:1290–7.

106. Wong WS, Rosenberg PA, Boylan RJ, et al. A comparison of the apical seals achieved using retrograde amalgam fillings and the Nd:YAG laser. J Endod 1994;20:595–7.

107. Ebihara A, Wadachi R, Sekine Y, et al. Application of Er:YAG laser to retrograde cavity preparation. J Japan Soci Laser Dent 1998;9:23–31.

108. Gouw-Soares S, Stabholz A, Lage-Marques JL, et al. Comparative study of dentine permeability after apicectomy and surface treatment with 9.6 micrometer TEA CO_2 and Er:YAG laser irradiation. J Clin Laser Med Surg 2004;22:129–39.

109. Paghdiwala AF. Root resection of endodontically treated teeth by Er:YAG laser radiation. J Endod 1993;19:91–4.

110. Komori T, Yokoyama K, Matsumoto Y, Matsumoto K. Er:YAG and Ho:YAG laser root resection of extracted human teeth. J Clin Laser Med Surg 1997;15:9–3.

111. Komori T, Yokoyama K, Takato T, Matsumoto K. Clinical application of the Er:YAG laser for apicoectomy. J Endod 1997;23:748–50.

112. Gouw-Soares S, Tanji E, Haypek P, et al. The use of Er:YAG, Nd:YAG and Ga-Al-As. Lasers in periapical surgery: a three year clinical study. J Clin Surg Med 2001;19:193–8.

113. Karlovic Z, Pezelj-Ribaric S, Miletic I, et al. Er-YAG laser versus ultrasonic in preparation of root-end cavities. J Endod 2005; 31:821–3.

114. Stabholz A, Sahar-Helft S, Moshonov J. Lasers in endodontics. Dent Clin N Am 2004;48:809–32.

CHAPTER 26F

F. VISUAL ENHANCEMENT

JAMES K. BAHCALL

Visualization during surgical and conventional endodontic treatment has historically been limited to two-dimensional dental radiography representative of a three-dimensional biologic system and what could be seen with the naked eye (perhaps enhanced by loupes). Today, endodontic treatment is to a large extent viewed as a microsurgical procedure. The principle upon which all microsurgery is based is the observation that the hand can perform remarkably intricate micromanipulations as long as the eye can see a magnified field and it can be interpreted by the mind.[1] Magnification affects vision by increasing the size of an image on the retina. "Visual image" is the basic parameter used to describe how large something appears, and is expressed in units of degree or cycles/degree.[2] The use of optical magnification instruments such as loupes, microscopes, endoscopes, and orascopes enables the endodontist to magnify a specified treatment field beyond that perceived by the naked eye.

Optical Definitions

Working Distance: The distance measured from the dentist's eye to the treatment field being viewed.
Depth of Field: The amount of distance between the nearest and furthest objects that appear in acceptably sharp focus.
Convergence Angle: The aligning of two oculars to be sure they are pointing at the identical distance and angle to the object or treatment field.
Field of View: The area that is visible through optical magnification.
Viewing Angle: The angular position of the optics allowing for a comfortable viewing position for the operator.

Loupes

Dental loupes are the most common magnification system used in dentistry. All loupes use convergent lenses to form a magnified image.[3] The simplest form of optical magnification is *single-lens loupes* (ie, jeweler's flip-down magnifiers). Single lenses have a fixed focal length and working distance.[4] The advantages of these types of loupes are low cost and light weight as they are made of plastic. The disadvantage of single-lens loupes is poor image resolution compared with multi-lens glass optics (telescopic loupes and microscopes).[5] Because single-lens loupes provide a set working distance, the dentist may find the ergonomics incorrect and may need to compensate with poor body posture, causing the possible neck and back strain.

In order to overcome the disadvantages of single-lens loupe optics, the use of *multi-lens optic* system is recommended. This type of glass multi-lens configuration is known as a Galilean optical system (Figure 1). It provides a higher level of magnification, improved depth of field and working distance, and higher optical resolution compared with single-lens optics.[4] Telescopic loupes use Galilean optics. Ideal magnification with telescopic loupes is ×2.5. This offers a good compromise between weight, optical performance, and cost. Galilean lens systems cannot offer magnification much greater than ×2.5 without incurring weight, size, and image resolution problems.[5] Silber recommends the use of ×2.5 operating loupes because magnification of loupes greater than ×2.5 limits the depth of field and working distance during treatment.[1] Any head movement of the operator, while using loupes with magnification greater than ×2.5, will move a treatment field in and out of focus, very distracting and irritating to the clinician. When need for higher magnification is required (up to ×6), *prism optics* are

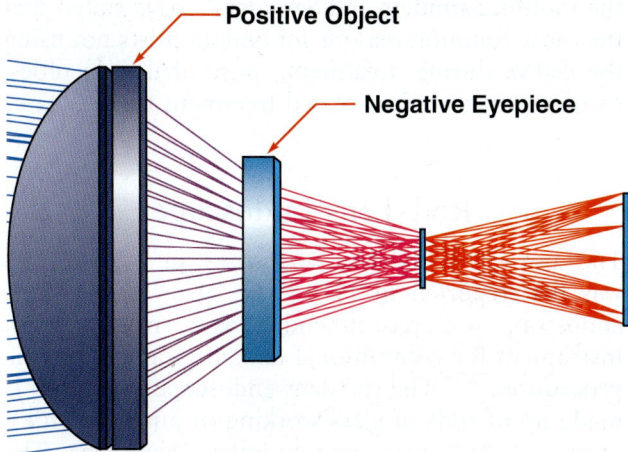

Figure 1 Diagram of Galilean optics. Illustration courtesy of Designs for Vision, Inc., Ronkonkoma, NY.

available. This optical system is based on the Keplarian astronomic telescope, which uses five lenses and two prisms. The advantages of this optical system are superior optical clarity and a flatter view from edge to edge. However, the disadvantages are expense and added weight to loupes.[5] And as the magnification in loupes increases, the need for more illumination is required.[6] Loupe manufacturers have designed portable clip-on light sources to accommodate demand for increased light.

Microscopes

Baumann[7] was the first to report the use and benefits of an operating microscope for conventional endodontics. Since then, the use of the *surgical operating microscope* (SOM) has evolved in the field of endodontics as an invaluable optical magnification instrument[8–10] (Figure 2). Today, this visual evolution in endodontics, from using loupes and headlamps to the use of the microscope, parallels a similar transition in medical specialties, such as ophthalmology and neurosurgery.[11] On January 1, 1998, the American Dental Association Accreditation Standards for Advanced Specialty Education Programs in Endodontics were revised; formal microscope training must be included in surgical and nonsurgical endodontic treatment.[11]

The magnification needs in endodontic treatment range from ×3 to ×30.[12] A SOM accommodates these magnification requirements. Although loupes can have a magnification as high as ×6, they are not able to provide the same depth of field at ×6 magnification compared with the microscope,[1] and fiber optic light source of the SOM provides two to three times the light emitted from a surgical headlamp.[13]

Similar to loupes, microscopes use the Galilean lens system. The magnification of the SOM is

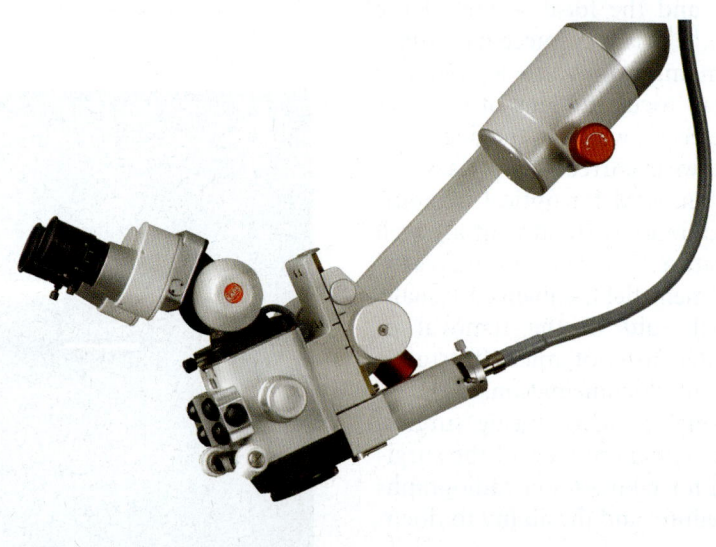

Figure 2 Clinical use of surgical operating microscope. Photo courtesy of Jedmed, St. Louis, MO.

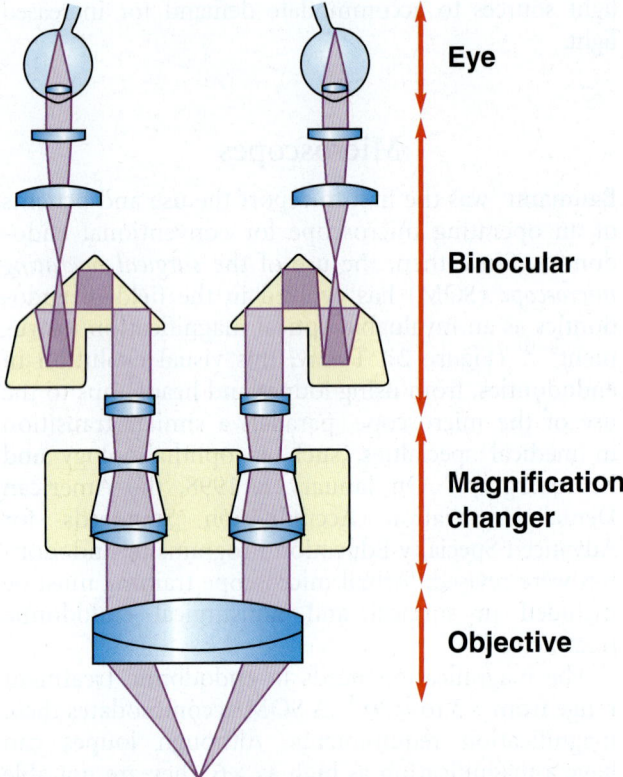

Figure 3 A schematic diagram of the surgical operating microscope. The eyepiece connected to binocular field glasses allows adequate focal length. The objective lens increases the magnification. The magnification changer adds to the flexibility of the microscope.

determined by the magnification power of the eyepiece, the focal length of the binoculars, the magnification changer factor, and the focal length of the objective lens (Figure 3).[12,14] The eyepiece has adjustable diopter settings ranging from –5 to +5. Diopter settings help the clinician focus the lens of the eyes and adjust for refractive error, which is the degree to which a person needs to wear corrective eyeglasses.[12]

The benefits of using an SOM for optical magnification in conventional endodontic treatment are well documented in the literature.[15–19] They are increased visualization of the treatment field, enhanced visualization in locating canals, aid in the removal of separated instruments, diagnosis of micro fractures, perforation repair, and case documentation.

The advantages of using an SOM during surgical endodontic treatment are enhanced view of the surgical treatment field, need for taking fewer radiographs during the surgical procedure, and the ability to document the treatment.[20]

When viewing an endodontic treatment field through a microscope, the use of a standard dental mirror or micromirror is usually required, in conjunction with the microscope, to overcome the angulation difficulties of certain tooth positions in the mouth. Saunders and Saunders[15] have stated that the most common reasons for endodontists not using the SOM during treatment: positional difficulties, inconvenience, and increased treatment time.

Rod–Lens Endoscope

The use of a *rod–lens endoscope* in endodontics was first reported in 1979.[21] In 1996, the rod–lens endoscope was recommended as a magnification instrument for conventional and surgical endodontic procedures.[22,23] The rod–lens endoscope (Figure 4) is made up of rods of glass working in junction with a camera, light source, and monitor (Figure 5). The option of a digital recorder (either streaming video or still capture) may be added to the system for documentation.

The rod–lens endoscope allows clinicians' greater magnification than that achieved with loupes or a microscope, with optical resolution comparable with that of microscopes and/or loupes. Although the endoscope can be used as a visualization instrument for conventional endodontic treatment, it can be bulky and difficult to maintain a fixed field of vision compared with a microscope. A fixed field of vision is defined as "viewing a treatment field from one single angle and distance."[24] The use of the endoscope is therefore recommended for visualization of surgical endodontic treatment.[22–27] The

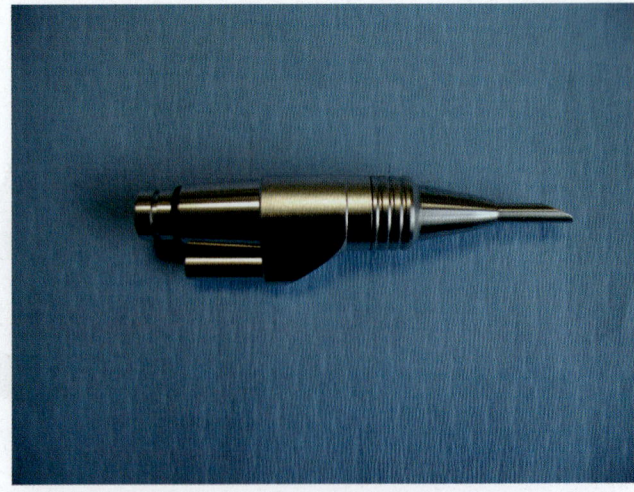

Figure 4 A rod–lens endoscope (Jedmed, St. Louis, MO).

Hemostasis of the surgical field must be obtained before the endoscope is used because the scope cannot provide a discernible image when placed in blood. The warmth of the blood can also create lens condensation and a blurred image. If this occurs, the use of suction and irrigation, or an antifogging agent, will eliminate the fogging effect. The tips of the endoscope should be placed on bone around the surgical crypt in order to stabilize the scope. Prior to usage, a protective metal sheath is placed over the endoscope to add rigidity and allow the endoscope to be held in a stable position. It is not recommended to use the endoscope to also retract gingival tissue while viewing a surgical treatment field. This will not allow free movement of the scope by the operator while also having difficulty keeping the gingival tissue out of the line of sight.

Orascope

An orascope is a *fiber optic endoscope* and like the rod–lens endoscope works in injunction with a camera, light source, and monitor. Fiber optics are made of plastics and therefore are small, lightweight, and flexible. It is important to note that image quality from fiber optic magnification has a direct correlation with the number of fibers and size of the lens used. The fiber optic endoscope is designed for intracanal visualization.[28] The orascope has a 0.8 mm tip diameter and 0° lens and the working portion is 15 mm in length (Figure 6). The orascope is

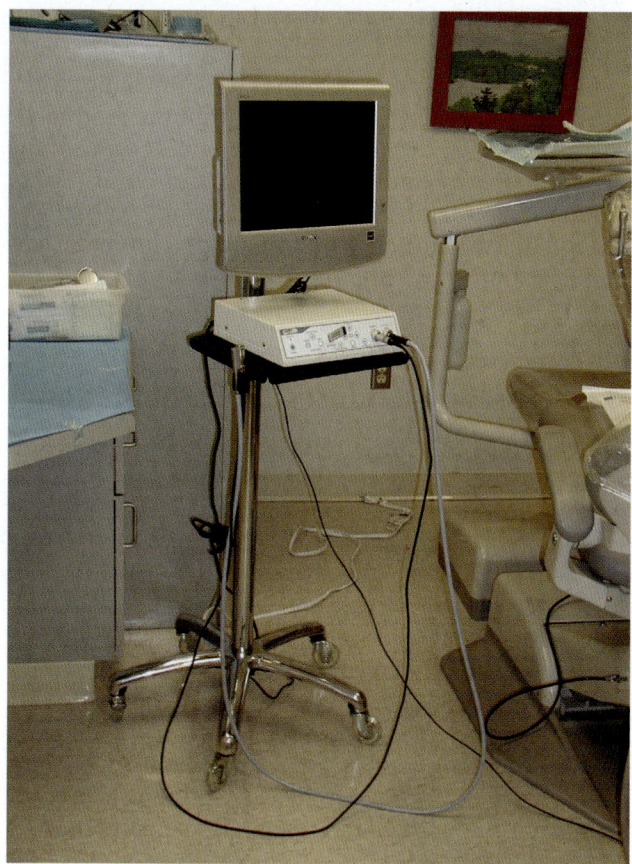

Figure 5 Endoscope visual system (EVS) (Jedmed, St. Louis, MO).

visualization advantage, in surgical endodontic treatment, the endoscope provides over the microscope, is the ability to view a surgical treatment field in a nonfixed field of vision. This is defined as the ability to view a treatment field at various angles and distances without losing depth of field and focus.[24]

The recommended rod–lens endoscope sizes, for endodontic surgical application, are a 2.7 mm lens diameter, 70° angulation, 3 cm length rod–lens, and a 4 mm lens diameter, 30° angulation, and 4 cm length rod–lens.[24] A pair of ×2 to ×2.5 loupes should be used for visualization prior to the use of the endoscope.[1,24] Loupes aid the endodontist during surgery when reflecting gingival tissue, removing cortical and medullary bone, and isolating root ends. The clinician should hold the endoscope while the assistant retracts gingival tissue and suctions.[24] This maintains good eye–hand coordination during examination or treatment. The clinician and the assistant(s) view the magnified image on the monitor.

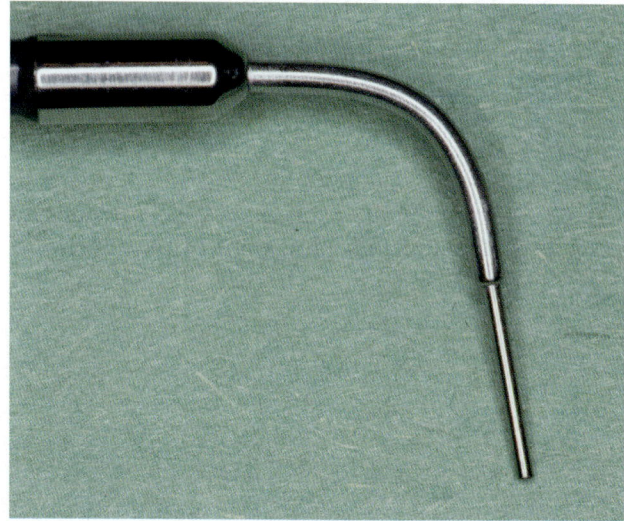

Figure 6 An orascope (Jedmed, St. Louis, MO).

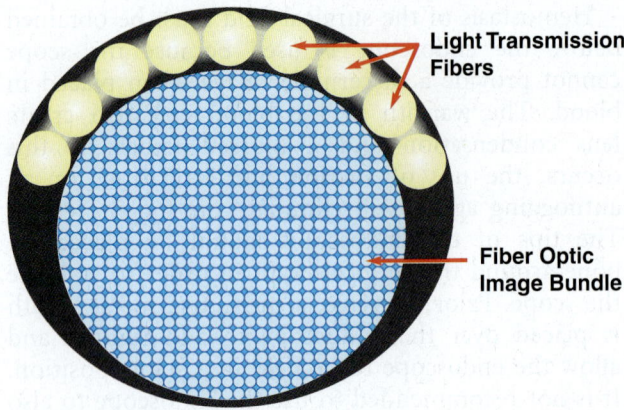

Figure 7 Cross-section of orascope probe showing the distribution of fiber optic image bundle and the light transmission fibers.

made up of 10,000 parallel visual fibers. Each visual fiber is between 3.7 and 5.0 μm in diameter. A ring of much larger light transmitting fibers surrounds the visual fibers for illumination of a treatment field (Figure 7).

Prior to the placement of the 0.8 mm fiber optic scope, it is recommended that ×2 to ×2.5 loupes or a SOM be used for conventional endodontic visualization during access to the canal(s). A canal must be prepared to a minimum size of a 90 file in the coronal 15 mm of the canal. If the canal is under-instrumented, a wedging of the orascope may damage some of the fiber optic bundles within the scope. The proper canal enlargement also allows the full 15 mm of the scope to penetrate within the canal. The canal must also be dried before the 0.8 mm fiber optic scope is placed. Although the scope will see through sodium hypochlorite, this solution has a high light-refractory index. This will cause greater amounts of light that will be reflected, thus making it difficult to see details of the canal.

The focus and depth of field of an orascope is from 0 mm to infinity. This allows the orascope to provide imaging of the apical third of the root without actually having to be placed in this region of the canal.

Similar to the endoscope, the endodontist holds the orascope while viewing the image from the monitor.[28] Temperature and humidity difference between the dental operatory and the canal can cause moisture to condense on the fiber optic lens, causing fogging. The use of a lens antifog solution helps eliminate lens condensation build-up.

Microscope–Endoscope Combination

In conventional and surgical endodontic treatment, there are different visualization parameters for each type of treatment, when magnification beyond loupes is required. Although both the microscope and rod–lens endoscope can be used for magnification for either type of endodontic treatment, the advantages for using a microscope for conventional endodontic treatment and a rod–lens endoscope for surgical visualization led to the development of a microscope coupler (Jedmed, St. Louis, MO) that enables the endodontists to combine both technologies (Figure 8). The combination unit also allows for the use of the orascope and digital documentation.

Magnification versus Differentiation

Magnification is defined as making an object or treatment field greater in size. *Differentiation* is defined as making something distinct or specialized.[29] The need to differentiate a magnified treatment field, when looking for a fracture in conventional endodontic therapy, or in surgical endodontic therapy when trying to identify the periodontal ligament space, an isthmus, or marginal leakage around a previous root-end filling, is important. Methylene blue, a nontoxic, biocompatible dye, can be used in conjunction with endodontic visualization instruments to help differentiate a treatment field in order to aid the endodontist in identifying etiology[30] (Figure 9).

Chapter 26 / Endodontics Instruments and Armamentarium / 875

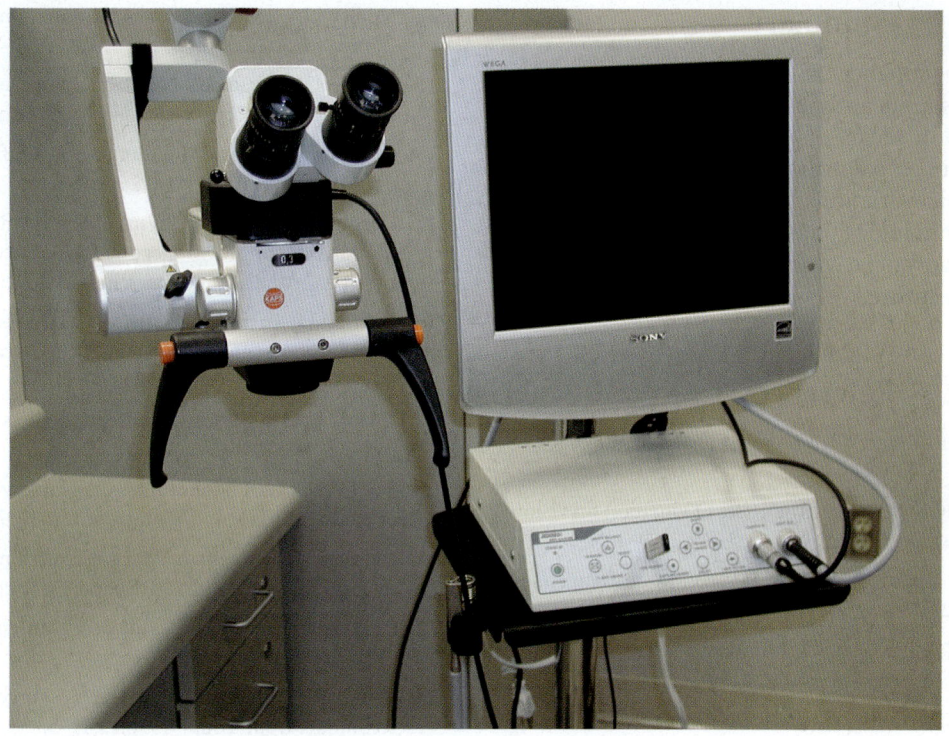

Figure 8 Combination microscope–endoscope visualization system (Jedmed, St. Louis, MO).

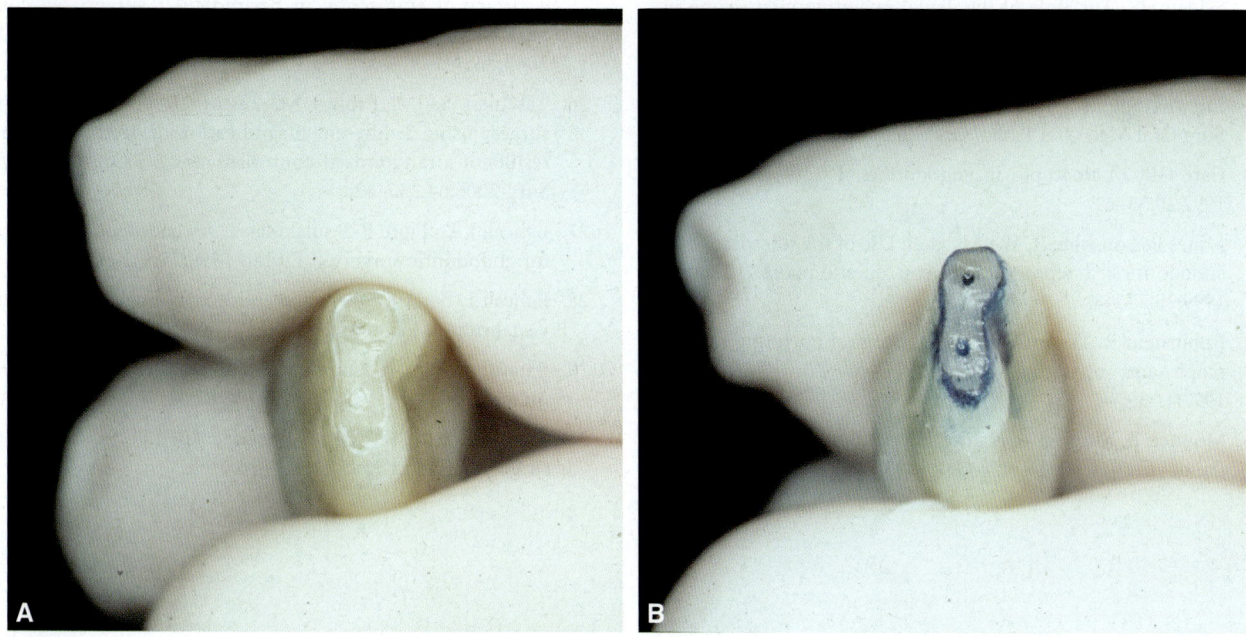

Figure 9 ***A,*** Magnification of a root end without differentiation. ***B,*** Magnification of a root end with methylene blue added for differentiation.

Summary

The ability to enhance vision during endodontic procedures has significantly increased the comfort level of endodontists in terms of identifying fracture lines, locating minuscule canal orifices, and confidently determining anatomic variations in teeth and supporting structures. Technological advances are continuously being made in advanced vision equipment, promising an even brighter future.

References

1. Silber S. Microsurgery. Baltimore: William & Wilkins Co; 1979. p. 1.
2. Kagan J, Gehly J, Wilson H. The effect of vibration on vision during microsurgery. Microsurgery 1983;4:209–14.
3. Shanelec DA. Optical principles of loupes. J Can Dent Assoc 1992;20:25–32.
4. Kanca J, Jordan PG. Magnification systems in clinical dentistry. J Can Dent Assoc 1995;61:851–6.
5. Millar BJ. Focus on loupes. Br Dent J 1998;185:504–8.
6. Caplan SA. Magnification in dentistry. J Esthet Dent 1990;2:17–21.
7. Baumann RR. How may the dentist benefit from the operating microscope? Quintessence Int 1977;5:17–18.
8. Selden HS. The Role of the dental operating microscope in endodontics. Penn Dent J 1986;53:36–7.
9. Selden HS. The role of a dental operating microscope in improved nonsurgical treatment of "calcified" canals. Oral Surg Oral Med Oral Pathol Oral Radiol Endod 1989;68:93–8.
10. Carr GB. Microscopes in endodontics. J Calif Dent Assoc 1992;20:55–61.
11. Mines P, Loushine R, West L, et al. Use of the microscope in endodontics: a report based on a questionnaire. J Endod 1999;25:755–8.
12. Rubinstein R. The anatomy of the surgical operating microscope and operating positions. Dent Clin North Am 1997;41:391–4.
13. Mounce R. Surgical operating microscopes in endodontics: the quantum leap. Dent Today 1993;12:88–91.
14. Nunley JA. Microscopes and microinstruments. Hand Clinics 1985;1(2):197–204.
15. Saunders WP, Saunders EM. Conventional endodontics and the operating microscope. Dent Clin North Am 1997;41:415–27.
16. Coelho de Carvalho MC, Zuolo ML. Orifice locating with a microscope. J Endod 2000;26:532–4.
17. Gorduysus MO, Gorduysus M, Friedman S. Operating Microscope improves negotiation of second mesiobuccal canals in maxillary molars. J Endod 2001;27:683–6.
18. Buhrley LJ, Barrows MJ, BeGole EA, Wenkus CS. Effect of magnification on locating the MB2 canal in maxillary molars. J Endod 2002;28:324–7.
19. Kim S. The microscope and endodontics. Dent Clin North Am 2004;48:11–18.
20. Rubinstein R. Endodontic microsurgery and the surgical operating microscope. Compendium 1997;18:659–72.
21. Detsch S, Cunningham W, Langloss J. Endoscopy as an aid to endodontic diagnosis. J Endod 1979;5:60–2.
22. Held S, Kao Y, Well D. Endoscope-an endodontic application. J Endod 1996;22:327–9.
23. Shulman B, Leung B. Endoscopic surgery: an alternative technique. Dent Today 1996;15:42–5.
24. Bahcall J, Barss J. Orascopic visualization technique for conventional and surgical endodontics. Int Endod J 2003;27:128–9.
25. von Arx T, Montagne D, Zwinggi C, Lussi A. Diagnostic accuracy of endoscopy in periradicular surgery—a comparison with scanning electron microscopy. Int Endod J 2003;36:691–9.
26. Taschieri S, Del Fabbro M, Testori T, et al. Endodontic surgery using 2 different magnification devices: preliminary results of a randomized controlled study. J Oral Maxillofac Surg 2006;64:235–42.
27. Bahcall J, Di Fiore P, Poulakidas T. An endoscopic technique for endodontic surgery. J Endod 1999;25:132–5.
28. Bahcall J, Barss J. Fiberoptic endoscope usage for intracanal visualization. J Endod 2001;27:128–9.
29. Bahcall J, Barss J. Orascopy: a vision for the new millennium, Part 2. Dent Today 1999;18:82–4.
30. Cambruzzi J. Methylene blue dye: an aid to endodontic surgery. J Endod 1985;11:311–14.

CHAPTER 27

PREPARATION OF CORONAL AND RADICULAR SPACES

OVE A. PETERS, RAVI S. KOKA

It has been well established over the past 30 years that endodontic disease, the presence of apical periodontitis, has a microbial pathogenesis.[1,2] Consequently, root canal treatment is performed to treat endodontic disease by eradicating bacteria from the root canal space. It is widely accepted that disinfection and subsequent obturation of the root canal space require mechanical enlargement of the main canals,[3] and the vast majority of techniques and instruments today are based on this objective. Therefore, this chapter will focus on the principles of preparation of coronal and radicular canal spaces; it breaks this down into two distinct steps: first, preparation of the coronal access cavity and second, radicular canal shaping.

Coronal Access Cavity Preparation

The objective of the coronal access preparation is to provide a smooth free-flowing tapered channel from the orifice to the apex that allows instruments, irrigants, and medicaments to attempt cleaning and shaping of the entire length and circumference of the canal, with as minimal a loss of structural integrity to the tooth as possible. The access preparation generally refers to that part of the cavity from the occlusal table to the canal orifice. However, its design is dependent on the position and curvature of the entire length of the canal, not just the position of the orifice, and is therefore not a simple cavity.

In this first section on coronal access cavity preparation, the section on principles is intended for all teeth in general. The following sections will deal with the individual nuances in access preparation for each tooth.

General Principles

"DO NO HARM"

No practitioner performs treatment with the intent to harm and yet substandard quality does occur. The problem seems to stem partially from a lack of awareness and knowledge. In addition, the daily stresses within the practice environment compound this issue, and the stage is set for inadvertently causing harm or damage to the tooth and ultimately the patient. To minimize the frequency of harm clinicians may cause, learning and awareness should be lifelong objectives. A "mindful practice" is the objective that continuously monitors and reevaluates results and techniques over time with introspection.

CONFIRMATION OF ETIOLOGY OF PULPAL PATHOSIS

Part of the objective of the access preparation is to confirm the etiology of pulpal breakdown assessed during diagnosis. The only proven etiological factors are bacterial contamination (via caries, coronal leakage under restorations, fractures) and trauma (e.g., resorption, thermal, mechanical, and physical). As the pulp chamber is entered, the clinician must visually inspect the state of its contents to check that it matches with the preoperative diagnosis. It is disconcerting to expose the vital tissue when a preoperative diagnosis of necrosis has been made. Also the etiology of the pulpal breakdown has to be discerned. At times, it is easy to confirm the etiology, for example, the presence of a carious lesion, but in the absence of obvious clinical evidence, the practitioner must make a conscious effort to search for the cause. Clinically, presentation of microleakage and cracks is extremely subtle and difficult to detect. Staining, high-power magnification under a microscope, transillumination may all help discover these sources.

ASSESSMENT OF RESTORABILITY

Although it is tempting to develop an "endodontics mode" mindset, once root canal treatment has been diagnosed, another major objective is to check the restorability of the tooth prior to root canal treatment. Existing restorations, caries, and unsupported enamel and dentin should be removed and the remaining tooth structure examined under a microscope. The operator should search for the presence of cracks, height, and thickness of the remaining dentinal walls for ferrule effect, the relationship of the remaining coronal tooth margins relative to the osseous crest, root length, location of the furcation, amount and quality of attached gingiva, and position of the tooth in the arch. This can result in several advantages:[4]

- Before root canal treatment is started, the patient can be forewarned of risks, benefits, and alternatives of any further procedures and/or costs to restore the tooth completed, for example, crown lengthening, gingivectomy, extrusion, or placement of orthodontic bands.
- A more educated opinion on long-term prognosis can be provided by the clinician to enable the patient to choose whether root canal treatment or implant therapy is more beneficial.
- Leakage of bacteria back into the root canal space under a preexisting defective restoration can be prevented.
- Cracks on the remaining tooth structure can be more readily assessed. This may change the clinician's decision to extract versus restore, to place build up immediately, to perform cuspal reduction or warn the patient more emphatically of the chance of fracture postoperatively.

However, in certain situations it can be argued that a portion of the restoration should be left in place until the root canal treatment is almost complete. This provides a circumferential matrix to enable a seal by the rubber dam or help hold the clamp in place (as long as no leakage can be seen under higher magnification).

A more difficult situation arises when an existing crown is present on the tooth that requires endodontic treatment. Accessing through a crown has several distinct disadvantages: the amount of remaining tooth structure, the quality of the build-up restoration, the extent of any decay, and the quality of the crown seal cannot be thoroughly assessed. In fact, Abbott[4] found that there was less than 60% chance to detect caries, fractures, and marginal breakdown, without complete removal of restorations. All of these factors have a profound effect on the long-term success of the root canal treatment, and longevity of the tooth. However, it is impractical to suggest removing all crowns prior to root canal treatment, and therefore a careful assessment of the integrity of the crown must be attempted through history-taking and clinical examination before and during treatment.

STRAIGHT-LINE ACCESS

It is well documented that to prepare the apical third of the canal circumferentially, a straight path for the cutting instrument from the orifice to the apex is imperative.[5,6] As the curvature of the canal increases, a file that enters into the canal is deflected at its tip by the force exerted by the dentin. However, according to Newton's Law, the file tip exerts back an equal and opposite reaction upon the dentin, that is, force on the outer dentinal surface of the canal as the file attempts to straighten back to its original dimension. If the dentin exerts a greater force than the file, the file bends, but this changes as the file size increases. Eventually, the file will cut the dentin rather than bend. At this point, the outer dentinal wall of the curvature is cut preferentially, known as gouging, which is the start of ledging and transportation. This effect is accentuated with cutting-tip files compared with noncutting tips and with a vertical filing motion versus rotational motion.

A concomitant problem develops as the file tip exerts a force back on the dentin. A fulcrum point develops, which is the most protuberant point of contact on the furcal dentinal surface. Therefore, preferential cutting occurs on the furcal surface also, the site of a most common procedural error, known as stripping that can lead to perforation.

The term "straight-line access" (SLA) describes a preparation that provides a straight or outwardly flared, unimpeded path from the occlusal surface to the apex. This allows the file to reach the apex with minimal deflection (Figure 1). The main corollary is that it has to be accomplished without compromising the furcal surface of the canal that could ultimately lead to strip perforation. Access is continually

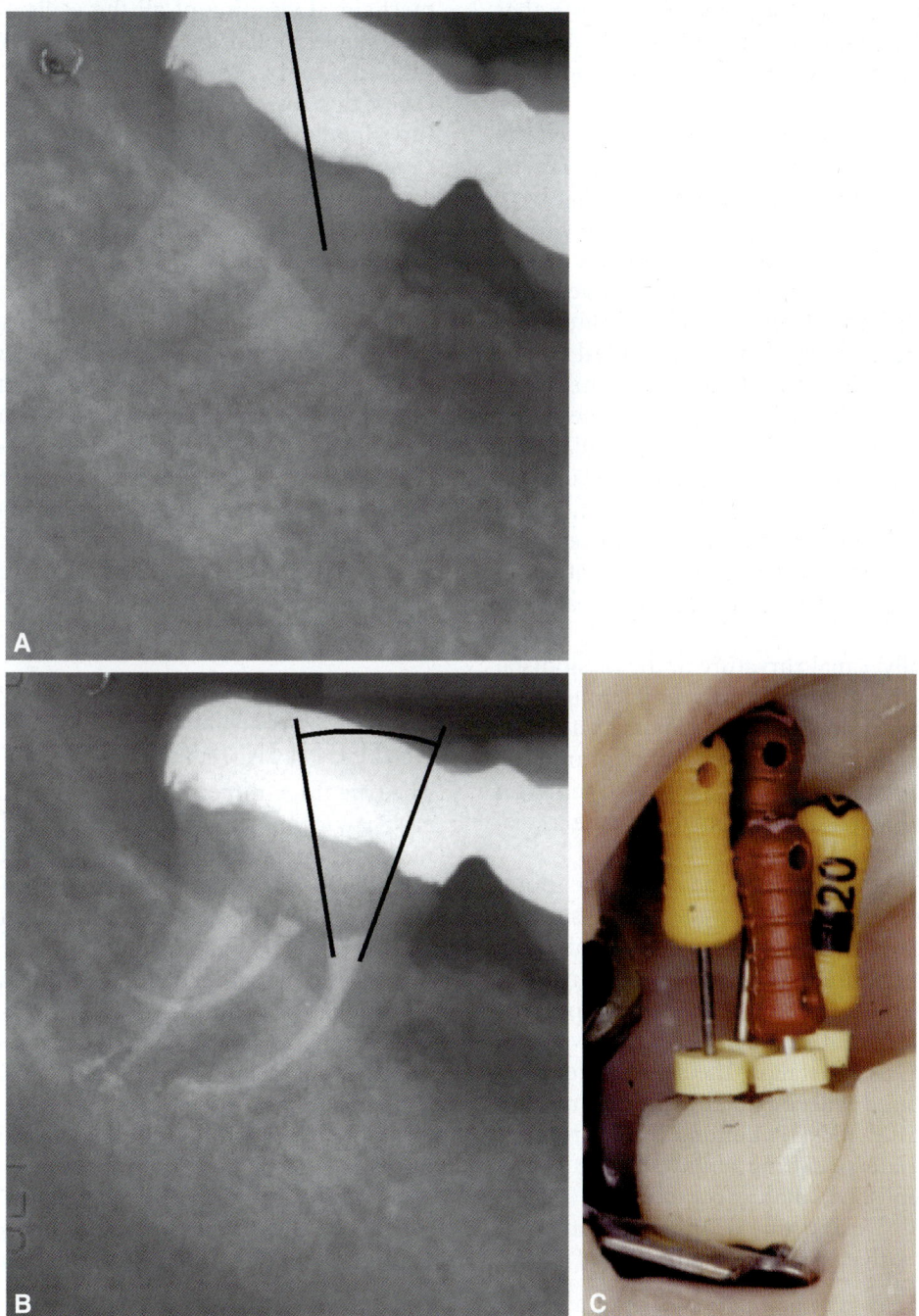

Figure 1 Straight line access in a mandibular third molar **A,** The orifice opening and path of insertion preoperatively is indicated by a black line. The mesial wall had to be cut to obtain a straight-line access **B,** The handles of the files are standing upright without crossing over each other indicating adequate Straight-line access **C,** However, often the distal canals are angled such that the file handles project out of the orifice mesially while still maintaining SLA.

adjusted until the selected master apical file (MAF) reaches the working length (WL) without undue stress upon it. A more aggressive SLA is required as the size of the file used and/or the degree of canal curvature increases. In this context, "aggressive" suggests that the orifice wall leading to the canal has to be moved and flared more obtusely toward the corresponding line angle.

The diameter of the apical preparation also effects the access preparation. To prepare a larger apical diameter, correspondingly larger, stiffer files that have a stronger tendency to straighten the canal have to be taken to the apex. In order to avoid stripping on the furcal surface or transporting the apex, one must achieve SLA beforehand. Unfortunately, the literature does not provide a consensus on the ideal apical diameter. However, in vitro studies have measured canal diameters.[7,8] Other studies[9–12] have measured canal cleanliness after a small versus larger diameter apical preparation and have shown better cleanliness with the larger diameters. One study, however, found that improvement gained with larger diameters was not statistically significant and concluded that small apical diameters were sufficient for adequate bacterial reduction.[13]

Radiographically, canal curvature in the mesiodistal plane can be directly observed; however, Cunningham and Senia[14] demonstrated that canals possess a three-dimensional curvature. Therefore to obtain an SLA, sometimes tooth structure must be removed more on the buccal or the lingual surface than just on the mesial or the distal surface.

SLA involves the selective removal of the outer canal tooth structure to protect the furcal surface. Various methods have been advocated for this. The so-called "anticurvature" filing (see below) involves cutting only on the outward stroke away from the furcal surface but is not effective beyond curvatures. Gates Glidden (GG) burs allow the selective removal of dentin when used with a laterally directed motion and similarly stiffer nickel–titanium (NiTi) rotaries have significant lateral cutting ability (Paque F and Peters OA, unpublished data).

Peters et al.,[15,16] using microcomputed tomography, have shown that significant portions of canals are not touched during instrumentation due to the irregularities and curvature of the canals. This reiterates the importance of achieving SLA.

Mannan et al.[5] tested whether SLA would allow mechanical cleaning of all the walls of the root canal in a single-rooted anterior tooth with a simple root canal anatomy. They prepared three types of access cavity designs: a "lingual cingulum" just coronal to the cingulum, a "lingual conventional" where the cavity was extended to within 2 mm of the incisal edge, and an access cavity involving the "incisal edge" but not the labial surface. They found that none of the cavity designs allowed complete planing of the root canal walls although the incisal edge design allowed a greater proportion of the root canal walls to be filed than the other two. This study, however, determined the MAF size as three sizes larger than the first file to bind, which had already been shown by other researchers to be an ineffective technique to properly clean the apical canal third.[8] Another possible deficiency was that they did not extend the access cavities onto the labial surface, which is often necessary for true SLA as shown earlier.[17,18] However, the study did emphasize that SLA provides the best chance of débridement of the entire canal.

THREE-DIMENSIONAL POSITION OF TEETH IN JAWS

The true three-dimensional position that teeth hold in each jaw cannot be assessed accurately by clinical or radiographic perspectives. Therefore, using the occlusal table of the tooth as a guide to the location of the chamber can be quite misleading. Figure 2 shows the lingual and mesial inclination of the mandibular molars, the mesial inclination of the maxillary molars, and the labial inclination of all the incisors.[19] Correspondingly, when accessing, the bur must be angled to mimic these inclinations in both mesiodistal and buccolingual planes. However, other factors that limit the ideal angulation come into consideration. A compromise is reached, for example, trying to avoid encroaching on the incisal edge when accessing anterior teeth, or trying to avoid breaking through a marginal ridge. Improper angulation results in the

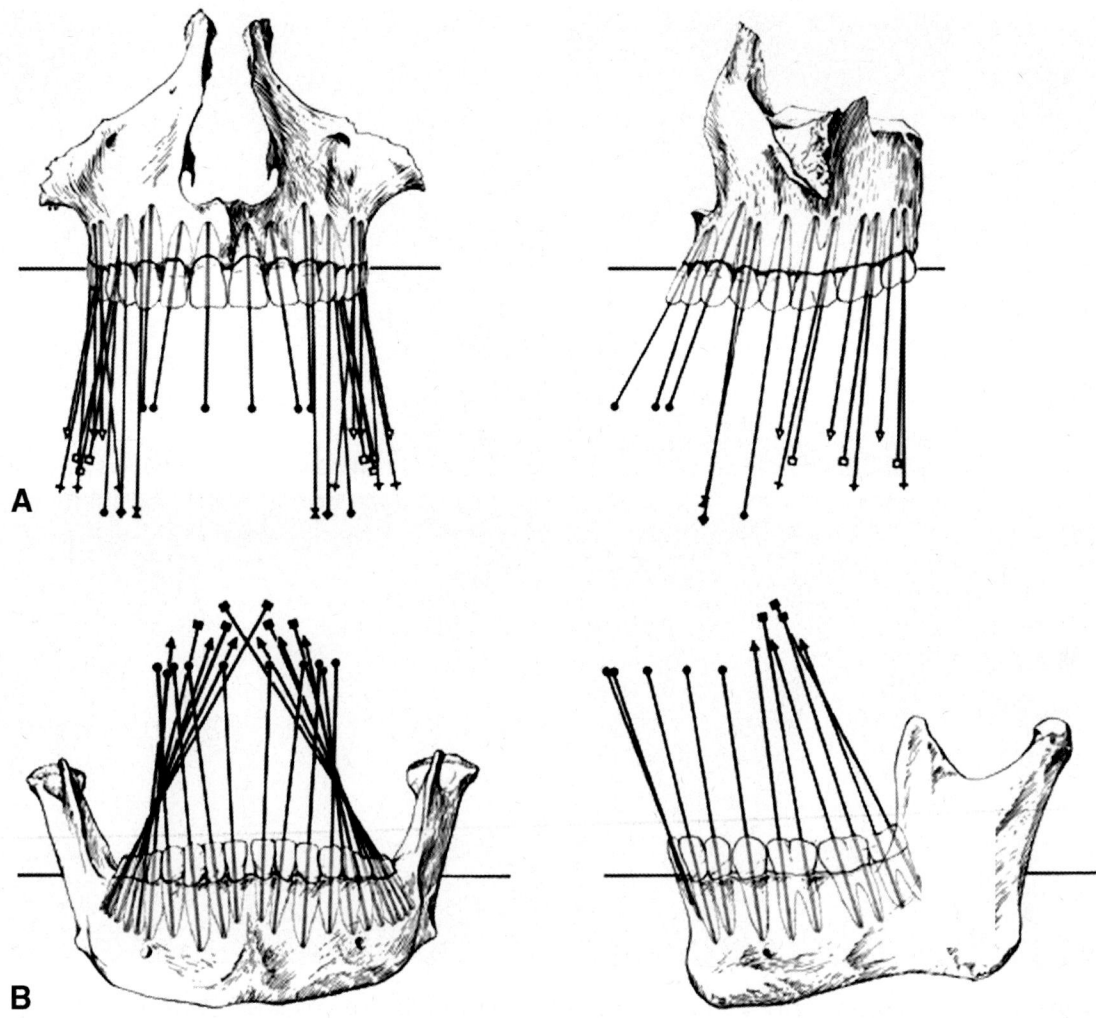

Figure 2 Schematic views of the three-dimensional positions of teeth in jaws in frontal and saggital views with long axes of the teeth displayed. It is prudent during access to mimic these angulations to avoid unnecessary gouging. Root types are indicated by symbols on arrows. ***A,*** Maxilla. Note the mesial and buccal angulation of the molars and proclination of the anteriors. ***B,*** Mandible. Note the mesial and lingual angulation of the molars and proclination of the anteriors. Adapted 2007 with permission from Dempster et al., J Am Dent Assoc 67:779, 1963, Copyright © American Dental Association.[19]

common occurrence of unnecessary gouging of the dentinal walls that weakens the remaining tooth structure and in extreme cases leads to external perforation (Figure 3).

Part of the reason that these angulations are hard to transfer to the clinical setting is that the operator usually sits in the 10, 11, or 12 O'clock position with the patient reclined. This can be disorienting. The tooth is not viewed from the perspective shown in the figure, and is not in line with any external horizontal or vertical plane landmarks.

The operator has to physically move to view the angle of the bur relative to the patient's vertical and horizontal planes. This is similar to taking a radiograph by the paralleling technique.

EXTERNAL ROOT SURFACE AS A GUIDE

External root anatomy is determined by the internal pulp. The mesenchymal pulp tissue gives rise to odontoblasts that in turn lay down the dentin. As

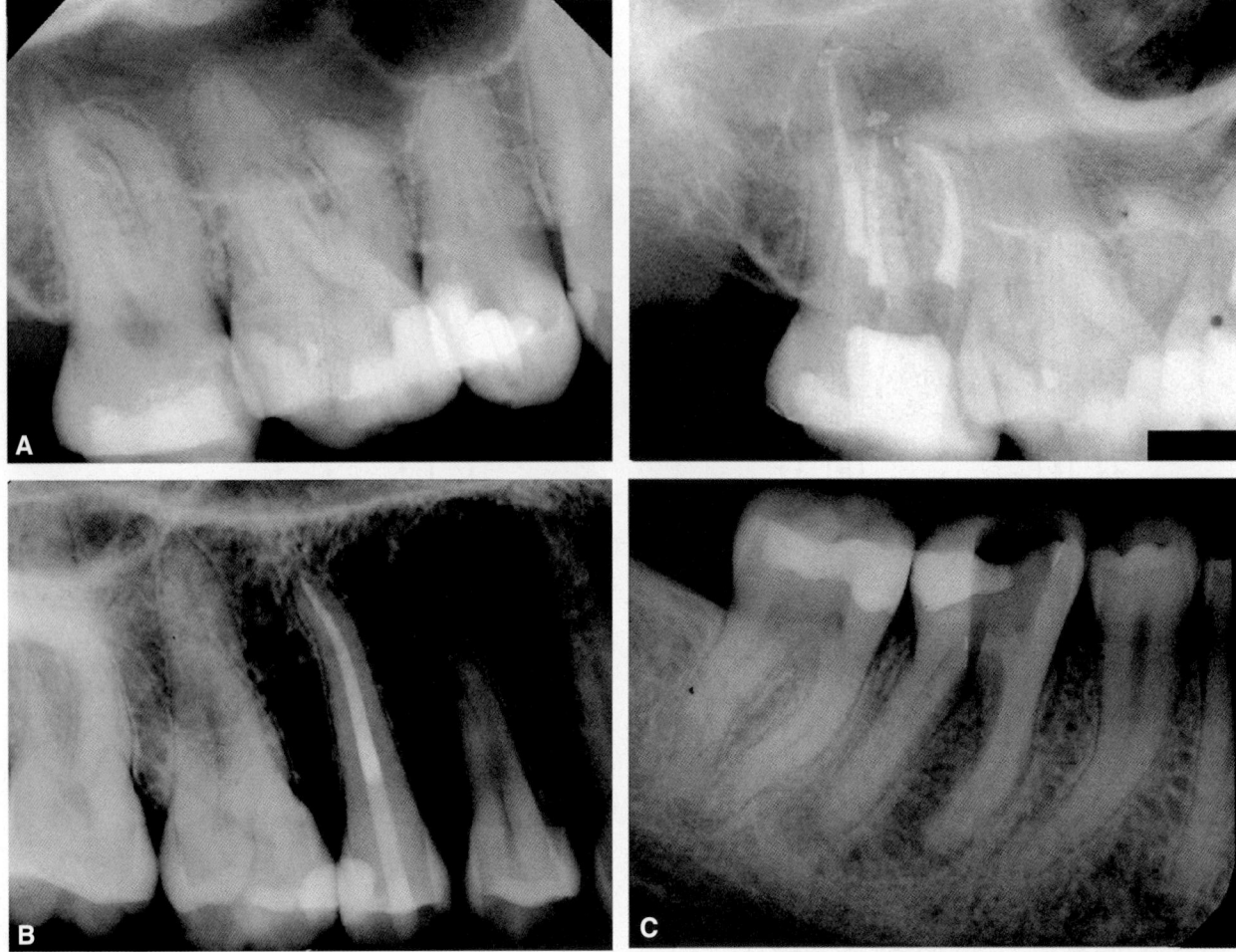

Figure 3 Examples of unnecessary gouging of axial or furcation dentin due to improper angulation of the bur during access preparation. **A,** Preoperative and postoperative radiographs showing gouging of furcal dentin in the entrance to the mesiobuccal canals due to underextension of the mesial wall during initial instrumentation. **B,** Proper angulation was maintained allowing minimal tooth structure loss. **C,** Vertical instead of distal angulation while searching for distal canals.

the long axis of the tooth cannot be seen in the clinical setting, the next best guide is the external root surface. Acosta and Trugeda[20] sequentially reduced the clinical crowns of 134 extracted maxillary molars and examined the pulp chamber at the level of the pulpal floor. They found the pulp chamber in the center of the tooth, closely matching its outer contour and maintaining the same distance from the mesial, distal, buccal, and lingual surfaces. This finding was confirmed more recently using mathematical models based on microtomography data.[21] It was noted that the shape of the pulp chamber was trapezoidal, and it was therefore recommended shaping the access preparation in the same way.[20]

In another study,[22] 500 teeth were used of which 400 were sectioned at the cementoenamel junction (CEJ), 50 buccolingually, and 50 mesiodistally. The

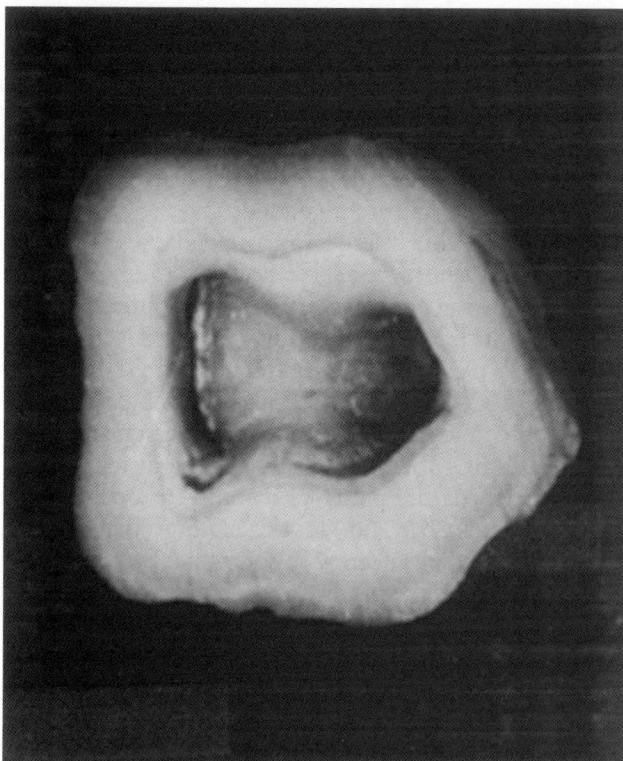

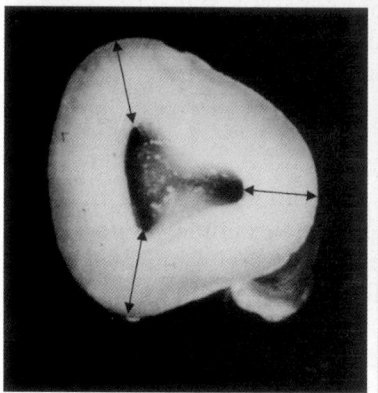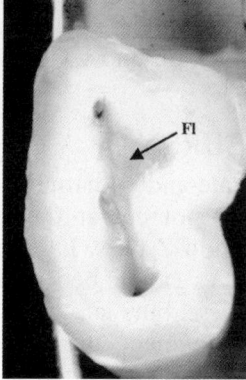

Figure 4 The pulp chamber is usually centered at the cementoenamel junction (CEJ) level allowing the use of external root surfaces as a guide for access. The distance from the pulp chamber to the outer contour indicated by arrows. Fl, floor of the pulp chamber. Reprinted with permission from Krasner P and Rankow HJ.[22]

patterns in orifice location, size, color, shape, and several conclusions were noted (Figure 4):

Law of Centrality: The floor of the pulp chamber is always located in the center of the tooth at the level of the CEJ.

Law of Concentricity: The walls of the pulp chamber are always concentric to the external surface of the tooth at the level of the CEJ, that is, the external root surface anatomy reflects the internal pulp chamber anatomy.

Law of the CEJ: The distance from the external surface of the clinical crown to the wall of the pulp chamber is the same throughout the circumference of the tooth at the level of the CEJ—the CEJ is the most consistent repeatable landmark for locating the position of the pulp chamber.

Law of Symmetry 1: Except for the maxillary molars, the orifices of the canals are equidistant from a line drawn in a mesial–distal direction, through the pulp chamber floor.

Law of Symmetry 2: Except for the maxillary molars, the orifices of the canals lie on a line perpendicular to a line drawn in a mesial–distal direction across the center of the floor of the pulp chamber.

Law of Color Change: The color of the pulp chamber floor is always darker than the walls.

Law of Orifice Location 1: The orifices of the root canals are always located at the junction of the walls and the floor.

Law of Orifice Location 2: The orifices of the root canals are located at the angles in the floor–wall junction.

Law of Orifice Location 3: The orifices of the root canals are located at the terminus of the root developmental fusion lines.

As the external root surface is a reliable guide, it can be quite frustrating to place the rubber dam, which completely obscures it. Therefore, in difficult cases, it is prudent to prepare the initial access shape and find the pulp chamber or at least one orifice prior to rubber dam placement. Alternatively, multiple teeth can be isolated by clamping one tooth more posterior so that the CEJ and the relationship of adjacent teeth are visible and palpable on the treated tooth. The Silker-Glickman clamp (Silk Pages Publishing, Deerwood, MN) was designed for this purpose. Otherwise, a single tooth clamp may be used and the dam flossed between the mesial contacts.

KNOWLEDGE OF PERCENTAGES FOR THE NUMBER OF CANALS WITHIN A ROOT

It has been known that roots contain multiple complex canal systems since at least 1925 as described by Hess and Zurcher.[23] Since then, research has focused on determining their classification and incidence. Data for canal numbers and configurations extracted from selected references are presented in Chapter 6, "Morphology of teeth and their root canal systems". Some factors that affect such data have been noted, for example, methods and materials, type of magnification, in vivo, ex vivo, but many factors have not been noted, for example, case report articles, ethnic groups, age groups, individual interpretation of classification systems by the various researchers.

From the material presented in Chapter 6, "Morphology of teeth and their root canal systems", it can be extrapolated that studies report the incidence of multiple canals from 0% to as high as 95% for certain roots. Therefore the clinician must, to increase chances of finding them, have a thorough knowledge of the number, incidence, location, and the variability of the canal systems of each tooth and root, in order to design the access cavity. Selective removal of otherwise solid tooth structure can be justified only when the operator is confident of the knowledge that further canal systems may exist more apically and that the subsequent weakening of the tooth is offset by the significant advantage to long-term prognosis in finding another canal system.

MINDSET

Knowing that roots can have multiple complex canal systems, how zealous should the clinician be in looking for them? Obviously, the downside in removing the tooth structure to look for canals without success is the decrease in structural integrity and reduced long-term prognosis. Also, clinicians are trained to conserve as much tooth structure as possible. A tooth should be entered under the assumption that every root has multiple canals. This assumption can be proved wrong only after adequate searching, defined by objective criteria, for example, troughing through the lighter-colored dentin of the walls compared to the darker dentin of the pulpal floor or drilling approximately 5 to 7 mm below the furcal floor. Clinicians can then regularly self-assess, by comparison to the actual figures presented in the various studies and by discussion with peers. There is a balance between selectively extending the access cavity to search for canals and unnecessary overextension—the art is in determining this line.

MAGNIFICATION/MICROSCOPE

Little controversy remains over the effectiveness of the dental operating microscope. Several studies have shown that it increases the dentist's ability to find canals, allows precise repair of perforations, aids in removing separated files, and improves surgical visibility (see Chapter 26F, Visual Enhancement for more details).

Clinical Armamentarium

Access preparation requires few standard hand instruments, but a wide range of equipment for differing situations. The basic requirements are a mirror, a DG16-type endodontic explorer (e.g., HuFriedy, Chicago, IL), high- and slow-speed handpieces, a range of burs, and a microscope. A standard set of burs (Figure 5) should include at least a #2 round diamond, a #1 round carbide, a transmetal bur (Dentsply Maillefer, Ballaigues, Switzerland), various cylindrical diamonds (e.g., 859–010, 859–012, 859–014, BrasselerUSA, Savannah, GA), and an EndoZ bur (Dentsply Maillefer).

The following are accessory items for differing situations or routine use depending on the practitioner's preference. Bendable and differently sized heads of mirrors (eie2, San Diego, CA) allow improved maneuverability and visibility but can be particularly helpful in cases of difficult access due to the distal location of the tooth or the patient's inability to open widely (see Figure 5). An endodontic explorer that is finer than the regular DG16 is also available, the Micro JW17 endodontic explorer (CK Dental, Orange, CA).

Some clinicians find the Micro-Openers and Micro-Debriders (Dentsply Maillefer) helpful. The former have 7 mm of K-type flutes in 0.04 and 0.06 tapers in ISO sizes #10 and #15, and the latter have 16 mm of Hedström-type cutting flutes in sizes #20 and #30. Both are mounted as a handheld instrument at a double angle and can be useful for initial orifice location and widening.

BURS

Safe-ended diamonds and tungsten carbide burs that do not cut at their tip, for example, Endo Access, Endo Z burs, LA Axxess burs (SybronEndo, Orange, CA), can be beneficial in avoiding gouging. However, these burs are wide and should be used for final refinement after precise extension has already been determined with thinner cylindrical diamonds. The Mueller bur (BrasselerUSA) is a latch-grip surgical length round carbide bur available in sizes 0.9, 1.0, 1.2, 1.4, 1.6, and 1.8 mm diameters. Similarly, Munce Discovery burs (CJM Engineering, Santa Barbara, CA) are 34-mm-long, narrow-shafted, nonflexible round carbide burs available in sizes 1/4 (0.5 mm diameter), 1/2 (0.6 mm), 1 (0.8 mm), 2 (1.0 mm), 3 (1.2 mm), and 4 (1.4 mm). The extended length of both these burs reduces the head of the handpiece blocking the operator's view. The Munce burs are not as flexible as the Mueller burs due to a slightly greater shaft diameter and are available in smaller sizes. Both these burs are useful for deep troughing to find canals, opening isthmuses, or reaching separated instruments and seem to leave an easier-to-read dentin surface than ultrasonics (see Figure 5).

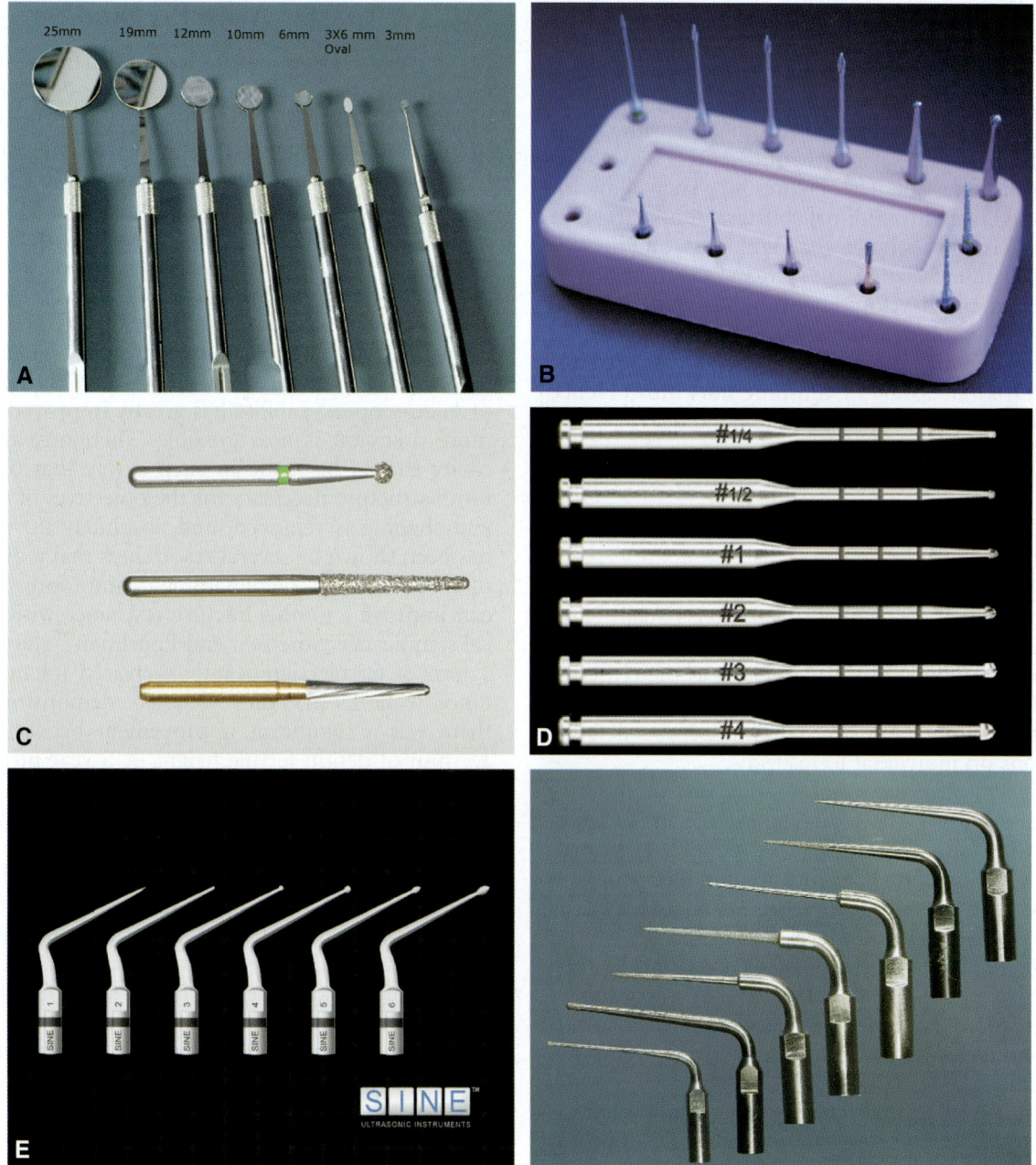

Figure 5 Examples of armamentarium for access and inspection of pulp chambers. *A,* Mirrors with variable head sizes and bendable shafts. *B,* Bur block used in the practice of one of the authors (R.K.). *C,* Additional typical burs used for access: #2 round diamond, tapered diamond, EndoZ bur. *D,* Munce Discovery burs. *E,* Various ultrasonic tips. Images courtesy of Dr. Gary Carr, Dr. Cliff Ruddle and C.J.M. Engineering, Solvang, CA, USA.

ROTARY INSTRUMENTS

For gaining SLA in the coronal portion of the canals, rotary instruments that selectively cut laterally are useful to minimize excess removal of the furcal dentin. GG drills (sizes 1 (ISO #50), 2 (#70), 3 (#90), 4 (#110), 5 (#130), and 6 (#150)) have been used for many years and are efficient and relatively inexpensive. Some of the stiffer NiTi rotaries also have lateral cutting ability.

ACCESSORY INSTRUMENTS

The Stropko Irrigator (Vista Dental Products, Racine, WI) is an adapter that connects to the air/water syringe and accepts standard Luer-lock needle tips for pinpoint irrigation or aeration. It regulates air or water flow to between 2 and 7 psi and provides a very precise delivery. It aids visibility at high-power magnification under a microscope.

Ultrasonically powered instruments with well-adapted tips from various manufacturers have now become indispensable (see Figure 5E). They allow for deep troughing with minimal collateral tooth structure removal. Visibility is better than with burs, and the tips can be diamond-coated to increase their efficiency. However, all tips develop significant heat and can cause necrosis of the surrounding bone if used without a coolant. Some practitioners finish their access preparations with sandblasting or finishing burs; this practice may have an impact on composite bonding.[24]

Clinical Guidelines

PREOPERATIVE CLINICAL GUIDELINES

Determination of the point of penetration: Usually entry is in the center of the occlusal table but in certain teeth (e.g., maxillary molars) it is deceiving, as the center of the occlusal table does not reflect the center of the pulp chamber. Anatomy and strategies for access is detailed in sections on individual teeth below.

Assessment of occlusal and external root form: Once the point of entry has been determined, the bur's angulation in three dimensions has to be mentally envisaged. This is determined by taking into account the angulation of the teeth in the jaws (see Figure 2) and assessing the external root surface at the level of the CEJ.

Radiographic measurement of the depth of the pulp chamber roof from the occlusal table: The initial bur in the high-speed handpiece is placed against a radiograph or a measurement determined from a calibrated digital image.

Assessment of complicating factors: Rotations/tipping of tooth, calcifications (stones, deep restorations, buccal/lingual restorations (mid-root calcification), root length, width, curvature) affect the angle of entry and the degree of extension of the access cavity in the horizontal and vertical dimensions.

Radiographic assessment: Angled views should be taken in an attempt to visualize the breadth of the roots and the centeredness of the canal within it. One also has to assess the angle at which the canal leaves the pulp chamber—the root may not seem curved but if there is a sharp angle between the chamber and the canal, SLA will require a significant reduction of the orifice walls. To aid in orientation, the access preparation can be started without rubber dam until the pulp chamber is located.

Access Cavity Preparation

Access cavity design has undergone changes throughout the years. Originally, it was thought that the cavities should be round in anterior teeth, oval in premolars, and triangular in molars. This gave way to triangular cavity shapes in anterior teeth and quadrilateral shapes in molars.[25]

It was considered acceptable to state "make access cavities large." Also, "make them like an inlay preparation," where circumferentially around the access cavity, every point coronal from the pulpal floor is wider. However, these protocols resulted in excessive, unnecessary tooth structure removal. With the advent of microscopes, visibility has greatly improved and far more precision is now possible. Therefore, an access cavity should be made in such a way that only that tooth structure necessary for the objectives of cleaning and shaping is removed, and absolutely no more. It has been shown by several researchers that a difference of 0.5 to 1 mm of the remaining dentin tooth structure can improve a tooth's fracture resistance with statistical significance. Sorensen and Engelman[26] showed that 1 mm of ferrule significantly increased fracture resistance, while Libman and Nicholls[27] demonstrated that there was a significant improvement between 1 and 1.5 mm of dentin ferrule height. A 5-year prospective clinical study[28] showed that the remaining dentin thickness and height affected survivability but found no difference in survivability among cast post and core, prefabricated post and core, and composite-only cores. Tan et al.[29] showed a significant difference between a uniform, circumferential 2-mm ferrule and a nonuniform ferrule with only 0.5 mm proximal but 2 mm buccal and lingual dentin height (see Chapter 40, Restoration of Endodontically treated Teeth).

It must be remembered that just having remaining outer tooth structure around the access preparation is not sufficient; the long-term prognosis is more accurately assessed after both access preparation and crown preparation are completed. A developing concern is that full porcelain crowns require more dentin removal to allow adequate strength to the crowns and are becoming more popular due to their improved esthetics. Therefore, the practitioner should not base the access cavity design on the ease of visibility, but only on removing what is absolutely necessary and no more. The common retort is that restricting the access cavity will jeopardize the success of the root canal treatment, as visibility will be impaired. However, it will be shown that all the objectives necessary for cleaning and shaping can be adequately met, without restriction of visibility or instrument access, as unnecessary tooth structure removal is avoided. If the access cavity has to be extended to facilitate visibility, it should be done with precision.

An access cavity should be considered specific and individual for each tooth and for each patient, as is a class II restorative cavity or crown preparation. The access cavity will vary according to the degree of curvature within the canal (i.e., the angle at which the canal leaves the pulp chamber may be very different from the root curvature), the position of the canal apex relative to its cusp tip, canal length, degree of calcification, size, shape, and position of the tooth in the jaw. It is suggested that only the initial entry point on the occlusal table should be based on a standardized protocol but once the pulp chamber has been found, the cavity should be "tailor-made."

The sequence of steps for access preparation will be discussed here and can also be followed in Figure 6. The *first objective* is to penetrate through the occlusal surface. Penetrating enamel or precious metal is predictable using a high-speed handpiece with a tungsten carbide bur. Porcelain and nonprecious metals, however, present more difficulties, in particular with chipping when a steel round bur is used. Diamond burs easily penetrate porcelain but are generally much less efficient with metal. Stokes and Tidmarsh[30] evaluated the cutting efficiency of diamond and tungsten carbide burs through metal crowns. They tested coarse grit round and dome-ended cylinder diamonds and six-bladed tungsten carbide cross-cut fissure or round burs. They found that for precious alloys, tungsten carbide burs were significantly quicker. For the

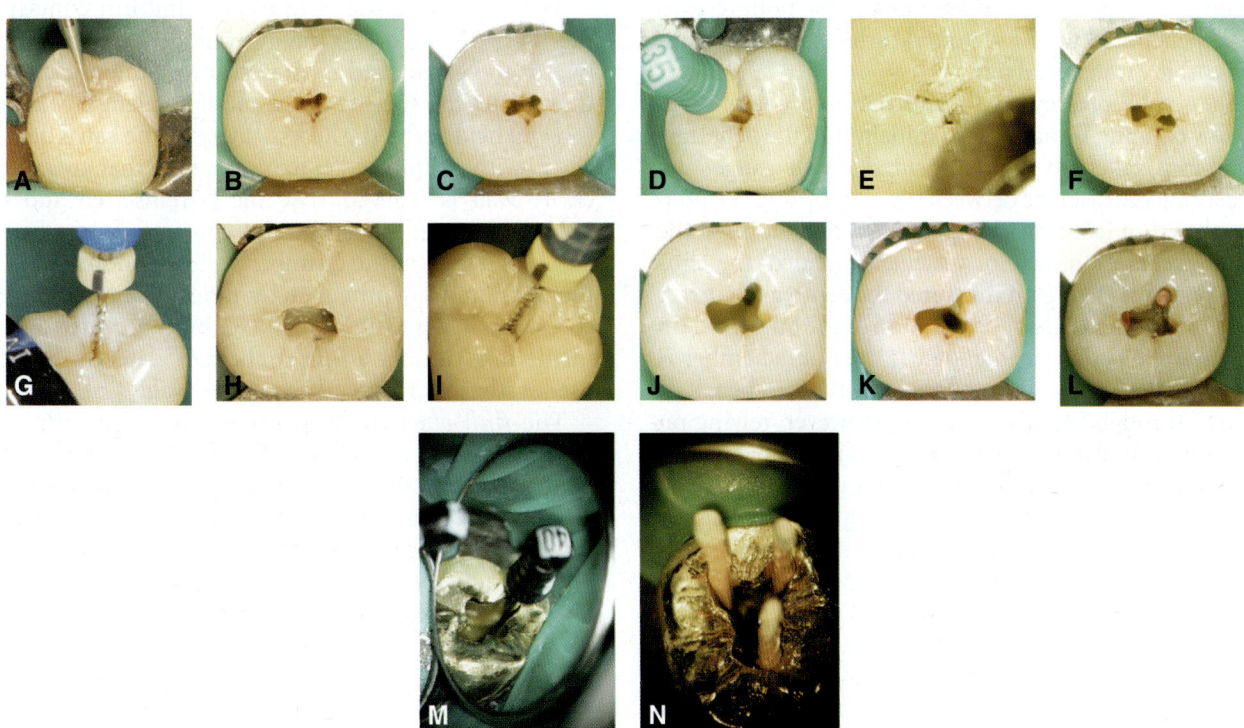

Figure 6 Sequential steps in endodontic access preparation on an extracted lower molar. Initial entry **A,** with bur is angled toward buccal and distal; narrow entry is sufficient to find the pulp chamber **B,** A K-file size #10 or #15 is then used to find the position of orifices to determine points of extension **C,** Further extension based on the position of orifices **D,** and a file is now placed into the coronal portion of the canal to determine the location of the restrictive dentin. The restriction can be seen under the microscope at the orifice level, and further extension of the occlusal surface is not warranted at this time. The buccal surface is undercut to remove the pulp chamber roof minimizing the removal of occlusal dentin/enamel **E,** Similar extension is done for lingual, mesial, and distal surfaces **F,** Large pulp stones are removed by sectioning, not widening the cavity **G,** Once the restrictive dentin at the orifice is removed, a file starts to contact the entire wall. Now only that slice of dentin contacted by the file from the occlusal surface to the orifice level is cut with a flared-out angle with a narrow tapered diamond bur **H,** so that a slot-shaped preparation starts to develop **I,** This is repeatedly extended after checking each time for location of dentinal contact with a file **J,** Completed access preparation shows straight-line access (SLA) into the mesiobuccal **K,** and mesiolingual canal **L,** after root canal filling. The fin between the mesiobuccal and mesiolingual canals can be identified under the microscope as blind-ended. In case of less than ideal visibility, the mesial wall would have to be straightened and flared for deeper access and visibility. **M,** A clinical example of a file placed at working length (WL) without undue strain from the outer wall and precisely in its slot. A similar clinical example shows gutta-percha cones prior to taking master cone radiograph **N.**

precious alloys, though no difference initially, after five cavity preparations, only the dome-ended cylinder diamond cuts significantly faster than other bur types. They found the diamond burs to be smoother with less "chatter" during cutting than the tungsten carbide burs. They concluded that cutting efficiency appears to relate not only to grit size but to bur shape as well. Teplitsky and Sutherland[31] showed that of the 56 porcelain crowns, none fractured after access preparation with diamond burs, whereas tungsten carbide burs dulled rapidly and were ineffective. Cohen and Wallace[32] showed that of the Dicor crowns cemented with zinc phosphate, porcelain chipped and the seal was lost after accessing. However, when a bondable cement was used (polycarboxylate), none of the crowns lost retention. When penetrating a porcelain-fused-to-metal crown, the porcelain should be removed with a dome-ended cylindrical or a #2 round diamond and the nonprecious metal penetrated with a #1 round carbide bur or a tungsten carbide transmetal bur.

The *second objective* is to find the pulp chamber. A narrow opening is maintained initially and the penetrating bur is taken to a premeasured depth gauged by measuring the distance between the cusp tip and the pulp chamber roof from the preoperative radiograph. As the access preparation has not yet been extended, the clinician relies on having premeasured the depth and correct judgment of the angle of penetration of the bur based on the parameters described above. If the pulp chamber is large and the angulation is correct, the bur can be felt to "drop" through into the chamber. However, relying on this feeling is dangerous for it is unpredictable. If the chamber is calcified or deep, the "drop" is often not discernable, and unnecessary gouging of the walls or floor or even perforation can occur, if the clinician is not exactly on target. Therefore, the bur should penetrate only to the premeasured distance, and if the chamber is not found, the access should be minimally extended into a narrow slot in the anticipated direction of the canals using the microscope with good illumination to look for signs of the chamber. Often a pulp horn may already be exposed or the cavity already overextended in certain spots. Extending the cavity without visualization usually results in unnecessary tooth structure loss, and therefore extreme care must be paid. When searching for the pulp chamber, tapered instruments should never be forced but be allowed to cut their own way with a light touch by the operator. When forced, they will act as a wedge. This may cause the enamel to "check" or "craze" and will materially weaken the tooth.

The *third objective* is to "unroof" the dentin that covers the pulp chamber. This is carefully done under the microscope with a thin needle diamond cylinder (e.g., #859–010, BrasselerUSA) so as to avoid unnecessary widening of the isthmus. The bur is angled to undercut the occlusal surface thereby maintaining as much tooth structure as possible. Ultrasonic tips can also be used very precisely to accomplish this. Round burs should be avoided during access preparation other than perhaps for initial penetration as they cause indiscriminate gouging of the walls. Safe-ended cutting burs can be used but their width is rather large for use at this time. In this step, the clinician depends mostly on the "feel" of the bur deep inside the tooth, against the roof and walls of the pulp chamber, to judge the extensions that are necessary.

The entire roof of the pulp chamber is removed. In this operation high-speed equipment should be operated with vision and is not generally employed in a blind area where reliance on tactile sensation is necessary.

The *fourth objective* is to obtain uniform contact of the file with the access cavity wall. A file is placed in one of the canals and is viewed under the microscope to evaluate the specific points along its length where it is being held up by the access cavity or the canal dentin. Then, with a thin needle diamond, only that area of the cavity wall is relieved. The file is reinserted and the process repeated until the file contacts dentin evenly along its length in the chamber without undue strain. If the restraining dentin is determined to be within the coronal portion of the canal, GG burs or other instruments that can cut a "relief channel" laterally may be used, rather than extend the entire wall.

The *fifth objective* is to obtain SLA. The clinician must assess the degree of taper to be imparted to the dentin access wall in the one line the file is uniformly contacting. A radiograph can be used to help assess. This single "slice" of dentin is then flared out to an obtuse angle relative to the pulp chamber floor, creating a slot-like extension. All other points of the walls are kept flared in or undercut or at as acute an angle as possible that allows complete visibility of the floor when viewed under a microscope. The floor and canals will not be visible in one view—the mirror has to be moved.

The diameter of the bur that cuts the slot extension should only be the maximum diameter of the largest file that is necessary at the canal orifice. A taper is not required for that part of the access preparation between the orifice and the occlusal table as compaction forces for obturation will not apply. The "010" suffix of cylinder and tapered diamond burs connotes the maximum cutting shaft diameter is 1 mm and of "012" is 1.2 mm, etc. It should be remembered that with natural hand movement, the diameter of the cut made by these burs would be still larger. Therefore, usually a #859–010 is large enough. The operator should also be aware of the maximum diameters of the files chosen, for example, GG4 (1.1 mm) and ProTaper (1.2 mm). A 35/0.06 Profile is 1.3 mm at D16, which will necessitate a larger access cavity than is usually required for cleaning and shaping. An orifice diameter can generally be maintained between 0.9 and 1.1 mm for adequate cleaning and shaping while minimizing the loss of root strength.

The canal access slot is continually moved to the outer surface to prevent cutting on the furcal surface during cleaning and shaping as the larger files that require more and more space are introduced.

The mesiodistal width of the access preparation can be kept as small as possible. It has been shown that the average dimensions between walls at the pulp chamber floor are 2.2 mm mesiodistally and 5.1 mm buccolingually.[20] Examples of basic access cavity preparations, before individual slot extensions for SLA, as well as plates covering common clinical errors, may be seen on the DVD accompanying this text.

Maxillary Central Incisors

ANATOMY AND MORPHOLOGY

The tip of the root and the incisal edge are on the midline from a proximal view (Figure 7).[33] It is very rare for these roots to have true second canals[34,35] but quite common to have lateral canals. The roots are straight and have the least incidence of dilacerations.[36] Kasahara et al.[37] used 510 extracted maxillary central incisors with no abnormalities and decalcified them in nitric acid for 48 hours. They suggested that over 60% showed accessory canals that were impossible to clean mechanically. Most lateral branches were small, 80% were size #10 reamer or less, and 3% were larger than a #40 reamer. Eighty percent of all apical foramina were located within 0.5 mm of the apex and 95% within 1 mm.

There are many case reports showing two canals (and one showing four canals) but usually the crowns and/or roots are unusually large, suggesting fusion, gemination, or presence of a dens-in-dente. However, case reports of maxillary centrals with two roots/canals and normal crowns have been reported.[38,39]

CLINICAL

Initial penetration should be approximately in the middle of the lingual surface of the tooth, just above the cingulum almost perpendicular to the lingual surface. After locating the canal, long tapered diamonds can be used to extend the access into a roughly triangular outline. However, this extension when carried out under the microscope can be made precisely to each tooth to only uncover the pulp chamber and horns and to provide continuous smooth walls down the chamber into the canal.

Even though it has been shown that a better SLA can be achieved through an incisal access cavity,[18] the lingual approach is used in order to maintain as much tooth structure on the labial surface as possible for esthetic reasons. The reciprocal compromise is that a lingual triangle is formed, which has to be removed to achieve SLA. In fact, LaTurno and Zillich[18] showed that only 10% of the 50 maxillary central canals examined projected solely onto the lingual surface with an SLA. Eighty-four percent of the configurations involved at least the incisal edge and 6% were solely on the buccal (Figure 8).

After initial penetration into the chamber, the access cavity has to be extended precisely in both the labiolingual and mesiodistal dimensions. In the labiolingual plane, there are two particular areas generally described as the lingual and labial triangles that have

890 / Endodontics

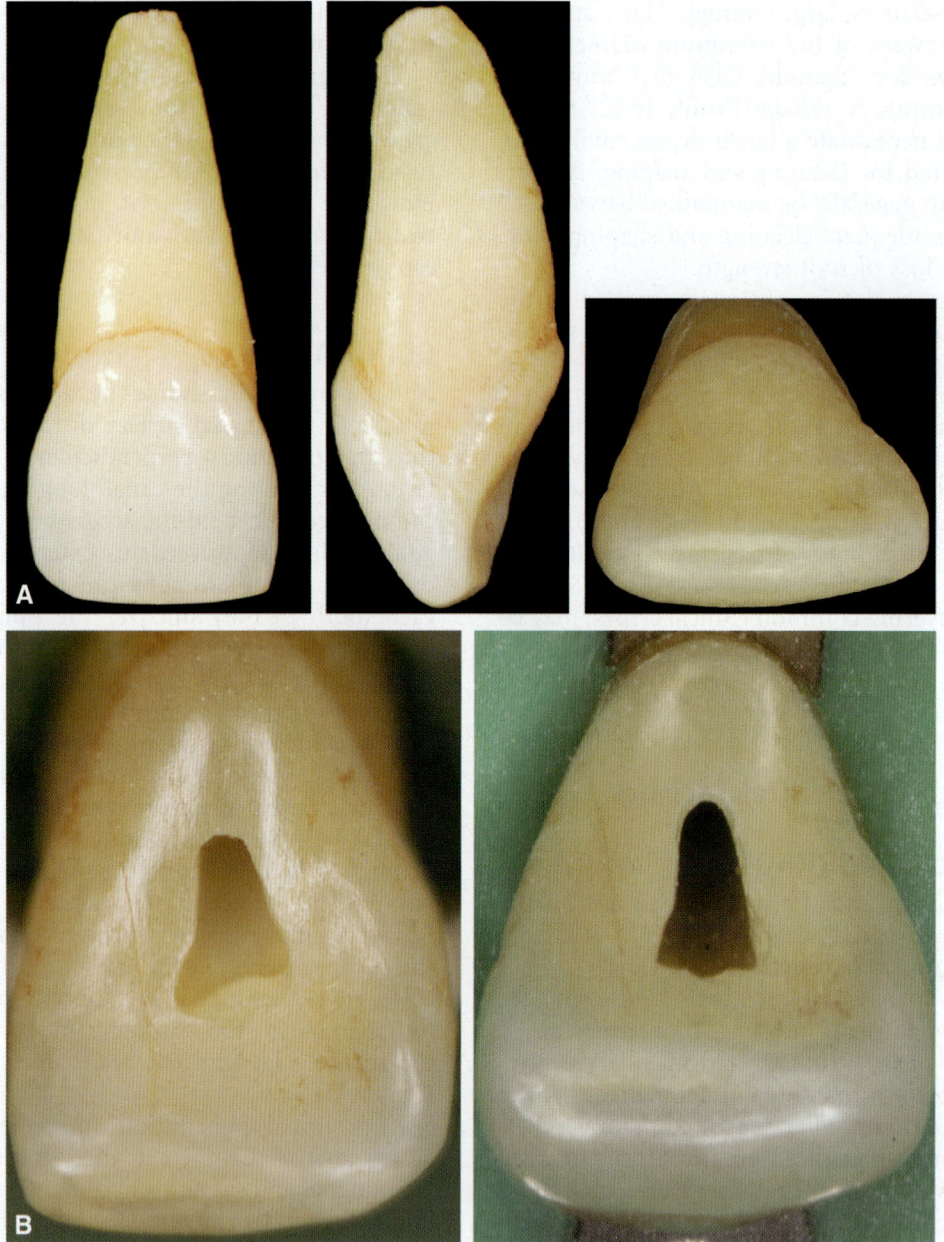

Figure 7 Example of a maxillary central incisor showing labial, mesial, and incisal views ***A,*** The access preparation can be assessed from a more incisal view and a lingual view ***B,*** The width of the preparation in the cingulum is 1.1 mm. Note also the extension of the mesial and distal incisal areas to open up the pulp horns.

to be removed to obtain an SLA. However, the labial triangle can often be a quadrilateral as shown in Figure 9.

With regard to mesiodistal extension, all access cavities should uncover the pulp horns, but special attention has to be paid to the maxillary incisors as the pulp horns are not in the direct line of vision of the access cavity. If even minute amounts of tissue remain in the pulp horns, they will subsequently discolor the remaining tooth structure over time. Complete extensions can be accomplished by feeling the extension of the pulp horns under each mesial and distal angle with a cowhorn explorer (HuFriedy). Fine extensions that require opening with a half-round

Due to the lingual approach, the points of restriction on the files are against the coronal portion of the lingual wall and the most incisal portion of the labial wall. Khademi[40] suggests notching the midpoint on the labial preemptively to accommodate the larger files more easily.

There is a debate as to how far the incisal extension should be taken. As we know that most anterior teeth have a better SLA from the buccal or the incisal surface, the operator has to assess on a case-by-case basis and sometimes the extension will be more aggressive than others.

Maxillary Lateral Incisors

ANATOMY AND MORPHOLOGY

These teeth have a function very similar to centrals and are therefore similar except for a smaller scale in all dimensions except root length. They have more rounded incisal angles and the root typically curves to the distal although some can be straight or curving to the mesial. There is often a deep developmental groove running along the cingulum on the lingual surface.[33]

Again it is very rare to find more than one canal,[34,35] but several case reports have shown more canals with separate apices.[41–44] The pulp horns may not be quite as pronounced, but the concept of lingual shelf removal and extending the pulp horns till it can be verified with a cowhorn explorer that the angles are smooth still holds.

Regarding SLA, LaTurno and Zillich[18] as well as Zillich and Jerome[17] showed that of the 131 teeth examined, only 0.8% of canals had a coronal projection that was entirely lingual and did not involve the incisal or buccal surfaces with 16% entirely on the buccal (see Figure 9). Therefore, the clinician should be more fastidious about the removal of the lingual triangle for these teeth. Compounding the difficulty of achieving SLA from a lingual approach is that these teeth tend to have a curvature to the distal.

It must also be noted that incisors can have many anomalies that severely increase the difficulty in treatment of these cases, for example, radicular palatal grooves, fusion with supernumerary teeth, gemination, dens invaginatus, dens evaginatus, incomplete apical closure; it is beyond the scope of this chapter to cover these treatment protocols.

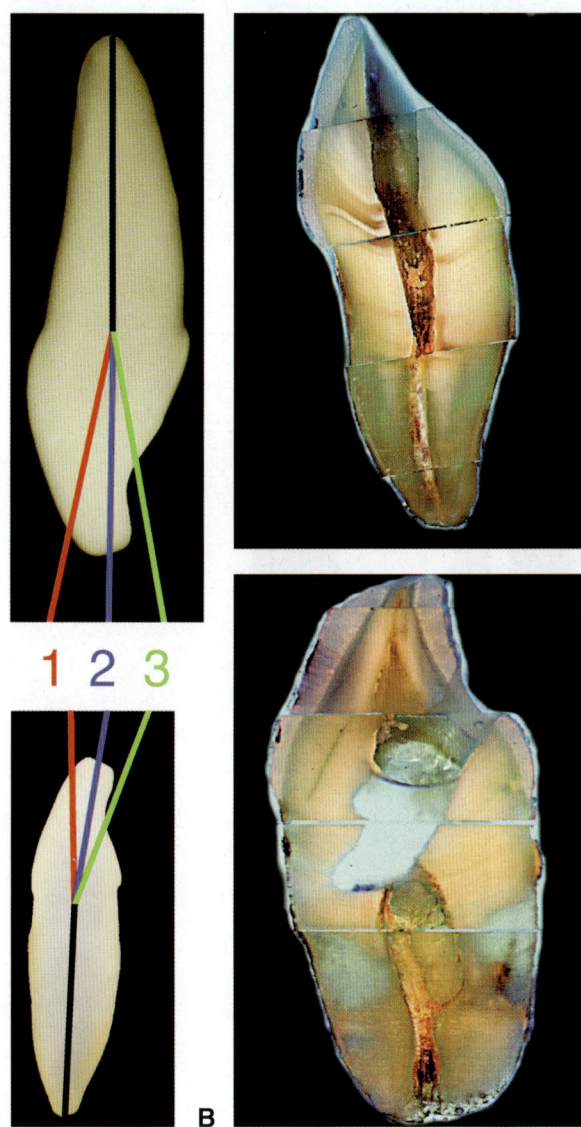

Figure 8 Impact of initial entry into pulp chambers of incisor teeth, from labial (1) to incisal (2) and the usual oral access (3). **A,** Schematic diagrams for maxillary and mandibular incisors. **B,** Original micrographs with access from incisal (top) and oral (bottom). Reprinted with permission from Sonntag D et al.[6]

carbide bur often occur. These extensions should be blended into the main access chamber so that residual debris, sealer, or gutta-percha does not become trapped and cause discoloration. Younger patients have more pronounced pulp horns and require particular care to remove the remaining potential tissue.

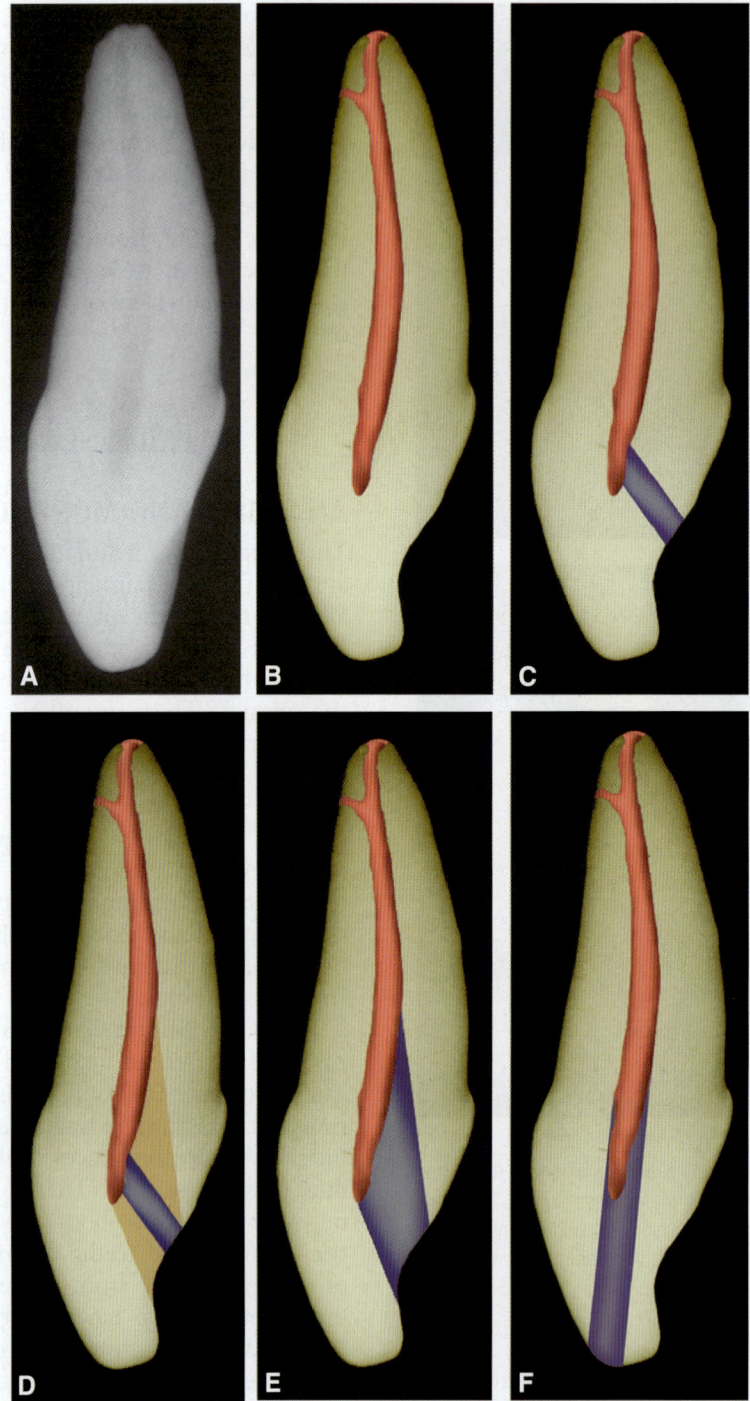

Figure 9 Potential design of access into a maxillary incisor with schematic drawings based on an original radiograph **A**, The preoperative relation of the canal within the root can be estimated **B**, note how the true straight-line access (SLA) is labial to the incisal edge **C**, The initial access entry site and angulation **D**, tan-colored highlights) show the restrictive dentin impeding SLA. The completed lingual access preparation with SLA **E**, can be compared to a completed access preparation done from a labial approach **F**, Note how far more tooth structure may be conserved with a labial access but at the cost of disrupting the labial esthetic surface.

Maxillary Canines

ANATOMY AND MORPHOLOGY

The labiolingual measurement of the crown is about 1 mm greater than that of the maxillary central incisor and the mesiodistal measurement is approximately 1 mm less (Figure 10). The position of the cusp tip relative to the long axis of the root is in line with the center of the root tip in the labial view but lies labial in the proximal view.[33] LaTurno and Zillich[18] showed that none of the 48 maxillary canines examined projected solely onto the lingual surface with an SLA. About 98% of the configurations involved the incisal edge (of which 43% involved incisal and lingual) and 2.1% were purely on the buccal. Usually one root

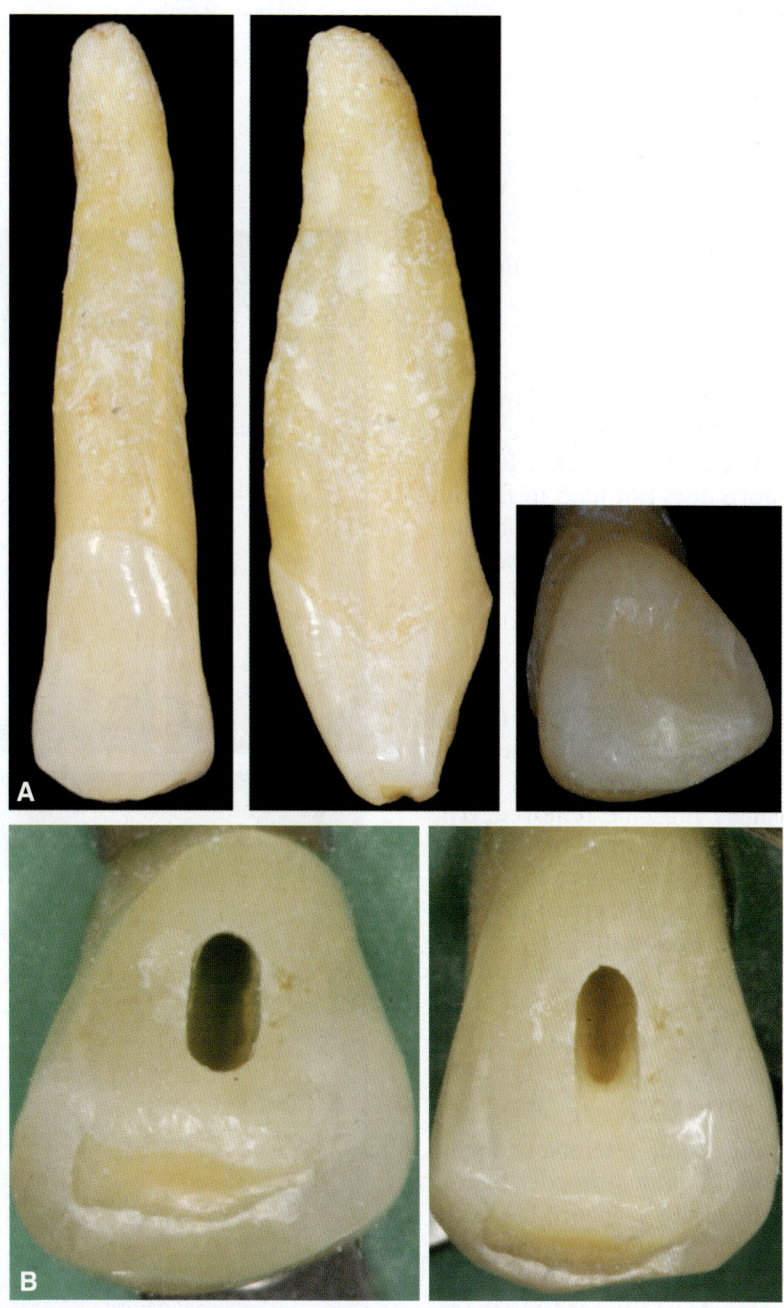

Figure 10 Example of a maxillary canine showing labial, mesial, and incisal views **A,** The access preparation can be assessed from a more incisal view and a lingual view **B.**

Author	Year	Number of Teeth	Method	One Coronal Canal	Two Coronal Canals	Three Coronal Canals	One Apical Foramen	Two Apical Foramina	Three Apical Foramina
Carns[46]	1973	100	Vacuum-drawn polyester cast resin, decalcified	9%	85%	6%	22%	72%	6%
Vertucci[47]	1979	400	Decalcified, dye injected, cast in resin, microscope	8%	87%	5%	26%	69%	5%
Walker[48]	1987	100	Radiographic in vitro	13%	87%	0%	36%	64%	0%
Pecora[49]	1991	240	Decalcified, India ink-dyed, gelatin injection	17.1%	80.4%	2.5%	Not specified	Not specified	Not specified
Caliskan[45]	1995	100	Dyed, decalcified, stereomicroscope x12	4%	97%	0%	10%	90%	0%
Kartal[50]	1998	300	Decalcified, ink dye, microscope x0.6–4	8.66%	89.64%	1.66%	9.66%	88.64%	1.66%
Pineda[34]	1972	259	Radiographic in vitro	26.2%	73.3%	0.5%	50.1%	49.4%	0.5%
Kerekes[51]	1977	20	Sectioned, microscope	10%	80%	10%	10%	80%	2%
Bellizzi[52]	1985	514	Radiographic in vivo	6.2%	90.5%	3.3%	Not examined	Not examined	Not examined
Green[53]	1973	50	Ground sections, microscope	8%	92%	0%	34%	66%	0%
Sert[54]	2004	200	Decalcified, dyed	10.5.%	85%	4.5%	28.5%	68.5%	3%

Table 1 Summary of Studies Detailing Root and Root Canal Anatomy of Maxillary First Premolars

canal is present,[34,35] but cases with two canals have also been reported[45] (see Figure 8).

CLINICAL

These teeth have a point of entry just about the cingulum with the tip of the bur aiming for the center point at the CEJ level. The occlusal outline form is oval as the single pulp horn does not tend to fan out to the mesial or distal; however it is broad labiolingually. Again, this is checked with a cowhorn explorer and is adjusted according to the individual tooth. The extension to the buccal or lingual is done only as necessary to clearly uncover the horns and to allow unheeded insertion of any file.

It is usually the longest tooth and the largest root in the mouth and is critical to the occlusion. The canal often curves apically. As with the central and lateral incisors, the lingual triangle must be removed. The main difficulty with these teeth is that they can be long—often over 30 mm. This will affect the access cavity in that to provide an adequate apical preparation size, SLA becomes more important.

Maxillary First Premolars

ANATOMY AND MORPHOLOGY

From the occlusal aspect, the tooth resembles roughly a hexagonal structure, and it is much broader buccolingually than mesiodistally (Table 1, Figure 11). As in all posterior maxillary teeth, the measurement from the buccal cusp tip to the lingual cusp tip is less than the buccolingual measurement of the root at its cervical level. As more of the buccal cusp is seen than the lingual, the access preparation is angled buccally into the cervical areas but not extended to the same degree on the occlusal table. There is a marked

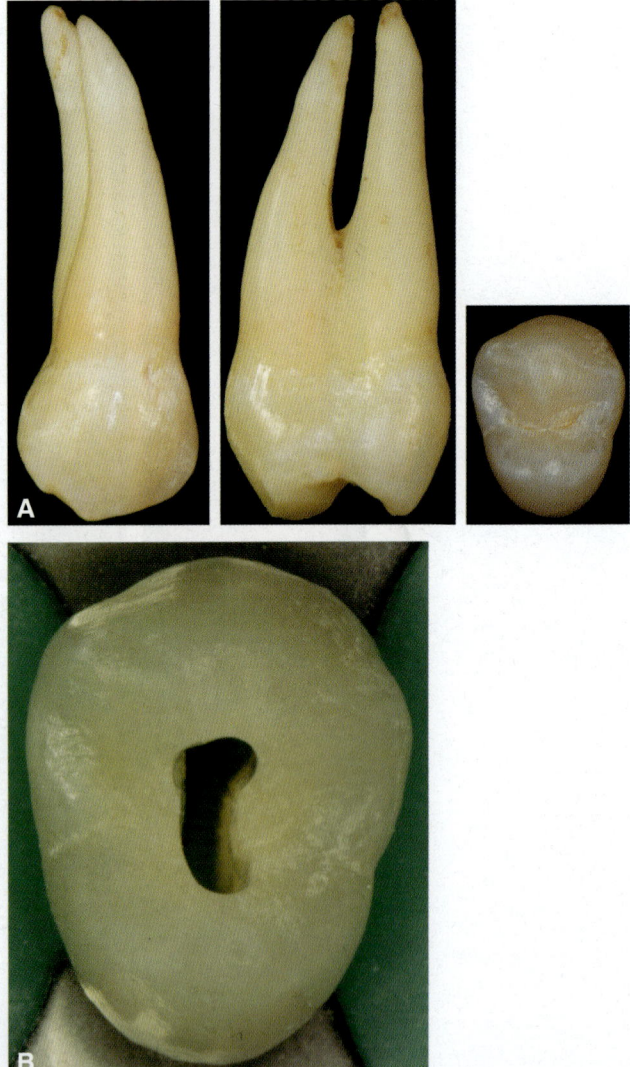

Figure 11 Example of a maxillary first premolar showing buccal, mesial, and occlusal views **A**, and a typical access preparation **B**, Note how the buccal part of the preparation has been extended mesiodistally to explore a potential second buccal canal.

developmental depression on the mesial surface that extends from just below the mesial contact point between the roots and ends at the bifurcation. There is also a well-defined developmental groove in the enamel of the mesial marginal ridge that runs into the central groove on the occlusal table. This can be deceiving during access as off-angulation of the bur can result in perforation. It must be assumed that at least two canals are present, and the third canal is shown to exist in high enough numbers that the access preparation must be designed to search for it (either mesiobuccal or distobuccal canals, abbreviated MB or DB). When three canals are present, the pulp chamber morphology resembles that of a maxillary molar, and they have been termed "mini-molars." The width of the access can be kept minimal between the canal orifices.

CLINICAL

The point of entry is centrally in the fossa, aiming at the center point at the CEJ. The outline is an elongated slot and can extend almost to the cusp tips depending on the angle. However, the operator must search for a third canal—usually the mesiobuccal canal. If three canals are found, the orientation is very similar to that of the maxillary molar (Figure 12).

Maxillary Second Premolar

ANATOMY AND MORPHOLOGY

The occlusal table is very similar to that of the first premolar (see Figure 11), presenting without a

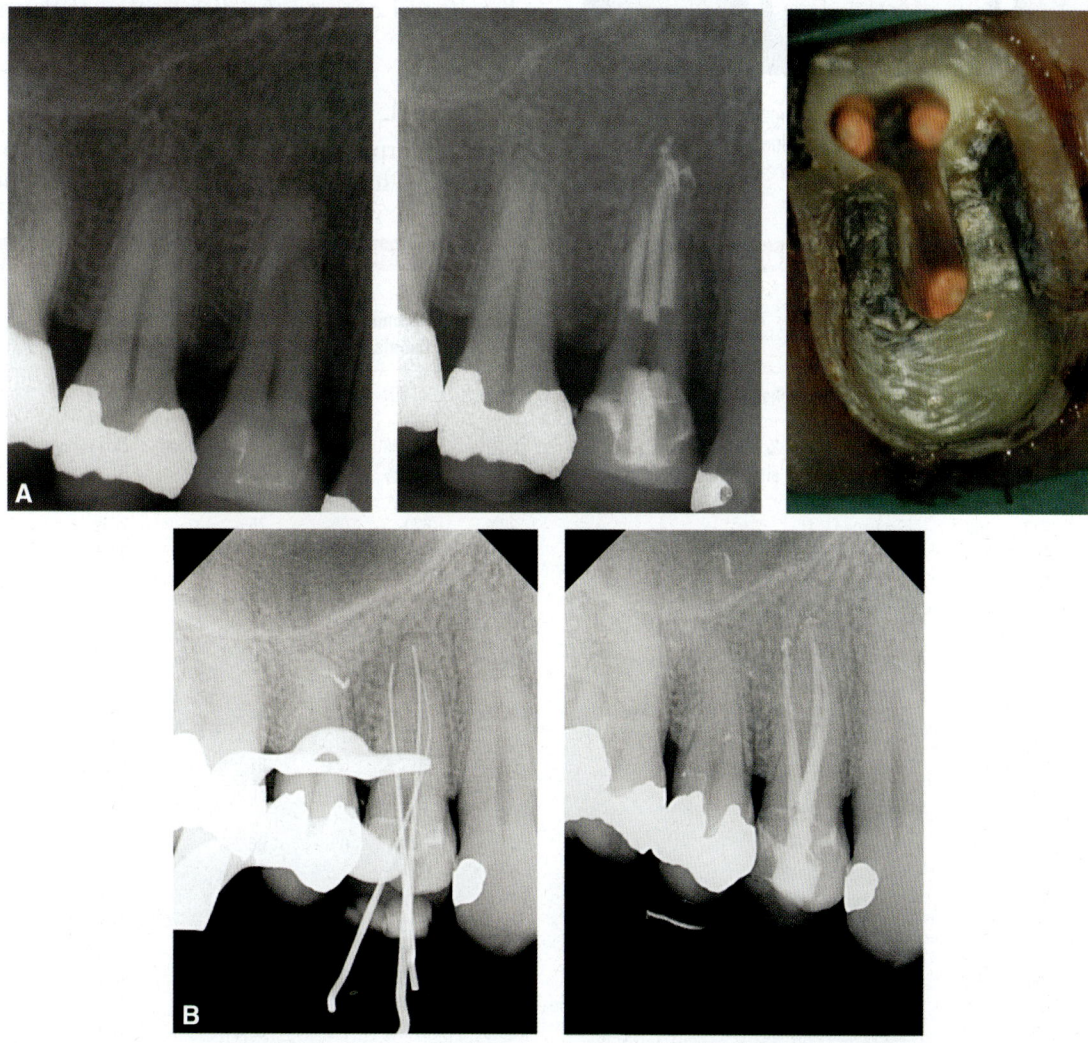

Figure 12 Two examples of maxillary first premolars with three canals that were endodontically treated. A clinical view of the access cavity is provided in **A**.

depression in the mesial root surface (Figure 13). It has a more rounded crown form and has a single root when compared with the first premolar. Internally, the incidence of two canals is significantly less but when present they are not spaced so far apart from each other.

Maxillary First Molar

ANATOMY AND MORPHOLOGY

It is the largest tooth in the maxillary arch with four well-defined cusps and a supplemental cusp of Carabelli of the mesiolingual cusp (Tables 2–4, Figure 14). From the occlusal view, it has a roughly rhomboidal outline. The distobuccal cusp becomes progressively smaller on the second and third maxillary molars. There are two major fossae (central fossa mesial to the oblique ridge and the distal fossa distal to the oblique ridge) and two minor fossae (the mesial and distal triangular fossae that lie just distal to the mesial marginal ridge and just mesial to the distal marginal ridge, respectively). The oblique ridge crosses the occlusal surface from the ridge of the distobuccal cusp to the distal ridge of the mesiolingual cusp.

CLINICAL

For the purpose of access cavities, the molars can be viewed as having a triangular arrangement of the

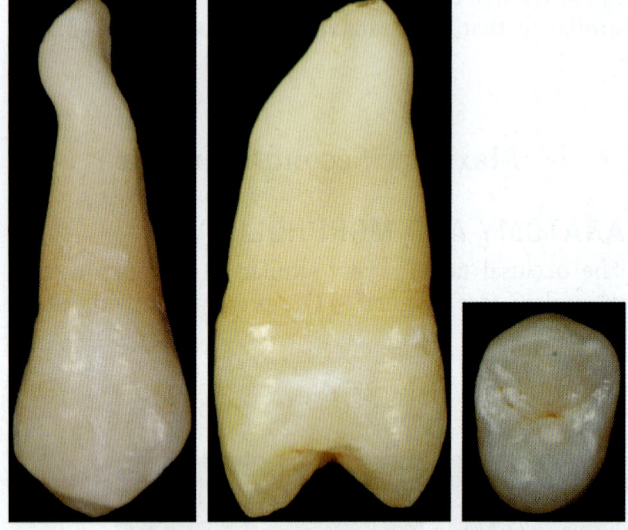

Figure 13 Example of a maxillary second premolar showing buccal, mesial, and occlusal views. The access preparation is virtually identical to the one of maxillary first premolar (see Figure 11).

Table 2 Summary of Studies Detailing Root and Root Canal Anatomy of the Mesiobuccal Root of First Maxillary Molars

Author	Year	Number of Teeth	Method	One Coronal Canal	Two Coronal Canals	Three Coronal Canals	One Apical Foramen	Two Apical Foramina	Three Apical Foramina
Gilles[55]	1990	21	SEM and decalcified, injected ink dye, microscope	9.5%	90.5%		61.9%	38.1%	
Buhrley[56]	2002	58	Clinically in vivo & Microscope	28.9%	71.1%		Not examined	Not examined	
Fogel[57]	1994	208	Clinically in vivo and loupes, headlamps	29.8%	71.2%		68.3%	31.7%	
Pomeranz[58]	1974	71	In vivo clinical	72%	28%	0%	89%	11%	0%
Seidberg[59]	1973	100	Sectioned	38%	62%	0%	75%	25%	0%
Thomas[60]	1993	216	Radiography ex vivo—radiopaque infusion of canals	26.4%	61.1%	12.5%	53.7%	33.8%	12.5%
Kulild[61]	1990	51	Ex vivo accessed, ground sections, microscope	3.9%%	96.1%	0%	54.2%	45.8%	
Al-Shalabi[62]	2000	83	Dye, decalcified, cleared, microscope x20 magnification	19.3%	79.5%	1.2%	34.9%	63.9%	1.2%
Vertucci[35]	1984	100	Decalcified, dye injected, cast in resin, microscope	45%	55%	0%	82%	18%	0%
Pineda[34]	1972	262	Radiographic ex vivo	39.3%	60.7%	0%	51.5%	48.5%	0%
Caliskan[45]	1995	100	Dyed, decalcified, stereomicroscope x12	34%	66%	0%	75%	25%	0%
Weine[63]	1999	300	Radiographic ex vivo	42%	58%	0%	66.2%	33.8%	0%
Alavi[64]	2002	52	Dyed, decalcified	32.7%	65.4%	1.9%	53.8%	46.2%	0%
Imura[65]	1998	42	Root canal treatment ex vivo, decalcified	19%	81%'	0%	28.6%	71.4%	0%
Sert[54]	2004	200	Decalcified, dyed	6.5%	92.5%	1%	61%	39%	0%
Weine[66]	1969	208	Sectioned	48.6%	51.4%	0%	86.1%	13.9%	0%
Stropko[67]	1999	168	Clinically in vivo (microscope only)	13.1%	86.9%	0%	54.8%	45.2%	0%
Wasti[68]	2001	30	Decalcified, ink dye, x10 dissecting microscope	33.3%	66.7%	0%	56.6%	43.4%	0%
Ng[69]	2001	90	Ink dye, decalcified	30%	67.8%	2.2%	57.8%	41.1%	1.1%

Table 3 Summary of Studies Detailing Root and Root Canal Anatomy of the Distobuccal Root of First Maxillary Molars

Author	Year	Number of Teeth	Method	One Canal Coronally	Two Canals Coronally	Three Canals Coronally	One Apical Foramen	Two Apical Foramina	Three Apical Foramen
Thomas[60]	1993	208	Radiography ex vivo, radiopaque infusion of canals	95.7%	2.4%	1.9%	96.2%	1.9%	1.9%
Al-Shalabi[62]	2000	81	Dye, decalcified, cleared, microscope x20 magnification	97.5%	2.5%	0%	97.5%	2.5%	0%
Vertucci[35]	1984	100	Decalcified, dye injected, cast in resin, microscope	100%	0%	0%	100%	0%	0%
Pienda[34]	1972	262	Radiographic ex vivo	96.4%	3.6%	0%	96.4%	3.6%	0%
Caliskan[45]	1995	100	Dyed, decalcified, stereomicroscope x12	98%	2%	0%	98%	2%	0%
Alavi[64]	2002	52	Dyed, decalcified	98.1%	1.9%	0%	100%	0%	0%
Sert[54]	2004	200	Dyed, decalcified	90.5%	9.5%	0%	97%	3%	0%
Wasti[68]	2001	30	Decalcified, ink dye, x10 dissecting microscope	83.3%	16.7%	0%	83.3%	16.7%	0%
Ng[69]	2001	90	Ink dye, decalcified	94.5%	4.4%	1.1%	97.8%	1.1%	1.1%

Table 4 Summary of Studies Detailing Root and Root Canal Anatomy of the Palatal Root of First Maxillary Molars

Author	Year	Number of Teeth	Method	One Canal Coronally	Two Canals Coronally	Three Canals Coronally	One Apical Foramen	Two Apical Foramina	Three Apical Foramen
Thomas[60]	1993	216	Radiography ex vivo, radiopaque infusion of canals	97.7%	2.3%	0%	98.2%	1.8%	0%
Al-Shalabi[62]	2000	82	Dye, decalcified, cleared, microscope x20 magnification	98.8%	1.2%	0%	98.8%	1.2%	0%
Vertucci[35]	1984	100	Decalcified, dye injected, cast in resin, microscope	100%	0%	0%	100%	0%	0%
Pineda[34]	1972	262	Radiographic ex vivo	100%	0%	0%	100%	0%	0%
Caliskan[45]	1995	100	Dyed, decalcified, stereomicroscope x12	93%	7%	0%	97%	3%	0%
Alavi[64]	2002	52	Dyed, decalcified	100%	0%	0%	100%	0%	0%
Sert[54]	2004	200	Dyed, decalcified	94.5%	4%	1.5%	96%	2.5%	1.5%
Wasti[68]	2001	30	Decalcified, ink dye, x10 dissecting microscope	66.7%	33.3%	0%	66.7%	33.3%	0%
Ng[69]	2001	90	Ink dye, decalcified	100%	0%	0%	100%	0%	0%

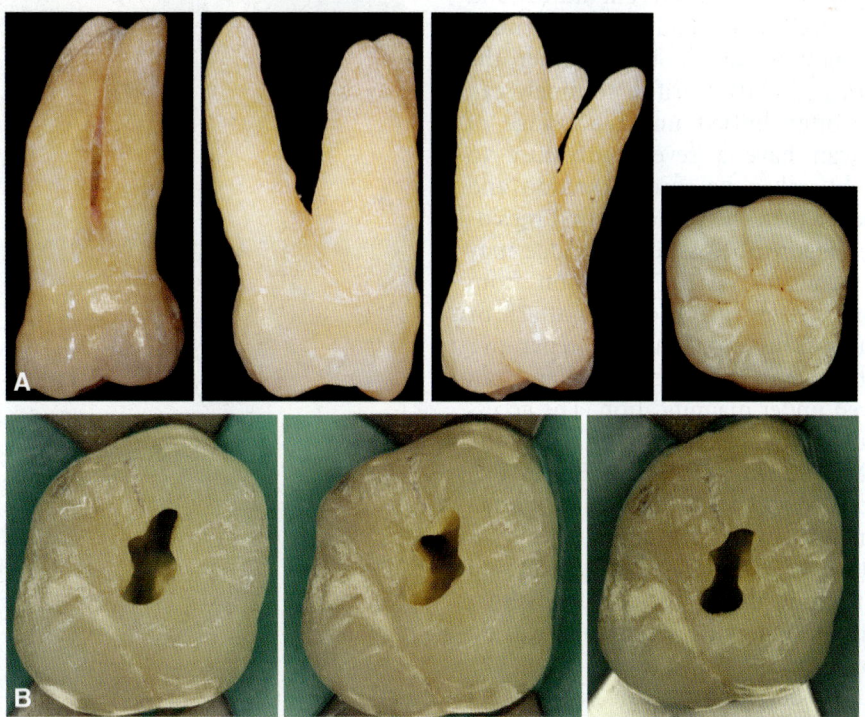

Figure 14 Example of a maxillary molar shown in buccal, mesial palatal and occlusal views. ***A***, Access into both mesiobuccal canals and distobuccal and palatal canals is gained ***B***, Note that the preparation has not been extended much on the occlusal table for the distobuccal canal as the canal projects distally naturally. All canals accept a size #40 or #50 hand file to working length (WL); access preparations may have to be extended further slightly to accommodate larger step-back files.

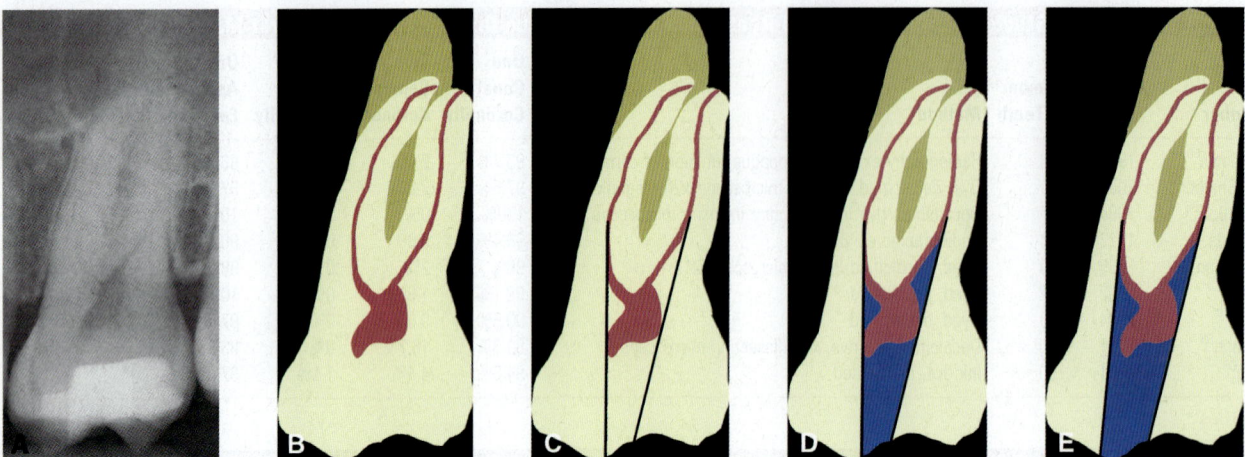

Figure 15 ***A, B,*** Schematic diagrams of maxillary molar access preparation based on the original radiograph ***C,*** Access penetration and angulation shows an initial narrow opening on the occlusal surface. ***D, E,*** Dentin (blue areas) is removed carefully so that a file can stand upright to show exactly where the access preparation must be extended further. Note how the distobuccal wall does not need to be extended significantly as it naturally projects distally.

cusps (without the distolingual cusp). In fact the access cavity is made without encroaching onto the distolingual cusp and is usually kept mesial to the oblique ridge.

Maxillary molars are widely recognized as being one of the most difficult teeth to treat endodontically. They can present with mild to severe curvatures and usually have two or three canals in any root (but most commonly in the mesiobuccal root). Locating the second mesiobuccal canal (MB2) orifice routinely can be difficult as it is often buried under a bridge of dentin. The canal can have a severe curvature to the mesial and the buccal in its coronal section and is usually much smaller than the principal first mesiobuccal canal (MB1) (Figure 15). A dentin bridge may occur due to the secondary dentin formation from aging and/or reparative dentin from carious attack or restorative procedures. This secondary or reparative dentin is usually whiter than the pulpal floor and can be selectively removed under magnification. The access shape should be quadrilateral to allow for troughing 2–3 mm lingual to MB1 to search for MB2 (Figure 16). The clinician should keep an eye on the mesial external root surface as a guide to avoid perforating furcally or mesially. Endodontists have reported troughing well over 4 mm below the pulpal floor before uncovering the MB2 orifice. In the following, each root will be described separately (Figure 17).

In principle, all maxillary molars can be accessed following a similar strategy. Entry should be in the mesial fossa and should be kept small initially. Under

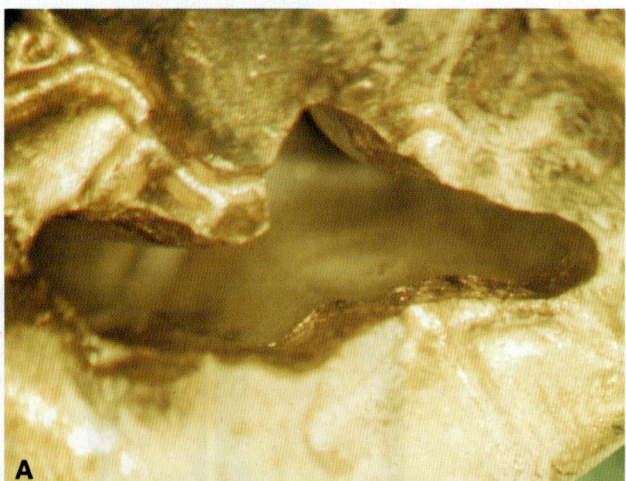
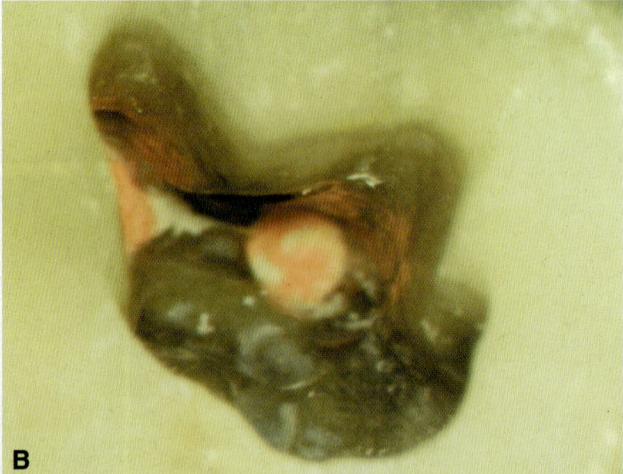

Figure 16 Variations in access cavity shapes in maxillary molars.

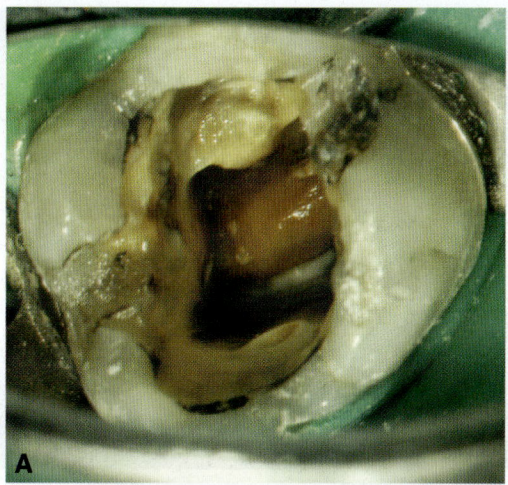

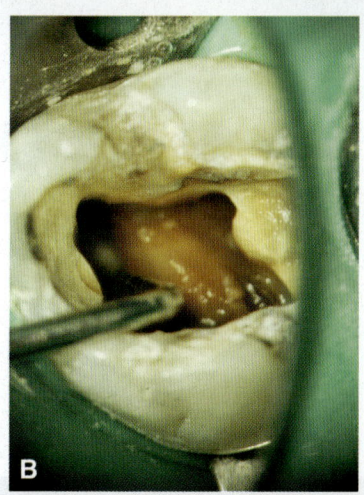

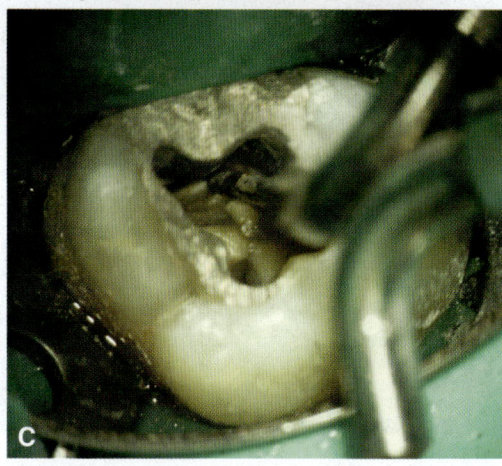

Figure 17 ***A***, The isthmus between the two mesiobuccal canals is troughed and no further fin or isthmus is evident. ***B***, Measurement of troughing depth with a periodontal probe gives the practitioner an objective perspective. ***C***, Incorrect angulation of ultrasonic tip during troughing due to inadequate extension of the mesial wall resulting in the removal of furcal dentin.

higher-power magnification, it can be extended selectively. Initial penetration may be aimed at the large palatal canal orifice. There is ample evidence to demonstrate that the mesiobuccal root has a second canal with such frequency that it must be accommodated for in the initial access and always searched for. In vivo, Stropko[67] reported finding two canals in 73.2% of first molars before using the microscope and 93% after; 90% of the MB2s were negotiable to the apex. He classified it as a canal if he could instrument 4 mm into it. Baldassari-Cruz et al.[70] located MB2 canals in 51% of the cases with the naked eye compared to 82% with the microscope.

Gilles and Reader[55] found that the mean distance of MB2 orifice from MB1 was 2.31 mm (range 0.7 to 3.75 mm). Kulild and Peters[61] found that the distance between MB1 and MB2 was on average 1.82 mm and the orifice was to the lingual of MB1. However, the MB2 orifice can sometimes be found close to or even in the palatal canal orifice (Figure 18). While two mesiobuccal orifices are most common, three can also be present (Figure 19).

The mesiobuccal canals have two separate apical foramina or, more commonly, join to exit at one foramen (Figure 20). In contrast, the distobuccal root is conical and usually straight but may have a slight curvature to the mesial. Although far more infrequent than the mesiobuccal root, the distobuccal root can also have a second canal that almost invariably joins the main (DB) canal to a common apex. It can be found lingually to the main canal and usually in a visible fin connecting the DB canal to the palatal canal. The incidence of two DB canals ranges from 2% to 9%.

The access preparation for the DB canals does not have to be extended as far toward its line angle as the mesial canals. The distal canal is distally inclined and so the file projects out of the orifice to the mesial naturally. Therefore, the transverse ridge can usually be preserved (see Figure 15).

The palatal root is broad mesiodistally and its canal mirrors it. Therefore the access should be extended mesiodistally. The extent to which it has to be extended palatally can be deceiving as the orifice coronally projects palatally naturally and therefore the file does not seem to contact the palatal wall toward the orifice. However, the apical third often curves to the buccal, and to reach the apex with large files, one needs to extend the palatal wall slot palatally and flare the coronal mid thirds of the canal. Again, a file is inserted and only that area of the dentin that contacts the file is removed to achieve SLA. This can also be accomplished using an ultrasonic tip.

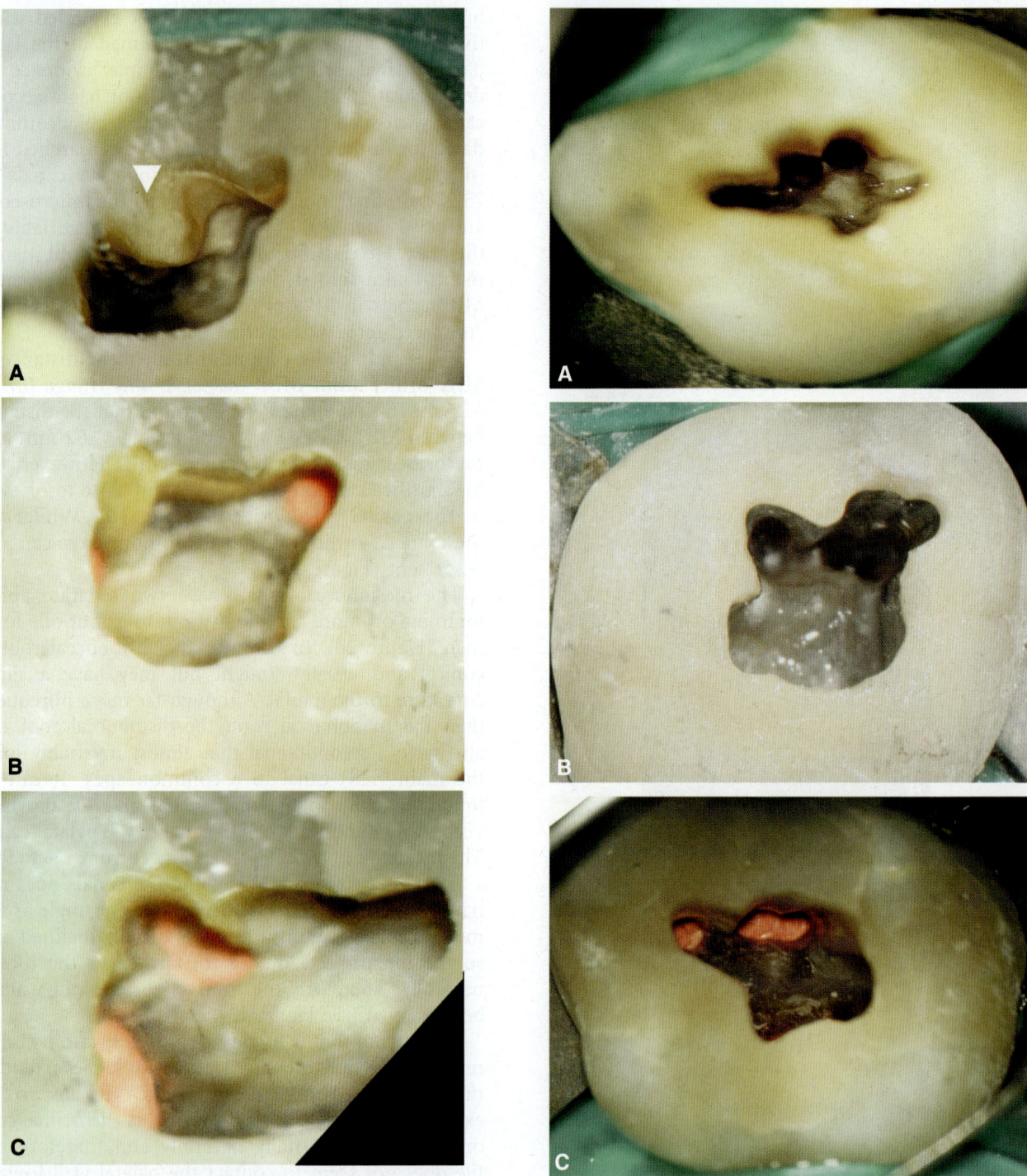

Figure 18 The MB2 canal can be located anywhere along the fin between the MB1 and palatal canals. ***A,*** Second mesiobuccal orifice was found in the entrance (arrowhead) to the palatal canal and shows how the customary extension was inadequate. ***B,*** Obturation and the distance between MB1 and MB2. ***C,*** Proximity of MB2 to the palatal orifice.

Figure 19 Clinical examples of maxillary molars with three mesiobuccal canal orifices.

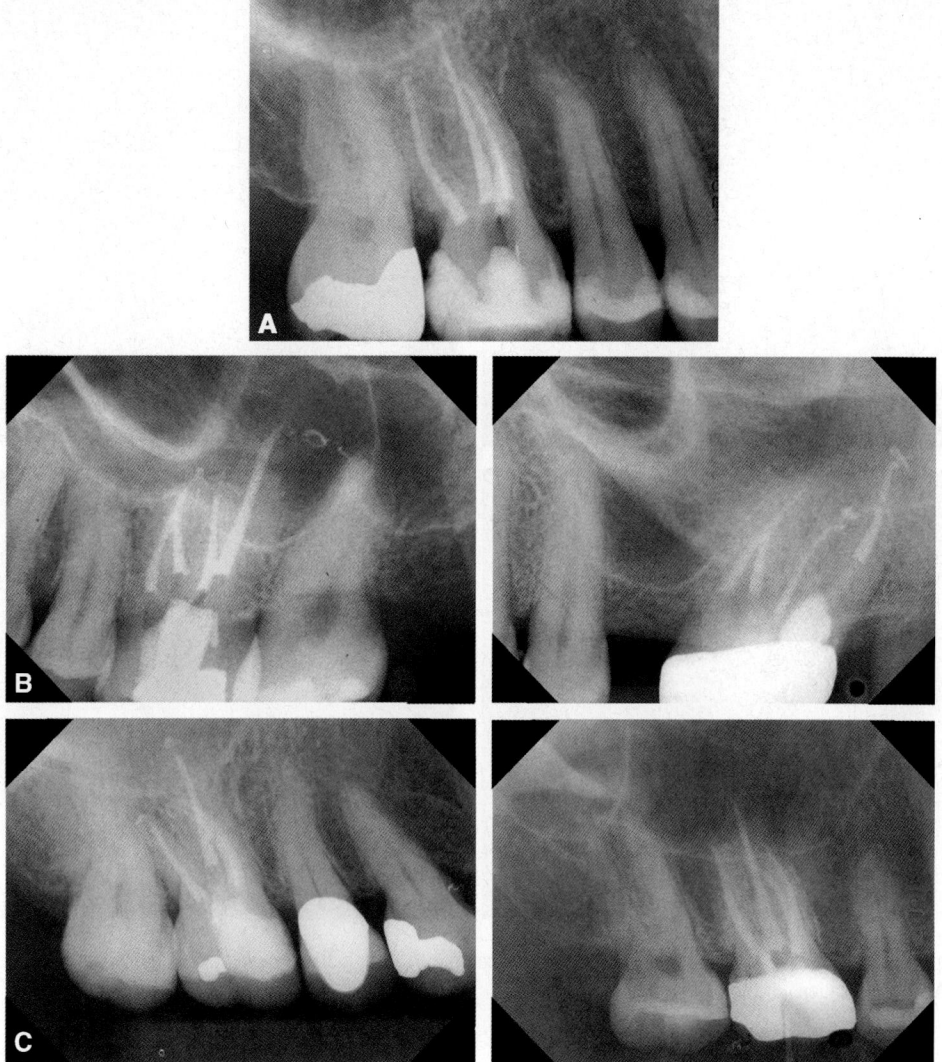

Figure 20 Radiographs illustrating possible variations in the anatomy of mesiobuccal root canal system of maxillary first molars. *A,* Two canals joining in the coronal root canal third. *B,* Widely separated canals but joining to a common apex. *C,* Separate apical foramina.

Also the palatal canal can split into two, and therefore the access preparation needs be extended mesiodistally (Figure 21). In such oval-shaped canals,[8] simple instrumentation with round cross-section files will not suffice for complete débridement of the canals (see Figure 14A).

Maxillary Second Molars

ANATOMY AND MORPHOLOGY

Maxillary second molars are very similar in form and function to the maxillary first molars with some variations (Table 5). The mesiobuccal and mesiolingual cusps are larger but the distobuccal and distolingual cusps are smaller. The cusp of Carabelli is usually absent. The buccolingual diameter of the crown is about equal to the first, but the mesiodistal diameter is approximately 1 mm less. There are two types of maxillary second molars when viewed from the occlusal aspect:

(1) *Rhomboidal:* four-cusp outline similar to the first molars but more rounded. This is the more common form.
(2) *Triangular:* three-cusp form more similar to the third molar form where the distolingual cusp is poorly developed.

The roots are usually closer together than the first molar's and can also have two or three fused roots. The canal system can vary from one large canal, two canals, or three or four canals. The palatal root can

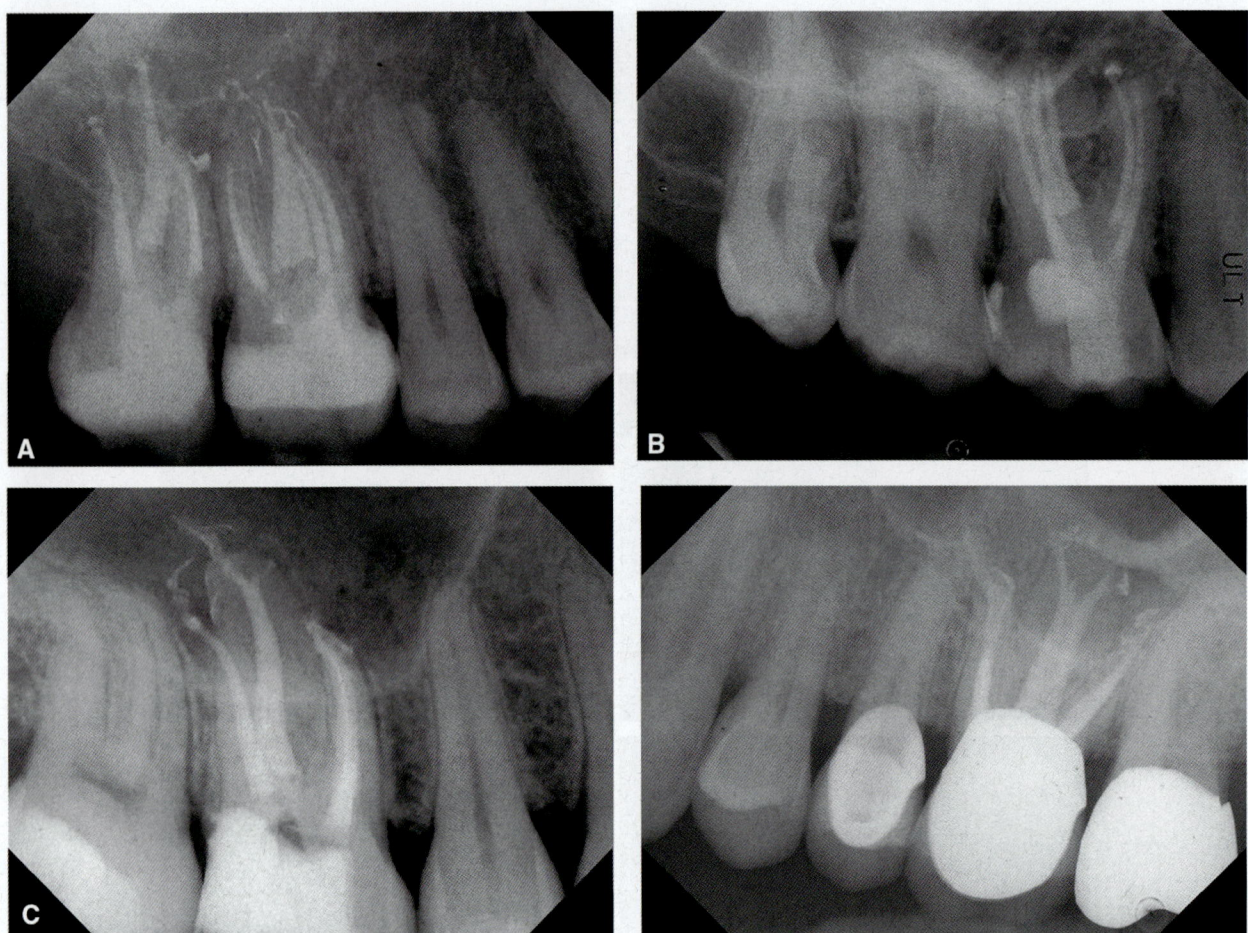

Figure 21 Radiographs illustrating variations in the palatal root canal anatomy. ***A,*** First molar showing one wide canal. ***B,*** Two canals in another first maxillary molar. ***C,*** Apical bifurcations in the palatal root.

Table 5 Summary of Studies Detailing Root and Root Canal Anatomy of the Mesiobuccal Root of Second Maxillary Molars									
Author	Year	Number of Teeth	Method	One Coronal Canal	Two Coronal Canals	Three Coronal Canals	One Apical Foramen	Two Apical Foramina	Three Apical Foramina
Vertucci[35]	1984	100		71%	57%	2%	76%	23%	1%
Pomeranz[58]	1974	29	Clinical in vivo	62%	38%	0%	76%	24%	0%
Caliskan[45] Sert[54]	2004	200	Decalcified, dyed	41%	57%	2%	76%	23.5%	0% (0.5% four foramina)
Pineda[34]	1972	294		64.6%	35.4%	0%	72.8%	27.2%	0%
Eskoz[71]	1995	67	Radiographic in vitro	59.7%	40.3%	0%	80.6%	19.4%	0%
Gilles[55]	1990	37	SEM and decalcified, injected ink dye, microscope	29.7%	70.2%	0%	62.1%	37.8%	0%
Kulild[61]	1990	32		6.3%	93.7%		54.2%	45.8%	
Buhrley[56]	2002	36	Clinically in vivo, microscope	63.9%	36.1%				
Alavi[64]	2002	65	Dyed, decalcified	41.5%	55.4%	3.1%%	53.8%	44.6%	1.5%
Imura[65]	1998	30	Root canal treatment ex vivo, sectioned, decalcified	33.3%	66.7%	0%	53.3%	46.7%	0%
Ng[69]	2001	77	Ink dye, decalcified	49.3%	48.1%	2.6%	74%	26%	0%

also have two separate roots with separate canals within each. The occlusal table is smaller.

CLINICAL

Access is more complicated due to the tooth being further back in the arch and more difficult to reach. Shorter length burs may sometimes be needed. Gilles and Reader[55] found that the mean diameter of the MB2 orifice in the second molars was 0.42 mm with a range of 0.15 to 1.00 mm. The mean distance from MB1 orifice to MB2 orifice was 2.6 mm (range 0.9 to 3.9 mm). The distobuccal canal can sometimes be hidden under a large shelf of dentin. The orifice appears on the same line joining the mesiobuccal and palatal canals. However, during cleaning and shaping, the shelf must be carefully removed so that the furcal surface is not encroached upon.

The palatal root usually has one canal, as described in vitro (see Table 6–18). Peikoff et al.[72] found in vivo that only 1.4% of maxillary second molars had two palatal roots and two palatal canals.

Maxillary Third Molars

ANATOMY AND MORPHOLOGY

From an occlusal viewpoint, this tooth usually presents with a heart-shaped triangular outline similar to the second molar. The distolingual cusp is typically small and often completely absent. Unlike the mandibular third molars, these teeth tend to have underdeveloped crowns. The roots are often fused forming one large root.

CLINICAL

Alavi et al.[64] found that 50.9% of third maxillary molars had three separate roots of which 45.5% had two

Table 6 Summary of Studies Detailing Root and Root Canal Anatomy of Mandibular Incisors

Author	Year	Tooth	Number of Teeth	Method	One Coronal Canal	Two Coronal Canals	Three Coronal Canals	One Apical Foramen	Two Apical Foramina	Three Apical Foramina
Rankine-Wilson[73]	1972	Both	111	Radiographic ex vivo	59.5%	40.5%		94.6%	5.4%	
Pineda[34]	1972	Central	179	Radiographic ex vivo	72.4%	26.6%		97.9%	2.1%	
		Lateral	184	Radiographic ex vivo	76.2%	23.8%		98.7%	1.3%	
Madeira[74]	1973	Central	683	Dyed, rendered transparent by clearing agents	88.7%	11.3%		99.7%	0.3%	
		Lateral	650	Dyed, rendered transparent by clearing agents	88.2%	11.9%		99.3%	0.8%	
Benjamin[75]	1974	Both	364	Radiographic ex vivo	58.6%	41.4%		98.7	1.3%	
Vertucci[35]	1984	Central	100	Decalcified, dye injected, cast in resin, microscope	70%	30%		97%	3%	
		Lateral	100	Decalcified, dye injected, cast in resin, microscope	75%	25%		98%	2%	
Caliskan[45]	1995	Central	100	Dyed, decalcified, stereomicroscope x12	69%	29%	2%	96%	2%	2%
		Lateral	100	Dyed, decalcified, stereomicroscope x12	69%	31%		98%	2%	
Kartal[76]	1992	Both	100	Dyed, decalcified, cleared, microscope	55%	44%	1%	92%	7%	1%
Miyashita[77]	1997	Both	1,085	Ink dye, decalcified, naked eye	87.6%	12.4%		98.3%	1.7%	
Sert[54]	2004	Central	200	Decalcified, ink dye	33.5%	65%	2.5%	87%	11%	2%
		Lateral	201	Decalcified, ink dye	36.8%	62.7%	0.5%	90%	9.5%	0.5%
Bellizzi[78]	1983	Central	254	Radiographic in vivo	83.1%	16.9%		Not examined	Not examined	
		Lateral	163	Radiographic in vivo	79.8%	20.2%		Not examined	Not examined	
Walker[79]	1988									
		Central	100	Radiographic ex vivo	78%	22%		99%	1%	
		Lateral	100	Radiographic ex vivo	68%	32%		99%	1%	
Green[53]	73	Both	500	Ground sections, microscope	79%	21%		96%	4%	
Al-Qudah[80]	06	Both	450	Decalcified, cleared, naked eye	73.8%	26.2%		91.4%	8.7%	

or more canals in the mesiobuccal root. About 45.7% had fused roots, 2% had C-shaped canals, and 2% had four separate roots. Therefore, modifications must be made in accessing these teeth compared to first and second molars to accommodate these anatomical variations.

Mandibular Central and Lateral Incisors

ANATOMY AND MORPHOLOGY

The mandibular central incisor is usually the smallest tooth in the mouth, having a little more than half the mesiodistal diameter of the maxillary central incisor; however, the labiolingual diameter is only about 1 mm less (Table 6, Figure 22). Bilateral symmetry is usually evident with central incisors.[33] There are slight differences between central and lateral incisors, but the most important with regard to access is that the crowns of lateral incisors are not as symmetrical as central incisors from the incisal view as they curve distally to accommodate the curvature of the arch and correspondingly the cingulum is displaced slightly to the distal. Lateral incisors are also slightly larger than the centrals; this is the reverse relationship found in the maxillary incisors.[33]

The incisal edge relative to the long axis of the root in the proximal view is lingually placed—this is clinically corroborated by LaTurno and Zillich's study.[18] However, this should have little bearing on the access preparation, and the two teeth can be approached with the same criteria. It is important to note that often the most bulbous or the broadest lingual aspect of the tooth is below the free gingival margin. Therefore, using the free gingival margin to determine the extent of lingual extension of the access cavity can leave it underextended. One has to use a probe to palpate the contour of the crown below the free gingival margin.

CLINICAL

According to LaTurno and Zillich,[18] incisors do not have SLA projections entirely on the lingual; all involved the incisal edge and/or the facial surface (6% projected completely onto the buccal) (see Figure 8). Mauger et al.[81] in a similar study found that an ideal SLA was at the incisal edge in 72.4% and in 27.6% was facial of the incisal edge. They also found that as the wear of the incisal edge increased, the ideal access moved from the facial toward the incisal. Similarly, Sonntag et al.[6] showed that a shift toward the incisal edge resulted in more adequate preparation and in fact less loss of hard tissue.

The entry point for access should be just above the cingulum with the bur angled perpendicularly to the surface of the entry point. As these teeth are narrow mesiodistally, the main concern is the width of the preparation. No more than a #1/2 round bur or a long thin cylindrical diamond is used to initiate the access, followed by a cylindrical diamond bur to extend only as a slot in a labiolingual dimension. The main point being that unnecessary extension toward the mesiodistal surface is avoided. Even the thinnest bur will provide an adequate width once collateral hand movement is taken into account. The disadvantage is of course that visibility is restricted and therefore the use of microscopes becomes paramount.

Once the chamber or the canal is found, the access can be precisely widened for each individual tooth according to its SLA projection. The other point is that 40% of mandibular incisors have two canals—buccal and lingual with only 2 to 3% having separate apical foramina (Figure 23). The lingual is by far the harder to locate because the angulation of these teeth in the jaws is proclined (see Figure 2). It is natural for the hand to angle the bur toward the buccal (thereby running the risk of gouging the labial wall). The lingual canal lies 1 to 3 mm away from the buccal, directly under the cingulum. Even when two canals are present, there is often a fin or a groove with pulp tissue between them (see Figure 23).

In summary, finding extra canals requires conviction that they are there and extending the access to look for them. Although the two canals seldom exit as separate apices, bacterial by-products from the necrotic tissue in the unfilled canal can communicate with the periodontal ligament via lateral canals or through a poor apical seal.

Mandibular Canines

ANATOMY AND MORPHOLOGY

These teeth are very similar to their maxillary counterparts and can be described in relation to them

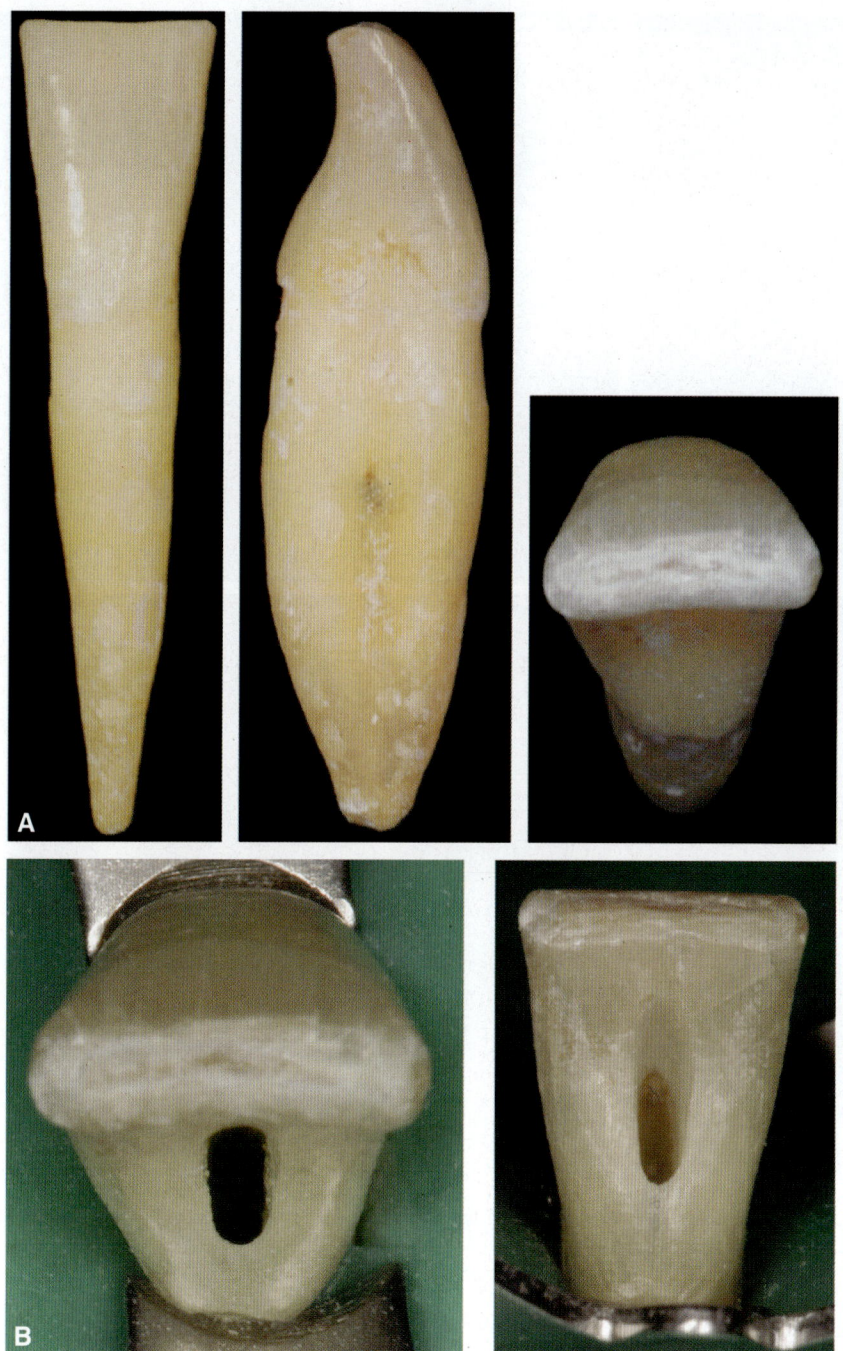

Figure 22 ***A,*** Example of a mandibular incisor showing labial, mesial, and incisal views. ***B,*** The access preparation can be assessed from a more incisal view and a lingual view. Note how the lingual extension of the access preparation extends well into the cingulum.

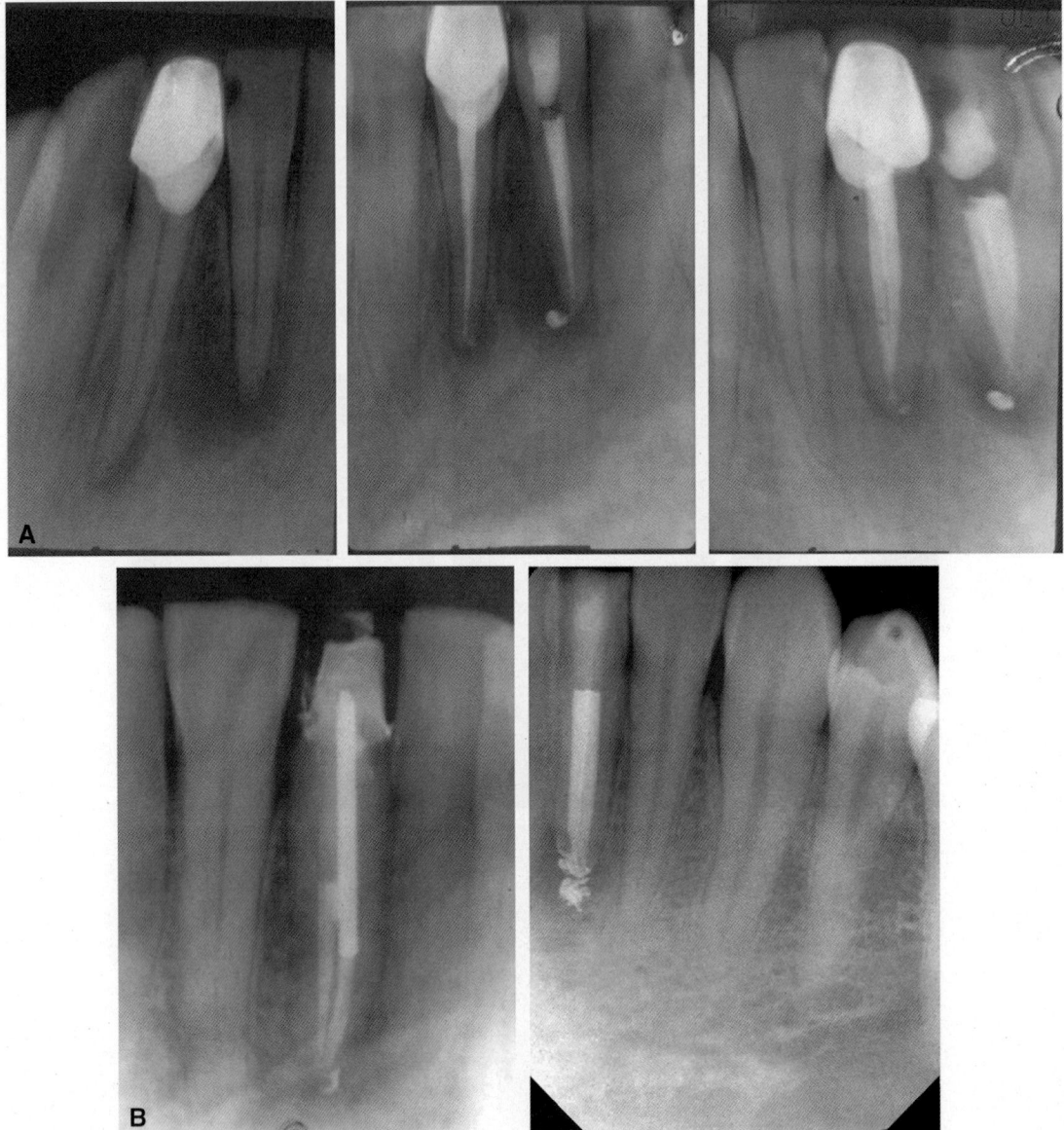

Figure 23 Radiographs illustrating variations of lower incisors with two canals. **A,** Although usually both canals exit from a common apex, they can, **B,** have two separate or a figure eight-shaped foramen.

(see Figure 18A). Mandibular canines are usually narrower than maxillary canines (approximately 1 mm) and shorter in root length by 1 to 2 mm (Figure 24). The mesial edge is almost straight and therefore the access cavity can be prepared more to the mesial of the center point of the lingual surface. Also the cusp tip is inclined more to the lingual, similar to the incisors.[33] According to LaTurno and Zillich,[18] none have SLA projections entirely to the lingual; 90% involved the incisal edge or incisal edge and buccal surface with 4% entirely on the buccal. Canine crowns are asymmetrical with a larger distal half. Therefore, the access preparation can be started just slightly to the mesial of the mid-point mesiodistally, and checked that it corresponds to the center point at the CEJ. Similar to their maxillary counterparts, mandibular canines extend buccolingually, albeit to a smaller extent.

Heling et al.[82] reported a mandibular canine with two roots and three canals but did not state whether two or three apical foramina were present. Orguneser and Kartal[83] reported a case of a three-canal mandibular canine with two apical foramina.

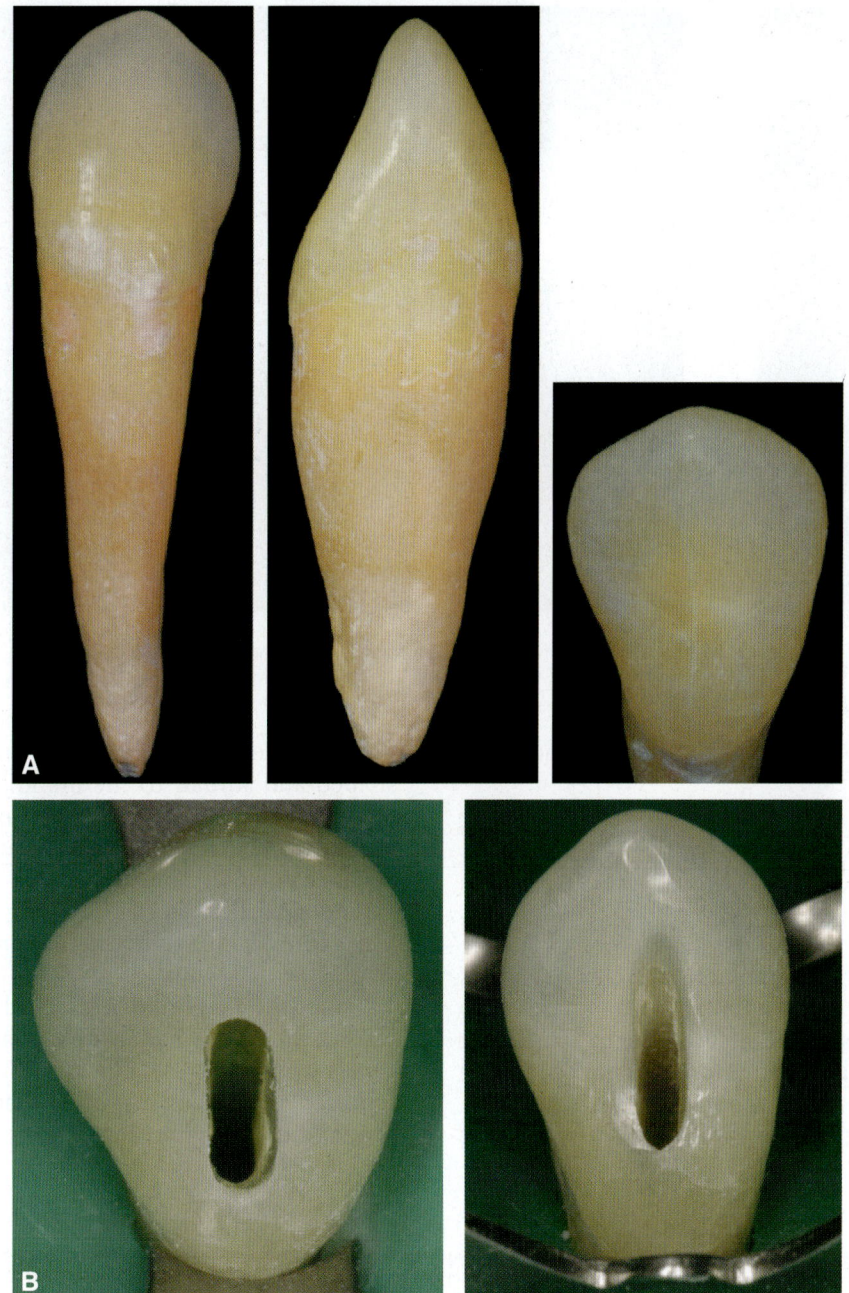

Figure 24 *A,* Example of a mandibular canine showing labial, mesial, and incisal views. *B,* The access preparation can be assessed from a more incisal view and a lingual view. Note that the access is extended lingually to look for a second, usually lingually located canal.

CLINICAL

The shape of the preparation ranges from an oval to a rounded slot depending on the size of the pulp chamber inside. As canines have large roots, the MAF (Box 1) is also large (size #40 to #60). Therefore, after creating a tapered preparation via step-back or rotary files, the

Box 1 Descriptors of Canal Shaping Procedures	
WL	Working length
WW	Working width
IAF (IAR)	Initial apical file/rotary
MAF (MAR)	Master apical file/rotary
FF (FR)	Final file/rotary

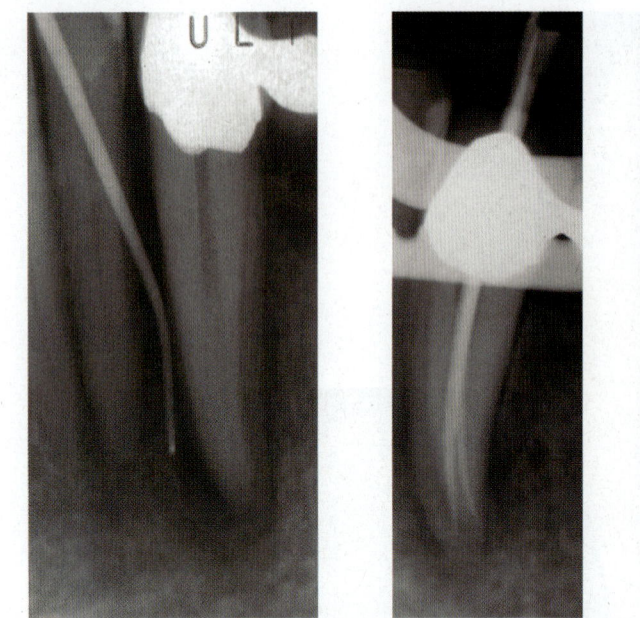

Figure 25 Radiographs of a treatment sequence illustrating two canals in a mandibular canine.

coronal orifice will be larger than for incisors mesiodistally (Figure 25).

Mandibular First Premolars

ANATOMY AND MORPHOLOGY

The mandibular first premolars have characteristics of a small canine because of a sharp buccal cusp (only occluding cusp) and a small lingual cusp that sometimes resemble a cingulum (Table 7, Figure 26). There is a characteristic mesiolingual developmental groove that makes the tooth asymmetrical. From the occlusal view, the outline is diamond-shaped and similar to the mandibular canine. These teeth have a variable root anatomy. The crown is lingually inclined that makes searching for a lingual canal difficult. Therefore, the access has to be extended further to the lingual to search for it. This feels counterintuitive, as the lingual cusp is very small.

Nallapati[88] reported a case where both first and second premolars had type V anatomy, that is, three canals with separate apices, while Baisden et al.[85] reported the possibility of C-shaped canal anatomy in mandibular premolars.

Table 7 Summary of Studies Detailing Root and Root Canal Anatomy of Mandibular First Premolars									
Author	Year	Number of Teeth	Method	One Coronal Canal	Two Coronal Canals	Three Coronal Canals	One Apical Foramen	Two Apical Foramina	Three Apical Foramina
Vertucci[35,84]	78/84	400	Decalcified, dye injected, cast in resin, microscope	70%	29.5%	0.5%	74%	25.5%	0.5%
Pineda[34]	72	202	Radiographic ex vivo	69.3%	29.8%	0.9%	74.2%	24.9%	0.9%
Baisden[85]	92	106	Serial sections, stereomicroscope x12	74%	26%		76%	24%	
Caliskan[45]	95	100	Dyed, decalcified, stereomicroscope x12	64%	30%	6%	75%	19%	6%
Zillich[86]	73	1,287	Radiographic ex vivo	75.1%	24.5%	0.4%	77.2%	22.5%	0.4%
Yoshioka[87]	04	139	Ink-dyed, demineralized	80.6%	15.1%	4.3% (three to four canals)	Not reported	Not reported	Not reported
Sert[54]	04	200	Decalcified, ink-dyed	60.5%	38.5%	1%	89.5%	9.5%	1%
Green[53]	73	50	Ground sections and microscope	86%	14%	0%	90%	10%	0%

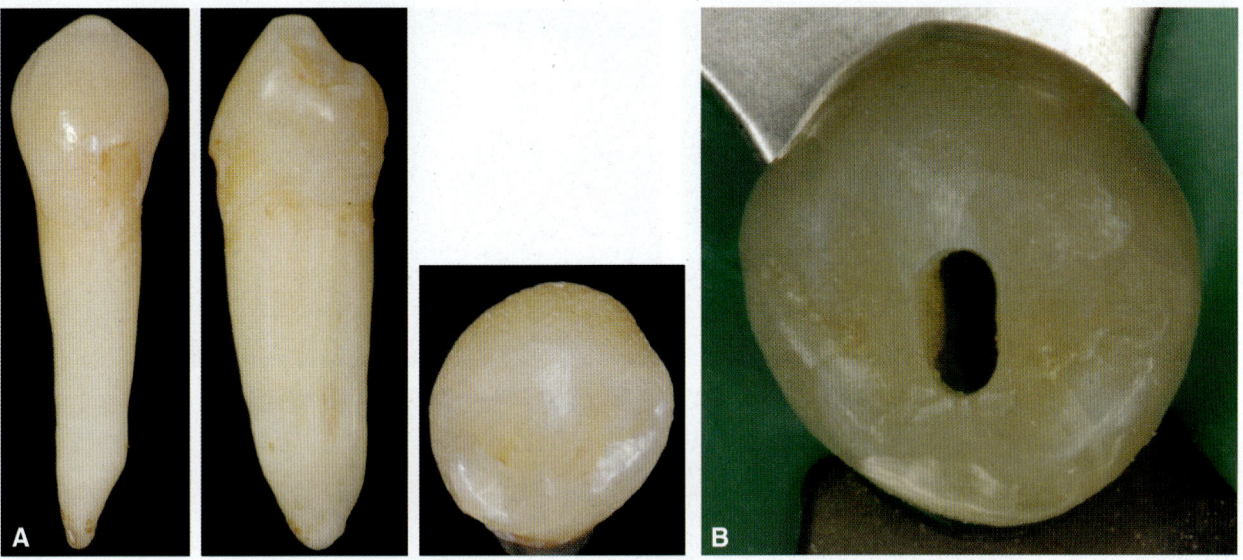

Figure 26 ***A,*** Example of a mandibular first premolar showing buccal, mesial, and occlusal views. ***B,*** The access preparation can be assessed from an occlusal view.

CLINICAL

The entry point is in the middle of the central groove, and the bur is directed to the buccal. Again, the access shape is an oval slot. As the crown is lingually inclined, the access cavity will result in the removal of more of the buccal cusp than the lingual (Figure 27).

Mandibular Second Premolar

ANATOMY AND MORPHOLOGY

Unlike the maxillary premolars, the mandibular second premolar is quite distinct from its neighboring first premolar (Figure 28). It resembles the first only from the buccal aspect but is otherwise larger. The tooth has two forms from the occlusal aspect, the more common three-cusp type and the two-cusp type. With the three-cusp type, the buccal cusp is the largest followed by the mesiolingual cusp and then the distolingual. The occlusal outline is square. The two-cusp form is more rounded and has a smaller occlusal table. Case reports detailing four[89–91] and five[92] coronal canals but only one showing four apical foramina have also been reported.[89]

CLINICAL

Access is similar to first mandibular premolars, taking overall dimensions into account.

Mandibular First Molars

ANATOMY AND MORPHOLOGY

The occlusal surface of mandibular first molars has one major (or central) and two minor (mesial and distal)

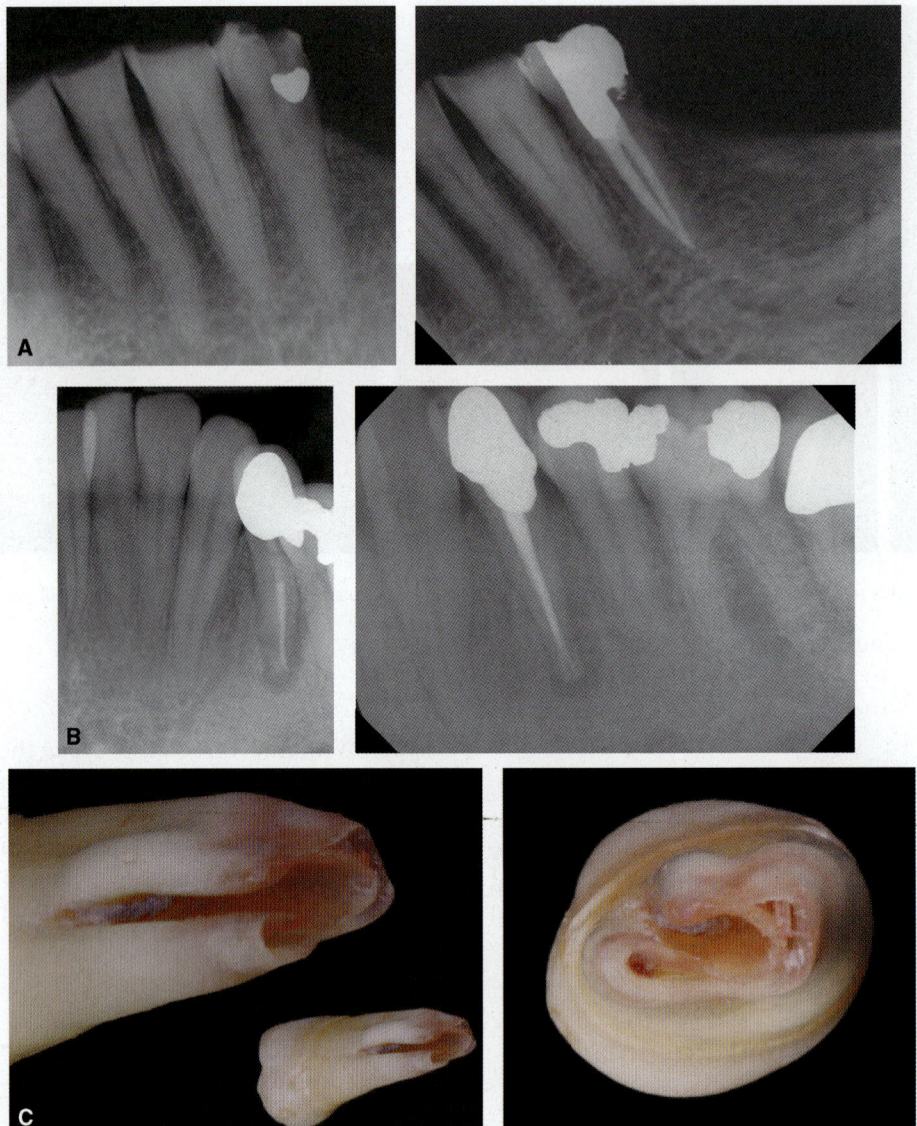

Figure 27 *A, B,* Two examples of lower first premolars with two canals. *C,* Photographs of an extracted tooth demonstrate a C-shaped root cross section and suggest the impossibility of adequately cleaning and shaping the entire canal system.

triangular fossae (Tables 8 and 9, Figure 29). These teeth usually have two distinct buccal and two lingual cusps and one distal cusp. The buccal cusp tips are located more to the midline on the occlusal table compared to the lingual cusp tips that are almost directly over the outer surface at the "neck" of the tooth. Therefore, access preparations often encroach on the buccal cusp tip (mesiobuccal) but rarely onto the lingual.

Mandibular molars are known to have complex anatomy and like their upper counterparts can be deceptively difficult to treat, as the radiographic canal anatomy can appear simple in two dimensions. There are usually four canals but three and five canals are well documented and one, two, and six canals have been reported. It is important to note that there is almost always a concavity on the furcal side of both the mesial and distal roots; therefore care must be taken during cleaning and shaping to avoid strip perforation. The roots start to bifurcate 3 mm below the CEJ. This gives a sense of the depth at which furcal perforation is possible. As the access cavity determines cleaning and shaping, the access cavity has to be designed to allow for protection of the furcal surfaces during instrumentation.

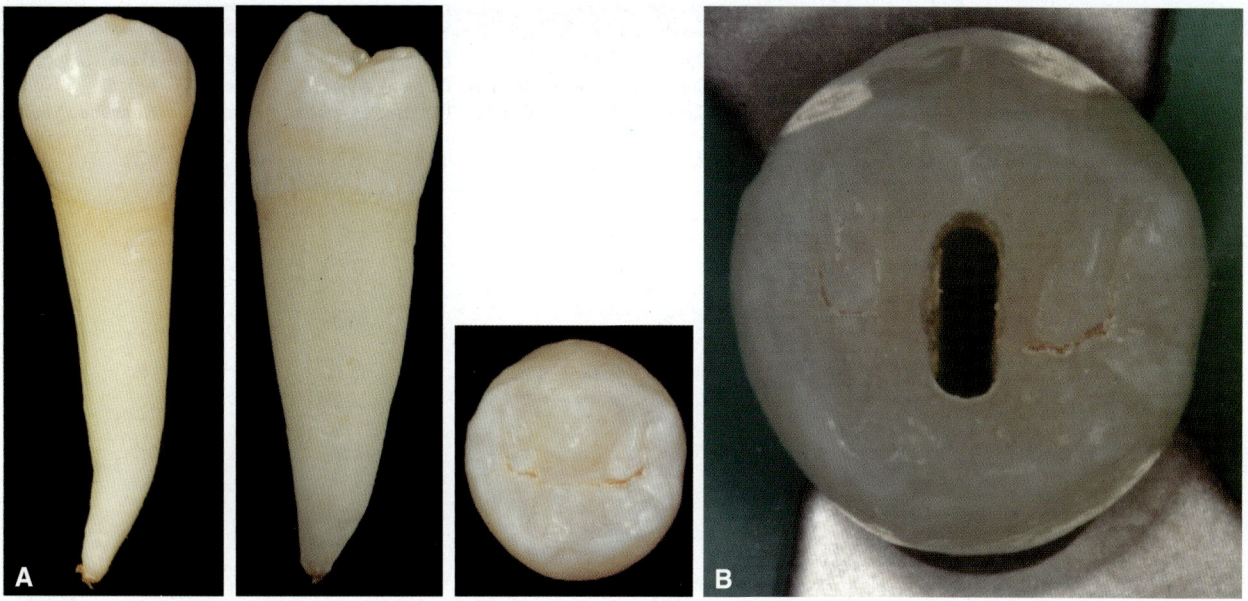

Figure 28 ***A***, Example of a mandibular second premolar showing buccal, mesial, and occlusal views. ***B***, The access preparation can be assessed from an occlusal view.

Table 8 Summary of Studies Detailing Root and Root Canal Anatomy of the Mesial Root of Mandibular First Molars											
Author	Year	Number of Teeth	Method	One Coronal Canal	Two Coronal Canals	Three Coronal Canals	Four Coronal Canals	One Apical Foramen	Two Apical Foramina	Three Apical Foramina	Four Apical Foramina
Gulabivala[93]	2002	118	Vacuum applied, dyed, decalcified, methyl salicylate	3.4%	89.8%	5.9%	0.8%	35.6%	60.2%	3.4%	0.8%
Sert[54]	2004	200	Decalcified and dyed	2%	94%	4%		51%	47.5%	1.5%	
Zaatar[94]	1998	49	Vacuum-drawn Duralay resin	6.2%	91.8%	2%		63.3%	36.7%	0%	
Skidmore[95]	1971	45	Vacuum-drawn polyester cast resin, decalcified	6.7%	93.3%			44.4%	55.6%		
Pineda[34]	1972	300	Radiographic ex vivo	12.8%	87.2%	0%		43%	57%	0%	
Vertucci[35]	1984	100	Decalcified, dye injected, cast in resin, microscope	12%	87%	1%		40%	59%	1%	
Caliskan[45]	1995	100	Dyed, decalcified, stereomicroscope x12	~4%	~96%	~3%		37%	56.6%	3.4%	
Walker[96]	1988	100	Radiographic ex vivo	3%	96%	1%		24%	75%	1%	
Wasti[68]	2001	30	Decalcified, ink-dyed, x10 dissecting microscope	0%	96.7%	3.3%		23%	73.7%	3.3%	
Pomeranz[97]	1981	61	Clinical in vivo	Not reported	Not reported	11.5%		Not reported	Not reported	1.6%	Not reported
Fabra-Campos[98]	1985	145	Radiographic clinical in vivo	0%	97.2%	2.8%		Not reported	Not reported	0%	
Da Costa[99]	1996	199	Decalcified, India ink-dyed gelatin injection	7.5%	92.7%		54.8%	45.4%			

Both mesial and distal roots are broad and usually have two canals and often have an interconnecting fin that can be extremely variable in its persistence at the apex. Mannocci et al.[100] found that of the 20 mesial roots observed with microcomputed tomography, 17 had isthmuses in one or more of the sectioned apical five

Table 9 Summary of Studies Detailing Root and Root Canal Anatomy of the Distal Root of Mandibular First Molars

Author	Year	Number of Teeth	Method	One Coronal Canal	Two Coronal Canals	Three Coronal Canals	Four Coronal Canals	One Apical Foramen	Two Apical Foramina	Three Apical Foramina	Four Apical Foramina
Gulabivala[93]	2002	118	Vacuum applied, dyed, decalcified, methyl salicylate	59.3%	34.7%	5.1%	0.8%	66.9%	28%	4.3%	0.8%
Sert[54]	2004	200	Decalcified and dyed	53.5%	45.5%	1%		87%	12%	1%	
Zaatar[94]	1998	49	Vacuum–drawn Duralay resin	8.2%%	91.8%	0%		83.7%	16.3%%	0%	
Skidmore[95]	1971	45	Vacuum-drawn polyester cast resin, decalcified	71.1%	28.9%			88.9%	11.1%		
Pineda[34]	1972	300	Decalcified, dye injected, cast in resin, microscope	70%	27%	0%		85.7%	14.3%	0%	
Vertucci[35]	1984	100	Decalcified, dye injected, cast in resin, microscope	70%	30%	0%		85%	15%	0%	
Caliskan[45]	1995	100	Dyed, decalcified, stereomicroscope x12	60%	52%	2%		81%	17%	2%	
Walker[96]	1988	100	Radiograpic in vitro	55%	45%	0%		72%	28%	0%	
Wasti[68]	2001	30	Decalcified, ink dye, x10 dissecting microscope	30%	70%	0%		56.7%	43.3%	0%	
Fabra-Campos[98]	1985	145	Radiographic clinical in vivo	50.34%	49.6%	0%		Not reported	Not reported	Not reported	
Da Costa[99]	1996	199	Decalcified, India ink-dyed gelatin injection	78.9%	21.1%			90.5%	9.5%		

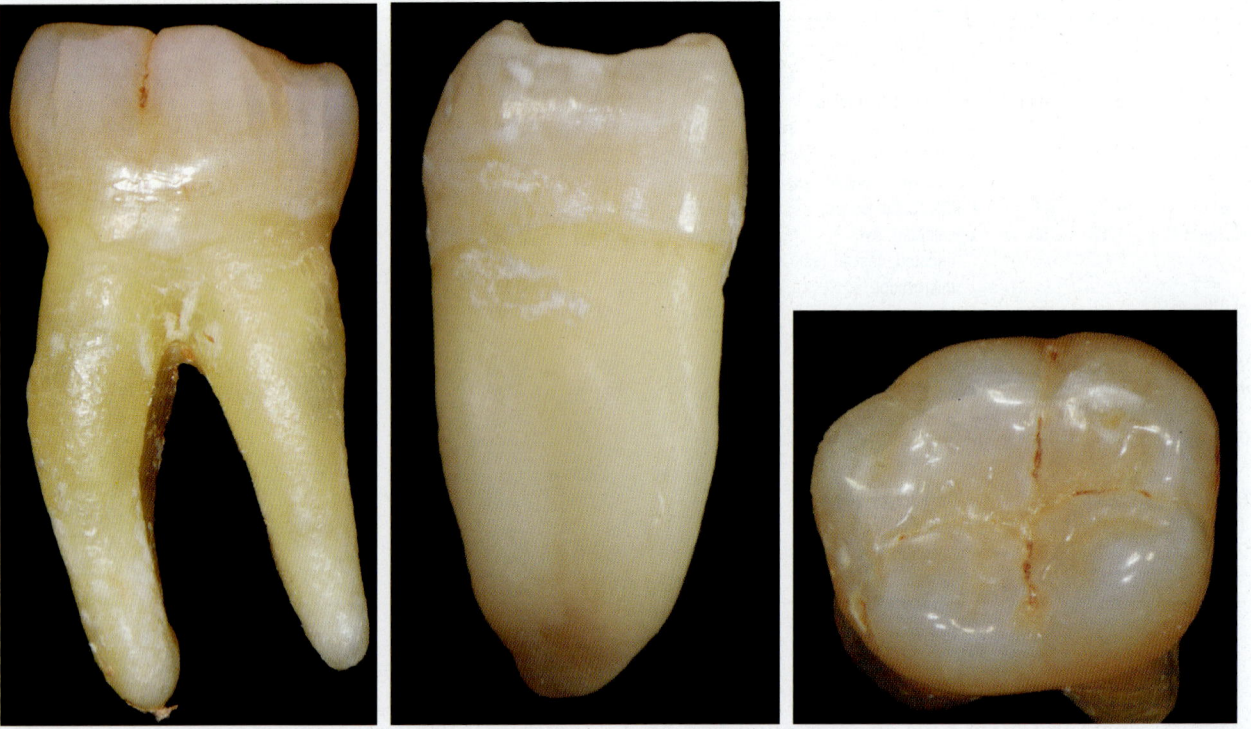

Figure 29 Example of a mandibular molar showing buccal mesial occlusal views. For access preparations, please see Figures 6 and 30.

millimeters. Only four of the 17 roots had an isthmus that was continuous from its coronal beginning to its apical end, the other 13 had sections with and without the isthmus. The third section from the apex had the highest incidence of isthmuses (50%). Two distal roots can occur but are rare—however, reported to be more prevalent in the South East Asian population.

CLINICAL

The important point to note with the mandibular molars is the degree to which they are lingually and mesially inclined.[19] To prevent unnecessary gouging of the axial walls of the access preparation, the bur should mimic this angulation of the tooth in the mandible.

The entry point is just mesial to the central pit. Initially, the access preparation should not be extended further distally as the distal canals project mesially toward the occlusal table. Once the angle of the canals has been determined with files, the decision can then be made to extend the access distally if needed. However, the access will be located largely in the mesial half of the tooth, as SLA for the mesial canals will dictate. Sometimes it is necessary to encroach on the mesiobuccal cusp tip to achieve SLA (Figure 30).

The groove between the mesiobuccal/mesiolingual and distobuccal/distolingual canals must always be troughed with a bur and/or ultrasonics and checked with files to search for mesial canals (Figure 31)—this can be best accomplished with a microscope.

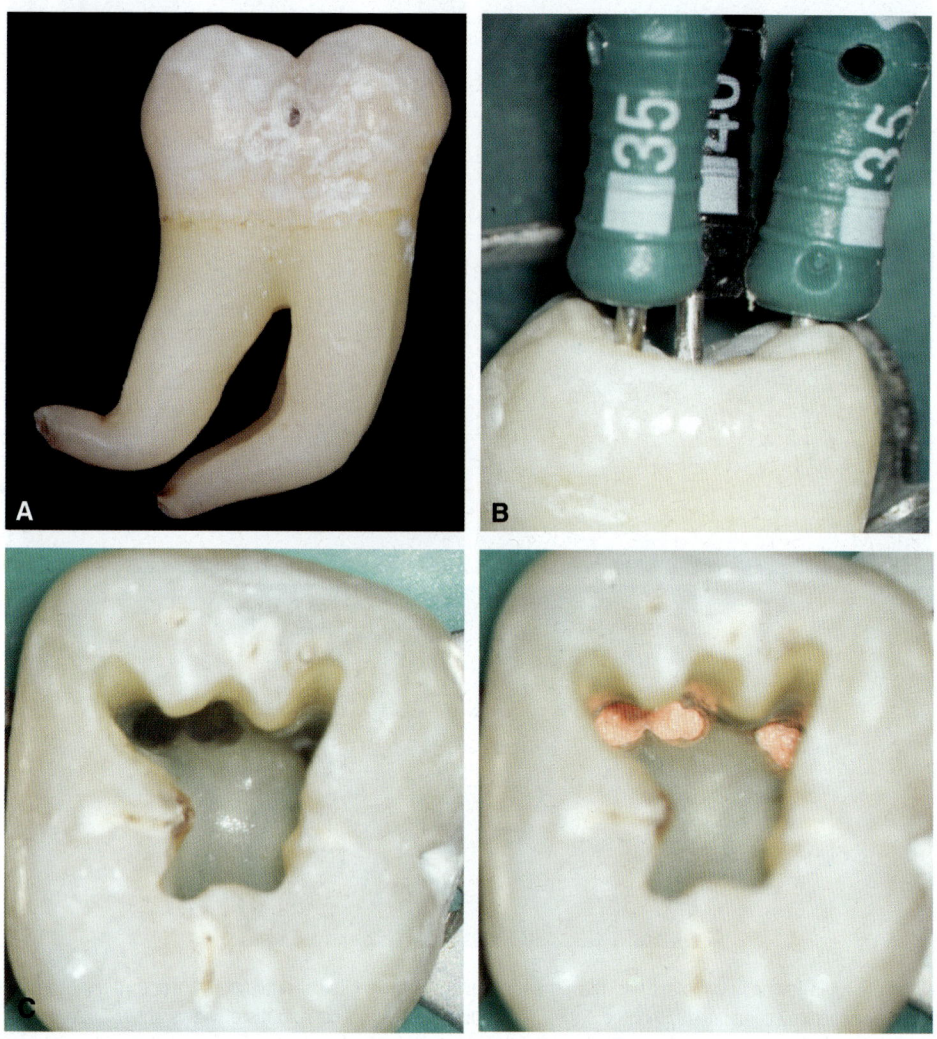

Figure 30 *A,* Access preparation in a mandibular molar with moderate/severe root curvature. *B,* Hand files can be placed to length in all three mesial canals after adequate access and canal preparation. *C,* However, the access preparation requires an extreme extension for the mesiobuccal and mesiolingual canals due to the root curvature.

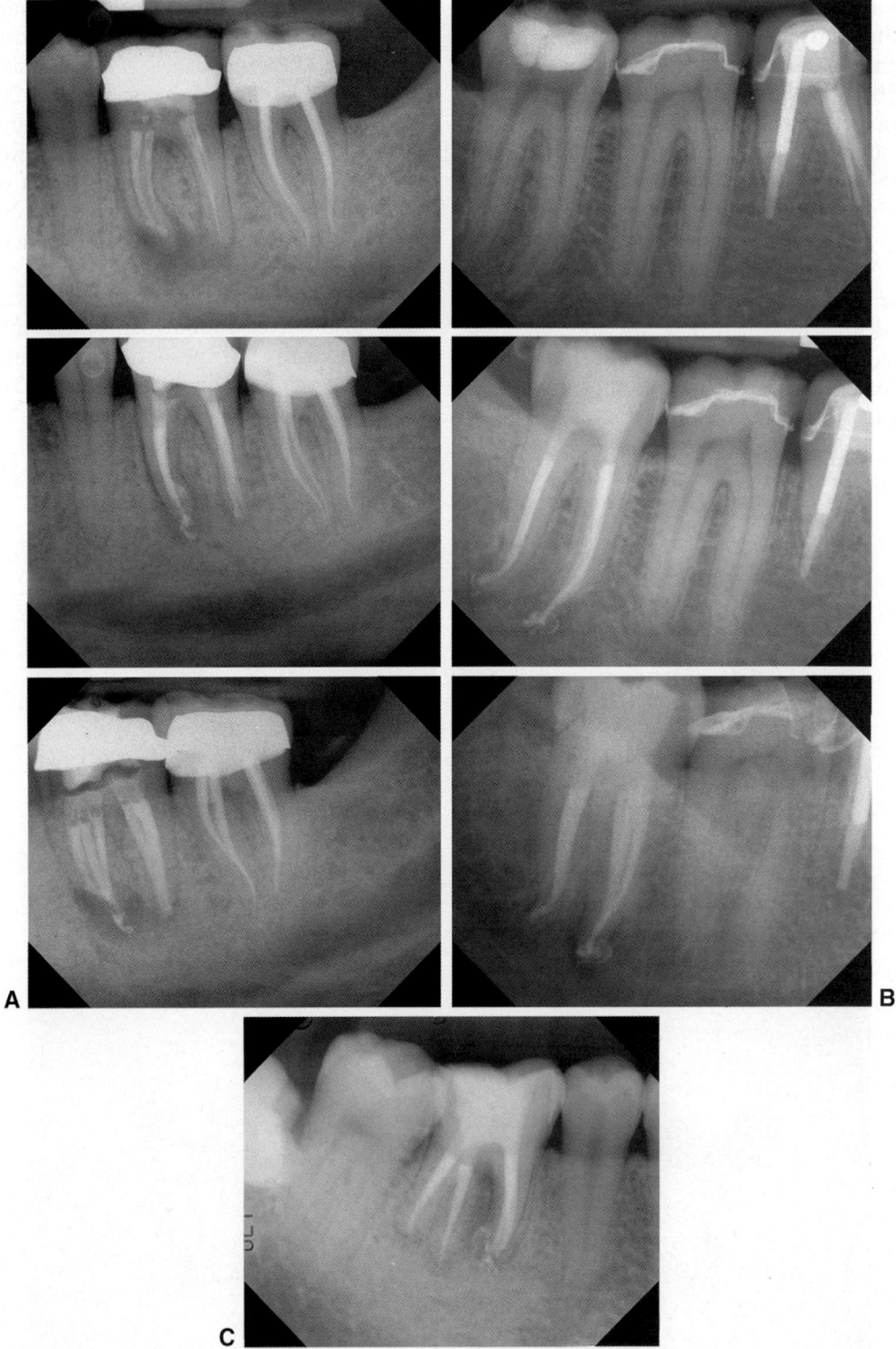

Figure 31 Anatomical variations in lower first molars and the potential for a negative clinical outcome. ***A***, Tooth diagnosed with a failing root canal treatment that had had an apicoectomy completed 8 months earlier. The postoperative buccal and distal views show three mesial canals with separate portals of exit, probably causing the persistent infection. ***B***, Mandibular third molar with preoperative view as well as straight and distal postoperative views. This tooth presented with three mesial canals; typically the middle mesial canal joins either the mesiobuccal or the mesiolingual canal early and is a more common form than the one in ***A***. ***C***, Tooth diagnosed with radix entomolaris. The distolingual root often has a significant curvature in the buccolingual plane and can therefore be deceptively difficult to treat.

The distal canal is ovoid or figure eight-shaped buccolingually if only one canal is present, and a microscope should be used to confirm this. There can be a second distal canal that bifurcates in the apical third—to minimize chances of missing these; the walls of the preparation should be divergent, and the clinician should be able to see the entire surface of the buccal and distal walls of the canal to the apex with a microscope. It is advisable to "feel" the wall of the canal with precurved files for areas in the middle and apical thirds of the canal where the instruments may stick.

It is easy to assume that the canals curve only to the mesial or the distal, but because these roots are so broad, they always have a curvature in the buccolingual dimension that cannot be assessed radiographically. Cunningham and Senia[14] showed that of the 100 mesial roots of mandibular molars, all demonstrated curvature in mesiobuccal and mesiolingual canals in both buccal and proximal view radiographs. They reported a reduction of canal curvature after coronal flaring. It is important to remember that the flaring will have to occur in both the mesial and buccal planes for mesiobuccal canals as well as in mesial and lingual planes for mesiolingual canals. Similar planes need to be addressed respectively for the distobuccal and distolingual canals. Fabra-Campos[101] found that 4 molars out of 145 had five canals that were confirmed radiographically—the extra canal was the middle mesial canal in the mesial root.

The presence and impact of furcation canals has been widely discussed. Vertucci and Williams,[102] using decalcification and staining, found that of the 100 mandibular first molars, 46% had furcation canals and 13% had a single lateral canal from the floor to the interradicular region. Of these, 57.1% extended from the center of the pulp floor, 28.5% arose from the mesial aspect of the floor, and 14.4% extended from the distal aspect. In 23%, lateral canals were found originating in the coronal third (distal root 80%, mesial 20%). Finally, in 10% of the cases, both lateral and furcation canals were found. Vertucci and Anthony[103] used scanning electron microscope (SEM) and found 32% of mandibular first molars and 24% of mandibular second molars, a total of 56% with accessory canals. Although relatively uncommon, mandibular first molars can also have C-shaped canals.[104,105] In a study on Burmese subjects, about 10.1% of observed teeth had an extra distal root on the lingual aspect (*radix entomolaris*).[106] Gulabivala et al.[93] found an additional distolingual root with one canal and one apical foramen 12.7% of the time (see Figure 31C).

Mandibular Second Molars

ANATOMY AND MORPHOLOGY

Generally, mandibular second molars differ from the first molars in their capacity for variation (Figure 32). Usually the crowns and roots of second molars are smaller than the first molars by less than a millimeter in all dimensions. The occlusal table is more symmetrical and rectangular with four equally apportioned cusps; a fifth cusp is not present. The roots of the second molars are inclined more distally, in relation to the occlusal table, than the first molars, but less than the third molars. Therefore, the access cavity may have to be extended more toward the mesial marginal ridge than for first molars. The roots, and therefore canals, are usually closer together and can be fused to a single conical root with varying internal anatomy or often C-shaped canal systems. Cooke and Cox[107] were the first to report C-shaped configurations in mandibular molars. Weine et al.[108] evaluated 811 endodontically treated second molars and reported 7.6% had C-shaped canal systems.

CLINICAL

The entry point of the access cavity should be mesial to the central pit similar to the first molars, but may not require the same degree of mesial extension if the roots are closer together. Otherwise, a similar preparation as for the first molar can be made. Cleaning C-shaped canals is unpredictable as there are many different types with several subtypes. The access cavity will follow the curvature of the canals.

According to Melton,[109] C-shaped canals can be divided into three categories:

Category I: The continuous C-shaped canal is any C-canal outline without any separation.
Category II: The "semicolon"-shaped canal—referred to canal configurations in which dentin separates one distinct canal from a buccal or a lingual C-shaped canal in the same section.
Category III: Simply with two or more discrete and separate canals.

Mandibular Third Molars

ANATOMY AND MORPHOLOGY

Third molars have significant variations and anomalies. They are usually less developed, with oversized crowns and undersized roots. Due to the lack of space in the jaws, they are often impacted and may have

916 / Endodontics

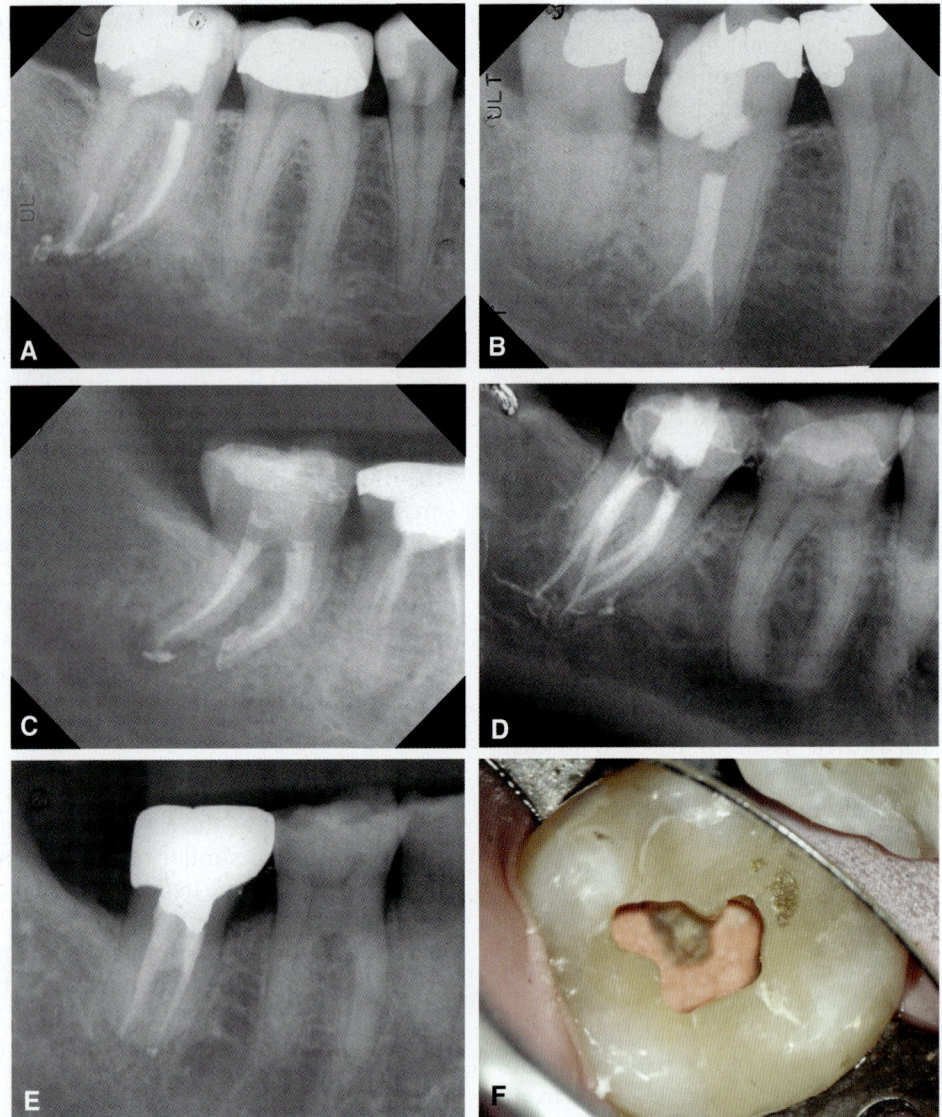

Figure 32 Variations in mandibular second molar anatomy. **A,** Common anatomy. **B,** Apical bifurcation. **C,** Dilacerated roots. **D,** Four separate apical foramina. **E, F,** C-shaped configuration.

very curved roots. They may have four or five cusps. Usually, when in good alignment and occlusion, the crown is likely to have four cusps and is similar to the second molar. Usually third molars have two roots—a mesial and a distal root that can be bifurcated or fused. When fully erupted and in functional occlusion, third molars provide excellent protection for the first and second molars by spreading the occlusal load. In such situations, keeping these teeth is beneficial and therefore knowledge of their anatomy and morphology is important.

CLINICAL

Similar to mandibular first molars, anatomical variations will require modifications compared to accessing first and second molars.

Procedural Mishaps

Successful endodontic treatment originates from a well-designed and executed access preparation. The opposite is also true; errors during root canal treatment can often be traced back to a problem originating from an inadequate access preparation. Errors generally stem from two access cavity characteristics: underextension and overextension.

UNDEREXTENSION

Not opening up the access cavity across the width of the root sufficiently can result in the operator missing canals. They can often be buried under calcified dentin. However, if the canal is found but the cavity is not extended away from the furcation sufficiently, the file will preferentially cut the furcal dentin causing a strip perforation. Another possibility, of not extending the access far enough, is that the coronal canal curvature is not removed. This will increase chances of instrument separation as the file tries to go around more than one curve, or transportation at the apex as the coronal canal curvature renders the file tip uncontrollable. Underextension of the access preparation also limits the final diameter of the apical preparation size. In anterior teeth, if the pulp horns are not adequately exposed and cleaned, the remaining pulpal tissue will cause coronal discoloration.

OVEREXTENSION

Generally, overextension will cause unnecessary removal of tooth structure that weakens the remaining crown and ultimately decreases the long-term prognosis of restoration, and therefore the tooth. With the acceptance of implants that have good long-term prognosis, remaining tooth structure will be the critical determinant between these two treatment choices.

Effect of Access Cavity Preparation on Structural Integrity

There is little debate that endodontic treatment weakens teeth resulting in an increased susceptibility to fracture (Figure 33).[110] But it has been widely stated that this may be due to endodontic treatment resulting in increased brittleness of the dentin.[111–114] However, it does not seem that root canal treatment changes the quality of the dentin, except some moisture loss,[115] and it is thought that weakening of the tooth is more a result of tooth structure loss.

Using strain gauges in extracted premolars, Reeh et al.[116] showed that endodontic procedures reduced the relative cuspal stiffness by only 5%. This was in contrast to an occlusal cavity preparation (20%), an MO/DO cavity (46%), and an MOD cavity preparation (63%). Howe and McKendry[117] examined 40 freshly extracted noncarious, unrestored human mandibular first and second molars, prepared endodontic access preparations and/or MOD amalgam cavities, and then subjected them to increasing occlusal load until fracture. They found that an endodontic access cavity, or a conservative MOD cavity, fractured at the same load (225.5 and 222.4 kg, respectively). On the other hand, an access cavity with both marginal ridges breached fractured with significantly less load (121.7 kg). Intact teeth fractured at significantly more force (341.4 kg) than all other groups. They suggested that when access cavities are kept conservative and proximal tooth structure remains intact, simple restoration of access cavities might suffice.

Sedgley and Messer[118] studied whether loss of pulp vitality resulted in changes in tooth structure as measured by biomechanical properties (punch shear strength, toughness, load to fracture, and microhardness). Twenty-three matched pairs of teeth were obtained where one tooth in each pair had endodontic treatment while the other was vital. Teeth were extracted and for comparison, data were collected immediately after extraction and after 3 months. The authors found no significant differences in punch shear strength, toughness, and load to fracture between groups. Vital dentin was 3.5% harder than the endodontically treated matched pair. They suggested that the dentin does not change in character but rather it is the cumulative loss of tooth structure from caries, restorative, and endodontic procedures that increases the susceptibility to fracture. Another possibility is that loss of pressoreception or an elevated pain threshold may allow larger loads without triggering a protective response.

In a study similar to experiments by Reeh et al.,[116] Panitvisai and Messer[119] measured actual cuspal deflection (rather than relative cuspal stiffness) and used more extensive cavity preparations (no tooth structure between access cavity and box preparation) to simulate clinical situations more closely. They used 13 extracted human mandibular molars and used a ramped load of 100 N to the mesial cusps. Increasingly extensive MO or MOD cavities were prepared, tested, and finally followed by an access preparation. They found that cuspal deflection increased with increasing cavity size, with the greatest deflection after access preparation when cuspal deflections of more than 10 μm were observed. They reiterated the importance of cuspal coverage to minimize marginal leakage and cuspal fracture.

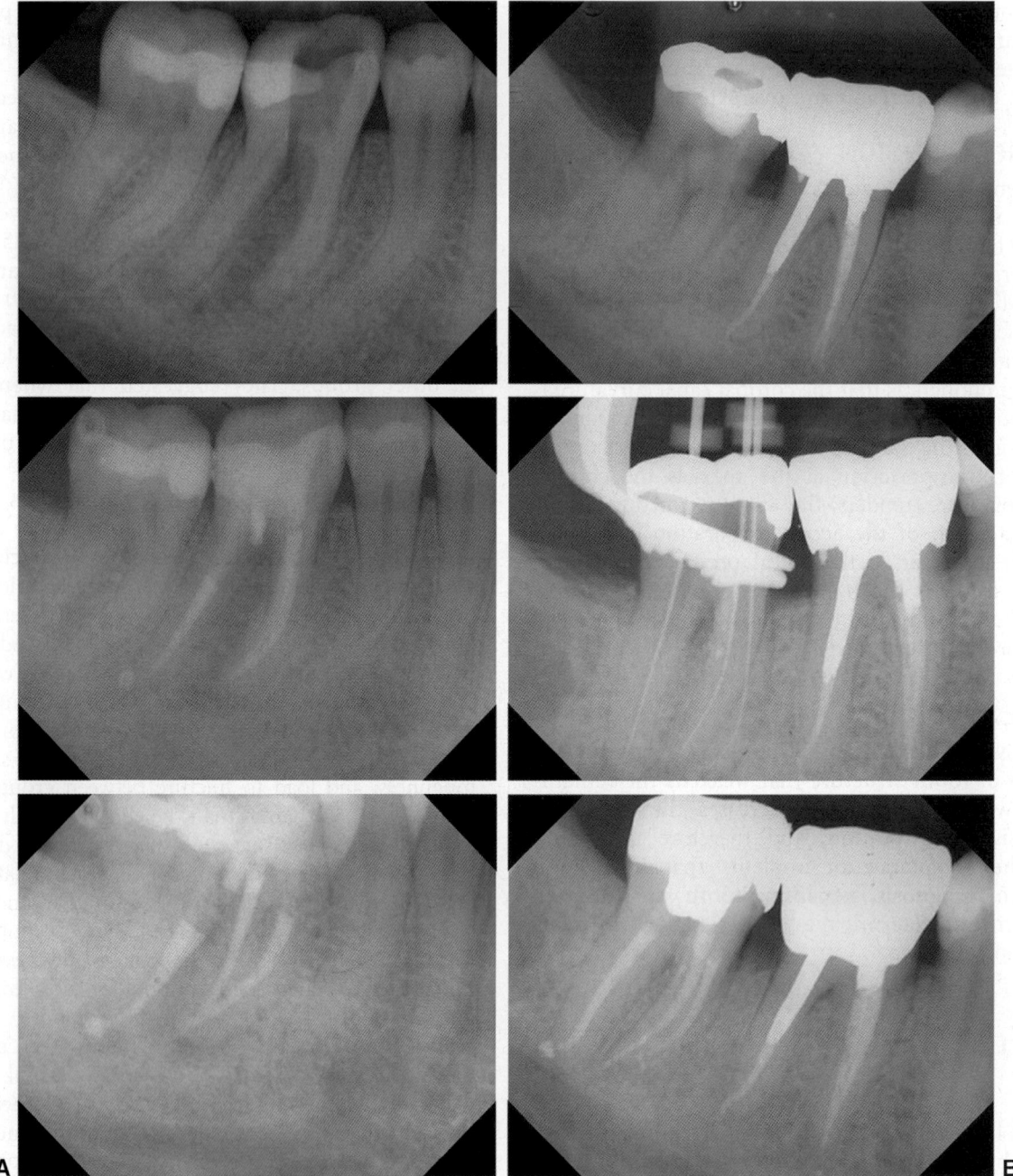

Figure 33 ***A***, Improper angulation of the bur resulted in furcal perforation. ***B***, Underextension of the mesial wall causing a strip perforation in the mesiolingual canal.

Radicular Preparations

OBJECTIVES

Upon the completion of the coronal access cavity and the identification of root canal orifices, preparation of the root canal system is initiated. Root canal preparation serves two main objectives: mechanical and chemical elimination of intracanal tissue and pathogens, aided by antimicrobial substances and by optimized root canal fillings.[120–122] A well-executed root canal preparation is a prerequisite for success (Figure 34).

Using anaerobic culturing, a reduction of intracanal bacteria after canal preparation has been demonstrated to a level of 10 to 100 CFU/mL,[9,123–127] but it is highly unlikely that any root canal is rendered sterile in a clinical setting. Both clinically successful and failing cases illustrate the presence of bacteria and immune cells.[128–130] However, in using stringent criteria for assessing healing of apical periodontitis, that is, the reconstitution of a lamina dura around the entire root perimeter[131] as well as the absence of inflammatory cells, only 6% of endodontically treated teeth were deemed successful.[128] The fate of bacteria initially remaining in inaccessible canal areas, regardless of the clinical technique,[132] has been a matter of speculation: do they die from starvation,[133] are they killed by sealer components[134] or can they survive and cause posttreatment disease?[135] On the other hand, a comparison of histological and clinical material

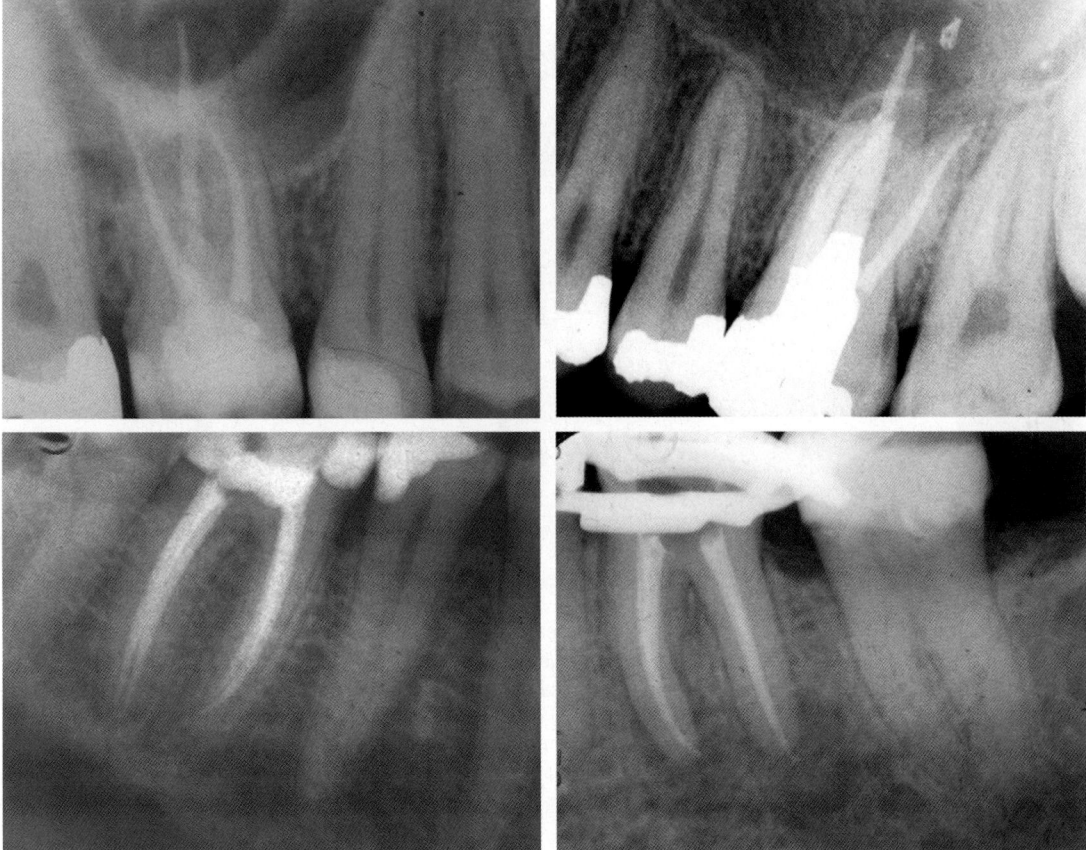

Figure 34 Examples of root canal-treated first maxillary and mandibular molars in which cleaning and shaping was done adhering to the principles laid out in this chapter. Radiographs represent situation immediately after root canal filling.

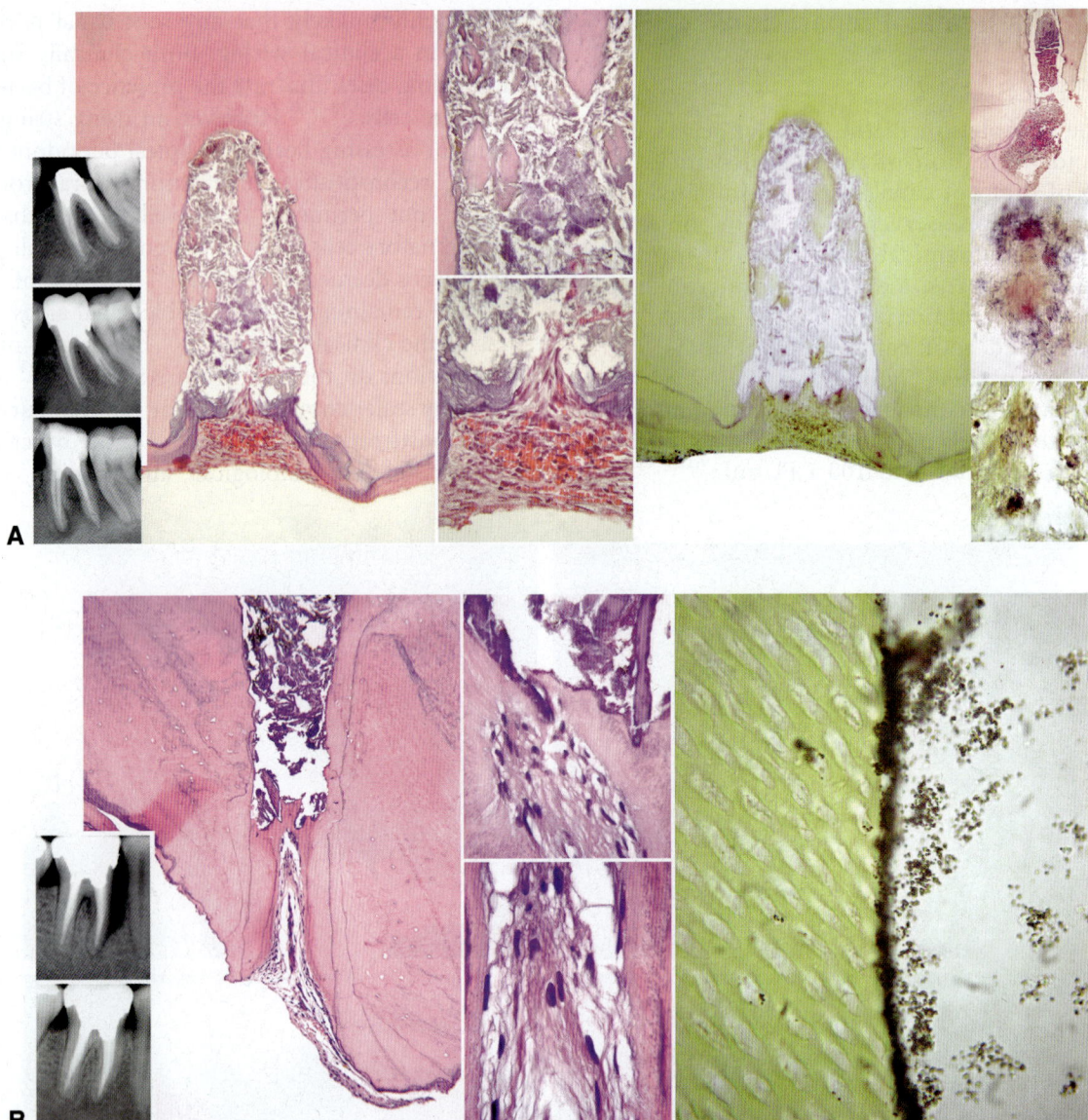

Figure 35 Healing is commonly detected by clinical and radiographic appearances and only occasionally it is possible to assess the outcome of root canal treatment histologically. Both cases shown here had preoperative diagnoses of chronic periapical periodontitis and were extracted for nonendodontic reasons. ***A,*** During the 13-year follow-up period of this case, the mesial root apex of this mandibular molar did not present complete healing of the original radiolucency, despite the absence of symptoms. The obvious reason was the presence of bacteria, as shown in the histological images. ***B,*** In this mandibular molar, the periapical region of the distal root exhibited radiographic healing, contrary to the mesial root, where a vertical fracture was the ultimate reason for extraction. Radiographic features of healing were confirmed by the histological picture, showing fibrous uninflamed tissue in the apical part of the root canal and calcified tissue. The latter did not completely obturate the lumen, as shown by serial sections. Images courtesy of Dr. Domenico Ricucci.

presented in Figure 35 demonstrates that histological success is present only if microbial contamination is absent.[136]

Furthermore, it was recently shown that well-filled and presumably well-shaped canals may still be associated with failing root canal treatments, mainly due to the fact that microorganisms remain in inaccessible areas of the root canal system.[137,138] Consequently, rather than "sterilizing" root canal systems, intracanal procedures are tailored to reduce microbial burden,

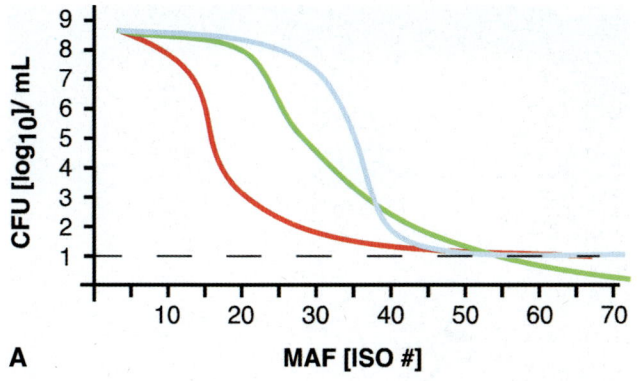

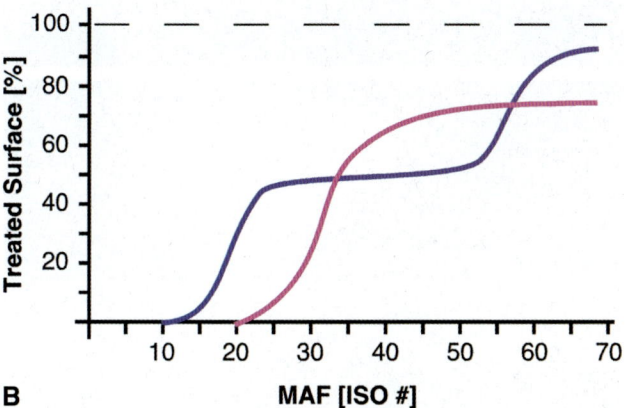

Figure 36 Proposed relationships between preparation size and elimination of bacteria as well as prepared canal surface. ***A,*** Based on bacterial sampling with a detection threshold of about 10 colony forming units (CFU), this threshold, essentially a canal with negative culture, may be reached on various pathways (colored lines in graph). ***B,*** Based on microcomputed tomography and analysis of cross sections, complete preparation of canal surface is unlikely. Again, values between 40 and 60% treated surface may be obtained with various canal shapes and apical sizes.

so that it becomes compatible with success, by creating conditions prohibiting regrowth and persistent infection.

Apparently, a threshold may be reached with different disinfection and preparation paradigms (Figure 36) that depend on numbers, virulence, and location of surviving microorganisms. The objective of root canal preparation, therefore, is to provide an environment in which periapical disease is prevented or the body's immune system achieves healing periapical disease.

A futuristic vision of ideal endodontic treatment is to replace necrotic or irreversibly inflamed pulp tissue with new healthy pulp tissue. Revascularization of empty pulp spaces in juvenile teeth may occur, but it is an ongoing topic of investigation and many open questions are yet to be solved.[139,140]

Because this ultimate goal is not yet obtainable, clinicians still have to deal with contaminated and inflamed pulp tissue. Rendering or keeping root canals bacteria-free during endodontic treatment is one of the most important goals to achieve successful healing or to maintain periapical health.[141] To reiterate, the prime condition under which medical professionals work, *nihil nocere* or "do not harm," should prevail in root canal treatments and canal preparation in particular, since obvious iatric errors are likely to decrease the prognosis of a case.

EVIDENCE AND STRATEGIES FOR SHAPING THE ROOT CANAL SYSTEM

The first objective, elimination of tissue and pathogens, is achieved by skillful instrumentation including copious irrigation and, if deemed necessary, interappointment medication. Mechanical instrumentation alone is effective in reducing bacterial load,[142,143] but should be complimented with irrigation to further eliminate microorganisms.[144,145] Some authors have differentiated between the mere flushing action of saline[142,146,147] and the added antimicrobial effect of the most widely used irrigant, sodium hypochlorite (NaOCl).[148,149] Both of those actions are dependent on canal size and shape,[10,150] but the latter depends also on factors such as NaOCl turnover, the amount of available chlorine, and contact time (for a more detailed review of endodontic irrigants, see Chapter 28, Irrigants and Intracanal Medicaments).

The accessibility of the contaminated root canal areas is key to disinfecting efficacy. Thus, overall canal anatomy and in particular canal dimensions (reviewed in detail in Chapter 6, Morphology of teeth and their root canal systems) play an integral role in radicular shaping (Figure 37). Two basic numerical concepts govern root canal shaping procedures (see Box 1): WL and apical size, recently also described as working width.[151]

Clinical experience has shown periapical bony lesions to heal predictably if the offending tooth is extracted, thus removing all intracanal and adhering microorganisms. This observation supports the notion that extraradicular bacteria play a minor role in supporting periapical disease, insofar as they colonize the periapical lesion.[152] Therefore, procedures

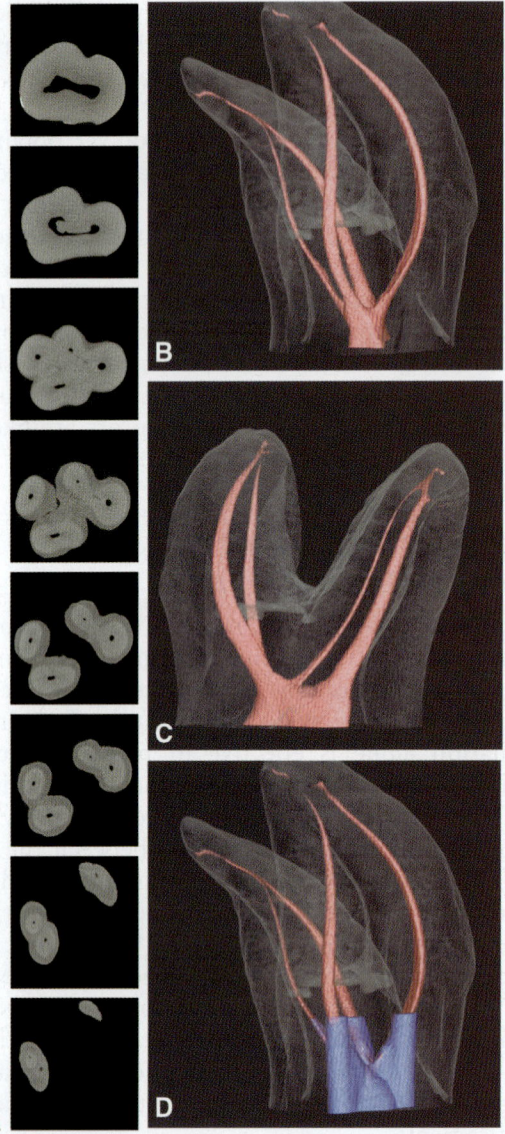

Figure 37 Relationship between cross sections of roots and root canals. Following the principles of dentinogenesis, the pulp space has a very similar outline as the outer root contour. ***A***, Sequence of microcomputed tomography slices (resolution 36 μm) of a second maxillary molar. ***B***, Clinical or buccolingual view of the reconstructed outer contour and root canal system. ***C***, Mesiodistal view clearly illustrating the existence of a fourth canal, in this case a second distobuccal canal that merges into the lingual (palatal). ***D***, Schematic illustration for the required amount of dentin removal in the coronal third for adequate access to middle and apical root canal thirds. Modified with permission from Peters OA. Pract Proced Aesthet Dent 2006;18:277.

confined to the root canal space[153–155] seem to be able to address most of the cases of endodontic treatment needs.

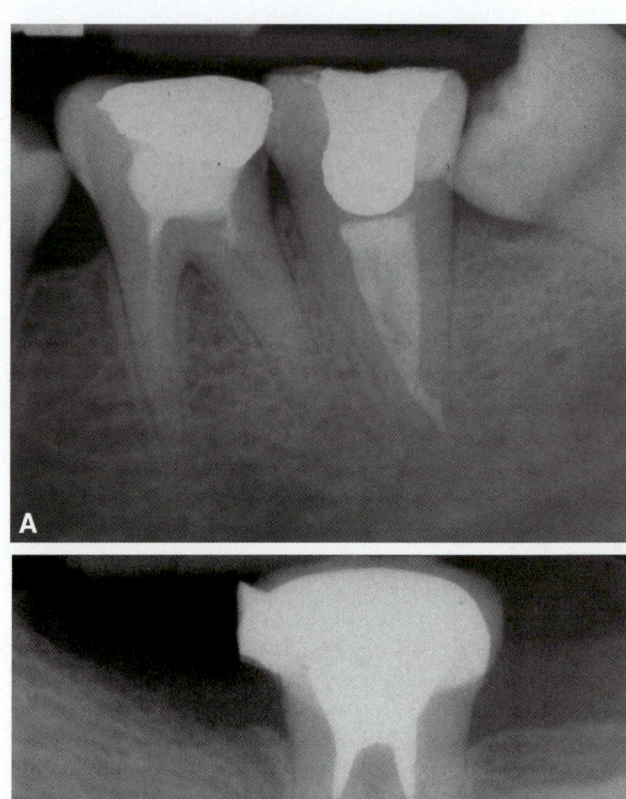

Figure 38 Examples of two cases in which incomplete shaping and short fills did not result in periapical pathosis. Patients indicated root canal treatments were performed ***A***, 10 years and ***B***, 27 years earlier.

Varying concepts have been proposed regarding WL,[155] partially depending on preoperative diagnoses. Clinical experience suggests that *vital cases* will be clinically successful despite apparent short fills (Figure 38). This may be explained by the absence of microorganisms in these cases, and a vital pulp stump may be beneficial for periapical health.[156,157] However, with existing periapical lesions and contaminated canal systems, WL definitions closer to the apex must be adopted. Classic studies suggest that a WL between 0 and 2 mm from the radiographic apex

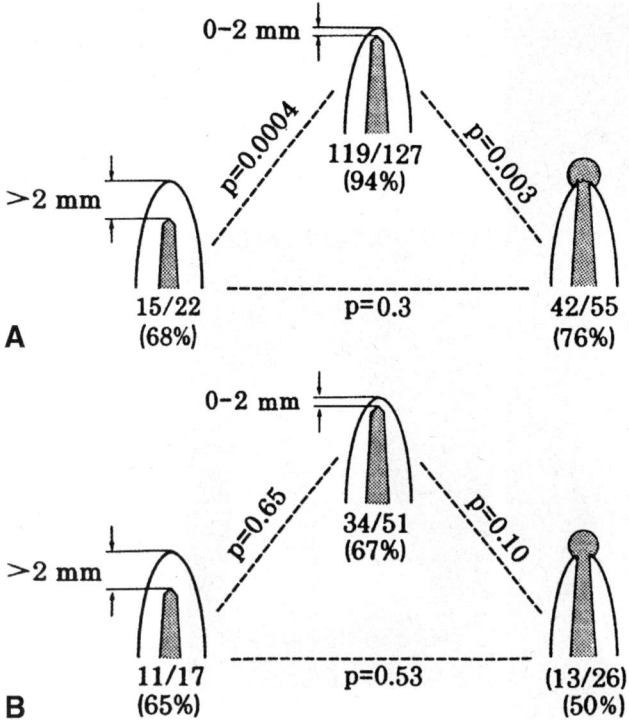

Figure 39 Relationship between the length of the fill and the presence and absence of periapical pathosis. **A,** Cases with a diagnosis of irreversible pulpitis. **B,** Cases with pulpal necrosis and periapical pathosis. Reprinted with permission from Sjögren U et al.[160]

results more often in success (healing of periapical lesions) than shorter or longer fills (Figure 39).

One school of thought recommends the use of a patency file, a small, that is, size #10, K-file that is gently just pushed through an apical foramen without actually enlarging it. The purported benefit is to "clean" a foramen and to avoid apical blockage; however, a clinical benefit of this approach has not been demonstrated so far. In fact, the patency technique is controversial and is not uniformly accepted or taught in all US dental schools.[158]

On the other hand, a deleterious effect that could have been brought about by mechanically injuring periapical tissues or by inoculating microorganisms[159] may be suspected but was not conclusively demonstrated.[160] This may be due to the fact that a contaminated file that passes through canal spaces filled with NaOCl is unlikely to carry any significant numbers of microorganisms past the foramen.[161] However, the extrusion of debris is more likely if the apical foramen is patent.[162,163] Certainly, cleaning the foramen, in the sense that the foramen is enlarged and debris is mechanically removed with a small file, is unlikely.[164]

It should be stressed that the use of a patency file is distinct from "apical clearing," which is defined as a technique to remove loose debris from the apical extent, and involves sequentially rotating files two to four sizes larger than the initial apical file at WL; the largest apical file is then again rotated after a final irrigation and drying.[165] This technique may be useful after hand instrumentation[166] but no effect has been shown after rotary instrumentation.

It is commonly held that the use of a patency file during preparation would minimize the blocking of canal space with dentin mud and thus improving shapes. However, Goldberg and Massone[167] showed canal transportation in more than half of their specimens shaped with stainless steel or NiTi K-files used as patency files. Confining shaping procedures to the canal space was already recommended by Schilder; he in fact stressed that the apical foramen should remain in its position and not be enlarged.[3]

The question then is where does the root canal end (Figure 40) and how close to that point can clinicians estimate their WL. Histological studies indicated the presence of the transition of the pulp to the periapical tissue as well as dentin and cementum in the area of constriction (Figure 41).[168] However, a constriction in the classic sense may be absent.[169] In fact, high-resolution tomographic studies suggest more complicated apical canal configurations than previously shown (Figure 42). Therefore, radiographic interpretation alone may not give the clinician a good estimate for WL determination.[170–172] Indeed, shaping to the radiographic apex, or even slightly short of it, will lead to frequent overinstrumentation.[171,173]

DETERMINATION OF WORKING LENGTH

The term "WL" (Figure 43 and Box 1) is defined in the Glossary of Endodontic Terms as "the distance from a coronal reference point to the point at which canal preparation and obturation should terminate."[174] The anatomical apex is the tip or the end of the root determined morphologically, whereas the radiographic apex is the tip or the end of the root determined radiographically.[174] It is well established that root morphology and radiographic distortion may cause the location of the radiographic apex to vary from the anatomical apex. The apical foramen is the main apical opening of the root canal. It is often eccentrically located away from the anatomical or the radiographic apex.[168,169,175,176] Kuttler's[168] investigation showed that this deviation occurred in 68 to 80%

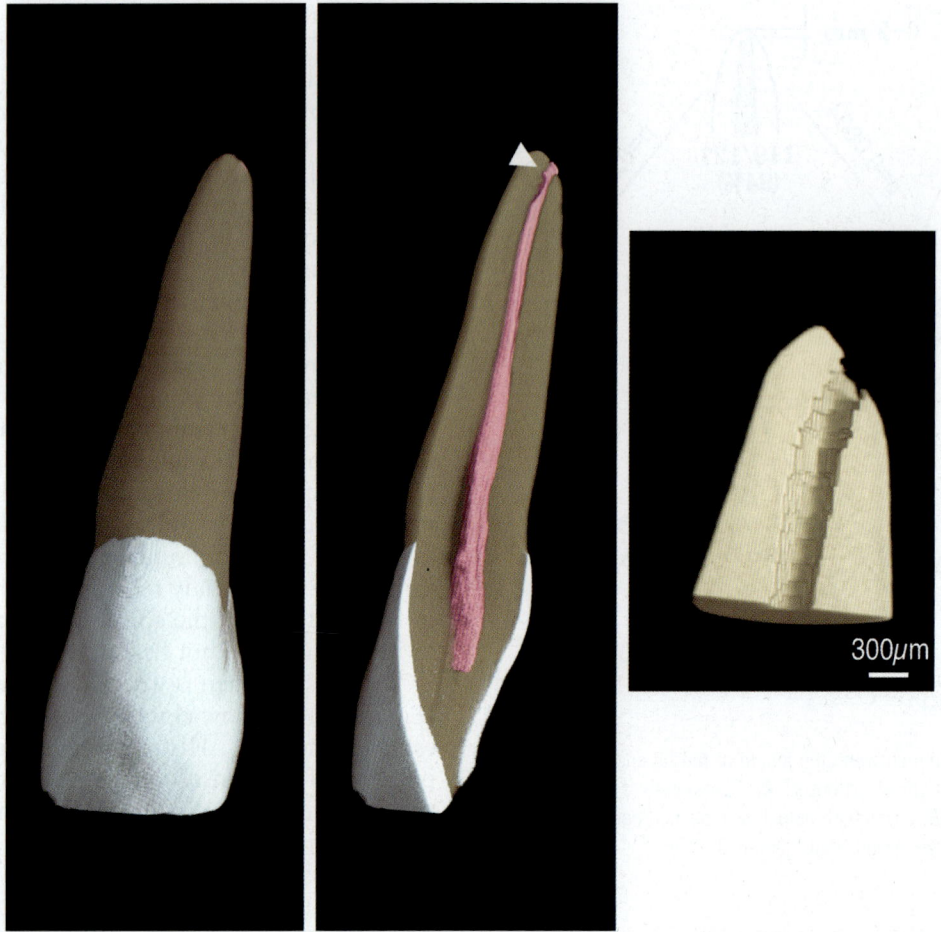

Figure 40 Microcomputed tomography reconstructions demonstrating external and internal anatomy of a maxillary anterior. The insert is a magnified view of an apical segment of 2 mm length showing no appreciable constriction (see arrowhead in larger image) and a cross-sectional diameter of the root canal of approximately 300 μm.

of teeth under investigation. An accessory foramen is an orifice on the surface of the root communicating with a lateral or an accessory canal.[174] They may be found as a single foramen or as multiple foramina. The apical constriction (minor apical diameter) (see Figures 40 and 43) is the apical portion of the root canal with the narrowest diameter. This position may vary but is often 0.5 to 1.0 mm short of the center of the apical foramen.[168,169] The constriction widens apically to the foramen (major diameter) and assumes a funnel shape.

Probably owing to its importance as a clinical entity, the apical third of the root canal and the foramen location have been the topic of numerous investigations.[7,168,169,175–183] Dummer et al.[169] reported four basic variations in the apical canal area that included about 50% of cases where a constriction was present. They also reported 6% of their cases where the constriction was probably blocked by cementum.[169] The cementodentinal junction is the region where the dentin and the cementum are united; this is the point at which the cemental surface terminates at or near the apex of a tooth.[174] Of course the cementodentinal junction is a histological landmark that cannot be located clinically or radiographically. Langeland[184] reported that the cementodentinal junction does not always coincide with the apical constriction. The location of the cementinodentinal junction also ranges from 0.5 to 3.0 mm short of the anatomical apex.[168,169,175,176] Therefore, it is generally accepted that the apical constriction is most frequently located 0.5 to 1.0 mm short of the radiographic apex. It has been pointed out by Ricucci[153] that significant anatomical variation makes difficult the direct clinical use of these average values as end points of canal preparation. Further problems exist in locating apical landmarks and in interpreting their positions on radiographs.

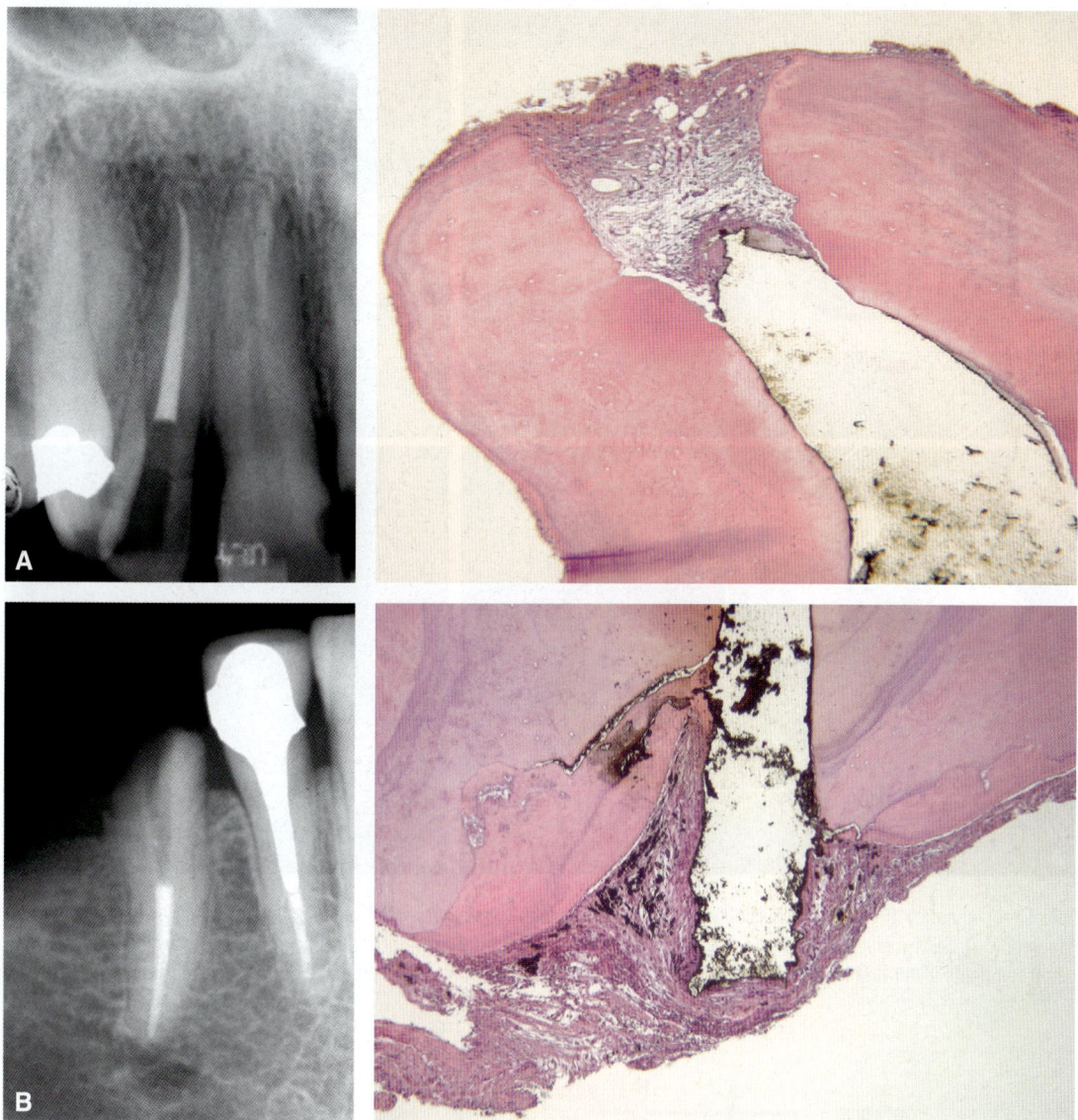

Figure 41 Comparison of radiographic and histological aspects of working length (WL). Teeth were extracted for nonendodontic reasons and processed for routine histological examination. *A,* Radiograph indicates adequate fill just short of the apex; light micrograph demonstrates short fill with connective tissue in the apical canal segment. *B,* Radiograph indicates adequate fill just short of the apex; light micrograph demonstrates overfill with some inflammatory cells surrounding the gutta-percha point. Images courtesy of Dr. Domenico Ricucci.

METHODOLOGICAL CONSIDERATIONS

Before determining a definitive WL, the coronal access to the pulp chamber must provide a straight-line pathway into the canal orifice. Modifications in access preparation may be required to permit the instrument to penetrate, unimpeded, into the apical constriction. Similarly, a crown-down preparation, including WL determination after initial shaping, will alleviate this problem. The loss of WL during cleaning and shaping can be a frustrating procedural error. Once the apical preparation is accomplished, it is useful to reassess the WL since the WL may shorten as a curved canal is straightened.[185–187] WL may also be lost owing to ledge formation or blockage of the canal.

As stated above, most dentists agree that the desired end point is the apical constriction. Failure to accurately determine and maintain WL may result in the length being too long and may lead to perforation through the apical constriction. Enlargement of the apical narrowing may lead to overfilling or overextension and subsequently to increased incidence of postoperative pain. In addition, one might expect a

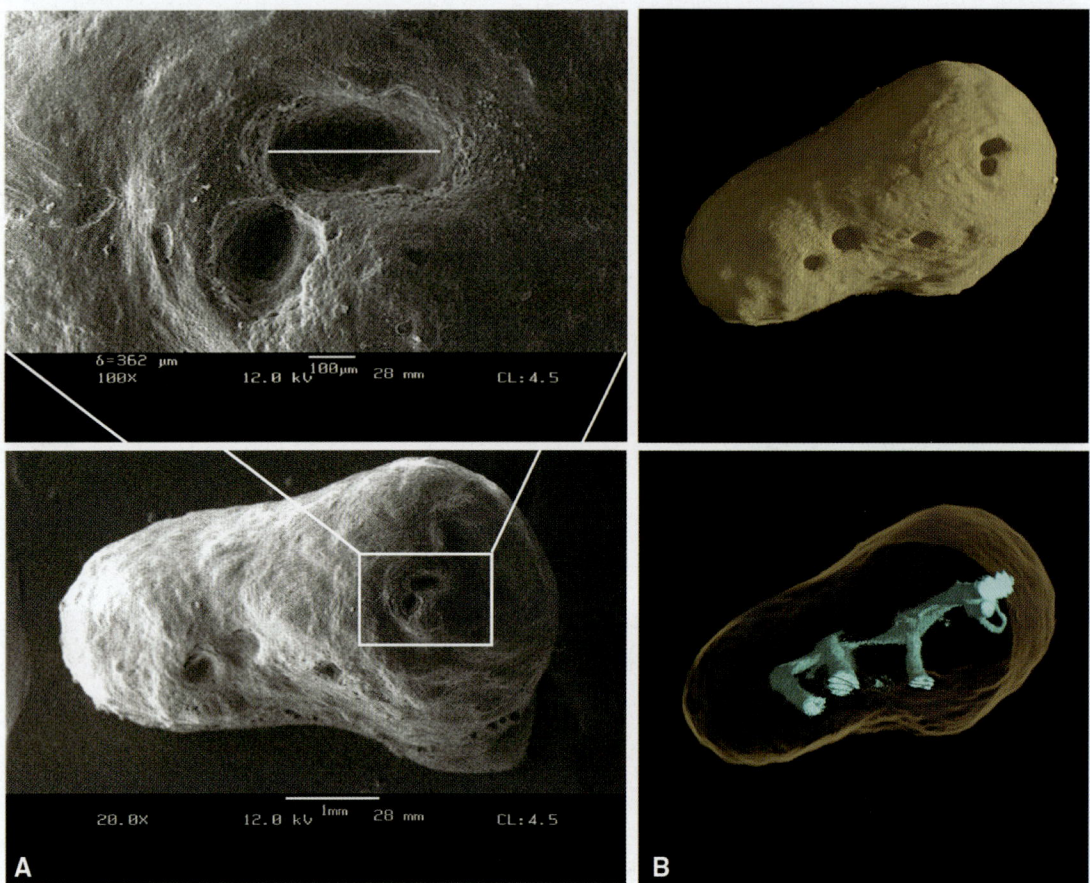

Figure 42 Apical root anatomy of the same mesiobuccal root of a maxillary molar assessed using scanning electron microscopy (SEM) and micro computed tomography. ***A,*** SEM pictures of multiple apical foramina at x20 and x100 magnification. Bar indicates long diameter of 0.35 mm. ***B,*** Outer contour and canal segments illustrated with μCT at a resolution of 9 μm. Note that all canals merge and connect. Images courtesy of Dr. Ephraim Radzik.

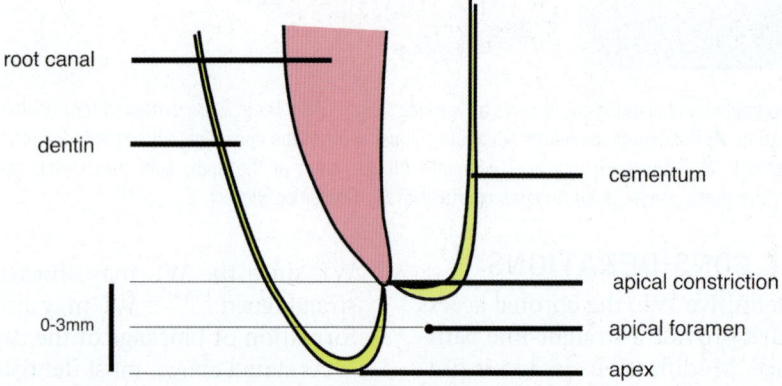

Figure 43 Schematic diagram of the root apex and anatomical landmarks. The distance between the anatomical apex and the narrowest point of the main root canal varies substantially and changes with cementum deposition during aging.

prolonged healing period and lower success rate.[153,155,188–190] Failure to determine and maintain WL accurately may also lead to shaping and cleaning short of the apical constriction. Incomplete cleaning and underfilling may cause persistent discomfort, may support the continued existence of viable bacteria, and thus contribute to a continued periapical lesion and ultimately a lowered rate of success.

In this era of improved illumination and magnification, WL determination should be to the nearest one-half millimeter, which is the maximum resolution of the naked eye in working distance. The measurement should be made from a secure reference point on the crown in close proximity to the straight-line path of the instrument, a point that can be identified and monitored accurately. The length adjustment of the stop attachments should be made against the edge of a sterile metric ruler or a gauge made specifically for endodontics (Figure 44). The requirements of an ideal clinical method for determining WL include rapid location of the apical constriction in all pulpal conditions and all canal contents; easy measurement, even when the relationship between the apical constriction and the radiographic apex is unusual; rapid periodic monitoring and confirmation; patient and clinician comfort; minimal radiation to the patient; ease of use in special patients such as those with severe gag reflex, reduced mouth opening, pregnancy; and

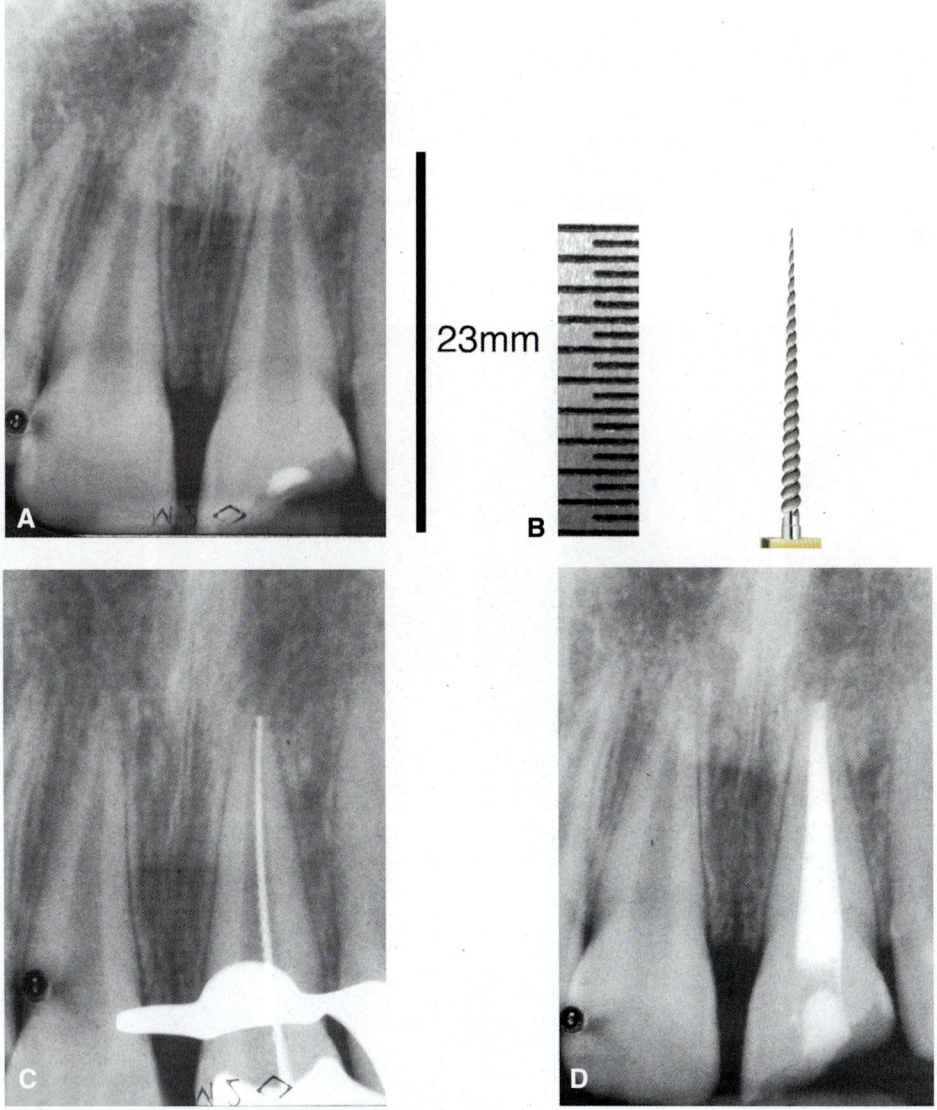

Figure 44 Sequence of steps in working length (WL) determination. ***A,*** Initial measurement. Tooth is measured on an orthogonal and diagnostic preoperative radiograph. In this case the tooth seems to be about 23 mm long. ***B,*** Tentative WL, as a safety measure during coronal pre-enlargement and crown-down, subtract 1 mm from tooth length and allow instruments to go to two-thirds of this length. ***C,*** After the coronal two-thirds of the canal have been prepared, advance the hand file to tentative full WL, using the electronic foramen locator, and expose the radiograph. ***D,*** Final radiograph after root canal filling and removal of rubber dam.

cost effectiveness.[172,191,192] To achieve the highest degree of accuracy in WL determination, a combination of several methods should be used. This is most important in canals for which WL determination is difficult.[193] The most common methods are radiographic methods, digital tactile sense, patients' response to a file introduced into the canal, or a point to which a paper point can be placed and removed dry.[194] However, current electrical foramen locators (see Chapter 26D, Electronic Apex Locators) greatly aid in determining the narrowest cross-sectional diameter and width and therefore in approximating WL.[195]

CLINICAL DETERMINATION OF WORKING LENGTH

Methods requiring formulas to determine WL have been largely abandoned. Bramante and Berbert[196] reported great variability in formulaic determination of WL, with only a small percentage of successful measurements. The following items are essential to perform radiographic WL estimation:

1. Good, undistorted, preoperative radiographs showing the total length and all roots of the involved tooth.
2. Adequate coronal access to all canals.
3. An endodontic millimeter ruler.
4. Working knowledge of the average length of all of the teeth.
5. A definite, repeatable plane of reference to an anatomical landmark on the tooth, a fact that should be noted on the patient's record.

To secure reproducible reference points, cusps severely weakened by caries or restoration may be reduced to a flattened surface, supported by dentin. Failure to do so may result in cusps or weak enamel walls being fractured between appointments (Figure 45). Thus the original site of reference is lost. If this fracture is not accounted for, then there is the

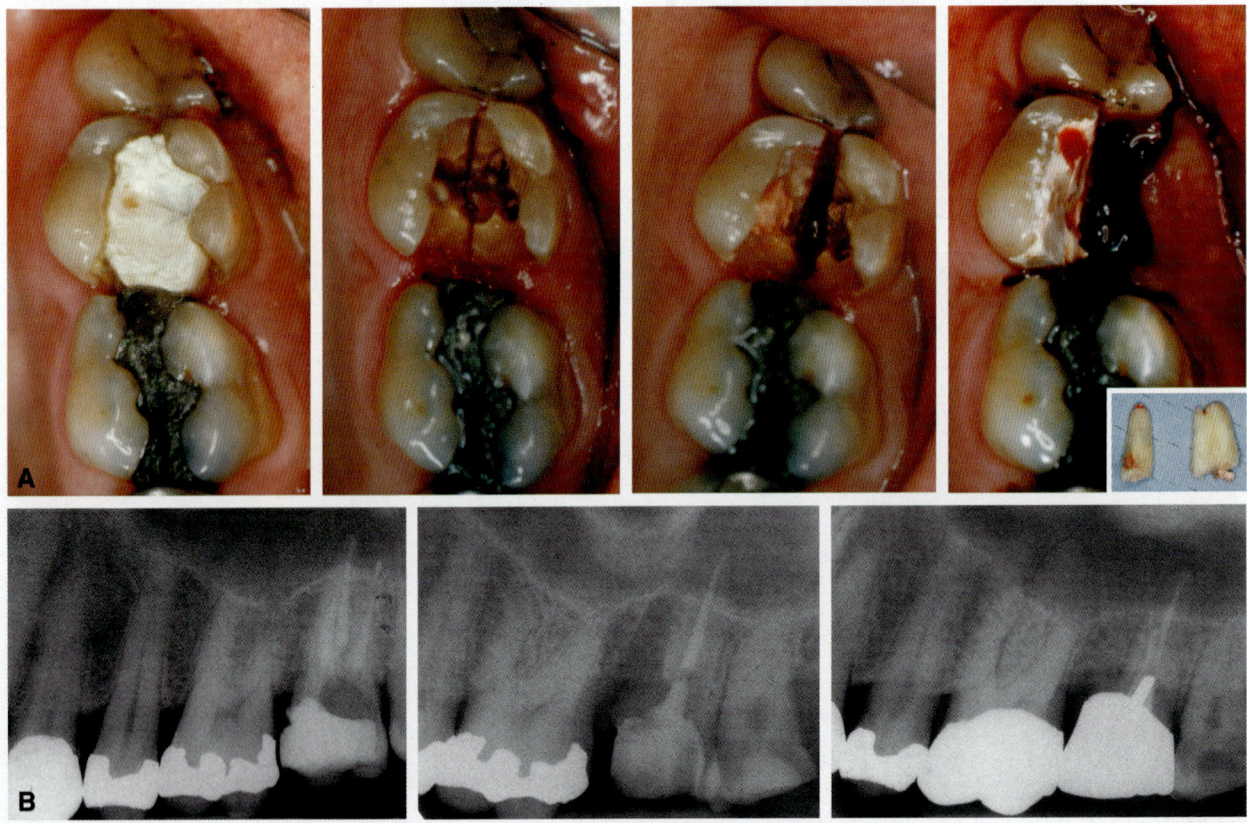

Figure 45 Example of a root canal-treated tooth that presented with a fracture prior to placement of the planned definitive restoration. In this case, the palatal root was preserved and crown was restored after placement of a post and core. **A,** Clinical sequence from temporized access to status after surgical extraction of the two buccal roots. **B,** Radiographs immediately after endodontic treatment, after surgery and at 1-year follow-up. Images courtesy of Dr. Craig Noblett.

probability of overinstrumentation and overfilling. To establish the length of the tooth, a K-file with an instrument stop on the shaft is needed. The exploring instrument size must be small enough to negotiate the total length of the canal but large enough not to be loose in the canal. A loose instrument may move in or out of the canal after the radiograph and may also cause errors in determining tooth lengths. Moreover, tips of fine instruments (size #08 and #10) are often difficult to see in a radiograph,[197] as are NiTi instruments.

Clinically, it is advisable to estimate canal lengths from a preoperative radiograph (see Figure 44). About 1.0 mm "safety allowance" for possible image distortion is deducted,[198,199] the endodontic ruler is set to this tentative WL, and the stop on the instrument adjusted at this level (see Figure 44). The instrument is placed in the canal until the stop is at the plane of reference unless pain is felt, in which case the instrument is left at this level and the rubber stop readjusted. An electric foramen locator (see Chapter 26D, Apex Locator) should be used to verify and potentially further adjust the rubber stop. A radiograph is exposed and the difference between the end of the instrument and the end of the root is determined.

Current apex locators are sufficiently precise[200] to allow WL determination, thus reducing the frequency of overinstrumentation when only radiographs are used.[173,201] Even in cases of apical resorption and wide-open apices after root-end resection, these apex locators are shown to be accurate.[202,203] Therefore, it seems warranted to focus on the electronically determined WL and to use the radiograph merely to avoid gross errors in case the apex locator does not appear to work correctly. This strategy eliminates approximation strategies such as shortening WL, as suggested by Weine,[204] to allow for apical resorption. Independent of the strategy, the final WL and the coronal point of reference are recorded on the patient's chart. When two canals located in the buccolingual plane appear to be superimposed, much confusion and time may be saved by several simple means. Occasionally, it is advantageous to take individual radiographs of each canal with its length-of-tooth instrument in place. A preferable method is to expose the radiograph from a mesial–horizontal angle. This causes the lingual canal to always be the more mesial one in the image (MLM, also known as Clark's rule). For any mesial- or distal-angulated radiographs, the SLOB ("same lingual, opposite buccal") rule, or the Ingle MBD Rule ("**S**hoot" from the **M**esial and the **B**uccal root will be **D**istal), may be applied to locate instruments.

Radiographic WL determination, using conventional films alone, is accurate less than 90% of the time,[176,205,206] and it is unclear if digital radiography is currently an improvement over conventional films regarding WL determination accuracy.[207] In fact, inferior[208] as well as superior[209,210] results were reported for phosphor plate systems. Sensor-based radiovisiography performed similar to films regarding accuracy in some studies[211–213] but was recently shown to be superior.[214]

Electronic foramen locators sometimes do not function accurately, for example, in cases where current may flow into the marginal gingiva or into metal restorations causing erroneous readings. Therefore, additional methods such as tactile assessment and detection of moisture on the tip of a paper point were recommended.[176] If the coronal portion of the canal is not constricted, an experienced clinician may also detect an increase in resistance as the file approaches the apical 2 to 3 mm. This detection is by tactile sense. In the apical region, the canal frequently features a constriction or a smaller diameter before exiting the root. There is also a tendency for the canal to deviate from the radiographic apex in this region,[7,168,175] and both these geometric features may be perceived by a clinician. However, Seidberg et al.[194] reported an accuracy in WL determination of just 64% using digital tactile sense. If the canals were preflared, it was possible for an expert to detect the apical constriction in about 75% of the cases.[215] If the canals were not preflared, determination of the apical constriction by tactile sensation was possible in only about one-third of the cases.[216] Preflaring and subsequently determining WL also reduce the amount and incidence of WL changes during the course of canal shaping procedures.[186]

All clinicians should be aware that this method, by itself, is often inexact. It is ineffective in root canals with an immature apex and is highly inaccurate if the canal is constricted throughout its entire length or if the canal has excessive curvature. Therefore, tactile detection should be considered as a supplementary to high-quality, carefully aligned, parallel WL radiographs and/or an apex locator. Consequently, a survey found that few general practice dentists and no endodontists trust the digital tactile sense method of determining WL by itself.[217] Even the most experienced specialist would be prudent to use two or more methods to determine accurate WLs in every canal.

In a root canal with an immature (i.e., wide open) apex, a relatively reliable means of determining WL is by gently passing the blunt end of a paper point into the canal after profound anesthesia has been achieved.

The moisture or blood on the portion of the paper point that passes beyond the apex may be an estimation of WL or the junction between the root apex and the bone. In cases in which the apical constriction has been lost owing to resorption or perforation, and in which there is no free bleeding or suppuration into the canal, the moisture or blood on the paper point is an estimate of the amount the preparation overextended. This paper point measurement method is also a supplementary one. As stated earlier, nonsurgical endodontic procedures should best be confined to the root canal. This is true for files also, or paper points, in the process of WL determination. WL determination should be painless. Advancing an instrument into a canal toward inflamed tissue may cause moderate to severe instantaneous pain. At the onset of the pain, the instrument tip may still be several millimeters short of the apical constriction. When pain is inflicted in this manner, little useful information can be gained and considerable damage is done to the patient's trust. When the canal contents are necrotic, however, the passage of an instrument into the canal and past the apical constriction may evoke only a mild awareness or possibly no reaction at all.

On the other hand, Langeland et al.[184,218] reported that vital pulp tissue with nerves and vessels may remain in the most apical part of the main canal even in the presence of a large periapical lesion. Finally, passing a file through necrotic canal contents may inoculate bacteria-contaminated dentin shavings into periapical tissues, thus supporting or causing apical periodontitis.[219,220] However, Izu et al.[161] showed that small files used as patency files are unlikely to carry bacteria past a reservoir of NaOCl.

CLINICAL DETERMINATION OF WORKING WIDTH

The second factor to be considered is apical width or preparation size. It is a matter of debate as to which apical enlargement and more specifically which shape would lead to an optimal reduction of the intracanal microbial load.[221] Baumgartner's group[10,150] has recently attempted to address this question in vitro, and they concluded that an apical preparation size #20 would be inferior to sizes #30 and #40 regarding canal débridement but that a larger taper (e.g., 0.10) may potentially compensate for smaller sizes. This notion is supported by an in vitro study on the efficacy of ultrasonically activated irrigation that demonstrated better débridement with 0.10 taper preparation.[222] Similarly, Mickel et al.,[12] based on microbiological assays, as well as Khademi et al.,[223] using SEM, found that apical preparation to size #30 is required to effectively clean root canals. Moreover, recent elegant analyses, using a thermal imaging system, revealed detailed relationships between MAF size, needle diameter, and insertion depth.[224] Taken together, these results indicate that sufficient apical preparation size and the use of a small-caliber irrigation needle are desirable to promote irrigation and hence antimicrobial efficacy.

In situ, however, even larger apical preparation sizes were favored by results from Trope's group,[9,125,127] in particular, when an interappointment dressing of calcium hydroxide was used. Interestingly, larger apical sizes (#40, taper 0.04 compared to #20, taper 0.10) facilitated the application of calcium hydroxide medication in vitro.[225]

Most clinical outcome studies incorporate the factor "apical preparation size" with often insufficient statistical power and with conflicting results.[226–228] A review of the technical aspects of root canal treatments[229] found that apical periodontitis was more frequent with inadequate root canal fillings; however, they did not find evidence that canal instrumentation methods, and in particular apical sizes, had any measurable effect on outcomes. Conversely, one result of the Toronto study[230] on endodontic outcomes seemed to favor smaller preparations in conjunction with tapered shapes and vertically compacted gutta-percha over step-back preparation to larger apical shapes (90% and 80% success, respectively). Again in contrast, using Periapical Index (PAI) scores determined from radiographs, Ørstavik et al.[231] did not find any significant impact of preparation size on outcomes.

It is not possible to determine canal diameters from radiographs;[151] however, μCT scans may be able to give more detailed information regarding root canal anatomy in vivo (Figure 46). The resolution of current systems is in the range of 100 μm, corresponding to a size #10 K-file, and hence not sufficient to determine canal diameters with precision. Clinically, canal width may be determined by passing a series of K-files to WL to gauge, as suggested by Ruddle.[232] This process may depend on the file type and the amount of preflaring.[8,233,234] Clearly, the first instrument that gives the clinician a sense of binding does not correspond to any canal diameter. Wu et al.[8] demonstrated that the diameter of the "binding" instrument was smaller than the canals' diameter in 90% of the cases with a difference of up to 0.19 mm. Unexpectedly,

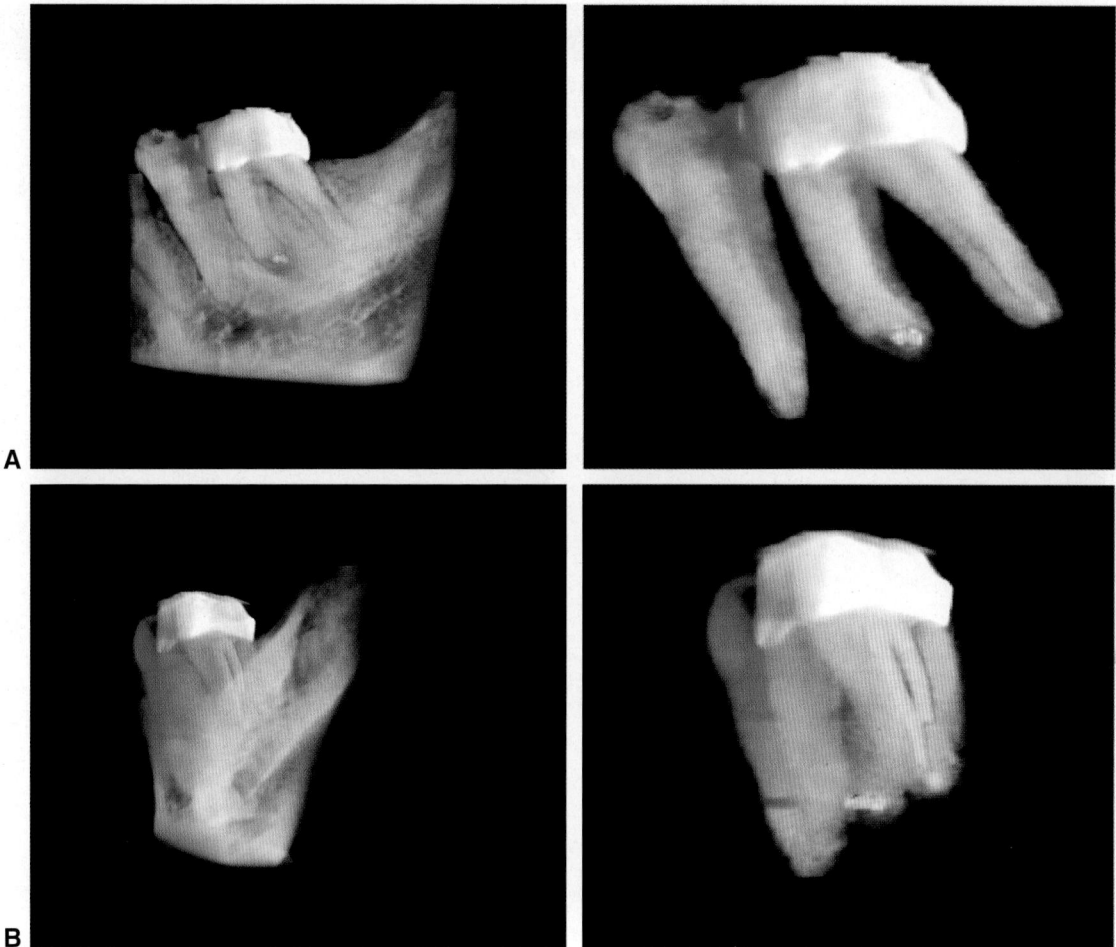

Figure 46 Potential of a clinically used high-resolution computed tomography to show root canal anatomy. Scans were done in vivo using an Accuitomo cone beam machine (Morita, Tokyo, Japan). **A,** Reconstructed jaw segment with three teeth is shown after apicoectomy and retrograde fill of mesial root of lower left first molar in clinical. **B,** Distally angled projection. Two teeth were segmented free from bone and are shown independently. Note incomplete fill of mesial root and two merging canals in the distal root of the molar.

LightSpeed (LS) instruments (Discus Dental, Culver City, CA) that possess a fine noncutting shaft did not perform better than K-files with 0.02 taper. Therefore, they concluded that it is uncertain that circumferential removal of dentin occurs based on the criterion that one should prepare three sizes larger than the first binding file;[8] this and also the criterion "clean dentin shavings" are not considered adequate to indicate sufficient apical preparation.[235]

It seems that preflaring, prior to any attempt at assessing canal diameter, is essential[233,234] since it allows the probing file to approach the apical area with less interferences. Tan and Messer[233] indeed found that K-files and LS instruments determined apical sizes about one ISO size larger after preflaring. In their study, LS instruments that were felt to bind at the apex were almost two ISO sizes larger than K-files.

After preoperative canal size is estimated, working width determination may be done. Jou et al.[151] suggested definitions based on variations in cross-sectional canal shape. Their goal was to allow clinicians to obtain a more complete shape regarding instrumented surface area; this strategy is in line with current guidelines.[236,237] However, this goal may be unattainable with current instrumentation techniques.[120] In conclusion, there may be no practical way to objectively determine a final file size that predictably allows complete instrumentation of canal walls. Consequently, all potential mechanisms to increase irrigation efficacy should be explored.

Table 10 Measured Apical Diameters and Suggested Preparation Sizes for Mandibular and Maxillary Teeth, Taken from Representative References over the Last 50 Years

Reference	Kuttler[168]	Green[177]	Kerekes[51,238,239]	Morfis[180]	Wu[182]	Briseno[183]	Grossman[240]	Sabala[241]	Tronstad[242]	Glickman[243]
Type	268 Teeth In Vitro	110 Teeth In Vitro	220 Teeth In Vitro	213 Teeth In Vitro	180 Teeth In Vitro	1,097 Teeth In Vitro	Suggestions	Review	Suggestion	Suggestion
Maxillary teeth										
Centrals	25–35		45	30	34		80–90	80	70–90	35–60
Laterals	25–35		60	30	45		70–80	80	60–80	25–40
Canines	25–35		45		31		60–90	80	50–70	30–50
First premolars	25–35	20	50	21	37		30–40	60	35–90	25–40
One canal			70		30			60		
Two canals			20		23					
Second premolars	25–35			21	37		50–55		35–90	25–40
One canal			70		30			80		
Two canals			35		23			45–60		
Molars	25–35						30–55			
Mesiobuccal		25	60	24	43	11–73		45	35–60	25–40
One canal			40		19	09–60				
Two canals			40		19	11–44				
Distobuccal		25	40	23	22	08–73		45	35–60	25–40
Palatal		35	40	30	29	08–69		60	80–100	25–40
Mandibular teeth										
Centrals	25–35		70	26	37		40–50	60	35–70	25–40
Laterals	25–35		70		37		40–50	60	35–70	25–40
Canines	25–35		70		47		50–55	80	50–70	30–50
First premolars	25–35		35	27	35		30–40		35–70	30–50
One canal					20			80		
Two canals					19			45–60		
Second premolars	25–35		40	27	35		50–55		35–70	30–50
One canal					20			80		
Two canals					13			45–60		
Molars	25–35						30–55			
Mesial root		25	60	26	38–45	10–64		45	35–45	25–40
Distal root		30	60	39	46	12–64		60	40–80	25–40

Table 10 presents an overview of anatomical studies detailing physiological foramen diameters. There is an apparent variation in these measurements, probably due to variation in experimental conditions. Consequently, there is also a great deal of variation in recommended apical sizes, as shown in the left segment of Table 10.

For example, apical sizes ranging from sizes #20 to #100 for maxillary molar roots have been recommended. Figure 47A illustrates apical dimensions before and after shaping with two rotary instrumentation paradigms.

A third as yet incompletely understood aspect of canal shape is taper. Some have expressed concerns that the importance of root canal taper should be seen only in conjunction with root canal filling techniques, most notably vertical compaction.[244] However, as stated before, there are some experimental evidences that taper may be connected to the ability to clean the root canal system by improving irrigant action.[10,150,222] Limited microbiological data are conflicting regarding the potential of smaller apical preparations with larger taper to disinfect root canal system.[13,127] Using the amount of instrumented canal area as a surrogate outcome for disinfecting capacity, no significant differences were found overall, comparing shapes with GT 20 0.10 taper to apical size #40 with smaller tapers.[245] However, there were significant differences when the apical canal segment was evaluated for instrumented canal surface area (Paque F, unpublished data).

Schilder[3] described five *design objectives* for cases to be filled with gutta-percha, which are as follows:

- The shape should be a continuously tapering funnel from the apex to the access cavity.

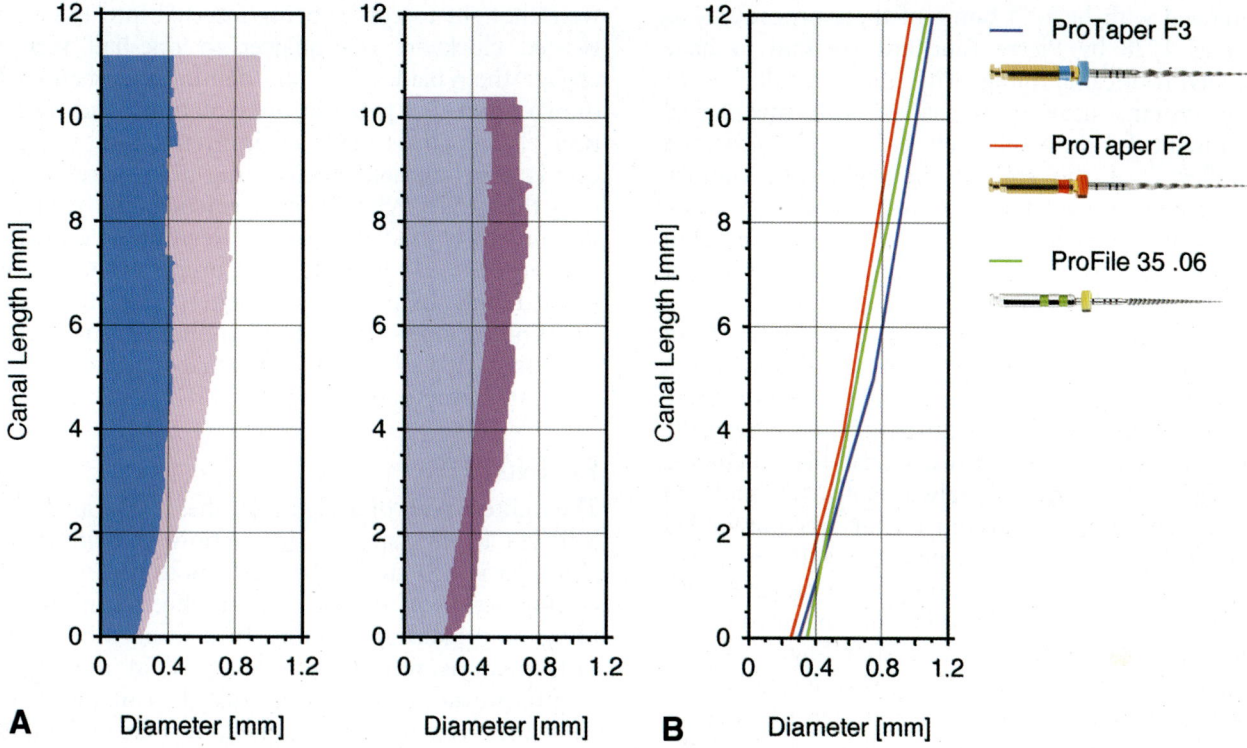

Figure 47 Pre- and postoperative canal diameters after shaping with common instrument types. Measurements are from microcomputed tomography reconstructions. **A,** Original data from 12 mesiobuccal canals shaped to an apical size #40 with FlexMaster (left panel, VDW) and ProTaper (right panel, Dentsply Maillefer). **B,** Dimension of selected rotary instruments for comparison.

- Cross-sectional diameters should be narrower at every point apically.
- The root canal preparation should flow with the shape of the original canal.
- The apical foramen should remain in its original position.
- The apical opening should be kept as small as practical.

There were also four important biological objectives that are as follows:

- Procedures should be confined to the roots themselves.
- Necrotic debris should not be forced beyond the foramina.
- All tissues should be removed from the root canal space.
- Sufficient space for intracanal medicaments and irrigation should be created.

These objectives form the basis for today's quality criteria[236,237] and also for the development of operational techniques that will be described below in detail. All of these techniques rely on the adaptation of geometric forms, of either handheld or engine-driven instruments to root canal anatomy, by way of particular instrumentation sequences and usage parameters. However, an experimental, noninstrumentation system for root canal cleaning has been tested in vitro and in vivo;[246,247] since neither this system nor potential alternatives are currently available for the clinic, mechanical preparation will be utilized to clean and shape root canals for the foreseeable future.

In conclusion, the current strategy in radicular preparation calls for the enlargement of root canals to a size sufficient to allow disinfection and subsequent root canal filling.[120] Available evidence to support a particular shape in direct connection with any given root canal filling technique is limited to Allison et al.,[248] who found a better seal when spreaders used for lateral compaction could penetrate close to WL. Consequently, efforts continue to determine the best possible root canal shape for management of intracanal infection by mechanical action, irrigant delivery, and placement of interappointment medicaments.

MEANS FOR RADICULAR SHAPING

Historically, painful teeth were opened and symptomatic pulps were treated with caustic substances or cauterized with heat.[249] Some of these procedures as early as 1728 by Pierre Fauchard are said to have included root canal fillings with lead or gold.[250] Root canal systems have been shaped with mechanical instruments for more than 200 years.[250–252] According to Lilley[251] at the end of the eighteenth century "... only primitive hand instruments and excavators, some iron cautery instruments and only very few thin and flexible instruments for endodontic treatment had been available...".

The development of the first endodontic hand instruments by Edwin Maynard involved notching a round wire (e.g., watch springs, piano wires) to create fine needles for pulp tissue extirpation and potentially shaping.[253] In 1852, Arthur used small files to enlarge and shape root canals.[254] Subsequently, textbooks in the middle of the nineteenth century recommended that root canals should be enlarged with broaches: "But the best method of forming these canals is with a three- or four-sided broach, tapering to a sharp point, and its inclination corresponding as far as possible with that of the fang. This instrument is employed to enlarge the canal and give it a regular shape".[122,252] In 1885, the GG drill and in 1904 the K-file were introduced, both of which are still in use to date. Standardization of instruments had been proposed by Trebitsch in 1929 and again by Ingle in 1958[122] but remains an issue today with NiTi rotary instruments.[255] For a detailed description of various instrument types and alloys, the reader is referred to Chapters 26B, "Introduction of Nickel-titanium Alloy to Endodontics" and Chapter 26C, "Instruments for Cleaning and Shaping".

Instrument Movements While Shaping

WATCH-WINDING
The least aggressive instrument action is most desirable in the early phases of root canal instrumentation. Many clinicians[232,256,257] recommend a "watch-winding" movement with rotations of a quarter turn using small (size #08 or #10) K-files to reach WL or to explore the canal prior to coronal flaring (see below). Importantly, copious irrigation and constant cleansing of the instrument with sterile gauze are necessary to clear the flutes and to prevent packing debris at or through the apical foramen.

REAMING
Reamers are instruments designed to enlarge or taper preexisting spaces. Traditionally, endodontic reamers were thought to cut by being inserted into the canal, twisted clockwise one-quarter to one-half turn to engage their blades into the dentin, and then withdrawn, that is, penetration, rotation, and retraction.[258] The cut is made during retraction. The process is then repeated, penetrating deeper and deeper into the canal. When WL is reached, the next size instrument is used, and so on. Reaming is a method that produces a round, tapered preparation, and this is used only in perfectly straight canals. In such a situation, reamers can be rotated one-half turn before retracting. In a slightly curved canal, a reamer should be rotated only one-quarter turn.

FILING
The tighter spiral of a file establishes a rake angle that achieves its primary cutting action on withdrawal, although it will cut in the push motion as well. The cutting action of the file can be effected in either a filing or a reaming motion. In a filing motion, the instrument is placed into the canal at the desired length, pressure is exerted against the canal wall, and while this pressure is maintained, the rake of the flutes rasps the wall as the instrument is withdrawn without turning. The file need not contact all walls simultaneously. For example, the entire length and circumference of large-diameter canals can be filed by inserting the instrument to the desired working distance and filing circumferentially around all of the walls. When using a file in a reaming action, the motion is obviously the same as for a reamer.[258] Withdrawing the file then cuts the engaged dentin. Filing is very efficiently done with Hedström files while K-files are the most popular instruments.[259] One the other hand, the often advocated technique of circumferential filing[260] has been shown to leave significant canal areas unprepared.[261] Finally, hand versions of current NiTi rotary instruments, such as ProSystem GT (Dentsply Tulsa Dental, Tulsa, OK) and ProTaper (Dentsply Maillefer), may be used in filing and reaming action.

ROTARY MOVEMENTS
Until the advent of NiTi alloy, continuous rotary movement was thought undesirable for shaping curved canals due to the danger of instrument fractures. Nevertheless, it has been recommended to use stainless steel GG drills into the apical third of straight root canals,[3,262] which have the potential of undesirable canal shapes (Figure 48) and instrument fracture. Furthermore, strip perforations may occur with indiscriminate use of GG or Peeso drills.[263,264] However, it has been clearly established that continuous rotary

movement with NiTi instruments with noncutting tips creates shapes with little or no incidence of preparation errors.[120]

POTENTIAL SHAPES

Figure 49 illustrates basic requirements for a radicular shape, with adequate WL and working width as well as a homogenous taper that attempts to recreate the original main canal shape in an enlarged form. Cases present clinicians with a variety of anatomical and other challenges but the principles for root canal shaping remain the same for straight and curved canals (see Figure 49). However, specific cases, such as wide apices found in incompletely formed roots or after apical root resorption, call for modified approaches due to thin dentin walls and difficulties in controlling the apical extent of the fill. Special procedures such as apexogenesis and apexification may be required to provide adequate obturation (see Chapter 30, Obturation of the Radicular Space).

Variations in apical shape have received special attention and varying recommendations. Names were given for the desired configuration (lower panel in Figure 49): "apical stop,"[265] "apical box,"[242] "apical capture or control zone."[266,267] The intent of all the described techniques is two-fold: (1) allow irrigant access to the apical root canal system and (2) prevent filling material from being extruded into the periapical space. As stated earlier, no conclusive evidence favors one apical shape over another regarding clinical outcomes; however, Kast'akova et al.[268] demonstrated that an apical stop, prepared to follow the recommendation to prepare three sizes larger than the first file to bind at WL, did not prevent sealer or gutta-percha extrusion.

Finally, the argument has been made that a tapered apical preparation would reduce the incidence of overpreparation that may occur following a length determination error and an apical stop preparation.[269] This idea derived its attraction from the well-supported notion that preparation errors should be avoided as they are associated with inferior outcomes.[270–275] Preparation errors and their development are discussed further below.

Several systems to prepare canal with hand or engine-driven instruments have been described, beginning with Ingle's standardized technique[276] (Table 11). There are two principally different approaches: the "apex first" and the "coronal first" techniques. The former approach advocates that WL is reached and the apical area is prepared first with increasingly larger instrument

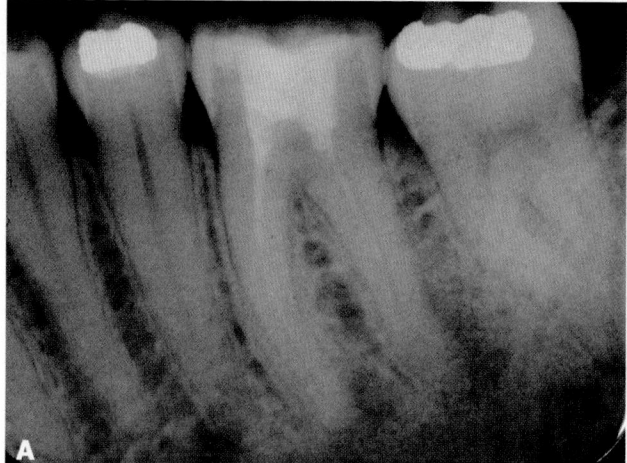
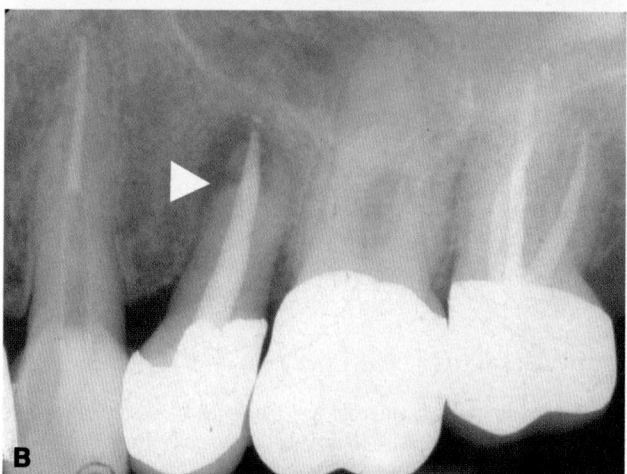
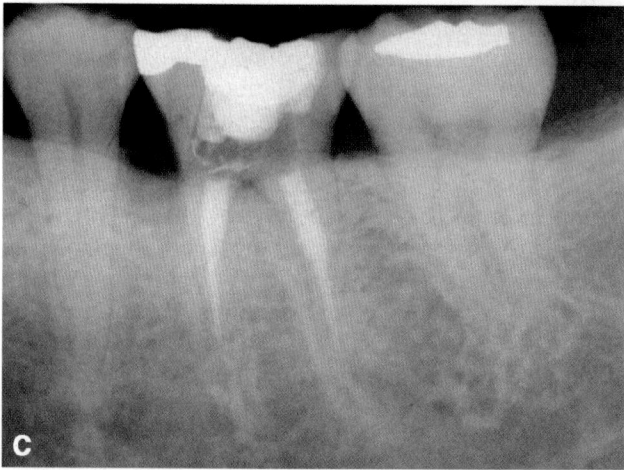

Figure 48 Clinical examples of root canal filled teeth that do not follow principles for an optimized shape. ***A,*** Very narrow shape that is not conducive to cleaning and irrigant access. ***B,*** Overenlargement that may predispose to vertical root fracture (arrowhead). ***C,*** The so-called "coke bottle" shape produced by overzealous action of Gates Glidden drills.

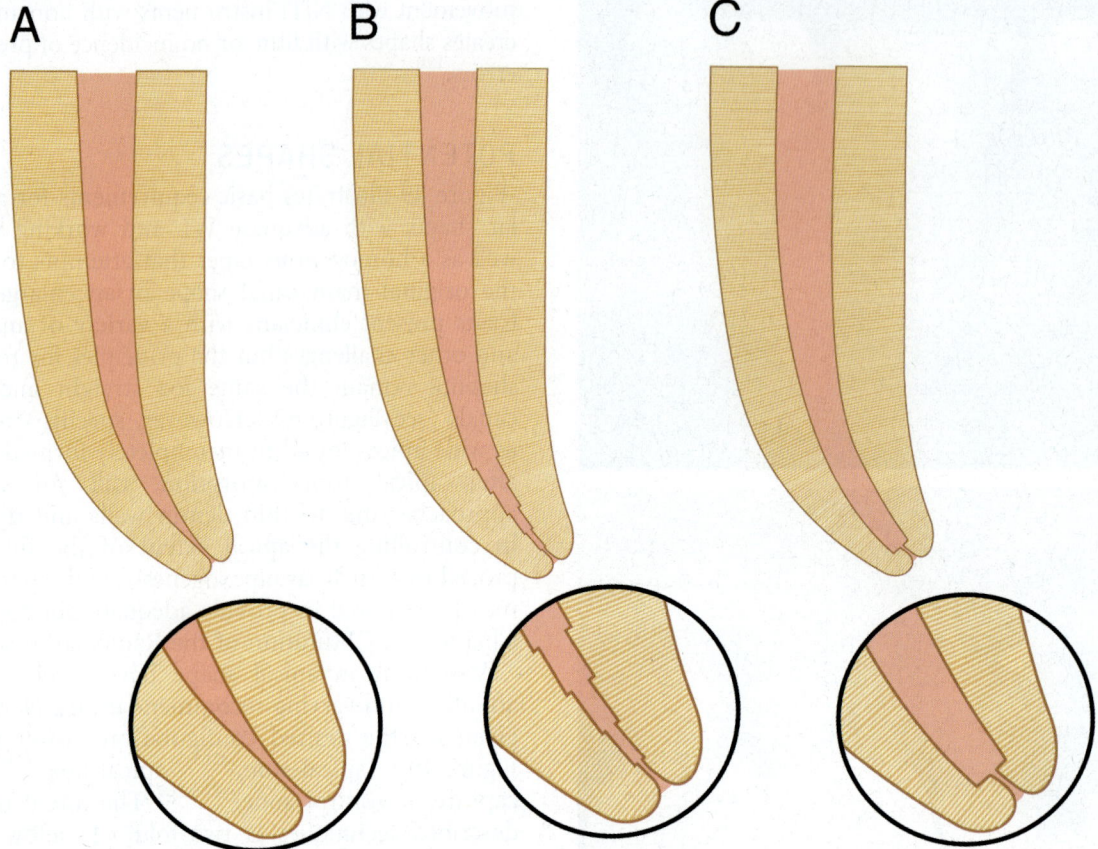

Figure 49 Schematic diagrams of potential root canal shapes after preparation. Depending on the instrument and the sequence used, the canal is enlarged into a tapered shape (***A**,* for example, rotary instrumentation), a taper with incremental size increase (***B**,* step-back preparation), or a slight taper with defined apical stop ***C***. The bottom panel shows magnified apical shapes produced.

sizes, whereas the latter uses descending instrument sizes to prepare coronal canal areas first and apical ones last. The following section will describe the basic techniques and some subaspects of them in more detail. As these techniques are generally independent of the instruments with which they are performed, the reader is referred to Chapter 26C, "Instruments for Cleaning and Shaping" for a detailed review of design and properties of handheld and engine-driven endodontic instruments. However, it needs to be kept in mind that the literature is replete with references to the superiority of one instrument or one method of preparation over all others.[288–290] The following statement may put expectations on any particular file type into perspective: "Regardless of the instrument type, none was able to reproduce ideal results; however, clinically acceptable results could be obtained with all of them."[291]

Preparation Techniques

STANDARDIZED

The standardized technique uses the same WL definition for all instruments introduced into a root canal

Table 11 Summary of Preparation Techniques Suggested for Hand and Rotary Instruments

Reference	Year	Technique
Ingle[276]	1961	Standardized instrumentation
Clem[277], Weine[278]	1969–1974	Step-back, serial preparation
Schilder[3]		
Abou-Rass[279]	1980	Anticurvature filing
Marshall[280,281]	1980	Crown-down pressureless
Goerig[262]	1982	Step-down
Fava[282,283]	1983/1992	Double flare, with modifications
Roane[284]	1985	Balanced force
Torabinejad[285,286]	1994	Passive step back
Siqueira[287]	2002	Alternate rotary motion

and therefore relies on the inherent shape of the instruments to impart the final shape to the canal. It can therefore also be called a "single-length technique," an approach that has recently gained popularity with the ProTaper (Dentsply Maillefer) and MTwo (Sweden and Martina, Padova, Italy) NiTi rotary instruments.

Negotiation of fine canals is initiated with fine files that are then advanced to WL and worked until a next larger instrument may be used. Conceptually, the final shape is predicted by the last-used instrument (also named MAF, see Box 1). A single matching gutta-percha point may then be used for root canal filling. In reality, this concept suffers from two factors of variation: first, canals (in particular those with curvatures), shaped with the standardized technique, end up wider than the instrument size would suggest,[292,293] and second, production quality is insufficient, both for instruments and for gutta-percha cones, leading to size variations.[294,295]

STEP-BACK

Realizing the importance of a shape larger than that produced with the standardized approach, Clem[277] and Weine[278] introduced the step-back technique, sometimes also called telescopic technique.[296] This paradigm relies on stepwise reduction of WL for larger files, typically in 1- or 0.5-mm steps, resulting in flared shapes with 0.05 and 0.10 taper, respectively. Incrementally reducing WL for larger and stiffer instruments in turn lessened the forces associated with aberrant preparations, in particular in curved canals (Figure 50).

Clem[277] originally described the step-back technique for curved canals in teeth of adolescents, as the creation of a single step, at the transition from the straight to the curved portion of the root. The resulting shape is somewhat similar to the "coke bottle" configurations that occur when inflexible engine-driven instruments such as GG or Peeso drills are advanced past the middle root canal third (see Figure 48). Taking GG and Peeso drills deep into canals carries the risk of fracture as they are not very resistant to fatigue occurring in curved canals.[297] Furthermore, overpreparation and subsequent strip perforations may occur,[263,264,298] and therefore these shapes are generally not desirable.

Subsequently, Schilder[3] suggested a "serial preparation" that included enlarging to a file size #30 or #35 and then serially reducing WL for the following instruments. Initially, he did not advocate a metrically defined step but rather a tactile feedback and cutting of dentin when initial wall contact was made. Thus,

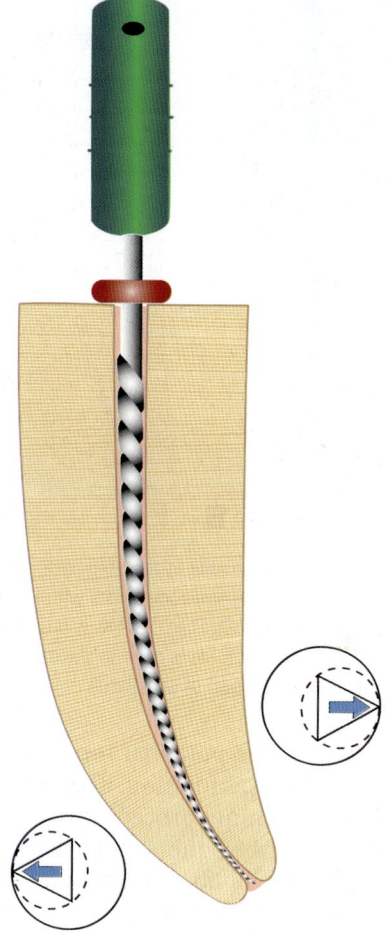

Figure 50 Principles of radicular dentin removal. In a curved canal, apical pressure leads to transportation toward the outer curvature. At the same time, the reactionary force builds up in the straightening instrument against the dentin coronal of the curvature and leads to transportation toward the inner curvature (e.g., furcation).

larger instruments would be used with decreasing WL and finally a smoothly tapered canal shape would result. The developed shape, however, may be very similar to what had been described as the outcome of a step-back procedure and in fact later, Schilder-type preparation was illustrated as involving regular predetermined steps.[258] Coffae and Brilliant,[299] for example, described a serial procedure that entailed the use of a #35 file to WL, stepwise reduction of WL for subsequent files up to size #60, and then the use of GG drills Nos. 2 and 3 approximately 16 and 14, respectively, into the canal (Figure 51). They describe superior débridement with serial preparation compared to standardized shapes.[299] Walton et al.[300] corroborated these results by histological evaluations. Clearly, coronal enlargement (flaring) appeared beneficial for cleaning and obturation.[248] However, there

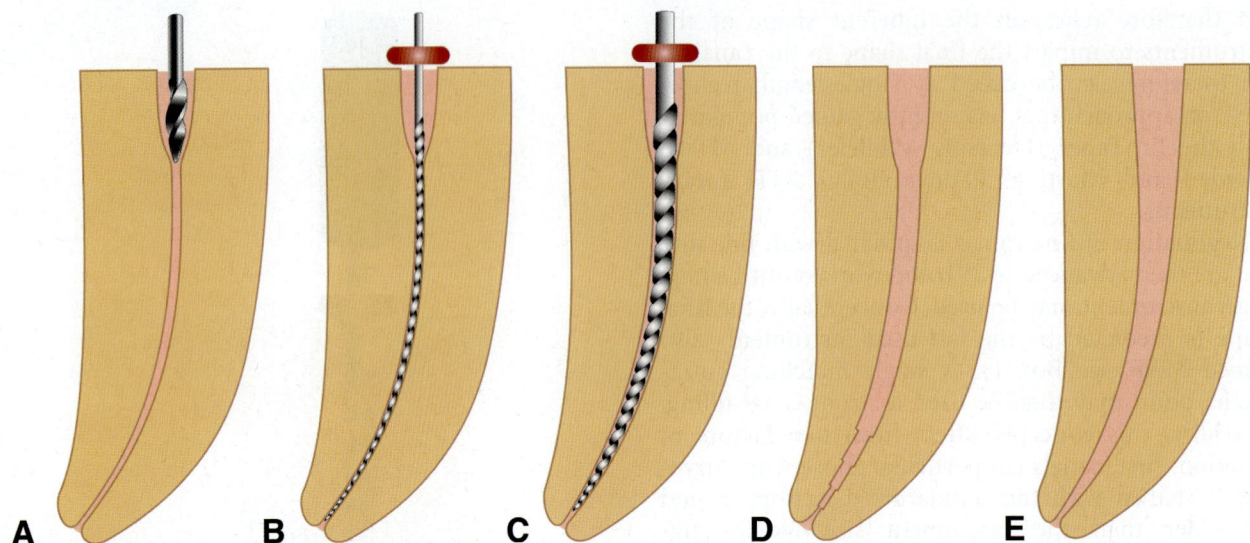

Figure 51 Sequence of instruments in the step-back procedure. After coronal preenlargement with Gates Glidden burs **A,** apical preparation to the desired master apical file (MAF) size commences with K-Files to determine working length (WL) **B** and then files of ascending size to the desired apical dimension (also called Phase I, **C**). Then, the WL is progressively decreased ("stepped-back") by 1 or 0.5 mm to create a more tapered shape (Phase IIa, **D**). Recapitulation with a small K-file is done to smooth canal walls and to ensure that the canal lumen is not blocked (Phase IIb, **E**). Frequent irrigation promotes disinfection and removal of soft tissue.

was concern about the potential for overinstrumentation and potential perforation. Development continued to modify shaping procedures.

Mullaney[301] described the step-back technique as particularly effective in fine canals. He divided the step-back preparation into two phases. Phase I is the apical preparation starting at the apical constriction. Phase II is the preparation of the remainder of the canal, gradually stepping back while increasing the instrument size. The completion of the preparation is the Refining Phase IIa and IIb to produce the continuing taper from the apex to the cervical (see Figure 51). To start Phase I instrumentation, the canal should have been explored with a fine instrument and the WL established. It is important that a lubricant is used at this point since fibrous pulp stumps may be compacted against the apical constriction and cause apical blockage.[302] In very fine canals, the irrigant that will reach this area may be insufficient to dissolve tissue. Lubrication is believed to emulsify tissue, allowing instrument tips to macerate and remove this tissue. It is only later, in canal filing, that dentin chips pack apically blocking the constriction. When the MAF size has been used to full WL, Phase I is considered complete and the 1.0- to 2.0-mm space back from the apical constriction should be clean of debris.

It must be emphasized here that irrigation between each instrument use as well as recapitulation with the previous smaller instrument carried to full depth is crucial. Then the step-back process (Phase II) begins with a file one size larger than the MAF. Its WL is set 1 mm short of the full WL, and it is carried down the canal to the new shortened depth. The same process is repeated with subsequent instruments again shortened by 1.0 or 0.5 mm from the MAF. Thus, the preparation steps back up the canal with either 1 or 0.5 mm and one larger instrument at a time. It has been recommended to end this step-back phase at size #60[3] or when the instrument has reached the wider straight portion of the root canal. In any case, frequent turnover of the irrigant and recapitulation with the MAF are necessary to promote canal disinfection and prevent blockage. The most coronal canal portion may then be carefully flared with GG drills or Hedström files. The refining Phase IIb is a return to the MAF, smoothing all around the walls to perfect the taper from the apical constriction to the cervical canal orifice, which would then be a larger replica of the original canal.[303]

Although the step-back technique was primarily designed to avoid preparation errors in curved canals, it applies to straight canal preparation as well. In fact, all root canals have some curvature.[14,304,305] Apparently straight canals are usually curved to some degree and canals that appear to curve in one direction often curve in other directions as well.[14] While it has been maintained that only curved instruments should be introduced into curved canals,[302] it seems in fact unlikely that one can successfully match canals' curvature with a precurved file. Moreover, rotary instruments are straight and should be introduced only into canal areas that a straight hand instrument, size #15 or #20, has explored ("glide path," see below).

A modification of the step-down approach using hand instruments has been described by Torabinejad.[285,286] He advocated insertion of progressively larger hand instruments as deep as they would passively go in order to gain insight into the canal anatomy and to provide some enlargement prior to reaching the WL. Subsequent use of GG drills or Peeso reamers will provide additional coronal enlargement and improve tactile feedback from the apical region as well as better access for irrigants.[306,307] The use of an ultrasonically activated size #15 K-file has been advocated to further blend canal irregularities.[286] A second, probably even more important, benefit is the ultrasonic or sonic activation of the irrigant placed in the root canal for 1 to 2 minutes, and is turned over every 30 seconds.[222,286]

ANTICURVATURE FILING

In this context, Abou Rass, Glick, and Frank[308] described a method called "anticurvature filing" to prevent excessive removal of dentin from thinner root sections in curved canals. The underlying observation was that the furcation side (danger zone) of cross sections of mesial roots of mandibular molars has less dentin thickness than the mesial side (safety zone).[34,309] The technique included the use of precurved hand files that were purposefully manipulated to file the canal away from the danger zone. It also incorporates coronal flaring with rotary instruments after the use of hand instruments, but it is stated that such instruments should not be introduced more than 3 mm into root canals.[308] The final use of a manual instrument to blend the apical and coronal segments was advocated.

Kessler et al.[310] as well as Lim and Stock[260] demonstrated that "anticurvature" filing in fact helped to reduce the risk of perforation. Later, Safety Hedström files (Kerr/Sybron, Romulus, MI) followed a similar concept, namely filing away from the danger zone. These files had cutting edges that were flattened and thus dulled at one side and were therefore believed to remove less material in one direction.[311] However, subsequent research showed that Safety Hedström files when used as engine-driven versions are in fact not safe but tend to create preparation errors.[312]

STEP-DOWN

A different approach was taken by Goerig et al.,[262] who advocated shaping the coronal aspect of a root canal first before apical instrumentation commenced. The authors list the following advantages: the technique permits straighter access to the apical region, it eliminates coronal interferences, it removes the bulk of tissue and microorganisms before apical shaping, it allows deeper penetration of irrigants, and the WL is less likely to change. Subsequently, several of these claims were investigated; it was found that shaping was subjectively easier but had no measurable effect on canal transportation.[313] Furthermore, there was a small but significant beneficial effect on WL retention.[186,314] The removal of coronal obstructions does allow a better determination of apical canal sizes;[233,234] however, it is not clear if better irrigant penetration occurs and if that has clinically measurable benefits.

Another primary purpose of this technique is to minimize or eliminate the amount of necrotic debris that could be extruded through the apical foramen during instrumentation. This would help prevent post-treatment discomfort, incomplete cleansing, and difficulty in achieving a biocompatible seal at the apical constriction.[280] One of the major advantages of step-down preparation is the freedom from the constraint of the apical enlarging instruments. By first flaring the coronal two-thirds of the canal, the final apical instruments are unimpeded through most of their length. This increased access allows greater control and less chance of zipping near the apical constriction.[315] In addition, it "provides a coronal escape way that reduces the piston in a cylinder effect"[204] responsible for debris extrusion from the apex. This is one possible reason for the finding that coronal preflaring reduced the amount of apically extruded debris.[316]

The procedure itself involves the preparation of two coronal root canal thirds using Hedström files of size #15, #20, and #25 to 16 to 18 mm or where they bind. Thereafter, GG drills Nos. 2 and 3, and then potentially No. 4, are used sequentially shorter, thus flaring the coronal segment of the main root canal. Then, apical instrumentation is initiated; it consists of negotiating the remainder of the canal with a small K-file, shaping an apical "seat," and combining the two parts, step-down and apical shape, by stepwise decreasing of WL of incrementally larger files. Frequent recapitulation with a #25 K-file to WL is advised to prevent blockage.

Numerous modifications of the original step-down technique have been used clinically but most include the use of a small initial penetrating instrument, mostly a stainless steel K-file exploring the apical constriction and establishing the WL. To ensure this penetration, one may have to enlarge the coronal third of the canal with progressively smaller GG drills or with other rotary instruments. At this point, and in the presence of NaOCl, step-down cleaning and shaping may begin with a variety of instruments. For example, starting with a size #50 K-file and working down the canal, the instruments are used until the apical constriction (or WL) is reached. When resistance is met for further penetration, the next smallest size is used. Irrigation should follow the use of each instrument and recapitulation after every other instrument. To properly enlarge the apical third and to round out ovoid shape and lateral canal orifices, a reverse order of instruments may be used starting with a size #20 (for example) and enlarging this region to a size #40 or #50 (for example). The tapered shape can be improved by stepping back up the canal with larger instruments, bearing in mind all the time the importance of irrigation and recapitulation.

BALANCED FORCE

After many years of experimentation, Roane et al.[284] introduced the "Balanced Force" concept of canal preparation in 1985. The concept came to fruition, they claimed, with the development and introduction of a new K-type file design, the Flex-R File[284,317] (originally manufactured by Moyco Union Broach, now Miltex, York, PA). The technique can be described as "positioning and preloading an instrument through a clockwise rotation and then shaping the canal with a counterclockwise rotation."[284] The authors evaluated the damaged instruments produced by the use of this technique and discovered that a greater risk of instrument damage was associated with clockwise movement.[318] For the best results with the "Balanced Force" technique, preparation is completed in a step-down approach. The coronal and mid-thirds of a canal are flared with GG drills, beginning with small sizes, and then shaping with hand instrument is carried out in the apical areas. Similar to techniques described above, increasing the diameter of the coronal and mid-thirds of a canal removes most of the contamination and provides access for a more passive movement of hand instruments into the apical third. Shaping becomes less difficult: the radius of curvature is increased as the arc is decreased. In other words, the canal becomes straighter and the apex is accessible with less flexing of the shaping instruments (see Figure 50).

After mechanical shaping with GG drills, Balanced Force hand instrumentation begins with the typical triad of movements: placing, cutting, and removing instruments using only rotary motions (Figure 52).

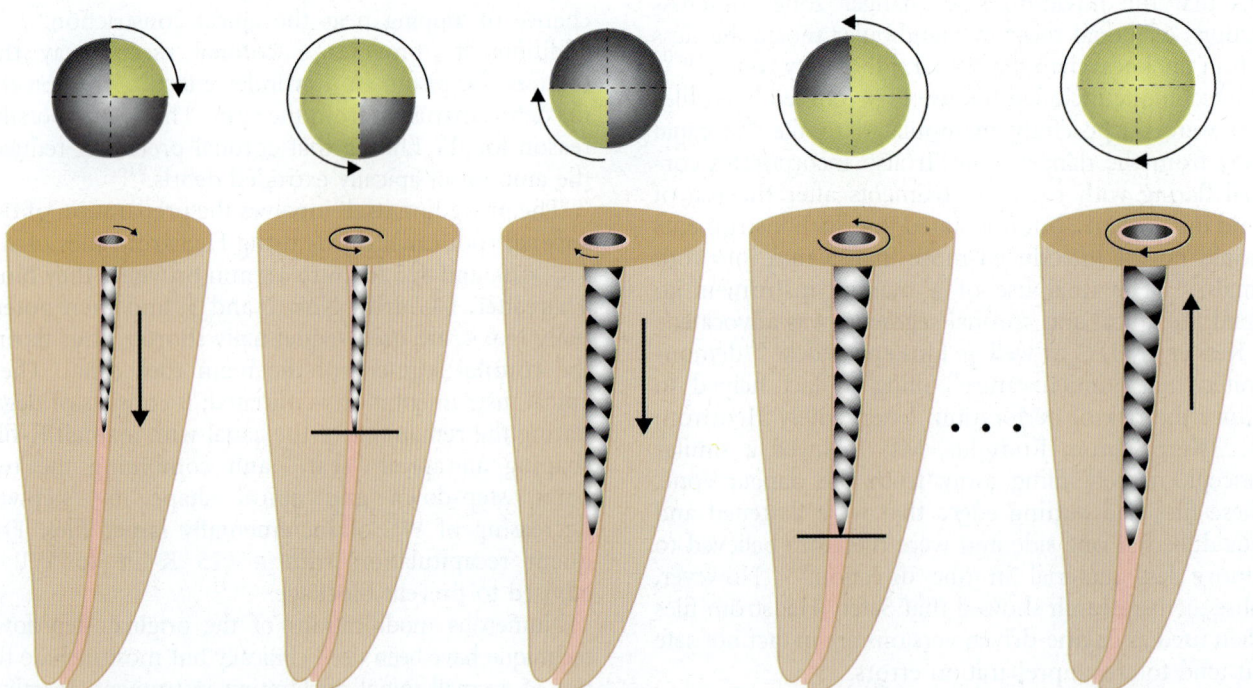

Figure 52 Principles of the Balanced Force technique. Instruments with a symmetrical triangular cross section and pilot tips (e.g., Flex-R files, Moyco Union Broach, Montgomeryville, PA) were originally suggested to be used in three steps in a rotational movement. A file may be advanced into the canal with a one-quarter clockwise rotation. The second movement involves adequate apical pressure to keep the instrument at this level of the canal while rotate counterclockwise for a half- to three-quarter turn. Currently, it is recommended to use the first two movements repeatedly, progressing more apically. Then the third movement pulls the instrument gently out of the canal with clockwise rotation.

Insertion is done by a quarter-turn clockwise rotation while slight or no apical pressure is applied. Cutting is then accomplished by counterclockwise rotation applying sufficient apical pressure to the instrument.

The amount of apical pressure must be adjusted to match the file size (i.e., very light for fine instruments to fairly heavy for large instruments).[284] Pressure should maintain the instrument at or near its clockwise insertion depth. Then counterclockwise rotation and apical pressure act together to enlarge and shape the canal to the diameter of the instrument. Counterclockwise motion should be 120° or greater. It must rotate the instrument sufficiently to move the next larger cutting edge into the location of the blade that preceded it in order to shape the full circumference of a canal. A greater degree of rotation is preferred and will more completely shape the canal to provide a diameter equal to or greater than that established by the counterclockwise instrument twisting during its manufacture. It is important to understand that clockwise rotation allows the instrument to engage dentin, and this motion should not exceed 90°. If excess clockwise rotation is used, the instrument tip can become locked into place and the file may unwind.[284] If continued, when twisted counterclockwise, the file may fail unexpectedly. The process is repeated (clockwise insertion and counterclockwise cutting) as the instrument is advanced toward the apex in shallow steps. After the working depth is obtained, the instrument is freed by one or more counterclockwise rotations made, while the depth is held constant. The file is then removed from the canal by a slow clockwise rotation that loads debris into the flutes and elevates it away from the apical foramen.[284] A more or less flared final shape may be obtained by stepping back in 0.5 or 1 mm increments.

Generous irrigation follows each shaping instrument, since residual debris will cause transportation of the shape. Debris applies supplemental pressures against the next shaping instrument and tends to cause straightening of the curvature. By repeating the previously described steps, the clinician gradually enlarges the apical third of the canal by advancing to larger and larger instruments. Working depths are changed between instruments to produce an apical taper. The working loads can and should be kept very light by limiting the clockwise motion and thereby reducing the amount of tooth structure removed by each counterclockwise shaping movement. This technique can and should be used with minimal force.

The Balanced Force technique may be used with any file with symmetrical cross section;[319] however, shaping and transportation control are considered optimal when a Flex-R file is used.[320] The Flex-R file design removes the transition angles inherent to the tip of standard K-files (see Chapter 26C, Instruments for Cleaning and Shaping). These angles may cut a ledge into the canal wall.[321–324] The specific tip design prevents Flex-R files from transporting the canal into the external wall of a curve.[325]

Balanced Force instrumentation initiated from the belief that the apical area should be shaped to sizes larger than were generally practiced (see Table 10). The original Balanced Force concept then refers to apical control zones by, for example, first using sizes #15 and #20 files to the periodontal ligament (i.e., through the apical foramen) and then reducing the working depth by 0.5 mm for subsequent sizes #25, #30, and #35. The apical shape is then completed 1 mm short using sizes #40 and #45 under continuing irrigation with NaOCl. Single-appointment preparation and obturation played an important role in the formation of these shaping concepts.

The success of this shaping technique and enlarging scheme has been closely evaluated in both clinical practice and student clinics, and it can be said that files used in "Balanced Force" motion generally lead to comparatively little canal transportation. However, subsequent research has indicated that the underlying mechanisms are different from what was originally envisaged.[326,327] Specifically, there is evidence that the force required to hold the instrument close to the position during counterclockwise rotation closely matches the amount of force required to bend an instrument into a curve similar to the main curve of the canal that is prepared.[326] Nevertheless, in vitro reports indicate that shapes created with the Balanced Force technique are of excellent quality[328] and are comparable to those with NiTi rotary instruments.[245,329,330] Furthermore, extrusion of material was less than with other techniques, such as the step-back filing technique and the CaviEndo ultrasonic method.[331] More recently, Siqueira et al.[287] tested a modification of the Balanced Forces technique they had earlier called alternated rotary movements. This approach did not recommend withdrawal of the instrument after each set of rotations but emphasized incremental apically directed movement and withdrawal only when the file, for example, a size #25 NitiFlex (Dentsply Maillefer) has reached the WL. Canals shaped to an apical size #40 had in vitro bacterial reduction similar to canals prepared with GT rotaries to size #20 0.12 taper.[287]

CROWN-DOWN PRESSURELESS

The first description of a crown-down preparation, in which larger files are first used in the coronal two-thirds of the canals and then progressively smaller files are used more apically, can be found in a Master's Thesis by John Pappin[332] and the endodontic technique manual of the Oregon Health & Science University.[281] They described the approach as follows (Figure 53):

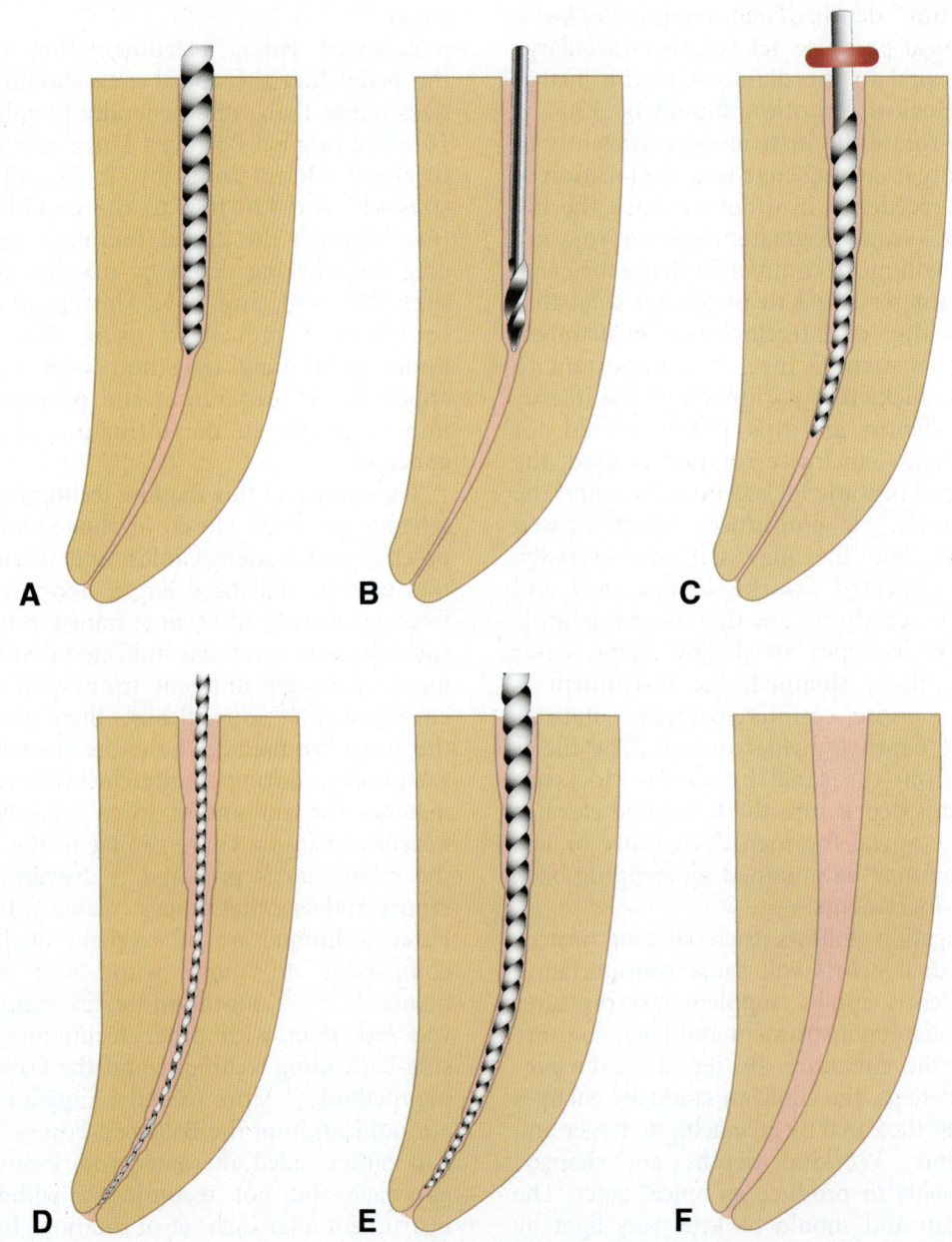

Figure 53 Sequence of instruments in the crown-down approach. Coronal preenlargement was originally suggested to commence after determination of a provisional working length (WL) with a size #35 hand file **A**, Then, Gates Glidden burs were used **B**, followed by hand files starting with a large file (e.g., size #60) and progressing apically with smaller sizes **C**, The definitive WL was determined as soon as the progress was made beyond the provisional WL **D**, Apical enlargement **E**, and recapitulation **F**, created a homogenous shape that may be similar to the one created with the step-back approach, provided that both techniques were performed with little or no procedural errors. Both step-back and crown-down techniques may be used in conjunction with hand and rotary instruments but in vitro evidence suggests that a crown-down approach is preferred for tapered rotary instruments.[335]

After completion of coronal access, a provisional WL is determined and a size #35 K-file is introduced into the root canal with no apically directed pressure. Then, a GG No. 2 is used, short of or to the length explored by the size #35 file. The GG No. 2 flares the coronal root canal and is followed by GG Nos. 3 and 4 with progressively shorter WLs. The next step is the core of what is now known as crown-down technique: a size #60 hand file is used with no apical force, and reaming is employed to enlarge the canal, followed by incrementally smaller instruments progressing deeper into the canal. A radiograph is taken when an instrument penetrates deeper than the provisional WL; after that, the apically directed procedure continues until an instrument reached the definitive WL.

The final step is to enlarge the apical area to three sizes larger than the first file that bound at WL. This is accomplished by going through the sequence of descending instrument sizes starting with a file one size larger than the starting size in the preceding series. Copious irrigation and recapitulation at the end of the procedure is advocated. Marshall in 1984 and 1987 amended the manual to include "Balanced Force" movements (Tinkle J, personal communication).

Morgan and Montgomery[333] described a slightly different method where both GG Nos. 2 and 3 were introduced to a straight portion of the canal and the "crown-down" process was started with a size #30 K-file. They showed superior ratings by experts judging canal shapes, but similar occurrence of preparation errors, compared to the step-back preparation.[333] However, a subsequent study found no differences in canal transportation when comparing "crown-down," "step-back," sonic instrumentation, and a NiTi rotary system.[334] Nevertheless, a crown-down approach is currently advocated for the majority of engine-driven rotary systems due to reduced contact areas and forces on the instruments.[335]

DOUBLE FLARE

Fava[282] presented a preparation technique that consisted of an exploratory action with a small file, a crown-down portion with K-files of descending sizes, and an apical enlargement to size #40 or similar. He recommended stepping back in 1 mm increments with ascending files sizes and frequent recapitulations with the MAF. Copious irrigation is considered mandatory. It is further emphasized that significant wall contact should be avoided in the crown-down phase to reduce hydrostatic pressure and the possibility of blockage. At this time, the double-flare technique was felt to be indicated for straight canals treated in one visit.[282] Later studies demonstrated better preparations in teeth with curved root canals shaped with a modified double-flare technique and Flex-R files compared to shapes prepared with K-files and step-back technique. A double-flare technique was also suggested for ProFile rotary instruments.[336]

Rotary Instrumentation

The introduction of NiTi alloy[337] for manufacturing hand files,[338] and later engine-driven instruments,[339] has altered canal shaping procedures drastically over the past two decades.[340] The endodontic literature is replete with accounts of shaping outcomes in vitro and descriptions of forces to which NiTi instruments are subjected (for review see references 120 and 122). NiTi rotary instruments and their design specifics are described in detail in Chapter 26B, "Introduction of Nickel-titanium Alloy to Endodontics" and Chapter 26C, "Instruments for Cleaning and Shaping". The following section is dedicated to their clinical use.

A major benefit of NiTi rotaries is their potential to avoid preparation errors.[341] This in turn may result in better clinical outcomes.[228,273] Moreover, through changes in instrument geometries, the creation of optimized canal shapes has been simplified. There is an ongoing debate over which shape is the most useful. In any event, shapes that are apically narrow and have a smooth taper can be safely prepared to become more parallel and apically larger. In achieving these designs, most manufacturers of rotary files recommend a strict crown-down sequence, with the exception of the LS instrument.[342] Several strategies have been recommended for this instrument, most of which represent a double-flare technique. Recently, other instruments (ProTaper, MTwo) have appeared on the market that are to be used in a single-length technique, somewhat similar to the standardized technique for hand instruments.

A main reason for recommending a crown-down approach is to avoid overloading rotating instruments with large frictional wall contact; this is believed to reduce the incidence of file fracture, in particular torsional fracture (Box 2).[343,344] One possible

Box 2 Fracture Mechanisms for Endodontic Instruments and Possible Mechanisms	
Torsional failure	Forcing the instrument into a narrow canal space and rotating it
Fatigue failure	Overusing an instrument by prolonged rotation in a curved canal
Corrosive failure	Combination of torsional and fatigue failure of an instrument with signs of corrosion

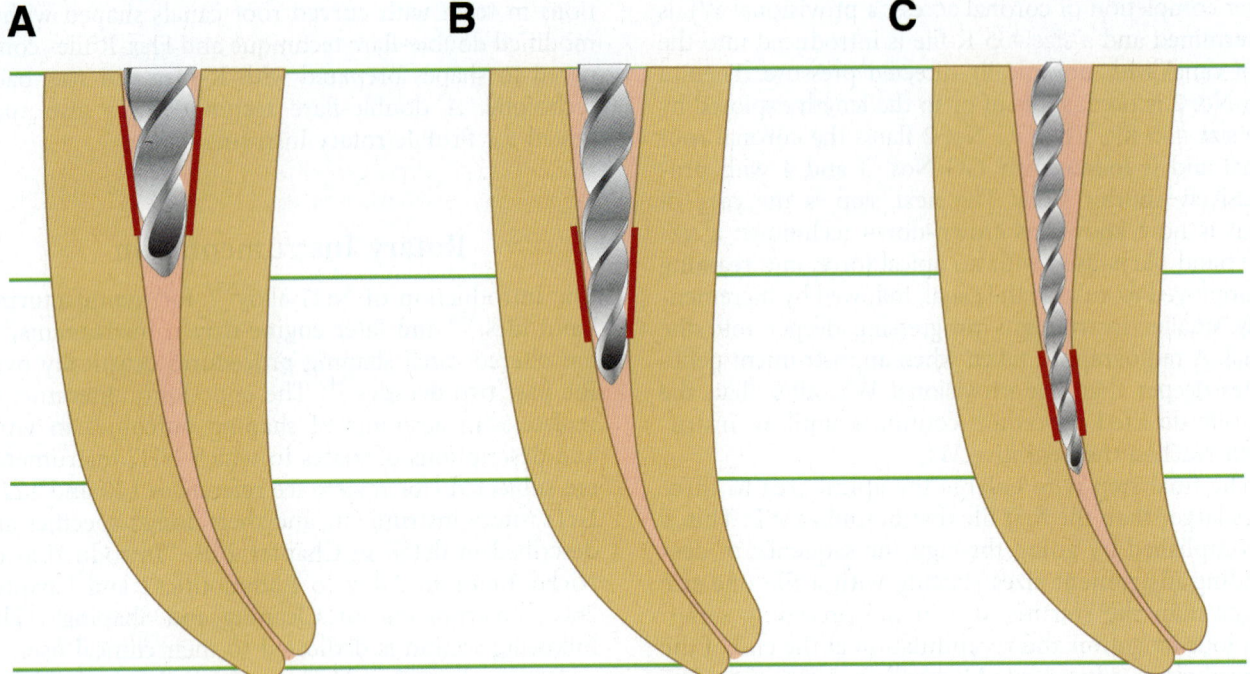

Figure 54 Rotary instruments may be subject to taper lock as soon as the canal taper approaches their dimension. Then, a large proportion of the instrument surface engages the canal wall (indicated by red bars), frictional resistance and hence torque increases, with a high risk of instrument fracture. This risk may be minimized by sequentially *A* to *C* using instruments with smaller tip sizes or taper, thus reducing contact areas and torque.[336]

mechanism for this type of fracture is an event known as "taper lock," illustrated in Figure 54.[345,346] Taper lock occurs when the shape of the tapered root canal being prepared becomes similar to the instrument in use. Instruments may then become locked into the canal, and the tip may fracture.[343] In a crown-down pattern, the next smaller instrument should be selected before taper lock can occur. Blum et al.[335] were convinced that ProFiles used this way experienced much less torque than when a step-back pattern was followed. This finding can be extended to most of the other rotaries that have a similar longitudinal design, for example, K3 (SybronEndo), EndoSequence (BrasselerUSA), HERO 642 (MicroMega, BesanÔon, France), and several others.

The distinctive design of LightSpeed instruments (Discus Dental) maximizes flexibility and allows larger apical preparations without unnecessary removal of dentin. The LightSpeed (LSX) has a noncutting shaft and a very short blade. After making SLA to about the mid-root, the coronal third is flared with the instrument of choice (not with the LSX). After flaring, at least #15 K-file is used to obtain patency to WL. A #20 LSX and sequentially larger sizes are used to prepare the apical third. The Final Apical instrument Size (FAS) is the blade size that encounters 4 mm or more of cutting resistance apically. A 4-mm step back with the next larger instrument (than the FAS) completes the apical preparation. The mid-root is then cleaned and tapered with the next two or three sequentially larger LSX sizes, blending mid-root instrumentation with the previously prepared coronal third. Recapitulation is usually necessary only once, with the FAS, at the end of canal preparation. The new LSX is to be used at 2500 rpm, and irrigation is required throughout the procedure.

Apical enlargement is sometimes done after crown-down has been accomplished. At this stage, different strategies are possible, that is, switching tapers or tip sizes, changing to different instruments. Torsional stresses that files are subjected to depend on the sequence employed.[347] Little is known of the incidence of fractures with single-length techniques,[348] particularly when the recommendations of the manufacturers are followed. In addition, it is not certain how important overall NiTi instrument fractures are for clinical outcomes.[349] Nevertheless, strict monitoring of instrument use should be instituted so that NiTi files can be periodically disposed of prior to failure.[350,351] In fact, single use in severely curved or calcified canals may be preferable due to problems of decontamination[352–355] and corrosion[356–358] in addition to the greater amount of stress that the instruments are subjected to in such situations.

Three different main handling paradigms have been described for the use of rotary instruments. Buchanan[359] recommends feeding the rotating file into a root canal with very slight apical force, until the instrument stalls, and then to immediately withdraw the file. At this point the file has done its cutting action and the flutes are loaded with debris that must be removed. The file is then reinserted. A similar movement has been recommended for RaCe files (FKG, La Chaux-de-Fonds, Switzerland), designed to avoid threading into the canal.

In contrast, the second recommendation for most other instruments is to use them in an up-and-down movement[342,360] with a very light touch to avoid taper lock and to distribute forces throughout the canal. This movement is continued until a certain resistance is met or WL is reached. Rotation in a curved canal leads to accumulation of cyclic fatigue, another potential reason for instrument fracture (see Box 2).[343,361–363] Fatigue occurs through cyclic compression and elongation of metal. The compounded amount of strain leads to fracture after a typical lifespan of up to 1,500 rotations in the most commonly used experimental configuration.[364,365] While the lifespan, calculated as rotations to fracture, is independent of the rotational speed,[366] the instrument undergoing fatigue will fracture in a shorter time period with higher rotations per minute.

Regarding hand movements, there is mixed evidence regarding the protective effect of up-and-down movements on the accumulation of cyclic fatigue,[360,363] but it does not appear to be harmful for the instrument brands tested.

The third instrument usage recommendation is specifically for ProTaper instruments and is termed "brushing".[367] Instead of feeding the file axially into the root canal, it is moved distinctly laterally in order to avoid threading in. Such lateral cutting occurs most effectively with a positive rake angle and a stiffer instrument. Regarding operational safety, it was recently established for MTwo instruments that the "brushing" motion extended fatigue life for larger size instruments.[368] This finding may be extended to other instruments using lateral cutting (Peters OA, Paque F, Boessler C, unpublished data). However, GG drills, used in this manner in the coronal third of the canal,[308,310] occasionally separate through fatigue. In this case, the GG shaft may be readily removed since fracture usually occurs on the transition from shaft to shank.

A guideline emphasized for ProTaper[367] that may be extended to other currently available instruments suggests determination of a "glide path." Specifically, prior to the use of any rotary instrument, root canals should be explored with #10, #15, or even #20 K-files to avoid overloading NiTi instrument tips with unexpected canal curves or excessive wall contact.[369] Special pathfinding files with specially designed geometry are available for this task (e.g., ProFinder, Dentsply Maillefer). Regardless of the design, it is important to use straight, not precurved, files to allow the subsequent rotary files to reach the same depth, without encountering acute bends or very narrow canal areas.

Finally, it has been recommended by manufacturers to use gel-based lubricants in conjunction with NiTi rotary files, or to fill the access cavity with NaOCl prior to instrument insertion.[232,359] The use of gel-based lubricants could potentially reduce frictional resistance and hence torsional load.[370] However, experimental evidence, using a dentin disk model, suggests otherwise.[371] In fact, the use of ethylenediaminetetraacetic acid (EDTA)-containing gels such as RC-Prep (Premier Dental Products, Norristown, PA) or Glyde (Dentsply Maillefer) may be detrimental, due to increased torque scores[371,372] and, more importantly, due to chemical interaction with its EDTA moiety and NaOCl action.[373]

Therefore, and despite reports of its corrosive potential,[374,375] frequently replenishing a reservoir of NaOCl[376] is presently advocated, providing lubrication and disinfection during canal shaping. After rotary instrumentation is complete, irrigation with EDTA and/or NaOCl may be done[377], with and without ultrasonic activation.[147,222,378]

The following ten principles apply to the successful use of currently available NiTi rotary files:

1. As with any type of instrument, poor access preparation will lead to procedural errors. While generally important in root canal preparation, it is crucial for the use of NiTi rotaries.
2. Files should never be forced, as NiTi instruments require a passive technique. If resistance is encountered, stop immediately and before continuing, increase the coronal taper and verify the "glide path" using small stainless steel hand files.
3. Canals representing difficult anatomy should be detected, analyzed, and carefully instrumented following specific rules (Figure 55, see below for more details).
4. Files should not be overused. Once only is the safest number but the actual stress level depends upon the case. Hence files may be used for more than one canal, but may have to be replaced when shaping a particularly difficult canal.

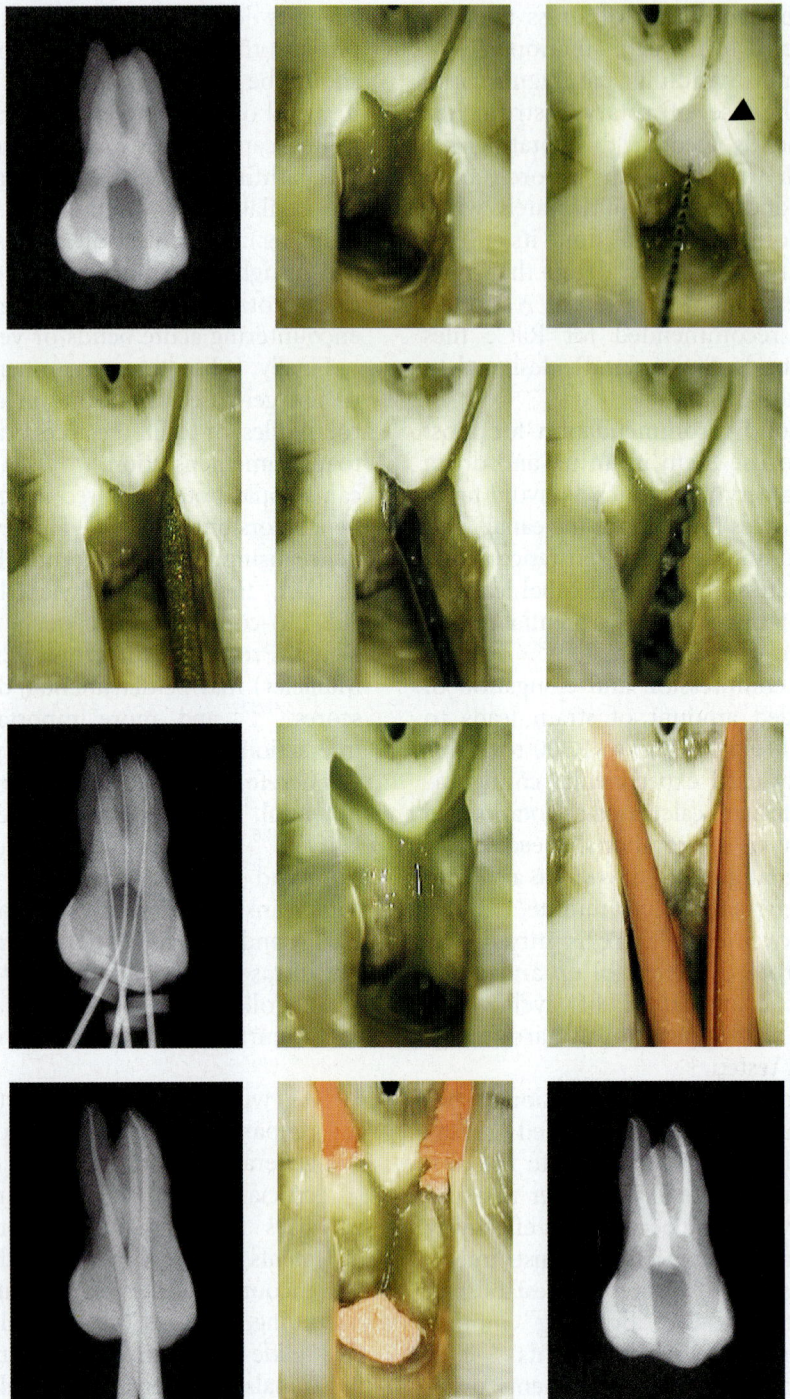

Figure 55 Example of a sequence of instruments to safely enlarge and shape the coronal part of the root canal system. This enables a complete shape of the apical third also. Shown are magnified buccal views into the access cavity of a maxillary molar and respective radiographs. After pathfinding with a lubricated (arrowhead) K-file, straight-line access (SLA) is created with ultrasonically powered and rotary instruments. This is often difficult but equally important in the second mesiobuccal canal (shown accessed here). Then working lengths (WLs) in all four canals are determined; subsequently canals are enlarged and filled.

5. Instrument breakage occurs more often during the initial stages of the learning curve. The clinician changing from stainless steel to NiTi should take continuing education courses with experienced clinicians and educators, followed by in vitro practice on plastic blocks and extracted teeth.

6. NiTi rotaries should not be used to bypass ledges. Confirmation of a glide path with a straight K-file is required prior to the use of any NiTi rotary.
7. Cutting with the entire length of the file blade should be avoided. This total or frictional fit of the file in the canal will cause the instrument to lock.
8. Sudden changes in the direction of an instrument caused by the operator (i.e., stopping and starting while inside the canal) must be avoided. A smooth gentle reaming or rotary motion is most efficient.
9. Inspection of instruments, particularly used instruments, by staff and doctor is essential. It should be remembered that NiTi has an excellent memory. The file should be straight. If any bend is present, the instrument is fatigued and should be replaced.
10. WL should be well established and controlled, as should the actual length of the file. If a file breaks without the clinician taking notice, a very sharp tipped instrument, upon the next insertion, will create procedural errors.

It is extremely important, for successful root canal preparation with rotary instruments, to carefully review the specific anatomy of each case (see earlier in this chapter and Chapter 6, Morphology of teeth and their root canal systems). Straight access into the root canal middle third should be created, with extended access cavities and early coronal flaring. When using rotary instruments, canals that curve, recurve, dilacerate, divide, or merge should be approached with extra care.[232] Figure 56 illustrates other problematic canal configurations. For example, very long narrow canals do not allow early coronal enlargement to the same extent as regular canals. The consequence is an increased frictional contact area and the potential for torsional overloading. There is no ideal solution to this problem except for extra careful flaring and potentially using hand instruments.

Acute bends, that is, those with a small radius of curvature, more coronally (see Figure 56B), puts a larger instrument cross section under cyclic fatigue and may cause breakage.[362] Here coronal flaring to the point of curvature and the use of rotary files with less taper to the WL are indicated. Ovoid canals that are wide buccolingually, such as distal canals of mandibular molars or some premolars, present a different problem. Instrument fracture is not very likely, but they can rarely be prepared to be round; hence débridement may be incomplete. It may be appropriate to approach these cases as if two canals existed buccally and lingually, and then merge the preparations by

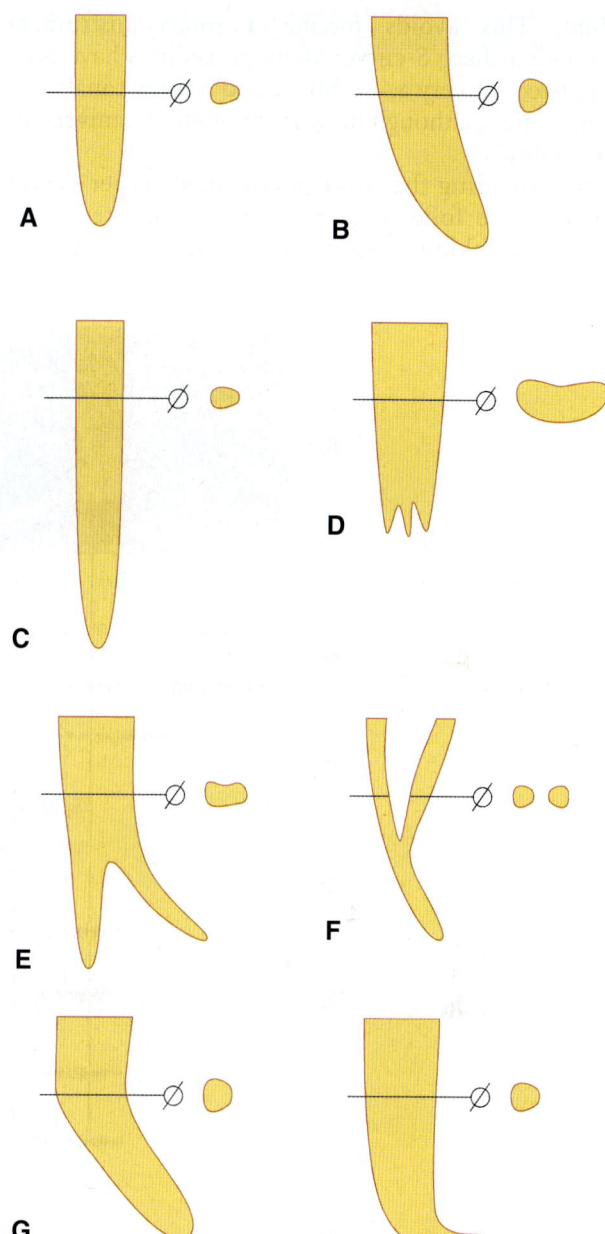

Figure 56 Schematic diagram of typical root canal anatomy with increasing degrees of difficulty for root canal preparation. Shown are basic canal shapes and cross sections at the middle root canal third (see text for more details). **A**, Short straight canal. **B**, Longer canal with moderate curvature. **C**, Very long canal. **D**, Canal that is wide buccolingually and may have multiple apical ramifications. **E**, Canal that splits apically in two main canals. **F**, Canals merging at the transition of middle and apical thirds. **G**, Acute curvature in coronal root canal third. **H**, Extreme curve in the apical 2 to 3 mm.

filing action with ultrasonic files or hand files. For merging canals, it is suggested to prepare the straighter canal to WL and the other canal to the merging point. This avoids forcing a rotary instrument through a sharp S-curve. Many procedures have been suggested for very acute curves and narrow canals (see Figure 56C), although none is certain to be universally successful.

By extending the strategies detailed earlier in this chapter, the following recommendations represent current thinking[379] for such a procedure. In part, these are different from earlier descriptions for hand instruments.[256,257] Coronal enlargement and creation of SLA are important to allow rotary instrument to work without undue stress. Moreover, this procedure reduces the danger of ledging and blocking. Figure 57 illustrates how this may be accomplished for a curved canal in a maxillary molar.

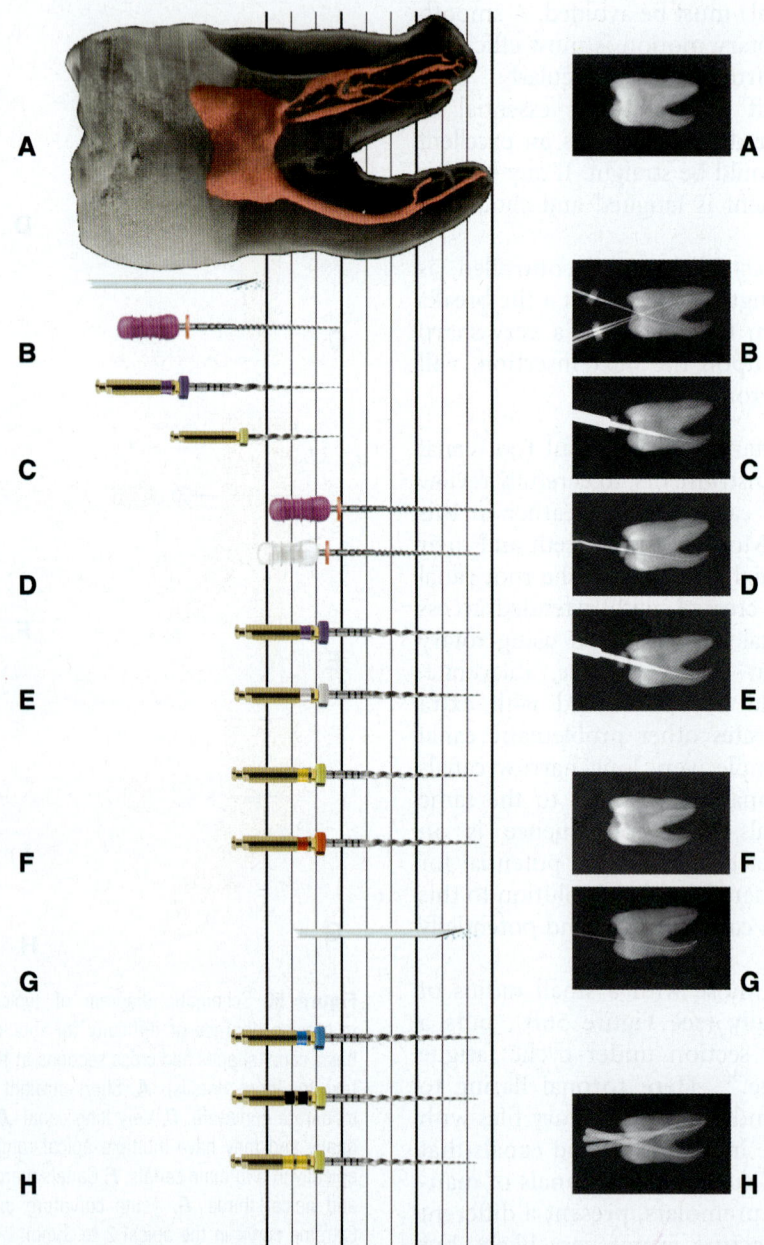

Figure 57 Example of a clinical sequence of instruments to safely enlarge and shape the apical two-thirds of curved root canal systems (palatal canal in **A**) using hand and rotary instruments. After pathfinding with small hand instruments **B**, and coronal preenlargement **C**, working length (WL) is determined. For a safe use of rotary instruments, a glide path is established with a series of hand instruments **D**, which rotary instruments can then follow **E**, Sufficient apical enlargement **F**, allows small irrigation needles to be passively inserted deep into the main canal **G**, and facilitates fitting of master cones **H**.

Calcifications occur nearest to the irritant to which the pulp is reacting. Since most irritants are in the coronal region of the pulp, the farther apical one goes into the canal, the more unlikely it is to be calcified. When files bind in these canals, it may be from small constrictions in the coronal part of the canal.

Obviously, before the canals can be entered, their orifices must be found. Knowledge of pulp anatomy is of first importance. Perseverance is the second requirement, followed by a calm determination not to become desperate and decimate the internal tooth when the expected orifice does not appear. The endodontic explorer is the greatest aid in finding a minute canal entrance (see Figures 18 and 55), feeling along the walls and into the floor of the chamber in the area where the orifices are expected to be.

A valuable aid in finding and enlarging canal orifices, particularly with magnification, is the Micro-Opener (Dentsply Maillefer) or the EndoHandle (Logan Dental, Logan, UT), with K-type flutes in 0.04 and 0.06 tapers.

Radiographs are indispensable in determining where and in which direction canals enter into the pulp chamber. The initial radiograph is one of the most important aids available to the clinician; a bitewing radiograph is helpful in providing an undistorted and metrically accurate view of the pulp chamber. The handpiece and the bur may be held up to the radiograph to estimate the correct depth of penetration and direction to the orifices. Color is another important aid in finding a canal orifice. The floor of the pulp chamber and the continuous anatomical line that connects the orifices (the so-called molar triangle) are dark gray or sometimes brown in contrast to the white or light yellow of the walls of the chamber (see Figure 55). Various ultrasonically powered tips are very helpful in relocating and enlarging orifices once their position has been determined (see Figure 55).

Current rotary instruments have noncutting tips and, with correct handling, pose relatively little risk of ledging the canal, certainly not in the coronal two-thirds. Provided that copious irrigation is used, apically directed transport of debris is less than with hand instruments and filing actions.[162,380,381] Verifying a glide path, as illustrated earlier, is particularly important when shaping narrow canals. This may be accomplished with a small (size #6, #8, or #10) K- or C-file (Dentsply Maillefer), lubricated and used in a watch-winding motion (see Figures 55 and 57).

An argument against using a straight instrument is that it tends to engage the wall at the curve or the pivot on a catch on the wall. Rotary instruments, however, are also straight. Therefore, the presence of a glide path has to be verified with a straight hand file. When the presence of sharp curves, debris, or very narrow canal areas is expected, precurving an exploratory file is indeed indicated (Figure 58). Most often, the pathfinding file can be advanced to WL with adequate hand movements, in particular gentle watch-winding. If this cannot be accomplished, coronal interferences must be removed by increasing the taper of the already explored coronal canal segment (see Figure 55).

When tentative WL is reached with a pathfinder file, the clinician may determine the direction of a major curvature by noting the direction of the tip of the file when it is withdrawn. This is a valuable clue, since the clinician understands the direction in which the canal curves and may guide the instrument accordingly. Valuable time may be saved when exploration is eliminated each time the instrument is

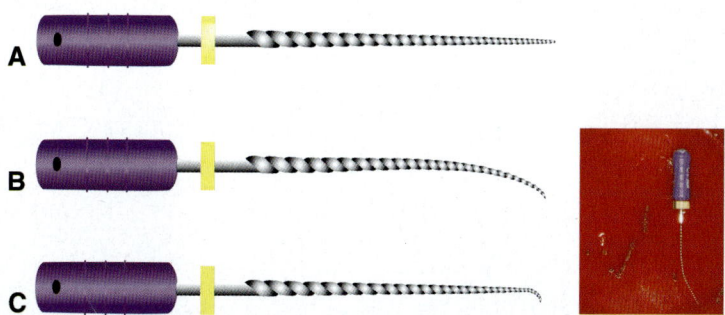

Figure 58 Flexible endodontic files may be used straight *A*, to initially scout and pathfind a root canal, since a subsequent rotary instrument can more safely be used in a canal area that a straight hand file negotiated ("glide path"). If an intracanal obstruction is encountered, an adequately precurved manual instrument should be used to conform more to overall canal anatomy *B*, A more acutely curved instrument can be utilized to bypass ledges or blockages *C*, Inset shows bacterial growth on blood agar after a K-file was bent using "clean" gloved fingertips.

placed in the canal. A pointed silicone stop will clearly show the direction of the file curvature. The WL may then be confirmed with a radiograph using a size #15 K-file. After determining the WL, a curved pathfinding file should be used if additional canals are suspected, for example, in mandibular incisors, mandibular premolars, the distal root of mandibular molars, or the mesiobuccal root of maxillary molars.

While ultrasonically powered inserts are routinely used under magnification to explore and refine access into canals, rarely do they need to be used into middle and even apical third of canals. However, when severe calcification is present, there is the option to locate a canal cross section that needs further shaping with hand or rotary files to WL (Figure 59).

Others have recommended the use of EDTA buffered to a pH of 7.3 to "dissolve" a pathway for exploring instruments.[382,383] When the mineral salts have been removed from the obstructing dentin by chelation, only the softened matrix remains.[384] However, this action has been disputed by others, since chelation does not readily occur in narrow parts of the canal, although softening can occur in the cervical and middle portions.[385,386] EDTA must be concentrated enough in an area to be effective.

Like in many other situations in root canal therapy, it is the obligation of an astute clinician to execute a cost-benefit evaluation, in order to determine if further progress without clear evidence of a canal cross section is indicated. Magnification and

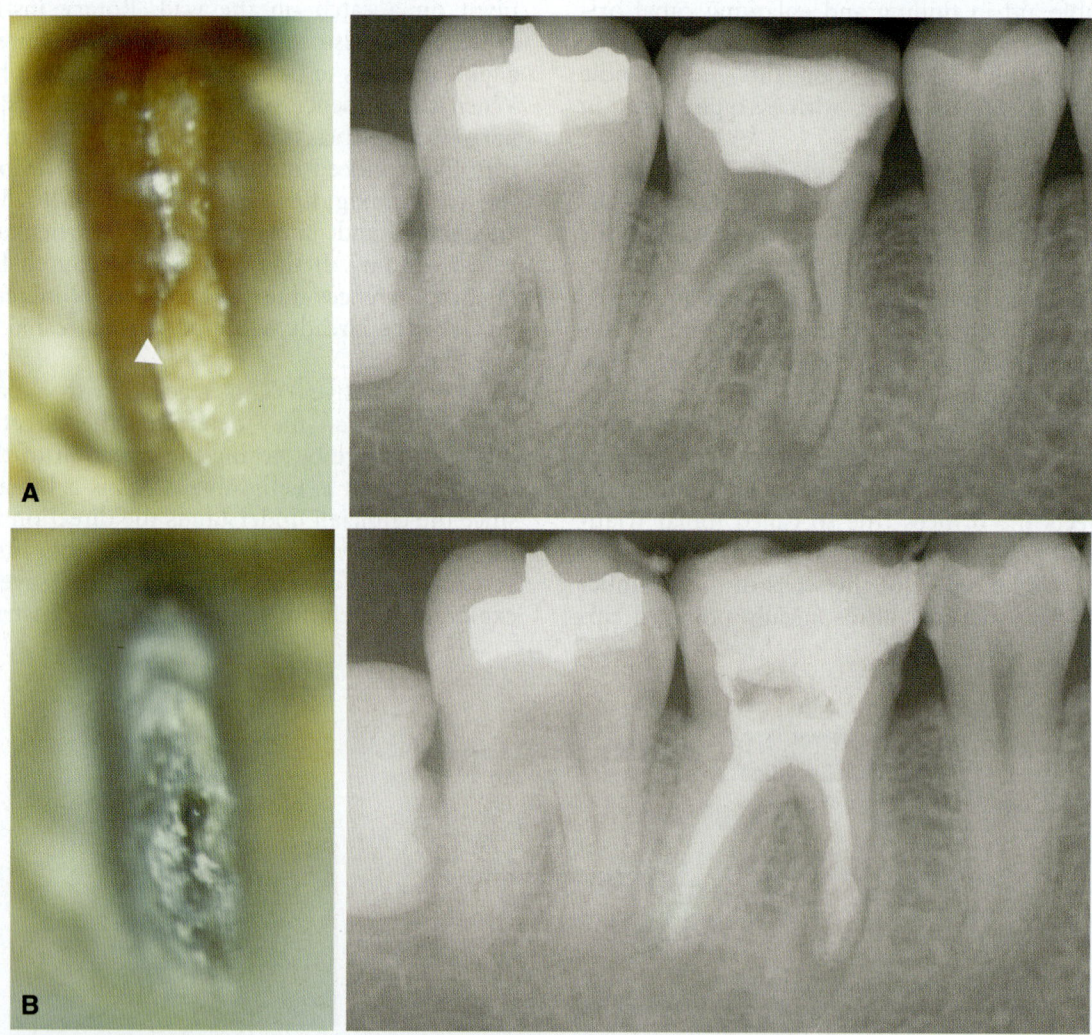

Figure 59 Occasionally, calcification may occur more apically than usual. In this case, ultrasonic instruments were used to remove the obstruction (arrowhead in **A**); both mesial and distal canals were shaped and filled to the desired working length (WL). **A,** View through the operating microscope before using ultrasonic tips and preoperative radiographs. **B,** Canal lumen exposed as seen in the operating microscope and postoperative radiograph. Images courtesy of Dr. Peter Velvart.

illumination are keys to this task and experience will help to guide the clinician here more than textbooks.

In conclusion, it needs to be emphasized that the suggested methods are by no means the only way to approach difficult root canals. Again, it is in the hands of an artful clinician to master all aspects of such a case.

Devices for Powered Canal Preparation

Engine-driven instruments have been used in root canal preparation for more than 100 years beginning with GG drills in 1885. These drills were mostly used in handpieces connected to belt drives and were pedal-powered, even though the first electric dental handpiece had been patented in 1875. Subsequently, many modifications, and specifically handpieces with various oscillating movements, were brought to the market, none of which provided superior preparation quality.[122] Currently, the newest major energy sources for root canal preparation are again electric motors for continuous rotary motion and ultrasonic/sonic units for vibration.

MOTORS FOR ROTARY INSTRUMENTATION

Engine-driven instruments can be used in three types of contra-angle handpieces: a full rotary handpiece, mostly latch grip, a reciprocating/quarter-turn handpiece, or a special handpiece that imparts a vertical stroke but with an added reciprocating quarter turn that "cuts in" when the instrument is stressed. These all are powered by electric or air-driven motors. While electric motors are more popular in Europe, air-powered motors are in much use in the United States. It is not clear if there are relevant differences between these two motor types regarding file breakage.[387] In addition to these two motors, there are battery-powered, slow-speed handpieces that may be combined with an apex locator, designed to simplify WL-control as well as torque-control motors (Figure 60).

As stated above, traditional handpieces with non-continuous movement such as the Giromatic (Micro-Mega) and M4 Safety handpiece (Kerr/Sybron) (see reference 122 for review) have been shown to lead to aberrant canal preparations. Some reports for these systems were favorable[388–390] while most others demonstrated problems, most notably a high incidence of preparation errors.[391–397] Consequently, these handpieces have lost popularity in the last years with the increased market share of NiTi rotaries.

An exception may be the Canal Finder system developed by Levy (currently marketed by SET, Olching, Germany) that uses a handpiece, either air-powered or electrically driven, that delivers a vertical stroke ranging from 0.3 to 1 mm. The more freely the instrument moves in the canal, the longer is the stroke. The handpiece also has a quarter-turn reciprocating motion that starts along with the vertical stroke when the canal instrument is under bind in a tight canal. If it is too tight, the motion ceases and the clinician switches to a smaller file.

More recently another handpiece with oscillating action was introduced (EndoEZE AET, Ultradent, South Jordan, UT) to more adequately prepare canals with oval cross sections. Unfortunately, this technique in its original configuration did not perform well in curved canals,[398] but with updates, in file type and alloy as well as instrument sequence, it may serve as an adjunct to address cases not suitable for rotary preparation alone.[399]

Recommended speeds for currently available NiTi rotaries are in the range of 150 to 600 rpm, with the exception of LS that works predominantly above 1,500 rpm. This range of speeds is typically reached with reduction gear handpieces (1:8 or 1:10). Higher speed is occasionally advocated for better efficacy and safety,[400] but the majority of authors maintain that lower speeds are beneficial, offering a better

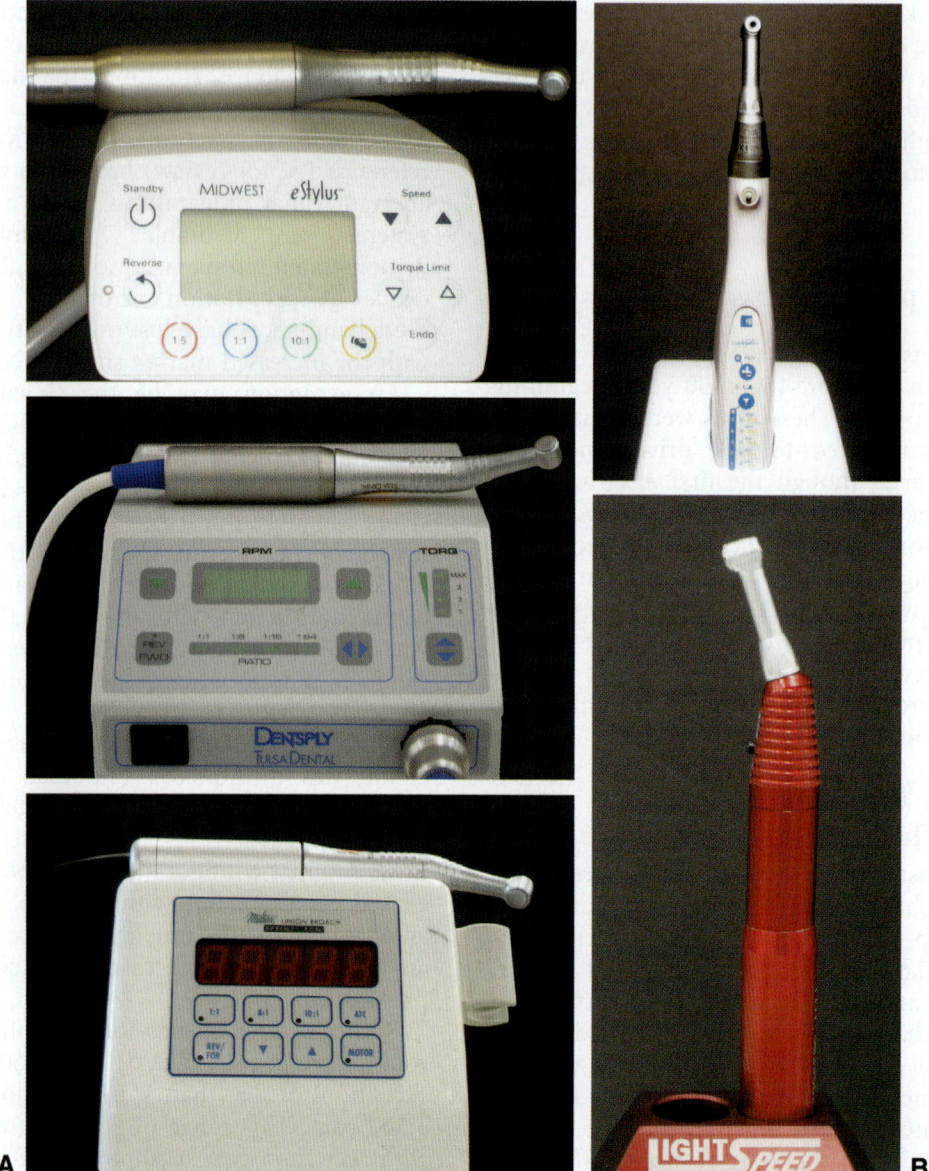

Figure 60 Selection of cable-bound **A**, and cordless **B**, motors intended for use with nickel–titanium (NiTi) rotary instruments.

compromise regarding fatigue lifespan[387,401,402] and occurrence of taper lock.[345,346,403,404]

For continuous rotary movement, electric motors offer several benefits over air-powered ones, such as stable preset rotations per minute. However, the most attention has been focused on the potential to preselect maximum torque in order to protect instrument tips from fracturing.[405] This is accomplished by setting a maximum current (DC motors) except for the so-called stepper motor that is software-controlled (EndoStepper, SET). There is some evidence that the use a of a torque-limiting motor reduces the overall load on NiTi files and hence increases their fatigue lifespan.[406,407] Moreover, these motors are seen as useful for beginners, to avoid forcing an instrument.[404] Various settings are possible for some torque-limited motors; for example, the motor can stop, go into reverse or into oscillations.

On the other hand, electronics inside motors and hence their torque limits are not very precise;[408–410] wear and friction inside the handpiece must also be further taken into account. Moreover, these motors depend on correct presets for the expected fracture limit. The limits are determined according to the

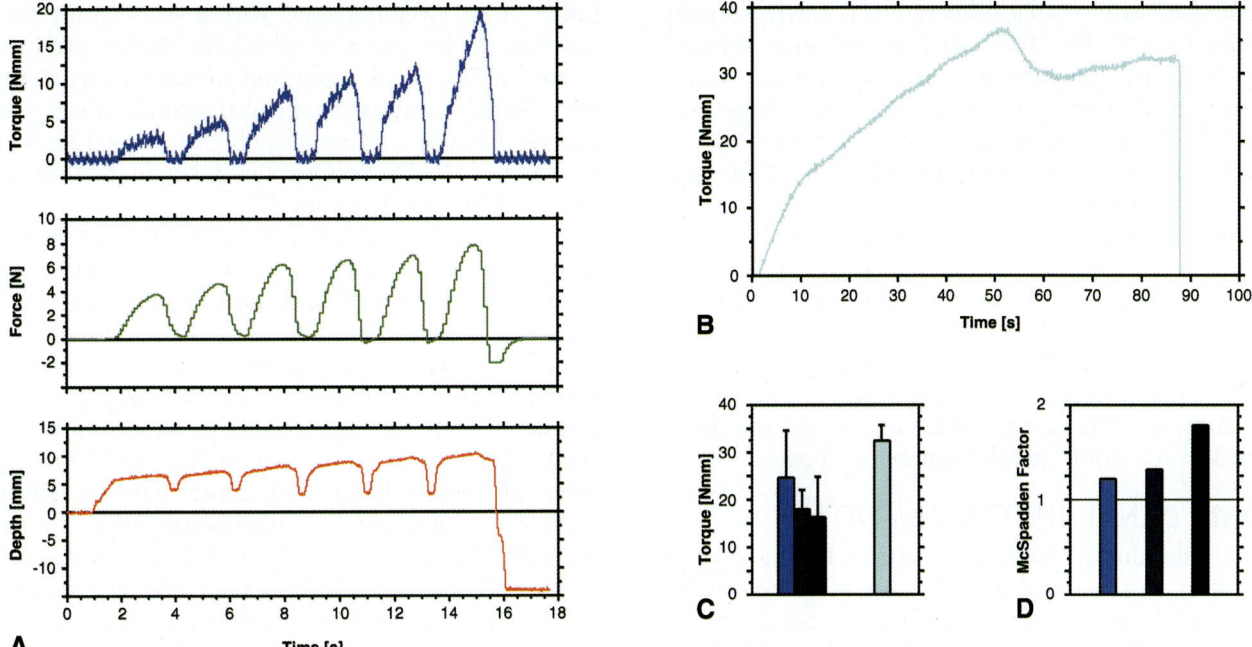

Figure 61 Relationship of torque during canal preparation and fracture load: The McSpadden Factor. **A,** Working torque (in blue), apically directed force (in green), and insertion depth (in red) into an extracted tooth simultaneously recorded during preparation with a ProFile 0.04 60 rotary using a testing platform. Note that total length of the instrument use was about 16 seconds. **B,** Determination of fracture load according to ISO 3630-1 at 2 rpm, determined at D3. **C,** Mean working torques (means SD, n = 10 each) in straight and curved plastic blocks or in extracted teeth (indicated by various shades of dark blue) and static fracture load (bright blue bar, n = 8). Modified with permission from Peters OA and Barbakow F.[363] **D,** Values of the McSpadden factors for ProFile 0.04 60 are above 1 in all tested conditions, indicating a very fracture-resistant instrument (bar shades correspond to panel C).

pertinent norms at D3, 3 mm from the tip of the file.[411] Hence, a short and less resistant segment of the file can still break even when the presets are correct.

A minimum torque is required for a rotary instrument to work against friction to prepare a canal (Figure 61). This torque level depends on instrument cross sections and hand movements employed. The relationship between fracture load at D3 and working torque has been referred to by J.T. McSpadden as the "safety quotient"; it is calculated by dividing fracture load by working torque.

If working torque is high and the fracture limit is a small torque value, the instrument's safety quotient is below 1. This indicates that the instruments may operate with imminent danger of fracturing. In contrast, if there is very little working torque and a high torque is required to fracture the instrument, the quotient is well above 1, and hence safety is considered high (see Figure 61). However, Blum et al.[412] have correctly pointed out that the quotient should refer to a specific instrument cross section rather than D3 alone to be more meaningful.

ULTRASONIC CANAL INSTRUMENTATION

The use of ultrasonic in endodontics is based on sound as an energy source (at 20 to 25 kHz) that activates an endodontic file. As a result, three-dimensional file movement in the surrounding medium of root canals may be enlarged.[413] The main débridement action of ultrasonics was initially thought to be by cavitation, a process by which bubbles formed from the action of the file become unstable, collapse, and cause an implosion. A combined shock, shear, and vacuum action resulted.[413] Ultrasonic handpieces typically use K-files as instruments for canal shaping. Before a size #15 file can fully function, however, the canal must be enlarged with hand instruments to at least a size #20 to allow the file to oscillate without constraint. Although Richman must be credited with the first report (1957) of the use of ultrasonics in endodontics,[414] Martin and Cunningham[415–420] were the first to develop a device, test it, and see it marketed in 1976. It was named the Cavitron Endodontic System by Dentsply Caulk and was followed by many other devices on the market. These instruments all deliver an irrigant/coolant, usually NaOCl, into the canal space while canal preparation is carried out by a vibrating K-file. The canal shapes and surfaces achieved, by preparation with ultrasonic units, have ranged from outstanding[419–424] to disappointing,[166,425–428] in particular regarding canal shapes,[289,429,430] and the use of ultrasonics to shape canals has fallen into disregard over the last decade.

Research into the potential mechanisms of ultrasonic action has continued and has revealed that it is not cavitation, but a different physical phenomenon, acoustic streaming, that is responsible for the débridement.[431–433] Clearly, acoustic streaming depends on the free displacement amplitude of the file, and if the vibrating file is at least partially constrained and dampened in its action, it will become ineffective.[434]

SONIC CANAL INSTRUMENTATION

Sonic endodontic handpieces attach to the regular airline at a pressure of 0.4 MPa. Air pressure may be varied with an adjustable ring on the handpiece to give an oscillatory range of 1.5 to 3 kHz. Tap water irrigant/coolant is delivered into the preparation from the handpiece. Walmsley et al.[434,435] studied the oscillatory pattern of sonically powered files. They found that out in the air, the sonic file oscillated in a large elliptical motion at the tip. However, when loaded, as in a canal, they found that the oscillatory motion changed to a longitudinal motion, up and down, "...a particularly efficient form of vibration for the preparation of root canals...."[435]

Similar to ultrasonic instrumentation, there is currently little support for the use of sonic vibration to prepare root canals, with the only exception of retrograde canal preparation during endodontic surgery (see Chapter 32, Endodontic treatment outcome: the potential for healing and retained function).

Today ultrasonically activated instruments are used for final canal débridement rather than canal preparation.[436] Passive sonic and ultrasonic irrigation is distinct from active irrigation; in the former, irrigant deposited in the canal is activated, whereas in the latter, a stream of solution is continuously delivered from the ultrasonic or sonic unit. Passive irrigation (after smear layer removal) with a size #15 file for 3 minutes in the presence of 5.25% NaOCl produced cleaner canals when compared to hand instrumentation alone.[437] Improvement in irrigation efficacy was also reported by authors using 5.25% NaOCl for 30 to 60 seconds,[438] 2% NaOCl for 3 minutes,[222] or 2% chlorhexidine for 1 minute.[439]

There has been concern that cutting instruments would in fact negatively impact canal surface and shape and therefore blunt noncutting inserts have been advocated. Figure 62 shows canal segments after passive ultrasonic irrigation, demonstrating no damage with either cutting or noncutting instruments.[378,440] It has also been of interest to see if NaOCl may be extruded out of the apical foramen from ultrasonic filing and cause harmful effects. Alacam[441] intentionally overinstrumented beyond the apex in a monkey study and then evaluated the tissue response when NaOCl was used with conventional filing versus ultrasonic filing/irrigation. He did not find any difference between the two methods and noted a low to moderate inflammatory response periapically.

Ultrasonically and sonically activated passive irrigation exerts its effects via acoustic streaming and increase in temperature[442,443] (Figure 63) rather than cavitations as previously thought. Using both mechanisms, 3 minutes of ultrasonic instrumentation with a size #15 file and 5.25% NaOCl improved canal cleanliness.[444] It is presently not clear which combination of file size and canal shape produces the best results. In one study, smaller files generated greater acoustic streaming and hence much cleaner canals.[432] As it had been shown that constraint of the activated insert in the apical canal third was an important factor,[434,445] a freely oscillating size #15 K-file was used for 5 minutes with a free flow of 1% NaOCl. The same authors found that root canals had to be enlarged to the size of a size #40 file to permit enough clearance for the free vibration of the size #15 file at full amplitude.[446] Others have also recommended a size #15 file;[378,427,447] however, van der Sluis et al.[440] recently speculated that the shape of the insert in

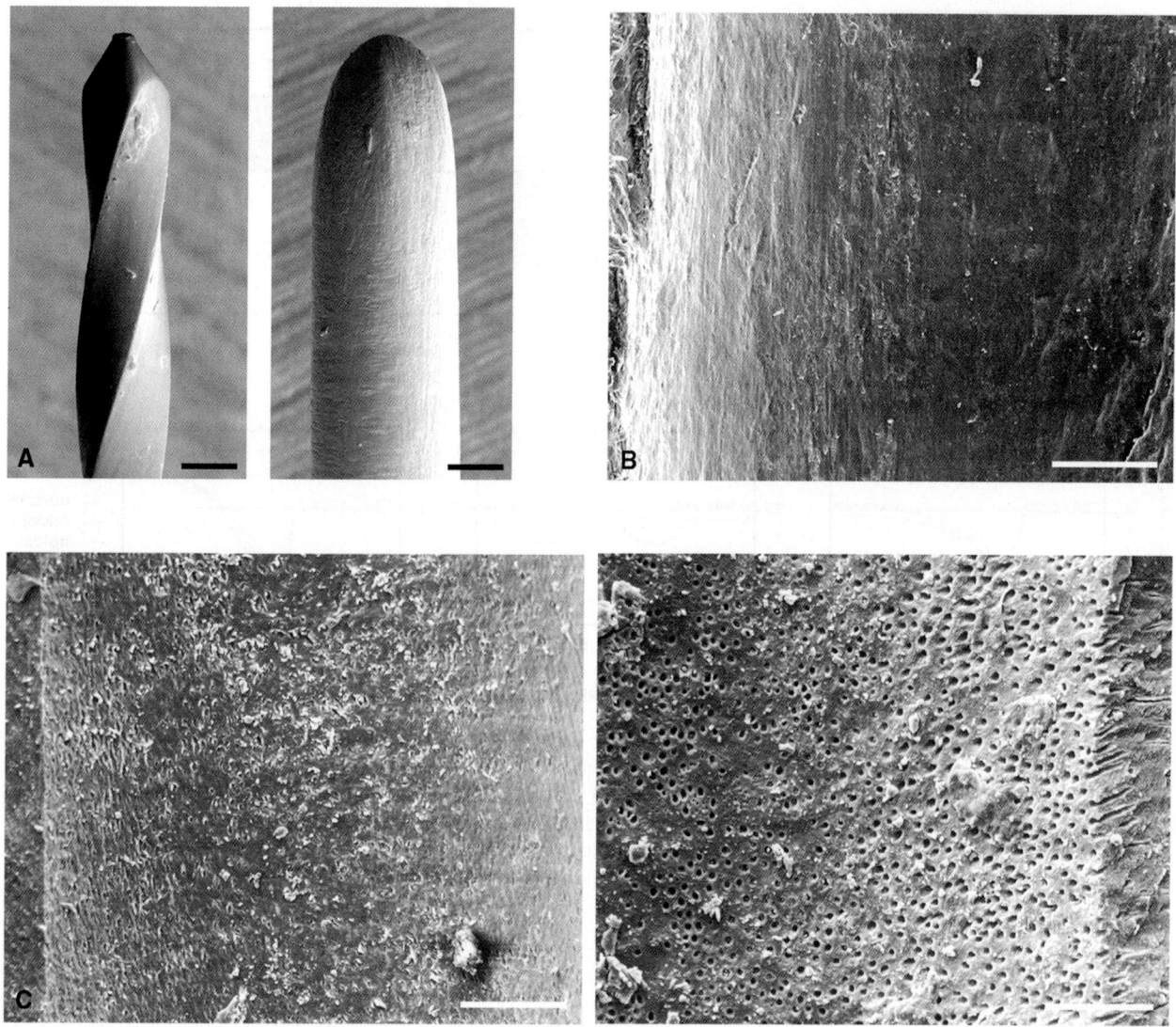

Figure 62 Varying effect of ultrasonic activation of deposited irrigation solution on apical canal wall morphology. In this experiment, both 5.25% sodium hypochlorite (NaOCl) and 17% ethylenediaminetetraacetic acid (EDTA) irrigation were activated with either K-file-type or prototype noncutting inserts after enlargement of single-rooted teeth to an apical size #45. ***A,*** Scanning electron micrographs of ultrasonic inserts, black bars are 300 μm. ***B,*** Canal surface with smear layer without the use of EDTA (control). ***C,*** Apical segments after irrigation with NaOCl and EDTA with ultrasonic activation, demonstrating thin continuous (left) or no smear layer with open dentinal tubules (right, white bars are 50 μm).

relation to the canal shape may play a role for its efficacy. Indeed, temperature changes during activation of irrigants vary with the geometry and the material of the insert, indicative of energy transfer (Paque F and Peters OA, unpublished data) (see Figure 63). While the majority of in vitro studies support improved débridement with the use of passive ultrasonic irrigation, potential clinical benefit is as yet unproven. In fact, ultrasonic inserts may fracture, representing an iatrogenic problem during canal shaping (Figure 64).

Evaluation of Canal Preparation Techniques

A variety of techniques have been used over the years to assess preparation quality (see references 120, 122 for review), and most of these investigations were done in vitro. Previously, two main parameters were addressed, mostly from a mechanistic viewpoint: canal shapes and appearance of canal surfaces, the latter also termed cleanliness.

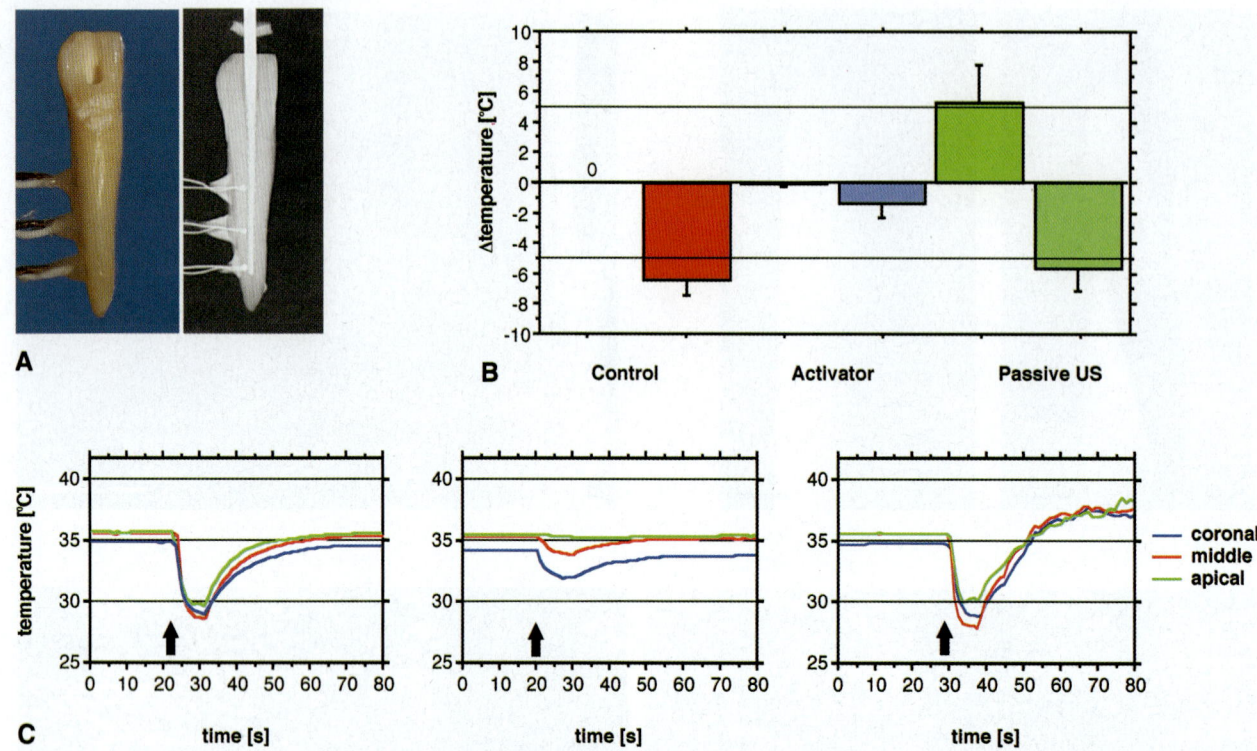

Figure 63 Effect of ultrasonic activation on intracanal temperature in vitro. Thermocouples were attached to single-rooted teeth and the assembly was placed in a water bath at 37°C. Irrigation solution was either added and activated or continuously deposited concurrent with ultrasonic activation using various inserts. **A,** Three thermocouples fitted into holes drilled in radicular dentin close to the intracanal surface. **B,** Bar diagrams showing maximum and minimum temperatures at the coronal, middle, and apical levels. Measurement duration 2.5 minutes, n=15. **C,** Original records of temperature over time with no ultrasonic activation (control, left), using an agitator at sonic frequency (prototype, middle) and a blunt nickel–titanium (NiTi) wire for passive ultrasonic agitation (right, EndoSoft, EMS, Nyon, Switzerland). Beginning of irrigation indicated by arrows.

The ability of an instrument or a technique to allow the prepared canal to stay centered in root cross sections is seen as beneficial (Figure 65). Conversely, canal transportation, or any deviation from the original canal path, is seen as negative and in particular the end points of transportation, namely preparation errors (Figure 66). The term "zip" was coined by Weine,[278] who described the appearance of a "zipped" apex when viewed directly in vitro. The formation of preparation errors is believed to be due to the interaction of canal curvature, file design, and file handling (see Figure 50). The tendency of a file to straighten

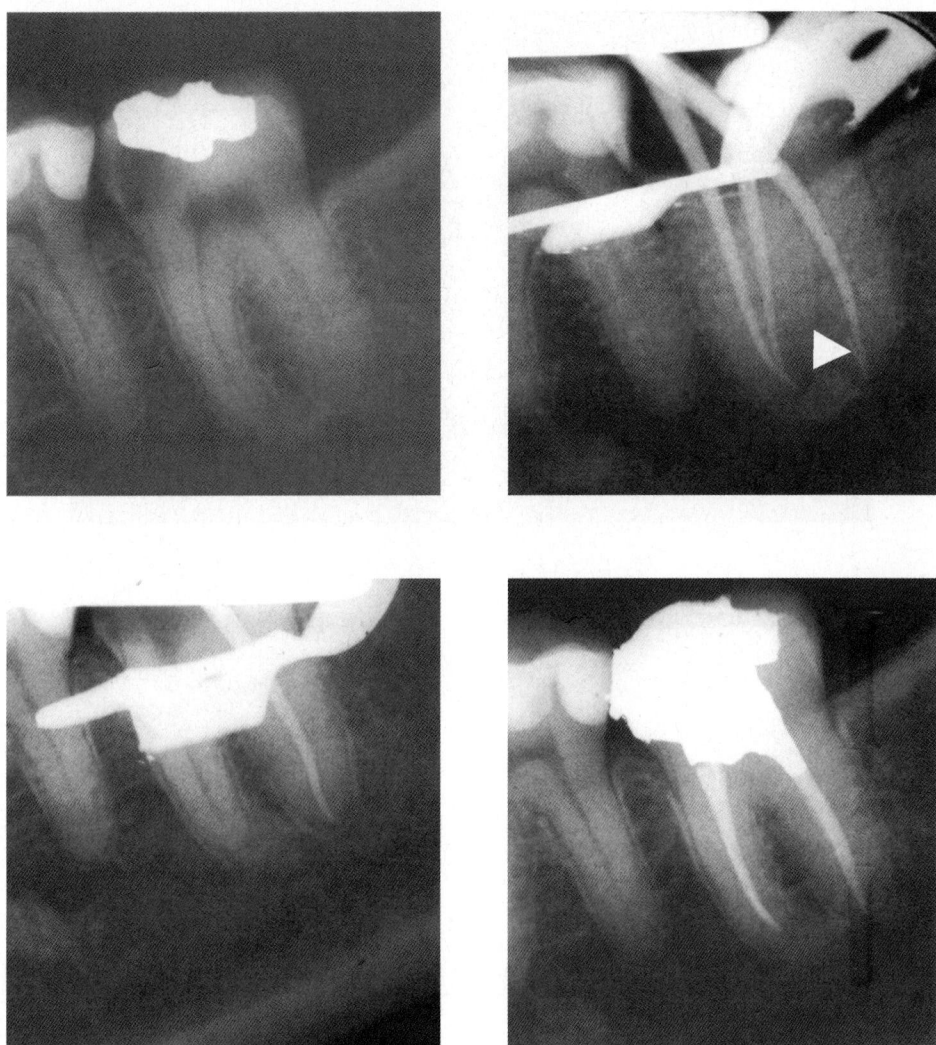

Figure 64 Use of activated irrigation in the clinical setting. A size #15 K-file was attached to an ultrasonic unit (middle power setting) and activated for 30 s. During cone fit, it was noted that a segment of the instrument had fractured. The fragment was removed and the root canal system filled with thermoplasticized gutta-percha.

itself cannot be completely overcome by precurving and leads to uneven distribution of forces and hence material removal.[284,448]

Moreover, the cutting action of instruments in the apical region, particularly when extended beyond the canal space, may create an apical zip with perforation.[449] The occurrence of such apical preparation errors has previously been linked to hand and rotary instruments with sharp tips.[450–452] Zip-and-elbow formation and other well-described preparation outcomes such as ledges, strip perforations, or excessive thinning of canal walls[453] may have clinical consequences such as incomplete débridement, problems with root canal filling, or eventual vertical root fracture (Figure 67). Preparation errors may decrease outcomes, most likely via reduced antimicrobial efficacy, but their clinical consequences are still a matter of debate.[270–274,454,455]

Generally, apical canal areas tend to be overprepared toward the outer curve or the convexity of the canal, while more coronal areas are transported toward the concavity or the furcation in multirooted teeth (see Figure 50). This results in an uneven preparation demonstrated in canal cross sections with large areas left unprepared.[456–460] This finding was validated by three-dimensional analyses (see Figure 66) using micro-computed tomography.[245,263,461–464] While the amount

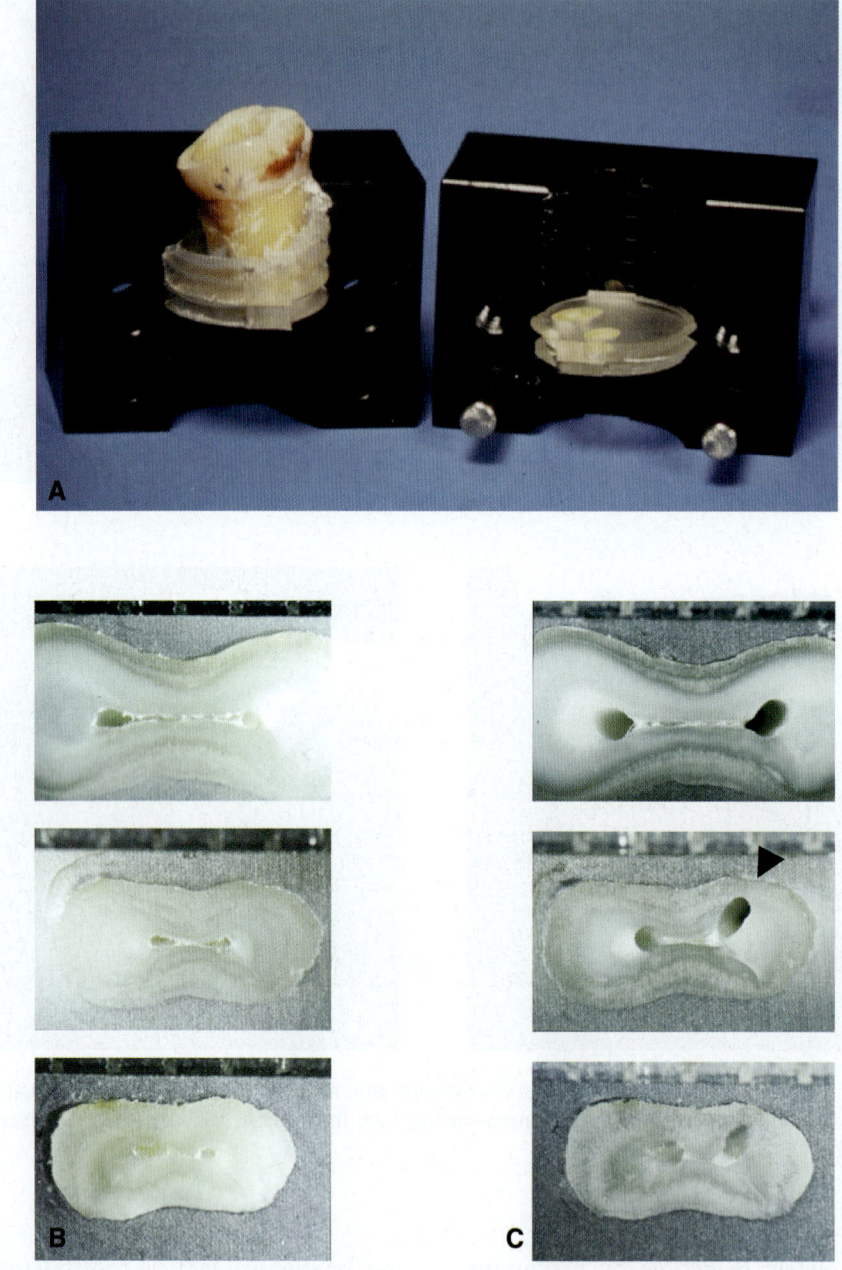

Figure 65 Canal cross sections before and after preparation can be assessed using a specially designed mold that allows sectioning of root, removal, and precise reposition of the resulting root disks ***A,*** Photographs can be taken and the effect of canal preparation numerically determined, for example, in the coronal, middle, and apical root thirds before ***B,*** and after preparation ***C,*** In this case shown, rotary preparation (left canals) resulted in round and centered shapes, while hand instrumentation produced canal transportation and thinning of root structure (arrowhead, ***C***). Gradation of bar is 0.5 mm.

of prepared canal surface seems to be independent of the instrument type, it was significantly affected by preoperative canal anatomy.[245,463,464] Sequential mechanical enlargement, as shown in Figure 68, may be indicated in order to increase prepared surface areas, in particular to remove tenacious biofilms present in retreatment cases.[465]

While the use of microcomputed tomography represents the latest available technology, there are numerous other ways to evaluate canal shapes, for

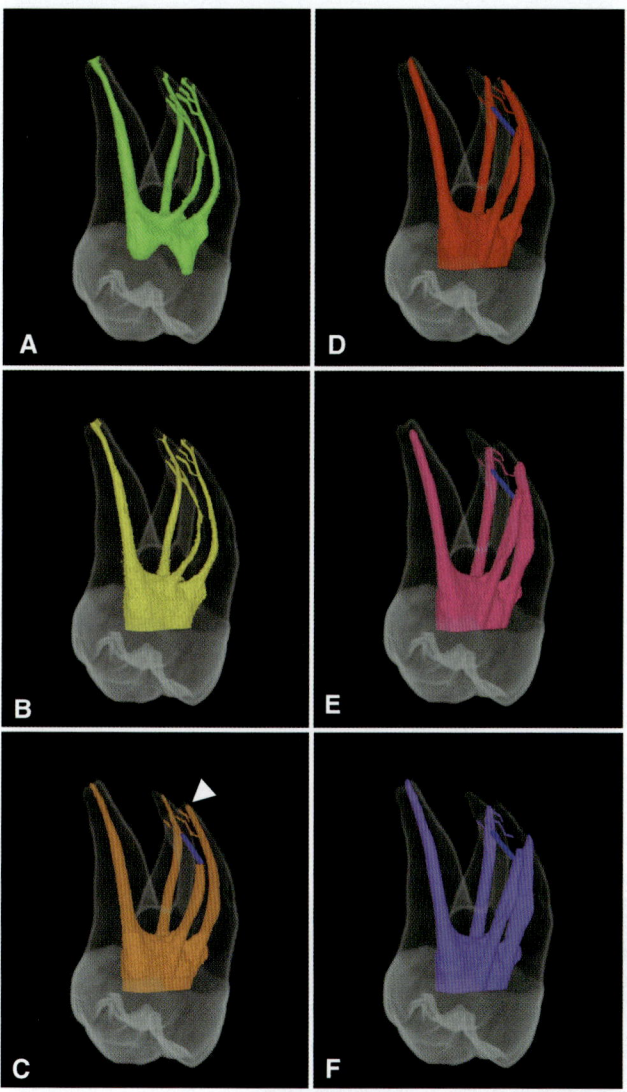

Figure 66 Root canal preparation errors develop more readily with increasing instrument size and hence stiffness. This panel of microcomputed tomography data shows canal straightening and perforation after shaping to size #25 in an experiment where quarter-turn pull motion was employed with stainless steel hand files. ***A***, Unprepared root canal system of a maxillary molar. ***B***, Accessed and coronal scouting with a size #15 file. ***C***, Enlargement to size #15 (buccal canals) and #25 (palatal canal) to working length (WL), note fractured instrument in second mesiobuccal canal (arrowhead). ***D***, Enlargement to size #30 (buccal canals) and #35 (palatal canal), note perforation in main mesiobuccal canal. ***E***, Enlargement to size #50 and #55 in buccal and palatal canals, respectively. ***F***, Enlargement to size #60 and #70 in buccal and palatal canals, respectively.

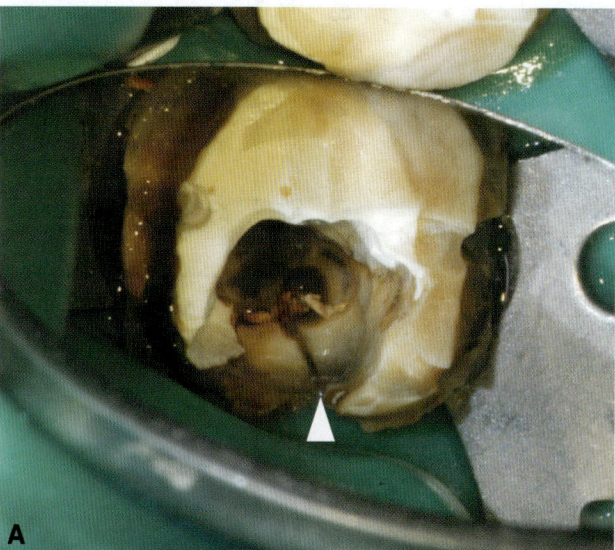

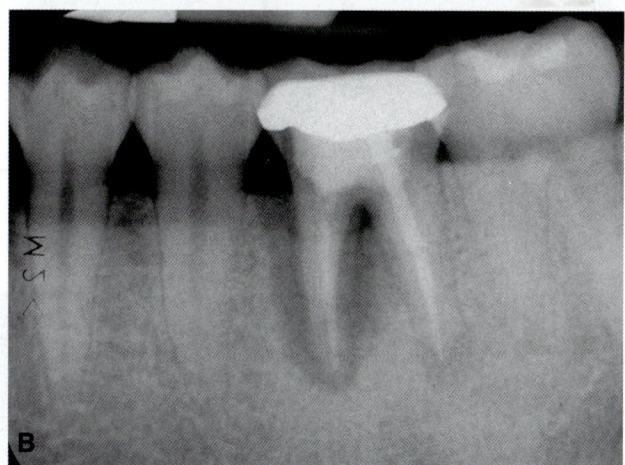

Figure 67 Relationship between vertical root fracture location, clinical, and radiographic appearance. A buccal swelling but not appreciable probing was present in this case. Only after the removal of the crown and the buildup material, a fracture line extending to the mesial was apparent (arrowhead in ***A***). A periodontal defect (probing depth 11 mm) was detected that corresponded to radiographically visible bone destruction ***B***, Images courtesy of Dr. Tri Huynh.

example, superimposing radiographs before and after shaping.[334,466–468] Bramante et al.[469] and later others[470–474] embedded teeth with their roots in a muffle system (see Figure 65). They were then cut and the cross sections evaluated before and after canal preparation. Center points of the canals were determined and movements of the canals' centers calculated.[472,474–480] Numerous studies evaluated shaping capabilities of specific instruments using canals of varying geometry in plastic blocks and extracted teeth. Various factors for canal transportation have been

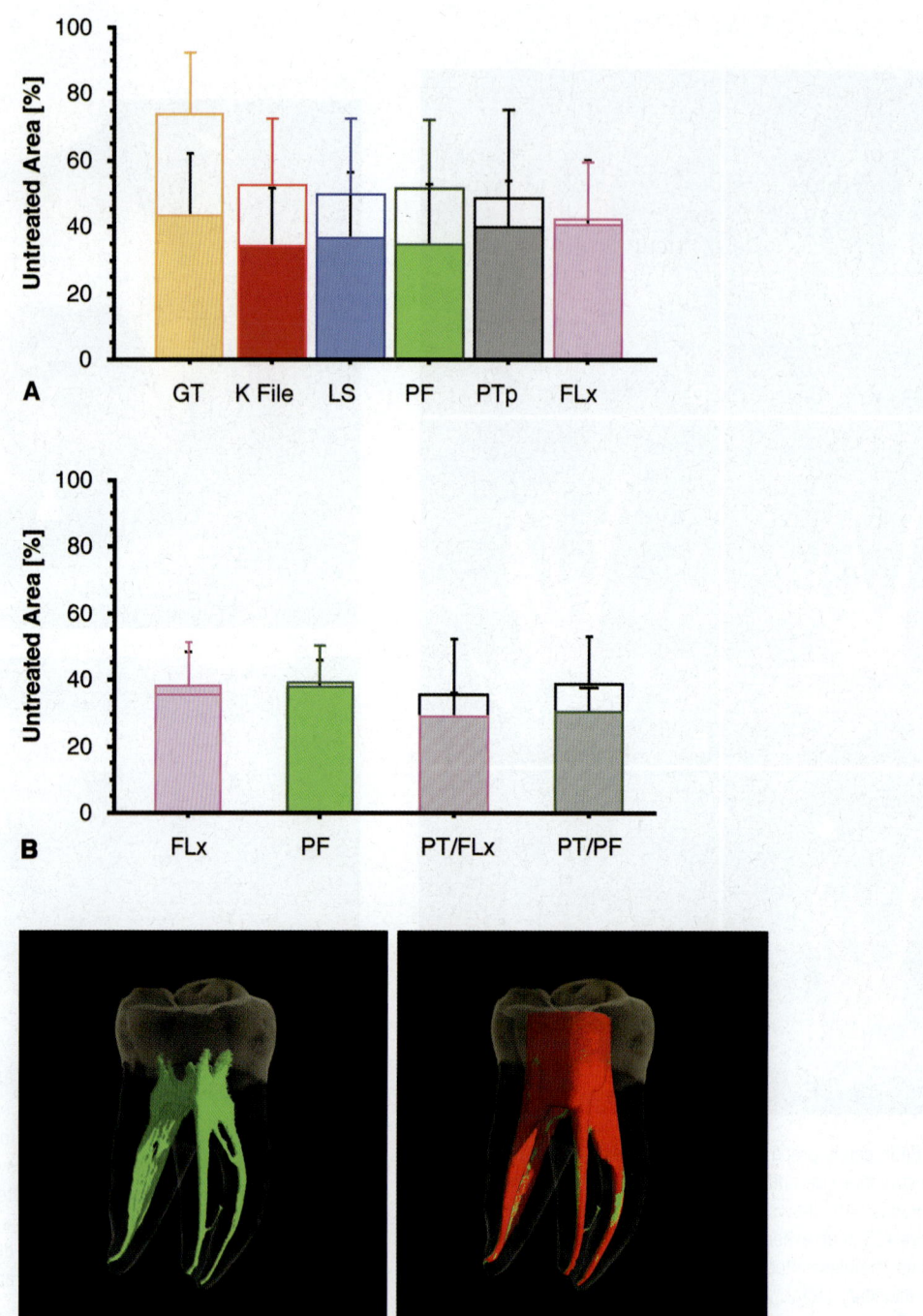

Figure 68 Dependence of instrumented canal surface on file geometry and usage. ***A,*** Bar diagram showing overall and apical fractions of instrumented canal surface. Data recalculated from Peters OA, et al.[245] ***B,*** Bar diagram showing increase of instrumented surface with increased apical sizes (Paqué F, Peters OA, unpublished data). ***C,*** Microcomputed tomography reconstructions of canals shaped with cutting and noncutting instruments used subsequently.

identified, such as canal anatomy, instrument type, cross-sectional and tip design, instrument taper, sequence, operator experience, rpm, and the use of irrigants or lubricants.[120]

The effect of canal anatomy on shaping outcome is well documented for LS, ProFile 0.4 and 0.06, Quantec LX and SC (Analytic Endodontics, Glendora, CA, USA), and HERO 642, in particular by experiments from Dummer's group[452,481–488] using plastic blocks. Taken together, these studies demonstrated an impact of canal geometry on outcome: the more severe the angle and radius of the curve, the more severe the canal transportation. On the other hand, there was no significant effect of canal shape on preparation times.

Furthermore, file design was crucial to avoid preparation errors: actively cutting tips such as with Quantec SC and LX[452,488] produced more aberrations than instruments with noncutting tips.[450,451,488–492]

The direction of apical canal transportation varied, but occurred mainly outward in relation to the canals' curve; the total amount of canal transportation varied significantly, again in relation to canal geometry, and ranged in most cases between 0.01 and 0.150 mm.[452,481–488]

Compared to stainless steel hand files, NiTi instruments were superior in their shaping ability.[493,494] Schäfer et al. reported that HERO 642,[495] FlexMaster (VDW, Munich, Germany),[496] and K3 instruments[497] maintained the original canal path in curved plastic blocks better compared to stainless steel hand instruments. They found little incidence of canal aberrations and material removal in excess of 0.15 mm in less than 50% of the levels analyzed for HERO, FlexMaster, and K3,[495–497] while hand instrumentation resulted in significantly greater material removal (up to 0.69 mm).[497]

ProTaper instruments prepared curved canals in plastic blocks in less time and with no definite canal aberrations, but with a larger amount of material removed, compared to GT Rotary, Quantec, and ProFile 0.04 and 0.06 instruments.[498] In a study using another brand of plastic blocks, Hata et al. found overly long preparation times (>250s) for ProFile 0.04 and 0.06, GT Rotary, and in particular for "Balanced Force" instrumentation.[330]

Instrument shaft design did not significantly modify shapes of similar apical sizes in one series of studies,[461,462] while it is generally held that a thin flexible shaft will allow larger apical shapes with less aberrations.[9,472] In contrast, ProFile 0.04 instruments alone removed more material compared to a combination of ProFile 0.04 and 0.06.[330]

Cutting blade design was modified lately from passive, so-called U-file designs to more actively cutting triangular ones in instruments such as ProTaper, FlexMaster, K3, HERO 642, and RaCe. However, while there is only limited evidence for each individual file,[462–464,495,496,499,500] the introduction of actively cutting cross sections does not appear to negatively affect centering abilities.

K-files used in most techniques, with the exception of "Balance forces," performed inferior to NiTi rotary in vitro.[290,292,501–503] Clearly, reaming produced rounder canal shapes in cross section,[504–506] which may be desirable as long as a canal may be reasonably prepared round.

Handpieces with noncontinuous rotation have also been extensively tested, and some are better in cutting efficiency, some in following narrow curved canals, some in producing smooth canals, and some in allowing irrigation and smear layer removal.[398,423,507–514] While all of the automated devices may be occasionally useful, none has proved to be outstanding; currently NiTi rotary instrumentation is widely believed to be a better choice for root canal preparation.

As stated earlier, rotary instrumentation is potentially associated with an increased risk of instrument breakage.[349,515–518] Substantial work has been done in vitro to elucidate the fracture mechanisms involved (see Box 2); however, the clinical impact of instrument fractures is less well documented and does not lend itself to assessment in prospective clinical studies.

Currently available evidence for outcome studies regarding the impact of file breakage, as recently reviewed by Parashos and Messer,[349] relates mainly to the pre-NiTi era, with few exceptions.[518,519] For example, Strindberg[131] using very stringent criteria in his comprehensive outcome study found a 19% higher incidence of failure when a file fragment was retained. He speculated that infection of the root canal apically of the retained fragment would render the prognosis poorer. On the other hand, a retrospective analysis by Crump and Natkin[454] of the outcomes of root canal treatments done by dental students revealed instrument fractures in 178 out of approximately 8,500 cases. Matched control cases of the same cohort without instrument fracture had statistically similar outcomes when cases were evaluated as "success," "failure," or "uncertain," based on clinical and radiographic criteria. In fact, the success rate was slightly higher in the cases with retained fragments (81.2% versus 73.6%, $p>0.05$).

In a retrospective assessment of 66 cases with broken instruments, Grossman[520] found over a recall period of up to 5 years, that out of cases without pre-existing apical periodontitis (47/66) about 90% stayed healthy and only 2 showed signs of a lesion. Of the 19 cases with a diagnosis of apical periodontitis, however, healing occurred only in 9 cases. Similar results were reported by Fox et al.[521] referring to 204 cases with accidentally broken files, out of which only 12 were scored as failures.

In a recent study on 8,460 cases, Spili et al.[518] found overall a 3.3% prevalence of instrument fractures but a prevalence of 5.1% after the introduction of NiTi rotaries (4.4% NiTi versus 0.7% stainless steel). However, success rates were similar for teeth with and without a retained instrument fragment (91.8% versus 94.5%). Moreover, if an instrument fractured in a tooth with existing apical periodontitis, the healing rate would be lower (86.7% versus 92.9%), but this difference was not significant. Similarly, Wolcott et al.[519] in an analysis of 4,652 cases found an overall fracture incidence of 2.4% using ProTaper instruments; however, they did not report on clinical outcomes of these cases.

From the described outcome studies, fractures that developed early compared to late during cleaning and shaping may be viewed differently, regarding the potential to remove microbes from the root canal space. Irrigant efficacy is affected by the amount of canal enlargement;[9,10,222] therefore, a fragment lodged in the canal before sufficient enlargement has taken place may render canal disinfection ineffective. In case of corrosion[356,358,522] of the retained fragment, changed ion concentrations in the microenvironment may inhibit microorganism growth.[523] At least this partially explains acceptable outcomes, even in the presence of retained instrument fragments.[349]

Opinions vary over the risk and incidence of rotary instrument fractures, but even without solid clinical data it is generally thought that NiTi rotary fracture incidence is higher when compared to stainless steel hand instruments. The impact of these fractures on healing probabilities[524] is not clear.[349] In fact, consequences of a retained or removed instrument fragment are part of a complex array of impact factors governing the spectrum of clinical outcomes. Therefore, an immediate attempt to remove a fractured root canal instrument is mainly indicated if the coronal aspect of the fragment is visible, aided by magnification, and if there is microbial contamination apical to the fragment. A fragment position apical to a major curve significantly decreases the potential of successful removal.[525,526]

In summary, available evidence from recall studies would suggest to take a conservative approach after a fracture of a root canal instrument: (1) when a preoperative diagnosis of irreversible pulpitis and hence a noncontaminated root canal system had been made; (2) if the instrument fractured very late in the procedure, after a sufficient attempt for canal disinfection had been done; and (3) if the instrument fractured apical to a significant curve. For a detailed account of techniques for instrument removal, the reader is referred to Chapter 31, "Retreatment of non-healing endodontic therapy and management of mishaps".

Nontraditional Techniques

Besides hand and rotary instruments, lasers have been proposed for root canal preparation for some time and is still contemplated by some authors today.[527] On the other hand, if no enlargement of the root canal system was required for disinfection and root canal filling, no preparation errors could be made; this may be possible with the so-called noninstrumentation technique.[528] Finally, ongoing research is aimed at changing the paradigm of root canal preparation for disinfection and filling altogether, with the potential of seeding stem cells or at least allowing local cell population to recolonize endodontic spaces.[529]

LASER-ASSISTED CANAL PREPARATION

Early studies of the effects of lasers on hard dental tissues were based simply on the empirical use of available lasers and an examination of the tissue modified by various techniques. Lasers emitting in the ultraviolet, visible (i.e., argon laser, wavelengths of 488 and 514 nm), and near infrared (i.e., neodymium:yttrium–aluminum-garnet laser, 1.064 μm) are weakly absorbed by dental hard tissues, such as enamel and dentin.[530,531] Nd:YAG laser energy, on the other hand, interacts well with dark tissues and is transmitted by water. Excimer lasers (193, 248, and 308 nm) and erbium lasers (~3.0 μm) are strongly absorbed by dental hard tissues.[530,531] Studies have been conducted evaluating the effects of laser irradiation inside root canals. The authors have discussed laser endodontic therapy, some as supplementary and others as a purely laser-assisted method.[532]

Applications of lasers in endodontic therapy have been aggressively investigated over the last two decades, and this is discussed in more detail in Chapter 26E, "Lasers". Briefly, there are three main areas in endodontics for the use of lasers: (1) hard tissue, (2) root canal surface, and (3) the periapex. Obviously, laser light travels straight; therefore, specific light-

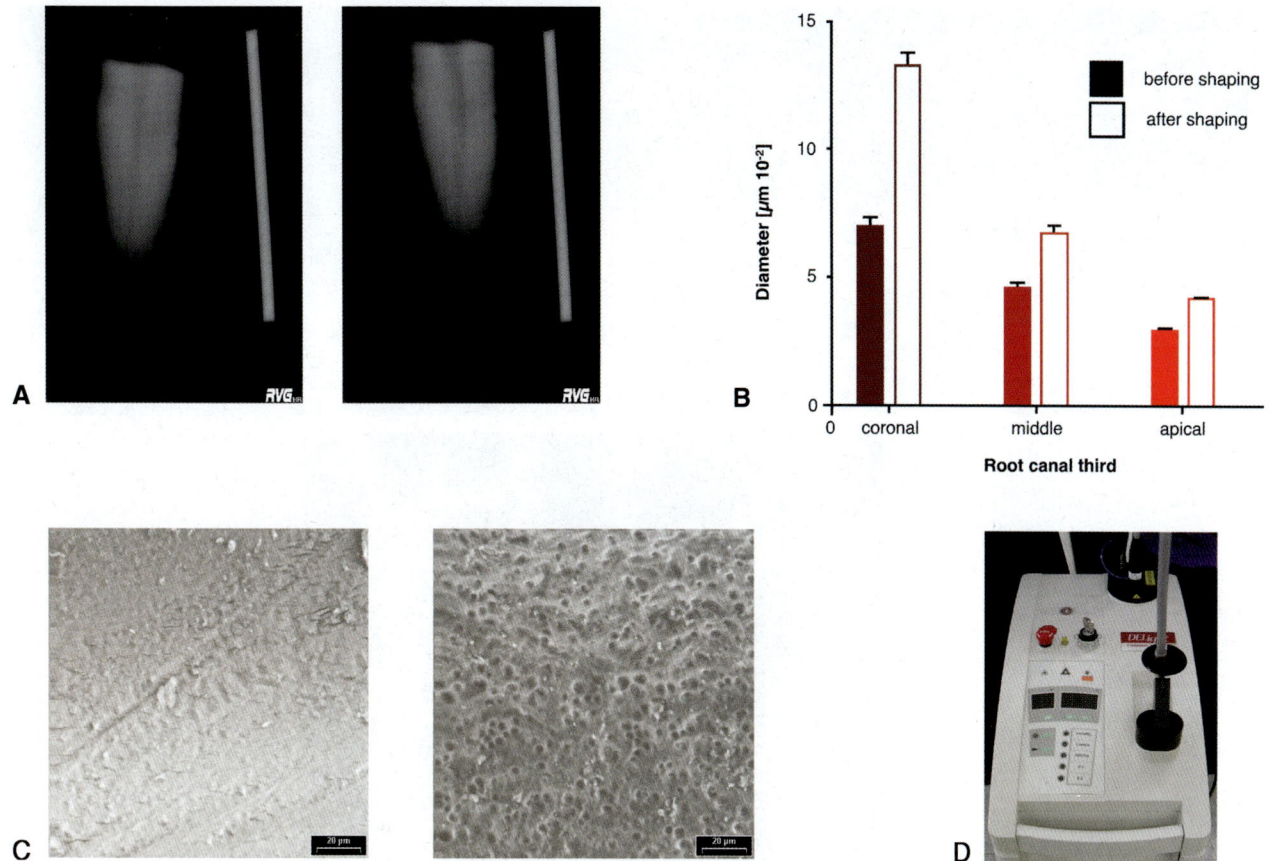

Figure 69 Shaping of single-rooted teeth in vitro using an Er:YAG laser. **A,** Canal diameters compared using standardized radiographs. **B,** Bar diagram showing mean (~ SD) canal diameters before and after shaping. **C,** Scanning electron micrographs of lased apical canal surface (left) and control after rotary instrumentation (right). **D,** Er:YAG laser used in the study. Images courtesy of Dr. Mark Roper.

emitting probes have been developed to direct laser energy not only into straight but also into curved root canals. Enlargement and cleaning of straight canals with an Er:YAG laser was found to be effective and in fact faster than with step-back preparation with K-files.[527] However, shaping curved root canals, independent of the probes used, has not been satisfactory (Figure 69).

Several authors have reported better removal of debris, for example, using an erbium:YAG laser,[533,534] although areas covered by residual debris could be found where the laser light did not get into contact with the root canal surface.[535] An erbium:YAG laser was more effective in debris removal (Figure 70), producing a cleaner surface with a greater number of open tubules when compared with a Nd:YAG laser and an unlased control without laser treatment.

Nd:YAG laser-irradiated samples presented not only with melted and recrystallized dentin and smear layer removal but also with charring in light microscopic images.[536] However, SEM evaluation showed specific patterns for erbium:YAG and Nd:YAG irradiation as a result of different mechanisms of laser–tissue interaction by these two wavelengths.[533–535,537]

Dederich et al.[532] used a Nd:YAG laser to irradiate the root canal walls and showed melted, recrystallized, and glazed surfaces. The process of melting and recrystallizing root canal surfaces was hoped to create a clean and less penetrable canal.[538] Laser energy transferred into canal surfaces, when sufficient to melt dentin, may overheat the periodontal ligament also. Bahcall et al.,[539] for example, investigated the use of the pulsed Nd:YAG laser to clean root canals. Their results showed that the Nd:YAG laser may cause harm to the bone and periodontal tissues by overheating, which was also suggested by others.[536,540,541] According to Hibst et al.,[542] the use of a highly absorbed laser light tends to localize heating to a thin layer at the sample surface, thus minimizing the absorption depth.

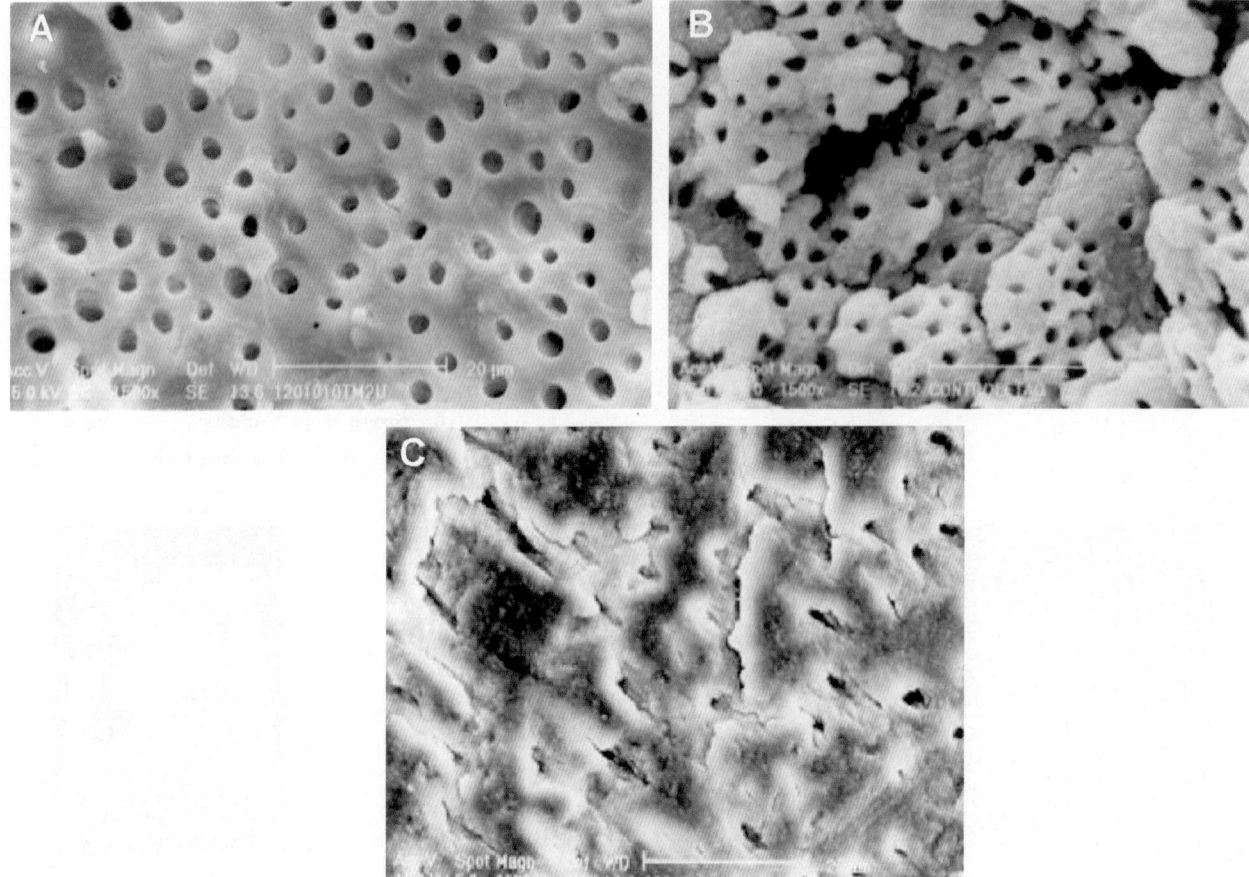

Figure 70 Intracanal dentin surfaces (apical third) under scanning electron microscope (SEM) (orig. mag. ×1500) after laser treatment. ***A,*** Dentin treated with erbium:YAG laser (100 mJ, 15 Hz). Note effective debris removal. ***B,*** Control, unlased dentin surface. ***C,*** Dentin surface treated with Nd:YAG laser (80 mJ, 10 Hz). Note melted and recrystallized dentin surface. Reproduced with permission from Cecchini SCM et al.[537]

Consequently, the risk of subsurface thermal damage may decrease since less energy is necessary to heat the surface.[543]

One of the limitations of the laser treatment was demonstrated in a study by Harashima et al.[544] Where the (argon) laser optic fiber had not touched or reached the canal walls, areas with clean root canal surfaces were interspersed with areas covered by residual debris. Access into severely curved roots and the cost of the equipment are other limitations. Finally, operator and patient safety are of concern in the application of lasers in endodontics; safety precautions include safety glasses specific for each wavelength, warning signs, and high-volume evacuation close to the treated area.

NONINSTRUMENTATION TECHNIQUE

Based on the premise that optimal cleansing of the root canal system is a prime prerequisite for long-term success in endodontics, Lussi et al.[246] introduced a minimally invasive approach for removing canal contents and accomplishing disinfection that did not involve the use of a file (the noninstrumentation technique or NIT). This system consists of a pump, a hose, a special valve, and a connector that needs to be cemented into the access cavity (Figure 71). Cleaning action is then provided by oscillations of the irrigation solution (1% to 3% NaOCl) at a reduced pressure. Cavitation likely loosens the debris and NaOCl dissolves viable and necrotic tissue components that are then removed by suction from the low pressure. It needs to be stressed that this system is different from other recently proposed active irrigation systems,[545–547] since the latter techniques still rely on mechanical shaping prior to the use of irrigation while a canal undergoing NIT is not enlarged.

The evolution of the technique over the years[548,549] has resulted in good cleaning ability in vitro. However, clinical moisture control and filling

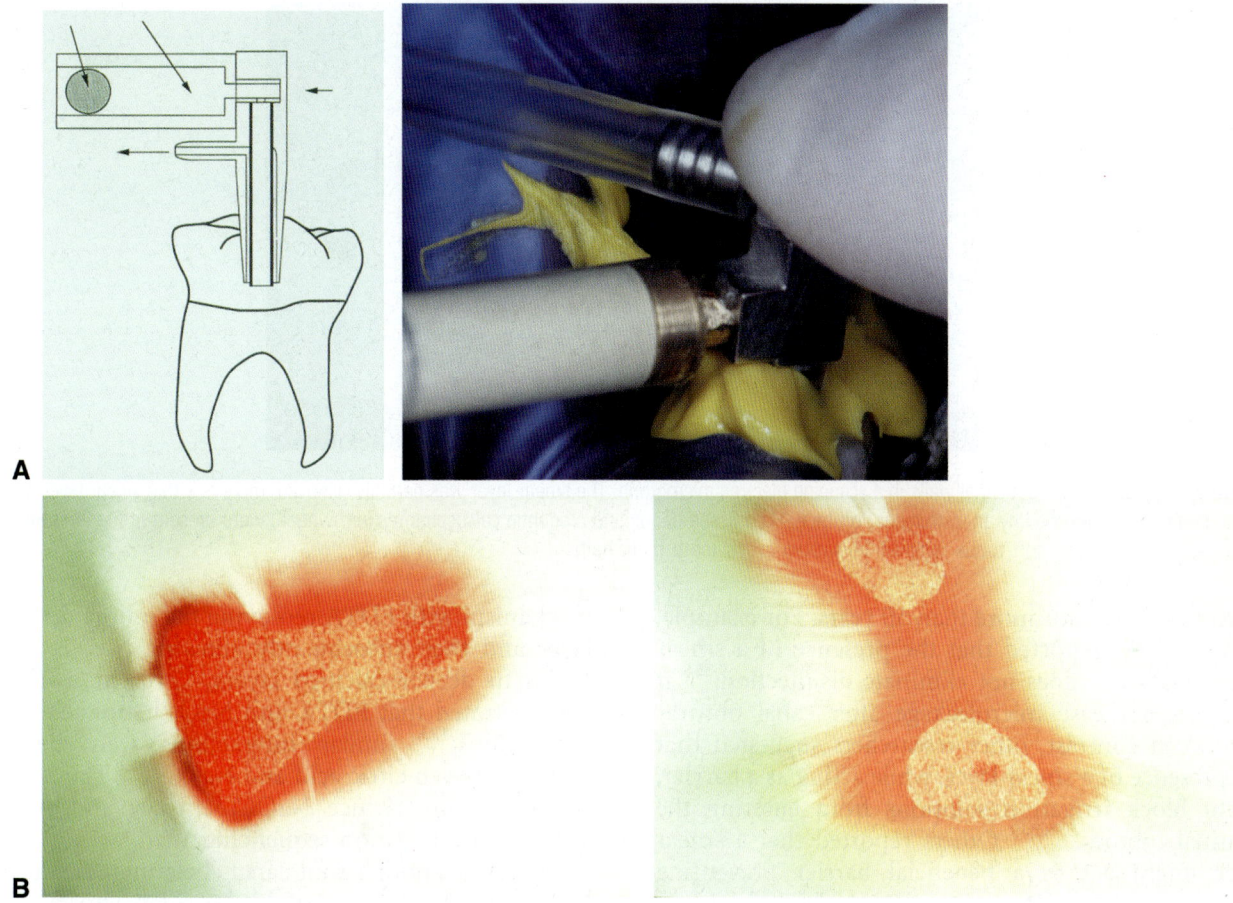

Figure 71 Application of the noninstrumentation technique for root canal cleaning and filling. **A,** Principle and clinical placement of the tubing system. The pump is connected to a tubing system and via a three-way valve to a cannula. This cannula is sealed into the access cavity with impression material to provide an air-tight system. **B,** After removal of the soft tissue with oscillating pressure waves of sodium hypochlorite (NaOCl), highly viscous sealer is delivered into the canal system at low pressure. Micrographs show adaptation of sealer at canal walls and also diffusion of sealer stained with red dye into the dentinal tubules. Images courtesy of Prof. Adrian Lussi.

root canal system, while possible,[550,551] is not straightforward. Moreover, preliminary in vivo results are mixed and the technique is currently not commercially available.[247]

Canal Surface Modification

It has been established that mechanical canal preparation[142] alone cannot predictably remove microbial canal contaminants and therefore irrigation with antimicrobial solutions is recommended. The effect of various irrigants and medicaments is described in Chapter 28, "Irrigants and Intracanal Medicaments" but some issues pertinent to canal preparation will be detailed below.

In addition to the removal of soft tissue and microorganisms, the canal surface is modified by irrigation solutions.[552] Canal surface after shaping with mechanical instruments is characterized by an irregularly distributed layer of soft and hard tissue debris that is smeared onto dentin surfaces (Figure 72).[553–555] This 1- to 5-μm-thin superficial structure consists of two separate layers: a loose superficial layer and an attached layer that also extends into dentinal tubules to form occluding plugs.[421] A smear layer consists of several components: dentin "mud," remnants of odontoblastic processes, pulp tissue, and microorganisms.[554] Its appearance and structure differs depending on the contacting instrument's cutting action: more actively cutting blades shear off dentin leaving thinner smear layer, while U-blade designs tend to burnish a thicker smear layer deeper into dentinal tubuli.[556,557]

The question as whether to leave the smear layer in situ on the canal walls or to remove it has been a

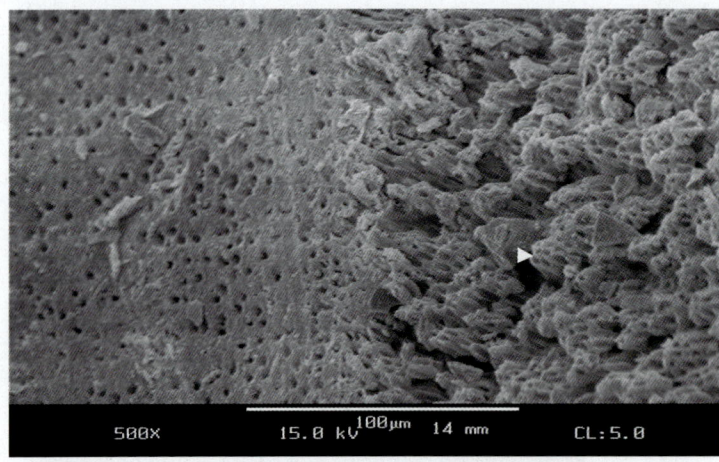

Figure 72 Appearance of root canal walls in a scanning electron micrograph. The smear layer was partially removed; there is a thin smear layer present in the area that was touched by an instrument (left half). Hard tissue debris and predentin calcospherites (arrowhead) were present in the area that was not instrumented but had soft tissue removed by sodium hypochlorite (right half).

matter of debate for more than 50 years. For example, some authors reported that the presence of a smear layer delays but does not eliminate disinfection;[558] it may also increase microleakage after canal obturation.[554] In contrast, other researchers suggested that the presence of a smear layer, while acting as a barrier, might block irrigation solutions from entering the dentinal tubules.[555,559] Others reported that a smear layer might act as a beneficial barrier preventing microorganisms from entering dentinal tubules when a root canal is contaminated between appointments. Their microbiological analyses of split root halves showed that the early removal of the smear layer may lead to significantly higher bacteria counts.[560]

Smear layer removal may be accomplished by various chemicals, as suggested over the last 50 years (Table 12), ranging from EDTA[382] to bisphosphonates.[552] Earlier studies had suggested a synergistic mechanism with EDTA removing the inorganic smear layer and then subsequently allowing NaOCl better access to deeper calcified layers;[145] recent work has demonstrated that EDTA and NaOCl show chemical interactions;[373] similar interactions were demonstrated between citric acid and NaOCl.[552] These interactions greatly reduce NaOCl efficacy and suggest attention to irrigation sequencing.

Salvizol is another root canal chelating irrigant that has a broad spectrum of bactericidal activity. This gives the product a cleansing potency while being biologically compatible.[570] Kaufman[567] reported the success of several cases using bis-dequalinium acetate as a disinfectant and chemotherapeutic agent. He cited its low toxicity, lubrication action, disinfecting ability, and low surface tension, as well as its chelating properties and low incidence of posttreatment pain. Salvizol, as well as several EDTA formulations,

Table 12 Available and Potential Solutions and Pastes for Smear Layer Removal.		
Reference	Year	Chemical
Baumgartner[561]	1984	Citric acid 10%
Wayman[562]	1979	Citric acid 20%
Tidmarsh[563]	1978	Citric acid 40%
Nygaard-Østby[382]	1957	EDTA (15%, ethylenediamineacetate)
Fehr[383]	1963	EDTAC (15% EDTA plus cetrimide)
Stewart[564]	1969	RC Prep (Premier Dental, Philadelphia, PA) (10% urea peroxide, 15% EDTA)*
Koskinen[565]	1975	Tubulicid (38% benzalkonium chloride, EDTA, 50% citric acid)
Koskinen[566]	1980	Largal Ultra (Septodont, Paris, France), 15% EDTA, cetrimide, NaOH)
Kaufman[567]	1981	Salvizol (Ravensberg, Konstanz, Germany), 5% aminoquinaldinium diacetate, propylene glycol
Berry[568]	1987	40% polyacrylic acid
Torabinejad[569]	2003	MTAD (Densply Tulsa Dental) (4.25% citric acid, 3% doxycycline, 0.5% Tween 80)
Zehnder[552]	2005	HEBP (7% 1-hydroxyethylidene-1,1-bisphosphonate)

*Other preparations are similar, for example, Glyde (Dentsply Maillefer), File Care (VDW), FileEze (Ultradent), except for the base that could be carbowax or glycerine.

contains surface-active substances that are supposed to increase wetting and hence chelating action. There are conflicting reports regarding the benefits of such surface-active components such as Tween 80.[571–574]

MTAD, commercially available as BioPure (Dentsply Tulsa Dental), contains citric acid and doxycycline as decalcifying substances and has been shown to effectively remove the smear layer;[569,575] moreover, it was shown to be effective against *Enterococcus faecalis*.[576,577] However, others report that 1.3% NaOCl/MTAD is less effective than 5.25% NaOCl/15% EDTA;[578] moreover, understanding of its effect on outcomes is limited at this point.[579]

Recently, substances such as bisphosphonates[580] and sodium triphosphate[552] have been investigated as potential chelators. While no significant interaction between these substances and NaOCl activity was found, the potential of these experimental chelators to remove the smear layer, measured both as smear layer scores and amount of dissolved calcium, is lower than that of EDTA and citric acid.[552] A gel-based formulation of a bisphosphonate, however, may offer advantages in the initial phase of root canal instrumentation with hand files.[372,580] Finally, the organic component of dentin undergoes modifications in contact with NaOCl,[581,582] while EDTA may lead to erosions.[575,583] Taken together, these results suggest that chelators and concentrated NaOCl do have beneficial effects but should be used with a clear understanding of potential harmful effects to the substrate.[584]

IRRIGATION DYNAMICS

As stated earlier, the relationship between prepared canal shapes and irrigation needle size is important for apical irrigation (Figure 73).[10,146,150,224] On the other hand, canal preparation itself produces dentin chips of various sizes[585] that need to be removed. These chips are part of what is described as unclean canals when observed in a SEM and should be removed by irrigation.

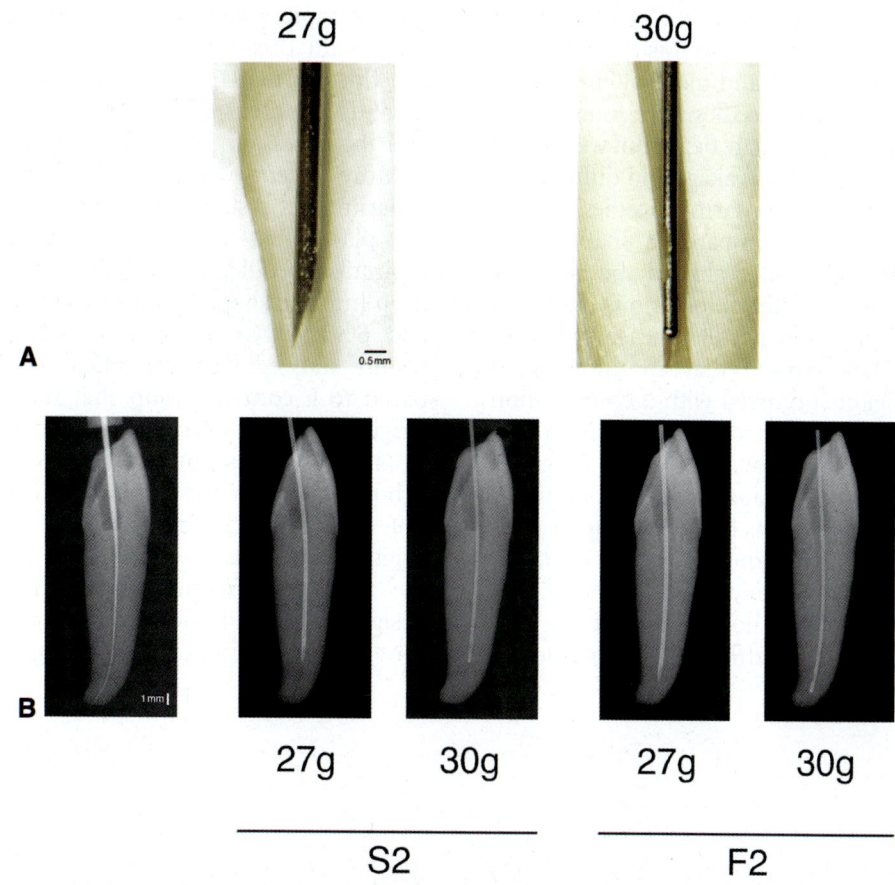

Figure 73 Effect of different irrigation needle sizes and canal diameters on needle position. *A*, Light micrographs of irrigation needles of size 27 and 30 gauge (0.4 and 0.31 mm). *B*, Mandibular canine shaped with ProTaper instrument S2 and then F2, corresponding to apical diameters of size #17 and #25. Shown are the insertion depths of both needles without binding in the canal.

Irrigation is commonly applied by a syringe and a needle, with needle sizes varying typically between 27 and 30 gauge (see Figure 73), 0.635 and 0.305 mm, respectively. With such a system, irrigation solutions will not travel apically more than 1 mm beyond the tip of the needle.[307,586] While it is therefore desirable to place the irrigation needle into the shaped root canals, the needle must not be locked in to avoid expressing the irrigation solution into periapical tissues. Serious incidents have been reported following NaOCl expressed into maxillary sinus or close to nerves.[587–590]

With careful use, the benefits of deep intracanal irrigation clearly seem to outweigh the risks.[591] In fact the proximity of the irrigation needle to the apex plays an important role in removing root canal debris.[592] Druttman and Stock[593] found that irrigation performance varied with the size of the needle and the volume of the irrigant, while Walton and Torabinejad[594] stated in their textbook that perhaps the most important factor is the delivery system and not the irrigating solution per se.

Canal size and shape are crucial to the penetration of the irrigant. The apical 5 mm are not flushed until they have been enlarged to size #30 and more often size #40 file.[146,595–597] Small-diameter needles were found to be more effective in reaching adequate depth but were more prone to problems of possible breakage and difficulty in expressing the irrigant from the narrow needles.[591]

Recently, Hsieh et al.[224] compared a shaped root canal to a "wind tunnel" and evaluated the behavior of irrigation solutions deposited into various depths of flared canals from irrigation needles measuring from 23 to 27 gauge. They showed that an undisturbed laminar flow of irrigants occurred with a combination of sufficiently enlarged canals, deep needle insertion, and small needle diameter, for example, a 27-gauge needle placed 3 mm from the apex in a canal prepared to size #30. Similar observations had been made earlier in experiments using radiopaque irrigation solutions (Machtou P, personal communication).

Several methods have been devised to increase irrigant turnover and overall efficacy. As mentioned earlier, the use of ultrasonic or sonic irrigation to remove dentin filings, debris, and bacteria from root canals has been well documented (Figure 62 and Figure 74).[123,147,222,351,417,598,599]

However, there are doubts that passive ultrasonically or sonically assisted irrigation can in fact remove all contaminants.[600,601] While the time frames and sequence of irrigation solutions is still a matter of debate,[149,602] the cleanest canals were produced by irrigating with ultrasonics and NaOCl after the canal has been fully prepared. Ultrasonics was shown to be superior to syringe irrigation alone when the canal was prepared to 0.3 mm (size #30 instrument).[603]

Several novel strategies have been proposed to increase irrigation efficacy. Gutarts et al.[546] evaluated the use of a 25-gauge irrigation needle, connected to an ultrasonic unit, through which 6% NaOCl was delivered for 1 minute at the conclusion of canal shaping. They reported significantly cleaner canals compared to a control group that did not receive ultrasonic irrigation.

Irrigation with positive pressure has also been tried, for example, with the system RinsEndo (Duerr, Bietigheim-Bissingen, Germany). However, reports for this particular device are sparse;[604] moreover, there is a potential for apical extrusion of NaOCl, and the necessary precautions should be taken.

More recently, Fukumoto et al.[547] described an experimental system that consisted of a washing needle, placed just into the root canal, and a 27-gauge aspiration needle, ground flat at the tip and placed deep into the shaped root canal. Irrigants, 14% EDTA and 6% NaOCl, were aspirated at ~20 kPa; their results showed superior smear layer removal compared to a control group that received conventional irrigation with a needle of the same diameter.

This system is similar to a patent submitted by Schoeffel[545] with the exception that his system does not include a constantly operating washing line (Figure 75). Irrigant is deposited into the access cavity; then, two sequentially operated and specially designed aspiration needles are placed into the shaped root canal. Preliminary data suggest good cleaning

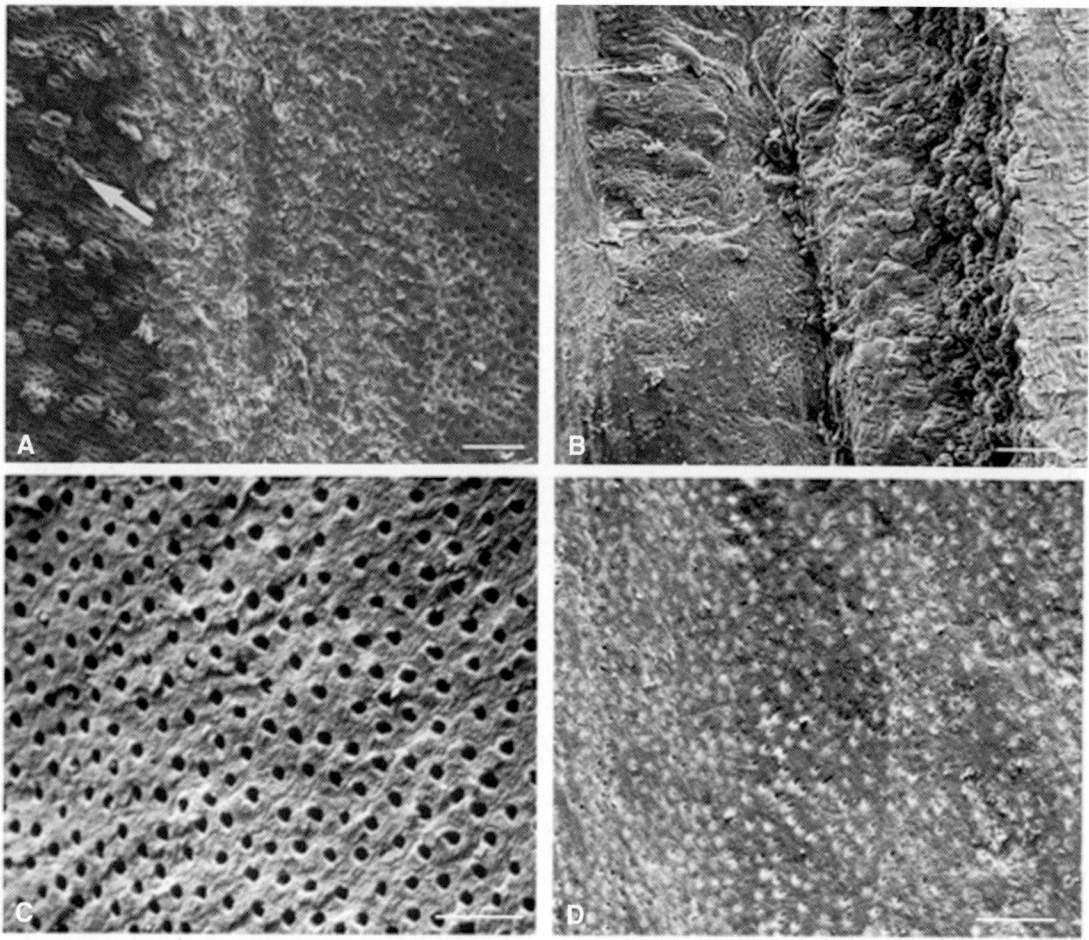

Figure 74 Canal surfaces as seen in scanning electron micrographs. ***A***, Typical appearance after cleaning and shaping with wall areas that has instrument contact and some smear layer removal as well as uninstrumented areas with calcospherites as part of the mineralization front in predentin (arrow). ***B***, Uninstrumented canal that was washed with 5.25% sodium hypochlorite (NaOCl). ***C***, Canal wall segment presenting with all dentinal tubules open. ***D***, Completely shaped canal wall area with a thin remaining smear layer. Bars are 30 μm.

capacity;[605] however, currently no published results are available regarding clinical outcomes using these new irrigation techniques.

Currently, ultrasonically activated passive irrigation seems to be the standard until more experimental techniques are scientifically evaluated and brought to the market. However, as mentioned earlier, using an ultrasonically activated insert deep in a root canal carries some risk (see Figure 63). Furthermore, more work is needed to clarify insert shapes and materials as well as activation times and power settings.

PHOTODYNAMIC THERAPY

While lasers are probably not a good alternative for mechanical root canal preparation, they have been

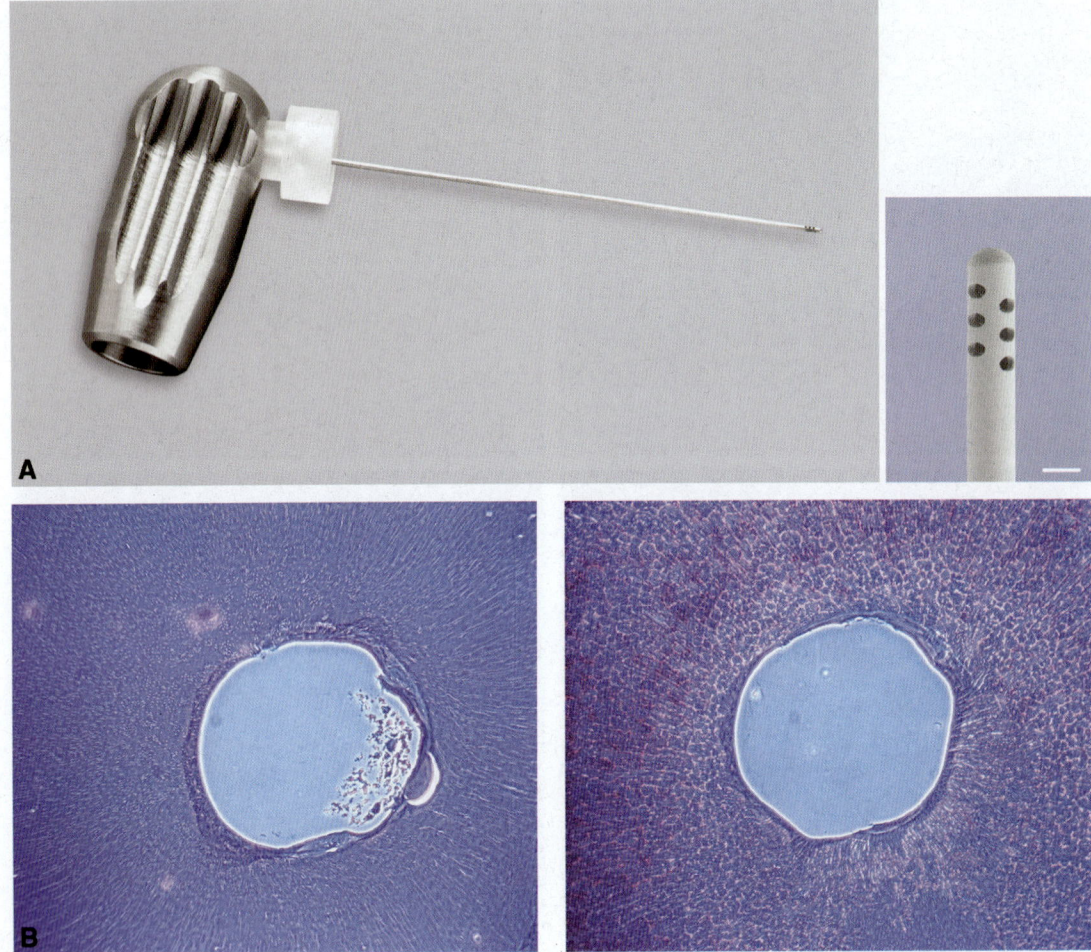

Figure 75 The EndoVac system (Discus Dental) for apical negative pressure irrigation. Recent in vitro results demonstrate better debridement compared to conventional syringe irrigation.[605] ***A,*** Overview of the micro cannula demonstrating a closed rounded tip and an array of 12 openings in the apical end (inset, bar is 250 μm). ***B,*** Light microscopic images of canals irrigated with conventional syringe (left) and with the EndoVac system (right). Orig. mag. x100. Images courtesy of Dr. John Schoeffel.

shown to be effective for canal disinfection and canal surface modification, as reviewed in detail in Chapter 26E, "Lasers". In this context, the use of lasers for photoactivated disinfection, also known as photodynamic therapy, has been promoted.[606–608] This technique does not provide canal enlargement but assists in the eradication of intracanal microorganisms. Photodynamic therapy is well known as a treatment for cancer and other diseases[609] and is based on the concept that a nontoxic photosensitizing agent can be preferentially localized in target tissues. The agent is then activated by light of appropriate wavelength to generate reactive molecules that in turn are toxic to cells of the target tissue.[609] Visible light can also kill bacteria in root canal systems after treatment with an appropriate agent (Kishen A, personal communication).

Such photoactivated disinfection has only recently been explored to treat bacterial infections in humans.[606] A wide range of oral bacteria could be killed by red light after sensitization with toluidine blue and methylene blue.[610] More than 400 photoactive substances are known that can be combined with lasers tailored to their specific wavelengths of absorption. Potentially one of these substances will be able to penetrate into the root canal system better than currently available irrigants. In fact, partial inactivation of *Streptococcus intermedius* biofilms in root canals of extracted teeth using toluidine blue and light applied at the orifice level has been recently reported.[611]

Clinically, the photoactivated agent is used as an irrigant after mechanical canal enlargement (Figure 76) and activation; root canal filling is accomplished

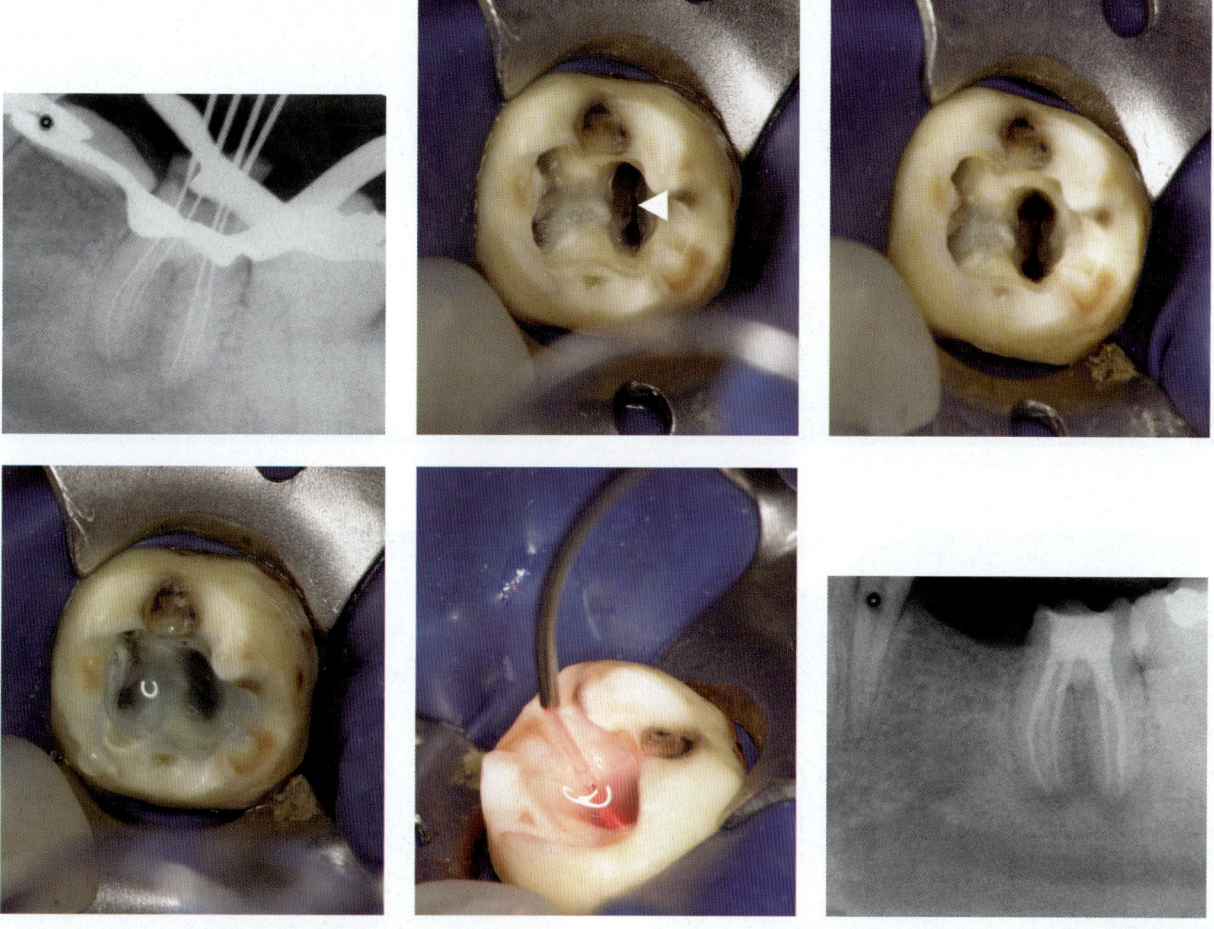

Figure 76 Use of photoactivated disinfection in a case of post-endodontic disease. The existing root canal filling was removed (Arrowhead) and the canals reshaped with ProFile instruments (upper panel). Then, tolonium chloride (also known as toluidine blue O) was placed in the root canal system and irradiated with a diode laser (lower panel, also showing root canal filling after retreatment). Images courtesy of Prof. Paul Lambrechts.

conventionally. This technique is experimental and its impact on clinical outcomes needs to be evaluated.

Conclusion

The past decade has brought significant changes to root canal preparation, for example, the use of rotary NiTi instruments and magnification. These techniques have allowed more complicated root canal treatment to be undertaken safely and successfully (Figure 77). The way educational content is delivered is also changing: private educational institutions are taking the lead in presenting information to clinicians. Moreover, electronic media and web-based content have gained more widespread acceptance. Using these

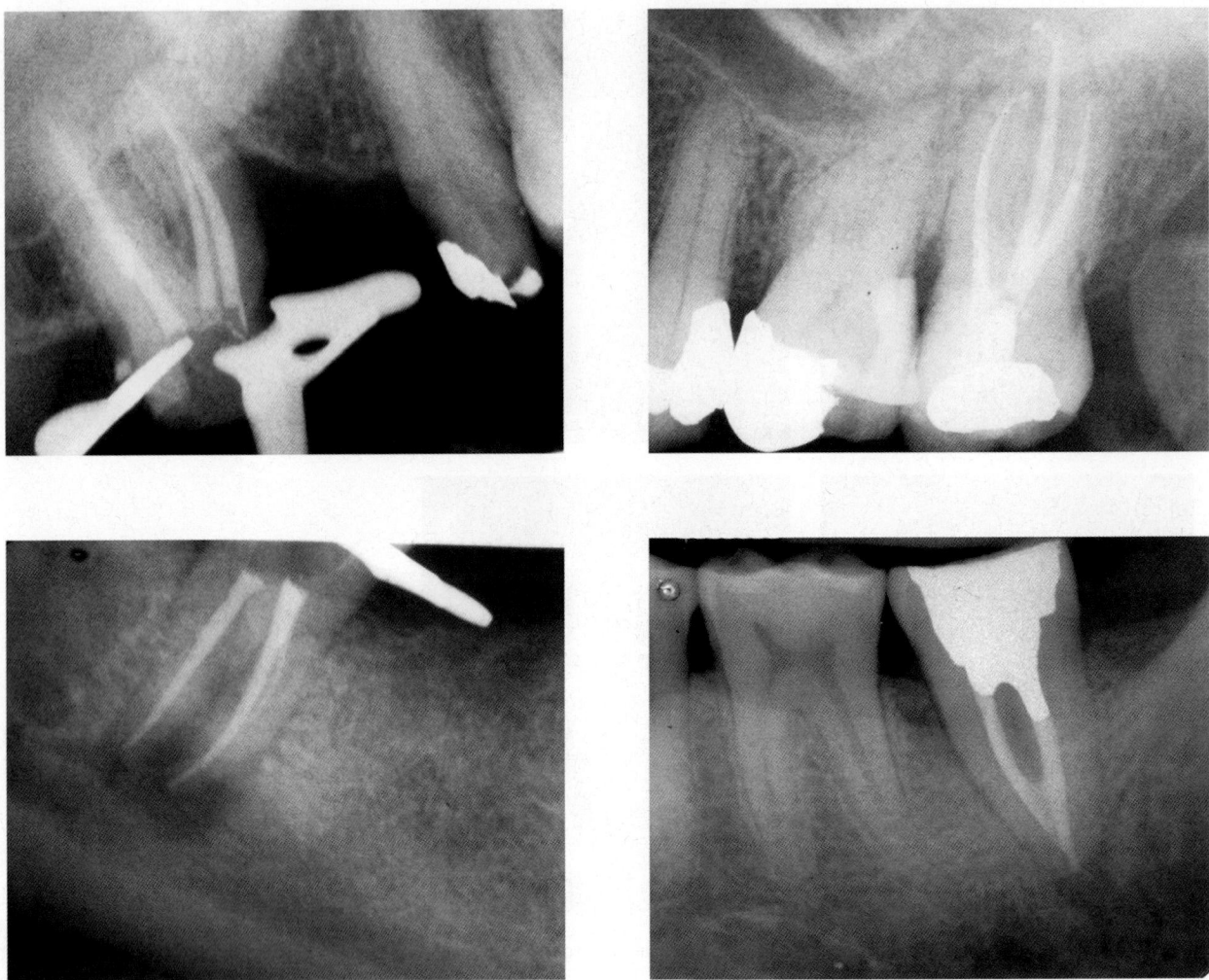

Figure 77 Routine cases of second maxillary and mandibular molars that had coronal and radicular preparation done adhering to the principles laid out in this chapter. Radiographs represent situation immediately after root canal filling.

avenues, evidence-based information will reach clinicians who at present have limited access to book, journals, or hands-on teaching.

Aseptic techniques are a prerequisite for successful endodontic therapy as they are in the goal of eradicating the causative microbial flora (Figure 78). Asked for any particular direction for development in the next decade, disinfection and systems to increase its efficacy are the most likely candidates. Seemingly exotic applications such as the use of ozone (e.g., Healozone, KaVo, Biberach, Germany) or high-frequency current (Endox, Lysis, Nova Milanese, Italy)[612] or photoactivated disinfection may be utilized more; however, it will be difficult to prove with statistical methods that any individual device will have significant and clinically relevant impact.

Regarding instrument and strategies, new materials may appear, such as more durable and flexible alloys or plastic materials, but the basic strategy will likely remain the same in the next decade: enlargement for subsequent disinfection and filling. The long-term goal is certainly to replace root canal therapy, as part of current repair methods, with tissue-engineering strategies that provide healing in the sense of a *restitutio ad integrum*.

ACKNOWLEDGMENT

The authors would like to express their special gratitude to Vickie Leow, Master Graphic Designer at the UCSF School of Dentistry, as well as Anjan Lall for their expert help with the schematic drawings used in this chapter.

References

1. Kakehashi S, Stanley HR, Fitzgerald RJ. The effects of surgical exposures of dental pulps in germ-free and conventional laboratory rats. Oral Surg Oral Med Oral Pathol Oral Radiol Endod 1965;20:340.
2. Möller AJ, Fabricius L, Dahlen G, et al. Influence on periapical tissues of indigenous oral bacteria and necrotic pulp tissue in monkeys. Scand J Dent Res 1981;89:475.
3. Schilder H. Cleaning and shaping the root canal. Dent Clin North Am 1974;18:269.
4. Abbott PV. Assessing restored teeth with pulp and periapical diseases for the presence of cracks, caries and marginal breakdown. Aust Dent J 2004;49:33.
5. Mannan G, Smallwood ER, Gulabivala K. Effects of access cavity location and design on degree and distribution of instrumented root canal surface in maxillary anterior teeth. Int Endod J 2001;34:176.
6. Sonntag D, Mollaakbari K, Kock K, Stachniss V. Einfluss der Zugangskavität auf Hartsubstanzverlust und Kanaldetektion bei humanen Frontzähnen. Dtsch Zahnärztl Z 2006;61:612.
7. Green D. A stereomicroscopic investigation of the root apices of 400 maxillary and mandibular anterior teeth. Oral Surg Oral Med Oral Pathol Oral Radiol Endod 1956;9:1224.
8. Wu M-K, Barkis D, Roris A, Wesselink PR. Does the first file to bind correspond to the diameter of the canal in the apical region. Int Endod J 2002;35:264.
9. Card SJ, Sigurdsson A, Ørstavik D, Trope M. The effectiveness of increased apical enlargement in reducing intracanal bacteria. J Endod 2002;28:779.
10. Usman N, Baumgartner JC, Marshall JG. Influence of instrument size on root canal debridement. J Endod 2004;30:110.
11. Nguy D, Sedgley C. The influence of canal curvature on the mechanical efficacy of root canal irrigation in vitro using real-time imaging of bioluminescent bacteria. J Endod 2006;32:1077.
12. Mickel AK, Chogle S, Liddle J, et al. The role of apical size determination and enlargement in the reduction of intracanal bacteria. J Endod 2007;33:21.

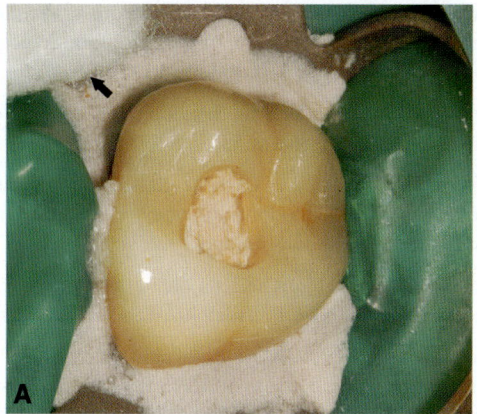
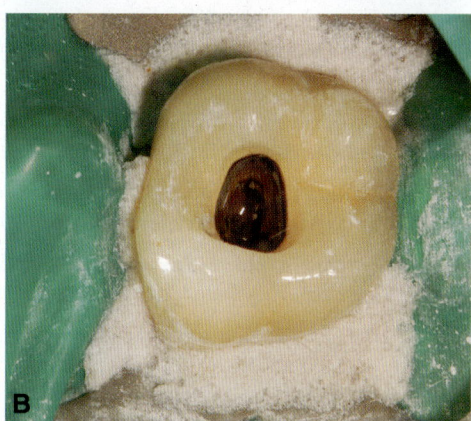
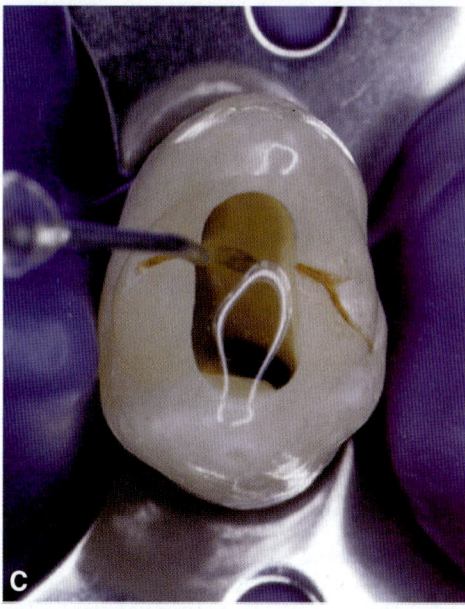

Figure 78 Aseptic techniques and disinfection of the root canal system. ***A***, Swabbing of the operation site, for example, with sodium hypochlorite (arrow), while marginal imperfections of the rubber dam seal are corrected with a caulking material (e.g., Oraseal, Ultradent). ***B***, Reservoir of sodium hypochlorite (NaOCl) is always present in the access cavity during hand and rotary instrumentation to promote disinfection and lubrication.

13. Coldero LG, McHugh S, MacKenzie D, Saunders WP. Reduction in intracanal bacteria during root canal preparation with and without apical enlargement. Int Endod J 2002;35:437.
14. Cunningham CJ, Senia ES. A three-dimensional study of canal curvatures in the mesial roots of mandibular molars. J Endod 1992;18:294.
15. Peters OA, Laib A, Göhring TN, Barbakow F. Changes in root canal geometry after preparation assessed by high-resolution computed tomography. J Endod 2001;27:1.
16. Peters OA, Peters CI, Schönenberger K, Barbakow F. ProTaper rotary root canal preparation: effects of canal anatomy on final shape analysed by micro CT. Int Endod J 2003;36:86.
17. Zillich RM, Jerome JK. Endodontic access to maxillary lateral incisors. Oral Surg Oral Med Oral Pathol Oral Radiol Endod 1981;52:443.
18. LaTurno SA, Zillich RM. Straight-line endodontic access to anterior teeth. Oral Surg Oral Med Oral Pathol Oral Radiol Endod 1985;59:418.
19. Dempster WT, Adams WJ, Duddles RA. Arrangement in the jaws of the roots of the teeth. J Am Dent Assoc 1963;67:779.
20. Acosta Vigouroux SA, Trugeda Bosaans SA. Anatomy of the pulp chamber floor of the permanent maxillary first molar. J Endod 1978;4:214.
21. Bjørndal L, Carlsen O, Thuesen G, Darvann T, Kreiborg S. External and internal macromorphology in 3D-reconstructed maxillary molars using computerized X-ray microtomography. Int Endod J 1999;32:3.
22. Krasner P, Rankow HJ. Anatomy of the pulp-chamber Floor. J Endod 2004;30:5.
23. Hess W, Zurcher E. The anatomy of root canals of the teeth of the permanent and deciduous dentitions. New York: William Wood; 1925.
24. Peters OA, Göhring TN, Lutz F. Effect of a eugenol-containing sealer on marginal adaptation of dentine-bonded resin fillings. Int Endod J 2000;33:53.
25. Janik JM. Access cavity preparation. Dent Clin North Am 1984;28:809.
26. Sorensen JA, Engelman MJ. Ferrule design and fracture resistance of endodontically treated teeth. J Prosthet Dent 1990;63:529.
27. Libman WJ, Nicholls JI. Load fatigue of teeth restored with cast posts and cores and complete crowns. Int J Prosthodont 1995;8:155.
28. Creugers NH. 5-year follow-up of a prospective clinical study on various types of core restorations. Int J Prosthodont 2005;18:34.
29. Tan PL, Aquilino SA, Gratton DG, Stanford CM, et al. In vitro fracture resistance of endodontically treated central incisors with varying ferrule heights and configurations. J Prosthet Dent 2005;93:331.
30. Stokes AN, Tidmarsh BG. A comparison of diamond and tungsten carbide burs for preparing endodontic access cavities through crowns. J Endod 1988;14:550.
31. Teplitsky PE, Sutherland JK. Endodontic access of Cerestore crowns. J Endod 1985;11:555.
32. Cohen BD, Wallace JA. Castable glass ceramic crowns and their reaction to endodontic therapy. Oral Surg Oral Med Oral Pathol Oral Radiol Endod 1991;72:108.
33. Ash MM, Nelson SJ. Wheeler's dental anatomy, physiology and occlusion. 8th ed. Philadelphia, PA: WB Saunders; 2003.
34. Pineda F, Kuttler Y. Mesiodistal and buccolingual roentgenographic investigation of 7,275 root canals. Oral Surg Oral Med Oral Pathol Oral Radiol Endod 1972;33:101.
35. Vertucci FJ. Root canal anatomy of the human permanent teeth. Oral Surg Oral Med Oral Pathol Oral Radiol Endod 1984;58:589.
36. Hamasa AA, Al-Khateeb T, Darwazeh A. Prevalence of dilaceration in Jordanian adults. Int Endod J 2002;35:910.
37. Kasahara E, Yasuda E, Yamamoto A, Anzai M. Root canal system of the maxillary central incisor. J Endod 1990;16:158.
38. Genovese FR, Marsico EM. Maxillary central incisor with two roots: a case report. J Endod 2003;29:220.
39. Lin WC, Yan SF, Pai SF. Non-surgical endodontic treatment of a two rooted maxillary central incisor. J Endod 2006;32:478.
40. Khademi J. Endodontic Access. In: Johnson WT, editor. Color atlas of endodontics. Philadelphia, PA: WB Saunders; 2002. p. 21.
41. Christie WH, Peikoff MD, Acheson DW. Endodontic treatment of two maxillary lateral incisors with anomalous root formation. J Endod 1981;7:528.
42. Fried IL, Winter AA. Diagnosis and treatment of a two-rooted maxillary lateral incisor. Periodont Case Rep 1984;6:40.
43. Yoshikawa M, Hosomi T, Sakiyama Y, Toda T. Endodontic therapy for a permanent maxillary lateral incisor having two roots. J Osaka Dent Univ 1987;21:87.
44. Hatton JF, Ferrillo PJ Jr. Successful treatment of a two-canaled maxillary lateral incisor. J Endod 1989;15:216.
45. Caliskan MK, Pehlivan Y, Sepetcioglu F, et al. Root canal morphology of human permanent teeth in a Turkish population. J Endod 1995;21:200.
46. Carns EJ, Skidmore AE. Configurations and deviations of root canals of maxillary first premolars. Oral Surg Oral Med Oral Pathol Oral Radiol Endod 1973;36:880.
47. Vertucci FJ, Gegauff A. Root canal morphology of the maxillary first premolar. J Am Dent Assoc 1979;99:194.
48. Walker RT. Root form and canal anatomy of maxillary first premolars in a southern Chinese population. Endod Dent Traumatol 1987;3:130.

49. Pecora JD, Saquy PC, Sousa Neto MD, Woelfel JB. Root form and canal anatomy of maxillary first premolars. Braz Dent J 1991;2:87.
50. Kartal N, Ozcelilk B, Cimilli H. Root canal morphology of maxillary premolars. J Endod 1998;24:417.
51. Kerekes K, Tronstad L. Morphometric observations on root canals of human premolars. J Endod 1977;3:74.
52. Bellizzi R, Hartwell G. Radiographic evaluation of root canal anatomy of in vivo endodontically treated maxillary premolars. J Endod 1985;11:37.
53. Green D. Double canals in single roots. Oral Surg Oral Med Oral Pathol Oral Radiol Endod 1973;35:689.
54. Sert S, Bayirli GS. Evaluation of the root canal configurations of the mandibular and maxillary permanent teeth by gender in the Turkish population. J Endod 2004;30:391.
55. Gilles J, Reader A. An SEM investigation of the mesiolingual canal in human maxillary first and second molars. Oral Surg Oral Med Oral Pathol Oral Radiol Endod 1990;70:638.
56. Buhrley LJ, Barrows MJ, BeGole E, Wenckus CS. Effect of magnification on locating the mb2 canal in maxillary molars. J Endod 2002;28:324.
57. Fogel HM, Peikoff MD, Christie WH. Canal configuration in the mesiobuccal root of the maxillary first molar: a clinical study. J Endod 1994;20:135.
58. Pomeranz HH, Fishelberg G. The secondary mesiobuccal canal of maxillary molars. J Am Dent Assoc 1974;88:119.
59. Seidberg BH, Altman M, Guttuso J, Suson M. Frequency of two mesiobuccal root canals in maxillary permanent first molars. J Am Dent Assoc 1973;87:852.
60. Thomas RP, Moule AJ, Bryant R. Root canal morphology of maxillary permanent first molar teeth at various ages. Int Endod J 1993;26:257.
61. Kulild JC, Peters DD. Incidence and configuration of canal systems in the mesiobuccal root of maxillary first and second molars. J Endod 1990;16:311.
62. Al-Shalabi RM, Omer OE, Glennon J, et al. Root canal anatomy of maxillary first and second permanent molars. Int Endod J 2000;33.
63. Weine FS, Hayami S, Hata G, Toda T. Canal configuration of the mesiobuccal root of the maxillary first molar of a Japanese sub-population. Int Endod J 1999;32:79.
64. Alavi AM, Opasanon A, Ng Y-L, Gulabivala K. Root and canal morphology of Thai maxillary molars. Int Endod J 2002;35:478.
65. Imura N, Hata GI, Toda T, et al. Two canals in mesiobuccal roots of maxillary molars. Int Endod J 1998;31:410.
66. Weine FS, Healey HJ, Gerstein H, Evanson L. Canal configuration in the mesiobuccal root of the maxillary first molar and its endodontic significance. Oral Surg Oral Med Oral Pathol Oral Radiol Endod 1969;28:419.
67. Stropko J. Canal Morphology of maxillary molars: clinical observations on canal configurations. J Endod 1999;25:446.
68. Wasti F, Shearer AC, Wilson NH. Root canal systems of the mandibular and maxillary first permanent molar teeth of south Asian Pakistanis. Int Endod J 2001;34:263.
69. Ng YL, Aung TH, Alavi A, Gulabivala K. Root and canal morphology of Burmese maxillary molars. Int Endod J 2001;34:620.
70. Baldassari-Cruz LA, Lilly JP, Rivera EM. The influence of dental operating microscope in locating the mesiolingual canal orifice. Oral Surg Oral Med Oral Pathol Oral Radiol Endod 2002;93:190.
71. Eskoz N, Weine FS. Canal configuration of the mesiobuccal root of the maxillary second molar. J Endod 1995;21:38.
72. Peikoff MD, Christie WH, Fogel HM. The maxillary second molar: variations in the number of roots and canals. Int Endod J 1996;29:365.
73. Rankine-Wilson RW, Henry PJ. The bifurcated root canal in lower anterior teeth. J Am Dent Assoc 1965;70:1162.
74. Madeira MC, Hetem S. Incidence of bifurcations in mandibular incisors. Oral Surg Oral Med Oral Pathol Oral Radiol Endod 1973;36:589.
75. Benjamin KA, Dowson J. Incidence of two root canals in human mandibular incisor teeth. Oral Surg Oral Med Oral Pathol Oral Radiol Endod 1974;38:122.
76. Kartal N, Yanikoglu FC. Root canal morphology of mandibular incisors. J Endod 1992;18:562.
77. Miyashita M, Kasahara E, Yasuda E, et al. Root canal system of the mandibular incisor. J Endod 1997;23:479.
78. Bellizzi R, Hartwell G. Clinical investigation of in vivo endodontically treated mandibular anterior teeth. J Endod 1983;9:246.
79. Walker RT. The root canal anatomy of mandibular incisors in a southern Chinese population. Int Endod J 1988;21:218.
80. Al-Qudah AA, Awawdeh LA. Root canal morphology of mandibular incisors in a Jordanian population. Int Endod J 2006;39:873.
81. Mauger MJ, Waite RM, Alexander JB, Schindler WG. Ideal endodontic access in mandibular incisors. J Endod 1999;25:206.
82. Heling I, Gottlieb-Dadon I, Chandler NP. Mandibular canine with two roots and three root canals. Endod Dent Traumatol 1995;11:301.
83. Orguneser A, Kartal N. Mandibular canine with two roots and three canals. Endod Dent Traumatol 1998;11:301.
84. Vertucci FJ. Root canal morphology of mandibular premolars. J Am Dent Assoc 1978;97:47.
85. Baisden MK, Kulild JC, Weller RN. Root canal configuration of the mandibular first premolar. J Endod 1992;18:505.

86. Zillich R, Dowson J. Root canal morphology of mandibular first and second premolars. Oral Surg Oral Med Oral Pathol Oral Radiol Endod 1973;36:738.

87. Yoshioka TV, Villegas JC, Kobayashi C, Suda H. Radiographic evaluation of root canal multiplicity in mandibular first premolars. J Endod 2004;30:73.

88. Nallapati S. Three canal mandibular first and second premolars: a treatment approach. A case report. J Endod 2005;31:474.

89. Bram SM, Fleisher R. Endodontic therapy in a mandibular second bicuspid with four canals. J Endod 1991;17:513.

90. Holtzman L. Root canal treatment of mandibular second premolar with four root canals: a case report. Int Endod J 1998;31:364.

91. Rhodes JS. A case of unusual anatomy: a mandibular second premolar with four canals. Int Endod J 2001;34:645.

92. Macri E, Zmener O. Five canals in a mandibular second premolar. J Endod 2000;26:304.

93. Gulabivala K, Opasanon A, Ng YL, Alavi A. Root and canal morphology of Thai mandibular molars. Int Endod J 2002;35:56.

94. Zaatar EI, Anizi SA, Al-Duwairi Y. A study of the dental pulp cavity of mandibular first permanent molars in the Kuwaiti population. J Endod 1998;24:125.

95. Skidmore AE, Bjorndal AM. Root canal morphology of the human mandibular first molar. Oral Surg Oral Med Oral Pathol Oral Radiol Endod 1971;32:778.

96. Walker RT. Root form and canal anatomy of mandibular first molars in a southern Chinese population. Endod Dent Traumatol 1988;4:19.

97. Pomeranz HH, Eidelman DL, Goldberg MG. Treatment considerations of the middle mesial canal of mandibular first and second molars. J Endod 1981;7:565.

98. Fabra-Campos H. Unusual root anatomy of mandibular first molars. J Endod 1985;11:568.

99. da Costa LF, Sousa Neto MD, Fidel SR, et al. External and internal anatomy of mandibular molars. Braz Dent J 1996;7:33.

100. Mannocci F, Peru M, Sheriff M, et al. The isthmuses of the mesial root of mandibular molars: a micro-computed tomographic study. Int Endod J 2005;38:558.

101. Fabra-Campos H. Three canals in the mesial root of mandibular first permanent molars: a clinical study. Int Endod J 1989;22:39.

102. Vertucci FJ, Williams RG. Furcation canals in the human mandibular first molar. Oral Surg Oral Med Oral Pathol Oral Radiol Endod 1974;38:308.

103. Vertucci FJ, Anthony RL. A scanning electron microscopic investigation of accessory foramina in the furcation and pulp chamber floor of molar teeth. Oral Surg Oral Med Oral Pathol Oral Radiol Endod 1986;62:319.

104. Rice RT, Gilbert BO Jr. An unusual canal configuration in a mandibular first molar. J Endod 1987;13:515.

105. Bolger WL, Schindler WG. A mandibular first molar with a C-shaped root configuration. J Endod 1988;14:515.

106. Gulabivala K, Aung TH, Alavi A, Ng YL. Root and canal morphology of Burmese mandibular molars. Int Endod J 2001;34:359.

107. Cooke HG III, Cox FL. C-shaped canal configurations in mandibular molars. J Am Dent Assoc 1979;99:836.

108. Weine FS. The C-shaped mandibular second molar: incidence and other considerations (with members of the Arizona Endodontic Association). J Endod 1998;24:372.

109. Melton DC, Krell KV, Fuller MW. Anatomical and histological features of C-shaped canals in mandibular second molars. J Endod 1991;17:384.

110. Sorensen JA, Martinoff JT. Intracoronal reinforcement and coronal coverage: a study of endodontically treated teeth. J Prosthet Dent 1984;51:780.

111. Rosen H. Operative procedures on mutilated endodontically treated teeth. J Prosthet Dent 1961;11:972.

112. Johnson JK, Schwartz NL, Blackwell RT. Evaluation and restoration of endodontically treated posterior teeth. J Am Dent Assoc 1976;93:597.

113. Greenfeld RS, Marshall FJ. Factors affecting dowel (post) selection and use in endodontically treated teeth. J Can Dent Assoc 1983;49:777.

114. Radke RA, Eissmann HF. Postendodontic restoration. In: Cohen S, Burns RC, editors. Pathways of the pulp. 5th ed. St. Louis, MO: CV Mosby; 1991.

115. Helfer AR, Melnick S, Schilder H. Determination of the moisture content of vital and pulpless teeth. Oral Surg Oral Med Oral Pathol Oral Radiol Endod 1972;34:661.

116. Reeh ES, Messer HH, Douglas WH. Reduction in tooth stiffness as a result of endodontic and restorative procedures. J Endod 1989;15:512.

117. Howe CA, McKendry DJ. Effect of endodontic access preparation on resistance to crown–root fracture. J Am Dent Assoc 1990;121:712.

118. Sedgley CM, Messer HH. Are endodontically treated teeth more brittle? J Endod 1992;18:332.

119. Panitvisai P, Messer HH. Cuspal deflection in molars in relation to endodontic and restorative procedures. J Endod 1995;21:57.

120. Peters OA. Current challenges and concepts in the preparation of root canal systems: a review. J Endod 2004;30:559.

121. Peters OA, Dummer PM. Infection control through root canal preparation: a review of cleaning and shaping procedures. In: Peters OA, Dummer PM, editors. Endodontic Topics. Copenhagen, Denmark: Blackwell Munksgaard; 2005.

122. Hülsmann M, Peters OA, Dummer PMH. Mechanical preparation of root canals: shaping goals, techniques and means. Endod Top 2005;10:30.

123. Sjögren U, Sundqvist G. Bacteriologic evaluation of ultrasonic root canal instrumentation. Oral Surg Oral Med Oral Pathol Oral Radiol Endod 1987;63:366.

124. Yared GM, Bou Dagher FE. Influence of apical enlargement on bacterial infection during treatment of apical periodontitis. J Endod 1994;20:535.

125. Dalton BC, Ørstavik D, Phillips C, et al. Bacterial reduction with nickel-titanium rotary instrumentation. J Endod 1998;24:763.

126. Peters LB, Wesselink PR. Periapical healing of endodontically treated teeth in one and two visits obturated in the presence or absence of detectable microorganisms. Int Endod J 2002;35:660.

127. McGurkin-Smith R, Trope M, Caplan D, Sigurdsson A. Reduction of intracanal bacteria using GT rotary instrumentation, 5.25% NaOCl, EDTA, and $Ca(OH)_2$. J Endod 2005;31:359.

128. Brynolf I. A histological and roentgenological study of the periapical region of human incisors. Odontol Revy 1967;18(Suppl 11).

129. Green TL, Walton RE, Taylor JK, Merrell P. Radiographic and histologic periapical findings of root canal treated teeth in cadaver. Oral Surg Oral Med Oral Pathol Oral Radiol Endod 1997;83:707.

130. Barthel CR, Zimmer S, Trope M. Relationship of radiologic and histologic signs of inflammation in human root-filled teeth. J Endod 2004;30:75.

131. Strindberg L. The dependence of the results of pulp therapy on certain factors. Acta Odontol Scand 1956;14(Suppl 21).

132. Nair PN, Henry S, Cano V, Vera J. Microbial status of apical root canal system of human mandibular first molars with primary apical periodontitis after "one-visit" endodontic treatment. Oral Surg Oral Med Oral Path Oral Radiol Endod 2005;99:231.

133. Peters LB, Wesselink PR, Moorer WR. The fate and the role of bacteria left in root dentinal tubules. Int Endod J 1995;28:95.

134. Saleh IM, Ruyter IE, Haapasalo M, Ørstavik D. Survival of *Enterococcus faecalis* in infected dentinal tubules after root canal filling with different root canal sealers in vitro. Int Endod J 2004;37:193.

135. Wu MK, Dummer PM, Wesselink PR. Consequences of and strategies to deal with residual post-treatment root canal infection. Int Endod J 2006;39:343.

136. Fabricius L, Dahlen G, Sundqvist G, et al. Influence of residual bacteria on periapical tissue healing after chemomechanical treatment and root filling of experimentally infected monkey teeth. Eur J Oral Sci 2006;114:278.

137. Siqueira JF. The etiology of root canal treatment failure: why well-treated teeth can fail. Int Endod J 2001;34:1.

138. Nair PN. On the causes of persistent apical periodontitis: a review. Int Endod J 2006;39:249.

139. Iwaya SI, Ikawa M, Kubota M. Revascularization of an immature permanent tooth with apical periodontitis and sinus tract. Endod Dent Traumatol 2001;17:185.

140. Banchs F, Trope M. Revascularization of immature permanent teeth with apical periodontitis: new treatment protocol? J Endod 2004;30:196.

141. Love RM. Clinical management of infected root canal dentin. Pract Periodont Aesthet Dent 1996;8:581.

142. Byström A, Sundqvist G. Bacteriologic evaluation of the efficacy of mechanical root canal instrumentation in endodontic therapy. Scand J Dent Res 1981;89:321.

143. Siqueira J, Lima K, Magalhaes F, et al. Mechanical reduction of the bacterial population in the root canal by three instrumentation techniques. J Endod 1999;25:332.

144. Byström A, Sundqvist G. Bacteriologic evaluation of the effect of 0.5 percent sodium hypochlorite in endodontic therapy. Oral Surg Oral Med Oral Pathol Oral Radiol Endod 1983;55:307.

145. Byström A, Sundqvist G. The antibacterial action of sodium hypochlorite and EDTA in 60 cases of endodontic therapy. Int Endod J 1985;18:35.

146. Falk KW, Sedgley CM. The influence of preparation size on the mechanical efficacy of root canal irrigation in vitro. J Endod 2005;31:742.

147. van der Sluis LW, Gambarini G, Wu MK, Wesselink PR. The influence of volume, type of irrigant and flushing method on removing artificially placed dentine debris from the apical root canal during passive ultrasonic irrigation. Int Endod J 2006;39:472.

148. Haapasalo M, Endal U, Zandi H, Coil JM. Eradication of endodontic infection by instrumentation and irrigation solutions. Endod Top 2005;10:77.

149. Zehnder M. Root canal irrigants. J Endod 2006;32:389.

150. Albrecht L, Baumgartner J, Marshall J. Evaluation of apical debris removal using various sizes and tapers of ProFile GT files. J Endod 2004;30:425.

151. Jou Y-T, Karabuchak B, Levin J, Liu D. Endodontic working width: current concepts and techniques. Dent Clin North Am 2004;48:323.

152. Nair PMR. Apical periodontitis: a dynamic encounter between root canal infection and host response. Periodontology 2000 2000;13:121.

153. Ricucci D. Apical limit of root canal instrumentation and obturation, part1. Literature review. Int Endod J 1998;31:384.

154. Certosimo FJ, Milos MF, Walker T. Endodontic working length determination—where does it end? Gen Dent 1999;47:281.

155. Wu MK, Wesselink PR, Walton RE. Apical terminus location of root canal treatment procedures. Oral Surg Oral Med Oral Pathol Oral Radiol Endod 2000;89:99.

156. Davis WJ. Pulpectomy vs pulp-extirpation. Dent Items Interest 1922;44:81.

157. Kerekes K, Tronstad L. Long-term results of endodontic treatment performed with a standardized technique. J Endod 1979;5:83.

158. Cailleteau JG, Mullaney TP. Prevalence of teaching apical patency and various instrumentation and obturation techniques in United States dental schools. J Endod 1997;23:394.

159. Holland R, Sant'Anna Junior A, Souza V, et al. Influence of apical patency and filling material on healing process of dog's teeth with vital pulp after root canal therapy. Braz Dent J 2005;19:9.

160. Sjögren U, Hagglund B, Sundqvist G, Wing K. Factors affecting the long-term results of endodontic treatment. J Endod 1990;16:498.

161. Izu KH, Thomas SJ, Zhang P, et al. Effectiveness of sodium hypochlorite in preventing inoculation of periapical tissue with contaminated patency files. J Endod 2004;30:92.

162. Beeson TJ, Hartwell GR, Thornton JD, Gunsolley JC. Comparison of debris extruded apically in straight canals: conventional filing versus ProFile .04 taper series 29. J Endod 1998;24:18.

163. Tinaz AC, Alacam T, Uzun O, et al. The effect of disruption of the apical constriction on periapical extrusion. J Endod 2005;31:533.

164. Souza RA. The importance of apical patency and cleaning the apical foramen on root canal preparation. Braz Dent J 2006;17:6.

165. Parris J, Wilcox L, Walton R. Effectiveness of apical clearing: histological and radiographical evaluation. J Endod 1994;20:219.

166. Heard F, Walton RE. Scanning electron microscope study comparing four root canal preparation techniques in small curved canals. Int Endod J 1997;30:323.

167. Goldberg F, Massone EJ. Patency file and apical transportation: an in vitro study. J Endod 2002;28:510.

168. Kuttler Y. Microscopic investigation of root apexes. J Am Dent Assoc 1955;50:544.

169. Dummer PMH, McGinn JH, Rees DG. The position and topography of the apical canal constriction and apical foramen. Int Endod J 1984;17:192.

170. Tidmarsh BG, Sherson W, Stalker NL. Establishing endodontic working length: a comparison of radiographic and electronic methods. N Z Dent J 1985;81:93.

171. Stein TJ, Corcoran JF. Radiographic "working length" revisited. Oral Surg Oral Med Oral Pathol Oral Radiol Endod 1992;74:796.

172. Gutmann JL, Leonard JE. Problem solving in endodontic working-length determination. Compend Contin Educ Dent 1995;16:288.

173. El Ayouti A, Weiger R, Löst C. Frequency of overinstrumentation with an acceptable radiographic working length. J Endod 2001;27:49.

174. Glossary of endodontic terms. 7th ed. Chicago, IL: American Association of Endodontists; 2003.

175. Palmer MJ, Weine FS, Healey HJ. Position of the apical foramen in relation to endodontic therapy. J Can Dent Assoc 1971;37:305.

176. Olson AK, Goerig AC, Cavataio RE, Luciano J. The ability of the radiograph to determine the location of the apical foramen. Int Endod J 1991;24:28.

177. Green EN. Microscopic investigation of root canal diameters. J Am Dent Assoc 1958;57:636.

178. Green D. Stereomicroscopic study of 700 root apices of maxillary and mandibular posterior teeth. Oral Surg Oral Med Oral Pathol Oral Radiol Endod 1960;13:728.

179. Chapman CE. A microscopic study of the apical region of human anterior teeth. J Br Endod Soc 1969;3:52.

180. Morfis A, Sylaras SN, Georgopoulou M, et al. Study of the apices of human permanent teeth with the use of a scanning electron microscope. Oral Surg Oral Med Oral Path Oral Radiol Endod 1994;77:172.

181. Guiterrez JH, Aguayo P. Apical foraminal openings in human teeth. Number and location. Oral Surg Oral Med Oral Path Oral Radiol Endod 1995;79:769.

182. Wu MK, R'Oris A, Barkis D, Wesselink PR. Prevalence and extent of long oval canals in the apical third. Oral Surg Oral Med Oral Pathol Oral Radiol Endod 2000;89:739.

183. Briseno Marroquin B, El-Sayed MAA, Willershausen-Zönnchen B. Morphology of the physiological foramen: I. Maxillary and mandibular molars. J Endod 2004;30:321.

184. Langeland K. The histopathologic basis in endodontic treatment. Dent Clin North Am 1967;Nov:491.

185. Caldwell JL. Change in working length following instrumentation of molar canals. Oral Surg Oral Med Oral Pathol Oral Radiol Endod 1976;41:114.

186. Davis RD, Marshall JG, Baumgartner JC. Effect of early coronal flaring on working length change in curved canals using rotary nickel–titanium versus stainless steel instruments. J Endod 2002;28:438.

187. Sonntag D, Stachniss-Carp S, Stachniss V. Determination of root canal curvatures before and after canal preparation (part 1): a literature review. Aust Endod J 2005;31:89.

188. Oguntebi B, Slee AM, Tanker JM, Langeland K. Predominant microflora associated with human dental periapical abscesses. J Clin Microbiol 1982;15:964.

189. Pascon EA, Introcaso JH, Langeland K. Development of predictable periapical lesion monitored by subtraction radiography. Endod Dent Traumatol 1987;3:192.

190. Ricucci D, Langeland K. Apical limit of root canal instrumentation and obturation, part 2. A histological study. Int Endod J 1998;31:394.

191. Katz A, Szajkis S, Tamse A, Tagger M. Standardization of endodontic instruments and materials: expectations and reality. Part 1: Development of the system. Refuat Ha-Shinayim 1984;2:18.

192. Steffen H, Splieth CH, Behr K. Comparison of measurements obtained with hand files or the Canal Leader attached to electronic apex locators: an in vitro study. Int Endod J 1999;32:103.

193. Simon JH. The apex: how critical is it? Gen Dent 1994;42:330.

194. Seidberg BH, Alibrandi BV, Fine H, Logue B. Clinical investigation of measuring working lengths of root canals with an electronic device and with digital-tactile sense. J Am Dent Assoc 1975;90:379.

195. Balto KA. Modern electronic apex locators are reliable for determining root canal working length. Evid Based Dent 2006;7:31.

196. Bramante CM, Berbert A. A critical evaluation of some methods of determining tooth length. Oral Surg Oral Med Oral Pathol Oral Radiol Endod 1974;37:463.

197. Dummer PM, Lewis JM. An evaluation of the Endometric Probe in root canal length estimation. Int Endod J 1987;20:25.

198. Ingle JI. Endodontics. 1st ed. Philadelphia, PA: Lea & Febiger; 1965.

199. Vande Voorde HE, Bjorndahl AM. Estimating endodontic "working length" with paralleling radiographs. Oral Surg Oral Med Oral Pathol Oral Radiol Endod 1969;27:106.

200. Hoer D, Attin T. The accuracy of electronic working length determination. Int Endod J 2004;37:125.

201. El Ayouti A, Weiger R, Lost C. The ability of root ZX apex locator to reduce the frequency of overestimated radiographic working length. J Endod 2002;28:116.

202. Nguyen HQ, Kaufman AY, Komorowski RC, Friedman S. Electronic length measurement using small and large files in enlarged canals. Int Endod J 1996;29:359.

203. El Ayouti A, Kimionis I, Chu AL, Löst C. Determining the apical terminus of root-end resected teeth using three modern apex locators: a comparative ex vivo study. Int Endod J 2005;38:827.

204. Weine FS. Endodontic therapy. 4th ed. St. Louis, MO: CV Mosby; 1989.

205. Von der Lehr WN, Marsh RA. A radiographic study of the point of endodontic egress. Oral Surg Oral Med Oral Pathol Oral Radiol Endod 1973;35:705.

206. Cox VS, Brown CE Jr, Bricker SL, Newton CW. Radiographic interpretation of endodontic file length. Oral Surg Oral Med Oral Pathol Oral Radiol Endod 1991;72:340.

207. Nair MK, Nair UP. Digital and advanced imaging in endodontics: a review. J Endod 2007;33:1.

208. Friedlander LT, Love RM, Chandler NP. A comparison of phosphor-plate digital images with conventional radiographs for the perceived clarity of fine endodontic files and apical lesions. Oral Surg Oral Med Oral Path Oral Radiol Endod 2002;93:321.

209. Borg E, Gröndahl HG. Endodontic measurements in digital radiographs acquired by a photostimulable, storage phosphor system. Endod Dent Traumatol 1996;12:20.

210. Cederberg RA, Tidwell E, Frederiksen NL, Benson BW. Endodontic working length assessment. Comparison of storage phosphor digital imaging and radiographic film. Oral Surg Oral Med Oral Pathol Oral Radiol Endod 1998;85:325.

211. Leddy BJ, Miles DA, Newton CW, Brown CE Jr. Interpretation of endodontic file lengths using RadioVisiography. J Endod 1994;20:542.

212. Sanderink GC, Huiskens R, van der Stelt PF, et al. Image quality of direct digital intraoral X-ray sensors in assessing root canal length. The RadioVisioGraphy, Visualix/VIXA, Sens-A-Ray, and Flash Dent systems compared with Ektaspeed films. Oral Surg Oral Med Oral Pathol Oral Radiol Endod 1994;78:125.

213. Woolhiser GA, Brand JW, Hoen MM, et al. Accuracy of film-based, digital, and enhanced digital images for endodontic length determination. Oral Surg Oral Med Oral Path Oral Radiol Endod 2005;99:499.

214. Radel RT, Goodell GG, McClanahan SB, Cohen ME. In vitro radiographic determination of distances from working length files to root ends comparing Kodak RVG 6000, Schick CDR, and Kodak insight film. J Endod 2006;32:566.

215. Stabholz A, Rotstein I, Torabinejad M. Effect of preflaring on tactile detection of the apical constriction. J Endod 1995;21:92.

216. Ounsi HF, Haddad G. In vitro evaluation of the reliability of the Endex electronic apex locator. J Endod 1998;24:120.

217. Clouse HR. Electronic methods of root canal measurement. Gen Dent 1991;39:432.

218. Lin L, Shovlin F, Skribner J, Langeland K. Pulp biopsies from the teeth associated with periapical radiolucency. J Endod 1984;10:436.

219. Yusuf H. The significance of the presence of foreign material periapically as a cause of failure of root treatment. Oral Surg Oral Med Oral Pathol Oral Radiol Endod 1982;54:566.

220. Walton RE. Current concepts of canal preparation. Dent Clin North Am 1992;36:309.

221. Baugh D, Wallace J. The role of apical instrumentation in root canal treatment: a review of the literature. J Endod 2005;31:333.

222. van der Sluis LW, Wu MK, Wesselink PR. The efficacy of ultrasonic irrigation to remove artificially placed dentine

debris from human root canals prepared using instruments of varying taper. Int Endod J 2005;38:764.

223. Khademi A, Yazdizadeh M, Feizianfard M. Determination of minimum instrumentation size for the penetration of irrigants to the apical third of root canal systems. J Endod 2006;32:417.

224. Hsieh YD, Gau CH, Kung Wu SF, et al. Dynamic recording of irrigation fluid distribution in root canals using thermal image analysis. Int Endod J 2007;40:11.

225. Peters CI, Koka RS, Highsmith S, Peters OA. Calcium hydroxide dressings using different preparation and application modes: density and dissolution by simulated tissue pressure. Int Endod J 2005;38:889.

226. Pekruhn RB. The incidence of failure following single-visit endodontic therapy. J Endod 1986;12:68.

227. Hoskinson SE, Ng YL, Hoskinson AE, et al. A retrospective comparison of outcome of root canal treatment using two different protocols. Oral Surg Oral Med Oral Pathol Oral Radiol Endod 2002;93:705.

228. Peters OA, Barbakow F, Peters CI. An analysis of endodontic treatment with three nickel–titanium rotary root canal preparation techniques. Int Endod J 2004;37:849.

229. Kirkevang LL, Hørsted-Bindslev P. Technical aspects of treatment in relation to treatment outcome. Endod Top 2002;2:89.

230. Farzaneh M, Abitbol S, Lawrence HP, Friedman S. Treatment outcome in endodontics-the Toronto study. Pahse II: initial treatment. J Endod 2004;30:302.

231. Ørstavik D, Qvist V, Stoltze K. A multivariate analysis of the outcome of endodontic treatment. Eur J Oral Sci 2004;112:224.

232. Ruddle C. Cleaning and shaping the root canal system. In: Cohen S, Burns RC, editors. Pathways of the pulp. 8th ed. St. Louis, MO: Mosby; 2002. p. 231.

233. Tan BT, Messer HH: The effect of instrument type and preflaring on apical file size determination. Int Endod J 2002;35:752.

234. Pecora JD, Capelli A, Guersoli DM, et al. Influence of cervical preflaring on apical file size determination. Int Endod J 2005;38.

235. Gutmann JL, Witherspoon DE. Obturation of the cleaned and shaped root canal system. In: Cohen S, Burns RC, editors. Pathways of the pulp. 8th ed. St. Louis, MO: Mosby; 2002. p. 293.

236. Guide to clinical endodontics. 4th ed. Chicago, IL: American Association of Endodontists; 2004.

237. European Society of Endodontology. Quality guidelines of endodontic treatment: consensus report of the European Society of Endodontology. Int Endod J 2006.

238. Kerekes K, Tronstad L. Morphometric observations on root canals of human anterior teeth. J Endod 1977;3:24.

239. Kerekes K, Tronstad L. Morphometric observations on the root canals of human molars. J Endod 1977;3:114.

240. Grossman L. Endodontic practice. 10th ed. Philadelphia, PA: Lea & Febiger; 1986.

241. Sabala CL, Biggs JT. A standard predetermined endodontic preparation concept. Compend Contin Educ Dent 1991;12:656.

242. Tronstad L. Endodontic techniques. In: Clinical endodontics. 1st ed. Stuttgart, New York: Thieme; 1991. p. 167.

243. Glickman GN, Dumsha TC. Problems in cleaning and shaping. In: Gutman J, Dumsha TC, Lovdahl PE, Hovland E, editors, Problem solving in endodontics. 3rd ed. St. Louis, MO: Mosby; 1997;

244. Spångberg L. The wonderful world of rotary root canal preparation. Oral Surg Oral Med Oral Pathol Oral Radiol Endod 2001;92:479.

245. Peters OA, Schönenberger K, Laib A. Effects of four NiTi preparation techniques on root canal geometry assessed by micro computed tomography. Int Endod J 2001;34:221.

246. Lussi A, Nussbacher U, Grosrey J. A novel noninstrumented technique for cleansing the root canal system. J Endod 1993;19:549.

247. Attin T, Buchalla W, Zirkel C, Lussi A. Clinical evaluation of the cleansing properties of the noninstrumental technique for cleaning root canals. Int Endod J 2002;35:929.

248. Allison DA, Weber CR, Walton RE. The influence of the method of canal preparation on the quality of apical and coronal obturation. J Endod 1979;5:298.

249. Grossman LI. Endodontics 1776–1976: a bicentennial history against the background of general dentistry. J Am Dent Assoc 1976;93:78.

250. Cruse WP, Bellizzi R. A historic review of endodontics, 1689–1963, part 1. J Endod 1980;6:495.

251. Lilley JD. Endodontic instrumentation before 1800. J Br Endod Soc 1976;9:67.

252. Hülsmann M. Zur Geschichte der Wurzelkanalaufbereitung. Endodontie 1996:97.

253. Bellizzi R, Cruse WP. A historic review of endodontics, 1689–1963, part III. J Endod 1980;6:576.

254. Anthony LP, Grossman LI. A brief history of root-canal therapy in the United States. J Am Med Assoc 1945;32:43.

255. Ehrmann EH. Wanted: a standard for the recognition of rotary instruments. Int Endod J 2002;35:215.

256. Mullaney TP. Instrumentation of finely curved canals. Dent Clin North Am 1979;23:575.

257. Taylor GN. Advanced techniques for intracanal preparation and filling in routine endodontic therapy. Dent Clin North Am 1984;28:819.

258. Ingle JI, Himel VT, Hawrish CE, et al. Endodontic cavity preparation. In: Ingle JI, Bakland LK, editors. Endodontics. 5th ed. Hamilton, ON: B.C. Decker; 2002.

259. Barbakow F. The status of root canal therapy in Switzerland in 1993. J Dent Assoc S Afr 1996;51:819.

260. Lim SS, Stock CJ. The risk of perforation in the curved canal: anticurvature filing compared with the stepback technique. Int Endod J 1987;20:33.

261. Wu M-K, van der Sluis LW, Wesselink PR. The capability of two hand instrumentation techniques to remove the inner layer of dentine in oval canals. Int Endod J 2003;36:218.

262. Goerig AC, Michelich RJ, Schultz HH. Instrumentation of root canals in molar using the step-down technique. J Endod 1982;8:550.

263. Gluskin AH, Brown DC, Buchanan LS. A reconstructed computerized tomographic comparison of Ni–Ti rotary GT files versus traditional instruments in canals shaped by novice operators. Int Endod J 2001;34:476.

264. Wu M-K, van der Sluis LW, Wesselink PR. The risk of furcal perforation in mandibular molars using Gates-Glidden drills with anticurvature pressure. Oral Surg Oral Med Oral Pathol Oral Radiol Endod 2005;99:378.

265. Guldener PH. [The filling technic in endodontics]. Schweiz Monatsschr Zahnmed 1971;81:311.

266. Roane JB. Balanced force, crown-down preparation, and inject-R Fill obturation. Compend Contin Educ Dent 1998;19:1137.

267. Serota KS, Nahmias Y, Barnett F, et al. Predictable endodontic success. The apical control zone. Dentistry Today 2003;22:90.

268. Kast'akova A, Wu MK, Wesselink PR. An in vitro experiment on the effect of an attempt to create an apical matrix during root canal preparation on coronal leakage and material extrusion. Oral Surg Oral Med Oral Pathol Oral Radiol Endod 2001;91:462.

269. Buchanan LS. The standardized-taper root canal preparation—Part 1. Concepts for variably tapered shaping instruments. Int Endod J 2000;33:516.

270. Stadler LE, Wennberg A, Olgart L. Instrumentation of the curved root canal using filing or reaming technique—a clinical study of technical complications. Swed Dent J 1986;10:37.

271. Greene KJ, Krell KV. Clinical factors associated with ledged canals in maxillary and mandibular molars. Oral Surg Oral Med Oral Pathol Oral Radiol Endod 1990;70:490.

272. Kapalas A, Lambrianidis T. Factors associated with root canal ledging during instrumentation. Endod Dent Traumatol 2000;16:229.

273. Pettiette MT, Delano EO, Trope M. Evaluation of success rate of endodontic treatment performed by students with stainless-steel K-files and nickel-titanium hand files. J Endod 2001;27:124.

274. Eleftheriades G, Lambrianidis T. Technical quality of root canal treatment and detection of iatrogenic errors in an undergraduate dental clinic. Int Endod J 2005;38:725.

275. Lin LM, Rosenberg PA, Lin J. Do procedural errors cause endodontic treatment failure? J Am Dent Assoc 2005;136:187.

276. Ingle JI. A standardized endodontic technique using newly development instruments and filling materials. Oral Surg Oral Med Oral Pathol Oral Radiol Endod 1961;14:83.

277. Clem WH. Endodontics: the adolescent patient. Dent Clin North Am 1969;13:482.

278. Weine FS, Healey HJ, Gerstein H, Evanson L. Pre-curved files and incremental instrumentation for root canal enlargement. J Can Dent Assoc 1970;36:155.

279. Abou-Rass M, Frank AL, Glick DH. The anticurvature filing method to prepare the curved root canal. J Am Dent Assoc 1980;101:792.

280. Marshall FJ, Pappin JB. A crown-down pressureless preparation root canal enlargement technique. Technique Manual. ed. Portland OR: Oregon Health Sciences University; 1980.

281. Froese WJ, Schechter DS. Sophomore Laboratory Manual. ed. Portland OR: Oregon Health Sciences University; 1981.

282. Fava LR. The double-flared technique: an alternative for biomechanical preparation. J Endod 1983;9:76.

283. Saunders WP, Saunders EM. Effect of noncutting tipped instruments on the quality of root canal preparation using a modified double-flared technique. J Endod 1992;18:32.

284. Roane JB, Sabala CL, Duncanson MG Jr. The "balanced force" concept for instrumentation of curved canals. J Endod 1985;11:203.

285. Torabinejad M. Passive step-back technique. Oral Surg Oral Med Oral Pathol Oral Radiol Endod 1994;77:398.

286. Torabinejad M. Passive step-back technique. A sequential use of ultrasonic and hand instruments. Oral Surg Oral Med Oral Pathol Oral Radiol Endod 1994;77:402.

287. Siqueira JF Jr, Rjcas IN, Santos SR, et al. Efficacy of instrumentation techniques and irrigation regimens in reducing the bacterial population within root canals. J Endod 2002;28:181.

288. Cimis GM, Boyer TJ, Pelleu GB Jr. Effect of three file types on the apical preparations of moderately curved canals. J Endod 1988;14:441.

289. Calhoun G, Montgomery S. The effects of four instrumentation techniques on root canal shape. J Endod 1988;14:273.

290. Alodeh MHA, Dummer PMH. A comparison of the ability of K-files and Hedstrom files to shape simulated root canals in resin blocks. Int Endod J 1989;22:226.

291. Briseno BM, Sonnabend E. The influence of different root canal instruments on root canal preparation: an in vitro study. Int Endod J 1991;24:15.

292. Alodeh MH, Doller R, Dummer PM. Shaping of simulated root canals in resin blocks using the step-back technique with K-files manipulated in a simple in/out filling motion. Int Endod J 1989;22:107.

293. Schäfer E, Tepel J, Hoppe W. Properties of endodontic hand instruments used in rotary motion. Part 2. Instrumentation of curved canals. J Endod 1995;21:493.

294. Stenman E, Spångberg LS. Root canal instruments are poorly standardized. J Endod 1993;19:327.

295. Moule AJ, Kellaway R, Clarkson R, et al. Variability of master gutta-percha cones. Aus Endod J 2002;28:38.

296. Martin H. A telescopic technique for endodontics. J Dist Columbia Dent Soc 1974;49:12.

297. Brantley WA, Luebke NH, Luebke FL, Mitchell JC. Performance of engine-driven rotary endodontic instruments with a superimposed bending deflection: V. Gates Glidden and Peeso drills. J Endod 1994;20:241.

298. Kuttler S, MacLean A, Dorn S, Fischzang A. The impact of post space preparation with Gates-Glidden drills on residual dentin thickness in distal roots of mandibular molars. J Am Dent Assoc 2004;135:903.

299. Coffae KP, Brilliant JD. The effect of serial preparation versus nonserial preparation on tissue removal in the root canals of extracted mandibular human molars. J Endod 1975;14:527.

300. Walton RE. Histologic evaluation of different methods of enlarging the pulp canal space. J Endod 1976;2:304.

301. Mullaney TP. Instrumentation of finely curved canals. Dent Clin North Am 1979;4:575.

302. Buchanan LS. Paradigm shifts in cleaning and shaping. J Calif Dent Assoc 1991;19:23.

303. Gutmann JL, Rakusin H. Perspectives on root canal obturation with thermoplasticized injectable gutta-percha. Int Endod J 1987;20:261.

304. Kartal N, Cimilli HK. The degrees and configurations of mesial canal curvatures of mandibular first molars. J Endod 1997;23:358.

305. Schäfer E, Diey C, Hoppe W, Tepel J. Roentgenographic investigation of frequency and degree of canal curvatures in human permanent teeth. J Endod 2002;28:211.

306. Baker NA, Eleazer PD, Averbach RE, Seltzer S. Scanning electron microscopic study of the efficacy of various irrigating solutions. J Endod 1975;1:127.

307. Ram Z. Effectiveness of root canal irrigation. Oral Surg Oral Med Oral Pathol Oral Radiol Endod 1977;44:306.

308. Abou Rass M, Jastrab RJ. The use of rotary instruments as auxiliary aids to root canal preparation of molars. J Endod 1982;8:78.

309. Vertucci F. Root canal morphology and its relationship to endodontic procedures. Endod Top 2005;10:3.

310. Kessler JR, Peters DD, Lorton L. Comparison of the relative risk of molar root perforations using various endodontic instrumentation techniques. J Endod 1983;9:439.

311. Lumley PJ. A comparison of dentine removal using safety or conventional Hedstrom files. Endod Dent Traumatol 1997;13:65.

312. Lloyd A, Jaunberzins A, Dhopatkar A, et al. Shaping of simulated root canals by the M4 handpiece and Safety Hedström files when oriented incorrectly. Braz Endod J 1997;2:7.

313. Swindle RB, Neaverth EJ, Pantera EA Jr, Ringle RD. Effect of coronal–radicular flaring on apical transportation. J Endod 1991;17:147.

314. Schroeder KP, Walton RE, Rivera EM. Straight line access and coronal flaring: effect on canal length. J Endod 2002;28:474.

315. Leeb J. Canal orifice enlargement as related to biomechanical preparation. J Endod 1983;9:463.

316. Fairbourn DR, McWalter GM, Montgomery S. The effect of four preparation techniques on the amount of apically extruded debris. J Endod 1987;13:102.

317. Roane JB, Powell SE. The optimal instrument design for canal preparation. J Am Dent Assoc 1986;113:596.

318. Roane JB, Sabala C. Clockwise or counterclockwise. J Endod 1984;10:349.

319. Southard DW, Oswald RJ, Natkin E. Instrumentation of curved molar root canals with the Roane technique. J Endod 1987;13:479.

320. Backman CA, Oswald RJ, Pitts DL. A radiographic comparison of two root canal instrumentation techniques. J Endod 1992;18:19.

321. Al-Omari MA, Dummer PM, Newcombe RG, Doller R. Comparison of six files to prepare simulated root canals. Part 2. Int Endod J 1992;25:67.

322. Al-Omari MA, Dummer PM, Newcombe RG. Comparison of six files to prepare simulated root canals. Part 1. Int Endod J 1992;25:57.

323. Dummer PMH, Al-Omari MAO, Bryant S. Comparison of the performance of four files with rounded tips during shaping of simulated root canals. J Endod 1998;24:364.

324. Ponce de Leon Del Bello T, Wang N, Roane JB. Crown-down tip design and shaping. J Endod 2003;29:513.

325. Sabala CL, Roane JB, Southard LZ. Instrumentation of curved canals using a modified tipped instrument: a comparison study. J Endod 1988;14:59.

326. Kyomen SM, Caputo AA, White SN. Critical analysis of the balanced force technique in endodontics. J Endod 1994;20:332.

327. Charles TJ, Charles JE. The 'balanced force' concept for instrumentation of curved canals revisited. Int Endod J 1998;31:166.

328. Schäfer E. Effects of four instrumentation techniques on curved canals: a comparison study. J Endod 1996;22:685.

329. Imura N, Kato AS, Novo NF, et al. A comparison of mesial molar root canal preparations using two engine-driven instruments and the balanced-force technique. J Endod 2001;27:627.

330. Hata G, Uemura M, Kato AS, et al. A comparison of shaping ability using ProFile, GT file, and Flex-R endodontic instruments in simulated canals. J Endod 2002;28:316.

331. McKendry DJ. Comparison of balanced forces, endosonic, and step-back filing instrumentation techniques: quantification of extruded apical debris. J Endod 1990;16:24.

332. Pappin JB. Biologic sealing of the apex in endodontically treated human teeth [Masters Thesis]. Portland OR: Oregon Health & Sciences University; 1982.

333. Morgan LF, Montgomery S: An evaluation of the crown-down pressureless technique. J Endod 1984;10:491.

334. Luiten DJ, Morgan LA, Baumgartner JC, Marshall JG. A comparison of four instrumentation techniques on apical canal transportation. J Endod 1995;1995:26.

335. Blum JY, Machtou P, Micallef JP. Location of contact areas on rotary Profile instruments in relationship to the forces developed during mechanical preparation on extracted teeth. Int Endod J 1999;32:108.

336. Schrader C, Ackermann M, Barbakow F. Step-by-step description of a rotary root canal preparation technique. Int Endod J 1999;32:312.

337. Thompson SA. An overview of nickel–titanium alloys used in dentistry. Int Endod J 2000;33:297.

338. Walia HM, Brantley WA, Gerstein H. An initial investigation of the bending and torsional properties of Nitinol root canal files. J Endod 1988;14:346.

339. Serene TP, Adams JD, Saxena A. Nickel–titanium instruments: applications in endodontics. St. Louis, MO: Ishiaku EuroAmerica; 1995.

340. Parashos P, Messer HH. The diffusion of innovation in dentistry: a review using rotary nickel–titanium technology as an example. Oral Surg Oral Med Oral Path Oral Radiol Endod 2006;101:395.

341. Pettiette MT, Metzger Z, Phillips C, Trope M. Endodontic complications of root canal therapy performed by dental students with stainless-steel K-files and nickel-titanium hand files. J Endod 1999;25:230.

342. Barbakow. The LightSpeed system. Dent Clin North Am 2004;48:113.

343. Sattapan B, Nervo GJ, Palamara JEA, Messer HH. Defects in rotary nickel–titanium files after clinical use. J Endod 2000;26:161.

344. Roland DD, Andelin WE, Browning DF, et al. The effect of preflaring on the rates of separation for 0.04 taper nickel titanium rotary instruments. J Endod 2002;28:543.

345. Yared GM, Bou Dagher FE, Machtou P, Kulkarni GK. Influence of rotational speed, torque and operator proficiency on failure of Greater Taper files. Int Endod J 2002;35:7.

346. Yared GM, Bou Dagher FE, Machtou P. Influence of rotational speed, torque and operator's proficiency on ProFile failures. Int Endod J 2001;34:47.

347. Schrader C, Peters OA. Analysis of torque and force during step-back with differently tapered rotary endodontic instruments in vitro. J Endod 2005;31:120.

348. Peng B, Shen Y, Cheung GS, Xia TJ. Defects in ProTaper S1 instruments after clinical use: longitudinal examination. Int Endod J 2005;38:550.

349. Parashos P, Messer HH. Rotary NiTi instrument fracture and its consequences. J Endod 2006;32:1031.

350. Zuolo ML, Walton RE. Instrument deterioration with usage: nickel–titanium versus stainless steel. Quintessence Int 1997;28:397.

351. Herold KS, Johnson BR, Wenckus CS. A scanning electron microscopy evaluation of microfractures, deformation and separation in EndoSequence and Profile Nickel-Titanium rotary files using an extracted molar tooth model. J Endod 2007;33:712.

352. Lemmer K, Mielke M, Pauli G, Beekes M. Decontamination of surgical instruments from prion proteins. in vitro studies on the detachment, destabilization and degradation of PrPSc bound to steel surfaces. J Gen Virol 2004;85:3805.

353. Aasim SA, Mellor AC, Qualtrough AJ. The effect of pre-soaking and time in the ultrasonic cleaner on the cleanliness of sterilized endodontic files. Int Endod J 2006;39:143.

354. Peretz D, Supattapone S, Giles K, et al. Inactivation of prions by acidic sodium dodecyl sulfate. J Virol 2006;80:322.

355. Sonntag D, Peters OA. Effect of prion decontamination protocols on nickel–titanium rotary surfaces. J Endod 2007;33.

356. O'Hoy PY, Messer HH, Palamara JE. The effect of cleaning procedures on fracture properties and corrosion of NiTi files. Int Endod J 2003;36:724.

357. Darabara M, Bourithis L, Zinelis S, Papadimitriou GD. Susceptibility to localized corrosion of stainless steel and NiTi endodontic instruments in irrigating solutions. Int Endod J 2004;37:705.

358. Peters OA, Roelicke JO, Baumann MA. Effect of immersion in sodium hypochlorite on torque and fatigue resistance of nickel–titanium instruments. J Endod 2007;33:589.

359. Buchanan LS. The standardized-taper root canal preparation—Part 1. Concepts for variably tapered shaping instruments. Int Endod J 2000;33:516.

360. Li UM, Lee BS, Shih CT, et al. Cyclic fatigue of endodontic nickel titanium rotary instruments: static and dynamic tests. J Endod 2002;28:448.

361. Rowan MB, Nicholls JI, Steiner J. Torsional properties of stainless steel and nickel–titanium endodontic files. J Endod 1996;22:341.

362. Pruett JP, Clement DJ, Carnes DL. Cyclic fatigue testing of nickel–titanium endodontic instruments. J Endod 1997;23:77.

363. Peters OA, Barbakow F. Dynamic torque and apical forces of ProFile .04 rotary instruments during preparation of curved canals. Int Endod J 2002;35:379.

364. Haikel Y, Serfaty R, Bateman G, et al. Dynamic and cyclic fatigue of engine-driven rotary nickel–titanium endodontic instruments. J Endod 1999;25:434.

365. Ullmann C, Peters OA. Effect of cyclic fatigue on static fracture loads in ProTaper nickel–titanium rotary instruments. J Endod 2005;31:183.

366. Kitchens GG, Liewehr FR, Moon PC. The effect of operational speed on the fracture of nickel–titanium rotary instruments. J Endod 2007;33:52.

367. Ruddle C. The Protaper technique. Endod Top 2005;10:187.

368. Plotino G, Grande NM, Sorci E, et al. Influence of a brushing working motion on the fatigue life of NiTi rotary instruments. Int Endod J 2007;40:45.

369. Patino PV, Biedma BM, Liebana CR, et al. The influence of a manual glide path on the separation of NiTi rotary instruments. J Endod 2005;31:114.

370. Anderson DN, Joyce AP, Roberts S, Runner R. A comparative photoelastic stress analysis of internal root stresses between RC Prep and saline when applied to the Profile/GT rotary instrumentation system. J Endod 2006;32:224.

371. Peters OA, Boessler C, Zehnder M. Effect of liquid and paste-type lubricants on torque values during simulated rotary root canal instrumentation. Int Endod J 2005;38:223.

372. Boessler C, Peters OA, Zehnder M. Impact of lubricant parameter on rotary instrument torque and force. J Endod 2007;33:280.

373. Grawehr M, Sener B, Waltimo T, Zehnder M. Interactions of ethylenediaminetetraacetic acid with sodium hypochlorite in aqueous solutions. Int Endod J 2003;36:411.

374. Berutti E, Angelini E, Rigolone M, et al. Influence of sodium hypochlorite on fracture properties and corrosion of ProTaper rotary instruments. Int Endod J 2006;39:693.

375. Castro Martins R, Bahia MGA, Buono VTL. The effect of sodium hypochlorite on the surface characteristics and fatigue resistance of ProFile nickel-titanium instruments. Oral Surg Oral Med Oral Path Oral Radiol Endod 2006;102:99.

376. Baumgartner JC, Cuenin PR. Efficacy of several concentrations of sodium hypochlorite for root canal irrigation. J Endod 1992;18:605.

377. Grandini S, Balleri P, Ferrari M. Evaluation of Glyde File Prep in combination with sodium hypochlorite as a root canal irrigant. J Endod 2002;28:300.

378. Mayer BE, Peters OA, Barbakow F. Effects of rotary instruments and ultrasonic irrigation on debris and smear layer scores: a scanning electron microscopic study. Int Endod J 2002;35:582.

379. Regan JD, Gutmann JL. Preparation of the root canal system. In: Pitt Ford TR, editors. Endodontics in clinical practice, 5th ed. Oxford: Elsevier; 2003. p. 77.

380. Al-Omari MA, Dummer PM. Canal blockage and debris extrusion with eight preparation techniques. J Endod 1995;21:154.

381. Reddy SA, Hicks ML. Apical extrusion of debris using two hand and two rotary instrumentation techniques. J Endod 1998;24:180.

382. Nygaard-Østby B. Chelation in endodontic therapy: ethylenediamineacetate acid for cleansing and widening of root canals. Odontologisk Tidskrift 1957;65:3.

383. Fehr F, Nygaard-Østby B. Effect of EDTAC and sulfuric acid on root canal dentin. Oral Surg Oral Med Oral Pathol Oral Radiol Endod 1963;12:99.

384. Goldberg F, Spielberg C. The effect of EDTAC and the variation of its working time analyzed with scanning electron microscopy. Oral Surg Oral Med Oral Pathol Oral Radiol Endod 1982;53:74.

385. Fraser JG. Chelating agents: their softening effect on root canal dentin. Oral Surg Oral Med Oral Pathol Oral Radiol Endod 1974;37:803.

386. Fraser JG, Laws AJ. Chelating agents: their effect on the permeability of root canal dentin. Oral Surg Oral Med Oral Pathol Oral Radiol Endod 1976;41:534.

387. Bortnick KL, Steiman HR, Ruskin A. Comparison of nickel–titanium file distortion using electric and air-driven handpieces. J Endod 2001;27:57.

388. Molven O. A comparison of the dentin-removing ability of five root canal instruments. Scand J Dent Res 1970;78:500.

389. O'Connell DT, Brayton SM. Evaluation of root canal preparation with two automated endodontic handpieces. Oral Surg Oral Med Oral Pathol Oral Radiol Endod 1975;39:298.

390. Klayman SM, Brilliant JD. A comparison of the efficacy of serial preparation versus Giromatic preparation. J Endod 1975;1:334.

391. Harty FJ, Stock C. The Giromatic system compared with hand instrumentation in endodontics. Br Dent J 1974;137:239.

392. Weine FS, Kelly RF, Bray KE. Effect of preparation with endodontic handpieces on original canal shape. J Endod 1976;2:298.

393. Felt RA, Moser JB, Heuer MA. Flute design of endodontic instruments: its influence on cutting efficiency. J Endod 1982;8:253.

394. Spyropoulos S, Eldeeb ME, Messer HH. The effect of Giromatic files on the preparation shape of severely curved canals. Int Endod J 1987;20:133.

395. Hülsmann M, Stryga F. Comparison of root canal preparation using different automated devices and hand instrumentation. J Endod 1993;19:141.

396. Schäfer E, Zapke K. A comparative scanning electron microscopic investigation of the efficacy of manual and automated instrumentation of root canals. J Endod 2000;26:660.

397. Tepel J. Experimentelle Untersuchungen über die maschinelle Wurzelkanalaufbereitung.Berlin, Germany: Quintessenz Verlags-GmbH; 2000.

398. Paque F, Barbakow F, Peters OA. Root canal preparation with Endo-Eze AET: changes in root canal shape assessed by micro-computed tomography. Int Endod J 2005;38:456.

399. Zmener O, Pamaijer CH, Banegas G. Effectiveness in cleaning oval-shaped root canals using Anatomic Endodontic Technology, ProFile and manual instrumentation: a scanning electron microscopic study. Int Endod J 2005;38:356.

400. Daugherty DW, Gound TG, Comer TL. Comparison of fracture rate, deformation rate, and efficiency between rotary endodontic instruments driven at 150 rpm and 350 rpm. J Endod 2001;27:93.

401. Gabel WP, Hoen M, Steiman HR, et al. Effect of rotational speed on nickel–titanium file distortion. J Endod 1999;25:752.

402. Dietz DB, Di Fiore PM, Bahcall JK, Lautenschlager EP. Effect of rotational speed on the breakage of nickel-titanium rotary files. J Endod 2000;26:68.

403. Yared GM. Behaviour of Hero NiTi instruments used by an experienced operator under access limitations. Aust Endod J 2002;28:64.

404. Yared G, Bou Dagher F, Kulkarni K. Influence of torque control motors and the operator's proficiency on ProTaper failures. Oral Surg Oral Med Oral Pathol Oral Radiol Endod 2003;96:229.

405. Gambarini G. Rationale for the use of low-torque endodontic motors in root canal instrumentation. Endod Dent Traumatol 2000;16:95.

406. Gambarini G. Cyclic fatigue of nickel–titanium rotary instruments after clinical use with low- and high-torque endodontic motors. J Endod 2001;27:772.

407. Gambarini G. Advantages and disadvantages of new torque-controlled endodontic motors and low-torque NiTi rotary instrumentation. Aust Endod J 2001;27:99.

408. Yared G, Kulkarni GK. Accuracy of the DTC torque control motor for nickel–titanium rotary instruments. Int Endod J 2004;37:399.

409. Yared G, Kuklarni GK. Accuracy of the TCM Endo III torque-control motor for nickel–titanium rotary instruments. J Endod 2004;30:644.

410. Yared G, Kulkarni GK. Accuracy of the Nouvag torque control motor for nickel-titanium rotary instruments. Oral Surg Oral Med Oral Path Oral Radiol Endod 2004;97:499.

411. Dental root-canal instruments—Part 1: Files, reamers, barbed broaches, rasps, paste carriers, explorers and cotton broaches. Geneva: International Organization for Standardization; 1992.

412. Blum JY, Machtou P, Ruddle C, Micallef JP. Analysis of mechanical preparations in extracted teeth using ProTaper rotary instruments: value of the safety quotient. J Endod 2003;29:567.

413. Johnson TA, Zelikow R. Ultrasonic endodontics: a clinical review. J Am Dent Assoc 1987;114:655.

414. Richman MJ. The use of ultrasonics in root canal therapy and root resection. J Dent Med 1957;12:12.

415. Martin H. Ultrasonic disinfection of the root canal. Oral Surg Oral Med Oral Pathol Oral Radiol Endod 1976;42:92.

416. Cunningham WT, Martin H. A scanning electron microscope evaluation of root canal debridement with the endosonic ultrasonic synergistic system. Oral Surg Oral Med Oral Pathol Oral Radiol Endod 1982;53:527.

417. Cunningham WT, Martin H, Forrest WR. Evaluation of root canal debridement by the endosonic ultrasonic synergistic system. Oral Surg Oral Med Oral Pathol Oral Radiol Endod 1982;53:401.

418. Cunningham WT, Martin H, Pelleu GB Jr, Stoops DE. A comparison of antimicrobial effectiveness of endosonic and hand root canal therapy. Oral Surg Oral Med Oral Pathol Oral Radiol Endod 1982;54:238.

419. Martin H, Cunningham W. Endosonic endodontics: the ultrasonic synergistic system. Int Dent J 1984;34:198.

420. Martin H, Cunningham W. Endosonics—the ultrasonic synergistic system of endodontics. Endod Dent Traumatol 1985;1:201.

421. Cameron JA. The use of ultrasonics in the removal of the smear layer: a scanning electron microscope study. J Endod 1983;9:289.

422. Barnett F, Trope M, Khoja M, Tronstad L. Bacteriologic status of the root canal after sonic, ultrasonic and hand instrumentation. Endod Dent Traumatol 1985;1:228.

423. Reynolds MA, Madison S, Walton RE, et al. An in vitro histological comparison of the step-back, sonic, and ultrasonic instrumentation techniques in small, curved root canals. J Endod 1987;13:307.

424. Yamaguchi M, Matsumori M, Ishikawa H, et al. The use of ultrasonic instrumentation in the cleansing and enlargement of the root canal. Oral Surg Oral Med Oral Pathol Oral Radiol Endod 1988;65:349.

425. Pedicord D, elDeeb ME, Messer HH. Hand versus ultrasonic instrumentation: its effect on canal shape and instrumentation time. J Endod 1986;12:375.

426. Baker MC, Ashrafi SH, Van Cura JE, Remeikis NA. Ultrasonic compared with hand instrumentation: a scanning electron microscopic study. J Endod 1988;14:435.

427. Chenail BL, Teplitsky PE. Endosonics in curved root canals. Part II. J Endod 1988;14:214.

428. Krell KV, Johnson RJ. Irrigation patterns of ultrasonic endodontic files. Part II. Diamond coated files. J Endod 1988;14:535.

429. Loushine RJ, Weller RN, Hartwell GR. Stereomicroscopic evaluation of canal shape following hand, sonic, and ultrasonic instrumentation. J Endod 1989;15:417.

430. Schulz-Bongert U, Weine FS, Schulz-Bongert J. Preparation of curved canals using a combined hand-filing, ultrasonic technique. Comp Cont Ed Dent 1995;16:270.

431. Ahmad M, Pitt Ford TR, Crum LA. Ultrasonic debridement of root canals: an insight into the mechanisms involved. J Endod 1987;13:93.

432. Ahmad M, Pitt Ford TR, Crum LA. Ultrasonic debridement of root canals: acoustic streaming and its possible role. J Endod 1987;13:490.

433. Ahmad M, Pitt Ford TR, Crum LA, Walton AJ. Ultrasonic debridement of root canals: acoustic cavitation and its relevance. J Endod 1988;14:486.

434. Walmsley AD, Williams AR. Effects of constraint on the oscillatory pattern of endosonic files. J Endod 1989;15:189.

435. Walmsley AD, Lumley PJ, Laird WRE. The oscillatory pattern of sonically powered endodontic files. Int Endod J 1989;22:125.

436. Burleson A, Nusstein J, Reader A, Beck M. The in vivo evaluation of hand/rotary/ultrasound instrumentation in necrotic, human mandibular molars. J Endod 2007;33:782.

437. Jensen SA, Walker TL, Hutter JW, Nicoll BK. Comparison of the cleaning efficacy of passive sonic activation and passive ultrasonic activation after hand instrumentation in molar root canals. J Endod 1999;25:735.

438. Sabins RA, Johnson JD, Hellstein JW. A comparison of the cleaning ability of short-term sonic and ultrasonic passive irrigation after hand instrumentation in molar root canals. J Endod 2003;29:674.

439. Weber CD, McClanahan SB, Miller GA, et al. The effect of passive ultrasonic activation of 2% chlorhexidine and of 5.25% sodium hypochlorite irrigant on residual microbial activity in root canals. J Endod 2003;29:562.

440. van der Sluis LW, Wu MK, Wesselink PR. A comparison between a smooth wire and a K-file in removing artificially placed dentine debris from root canals in resin blocks during ultrasonic irrigation. Int Endod J 2005;38:593.

441. Alacam T. Scanning electron microscope study comparing the efficacy of endodontic irrigating systems. Int Endod J 1987;20:287.

442. Cunningham WT, Balekjian AY. Effect of temperature on collagen-dissolving ability of sodium hypochlorite endodontic irrigant. Oral Surg Oral Med Oral Pathol Oral Radiol Endod 1980;49:175.

443. Cameron JA. The effect of ultrasonic endodontics on the temperature of the root canal wall. J Endod 1988;14:554.

444. Archer R, Reader A, Nist R, et al. An in vivo evaluation of the efficacy of ultrasound after step-back preparation in mandibular molars. J Endod 1992;18:549.

445. Krell KV, Johnson RJ, Madison S. Irrigation patterns during ultrasonic canal instrumentation. Part I. K-type files. J Endod 1988;14:65.

446. Ahmad M, Ford TR, Crum LA, Walton AJ. Ultrasonic debridement of root canals: acoustic cavitation and its relevance. J Endod 1988;14:486.

447. Martin H, Cunningham WT, Norris JP, Cotton WR. Ultrasonic versus hand filing of dentin: a quantitative study. Oral Surg Oral Med Oral Pathol Oral Radiol Endod 1980;49:79.

448. Wildey WL, Senia ES, Montgomery S. Another look at root canal instrumentation. Oral Surg Oral Med Oral Pathol Oral Radiol Endod 1992;74:499.

449. Lam TV, Lewis DJ. Changes in root canal morphology in simulated curved canals over-instrumented with a variety of stainless steel and nickel titanium files. Aust Dent J 1999;44(1):12.

450. Powell SE, Simon JH, Maze BB. A comparison of the effect of modified and nonmodified instrument tips on apical canal configuration. J Endod 1986;12:293.

451. Dummer PM, Al-Omari MA, Bryant S. Comparison of the performance of four files with rounded tips during shaping of simulated root canals. J Endod 1998;24:364.

452. Griffiths IT, Bryant ST, Dummer PMH. Canal shapes produced sequentially during instrumentation with Quantec LX rotary nickel–titanium instruments: a study in simulated canals. Int Endod J 2000;33:346.

453. Garala M, Kuttler S, Hardigan P, et al. A comparison of the minimum canal wall thickness remaining following preparation using two nickel–titanium rotary systems. Int Endod J 2003;36:636.

454. Crump MC, Natkin E. Relationship of broken root canal instruments to endodontic case prognosis: a clinical investigation. J Am Dent Assoc 1970;80:1341.

455. Weine FS, Kelly RF, Lio PJ. The effect of preparation procedures on original shape and on apical foramen shape. J Endod 1975;1:255.

456. Tucker DM, Wenckus CS, Bentkover SK. Canal wall planning by engine-driven nickel–titanium instruments, compared with stainless-steel hand instrumentation. J Endod 1997;23:170.

457. Wu MK, Wesselink PR. A primary observation on the preparation and obturation of oval canals. Int Endod J 2001;34:137.

458. Tan BT, Messer HH. The quality of apical canal preparation using hand and rotary instruments with specific criteria for enlargement based on initial apical file size. J Endod 2002;28:658.

459. Rödig T, Hülsmann M, Muhge M, Schäfers F. Quality of preparation of oval distal root canals in mandibular molars using nickel–titanium instruments. Int Endod J 2002;35:919.

460. Weiger R, El Ayouti A, Löst C. Efficiency of hand and rotary instruments in shaping oval root canals. J Endod 2002;28:580.

461. Bergmans L, Van Cleynenbreugel J, Beullens M, et al. Smooth flexible versus active tapered shaft design using NiTi rotary instruments. Int Endod J 2002;35:820.

462. Bergmans L, Van Cleynenbreugel J, Beullens M, et al. Progressive versus constant tapered shaft design using NiTi rotary instruments. Int Endod J 2003;36:288.

463. Peters OA, Peters CI, Schönenberger K, Barbakow F. ProTaper rotary root canal preparation: assessment of torque and force in relation to canal anatomy. Int Endod J 2003;36:93.

464. Hübscher W, Barbakow F, Peters OA. Root canal preparation with FlexMaster: canal shapes analysed by microcomputed tomography. Int Endod J 2003;36:740.

465. Stuart CH, Schwartz SA, Beeson TJ, Owatz CB. *Enterococcus faecalis*: its role in root canal treatment failure and current concepts in retreatment. J Endod 2006;32:93.

466. Pertot WJ, Camps J, Damiani MG. Transportation of curved canals prepared with Canal Master-U, Canal Master-U-NiTi, and stainless steel K-type files. Oral Surg Oral Med Oral Path Oral Radiol Endod 1995;79:504.

467. Jardine SJ, Gulabivala K. An in vitro comparison of canal preparation using two automated rotary nickel–titanium instrumentation techniques. Int Endod J 2000;33:381.

468. Iqbal MK, Maggiore F, Suh B, et al. Comparison of apical transportation in four Ni–Ti rotary instrumentation techniques. J Endod 2003;29:587.

469. Bramante CM, Berbert A, Borges RP. A methodology for evaluation of root canal instrumentation. J Endod 1987;13:243.

470. McCann JT, Keller DL, LaBounty GL. A modification of the muffle model system to study root canal morphology. J Endod 1990;16:114.

471. Tamse A, Pilo R. A new muffle model system to study root canal morphology and instrumentation techniques. J Endod 1998;24:540.

472. Portenier I, Lutz F, Barbakow F. Preparation of the apical part of the root canal by the Lightspeed and step-back techniques. Int Endod J 1998;31:103.

473. Kuttler S, Garala M, Perez R, Dorn SO. The endodontic cube: a system designed for evaluation of root canal anatomy and canal preparation. J Endod 2001;27:533.

474. Deplazes P, Peters O, Barbakow F. Comparing apical preparations of root canals shaped by nickel titanium rotary and nickel titanium hand instruments. J Endod 2001;27:196.

475. Leseberg DA, Montgomery S. The effects of Canal Master, Flex-R, and K-Flex instrumentation on root canal configuration. J Endod 1991;17:59.

476. Coleman CL, Svec TA. Analysis of Ni-Ti versus stainless steel instrumentation in resin simulated canals. J Endod 1997;23:232.

477. Short JA, Morgan LA, Baumgartner JC. A comparison of canal centering ability of four instrumentation techniques. J Endod 1997;23:503.

478. Shadid DB, Nicholls JI, Steiner JC. A comparison of curved canal transportation with balanced force versus lightspeed. J Endod 1998;24:651.

479. Kosa D, Marshall G, Baumgartner J. An analysis of canal centering using mechanical instrumentation techniques. J Endod 1999;25:441.

480. Porto Carvalho LA, Bonetti I, Gagliardi Borges MA. A comparison of molar root canal preparation using stainless steel and nickel–titanium instruments. J Endod 1999;25:807.

481. Thompson SA, Dummer PM. Shaping ability of Lightspeed rotary nickel–titanium instruments in simulated root canals. Part 1. J Endod 1997;23:698.

482. Thompson SA, Dummer PM. Shaping ability of Lightspeed rotary nickel–titanium instruments in simulated root canals. Part 2. J Endod 1997;23:742.

483. Bryant ST, Thompson SA, Al-Omari MAO, Dummer PMH. Shaping ability of ProFile rotary nickel–titanium instruments with ISO sized tips in simulated root canals: Part 1. Int Endod J 1998;31:275.

484. Bryant ST, Thompson SA, Al-Omari MAO, Dummer PMH. Shaping ability of ProFile rotary nickel–titanium instruments with ISO sized tips in simulated root canals: Part 2. Int Endod J 1998;31:282.

485. Bryant ST, Dummer PM, Pitoni C, et al. Shaping ability of .04 and .06 taper ProFile rotary nickel–titanium instruments in simulated root canals. Int Endod J 1999;32:155.

486. Thompson SA, Dummer PM. Shaping ability of Hero 642 rotary nickel–titanium instruments in simulated root canals: Part 2. Int Endod J 2000;33:255.

487. Thompson SA, Dummer PM. Shaping ability of Hero 642 rotary nickel–titanium instruments in simulated root canals: Part 1. Int Endod J 2000;33:248.

488. Griffiths IT, Chassot AL, Nascimento MF, et al. Canal shapes produced sequentially during instrumentation with Quantec SC rotary nickel–titanium instruments: a study in simulated canals. Int Endod J 2001;34:107.

489. Powell SE, Wong PD, Simon JH. A comparison of the effect of modified and nonmodified instrument tips on apical canal configuration. Part II. J Endod 1988;14:224.

490. Kuhn WG, Carnes DL Jr, Clement DJ, Walker WA III. Effect of tip design of nickel–titanium and stainless steel files on root canal preparation. J Endod 1997;23:735.

491. Hülsmann M, Schade M, Schäfers F. A comparative study of root canal preparation with HERO 642 and Quantec SC rotary Ni–Ti instruments. Int Endod J 2001;34:538.

492. Hülsmann M, Herbst U, Schäfers F. Comparative study of root-canal preparation using Lightspeed and Quantec SC rotary NiTi instruments. Int Endod J 2003;36:748.

493. Al-Omari MA, Bryant S, Dummer PM. Comparison of two stainless steel files to shape simulated root canals. Int Endod J 1997;30:35.

494. Bishop K, Dummer PM. A comparison of stainless steel Flexofiles and nickel-titanium NiTiFlex files during the shaping of simulated canals. Int Endod J 1997;30:25.

495. Schäfer E. Shaping ability of Hero 642 rotary nickel-titanium instruments and stainless steel hand K-Flexofiles in simulated curved root canals. Oral Surg Oral Med Oral Pathol Oral Radiol Endod 2001;92:215.

496. Schäfer E, Lohmann D. Efficiency of rotary nickel–titanium FlexMaster instruments compared with stainless steel hand K-Flexofile—Part 1. Shaping ability in simulated curved canals. Int Endod J 2002;35:505.

497. Schäfer E, Florek H. Efficiency of rotary nickel–titanium K3 instruments compared with stainless steel hand K-flexofile. Part 1. Shaping ability in simulated curved canals. Int Endod J 2003;36:199.

498. Yun HH, Kim SK. A comparison of the shaping abilities of 4 nickel–titanium rotary instruments in simulated root canals. Oral Surg Oral Med Oral Pathol Oral Radiol Endod 2003;95:228.

499. Hülsmann M, Gressmann G, Schäfers F. A comparative study of root canal preparation using FlexMaster and HERO 642 rotary Ni–Ti instruments. Int Endod J 2003;36:358.

500. Schäfer E, Schlingemann R. Efficiency of rotary nickel–titanium K3 instruments compared with stainless steel hand K-Flexofile. Part 2. Cleaning effectiveness and shaping ability in severely curved root canals of extracted teeth. Int Endod J 2003;36:208.

501. Lim KC, Webber J. The validity of simulated root canals for the investigation of the prepared root canal shape. Int Endod J 1985;18:240.

502. Lim KC, Webber J. The effect of root canal preparation on the shape of the curved root canal. Int Endod J 1985;18:233.

503. Ciucchi B, Cergneux M, Holz J. Comparison of curved canal shape using filing and rotational instrumentation techniques. Int Endod J 1990;23:139.

504. Haga CS. Microscopic measurements of root canal preparations following instrumentation. J Br Endod Soc 1968;2:41.

505. Vessey R. The effect of filing versus reaming on the shape of the prepared root canal. Oral Surg Oral Med Oral Pathol Oral Radiol Endod 1969;27:544.

506. Jungmann CL, Uchin RA, Bucher JF. Effect of instrumentation on the shape of the root canal. J Endod 1975;1:66.

507. Tronstad L, Niemczyk SP. Efficacy and safety tests of six automated devices for root canal instrumentation. Endod Dent Traumatol 1986;2:270.

508. Kielt LW, Montgomery S. The effect of endosonic instrumentation in simulated curved root canals. J Endod 1987;13:215.

509. Lev R, Reader A, Beck M, Meyers W. An in vitro comparison of the step-back technique versus a step-back/ultrasonic technique for 1 and 3 minutes. J Endod 1987;13:523.

510. Bolanos OR, Sinai IH, Gonsky R, Srinivasan R. A comparison of engine and air-driven instrumentation methods with hand instrumentation. J Endod 1988;14:392.

511. Miserendino LJ, Miserendino CA, Moser JB, et al. Cutting efficiency of endodontic instruments. Part III. Comparison of sonic and ultrasonic instrument systems. J Endod 1988;14:24.

512. Walker TL, del Rio CE. Histological evaluation of ultrasonic and sonic instrumentation of curved root canals. J Endod 1989;15:49.

513. Yahya AS, ElDeeb ME. Effect of sonic versus ultrasonic instrumentation on canal preparation. J Endod 1989;15:235.

514. Lloyd A, Jaunberzins A, Dhopatkar A, et al. Shaping ability of the M4 handpiece and Safety Hedstrom files in simulated root canals. Int Endod J 1997;30:16.

515. Barbakow F, Lutz F. The 'Lightspeed' preparation technique evaluated by Swiss clinicians after attending continuing education courses. Int Endod J 1997;30:46.

516. Mandel E, Adib-Yazdi M, Benhamou L-M, et al. Rotary Ni–Ti ProFile systems for preparing curved canals in resin blocks: influence of operator on instrument breakage. Int Endod J 1999;32:436.

517. Al-Fouzan KS. Incidence of rotary ProFile instrument fracture and the potential for bypassing in vivo. Int Endod J 2003;36:864.

518. Spili P, Parahos P, Messer HH. The impact of instrument fracture on outcome of endodontic treatment. J Endod 2005;31:845.

519. Wolcott S, Wolcott J, Ishley D, et al. Separation incidence of ProTaper rotary instruments: a large cohort clinical investigation. J Endod 2006;12:1139.

520. Grossman LI. Fate of endodontically treated teeth with fractured root canal instruments. J Br Endod Soc 1968;2:35.

521. Fox J, Moodnik RM, Greenfield E, Atkinson JS. Filing root canals with files radiographic evaluation of 304 cases. N Y State Dent J 1972;38:154.

522. Sonntag D, Heithecker K. Korrosion von Nickel-Titan-Instrumenten. Endodontie 2006;15:23.

523. Borkow G, Gabbay J. Copper as biocidal tool. Curr Med Chem 2004;12:2163.

524. Thoden van Velzen SK, Duivenvoorden HJ, Schuurs AH. Probabilities of success and failure in endodontic treatment: a Bayesian approach. Oral Surg Oral Med Oral Pathol Oral Radiol Endod 1981;52:85.

525. Ward JR, Parashos P, Messer HH. Evaluation of an ultrasonic technique to remove fractured rotary nickel–titanium endodontic instruments from root canals: an experimental study. J Endod 2003;29:756.

526. Ward JR, Parashos P, Messer HH. Evaluation of an ultrasonic technique to remove fractured rotary nickel–titanium endodontic instruments from root canals: clinical cases. J Endod 2003;29:764.

527. Kesler G, Gal R, Kesler A, Koren R. Histological and scanning electron microscope examination of root canal after preparation with Er:YAG laser microprobe: a preliminary in vitro study. J Clin Laser Med Surg 2002;20:269.

528. Lussi A, Messerli L, Hotz P, Grosrey J. A new non-instrumental technique for cleaning and filling root canals. Int Endod J 1995;28:1.

529. Nakashima M, Akamine A. The application of tissue engineering to regeneration of pulp and dentin in endodontics. J Endod 2005;31:711.

530. Matsumoto K. Lasers in endodontics. Dent Clin North Am 1990;44:889.

531. Stabholz A, Sahar-Helft S, Moshonov J. Lasers in endodontics. Dent Clin North Am 2004;48:809.

532. Dederich DN, Zakariasen KL, Tulip J. Scanning electron microscopic analysis of canal wall dentin following neodymium–yttrium–aluminum–garnet laser irradiation. J Endod 1984;10:428.

533. Takeda FH, Harashima T, Eto JN, et al. Effect of Er:YAG laser treatment on the root canal walls of human teeth: an SEM study. Endod Dent Traumatol 1998;14:270.

534. Takeda FH, Harashima T, Kimura Y, Matsumoto K. Efficacy of Er:YAG laser irradiation in removing debris and smear layer on root canal walls. J Endod 1998;24:548.

535. Harashima T, Takeda FH, Kimura Y, Matsumoto K. Effect of Nd:YAG laser irradiation for removal of intracanal debris and smear layer in extracted human teeth. J Clin Laser Med Surg 1997;15:131.

536. Barbakow F, Peters O, Havranek L. Effects of Nd: YAG lasers on root canal walls: A light and scanning electron microscopic study. Quintessence Int 1999;30:837.

537. Cecchini SCM, Zezell DM, Bachmann L. Evaluation of two laser systems for intracanal irradiation. In: Featherstone JDB, Rechmann P, Fried D, editors, Lasers in dentistry V. Proc SPIEE; 1999. p. 31.

538. Liu HC, Lin CP, Lan WH. Sealing depth of Nd:YAG laser on human dentinal tubules. J Endod 1997;23:691.

539. Bahcall JK, Miserendino CA, Walia H, Belardi DW. Scanning electron microscopic comparison of canal preparation with Nd:YAG laser and hand instrumentation: a preliminary study. Gen Dent 1993;41:45.

540. Anic I, Dzubur A, Vidovic D, Tudja M. Temperature and surface changes of dentine and cementum induced by CO_2 laser exposure. Int Endod J 1993;26:284.

541. Ramskold LO, Fong CD, Stromberg T. Thermal effects and antibacterial properties of energy levels required to sterilize stained root canals with an Nd:YAG laser. J Endod 1997;23:96.

542. Hibst R, Stock K, Gall R, Keller U. ErYAG laser for endodontics efficiency and safety. In: Altshuler GB, Bringruber R, Dal Fante M, et al., editors, Medical applications of lasers in dermatology, ophthalmology, dentistry, and endoscopy. Proc SPIEE, Vol 3192; 1997. p. 14.

543. da Costa Ribeiro A, Nogueira GEC, Antoniazzi JH, et al. Effects of a diode laser (810 nm) irradiation on root canal walls: thermographic and morphological studies. J Endod 2006;33:252.

544. Harashima T, Takeda FH, Zhang C, et al. Effect of argon laser irradiation on instrumented root canal walls. Endod Dent Traumatol 1998;14:26.

545. Schoeffel GJ. Apparatus for evacuation of root canal; 2004.

546. Gutarts R, Nusstein J, Reader A, Beck M. In vivo debridement efficacy of ultrasonic irrigation following hand-rotary instrumentation in human mandibular molars. J Endod 2005;31:166.

547. Fukumoto Y, Kikuchi I, Yoshioka T, et al. An ex vivo evaluation of a new root canal irrigation technique with intracanal aspiration. Int Endod J 2006;39:93.

548. Lussi A, Portmann P, Nussbacher U, et al. Comparison of two devices for root canal cleansing by the noninstrumentation technology. J Endod 1999;25:9.

549. Lussi A. Die Reinigung und Obturation des Wurzelkanalsystems ohne konventionelle Instrumente-eine Standortbestimmung. Schweizerische Monatsschrift für Zahnmedizin 2000;110:249.

550. Lussi A, Suter B, Grosrey J. Obturation of root canals in vivo with a new vacuum technique. J Endod 1997;23:629.

551. Lussi A, Imwinkelried S, Stich H. Obturation of root canals with different sealers using non-instrumentation technology. Int Endod J 1999;32:17.

552. Zehnder M, Schmidlin P, Sener B, Waltimo T. Chelation in root canal therapy reconsidered. J Endod 2005;31:817.

553. Mader CL, Baumgartner JC, Peters DD. Scanning electron microscopic investigation of the smeared layer on root canal walls. J Endod 1984;10:477.

554. Sen BH, Wesselink PR, Türkün M. The smear layer: a phenomenon in root canal therapy. Int Endod J 1995;28:141.

555. Torabinejad M, Handysides R, Khademi AA, Bakland LK. Clinical implications of the smear layer in endodontics: a review. Oral Surg Oral Med Oral Path Oral Radiol Endod 2002;94:658.

556. Jeon IS, Spångberg LS, Yoon TC, et al. Smear layer production by 3 rotary reamers with different cutting blade designs in straight root canals: a scanning electron microscopic study. Oral Surg Oral Med Oral Path Oral Radiol Endod 2003;96:601.

557. Kum K-Y, Kazemi RB, Cha BY, Zhu Q. Smear layer production of K3 and ProFile Ni–Ti rotary instruments in curved root canals: a comparative SEM study. Oral Surg Oral Med Oral Path Oral Radiol Endod 2006;101:536.

558. Ørstavik D, Haapasalo M. Disinfection by endodontic irrigants and dressings of experimentally infected dentinal tubules. Endod Dent Traumatol 1990;6:142.

559. Kokkas AB, Boutsioukis A, Vassiliades LP, Stavrianos CK. The influence of the smear layer on dentinal tubule penetration depth by three different root canal sealers: an in vitro study. J Endod 2004;30:100.

560. Drake DR, Wiemann AH. Bacterial retention in canal walls in vitro: effect of smear layer. J Endod 1994;20, 2:78.

561. Baumgartner JC, Brown CM, Mader CL, et al. A scanning electron microscopic evaluation of root canal debridement using saline, sodium hypochlorite, and citric acid. J Endod 1984;10:525.

562. Wayman BE, Kopp WM, Pinero GJ, Lazzari EP. Citric and lactic acids as root canal irrigants in vitro. J Endod 1979;5:258.

563. Tidmarsh BG. Acid-cleansed and resin-sealed root canals. J Endod 1978;4:117.

564. Stewart GG, Kapsimalas P, Rappaport H. EDTA and urea peroxide for root canal preparation. J Am Dent Assoc 1969;78:335.

565. Koskinen KP, Rahkamo A, Hakala PE. Antimicrobial effect of some endodontic medicaments in vitro. Proc Finn Dent Soc 1975;71:132.

566. Koskinen KP, Meurman JH, Stenvall H. Appearance of chemically treated root canal walls in the scanning electron microscope. Scand J Dent Res 1980;88:505.

567. Kaufman AY. The use of dequalinium acetate as a disinfectant and chemotherapeutic agent in endodontics. Oral Surg Oral Med Oral Pathol Oral Radiol Endod 1981;51:434.

568. Berry EA, von der Lehr WN, Herrin HK. Dentin surface treatments for the removal of the smear layer: an SEM study. J Am Dent Assoc 1987;115:65.

569. Torabinejad M, Khademi AA, Babagoli J, et al. A new solution for the removal of the smear layer. J Endod 2003;29:170.

570. Kaufman AY. Accidental ingestion of an endodontic instrument. Quintessence Int 1978;9:83.

571. Abou-Rass M, Patonai FJ Jr. The effects of decreasing surface tension on the flow of irrigating solutions in narrow root canals. Oral Surg Oral Med Oral Pathol Oral Radiol Endod 1982;53:524.

572. Cameron JA. The effect of a fluorocarbon surfactant on the surface tension of the endodontic irrigant, sodium hypochlorite. A preliminary report. Aust Dent J 1986;31:364.

573. Tasman F, Cehreli ZC, Ogan C, Etikan I. Surface tension of root canal irrigants. J Endod 2000;26:586.

574. Zehnder M, Schicht O, Sener B, Schmidlin P. Reducing surface tension in endodontic chelator solutions has no effect on their ability to remove calcium from instrumented root canals. J Endod 2005;31:590.

575. Torabinejad M, Cho Y, Khademi AA, et al. The effect of various concentrations of sodium hypochlorite on the ability of MTAD to remove the smear layer. J Endod 2003;29:233.

576. Portenier I, Waltimo T, Ørstavik D, Haapasalo H. Killing of *Enterococcus faecalis* by MTAD and chlorhexidine digluconate with or without cetrimide in the presence or absence of dentine powder or BSA. J Endod 2006;32:138.

577. Krause TA, Liewehr FR, Hahn CL. The antimicrobial effect of MTAD, sodium hypochlorite, doxycycline, and citric acid on *Enterococcus faecalis*. J Endod 2007;33:28.

578. Baumgartner CJ, Johal S, Marshall JG. Comparison of the antimicrobial efficacy of 1.3% NaOCl/BioPure MTAD to 5.25% NaOCl/15% EDTA for root canal irrigation. J Endod 2007;33:48.

579. Torabinejad M, Shabahang S, Bahjri K. Effect of MTAD on postoperative discomfort: a randomized clinical trial. J Endod 2005;31:171.

580. Girard S, Paque F, Badertscher M, et al. Assessment of a gel-type chelating preparation containing 1-hydroxyethylidene-1, 1-bisphosphonate. Int Endod J 2005;38:810.

581. Sim TP, Knowles JC, Ng YL, et al. Effect of sodium hypochlorite on mechanical properties of dentine and tooth surface strain. Int Endod J 2001;34:120.

582. Grigoratos D, Knowles J, Ng YL, Gulabivala K. Effect of exposing dentine to sodium hypochlorite and calcium hydroxide on its flexural strength and elastic modulus. Int Endod J 2001;34:113.

583. Calt S, Serper A. Time-dependent effects of EDTA on dentin structures. J Endod 2002;28:17.

584. Sum CP, Neo J, Kishen A. What we leave behind in root canals after endodontic treatment: some issues and concerns. Aus Endod J 2005;31:94.

585. Guppy DR, Curtis RV, Ford TR. Dentine chips produced by nickel–titanium rotary instruments. Endod Dent Traumatol 2000;16:258.

586. Chow TW. Mechanical effectiveness of root canal irrigation. J Endod 1983;9:475.

587. Kaufman AY. Facial emphysema caused by hydrogen peroxide irrigation: report of a case. J Endod 1981;7:470.

588. Hülsmann M, Hahn W. Complications during root canal irrigation—literature review and case reports. Int Endod J 2000;33:186.

589. Witton R, Brennan PA. Severe tissue damage and neurological deficit following extravasation of sodium hypochlorite solution during routine endodontic treatment. Br Dent J 2005;198:749.

590. Bowden JR, Ethunanadan M, Brennan PA. Life-threatening airway obstruction secondary to hypochlorite extrusion during root canal treatment. Oral Surg Oral Med Oral Path Oral Radiol Endod 2006;101:402.

591. Abou-Rass M, Piccinino MV. The effectiveness of four clinical irrigation methods on the removal of root canal debris. Oral Surg Oral Med Oral Pathol Oral Radiol Endod 1982;54:323.

592. Moser JB, Heuer MA. Forces and efficacy in endodontic irrigation systems. Oral Surg Oral Med Oral Pathol Oral Radiol Endod 1982;53:425.
593. Druttman AC, Stock CJ. An in vitro comparison of ultrasonic and conventional methods of irrigant replacement. Int Endod J 1989;22:174.
594. Walton RE, Torabinejad M. Principles and practice of endodontics. Philadelphia, PA: WB Saunders; 2001.
595. Senia ES, Marshall FJ, Rosen S. The solvent action of sodium hypochlorite on pulp tissue of extracted teeth. Oral Surg Oral Med Oral Pathol Oral Radiol Endod 1971;31:96.
596. Salzgeber RM, Brilliant JD. An in vivo evaluation of the penetration of an irrigating solution in root canals. J Endod 1977;3:394.
597. Sedgley C, Applegate B, Agel A, Hall D. Real-time imaging and quantification of bioluminescent bacteria in root canals in vitro. J Endod 2004;30:893.
598. Cameron JA. The synergistic relationship between ultrasound and sodium hypochlorite: a scanning electron microscope evaluation. J Endod 1987;13:541.
599. Griffiths BM, Stock CJ. The efficiency of irrigants in removing root canal debris when used with ultrasonic preparation technique. Int Endod J 1986;19:277.
600. Cameron JA. The use of sodium hypochlorite activated by ultrasound for the debridement of infected, immature root canals. J Endod 1986;12:550.
601. Walker TL, del Rio CE. Histological evaluation of ultrasonic debridement comparing sodium hypochlorite and water. J Endod 1991;17:66.
602. Hülsmann M, Heckendorff M, Lennon A. Chelating agents in root canal treatment: mode of action and indications for their use. Int Endod J 2003;36:810.
603. Teplitsky PE, Chenail BL, Mack B, Machnee CH. Endodontic irrigation—a comparison of endosonic and syringe delivery systems. Int Endod J 1987;20:233.
604. Braun A, Kappes D, Kruse F, Jepsen S. Efficiency of a novel rinsing device for the removal of pulp tissue in vitro. Int Endod J 2005;38:8.
605. Nielsen BA, Baumgartner JC. Comparison of the EndoVac system to needle irrigation of root canals. J Endod 2007;33:611.
606. Lee MT, Bird PS, Walsh LJ. Photo-activated disinfection of the root canal: a new role for lasers in endodontics. Aus Endod J 2004;30:93.
607. Bonsor SJ, Nichol R, Reid TM, Pearson GJ. An alternative regimen for root canal disinfection. Br Dent J 2006;22:101.
608. Soukos NS, Chen PS, Morris JT, et al. Photodynamic therapy for endodontic disinfection. J Endod 2006;32:979.
609. Dougherty TJ, Gomer CJ, Henderson BW, et al. Photodynamic therapy. J Nat Canc Inst 1998;90:889.
610. Soukos NS, Mulholland SE, Socransky SS, Doukas AG. Photodestruction of human dental plaque bacteria: enhancement of the photodynamic effect by photomechanical waves in an oral biofilm model. Lasers Surg Med 2003;33:161.
611. Seal GJ, Ng Y-L, Spratt DA, et al. An in vitro comparison of the bactericidal efficacy of lethal photosensitization or sodium hypochlorite irrigation on *Streptococcus intermedius* biofilms in root canals. Int Endod J 2002;35:268.
612. Lendini M, Alamano E, Migliaretti G, Berutti E. The effect of high-frequency electrical pulses on organic tissue in root canals. Int Endod J 2005;38:531.

CHAPTER 28

IRRIGANTS AND INTRACANAL MEDICAMENTS

MARKUS HAAPASALO, WEI QIAN

Infection Control in the Human Body

Successful elimination of opportunistic infections in most parts of the human body usually requires only involvement of normal host defense mechanisms. Occasionally, a systemic antibiotic therapy or manipulative treatment (such as drainage of pus) is applied in addition in order to resolve the infection. Elimination of endodontic infection, however, follows a different pathway. Host measures that are sufficient to eliminate the infective microorganisms in other sites are unable to completely eliminate endodontic infections. Because of the special anatomical challenges, control of an endodontic infection must be built on a joint effort by a number of host and treatment factors.[1–3] Success in all parts of treatment will be needed for elimination of infection and healing of periapical pathosis. The sequence of events and procedures in the control of endodontic infections are host defense system, systemic antibiotic therapy (rarely used with specific indications only), instrumentation and irrigation ("cleaning and shaping"), intracanal medicaments used between appointments, permanent root filling, and coronal restoration.[1–3]

Host defense is responsible for the prevention of spreading canal infections to the bone and to other parts of the body. The body defense is usually successful in stabilizing the lesion size and preventing its expansion after the initial growth period. However, because of the lack of circulation, host defense mechanisms cannot effectively reach the microbes residing inside the tooth in the necrotic root canal system. Mechanical instrumentation removes a portion of the microbes from the main root canal space, but its main purpose is to enhance irrigation and the placement of medication and the root filling. Irrigation supports mechanical instrumentation, by reducing friction and removing dead and living microbes from the root canal. In addition, many irrigating solutions have antimicrobial activity that effectively kill residual microbes in the canal. Intracanal antimicrobial medicaments, on the other hand, are used in multi-appointment endodontic treatments to complete the work started by instrumentation and irrigation and, optimally, to render the root canal system bacteria-free.

The classical study by Sjögren and his colleagues[4] and by others indicated that a bacteria-free canal at the time of filling is a prerequisite for high success rate and that calcium hydroxide [$Ca(OH)_2$] as an intracanal medicament will predictably help reach this goal.[5–7] A number of other studies, however, have challenged these results, and at present, there is no clear consensus regarding the use of intracanal medicaments, or the microbiological and other advantages from their use.[8–10]

In this chapter, the focus is on the role of irrigation and intracanal medication in killing and reducing the number of bacteria in the root canal system. It is important, however, to understand that irrigation and local antibacterial dressings in the root canal are part of a concerted effort to control endodontic infections. Alone they cannot guarantee success if there are problems in quality of some other parts of the treatment.

Complete Elimination of Microbes in the Root Canal System

Pulpitis is caused by microbial antigens entering the pulp from a carious lesion or a leaking filling through dentinal tubules. As long as the pulp remains vital, the number of bacteria in the pulp is considered minimal and of no clinical significance. However, with proceeding infection, necrosis and apical periodontitis, the entire root canal system becomes invaded by bacteria. It has been shown beyond doubt that microorganisms are the etiological factor of apical periodontitis (Figure 1).[11–13] It has been suggested that, in a small

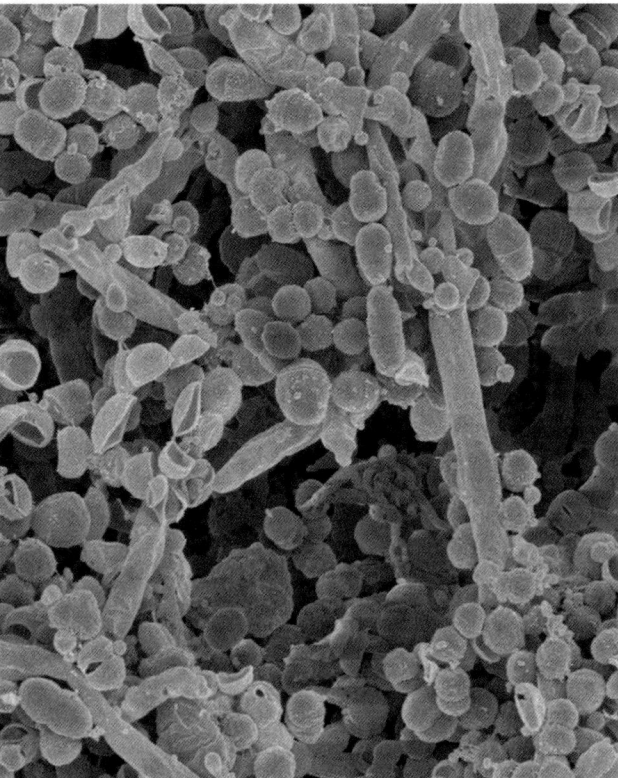

Figure 1 Bacteria are the etiological factor of apical periodontitis. Six-week-old biofilm on the main root canal wall created by a mixed culture of oral bacteria under anaerobic conditions. Notice that several cells have died (hollow cells) because of limited availability of nutrients.

number of cases, non-microbial factors are responsible for the persistence of the lesion after treatment.[14,15] Nevertheless, there is general consensus that, in an optimal situation, the goal of endodontic treatment is to remove and kill all microorganisms in the root canal and to neutralize any antigens that may be left in the canal after killing the microbes. Reaching this goal is expected to guarantee healing of periapical lesions. It has become obvious that complete destruction of root canal microbes is a particularly difficult challenge. On the other hand, in a high number of cases, high quality treatment is followed by complete healing.[16–18] It has also been shown that a majority of cases harboring living bacteria at the time of filling healed completely.[4] It is clear, therefore, that although destroying 100% of the infective flora is the optimal goal, complete clinical and radiographic healing can also occur when the microbiological goal of treatment has not been fully realized. The situation may be compared to marginal periodontitis and gingivitis, where it is not possible to gain a totally bacteria-free environment in the gingival crevice area. Periodontal treatment of good quality, however, results in healing of the periodontal disease.

The Goal of Endodontic Treatment

The goal, with the great majority of teeth requiring root canal treatment, is either the prevention or treatment of apical periodontitis.[19] In other words, the goal is prevention or elimination of a microbial infection in the root canal system. In some special situations, such as resorptions and endodontic complications, there may be a variety of intermediate goals of a more "technical" nature. Even then, the final success is dependent on successful infection control. There is a widely accepted view that cleaning and shaping of the root canal system is the most important step toward a sterile canal free from a microbial presence.

Instrumentation of the Root Canal

The goal of hand and rotary instrumentation and irrigation is to remove all necrotic and vital organic tissue, as well as some hard tissue including dentin chips created by instrumentation, from the root canal system and give the canal system a shape that facilitates optimal irrigation, débridement and placement of local medicaments, and permanent root filling. From a biological point of view, the goal of instrumentation and irrigation is to remove and eradicate the microorganisms residing in the necrotic root canal system. Furthermore, the goal is to neutralize any residual antigenic material remaining in the canal after instrumentation and irrigation.

The Effect of Instrumentation on the Root Canal Microbes

Instrumentation has a key role in the cascade of treatment procedures to eradicate microbes in the root canal system. Instrumentation removes a great number of microbes from the accessible parts of the main root canal by direct mechanical cleaning action. Moreover, instrumentation shapes the root canal in such a way that effective irrigation becomes possible. In other words, instrumentation is a way of mechanically removing microbes from the root canal. In addition, it supports and facilitates mechanical removal and chemical eradication of the infection by irrigation during and following instrumentation.

The classical studies from Umeå, Sweden have greatly influenced our understanding of the effects of instrumentation and irrigation of the intracanal microflora.[20] In a series of studies on teeth with apical periodontitis, the authors demonstrated that thorough mechanical instrumentation with hand stainless steel instruments, together with irrigation with either physiological saline, ethylenediamine-tetra-acetic acid (EDTA), or EDTA and sodium hypochlorite (NaOCl), they were unable to predictably produce sterile root canals. Fifteen root canals were instrumented at five sequential appointments and sampled at the beginning and end of each appointment. The access cavity was sealed with a bacteria-tight temporary filling, but the canals were left empty between the appointments. This procedure resulted in a 100- to 1000-fold reduction in bacterial numbers, but it was difficult to obtain completely bacteria-free root canals. Corresponding results were also reported by Ørstavik et al.[21] and Cvek et al.[22] in teeth with closed and immature apices. The antibacterial effect of mechanical cleansing with sterile saline was reported to be very low and limited to the teeth with fully developed roots. NaOCl increased the antibacterial effect as compared with saline irrigation. Interestingly, no statistical difference was found in the antibacterial effect between 0.5% and 5.0% NaOCl solutions.[22]

The effects of instrumentation and irrigation were investigated in an excellent series of studies by Dalton et al.[23] They measured reduction in microbial counts in 48 patients, on teeth instrumented with 0.04 taper nickel–titanium (NiTi) rotary instruments or with stainless steel K-files using the step back technique with saline for irrigation. Bacteriological samples were obtained before, during, and after instrumentation. All teeth with apical periodontitis yielded positive growth at the beginning, whereas control teeth with vital pulp and irreversible pulpitis were sterile. A reduction in bacterial counts was detected with progressive enlargement of the root canals with both techniques. However, only 28% of the teeth became bacteria-free following instrumentation.

Similar observations were reported by Siqueira et al.[24] when saline was used in irrigation. Interestingly, this study showed that increasing the size of apical preparation from #30 to #40 resulted in a significant reduction in microbial counts. Ex vivo studies by Pataky et al.,[25] using 40 human first maxillary premolars extracted for orthodontic reasons, also verified the difficulty of obtaining sterility of the infected canal space by instrumentation and saline irrigation. Although a considerable reduction in bacterial counts was detected after instrumentation, none of the teeth became bacteria-free. It should be mentioned, however, that the size of the master apical file in some of the studies was quite small, #25, and that may increase the possibility of positive cultures.[25] It can be concluded that instrumentation and irrigation with saline alone cannot predictably eliminate all bacteria from infected root canals. Therefore, it is not surprising that the focus of activity in root canal disinfection is placed on the development and use of irrigating solutions and other intracanal disinfecting agents with strong antibacterial activity. In addition, there is growing interest in the combined effect of ultrasonic energy and irrigating solutions as well as other new ways of mechanical irrigation.

Root Canal Disinfection by Chemical Means

THE CHALLENGES AND PITFALLS IN STUDYING THE ANTIMICROBIAL EFFECTIVENESS OF ENDODONTIC IRRIGATING SOLUTIONS AND INTRACANAL MEDICAMENTS

In Vitro Models

The testing of the antimicrobial activity of various chemical compounds may appear to be straightforward and simple procedure. In theory, this may be true—the microbes of interest are exposed to the antimicrobial agent to be examined. At certain time intervals, microbiological samples are collected and cultured on suitable media. The results are then expressed as the length of time required to kill all microbes. In reality, regarding endodontic disinfecting agents, it is, however, quite different. Research focusing on the antimicrobial effectiveness of irrigating solutions and temporarily used intracanal medicaments has in many occasions adopted techniques originally designed for some other context, for example, antibiotic susceptibility using agar plates. Testing of systemically used antibiotics is based on tens of years of international standardization.[26-30] The chemical composition of both the antibiotic discs and the culture media used in testing are defined in detail in order to secure predictable diffusion of the active ingredient of the antibiotic and the absence of chemical reactions between the agar plate ingredients and the antibiotic. Zones of inhibition of growth around the antibiotic disc have been compared through clinical studies to the serum and tissue concentrations that are possible to reach with safe dosages of low toxicity, as well as the clinical effectiveness of the antibiotics. In addition, reference strains from culture collections with known antibiotic susceptibilities are used as internal standards for quality testing of each new batch of plates. Most aerobic and facultative bacteria can be reliably tested using the disc diffusion method. However, despite years of extensive research, there is still no generally accepted standard for susceptibility testing anaerobic bacteria using the disc diffusion method.[31]

The use of agar diffusion method in endodontics, despite good intentions, is not based on any kind of standardization of the media or the tested materials. Chemical interactions between the media and the disinfecting agents are largely unknown. Furthermore, there are no true comparative studies helping to draw conclusions from the zones of inhibition to the performance of the disinfectants in vivo. The antimicrobial effect of some endodontic medicaments is based on the pH effect; therefore, the buffering capacity of the agar plate is in key position in determining the diameter of the growth inhibition zone. Another example is EDTA, that causes a zone of inhibition on an agar plate, but fails to reduce the number of viable microbes even after 24-hour incubation in a test tube. The growth inhibition on agar plates is based on removal of important ingredients from the media by EDTA, that makes the medium unsuitable for growth of many species. Such bacteria, even if alive, cannot multiply on the plate which has been nutritionally altered by EDTA. In conclusion, the information obtained from agar diffusion studies is at best of limited value and should not be used to compare and select disinfecting agents for clinical use.

Another matter of importance in susceptibility testing is understanding the difference between bacteriostatic and bactericidal activities. Bacteriostatic means prevention of growth of the microbial cells. However, they are not killed, unlike when the medicament has bactericidal activity. In endodontic studies, this difference is not always clearly addressed, and the results are often reported as "antibacterial activity." The agar diffusion test, when properly used, is an example of measuring bacteriostatic activity. In endodontics, a bactericidal effect of a disinfecting agent is more important than a bacteriostatic effect. In the necrotic root canal system, a temporary prevention of bacterial growth (as long as the disinfecting agent remains in the canal) is of limited value, because the microbes may still grow in numbers afterwards causing a new challenge to the host defense.

Testing endodontic disinfecting agents in vitro can be done in test tubes using a mixture of the microbes (suspended in sterile water) and the medicament. The presence of a culture medium in the mixture is commonly seen in endodontic literature. However, culture medium or other organic material is a confounding factor: the disinfecting agents vary in their susceptibility to the inactivating effect of the various organic substances.[32] Experiments done under such conditions do not give a reliable picture of the characteristics and activity of the medicament/disinfectant against the tested microbe.

"Carry-over effect" means that the medicament, in active form, follows along with the sample into the dilution series and even to the culture plate (or liquid culture), where surviving microbes are calculated [e.g., "percentage of colony forming units (CFU) surviving"]. A high enough concentration of the disinfectant, in such a situation, can cause a false-negative result: the microbes are not killed, but residual medicament in the culture media prevents their growth by a bacteriostatic effect. Thus, carry-over, if undetected, gives a too positive picture of the antibacterial effectiveness of the medicament. Endodontic irrigants and disinfecting agents, containing local antibiotics, are at particularly high risk of causing false-negative results. Effective inactivators are not available for many antibiotics. If they are used in high concentration, carry-over effect is possible even after several 10-fold dilutions.[32]

Various inactivating agents are used to prevent the effects of carry-over. Citric acid has been used in the root canal to neutralize $Ca(OH)_2$, sodium thiosulfate neutralizes NaOCl,[33] and a mixture of Tween 80 and alpha-lecithin inactivates chlorhexidine (CHX).[34] Inactivation, however, is dependent on the concentration of the medicaments. When they are used in high concentration, inactivation may not be complete. A good example of this is CHX that cannot be effectively inactivated with Tween and alpha-lecithin if CHX concentrations of 1% or more are used (Figure 2A). The importance of the careful design of the experiments and proper controls cannot be overestimated, in order to avoid the possibility of false negative results.

Ex Vivo and In Vivo Models

In vitro models give valuable information about the spectrum and antimicrobial potential of endodontic disinfecting agents. However, information from such experiments alone is not enough to predict their performance in a clinical situation in the root canal. The effectiveness of the medicament in vivo can be reduced by a variety of factors. These include problems in delivery, low

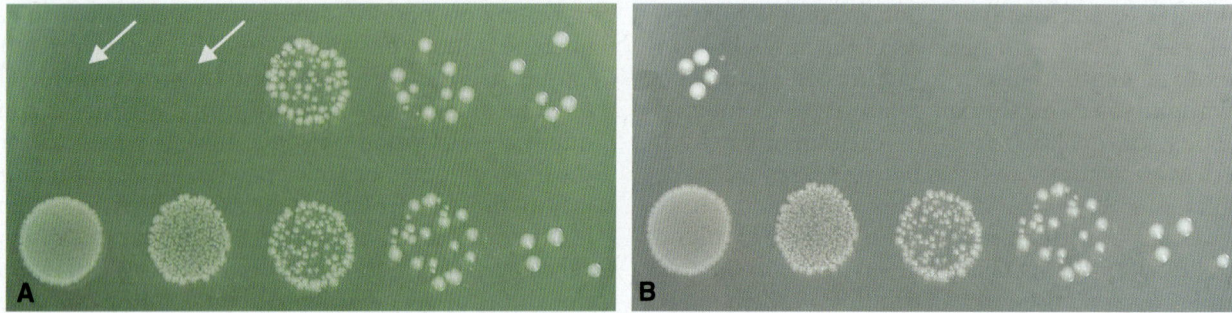

Figure 2 *A,* Samples of *Enterococcus faecalis* from 10-fold dilution series after a brief contact with 2% chlorhexidine. Because of short contact time (2 seconds), no killing has taken place. Chlorhexidine (CHX) "carry-over" has prevented growth of the first two samples (arrows) on the plate (upper row, left) despite the presence of Tween-lecithin inactivator in the dilution series. Lower row: control sample with no CHX. If only the first two dilutions had been made, the result would have indicated complete killing of the microbes in just 2 seconds. *B,* The size of the initial inoculum and the length of the dilution series determine the depth of measurement of the colony forming units. In this example, killing effectiveness can by calculated to a level of about 99.99%. Upper row: medicament; lower row: control.

overall volume, poor/incomplete penetration in the main root canal system, poor penetration into dentin, short contact time, or inactivation of the activity of the disinfecting agent by one or more of the chemical compounds present in the necrotic root canal. Therefore, a number of ex vivo and in vivo models have been developed in order to meet the challenge by the various confounding factors of the root canal and to improve the correlation between the test results and clinical performance. The ex vivo and in vivo models include the dentin block model,[35,36] dentin powder model,[37–39] and several modifications using roots/root canals from extracted teeth.[40,41] More studies are also made in vivo during the treatment of endodontic infections.[42,43]

The dentin powder model, with its modifications, makes it possible to obtain information about the inhibition of the medicament activity by dentin and other compounds (biomolecules, microbial biomass, etc.) in various concentrations.[37] It also allows standardization of the experimental conditions for large series of tests. Prolonged incubation time to create dentin infection is not required because the dentin is powdered. The downsides of the powder model include partial loss of the microanatomical structure of the tooth and the difficulty to use/create microbial biofilms. In short, the dentin powder model is an effort to simulate the chemical environment of the tooth.

The dentin block model has been widely used for testing endodontic medicaments.[35] The benefits of the model include simulation of the chemical and microanatomical environment of the tooth and the root canal system. The root canal is usually standardized in size, making it easier to obtain comparable samples of dentin in different blocks. It also allows the use of microbial biofilms in the experiments. On the other hand, the dentin block model is quite laborious in use; it cannot be fully standardized as different blocks may vary in thickness and dentin microstructure. Handling of the block presents some challenges which may increase the risk for false-positive results (contaminations from outside the sampling area). Despite its limitations, the dentin block model has greatly contributed to our understanding of dentin disinfection, and it is still frequently used in endodontic research.

Newer ex vivo and in vivo models use "natural" root canals either in extracted teeth or directly in vivo. The obvious benefit of these experiments is the more complete simulation of the clinical situation; the results obtained with the various materials may best reflect their true activity clinically. However, in addition to the well-known difficulty to organize controlled clinical studies, and to gather patients for such studies, there are also other potential pitfalls that may weaken the usefulness of the results. These include the difficulty to standardize the size of the apical preparation because of the great natural variation in canal sizes, different total volume of the canals, variations in the microanatomy of the root canals, and differences in the quality and quantity of the microbial infection. In addition to this kind of natural variation, there does not seem to be any standard way of dealing with the smear layer or taking the microbiological samples. According to the treatment protocols, the smear layer has not been removed in a great number of the studies. This is likely to have an effect on the ability of several sampling methods to collect viable microorganisms left in the dentinal tubules or lateral canals behind the smear layer. In quantitative studies where dentin is sampled, it is difficult to collect equal amounts of dentin (sample) because of the natural variations in canal sizes and shapes and different types of instruments used.

QUALITATIVE OR QUANTITATIVE RESULTS; DETECTION LEVEL: MORE CHALLENGES?

Optimally, the goal of endodontic disinfection is complete eradication of the microbes from the root canal system of the affected tooth. Although difficult to achieve, this noble goal may have affected the study design of several studies as the results are often expressed qualitatively, only as "growth" or "no growth." This approach may in some cases hide differences in the effectiveness of different treatment protocols and chemicals used for disinfection. For example, two different treatments that cause 10% and 99.95% reduction in bacterial counts per canal, respectively, are reported as equal ("growth"), unless the overall number of "no growth" cases is higher with one of the methods. It is possible that some of the recent poor results with $Ca(OH)_2$ as a disinfecting agent can be partly explained by the fact that qualitative rather than quantitative approach has been used to measure the effectiveness of the disinfection. Quantitative measurement of the effect by endodontic disinfecting agents should therefore be preferred over qualitative approach. Accordingly, quantitative reporting has been used in some studies.[32,44]

However, there are a number of factors that create challenges for accurate and comparable counting of microbes in the samples. Residual medicament in dentin may result in a very low number of CFU per sample unless neutralizing agents are properly used. Dispersing the sample effectively may be required to detach the viable cells from the dentin chips, to increase the CFU numbers to correctly reflect the true number of microbes in the sample. Collection of small dentin samples is technically demanding and requires great care to secure a standardized yield from all samples. When the overall number of CFU in the sample is low, which is often the situation in infected and medicated dentin, it is also important not to lose the microbes during too vigorous dilution process.

Success in both qualitative and quantitative measurement of (surviving) microbes is dependent, among other factors mentioned above, on the design of the microbiological procedures that determine the detection level of the method. Detection level dictates whether the most effective killing can be announced, for example, on the level of 99%, 99.9% or 99.99% (see Figure 2B). In other words, detection level tells how many cells in the test mixture must be alive so that growth can be detected by the culturing. Detection level is mainly dependent on the total number of cells in the initial reaction mixture/sample, proportion of the initial sample transferred into the dilution series, and the proportion of the mixture plated from each dilution. Theoretically, the detection limit can be easily calculated from the above numbers. In practice, detection limit is often reduced by carry-over of strong medicaments such as CHX or MTAD that may cause false-negative results at the beginning of the dilution series. Detection limit gives important information about the design and quality of the methods in studies of endodontic disinfecting agents. Unfortunately, detection limits are only rarely reported, making it more difficult to compare the results from different studies. One would hope that in the future, reporting the detection limit will be a routine requirement for studies on endodontic disinfection.

ANTIBACTERIAL IRRIGATING SOLUTIONS

The use of irrigating solutions is an important part of endodontic treatment. The irrigants facilitate removal of necrotic tissue, microorganisms and dentin chips from the root canal by a flushing action. Irrigants can also help prevent packing infected hard and soft tissue apically in the root canal and into the periapical area. Some irrigating solutions dissolve either organic or inorganic tissue. Finally, several irrigating solutions exhibit antimicrobial activity by actively killing bacteria and yeasts when in direct contact with the microorganisms. On the negative side, many irrigating solutions have shown cytotoxic activity and may cause severe pain reaction if they gain access into the periapical tissues.[45]

An optimal irrigant should have all or most of the positive characteristics listed above, but none of the negative or harmful properties. Presently, none of the available irrigating solutions can be regarded as optimal. However, with a combined use of selected products, irrigation will greatly contribute to successful outcome of treatment.

NaOCl

NaOCl is the most widely used irrigating solution. In water, NaOCl ionizes to produce Na^+ and the hypochlorite ion, OCl^-, that establishes an equilibrium with hypochlorous acid, HOCl. Between pH 4 and 7,

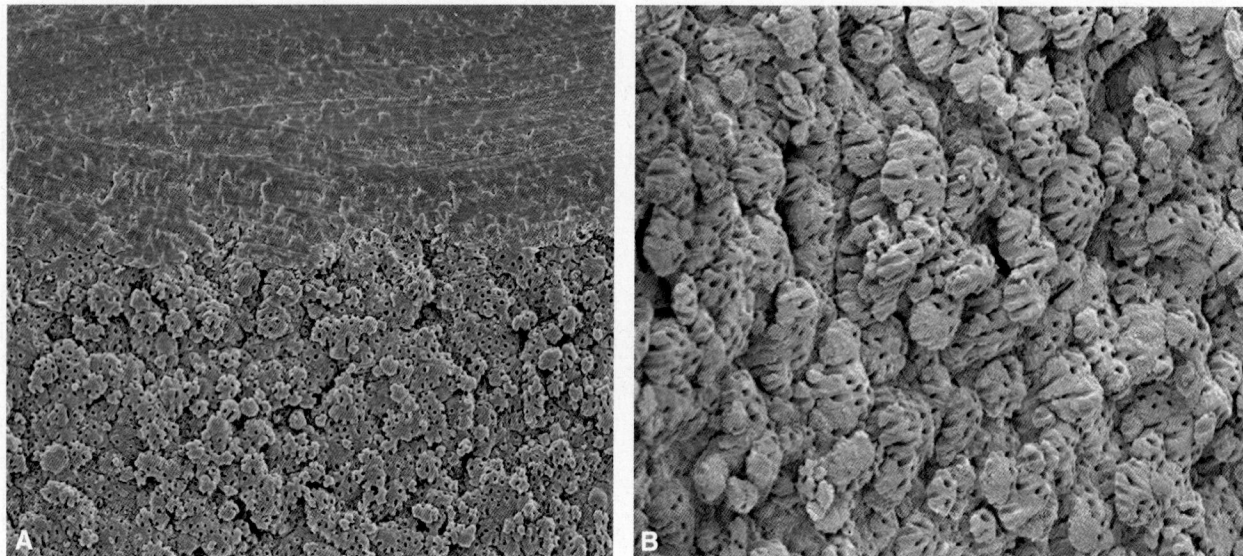

Figure 3 ***A***, Instrumented (upper part of the picture) and uninstrumented (lower part) root canal wall after irrigation with 5% sodium hypochlorite (NaOCl) for 10 minutes. Pulpal remnants and predentin have been effectively removed with NaOCl while the instrumented part (smear layer) seems relatively unaffected. Notice the typical calcospherites at the lower part of the image. ***B***, Calcospherites on the uninstrumented canal wall after irrigation for 10 minutes with 2.6% NaOCl.

chlorine exists predominantly as HClO, the active moiety, whereas above pH 9, OCl⁻ predominates.[46] It is the hypochlorous acid that is responsible for bacteria inactivation, the OCl⁻ ion being less effective than the undisassociated HOCl. Hypochlorous acid disrupts oxidative phosphorylation and other membrane-associated activities as well as DNA synthesis.[47,48]

NaOCl is used in concentrations varying from 0.5 to 7%. It is a very potent antimicrobial agent and effectively dissolves pulpal remnants and organic components of dentin (Figure 3). It is used both as an unbuffered solution at pH 11 in concentrations mentioned above and buffered with a bicarbonate buffer (pH 9.0) usually as a 0.5% (Dakin's solution) or 1% solution.[46] Contradicting earlier statements, Zehnder et al.[49] reported that buffering had little effect on tissue dissolution, and Dakin's solution was equally effective on decayed (necrotic) and fresh tissues. In addition, no differences were recorded for the antibacterial properties of Dakin's solution with an equivalent unbuffered hypochlorite solution.[49]

NaOCl is best known for its strong antibacterial activity; it kills bacteria very rapidly even at low concentrations. Waltimo et al.[50] showed that the resistant microorganism, *Candida albicans*, was killed in vitro in 30 seconds by both 5% and 0.5% NaOCl, whereas concentrations 0.05% and 0.005% were too weak to kill the yeast even after 24 hours of incubation. The high susceptibility of *C. albicans* to NaOCl was recently also verified by Radcliffe et al.[33] Later, Vianna et al.[51] contrasted these results partly, as 0.5% NaOCl required 30 minutes to kill *C. albicans*, whereas 5.25% solution killed all yeast cells in 15 seconds. In the latter study, however, organic material from the broth culture medium may have been present during the incubation with NaOCl which would explain delayed killing. Gomes et al.[52] tested in vitro the effect of various concentrations of NaOCl against enterococcus. *Enterococcus faecalis* (Figure 4) was killed within 30 seconds by the 5.25% solution, while 10 and 30 minutes was required for killing all bacteria by 2.5 and 0.5% solutions, respectively. The higher resistance of *E. faecalis* to hypochlorite as compared with the yeast *C. albicans* was suggested also by Radcliffe et al.[33] However, both of these studies are in contrast to the results reported by Haapasalo et al.[37] who demonstrated rapid killing of *E. faecalis* by 0.3% NaOCl and by Portenier et al.[53] who were able to show rapid killing of *E. faecalis* strains in logarithmic and stationary growth phase by even 0.001% NaOCl.

Experiments with Gram-negative anaerobic rods *Porphyromonas gingivalis*, *Porphyromonas endodontalis*, and *Prevotella intermedia*, often isolated from apical periodontitis, demonstrated high susceptibility to

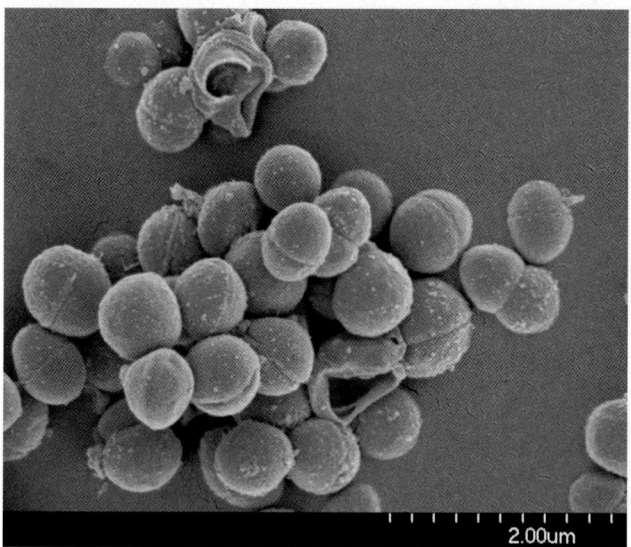

Figure 4 A scanning electron micrograph of growing *Enterococcus faecalis* cells.

NaOCl, and all three species were killed within 15 seconds with 0.5 to 5% concentrations of NaOCl.[51]

The differences between in vitro and in vivo studies include the volume of the medicament available for killing, access to all microbes, and absence of other materials in the in vitro experiments that potentially protect bacteria in vivo. Many of the in vivo studies have failed to show a better antibacterial effect in the root canal by high concentrations of NaOCl as compared to low concentrations. Byström and Sundqvist[54,55] studied root canals naturally infected, mainly with a mixture of anaerobic bacteria, and showed that although 0.5% NaOCl, with or without EDTA, improved the antibacterial efficiency of preparations compared with saline irrigation, all canals were not bacteria free even after several appointments. No significant difference in antibacterial efficiency in vivo between 0.5 and 5% NaOCl solutions was found in the study. Siqueira et al.[56] using *E. faecalis*-infected root canals demonstrated the superior antibacterial affect against root canal bacteria of hypochlorite in comparison with physiological saline. However, no difference was detected between 1, 2.5, and 5% NaOCl solutions.

Many of the studies about the antibacterial effect of NaOCl against root canal bacteria are in vitro studies, in either "neutral" test tube conditions, in the root canals of extracted teeth, or in dentin blocks infected with a pure culture of one organism at a time. The in vivo studies, on the other hand, have focused on the eradication of bacteria from the root canals of teeth with primary apical periodontitis.

Peciuliene et al.[57] studied the effect of instrumentation and NaOCl irrigation in failed, previously root-filled teeth with apical periodontitis. Old root fillings were removed with hand instruments, and the first sample was taken. No chloroform was used to avoid false-negative cultures. Bacteria were isolated in 33 of the 40 teeth before further instrumentation. *E. faecalis* was found in 21 teeth (in 11 as a pure culture), the yeast *C. albicans* in 6 teeth, Gram-negative enteric rods in 3 teeth, and other microbes in 17 teeth. The canals were then hand instrumented to size #40 or larger and irrigated with 2.5% NaOCl (10 mL per canal) and 17% buffered EDTA (pH 7 and 5 mL per canal). After instrumentation and irrigation, *E. faecalis* was still detected in six canals. Other microbes persisted in five canals after preparation. Enteric Gram-negative rods were no longer present in the second sample.

The disappearance of yeasts but not *E. faecalis* in the root canals may reflect their different susceptibilities to the described chemomechanical instrumentation or it may be a result of different biofilm characteristics and dentin penetration by these species.

The weaknesses of NaOCl include unpleasant taste, toxicity, and its inability to remove smear layer because of its lack of effect on inorganic material.[58,59] The poorer antimicrobial effectiveness of NaOCl in vivo than in vitro is also somewhat disappointing. There are several possible reasons for the reduced in vivo performance. Root canal anatomy, particularly the difficulty to effectively irrigate the most apical region of the canal, is generally acknowledged as one of the main challenges. In addition, the chemical milieu in the canal is different from a test tube. Haapasalo et al.[37] showed that the presence of dentin caused marked delays in the killing of *E. faecalis* by 1% NaOCl. The effect of other materials present in the necrotic or previously treated root canal, to the antimicrobial potential of NaOCl, has not been studied.

Studies measuring NaOCl cytotoxicity have indicated greater cytotoxicity and caustic effects on healthy tissue with 5.25% NaOCl than with 1.0 and 0.5% solutions.[60,61] The fear of toxic and chemical complications is the main reason for that low concentrations 0.5 to 1% NaOCl solutions are used for canal irrigation instead of the 5.25% solution in many countries.[45] However, more in vivo studies on persistent endodontic infections and retreatment are necessary for a deeper understanding of the relationship between NaOCl concentration and its antimicrobial activity against specific microorganisms, before final

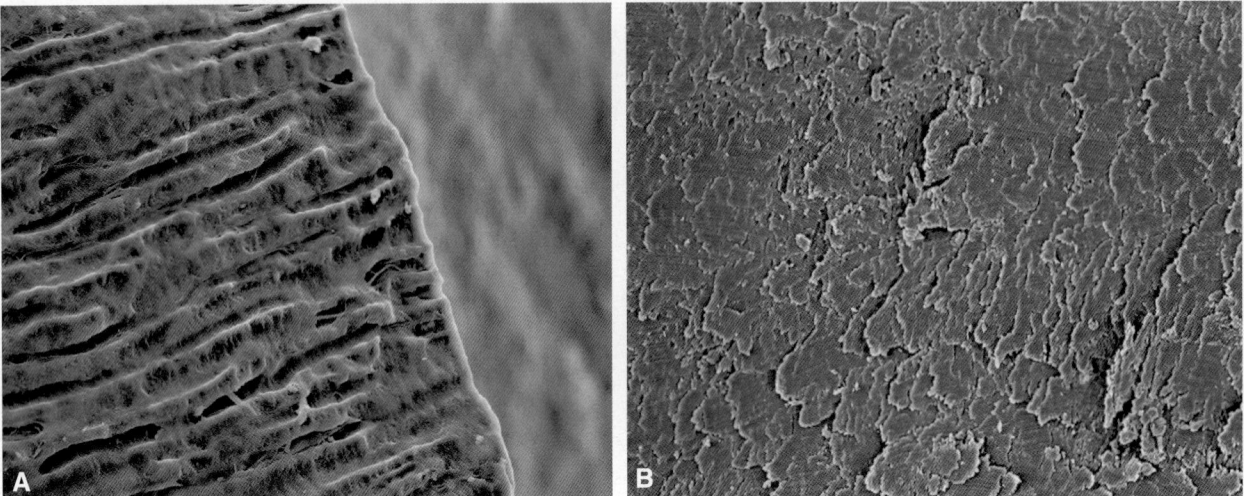

Figure 5 ***A***, Smear layer on the surface of the root canal wall after hand instrumentation with H-files. ***B***, Smear layer after instrumentation of the root canal before ethylenediamine-tetra-acetic acid irrigation.

conclusions can be drawn regarding the optimal NaOCl concentration.

EDTA, Citric Acid and Other Acids

EDTA (17%, disodium salt, pH 7) has little if any antibacterial activity. On direct exposure for extended time, EDTA releases some of the bacteria's surface proteins by combining with metal ions from the cell envelope. This can cause even bacterial death. More importantly, EDTA is an effective chelating agent in the root canal.[62,63] It removes smear layer (Figure 5) when used together (but not simultaneously) with NaOCl by acting on the inorganic component of the dentin (Figure 6). Therefore, by facilitating cleaning and removal of infected tissue, EDTA contributes to the elimination of bacteria in the root canal. It has also been shown that removal of the smear layer by EDTA (or citric acid) improves the antibacterial effect of locally used disinfecting agents in deeper layers of dentin.[35,36] Niu et al.[64] studied the ultrastructure on canal walls after EDTA and EDTA plus NaOCl irrigation by scanning electron microscopy (SEM): more debris was removed by irrigation with EDTA followed by NaOCl than with EDTA alone (Figure 7).

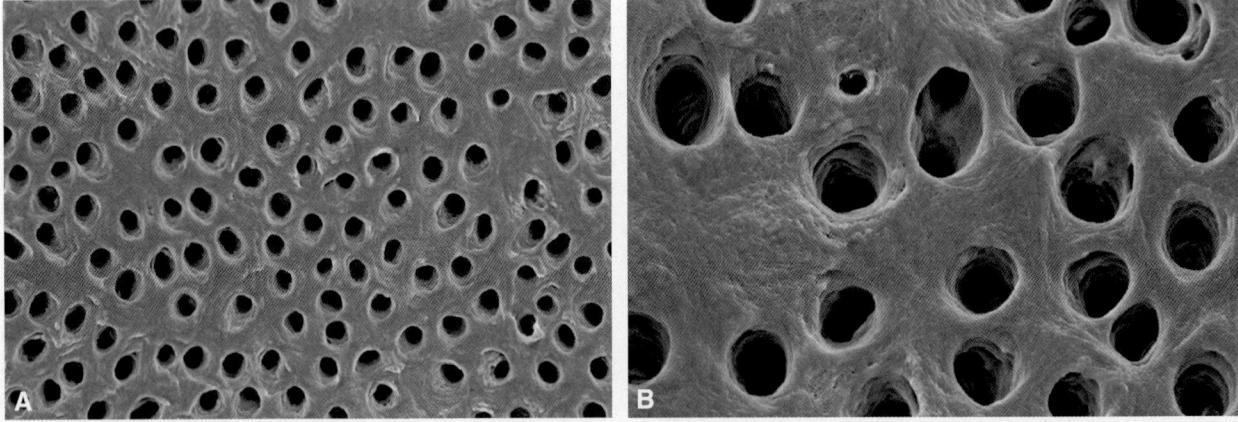

Figure 6 ***A***, Instrumented root canal wall after irrigation with 5% sodium hypochlorite (NaOCl) and 17% ethylenediamine-tetra-acetic acid (EDTA), each for 5 minutes. Smear layer has been completely removed. ***B***, Close-up scanning electron micrograph of the root canal wall after removal of smear layer with NaOCl and EDTA.

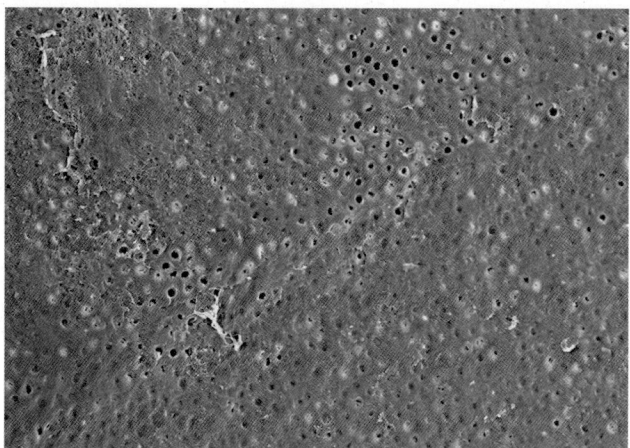

Figure 7 Partial removal of smear layer by irrigation for 10 minutes with 17% ethylenediamine-tetra-acetic acid only. Mainly organic material has been left covering the surface.

Citric acid can also be used for irrigation of the root canal and for removal of the smear layer.[62,65,66] Similar to EDTA, complete removal of smear layer requires also irrigation with NaOCl before or after citric acid irrigation (Figure 8). Concentrations ranging from 1 to 50% have been used.[65] In comparison with ultrasound, 10% citric acid has been shown to remove the smear layer more effectively from apical root-end cavities than ultrasound.[67] In another study, powdered dentin–resin mixture was more soluble in a 0.5, 1, and 2 M citric acid than in 0.5 M EDTA.[68] Contrary to this, Liolios et al.[69] reported better removal of smear layer by commercial EDTA preparations than with 50% citric acid, while other studies have found only small or no difference between citric acid and 15% EDTA in their capacity to remove the smear layer.[70,71] A comparative study showed that 10% citric acid was more effective than 1% citric acid, which was more effective than EDTA in demineralizing dentin.[72] Takeda et al.[73] reported that irrigation with 17% EDTA, 6% phosphoric acid, and 6% citric acid did not remove the entire smear layer from the root canal system. This is not unexpected, however, as it is known that NaOCl is also required for complete removal of the smear layer. The acids demineralized the intertubular dentin making the tubular openings larger than by EDTA. The authors also showed that CO_2 laser was useful in removing the smear layer and that the Er:YAG laser was even more effective than the CO_2 laser in smear layer removal.

Smear layer removal facilitates penetration of sealers into the dentinal tubules. It also enhances disinfection of the root canal wall and deeper layers of dentin. Both EDTA and citric acid can effectively remove the smear layer when used together with NaOCl. Citric acid and EDTA may have weak antimicrobial activity as stand-alone products. However, their antimicrobial effectiveness has not been extensively documented and appears to be of minor importance.

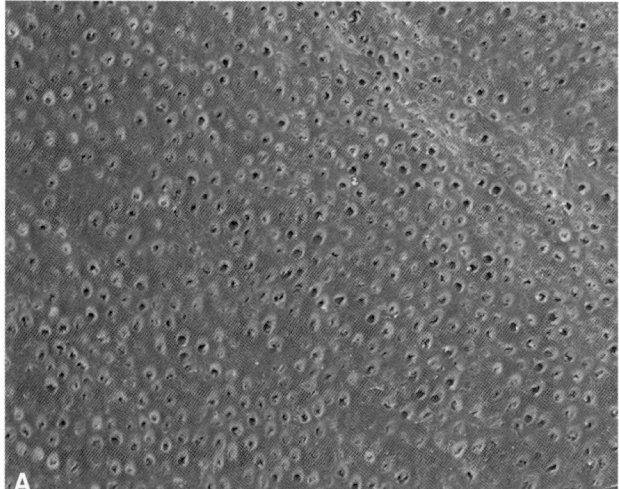
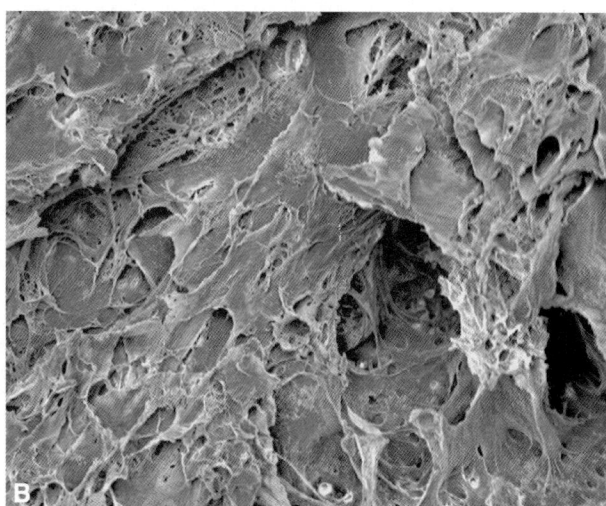

Figure 8 ***A***, Instrumented root canal wall after irrigation for 10 minutes with 50% citric acid only. Similar to ethylenediamine-tetra-acetic acid, sodium hypochlorite irrigation is needed in addition for complete removal of the smear layer. ***B***, Uninstrumented part of the root canal wall after irrigation for 10 minutes with 50% citric acid. Citric acid alone cannot dissolve the organic tissue within a reasonable time.

Hydrogen Peroxide

Hydrogen peroxide (H_2O_2) is a biocide that has been widely used for disinfection and sterilization.[46] However, in endodontics, H_2O_2 has not been very popular, and presently its use is generally in decline. H_2O_2 is a clear and colorless liquid. Concentrations from 1 to 30% have been used. H_2O_2 produces hydroxyl-free radicals ($HO^{\cdot}$) that attack microbial components such as proteins and DNA.[46] H_2O_2 is nonproblematic from an environmental point of view because it degrades into water and oxygen. H_2O_2 is relatively stable in solution, but many products contain stabilizers to prevent decomposition. H_2O_2 has antimicrobial activity against various microorganisms including viruses, bacteria, yeasts, and even bacterial spores.[74] It is more effective against Gram-positive than Gram-negative bacteria. Catalase or superoxide dismutase produced by several bacteria can provide them partial protection against H_2O_2.

Use of H_2O_2 in endodontics has been based on its antimicrobial and cleansing properties. Thirty percent H_2O_2 (Superoxol) has been recommended as the first step in tooth surface disinfection after mechanical cleaning.[75] H_2O_2 acts on the organic matter on the tooth making other disinfectants, such as iodine, more effective. It has been widely used earlier for cleaning the pulp chamber from blood and tissue remnants. It has also been used in canal irrigation, but evidence supporting the effectiveness of H_2O_2 as a root canal irrigant is scarce. On the contrary, Siqueira et al.[76] reported that a combination of NaOCl and H_2O_2 gave no advantage over NaOCl alone against E. faecalis in contaminated root canals ex vivo. Heling and Chandler[77] found strong synergism between H_2O_2 and Chlorhexidine (CHX) in disinfection of infected dentin: a combination of the two medicaments at low concentration was far more effective in sterilizing dentin than these or any other medicament alone. The synergistic mode of action between CHX and H_2O_2 was later documented also by Steinberg et al.[78] In a recent study, 10% H_2O_2 was used as part of the irrigating protocol in monkey teeth.[79] A total of 186 root canals in 176 teeth were inoculated with a known mixture of bacteria for several months. One group consisted of anaerobic bacteria and streptococci; the second group was identical to group one except with added E. faecalis. The root canals were sampled and instrumented manually to size #40 to #60 and irrigated with buffered 1% NaOCl, followed by 10% H_2O_2. Final irrigation was with NaOCl. Sodium thiosulpfate was used to inactivate hypochlorite before sampling, and a second bacteriological sample was taken. In group 1 (160 canals), bacteria were found in 98% and 68% of the canals in samples 1 and 2, respectively. In group 2, with E. faecalis, the corresponding frequencies were 100% and 88%. Although the bacterial counts were greatly reduced, the study indicated the difficulty to completely eradicate bacteria from infected root canals in monkey teeth.[79]

Despite the long history of use of H_2O_2 in endodontics, evidence supporting its use is at best weak. However, it still has a role as part of the tooth surface disinfection protocol. Furthermore, the potential benefit of the suggested synergistic effect with CHX in deep dentin disinfection remains to be evaluated clinically.

CHX

Chlorhexidine digluconate (CHX) is widely used in disinfection because of its excellent antimicrobial activity.[80–82] It has gained increased popularity in endodontics as an irrigating solution and as an intracanal medicament. Unlike NaOCl, CHX does not have bad smell, it is not equally irritating to periapical tissues, and neither does it cause dramatic spot bleaching of the patients clothes. Its antimicrobial effectiveness is well documented in endodontics. However, it completely lacks tissue dissolving capability, an important reason for the popularity of NaOCl (Figure 9).

CHX is perhaps the most widely used antimicrobial agent in antiseptic products. It permeates the cell wall or outer membrane (Gram-negative cells) and attacks the bacterial cytoplasmic or inner membrane of the yeast plasma membrane. In high concentrations, CHX causes coagulation of intracellular components.[46] CHX gluconate has been in use for some time in dentistry because of its antimicrobial properties, its substantivity (long-term continued effect), and its relatively low toxicity compared to some other agents. However, the activity of CHX is dependent on the pH and is greatly reduced also in the presence of organic matter.[82]

CHX is effective against both Gram-positive and Gram-negative bacteria as well as yeasts, although activity against Gram-negative bacteria is not as good as against Gram-positive bacteria.[83–85] Mycobacteria and bacterial spores are resistant to CHX.[80,81] Therefore, CHX is not as suited to chairside sterilization of gutta-percha cones as NaOCl.[86,87] Studies indicating equally good performance by CHX and NaOCl in gutta-percha disinfection have not used bacterial spores in testing.[88] CHX is not very effective against viruses, its activity being limited to viruses with a lipid envelope.[89] CHX is cytotoxic in direct contact with

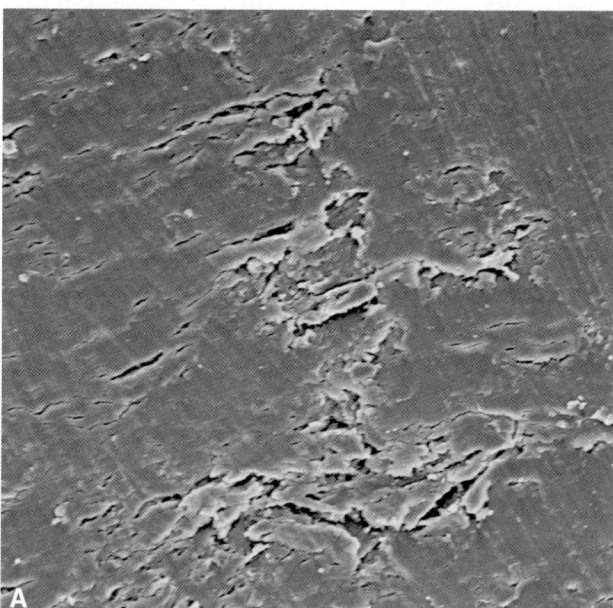 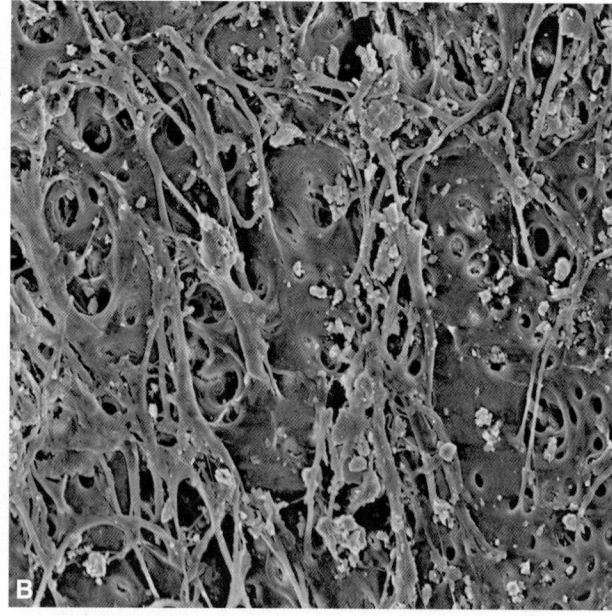

Figure 9 ***A,*** Instrumentation smear layer seems intact after irrigation for 10 minutes with 2% chlorhexidine. ***B,*** Uninstrumented area in the root canal after irrigation with 2% chlorhexidine only. Chlorhexidine has no tissue dissolving capability.

human cells. A study using fluorescence assay on human periodontal ligament (PDL) cells showed no difference in cytotoxicity by 0.4% NaOCl and 0.1% CHX.[61] The potential benefits of using CHX in endodontics have been under active research over the last several years. Several studies have compared the antibacterial effect of NaOCl and CHX against intracanal infection.

While many studies show little or no difference between their antimicrobial effectiveness,[77,90–92] their mode of action may indicate important differences. The effects of 15 minutes of irrigation of experimental biofilms by mixtures of endodontic bacteria on dentin blocks have been evaluated by SEM and by culturing.[93] Six percent NaOCl was the only irrigant that completely eliminated (removed) the biofilm as verified by SEM observations and killed all bacteria. Two percent CHX was equally effective in bacterial killing, and no growth was detected in any of the samples after the CHX treatment. However, an important difference was observed in how the biofilm was structurally affected by irrigation with these two solutions: 6% hypochlorite completely removed the biofilm while the CHX solution had no effect on the biofilm structure.[93] Although the bacteria were killed, the result indicates that as the biofilm remains in the canal after CHX irrigation, it may continue to express its antigenic potential if allowed the possibility to communicate with living periapical tissue. Moreover, such residual organic tissue may have a negative impact on the quality of the seal of the permanent root filling. Different types of biofilm are shown in Figure 10.

Some studies have indicated differences in the killing of certain endodontic microbes by hypochlorite and CHX. An in vitro study demonstrated differences in the killing of enterococci by CHX and NaOCl. While 5.25% NaOCl killed *E. faecalis* within 30 seconds, lower concentration (4.0 to 0.5%) of hypochlorite required 5 to 30 minutes for complete killing of the bacteria.[52] In the same study, 0.2 to 2% CHX killed the *E. faecalis* cells in 30 seconds or less in all concentrations tested. The result was later supported by two other studies using *E. faecalis* and *Staphylococcus aureus* as test organisms.[51,94] However, the results of these studies have been contradicted by some other studies with regard to the effectiveness of NaOCl.[37,53]

The antifungal effectiveness of CHX has been shown in several studies.[50,95–97] In a study of the effectiveness of various endodontic disinfecting agents, it was found that combinations of disinfectants were equally or less effective against fungi than the more effective component alone.[50]

An interesting, but not yet fully understood synergism has been reported between CHX and H_2O_2.[77] In

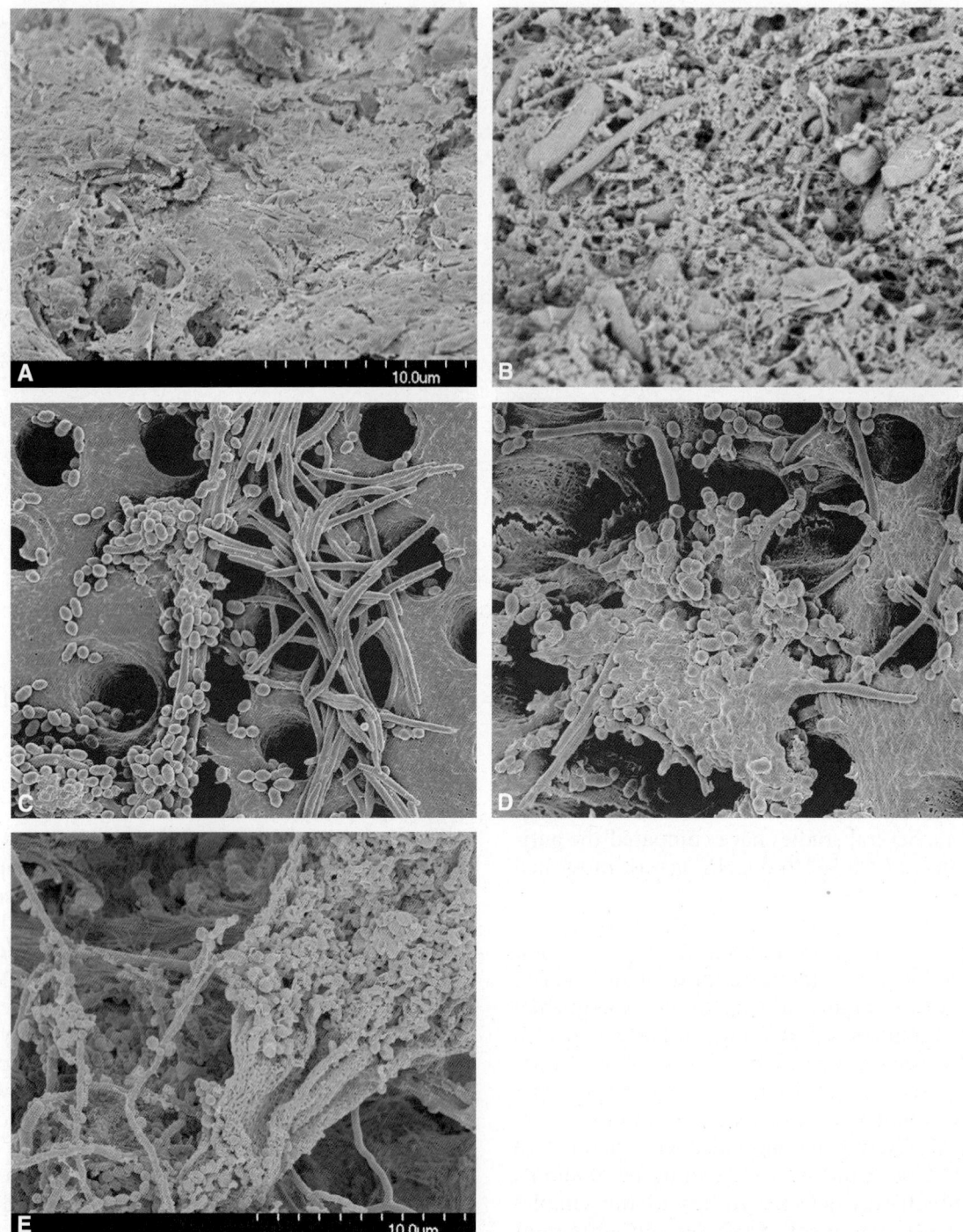

Figure 10 *A,* Densely packed natural biofilm (in vivo) on the root canal wall of a tooth with apical periodontitis. The film consists of bacteria of different types and shapes and remnants of necrotic pulp tissue. *B,* Cocci and rod-shaped bacteria in necrotic pulp tissue of a tooth with apical periodontitis. *C,* Early stages of biofilm formation in vitro on root dentin by a mixture of oral bacteria. Binding of coccoid cells on long rod-shaped bacteria can be seen. *D,* More advanced stage of biofilm formation in vitro on root dentin by a mixture of oral bacteria. Many of the bacterial cells in the larger aggregate are embedded in extracellular matrix. *E,* Biofilm by a mixture of oral bacteria grown under increased CO_2 atmosphere *in vitro* on root dentin.

vitro studies using the dentin block model indicated strong synergism between these two agents against *E. faecalis* infection in dentinal tubules. Complementary in vitro experiments by Steinberg et al.[78] demonstrated that the combination of CHX and H_2O_2 completely eradicated *E. faecalis* in concentrations clearly lower than required when the compounds were used alone. It is possible that CHX, as a membrane active agent, makes the bacterial membranes more permeable to H_2O_2, that can more easily penetrate the cells and cause damage to the intracellular organelles.[78] Although NaOCl and H_2O_2 are occasionally used together in root canal irrigation, such synergistic effect has not been detected between them in the dentin block model.[77] The CHX–H_2O_2 synergism has been demonstrated also in a study of antiplaque mouth rinse.[98] Surprisingly, so far there are no published studies of the clinical performance of the combinations of CHX and H_2O_2. Combinations of CHX and carbamide peroxide have been shown to be additive in their cytotoxicity,[99] but corresponding experiments with CHX and H_2O_2 are lacking.

Inhibition of the antimicrobial activity of endodontic irrigants, by substances present in the root canal, has recently been discussed in a number of studies.[37–39] Haapasalo et al.[37] showed in an in vitro study that the effect of CHX is reduced or delayed, by the presence of dentin. In following studies by the same group, Portenier et al.[38] detected loss of CHX antimicrobial activity by high concentration (18%, v/w) of bovine serum albumin. In a clinical situation, inflammatory exudate rich in proteins may thus have a negative impact on the effectiveness of CHX. A subsequent study showed that organic dentin matrix and heat-killed microbial cells were effective inhibitors of CHX activity.[39] In a study by Sassone et al.,[100] CHX was incubated together with low concentration (0.5%, v/w) albumin, and no inhibition of the CHX activity could be detected. Albumin concentration in human serum is approximately 2 to 3% and the total protein concentration is approximately 7%.[101]

During the last few years, several studies have measured the activity of CHX gel against root canal bacteria. Vianna et al.[51] found that CHX in a gel form required a longer time to kill *E. faecalis* than the corresponding concentration in a liquid. Oliveira et al.[102] reported that 2% CHX gel and 5.25% NaOCl showed excellent activity against *E. faecalis*. When diluted to 1.5% solution, NaOCl reduced the *E. faecalis* counts initially, but the bacterial counts increased during the 7-day follow-up period to the level comparable to the control group.

Because CHX lacks the tissue dissolving activity of NaOCl, there have been efforts to simplify the clinical work by combining the two solutions to obtain combined benefits from both. However, CHX and NaOCl are not soluble in each other and a brownish-orange precipitate is formed (Figure 11). Although the antimicrobial and other characteristics of the precipitate and the liquid phase have not been thoroughly examined, the precipitate prevents clinical use of the mixture. Marchesan et al.[103] showed that the precipitate was soluble to 0.1 mol/L acetic acid, but the brown/orange color of the solution remained. Atomic absorption spectrophotometry indicated that the precipitate contained iron which may be the reason for the color.

Despite of some shortcomings, there is increasing evidence that CHX gluconate, as a 2% solution (liquid or gel), may offer a good alternative for root canal

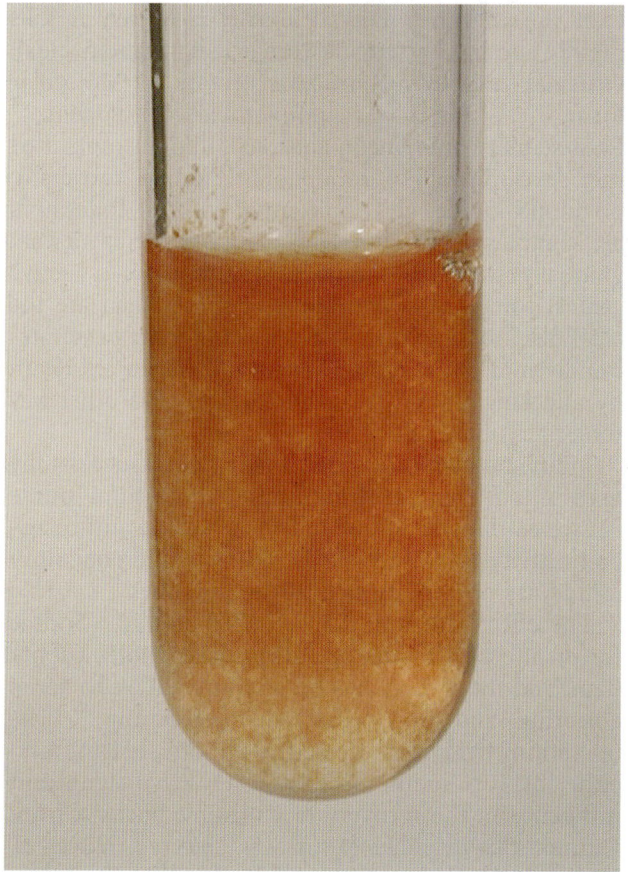

Figure 11 Mixing sodium hypochlorite with chlorhexidine causes a brown/orange precipitate. The color may be due to iron impurities in hypochlorite. The mixture should not be used for irrigation of the root canals.

irrigation. However, one should bear in mind that the majority of the research on the use of CHX in endodontics is done using in vitro and ex vivo models and Gram-positive test organisms, mostly E. faecalis. The possibility cannot be excluded that the experimental designs give a biased (too positive) picture of the usefulness of CHX as an antimicrobial agent in endodontics. More research is needed to identify the optimal irrigation regimen for various types of endodontic treatments. CHX is presently marketed as a water-based solution, as a gel (with Natrosol), and as a liquid mixture with surface active agents. Future studies of the various CHX preparations will establish the comparative effectiveness of the various CHX combinations in vivo.

Iodine Potassium Iodide (IPI)

Iodine compounds are among the oldest disinfectants still actively used. They are best known for their use on surfaces, skin, and operation fields. Iodine is less reactive than the chlorine in hypochlorite. However, it kills rapidly and has bactericidal, fungicidal, tuberculocidal, virucidal, and even sporicidal activity.[101] Molecular form, I_2, is the active antimicrobial component.[104] Poor stability of iodine in aqueous solutions motivated the development of iodophors ("iodine carriers"): povidone–iodine and poloxamer–iodine. Iodophors are complexes of iodine and a solubilizing agent that gradually releases the iodine.[104] Iodophors are less active against some yeasts and bacterial spores than are the alcoholic iodine solutions (tinctures). Iodine penetrates rapidly into the microorganisms and causes cell death by attacking the proteins, nucleotides, and other key molecules of the cell.[104,105]

Iodine potassium iodide (IPI) has been successfully used in tooth surface disinfection.[75] Potassium iodide is used to dissolve iodine in water, but the antimicrobial activity is carried by the iodine, while potassium iodide has no activity against the microbes.

The effectiveness of 2.5% NaOCl and 10% iodine for disinfection of the operation field (tooth, rubber dam, and the clamp) has been compared by bacterial culturing and polymerase chain reaction.[106] The operation field was treated with 30% H_2O_2 and either by 10% iodine or 2.5% NaOCl. No significant difference in the recovery of cultivable bacteria from various sites in either group was detected. However, bacterial DNA was detected significantly more frequently from the tooth surfaces after iodine treatment (45%) than after NaOCl (13%) treatment.[106]

Molander et al.[107] suggested that irrigation with 5% IPI before $Ca(OH)_2$ medication did not have an effect on the overall antimicrobial power. However, it is possible that IPI reduces the frequency of persisting strains of E. faecalis. Peciuliene et al.[57] studied the effect of iodine irrigation in 20 teeth with previously root-filled canals and apical periodontitis. The results showed that when used after normal chemomechanical preparation, IPI increased the number of culture negative canals.

In the root canal, iodine compounds come in contact with a variety of substances such as dentin and various proteins. Studies of the interaction of IPI with the chemical environment of the necrotic root canal have shown that dentin can reduce or even abolish the effect of 0.2/0.4% IPI against E. faecalis.[37,38] However, pure hydroxyl apatite or bovine serum albumin had little or no effect on the antibacterial activity of IPI. Portenier et al.[39] have shown that dentin matrix (mostly dentin collagen) and heat-killed cells of E. faecalis and C. albicans inhibit the antibacterial activity of IPI. These studies indicate that inactivation of iodine compounds is one factor explaining the difficulty in obtaining sterile root canals.

ANTIBIOTIC-CONTAINING IRRIGATION SOLUTIONS

MTAD and Tetraclean

MTAD [a mixture of tetracycline isomer, acid, and detergent (Biopure, Dentsply, Tulsa, OK)] is a new generation combination product for root canal irrigation.[105,106] Tetraclean (Ogna Laboratori Farmaceutici, Muggiò, Italy) is another combination product similar or close to MTAD.[108] MTAD has a low pH (2.15) because it contains citric acid, it removes smear layer after NaOCl irrigation, and it has antibacterial activity against endodontic microbes. The main potential benefits of MTAD are that it makes irrigation simpler by combining smear layer removal activity with antimicrobial effect and that it may be "gentler" with dentin than EDTA.[109] The authors who introduced MTAD have recommended the use of 1.3% NaOCl during instrumentation, followed by MTAD to remove the smear layer.[110] However, 1.3% NaOCl may not be strong enough to completely clean the uninstrumented parts of the root canal (Figure 12). Beltz et al.[111] found that MTAD solubilizes dentin, whereas organic pulp tissue is unaffected by it. Zhang et al.[112] showed that MTAD is less cytotoxic than eugenol, 3% H_2O_2, $Ca(OH)_2$ paste, 5.25% NaOCl and EDTA, but more cytotoxic than 2.63% NaOCl.

The antibacterial activity of MTAD is of particular interest as it contains doxycycline (tetracycline) in

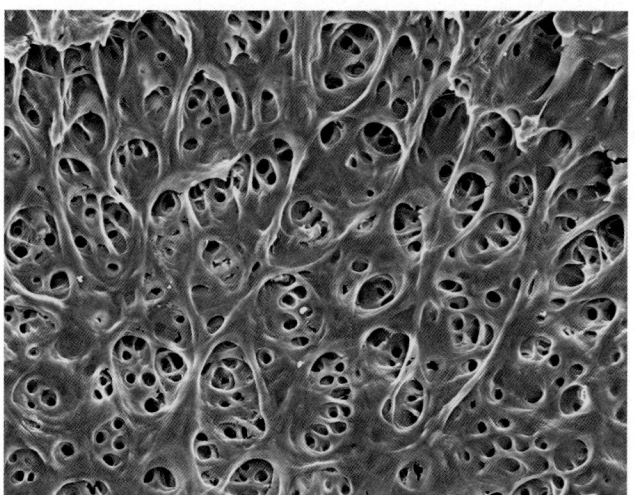

Figure 12 Uninstrumented root canal wall irrigated for 5 minutes with 1.3% sodium hypochlorite (NaOCl) followed by 5-minute irrigation with MTAD (a mixture of tetracycline isomer, acid, and detergent). Although this combination produces excellently clean canal walls in the instrumented areas (smear layer), the low concentration NaOCl may be too mild to thoroughly clean the uninstrumented areas if the irrigation time is not long enough. In this figure, some of the predentin is still left to cover the mineralized dentin and the calcospherites.

high concentration. Shabahang et al.[113] and Shabahang and Torabinejad[114] investigated the effect of MTAD on root canals contaminated with either whole saliva or *E. faecalis* of extracted human teeth and reported good antibacterial activity. Portenier et al.[32] showed that MTAD killed *E. faecalis* in vitro in less than 5 minutes. In an ex vivo study, Kho and Baumgartner[115] compared the antimicrobial effectiveness of NaOCl/EDTA and NaOCl/MTAD in extracted roots infected for 4 weeks with *E. faecalis*. After chemomechanical preparation and irrigation, the roots were pulverized in liquid nitrogen and viable bacteria were counted. No difference was measured between the two irrigation regimens. Another ex vivo study using roots of 26 matched pairs of teeth compared the same irrigation regimens with a different type of sampling procedure.[116] In this study, NaOCl/EDTA (5.25%/15%) irrigation resulted in 0/20 culture positive samples in both sample 1 (directly after irrigation) and sample 2 (after instrumenting the canals 2 instrument sizes wider) using a sensitive sampling protocol. However, in the other experimental group of 1.3% NaOCl/MTAD, the corresponding number of culture positive samples was 8 and 10 out of the total of 20 samples in each group. It should be noted that in the absence of negative control (e.g. water irrigation), it is not possible to know what may have been the reduction of bacterial CFU in the NaOCl/MTAD group. Nevertheless, the result indicates better performance by NaOCl/EDTA than by NaOCl/MTAD irrigation. The result is interesting because EDTA alone lacks antimicrobial activity against *E. faecalis*. The mechanisms of action of sequential use of NaOCl and EDTA on bacterial viability have not been thoroughly studied. There are no reports so far on the antibacterial effectiveness of Tetraclean.

The antibacterial effect of MTAD may be based not only on the antibiotic component (doxycycline) but also on the combined effect of doxycycline and the other ingredients (Tween 80, citric acid) on the integrity and stability of the microbial cell wall. However, there is no specific information available on such effects regarding MTAD.

Physical Means of Canal Cleaning and Disinfection

ULTRASONIC CLEANING

Endodontic ultrasound has become an important tool in modern endodontic work. Ultrasound is used in a variety of tasks including finishing access cavity preparation, removing pulp stones, locating canal orifices, opening calcified canals, fractured instrument removal, placing cements and root filling materials, and retro canal preparation during surgical procedures.[117] The use of ultrasonic energy for cleaning of the root canal and to facilitate disinfection has a long history in endodontics. The comparative effectiveness of ultrasonics and hand instrumentation techniques has been evaluated in a number of earlier studies.[117–121] The majority of these studies concluded that the ultrasonics, together with an irrigant, contributed to a better cleaning of the root canal system than irrigation and hand instrumentation alone. Cavitation and acoustic streaming of the irrigant contribute to the biological chemical activity for maximum effectiveness.[122] Analysis of the physical mechanisms of the hydrodynamic response of an oscillating ultrasonic file suggested that stable and transient cavitation of a file, steady streaming, and cavitation microstreaming all contribute to the cleaning of the root canal.[123]

Several different methods have been used to study the effect of ultrasound on the cleanliness of the canal. These include bacteriological, histological, and microscopic techniques.[124–128] Studies focusing on the ability of ultrasound to remove smear layer have shown contradictory results. This is not, in fact, surprising because it is generally known that smear layer can be removed primarily by chemical means only, or by appropriate laser treatment.[129,130] It has also been shown that to work effectively, ultrasonic files must be free in the canal without contact with the canal walls.[131]

Among the areas that are particularly difficult to clean are anastomoses between double canals, isthmuses and fins. Several studies have indicated the importance of ultrasonic preparation for optimal debridement of the root canals and isthmuses.[130,132–134] Ultrasonics also eliminated bacteria from canals more effectively than hand instrumentation.[134–136] However, not all studies have supported this finding.[137] It has been proposed that canal anatomy is more important than ultrasound for effectiveness of the cleaning procedures.[138]

The direct bactericidal effect by ultrasonic energy seems to be very limited at best.[139,140] Ultrasonics seems to exert its antimicrobial effect when used together with irrigants, perhaps via the physical mechanisms of cavitation and acoustic streaming. It is also possible that ultrasonics helps irrigants penetrate into areas, in complex canal systems, not easily reached by normal irrigation.

In a series of studies on the effect of canal shape (taper) and instrument design, Lee et al.[141] demonstrated in simulated plastic root canals that the diameter and taper of root canal influenced the effectiveness of ultrasonic irrigation to remove artificially placed dentin debris. After ultrasonic irrigation, the amount of debris in the #20/04 taper group was significantly higher than that for the size #20/06 group and the size #20/08 group. Van der Sluis et al.[142] using roots from human teeth ex vivo reported that there was a tendency for ultrasonic irrigation to be more effective in removing artificially placed dentin debris from simulated canal extensions from canals with greater tapers.

A study using a split tooth technique found that ultrasonic irrigation ex vivo was more effective than syringe irrigation in removing artificially created dentin debris placed in simulated uninstrumented extensions and irregularities in straight, wide root canals.[141] In another study, passive ultrasonic irrigation with 2% NaOCl was more effective in removing Ca(OH)$_2$ paste from artificial root canal grooves than syringe delivery of 2% NaOCl or water as an irrigant.[143]

Ultrasonic instrumentation can also have an impact on canal dimensions and in some cases can cause unwanted complications such as straightening of the canal (transportation), perforations, and extrusion of infectious material beyond the apex.[131,144–147] A histobacteriological study of teeth with non-vital pulps showed compacted debris and bacteria in the apical region and in the dentinal tubules after ultrasonic instrumentation.[148] In one study, the step preparation technique was shown to cause more extrusion than the standard technique, whereas the least extrusion was detected with the crown down and ultrasound techniques.[149] Interestingly, Van der Sluis et al.[142] suggested that a smooth wire during ultrasonic irrigation is as effective as a size 15 K-file in removal of artificially placed dentin debris in grooves in simulated root canals in resin blocks. It is possible that using an ultrasonic tip with a smooth, inactive surface, preparation complications are less likely to occur.

Recently, serious damage to paradental tissues was reported in a case where dental cement, used for cementing a post, was removed by ultrasound from a maxillary incisor.[150] After "several minutes" of ultrasound treatment, the patient complained of discomfort. During the following days and weeks, a large necrotic zone developed, affecting the bone and soft tissue around the tooth, resulting in the loss of the tooth. In controlled use, ultrasound together with irrigation, however, is not likely to cause harmful temperature rise.[151]

LASERS

Lasers in endodontics are dealt with in Chapter 26E, "Laser in Endodontics". However, their role in endodontic disinfection will be summarized briefly in the following sections. The potential of different endodontic lasers in eradicating root canal microbes has been a focus of interest for many years. Early comparative studies indicated, however, that the antibacterial effectiveness of lasers in the root canal was inferior to NaOCl irrigation.[152–154] Excellent antibacterial efficiency against *E. faecalis* was reported by Gutknecht et al.;[155] using a holmium:yttrium–aluminum–garnet (Ho:YAG) laser on root canals infected with this species in vitro, 99.98% of the bacteria were eliminated. However, Le Goff et al.[156] obtained only an 85% decrease in the bacterial counts by a CO_2 laser, clearly less than by irrigation with 3% NaOCl. Contrary to the main stream of results with laser treatment, Kesler et al.[157] indicated that complete sterility of the root canal can be obtained with a CO_2 laser microprobe coupled onto a special hand piece attached to the delivery fiber. Schoop et al.[158] in subsequent studies indicated that the effect of laser is dependent on the applied output power and specific for different bacteria. Complete sterility still seems to remain a challenge with laser treatment.[159,160] Another important aspect of laser radiation in endodontics is the effect of lasers on the smear layer, which may also facilitate effective disinfection of the canal.

New Developments in Root Canal Disinfection

Several new technologies have been introduced during the last few years to improve the effectiveness of root canal disinfection. Increasing attention has been focused on the use of ozone, photoactivated disinfection with low-energy laser, electrochemically activated water, and electric current.[161–165] In a comparative study, 3% NaOCl was more effective than electrochemically activated water in eradicating E. faecalis in an ex vivo model.[162] Nagayoshi et al.[164] reported relatively equal effectiveness in killing E. faecalis with ozonated water and 2.5% NaOCl, when the specimen was irrigated with sonication. However, NaOCl was superior to ozonated water in killing E. faecalis in broth culture and in biofilms.[166] Estrela et al.[167] studied root blocks infected for 60 days with a strain of E. faecalis and were unable to eradicate all bacteria with any of the methods used, including ozonated water, gaseous ozone, 2.5% NaOCl, and 2% CHX. Many of the new methods offer a biological approach to canal disinfection. However, available evidence so far has failed to show that these methods would be superior or sometimes even equal to existing ones with regard to their antimicrobial effectiveness in the infected root canal.

One of the latest new developments for canal disinfection are bioactive materials such as bio(active) glass.[168] In vitro studies have shown that bioglass has antimicrobial activity against a range of microbes and that this activity is, surprisingly, potentiated by dentin.[169,170] However, studies demonstrating better antimicrobial effect when compared to $Ca(OH)_2$ in vivo so far are lacking. Recent experiments with nanometric bioactive glass indicated excellent antimicrobial effect in a human dentin model.[171] More research will be needed to evaluate the value of bioglass in root canal disinfection.

Intracanal Interappointment Medicaments

In the treatment of teeth with a vital pulp, there is no need for intracanal medication. However, if time does not allow completion of the treatment in one appointment, it is generally recommended that the root canal should be filled between appointments with an antibacterial dressing, for example, $Ca(OH)_2$, to provide sterility in the canal space until a permanent root filling is placed. However, there are no studies comparing the bacteriological status of the root canals following pulpectomy, when the canals have been left empty or filled with an antibacterial dressing.

The question of the role of intracanal medicaments becomes more relevant, and complex, in the treatment of pulpal necrosis and apical periodontitis. There is overwhelming evidence in the literature that many if not most root canals contain viable microorganisms after the completion of the chemomechanical preparation at the end of the first appointment.[8–10,54,55,57,172–175] Therefore, a variety of intracanal medicaments have been used between appointments to complete disinfection of the root canal. In addition to killing bacteria, intracanal medicaments may have other beneficial functions. $Ca(OH)_2$ neutralizes the biological activity of bacterial lipopolysaccharide[176,177] and makes necrotic tissue more susceptible to the solubilizing action of NaOCl at the next appointment. Another aspect in using intracanal medicaments may be that a more thorough instrumentation is achieved because of the longer overall time used for the treatment. On the other hand, several appointments can also increase the risk for aseptic complications, for instance, through a leaking temporary filling and poor patient compliance.[178]

Several studies have indicated a poorer prognosis of the treatment of apical periodontitis if viable bacteria are residing in the root canal system at the time of filling.[5–7] Other studies, however, have contradicted these results and reported no significant differences in healing between teeth filled after positive or negative cultures from the root canal,[8] or between treatments performed in one or two appointments.[8,9] It has also been suggested that "intracanal sampling techniques suffer from deficiencies that limit their predictive value."[179] A permanent root filling of high quality using endodontic cements with antibacterial activity can effectively seal and entomb residual microorganisms in the canal and prevent communication with periradicular tissues. Continued killing of the microorganisms could take place due to the antibacterial activity of the root-filling materials[44,180] and unavailability of nutrients.

$Ca(OH)_2$

$Ca(OH)_2$ has a special position in endodontics. Indications for the use of $Ca(OH)_2$ in the prevention and treatment of various pulpal and periapical conditions have been numerous. In addition to endodontic infections, use of $Ca(OH)_2$ has been widely advocated in dental traumatology and in the treatment of resorptions. The classical studies in the 1970s and 1980s at the university of Umeå, Sweden, were a strong stimulus for the wide spread use of $Ca(OH)_2$ as a local disinfecting medicament in the root canal for the treatment of apical periodontitis. Byström et al.[6] reported that $Ca(OH)_2$ was an effective intracanal medicament, rendering 34 out of 35 canals bacteria free after a 4-week period. The effectiveness of interappointment $Ca(OH)_2$ was also reported by Sjögren et al.,[181] who demonstrated that a 7-day dressing with $Ca(OH)_2$ eliminated all bacteria in the root canal. However, these pioneer studies have been challenged by others who reported a residual flora in 7 to 35% of teeth after 1 or more weeks with $Ca(OH)_2$ in the canal.[21,182–184] Kvist et al.[185] reported the antimicrobial efficacy of endodontic procedures performed in a single visit (with 10-minute iodine irrigation), compared with a two-visit procedure, including an interappointment dressing with a $Ca(OH)_2$ paste. Residual microorganisms were detected in 29% of the one-visit teeth and in 36% of the two-visit-treated teeth, with no statistically significant differences between the groups.

Zerella et al.[42] compared the antibacterial activity of $Ca(OH)_2$ mixed either with water or with 2% CHX in vivo. Pure $Ca(OH)_2$ completely disinfected 12 out of 20 teeth, while the $Ca(OH)_2$–CHX paste disinfected 16 of 20 teeth. The difference, however, was not statistically significant because of small sample size. Siqueira et al.[186] examined bacterial reduction in teeth with apical periodontitis, after instrumentation and irrigation with 0.12% CHX solution and after 7 days of intracanal medicament with a $Ca(OH)_2$–CHX (0.12%) mixture. After finishing the chemomechanical preparation, 7 of the 13 cases still showed growth, while after the $Ca(OH)_2$–CHX treatment only one of 13 teeth was culture positive.

Vivacqua-Gomes et al.[40] examined the benefit of interappointment $Ca(OH)_2$ medicament in root canals in an ex vivo model. The premolar teeth were infected with E. faecalis for 60 days, and the canals were instrumented using rotary instruments. Irrigation, interappointment medication, and root filling were performed following five different protocols, either in single visit or in multiple visits. A second bacteriological sample was obtained 60 days after the root filling (the root fillings were removed and samples taken). Bacteria were found in 3 of 15 teeth (20%) irrigated with 2% CHX gel and filled in single visit and in 4 of 15 teeth (25%) irrigated with CHX and filled with $Ca(OH)_2$ for 14 days before the gutta-percha/sealer root filling was placed. Teeth that were left empty for 1 week after irrigation and before root filling, or irrigated with saline only instead of CHX, or filled without sealer showed bacteria in 40 to 100% of the teeth 60 days after the root filling was placed. Because of the small size of the experimental groups, far-reaching conclusions cannot be made. However, the result supports the finding of other studies indicating that interappointment $Ca(OH)_2$ may not add to the antibacterial effectiveness of the treatment. Moreover, the results emphasize the importance of not leaving the root canal empty (no medicament, no root filling) as well the role of sealer in the joined effort to combat infection.

CHLORHEXIDINE DIGLUCONATE

CHX is used as an irrigating solution during or at the end of instrumentation. However, CHX has also been used as an intracanal medicament between the appointments. Recently, interest has been focused on the effectiveness of CHX in gel form or as a mixture with $Ca(OH)_2$ as an intracanal interappointment dressing.[187,188] The information available is based mostly on in vitro and ex vivo experiments in which several intracanal medicaments have been compared for their activity against induced dentin infection. Siren et al.[188] using a bovine dentin block model reported that $Ca(OH)_2$ mixed with CHX was much more effective in disinfecting dentin infected with E. faecalis that pure $Ca(OH)_2$. Ercan et al.[187] reported 2% CHX gel was significantly more effective than $Ca(OH)_2$ combined with 2% CHX, or $Ca(OH)_2$ alone, against root dentin infected with E. faecalis and the yeast C. albicans after 7, 15, and 30 days of incubation. Similarly, it has been reported that 2% CHX gel alone completely inhibited the growth of E. faecalis after 1, 2, 7, and 15 days in the root canal whereas $Ca(OH)_2$ allowed some microbial growth at all experimental times.[41] Interestingly, in this study, the combination of the CHX gel and $Ca(OH)_2$ had killed all bacteria in the 1- and 2-day samples, but failed to secure sterility in the 7- and 15-day samples. The antibacterial efficacy of intracanal medication with $Ca(OH)_2$, 2% CHX gel, and a combination of both was assessed in a clinical study in teeth with chronic apical periodontitis.[43] Bacterial samples were taken before and 7 days after filling the canals temporarily with the medicaments. CHX and

Ca(OH)$_2$, alone as well as their mixture, all performed equally well, and no statistically significant differences could be detected in their antibacterial effectiveness.

OTHER ALTERNATIVES FOR INTERAPPOINTMENT MEDICAMENTS

Intracanal Medicaments Containing Antibiotics

Throughout the history of endodontics, there have been time periods with increased interest in the use of local antibiotics as temporary canal dressings for root canal disinfection.[189–196] Locally used antibiotics have not, however, become an established part of root canal disinfection and eradication of the infection. The reasons for the failure of antibiotics to overtake endodontic infection control are many. Many of the antibiotics tested are bacteriostatic, which may not be a good strategy for treating endodontic infections. Generally, bacteriostatic antibiotics prevent the growth of the microorganisms without killing them, giving the host defense a possibility to deal with the infection. In the necrotic root canal, however, there is no host defense because of the lack of the circulation. Therefore, the antibacterial effect of such antibiotics in the root canal may be only temporary. On the other hand, it is possible that some bacteriostatic antibiotics can have a bactericidal effect when used in high concentrations, usually the case with locally used antibiotics. However, information about this is scarce and presently there is no direct evidence of bacteriostatic antibiotics used in the root canal, although one study indicated that mixing erythromycin with Ca(OH)$_2$ improved the effectiveness against *E. faecalis* as compared to Ca(OH)$_2$ alone.[197]

With bactericidal antibiotics, the potential problem in the root canal may be the metabolic and physiological state of the microorganisms. Many bactericidal antibiotics are most effective when the microbial cells are in active growth phase, which may not be the case in the necrotic root canal with only limited nutrients available. In general, specific information about the effectiveness of intracanal antibiotics in infection control in endodontics is limited. Recently, an interesting new development has taken place with the use of antibiotic cocktails in the treatment of teeth with immature apex and apical periodontitis.[198,199] It is possible that better circulation and survival of some pulpal cells in the apical root canal are among the key factors for the promising results reported so far. Future research will show whether this approach can be extended to the treatment of teeth with closed apex and apical periodontitis.

Phenol Compounds.

Chemicals of the phenol group such as phenol, formocreosol, cresatin, parachlorophenol (monoparachlorophenol), camphorated phenol, and camphorated parachlorophenol have a long history in endodontics as locally used root canal disinfecting agents. They have been applied into the pulp chamber in a moist cotton pellet (vapor effect), or the whole canal has been filled with liquid with various concentrations of the phenol compound.[200–208] The rationale of using phenol compounds for root canal disinfection has its roots in their role as general disinfecting agents in the past. However, emphasis of safety in addition to effectiveness has resulted in dramatic decline in their use generally. Also in endodontics, concerns have been raised regarding the toxicity and possible mutagenicity of the disinfecting agents of the phenol group.[209–213] There are several demonstrations of their cytotoxicity,[209,214,215] however, recent studies indicate that the risk of genotoxicity by the various phenol compounds used in endodontics is small.[211–213] Comparative studies of the antimicrobial effectiveness of the phenol compounds have not been able to show superiority of the substances over the other. On the contrary,[200,203,205,208,209] Byström et al.[203] reported that Ca(OH)$_2$ was superior to camphorated parachlorophenol (CMCP) by its antibacterial potential when used for 4 weeks as the local intracanal medicament. Several studies have indicated relatively rapid loss of activity of CMCP in the canal, although the results show variation.[206,216] In the balance of the benefits and the demonstrated and potential weaknesses of phenol compounds, it can be predicted that they will be increasingly replaced by other, more biological disinfecting agents.

References

1. Spångberg LZ, Haapasalo M. Rationale and efficacy of root canal medicaments and filling materials with emphasis on treatment outcome. Endod Topics 2002;2:35–58.

2. Haapasalo M, Udnæs T, Endal U. Persistent, recurrent and acquired infection of the root canal system post-treatment. Endod Topics 2003;6:29–56.

3. Haapasalo M, Endal U, Zandi H, Coil J. Eradication of endodontic infection by instrumentation and irrigation solutions. Endod Topics 2005;10:72–102.

4. Sjögren U, Figdor D, Persson S, Sundqvist G. Influence of infection at the time of root filling on the outcome of

endodontic treatment of teeth with apical periodontitis. Int Endod J 1997;30:297–306.

5. Engström B. The significance of enterococci in root canal treatment. Odontol Revy 1964;15:87–106.

6. Byström A, Claesson R, Sundqvist G. The antibacterial effect of camphorated paramonochlorophenol, camphorated phenol and calcium hydroxide in the treatment of infected root canals. Endod Dent Traumatol 1985;1:170–5.

7. Katebzadeh N, Sigurdsson A, Trope M. Radiographic evaluation of periapical healing after obturation of infected root canals: an in vivo study. Int Endod J 2000;33:60–6.

8. Peters LB, Wesselink PR. Periapical healing of endodontically treated teeth in one and two visits obturated in the presence or absence of detectable microorganisms. Int Endod J 2002;35:660–7.

9. Weiger R, Rosendahl R, Löst C. Influence of calcium hydroxide intracanal dressings on the prognosis of teeth with endodontically induced periapical lesions. Int Endod J 2000;33:219–26.

10. Sathorn C, Parashos P, Messer H. Antibacterial efficacy of calcium hydroxide intracanal dressing: a systematic review and meta-analysis. Int Endod J 2007;40:2–10.

11. Kakehashi S, Stanley HR, Fitzgerald RJ. The effects of surgical exposures of dental pulps in germfree and conventional laboratory rats. J Southern Calif Dent Assoc 1966: 34: 449–51.

12. Bergenholtz G. Micro-organisms from necrotic pulp of traumatized teeth. Odontol Revy 1974;25:347–58.

13. Sundqvist G. Bacteriological studies of necrotic dental pulps. [Umeå University Odontological Dissertation No. 7]. Umeå, Sweden: University of Umeå; 1976.

14. Nair PN. On the causes of persistent apical periodontitis: a review. Int Endod J 2006;39:249–81.

15. Nair PN. Pathogenesis of apical periodontitis and the causes of endodontic failures. Crit Rev Oral Biol Med 2004 Nov 1;15:348–81.

16. Friedman S. Treatment outcome and prognosis of endodontic therapy. In: Ørstavik D, Pitt Ford TR, editors. Essential endodontics. Osney Mead, Oxford: Blackwell Science Ltd; 1998, pp. 367–91.

17. Shetty K, Garcia J, Leigh J. Success of root canal therapy in HIV-positive patients. Gen Dent 2006;54:397–402.

18. Taschieri S, Del Fabbro M, Testori T, et al. Endodontic surgery with ultrasonic retrotips: one-year follow-up. Oral Surg Oral Med Oral Pathol Oral Radiol Endod 2005;100:380–7.

19. Ørstavik D, Pitt Ford TR. Essential endodontology: prevention and treatment of apical periodontitis. Oxford: Blackwell Science; 1998.

20. Byström A, Sundqvist G. Bacteriologic evaluation of the efficacy of mechanical root canal instrumentation in endodontic therapy. Scand J Dent Res 1981;89:321–8.

21. Ørstavik D, Kerekes K, Molven O. Effects of extensive apical reaming and calcium hydroxide dressing on bacterial infection during treatment of apical periodontitis: a pilot study. Int Endod J 1991;24:1–7.

22. Cvek M, Nord CE, Hollender L. Antimicrobial effect of root canal debridement in teeth with immature root. A clinical and microbiologic study. Odontol Revy 1976;27:1–10.

23. Dalton BC, Ørstavik D, Phillips C, et al. Bacterial reduction with nickel-titanium rotary instrumentation. J Endod 1998;24:763–7.

24. Siqueira JF Jr, Lima KC, Magalhaes FA, et al. Mechanical reduction of the bacterial population in the root canal by three instrumentation techniques. J Endod 1999;25:332–5.

25. Pataky L, Ivanyi I, Grigar A, Fazekas A. Antimicrobial efficacy of various root canal preparation techniques: an in vitro comparative study. J Endod 2002;28:603–5.

26. Baquero F. European standards for antibiotic susceptibility testing: towards a theoretical consensus. Eur J Clin Microbiol Infect Dis 1990;9:492–5.

27. Kronvall G, Ringertz S. Antibiotic disk diffusion testing revisited. Single strain regression analysis. Review article. APMIS 1991;99:295–306.

28. Oakes AR, Badger R, Grove DI. Comparison of direct and standardized testing of infected urine for antimicrobial susceptibilities by disk diffusion. J Clin Microbiol 1994;32:40–5.

29. Dowzicky MJ, Nadler HL, Sheikh W. Comparison of sensititre broth microdilution and agar dilution susceptibility testing techniques for meropenem to determine accuracy, reproducibility, and predictive values. J Clin Microbiol 1994;32:2204–7.

30. Espinel-Ingroff A, Chaturvedi V, Fothergill A, Rinaldi MG. Optimal testing conditions for determining MICs and minimum fungicidal concentrations of new and established antifungal agents for uncommon molds: NCCLS collaborative study. J Clin Microbiol 2002;40(10):3776–81.

31. Dubreuil L, Houcke I, Singer E. Susceptibility testing of anaerobic bacteria: evaluation of the redesigned (Version 96) bioMerieux ATB ANA device. J Clin Microbiol 1999;37:1824–8.

32. Portenier I, Waltimo T, Ørstavik D, Haapasalo M. Killing of *Enterococcus faecalis* by MTAD and chlorhexidine digluconate with or without cetrimide in the presence or absence of dentine powder or BSA. J Endod 2006;32:138–41.

33. Radcliffe CE, Potouridou L, Qureshi R, et al. Antimicrobial activity of varying concentrations of sodium hypochlorite on the endodontic microorganisms Actinomyces israelii, A. naeslundii, Candida albicans and Enterococcus faecalis. Int Endod J 2004;37:438–46.

34. Zamany A, Spångberg LS. An effective method of inactivating chlorhexidine. Oral Surg Oral Med Oral Pathol Oral Radiol Endod 2002;93:617–20.

35. Haapasalo M, Ørstavik D. In vitro infection and disinfection of dentinal tubules. J Dent Res 1987;66:1375–9.
36. Ørstavik D, Haapasalo M. Disinfection by endodontic irrigants and dressings of experimentally infected dentinal tubules. Endod Dent Traumatol 1990;6:142–9.
37. Haapasalo HK, Siren EK, Waltimo TM, et al. Inactivation of local root canal medicaments by dentine: an *in vitro* study. Int Endod J 2000;33:126–31.
38. Portenier I, Haapasalo H, Rye A, et al. Inactivation of root canal medicaments by dentine, hydroxylapatite and bovine serum albumin. Int Endod J 2001;34:184–8.
39. Portenier I, Haapasalo H, Ørstavik D, et al. Inactivation of the antibacterial activity of iodine potassium iodide and chlorhexidine digluconate against *Enterococcus faecalis* by dentin, dentin matrix, type-I collagen, and heat-killed microbial whole cells. J Endod 2002;28:634–7.
40. Vivacqua-Gomes N, Gurgel-Filho ED, Gomes BP, et al. Recovery of *Enterococcus faecalis* after single- or multiple-visit root canal treatments carried out in infected teeth ex vivo. Int Endod J 2005;38:697–704.
41. Gomes BP, Souza SF, Ferraz CC, et al. Effectiveness of 2% chlorhexidine gel and calcium hydroxide against *Enterococcus faecalis* in bovine root dentine in vitro. Int Endod J 2003;36:267–75.
42. Zerella JA, Fouad AF, Spångberg LS. Effectiveness of a calcium hydroxide and chlorhexidine digluconate mixture as disinfectant during retreatment of failed endodontic cases. Oral Surg Oral Med Oral Pathol Oral Radiol Endod 2005;100:756–61.
43. Manzur A, Gonzalez AM, Pozos A, et al. Bacterial quantification in teeth with apical periodontitis related to instrumentation and different intracanal medications: a randomized clinical trial. J Endod 2007;33:114–18.
44. Saleh IM, Ruyter IE, Haapasalo M, Ørstavik D. Survival of *Enterococcus faecalis* in infected dentinal tubules after root canal filling with different root canal sealers in vitro. Int Endod J 2004;37:193–8.
45. Hulsmann M, Hahn W. Complications during root canal irrigation: literature review and case reports. Int Endod J 2000;33:186–93.
46. Mcdonnell G, Russell D. Antiseptics and disinfectants: activity, action, and resistance. Clin Microbiol Rev 1999;12:147–79.
47. Barrette WC Jr, Hannum DM, Wheeler WD, Hurst JK. General mechanism for the bacterial toxicity of hypochlorous acid: abolition of ATP production. Biochemistry 1989;28:9172–8.
48. McKenna SM, Davies KJA. The inhibition of bacterial growth by hypochlorous acid. Biochem J 1988;254:685–92.
49. Zehnder M, Kosicki D, Luder H, et al. Tissue-dissolving capacity and antibacterial effect of buffered and unbuffered hypochlorite solutions. Oral Surg Oral Med Oral Pathol Oral Radiol Endod 2002;94:756–62.
50. Waltimo TM, Ørstavik D, Siren EK, Haapasalo MP. *In vitro* susceptibility of Candida albicans to four disinfectants and their combinations. Int Endod J 1999;32:421–9.
51. Vianna ME, Gomes BP, Berber VB, et al. *In vitro* evaluation of the antimicrobial activity of chlorhexidine and sodium hypochlorite. Oral Surg Oral Med Oral Pathol Oral Radiol Endod 2004;97:79–84.
52. Gomes BP, Ferraz CC, Vianna ME, et al. *In vitro* antimicrobial activity of several concentrations of sodium hypochlorite and chlorhexidine gluconate in the elimination of *Enterococcus faecalis*. Int Endod J 2001;34:424–8.
53. Portenier I, Waltimo T, Ørstavik D, Haapasalo M. The susceptibility of starved, stationary phase, and growing cells of *Enterococcus faecalis* to endodontic medicaments. J Endod 2005;31:380–6.
54. Byström A, Sundqvist G. Bacteriologic evaluation of the effect of 0.5 percent sodium hypochlorite in endodontic therapy. Oral Surg Oral Med Oral Pathol Oral Radiol Endod 1983;55:307–12.
55. Byström A, Sundqvist G. The antibacterial action of sodium hypochlorite and EDTA in 60 cases of endodontic therapy. Int Endod J 1985;18: 35–40.
56. Siqueira JF Jr, Rocas IN, Santos SR, et al. Efficacy of instrumentation techniques and irrigation regimens in reducing the bacterial population within root canals. J Endod 2002;28:181–4.
57. Peciuliene V, Reynaud A, Balciuniene I, Haapasalo M. Isolation of yeasts and enteric bacteria in root-filled teeth with chronic apical periodontitis. Int Endod J 2001;34:429–34.
58. Spångberg L, Engström B, Langeland K. Biologic effects of dental materials. 3. Toxicity and antimicrobial effect of endodontic antiseptics in vitro. Oral Surg Oral Med Oral Pathol Oral Radiol Endod 1973;36:856–71.
59. McComb D, Smith DC, Beagrie GS. The results of in vivo endodontic chemomechanical instrumentation: a scanning electron microscopic study. J Br Endod Soc 1976;9:11–18.
60. Pashley EL, Birdsong NL, Bowman K, Pashley DH. Cytotoxic effects of NaOCl on vital tissue. J Endod 1985;11:525–8.
61. Chang YC, Huang FM, Tai KW, Chou MY. The effect of sodium hypochlorite and chlorhexidine on cultured human periodontal ligament cells. Oral Surg Oral Med Oral Pathol Oral Radiol Endod 2001;92:446–50.
62. Czonstkowsky M, Wilson EG, Holstein FA. The smear layer in endodontics. Dent Clin North Am 1990;34:13–25.
63. Baumgartner JC, Mader CL. A scanning electron microscopic evaluation of four root canal irrigation regimens. J Endod 1987;13:147–57.
64. Niu W, Yoshioka T, Kobayashi C, Suda H. A scanning electron microscopic study of dentinal erosion by final irrigation with EDTA and NaOCl solutions. Int Endod J 2002;35:934–9.

65. Loel DA. Use of acid cleanser in endodontic therapy. J Am Dent Assoc 1975;90:148–51.

66. Baumgartner JC, Brown CM, Mader CL, et al. A scanning electron microscopic evaluation of root canal debridement using saline, sodium hypochlorite, and citric acid. J Endod 1984;10:525–31.

67. Gutmann JL, Saunders WP, Nguyen L, et al. Ultrasonic root-end preparation. Part 1. SEM analysis. Int Endod J 1994;27:318–24.

68. Yamaguchi M, Yoshida K, Suzuki R, Nakamura H. Root canal irrigation with citric acid solution. J Endod 1996;22:27–9.

69. Liolios E, Economides N, Parissis-Messimeris S, Boutsioukis A. The effectiveness of three irrigating solutions on root canal cleaning after hand and mechanical preparation. Int Endod J 1997;30:51–7.

70. Di Lenarda R, Cadenaro M, Sbaizero O. Effectiveness of 1 mol L-1 citric acid and 15% EDTA irrigation on smear layer removal. Int Endod J 2000;33:46–52.

71. Scelza MF, Teixeira AM, Scelza P. Decalcifying effect of EDTA-T, 10% citric acid, and 17% EDTA on root canal dentin. Oral Surg Oral Med Oral Pathol Oral Radiol Endod 2003;95:234–6.

72. Machado-Silveiro LF, Gonzalez-Lopez S, Gonzalez-Rodriguez MP. Decalcification of root canal dentine by citric acid, EDTA and sodium citrate. Int Endod J 2004;37:365–9.

73. Takeda FH, Harashima T, Kimura Y, Matsumoto K. A comparative study of the removal of smear layer by three endodontic irrigants and two types of laser. Int Endod J 1999;32:32–9.

74. Block SS. Peroxygen compounds. In: Block SS, editor. Disinfection, sterilization, and preservation. 4th ed. Philadelphia, PA: Lea & Febiger; 1991, pp. 167–81.

75. Möller AJ. Microbiological examination of root canals and periapical tissues of human teeth Methodological studies (thesis). Odontol Tidskr 1966;74:1–380.

76. Siqueira JF Jr, Machado AG, Silveira RM, et al. Evaluation of the effectiveness of sodium hypochlorite used with three irrigation methods in the elimination of *Enterococcus faecalis* from the root canal, in vitro. Int Endod J 1997;30:279–82.

77. Heling I, Chandler NP. Antimicrobial effect of irrigant combinations within dentinal tubules. Int Endod J 1998;31:8–14.

78. Steinberg D, Heling I, Daniel I, Ginsburg I. Antibacterial synergistic effect of chlorhexidine and hydrogen peroxide against *Streptococcus sobrinus*, *Streptococcus faecalis* and *Staphylococcus aureus*. J Oral Rehabil 1999;26:151–6.

79. Möller AJ, Fabricius L, Dahlen G, et al. Apical periodontitis development and bacterial response to endodontic treatment. Experimental root canal infections in monkeys with selected bacterial strains. Eur J Oral Sci 2004;112:207–15.

80. Russell AD. Activity of biocides against mycobacteria. J Appl Bacteriol Symp 1996;81(Suppl):87S–101S.

81. Shaker LA, Dancer BN, Russell AD, Furr JR. Emergence and development of chlorhexidine resistance during sporulation of *Bacillus subtilis* 168. FEMS Microbiol Lett 1988;51:73–6.

82. Russell AD, Day MJ. Antibacterial activity of chlorhexidine. J Hosp Infect 1993;25:229–38.

83. Davies GE, Francis J, Martin AR, et al. 1:6-Di-4'-chlorophenyl-diguanidohexane (hibitane); laboratory investigation of a new antibacterial agent of high potency. Br J Pharmacol Chemother 1954;9:192–6.

84. Hennessey TS. Some antibacterial properties of chlorhexidine. J Periodontal Res Suppl 1973;12:61–7.

85. Emilson CG. Susceptibility of various microorganisms to chlorhexidine. Scand J Dent Res 1977;85:255–65.

86. Siqueira JF Jr, da Silva CH, Cerqueira M das D, et al. Effectiveness of four chemical solutions in eliminating *Bacillus subtilis* spores on gutta-percha cones. Endod Dent Traumatol 1998;14:124–6.

87. Gomes BP, Vianna ME, Matsumoto CU, et al. Disinfection of gutta-percha cones with chlorhexidine and sodium hypochlorite. Oral Surg Oral Med Oral Pathol Oral Radiol Endod 2005;100:512–17.

88. Royal MJ, Williamson AE, Drake DR. Comparison of 5.25% sodium hypochlorite, MTAD, and 2% chlorhexidine in the rapid disinfection of polycaprolactone-based root canal filling material. J Endod. 2007;33:42–4.

89. Park JB, Park NH. Effect of chlorhexidine on the in vitro and in vivo herpes simplex virus infection. Oral Surg Oral Med Oral Pathol Oral Radiol Endod 1989;67:149–53.

90. Vahdaty A, Pitt Ford TR, Wilson RF. Efficacy of chlorhexidine in disinfecting dentinal tubules in vitro. Endod Dent Traumatol 1993;9:243–8.

91. Buck RA, Eleazer PD, Staat RH, Scheetz JP. Effectiveness of three endodontic irrigants at various tubular depths in human dentin. J Endod 2001;27:206–8.

92. Jeansonne MJ, White RR. A comparison of 2.0% chlorhexidine gluconate and 5.25% sodium hypochlorite as antimicrobial endodontic irrigants. J Endod 1994;20:276–8.

93. Clegg MS, Vertucci FJ, Walker C, et al. The effect of exposure to irrigant solutions on apical dentin biofilms in vitro. J Endod 2006;32:434–7.

94. Oncag O, Hosgor M, Hilmioglu S, et al. Comparison of antibacterial and toxic effects of various root canal irrigants. Int Endod J 2003;36:423–32.

95. Barkvoll P, Attramadal A. Effect of nystatin and chlorhexidine digluconate on Candida albicans. Oral Surg Oral Med Oral Pathol 1989;67:279–81.

96. Hamers AD, Shay K, Hahn BL, Sohnle PG. Use of a microtiter plate assay to detect the rate of killing of adherent Candida albicans by antifungal agents. Oral Surg Oral Med Oral Pathol Oral Radiol Endod 1996;81:44–9.

97. Hiom SJ, Furr JR, Russell AD, Dickinson JR. Effects of chlorhexidine diacetate on *Candida albicans, C. glabrata* and *Saccharomyces cerevisiae*. J Appl Bacteriol 1992; 72:335–40.

98. Dona BL, Grundemann LJ, Steinfort J, et al. The inhibitory effect of combining chlorhexidine and hydrogen peroxide on 3-day plaque accumulation. J Clin Periodontol 1998;25:879–83.

99. Babich H, Wurzburger BJ, Rubin YL, et al. An *in vitro* study on the cytotoxicity of chlorhexidine digluconate to human gingival cells. Cell Biol Toxicol 1995;11:79–88.

100. Sassone LM, Fidel R, Fidel S, et al. The influence of organic load on the antimicrobial activity of different concentrations of NaOCl and chlorhexidine in vitro. Int Endod J 2003;36(12):848–52.

101. Hoefs JC. Serum protein concentration and portal pressure determine the ascitic fluid protein concentration in patients with chronic liver disease. J Lab Clin Med 1983;102:260–73.

102. Oliveira DP, Barbizam JV, Trope M, Teixeira FB. In vitro antibacterial efficacy of endodontic irrigants against *Enterococcus faecalis*. Oral Surg Oral Med Oral Pathol Oral Radiol Endod 2007;103:702–6.

103. Marchesan MA, Pasternak B Jr, Afonso MM, et al. Chemical analysis of the flocculate formed by the association of sodium hypochlorite and chlorhexidine. Oral Surg Oral Med Oral Pathol Oral Radiol Endod 2007;103:103–5.

104. Gottardi W. Iodine and iodine compounds. In: Block SS, editor. Disinfection, sterilization, and preservation. 4th ed. Philadelphia, PA: Lea & Febiger; 1991, pp. 152–66.

105. Chang SL. Modern concept of disinfection. J Sanit Eng Div Proc ASCE 1971;97:689.

106. Ng YL, Spratt D, Sriskantharajah S, Gulabivala K. Evaluation of protocols for field decontamination before bacterial sampling of root canals for contemporary microbiology techniques. J Endod 2003;29:317–20.

107. Molander A, Reit C, Dahlen G. The antimicrobial effect of calcium hydroxide in root canals pretreated with 5% iodine potassium iodide. Endod Dent Traumatol 1999;15:205–9.

108. Giardino L, Ambu E, Becce C, et al. Surface tension comparison of four common root canal irrigants and two new irrigants containing antibiotic. J Endod 2006;32:1091–3.

109. Torabinejad M, Khademi AA, Babagoli J, et al. A new solution for the removal of the smear layer. J Endod 2003;29:170–5.

110. Torabinejad M, Cho Y, Khademi AA, et al. The effect of various concentrations of sodium hypochlorite on the ability of MTAD to remove the smear layer. J Endod 2003;29:233–9.

111. Beltz RE, Torabinejad M, Pouresmail M. Quantitative analysis of the solubilizing action of MTAD, sodium hypochlorite, and EDTA on bovine pulp and dentin. J Endod 2003;29:334–7.

112. Zhang W, Torabinejad M, Li Y. Evaluation of cytotoxicity of MTAD using the MTT-tetrazolium method. J Endod 2003;29:654–7.

113. Shabahang S, Pouresmail M, Torabinejad M. *In vitro* antimicrobial efficacy of MTAD and sodium. J Endod 2003;29:450–2.

114. Shabahang S, Torabinejad M. Effect of MTAD on *Enterococcus faecalis*-contaminated root canals of extracted human teeth. J Endod 2003;29:576–9.

115. Kho P, Baumgartner JC. A comparison of the antimicrobial efficacy of NaOCl/Biopure MTAD versus NaOCl/EDTA against *Enterococcus faecalis*. J Endod 2006;32:652–5.

116. Baumgartner JC, Johal S, Marshall JG. Comparison of the antimicrobial efficacy of 1.3% NaOCl/BioPure MTAD to 5.25% NaOCl/15% EDTA for root canal irrigation. J Endod 2007;33:48–51.

117. Plotino G, Pameijer CH, Grande NM, Somma F. Ultrasonics in endodontics: a review of the literature. J Endod 2007;33:81–95.

118. Martin H. Ultrasonic disinfection of the root canal. Oral Surg Oral Med Oral Pathol Oral Radiol Endod 1976;42:92–9.

119. Cunningham W, Martin H, Forrest W. Evaluation of root canal debridement by the endosonic ultrasonic synergistic system. Oral Surg Oral Med Oral Pathol Oral Radiol Endod 1982;53:401–4.

120. Cunningham W, Martin H. A scanning electron microscope evaluation of root canal debridement with the endosonic ultrasonic synergistic system. Oral Surg Oral Med Oral Pathol Oral Radiol Endod 1982;53:527–31.

121. Cunningham W, Martin H, Pelleu G, Stoops D. A conmparison of antimicrobial effectiveness of endosonic and hand root canal therapy. Oral Surg Oral Med Oral Pathol Oral Radiol Endod 1982;54:238–41.

122. Martin H, CunninghamW. Endosonics – the ultrasonic synergistic system of endodontics. Endod Dent Traumatol 1985;1:201–6.

123. Roy RA, Ahmad M, Crum LA. Physical mechanisms governing the hydrodynamic response of an oscillating ultrasonic file. Int Endod J 1994;27:197–207.

124. Reynolds MA, Madison S, Walton RE, et al. An in vitro histological comparison of the step-back, sonic, and ultrasonic instrumentation techniques in small, curved root canals. J Endod 1987;13:307–14.

125. Heard F, Walton RE. Scanning electron microscope study comparing four root canal pereparation techniques in small curved canals. Int Endod J 1997;30:323–31.

126. Lumley PJ, Walmsley AD, Walton RE, Rippin JW. Cleaning of oval canals using ultrasonic or sonic instrumentation. J Endod 1993;19:453–7.

127. Cheung GS, Stock CJ. In vitro cleaning ability of root canal irrigants with and without endosonics. Int Endod J 1993;26:334–43.

128. Hülsmann M, Rümmelin C, Schäfers F. Root canal cleanliness after preparation with different endodontic handpieces

and hand instruments: a comparative SEM investigation. J Endod 1997;23:301–6.
129. Cameron JA. Factors affecting the clinical efficiency of ultrasonic endodontics: a scanning electron microscopy study. Int Endod J 1995;28:47–53.
130. Cameron JA. The choice of irrigant during hand instrumentation and ultrasonic irrigation of the root canal: a scanning electron microscope study. Aust Dent J 1995;40:85–90.
131. Lumley PJ, Walmsley AD, Walton RE, Rippin JW. Effect of pre-curving endosonic files on the amount of debris and smear layer remaining in curved root canals. J Endod 1992;18:616–19.
132. Goodman A, Reader A, Beck M, et al. An *in vitro* comparison of the efficacy of the step-back technique versus a step-back ultrasonic technique in humanmandibularmolars. J Endod 1985;11:249–56.
133. Archer R, Reader A, Nist R, et al. An in vivo evaluation of the efficacy of ultrasound after stepback preparation in mandibular molars. J Endod 1992;18:549–52.
134. Sjögren U, Sundqvist G. Bacteriologic evaluation of ultrasonic root canal instrumentation. Oral Surg Oral Med Oral Pathol Oral Radiol Endod 1987;63:366–70.
135. Spoleti P, Siragusa M, Spoleti MJ. Bacteriological evaluation of passive ultrasonic activation. J Endod 2002;29:12–14.
136. Sabins RA, Johnson JD, Hellstein JW. A comparison of the cleaning efficacy of short term sonic and ultrasonic passive irrigation after hand instrumentation in molar root canals. J Endod 2003;29:674–8.
137. DeNunzio MS, Hicks ML, Pelleu GB Jr, et al. Bacteriological comparison of ultrasonic and hand instrumentation of root canals in dogs. J Endod 1989;15:290–3.
138. Biffi JC, Rodrigues HH. Ultrasound in endodontics: a quantitative and histological assessment using human teeth. Endod Dent Traumatol 1989;5:55–62.
139. Ahmad M. Effect of ultrasonic instrumentation on Bacteriodes intermedius. Endod Dent Traumatol 1989;5:83–6.
140. Ahmad M, Pitt Ford TR, Crum LA, Wilson RF. Effectiveness of ultrasonic files in the disruption of root canal bacteria. Oral Surg Oral Med Oral Pathol Oral Radiol Endod 1990;70:328–32.
141. Lee SJ, Wu MK, Wesselink PR. The effectiveness of syringe irrigation and ultrasonics to remove debris from simulated irregularities within prepared root canal walls. Int Endod J 2004;37:672–8.
142. Van der Sluis LW, Wu MK, Wesselink PR. A comparison between a smooth wire and a K-file in removing artificially placed dentine debris from root canals in resin blocks during ultrasonic irrigation. Int Endod J. 2005;38:593–6.
143. Van der Sluis LW, Wu MK, Wesselink PR. The evaluation of removal of calcium hydroxide paste from an artificial standardized groove in the apical root canal using different irrigation methodologies. Int Endod J 2007;40:52–7.
144. Calhoun G, Montgomery S. The effects of four instrumentation techniques on root canal shape. J Endod 1988;14:273–7.
145. Schulz-Bongert U, Weine FS, Schulz-Bongert J. Preparation of curved canals using a combined hand-filing, ultrasonic technique. Compend Contin Educ Dent 1995;16:272–4.
146. McCann JT, Keller DL, LaBounty GL. Remaining dentin/cementum thickness after hand or ultrasonic instrumentation. J Endod 1990;16:109–13.
147. McKendry DJ. Comparison of balanced forces, endosonic, and step-back filing instrumentation techniqaues: quantification of extruded apical debris. J Endod 1990;16:24–7.
148. Rodrigues HH, Biffi JC. A histobacteriological assessment of nonvitgal teeth after ultrasonic root canal instrumentation. Endod Dent Traumatol 1989;5:182–7.
149. Vansan LP, Pecora JD, Costa WF, et al. Effects of various irrigating solutions on the cleaning of the root canal with ultrasonic instrumentation. Braz Dent J 1990;1:37–44.
150. Walters JD, Rawal SY. Severe periodontal damage by an ultrasonic endodontic device: a case report. Dent Traumatol 2007;23:123–7.
151. Ahmad M. Measurements of temperature generated by ultrasonic file in vitro. Endod Dent Traumatol 1990;6:230–1.
152. Fegan SE, Steiman HR. Comparative evaluation of the antibacterial effects of intracanal Nd:YAG laser irradiation: an in vitro study. J Endod 1995;21:415–17.
153. Moshonov J, Ørstavik D, Yamauchi S, et al. Nd:YAG laser irradiation in root canal disinfection. Endod Dent Traumatol 1995;11:220–4.
154. Blum JY, Michailesco P, Abadie MJ. An evaluation of the bactericidal effect of the Nd:YAP laser. J Endod 1997; 23:583–5.
155. Gutknecht N, Nuebler-Moritz M, Burghardt SF, Lampert F. The efficiency of root canal disinfection using a holmium:yttrium–aluminum–garnet laser in vitro. J Clin Laser Med Surg 1997;15:75–8.
156. Le Goff A, Dautel-Morazin A, Guigand M, et al. An evaluation of the CO_2 laser for endodontic disinfection. J Endod 1999;25:105–8.
157. Kesler G, Koren R, Kesler A, et al. Histological changes induced by CO_2 laser microprobe specially designed for root canal sterilization: in vivo study. J Clin Laser Med Surg 1998;16:263–7.
158. Schoop U, Moritz A, Kluger W, et al. The Er:YAG laser in endodontics: results of an *in vitro* study. Lasers Surg Med 2002;30:360–4.
159. Piccolomini R, D'Arcangelo C, D'Ercole S, et al. Bacteriologic evaluation of the effect of Nd:YAG laser irradiation in experimental infected root canals. J Endod 2002;28:276–8.
160. Mehl A, Folwaczny M, Haffner C, Hickel R. Bactericidal effects of 2.94 microns Er:YAG-laser radiation in dental root canals. J Endod 1999;25:490–3.

161. Lee MT, Bird PS, Walsh LJ. Photo-activated disinfection of the root canal: a new role for lasers in endodontics. Aust Endod J 2004;30:93–8.

162. Gulabivala K, Stock CJ, Lewsey JD, et al. Effectiveness of electrochemically activated water as an irrigant in an infected tooth model. Int Endod J 2004;37:624–31.

163. Solovyeva AM, Dummer PM. Cleaning effectiveness of root canal irrigation with electrochemically activated anolyte and catholyte solutions: a pilot study. Int Endod J 2000;33:494–504.

164. Nagayoshi M, Kitamura C, Fukuizumi T, et al. Antimicrobial effect of ozonated water on bacteria invading dentinal tubules. J Endod 2004;30:778–81.

165. Millar BJ, Hodson N. Assessment of the safety of two ozone delivery devices. J Dent 2007;35:195–200.

166. Hems RS, Gulabivala K, Ng YL, et al. An in vitro evaluation of the ability of ozone to kill a strain of *Enterococcus faecalis*. Int Endod J 2005;38:22–9.

167. Estrela C, Estrela CR, Decurcio DA, et al. Antimicrobial efficacy of ozonated water, gaseous ozone, sodium hypochlorite and chlorhexidine in infected human root canals. Int Endod J 2007;40:85–93.

168. Stoor P, Soderling E, Salonen JI. Antibacterial effects of a bioactive glass paste on oral microorganisms. Acta Odontol Scand 1998;56:161–5.

169. Zehnder M, Soderling E, Salonen J, Waltimo T. Preliminary evaluation of bioactive glass S53P4 as an endodontic medication in vitro. J Endod 2004;30:220–4.

170. Zehnder M, Waltimo T, Sener B, Söderling E. Dentin enhances the effectiveness of bioactive glass S53P4 against a strain of *Enterococcus faecalis*. Oral Surg Oral Med Oral Pathol Oral Radiol Endod 2006;101:530–5.

171. Waltimo T, Brunner T, Wendelin A, Zehnder M. Antimicrobial effect of nanometric bioactive glass 45S5. J Dent Res, 2007;86:754–7.

172. Chugal NM, Clive JM, Spångberg LS. A prognostic model for assessment of the outcome of endodontic treatment: effect of biologic and diagnostic variables. Oral Surg Oral Med Oral Pathol Oral Radiol Endod 2001;91:342–52.

173. Coldero LG, McHugh S, Mackenzie D, Saunders WP. Reduction in intracanal bacteria during root canal preparation with and without apical enlargement. Int Endod J 2002;35:437–46.

174. Rollison S, Barnett F, Stevens RH. Efficacy of bacterial removal from instrumented root canals in vitro related to instrumentation technique and size. Oral Surg Oral Med Oral Pathol Oral Radiol Endod 2002;94:366–71.

175. Card SJ, Sigurdsson A, Ørstavik D, Trope M. The effectiveness of increased apical enlargement in reducing intracanal bacteria. J Endod 2002;28:779–83.

176. Safavi KE, Nichols FC. Effect of calcium hydroxide on bacterial lipopolysaccharide. J Endod 1993;19:76–8.

177. Tanomaru JM, Leonardo MR, Tanomaru Filho M, et al. Effect of different irrigation solutions and calcium hydroxide on bacterial LPS. Int Endod J 2003;36:733–9.

178. Siren EK, Haapasalo MP, Ranta K, et al. Microbiological findings and clinical treatment procedures in endodontic cases selected for microbiological investigation. Int Endod J 1997;30:91–5.

179. Sathorn C, Parashos P, Messer HH. How useful is root canal culturing in predicting treatment outcome? J Endod 2007;33:220–5.

180. Ørstavik D. Antibacterial properties of endodontic materials. Int Endod J 1988;21:161–9.

181. Sjögren U, Figdor D, Spångberg L, Sundqvist G. The antimicrobial effect of calcium hydroxide as a short term intracanal dressing. Int Endod J 1991;24:119–25.

182. Reit C, Molander A, Dahlen G. The diagnostic accuracy of microbiologic root canal sampling and the influence of antimicrobial dressings. Endod Dent Traumatol 1999;15:278–83.

183. Shuping GB, Ørstavik D, Sigurdsson A, Trope M. Reduction of intracanal bacteria using nickel-titanium rotary instrumentation and various medications. J Endod 2000;26:751–5.

184. Peters LB, Van Winkelhoff AJ, Buijs JF, Wesselink PR. Effects of instrumentation, irrigation and dressing with calcium hydroxide on infection in pulpless teeth with periapical bone lesions. Int Endod J 2002;35:13–21.

185. Kvist T, Molander A, Dahlen G, Reit C. Microbiological evaluation of one- and two-visit endodontic treatment of teeth with apical periodontitis: a randomized, clinical trial. J Endod 2004;30:572–6.

186. Siqueira JF Jr, Paiva SS, Rocas IN. Reduction in the cultivable bacterial populations in infected root canals by a chlorhexidine-based antimicrobial protocol. J Endod 2007;33:541–7.

187. Ercan E, Dalli M, Dulgergil CT. In vitro assessment of the effectiveness of chlorhexidine gel and calcium hydroxide paste with chlorhexidine against *Enterococcus faecalis* and *Candida albicans*. Oral Surg Oral Med Oral Pathol Oral Radiol Endod 2006;102:27–31.

188. Siren EK, Haapasalo MP, Waltimo TM, Ørstavik D. In vitro antibacterial effect of calcium hydroxide combined with chlorhexidine or iodine potassium iodide on *Enterococcus faecalis*. Eur J Oral Sci 2004;112:326–31.

189. Grossman LI. Polyantibiotic treatment of pulpless teeth. J Am Dent Assoc 1951;43:265–78.

190. Bender IB, Seltzer S. Combination of antibiotics and fungicides used in treatment of the infected pulpless tooth. J Am Dent Assoc 1952;45:293–300.

191. Rubbo SD, Reich J, Dixson S. The use of a combination of neomycin, bacitracin, and polymyxin in endodontia. Oral Surg Oral Med Oral Pathol Oral Radiol Endod 1958;11:878–96.

192. Baker GR, Mitchell DF. Topical antibiotic treatment of infected dental pulps of monkeys. J Dent Res 1969 May–June;48:351–5.

193. Hoshino E, Iwaku M, Sato M, et al. Bactericidal efficacy of metronidazole against bacteria of human carious dentin *in vivo*. Caries Res 1989;23:78–80.

194. Hoshino E, Kurihara-Ando N, Sato I, et al. In-vitro antibacterial susceptibility of bacteria taken from infected root dentine to a mixture of ciprofloxacin, metronidazole and minocycline. Int Endod J 1996 Mar;29:125–30.

195. Sato I, Ando-Kurihara N, Kota K, et al. Sterilization of infected root-canal dentine by topical application of a mixture of ciprofloxacin, metronidazole and minocycline in situ. Int Endod J 1996;29:118–24.

196. Molander A, Reit C, Dahlen G. Microbiological evaluation of clindamycin as a root canal dressing in teeth with apical periodontitis. Int Endod J 1990;23:113–18.

197. Molander A, Dahlen G. Evaluation of the antibacterial potential of tetracycline or erythromycin mixed with calcium hydroxide as intracanal dressing against Enterococcus faecalis in vivo. Oral Surg Oral Med Oral Pathol Oral Radiol Endod 2003;96:744–50.

198. Banchs F, Trope M. Revascularization of immature permanent teeth with apical periodontitis: new treatment protocol? J Endod 2004;30:196–200.

199. Windley W III, Teixeira F, Levin L, et al. Disinfection of immature teeth with a triple antibiotic paste. J Endod 2005;31:439–43.

200. Harrison JW, Madonia JV. Antimicrobial effectiveness of parachlorophenol. Oral Surg Oral Med Oral Pathol Oral Radiol Endod 1970;30:267–75.

201. Harrison JW, Madonia JV. The toxicity of parachlorophenol. Oral Surg Oral Med Oral Patho Oral Radiol Endod 1971;32:90–9.

202. Taylor GN, Madonia JV, Wood NK, Heuer MA. In vivo autoradiographic study of relative penetrating abilities of aqueous 2% parachlorophenol and cambhorated 35% parachlorophenol. J Endod 1976;2:81–6.

203. Byström A, Claesson R, Sundqvist G. The antibacterial effect of camphorated paramonochlorophenol, camphorated phenol and calcium hydroxide in the treatment of infected root canals. Endod Dent Traumatol 1985;1:170–5.

204. Fager FK, Messer HH. Systemic distribution of camphorated monochlorophenol from cotton pellets sealed in pulp chambers. J Endod 1986;12:225–30.

205. Koontongkaew S, Silapichit R, Thaweboon B. Clinical and laboratory assessments of camphorated monochlorophenol in endodontic therapy. Oral Surg Oral Med Oral Pathol Oral Radiol Endod 1988;65:757–62.

206. Alencar AH, Leonardo MR, Silva LA, et al. Determination of the p-monochlorophenol residue in the calcium hydroxide + P-monochlorophenol combination used as an intracanal dressing in pulpless teeth of dogs with induced chronic periapical lesion. J Endod 1997;23:522–4.

207. Siqueira JF Jr, Rocas IN, Favieri A, et al. Incidence of postoperative pain after intracanal procedures based on an antimicrobial strategy. J Endod 2002;28:457–60.

208. Ferrari PH, Cai S, Bombana AC. Effect of endodontic procedures on enterococci, enteric bacteria and yeasts in primary endodontic infections. Int Endod J 2005;38:372–80.

209. Messer HH, Feigal RJ. A comparison of the antibacterial and cytotoxic effects of parachlorophenol. J Dent Res 1985;64:818–21.

210. Fager FK, Messer HH. Systemic distribution of camphorated monochlorophenol from cotton pellets sealed in pulp chambers. J Endod 1986;12:225–30.

211. Ribeiro DA, Marques ME, Salvadori DM. Antimicrobial endodontic compounds do not modulate alkylation-induced genotoxicity and oxidative stress in vitro. Oral Surg Oral Med Oral Pathol Oral Radiol Endod 2006;102:32–6.

212. Hagiwara M, Watanabe E, Barrett JC, Tsutsui T. Assessment of genotoxicity of 14 chemical agents used in dental practice: ability to induce chromosome aberrations in Syrian hamster embryo cells. Mutat Res 2006;603:111–20.

213. Ribeiro DA, Scolastici C, De Lima PL, et al. Genotoxicity of antimicrobial endodontic compounds by single cell gel (comet) assay in Chinese hamster ovary (CHO) cells. Oral Surg Oral Med Oral Pathol Oral Radiol Endod 2005;99:637–40.

214. Breault LG, Schuster GS, Billman MA, et al. The effects of intracanal medicaments, fillers, and sealers on the attachment of human gingival fibroblasts to an exposed dentin surface free of a smear layer. J Periodontol 1995;66:545–51.

215. Chang YC, Tai KW, Chou LS, Chou MY. Effects of camphorated parachlorophenol on human periodontal ligament cells in vitro. J Endod 1999;25:779–81.

216. Messer HH, Chen RS. The duration of effectiveness of root canal medicaments. J Endod 1984;10:240–5.

CHAPTER 29

Root Canal Filling Materials

James David Johnson

Historically, many materials have been used to fill root canals. In the 1800s and before, materials ranging from tin foil, lead foil, gold foil, cotton pellets with various medicaments, wood, spunk, plaster of Paris, oxychloride of zinc, oxyphosphate of zinc, zinc oxide, paraffin, copper points, and various other concoctions were used to fill root canals. Sometimes canals were not filled at all, and only a mixture of Hill's stopping was placed over canals.[1] With Asa Hill's development of Hill's stopping in 1847, which consisted of bleached gutta-percha and carbonate of lime and quartz, the advent of gutta-percha as a root canal filling material in endodontics began.[2] In 1867, G. A. Bowman of St. Louis was credited with using gutta-percha points to obturate root canals.[1] The S. S. White Company began to market gutta-percha points to the profession in 1887.[3] Gutta-percha, as an obturating material, has survived, and today exists in many forms, and is still the most widely used material to obturate root canals.

Requirements for an Ideal Root Canal Filling Material

Grossman[4] modified Brownlee's[5] criteria for the ideal root canal filling material and listed the following criteria for an ideal root canal filling material:

1. It should be easily introduced into the root canal.
2. It should seal the canal laterally as well as apically.
3. It should not shrink after being inserted.
4. It should be impervious to moisture.
5. It should be bacteriostatic or at least not encourage bacterial growth.
6. It should be radiopaque.
7. It should not stain tooth structure.
8. It should not irritate periradicular tissues.
9. It should be sterile, or easily and quickly sterilized, immediately before insertion.
10. It should be removed easily from the root canal, if necessary.

Root canal filling materials have been classified as solid-core filling materials, semisolid-core filling materials, and paste filling materials. Silver points are an example of solid-core filling materials. Gutta-percha is the most widely used semisolid-core material. Various paste systems have been used over the years, such as zinc oxide-containing pastes.

Solid-Core Filling Materials

HISTORICAL ROOT CANAL FILLING MATERIALS (SILVER POINTS)

Silver points, having the same diameter and taper as files and reamers, were introduced by Jasper in 1933.[2] Silver points were widely used in the 1930s to the 1960s, particularly in smaller canals. They were fabricated to the same size as instruments used in the preparation of the canal. Silver points had the advantages of being easy to insert, and length control was easier. Although silver points fulfilled many of Grossman's requirements, the main drawback of silver points is that they do not seal well laterally or apically because of their lack of plasticity. Silver points cannot adequately fill all the canal space and cannot be compacted into spaces or voids within the root canal system. They maintain their round shape and no canal is perfectly round in shape, even after instrumentation. This leaves too much space to be filled by sealer or cement, thus leading to leakage. The leakage allows corrosion of the silver points and the formation of silver salts. These products were found to be cytotoxic. Seltzer et al.[6] found such products as silver amine sulfate amide hydrate, silver sulfides, and silver sulfates from silver points removed from canals that were obturated with silver points. Brady and Del Rio[7] found corrosion products of sulfur and chlorides by microanalysis of failed silver points. Goldberg[8] found that corrosion was present microscopically in cases obturated with silver points that were deemed successful clinically and radiographically. Gutierrez et al.[9] reported that canal irrigants could corrode silver points. Kehoe[10] reported a case of localized argyria leading to "tattooing" of the alveolar mucosa associated with corroding of a silver point in a maxillary premolar.

Silver points used in smaller canals were very successful in their era. The inappropriate use of silver points in larger canals helped to give rise to their reputation as an inferior obturation method. With the advent of different instrumentation techniques that allowed for successful obturation of smaller canals with gutta-percha, the use of silver points has declined because of their inherent disadvantages. The use of silver points in modern endodontic therapy is extremely limited, and there seems to be no indications or justification for their use today.

Semisolid-Core Filling Materials

Gutta-percha is by far the most popular and commonly used root canal filling material. Although it does not meet all the criteria for an ideal filling material, it satisfies most of them. The major disadvantage of gutta-percha as a root canal filling material is its lack of rigidity. Gutta-percha, particularly the smaller sizes, will bend easily under lateral pressure.

Gutta-percha, known as "mazer wood," was introduced to England from Asia in the 1600s and existed as little more than a curiosity of the East for nearly 200 years.[11] It was not until 1848 that Ernst Werner von Siemans used gutta-percha as insulation for underwater cable. With its many desirable properties, gutta-percha soon was being used in many different ways and in many different products. Patents were applied for new products using gutta-percha, which included "corks, cements, thread, surgical instruments, garments, pipes, musical instruments, candelabras, gaiters, garters, suspenders, window shades, carpets, gloves, mattresses, pillows, tents, umbrellas, and sheathing for ships."[11] Perhaps the best known use of gutta-percha was in golf balls, introduced in the later part of the nineteenth century and used until 1920. These golf balls were called "gutties."[11]

Natural gutta-percha has been described as the product of various species of rubber trees from Malaysia, Borneo, Indonesia, and South America, mainly Brazil. Some of the species mentioned as sources of natural gutta-percha are *Palaquium gutta*, *Mimusops globsa*, and *Manilkara bidentata*, and are of the same botanical family as the natural rubber tree *Hevea brasiliensis*. Raw gutta-percha is the flexible hardened juice of these tropical trees.

Gutta-balata is identical in chemical structure and physical properties to gutta-percha and has long been used as gutta-percha, or added to gutta-percha in commercial brands. Additionally, synthetic *trans*-polyisoprene may be added to commercial gutta-percha. Raw gutta-percha from the tree undergoes a rigorous process to convert it into commercial grade gutta-percha. This process involves purification, dissolving of resins, and denaturing of proteins.[12]

Friedman et al.[13] investigated the ingredients of five commercial brands of gutta-percha points. They found the composition of these commercially available gutta-percha points, as seen in Table 1, to consist of 18 to 22% gutta-percha, 59 to 76% zinc oxide, 1 to 4% waxes and resins, and 1 to 18% metal sulfates. Although gutta-percha is not the major ingredient, it serves as the matrix. Zinc oxide acts as the filler, whereas the waxes and resins serve as plasticizers. Metal sulfates, such as barium sulfate, provide the radiopacity to identify the material radiographically.

Evidence of slight antibacterial activity from gutta-percha points exists, presumably from the zinc oxide in commercially available gutta-percha[14]; however, it is too weak to be an effective microbiocide. As the destruction of bacteria is key to endodontic success, a new formulation of gutta-percha that contains iodoform, medicated gutta-percha (MGP) (Medidenta International, Inc., Woodside, NY), has been developed by Martin and Martin.[15] Within the filled root canal, the iodine/iodoform depot in the MGP point is a biologically active source for inhibiting microbial growth. The iodoform is centrally located within the gutta-percha and takes about 24 hours to leach to the surface. "The iodoform remains inert until it comes in

Table 1 Composition of Gutta-Percha Endodontic Filling Materials (Mean Percentage ± SD)

Sample	Gutta-Percha	Wax and/or Resin	Heavy Metal Sulfates	Zinc Oxide
Premier	18.9 ± 0.1	4.1 ± 0.2	14.5 ± 0.4	61.5 ± 0.5
Mynol	19.9 ± 0.1	3.9 ± 0.02	16.2 ± 1.8	59.1 ± 2.0
Union Broach	21.8 ± 0.2	1.0 ± 0.02	17.3 ± 0.3	59.6 ± 0.1
Schwed	19.9 ± 0.2	2.8 ± 0.2	1.5 ± 0.3	75.3 ± 0.5
Star Dental	20.6 ± 1.4	2.9 ± 0.2	3.4 ± 2.1	73.4 ± 2.0

Adapted and reproduced with permission from Friedman et al (1975).[13] Composition of commercially available gutta-percha by quantitative analysis as performed by Friedman, Sandrik, Heuer, and Rapp.

contact with tissue fluids that activate the free iodine."[15] A canal filled with MGP gutta-percha could serve as a protection against bacterial contamination from coronal microleakage reaching the apical tissue. The use of heat during obturation does not affect either the release of iodoform or its chemical composition.[16] Presumably, the use of iodine containing gutta-percha points would be contraindicated in a patient with a history of allergy to iodine.

An in vitro assessment of iodoform containing gutta-percha tested the ability of the iodoform containing gutta-percha to delay the infiltration of *Enterococcus faecalis* using a bacterial microleakage model.[17] The results showed no difference between regular gutta-percha points and iodoform-containing gutta-percha points, both with Roth's 801 sealer, in their ability to delay microleakage of *E. faecalis*.

Gutta-percha points have also been introduced that contain a high percentage of calcium hydroxide (40–60%) (Roeko/Coltene/Whaledent, Langenau, Germany). This permits a simple placement of the medicament within the canal space between appointments. Calcium hydroxide points combine the efficacy of calcium hydroxide in a matrix of 42% bio-inert gutta-percha. Once the calcium hydroxide has leached out, the point is no longer useful as a filling material and must be removed. Holland et al.[18] have reported on the use of an experimental calcium hydroxide containing gutta-percha point that can be used for root canal filling. Their results indicate that these points produced an improvement in the apical sealing quality of the root canal filling.

There are also gutta-percha points available that contain chlorhexidine (Activ Point) (Roeko/Coltene/ Whaledent) that have a slow release of the chlorhexidine, and are used in a similar manner as the calcium hydroxide-containing gutta-percha. Some studies have shown that the points containing chlorhexidine had a better antibacterial effect than the calcium hydroxide containing gutta-percha points.[19]

Podbielski et al.[20] tested gutta-percha points containing calcium hydroxide and zinc oxide, points containing zinc oxide and chlorhexidine, points containing iodine–polyvinylpyrrolidone, and gutta-percha points containing a mixture of chlorhexidine and iodine–polyvinylpyrrolidone for their ability to inhibit growth of pure cultures of bacterial species commonly involved in endodontic infections. The calcium hydroxide-containing gutta-percha points proved to possess the strongest antibacterial activity, compared with the other three of the four types, for all bacteria tested, with the exception *Peptostreptococcus micros*.

One study investigated the antimicrobial efficacy of medicated filling materials, including standard gutta-percha, iodoform gutta-percha (MGP), and gutta-percha with tetracycline.[21] These medicated filling materials were tested against several strains of bacteria including *Actinomyces israelii*, *Actinomyces naeslundii*, *E. faecalis*, and *Fusobacterium nucleatum*. Standard gutta-percha and the iodoform-containing gutta-percha weakly inhibited *F. nucleatum* and *A. naeslundii*. In addition, the iodoform gutta-percha also inhibited *A. israelii*. Only the tetracycline-containing gutta-percha inhibited all bacterial strains, including *E. faecalis*.

In 1942, Bunn[22] discovered that natural gutta-percha existed in a 1,4-*trans*-polyisoprene stereochemical structure. Natural rubber has a 1,4-*cis*-polyisoprene stereochemical structure. Both gutta-percha and natural rubber are high-molecular-weight stereo-isomers of polyisoprene. In the *cis* form of natural rubber, the CH_2 group is on the same side of the double bond, whereas in the *trans* form of polyisoprene (gutta-percha) the CH_2 groups are on the opposite side of the double bond as shown in Figure 1. The *cis* configuration of natural rubber allows for mobility of one chain past another and gives rise to the elastic nature of rubber, whereas the *trans* configuration of gutta-percha is more linear and crystallizes more readily making gutta-percha harder, more brittle, and less elastic than natural rubber.[11,23] The scientific methods available to Bunn in 1942 did not allow for 100% identification of the 1,4-polyisoprene configuration, as he could not rule out the presence of a minority *cis* form.[24] In 1993, Marciano et al.,[24] using nuclear

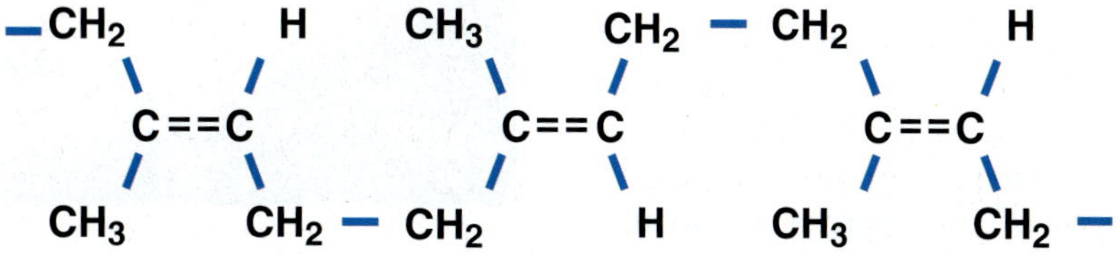

Figure 1 Stereochemical structure of gutta-percha, 1,4-*trans*-polyisoprene isomer (natural gutta-percha). CH_2 groups are on opposite sides of the double bond for each successive monomer. Adapted and reproduced with permission from Marciano J et al (1993).[24]

magnetic resonance, were able to confirm that both natural and commercial gutta-percha mainly have a 1,4 trans stereochemical structure and that the coloring agent in commercial gutta-percha is erythrosine. Less than 1% of the sample had the 1,4 cis stereochemical structure.

Gutta-percha exists in two distinct crystalline forms, alpha and beta.[22] Raw gutta-percha, as it comes directly from the tree, is in the alpha form. Once purified, gutta-percha, as it appears commercially in manufactured gutta-percha products, is in the beta crystalline form. There are few differences in physical properties between the two forms, merely a difference in the crystalline lattice depending on the annealing and/or drawing process used when manufacturing the final product.[25] Although there is apparently no difference in the mechanical properties of the two crystalline forms, there are thermal and volumetric differences.[11] Unlike many materials, there are volumetric changes associated with temperature changes in gutta-percha, which has clinical implications.

If the natural alpha form which comes from the tree is heated above 65°C, it will melt and become amorphous. If it is very slowly cooled at a rate of 0.5° per hour, the original alpha form will recrystallize. However, if the heated amorphous form cools normally, the beta form will crystallize.[11] Schilder et al.[26] investigated the temperatures at which the crystalline phase transitions occurred. They found that, when dental gutta-percha in the beta crystalline form was heated, a crystalline phase transition to the alpha form took place between 42° and 49°C, depending on the specific compound being tested. The alpha-to-amorphous phase transition occurred at a higher temperature of between 53° and 59°C, again depending on the make up of the specific compound being tested. This information is useful clinically, when the clinician needs the amorphous form of gutta-percha in order to flow gutta-percha into all parts of the canal and to utilize thermoplastic techniques.

In a study on the thermomechanical properties of gutta-percha, Schilder et al.[27] found that compaction, as opposed to compression, is what occurs in clinical situations with gutta-percha. Additionally, the reduction in volume that takes place with mechanical manipulation of gutta-percha is due to the consolidation and collapse of internal voids in gutta-percha, and this occurs within compaction forces. Finally, there is no molecular spring back after compaction of gutta-percha that would aid in the seal of gutta-percha within the root canal system. To overcome the shrinkage of gutta-percha as it cools, it is necessary to put pressure on the gutta-percha with a plugger.

Traditionally, the beta form of gutta-percha was used to manufacture endodontic gutta-percha points to achieve an improved stability and hardness and to reduce stickiness. However, through special processing and/or modifications to the formulation of the gutta-percha compound, more alpha-like forms of gutta-percha have been introduced, resulting in changes in the melting point, viscosity, and tackiness of the gutta-percha. Gutta-percha with low viscosity will flow with less pressure or stress,[25] whereas an increase in tackiness will help create a more homogeneous filling. Various manufacturers have introduced products to take advantage of these properties (e.g., Themafil, Densfil, MicroSeal).[16]

Gutta-percha points come in the standardized ISO (International Standards Organization) sizes to correspond to endodontic instruments. Initially, the ISO-sized gutta-percha points came in the standard 0.02 taper to match the instruments available in that era. Now gutta-percha points are available in the increased taper sizes of 0.04, 0.06, etc to match the endodontic instruments that have these greater tapers. Color coding to match the ISO size is available on most gutta-percha points marketed today (Figure 2).

The traditional configuration of gutta-percha points is manufactured in a form that does not correspond to

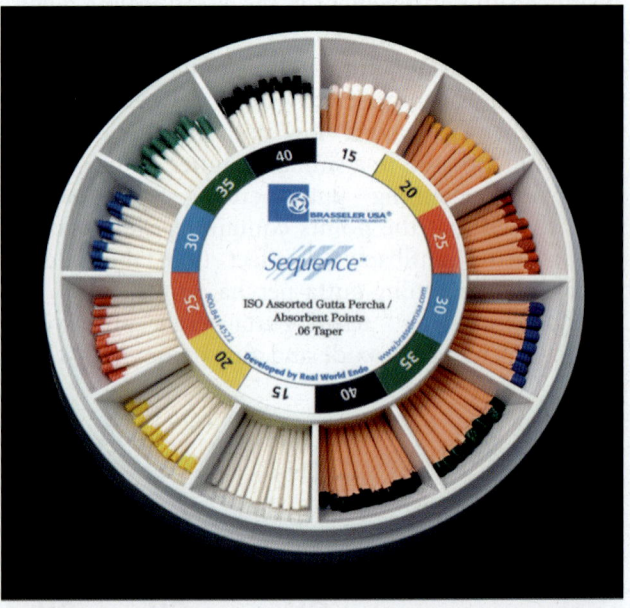

Figure 2 Assorted gutta-percha points and absorbent paper points with 0.06 taper are shown here, with color coded ends for easy identification of the size of the point. Reproduced with permission of Brasseler USA.

ISO sizes but has tapers that closely match the final instrumented size of canals. These traditional sizes (extra-fine, fine-fine, medium-fine, fine, fine-medium, medium, medium-large, large, and extra-large) have long been used in warm vertical obturation techniques and also match spreader sizes used in lateral compaction techniques.

With the thermoplasticized injectable techniques of gutta-percha placement and obturation of canals, the gutta-percha is produced in pellet form that may be loaded into the heating devise (Obtura III) or as prepackaged cannulas or cartridges (UltraFil, Calamus, Elements). Carrier-based gutta-percha products have gutta-percha surrounding a carrier made of metal or plastic.

Gutta-percha that has been stored for extended periods of time can become brittle with aging. Sorin et al.[28] presented a method to rejuvenate aged and brittle gutta-percha by immersing it in hot tap water (above 55°C) until the grasping forceps indents the now softened gutta-percha. The gutta-percha is then removed from the hot water and immediately quenched in cold tap water (less than 20°C) for several seconds. The gutta-percha point can now be sterilized and used to obturate the canal.

Gutta-percha should be stored in a cool location with low humidity. Kolokruis et al.[29] investigated the effects of moisture and aging on gutta-percha. They found that high humidity causes the absorption of water by the gutta-percha points, which lowers the values for tensile strength and torsional strain resistance, increases the value for elongation, and has a plasticizing effect on the gutta-percha cones. The plasticizing effect is due to the insertion of water molecules in the polymer chains.

Senia et al.[30] suggested sterilizing gutta-percha prior to insertion into the canal by immersion into 5.25% sodium hypochlorite for at least 1 minute to kill bacteria and spores on gutta-percha. Examination with a dissecting microscope showed no adverse effects on the gutta-percha points that were immersed for 5 minutes in 5.25% sodium hypochlorite.

In a scanning electron microscope (SEM) study, Short et al.[31] examined the affect of the sodium hypochlorite on gutta-percha points and determined that gutta-percha fresh from the box had no crystals on its surface. All the gutta-percha points placed in sodium hypochlorite had sodium chloride crystals present after the rapid-sterilization technique using 5.25 and 2.5% sodium hypochlorite. However, the sodium chloride crystals could be removed from the gutta-percha surface by 96% ethyl alcohol, 70% isopropyl alcohol, or distilled water.

The structural effects of sodium hypochlorite solutions on gutta-percha points were examined in an atomic force microscopy study by Valois et al.[32] They found aggressive deteriorating effects on the gutta-percha points that had been placed in 5.25% sodium hypochlorite for 1 minute. After 5 minutes in either 2.5% or 5.25% sodium hypochlorite, there were topographic changes. However, a 0.5% solution of sodium hypochlorite did not cause any alteration in the topography or elasticity of gutta-percha points. They concluded that a 0.5% solution of sodium hypochlorite would be a safe alternative for rapid decontamination of gutta-percha points.

As another alternative for the disinfection of gutta-percha points, Gomes et al.[33] looked at the effectiveness of chlorhexidine and sodium hypochlorite as solutions for the disinfection of gutta-percha points. In their boxes, gutta-percha points had a contamination rate of 5.5%. Microbes found most frequently, after intentional contamination with gloves, were Staphylococcus organisms. Chlorhexidine was not effective in eliminating *Bacillus subtilis* spores on gutta-percha, whereas 5.25% sodium hypochlorite eliminated spores on gutta-percha after 1 minute of disinfection.

THERMOPLASTICIZED GUTTA-PERCHA

Yee et al.[34] introduced the concept of obturating root canals using injection-molded thermoplasticized dental gutta-percha. They developed a prototype devise (PAC-160) where gutta-percha points were loaded into a pressure syringe and heated to 160°C. They injected the heated and softened gutta-percha into prepared canals, with and without sealer. They found injected thermoplasticized gutta-percha could produce an effective apical seal, especially when used with sealer. They introduced what would become the Obtura unit.

Injectable thermoplasticized gutta-percha may be used as a primary obturation technique, or, as it is used most often today, as a back-filling technique to fill the coronal aspects of the canal after the initial placement and compaction of gutta-percha by other techniques in the apical portion of the canal. The thermoplasticized gutta-percha injection techniques are classified as high-temperature and low-temperature thermoplasticized gutta-percha injection systems. These systems have made obturation quicker with the back-filling technique.

The first commercially available thermoplasticized gutta-percha system was the *Obtura system*. The Obtura

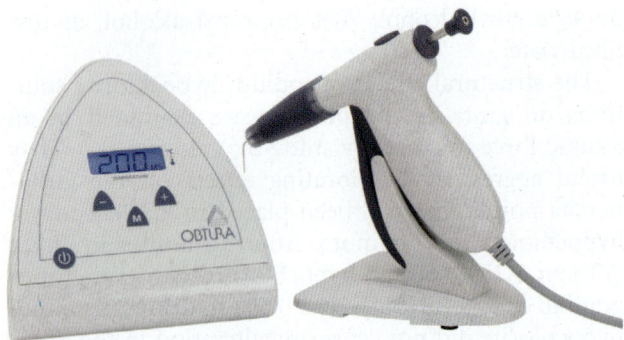

Figure 3 Obtura III Thermoplasticized gutta-percha delivery system by Obtura Spartan. Reproduced with permission from Obtura Spartan.

III Unit (Obtura/Spartan Corp., Fenton, MO) (Figure 3) is a high-temperature thermoplasticized gutta-percha system that requires gutta-percha pellets to be inserted into a delivery system gun, and then the gutta-percha pellet is heated to 150° to 200°C prior to delivery into the canal system. The warmed and softened gutta-percha is then delivered through 20-, 23-, or 25-gauge needles. Obtura gutta-percha also comes in the Flow-150 pellets, which is lower temperature thermoplasticized gutta-percha, and requires heating only to 150°C. The Obtura III also can be used with Resilon pellets, and lower temperatures are required to thermally soften the Resilon.

In a clinical study using the Obtura II system, Tani-Ishii and Teranaka[35] reported an overall success rate of 96% with a 1-year follow-up with cases obturated only with the Obtura II thermoplasticized injection technique.

Several studies have evaluated the safety of the temperatures used with injectable thermoplasticized systems and, for the most part, found them to be well below the critical 10°C rise in temperature that will cause damage to the periodontal ligament and bone.[36–39] According to a study by Lipski,[40] high-temperature thermoplasticized injectable gutta-percha in mandibular incisors may show an increase in temperature above the 10°C rise that is crucial if damage to the attachment apparatus is to be prevented. Maxillary incisors, however, did not show an external temperature rise above 10°C.

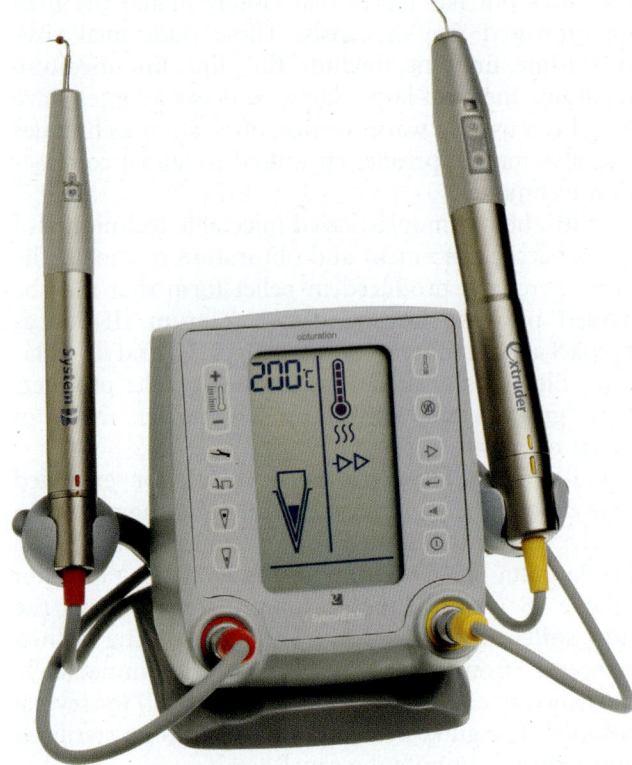

Figure 4 Elements thermoplasticized gutta-percha delivery system with System B heat source by Sybron Endo. Reproduced with permission from Sybron Endo.

The *Elements system* (Sybron Endo, Orange, CA) is a high-temperature thermoplasticized gutta-percha system that uses preloaded gutta-percha cartridges that are heated prior to delivery through the unit by an activation button. The gutta-percha is heated to 200°C. The gutta-percha is delivered through a 45° pre-bent needle that comes in sizes 20, 23, or 25 gauges (Figure 4).

The *Calamus system* is manufactured by (Tulsa Dental Products, Tulsa, OK). The high-temperature system heats the gutta-percha cannulas from 60° to 200°C. The delivery system may be activated by finger pressure on a blue ring with multiple positions. Besides the temperature control, the flow rate may be controlled by the operator as well. The flow rate of the softened and heated gutta-percha may be

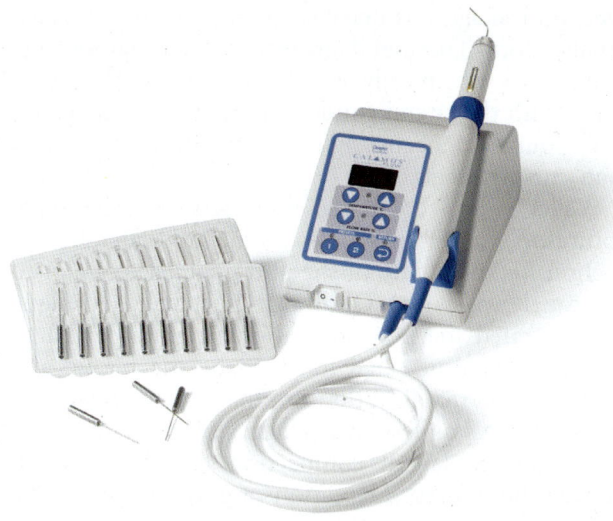

Figure 5 Calamus thermoplasticized gutta-percha delivery system by Tulsa Dentsply. Reproduced with permission of Tulsa Dentsply.

regulated from 20, 40, 60, 80, and 100%. The Calamus unit only comes with needle sizes of 20 and 23 gauges (Figure 5).

UltraFil (Hygienic Corp., Akron, OH) is a low-temperature thermoplasticized gutta-percha delivery system that has prepackaged cannulas with attached 22-gauge needles. The gutta-percha is prepared in the alpha phase form so that it softens at a temperature of 70° to 90°C in the heating unit. Once heated, the cannulas are then placed in the injection syringe and the softened thermoplasticized gutta-percha is ready for injection into canal.

Michanowicz and Czonstkowsky[41] in a dye study using a low-temperature injection system (70°C) found that when sealer was used, there was very little leakage. They used no compaction with this technique. Lipski[42] found temperatures transmitted to the periodontal ligament with the Ultra-Fil system were below levels causing damage or injury.

Thermomechanical Compaction of Gutta-Percha

Several thermomechanical compaction methods and products have been marketed. McSpadden first introduced the McSpadden Compactor, which resembled a reverse Hedstrom file, which was rotated at up to 20,000 rpm. Heat generated by friction softened gutta-percha, and the blade design pushed material apically.

The *MicroSeal System* (Sybron Endo) was also developed by John McSpadden. He redesigned the Compactor into the NT Condenser that is used with the *Microseal System*. The NT Condenser rotates at slower speeds (1,000 to 4,000 rpm) than the original McSpadden Compactor and utilizes nickel–titanium instruments.

The system uses MicroSeal gutta-percha master cones, and specially formulated gutta-percha, termed low-fusing or ultra-low-fusing gutta-percha, in a cartridge that is heated in the MicroSeal heater. This specially formulated low-fusing gutta-percha is advertised to be alpha phase gutta-percha, as are the points. A rotating mechanical condenser in a handpiece is coated with the heated gutta-percha and inserted into the canal. This rotating condenser creates heat from friction that thermally softens the single gutta-percha master point previously seated in the canal. It also flows laterally, by centrifugal force, the low-fusing or ultra-low-fusing gutta-percha coated on the condenser into all aspects of the canal.[43]

Cathro and Love[44] compared MicroSeal with a technique using the System B with Obtura II backfill obturation. The MicroSeal technique produced a dense homogenous gutta-percha fill at the apical 1 and 2 mm similar to the System B/Obtura II technique. Further coronally, the sealer became mixed into the MicroFlow gutta-percha, producing a heterogeneous mass with less solid gutta-percha compared with the System B/Obtura II technique.

Carrier-Based Gutta-Percha

The concept of a carrier-based thermoplasticized gutta-percha obturation method was introduced by Johnson in 1978.[45] These products are marketed today as *ThermaFil Plus Obturators* (Tulsa Dental Products) (Figure 6), GT Obturators (Tulsa Dental Products), ProTaper Obturators (Tulsa Dental Products), Densfil

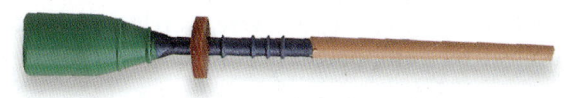

Figure 6 ThermaFil Plus Obturator by Tulsa Dentsply. Reproduced with permission of Tulsa Dentsply.

(Dentsply Tulsa, Tulsa, OK), and Soft-Core (Soft-Core System, Inc., CMS Dental, Copenhagen, Denmark).

The original ThermaFil obturators had a metal carrier, now replaced with a grooved plastic carrier. Gutta-percha, which coats the carrier, is said to be alpha phase gutta-percha, and certainly after heating in the ThermaFil oven, the gutta-percha is in the alpha or amorphous phase.

Gutmann et al.[46] compared lateral compaction with ThermaFil obturation and found that curved canals, treated with ThermaFil, resulted in a denser, better-adapted obturation on radiographic examination than those obturated with lateral compaction. However, both showed acceptable root canal fills in the apical one third, and ThermaFil extruded more material beyond the apex. In the second part of the study, no significant difference was seen in dye leakage after obturation with lateral compaction or ThermaFil. Both demonstrated dye leakage over a 5-month period.[47]

Becker and Donnelly[48] in a literature review of ThermaFil obturation made these observations. ThermaFil appears to seal the apical foramen as well as other thermoplasticized techniques, lateral compaction techniques, or vertical compaction techniques.[47,49–60] ThermaFil appears to adapt well to canal walls, but the long-term seal may be affected by exposed (bare) carrier.[61] Corrosion of metal carriers should not cause concern. There is significantly more extrusion of gutta-percha compared with lateral compaction.[46,56,60] Coronal leakage varies by study, but ThermaFil appears to allow significantly more leakage.[62–64] The effect of post-space preparation on the apical leakage of ThermaFil obturators varied depending on the particular study.[65–72] Re-treatment may be more difficult, especially with metal carriers and if the canal has been prepared for a post.[72–76] Metal carriers may limit the ability to perform root-end resection.[77,78]

Felstead et al.[52] examined apical leakage and found no statistically significant difference among teeth obturated with ThermaFil when heated to 100°, 120°, or 144°C, but there was a trend toward less leakage with lower temperatures. There was no significant leakage difference between teeth obturated with ThermaFil or lateral condensation.

Clark and El Deeb[56] investigated the sealing ability of plastic versus metal carriers in ThermaFil obturators. Both carrier types were rarely completely entombed by gutta-percha in the apical third; however, no leakage was detected in any of the obturated canals. Both ThermaFil groups yielded significantly more cases of apically extruded gutta-percha compared with the lateral condensation group. Extrusions were found to occur significantly more in straight than curved canals.

Weller et al.[79] compared three types of ThermaFil obturators, the Obtura II technique, and lateral compaction for the ability of the gutta-percha to adapt to the canal walls. The Obtura II injectable technique demonstrated the best adaptation of gutta-percha to the prepared root canal followed by the plastic and titanium ThermaFil obturators that were similar, followed by the stainless steel ThermaFil obturators, and finally by the lateral compaction technique, which showed the poorest adaptation of gutta-percha to the canal walls.

GT Obturators are designed to be used after preparation with GT files (Tulsa Dental Products), and ProTaper obturators after preparing a canal with ProTaper files (Tulsa Dental Products).

Robinson et al.[80] compared extrusion of gutta-percha in teeth instrumented with ProFile 0.06 or ProFile GT and obturated with ThermaFil Plus obturators or ThermaFil GT obturators, respectively, or with warm vertical condensation. Extrusion of gutta-percha was seen more often in the teeth obturated with ThermaFil GT obturators, followed by teeth obturated with ThermaFil Plus obturators, with the least amount of extrusion occurring with the warm vertical condensation technique with either instrumentation method.

In one study, the percentage of gutta-percha-filled area in the apical third of root canals obturated with either lateral condensation technique, System B technique, or ThermaFil technique was examined. There was no significant difference between the percentages of gutta-percha-filled area for lateral condensation or System B technique, but the coated carrier gutta-percha system (ThermaFil) produced a significantly higher percentage of gutta-percha-filled area than the other two techniques.[81]

Temperatures produced by heated carrier-based gutta-percha have been found to be at levels safe for bone and periodontal ligament.[40,82]

Densfil (Maillefer/Dentsply International, York, PA) is a carrier-based gutta-percha system with both plastic and titanium carriers, a spin-off of ThermaFil.

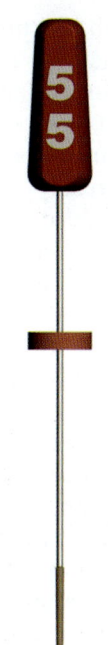

Figure 7 SimpliFil has a metal carrier that comes in ISO sizes 35 to 130 with a 5 mm plug of gutta-percha or Resilon on the end. Reproduced with permission of LightSpeed.

SimpliFil (LightSpeedUSA, San Antonio, TX) (Figure 7) is a 5 mm apical plug of gutta-percha or Resilon on the end of a file and is used similar to a carrier-based system. It has the advantage of not leaving the carrier in the canal, as it is twisted off of the apical plug.

Jarrett et al.[83] compared the apical density of gutta-percha in palatal roots of maxillary molars when filled with SimpliFil, as recommended by the manufacturer; ThermaFil; warm vertical condensation Schilder technique; warm vertical continuous wave technique; mechanical lateral technique; cold lateral condensation technique; and a modified SimpliFil technique. SimpliFil, as recommended, and ThermaFil had the greatest mean obturated area, but neither was statistically better than mechanical lateral or warm vertical condensation (Schilder) technique. SimpliFil, as recommended, and ThermaFil were statistically better than cold lateral condensation technique, warm vertical condensation (continuous wave) technique, and the modified SimpliFil group. Mechanical lateral and warm vertical condensation (Schilder) techniques had statistically more obturated area than warm vertical condensation (continuous wave) and modified SimpliFil techniques. Cold lateral and warm vertical condensation (continuous wave) had significantly more obturated area than modified SimpliFil.

Shipper and Trope[84] compared microbial leakage in canals obturated with one of the following techniques: lateral compaction, vertical compaction, Obtura II thermoplasticized injection technique, SimpliFil with Obtura II, FibreFil (Pentron Clinical Technologies, Wallingford, CT), or a combination of FibreFil and SimpliFil. Microbial leakage occurred more quickly in the lateral and vertical compaction techniques compared with SimpliFil and FibreFil techniques. A combination of an apical plug of gutta-percha with SimpliFil and a FibreFil coronal seal provided the best obturation.

SuccessFil is a carrier-based gutta-percha system combined with the UltraFil thermoplasticizied injection system to create what is marketed as the Trifecta System (Hygienic/Coltene/Whaledent). Goldberg et al.[85] compared the sealing ability of Trifecta, lateral condensation and SuccessFil with lateral condensation. No statistically significant differences in leakage were seen between the groups.

JS Quick-Fill (JS Dental Manufacturing, Inc., Ridgefield, CT) is an alpha phase gutta-percha-coated titanium core in ISO sizes 15 to 60. The carrier-based material is spun into the canal at low speed, and the core may be left in the canal or slowly removed.

Properties of Gutta-Percha

Gutta-percha is generally regarded as a very acceptable material with good biocompatibility with the periapical tissues. This has, for the most part, been verified in several studies, with the exception that some formulations of gutta-percha have produced localized severe inflammatory reactions in animals.[86] Wolfson and Seltzer,[87] in a 1975 study, found severe tissue reaction to eight brands of gutta-percha they injected into the skin of rats.

Tavares et al.[88] looked at the reaction of rat subcutaneous tissue to implants of different commercially available gutta-percha compared with Teflon control cylinders. Studies were conducted on Kerr and Hygenic brands of gutta-percha, and cylinders used with the UltraFil thermoplastic injectable gutta-percha from Hygenic Corp. The Kerr points gave mild reactions throughout all experimental periods, and the UltraFil cylinders initially produced a foreign body reaction caused by the dispersion of filling material particles mediated by macrophages and giant cells, but this response decreased with time and thus was considered biologically acceptable. The Hygenic gutta-percha points caused a severe initial inflammatory tissue reaction suggestive of bioincompatibility.

The ingredients of gutta-percha, such as zinc oxide, may contribute to the cytotoxic effects of some commercial gutta-percha.[89] However, other studies have suggested that the zinc oxide component may reduce the toxicity of other ingredients, especially rosin and resin acids.[90]

The tissue toxicity exerted by gutta-percha is more evident in the advent of an overfill or overextension of gutta-percha into the periapical area. Sjögren et al.[91] demonstrated that the size of gutta-percha particle may make a difference in the intensity of the inflammatory response. Large gutta-percha particles had very little inflammation around them, and appeared to be well encapsulated, whereas the smaller particles of gutta-percha caused a more intense localized response. Additionally, they found that gutta-percha with a rosin and chloroform component invoked a response considered severe.

In a study by Holland et al.,[92] one brand or formulation of gutta-percha caused a severe inflammatory response in rat connective tissue with a fibrous capsule formation, whereas another brand was well tolerated.

Serene et al.[93] looked at the activation of complement to examine the inflammatory response of four different commercially available brands of gutta-percha, and the ingredients in one of the brands. This in vitro study showed that each of the four brands of commercially available gutta-percha and each of the ingredients could cause activation of the complement system.

Although some gutta-percha has been shown to be cytotoxic, invoking inflammatory reactions in connective tissue, the most toxic portion of the sealer–gutta-percha obturation is the sealer.[86]

Because gutta-percha and gutta-balata are derived from the *Paliquium gutta* and *M. globsa* trees, which are of the same botanical family of trees as the natural rubber latex tree, *H. brasiliensis*, there was concern about the possible cross-reactivity between gutta-percha and natural rubber latex in individuals who may have immediate-type hypersensitivity to natural rubber latex. There have been case reports suggesting that gutta-percha may release proteins that induce reactions in latex-allergic individuals.[94,95] In these cases, the symptoms were uncharacteristic of those routinely experienced by patients with latex allergies. Other causes, more directly related to the quality of the endodontic treatment itself, may have been the reason for the patients' symptoms. These case reports did not prove the cross-reactivity between *Hevea* latex and gutta-percha. On the other hand, Knowles et al.[96] and Kleier and Shibilski[97] presented case reports where gutta-percha was successfully used to obturate canals in patients with documented IgE antibody-mediated allergy to natural rubber latex.[12] Studies by Costa et al.[12] and Hamann et al.[98] using the radioallergosorbent test (RAST) inhibition and enzyme-linked immunosorbent assay (ELISA)[98] showed that commercially available gutta-percha alone is not likely to induce symptoms in the patient with type I natural rubber latex allergy and that commercially available gutta-percha can safely be used in these patients. The refining process for gutta-percha is so severe that most proteins would be denatured by the process. Raw gutta-balata was the only substance that showed cross-reactivity with natural rubber latex.[12] None of the processed gutta-percha products, or natural raw gutta-percha, showed any cross-reactivity with natural rubber latex.[12] Nevertheless, it is always prudent to investigate natural rubber latex allergies in patients because it is very common, particularly among health care workers (17%) and spina bifida patients (67%).[99–101]

Newer Solid-Core Filling Materials

Resilon (Pentron Clinical Technologies), and RealSeal (Sybron Endo), is a polycaprolactone core material with difunctional methacrylate resin, bioactive glass, bismuth and barium salts as fillers, and pigments, which is used with a resin sealer (Epiphany or Real-Seal) that is packaged with the core filling material (Figures 8). The rational behind the product is to create a "monoblock" consisting of a resin sealer with

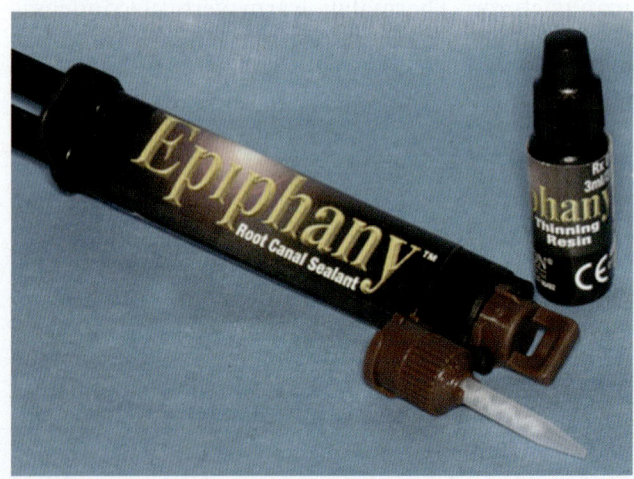

Figure 8 Epiphany sealer is a resin type of sealer used with polycaprolactone core materials such as Resilon core material. Courtesy, James David Johnson.

resin tags that enter into and bond to dentinal tubules, and to the dentin on the canal wall, as well as adhesively bonding to the core material, and which can also be light cured and sealed coronally as well. The Resilon system consists of a primer, a sealer, and synthetic polymer points or pellets.

Whereas the sealer used with Resilon is discussed under the discussion on sealers later in this chapter, the Resilon system, core material and sealer, has to be used together, as it is one system, and each part relies on the other parts to be successful.

The polyester core material is marketed in ISO-sized points with accessory points for lateral compaction and warm vertical techniques, or pellets for use in thermoplasticized techniques.[101] The temperatures used in the thermoplasticized techniques for the polyester resin core materials are lower than those used for gutta-percha techniques (150°C, compared to 200°C), but otherwise has handling characteristics that are similar to gutta-percha and allows for lateral compaction or warm vertical obturation techniques. In the case of using Resilon with the System B unit, the temperature is set at 150°C and the power is set at 10. If Resilon is used with the Obtura III thermoplasticizing unit with 25-gauge needles, the temperature is set at 160°C; with 23-gauge needles, the temperature is set at 140°C; and for use with 20-gauge needles, the temperature is set at 120° to 130°C.

One study compared Resilon with gutta-percha in terms of the melting point, specific heat capacity, enthalpy change with melting, and heat transfer. It was found that there was no difference in the melting point temperatures for the two materials, but Resilon had a significantly greater specific heat capacity and endothermic enthalpy change. There was a significant difference in the heat transfer test in the temperature increase between gutta-percha and Resilon within 3 mm of the heat source, with gutta-percha having a greater temperature change. They concluded that Resilon may not be thermoplasticized the same as gutta-percha because there is a higher specific heat, higher enthalpy change with melting, and less heat transfer.[102]

Nielsen and Baumgartner[103] examined the depth of nickel–titanium spreader penetration in root canals having a 0.04 preparation size taper using 0.02 and 0.04 tapered master gutta-percha or Resilon points. A significant difference in penetration depth was found for both taper of the point and the material used. The depth of spreader penetration was greatest for 0.02 tapered Resilon, followed by 0.02 gutta-percha, followed by 0.04 tapered Resilon, and the least spreader penetration occurred with the 0.04 gutta-percha.

Shipper et al.[104] investigated the resistance to bacterial penetration of gutta-percha with AH 26 sealer, gutta-percha with Epiphany sealer, and Resilon with Epiphany sealer. Each combination of core material and sealer was obturated with both lateral and vertical condensation techniques. The Resilon groups were found to have less leakage than the gutta-percha groups with respect to the number and rate of the specimens in each group that leaked. All Resilon and Epiphany sealer groups leaked significantly less than all groups in which AH 26 was used as a sealer.

By contrast, other investigators[105] performed an ultrastructural evaluation of the apical seal in roots filled with a polycaprolactone-based root canal filling material. This study compared the ultrastructural quality of the apical seal achieved with Resilon and Epiphany sealer with that produced by gutta-percha and AH Plus sealer. The SEM revealed both gap-free regions and gap-containing regions in canals filled with both materials. The transmission electron microscope revealed the presence of silver deposits along the sealer-hybrid layer interface in the Resilon/Epiphany samples and between the sealer and gutta-percha samples. They concluded that a complete apical seal cannot be achieved with either combination of root canal filling material and sealer.

The susceptibility of a polycaprolactone-based root canal filling material (Resilon) to degradation has been investigated. Tay et al.[106] examined what effect alkaline hydrolysis would have on disks of Resilon or gutta-percha using scanning electron microscopy and energy dispersive X-ray analysis. They found that for Resilon, the surface resinous component was hydrolyzed after 20 minutes of immersion in sodium ethoxide, which exposed the spherulitic polymer structure and subsurface glass and bismuth oxychloride fillers. Gutta-percha did not undergo alkaline hydrolysis when immersed in sodium ethoxide.

Tay et al.[107] evaluated the susceptibility of Resilon, gutta-percha, and polycaprolactone disks to hydrolytic enzymes present in saliva or secreted by endodontically-relevant bacteria. All three materials had slight weight gains when incubated in phosphate-buffered saline. Gutta-percha showed similar weight gains with the enzymes, lipase polysaccharide, and cholesterol esterase, but Resilon and polycaprolactone exhibited extensive surface thinning and weight loss after incubation in lipase polysaccharide and cholesterol esterase. Glass filler particles in Resilon were exposed following surface dissolution of the polymer matrix, which created a rough surface topography. They concluded that biodegradation of Resilon by bacterial and salivary enzymes warrants further investigation.

The interfacial strengths of Resilon with Epiphany sealer have been compared with those of gutta-percha with AH Plus sealer by Gesi et al.[108] The gutta-percha/AH Plus testing group exhibited significantly higher interfacial strength than did the Resilon/Epiphany group, when premature failures that occurred in Resilon root slices were included. The gutta-percha root slices failed exclusively along the gutta-percha/sealer interface. The Resilon root slices failed predominantly along the sealer/dentin interface with recognizable, fractured resin tags. Detachment of Resilon from the Epiphany sealer was also observed in some specimens. The relatively low interfacial strengths of materials, gutta-percha/AH Plus, and Resilon/Epiphany seemed to challenge the concept that root strengthening is accomplished with either material.

Stratton et al.[109] looked at the sealing ability of Resilon and Epiphany sealer versus that of gutta-percha and AH Plus sealer, by means of fluid filtration testing. They found significantly less leakage using Resilon and Epiphany as compared with the gutta-percha and AH Plus sealer.

Another study found Resilon with Epiphany sealer had less leakage after 30 days than gutta-percha and sealer. All canals obturated with gutta-percha and sealer, and those obturated with Resilon or gutta-percha without sealer leaked within 30 days.[110]

Wang et al.[111] investigated the effects of calcium hydroxide medication on the sealing ability of Resilon and found that calcium hydroxide did not adversely affect the seal of the root canal system that was subsequently filled with Resilon.

In an investigation comparing the completeness of root canal obturation with gutta-percha techniques versus Resilon with Epiphany sealer, using lateral compaction and continuous wave obturation, results showed that lateral compaction of gutta-percha was the only group with significantly more voids than gutta-percha with the continuous wave obturation, or Resilon with Epiphany sealer using either obturation technique.[112]

Resilon has been reported to reinforce the root canal system because of its adhesion to the canal wall and integration of the core material.[113] On the other hand, another study compared cohesive strength and the stiffness of Resilon and gutta-percha under dry conditions and after 1 month of water storage, to determine whether they are stiff enough to reinforce roots. They found that both Resilon and gutta-percha had relatively low cohesive strength and modulus of elasticity, and did not have enough stiffness to reinforce roots after endodontic therapy.[114]

Long-term results and clinical trials will be useful in the evaluation of Resilon as compared with gutta-percha, and the evolution of newer generations of Resilon may further improve the material.

Paste Filling Materials

Zinc oxide is a major component of many paste materials used in endodontics. It is the other ingredients in many zinc oxide paste materials that are responsible for other properties and potential toxicity. These pastes will be discussed under the pastes containing other ingredients. Because of the solubility of zinc oxide, they do not make effective core filling materials.

A paste filling material that has been widely used in Eastern European countries and some Asian and Pacific Rim nations is a resin type of material known as "Russian Red."[115] This is resorcin–formaldehyde paste, a type of phenol–formaldehyde or Bakelite resin.[101] Ørstavik[101] reported it is strongly antimicrobial, but with the disadvantage of shrinkage in the canal once placed, and that it often stains tooth structure a dark red. Sometimes re-treatments can be difficult, if the resin sets completely and there is sufficient bulk to the material.[115]

Trailement SPAD is another resin-based type of paste material that has been used in Europe.

Mineral Trioxide Aggregate

Mineral trioxide aggregate (MTA) has many uses in endodontics (Figure 9). MTA is used as a pulp-capping material,[116–118] as a perforation repair agent,[119–122] as a root-end filling material,[123–125] as an apical barrier,[126–128] and as an intraorifice barrier,[129] and

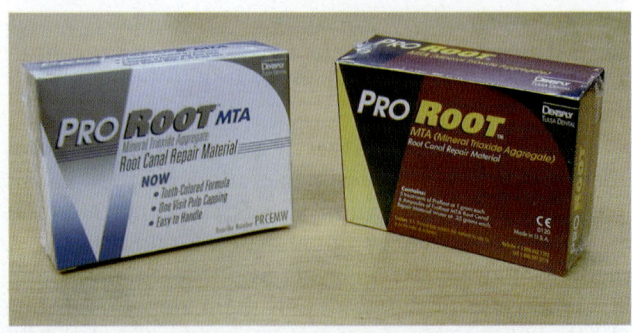

Figure 9 White and gray ProRoot mineral trioxide aggregate (MTA) by Tulsa Dentsply. Reproduced with permission of Tulsa Dentsply.

may be considered as a paste filling material for the obturation of root canals. Because of its sealing ability, biocompatibility, and other desirable properties, it would seem to be a paste filling material that is indicated when more conventional core filling materials cannot be used. The major drawbacks of MTA are its somewhat difficult handling characteristics, which may be overcome with experience, and its extended setting time of at least 3 hours or more. Its many favorable properties and characteristics make it a valuable material in many aspects of endodontics.

ProRoot MTA (Tulsa Dental Products, Tulsa, OK) was introduced by Torabinejad et al.[123] in 1993 as a root-end filling material and as a root perforation repair material.[119] They reported the ingredients as tricalcium silicate, tricalcium aluminate, tricalcium oxide, and silicate oxide, with some other mineral oxides that were responsible for the chemical and physical properties of the aggregate. The powder consists of fine hydrophilic particles that set in the presence of moisture. The hydration of the powder results in a colloidal gel with a pH of 12.5 that will set in approximately 4 hours.[130]

Several studies have stated that MTA is very similar in nature to commercial Portland cement.[131–135] Wucherpfenning and Green[132] analyzed MTA and Portland cement by X-ray diffraction and reported that they were similar macroscopically and microscopically. Estrela et al.[133] showed that Portland cement contains the same chemical elements as MTA, with the exception of bismuth oxide, which is added to MTA to increase its radiopacity. Duarte et al.[136] reported that MTA Angelus is 80% Portland cement and 20% bismuth oxide. Sarkar et al.[137] stated that MTA is a mechanical mixture of three powder ingredients, which are Portland cement (75%), bismuth oxide (20%), and gypsum (5%), with trace amounts of SiO_2, CaO, MgO, K_2SO_4, and Na_2SO_4. They also listed the ingredients of the major component, Portland cement, as dicalcium silicate, tricalcium silicate, tricalcium aluminate, and tetracalcium aluminoferrite.

One of the very favorable properties of MTA is its outstanding sealing ability. This has been verified in many studies using MTA as a root-end filling material and for sealing perforations in both dye leakage and bacterial leakage models. Torabinejad et al.[123] using an aqueous solution of rhodamine B fluorescent dye found MTA leaked significantly less than amalgam or ethoxybenzoic acid (Super EBA) as a root-end filling material. In another dye study, Torabinejad et al.[138] found MTA sealed better as a root-end filling material than amalgam, Intermediate Restorative Material (IRM), or Super EBA, even in the presence of blood contamination. Gondim et al.[139] demonstrated, with a dye study, that MTA leaked significantly less than Super EBA or IRM, regardless of the finishing technique employed. In a bacterial leakage investigation of root-end filling materials, Torabinejad et al.[140] showed that MTA leaked significantly less than the other root-end filling materials tested. MTA was also found to allow less leakage of endotoxin in a study by Tang et al.[141] Tselnik et al.[129] examined bacterial leakage with MTA or a resin-modified glass ionomer as a coronal barrier. They found both gray and white MTA, when used as a coronal barrier, prevented microbial leakage for over 90 days. Nakata and coworkers[121] found that MTA provided a better seal than amalgam to prevent the leakage of *F. nucleatum* into furcation perforations.

In a SEM study, Torabinejad et al.[142] showed that MTA had better marginal adaptation than amalgam, Super EBA or IRM. Other studies using the SEM have agreed with these findings with regard to MTA adaptation.[143,144] Xavier et al.[145] examined both dye leakage and marginal adaptation as viewed under the SEM and found that MTA Angelus leaked significantly less than a glass ionomer, but statistically more than Super EBA. They found that MTA Angelus had much better marginal adaptation than EBA, or the glass ionomer when viewed under the SEM. Mangin et al.[146] found no difference in leakage of radioactive labeled bacteria between hydroxyapatite cement, MTA, and Super EBA when used as root-end filling materials.

In a fluid filtration model, Bates et al.[147] found MTA was comparable with Super EBA in the prevention of leakage, but Wu et al.[148] reported MTA leaked significantly less than Super EBA. DeBruyne et al.[149] using a fluid transport and capillary flow porometry technique found that after 1 day, and after 1 month there was no statistical significant difference in leakage between a reinforced glass ionomer cement and white MTA in root-end fillings. At 6 months, however, the glass ionomer leaked significantly less than MTA. There were no significant differences observed with flow porometry between pore diameters of the materials tested.

The effects of the thickness and of resection of MTA have been investigated. Andelin et al.[150] examined leakage after the resection of MTA placed in canals before the root end was resected and found that the resection of set MTA did not affect its sealing ability. Lamb et al.[151] had similar findings, as long as at least 3 mm of MTA remained. Valois et al.[152] examined the influence of thickness of MTA on the sealing ability of the material and showed that a 4 mm thickness of MTA was significantly more effective in preventing protein leakage than lesser thicknesses of MTA. Matt et al.[153] found that for an apical barrier, 5 mm of MTA was significantly harder than a 2 mm barrier, and allowed significantly less leakage. These dimensions may be important, not only in the depth of root-end fillings with MTA but when it is used as an apical barrier, or as a perforation repair material, or for other purposes.

MTA has been studied extensively for its biocompatibility with its application as a root-end filling material in root-end endodontic surgery. Cell culture studies have demonstrated that the cytotoxicity of MTA was significantly less than that of IRM or Super EBA.[154] Implantation of MTA into tibias and mandibles of guinea pigs resulted in a tissue reaction considered favorable and slightly milder than that of Super EBA.[155] Koh et al.[156] found favorable biologic responses to MTA from human osteoblasts, and favorable cellular response to MTA.[157]

Haglund et al.[158] compared MTA, amalgam, IRM, and a composite resin for their effects on mouse fibroblasts and macrophages. They found all four materials inhibited cell growth. There were significantly fewer cells cultured with the fresh IRM and composite groups compared with the MTA and amalgam groups, and there was no difference between a fresh mix of MTA and a fresh mix of amalgam. For set materials, there was no significant differences in the fibroblast cell growth between MTA, amalgam, and the composite resin. In the fibroblast cell line, set IRM had significalntly fewer surviving cells than the other set materials. There was a significant difference in the survival of cells in the macrophage cell line in the presence of the set materials between the composite resin group and MTA, and between the composite resin group and amalgam, with fewer macrophages surviving in the presence of the composite resin set material. Set IRM had significantly fewer cells survive than the other set material in the macrophage cell line also. DeDeus et al.[159] compared the cytotoxicity of ProRoot MTA, MTA Angelus, and Portland cement and found no significant difference between the three materials in terms of cytotoxicity and that all three initially showed similar elevated cytotoxic effects that decreased gradually with time, allowing the cell culture to become reestablished.

Hernandez et al.[160] studied the effect of mixing chlorhexidine with MTA versus MTA mixed with water on the apoptosis and cell cycle of fibroblasts and macrophages. They found that mixing MTA with chlorhexidine induced apoptosis of fibroblasts and macrophages and decreased the percentage of both cell types in the S phase (DNA synthesis) of cell cycles. Thus, mixing sterile water with MTA was determined to be less cytotoxic than mixing MTA with chlorhexidine. Melegari et al.[161] studied the production of prostaglandin E_2 (PGE_2) and the viability of cells cultured in contact with freshly mixed Roth's 801 sealer, Sealapex sealer, and MTA. It was found that none of the materials stimulated the release of PGE_2.

MTA is also reported to have qualities that may provide an environment for repair and regeneration of periapical tissues. MTA has shown an inductive effect on cementoblasts in dogs and monkeys.[124,125] Zhu et al.[162] showed osteoblasts attaching and spreading on MTA. Regan et al.[163] demonstrated that both MTA and Diaket can support almost complete regeneration of the periradicular periodontium when used as a root-end filling material on teeth that are not infected. Baek et al.[164] found that MTA showed the most favorable periapical tissue response and that there was neoformation of cemental coverage over MTA.

There is conflicting information as to whether gray and white MTA have the same physical properties and biocompatibility. Holland et al.[135,165,166] have shown that both white and gray formulations are biocompatible when implanted into rat connective tissue. Perez et al.[167] demonstrated that white MTA was less biocompatible than gray MTA. Camilleri et al.[168] showed no difference between the gray and white formulations of MTA. Ribeiro et al.[169] showed no difference in cytotoxic effects for gray MTA, white MTA, or Portland cement. The same group found no difference in genotoxicity or cytotoxicity between gray or white MTA.[170] Asgary et al.[171] by electron probe microanalysis observed that the concentrations of Al_2O_3, MgO, and particularly FeO in white MTA are considerably lower than those found in gray MTA. The FeO is thought to be the primary ingredient responsible for the color differences between white and gray MTA. Oviir et al.[172] investigated the proliferation of oral keratinocytes and cementoblasts on gray and white MTA. They found both cell types grew significantly better on the surface of white MTA compared with gray MTA. In addition, both cell types showed significantly higher proliferation when grown on 12-day-cured gray MTA compared with 24-hour-cured gray MTA. Matt et al.[153] found that white MTA leaked significantly more than did gray MTA and that a two-step technique, where a moist cotton pellet is placed over the MTA for 24 hours to allow it to set, showed less leakage than a one-step technique for placing an apical barrier.

There is some conflicting opinion as to whether a moist cotton pellet is needed to allow the MTA to set properly when used within the root canal system, other than as a root-end filling material where it is in contact with moisture. This step adds another appointment to the treatment when MTA is used as a perforation repair material, as an apical barrier, or as an intraorifice barrier. There have been case reports where a moist cotton pellet is used between appointments to allow for the MTA to set.[126–128] On the other hand, Sluyk et al.[173] showed that the retention characteristics of MTA used as a perforation repair material was not altered by the placement of either a dry or a moist cotton pellet over the MTA, and the moisture from the periradicular tissues may provide adequate moisture to allow the MTA to set properly. Matt et al.[153] did show, however, that the application of a moist cotton pellet significantly reduced leakage of MTA used as an apical barrier.

The long-term solubility of MTA was investigated by Fridland et al.[174] Their results showed that MTA is capable of partially releasing its soluble fraction into an aqueous environment over a long period of time and it still maintains its high pH level of 11 to 12 over at least 78 days, while also maintaining its insoluble matrix of silica which produces MTA's structural integrity even while in contact with water. This soluble fraction is mainly composed of calcium hydroxide, which may provide the alkalinity favorable for cell division and matrix formation for healing of periradicular tissues and for antimicrobial activity. Sarkar et al.[137] speculated that after placement of MTA in root canals and its gradual dissolution, hydroxyapatite crystals nucleate and grow, filling the microscopic space between MTA and the dentinal wall. This seal is first mechanical, but then they envision a reaction between the apatite layer and the dentin in the form of a chemical bond, and a seal between MTA and dentin.

Some investigators are looking into modifications of Portland type cements to alter the setting properties and handling characteristics. One of the main disadvantages of using MTA is its extended setting time. In industrial uses of Portland cement, the setting time may be increased by adding gypsum or reduced to a flash set by removing gypsum. Camilleri et al.[175] investigated a new accelerated Portland cement. The setting time of the Portland cement was reduced by excluding gypsum in the last stage of the manufacturing process. The biocompatibility testing of this accelerated Portland cement was not altered by adding bismuth oxide for radiopacity and had similar biocompatibility as gray MTA, white MTA, and white Portland cement. Future research will have to determine whether altering the undesirable aspects of MTA can be accomplished without affecting its very desirable properties of sealing, biocompatibility, and favorable conditions for repair and regeneration of periradicular tissues.

Paraformaldehyde Pastes

Paraformaldehyde pastes may also be considered as sealers, and are used as sealers by some. The addition of paraformaldehyde is for its antimicrobial and mummifying effects, but unfortunately its severe toxicity to host tissues outweighs any antimicrobial effects it may possess as an ingredient in endodontic materials.

N2 paste (Indrag-Agsa, Losone, Switzerland) and its US counterpart, RC2B, is a liquid and powder paste. The powder contains zinc oxide, bismuth nitrate, bismuth carbonate, paraformaldehyde, and titanium oxide. The liquid consists of eugenol, peanut oil, and rose oil.[176] The contents of N2 have changed over the years in response to studies identifying toxic substances, such as lead oxide and organic mercury.[177] It still contains large amounts of paraformaldehyde (4–8%).[86] N2 has been found to be extremely toxic.[178,179] Furthermore, because it is used as a paste, the extrusion of this toxic material is easier and has caused severe neurological damage in reported cases.[180–183] The Food and Drug Administration (FDA) lists N2 or RC2B as an unapproved new drug not legally imported or shipped across interstate lines.[184] The American Dental Association (ADA) Council of Dental Therapeutics does not approve the use of paraformaldehyde pastes or sealers. A case report of a dentist who was found liable for a patient's permanent disability as a result of root canal therapy with N2 (Sargenti's) paste was presented in the status report. The canal was obturated with N2, which reportedly extruded into the mandibular canal causing nerve damage, facial dysesthesia, and pain. The patient was awarded $250,000 (US) for injury.[185]

The American Association of Endodontists has issued a position paper on the use of paraformaldehyde-containing endodontic materials, recommending against their use.[186] Some states, including Florida, have banned the use of paraformaldehyde pastes.[187] Because of the toxicity, legal issues, risks to patients, and the fact there are numerous other obturating materials available that provide a better outcome, without risk to the patient, the use of these materials in modern-day endodontics cannot be supported.

Endomethasone (Septodont, Paris, France) is a liquid-powder sealer used in Europe. The powder contains dexamethasone, hydrocortisone acetate, thymol iodide, paraformaldehyde, and a radiopaque excipient, whereas the liquid contains eugenol, peppermint oil, and Anise oil.[176] The difference between Endomethasone and other paraformaldehyde-containing sealers is the addition of the hydrocortisone. The toxicity of the paraformaldehyde still remains.

Riebler's paste (Amubarut; Wera Karl, Biesingen, Germany) is another paraformaldehyde-containing paste as is *Trailement SPAD*, another resin-based type of paste material that has been used in Europe.

Sealers

REQUIREMENTS FOR AN IDEAL ROOT CANAL SEALING MATERIAL

In addition to the basic requirements for core filling materials, Grossman also listed the following 11 requirements for a root canal sealer:[188,189]

1. It should be tacky when mixed to provide good adhesion between it and the canal wall when set.
2. It should make a hermetic seal.
3. It should be radiopaque so it can be visualized in the radiograph.
4. The particles of powder should be very fine so they can mix easily with the liquid.
5. It should not shrink upon setting.
6. It should not stain tooth structure.
7. It should be bacteriostatic or at least not encourage bacterial growth.
8. It should set slowly.
9. It should be insoluble in tissue fluids.
10. It should be tissue tolerant, that is, nonirritating to periradicular tissues.
11. It should be soluble in a common solvent, if it is necessary to remove the root canal filling.

One might add the following to Grossman's original basic requirements:

12. It should not provoke an immune response in periradicular tissues.[190–193]
13. It should be neither mutagenic nor carcinogenic.[194,195]

Zinc Oxide-Containing Sealers

For many years, zinc oxide-containing sealers have been the most popular and widely used sealers. There are many formulations and brands of sealers that have zinc oxide as the primary ingredient, differing only by other components added to the sealers.

Zinc oxide sealers allow for addition of other chemicals, such as paraformaldehyde, rosin, Canada balsam, and others, all of which may increase their toxicity.[86] Zinc oxide-containing sealers that have other ingredients will be discussed under those sections.

Grossman's original formula contained zinc oxide, staybelite resin, bismuth subcarbonate, barium sulfate, and sodium borate (anhydrous) with eugenol as the liquid component.[188] It has been marketed as Procosol sealer, as well as other product names.

Roth's 801 sealer (Roth's Pharmacy, Chicago, IL) is essentially the same as Grossman's original formulation, with the substitution of bismuth subnitrate for bismuth subcarbonate. Eugenol is used as the liquid of the sealer (Figure 10).

Rickert's formula was an early zinc oxide-containing sealer. It has long been an acceptable standard, meeting most of Grossman's requirements for an ideal sealer. Its major drawback was the staining of tooth structure from the silver that was used for radiopacity.[16] Rickert's formula was marketed as Kerr's Pulp Canal Sealer (Sybron Endo/Kerr, Orange, CA). Pulp Canal Sealer has been popularized by clinicians using the warm vertical obturation techniques. A major disadvantage of Pulp Canal Sealer was its rapid setting time, especially with heat and in regions with high temperatures and high humidity.[16] To overcome this disadvantage, researchers formulated Pulp Canal Sealer EWT (Extended Working Time) (Sybron

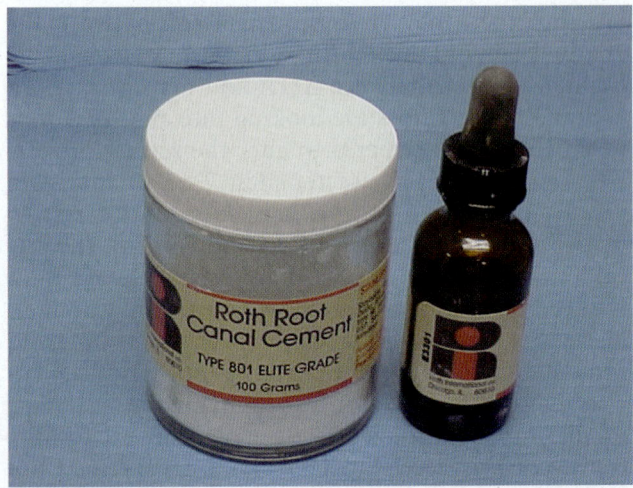

Figure 10 Roth Root Canal Cement is an example of a zinc oxide and eugenol sealer. Courtesy, James David Johnson.

Endo/Kerr) which reportedly has a working time of 6 hours.[16]

Tubli-Seal (Sybron Endo/Kerr) is a two-paste system contained in two separate tubes. Developed as a nonstaining alternative to the silver-containing Pulp Canal Sealer, Tubli-Seal is a zinc oxide-base paste with barium sulfate for radiopacity, and mineral oil, cornstarch, and lecithin. The catalyst tube has polypale resin, eugenol, and thymol iodide. Tubli-Seal is easy to mix but has the disadvantage of rapid setting time.[16] Tubli-Seal EWT has the same properties as the regular setting Tubli-Seal but has an extended working time.

Wach's cement (Roth International Inc., Chicago, IL) consists of a powder of zinc oxide, bismuth subnitrate, bismuth subiodide, magnesium oxide, and calcium phosphate. The liquid contains oil of cloves, eucalyptol, Canada balsam, and beechwood creosote. The liquid gives Wach's cement a rather distinctive odor of an old-time dental office.[16] It has the advantage of having a smooth consistency, and the Canada balsam makes the sealer tacky.

Nogenol (GC America, Inc., Alsip, IL) was developed to overcome the irritating effects of eugenol.[196] This product is an extension of the noneugenol periodontal dressings. It is a two-tube, base and catalyst system with a base of zinc oxide, barium sulfate, bismuth oxychloride, and vegetable oil. Hydrogenated rosin, methyl abietate, lauric acid, chlorothymol, and salicylic acid in the catalyst accelerate the setting time.[16]

Medicated Canal Sealer (Medidenta International, Inc.) was developed by Martin.[15] This sealer contains iodoform for antibacterial purposes and is to be used with MGP gutta-percha, which also contains 10% iodoform.[16]

Calcium Hydroxide-Containing Sealers

Sealapex (Sybron Endo/Kerr) is a calcium hydroxide-containing noneugenol polymeric sealer that is packaged as two tubes. Sealapex has zinc oxide in the base along with calcium hydroxide and also contains butyl benzene, sulfonamide, and zinc stearate. The catalyst tube has barium sulfate and titanium dioxide for radiopacity, and a proprietary resin, isobutyl salicylate, and aerocil R792.[16] Sealapex had no greater dissolution than Tubli-Seal at both 2 and 32 weeks. It appears that Sealapex had a sealing ability comparable with Tubli-Seal and could withstand long-term leakage.[197]

Holland and De Souza[198] studied Sealapex sealer to see if it could induce hard tissue formation. Sealapex with calcium hydroxide did encourage apical closure by cementum deposition. Closure was also observed in the control groups (5%) and in Kerr Pulp Canal Sealer groups (10%), but was associated with dentin chips that also stimulate cementum formation. Both Sealapex and Kerr Pulp Canal Sealer, when overextended, provoke a chronic inflammatory reaction in the periodontal ligament (PDL).

Apexit (Ivoclar Vivadent, Schaan, Liechtenstein) is a calcium hydroxide sealer with salicylates also incorporated into the formula.

CRCS (Calciobiotic Root Canal Sealer; Coltene/Whaledent/Hygenic, Mahwah, NJ) is a calcium hydroxide-containing sealer with a zinc oxide–eugenol–eucalyptol base. CRCS is a rather slow setting sealer, especially in dry or in humid climates. It may require up to 3 days to fully set.[16] The set sealer is quite stable, which improves its sealing qualities, but may mean that calcium hydroxide is not as readily released, and the stimulation of cementum and bone formation may be severely limited.

Beltes et al.[199] did an in vitro evaluation of cytotoxicity of calcium hydroxide-based root canal sealers. Sealapex was the most cytotoxic, followed by CRCS, with Apexit being the least cytotoxic with the least decrease in cell density.

Siqueira et al.[200] investigated the sealing ability, pH, and flow rate of three calcium hydroxide-based sealers (Sealapex, Sealer 26, and Apexit). There was no significant difference found between apical sealing ability and dye penetration. All calcium hydroxide sealers alkalinized adjacent tissues. Sealer 26 had significantly superior flow characteristics. They concluded calcium hydroxide sealers compare favorably with zinc oxide and eugenol (ZOE) cements for use in obturation.

Vitapex (NEO Dental International, Inc, Federal Way, WA) is a sealer, which was developed in Japan, and contains, not only calcium hydroxide, but also 40% iodoform and silicone oil among other ingredients.

Resin Sealers

Epoxy resin sealers have an established record in endodontics, especially in the form of AH 26 and its successor AH Plus (Dentsply International, York, PA).

AH 26 (Dentsply International/Maillefer) is a bisphenol epoxy resin sealer that uses hexamethylenetetramine (methenamine) for polymerization and has been used for many years as a sealer.[101,201] The methenamine will give off some formaldehyde as it sets, and this has been one of its major drawbacks. The highest amount of formaldehyde release is in the freshly mixed sealer, and the amount of formaldehyde

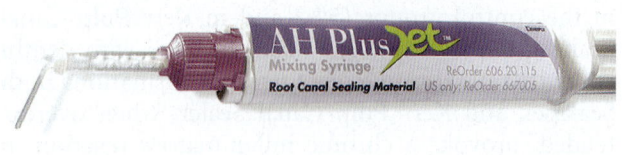

Figure 11 AH Plus Root Canal Sealer by Tulsa Dentsply is a resin type sealer shown here in a mixing syringe. Reproduced with permission of Tulsa Dentsply.

released goes down after 48 hours, and after 2 weeks the amount released is insignificant.[202] The amount of formaldehyde produced during the setting process has been reported to be several thousand times lower than the long-term release from formaldehyde-containing sealers such as N2.[86,201] Other disadvantages are staining and an extended working time. On the other hand, AH 26 does not seem to be affected by moisture, and will even set under water.[16]

AH Plus and ThermaSeal Plus (Dentsply International) (Figure 11) were formulated with a mixture of amines that would allow for polymerization without the unwanted formation of formaldehyde,[201,203] but with all the advantages of AH 26, such as increased radiopacity, low solubility, slight shrinkage, and tissue compatibility. AH Plus is an epoxy–bis-phenol resin that also contains adamantine.[101] AH Plus comes as a two-paste system, unlike the liquid-powder system of AH 26. AH Plus has a working time of 4 hours and a setting time of 8 hours. Other improvements over the older AH 26 formulation are the thinner film thickness and the decreased solubility of AH Plus, both about half that of AH 26. AH Plus has been shown to be less cytotoxic than AH 26, but both caused a dose-dependent increase in genotoxicity.[176]

Epiphany (Pentron Clinical Technologies) or Real-Seal (Sybron Endo) is a sealer that contains urethane dimethacrylate (UDMA), Poly(ethylene glycol) dimethacrylates (PEGDMA), ethoxylated bisphenol A-dimethacrylate (EBPADMA), Bisphenol-A-glycidyl-dimethacrylate (BisGMA) resins designed for use with the polycaprolactone core materials. Additionally, these sealers contain silane-treated barium borosilicate glass, barium sulfate, silica, calcium hydroxide, bismuth oxychloride with amines, peroxide, a photo inhibitor, and pigments. Epiphany sealer is a dual-cure dental resin composite sealer that self-cures in about 25 minutes. It comes with a self-etch primer with sulfonic acid-terminated functional monomer, Hydroxyethylmethacrylate (HEMA), water, and polymerization initiator. Sodium hypochlorite may negatively affect bond strength of the primer, so after using sodium hypochlorite for irrigation, one should irrigate with ethylenediaminetetraacetic acid (EDTA) and sterile water. Peroxide-containing lubricants might also have a retarding effect on the resins, so a final rinse with EDTA and sterile water is recommended after using these lubricants. Chlorhexidine does not affect the bond strength. When obturation is completed, the coronal surface may be light-cured for 40 seconds to create a coronal seal.

In a study comparing Epiphany sealer with AH Plus and EndoREZ sealers for intraosseous biocompatibility for 4 and 12 weeks, as recommended by the Technical Report 9 of the Federation Dentaire Internationale (FDI), Sousa et al.[204] found the inflammatory tissue reaction to EndoREZ was severe and the AH Plus inflammatory reaction went from severe to moderate with time, whereas Epiphany showed biological compataibility in regard to bone formation, and it also produced either no, or very slight inflammation.

In a direct comparison of physical and chemical properties of AH Plus and Epiphany sealers, Versiani et al.[205] found there was no significant difference in flow or film thickness between AH Plus and Epiphany sealers. There was a statistical difference between the two with the solubility of Epiphany being 3.41% versus 0.21% for AH Plus, and for dimensional stability, there was also a statistical difference with AH Plus expanding 1.3% on setting and Epiphany expanding 8.1% following setting. The setting time, flow, and film thickness tests for both cements conformed to American National Standards Institute (ANSI)/ADA standards. Dimensional alteration tests for both sealers were greater than values considered acceptable by ANSI/ADA standards, and the values for Epiphany sealer with regard to solubility were also greater than values considered acceptable by ANSI/ADA.

Ungor et al.[206] evaluated the push-out bond strength of the Epiphany–Resilon root canal filling system with the bond strengths of different pairings of AH Plus, gutta-percha, Epiphany, and Resilon. Their results showed that Epiphany with gutta-percha had significantly greater bond strength than all the other groups. There was no significant difference between the Epiphany with Resilon combination and the AH Plus with gutta-percha. Inspection of the surfaces revealed the bond failure to be mainly adhesive to dentin for all groups.

Diaket (3M/ESPE, Minneapolis, MN) has been a popular sealer in Europe for many years and is a polyketone compound containing vinyl polymers mixed with zinc oxide and bismuth phosphate.[86] Diaket is a sealer that sets by chelation, but it contains polyvinyl chloride in polymer form as a main ingredient.[101] It has a liquid component of B-diketone. It is a tacky material that contracts upon setting, but this is offset by its absorption of water.[16] It has done well in in-vitro tests, including biocompatibility studies.[101] Studies have shown that after initial mild tissue reactions, and after longer times of 2 weeks or more, there seems to be a decrease in tissue irritation.[207–209] Ørstavik and Mjör[210] reported that Diaket demonstrated good biocompatibility compared with other sealers.

Eldeniz et al.[211] evaluated the shear bond strength of three resin-based sealers (Diaket, AH Plus, and EndoREZ) to dentin with and without the smear layer. Bond strength of root canal sealers to dentin is an important property for the integrity of the sealing of root canals. A significant difference was found among the bond strength of the sealers, smear layer, and control groups. AH Plus sealer showed the highest bond strength in smear layer-free surfaces, and had the strongest bond to dentin with the smear layer intact.

Glass Ionomer-Based Sealers

There are currently no glass ionomer sealers being marketed. Ketac-Endo (3M, Minneapolis, MN) is mentioned here because it appears in many studies as a comparative sealer.

Silicone-Based Sealers

Silicone-based sealers utilize the same qualities as caulking compounds used in household construction around kitchen and bathroom structures providing adhesion, a moisture-resistant seal, and stability.[101]

Lee Endo-Fill (Lee Pharmaceuticals, El Monte, CA) is an example of a silicone-based root canal sealer.

RoekoSeal (Roeko/Coltene/Whaledent, Langenau, Germany) is a polyvinylsiloxane that is a white paste-like sealer.[212] RoekoSeal is reported to polymerize without shrinkage and utilizes platinum as a catalyzing agent.[101]

Wu et al.[213] reported a 1-year follow-up study on leakage, using a fluid transport model, of single-cone fillings with RoekoRSA sealer. The apical filling in all roots did not show leakage either at 1 week or at 1 year.

GuttaFlow (Roeko/Coltene/Whaledent) is a polyvinylsiloxane with finely milled gutta-percha particles added to the RoekoSeal sealer. GuttaFlow also contains silicone oil, paraffin oil, platin catalyst, zirconium dioxide, nano-silver as a preservative, and a coloring agent. It is eugenol free. It is a cold flowable gutta-percha filling system for the obturation of root canals. GuttaFlow is triturated in its cannula and passively injected into the canal and then used with single or multiple gutta-percha points.

Solvent-Based Sealers

The use of chloroform or solvent-based sealers was popularized by Johnston and Callahan.[214] The technique is still practiced today with various types of chloroform sealers, including chloropercha and Kloropercha N-Ø. Gutta-percha particles are added to the chloroform to produce a sealer, which has the same color as gutta-percha. The mixture can then be used as a sealer with gutta-percha points for obturation of the canal. There is more shrinkage with the chloroform solvent techniques, and this often translates into leakage, with the material pulling away from the canal walls as it shrinks creating voids through which leakage may occur.[215]

Chlororosin lateral condensation uses 5% to 8% rosin in chloroform, which leaves a very adhesive residue.

Chloropercha is white gutta-percha with chloroform and has no adhesive properties.

Kloropercha N-Ø contains additional resin, plus Canada balsam, that adds adhesive property to the material.

Urethane Methacrylate Sealers

EndoRez (Ultradent, South Jordon, UT) is a hydrophilic UDMA resin sealer that reportedly has good canal wetting and flow into dentinal tubules.[212] The hydrophilic property improves its sealing abilities, if some moisture is still in the canal at obturation.[101] EndoRez is introduced into the canal with a narrow 30-gauge Navitip needle (Ultradent). A single gutta-percha point technique or the lateral compaction obturation technique may be used.

EndoRez resin-coated gutta-percha is also marketed, which reportedly chemically bonds to the EndoRez sealer and works with all resin-based sealers. EndoRez points come in ISO standard sizes.

Tay et al.[216] investigated the effectiveness of obturating root canals with the polybutadiene–diisocyanate–methacrylate resin-coated gutta-percha (EndoREZ). This enables the polyisoprene in the gutta-percha to chemically couple with the methacrylate-based resin sealer (EndoREZ). This study examined the effectiveness of using passively fitting resin-coated gutta-percha points with the dual-cured version of EndoREZ sealer. It was found that the hydrophilic nature of the sealer enabled the creation of an extensive network of 800 to 1200 μm long sealer resin tags after removal of the endodontic smear layer. Still there were interfacial gaps and silver leakage could be observed along the sealer–dentin interfaces. This was primarily attributed to polymerization shrinkage of the sealer. Gaps and silver leakage was also seen between the resin-coated gutta-percha and the sealer.

The shear strength of EndoREZ to resin-coated gutta-percha was examined, and it was also examined whether shear strength is improved by creating an oxygen inhibition resin layer via the application of a dual-cured dentin adhesive to resin-coated gutta-percha.[217] The authors concluded that in-situ dentin adhesive application may be valuable in enhancing the coupling of resin-coated gutta-percha to methacrylate sealers.

A study of bone response to the methacrylate-based sealer, EndoREZ, revealed, that at 10 days after placement, the amount of reactionary bone formation in direct contact with EndoREZ was significantly less than that observed with the controls, and the number of inflammatory cells next to the EndoREZ sealer was significantly higher than the controls. However, after 60 days, no differences were noted between the experimental and control groups. This indicated that the sealer produces a response similar to that of many sealers.[218] Zmener et al.[219] looked at the apical seal produced with the methacrylate-based sealer (EndoREZ) and Grossman's sealer. Three groups were evaluated. The first combination of materials and techniques was a single gutta-percha point with the methacrylate sealer, the second was lateral compaction with the methacrylate sealer, and the third technique was gutta-percha with Grossman's sealer. The results demonstrated that the dye penetration in the two methacrylate sealer groups occurred at the sealer–dentin or sealer–gutta-percha interface. In the Grossman's sealer group, the dye leakage occurred at both interfaces, and throughout the mass.

EZ Fill (Essential Dental Systems, South Hackensack, NJ) is a noneugenol epoxy resin sealer that is placed with a bidirectional spiral, rotating in a handpiece, and used with a single gutta-percha point tech-

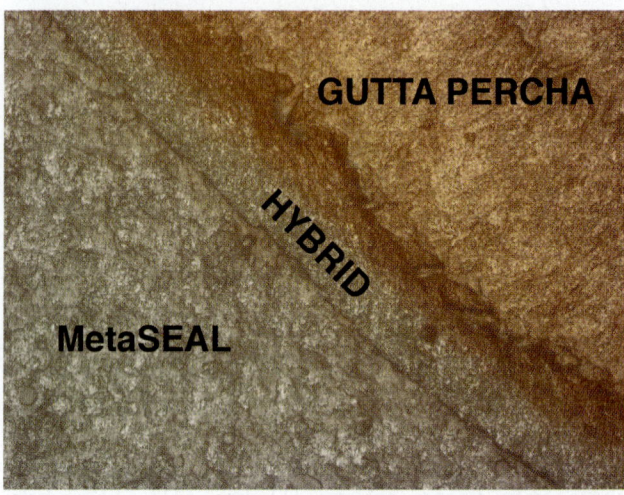

Figure 12 Micrograph showing hybrid bond between MetaSEAL and gutta-percha by penetration of the gutta-percha. Courtesy, Parkell.

nique. The spiral is designed to spread the sealer laterally in the apical region of the canal. It is reportedly nonshrinking on setting and is hydrophobic in nature, making it resistant to fluid degradation. One study has shown EZ fill to seal as well as other techniques.[220] Favorable clinical outcomes have also been reported.[212,222]

MetaSEAL (Parkell, Inc., Edgewood, NY) marketed in the United States and Canada is a thinner version of 4-Meta, used for years as a restorative sealer. Belli et al.[223] compared MetaSEAL for leakage against Epiphany/Real Seal and AH Plus and found it to show significantly lower leakage after the first week. After 4 and 12 weeks, there was no significant difference among the groups. MetaSEAL's self-etching formula hybridizes the canal wall preventing leakage and bonds to gutta-percha (Figure 12) and Resilon.

Paraformaldehyde-Containing Sealers (Riebler's)

Reibler's paste is a paraformaldehyde-containing sealer and was discussed earlier under paraformaldehyde-containing paste materials.

Evaluation and Comparison of Sealers

Ørstavik[101,224] has listed the various evaluation parameters for testing endodontic sealers. They include technologic tests standardized by the ADA/ANSI in the United States, and the ISO internationally. These technologic tests include flow, working time, setting time, radiopacity, solubility and disintegration, and dimensional change following setting. Additionally, biologic tests, usage testing, and antibacterial testing are useful. Clinical testing should be included to establish outcomes of treatment.

LEAKAGE

The influence of root canal shape (curved or straight) on the sealing ability of sealers has been studied in a fluid transport model.[225] Canals were laterally compacted with gutta-percha with either Pulp Canal Sealer or Sealapex sealer. It was found that Sealapex allowed more leakage than Pulp Canal Sealer at 1 year. The authors concluded that canal form affects sealing ability at 1 month, but the sealer affects the quality of seal at 1 year.

The sealing ability of four sealers was evaluated quantitatively by Cobankara et al.[226] The sealers tested were Rocanal, a zinc oxide–eugenol powder-liquid system; AH Plus, an epoxy resin-based sealer; Sealapex, a calcium hydroxide-based sealer; and RC Sealer, an adhesive resin sealer. Apical leakage decreased gradually for all sealers from 7 to 21 days. Sealapex demonstrated better apical sealing than the other sealers, and AH Plus, RC Sealer, and Rocanal all showed similar apical leakage at every time period.

Another in vitro study evaluated the apical leakage, by a fluid filtration meter, of three root canal sealers, AH Plus, Diaket, and EndoREZ.[227] Statistical analysis indicated that root canal fillings with Diaket in combination with the cold lateral compaction technique showed less apical leakage than the other two sealers.

Saleh et al.[228] used the SEM and energy dispersive spectroscopy to evaluate the adhesion of sealers. The microscopic details of the debonded interfaces between endodontic sealers and dentin or gutta-percha were assessed in this study. Grossman's sealer, Apexit, Ketac-Endo, AH Plus, RoekoSeal Automix, and RoekoSeal Automix with an experimental primer were examined. After tensile bond strength testing, the morphologic aspects of the fractured surfaces were assessed. The energy-dispersive spectroscopy successfully traced sealer components to the debonded surfaces. Some of the sealers penetrated into the dentinal tubules when the dentin surface had been pretreated with acids. However, these sealer tags remained, occluding the tubules after bond failure in some instances only (Grossman's sealer, RoekoSeal Automix with an experimental primer, AH Plus/EDTA). Penetration of the endodontic sealers into the dentinal tubules, when the smear layer was removed, was not associated with higher bond strength.

Pommel et al.[229] examined the efficacy of four types of sealers in obtaining an impervious apical seal, and to correlate those seals with their adhesive properties. Pulp Canal Sealer, Sealapex, AH 26, and Ketac-Endo were the sealers evaluated. The results showed that teeth filled with Sealapex displayed higher apical leakage than the other sealers. No statistically significant difference was found between AH 26, Pulp Canal Sealer, and Ketac-Endo. No correlation was found between the sealing efficiency of the four sealers and their adhesive properties.

Lee et al.[230] investigated the adhesion of endodontic sealers to dentin and gutta-percha. The bond strength to the dentin of the four sealers gave the following order from lowest to highest: Kerr Sealer < Sealapex < Ketac-Endo < AH 26. The bond strengths to gutta-percha gave the following order from lowest to highest: Ketac-Endo < Sealapex < Kerr < AH 26. The bond between the Kerr Sealer and dentin all failed adhesively, whereas the Sealapex bonds failed cohesively (80%). AH 26 demonstrated no adhesive failures. The AH 26 gave the highest bond strength values to both dentin and gutta-percha. These finding suggest that the resin may not only react with the collagen to form bonds but react with gutta-percha as well.

In another study, Tagger et al.[231] showed AH 26 had a significantly stronger bond to gutta-percha than the remaining five sealers, including Roth's 801 and Sealapex.

TISSUE TOLERANCE

The cytotoxicity of RoekoSeal Automix and AH Plus was evaluated using human cervical carcinoma cells and mouse skin fibroblasts.[232] AH Plus was significantly more cytotoxic for both cell lines after 1 hour, 24 hours, and 48 hours, compared with the 7-day and 1-month setting periods. RoekoSeal had no cytotoxic effects on either cell line at any setting time.

Spångberg and Pascon[233] examined the cytotoxicity of seven endodontic sealers (Wach's, Grossman's, Tubli-Seal, AH 26, Nogenol, Diaket, and Endo-Fill). Evaluated as solid materials, Wach's Sealer, Grossman's Sealer, Tubli-Seal, and Diaket were the most toxic. Nogenol was less toxic and the least toxic materials were AH 26 and Lee Endo-Fill. When solubilized, however, Grossman's sealer, Tubli-Seal, and Endo-Fill had very low toxicity, Nogenol had low to medium toxicity, and AH 26, Diaket, and Wach's sealers were very toxic as liquids.

Economides et al.[234] investigated the biocompatibility of four root canal sealers (AH 26, Roth's 811, CRCS, and Sealapex). Sealapex and Roth's 811 sealers caused moderate to severe inflammation reactions, whereas CRCS caused a mild to moderate reaction. AH 26 caused the greatest irritation initially, but this inflammatory reaction decreased with time.

Bernath and Szabo[235] examined tissue reaction initiated by different sealers. The aim of this study was to analyze the tissue reactions of the calcium hydroxide sealer, Apexit, and to compare it with the reactions of sealers with different chemical compositions (Endomethasone, AH 26, and Grossman's sealer). When filled within the root, AH 26 and Endomethasone initiated a mild lymphocytic/plasmocytic reaction in some cases. In the group of overfilled canals, all four sealers initiated an inflammatory response: Endomethasone initiated a foreign body-type granulamatous reaction; AH 26 particles were engulfed by macrophages; Apexit and Grossman's sealers initiated only a lymphocytic/plasmocytic reaction.

Huumonen and coworkers[236] evaluated the healing of patients with apical periodontitis after endodontic treatment by comparing a silicone-based sealer (RoekoSeal Automix) and a zinc oxide-based sealer. After a 1-year follow-up, 199 teeth were assessed to evaluate their periapical status. The results of the study showed that there was no statistical difference between the success rates of the two study groups. The overall success rate at 12 months was 76%.

FLOW

Ørstavik[224] rated the flow for Tubli-Seal to be greater than that of Kerr's PCS, which was better than Diaket and Kloroperka NØ. He also stated that flow properties may be affected by changes in the powder-to-liquid ratio.

The rheologic properties of Apexit, Tubli-Seal EWT, Grossman's sealer, and Ketac-Endo were tested in a capillary system by Lacey and coworkers.[237] Tubli-Seal EWT had a thinner film thickness than the other sealers. Tubli-Seal EWT had lower viscosity and better flow than the other sealers. Increased strain rate gave a significant increase in the flow rate of all sealers. The reduction in powder-to-liquid ratio for Grossman's sealer significantly increased flow in narrow tubes, and at a higher strain rate. Increasing the rate of insertion gave increased volumetric flow and therefore a reduced viscosity for all sealers. As the internal width of the canals was reduced, there was a reduction in volumetric flow and therefore an increased viscosity.

McMichen et al.[238] did a comparative study of selected physical properties of five root canal sealers. This study sought to investigate the physical properties of five sealers: Roth's 801, Tubi-Seal EWT, AH Plus, Apexit, and Endion. Solubility in water, film thickness, flow, working time, and setting time were tested. AH Plus had the greatest stability in solution. But AH Plus also had the greatest film thickness. Flow rates were similar, and the working times for all were greater than 50 minutes. Setting time for Roth's 801 was 8 days.

Tagger et al.[239] studied the interaction between sealers and gutta-percha cones. AH 26 silver-free had a notable softening effect on most gutta-percha brands, resulting in increased flow. Liquid (bisphenol epoxy resin) and chemical-bond formation could act as partial solvent effect of the resin. Eugenol has a solvent effect on gutta-percha. The combination of Apexit and UDM gutta-percha cones (United Dental Manufacturers, Zipperer, VDW, Munich, Germany) gave the greatest penetration in lateral canals. Understanding the interaction between gutta-percha and sealers may serve as a guide for using the most suitable combination for specific clinical cases. A tooth with a wide apical foramen should be filled with a combination that provides little flow; conversely, canals with very fine apical foramina and internal irregularities should be filled with a more fluid combination.

SETTING TIME

The setting time for 11 sealers was determined in both aerobic and anaerobic environments by Nielsen et al.[240] Kerr Tubli-Seal and Ketac-Endo were the fastest sealers to set under aerobic environments, and Ketac-Endo and Resilon sealer (Epiphany) were the fastest sealers to set under anaerobic environments. Roth's 801 and Roth's 811 sealers were the slowest sealers to set under both aerobic and anaerobic environments, taking over 3 weeks to set. Resilon sealer (Epiphany) set in 30 minutes under anaerobic conditions, but in the presence of air, Resilon sealer (Epiphany) took a week to set, and an uncured layer remained on its surface.

WORKING TIME

Ørstavik[224] stated that the assessment of working time is preferably done with measurements of flow as a function of time. It is the time from the start of mixing to the point at which the flow has been reduced to 90% of the initial flow measurement. The working time for zinc oxide–eugenol sealers demonstrated an initial increase in flow, followed by a later reduction in flow.

SOLUBILITY

The zinc oxide sealers and the calcium hydroxide sealers appear to have greater solubility than other sealers.[197,241–243]

Schafer and Zandbiglari[244] studied the solubility of root canal sealers in water and artificial saliva. The sealers examined were (epoxy resin [AH 26, AH Plus], silicone [RSA RoekoSeal], calcium hydroxide [Apexit, Sealapex], zinc oxide–eugenol [Aptal-Harz], glass ionomer [Ketac-Endo], and a polyketone-based sealer [Diaket]). Most sealers were of low solubility, although Sealapex, Aptal-Harz, and Ketac-Endo showed a marked weight loss in all liquids. Even after 28 days of storage in water, AH 26, AH Plus, RSA RoekoSeal, and Diaket showed less than 3% weight loss. AH Plus showed the least weight loss of all sealers tested, independent of the solubility medium used. Sealapex, Aptal-Harz, and Ketac-Endo had a marked weight loss in all liquids.

DIMENSIONAL CHANGE FOLLOWING SETTING

Kazemi et al.[245] examined the long-term comparison of the dimensional changes of four sealers, ZnOE, AH 26, Endo-Fill, and Endomethasone. The two zinc oxide and eugenol sealers started to shrink within hours after mixing. The first volumetric loss for AH 26 and Endo-Fill was recorded after 30 days. The least dimensional change at any time period was observed for Endo-Fill. Significant dimensional change and continued volume loss can occur in some endodontic sealers. The setting times for Endo-Fill, ZnOE, Endomethasone, and AH 26 were 2.5, 4, 9, and 12 hours, respectively. Endo-Fill and AH 26 had lower rates of solubility, water sorption, and dimensional change than ZnOE and Endomethasone over 180 days.

ANTIBACTERIAL ACTIVITY

The *in vitro* antibacterial activity of Fill Canal (zinc oxide based sealer), Sealapex, Sealer 26, Apexit, and calcium hydroxide against various species of microorganisms was studied.[246] Fill Canal demonstrated large zones of inhibition against all bacteria tested. Sealer 26 was not effective against *Porphyromonas endodontalis* or *Porhyromonas gingivalis*. Sealapex and calcium hydroxide showed similar effects against the various bacteria, being effective against *Actinomyces israelii*, and *Actinomyces naeslundii*. Sealapex was not effective against *Staphylococcus aureus*, but calcium hydroxide was effective against *Staphylococcus aureus*. Apexit was not effective against any of the microorganisms tested.

An in vitro antibacterial activity study of four root canal sealers tested AH Plus, Endomethasone, Pulp Canal Sealer, and Vcanalare, a zinc oxide and ortho-phenylphenol containing sealer.[247] All of the freshly mixed sealers showed complete inhibition of bacterial growth. Similar results were obtained after 24 hours, with the exception of AH Plus. Vcanalare was the only sealer still inhibiting bacterial growth 7 days after mixing.

The amount of bacterial endotoxin penetration through root canals obturated either with cold lateral compaction or with a continuous wave technique with backfill of thermoplasticized gutta-percha, with either Roth's 801 sealer or AH 26 sealer, was evaluated by Williamson et al.[248] The groups differed significantly. Thermoplasticized gutta-percha with Roth's 801 sealer permitted the least amount of endotoxin penetration, suggesting that the Roth's 801 sealer may have a role in inhibiting endotoxin penetration into obturated root canals.

Siqueira and Goncalves[249] found that zinc oxide–eugenol sealers inhibited all the bacteria tested in their study. Sealer 26, the epoxy resin containing calcium hydroxide, was inhibitory on most strains of bacteria tested, but not against *Porphyromonas endodontalis* and *Porphyromonas gingivalis*. Sealapex had low antibacterial activity.

Leonardo et al.[250] examined the antimicrobial activity of four root canal sealers (AH plus, Sealapex, Ketac-Endo, and Fill Canal), two calcium hydroxide pastes (Calen and Calasept), and a zinc oxide paste against seven bacterial strains. All sealers and pastes presented in vitro antimicrobial activity for all bacterial strains after a 24-hour incubation period at 37°C.

Kayaoglu et al.[251] tested short-term antibacterial activity of root canal sealers toward *E. faecalis*. *E. faecalis* suspensions were exposed to freshly mixed sealers (MCS [Medidenta International, Inc.], AH Plus, Grossman's, Sealapex, Apexit). MCS contains iodoform. MCS, AH Plus, and Grossman's sealer significantly reduced the number of viable bacteria in both tests. Sealapex and Apexit were not statistically different from the controls. MCS, AH Plus, and Grossman's sealer were effective in reducing the number of cultivable cells of *E. faecalis*. Calcium hydroxide-based sealers, Sealapex and Apexit, were ineffective in this short-term experiment.

Intraorifice Barriers

The prevention of coronal bacterial leakage back into the root canal system is crucial for the ultimate success of endodontic therapy. Several studies have shown that leakage can occur through the obturated root canal system in a relatively short time period.[252–255] The issue of coronal leakage and its effect on endodontic outcomes has been investigated. Whereas some authors feel that the quality of the endodontic obturation is a more important factor than the quality of the coronal restoration,[256–258] others feel that preventing coronal microleakage can play a significant role in the success of endodontic therapy.[259] In any event, the placement of another barrier to the penetration of microorganisms into the obturated root canal system would seem to prevent leakage due to delay in placement of a permanent restoration or leakage from failed or inadequate coronal restorations. Several studies have looked at materials that may be used as intraorifice barriers placed 1 to 2 mm into the orifice of canals, or on the pulpal floor, to add another layer to prevent microleakage.[129,260–268]

COMPOSITE RESINS

Yamauchi et al.,[269] in a dog study, examined the effect of an orifice plug of 2 mm of IRM or a dentin bonding/composite resin on coronal leakage of teeth that had canals obturated with gutta-percha and the access cavities left open for 8 months. Periapical inflammation was observed in 89% of the group without plugs, but in those with composite plugs only 39% had periapical inflammation and only 38% in the IRM-plugged group.

An investigation, comparing Cavit, against a flowable light-cured composite resin (Tetric), and MTA (ProRoot) as intraorifice barriers at 1, 2, 3, or 4 mm in canals obturated with gutta-percha, demonstrated a better seal with the flowable composite than with either MTA or Cavit.[270]

GLASS IONOMERS

Chailertvanitkul et al.[261] investigated coronal bacterial leakage, through coronal access using Vitrebond (3M), a resin-modified glass ionomer liner, as a barrier on the pulpal floor. The teeth with the Vitrebond liner that had been placed on the pulpal floor showed no leakage of bacteria, whereas 60% of the specimens without a Vitrebond liner showed leakage after 60 days. Wolcott et al.[260] found that there was no significant difference between Vitrebond, a colored trial GC America glass ionomer, and Ketac-Bond. There was significantly less coronal leakage when the glass ionomers were used than when no barrier was placed.

Maloney et al.[267] found that thermocycling Triage (GC America, Inc.), a colored resin-modified glass ionomer, had no effect on the seal produced by Triage, when it was used as an intraorifice barrier at depths of 1 or 2 mm. The 1 and 2 mm intracoronal barrier significantly reduced coronal microleakage compared with no barrier placement.

Mavec et al.[271] investigated the use of a glass ionomer barrier against bacterial leakage a when post space is required. They found that a 1 mm barrier of glass ionomer over as little as 2 or 3 mm of gutta-percha could reduce the risk of recontamination of the apical gutta-percha. This could be beneficial in cases where there is a minimum amount of root length for a post.

OTHER MATERIALS

Pisano et al.[262] compared Cavit, IRM, and Super EBA as intraorifice barriers to prevent coronal microleakage and found that all three groups leaked less than those obturated canals that did not receive a barrier.

Wolanek et al.[265] tested the effectiveness of a dentin-bonding agent used as an intraorifice barrier and found that it reduced coronal bacterial leakage.

Galvan et al.[264] evaluated Amalgbond Plus, C&B Metabond, One-Step Adhesive with Eliteflo composite, One-Step Dentin Adhesive with Palfique composite, and IRM as intracoronal barriers. At 7 days, the IRM, AEliteflo, and Palfique composite leaked significantly more than Amalgabond or C&B Metabond. Amalgabond consistently produced the best seal through all time periods.

Temporary Filling Materials

The problem of coronal leakage is also important in the choice of an interim restoration material to seal off the access preparation, either between appointments or before the endodontically treated tooth receives a permanent restoration.

Cavit (ESPE, Seefeld, Germany), in a number of studies, has been found to prevent leakage, when used as a temporary filling material to close access preparations, either as an interim filling material or after final obturation before a permanent restoration is placed.[272–280] Cavit is premixed and is easily introduced into the access cavity, as well as being easy to remove from the access cavity at the subsequent appointment. The ingredients in Cavit are zinc oxide, calcium sulfate, zinc sulfate, glycoacetate, polyvinylacetate resin, polyvinylchloride-acetate, triethanolamine, and red pigment.[272] The calcium sulfate is hydrophilic and causes hydroscopic expansion of

Cavit. This absorption of moisture and subsequent expansion cause Cavit to seal very well as it sets in a moist environment.

In a survey of Diplomates of the American Board of Endodontics, Vail and Steffel[281] found that Cavit was the temporary restoration of choice for both anterior and posterior teeth.

Webber et al.[282] found that to seal adequately, Cavit must have a depth of at least 3.5 mm.

The ability of Cavit to prevent bacterial penetration into root canals containing four medicaments was evaluated.[283] The medicaments were calcium hydroxide, chlorhexidine, an antibiotic-corticoid compound (Ledermix), and chloromono-campherphenolic compound (ChKM). The authors found that Cavit prolonged the protection of all the medicaments from 13 to 18 days but that an adequate seal could not be provided for more than 1 month.

Balto[274] assessed microbial leakage of three temporary filling materials (Cavit, IRM, and Dyract). IRM began to leak after 10 days, whereas Cavit and Dyract did not leak until after 2 weeks.

After 3 weeks, Beach et al.[273] found that 4 of 14 TERM samples and 1 of 18 IRM samples leaked and showed positive bacterial growth. None of the Cavit samples in the study leaked. It was shown that Cavit provided a significantly better seal than the other temporary filling materials.

Kazemi and coworkers[277] found that Tempit (Centrix, Milford, CT) and IRM (Dentsply International/L.D. Caulk Division, Milford, DE) seemed less appropriate as an interim endodontic restoration than Cavit based on an assessment of marginal stability and permeability to dye penetration.

IRM is a temporary filling material that comes in a liquid-powder form that requires mixing. It is a polymer-resin-reinforced zinc oxide–eugenol material. Although many studies show it has inferior sealing abilities compared with Cavit, in clinical situations, however, which require greater bulk and resistance to occlusal forces, IRM may be used as a temporary restorative material. Zinc oxide and eugenol materials, such as IRM, possess about double the compressive strength value of Cavit.[284] Glass ionomer cements or composite resins may also be used in these situations and may have better sealing ability and greater compressive strength.

The antibacterial properties of several temporary filling materials were examined. Revoltek LC (GC Corporation, Tokyo, Japan), Tempit (Centrix), Systemp inlay (Vivadent, Schaan, Liechtenstein), and IRM were tested against *Streptococcus mutans* and *E. faecalis*. Systemp inlay exhibited antibacterial properties when in contact with *S. mutans* for at least 7 days, whereas Tempit and IRM sustained this ability for at least 14 days. When in contact with *E. faecalis*, Tempit and IRM were antibacterial immediately after setting, and IRM sustained this activity for at least 1 day.[285]

Zmener et al.[286] found no statistically significant difference in the marginal leakage between Cavit, IRM, and Ultratemp Firm after thermocycling. All of the materials leaked at the interface of the material with the dentin, and some of the IRM specimens absorbed the dye into the bulk of the material.

Orahood et al.[287] found there was no difference in marginal leakage between Cavit and ZOE when used to seal access preparations through either alloy or composite restorations. One study found IRM more watertight than Fermit-N or Cavit G intermediate restorative materials.[288]

TERM (Dentsply International/L.D. Caulk Division) is a composite resin interim restorative material for endodontics. It is a visible-light-cured resin containing UDMA polymers, inorganic radiopaque filler, pigments, and initiators.[272]

Seiler[289] studied bacterial leakage of three glass ionomers, IRM, and Cavit as used as a temporary endodontic restorative material. Cavit provided a slightly better seal than IRM; however, the glass ionomer and resin-modified glass ionomer materials provided better seals against bacteria than either IRM or Cavit. If 3.5 mm of space does not exist for a temporary filling material, Hansen and Montgomery[290] found that TERM may provide a superior temporary restoration. They found that TERM provides an adequate seal at 1, 2, 3, and 4 mm.

Summary

As new materials are introduced to fill the root canal system, it is important to remember Grossman's tenets and to remember the proven success of many of the materials currently in use. However, there still is a need to constantly improve what we can offer our patients, and to improve the outcome of endodontic treatment, in order to preserve the natural dentition. Long-term randomized clinical trials are needed on all the materials, new and time tested, which are used in modern-day endodontics.

With advances in materials and other aspects of endodontics, one cannot imagine materials that will be available to use in root canal systems in the future. They, no doubt, will be much more biocompatible and, one might hope, may promote regeneration of tissues within the tooth and bone.

References

1. Grossman LI. Endodontics 1776–1976: a bicentennial history against the background of general dentistry. J Am Dent Assoc 1976;93:78–87.
2. Milas VB. History. In: Cohen S, Burns RC, editors. Pathways of the pulp. 2nd ed. St. Louis: C V Mosby Company; 1980, pp. 687–701.
3. Keane HC. A century of service to dentistry. Philadelphia: S.S. White Dental Manufacturing Co.; 1944.
4. Grossman LI. Root canal therapy. Philadelphia: Lea & Febiger; 1940.
5. Brownlee WA. Filling of root canals in recently devitalized teeth. Dominion Dent J 1900;12(8):254.
6. Seltzer S, Green DB, Weiner N, DeRensis F. A scanning EM examination of silver cones removed from endodontically treated teeth. Oral Surg Oral Med Oral Pathol Oral Radiol Endod 1972;33:589–605.
7. Brady JM, Del Rio CE. Corrosion of endodontic silver cones in humans: a scanning electron microscope and x-ray microprobe study. J Endod 1975;1:205–10.
8. Goldberg F. Relationship between corroded silver points and endodontic failure. J Endod 1981;7:224–7.
9. Gutierrez JH, Villena F, Gigoux C, Mujica F. Microscope and scanning electron microscope examination of silver points corrosion caused by endodontic materials. J Endod 1982;8:301–11.
10. Kehoe JC. Intracanal corrosion of a silver cone producing localized argyria. J Endod 1984;10:199–201.
11. Goodman A, Schilder H, Aldrich W. The thermomechanical properties of gutta-percha. II. The history and molecular chemistry of gutta-percha. Oral Surg Oral Med Oral Pathol Oral Radiol Endod 1974;37(6):954–61.
12. Costa GE, Johnson JD, Hamilton RG. Cross-reactivity studies of gutta-percha, gutta-balata, and natural rubber latex (Hevea brasiliensis). J Endod 2001;27(9):584–7.
13. Friedman CM, Sandrik JL, Heuer MA, Rapp GW. Composition and mechanical properties of gutta-percha endodontic points. J Dent Res 1975;54(5):921–5.
14. Moorer WR, Genet JM. Evidence for antibacterial activity of endodontic gutta-percha cones. Oral Surg Oral Med Oral Pathol Oral Radiol Endod 1982;53:503–7.
15. Martin H, Martin TR. Iodoform gutta-percha: MGP a new endodontic paradigm. Dent Today 1999;18:76.
16. Ingle JI, Newton CW, West JD, et al, editors. Obturation of the radicular space. In: Ingle JI, Bakland LK, editors. Endodontics. 5th ed. Hamilton, London: BC Decker, Inc.; 2002, pp. 571–668.
17. Chogle S, Mickel AK, Huffaker SK, Neibaur B. An in vitro assessment of iodoform gutta-percha. J Endod 2005;31:814–16.
18. Holland R, Murata SS, Dezan E, Garlipp O. Apical leakage after root canal filling with an experimental calcium hydroxide gutta-percha point. J Endod 1996;22:71–3.
19. Lin S, Levin L, Weiss EI, et al. In vitro antibacterial efficacy of a new chlorhexidine slow-release device. Quintessence Int 2006;37(5):391–4.
20. Podbielski A, Boeckh C, Haller B. Growth inhibitory activity of gutta-percha points containing root canal medications on common endodontic bacterial pathogens as determined by an optimized in vitro assay. J Endod 2000;26:398–403.
21. Melker KB, Vertucci FJ, Rojas MF, et al. Antimicrobial efficacy of medicated root canal filling materials. J Endod 2006;32(2):148–51.
22. Bunn CW. Molecular structure of rubber-like elasticity. Part I: The crystal structure of gutta-percha, rubber and polychloroprene. Proc R Soc Lond B Biol Sci 1942;80:40.
23. Baterman L. The chemistry and physics of rubber-like substances. London: McLaren & Sons, Ltd; 1963.
24. Marciano J, Michailesco P, Abadie MJ. Stereochemical structure characterization of dental gutta-percha. J Endod 1993;19(1):31–4.
25. Arvanitoyannis I, Kokokuris I, Blanshard JMV, Robinson C. Study of the effect of annealing, draw ratio, and moisture upon the crystallinity of native and commercial gutta-percha (transpolyisoprene) with DSC, DMTA, and x-rays: determination of the activation energies of T. Appl Polymer Sci 1993;48:987.
26. Schilder H, Goodman A, Aldrich W. The thermomechanical properties of gutta-percha. 3. Determination of phase transition temperatures for gutta-percha. Oral Surg Oral Med Oral Pathol Oral Radiol Endod 1974;38(1):109–14.
27. Schilder H, Goodman A, Aldrich W. The thermomechanical properties of gutta-percha. I. The compressibility of gutta-percha. Oral Surg Oral Med Oral Pathol Oral Radiol Endod 1974;37(6):946–53.
28. Sorin SM, Oliet S, Pearlstein F. Rejuvenation of aged (brittle) endodontic gutta-percha cones. J Endod 1979;5(8):233–8.
29. Kolokruis I, Arvanitoyannis I, Robinson C, Blanchard JM. Effects of moisture and aging on gutta-percha. J Endod 1992;18:583–8.
30. Senia ES, Marraro RV, Mitchell JL, et al. Rapid sterilization of gutta-percha cones with 5.25% sodium hypochlorite. J Endod 1975;1(4):136–40.
31. Short RD, Dorn SO, Kuttler S. The crystallization of sodium hypochlorite on gutta-percha cones after the rapid-sterilization technique: an SEM study. J Endod 2003;29(10):670–3.
32. Valois CR, Silva LP, Azevedo RB. Structural effects of sodium hypochlorite solutions on gutta-percha cones: atomic force microscopy. J Endod 2005;31:749–51.
33. Gomes BP, Vianna ME, Matsumoto CU, et al. Disinfection of gutta-percha cones with chlorhexidine and sodium

hypochlorite. Oral Surg Oral Med Oral Pathol Oral Radiol Endod 2005;100:512–17.

34. Yee FS, Marlin J, Krakow AA, Gron P. Three dimensional obturation of the root canal using injection-molded thermoplasticized dental gutta-percha. J Endod 1977;3:168–74.

35. Tani-Ishii N, Teranaka T. Clinical and radiographic evaluation of root-canal obturation with Obtura II. J Endod 2003;29:739–42.

36. Eriksson AR, Albrektsson T. Temperature threshold levels for heat-induced bone tissue injury: A vital-microscopic study in the rabbit. J Prosthet 1983;50:101–7.

37. Weller RN, Koch KA. In vitro radicular temperature produced by injectable-thermoplasticized gutta-percha. Int Endod J 1995;28:86–90.

38. Gutmann JL, Rakusin H, Powe R, Bowles WH. Evaluation of heat transfer during root canal obturation with thermoplasticized gutta-percha. Part II: In vivo response to heat levels generated. J Endod 1987;13:441–8.

39. Sweatman TL, Baumgartner JC, Sakaguchi RL. Radicular temperature associated with thermoplasticized gutta-percha. J Endod 2001;27:512–15.

40. Lipski M. In vitro infrared thermographic assessment of root surface temperatures generated by high-temperature thermoplasticized injectable gutta-percha obturation technique. J Endod 2006;32:438–41.

41. Michanowicz A, Czonstkowsky M. Sealing properties of an injection-thermoplasticized low-temperature (70°C) gutta-percha: a preliminary study. J Endod 1984;10:563–6.

42. Lipski M. Root surface temperature rises in vitro during root canal obturation using hybrid and Microseal techniques. J Endod 2005;31:297–300.

43. Maggiore F. MicroSeal systems and modified technique. Dent Clin North Am 2004;48:217–64.

44. Cathro PR, Love RM. Comparison of MicroSeal and System B/Obtura II obturation techniques. Int Endod J 2003;36:876–82.

45. Johnson WB. A new gutta-percha filling technique. J Endod 1978;4:184.

46. Gutmann JL, Saunders WP, Saunders EM, Nguyen L. An assessment of the plastic thermafil obturation technique. Part 1: Radiographic evaluation of adaptation and placement. Int Endod J 1993;26:173–8.

47. Gutmann JL, Saunders WP, Saunders EM, Nguyen L. An assessment of the plastic thermafil obturation technique. Part 2: Material adaptation and sealability. Int Endod J 1993;26:179–83.

48. Becker TA, Donnelly JC. Thermafil obturation: a literature review. Gen Dent 1997;45:46–54.

49. Bhambhani SM, Sprechman K. Microleakage comparison of Thermafil vs vertical condensation using two different sealers. Oral Surg Oral Med Oral Pathol Oral Radiol Endod 1994;78:105–8.

50. Dalat DM, Spangberg LSW. Comparison of apical leakage in root canals obturated with various gutta-percha techniques using a dye vacuum tracing method. J Endod 1994;20:315–19.

51. Dummer PMH, Lyle L, Rawle J, Kennedy JK. A laboratory study of root fillings in teeth obturated by lateral condensation of gutta-percha or Thermafil obturators. Int Endod J 1994;27:32–8.

52. Felstead AM, Lumley PJ, Harrington E. An in vitro investigation of Thermafil obturation at different temperatures. Endod Dent Traumatol 1994;10:141–3.

53. Hata G, Kawazoe S, Toda T. Sealing ability of various thermoplastic techniques. J Endod 1993;19:207–10.

54. Hata G, Kawazoe S, Toda T, Weine FW. Sealing ability of Thermafil with and without sealer. J Endod 1992;18:322–6.

55. Lares C, ElDeeb ME. The sealing ability of the Thermafil obturation technique. J Endod 1990;16:474–9.

56. Clark DS, ElDeeb ME. Apical sealing ability of metal versus plastic carrier Thermafil obturators. J Endod 1993;19:4–9.

57. Fabra-Campos H. Experimental apical sealing with a new canal obturation system. J Endod 1993;19:71–5.

58. McMurtrey LG, Krell KV, Wilcox LR. A comparison between Thermafil and lateral condensation in highly curved canals. J Endod 1992;18:68–71.

59. Dummer PMH, Kelly T, Meghji A, et al. An in vitro study of the quality of root fillings in teeth obturated by lateral condensation of gutta-percha or Thermafil obturators. Int Endod J 1993;29:99–105.

60. Scott AC, Vire DE, Swanson R. An evaluation of the Thermafil endodontic obturation technique. J Endod 1992;18:340–3.

61. Juhlin JJ, Walton RE, Dovgan JS. Adaptation of Thermafil components to canal walls. J Endod 1993;19:130–5.

62. Taylor JK, Baumgardner KR, Walton RE. Comparison of the coronal leakage in lateral condensation and Thermafil obturations [abstract]. J Endod 1991;17:195.

63. Baumgardner KR, Taylor J, Walton RE. Canal adaptation and coronal leakage: lateral condensation compared to Thermafil. J Am Dent Assoc 1995;126(3):351–6.

64. Saunders WP, Saunders EM. Influence of smear layer on the coronal leakage of Thermafil and laterally condensed root fillings with a glass ionomer sealer. J Endod 1994;20:155–8.

65. Dalat DM, Spangberg LS. Effect of post preparation on the apical seal of teeth obturated with plastic Thermafil obturators. Oral Surg Oral Med Oral Pathol Oral Radiol Endod 1993;76:760–5.

66. Ravanshad S, Torabinejad M. Coronal dye penetration of the apical filling materials after post preparation. Oral Surg Oral Med Oral Pathol Oral Radiol Endod 1992;74:644–7.

67. Mattison GD, Hwang CL, Cunningham C, Pink FE. The effect of the post preparation on the apical seal in teeth filled with Thermafil [abstract]. J Dent Res 1992;72:600.

68. McGinnity TL, Mueninghoff LA, Brandt RE. Obturation efficiency after post-space preparation: effect of obturation diameter. J Dent Res 1990;69(176): Abstract 542.
69. Ricci ER, Kessler JR. Apical seal of teeth obturated by the lateral condensed gutta-percha, the Thermafil plastic, and Thermafil metal obturator techniques after post-space preparation. J Endod 1994;20:123–6.
70. Rybicki R, Zillich R. Apical sealing ability of Thermafil following immediate and delayed post-space preparations. J Endod 1994;20:64–6.
71. Saunders WP, Saunders EM, Gutmann JL, Gutmann ML. An assessment of the plastic Thermafil obturation technique. Part 3: The effect of post-space preparation on the apical seal. Int Endod J 1993;26:184–9.
72. Zuolo ML, Imura N, Fernandes Ferreira MO. Endodontic retreatment of Thermafil or lateral condensation obturations in post-space prepared teeth. J Endod 1994;20:9–12.
73. Imura N, Zuolo ML, Kherlakian D. Comparison of endodontic retreatment of laterally condensed gutta-percha and Thermafil with plastic carriers. J Endod 1993;19:609–12.
74. Ibarrola JL, Knowles KI, Ludlow MO. Retrievability of Thermafil plastic cores using organic solvents. J Endod 1993;19:417–18.
75. Wilcox LR. Thermafil retreatment with and without chloroform solvent. J Endod 1993;19:563–6.
76. Wilcox LR, Juhlin JJ. Endodontic retreatment of Thermafil vs. lateral condensation gutta-percha. J Endod 1994;20:115–17.
77. Baker PS, Oguntebi BR. Effect of apical resection and reverse fillings on Thermafil root canal obturations. J Endod 1990;16:227–9.
78. Mock ES, Olson AK, DeWald EJ, Radke PK. Apicoectomy and retrofilling preparation of Thermafil obturators. Gen Dent 1993;41:471–3.
79. Weller RN, Kimbrough WF, Anderson RW. A comparison of thermoplastic obturation techniques: adaptation to the canal walls. J Endod 1997;23:703–6.
80. Robinson MJ, McDonald NJ, Mullally PJ. Apical extrusion of thermoplasticized obturating material in canals instrumented with Profile 0.06 or Profile GT. J Endod 2004;30:418–21.
81. De-Deus G, Gurgel-Filho ED, Magalhaes KM, Coutinho-Filho T. A laboratory analysis of gutta-percha-filled area obtained using Thermafil, System B and lateral condensation. Int Endod J 2006;39:378–83.
82. Lipski M. Root surface temperature rises in vitro during root canal obturation with thermoplasticized gutta-percha on a carrier or by injection. J Endod 2004;30:441–3.
83. Jarrett IS, Marx D, Covey D, et al. Percentage of canals filled in apical cross sections—an in vitro study of seven obturation techniques. Int Endod J 2004;37:392–8.
84. Shipper G, Trope M. An vitro microbial leakage of endodontically treated teeth using new and standard obturation techniques. J Endod 2004;30:154–8.
85. Goldberg F, Massone EJ, Artaza LP. Comparison of the sealing capacity of three endodontic filling techniques. J Endod 1995;21:1–3.
86. Hauman CH, Love RM. Biocompatability of dental materials used in contemporary endodontic therapy: a review. Part 2: Root canal filling materials. Int Endod J 2003;36(3):147–60.
87. Wolfson EM, Seltzer S. Reaction of rat connective tissue to some gutta-percha formulations. J Endod 1975;1:395–402.
88. Tavares T, Soares IJ, Silveira NL. Reaction of rat subcutaneous tissue to implants of gutta-percha for endodontic use. Endod Dent Traumatol 1994;10(4):174–8.
89. Pascon EA, Spangberg LS. *In vitro* cytotoxicity of root-canal-filling materials. Part 1: Gutta-percha. J Endod 1990;16:429–33.
90. Munaco FS, Miller WA, Everett MM. A study of long-term toxicity of endodontic materials with use of an *in vitro* model. J Endod 1978;4:151–7.
91. Sjögren U, Sundquist G, Nair PNR. Tissue reaction to gutta-percha particles of various sizes when implanted subcutaneously in guinea pigs. Eur J Oral Sci 1995;103:313–21.
92. Holland R, DeSouza V, Nery MJ, et al. Reaction of rat connective tissue to gutta-percha and silver points. A long-term histological study. Aust Dent J 1982;27:224–6.
93. Serene TP, Vesely J, Boackle R. Complement activation as a possible *in vitro* indication of the inflammatory potential of endodontic materials. Oral Surg Oral Med Oral Pathol Oral Radiol Endod 1988;65:354–7.
94. Gazelius B, Olgart L, Wrangsjo K. Unexpected symptoms to root filling with gutta-percha. A case report. Int Endod J 1986;19:202–4.
95. Boxer MB, Grammer LC, Orfan N. Gutta-percha allergy in a healthcare worker with latex allergy. J Allergy Clin Immunol 1994;93:943–4.
96. Knowles II, Ibarrola JL, Ludlow MO, et al. Rubber latex allergy and the endodontic patient. J Endod 1994;24:760–2.
97. Kleier D, Shibilski K. Management of the latex hypersensitive patient in the endodontic office. J Endod 1999;25:825–8.
98. Hamann C, Rodgers PA, Alenius H, et al. Cross-reactivity between gutta-percha and natural latex: assumption vs. reality. J Am Dent Assoc 2002;133:1357–67.
99. Charous BL, Hamilton RG, Yunginger JW. Occupational latex exposure: characteristics of contact and systemic reactions in 47 workers. J Allergy Clin Immunol 1994;94:12–18.
100. Yunginger JW. Natural rubber latex allergy. In: Middleton EM, Jr., Ellis EF, Yunginger JW, et al, editors. Allergy: principles and practice. 5th ed. St Louis: Mosby Year Book; 1998, pp. 1073–18.
101. Ørstavik D. Materials used for root canal obturation: technical, biological and clinical testing. Endod Topics 2005; 12:25–38.
102. Miner MR, Berzins DW, Bahcall JK. A comparison of thermal properties between gutta-percha and a synthetic

polymer based root canal filling material (Resilon). J Endod 2006;32:683–6.

103. Nielsen BA, Baumgartner JC. Spreader penetration during lateral compaction of Resilon and gutta-percha. J Endod 2006;32:52–4.

104. Shipper G, Ørstavik D, Teixeira FB, Trope M. An evaluation of microbial leakage in roots filled with a thermoplastic synthetic polymer-based root canal filling material (Resilon). J Endod 2004;30:342–7.

105. Tay FR, Loushine RJ, Weller RN, et al. Ultrastructural evaluation of the apical seal in roots filled with a polycaprolactone-based root canal filling material. J Endod 2005;31:514–19.

106. Tay FR, Pashley DH, Williams MC, et al. Susceptibility of a polycaprolactone-based root canal filling material to degradation. I. Alkaline hydrolysis. J Endod 2005;31(8):593–8.

107. Tay FR, Pashley DH, Yiu CK, et al. Susceptibility of a polycaprolactone-based root canal filling material to degradation. II. Gravimetric evaluation of enzymatic hydrolysis. J Endod 2005;31:737–41.

108. Gesi A, Raffaelli O, Goracci C, et al. Interfacial strength of resilon and gutta-percha to intraradicular dentin. J Endod 2005;31:809–13.

109. Stratton RK, Apicella MJ, Mines P. A fluid filtration comparison of gutta-percha versus Resilon, a new soft resin endodontic obturation system. J Endod 2006;32:642–5.

110. Von Fraunhofer JA, Kurtzman GM, Norby CE. Resin-based sealing of root canals in endodontic therapy. Gen Dent 2006;54:243–6.

111. Wang CS, Debelian GJ, Teixeira FB. Effect of intracanal medicament on the sealing ability of root canals filled with Resilon. J Endod 2006;32:532–6.

112. Epley SR, Fleischman J, Hartwell G, Cicalese C. Completeness of root canal obturations: Epiphany techniques versus gutta-percha techniques. J Endod 2006;32:541–4.

113. Teixeira FB, Teixeira EC, Thompson JY, Trope M. Fracture resistance of roots endodontically treated with a new resin filling material. J Am Dent Assoc 2004;135:646–52.

114. Williams C, Loushine RJ, Weller RN, et al. A comparison of cohesive strength and stiffness of Resilon and gutta-percha. J Endod 2006;32(6):553–5.

115. Schwandt NW, Gound TG. Resourcinol-formaldehyde resin "Russian Red" endodontic therapy. J Endod 2003;29:435–7.

116. Pitt Ford TR, Torabinejad M, Abedi HR, et al. Mineral trioxide aggregate as a pulp capping material. J Am Dent Assoc 1996;127:1491–4.

117. Andelin WE, Shabahang S, Wright K, Torabinejad M. Identification of hard tissue using dentin sialoprotein (DSP) as a marker. J Endod 2003;29:646–50.

118. Bakland LK. Management of traumatically injured pulps in immature teeth using MTA. Calif Dent Assoc J 2000:855–8.

119. Lee SJ, Monsef M, Torabinejad M. Sealing ability of a mineral trioxide aggregate for repair of lateral root perforations. J Endod 1993;19:541–4.

120. Pitt Ford TR, Torabinejad M, Hong CU, Kariyawasam SP. Use of mineral trioxide aggregate for repair of furcal perforations. Oral Surg Oral Med Oral Pathol Endod 1995;79:756–63.

121. Nakata TT, Bae KS, Baumgartner JC. Perforation repair comparing mineral trioxide aggregate and amalgam using an anaerobic bacterial leakage model. J Endod 1998;24:184–6.

122. Main C, Mirzayan N, Shabahang S, Torabinejad M. Repair of root perforations using mineral trioxide aggregate: a long-term study. J Endod 2004;30:80–3.

123. Torabinejad M, Watson TF, Pitt Ford TR. Sealing ability of a mineral trioxide aggregate when used as a root-end filling material. J Endod 1993;19:591–5.

124. Torabinejad M, Hong CU, Lee SJ, et al. Investigation of mineral trioxide aggregate for root end fillings in dogs. J Endod 1995;21:603–8.

125. Torabinejad M, Pitt Ford TR, McKendry DJ, et al. Histologic assessment of MTA as a root end filling in monkeys. J Endod 1997;23:225–8.

126. Torabinejad M, Chivian N. Clinical applications of mineral trioxide aggregate. J Endod 1999;25:197–205.

127. Shabahang S, Torabinejad M. Treatment of teeth with open apices using mineral trioxide aggregate. Pract Periodontics Aesthet Dent 2000;12:315–20.

128. Hayashi M, Shimizu A, Ebisu S. MTA for obturation of mandibular central incisors with open apices: case report. J Endod 2004;30:120–2.

129. Tselnik M, Baumgartner JC, Marshall JG. Bacterial leakage with mineral trioxide aggregate or a resin-modified glass ionomer used as a coronal barrier. J Endod 2004;30(11):782–4.

130. Torabinejad M, Hong CU, Pitt Ford TR. Physical properties of a new root end filling material. J Endod 1995;21:349–53.

131. Holland R, de Souza V, Nery MJ, et al. Reaction of dog's teeth to root canal filling with mineral trioxide aggregate or a glass ionomer sealer. J Endod 1999;25:728–30.

132. Wucherpfenning AL, Green DB. Mineral trioxide vs. Portland cement: two biocompatible materials. J Endod 1999;25:308.

133. Estrela C, Bammann LL, Estrela CRA, et al. Antimicrobial and chemical study of MTA, Portland cement, calcium hydroxide paste, Sealapex, and Dycal. Braz Dent J 2000;11:3–9.

134. Holland R, Souza V, Nery MJ, et al. Reaction of rat connective tissue to implanted dentin tube filled with mineral trioxide aggregate, Portland cement or calcium hydroxide. Braz Dent J 2001;12:3–8.

135. Holland R, de Souza V, Murata SS, et al. Healing process of dog dental pulp after pulpotomy and pulp covering with

mineral trioxide aggregate or Portland cement. Braz Dent J 2001;12:109–13.
136. Duarte MAH, Demarchi ACCO, Yamashita JC, et al. pH and calcium ion release of 2 root-filling materials. Oral Surg Oral Med Oral Pathol Oral Radiol Endod 2003;95:245–7.
137. Sarkar NK, Caicedo R, Ritwik P, et al. Physicochemical basis of the biologic properties of mineral trioxide aggregate. J Endod 2005;31(2):97–100.
138. Torabinejad M, Higa RK, McKendry DJ, Pitt Ford TR. Dye leakage of four root end filling materials: effects of blood contamination. J Endod 1994;20(4):159–63.
139. Gondim EJ, Kim S, Souza Filho FJ. An investigation of microleakage from root-end fillings in ultrasonic retrograde cavities with or without finishing: a quantitative analysis. Oral Surg Oral Med Oral Pathol Oral Radiol Endod 2005;99(6):755–9.
140. Torabinejad M, Rastegar AF, Kettering JD, Pitt Ford TR. Bacterial leakage of mineral trioxide aggregate as a root-end filling material. J Endod 1995;21(3):109–12.
141. Tang HM, Torabinejad M, Kettering JD. Leakage evaluation of root end filling materials using endotoxin. J Endod 2002;28(1):5–7.
142. Torabinejad M, Smith PW, Kettering JD, Pitt Ford TR. Comparative investigation of marginal adaptation of mineral trioxide aggregate and other commonly used root-end filling materials. J Endod 1995;21(6):295–9.
143. Peters CI, Peters OA. Occlusal loading of EBA and MTA root-end fillings in a computer-controlled masticator: a scanning electron microscope study. Int Endod J 2002;35:22–9.
144. Gondim EJ, Zaia AA, Gomes BA, et al. Investigation of the marginal adaptation of root-end filling materials in root-end cavities prepared with ultrasonic tips. Int Endod J 2003;36:491–9.
145. Xavier CB, Weismann R, de Oliveira MG, et al. Root-end filling materials: apical microleakage and marginal adaptation. J Endod 2005;31(7):539–42.
146. Mangin C, Yesilsoy C, Nissan R, Stevens R. The comparative sealing ability of hydroxyapatite cement, mineral trioxide aggregate, and super ethoxybenzoic acid as root-end filling materials. J Endod 2003;29(4):261–4.
147. Bates CF, Carnes DL, Del Rio CE. Longitudinal sealing ability of mineral trioxide aggregate as a root-end filling material. J Endod 1996;22:575–8.
148. Wu MK, Kontakiotis EG, Wesselink PR. Long-term seal provided by some root-end filling materials. J Endod 1998;24:557–60.
149. DeBruyne MAA, DeBruyne RJE, Rosiers L, DeMoor RJG. Longitudinal study on microleakage of three root-end filling materials by the fluid transport method and by capillary flow porometry. Int Endod J 2005;38:129–36.
150. Andelin WE, Browning DF, Hsu G-HR, et al. Microleakage of resected MTA. J Endod 2002;28(8):573–4.

151. Lamb EL, Loushine RJ, Weller RN, et al. Effect of root resection on the apical sealing ability of mineral trioxide aggregate. Oral Surg Oral Med Oral Pathol Oral Radiol Endod 2003;95(6):732–5.
152. Valois CRA, Costa EDJ. Influence of the thickness of mineral trioxide aggregate on sealing ability of root-end fillings in vitro. Oral Surg Oral Med Oral Pathol Oral Radiol Endod 2004;97(1):108–11.
153. Matt GD, Thorpe JR, Strother JM, McClanahan SB. Comparative study of white and gray mineral trioxide aggregate (MTA) simulating a one- or two-step apical barrier technique. J Endod 2004;30(12):876–9.
154. Torabinejad M, Hong CU, Pitt Ford TR, Kettering JD. Cytotoxicity of four root end filling materials. J Endod 1995;21:489–92.
155. Torabinejad M, Pitt Ford TR, Abedi HR, et al. Tissue reaction to implanted potential root-end filling materials in the tibia and mandible of guinea pigs. J Endod 1998;24:568–71.
156. Koh ET, Torabinejad M, Pitt Ford TR, et al. Mineral trioxide aggregate stimulates a biological response in human osteoblasts. J Biomed Mater Res 1997;37:432–9.
157. Koh ET, McDonald F, Pitt Ford TR, Torabinejad M. Cellular response to mineral trioxide aggregate. J Endod 1998;24:543–7.
158. Haglund R, He J, Jarvis J, et al. Effects of root-end filling materials on fibroblasts and macrophages in vitro. Oral Surg Oral Med Oral Pathol Oral Radiol Endod 2003;95:739–45.
159. DeDeus G, Ximenes R, Gurgel-Filho ED, et al. Cytotoxicity of MTA and Portland cement on human ECV 304 endothelial cells. Int Endod J 2005;38:604–9.
160. Hernandez EP, Botero TM, Mantellini MG, et al. Effect of ProRoot MTA mixed with chlorhexidine on apoptosis and cell cycle of fibroblasts and macrophages *in vitro*. Int Endod J 2005;38:137–43.
161. Melegari KK, Botero TM, Holland GR. Prostaglandin E production and viability of cells cultured in contact with freshly mixed endodontic materials. Int Endod J 2006;39:357–62.
162. Zhu Q, Haglund R, Safavi KE, Spangberg LSW. Adhesion of human osteoblasts on root-end filling materials. J Endod 2000;26(7):404–6.
163. Regan JD, Gutmann JL, Witherspoon DE. Comparison of Diaket and MTA when used as root-end filling materials to support regeneration of the periradicular tissues. Int Endod J 2002;35:840–7.
164. Baek S-H, Plenk HJ, Kim S. Periapical tissue responses and cementum regeneration with amalgam, Super EBA, and MTA as root-end filling materials. J Endod 2005;31(6):444–9.
165. Holland R, deSouza V, Nery MJ, et al. Reaction of rat connective tissue to implanted dentin tubes filled with mineral trioxide aggregate or calcium hydroxide. J Endod 1999;25:161–6.

canal sealers and their influence on the zinc and calcium content of several tissues. J Endod 1995;21(3):122–7.

235. Bernath M, Szabo J. Tissue reaction initiated by different sealers. Int Endod J 2003;36:256–61.

236. Huumonen S, Lenander-Lumikari M, Sigurdsson A, Ørstavik D. Healing of apical periodontitis after endodontic treatment: a comparison between a silicone-based and a zinc oxide based sealer. Int Endod J 2003;36:295–301.

237. Lacey S, Pitt Ford TR, Watson TF, Sherriff M. A study of the rheological properties of endodontic sealers. Int Endod J 2005;38(8):499–504.

238. McMichen FR, Pearson G, Rahbaran S, et al. A comparative study of selected physical properties of five root-canal sealers. Int Endod J 2003;36(9):629–35.

239. Tagger M, Greenberg B, Sela G. Interaction between sealers and gutta-percha cones. J Endod 2003;29(12):835–7.

240. Nielsen BA, Beeler WJ, Vy C, Baumgartner JC. Setting times of Resilon and other sealers in aerobic and anaerobic environments. J Endod 2006;32(2):130–2.

241. Peters DP. Two year in vitro solubility evaluation of four gutta-percha sealer obturation techniques. J Endod 1986;12:139–45.

242. Crane DL, Heuer MA, Kaminski EJ, Moser JB. Biological and physical properties of an experimental root canal sealer without eugenol. J Endod 1980;6:438–45.

243. Caicedo R, von Fraunhofer JA. The properties of endodontic sealers. J Endod 1988;14:527–34.

244. Schafer E, Zandbiglari T. Solubility of root-canal sealers in water and artificial saliva. Int Endod J 2003;36(10):660–9.

245. Kazemi RB, Safavi KE, Spangberg LS. Dimensional changes of endodontic sealers. Oral Surg Oral Med Oral Pathol Oral Radiol Endod 1993;76(6):766–71.

246. Sipert CR, Hussne RP, Nishiyama CK, Torres SA. In vitro antimicrobial activity of Fill Canal, Sealapex, Mineral Trioxide Aggregate, Portland cement and EndoRez. Int Endod J 2005;38(8):539–43.

247. Pizzo G, Giammanco GM, Cumbo E, et al. In vitro antibacterial activity of endodontic sealers. J Dent 2006;34(1):35–40.

248. Williamson AE, Dawson DV, Drake DR, et al. Effect of root canal filling/sealer systems on apical endotoxin penetration: a coronal leakage evaluation. J Endod 2005;31(8):599–604.

249. Siqueira FJ, Jr., Goncalves RB. Antibacterial activities of root canal sealers against selected anaerobic bacteria. J Endod 1996;22(2):79–80.

250. Leonardo MR, da Silva LAB, Filho MT, et al. In vitro evaluation of antimicrobial activity of sealers and pastes used in endodontics. J Endod 2000;26:391–4.

251. Kayaoglu G, Erten H, Alacam T, Ørstavik D. Short-term antibacterial activity of root canal sealers towards Enterococcus faecalis. Int Endod J 2005;38(7):483–8.

252. Swanson K, Madison S. An evaluation of coronal microleakage in endodontically treated teeth. Part I: Time periods. J Endod 1987;13:56–9.

253. Torabinejad M, Ung B, Kettering JD. In vitro bacterial penetration of coronally unsealed endodontically treated teeth. J Endod 1990;16:556–9.

254. Magura ME, Kafrawy AH, Brown CE, Newton CW. Human saliva coronal microleakage in obturated root canals: an in vitro study. J Endod 1991;17:324–31.

255. Khayat A, Lee SJ, Torabinejad M. Human saliva penetration of coronally unsealed obturated root canals. J Endod 1993;19:458–61.

256. Tronstad L, Asbjornsen K, Doving L, et al. Influence of coronal restorations on the periapical health of endodontically treated teeth. Endod Dent Traumatol 2000;16:218–21.

257. Ricucci D, Grondahl K, Bergenholtz G. Periapical status of root-filled exposed to the oral environment by loss of restoration or caries. Oral Surg Oral Med Oral Pathol Oral Radiol Endod 2000;90:254–9.

258. Ricucci D, Bergenholtz G. Bacterial status in root-filled teeth exposed to the oral environment by loss of restoration and fracture or caries—a histobacteriological study of treated cases. Int Endod J 2003;36:787–802.

259. Saunders WP, Saunders EM. Coronal leakage as a cause of failure in root-canal therapy: a review. Endod Dent Traumatol 1994;10:105–8.

260. Wolcott JF, Hicks ML, Himel VT. Evaluation of pigmented intraorifice barriers in endodontically treated teeth. J Endod 1999;25:589–92.

261. Chailertvanitkul P, Saunders WP, Saunders EM, MacKenzie D. An evaluation of microbial coronal leakage in the restored pulp chamber of root-canal treated multirooted teeth. Int Endod J 1997;30:18–22.

262. Pisano DM, DiFiore PM, McClanahan SB, et al. Intraorifice sealing of gutta-percha obturated root canals to prevent coronal microleakage. J Endod 1998;24:659–62.

263. Beckham BM, Anderson RW, Morris CF. An evaluation of three materials as barriers to coronal microleakage in endodontically treated teeth. J Endod 1993;19:388–91.

264. Galvan RR, West LA, Liewehr FR, Pashley DH. Coronal microleakage of five materials used to create an intraoral seal in endodontically treated teeth. J Endod 2002;28:59–61.

265. Wolanek GA, Loushine RJ, Weller RN, et al. In vitro bacterial penetration of endodontically treated teeth coronally sealed with a dentin bonding agent. J Endod 2001;27:354–7.

266. Schwartz RS, Fransman R. Adhesive dentistry and endodontics: materials, clinical strategies and procedures for restoration of access cavities: a review. J Endod 2005;31(5):151–65.

267. Maloney SM, McClanahan SB, Goodell GG. The effect of thermocycling on a colored glass ionomer intracoronal barrier. J Endod 2005;31(7):526–8.

268. Hommez GMG, Coppens CRM, DeMoor RJG. Periapical health related to the quality of coronal restorations and root fillings. Int Endod J 2002;35:680–9.

269. Yamauchi S, Shipper G, Buttke T, et al. Effect of orifice plugs on periapical inflammation in dogs. J Endod 2006;32(6):524–6.

270. Jenkins S, Kulild J, Williams K, et al. Sealing ability of three materials in the orifice of root canal systems obturated with gutta-percha. J Endod 2006;32(3):225–7.

271. Mavec JC, McClanahan SB, Minah GE, et al. Effects of an intracanal glass ionomer barrier on coronal microleakage in teeth with post space. J Endod 2006;32(2):120–22.

272. Barkhordar RA, Stark MM. Sealing ability of intermediate restorations and cavity design used in endodontics. Oral Surg Oral Med Oral Pathol Oral Radiol Endod 1990;69(1):99–101.

273. Beach CW, Calhoun JC, Bramwell JD, et al. Clinical evaluation of bacterial leakage of endodontic temporary filling materials. J Endod 1996;22(9):459–62.

274. Balto H. An assessment of microbial coronal leakge of temporary filling materials in endodontically treated teeth. J Endod 2002;28:762–4.

275. Lee YC, Yang SF, Hwang YF, et al. Microleakage of endodontic temporary restorative materials. J Endod 1993;19(10):516–20.

276. Noguera AP, McDonald NJ. A comparative in vitro coronal microleakage study of new endodontic restorative materials. J Endod 1990;16:523–7.

277. Kazemi RB, Safavi KE, Spangberg LS. Assessment of marginal stability and permeability of an interim restorative endodontic material. Oral Surg Oral Med Oral Pathol Oral Radiol Endod 1994;78(6):788–96.

278. Mayer T, Eickholz P. Microleakage of temporary restorations after thermocycling and mechanical loading. J Endod 1997;23(5):320–2.

279. Teplitsky PE, Meimaris IT. Sealing ability of Cavit and TERM as intermediate restorative materials. J Endod 1988;14:278–82.

280. Paris L, Kapsimalis P. The effect of temperature change on the sealing properties of temporary filling materials: Part 1. Oral Surg Oral Med Oral Pathol Oral Radiol Endod 1960;13:982–9.

281. Vail MM, Steffel CL. Preference of temporary restorations and spacers: a survey of Diplomates of the American Board of Endodontics. J Endod 2006;32:513–15.

282. Webber RT, del Rio CE, Brady JM, Segall RO. Sealing quality of a temporary filling material. Oral Surg Oral Med Oral Pathol Oral Radiol Endod 1978;46(1):123–30.

283. Barthel CR, Zaritzki FF, Raab WH, Zimmer S. Bacterial leakage in roots filled with different medicaments and sealed with Cavit. J Endod 2006;32(2):127–9.

284. Wilderman FH, Eames WB, Serene TP. The physical and biologic properties of Cavit. J Am Dent Assoc 1971;82(2):378–82.

285. Slutzky H, Slutzky-Goldberg I, Weiss EI, Matalon S. Antibacterial properties of temporary filling materials. J Endod 2006;32(3):214–17.

286. Zmener O, Banegas G, Pameijer CH. Coronal microleakage of three temporary restorative materials: an in vitro study. J Endod 2004;30(8):582–4.

287. Orahood JP, Cochran MA, Swartz M, Newton CW. In vitro study of marginal leakage between temporary sealing materials and recently placed restorative materials. J Endod 1986;12(11):523–7.

288. Jacquot BM, Panighi MM, Steinmetz P, G'Sell C. Evaluation of temporary restorations' microleakage by means of electrochemical impedance measurements. J Endod 1996;22(11):586–9.

289. Seiler KB. An evaluation of glass ionomer–based restorative materials as temporary restorations in endodontics. Gen Dent 2006;54(1):33–6.

290. Hansen SR, Montgomery S. Effect of restoration thickness on the sealing ability of TERM. J Endod 1993;19(9):448–52.

CHAPTER 30

OBTURATION OF THE RADICULAR SPACE

FRED W. BENENATI

It has been four decades since the late Dr. Herbert Schilder published his classic article on filling the root canal space in three dimensions.[1] Ironically, it came 7 years before his treatise on cleaning and shaping the root canal system.[2] One might extrapolate from this fact that closing off or obturating a cleaned and shaped radicular space has considerable importance.

Rationale of Obturation

HISTORICAL PERSPECTIVE

Obturation of the radicular space has been described in various ways for well over 100 years, including Edward Hudson's 1825 report of filling with gold foil.[3] Controlled length obturation of the root canal system was not verified until Edmund Kells produced the first endodontic radiograph in 1899.

Root canal therapy, including obturation, experienced a setback in 1910 when William Hunter delivered his address entitled "the role of sepsis and asepsis." Chivian[3] stated that Hunter's thesis regarding focal infection was "misinterpreted to include periapical lesions and root canal therapy in general." This likely led to, as the modern-day challenge against amalgam has, more careful practice and a rebirth of research and development in the specialty of endodontics. Perhaps one could view this as a *déjà vu* impetus for the modern-day call for evidence-based endodontics!

In 1967 Grossman[4] described the reasons for the growth and acceptance of endodontics in spite of the focal infection theory. These included better research methods, minimal health risks, and the demand for restorative dentistry. His principles may be considered classic, including his "Principle 9," having to do with obturation, or as he termed it "hermetic seal of the canal" terminating at the dentinocemental junction. Principle 10 dealt with the acceptability of the filling material. The term "hermetic seal" is now considered inaccurate. "Hermetic" is defined as "airtight by fusion or sealing." The concern in closing or obturating the canal space is not related to air; it is about fluid leakage at the apex or the coronal level. An "impermeable seal" is a more accurate term.[5]

OBJECTIVE OF OBTURATION

Schilder[1] describes the final objective of endodontic procedures as being "the total obturation of the root canal space." He also stated "in the final analysis, it is the sealing of the complex root canal system from the periodontal bone that ensures the health of the attachment apparatus against breakdown of endodontic origin." Nearly a decade later, Dubrow[6] questioned the validity of a "hermetic seal" produced by silver points or gutta-percha and sealer. He described cases that healed after instrumentation, medication, and a coronal seal, but no obturation. The question has not been answered, however: will this last, and for how long, without full canal length obturation?

In the previous edition of this text, the authors of the chapter on obturation of the root canal space described bacteria and bacterial toxin ingress as the major cause of tissue irritation. Even in bacterial absence, degraded serum may serve as a periapical tissue irritant. They pointed out that "bacteria are the primary source of persistent periradicular inflammation and endodontic failure."[7] Thus, it may be deduced that following total débridement of the radicular space, "the development of a fluid-tight seal of the apical foramen and the total obliteration of the root canal" must follow to ensure the best chance of long-term success (Figure 1). The present-day knowledge of the importance of a coronal seal cannot be overlooked as well.

WHEN IS THE CANAL READY TO OBTURATE?

Radicular space obturation is ideally accomplished after cleaning and shaping has been completed to an optimum

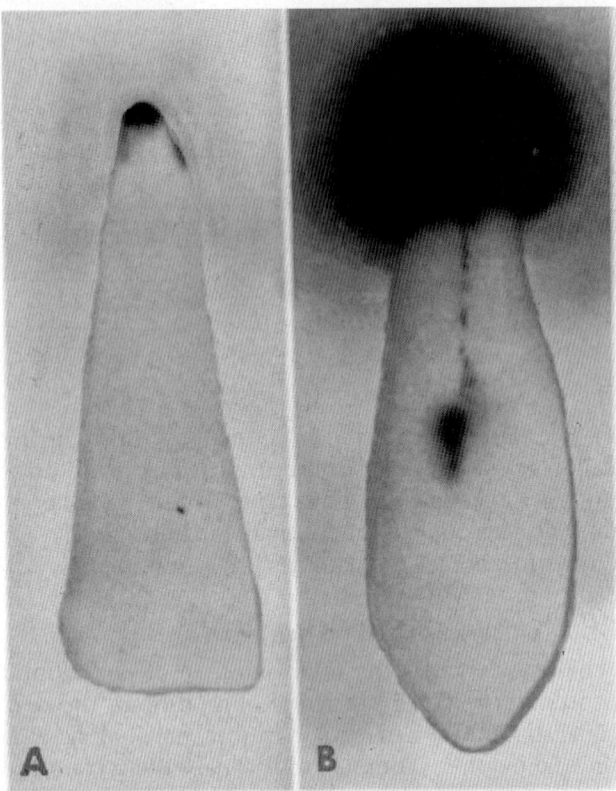

Figure 1 **A,** Failure of reactive iodine (131 I) to penetrate into well obturated root canal. Only periapical cementum that was not coated with sticky wax has absorbed isotope. **B,** Massive reaction to penetration of radioactive iodine (131 I) into poorly filled canal. Violent response at periapex is comparable to *in vivo* response to toxic and/or infective canal products. Reproduced with permission from Dow PR. Ingle JI.[22]

size.[7] Although there is no universal agreement on what constitutes an optimal size, it seems that the canal(s) should be dry, with no "weeping" of fluids into the radicular space.[7]

The tooth should ideally be asymptomatic, although those completely instrumented, yet with mild symptoms or even significant symptoms, have been shown to become asymptomatic upon obturation.[7,8] There are also reports showing the importance of obturating canals following negative bacterial cultures.[9,10] Sjogren et al.[10] found that upon a 5-year recall, 94% of cases exhibiting negative cultures were found to be successful, whereas only 68% of those filled with positive cultures were successful.

APICAL EXTENT OF OBTURATION: WHERE AND WHY?

As early as 1930 and again in 1967, Grossman[4] remarked that there was no general agreement on where a canal filling should end. However, the consensus was that it should be the dentinocemental junction. The trend at the time was to obturate a canal "even with the root apex or just short of it, rather than to overfill the canal." Today, we recognize a difference in semantics between *overfilling* and *overextension*. Overfilling actually denotes "total obturation of the root canal space with excess material extruding beyond the apical foramen."[11] Overextension also denotes filling material beyond the apex, but the canal may not have been filled adequately within its confines.

The dentinocemental junction has been described by Kuttler[12] as an average of approximately 0.5 to 0.7 mm from the external surface of the apical foramen (Figure 2). Thus, it could be construed that filling to the radiographic

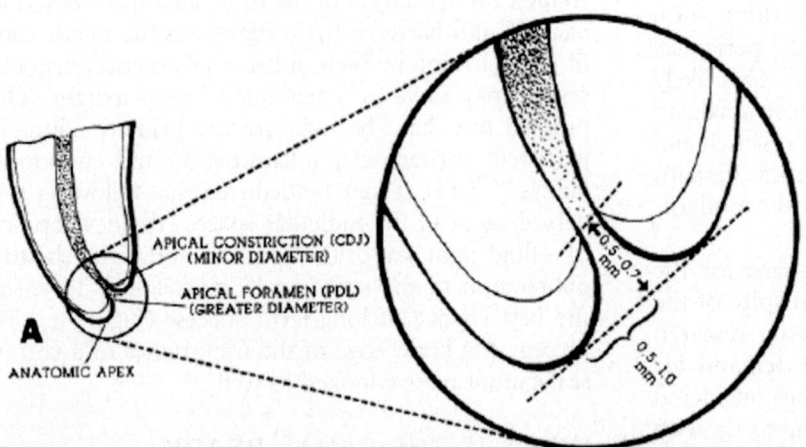
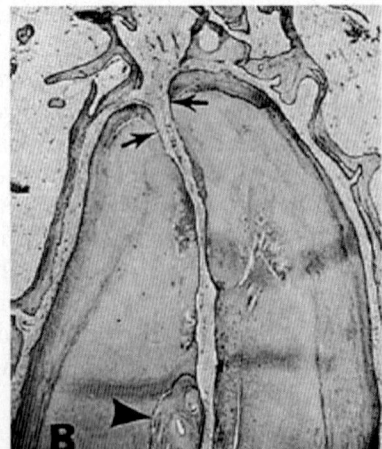

Figure 2 Ideal termination of canal preparation and obturation. **A,** Apical constriction at cementodentinal junction marks end of root canal. From this point to anatomic apex (0.5 to 0.7mm), tissue is periodontal. **B,** Photomicrograph of periapex. Small arrows at cementodentinal junction. Large arrow (bottom) at denticle inclusion. **A,** Reproduced with permission from Goerig AC in Besner E, Practical Endodontics CV Mosby; 1993. **B,** Permission from Brynolf I in Odontol Revy; 1967.

apex is actually overfilling. Blayney[13] advocated filling just short of the radiographic apex, while Morse and coworkers[14] had better clinical success with radiographically flush fillings than with fillings short of the radiographic apex. More recently, using optical microscopy, Ponce and Fernandez[15] found great variation in the measurements of the extension of the cementum into the root canal, suggesting that precise measurement of such is even more inconsistent. Wu et al.[16] advocated different positions for the extent of apical obturation based on the pulpal status, with vital pulp root canals faring better with obturations 2 to 3 mm short of the radiographic apex. They also found that better success in nonvital cases was achieved when filled within 2 mm of the radiographic apex. Schaeffer and associates[17] recently presented an analysis of several success/failure studies based on different obturation lengths. Their findings are presented in Tables 1 and 2 and indicate a better success rate when obturation is short of the radiographic apex.

DESIRED PROPERTIES OF OBTURATING MATERIALS

Grossman's description of ideal properties of obturating materials is a classic benchmark and has stood the test of several decades of time.[18] The desired properties of both core and sealer materials are more extensively discussed in Chapter 29, "Root Canal Filling Materials."

Table 1 Comparison of the Four Studies that were Used in the Meta-analysis. Reproduced with permission from Schaeffer MA et al.[17]

Study	Method	Participants	No. of teeth	Treated by	Results
Harty et al. (1970)	Does not state who read the radiographs. Retrospective study	All patients accepted for RCT on upper and lower incisor and canine teeth between 1954 and 1963 at the Department of Conservative Dentistry, Institute of Dental Surgery (London, England)	1025 teeth	Post-graduate students and staff at the Department of Conservative Dentistry, Institute of Dental Surgery	The teeth obturated between 0 and 1 mm (acceptable) were more successful (92.6%) than short (87.82%) or long (86.81%)
Kerekes et al. (1979)	Interpretation of the radiographs was done independently by two endodontists. Prospective study	All patients accepted for RCT and treated by undergraduate students at the University of Oslo (Norway) in 1971 and who participated in regular clinical and radiographic follow-up exams	501 of 647 teeth were evaluated	Undergraduate students at the University of Oslo (Norway)	In vital teeth, roots that were short of the apex > 1 mm had a higher success rate (96%) than at the apex (0–1 mm) (92%). In necrotic teeth, roots that were short of the apex > 1 mm had a lower success rate (85%) than those at the apex (93%)
Matsumoto et al. (1987)	Does not state who read the radiographs Prospective study 62% loss to follow-up (85 of 223 evaluated)	Patients were treated at the School of Dentistry, AichiGakuin University in Nagoya, Japan	85 of 223 teeth were eval for the minimum 2–3 year follow-up exam	Members of the endodontic staff at the School	The teeth obturated between 1.1 and 2.0 mm underextended (100%) were more successful than 0.5–1.0 mm underextended (88%) or 0–0.4 mm underextended (61.5%) or overextended (40%)
Kerekes et al. (1978)	The interpretation of the radiographs was done independently by two endodontists Retrospective study Clinical exam	Two retrospective studies were done. The first survey evaluated 188 root canals treated by undergraduate students (US) at the University of Oslo in 1969 and had been followed for 3–5 years. The second survey consisted of 379 root canals treated by general dentists (GP)	188 teeth done by undergrads at University of Oslo and 379 teeth done by general dentists (GP) in Norway	RCT done by Undergraduate students at the University of Oslo (Norway) in 1969. Second group of RCT done by general dentists (GP) in Norway in 1968	Those root canals done by US short of apex 1–3 mm were more successful (88%) than at the apex 0–1 mm (84%), than overfilled (79%), than short of apex > 3 mm (79%) Those root canals done by GP at the apex (0–1 mm) were more successful (73%) than short of apex 1–3 mm (71%), than short of apex > 3 mm (54%) than overfilled (44%)

Table 2 Success/Failure of Root Canal Therapy in the Four Studies in Relation to their Length. Reproduced with Permission from Schaeffer MA et al.[17]

Length	Successful	Failed	Uncertain	Total
Harty et al. (1970)				
Group A	525 (92.60%)	42 (7.40%)	—	567 (49.78%)
Group B	173 (87.82%)	24 (12.18%)	—	197 (17.24%)
Group C	316 (86.81%)	48 (13.19%)	—	364 (31.98%)
Total	1025 (90.0%)	114 (10.0%)	—	1139 (100%)
Kerekes et al. (1979)				
Group A	286 (91.96%)	10 (3.22%)	15 (4.82%)	311 (62.08%)
Group B	155 (90.12%)	13 (7.56%)	4 (2.33%)	172 (34.33%)
Group C	12 (66.67%)	3 (16.67%)	3 (16.67%)	18 (3.6%)
Total	453 (90.42%)	26 (5.19%)	22 (4.39%)	501 (100%)
Matsumoto et al. (1987)				
Group A	30 (78.9%)	8 (21.1%)	—	38 (80.9%)
Group B	4 (100%)	0 (0%)	—	4 (8.5%)
Group C	2 (40%)	3 (60%)	—	5 (10.6%)
Total	36 (76.6%)	11 (23.4%)	—	47 (100%)
Kerekes et al. (1978)				
Group A	122 (80.26%)	30 (19.74%)	—	152 (26.81%)
Group B	203 (63.44%)	117 (36.56%)	—	320 (56.44%)
Group C	22 (23.16%)	73 (76.84%)	—	95 (16.75%)
Total	347 (61.20%)	220 (38.80%)	—	567 (100%)

Criteria for Evaluation of Obturating Materials and Sealers

It is well known that most obturating materials do not completely fill the root canal system. This has been confirmed by several methods of microleakage evaluation, including dye penetration, radioisotopes, electrochemical, fluorometrics, scanning electron microscopic examination, root clarification (Figure 3), fluid filtration, and fluid transport.[19-29] The limitation of these methods is of course that they do not precisely duplicate the clinical situation of the periapical tissue and the fluid environment, although Friedman et al.[30] developed an in vivo model to assess the efficacy of obturation.

VOIDS IN OBTURATING MATERIALS

A concern when using gutta-percha (or other core materials) to obturate canals is its potential of creating voids in the root canal filling. Eguchi et al.[31] compared four different methods of gutta-percha and sealer techniques, viewing three sections at different levels of obturation. Voids were found in the apical third with at least one of the techniques (lateral condensation). They cautioned that using different condensation techniques and different sealers would likely produce more sealer (and less gutta-percha) in some areas of the canal than in others and that the obturating techniques producing the most mass of core filling material (least voids) would require much sealer for an adequate canal seal.

TISSUE TOXICITY

Obturating materials are currently evaluated for tissue toxicity by four methods: (1) cytotoxicity evaluation, (2) subcutaneous implantation, (3) intraosseous implantation, and (4) in vivo periapical reactions.[18] Despite some materials exhibiting tissue toxicity, they have been used successfully for many years in the practice of clinical endodontics. For example, over 130 years ago, Chisholm introduced zinc oxide and oil of cloves to dentistry.[32] Surprisingly, eugenol (refined oil of cloves) is quite cytotoxic but still stands as a commonly used component of sealers.[33,34] This is one example of a material that in spite of its cytotoxicity has stood the test of time in clinical endodontics with a proven track record. For a more in-depth discussion of toxicity of obturating materials, the reader is referred to Chapter 29, "Root Canal Filling Materials."

Techniques of Obturation: Semisolid and Solid Core Materials

Gutta-Percha: The use of gutta-percha for obturation of canals has been enhanced by its ability to change volumetrically upon heating. Force applied to gutta-percha causes it to become *compacted*, not

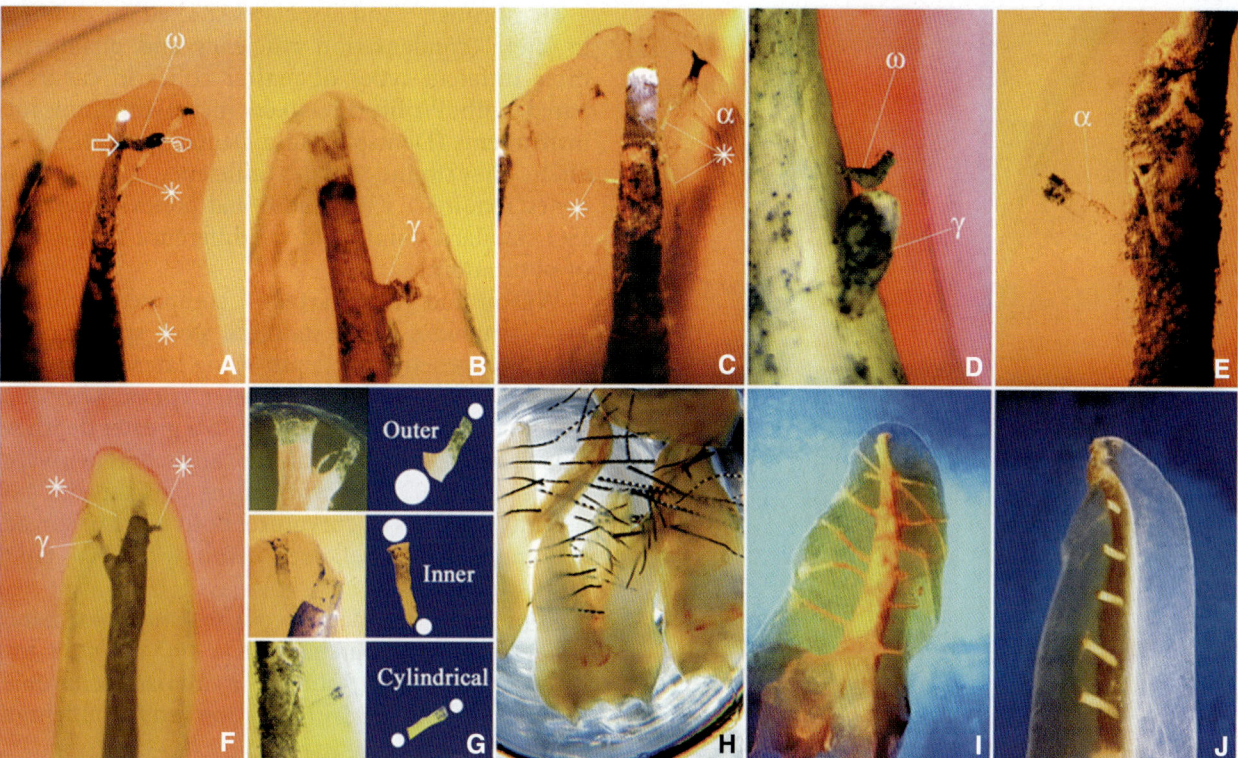

Figure 3 *A–F,* Stereomicroscopic images of human cleared roots. Inner diameter of the ramifications was measure in proximity to the endodontic main canal (a, arrow), outer diameter was measured in proximity to the external surface of the root (a, pointing hand). *A,C,F,* Asterisks: lateral canals in the apical third with inner diameter smaller than 50μm. *B,D,F,* γ: lateral canals showing cylindrical shape. *G,* Diagram of each type of lateral canals described in the study. *H–J,* Stereomicroscopic images of artificial lateral canals. *H,* Specimens with the instruments inserted immersed in methyl-salicylate for hardening. *I,* Specimen after final clearing showing the filling of the artificial lateral canals obtained at different distances from the apex (1,2,3, 4.5 and 6mm). *J,* Specimen showing a regular line of lateral canal. Reproduced with permission from Venturi M, DiLenarda R, Prati C et al.[29]

compressed as originally thought.[35] It has also been used in its cold (unheated) state with condensation pressures laterally, resulting in minimal deformation.[36] In contrast to this, Camps et al.[37] reported that warm gutta-percha compaction was maximized by plugger advancement apically to produce the best permanent deformation with compaction. An important concept in the use of gutta-percha for obturation is that it does not seal purely by itself. Sealing agents are necessary to accomplish this, since gutta-percha does not adhere to the dentinal wall.[38–40]

No matter what technique is used for the placement of gutta-percha in the canal, a good aseptic technique dictates that it should be disinfected. Sequira et al.[41] found that a simple immersion in 5.25% sodium hypochlorite eliminated *Bacillus subtilis* spores after just 1 minute of contact. Melker et al.[42] found that tetracycline-containing gutta-percha inhibited the growth of four common oral cavity bacterial inhabitants.

LATERAL COMPACTION

The most widely taught method of obturating root canals in dental schools is lateral compaction of cold gutta-percha and sealer, although compaction of heated gutta-percha is overtaking it.[43] This method is most optimally accomplished following meticulous canal preparation with a continuous tapered shape. The spreader used for lateral compaction should be placed within 1 to 2 mm of the working length when an apical stop has been created.[44] Criteria for the use of lateral

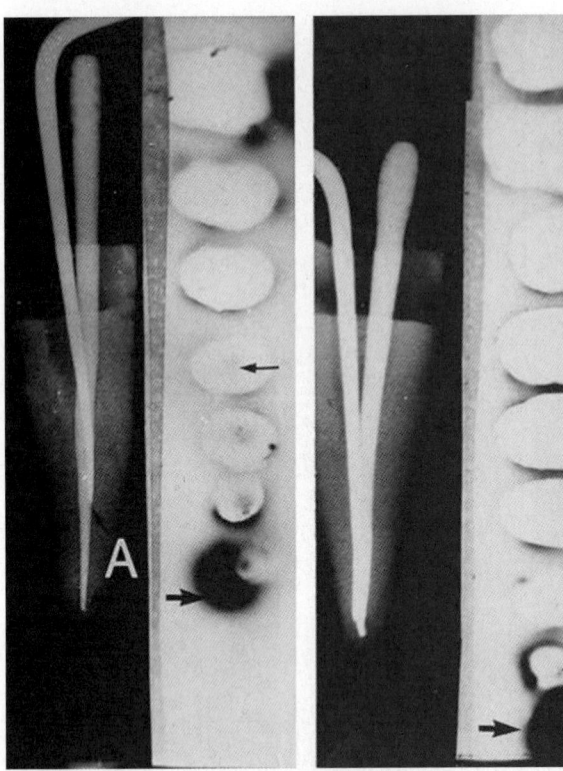

Figure 4 Microleakage into obturated canals related to flare of cavity preparation and depth of spreader penetration. **Left,** Final depth of spreader, A, is 5mm short of prepared length of canal. Radioisotope leakage is 4.8mm (**between arrows**) into canal. **Right,** Canal with flared preparation allows spreader depth to within 1mm of primary point length. Radioisotope leakage (**between arrows**) only 0.8mm into canal. Reproduced with permission from Allison DA, Weber CR, Walton RE.[45]

condensation should include the shape and size of the preparation, the sealer used, and the spreader size (Figure 4) required to be placed within the apical 2 mm. This "deep spreader penetration" assures the best likelihood to minimize apical leakage or percolation.[45]

More recent popularity of wider-flared canal preparations prompted Bal et al.[46] to compare the quality of seals in canals prepared with 0.06 and 0.02 tapered instruments and filled by lateral condensation with like tapered master cones. They noted spreader penetration to greater depth with 0.02 tapered preparations and cones.

Hembrough[47] and associates studied the differences in lateral condensation efficiency and quality using three different types of master cones in canals prepared with Profile ISO 0.06 nickel–titanium rotary instruments (Dentsply Tulsa Dental Specialties, Tulsa, OK). They found greater efficiency (less accessory cones required) with traditional cones compared to ISO standard points, but no difference in the quality of obturation.

Wilson and Baumgartner[48] compared similar size nickel–titanium with stainless steel spreaders with regard to penetration depth using lateral compaction of 0.02 and 0.04 tapered master cones. They found that NiTi spreaders penetrated to a greater depth with 0.02 tapered gutta-percha in canals with curvatures greater than 20° than when using 0.04 tapered gutta-percha regardless of curvature. Both types of spreaders penetrated to a shallower depth with 0.04 tapered gutta-percha.

Pomeranz[49] has described a technique for laterally condensing gutta-percha with a #10 file after initial spreader placement, solving a myriad of problems related to both instrumentation and condensation errors.

Although lateral compaction has worked well as a standard, it has been challenged with the more recent popularity of vertical compaction of heated gutta-percha. Gilhooly et al.[50] found more apical leakage to dye with in vitro teeth obturated with lateral condensation rather than with heated multi-phase gutta-percha obturation. Interestingly enough, they also found that lateral condensation yielded better radiographic quality than did the multi-phase obturation.

DaSilva et al.[51] using plastic blocks, compared the quality of obturations accomplished by lateral compaction, ThermaFil, and a new backfilling technique with the emphasis on length control. Although lateral compaction and ThermaFil backfill techniques yielded fewer overfills, blocks obturated by ThermaFil had no voids, while the other techniques demonstrated small voids.

Other studies regarding density and fill by weight of obturations showed heat-related techniques of compacting gutta-percha to have advantages over lateral

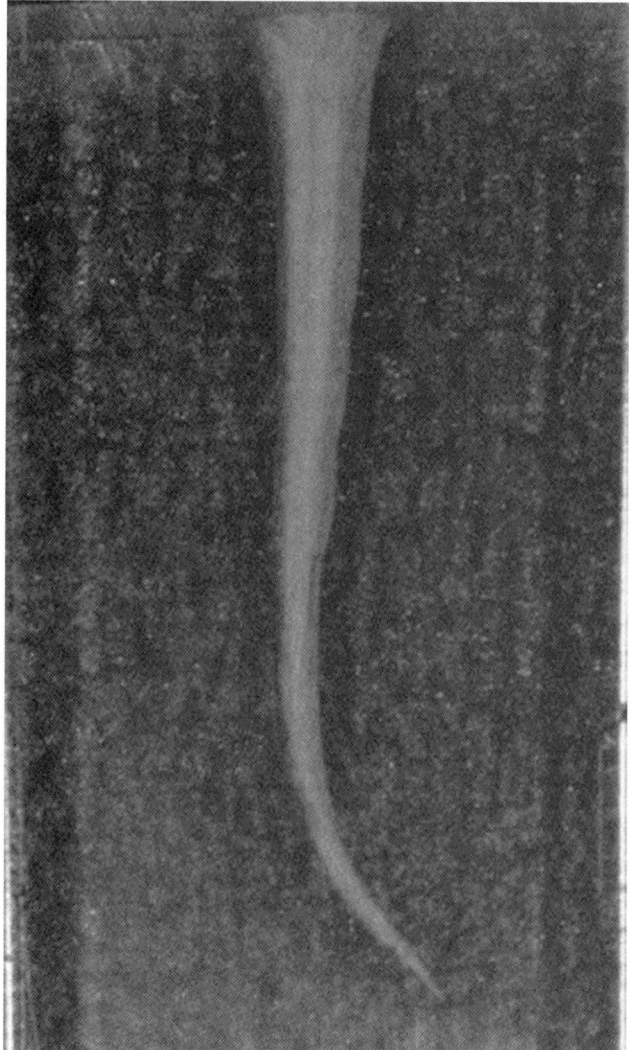

Figure 5 Obturated transparent resin block by cold lateral compaction. Reproduced with permission from Lea CS, Apicella MJ, Mines P et al.[53]

compaction (Figures 5 and 6) as well as gutta-percha to sealer ratio.[52,53] More recently, Collins et al.[54] used a split tooth model to assess the ability of cold lateral, warm lateral, and warm vertical compaction methods to replicate intracanal wall defects. They found a statistically better result with warm techniques over cold lateral compaction, but no significant difference between the two warm techniques.

VERTICAL COMPACTION

Arguably the most classic article describing this technique is Schilder's[2] treatise that describes in detail the technique offering an alternative to lateral compaction. This technique was based on a single cone adaptation and compaction, followed by additional

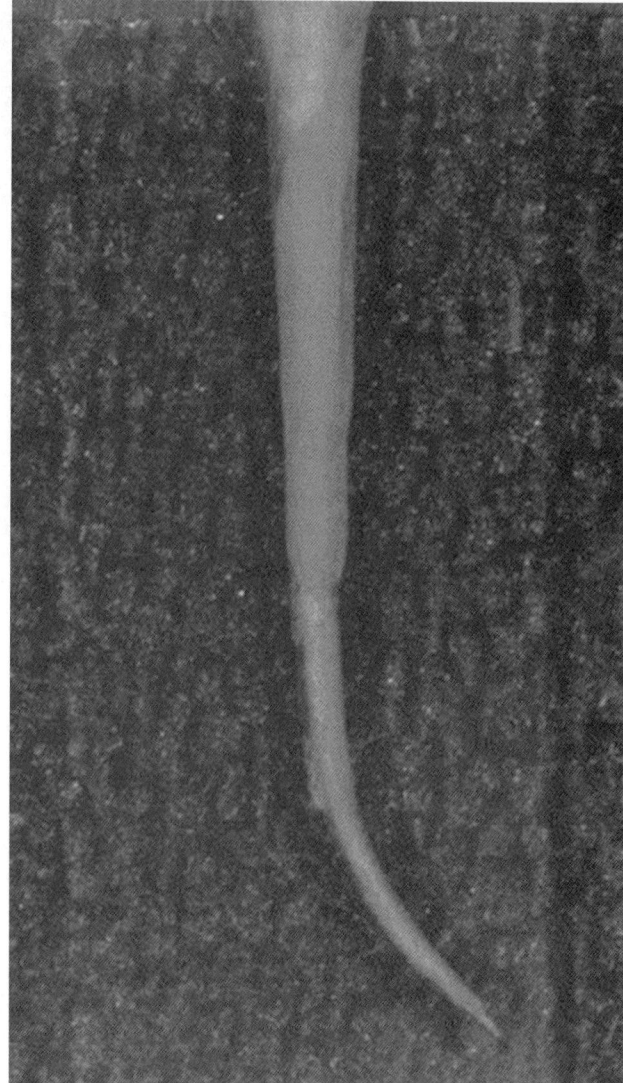

Figure 6 Obturated transparent resin block by warm vertical compaction. Reproduced with permission from Lea CS, Apicella MJ, Mines P et al.[53]

segments of gutta-percha, a technique previously described by Berg.[55] Historically, a single cone technique was also described in 1961 by Marshall and Massler.[56] This technique was touted as ensuring that potentially more than one portal of exit, lateral, and accessory canals may be filled over 40% of the time.[57]

An ongoing comparison of canal wall adaptability and microleakage studies has existed between lateral compaction and warm gutta-percha/vertical compaction. Brothman[58] found "no statistically significant difference in filling efficiency," but found that more accessory canals were filled with sealer using vertical compaction. He also concluded, however, that lateral

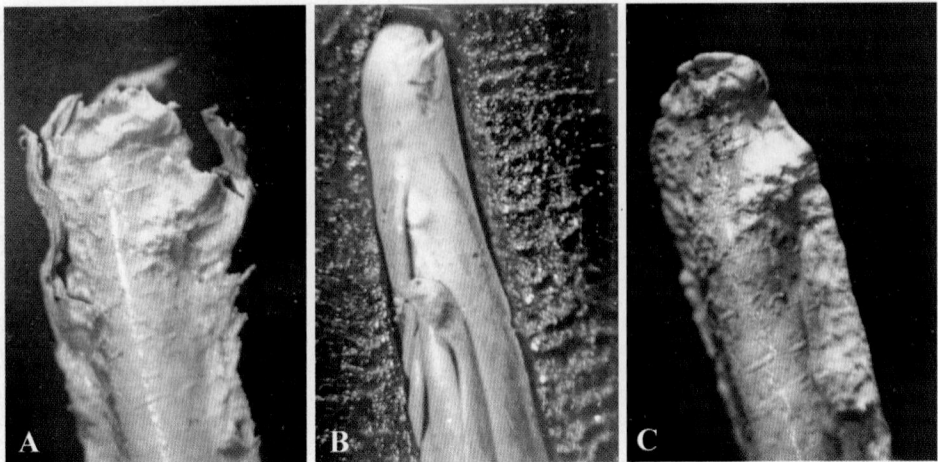

Figure 7 Compaction results from three methods of obturation purposely done without sealer. **A,** Chloropercha filling presents best immediate appearance. Unfortunately, a 12.4% shrinkage follows, leading to massive leakage. **B,** Lateral compaction –cold gutta-percha showing coalescence of primary and accessory points at apex but separating mid-canal. **C,** Warm gutta-percha/vertical compaction. Filling is homogeneous; replication is excellent. Reproduced with permission from Wong M et al.

compaction was more appropriate for ribbon-shaped canals, whereas vertical compaction was better suited for centric canals. Torabinejad and coworkers[59] compared multiple obturation techniques and found that all gave favorable results, but the vertical method resulted in closer adaptation to the canal walls in the middle and apical thirds. Wong et al.[60] compared homogeneity/replication of canal walls using chloropercha, lateral compaction, and warm gutta-percha vertical compaction without sealer and found the best results with the latter technique (Figure 7). With regard to microleakage, Benner et al.[61] used radioisotopes to study the difference in three obturation methods, including warm gutta-percha/vertical compaction and found no significant differences. Perhaps of more significance is a study by a Toronto group[62] who found a 10% higher rate of clinical success with warm vertical compaction versus cold lateral compaction in cases with apical periodontitis.

Since Schilder's description of vertical compaction, there have been criteria expressed by Glickman and Gutmann[63] that could apply to all subsequent techniques of gutta-percha placement utilizing heat. These relate to tapered shaped cones, cone selection, sealer amounts, and full-length softening and condensing instruments used.

THERMOMECHANICAL COMPACTION OF GUTTA-PERCHA

A different method of softening and compacting gutta-percha was introduced in 1979 by McSpadden.[64] After some difficulties with instrumentation, he was able to improve compaction, as well as length control. The technique has enjoyed more popularity in Europe, and a hybrid method was introduced by Tagger and associates in Israel.[65] They promoted placement of a master cone with sealer, lateral action with a finger spreader, and placement of an accessory cone. This was followed by rotary compaction that resulted in less apical leakage than lateral compaction alone. Fuss et al.[66] agreed that there was no difference in apical leakage between the two techniques. However, Budd and coworkers[67] found that thermomechanical compaction resulted in a better apical seal. Saunders[68] added a note of caution with this technique, as the heat generated in his in vitro study resulted in 25% of ferrets in an in vivo study developing root resorption or ankylosis.

THERMOMECHANICAL SOLID CORE GUTTA-PERCHA OBTURATION

This system, employing a titanium core/carrier coated with alpha-phase gutta-percha, can be used with core retention or removal, followed by hand plugger compaction. Pallares and Fuss[69] found no difference in apical leakage with this system compared to lateral compaction. Canalda-Sahil et al.[70] also found good results in attempting to seal canals in teeth with large, straight canals.

ULTRASONIC PLASTICIZED GUTTA-PERCHA

The use of an ultrasonic instrument to plasticize gutta-percha was first described by Moreno.[71] He

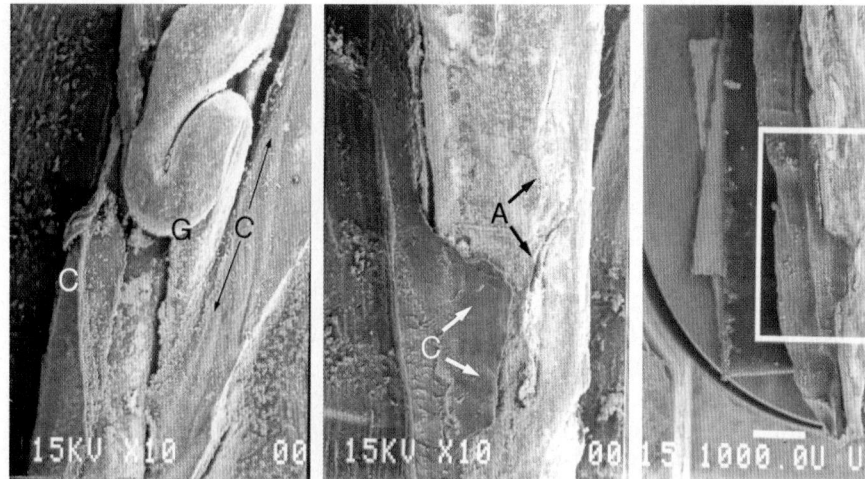

Figure 8 Comparison in obturation between hand-lateral compaction and **ultrasonic compaction**. **Left,** Accessory point folded in canal during lateral compaction following finger spreading. G, individual gutta-percha points. *C,* canal wall. High power (x320 original magnification). **Center,** Gutta-percha compacted by **Enac ultrasonic** spreader tips (no fluid coolant). Note uniformity of gutta-percha mass with only two "crevice marks" at (A). C denotes canal walls. High power (x320 original magnification). **Right,** Low power (x10 original magnification) of apical third obturation by ultrasonic. B marks well-filled foramen. Rectangular area is seen at high power in center panel. Reproduced with permission from Baumgardner KR, Krell KV.

employed its friction plus hand or finger pluggers for condensation. Joiner et al.[72] studied the effect of heat generated by this technique and concluded that it was safe. Baumgardner and Krell[73] attached an Enac ultrasonic point (Osada, Los Angeles, CA) to a spreader to penetrate the gutta-percha mass and found more homogeneous compaction and less apical microleakage than hand lateral compaction (Figure 8).

THERMOPLASTICIZED INJECTABLE GUTTA-PERCHA

A group at Harvard/Forsythe Institute[74] developed an injection device in 1977 to deliver heat-softened gutta-percha to the canal space. Currently, the latest model of this system, Obtura II Heated Gutta-Percha System (Obtura Spartan, Fenton, MD), uses temperatures up to 200°C and beta-phase gutta-percha or less viscous Easy Flow gutta-percha (Charles B. Schwed Co., Kew Gardens, NY). Gutmann and Raskin[75] stressed the importance of a meticulously tapered preparation with this system to minimize flow and containment of the gutta-percha. Lambrianidis et al.[76] found in their 1990 study that no matter what was the distance of the needle tip to the foramen, there was no significant difference in linear dye leakage using Obtura II in canals.

A question may be raised about the safety of heat generated and delivered to canals by the above method. Gutmann and associates[77] found in their in vitro study that the temperature of gutta-percha emerging from the needle was 71.2°C in a body temperature environment. Their in vivo study in dogs concluded that it was safe with only a 1.1°C rise in temperature over 60 seconds, in the overlying bone.

Hardie[78] reported much higher temperatures in the canal (137.8°C) and a rise of 9.65°C on the root surface. If maintained for 1 minute, this is reported to cause injury.[79] Weller and Koch[80] reported safe (less than 10°C) temperature rises when using gutta-percha thermoplasticized to 200°C. More recently, Sweatman et al.[81] have verified these findings. It is also documented that these injectable gutta-percha techniques still require a sealer to avoid microleakage.[82] Care in apical preparation design is emphasized, as more studies have indicated overextensions or extrusions of material with inadequate apical taper.[83,84] Tan-Ishii and Teranaka[85] followed 236 obturated canals filled with the Obtura II system, achieving a 96% success rate. They also found that "root filling excess had no impact on the healing process."

SYSTEM B PLUGGER TECHNIQUE

An additional heat-assisted gutta-percha compaction technique was introduced by Buchanan in 1996 and was marketed by Analytic Technology (Sybron Endo, Orange, CA) as System B.[86] This was an upgrade or improvement to their 1982 Touch 'n Heat and was reported to be more rapid, simple, and more effective. Pommel and Camps[87] studied its ability to resist leakage in vitro and found that initially it was more resistant than lateral compaction or single cone technique. After 1 month, however, there was no difference. It was also found to be as effective in initial resistance to apical leakage as warm vertical condensation and ThermaFil.

Guess et al.[88] studied the in vitro influence of System B plugger depth on gutta-percha filling adaptation to the canal wall using single cone continuous wave technique in one group and lateral compaction followed by continuous wave downpack in the other. They found no significant difference in adaptability, and the best results were obtained with plugger depth 3 to 4.5 mm from the working length. Jung and associates[89] compared gutta-percha filled areas in plastic blocks, with varying temperatures and plugger depths for System B-assisted obturation. They found no significant differences with temperature variation, but better adaptability with deeper plugger depth placement.

Villegas et al.[90] in 2004 used Obtura II to backfill extracted teeth filled by single versus multiple positioned System B pluggers and compared each to assess gutta-percha mass adaptability to the canal wall. They found that there was better adaptation of this mass (Figure 9) when the System B plugger was used in three steps instead of one insertion at 3 mm short of working length.

LATERAL/VERTICAL COMPACTION OF WARM GUTTA-PERCHA HYBRID TECHNIQUE

Considering the ease and speed of lateral compaction, as well as the superior density achieved with vertical compaction of warm gutta-percha, Martin[91] developed a device that incorporates the qualities of both techniques. The Endotec II (Medidenta, Woodside, NY) is a battery-powered, heat-controlled spreader/plugger. Similar units are marketed as Thermique (Parkell, Edgewood, NY) and as DownPak (Hu Friedy, Chicago, IL). Several studies[92–94] found the technique to be better than other methods tested for preventing leakage and for filling canal irregularities. Jurcak et al.,[95] concerned about possible ill effects of warm gutta-percha on vital tissues, found that heating a mass of gutta-percha to 102°C "would not be of significant magnitude to cause damage to the periodontal tissues."

INJECT-R FILL

This system is marketed by Miltex Corporation (Troy, PA) and consists of a small metal tube filled with gutta-percha and a plugger/plunger attached. It is heated

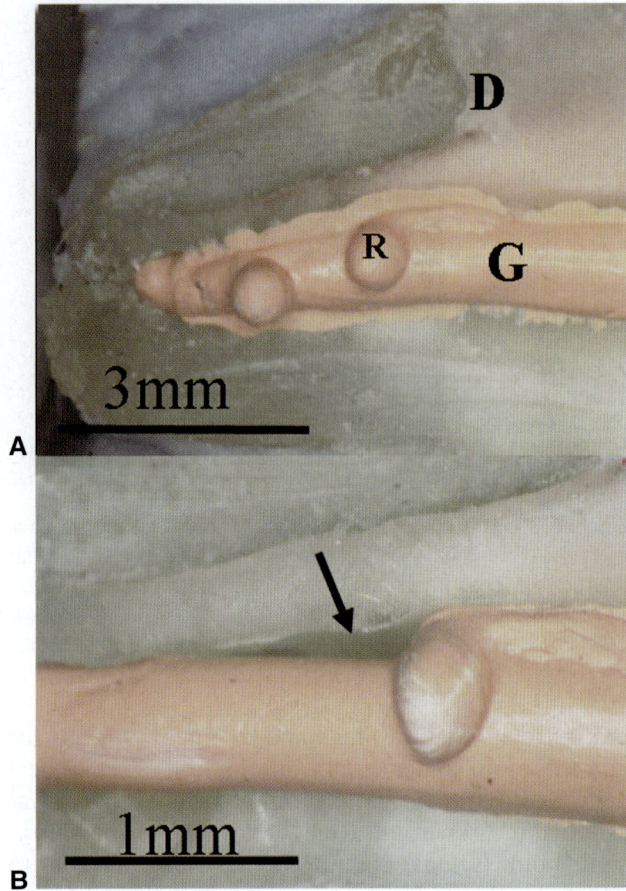

Figure 9 *A*, Representative Group A gutta-percha root filling in the split tooth model with a straight and round canal. Note the good adaptation of gutta-percha to the root canal walls within the apical 3mm and replication of the artificial depressions. D, dentine; G, gutta-percha mass; R, artificial round depression replication. *B*, Representative Group B GP root filling in the split-tooth model with a straight and round canal. Note space between gutta-percha mass and root canal wall (arrow) within the apical 3mm. Reproduced with permission from Villegas, JC et al.[92]

either by a flame or an electric warmer/container and produces a result similar to vertical compaction, when injected and compacted upon a preexisting downpack of gutta-percha, according to Roane.[96]

CONDENSATION FORCES: VERTICAL VERSUS LATERAL

A concern was expressed in the early 1980s about the forces generated during vertical compaction and their possible transference, inducing vertical cracks in roots. Gimlin and associates[97] studied both lateral and vertical "condensation forces" using a mathematical model. Their results suggested that lateral condensation was

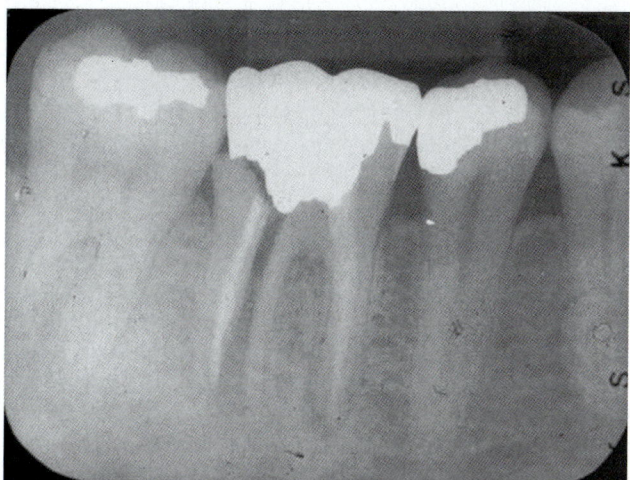

Figure 10 Root fracture occurs when the wedging force is absorbed by the canal walls. Premeasuring the spreader depth can reduce the risk of fracture.

more likely to produce undesirable stress concentration (near the apex) than was vertical condensation (for gutta-percha compaction) (Figure 10).

Solid Core Carriers with Manual Placement Techniques

The previously mentioned techniques for condensing or compacting gutta-percha aimed at minimizing sealer or maximizing gutta-percha content. The past two decades have seen an increase in the use of carrier-based gutta-percha techniques to accomplish this task. A discussion of these systems follows, including their advantages and limitations.

THERMAFIL

A new concept in delivering gutta-percha to the radicular space was introduced in 1978 by Johnson.[98] It consisted of alpha-phase gutta-percha on a fluted metal instrument, while the current version has the gutta-percha on a plastic carrier. There are additional similar systems, namely Densfil (Dentsply Maillefer, Tulsa, OK), Soft-Core (Axis Dental Corp., Irving, TX), and Three Dee GP (Deproco Ltd., Dorking, UK). The ThermaFil technique was found to exert less strain on the root when placing and compacting its gutta-percha core when compared to Obtura or lateral compaction.[99]

The importance of a good apical stop or constriction when using ThermaFil was stressed by Scott and Vire[100] when compared with other techniques, in avoiding extrusion of filling material. Gutmann et al.[101] reported that ThermaFil placement was at least

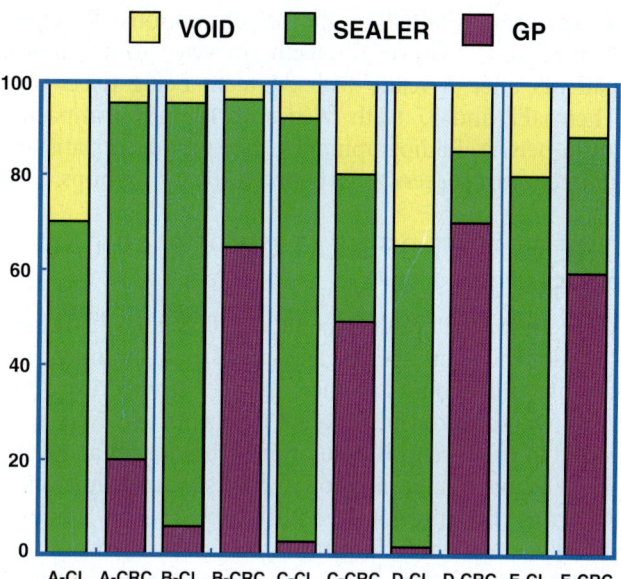

Figure 11 Each pair of columns represents lateral canals A to E with each left hand column representing obturation with cold lateral (CL) and each right hand column representing obturation with the coated rigid carrier (CRC). Reproduced and adapted with permission from Wolcott J, Himel VT, Powell W et al.[100]

comparable to lateral compaction when filling irregularities of any type in a canal space. A similar study by Kytridou et al.[102] showed equivalent results for ThermaFil when comparing it with the System B technique. When comparing adaptation to the canal wall, Wolcott et al.[103] found that ThermaFil gutta-percha and sealer moved into lateral canals as well as did lateral compaction; however, ThermaFil surpassed it in this regard in the main canal (Figure 11).

Gutmann et al.[101] found similar microleakage between contemporary (plastic core) ThermaFil and lateral compaction after 3 to 5 months. Fabra-Campos[104] reported similar findings in his 1993 study. Another study by Valli et al.[105] found more in vitro depth of coronal leakage in lateral compaction than with Densfil. In 2001, Abarca et al.[106] investigated apical linear leakage and apical extrusion in mesial roots of mandibular molars obturated with lateral compaction and ThermaFil. There were no statistically different findings for either technique in both areas studied. ThermaFil did not fare as well as System B in a 1999 study by Kytridou et al.[107] in which they found greater apical leakage with ThermaFil after 67 days when both groups of teeth were stored in Hanks Balanced Salt Solution.

Levitan et al.[108] studied the effect of insertion rate of ThermaFil Plus on apical extension and found that the faster insertion resulted in more overextension, while slower rates resulted in shorter obturations. Recently, Chu et al.[109] followed 71 teeth (in vivo) in 64 clinical patients after 3 years, with 34 teeth being filled with ThermaFil and 37 teeth filled with laterally compacted gutta-percha. Radiographically, they found no statistical difference in success rates between the two groups.

THE EFFECT OF HEAT ON PERIAPICAL TISSUES

Concern for the health of periodontal tissues, when using heat-softened gutta-percha techniques, has continued into the new millennium. Romero et al.[110] studied extracted teeth with artificial periodontal ligaments that were subjected to the System B obturation technique set at 200°C. They found significantly lower root surface temperature increases than previously reported by Hardie.[78] Subsequent studies have confirmed root surface temperature changes of less than 10°C, concluding no detriment to periodontal tissue adjacent to root surfaces.[111,112]

RESIN-BASED CORE (RESILON)

Resilon, a thermoplastic synthetic (polycaprolactone) polymer-based obturating material (Resilon Research LLC, Madison, CT), has gained considerable popularity in the past few years. Studies regarding its attributes began to appear in 2004 when Shipper et al.[113] discussed its ability to resist microbial leakage. They compared laterally and vertically compacted gutta-percha and sealer groups with Resilon and its sealer and their resistance to leakage with *Streptococcus mutans* and *Enterococcus faecalis* and found that the Resilon groups were "superior to gutta-percha groups" in amounts of leakage allowed (Figures 12 and 13). Teixeira et al.[114] studied the fracture resistance under load in vitro of teeth obturated with lateral and vertical compaction of gutta-percha and that of those obturated with Resilon. They found that filling canals with Resilon increased the resistance to root fracture.

Using both scanning electron microscope (SEM) and transmission electron microscope (TEM), Tay et al.[115] studied the quality of apical seal between Resilon/Epiphany sealer and gutta-percha/AH Plus. They looked for gaps along the canal walls with an SEM (Figure 14) and for apical leakage with a TEM and concluded that "a complete hermetic (sic) apical seal cannot be achieved with either root filling material."

The implied increased resistance to root fracture as a result of the Teixeira et al.[114] study was challenged in 2005 by Gesi et al.[116] when studying interfacial strength and dislocation resistance between gutta-percha/sealer and Resilon/sealer, and intraradicular

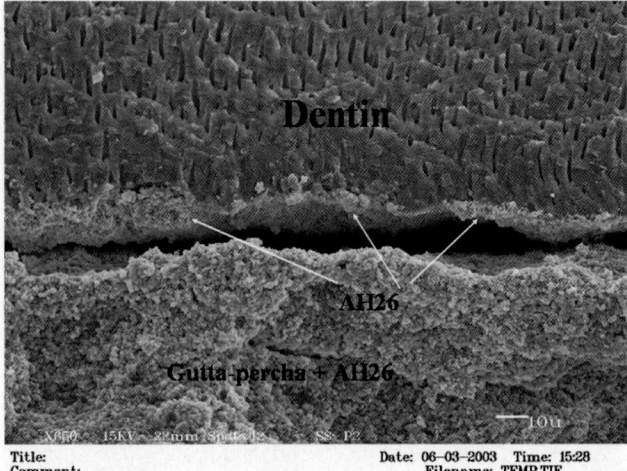

Figure 12 High power SEM (650x) micrograph of a longitudinal section of a root filled with gutta-percha. The resin tags of the sealer penetrated the dentin, but a gap is evident between the sealer-dentin interface and the gutta-percha filling. Reproduced with permission from Shipper G, Ørstavik D, Teixeira FB et al.[110]

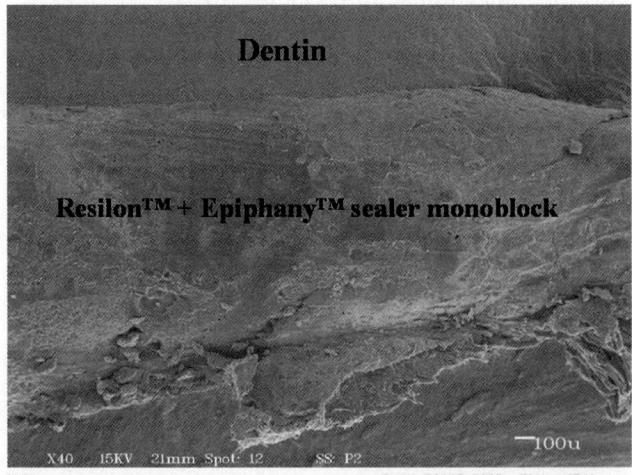

Figure 13 Low-power SE (40x) micrograph of a longitudinal section of a root filled with Resilon™. No gap is evident between the Resilon™ filling and the dentin. Reproduced with permission from Shipper G, Ørstavik D, Teixeira FB et al.[110]

dentin using a thin slice push-out test design. Their results indicated a higher interfacial strength for gutta-percha, with more failure along the sealer/dentin interface with Resilon.

Nielsen and Baumgartner[117] studied the penetration depth of a nickel–titanium spreader in 0.04 taper prepared canals against 0.02 and 0.04 tapered gutta-percha and Resilon master cones and found significant differences in penetration depth, with 0.02 tapered Resilon permitting the deepest penetration, followed by 0.02 tapered gutta-

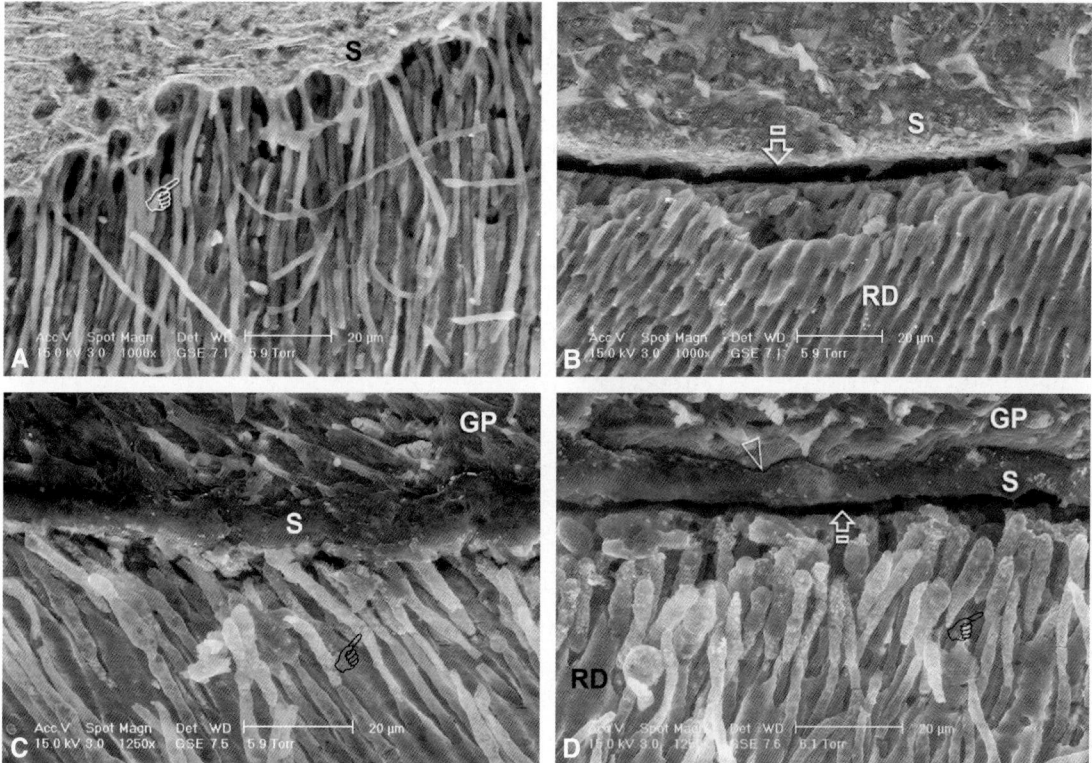

Figure 14 Fe-ESEM micrographs of wet, non-dehydrated sectioned specimens of vertical condensation filled roots, showing the variability of gap formation. ***A,*** Specimen that was filled with Resilon bonded with the self-etching resin system Epiphany, taken at a level 4mm from the apex. No gap could be seen between the filled resin sealer (S) and the root dentin. Numerous resin tags (pointer) extended into the dentinal tubules. ***B,*** Another region from the opposite side of the Resilon/Epiphany-filled root canal, taken 4mm from the apex. A gap (arrow) could be seen between the S and the root dentin (RD). No resin tags could be identified in dentinal tubules. ***C,*** Control specimen that was filled with gutta-percha (GP) and AH Plus, taken at a level 4mm from the apex. No gap could be discerned between the sealer (S) and root dentin. Numerous resin tags (pointer) were present. ***D,*** Another region from the same tooth, showing separation of the GP from the sealer (S), and the presence of a gap (arrow) between the sealer and the RD, despite the presence of resin tags (pointer). Reproduced with permission from Tay FR, Loushine RJ, Weller RN et al.[112]

percha, 0.04 tapered Resilon, and 0.04 tapered gutta-percha.

The adhesive strength of a methacrylate-based sealer (Real Seal) to Resilon was evaluated by Tay et al.[118] using a modified microshear bond testing design. A composite control was used to compare results. There was phase separation of the polymeric components in Resilon, suggesting that the amount of dimethacrylate in it may not be optimal for coupling to Real Seal. Another study by Nielsen et al.[119] addressed the differences in setting time between 11 sealers in both aerobic and anaerobic environments. There were several conditions used for observation, including aerobic and anaerobic incubators and buffering solutions. Ketac-Endo and Resilon were found to set the quickest in anaerobic environments. However, when exposed to air, Resilon took 7 days to set and when placed in phosphate buffer solution, "an uncured layer remained on the surface."

Recently, Stratton et al.[120] compared the sealing ability of gutta-percha with AH Plus sealer versus Resilon and Epiphany Resilon Sealer. Using a fluid filtration system, they found significantly less leakage in canals filled with Resilon and Epiphany Sealer using the continuous wave obturation method. Because of the very recent introduction of Resilon, further studies are certainly warranted to assess its long-term effectiveness in clinical usage.

SILVER POINTS

This solid core material is becoming more and more of historical significance. It was commonly used in previous times when less efficiently designed instruments and lesser quality metallurgy prevented larger, more accurate preparation of the canal space. Silver points were machined round in cross section and were

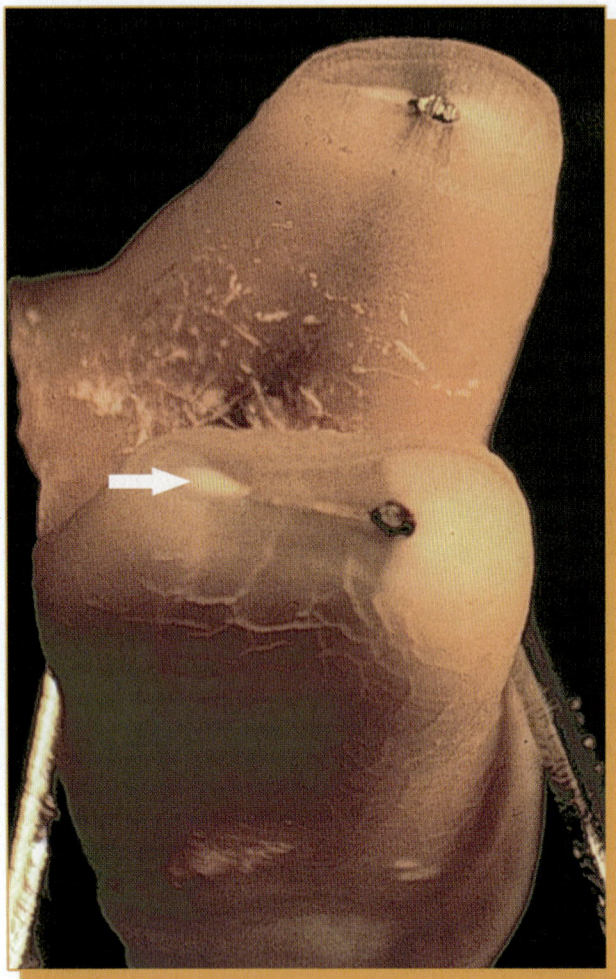

Figure 15 Cross section of extracted maxillary molar showing inadequately enlarged canals, and the disparity between the circular silver points and ribbon or oval shaped canals and lack of adaptation. Note undetected second mesio-buccal canal (white arrow). (Courtesy Dr. Fred Benenati)

sometimes placed into canals more often ovoid than round (Figure 15). Not surprisingly, long-term success rates may not be as high in these situations.

Siskin[121] published a classic article in 1957 that included the use of silver points in straight, round-shaped canals and credited Jaspers for introducing them. Using the SEM, Seltzer et al.[122] showed the appearance of corrosion on silver points from extracted endodontically treated teeth. Another SEM study of silver points placed in bones showed sulfur and chlorine corrosive products on their surfaces.[123] A report by Timpawat and coworkers[124] in 1983 involved an in vitro study of gutta-percha cones, stainless steel files, and silver points filling curved canals. They found that canals filled with silver cones actually resisted dye penetration better than gutta-percha.

Present-day instrumentation allows larger and more accurate canal preparations, and to accommodate these preparations often with many irregularities, gutta-percha as a core material appears better suited than the round silver points.

Cements and Pastes as Root Canal Filling Materials

N2/SARGENTI PASTE

Although first used in Europe, N2 paste has been produced in the United States as RC2B. The constituent of most concern in the paste is paraformaldehyde (6.5% concentration), which is quite toxic.[125] Several other reports have produced negative connotations for it, including a position by the American Association of Endodontists condemning its use.[126–130]

Two well-known in vivo studies regarding the effects of paraformaldehyde, which Sargenti refused to remove from his paste, were conducted at the University of Indiana[131,132] and showed severe inflammation of the pulp when RC2B was applied against it (Figure 16). An additional study even showed evidence of osteomyelitis in the apical tissue from teeth filled with RC2B.[133]

Two other common problems with Sargenti paste, or RC2B in the United States, were overextension (even 15% of the cases submitted for Fellowship in the American Endodontic Society had overextensions) and required cortical trephinations 20.5% of the time in a survey conducted by the American Endodontic Society (supporters of the Sargenti technique).[134,135] Perhaps of more magnitude of concern are the cases of persistent paresthesia from the misuse of these paraformaldehyde cements, unlike the temporary effects of such from other cements (J. Weichman, D.D.S., J.D., personal communication, June 1982).[136,137,138] This type of cement or paste filling has not gained favor with organized dentistry or its component regulatory systems as a result of the above-described problems.

CALCIUM PHOSPHATE CEMENT

Based on the earlier experience with calcium phosphate gels, tricalcium phosphate has been suggested by Harbert[139] for use as an apical plug. In 1985, calcium phosphate cement (CPC) was advocated for use as a complete canal obturation material.[140] A blend of cements—one acidic and one basic—are combined to set as hydroxyapatite. It is nearly insoluble, except in the presence of strong acids.[141] A dye leakage study conducted

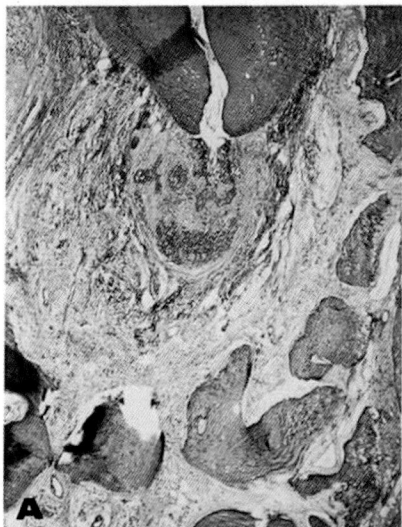 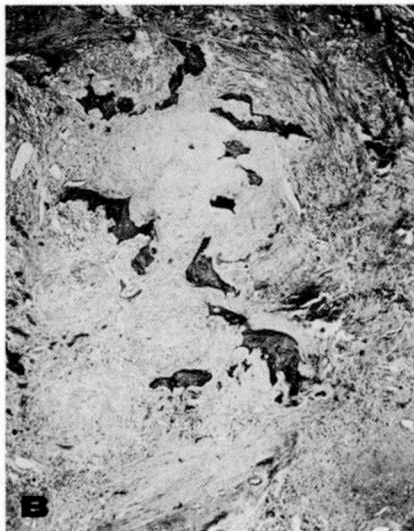 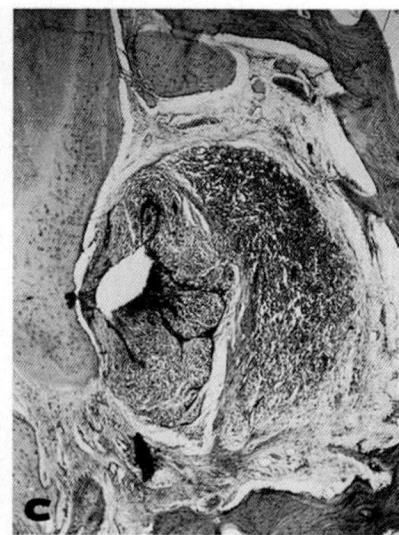

Figure 16 N2/RC2B formalin cement study. ***A,* Control** specimen, pulp necrosis 3 months standing. Apical periodontitis with epithelial proliferation. ***B,*** Osteomyelitis 6 months after treatment of necrotic canal with RC2B. Areas of necrotic bone within dense inflammatory infiltrate. ***C,*** Apical cyst developing 6 months after treatment of necrotic canal with RC2B. Note epithelial lining within dense inflammatory infiltrate. Reproduced with permission from Newton CW et al.

against it was impressive from the standpoint that there was only 0.15 mm penetration in vitro.[142] The resistance to dye penetration was so impressive that it prompted Goodell et al.[143] to recommend CPC as a replacement for calcium hydroxide in apexification cases.

RESIN CEMENTS

There have been few studies that have addressed resin as a complete root canal filling material.[144,145,146] The problem lies with its inability to bond with gutta-percha and to wet dentin walls. Kanca[147] commended All Bond 2 since it adheres to both wet and dry dentin.

CALCIUM HYDROXIDE

This compound has been called the endodontic panacea and an ultimate medicament.[148] Its use as a permanent obturating material has been mostly confined to the apical portion of the canal. Calcium hydroxide has been shown to encourage cementogenesis and osteogenesis and promotes apexification after thorough cleaning and shaping (Figure 17).[149,150] Due to its solubility, calcium hydroxide has been used mainly as an apical obturation or a dentinal plug.[151] Weisenseel et al.[152] found less apical leakage with calcium hydroxide plugs and laterally compacted gutta-percha than without apical plugs. Schumacher and Rutledge[153] endorsed a technique for placing calcium hydroxide as an apical barrier followed by immediate obturation with gutta-percha and sealer in open apex cases, suggesting an end or an alternative to the laborious traditional multiple appointment apexification technique.

More recently, the placement of calcium hydroxide has been studied, and Torres et al.[154] found that placement of calcium hydroxide with a Lentulo spiral was more effective than with an Ultradent tip. Robert et al.[155] used an in vitro agar model to study three calcium hydroxide medicaments of varying viscosity through simulated root canals with various sizes of apical foramina. They found that a "thinner mix of 10% calcium hydroxide in sterile water can produce a higher pH and calcium ion concentration in an agar environment and could similarly produce both a higher pH and calcium levels in a periapical lesion than Pulpdent or calcium hydroxide and sterile water mixed to a similar consistency."

Haenni et al.[156] compared conventional calcium hydroxide/saline paste to calcium hydroxide mixed with chlorhexidine, with sodium hypochlorite, or with iodine potassium iodide solutions. Each was exposed to *E. faecalis* and *Candida albicans* in a diffusion assay. They found that none of these mixtures provided a better antimicrobial effect than conventional calcium hydroxide and saline.

DENTIN CHIP APICAL OBTURATION

Dentin chips or dentinal debris often occupy the apical portions of prepared and even sealed canals.[157] It has been well established that dentin filings stimulate both

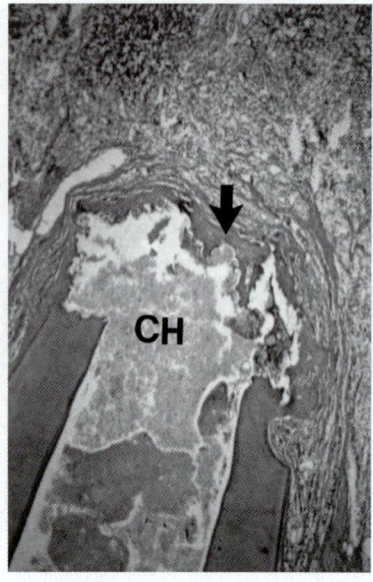 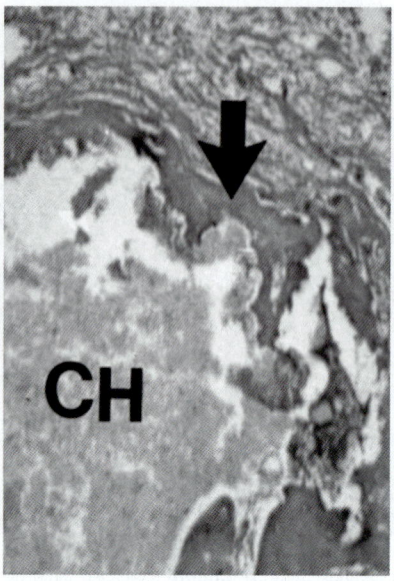

Figure 17 Periapical repair following intracanal application of calcium hydroxide. **A,** Low-power view of periapex. Acute inflammatory resorption of dentin and cementum following pulpectomy. Canal filled with calcium hydroxide mixture (CH). New hard tissue forming across apex in response to Ca(OH)2. **B,** Higher-power view of repair leading to "apical stop" **(arrow)**. Reproduced with permission from Jeansonne BG.

osteo- and cementogenesis.[158,159] El Deeb et al.[160] and Oswald et al.[161] all concluded that dentin chips, acting as an apical barrier, confined materials to the canal space and led to quicker healing, minimal inflammation, and cementum deposition (Figure 18). A study by Torneck et al.[162] contradicted the previous studies, finding that some dentin chips could interfere with repair.

A study by Holland et al.[163] mentioned a previous finding that infected dentin chips could impede healing and compared cementogenesis and inflammation between dentin chips and calcium hydroxide in ferrets. They found thicker cementum formation with dentin chips but no overall difference between the materials. Based upon these findings and the previous study by Pitts et al.[151] this technique has been endorsed as a "new technique," and a "biologic seal" and should be considered for wider use.[164,165]

Endodontic Sealers and Apical Leakage

RATIONALE FOR THE USE OF SEALERS

The importance of filling the prepared root canal system with a sealer and a protective core has been

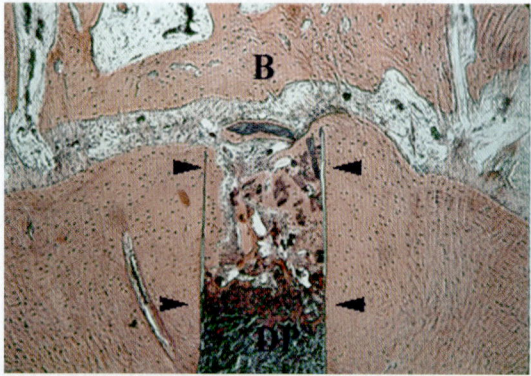 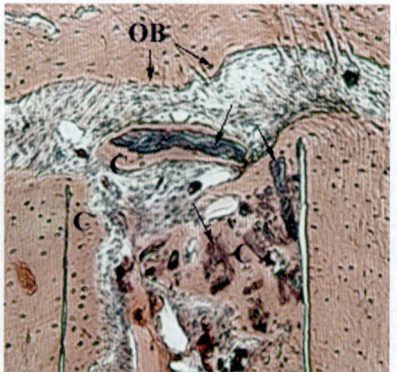

Figure 18 Dentin chip root canal plug after 3 months. **Left,** Periapical area, B, bone, C cementum, DP, dentin plug. **Arrows** indicate canal wall. **Right,** High-power view of same periapical area. C, cementum within canal around dentin chips **(arrows)**. OB, new bone cells. Reproduced with permission from Oswald RJ, Friedman CF.

previously discussed.[4] Friedman et al.[166] reiterated that importance and addressed the assessment of leakage of sealers. Wu, Fan and Wesselink[167] investigated the long-term success of gutta-percha with and without the use of a sealer and concluded that the "long-term seal of root fillings is affected by the volume change of both gutta-percha and sealer." They found that leakage up to 6 months was always worse in canals filled with gutta-percha alone compared to those with gutta-percha and sealer. After 6 months, leakage amounts in both groups were similar. This may have been due to the ability of gutta-percha to flow and approximate canal walls. On the other hand, a solubility study by Peters[168] found that after 2 years, canals filled only with zinc oxide were completely free of the material. This should dispel the notion of core material being optional or unnecessary.

The properties of sealers are discussed in Chapter 29, "Root Canal Filling Materials," so the following will emphasize how they perform in the canal space as well as their comparative abilities to resist apical microleakage. Coronal microleakage will be discussed separately.

MICROLEAKAGE AND ITS EVALUATION

Microleakage and how it is evaluated are important issues in endodontics. Clinical studies addressing the causes of endodontic failure found that incomplete obturation accounted for many of them, and an in vitro study indicated that incomplete obturation caused microleakage.[169,170] These studies agree that an "evaluation of the apical leakage of particles or solutions between a root canal filling and the root canal walls is a proper method to establish the quality of an endodontic obturation."

The most common method for the evaluation of microleakage has been the linear measurement of tracer dye penetration.[171,172] These include eosin, methylene blue, India ink, radioisotopes, and even bacteria. They have been measured by longitudinal splitting, cross sectioning or decalcification, and clearing of the root.

Recently, Lyroudia et al.[173] evaluated a method involving computer-aided three-dimensional construction to measure and study apical microleakage. They used collaged stereoscopic microscope photos, after immersion in India ink, to reconstruct the roots three dimensionally via computer imaging, photorealistic effects, color and texture addition, light, and shading (Figure 19). Other recent methods of testing apical leakage include a vacuum technique, fluid filtration, and movement of an air bubble in a glass tube.[174–176]

ZINC OXIDE–EUGENOL-CONTAINING SEALERS

Early zinc oxide–eugenol (ZOE)-containing sealers included Rickert's Kerr Pulp Canal Sealer and Procosol (Grossman's sealer). They were reported upon by Marshall and Massler,[56] who studied their resistance to leakage to radioisotopes in human teeth. They found that the Kerr formula was better than Procosol in this regard. A more recent study showed the current formula, Kerr EWT (Extended Working Time), to surpass Roth 801 and AH 26 at 24 weeks.[177] Other ZOE sealers include Wach's cement and Nogenol, neither of which shows a long-lasting seal against liquid exposure.[178]

ROTH'S 801

This modern-day Grossman's formula has been shown to inhibit bacterial growth.[179] A newer version of this sealer has been produced as Roth's 811.

KERR PULP CANAL SEALER EWT

Perhaps the longest surviving ZOE sealer, it has been compared with the more current calcium hydroxide-containing sealers and resin-based sealers, with regard to apical leakage. The results of these comparisons will be discussed with each of those sealers.

CALCIOBIOTIC ROOT CANAL SEALER

This ZOE/eucalyptol sealer with calcium hydroxide has shown some promise in minimal water sorption; however, if the calcium hydroxide is bound to other ingredients, it would be difficult to exert its purported osteogenic effect.[180,181]

SEALAPEX

This calcium hydroxide sealer has been noted to have minimal dissolution at the apex in one study.[182] In contrast to this, Gutmann and Fava[183] found in an in vivo study that this material had disappeared from periapical tissues and may do the same in the canal system.

In a previously mentioned study, Pommel et al.[175] used a fluid filtration method to compare apical leakage between SealApex, Kerr Pulp Canal Sealer, AH 26, and Ketac-Endo and found SealApex to leak significantly more than the others. There was no significant leakage difference between the other sealers. On the other hand, Cobankara et al.[184] used the same method to evaluate leakage between SealApex, RC Sealer,

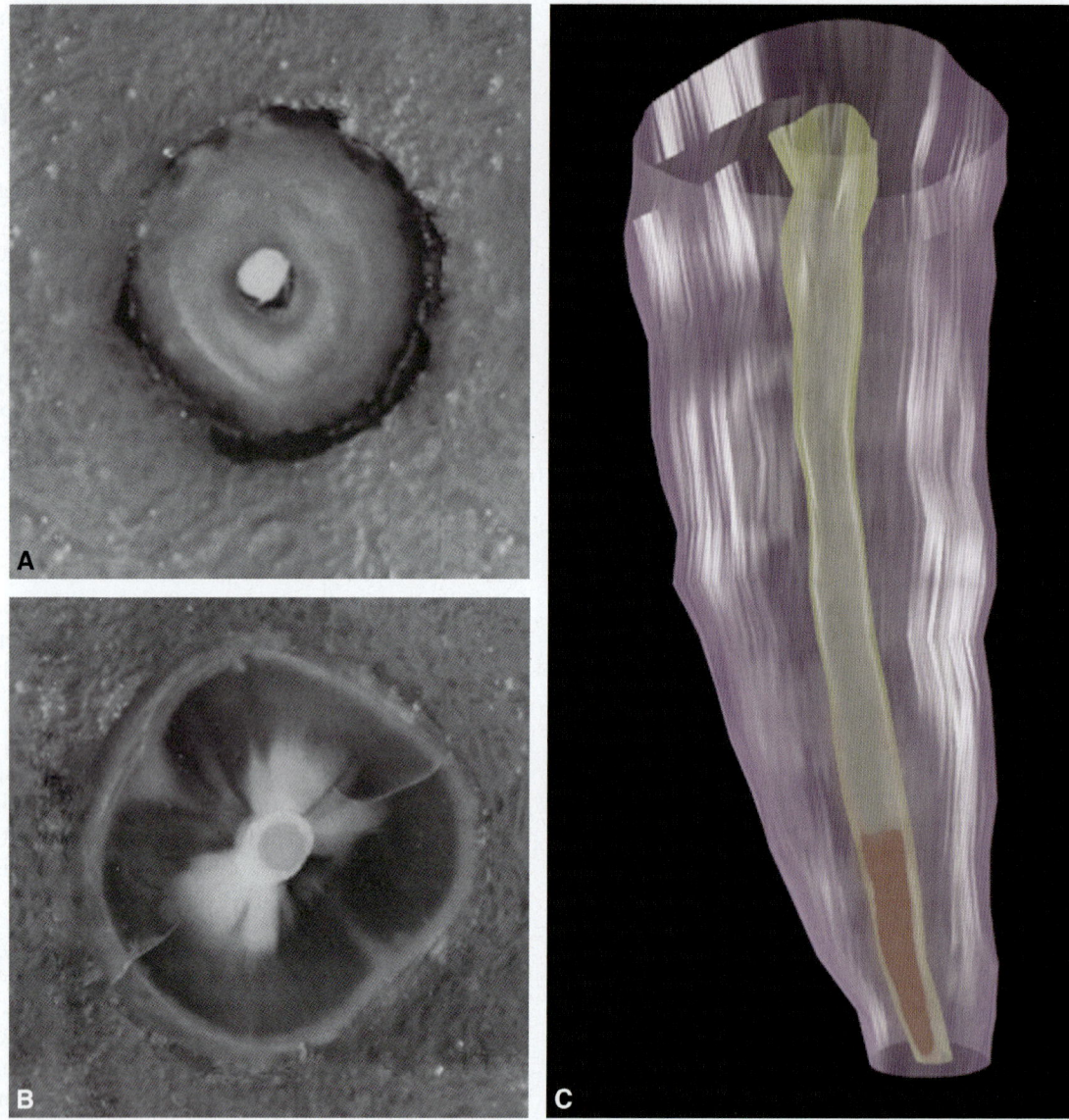

Figure 19 *A,* Cross-section of the apical third of the treated tooth. Microleakage is obvious in almost half of the perimeter of the root canal. *B,* Cross-section of the coronal third of the treated root. *C,* Three-dimensional reconstruction of the case. The external surface of the tooth is shown as purple, the root canal as yellow, and apical microleakage as cherry red. Reproduced by permission from Lyroudia K, Pantelidou O, Mikrogeorgis G et al.[170]

AH Plus, and Rocanal 2 and found that SealApex had less leakage than the others.

APEXIT

This additional calcium hydroxide-based sealer was found to seal better than SealApex in a 1991 study by Limkangwalmongkol et al.[185]. However, in 2002, Miletic et al.[186] used the measurement of an air bubble in a tube to compare apical leakage among five sealers and concluded that "Apexit showed significantly more leakage than AH Plus and Ketac-Endo. Leakage of AH 26 and Diaket sealers was not significantly different from that of AH 26 and Ketac-Endo, which showed the least leakage, or from Apexit, which showed the most" (Table 3).

VITAPEX

Developed for its potential bactericidal and osteogenic activity, no mention was given to this material's sealing ability in a report by Kawakami and associates.[187]

Table 3 Mean Leakage Values and Standard Deviation for Each Tested Sealer. Reproduced with permission from Miletic I et al.[186]

Sealer	Mean ± SD Value (μL)
Ketac-Endo	0.357 ± 0.082
AH Plus	0.378 ± 0.076
AH26	0.390 ± 0.071
Diaket	0.429 ± 0.152
Apexit	0.490 ± 0.137

Plastic- and Resin-Based Sealers

DIAKET

Although first introduced in the 1950s, little has been written about its sealing abilities. A report by Ozata et al.[188] in 1999 indicated that it had similar sealing abilities to Apexit, but better than Ketac-Endo when resisting dye penetration.

AH 26 (THERMASEAL)

This slow-setting resin sealer, when tested for tensile strength and bonding to dentin, performed better than Kerr Pulp Canal Sealer, SealApex, and Ketac-Endo.[189] It was the precursor to the current product, AH Plus. When comparing AH Plus to Ketac-Endo and Fill Canal, De Almeida et al.[190] found it to be superior in dye-leakage resistance. Recently, Wuerch et al.[191] studied the effect of intracanal medicaments, chlorhexidine gel, and calcium hydroxide on the sealing ability of AH Plus. Using the "fluid conductance model" (Figure 20), they found that neither impeded the apical seal when using AH Plus as a sealer.

McMichen et al.[192] investigated several properties, including solubility, regarding AH Plus versus Tubliseal, Kerr Pulp Canal Sealer EWT, Roth 801, Apexit, and Endion. Using weight change of the roots in water over a 3-month period, they found AH Plus to be the least soluble. Another study by Schafer and Zandbiglari[193] addressed solubility by comparing the weight loss of ring molds filled with eight different sealers immersed in water. AH Plus had the least weight loss, with SealApex and Ketac-Endo showing the most weight loss. Eldeniz et al.[194] compared the shear bond strength to dentin with AH Plus, Diaket, and Endo-Rez and found AH Plus to be superior to both.

KETAC-ENDO

Ketac-Endo is a glass ionomer cement with properties similar in behavior to resin or plastic sealers. It has been discontinued but is discussed here because it has

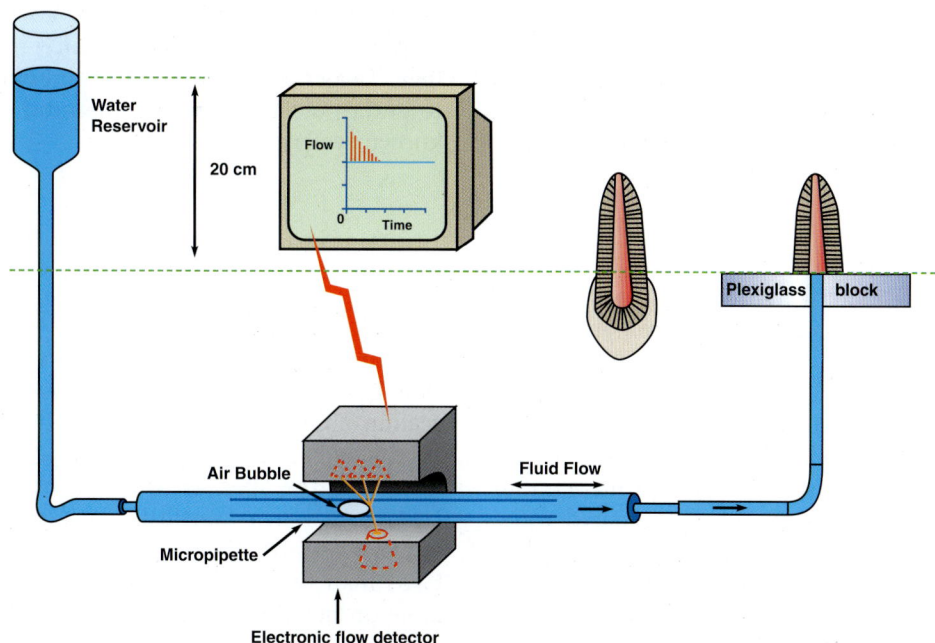

Figure 20 Schematic illustrating the device developed by Dr. David Pashley at Medical College of Georgia and used to measure fluid flow around root canal fillings. The root cemented to a block of Plexiglas penetrated by an 18-gauge stainless steel tube, the entire system filled with water at a hydrostatic pressure of 20cm H_2O. Reproduced with permission from Wuerch RM, Apicella MJ, Mines P et al.[188]

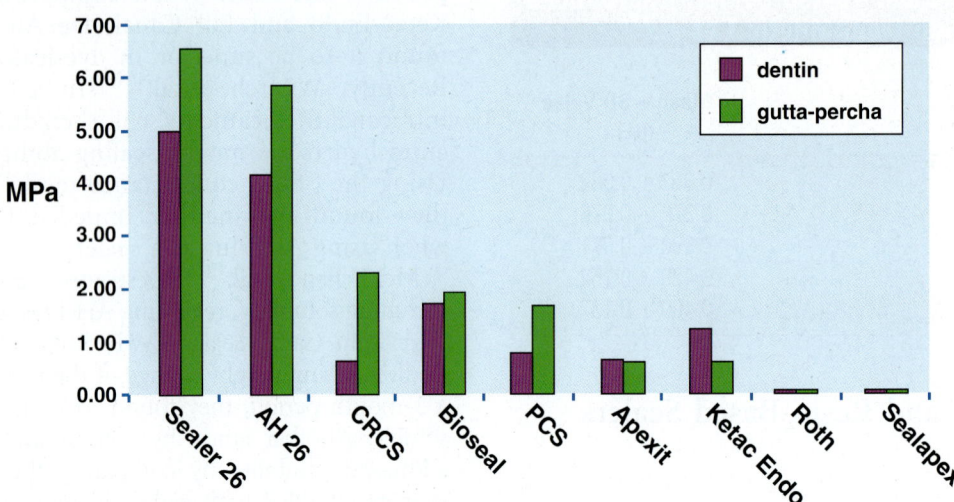

Figure 21 Bonding of endodontic sealers to gutta-percha and dentin. Reproduced with permission from Tagger M, Tagger E, Tjan AHL et al.[202]

been included in so many studies. Although somewhat difficult to remove from the canal, it is possible to do so.[195] Regarding microleakage, Ketac-Endo did not perform as well as Roth's 801 and AH 26 in a study by Rohde et al.[196]. Another study by Dalat and Onai[197] confirmed these findings when comparing Ketac-Endo to AH 26. However, a report by Wu et al.[198] found the opposite, that is, "AH 26 leaked more than Ketac-Endo." When testing the antibacterial properties of five sealers including Ketac-Endo, Cobankara et al.[199] found that Ketac-Endo had less antibacterial effect against *E. faecalis* than did AH Plus, SealApex, and Sultan (Roeko-Seal) had none at all.

ROEKO-SEAL AUTOMIX

This silicone-based material, a relatively new sealer, was compared clinically with other cases obturated with Grossman's sealer and evaluated up to 12 months after treatment.[200] No difference in success rates was noted. Lucena-Martin and associates[201] compared leakage to black ink between Roeko-Seal, Top Seal, and Endomethasone and found no significant differences between them. When compared with the more commonly used AH Plus and Ketac-Endo, Cobankara et al.[202] found Roeko-Seal to have better resistance to leakage than both of the others when subjected to fluid filtration. Using fluid filtration, Wu et al.[203] compared the leakage in root canal fillings in extracted teeth filled vertically and laterally using gutta-percha and Roeko-Seal, Kerr Pulp Canal Sealer. They found that Roeko-Seal leaked less than Kerr Sealer.

SEALER 26

This epoxy-based resin has been shown to have better adherence to dentin than zinc oxide-based sealers, when used with and without laser application.[204] Apparently its bond strength ability is its main advantage. Tagger et al.[205] showed it to bond more strongly to gutta-percha and dentin than did eight other well-known sealers (Figure 21).

Methacrylate Resin Sealers

ENDO-REZ

This urethane-based resin sealer was compared to AH Plus by Kardon et al.,[206] assessing the differences in sealing ability by the fluid filtration method. Their results indicated that Endo-Rez was not as effective at sealing the apex as AH Plus when using a single cone or warm vertical condensation. However, another study found more apical leakage with Grossman's sealer than with Endo-Rez in either single cone or lateral compaction methods of obturation.[207] Two more recent studies by the same group showed the sealing ability of Endo-Rez to be enhanced by the use of a self-etching adhesive.[208,209]

EPIPHANY

This recently developed curable resin composite sealer was analyzed in 2005 in a previously mentioned study using an SEM to compare the ultrastructural quality of its apical seal (combined with Resilon) with that of gutta-percha and AH Plus.[114] Neither sealer achieved a complete apical seal as previously mentioned. An in vitro study by Tunga and Bodrumlu[210] addressed leakage allowed via fluid transport in human anterior teeth after instrumentation, smear layer removal, and obturation with either laterally compacted gutta-percha and AH 26 or AH Plus sealers or Epiphany sealer and Resilon. Teeth filled with AH 26 and gutta-percha exhibited the most leakage, while the least leakage was observed with Epiphany and Resilon. Biggs and associates[211] compared the sealing abilities of gutta-percha/Roth 801 and gutta-percha/AH Plus to Resilon/Epiphany and found no differences in sealing abilities. Because of the rising popularity of the Resilon/Epiphany combination for obturating canals, much remains to be seen regarding the future performance of Epiphany as a sealer.

FIBREFILL

Another methacrylate resin sealer, its shear bond strength was analyzed by Gogos et al.[212] and compared Endion, calciobiotic root canal sealer (CRCS), and Topseal (an epoxy resin). Fibrefill was found to have the bond strength of these four sealers. The apical leakage associated with Fibrefill with and without the presence of a smear layer was compared to that of CRCS in a study in Greece.[213] The findings indicated that Fibrefill leaked significantly less than CRCS with or without a smear layer, but especially without the smear layer.

METASEAL

MetaSEAL (Parkell, Edgewood, NY) is the latest resin root canal sealer. MetaSEAL is the endodontic version of 4-Meta, a long-standing restorative sealer. Its self-etch formula hybridizes the dentin wall of the canal to prevent leakage. It bonds to both Resilon and gutta-percha. Belli et al.[214] compared MetaSEAL with Epiphany/Real Seal and AH Plus with gutta-percha and found less leakage with MetaSEAL after 1 week, but no difference among the sealer groups at 4- and 12-weeks time periods.

The Smear Layer and Apical Leakage

The question of the presence of the smear layer and its effect on apical seal continues to be addressed. Yamada et al.[215] have extolled the virtue of its removal and how it promotes a better apical seal with the filling material via dentinal tubule penetration. Cobankara and associates[216] studied the effects of the presence or the absence of the smear layer on root fracture resistance in vitro and found no difference whether it was present or absent. They also found no difference whether AH 26 or Ketac-Endo was used as a sealer.

An SEM study compared intact smear layers in prepared canals and those with removed smear layers and the ability of AH Plus, Apexit, and Roth 811 to penetrate dentinal tubules.[217] The authors found that the presence of a smear layer obstructed all sealers from penetration; however, all three sealers penetrated the tubules with the removal of the smear layer (Figure 22). They concluded that the "smear layer plays an important role in sealer penetration into the dentinal tubules, as well as in the potential clinical implications."

Eldeniz et al.[218] tested the shear bond strength of Diaket, AH Plus, and Endo-Rez with and without the presence of a smear layer. AH Plus was found to have the highest shear bond strength of any of these in either condition, and higher with no smear layer. Another study evaluated the effects of final irrigants on apical leakage in smear layer-free canals using fluid filtration measurements.[219] Although the authors used only one sealer (Roth 801), whether the final irrigant was 70% isopropyl alcohol, NaOCl, or Peridex, no significant difference was noted for sealer penetration or microleakage. Additional investigations are needed, using current sealers, to study the effects of the presence or the absence of the smear layer on sealer penetration and microleakage in filled canals.

Lasers and Apical Microleakage

The advent of laser use in dentistry has expanded its applications in hard tissue, specifically to include intracanal use. Kimura et al.[220] evaluated the amount of apical leakage in vitro after root canal preparation using Er:YAG laser irradiation versus a control group without irradiation. They found no significant difference in the amount of leakage between the two groups. Another in vitro investigation by Goy et al.[221] involved instrumented teeth that were lased with

1074 / Endodontics

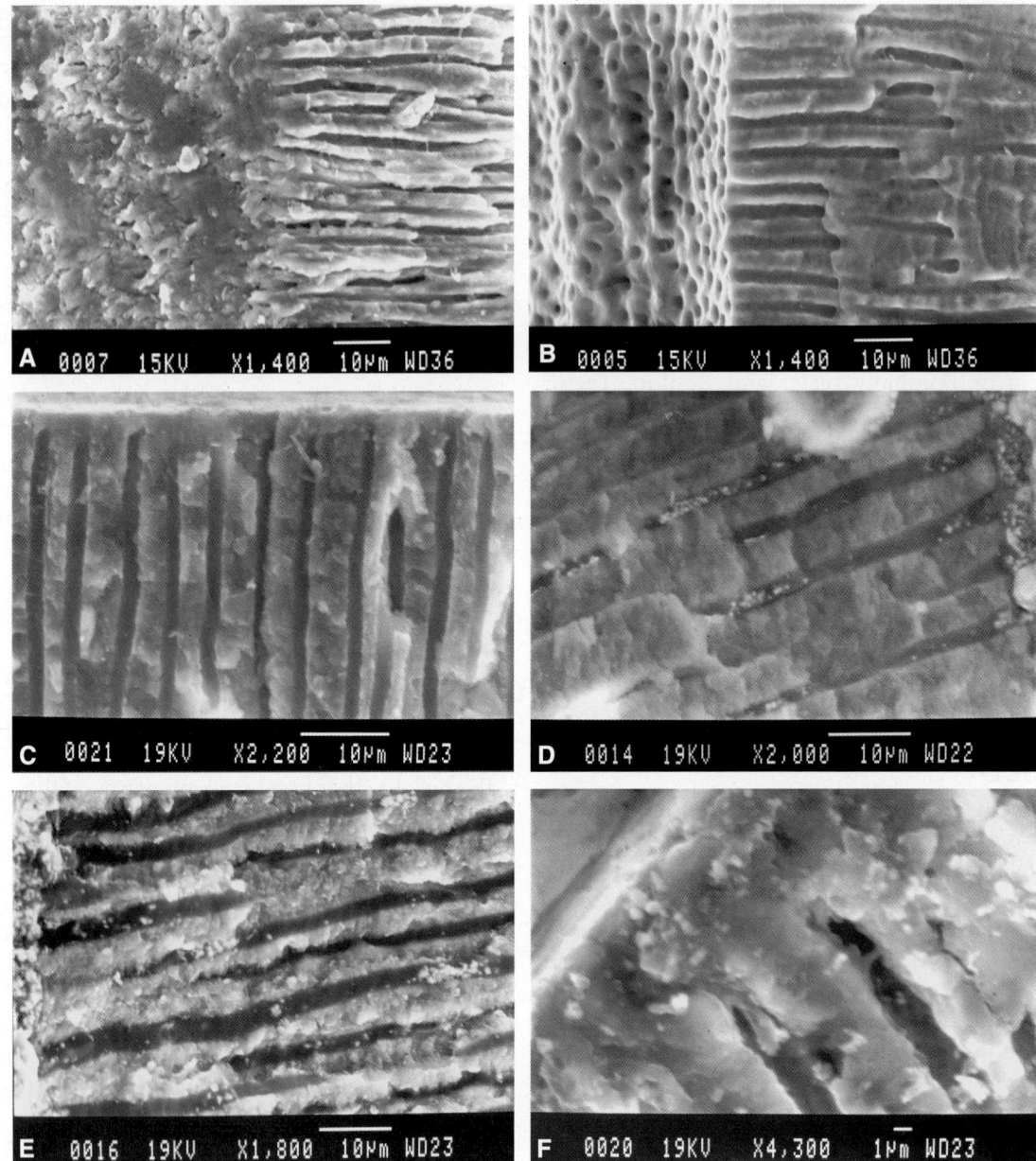

Figure 22 Appearance of experimental groups: **A,** Smear layer covering the root canal walls. **B,** Smear layer-free root canal walls. **C,** Smear layer inhibited Apexit from penetrating dentinal tubules. **D,** Area between root canal walls and maximum penetration depth in smear layer-free root canal walls for AH Plus; **E,** Apexit; and **F,** Roth 811. Reproduced with permission from Kokkas AB, Boutsioukis AC, Vassiliadis LP et al.[213]

Nd:YAG irradiation, followed by black ink application in one group and without black ink as a control. The canals were filled and then evaluated by stereoscopy or SEM. They concluded that laser irradiation following black ink application increased smear layer removal and significantly reduced apical leakage after obturation.

Similar findings were reported by Park et al.[222] They also used Nd:YAG laser following rotary instrumentation or hand instrumentation, with teeth likewise instrumented, without irradiation. All teeth were sealed with Kerr Pulp Canal Sealer and gutta-percha. They concluded that laser irradiation immediately following canal preparation reduced apical leakage after obturation.

More studies on the effect of laser irradiation will certainly be forthcoming. It appears that lasers are at least nondetrimental to preparation and obturation,

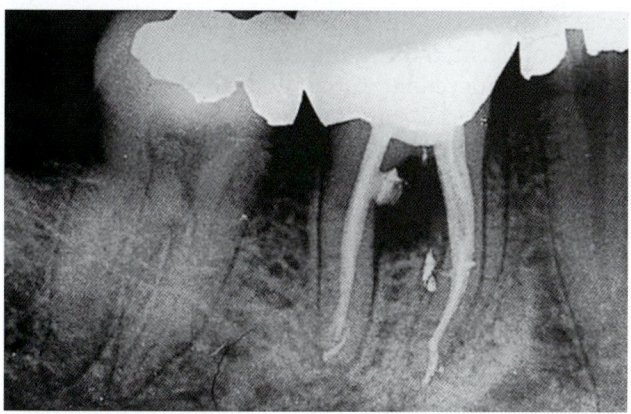

Figure 23 Furcal accessory canal and lateral canal, mesial root filled by vertical compaction of warm gutta-percha. Reproduced with permission from West JD.

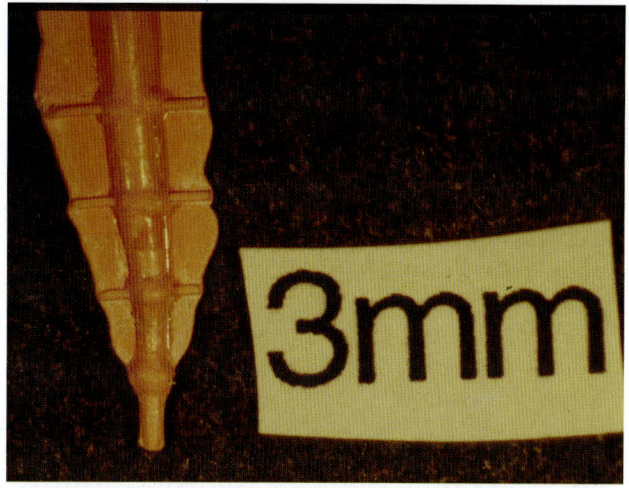

Figure 24 Gutta-percha replication of lateral grooves and depressions when the System B Fine heat plugger was inserted to a depth of 3mm (group C) from working length. Group A (not shown) had the System B Fine heat plugger inserted to a depth of 5mm from the WL, and group B (not shown) had the System B Fine heat plugger inserted to a depth of 4mm from the WL. Group C had statistically better movement of gutta-percha into the 1mm dentin depression than either group A or group B and better movement of gutta-percha into the 3mm dentin depression than group A. Group C also demonstrated statistically better movement of gutta-percha into the lateral grooves at 3mm from the WL than either group A or group B. Reproduced with permission from Bowman, CJ and Baumgartner, JC. [223]

and at most, appear to somewhat enhance them. See Chapter 26E, "Endodontics Instruments and Armamentarium," for more information on the use of lasers in endodontics.

Filling Lateral and Accessory Canals

Historically, the question of the significance of filling lateral canals (Figure 23) has persisted for nearly four decades. Kitagawa[223] espoused the greater lack of bacteria in dentin around lateral canals than in the main canal(s). In somewhat contradistinction, Fox et al.[224] remarked that the periodontal ligament adjacent to occluded lateral canals remained noninflamed regardless of the pulpal condition and that due to instrumentation, the orifices to such canals were frequently blocked.

Weine's[225] classic article in 1984 addressed the significance of filling lateral canals (a branch of the main canal coronal to the apical region) and accessory canals (going from the secondary branching of the canal) in the apical region. He refuted the assertion that vertically compacted gutta-percha and sealer close off more lateral canals than other methods of obturation. He also stated that lateral canals may cause pain during treatment and may even lead to failure if not adequately cleaned and sealed.

A study in 2001 by Goldberg et al.[226] evaluated the ability of lateral compaction of gutta-percha and of five thermoplasticized gutta-percha filling techniques to obturate simulated (artificial) lateral canals. More lateral canals were filled with Ultrafil, ThermaFil, and System B plus Obtura II than with Obura II alone or with lateral compaction. Bowman and Baumgartner[227] used a split tooth plastic model to evaluate the movement of gutta-percha into lateral grooves and depressions in the apical 7 mm, using System B Heat Source and Obtura II for backfill. Only when the System B plugger reached 3 mm from the apex, gutta-percha was observed in the lateral grooves (Figure 24).

Villegas et al.[228] evaluated accessory canal obturations in vitro after using no irrigation, distilled water, sodium hypochlorite, or sodium hypochlorite in conjunction with ethylenediaminetetraacetic acid (EDTA). They measured gutta-percha penetration into accessory canals and concluded that sodium hypochlorite alone or in conjunction with EDTA in final irrigation may facilitate obturation material flow into accessory canals.

The importance of lateral and accessory canal obturation is still under investigation, and further studies would seem to be appropriate to continue to address this issue.[28]

Coronal Protection of the Obturation

RATIONALE FOR A CORONAL SEAL

The importance of a coronal restoration placed over a canal obturation to prevent microleakage is emphasized by the findings of Torabinejad et al.[229] They found that without a coronal protection seal of the canal obturation(s), it took only 19 days for Staphylococcus organisms placed in a coronal access cavity to reach the apex in half of their test cases and 42 days for the same percentage of Proteus samples. Alves et al.[230] found that bacterial endotoxins could reach the apex of obturated canals in as little as 20 days if not protected by a coronal seal.

METHODS OF EVALUATING CORONAL LEAKAGE

Not surprisingly, techniques used to study coronal leakage are similar to those employed to evaluate apical microleakage. Wimonchit et al.[231] mention methods including vacuum dye penetration, fluid filtration, and passive dye penetration, with the vacuum dye method allowing significantly more penetration. Lyroudia et al.[232] have described the use of a 3D computer-assisted reconstruction of a tooth and a root canal in order to study coronal leakage.

TEMPORARY CORONAL CLOSURE MATERIALS

For the reasons mentioned above, canal obturations require protective seals. Restorative requirements may sometimes necessitate the use of temporary filling materials (cements) to accomplish this. The knowledge that *Streptococcus sanguis* bacteria are 500 times larger than aniline blue dye prompted Deveaux et al.[233] to study the ability of *S. sanguis* to penetrate 4 mm of Cavit, TERM, and IRM cements before and after thermocycling. Cavit and IRM succeeded in denying bacterial passage, but after thermocycling, 60% of the TERM fillings allowed bacterial penetration.

There are other reports that found favor with or conflicted with the above study. Some found Cavit to be among the best temporary filling materials regarding sealability (although quite soluble).[234,235] Other studies concluded that it was inferior to IRM and ZOE.[236,237] Acid-containing cements (zinc phosphate and polycarboxylate) did not fare as well against bacterial leakage. However, when dentinal walls were etched, KetacFil was adequate.[238]

Barthel et al.[239] suggested that a double seal of IRM and glass ionomer cement may prevent bacterial penetration. When considering Amalgambond (Parkell) as an interim material, in a leakage study by Galvan and associates,[240] it was found to outperform IRM and even C&B Metabond. In a more recent study involving methylene blue dye penetration, there was no significant difference in marginal leakage between Cavit, IRM, and Ultratemp Firm.[241] Cruz et al.[242] evaluated two lesser-known cements, Fermin and Canseal against Cavit and Caviton, and found that Fermin resisted methylene blue dye penetration better than the other cements.

PERMANENT CORONAL CLOSURE MATERIALS

It is disconcerting to find that with permanent filling materials and bases placed over endodontic access cavities, bacterial leakage still occurs.[243] Even full coverage, the ultimate protection of endodontic accesses, is a restoration that can allow leakage to the obturation level.[244,245] The latter of these two studies showed that both amalgam and composites can leak, even under a cast metal crown.

Today's restorative world includes materials such as Ketac-Fil glass ionomer, Herculite composite resin, and etchant agents including GLUMA. After thermocycling, Wilcox and Diaz-Arnold[243] found that all of them leaked (Figure 25). However, Tjan et al.[246,247] found that when using Amalgambond to line prepared dentin and enamel, a newly placed amalgam restoration was leakproof (Figure 26). In the same studies, teeth lined with Copalite did not fare as well and leaked to the pulpal level. Wolcott et al.[248] found that a glass ionomer intraorifice barrier inhibited the leakage considerably more

250. Madison S, Wilcox LR. An evaluation of coronal microleakage in endodontically treated teeth. Part III. *In vitro* study. J Endod 1988;14:455.

251. Bourgeois RS, Lemon RR. Dowel space preparation and apical leakage. J Endod 1981;7(2):66.

252. Dickey DJ, Harris GZ, Lemon RR, et al. Effect of post space preparation on apical seal using solvent techniques and peezo reamers. J Endod 1982;8:351.

253. Mattison GD, Delivanis PD, Thacker RW, et al. Effect of post preparation on the apical seal. J Prosthet Dent 1984;51:785.

254. Fan B, Wu MK, Wesselink PR. Coronal leakage along apical root fillings after immediate and delayed post space preparation. Endod Dent Traumatol 1999;15:124.

255. Abramovitz I, Tagger M, Tamse A, et al. The effect of immediate vs. delayed post space preparation on the apical seal of a root canal filling: a study in an increased-sensitivity pressure-driven system. J Endod 2000;26:435.

256. DeNys M, Martens L, De Coster W, et al. Evaluation of dowel space preparation on the apical seal using an image processing system. Int Endod J 1999;22:240.

257. Goodacre CJ, Spolnik KJ. The prosthodontic management of endodontically treated teeth: a literature review. Part III. Teeth preparation considerations. J Prosthodont 1995;4:122.

258. Abramovitz L, Lev R, Fuss Z, et al. The unpredictability of seal after post space preparation: a fluid transport study. J Endod 2001;27(4):292.

259. Ravanshad S, Torabinejad M. Coronal dye penetration of the apical filling materials after post space preparation. Oral Surg Oral Med Oral Pathol Oral Radiol Endod 1992;74:644.

260. Mattison G. The effect of post space preparation of the apical seal in teeth filled with ThermaFil: a volumetric analysis (abstract). IADR meeting; 1992 July 1–4; Scotland: Glascow.

261. Solano F, Hartwell G, Appelstein C. Comparison of apical leakage between immediate versus delayed post space preparation using AH Plus sealer. J Endod 2005;31(10):752.

262. Kvist T, Rydin E, Reit C. The relative frequency of periradicular lesions in teeth with root canal-retained posts. J Endod 1989;15:578.

263. Schwartz RS, Robbins JW. Post placement and restoration of endodontically treated teeth. J Endod 2004;30(5):289.

CHAPTER 31

RETREATMENT OF NON-HEALING ENDODONTIC THERAPY AND MANAGEMENT OF MISHAPS

ALAN H. GLUSKIN, CHRISTINE I. PETERS, RALAN DAI MING WONG, CLIFFORD J. RUDDLE

In recent years, significant refinements in the delivery of endodontic services have increased both professional and public expectations for the successful retention of the natural dentition. Along with the salvation of those many millions of teeth every year comes the inevitable percentage of non-healed and unsuccessful treatments. The literature concerning non-healed endodontically treated cases and available retreatment options to return periapical pathosis to health offers a scarcity of prospective randomized controlled trials dealing with non-surgical retreatment and surgical revision. This lack of literature involving the highest level of evidence is not only true for the endodontic field but is similarly true for other areas of dentistry, including implant studies.[1] Best available evidence apart from randomized controlled clinical trials may include non-randomized controlled clinical trials, cohort and case control studies, cross-over, cross-sectional and case studies, or consensus opinions of experts in the field.[2] Many factors including microbial challenge, location of the infection, and host defense play a role in the decision whether to retreat a case non-surgically, address the problem surgically, or to extract and place an implant (Figure 1). The skills and preferences of the clinician treating the patient are also significant considerations. When comparable criteria are applied to outcomes, the survival rates of endodontic treatment and or extraction and implant placement are similar.[3] However, an endodontic procedure is less expensive, significantly less time consuming and allows the patient to preserve their natural dentition.[1,4]

Post-Treatment Infection of the Root Canal System

DISEASE FACTORS

The treatment of chronic apical periodontitis has an unexpectedly high degree of success considering the fact that the root canal system is infected[5–9] and that a high percentage of areas within the root canal system are neither touched by instruments nor effectively cleaned using mechanical and chemical antimicrobial strategies.[10–12] As a consequence of infection, endodontic treatment can fail when root canal treatment has not adequately eliminated or reduced the intraradicular bioburden. Failures occur even when the highest standards and the most conscientious procedures are adhered to because there are root canal complexities that cannot be cleaned and/or obturated with current technologies. Therefore, infection can persist or quickly reestablish itself.[13–15] In rare cases, factors located outside the tooth within the inflamed periapical area can impede healing of apical periodontitis after a tooth has been treated endodontically. Nair[16–19] has identified six biological factors that lead to recalcitrant asymptomatic radiolucencies: (1) continued intraradicular infection inside the root canal system; (2) extraradicular infection, such as periapical actinomycosis; (3) foreign body reaction due to extrusion of endodontic materials; (4) accumulation of endogenous cholesterol crystals that cause inflammation of periapical tissues; (5) true cysts with no connection to the root canal

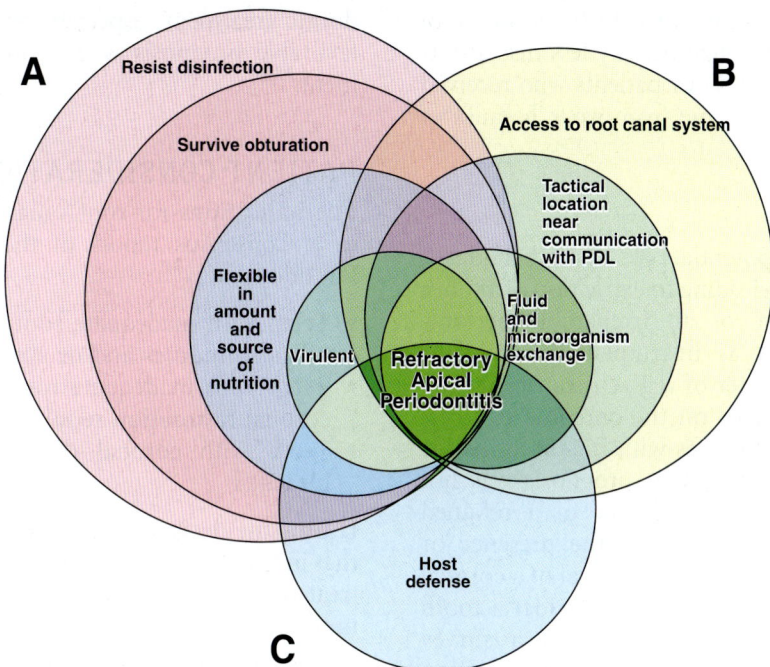

Figure 1 Interaction and characteristics of an endodontic infection. **A,** Microbial challenge. **B,** Location of the infection. **C,** Host defense in inflammation and persistence of disease after endodontic treatment. Adapted from Sundqvist G, Figdor D. Life as an endodontic pathogen. Ecological differences between the untreated and root-filled root canals. Endod Topics 2003;6:3–28.

space, and (6) scar tissue remaining after the healing of a lesion. Specific factors affecting the success of endodontic treatment are covered in Chapter 32, "Endodontic Treatment Outcome."

PREVIOUS ROOT CANAL TREATMENT

In general, the fact that previously treated teeth have been instrumented and may have been subjected to procedural errors and unwanted changes in the original canal geometry, as well as possible contamination, results in lower success rates: healing of lesions in retreatment cases ranges from 56% to 84%, whereas initial treatment of apical periodontitis is 83 to 100%.[20,21] In addition, when samples are taken from root canals during retreatment, there is a difference in the microbial flora between inadequately treated teeth and well-treated teeth that may contain microorganisms difficult to eradicate.[22]

Case Selection Criteria: Risks versus Benefits

Root-filled teeth displaying apical periodontitis often embody multi-factorial difficulties over teeth with primary apical periodontitis and no prior treatment.[23]

Ironically, in an effort to accomplish infection control and to prevent re-contamination, clinicians use methods, devices, and materials that may instigate and promote damage to periapical tissues.[24] When initial treatments do not lead to healing, a clinician may decide to retreat, to intentionally replant, to perform endodontic surgery, or to extract the tooth.[23]

BENEFITS

While acknowledging extraction as valid treatment, albeit a terminal step, repeating root canal therapy offers benefits over apical surgery. Most cases that continue to display apical rarefactions are infected inside the root canal system. Retreatment presents an effort to eliminate microorganisms, while the focus of apical surgery is to restrict microorganisms from egress beyond the root canal system.[25] In the scenario of intracanal infection, retreatment has the benefit of potentially disinfecting the root canal. Due to a lack of higher evidence, the proof of a better retreatment outcome over a surgical outcome still needs to be determined.[25] Kvist and Reit[26] compared the results of surgical and non-surgical treatment. After 1 year, the surgically treated cases had healed more quickly, but after 4 years the slower healing of the non-surgical cases had "caught up" and there were some failures in the surgical group, resulting in no difference. When directly compared to the sequelae of periapical surgery, there is significantly less discomfort and pain after retreatment. Only patients who received surgical treatment stayed home from work because of postoperative symptoms.

RISKS

Every treatment carries potential risks versus benefits. A significant complication leading to extraction of a tooth would be root fracture or an irreparable perforation.[27,28] Mishaps such as instrument breakage or transportation of the center of a given root canal can also have a negative impact on the outcome of treatment.[25,29] Spili[30] followed cases with fractured instruments for 1 year and found that prognosis was not significantly affected by the presence of a retained instrument fragment but rather by the presence or absence of a periapical lesion. The removal of a coronal restoration and buildup materials may render a tooth non-restorable. Al-Ali et al.[31] conducted a survey among students about endodontic retreatment decision making. They noticed that cases of teeth with posts led the clinician to favor apical surgery over non-invasive measures. Post removal has become a predictable procedure if appropriate armamentarium is used with adequate skill. The risk of root fracture is very small. In Abbott's study[32] of techniques used for post removal, only 1 of the 1600 teeth (0.06%) developed a root fracture during post removal. If a previously filled root canal is not accessible due to hard setting materials or other obstacles, the risk of perforating the root increases as the clinician approaches the apical portion of the canal. However, the use of materials with good marginal adaptation such as mineral trioxide aggregate (MTA) to repair root perforations has made this complication much more manageable.[33–35]

SPECIAL CONCERNS IN ENDODONTIC RETREATMENT

Although continuing periapical radiolucency is a clear sign of pathosis, many dentists do not automatically retreat the associated teeth.[31,36] While Friedman[25] describes apical surgery as a compromise after unsuccessful or unfeasible retreatment, apical surgery appears to be more frequently preferred than non-surgical retreatment.[25,37] Large and/or recently incorporated or expensive restorations may require replacement after retreatment. Obturation and restorative materials must be removed from the root canals, a step that may lead to procedural errors.[38] Technical problems due to previous treatment may be encountered.[39] Hence, patients and clinicians may be less willing to repeat the endodontic treatment, especially when considering a less favorable prognosis when compared to initial treatment.[38,40]

PATIENT CONSIDERATIONS

The indications for root canal retreatment are stated in a Consensus report of the European Society of Endodontology[41]:

- Teeth with inadequate root canal filling with radiological findings and/or symptoms
- Teeth with inadequate root canal filling when the coronal restoration requires replacement
- Teeth with coronal dental tissue that is to be bleached

During the decision-making process it may be decided that in the absence of apical pathosis, an endodontically treated tooth with inadequate obturation may only be monitored but not retreated. Further radiographic monitoring and non-intervention were favored by a majority of general practitioners.[42] However, treatment is recommended in cases of periapical radiolucency and discomfort or pain.

A reliable and effective alternative to deal with a painful root-treated tooth is extraction of the tooth in question,[43] a step that might entail additional dental treatment and costs. Large non-healing lesions lead to higher frequencies of therapeutic intervention than do smaller persistent lesions.[44] Reit and Grondahl[36,45] found large inter-individual variations among general dental practitioners in attitudes to treatment of asymptomatic periapical lesions. The important decision whether or not to retreat a tooth is further influenced by ethnic values and financial considerations, as well as by the technical quality of the primary treatment.[46] In cases where endodontic surgery is planned, orthograde retreatment should be attempted prior to surgery, because renewed disinfection and obturation improves the surgical success rate considerably.[47] Grung et al.[48] investigated 477 teeth that underwent apicoectomy and found that if teeth were retreated conventionally before periapical surgery, there was a 24% higher success rate than in teeth with periapical surgery alone.

The Praxis Concept theory according to Kvist et al.[46] hypothesized that dentists do not view periapical health and disease as two different entities, but rather as on a sliding scale. The investigators found that dentists regard the size of periapical lesions as corresponding to an increasingly more severe disease on a continuous scale. The personal threshold of each clinician seems to dictate when intervention is

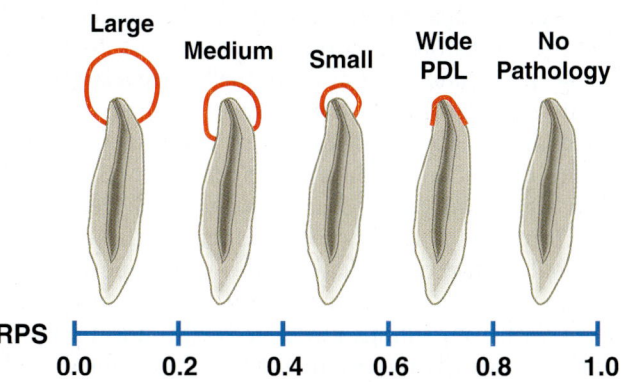

Figure 2 Calculation of the "retreatment preference score" (RPS) between 0.0 and 1.0: Clinicians assessed five periapical conditions and chose a periapical situation as their cut-off point for retreatment. The mean score chosen was a cut-off point very close to "medium-sized lesion" (RPS = 0.38). Adapted from Kvist and Reit C.[50]

considered necessary.[44,49,50] In a study by Kvist et al.,[44] dentists reviewed six cases with five different periapical conditions. For each case, a cut-off point indicating that retreatment was necessary was identified. A "retreatment preference score" (RPS) was constructed to correspond to different cut-off points and to vary between 0.0 and 1.0 (Figure 2). The mean RPS was 0.38, representative of therapeutic intervention in cases of medium sized lesions. The decision to retreat a tooth was significantly more frequent if defective root fillings were present and in the absence of any crown and post that would require removal. There were large variations between practitioners as to the cut-off point at which retreatment was felt to be appropriate. Differing cultural ethics and dental attitudes, prevailing level of educational background, and health care disparities may also play an important role in decision making.[4,51–53]

Coronal Leakage and Prognosis for Healing

A significant factor in endodontic failures is coronal microleakage. As far back as 1961, coronal leakage was investigated to determine its role in the success of endodontics.[54] However, in recent years, the role of coronal leakage in restorative dentistry has now become a research niche in an attempt to account for endodontic treatment failures.[55–58] In fact most of the emphasis today has been placed on the quality and integrity of the interface between the final restoration and dentinal surface sealing the root canal. Coronal leakage has become a clinical focus as a major factor in the overall success of root canal therapy.[59–62] Numerous studies have confirmed that sealing the coronal aspect of the tooth is of paramount importance for the overall success of root canal therapy.[63–66] Coronal leakage has been shown to be responsible for a constant source of microorganisms and nutrients that can initiate and maintain periapical inflammation[67] (Figure 3). In addition, the fact that gutta-percha and root canal sealers are not effective barriers to the oral environment was

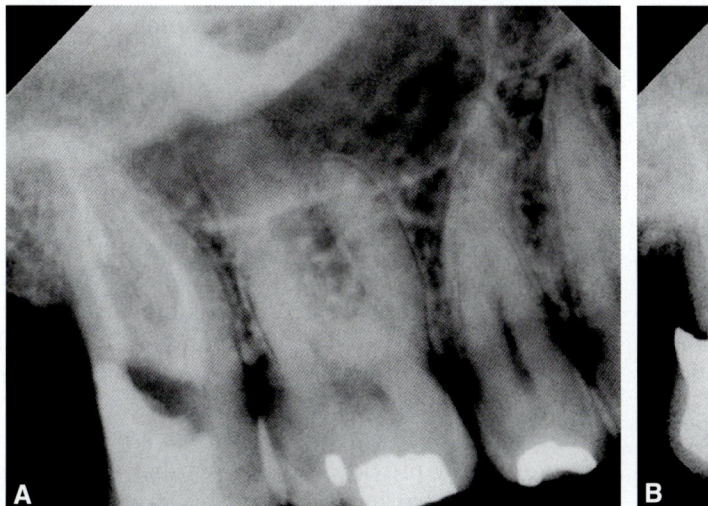
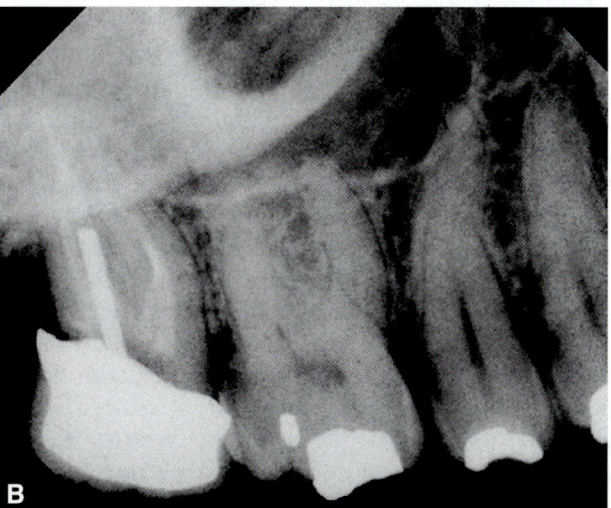

Figure 3 *A,* Postoperative radiograph of a completed root canal treatment on maxillary second molar with a bonded resin temporary filling. *B,* Three-month recall radiograph shows open crown margins that can result in bacterial invasion and eventual treatment failure.

shown in 1987.[68,69] It has also been demonstrated that all crowns display some amount of leakage even though it may not be detectable clinically.[70]

The microleakage associated with restorative materials has been studied in vitro as far back as 1990 for its role in failure rates of endodontic therapy. Root canals and pulp chambers of 69 extracted teeth were prepared and sealed using cold lateral condensation. Gutta-percha was removed from the pulp chambers of 3 of the groups of 15 teeth and filled with one of three materials. Results demonstrated that those teeth with no filling in the pulp chamber showed extensive leakage. The gutta-percha-filled-chamber group demonstrated greater leakage than did the groups in which other restorative materials had been employed. Therefore, it was recommended that the pulp chamber of molars be restored with a definitive restorative filling material following root canal treatment.[71]

Amount of leakage and percolation from saliva were evaluated to mimic the clinical setting. At 2, 7, 14, 28, and 90 days, salivary penetration was assessed in histological sections. The results strongly suggested that obturated root canals that have been exposed to the oral cavity for at least 3 months should be retreated due to the level of contamination.[72] Leaking coronal restorations, and their relation to root canal failure rates, were further corroborated by investigations to determine the amount of time needed for bacteria in natural saliva to contaminate the entire length of sealed root canals. Observed results showed that all root canals were recontaminated in less than 30 days.[73] Similar tests results were obtained by other investigators that indicated specimens were contaminated in 30 and 60 days.[74] Attempts to evaluate amounts of bacteria present when coronal restorations were defective were also undertaken. Freshly extracted teeth were used for this study. Results demonstrated that the amount of bacteria present was just as important as the salivary contamination. A total of 252 bacterial strains were isolated from all the teeth. The predominant group of bacteria in root-filled teeth with persistent apical periodontitis and coronal leakage was Gram-positive facultative anaerobes of which staphylococci followed by streptococci and enterococci were the most prevalent.[75]

Post-obturation bacterial contact was viewed to be of paramount importance for success of endodontics. One study reported that over 50% of unrestored and uncovered root canals in the test groups were completely contaminated after a 19-day exposure to *Staphylococcus epidermidis*. Furthermore, 50% of the root canals were completely contaminated when the coronal surfaces of their fillings were exposed to *Proteus vulgaris* for 42 days.[76] Similarly, Barrieshi et al.[77] examined bacterial leakage of a mixed anaerobic community of organisms in obturated canals after post space preparation. They reported that 80% of the teeth demonstrating coronal leakage lost their seal between 48 and 84 days. In further investigations, results demonstrated that leakage reached the apex through the obturated canals of experimental teeth at the earliest in 17 days and at latest by 88 days.[78] This study was corroborated in the work performed by Hommez et al.[79] who investigated the effect of coronal restoration quality on the composition of the root canal flora of teeth with necrotic pulps and teeth with root fillings associated with apical periodontitis. They discovered that only in root-filled teeth did defective coronal restorations have a statistically significant influence on the mean numbers of detected bacteria in their samples.

Bacteria and their by-products have also been shown to penetrate root canal obturating materials and influence periapical tissues and outcomes for success. Endotoxin, a component of the cell membrane of Gram-negative bacteria, is a potent inflammatory agent that, due to its smaller size, may be able to penetrate obturating materials faster than bacteria. For that reason, the evaluation of bacterial endotoxin to pass through obturated root canals was also observed. Endotoxins demonstrated contamination in all teeth within 21 days.[80] A similar in vitro study examined the possible penetration of post-prepared canals by endotoxin and bacteria. Results showed that both bacteria and endotoxins were able to penetrate the obturating materials in post-prepared canals; however, endotoxin penetration was faster than bacterial. A conclusion was made that the need for an immediate and proper coronal restoration after root canal treatment was optimum.[81]

Several groups have reported that root canals with post space preparations only need 30 days to be recontaminated and that dowel-space preparations had a negative influence on the sealing ability of the remaining root canal-filling material.[82–84] This finding was supported with a case report of a tooth that was restored coronally with a post space left empty, and 14 months later, pain and furcal radiolucency developed. Cleaning, shaping, medicating, and filling the post space resulted in the resolution of symptoms and healing of the radiolucency.[85]

Early studies in coronal leakage were performed in vitro and only provided a sense of what was happening clinically. An in vivo study by Ray and Trope[86] evaluated the relationship of the quality of the coronal restoration and the root canal obturation on the periapical status of endodontically treated teeth. The conclusion reported that the condition of the coronal restoration was more important than the quality of the endodontic treatment. It was observed that poor restorations in combination with good root canal therapy had negative results. The findings suggested that leakage of bacteria and their products along the margins of the restoration and the root filling will induce or maintain apical inflammatory lesions. When both the coronal restorations and endodontic fillings were inadequate, failure rates rose.

Tronstad et al.[65] found that the technical quality of endodontic therapy was significantly more important than the condition of the coronal restoration when the periapical status of endodontically treated teeth was evaluated. Their research highlighted the importance of the coronal restoration in cases where the endodontic treatment appeared satisfactory. However, if the quality of the endodontic treatment was poor, the quality of the restoration was of no significance. This study was corroborated when Hommez et al.[66] found that a good coronal restoration, as well as a good root canal filling, should be emphasized as the most influential factors on the periapical status. In another corroborating study, while the coronal restoration had a significant impact on periapical health, the quality of the root canal filling was found to be the most critical factor in this regard.[24]

The majority conclusion appears to be that no matter what clinicians use to obturate root canal systems, if the coronal portion of the canal is left unsealed, dissolution of the cement will occur and bacterial by-products will migrate down the canal walls contributing to an endodontic failure.[87–91]

While these studies have all concluded that sealing the interface of the coronal restoration and dentinal walls of the root canal system is of paramount importance, it is not clear if these studies measured the true interrelationship between the coronal restoration and periapical health. When inferior root canal therapy is present, the issue of coronal microleakage is a mute point.[55]

Bergenholtz and Spångberg[55] evaluated the quality of root canal therapy as well as the quality of the coronal restoration with respect to endodontic failures. The data suggested that the problem of coronal leakage might not be of such a great clinical importance as implied by numerous in vitro studies, provided instrumentation and root fillings were carefully performed. There was however a 3-fold increase in the likelihood for radiographic periapical lesions to occur in teeth with a poor coronal seal or lack of a seal.[92] This is in agreement with other researchers who support the premise that success stems from good endodontic therapy plus a good coronal restoration as an important secondary factor.[64,65,93,94] Thus, it appears to be the majority finding that once the endodontic therapy is complete, the best unequivocal recommendation to avoid re-infection of the root canal system is to restore the tooth immediately with either an immediate coronal restoration or a prefabricated post and composite system.[81,83,95–98]

When sealing the coronal access opening after endodontic therapy, amalgam has been a material of choice. A bonded amalgam filling has been shown to produce significantly less leakage than non-bonded.[89] The technique has been shown to prevent re-infection of an endodontically treated molar through utilization of a bonded amalgam buildup.[99] Other long-term leakage studies have demonstrated resistance to salivary contamination improves by performing core buildups with adhesive materials.[89] Fabricating buildups with a glass ionomer base and an overlaying composite resin restoration demonstrated less leakage due to the composite resin protecting the glass ionomer from dissolution by saliva over time.[100]

However, the clinician cannot always restore the tooth with a permanent restoration immediately following endodontic therapy. The restoring dentist and endodontist alike must be sure to communicate to the patient the need for a sealed temporary restoration and a minimum time interval prior to a permanent restoration. A major goal in restoration of the tooth after root canal treatment should be to prevent recontamination of the root canal system.[98] Grossman[101] first emphasized the importance of achieving a bacteria-tight seal between visits with the use of temporary restorations. Lack of satisfactory temporary restorations during endodontic therapy ranked as the second leading contributing factor in continuing pain after commencement of treatment.[41] Consequently, temporary restorative materials must then provide an adequate seal to prevent bacteria, fluids, and saliva from the oral cavity to recontaminate the obturated root canal system. To achieve effective temporization, it is essential to have adequate knowledge of the materials and their properties in order to select the proper temporary for the particular clinical circumstance.

TEMPORARY CORONAL RESTORATIONS

Temporary restorations have been available for decades, and manufacturers are continually developing new ones. The most common temporary restorations used in endodontics are zinc oxide–eugenol (ZOE) compounds such as intermediate restorative material (IRM) and zinc oxide and calcium sulfate mixtures such as Cavit. Adhesive dentistry has impacted endodontics, and resin-based materials including composites such as TERM and modified glass ionomer materials such as Ketac, Vitrebond, and FUJI are increasing in popularity.[102] Temporary restorations for use during and after non-surgical endodontic treatment have received a great deal of basic research and clinical evaluation (see Chapter 29, Root Canal Filling Materials). Studies have evaluated the materials for sealing ability, resistance to dissolution, radiopacity, and strength.[98–142]

The placements of orifice plugs have also been suggested to augment the seal of conventional root canal fillings. Utilizing an in vivo model, the efficacy of white MTA plugs in preventing periapical inflammation subsequent to coronal inoculation of root-filled teeth was investigated. None of the roots revealed radiographic or histological evidence of severe inflammation after inoculation. Therefore, it was equivocal if MTA should be used as a barrier to improve resistance to leakage.[23] Further investigations evaluated gray and white MTA as well as Fuji II LC cement as coronal barriers to bacterial leakage. Results suggest that either gray or white MTA or Fuji II could be recommended as a coronal barrier for up to 3 months.[143] Glass ionomer cement was shown to prevent microleakage in teeth with post spaces when the glass ionomer was used as a plug over the remaining gutta-percha.[144]

THE TECHNOLOGY OF RETREATMENT

With so much potential for endodontic success, the fact remains clinicians are confronted with post-treatment disease.[145,146] Before commencing with any treatment, it is wise to fully consider all the various treatment options.[27,147] When the choice is non-surgical endodontic retreatment, then the goal is to access the pulp chamber and remove materials from the root canal space and if present address deficiencies or repair defects that are pathologic or iatrogenic in origin[148,149] (Figure 4). Furthermore, endodontic access provides the opportunity to diagnostically evaluate teeth for coronal leakage, fractures, and missed canals.[150] Importantly, following disassembly procedures, the root canals can be re-shaped and disinfected and obturated in a manner that allows periapical healing.[151–153]

This section of the chapter will focus on the science, strategies, techniques, and technology that can produce successful results in non-surgical retreatment. In the last decade alone, significant procedural refinements have led to more predictable results. Properly

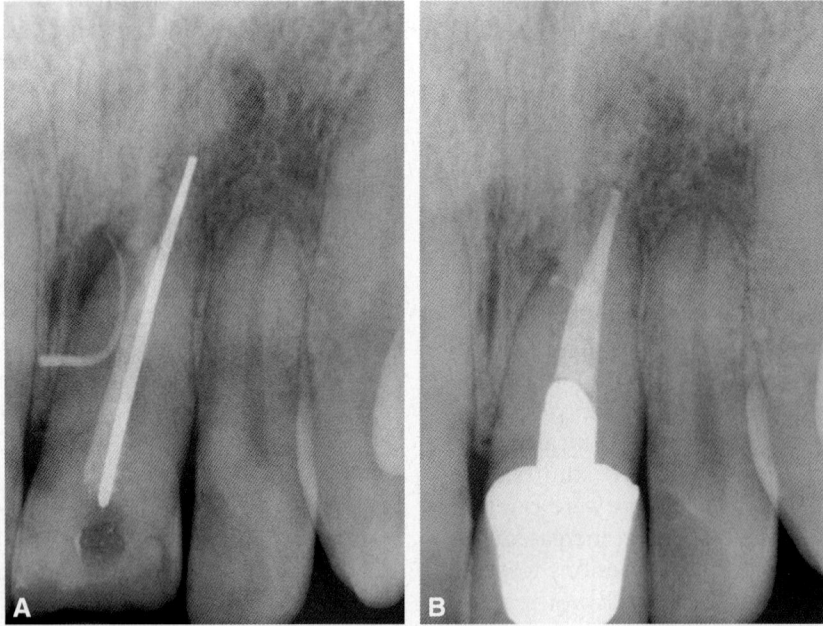

Figure 4 ***A***, Preoperative radiograph of an endodontically treated, non-healing maxillary central incisor. A gutta-percha point traces a sinus tract to a large lateral periapical lesion. ***B***, Five-year recall radiograph demonstrates osseous repair following cleaning, shaping, and obturation. Note that the lateral lesion was associated with a lateral canal.

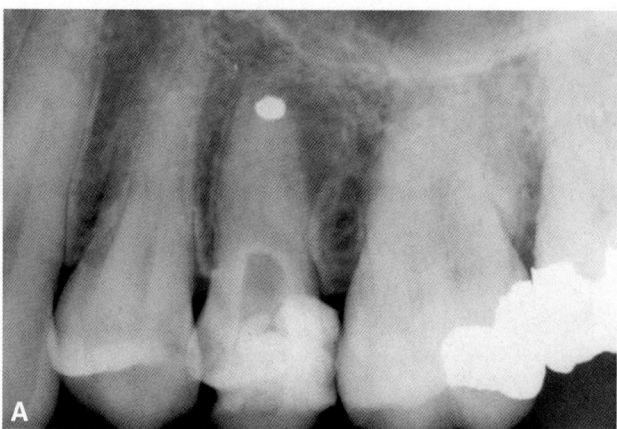 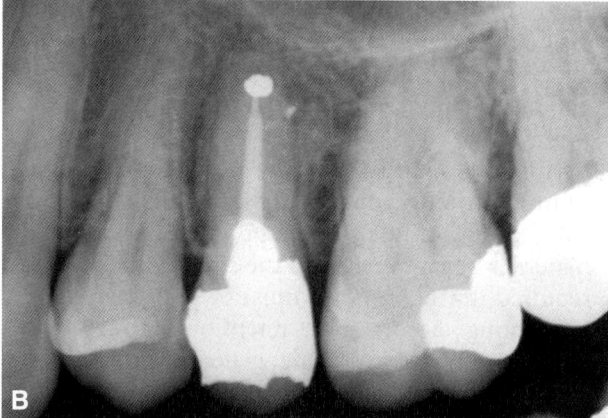

Figure 5 ***A,*** Preoperative radiograph shows a failing surgical treatment of a maxillary premolar with a laterally positioned lesion of endodontic origin. Note the "mineralized" canal and history of surgery. ***B,*** The tooth was successfully treated endodontically, and the 1-year recall radiograph demonstrates healing.

performed with advanced techniques, non-surgical endodontic retreatment is a strategic cornerstone of restorative and reconstructive dental procedures.

NON-SURGICAL VERSUS SURGICAL RETREATMENT

Endodontic revision must be carefully evaluated so a decision can be made among non-surgical retreatment (NSRCT), surgical retreatment (SRCT), or extraction.[154,155] NSRCT are disassembly and corrective procedures which are performed to potentially enable the clinician to properly clean, shape, and seal the root canal system.[156] Historically, endodontic surgery has been selected as the primary approach in resolving treatment outcomes that do not heal and sometimes in situations in which root canals have been mistakenly assumed to be "mineralized" and not treatable (Figure 5). Even with the vast improvements achieved in surgical endodontics in recent years, surgical techniques are restricted in their ability to eliminate pulp tissue, microorganisms, and related irritants from the root canal system.[157–159]

Infrequently, but on occasion after revision, surgery may still be necessary. However, higher success rates can be achieved if the root canal space has been adequately addressed prior to a surgical intervention. Consultation with the patient should be directed toward communicating the critical importance of retreatment, the cost of this approach compared to potentially less effective treatment choices, and the fact that this modality generally improves long-term results. Today, endodontic success can approach 100%.[152] This significant improvement is related to a large number of factors. Clinicians now have a better understanding of biological principles and a greater knowledge, appreciation, and respect for root canal system anatomy and the role it plays in success and healing. Better training, advanced techniques, relevant new technologies, and attention to restorative excellence improve the potential for long-term success.

CORONAL DISASSEMBLY

Clinicians typically access the pulp chamber through the existing restoration if it is judged to be functionally designed, well fitting, and esthetically pleasing. Endodontically, the decision to remove any restoration is based primarily on whether additional access is required to facilitate disassembly and retreatment.[156,160] If the restorative is deemed inadequate and/or additional access is required, the restoration should be sacrificed. However, on specific occasions, it is desirable to preserve and remove the existing restorative dentistry.[161] A variety of new technologies allow clinicians to more predictably eliminate coronal restorations.

FACTORS INFLUENCING RESTORATIVE REMOVAL

The removal of a restorative is dramatically enhanced when there is knowledge, respect, and appreciation for the concepts, materials, and techniques used in restorative and reconstructive dentistry. The safe dislodgment of a restorative is dependent on five factors that must be considered:

1. Preparation type: Preparations vary in retention depending on the total surface area of the tooth covered and the height, diameter, and degree of taper of the axial walls.

2. Restoration design and strength: The design and ultimate strength of a restorative is dependent on its physical properties, thickness of material(s), and the quality and techniques of the laboratory technician.
3. Restorative material(s): The composition of a restoration ranges from different metals to tooth colored restoratives such as porcelain. How these materials behave related to the stresses and strains required during removal must be appreciated.
4. Cementing agent: The retention of cements ranges from weak to strong, generally progressing from ZOE, polycarboxylate, silico-phosphate, zinc phosphate, glass ionomers, resin-modified glass ionomers to bonded resins.[162] Clearly, the new generation bonding materials, in conjunction with well-designed and retentive preparations, have made restorative removal more difficult and, at times, unwise.
5. Removal devices: The safe and successful dislodgment of prosthetic dentistry requires knowledge in the selection and use of a variety of devices. Clinicians need to identify and become familiar with each device, its safe application, effectiveness, limitations, and costs.[156]

A clinician must obtain a careful case history, confer with the original treating dentist if possible, and then consult with their patient to clearly define the risk versus benefit when entertaining the intact removal of an existing restorative.

CORONAL DISASSEMBLY DEVICES

Although there are many instruments available for coronal disassembly, the following represent a consensus of preferred instruments for the removal of various restorations. The tools used for disassembly have been arbitrarily divided into three categories. They can be used solely; however, it is useful to appreciate that they may be used in combination to synergistically attain removal success.[163]

Grasping Instruments

In general, this class of hand instruments works by applying inward pressure on two opposing handles. Increasing the handle pressure proportionally increases the instrument's ability to grip a restoration. The actual grasping instrument selected should protect the restoration and provide a strong purchase while reducing dangerous slippage. These grasping devices are best used in removing temporary restorations and include K.Y. Pliers (G.C. America, Alsip, IL), the Wynman Crown Gripper (Miltex Instrument Company,

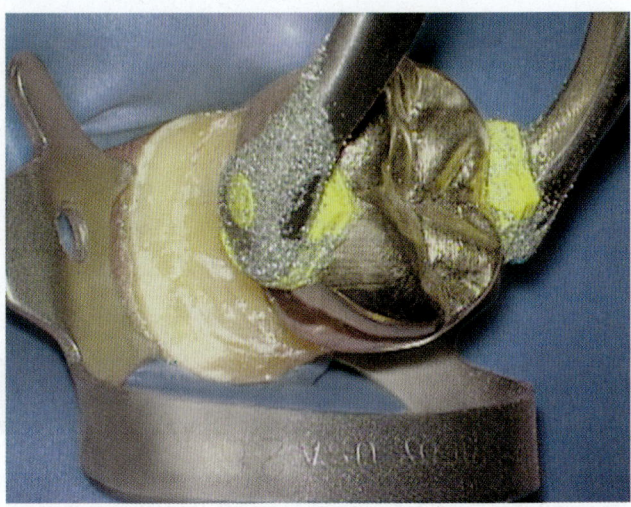

Figure 6 Removal of a crown using the K.Y. Pliers. Note the grasping pads have been dipped in emery powder to reduce slippage.

Lake Success, NY), and the Trident Crown Placer-Remover (Trident Dental Inc., Hendersonville, NC). An example of one of these grasping instruments is shown in (Figure 6).

Percussive Instruments

This method of prosthetic disassembly involves utilizing a selected and controlled, percussive removal force. This family of instruments delivers an impact either directly to a restorative or indirectly to another securely engaged prosthetic removal device. Although these devices are valuable removal instruments, caution must be exercised when considering the disassembly of tooth colored restoratives. Examples of percussive devices include Crown-A-Matic (Peerless International Inc., North Easton, MA) and the Coronaflex (Kavo America, Lake Zurich, IL), both of which are used to remove both temporary and permanently cemented prostheses.

Active Instruments

The instruments in this category actively engage restorations, enabling a specific dislodgment force to potentially lift off the prosthesis. These devices require a small access window to be cut through the restorative to facilitate the mechanical action of the instrument. In this method of removal, the downside of making and then repairing the access hole is significantly offset by the upside of saving the patient's existing restorative dentistry. Active devices among the most effective for removing permanently placed restorations intact are the Metalift (Classic Practice

Resources, Baton Rouge, LA), the WAMkey Removal Keys (Dentsply Maillefer, Ballaigues, Switzerland), the Kline Crown Remover (Brasseler, Savanna, GA), and the Higa Bridge Remover (Higa Manufacturing, West Vancouver, B.C.). An example of one of these active instruments is shown in Figure 7.

ARMAMENTARIA AND TECHNIQUES ASSOCIATED WITH MISSED CANALS

The etiology of endodontic failure is multi-faceted, but a significant percentage of failures are related to inadequate débridement of root canal systems. Missed canals contain tissue, as well as bacteria and other irritants that inevitably contribute to clinical symptoms and lesions of endodontic origin (Figure 8).[164–166] Historically, and all too often, surgical treatment has been directed toward "corking" the end of the canal with the

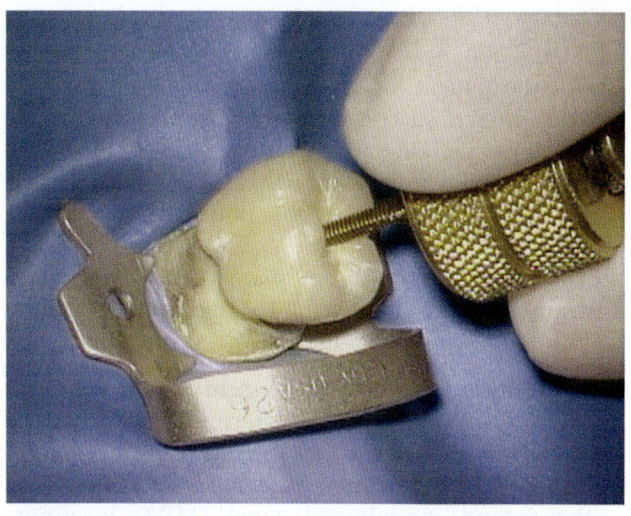

Figure 7 Removal of a Pocelain fused to metal (PFM) crown using the Metalift. This system applies a force between the crown and the tooth.

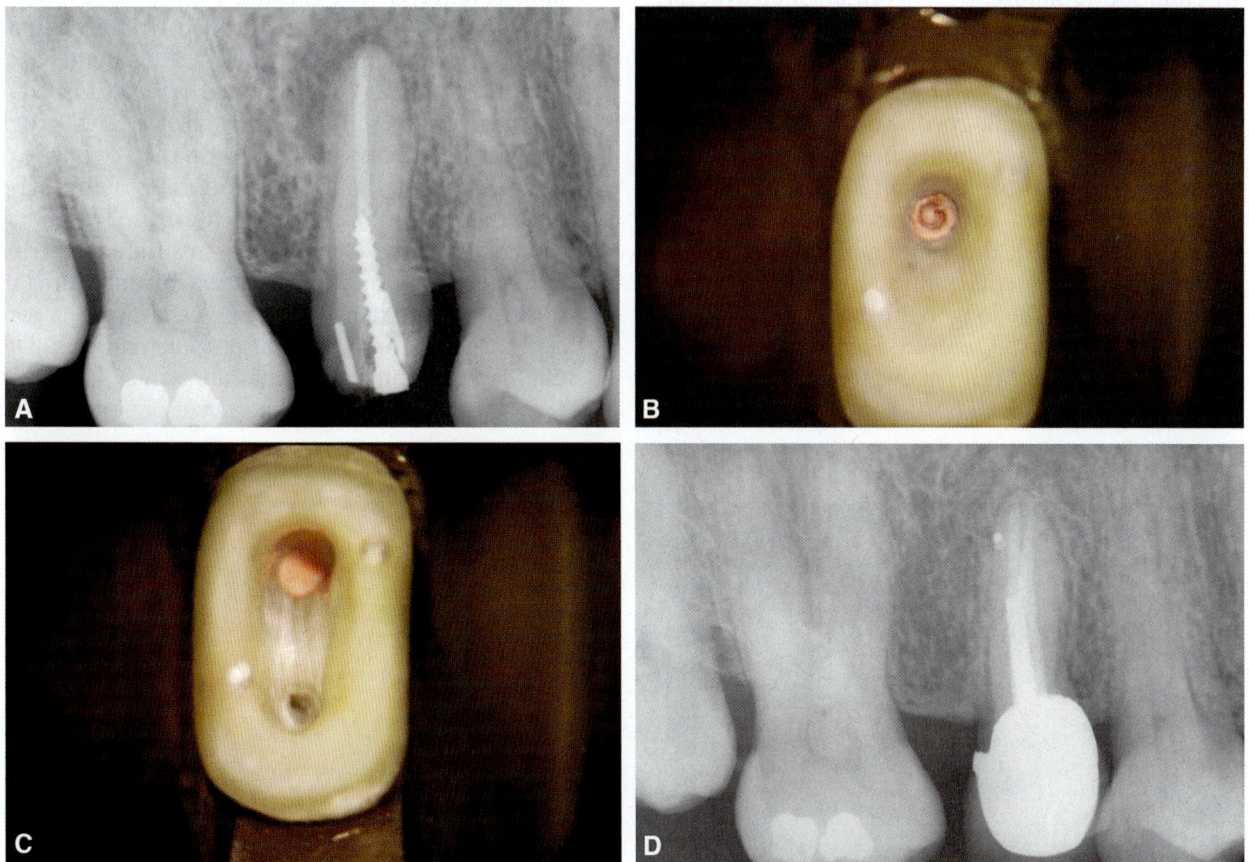

Figure 8 *A*, Radiograph of a maxillary right second premolar reveals pins, a post, insufficient endodontic treatment and an asymmetrical apical lesion. *B*, Photograph (×12 original magnification) after removal of the post from the buccal canal. The palatal canal had not been treated. *C*, Photograph (×12 original magnification) of completed access and palatal canal preparation. *D*, Ten-year recall radiograph shows osseous repair, demonstrating the importance of correct endodontic treatment, and a well-designed prosthesis.

hopes that the retrograde filling material will incarcerate biological irritants within the root canal system over the life of the patient.[156–159] Although this scenario may provide clinical success, it is not nearly as predictable for healing as non-surgical retreatment. Endodontic prognosis is maximized in teeth whose root canal systems are cleaned, shaped, and obturated in all their dimensions.[160,167]

There are multiple concepts, armamentaria, and instruments that are useful to find missed canals, and the following represent the most important.

- Anatomical familiarity. It is essential before preparing the access cavity or re-entering a tooth that has had prior endodontic treatment.[168] For example, one can appreciate in the maxillary first molar that the second mesiobuccal canal (MB2) is almost never on the imaginary line between the MB1 and the palatal orifices. This canal is typically mesial to that imaginary line.
- Radiographic analysis. It is critical when evaluating an endodontic failure.[169,170] Well-angulated periapical films should be taken with the cone directed straight-on, mesio-oblique, and disto-oblique. This technique oftentimes reveals and clarifies the three-dimensional morphology of the tooth. In teeth where complete endodontic treatment has been performed, obturation materials are seen radiographically as centered within the root regardless of the selected angle of the radiograph. Conversely, if the obturation materials appear positioned asymmetrically within the long axis of the root, a missed canal should be suspected (see Figure 8).[170] Digital radiography and other imaging technologies mentioned in this chapter afford a variety of software features significantly enhancing radiographic diagnostics in identifying hidden, calcified, or untreated canals.
- Vision. It is enhanced with magnification glasses, headlamps, and transilluminating devices. A dental operating microscope affords extraordinary light and magnification and gives the clinician unsurpassed vision, control, and confidence in identifying or chasing extra canals.[151] Operating microscopes typically have a range of magnification from about ×2.5 to around ×20. Magnification plus improved lighting equals significantly enhanced vision. Surgical length burs enhance direct vision by importantly moving the head of the handpiece further away from the occlusal table and improving the line of sight along the shaft of the bur.
- Access cavities. These should be prepared and expanded so their smallest dimensions are dictated by the separation of the orifices on the pulpal floor and their widest dimensions are at the occlusal table (Figure 9). The isthmus areas and/or developmental grooves are firmly probed with an explorer in an effort to find a "catch." In general, access cavities should be expanded and finished to enhance vision, improve diagnostics, and provide straight-line access to the orifice(s).[171]
- Piezoelectric ultrasonics. It provides a breakthrough for exploring and identifying missed canals. The clinician should recognize that ultrasonic instruments perform optimally when they are designed, manufactured and tuned for a specific generator. Synergistically, a piezoelectric generator (P5, Dentsply International, Tulsa, OK) in conjunction with ultrasonic instruments (ProUltra ENDO Instruments, Dentsply International)

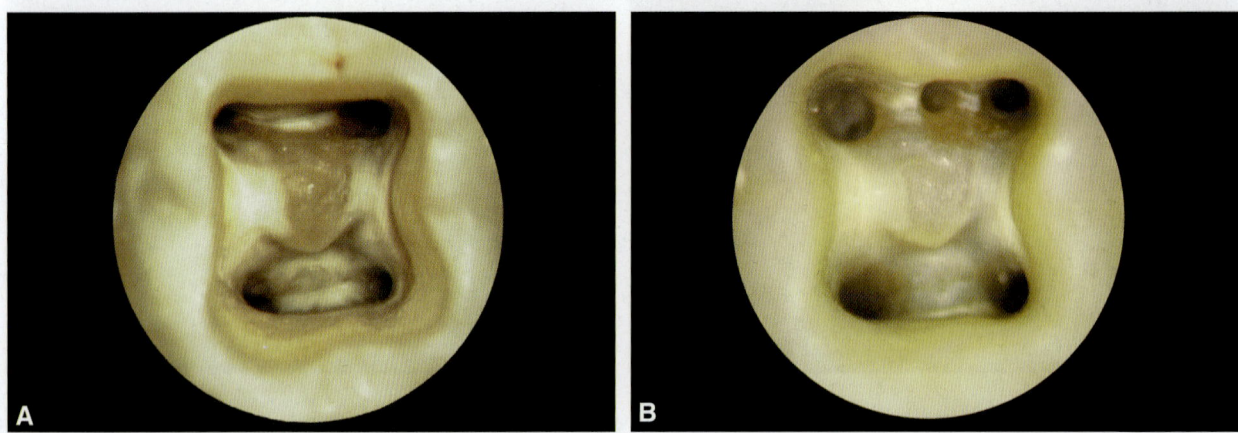

Figure 9 ***A,*** Magnified view into the access cavity in a mandibular first molar shows the four orifices to the root canal system. ***B,*** Photograph showing a third mesial orifice in another mandibular molar. It is important to explore the isthmus connecting the mesiobuccal and mesiolingual orifices.

are used to transfer energy and perform a variety of clinical procedures (Figure 10).[172–174] Ultrasonic systems importantly eliminate the bulky head of the conventional handpiece that frequently obstructs vision. The working ends of specific ultrasonic instruments are 10 times smaller than the smallest manufactured round burs, and their abrasive coatings allow them to precisely prepare away dentin when exploring for missed canals.

- Micro-Openers (Dentsply International). These are flexible, stainless steel hand instruments that feature ergonomically designed off-set handles. Micro-Openers have limited length cutting blades which, in conjunction with their 0.04 and 0.06 tapers, enhance tensile strength, making it easier to locate, penetrate, and perform initial canal enlargement procedures. These instruments provide unobstructed vision when operating in difficult teeth with limited access.

- Dyes. Various dyes like methylene blue can be irrigated into the pulp chambers of teeth to aid in diagnosis. The chamber is subsequently rinsed thoroughly with water, dried, and visualized. Frequently the dye will be absorbed into orifices, fins, and isthmus areas and serves to "roadmap" the anatomy. This technique can aid in the identification and treatment of missed canals and enhance diagnostics, including the visualization of fractures.

- Sodium hypochlorite (NaOCl). NaOCl can aid in the diagnosis of missed or hidden canals.[151,161] Following cleaning and shaping procedures, the access cavity is flooded with NaOCl and the solution is observed to see if bubbles emanate toward the occlusal table. A positive "bubble" reaction signifies that NaOCl is either reacting with residual tissue within a missed canal or with residual chelator still present within a canal being prepared.

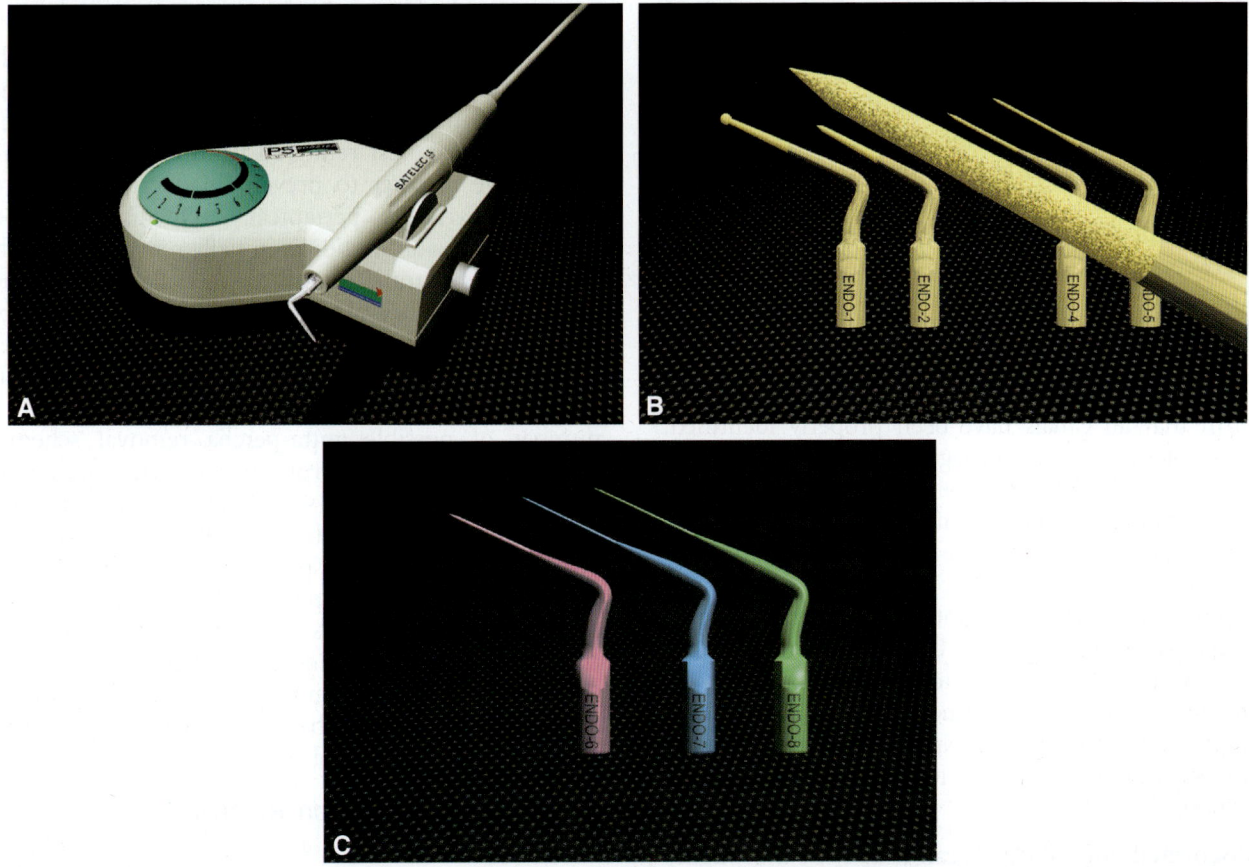

Figure 10 Ultrasonic instruments. **A,** The Satellec P5 ultrasonic unit. **B,** The ProUltra ENDO 1-5 ultrasonic instruments have an abrasive zirconium nitride coating to improve efficiency, precision, and clinical performance. **C,** The ProUltra ENDO-6, 7, and 8 titanium ultrasonic instruments provide longer lengths and smaller diameters and are used when space is restrictive.

- Transillumination. It is accomplished by positioning a fiber optic wand either above or below the rubber dam and directing light buccal to lingual. Diagnostics are, at times, improved by turning off the overhead or microscope light source to achieve a different optical effect.
- Explorer pressure. It can help to identify a missed canal. Firm explorer pressure is used to punch through a thin layer of secondary dentin.
- White line test. Oftentimes, a shelf of dentin meets the pulpal floor and forms a groove. It is important to recognize that extra canals can be more readily identified by progressively preparing away this shelf of dentin with abrasively coated ultrasonic instruments. During ultrasonic procedures in necrotic canals, dentinal dust moves into available anatomical space, such as the isthmus, and forms a visible white line. The white line test is a visible road map that can be followed and diagnostically aid in identifying, as an example, an MB2 orifice/canal.
- Red line test. In vital cases, blood frequently moves into an isthmus area. Like a dye, blood absorbs into orifices, fins, and isthmuses, which serves to roadmap and aid in the identification of the underlying anatomy.
- Restorative disassembly. It provides better orientation to the underlying tooth structure and improves safe access to the pulp chamber.
- Perio-probing. It is another important adjunct for locating canals. Probing the sulcus can provide important information as to the relationship between the long axis of the clinical crown and the underlying root as well as indicate possible root fracture.
- Symmetry. It is an important visual test that can encourage looking for another orifice/canal or confirm that all canals have been properly identified. The rules of symmetry suggest that if any given root contains only one canal, then regardless of its anatomical configuration, the orifice should be positioned an equal distance from the external cavo-surface of the root.
- Color. Color changes indicate developmental grooves n the pulpal chamber floor. Oftentimes, a dark groove on the pulpal floor of a multi-canal tooth can be followed and will lead to another canal orifice. Additionally, orifices frequently appear a darker color than the surrounding dentin in teeth exhibiting mineralization.

If discovered, missed canals can usually be thoroughly cleaned, shaped, and sealed. However, if a missed canal is suspected but cannot be readily identified, then an endodontic referral may be prudent to avoid further complications. Caution should be exercised when contemplating surgery due to the aforementioned concerns, but at times, surgery may be necessary in the hopes of salvaging the tooth.

Removal of Obturation Materials

The obturation materials most frequently found in the root canal space generally reflect a past era of knowledge, a current school of thought, or a personal philosophy of treatment. There are some commonly encountered materials found in obturated root canal systems: gutta-percha, carrier-based obturators, silver points, and paste fillers. In addition, new obturation materials based on resin fillers and sealers have recently been recommended for obturation of root canal systems. Resin-based materials can generally be removed using the same technique described for the removal of gutta-percha. Frequently, it is necessary to partially or totally remove an obturation material to achieve endodontic retreatment success or to facilitate placing a post for restorative reasons.

GUTTA-PERCHA REMOVAL

The relative difficulty in removing gutta-percha varies according to the canal's length, cross-sectional diameter, and curvature. Regardless of technique, gutta-percha is best removed from a root canal in a progressive manner to prevent inadvertent displacement of irritants periapically. Dividing the root into thirds, the obturation is initially removed from the canal in the coronal one-third, then the middle one-third, and finally eliminated from the apical one-third. In canals that are relatively large and straight, loosely fitting cones can, at times, be removed with one instrument in one motion. For other canals, there are a number of possible gutta-percha removal schemes. The techniques include rotary files, ultrasonic instruments, heat, hand files with heat or chemicals, and paper points with chemicals.[175] Of these options, the best technique(s) for a specific case is selected based on preoperative radiographs and clinically assessing the diameter of the orifices after re-entering the pulp chamber. Often, a combination of methods is required to achieve a safe, efficient, and potentially complete elimination of gutta-percha and sealer from the internal anatomy of the root canal system.

Rotary Instrumentation Removal of Gutta-Percha

Rotary instrumentation is the most efficient method for removing gutta-percha from a previously treated root canal (Figure 11). The ProTaper Retreatment Kit

(Dentsply International) is an example of a system that is useful in the retreatment of gutta-percha-filled root canals. However, to avoid instrument fracture, rotary instruments should be used with caution in under-prepared canals and are generally not selected for removal of gutta-percha in canals that do not have a glide path that allows the instrument to cut passively. When attempting gutta-percha removal, it may be useful to divide the root into thirds and then select two or three appropriately sized rotary instruments that will fit

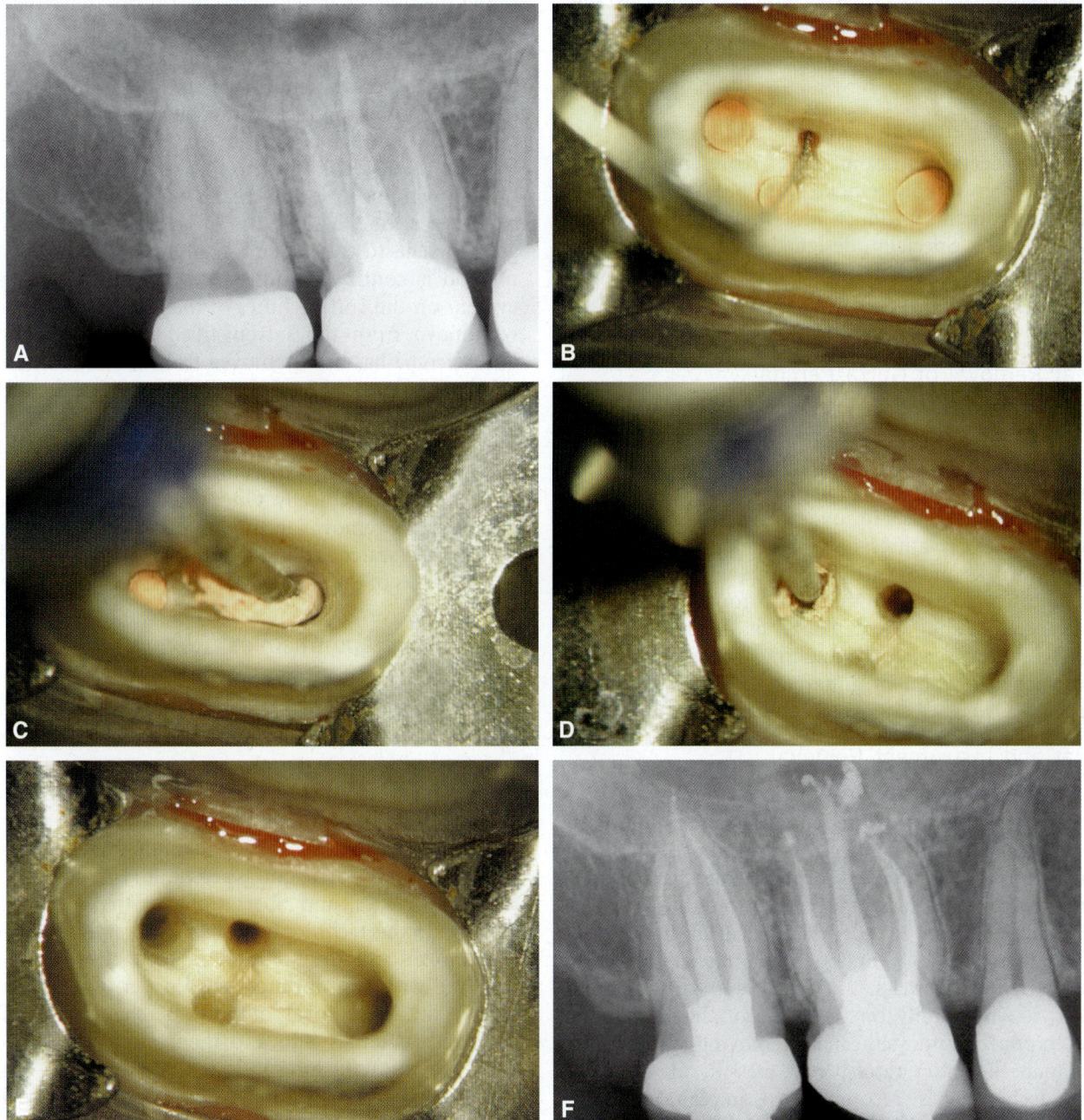

Figure 11 ***A,*** Radiograph of an endodontically treated, failing maxillary right first molar. Note the inadequate treatment resulting in an apical lesion. ***B,*** Photograph (×15 original magnification) after crown removal, adequate access, and the identification of an MB2 root canal orifice. ***C,*** Photograph (×15 original magnification) demonstrates the removal of gutta-percha from the palatal canal with a 0.06 tapered NiTi rotary profile. ***D,*** Photograph (×15 original magnification) demonstrates the removal of gutta-percha from the mesiobuccal canal with a smaller sized 0.06 tapered NiTi rotary profile. ***E,*** Photograph (×15 original magnification) shows the pulpal floor and orifices following canal preparation procedures. ***F,*** Postoperative radiograph after completion of retreatment.

passively within these progressively narrower regions. To mechanically soften and effectively remove gutta-percha, rotary instruments should turn at speeds ranging between 900 and 1200 rpm. Ultimately, the rotational speed has an effect on the amount of frictional heat generated to mechanically soften and effectively auger gutta-percha coronally. Coronal removal of gutta-percha allows the early introduction of solvents into the canal(s) and facilitates subsequent cleaning and shaping procedures.

Ultrasonic Removal of Gutta-Percha

The piezoelectric ultrasonic effect represents a useful technology to rapidly remove gutta-percha. The energized instruments produce heat that thermo-softens gutta-percha. Specially designed ultrasonic instruments may be carried into shaped canals and will displace gutta-percha coronally into the pulp chamber where it subsequently can be removed.

Heat Removal of Gutta-Percha

A power source in conjunction with specific electric heat carrier instruments may be used to thermo-soften and remove increments of gutta-percha from root canal systems.[152] The cross-sectional diameter of the heat carrier limits its use in under-prepared canals and around canal curvatures; however, in larger canals, this method works quite well. The technique involves guiding a heated plugger into the most coronal aspect of the gutta-percha. The heated plugger is then deactivated and withdrawn, generally resulting in the removal of an attached portion of gutta-percha. This process is repeated as long as it continues to be productive.

Heat and Instrument Removal of Gutta-Percha

Another technique to remove gutta-percha employs heat and Hedström files. In this method of removal, a hot instrument is plunged into the gutta-percha and immediately withdrawn in order to only heat-soften the material. A size 35, 40, or 45 Hedström file is then selected and quickly and gently screwed into the thermo-softened mass.[148] When the gutta-percha cools, it will solidify on the flutes of the Hedström file. In poorly obturated canals, removing the file may eliminate the entire gutta-percha mass in one motion. This technique is recommended in canals where gutta-percha extends beyond the apical foramen. After removing as much of the gutta-percha as possible, the clinician must verify whether residual gutta-percha and sealer are entrapped within the canal system. Chemical removal techniques are then used in conjunction with the described technique.

File and Chemical Removal of Gutta-Percha

The file and chemical removal technique is best used to remove gutta-percha from small and/or more curved canals. Chloroform is the most frequently used solvent and plays an important role in chemically softening gutta-percha.[176–179] This sequential technique involves filling the pulp chamber with chloroform, selecting an appropriately sized K-type file, and then carefully preparing the canal while removing the chemically softened gutta-percha. Initially, a size 10 or 15 stainless steel file is used to "pick" into the gutta-percha occupying the coronal one-third of the canal. Frequent irrigation with chloroform in combination with a "watch-winding" motion creates a pilot hole and sufficient space for the serial use of larger files to remove gutta-percha in this specific region of the canal. This method is continued until gutta-percha is no longer evident on the cutting flutes of the files when they are withdrawn from the solvent-filled canal. Only after gutta-percha has been removed from the coronal one-third of the canal should the clinician repeat the technique in the middle one-third and finally in the apical one-third. This progressive removal technique helps prevent the needless extrusion of chemically softened gutta-percha periapically. Once the "file and chemical" gutta-percha removal technique has been completed, the residual sealer and gutta-percha that remain in the irregularities of the root canal system need to removed.

Paper Point and Chemical Removal of Gutta-Percha

Gutta-percha and most sealers are miscible in chloroform and, once in solution, can be absorbed and removed with appropriately sized paper points. Drying solvent-filled canals with paper points is known as "wicking" and should always be the final step during gutta-percha removal.[148] The wicking action is essential in removing residual gutta-percha and sealer out of fins, cul-de-sacs, and aberrations of the root canal systems. In this technique, the canal is first flushed with chloroform and the solution is then absorbed and removed with appropriately sized paper points. Paper points aid in removal of gutta-percha by drawing dissolved materials into and then out of the shaped canal. Chemical flushing and wicking procedures more effectively liberate residual gutta-percha and sealer from the root canal system. This process is repeated as long as it continues to be visibly productive.

Even when paper points come out of the canal clean, white, and dry, the clinician should assume residual gutta-percha and sealer are still present. At this point, the chamber is again flooded with chloroform, but it is now introduced with more of an irrigation and vacuum "flushing action." The irrigating canula is placed below the orifice and the solvent is passively and repeatedly irrigated, then aspirated. This alternating method of irrigating then aspirating creates a vigorous back and forth turbulence that will promote the elimination of the root canal filling materials. Following chloroform wicking procedures, the canal is liberally flushed with 70% isopropyl alcohol and dried to further encourage the elimination of chemically softened gutta-percha residues. Removal of all residual material in this manner enhances the efficacy of NaOCl when it is used during subsequent cleaning and shaping procedures.

REMOVAL OF RESILON

Recently, a new root filling material, Resilon (Resilon Research LLC, Madison, CT), was introduced. Derived from polymers of polyester, it contains bioactive glass and radiopaque fillers. It has the same handling properties as gutta-percha. The Resilon core materials, similar to gutta-percha cones, are available in ISO sizes with 0.02, 0.04 and 0.06 tapers. Additionally, pellets of this material (Epiphany Pellets; Pentron Clinical Technologies LLC, Wallingford, CT) are available for use with the Obtura II delivery system (Obtura Spartan, Fenton, MO). Resilon is recommended for use in combination with a new dual curable dental resin composite sealer Epiphany Root Canal Sealant (Pentron Clinical Technologies LLC). There have been only a few reports concerning retreatment of teeth filled using Resilon and Epiphany sealer. Often in these types of studies, the hypothesis is tested that root canals filled with these materials can be retreated using hand and rotary instrumentation combinations in the same manner as canals filled with gutta-percha and conventional sealer. In three recent studies of Resilon and Epiphany sealer, they were removed more effectively from treated root canal systems compared to gutta-percha.[180–182] In two investigations, the most effective removal techniques involved a combination of rotary instrumentation and chloroform dissolution.[181,182] When no solvent was used in retreatment, Resilon and Epiphany sealer was removed most effectively with Gates Glidden (GG) burs and Hedström files compared to rotary only instrumentation.[180]

REMOVAL OF SILVER POINTS

The relative ease of removing failing silver points is based on the fact that chronic leakage and corrosion greatly reduce the seal, and hence, the lateral retention of the cone. Before any given silver point retrieval technique is selected, it is useful to recall the canal preparation prescribed for this method of obturation. Typically, the apical 2 to 3 mm of the canal was prepared relatively parallel and then flared coronal to this apical zone. When clinicians evaluate silver point failures and subsequent retreatment strategies, they should recognize that the silver point is slightly tapered over its length. In a coronally shaped canal, one may take advantage of this available space when approaching retreatment.[183]

Many techniques have been developed for removing silver points primarily addressing their varying lengths, diameters, and positions within the root canal space.[151,184,185] Certain removal techniques evolved to address silver points that bind in unshaped canals over a greater length. Other techniques have arisen to remove silver points with large cross-sections, resembling small diameter posts. Finally, other techniques are necessary to remove the split cone or intentionally sectioned silver points lying deep within the root canal space.

Access to Silver Points

Typically, the coronal portions of silver points are within pulp chambers and may be imbedded in cements, composites, or amalgam cores. Access preparations should be thoughtfully planned and prepared in order to minimize the risk of inadvertently shortening the silver points. Initial access is accomplished with high speed, surgical length cutting tools. Subsequently, ultrasonic instruments may be carefully used within the pulp chamber to "brush-cut" away restorative materials and progressively expose the silver point while avoiding direct contact of the silver point with the ultrasonic tip.

Pliers to Remove Silver Points

After completing access and fully exposing the coronal portion of the silver point inside the pulp chamber, a suitable grasping instrument (Stieglitz Forceps, Hu-Friedy; Chicago, IL) is selected. To identify the best removal strategy, a strong hold is obtained on the silver point and a gentle pull is exercised to confirm its relative tightness. A second lock on the grasping instrument by means of a hemostat can often enhance a tenuous grip.[184] Oftentimes, dentists make the mistake of over-manipulating the head of the silver point and needlessly shortening it, making subsequent retrieval efforts difficult, if not impossible. When grasping a silver point, rather than trying to pull it straight out of the canal, the pliers may be rotated and levered, using fulcrum mechanics, against the restoration or tooth structure to enhance removal efforts[151] (Figure 12).

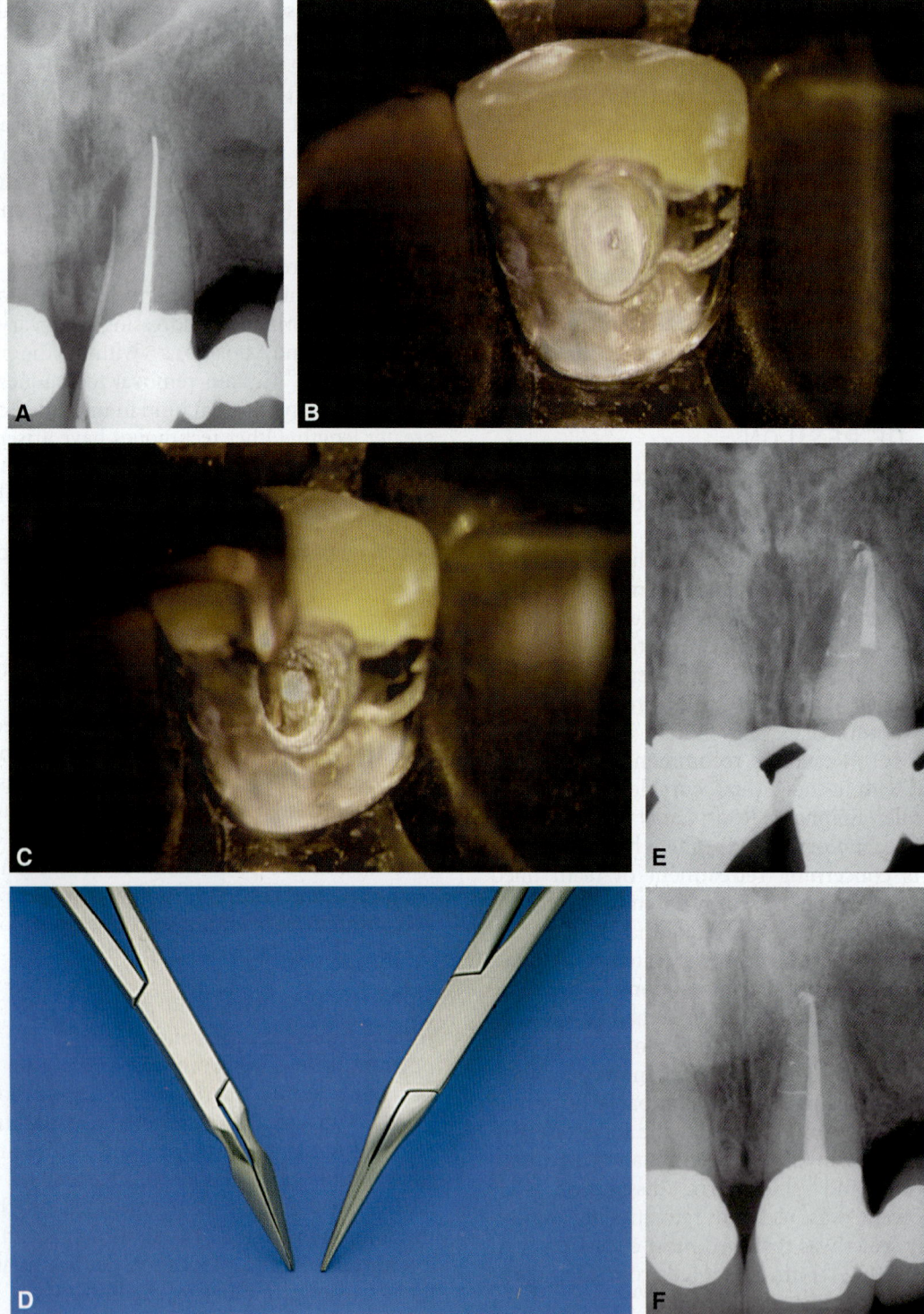

Figure 12 *A,* Preoperative radiograph of a failing endodontically treated maxillary central incisor bridge abutment; a gutta-percha point is tracing a sinus tract to a large lateral periapical lesion. Note the poorly filled root canal. *B,* Photograph (×15 magnification) reveals lingual access and restorative buildup around the coronal most aspect of the exposed silver point. *C,* Photograph (×15 magnification) demonstrates the ProUltra ENDO-3 ultrasonic instrument removing material lateral to the silver point. *D,* The left image shows the Stieglitz pliers used for grasping intracanal obstructions. The right image shows the "modified" Stieglitz pliers which working end has been altered to enhance access. *E,* Working radiograph during the down-pack phase of thermoplastic obturation reveals extensions apically and laterally. Note the thermosoftened and compacted gutta-percha is apical to the most coronally positioned lateral canal. *F,* Five-year review demonstrates that thorough endodontic treatment promotes healing.

Indirect Ultrasonics to Remove Silver Points

When a segment of a silver point is present below the canal orifice and space is restricted, an appropriate ultrasonic tip should be selected (e.g., ProUltra ENDO-3, 4, and 5, Dentsply International). These ultrasonic tips have parallel walls and provide progressively longer lengths and smaller diameters. The appropriate instrument is selected based on its anticipated depth of use and the available canal diameter. The ultrasonic instruments are used to trephine circumferentially around the obstruction, disintegrate the cement interface, and safely expose as much of the silver point as possible. Caution should be exercised not to use ultrasonic instruments directly on silver points because they rapidly erode during mechanical manipulation. Once the surrounding material is removed, ultrasonic energy may then be transmitted directly to the grasping pliers. This form of "indirect" ultrasonics advantageously transfers energy along the silver point, breaks up the interface deep within the canal, and enhances removal efforts.[184]

Files, Solvents, and Chelators to Remove Silver Points

If grasping techniques and/or indirect ultrasonics are unsuccessful, then the clinician should make use of the fact that silver points are perfectly round and root canal systems are typically irregular in their cross-sectional shapes. This discrepancy provides the clinician with an opportunity to use solvents and a size 10 or 15 stainless steel file alongside the silver point. In a solvent-filled chamber, files are used lateral to the silver point to loosen cements and to undermine and loosen the point for removal. In under-prepared canals, chelators may be more effective than solvents by lubricating the instrument. If space exists or can be created between the silver point and the canal wall, a 35, 40, or 45 Hedström file can be inserted into this space. The Hedström instrument promotes the removal process as its positive rake angle engages and establishes a strong purchase on the soft silver.

MICROTUBE REMOVAL OPTIONS

Several microtube removal methods exist that are designed to mechanically remove an intracanal obstruction such as a silver point or separated instrument. However, it should be remembered that many of these microtube removal methods require excessive removal of dentin and may not be effective. For clinicians, the critical dimension when considering microtube removal methods is not the inside diameter of the device but, importantly, it is the outside diameter, that defines how deeply it can be safely introduced into a given canal. The following list includes some of the various microtube removal methods and techniques.

- Lasso and anchor: In this removal method, an appropriately sized microtube is selected and a wire passed through the tube, then looped at one end and passed back through the tube. This loop can potentially lasso a coronally exposed obstruction and, when successful, form a purchase by pushing the tube apically while simultaneously pulling the wire ends coronally.[186] Although reported in the literature, this removal method has been essentially replaced with more practical techniques.[187]

- Tube and glue: The Cancellier Extractor Kit (SybronEndo, Orange, CA) contains four different sized microtubes with outside diameters of approximately 0.5, 0.6, 0.7, and 0.8 mm. An ultrasonic instrument may be used to trephine around and ideally expose the coronal 3 mm of an obstruction. A microtube is prefit to ensure its internal diameter can just fit over the coronally exposed obstruction. The prefit microtube may now be bonded onto the obstruction with an adhesive, such as core paste[148,161] or cyanoacrylate cement.[184] The diameters of Cancellier microtubes are safely scaled for progressively deeper placement into canals of posterior roots. This removal method may be effective for retrieving silver points, a fractured root canal instrument, or in cases of retrieval of a separated file that is already loose. Caution should be exercised to not use too much adhesive which could inadvertently block a canal.

- Tap and thread: The Post Removal System (PRS) kit (SybronEndo) contains five microtubular taps. The smallest PRS tap can be used to internally form threads and mechanically engage the most coronal aspect of any obstruction whose diameter is 0.6 mm or greater.[148] These microtubular taps contain a reverse thread and engage an obstruction by turning in a counterclockwise (CCW) motion. Because intracanal space is often restrictive, this system is generally used for removal of instruments or posts that extend into the pulp chamber (Figure 13). The PRS will be discussed in greater detail in the "Post Removal" section later in this chapter.

- Masserann: The Masserann kit (Micromega, Besançon, France) represents a time-honored method to remove a broken instrument.[188] Its smallest tubular extractors have outside diameters of 1.2 and 1.5 mm, limiting their safe use to larger canals in anterior teeth.

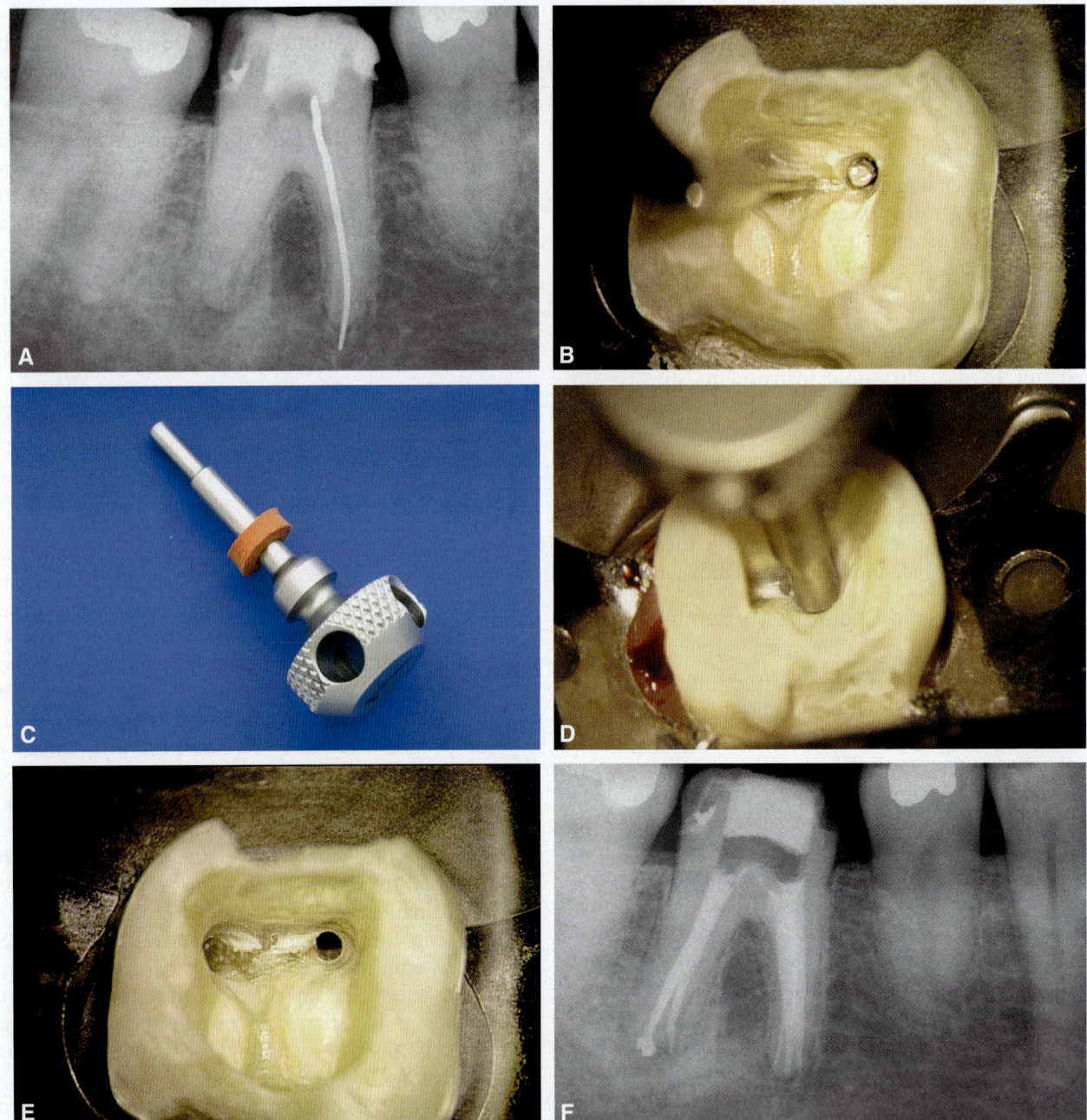

Figure 13 *A,* Radiograph of a mandibular right first molar with a silver point in the mesial root. *B,* Photograph (×15 original magnification) shows a ProUltra ENDO-3 ultrasonic instrument brush cutting the pulp chamber roof and improving access to the silver point. *C,* Microtubular tap from the Post Removal System kit. The tap may be used to engage an obstruction, and the rubber cushion protects the tooth during the extracting forces. *D,* Microtubular tap engages the silver point by turning the instrument counterclockwise. Care is exercised not to over-thread and shear off the point within the tap. *E,* Photograph (×15, original magnification) shows the elimination of the silver point. *F,* Postoperative radiograph shows non-surgical retreatment, including a filled third mesial canal.

- Spinal tap needle (STN): A STN (Ranfac, Avon, MA) in conjunction with its metal insert plunger or a Hedström file is another technique advocated to remove broken instruments.[148] With limitations, this method of removal involves sizing the correct microtube so it can be placed over an ultrasonically exposed obstruction. Microtube sizes that are clinically relevant are 19-, 21-, and 23-gauge needles

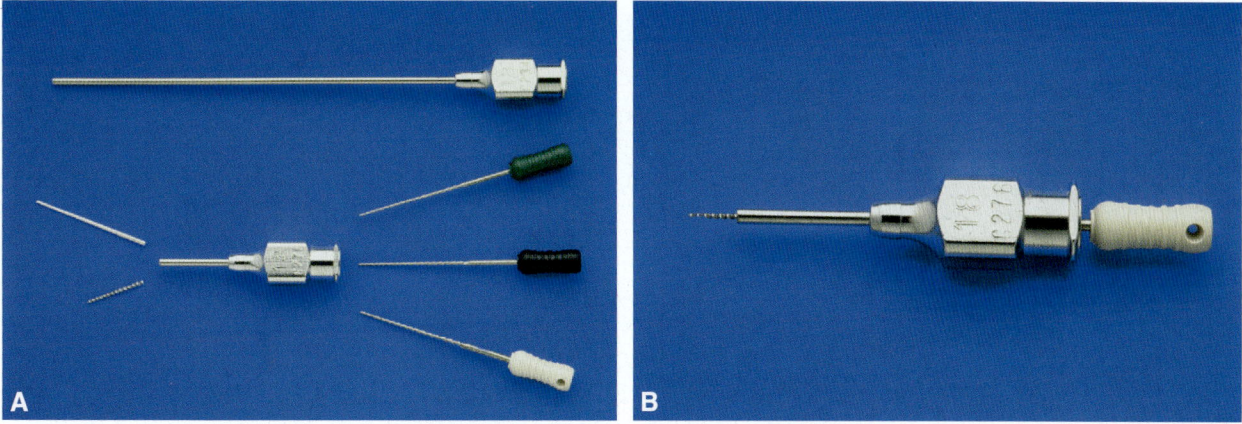

Figure 14 ***A,*** Full-length spinal tap needle (STN) (top). The STN is shortened and placed over a coronally exposed object, and Hedström files are passed through the proximal end of the STN to engage an obstruction. ***B,*** Assembled STN with a #45 Hedström file to engage a fractured file segment.

corresponding to outside tube diameters of approximately 1.0, 0.8, and 0.6 mm, respectively. Because of their unique threading effect, smaller sized Hedström files may be selected and inserted into the coronal most aspect of the microtube.[148,189] The Hedström is passed down the length of the tube until it wedges tightly between the obstruction and the internal lumen of the microtube (Figure 14). However, because ISO files increase by 0.32 mm over 16 mm of cutting blade, the taper of the file may restrict its placement through a smaller sized parallel microtube. In this instance, the STN's metal insert plunger may be used to potentially wedge the obstruction. This method is effective when removing obstructions from larger canals.

- Endo extractor/Meisinger Meitrac: The Endo Extractor System (Roydent Dental Products, Johnson City, TN) and the recently released Meisinger Meitrac Instrument System (Hager & Meisinger GmbH, Neuss, Germany) are techniques used for the removal of silver points or a separated instrument. However, the smallest Meitrac I trephine and extractor have outside diameters of approximately 1.5 mm. This diameter limits the practical use of this instrument to the coronal aspects of larger canals.
- Instrument Removal System (iRS): The iRS (Dentsply Maillefer) provides another mechanical method for the removal of intracanal obstructions such as silver points, carrier-based obturators, or broken file segments (Figure 15).[148] The iRS is indicated when ultrasonic efforts prove to be unsuccessful and may be used to remove fractured instruments that are lodged in the straight portions of the root or partially around the canal curvature. For method of use of this device, see the "Fractured Instrument Removal" section later in this chapter.

CARRIER-BASED GUTTA-PERCHA REMOVAL

The techniques for removing carrier-based gutta-percha are the same methods previously described separately for gutta-percha and silver point removal. Carrier-based obturators were originally metal and file-like; yet over the past several years, they have been manufactured from easier-to-remove plastic materials. Metal carriers, although no longer distributed, are occasionally encountered clinically and are more difficult to remove than silver points because their retention flutes may engage dentin walls.[190]

Following careful access and complete circumferential exposure of the carrier, suitable grasping pliers are selected and a grasp is obtained on the carrier. The relative tightness of the carrier within the canal can then be tested utilizing pliers. Successful removal in these cases is enhanced by recognizing that the carrier is embedded in gutta-percha. With this in mind, the following techniques are used to remove carriers:

- The carrier is grasped with the pliers and extrication is attempted using fulcrum mechanics rather than a straight pull out of the tooth.
- If enough canal width exists, an ultrasonic instrument can be used alongside the carrier to produce heat and thermo-soften the gutta-percha. The activated ultrasonic instrument is gently moved apically and the carrier may be displaced coronally.

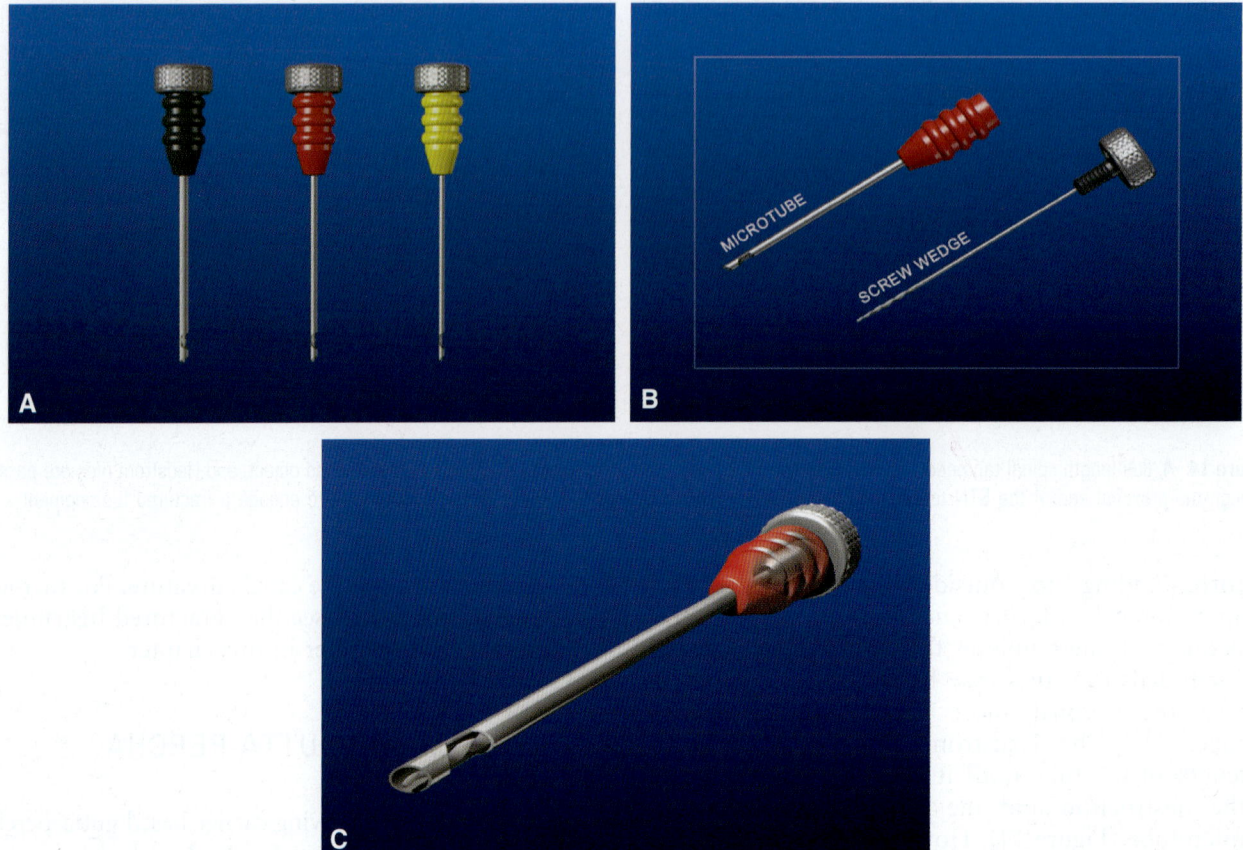

Figure 15 ***A,*** The Instrument Removal System (iRS) is a set of devices used for removing fractured instruments or other intracanal obstructions. ***B,*** Each iRS instrument is comprised of a microtube and an internal screw wedge designed to mechanically engage and remove intracanal obstructions. ***C,*** Close-up of the assembled iRS.

- Indirect ultrasonics can be performed by grasping the exposed carrier with pliers and then placing an ultrasonic instrument against the pliers.
- Rotary instrumentation can be used to remove a plastic carrier out of a canal. This should only be attempted if there is sufficient space to passively accommodate the rotary instrument without engaging lateral dentin.
- The iRS, as previously mentioned regarding silver point removal, may be considered, in certain cases, to remove a carrier. This method of removal is especially appropriate if the core of the carrier is metal and has retention flutes engaging lateral dentin.
- Solvents will chemically soften gutta-percha and allow small files to work deeper, circumferentially and laterally, while loosening a carrier for removal.

If any of these efforts are successful, a carrier will be extracted from the canal. The canal can then be retreated using any of the gutta-percha removal strategies followed by chemical solvents and paper point wicking procedures.

PASTE REMOVAL

A great variety of paste types exist. Originally, paste use was intended to simplify root canal treatment and reduce the cost to patients hoping to overcome deficiencies in the removal of tissue, bacterial by-products, and related irritants during canal preparation. This was often addressed by adding toxic ingredients and chemical formulations to the paste.

When evaluating a tooth obturated with paste for retreatment, it is useful to recall that pastes can generally be divided into soft, penetrable, and removable versus hard, impenetrable, and at times, non-removable formulations.[150,191] Hard setting whitish-colored paste often used in Russia and the reddish-brown resin paste commonly used in Eastern Europe and the Pacific Rim is very difficult to remove.[191] However, it is important to understand that, due to the

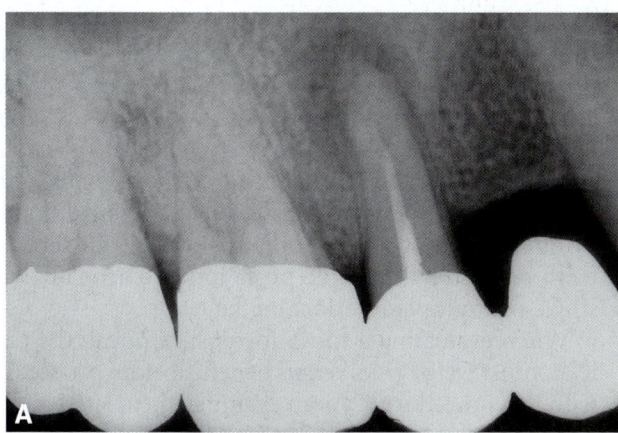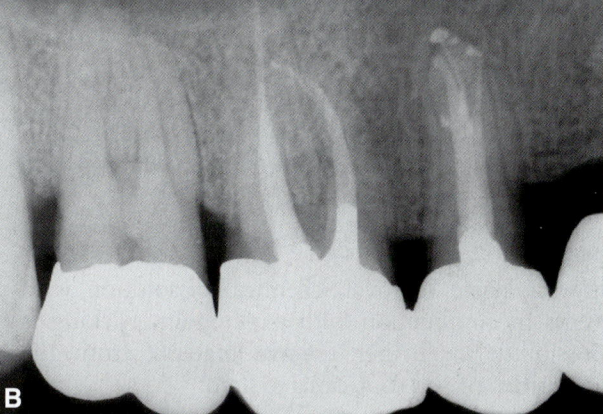

Figure 16 ***A,*** Maxillary premolar with the root canal system treated with a paste material. Note the large periapical lesion indicating bacterial contamination of the root canal system. ***B,*** Ten-year recall radiograph shows the result of complete endodontic treatment.

method of placement (e.g., packing or a rotary spiral), the densest portion of the paste in the canal is coronal and the material is progressively less dense moving apically. In addition, mineralization and resorption may be associated with paste-filled roots (Figure 16).

Ultrasonic Energy for Paste Removal

Ultrasonic instruments, in conjunction with the microscope, afford superior control in removing paste from the straight portions of a root canal.[192–194] Specially coated ultrasonic instruments may be used below the orifice to remove brick-hard resin-type pastes. To remove filling materials apical to a curvature, small-sized hand files should be used first to negotiate this region of the canal. Once a glide path has been created, then an appropriately sized precurved file may be attached to a specially designed adapter (File Adapter 11, SybronEndo) that mounts on, and is activated by, the ultrasonic handpiece.

Heat for Paste Removal

Certain resin pastes soften with heat. Heat carriers can be selected if this modality of removal is chosen.

Rotary Instruments for Paste Removal

Stainless steel 0.02 tapered hand files may be used to negotiate paste-filled root canals. These files are used to create a pilot hole for safe-ended NiTi rotary instruments which do not cut at the tip to follow and effectively remove the material coronally. At times helpful are end-cutting NiTi rotary instruments to penetrate paste. These instruments are more active apically and hence more prone to preparation error should they be used too aggressively.

Solvents and Hand Files for Paste Removal

Reagents like Endosolv "R" and Endosolv "E" (Endoco; Memphis, TN) may be helpful in chemically softening hard paste.[191] The "R" designates the solution of choice for the removal of resin-based pastes and the "E" is the solution for the softening of eugenol-based pastes (Figure 17). These solutions may be placed between appointments against a paste-type material via paper points or cotton pellets to promote subsequent removal.

Micro-Debriders for Paste Removal

After removing the paste filling and shaping the root canal, it should be remembered that residual paste will still be contained within the irregularities of the root

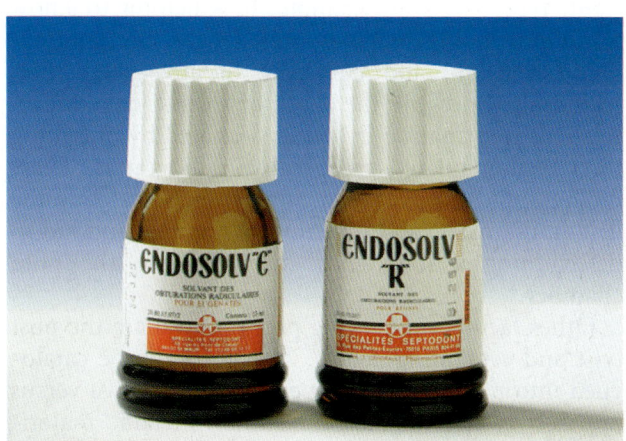

Figure 17 Endosolv "E" is a solvent for eugenol-based pastes whereas Endosolv "R" is for resin-based pastes.

canal system. Micro-Debriders (Dentsply International) are specially designed instruments to remove residual paste materials from a root canal system. These stainless steel instruments enhance vision due to their offset handles, have tip diameters of 0.2 and 0.3 mm, and are available in 0.02 tapers with 16 mm of efficient Hedström-type cutting blades.

Solvents and Paper Points for Paste Removal

Following paste removal, chemical dissolution with solvents in conjunction with paper point wicking is a possibility to further remove material from the irregularities of the root canal system.

Post Removal

It is common to encounter endodontically treated teeth containing posts. When endodontic treatment fails to achieve healing, the need may arise to remove a post in order to gain access and allow retreatment. In other instances, the endodontic treatment may be judged successful, but restorative needs require the removal of an existing post to improve the design, mechanics, or esthetics of a new restoration. Over time, many techniques have been advocated for the removal of posts and other large intracanal obstructions.[37,188,195]

FACTORS INFLUENCING POST REMOVAL

There are many factors that influence post removal such as operator judgment, training, experience, and choice of technologies and techniques.[148,184] Furthermore, clinicians should have knowledge of the anatomy of the teeth being treated and be familiar with the typical range of variation associated with each tooth type.[196] As an example, it is helpful to know tooth morphology, including the length, circumferential dimension, and curvature of any given root, including, if present, the depth of an external concavity. This information is best appreciated by obtaining three well-angulated preoperative radiographs. These radiographs also assist the clinician in visualizing the length, diameter, and direction of the post and aid in determining if it extends coronally into the pulp chamber.[172]

Other factors influencing post removal are the post type and cementing agent.[197,198] Posts can be catalogued into parallel versus tapered shapes, active versus non-active, and metallic versus non-metallic materials.[199,200] Posts retained with the classic cements such as zinc phosphate can generally be removed more predictably; however, posts bonded into the root canal space with composite resins or glass ionomers may be more difficult to remove.[173] Additional factors that impact post removal are the available inter-occlusal space, existing restoration, and whether the most coronal aspect of the post is supracrestal or subcrestal. In general, post removal becomes more challenging moving from anterior to posterior teeth. The difficulty in removing a post substantially increases in furcated teeth containing multiple posts joined coronally with single or multiple interlocking keyways.

When evaluating a tooth for post removal, the clinician must weigh risks versus benefits before proceeding with this procedure.[32] As an example, the relative radiodensity between titanium or a titanium alloy post can appear very similar, or even identical, to gutta-percha when viewed radiographically. As such, when considering non-surgical retreatment, clinicians need to be familiar with the radiographic characteristics of these metallic and non-metallic posts.[201] A root can be structurally weakened, perforated or fractured during any phase of retreatment ranging from radicular disassembly to subsequent shaping and filling procedures. In some instances, it may be wise to consider a surgical approach to resolve an endodontic failure.

TECHNIQUES FOR ACCESS FOR POST REMOVAL

Successful post removal requires eliminating all circumferential restorative materials from the pulp chamber. Once straight-line access into the pulp chamber is established, the restorative materials circumferential to the post are removed. Surgical length burs are useful to section and eliminate cores because their added lengths improve vision during re-entry into the pulp chamber. Removing the greatest bulk of restorative materials that commonly surround various post head configurations will expose the coronal aspect of a post.

Ultrasonic energy in conjunction with appropriate ultrasonic instruments provides important advantages when performing access refinement procedures. Advantageously, small-sized ultrasonic instruments afford continuous and improved vision into the field of operation (see Figure 10). On the contrary, a rotating bur in a dental handpiece is oftentimes difficult to see because even a small handpiece head may block the line of sight. Strategically, contra-angled, parallel-sided, and abrasively coated stainless steel ultrasonic instruments enhance access, vision, and cutting precision when progressively removing various materials. In general, ultrasonic instruments are used at the lowest power settings that will efficiently accomplish the clinical task. Thinner and more parallel-sided ultrasonic instruments are designed to work in smaller spaces, such as between a post and an axial wall. Importantly, a parallel-sided ultrasonic instrument may be safely used below the orifice and lateral to a post, especially in an irregularly shaped canal.[156]

If space is restrictive within the field of operation, then an appropriately sized titanium ultrasonic instrument may be selected and is generally used at a lower intensity. These instruments provide the clinician with thinner diameters and longer lengths as compared to abrasively coated or non-coated stainless steel ultrasonic instruments (see Figure 10C). Ultrasonic instruments are best used with a light brush-cutting motion and on the peripheral edge of a sectioned core to chip, break up, and "sand away" materials such as cement, composite, or amalgam. Eliminating these materials from the pulp chamber serves to undermine the retention of a post. To optimize vision, virtually all non-surgical ultrasonic procedures are performed under air stream. When an abrasively coated ultrasonic instrument removes dentin or a restorative material, the by-product of this ultrasonic action is dust. The dental assistant may use compressed air to clear the field of vision by utilizing the Stropko three-way adapter with the White Mac tip (Ultradent, South Jordan, UT) to direct and control a continuous stream of air into the field. Debris is blown away and, importantly, allows the clinician to maintain visual contact with the energized tip of the instrument.[148]

Water port technology in non-surgical ultrasonic instruments is not recommended for four important reasons: (1) water flowing through an ultrasonic instrument dampens movement and decreases tip performance; (2) small diameter ultrasonic instruments are weakened and more predisposed to expensive breakage when they are machined for internal water flow; (3) there is an undesirable aerosol effect regardless of where the water port is positioned on an ultrasonic instrument; (4) and most important, water in combination with dentinal dust, creates mud, reduces vision, and increases the potential for iatrogenic outcomes. In summary, clinical experience supports the strategy that the vast majority of all non-surgical ultrasonic procedures may be performed under air stream and at the lowest power setting that will safely accomplish the clinical task. However, if ultrasonic procedures are performed at higher energy levels, for longer periods of time, and against larger, conductive objects, such as a metal post, then it is critically essential that the dental assistant use a triplex syringe with an intermittent water spray to reduce heat buildup and heat transfer to the periodontal tissues.[202] Fortunately, heat does not conduct well through dentin and is further rapidly dissipated due to the moisture content in the attachment apparatus.[203–205] However, later in the section titled "Thermal Injury with the Use of Ultrasonics," the sequelae of inappropriate heat transfer to the attachment and bone through vibratory energy to metallic posts will be discussed.[202]

TECHNIQUES FOR POST REMOVAL

Once straight-line access into the pulp chamber has been accomplished, all core materials eliminated, and the post has been fully exposed, then a variety of techniques have been advocated to finally remove a post.[174,195,206,207] No single method always produces a successful result. It is important to be familiar with a variety of techniques to maximize success.

Rotosonic Vibration for Post Removal

Rotosonics is a method to potentially loosen and remove a fully exposed post. The Regular Tip Roto-Pro bur (Ellman International, Hewlett, NY) is a high-speed, friction grip bur whose six sides utilize six edges which when rotated in one revolution produce six vibrations per revolution. When the instrument is rotated at 200,000 rpm, it produces 1.2 million vibrations per minute or 20,000 vibrations per second. This instrument provides an inexpensive method to remove certain posts especially those secured with zinc phosphate cement. The bur is kept in intimate contact with the obstruction and is generally moved CCW around the post.

Ultrasonic Energy for Post Removal

The active distal end of an appropriately designed ultrasonic instrument may be kept in intimate contact with the post to maximize energy transfer and promote cement/bond failure (Figure 18A). The selected ultrasonic instrument is energized and moved around the post circumferentially and up and down along its exposed length.[208] Again, it must be stressed that the by-product of ultrasonic energy is heat (see Figure 18B). When performing ultrasonic procedures for extended periods of time in cases of larger conductive metal posts, the operating field should be cooled with water to decrease heat buildup and the potential for dangerous heat transfer to the periodontal tissues (see Figure 18C).[202–204] Experience suggests that after removing all circumferential restorative materials, the majority of posts can be safely and successfully removed within approximately 10 minutes (see Figure 18D).[197,209] Certain posts resist removal even after ultrasonic efforts using the

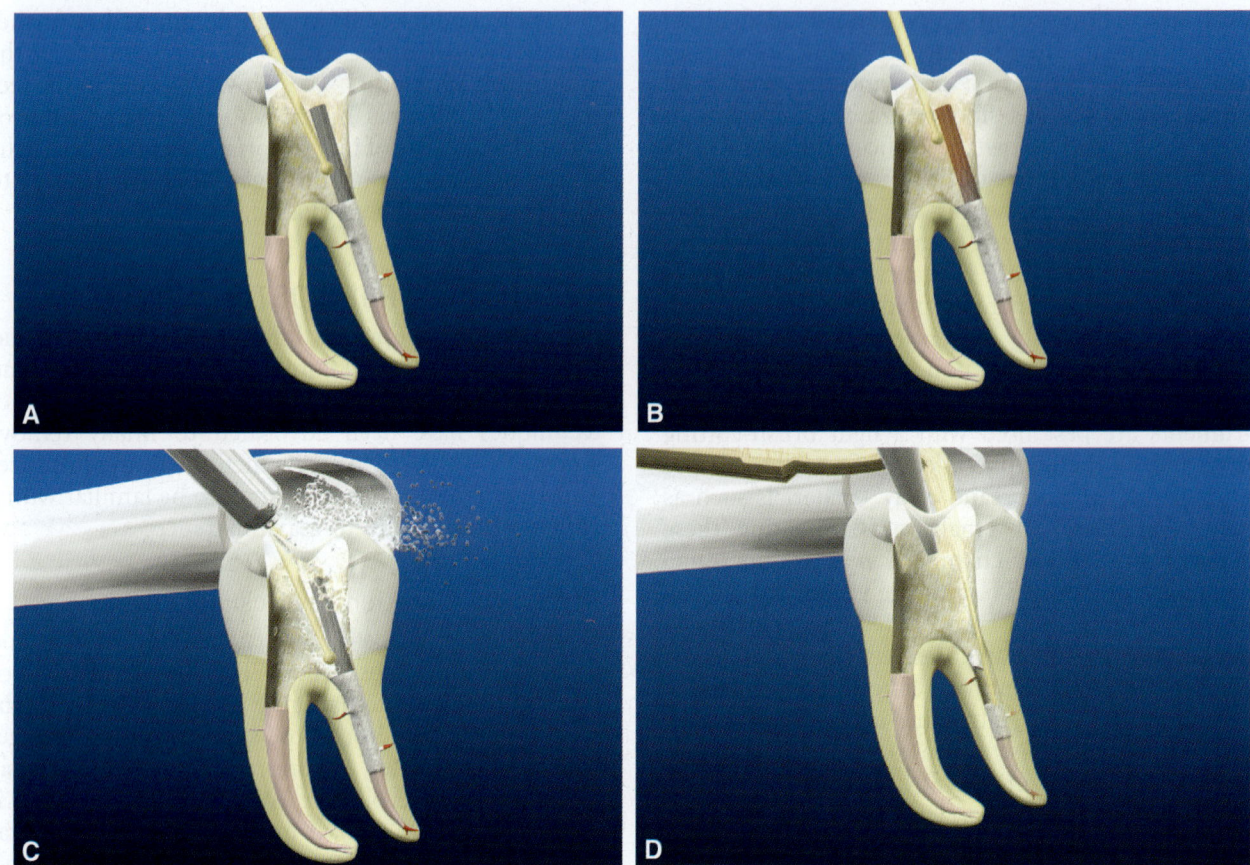

Figure 18 ***A****,* The ProUltra ENDO-1 is activated and used to vibrate against all aspects of the exposed post. ***B****,* Illustration of how ultrasonic procedures generate heat, particularly when removing larger, more conductive metal posts. ***C****,* A graphic representation demonstrating the importance of using an external water source to reduce temperature and eliminate heat transfer. ***D****,* Following post removal, an ultrasonic instrument loosens intracanal cement and a White Mac Tip collimates air and blows out debris.

"10-Minute Rule." Caution is important for safe and efficient alternative strategy to loosen these posts.[210]

MECHANICAL DEVICES FOR POST REMOVAL

Many of the available mechanical devices, such as the Masserann kit (Micromega) and the Post Puller (Brasseler), have had limited success because they may frequently require excessive removal of tooth structure, which predisposes to ledges, perforations, or root fractures. The Gonon post extractor (EFDM-Pneumat, Bourge, France) represents a definite improvement over the Masserann and the Post Puller devices in that it is less invasive and requires less removal of tooth structure.[37,195] The PRS kit (Sybron-Endo) (Figure 19) was designed to mechanically engage and remove different kinds of post types or other intracanal obstructions whose cross-sectional diameters are 0.6 mm or greater.[148] The PRS kit contains extracting pliers, a transmetal bur, five trephines of varying internal diameters, five corresponding

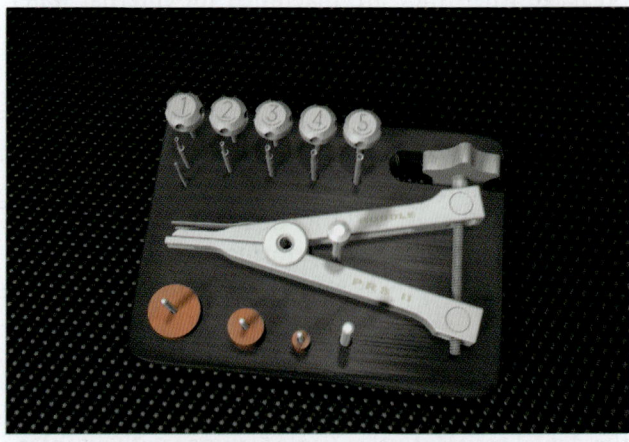

Figure 19 The Post Removal System is a kit designed to mechanically engage and remove many different types of posts.

tubular taps whose internal diameters range from 0.6 to 1.6 mm, a torque bar, tube spacers, and a selection of rubber cushions. The preparatory procedures before utilizing the PRS require straight-line access and complete circumferential visualization of the post within the pulp chamber.

A transmetal bur is used to round-off or taper the coronal most aspect of the post (Figure 20A).

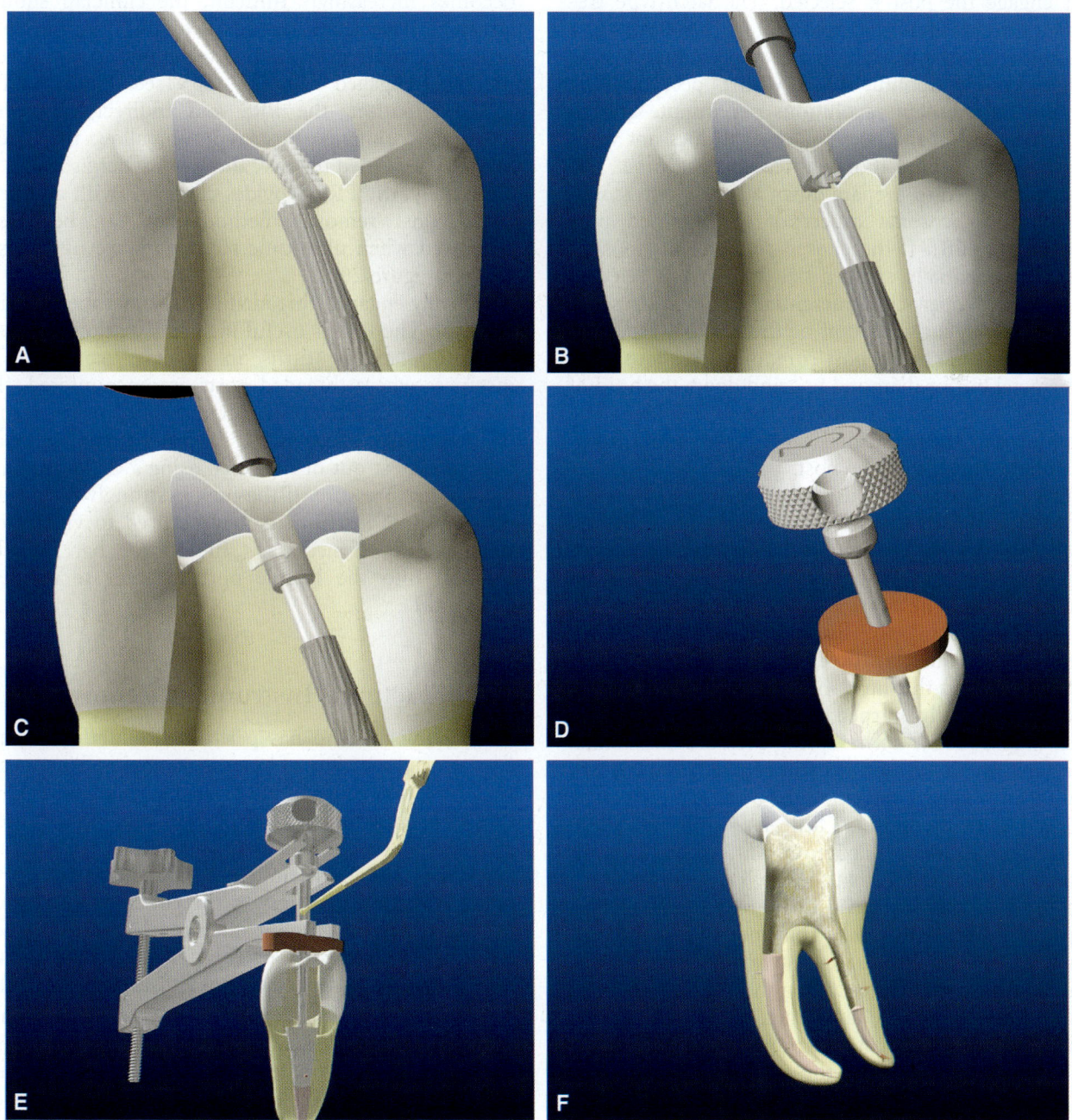

Figure 20 ***A***, Graphic representation depicting a transmetal bur efficiently doming the post head. ***B***, The no. 3 trephine has precisely machined down the coronal 3 mm of the post. ***C***, The tubular tap is turned counterclockwise to form threads, draw down, and strongly engage the post. ***D***, Once the tap is securely engaged to the post, then the rubber bumper is seated against the occlusal surface to protect the tooth. ***E***, Graphic representation of the mounted and activated Post Removal System extracting pliers. Note the energized ProUltra ENDO-1 may advantageously be placed against the post-engaged tap to synergistically facilitate the removal effort. ***F***, Completed post removal.

"Doming" the head of the post will serve to effectively guide subsequent instruments over the post. A chelator, such as RC Prep, Glyde or ProLube, may be placed on the head of the post to act as a lubricant to facilitate the machining process. In order to ensure circumferential milling, the largest trephine that will just engage the post is selected. The latch-type trephines should rotate at approximately 15,000 rpm in a clockwise (CW) direction, in a slowspeed, high torque handpiece. The trephine is used with a "peck" drilling motion to maintain revolutions per minute and to keep the head of the post cooler so it does not work harden and become more difficult to machine. The trephine is used to prepare down a 2 to 3 mm length of the most coronal aspect of the exposed post (see Figure 20B). If the chosen trephine fits loosely, then a sequentially smaller size trephine is selected to ensure proper circumferential milling. In some instances, the configuration of the coronal aspect of the post, such as a cast post/core, dictates the use of a transmetal bur or diamond to grind down the head of the post to create a relatively round cylinder. The trephine can then machine a precisely round cross-sectional diameter on the post.

In general, trephines used for machining the post dictate the subsequent selection of a correspondingly sized tubular tap. An appropriately sized protective rubber cushion is selected and inserted over the distal end of the tap. The cushion serves to act as a bumper, evenly distributing the loads to protect the tooth during the removal procedure. The tubular tap is pushed against the head of the milled down post and is manually turned CCW to form threads (see Figure 20C). Firm apical pressure and small quarter-turn CCW motions will generally draw down and securely engage the tap to the post. The tap can be screwed over the post as little as 1 mm or, more optimally, up to a maximum of 3 mm. Caution should be exercised so that the tap is not drawn down too far over the post because its maximum internal depth is 4 mm. If the tap bottoms out against the post head, it can predispose to stripping the threads, breaking the wall of the tap, or shearing off the post inside the lumen of the tap. When the tubular tap has snugly engaged the post, the protective rubber cushion is pushed down onto the occlusal surface of the tooth (see Figure 20D).

The post removal pliers are then selected and the extracting jaws are mounted onto the tubular tap. The instrument is held securely with one hand, while the fingers of the other hand begin opening the jaws by turning the screw knob CW. As the jaws slowly begin to open, increasing pressure will be noted on the screw knob. The clinician should repeatedly verify that the compressing rubber cushion is properly protecting the tooth. Furthermore, when utilizing this removal method, the clinician should visually confirm the post is being safely withdrawn along the long axis of the root canal. If turning the screw knob becomes increasingly difficult, the clinician should either hesitate a few seconds before continuing and/or use the indirect ultrasonic technique to vibrate on the post-engaged tubular tap (see Figure 20E). In combination, the PRS and indirect ultrasonic techniques enhance post removal, allow the screw knob to be turned further, and work synergistically.[210] Ultimately, the PRS provides clinicians with an alternative post removal method that can be safely employed when ultrasonic techniques are unsuccessful (see Figure 20F).

Actively engaged threaded posts sometimes require removal. The PRS is useful in such situations because each tubular tap turns in a CCW rotation. In instances where threaded posts are encountered, the use of the extracting pliers is contra-indicated because of the active engagement. Typically, the clinician backs the post out of the canal using a CCW rotation with finger pressure. If the post is strongly anchored, an ultrasonic instrument may be used to vibrate on the tap and, if necessary, the torque bar may be inserted into the handle port to increase leverage (Figure 21).

Fractured Instrument Removal

Every clinician who has performed endodontics has experienced a variety of outcomes ranging from a case well done to a procedural accident such as the separation of an instrument. During root canal preparation procedures, the risk of instrument breakage or fracture exists. When instrument breakage occurs, it provokes considerable stress to the clinician.[211] In fact, the fractured instrument dilemma has caused such emotional distress that this event is frequently referred to as a "separated" or "disarticulated" file.

Many clinicians associate a "broken instrument" with a separated file, but the term could also apply to a sectioned silver point, a segment of a Lentulo instrument, a GG drill, a portion of a carrier-based obturator, or any other device obstructing the canal.[212,213] With the advent of rotary NiTi files, there has been an increase in the occurrence of fractured instruments.[214,215] The prognosis of leaving, versus removing broken instruments from the canal have been discussed in the literature.[39,216] Over the years,

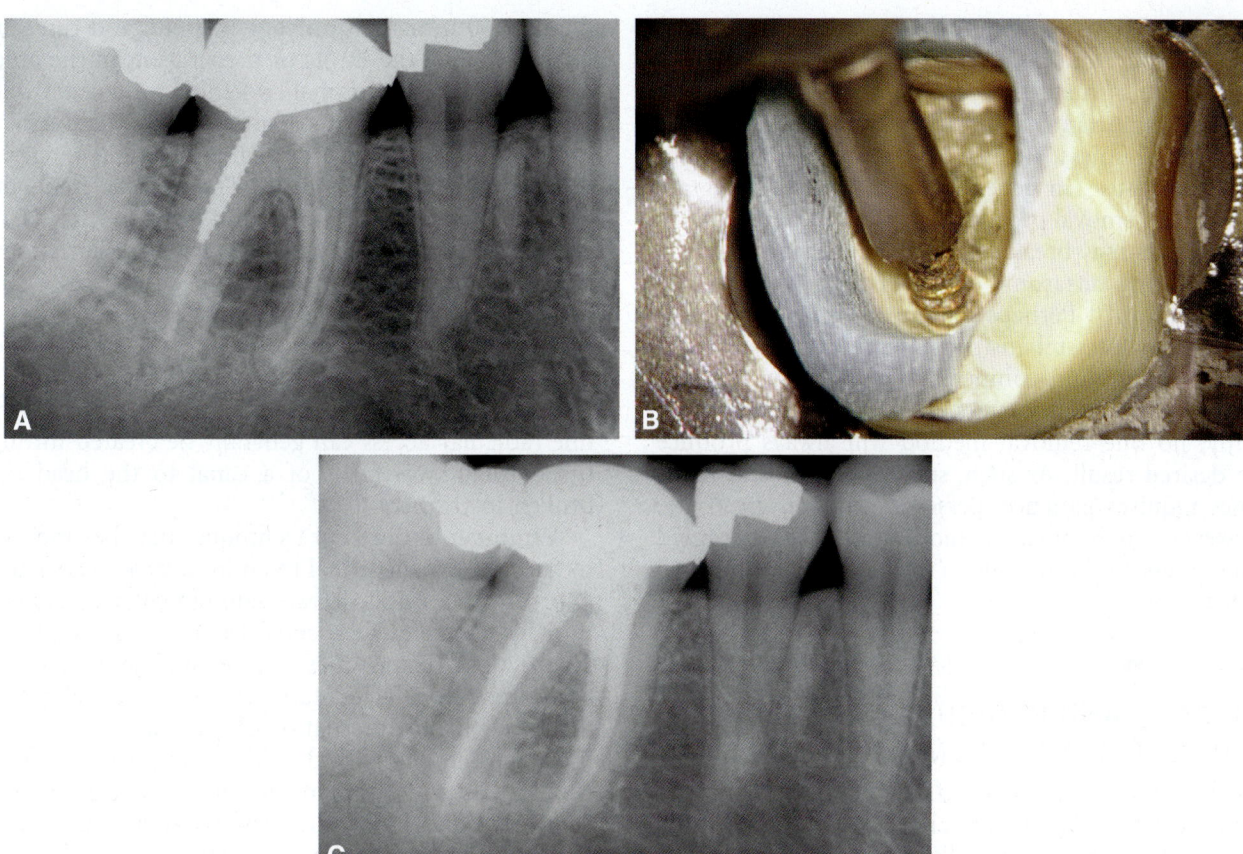

Figure 21 ***A,*** Radiograph of a mandibular right first molar with a crown, a screw post, and inadequate endodontic treatment. ***B,*** Clinical photograph demonstrates a tap forming threads and being drawn down to tightly engage the post. ***C,*** Postoperative radiograph of completed retreatment.

a variety of approaches for managing broken instruments have been presented.[42,188,217]

Today, separated instruments can usually be removed due to technological advancements in vision, ultrasonic instrumentation, and microtube delivery methods.[148,218] Specifically, the increasing integration of the dental operating microscope into clinical practice allows clinicians to visualize the coronal portion of most fractured instruments.[219] In combination, the microscope and ultrasonic instrumentation have created "microsonic" strategies which have greatly improved the potential and safety of removing broken instruments.[148,220,221]

FACTORS INFLUENCING FRACTURED INSTRUMENT REMOVAL

The factors influencing non-surgical access and removal of a fractured instrument include the diameter, length, and position of the obstruction within a canal.[184,222] Additionally, the chosen approach to safely remove a broken instrument is guided by anatomy, including the diameter, length, and curvature of the canal. Limiting factors include the circumferential dimensions and thickness of dentin and the depth of an external concavity.[223,224] In most instances, if one-third of the overall length of an obstruction can be exposed, it can usually be removed. Instruments that lie in the straight, more coronal portions of the canal can be removed more readily than separated instruments that lie partially around canal curvatures. In these cases, an attempt to establish straight-line access to their most coronal extents may prove successful.[148,221,225] If the fractured instrument segment is apical to the curvature of a canal and access without compromising the structural integrity of the root cannot be accomplished, then removal is not feasible, and in the presence of signs or symptoms, surgery or an extraction may be required.

The type of material comprising an obstruction is another important factor to be considered. As an example, stainless steel files tend to be easier to remove because, in general, they do not disintegrate during the removal process. Separated nickel-titanium instruments may break again, albeit deeper within the canal, during ultrasonic efforts. This may be due to heat buildup.[161] Perhaps, the most important factors central to successful instrument removal are knowledge, training, and competency in selecting the best contemporary technologies and techniques. Importantly, no one removal method will always produce the desired result. As such, successful removal oftentimes requires patience, perseverance, and creativity. However, no removal method should be attempted until access has been made to the head of an intracanal obstruction.

CORONAL AND RADICULAR ACCESS FOR INSTRUMENT REMOVAL

Prior to the initiation of efforts to remove a fractured instrument, the clinician should thoughtfully observe different horizontally angulated preoperative radiographs. Coronal access is the first step in the removal of a fragment. Surgical length burs are selected to create straight-line access to all canal orifices. Flaring the canal wall alongside the instrument aids in efforts to provide space for subsequent treatment steps.

Radicular access is the next step in the attempted removal of a broken instrument. However, before commencing with radicular access, some basic morphological data must guide one's clinical actions. With exceptions, the vast majority of teeth range from 19 to 25 mm in overall length. Most clinical crowns are about 10 mm and most roots range from 9 to 15 mm in length. If the root is divided into coronal, middle, and apical one-thirds, then each third is between 3 and 5 mm in length. An important concept in retreatment strategy is how wide a canal can be optimally flared without creating a problem. The answer is to review the dimensions of a typical preparation in a longer, thinner, and more curved root form.[152,226] An ISO size 20 apical preparation in conjunction with 1/2 mm increment stepback technique leads to a taper of 10%. In this specific example, the diameter of the canal 4 mm coronal to the apical end point of the preparation would be equivalent to a 60 file or 0.60 mm. This analogy is useful and can serve to safely guide the limits of preparation in the apical one-third and the coronal two-thirds of a canal when there is a separated instrument.[227] The majority of broken files separate toward their terminal extents at between D_3, D_4, or D_5.[228,229] Files most frequently break in the apical 3 to 5 mm because this is the region where a canal usually has its smallest diameter and exhibits its greatest degree of curvature or propensity to divide.[230] Even if a file fracture occurs at the working length, the position of the cross-section of the instrument typically lies at the junction of the middle and apical one-thirds. Fortuitously, straight-line radicular access can generally be created through the coronal two-thirds of a canal to the head of a broken instrument.[148,225]

A number of different techniques may be employed to flare the canal coronal to an intracanal obstruction. A predictable way to create safe radicular access is to initially use hand files, small to large, coronal to the obstruction. Hand files create sufficient space to accommodate NiTi rotary files or, preferably, GG drills (Dentsply International). GG sizes 1 to 4 are most typically employed in the coronal one-third of root canals and have maximum diameters of 0.50, 0.70, 0.90, and 1.10 mm, respectively. In many cases, GGs are used to create radicular access and a uniform tapering funnel to the obstruction. GGs are more safely rotated at speeds of about 750 rpm and, importantly, are safely used with a "brushing motion" to create a tapered shape and maximize visibility.[225] Increasingly, larger GGs are uniformly stepped out of the canal to create a smooth flowing funnel that is largest at the orifice and narrowest at the obstruction. To avoid strip perforations, GG drills should be limited to the straightaway portions of the canal. However, in the case of a fractured instrument, a GG-1 or GG-2 can be carried to the depth of the head of a separated instrument. The GGs are used cautiously approximating the obstruction with attention to brush-cutting out of the canal and away from the furcal direction. Deliberately relocating the coronal one-third of a canal away from the furcation maximizes remaining dentin, produces a more centered preparation, and improves straight-line radicular access.[225] The GG-3 is carried short of the level where the GG-2 was used and, in furcated teeth, the GG-4 is confined to a depth of no more than one length of the cutting portion below the orifice. Ideally, radicular access would be performed in a way that the canal is pre-enlarged and shaped to the same diameter than it would otherwise be prepared if there was no broken instrument obstructing the canal.

CREATING A STAGING PLATFORM

When the canal has been shaped, microsonic techniques are usually the first step selected to remove a broken file segment. When an ultrasonic instrument is introduced into a pre-enlarged canal, often its activated tip does not have enough space, lateral to the broken file segment, for the amplitude of vibration to effectively trephine. If more lateral space is required, then the cutting head of a GG can be modified and used to create a circumferential "staging platform".[148,161] The staging platform is made by selecting a GG drill whose maximum cross-sectional diameter is slightly larger than the visualized instrument. The cutting portion of the GG drill is altered by cutting it perpendicular to its long axis at its maximum cross-sectional diameter (Figure 22). This modified GG drill is carried into the pre-enlarged canal, rotated at a reduced speed of approximately 300 rpm, and directed apically until it lightly contacts the most coronal aspect of the obstruction. This clinical step creates a small platform that facilitates the introduction of an ultrasonic instrument. If properly performed, straight-line coronal and radicular access, in conjunction with magnification and lighting, should enable the clinician to fully visualize the coronal most aspect of a broken instrument. To facilitate excellent vision to the intra-radicular obstruction, the canal should be thoroughly irrigated and thoroughly dried prior to beginning ultrasonic procedures.

TECHNIQUES FOR REMOVING FRACTURED INSTRUMENTS

A number of devices, technologies, and techniques have been reported to remove an intracanal obstruction such as a separated instrument.[231–233] However, many of the removal techniques described in the early literature did not make use of the operating microscope. Today, most fractured instruments can be retrieved if straight-line access can be safely made to the coronal most extent of a broken instrument.[148,221,225] The most predictable and safe removal schemes utilize a microscope in conjunction with optimally designed ultrasonic instruments and/or a microtube method.[161,225,234]

ULTRASONIC TECHNIQUES FOR REMOVING FRACTURED INSTRUMENTS

Prior to performing any radicular removal techniques, it is wise to place cotton pellets into other canal orifices, if present, to prevent the nuisance re-entry of the fragment into another canal. The first option to remove a broken instrument is to utilize piezoelectric ultrasonic technology and specific ultrasonic instruments. An ultrasonic generator should provide a broad range of power, precise adjustment within the lower settings, and electrical feedback to regulate amplitude and safe tip movement. Ideally, ultrasonic instruments should have a contra-angled design to provide access into all regions of the mouth, parallel-sided walls to create a line of sight between the instrument and the tapered canal, and non-aggressive coatings, such as zirconium nitride, to precisely remove dentin during trephination. Furthermore, an ultrasonic instrument of appropriate length should be chosen that allows contact with the

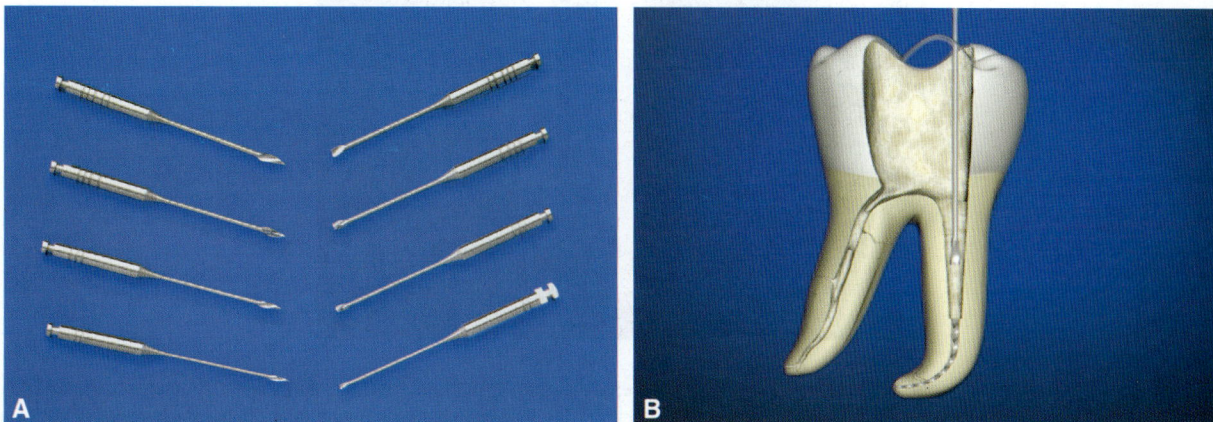

Figure 22 ***A***, Selected Gates Glidden drills (left) and their subsequent modification (right). ***B***, Graphic representation of a staging platform.

instrument fragment and affords an unobstructed line of sight into the canal. The tip of this ultrasonic instrument is placed in direct contact with the obstruction and is activated within the lower power settings (Figure 23A). One should choose the lowest power setting that will efficiently and safely accomplish the clinical task. All ultrasonic preparation below the orifice is conducted with a compressed air stream so visualization of the energized tip against the broken instrument is possible. To maintain vision, the dental assistant may utilize a Stropko three-way adapter with an appropriate luer lock tip to collimate and direct the continuous stream of air and water to remove dentinal dust. Microsonic techniques during removal of fractured instruments do not generate sufficient heat to become harmful to the attachment apparatus if they are used correctly and are cooled using water and air.

The selected ultrasonic instrument is moved lightly, in a CCW direction, removing dentin around the obstruction. An exception is made when removing a file that has a left-handed thread in which case the direction would be CW. This ultrasonic action trephines, precisely prepares dentin, and thus exposes the coronal millimeters of the obstruction (see Figure 23B). Often, during ultrasonic use, the obstruction begins to loosen, unwind, and then spin around its long axis. Gently wedging the energized tip between the tapered file and canal wall may cause the broken instrument to suddenly move in the coronal direction.

In the circumstance where a separated file tip is located further apically in a slender root morphology, ultrasonic procedures are then restricted to a smaller space. A longer length and smaller diameter, abrasively coated, ultrasonic instrument may be useful in promoting safe retrieval. In longer roots, or when space is even more restrictive, an appropriately sized titanium instrument may be chosen. Titanium instruments provide a less aggressive cutting action when trephining

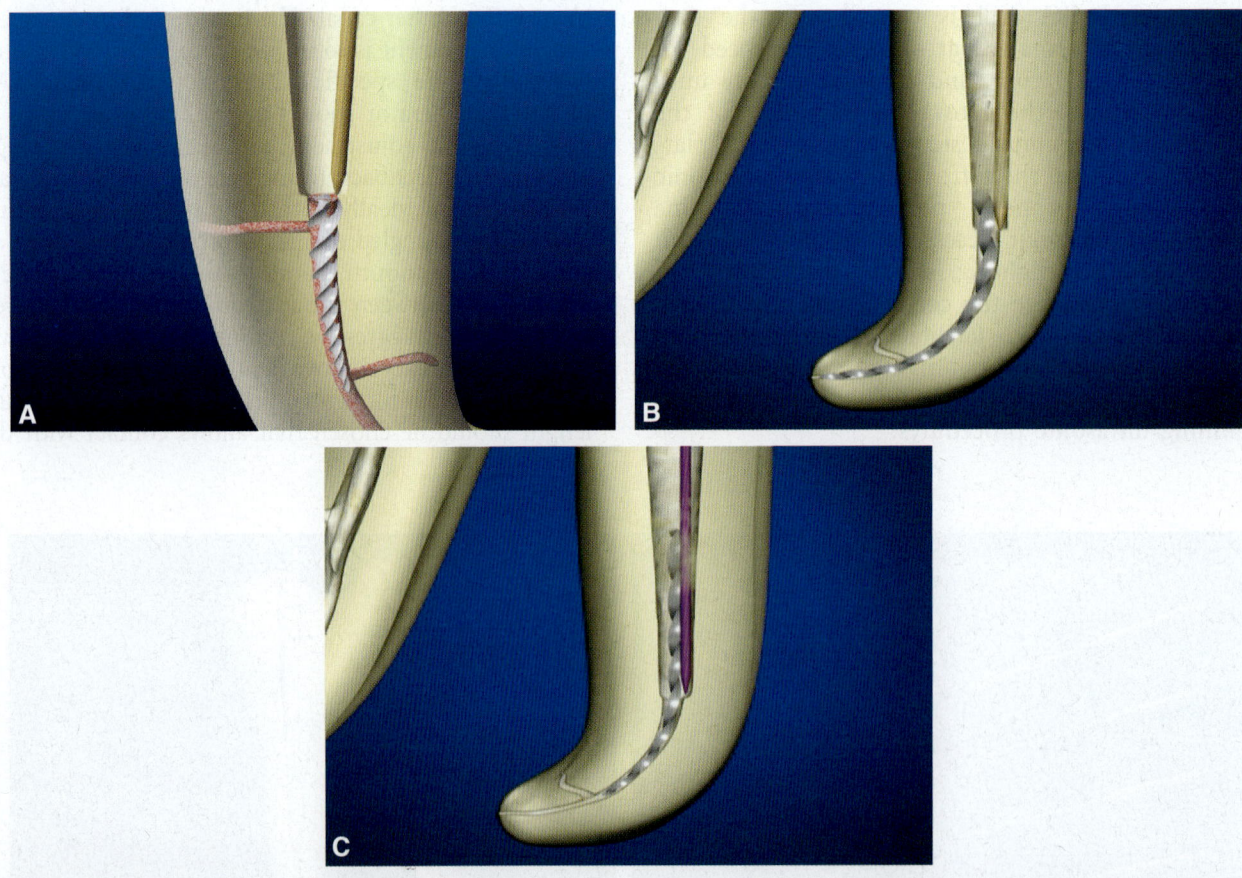

Figure 23 *A,* Illustration of the importance of coronal and radicular access, the staging platform, and the ultrasonic instrument just lateral to the fractured file. *B,* The ultrasonic instrument maintains contact with the fractured file, precisely removes dentin, and progressively exposes the coronal aspect of the fractured file. *C,* Longer length and smaller diameter titanium instrument is selected to conserve dentin and successfully displace the fractured instrument.

deeper within a canal (see Figure 23C). At times, weighing risk versus benefit, ultrasonic trephining procedures may have to be aborted. In these instances, manual use of the sharp cutting edges of a hypodermic needle may allow further exposure of the head of a file fragment.[235] Exposing 2 to 3 mm of the coronal most aspect of an obstruction, or about one-third of its overall length, will generally produce the desired result. On occasion, despite sufficient coronal and radicular access, exposure of the separated instrument and ultrasonic trephining procedures, it may be impossible to loosen and extract the instrument from the canal. Lack of vision or anatomical restrictions may render further efforts unsafe. In this instance, small hand files may be used with an aqueous or viscous chelator, to partially or completely bypass or remove an instrument fragment. Even when this tedious removal method is unsuccessful, space can be created along a portion of the overall length of a retained instrument. To maximize efficiency and success, the handle from a stainless steel hand file can be removed intentionally and the shaft of the instrument inserted into a special device, for example, a File Adapter. The File Adapter attaches to the ultrasonic handpiece and its chuck will retain a 0.02 tapered hand file. Small, stainless steel hand files can be precurved, and if indicated, inserted into available space, and used at low power in an ultrasonic effort to remove a broken instrument. This technique may be useful when the root is thin or a portion of the file lies apical to a canal curvature.[236] Another clinical challenge is encountered when trying to remove a broken NiTi file that lies partially around a canal curvature. In these situations, the mechanical reality is that the head of a broken NiTi file will always lie against the outer wall even after optimal ultrasonic trephining procedures. Even when loose, the angle formed between the coronally flared canal and the head of the broken instrument oftentimes precludes its removal. This situation is best managed using a microtube removal method (Figure 24).[148,225]

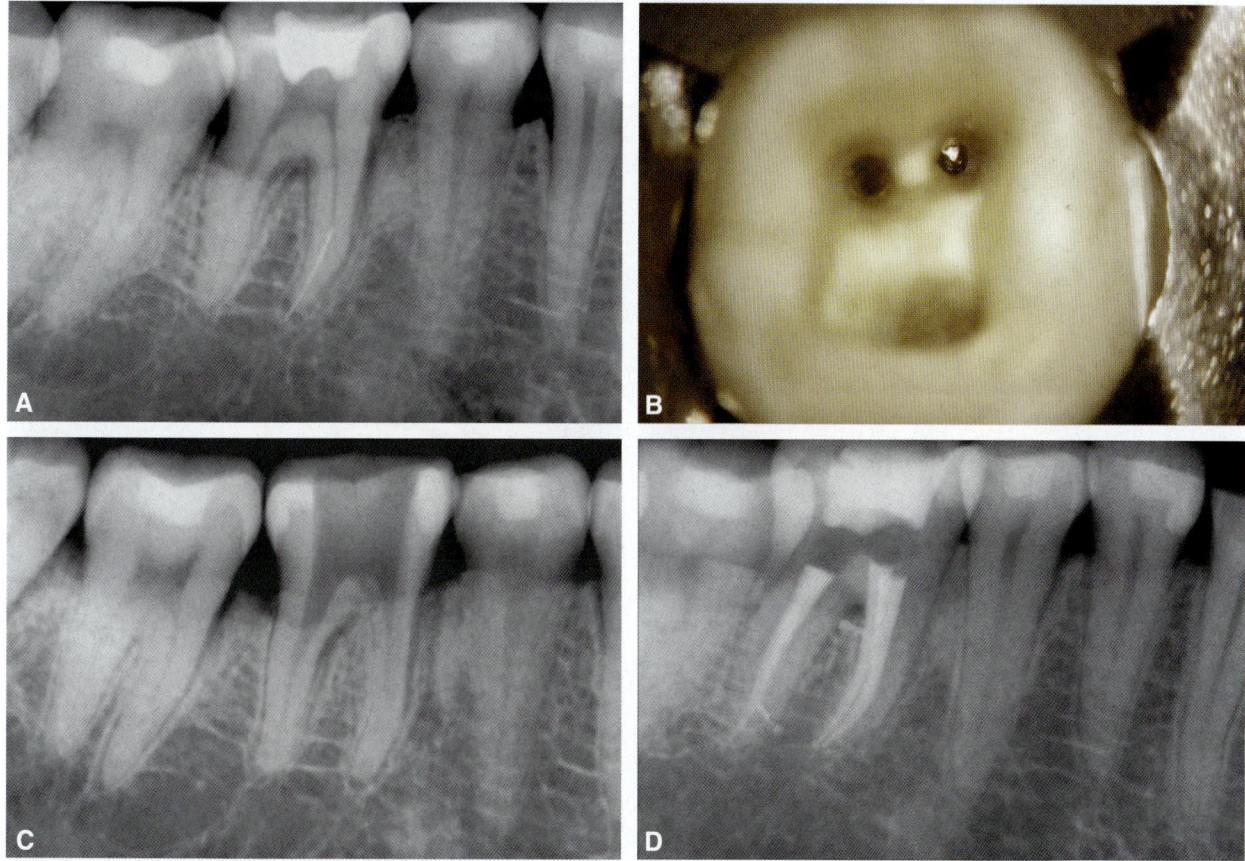

Figure 24 ***A***, Preoperative radiograph of a mandibular left first molar with a fractured instrument in the apical one-third of the mesial root. ***B***, After refining access and completing ultrasonic procedures, photograph shows the head of the fractured NiTi file leaning against the outer canal wall. ***C***, Radiograph confirms straight-line access and removal of the separated file. ***D***, Post-treatment radiograph demonstrates a furcal canal and that the distal system bifurcates apically.

REMOVAL OF FRACTURED INSTRUMENTS USING A MICROTUBE SYSTEM

As previously mentioned in the section concerning "Silver Point Removal," there are several microtube removal methods designed to mechanically engage an intracanal obstruction. The iRS provides a conservative advantage in the retrieval of broken instruments lodged deep within the root canal space. The iRS is composed of variously sized microtubes and insert wedges that are scaled to fit and work deep within the root canal space (see Figure 15A). The iRS is indicated when ultrasonic efforts prove to be unsuccessful and may be used to remove broken instruments that are lodged in straight portions of the root or partially inside a canal curvature. The black instrument has an outside diameter of 1.00 mm and is designed to work in the coronal one-third of larger canals, whereas the red and yellow instruments have outside diameters of 0.80 and 0.60 mm, respectively, and may be placed deeper into more narrow canals. Each complete instrument is comprised of a color coordinated microtube and screw wedge (see Figure 15B). Each microtube has a small-sized plastic handle to enhance vision during placement, a side window to improve mechanics, and a 45° beveled end to "scoop up" the coronal end of a broken instrument. Each screw wedge has a knurled metal handle, a left-handed screw mechanism proximally, and a solid cylinder that transitions into 0.02 tapered K-type file blades toward its distal end to facilitate engaging an obstruction.

As has been emphasized for any removal technique, straight-line coronal and radicular access is required to expose and subsequently visualize the coronal most end of the broken instrument. However, ultrasonic instruments can only circumferentially trephine dentin and expose the portion of the obstruction that lies in the straight portion of a canal. Therefore, in order to create the potential for instrument retrieval, the goal is to expose 2 to 3 mm, or about one-third of the total length, of a separated instrument (Figure 25A).

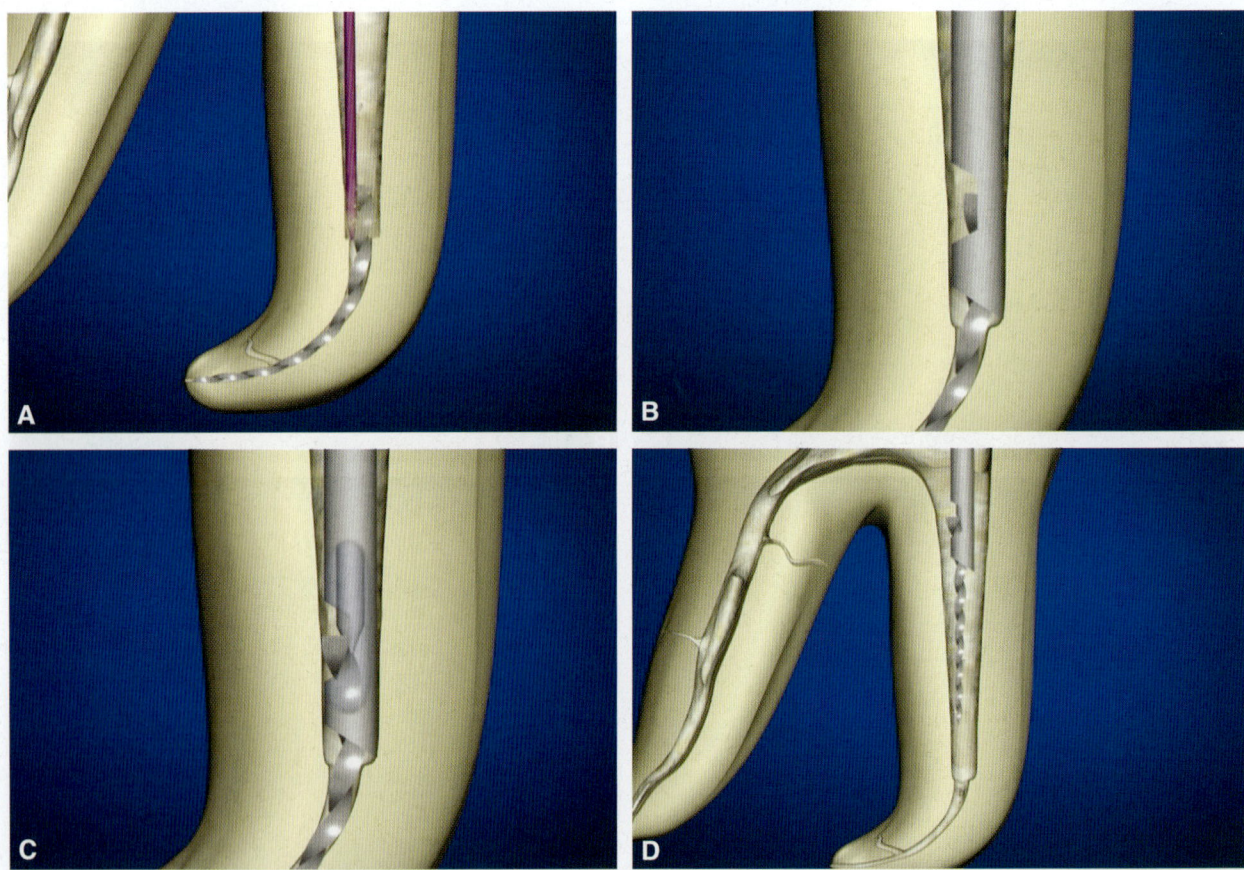

Figure 25 *A*, Graphic representation demonstrates a titanium ProUltra ENDO-6 tip trephining deep around the coronal aspect of the fractured file. *B*, When ultrasonic procedures prove ineffective, the beveled end of an Instrument Removal System (iRS) microtube is designed to "scoop up" the head of a fractured file. *C*, Illustration shows the introduction of the screw wedge which is rotated counterclockwise to engage and potentially displace the head of the file out the side window. *D*, The iRS can strongly grip, unwind, and remove a fractured instrument.

An iRS microtube is selected that can passively move through the pre-enlarged canal and over the exposed broken instrument. As previously mentioned, in a curved canal, the head of a fractured file will usually lay against the outer dentin wall. In these instances, the microtube is inserted into the canal with the long part of its beveled end oriented to the outer wall of the canal to scoop up the head of the broken instrument and guide it into the microtube (see Figure 25B). Once the microtube has been positioned, the same color-coded screw wedge is inserted through the microtube's length until it contacts the obstruction. The obstruction is engaged by gently turning the screw wedge handle CCW. A few degrees of rotation will serve to tighten, wedge, and, oftentimes, displace the head of the obstruction through the microtube window (see Figure 25C). Several color-coded screw wedges may be tried to improve engagement and successful removal. When engaged, the obstruction can be potentially unwound and removed by rotating the microtube and screw wedge assembly CCW (see Figure 25D). The removal direction of rotation, in the instance of a broken file, is generally CCW, but ultimately should be appropriate to the thread design of the obstruction. If difficulty is encountered when rotating the microtube and screw wedge assembly CCW, then proceed with a limited CW rotation of 3° to 5° that will promote continued engagement, followed by turning the assembly CCW as feasible. This repeated reciprocating handle motion will serve to loosen and facilitate the removal process. Placing an activated ultrasonic instrument on the engaged assembly is another adjunct that will possibly facilitate removal. If a microtube cannot be placed over a broken instrument such that the head of the obstruction lies within the side window, then, in these instances, the microtube's beveled end may be reduced or eliminated to achieve better mechanics. A clinical case utilizing the iRS option is shown in Figure 26.

The best way to avoid a fractured file is prevention. Adhering to proven concepts and utilizing safe techniques during root canal preparation procedures will eliminate most instrument fractures.[148,227] Prevention may also be facilitated by using negotiating and shaping instruments as single-use items. Simply discarding all instruments after the completion of each endodontic case will reduce fractures, lost clinical time, and stress for clinician and patient. However, on occasion, an instrument may break and the treating dentist must decide on the best treatment strategy.[155] Weighing risk versus benefit, certain broken file segments may not be retrievable. In these cases, and in the presence of clinical symptoms and/or radiographic pathosis, surgery or extraction may be the best treatment option.

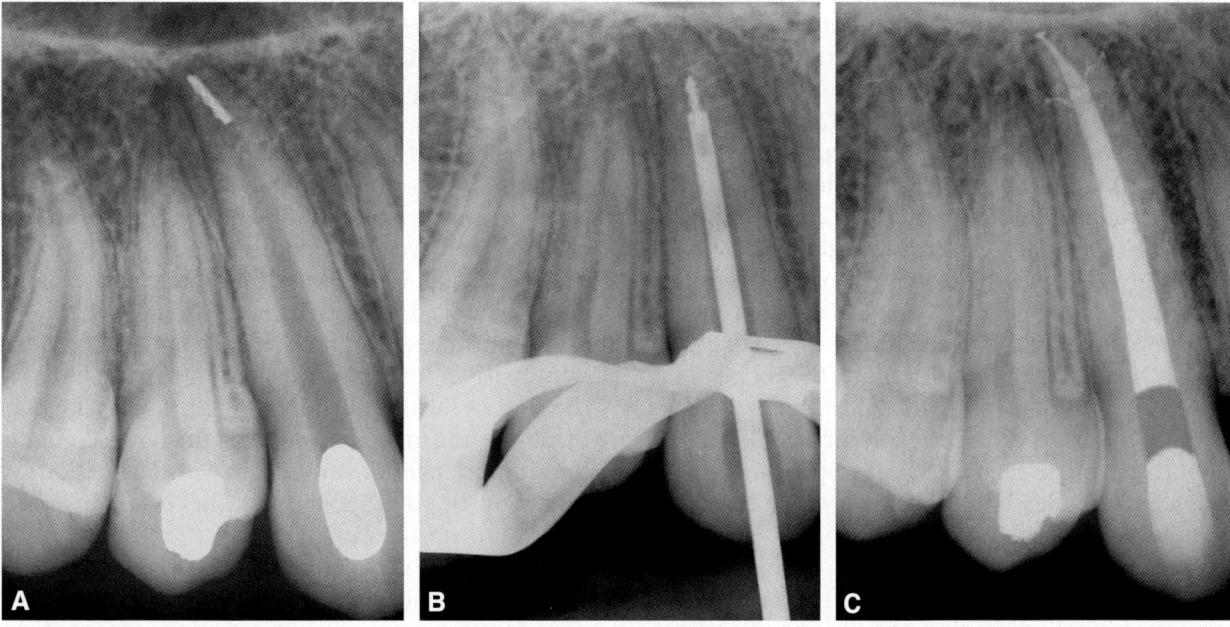

Figure 26 *A,* Preoperative radiograph of a maxillary cuspid with an instrument fractured deep into the apical one-third of the canal. *B,* Working radiograph shows that the 21-gauge Instrument Removal System has successfully engaged and partially elevated the deeply positioned file segment. *C,* Postoperative radiograph.

Blocks, Ledges, and Apical Transportations

It is important to understand the biological and mechanical objectives for shaping canals and cleaning root canal systems.[227,237] Failure to adhere to these objectives predisposes to needless complications such as blocks, ledges, apical transportations, and, potentially, perforations. Regrettably, these events are clinically encountered. Perhaps, the most overlooked and unstated method to negotiate a blocked canal, bypass the ledge, or manage transportation is determination, perseverance, and patience.

TECHNIQUES FOR MANAGING BLOCKED CANALS

When encountering a blocked canal, the canal should not be dry but irrigated with NaOCl as a lubricant. Well-angulated radiographs are necessary to determine the root curvature and apical pathosis. The clinician should appreciate that disease flow in a root canal system occurs in a coronal to apical direction. Consequently, lesions of endodontic origin form adjacent to portals of exit from the canal system onto the root surface. As such, and if applicable, files are directed toward apical lesions.

Generally, when managing blocked and/or ledged canals, the shortest file to reach working length should be chosen. Shorter instruments provide more stiffness and move the clinician's fingers closer to the tip of the instrument, resulting in greater tactile control. Appreciate that canals are frequently more curved than the roots that hold them. An ISO (0.02) size 10 file is precurved to simulate the expected curvature of the canal, and a marked rubber stop is oriented to match the file curvature. An attempt is then made to gently slide the file to length. If unsuccessful, the canal should be pre-enlarged above the stopping point to facilitate moving it to length. If an obstruction is encountered, the precurved file is used in an apically directed, gentle pecking action. During this procedure, the rubber stop should be continuously re-oriented which will re-direct the apical aspect of the precurved file in the attempt to negotiate the remainder of the canal.

A small-sized file should be used with very short amplitude, light pecking strokes in efforts to negotiate the canal terminus. Short amplitudes of this motion ensure safety, carry irrigant deeper, and increase the possibility of canal negotiation of a file's handle whose tip is engaged, should never be excessively rotated. The torsional loads over length will predispose the instrument to separation. If the apical extent of the file "sticks" or engages, then the handle motion should be a minimal back and forth reciprocating movement. If a #10 file begins to move apically, it may be useful to move to a smaller instrument whose tip diameter is 0.08 or 0.06 mm. A working radiograph or frequently removing the file helps to verify if its curve is following the expected root canal morphology. Depending on the severity of the blockage, these efforts may allow the clinician to passively reach the foramen and establish patency.

If no progress is made after diligent efforts over a time frame of approximately 2 to 3 minutes, then the NaOCl is removed from the root canal system and replaced with a viscous chelator, such as RC Prep, Glyde, or ProLube. The same techniques as described above are then used, recognizing that it takes a few minutes for the chelator to penetrate deep into the canal and soften superficial dentin. If a #10 file does not negotiate through the debris, then a smaller instrument such as a #08 file may be appropriate.

When the instrument reaches working length, its tip is gently moved to and minutely through the foramen. Pushing the instrument to length carries more chelator deeper into the canal, keeps debris into suspension, and lubricates the file so it will more readily reach the desired length. The clinician should continue with short amplitude push/pull strokes and move the file gently and subtly over a range of 1 to 2 mm. When the instrument moves freely, slightly longer 2 to 3mm amplitude strokes are taken. Finally, strokes of 3 to 4 mm are used until the file can be moved to the terminus with ease and predictability. These steps require time and patience.

Occasionally, clinical situations arise where the aforementioned techniques have been carefully attempted, but either the file is not progressing apically or is not maintaining the true pathway of the canal. Corrective steps require a thoughtful treatment decision. If the tooth is asymptomatic and symptoms are not masked by a pharmaceutical, and if the periodontium is healthy and there are no lesions of endodontic origin, then the preparation may be finished to the level of the obstruction and obturated. The patient must be informed of this less than ideal outcome, the importance of monitoring the situation with follow-up appointments, and the possible need for future surgery.

If a blocked canal is not negotiable and if clinical symptoms, periodontal breakdown, and/or a lesion of endodontic origin are present, then the root canal system should be treated and obturated as efficiently as possible, for at times postoperative radiographs may demonstrate that the hydraulics of a thermoplastic obturation has moved material into untreated areas of the root canal. The patient needs to be advised of the importance of follow-up visits and that future treatment options may include surgery, replantation, or extraction.

TECHNIQUES FOR MANAGING CANAL LEDGES

An internal transportation of the canal is termed a "ledge" and is a result of over-enlarging a curved canal and working short of full canal length. Many ledges may successfully be bypassed using the techniques described for blocks.[148] Once the tip of an instrument is apical to a ledge, it is moved in vertical amplitude utilizing very short push-pull movements while remaining apical to the defect. When the file moves freely, slightly longer push-pull strokes are used to reduce the ledge and confirm the presence or absence of any residual internal canal irregularities. Once the file reaches working length easily, it is turned CW upon withdrawal in an effort to rasp, reduce, smooth, or eliminate the ledge, which is typically on the outer wall of a canal curvature. During these correcting procedures, the file should be kept coronal to the full working length in order to prevent enlargement of the apical foramen. Once a ledge can be predictably bypassed, then efforts are directed toward establishing patency with a #10 file. Gently passing a 0.02 tapered #10 file 1 mm through the foramen increases its diameter to 0.12 mm and paves the way for the #15 file.

Root canal enlargement after ledge management may be accomplished by using nickel-titanium hand files, for example, ProTaper (Dentsply International). The major advantage of using NiTi files with larger taper to remove a ledge is their tapers are three to six times larger than conventional 0.02 tapered files, and thus, their ability to shape the canal more efficiently. Once a precurved NiTi hand file has been inserted into the canal and its precurved tip has successfully bypassed the ledge, then its larger taper oftentimes eliminates or reduces the extent of the ledge while using a minimum number of files.

NiTi files should not be introduced into the canal until the ledge has been bypassed, the canal negotiated, and patency established. Bypassing the ledge and preparing the canal up to a size 15, and if necessary a 20 K-file, creates a glide path that allows the tip of the NiTi instrument to passively reach the desired length. To move the apical extent of a NiTi file past a ledge, the instrument must be precurved, preferably with Bird Beak Pliers (Hu-Friedy). To successfully pre-curve a NiTi instrument, the working end of the NiTi file is securely grasped between the jaws of the pliers and the handle is pulled through a radius of between 180 and 270°. Nickel titanium has shape memory, and efforts to bend it must be exaggerated so that when the instrument is released from the pliers, it will have the desired curvature in its apical extent. A rubber stop on a manual NiTi instrument is oriented in a way that allows control of the file's precurved working end to bypass and move apical to the ledge. Following the use of NiTi hand files, the 10 file is used to verify ledge reduction or elimination. The canal then needs to be further enlarged to its final size and taper.[234]

In difficult cases and based on preoperative radiographs, a clinician occasionally must make a decision whether to continue shaping procedures in hopes of eliminating the ledge or to abort if continued efforts will weaken or perforate the root. Not all ledges can or should be removed. Clinicians must weigh risk versus benefit and make every effort to maximize remaining dentin.[227,237]

In cases where a ledge cannot be removed, fitting the master gutta-percha cone may be difficult. In these cases, a master cone is cut back from the tip so that its narrowest diameter equals the D_0 diameter of the file that fit tightly at length. The cone can then be precurved to simulate the curvature of the canal and its tip placed in a dappen dish of 70% isopropyl alcohol. The master cone is removed after a few seconds and the clinician will notice a significant increase in its rigidity. An orientation mark can be placed on the end of the master cone to identify working length and the direction of the cone's curvature. This technique greatly facilitates the placement of the master cone during obturation.

TECHNIQUES FOR MANAGING APICAL TRANSPORTATIONS

Moving the position of the canal's physiologic terminus to a new iatrogenic location on the external root surface equates to a transportation of the foramen.[153] Apical zipping or tearing is caused by using progressively larger and stiffer files to working length.[153,238] If apical transportation has occurred, then the canal exhibits a so-called elbow preparation with a reversed apical shape. This shape fails to provide a resistance form to condense gutta-percha. This leads to poorly packed cases that are vertically overextended but at the same time internally underfilled.[145,152] In general, apical transportations can be categorized into three types, each differing in the specific treatment strategy.

Type I Transportation

A Type I transportation represents a minor movement of the position of the physiologic foramen, resulting in its iatrogenic relocation. In this instance, the clinician must select the right technique trying to create positive apical canal architecture. Generating the correct shape coronal to the foramen will require additional removal of dentin and could predispose to root weakening or to a lateral strip perforation. If sufficient residual dentin can be maintained and the preparation above the foramen can be corrected, then some of these initially transported cases may be thoroughly cleaned, shaped, and filled.[148] Regretfully, many canals whose foramina have been significantly transported are not amenable to a Type I-related treatment approach and will require additional steps.

Type II Transportation

A Type II transportation represents a moderate movement of the physiologic position of the foramen, resulting in a considerable iatrogenic relocation on the external root surface. Apical zipping or tearing is more pronounced than in a Type I transportation. In these cases, a larger communication with the periapical space exists, and attempting to create additional coronal shape would risk weakening and/or perforating the root. In treating these canals, a barrier is selected to control bleeding and provide a matrix to condense against during subsequent obturation procedures.[148]

The barrier of choice for a Type II transportation is MTA (ProRoot, Dentsply International) (Figure 27A).[239–241] MTA is a biocompatible material for managing radicular repairs and can be used in canals which exhibit apical transportation as well as in immature roots and in Type II transportations. Additionally, MTA is used for non-surgical and surgical perforation repairs or as a surgical root end-filling material. Remarkably, cementum grows adjacent and onto this non-absorbable and radiopaque material, thus allowing for a normal periodontal attachment apparatus.[239] Although a dry field facilitates visual control, MTA is apparently not compromised by slight moisture and typically sets hard within 4 to 6 hours with slight expansion, creating a marginal adaptation as good as or better than the best materials used today.[34,239,240] A more comprehensive discussion of MTA will occur in the section "Perforation and Prognosis for Healing."

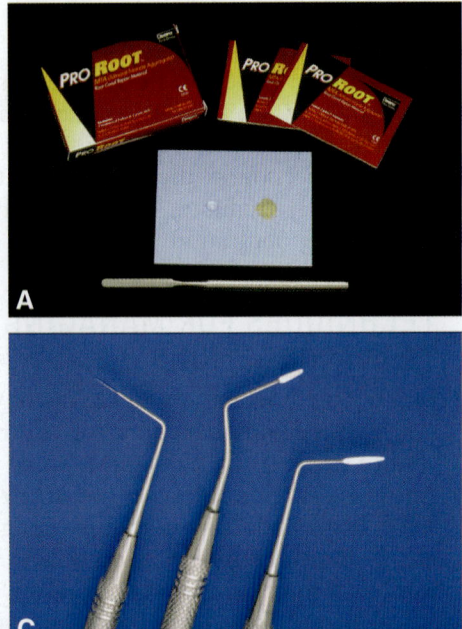
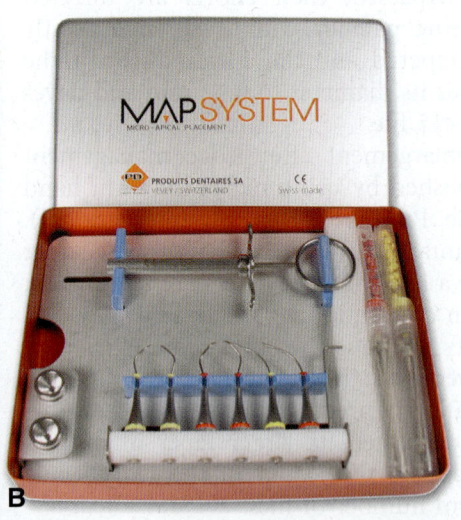

Figure 27 ***A***, ProRoot, or mineral trioxide aggregate (MTA), is packaged in a powder form and then mixed with sterile water to a heavy "cake-like" consistency. Photo shows gray MTA; white MTA is also available. ***B***, The MAP System (Micro-apical placement, Produits Dentaires SA, Vevey, Switzerland) offers one of many options to place MTA at the apex or within the canal space. ***C***, The West Perf Repair Instruments provide thin, flexible trowels angled at different orientations.

MTA powder is mixed with anesthetic solution, or sterile water, to a heavy viscous consistency. Fiberless 2 × 2 gauze may be used to absorb surplus moisture and achieve the ideal viscosity. A small aliquot of the MTA is introduced into the prepared canal with a microtube carrying device or on the side of a West Perf Repair Instrument (SybronEndo) (see Figure 27B,C). MTA is then gently tamped down the canal to approximate length using a customized non-standard gutta-percha cone as a flexible plugger. The gutta-percha cone should be trimmed apically to have sufficient diameter to effectively condense MTA. In straighter canals, MTA can be vibrated and moved into the defect and to length with an ultrasonic tip. The instrument chosen should be selected according to the length and diameter of the canal, inserted into the MTA mixture, and activated at the lowest energy. Direct ultrasonic energy will vibrate and generate a wave-like motion which facilitates moving and adapting the cement into the apical extent of the canal. Prior to initiating subsequent procedures, a dense 4- to 5-mm zone of MTA in the apical one-third of the canal should be confirmed radiographically.

In case the defect is located apical to a canal curvature, a 4- to 5-mm column of MTA is first pushed apically beyond the curvature with a flexible gutta-percha plugger. A precurved #15 or #20 stainless steel file is then inserted past the canal curvature, into the MTA and to within 1 to 2 mm of the working length. Indirect ultrasonics with an ultrasonic tip is then used on the shaft of the file. This vibratory energy will cause MTA to liquefy, move, and adapt to the configurations of the canal laterally as well as control its movement toward periapical tissues. Again, a dense 4- to 5-mm fill zone of MTA in the apical extent of the canal should be confirmed radiographically.

MTA sets when it comes into contact with moisture. Fluids present in periapical tissues external to the canal will provide sufficient moisture for the apical aspect of the positioned MTA to set. In addition, a pre-sized cotton pellet moistened with water must be placed against the coronal most aspect of the MTA within the canal. The tooth is then temporized and the patient dismissed. At a subsequent appointment, the temporary filling is taken out and the wet cotton pellet removed. The MTA cement is probed with a sharp explorer to determine its hardness. Typically, the material has set hard and the clinician can then obturate against this barrier. If the material is soft, it should be removed, the area irrigated, dried, and a new mix of MTA placed. Upon subsequent re-entry, a hard barrier should exist which will provide a matrix against which to condense the root canal filling. The clinical steps for managing a Type II transportation are illustrated in Figure 28.

Type III Transportation

A Type III transportation represents a severe movement of the physiologic position of the canal, resulting in a significant iatrogenic relocation of the physiologic foramen. In this situation, a barrier technique is usually not feasible and hence, thermoplastic obturation is impossible. If a tooth with a Type III transportation is to be retained, it requires obturation as best as possible followed by corrective surgery. Severe foramina transportations that cannot be treated surgically result in tooth removal as the only alternative.

Perforation and Prognosis for Healing

Because endodontic therapy can often be complex and challenging, some procedures carry an inherent risk for complications or procedural accidents. The access opening to initiate therapy and the shaping and debridement steps are unquestionably those types of procedures.

An endodontic perforation is an artificial opening in the tooth or its root, created by the clinician during entry to the canal system or by a biologic event such as pathologic resorption or caries that results in a communication between the root canal and the periodontal tissues.[242] A furcation perforation refers to a mid-curvature opening into the periodontal ligament space and is a worst possible outcome in root canal treatment.[243] A post space perforation is defined as a communication between the lateral root surface and the surrounding periodontal structures due to misdirection or an excessively large post enlargement.[244] Except for resorptive defects or caries, furcation or root perforations are iatrogenic in nature and are a key cause of endodontic failure. It has been reported that root perforations were the second greatest cause of failure accounting for 9.62% of all unsuccessful cases.[245] Seltzer et al.[246] also attributed 3.52% of all endodontic failures to perforation. However, these perforations were often created without the knowledge of the clinician.

TIMING OF PERFORATION REPAIR

The main complication arising from perforation is the potential for secondary inflammation of the periodontal attachment with eventual infection and ultimately tooth loss if untreatable.[28,242,246–251] When aseptic perforations were induced in dog canine teeth, attachment reactions were observed with granulation tissue formation, resulting in epithelialized polyps at the gingival margin.[252] In 1925, Euler[252] demonstrated that infected perforations would lead to marked

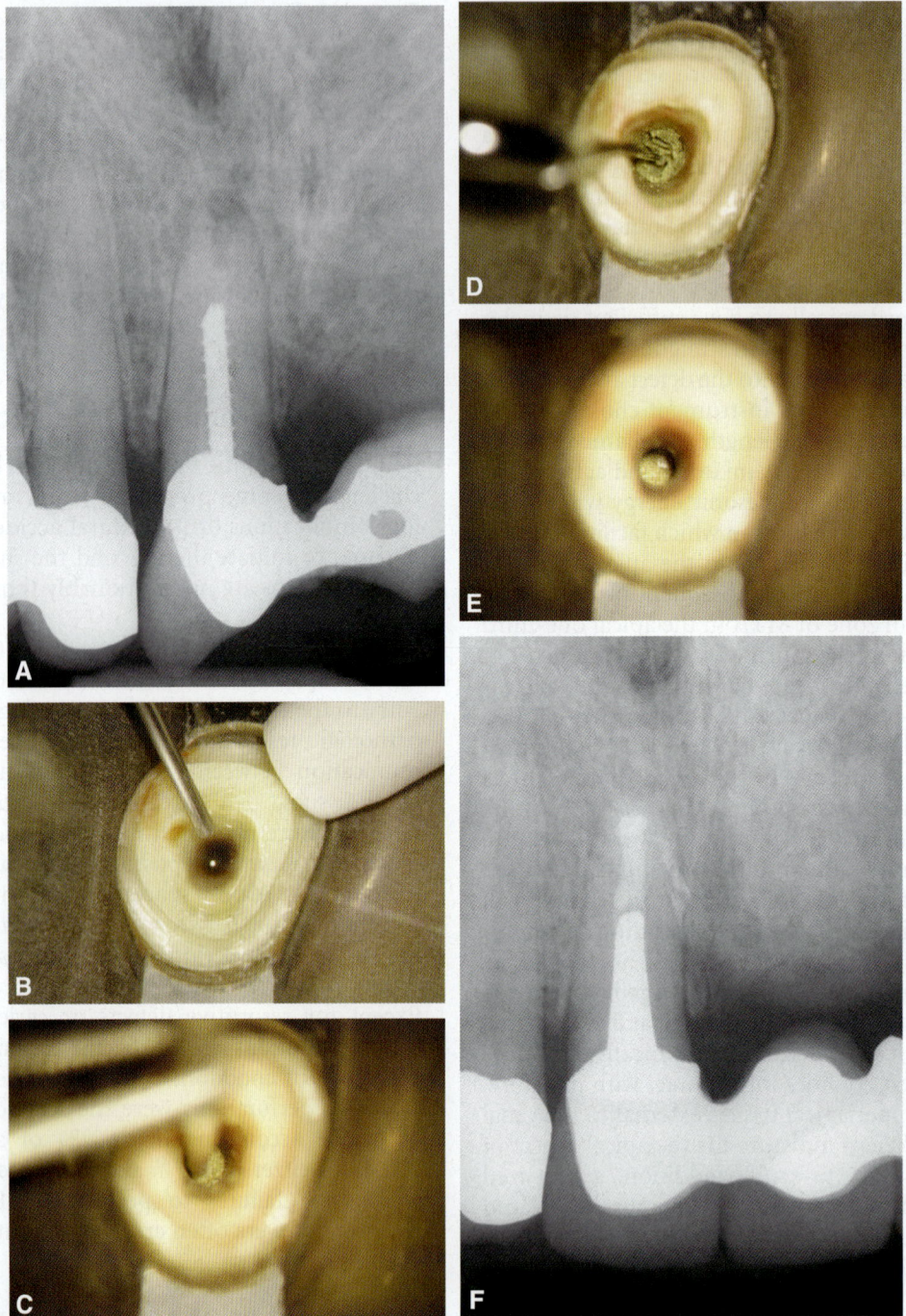

Figure 28 ***A,*** Preoperative radiograph of a maxillary right central incisor bridge abutment with a post and an apparently empty apical root canal system. It appears that the apical opening has been transported. ***B,*** Photograph (×8 original magnification) confirms post removal. The apical foramen is visible following cleaning and shaping procedures. ***C,*** Photograph shows tamping mineral trioxide aggregate (MTA) into the apical one-third with a gutta-percha cone used as a flexible plugger. ***D,*** Photograph shows the ProUltra ENDO-5 ultrasonic instrument vibrating MTA densely into the apical one-third of the canal. ***E,*** Photograph taken on a subsequent appointment shows set MTA. ***F,*** A 6-year recall radiograph demonstrates a new bridge, a post, non-surgical treatment, and osseous repair.

inflammation, poor organization of fibrous connective tissue, and abscess formation with subsequent proliferation of the crevicular epithelium. Similar results were observed when periodontal tissue reactions were investigated after aseptic and septic perforations in humans and dogs. In later stages, some repair and regeneration of the bone occurred in aseptic perforation sites whereas the infected perforations resulted only in abscess formation.[253] Similarly, aseptically induced perforations that were left open to the oral cavity would result in progressive destruction of the periodontal tissues.[250]

In consideration of the declining nature of an open perforation defect, repair of the unintended communication between the root canal system and periodontal attachment was strongly advocated.[254] Endodontic perforations in humans were examined by Kauffman[255] in 1944. Results showed formation of granulation tissue in most cases; yet on occasion, there was a closure of the defect with cementum. Favorable healing of the periodontal tissues occurred when the defects were closed as compared to those left open.[250] This also corroborated others findings, demonstrating that sealed perforations result in less inflammation than unsealed ones, even when those perforations were not immediately repaired.[256]

Therefore, the time lapsed between seal of the perforation and its inception plays an important role in determining the prognosis of periodontal repair. The timing of repair was categorized into immediate or delayed. The literature strongly advocates immediately closing the communication between the periodontal tissues and the root canal system to promote a superior healing potential.[241,246,248,257–261] Benenati et al.[262] evaluated perforation defects in dogs created under aseptic conditions and repaired either immediately or after 1 to 230 days postoperatively. Their results demonstrated favorable healing in response to immediate repair of the perforation. However, even in the delayed repair, a favorable prognosis was possible in aseptic perforations.

LOCATION OF PERFORATION

In addition to time intervals prior to repair, another criterion that strongly influences the prognosis of the perforated tooth is the location of the defect. Periodontal status is therefore a major contributing factor that determines the success or failure of perforation repair. Once perforations exhibit the formation of osseous defects, the prognosis is compromised significantly.[249,263] A study evaluating human root perforations indicated decreased success in cases where furcation perforations occurred. In those cases, epithelial proliferation and periodontitis increased, markedly influencing the prognosis of the tooth.[264] Many studies have identified that the position of the defect, with respect to the marginal gingival or junctional epithelium, is a definite determinant in the healing potential. Any perforation located near the gingival sulcus promoted inflammation and loss of epithelial attachment, resulting in periodontal pocket formation.[241,242,246,265,266] This was further corroborated by the fact that a perforation located away from the gingival sulcus in an otherwise healthy periodontium usually offers a fair prognosis.[267] Accordingly, perforations encountered clinically, well within the bony structures, were much more predictable following repair, than those in close proximity to the crestal bone.[248] Similarly observed were apical and midroot perforations without communication to the oral cavity. These had a good prognosis provided an immediate seal was obtained.[250] In a clinical assessment of perforation in humans, only 4 out of 48 perforations failed due to epithelial migration and communication with the oral cavity.[251]

Perforations can be categorized by location: subgingival, midroot, or apical.

Subgingival perforations occur most often during the access cavity preparation and the search for canal orifices. Careful attention should be paid to the three-dimensional spatial orientation of the tooth to be accessed. Three clear preoperative radiographs, two periapical views and one bitewing, should be taken to aid in proper access. Accurate film images reveal a wealth of pre-access information, such as the degree of cervical constriction, coronal asymmetry, disparities between the long axis of the root and the crown, and the presence of extra roots, canals, or both. A bitewing radiograph provides even more accurate information about the vertical dimension of the pulp chamber than a periapical projection.[268] With the advent of three-dimensional cone beam imaging and a surgical operating microscope, more accurate information is available to evaluate any tooth in all three spatial dimensions. Valuable clinical information can also be obtained before access. Palpation and periodontal probing of the root surfaces provides localization of the long axis of the root. This is most helpful when accessing through prosthetic crowns and in the presence of malposition of the teeth. Also, probing the cervical areas to provide the width and circumference of the furcation areas tells the clinician where the narrowest areas of invaginated tooth structure exist.

Midroot perforations occur mainly during post space preparation as well as during aggressive cleaning and shaping the midroot area of the canal. Careful preparation of the post space must follow the long axis of the root. Safe removal of coronal gutta-percha with heat and hand instruments provides a pilot track that keeps post drills centered in the canal.[250] This reduces their aggressive cutting nature and prevents the instruments from making their own canal. Post size selection is also an important factor. The post size should be no larger than one-third the mesial distal width of the tooth and should follow the canal anatomy.[269]

Apical perforation usually occurs during instrumentation, as a result of using large inflexible files in curved canals and by violating the apical constricture.[249,268] These perforations are often managed with the obturation material or by surgical correction.

SIZE OF PERFORATION

After duration and location, another criterion impacting the successful repair of perforations is the size of the defect. Small perforations of the canal space promote a direct and immediate restoration of the defect.[270] This offers fewer chances for periodontal breakdown and epithelial proliferation within the perforation site. Investigators have demonstrated that perforation size has a clinical significance for the success of perforation repairs.[249] A clinical report evaluated 55 root perforations and found that 12 of those cases were too large to repair and had to be extracted.[28] The smaller defect was also less likely to result in an overfill of repair material.[267] Conversely, the larger the perforation the more difficult to place a well-condensed properly shaped, uncontaminated seal.[271] In addition, prognosis is uncertain due to the large contact surface area of the restorative material with the periodontium that can allow inflammatory irritants to continuously diffuse into the surrounding vital tissues. Marginal adaptation also decreases with increased defect circumference.[272]

PERFORATION REPAIR MATERIALS

A final influencing criterion and one receiving the most investigative scrutiny in recent years is the material used to restore a perforation defect.[249,272,273] If the clinician's only criterion is adequate sealing of the perforation margins alone, a fair to poor prognosis for the repair will be the result.[271-273] The ideal repair material for furcation and root perforations should be antimicrobial, non-toxic, capable of providing an adequate seal, non-absorbable, radio-opaque, non-carcinogenic, and promote osteogenesis and cementogenesis. It should also be easily attainable and relatively inexpensive. Additionally, it should be stable during the repair process to allow new bone to repair against it and act as a matrix, against which, root canal obturating or restorative materials can be condensed.[249,267]

Many different restorative materials have been developed and used for non-surgical and surgical repair of iatrogenic perforation defects. Chloroform-rosin and gutta-percha cones with phosphate cement were first introduced in 1967.[250] ZOE cements were also used to repair perforations. This, however, always resulted in a chronic inflammatory response indicating a continuous destructive process.[246] Calcium hydroxide was introduced into the perforation defect in the hope of a positive attachment response and a possible hard tissue barrier to form. The root canal obturating materials could then be placed into the canals.[248,258] Calcium hydroxide was further investigated and reported to form a physical barrier to prevent overfilling of obturation materials into the defect and periodontal ligament space.[259] Beavers et al.[251] showed calcium hydroxide prevented in-growth of granulation tissue into the perforation defect. Root perforations repaired with calcium hydroxide were also compared with ZOE. These data demonstrated necrosis of the periodontal tissues adjacent to the perforation repair with calcium hydroxide. ZOE produced inflammatory reactions with abscess formation and resorption of the alveolar crest.[266] In a clinical and radiographic study, Cavit was investigated as a restorative material for endodontic perforations. In one study, there was a favorable response in approximately 89% of cases.[274] However, when Cavit was used in restoration of furcal perforations in dogs, a mild to moderate inflammatory response was seen histologically.[242] ElDeeb et al.[273] compared Cavit, calcium hydroxide, and amalgam as furcal repair materials. The conclusions followed that amalgam was the material of choice when assessing healing potential. Amalgam was also found to be superior to gutta-percha when reevaluating iatrogenic root perforations.[262,275]

Super EBA was introduced in 1985 to restore endodontic perforations after first being used as a retrograde filling material.[276,277] This material, however, provided a poorer seal than amalgam in root perforations.[278] In other investigations, Super EBA adapted better to the perforation site than amalgam and did not expand.[279-281] Several investigators have shown that Super EBA had a success rate of 95% from a period of 6 months to 10 years when used as a retro filling material.[282,283]

Glass ionomer cements were introduced in 1990 to restore lateral root perforations.[284] The sealing potential of glass ionomers and amalgam had no statistically significant difference.[285-288] Glass ionomers provoked an inflammatory response that was less severe than gutta-percha.[289,290]

MTA FOR PERFORATION REPAIR

MTA was introduced in the 1990s and investigated for repair of furcal perforation defects.[241] The composition of MTA includes calcium and phosphorus ions with a pH of 10.2.[291] MTA was reported to be the least toxic repair material when compared with amalgam Super EBA and IRM[292] a fact corroborated by several studies of the new material. For the first time, this material had demonstrated a biologic compatibility, growth of a cementum-like substance on the surface of the material that was either calcified or in its immature matrix form.[33,293–303] It was also noted that over time, MTA provoked less inflammatory infiltrative cells than other materials. Further investigations evaluated its marginal adaptation to dentin demonstrating a better adaptation to surrounding dentin than amalgam, Super EBA, or IRM.[240,304,305] Moreover, MTA was shown to leak significantly less than amalgam in the repair of lateral root perforations in extracted molars.[73,306] Clinically, the material leaked significantly less than glass ionomers.[307,308] MTA is technique sensitive. The consistency of the material and delivery are difficult. However in the presence of blood contamination, MTA was reported to be superior to amalgam, Super EBA, and IRM in resisting leakage.[309] This is a desirable property for a material, as placement often occurs in contact with periradicular fluids.

MTA has been used for the past 8 to 10 years with promising success. MTA has been reported to be the material of choice for furcal and root perforations.[310] In in vivo studies with patient follow-up, MTA demonstrated normal tissue healing and no pathologic changes adjacent to perforated sites.[35,311] Further studies have identified MTA as an excellent material for repair and reconstitution of the supporting structures.[312,313]

However, as no currently available material meets all the requirements of an ideal restorative material, improvements continue to enhance the properties of MTA, for example, to be more radiopaque and seal better against fluid leakage as well as bacterial contamination, be less technique sensitive, but still maintain all the biologic qualities that the original material has shown. MTA is currently the material of choice for perforation repair.[303,314–317]

CLINICAL CONSIDERATIONS INFLUENCING PERFORATION REPAIR BASED ON EVIDENCE

When evaluating a perforated tooth, the four variables mentioned above must be considered individually and collectively to properly guide treatment and understand how each of these entities critically affects treatment selection and prognosis.[148] Microscopes, paper points, electronic apex locators, and a diagnostic radiopaque contrast solution (e.g., Hypaque, available through pharmaceutical companies) are useful in determining the level, location, and extent of a perforation and the potential for successful management.[148] The following four defining characteristics of a perforation always occur in combination, which synergistically complicates treatment outcomes.

- Level: Perforations may occur in the subgingival, middle, and apical one-thirds of roots. Furcal perforations have similar considerations as coronal one-third perforations. Perforations at this level threaten the sulcular attachment and pose different treatment challenges than more apically occurring perforations due to communication with oral flora.
- Location: Perforations may be on the buccal, lingual, mesial, or distal aspects of roots. The location of the perforation is less important when non-surgical treatment is selected, and more so if surgery is considered.
- Size: Perforation size greatly affects the clinician's ability to establish a biologic seal. The area of a circular perforation can be mathematically described as πr^2. Therefore, doubling the perforation size increases the surface area to seal four-fold. Many perforations are ovoid in shape due to the nature of occurrence and represent large surface areas to effectively seal.
- Time: Regardless of etiology, a perforation should be repaired as soon as possible to discourage further loss of attachment and prevent periodontal pocket formation. Chronic perforations exhibiting a loss of sulcular attachment pose treatment challenges that potentially require surgical correction and efforts directed toward guided tissue regeneration procedures.[159,318,319]

PERIODONTAL CONDITION AND PERFORATION REPAIR

Teeth that have been perforated must be thoroughly examined periodontally. The sulci of these teeth must be carefully probed.[320,321,322] If the attachment apparatus is intact, then timing is critical, and the treatment is ideally directed toward non-surgical repair of the defect. However, if there is periodontal disease with resultant loss of attachment, then interdisciplinary consultations, including orthodontics, periodontics, endodontics, and restorative, should guide treatment planning, sequencing, and prognosis. In these instances, a decision must be made between a non-surgical repair and surgical correction, recognizing that at times combined treatment may be required to retain the tooth. Importantly, extraction may be a wise decision in some cases and a fixed bridge or restored implant considered.

ESTHETICS AND PERFORATION REPAIR

Perforations in the anterior region can undeniably impact esthetics. Patients that exhibit a high lip line may be esthetically compromised by soft tissue defects such as clefts, recessions, or discrepancies in the inciso-gingival dimensions of a crown as compared to the adjacent teeth.[322–324] Tooth colored restorations are chosen in areas that demand esthetics.[162] In the past, certain traditional materials have contributed to tooth discoloration, soft tissue tattoos, and a compromise in esthetics.

VISION AND PERFORATION REPAIR

Magnification loupes, headlamps, and transilluminating devices along with the dental operating microscope and Oroscope facilitate vision and are important adjuncts in addressing perforations (see Chapter 25E). They may be used to more predictably repair perforation defects non-surgically, thus reducing the need for surgical intervention and its associated risks.[151]

TREATMENT SEQUENCE FOR PERFORATION REPAIR

When there is a perforation and the canal has not been fully prepared, the defect should be repaired prior to proceeding with definitive endodontic treatment. Repairing the perforation will allow control of bleeding into the canal, confine irrigation, and facilitate obturation. However, any given perforated canal should be optimally enlarged and prepared, when necessary, to improve access to the defect, enhance visualization, and to minimize post-repair instrumentation. When repairing a perforation, it is necessary to maintain the pathway to the canal because the barriers and restorative materials used could inadvertently block the canal. A gutta-percha segment or a collagen plug may be placed apical to the defect to prevent canal blockage during the perforation repair procedures. In failing endodontic cases exhibiting a perforation, the existing obturation material may be used to hold the position of the canal. This allows the clinician to first repair the perforation before proceeding with endodontic retreatment efforts. However, in this sequence of treatment, caution must then be exercised not to disrupt the perforation repair material during subsequent disassembly, canal preparation, and obturation procedures.

HEMOSTATICS FOR PERFORATION REPAIR

Many perforation defects exhibit considerable hemorrhage due to granulomatous tissue in situ upon re-entry. Clinicians need to be familiar with a few hemostatic agents and materials that can predictably arrest bleeding.[325] A dry field enhances vision while creating an environment for the predictable placement of a restorative agent. Calcium hydroxide, a well-regarded material, may be passively syringed into the canal, hydraulically moved to place, and allowed to remain in the canal/defect for 4 to 5 minutes or longer. The calcium hydroxide is then flushed from the field using NaOCl. Two or three applications of placing and then removing calcium hydroxide usually control the bleeding. When hemostasis cannot be obtained, calcium hydroxide can be advantageously left in the canal until a future appointment.[326] Other increasingly important materials that can be used to achieve hemostasis by various mechanisms include collagen, calcium sulfate, freeze-dried bone, and MTA.[318,319,325,311] Other hemostatics exist but they are not generally selected due to factors such as cost, ease of handling and placement, or their by-products. Ironically, some of the most effective hemostatics, like ferric sulfate, leave a coagulum behind which may promote bacterial growth, compromise the seal at the tooth-restorative interface, and jeopardize the prognosis.[327]

BARRIER MATERIALS FOR PERFORATION REPAIR

The two main challenges a clinician faces when attempting to repair a perforation are hemostasis and the controlled placement of a restorative material. Barriers help produce a "dry field" and also provide an internal matrix or "back stop" against which to condense restorative materials.[148]

In general, barriers may be divided into absorbable and non-absorbable; however, it is important to note that the restorative material used oftentimes dictates the barrier that is selected.

Absorbable Barriers

Hemorrhage into the tooth must be arrested in order to successfully manage perforations. Hemostasis may be accomplished by introducing an absorbable barrier non-surgically through the access cavity, internally through the perforation defect, and ideally into a three-walled osseous defect.[148] Absorbable barrier materials are intended to be placed within the bone and not left inside tooth structure. The barrier should conform to the anatomy of the furcation or root surface involved. Although a variety of absorbable barriers exist, collagen and calcium sulfate materials are best employed due to supporting research, ease of handling, and observed clinical results.

- Collagen materials, such as CollaCote (Sulzer/Zimmer Dental, Carlsbad, CA), exhibit working properties that provides complete hemostasis.[325] CollaCote is biocompatible, supportive of new tissue growth, absorbable in 10 to 14 days, when left in situ.[311,318,328] Based on the size of the defect and the available access, pieces of CollaCote are cut to appropriate sizes and carried into the access cavity. The material is incrementally placed through the tooth and into the osseous defect until a solid barrier is established at the cavosurface of the root. Hemostasis is typically achieved in 2 to 5 minutes. Collagen barriers have been widely used in conjunction with amalgam, Super EBA, and other non-bonded restoratives.[328] CollaCote is contraindicated as a barrier if adhesion dentistry is contemplated as it absorbs moisture and will contaminate the restorative material.
- Calcium sulfate, marketed as Capset (Life Core Biomedical, Chaska, MN), can be used as both a barrier and hemostatic material in perforation management.[319,328,329] Calcium sulfate creates a tamponade effect, mechanically plugging vascular channels once it sets. Capset is biocompatible, does not promote inflammation, and is absorbable in 2 to 4 weeks. This material is syringed through the tooth and into the osseous defect utilizing a microtube delivery system. During its placement, calcium sulfate will fill the osseous defect and a portion of the space within the root defect. Calcium sulfate rapidly sets hard and may be prepared flush to the external root surface with ultrasonic instruments. Calcium sulfate is the barrier of choice when utilizing the techniques of adhesive bonding.[162,328,330] Importantly, the perforation defect can be rinsed of contaminants in preparation for adhesion dentistry.

Non-absorbable Barriers

MTA exhibits superior tissue biocompatibility and can be used both as a non-absorbable barrier and restorative material.[331] MTA has many clinical applications and represents an extraordinary breakthrough for managing radicular repairs.[239–241] MTA is the barrier of choice when there is potential moisture contamination or when there are restrictions in access and visibility. Furthermore, MTA can be used as the sole radicular filling material or as a barrier against which to condense another material. The mixing and use of MTA was previously discussed in the sections "Perforation and Prognosis for Healing" and "Techniques for Managing Apical Transportations".

RESTORATIVE MATERIALS IN PERFORATION REPAIR

Central to success when repairing a perforation is to select a restorative material that is easy to use, non-absorbable, biocompatible, esthetically pleasing, and one that provides a fluid-tight biologic seal. The materials widely employed to repair perforations include amalgam (no longer recommended), Super EBA resin cement (Henry J. Bosworth, Skokie, IL), composite bonded restoratives (Geristore, DenMat Corporation, Santa Maria, CA), calcium phosphate cement, and MTA.[306,281,332] The choice of the restorative repair material is based on the technical access to the defect, the ability to control moisture, and esthetic considerations.

TECHNIQUES FOR PERFORATION REPAIR

The barrier material and restoration selected to seal a perforation site should be based on sound research, judgment, experience, training, esthetics, ease of handling, and the advantages or disadvantages of a particular material in a specific clinical application. This section describes the armamentarium, materials, and techniques required to repair perforations.

Management of Coronal One-third and Furcal Perforations

The major difference between coronal one-third and furcation floor perforations is the shape of the resultant root defect. Mechanical perforations that occur in the furcal floor are generally round while those occurring in the lateral aspects of roots are ovoid by nature of occurrence. When managing these perforations, the clinician must first isolate the perforation site. Generally, if the perforation is mechanical and has just occurred, it is non-infected and hence clean. In this situation and if hemostasis is achieved, the defect should be repaired immediately. However, if the perforation is long-standing and exhibits microleakage, then the defect needs to be disinfected and prepared before receiving the restorative. Ultrasonic instruments are ideal for preparing perforation sites because of their geometries and coatings and because they afford direct vision.

Once the defect has been properly prepared, an appropriate barrier material and restorative are selected based on the following considerations:

- In a coronal one-third perforation where esthetics is a concern, a calcium sulfate barrier in conjunction with adhesive dentistry and a tooth-colored restoration is generally used.[330]
- Historically, amalgam and more recently Super EBA have been used to repair coronal one-

third perforations when esthetics was not an issue. Presently, MTA is rapidly becoming the barrier/restorative of choice for repairing non-esthetic coronal one-third defects because of its many desirable attributes. The choice to use MTA should only be made when there is no sulcular communication.

Following perforation repair, the tooth may be cleaned, shaped, and obturated if this has not already been accomplished (Figure 29).

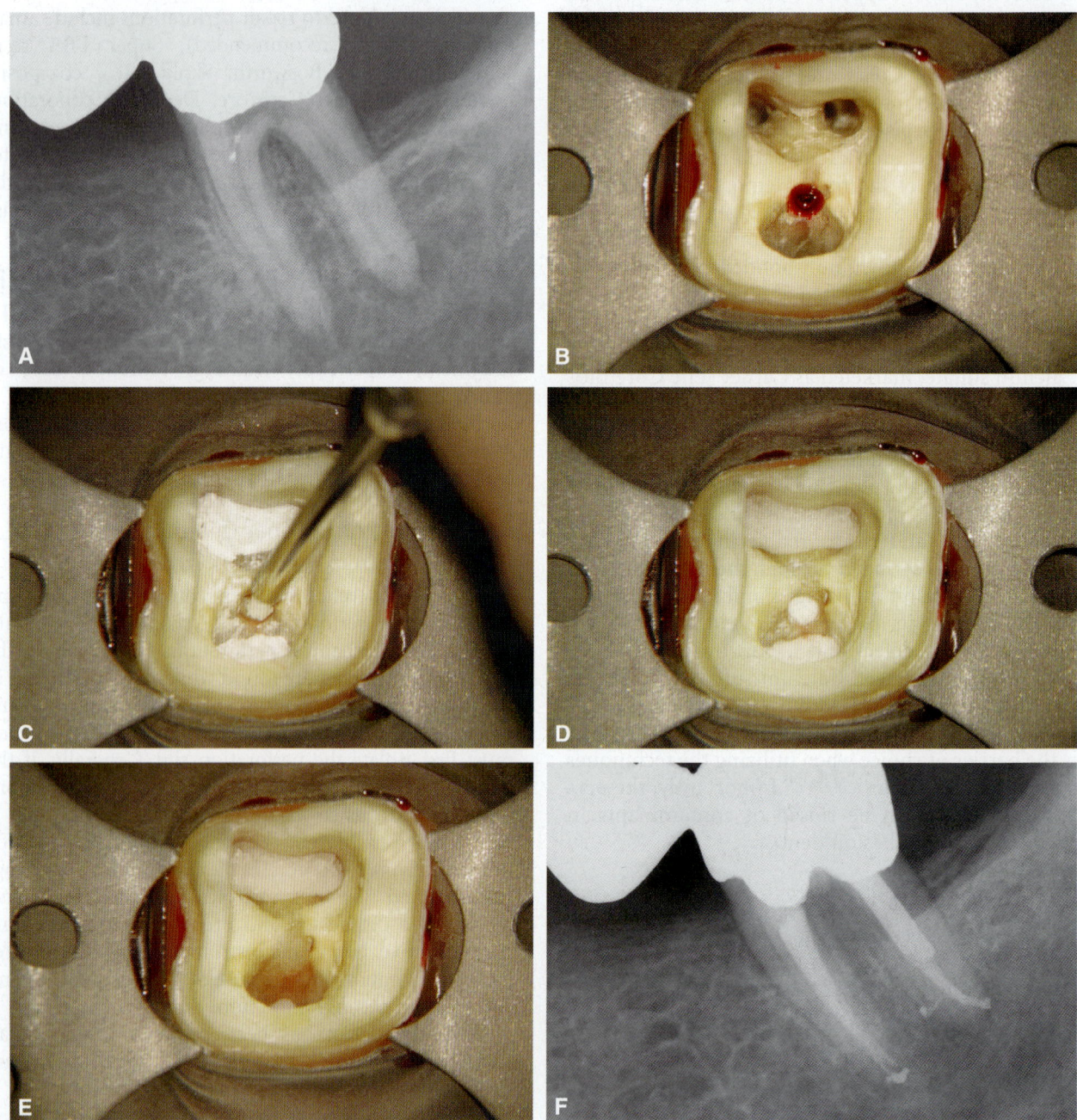

Figure 29 ***A,*** Preoperative radiograph showing periapical pathosis associated with a mandibular left second molar bridge abutment. Note the previous access and possible pulp chamber floor perforation. ***B,*** Photograph shows the canal orifices and an open furcal floor perforation. ***C,*** Photograph showing pieces of CollaCote sponge protecting the canal orifices and calcium sulfate being introduced into the perforation. ***D,*** The absorbable barrier is finished flush to the external root surface. ***E,*** The photograph shows the perforation repair with a dual cured composite material. ***F,*** A 5-year recall radiograph shows a new bridge and osseous repair in the furcation and apically.

Management of Perforations in the Middle One-third

Iatrogenic perforations in the *middle one-third* of roots are often caused by endodontic files, GG drills, or large misdirected post preparations. By the nature of their occurrence, these defects are ovoid in shape and typically represent relatively large surface areas to seal.

Middle one-third or strip perforations have the same technical considerations as coronal one-third perforations except the clinician is now dealing with defects located deeper and further away from the occlusal table. The factors that must be addressed in order to successfully treat these more apically positioned perforations are hemostasis, access, utilization of micro-instrumentation techniques, and the selection of suitable materials in a difficult environment. When managing deeper defects that are positioned on the lateral walls of canals, vision is enhanced when direct access exists or can be safely created. In some instances, direct access may not be possible without irreversibly compromising the structural integrity of the tooth and indirect repair techniques are required. Generally, perforations that occur secondary to overzealous canal instrumentation are sterile and do not require further modification. These should be sealed immediately. However, failing endodontic cases are associated with microleakage and microbial infection and may require ultrasonic instrumentation to clean and modify the defect in preparation for repair.

When the middle one-third perforation is a small defect, if the hemorrhage can be arrested and a dry working field obtained, then the perforation can be sealed and repaired during obturation. However, if the defect is large and the canal cannot be definitively dried, then the perforation must be repaired first before obturation. It is wise to finish the root canal preparation prior to initiating the perforation repair procedures. To prevent obstructing the root canal space during repair procedures, any readily retrievable material is placed in the canal as a space holder apical to the defect, before the perforation is repaired.

In these teeth, due to the difficult access, limited visibility, and the uncertainty of a moisture-free environment, the restorative/barrier material of choice is MTA. MTA is mixed and placed into the perforation site in accordance with the techniques discussed earlier in this chapter. After 4–6 hours, MTA will set hard and the clinician can proceed with the required treatment (Figure 30).

Management of Perforations in the Apical One-third

Perforations occurring in the apical one-third of roots primarily result from iatrogenic shaping procedures. Blocks and ledges lead to apical perforations and result from inadequate irrigation, inappropriate instrumentation, and failure to maintain patency. It is quite common that a root perforated in its apical one-third contains a canal that is both blocked and ledged. Recognizing the etiology of this type of perforation has led to surgical correction utilizing apicoectomy and retrograde-type procedures. However, it is generally recommended to first attempt non-surgical retreatment to enhance the existing endodontic treatment and, if present, to identify and treat missed canals.

The clinician should attempt to negotiate the full length of the root canal system with the concepts, instruments, and techniques previously discussed under "Techniques for Managing Blocked Canals" and "Techniques for Managing Canal Ledges." Occasionally, the apical extent of the file will engage the original canal path and the instrument will begin to track along the true canal position. The file is gently rotated to negotiate the physiologic pathway, establish patency, and pave the way for the next successively larger instrument. The next sequentially larger pre-curved file is then inserted and carried apical to the perforation, but not necessarily to length. This "holding file" maintains the pathway of the true canal and prevents it from being blocked during subsequent repair.

MTA is the material of choice for repairing deep perforations, especially when a dry environment is not possible. MTA is placed as has been previously described. To prevent the "holding file" from being cemented into MTA as it hardens, the instrument is grasped with Stieglitz pliers and moved up and down in short, 1- to 2-mm amplitude strokes. The loosened holding file is then sectioned so its coronal most aspect is below the occlusal table but well above the canal orifice. A radiograph should be taken to confirm the position of the MTA and the quality of the repair. A moist cotton pellet is placed within the pulp chamber and in contact with the MTA and the tooth is closed with a temporary filling until the following visit. Upon re-entry, the holding file is removed, and if the MTA is hard, copiously irrigated, and the preparation finalized. A gutta-percha master cone is then fit and the root canal system is obturated. It is wise to monitor these cases periodically to observe healing before placing a

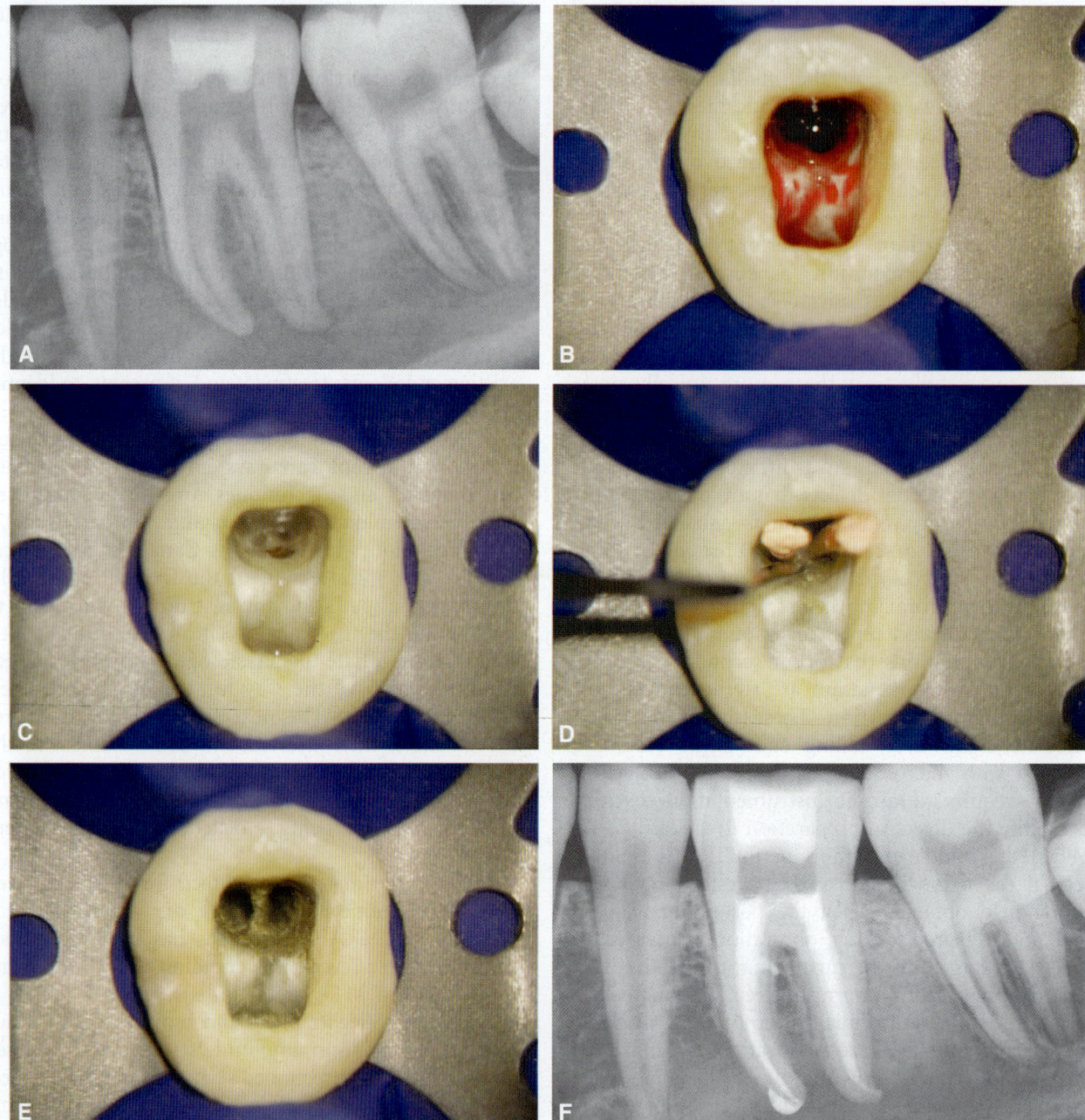

Figure 30 *A,* Preoperative radiograph of a mandibular left first molar with a periapical lesion. Note the previously over-enlarged mesial root canals. *B,* Photograph taken upon re-entry shows significant bleeding from the mesial root canals. *C,* The photograph demonstrates hemostasis and identifies the existence and position of a strip perforation. *D,* Gutta-percha cones in the mesiobuccal (MB)/mesiolingual (ML) root canals prevent their blockage. Mineral trioxide aggregate is being vibrated ultrasonically to make the material flow into the perforation defect. *E,* Photograph at a subsequent visit shows removal of the gutta-percha cones, perforation repair, and the canals ready to be obturated. *F,* Postoperative radiograph shows the repair of the perforation.

definitive restoration. It is also important to acknowledge that not all perforations can be corrected non-surgically, even when the best technologies are used in the hands of the most skilled practitioners. Some teeth will still require surgical treatment or extraction.

Mishaps and Serious Complications of Endodontic Therapy

THERMAL INJURY WITH THE USE OF ULTRASONICS

As described earlier, the use of vibratory energy has evolved as a highly efficient method for removal of obstructions and cements within the root canal space when retreatment or rehabilitation of that space is planned. In less than a decade, ultrasonic therapies have gained rapid and widespread acceptance within the community of practitioners as an adjunctive technique in overcoming a heretofore, formidable challenge. This has occurred because the ultimate goal in recovery of the root canal space is to ensure that the remaining dentin is sound and able to structurally support the subsequent restoration providing a restorative complex that is functionally healthy.[184] The use of ultrasonic devices has allowed dentists to embrace this important strategy.

Because conventional retreatment is the choice a prudent practitioner would first consider before turning to a surgical option, more and more clinicians are finding that ultrasonic technology is becoming indispensable in a modern dental practice. Ultrasonic energy is derived from one of two sources: magnetic resonance such as that used by devices such as the Cavitron or Cavi-endo units, or piezoelectric energy, such as that used by the Enac, Satelec's Suprasson P5 Booster, Analytic's MiniEndo II, and the Spartan MTS from Obtura Spartan. While it is recognized that piezoelectric devices operate in energy ranges that are higher than magneto-restrictive devices, most units used for post removal are within the higher ranges of operation.

Only a small number of investigators and authors have cautioned that ultrasonic energy can be harmful as intense heat can be generated within a metallic object that has its distal end millimeters away from any cooling effects created by the operator or the device itself.[204,203,333] The use of heat and the potential for injurious heat transfer to dentin and bone has been investigated for a number of different devices used in endodontics and associated restorative procedures.[334-339] It is generally accepted that external root temperature increases that exceed 10°C produce irreversible bone and attachment damage as well as dehydration effects on dentin often resulting in resorption.[340] Investigations of this kind have been in the literature for over two decades, and many investigators have used the 10°C threshold to examine devices that produce heat in dentistry. Heat transferred to the pulp through conventional cavity preparations and restorative procedures have been well documented in the literature.[341,342] Newer technologies such as laser use on dentin have also been investigated for intrapulpal heat transfer. Lasers may jeopardize pulp vitality through heat transfer. In recent research, temperature elevations between 0.5 and 32.0°C were registered in an energy- and time-dependent manner. Thinner dentin in the site of laser usage resulted in higher temperature elevations within the pulp. The time of application was a critical variable that mandated a "Caveat" to monitor time limits in usage.[339]

When investigating devices that create heat within the root canal space, the System B obturation system, when used according to the manufacturer's specifications, produces heat transfer to the attachment that falls below the critical threshold for irreversible injury.[204] Other researchers investigating different thermoplasticizing techniques have found similar results. Specifically, that generated temperature increases on the root surface are not sufficiently high to cause damage to the tooth-supporting tissues or exceed the critical 10°C.[336,337] In an assessment of heat transfer to the root surface during post preparation with Peeso reamers and Parapost drills, large temperatures were generated on the root surface by these engine-driven drills through frictional heating.[335,338]

There is very little evidence in published research for the considerable heat transfer that occurs during ultrasonic vibratory motion of devices during removal of posts, pastes, and separated instruments in teeth. A number of studies over the past few years have cautioned the practitioner regarding adequate coolant and the need to counter heat buildup.[203,333] There are far less published recommendations for how to accomplish this goal. Often, even the manufacturers are generic in their admonitions for usage and methods for cooling. Research studies of time intervals for application of energy consistently recognize that temperatures can rise to destructive levels within a few minutes without adequate and sufficient coolant.[203,333-344]

The general recommendation from this research is that care should be taken not to continue ultrasonic vibration over prolonged time periods. In addition, clinical protocols are needed to safely remove posts without causing thermal damage to the adjacent periodontal tissues. A recent study of ultrasonic heat transfer through ceramic and metallic posts reported that 75% of samples in both ceramic and stainless steel groups showed external root temperatures that exceeded the critical 10°C threshold of samples within the first 5 minutes. All samples were vibrated with a water spray coolant directed to the ultrasonic tip. There were no significant differences comparing the effects of heat generated by ceramic or stainless steel posts during removal.[203]

These authors cautioned against extrapolating in vitro data of root temperature rises to the in vivo clinical situation of a circulatory system within the attachment apparatus capable of dissipating heat. However, the results of this study showed temperature rises that would have greatly exceeded the dissipation effects of the periodontal vasculature. Accordingly, the authors warn the reader to maximize coolant and minimize application time.

The safe usage of ultrasonic devices is paramount. Thus, expediency should not compromise proper procedural design to protect the patient's safety and welfare. Because dentists are taught to be cautious with heat-generating devices contacting hard and/or soft tissue, a reasonably careful (and prudent) dentist should always be mindful of excessive heat potential with ultrasonic devices despite water coolants. Ultrasonic device usage should be coupled with monitoring intervals to assess overheating and to permit post cooling (Figure 31).

FACTORS INFLUENCING POST REMOVAL AND HEAT TRANSFER

Many factors that influence successful post removal were discussed in prior sections of this chapter. Individually and in combination, these factors should be carefully considered before commencing with any treatment.[145] There are several factors that serve to influence heat transfer and the potential for thermal injury. Specifically, there is virtually no research information available quantifying the optimal magnitude of energy, for any given ultrasonic device, that maximizes clinical efficiency yet mitigates dangerous heat transfer. Additionally, at any given ultrasonic power setting, little is reported regarding the length of time an instrument can vibrate against a post without causing thermal injury. Furthermore, protocols need to be developed to measure heat transfer based on the length, diameter, and configuration of a post

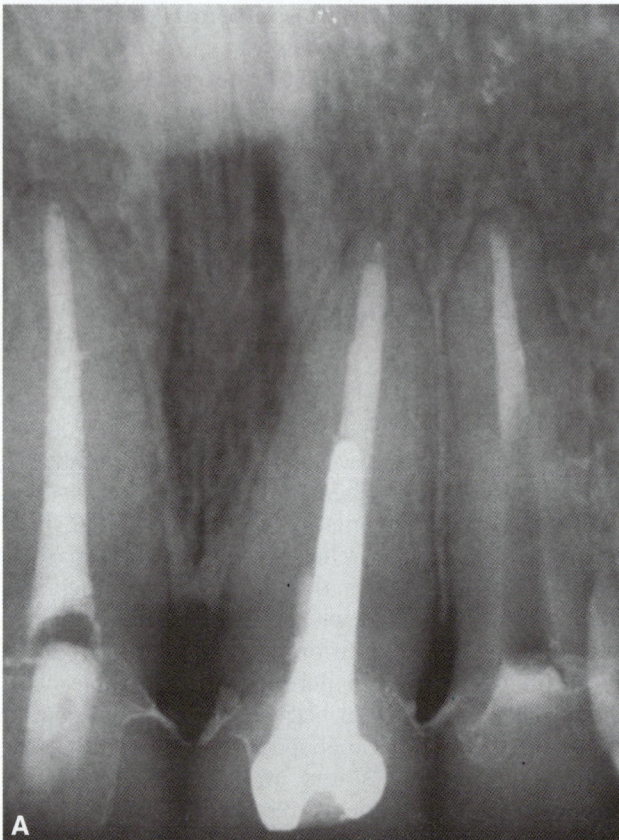

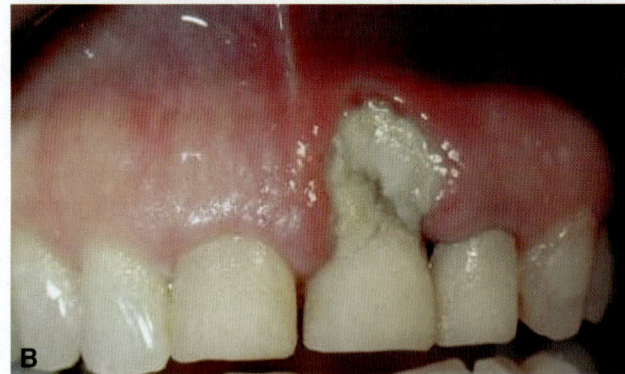

Figure 31 *A*, Preoperative radiograph of a maxillary left central incisor with a metal post. Ultrasonic vibration was used to remove the post. *B*, Postoperative appearance of the burn after post removal. The tooth was later extracted and the bone loss was severe.

and the type of material from which it is constructed. Another factor influencing heat transfer, when attempting to remove a post using the ultrasonic option, is the thickness of the remaining dentin. As an example, many posts observed radiographically to be centered within a root are oftentimes extremely close to the external root surface due to surface concavities. A recent investigation showed that when a #4 GG drill is used to prepare a post space in the distal root of mandibular molars, in 82% of cases the residual dentin thickness was less than 1 mm.[345]

Fortunately, adequate water coolant can safely reduce heat transfer and virtually eliminate the risk of thermal injury. However, the literature does not provide sufficient guidelines for how often a clinician should irrigate the tooth to dissipate the heat, how long ultrasonic energy should be applied and whether cool-down intervals are necessary to prevent cumulative damage. Also unknown is what volume of coolant is effective in maintaining a safe physiological temperature. Additional research needs to be performed and data gathered and published to clarify how each factor, or combination of factors, influences heat transfer.

Based on the best available evidence, the following recommendations can be made to provide safe and effective therapy using ultrasonic devices in intraradicular obstruction removal.

- Attempt to radiographically image residual dentin thickness for the working level within the root. This will help judge heat transmission rates to the attachment. Thicknesses below 1 mm in combination with metallic or ceramic posts will transmit heat rapidly.
- Use devices that allow water to reach the working end of the ultrasonic tip. This provides maximum cooling effect.
- Use copious water spray and effective suction at a continuous rate. There is ample evidence that when the working end of any ultrasonic device is deep within the root, heat generation occurs rapidly.
- Monitor the post temperature at 1- to 2-minute intervals. This seems to be the most prudent standard given the evidence that extreme temperatures on the root surface, even while using coolant, can be reached in 5 minutes.
- Where possible, monitor heat buildup in the post by touching it. A gloved finger will be able to sense a post overheating.
- Allow reasonable intervals between applications of ultrasonic energy. If post removal attempts are continued beyond 10 minutes, rest intervals between ultrasonic device applications should be at least 2 minutes. Timers with beepers should be considered to monitor time intervals; heat buildup appears to be dissipated in stages and recovery of physiologic temperatures occurs very slowly.
- Incorporate refrigerants (ethyl chloride or Endo Ice) applied to a cotton swab or ice sticks to cool the post down if necessary. The expansion/contraction effects of this strategy are minimal compared to the severe outcomes of a burn injury.
- Use post pullers and other vise-like devices as adjuncts to ultrasonic energy.

Each dental procedure has a variable degree of inherent risk. The practitioner is required to avoid unreasonable risks that may harm the patient. Treatment is deemed negligent when a reasonably careful clinician should have foreseen and prevented unreasonable risk of harm to the patient. Failure to follow the dictates of sound biologic practice increases the risk of negligently induced deleterious results.

Obturation and Irrigation Mishaps

Unfortunately, there are numerous examples reported in the literature that cite and document many disabling complications to the alveolar bone, neurovascular bundle, and maxillary sinus following inadvertent overextension of root canal filling materials and irrigants. These injuries require a thoughtful strategy for prevention during endodontic procedures as well as a responsible systematic approach to management, should the outcome of endodontic therapy produce an injury.

It is important to focus on measures that can prevent and/or minimize accidents that can occur under the most vulnerable of circumstances. The identification of those principal factors that can affect prognosis after injury will also be an important consideration in the remainder of this chapter. Many of the root-filling materials used today are either chemically neurotoxic or can be mechanically destructive to surrounding structures via compression injury. In addition, over-instrumentation errors in shaping root canal spaces may produce an abnormal over-enlargement of the apical constriction allowing overfill or instrument damage to structures through direct manipulation or rotation that severs susceptible tissues. With the use of rotation during instrumentation and heated obturation devices becoming increasingly available to all practitioners in the last decade, the introduction of endodontic filling materials into periapical tissues is quite common. This is of major concern when the teeth being treated are in close proximity to anatomically important structures such as the maxillary sinus or inferior alveolar canal. Overextension of the root canal-filling materials and/or irrigants risk injurious

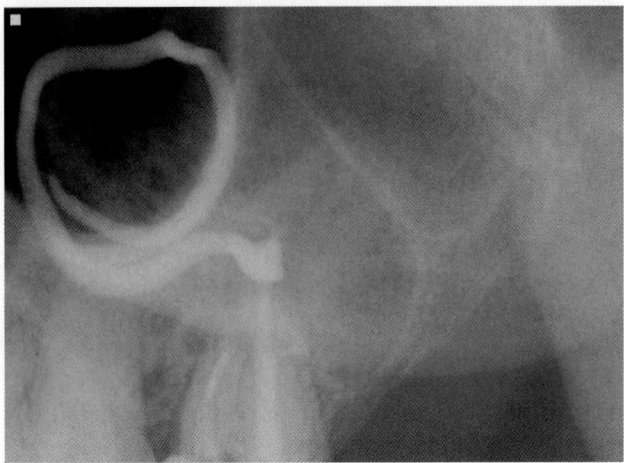

Figure 32 Extreme overfill into the sinus resulting from the combination of an over-instrumented apex and an automated thermoplastic technique.

consequences if the underlying inferior alveolar nerve or sinus structures are initially penetrated with files. A pathway of entry into the inferior alveolar nerve or sinus space can more likely result when the pathway is created by over-instrumentation or an open apex (Figure 32).

THE IMPORTANCE OF ACCURATE RADIOGRAPHIC IMAGING

While this is a common admonition by educators to many students in the medical sciences, as they are learning the principles and practice of diagnostic assessment, it is a fundamental truth. "You don't know ... what you don't know." For the practitioner embarking on endodontic therapy for a molar or premolar tooth in the anatomical vicinity of the maxillary sinus, mental foramen, or inferior alveolar nerve, this caveat is critical. It is a common understanding that both large and small pathoses as well as anatomic entities are routinely missed in radiographic surveys both by the operator and by the limitations of the technology when encountering differences in anatomic variation.[346]

ANATOMIC AND IMAGING CHARACTERISTICS OF THE MAXILLARY SINUS

The maxillary sinus or antrum is an air-filled cavity lined by respiratory mucosa. The inferior border of the sinus lies in the alveolar process of the maxilla and is situated above or often between the apices of the maxillary posterior teeth. The sinus may also be separated by bony walls into several compartments. Proper visualization of the maxillary sinuses is critical for interpretation of location and distances of root apices from the sinus space[347] (see Chapter 17).

A standard panoramic projection provides very good information about the dimensions of the sinus space notwithstanding the superimposition of the nasal and zygomatic structures in a panographic image. The size and configurations of the sinuses vary greatly; in some individuals, there is considerable bone between the apices of the teeth and the sinus cavity, whereas in others the roots directly project into the sinus with minimal or no bony covering.[348–352] Information derived from cone beam computed tomography (CT) was reported very useful in a case involving surgical access to a maxillary molar. The course of the sinus and its relationship to the roots of the first molar as well as potential sinus pathology were assessed.[353]

Neural distribution to the sinus is diagnostically important. The nerve supply is from the maxillary division of the trigeminal nerve, with branches coming from the posterior, middle, and anterior–superior portions. The inflammatory effects of overfilled endodontic materials as well as dental sepsis can affect the differential diagnosis of pain localized to the sinuses. High-contrast three-dimensional CT will greatly facilitate the evaluation of the sinuses and determine the position of foreign materials and their relation to the apices of teeth.[347] The inflammatory effects induced by irrigants, medicaments, and endodontic filling materials will extend a pathway to the sinus if proximity allows; great caution and care in the use of these products is indicated in root canals that adjoin the sinus.[348,349]

ANATOMIC AND IMAGING CHARACTERISTICS OF THE INFERIOR ALVEOLAR CANAL

The inferior alveolar canal starts at the mandibular foramen on the inner aspect of the ramus and passes in a downward and forward direction through the mandible. As it passes forward, it also moves from the lingual side of the body of the mandible in the third molar area to the buccal side in the premolar area. In traditional radiography and panographic films as well as digital images, it appears as a narrow, radiolucent ribbon between two radiopaque lines representing the canal walls. It has been reported that CT imaging was highly reliable when attempting to determine the relation between periapical lesions and the mandibular canal prior to endodontic surgery.[354]

In the region of the mental foramen, the mandibular nerve bifurcates into its two branches, the incisive and mental nerves. The exact location of the inferior alveolar canal and its mental branch is important in the placement of implants, surgical extractions, and endodontic therapy of roots within close proximity.[355] In a series of investigations on 75 human skulls to identify the radiographic position of the mental foramen on periapical and panographic film, the authors found that the foramen could be seen on only 75% of the horizontal periapical radiographs.[356] Visualization of the mental foramen was increased and enhanced when a panoramic radiograph was available due to a 23% magnification factor that occurs in a panographic film.[357]

Interruptions in the protective wall of the canal by dental manipulations can have serious and calamitous effects on the patient's sensibility in the distribution of the nerve.[358,359] In research that assessed the spatial relationship between the posterior teeth and the mandibular canal using 22 mature dried human skulls accounting for 264 specimen sections, second premolars and second molars had the closest distances to the canal with a mean distance of 4.7 and 3.7 mm respectively. The mandibular canal was directly inferior to the root apices of the posterior teeth 5% of the time. The data also determined that as the mandibular height decreased, the distance between the canal and root apices also decreased.[360] In prior studies, investigators have found that 60% of mandible specimens contained canals while 40% of the dissection samples had no distinct canals. Often, branches of the nerve showed significant morphologic variability and occupied only a space in the bone as opposed to residing within a distinct tunnel-like structure.[361] These findings have significant implications regarding the effects of endodontic medicaments, sealers and materials on bone, connective tissue, and specifically the neurovascular elements found in the antrum and inferior alveolar canal.

Endodontic filling materials and sealers are reviewed in Chapter 25. Biocompatibility of endodontic obturation materials have been investigated in great detail.[362–403] Biocompatibility studies have included tissue and cell culture studies,[366–368] bone and soft tissue reactions to set and unset implanted materials in experimental animals,[369–371] experimental and clinical studies on animals and humans,[372–374] and new assessments involving histochemical analysis and X-ray microanalysis.[374–376]

Length Determination Controversies in Endodontics

One of the major controversies in root canal treatment is the apical end point of the working length. It is a paradigm in modern endodontics that instrumentation beyond the apical foramen should be avoided because it is so often associated with a reduced success rate[404–408] and exposes the patient to the potential for injury.[409]

Generally, as discussed in here and prior chapters, most clinicians prefer to end the biomechanical instrumentation at the apical constriction (narrowest point in the canal at approximately the dentin–cemental junction),[410] where the contact between root canal filling material and the apical tissues is minimal. In addition, many dentists practice apical patency with small files in order to maintain communication with the apical tissues and prevent canal blockage and ledging coronal to the determined end point.

Despite the limited three-dimensional information provided by a conventional radiograph, a periapical radiograph remains the commonly used standard for working length determination.[411,412] However, the acceptance of apex locators is widely increasing with the introduction of devices well into their fourth generation. In addition, many clinicians use paper points to help determine the juncture of the canal confines from the serum of periapical tissues. Generally, a distance of 0 to 2 mm between radiographic apex and the obturation material marking the end point of root canal instrumentation has been designated as acceptable when evaluating postoperative radiographs. Accordingly, in a retrospective study that investigated the influence of the level of apical obturation on the treatment outcome,[406] a root canal filling was considered satisfactory, if among other factors its apical level was 0 to 2 mm short of the radiographic apex, this apical level contributing to the highest success rates.

Stein and Corcoran[413] discussed the possibility of unintentional over-instrumentation when radiographs alone were used for working length determination. They reported that the position of a file placed for working length determination appeared radiographically 0.7 mm shorter than its actual position. The results of another investigation suggest that a working length that ends radiographically 0 to 2 mm short of the radiographic apex does not guarantee that instrumentation beyond the apical foramen will be avoided in premolars and molars. The authors conclude that radiographic measurements should be combined with electronic working length determination using modern apex locators to better help identify the apical end point of root canal preparation and avoid over-instrumentation.[414]

In a recent review of the literature on the role of apical instrumentation in root canal treatment, Baugh and Wallace[410] concluded that because the apical dimensions of root canals range from very large to very small, the clinician should seek instruments and techniques that can help determine when instrumentation to the correct apical size has been achieved and that additional research was necessary given the controversy that still lingers regarding final apical size. Other researchers have shown the importance of combining therapies such as rotary instrumentation using larger apical sizes with the use of calcium hydroxide to reduce the numbers of bacteria in root canals and increase long-term success.[415] In a recent meta-analysis of studies done over the last three decades on optimal obturation length, the results demonstrated that obturating materials extruding beyond the radiographic apex correlated with a decreased prognosis for repair.[416] When faced with the possibility of inadvertent over-instrumentation into neurovascular anatomy, the research provides a substantial number of appropriate caveats.

Techniques for Obturation Control When Neurovascular Proximity Exists

There are a number of contributions to the literature that assess techniques for apical control of obturation materials. Tronstad[417] assessed the apical plug of dentin chips in monkeys and showed that a plug of clean dentin fillings could provide an apical matrix that was well tolerated by the tissues and would provide an apical barrier that would allow the canals to be well sealed yet protected against impingement of filling materials on the periodontal tissues. Others have found that a dentinal plug serves as an effective means of preventing extrusion when using thermoplasticized techniques[418,419] or to confine irrigating solutions.[420] In a comprehensive study comparing the apical plugs of dentin versus calcium hydroxide to prevent overfilling, when the apical foramen had been intentionally over-instrumented in cats, the investigators found plugs of calcium hydroxide or dentin to work equally well.[421] However, the calcium hydroxide plugs were less durable and produced foramina mineralization that was less complete than the dentinal plugs. Periapical healing was similar for both calcium hydroxide and dentin. In another study that looked at foramen size as it affected apical extrusion of thermoplasticized gutta-percha, it was noted that overfills and the extrusion of material occurred proportionately to the area of the apical opening. An opening the size of a #40 file (0.40 mm diameter) was found to be twice as likely to allow extrusion of material than an apical diameter sized at #20 (0.20 mm).[422] When the sealing ability of laterally condensed gutta-percha was compared to injection molded thermoplasticized gutta-percha in straight and curved canals, only the thermoplasticized technique produced overextensions.[423] It has also been shown that great differences in flowability exist between gutta-percha brands when used in a thermocompaction technique.[424] The recommendation to consider a hybrid technique when using thermoplasticized materials has often involved a cold condensation of gutta-percha apically followed by a thermomechanical compaction, providing a safer barrier for limiting the extrusion of material.[422]

Thermoplasticized Gutta-Percha and the Effects of Heat

Previously discussed in this chapter were a series of investigations in vitro[425] and on dogs,[426] wherein the heat of thermoplasticized gutta-percha was assessed for its potential injurious effects. Levels of heat generated by the plasticized gutta-percha did not appear to be at clinically deleterious levels and no apparent irreversible tissue destruction was evident.[426] Similar results have been obtained in other in vitro and in vivo studies when manufacturers' protocols for usage have been followed.[204,336,337,427,428] Where deleterious effects are seen either experimentally or in clinical situations, the lessons require heeding. Bailey et al.[333] in a study utilizing ultrasonic condensation of gutta-percha found that the combination of a high power setting and a 15-second application of activation energy resulted in temperature rise on the root surface beyond the recognized deleterious threshold of 10°C. Clinical case reports involving overfill with heat softened gutta-percha are increasing in the literature.[429,430] The current practice of maintaining apical patency and the popularity of thermoplastic gutta-percha filling techniques have increased the likelihood that overfills can involve the neurovascular anatomy. Fanibunda et al.[430] warn of the lesser known danger of thermal and mechanical insult from chemically "safer" materials other than paraformaldehyde, being extruded into the inferior alveolar canal. They report a case of thermally compacted gutta-percha having a severe affect on patient sensory loss after gross overfill into the mandibular canal. In this case, they identified a mechanical (compression), chemical (calcium hydroxide sealer), and thermal insult (molten gutta-percha) to the nerve.[430] A similar outcome for thermoplastic over-extension was reported by Blanas et al.[431].

Carrier-Based Gutta-Percha

Carrier-based gutta-percha was first introduced as Thermafil (Dentsply Tulsa Dental Specialties).[432] The Thermafil obturator currently consists of a plastic carrier and is covered in a uniform layer of gutta-percha. The carrier is constructed from a special radiopaque plastic similar to a manual or rotary endodontic instrument. The obturator is heated in a special oven where the gutta-percha it carries assumes a softened state with unique adhesive and flow characteristics. The ideal canal preparation for a carrier-based obturator must allow sufficient space for the flow of cement and gutta-percha.[433] Carrier-based obturators use techniques that caution against the use of excess cement because of the increased likelihood of overfilling due to the piston-like effect of the obturator during placement. Because the risk of overfilling is considered the only true limitation of carrier-based obturators, authors and manufacturers caution against the following major errors in technique:

- Incorrect canal preparation including over-instrumentation and laceration of the apical terminus.
- Excessive cement or gutta-percha.
- Excessive force and velocity during insertion.
- Improper obturator selection.[433]

Damage to the Neurovascular Anatomy: Causes and Outcomes

Reports in the literature involving serious injury to the inferior alveolar nerve have included paresthesia or anesthesia associated with overfill of N2 and similar paraformaldehyde pastes,[385,386,388–391] (Figure 33), Endomethasone,[387,399] AH26,[434,435–437] calcium hydroxide,[430,438] ZOE, and gutta-percha.[409,436] There is almost no current obturation material that has not been reported in the literature to produce paresthesia when overfilled into the neurovascular anatomy. If a new material is not currently cited, it is almost assured the mishap of overfill will eventually find itself in the literature.

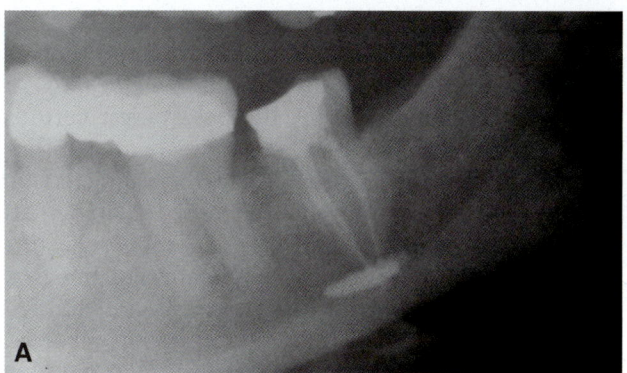
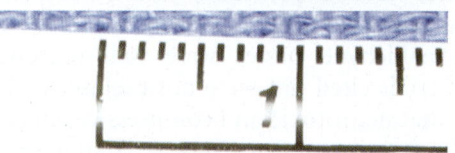
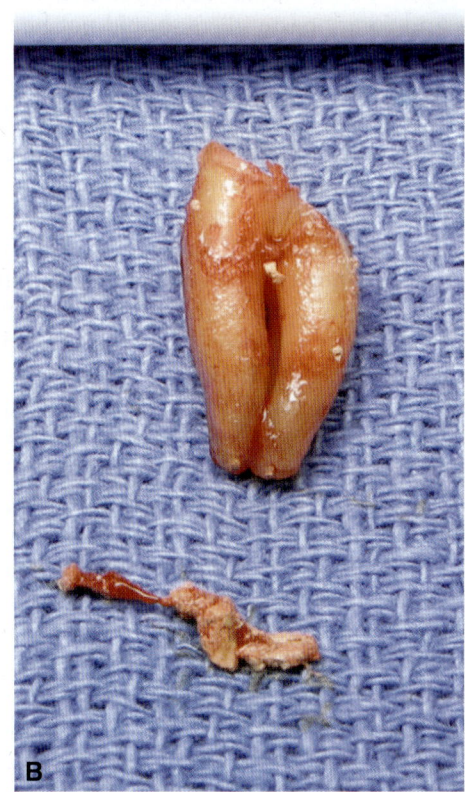

Figure 33 A, Postoperative radiograph of a paraformaldehyde paste overfill of a mandibular left second molar. The patient developed paresthesia that prompted surgical intervention weeks later. **B,** After extraction and removal of the extruded paste material, the patient continued to have a burning pain and anesthesia.

Ørstavik et al.[374] described 24 published cases of paresthesia involving the mandibular nerve. It was reported that there was no indication of healing in 14 of the 24 patients during the observation periods which ranged from 3 months to 18 years after initiation of the injury. They described the characteristic deficits of the inferior alveolar nerve as unilateral loss of sensitivity of the lip and gums, numbness, a tingling sensation, and dryness of the affected mucosa, often preceded by intense pain in the affected area.[374] All of the reported cases were molars or involved the lower second premolar. There were numerous materials involved, all of which are cited in here. Paraformaldehyde pastes were well represented in the materials cited but were not exclusive. They concluded that neurotoxic and compressive effects are the most frequent causes of paresthesia after endodontic overfill into the mandibular canal and that the use of syringes and rotary paste fillers should not be used to insert root-filling pastes or cements in teeth in areas susceptible to neurovascular damage.

A serious case of calcium hydroxide overfill has been reported through a lower second molar causing severe vasospasm and a resulting facial ischemia.[439] The ischemia caused cyanosis and necrosis on the face as well as a total absence of function in the mandibular and mental nerve. Again, the authors cautioned in this case report against the use of a syringe in applying the calcium hydroxide with a known level of toxicity and a high pH (12.4).[439]

It is difficult to ascertain with absolute certainty the primary etiology for paresthesia when assessing the sequelae and future prognosis for repair from overfill into neurovascular tissue. The clinician, therefore, must consider the following critical factors in all cases of overfill: the chemical neurotoxicity of the materials involved, the possibility of direct damage of files (crushing and mechanical injury),[386,436] the compression damage of solid materials such as gutta-percha (the pressure on the nerve bundle is directly proportional to the amount of material pushed into the canal),[430,436] and the possibility of epineural fibrosis resulting in neuroma.[388] In a clinical report that suggests the use of corticosteroids may be helpful in countering the injurious compression effects resulting in epineural and intraneural edema, Gatot and Tovi[440] have reported that prednisone therapy may limit the severity of injury as well as aid in the prevention of fibrosis. Others also report the pharmacologic use of corticosteroids in the treatment of paresthesia related to overfill.[441]

Inflammatory edema with resulting ischemia, that compresses and compromises blood supply to soft tissues and nerves in confined spaces such as the inferior alveolar canal, is termed compartment syndrome.[442] Compartment syndromes are a group of conditions that result from increased pressure within a limited anatomic space, acutely compromising the circulation, and ultimately threatening the function of the tissue within that space. Compartment syndrome occurs from an elevation of the interstitial pressure in a closed osseous compartment that results in microvascular compromise. The pathophysiology of compartment syndrome is an insult to normal local tissue homeostasis that results in increased tissue pressure, decreased capillary blood flow, and local tissue necrosis caused by oxygen deprivation. Compartment syndrome is caused by localized hemorrhage or post-ischemic swelling resulting in fibrosis that obstructs axonal regeneration. The clinician should have a high index of suspicion whenever a closed bony nerve compartment has the potential for bleeding or swelling. Compartment syndromes are characterized by pain beyond what should be experienced from the initial injury. Also, diminished sensation may be noted in the distribution of the nerve within a compartment that is being compressed.[442]

DIAGNOSIS AND MANAGEMENT OF INFERIOR ALVEOLAR NERVE INJURY

Nerve recovery subsequent to an endodontic mishap is unpredictable. Because of this unpredictability, the clinician is responsible for making a timely diagnosis and monitoring neurosensory changes. Careful follow-up evaluations and appropriate referral is our responsibility to the patient.[443–446]

Neurosensory function can be divided into two basic categories based on the specific receptors that are either stimulated or injured: mechanoreceptive and nociceptive. The mechanoreceptive aspect of sensory perception can be further divided into two-point discrimination and brush directional stroke. The nociceptive path can be subdivided into pinprick and thermal discrimination. Each type of nerve fiber varies with respect to diameter, conduction speed, and physiologic function. Each afferent nerve end offers a distinct receptor terminal that is specific for warmth, cold, pain, and touch. The first phase of any peripheral nerve regeneration is the degeneration of the axon and its myelin sheath along the nerve fiber at the site of injury. These changes along the nerve are known as Wallerian degeneration and lead to degeneration of the entire axon terminal over several weeks following a severe injury. Neural injuries are most commonly classified using the Seddon classification system.[447] Seddon's classification is derived from the extent of nerve injury. Neurotemesis is the most severe nerve injury because conduction is completely disrupted resulting in the loss of anatomic integrity of the endoneurium, perineurium, and epineurium. Axonotemesis, a less severe injury, results in damage to the axons, but the endoneurial and epineurial sheaths are preserved. Neuropraxia occurs when a nerve is injured and conduction is blocked, but this does not lead to Wallerian degeneration.

Clinically, neurotemesis leads to anesthesia with a loss of feeling or sensation. It can also produce dysesthesia, an abnormal unpleasant sensation often burning in character. Recovery is unlikely or limited. Axonotemesis causes paresthesia, an abnormal altered sensation that can show some degree of sensory recovery after several months. Neuropraxia is usually a transient paresthesia where recovery is complete from days to weeks.

The clinical evaluation of a patient who suffers a sensory loss in the oral or maxillofacial region subsequent to an endodontic obturation should begin by identifying the patient's subjective assessment of these alterations. The clinician should distinguish between anesthesia, dysesthesia, and paresthesia. Often considerable variability will exist within the descriptions outlined above, and few patients will fit perfectly within the Seddon categories.[443] However, it is important that any patient with anesthesia or a painful dysesthesia be evaluated in a systematic fashion.[443,444] The dentist should assess the chronologic history of the area even if that history has only been in the last several hours and note the patient's chief complaint—the nature, frequency, and severity of the symptoms and how they might be changing for better or worse as well as the loss of function that is occurring. If the initial symptom is anesthesia, the area of anesthesia should be mapped and placed in the patient's record. Any return of sensation should be noted.[445]

The physical evaluation should also include pinprick for deep pain (small myelinated A-delta fibers), brush stroke for directional discrimination (mediated by large myelinated A-alpha nerve fibers), and two-point discrimination for proprioception (large myelinated A-alpha fibers). The small myelinated fibers of the A-delta group and the smaller unmyelinated axons of the C group are responsible for sensations of temperature.[443]

Should anesthesia and painful dysesthesia be consequences of overfilling, the practitioner must understand when the referral to a surgeon (oral-maxillofacial or neurosurgeon), who is experienced in the surgical therapies for relief and healing, may be required to resolve the patient's problem.[446] The final management of such a case depends on several factors. Even the most acceptable materials can cause serious injury if extruded in large volumes into sensitive structures. Pastes and sealers that contain paraformaldehyde or known safer materials are difficult to control and may moreover create injuries to the maxillary division of the trigeminal nerve when extruded through maxillary teeth or into the sinus membranes.[448] In addition, maxillary root-treated teeth with overextensions of the root canal sealer or solid materials such as gutta-percha or silver cones into the sinus might be the main etiological factor for aspergillosis of the maxillary sinus in healthy patients. Root-filling materials based on ZOE are considered to be a growth factor for aspergillus.[449,450]

While paraformaldehyde-containing materials should never be used because of the dangers of chemical injury they present, all obturation materials should be used with extreme caution in all circumstances, especially in teeth intimately related to the inferior alveolar canal.

When presented with the extrusion of endodontic obturation materials into the neurovascular tissues, and after careful and systematic assessment of the nature and course of the injury and its effects, a decision to intervene surgically or delay and observe has to be made (Figure 34).

MANAGEMENT OF INFERIOR ALVEOLAR NERVE INJURIES

The oral surgery literature describes most inferior alveolar nerve injuries as neuropraxias and thus they resolve spontaneously within a 6-month time frame. These are often lingual nerve injuries as well as mandibular trauma subsequent to tooth removal. It is reported that inferior alveolar nerve injuries heal better than lingual nerve injuries due to the guidance provided by the bony mandibular canal.[445] This fact has relevance if oral surgical procedures are likely and decortication procedures and removal of overfill are contemplated. The clinical examination that results in a diagnosis of anesthesia or increasing painful dysesthesia unresponsive to non-surgical therapy should help guide this decision.[443,444] It is suggested that the decision to intervene surgically should include the high suspicion of injury resulting in the loss of conduction within the nerve due to suspected chemical toxicity and mechanical compression.

There are several recent reports in the literature of surgical intervention to provide decompression and removal of chemically toxic materials that demonstrate successful outcomes.[451,452] However, when the practitioner takes a "wait and observe"

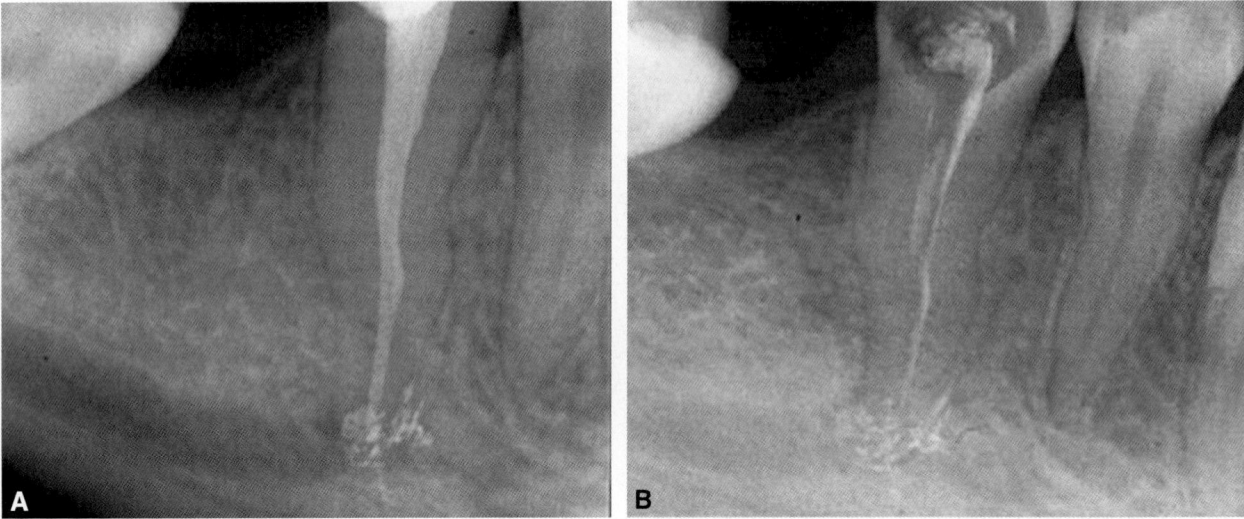

Figure 34 ***A,*** Radiograph shows zinc oxide–eugenol sealer extruded into the mental foramen from the canal of a mandibular second premolar. The patient experienced anesthesia in the distribution of the mental nerve 24 hours after injection of the sealer, and the decision was made to remove as much material as possible through the root canal space in an attempt to reduce the pressure on the neurovascular bundle. ***B,*** Patient exhibited signs of anesthesia for approximately 30 more days. After 60 days, the first signs of recovery appeared. The patient was symptom-free after 6 months.

approach, the favorable potential for long-term spontaneous recovery requires thoughtful consideration. When a peripheral nerve is injured, a non-surgical management that supports spontaneous neurosensory recovery and promotes patient tolerance of the sensory loss is a viable option.[445] The most compelling reason to wait is that a majority of injuries are known to recover spontaneously to some degree. Higher levels of recovery can also be expected when the patient is young and healthy. In addition, a "recovering patient profile" with improving levels of function, detection abilities, and sensory symptoms argues for restraint in management.[443,445]

In the final analysis, the decision of whether and when to intervene surgically in the removal of overfill should be based on objective criteria and a comprehensive assessment of each individual patient. The current guidelines for intervention are unfortunately not based on satisfactory evidence-based science, and this leaves a troublesome vacuum in our knowledge of effective therapies, making prevention of this injury critical to treatment planning prior to initiating root canal therapy.

Prevention of Obturation Mishaps

This chapter has offered a number of remedies to provide a safe and prudent approach to the obturation of posterior teeth in close proximity to the vulnerable tissues of the sinus or inferior alveolar nerve. In summary, the following recommendations are made.

- It is essential to image and identify radiographically the sensitive neural structures of the jaws and the sinuses in order to clearly understand the proximal risk.
- It is critical to use obturation materials that are well tolerated by the body after therapy, rather than paraformaldehyde formulations that can cause irreversible sensory nerve damage and should not be used in the good and safe practice of endodontics.
- The clinician must practice careful and judicious shaping strategies that use multiple confirmations of working length and take serious precaution against over-instrumentation.
- It is important to use "resistance form" in controlling overfills. This "resistance form" can be imparted during canal preparation by producing funnel-form, tapered preparations and by selecting gutta-percha cones to match those canal shapes that will resist the obturation forces which promote extrusion.
- When using thermoplastic techniques, it is important to respect the flow characteristics of the materials and the heat energy used.
- The use of paste fillers and syringes for applying endodontic sealers should be cautioned when there is close proximity to neural structures and control is compromised.

- In cases of extreme proximity to the neurovascular anatomy, the importance of creating a clean dentin plug or material barrier at the patent apical terminus should be carefully planned when the risk of extrusion is considerable.

NaOCl Accident

Accidental injection of NaOCl into the periapical tissues is an experience that neither the patient nor the practitioner will soon forget. The literature contains numerous case reports describing the morbidity associated with such occurrences.[453–457] A NaOCl accident refers to any event in which NaOCl is expressed beyond the apex of a tooth and the patient immediately manifests some combination of the following symptoms:

- Severe pain, even in areas that were previously anesthetized for dental treatment.
- Swelling.
- Profuse bleeding, both interstitially and through the tooth.

CAUSES OF NaOCl ACCIDENT

- Some of the reasons that a hypochlorite accident may occur include forceful injection of the irrigating solution, having an irrigating needle wedged into a root canal, and irrigating a tooth that has a large apical foramen, apical resorption, or an immature apex. Considering its excellent tissue-dissolving properties, a large volume of the irrigant under pressure will lead to immediate strong reactions.[458] Some patients have several days of increasing edema and ecchymosis, accompanied by tissue necrosis, paresthesia, and secondary infection (Figure 35). Although most patients recover within 1 to 2 weeks, long-term paresthesia and scarring have been reported,[456,457] as well as an incident that described the injection of NaOCl into the maxillary sinus resulting in hospitalization and surgical intervention.[459]

MANAGEMENT OF NaOCl ACCIDENT

- Recognize that a hypochlorite accident has occurred. NaOCl has immediate toxic effects on vital structures resulting in hemolysis, ulceration, and necrosis.[454,458]
- Attend to the immediate problem of pain and swelling. Administer a regional block with a long-acting

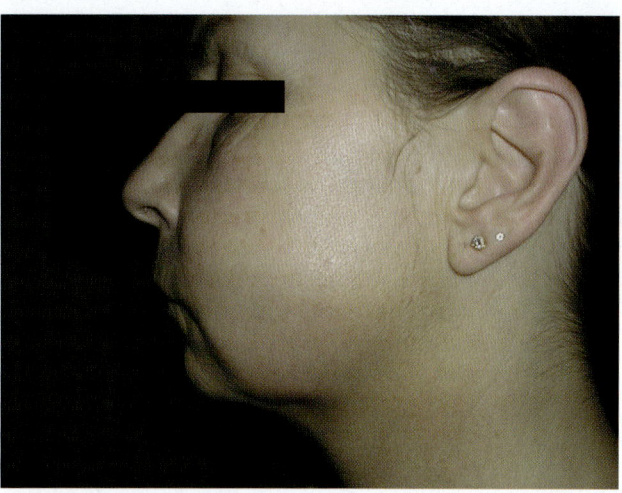

Figure 35 The situation several hours after 2.5% sodium hypochlorite solution was expressed through the roots of a maxillary premolar. The patient experienced immediate severe pain and swelling subsequent to the accident.

anesthetic solution. With the irrigant spreading rapidly over a wide region, pain management is difficult because symptoms from distant anatomic structures will continue to cause discomfort. This also explains the extreme pain felt during the accident despite establishment of adequate local anesthesia before treatment was begun. A reported incident describes flushing the palatal canal of a maxillary molar with sterile water to dilute the effects of the hypochlorite that was expressed into the sinus through the same route.[460]
- Reassure and calm the patient. The reaction, although alarmingly fast, is still a localized phenomenon and will resolve with time. If available, nitrous oxide sedation can help the patient cope throughout the remainder of this emergency.
- Monitor the tooth over the next half an hour. A bloody exudate may discharge into the canal. This bleeding is the body's reaction to the irrigant. Remove the fluid with high-volume evacuation to encourage further drainage from the periapical tissues. If drainage is persistent, consider leaving the tooth open over the next 24 hours.
- Consider antibiotic coverage. If the treated tooth is pulpless and cleansing and shaping procedures have not been completed, consider prescribing amoxicillin, 500 mg, four times a day, over the next 5 days.
- Consider administering an analgesic. Because of possible bleeding complications with aspirin and

other nonsteroidal anti-inflammatory drugs, an acetaminophen-narcotic analgesic combination may be more appropriate. If swelling is extensive, it is best to caution the patient to expect bruising or pooling of blood as it subsides.
- Consider prescribing a corticosteroid or antihistamines which can help minimize the ensuing inflammatory process.[453,458]
- Give the patient home care instructions. For the first 6 hours, the patient should use cold compresses to minimize pain and swelling. Subsequently, warm compresses should be used to encourage a healthy healing response.
- Consider referring the patient. If the patient continues to be apprehensive or needs additional reassurance or develops complications, referral to the endodontist or oral surgeon is appropriate. Informing the specialist about the patient and the nature of the problem will ensure a smooth transition between offices for the patient.

PREVENTION OF NaOCl ACCIDENT

A hypochlorite accident is completely avoidable. As an endodontic irrigant, hypochlorite solution is meant to flush debris from the root canal system. Part of the efficacy of hypochlorite depends on the volume of irrigation and the depth of penetration of the irrigating needle. Even so, the solution must be delivered in a passive manner to avoid apical extrusion. Because root canals are coronally flared during the cleansing and shaping process, the irrigating needle can penetrate deeper into the canal and still not bind against the walls.

The following measures are recommended to prevent a hypochlorite accident:

1. Side-vented needles will add a measure of safety to prevent binding and decrease intracanal pressures.[461]
2. Bend the irrigating needle as needed to confine the tip of the needle to higher levels in the root canal and to facilitate direct access to all teeth regardless of angulation.
3. Never place the needles so deeply into the canal that it binds against the walls.
4. Oscillate the needle in and out of the canal to ensure that the tip is free to express irrigant without resistance.
5. Express the irrigant slowly and gently.
6. Stop irrigating if the needle jams or if there is any detectable resistance when pressing against the plunger of the syringe.
7. Check the hub of the needle for a tight fit to prevent inadvertent separation and accidental exposure of the irrigant to the patient's eyes.

Although a hypochlorite accident requires immediate management, the definite assessment and accurate identification of this dental emergency must follow a prioritized process of recognition and response.

Air Emphysema

The dangers of air emphysema from compressed air are well known. Subsequent to surgical procedures in dentistry, there are reports of impingement on the airway as well as vision affects and cardiac complications.[462–464] Additionally, air introduced into periapical tissues during invasive root canal therapy has the potential to do great harm. While this phenomenon is a rare occurrence during endodontics, the risk is present and has been reported in animals to cause serious clinical complications.[465] Shovelton[462] reviewed 13 reports of air emphysema and found their etiology to range from pressurized air forced into the root canal to oxygen gas emphysema caused by irrigation past the apex with hydrogen peroxide. The patients in his review demonstrated signs of emphysema in the face, the neck, and suborbital regions. In an animal study in dogs, Rickles and Joshi[465] could not rule out air emphysema as the cause of death in four of seven dogs. When air dissects along fascial planes to produce emphysema, there may be impingement upon critical anatomical structures. Moreover, infection can be carried deeper into tissue spaces. The main symptom of emphysema is a crepitus of the swollen tissues (Figure 36).

In a study done on pigs, the investigators detected significant pressures during air-drying beyond the apex of the roots especially with apical root diameters of file sizes larger than #20. The authors concluded that compressed air should never be a component in the drying of a root canal that is open to the periapical tissues.[466]

The mishaps described in this chapter that could potentially cause permanent injury to a patient are disconcerting for any practitioner to consider. We recognize that knowledge of these injuries must encourage reflection on the safe and prudent practice of endodontics. Our ethical obligation to protect patients from harm is met when we as a profession can provide advanced and sophisticated therapies in a controlled manner with patient welfare as an overriding priority.

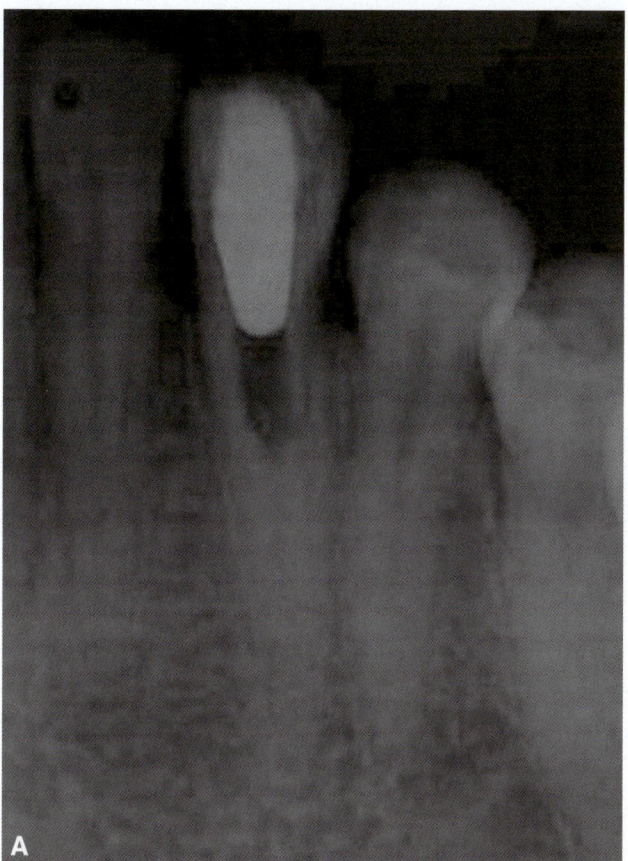
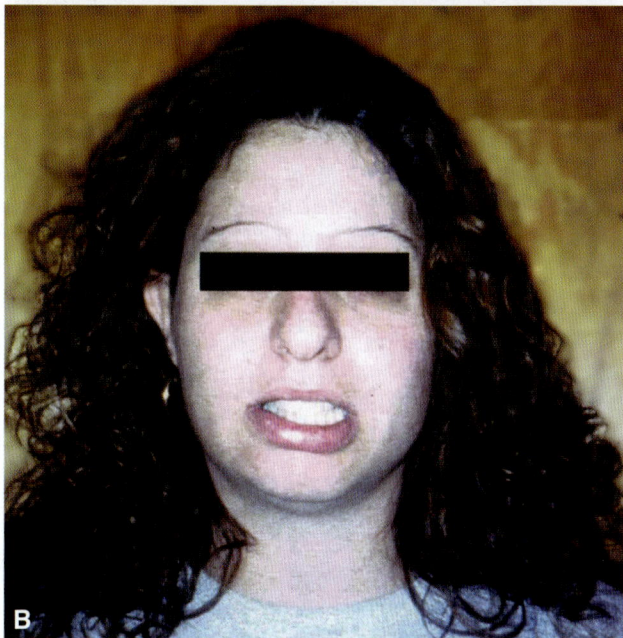

Figure 36 ***A,*** Radiograph of a lower left canine. The tooth was perforated during an attempt to locate the root canal space. An air emphysema complication occurred when air was blown into the access in an attempt to improve vision. ***B,*** The patient immediately experienced swelling and the characteristic air crepitus of the swollen tissues.

References

1. Cohn SA. Treatment choices for negative outcomes with non-surgical root canal treatment: non-surgical retreatment vs. surgical retreatment vs. implants. Endod Topics 2005;11(1):4–24.
2. Paik S, Sechrist C, Torabinejad M. Levels of evidence for the outcome of endodontic retreatment. J Endod 2004;30(11):745–50.
3. Doyle SL, Hodges JS, Pesun IJ, et al. Retrospective cross sectional comparison of initial nonsurgical endodontic treatment and single-tooth implants. J Endod 2006;32(9):822–7.
4. Torabinejad M, Goodacre CJ. Endodontic or dental implant therapy: The factors affecting treatment planning. J Am Dent Assoc 2006;137(7):973–7.
5. Kakehashi S, Stanley HR, Fitzgerald RJ. The effects of surgical exposures of dental pulps in germ-free and conventional laboratory rats. Oral Surg Oral Med Oral Pathol Oral Radiol Endod 1965;20:340–9.
6. Kakehashi S, Stanley HR, Fitzgerald RJ. The effects of surgical exposures of dental pulps in germfree and conventional laboratory rats. J South Calif Dent Assoc 1966;34(9):449–51.
7. Moller AJ, Fabricius L, Dahlen G, et al. Influence on periapical tissues of indigenous oral bacteria and necrotic pulp tissue in monkeys. Scand J Dent Res 1981;89(6):475–84.
8. Peciuliene V, Balciuniene I, Eriksen HM, Haapasalo M. Isolation of Enterococcus faecalis in previously root-filled canals in a Lithuanian population. J Endod 2000;26(10):593–5.
9. Peciuliene V, Reynaud AH, Balciuniene I, Haapasalo M. Isolation of yeasts and enteric bacteria in root-filled teeth with chronic apical periodontitis. Int Endod J 2001;34(6):429–34.
10. Nair PN. Pathogenesis of apical periodontitis and the causes of endodontic failures. Crit Rev Oral Biol Med 2004;15(6):348–81.
11. Peters OA, Laib A, Gohring TN, Barbakow F. Changes in root canal geometry after preparation assessed by high-resolution computed tomography. J Endod 2001;27(1):1–6.
12. Peters OA, Laib A, Ruegsegger P, Barbakow F. Three-dimensional analysis of root canal geometry by high-resolution computed tomography. J Dent Res 2000;79(6):1405–9.
13. Molander A, Reit C, Dahlen G, Kvist T. Microbiological status of root-filled teeth with apical periodontitis. Int Endod J 1998;31(1):1–7.
14. Hancock HH, 3rd, Sigurdsson A, Trope M, Moiseiwitsch J. Bacteria isolated after unsuccessful endodontic treatment in a North American population. Oral Surg Oral Med Oral Pathol Oral Radiol Endod 2001;91(5):579–86.
15. Chavez De Paz LE, Dahlen G, Molander A, et al. Bacteria recovered from teeth with apical periodontitis after antimicrobial endodontic treatment. Int Endod J 2003;36(7):500–8.

16. Nair PN, Sjogren U, Schumacher E, Sundqvist G. Radicular cyst affecting a root-filled human tooth: a long-term post-treatment follow-up. Int Endod J 1993;26(4):225–33.

17. Nair PN, Sjogren U, Sundqvist G. Cholesterol crystals as an etiological factor in non-resolving chronic inflammation: an experimental study in guinea pigs. Eur J Oral Sci 1998;106(2 Pt 1):644–50.

18. Nair PN, Sjogren U, Figdor D, Sundqvist G. Persistent periapical radiolucencies of root-filled human teeth, failed endodontic treatments, and periapical scars. Oral Surg Oral Med Oral Pathol Oral Radiol Endod 1999;87(5):617–27.

19. Nair PN. On the causes of persistent apical periodontitis: a review. Int Endod J 2006;39(4):249–81.

20. Sundqvist G, Figdor D. Endodontic treatment of apical periodontitis. In: Ørstavik D, Pitt Ford TR, editors. Essential endodontology. 2nd ed. Oxford: Blackwell Science; 1998. pp. 242–70.

21. Gorni FG, Gagliani MM. The outcome of endodontic retreatment: a 2-yr follow-up. J Endod 2004;30(1):1–4.

22. Pinheiro ET, Gomes BP, Ferraz CC, et al. Microorganisms from canals of root-filled teeth with periapical lesions. Int Endod J 2003;36(1):1–11.

23. Mah T, Basrani B, Santos JM, et al. Periapical inflammation affecting coronally-inoculated dog teeth with root fillings augmented by white MTA orifice plugs. J Endod 2003;29(7):442–6.

24. Siqueira JF, Jr., Rocas IN, Alves FR, Campos LC. Periradicular status related to the quality of coronal restorations and root canal fillings in a Brazilian population. Oral Surg Oral Med Oral Pathol Oral Radiol Endod 2005;100(3):369–74.

25. Friedman S. Considerations and concepts of case selection in the management of post-treatment endodontic disease (treatment failure). Endod Topics 2002(1):54–78.

26. Kvist T, Reit C. Postoperative discomfort associated with surgical and nonsurgical endodontic retreatment. Endod Dent Traumatol 2000;16(2):71–4.

27. Stabholz A, Friedman S. Endodontic retreatment–case selection and technique. Part 2: Treatment planning for retreatment. J Endod 1988;14(12):607–14.

28. Kvinnsland I, Oswald RJ, Halse A, Gronningsaeter AG. A clinical and roentgenological study of 55 cases of root perforation. Int Endod J 1989;22(2):75–84.

29. Suter B, Lussi A, Sequeira P. Probability of removing fractured instruments from root canals. Int Endod J 2005;38(2):112–23.

30. Spili P, Parashos P, Messer HH. The impact of instrument fracture on outcome of endodontic treatment. J Endod 2005;31(12):845–50.

31. Al-Ali K, Marghalani H, Al-Yahya A, Omar R. An assessment of endodontic re-treatment decision-making in an educational setting. Int Endod J 2005;38(7):470–6.

32. Abbott PV. Incidence of root fractures and methods used for post removal. Int Endod J 2002;35(1):63–7.

33. Torabinejad M, Chivian N. Clinical applications of mineral trioxide aggregate. J Endod 1999;25(3):197–205.

34. Peters CI, Peters OA. Occlusal loading of EBA and MTA root-end fillings in a computer-controlled masticator: a scanning electron microscopic study. Int Endod J 2002;35(1):22–9.

35. Main C, Mirzayan N, Shabahang S, Torabinejad M. Repair of root perforations using mineral trioxide aggregate: a long-term study. J Endod 2004;30(2):80–3.

36. Reit C, Grondahl HG. Endodontic retreatment decision making among a group of general practitioners. Scand J Dent Res 1988;96(2):112–17.

37. Stamos DE, Gutmann JL. Survey of endodontic retreatment methods used to remove intraradicular posts. J Endod 1993;19(7):366–9.

38. Friedman S. Prognosis of initial endodontic therapy. Endod Topics 2002;2:59–88.

39. Gorni FGM, Gaglinai MM. The outcome of endodontic retreatment: A 2-yr follow-up. J Endod 2004;30:1–4.

40. Friedman S. Treatment outcome and prognosis of endodontic therapy. Oxford: Blackwell Science Ltd.; 1998.

41. Abbott PV. Factors associated with continuing pain in endodontics. Aust Dent J 1994;39(3):157–61.

42. Hülsmann M. Removal of fractured instruments using a combined automated/ultrasonic technique. J Endod 1994;20(3):144–7.

43. Wu MK, Dummer PM, Wesselink PR. Consequences of and strategies to deal with residual post-treatment root canal infection. Int Endod J 2006;39(5):343–56.

44. Kvist T, Heden G, Reit C. Endodontic retreatment strategies used by general dental practitioners. Oral Surg Oral Med Oral Pathol Oral Radiol Endod 2004;97(4):502–7.

45. Reit C, Grondahl HG. Management of periapical lesions in endodontically treated teeth. A study on clinical decision making. Swed Dent J 1984;8(1):1–7.

46. Kvist T, Reit C, Esposito M, et al. Prescribing endodontic retreatment: towards a theory of dentist behaviour. Int Endod J 1994;27(6):285–90.

47. von Arx T. Failed root canals: the case for apicoectomy (periradicular surgery). J Oral Maxillofac Surg 2005;63(6):832–7.

48. Grung B, Molven O, Halse A. Periapical surgery in a Norwegian county hospital: follow-up findings of 477 teeth. J Endod 1990;16(9):411–17.

49. Reit C, Kvist T. Endodontic retreatment behaviour: the influence of disease concepts and personal values. Int Endod J 1998;31(5):358–63.

50. Kvist T, Reit C. The perceived benefit of endodontic retreatment. Int Endod J 2002;35(4):359–65.

51. Scott BJ, Leung KC, McMillan AS, et al. A transcultural perspective on the emotional effect of tooth loss in complete denture wearers. Int J Prosthodont 2001;14(5):461–5.

52. Gilbert GH, Duncan RP, Shelton BJ. Social determinants of tooth loss. Health Serv Res 2003;38(6 Pt 2):1843–62.

53. Omar R, Tashkandi E, Abduljabbar T, et al. Sentiments expressed in relation to tooth loss: a qualitative study among edentulous Saudis. Int J Prosthodont 2003;16(5):515–20.

54. Marshall FJ, Massler M. The sealing of pulpless teeth evaluated with radioisotopes. J Dent Med 1961;16:172–84.

55. Bergenholtz G, Spangberg L. Controversies in Endodontics. Crit Rev Oral Biol Med 2004;15(2):99–114.

56. Chailertvanitkul P, Saunders WP, Saunders EM, MacKenzie D. An evaluation of microbial coronal leakage in the restored pulp chamber of root-canal treated multirooted teeth. Int Endod J 1997;30(5):318–22.

57. De Moor R, Hommez G. [The importance of apical and coronal leakage in the success or failure of endodontic treatment]. Rev Belge Med Dent 2000;55(4):334–44.

58. Siqueira JF. The etiology of root canal treatment failure: Why well treated teeth can fail. Int Endod J 2001;34:1–10.

59. Sritharan A. Discuss that the coronal seal is more important than the apical seal for endodontic success. Aust Endod J 2002;28(3):112–15.

60. Kurtzman G. Restoring teeth with severe coronal breakdown as a prelude to endodontic therapy. Endod Therapy 2004;4:21–2.

61. Wu MK, Pehlivan Y, Kontakiotis EG, Wesselink PR. Microleakage along apical root fillings and cemented posts. The The J Prosthet Dent 1998;79(3):264–9.

62. Travassos RM, Caldas Ade F, de Albuquerque DS. Cohort study of endodontic therapy success. Braz Dent J 2003;14(2):109–13.

63. Begotka BA, Hartwell GR. The importance of the coronal seal following root canal treatment. Va Dent J 1996;73(4):8–10.

64. Kirkevang LL, Vaeth M, Horsted-Bindslev P, Wenzel A. Longitudinal study of periapical and endodontic status in a Danish population. Int Endod J 2006;39(2):100–7.

65. Tronstad L, Asbjornsen K, Doving L, et al. Influence of coronal restorations on the periapical health of endodontically treated teeth. Endod Dent Traumatol 2000;16(5):218–21.

66. Hommez GM, Coppens CR, De Moor RJ. Periapical health related to the quality of coronal restorations and root fillings. Int Endod J 2002;35(8):680–9.

67. Leonard JE, Gutmann JL, Guo IY. Apical and coronal seal of roots obturated with a dentine bonding agent and resin. Int Endod J 1996;29:76–83.

68. Swanson K, Madison S. An evaluation of coronal microleakage in endodontically treated teeth. Part I. Time periods. J Endod 1987;13(2):56–9.

69. Madison S, Swanson K, Chiles SA. An evaluation of coronal microleakage in endodontically treated teeth. Part II. Sealer types. J Endod 1987;13(3):109–12.

70. Goldman M, Laosonthorn P, White RR. Microleakage–full crowns and the dental pulp. J Endod 1992;18(10):473–5.

71. Saunders WP, Saunders EM. Assessment of leakage in the restored pulp chamber of endodontically treated multirooted teeth. Int Endod J 1990;23(1):28–33.

72. Magura ME, Kafrawy AH, Brown CE, Jr., Newton CW. Human saliva coronal microleakage in obturated root canals: an in vitro study. J Endod 1991;17(7):324–31.

73. Khayat A, Lee SJ, Torabinejad M. Human saliva penetration of coronally unsealed obturated root canals. J Endod 1993;19(9):458–61.

74. Siqueira JF, Jr., Rocas IN, Favieri A, et al. Bacterial leakage in coronally unsealed root canals obturated with 3 different techniques. Oral Surg Oral Med Oral Pathol Oral Radiol Endod 2000;90(5):647–50.

75. Adib V, Spratt D, Ng YL, Gulabivala K. Cultivable microbial flora associated with persistent periapical disease and coronal leakage after root canal treatment: a preliminary study. Int Endod J 2004;37(8):542–51.

76. Torabinejad M, Ung B, Kettering JD. In vitro bacterial penetration of coronally unsealed endodontically treated teeth. J Endod 1990;16(12):566–9.

77. Barrieshi KM, Walton RE, Johnson WT, Drake DR. Coronal leakage of mixed anaerobic bacteria after obturation and post space preparation. Oral Surg, Oral Med, Oral Pathol, Oral Radiol, and Endod 1997;84(3):310–14.

78. Chailertvanitkul P, Saunders WP, MacKenzie D. Coronal leakage of obturated root canals after long-term storage using a polymicrobial marker. J Endod 1997;23(10):610–13.

79. Hommez GM, Verhelst R, Claeys G, et al. Investigation of the effect of the coronal restoration quality on the composition of the root canal microflora in teeth with apical periodontitis by means of T-RFLP analysis. Int Endod J 2004;37(12):819–27.

80. Trope M, Chow E, Nissan R. In vitro endotoxin penetration of coronally unsealed endodontically treated teeth. Endod Dent Traumatol 1995;11(2):90–4.

81. Alves J, Walton R, Drake D. Coronal Leakage: Endotoxin from mixed bacterial communities through obturated, post-prepared root canals. J Endod 1998;24:587–91.

82. Metzger Z, Abramovitz R, Abramovitz L, Tagger M. Correlation between remaining length of root canal fillings after immediate post space preparation and coronal leakage. J Endod 2000;26(12):724–8.

83. Balto H, Al-Nazhan S, Al-Mansour K, et al. Microbial leakage of Cavit, IRM, and Temp Bond in post-prepared root canals using two methods of gutta-percha removal: an in vitro study. J Contemp Dent Pract 2005;6(3):53–61.

84. Pappen AF, Bravo M, Gonzalez-Lopez S, Gonzalez-Rodriguez MP. An in vitro study of coronal leakage after intraradicular preparation of cast-dowel space. J Prosthet Dent 2005;94(3):214–18.
85. Fishelberg G. Clinical response to a vacant post space. Int Endod J 2004;37(3):199–204.
86. Ray HA, Trope M. Periapical status of endodontically treated teeth in relation to the technical quality of the root filling and the coronal restoration. Int Endod J 1995;28(1):12–18.
87. Gutmann JL, Witherspoon DE. Obturation of the Cleaned and Shaped Root Canal System. In: Cohen S, Burns RC, editors. Pathways of the pulp. 8th ed. Saint Louis: Mosby Inc.;2002. pp. 293–364.
88. Britto LR, Grimaudo NJ, Vertucci FJ. Coronal microleakage assessed by polymicrobial markers. J Contemp Dent Pract 2003;4(3):1–10.
89. Kurtzman G. Improving Endodontic Success through Coronal Leakage Prevention. Inside Dent 2005;12:62–7.
90. Pisano DM, DiFiore PM, McClanahan SB, et al. Intraorifice sealing of gutta-percha obturated root canals to prevent coronal microleakage. J Endod 1998;24(10):659–62.
91. Kopper PM, Figueiredo JA, Della Bona A, et al. Comparative in vivo analysis of the sealing ability of three endodontic sealers in post-prepared root canals. Int Endod J 2003;36(12):857–63.
92. Ricucci D, Bergenholtz G. Bacterial status in root-filled teeth exposed to the oral environment by loss of restoration and fracture or caries–a histobacteriological study of treated cases. Int Endod J 2003;36(11):787–802.
93. Sidaravicius B, Aleksejuniene J, Eriksen HM. Endodontic treatment and prevalence of apical periodontitis in an adult population of Vilnius, Lithuania. Endod Dent Traumatol 1999;15(5):210–15.
94. Boucher Y, Matossian L, Rilliard F, Machtou P. Radiographic evaluation of the prevalence and technical quality of root canal treatment in a French subpopulation. Int Endod J 2002;35(3):229–38.
95. Fox K, Gutteridge DL. An in vitro study of coronal microleakage in root-canal-treated teeth restored by the post and core technique. Int Endod J 1997;30(6):361–8.
96. Demarchi MG, Sato EF. Leakage of interim post and cores used during laboratory fabrication of custom posts. J Endod 2002;28(4):328–9.
97. de Souza FD, Pecora JD, Silva RG. The effect on coronal leakage of liquid adhesive application over root fillings after smear layer removal with EDTA or Er:YAG laser. Oral Surg Oral Med Oral Pathol Oral Radiol Endod 2005;99(1):125–8.
98. Naoum HJ, Chandler NP. Temporization for endodontics. Int Endod J 2002;35(12):964–78.
99. Howdle MD, Fox K, Youngson CC. An in vitro study of coronal microleakage around bonded amalgam coronal-radicular cores in endodontically treated molar teeth. Quintessence Int 2002;33(1):22–9.
100. Kleitches AJ, Lemon RR, Jeansonne BG. Coronal microleakage in conservatively restored endodontic access preparations. J Tenn Dent Assoc 1995;75(1):31–4.
101. Grossman L. A study of temporary fillings as hermetic sealing agents. J Dent Res 1939;18:67–71.
102. Schwartz RS, Fransman R. Adhesive dentistry and endodontics: materials, clinical strategies and procedures for restoration of access cavities: a review. J Endod 2005;31(3):151–65.
103. Vail MM, Steffel CL. Preference of temporary restorations and spacers: a survey of Diplomates of the American Board of Endodontists. J Endod 2006;32(6):513–15.
104. Webber RT, del Rio CE, Brady JM, Segall RO. Sealing quality of a temporary filling material. Oral Surg Oral Med Oral Pathol Oral Radiol Endod 1978;46(1):123–30.
105. Blaney TD, Peters DD, Setterstrom J, Bernier WE. Marginal sealing quality of IRM and Cavit as assessed by microbiol penetration. J Endod 1981;7(10):453–7.
106. Anderson RW, Powell BJ, Pashley DH. Microleakage of IRM used to restore endodontic access preparations. Endod Dent Traumatol 1990;6(4):137–41.
107. Deveaux E, Hildelbert P, Neut C, et al. Bacterial microleakage of Cavit, IRM, and TERM. Oral Surg Oral Med Oral Pathol 1992;74(5):634–43.
108. Friedman S. Application of Glass-Ionomer in Endodontics. In: Davidson C, Mjor I, editors. Advances in glass-ionomer cements. Chicago: Quintessence Books; 1999. pp. 183–200.
109. Watson T. Bonding Glass-Ionomer Cements to Tooth Structure. In: Davidson C, Mjor I, editors. Advances in glass-ionomer cements. Chicago: Quintessence Books; 1999. pp. 121–35.
110. Tobias RS, Browne RM, Wilson CA. Antibacterial activity of dental restorative materials. Int Endod J 1985;18(3):161–71.
111. Chong BS, Owadally ID, Pitt Ford TR, Wilson RF. Antibacterial activity of potential retrograde root filling materials. Endod Dent Traumatol 1994;10(2):66–70.
112. Heling I, Chandler NP. The antimicrobial effect within dentinal tubules of four root canal sealers. J Endod 1996;22(5):257–9.
113. Herrera M, Castillo A, Baca P, Carrion P. Antibacterial activity of glass-ionomer restorative cements exposed to cavity-producing microorganisms. Oper Dent 1999;24(5):286–91.
114. Jacquot BM, Panighi MM, Steinmetz P, G'Sell C. Microleakage of Cavit, CavitW, CavitG and IRM by impedance spectroscopy. Int Endod J 1996;29(4):256–61.
115. Zmener O, Banegas G, Pameijer CH. Coronal microleakage of three temporary restorative materials: an in vitro study. J Endod 2004;30(8):582–4.
116. Sauaia TS, Gomes BP, Pinheiro ET, et al. Microleakage evaluation of intraorifice sealing materials in endodontically

treated teeth. Oral Surg Oral Med Oral Pathol Oral Radiol Endod 2006;102(2):242–6.

117. Cruz EV, Shigetani Y, Ishikawa K, et al. A laboratory study of coronal microleakage using four temporary restorative materials. Int Endod J 2002;35(4):315–20.

118. Barkhordar RA, Stark MM. Sealing ability of intermediate restorations and cavity design used in endodontics. Oral Surg Oral Med Oral Pathol Oral Radiol Endod 1990;69(1):99–101.

119. Lee YC, Yang SF, Hwang YF, et al. Microleakage of endodontic temporary restorative materials. J Endod 1993;19(10):516–20.

120. Hagemeier MK, Cooley RL, Hicks JL. Microleakage of five temporary endodontic restorative materials. J Esthet Dent 1990;2(6):166–9.

121. Turner JE, Anderson RW, Pashley DH, Pantera EA, Jr. Microleakage of temporary endodontic restorations in teeth restored with amalgam. J Endod 1990;16(1):1–4.

122. Anderson RW, Powell BJ, Pashley DH. Microleakage of temporary restorations in complex endodontic access preparations. J Endod 1989;15(11):526–9.

123. Shindo K, Kakuma Y, Ishikawa H, et al. The influence of orifice sealing with various filling materials on coronal leakage. Dent Mater J 2004;23(3):419–23.

124. Uranga A, Blum JY, Esber S, et al. A comparative study of four coronal obturation materials in endodontic treatment. J Endod 1999;25(3):178–80.

125. Nup C, Boylan R, Bhagat R, et al. An evaluation of resin-ionomers to prevent coronal microleakage in endodontically treated teeth. J Clin Dent 2000;11(1):16–19.

126. Jacquot BM, Panighi MM, Steinmetz P, G'Sell C. Evaluation of temporary restorations' microleakage by means of electrochemical impedance measurements. J Endod 1996;22(11):586–9.

127. Imura N, Otani SM, Campos MJ, et al. Bacterial penetration through temporary restorative materials in root-canal-treated teeth in vitro. Int Endod J 1997;30(6):381–5.

128. Scotti R, Ciocca L, Baldissara P. Microleakage of temporary endodontic restorations in overdenture tooth abutments. Int J Prosthodont 2002;15(5):479–82.

129. Kazemi RB, Safavi KE, Spangberg LS. Assessment of marginal stability and permeability of an interim restorative endodontic material. Oral Surg Oral Med Oral Pathol Oral Radiol Endod 1994;78(6):788–96.

130. Bobotis HG, Anderson RW, Pashley DH. A microleakage study of temporary restorative materials used in endodontics. J Endod 1989;15:569–72.

131. Balto H. An assessment of microbial coronal leakage of temporary filling materials in endodontically treated teeth. J Endod 2002;28(11):762–4.

132. Beach CW, Calhoun JC, Bramwell JD, et al. Clinical evaluation of bacterial leakage of endodontic temporary filling materials. J Endod 1996;22(9):459–62.

133. Barthel C, Strobach A, Briedigkeit H, et al. Leakage in Roots Coronally Sealed with Different Temporary Fillings. J Endod 1999;25(11):731–4.

134. Barthel CR, Zimmer S, Wussogk R, Roulet JF. Long-Term bacterial leakage along obturated roots restored with temporary and adhesive fillings. J Endod 2001;27(9):559–62.

135. Seiler KB. An evaluation of glass ionomer-based restorative materials as temporary restorations in endodontics. Gen Dent 2006;54(1):33–6.

136. Mayer T, Eickholz P. Microleakage of temporary restorations after thermocycling and mechanical loading. J Endod 1997;23(5):320–2.

137. Liberman R, Ben-Amar A, Frayberg E, et al. Effect of repeated vertical loads on microleakage of IRM and calcium sulfate-based temporary fillings. J Endod 2001;27(12):724–9.

138. Deveaux E, Hilderbert P, Neut C, Romond C. Bacterial Microleakage of Cavit, IRM, TERM, and Fermit: A 21-day In Vitro Study. J Endod 1999;25(10):653–9.

139. DuBois DJ, Reichl RB, Hondrum SO. The comparative radiopacity of Fuji IX-GP, an intermediate restorative material. Mil Med 2000;165(4):278–82.

140. Zaia AA, Nakagawa R, De Quadros I, et al. An in vitro evaluation of four materials as barriers to coronal microleakage in root-filled teeth. Int Endod J 2002;35(9):729–34.

141. Belli S, Zhang Y, Pereira PN, Pashley DH. Adhesive sealing of the pulp chamber. J Endod 2001;27(8):521–6.

142. Wolanek GA, Loushine RJ, Weller RN, et al. In vitro bacterial penetration of endodontically treated teeth coronally sealed with a dentin bonding agent. J Endod 2001;27(5):354–7.

143. Tselnik M, Baumgartner JC, Marshall JG. Bacterial leakage with mineral trioxide aggregate or a resin-modified glass ionomer used as a coronal barrier. J Endod 2004;30(11):782–4.

144. Mavec JC, McClanahan SB, Minah GE, et al. Effects of an intracanal glass ionomer barrier on coronal microleakage in teeth with post space. J Endod 2006;32(2):120–2.

145. Ruddle CJ. Nonsurgical retreatment. J Endod 2004;30(12):827–45.

146. Friedman S, Stabholz A. Endodontic retreatment–case selection and technique. Part 1: Criteria for case selection. J Endod 1986;12(1):28–33.

147. Friedman S, Stabholz A, Tamse A. Endodontic retreatment–case selection and technique. 3. Retreatment techniques. J Endod 1990;16(11):543–9.

148. Ruddle CJ. Nonsurgical endodontic retreatment. In: Cohen S, Burns RC, editors. Pathways of the pulp. St. Louis: Mosby; 2002. pp. 875–929.

149. Hoen MM, Pink FE. Contemporary endodontic retreatments: an analysis based on clinical treatment findings. J Endod 2002;28(12):834–6.

150. Wolcott J, Ishley D, Kennedy W, et al. Clinical investigation of second mesiobuccal canals in endodontically treated and retreated maxillary molars. J Endod 2002;28(6): 477–79.

151. Ruddle CJ. Microendodontic nonsurgical retreatment. In: Dent Clin North Am. Philadelphia: W.B. Saunders; 1997. pp. 429–54.

152. Schilder H. Filling root canals in three dimensions. Dent Clin North Am 1967:723–44.

153. Schilder H. Cleaning and shaping the root canal. Dent Clin North Am 1974;18(2):269–96.

154. Allen RK, Newton CW, Brown CE, Jr. A statistical analysis of surgical and nonsurgical endodontic retreatment cases. J Endod 1989;15(6):261–6.

155. Kvist T, Reit C. Results of endodontic retreatment: a randomized clinical study comparing surgical and nonsurgical procedures. J Endod 1999;25(12):814–17.

156. Ruddle C. Nonsurgical endodontic retreatment. J Calif Dent Assoc 1997;25(11):765–800.

157. Carr GB. Surgical endodontics. In: Cohen S, Burns RC, editors. Pathways of the pulp. 6th ed. St. Louis, Missouri, USA: Mosby–Year Book Inc.; 1994. pp. 531–67.

158. Ruddle CJ. Surgical endodontic retreatment. J Calif Dent Assoc 1991;19(5):61–7.

159. Kim S. Principles of endodontic microsurgery. Dent Clin North Am 1997;41(3):481–97.

160. Scianamblo MG. [Principal causes of endodontic failure]. Revue d Odonto-Stomatologie 1988;17(5):409–23.

161. Carr GB. Retreatment. In: Cohen S, Burns RC, editors. Pathways of the pulp. St. Louis: Mosby Co.; 1998. pp. 791–834.

162. Albers H. Tooth-Colored Restoratives. 8th ed. Santa Rosa, California: Alto Books; 1996.

163. Parreira FR, O'Connor RP, Hutter JW. Cast prosthesis removal using ultrasonics and a thermoplastic resin adhesive. J Endod 1994;20(3):141–3.

164. Barkhordar RA, Stewart GG. The potential of periodontal pocket formation associated with untreated accessory root canals. Oral Surg Oral Med Oral Pathol Oral Radiol Endod 1990;70(6):769–72.

165. Hess JC, Culieras MJ, Lambiable N. A scanning electron microscopic investigation of principal and accessory foramina on the root surfaces of human teeth: thoughts about endodontic pathology and therapeutics. J Endod 1983;9(7):275–81.

166. De Deus Q. Frequency, location and direction of the lateral, secondary, and accessory canals. J Endod 1975;1( ):361–6.

167. Ruddle CJ. Three-dimensional obturation: the rationale and application of warm gutta percha with vertical condensation. In: Cohen S, Burns RC, editors. Pathways of the pulp. St. Louis: Mosby Yearbook Co.; 1994.

168. Burns RC, Herbranson EJ. Tooth morphology and cavity preparations. In: Cohen S, Burns RC, editors. Pathways of the pulp. 7th ed. St. Louis Mosby Co.; 1998.

169. Pineda F, Kuttler Y. Mesiodistal and buccolingual roentgenographic investigation of 7,275 root canals. Oral Surg Oral Med Oral Pathol Oral Radiol Endod 1972;33(1):101–10.

170. Kersten HW, Wesselink PR, Thoden van Velzen SK. The diagnostic reliability of the buccal radiograph after root canal filling. Int Endod J 1987;20(1):20–4.

171. Mannan G, Smallwood ER, Gulabivala K. Effects of access cavity location and design on degree and distribution of instrumented root canal surface in maxillary anterior teeth. Int Endod J 2001;34:176–83.

172. Smith B. Removal of fractured posts using ultrasonic vibration: an in vivo study. J Endod 2001;27:632–4.

173. Gomes AP, Kubo CH, Santos RA, et al. The influence of ultrasound on the retention of cast posts cemented with different agents. Int Endod J 2001;34(2):93–9.

174. Johnson WT, Leary JM, Boyer DB. Effect of ultrasonic vibration on post removal in extracted human premolar teeth. J Endod 1996;22(9):487–8.

175. Wilcox LR, Krell KV, Madison S, Rittman B. Endodontic retreatment: evaluation of gutta-percha and sealer removal and canal reinstrumentation. J Endod 1987;13(9):453–7.

176. Tamse A, Unger U, Metzger Z, Rosenberg M. Gutta-percha solvents–a comparative study. J Endod 1986;12(8):337–9.

177. Barbosa SV, Burkard DH, Spangberg LS. Cytotoxic effects of gutta-percha solvents. J Endod 1994;20(1):6–8.

178. Kaplowitz GJ. Evaluation of Gutta-percha solvents. J Endod 1990;16(11):539–40.

179. Wilcox LR. Endodontic retreatment with halothane versus chloroform solvent. J Endod 1995;21(6):305–7.

180. Schirrmeister JF, Meyer KM, Hermanns P, et al. Effectiveness of hand and rotary instrumentation for removing a new synthetic polymer-based root canal obturation material (Epiphany) during retreatment. Int Endod J 2006;39(2):150–6.

181. Ezzie E, Fleury A, Solomon E, et al. Efficacy of retreatment techniques for a resin-based root canal obturation material. J Endod 2006;32(4):341–4.

182. Pinto de Oliveira D, Vicente Baroni Barbizam J, Trope M, Teixeira FB. Comparison between gutta-percha and resilon removal using two different techniques in endodontic retreatment. J Endod 2006;32(4):362–4.

183. Weine FS, Rice RT. Handling previously treated silver point cases: removal, retreatment, and tooth retention. Compend Contin Educ Dent 1986;7(9):652, 654–6, 658.

184. Goon WW. Managing the obstructed root canal space: rationale and techniques. Ensuring the soundness of the remaining tooth structure. J Calif Dent Assoc 1991;19(5):51–60.

185. Glick DH, Frank AL. Removal of silver points and fractured posts by ultrasonics. J Prosthet Dent 1986;55(2):212–15.
186. Roig-Greene JL. The retrieval of foreign objects from root canals: a simple aid. J Endod 1983;9(9):394–7.
187. Terauchi Y, O'Leary L, Suda H. Removal of separated files from root canals with a new file-removal system: Case Reports J Endod 2006;32:789–97.
188. Masserann J. [New method for extracting metallic fragments from canals]. Inf Dent 1972;54(43):3987–4005.
189. Suter B. A new method for retrieving silver points and separated instruments from root canals. J Endod 1998;24(6):446–8.
190. Bertrand MF, Pellegrino JC, Rocca JP, et al. Removal of Thermafil root canal filling material. J Endod 1997;23(1):54–7.
191. Vranas RN, Hartwell GR, Moon PC. The effect of endodontic solutions on resorcinol-formalin paste. J Endod 2003;29(1):69–72.
192. Wilcox LR. Endodontic retreatment: ultrasonics and chloroform as the final step in reinstrumentation. J Endod 1989;15(3):125–8.
193. Krell KV, Neo J. The use of ultrasonic endodontic instrumentation in the re-treatment of a paste-filled endodontic tooth. Oral Surg Oral Med Oral Pathol 1985;60(1):100–2.
194. Jeng HW, ElDeeb ME. Removal of hard paste fillings from the root canal by ultrasonic instrumentation. J Endod 1987;13(6):295–8.
195. Machtou P, Sarfati P, Cohen AG. Post removal prior to retreatment. J Endod 1989;15(11):552–4.
196. Hess W, Zurcher E. The Anatomy of the Root Canals of the Teeth of the Permanent and Deciduous Dentition. New York: William Wood & Co.; 1925.
197. Yoshida T, Gomyo S, Itoh T, et al. An experimental study of the removal of cemented dowel-retained cast cores by ultrasonic vibration. J Endod 1997;23(4):239–41.
198. Bergeron BE, Murchison DF, Schindler WG, Walker WA, 3rd. Effect of ultrasonic vibration and various sealer and cement combinations on titanium post removal. J Endod 2001;27(1):13–17.
199. Gluskin AH, Ahmed I, Herrero DB. The aesthetic post and core: unifying radicular form and structure. Pract Proced Aesthet Dent 2002;14(4):313–21; quiz 322.
200. Schwartz RS, Robbins JW. Post placement and restoration of endodontically treated teeth: a literature review. J Endod 2004;30(5):289–301.
201. Kleier DJ, Shibilski K, Averbach RE. Radiographic appearance of titanium posts in endodontically treated teeth. J Endod 1999;25(2):128–31.
202. Gluskin AH, Ruddle CJ, Zinman EJ. Thermal injury through intraradicular heat transfer using ultrasonic devices: precautions and practical preventive strategies. J Am Dent Assoc 2005;136(9):1286–93.
203. Satterthwaite JD, Stokes AN, Frankel NT. Potential for temperature change during application of ultrasonic vibration to intra-radicular posts. Eur J Prosthodont Restor Dent 2003;11(2):51–6.
204. Romero AD, Green DB, Wucherpfennig AL. Heat transfer to the periodontal ligament during root obturation procedures using an in vitro model. J Endod 2000;26(2):85–7.
205. Sweatman TL, Baumgartner JC, Sakaguchi RL. Radicular temperatures associated with thermoplasticized gutta-percha. J Endod 2001;27(8):512–15.
206. Gesi A, Magnolfi S, Goracci C, Ferrari M. Comparison of two techniques for removing fiber posts. J Endod 2003;29(9):580–2.
207. Gettleman BH, Spriggs KA, ElDeeb ME, Messer HH. Removal of canal obstructions with the Endo Extractor. J Endod 1991;17(12):608–11.
208. Dixon EB, Kaczkowski PJ, Nicholls JI, Harrington GW. Comparison of two ultrasonic instruments for post removal. J Endod 2002;28(2):111–15.
209. Buoncristiani J, Seto BG, Caputo AA. Evaluation of ultrasonic and sonic instruments for intraradicular post removal. J Endod 1994;20(10):486–9.
210. Altshul JH, Marshall G, Morgan LA, Baumgartner JC. Comparison of dentinal crack incidence and of post removal time resulting from post removal by ultrasonic or mechanical force. J Endod 1997;23(11):683–6.
211. Frank AL. The dilemma of the fractured instrument [editorial]. J Endod 1983;9(12):515–16.
212. Fors UG, Berg JO. Endodontic treatment of root canals obstructed by foreign objects. Int Endod J 1986;19(1):2–10.
213. Chenail BL, Teplitsky PE. Orthograde ultrasonic retrieval of root canal obstructions. J Endod 1987;13(4):186–90.
214. Berutti E, Chiandussi G, Gaviglio I, Ibba A. Comparative analysis of torsional and bending stresses in two mathematical models of nickel-titanium rotary instruments: ProTaper versus ProFile. J Endod 2003;29(1):15–19.
215. Wong R, Cho F. Microscopic management of procedural errors. Dent Clin North Am 1997;41(3):455–79.
216. Crump MC, Natkin E. Relationship of broken root canal instruments to endodontic case prognosis: a clinical investigation. J Am Dent Assoc 1970;80(6):1341–7.
217. Nagai O, Tani N, Kayaba Y, et al. Ultrasonic removal of broken instruments in root canals. Int Endod J 1986;19(6):298–304.
218. Baumgartner JC. Advanced Endodontics: Ruddle on Retreatment. J Endod 2002;28:413.
219. Mines P, Loushine R, West L, et al. Use of the microscope in endodontics: a report based questionnaire. J Endod 1999;25(11):755–8.

220. Ward JR, Parashos P, Messer HH. Evaluation of an ultrasonic technique to remove fractured rotary nickel-titanium endodontic instruments from root canals: an experimental study. J Endod 2003;29(11):756–63.

221. Ward JR, Parashos P, Messer HH. Evaluation of an ultrasonic technique to remove fractured rotary nickel-titanium endodontic instruments from root canals: clinical cases. J Endod 2003;29(11):764–7.

222. Hülsmann M, Schinkel I. Influence of several factors on the success or failure of removal of fractures instruments from the root canal. Endod Dent Traumatol 1999;15:252–8.

223. Peters OA, Laib A, Rüegsegger P, Barbakow F. Three dimensional analysis of root canal geometry using high resolution computed tomography. J Dent Res 2000;79:1405–9.

224. Rhodes JS, Pitt Ford TR, Lynch PJ, et al. Micro-computed tomograpy: a new tool for experimental endodontology. Int Endod J 1999;32:165–70.

225. Gorni FGM. The removal of broken instruments. Endod Prac 2001;4(3):21–6.

226. Vertucci F. Root canal morphology and its relationship to endodontic procedures. Endod Topics2005;10(1):3–29.

227. Ruddle C. Cleaning and shaping the root canal system. In: Cohen S, Burns RC, editors. Pathways of the pulp. 8th ed. St. Louis MO: Mosby; 2002. pp. 231–92.

228. Parashos P, Messer HH. Questionnaire survey on the use of rotary nickel-titanium endodontic instrument by Australian dentists. Int Endod J 2004;37:249–59.

229. Peng B, Shen Y, Cheung GS, Xia TJ. Defects in ProTaper S1 instruments after clinical use: longitudinal examination. Int Endod J 2005;38:550–7.

230. Sattapan B, Nervo GJ, Palamara JE, Messer HH. Defects in rotary Nickel-Titanium files after clinical use. J Endod 2000;26:161–5.

231. Nehme W. A new approach for the retrieval of broken instruments. J Endod 1999;25(9):633–5.

232. Fors UG, Berg JO. A method for the removal of broken endodontic instruments from root canals. J Endod 1983;9(4):156–9.

233. Hülsmann M. Removal of silver cones and fractured instruments using the Canal Finder System. J Endod 1990;16(12):596–600.

234. Ruddle C. Finishing the apical one-third. Endod Prac 2002;5(3):15–26.

235. Eleazer PD, O'Connor RP. Innovative uses for hypodermic needles in endodontics. J Endod 1999;25(3):190–1.

236. D'Arcangelo C, Varvara G, De Fazio P. Broken instrument removal–two cases. J Endod 2000;26(6):368–70.

237. Ruddle CJ. The Protaper Technique. Endod Topics2005;10:187–90.

238. Briseno BM, Sonnabend E. The influence of different root canal instruments on root canal preparation: an in vitro study. Int Endod J 1991;24(1):15–23.

239. Lee SJ, Monsef M, Torabinejad M. Sealing ability of a mineral trioxide aggregate for repair of lateral root perforations. J Endod 1993;19(11):541–4.

240. Torabinejad M, Watson TF, Pitt Ford TR. Sealing ability of a mineral trioxide aggregate when used as a root end filling material. J Endod 1993;19(12):591–5.

241. Pitt Ford TR, Torabinejad M, McKendry DJ, et al. Use of mineral trioxide aggregate for repair of furcal perforations. Oral Surg Oral Med Oral Pathol Oral Radiol Endod 1995;79(6):756–63.

242. Jew RC, Weine FS, Keene JJ, Jr., Smulson MH. A histologic evaluation of periodontal tissues adjacent to root perforations filled with Cavit. Oral Surg Oral Med Oral Pathol Oral Radiol Endod 1982;54(1):124–35.

243. West J, Roane J, Goerig A. Cleaning and shaping the root canal system. In: Cohen S, Burns R, editors. Pathways of the pulp. 6th ed. Saint Louis: Mosby-Yearbook Inc.; 1994. pp. 179–218.

244. Zinman E. Records and legal resposibilities. In: Cohen S, Burns R, editors. Pathways of the pulp. 6th ed. Saint Louis: Mosby-Yearbook Inc.; 1994. pp. 272–94.

245. Seltzer S, Bender IB, Smith J, et al. Endodontic failures—an analysis based on clinical, roentgenographic, and histologic findings. II. Oral Surg Oral Med Oral Pathol Oral Radiol Endod 1967;23(4):517–30.

246. Seltzer S, Sinai I, August D. Periodontal effects of root perforations before and during endodontic procedures. J Dent Res 1970;49(2):332–9.

247. Duggins LD, Clay JR, Himel VT, Dean JW. A combined endodontic retrofill and periodontal guided tissue regeneration technique for the repair of molar endodontic furcation perforations: report of a case. Quintessence Int 1994;25(2):109–14.

248. Frank AL. Resorption, perforations, and fractures. Dent Clin North Am 1974;18(2):465–87.

249. Himel VT, Brady J, Jr., Weir J, Jr. Evaluation of repair of mechanical perforations of the pulp chamber floor using biodegradable tricalcium phosphate or calcium hydroxide. J Endod 1985;11(4):161–5.

250. Lantz B, Persson PA. Periodontal tissue reactions after root perforations in dog's teeth. A histologic study. Odontol Tidskr 1967;75(3):209–37.

251. Beavers RA, Bergenholtz G, Cox CF. Periodontal wound healing following intentional root perforations in permanent teeth of Macaca mulatta. Int Endod J 1986;19(1):36–44.

252. Euler H. Perforation und Parodontium. Deutsche Medizinische Zahnheilkunde 1925;44(4):801–11.

253. Kübler A. Heilungsvorgänge nach Wurzelperforationen. Deutsche Medizinische Zahnheilkunde 1934;44(4):413–54.

254. Ruchenstein H. Perforations Radiculariers Traitees au Calxyl. Deutsche Medizinische Zahnheilk 1994;13(5):48–53.

255. Kauffman J. Untersuchungen am Parodontium der traumatisch perforierten Zahnwurzel. Deutsche Medizinische Zahnheilkunde 1944;54(5):387.

256. Bhaskar SN, Rappaport HM. Histologic evaluation of endodontic procedures in dogs. Oral Surg Oral Med Oral Pathol Oral Radiol Endod 1971;31(4):526–35.

257. Sinai IH. Endodontic perforations: their prognosis and treatment. J Am Dent Assoc 1977;95(1):90–5.

258. Oswald RJ. Procedural accidents and their repair. Dent Clin North Am 1979;23(4):593–616.

259. Martin LR, Gilbert B, Dickerson AWD. Management of endodontic perforations. Oral Surg Oral Med Oral Pathol Oral Radiol Endod 1982;54(6):668–77.

260. Aguirre R, elDeeb ME. Evaluation of the repair of mechanical furcation perforations using amalgam, gutta-percha, or indium foil. J Endod 1986;12(6):249–56.

261. Biggs JT, Benenati FW, Sabala CL. Treatment of iatrogenic root perforations with associated osseous lesions. J Endod 1988;14(12):620–4.

262. Benenati FW, Roane JB, Biggs JT, Simon JH. Recall evaluation of iatrogenic root perforations repaired with amalgam and gutta-percha. J Endod 1986;12(4):161–6.

263. Meister F, Jr., Lommel TJ, Gerstein H, Davies EE. Endodontic perforations which resulted in alveolar bone loss. Report of five cases. Oral Surg Oral Med Oral Pathol Oral Radiol Endod 1979;47(5):463–70.

264. Stromberg T, Hasselgren G, Bergstedt H. Endodontic treatment of resorptive periapical osteitis with fistula. A clinical and roentgenological follow-up study. Svensk Tandlakaretidskrift 1972;65(9):467–74.

265. Petersson K, Hasselgren G, Tronstad L. Endodontic treatment of experimental root perforations in dog teeth. Endod Dent Traumatol 1985;1(1):22–8.

266. Bramante CM, Berbert A. Root perforations dressed with calcium hydroxide or zinc oxide and eugenol. J Endod 1987;13(8):392–5.

267. Alhadainy HA. Root perforations. A review of literature. Oral Surg Oral Med Oral Pathol Oral Radiol Endod 1994;78(3):368–74.

268. Moreinis SA. Avoiding perforation during endodontic access. J Am Dent Assoc 1979;98(5):707–12.

269. Ingle JI, Glick DH. Modern endodontic therapy. In: Ingle JI, editor. Endodontics. Philadelphia: Lea & Febiger; 1965. pp. 35–77.

270. Nicholls E. Treatment of traumatic perforations of the pulp cavity. Oral Surg Oral Med Oral Pathol 1962;15:603–12.

271. Barnes IE. Surgical endodontics. 7. The repair of perforations. Dent Update 1981;8(7):503–5, 508–13.

272. Balla R, LoMonaco CJ, Skribner J, Lin LM. Histological study of furcation perforations treated with tricalcium phosphate, hydroxylapatite, amalgam, and Life. J Endod 1991;17(5):234–8.

273. ElDeeb ME, ElDeeb M, Tabibi A, Jensen JR. An evaluation of the use of amalgam, Cavit, and calcium hydroxide in the repair of furcation perforations. J Endod 1982;8(10):459–66.

274. Harris WE. A simplified method of treatment for endodontic perforations. J Endod 1976;2(5):126–34.

275. Roane JB, Benenati FW. Successful management of a perforated mandibular molar using amalgam and hydroxylapatite. J Endod 1987;13(8):400–4.

276. Oynick J, Oynick T. A study of a new material for retrograde fillings. J Endod 1978;4(7):203–6.

277. Oynick J, Oynick T. Treatment of endodontic perforations. J Endod 1985;11(4):191–2.

278. Tuggle ST, Anderson RW, Pantera EA, Jr., Neaverth EJ. A dye penetration study of retrofilling materials. J Endod 1989;15(3):122–4.

279. Szeremeta-Browar TL, VanCura JE, Zaki AE. A comparison of the sealing properties of different retrograde techniques: an autoradiographic study. Oral Surg Oral Med Oral Pathol Oral Radiol Endod 1985;59(1):82–7.

280. Owadally ID, Chong BS, Pitt Ford TR, Wilson RF. Biological properties of IRM with the addition of hydroxyapatite as a retrograde root filling material. Endod Dent Traumatol 1994;10(5):228–32.

281. Moloney LG, Feik SA, Ellender G. Sealing ability of three materials used to repair lateral root perforations. J Endod 1993;19(2):59–62.

282. Pitt Ford TR, Andreasen JO, Dorn SO, Kariyawasam SP. Effect of various zinc oxide materials as root-end fillings on healing after replantation. Int Endod J 1995;28(6):273–8.

283. Dorn SO, Gartner AH. Retrograde filling materials: a retrospective success-failure study of amalgam, EBA, and IRM. J Endod 1990;16(8):391–3.

284. Chong BS, Owadally ID, Pitt Ford TR, Wilson RF. Cytotoxicity of potential retrograde root-filling materials. Endod Dent Traumatol 1994;10(3):129–33.

285. Dazey S, Senia ES. An in vitro comparison of the sealing ability of materials placed in lateral root perforations. J Endod 1990;16(1):19–23.

286. Al-Ajam AD, McGregor AJ. Comparison of the sealing capabilities of Ketac-silver and extra high copper alloy amalgam when used as retrograde root canal filling. J Endod 1993;19(7):353–6.

287. Alhadainy HA, Himel VT. Comparative study of the sealing ability of light-cured versus chemically cured materials placed into furcation perforations. Oral Surg Oral Med Oral Pathol Oral Radiol Endod 1993;76(3):338–42.

288. Alhadainy HA, Himel VT. Evaluation of the sealing ability of amalgam, Cavit, and glass ionomer cement in the repair of furcation perforations. Oral Surg Oral Med Oral Pathol Oral Radiol Endod 1993;75(3):362–6.

289. Callis PD, Santini A. Tissue response to retrograde root fillings in the ferret canine: a comparison of a glass ionomer cement and gutta-percha with sealer. Oral Surg Oral Med Oral Pathol Oral Radiol Endod 1987;64(4):475–9.

290. Pitt Ford TR, Roberts GJ. Tissue response to glass ionomer retrograde root fillings. Int Endod J 1990;23(5):233–8.

291. Torabinejad M, Hong CU, McDonald F, Pitt Ford TR. Physical and chemical properties of a new root-end filling material. J Endod 1995;21(7):349–53.

292. Pitt Ford TR, Andreasen JO, Dorn SO, Kariyawasam SP. Effect of super-EBA as a root end filling on healing after replantation. J Endod 1995;21(1):13–15.

293. Torabinejad M, Hong CU, Pitt Ford TR, Kettering JD. Antibacterial effects of some root end filling materials. J Endod 1995;21(8):403–6.

294. Torabinejad M, Hong CU, Pitt Ford TR, Kettering JD. Cytotoxicity of four root end filling materials. J Endod 1995;21(10):489–92.

295. Torabinejad M, Hong CU, Pitt Ford TR, Kaiyawasam SP. Tissue reaction to implanted super-EBA and mineral trioxide aggregate in the mandible of guinea pigs: a preliminary report. J Endod 1995;21(11):569–71.

296. Torabinejad M, Hong CU, Lee SJ, et al. Investigation of mineral trioxide aggregate for root-end filling in dogs. J Endod 1995;21(12):603–8.

297. Souza NJ, Justo GZ, Oliveira CR, et al. Cytotoxicity of materials used in perforation repair tested using the V79 fibroblast cell line and the granulocyte-macrophage progenitor cells. Int Endod J 2006;39(1):40–7.

298. Chng HK, Islam I, Yap AU, et al. Properties of a new root-end filling material. J Endod 2005;31(9):665–8.

299. Yildirim T, Gencoglu N, Firat I, et al. Histologic study of furcation perforations treated with MTA or Super EBA in dogs' teeth. Oral Surg Oral Med Oral Pathol Oral Radiol Endod 2005;100(1):120–4.

300. Baek SH, Plenk H, Jr., Kim S. Periapical tissue responses and cementum regeneration with amalgam, SuperEBA, and MTA as root-end filling materials. J Endod 2005;31(6):444–9.

301. Hauman CH, Love RM. Biocompatibility of dental materials used in contemporary endodontic therapy: a review. Part 2. Root-canal-filling materials. Int Endod J 2003;36(3):147–60.

302. Holland R, Filho JA, de Souza V, et al. Mineral trioxide aggregate repair of lateral root perforations. J Endod 2001;27(4):281–4.

303. De Deus G, Ximenes R, Gurgel-Filho ED, et al. Cytotoxicity of MTA and Portland cement on human ECV 304 endothelial cells. Int Endod J 2005;38(9):604–9.

304. Torabinejad M, Smith PW, Kettering JD, Pitt Ford TR. Comparative investigation of marginal adaptation of mineral trioxide aggregate and other commonly used root-end filling materials. J Endod 1995;21(6):295–9.

305. Torabinejad M, Rastegar AF, Kettering JD, Pitt Ford TR. Bacterial leakage of mineral trioxide aggregate as a root-end filling material. J Endod 1995;21(3):109–12.

306. Nakata TT, Bae KS, Baumgartner JC. Perforation repair comparing mineral trioxide aggregate and amalgam using an anaerobic bacterial leakage model. J Endod 1998;24(3):184–6.

307. Tsatsas DV, Meliou HA, Kerezoudis NP. Sealing effectiveness of materials used in furcation perforation in vitro. Int Dent J 2005;55(3):133–41.

308. Daoudi MF, Saunders WP. In vitro evaluation of furcal perforation repair using mineral trioxide aggregate or resin modified glass Ionomer cement with and without the use of the operating microscope. J Endod 2002;28(7):512–15.

309. Torabinejad M, Higa RK, McKendry DJ, Pitt Ford TR. Dye leakage of four root end filling materials: effects of blood contamination. J Endod 1994;20(4):159–63.

310. Menezes R, da Silva Neto UX, Carneiro E, et al. MTA repair of a supracrestal perforation: a case report. J Endod 2005;31(3):212–14.

311. Arens DE, Torabinejad M. Repair of furcal perforations with mineral trioxide aggregate: two case reports. Oral Surg, Oral Med, Oral Pathol, Oral Radiol, Endod 1996;82(1):84–8.

312. Bargholz C. Perforation repair with mineral trioxide aggregate: a modified matrix concept. Int Endod J 2005;38(1):59–69.

313. Weldon JK, Jr., Pashley DH, Loushine RJ, et al. Sealing ability of mineral trioxide aggregate and super-EBA when used as furcation repair materials: a longitudinal study. J Endod 2002;28(6):467–70.

314. de Morais CA, Bernardineli N, Garcia RB, et al. Evaluation of tissue response to MTA and Portland cement with iodoform. Oral Surg Oral Med Oral Pathol Oral Radiol Endod 2006;102(3):417–21.

315. Islam I, Chng HK, Yap AU. X-ray diffraction analysis of mineral trioxide aggregate and Portland cement. Int Endod J 2006;39(3):220–5.

316. De Deus G, Petruccelli V, Gurgel-Filho E, Coutinho-Filho T. MTA versus Portland cement as repair material for furcal perforations: a laboratory study using a polymicrobial leakage model. Int Endod J 2006;39(4):293–8.

317. Ferris DM, Baumgartner JC. Perforation repair comparing two types of mineral trioxide aggregate. J Endod 2004;30(6):422–4.

318. Blumenthal NM. The use of collagen membranes for guided tissue regeneration. Compend Contin Educ Dent 1992;13(3):214, 216, 218 passim.

319. Sottosanti J. Calcium sulfate: a biodegradable and biocompatible barrier for guided tissue regeneration. Compend Contin Educ Dent 1992;13(3):226–8, 230, 232–34.
320. Simon JH, Glick DH, Frank AL. The relationship of endodontic-periodontal lesions. J Periodontol 1972;43(4):202–8.
321. Hiatt WH. Pulpal periodontal disease. J Periodontol 1977;48(9):598–609.
322. Nevins M, Mellonig JT. Periodontal therapy, clinical approaches and evidence of success. Chicago: Quintessence Publishing Co.; 1998.
323. Kois JC. The restorative-periodontal interface: biological parameters. Periodontol 2000 1996;11:29–38.
324. Shanelec DA, Tibbetts LS. A perspective on the future of periodontal microsurgery. Periodontol 2000 1996;11:58–64.
325. Kim S, Rethnam S. Hemostasis in endodontic microsurgery. Dent Clin North Am 1997;41(3):499–511.
326. Hammarstrom LE, Blomlof LB, Feiglin B, Lindskog SF. Effect of calcium hydroxide treatment on periodontal repair and root resorption. Endod Dent Traumatol 1986;2(5):184–9.
327. Lemon RR, Steele PJ, Jeansonne BG. Ferric sulfate hemostasis: effect on osseous wound healing. Left in situ for maximum exposure. J Endod 1993;19(4):170–3.
328. Pecora G, Baek SH, Rethnam S, Kim S. Barrier membrane techniques in endodontic microsurgery. Dent Clin North Am 1997;41(3):585–602.
329. Alhadainy HA, Abdalla AI. Artificial floor technique used for the repair of furcation perforations: a microleakage study. J Endod 1998;24(1):33–5.
330. Himel VT, Alhadainy HA. Effect of dentin preparation and acid etching on the sealing ability of glass ionomer and composite resin when used to repair furcation perforations over plaster of Paris barriers. J Endod 1995;21(3):142–5.
331. Koh ET, McDonald F, Pitt Ford TR, Torabinejad M. Cellular response to mineral trioxide aggregate. J Endod 1998;24:543–7.
332. Chau JY, Hutter JW, Mork TO, Nicoll BK. An in vitro study of furcation perforation repair using calcium phosphate cement. J Endod 1997;23(9):588–92.
333. Bailey GC, Cunnington SA, Ng YL, et al. Ultrasonic condensation of gutta-percha: the effect of power setting and activation time on temperature rise at the root surface - an in vitro study. Int Endod J 2004;37(7):447–54.
334. Atrizadeh F, Kennedy J, Zander H. Ankylosis of teeth following thermal injury. Journal of periodontal research 1971;6(3):159–67.
335. Saunders EM, Saunders WP. The heat generated on the external root surface during post space preparation. Int Endod J 1989;22(4):169–73.
336. Barkhordar RA, Goodis HE, Watanabe L, Koumdjian J. Evaluation of temperature rise on the outer surface of teeth during root canal obturation techniques. Quintessence International 1990;21(7):585–8.
337. Weller RN, Koch KA. In vitro radicular temperatures produced by injectable thermoplasticized gutta-percha. Int Endod J 1995;28(2):86–90.
338. Hussey DL, Biagioni PA, McCullagh JJ, Lamey PJ. Thermographic assessment of heat generated on the root surface during post space preparation. Int Endod J 1997;30(3):187–90.
339. Kreisler M, Al-Haj H, D'Hoedt B. Intrapulpal temperature changes during root surface irradiation with an 809-nm GaAlAs laser. Oral Surg Oral Med Oral Pathol Oral Radiol Endod 2002;93(6):730–5.
340. Eriksson AR, Albrektsson T. Temperature threshold levels for heat-induced bone tissue injury: a vital-microscopic study in the rabbit. J Prosthet Dent 1983;50(1):101–7.
341. Abrams H, Barkmeier WW, Cooley RL. Temperature changes in the pulp chamber produced by ultrasonic instrumentation. Gen Dent 1979;27(5):62–4.
342. Zach L, Cohen G. Pulp response to externally applied heat. Oral Surg Oral Med Oral Pathol Oral Radiol Endod 1965;19(4):515–30.
343. Budd JC, Gekelman D, White JM. Temperature rise of the post and on the root surface during ultrasonic post removal. Int Endod J 2005;38(10):705–11.
344. Huttula AS Tordik PA, Imamura G, et al. The effect of ultrasonic vibration on root surface temperature. J Endod 2006;32:247.
345. Kuttler S, McLean A, Dorn S, Fischzang A. The impact of post space preparation with Gates-Glidden drills on residual dentin thickness in distal roots of mandibular molars. J Am Dent Assoc 2004;135(7):903–9.
346. Langlais RP, Rodriguez IE, Maselle I. Principles of radiographic selection and interpretation. Dent Clin North Am 1994;38:1–12.
347. Van Dis ML, Miles DA. Disorders of the maxillary sinus. Dent Clin North Am 1994;38(1):155–66.
348. Selden HS. The interrelationship between the maxillary sinus and endodontics. Oral Surg Oral Med Oral Pathol Oral Radiol Endod 1974;38(4):623–9.
349. Watzek G, Bernhart T, Ulm C. Complications of sinus perforations and their management in endodontics. Dent Clin North Am 1997;41(3):563–83.
350. Dodd RB, Dodds RN, Hocomb JB. An endodontically induced maxillary sinusitis. J Endod 1984;10(10):504–6.
351. Selden HS. Endo-Antral syndrome and various endodontic complications. J Endod 1999;25(5):389–93.
352. Selden HS. The endo-antral syndrome: an endodontic complication. J Am Dent Assoc 1989;119(3):397–8, 401–392.
353. Rigolone M, Pasqualini D, Bianchi L, et al. Vestibular surgical access to the palatine root of the superior first molar:

"low-dose cone-beam" CT analysis of the pathway and its anatomic variations. J Endod 2003;29(11):773–5.

354. Velvart P, Hecker H, Tillinger G. Detection of the apical lesion and the mandibular canal in conventional radiography and computed tomography. Oral Surg Oral Med Oral Pathol Oral Radiol Endod 2001;92(6):682–8.

355. Phillips JL, Weller RN, Kulild JC. The mental foramen: 1. Size, orientation, and positional relationship to the mandibular second premolar. J Endod 1990;16(5):221–3.

356. Phillips JL, Weller RN, Kulild JC. The mental foramen: 2. Radiographic position in relation to the mandibular second premolar. J Endod 1992;18(6):271–4.

357. Phillips JL, Weller RN, Kulild JC. The mental foramen: 3. Size and position on panoramic radiographs. J Endod 1992;18(8):383–6.

358. Martini FH Timmons MJ, McKinley MP. Human Anatomy. 3rd ed. New Jersey: Prentice Hall; 2000.

359. Young B, Heath JW. Wheater's Functional Histology, a text and colour atlas. 4th ed. Edinburgh: Churchill Livingston; 2000.

360. Denio D, Torabinejad M, Bakland LK. Anatomical relationship of the mandibular canal to its surrounding structures in mature mandibles. J Endod 1992;18(4):161–5.

361. Carter RB, Keen EN. The intramandibular course of the inferior alveolar nerve. J Anat 1971;108(Pt 3):433–40.

362. Langeland K. Root canal sealants and pastes. Dent Clin North Am 1974;18(2):309–27.

363. Block RM, Lewis RD, Hirsch J, et al. Systemic distribution of 14C-labeled Paraformaldehyde incorporated within Formocresol following pulpotomies in dogs. J Endod 1983;9(5):176–89.

364. Branstetter J, von Fraunhofer JA. The physical properties and sealing action of endodontic sealer cements: a review of the literature. J Endod 1982;8(7):312–16.

365. Nair PN, Sjogren U, Krey G, Sundqvist G. Therapy-resistant foreign body giant cell granuloma at the periapex of a root-filled human tooth. J Endod 1990;16(12):589–95.

366. Briseno BM, Willershausen B. Root canal sealer cytotoxicity on human gingival fibroblasts. 1. Zinc oxide-eugenol-based sealers. J Endod 1990;16(8):383–6.

367. Briseno BM, Willershausen B. Root canal sealer cytotoxicity on human gingival fibroblasts: 2. Silicone- and resin-based sealers. J Endod 1991;17(11):537–40.

368. Briseno BM, Willershausen B. Root Canal Sealer Cytotoxicity with Human Gingival Fibroblasts. 3. Calcium hydroxide-based sealers. J Endod 1992;18:110–13.

369. Friend LA, Browne RM. Tissue reactions to some root filling materials. Br Dent J 1968;125(7):291–8.

370. Curson I, Kirk EE. An assessment of root canal-sealing cements. Oral Surg Oral Med Oral Pathol Oral Radiol Endod 1968;26(2):229–36.

371. Zmener O. Tissue response to a new methacrylate-based root canal sealer: preliminary observations in the subcutaneous connective tissue of rats. J Endod 2004;30(5):348–51.

372. Murazabal M, Erausquin J, Devoto FH. A study of periapical overfilling root canal treatment in the molar of the rat. Archives of oral biology 1966;11(4):373–83.

373. Rowe AH. Effect of root filling materials on the periapical tissues. Br Dent J 1967;122(3):98–102.

374. Ørstavik D, Brodin P, Aas E. Paraesthesia following endodontic treatment: survey of the literature and report of a case. Int Endod J 1983;16(4):167–72.

375. Kawakami T, Nakamura C, Eda S. Effects of the penetration of a root canal filling material into the mandibular canal. 1. Tissue reaction to the material. Endod Dent Traumatol 1991;7(1):36–41.

376. Kawakami T, Nakamura C, Eda S. Effects of the penetration of a root canal filling material into the mandibular canal. 2. Changes in the alveolar nerve tissue. Endod Dent Traumatol 1991;7(1):42–7.

377. Ørstavik D, Mjor IA. Histopathology and x-ray microanalysis of the subcutaneous tissue response to endodontic sealers. J Endod 1988;14(1):13–23.

378. Spångberg LS. Biological effects of root canal filling materials. 7. Reaction of bony tissue to implanted root canal filling material in guinea pigs. Odontol Tidskr 1969;77(2):133–59.

379. Kozam G. The effect of eugenol on nerve transmission. Oral Surg Oral Med Oral Pathol 1977;44(5):799–805.

380. Holland GR. A histological comparison of periapical inflammatory and neural responses to two endodontic sealers in the ferret. Arch Oral Biol 1994;39(7):539–44.

381. Boiesen J, Brodin P. Neurotoxic effect of two root canal sealers with calcium hydroxide on rat phrenic nerve in vitro. Endod Dent Traumatol 1991;7(6):242–5.

382. Serper A, Uncer O, Onur R, Etikan I. Comparative neurotoxic effects of root canal filling material on rat sciatic nerve. J Endod 1998;24:592–4.

383. Seidler B. Irrationalized endodontics: N2 and us too. J Am Dent Assoc 1974;89(6):1318–31.

384. Sargenti A, Richter S. Rationalized root canal treatment New York: AGSA Scientific Publications; 1959.

385. Montgomery S. Paresthesia following endodontic treatment. J Endod 1976;2(11):345–7.

386. Forman GH, Rood JP. Successful retrieval of endodontic material from the inferior alveolar nerve. J Dent 1977;5(1):47–50.

387. Kaufman AY, Rosenberg L. Paresthesia caused by endomethasone. J Endod 1980;6(4):529–31.

388. LaBlanc JP, Epker BN. Serious inferior alveolar nerve dysesthesia after endodontic procedure: report of three cases. JADA 1984;108:605–7.

389. Fanibunda KB. Adverse response to endodontic material containing paraformaldehyde. Br Dent J 1984;157(7):231–5.

390. Allard KU. Paraesthesia—a consequence of a controversial root-filling material? A case report. Int Endod J 1986;19(4):205–8.

391. Kleier DJ, Averbach RE. Painful dysesthesia of the inferior alveolar nerve following use of a paraformaldehyde-containing root canal sealer. Endod Dent Traumatol 1988;4(1):46–8.

392. Brodin P. Neurotoxic and analgesic effects of root canal cements and pulp-protecting dental materials. Endod Dent Traumatol 1988;4(1):1–11.

393. Barker BC, Lockett BC. Periapical response to N2 and other paraformaldehyde compounds confined within or extruded beyond the apices of dog root canals. Dent Pract Dent Rec 1972;22(10):370–9.

394. Cohler CM, Newton CW, Patterson SS, Kafrawy AH. Studies of Sargenti's technique of endodontic treatment: short-term response in monkeys. J Endod 1980;6(3):473–8.

395. Newton CW, Patterson SS, Kafrawy AH. Studies of Sargenti's technique of endodontic treatment: six-month and one-year responses. J Endod 1980;6(4):509–17.

396. Lewis BB, Chestner SB. Formaldehyde in dentistry: a review of mutagenic and carcinogenic potential. J Am Dent Assoc 1981;103(3):429–34.

397. Tagger E, Tagger M. Pulpal and periapical reactions to glutaraldehyde and paraformaldehyde pulpotomy dressing in monkeys. J Endod 1984;10(8):364–71.

398. Brodin P, Roed A, Aars H, Ørstavik D. Neurotoxic effects of root filling materials on rat phrenic nerve in vitro. J Dent Res 1982;61(8):1020–3.

399. Rowe AH. Damage to the inferior dental nerve during or following endodontic treatment. Br Dent J 1983;155(9):306–7.

400. Spångberg LS, Barbosa SV, Lavigne GD. AH 26 releases formaldehyde. J Endod 1993;19(12):596–8.

401. Sousa CJA, Montes CRM, Pascon EA, et al. Comparison of the intraosseous biocompatibility of AH Plus, EndoREZ, and Epiphany root canal sealers. J Endod 2006;32(7):656–62.

402. Key JE, Rahemtulla FG, Eleazer PD. Cytotoxicity of a new root canal filling material on human gingival fibroblasts. J Endod 2006;32(8):756–8.

403. Schwandt NW, Gound TG. Resorcinol-formaldehyde resin "Russian Red" endodontic therapy. J Endod 2003;29(7):435–7.

404. Seltzer S, Soltanoff W, Sinai I, et al. Biologic aspects of endodontics. 3. Periapical tissue reactions to root canal instrumentation. Oral Surg Oral Med Oral Pathol Oral Radiol Endod 1968;26(5):694–705.

405. Seltzer S, Soltanoff W, Sinai I, Smith J. Biologic aspects of endodontics. IV. Periapical tissue reactions to root-filled teeth whose canals had been instrumented short of their apices. Oral Surg Oral Med Oral Pathol Oral Radiol Endod 1969;28(5):724–38.

406. Sjögren U, Hagglund B, Sundqvist G, Wing K. Factors affecting the long-term results of endodontic treatment. J Endod 1990;16:498–504.

407. Smith CS, Setchell DJ, Harty FJ. Factors influencing the success of conventional root canal therapy–a five-year retrospective study. Int Endod J 1993;26(6):321–33.

408. Ricucci D, Langeland K. Apical limit of root canal instrumentation and obturation, part 2. A histological study. Int Endod J 1998;31(6):394–409.

409. Neaverth EJ. Disabling complications following inadvertent overextension of a root canal filling material. J Endod 1989;15(3):135–9.

410. Baugh D, Wallace J. The role of apical instrumentation in root canal treatment: a review of the literature. J Endod 2005;31:333–40.

411. Olson AK, Goerig AC, Cavataio RE, Luciano J. The ability of the radiograph to determine the location of the apical foramen. Int Endod J 1991;24(1):28–35.

412. Powell-Cullingford AW, Pitt Ford TR. The use of E-speed film for root canal length determination. Int Endod J 1993;26(5):268–72.

413. Stein TJ, Corcoran JF. Radiographic "working length" revisited. Oral Surg Oral Med Oral Pathol 1992;74(6):796–800.

414. ElAyouti A, Weiger R, Lost C. Frequency of overinstrumentation with an acceptable radiographic working length. J Endod 2001;27(1):49–52.

415. McGurkin-Smith R, Trope M, Caplan D, Sigurdsson A. Reduction of intracanal bacteria using GT rotary instrumentation, 5.25% NaOCl, EDTA, and Ca(OH)$_2$. J Endod 2005;31:359–63.

416. Schaeffer MA, White RR, Walton RE. Determining the optimal obturation length: a meta-analysis of literature. J Endod 2005;31(4):271–4.

417. Tronstad L. Tissue reactions following apical plugging of the root canal with dentin chips in monkey teeth subjected to pulpectomy. Oral Surg Oral Med Oral Pathol Oral Radiol Endod 1978;45(2):297–304.

418. Scott A, Vire D. An evaluation of the ability of a dentin plug to control extrusion of thermoplasticized gutta-percha. J Endod 1992;18(52–7).

419. Kast'akova A, Wu MK, Wesselink PR. An in vitro experiment on the effect of an attempt to create an apical matrix during root canal preparation on coronal leakage and material extrusion. Oral Surg Oral Med, Oral Pathol Oral Radiol Endod 2001;91(4):462–7.

420. ElDeeb ME, Thuc-Quyen NT, Jensen JR. The dentinal plug: its effect on confining substances to the canal and on the apical seal. J Endod 1983;9(9):355–9.

421. Pitts DL, Jones JE, Oswald RJ. A histological comparison of calcium hydroxide plugs and dentin plugs used for the

421. control of Gutta-percha root canal filling material. J Endod 1984;10(7):283–93.
422. Ritchie GM, Anderson DM, Sakumura JS. Apical extrusion of thermoplasticized Gutta-percha used as a root canal filling. J Endod 1988;14(3):128–32.
423. Mann SR, McWalter GM. Evaluation of apical seal and placement control in straight and curved canals obturated by laterally condensed and thermoplasticized gutta-percha. J Endod 1987;13(1):10–17.
424. Tagger M, Gold A. Flow of various brands of Gutta-percha cones under in vitro thermomechanical compaction. J Endod 1988;14(3):115–20.
425. Gutmann JL, Creel DC, Bowles WH. Evaluation of heat transfer during root canal obturation with thermoplasticized gutta-percha. Part I. In vitro heat levels during extrusion. J Endod 1987;13(8):378–83.
426. Gutmann JL, Rakusin H, Powe R, Bowles WH. Evaluation of heat transfer during root canal obturation with thermoplasticized gutta-percha. Part II. In vivo response to heat levels generated. J Endod 1987;13(9):441–8.
427. Saunders EM. In vivo findings associated with heat generation during thermomechanical compaction of gutta-percha. 1. Temperature levels at the external surface of the root. Int Endod J 1990;23(5):263–7.
428. Saunders EM. In vivo findings associated with heat generation during thermomechanical compaction of gutta-percha. 2. Histological response to temperature elevation on the external surface of the root. Int Endod J 1990;23(5):268–74.
429. Blanas N, Kienle F, Sandor GK. Injury to the inferior alveolar nerve due to thermoplastic gutta percha. J Oral Maxillofac Surg 2002;60(5):574–6.
430. Fanibunda K, Whitworth J, Steele J. The management of thermomechanically compacted gutta percha extrusion in the inferior dental canal. Br Dent J 1998;184(7):330–2.
431. Blanas N, Kienle F, Sandor GK. Inferior alveolar nerve injury caused by thermoplastic gutta-percha overextension. J Can Dent Assoc 2004;70(6):384–7.
432. Johnson WB. A new gutta-percha technique. J Endod 1978;4(6):184–8.
433. Cantatore G, Johnson WB. The Thermafil system. In: Castellucci A, editor. Endodontics, Vol. II. florence: Tridente S.r.l; 2006. p. 702.
434. Spielman A, Gutman D, Laufer D. Anesthesia following endodontic overfilling with AH26. Report of a case. Oral Surg Oral Med Oral Pathol Oral Radiol Endod 1981;52(5):554–6.
435. Tamse A, Kaffe I, Littner MM, Kozlovsky A. Paresthesia following overextension of AH-26: report of two cases and review of the literature. J Endod 1982;8(2):88–90.
436. Nitzan DW, Stabholz A, Azaz B. Concepts of accidental overfilling and overinstrumentation in the mandibular canal during root canal treatment. J Endod 1983;9(2):81–5.
437. Barkhordar RA, Nguyen NT. Paresthesia of the mental nerve after overextension with AH26 and gutta-percha: report of case. J Am Dent Assoc 1985;110(2):202–3.
438. Ahlgren FK, Johannessen AC, Hellem S. Displaced calcium hydroxide paste causing inferior alveolar nerve paraesthesia: report of a case. Oral Surg Oral Med Oral Pathol Oral Radiol Endod 2003;96(6):734–7.
439. Lindgren P, Eriksson KF, Ringberg A. Severe facial ischemia after endodontic treatment. J Oral Maxillofac Surg 2002;60(5):576–9.
440. Gatot A, Tovi F. Prednisone treatment for injury and compression of inferior alveolar nerve: report of a case of anesthesia following endodontic overfilling. Oral Surg Oral Med Oral Pathol Oral Radiol Endod 1986;62(6):704–6.
441. Morse DR. Endodontic-related inferior alveolar nerve and mental foramen paresthesia. Compend Contin Educ Dent 1997;18(10):963–87.
442. Schwartz S, Shires G, Spencer F. Principles of surgery. 7th ed. New York: McGraw-Hill; 1999.
443. Fleisher KE, Stevens MR. Diagnosis and management of inferior alveolar nerve injury. Compend Contin Educ Dent 1995;16(10):1028, 1031–22, 1034–40.
444. Donoff RB. Surgical management of inferior alveolar nerve injuries (Part I): The case for early repair. J Oral Maxillofac Surg 1995;53(11):1327–9.
445. Gregg JM. Surgical management of inferior alveolar nerve injuries (Part II): The case for delayed management. J Oral Maxillofac Surg 1995;53(11):1330–3.
446. Pogrel MA, Thamby S. The etiology of altered sensation in the inferior alveolar, lingual, and mental nerves as a result of dental treatment. J Calif Dent Assoc 1999;27(7):531, 534–8.
447. Seddon H. Three types of nerve injuries. Brain 1943;66:237–88.
448. Yaltirik M, Kocak Berberoglu H, Koray M, et al. Orbital pain and headache secondary to overfilling of a root canal. J Endod 2003;29(11):771–2.
449. Giardino L, Pontieri F, Savoldi E, Tallarigo F. Aspergillus mycetoma of the Maxillary Sinus Secondary to Overfilling of a Root Canal. J Endod 2006;32(7):692–4.
450. Khongkhunthian P, Reichart PA. Aspergillosis of the maxillary sinus as a complication of overfilling root canal material into the sinus: report of two cases. J Endod 2001;27(7):476–8.
451. Scolozzi P, Lombardi T, Jaques B. Successful inferior alveolar nerve decompression for dysesthesia following endodontic treatment: report of 4 cases treated by mandibular sagittal osteotomy. Oral Surg Oral Med Oral Pathol Oral Radiol Endod 2004;97(5):625–31.
452. Koseoglu BG, Tanrikulu S, Subay RK, Sencer S. Anesthesia following overfilling of a root canal sealer into the mandibular canal: a case report. Oral Surg Oral Med Oral Pathol Oral Radiol Endod 2006;101(6):803–6.

453. Gatot A, Arbelle J, Leiberman A, Yanai-Inbar I. Effects of sodium hypochlorite on soft tissues after its inadvertent injection beyond the root apex. J Endod 1991;17(11):573–4.

454. Hülsmann M, Hahn W. Complications during root canal irrigation–literature review and case reports. Int Endod J 2000;33(3):186–93.

455. Becker GL, Cohen S, Borer R. The sequelae of accidentally injecting sodium hypochlorite beyond the root apex. Report of a case. Oral Surg Oral Med Oral Pathol Oral Radiol Endod 1974;38(4):633–8.

456. Reeh ES, Messer HH. Long-term paresthesia following inadvertent forcing of sodium hypochlorite through perforation in maxillary incisor. Endod Dent Traumatol 1989;5(4):200–3.

457. Witton R, Henthorn K, Ethunandan M, et al. Neurological complications following extrusion of sodium hypochlorite solution during root canal treatment. Int Endod J 2005;38(11):843–8.

458. Bowden JR, Ethunandan M, Brennan PA. Life-threatening airway obstruction secondary to hypochlorite extrusion during root canal treatment. Oral Surg Oral Med Oral Pathol Oral Radiol Endod 2006;101(3):402–4.

459. Kavanagh CP, Taylor J. Inadvertent injection of sodium hypochlorite into the maxillary sinus. Br Dent J 1998;185(7):336–7.

460. Ehrich DG, Brian J, Walker WA. Sodium hypochlorite accident: inadvertent injection into the maxillary sinus. J Endod 1993;19(4):180–2.

461. Bradford CE, Eleazer PD, Downs KE, Scheetz JP. Apical pressures developed by needles for canal irrigation. J Endod 2002;28(4):333–5.

462. Shovelton D. Surgical emphysema as a complication of dental operations. Br Dent J 1957;102:397–404.

463. Lloyd RE. Surgical emphysema as a complication in endodontics. Br Dent J 1975;138(10):393–4.

464. Falomo OO. Surgical emphysema following root canal therapy. Report of a case. Oral Surg Oral Med Oral Pathol Oral Radiol Endod 1984;58(1):101–2.

465. Rickles NH, Joshi BA. A Possible case in a human and an investigation in dogs of death from air embolism during root canal therapy. J Am Dent Assoc 1963;67:397–404.

466. Eleazer PD, Eleazer KR. Air pressures developed beyond the apex from drying root canals with pressurized air. J Endod 1998;24(12):833–6.

CHAPTER 32

TREATMENT OUTCOME: THE POTENTIAL FOR HEALING AND RETAINED FUNCTION

SHIMON FRIEDMAN

Definitions and Classification

When attempting to review the outcome of studies on nonsurgical endodontic treatment (*initial* root canal treatment,[1-80] orthograde *re-treatment*,[1,2,6,16,34,41,43,50,57,81-92]) and surgical endodontic treatment (apical surgery,[82,84,88,89,93-151] intentional *replantation*[152-161]), it quickly becomes apparent that outcome definitions and classification have been inconsistent. This has resulted in considerable variability of the reported "success" rates.[162] Much of the confusion is created by the definition of outcomes using nonspecific ambiguous terms, such as "success" and "failure." The frequent lack of calibration in outcome assessment, particularly differences in observer strategies for recording of radiographic findings, has amplified the inconsistency of reported outcomes.

In the majority of endodontic outcome studies, the outcome assessment is based on clinical and radiographic measures. Nevertheless, in many studies on nonsurgical treatment,[3,11,12,16,22,28,37,41,45,47,48,52,54,56,58,60,66,71,75,163] and in at least one apical surgery study,[121] the radiographic appearance is used as the only outcome measure. This strategy may overstate the "success" rate by not noting teeth that could be radiographically normal but symptomatic.[164]

Radiographic Outcome Assessment

Assessment of radiographic images has been shown to be highly inconsistent.[165-169] The consistency of assessment can be significantly improved when structured observer and calibration strategies are applied, as suggested for endodontic treatment.[167,169-175] However, the suggested strategies have not been frequently applied in endodontic outcome studies.

To improve consistency of radiographic assessment, the Periapical Index (PAI)[176] has been used with increasing frequency. The PAI system includes a calibration kit of 100 radiographic images of root-filled teeth for determining a level of sufficient consistency. Assessed radiographs are compared with a set of five radiographic images (see Figure 1 in Chapter 16, "Radiographic Interpretation") derived from Brynolf's histologic–radiographic correlation study,[177] representing a healthy periapex (scores 1 and 2), and increasing extent and severity of apical periodontitis (scores 3 to 5). Radiographs are assessed independently in a "blind" manner, by assigning a score according to which of the five reference images it appears to match. This results in improved reproducibility and sensitivity of the assessment.[72,176] The PAI has been used mainly for outcome assessment after nonsurgical treatment.[48,52,54, 56,66,67,70-72,75,76,78,79,90] Although it has not been validated for outcome assessment after apical surgery,[144] the PAI was used in one apical surgery study[148] to assist in unbiased outcome assessment and to promote comparisons with studies on nonsurgical endodontic treatment reported by the same group of researchers.[67,70,78,90] Results obtained with the PAI scores cannot be directly interpreted as measures of "success" or "failure"; however, PAI scores have been dichotomized with scores 1 and 2 representing "healthy" periapical tissues and scores of 3 and above representing "disease."[54,56,66,67, 70,71,76,78,90,178-180]

AMBIGUITY OF OUTCOME DEFINITION AS "SUCCESS" AND "FAILURE"

The main confusion in reported outcomes results from differences among studies in the definition of a successful outcome when using "strict" or "lenient" classifications of "success."

Strict Definition of "Success"

In the majority of the studies, a successful outcome is strictly defined by complete absence of radiolucency and absence of clinical signs and symptoms. After nonsurgical treatment, complete normalcy has been named "success." However, a small radiolucency may be accepted around extruded root filling materials,[1,6,43,53,86] but any other remaining radiolucency is excluded, even if its size is decreased; unchanged radiolucencies represent "failure". A smaller radiolucency, in the presence of clinical normalcy, is usually considered as "incomplete healing."[50] This combination is not considered as a successful outcome, but rather as an interim outcome requiring further observation.

In studies on apical surgery, complete normalcy is often named "complete healing" and occasionally "success." A typical radiographic appearance of a periapical scar (Figure 1), named "incomplete healing" or "cicatrice," has also been considered a successful outcome.[96,174,181-183] A reduction in size of a radiolucency coupled with clinical normalcy is usually considered "uncertain healing." It appears that the "complete" healing category has been subject to considerable observer variation,[173] whereas the "incomplete healing" category has been subject to interpretation errors.[183]

Lenient Definition of "Success"

In some studies of nonsurgical treatment, "success" is defined as the absence of clinical signs and symptoms. Clinical normalcy may be accompanied by a residual radiolucency, either decreased[3,16,29-31,36,47,59,60,85] or unchanged in size,[11,33,42] but not increased. These lenient definitions contrast sharply with the strict one outlined above.

In studies on apical surgery, further confusion has been caused by misinterpretation or misuse of the "incomplete healing" category. Although teeth classified as "incomplete healing" are originally defined as healed by scar formation, researchers may erroneously include teeth with persistent disease in this category.[183] Furthermore, "incomplete healing" has been used to describe decreased radiolucency rather than scars, yet still considered a successful outcome. A successful outcome is occasionally defined primarily by the normal clinical presentation, even if it is accompanied by different degrees of residual radiolucency.[113,131]

Clearly, use of "lenient" outcome criteria that do not require radiographic normalcy increases the "success" rate in comparison with use of "strict" criteria that do require radiographic normalcy. Friedman et al.[50] reported 78% complete healing and 16% incomplete healing after nonsurgical treatment. This would be 94% by the "lenient" criteria. The discrepancy would be even larger if unchanged radiolucencies were included in the criteria for success. Wang et al.[148] reported that 74% of the teeth healed after apical surgery using "strict" criteria. However, they also report that 15% of the teeth presented with a decrease in size of the radiolucencies and only 9% had clinical signs and symptoms. By the "lenient" criteria, their success would be 89% if reduction of radiolucency was required or 91% if only clinical "normalcy" was required.

The debate regarding the use of strict versus lenient criteria for outcome assessment after endodontic treatment is specific to teeth affected by preoperative apical periodontitis. It is noteworthy that apical periodontitis is frequently asymptomatic, both before treatment and when persisting after treatment.[34,55,62,65,67,70,77,78,90,184-187] Notwithstanding the frequent absence of symptoms, apical periodontitis is universally considered a disease requiring therapy. Thus, persisting apical periodontitis after therapy cannot be regarded as "success" only because it is asymptomatic, and treatment is still indicated.

Outcome Definition as "Uncertain," "Questionable," "Doubtful," or "Improved"

The terms "uncertain," "questionable," "doubtful," or "improved" were originally introduced to imply uncertainty of the outcome. They have also been used to define improved outcomes. When used strictly, these terms described cases that could not be assessed because of insufficient radiographic information and thus were not included in either the successful or unsuccessful outcome categories.[1,2,6,22-24,28,57,62] Exclusion of these cases from the study sample usually lowered the success rate by approximately 5%, as demonstrated by recalculation of success rates in several of the relevant studies.[2,6,22,57] By contrast, the same terms have been used to describe cases with a decrease in size of the radiolucencies and considered either as a successful or as an uncertain outcome for nonsurgical treatment[7,17,19,40,41,50,51,55,61] and apical surgery.[82,93,96,98,100,101,103,107,109,118,127,137-139,141,146,147,150,151,163,188] Use of this modified classification lowered the failure rate in comparison with the strict classification. In many other studies on apical surgery,[84,89,99,112,116,117,120,122,130,133,136,138,140,145,183,189-191] "uncertain healing" has been used for a decrease in size of a radiolucency that appears different from "incomplete healing." In 'these studies, if "uncertain healing" persists for 4 years or longer, it is considered to be an unsuccessful outcome.

Consequences of Using the Terms "Success" and "Failure"

Clearly, the ambiguity of the term "success" confuses communication with patients. Of particular concern

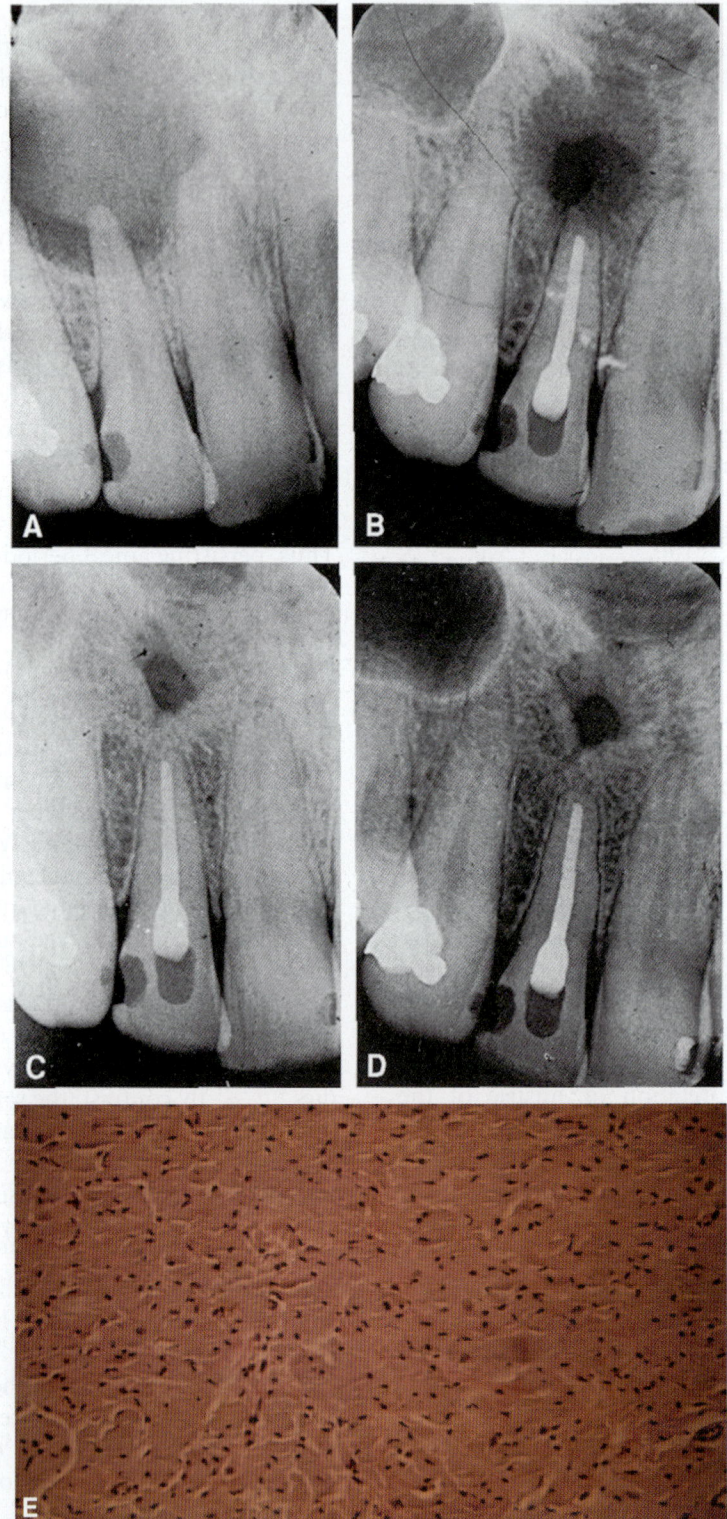

Figure 1 Progressive development of apical scar. This permanent artifact frequently follows through-and-through osseous destruction of both labial and palatal cortical plates. *A,* Before cyst enucleation. *B,* Six months following surgery. *C,* One year following surgery. *D,* Two years following surgery; scar is permanent. *E,* A similar nonpathologic radiolucent area was removed and examined; it is filled with fibrous connective tissue, no inflammatory cells. (*A–D,* Photos courtesy of Dr. M. Krasnoff; *E,* Photos courtesy of Dr. S.N. Bhaskar)

is the use of "success" for single-tooth implants, based on different criteria than those used in endodontics.[192,193] The very high "success" rates reported for single-tooth implants[193–197] may mislead patients who are weighing endodontic treatment against replacement of the tooth with an implant. Being unaware of the differences in the definition of "success," the patient may opt for the better chance of "success," and have a tooth removed that could remain functional for many years.

Classification of an unfavorable outcome as "failure," used in many endodontic treatment outcome studies, is also a concern. This term does not imply the necessity to pursue any course of action, and in addition, it has a negative connotation.[198] It has been suggested[52] that communication with patients can be improved by replacing the value-laden terms "success" and "failure" with neutral expressions, such as "chance of healing" and "risk of inflammation." It is advisable, therefore, to avoid the terms "success" and "failure" in defining the *outcome* of endodontic treatment.

USE OF THE TERMS HEALING/DISEASE/ FUNCTION FOR IMPROVED CLARITY

The general definition of success is "the accomplishment of an aim or purpose" (Oxford Dictionary), suggesting that the outcome is best defined in direct relation to the specific aim. In the context of endodontic treatment, the aim is to prevent or cure apical periodontitis.[199] Thus, the outcome of endodontic treatment should be related to "healing."[35,52,164,200,201] Although Rud et al.[174] introduced a classification for outcome assessment after apical surgery that referred to healing (complete, incomplete, uncertain, unsatisfactory), it was construed by others to represent "success" and "failure."[116,120, 138,143,150,151]
Rather than depending on interpretations of "success" and "failure," the terms "healed," "healing," and "disease" should be used to clearly describe the actual observation, as follows:

- Healed: Complete clinical and radiographic normalcy (no signs, symptoms, residual radiolucency) (Figure 2). This category also includes the typical appearance of a scar after apical surgery[116,120,173,174, 181–183] (see Figure 1).
- Healing (in progress): Decrease in size of a radiolucency and clinical normalcy after a follow-up period shorter than 4 years (Figure 3).
- Disease (refractory/recurrent/emerged apical periodontitis): Presence of radiolucency (new, increased, unchanged, or reduced after observation exceeding 4 years) regardless of clinical presentation (Figure 4), or presence of symptoms regardless of radiographic appearance.

Use of these aim-related terms, to define the outcome of treatment, can greatly improve communication with patients. Patients pursuing treatment should be encouraged to identify specific aims and thus define their expected outcome that can be considered a success. The majority of patients may expect healing; however, individual patients may be satisfied with just elimination of clinical signs and symptoms. This may be particularly relevant when clinical conditions suggest a compromised prognosis, such as an extensive loss of supporting bone prior to apical surgery.[110] In these circumstances, if a patient is still motivated to attempt treatment although healing is unlikely to occur, the aim of treatment is retention of the tooth in "asymptomatic function," and the outcome is defined as follows:

- Asymptomatic function: Clinical normalcy with or without a persistent radiolucency, decreased or unchanged (Figure 5).

THE EVIDENCE-BASE FOR THE OUTCOME OF ENDODONTIC TREATMENT

Like all health care providers in the past, endodontists had been expected to make clinical decisions and prescribe treatment for individual patients

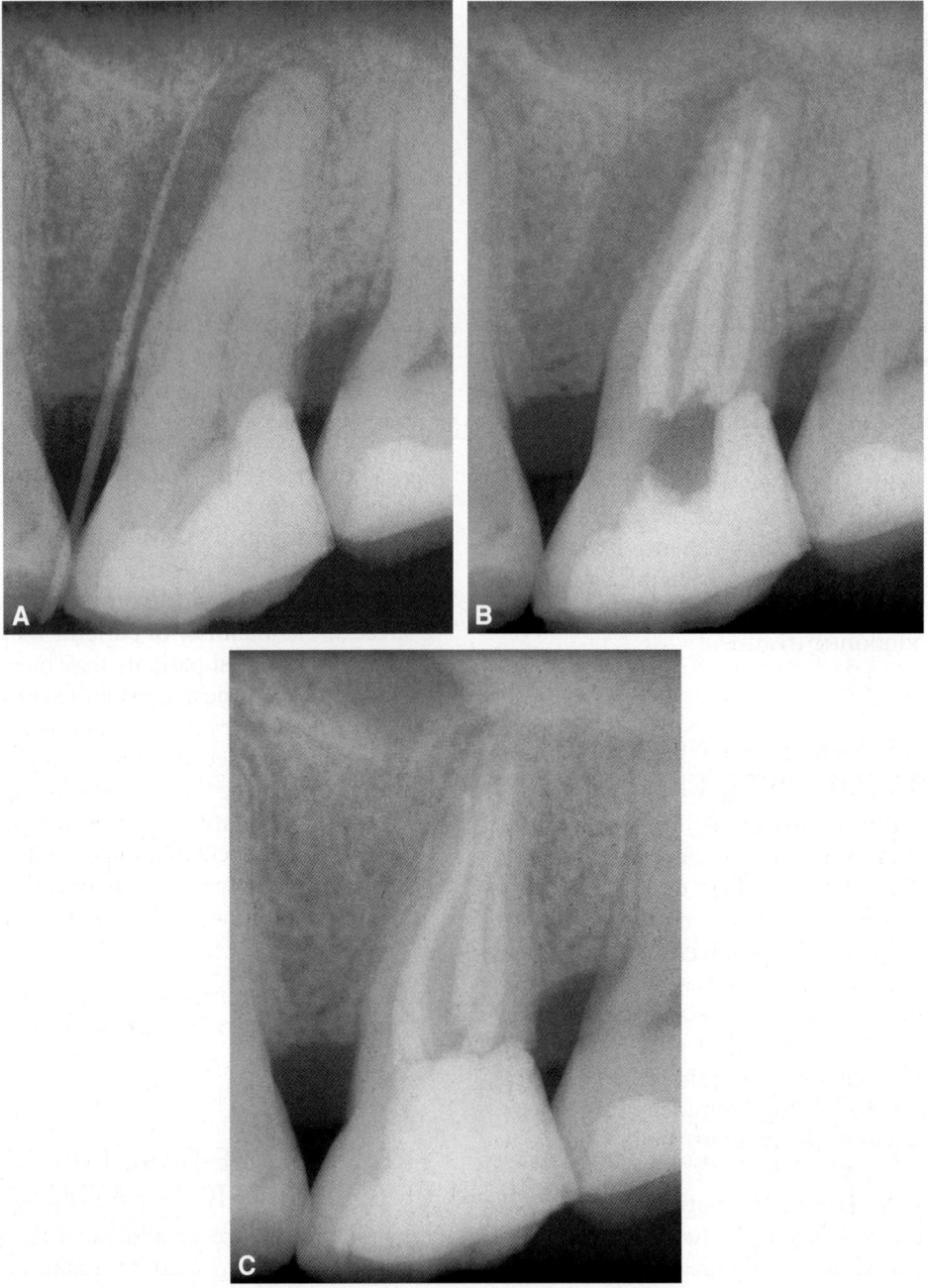

Figure 2 Outcome classification labeled as "healed" after initial treatment. **A,** Maxillary second molar with apical periodontitis extending along the mesial root surface, and associated sinus tract (traced with a gutta-percha cone). **B,** Completed treatment. **C,** At 1 year, the radiolucency is completely resolved and the tooth is symptom free, indicating the lesion has healed. (Reprinted with permission from Friedman 2002.[164])

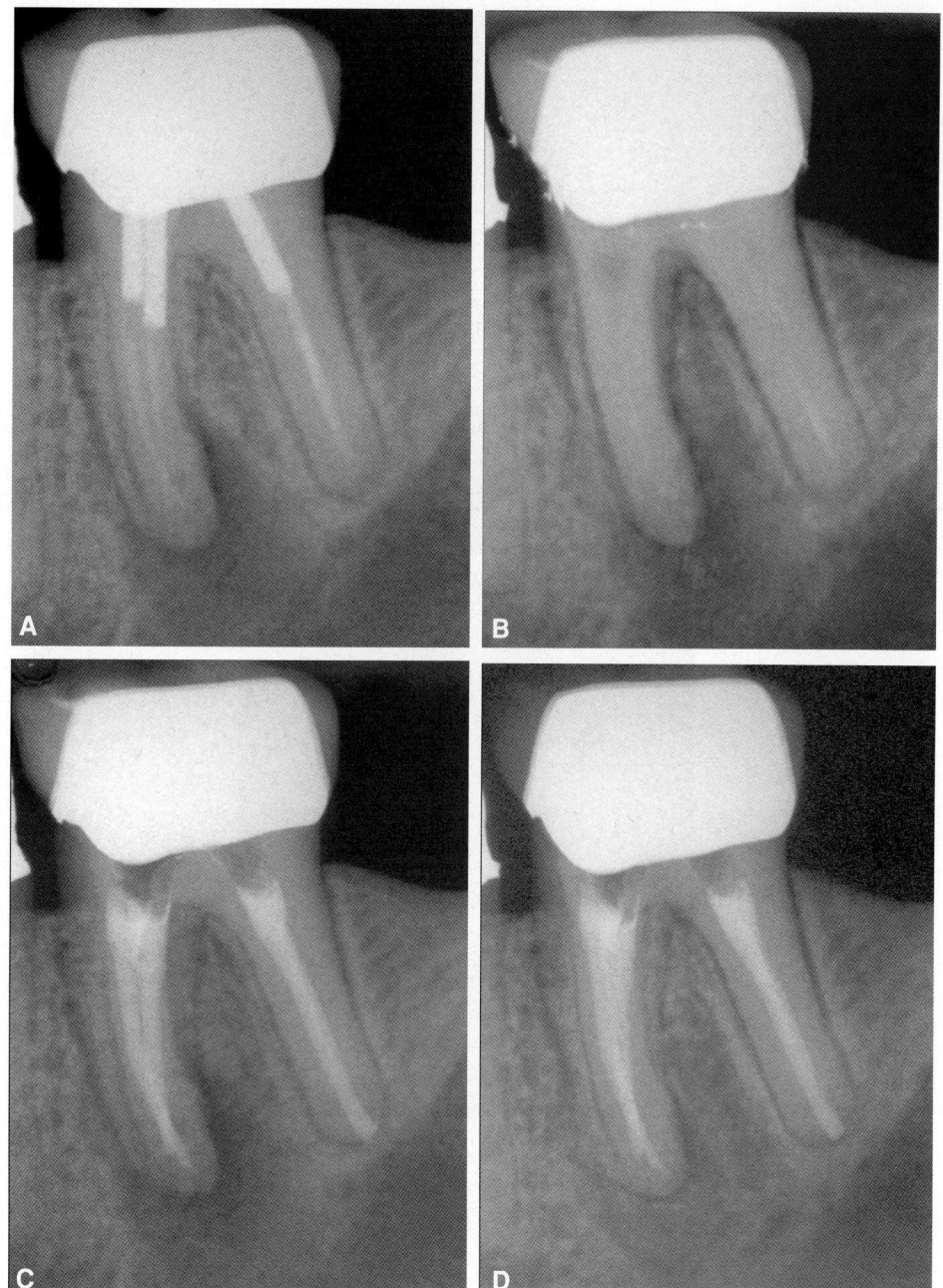

Figure 3 Outcome classification labeled as "healing" after orthograde re-treatment. ***A,*** Three prefabricated posts in mandibular molar with post-treatment disease. ***B,*** Access was prepared through the crown and posts were removed; canals were dressed with calcium hydroxide. ***C,*** Completed root canal re-treatment. ***D,*** At 6 months, the lesion is reduced and the tooth is symptom free, indicating that healing is in progress. Regrettably, the access cavity was not properly restored. (Reprinted with permission from Friedman 2002.[223])

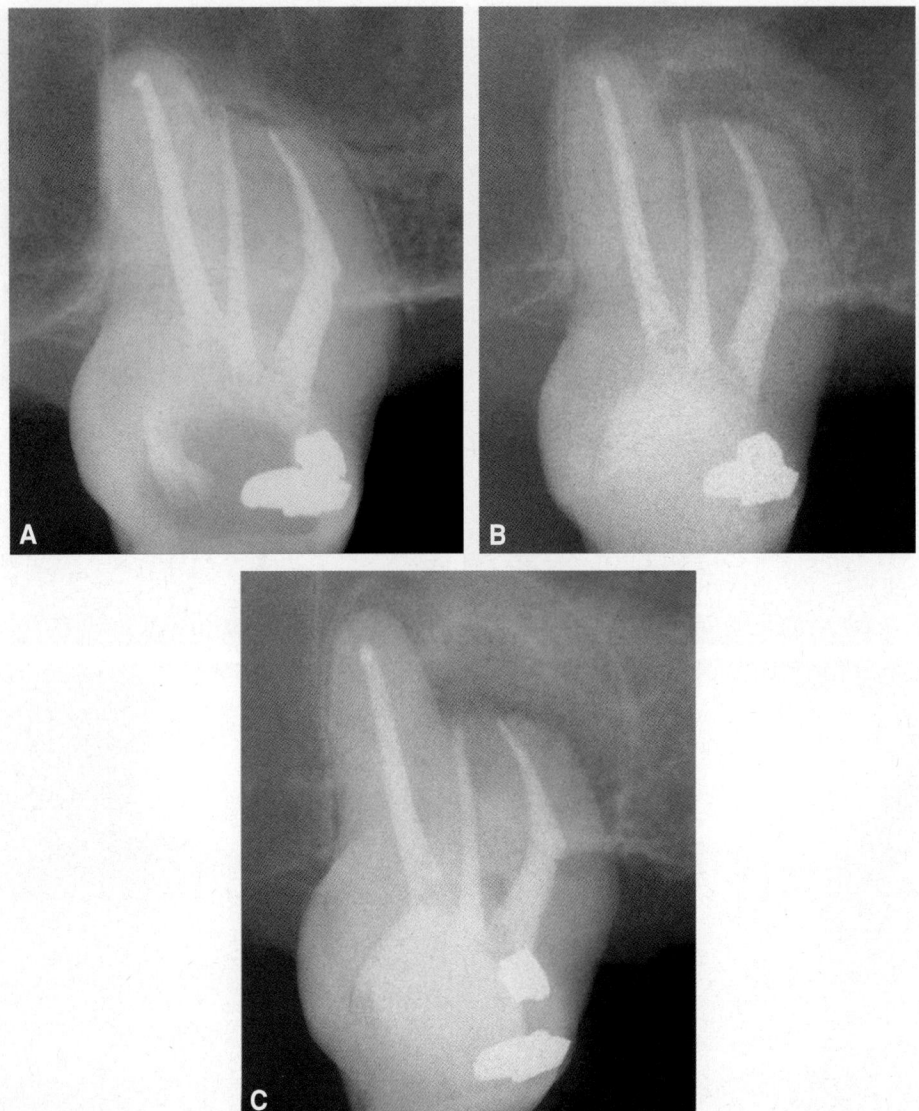

Figure 4 Outcome classification labeled as "emerged disease" after initial treatment. ***A,*** Immediate postoperative radiograph of maxillary second molar with no evidence of apical periodontitis. ***B,*** Emerged disease at 3 years. ***C,*** Further expansion of disease at 6 years. In spite of the presence of disease, the tooth is symptom free. (Reprinted with permission from Friedman 2002.[223])

based on their knowledge and experience. Currently, health care providers are expected to base clinical decisions on evidence derived from clinical trials. Furthermore, they are required to share the evidence-base information with patients, and to encourage them to participate in the clinical decision-making process, in accordance with the concept of "patient autonomy."[202–206] Thus, endodontists should inform patients about the benefits and risks of available treatment alternatives and then allow patients to select specific treatments. To be able to do so, endodontists must be well versed in the evidence, primarily the current knowledge about treatment outcomes, supporting the treatment procedures they suggest to patients.

As different forms of endodontic treatment have been used clinically for over 100 years, numerous studies have been published where information can be gleaned on the outcome of endodontic treatment encompassing data from over 20,000 treated teeth. As a whole, this extensive body of literature is characterized by great diversity of the reported outcomes. This

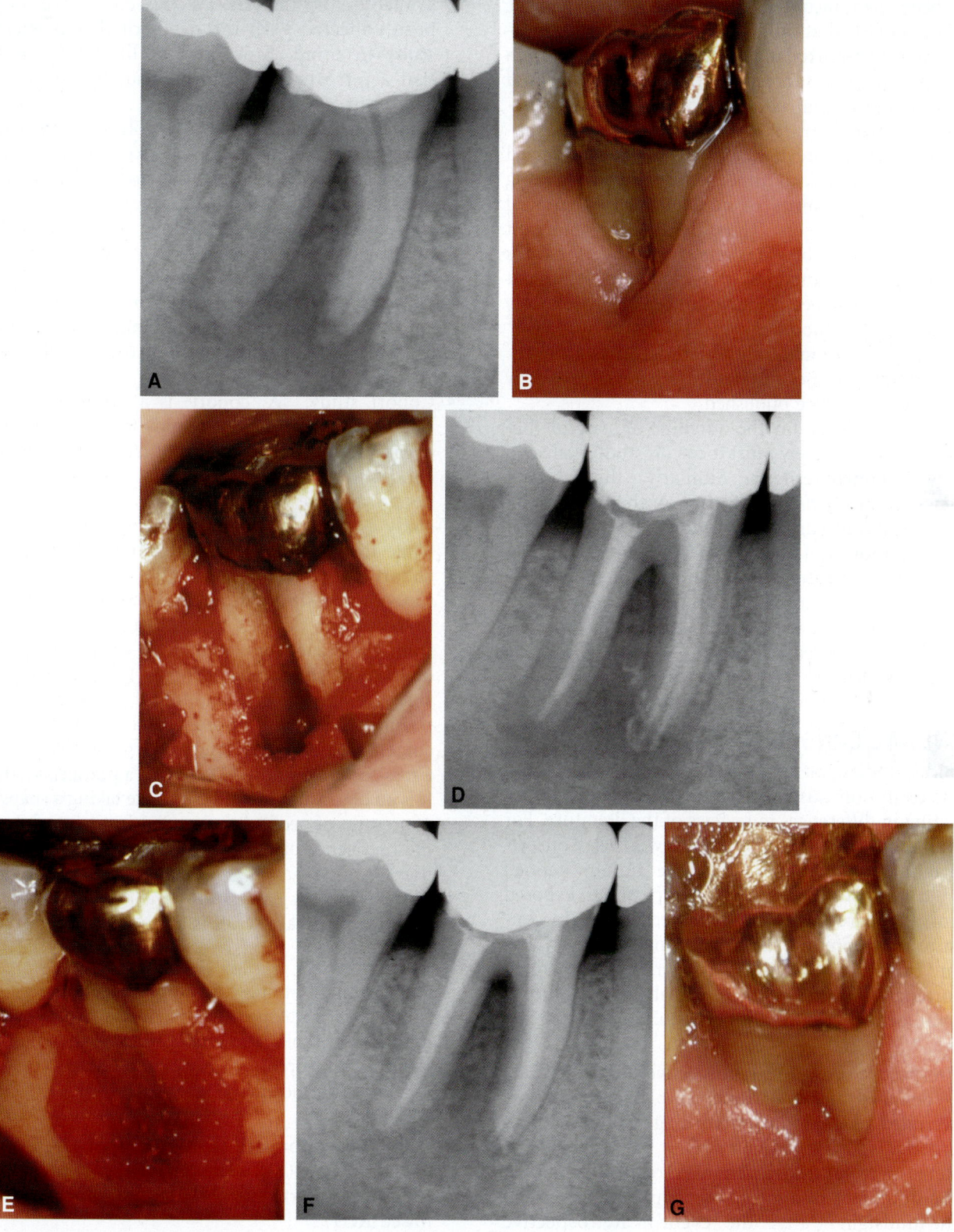

Figure 5 Outcome classification labeled as "functional" after initial treatment. **A–C,** Mandibular first molar with apical periodontitis, associated with gingival recession, probing depth beyond the apex, and extensive bone loss on the buccal aspect. The patient was advised of poor prognosis, but decided to proceed with treatment in an attempt to retain the tooth in function as long as possible. **D, E,** Completed root canal treatment and application of a resorbable guided tissue regeneration membrane. **F, G,** At 6 months, the radiolucency has been considerably decreased and the gingival tissue appears healthy. Although the prognosis remains poor, the patient's goal has been achieved. Replacement of the defective crown has been deferred by the patient. (Reprinted with permission from Friedman 2002.[164])

has been demonstrated in several comprehensive reviews published at different junctures, on nonsurgical treatment reported in the first half of the twentieth century,[1] on apical surgery reported up to 1970,[99] and on both nonsurgical and surgical endodontic treatments reported from 1956 to 1997.[162] These and subsequent narrative reviews[164,200,201,207] have revealed inconsistencies and, at times, contradictions among the reported outcomes of nonsurgical and surgical endodontic treatments. Thus, despite the abundant information available, answers to many questions concerning the outcome of endodontic treatment procedures have been equivocal because of poorly standardized methodology of the many studies.[162] The rapid evolution of clinical procedures has rendered results of specific studies less relevant today than when they were published.

To seek evidence for the outcome of state-of-the-art treatment, a review must focus on studies selected on well-defined criteria. Similarly, this chapter reviews *selected articles* reporting on the outcome of nonsurgical and surgical endodontic treatments for the prevention and therapy of apical periodontitis, to define the treatment outcomes, and to identify the predictors of outcome. The nonsurgical treatments, initial root canal treatment and orthograde re-treatment, are reviewed first, followed by surgical treatments.

GENERAL CONSIDERATIONS

Clinical studies fall into different design categories. Some confusion exists with regard to these categories, resulting in differences in reviews of the literature. For example, in a recent series of review articles on evidence-based endodontics,[208–211] the authors defined the "cohort study" as a follow-up of an exposed cohort compared with an unexposed cohort, in contrast to the definition suggested below.

In this chapter, study categories are defined according to the Cochrane Collaboration (http://www.informedhealthonline.org/item.aspx?tabid=15):

- Prospective study: "In a prospective study, the study is designed ahead of time, and people are then recruited and studied according to the study's criteria."
- Retrospective study: "In a retrospective study, the outcomes of a group of people are examined in hindsight ('after the event'). Retrospective studies are generally more limited in the data available for analysis, as the data have rarely been collected with the needs of that particular study in mind. This kind of limitation means that a retrospective study is usually less reliable than a prospective study."
- Clinical trial: "A clinical trial involves administering a treatment to test it. It is an experiment. Clinical trial is an umbrella term for a variety of health care trials... Types include uncontrolled trials, controlled clinical trials (CCT), community trials, and randomized controlled trials (RCT). A randomized controlled trial is always prospective."
- Observational study: "A survey or nonexperimental study. The researchers are examining and reporting on what is happening, without deliberately intervening in the course of events."
- Cohort study: "A 'cohort' is a group of people clearly identified; a cohort study follows that group over time, and reports on what happens to them. A cohort study is an observational study, and it can be prospective or retrospective." [A prospective study is also named "concurrent cohort study," while the retrospective study is named "historical cohort study."[212]]
- Case–control study: "Compares people with a disease or condition ('cases') to another group of people from the same population who do not have that disease or condition ('controls'). A case–control study can identify risks and trends, and suggest some possible causes for disease, or for particular outcomes. A case–control study is retrospective."
- Cross-sectional study: "Also called a prevalence study. It is an observational study. It is like taking a snapshot of a group of people at one point in time and seeing the prevalence of diseases or actions in that population."
- Case series: "A case study is a report of a single experience. A case series is a description of a number of 'cases.'"

One common strategy for appraisal of clinical studies has been developed for systematic reviews of the literature.[213] It ranks studies according to the following descending hierarchy of evidence, based on the research design and methodological rigor:

- Rigorous randomized controlled trial (RCT); systematic review (SR) or meta-analysis of the same.
- Rigorous cohort study; SR of the same; compromised RCT.
- Rigorous case–control study; SR of the same.

- Compromised cohort or case–control study; cross-sectional study; case series.
- Expert opinion; case report; narrative literature review.

The different designs of clinical studies may be best suited for different aims, focusing on effectiveness of different interventions, prognosis after a specific intervention, or risks associated with the intervention. Importantly, studies designed to assess prognosis should be differentiated from those designed to assess risk, because the prognostic factors identified by the former can be different from the risk factors identified by the latter.[212] Accordingly, a review geared to answer specific questions should focus on reviewing studies with matched design.[212] For example, the suggested design for questions regarding the prognosis is a cohort study, whereas the suggested design for questions regarding the benefits of different treatments is an RCT.[212,214]

Evidence-based practice is defined as "...the conscientious, explicit and judicious use of current best evidence in making decisions about the care of individual patients."[215] Thus, reviews should focus on the best evidence available, even if it does not comply with the highest level. In this context, the methodological rigor of a clinical study is a crucial consideration,[216] as rigorous cohort studies can outweigh compromised RCTs. Also, it has been suggested that structured reviews of well-designed observational studies can yield consistent conclusions with those of systematic reviews and meta-analyses of RCTs.[217,218] Therefore, to address the primary focus of this chapter—the prognosis of endodontic treatment—cohort studies that appear to be methodologically adequate are included in the appraisal process.

APPRAISAL OF ENDODONTIC OUTCOME STUDIES

A primary concern in the review of clinical studies is their validity and relevance.[213] Different forms of bias, frequently encountered in cohort studies, may distort their conclusions so that differences are demonstrated between groups that may not really exist, whereas existing differences may not be shown.[212] Bias can potentially occur during assembly of the study cohort when groups of subjects differ in regard to other prognostic factors than the studied ones, and these extraneous factors may influence the outcome of the study.[212] Thus, differences in outcome may be attributed to the assessed variables, although in reality they may result from inherent differences at the beginning of the study. In endodontic cohort studies, assembly bias can occur if subjects differ in preoperative characteristics, such as presence or absence of apical periodontitis in studies on nonsurgical treatment, or prior treatment history before apical surgery, i.e., only initial treatment or also re-treatment. Bias can also occur if assembled subjects have a preferential capacity to heal. For example, the majority of subjects may be healthy, whereas the healing capacity of others may be impaired because of compromised systemic health. In studies on apical surgery, occasional teeth treated without apical periodontitis[139,147] have a much better capacity to heal after surgery than the majority of the teeth affected by apical periodontitis. Another stage when bias can occur is during assessment of the outcome (measurement bias), when subjects differ in the chance of having a specific outcome detected.[212] In the endodontic cohort studies, the clinical signs and symptoms may not be detected. A particular concern is examination of the outcome by the providers of treatment, whose interpretation of follow-up radiographs may be biased toward more favorable assessment.[165]

To minimize bias in appraisal of studies on prognosis, the following checklist is suggested:[212,215,219–221]

- Was the study cohort defined, assembled at the inception of the study, described in detail, entered at a similar point in the course of the disease?
- Was the referral pattern described?
- Were baseline features measured reproducibly?
- Was the follow-up achieved in at least 80% of the inception cohort, the follow-up period described, and long enough for the outcome to occur?
- Were the criteria used for outcome assessment described, objective, clinically important, and reproducibly measured?
- Was the outcome assessment blind?
- Was adjustment for extraneous prognostic factors carried out?

The criteria included in the checklist above can be grouped into four general categories, used as the basis for appraisal of the endodontic outcome studies. This extensive body of literature is characterized by great diversity of reported outcomes, caused by differences among the studies in the composition of study materials, treatment procedures, and methodology. Examples of these differences are highlighted below, from studies on nonsurgical and surgical treatments.

Cohort, at Inception and Endpoint of the Study

Prospective studies, where the cohort is defined before the onset of the study and observed over time, provide the best evidence. To avoid biased interpretations, the inception cohort should be clearly characterized, including data about the subjects' age, gender, and health status, types of teeth treated, proportion of teeth with apical periodontitis, and previous endodontic treatment history. All these variables can potentially influence the outcome. In fact, the considerable variation in cohort characteristics of the endodontic studies may have contributed to the great diversity of reported outcomes, as can be observed in the following examples:

- Tooth location, number of roots: The minority of studies on nonsurgical endodontic treatment include only anterior or single-rooted teeth,[5,11,13–15,17,26,35,43,46,53,54,61,86,88,222] whereas the majority combine single- and multi-rooted teeth. By contrast, the majority of studies on apical surgery include primarily anterior or single-rooted teeth, fewer studies include a substantial proportion of multi-rooted teeth,[84,100,121,122,129–131,133–137,139,145,148,190] and only a few studies include primarily multi-rooted teeth.[102,107,108,117,118,140,141,147,191] Differences in complexity of treatment between single- and multi-rooted teeth may be reflected in the reported outcomes, particularly for apical surgery where access to the multi-rooted, posterior teeth is generally more restricted than to the anterior, single-rooted ones. Furthermore, in studies where each root is evaluated as an independent unit,[2,19,22,37,39–41,43,52,56,57,61,74,81] the contribution of multi-rooted teeth to the total study sample is multiplied because they contribute two or three units each, as opposed to the single unit contributed by each single-rooted tooth. Also, when multi-rooted teeth are evaluated as whole units and assessed by the worst appearing root, the risk of observing refractory apical periodontitis after treatment is multiplied[50] (Figure 6). Thus, the outcome recorded is poorer than what would be recorded if each root of the multi-rooted tooth were evaluated independently.

- Proportion of teeth with apical periodontitis: The proportion of teeth with preoperative apical periodontitis ranges from less than 30[2,7,8,15,21,37,40,57,65,69,72,80] to 100%,[13,24,26,28,35,39,42,45,51,53–55,61,66,76,86,88,222] and it is not even specified in many other studies.[4,20,25,29–32,49,52,56,62,79] It is well established that the presence of apical periodontitis has a negative influence on the outcome of nonsurgical endodontic treatment.[200] Therefore, the proportion of the affected teeth included in the cohorts of different studies may have influenced the reported outcomes; the more such teeth included, the poorer may be the overall outcome reported.

- Previous treatment history—initial treatment or re-treatment—before apical surgery: The majority of teeth included in studies on apical surgery have had only initial root canal treatment performed previously; refractory apical periodontitis in these teeth is likely to be sustained by bacteria harbored within the root canal system. Because containing the intra-canal bacteria by means of a root-end filling may be ineffective, the outcome of the surgical procedure may be compromised.[148,223] In one study, however, all the teeth had "at least one nonsurgical re-treatment to enhance canal debridement,"[138] and 91% of them healed. In another study[144] where 90% of the teeth healed, the authors state that "...if an existing root filling was deemed inadequate, it was replaced" indicating that an unknown proportion of teeth had re-treatment performed before surgery. Persistent disease after orthograde re-treatment is likely to be sustained by bacteria colonizing an inaccessible, possibly extra-radicular site (Figure 7). Because such sites can be eradicated by the surgical procedure, a healing rate in the range of 90% can be expected.[148,223] Thus, the previous treatment history of the teeth included in studies on apical surgery is expected to influence the reported outcome.

Among the characteristics specified, the pattern of referral of the treated cohort should be described, including type of patients treated and case selection criteria used. These data help determine the external

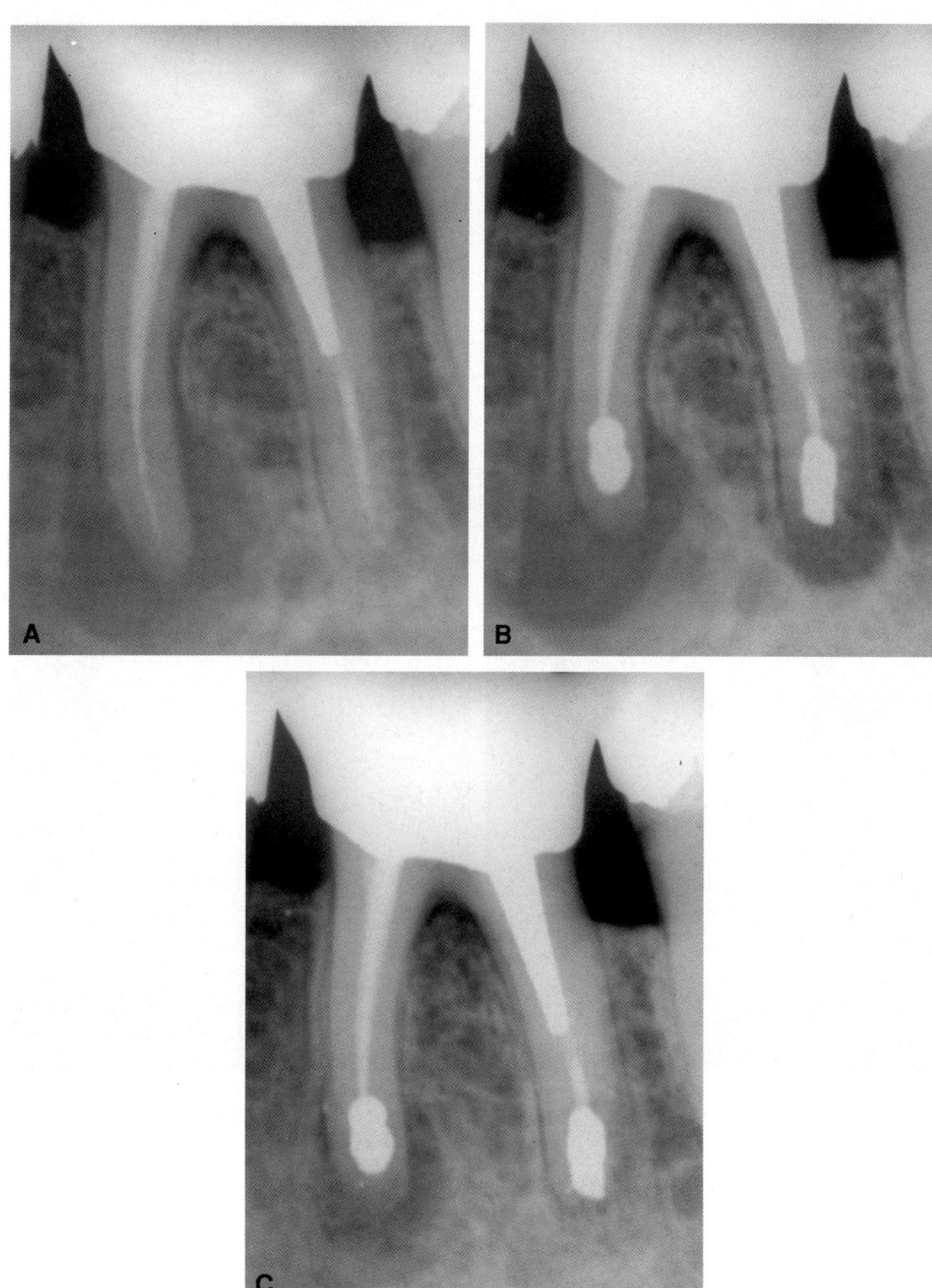

Figure 6 Outcome assessment of a multi-rooted tooth after apical surgery. **A,** Root-filled mandibular first molar with persistent apical periodontitis; the mesial lesion is considerably larger than the distal one. **B,** Completed surgery, including root-end fillings with amalgam and varnish. **C,** At 2.5 years, the distal radiolucency is resolved, but the mesial remains. Presence of symptoms suggests persistence of apical periodontitis. The tooth was then evaluated as one unit in a clinical study,[117] and being recorded as persistent disease. By contrast, if the roots were evaluated independently, the tooth would contribute two units, one healed and the other having persistent disease. (Reprinted with permission from Friedman 2006.[201])

validity (applicability to the population at large) of the reported results.[212] Case selection is likely to determine the results of a clinical study,[49] as potential study subjects are included or excluded according to prognosis. Inspection of the endodontic outcome studies reveals drastic differences in case selection criteria, as follows:

- Case selection criteria: Among studies on nonsurgical treatment, cases judged to have an unfavorable prognosis or subjects with a compromised immune system were excluded in specific studies.[11,29–31,54,66,71] By contrast, one study[40] included only teeth with obstructed canals in which the ability to fulfill

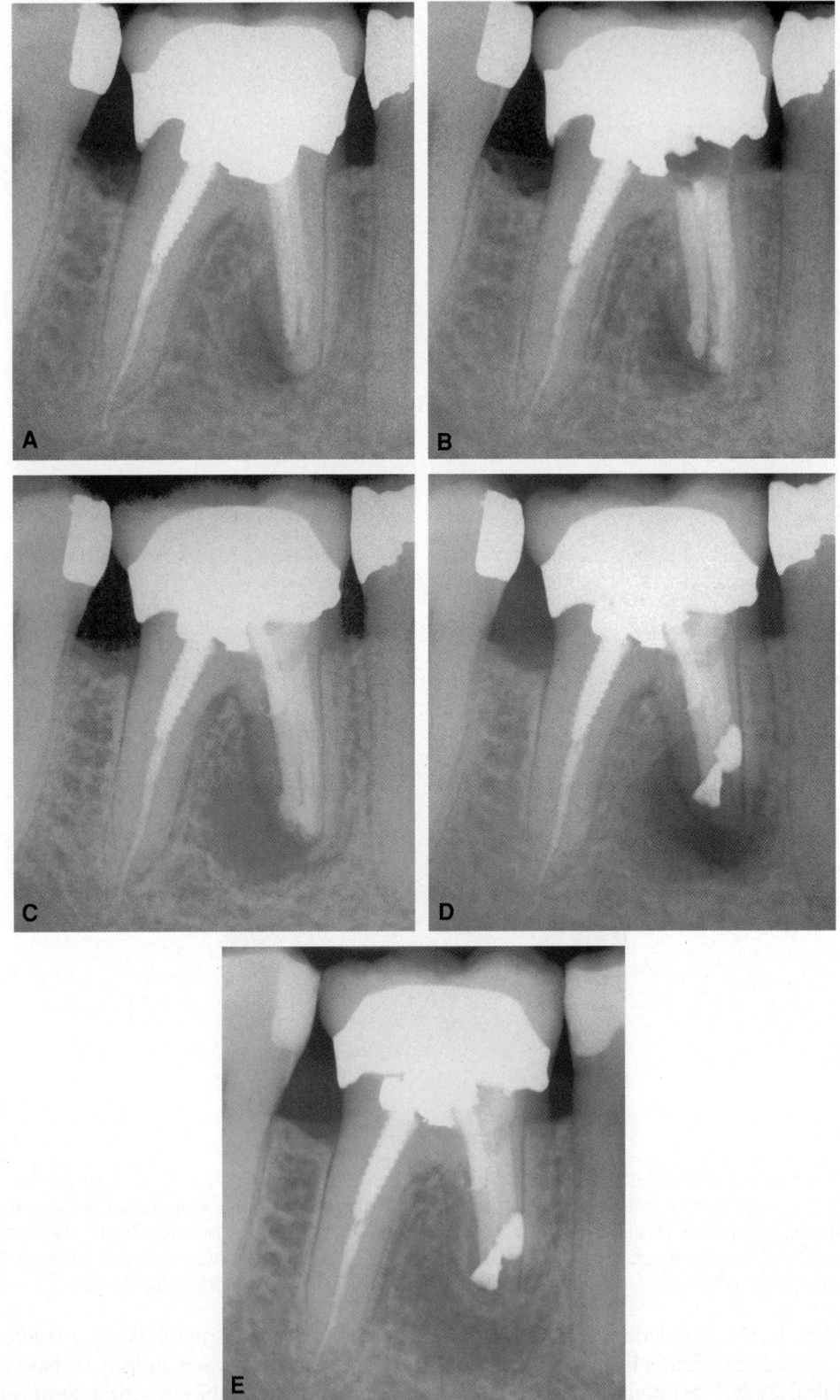

Figure 7 Persistent disease after previous re-treatment suggests probability of extra-radicular infection. **A,** Root-filled mandibular first molar with persistent apical periodontitis affecting the mesial root. **B,** Completed orthograde re-treatment of the mesial canals. **C,** At 1 year, the expanded lesion indicates persistence of apical periodontitis. As the previous re-treatment may have eliminated intra-canal bacteria, the infection may be sustained by extra-radicular bacteria. **D,** Completed surgery, including root-end filling with Super EBA. **E,** At 1 year after surgery, the lesion is healed. (Apical surgery and follow-up courtesy of Dr. Steven Cohen, Toronto, Canada; Reprinted with permission from Friedman 2006.[201])

the technical objectives of treatment was doubtful, whereas in other studies[50,67,70,78,90] teeth were included even if they were compromised by advanced periodontal disease or procedural errors, without specific exclusion criteria. Among studies on apical surgery, teeth with deep periodontal defects, that could impair the prognosis, were frequently excluded.[88,135,138,143,144,149,150] By contrast, one study[110] included only teeth affected by loss of the buccal bone plate, whereas in the majority of studies, consecutive cases were included without specific exclusion criteria. Thus, the reported outcomes in specific studies may have been influenced by inclusion of teeth with poor prognosis in the study sample.

Availability of the entire study cohort for outcome assessment at the endpoint of the study is subject to population mobility, particularly in long-term studies. The outcome of treatment in the unavailable subjects is unknown. In the best-case scenario (if all missing subjects experienced a favorable outcome), the reported outcome would be better, whereas in the worst-case scenario (if all missing subjects experienced an unfavorable outcome), the reported outcome would be poorer. For example, in a study on apical surgery,[148] the recall rate was 85%, and 74% of the teeth have healed. The authors calculated that in the best-case scenario 80% of the teeth would be healed, whereas in the worst-case scenario 57% would be healed. Because the overall "healed" rate is further from the lower value than from the upper one, it appears to be overestimated.[148] Thus, when a large proportion of the inception cohort is unavailable, the results of the study may be considerably skewed and subject to speculation.[1,212] The results may be considered invalid, unless the unavailable subjects are deceased or cannot be reached, suggesting that their absence is not related to the outcome.[1,212] For this reason, at least 80% of the treated subjects should be examined at the endpoint of the study for a high level of evidence to be achieved.[219–221] The rest of the inception cohort must be accounted for, so that "dropouts" (subjects who do not present for follow-up at their own volition; their absence may be related to the outcome of interest) and "discontinuers" (subjects who are excluded from the study by the investigator for accountable reasons, e.g., death or relocation; their absence is not related to the outcome of interest) are identified, allowing accurate calculation of the recall rate. The recall rates in the majority of the endodontic outcome studies fall below the requirements of a good level of evidence, as outlined below:

- Recall rate: The reported recall rates in the different studies on nonsurgical endodontic treatment have varied from under 20[16,18,57] to over 90%.[9,45,51,53,55,61,68,80,86,88] Similarly, in the studies on apical surgery, the recall rates varied from less than 20[129] to over 90%.[84,88,89,100,101,103,107,109–111,113,114,118,122–124,128,131,132,137,138,141,147,150,151] Moreover, the recall rate is not even reported in many of the studies on nonsurgical treatment[5,7,10,13,17,20,25,26,33,79,82] and on apical surgery.[82,104,112,115,119,120,125,126,224] This may be one reason for the inconsistent outcomes reported among all the studies.

Finally, the size of the sample included in the clinical study may be required to exceed a predetermined threshold. The sample size is one of the determinants of the study's internal and external validity.[214] It also determines the power of the statistical analysis, when assessing the effect of different variables on the outcome of treatment. The smaller the difference in outcome, the larger is the sample required in each group to achieve sufficient power for significance to be established,[214] as can be demonstrated in the following examples from endodontic outcome studies:

- Sample size: In a study of 86 teeth with apical periodontitis,[54] the difference in outcome of treatment in one session (64% healed, adjusted calculation) and two sessions (74% healed, adjusted calculation) was not significant. The authors' power analysis suggested that 354 teeth would be required in each group to statistically substantiate the 10% difference in healing (with 80% power). Similarly, in an apical surgery study,[148] the difference in outcome of treatment in 58 teeth with persistent disease after initial root canal treatment (74% healed) and 32 teeth with persistent disease after root canal re-treatment (84% healed) was not significant. The authors' power analysis suggested that 400 teeth would be required in the former group and 220 teeth in the latter group for the difference in their outcomes to be significant (with 80% power). Thus, in relatively small studies on nonsurgical treatment[4,13,15,26,35,36,40,42,44,45,53–55,60,61,67,73–77,84–86,88,89] and apical surgery,[84,88,89,102,104,107,110,111,113,114,118,123,126–129,135,137,141–143,148,150] specific variables may not have a significant association with the outcome, whereas in studies with large samples the same variables may emerge as significant outcome predictors.

Exposure (Treatment, Intervention)

The treatment procedures performed in the study should be explicitly described, so they can be related to the outcome without interpretation or guesswork.

Inspection of the endodontic outcome studies reveals a great variation in treatment procedures, as shown in the examples below:

- Asepsis (in nonsurgical treatment): In at least two of the studies,[19,24] treatment was routinely performed without rubber dam. It can be assumed that in these and several other studies, asepsis was not strictly observed; compromised asepsis would impair the outcome in a given study.
- Root canal preparation and filling (in nonsurgical treatment): Specific preparation techniques, such as serial filing,[22] and root filling materials, such as Kloroperka N-Ø and rosin-chloroform,[37,41] offer a poorer outcome than alternative techniques and materials. Those reportedly ineffective procedures have been used in specific studies.[1,19,20,22,28,35,40,41,43,47,53,86,88,225] By contrast, procedures alleged to be most effective, such as the "Schilder technique," have been used in other studies, exclusively[34] or in part of the sample.[67,70,78,79,90]
- Intra-canal medication (in nonsurgical treatment): Intra-canal medication may be critical for controlling root canal infection,[35,226–231] but not all agents used are effective and beneficial. For example, arsenic and formaldehyde—both extremely toxic and no longer used as intra-canal medication—were used in at least one study.[1] Medications commonly used in the past, such as camphorated phenol and paramonochlorophenol, iodine potassium iodide (IKI), and formocresol, may be insufficient for disinfection of canals associated with apical periodontitis[226] because their antimicrobial efficacy is short-lived.[232–234] These medications have been used frequently, and may have compromised the results, in older studies,[2,10–12,14,17,18,22–24,29–31] whereas the more effective calcium hydroxide dressing was used in more recent studies.[35,37,39,43,50–52,54,55,57,61,62,66,67,70,71,75,78,80,86,88,90] By contrast, in specific studies[21,32,34,53,69] treatment was invariably completed in one session, without the use of any intra-canal medication.
- Bacterial culturing of canals (in nonsurgical treatment): In several studies, absence of bacterial growth in root canal samples (negative culture) was a prerequisite for root filling.[6,28,35,43] Negative cultures are an indication of effective disinfection and have been associated with an improved prognosis relative to teeth with positive cultures.[6,53,86]
- Root-end management (in apical surgery): Round burs, commonly used in the past for root-end cavity preparation, are inferior to the currently used ultrasonic tips.[137,235–240] Likewise, previously highly prevalent root-end filling with amalgam has been shown to be inferior to the currently used materials, such as intermediate restorative material (IRM), ethoxybenzoic acid (EBA) cements, or mineral trioxide aggregate (MTA).[241–245] The reportedly less effective strategies have been used in the majority of studies in the past and in several recent ones,[84,88,89,132,134,136,145–147] whereas the current strategies, assumed to be more effective, have been used in other recent studies.[131,134–139,141,142,144,148,150,151] Furthermore, in specific studies[122,130,133,140,143,190,191,246] a root-end cavity was not prepared and the root-end was completely covered with bonded composite resin (Figure 8).
- Concurrent orthograde surgical treatment: There is a considerable difference in outcome between apical surgery performed alone on teeth where disease persisted after previous root canal treatment, and concurrent surgical and root canal treatments, consistent with the historic management of teeth with large lesions.[224] The latter had been commonly applied in the past and therefore represented the majority of the samples in specific studies.[94,98,99,102,108,109,112,114,116] In those studies, outcomes were often summarized for the entire study cohort, resulting in better outcomes reported than what should be expected if only apical surgery is performed.[224] Thus, in many studies, the proportion of teeth that received not just apical surgery but also concurrent root canal treatment determined the reported outcomes.
- Pre- and postoperative restoration: The influence of the type and timing of a definitive restoration on the outcome of nonsurgical endodontic treatment is equivocal. However, it has been shown that absence of a sound restoration may impair the prognosis of nonsurgical treatment[18,33,90] and apical surgery[121,139,148] (Figure 9). In several studies,[12,18,70,78,90] a proportion of the teeth had not

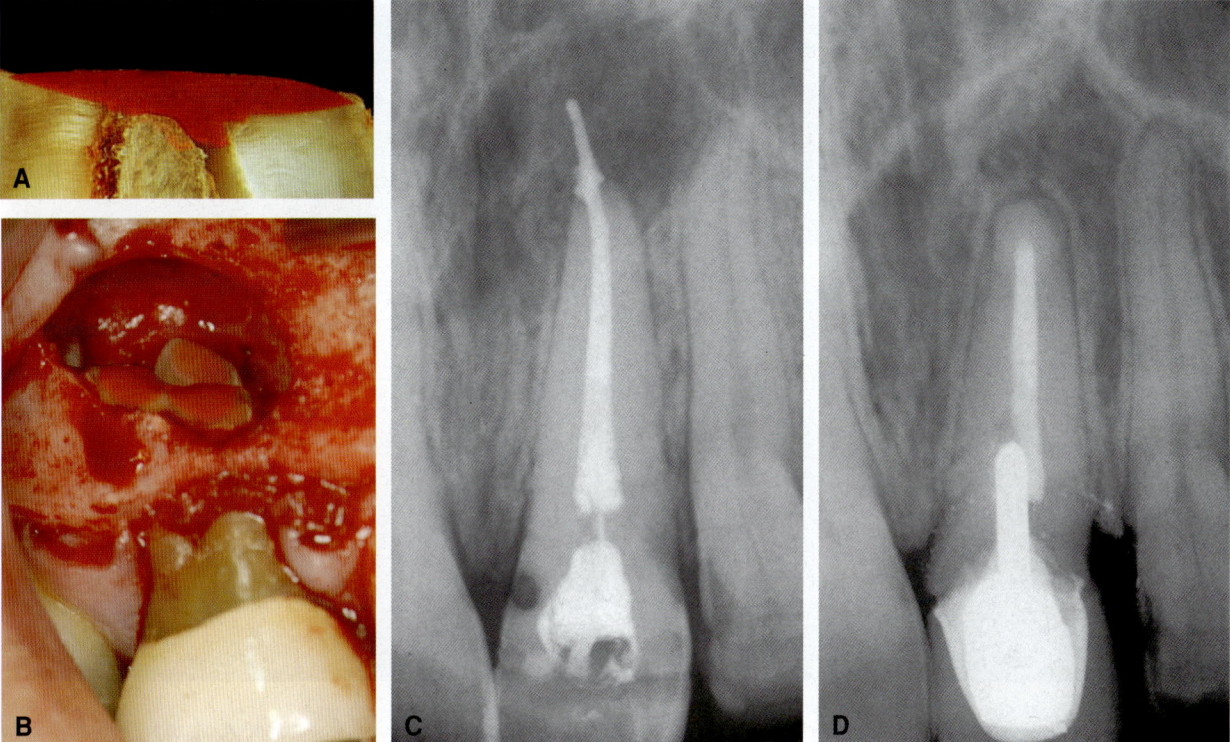

Figure 8 Root-end management with bonded composite resin. **A,** Vertical section through a root end with a bonded Retroplast "cap" (Retroplast Trading, Rörvig, Denmark). The cut root surface was prepared with a round bur to accommodate the resin. The bonded "cap" is sealing the main canal and an accessory one. **B,** Clinical view of a maxillary first molar with Retroplast bonded to the three root apexes. **C,** Root-filled maxillary central incisor with extruded root filling and persistent apical periodontitis. **D,** At 9 years after surgery with bonded Retroplast at the root end, the lesion is healed. Originally, Retroplast was only slightly radiopaque; the current generation is fully radiopaque. (Photos courtesy of Dr. Vibe Rud, Copenhagen, Denmark; Reprinted with permission from Friedman 2006.[201])

been restored, possibly adversely influencing the outcome in these studies. The majority of studies have not provided detailed information about the restorative status of the treated teeth, but it is likely that in many studies the reported outcomes were influenced by inclusion of teeth with defective or missing restorations.

The treatment providers' expertise may determine the outcomes of studies, as skillful operators are less likely to perform procedural errors that might impair the outcome.[49] Therefore, the treatment providers (students, general dentists, residents, specialists) should be characterized to establish the external validity of the results.[212] Examination of the endodontic studies reveals differences in the experience and qualifications of treatment providers that may be particularly important in studies on apical surgery:

- Treatment providers: Historically, apical surgery has been predominantly performed by oral surgeons, but over the years, it has been performed with increasing frequency by endodontists. Endodontists have significantly modified the procedure, routinely using operating microscopes and microsurgical instruments, ultrasonic cavity preparation devices, novel materials for root-end filling, and improved strategies for hemostasis and suturing. It appears that until recently, the majority of oral surgeons have not kept up with these modified procedures[146] and their treatment outcomes may have fallen behind those of endodontists.[139] Providers of treatment in the different studies on apical surgery included oral surgeons,[84,89,93,95–103,105–109,112,116,117,119,120,122,124,126–128,130–132, 134,136,137,140,141,145–147,150,151,183,188,190,191] endodontists,[82,88,117,119,121,125,129,135,138,142,144,149] and resident students.[82,121,139,143,148] In studies on nonsurgical endodontic treatment, providers of treatment varied from undergraduate students[2,6–8,10,12,18,19,22,28,33,35,37,39,41,43,48,49,52,56,63,66,74,81] to qualified endodontists.[1,3–5,9,16,20,21,25,29–32,34,36,49–51,54,55,61,62,69,71,75,79,80, 86,88,92]

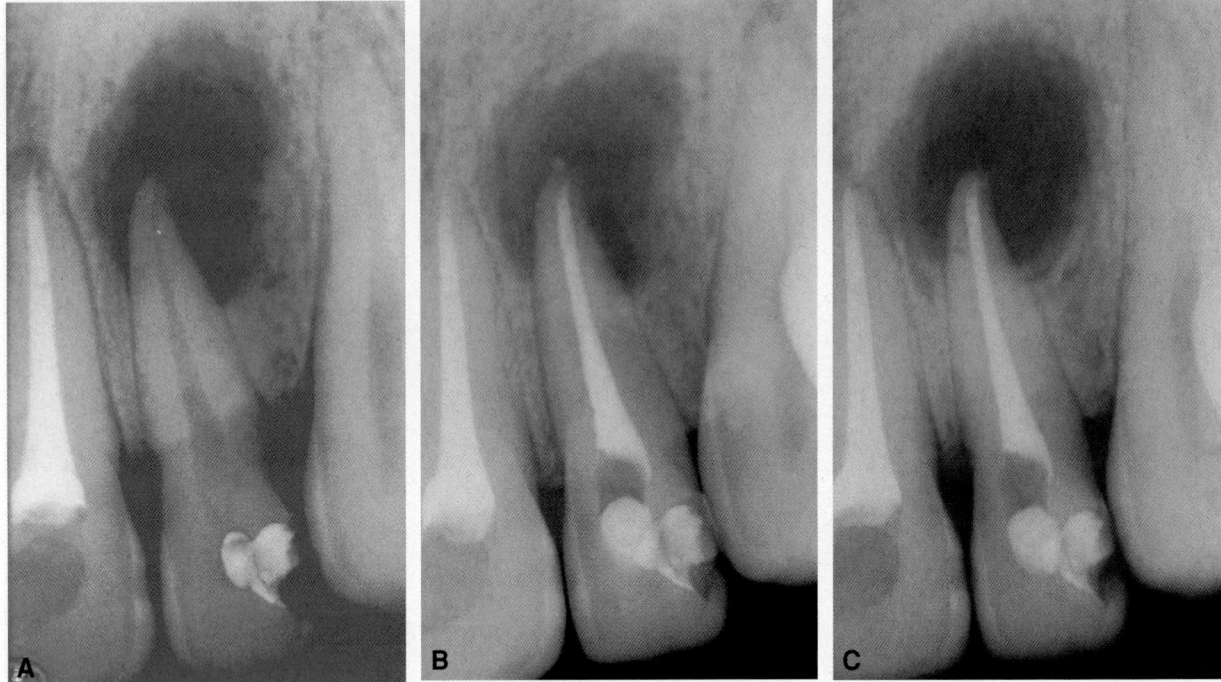

Figure 9 Lack of definitive restoration and outcome classification labeled as "persistent disease" after initial treatment. ***A,*** Maxillary lateral incisor with extensive apical periodontitis. ***B,*** Completed treatment. Access cavity is temporarily restored with reinforced zinc-oxide eugenol (IRM). ***C,*** At 3 years, disease persists. This unfavorable outcome may have been caused by the failure to place a definitive restoration. (Reprinted with permission from Friedman 2002.[164])

Finally, studies may be excluded if the treatment procedures described are considered irrelevant to the review or unacceptable. This consideration can be demonstrated with the following two examples from endodontic studies:

- Acceptable, relevant procedures: In one study on nonsurgical treatment,[29-31] roots associated with apical periodontitis were instrumented "to the approximate center of the lesion." In one study on apical surgery,[118] a specific "bony lid approach" has been described. Reviews concerned with typical forms of treatment may exclude both these studies.

Outcome Assessment

Strict rules should be followed when clinical outcomes are assessed, in order to minimize measurement bias.[212] Outcome dimensions and measures should be clearly defined. Of the four dimensions of dental outcomes,[247] the endodontic studies usually assess the physical/physiologic (pathosis, pain, and function) and the longevity/survival (tooth loss and time until repeat treatment for same or new condition) outcomes, but seldom the psychological (perceived esthetics, level of oral health, and satisfaction with oral health status) and economic (direct and indirect cost) outcomes. Outcome measures used to assess these dimensions should be objective and applied consistently in a blinded manner. Therefore, examiners who assess the outcome should be different from the provider(s) of treatment, and they should be properly calibrated with their reliability established. Also, direct comparisons of preoperative and follow-up radiographs must be avoided. Of particular concern in endodontic studies is the interpretation of radiographs and the inconsistency of criteria used for outcome assessment, as explained below:

- Interpretation of radiographs: Radiographs have been used invariably as the principal outcome measure in follow-up studies after endodontic treatment; however, radiographs are poorly standardized, being subject to changes in angulation and contrast, and they do not capture subtle inflammatory changes in the periapical tissues.[177]

Importantly, interpretation of radiographs is subject to bias.[165–169] Those limitations of radiographs may undermine the reliability of the results; therefore, bias and inconsistency can be minimized by assessment made by blinded examiners who are calibrated for standardized interpretation.[37,167,169–173] This requirement has not been fulfilled in the majority of studies; thus, the reported outcomes are likely to reflect differences in radiographic interpretations.

- Inconsistency of criteria: The main cause for the diverse outcomes reported in clinical studies in endodontics is the inconsistency of the criteria used. There tends to be an overestimation of the healing potential in specific studies where healed and reduced lesions are grouped together.[3,5,11,16,29–31,36,42,47,58,113,131]

To avoid ambiguity of reported outcomes, the follow-up period in clinical studies should be long enough to capture the outcome of interest. This requirement is particularly important in endodontic studies, where the conclusion of the dynamic healing processes must be captured in the majority of the study sample. Considerations specific to endodontic studies are outlined below:

- Follow-up period: One year has been suggested as an adequate follow-up period after nonsurgical and surgical endodontic treatments.[52,116,120,189] Indeed, a short-term observation after nonsurgical treatment of teeth with apical periodontitis may demonstrate signs of healing[1,45,50] and even reveal meaningful changes.[52,66,248] Nevertheless, sufficient time is required to observe completion of the healing process.[1,22,35,37,52,63,92,180] Thus, studies on nonsurgical treatment extending 1 year or less[3,16,29–31,33,34,50,54,66,82] may considerably underestimate the healing potential.[49,249] To record a stable treatment outcome, follow-up of 4 years or longer may be required.[1,22,35,37,52,63,92] In studies on apical surgery, a particular concern is recurrence of disease (Figure 10), shown to occur in 5 to 42% of healed teeth after periods of 4 years or longer.[88,96,103,125,128,142,147,189] For example, Kvist and Reit[88] report recurrence of disease at the 4-year follow-up, in 4 of 45 teeth (9%) recorded as healed at the 1-year follow-up. Therefore, short-term apical surgery studies[82,84,89,101,107,115,118,122,124,130,134,135,137,141,143,146,150,151] may overestimate the healing potential, and the follow-up period should extend at least 4 years. For the purpose of this chapter, the minimum follow-up of 1 year was required. Furthermore, because all root-filled teeth may in time become subject to adverse effects of periodontal and restorative deterioration, extensive follow-up periods are more likely to reveal the influence of those effects on the outcome. Indeed, long-term changes in outcome have been reported in several studies.[1,63,92,180] The many studies vary considerably in the extent of follow-up periods; therefore, their reported outcomes are likely to reflect this variability.

Reporting of Data and Analysis

Clinical studies should be reported in sufficient detail for a reader to be able to identify potential bias and assess the validity of the study. Thus, all data pertaining to the study cohort, the exposure, outcome assessment, and analysis, should be clearly provided in the report. Examples are abundant in the endodontic studies where essential details are not reported. The results of such studies cannot be used as the basis for estimating the outcome in specific clinical conditions.

Statistical analyses are used in clinical studies mainly to examine associations between the outcome and different variables. This issue can be considerably confused by the nature of the analysis, or the lack thereof. Therefore, the statistical analysis should be designed so as to minimize potential bias. The analysis should take into account extraneous factors and the potential confounding effects of different prognostic factors. In observational studies where the prognostic factors cannot be controlled by the investigators, they should be observed and recorded to allow judicious analysis of the outcomes. Preferably, multivariate analyses should be used to account for all the variables. Confounding effects of different variables can be found in the endodontic studies, as demonstrated by the following examples:

- Analysis and confounding effects: In the vast majority of studies on both nonsurgical and surgical treatments, only bivariate analyses have been used that ignore potential confounding effects of multiple variables.[1] For example, one study on nonsurgical treatment[225] offers two conclusions: (1) teeth in which overfilling occurred have a poorer outcome than teeth filled without overfilling, and (2) presence of apical periodontitis at the time of treatment has a strong negative influence on the outcome. The report reveals that overfilling occurred more frequently in teeth with apical periodontitis, suggesting that the poor outcome in

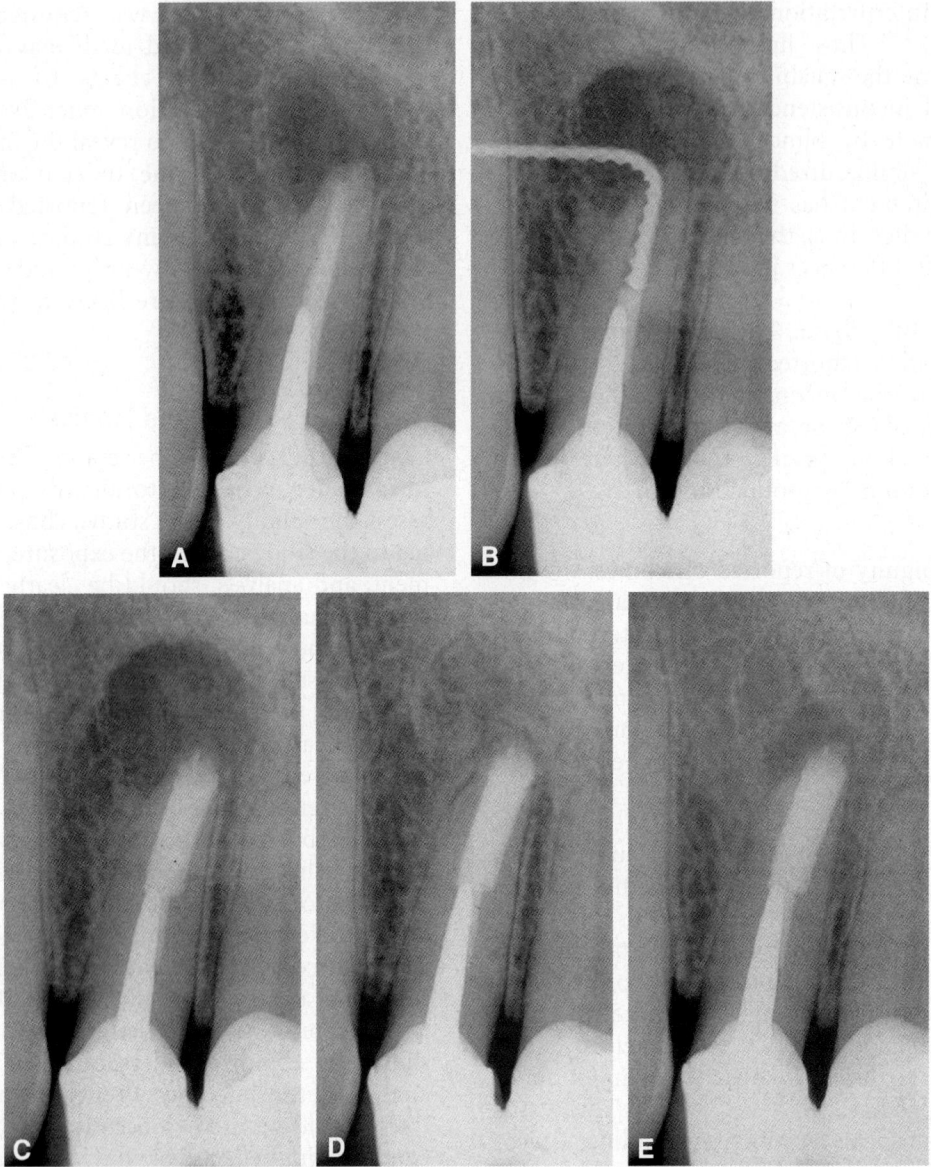

Figure 10 Recurrence of disease after confirmed healing following apical surgery. *A*, Root-filled maxillary lateral incisor with persistent apical periodontitis. *B*, Instrument film indicates extent of retrograde re-treatment carried out. *C*, Completed surgery, including a root filling with sealer and injectable gutta-percha. *D*, At 6 months, the lesion is healed. *E*, At 2.5 years, renewed radiolucency demonstrates recurrence of disease. (Reprinted with permission from Friedman 2006.[201])

overfilled teeth can be "blamed" on the presence of apical periodontitis. In studies on apical surgery, the presence or absence of a root-end filling has often been compared disregarding the fact that some teeth received root canal treatment in conjunction with surgery, whereas others did not. When performed, concurrent orthograde treatment had a strong positive impact on the outcome.[116,120] Because root-end fillings were usually absent in these teeth, researchers concluded that teeth without root-end filings had a better outcome than teeth with root-end fillings.[224] Thus, exclusive use of bivariate analysis may misrepresent the influence of specific variables on the outcome.

A specific concern in endodontic studies is the possibility to record the outcome for each root or for each tooth. Evaluating roots as individual units raises concerns in regard to multi-rooted teeth.[164] When the root is the evaluated unit, more weight is assigned to studies with a large proportion of multi-rooted teeth than to studies that include primarily single-rooted teeth. Also, the outcome is better than if whole teeth are evaluated as units[1,6,29–31,33,50,164] (see Figures 6). This can be demonstrated in the following examples:

- Unit of evaluation: In one follow-up study,[6] healing was observed in 78% of teeth and in 83% of roots. Similarly, in a cross-sectional study of root-filled teeth in a specific population,[178] apical periodontitis was observed in 30% of the teeth but only 24% of the roots. Although the majority of the studies have considered the tooth as the evaluated unit, the individual roots have been evaluated as independent units in many of the studies on nonsurgical treatment[1,2,19,22,37,40,41,43,52,63,72,81,92,248] and on apical surgery.[102,108,117,119,130,133,140,149,190]

SELECTED STUDIES COMPRISING THE "BEST" EVIDENCE

Studies that have reported on the outcome of initial root canal treatment, orthograde re-treatment, apical surgery, and intentional replantation in the past 40 years are listed in Tables 1, 2, 3, and 4, respectively. Studies on surgical treatment are summarized in Tables 5–7. The outcomes in the tables are construed from the original reports, so that combined clinical and radiographic normalcy is classified as "healed," reduced radiolucency combined with clinical normalcy is classified as "healing," and absence of signs and symptoms is classified as "functional"—for several studies this is simply the sum of "healed" and "healing" (when both are available), whereas for others it includes also teeth where the radiolucency persisted.

True "survival" is not used as an outcome category, because in the majority of studies the outcome is calculated after extracted teeth are excluded from the sample. Data on the long-term survival of teeth after nonsurgical and surgical endodontic treatments are available from several specific studies.[163,250–258] Typically, however, survival analyses of endodontically treated teeth are subject to bias. The "surviving" teeth do not necessarily represent all the teeth with a favorable endodontic treatment outcome;[254] thus, the potential for healing may be overestimated. On the other hand, treatment-planning considerations occasionally lead to extraction of functional and periapically healthy teeth, particularly when such teeth require further restorative or periodontal treatment and the patients select to forego this treatment and extract the tooth.[254] Thus, the potential for healing may be underestimated. In recent years, researchers have modified the format of survival analyses, by using reviews of either patient charts or electronic databases of dental insurance providers to record untoward events, such as tooth extraction, orthograde re-treatment, or apical surgery in the long term after initial root canal treatment.[253,255,256,259] This type of analysis also is subject to bias, and it appears to overestimate the healing potential after endodontic treatment.

Notation is made in the tables of the general compliance of the studies with the appraisal criteria outlined above. Studies that comply with any three of the four criteria—cohort, intervention, assessment, analysis/reporting—have been selected as methodologically adequate (insistence on strict compliance with all four criteria would result in a very narrow evidence base).

Table 1 includes 23 studies on initial root canal treatment.[1,6,22,35,37,43,48,52–55,61,62,66,67,70–72,75,76,78,80,248] The samples of two of these studies[37,54] have been repeated in later studies,[39,72,76] and the samples from the Toronto Study series have been added up from the first study[67] throughout the successive ones.[70,78] To avoid confounding of the analysis by repeated samples, only the most recent studies from these three clusters of studies are included in Table 5 reducing the number of selected studies to 18.

Additional six studies were selected on orthograde re-treatment[1,6,43,86,88,90] and nine studies on apical surgery.[88,138,139,143,144,148–151] None of the studies on intentional replantation meet the selection criteria; thus, the level of evidence to support the prognosis of this specific treatment modality is the lowest.

The methodology of the selected studies is rather uniform, but considerable differences still exist in case selection and composition of study materials. The selected studies represent the best available evidence for estimating the potential for healing after endodontic treatment. They also serve as reference for identifying significant outcome predictors (Tables 2–7).

Potential for Healing and Retained Function after NonSurgical Treatment (Tables 5, 6)

Initial root canal treatment and orthograde re-treatment share the same etiology and basic treatment procedures. It is appropriate, therefore, to lump them together into one category—nonsurgical treatment—when reviewing both their prognosis and outcome predictors.

Table 1 Follow-Up Studies on the Outcome of Initial Root Canal Treatment, Appraised for Inclusion/Exclusion in This Chapter Review

Study	Examined Sample (Teeth)	Follow-Up (Years)	Appraisal Categories				Outcome (%)		
			Cohort	Exposure	Assessment	Analysis	Healed	Healing	Functional*
Strindberg (1956)[1]	479	0.5–10	Y	Y	N	Y	90 [d]	–	≥90
Grahnén and Hansson (1961)[2]	1,277 [c]	4–5	Y	N	N	Y	86 [d]	–	–
Seltzer et al (1963)[3]	2,335	0.5	N	N	N	N	–	84	–
Zeldow and Ingle (1963)[4]	57	≥ 2	N	N	N	N	86	–	–
Bender and Seltzer (1964)[5]	706 [b]	2	N	N	N	N	–	82 [f]	–
Grossman et al (1964)[7]	432	1–5	N	N	N	N	90	–	–
Engström et al (1964)[6]	306	4–5	Y	Y	N	Y	82 [d]	–	–
Engström and Lundberg (1965)[8]	129	3.5–4	Y	Y	N	N	78 [a,d]	–	–
Oliet and Sorin (1969)[9]	398	–	N	N	N	N	79	13	≥92
Storms (1969)[10]	158	1	N	N	N	N	81	6	≥87
Harty et al (1970)[11]	1,139	0.5–2	N	N	N	N	90	–	–
Heling and Tamshe (1970)[12]	213	1–5	N	N	N	N	70	–	–
Cvek (1972)[13]	55	0.5–2.5	Y	Y	N	N	91	–	–
Tamse and Heling (1973)[14]	122	1–6	N	Y	N	N	84	–	–
Lambjerg-Hansen (1974)[15]	54	≤ 1.2	Y	Y	N	N	80	4	≥ 84
Selden (1974)[16]	504	0.5–1.5	N	N	N	N	–	93 [a]	–
Adenubi and Rule (1976)[17]	870	0.5–7	N	N	N	Y	88	8	≥ 96
Cvek et al (1976)[22]	131	0.5	Y	Y	N	N	46	49	≥ 95
Heling and Shapira (1978)[18]	118	1–5	N	Y	N	Y	78	–	–
Jokinen et al (1978)[19]	2,459 [c]	2–7	N	N	N	N	53	13	≥66
Soltanoff (1978)[20]	185	≤ 20	N	N	N	N	–	86	–
Ashkenaz (1979)[21]	145	1–2	N	Y	N	N	97	–	–
Kerekes and Tronstad (1979)[22]	501 [c]	3–5	Y	Y	N	Y	95 [d]	–	–
Barbakow et al (1980)[23]	554	≥ 1	N	N	N	N	79	11	≥90
Barbakow et al (1981)[24]	124 [b]	1–9	N	N	N	Y	59	29	≥88
Hession (1981)[25]	151 [c]	0.5–20	N	Y	N	N	99	–	–
Rudner and Oliet (1981) [Q1]	283	0.5–>2	N	N	N	N	89	–	–
Nelson (1982)[27]	299	2–30	N	N	N	N	–	82	–
Cvek et al (1982)[26]	54	4	Y	N	N	N	88 [e,g,i]	–	–
Oliet (1983)[32]	338	≥ 1.5	N	Y	N	N	–	89	–
Klevant and Eggink (1983)[28]	336	2	N	N	N	N	48 [f]	15	≥63
Morse et al (1983) [Q2]	220	1	N	N	N	Y	–	95	–
Swartz et al (1983)[33]	1,007	≥ 1	N	N	N	N	–	88	–
Pekruhn (1986)[34]	889	1	N	Y	N	N	95	–	–
Halse and Molven (1987)[225]	550	10–17	N	N	Y	Y	85	–	–
Safavi et al (1987)[38]	464	0.5–2	N	Y	Y	N	58	–	–
Byström et al (1987)[35]	79 [c]	2–5	Y	Y	Y	N	85	9	≥94
Matsumoto et al (1987)[36]	85	2–3	N	Y	N	N	–	75	–
Ørstavik et al (1987)[37]	546 [c]	1–4	N	Y	Y	Y	87 [i]	–	–
Eriksen et al (1988)[39]	121 [b,c]	3	N	Y	Y	Y	82	9	≥91
Åkerblom and Hasselgren (1988)[40]	64 [c]	2–12	N	Y	N	N	89 [g]	–	–
Molven and Halse (1988)[41]	220 [b,c]	10–17	N	N	Y	Y	80	–	–
Shah (1988)[42]	93	0.5–2	N	N	N	N	–	–	84
Augsburger and Peters (1990)[44]	67	0.3–6.5	N	Y	N	N	–	97	–
Sjögren et al (1990)[43]	849 [c]	8–10	Y	Y	Y	Y	91	–	–
Murphy et al (1991)[45]	89	0.3–2	N	N	N	N	46	48	94
Cvek (1992)[46]	885	4	Y	Y	N	N	91	–	–
Ørstavik and Hörsted-Bindslev (1993)[48]	282	1–4	N	Y	Y	Y	Not interpretable		
Smith et al (1993)[47]	821	2–5	N	N	N	N	–	81	–
Ingle et al (1994)	870	2–5	N	N	N	N	–	88	–

Table 1 Continued on Page 1183

Table 1 Continued from Page 1182

Study	N	Years					%	%	%
Friedman et al (1995)[50]	378	0.5–1.5	Y	Y	N	N	78	16	94
Caliskan and Sen (1996)[51]	172	2–5	Y	Y	N	N	81	8	89
Ørstavik (1996)[52]	**599** [b,c]	**4**	**N**	**Y**	**Y**	**Y**	**90**	**3**	**≥ 93**
Sjögren et al (1997)[53]	**53**	**≤ 5**	**Y**	**Y**	**Y**	**y**	**83**	**–**	**–**
Trope et al (1999)[54]	**76**	**1**	**N**	**Y**	**Y**	**Y**	**80** [h]	**–**	**–**
Weiger et al (2000)[55]	**67**	**1–5**	**Y**	**Y**	**N**	**Y**	**78**	**16**	**94**
Ricucci et al (2000) [Q3]	110	3–15	N	Y	N	N	85 [d]	–	–
Waltimo et al (2001)[56]	204	1–4	N	Y	Y	N	72	–	–
Chugal et al (2001)[57]	407	4	N	N	N	Y	78	78	–
Peak et al (2001)[59]	406	≤ 1	N	N	N	N	57	28	–
Pettiette et al (2001)[66]	40	1	N	Y	N	N	60	–	–
Heling et al (2001)[58]	319	1–12	N	Y	Y	N	–	65	–
Molven et al (2002)[63]	265 [b,c]	20–27	Y	N	Y	N	89	–	–
Benenati and Khajotia (2002)	894	0.5–6	N	N	N	N	62	29	–
Peters and Wesselink (2002)[61]	**38**	**1–4.5**	**Y**	**Y**	**Y**	**Y**	**76**	**21**	**97**
Hoskinson et al (2002)[62]	**200**	**4–5**	**Y**	**Y**	**N**	**Y**	**77**	**–**	**97**
Friedman et al (2003)[67]	**72** [a]	**4–6**	**Y**	**N**	**Y**	**Y**	**74**	**4**	**96**
Chugal et al (2003)[68]	200 [b]	4	N	N	Y	Y	not reported		
Fouad and Burlesson (2003)[65]	540	≥ 2	N	N	N	N	68	–	–
Huumonen et al (2003)[66]	**156**	**1**	**Y**	**Y**	**Y**	**N**	**76**	**2**	**–**
Field et al (2004)[69]	223	0.5–4	N	N	N	N	89	–	–
Peters et al (2004)[71]	**233**	**1–3**	**Y**	**Y**	**Y**	**Y**	**87**	**–**	**–**
Farzaneh et al (2004)[70]	**242** [b]	**4–6**	**Y**	**N**	**Y**	**Y**	**85**	**7**	**95**
Ørstavik et al (2004)[72]	**675** [b,c]	**3**	**N**	**Y**	**Y**	**Y**	**90**	**–**	**–**
Caliskan (2004)[73]	42	2–10	N	Y	Y	N	74	10	≥ 84
Moshonov et al (2005)[74]	94	1–5	N	N	N	N	39	–	–
Marending et al (2005)[75]	**66**	**≥ 2.5**	**Y**	**Y**	**Y**	**Y**	**88**	**–**	**–**
Waltimo et al (2005)[76]	**50** [b]	**1**	**N**	**Y**	**Y**	**Y**	**not interpretable**		
Chu et al (2005)[77]	71	3–4	N	Y	N	Y	80	–	85
Marquis et al (2006)[78]	**373** [b]	**4–6**	**Y**	**N**	**Y**	**Y**	**85**	**–**	**95**
Aqrabawi (2006)[79]	340	5	N	Y	Y	N	80	–	–
Gesi et al (2006) [Q4]	**244** [a]	**1–3**	**Y**	**Y**	**Y**	**Y**	**93**	**–**	**98**

Studies selected for review are in boldface.
*Asymptomatic, without or with residual radiolucency (≥ not reported; rate is sum of healed and healing).
[a] Results recorded at the final observation.
[b] Includes repeated material.
[c] Roots considered as unit of evaluation, rather than teeth.
[d] Recalculated after exclusion of cases classified as "uncertain."
[e] Cases with procedural errors excluded.
[f] Results recorded at 2-year observation.
[g] All canals obliterated to some extent.
[h] Teeth treated in two sessions without intracanal medication excluded.
[i] Results recorded at 4-year observation.
[y] Satisfies criteria of acceptable quality.
[n] Does not satisfy criteria of acceptable quality.

Teeth Treated Without Associated Apical Periodontitis

Frequently, endodontic treatment is performed in teeth not associated with apical periodontitis. These teeth may undergo initial treatment, if the pulp is vital—intact (elective treatment) or irreversibly inflamed—or if it is necrotic but not infected. Root-filled teeth may also undergo orthograde re-treatment even if they are not associated with apical periodontitis, if the root filling is suspected of becoming infected subsequent to placement of a new post/core and crown restoration. Distinct groups of teeth without apical periodontitis have been identified in the study samples of several of the selected studies on

Table 2 Follow-Up Studies on the Outcome of Orthograde Re-treatment, Appraised for Inclusion/Exclusion in This Chapter Review

Study	Examined Sample	Follow-Up (Years)	Appraisal Categories				Outcome (%)		
			Cohort	Exposure	Assessment	Analysis	Healed	Healing	Functional*
Strindberg (1956)[1]	**187**	**0.5–10**	**Y**	**Y**	**N**	**Y**	**88 [e]**	**–**	**–**
Grahnén and Hansson (1961)[2]	502 [c]	4–5	Y	N	N	Y	90 [d]	–	–
Engström et al (1964)[6]	**180**	**4–5**	**Y**	**Y**	**N**	**Y**	**85**	**–**	**–**
Selden (1974)[16]	52	0.5–1.5	N	N	N	N	–	88 [a]	–
Bergenholtz et al (1979)[81]	556 [c]	2	Y	Y	N	N	75	12	≥87
Pekruhn (1986)[34]	36	1	N	Y	N	N	83	–	–
Molven and Halse (1988)[41]	174 [c]	10–17	N	N	Y	Y	79 [d]	–	–
Allen et al (1989)[82]	315	≥0.5	N	N	N	N	73	12	≥85
Sjögren et al (1990)[43]	**267 [c]**	**8–10**	**Y**	**Y**	**Y**	**Y**	**85**	**–**	**–**
Van Nieuwenhuysen et al (1994)[83]	561 [c]	≥0.5	N	N	N	Y	78	–	–
Friedman et al (1995)[50]	128	0.5–1.5	Y	Y	Y	N	70	23	93
Danin et al (1996)[84]	18	1	N	Y	N	N	28	28	≥56
Sundqvist et al (1998)[86]	54	4	N	Y	Y	Y	74	–	–
Piatowska et al (1997) [Q5]	60	–	N	Y	N	N	43	42	≥85
Abbott (1999)[87]	432	0.3–4	N	N	N	N	98	1	–
Kvist and Reit (1999)[88]	**47**	**4**	**Y**	**Y**	**Y**	**N**	**58 [f]**	**–**	**–**
Chugal et al (2001)[57]	85 [c]	4	N	N	Y	Y	79	–	–
Hoskinson et al (2002)[g62]	76	4–5	N	Y	N	Y	78	–	–
Farzaneh et al (2004)[70]	**103**	**4–6**	**Y**	**N**	**Y**	**Y**	**81**	**5**	**93**
Gorni and Gagliani (2004)[91]	452	2	Y	N	N	N	65	4	–
Fristad et al (2004)[92]	112 [b,c]	20–27	N	N	Y	Y	96	–	–

Studies selected for review are in boldface.
*Asymptomatic, without or with residual radiolucency (≥ not reported; rate is sum of healed and healing).
[a] Results recorded at the final observation.
[b] Includes repeated material.
[c] Roots considered as unit of evaluation, rather than teeth.
[d] Cases classified as "uncertain" excluded.
[e] Results recorded at 4-year observation.
[f] Approximate figure deducted from graph.
[g] Study selected for initial treatment, but lacking detail in regards to re-treatment.
[Y] Satisfies criteria of acceptable quality.
[n] Does not satisfy criteria of acceptable quality.

nonsurgical treatment (Tables 5, 6). The reported outcomes in these teeth are rather consistent among these nine studies.

HEALED TEETH

The proportion of teeth that remained healed after initial treatment ranges from 88[6,62] to 97%,[43] and after re-treatment, from 94[6] to 98%.[43] The outcome in the two former studies (88%) appears to fall considerably below those of the other six studies (93–97%), and may be considered an outlier. As expected from the selected studies that are rather uniform methodologically, the range of their outcomes is considerably smaller than that observed across all studies (67–97%). Thus, the potential of teeth to remain free of apical periodontitis after nonsurgical treatment is 93 to 98%.

FUNCTIONAL TEETH

According to two studies[78,90] that specifically address this outcome, the proportion of functional teeth after nonsurgical treatment is 93 to 95%. This figure represents both teeth *without and with* apical periodontitis at the time of treatment. *Thus, the potential of teeth to remain asymptomatic and functional after nonsurgical treatment is at least 93%.*

DYNAMICS OF DEVELOPING DISEASE

Development of apical periodontitis subsequent to initial treatment is usually quick; of all the affected

Table 3 Follow-Up Studies Reporting on the Outcome of Apical Surgery, Appraised for Inclusion/Exclusion in This Chapter Review

Study	Examined Sample (Teeth)	Follow-Up (Years)	Cohort	Exposure	Assessment	Analysis	Orthograde and Surgery	Surgery	Healed	Healing	Functional*
Mattila and Altonen (1968)[93]	164	0.8–5	Yes	No	Yes	No	39		63	11	≥ 74
								61	49	17	≥ 66
Harty et al (1970)[94]	1,016	5	Yes	No	Yes	No	83		90	–	–
								17	89	–	–
Nord (1970)[95]	354	0.5–6.5	No	Yes	No	No		100	60	13	≥ 73
Nordenram and Svårdström (1970)[96]	697	0.6–6	No	Yes	No	Yes	15		82	11	≥ 93
								85	60	16	≥ 76
Lehtinen and Aitasalo (1972)[98]	460 [p]	n/a	No	No	No	No	n/a	78	11	≥ 89	
Rud et al (1972)[99]	1,000	1–15	No	No	Yes	Yes	100		90	6	≥ 96
Ericson et al (1974)[100]	314	0.5–12	No	No	No	No		100	54	25	≥ 79
Persson et al (1974)[101]	220	1	Yes	Yes	No	No		100	41	36	≥ 77
Altonen and Mattila (1976)[102]	46	1–6	No	No	No	No	69 [rt]		84	8	≥ 92
								31 [rt]	65	6	≥ 71
Finne et al (1977) [a103]	218	3	Yes	Yes	No	No		100	50	19	≥ 69
Tay et al (1978) [b104]	86	n/a	No	No	No	No	n/a	78	–	–	
Hirsch et al (1979)[105]	572	0.5–3	No	No	No	Yes	87	13	47	48	≥ 95
Malmström et al (1982)[106]	154	2.4	No	Yes	No	No	57 [1]		74	24	≥ 98
								43	54	33	≥ 87
Persson (1982)[107]	26	1	Yes	Yes	No	No		100	73	15	≥ 88
Ioannides and Borstlap (1983)[108]	182 [rt]	0.5–5	No	Yes	No	No	75		72	18	≥ 90
								25	73	11	≥ 84
Mikkonen et al (1983)[109]	174	1–2	Yes	Yes	No	No	93		56	28	≥ 84
								7	75	17	≥ 92
Skoglund and Persson (1985)[110]	27	0.5–7	No	Yes	No	No		100	37	33	≥ 70
Reit and Hirsch (1986)[111]	35	1–≥4	Yes	Yes	No	No		100 [r]	71	26	≥ 97
Forssell et al (1988)[112]	358	1–4	No	No	Yes	No	71		68	21	≥ 89
								29	69	7	≥ 76
Allen et al (1989)[82]ss	695	≥ 0.5	No	No	No	No		100	60	27	≥ 87
Amagasa et al (1989)[113]	64	1–7.5	Yes	Yes	No	No		100 [r]	–	–	95
Crosher et al (1989)[114]	85	2	No	Yes	No	No	100		92	–	–
Dorn and Gartner (1990)[115]	488	0.5	No	No	No	No	n/a	63	18	≥ 81	
Grung et al (1990)[116]	473	1–8	Yes	No	Yes	No	66		96	3	≥ 99
								34	72	12	≥ 84
Friedman et al (1991)[117]	136 [rt]	0.5–8	No	No	Yes	Yes		100	44	23	≥ 67
Lasaridis et al (1991)[118]	24	≥ 0.5	Yes	Yes	No	No	100		79	17	≥ 96
Lustmann et al (1991) [c119]	134 [rt]	0.5–8	No	No	Y	Y	7		70	30	≥ 100
								93	43	22	≥ 65
Molven et al (1991) [d120]	222	1–8	Yes	No	Yes	No	50		96	3	≥ 99
								50	73	14	≥ 87
Rapp et al (1991) [e121]	428	0.5–≥2	No	No	No	No		94	66	29	≥ 95
							6 [2]		56	33s	≥ 89
Rud et al (1991)[122]	388	0.5–1	No	Yes	Yes	No		100	78	15	≥ 93
Waikakul and Punwutikorn (1991)[123]	62	0.5 -2	Yes	Yes	No	No		100	81	17	≥ 96
Zetterqvist et al (1991)[124]	105	1	Yes	Yes	No	No		100	61	31	≥ 92
Frank et al (1992)[125]	104	≥ 10	No	No	No	No	n/a	58	–	–	
Cheung and Lam (1993)[126]	32	≥ 2	No	No	No	No	n/a	62	22	≥ 84	
Pantschev et al (1994)[127]	79	3	No	Yes	Yes	No		100	54	21	≥ 75
Jesslén et al (1995)[128]	93	5	Yes	Yes	No	No		100	59	28	≥ 87

Table 3 Continued on Page 1186

Table 3 Continued from Page 1185

Study	N	Years								
August (1996)[129]	39	10–23	No	No	No	No		74	15	≥ 89
Danin et al (1996)[84]	19	1	No	Yes	Yes	No	100	58	26	≥ 84
Rud et al (1996)[130]	351 rt	0.5–1.5	No	Yes	Yes	No	100	82	12	≥ 94
Sumi et al (1996)[131]	157	0.5–3	Yes	Yes	No	No	100	–	–	92
Jansson et al (1997)[132]	62	0.9–1.3	Yes	Yes	No	No	100	31	55	≥ 86
Rud et al (1997) f[133]	551 rt	0.5–1.5	No	Yes	Yes	No	100	79	16	≥ 95
Bader and Lejeune (1998)[134]	254	1	No	Yes	No	No	100	–	–	81
Danin et al (1999)[89]	10	1	No	Yes	Yes	No	100	50	50	≥ 100
Kvist and Reit (1999)[88]	**45**	**4**	**Yes**	**Yes**	**No**	**Yes**	**100**	**60**	**–**	**–**
Rubinstein and Kim (1999)[135]	94	1.2	No	Yes	No	No	100	97	–	–
Testori et al (1999)[136]	134	1–6	No	Yes	No	No	100	78	9	≥ 87
von Arx and Kurt (1999)[137]	43	1	Yes	Yes	No	No	100	82	14	≥ 96
Zuolo et al (2000)[138]	**102**	**1–4**	**Yes**	**Yes**	**Yes**	**No**	**100** [2]	**91**	**–**	**92**
Rahbaran et al (2001)[139]	**129** en	**≥ 4**	**Yes**	**Yes**	**Yes**	**Yes**	**100** [3]	**37**	**33**	**≥ 80**
Rud et al (2001)[140]	834 rt	0.5–12.5	No	Yes	Yes	No	100	92	1	≥ 93
von Arx and Kurt (2001)[141]	25	1	Yes	Yes	No	No	100	88	8	≥ 96
Rubinstein and Kim (2002) g[142]	59	5–7	Yes	Yes	No	No	100	92	–	–
Jensen et al (2002)[143]	**60** Rp	**1**	**Yes**	**Yes**	**No**	**Yes**	**100**	**73**	**17**	**≥ 90**
Chong et al (2003)[144]	**108**	**2**	**No**	**Yes**	**Yes**	**Yes**	**100**	**90**	**6**	**≥ 96**
Wesson and Gale (2003)[147]	790	5	Yes	Yes	No	No	100	57	5	≥ 62
Maddalone and Gagliani (2003)[145]	120	0.3–3	No	Yes	Yes	No	100	93	3	≥ 96
Schwartz-Arad et al (2003)[146]	262	0.5–0.9	No	Yes	No	Yes	100	44	21	≥ 65
Wang et al (2004)[148]	**94**	**4–8**	**Yes**	**Yes**	**Yes**	**Yes**	**100** [4]	**74**	**–**	**91**
Gagliani et al (2005)[149]	**231** rt	**5**	**Yes**	**Yes**	**No**	**Yes**	**100**	**78**	**10**	**89**
Lindeboom et al (2005)[150]	**100**	**1**	**Yes**	**Yes**	**No**	**Yes**	**100**	**89**	**10**	**99**
Von Arx et al (2007)[151]	**191**	**1**	**Yes**	**Yes**	**No**	**Yes**	**100**	**84**	**10**	**≥ 94**

Studies selected for review are in boldface.
*Asymptomatic, without or with residual radiolucency (≥ = not reported; rate is sum of healed and healing).
n/a = not available. P = Patients (as opposed to teeth), rt = roots (as opposed to teeth).
enOnly teeth treated in the endodontic clinic included. fRetrograde re-treatment.
RpOnly teeth treated with Retroplast included.
[1]31% of cases treated for persistent disease after orthograde re-treatment.
[2]Treated for persistent disease after orthograde retreatment.
[3]39% of cases treated for persistent disease after orthograde re-treatment.
[4]37% of cases treated for persistent disease after orthograde re-treatment.
aSample as in Persson et al. 1974.
bSample as in Harty et al. 1970.
cSample as in Friedman et al. 1991.
dSample as in Grung et al. 1990.
eSample as in Allen et al. 1989.
fSample as in Rud et al. 1991 and Rud et al 1996.
gSample as in Rubinstein et al. 1999.

teeth, approximately 75% show signs of the disease within the first year after treatment.[52,80] In the following years, the risk of developing disease is not increased[52] and late emergence of the disease is infrequent, suggesting that follow-up beyond 1 year may not be necessary.[52] Occasionally, however, a lesion that was observed to develop within 4 years after treatment may later disappear,[1] or a lesion may develop many years after treatment.[63,92] Even though these late developments are uncommon, their occurrence suggests that long-term follow-up of the treated teeth may be beneficial.

Table 4 Follow-Up Studies on the Outcome of Intentional Replantation

Study	Examined Sample (Teeth)	Follow-Up (Years)	Treatment Outcome (%)					
			Survival	Success	RR	IR	RES	AP
Schmidt (1954)*	500	5	–	77			–	–
Tombeur (1953)*	188	–	–	62			–	–
Bielas et al (1959)*	943	5	–	59			–	–
La Forgia (1955)*	60	–	–	55			–	–
Emmertsen and Andreasen (1966)[152]	100	1–13	80	34	4	27	31	50
Grossman and Chacker (1968)	61	3–11	100	57	–	–	18	27
Deeb (1968)[154]	117	0.5–2	93	67	–	–	–	–
Kingsbury and Wiesebaugh (1971)[156]	151	1–3	95	93	–	–	33	–
Will (1974)[157]	158	5–7	96	–	–	–	2	–
Koenig et al (1988)[158]	177	0.5–4	82	82	0	5	5	11
Kahnberg (1988)[159]	58	2–7	71	71	–	–	0	29
Keller (1990)[160]	34	3	91	91	–	–	0	9
Bender and Rossman (1993)[161]	31	0–22	81	81	–	–	6	10

*Cited by Grossman and Chacker (1968)[153]
RR = replacement resorption;
IR = inflammatory resorption;
RES = resorption of any kind;
AP = apical periodontitis.

Teeth Treated with Associated Apical Periodontitis

Teeth associated with apical periodontitis may undergo initial treatment for a primary infection of a necrotic pulp. Root-filled teeth may undergo orthograde re-treatment for a persistent or newly developed infection after a previous treatment. Distinct groups of teeth with apical periodontitis have been identified in 17 of the selected studies on initial treatment[1,6,22,35,43,48,52–55,61,62,66,71,72,75,78] and the 6 studies on re-treatment.[1,6,43,86,88,90] The outcomes reported in these studies still vary considerably, although the studies are methodologically compatible (Tables 5, 6).

HEALED TEETH

The proportion of teeth that healed completely after initial treatment ranges from 73[6] to 90%,[22] and after re-treatment, from 56[88] to 86% (in teeth without perforation).[90] These ranges are smaller than those observed across all studies on initial treatment (46–97%) and re-treatment (28–98%), as expected from the methodologically uniform selected studies. Furthermore, the outcomes of two studies on re-treatment[43,88]—56% (approximate; the exact rate was not provided) and 62%—fall considerably below those reported in the other studies, whereas the 90% outcome of initial treatment[22] falls above the reported range. These atypically low and high outcomes may be considered as outliers. *Thus, the potential of teeth with apical periodontitis to heal after nonsurgical treatment is 73 to 86%.*

Considering the uniformity of outcome criteria among the selected studies, the reported outcomes may have varied because of the following factors:

- Differences in tooth types or in definition of the evaluated unit—tooth or root:[164] The better outcomes are reported in studies that either included only single-rooted teeth[35,53] or calculated the outcome for each root.[43,260] Use of the root as the evaluated unit in studies with multi-rooted teeth usually improves the outcome compared with the use of the whole tooth as the evaluated unit.[164] It should be noted, however, that lower outcomes have been reported in several other selected studies where roots were assessed as the evaluated units.[39,52,54]
- Differences in case selection:[49] Cases treated by undergraduate students in several studies[6,22,35,39,43] may have been uncomplicated. By contrast, cases complicated by anatomy, advanced periodontal disease, or procedural errors (that occurred before referral for treatment) were occasionally included in one series of studies.[78,90]
- Prerequisite of a no-growth (negative) bacterial culture before root filling:[22,35,43] A significantly higher outcome of initial treatment has been reported when canals were filled after a negative culture (94% healed) than after a positive culture (68%).[53] An even greater difference in

outcome has been demonstrated in re-treated teeth filled after negative (80%) and positive (33%) cultures.[86]
- Differences in restoration: In the studies reported by the Umeå, Sweden group,[35,43,53,86] all teeth were restored immediately after endodontic treatment (personal communication), using a layer of zinc-oxide eugenol to seal the canal orifices.[53] Also in the study by Peters and Wesselink,[61] all the teeth were reportedly well restored. By contrast, 5 to 10% of the teeth in the Toronto Study series[78,90] were not definitively restored 4 to 6 years after treatment. Absence of a definitive restoration may allow microbial ingress into the filled canals[261] and consequent persistence of apical periodontitis.

HEALING IN PROGRESS

The proportion of teeth that demonstrate progressive or incomplete healing has not been frequently reported in the selected studies. When reported, progressive healing ranges from 9[35] to 21%.[61] Typically, the proportion of incomplete healing is inversely proportional to the follow-up period, because the completion of the healing process cannot be captured after a short follow-up;[164] however, this typical pattern is not evident in the selected studies. *Thus, the potential of teeth with apical periodontitis to demonstrate incomplete healing after nonsurgical treatment is approximately 10 to 20%.*

FUNCTIONAL TEETH

From six studies on initial treatment[35,39,52,55,61,78] and one study on re-treatment,[90] it appears that the proportion of functional teeth after nonsurgical treatment ranges from 88[52] to 96%.[62] Additional information can be gathered from the nonselected studies (see Tables 1 and 2). In these tables, asymptomatic function was noted only for healed and healing teeth, where symptoms were absent by definition. It can be assumed that additional asymptomatic teeth were present but not reported in the studies, because they did not show radiographic improvement. It appears, therefore, that the proportion of the functional teeth approaches or even exceeds 95%. It is also noteworthy that the reported survival rates—80% survival after initial treatment of teeth with apical periodontitis,[163] 86% general 5-year survival,[254] and at least 93% survival in chart/database reviews[253,255,256,259]—have been rather high. *Thus, the potential of teeth with apical periodontitis to remain functional after nonsurgical treatment may approximate 95%.*

This excellent potential for retained asymptomatic function *definitely justifies conservative endodontic treatment in teeth with primary or refractory apical periodontitis and reasonable restorative and periodontal prognosis. If initial treatment or re-treatment is considered feasible and acceptable to the patient, tooth extraction and replacement should not be contemplated.*

DYNAMICS OF HEALING

Healing of apical periodontitis ensues within the first year after nonsurgical treatment,[88,249] so that signs of healing are evident in nearly 90% of the teeth that heal eventually.[52] Completion of the healing process, however, often requires a longer time. Therefore, of all the teeth that heal eventually, only about 50% appear completely healed by 1 year,[17] the majority appear healed after 2 years,[35,37] and a small percentage appear healed only after 4 to 5 years,[17,35,37,43,52,88] or even longer.[1,63,92] In the interim follow-up periods, additional teeth demonstrate further reduction of the radiolucency.[28,35,37,43,52] For example, at 4 years about 13% of the teeth showed radiographic improvement,[52] whereas closer to 6 years nearly 7% of the teeth showed improvement.[70,78,90] Two studies with uniquely long follow-up periods offer an insight into the long-term healing dynamics after initial treatment[63] and re-treatment.[63,92] Over 6% of the initially treated teeth, and as many as 50% of the re-treated teeth were observed to still have disease 10 to 17 years after treatment but were completely healed a decade later, resulting in an improved outcome in the long term. The late healing was mainly characteristic of teeth with surplus root filling material.[92] Taking the healing dynamics into consideration, a demonstrated continuous reduction of the radiolucency (comparing at least two follow-up examinations) may be considered as a forecast of complete healing at a later time.[35]

Reversal of the healing process after nonsurgical treatment (Figure 11) is uncommon,[1,52,88] prompting the suggestion that extended follow-up of teeth that demonstrate signs of healing after 1 year may be unnecessary.[52] Notwithstanding the progressive nature of the healing process, all root-filled teeth remain constantly challenged by intra-oral microorganisms, placing them at risk of recurrent apical periodontitis in the long term, even if they are completely healed in a short term after therapy. For example, over 1% of teeth were observed to be healed 10 to 17 years after treatment but were reverted to disease a decade later.[63] To address the possibility of long-term changes, periodic follow-up of root-filled teeth is advocated as a viable routine.

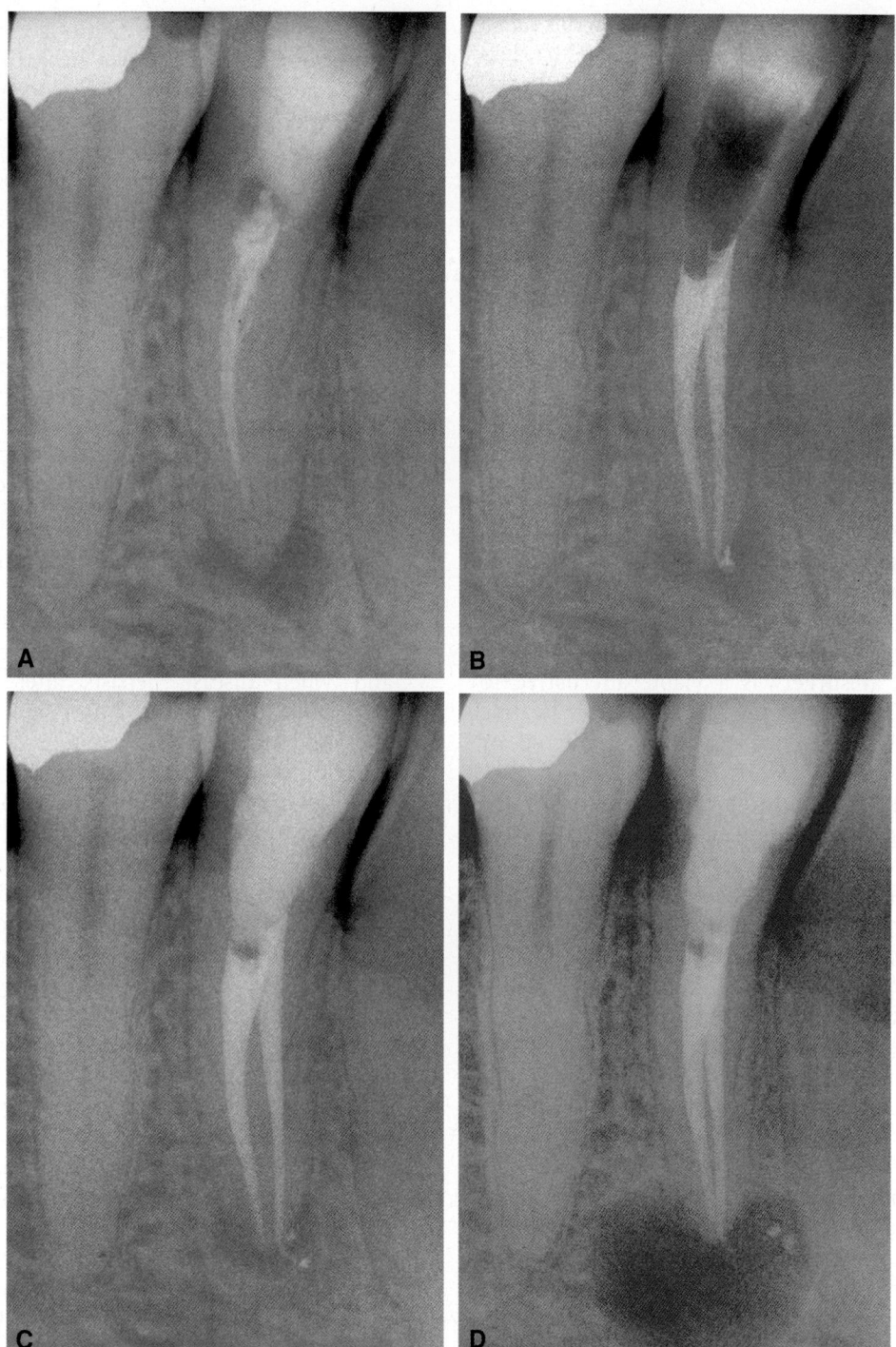

Figure 11 Reversal or regression in healing of apical periodontitis after re-treatment. ***A,*** Failing root canal treatment in mandibular premolar. ***B,*** Immediate postoperative radiograph of mandibular first premolar with apical periodontitis. ***C,*** At 7 months, the clearly reduced radiolucency is indicative of healing in progress. ***D,*** At 2 years, the radiolucency has grown larger again beyond its original size, indicative of reversal of the healing process. (Reprinted with permission from Friedman 2002.[164])

Teeth treated by apexification appear to demonstrate a different pattern of healing dynamics. Of those that had not shown signs of healing during apexification, approximately 66% healed after conclusion of treatment with a definitive root filling, whereas of those that appeared healed during the apexification process, approximately 8% reverted to disease 2 to 3 years after definitive root filling.[46]

In the long term, apical periodontitis lesions are expected to heal completely;[1,41,249] however, infrequently very extensive lesions can heal without total resolution of the radiolucency. In such cases, the residual radiolucency represents a fibrous periapical tissue (apical scar), rather than a pathologic lesion[35,262–265] (see Figure 1).

Potential for Healing and Retained Function after Apical Surgery

Patients deliberating different options for management of refractory apical periodontitis should consider the benefit—primarily the potential for healing—and risks associated with each treatment alternative. Apical surgery is a viable alternative to orthograde re-treatment; the potential for healing it offers should be weighed against that offered by re-treatment.

In contrast to the uniform characteristics of the selected studies on nonsurgical treatment, the nine selected studies on apical surgery[88,138,139,143,144,148–151] differ considerably in their cohort (population) and exposure (intervention) characteristics (Table 7). An important difference can be observed in regard to the treatment history before surgery, including only initial treatment, orthograde re-treatment, or apical surgery. For example, teeth that received previous orthograde re-treatment comprised 100% of the sample in one study,[138] an unknown proportion of the sample in another study[144] (personal communication), and close to 40% of the samples in two other studies,[139,148] whereas the remaining studies[88,143,149–151] did not mention the previous treatment history of their cohorts. The outcome of apical surgery is expected to be better when it is preceded by orthograde re-treatment, as highlighted below. Also, the proportions of teeth that received previous apical surgery varied, comprising 44,[139] 33,[149] and close to 10%[148,151] of the study cohorts. By contrast, only first-time surgery was included in one study,[143] whereas the remaining three studies[88,144,150] do not characterize their cohorts in regard to previous surgery. The outcome of repeat surgery is expected to be poorer than that of first-time surgery. These and other differences among the selected studies result in a considerable inconsistency in the reported outcomes.

HEALED TEETH

The proportion of teeth that healed completely after apical surgery ranges from 37%[139] to 91%.[138] Contrary to the expectation from the selected studies that are rather uniform methodologically, the range of their outcomes is almost as large as that observed across all studies (31%–98%) (Table 3). The highest two outcomes of 90%[144] and 91%[138] may have been affected by previous orthograde re-treatment, whereas the lowest outcome of 37%[139] appears to fall considerably below the range reported in the remaining four studies (60%–89%); these atypically high and low outcomes may be considered as outliers. *Thus, the potential for teeth to heal completely after apical surgery is 60% to 89%.* Considering the uniformity of outcome criteria among the selected studies, the reported outcomes may have varied because of the following factors:

- Assembly bias, particularly from inclusion of previously re-treated teeth in the study sample: The site where persistent bacteria colonize may differ in the case of persistent disease after initial treatment and when disease persists after orthograde re-treatment.[148,223] In the latter, "intra-canal irritants and contamination" were reduced[138] suggesting that infection is sustained by bacteria located in inaccessible sites: canal ramifications close to the apex,[265–267] the outer surface of the root tip,[268,269] or the periapical tissue.[270–287] Bacteria harbored in all these sites would be eradicated by the resection of the root tip and periapical curettage; therefore, the potential for healing is excellent, as demonstrated in two studies where 84[148] and 91%[138] of previously re-treated teeth healed after subsequent surgery. By contrast, when disease persists after initial treatment, bacteria are more likely to be located within the root canal.[86,184,186,187,266,288–303] The surgical procedure does not eliminate these bacteria, but rather an attempt is made to enclose them with a root-end filling. The proportion of previously re-treated teeth in the study sample has been specified in only three of the studies.[138,139,148]

- Differences in treatment procedures: In one of the selected studies,[88] less current techniques and materials were used than those used in the more recent studies.[138,139,143,144,148–151] First, the root-end cavities in the former study were prepared with round burs, as opposed to the ultrasonic cavity preparation (Figure 10B) in the recent studies, that results in deeper, cleaner, and better-aligned root-end cavities with less risk of lingual perforation.[235,237,238,240,304,305] Second, amalgam was used for root-end filling in the former study,[88] whereas IRM, Super EBA cement, MTA, or a dentin-bonded composite resin was used in the recent studies, with the expectation of improved clinical performance based on favorable outcomes in animal studies.[241–246] In addition, in five of the recent studies also magnification and micro-instruments were used[144,148–151] that facilitate visualization and treatment of accessory canals and isthmuses, as well as detection of root cracks.[238,304–307] Use of these modern tools allows the clinician to keep the bony crypt small and to reduce the apical bevel, so that fewer dentinal tubules become exposed.[235,237,238,240,305,308] Collectively, these current procedures may have improved the outcome in most of the recent studies,[138,143,144,148–151] compared with the study where these techniques were not used.[88]

HEALING IN PROGRESS

Progressive healing appears to range from 6%[144] to 33%.[139] Similarly to nonsurgical treatment, a high proportion of progressive healing captured in a study is typical of a short follow-up period;[164] therefore, the reporting of the highest proportion of progressive healing in a study with a follow-up of 4 years or longer[139] is surprising. This atypical pattern could possibly be explained if the study cohort included many large lesions that healed by formation of a fibrous scar and were classified as "uncertain healing" (consistent with this chapter's definition of "healing in progress"); by contrast, in the other selected studies scars were classified as "incomplete healing" (consistent with this chapter's definition of "healed"). *Thus, the potential of teeth to demonstrate incomplete healing after apical surgery is approximately 5% to 30%, depending on the case selection and outcome classification used.*

FUNCTIONAL TEETH

From eight studies,[138,143,144,148–151] it appears that the proportion of functional teeth after apical surgery exceeds 89%. This outcome does not take into account all lost teeth; therefore, it overestimates the chances of teeth to be retained after apical surgery. Also, it is not synonymous with the lower "survival" rate reported in another study;[257] however, it is noteworthy that typically, a survival analysis may underestimate the potential for tooth survival, when functional teeth without disease are extracted for reasons unrelated to the endodontic outcome. *Thus, the potential of teeth to remain functional after apical surgery may approximate or exceed 90%.*

This good potential for retained asymptomatic function *justifies conservative surgical treatment in teeth with primary or refractory apical periodontitis and reasonable restorative and periodontal prognosis.* If apical surgery is considered feasible and acceptable to the patient, tooth extraction and replacement should not be contemplated.

DYNAMICS OF HEALING

Healing progresses within the first year after apical surgery,[88,189] so that of all the teeth that heal eventually, 35% to 60% appear healed by 1 year.[105,106,116,145,147,183,189] About half of the teeth that show signs of healing at 1 year continue to heal, whereas about one quarter revert to disease; therefore, of the teeth that heal eventually, approximately 85% appear healed by 3 years.[96,116,189] Definitive outcomes (healed or diseased) observed at 1 year have been suggested to remain stable up to 3 to 5 years,[96,103,105,142,189] supporting the suggestion that the 1 year follow-up may be considered conclusive, except for teeth that show healing in progress.[183,189]

Notwithstanding the suggested stability of the outcome observed at 1 year, 5 to over 40% of healed teeth have been shown to revert to disease in the long term[88,96,103,125,128,142,147,189] (see Figure 4). Thus, recurrence of apical periodontitis is more prevalent after apical surgery than after nonsurgical treatment. To address the risk of recurrent disease in the long term, it is advisable to extend the follow-up and periodically examine the treated teeth.

Whereas apical scar formation after nonsurgical treatment is infrequent, healing by a fibrous scar rather than deposition of bone is quite common after apical surgery[173,174,181–183] (see Figure 1). Apical scars form particularly when both the buccal and lingual bone plates are perforated at the conclusion of the surgical procedure.[116,120] Post-surgery apical scars appear to remain stable over time;[183] therefore, they are considered a surrogate for a healed site.[173,174,183]

Etiology of Refractory Apical Periodontitis after Treatment

As highlighted in the previous sections of this chapter, persistence of apical periodontitis after endodontic treatment is not highly prevalent, but it is not uncommon either. Thorough comprehension of the etiologic factors of disease persistence is required for clinicians to devise strategies for preventing and for managing this unfavorable and frustrating occurrence. For the major part, persistent apical periodontitis is sustained by persistent or recurrent infection; however, the sites colonized by bacteria and the pathways of bacteria–host interactions may differ in nonsurgically and surgically treated teeth.

REFRACTORY INFECTION AFTER NONSURGICAL TREATMENT

Refractory apical periodontitis after initial treatment has been shown to occur in selected cases in response to nonmicrobial factors, including foreign materials and true cysts.[309–312] It appears this is not a common occurrence; it has been demonstrated in three out of nine specimens (33%) where disease persisted despite verified reduction of intra-canal bacteria before root filling, to a level below detection.[43] However, routine endodontic cases do not employ strict bacteriologic monitoring to verify bacterial elimination before root filling; therefore, if disease persists after routine treatment, a higher proportion of infective etiology and a lower proportion of nonmicrobial etiology are expected.

Indeed, evidence of microbial etiology of refractory apical periodontitis after nonsurgical treatment is consistent and undisputed.[223,296] Bacteria sustaining the disease process can colonize the following sites:

- The root canal system: This is the most frequently documented site of bacteria in teeth with refractory apical periodontitis.[86,184,186,187,265–267,288–303,313]
  The bacteria have either survived the root canal treatment procedures[53] or invaded the filled canal space after treatment, possibly through a coronal pathway.[261]
- The periapical tissues: Ample evidence has been accumulated demonstrating specific bacteria, particularly *Actinomyces israelii* and *Propionibacterium propionicum*, established in the periapical tissues of root-filled teeth with persistent disease, even after elimination of root canal bacteria.[271–282,302] These bacteria have either penetrated the host tissues during a long-term infection of the root canal system or were inoculated periapically during treatment. Refractory apical periodontitis caused by bacteria established outside the root canal system is referred to as "extra-radicular" infection.
- Other extra-radicular sites and bacteria: Different bacterial species, other than *Actinomyces*, have been identified outside the root canal space and implied in extra-radicular infection.[270,283–287] Bacteria were shown colonizing the root surface in cementum lacunae,[314,315] forming plaque-like biofilms surrounding the apical foramina,[268–270,316–319] and lodged in dentin debris inadvertently extruded periapically during treatment.[320] Notwithstanding the current evidence, the role of these demonstrated extra-radicular bacteria in the etiology of refractory apical periodontitis has not been sufficiently elucidated. Whether these bacteria sustain infection without dependence on presence of root canal bacteria still requires clarification; an unequivocal answer will have an important impact on strategies for management of refractory apical periodontitis. Until such answer is available, current knowledge suggests that refractory apical periodontitis is predominantly caused by root canal infection, with extra-radicular infection per se affecting a small percentage of cases.[223]

Even though repeated root canal disinfection during orthograde re-treatment specifically targets intra-canal bacteria, bacteria can still survive and sustain persistent apical periodontitis after re-treatment.[86,294,301] Nevertheless, the persistence of disease despite re-treatment increases the probability of the other etiologic factors highlighted above, including foreign body reaction and true cysts,[309,310] or extra-radicular infection.[268–316,270–287,314–320] This increased probability provides the rationale for apical surgery, as the treatment of choice for refractory apical periodontitis after orthograde re-treatment. The surgical procedure is well suited to address the likely etiologic factors.

REFRACTORY INFECTION AFTER APICAL SURGERY

Typical apical surgery comprises an attempt to seal an infected canal with a root-end filling. Persistence of apical periodontitis after surgery usually suggests that the bacteria are not effectively contained within the canal space.[224] Placement of a root-end filling is a technique-sensitive procedure, because of restricted accessibility and the challenge in preparing a well-centered root-end cavity of sufficient depth that is aligned with the long axis of the canal and seals all possible foramina and isthmuses. Considering the intricacy of the procedure, several pathways may allow continued interaction of root canal bacteria with the host tissues, resulting in persistence or recurrence of apical periodontitis:

- Communication through the margins of the root-end filling: Failure of the root-end filling to effectively seal the canal may result from poor

placement, poor adaptation to the canal walls, or poor sealing ability of the filling material.[224]
- Communication through accessory canals or isthmuses: Root canals in the apical third often diverge into multiple foramina, and in specific teeth, isthmuses are consistently present between canals. A root-end filling may fail to seal accessory foramina or isthmuses, particularly when it is placed without magnification and illumination aids.[238,321]
- Communication through exposed dentinal tubules: Apical resection is typically performed with a bevel, leaving open dentinal tubules at the cut surface. The number of opened tubules corresponds to the angle of the bevel;[322] at times, the angle is so acute that a shallow root-end filling does not internally seal all the tubules that open on the surface. The remaining open tubules communicate between the root canal space and periapical tissues.[322–324]

The typical apical surgery procedure targets the secondary etiologic factors, nonmicrobial and extraradicular infection, in addition to the attempted seal of the primary etiologic factor, intra-canal infection. Considering the bacterial pathways outlined above, persistence of disease after apical surgery is likely to be sustained by persistent root canal infection.[224] This probability provides the rationale for orthograde re-treatment, as the treatment of choice for refractory apical periodontitis after apical surgery. The re-treatment procedure may eliminate the likely etiologic factor. In selected cases, however, re-treatment may not be feasible. In such cases, the apical surgery procedure should be repeated, with an emphasis on effective sealing of the infected root canal.

Factors Influencing Healing after Endodontic Treatment (Tables 3, 5, 6, 7)

In the current structure of the clinical decision-making process, clinicians are expected to advise patients of the prognosis of available treatment alternatives. Furthermore, it is incumbent upon every clinician, once a treatment option is selected, to maximize the prognosis by using treatment methods based on solid evidence. In view of these requirements, this section focuses primarily on the selected studies that comprise the best evidence for initial treatment,[1,6,22,35,43,48,52–55,61,62,66,71,72,75,78,80] orthograde re-treatment,[1,6,43,86,88,90] and apical surgery.[88,138,139,143,144,148–151] Additional studies whose samples are included in specific selected studies[37,67,70,76,248] are also cited when appropriate. The nonselected studies are cited only where selected studies are not available as reference. The factors listed are divided into pre-, per-, and post-treatment categories.

The pretreatment variables should be recognized and duly considered at the stage when different treatment alternatives are weighed, for example, when selection has to be made between orthograde re-treatment, apical surgery or extraction and replacement. They form the basis for projecting the potential for healing, representing the expected benefit of treatment. The per-treatment variables should be recognized and duly considered at the stage when treatment is planned and executed, particularly when treatment strategies and techniques are selected. They can be instrumental in improving the outcome of endodontic treatment and thus maximizing the patient's benefit. The only post-treatment variable related to nonsurgical treatment is the definitive restoration, considering the common division of labor in nonsurgical treatment, whereby the restoration procedure is performed after completion of the root canal treatment procedures. However, it cannot be overemphasized that the restoration procedure is an inseparable component of the endodontic treatment continuum,[325] and may as well be considered a per-treatment variable. The only post-treatment variable related to apical surgery procedure is the results of a periapical tissue biopsy obtained during treatment. It may be considered when the follow-up schedule is devised.

Factors Influencing Healing after Nonsurgical Treatment

The similarities between initial treatment and orthograde re-treatment justify the consideration of the same pre-, per-, and post-treatment variables as outcome predictors. It is noteworthy that the evidence base for re-treatment is limited to only a few selected studies that do not allow conclusive assessment of the influence of many factors on the outcome. Also, specifically for re-treatment, characteristics of the previous root canal treatment history also have to be considered in the pretreatment category. These include the previous root filling, a perforation that may be present in a minority of re-treated teeth, and the time elapsed since initial treatment. As a conclusion to this review of outcome predictors in nonsurgical treatment, a specific section is dedicated to elimination of root canal bacteria, in recognition of their critical role in the etiology of refractory apical periodontitis.

PRETREATMENT VARIABLES

Age and Gender of the Patient

Except for one selected study[72] reporting a better outcome of initial treatment in older patients, age and gender have not been significantly associated with the outcome in the majority of the selected studies on initial treatment[22,43,48,61,62,78] and in the only re-treatment study that examined these factors.[90] Thus, the patient's age and gender do not appear to influence the potential for healing after nonsurgical endodontic treatment.

Systemic Health

The first selected study that examined the patient's health as a variable reported no significant association with the outcome.[1] Until recently, no other studies have addressed systemic health as a potential outcome predictor. A recent selected study[75] suggests that a compromised nonspecific immune system impairs the outcome of nonsurgical treatment in teeth with apical periodontitis. Similarly, a poorer outcome is reported in diabetic patients in a nonselected study.[65] Even though further evidence is required to confirm the association between the patient's systemic health and healing after nonsurgical treatment of teeth with apical periodontitis, the potential for healing appears to be poorer in immune-compromised patients in general, and diabetics in particular. The poorer prognosis, however, does not preclude treatment, as healing is still possible in these patients

Tooth Location

A better outcome is reported in mandibular teeth than in the maxilla in one selected study,[72] whereas in another selected study[22] a better outcome is reported in specific teeth (maxillary canines and second premolars, mandibular canines) without significant differences observed for anterior, posterior, maxillary, and mandibular teeth. Other selected studies have shown no association between tooth location and the outcome of initial treatment[48,55,61,62,78] and re-treatment.[90] Multi-rooted teeth have been shown to have a better outcome than single-rooted teeth in two selected studies,[1,6] but the opposite has been shown in two recent selected studies,[78,90] possibly reflecting the use of teeth (as opposed to roots) as the evaluated units, multiplying the chances of persistent disease by the number of roots.[78,90] Thus, the location and type of the tooth do not appear to influence the potential for healing after nonsurgical endodontic treatment.

Clinical Signs and Symptoms

Several selected studies have reported comparable treatment outcomes in asymptomatic teeth and in teeth presenting with pretreatment symptoms, after initial treatment[35,43,48,55,72,78] and re-treatment.[90] Thus, presence or absence of symptoms does not appear to influence the potential of healing after nonsurgical endodontic treatment.

Pulp Vitality or Necrosis (in Initial Treatment)

From two selected studies,[62,78] it appears that the outcome is better in teeth with vital than with necrotic pulps. This finding, however, is confounded by the presence or absence of apical periodontitis; therefore, the assessment should be limited to teeth without apical periodontitis. In the absence of apical periodontitis, the pulp status is not significantly associated with the outcome of treatment.[22,43,72,78] Thus, the pulp status does not appear to influence the potential of healing after initial endodontic treatment in teeth without apical periodontitis.

Presence or Absence of Radiolucency

The majority of the selected studies on initial treatment[1,6,52,62,71,72,75,78] have demonstrated a significantly poorer outcome (10%–15% difference) in teeth affected by apical periodontitis than in unaffected teeth. A similar difference (10%–20%) has been reported in selected studies on re-treatment.[1,6,43,90] In teeth with apical periodontitis, there may be difficulties in the repair process of the periapical tissues, and the ability to disinfect the root canal system is limited[1] (see Antibacterial Efficacy of Intra-Canal Procedures). Pretreatment apical periodontitis has a strong negative influence on the potential for healing after nonsurgical endodontic treatment.

Size of Radiolucency

Several selected studies have reported better outcomes in teeth with small lesions (≤ 5 mm in diameter) than in larger lesions, after initial treatment[1,6,55,62,72] and re-treatment.[86] A smaller number of root canal bacteria found in teeth with smaller lesions appeared to explain the clinical findings;[35] however, comparable outcomes have been reported for small and large lesions in other selected studies on initial treatment[35,43,48,53,61,78] and re-treatment.[90] Thus, the size of the radiolucency does not appear to influence the potential for healing after nonsurgical endodontic treatment.

Periodontal Support

Only few studies have examined the periodontal condition as a variable in nonsurgical treatment. A better outcome in teeth with better marginal support is reported in one selected study,[72] but in other selected studies[43,78,90] the periodontal status has not been significantly associated with the outcome. Periodontal defects present at the time of treatment are a sign of advanced periodontal disease that in time may necessitate extraction of the affected teeth. Indeed, in one selected study[67] over 50% of teeth extracted 4 to 6 years after initial treatment were lost because of periodontal disease, and in a survival analysis of root-filled teeth with periodontal disease,[251] the proportion of periodontal-driven extractions was 66% of all lost teeth over a 9-year period. Thus, periodontal defects do not appear to influence the potential for healing after nonsurgical endodontic treatment; however, advancing periodontal disease may cause loss of affected teeth over time.

Apparent Quality of Previous Root Filling (in Re-treatment)

One selected study on re-treatment[90] reports a significantly better outcome (15% difference) in teeth with apical periodontitis that have inadequate length or density of the previous root filling, compared with teeth with apparently adequate root fillings. In addition, one nonselected study[91] reports a poorer outcome in teeth where the previous root filling deviates from the pathway of the canal, than in teeth with unaltered morphology. The inadequately filled canals "constituted the infected sites, which, when re-treated, could be effectively disinfected and sealed, leading to healing."[90] By contrast, adequately filled canals may host root canal bacteria not susceptible to re-treatment procedures, or they may be free of bacteria when the disease is sustained by extra-radicular infection, cysts, or a foreign body.[90] Such extra-radicular etiologic factors do not respond to re-treatment. Thus, an apparent poor quality of the root filling in previously treated teeth with apical periodontitis has a positive influence on the potential for healing after re-treatment.

Previous Perforation (in Re-treatment)

Very little information is available on the outcome of teeth in which a root or chamber perforation occurred. In the first nonselected study that examined this variable,[326] healing is reported around 58% of perforations repaired with amalgam or gutta-percha. In a more recent selected study,[90] complete healing is reported in only 36% of teeth with apical periodontitis and perforations repaired with resin-modified glass ionomer cement, prompting the authors to speculate that "possibly, the use of MTA could have been beneficial." MTA was used for perforation repair in a case series study,[327] and all 16 treated teeth appeared to be healed 1 year or longer after treatment (Figure 12). Thus, a previous perforation may have a negative influence on the potential for healing after re-treatment, depending on the material used to seal the perforation.

Elapsed Time after Previous Treatment (in Re-treatment)

This variable has been examined in only one selected study,[90] where a comparable outcome is reported in teeth re-treated within 1 year or longer after initial treatment. Thus, the time elapsed since previous treatment does not appear to influence the potential for healing after re-treatment.

PER-TREATMENT VARIABLES

Based on the information gleaned from the selected studies, the per-treatment variables are clearly more critical in teeth with apical periodontitis than in teeth with intact periapical tissues.

Length of Canal Preparation and Filling

Several selected studies[1,6,72] qualify that the length of canal preparation should be distinguished from the length of the root filling; however, most frequently only the length of the root filling is addressed. In five of the selected studies,[1,6,43,48,72] the length of the root filling has been significantly associated with the outcome of initial treatment, whereas no such association has been reported in eight selected studies.[35,55,61,62,66,71,75,78] Similar inconsistency exists in studies on re-treatment, where one selected study[90] reports a poorer outcome in teeth with

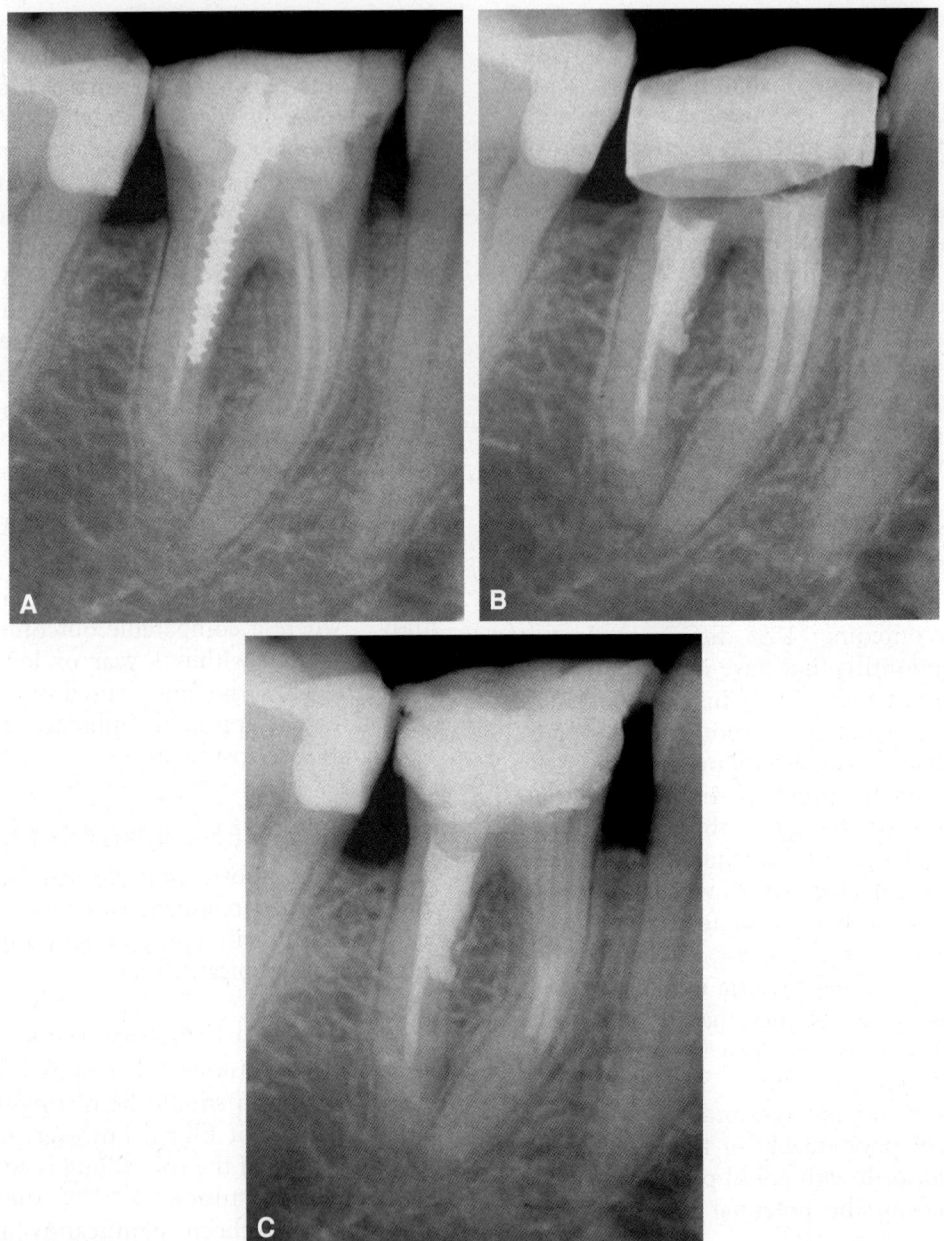

Figure 12 Re-treatment in conjunction with an internal perforation repair. ***A,*** Mandibular molar with a distal root perforation into the furcation and associated bone loss. ***B,*** Completed re-treatment and perforation seal with mineral trioxide aggregate (MTA) (ProRoot MTA; Tulsa Dental, Tulsa, OK). ***C,*** At 1.5 year, the bone in the furcation area is healed. Regrettably, the tooth has not been properly restored.

inadequate (too long or too short) root fillings, whereas two selected studies[43,86] do not corroborate this finding.

Impaired healing in teeth with extruded root fillings, particularly in the presence of apical periodontitis, has been shown in several selected studies.[1,6,43,48] The damage may have resulted from over-instrumentation and inoculation of the periapical tissues with infected debris, rather than from the extruded root filling[43,320] (Figure 13). Possibly, extruded root filling materials slow down healing of apical periodontitis and delay it as long as to the third decade after treatment,[92] even though they can be totally or partially removed during the healing process.[1,44,225]

One selected study[43] reports impaired healing in teeth with apical periodontitis, where canals

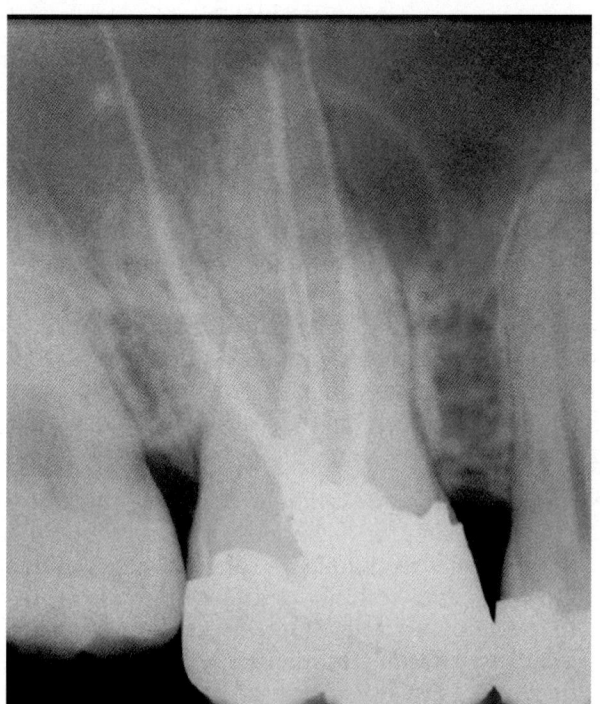

Figure 13 Periapically extruded root filling. Maxillary first molar with 2 gutta-percha cones extruded at least 10 mm beyond the terminus of both the buccal apexes. Although the same conditions apparently exist in both roots, the mesiobuccal root is associated with apical periodontitis whereas the distobuccal root is not, suggesting that the cause of apical periodontitis is not the extruded gutta-percha. (Reprinted with permission from Friedman 2002.[164])

were prepared and filled excessively short (2 mm or shorter); however, an earlier selected study reported by the same group[35] does not support this finding. Thus, the root filling length does not appear to influence the healing potential after nonsurgical endodontic treatment in teeth without apical periodontitis. With apical periodontitis present, the healing potential may be better if the canal is filled 0 to 2 mm short of the root end.

Apical Enlargement

Intra-canal bacteria can penetrate the dentin of teeth with apical periodontitis[315,328] to a depth of 150 to 250 μm[329–331] and remain protected from the antibacterial action of irrigants and medications.[332] It appears that the infected dentin can only be removed by enlargement of the canal by 300 to 500 μm, e.g., to ISO size 50 to 70 if the first file that binds is size 20. Because such extensive apical enlargement may enhance disinfection in the apical portion of the canal,[333–335] it should also improve the outcome of treatment. However, apical enlargement has not been significantly associated with the outcome of initial treatment in four selected studies,[22,61,62,72] whereas in a fifth selected study,[1] it appeared to impair the outcome. There is, therefore, no clinical evidence to support extensive apical enlargement in teeth with apical periodontitis. Possibly, this is due to problems associated with both extensive and minimal apical enlargement. Extensive enlargement can result in canal transportation if not carried out skillfully, whereas minimal enlargement may not remove infected dentin. Both effects would compromise healing.[164]

Most importantly, however, it should be noted that the true extent of apical enlargement cannot be assessed because the pretreatment canal dimensions in all the studies are unknown. Thus, there is insufficient data available to assess the influence of apical enlargement on the healing potential after initial endodontic treatment, and no data at all on apical enlargement in re-treatment.

Bacterial Culture Before Root Filling

Bacteriologic root canal sample without bacterial growth (negative culture) obtained before root filling was first associated with a better outcome by Engström et al.;[6] however, the microbiologic techniques utilized in this selected study did not adequately address the anaerobic endodontic pathogens.[53] Three decades later Sjögren et al.,[53] in one of the selected studies using an advanced anaerobic bacteriologic technique during initial treatment, reported healing in 94% of teeth that had a negative culture before root filling, in contrast to only 68% in teeth with positive cultures. In a parallel selected study on re-treatment,[86] 80% of teeth with negative cultures before root filling healed, compared with 33% of teeth with positive cultures. In a recent selected study,[76] a better outcome is reported in teeth treated in two sessions, where negative cultures were obtained at the beginning of the second session after dressing with calcium hydroxide, compared with teeth with positive cultures. Furthermore, the bacterial species recovered from the canal also may influence the prognosis.[53] All these findings, clearly demonstrating a significant association between negative cultures obtained with reliable culturing methods and the potential of healing after nonsurgical endodontic treatment, are apparently disputed by another selected study.[61] Significant or not, state-of-the-art techniques for obtaining bacteriologic samples from root canals are not readily available for use in the day-to-day endodontic practice.[53] Therefore, their usage should be directed mainly toward research to assess the efficacy of root canal treatment regimens. Thus, results of bacterial cultures obtained from root canals before root filling do not appear to influence the healing potential after nonsurgical endodontic treatment.

Number of Treatment Sessions

In recent years, considerable research efforts have been made to study the potential for healing after treatment in one session or two. In teeth without apical periodontitis, there is no difference in healing related to one or two treatment sessions[80] as the canals are not infected. In infected canals, however, root canal bacteria cannot be effectively eliminated in a single treatment session.[53] This and other studies[226–229,231,333,334,336] emphasize the need for intra-canal medication in order to maximize disinfection, suggesting a better outcome when treatment is performed in two sessions with an effective intra-canal medication used. However, this premise is not supported by the selected studies on initial treatment[54,55,61,78] and re-treatment,[90] that report nonsignificant inconsistent differences in healing in the range of 10%, after treatment in one or two sessions. As all these studies are underpowered—their samples are too small to show significance of the observed differences—this may have been the main reason for the lack of significance reported.

The number of sessions in multi-session treatment does not appear to influence the outcome in one of the selected studies.[22] However, it appears that efforts should be made to avoid prolongation of treatment, as teeth treated in one or two sessions have been shown to survive longer than teeth treated in three sessions or more.[163] Sirén et al.[337] suggest that teeth treated in multiple visits are at a greater risk of becoming infected with *E. faecalis* and developing refractory apical periodontitis.

As shown by one of the selected studies,[53] the potential for healing after treatment in one session is good. In fact, a systematic review of the pertinent literature concludes that "the biological benefit of multi-session treatment has not been supported by clinical evidence."[338] Thus, there is insufficient data available to assess the influence of the number of treatment sessions (one or two) on the healing potential after nonsurgical endodontic treatment in teeth with apical periodontitis. However, prolongation of treatment for more than two sessions should be avoided.

Flare-Up During Treatment

In several of the selected studies, there has been no significant association between flare-ups and the outcome of initial treatment[1,22,35,43,61,78] and re-treatment.[90] Thus, occurrence of flare-up or pain in the course of treatment does not appear to influence the healing potential after nonsurgical endodontic treatment.

Materials and Techniques

In contrast to the frequent occupation of the profession with endodontic techniques and materials, and the multitude of in vitro studies focused on comparing them, there is only limited information available in the selected studies on the influence of specific treatment regimens on the potential for healing. Only few aspects of materials and techniques have been examined, as follows:

- Instrumentation technique: A better outcome is reported using the "standardized" technique than the "serial" technique in one selected study;[22] however, both techniques are seldom used today. In recent selected studies examining current canal preparation techniques in initial treatment, there has been no significant association between the outcome and the use of hand or engine-driven instruments,[75] different engine-driven instrument systems,[71] and the degree of taper.[62] Thus, the instrumentation technique does not appear to influence the healing potential after initial treatment, and by extension, also after re-treatment.

- Intra-canal medication: A survival analysis study[163] suggests a better potential for survival of teeth where canals were dressed with calcium hydroxide than teeth dressed with other medications or with canals left empty between treatment sessions. In the absence of data from follow-up studies, there is insufficient data available to assess the influence of the type of intra-canal medication on the healing potential after nonsurgical endodontic treatment in teeth with apical periodontitis.

- Sealer: One sealer, Kloroperka N-Ø, is identified as adversely influencing the outcome in a selected study with a mixed sample of teeth without and with apical periodontitis.[72] The researchers suggest that the choice of sealer may influence the prognosis, but only in teeth without apical periodontitis. Indeed, in a subsample of teeth with apical periodontitis[39] and in three subsequent selected studies of larger populations reported by the same group,[48,56,66] the outcomes have been comparable for different sealer types. Thus, with the exception of Kloroperka N-Ø, the type of sealer does not appear to influence the healing potential after nonsurgical endodontic treatment.

- Root filling technique: In two selected studies that have examined different root filling techniques in initial treatment, comparable outcomes have been reported for hybrid and vertical compaction,[62] and for lateral and vertical compaction.[71] Thus, the technique used for root filling does not appear to influence the healing potential after initial treatment and, by extension, also after re-treatment.
- Comprehensive technique: In the recent selected Toronto Study series,[78] the proportion of healed teeth with apical periodontitis treated with the classic Schilder technique—flared canal preparation with ample irrigation and root filling with vertically-compacted warm gutta-percha—is significantly higher (10% difference) than in teeth treated with step-back or modified step-back instrumentation and lateral compaction of gutta-percha. Notwithstanding the demonstrated significance, the difference between the techniques requires validation from a RCT, because the Toronto Study was not randomized and controlled to assess the influence of a single variable on the outcome. Notably, in the re-treatment study of the Toronto Study series,[90] the difference healing between the same two techniques was smaller and not significant. Thus, in spite of the indication of the superiority of the Schilder technique, there is insufficient data available to assess the influence of this comprehensive treatment technique or others on the healing potential after nonsurgical endodontic treatment in teeth with apical periodontitis.

Complications

In one selected study,[72] there is no significant association between mid-treatment complications and healing. However, in several other selected studies,[1,22,43,78] healing has been impaired by complications, including perforation of the pulp chamber or root, file breakage at a stage that prevents cleaning of the canal, and massive extrusion of filling materials. It is noteworthy that endodontists currently may successfully manage these complications; for example, a recent review[339] concludes that "in the hands of skilled endodontists prognosis was not significantly affected by the presence of a retained fractured instrument," in contrast to early selected studies[1,22] that reported poorer outcomes in teeth with broken instruments. Likewise, a recent case series study[327] reports complete healing of all 16 teeth in which perforations were repaired with MTA. In regard to re-treatment, a recent selected study[90] reports a comparable outcome in teeth with and without mid-treatment complications. Thus, the negative influence of mid-treatment complications on the healing potential after nonsurgical treatment may be offset by current management strategies. Nevertheless, complications should be avoided, as depending on their severity they may impair healing of the affected teeth.

POST-TREATMENT VARIABLES

Restoration

When bacteria become established in the pulp chamber, they can penetrate the filled root canal, as shown in vitro,[340–351] and apical periodontitis can develop subsequently, as shown in an animal model.[261,352] Indeed, in one selected study,[90] impaired healing is reported in teeth that had not been definitively restored after re-treatment. The type of the restoration (temporary, definitive, filling, cast) has not been significantly associated with healing after initial treatment[53,78] and re-treatment.[90] However, one selected study[43] reports less healing in teeth restored with crowns and those serving as bridge abutments, than in teeth restored with fillings.

The restoration has also been examined in several cross-sectional studies, with conflicting results. In one study,[353] presence or absence of posts is not associated with healing, if at least 3 mm of the root filling remains under the post. In two other studies,[178,354] posts have been associated with an increased prevalence of apical periodontitis, whereas the opposite was reported in a third study.[355] It is noteworthy that cross-sectional studies provide a low level of evidence. In the selected studies,[43,78,90] there has been no significant association between the presence or absence of posts and the outcome of initial treatment and re-treatment. Thus, the type of the intra-radicular, intra-coronal, and extra-coronal restoration does not appear to influence the healing potential after nonsurgical endodontic treatment, as long as the tooth is definitively restored in a timely manner.

Nevertheless, the survival or loss of root-filled teeth clearly depends on the restoration, and

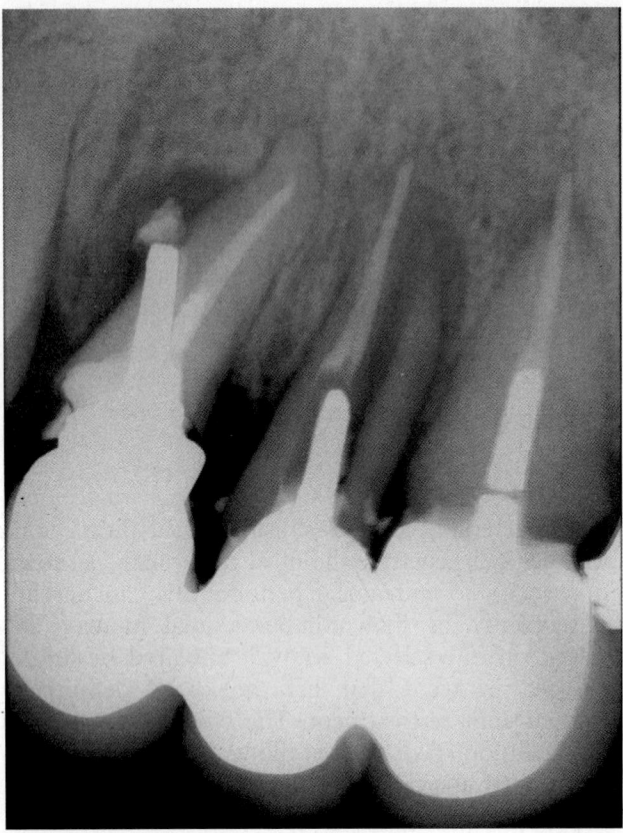

Figure 14 Risks associated with post-retained restorations of endodontically treated teeth (from left to right)—perforation, root fracture, and post fracture. (Reprinted with permission from Friedman 2002.[164])

particularly restorative failure.[356] For example, in the selected Toronto Study series,[67,70,78,90] over 35% of the 87 teeth extracted 4 to 6 years after treatment were lost because of restorative considerations. In a survival analysis after endodontic treatment,[163] 53% of extracted teeth were lost because of fracture (root or crown is not specified), with additional teeth extracted because of a "prosthetic need." In addition, posts have been implicated in vertical root fracture and tooth loss in approximately 9% of cases,[356] as well as in root perforations that impair healing.[357] Clearly, posts present a risk to root-filled teeth (Figure 14); they should be used sparingly and with caution.

ANTIBACTERIAL EFFICACY OF INTRA-CANAL PROCEDURES

Pretreatment presence of apical periodontitis is the dominant variable influencing the potential for healing after nonsurgical treatment. Apical periodontitis is sustained by root canal infection; therefore, "the bacteriological status of the root canal at the time of root filling is a critical factor in determining the outcome of endodontic treatment,"[53] suggesting that improved bacterial elimination may be considered as a surrogate measure for improved outcomes. The antibacterial efficacy of intra-canal procedures, measured by the proportion of bacteriological samples below the level of bacterial detection (negative culture) and by the number (density) of bacteria in the samples, is briefly reviewed below.

Irrigation

Root canal preparation coupled with inactive irrigants does not predictably eliminate bacteria, resulting in less than 50% negative cultures, regardless of the use of stainless-steel hand instruments or nickel–titanium engine-driven ones.[227,230,333] By contrast, irrigation with ≥0.5% sodium hypochlorite considerably improves bacterial elimination, resulting in 50 to 80% negative cultures, and over 99% reduction in bacterial counts, from an order of 10^5 to 10^2.[53,76,228,229,231,336,358–365] Subsequent irrigation with IKI may not improve bacterial elimination, resulting in over 70% negative cultures.[360] A similar result over 70% negative cultures may be expected after use of a new immersion-irrigating agent, MTAD, without significant improvement in bacterial elimination.[365]

Bacterial elimination during re-treatment has been evaluated considerably less than in initial treatment. Instrumentation and irrigation with sodium hypochlorite have resulted in 70% to 77% negative cultures,[294,301] a comparable efficacy to that reported for initial treatment. Further irrigation with IKI may improve bacterial elimination, resulting in 95% negative cultures.[294]

Dressing with Medication

The efficacy of antibacterial dressing between subsequent treatment sessions has met with much controversy. Initially, a superior efficacy of intra-canal dressing with calcium hydroxide has been clearly demonstrated,[35,226] and corroborated in more recent studies,[231,358,361] resulting in over 85% negative cultures and reduction of bacterial counts to the order of 10^1. In other studies,[333,334,363,366] bacterial elimination was not as dramatic, resulting in only 60 to 80% negative cultures. In stark contrast, a decline in negative cultures to 70% or less and an increase in bacterial counts have been reported in three recent studies.[76,359,360] Considerable differences in root canal culturing methodology make it difficult to reconcile these contrary findings, as the methodology itself has been questioned.[367] Nevertheless, the available data suggest that "calcium hydroxide has limited effectiveness in eliminating bacteria from human root canal when assessed by culture techniques."[368]

In regard to alternative intra-canal medications, dressing with clindamycin results in 76% negative cultures, similar to that achieved with calcium hydroxide.[336] Dressing with 2% chlorhexidine-gluconate liquid results in a decline in negative cultures—from 68 to 45%—and in increase in bacterial counts from the order of 10^2 to 10^3.[362] A 2% chlorhexidine gel appears to be more effective than the liquid; the proportion of negative cultures may remain stable with slightly reduced bacterial counts.[363,365]

The efficacy of intra-canal dressing with calcium hydroxide during re-treatment appears to be limited.[301] The authors report a decrease in negative cultures, from 77% after canal preparation to 57% after dressing with calcium hydroxide alone or mixed with chlorhexidine. After further canal preparation in the second treatment session negative cultures increased to 87%, but fell again to 70% after subsequent dressing.[301]

Clearly, more research is required to unequivocally establish the critical role of intra-canal dressing, with calcium hydroxide or another effective medication, in the elimination of root canal bacteria in nonsurgical endodontic treatment. However, notwithstanding the recent data challenging the efficacy of intra-canal medication, it is noteworthy that the proportion of negative cultures appears to increase, and the bacterial counts appear to decrease at the end of the second treatment session, compared with the end of the first session.[76,333,359,362,365,301] Thus, the two-session treatment with interim dressing appears to improve bacterial elimination beyond what can be achieved in one treatment session.

Apical Enlargement

Progressive enlargement of the root canal in early studies[333,334] has not significantly improved bacterial elimination. In a more recent study,[230] bacterial counts are somewhat reduced when the apical portion of the canal is enlarged from ISO size 45 (size 25 in curved canals) to size 50 and 60 (size 30 and 35 in curved canals). The bacterial reduction is even more pronounced when sodium hypochlorite is used,[231] and a further reduction is reported when the canal is enlarged with nickel–titanium instruments to very large sizes.[335]

The antibacterial efficacy of apical enlargement in re-treatment has not been assessed. When re-treatment is performed with any technique, a considerable amount of root filling residue remains attached to the canal walls.[369–386] Such residue may interfere with bacterial elimination, as it may shelter subjacent bacterial colonies. A recent in vitro study[386] indicates that the amount of residue can be reduced by further enlargement of the canal beyond its dimensions before re-treatment. Thus, bacterial elimination may also be improved by progressive apical enlargement during re-treatment.

In summary, copious irrigation with sodium hypochlorite delivered deep apically by means of a small gauge needle and substantial apical enlargement to sizes approximating those listed in a series of morphometric studies[260,387,388] are the critical basic steps in the elimination of root canal bacteria. The additional efficacy of root canal dressing with calcium hydroxide, chlorhexidine, or other medications has been cast into doubt and requires clarification. Because bacteria are the primary cause of refractory apical periodontitis, their maximal elimination by meticulously applying the aforementioned combination of therapeutic means improves the potential for healing after nonsurgical endodontic treatment.

Factors Influencing Healing after Apical Surgery

The majority of the selected studies on apical surgery have attempted to associate observed outcomes with different variables. For the major part, these variables are different from those that have been examined in relation to nonsurgical treatment.

PRETREATMENT VARIABLES

Age, Gender, and Systemic Health of the Patient

Age and gender have not been significantly associated with the outcome in the selected studies.[138,139,148,151] Systemic health has not been examined as a variable in any of the studies. Thus, the patient's age, gender, and systemic health do not appear to influence the potential for healing after nonsurgical endodontic treatment.

Tooth Location

Comparable outcomes have been reported for different tooth types in both the maxilla and the mandible in several selected studies.[138,139,148,149,151] The only exception is the frequent healing by scar tissue—consistent with complete healing—observed in maxillary lateral incisors.[116,120] Apparently, convenience of access and the specific root anatomy influence the potential for healing after apical surgery to a greater extent than the location of the tooth.

Clinical Signs and Symptoms

Teeth with signs and symptoms appear to demonstrate less healing, as suggested by one selected study[151] and one nonselected study.[112] However, in two selected studies,[139,148] there have been no significant association between the outcome and absence or presence of pretreatment symptoms. Thus, presence or absence of symptoms does not appear to influence the potential for healing after apical surgery.

Size of Radiolucency

One selected study[139] suggests that the lesion size has no significant influence on healing. However, another selected study[148] reports a significantly better outcome in teeth with small lesions (≤ 5 mm in diameter) than in teeth with larger lesions. A similar pattern is reported in a recent study, but without statistical significance.[151] Wang et al.[148] suggest that small lesions are completely eradicated when the crypt is surgically enlarged to gain adequate access, resulting in creation of an excisional wound in the surrounding bone.[389] Curettage of large lesions may be incomplete and an excisional wound is not created, as the access is adequate and the crypt is not enlarged to avoid injury to adjacent anatomic structures. When the lesion is very large (≤ 10 mm in diameter), healing by scar tissue frequently occurs, as shown in nonselected studies.[116,120] Thus, teeth with lesions not exceeding 5 mm appear to have a better potential for healing after apical surgery.

Supporting Bone Loss

Several nonselected studies[99,103,105,110,112,147] have suggested a poor prognosis for teeth with considerable vertical or marginal bone loss. Such bone loss can compromise periodontal reattachment by apical migration of gingival epithelium, possibly enabling bacteria present in the periodontal pocket to invade the periapical site and prevent healing. Thus, considerable attachment loss of the treated tooth may have a negative influence on the potential for healing after apical surgery.

Restoration

Frequently in apical surgery, the restoration type is a pretreatment variable, because the teeth are already restored at the time of treatment. A poorer outcome in teeth with a defective restoration or with a post is reported in one selected study,[139] but this finding is not supported by two other selected studies.[148,151] Nevertheless, defective restorations can impair the survival of root-filled teeth[356] (see Figure 9); indeed, in one selected study,[148] 7 of the 10 teeth extracted 4 to 8 years after treatment were lost because of restorative considerations, whereas 2 teeth were extracted because of fracture, and 1 tooth because of refractory apical periodontitis. Thus, there is insufficient data available to assess the influence of the type of the restoration on the potential for healing after apical surgery, as long as the tooth is adequately restored.

Apparent Quality of Previous Root Filling

The previous root fillings can be characterized by their material, density, and length. According to two selected studies,[139,148] the type of the filling material and the filling density—absence (see Figure 4) or presence (see Figure 7) of voids—are not associated with the outcome. In one selected study,[148] a significantly better outcome is reported when the filling is too short (≥ 2 mm from the root end) or too long (extruded beyond the root end) than when its length is adequate; however, this finding is not supported by two other selected studies.[139,151] Thus, there is insufficient data available to assess the influence of the length of the filling, whereas the type and density of the existing root filling do not appear to influence the potential for healing after apical surgery.

Second-Time Surgery

One selected study focusing on second-time surgery,[149] a nonselected study,[188] and a systematic review of several nonselected studies[390] have concluded that the outcome of second-time surgery is poorer than that of first-time surgery. This conclusion is not supported by three selected studies.[139,148,151] In one of these studies,[148] the difference in the proportion of healed teeth between first-time (79%) surgery and second-time (62%) surgery is not significant; however, with only eight teeth included in the second-time surgery group, this analysis is underpowered. Nevertheless, the authors suggest that modified case selection criteria and techniques may have improved the outcome of second-time surgery in their study compared with previous studies; typically, second-time surgery uses the same case selection criteria and techniques as the first-time surgery, whereas they routinely preferred root canal re-treatment over second-time surgery (Figure 15), and when surgery was selected, the technique differed from

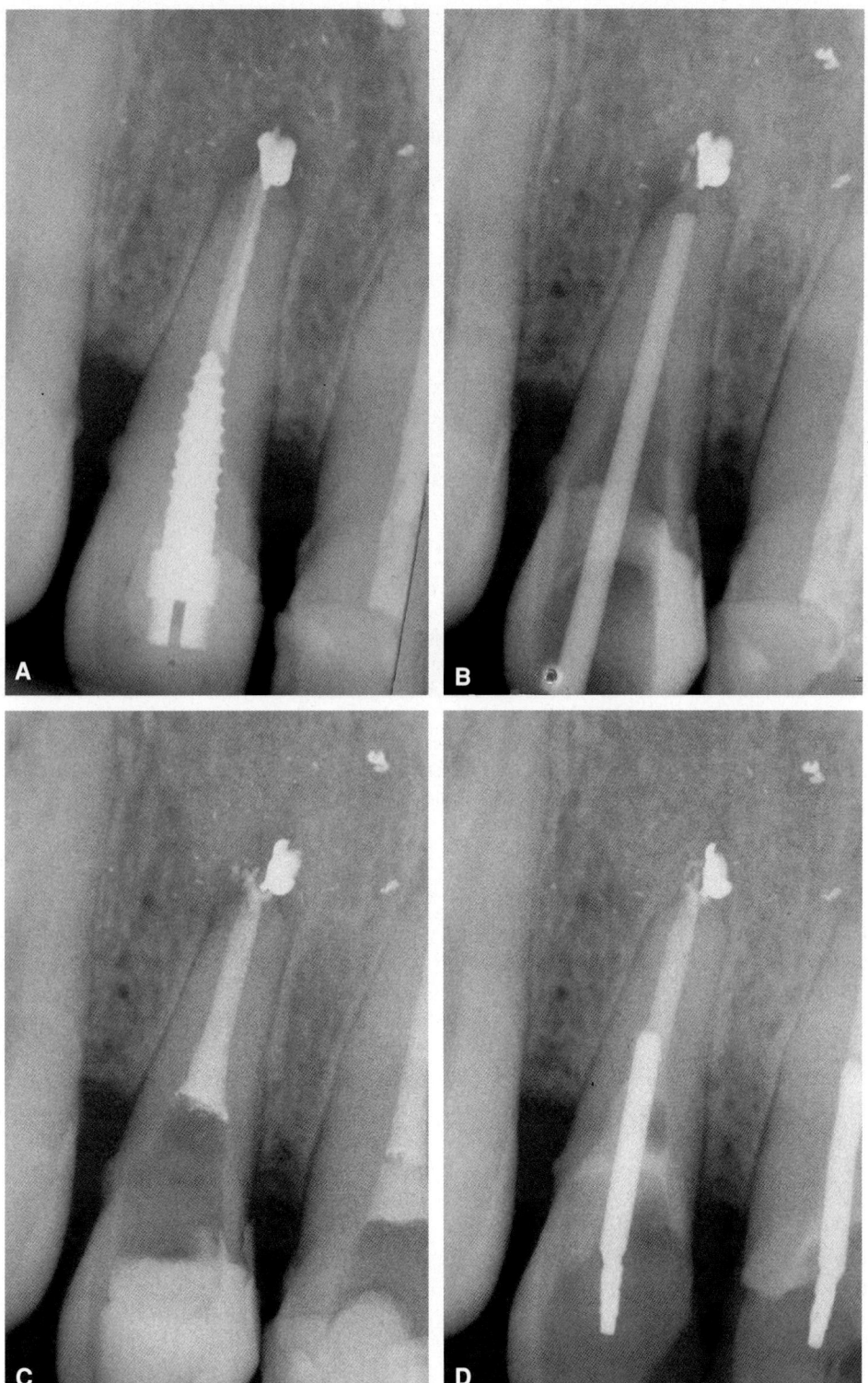

Figure 15 Persistent disease after apical surgery—treated by orthograde re-treatment. ***A,*** Root-filled and previously surgically-treated maxillary lateral incisor, with a broken file, poorly placed root-end filling, and persistent apical periodontitis. ***B,*** The film shows fit of the master cone during orthograde re-treatment. All restorative material was removed from the coronal portion of the tooth, revealing an extensive cavity. ***C,*** Completed root canal re-treatment. The root-end amalgam was displaced outside the canal. ***D,*** At 2 years, the lesion is healed. (Reprinted with permission from Friedman 2006.[201])

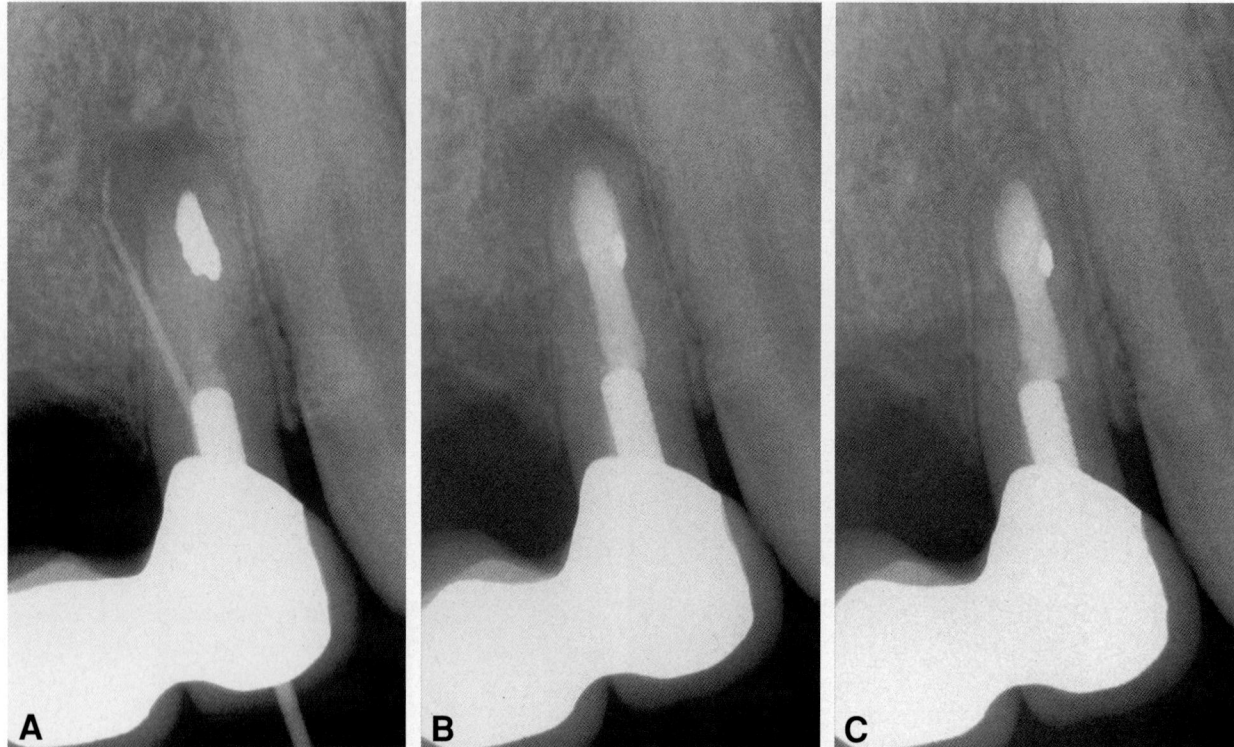

Figure 16 Repeat (second-time) surgery. ***A,*** Root-filled and previously surgically-treated maxillary lateral incisor with persistent apical periodontitis, and a gutta-percha cone tracing the sinus tract. ***B,*** Completed repeat surgery, comprising retrograde re-treatment and filled with mineral trioxide aggregate (MTA). ***C,*** At 3 years, the lesion is healed. (Reprinted with permission from Friedman 2002.[223])

that of the first-time surgery[148] (Figure 16). Thus, the second-time surgery may offer a poorer potential for healing than first-time surgery, unless an improved strategy is used.

PER-TREATMENT VARIABLES

Level of Apical Resection and Degree of Beveling

A better outcome is reported after resection at the mid-root level than at a more apical level in one nonselected study.[102] A more conservative resection may expose canal ramifications that can allow intra-canal bacteria to sustain disease after surgery.[238] Therefore, the root should be resected approximately 3 mm from the apex, where ramifications are fewer.[305,391] Furthermore, a more coronal resection level facilitates preparation of the root-end cavity and filling. Thus, a more coronal level of resection may have a positive influence on the potential for healing after apical surgery.

The degree of bevel should be minimal to avoid the risk of missing canals emerging at the lingual aspect of the root.[238,305] Furthermore, a minimal bevel also reduces the number of exposed dentinal tubules on the cut root surface, minimizing the pathway available for root canal bacteria to sustain disease after surgery[141,305,322,324] (Figure 17).

Presence or Absence of a Root-End Filling

A root-end filling is placed to establish an effective barrier against interaction of intra-canal bacteria with the periapical tissues.[224] This rationale applies in all teeth where apical periodontitis is presumably sustained by persistent intra-canal infection.[224] When

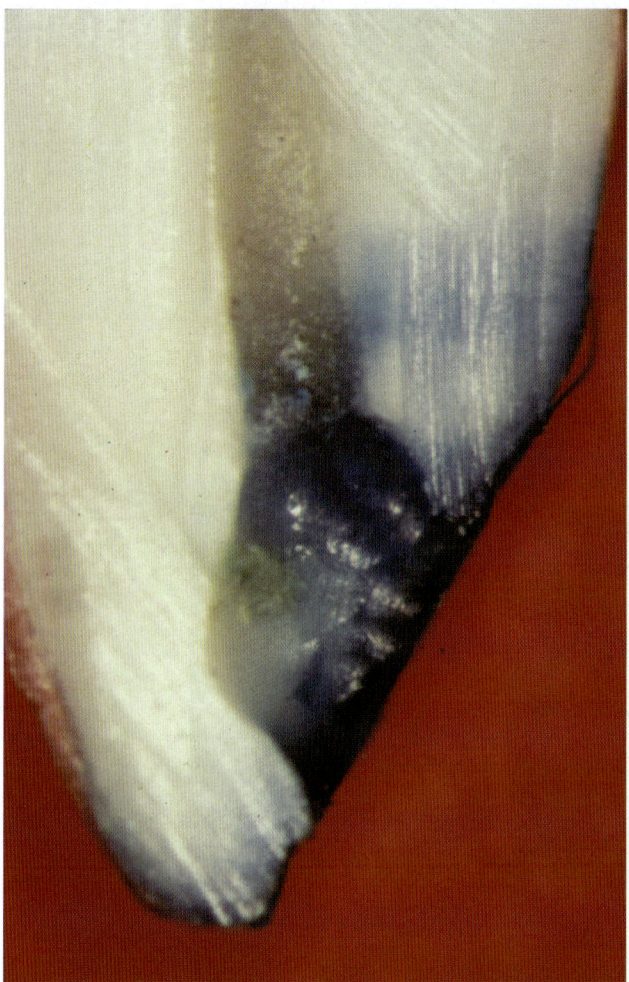

Figure 17 Patent dentinal tubules at the cut apical root surface. A specimen, taken 6 months after apical surgery on a dog, then subjected to dye leakage and sectioned vertically. The root-end filling was dislodged to allow assessment of dye penetration. Note the beveled cut surface and dye penetration through the dentinal tubules, demonstrating the communication between the root canal and apical environment. The dentinal tubules can provide a pathway for intra-canal bacteria to bypass the root-end filling and sustain the disease process. (Reprinted with permission from Friedman 2006.[201])

extra-radicular infection is suspected, a root-end filling may be superfluous[148,224] (Figure 18); indeed, in one selected study,[148] seven of eight teeth (88%) suspected for extra-radicular infection healed without receiving a root-end filling.

Many nonselected studies published over the years[93,96,98,102,106,108,112,116,120] have suggested that presence of a root-end filling impairs the prognosis. As stated in one of these studies,[116] "retrofills have a strong negative effect on the end results." It is noteworthy that in these studies, root-end fillings were placed only in the teeth treated exclusively by apical surgery, but not in teeth where orthograde treatment was performed in conjunction with surgery. Therefore, comparison of teeth without and with root-end fillings was confounded by orthograde treatment, performed concurrently with the former but not with the latter.[224] However, when only surgically treated teeth are analyzed in the same studies and others, better outcomes can be observed with root-end fillings than without.[93,102,105,117,121] Thus, placement of a root-end filling may have a positive influence on the potential for healing after apical surgery, particularly when persistent root canal infection is presumably the cause of persistent disease.

Root-End Cavity Design

The classical root-end cavity drilled with a small round bur has been replaced in the past two decades with two main modifications. Rud et al.[122,246,392] bonded a "cap" of composite resin—Retroplast—over the cut root surface to seal all possible bacterial pathways, including the main canal, accessory canals, isthmuses, and exposed dentinal tubules (see Figure 8). To avoid adverse effects of shrinkage, Retroplast is placed as a thin layer into a concavity created in the resected surface with a large round bur. In two selected studies,[143,151] the proportions of "healed" and "healing" teeth 1 year after apical surgery with Retroplast are 73% and 85%, respectively. The outcomes in these studies and several nonselected ones where Retroplast was used[122,130,133,140,190,246] appear to surpass the outcomes reported in studies where root-end cavities have been prepared and filled with a variety of materials (Tables 3, 7). Other composite resins, such as Geristore[393,394] and OptiBond,[238] can possibly be used as alternatives to Retroplast; however, their clinical effectiveness in this application has not been reported.

Thus, there is no strong evidence to suggest that both modifications of the classical root-end cavity—bonded apical "cap" and ultrasonic preparation—offer a better potential for healing after apical surgery; however, there is a sound clinical rationale for using both approaches. Both approaches also offer greater ease and consistency of application than the outdated drilling of the root-end cavity with small round burs.

Carr[238,304] developed special angled tips for ultrasonic use that significantly modified the form of the root-end cavity. These tips can be used with less beveling of the cut root surface and in smaller crypts than burs.[141,237,238,240,305] Most importantly, the

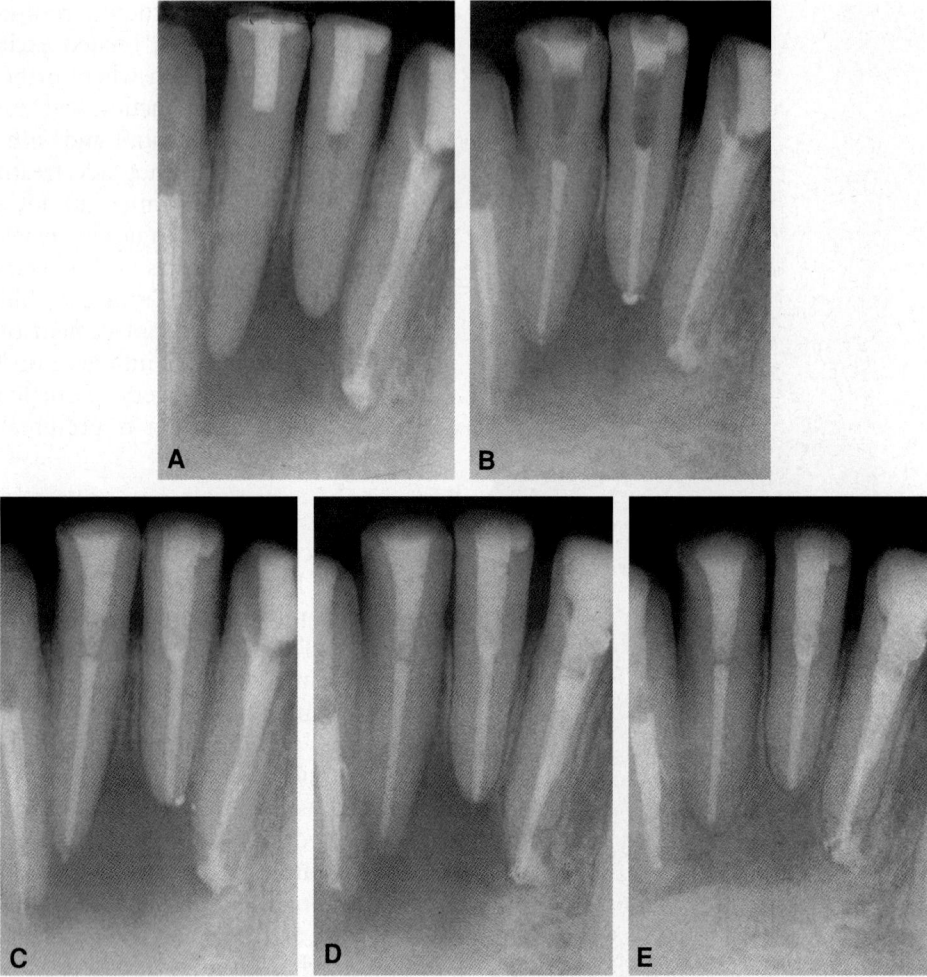

Figure 18 Suspected extra-radicular infection—placement of root-end fillings may be superfluous. *A,* Mandibular central incisors with extensive apical periodontitis. *B,* Completed root canal therapy. *C,* At 2 years, the lesion is enlarged suggesting persistence of the disease, possibly because of extra-radicular infection. *D,* Completed surgery consisting of only periapical curettage. *E,* At 1 year after surgery, the lesion is healed. (Reprinted with permission from Friedman 2006.[201])

created cavities are deeper, allowing the root-end filling to seal exposed dentinal tubules from within the canal.[235,237,240] Furthermore, the cavities are cleaner and better aligned with the long axis of the canal, reducing the risk of root perforation on the lingual aspect.[236,239,240] A better outcome after ultrasonic root-end cavity preparation than after use of burs has been reported in two nonselected studies;[134,136] however, the analyses in both studies were confounded by extraneous factors, undermining their conclusions. It is noteworthy that the "healed" rates reported in the selected studies in which root-end cavities were prepared with ultrasonic tips range from 37 to 91%;[138,139,144,148–151] this wide range is not different from that of studies where root-end cavities were drilled with burs.

Quality and Depth of Root-End Filling

Only one selected study[139] highlights the significance of the quality of the root-end filling, particularly its correct placement, whereas another selected study[148] reports comparable outcomes for root-end fillings extending ≥2 mm into the canal space. However, the frequent beveling of the apical surface of the root precludes reliable radiographic assessment of the depth of the root-end filling.[139] Thus, there is insufficient data available to assess the influence of the root-end filling depth, ranging from 1 to 4 mm, on the potential for healing after apical surgery. Nevertheless, the potential for healing is certainly improved after accurate placement of the root-end filling.

Root-End Filling Material

A plethora of restorative and endodontic materials have been suggested over the years for root-end filling, including amalgam (with or without varnish), zinc-oxide eugenol cement (plain or reinforced), EBA and Super EBA cement, polycarboxylate cement, glass ionomer cement, gutta-percha (burnished or injectable), composite resin, cyanoacrylate glue, Teflon, gold foil, titanium screws, and Cavit. In the past decade, MTA has gained popularity as a root-end filling material.[244,395] This plethora of materials has primarily been assessed using in vitro models with highly inconsistent results.[224,396] To better simulate clinical conditions, Friedman et al.[397] developed an in vivo model (Figure 19) that has been used with some variations in several studies.[241–245,398] In these animal studies, IRM,[241,242] Super EBA,[243,245] MTA,[244] and Diaket[398] have performed better than other materials. However, animal studies do not provide the evidence-base required for supporting the clinical effectiveness of these root-end filling materials.

Several nonselected studies, primarily nonrandomized clinical trials, have assessed different root-end filling materials, including Biobond,[97] Cavit,[101,103] glass ionomer cement,[124,128,399] Retroplast,[246] IRM,[115,121,146] EBA,[115,121,127] gold leaf,[123] and titanium inlay.[400] Amalgam has been frequently used as the "gold standard" control in these studies. The conclusions of all these studies are undermined by their methodological inadequacies. For example, amalgam and EBA cement can be compared in three studies: EBA cement is significantly superior in one study (95% vs. 51% success, respectively),[115] marginally superior in the second study (57% vs. 52%, respectively),[127] and marginally inferior in a third study (65% vs. 71%, respectively).[121] Better evidence is available in recent selected RCTs[143,144,150] and

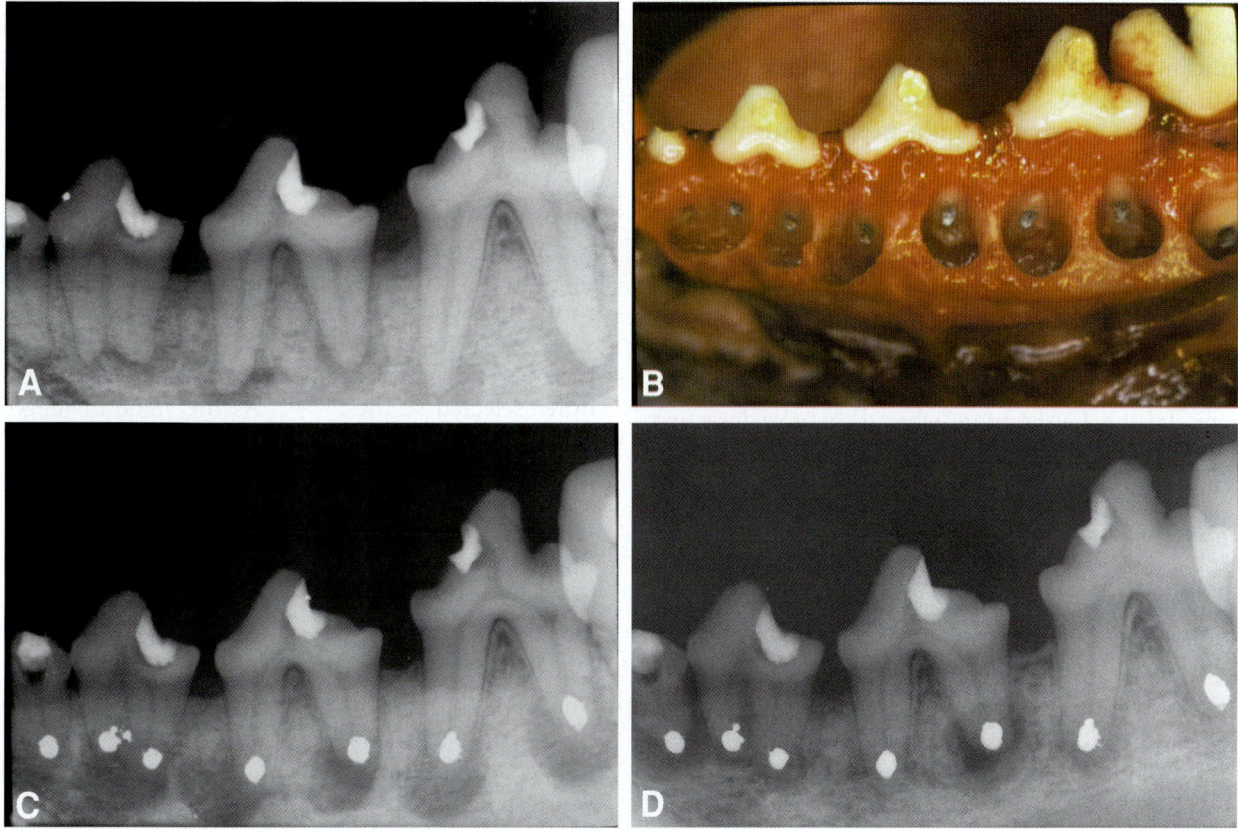

Figure 19 An animal model for assessing the efficacy of root-end filling materials. **A,** Mandibular premolars in a dog, with apical periodontitis induced by inoculation of the canals with plaque. **B,** Clinical view of the crypts and root-end fillings with amalgam and varnish in all the canals of the four premolars. **C,** Radiographic view of completed surgery. **D,** At 6 months, some of the lesions are healed and others are not. Healing is the measure of the sealing efficacy of the root-end fillings. (Reprinted with permission from Friedman 2006.[201])

a selected nonrandomized trial.[151] Retroplast is significantly better for apical "cap" bonding than glass ionomer cement (observed to detach in several teeth).[143] Apical bonding with Retroplast is apparently comparable with root-end filling with MTA.[151] When root-end fillings are used, MTA appears to be equally effective to IRM.[144,150] Healing may be poorer when using Super EBA than MTA.[151] Thus, for the apical bonded "cap" approach, Retroplast offers a better potential for healing, whereas for the intra-canal root-end cavity approach, the potential for healing does not appear to be influenced by use of IRM or MTA, but may be somewhat compromised by use of EBA cements.

Hemostasis

Different hemostatic agents, including epinephrine-saturated pellets, ferric sulfate, bone wax, thrombin, calcium sulfate, Gelfoam, Surgicel, and collagen wound dressing, have been routinely used for crypt control by many clinicians.[238,305,401,402] Good hemostasis is critically important for the quality of the root-end filling[238] and bonding of an apical "cap."[143] However, in a recent selected study,[148] there was no significant association between the outcome and the use of hemostatic agents. Thus, use of hemostatic agents does not appear to influence the potential for healing after apical surgery.

Concurrent Surgical and Orthograde Treatment

Concurrent apical surgery and initial treatment or re-treatment addresses all possible bacterial sites, including root canal ramifications, the apical root surface, and the periapical tissue. Furthermore, when these procedures are performed concurrently "infection is eliminated and re-infection is prevented."[120] Therefore, the outcome is usually better in studies combining both procedures in the majority of the sample than in studies where only apical surgery was performed.[207,224] The difference between the two approaches is also evident in specific nonselected studies.[93,96,98,99,102,106,116] It confirms that root canal bacteria are the predominant cause of refractory apical periodontitis,[302,303] and that they may still sustain the disease process in spite of the root-end filling. Currently, however, apical surgery is not considered imminent when the root canal is accessible from the coronal pathway; rather, it is performed alone as an alternative to orthograde re-treatment. Thus, the better potential for healing offered by performing concurrent apical surgery and orthograde treatment is merely of academic interest.

Retrograde Root Canal Re-treatment

An alternative to the typical root-end filling is an attempt to instrument, irrigate, and fill the root canal as far coronally as can be reached from the apical end.[111,113,403–407] Studies on retrograde re-treatment have reported complete healing in 71% to 100% of the teeth, with persistent disease not exceeding 16%.[111,113,148,408] The deeper barrier placed using this approach, between intra-canal bacteria and the periapical tissue, offers an advantage over the standard root-end filling. Nevertheless, continued bacterial ingress into the canal, under the restoration and along the post, may result in recurrence of disease (see Figure 10). Thus, even though retrograde re-treatment may not prevent recurrence of disease, it can enhance the outcome of apical surgery.

Magnification and Illumination

The use of aids to enhance visualization during apical surgery has become more common among clinicians than in the past. Magnification aids include loupes,[150] operating microscopes,[304,409,410] and endoscopes.[411,412] The latter two also greatly enhance illumination. These aids improve operator convenience, while also facilitating identification of root and canal anatomy and improving control of all aspects of the surgical procedure by improving the view of the surgical field.[238,304–308,411–413] One nonselected study[135] reports 97% "success" and implies that the outcome of apical surgery can be improved by use of the operating microscope and Super EBA cement as the root-end filling. In several selected studies, loupes were used to enhance visualization,[148–150] whereas the operating microscope or endoscope were used in other selected studies.[144,151] As the value of magnification and illumination has not been assessed at an adequate level of evidence, there is no data available to assess their influence on healing after apical surgery. Nevertheless, there is a sound rationale for use of these aids to improve the quality of the surgical procedure.

Laser Irradiation

The rationale for laser irradiation of the resected root surface and crypt in apical surgery is the potential for sterilization, hemostasis,[414–416] and the prevention of dentin permeability on the cut root surface.[417–421] Notwithstanding the theoretical benefits of laser irradiation, healing after apical surgery does not appear to be influenced, as shown in animal studies[397,422] and in a clinical trial.[134] Thus, healing after apical surgery is unlikely to be affected by use of laser irradiation in different steps of the procedure.

Barriers and Bone Grafting Substances
Incorporation of guided regeneration barriers[423,424] and various bone grafting substances[425–429] has been advocated in apical surgery. The handful of case series reports[424,430–433] do not provide evidence to support the routine use of these procedures. Thus, healing after apical surgery is unlikely to be enhanced by use of barriers and bone grafting substances. When such are applied, care must be taken to avoid infection.

Operator's Skill
The individual operator's skill has been suggested to influence the potential for healing in two nonselected studies.[102,119] Among the selected studies, resident students were the treatment providers in three studies,[139,143,148] whereas specialists, either oral surgeons or endodontists, performed the treatment in the remaining six studies.[138,144,149–151,434] Therefore, reference to operator skill in the selected studies is scarce. Thus, even though it is likely that the operator's skill may influence the potential for healing after apical surgery, there is insufficient data available to assess the extent of this influence.

Complications
Complications that may occur during apical surgery include a perforation in the opposing (lingual or palatal) aspect of the root or cortical bone plate, maxillary sinus exposure, or paresthesia of the inferior alveolar nerve. Information on the relation of these complications to healing is scarce. Perforation of the opposing bone plate may not influence healing beyond an increased rate scar tissue.[116,120,148] Healing also appears to be unaffected by perforation into the sinus.[100,107,191] Paresthesia has been reported in as many as 20% of patients after apical surgery in mandibular molars.[147] The majority of these patients regained normal sensation within 3 months after surgery, in 1% the sensory deficit lingered for 2 years, and in 1% it lingered beyond 2 years.[147] There was no association of the sensory deficit with periapical healing. Thus, healing after apical surgery does not appear to be affected by procedural complications. Sensory deficit, although not related to healing, must be considered as a risk when mandibular molars are treated.

Antibiotics
The rationale for prescribing antibiotics after apical surgery is to prevent infection of a postoperative hematoma. According to three selected studies,[139,148,151] a course of systemic antibiotics starting before and continuing after treatment does not influence healing. Thus, the use of systemic antibiotics is unlikely to influence healing after apical surgery.

POST-TREATMENT VARIABLE

Results of Biopsy
The periapical pathologic tissue is frequently removed during apical surgery and submitted to histopathologic examination. Theoretically, the biopsy results defining the pathologic lesion—apical periodontitis or cyst—might be used as indicators of the potential for healing. A significant association between the biopsy results and healing has been reported in one selected study[143] but not in two other selected studies.[138,148] These conflicting reports may be the result of differences in processing of biopsy specimens. Routine biopsies are seldom subjected to serial sections and therefore may not accurately reflect the nature of the pathologic lesion. Thus, a biopsy report on the nature of the lesion removed during apical surgery should not be used to project the potential for healing.

Potential for Healing and Retained Function after Intentional Replantation
Intentional replantation as an endodontic treatment modality has been used over the years as an alternative to difficult endodontic treatment,[156] apical surgery, and root canal re-treatment,[435] and even to prevent "predictable failures."[436] In accordance with current concepts, intentional replantation may be used as an alternative to extraction, when both re-treatment and apical surgery are not feasible in situ[152,154,437,438] (Figure 20). The expected goal is survival of the replanted tooth, considered as success[155] even if pathologic processes persist. Therefore, direct comparison of success and failure between intentional replantation and root canal re-treatment or apical surgery is not appropriate.

A replanted tooth requires healing of the attachment apparatus without root resorption. Periapical healing appears to be determined by survival of the periodontal ligament and cementum along the root surface,[439,440] and by infection of the root canal[441] and the socket.[442] Reattachment without resorption is affected by the trauma associated with exarticulation,

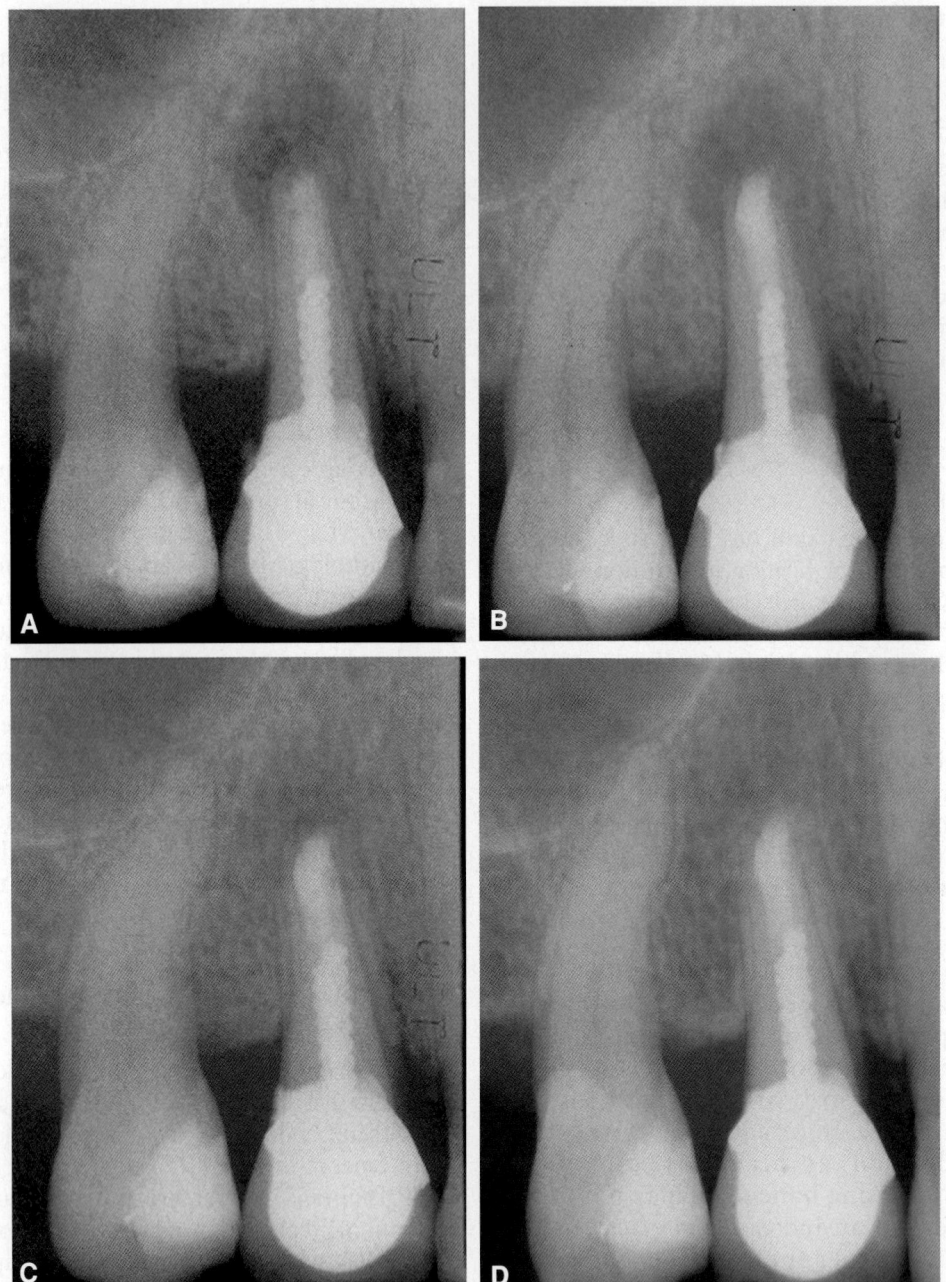

Figure 20 Intentional replantation when conventional treatment (orthograde re-treatment and apical surgery) is not feasible. *A,* Root-filled, previously surgically-treated, maxillary first premolar with persistent apical periodontitis and deep probing to the apex on the distal aspect. *B,* Completed intentional replantation that included two root-end fillings with MTA. *C,* At 3 months, the lesion is considerably decreased. *D,* At 2 years, the treated tooth is completely healed. The probing depth at the distal aspect is reduced to 4 mm.

extraoral manipulation and replantation, the extraoral time and environment, and the type and duration of splinting.[443,444] The optimal conditions for healing after intentional replantation include: (1) gentle extraction and reinsertion; (2) careful extraoral manipulation of the root, keeping it moist; (3) retrograde cleaning and filling of the root canal as far coronally as possible; (4) replantation within 15 minutes; (5) flexible splinting for 7 to 14 days and elimination of occlusal contacts; (6) pre- and postoperative antibiotic regimen; and (7) pre- and postoperative antiseptic mouth rinsing.

The majority of the studies on healing after intentional replantation (Table 4) have been reported over 20 years ago, and no current studies are available. According to the available studies, the "success" rate of intentional replantation ranges from 34%[152] to 93%,[156] whereas the survival rate appears to exceed 80%, but the evaluation criteria are often vague. Although the treatment procedures in the studies listed in Table 4 differ considerably, their clinical protocols seldom meet the currently recognized requirements for successful replantation of teeth. For example, Grossman and Chacker[153] did not place root-end fillings in 28 replanted root-filled teeth with refractory apical periodontitis; this was likely the cause of refractory infection observed in 27% of their material. Emmertsen and Andreasen[152] replanted the teeth after 30 to 60 minutes and tapered some roots by grinding to facilitate replantation; both factors compromise the tissues on the root surface, increasing the risk of resorption. When root fillings were performed, the inefficient method of gutta-percha and Kloroperka N-Ø was frequently used. Many roots were only sealed apically by root-end filling without a root filling; these roots were frequently associated with inflammatory root resorption, probably caused by persisting intra-canal bacteria that propagated through the dentinal tubules and infected the root surface.[445] A similar technique was used in all or part of the sample in two more recent studies.[158,160] Deeb[154] performed the root canal treatment and occasionally also the coronal restoration outside the mouth, probably extending the extraoral period over 15 minutes.

The realistic treatment outcome of proper intentional replantation cannot be assessed on the basis of the published studies, because of their procedural inadequacy. Projection from reported outcomes after replantation of traumatically avulsed teeth is inappropriate, because intentional replantation affords superior control over most of the factors influencing healing. In the absence of suitable clinical studies, clues about the potential for healing may be obtained from animal studies on replantation and root resorption, where intentional replantation was the actual experimental procedure. These studies suggest that development of progressive root resorption may be minimized to 4% or below, when the optimal conditions for replantation are present.[443] Indeed, three of the clinical studies on intentional replantation have reported root resorption in only 2% to 5% of the replanted teeth (see Table 4). Replacement resorption should not occur at all[158] because of the optimal extraoral time and environment. Indeed, in spite of the compromised protocol in one study,[152] replacement resorption occurred in only 4% of the teeth. Beyond the prevention of resorption, healing of apical periodontitis may be achieved rather predictably, because the infected root canal can be effectively sealed when the root-end filling is carried out extraorally. The low incidence of resorption and persistent infection after intentional replantation is corroborated by many case reports.[435–437,446–456] These reports have demonstrated the predictable healing potential after intentional replantation performed in well-controlled conditions, albeit at the lowest level of evidence.

Dynamics of Resorption

When resorption develops after intentional replantation, in the majority of the teeth it is discernible within 1 year.[152] This is definitely true regarding inflammatory resorption. Replacement resorption may be first observed radiographically several years after replantation.[440] However, it may be indicated clinically much earlier than radiographically, by a specific sound pitch upon percussion.

Realistic Outcome of Endodontic Treatment in the Population

The prevalence of apical periodontitis in the general population in different countries has been reported in many cross-sectional studies.[178–180,354,355,457–492] These studies have highlighted an alarmingly high prevalence of apical periodontitis among root-filled teeth (Table 8), ranging from 20% to over 60%, and they reflect the realistic outcome of endodontic treatment in the general population. The reported prevalence is lower in some of the studies because those populations have less remaining teeth than populations of other studies. Less remaining teeth suggests that teeth affected by refractory apical periodontitis after endodontic treatment may have been extracted, and thus not accounted in the respective studies.[477]

Table 5 Methodological Characteristics and Specific Outcomes of Selected Follow-up Studies on the Outcome of Initial Root Canal Treatment

Study	Recall rate (%)	Proportion of AP (%)	Tooth types	Treatment providers	Root filling	Intracanal medication	Healed (%) - AP	Healed (%) + AP
Strindberg 1956	74	42	mix	en	lc	f	93	88
Engström et al. 1964	72	53	mix	us	–	–	88	76
Kerekes & Tronstad 1979	77	34	mix	us	lc	ct, f	97	91
Byström et al. 1987	56	100	sr	us	lc	ch	–	85
Ørstavik et al. 1987	67	29	mix	us	lc	–	–	–
Eriksen et al. 1988	52	100	mix	us	lc	ch	–	82
Sjögren et al. 1990	46	31	mix	us	lc	ch	97	86
Ørstavik & Hörsted-Bindslev 1993	–	67	mix	us	lc	–	not interpretable	
Ørstavik 1996	82	–	mix	s	lc	ch	94	75
Sjögren et al. 1997	96	100	mix	en	lc	ch, os	–	83
Trope et al. 1999	100 ?	100 ?	sr	en	lc	ch, os	–	80
Weiger et al. 2000	92	100	–	en	lc	ch	–	78
Peters & Wesselink 2002	100	100	sr	en	wl	ch	–	76
Hoskinson et al. 2002	42	70	mix	en	hc, wv	ch, os	88	74
Friedman et al. 2003	sample included in Marquis et al. 2006							
Huumonen et al. 2003	78	–	mix	us, gs, en	lc	ch	–	–
Peters et al. 2004	89	44	mix	en	lc, sb	ch, os	95	76
Farzaneh et al. 2004	sample included in Marquis et al. 2006							
Ørstavik et al. 2004	same sample as Ørstavik, et al. 1987						94	79
Marending et al. 2005	79	52	mix	en	lc	ch, os	–	–
Waltimo et al. 2005	same sample as Trope et al. 1999							
Marquis et al. 2006	50	57	mix	gs	lc, wv	ch, os	93	80
Gesi et al. 2006	90	0	mix	en	lc	ch, os	93	–

mix all tooth types included
sr   single-rooted teeth, or single roots from multi-rooted teeth included
en   endodontist(s)
us   undergraduate students
gs   graduate students
lc   cold lateral compaction of gutta-percha
wv   vertical compaction of warm gutta-percha
hc   hybrid thermo-compaction of gutta-percha
wl   warm lateral compaction of gutta-percha
f   formalin (and other medications in fewer cases)
ct   chloramine T
ch   calcium hydroxide
os   one-session treatment

Because the cross-sectional study methodology does not allow collection of all the data regarding the treatment histories of the observed root-filled teeth, the reported "snapshot" data of the percentage of teeth presenting with periapical radiolucency is subject to interpretation.[493] Some of the radiolucencies captured may have been reduced from their original size and healing, if the teeth have been captured shortly after treatment. Thus, the proportion of root-filled teeth with refractory apical periodontitis may be overestimated. However, when specific populations were re-examined 6 to 11 years after their first account in a cross-sectional

Table 6 Methodological Characteristics and Specific Outcomes of Selected Follow-up Studies on the Outcome of Orthograde Retreatment

Study	Recall rate (%)	Proportion of AP (%)	Tooth types	Treatment providers	Root filling	Intracanal medication	Healed (%) without AP	Healed (%) with AP
Strindberg 1956	74	42	mix	en	lc	f	95	84
Engström et al. 1964	72	53	mix	us	-	-	93	74
Sjögren et al. 1990	46	31	mix	us	lc	ch	98	62
Sundqvist et al. 1998	100	100	sr	en	lc	ch	-	74
Kvist & Reit 1999	100	100	sr	en	lc	ch	-	58
Farzaneh et al. 2004	34	71	mix	gs	lc, wv	ch	97	78

AP   apical periodontitis
mix all tooth types included
sr   single-rooted teeth (5 two-rooted teeth also included)
en   endodontist(s)
us   undergraduate students
gs   graduate students
lc   cold lateral compaction of gutta-percha
wv   vertical compaction of warm gutta-percha
f   formalin (and other medications in fewer cases)
ch   calcium hydroxide

study, those lesions that were observed to heal were offset by a comparable number of new lesions that had developed.[180,482,494,495]

Attempts to use the cross-sectional data to explore relationships between healing and specific clinical variables, notably the apparent quality of the restoration and root filling, have been contradictory. One study[472] suggests that the quality of the restoration influences healing more than the quality of the root filling, whereas other studies suggest the opposite[441] or report no difference.[179,355,478,480,483] These contradictions arise from the limitations of the cross-sectional methodology, that is unsuitable for investigating such relationships.[212] Thus, the influence on healing of the quality of the restoration or the root filling cited in these studies is not valid.

Expansion of the data collected in cross-sectional studies has been attempted in recent years by interviewing the subjects included in the studies and ascertaining that recently treated teeth are excluded.[179,476,478,483] Nevertheless, even with the improved methodology, vital information on the pretreatment diagnosis and treatment methods is still unavailable. One observation, however, is consistent throughout the cross-sectional studies—the apparent quality of the root fillings is poor in the majority of the treated teeth (see Table 8) and possibly correlated with the poor outcome observed in the studies.[355,480]

Comments on Case Selection

Selection of cases for endodontic treatment takes into consideration the potential for healing and retained function, but also health and socioeconomic factors. Contraindications to treatment include nonrestorable and periodontally hopeless teeth, patients with extensive dental problems and restricted resources (that should be selectively utilized to benefit as many teeth as possible), and medically compromised patients at high-risk of infection or, for surgical procedures, those with bleeding disorders.

From the endodontic perspective, none of the preoperative clinical variables truly contraindicates therapy. The potential for healing after endodontic therapy of apical periodontitis is good, and the chance to retain a well-restored tooth in symptom-free function over time is excellent. Therefore, whenever it is feasible, either nonsurgical or surgical

Table 7 Methodological Characteristics of Selected Follow-up Studies on the Outcome of Apical Surgery

Methodological considerations		Kvist & Reit 1999	Zuolo et al. 2000	Rahbaran et al. 2001	Jensen et al. 2002	Chong et al. 2003	Wang et al. 2004	Gagliani et al. 2005	Lindeboom et al. 2005	Von Arx et al. 2007
Type of study	Direction	Prospective	Prospective ?	Retrospective	Prospective	Prospective	Prospective	Prospective ?	Prospective	Prospective
	Design	RCT	Cohort	Cohort	RCT	RCT	Cohort	Cohort	RCT	Cohort
Cohort	Tooth type	Anteriors	Anteriors 38% Premolars 24% Molars 38%	Anteriors 73% Premolars 19% Molars 8%	Anteriors 25% Premolars 33% Molars 42%	Single-rooted Molars (M roots)	Anteriors 39% Posterior 61%	Anteriors 17% Premolars 33% Molars 50%	Anteriors 58% Premolars 42%	Anteriors 31% Premolars 29% Molars 40%
	Inclusion criteria	AP present	AP present 1 tooth/subject At least 1 retreat Good restoration	20% w/o AP No probing Good root filling Good restoration	1 tooth/subject	AP present 1 tooth/subject No probing Good root filling Good restoration	All included	No probing Good root filling Lesion <10mm	AP present Root filling present Single rooted	Root-end filled AP present at apex
	Exclusion criteria	Recent retreatment Probing to apex	Fracture Perforation Resorption Trauma Probing >7mm Loss of bone plate		Previous surgery		None		Perforation present Probing > 5 mm Fracture Lesion >10 mm	Combined endo-perio lesions
	Previous retreatment		100%	39%		Yes; ?%	37%			
	Previous surgery		None	44%	None		10%	32%		
Intervention	Operators	Endodontist	Endodontist	Endodontics residents	4 Oral surgery residents	Endodontist	Endodontics residents	Endodontist	Oral surgeons	Oral surgeon
	Resection level	1–2 mm	2–4 mm		2–3 mm			3 mm	3 mm	3 mm
			Bevel			No bevel		Little bevel	10–25°	
	Hemostasis				Epinephrin		Epinephrin Ferric sulfate	Ferric sulfate	Pressure Hemostatic agents	Aluminum chloride Ferric sulfate
	Cavity preparation	Bur	Ultrasonic	Bur or ultrasonic	Scooped	Ultrasonic	Ultrasonic 7% R-rtx	Ultrasonic	Ultrasonic	Sonic
	Root-end filling material	34% R-rtx GP softened with chloroform or heat	IRM	S-EBA, amalgam, IRM, GP, none	Retroplast GIC	IRM MTA	Amalgam, IRM s-EBA, CR, MTA, none	ZOE with EBA	IRM MTA	Super EBA MTA Retroplast
	Magnification					Microscope	Loops	Loops × 4.5	Loops × 3.5	Rigid endoscope
	Sutures		Monofilament 5x0 3–4 days		Vicryl 4x0			Silk		
	Antibiotics		7 days Steroid	4–7 days	Only when sinus invaded	4–7 days	44% of teeth			Minority of teeth NSAID
	Anti-inflammatories			45% of teeth						
	Antiseptic rinse		4 days	7 days	None used	Used	7 days			10 days
Assessment	Radiographic aids	Stents				Stents	Parallel device PAI 1, 2	Parallel device	Long cone	
	Radiographic criteria	"Strict definition of healing/disease"	CH = success IH = success UH = failure >4 years US = failure	CH = success UH = uncertain Failure	CH = success IH = success UH = doubtful US = failure	CH = success IH = success UH = failure US = failure		CH = success IH = improvement Failure	CH IH UH US = failure	CH = success IH = success UH = doubtful US = failure

Table 7 Continued on page 1215

Table 7 Continued on page 1214

Calibration		Yes	Yes	No	Yes	Yes	Yes	No	No
Binding			Yes	No	Yes	Yes	Yes		
Observers	2	2	3	3	2	1	2	2	3
Conflicts resolved	Joint assessment	Joint assessment	Joint assessment	Concensus or majority	Joint assessment	N/a	Worst accepted	Third examiner	Majority
Follow-up	6, 12, 24, 48 months	1–4 years	1, 2, 4 years	1 year	1, 2 years	4–8 years	5 years	1 year	1 year
		Successful not followed further							
Analysis									
Evaluated unit	Tooth	Tooth	Tooth	Tooth	Root and tooth	Tooth	Root	Tooth	Tooth
Bivariate tests	Used	Used	Not used	Used	Used	Used	Used	Used	Used
Multivariate tests	N/a	Not used	Used	Used	N/a	Used	N/a	N/a	Used

AP = apical periodontitis
R-rtx = retrograde retreatment
GP = gutta-percha
GIC = glass-ionomer cement
CR = composite resin
ZOE = zinc oxide eugenol
CH = complete healing
IH = incomplete healing
UH = uncertain healing
US = unsatisfactory healing
N/a = not applicable

Table 8 Cross-Sectional Studies Reporting on the Prevalence of Apical Periodontitis and Inadequate Root Fillings in Root-Filled Teeth

Study	Country	Subjects	Ages(years)	Apical periodontitis	Inadequate root filling
Hansen & Johansen 1976	Sweden	111	35	20%	–
Hugoson & Koch 1979	Sweden	1000	20–70	22–29%	–
Hugoson et al. 1986	Sweden	1000	20–80	23–44%	–
Allard & Palmqvist 1986	Sweden	500	≥65	27%	69%
Petersson et al. 1986	Sweden	861	20–60	31%	60%
Bergström et al.1987	Sweden	250	21–60	29%	–
Eckerbom et al. 1987	Sweden	200	20–60+	26%	55%
Eriksen et al. 1988	Norway	141	35	26%	59%
Eckerbom et al. 1989	Sweden	200	20–60+	22%	49%
Petersson et al. 1989	Sweden	567	20–70+	21%[nst] 65%[st]	63%
Ødesjö et al. 1990	Sweden	751	20–80+	25%	70%
Eriksen & Bjertness 1991	Norway	119	50	37%	51%
Imfeld 1991	Switzerland	143	66	31%	64%
Eckerbom et al. 1991	Sweden	200	20–60+	26%	–
De Cleen et al. 1993	Netherlands	184	20–60+	39%	51%
Petersson 1993	Sweden	586	20–60	31%	50%
Ray & Trope 1995	U.S.A.	985[teeth]		39%	50%
Buckley & Spångberg 1995	U.S.A.	208	−20–80+	31%	58%
Eriksen et al. 1995	Norway	121	35	38%	33%
Soikonen 1995	Finland	133	76, 81, 86	16%	75%
Saunders et al. 1997	UK	340	20–59+	58%	58%
Weiger et al. 1997	Germany	323	12–89	61%	86%
Marques et al. 1998	Portugal	179	30–39	22%	54%
Sidaravicius et al. 1999	Lithuania	147	35–44	35%[a]	87%
De Moor et al. 2000	Belgium	206	18–59	40%	57%
Tronstad et al. 2000	Norway	1001[teeth]	–	37%	49%
Kirkevang et al. 2000	Denmark	614	20–60+	52%	74%
Kirkevang et al. 2001	Denmark	602	20–60+	51%[c] 58%[d]	73% 74%
Kirkevang et al. 2001	Denmark	614[b]	20–60+	52%	–
Boucher et al. 2002	France	208	18–70	30%	79%
Lupi-Pegurier et al. 2002	France	344	33–65	32%	69%
Hommez et al. 2002	Belgium	745[teeth]	–	33%	66%
Dugas et al. 2003	Canada	610	25–40	45%	61%
Boltacz-Rzepkowska & Pawlicka 2003	Poland	236	15–76	25%	51%
Segura-Egea et al. 2004	Spain	180	31–53	65%	66%
Loftus, et al. 2005	Ireland	302	16–98	25%	53%
Georgopolou et al. 2005	Greece	320	16–77	60%	–
Kabak & Abbott 2005	Belarus	1423	15–65+	45%	48%
Kirkevang et al. 2006	Denmark	473[b]	20–60+	44%	–
Sunay et al. 2007	Turkey	375	16–82	54%	58%
Chen et al. 2007	U.S.A.	206	55–97	37%	74%

nst – non-surgically treated
st – surgically treated
a   pulp amputated teeth excluded
b   repeated sample
c   treated in 1974–75
d   treated in 1997–78

endodontic treatment should be attempted before considering tooth extraction and replacement.

References

1. Strindberg LZ. The dependence of the results of pulp therapy on certain factors. An analytic study based on radiographic and clinical follow-up examination. Acta Odontol Scand 1956;14:21.
2. Grahnén H, Hansson L. The prognosis of pulp and root canal therapy. Odontol Revy 1961;12:146–65.
3. Seltzer S, Bender IB, Turkenkopf S. Factors affecting successful repair after root canal therapy. J Am Dent Assoc 1963;52:651–62.
4. Zeldow B, Ingle JI. Correlation of the positive culture to the prognosis of endodontically treated teeth: a clinical study. J Am Dent Assoc 1963;66:23–7.
5. Bender IB, Seltzer S. To culture or not to culture? Oral Surg Oral Med Oral Pathol Oral Radiol Endod 1964;18:527–40.
6. Engström B, Hard AF, Segerstad L, et al. Correlation of postive cultures with the prognosis for root canal treatment. Odontol Revy 1964;15:257–70.
7. Grossman LI, Shepard LI, Pearson LA. Roentgenologic and clinical evaluation of endodontically treated teeth. Oral Surg Oral Med Oral Pathol Oral Radiol Endod 1964;17:368–74.
8. Engström B, Lundberg M. The correlation between positive culture and the prognosis of root canal therapy after pulpectomy. Odontol Revy 1965;16:193–203.
9. Oliet S, Sorin SM. Evaluation of clinical results based upon culturing root canals. J Br Endod Soc 1969;3:3–6.
10. Storms JL. Factors that influence the success of endodontic treatment. J Can Dent Assoc 1969;35:83–97.
11. Harty FJ, Parkins BJ, Wengraf AM. Success rate in root canal therapy. A retrospective study of conventional cases. Br Dent J 1970;128:65–70.
12. Heling B, Tamshe A. Evaluation of the success of endodontically treated teeth. Oral Surg Oral Med Oral Pathol Radiol Endod 1970;30:533–6.
13. Cvek M. Treatment of non-vital permanent incisors with calcium hydroxide. I. Follow-up of periapical repair and apical closure of immature roots. Odontol Revy 1972;23:27–44.
14. Tamse A, Heling B. Success of endodontically treated anterior teeth in young and adult patients. Ann Dent 1973;32:20–6.
15. Lambjerg-Hansen H. Vital and mortal pulpectomy on permanent human teeth. An experimental comparative histologic investigation. Scand J Dent Res 1974;82:243–332.
16. Selden HS. Pulpoperiapical disease: diagnosis and healing. A clinical endodontic study. Oral Surg Oral Med Oral Pathol Radiol Endod 1974;37:271–83.
17. Adenubi JO, Rule DC. Success rate for root fillings in young patients. A retrospective analysis of treated cases. Br Dent J 1976;141:237–41.
18. Heling B, Shapira J. Roentgenologic and clinical evaluation of endodontically treated teeth, with or without negative culture. Quintessence Int 1978;9:79–84.
19. Jokinen MA, Kotilainen R, Poikkeus P, et al. Clinical and radiographic study of pulpectomy and root canal therapy. Scand J Dent Res 1978;86:366–73.
20. Soltanoff W. A comparative study of the single-visit and the multiple-visit edodontic procedure. J Endod 1978;4:278–81.
21. Ashkenaz PJ. One-visit endodontics—a preliminary report. Dent. Surv 1979;55:62–7.
22. Kerekes K, Tronstad L. Long-term results of endodontic treatment performed with a standardized technique. J Endod 1979;5:83–90.
23. Barbakow FH, Cleaton-Jones P, Friedman D. An evaluation of 566 cases of root canal therapy in general dental practice. 2. Postoperative observations. J Endod 1980;6:485–9.
24. Barbakow FH, Cleaton-Jones PE, Friedman D. Endodontic treatment of teeth with periapical radiolucent areas in a general dental practice. Oral Surg Oral Med Oral Pathol Radiol Endod 1981;51:552–9.
25. Hession RW. Long-term evaluation of endodontic treatment: anatomy, instrumentation, obturation—the endodontic practice triad. Int Endod J 1981;14:179–84.
26. Cvek M, Granath L, Lundberg M. Failures and healing in endodontically treated non-vital anterior teeth with post-traumatically reduced pulpal lumen. Acta Odontol Scand 1982;40:223–8.
27. Nelson IA. Endodontics in general practice—a retrospective survey. Int Endod J 1982;15:168–72.
28. Klevant FJ, Eggink CO. The effect of canal preparation on periapical disease. Int Endod J 1983;16:68–75.
29. Morse DR, Esposito JV, Pike C, Furst ML. A radiographic evaluation of the periapical status of teeth treated by the gutta-percha-eucapercha endodontic method: a one-year follow-up study of 458 root canals. Part III. Oral Surg Oral Med Oral Pathol Radiol Endod 1983;56:190–7.
30. Morse DR, Esposito JV, Pike C, Furst ML. A radiographic evaluation of the periapical status of teeth treated by the gutta-percha—eucapercha endodontic method: a one-year follow-up study of 458 root canals. Part II. Oral Surg Oral Med Oral Pathol Radiol Endod 1983;56:89–96.
31. Morse DR, Esposito JV, Pike C, Furst ML. A radiographic evaluation of the periapical status of teeth treated by the

gutta-percha—eucapercha endodontic method: a one-year follow-up study of 458 root canals. Part I. Oral Surg Oral Med Oral Pathol Radiol Endod 1983;55:607–10.
32. Oliet S. Single-visit endodontics: a clinical study. J Endod 1983;9:147–52.
33. Swartz DB, Skidmore AE, Griffin JA Jr. Twenty years of endodontic success and failure. J Endod 1983;9:198–202.
34. Pekruhn RB. The incidence of failure following single-visit endodontic therapy. J Endod 1986;12:68–72.
35. Bystrom A, Happonen RP, Sjögren U, Sundqvist G. Healing of periapical lesions of pulpless teeth after endodontic treatment with controlled asepsis. Endod Dent Traumatol 1987;3:58–63.
36. Matsumoto T, Nagai T, Ida K, et al. Factors affecting successful prognosis of root canal treatment. J Endod 1987;13:239–42.
37. Ørstavik D, Kerekes K, Eriksen HM. Clinical performance of three endodontic sealers. Endod Dent Traumatol 1987;3:178–86.
38. Safavi KE, Dowden WE, Langeland K. Influence of delayed coronal permanent restoration on endodontic prognosis. Endod Dent Traumatol 1987;3:187–91.
39. Eriksen HM, Orstavik D, Kerekes K. Healing of apical periodontitis after endodontic treatment using three different root canal sealers. Endod Dent Traumatol 1988;4:114–17.
40. Åkerblom A, Hasselgren G. The prognosis for endodontic treatment of obliterated root canals. J Endod 1988;14:565–7.
41. Molven O, Halse A. Success rates for gutta-percha and Kloroperka N-0 root fillings made by undergraduate students: radiographic findings after 10-17 years. Int Endod J 1988;21:243–50.
42. Shah N. Nonsurgical management of periapical lesions: a prospective study. Oral Surg Oral Med Oral Pathol Radiol Endod 1988;66:365–71.
43. Sjögren U, Hagglund B, Sundqvist G, Wing K. Factors affecting the long-term results of endodontic treatment. J Endod 1990;16:498–504.
44. Augsburger RA, Peters DD. Radiographic evaluation of extruded obturation materials. J Endod 1990;16:492–7.
45. Murphy WK, Kaugars GE, Collett WK, Dodds RN. Healing of periapical radiolucencies after nonsurgical endodontic therapy. Oral Surg Oral Med Oral Pathol Radiol Endod 1991;71:620–4.
46. Cvek M. Prognosis of luxated non-vital maxillary incisors treated with calcium hydroxide and filled with gutta-percha. A retrospective clinical study. Endod Dent Traumatol 1992;8:45–55.
47. Smith CS, Setchell DJ, Harty FJ. Factors influencing the success of conventional root canal therapy—a five-year retrospective study. Int Endod J 1993;26:321–33.
48. Ørstavik D, Hörsted-Bindslev P. A comparison of endodontic treatment results at two dental schools. Int Endod J 1993;26:348–54.
49. Ingle JI, Beveridge EE, Glick DH, Weichman JA. Modern endodontic therapy. In: Ingle JI, Bakland LK, editors. Endodontics. 4th ed. Baltimore: Williams & Wilkins; 1994. pp. 27–53.
50. Friedman S, Löst C, Zarrabian M, Trope M. Evaluation of success and failure after endodontic therapy using a glass ionomer cement sealer. J Endod 1995;21:384–90.
51. Caliskan MK, Sen BH. Endodontic treatment of teeth with apical periodontitis using calcium hydroxide: a long-term study. Endod Dent Traumatol 1996;12:215–21.
52. Ørstavik D. Time-course and risk analyses of the development and healing of chronic apical periodontitis in man. Int Endod J 1996;29:150–5.
53. Sjögren U, Figdor D, Persson S, Sundqvist G. Influence of infection at the time of root filling on the outcome of endodontic treatment of teeth with apical periodontitis. Int Endod J 1997;30:297–306.
54. Trope M, Delano EO, Ørstavik D. Endodontic treatment of teeth with apical periodontitis: single vs. multivisit treatment. J Endod 1999;25:345–50.
55. Weiger R, Rosendahl R, Löst C. Influence of calcium hydroxide intracanal dressings on the prognosis of teeth with endodontically induced periapical lesions. Int Endod J 2000;33:219–26.
56. Waltimo T, Boiesen J, Eriksen HM, Ørstavik D. Clinical performance of 3 endodontic sealers. Oral Surg, Oral Med, Oral Pathol, Oral Radiol, Endod 2001;92:89–92.
57. Chugal NM, Clive JM, Spangberg LS. A prognostic model for assessment of the outcome of endodontic treatment: Effect of biologic and diagnostic variables. Oral Surg Oral Med Oral Pathol Oral Radiol Endod 2001;91:342–52.
58. Heling I, Bialla-Shenkman S, Turetzky A, et al. The outcome of teeth with periapical periodontitis treated with nonsurgical endodontic treatment: a computerized morphometric study. Quintessence Int 2001;32:397–400.
59. Peak JD, Hayes SJ, Bryant ST, Dummer PM. The outcome of root canal treatment. A retrospective study within the armed forces (Royal Air Force). Br Dent J 2001;190:140–4.
60. Pettiette MT, Delano EO, Trope M. Evaluation of success rate of endodontic treatment performed by students with stainless-steel K-files and nickel-titanium hand files. J Endod 2001;27:124–7.
61. Peters LB, Wesselink PR. Periapical healing of endodontically treated teeth in one and two visits obturated in the presence or absence of detectable microorganisms. Int Endod J 2002;35:660–7.
62. Hoskinson SE, Ng YL, Hoskinson AE, et al. A retrospective comparison of outcome of root canal treatment using two

different protocols. Oral Surg Oral Med Oral Pathol Oral Radiol Endod 2002;93:705–15.

63. Molven O, Halse A, Fristad I, MacDonald-Jankowksi D. Periapical changes following root-canal treatment observed 20–27 years postoperatively. Int Endod J 2002;35:784–90.

64. Benenati FW, Khajotia SS. A radiographic recall evaluation of 894 endodontic cases treated in a dental school setting. J Endod 2002;28:391–5.

65. Fouad A, Burleson J. The effect of diabetes mellitus on endodontic treatment outcome: data from an electronic patient record. J Am Dent Assoc 2003;134:43–51.

66. Huumonen S, Lenander-Lumikari M, Sigurdsson A, Orstavik D. Healing of apical periodontitis after endodontic treatment: a comparison between a silicone-based and a zinc oxide-eugenol-based sealer. Int Endod J 2003;36:296–301.

67. Friedman S, Abitbol S, Lawrence HP. Treatment outcome in endodontics: the Toronto Study. Phase 1: initial treatment. J Endod 2003;29:787–93.

68. Chugal NM, Clive JM, Spangberg LS. Endodontic infection: some biologic and treatment factors associated with outcome. Oral Surg Oral Med Oral Pathol Oral Radiol Endod 2003;96:81–90.

69. Field JW, Gutmann JL, Solomon ES, Rakusin H. A clinical radiographic retrospective assessment of the success rate of single-visit root canal treatment. Int Endod J 2004;37:70–82.

70. Farzaneh M, Abitbol S, Lawrence HP, Friedman S. Treatment outcome in endodontics-the Toronto Study. Phase II: initial treatment. J Endod 2004;30:302–9.

71. Peters OA, Barbakow F, Peters CI. An analysis of endodontic treatment with three nickel-titanium rotary root canal preparation techniques. Int Endod J 2004;37:849–59.

72. Orstavik D, Qvist V, Stoltze K. A mutlivariate analysis of the outcome of endodontic treatment. Eur J Oral Sci 2004;112:224–30.

73. Caliskan MK. Prognosis of large cyst-like periapical lesions following nonsurgical root canal treatment: a clinical review. Int Endod J 2004;37:408–16.

74. Moshonov J, Slutzky-Goldberg I, Gottlieb A, Peretz B. The effect of the distance between post and residual gutta-percha on the clinical outcome of endodontic treatment. J Endod 2005;31:177–9.

75. Marending M, Peters OA, Zehnder M. Factors affecting the outcome of orthograde root canal therapy in a general dentistry hospital practice. Oral Surg Oral Med Oral Pathol Oral Radiol Endod 2005;99:119–24.

76. Waltimo T, Trope M, Haapasalo M, Ørstavik D. Clinical efficacy of treatment procedures in Endodontic infection control and one year follow-up of periapical healing. J Endod 2005;31:863–6.

77. Chu C, Lo ECM, Cheung GSP. Outcome of root canal treatment using Thermafil and cold latyeral condensation filling techniques. Int Endod J 2005;38:179–85.

78. Marquis V, Dao T, Farzaneh M, et al. Treatment outcome in Endodontics: The Toronto Study. Phase III: Initial treatment. J Endod 2006;32:299–306.

79. Aqrabawi JA. Outcome of endodontic treatment of teeth filled using lateral condensation versus vertical compaction (Schilder's technique). J Contemp Dent Pract 2006;7:17–24.

80. Gesi A, Hakeberg M, Warfvinge J, Bergenholtz G. Incidence of periapical lesions and clinical symptoms after pulpectomy—a clinical and radiographic evaluation of 1- versus 2-session treatment. Oral Surg Oral Med Oral Pathol Oral Radiol Endod 2006;101:379–88.

81. Bergenholtz G, Lekholm U, Milthon R, et al. Retreatment of endodontic fillings. Scand J Dent Res 1979;87:217–24.

82. Allen RK, Newton CW, Brown CE Jr. A statistical analysis of surgical and nonsurgical endodontic retreatment cases. J Endod 1989;15:261–6.

83. Van Nieuwenhuysen JP, Aouar M, D'Hoore W. Retreatment or radiographic monitoring in endodontics. Int Endod J 1994;27:75–81.

84. Danin J, Stromberg T, Forsgren H, et al. Clinical management of nonhealing periradicular pathosis. Surgery versus endodontic retreatment. Oral Surg Oral Med Oral Pathol Oral Radiol Endod 1996;82:213–17.

85. Piatowska D, Pawlicka H, Laskiewicz J, et al. Evaluation of endodontic re-treatment. Czas Stomat 1997;L:451–8.

86. Sundqvist G, Figdor D, Persson S, Sjögren U. Microbiologic analysis of teeth with failed endodontic treatment and the outcome of conservative re-treatment. Oral Surg Oral Med Oral Pathol Oral Radiol Endod 1998;85:86–93.

87. Abbott P. A retrospective analysis of the resons for, and the outcome of, conservative endodontic re-treatment and periradicular surgery. Aust Dent J 1999;44:3–4.

88. Kvist T, Reit C. Results of endodontic retreatment: a randomized clinical study comparing surgical and nonsurgical procedures. J Endod 1999;25:814–17.

89. Danin J, Linder LE, Lundqvist G, et al. Outcomes of periradicular surgery in cases with apical pathosis and untreated canals. Oral Surg Oral Med Oral Pathol Oral Radiol Endod 1999;87:227–32.

90. Farzaneh M, Abitbol S, Friedman S. Treatment outcome in endodontics: the Toronto study. Phases I and II: Orthograde retreatment. J Endod 2004;30:627–33.

91. Gorni F, Gagliani MM. The outcome of Endodontic Retreatment: a 2-yr follow-up. J Endod 2004;30:1–4.

92. Fristad I, Molven O, Halse A. Nonsurgically retreated root-filled teeth—radiographic findings after 20–27 years. Int Endod J 2004;37:12–18.

93. Mattila K, Altonen M. A clinical and roentgenological study of apicoectomized teeth. Odont Tidskr 1968;76:389–408.
94. Harty FJ, Parkins BJ, Wengraf AM. The success rate of apicectomy. A retrospective study of 1,016 cases. Br Dent J 1970;129:407–13.
95. Nord PG. Retrograde rootfilling with Cavit: a clinical and roentgenological study. Svensk Tandlakaretidskrift 1970; 63:261–73.
96. Nordenram A, Svardstrom G. Results of apicectomy. Svensk Tandlakaretidskrift 1970;63:593–604.
97. Nordenram A. Biobond for retrograde root filling in apicoectomy. Scand J Dent Res 1970;78:251–5.
98. Lehtinen R, Aitasalo K. Comparison of the clinical and roentgenological state at the re-examination of root resections. Proc Finn Dent Soc 1972;68:209–11.
99. Rud J, Andreasen JO, Jensen JE. A follow-up study of 1,000 cases treated by endodontic surgery. Int J Oral Surg 1972;1:215–28.
100. Ericson S, Finne K, Persson G. Results of apicoectomy of maxillary canines, premolars and molars with special reference to oroantral communication as a prognostic factor. Int J Oral Surg 1974;3:386–93.
101. Persson G, Lennartson B, Lundstrom I. Results of retrograde root-filling with special reference to amalgam and Cavit as root-filling materials. Svensk Tandlakaretidskrift 1974; 67:123–43.
102. Altonen M, Mattila K. Follow-up study of apicoectomized molars. Int J Oral Surg 1976;5:33–40.
103. Finne K, Nord PG, Persson G, Lennartsson B. Retrograde root filling with amalgam and Cavit. Oral Surg Oral Med Oral Pathol Oral Radiol Endod 1977;43:621–6.
104. Tay WM, Gale KM, Harty FJ. The influence of periapical radiolucencies on the success or failure of apicoectomies. J Br Endod Soc 1978;11:3–6.
105. Hirsch JM, Ahlstrom U, Henrikson PA, et al. Periapical surgery. Int J Oral Surg 1979;8:173–85.
106. Malmstrom M, Perkki K, Lindquist K. Apicectomy. A retrospective study. Proc Finn Dent Soc 1982;78:26–31.
107. Persson G. Periapical surgery of molars. Int J Oral Surg 1982;11:96–100.
108. Ioannides C, Borstlap WA. Apicoectomy on molars: a clinical and radiographical study. Int J Oral Surg 1983;12:73–9.
109. Mikkonen M, Kullaa-Mikkonen A, Kotilainen R. Clinical and radiologic re-examination of apicoectomized teeth. Oral Surg Oral Med Oral Pathol Oral Radiol Endod 1983;55:302–6.
110. Skoglund A, Persson G. A follow-up study of apicoectomized teeth with total loss of the buccal bone plate. Oral Surg Oral Med Oral Pathol Oral Radiol Endod 1985; 59:78–81.
111. Reit C, Hirsch J. Surgical endodontic retreatment. Int Endod J 1986;19:107–12.
112. Forssell H, Tammisalo T, Forssell K. A follow-up study of apicectomized teeth. Proc Finn Den Soc 1988;84:85–93.
113. Amagasa T, Nagase M, Sato T, Shioda S. Apicoectomy with retrograde gutta-percha root filling. Oral Surg Oral Med Oral Pathol Oral Radiol Endod 1989;68:339–42.
114. Crosher RF, Dinsdale RC, Holmes A. One visit apicectomy technique using calcium hydroxide cement as the canal filling material combined with retrograde amalgam. Int Endod J 1989;22:283–9.
115. Dorn SO, Gartner AH. Retrograde filling materials: a retrospective success-failure study of amalgam, EBA, and IRM. J Endod 1990;16:391–3.
116. Grung B, Molven O, Halse A. Periapical surgery in a Norwegian county hospital: follow-up findings of 477 teeth. J Endod 1990;16:411–17.
117. Friedman S, Lustmann J, Shaharabany V. Treatment results of apical surgery in premolar and molar teeth. J Endod 1991;17:30–3.
118. Lasaridis N, Zouloumis L, Antoniadis K. Bony lid approach for apicoectomy of mandibular molars. Aust Dent J 1991;36:366–8.
119. Lustmann J, Friedman S, Shaharabany V. Relation of pre- and intraoperative factors to prognosis of posterior apical surgery. J Endod 1991;17:239–41.
120. Molven O, Halse A, Grung B. Surgical management of endodontic failures: indications and treatment results. Int Dent J 1991;41:33–42.
121. Rapp EL, Brown CE Jr, Newton CW. An analysis of success and failure of apicoectomies. J Endod 1991;17:508–12.
122. Rud J, Munksgaard EC, Andreasen JO, Rud V. Retrograde root filling with composite and a dentin-bonding agent. 2. Endod Dent Traumatol 1991;7:126–31.
123. Waikakul A, Punwutikorn J. Clinical study of retrograde filling with gold leaf: comparison with amalgam. Oral Surg Oral Med Oral Pathol Oral Radiol Endod 1991; 71:228–31.
124. Zetterqvist L, Hall G, Holmlund A. Apicectomy: a comparative clinical study of amalgam and glass ionomer cement as apical sealants. Oral Surg Oral Med Oral Pathol Oral Radiol Endod 1991;71:489–91.
125. Frank AL, Glick DH, Patterson SS, Weine FS. Long-term evaluation of surgically placed amalgam fillings. J Endod 1992;18:391–8.
126. Cheung LK, Lam J. Apicectomy of posterior teeth—a clinical study. Aust Dent J 1993;38:17–21.
127. Pantschev A, Carlsson AP, Andersson L. Retrograde root filling with EBA cement or amalgam. A comparative clinical study. Oral Surg Oral Med Oral Pathol Oral Radiol Endod 1994;78:101–4.

128. Jesslen P, Zetterqvist L, Heimdahl A. Long-term results of amalgam versus glass ionomer cement as apical sealant after apicectomy. Oral Surg Oral Med Oral Pathol Oral Radiol Endod 1995;79:101–3.

129. August DS. Long-term, postsurgical results on teeth with periapical radiolucencies. J Endod 1996;22:380–3.

130. Rud J, Rud V, Munksgaard EC. Retrograde root filling with dentin-bonded modified resin composite. J Endod 1996;22:477–80.

131. Sumi Y, Hattori H, Hayashi K, Ueda M. Ultrasonic root-end preparation: clinical and radiographic evaluation of results. J Oral Maxillofac Surg 1996;54:590–3.

132. Jansson L, Sandstedt P, Laftman AC, Skoglund A. Relationship between apical and marginal healing in periradicular surgery. Oral Surg Oral Med Oral Pathol Oral Radiol Endod 1997;83:596–601.

133. Rud J, Rud V, Munksgaard EC. Effect of root canal contents on healing of teeth with dentin-bonded resin composite retrograde seal. J Endod 1997;23:535–41.

134. Bader G, Lejeune S. Prospective study of two retrograde endodontic apical preparations with and without the use of CO2 laser. Endod Dent Traumatol 1998;14:75–8.

135. Rubinstein RA, Kim S. Short-term observation of the results of endodontic surgery with the use of a surgical operation microscope and Super-EBA as root-end filling material. J Endod 1999;25:43–8.

136. Testori T, Capelli M, Milani S, Weinstein RL. Success and failure in periradicular surgery: a longitudinal retrospective analysis. Oral Surg Oral Med Oral Pathol Oral Radiol Endod 1999;87:493–8.

137. von Arx T, Kurt B. Root-end cavity preparation after apicoectomy using a new type of sonic and diamond-surfaced retrotip: a 1-year follow-up study. J Oral Maxillofac Surg 1999;57:656–61.

138. Zuolo ML, Ferreira MO, Gutmann JL. Prognosis in periradicular surgery: a clinical prospective study. Int Endod J 2000;33:91–8.

139. Rahbaran S, Gilthorpe MS, Harrison SD, Gulabivala K. Comparison of clinical outcome of periapical surgery in endodontic and oral surgery units of a teaching dental hospital: a retrospective study. Oral Surg Oral Med Oral Pathol Oral Radiol Endod 2001;91:700–9.

140. Rud J, Rud V, Munksgaard EC. Periapical healing of mandibular molars after root-end sealing with dentine-bonded composite. Int Endod J 2001;34:285–92.

141. von Arx T, Gerber C, Hardt N. Periradicular surgery of molars: a prospective clinical study with a one-year follow-up. Int Endod J 2001;34:520–5.

142. Rubinstein RA, Kim S. Long-term follow-up of cases considered healed one year after apical microsurgery. J Endod 2002;28:378–83.

143. Jensen SS, Nattestad A, Egdo P, et al. A prospective, randomized, comparative clinical study of resin composite and glass ionomer cement for retrograde root filling. Clin Oral Investig 2002;6:236–43.

144. Chong BS, Pitt Ford TR, Hudson MB. A prospective clinical study of Mineral Trioxide Aggregate and IRM when used as root-end filling materials in endodontic surgery. Int Endod J 2003;36:520–6.

145. Maddalone M, Gagliani M. Periapical endodontic surgery: a 3-year follow-up study. Int Endod J 2003;36:193–8.

146. Schwartz-Arad D, Yaorm N, Lustig JP, Kaffe I. A retrospective radiographic study of root-end surgery with amalgam and intermediate restorative material. Oral Surg Oral Med Oral Pathol Oral Radiol Endod 2003;96:472–7.

147. Wesson CM, Gale TM. Molar apicectomy with amalgam root-end filling: results of a prospective study in two district general hospitals. Br Dent J 2003;195:707–14; discussion 698.

148. Wang N, Knight K, Dao T, Friedman S. Treatment outcome in endodontics-The Toronto Study. Phases I and II: apical surgery. J Endod 2004;30:751–61.

149. Gagliani MM, Gorni FGM, Strohmenger L. Periapcial resurgery versus periapical surgery: a 5-year longitudinal comparison. Int Endod J 2005;38:320–7.

150. Lindeboom JA, Frenken JW, Kroon FH, van den Akker HP. A comparative prospective randomized clinical study of MTA and IRM as root-end filling materials in single-rooted teeth in endodontic surgery. Oral Surg Oral Med Oral Pathol Oral Radiol Endod 2005;100:495–500.

151. von Arx T, Jensen SS, Hanni S. Clinical and radiographic assessment of various predictors for healing outcome 1 year after periapical surgery. J Endod 2007;33:123–8.

152. Emmertsen E, Andreasen JO. Replantation of extracted molars. A radiographic and histological study. Acta Odontol Scand 1966;24:327–46.

153. Grossman L, Chacker F. Clinical evaluation and histologic study of intentionally replanted teeth. Transaction, Fourth International Conference on Endodontics: American Association of Endodontics; 1968. p. 127–44.

154. Deeb E. Intentional replantation of endodontically treated teeth. Transaction, Fourth International Conference on Endodontics: American Association of Endodontics; 1968. p. 147–57.

155. Grossman LI. Intentional replantation of teeth: a clinical evaluation. J Am Dent Assoc 1982;104:633–9.

156. Kingsbury BC Jr, Wiesenbaugh JM Jr. Intentional replantation of mandibular premolars and molars. J Am Dent Assoc 1971;83:1053–7.

157. Will R. Reimplantation—a form of therapy. Quintessence Int 1974;5:13–7.

158. Koenig KH, Nguyen NT, Barkhordar RA. Intentional replantation: a report of 192 cases. Gen Dent 1988;36:327–31.

159. Kahnberg KE. Surgical extrusion of root-fractured teeth—a follow-up study of two surgical methods. Endod Dent Traumatol 1988;4:85–9.
160. Keller U. A new method of tooth replantation and autotransplantation: aluminum oxide ceramic for extraoral retrograde root filling. Oral Surg Oral Med Oral Pathol Oral Radiol Endod 1990;70:341–4.
161. Bender IB, Rossman LE. Intentional replantation of endodontically treated teeth. Oral Surg Oral Med Oral Pathol Oral Radiol Endod 1993;76:623–30.
162. Friedman S. Treatment outcome and prognosis of endodontic therapy. In: Ørstavik D, Pitt Ford TR, editors. Essential endodontology: prevention and treatment of apical periodontitis: Oxford: Blackwell Science; 1998.
163. Cheung GS. Survival of first-time nonsurgical root canal treatment performed in a dental teaching hospital. Oral Surg Oral Med Oral Pathol Oral Radiol Endod 2002;93:596–604.
164. Friedman S. Prognosis of initial endodontic therapy. Endod Topics 2002;2:59–88.
165. Goldman M, Pearson AH, Darzenta N. Endodontic success—who's reading the radiograph? Oral Surg Oral Med Oral Pathol Oral Radiol Endod 1972;33:432–7.
166. Goldman M, Pearson AH, Darzenta N. Reliability of radiographic interpretations. Oral Surg Oral Med Oral Pathol Oral Radiol Endod 1974;38:287–93.
167. Reit C, Hollender L. Radiographic evaluation of endodontic therapy and the influence of observer variation. Scand J Dent Res 1983;91:205–12.
168. Zakariasen KL, Scott DA, Jensen JR. Endodontic recall radiographs: how reliable is our interpretation of endodontic success or failure and what factors affect our reliability? Oral Surg Oral Med Oral Pathol Oral Radiol Endod 1984;57:343–7.
169. Eckerbom M, Andersson JE, Magnusson T. Interobserver variation in radiographic examination of endodontic variables. Endod Dent Traumatol 1986;2:243–6.
170. Lambrianidis T. Observer variations in radiographic evaluation of endodontic therapy. Endod Dent Traumatol 1985; 1: 235–41.
171. Halse A, Molven O. A strategy for the diagnosis of periapical pathosis. J Endod 1986;12:534–8.
172. Reit C. The influence of observer calibration on radiographic periapical diagnosis. Int Endod J 1987;20:75–81.
173. Molven O, Halse A, Grung B. Observer strategy and the radiographic classification of healing after endodontic surgery. Int J Oral Maxillofac Surg 1987;16:432–9.
174. Rud J, Andreasen JO, Jensen JE. Radiographic criteria for the assessment of healing after endodontic surgery. Int J Oral Surg 1972;1:195–214.
175. Molven O, Halse A, Fristad I. Long-term reliability and observer comparisons in the radiographic diagnosis of periapical disease. Int Endod J 2002;35:142–7.
176. Orstavik D, Kerekes K, Eriksen HM. The periapical index: a scoring system for radiographic assessment of apical periodontitis. Endod Dent Traumatol 1986;2:20–34.
177. Brynolf L. Histological and roentgenological study of periapical region of human upper incisors. Odontol Revy 1967; 18:(Suppl. 11):1–168.
178. Boucher Y, Matossian L, Rilliard F, Machtou P. Radiographic evaluation of the prevalence and technical quality of root canal treatment in a French subpopulation. Int Endod J 2002;35:229–38.
179. Dugas NN, Lawrence HP, Teplitsky PE, et al. Periapical health and treatment quality assessment of root-filled teeth in two Canadian populations. Int Endod J 2003;36:181–92.
180. Kirkevang L-L, Vaeth M, Horsted-Bindslev P, Wenzel A. Longitudinal study of periapical and endodontic status in a Danish population. Int Endod J 2006;39:100–7.
181. Andreasen JO, Rud J. Modes of healing histologically after endodontic surgery in 70 cases. Int JOral Surg 1972;1:148–60.
182. Andreasen JO, Rud J. Correlation between histology and radiography in the assessment of healing after endodontic surgery. Int J Oral Surg 1972;1:161–73.
183. Molven O, Halse A, Grung B. Incomplete healing (scar tissue) after periapical surgery—radiographic findings 8 to 12 years after treatment. J Endod 1996;22:264–8.
184. Lin LM, Pascon EA, Skribner J, et al. Clinical, radiographic, and histologic study of endodontic treatment failures. Oral Surg Oral Med Oral Pathol Oral Radiol Endod 1991; 71:603–11.
185. Hoen MM, Pink FE. Contemporary endodontic retreatments: an analysis based on clinical treatment findings. J Endod 2002;28:834–6.
186. Pinheiro ET, Gomes BP, Ferraz CC, et al. Microorganisms from canals of root-filled teeth with periapical lesions. Int Endod J 2003;36:1–11.
187. Pinheiro ET, Gomes BP, Ferraz CC, et al. Evaluation of root canal microorganisms isolated from teeth with endodontic failure and their antimicrobial susceptibility. Oral Microbiol Immunol 2003;18:100–3.
188. Persson G. Prognosis of reoperation after apicectomy. A clinical-radiological investigation. Svensk Tandlakaretidskrift 1973;66:49–68.
189. Halse A, Molven O, Grung B. Follow-up after periapical surgery: the value of the one-year control. Endod Dent Traumatol 1991;7:246–50.
190. Rud J, Rud V, Munksgaard EC. Long-term evaluation of retrograde root filling with dentin-bonded resin composite. J Endod 1996;22:90–3.
191. Rud J, Rud V. Surgical endodontics of upper molars: relation to the maxillary sinus and operation in acute state of infection. J Endod 1998;24:260–1.
192. Smith DE, Zarb GA. Criteria for success of osseointegrated endosseous implants. J Prosthet Dent 1989;62:567–72.

193. Avivi-Arber L, Zarb GA. Clinical effectiveness of implant-supported single-tooth replacement: the Toronto Study. Int J Oral Maxillofac Implants 1996;11:311–21.

194. Priest G. Single-tooth implants and their role in preserving remaining teeth: a 10-year survival study. Int J Oral Maxillofac Implants 1999;14:181–8.

195. Thilander B, Odman J, Jemt T. Single implants in the upper incisor region and their relationship to the adjacent teeth. An 8-year follow-up study. Clin Oral Implants Res 1999;10:346–55.

196. Creugers NH, Kreulen CM, Snoek PA, de Kanter RJ. A systematic review of single-tooth restorations supported by implants. J Dent 2000;28:209–17.

197. Haas R, Polak C, Furhauser R, et al. A long-term follow-up of 76 Branemark single-tooth implants. Clin Oral Implants Res 2002;13:38–43.

198. Taintor JF, Ingle JI, Fahid A. Retreatment versus further treatment. Clin Prev Dent 1983;5:8–14.

199. Ørstavik D, Pitt Ford TR. Apical periodontitis: Microbial infection and host responses. In: Ørstavik D, Pitt Ford TR, editors. Essential endodontology: prevention of treatment of apical periodontitis. Oxford: Blackwell Science; 1998.

200. Friedman S, Mor C. The success of endodontic therapy—healing and functionality. Calif Dent Assoc J 2004;32:493–503.

201. Friedman S. The prognosis and expected outcome of apical surgery. Endod Topics 2006;11:219–62.

202. Pellegrino ED. Patient autonomy and the physician's ethics. Ann R Coll Physicians Surg Can 1994;27:171–3.

203. Ambrosio E, Walkerley S. Broadening the ethical focus: a community perspective on patient autonomy. Hum Health Care Int 1996;12:E10.

204. Wertz DC. Patient and professional views on autonomy: a survey in the United States and Canada. Health Law Rev 1998;7:9–10.

205. Fournier V. The balance between beneficence and respect for patient autonomy in clinical medical ethics in France. Camb Q Healthc Ethics 2005;14:281–6.

206. Schattner A, Tal M. Truth telling and patient autonomy: the patient's point of view. Am J Med 2002;113:66–9.

207. Hepworth MJ, Friedman S. Treatment outcome of surgical and non-surgical management of endodontic failures. J Can Dent Assoc 1997;63:364–71.

208. Paik S, Sechrist C, Torabinejad M. Levels of evidence for the outcome of endodontic retreatment. J Endod 2004;30:745–50.

209. Torabinejad M, Bahjri K. Essential elements of evidenced-based endodontics: steps involved in conducting clinical research. J Endod 2005;31:563–9.

210. Torabinejad M, Kutsenko D, Machnick TK, et al. Levels of evidence for the outcome of nonsurgical endodontic treatment. J Endod 2005;31:637–46.

211. Mead C, Javidan-Nejad S, Mego ME, et al. Levels of evidence for the outcome of endodontic surgery. J Endod 2005;31:19–24.

212. Fletcher RH, Fletcher SW, Wagner EH. Clinical epidemiology: the essentials. 3rd ed. Baltimore: Williams & Wilkins; 1996.

213. Oxman AD. Checklists for review articles. Bmj. 1994;309:648–51.

214. Green SB, Byar DP. Using observational data from registries to compare treatments: the fallacy of omnimetrics. Stat Med 1984;3:361–73.

215. Sackett DL, Haynes RB, Guyatt GH, Tugwell P. In: Clinical epidemiology: a basic science of clinical medicine. 2nd ed. Boston: Little, Brown; 1991.

216. Barton S. Which clinical studies provide the best evidence? [editorial] Br Med J 2000;321:255–6.

217. Benson K, Hartz AJ. A comparison of observational studies and randomized, controlled trials. N Engl J Med 2000;342:1878–86.

218. Concato J, Shah N, Horwitz RI. Randomized, controlled trials, observational studies, and the hierarchy of research designs. N Engl J Med 2000;342:1887–92.

219. Department of Clinical Epidemiology and Biostatistics MUHSC. How to read clinical journals: III. To learn the clinical course and prognosis of disease. Canad Med Assoc J 1981;124:869–72.

220. Laupacis A, Wells G, Richardson WS, Tugwell P. Users' guides to the medical literature. V. How to use an article about prognosis. Evidence-Based Medicine Working Group. J Am Dent Assoc 1994;272:234–7.

221. Sutherland SE. Evidence-based dentistry: Part VI. Critical appraisal of the dental literature: papers about diagnosis, etiology and prognosis. J Can Dent Assoc 2001;67:582–5.

222. Cvek M, Hollender L, Nord CE. Treatment of non-vital permanent incisors with calcium hydroxide. VI. A clinical, microbiological and radiological evaluation of treatment in one sitting of teeth with mature or immature root. Odontol Revy 1976;27:93–108.

223. Friedman S. Considerations and concepts of case selection in the management of post-treatment endodontic disease (treatment failure). Endod Topics 2002;1:54–78.

224. Friedman S. Retrograde approaches in endodontic therapy. Endod Dent Traumatol 1991;7:97–107.

225. Halse A, Molven O. Overextended gutta-percha and Kloroperka N-O root canal fillings. Radiographic findings after 10–17 years. Acta Odontol Scand 1987;45:171–7.

226. Byström A, Claesson R, Sundqvist G. The antibacterial effect of camphorated paramonochlorophenol, camphorated phenol

and calcium hydroxide in the treatment of infected root canals. Endod Dent Traumatol 1985;1:170–5.

227. Byström A, Sundqvist G. Bacteriologic evaluation of the efficacy of mechanical root canal instrumentation in endodontic therapy. Scand J Dent Res 1981;89:321–8.

228. Byström A, Sundqvist G. Bacteriologic evaluation of the effect of 0.5 percent sodium hypochlorite in endodontic therapy. Oral Surg Oral Med Oral Pathol Oral Radiol Endod 1983;55:307–12.

229. Byström A, Sundqvist G. The antibacterial action of sodium hypochlorite and EDTA in 60 cases of endodontic therapy. Int Endod J 1985;18:35–40.

230. Dalton BC, Ørstavik D, Phillips C, et al. Bacterial reduction with nickel-titanium rotary instrumentation. J Endod 1998; 24:763–7.

231. Shuping GB, Ørstavik D, Sigurdsson A, Trope M. Reduction of intracanal bacteria using nickel-titanium rotary instrumentation and various medications. J Endod 2000;26:751–5.

232. Messer HH, Chen RS. The duration of effectiveness of root canal medicaments. J Endod 1984;10:240–5.

233. Tronstad L, Yang ZP, Trope M, et al. Controlled release of medicaments in endodontic therapy. Endod Dent Traumatol 1985;1:130–4.

234. Fager FK, Messer HH. Systemic distribution of camphorated monochlorophenol from cotton pellets sealed in pulp chambers. J Endod 1986;12:225–30.

235. Wuchenich G, Meadows D, Torabinejad M. A comparison between two root end preparation techniques in human cadavers. J Endod 1994;20:279–82.

236. Gorman MC, Steiman HR, Gartner AH. Scanning electron microscopic evaluation of root-end preparations. J Endod 1995;21:113–17.

237. Mehlhaff DS, Marshall JG, Baumgartner JC. Comparison of ultrasonic and high-speed-bur root-end preparations using bilaterally matched teeth. J Endod 1997;23:448–52.

238. Carr GB, Bentkover SK. Surgical endodontics. In: Cohen S, Burns RC, editors. Pathways of the pulp, Mosby, St. Louis. 1998:608–56.

239. Lin CP, Chou HG, Kuo JC, Lan WH. The quality of ultrasonic root-end preparation: a quantitative study. J Endod 1998;24:666–70.

240. von Arx T, Walker WA III. Microsurgical instruments for root-end cavity preparation following apicoectomy: a literature review. Endod Dent Traumatol 2000;16:47–62.

241. Andreasen JO, Pitt Ford TR. A radiographic study of the effect of various retrograde fillings on periapical healing after replantation. Endod Dent Traumatol 1994;10:276–81.

242. Pitt Ford TR, Andreasen JO, Dorn SO, Kariyawasam SP. Effect of IRM root end fillings on healing after replantation. J Endod 1994;20:381–5.

243. Pitt Ford TR, Andreasen JO, Dorn SO, Kariyawasam SP. Effect of super-EBA as a root end filling on healing after replantation. J Endod 1995;21:13–15.

244. Torabinejad M, Hong CU, Lee SJ, et al. Investigation of mineral trioxide aggregate for root-end filling in dogs. J Endod 1995;21:603–8.

245. Trope M, Löst C, Schmitz HJ, Friedman S. Healing of apical periodontitis in dogs after apicoectomy and retrofilling with various filling materials. Oral Surg Oral Med Oral Pathol Oral Radiol Endod 1996;81:221–8.

246. Rud J, Munksgaard EC, Andreasen JO, et al. Retrograde root filling with composite and a dentin-bonding agent. 1. Endod Dent Traumatol 1991;7:118–25.

247. Bader JD, Shugars DA. Variation, treatment outcomes, and practice guidelines in dental practice. J Dent Educ 1995;59: 61–95.

248. Eriksen HM. Epidemiology of apical periodontitis. In: Orstavik D, Pitt Ford TR, editors. Essential endodontology: prevention and treatment of apical periodontitis. Oxford: Blackwell Science; 1998.

249. Reit C. Decision strategies in endodontics: on the design of a recall program. Endod Dent Traumatol 1987;3:233–9.

250. Meeuwissen R, Eschen S. Twenty years of endodontic treatment. J Endod 1983;9:390–3.

251. Jaoui L, Machtou P, Ouhayoun JP. Long-term evaluation of endodontic and periodontal treatment. Int Endod J 1995; 28:249–54.

252. Caplan DJ, Weintraub JA. Factors related to loss of root canal filled teeth. J Public Health Dent 1997;57:31–9.

253. Lazarski MP, Walker WA III, Flores CM, et al. Epidemiological evaluation of the outcomes of nonsurgical root canal treatment in a large cohort of insured dental patients. J Endod 2001;27:791–6.

254. Caplan DJ, Kolker J, Rivera EM, Walton RE. Relationship between number of proximal contacts and survival of root canal treated teeth. Int Endod J 2002;35:193–9.

255. Alley BS, Kitchens GG, Alley LW, Eleazer PD. A comparison of survival of teeth following endodontic treatment performed by general dentists or by specialists. Oral Surg Oral Med Oral Pathol Oral Radiol Endod 2004;98:115–18.

256. Salehrabi R, Rotstein I. Endodontic treatment outcomes in a large patient population in the USA: an epidemiological study. J Endod 2004;30:846–50.

257. Wang Q, Cheung GS, Ng RP. Survival of surgical endodontic treatment performed in a dental teaching hospital: a cohort study. Int Endod J 2004;37:764–75.

258. Doyle SL, Hodges JS, Pesun IJ, et al. Retrospective cross sectional comparison of initial nonsurgical endodontic treatment and single-tooth implants. J Endod 2006;32:822–7.

259. Chen SC, Chueh LH, Kate Hsiao C, et al. An epidemiologic study of tooth retention after nonsurgical endodontic

treatment in a large population in Taiwan. J Endod 2007; 33:226–9.

260. Kerekes K, Tronstad L. Morphometric observations on the root canals of human molars. J Endod 1977;3:114–18.

261. Friedman S, Komorowski R, Maillet W, et al. In vivo resistance of coronally induced bacterial ingress by an experimental glass ionomer cement root canal sealer. J Endod 2000;26:1–5.

262. Penick EC. Periapical repair by dense fibrous connective tissue following conservative endodontic therapy. Oral Surg Oral Med Oral Pathol Oral Radiol Endod. 1961; 14:239–42.

263. Bhaskar SN. Oral surgery—oral pathology conference No. 17, Walter Reed Army Medical Center. Periapical lesions—types, incidence, and clinical features. Oral Surg Oral Med Oral Pathol Oral Radiol Endod 1966;21:657–71.

264. Selden HS. Periradicular scars: a sometime diagnostic conundrum. J Endod 1999;25:829–30.

265. Nair PN, Sjögren U, Figdor D, Sundqvist G. Persistent periapical radiolucencies of root-filled human teeth, failed endodontic treatments, and periapical scars. Oral Surg Oral Med Oral Pathol Oral Radiol Endod 1999;87:617–27.

266. Nair PN, Sjögren U, Krey G, et al. Intraradicular bacteria and fungi in root-filled, asymptomatic human teeth with therapy-resistant periapical lesions: a long-term light and electron microscopic follow-up study. J Endod 1990;16:580–8.

267. Nair P. Pathogenesis of apical periodontitis and the causes of endodontic failures. Crit Rev in Oral Biol Med 2004; 15:348–81.

268. Tronstad L, Barnett F, Riso K, Slots J. Extraradicular endodontic infections. Endod Dent Traumatol 1987;3:86–90.

269. Tronstad L, Kreshtool D, Barnett F. Microbiological monitoring and results of treatment of extraradicular endodontic infection. Endod Dent Traumatol 1990;6:129–36.

270. Tronstad L, Sunde PT. The evolving new understanding of endodontic infections. Endod Topics 2003;6:57–77.

271. Sundqvist G, Reuterving CO. Isolation of Actinomyces israelii from periapical lesion. J Endod 1980;6:602–6.

272. Nair PN, Shroeder JH. Periapical actinomycosis. J Endod 1984;10:567–70.

273. Happonen RP, Soderling E, Viander M, et al. Immunocytochemical demonstration of Actinomyces species and Arachnia propionica in periapical infections. J Oral Pathol 1985;14:405–13.

274. Happonen RP. Periapical actinomycosis: a follow-up study of 16 surgically treated cases. Endod Dent Traumatol 1986; 2:205–9.

275. Haapasalo M, Ranta K, Ranta H. Mixed anaerobic periapical infection with sinus tract. Endod Dent Traumatol 1987; 3:83–5.

276. O'Grady JF, Reade PC. Periapical actinomycosis involving Actinomyces israelii. J Endod 1988;14:147–9.

277. Sjögren U, Happonen RP, Kahnberg KE, Sundqvist G. Survival of Arachnia propionica in periapical tissue. Int Endod J 1988;21:277–82.

278. Figures KH, Douglas CW. Actinomycosis associated with a root-treated tooth: report of a case. Int Endod J 1991;24: 326–9.

279. Sakellariou PL. Periapical actinomycosis: report of a case and review of the literature. Endod Dent Traumatol 1996; 12:151–4.

280. Kalfas S, Figdor D, Sundqvist G. A new bacterial species associated with failed endodontic treatment: identification and description of Actinomyces radicidentis. Oral Surg Oral Med Oral Pathol Oral Radiol Endod 2001;92:208–14.

281. Siqueira J. Periapical actinomycosis and infection with *Propionibacterium Propionicum*. Endod Topics 2003;6:78–95.

282. Figdor D. Microbial aetiology of endodontic treatment failure and pathogenic properties of selected species. Aust Endod J 2004;30:11–14.

283. Gatti JJ, Dobeck JM, Smith C, et al. Bacteria of asymptomatic periradicular endodontic lesions identified by DNA-DNA hybridization. Endod Dent Traumatol 2000;16: 197–204.

284. Sunde PT, Olsen I, Lind PO, Tronstad L. Extraradicular infection: a methodological study. Endod Dent Traumatol 2000;16:84–90.

285. Sunde PT, Tronstad L, Eribe ER, et al. Assessment of periradicular microbiota by DNA-DNA hybridization. Endod Dent Traumatol 2000;16:191–6.

286. Sunde PT, Olsen I, Debelian GJ, Tronstad L. Microbiota of periapical lesions refractory to endodontic therapy. J Endod 2002;28:304–10.

287. Sunde PT, Olsen I, Gobel UB, et al. Fluorescence in situ hybridization (FISH) for direct visualization of bacteria in periapical lesions of asymptomatic root-filled teeth. Microbiology 2003;149:1095–102.

288. Borssen E, Sundqvist G. Actinomyces of infected dental root canals. Oral Surg Oral Med Oral Pathol Oral Radiol Endod 1981;51:643–8.

289. Fukushima H, Yamamoto K, Hirohata K, et al. Localization and identification of root canal bacteria in clinically asymptomatic periapical pathosis. J Endod 1990;16: 534–8.

290. Baumgartner JC, Falkler WA Jr. Bacteria in the apical 5 mm of infected root canals. J Endod 1991;17:380–3.

291. Lin LM, Skribner JE, Gaengler P. Factors associated with endodontic treatment failures. J Endod 1992;18:625–7.

292. Molander A, Reit C, Dahlen G, Kvist T. Microbiological status of root-filled teeth with apical periodontitis. Int Endod J 1998; 31:1–7.

293. Peciuliene V, Balciuniene I, Eriksen HM, Haapasalo M. Isolation of Enterococcus faecalis in previously root-filled canals in a Lithuanian population. J Endod 2000;26:593–5.

294. Peciuliene V, Reynaud AH, Balciuniene I, Haapasalo M. Isolation of yeasts and enteric bacteria in root-filled teeth with chronic apical periodontitis. Int Endod J 2001; 34:429–34.

295. Cheung GS, Ho MW. Microbial flora of root canal-treated teeth associated with asymptomatic periapical radiolucent lesions. Oral Microbiol Immunol 2001;16:332–7.

296. Siqueira Junior JF. Aetiology of root canal treatment failure: why well-treated teeth can fail. Int Endod J 2001;34:1–10.

297. Rolph HJ, Lennon A, Riggio MP, et al. Molecular identification of microorganisms from endodontic infections. J Clin Microbiol 2001;39:3282–9.

298. Hancock HH III, Sigurdsson A, Trope M, Moiseiwitsch J. Bacteria isolated after unsuccessful endodontic treatment in a North American population. Oral Surg Oral Med Oral Pathol Oral Radiol Endod 2001;91:579–86.

299. Fouad AF, Zerella J, Barry J, Spangberg LS. Molecular detection of Enterococcus species in root canals of therapy-resistant endodontic infections. Oral Surg Oral Med Oral Pathol Oral Radiol Endod 2005;99:112–18.

300. Kaufman B, Spangberg L, Barry J, Fouad AF. Enterococcus spp. in endodontically treated teeth with and without periradicular lesions. J Endod 2005;31:851–6.

301. Zerella JA, Fouad AF, Spangberg LS. Effectiveness of a calcium hydroxide and chlorhexidine digluconate mixture as disinfectant during retreatment of failed endodontic cases. Oral Surg Oral Med Oral Pathol Oral Radiol Endod 2005; 100:756–61.

302. Sundqvist G, Figdor D. Life as an endodontic pathogen. Ecological differences between the untreated and the root-filled root canals. Endod Topics 2003;6:3–28.

303. Haapasalo M, Udnaes T, Endal U. Persistent, recurrent, and acquired infection of the root canal system post-treatment. Endod Topics 2003;6:29–56.

304. Carr GB. Microscopes in endodontics. J Calif Dent Assoc 1992;20:55–61.

305. Kim S, Kratchman S. Modern endodontic surgery concepts and practice: a review. J Endod 2006;32:601–23.

306. Pecora G, Andreana S. Use of dental operating microscope in endodontic surgery. Oral Surg Oral Med Oral Pathol Oral Radiol Endod 1993;75:751–8.

307. Kim S, Baek S. The microscope and endodontics. Dent Clin North Am 2004;48:11–18.

308. Kim S. Principles of endodontic microsurgery. Dent Clin North Am 1997;41:481–97.

309. Nair PN, Sjögren U, Krey G, Sundqvist G. Therapy-resistant foreign body giant cell granuloma at the periapex of a root-filled human tooth. J Endod 1990;16:589–95.

310. Nair PN, Sjögren U, Schumacher E, Sundqvist G. Radicular cyst affecting a root-filled human tooth: a long-term post-treatment follow-up. Int Endod J 1993;26:225–33.

311. Nair P. Non-microbial etiology: foreign body reaction maintaining post-treatment apical periodontitis. Endod Topics 2003;6:114–34.

312. Nair P. Non-microbial etiology: periapical cysts sustain post-treatment apical periododontitis. Endod Topics 2003; 6:96–113.

313. Gomes BP, Jacinto RC, Pinheiro ET, et al. Molecular analysis of Filifactor alocis, Tannerella forsythia, and treponema denticola associated with primary endodontic infections and failed endodontic treatment. J Endod 2006;32:937–40.

314. Pitt Ford TR. The effects on the periapical tissues of bacterial contamination of the filled root canal. Int Endod J 1982; 15:16–22.

315. Nair PN. Light and electron microscopic studies of root canal flora and periapical lesions. J Endod 1987;13:29–39.

316. Siqueira JF, Lopes HP. Bacteria on the apical root surfaces of untreated teeth with periradicular lesions: a scanning electron microscopy study. Int Endod J 2001;34:216–20.

317. Leonardo MR, Rossi MA, Silva LA, et al. EM evaluation of bacterial biofilm and microorganisms on the apical external root surface of human teeth. J Endod 2002;28:815–18.

318. Noiri Y, Ehara A, Kawahara T, et al. Participation of bacterial biofilms in refractory and chronic periapical periodontitis. J Endod 2002;28:679–83.

319. Tronstad L, Barnett F, Cervone F. Periapical bacterial plaque in teeth refractory to endodontic treatment. Endod Dent Traumatol 1990;6:73–7.

320. Yusuf H. The significance of the presence of foreign material periapically as a cause of failure of root treatment. Oral Surg Oral Med Oral Pathol Oral Radiol Endod 1982;54:566–74.

321. Hsu YY, Kim S. The resected root surface. The issue of canal isthmuses. Dent Clin North Am 1997;41:529–40.

322. Gilheany PA, Figdor D, Tyas MJ. Apical dentin permeability and microleakage associated with root end resection and retrograde filling. J Endod 1994;20:22–6.

323. Vertucci FJ, Beatty RG. Apical leakage associated with retrofilling techniques: a dye study. J Endod 1986;12:331–6.

324. Tidmarsh BG, Arrowsmith MG. Dentinal tubules at the root ends of apicected teeth: a scanning electron microscopic study. Int Endod J 1989;22:184–9.

325. Saunders WP, Saunders EM. The root filling and restoration continuum—prevention of long-term endodontic failures. Alpha Omegan 1997;90:40–6.

326. Benenati FW, Roane JB, Biggs JT, Simon JH. Recall evaluation of iatrogenic root perforations repaired with amalgam and gutta-percha. J Endod 1986;12:161–6.

327. Main C, Mirzayan N, Shabahang S, Torabinejad M. Repair of root perforations using mineral trioxide aggregate: a long-term study. J Endod 2004;30:80–3.

328. Peters LB, Wesselink PR, Buijs JF, van Winkelhoff AJ. Viable bacteria in root dentinal tubules of teeth with apical periodontitis. J Endod 2001;27:76–81.

329. Gutierrez JH, Jofre A, Villena F. Scanning electron microscope study on the action of endodontic irrigants on bacteria invading the dentinal tubules. Oral Surg Oral Med Oral Pathol Oral Radiol Endod 1990;69:491–501.

330. Sen BH, Piskin B, Demirci T. Observation of bacteria and fungi in infected root canals and dentinal tubules by SEM. Endod Dent Traumatol 1995;11:6–9.

331. Love RM. Regional variation in root dentinal tubule infection by Streptococcus gordonii. J Endod 1996;22:290–3.

332. Oguntebi BR. Dentine tubule infection and endodontic therapy implications. Int Endod J 1994;27:218–22.

333. Orstavik D, Kerekes K, Molven O. Effects of extensive apical reaming and calcium hydroxide dressing on bacterial infection during treatment of apical periodontitis: a pilot study. Int Endod J 1991;24:1–7.

334. Yared GM, Dagher FE. Influence of apical enlargement on bacterial infection during treatment of apical periodontitis. J Endod 1994;20:535–7.

335. Card SJ, Sigurdsson A, Orstavik D, Trope M. The effectiveness of increased apical enlargement in reducing intracanal bacteria. J Endod 2002;28:779–83.

336. Molander A, Reit C, Dahlen G. Microbiological evaluation of clindamycin as a root canal dressing in teeth with apical periodontitis. Int Endod J 1990;23:113–18.

337. Sirén EK, Haapasalo MP, Ranta K, et al. Microbiological findings and clinical treatment procedures in endodontic cases selected for microbiological investigation. Int Endod J 1997;30:91–5.

338. Sathorn C, Parashos P, Messer HH. Effectiveness of single- versus multiple-visit endodontic treatment of teeth with apical periodontitis: a systematic review and meta-analysis. Int Endod J 2005;38:347–55.

339. Spili P, Parashos P, Messer HH. The impact of instrument fracture on outcome of endodontic treatment. J Endod 2005;31:845–50.

340. Swanson K, Madison S. An evaluation of coronal microleakage in endodontically treated teeth. Part I. Time periods. J Endod 1987;13:56–9.

341. Madison S, Swanson K, Chiles SA. An evaluation of coronal microleakage in endodontically treated teeth. Part II. Sealer types. J Endod 1987;13:109–12.

342. Madison S, Wilcox LR. An evaluation of coronal microleakage in endodontically treated teeth. Part III. In vivo study. J Endod 1988;14:455–8.

343. Torabinejad M, Ung B, Kettering JD. In vitro bacterial penetration of coronally unsealed endodontically treated teeth. J Endod 1990;16:566–9.

344. Magura ME, Kafrawy AH, Brown CE Jr, Newton CW. Human saliva coronal microleakage in obturated root canals: an in vitro study. J Endod 1991;17:324–31.

345. Beckham BM, Anderson RW, Morris CF. An evaluation of three materials as barriers to coronal microleakage in endodontically treated teeth. J Endod 1993;19:388–91.

346. Khayat A, Lee SJ, Torabinejad M. Human saliva penetration of coronally unsealed obturated root canals. J Endod 1993;19:458–61.

347. Gish SP, Drake DR, Walton RE, Wilcox L. Coronal leakage: bacterial penetration through obturated canals following post preparation. J Am Dent Assoc 1994;125:1369–72.

348. Chailertvanitkul P, Saunders WP, Mackenzie D. An assessment of microbial coronal leakage in teeth root filled with gutta-percha and three different sealers. Int Endod J 1996;29:387–92.

349. Chailertvanitkul P, Saunders WP, MacKenzie D. The effect of smear layer on microbial coronal leakage of gutta-percha root fillings. Int Endod J 1996;29:242–8.

350. Chailertvanitkul P, Saunders WP, MacKenzie D, Weetman DA. An in vitro study of the coronal leakage of two root canal sealers using an obligate anaerobe microbial marker. Int Endod J 1996;29:249–55.

351. Barrieshi KM, Walton RE, Johnson WT, Drake DR. Coronal leakage of mixed anaerobic bacteria after obturation and post space preparation. Oral Surg Oral Med Oral Pathol Oral Radiol Endod 1997;84:310–14.

352. Friedman S, Torneck CD, Komorowski R, et al. In vivo model for assessing the functional efficacy of endodontic filling materials and techniques. J Endod 1997;23:557–61.

353. Kvist T, Rydin E, Reit C. The relative frequency of periapical lesions in teeth with root canal-retained posts. J Endod 1989;15:578–80.

354. Saunders WP, Saunders EM, Sadiq J, Cruickshank E. Technical standard of root canal treatment in an adult Scottish sub-population. Br Dent J 1997;182:382–6.

355. Tronstad L, Asbjornsen K, Doving L, et al. Influence of coronal restorations on the periapical health of endodontically treated teeth. Endod Dent Traumatol 2000;16:218–21.

356. Vire DE. Failure of endodontically treated teeth: classification and evaluation. J Endod 1991;17:338–42.

357. Kvinnsland I, Oswald RJ, Halse A, Gronningsaeter AG. A clinical and roentgenological study of 55 cases of root perforation. Int Endod J 1989;22:75–84.

358. Sjögren U, Figdor D, Spangberg L, Sundqvist G. The antimicrobial effect of calcium hydroxide as a short-term intracanal dressing. Int Endod J 1991;24:119–25.

359. Peters LB, van Winkelhoff AJ, Buijs JF, Wesselink PR. Effects of instrumentation, irrigation and dressing with calcium hydroxide on infection in pulpless teeth with periapical bone lesions. Int Endod J 2002;35:13–21.

360. Kvist T, Molander A, Dahlen G, Reit C. Microbiological evaluation of one- and two-visit endodontic treatment of teeth with apical periodontitis: a randomized, clinical trial. J Endod 2004;30:572–6.

361. McGurkin-Smith R, Trope M, Caplan D, Sigurdsson A. Reduction of intracanal bacteria using GT rotary instrumentation, 5.25% NaOCl, EDTA, and Ca(OH)2. J Endod 2005; 31:359–63.

362. Paquette L, Legner M, Fillery ED, Friedman S. Antibacterial efficacy of chlorhexidine gluconate intracanal medication in vivo. J Endod. 2006;33:788–95.

363. Manzur A, Gonzalez AM, Pozos A, et al. Bacterial quantification in teeth with apical periodontitis related to instrumentation and different intracanal medications: a randomized clinical trial. J Endod 2007;33:114–18.

364. Vianna ME, Horz HP, Gomes BP, Conrads G. In vivo evaluation of microbial reduction after chemo-mechanical preparation of human root canals containing necrotic pulp tissue. Int Endod J 2006;39:484–92.

365. Malkhassian G, Manzur A, Legner M, Friedman S, et al. Antibacterial effectiveness of a final rinse with MTAD and intracanal medication with 2% chlorhexidine gel in teeth with apical periodontitis. J Endod 2007;33:334.

366. Molander A, Reit C, Dahlen G. The antimicrobial effect of calcium hydroxide in root canals pretreated with 5% iodine potassium iodide. Endod Dent Traumatol 1999;15: 205–9.

367. Sathorn C, Parashos P, Messer HH. How useful is root canal culturing in predicting treatment outcome? J Endod 2007; 33:220–5.

368. Sathorn C, Parashos P, Messer H. Antibacterial efficacy of calcium hydroxide intracanal dressing: a systematic review and meta-analysis. Int Endod J 2007;40:2–10.

369. Wilcox LR. Endodontic retreatment with halothane versus chloroform solvent. J Endod 1995;21:305–7.

370. Wilcox LR. Endodontic retreatment: ultrasonics and chloroform as the final step in reinstrumentation. J Endod 1989; 15:125–8.

371. Wilcox LR. Thermafil retreatment with and without chloroform solvent. J Endod 1993;19:563–6.

372. Wilcox LR, Juhlin JJ. Endodontic retreatment of Thermafil versus laterally condensed gutta-percha. J Endod 1994;20: 115–17.

373. Wilcox LR, Krell KV, Madison S, Rittman B. Endodontic retreatment: evaluation of gutta-percha and sealer removal and canal reinstrumentation. J Endod 1987;13:453–7.

374. Wilcox LR, Swift ML. Endodontic retreatment in small and large curved canals. J Endod 1991;17:313–15.

375. Wilcox LR, Van Surksum R. Endodontic retreatment in large and small straight canals. J Endod 1991;17:119–21.

376. Baldassari-Cruz LA, Wilcox LR. Effectiveness of gutta-percha removal with and without the microscope. J Endod 1999; 25:627–8.

377. Ladley RW, Campbell AD, Hicks ML, Li SH. Effectiveness of halothane used with ultrasonic or hand instrumentation to remove gutta-percha from the root canal. J Endod 1991; 17:221–4.

378. Teplitsky PE, Rayner D, Chin I, Markowsky R. Gutta percha removal utilizing GPX instrumentation. J Can Dent Assoc 1992;58:53–8.

379. Friedman S, Moshonov J, Trope M. Efficacy of removing glass ionomer cement, zinc oxide eugenol, and epoxy resin sealers from retreated root canals. Oral Surg Oral Med Oral Pathol Oral Radiol Endod 1992;73:609–12.

380. Friedman S, Moshonov J, Trope M. Residue of gutta-percha and a glass ionomer cement sealer following root canal retreatment. Int Endod J 1993;26:169–72.

381. Sae-Lim V, Rajamanickam I, Lim BK, Lee HL. Effectiveness of ProFile.04 taper rotary instruments in endodontic retreatment. J Endod 2000;26:100–4.

382. Ferreira JJ, Rhodes JS, Ford TR. The efficacy of gutta-percha removal using ProFiles. Int Endod J 2001;34:267–74.

383. Hulsmann M, Bluhm V. Efficacy, cleaning ability and safety of different rotary NiTi instruments in root canal retreatment. Int Endod J 2004;37:468–76.

384. Kosti E, Lambrianidis T, Economides N, Neofitou C. Ex vivo study of the efficacy of H-files and rotary Ni-Ti instruments to remove gutta-percha and four types of sealer. Int Endod J 2006;39:48–54.

385. Schirrmeister JF, Meyer KM, Hermanns P, et al. Effectiveness of hand and rotary instrumentation for removing a new synthetic polymer-based root canal obturation material (Epiphany) during retreatment. Int Endod J 2006;39: 150–6.

386. Hassanloo A, Finer Y, Watson P, Friedman S. Retreatment efficacy of Epiphany Resin Percha Obturating System. Int Endod J 2007;44:633-43.

387. Kerekes K, Tronstad L. Morphometric observations on root canals of human anterior teeth. J Endod 1977;3:24–9.

388. Kerekes K, Tronstad L. Morphometric observations on root canals of human premolars. J Endod 1977;3:74–9.

389. Harrison J, Jurosky K. Wound healing in the tissues of the periodontium following periradicular surgery. 3. The excisional wound. J Endod 1992;18:76–81.

390. Peterson J, Gutmann JL. The outcome of endodontic resurgery: a systematic review. Int Endod J 2001;34:169–75.

391. Kim S. Endodontic microsurgery. In: Cohen S, Burns RC, editors. Pathways of the pulp. Eighth edition ed. St. Louis: Mosby; 2002. pp. 683–725.

392. Andreasen JO, Munksgaard L., Rud J. Periodontal tissue regeneration including cementogenesis adjacent to dentin-bonded retrograde composite fillings in humans. J Endod 1993;19:151–3.

393. Dragoo MR. Resin-ionomer and hybrid-ionomer cements: Part I. Comparison of three materials for the treatment of subgingival root lesions. Int J Periodontics Restorative Dent 1996;16:594–601.

394. Dragoo MR, Wheeler BG. Clinical evaluation of subgingival debridement with ultrasonic instruments used by trained and untrained operators. Gen Dent 1996;44:234–7.

395. Torabinejad M, Chivian N. Clinical applications of mineral trioxide aggregate. J Endod 1999;25:197–205.

396. Theodosopoulou JN, Niederman R. A systematic review of in vitro retrograde obturation materials. J Endod 2005;31: 341–9.

397. Friedman S, Rotstein I, Mahamid A. In vivo efficacy of various retrofills and of CO_2 laser in apical surgery. Endod Dent Traumatol 1991;7:19–25.

398. Witherspoon DE, Gutmann JL. Analysis of the healing response to gutta-percha and Diaket when used as root-end filling materials in periradicular surgery. Int Endod J 2000; 33:37–45.

399. Dalal MB, Gohil KS. Comparison of silver amalgam, glass ionomer cement & gutta percha as retrofilling materials, an in vivo & an in vitro study. J Indian Dent Assoc 1983;55: 153–8.

400. Sumi Y, Hattori H, Hayashi K, Ueda M. Titanium-inlay—a new root-end filling material. J Endod 1997;23:121–3.

401. Jeansonne BG, Boggs WS, Lemon RR. Ferric sulfate hemostasis: effect on osseous wound healing. II. With curettage and irrigation. J Endod 1993;19:174–6.

402. Kim S, Rethnam S. Hemostasis in endodontic microsurgery. Dent Clin North Am 1997;41:499–511.

403. Nygaard-Ostby B. Introduction to endodontics; 1971.

404. Storms JL. Root canal therapy via the apical foramen—radical or conservative? Oral Health 1978;68:60–5.

405. Serota KS, Krakow AA. Retrograde instrumentation and obturation of the root canal space. J Endod 1983;9:448–51.

406. Flath RK, Hicks ML. Retrograde instrumentation and obturation with new devices. J Endod 1987;13:546–9.

407. Goldberg F, Torres MD, Bottero C. Thermoplasticized gutta-percha in endodontic surgical procedures. Endod Dent Traumatol 1990;6:109–13.

408. Goldberg F, Torres MD, Bottero C, Alvarez AF. The use of thermoplasticized gutta-percha as a retrograde filling material. Endodontology 1991;3:1–6.

409. Mines P, Loushine RJ, West LA, et al. Use of the microscope in endodontics: a report based on a questionnaire. J Endod 1999;25:755–8.

410. Rubinstein R. The anatomy of the surgical operating microscope and operating positions. Dent Clin North Am 1997;41: 391–413.

411. von Arx T, Montagne D, Zwinggi C, Lussi A. Diagnostic accuracy of endoscopy in periradicular surgery—a comparison with scanning electron microscopy. Int Endod J 2003; 36:691–9.

412. von Arx T. Frequency and type of canal isthmuses in first molars detected by endoscopic inspection during periradicular surgery. Int Endod J 2005;38:160–8.

413. Velvart P, Peters CI. Soft tissue management in endodontic surgery. J Endod 2005;31:4–16.

414. Melcer J. Latest treatment in dentistry by means of the CO_2 laser beam. Las Surg Med 1986;6:396–8.

415. Miserendino LJ. The laser apicoectomy: endodontic application of the CO_2 laser for periapical surgery. Oral Surg Oral Med Oral Pathol Oral Radiol Endod 1988;66:615–19.

416. Komori T, Yokoyama K, Takato T, Matsumoto K. Clinical application of the erbium: YAG laser for apicoectomy. J Endod 1997;23:748–50.

417. Stabholz A, Khayat A, Ravanshad SH, et al. Effects of Nd: YAG laser on apical seal of teeth after apicoectomy and retrofill. J Endod 1992;18:371–5.

418. Stabholz A, Khayat A, Weeks DA, et al. Scanning electron microscopic study of the apical dentine surfaces lased with ND: YAG laser following apicectomy and retrofill. Int Endod J 1992;25:288–91.

419. Paghdiwala AF. Root resection of endodontically treated teeth by erbium: YAG laser radiation. J Endod 1993;19: 91–4.

420. Arens DL, Levy GC, Rizoiu IM. A comparison of dentin permeability after bur and laser apicoectomies. Compendium 1993;14:1290, 1292, 1294 passim; quiz 1298.

421. Wong SW, Rosenberg PA, Boylan RJ, Schulman A. A comparison of the apical seal achieved using retrograde amalgam fillings and the Nd: YAG laser. J Endod 1994;20:595–7.

422. Takeda A. An experimental study upon the application of Nd:YAG laser to surgical endodontics. Japan J Conserv Dent 1989;32:541–53.

423. Pecora G, Baek SH, Rethnam S, Kim S. Barrier membrane techniques in endodontic microsurgery. Dent Clin North Am 1997;41:585–602.

424. Pecora G, Kim S, Celletti R, Davarpanah M. The guided tissue regeneration principle in endodontic surgery: one-year postoperative results of large periapical lesions. Int Endod J 1995;28:41–6.

425. Sikri K, Dua SS, Kapur R. Use of tricalcium phosphate ceramic in apicoectomized teeth and in their peri-apical areas—clinical and radiological evaluation. J Indian Dent Assoc 1986; 58:441–7.

426. Pecora G, Andreana S, Margarone JE III, et al. Bone regeneration with a calcium sulfate barrier. Oral Surg Oral Med Oral Pathol Oral Radiol Endod 1997;84:424–9.

427. Pecora G, De Leonardis D, Ibrahim N, et al. The use of calcium sulphate in the surgical treatment of a 'through and through' periradicular lesion. Int Endod J 2001;34: 189–97.

428. Murashima Y, Yoshikawa G, Wadachi R, et al. Calcium sulfate as a bone substitute for various osseous defects in conjunction with apicectomy. Int Endod J 2002;35:768–74.

429. Yoshikawa G, Murashima Y, Wadachi R, et al. Guided bone regeneration (GBR) using membranes and calcium sulphate after apicectomy: a comparative histomorphometrical study. Int Endod J 2002;35:255–64.

430. Saad AY, Abdellatief E-SM. Healing assessment of osseous defects of periapical lesions associated with failed endodontically treated teeth with use of freeze-dried bone allograft. Oral Surg Oral Med Oral Pathol Oral Radiol Endod 1991; 71:612–17.

431. Grimes EW. A use of freeze-dried bone in endodontics. J Endod 1994;20:355–6.

432. Rankow HJ, Krasner PR. Endodontic applications of guided tissue regeneration in endodontic surgery. Oral Health 1996; 86:33–35, 37–40, 43.

433. Tobon SI, Arismendi JA, Marin ML, et al. Comparison between a conventional technique and two bone regeneration techniques in periradicular surgery. Int Endod J 2002;35:635–41.

434. Kvist T. Endodontic retreatment. Aspects of decision making and clinical outcome. Swed Dent J Suppl 2001;1–57.

435. Rosenberg ES, Rossman LE, Sandler AB. Intentional replantation: a case report. J Endod 1980;6:610–3.

436. Nosonowitz DM, Stanley HR. Intentional replantation to prevent predictable endodontic failures. Oral Surg Oral Med Oral Pathol Oral Radiol Endod 1984;57:423–32.

437. Guy SC, Goerig AC. Intentional replantation: technique and rationale. Quintessence Int 1984;15:595–603.

438. Dumsha TC, Gutmann JL. Clinical guidelines for intentional replantation. Compend Contin Educ Dent 1985;6:604.

439. Andreasen JO. External root resorption: its implication in dental traumatology, paedodontics, periodontics, orthodontics and endodontics. Int Endod J 1985;18:109–18.

440. Andreasen JO, Borum MK, Jacobsen HL, Andreasen FM. Replantation of 400 avulsed permanent incisors. 4. Factors related to periodontal ligament healing. Endod Dent Traumatol 1995;11:76–89.

441. Tronstad L. Root resorption—etiology, terminology and clinical manifestations. Endod Dent Traumatol 1988; 4:241–52.

442. Trope M, Friedman S. Periodontal healing of replanted dog teeth stored in Viaspan, milk and Hank's balanced salt solution. Endod Dent Traumatol 1992;8:183–8.

443. Hammarstrom L, Pierce A, Blomlof L, et al. Tooth avulsion and replantation—a review. Endod Dent Traumatol 1986; 2:1–8.

444. Oikarinen K. Dental tissues involved in exarticulation, root resorption and factors influencing prognosis in relation to replanted teeth. A review. Proc Finn Dent Soc 1993;89: 29–44.

445. Ehnevid H, Jansson L, Lindskog S, et al. Endodontic pathogens: propagation of infection through patent dentinal tubules in traumatized monkey teeth. Endod Dent Traumatol 1995;11:229–34.

446. Feldman G, Solomon C, Notaro P, Moskowitz E. Intentional replantation of a molar tooth. N Y J Dent 1971;41:352–3.

447. Solomon CS, Abelson J. Intentional replantation: report of case. J Endod 1981;7:317–19.

448. Stroner WF, Laskin DM. Replantation of a mandibular molar: report of case. J Am Dent Assoc 1981;103:730–1.

449. Kaufman AY. Intentional replantation of a maxillary molar. A 4-year follow-up. Oral Surg Oral Med Oral Pathol Oral Radiol Endod 1982;54:686–8.

450. Lubin H. Intentional reimplantation: report of case. J Am Dent Assoc 1982;104:858–9.

451. Ross WJ. Intentional replantation: an alternative. Compend Contin Educ Dent 1985;6:734.

452. Lindeberg RW, Girardi AF, Troxell JB. Intentional replantation: management in contraindicated situations. Compend Contin Educ Dent 1986;7:248.

453. Lu DP. Intentional replantation of periodontally involved and endodontically mistreated tooth. Oral Surg Oral Med Oral Pathol Oral Radiol Endod 1986;61:508–13.

454. Madison S. Intentional replantation. Oral Surg Oral Med Oral Pathol Oral Radiol Endod 1986;62:707–9.

455. Dryden JA. Ten-year follow-up of intentionally replanted mandibular second molar. J Endod 1986;12:265–7.

456. Messkoub M. Intentional replantation: a successful alternative for hopeless teeth. Oral Surg Oral Med Oral Pathol Oral Radiol Endod 1991;71:743–7.

457. Hansen BF, Johansen JR. Oral roentgenologic findings in a Norwegian urban population. Oral Surg Oral Med Oral Pathol Oral Radiol Endod 1976;41:261–6.

458. Hugoson A, Koch G. Oral health in 1000 individuals aged 3–70 years in the community of Jonkoping, Sweden. A review. Swed Den J 1979;3:69–87.

459. Hugoson A, Koch G, Bergendal T, et al. Oral health of individuals aged 3–80 years in Jonkoping, Sweden, in 1973 and 1983. II. A review of clinical and radiographic findings. Swed Dent J 1986;10:175–94.

460. Allard U, Palmqvist S. A radiographic survey of periapical conditions in elderly people in a Swedish county population. Endod Dent Traumatol 1986;2:103–8.

461. Petersson K, Petersson A, Olsson B, et al. Technical quality of root fillings in an adult Swedish population. Endod Dent Traumatol 1986;2:99–102.

462. Bergstrom J, Eliasson S, Ahlberg KF. Periapical status in subjects with regular dental care habits. Community Dentistry & Oral Epidemiology 1987;15:236–9.
463. Eckerbom M, Andersson JE, Magnusson T. Frequency and technical standard of endodontic treatment in a Swedish population. Endod Dent Traumatol 1987;3:245–8.
464. Eriksen HM, Bjertness E, Ørstavik D. Prevalence and quality of endodontic treatment in an urban adult population in Norway. Endod Dent Traumatol 1988;4:122–6.
465. Petersson K, Lewin B, Hakansson J, et al. Endodontic status and suggested treatment in a population requiring substantial dental care. Endod Dent Traumatol 1989;5:153–8.
466. Odesjo B, Hellden L, Salonen L, Langeland K. Prevalence of previous endodontic treatment, technical standard and occurrence of periapical lesions in a randomly selected adult, general population. Endod Dent Traumatol 1990;6:265–72.
467. Eriksen HM, Bjertness E. Prevalence of apical periodontitis and results of endodontic treatment in middle-aged adults in Norway. Endod Dent Traumatol 1991;7:1–4.
468. Imfeld TN. Prevalence and quality of endodontic treatment in an elderly urban population of Switzerland. J Endod 1991;17:604–7.
469. Eckerbom M, Magnusson T, Martinsson T. Prevalence of apical periodontitis, crowned teeth and teeth with posts in a Swedish population. Endod Dent Traumatol 1991;7:214–20.
470. De Cleen MJ, Schuurs AH, Wesselink PR, Wu MK. Periapical status and prevalence of endodontic treatment in an adult Dutch population. Int Endod J 1993;26:112–19.
471. Petersson K. Endodontic status of mandibular premolars and molars in an adult Swedish population. A longitudinal study 1974–1985. Endod Dent Traumatol 1993;9:13–18.
472. Ray HA, Trope M. Periapical status of endodontically treated teeth in relation to the technical quality of the root filling and the coronal restoration. Int Endod J 1995;28:12–18.
473. Buckley M, Spangberg LS. The prevalence and technical quality of endodontic treatment in an American subpopulation. Oral Surg Oral Med Oral Pathol Oral Radiol Endod 1995;79:92–100.
474. Eriksen HM, Berset GP, Hansen BF, Bjertness E. Changes in endodontic status 1973–1993 among 35-year-olds in Oslo, Norway. Int Endod J 1995;28:12932.
475. Soikkonen K. Endodontically treated teeth and periapical findings in the elderly. Int Endod J 1995;28:200–3.
476. Weiger R, Hitzler S, Hermle G, Lost C. Periapical status, quality of root canal fillings and estimated endodontic treatment needs in an urban German population. Endod Dent Traumatol 1997;13:69–74.
477. Marques MD, Moreira B, Eriksen HM. Prevalence of apical periodontitis and results of endodontic treatment in an adult, Portuguese population. Int Endod J 1998;31:161–5.
478. Sidaravicius B, Aleksejuniene J, Eriksen HM. Endodontic treatment and prevalence of apical periodontitis in an adult population of Vilnius, Lithuania. Endod Dent Traumatol 1999;15:210–15.
479. De Moor RJ, Hommez GM, De Boever JG, et al. Periapical health related to the quality of root canal treatment in a Belgian population. Int Endod J 2000;33:113–20.
480. Kirkevang LL, Ørstavik D, Horsted-Bindslev P, Wenzel A. Periapical status and quality of root fillings and coronal restorations in a Danish population. Int Endod J 2000;33:509–15.
481. Kirkevang LL, Horsted-Bindslev P, Ørstavik D, Wenzel A. Frequency and distribution of endodontically treated teeth and apical periodontitis in an urban Danish population. Int Endod J 2001;34:198–205.
482. Kirkevang L-L, Horsted-Bindslev P, Ørstavik D, Wenzel A. A comparison of the quality of root canal treatment in two Danish subpopulations examined 1974–75 and 1997–98. Int Endod J 2001;34:607–12.
483. Hommez G, Coppens CRM, DeMoor RJG. Periapical health related to the quality of coronal restorations and root fillings. Int Endod J 2002;35:680–9.
484. Lupi-Pegurier L, Bertrand, M-F, Muller-Bolla M, et al. Periapical status, prevalence and quality of endodontic treatment in an adult French population. Int Endod J 2002;35:690–7.
485. Boltacz-Rzepkowska E, Pawlicka H. Radiographic features and outcome of root canal treatment carried out in the Lodz region of Poland. Int Endod J 2003;36:27–32.
486. Jimenez-Pinzon A, Segura-Egea JJ, Poyato-Ferrera M, et al. Prevalence of apical periodontitis and frequency of root-filled teeth in an adult Spanish population. Int Endod J 2004;37:167–73.
487. Segura-Egea JJ, Jimenez-Pinzon A, Poyato-Ferrera M, et al. Periapical status and quality of root fillings and coronal restorations in an adult Spanish population. Int Endod J 2004;37:525–30.
488. Kabak Y, Abbott PV. Prevalence of apical periodontitis and the quality of endodontic treatment in an adult Belarusian population. Int Endod J 2005;38:238–45.
489. Georgopoulou MK, Spanaki-Voreadi AP, Pantazis N, Kontakiotis EG. Frequency and distribution of root filled teeth and apical periodontitis in a Greek population. Int Endod J 2005;38:105–11.
490. Loftus JJ, Keating AP, McCartan BE. Periapical status and quality of endodontic treatment in an adult Irish population. Int Endod J 2005;38:81–6.
491. Sunay H, Tanalp J, Dikbas I, Bayirli G. Cross-sectional evaluation of the periapical status and quality of root canal

treatment in a selected population of urban Turkish adults. Int Endod J 2007;40:139–45.

492. Chen CY, Hasselgren G, Serman N, et al. Prevalence and quality of endodontic treatment in the northern Manhattan elderly. J Endod 2007;33:230–4.

493. Eriksen HM. Endodontology—epidemiologic considerations. Endod Dent Traumatol 1991;7:189–95.

494. Eckerbom M, Andersson JE, Magnusson T. A longitudinal study of changes in frequency and technical standard of endodontic treatment in a Swedish population. Endod Dent Traumatol 1989;5:27–31.

495. Petersson K, Hakansson R, Hakansson J, et al. Follow-up study of endodontic status in an adult Swedish population. Endod Dent Traumatol 1991;7:221–5.

SURGICAL PROCEDURES IN ENDODONTICS

CHAPTER 33

ENDODONTIC SURGERY

GERALD N. GLICKMAN, GARY R. HARTWELL

Historical Perspectives

Endodontic surgery, once thought to be a therapy of last resort, has advanced in recent years to increase the clinician's ability to achieve more predictably successful clinical outcomes. Advances in technology including specially designed instruments, improved root-end filling materials, and better visualization with microscopes, along with a more thorough understanding of the biology of wound healing, have all contributed to the contemporary concept of "microsurgical endodontics." In fact, patient misconceptions about endodontic surgery were negated in a recent study by Iqbal et al.[1] in 2007 who demonstrated that patients, following "microsurgical endodontics," claimed the procedure was better than expected and reported less or equal postoperative discomfort compared to nonsurgical endodontic treatment.

Despite these recent advances, endodontic surgery is not new to contemporary dentistry. The first recorded endodontic surgical procedure was the incision and drainage of an acute endodontic abscess performed over 1500 years ago.[2] Since that time, endodontic surgical procedures have continuously evolved as a result of the valuable contributions of many pioneers in dentistry including Abulcasis, Farrar, Fauchard, Hullihan, Martin, Partsch, and Black.[3]

In 1910, William Hunter's classic presentation, "*An Address on the Role of Sepsis and Antisepsis in Medicine,*" was delivered to the Faculty of Medicine of McGill University in Montreal; it had a major impact on dentistry and initiated the concept of "focal infection," the ramifications of which still remain today. Consequently, the development of endodontic surgery was best characterized as both progressive and regressive—progressive because of the advancements in flap design and root-end management techniques and regressive because advocates of focal infection considered pulpless teeth to be foci of infection and ultimately responsible for arthritis, nephritis, and other systemic diseases. While tremendous strides were made in the development and application of endodontic surgical techniques, the concepts involved in endodontic surgery were unjustly being attacked by the medical profession.[3]

While Hunter's presentation initiated a major conflict, it turned out to be the stimulus for the development of endodontics and endodontic surgery.

The results of scientific investigation and the clinical application of the techniques and concepts developed during the second half of the twentieth century represent the foundation of what is known and will be practiced into the twenty-first century. However, endodontic surgery is dynamic and it is imperative that scientific investigation continues; concepts, techniques, and materials used in "microsurgical endodontics" must be continually evaluated and modified and more emphasis must be placed on the assessment of long-term clinical outcomes with a better understanding of the molecular basis for surgical wound healing.

Indications, Contraindications, and Classification

During the last 20 years, endodontics has seen a dramatic shift in the application of periradicular surgery. Previously, periradicular surgery was commonly considered the treatment of choice when nonsurgical treatment had failed or if existing restorative or prosthetic treatment would be endangered by orthograde treatment.[4] Grossman et al.[5] provided a list of indications for endodontic surgery including the presence of large and intruding periapical lesions, overfilled canals, incomplete apical root formation, and destruction of the apical constriction by over-instrumentation amongst others. In addition, the dental literature contains an abundance of clinical articles, scientific reports, and textbook chapters that provide extensive lists of indications for periradicular surgery. However, many of the previously accepted indications are no longer valid in light of current concepts of the biological basis for endodontic treatment. Therefore, it must be recognized that periradicular surgery has become very selective in contemporary endodontic practice.

The emphasis on nonsurgical retreatment of endodontic failures has probably had the single greatest impact on the indications for surgical intervention in the treatment of endodontic pathosis. Studies reporting the success rate for nonsurgical retreatment indicate success rates as low as 62% to as high as 98% depending on the clinical status of the case.[6-10] With the advent of the microscope and microsurgical tools, nonsurgical retreatment has become more predictable. Given these success rates and improved technology, there are specific indications for periradicular surgery today. These are (1) failure of nonsurgical retreatment (treatment has been rendered at least two times), (2) failure of nonsurgical (initial) treatment and retreatment is not possible or practical or would not achieve a better result, or (3) when a biopsy is necessary. It is paramount that these indications must be in the best interests of the patient, within the skills of the clinician, and reflective of biological principles of endodontic therapy.

Few absolute contraindications to endodontic surgery exist. Most contraindications are relative and they are usually limited to three areas: (1) the patient's medical status, (2) anatomical considerations, and (3) the practitioner's skills and experience. When considering performing any surgical procedure on a patient who reports a major system disorder (cardiovascular, respiratory, digestive, hepatic, renal, immune, or skeleton-muscular), a thorough medical history is mandatory. Following the identification of all potential medical complications and a review of the patient's current drug regimen, a consultation with the primary care physician or specialist may be in order. The dentist should explain to the physician the needed endodontic surgical treatment, including a brief description of the procedure, anesthetic agents and other drugs to be used, the approximate length of time required for the procedure, and the expected length of recovery. In this way, the physician can more adequately assess the medical risks involved and can assist the endodontist in determining the appropriate treatment modifications. These modifications may be preoperative (alteration of drug therapy, sedative or hypnotic, and systemic antibiotics), intra-operative (N_2O_2 and intravenous sedation), or postoperative (re-establishment of drug therapy, sedatives, and analgesics).

Although anatomical considerations will be addressed later in this chapter, it should be emphasized that the majority of these present contraindications that must be addressed as they relate to each individual patient. The major anatomical considerations of importance to endodontic surgery involve (1) the nasal floor, (2) the maxillary sinus, (3) the mandibular canal and its neurovascular bundle, (4) the mental foramen and its neurovascular bundle, and (5) anatomical limitations to adequate visual and mechanical access to the surgical site. A skilled surgeon with the needed microsurgical armamentarium is usually able to circumvent these anatomical limitations and accomplish successful endodontic surgery.[11]

It is imperative that dental professionals keep in mind that all treatment rendered by them to their patients must be in the patients' best interests and at the highest quality of care. As a professional, one has an obligation to know one's limitations of clinical skills and to perform treatment procedures consistent with those limitations. The majority of endodontic surgical procedures should be performed by trained endodontic specialists. When receiving care of a specialized nature, patients need and deserve treatment that meets the standard of care delivered by competent practitioners trained as specialists.[12]

A contemporary classification of endodontic surgery is as follows:[3]

1. Fistulative surgery
   a. Incision and drainage (I&D)
   b. Cortical trephination
   c. Decompression procedures
2. Periradicular surgery (primary focus of this chapter)
   a. Curettage
   b. Root-end resection
   c. Root-end preparation
   d. Root-end filling
3. Corrective surgery
   a. Perforation repair
      i. Mechanical (iatrogenic)
      ii. Resorptive
   b. Periodontal management
      i. Root resection
      ii. Tooth resection
   c. Intentional replantation

Treatment Planning for Periradicular Surgery

As was previously discussed, the indications for and the application of periradicular endodontic surgery have undergone dramatic changes in the last two decades. These changes have been evident especially when dealing with the treatment of failed nonsurgical endodontic treatments. The most important principle of endodontic diagnosis and treatment planning is that the primary modality for endodontic treatment failure should be nonsurgical endodontic retreatment whenever possible.[3,4,9,13–17] The importance of thorough and meticulous presurgical planning cannot be over-emphasized. Not only must the practitioner and staff be thoroughly trained, but also all necessary instruments, equipment, and supplies must be readily available in the treatment room. This requires that every step of the procedure be carefully planned and analyzed. The potential for possible complications must be anticipated and incorporated into the presurgical planning.

Good patient communication is essential for thorough surgical preparation. It is important that the patient understands the reason surgery is needed as well as other treatment options available. The patient must be informed of the prognosis for a successful outcome and the risks involved in the surgical procedure in addition to the benefits. It is also important that the patient is informed of the possible short-term effects of the surgery such as pain, swelling, discoloration, and infection. Signed consent forms are essential.

A presurgical mouth rinse will improve the surgical environment by decreasing the tissue surface bacterial contamination and thereby reducing the inoculation of microorganisms into the surgical wound. Chlorhexidine gluconate (Peridex) has been shown to decrease salivary bacterial counts by 80% to 90% with a return to normal within 48 hours.[18] Gutmann and Harrison recommend that chlorhexidine gluconate oral rinses should be started the day prior to surgery, immediately before surgery and continued for 4 to 5 days following surgery. The reduction in numbers of oral bacteria prior to and during the early postsurgical period and the inhibition of plaque formation produce a markedly improved environment for the wound healing.[3]

Most periradicular surgical procedures, regardless of their indication, share a number of concepts and principles in common: (1) need for profound local anesthesia and hemostasis; (2) management of soft tissues; (3) management of hard tissues; (4) surgical access, both visual and operative; (5) access to root structure; (6) periradicular curettage; (7) root-end resection; (8) root-end preparation; (9) root-end filling; (10) soft tissue repositioning and suturing; and (11) postsurgical care. All of these concepts and principles may not be employed in any given surgery. However, an in-depth knowledge and understanding of these principles, and the manner in which they relate to the biology and physiology of the tissues involved, is of major importance. The strict adherence to and application of these principles will greatly influence the success of the surgical treatment and minimize patient morbidity.

Anatomical Considerations

Anatomical structures that may be of importance during endodontic surgery include the neurovascular bundle associated with the greater palatine foramen, the mandibular canal, and the mental foramen; the floor of the nose; the maxillary sinus; and any other anatomical structures that limit or compromise visualization and access to the surgical site. One must also be cognizant of individual root anatomy where more than one root canal system is present within a single root and an isthmus exists between the canals. An endodontist or other surgeon with the appropriate training, experience, skill level, and armamentarium can usually circumvent these anatomical limitations and accomplish endodontic surgery in a predictable and successful manner.

During surgical procedures on maxillary incisors, the floor of the nose will infrequently be encountered unless the roots of the incisors are extremely long or the periradicular lesion extends superiorly and has eroded through the bony floor of the nose. The greater palatine foramen (Figure 1) is most frequently located between the maxillary second and third molars in a position approximately 1 cm from the margin of the palatal gingiva toward the midline of the palate.[19] The greater palatine foramen and its

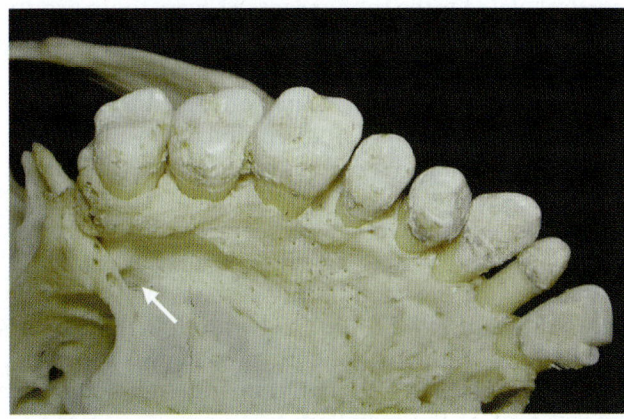

Figure 1 Opening of greater palatine foramen (arrow). Note location of groove where neurovascular bundle courses in posterior portion of the palate.

contents generally do not pose a problem because very few apical surgical procedures are performed on the palatal root of maxillary second and third molars.

Exposure of the maxillary sinus may occur when apical surgical procedures are performed on the roots of any of the teeth located in the maxillary posterior quadrants. It has been reported by Eberhardt et al.[20] that the apex of the mesiobuccal root of the maxillary second molar is closest to the floor of the maxillary sinus (mean = 0.83 mm) and that the apex of the buccal root of the maxillary first premolar is furthest away (mean = 7.05 mm). The root apices of the maxillary second premolar, mesiobuccal, and distobuccal roots of the maxillary first molar were all approximately 2.8 mm from the floor of the sinus. Twelve autopsy specimens and 38 human patients were subjected to computed tomography to arrive at these means.

Ericson et al.[21] noted in 314 apical surgical procedures performed on maxillary canines, premolars, and molars in 276 patients that oroantral communication was noted in 41 cases (13%). They found in this clinical study that the sinus communication did not impair healing, as there was no difference in the success rate between those cases with or without sinus exposure. In another clinical study reported by Rud and Rud,[22] a sinus perforation occurred in 50% of 200 maxillary first molars treated with an apical surgical procedure. Of the cases with a sinus exposure, only two developed a postoperative sinusitis.

When performing surgical procedures on teeth in situations where the apical lesion has not penetrated the cortical plate, the surgeon should be aware of the mean thickness of bone that must be penetrated to reach the root apices. Jin et al.[23] calculated the mean distance from the root apices to the buccal or palatal cortical plate for the root or roots of every tooth group except third molars. One thousand eight hundred and six teeth were evaluated using computed tomography in a population of 66 Asian patients. In a similar computed tomography study conducted by Eberhardt et al.,[20] only maxillary premolars and the maxillary first and second molars were studied. The greatest mean distance between a root apex and the buccal cortical plate reported in the two studies was for the distal root of the mandibular second molar with a mean distance of 8.51 mm.[23] The tooth with the root apex closest to the buccal cortical plate was the maxillary canine (mean = 1.64 mm) in one study[23] and the buccal root of the maxillary first premolar (mean = 1.63mm) in the second study.[20]

When performing apical surgery on mandibular premolars and molars, it is not only important to know the location of the root apices in relationship to the buccal cortical plate but also to the relationship of the root apices to the mandibular canal. The distal root of the mandibular second molar is located furthest from the buccal cortical plate, and as one progresses forward in the arch, the root apices of each succeeding tooth become progressively closer to the buccal cortical plate.[23,24] The mandibular canal follows an "S-shaped" pathway as it moves from a position inferior and buccal to the distal root apex of the mandibular second molar to a more lingual position inferior to the mesial root apex of the mandibular second molar and the apices of both roots of the mandibular first molar. The canal then crosses back to a more buccal position beneath the apex of the mandibular second premolar.[25,26] Denio et al.[26] found that the root apices of the mandibular second molar (mean = 3.7 mm) and the mandibular second premolar (mean = 4.7 mm) were closest to the mandibular canal. The mesial root apex of the mandibular first molar was found to be furthest from the canal (mean = 6.9 mm). Similar results were noted in the study by Littner et al.[25]

The anatomy and location of the mental foramen has been studied by multiple investigators.[27–34] According to the studies,[27–30,34] the mental foramen may be located anywhere between the apex of the mandibular first premolar and the mesial root of the mandibular first molar. In two reports[27,28] where 100 adult mandibles were studied, the most frequent location was apical to the mandibular second premolar (Figure 2). This was also the most frequent location in another study[30] which looked at 75 dry mandibles. In a study[34] of 105

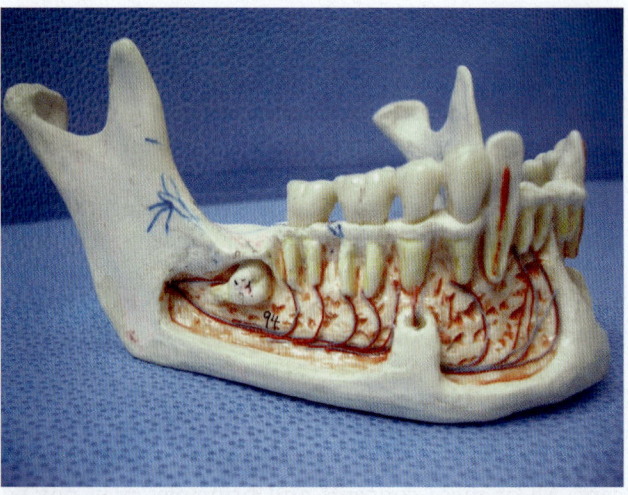

Figure 2 Most frequent location of mental foramen is inferior to the apex of the root of the mandibular second premolar.

cadaver specimens, the most frequent location was found to be between the apices of the mandibular first and second premolars. In another study[29] that reviewed 1,000 full mouth series of radiographs, 70% were found to be located between the apices of the two premolars. It is obvious that this foramen can be quite variable in location for different individuals.

Phillips et al.[30–32] compared the size of the mental foramen as measured on dry mandibles with the size measured on periapical and panoramic radiographs. The mean horizontal measurement on the 75 dry mandibles was 4.6 mm and the mean vertical measurement was 3.4 mm. The periapical radiographic measurement was smaller with a mean of 2.6 mm for the horizontal and 2.3 mm for the vertical. The measurements from the panoramic film were slightly larger than those obtained from the periapical radiographs (horizontal mean = 2.9 mm and vertical mean = 2.5 mm). In two-thirds of the 75 dry specimens, the foramen was found to exit in a posterior and superior direction.[30]

When performing apical surgery on a root containing more than one root canal system, the surgeon must be aware that an isthmus may exist between the canals. Weller et al.[35] were one of the first to point out the significance of the isthmus in surgical endodontics. In mesiobuccal roots of the maxillary first molar with two root canal systems, they reported the highest incidence of an isthmus occurred in the apical 3 to 5 mm and that an isthmus was present 100% of the time at the 4 mm level. In a more recent clinical study,[36] an isthmus was found in 76% of mesiobuccal roots of maxillary first molars with a 3 to 4 mm apical root resection. In a micro-computed tomographic study,[37] an isthmus was found to be present in 85% of the time in the mesial root of the mandibular first molars evaluated. This incidence of isthmuses in the mesial root of mandibular first molars is very close to the 83% reported in a clinical surgical study.[36] In von Arx's [36] clinical study, an isthmus was found 36% of the time when the distal root of mandibular first molars presented with two canals.

Anesthesia and Hemostasis

The injection of a local anesthetic agent that contains a vasoconstrictor has two equally important objectives: (1) to obtain profound and prolonged anesthesia and (2) to provide good hemostasis both during and after the surgical procedure. Failure to obtain profound surgical anesthesia will result in needless pain and anxiety for the patient. Inadequate hemostasis will result in poor visibility of the surgical site thus prolonging the procedure, resulting in increased patient morbidity. With the proper handling of any medical condition, with which the patient may present, and the selection of an appropriate anesthetic agent and vasoconstrictor, it is possible to accomplish both objectives.

The selection of an appropriate anesthetic agent should always be based on the medical status of the patient and the desired duration of anesthesia needed. The two major groups of local anesthetic agents are the esters and amides. The important difference between these groups is not in their ability to produce profound anesthesia but in the manner in which they are metabolized and the potential for allergic reactions. Esters have a much higher allergic potential than amides.[38] The only ester local anesthetic available in dental cartridges in the United States is a combination of propoxycaine and procaine (Ravocaine).

The amide group of local anesthetics, which include lidocaine (Xylocaine), mepivacaine (Carbocaine), prilocaine (Citanest), bupivacaine (Marcaine), etidocaine (Duranest), and articaine (Ultracaine), undergo a complex metabolic breakdown in the liver. Patients with a known liver dysfunction should be administered amide local anesthetic agents with caution due to the potential for a high systemic blood concentration of the drug. Patients with severe renal impairment may be unable to remove the anesthetic agent from the blood, which may result in an increased potential for toxicity due to elevated blood levels of the drug. Therefore, significant renal dysfunction presents a relative contraindication, and dosage limits should be lowered.[39,40]

The high clinical success rate in producing profound and prolonged local anesthesia along with its low potential for allergic reactions makes lidocaine (Xylocaine) the anesthetic agent of choice for periradicular surgery. Selection of another anesthetic agent is indicated only in the presence of a true documented contraindication. If the use of an amide anesthetic agent (lidocaine) is absolutely contraindicated, the ester agents, procaine-propoxycaine with levonordefrin (Ravocaine with Neo-Cobefrin) is presently the only choice.[39]

The choice of vasoconstrictor in the local anesthetic will have an effect on both the duration of anesthesia and the quality of hemorrhage control at the surgical site.[39–42] Vasopressor agents used in dentistry are direct acting, sympathomimetic (adrenergic) amines that exert their action by stimulating special receptors (alpha- and beta-adrenergic receptors) on the smooth muscle cells in the microcirculation of various tissues. These agents include epinephrine (Adrenalin), levonordefrin (Neo-Cobefrin), and levarterenol

(Levophed, Noradrenaline, and norepinephrine).[38] For the purpose of hemostasis, there is little or no justification for the use of levarterenol. The degree of hemostasis required for most periradicular surgical procedures cannot be produced safely by levarterenol.[38]

There are two types of adrenergic receptors in tissues, alpha and beta, that respond differently when stimulated. However, depending on the specific tissue, one will usually predominate. Gage[43] demonstrated that the action of a vasopressor drug on the microvasculature is dependent upon (1) the predominant receptor type and (2) the receptor selectivity of the vasopressor drug. Alpha receptors predominate in the oral mucosa and gingival tissues while beta receptors predominate in skeletal muscle.[40,44] Epinephrine receptor selectivity is approximately equal for alpha and beta receptors. Levonordefrin receptor selectivity, however, is primarily for alpha-adrenergic receptors. Stimulation of the alpha-adrenergic receptors will result in contraction of the smooth muscle cells in the microvasculature with a subsequent reduction of blood flow through the vascular bed. Stimulation of the beta-adrenergic receptors will result in a relaxation of the smooth muscle cells in the microvasculature with a subsequent increased blood flow through the vascular bed. As epinephrine selectivity is equal for alpha and beta receptors, and beta receptors predominate in skeletal muscle, it is important not to inject epinephrine into skeletal muscles in the area of endodontic surgery or a vasodilation with increased blood flow will result.[40,43]

Epinephrine is the most effective and most widely used vasoconstrictor agent in dental anesthetics.[38,45–47] The other vasopressors available are less effective. Even though they are used in higher concentrations in an effort to compensate for their lower effectiveness, the difference in the degree of clinical effect is readily observable. Many studies have been reported measuring the plasma catecholamine levels and the clinical effects of the injection of epinephrine containing local anesthetics for dental treatment.[48–52] The results of these studies indicate that even though the plasma level of catecholamines increases following the injection, this increase does not generally appear to be associated with any significant cardiovascular effects in healthy patients or those with mild to moderate heart disease. Pallasch[53] has stated that the hemodynamic alterations seen with elevated plasma epinephrine are usually quite short in duration, probably because of the very short plasma half-life of epinephrine, usually less than 1 minute. He also stated that the good achieved by the inclusion of vasoconstrictors in dental local anesthetics greatly outweighs any potential deleterious effects of these agents.

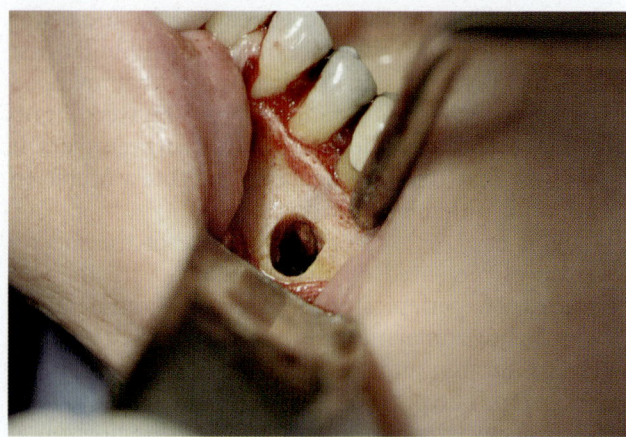

Figure 3 Osteotomy on mandibular molar. Note excellent hemorrhage control following reflection of a full mucoperiosteal flap. Collagen was used as a hemostatic agent during root-end filling.

For periradicular surgery, it is imperative that profound prolonged anesthesia and maximum hemostasis be achieved (Figure 3). In addition to the choice of anesthetic and vasopressor agents, the sites and technique of injection are important factors as well. It is significant to note that nerve block anesthesia involves injection in close proximity to a main nerve trunk that is usually located some distance from the surgical site. Thus, the vasopressor agent in the anesthetic preparation used in nerve block anesthesia will not significantly affect the blood flow at the surgical site. Profound nerve block anesthesia can be achieved with a local anesthetic containing dilute (1:100,000 or 1:200,000) epinephrine.[40]

Hemostasis, unlike anesthesia, however, cannot be achieved by injecting into distant sites.[45] Larger vascular channels are not affected by the injected vasopressor, only the small vessels of the microvasculature. An inferior alveolar nerve block injection effectively blocks pain transmission from the surgical site; however, the vasopressor injected has no effect on the inferior alveolar artery and normal blood flow continues to the peripheral surgical site. Therefore, additional injections must be administered in the soft tissue in the immediate area of the surgery. This is accomplished by local infiltration using a higher concentration of epinephrine (1:50,000) in the anesthetic solution. In the maxilla, infiltration anesthesia can simultaneously achieve anesthesia and hemostasis. It is important to note that whatever technique is used to obtain anesthesia, infiltration in the surgical site is always required to obtain hemostasis.[54]

The infiltration sites of injection for periradicular surgery are always multiple and involve deposition of anesthetics throughout the entire surgical field in the alveolar mucosa just superficial to the periosteum at the level of the root apices. Following block anesthesia, using a 30-gauge needle with the bevel toward bone, a small amount of solution (0.25 to 0.50 mL) should be slowly deposited. The needle tip is then moved peripherally (mesially and distally) and similar small amounts are slowly injected in adjacent areas.[45] The rate of injection in the target sites directly affects the degree of hemostasis. The recommended injection rate is 1 mL/min, with a maximum safe rate of 2 mL/min. Rapid injection produces localized pooling of solution in the injected tissues, resulting in delayed and limited diffusion into adjacent tissues. This results in minimal surface contact with the microvascular bed and less than optimal hemostasis.

The amount of anesthetic solution needed varies and is dependent upon the size of the surgical site. In a small surgical site involving only a few teeth, one cartridge (1.8 cc) of solution containing 1:50,000 epinephrine is usually sufficient to obtain adequate hemostasis. For more extensive surgery involving multiple teeth, it is rarely necessary to inject more than two cartridges (3.6 cc) of anesthetic (1:50,000 epinephrine) to achieve both anesthesia and hemostasis.

It is important that the endodontic surgeon be aware of the delayed beta-adrenergic effect that follows the hemostasis produced by the injection of vasopressor amines. A rebound occurs from an alpha (vasoconstriction) to a beta (vasodilation) response and is termed reactive hyperemia or the rebound phenomenon.[55] Following the injection of a vasopressor amine, tissue concentration of the vasopressor gradually decreases to a level that no longer produces an alpha-adrenergic vasoconstriction. The restricted blood flow slowly returns to normal but then rapidly increases far beyond normal, as a beta-adrenergic dilation occurs.[40,55] This rebound phenomenon is not the result of beta-receptor activity but results from localized tissue hypoxia and acidosis caused by the prolonged vasoconstriction.[44] Once this reactive hyperemia occurs, it is usually impossible to reestablish hemostasis by additional injections. Therefore, if a long surgical procedure is planned (multiple roots or procedures), the more complicated and hemostasis-dependent procedures (root-end resection, root-end preparation and filling) should be done first. The procedures that are least dependent on hemostasis, such as periradicular curettage, biopsy, or root amputation, should be reserved for last. The rebound phenomenon has another important clinical implication, postsurgical hemorrhage and hematoma. These possible postsurgical sequelae are best minimized by proper soft tissue repositioning and postsurgical care, to be covered in more detail later in this chapter.

Soft Tissue Management and Flap Design

Optimal surgical access, both visual and operative, is a requirement for all surgical procedures. Visual access enables the endodontic surgeon to see the entire surgical field while operative access allows the clinician to perform the requisite surgical procedures with the highest quality and in the shortest period of time. This will result in the least amount of surgical trauma and a reduction in postsurgical morbidity. Surgical procedures require the intentional wounding of specific tissues, and the subsequent wound healing depends on the type of tissues wounded and the type of wound inflicted. The clinician's goal must always be to minimize trauma to both the soft and hard tissues involved in the surgical procedure. Periradicular surgical procedures will require reflecting a mucoperiosteal flap.

Good surgical access is fundamentally dependent on the selection of an appropriate flap design. Numerous flap designs have been proposed for periradicular surgery. Although no single flap design is suitable for all surgical situations, the full mucoperiosteal triangular flap is the design most frequently indicated. However, it is still incumbent upon the clinician to know the advantages and disadvantages of each flap design.

Regardless of the design of the surgical flap, there are a number of principles and guidelines that apply to the location and extent of incisions. The adherence to these principles and guidelines will ensure that the reflected soft tissues will fit snugly in their original position, will properly cover the osseous wound site, and provide an adequate vascular bed for healing.

1. Avoid horizontal and severely angled vertical incisions. The gingival blood supply is primarily from the same vessels supplying the alveolar mucosa. As these vessels enter into the gingiva, they assume a vertical course parallel to the long axis of the teeth and are positioned in the reticular layer superficial to the periosteum. They are known as the supraperiosteal vessels.[56,57]

    They are arterioles with a diameter of about 100 μm and are the terminal branches of the buccal, lingual, greater palatine, inferior alveolar, and superior alveolar arteries.[58] Collagen fibers of the gingiva and alveolar mucosa provide structural strength to these tissues. Collectively, these fibers are termed the gingival ligament. This ligament consists of a number of fiber groups that form attachments from crestal bone and supracrestal cementum to the gingiva and the periosteum on the buccal and lingual radicular bone. The collagen fibers that attach to the periosteum course over the crestal radicular bone in a direction parallel to the long axis of the teeth.[59]

Horizontal and severely angled incisions, such as used in semilunar flaps and in broad-based rectangular flaps, shrink excessively during surgery as a result of contraction of the cut collagen fibers that run perpendicular to the line of incision. As a result of this shrinkage, it is often difficult to return the flap edges to their original position without placing excessive tension on the soft tissues. This often results in tearing-out of the sutures and subsequent scar formation from healing by secondary intention. Horizontal or severely angled incisions may also result in interference of the blood supply to the non-reflected gingival tissues due to severance of the gingival blood vessels that run perpendicular to the line of incision. The initial portion of the vertical incision should be placed perpendicular to the gingival margin toward the midsection of the papilla and gradually turning the incision parallel to the tooth axis.

2. Avoid incisions over radicular eminences. Radicular eminences, such as the canine, maxillary first premolar and first molar mesiobuccal root prominences, often fenestrate through the cortical bone or are covered by very thin bone with a poor blood supply. These bony defects may lead to soft tissue fenestrations if incisions are made over them. Vertical (releasing) incisions should be made parallel to the long axis of the teeth and placed between the adjacent teeth over solid interdental bone, never over radicular bone.

3. Incisions should be placed and flaps repositioned over solid bone. Incisions should never be placed over areas of periodontal bone loss or periradicular lesions. Without good solid bone to support the repositioned edges of the mucoperiosteal flap, inadequate blood supply results in necrosis and sloughing of the soft tissue. The endodontic surgeon must take into consideration the extent of osseous bone removal necessary to accomplish the intended periradicular surgery when designing the flap so the repositioned flap margins will be supported by solid bone. Hooley and Whitacre[60] suggest that a minimum of 5 mm of bone should exist between the edge of a bony defect and the incision line.

4. Avoid incisions across major muscle attachments. Incisions across major muscle attachments (frena) make repositioning of the flap and subsequent healing much more difficult. Healing and scar tissue formation by secondary intention healing often results. This can be circumvented by laterally extending the horizontal incision so the vertical incision bypasses the muscle attachment and it is included within the flap.

5. Tissue retractor should rest on solid bone. The extension of the vertical incision should be sufficient to allow the tissue retractor to seat on solid bone, thereby leaving the root apex well exposed. If the vertical incisions are not adequately extended, there will be a tendency for the retractor to traumatize the mucosal tissue in the fold at the base of the flap. This may affect the blood supply to these tissues and will result in increased postsurgical morbidity.

6. Extent of the horizontal incision should be adequate to provide visual and operative access with minimal soft tissue trauma. In general, the horizontal incision for mucoperiosteal flaps in periradicular surgery should extend at least one to two teeth lateral to the tooth to be treated. This will allow for adequate surgical access and minimize tension and stretching of the soft tissue. A time-tested axiom regarding the length of an incision is that more trauma results from too short an incision rather than too long, and incisions heal from side-to-side, not end-to-end.

7. The junction of the horizontal sulcular and vertical incisions should either include or exclude the involved interdental papilla. Vertical releasing incisions should be made parallel to the long axis of the teeth and placed between the adjacent teeth over solid interdental bone, never over radicular bone. The vertical incision should intersect the horizontal incision and terminate in the intrasulcular area at the mesial or distal line angle of the tooth. The involved interdental papilla should never be split by the vertical incision or intersect the horizontal incision in the mid-root area.

8. The flap should include the entire mucoperiosteum (full thickness): marginal, interdental and attached gingiva, alveolar mucosa, and periosteum. Full-thickness flaps result in less surgical trauma to the soft tissues and better surgical hemostasis than split-thickness flaps. The major advantages of full-thickness flaps are derived from the maintenance of the supraperiosteal blood vessels that supply these tissues.

According to Gutmann and Harrison,[57] the two major categories of periradicular surgical flaps are the full mucoperiosteal flaps and the limited mucoperiosteal flaps. The location of the horizontal component of the incision is the distinguishing characteristic between the two categories of surgical flaps. All full mucoperiosteal flaps involve an intrasulcular horizontal incision with reflection of the marginal and interdental (papillary)

Table 1 Classification of Surgical Flaps

1. Full mucoperiosteal flaps
   A. Triangular (one vertical releasing incision)
   B. Rectangular (two vertical releasing incisions)
   C. Trapezoidal (broad-based rectangular)
   D. Horizontal (no vertical releasing incision)
   E. Papilla-base flap
2. Limited mucoperiosteal flaps
   A. Submarginal curved (semilunar)
   B. Submarginal scalloped rectangular (Luebke-Ochsenbein)

gingival tissues as part of the flap. Limited mucoperiosteal flaps have a submarginal (subsulcular) horizontal, or horizontally orientated, incision, and the flap does not include the marginal or interdental tissues. The addition of plane geometric terms to describe flap designs, as suggested by Luebke and Ingle,[61] provides for an easily identifiable classification of periradicular surgical flap designs. The classification of periradicular surgical flaps is summarized in Table 1, and a description of these flaps and their application in endodontic surgery follows.

The triangular flap is formed by a horizontal, intrasulcular incision, and one vertical releasing incision (Figure 4). The primary advantages of this flap design are that it affords good wound healing, which is a result of a minimal disruption of the vascular supply to the flapped tissue, and ease of flap re-approximation with a minimal number of sutures required. The major disadvantage of this flap design is the somewhat limited surgical access it provides due to the single vertical releasing incision. This limited surgical access often makes it difficult to expose the root apexes of long teeth (e.g., maxillary cuspids) and mandibular anterior teeth. In posterior surgery, both maxillary (Figure 5) and mandibular (Figure 6), the vertical releasing incision is placed at the mesial extent of the horizontal incision. This affords the surgeon the maximum visual and operative access with minimum soft tissue trauma. For anterior surgery, the vertical releasing incision should be placed at the extent of the horizontal incision closest to the surgeon and is therefore dependent on the surgeon's position to the right or left of the patient. After reflecting a triangular flap, sometimes the surgeon may find it necessary to obtain additional access. This can be easily obtained by placement of a distal relaxing incision. A relaxing incision is a short vertical incision placed in the marginal and attached gingiva and located at the extent of the horizontal incision opposite the vertical releasing incision. This

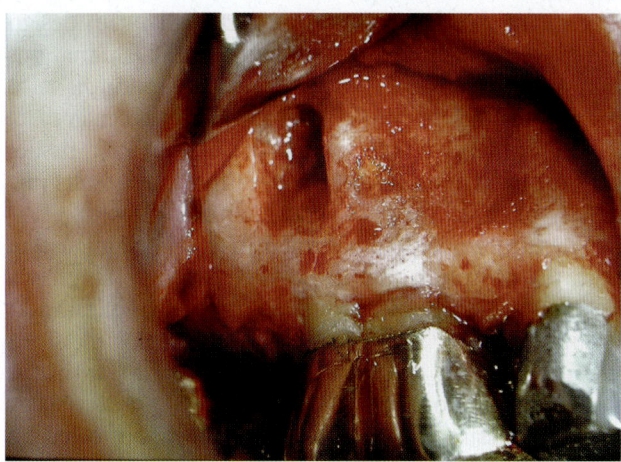

Figure 5 Triangular flap to perform periapical surgery on the distobuccal root of a maxillary molar.

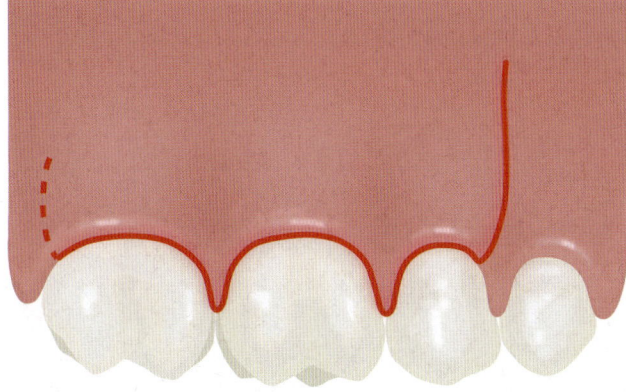

Figure 4 Full mucoperiosteal triangular flap with one vertical incision and a horizontal intrasulcular incision. A distal vertical relaxing incision (dotted line) is often used to relieve tension on soft tissues during flap reflection and increases visibility for a maxillary first molar.

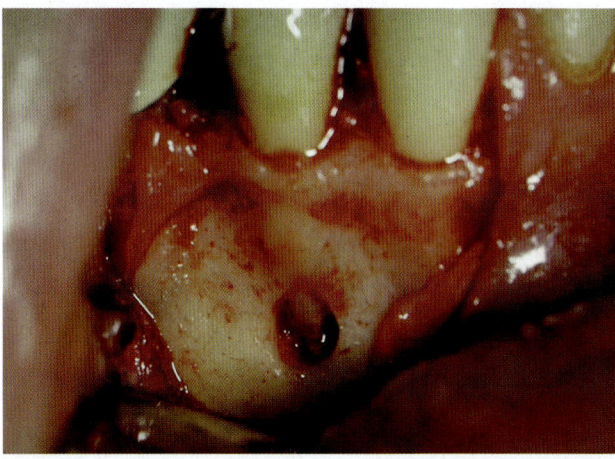

Figure 6 Triangular flap to perform periapical surgery on a mandibular second premolar.

incision is also good for relieving flap retraction tension while achieving adequate surgical access. Due to the excellent wound healing potential of this flap design and the generally favorable surgical access it provides, use of the triangular mucoperiosteal flap is recommended whenever possible. It is recommended for maxillary incisors and posterior teeth. It is the only recommended flap design for mandibular posterior teeth because of anatomic structures contraindicating other flap designs.[57]

The rectangular flap is formed by an intrasulcular, horizontal incision and two vertical releasing incisions (Figure 7). The major advantage of this flap design is increased surgical access to the root apex (Figure 8). This flap design is especially useful for mandibular anterior teeth, when multiple teeth are involved in the surgery, and for teeth with long roots such as maxillary canines. The major disadvantages of the rectangular flap design are the difficulty in re-approximation of the flap margins and wound closure. Postsurgical stabilization is also more difficult with this design than the triangular flap. This is primarily due to the fact that the reflected tissues are held in position solely by the sutures. This results in a greater potential for postsurgical flap dislodgment.

The trapezoidal flap is similar to the rectangular flap with the exception that the two vertical releasing incisions intersect the horizontal, intrasulcular incision at an obtuse angle. The angled vertical releasing incisions are designed to create a broad-based flap with the vestibular portion being wider than the sulcular portion. The desirability of this flap design is predicated on the assumption that this will provide a better blood supply to the flapped tissues. While this concept is valid in other tissues, such as the skin, its application

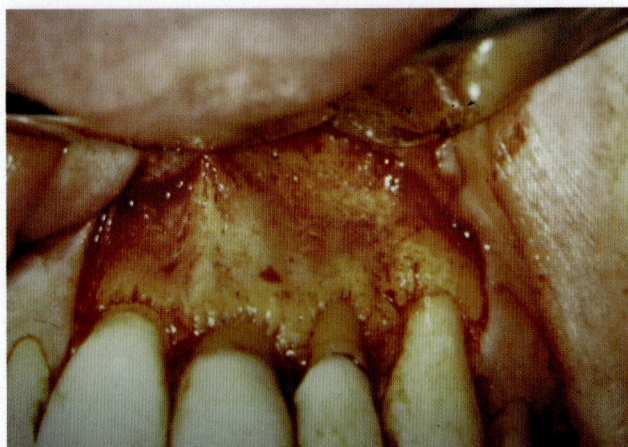

Figure 8 Rectangular flap to perform periapical surgery on maxillary central and lateral incisors.

is unfounded to periradicular surgery.[62] The blood vessels and collagen fibers in the mucoperiosteal tissues are oriented in a vertical direction so the angled vertical releasing incisions will sever more of these vital structures. This will result in more bleeding, a disruption of the vascular supply to the non-flapped tissues, and shrinkage of the flapped tissues. The trapezoidal flap is contraindicated in periradicular surgery.[62]

The papilla-base flap is designed to prevent recession of the papilla following endodontic surgery as it essentially excludes the papillae (Figure 9). The technique involves two different incisions at the papillary base: a shallow first incision at the base followed by a second incision directed toward the crestal bone. Once the papillae are incised, a full thickness mucoperiosteal flap is elevated. Although this flap design is

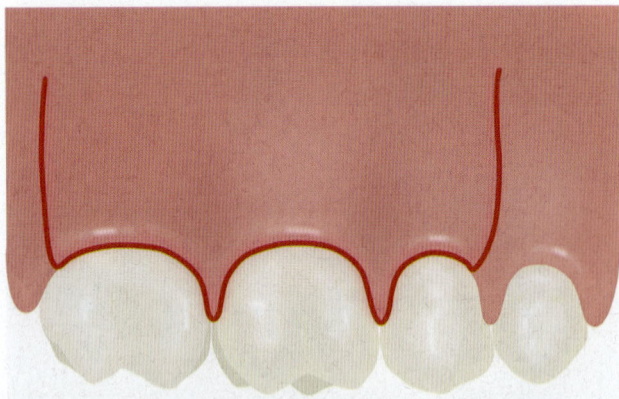

Figure 7 Full mucoperiosteal rectangular flap with two vertical releasing incisions and a horizontal intrasulcular incision. Rectangular flaps are frequently used in the mandibular anterior region or when multiple teeth require endodontic surgery.

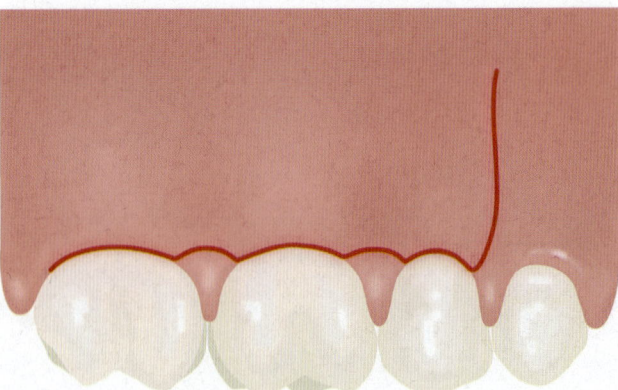

Figure 9 Papilla-based flap consists of at least one vertical incision connected by the papilla-based incision and intrasulcular incision in the cervical area of the teeth. This flap is designed to preserve the papilla and prevent recession.

more challenging to master, if properly executed, it can produce excellent results.[63]

The horizontal or envelope flap is created by a horizontal, intrasulcular incision with no vertical releasing incisions. This flap design has very limited application in periradicular surgery due to the limited surgical access it provides. Its major applications in endodontic surgery are limited to repair of cervical defects (root perforations, resorption, caries, etc) and hemisections and root amputations.

The submarginal curved or semilunar flap is formed by a curved incision in the alveolar mucosa and the attached gingiva. The incision begins in the alveolar mucosa extending into the attached gingiva and then curves back into the alveolar mucosa. There are no advantages to this flap design, and its disadvantages are many including poor surgical access and poor wound healing which results in scarring (Figure 10). This flap design is not recommended for periradicular surgery.

The submarginal scalloped rectangular flap is a modification of the rectangular flap discussed previously in that the horizontal incision is not placed in the gingival sulcus but in the buccal or labial attached gingiva (Figure 11). The horizontal incision is scalloped and follows the contour of the marginal gingiva above the free gingival groove. The major advantages of this flap design are that it does not involve the marginal or interdental gingiva and the crestal bone is not exposed. The primary disadvantages are that the vertically oriented blood vessels and collagen fibers are severed. The result is more bleeding and a greater potential for flap shrinkage, delayed

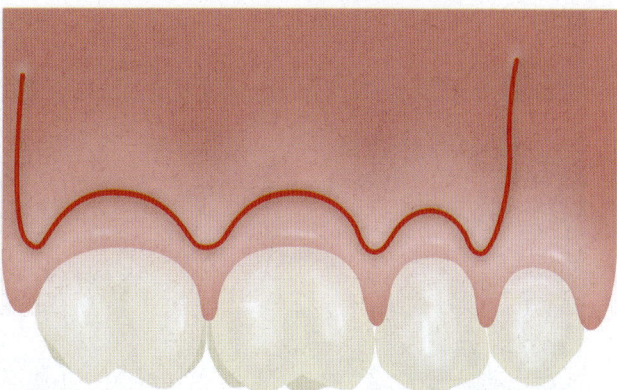

Figure 11 Limited mucoperiostal Luebke-Ochsenbein flap with two vertical incisions connected by a scalloped submarginal horizonal incision in the attached gingiva. This design is essentially limited to the maxilla with a sufficient amount of attached gingiva.

healing, and scar formation (Figure 12A&B). When considering the use of this flap design, the endodontic surgeon must keep in mind that the horizontal, scalloped incision must be placed and the flap repositioned over solid bone. Careful evaluation of any buccal or labial periodontal pockets must also be made in order to minimize the possibility of leaving non-flapped gingival tissue without bony support. The importance of properly angled diagnostic radiographs cannot be overemphasized when considering the use of this flap design. The size and position of any periradicular inflammatory bone loss must also be considered when placing the horizontal incision to ensure that the margins of the flap, when re-approximated, will be adequately supported by solid bone. Proponents of this flap design stress the importance of not involving the marginal gingiva and the gingival sulcus in the horizontal incision that may result in an alteration of the soft tissue attachment and crestal bone levels. It has been reported, however, that with proper re-approximation of the reflected tissues and good soft tissue management, the gingival attachment level is minimally altered or unchanged when full mucoperiosteal flaps are employed.

The key element in preventing loss of soft tissue attachment level is ensuring that the root-attached tissues are not damaged or removed during surgery.[62,64,65] It has also been reported that crestal bone loss is minimal (about 0.5 mm) when full mucoperiosteal flaps are used in periodontal surgery. These procedures may involve apical positioning of flaps, excision of marginal gingiva, and root planning that must rely on new attachment of soft tissue to cementum. Unlike periodontal surgery, endodontic surgery

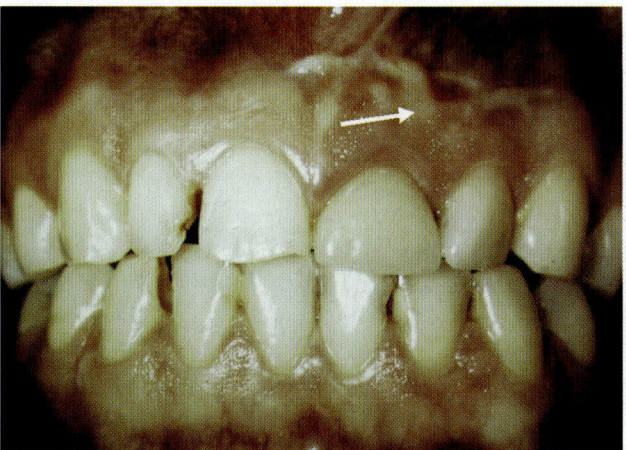

Figure 10 Scar (arrow) in the gingival tissues resulting from the use of a semilunar flap for periapical surgery.

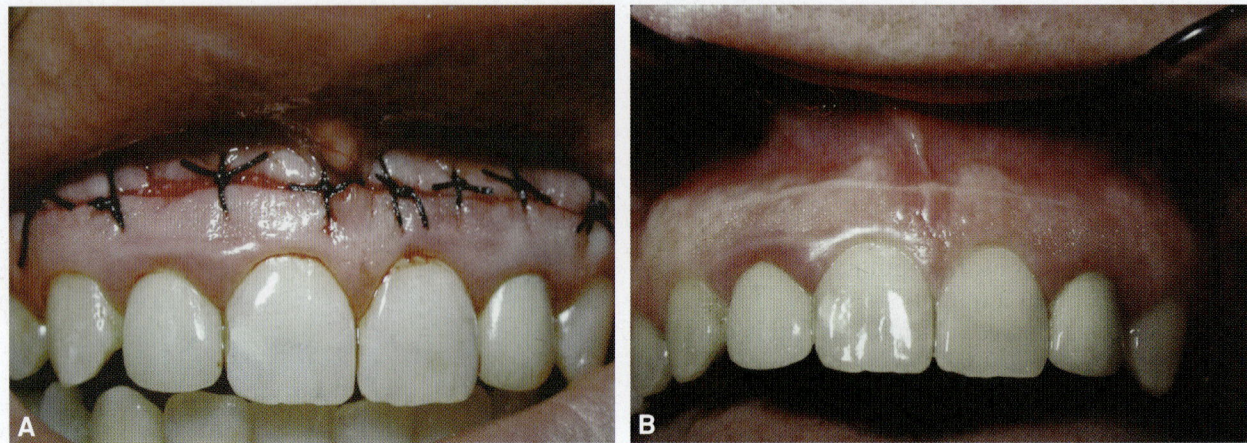

Figure 12 ***A,*** Submarginal flap at the time of suture placement; ***B,*** Submarginal flap 3 months postsurgery. Note scarring along submarginal incision line.

can accomplish reattachment that results in little or no crestal bone loss. Harrison and Jurosky[65] reported that crestal bone showed complete osseous repair of resorptive defects and no alteration of crestal height following periradicular surgery using a triangular (full mucoperiosteal) flap. In the absence of periodontal disease, a complete return to anatomic and functional normalcy can be expected following periradicular surgery using triangular or rectangular flap designs.[57]

Periradicular surgery from a palatal approach is more difficult due to the clinician's limited visual and operative access to this area. The only flap designs indicated for palatal approach surgery are the horizontal (envelope) and the triangular, with the latter being preferred. The palatal surgical approach should be limited to the posterior teeth (Figure 13A&B). Anterior teeth should be approached from the labial except when radicular pathosis dictates a palatal approach, for example, curettement of a cyst located toward the palate. The horizontal intrasulcular incision for the triangular flap should extend anteriorly to the mesial of the first premolar or, for the horizontal (envelope) flap, to the midline. It should extend distally as far as needed to afford access to the involved palatal root. A distal relaxing incision extending a few millimeters from the marginal gingiva toward the midline or over the tuberosity area can be added to achieve better access and to relieve tension on the distal extent of the flap. The vertical releasing incision for the triangular flap should extend from a point near the midline and join the anterior extent of the horizontal incision mesial to the first premolar. There is no validity to concerns regarding a potential hemorrhage problem with vertical incisions in the palatal mucosa in the

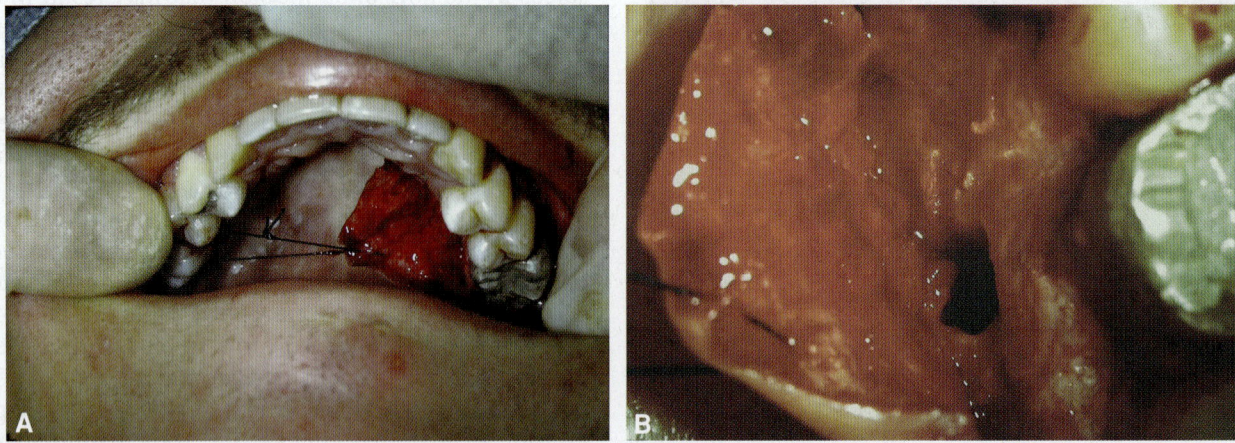

Figure 13 ***A,*** Palatal flap reflected and sutured to opposite side of arch to afford better access and visualization; ***B,*** Bony defect and palatal root apex of maxillary first molar exposed.

premolar area. The greater palatine artery branches rapidly as it courses anteriorly, and an incision in the premolar area results in a minimal disruption to the vascular supply.

The palatal mucosa is tough and fibrous, and flap reflection and retraction can be difficult in this area. Placement of a sling suture in the flapped tissue attached to a tooth or a bite block on the opposite side of the maxillary arch (see Figure 13A) may aid the surgeon in improving visual and operative access by eliminating the need to manually retract the flap while performing this potentially difficult surgical procedure.

Following the selection of the flap design, it is important to select the proper scalpel blade to accomplish the delicate task of making smooth, clean atraumatic incisions. Incisions for the majority of mucoperiosteal flaps for periradicular surgery can be accomplished by using one or more of four scalpel blades, No. 11, No. 12, No. 15, and No. 15-C. The horizontal incision should be made first, followed by the vertical releasing incisions to complete the perimeters of the flap design. The horizontal incision for a full mucoperiosteal flap (Figure 14) begins in the gingival sulcus and should extend through the fibers of the gingival attachment to the crestal bone. Care should be exercised to ensure that the interdental papilla be incised through the mid-col area, separating the buccal and lingual papilla and incising the fibers of the epithelial attachment to crestal bone. Because these tissues are extremely delicate and space is very limited, this important incision is best made with a small scalpel blade, such as No. 11 or No. 15C. By holding the scalpel handle in a pen grasp and using finger rests on the teeth, the surgeon can achieve maximum control and stability when performing these delicate incision strokes. An attempt should be made to accomplish the horizontal incision using as few incision strokes as necessary in order to minimize trauma to the marginal gingiva.

The horizontal incision for a limited mucoperiosteal flap should begin in the attached gingiva and be placed about 2 mm coronal to the mucogingival junction. The incision should be scalloped following the contour of the marginal gingiva. It is important that the horizontal incision never be placed coronal to the depth of the gingival sulcus. The depth of the gingival sulcus must be measured prior to placement of this flap design. The No. 15 or No. 15-C scalpel blade is recommended for this incision. An attempt should be made to incise through the gingiva and periosteum to the cortical bone using firm pressure and a single, smooth stroke. Multiple incision strokes will result in increased trauma to the gingival tissue, which may contribute to retarded healing and scar formation.

Vertical releasing incisions, whether for full or limited mucoperiosteal flaps, should always be vertical and placed between adjacent teeth over interdental bone (Figure 15). They should never be placed over radicular bone. The incision should penetrate through the periosteum so that it can be included in the flap. The incision stroke should begin in the alveolar mucosa and proceed in a coronal direction until it intersects the horizontal incision. Contrary to an often, well-ingrained surgical axiom, however, it is not necessary to accomplish this incision in a single stroke.[57] It is often difficult to accomplish penetration completely through the gingiva, mucosa, submucosa, and periosteum in a single stroke of the scalpel. An initial

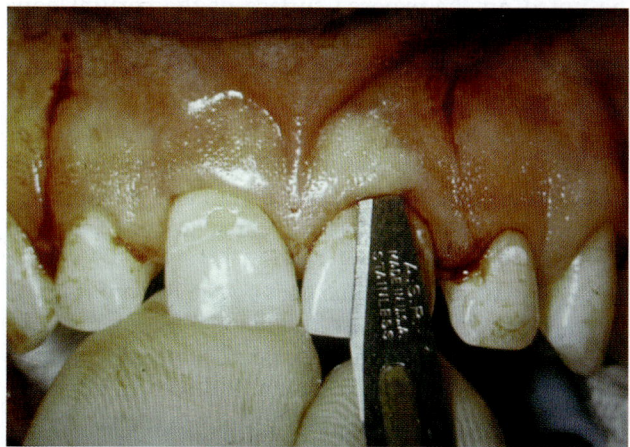

Figure 14 Horizontal sulcular incision with a No. 11 Bard Parker scapel blade.

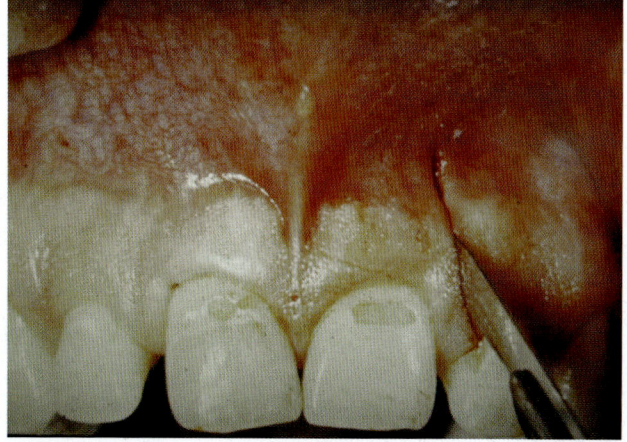

Figure 15 Vertical incision with a No. 15 Bard Parker scapel blade.

incision stroke that penetrates the mucosa and gingiva can be followed by a second that penetrates through the periosteum to the surface of the cortical bone. More accurate placement of the vertical releasing incision will often result from this two-stroke incision technique because less pressure is required on the initial stroke, affording the surgeon more control over the direction of the scalpel blade. It may be necessary to replace the scalpel blade with a fresh, sharp one in order to produce clean, sharp incision lines.

Reflection of soft tissues for full or limited mucoperiosteal flaps is a very critical process in the effort to reduce surgical trauma and postsurgical morbidity. Marginal gingiva is very delicate and easily injured. It is, therefore, not appropriate to begin the reflective process in the horizontal incision for full mucoperiosteal flaps (Figure 16). The supracrestal root attachment fibers are of even greater clinical significance than the marginal gingiva. These root attachment fibers are easily damaged or destroyed by direct reflective forces. Damage to these tissues may result in the loss of their viability, allowing for apical epithelial down growth along the root surface. This epithelial down growth will result in increased sulcular depth and loss of soft tissue attachment level.[57,66] Maintenance of the viability of these root attachment fibers, however, will likely result in the soft tissue attachment levels being unaltered following surgery.[64,67]

Initiating the flap reflective process in the horizontal incision for submarginal flaps is not as injurious to the soft tissues as in the full flap design as the horizontal incision for the former is placed in attached gingiva. This will, however, result in damaging forces being applied to a critical wound edge and should be avoided whenever possible. The horizontal incision is more subject to delayed wound healing than the vertical incisions in this flap design. Additional trauma to the attached gingival tissues during flap reflection may result in tissue shrinkage and healing by secondary intention, which results in increased scar tissue formation. The reflective procedure for the limited mucoperiosteal flap should begin in the attached gingiva of the vertical incision whenever possible.

Flap reflection is the process of separating the soft tissues (gingiva, mucosa, and periosteum) from the surface of the alveolar bone. This process should begin in the vertical incision a few millimeters apical to the junction of the horizontal and vertical incisions. The periosteal elevator of choice should be used to gently elevate the periosteum and its superficial tissues from the cortical plate (Figure 17A). Once these tissues have been lifted from the cortical plate and the periosteal elevator can be inserted between them and the bone, the elevator is then directed coronally. This allows the marginal and interdental gingiva to be separated from the underlying bone and the opposing incisional wound edge without direct application of dissectional forces. This technique allows for all of the direct reflective forces to be applied to the periosteum and the bone. This approach to flap reflection is referred to as "undermining elevation."[57] This "undermining elevation" should continue until the attached gingival tissues (marginal and interdental) have been lifted from the underlying bone to the full extent of the horizontal incision (see Figure 17B). After reflection of these tissues, soft tissue elevation is continued in an apical direction, lifting the alveolar mucosa, along with the underlying periosteum, from the cortical bone until adequate surgical access to the intended surgical area has been achieved. Small bleeding tissue tags will often be noted on the exposed surface of the cortical bone once the flap is fully reflected (see Figure 17C), especially in the interradicular depressed areas. Bleeding from these tissue tags will stop in a few minutes and they should not be damaged or removed. Research evidence strongly suggests that these bleeding tissue tags are cortical retained periosteal tissues and may play an important role in healing and reattachment of the flap to the cortical bone.[65]

In posterior mandibular surgery, it is important to be aware of the presence of the mental foramen and its associated neurovascular bundle. The most common location of the mental foramen is directly inferior to the crown of the second premolar and mesial to and inferior to its root apex (see Figure 2); however,

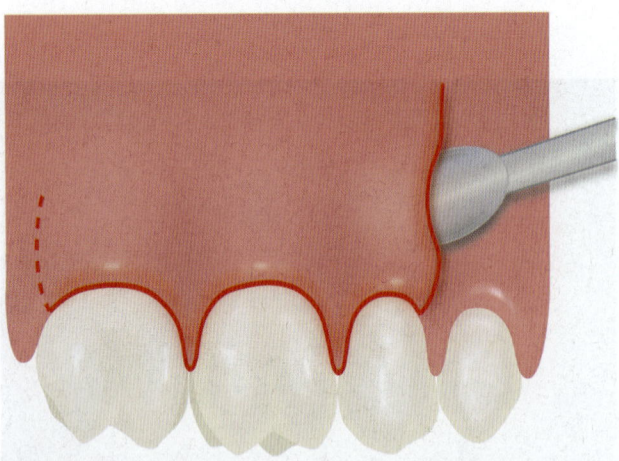

Figure 16 Initial undermining elevation of the flap should begin in the vertical incision in attached gingiva.

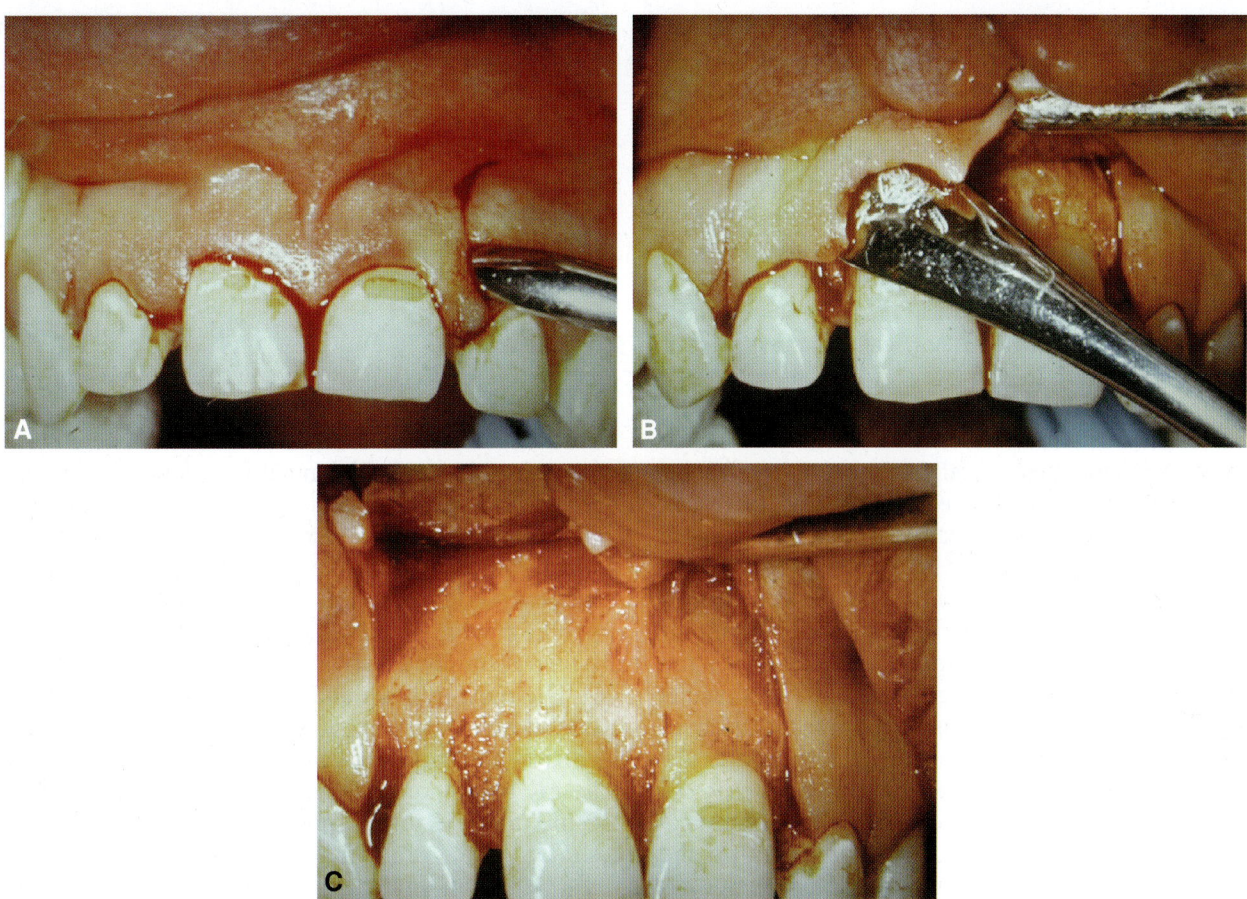

Figure 17 *A,* Initial elevation of flap; *B,* Flap partially reflected; *C,* Flap completely reflected.

anatomical variances can occur (Figure 18). The mental foramen is visible approximately 75% of the time on periapical radiographs. When it is not visible on the radiograph, it is usually below the border of the film.[30,31] During flap reflection in the mandibular premolar area, the surgeon must be alert to subtle changes in the resistance of the periosteum to separation from the cortical bone. The resistance of Sharpey's fibers, which attach the periosteum to the bone, to separation results in a thin, white band at the junction of the flapped soft tissues and the cortical bone. Because there are no Sharpey's fibers attaching the periosteum to the border of the mental foramen, this thin, white band will disappear when the border of the mental foramen has been reached. Further reflection of the soft tissues in this area will result in the identification of the neurovascular bundle as it exits from the foramen. Maximum protection to the neurovascular bundle will

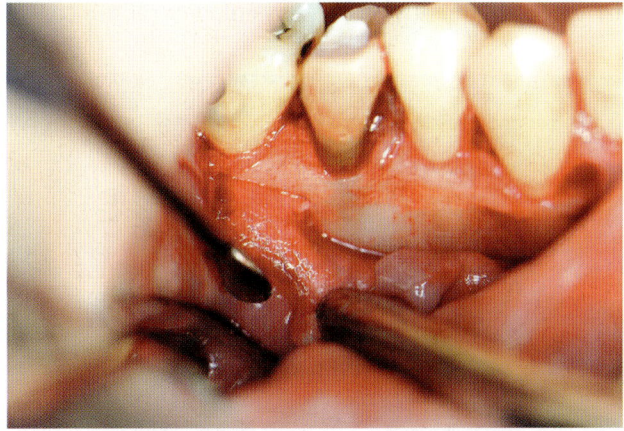

Figure 18 Neurovascular bundle exiting from mental foramen. The endodontic surgeon must be cognizant of anatomic variances so as to avoid injury during surgery.

be best achieved by its early identification during the flap reflective process. This will allow the surgeon to avoid injury to these important anatomic structures during the remainder of the surgical procedure.

Flap retraction is the process of holding in position the reflected soft tissues. Proper retraction depends on adequate extension of the flap incisions and proper reflection of the mucoperiosteum. It is necessary to provide both visual and operative access to the periradicular and radicular tissues. The tissue retractor must always rest on solid cortical bone with light but firm pressure. In this way, it acts as a passive mechanical barrier to the reflected soft tissues. If the retractor inadvertently rests on the soft tissue at the base of the flap, mechanical trauma to the alveolar mucosa may result in delayed healing and increased postsurgical morbidity. Selection of the proper size and shape of the retractor (Figure 19) is important in minimizing soft tissue trauma. If the retractor is too large, it may traumatize the surrounding tissue. If the retractor is too small, flapped tissue falls over the retractor and impairs the surgeon's access. This results not only in increased soft tissue trauma but also in extending the length of the surgical procedure. An axiomatic principle of endodontic surgery is that the longer the flap is retracted, the greater the postsurgical morbidity. This is a logical conclusion based on the probability that blood flow to the flapped tissues is impeded during flap retraction. In time, this will result in hypoxia and acidosis with a resulting delay in wound healing.[57]

Regardless of whether the retraction time is short or long, the periosteal surface of the flap should be irrigated frequently with physiologic saline (0.9%

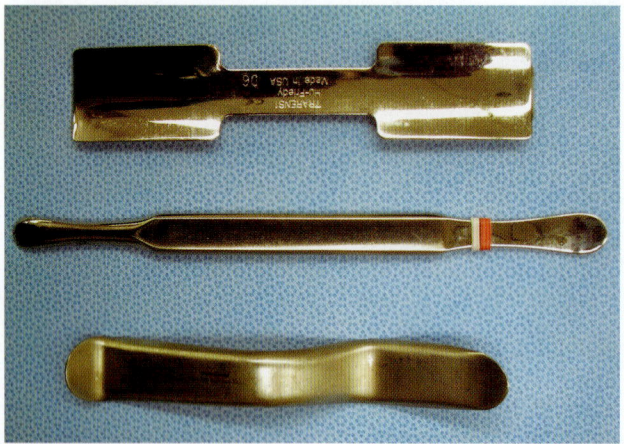

Figure 19 Examples of endodontic tissue retractors (Top—Arens Tissue Retractor; Middle—Selden retractor; Bottom—University of Minnesota retractor).

sodium chloride) solution. Saline should be used, rather than water, because the latter is hypotonic to tissue fluids. It is not necessary to irrigate the superficial surface of the flap because the stratified squamous epithelium prevents dehydration from this surface. Limited mucoperiosteal flaps are more susceptible to dehydration and may require more frequent irrigation than full mucoperiosteal flaps.[57]

Hard Tissue Management and Curettage

Following reflection and retraction of the mucoperiosteal flap, surgical access must be made through the cortical bone to the roots of the teeth. Where cortical bone is thin, as in the maxilla, a large periradicular lesion may result in the loss of buccal or labial cortical plate, or if a natural root fenestration is present, the tooth root may be visible through the cortical plate. In other cases, the cortical bone may be very thin, and probing with a small sharp curette will allow the penetration of the cortical plate.

The most difficult and challenging situation for the endodontic surgeon is when several millimeters of cortical and cancellous bone must be removed to gain access to the root, especially when no periradicular radiolucent lesion is present. A number of factors should be considered to determine the location of the bony window in this clinical situation. The angle of the crown of the tooth to the root should be assessed. Often the long axis of the crown and its root are not the same, especially when a prosthetic crown has been placed. When a root prominence or eminence in the cortical plate is present, the root angulation and position is more easily determined. Measurement of the entire tooth length can be obtained from a well-angled radiograph and transferred to the surgical site by the use of a measured sterile file or ruler. After a small defect has been created on the surface of the cortical plate, a radiopaque marker, such as a small piece of lead foil from a radiographic film packet or a small piece of gutta-percha, can be placed in the bony defect and a direct (not angled) image exposed. The radiopaque object will provide guidance for the position of the root apex. When the cortical plate is intact, another method to locate the root apex is to first locate the body of the root coronal to the apex where the bone covering the root is thinner. Once the root has been located and identified, the bone covering the root is slowly and carefully removed with light brush strokes, working in an apical direction until the root apex is identified (Figure 20). The root surface can be distinguished from the surrounding osseous tissue in four

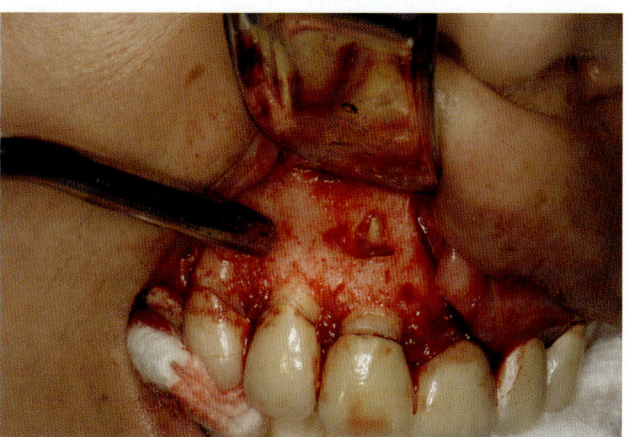

Figure 20 Root end located following careful osseous removal.

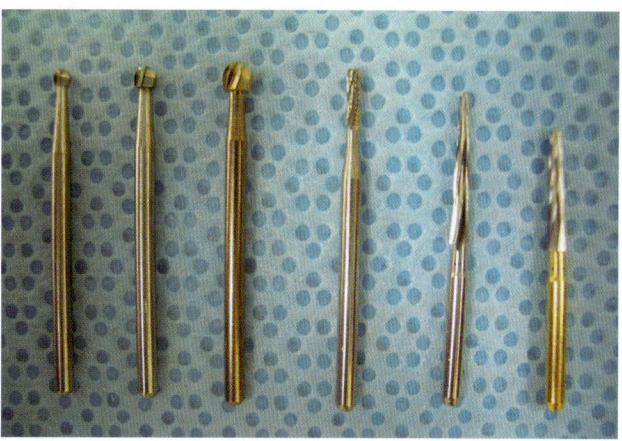

Figure 21 Burs for gaining access to the bony crypt and for resection of the root apex (From left to right: No. 4 round bur; No. 6 round bur; No. 8 round bur; No. 57 fissure bur; multi-purpose bur; Endo-Z bur).

ways: (1) root structure generally has a yellowish color, (2) roots do not bleed when probed, (3) root texture is smooth and hard as opposed to the granular and porous nature of bone, and (4) it is surrounded by the periodontal ligament. Under some clinical conditions, the root may be very difficult to distinguish from the surrounding osseous tissue. Some authors advocate the use of methylene blue dye to aid in the identification of the periodontal ligament. A small amount of the dye is painted on the area in question and left for 1 to 2 minutes. When the dye is washed off with saline, the periodontal ligament will be stained with the dye making it easier to identify the location of the root.

Osseous tissue response to surgical removal is complicated and depends on a number of variables. One important factor is that bone in the surgical site has a temporary decrease in vascular supply due to the local anesthetic vasoconstrictor. This results in the osseous tissue being more heat sensitive and less resistant to injury. Of major importance in osseous tissue removal by burs is the generation of heat. Variables such as bur sharpness, rotary speed, flute design, and pressure applied will all have direct influence on heat generation.

The use of a liquid coolant is indispensable in controlling temperature increase during bone removal by dissipating the heat generated and by keeping the cutting flutes of the instruments free of debris. Osseous temperatures higher than 100°C have been recorded during bone removal with burs even when a liquid coolant is used.[68] Animal studies have shown that vascular changes occur in bone when temperatures exceed 40°C. Heating bone tissue in excess of 60°C results in inactivation of alkaline phosphatase, interruption of blood flow, and tissue necrosis.[69–72] The coolant will be most effective when it is directed on the head of the bur in order to prevent tissue debris from clogging the flutes.

The shape of the bur used for bone removal and the design of its flutes play a significant role in postsurgical healing. Cutting of osseous tissue with a #6 or #8 round bur (Figure 21) produces less inflammation, results in a smoother cut surface, and a shorter healing time than when a fissure bur or diamond bur is used.[73,74] Burs with the ability to cut sharply and cleanly, with the largest space between cutting flutes, regardless of the speed of rotation, leave defects that heal in the shortest postsurgical time.[75,76] The amount of pressure applied to the bone by burs during osseous tissue removal will have a direct effect on the frictional heat generated during the cutting process. Light "brush strokes" with short, multiple periods of osseous cutting will maximize cutting efficiency and minimize the generation of frictional heat.

No studies presently exist which support a biologic basis for the use of low speed over the proper use of a high speed handpiece for bone removal.[69] In most areas of the mouth, visual access is adequate while using a high speed handpiece and surgical length burs. In areas of restricted visibility, the use of a high speed handpiece with a 45° angled head significantly increases visibility. The Impact Air 45° high speed handpiece (Figure 22) offers the added advantage that the air is exhausted to the rear of the turbine rather than toward the bur and the surgical site. Case reports of surgical emphysema resulting in subcutaneous emphysema of the face including fatal descending necrotizing mediastinitis from the use of a high speed dental handpiece have been published.[77] Clinicians should be aware of the spectrum of this potential

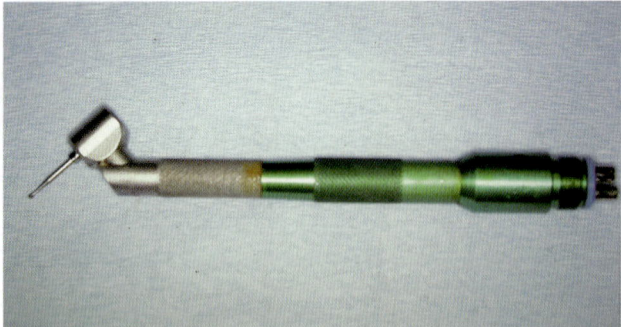

Figure 22 Air Impact 45 Handpiece.

problem and specifically of the potential hazards of pressurized nonsterile air blown into open surgical sites by the dental drill.[78]

When performing periradicular surgery, inexperienced endodontic surgeons, in their attempt to be conservative in the removal of osseous tissue, often create too small a window through the cortical plate to expose the tooth root. As a result, both visual and operative access is impaired for the most delicate and critical part of the surgery—root-end resection and root-end filling. While it is advisable to limit osseous tissue removal to no more than is necessary, failure to achieve sufficient visual and operative access results in extending the time required for the surgical procedure, increasing the stress level of the surgeon, trauma to adjacent tissues, and postsurgical patient morbidity.

Once the root and the root apex have been identified and the surgical window through the cortical and medullary bone has been properly established (Figure 23), any diseased tissue should be removed from the periradicular bony lesion (Figure 24). This removal of periradicular inflammatory tissue is best

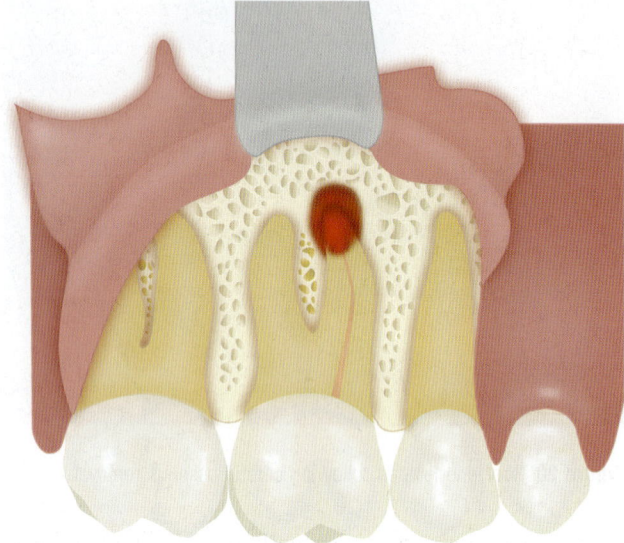

Figure 24 Soft tissue lesion on mesiobuccal root of maxillary first molar after reflection of a full thickness mucoperiosteal flap.

accomplished by using various sizes and shapes of sharp surgical bone curettes and angled periodontal curettes (Figure 25). The choice of specific curettes is very subjective, and endodontic surgeons will develop a preference for curettes that work best for them. It is advisable, however, to have a wide assortment of curettes available in the sterile surgery pack to use should the need arise.

Prior to periradicular curettage, it is advisable to inject a local anesthetic solution containing a vasoconstrictor into the soft tissue mass. This will reduce the

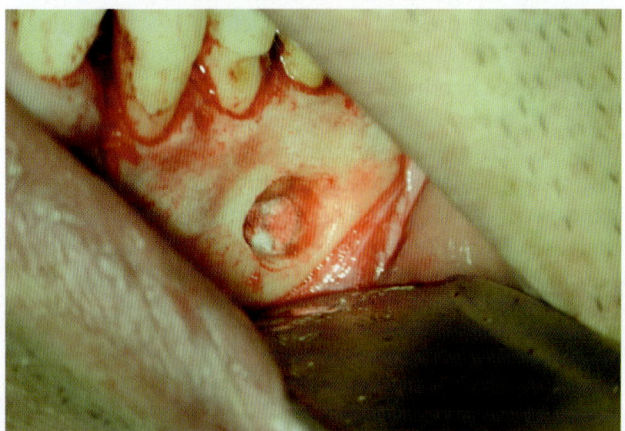

Figure 23 Bony window of adequate size to perform periapical surgery on a mandibular premolar.

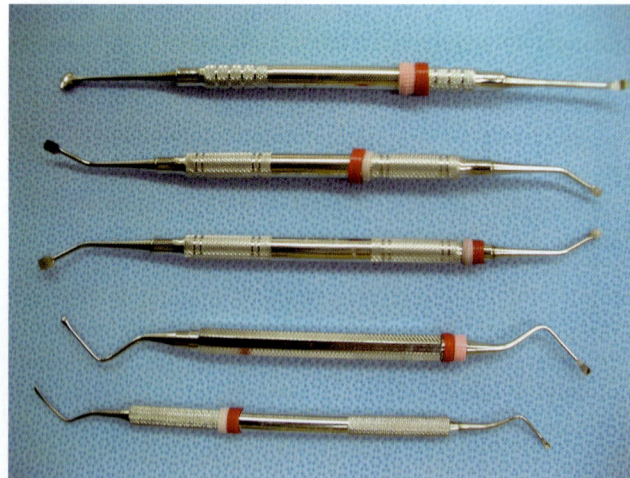

Figure 25 Variety of spoon excavators and curettes for removal of soft tissue from the bony crypt.

possibility of discomfort to the patient during the debridement process and will also serve as hemorrhage control at the surgical site. Additional injections of local anesthetic solution may be necessary if the amount of soft tissue needing to be removed is extensive and hemorrhage control is a problem.

Curettage of the inflammatory soft tissue will be facilitated if the tissue mass can be removed in one piece. Penetration of the soft tissue mass with a curette will result in increased hemorrhage, and shredding the tissue will result in more difficult removal. To accomplish removal of the entire tissue mass, the largest bone curette, consistent with the size of the lesion, is placed between the soft tissue mass and the lateral wall of the bony crypt with the concave surface of the curette facing the bone. Pressure should be applied against the bone as the curette is inserted between the soft tissue mass and the bone around the lateral margins of the lesion. Once the soft tissue has been freed along the periphery of the lesion, the bone curette should be turned with the concave portion toward the soft tissue and used in a scraping fashion to free the tissue from the deep walls of the bony crypt (Figure 26A,B,C,D). Once the tissue has been detached from the walls of the crypt, it can then be easily removed by grasping it with a pair of tissue forceps. The tissue should be

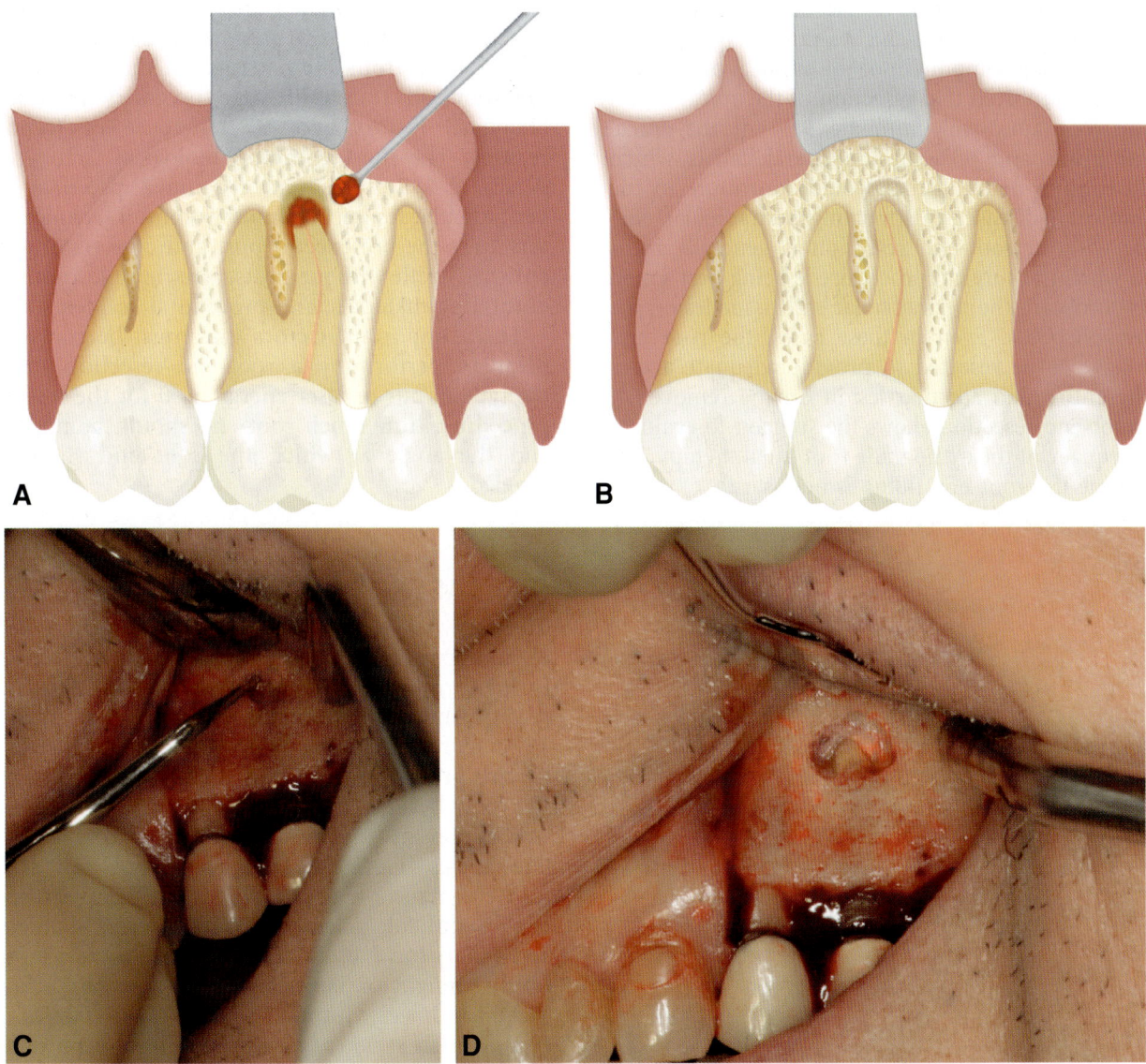

Figure 26 *A*, Curettage of soft tissue lesion allows for visualization of mesiobuccal root apex. Tissue removed should be submitted for biopsy; *B*, Root end exposed and more visible following curettage; *C*, Soft tissue lesion overlying apex; *D*, Root-end exposed following curettage and osseous removal.

immediately placed in a bottle containing 10% buffered formalin solution and submitted for biopsy. While the majority of periradicular lesions of pulpal origin are granulomas, radicular cysts, or abscesses, all tissue removed during periradicular curettage should be sent for histopathologic examination to ensure that no potentially serious pathologic condition exists.[79] Lin and Gaengler[80] state that it is not always necessary to completely curette all of the inflammatory tissues so long as the etiology is apparent and eliminated.

Root-End Resection

When endodontic surgery is performed in the area around a root apex, root-end resection (Figure 27) is almost always a component of the surgical procedure. It has been reported that resection of the apical 3 mm of the root apex will eliminate 98% of the apical ramifications and 93% of the lateral canals which could contain material that would contribute to the periradicular disease.[11] Performing periradicular curettage without root-end resection is generally indicated when the surgical procedure is being performed solely to obtain the periradicular soft tissue lesion for biopsy purposes. Even in these cases, the root end may have to be resected to provide adequate access so the entire periradicular lesion can be removed.[57] The root-end resection allows the surgeon to evaluate the adequacy of the orthograde root canal therapy and determine if a root-end filling is necessary.[57]

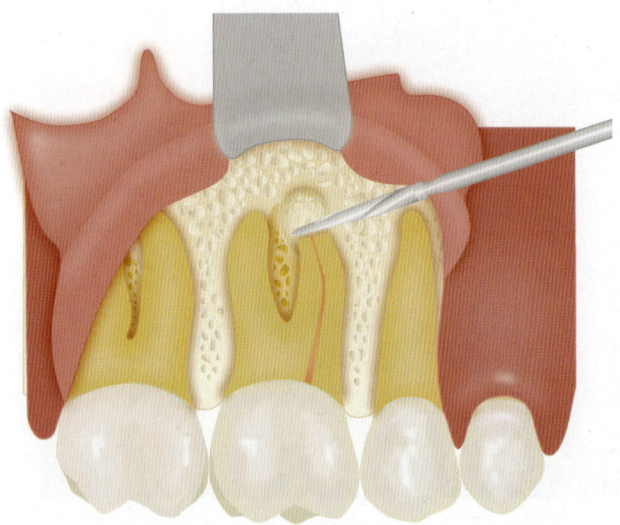

Figure 27 Root-end resection with a plain fissure or multi-purpose bur.

INDICATIONS

Root end resection is indicated for different reasons. Removal of the root apex will aid in eliminating anatomical variations, resorptive defects, ledges, perforation defects, canal obstructions, and separated instruments that may be present in this area of the root.[11,57] Removal of the root apex also will allow the operator to better visualize the seal created by the orthograde obturating material, the need for a root-end seal, and to gain access for the removal of pathologic tissue that may be trapped along the lingual surface of the root.[57]

El-Swiah and Walker[81] classified the indications as being either biological or technical. In their retrospective study, they evaluated the clinical factors involved in deciding the need to perform root-end resections on 517 teeth from 392 patients. Of the total, 60% of the root-end resections were necessary because of biological factors and 40% because of technical reasons. The most common biological factors were persistent symptoms and continued presence of a periradicular lesion. The most common technical factors were the presence of post and core restorations, crowned teeth without posts, irretrievable root canal obturating materials, and procedural accidents.

Three important factors that must be considered prior to performing a root-end resection include the type of bur or laser energy used for the resection procedure, how much root end should be removed, and the angle at which the root end should be beveled.

BUR/LASER SELECTION

The bur type (see Figure 21) and choice of either a high or slow speed handpiece are important considerations in performing root-end resections. Ingle et al.[82] recommended using a #702 tapered fissure bur or a #6 or #8 round bur in a slo-speed straight handpiece for this procedure. They stated that a large round bur was best because it could be easily controlled and would prevent gouging and the formation of sharp line angles. Gutmann and Harrison[57] stated that root-end resection with a slo-speed handpiece could be very difficult unless a good finger rest is obtained and a sharp bur is used. They suggested using a surgical length straight or tapered plain fissure bur in a hi-speed handpiece. Gutmann and Pitt Ford[83] stated that even though various types of burs have been recommended for root-end resections, there is no evidence to support any advantage of one bur type over another with regard to tissue healing response. In spite of this, clinicians continue to favor a smooth, flat resected root surface.

In an ex vivo study, Nedderman et al.[84] used the scanning electron microscope (SEM) to examine the resected root face and gutta-percha fillings following root-end resection with a variety of bur types using both hi- and slo-speed handpieces. They reported that the use of round burs at both speeds resulted in scooping or ditching of the resected root surface. Crosscut fissure burs at both speeds produced the roughest and most irregular resected root surfaces with the gutta-percha being smeared across the root face. The plain fissure bur, both at high or slow speed, produced the smoothest resected root surface, and the plain fissure bur at slo-speed resulted in the least distortion of the gutta-percha.

Morgan and Marshall[85] compared the topography of resected root surfaces using a #57 fissure, Lindeman, or Multi-purpose burs. Additional comparisons were made after refinements to the cut root surface were made with either a multi-fluted carbide or an ultra fine diamond-coated finishing bur. The resected root surfaces were examined for smoothness and irregularities using a stereomicroscope at ×20 magnification. Their results indicated that the surface produced by multi-purpose bur was smoother and more uniplanar than that produced by the #5 fissure bur, but it was not significantly different from the surface produced by the Lindeman bur. There was less damage to the root with the multi-purpose bur as compared to either the #57 fissure or Lindeman burs. The resected root surface smoothness was improved when multi-fluted carbide was used while the ultra fine diamond tended to roughen the surface.

Many investigators[86–91] have studied or reported on the ex vivo and in vivo effects of the application of laser energy to perform root-end resections. Investigators[86] from the Tokyo Medical and Dental University in Japan reported the results of an ex vivo study using the Er:YAG laser for root-end resections. They reported that there was no smear layer or debris left on the resected root surfaces prepared using the Er:YAG laser. A smear layer and debris were left on the root surfaces of the group where the root end was prepared with a fissure bur.

Komori and associates[87] studied root ends resected with Er:YAG and the Ho:YAG lasers. They reported that the Er:YAG laser produced smooth, clean resected root surfaces free of any signs of thermal damage while the Ho:YAG laser produced signs of thermal damage to the cut root surface and large voids between the gutta-percha root canal filling and the root canal walls.

In an evaluation of the carbon dioxide (CO_2) laser, Moritz et al.[88] reported that the use of the CO_2 laser as an adjunct following root-end resection with a fissure bur resulted in decreased dentin permeability. The dentin permeability was measured by dye penetration, and sealing of dentinal tubules was determined by SEM examination. They concluded that the CO_2 laser treatment optimally prepared the resected root surface by sealing the dentinal tubules, eliminating the niches for bacterial growth and sterilizing the root surface.

The connective tissue healing response adjacent to the surface of dentin cut by a Nd:YAG laser was compared to dentin cut with a fissure bur by Maillet and associates.[89] Disks of human root dentin 3.5 mm thick were prepared by the two techniques and then implanted in the dorsal subcutaneous tissue of rats for 90 days. The disks and surrounding soft tissue were recovered at various periods of time. Using light microscopy, the tissue adjacent to the prepared dentin surfaces was assessed for inflammation and fibrous capsule thickness. The results indicated a statistically significant increase in inflammation and fibrous capsule thickness adjacent to the dentin surfaces cut with the Nd:YAG laser as compared to the surfaces cut with the fissure bur.

Reports on the clinical use of lasers for root-end resection is very limited. In a case report by Miserendino,[90] a CO_2 laser was used to perform a root-end resection and to sterilize the unfilled apical portion of the root canal space. He stated that the rationale for laser use were improved hemostasis which improves visualization of the operative field, potential to sterilize the contaminated root apex, a potential reduction in permeability of cut root surface dentin, reduction of postoperative pain, and a reduced risk of contamination of the surgical site through the elimination of a need for aerosol-producing air turbine handpieces. He concluded that the initial results of the clinical use of the CO_2 laser for endodontic periradicular surgery confirmed the previous ex vivo findings but that further clinical studies of the application of lasers for microsurgical procedures in endodontics is needed. Komori and associates[91] reported on 8 patients with 13 teeth in which the Er:YAG laser was used for root-end resections. All of the procedures were performed without the use of a hi- or slo-speed dental handpiece and even though the cutting speed of the laser was slightly slower than the use of burs, the advantages of the laser use included the absence of discomfort and vibrations, less chance for contamination of the surgical site, and reduced risk of trauma to adjacent tissue.

Regardless of the technique used for root-end resection, the cut root surface must be carefully examined for possible cracks, anatomical variations, and the adequacy of the orthograde obturating material.[11,57,92,93] Kim and Kratchman[11] noted that the only way that the anatomical detail of the resected root apex can be accurately assessed is with the operating microscope at a high power of magnification and the root end stained with methylene blue dye. In an ex vivo study,[92] cracks were artificially created in the root face of 50 maxillary central incisors after 3 mm was resected from the root end. The Orascope at a magnification of ×35 was found to be superior in identifying the cracks when compared to the operating microscope at ×10 power, loupes at ×3.3 power, and unaided/corrected vision. In another study,[93] a combination of different dyes, transillumination, and the operating microscope at ×8 power were used, and the best discrimination of cracks in the cut root surface was found with a combination of methylene blue dye, transillumination, and the operating microscope. All of the techniques and combinations were more effective than a random chance of detecting the cracks.

EXTENT OF THE ROOT-END RESECTION:

There is no agreement on how much of the root end should be resected.[11] The extent of root end resection will be related to what is to be accomplished with the surgical procedure and a number of variable factors that must be evaluated on an individual case-by-case basis.[57] There is no predetermined amount of root-end removal that will be appropriate for all clinical situations. Routinely removing the entire root end apical to the most coronal extent of the bony crypt is not valid.[57] In some instances, more of the root end may have to be sacrificed in order to visualize and gain access to roots and other structures that lie lingual to the root in question (Figure 28A,B,C,D). The shape of the root and the number and location of canals within the root may dictate the amount of root resection. When a root-end filling is required, enough of the root end must be resected so that the root-end filling material is surrounded by sound dentin. The amount to be resected may also be dictated by the location of perforation defects, ledges, separated instruments, and the apical extent of posts and orthograde obturating materials. The level of the crestal bone and the presence of periodontal defects will be major factors in determining how much root end can or should be resected. The conservation of root length should not compromise the goals of the surgical procedure.

ANGLE OF ROOT-END RESECTION

Historically, endodontic text books and other literature have recommended that the angle of root-end resections, when used in periradicular surgery, should be 30° to 45° from the long axis of the root facing toward the buccal or facial aspect of the root. The purpose for the angled root-end resections was to provide enhanced visibility to the resected root end and operative access to enable the surgeon to accomplish a root-end preparation with a bur in a slo-speed handpiece.[11,57,83,3,4,94–98] Kim and Kratchman[1] noted that there is no biological justification for creating a steep bevel on the resected root end. They noted that the steeper the bevel, the more potential there is for damage to the buccal supporting bone. In the past, the bevel was placed strictly for the convenience of the surgeon, but with modern microsurgical instruments and use of the surgical operating microscope, this need is no longer justified.[11,57]

Several authors[99–104] have presented evidence indicating that beveling of the root-end results in opening of dentinal tubules on the resected root surface that may communicate with the root canal space and result in apical leakage, even when a root-end filling has been placed. Ichesco and associates,[100] using a spectrophotometric analysis of dye penetration, concluded that the resected root end of an endodontically treated tooth exhibited more apical leakage than one without root-end resection. Beatty,[101] using a similar dye penetration analysis, examined apical leakage at different root-end resection angles. He reported that significantly more leakage occurred in those roots where the root-end filling did not extend into the prepared root-end preparation to the height of the bevel. If infection were to persist within the root canal system in an area not sealed by the root-end filling, the likelihood of bacteria and/or bacterial byproducts spreading outside of the root canal system is likely to occur.[102] In another study[27] using the fluid filtration method to determine leakage, it was found that there was a significant increase in leakage as the angle of the bevel increased.

Dye penetration was measured in another apical leakage study[105] using extracted teeth with root-end resections at 45° and 90° angles from the long axis of the root. There was a statistically significant increase in leakage extending to the root canal space through

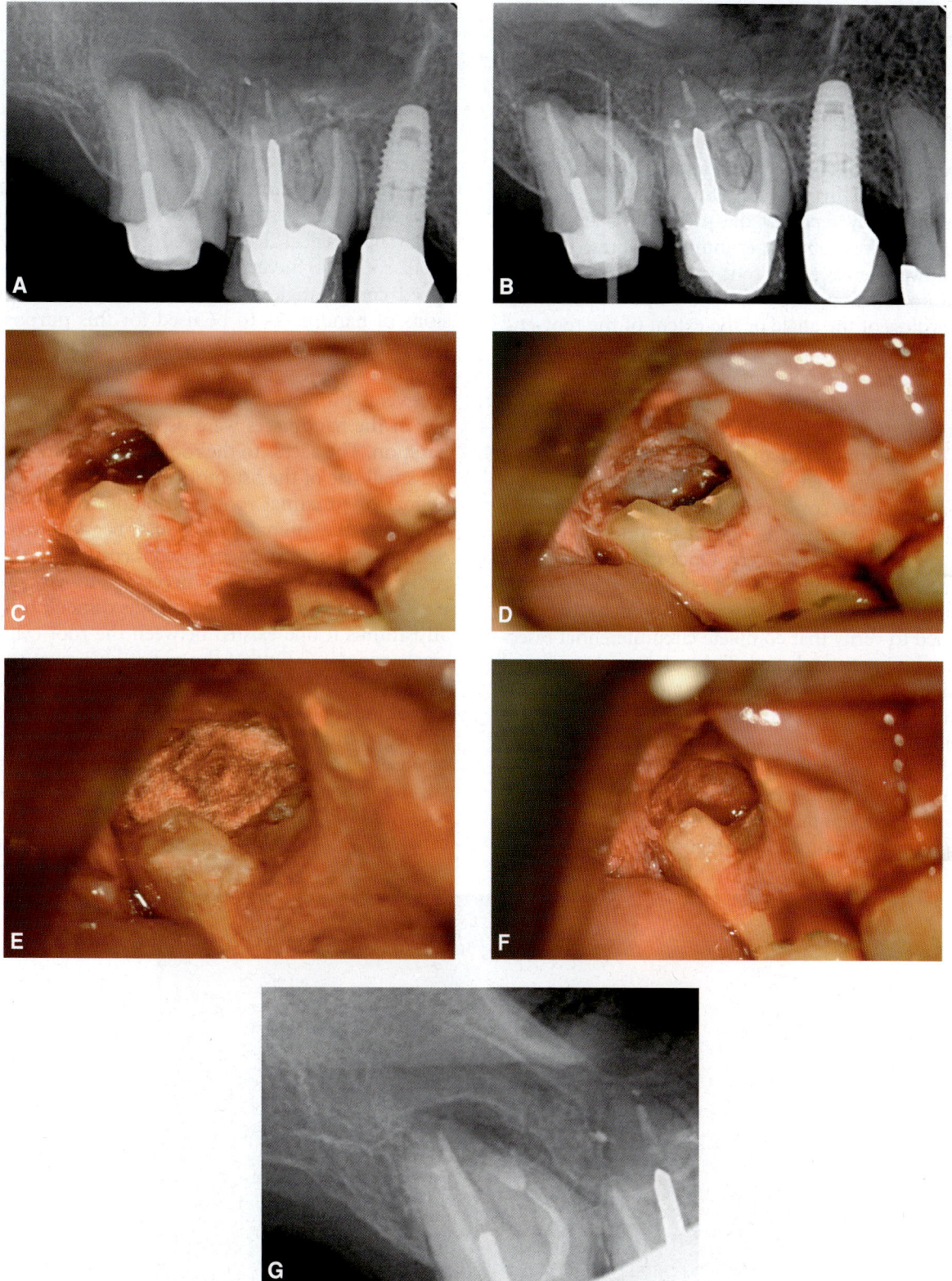

Figure 28 *A,* Pretreatment radiograph of a maxillary right second molar. Tooth was symptomatic with evidence of a large periapical radiolucency associated with the mesiobuccal and distobuccal root apices; *B,* Sinus tract traced with a gutta-percha point; *C,* Initial resection of both buccal root apicies exposing soft tissue lingual to the roots; *D,* Buccal roots resected further to expose the gutta-percha obturations and facilitate the removal of all the tissue lingual to the buccal roots; *E,* Root-end preparations in both buccal roots; *F,* Root-end preparations filled with Super-EBA cement; *G,* Radiograph with root-end fillings in place.

dentinal tubules in those teeth with 45° angled root-end resections as compared to those with 90° bevels. They concluded that by increasing the angle of the root-end resection, the number of exposed dentinal tubules would also increase. Tidmarsh and Arrowsmith[104] examined the root surface following root-end resections at angles between 45° and 60° approximately 3 mm from the root apex. Using scanning electron microscopy, they reported the presence of an average of 27,000 dentinal tubules per mm^2 on the resected root face midway between the root canal and the dentinocementum junction.

Regardless of the angle or the extent of the root-end resection, it is extremely important that the resection is complete and that no segment of root is left unresected. The potential for incomplete root end resection is especially high in cases where the root is broad in its labial-lingual dimension and where surgical access and visibility are impaired.[11,57] Carr and Bentkover[106] stated that failure to completely cut through a root in a buccal-lingual direction is one of the most common errors in periradicular surgery. Once the desired extent and bevel of root-end resection has been achieved, the face of the resected root surface should be carefully examined to verify that complete circumferential resection has been accomplished. This can be accomplished by using a fine, sharp explorer guided around the periphery of the resected root surface.[57] If complete resection is in doubt, a small amount of methylene blue dye can be applied to the root surface for 5 to 10 seconds. After the area is then irrigated with sterile saline, the periodontal ligament will appear dark blue, highlighting the root outline (Figure 29).

Root-End Preparation

The purpose of a root-end preparation in periradicular surgery is to create a space into which a root-end filling can be placed (see Figure 28E,F,G). Root-end preparations were originally made with sections of hand files held in hemostats or specially designed root-end preparation file holders.[107] The next procedure employed a small round but in straight, slo-speed handpiece. The procedure improved when a small round or inverted cone bur was used in a slo-speed contra-angle handpiece. The most recent versions of handpieces to be used for this purpose were the miniature surgical slo-speed contra-angle or the hi-speed with a pediatric size contra-angle head.[11,57]

Several problems were noted when rotary burs in any of the handpieces were used for the root-end preparation. The access to the root end was difficult due to the small size of the osteotomy, there was a high risk of lingual or proximal root perforation, only a minimal depth of the preparation could be achieved, more dentinal tubules were exposed because of the large root-end bevel that was necessary to visualize and perform the preparation, and it was difficult to remove an isthmus if one existed between the root canals in a single root.[11,108] One of the major objectives of a root end preparation is that it be placed parallel to the long axis of the root. It is rare that sufficient access is present to allow a bur in a contra angle or straight handpiece to be inserted down the long axis of a root. These preparations are almost always placed obliquely into the root and do not follow the direction of the root canal.[11,57,108–110] Mehlhaff et al.[109] found that the

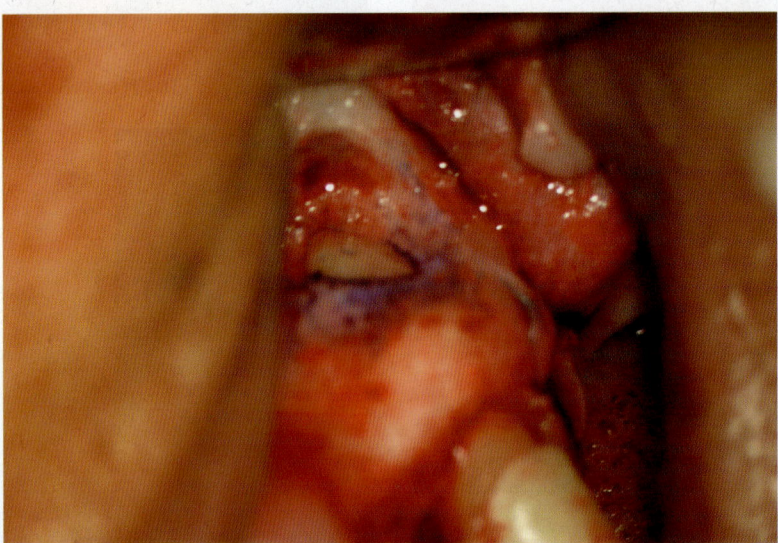

Figure 29 Methylene blue dye used to stain PDL of resected root end.

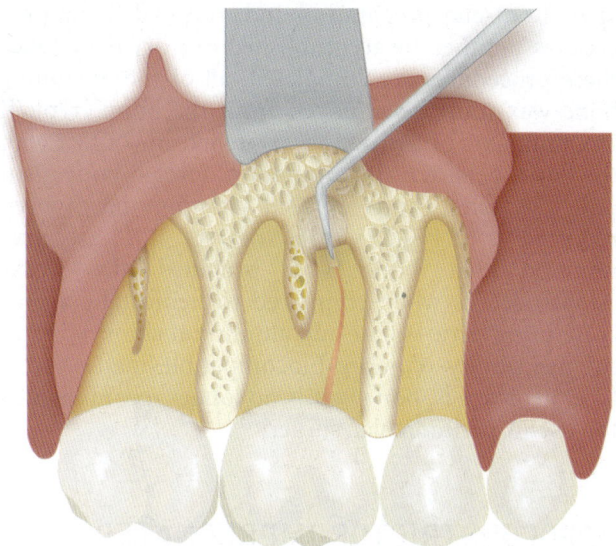

Figure 30 Ultrasonic root-end preparation illustration.

average root-end bevel required when using rotary burs was 35.1°. Two other studies[102,103] demonstrated that as the root-end bevel increased, the depth of leakage around the root-end filling also increased.

One of the most significant advances in periradicular surgery was the introduction of ultrasonic microsurgical tips for the root-end preparation (Figure 30). The need for creating severe root-end beveling was eliminated; the tip was able to stay centered in the root and follow the original root canal space thus decreasing the possibility of lingual or lateral root perforations and conserving a greater thickness of the remaining root canal wall; a smaller osteotomy was required to accommodate the ultrasonic tips; a deeper root-end preparation could be achieved; and less dentinal tubles were exposed decreasing the chances of leakage around the root-end filling material (Figure 31A,B).[11,102,108–112]

Several studies[110–114] have also reported that the root-end cavity is much cleaner when ultrasonic tip preparations are compared to bur preparations. Zuolo et al.[111] found the walls of the preparation were smoother, contained less debris and smear layer when the root-end preparation was accomplished with a smooth ultrasonic tip versus a diamond-coated tip. Diamond tips cut faster than noncoated tips but also create a larger preparation because of the diamond coating.[11] Newer zirconium tips create a smaller space because the zirconium nitride is processed into the metal thus making it narrower in diameter. A reported drawback to the zirconium tips is their inability to remove gutta-percha.[11] Navarre and Steiman[115] found that zirconium tips removed gutta-percha from the axial walls and created the apical preparation faster than stainless steel tips.

Controversy exists if microfractures are created in the dentin walls when ultrasonic tips are used to develop the root-end preparation.[108,116–122] In an ex vivo study using extracted teeth, Abedi et al.[116] found a significantly higher incidence of microfractures in root ends prepared with two ultrasonic units than those prepared with burs. In another study,[117] the highest incidence of microfractures occurred when the ultrasonic unit was used at a high setting. There were significantly fewer infractions when the unit was set at a medium setting. In a matched pair ex vivo study[118] where the ultrasonic energy was used at a low setting, no difference in crack formation was noted

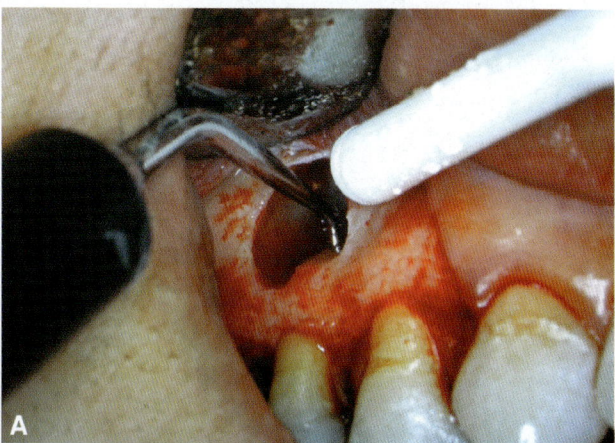
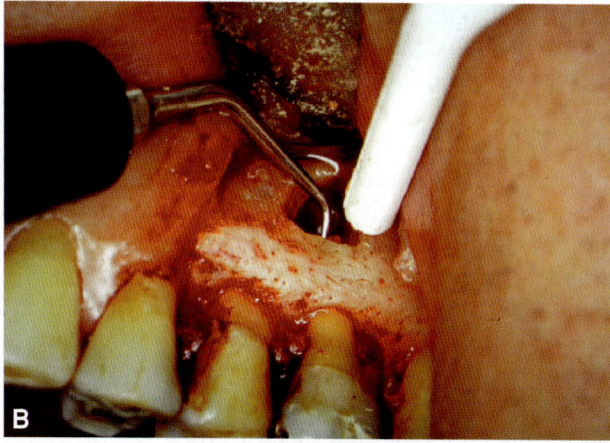

Figure 31 ***A,*** Ultrasonic tip used for root-end preparation on maxillary second premolar; ***B,*** Ultrasonic tip used for root-end preparation on mesiobuccal root of a maxillary first molar. Note how the ultrasonic tip in each case follows the long axis of the root being prepared.

from those root ends that had just received a root-end resection. The same group[119] also evaluated diamond-coated tips and found that their use did not result in significant root-end cracking. Rainwater et al.[120] also found no significant difference in microcrack formation between stainless steel and diamond tips used at low energy settings compared to preparations with a hi-speed #2 round bur. Calzonetti et al.[121] used cadaver specimens and found that the ultrasonic root-end preparations did not cause any microfractures. A clinical study[122] using human patients reported only one incomplete canal fracture in 25 teeth treated with both stainless steel and diamond-coated tips using the lowest ultrasonic unit energy setting, water spray and a light touch.

Topical/Local Hemostasis

Good visualization of the surgical field and of the resected root surface is essential in determining the optimum placement of the root-end preparation. The ability to visualize the fine detail of the anatomy on the resected root surface is dependent upon obtaining hemostasis within the bony crypt to provide a clean, dry surgical site.[123] Hemostasis provided by the presurgical local anesthetic solutions and vasoconstrictors was discussed earlier in this chapter, and their importance cannot be overemphasized. Frequently there is the need for additional hemostasis within the bony surgical site once the crypt has been curetted and the root end resected. The type of hemostasis required in this area is best achieved by using a variety of topical hemostatic agents.[13,11,123–135] Ideally, these hemostatic agents should be placed into contact with the bone after root-end resection and prior to the root-end preparation and filling.[3] These topical hemostatic agents have been broadly classified as either non-collagen-based or collagen-based agents.[123]

BONE WAX

Bone wax was introduced as a hemostatic agent by Horsley in 1892.[11,124] It is a nonresorbable material composed of approximately 88% highly purified beeswax and 12% isopropyl palmitate. The latter acts as a softening and conditioning agent.[11,123,125] It plugs the vascular openings by a mechanical or tamponade mechanism of action when it is packed firmly into contact with the bone surface. It does not have any effect on the blood clotting mechanism.[11,125]

When using bone wax the entire bony crypt is filled with the material under firm pressure. The excess wax is then removed with a curette to expose the root apex. Root-end preparation and root-end filling procedures can then be accomplished in a dry field. Once these procedures are completed, all of the remaining bone wax must be removed from the bony crypt. If any remnants of the bone wax are left in contact with the bone, persistent inflammation, foreign body giant cell reactions, and delayed healing have been reported.[11,123,125–128] von Arx et al.[129] recently reported that bone wax provided the weakest hemostasis when compared to hemostatic agents containing ferric sulfate and aluminum chloride. With the availability of more biocompatible materials for local hemostasis, bone wax is no longer recommended for use in periradicular surgery.[3,11,123,126]

VASOCONSTRICTOR-IMPREGNATED COTTON PELLETS/SPONGES

Vasoconstrictors have been recommended as topical agents for hemorrhage control during periradicular surgery. Of these agents, epinephrine has been shown to be the most effective and the most often recommended.[3,11] Cotton pellets containing racemic epinephrine hydrochloride (Epidri, Racellet, and Radri) are available commercially (Figure 32). The amount of epinephrine hydrochloride in each pellet varies. For example, each Epidri pellet contains an average of 1.9 mg of racemic epinephrine. Each Racellet #2 pellet contains an average of 1.15 mg and each Racellet #3 pellet contains an average of 0.55 mg of epinephrine. Radri pellets contain a combination of a vasoconstrictor and an astringent. Each Radri pellet contains an

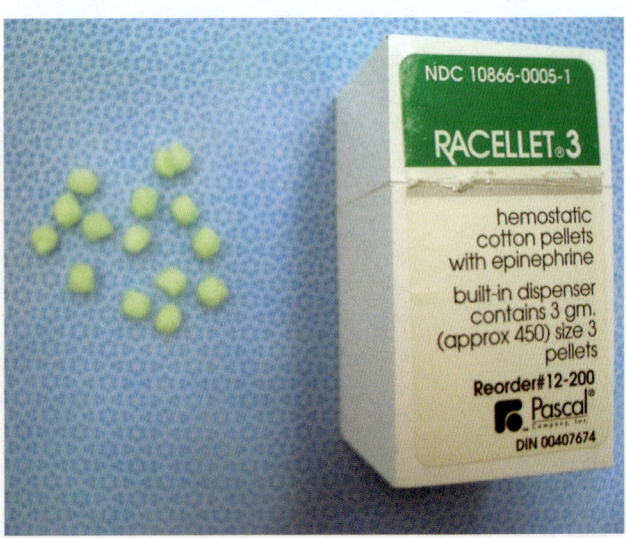

Figure 32 Racellet container and pellets.

average of 0.45 mg of epinephrine hydrochloride and an average of 1.85 mg of zinc phenol sulfonate.[11]

An impregnated pellet is placed into the bony crypt. Additional non-impregnated pellets are then placed on top of the first pellet and held under pressure for 2 to 4 minutes (see Figure 28E). All of the non-impregnated pellets are then removed, and the site is evaluated to determine if adequate hemostasis has been obtained. The process is repeated until hemostasis is achieved (see Figure 23). Once a dry field is obtained, the required root-end procedures can be performed. The impregnated pellets work both by mechanical and chemical actions. The pressure provides the mechanical action, and the epinephrine hydrochloride provides the chemical effect by causing immediate, local vasoconstriction of the blood vessels. The epinephrine hydrochloride acts on the α-1 receptors in the blood vessel wall to cause the vasoconstriction. The blood vessel wall contains approximately 95% α receptors and 5% β receptors.[11] In a study[130] of 39 ASA type I or II patients, #3 Racellet pellets were compared to 20% ferric chloride for adequacy of providing local hemostasis during periradicular surgery. Both methods were found to be equally effective in providing hemostasis. Another study[131] found that in only 1 of 42 patients was there a failure to achieve local hemostasis when collagen pellets soaked with 2.25% epinephrine were used for local hemostasis. This compared to 5 of 6 cases where local hemostasis was not achieved when the collagen pellets were soaked with saline.

There are two areas of concern when using epinephrine-impregnated cotton pellets for topical hemostasis. The first is the potential for leaving cotton fibers in the surgical site and the second is the possible effect topical epinephrine hypochloride might have on the patient's cardiovascular system. Gutmann and Harrison[3] state that loose cotton fibers left in the surgical site may affect the root-end seal by becoming trapped between the root-end cavity preparation and the root-end filling material. They also note that cotton fibers may serve as foreign bodies in the surgical site and result in impaired or delayed wound healing. Sterile Telfa pads or collagen sponges cut into small squares and saturated with epinephrine hydrochloride can be placed into and easily adapted to the shape of the crypt. They may be used in the place of the cotton products as they contain no loose fibers.[3,131]

The concern about the topical use of epinephrine in periradicular surgical procedures causing systemic cardiovascular changes has been addressed by several studies.[130–132] Besner[132] reported that the pulse rate of the patient did not change when a #2 Racellet pellet containing an average of 1.15 mg of epinephrine hydrochloride was used during periradicular surgery. This finding was confirmed in another study[130] where 1 to 7 #3 Racellet pellets (average of 0.55 mg epinephrine hydrochloride per pellet) were left in place for 2 to 4 minutes. The blood pressure and pulse rate taken at five different intervals in 39 patients treated in this study did not vary significantly at any of the evaluation points. Vy et al.[131] also found that the blood pressure and pulse rate did not change in 42 patients where collagen sponges were saturated with 2.25% racemic epinephrine and used for local hemostasis during periradicular surgery. Kim and Kratchman[11] state that when epinephrine is used topically it causes immediate local vasoconstriction; therefore, there is little absorption into the systemic circulation, reducing the chance of having an effect on the cardiovascular system.

FERRIC SULFATE

Ferric sulfate is a chemical that has been used as a hemostatic agent since it was first introduced as Monsel's solution (20% ferric subsulfate) in 1857.[11] It is a necrotizing agent with an extremely low pH (0.8 to 1.6).[123] Its mode of action results from a chemical reaction of blood with the iron and sulfate ions to form an agglutination of blood proteins. The coagulum that is formed plugs the capillary openings to create the resulting hemostasis.[11,123]

Ferric sulfate is directly applied to the bone surface with hemostasis being achieved almost immediately. This agent is known to be cytotoxic and if not completely removed from the bone surface at the end of the procedure will result in severe inflammation and delayed healing of the surgical site.[11,123,133,134] Lemon and associates,[133] using standardized osseous defects created in rabbit mandibles, reported a significant adverse effect on osseous healing when ferric sulfate was left in situ for the duration of the experiment. In a follow-up study[134] using the same rabbit model, there was no significant difference in healing between the experimental and untreated control groups when the surgical site was curetted and irrigated with saline following a 5 minute application of ferric sulfate. The surgical site was then thoroughly curetted and irrigated with sterile saline with the result being that there was no significant difference in osseous healing between this experimental group and the untreated controls. Ferric sulfate solutions appear to be safe hemostatic agents as long as they are used in limited quantities, and care is taken to thoroughly remove them from the surgical site prior to suturing.[11,123,134,135]

THROMBIN

Topical thrombin was developed to provide hemostasis when wounds are oozing blood from small capillaries and venules. Thrombin acts to initiate the extrinsic and intrinsic clotting pathways and acts rapidly to clot blood fibrinogen directly.[11] It is designed only for topical application and may be life threatening if injected. Topical thrombin has been investigated as a hemostatic agent in abating bleeding in cancellous bone. While there was less bleeding than the control, thrombin was less effective than other topical hemostatic agents.[123] Even though topical thrombin has been used successfully in neurosurgery, cardiovascular surgery, and burn surgery, it is not being used in conjunction with periradicular surgery at this time. The main disadvantages in using the topical thrombin powder are difficult handling characteristics and high cost.[11,123]

CALCIUM SULFATE

Even though calcium sulfate (plaster of Paris) has been used primarily in dentistry to fill large surgical bone defects, as a barrier material in guided tissue regenerative procedures and repair of furcation defects, it can also be used for hemostasis during periradicular surgery.[136,137] It is a resorbable material that consists of powder and liquid components which can be mixed into a thick putty-like consistency and placed in the bony crypt using wet cotton pellets to press it against the walls. The mechanism of action is similar to bone wax in that it acts as a mechanical barrier to plug the vascular channels. In contrast to bone wax, calcium sulfate is biocompatible, completely resorbs in 2 to 4 weeks, and does not cause a long-term inflammatory response. It also has the advantage of being relatively inexpensive.[137]

GELFOAM AND SPONGOSTAN

Gelfoam and Spongostan are gelatin-based sponges that are water insoluble and biologically resorbable.[123,125,137] They are made of purified animal skin and become soft on contact with blood.[135] Gelatin sponges are thought to act intrinsically by promoting the disintegration of platelets with the subsequent release of thromboplastin and plastin. This, in turn, stimulates the formation of thrombin and supports fibrin strands infiltration of the interstices of the sponge.[123,125,137]

When these gelatin-based sponges are used to control bleeding during periradicular surgery, they swell and form a soft, gelatinous mass. This swollen, soft gelatinous mass may visually obscure the surgical site making it difficult to complete the root-end preparation and root-end filling procedures. Because they become so soft, it is difficult to put pressure on the sponges without displacing them with the result being a continuation of bleeding. The primary use for gelatin-based sponges in periradicular surgery is placement into the bony crypt, after root-end resection and root-end filling have been completed, just prior to wound closure. Because they promote the formation of thrombin, they may be beneficial in the initial stages of clot formation.

Gelatin-based sponge material left in situ may result in a decrease in the osseous healing rate, but the inflammatory response seems to be minimal. The net result is a material that is totally resorbed and well tolerated by the surrounding tissues.[123] The study by Ibarrola et al.[125] compared the response of rat tibias to bone wax, Surgicel and Gelfoam. They found the best histological response was obtained in those sites where Gelfoam was used. At the end of the 120-day experiment, the Gelfoam was usually completely resorbed, and healing of the bone defects was complete. Other studies[138,139] have reported on the use of Gelfoam in extraction sockets and the results have been varied. The Ibarrola study most closely relates to the type of clinical situation that would be encountered in periradicular surgery.

COLLAGEN PRODUCTS

Collagen-based products consist primarily of collagen of differing microstructures and densities and have been used extensively as surgical hemostatic agents. These products are believed to have four principal mechanisms of action involved in hemostasis: (1) stimulation of platelet adhesion, aggregation, and release; (2) activation of Factor VIII (Hageman Factor); (3) mechanical tamponade action; and (4) the release of serotonin.[123,135,140–143] The collagen used for surgical hemostasis is obtained from bovine sources and is supplied in sheets and sponge pads. Both forms are applied dry, directly to the bleeding site while using pressure. Hemostasis is usually achieved in 2 to 5 minutes.[137]

MICROFIBRILLAR COLLAGEN HEMOSTAT

Avitene and Instat are two popular forms of microfibrillar collagen. These products are derived from purified bovine dermal collagen, which is shredded into fibrils and then converted into a fine powder as an insoluble partial hydrochloric acid salt. They provide topical hemostasis by forming a collagen framework for platelet adhesion. This process initiates platelet aggregation and adhesion with the result being the formation of a platelet plug.[123,135] Haasch et al.[144] reported on their potential use in periradicular surgery. Another study,[145] using Avitene, found that new bone formation proceeded uneventfully without a foreign body reaction to the material.

The handling characteristics of these microfibrillar collagen products are not ideal. The materials have an affinity for wet surfaces and as such readily adhere to instruments and gloves. It has been recommended that they be applied to the surgical site using a spray technique that allows direct application of the agents to the bleeding points.[146] Other disadvantages of these products include being inactivated by autoclaving, increasing the chance of infection when used in contaminated wounds, and being much more expensive compared to other topical hemostatic agents.[137]

SURGICEL

Surgicel is a material that resembles surgical gauze and is prepared by the oxidation of regenerated α-cellulose (oxycellulose).[123,125] The preparation is spun into threads and then woven into gauze that is chemically sterilized with formaldehyde. Its mode of action is principally mechanical as it does not have an affect on the clotting cascade.[123,125] When the gauze is initially placed into contact with surgical site it acts as a physical barrier to any bleeding points. As blood becomes entrapped in the gauze, the mixture becomes tacky and forms an artificial coagulum or plug to provide hemostasis.[123,125]

In an animal study[125] that compared the osseous response of three different hemostatic agents, Surgicel, when left in situ, retarded the rate of healing and caused the most intense inflammatory reaction of any of the materials. The same study also noted that due to the difficulty in removing all of the Surgicel from bony wounds, the small fragments left behind resulted in a prolonged inflammatory response and foreign body reaction. The implantation of Surgicel into a surgical wound is not recommended.[123,125]

ROOT-END FILLING MATERIALS

The purpose of a root-end filling is to establish a seal between the root canal space and the periradicular tissues. An ideal root-end filling material should be (1) able to prevent leakage of bacteria and their byproducts into the periradicular tissues, (2) non-toxic, (3) non-carcinogenic, (4) biocompatible with the host tissues, (5) insoluble in tissue fluids, (6) dimensionally stable, (7) unaffected by moisture during setting, (8) easy to use, (9) radiopaque, (10) nonstaining, and (11) bioinductive (promote cementogenesis).[147] Numerous materials have been suggested for use as root-end fillings including gutta-percha, amalgam, Cavit, intermediate restorative material (IRM), Super-EBA, Diaket (Figure 33A,B,C), glass ionomers, composite resins,

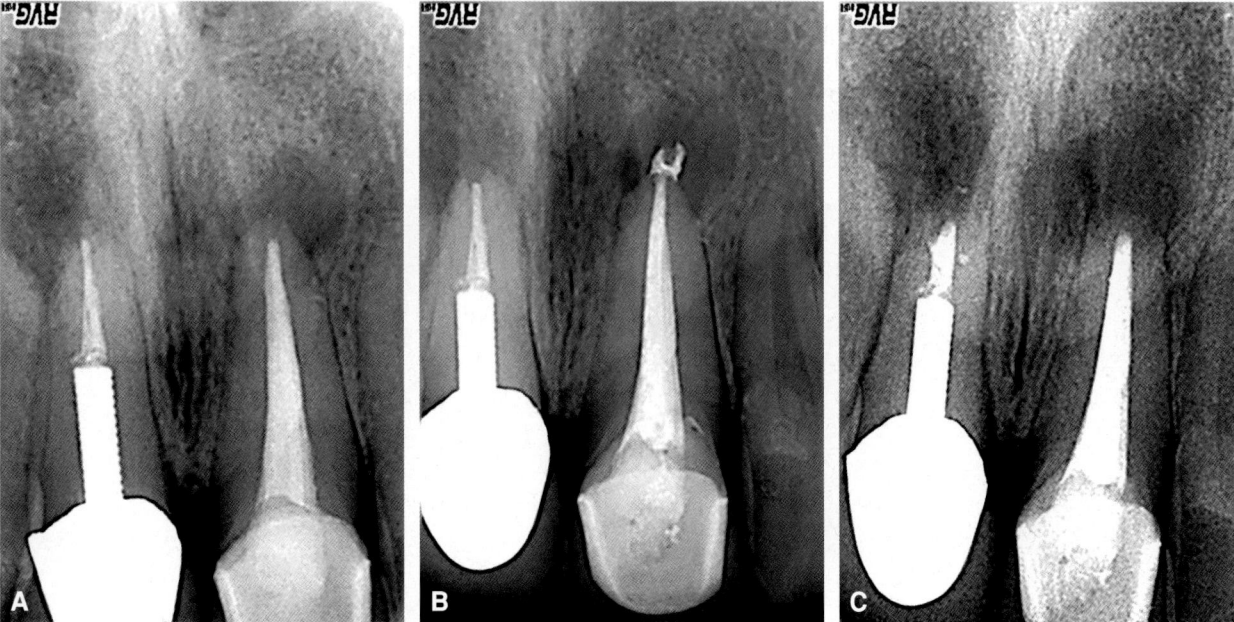

Figure 33 *A,* Preop digital radiograph showing apical radiolucencies on both maxillary central incisors. *B,* Postop digital radiograph after nonsurgical retreatment on the maxillary left central incisor. *C,* Postop digital radiograph demonstrating root-end resections on both teeth and Diaket root-end filling on the right central incisor.

carboxylate cements, zinc phosphate cements, zinc oxide eugenol cements, and mineral trioxide aggregate (MTA). The suitability of these various materials has been tested by evaluating their microleakage (dye, radioisotope, bacterial penetration, and fluid filtration), marginal adaptation, cytotoxicity, and clinical testing in experimental animals and humans.

A large number of in vitro studies dealing with the marginal adaptation and sealing ability (leakage) of various root-end filling materials have been published. The results of these studies have often been inconsistent, contradictory and confusing, and have been questioned as to their clinical relevance. Factors such as the choice of storage solutions, the molecular size of the dye particles, and other variables can influence the outcome of in vitro studies.[148]

In vitro cytotoxicity and biocompatibility studies using cell cultures have also been published. Owadally and associates reported on an in vitro antibacterial and cytotoxicity study comparing IRM and amalgam. Their results indicated that IRM was significantly more antibacterial than amalgam at all time periods of exposure, and amalgam was significantly more cytotoxic than IRM.[149] Makkawy et al. evaluated the cytotoxicity of resin-reinforced glass ionomer cements compared to amalgam using human periodontal ligament cells. Their results indicated that at 24 hours amalgam significantly inhibited cell viability as compared to resin-reinforced glass ionomer cement and the controls. At 48 and 72 hours, however, all materials tested exhibited a similar slightly inhibitory effect on cell viability.[150] Chong et al. compared the cytotoxicity of a glass ionomer cement (Vitrebond), Kalzinol, IRM and EBA cements, and amalgam. Their results indicated that fresh IRM cement exhibited the most pronounced cytotoxic effect of all materials tested. Aged Kalzinol was the second most cytotoxic material with no significant difference being reported between Vitrebond, EBA cement and amalgam.[151]

Zhu, Safavi, and Spangberg evaluated the cytotoxicity of amalgam, IRM, and Super-EBA cements in cultures of human periodontal ligament cells and human osteoblast-like cells. Their results indicated that amalgam was the most cytotoxic of the materials tested and showed a reduction in total cell numbers for both cell types. IRM and Super-EBA, however, were significantly less cytotoxic than amalgam and demonstrated no reduction in total cell numbers for both periodontal ligament and osteoblast-like cells (Figure 34A,B).[152]

Several authors have published results of in vivo tissue compatibility studies of various root-end filling materials using an experimental animal model. Harrison and Johnson reported on a study designed to determine the excisional wound healing responses of the periradicular tissues to IRM, amalgam, and gutta-percha using a dog model. Healing responses were evaluated microscopically and radiographically at 10 and 45 days postsurgically. They reported no evidence of inhibition of dentoalveolar or osseous wound healing associated with amalgam, gutta-percha, or IRM. Statistical analysis showed no difference in wound healing between the three materials tested.[153]

Pitt Ford, Andreasen et al. examined the effects of IRM, Super-EBA, and amalgam as root-end filling materials in the roots of mandibular molars of monkeys.

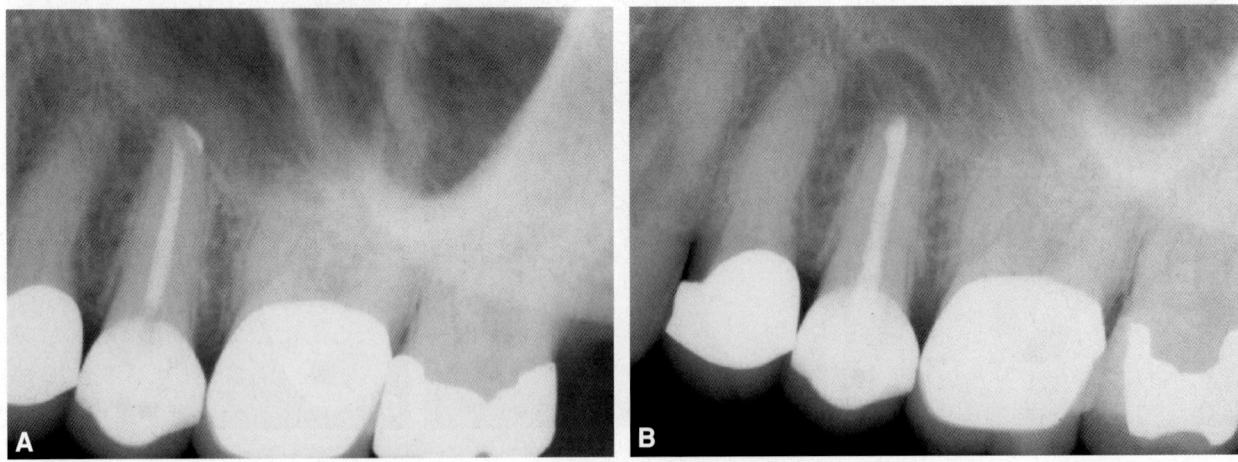

Figure 34 ***A,*** Preop digital image of maxillary premolar following nonsurgical retreatment; lesion still persists after one year. ***B,*** Postop digital image following curettage, root-end resection, and root-end filling with Super-EBA.

They reported that the tissue response to IRM and Super-EBA was less severe than that to amalgam. No inflammation was evident in the bone marrow spaces adjacent to root-end fillings of IRM and Super-EBA. In contrast, however, inflammation was present in the alveolar bone marrow spaces with every root end filled with amalgam.[154,155]

Maeda et al. reported the results of a histological study comparing the effects of various root-end filling materials including a 4-META-TBB resin (C&B Metabond) using a rat model. The materials tested were amalgam, light-cured glass ionomer cement, IRM, a 4-META-TBB resin, and light-cured composite resin. The 4-META-TBB resin and light-cured composite resin root-end fillings showed the most favorable histological response among the materials tested. These materials did not provoke inflammation and did not appear to inhibit new bone formation as seen with the other materials.[156]

Torabinejad and others developed MTA (ProRoot) at Loma Linda University. The main molecules present in MTA are calcium and phosphorous ions, derived primarily from tricalcium silicate, tricalcium aluminate, tricalcium oxide, and silicate oxide. Its pH, when set, is 12.5 and its setting time is 2 hours and 45 minutes. The compressive strength of MTA is reported to be 40 MPa immediately after setting and increases to 70 MPa after 21 days. The results of solubility testing of MTA (ADA specification #30) indicated an insignificant weight loss following testing.[157]

Another study by Torabinejad et al. was designed to examine and compare the tissue reaction to several commonly used root-end filling materials and MTA. Their study involved the implantation of amalgam, IRM, Super-EBA, and MTA in the tibias and mandibles of guinea pigs. The presence of inflammation, predominant cell type, and thickness of fibrous connective tissue adjacent to each implanted material were evaluated. The tissue reaction to implanted MTA was the most favorable observed at both implantation sites; in every specimen, it was free of inflammation. MTA was also the material most often observed with direct bone apposition (Figure 35A,B).[158]

MTA has been extensively evaluated for microleakage (dye penetration, fluid filtration, and bacterial leakage), marginal adaptation (SEM), and biocompatibility (cytotoxicity, tissue implantation, and in vivo animal histology). The sealing ability of MTA has been shown to be superior to that of Super-EBA and was not adversely affected by blood contamination. Its marginal adaptation was shown to be better than amalgam, IRM, or Super-EBA. MTA has also been shown to be less cytotoxic than amalgam, IRM, or Super-EBA. Animal usage tests in which MTA and other commonly used root-end filling material were compared have resulted in less observed inflammation and better healing with MTA. In addition, with MTA, new cementum was observed being deposited on the surface of the material.[159–170]

Many prospective and retrospective human clinical usage studies have been reported assessing the outcome of periradicular surgery involving the placement of various root-end filling materials. It is difficult to compare the results of these studies because the authors have used differing evaluation criteria and observations periods. It is important, however, to

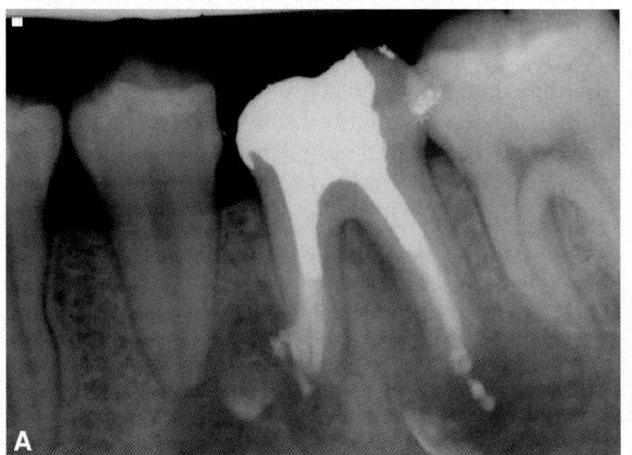 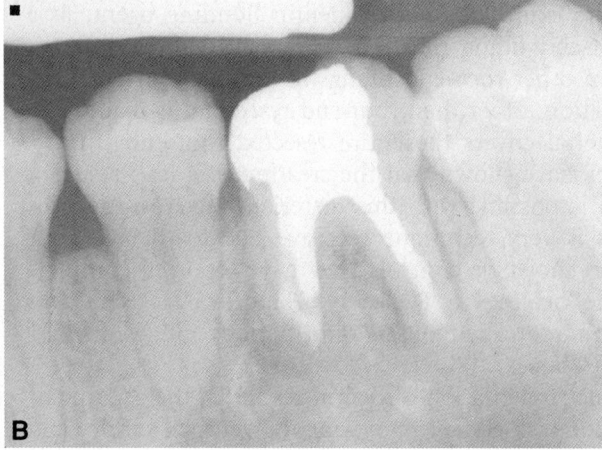

Figure 35 *A,* Preop digital image of mandibular molar following nonsurgical retreatment; extrusion of filling material occurred on both roots. *B,* Postop digital image following curettage, root-end resection, and root-end fillings with MTA.

consider some of the more significant of these clinical usage reports.

In 1978, Oynick and Oynick reported on the clinical use of a resin and silicone reinforced zinc oxide and eugenol cement (Stailine Super-EBA, Staines, England) as a root-end filling material in 200 cases over a period of 14 years. Radiographic evaluations following periradicular surgical procedures using Stailine indicated favorable healing. Histological and SEM evaluations of the root apex and adjacent periradicular bone, taken by block section, revealed newly formed bone in areas of previous resorption and collagen fibers growing into the filling material.[171]

Dorn and Gartner reported on a retrospective study of 488 periradicular surgical treatments in which three different root-end filling materials were used, IRM, Super-EBA, and amalgam. The evaluation period was from 6 months to 10 years. Outcomes assessment was conducted by evaluation of the most recent recall radiograph as compared to the immediate postsurgical radiograph. Analysis of the data indicated there was no significant difference in the outcome of healing rates between IRM and Super-EBA. There was a significant difference, however, in the outcome between IRM, Super-EBA, and amalgam, the latter being the worst.[172] Pantschev and associates, however, reported on a prospective clinical study evaluating the outcome of periradicular surgical procedures using either EBA cement or amalgam. The minimum evaluation period was 3 years, and healing was based on clinical and radiographic analysis. Their data indicated no significant difference in the outcome between the two materials evaluated.[173]

Rud et al. have reported on several prospective and retrospective human usage studies in an attempt to evaluate the acceptability of a composite resin (Retroplast), combined with a dentin bonding agent, as a root-end filling material. The placement is different from other root-end fillings in that no root-end preparation, other than root-end resection, is made. The material covers the entire resected root-end surface. They have shown that the creation of a leak-resistant seal is possible with this material; however, the process is very technique sensitive due to the need for strict moisture control. They have reported complete bone healing in 80% to 92% of cases using this technique. Their observation periods ranged from 1 to 9 years.[174-178]

Instrumentation of dentin results in the accumulation of a smear layer covering the dentinal surface and occluding the dentinal tubules. It has been shown that bacteria may colonize in the smear layer and penetrate the dentinal tubules.[179] Removal of this smear layer seems desirable in the situation of root-end fillings that are placed in a bacterially contaminated root apex. Irrigation with tetracycline has been shown to remove the smear layer.[180] Smear layer removal from resected root ends and dentin demineralization by citric acid has been shown to be associated with more rapid healing and deposition of cementum on the resected root end.[181]

Tetracyclines have a number of properties of interest to endodontists; they are antimicrobial agents, effective against periodontal pathogens, they bind strongly to dentin, and when released are still biologically active. Root surfaces exposed to anaerobic bacteria accumulate endotoxin and exhibit collagen loss, which may suppress fibroblast migration and proliferation, thus interfering with healing. Root surface conditioning with acidic agents, such as tetracycline, not only removes the smear layer but it also removes endotoxin from contaminated root surfaces.[182] Barkhordar and Russel reported on an in vitro study that examined the effect of irrigation with doxycycline hydrochloride, a hydroxy derivative of tetracycline, on the sealing ability of IRM and amalgam when used as root-end fillings. Their results indicated significantly less microleakage following irrigation with doxycycline involving both IRM and amalgam compared to the control irrigation with saline. They also suggested that, due to the long-lasting substantivity of doxycycline on root surfaces and its slow release in a biologically active state, their results support its use for dentin conditioning prior to placement of a root-end filling in periradicular surgery.[183]

Based on a review of the currently available literature, there does not appear to be an "ideal" root-end filling material. MTA appears to be the currently available material that most closely meets the requirements, both physical and biological, for a root-end filling material, especially due to its regenerative potential. Its primary disadvantage is its handling characteristics, and multiple devices have been designed to assist in its delivery. In a 2003 prospective human clinical trial, Chong, Pitt-Ford, and Hudson demonstrated a high success rate with MTA over a 2-year period. Retroplast appears to be a "second-best" root-end material but is not yet available in the United States.[184]

The method for placement of the root-end filling material will vary depending on the type of filling material used. Amalgam may be carried to the root-end preparation with a small K-G carrier that is sized for root-end preparations. Deeper lying apices may be more easily reached by using a messing gun. Zinc oxide–eugenol cements (IRM and Super-EBA) are best mixed to a thick clay-like consistency, shaped into a small cone, and attached to the back side of a spoon excavator or the tip of a plastic instrument or Hollenback carver and placed into the root-end preparation.

MTA is a unique root-end filling material with physical properties much different than other materials. It is a very fine, gray colored powder that is mixed with a sterile liquid, such as saline or local anesthetic solution, on a sterile glass slab. It cannot be mixed to a clay-like consistency, similar to IRM or Super-EBA, because, as more powder is added to the liquid, the mix becomes dry and crumbly. If the mix is too wet, it is runny and very difficult to handle due to its lack of form. The surgical area must be kept very dry during its placement, and care must be taken not to wash out the filling material by irrigation prior to closure of the soft tissue. The setting time of MTA is 2.5 to 3 hours. Properly mixed, MTA should be free of excess moisture, firm, but not crumbly. It can be delivered to the root-end preparation by placing a small amount on the backside of a small spoon excavator or by using a small amalgam-type carrier or the MAP system (Roydent), a micro-apical placement system very similar to a miniature messing gun (Figure 36 & 37). Recently introduced is white MTA with less potential for staining;

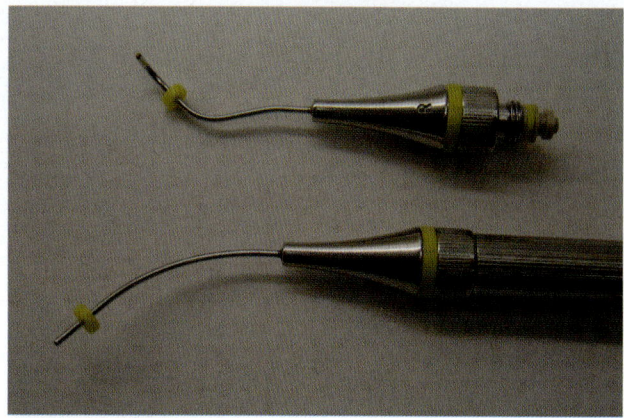

Figure 37 Microapical placement carriers used for placement of mineral trioxide aggregate into root-end preparations.

most of the research suggests that the gray and white have similar properties.[185]

Root-end preparations using ultrasonic tips tend to be smaller in diameter and extend deeper into the root canal than those prepared with a bur. As a result, the need for specially designed root-end filling condensers has resulted in their availability from many different manufactures in various styles and shapes. It is important that the endodontic surgeon becomes familiar with the different shapes and styles of condensers to enable one to properly condense the root-end filling material to the full extent of the root-end preparation. The condenser should be small enough in diameter that it does not bind on the walls of the root-end preparation during condensation, resulting in the possibility of root-end fractures. It is also important that the condenser is long enough to properly condense the filling material into the deepest part of the root-end preparation.

Various techniques have been advocated for finishing root-end fillings in periradicular surgery. Fitzpatrick and Steiman reported on an in vitro study designed to evaluate the marginal interfaces between the dentin and root-end fillings of IRM and Super-EBA. Following placement of the root-end fillings, they were finished by either burnishing with a ball burnisher, a moistened cotton pellet, or with a carbide-finishing bur in a high speed handpiece with air/water spray. Their results indicated that root-end fillings finished with a finishing bur displayed significantly better marginal adaptation, with little evidence of flash, when compared to the other methods (Figure 38). There was no significant

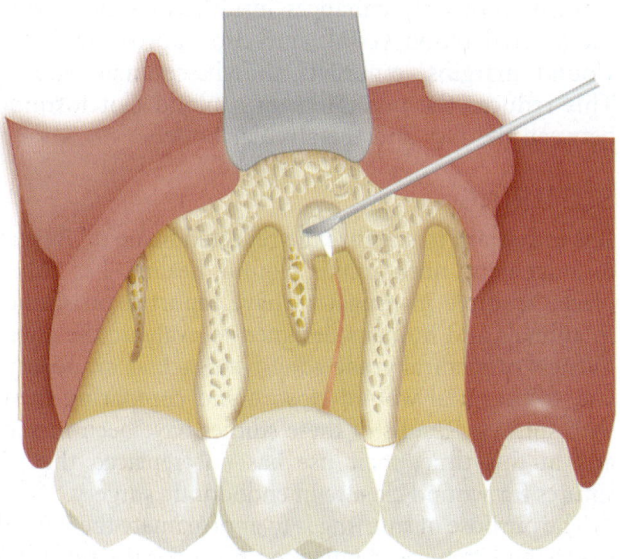

Figure 36 Placement of root-end filling material into preparation.

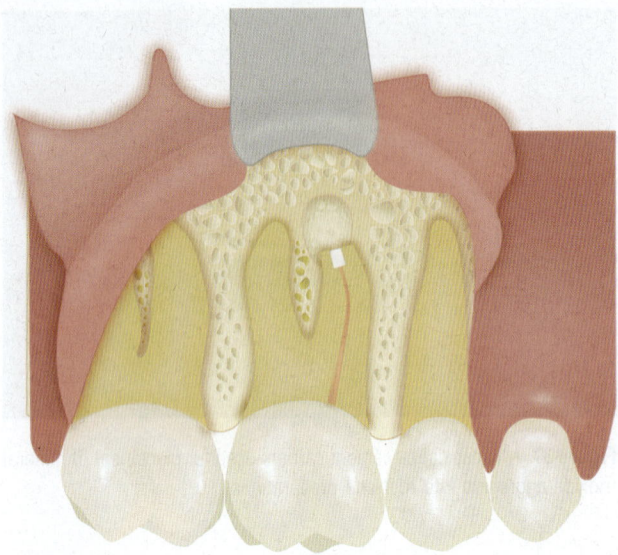

Figure 38 Root-end preparation filled with root-end filling material.

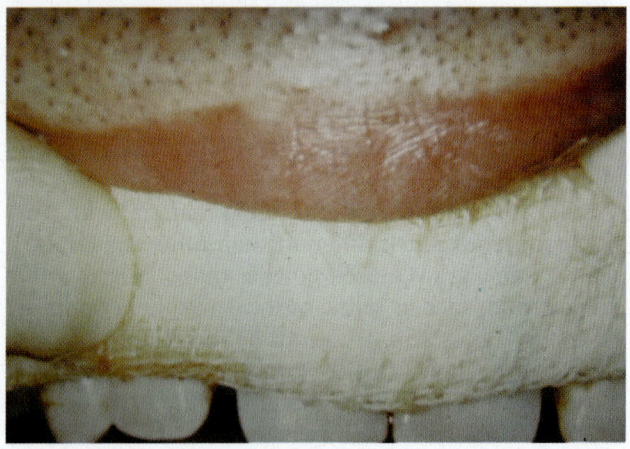

Figure 39 Gauze sponge moistened with saline and applied to flap both before and after suturing.

difference between the other finishing techniques or between the materials tested.[186]

Forte and associates reported on an in vitro study designed to compare microleakage, by the fluid filtration method, of root-end fillings of Super-EBA either unfinished or finished with a 30-flute high speed finishing bur. Their results indicated no significant difference in microleakage after 180 days between root-end fillings of Super-EBA, finished or unfinished.[187]

Soft Tissue Management, Suturing, and Postoperative Care

After final inspection of the root-end filling and removal of all visible excess filling material and any surgical packing, a radiograph should be taken to evaluate the placement of the root-end filling and to check for the presence of any root fragments or excess root-end filling material. Thorough examination of the underside of the flap and in the depth of the fold between the mucoperiosteum and the alveolar bone should be done prior to repositioning the flap in order to remove any debris or foreign material that may be present. The final steps in the periradicular surgical procedure are wound closure and soft tissue stabilization.

REPOSITIONING AND COMPRESSION

The elevated mucoperiosteal tissue should be gently replaced to its original position with the incision lines approximated as closely as possible. The type of flap design will affect the ease of repositioning, with full mucoperiosteal flaps generally providing less resistance to repositioning than limited mucoperiosteal flaps. Using surgical gauze, slightly moistened with sterile saline, gentle but firm pressure should be applied to the flapped tissue for 2 to 3 minutes (5 minutes for palatal tissue) prior to suturing (Figure 39). Tissue compression, both before and after suturing, not only enhances intravascular clotting in the severed blood vessels but also approximates the wound margins, especially the dissectional wound. This reduces the possibility of a blood clot forming between the flap and the alveolar bone.

SUTURING

It is important to stabilize the reflected tissue to prevent dislodgement until initial wound healing has taken place. Multiple investigators have reported on studies in animals and humans designed to evaluate the effectiveness of medical grade adhesives, such as cyanoacrylate, for surgical wound closure and comparing them with sutures. Results of these studies have been mixed, and at this time, their use has not replaced that of sutures for wound closure in endodontic surgery.[188–194]

The purpose of suturing is to approximate the incised tissues and stabilize the flapped mucoperiosteum until reattachment occurs (Figure 40A,B,C). The placement of sutures in oral tissues, however, creates unique problems. It is evident that incisional wounds in oral tissues heal more rapidly than in skin. However, sutures are better tolerated and interfere less with postsurgical healing in the skin. The major problem in oral tissues is the constant bathing of the suture material and suture tract with saliva containing a high concentration of microorganisms that may gain entrance to underlying tissues.

Sutures are available in many different materials, the most common being synthetic fibers [nylon, polyester, polyglactin (PG), and polyglycolic acid (PGA)], collagen, gut, and silk. Sutures are classified as absorbable or nonabsorbable, by size according to the manufacturer's minimum diameter, and by physical design as monofilament, multifilament, twisted, or braided. The classification of suture size is complicated by the existence of two standards, the United States Pharmacopeia (USP) and the European Pharmacopeia (EP). The USP size is designated by two Arabic numbers, one a zero, being separated by a hyphen (3-0, 4-0, 5-0, etc). The higher the first number, the smaller the diameter of the suture material. The EP system is a number that represents the manufacturer's minimum diameter tolerance, in millimeters (1 = 0.10 mm, 1.5 = 0.15 mm, etc.) of the suture.

SILK

Silk sutures are made of protein fibers (fibroin) bound together with biological glue (sericin), similar to fibronectin, produced by silkworms. Silk sutures are nonabsorbable, multifilamentous, and braided (Figure 41). They have a high capillary action effect that enhances

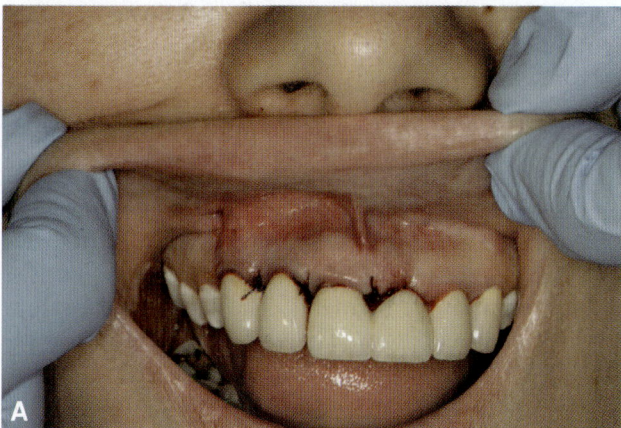
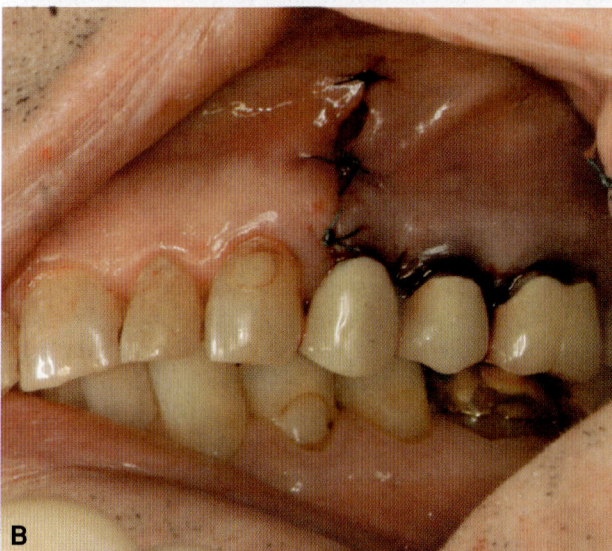
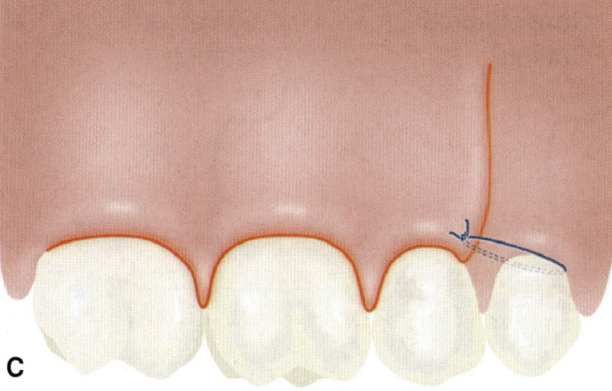

Figure 40 ***A,*** Proper flap repositioning and suturing. ***B,*** Large gap in vertical incision after suturing; another interrupted suture should have been placed. ***C,*** In cases of gapping, anchor sutures can be used to help pull repositioned flapped tissue towards the unreflected tissue by using a nearby tooth as an anchor.

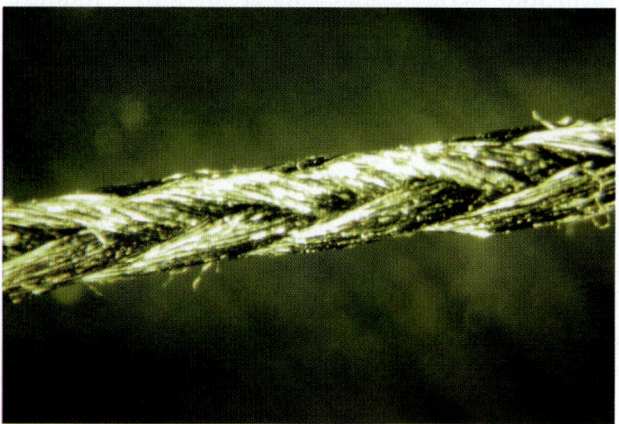

Figure 41 High power view of a silk suture demonstrating that it is a multifilament and braided material.

the movement of fluids between the fibers ("wicking" action), resulting in severe oral tissue reactions.[195–197] This tissue reaction results from the accumulation of plaque on the fibers that occurs within a few hours following insertion into the tissues.[198] Silk's advantage is limited to its ease of manipulation. Due to the severe tissue reaction to silk, it is not the suture material of choice for endodontic surgery today.[189] If silk sutures are used, however, the patient should rinse with chlorhexidine during the postoperative period.

GUT

Collagen is the basic component of plain gut suture material and is derived from sheep or bovine intestines. The collagen is treated with diluted formaldehyde to increase its strength and is then shaped into the appropriate monofilament size. Gut sutures are absorbable; however, the absorption rate is variable and can take up to 10 days. Because of the unpredictability of gut suture absorption in oral tissues, a scheduled suture removal appointment should be made. Chromic gut sutures consist of plain gut that has been treated with chromium trioxide. This results in a delay in the absorption rate. Because retention of sutures beyond a few days is not recommended in endodontic surgery, the use of chromic gut sutures offers no advantage. In addition, evidence indicates that plain gut is more biocompatible with oral soft tissues than chromic gut.[195–197] Gut suture material is marketed in sterile packets containing isopropyl alcohol. When removed from the packet, the suture is hard and non-pliable due to its dehydration. Prior to using, gut sutures should be hydrated by placing them into sterile, distilled water for 3 to 5 minutes. After hydration, the gut suture material will be smooth and pliable with manipulative properties similar to silk.[199]

COLLAGEN

Reconstituted collagen sutures are made from bovine tendon after it has been treated with cyanoacetic acid and then coagulated with acetone and dried. Collagen sutures offer no advantage over gut for endodontic surgery as their absorption rate and tissue response is similar. They are available only in small sizes and used almost exclusively in microsurgery.

PGA

Sutures made from fibers of polymerized glycolic acid are absorbable in mammalian tissue. The rate of absorption is about 16 to 20 days. PGA sutures consist of multiple filaments that are braided and share handling characteristics similar to silk. PGA was the first synthetic absorbable suture and it is manufactured as Dexon.

PG

In 1975, Craig and coworkers[200] reported the development of a copolymer of lactic acid and glycolic acid called PG 910 (90 parts glycolic acid and 10 parts lactic acid). Sutures of PG are absorbable and consist of braided multiple filaments. Their absorption rate is similar to that of PGA. They are commercially available as Vicryl.

Many studies have been reported evaluating the response of the oral soft tissues to gut, collagen, PGA, and PG sutures, with conflicting results. As a result, there is insufficient evidence at this time to make a strong recommendation between these materials. The important factor to remember regarding sutures, regardless of the material, is that they should be removed as early as the clinical situation will permit.

NEEDLE SELECTION

Surgical needles are designed to carry the suture material through the tissues with minimal trauma. For that reason, a needle with a reverse cutting edge (the cutting edge is on the outside of the curve) is preferable (Figure 42). The arc of the surgical needle selected should match the optimum curvature needed to penetrate the tissues in and out on both sides of the incision, 2 to 3 mm from the wound margins. Suture

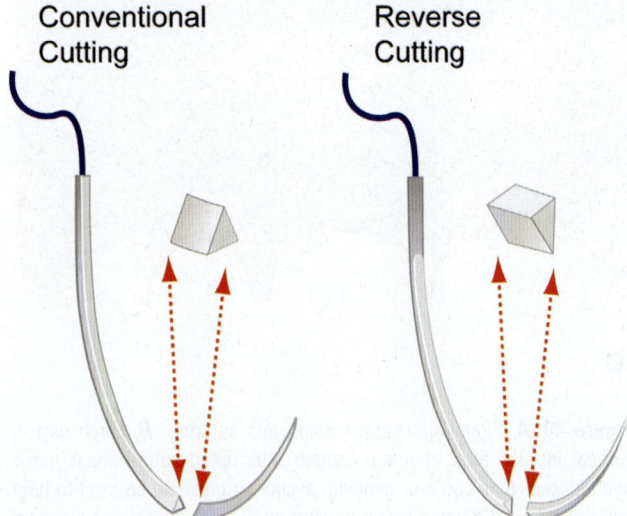

Figure 42 Conventional cutting needles are not recommended because the cutting edge on the inside curvature tends to pull through the flap edge; reverse cutting suture needles prevent suture material from tearing through surgical flaps.

needles are available in arcs of one-fourth, three-eighths, one-half, and five-eighths of a circle, with the most useful being the three-eighths and one-half circle. The radius of the arch of the needle is also an important consideration. The smaller the radius of the arch, the more conducive the needle is to quick turnout. For vertical incision lines and anterior embrasure suturing, a relatively tight arc is necessary to allow for quick needle turnout. Suturing in posterior areas, however, requires less curvature and a longer needle to reach through the embrasure. The final selection of an appropriate surgical needle is based on a combination of factors including the location of the incision, the size and shape of the interdental embrasure, the flap design, and the suture technique planned.

SUTURING TECHNIQUES

There is a wide variety of suture techniques designed to accomplish the goals of closure and stabilization of flaps involving oral mucoperiosteal tissues. All suturing techniques should be evaluated on the basis of their ability to accomplish these goals. Several authors have compared the effects of continuous and interrupted suture techniques. Their findings indicate that the interrupted suturing technique provides for better flap adaptation than the continuous and, therefore, is the recommended technique, and the most commonly used, for endodontic surgery.[201,202] Sutures are holding mechanisms and should not pull or stretch the tissue as a tear in the flap margin may result. Sutures that close an incision too tightly compromise circulation and increase chances for the sutures to tear loose upon swelling. Before placing sutures, bleeding should be controlled to prevent the formation of a hematoma under the flap. A hematoma will prevent the direct apposition of the flap to the bone and can act as a culture medium for bacterial growth. The suturing techniques that are most conducive to rapid surgical wound healing are the single interrupted suture, the interrupted loop (interdental) suture, the vertical mattress suture, and the single sling suture.

SINGLE INTERRUPTED SUTURE

The single interrupted suture is used primarily for closure and stabilization of vertical releasing and relaxing incisions in full mucoperiosteal flaps and horizontal incisions in limited mucoperiosteal flap designs (Figure 43). The initial needle penetration should be through the independent (movable) tissue. The point of needle entry should be from the buccal or facial and 2 to 3 mm from the incision margin in order to provide sufficient tissue to minimize suture tear-out.

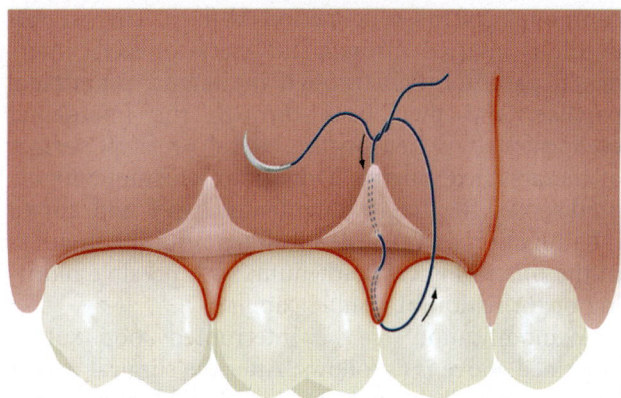

Figure 43 Single interrupted sutures can be used for both the horizontal incision and the vertical incision.

The needle should then enter the under surface of the mucoperiosteum of the dependent (immovable) tissue and penetrate through the mucoperiosteum at a point 2 to 3 mm from the incision margin. In order to accomplish this, it is often necessary to elevate the attached mucoperiosteum from the underlying bone for a distance of a few millimeters at the point of needle insertion. It is important that the periosteum is included with the tissue bite otherwise the suture will most likely tear out of the fragile attached gingiva.

After the suture needle has been passed through the mucoperiosteum on both sides of the incision, the suture material should be drawn through the tissue until the end opposite the needle is approximately 1 to 2 inches from the tissue. The suture should be tied with a secure knot. A surgical knot is the most effective and least likely to slip. The surgeon's knot is best tied by wrapping double loops or throws of the long end (end with the needle attached) of the suture around the needle holder. By then grasping the short end of the suture with the needle holder and slipping the throws off, the first half of the surgical knot is tied. After adjusting the tissue tension, the second half of the knot is tied by repeating the same process, only wrapping the loops of suture around the needle holder in the opposite direction from the first tie, like a square knot. Suture knots should be placed to the side of the incision. Suture knots collect food, plaque, and bacteria, thus resulting in localized infection and a delay in healing when placed directly over the incision.

INTERRUPTED LOOP (INTERDENTAL) SUTURE

The interrupted loop, or interdental suture, is used primarily to secure and stabilize the horizontal component of full mucoperiosteal flaps. The surgical needle is inserted through the buccal or facial interdental papillae, then through the lingual interdental papillae, and then back through the interdental embrasure. It is tied on the buccal or facial surface of the attached gingiva. This suture technique highly predisposes the fragile interdental tissue and col to inflammation and retarded healing, resulting in a loss of the outer gingival epithelium, with possible blunting or formation of double papillae.

A modification of the interrupted loop suture described above is as follows. After the surgical needle has been passed through the buccal and lingual papillary gingiva, the suture is passed over the interdental contact and secured with a surgeon's knot. This modification eliminates the presence of suture material in the interdental embrasure, thus reducing postsurgical inflammation to this delicate tissue. In clinical situations where the horizontal component of a full mucoperiosteal flap involves a tooth or teeth with full coverage crowns, this modification allows for a slight incisal or occlusal repositioning of the mucoperiosteal flap. This can be accomplished by placing slight tension on the suture over the interdental contact and may compensate for a loss of gingival height resulting from the sulcular incision.

VERTICAL MATTRESS SUTURE

The vertical mattress suture has the advantage that it does not require needle penetration or suture material being passed through tissue involved in the incisional wound (Figure 44). The surgical needle enters and exits the flapped mucoperiosteum some distance apical from the incision line. The suture is then passed through the interdental embrasure, directed to the lingual of the adjacent tooth, and passed back through the opposite interdental embrasure. The needle then enters and exits the flapped mucoperiosteum again, is passed through the embrasure and again, lingual to the tooth and through the opposite interdental embrasure to be tied on the buccal surface with a surgeon's knot. This suture technique also provides for the opportunity to return the flapped tissue to a slightly incisal or occlusal position from its original in order to compensate for a loss of gingival height.

SINGLE SLING SUTURE

The single sling suture is similar to the vertical mattress suture (Figure 45A,B). The surgical needle is passed through the attached gingiva of the flap, through the interdental embrasure but not through the lingual soft tissue. It is then directed lingual to the tooth and passed through the opposite interdental embrasure and over the incisal or occlusal margin of the flap. The needle is then passed through the attached gingiva of the flap, from the buccal or facial, back through the embrasure, passed lingual to the tooth, through the opposite embrasure, passed over the flap margin and tied with a surgeon's knot (Figure 46A,B). This suture technique is particularly effective for achieving the maximum incisal or occlusal level when repositioning the flap. Because the lingual anchor is the lingual surface of the tooth and not the fragile lingual tissue, tension can be placed on the flapped tissue to adjust the height of the flap margin.

POSTOPERATIVE CARE

Postsurgical management of the patient is equally as important as the surgical procedure itself. An important component of postsurgical care is a genuine expression of concern and reassurance to the patient regarding both their physical and emotional experience. It is well known that the emotional state of a patient has a direct relationship on the level of morbidity following a surgical procedure. The patient's awareness that the surgeon cares and that he/she is readily available, should they have a problem, is a priceless adjunct to healing. A telephone call to the patient, the evening following or the morning after endodontic surgery, is very reassuring and helps to build a strong doctor–patient relationship. This also allows any patient anxieties to be dealt with before they become major concerns.

Another important component of postsurgical care is good patient communication. It is the endodontic surgeon's responsibility to properly communicate to

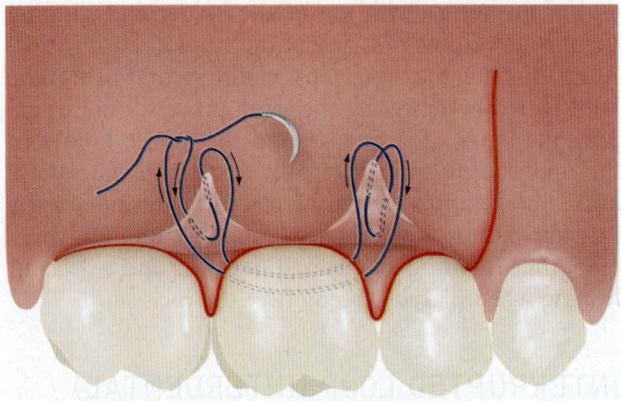

Figure 44 Vertical mattress suture avoids penetration of tissues in the incisional wound and supports the interdental papilla in a coronal direction.

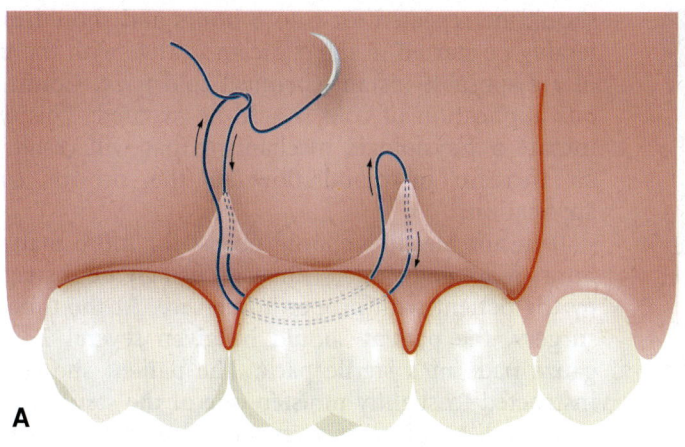
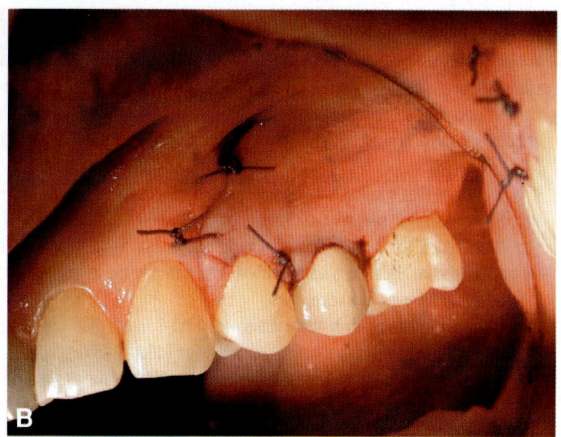

Figure 45 *A,* Sling suturing technique; *B,* Single sling suture used following surgery on a maxillary second premolar.

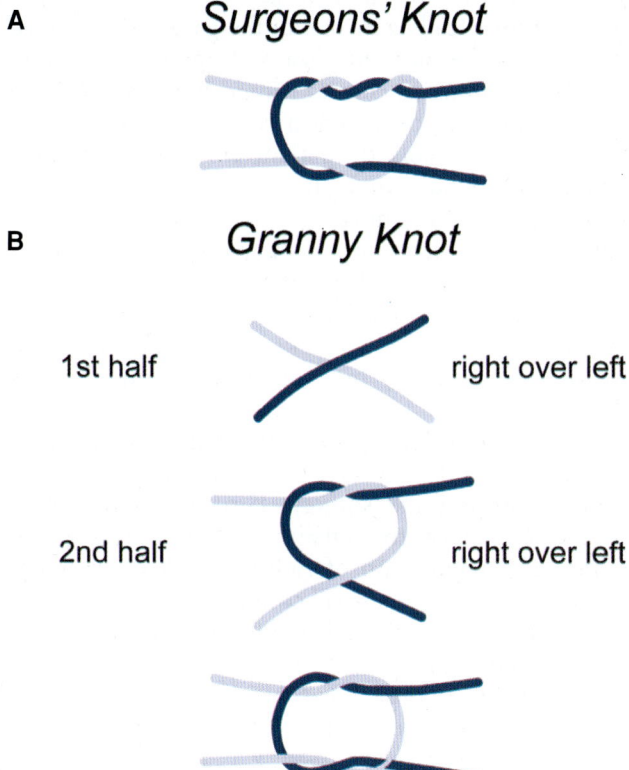

Figure 46 *A,* Surgeons' knot is a modified square knot in which the first overhand knot is doubled; the doubling prevents slippage especially when flaps are under tension; *B,* Granny knots result when a throw (complete twist of two strands) is followed by another throw in the same sequence. Granny knots result in knot slippage with less security than a surgeon's knot.

the patient the expected and normal postsurgical sequelae as well as detailed home care instructions. These are best conveyed both verbally and in writing.

Alexander stated that without written reinforcement, the understanding and retention of verbal instructions could not be assured. He also advised that written materials should be presented after oral instructions have been given rather than before. Because up to 20% of Americans are functionally illiterate, written instructions should use simple words (preferably 1 to 2 syllables) and short sentences of no more than 10 words.[105] Normal postsurgical sequelae include the possibility of slight bleeding from the surgical area for a few hours, pain that may persist for a few days, and swelling and soft tissue discoloration (ecchymosis) in the surgical area that may be evident for as much as 8 to 10 days. An example of written postsurgical instructions, which should be reviewed verbally with the patient before they are dismissed, is provided in Table 2.

Bleeding, swelling, discoloration, pain, and infection are the most likely untoward sequelae following endodontic surgery. These should be thoroughly discussed with the patient during the presurgical consultation and should be reinforced at the time of surgery, prior to dismissal of the patient.

BLEEDING AND SWELLING

Slight oozing of blood from severed microvessels may be evident for several hours following surgery. When a little blood is mixed with saliva, it often appears to the patient as a lot of blood. If the patient is forewarned of this possibility, it goes a long way to reducing their anxiety. Slight swelling of the intraoral and extraoral tissues is a normal consequence of surgical trauma and leakage of blood from the severed microvessels. Proper compression of the surgical flap both before

Table 2 Sample Instructions for Postoperative Care Following Endodontic Surgery

1. Limit physical activity for the first 24 hours. Easy activity is OK but be careful and do not bump your face where the surgery was done. You should not drink any alcohol or use any tobacco (smoke or chew) for the next 3 days.
2. It is important that you have a good diet and drink plenty of liquids for the first few days after surgery. Juices, soups, and other soft foods, like yogurt and puddings, are suggested. Liquid meals, like Sego, Slender, and Carnation Instant Breakfast, can be used. You can buy these at most food stores. Avoid carbonated beverages.
3. Do not brush in the area of the incision for first 3 days, then use a soft brush very carefully; use warm salt water rinses (dilute 1/8 teaspoon salt per 8 oz glass of water) and rinse for 1 minute swishing the surgical area every 2 hours during the day. Continue rinses until 2 days after sutures removed.
4. Do not lift up your lip or pull back your cheek to look where the surgery was done. This may loosen the stitches, causing them to tear the gum tissue and start bleeding.
5. A little bleeding from where the surgery was done is normal. This should only last for a few hours. You may also have a little swelling and bruising of your face. This should only last for a few days.
6. Place an ice bag (cold) on your face where the surgery was done. You should leave it on for 20 minutes and take it off for 20 minutes. You should do this for 6 to 8 hours. After 8 hours, the ice bag (cold) should not be used. The next day after surgery, you can put a soft, wet, hot towel on your face where the surgery was done. Do this as often as you can for the next 2 to 3 days.
7. Discomfort after the surgery should not be bad but the area will be sore. You should use the pain medicine you were given or recommended to you, as needed.
8. Rinse your mouth with one tablespoon of the chlorhexidine mouthwash (Peridex) you were given or prescribed. This should be done two times a day (once in the morning and once at night before going to bed). You should do this for 5 days.
9. The stitches that were placed need to be taken out in a few days. You will be told when to return. It is important that you come in to have this done!!
10. You will be coming back to the office several times during the next few months so we can evaluate how you are healing. These are very important visits and you should come in even if everything feels OK.
11. If you have any problems or if you have any questions, you should call the office. The office phone number is xxx-xxxx. If you call after regular office hours or on the weekend, you will be given instructions on how to page the doctor on call.

and after suturing greatly reduces postoperative bleeding and swelling (Figure 39).

Additional supportive therapy is the application of an ice pack, with firm pressure, to the facial area over the surgical site. Pressure and reduction of temperature slows the flow of blood and helps to counteract the rebound phenomenon, which occurs following the use of a vasoconstrictor in the local anesthetic. Application of cold also acts as an effective analgesic due to its reduction in sensitivity of the peripheral nerve endings. The ice pack should be applied in a 20 minutes on and 20 minutes off cycle. This regimen should be repeated for 6 to 8 hours and should preferably be started in the clinician's office with the use of a disposable instant chemical cold pack. Continuous application of cold should be avoided. This will initiate a physiologic mechanism that will result in an increase in blood flow to the site of cold application.[203]

If minor bleeding should persist for more than 12 hours following surgery, this can usually be managed by the patient with proper home care. At the time of surgery, the patient should be given several 2 × 2 gauze pads in a sterile pack. The patient should be instructed to slightly moisten one of the sterile gauze pads and to place it over the bleeding site while applying firm pressure. Pressure should be applied to the area for 10 to 15 minutes. Should the bleeding problem persist, the patient should be instructed to place a moist tea bag or one of the gauze pads soaked in tea over the bleeding area and appliy pressure in the same manner as before. Tannic acid, contained in tea, is known to be an effective hemostatic agent. If home treatment fails, the patient should be seen in the dental office where the dentist can inject a local anesthetic agent containing 1:50,000 epinephrine and apply tissue compression to the bleeding area. Unless there is an undisclosed or undiagnosed bleeding disorder, this should resolve the problem. The patient should be warned not to take aspirin for pain prior to surgery or after, but rather acetaminophen or ibuprofen.

Application of moist heat over the surgical site is recommended; however, it should not begin until 24 hours following the surgery. Heat promotes blood flow and enhances the inflammatory and healing processes. The application of moist heat is best accomplished by the use of a small cotton towel that has been wet with hot tap water. The hot, moist towel should be applied to the surface of the face over the surgical area for about 30 minutes. The towel should be re-heated with hot tap water every 5 to 10 minutes to maintain the temperature.

Discoloration of the mucoperiosteal and/or facial tissues following surgery is the result of the breakdown of blood that has leaked into the surrounding tissues. The patients should be made aware of the potential for postsurgical discoloration at the presurgical consultation visit and again reinforced at the time of surgery. This ecchymosis can last for up to 2 weeks and is observed more in the elderly and fair-complexioned patients (Figure 47). This is an esthetic problem only and requires no special treatment. In patients with ecchymosis, applications of moist heat may be beneficial for up to 2 weeks following surgery.

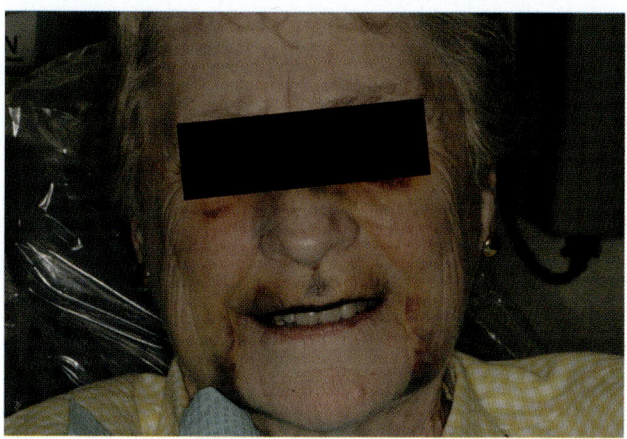

Figure 47 Bilateral ecchymosis following endodontic surgery on multiple maxillary anterior teeth.

Heat promotes fluid exchange and speeds resorption of discoloring agents from the tissues.

In the majority of patients, pain following periradicular surgery is surprisingly minimal. Postsurgical pain is usually of short duration and most often reaches its maximum intensity about 6 to 8 hours following surgery. A significant reduction in pain can usually be expected on the first postoperative day followed by a steady decrease in discomfort each day following surgery. It is unusual for a patient to experience pain that cannot be managed by mild to moderate analgesics.[204]

Another method of postsurgical pain control is the use of long-acting local anesthetic agents, such as bupivacaine (Marcaine) or etidocaine (Duranest), which provide 6 to 8 hours of local anesthesia and up to 10 hours of local analgesia.[205,206] Because these long-acting anesthetic agents contain a low concentration of vasoconstrictor (1:200,000), they are not suitable to be used alone in periradicular surgery. They can either be used prior to surgery, in conjunction with lidocaine containing 1:50,000 epinephrine or at the conclusion of the surgical procedure prior to dismissal of the patient. The return of sensation is more gradual with the long-acting anesthetics than with the short acting; therefore, the onset of discomfort is less sudden.

Endodontic surgery is performed in an area that is heavily populated with microorganisms; however, postsurgical infections are rare. For this reason, peritreatment systemic antibiotic therapy is seldom required and is not considered part of routine postsurgical care in healthy patients. The most common causes of postsurgical infections following periradicular surgery are the result of inadequate aseptic techniques and improper soft tissue reapproximation and stabilization. These are under the direct control of the endodontic surgeon. The clinical signs and symptoms of a postsurgical infection are usually evident 36 to 48 hours after surgery. The most common indications are progressively increasing pain and swelling. Suppuration, elevated temperature, and lymphadenopathy may or may not be present. Systemic antibiotic therapy should be initiated promptly when indicated. The antibiotic of choice is penicillin V, and the recommended dosage is 1 gram as an initial dose followed by a maintenance dose of 500 milligrams. The dosing interval should be every 3 to 4 hours, preferably without food. In patients allergic to penicillin, the antibiotic of choice is clindamycin with an initial dose of 600 milligrams followed by a maintenance dose of 150 to 300 milligrams depending on the age and weight of the patient. The dosing interval should be every 8 hours, preferably without food. The patient should be monitored every 24 hours and antibiotic therapy withdrawn as soon as the clinical condition indicates that the patient's host defenses have regained control of the infection and that the infection is resolving or has resolved.

Oral hygiene often presents a postsurgical problem for many patients. A toothbrush should not be used as an aid to oral hygiene in the area of surgery until the day following surgery and then only on the occlusal or incisal surfaces of the teeth. Use of a toothbrush in the surgical area may dislodge the mucoperiosteal flap and lead to serious postsurgical complications. A cotton swab soaked with chlorhexidine oral rinse (Peridex) or 3% hydrogen peroxide may be used to gently remove oral debris from the surgical area. A regimen of twice daily (morning and evening) rinsing with chlorhexidine oral rinse will provide an effective means for reduction of debris, decreasing the population of the oral microbial flora, and inhibiting plaque formation. Chlorhexidine oral rinses should continue for 4 to 6 days following surgery (2 to 3 days following suture removal).

According to Gutmann and Harrison,[3] the key to preventing sutures from having a negative effect on wound healing following surgery is their early removal. The primary purpose for placing sutures following endodontic surgery is to approximate the edges of the incisional wound and provide stabilization until the epithelium and myofibroblast–fibronectin network provides a sufficient barrier to dislodgment of the flapped tissues. This usually occurs within 48 hours following surgery. It has been recommended that sutures should not be allowed to remain longer than 96 hours. A suture removal kit should contain a cotton swab, 2" × 2" gauze sponges, suture scissors, cotton pliers, and a mouth mirror. The sutures and surrounding mucosa should be cleaned with a cotton swab containing a mild disinfectant followed by hydrogen peroxide. This helps to destroy bacteria and remove plaque and debris that have accumulated on the sutures, thus reducing the inoculation of bacteria into the underlying tissues as the suture is pulled through. A topical anesthetic should also be applied with a swab to the surgical site. This greatly reduces the discomfort associated with the placement of the scissors blade under the suture, a procedure that is particularly painful in areas of persistent swelling and edema, commonly seen in the mucobuccal fold. Sharp-pointed scissors are used to cut the suture material followed by grasping the knotted portion with cotton pliers and removing the suture. Various designs of scissors are available and can be selected according to specific access needs in different areas of the mouth. It has been suggested that a No. 12 scalpel blade be used to sever the suture. The advantages are stated to be a predictably sharp cutting edge and less "tug" on the suture.[207]

Corrective Surgery

Corrective surgery can be defined as the surgical procedure required to repair defects that occur in root or furcation areas as a result of therapeutic misadventures or pathologic processes. These defects are located in areas of the root other than the apex and are not amenable to nonsurgical repair. When a periodontal pocket is associated with a defect located in the cervical one-half of the root, it will be necessary to reflect a mucoperiosteal flap to insure proper repair of the root defect and correction of the periodontal defect. Furcation defects are generally repaired nonsurgically, but there are situations where a periodontal component is present and can only be corrected via a surgical approach. Therapeutic misadventures requiring corrective procedures include, but are not limited to, perforations that occur during complicated endodontic access, root canal location, and preparation procedures or as a result of misdirection of burs during the preparation of post space. Pathological processes that may cause some of these defects include caries, periodontal lesions, external resorption, and perforating internal resorption. Traumatic injuries that result in fractures of the root may require a surgical approach to treatment in order to retain the remaining root or combination of root and crown structures. Corrective surgical procedures include periradicular surgery where access is gained through a flap procedure to repair the root and periodontal defects. Root amputation is also a possibility when a defect can only be corrected if an entire root of a multirooted tooth is removed and the remaining crown of the tooth is recontoured and retained. In mandibular molars, a hemisection procedure may be required to remove the entire crown and root on the side of the tooth where the defect is present. An intentional replantation procedure is only a treatment option when all other nonsurgical and surgical procedures have already been attempted and failed or have been deemed impossible to perform.[208] In these cases the tooth is extracted, the defect repaired, and the tooth repositioned back into its original socket.

PERFORATION REPAIR

Perforations in the floor of the pulp chamber in multirooted teeth may occur during endodontic access preparation, post space preparation, or in conjunction with extensive caries or resorption lesions. The multirooted teeth with the greatest potential for furcation perforations are the maxillary and mandibular molars. When a perforation occurs in this area of the tooth, the initial attempt at repair should be from an internal, nonsurgical approach. Corrective surgery is reserved for those teeth where nonsurgical repair is not a treatment option or the attempted nonsurgical repair has failed. When surgery is necessary, a buccal mucoperiosteal flap is reflected, the furcation bony defect is curetted to remove any pathologic tissue, and the perforation site is repaired.

In an animal study by Dean et al.,[209] it was reported that when the perforation defect was repaired surgically, the associated bone defect filled with decalcified freeze-dried bone and the window in the bone was covered with a periodontal membrane, the percentage of osseous healing was 75% to 100%. In those cases where the perforation was repaired, the bone defect was allowed to fill with blood and the bone window was covered with a periodontal membrane, the percentage of osseous healing was 92% to 100%. When only the perforation was repaired and the other two procedures were not done, the osseous healing was only 52% to 70%. In the remaining three groups, the same blood clot, membrane and osseous fill were performed on the bone defect, but none of the perforations in these three groups was repaired. The amount of osseous repair for these three groups ranged from 0% to 15%. The results suggest that, in this particular model, repair and sealing of the perforation site was necessary to achieve significant osseous healing.

Strip perforations in the cervical one-third of the root occur most frequently in the thin distal aspects of the mesial roots of mandibular molars and the mesiobuccal roots of maxillary molars. Nonsurgical repair should be the first treatment option in these cases. If surgical repair is deemed necessary, the perforation must be accessed and visualized through a window created in the buccal bone. In many cases, surgical repair will be very difficult, if not impossible, and the bony window may be so large that a periodontal defect is created. If neither the nonsurgical nor surgical options are feasible, other possible treatment options include root amputation, hemisection, intentional replantation, or extraction followed by the placement of a bridge or osseointegrated implant.

If an external cervical root defect is present as a result of root caries or external resorption, the treatment approach may be different from that proposed for a perforation defect in the same area. If the carious or resorptive defect does not penetrate into the pulp canal space, a surgical approach to treatment is the first choice. A limited envelope soft tissue flap is generally adequate to visualize, cleanse, and repair the affected area. If the defect is in a cosmetic area, an appropriate composite resin or glass ionomer material will be the material of choice. Amalgam, MTA, and Ketac materials might also be choices if the defect is in an area where cosmetics are not an issue. Periodontal pocketing is often associated with these cervical defects so crown lengthening or vertical root extrusion may also have to be performed in order for the area to be properly restored and cleansed.

Perforations occurring at the mid-root level are usually the result of burs being misdirected or overthinning of the root canal walls during post space preparation. If possible, these defects should be immediately sealed via an internal approach. If surgery is necessary (Figure 48A,B,C,D), the same steps are followed as for the other areas that require surgical repair. If there is cortical bone covering the root surface coronal to the level of the mid-root repair site, there will be less chance of creating a chronic periodontal problem. A perforation located in the apical third of the root is treated surgically by removing that portion of the root apical to the perforation site and, if necessary, placement of a root-end filling.

The management of external root resorption lesions located apical to the cervical area will depend on whether the defect communicates or does not communicate with the pulp canal space. Those lesions that do not communicate with the pulp canal space will need to be corrected surgically in order to arrest the active resorptive process. The location of the resorptive defect on the root surface will be a key factor in determining whether a successful surgical repair can be accomplished. If the lesion is located on the distal of lingual surface of the root, it may be impossible to visualize and correct the defect from a surgical approach. In these situations, intentional replantation for a single-rooted tooth or root amputation or hemisection may be the only treatment choices if an attempt is to be made to retain the tooth. Otherwise, extraction may be the only option.

When these external resorptive defects are approached surgically, a full thickness mucoperiosteal flap is reflected, the bony window over the defect site is enlarged for visualization, the resorptive defect is curetted, and the site is repaired with MTA or an appropriate bonded resin material. If there is no bone covering the root surface coronal to the defect, a periodontal regenerative procedure may also be performed in conjunction with the corrective surgical procedure.

When an external root resorptive defect communicates with the pulp canal space or an internal resorptive defect communicates with the external root surface, a combination of nonsurgical and surgical approach to treatment may be required. The first step in either of these situations is to cleanse and shape the root canal system and place an internal dressing of calcium hydroxide. At a subsequent visit the calcium hydroxide is removed, the root canal dried, and that portion of the root canal system apical to the perforating defect is obturated with an appropriate obturating material. The external portion of perforation defect is then packed with a matrix/barrier material, and the repair site is repaired internally. If it is impossible to adequately dry the root canal system so that root canal obturation can be performed or the external resorptive process remains active, then a combination treatment must be performed.

With a combination treatment a mucoperiosteal soft tissue flap is reflected, the pathologic defect on the root surface is curetted, the root canal space can then be dried, and the portion of the root canal space apical to the defect can be obturated. The perforation defect on the root surface and into the root canal space is then repaired with an appropriate repair material. Another technique which has been suggested is to place a tight fitting gutta-percha cone into the root canal space without sealer, repair the external defect, and let the repair material set and then remove the gutta-percha cone and proceed with the internal root canal obturation procedure. The inherent danger with this latter

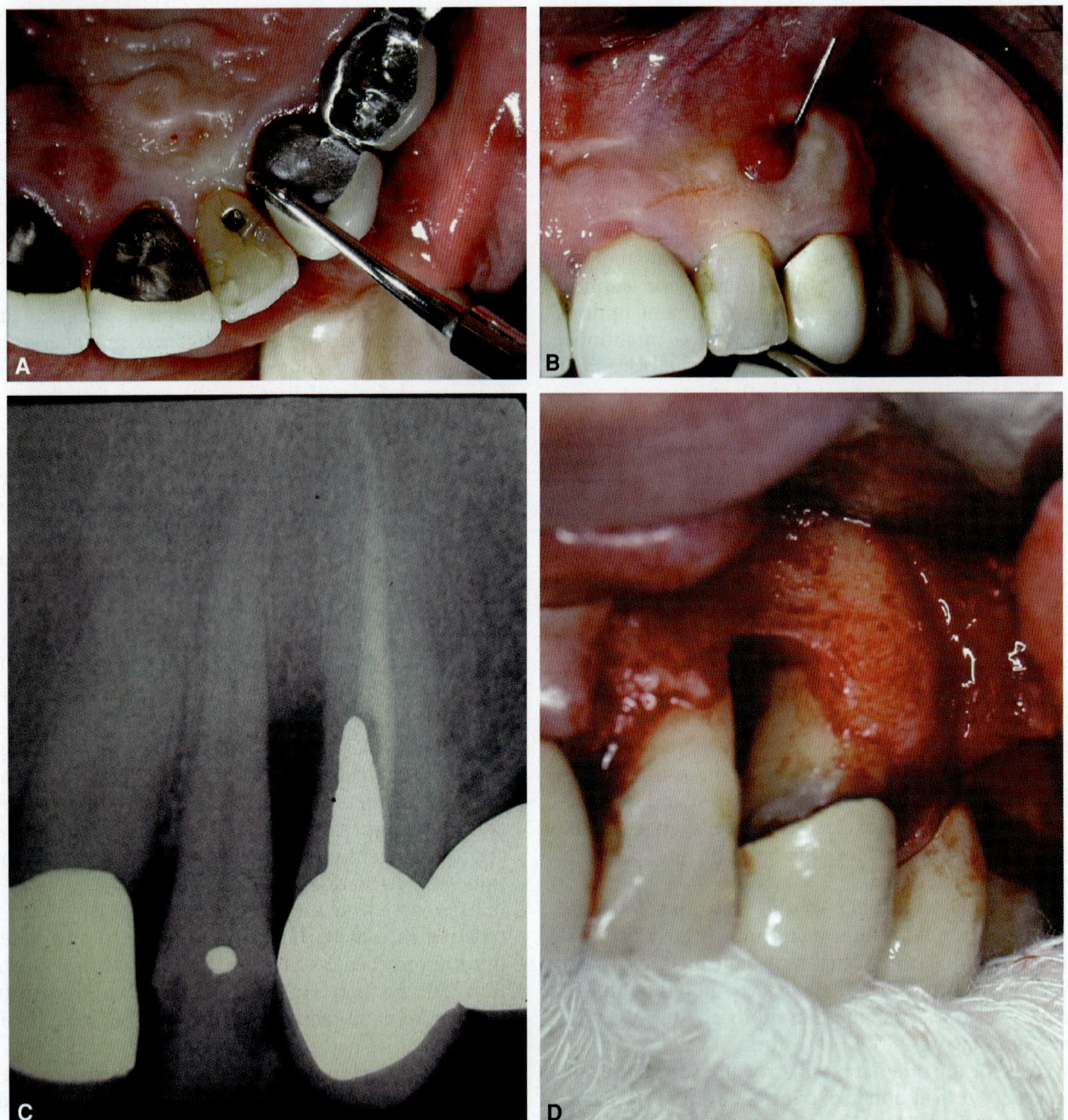

Figure 48 ***A,*** Periodontal probe placed into lingual defect; ***B,*** Point of periodontal probe exits via sinus tract on the buccal gingival tissues; ***C,*** Radiograph depicts perforation of post at mid-root level on mesial surface of root; ***D,*** Flap reflected to demonstrate root and bony defects that required sealing the perforation site and then periodontal bone grafting and membrane placement to resolve the problem and retain the tooth.

technique is that the compacting forces required to perform the obturation procedure may displace the external repair material. Once the soft tissue flap is sutured, the access opening is closed with a temporary sealing material. Any additional nonsurgical treatment can be completed at a subsequent visit after the soft tissue flap has healed. If there is extensive bone loss over the external root surface, a periodontal regenerative procedure may also be required. If the defect is found to be so extensive that the root cannot be retained, one of the alternative treatment options noted above must be considered.

TRAUMATIC ROOT FRACTURE REPAIR

The clinical management of teeth with traumatic root fractures will be discussed in detail in Chapter 31, "Endodontic Treatment Outcome: The Potential for Healing and Retained Function." Corrective surgical procedures will only be required in those cases where periradicular pathology develops at the fracture site and the apical segment of the root must be removed surgically.

ROOT AMPUTATION

Root amputation procedures may be indicated when a mutirooted tooth has one root that cannot be retained and the other roots have adequate periodontal support and the remaining crown structure can be restored (Figure 49). These procedures are most frequently indicated when one root of a maxillary molar must be eliminated. This is considered a corrective endodontic surgical procedure when the root that must be sacrificed is the result of a vertical root fracture, a pathologic resorptive or dentistogenic defect that cannot be repaired. If the root to be removed has inadequate bone support as a result of chronic periodontal disease, the root amputation procedure may be one of the treatment options considered by the dentist performing the periodontal therapy. The root removal must allow access for proper home care and plaque control so that a chronic periodontal problem is not created. Retention of the remaining tooth structure may also be necessary for prosthetic reasons such as to retain an abutment tooth for a long-span fixed or removable partial denture. Case selection is an important factor in success because the strategic value of the tooth must be critical to the patient's overall dental treatment plan. Because the prognosis for long-term retention of teeth with root amputations is guarded, there is a tendency in today's dental practice to extract these teeth and replace them with osseointegrated implants. A root amputation procedure may also be contraindicated if the

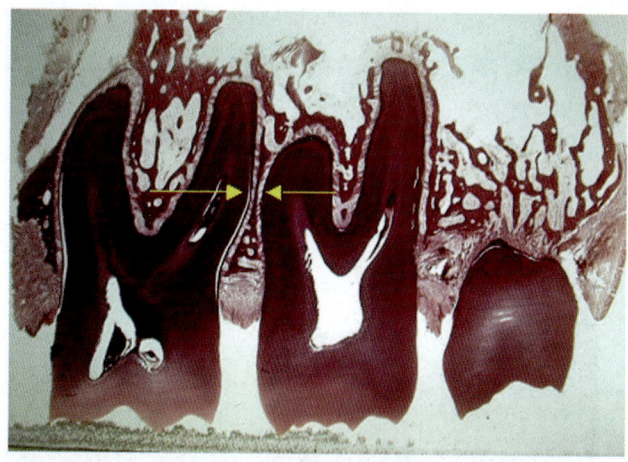

Figure 49 If the space between the roots of two maxillary molars is so narrow (illustrated by the two arrows), new bone cannot be regenerated in this area if a periodontal pocket develops between the two roots.

remaining roots do not have adequate periodontal osseous support, the root to be removed is fused to an adjacent root, the remaining roots cannot be successfully treated endodontically, or the patient has poor home care and oral hygiene.

Nonsurgical root canal therapy should be completed on the roots to be retained before performing the amputation procedure (Figure 50A,B,C). The root canal system in the root to be amputated should be cleansed and shaped in the usual manner. The apical half of this root may or may not be obturated with gutta-percha. The entire root canal or at least the coronal one-half should be filled with either amalgam or MTA. A bonded core or post and core restoration is placed into the pulp chamber and the occlusion is adjusted to eliminate any excessive forces during lateral excursive movements. Once the restorative materials have set, the surgical procedure can be performed.

Before reflecting a soft tissue flap, the amputation procedure is started by recontouring the crown of the tooth to provide for cleansing and good home care of the resected area, to direct occlusal forces along the long axis of the remaining roots, and to expose the coronal portion of the root that is to be removed. This technique was recommended by Kirchoff and

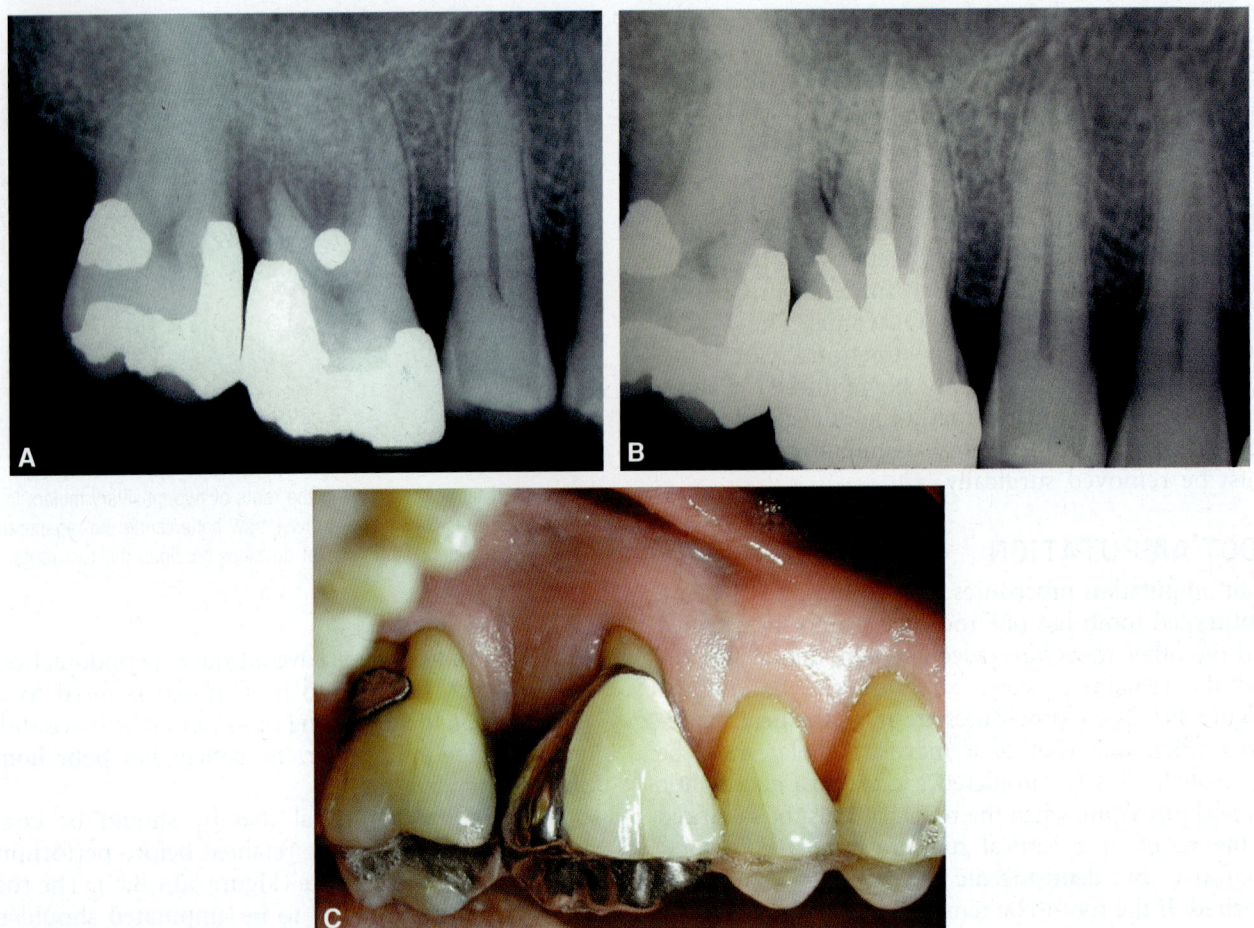

Figure 50 ***A,*** Radiograph depicts a defect between the distobuccal root of a maxillary first molar and the mesiobuccal root of the maxillary second molar; ***B,*** Root canal therapy is completed and an amalgam core is placed into the root to be amputated; ***C,*** The same case 4 years after the amputation procedure, note the presence of a well-contoured crown and the health of the interproximal periodontal tissues.

Gerstein[210] and is best performed by using a combination of smooth fissure and diamond burs. A surgical length bur may be required for the resection of the mesiobuccal root of a maxillary molar because this root is generally very broad in a buccolingual dimension and may extend one-half the distance to the palatal root. The distobuccal root is generally conical in shape and may be resected with a normal length bur. Palatal root amputations are rarely performed because of the poor prognosis of retention of these teeth with just the two retained buccal roots. It is also rare that both buccal roots will be amputated to leave a single palatal root to provide all of the support for the remaining coronal tooth structure.

Performing the majority of the root amputation and crown contouring prior to extraction of the root will prevent debris from collecting in the open extraction socket. Either a limited or full mucoperiosteal flap is then reflected to facilitate completion of the amputation procedure (Figure 51A,B), removal of the resected root, and to allow for recontouring of the bone in the area where the root was removed. A limited lingual flap may also be required to complete the osseous recontouring. After these procedures are completed, the flap is repositioned and sutured. At a subsequent visit after the coronal portion of the socket has healed, any refinement to the contour of the remaining coronal tooth structure can be accomplished and the appropriate final restorative procedure can be completed (see Figure 50C).

Root amputation is not the treatment of choice when only a portion of a mandibular molar must be removed.

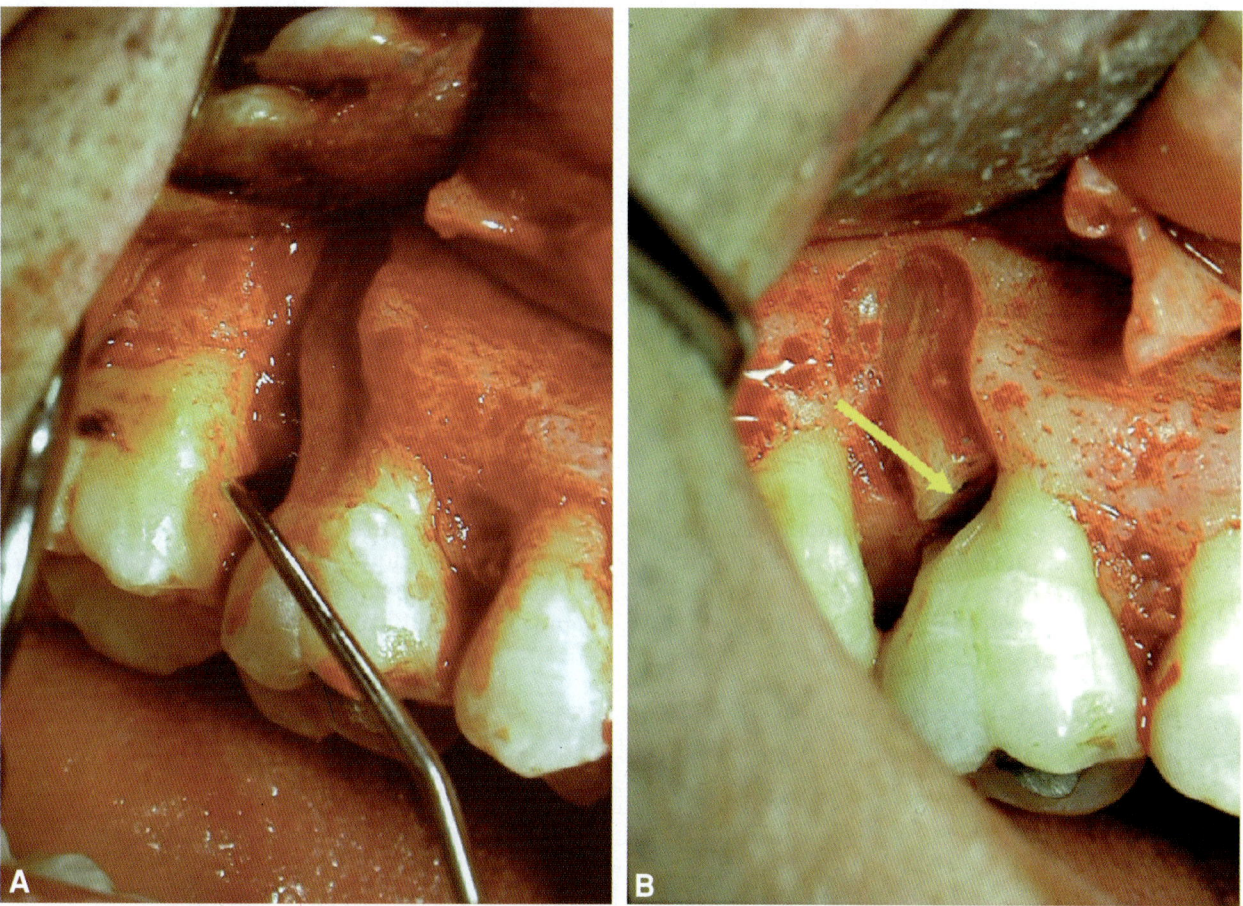

Figure 51 ***A***, Curved periodontal probe illustrates the periodontal defect that exists between the distobuccal and palatal roots of this maxillary first molar; ***B***, The root amputation procedure has been completed and the distobuccal root is now ready for extraction. The arrow notes the presence of the amalgam core in the distobuccal root canal.

This procedure is normally only indicated in mandibular molars when the tooth is acting as an abutment for a well-fitting, serviceable fixed partial denture or a single crown with good proximal contact with the adjacent tooth. As with the maxillary molar, the majority of the crown contouring and amputation procedure must be accomplished with surgical length fissure or diamond burs prior to reflection of the soft tissue flap. The recontoured portion of the tooth should resemble a sanitary pontic. This will allow the patient to be able to adequately clean the undersurface of that portion of the crown in the area where the root was amputated. Delivery of the resected root in mandibular molars is much more difficult than for maxillary molars because the root is as broad as the tooth in a buccolingual dimension. After reflection of a limited soft tissue flap, the resected root will be reduced in length in a coronal to apical direction so that it can be removed from the socket without compromising the stability of the remaining root and coronal tooth structure. Once the root is removed, the bone surrounding the socket will be smoothed and the soft tissue flap will be sutured. Once the coronal portion of the socket is adequately healed, the final recontouring and polishing of the crown can be completed.

HEMISECTION

When root removal is indicated in a mandibular molar because of a vertical root fracture, therapeutic misadventure, or pathologic resorptive process, hemisection is usually the treatment of choice. Due to the difficulties noted above in attempting to perform a root amputation procedure on mandibular molars, removal of one-half the tooth is a more predictable treatment procedure. This procedure is also falling out of favor as a treatment procedure today because the prognosis for success with osseointegrated implants is much better than that for hemisected teeth. The ideal situation for performing a hemisection procedure is when one-half of a mandibular second molar can be retained to occlude with and prevent the supereruption of a maxillary second molar. The root and crown structure that is retained can be restored as a premolar. This procedure is only indicated if the remaining root has adequate periodontal support and the crown can be restored. The mesial root of a mandibular molar has more surface area so it will be more stable periodontally, but because there is generally a concavity present on the distal surface of this root, it is more difficult to restore and cleanse with dental floss and a toothbrush. The distal root is generally more conical in shape and is easier to restore and maintain. The procedure is contraindicated if the roots are fused; there will be inadequate bone support for the remaining root or if the tooth cannot be adequately restored.

As with a tooth being prepared for root amputation, nonsurgical endodontic therapy is completed first and then core material or a post and core restoration is placed into the coronal aspect of the root to be retained and pulp chamber (Figure 52A,B). Once the core material is set, the location of the buccal and lingual furcations is identified and selective occlusal adjustments are made so that the retained portion of tooth will not be in occlusion. The majority of the sectioning procedure is accomplished with a surgical length fissure bur using rubber dam isolation. This prevents debris from accumulating in the mucobuccal fold and possibly getting under the soft tissue flap once it is reflected or into the open extraction socket. The initial resection should begin on the buccal surface and move in a lingual and apical direction until the furcation area is reached. The sectioning should be accomplished at the expense of that portion of the crown that is scheduled for removal. A sufficient amount of tooth structure

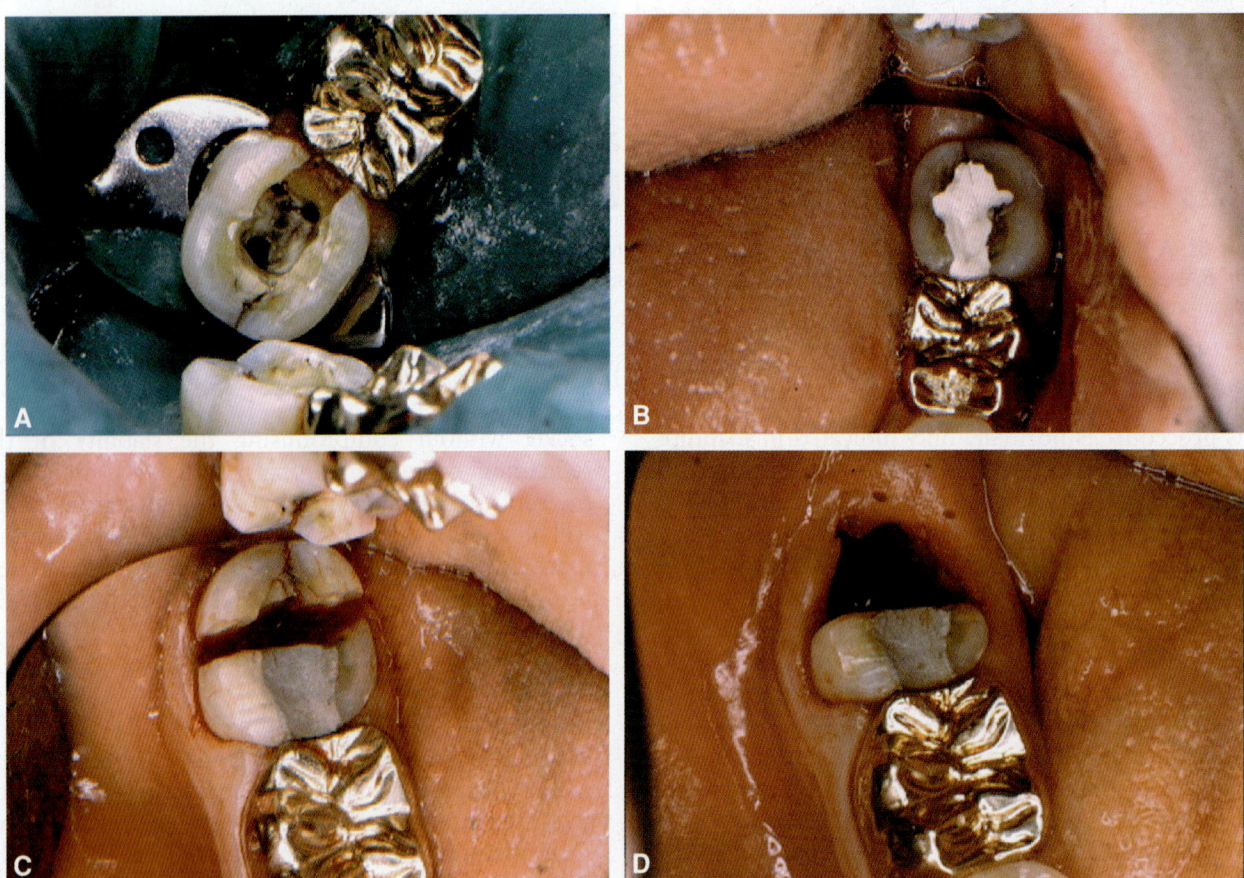

Figure 52 *A,* Mandibular second molar with a fracture across the distal marginal ridge extending to the midroot level; *B,* Amalgam core has been placed; *C,* Hemisection procedure has been completed and the distal root is ready for extraction; *D,* Mesial half of the tooth has been retained as a bicuspid to form an occlusal stop to prevent the extrusion of the opposing maxillary molar.

should be left in the furca area of the portion of the tooth that is to be retained so that a restorative finish line can be established in that area of the tooth. Once the resection has reached the furcation area, the rubber dam is removed and the final separation of the roots is completed with a fissure or tapered diamond bur (see Figure 52C).

The gingival tissue attached to the portion of the tooth to be extracted is loosened. A limited soft tissue envelope-type flap may also be reflected to facilitate removal of the root. The portion of the tooth to be removed should be gently elevated so that the retained root is not disturbed. Using the appropriate forcep, hemostat or ronguer, the loosened root is removed from the socket (see Figure 52D). The socket walls are compressed, the bone margins smoothed, and the soft tissue is repositioned and sutured. If any additional contouring of the remaining tooth is required at this time, the socket should be covered with sterile gauze to prevent particles of tooth and restorative materials from falling into the open extraction socket. Once the healing of the socket has progressed to a point that the coronal portion of the socket is completely covered, restorative procedures can be initiated.

Bicuspidization refers to a procedure that was once recommended for mandibular molars when a hemisection procedure was performed but both roots were to be retained. The purpose of this procedure was to create a situation in a molar tooth with a furcation defect that would be more favorable for cleansing and maintenance. The procedure was found to have a very poor long-term prognosis and is rarely recommended as a treatment option today.

The results of several studies[211–220] report success rates ranging from 62% to 100% with follow-up periods of 1 to 23 years. The combined data from these studies indicates an overall success rate of approximately 88% can be expected when these procedures are performed. The long-term prognosis for teeth with roots amputations or hemisections will depend on a number of factors: the quality of the root canal therapy in the retained root or roots, the contouring and quality of the final restoration, and the ability to maintain the health of the supporting periodontal soft and hard tissues. Any one, or combination, of these factors may result in failure of the case.

PERIODONTAL REGENERATIVE PROCEDURES

In the previous sections dealing with corrective surgical procedures, it was noted that situations might be encountered that will require periodontal regenerative procedures in addition to the corrective root surgery. These regenerative procedures may include, but are not limited to, placement of decalcified freeze-dried bone allograft or calcium sulfate materials[209,221,222] into large bone defects and guided tissue procedures[223–233] using either resorbable or nonresorbable membranes. It is beyond the scope of this chapter to detail every periodontal regenerative procedure. A selected bibiography[209,221–223] dealing with the utilization of these procedures in conjunction with endodontic procedures is provided. For more detail about the clinical techniques involved in the utilization and placement of these materials, the reader is referred to any number of excellent periodontal textbooks.

INTENTIONAL REPLANTATION

Intentional replantation may be defined as the purposeful extraction of a tooth to repair a defect or cause of a treatment failure and then returning the tooth to its original socket.[234,235] The individual first credited with the principle of extraction and replantation was an Arabian physician by the name of Abulcasis who practiced in the eleventh century.[236] Since that time there have been many published reports of studies and case reports dealing with the technique and results of the intentional replantation procedure.[234–245]

Weine[245] has stated that intentional replantation is only indicated when all other endodontic nonsurgical and surgical treatments have been performed and failed or were deemed impossible to perform. This procedure is generally an acceptable treatment alternative when periradicular surgery will not allow visualization of the area on the root to be repaired or there is danger of damaging adjacent vital structures such as the contents of the mandibular canal or mental foramen.[234,235] Specific indications[234,235,239] may include but are not limited to the following situations where nonsurgical and surgical endodontic procedures have been deemed impossible and the patient desires all possible efforts be made to retain the natural tooth: limited mandibular opening that prevents the performance of nonsurgical or periradicular surgical endodontic procedures; root canal obstructions; nonsurgical and surgical treatments have failed and symptoms and/or periradicular disease persists; resorptive or perforation root defects that exist on areas that are not accessible via the usual surgical approach without excessive loss of root length or alveolar bone; and to allow thorough examination of all surfaces of the root in order to identify or rule out the presence of a root defect, such as a crack or root perforation.

Contraindications[234,235,245] may include the following: teeth with long, curved roots that require a surgical extraction procedure for removal from the socket; advanced periodontal disease that has resulted in poor periodontal support and mobility of the tooth; mutirooted teeth with roots that diverge making extraction and replantation impossible; teeth with nonrestorable caries; and teeth that are amenable to additional nonsurgical and surgical endodontic procedures.

To provide the best long-term prognosis for a tooth intentionally reimplanted, the tooth should be kept out of the socket for the shortest time possible, the periodontal ligament attached to the root surface should be kept in moist saline or in Hanks Balanced Salt Solution during entire time the tooth is out of the socket, and the extraction of the tooth should be accomplished as atraumatically as possible to minimize damage to the cementum and periodontal ligament.[234,235] Part of the success of the procedure will also depend on the ability to extract the involved tooth without fracturing the root or roots (Figure 53). The patient should always be advised that fracture of the tooth is possible during the extraction procedure, and if this occurs, the pieces of the tooth will be removed and discarded.

Kingsbury and Wiesenbaugh[240] reported a 95% success rate with 151 mandibular premolar and molar teeth that were intentionally reimplanted over a 3-year period. In another study[241] involving 192 intentionally reimplanted teeth with evaluation periods of between 6 and 51 months, a success rate of 82% was reported. In a more recent report, Bender and Rossman[235] had 80.6% success with 31 intentional reimplantation cases with observation periods of up to 22 years. Raghoebar and Vissink[242] had only 72% success in 29 cases after a 5-year observation period. Intentional replantation is not a completely predictable procedure, but under favorable conditions, some fairly acceptable success have been reported.[239–244]

Once the decision has been made and accepted by the patient to perform the intentional replantation procedure, any nonsurgical endodontic procedures should be completed to the best degree possible (Figure 54A). The pulp chamber and coronal access are then restored to help stabilize and reinforce the coronal tooth structure during the extraction procedure. Intentional replantation is best accomplished as a team effort because each member of the team will be assigned, trained, and skilled to perform a specific function. This team approach will minimize the extra-oral time for the tooth, facilitate the removal of any diseased tissue from the apical portion of the socket, and accelerate the repair of the root surface defect or the placement of a root-end filling. Another method to minimize the time the tooth is out of the socket is to plan so that all necessary instruments and materials necessary to accomplish the entire procedure are out and readily available in the operating area.

Once adequate local anesthesia is obtained, the periodontal fibers in the gingival crevice area are detached with a scalpel blade of an appropriate size in order to loosen the gingival tissues attached to the tooth in this area. A surgical elevator should either not be used or used only minimally to loosen the tooth in the socket. If the use of the elevator results in damage to the cementum or periodontal ligament on the root surface, it may compromise the success of the case. If possible all the loosening of the tooth should be accomplished with the extraction forcep as the tooth is slowly and gently loosened

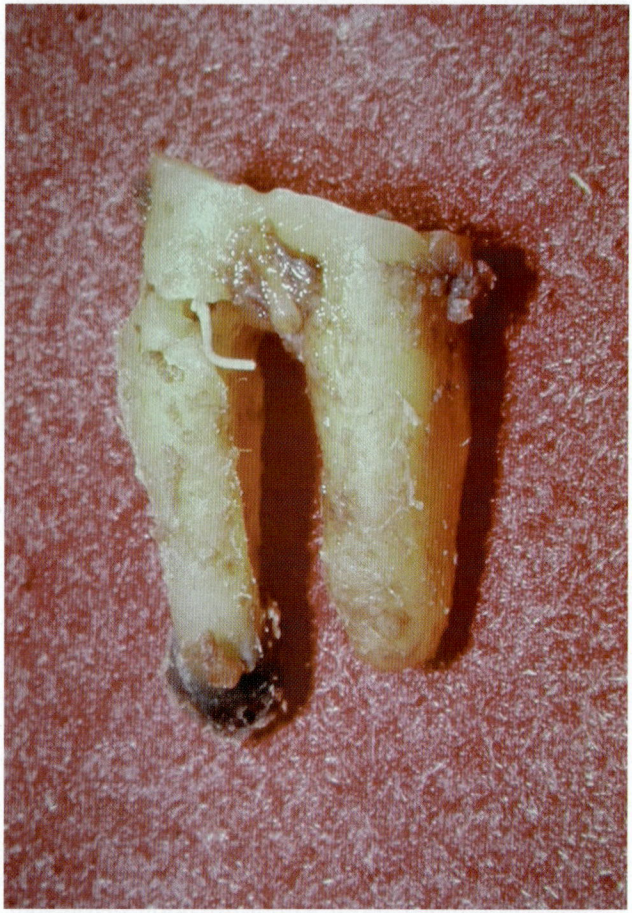

Figure 53 An attempt to perform an intentional replantation on a mandibular second molar failed because the tooth fractured during the extraction process.

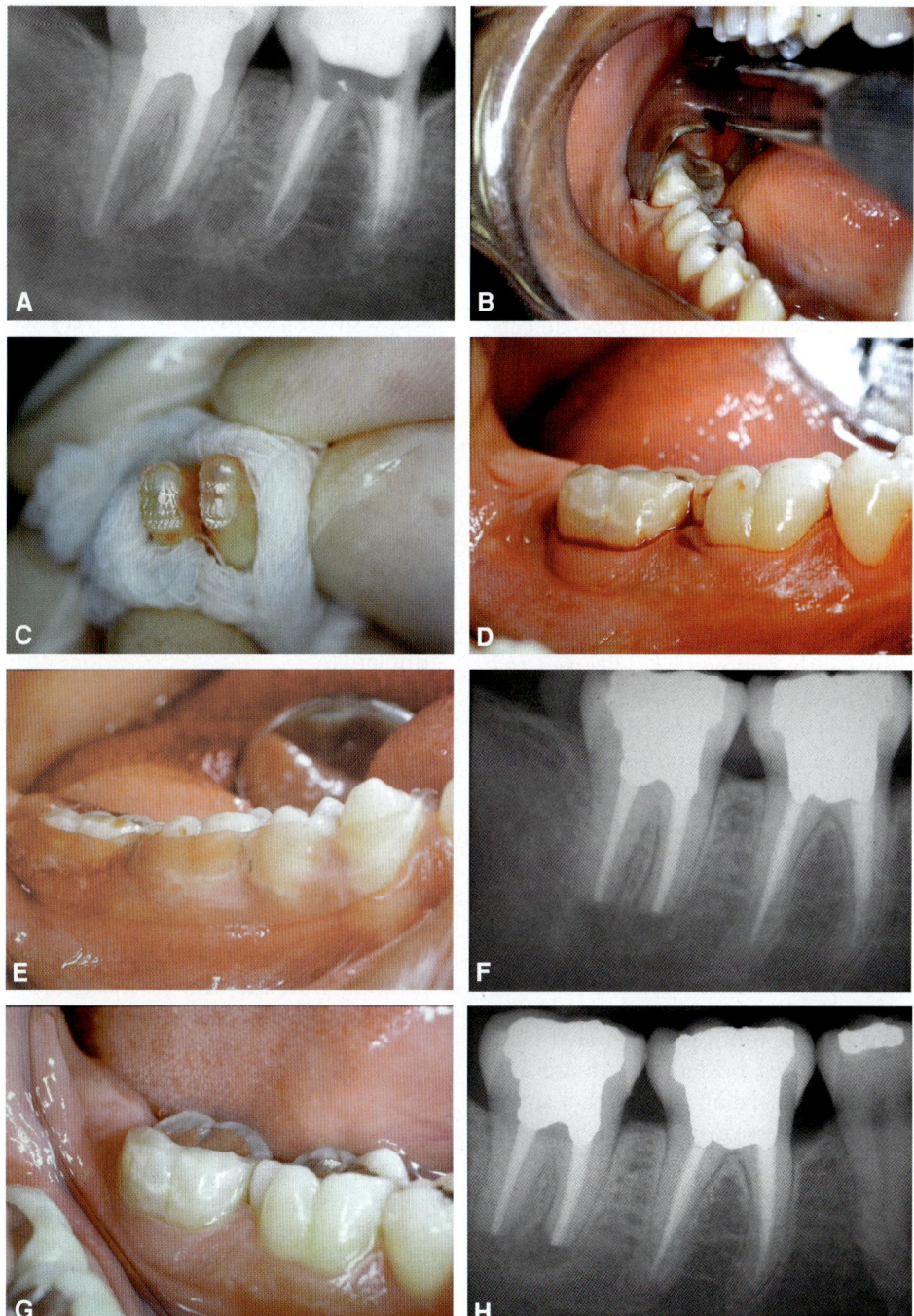

Figure 54 *A*, The mandibular second molar remained symptomatic after an unsuccessful attempt was made to negotiate the apical portion of both mesial canals and to retrieve the separated instrument from one of the canals. Due to the close proximity of the mandibular canal to the apices of the roots of the second molar, an intentional replantation procedure was recommended rather than periapical surgery; *B*, Forcep extraction; *C*, Root ends resected; *D*, Tooth reimplanted; *E*, Acrylic splint placed; *F*, Immediate postoperative radiograph; *G*, Soft tissues are healthy and tooth is asymptomatic at the 6-month follow-up; *H*, There has been a reduction in the size of the periapical radiolucent defect on the 6-month follow-up radiograph.

and removed from the socket (see Figure 54B). It is crucial to remove the tooth and roots in one piece.

Following extraction, the crown of the tooth should be wrapped in gauze moistened with saline or Hanks Balanced Salt Solution and held with the beaks of the forceps. It is also extremely important that the root surfaces be constantly bathed with one of these solutions during the entire extra-oral time. The roots are then thoroughly examined with magnification and a fiber optic light to evaluate for the presence of root fractures or periradicular perforation or resorptive defects. Sterile methylene blue dye may be applied to the root surfaces in order to enhance the visualization of root defects.

If no root fractures are found and the prognosis for replantation appears to be positive, any root defects noted should be repaired with an appropriate material. If root-end resection is indicated, it should be accomplished perpendicular to the long axis of the root with the same bur and in the same manner as if the tooth was still in the socket (see Figure 54C). After root-end resection, the appropriate ultrasonic tip is used to create the small 3-mm-deep Class I root-end preparation. An appropriate root-end filling material will then be placed. If a team approach is being used, one operator repairs the root defect while the second operator gently removes any diseased tissue from the extraction socket. Once the repair/root-end filling material is placed, the extraction socket is irrigated with normal saline and gently suctioned to remove any blood clot that may have formed. The tooth is then carefully reinserted back into its socket (see Figure 54D). Reinsertion of the tooth into the socket may be difficult at times so care must be taken to assure the tooth is returned to the socket in its proper orientation.

After the tooth has been inserted back into the socket, the patient is asked to bite so that the occlusion can be checked to assure the tooth is fully seated back into the socket. In some cases, posterior teeth are well retained in their sockets and stabilization with a splint may not be required. If excessive mobility is present, splinting will be necessary (see Figure 54E). The recommended splinting type and length of time are the same as those for replantation of the traumatically avulsed tooth as discussed in Chapter 31, "Endodontic Treatment Outcome: The Potential for Healing and Retained Function." In the case of a posterior tooth, stabilization may be achieved by placing a figure-8 suture over the occlusal surface of the tooth or by using a prefabricated acrylic splint. Stabilization may also be achieved by using a flexible wire or monofilament line bonded to adjacent teeth with an acid-etch composite resin system.[234,235]

The patient should be re-evaluated 7 to 14 days following the intentional replantation to remove any stabilization that was placed and to evaluate tooth mobility. Other follow-up visits should be scheduled 1, 3, 6, and 12 months following the procedure (see 54F,G,H).

Implant Surgery

OSSEOINTEGRATED IMPLANTS

It is important to emphasize that while the surgical placement of osseointegrated implants is within the scope of endodontics, it is a very technique-sensitive procedure. Attention to detail is required in the alignment of the implant so that it can be properly restored and maintain the health of the supporting periodontal tissues. Dentists who plan to incorporate this procedure into their practice should participate in advanced training programs in order to gain knowledge in diagnosis, treatment planning, and placement of osseointegrated implants prior to implementing their use in clinical practice. This topic is covered in detail in Chapter 34, "Osseointegrated Dental Implants."

ENDODONTIC ENDOSSEOUS IMPLANTS

This type of implant is rarely ever used in today's practice of dentistry and will only be mentioned from a historical perspective. It seemed like a good idea when the procedure was introduced because the rigid implant would be contained within the confines of the root canal system, extend into the apical bone to stabilize the tooth, and not have any direct communication with the oral cavity. Orlay[246] was one of the first to use and advocate this type of implant. Al Frank[247,248] is credited with developing the instruments and matching implants along with standardizing the clinical nonsurgical and surgical techniques. It was reported[249] that these implants were accepted by the periradicular tissue and that healthy fibrous connective tissue surrounded the metal implant and separated it from the alveolar bone. In 1993 Weine and Frank[250] reported that while many of the cases they had placed over a 10-year period failed, some had resulted in long-term successes. Their recommendation was that endodontic endosseous implants be used only in carefully selected cases. With the advent of the true osseointegrated implants, the endodontic implant is no longer considered a treatment option.

Emergency Surgical Procedures

Emergency surgical procedures are indicated when drainage must be established to evacuate purulent and/or hemorrhagic exudate that has formed within the soft tissue or the alveolar bone as a result of a periradicular abscess. These procedures decrease the pressure and pain that result from the buildup of byproducts of the inflammatory and infective process present within the area of the abscess. The length of the morbidity will also be decreased resulting in more rapid healing. If swelling is present in the soft tissues, an incision and drainage procedure will be the treatment of choice. The result of the incision and drainage procedure will be most dramatic if the swelling is fluctuant and the incision results in a productive flow of purulent exudate. If severe pain is present and there is no soft tissue swelling, a cortical trephination procedure may be required to establish drainage and relief of the painful symptoms. The clinical techniques for performing these two procedures are discussed in more detail in Chapter 21, "Treatment of Endodontic Infections, Cysts, and Flare-ups."

Surgical Outcomes (Success/Failure)

Outcomes assessment of endodontic surgical procedures must be addressed from a historical prospective. The techniques, armamentarium, and materials used when performing endodontic surgical procedures today are dramatically different from those being used when some of the early modern era endodontic surgical outcomes studies[251–253] were published. Today the surgeon is able to visualize the surgical field with a surgical operating microscope equipped with an excellent light source. Ultrasonic surgical tips used to prepare the resected root for a root-end filling decrease the need for creating severe beveling of the root end and conserve a greater thickness of dentin and cementum of the root canal walls. This results in greater strength to the remaining root structure. Root-end filling materials used today have proven to be more biocompatible and to have better sealing capability than some of those used in the past. Not only will new cementum cover the resected root end, but it will also grow into contact with certain of these materials so that the entire root end and material is capable of being covered with new cementum.

The results of the studies dealing with outcomes of endodontic surgical treatment are based upon clinical signs and symptoms along with radiographic interpretation at varying follow-up periods of time. The criteria and classification generally used for reporting surgical outcomes are either those proposed by Rud et al.[251,252] or some modification of their original suggestions. Their four classifications for outcomes included a category of "complete healing" which denoted complete radiographic bone fill of the surgical crypt. The second classification was "incomplete healing" which indicated that the surgical crypt had healed with fibrous connective tissue (scar). Radiographically the surgical defect would have significantly reduced in size, but a small radiolucency would still be present. Some studies combine these two categories into one "healing" classification as they both would note a successful result as long as there were no signs and symptoms still associated with the case. The "uncertain healing" category notes there has been little, if any, reduction in the size of the radiolucent surgical defect but that there are no adverse signs or symptoms present at the time of the follow-up. With a longer follow-up period, cases in this category could either end up in one of the healing classifications or in the "unsatisfactory healing" category. This latter category denotes failure of the treatment. In the "failure" category, there will either be no evidence of any reduction in the size of the radiographic surgical defect or the radiographic defect will have enlarged in size. The presence of adverse clinical signs and symptoms can also denote failure even though there are no significant changes radiographically.

Using their established criteria, Rud et al.[251] reported complete healing in 18%, incomplete healing in 23%, and uncertain healing and unsatisfactory healing in 36% of 120 surgical cases with a minimum of a 1-year follow-up period. In a more extensive study[252] of 1,000 surgical cases, they reported on the outcomes at 1 year and then at longer follow-up times. They noted that with the longer follow-up periods there were increases in the complete (66% to 81%) and unsatisfactory categories (2% to 4%) and a decrease in the incomplete (15% to 9%) and uncertain categories (17% to 6%). In another study[253] from this same time period, the complete healing results of 71% were very similar to those reported in the second Rud et al. study[252].

In the 1980s, some changes began to take place with regard to the type of materials being used for root-end fillings. In 1990, Dorn and Gartner[172] reported that in a clinical study of 488 cases, the success rate obtained with Super-EBA cement as a root-end filling material was 95% and 91% for IRM root-end fillings. The results obtained when these two materials were used were significantly better than the 75% success they reported for the cases with amalgam root-end fillings. Frank et al.[254] in 1992 reported on the success of 104 surgical cases with a minimum of a 10-year follow-up period. All 104 teeth had amalgam root-end fillings placed at the time of surgery and had been considered as treatment successes at earlier follow-up evaluations. The success rate in the long-term cases was only 57.7%, suggesting that cases with amalgam root-end fillings would result in short-term successes but might not result in long-term successes. In other reports[255,256] from the early 1990s, the reported surgical success rates are not significantly different from those reported in the 1970s.

The 1990s brought about a revolution in the management of endodontic surgical cases. With the introduction of the surgical operating microscope to endodontics, the ability to better visualize and illuminate the surgical site was changed. Microsurgical instruments were developed and surgical tips were designed for ultrasonic and sonic units. MTA and a dentin-bonded resin composite material (Retroplast) were introduced as potential root-end filling materials. The primary goal of all of these changes was to improve the chances of obtaining a successful outcome for patients requiring endodontic surgical procedures.

Rud et al.[176] reported 97% success in 33 of 34 cases with an 8- or 9-year follow-up where a dentin-bonded resin composite had been used as the root-end filling material. They[178] then reported complete healing in 92% of 551 infected roots treated with the same material and followed for 2 to 4 years. In a 2001 report[257] using the same material, they noted complete healing in 92% of 834 roots after follow-up periods of 6 months to 12.5 years.

Rubinstein and Kim[258] were one of the first to report on success when the endodontic surgical procedure had been performed using the operating microscope. At the 1-year and 2-month follow-up evaluation of 94 cases treated with the microscope and root end filled with Super-EBA cement, they reported a success rate of 96.8%. Of the cases that were considered to be healed after 5 to 7 years, 59 cases were available for follow-up evaluations and the success rate was still very high (91.5%).[259] In another study of 120 teeth treated using the microscope, ultrasonic root-end preparation and Super-EBA root-end filling, an overall success of 92.5% was obtained at the 3-year follow-up evaluation.[260] Von Arx et al.[261] reported an overall success of 83.8% for 191 teeth with a short-term, 1-year follow-up period. Their clinical technique varied in that an endoscope was used rather than an operating microscope, sonic rather than ultrasonic root-end preparation, and three different root-end filling materials were selected for use in an nonrandomized, uncontrolled manner. In a prospective clinical study[262] that specifically assessed surgical success when root-end preparations were accomplished with ultrasonic surgical tips, 42 of 46 cases (91.3%) were judged to be successful at the end of 1 year.

Several prospective clinical studies[184,261,263] have compared success rates when different root-end filling materials have been used. Chong et al.[184] compared MTA and IRM when used as root-end filling materials and reported no statistically significant difference in success between MTA (92%) and IRM (87%) after a 2-year follow-up period. In a study[263] comparing the same two materials, complete healing was found to occur in 64% and incomplete healing in 28% of the 50 teeth root-end filled with MTA after just a 1-year follow-up. In the 50 teeth in this study with IRM root-end fillings, 50% of the teeth were judged to have complete healing and 36% with incomplete healing. If the two healing categories were to be combined, the reported success would be almost identical to that of Chong et al.[184] The success with MTA (90.2%), Retroplast (84.7%), and Super-EBA (76.4%) were compared, but this prospective clinical study[261] failed to control the randomization usage of the three root-end filling materials.

In a systematic review[264] of the endodontic literature, it was found that 330 of 2,788 teeth in 2375 patients required a resurgery procedure. Of these 330 teeth, only 35.7% were found to have successfully healed at the end of 1 year. Thirty-eight percent were determined to be failures and 26.3% were classified in the uncertain healing category at this same time period. In a longitudinal 5-year study[265] first-time versus resurgery cases, the success at 5 years for the resurgery cases was only 59% compared to an 86% success for the first-time surgery cases. A much higher success rate of 77.8% for resurgery cases evaluated at the end of 1 year was reported by von Arx et al.[261] The predictability of achieving successful healing with resurgery cases is significantly less than what we have come to expect with first-time surgery using modern armamentarium, techniques, and materials.

Carbocaine (AstraZeneca Pharmaceuticals, Wilmington DE)
Cavit (3M ESPE, St. Paul MN)
Citanest (AstraZeneca Pharmaceuticals, Wilmington DE)
Duranest (AstraZeneca Pharmaceuticals, Wilmington DE)
IRM (Dentsply Caulk, York PA)
Marcaine (AstraZeneca Pharmaceuticals, Wilmington DE)
MTA (Dentsply Tulsa Dental, Tulsa OK)

Peridex (Zila Pharmaceuticals, 3M, St. Paul MN)
Ravocaine (Cook-Waite, Rochester NY)
Scalpel blades (Becton Dickinson & Co, Franklin Lakes NJ)
Super EBA (Harry J. Bosworth, Skokie IL)
Suture materials (Ethicon, Johnson Johnson, Arlington, TX)
Gelfoam (Pharmacia Canada Inc., Mississauga, Ontario)
Septocaine (Ultracaine) (Septodont, New Castle DE)
Xylocaine (AstraZeneca Pharmaceuticals, Wilmington DE)
Physiologic Saline (Baxter Healthcare Corp., Deerfield, IL)
Arens Tissue Retractor (Hu-Friedy, Chicago, IL)
Seldin Retractor (Hu-Friedy, Chicago, IL)
University of Minnesota Retractor (Hu-Friedy, Chicago, Il)
Multi-Purpose Bur (Caulk Dentsply, Johnson City, TN)
Endo-Z Bur (Caulk Dentsply, Johnson City, TN)
Air Impact Handpiece (Brasseler, Savannah, GA)
Methylene Blue Dye (Roydent, Johnson City, TN)
Surgical Ultrasonic Tips (Dentsply Tulsa Dental, Tulsa, OK)
MAP Delivery System (Roydent, Johnson City, TN)
Racellete Pellets (Pascal Co. Inc., Bellevue, WA)
Surgical Burs (Brasseler, Savannah, GA)
Endodontic and Periodontal Surgical Curettes (Hu-Friedy, Chicago, IL)
Surgicel (Ethicon Inc., Sommerville, NJ)
Sterile Telfa Pads (Johnson & Johnson, Arlington, TX)
Gelfoam (Pharmacia Canada Inc., Mississauga, Ontario)
Ketac (ESPE. Germany)

References

1. Iqbal M, Kratchman SI, Guess GM, et al. Microscopic periradicular surgery:perioperative predictors for postoperative clinical outcomes and quality of life assessment. J Endod 2007;33:239–44.
2. Guerini V. A History of dentistry. Philadelphia, Lea & Febiger, p. 117, 1909.
3. Gutmann JL, Harrison JW. Surgical endodontics. St. Louis (MO): Ishiyaku EuroAmerica;1994.
4. Frank A, Simon J, Abou-Rass M, Glick D. Clinical and surgical endodontics: concepts in practice, Philadelphia:JB Lippincott;1983.
5. Grossman L, Oliet S, Del Rio C. Endodontic practice 11th ed. Philadelphia: Lea & Febiger;1988.
6. Friedman S. Retreatment of failures. In: Principles and practice of endodontics. 2nd ed. Philadelphia:WB Saunders;1996.
7. Bergenholtz G, Lekholm U, Milthon R. Retreatment of endodontic fillings. Scand J Dent Res 1979;87:217.
8. Allen RK, Newton CW, Brown CE. A statistical analysis of surgical and nonsurgical retreatment cases. J Endod 1989;15:261.
9. Van Nieuwenhuysen JP, Aouar M, D'Hoore W. Retreatment or radiographic monitoring in endodontics. Int Endod J 1964;27:75.
10. Hepworth MJ, Friedman S. Treatment outcome of surgical and nonsurgical management of endodontic failures. J Can Dent Assoc 1997;63:364.
11. Kim S, Kratchman S. Modern endodontic surgery concepts and practice: a review. J Endod 2006;32:601.
12. Luebke RG, Glick DH, Ingle JI. Indications and contraindications for endodontic surgery. Oral Surg 1964;18:97.
13. McDonald NJ, Hovland EJ. Surgical endodontics. In: Walton R, Torabinejad M. editors. Principles and practice of endodontics. 2nd ed. Philadelphia: WB Saunders;1996.
14. Lovdahl PE. Endodontic retreatment. Dent Clin North Am 1992:36:473.
15. Weine FS. Nonsurgical retreatment of endodontic failures. Compend Cont Educ Dent 1995;16:324.
16. Cheung GS. Endodontic failures-changing the approach. Int Dent J 1996;46:131.
17. Moiseiwitsch JR, Trope M. Nonsurgical root canal therapy with apparent indications for root-end surgery. Oral Surg 1998;3:335.
18. Schiott CR, Loe H, Borglum-Jensen S, et al. The effects of chlorhexidine mouth rinses on the human oral flora. J Peridont Res 1970;5:84.
19. Lin L, Chance K, Skribner J, Langeland K. Oroantral communication in periapical surgery of maxillary posterior teeth. J Endod 1985;11:40.
20. Eberhardt JA, Torabinejad M, Christiansen EL. A computed tomographic study of the distances between the maxillary sinus floor and the apicies of the maxillary posterior teeth. Oral Surg Oral Med Oral Pathol Oral Radiol Endod 1992;73:345.
21. Ericson S, Finne K, Persson G. Results of apicoectomy of maxillary canines, premolars and molars with special reference to oroantral communication as a prognostic factor. Int J Oral Surg 1974;3:386.
22. Rud J, Rud V. Surgical endodontics of upper molars: relation to the maxillary sinus and operation in acute state of infection. J Endod 1998:24:260.

23. Jin G-C, Kim K-D, Roh B-D, et al. Buccal bone plate thickness of the Asian people. J Endod 2005;31:430.

24. Frankle KT, Seibel W, Dumsha TC. An anatomical study of the position of the mesial roots of mandibular molars. J Endod 1990;16:480.

25. Littner MM, Kaffe I, Tamse A, Dicapua P. Relationship between the apicies of the lower molars and the mandibular canal – A radiographic study. Oral Surg Oral Med Oral Pathol Oral Radiol Endod 1986;62:595.

26. Denio D, Torabinejad M, Bakland LK. Anatomical relationship of the mandibular canal to its surrounding structures in mature mandibles. J Endod 1992;18:161.

27. Tebo HG, Telford IR. An analysis of the relative positions of the mental foramen, Anat Record 1950;106:254.

28. Tebo HG. Variations in the position of the mental foramen. Dent items of interest 1951;73:52.

29. Fishel D, Buchner A, Hershkowith A, Kaffe I. Roentgenologic study of the mental foramen. Oral Surg Oral Med Oral Pathol Oral Radiol Endod 1976;41:682.

30. Phillips JL, Weller RN, Kulild JC. The mental foramen: Part I. Size, orientation, and positional relationship to the mandibular second premolar. J Endod 1990;16:221.

31. Phillips JL, Weller RN, Kulild JC. The mental foramen: Part II. Radiographic position in relation to the mandibular second premolar. J Endod 1992;18:271.

32. Phillips JL, Weller RN, Kulild JC. The mental foramen: Part III. Size and position on panoramic radiographs. J Endod 1992;18:383.

33. Moiseiwitsch JRD. Avoiding the mental foramen during periapical surgery. J Endod 1995;21:340.

34. Moiseiwitsch JRD. Position of the mental foramen in a North American, whit population. Oral Surg Oral Med Oral Pathol Oral Radiol Endod 1998;85:457.

35. Weller RN, Niemczyk SP, Kim S. Incidence and position of the canal isthmus. Part1. Mesiobuccal root of the maxillary first molar. J Endod 1995;21:380.

36. von Arx T. Frequency and type of canal isthmuses in first molars detected by endoscopic inspection during periradicular surgery. Int Endod J 2005;38:160.

37. Mannocci F, Peru M, Sherriff M, et al. The isthmuses of the mesial root of mandibular molars: A micro-computed tomographic study. Int Endod J 2005;38:558.

38. Malamed SF. Handbook of local anesthetics. 2nd ed St. Louis (MO): Mosby;1986.

39. Jastak JT, Yagiela JA. Regional anesthesia of the oral cavity. St. Louis (MO): Mosby;1981.

40. Milam SB, Giovannitti JA. Local anesthetics in dental practice. Dent Clin North Am. 1984;28:493.

41. Simard-Savoie S. New method for comparing the activity of local anesthetics used in dentistry. J Dent Res 1975;54:978.

42. Sisk AL. Vasoconstrictors in local anesthesia for dentistry. Anesth Prog 1993;39:187.

43. Gage TW. Pharmacology of the autonomic nervous system. In: Holroyd SV, Wynn RL, Requa-Clark B: Clinical pharmacology in dental practice. 4th ed. St. Louis (MO);Mosby:1988.

44. Weiner N. Norepinephrine, epinephrine, and the sympathomimetic amines. In: Gilman AF, Goodman LS, Gilman A, editors. Goodman and Gilman's the pharmacologic basis of therapeutics. 6th ed. New York: Macmillan Publishing;1980.

45. Bennett CR. Monheim's local anesthesia and pain control in dental practice, 7th ed. St. Louis (MO):Mosby;1984.

46. Council on Dental Therapeutics of the American Dental Association. Accepted dental therapeutics. 40th ed. Chicago: American Dental Association;1984.

47. Neidle EA. Introduction to autonomic nervous system drugs. In: Neidle EA, Kroeger, DC, Yageila JA, editors. Pharmacology and therapeutics for dentistry. 2nd ed. St. Louis (MO): Mosby;1985.

48. Tolas AG, Pflug AD, Halter JB. Arterial plasma epinephrine concentrations and hemodynamic response after dental injection of local anesthetic with epinephrine. J Am Dent Assoc 1982;104:41.

49. Chernow B, Balestrieri F, Ferguson DD, et al. Local anesthesia with epinephrine: Minimal effects on the sympathetic nervous system or on hemodynamic variables. Arch Intern Med 1983;143:2141.

50. Davenport RE, Porcelli RJ, Iaacono VJ, et al. Effects of anesthetics containing epinephrine on catecholamine levels during periodontal surgery. J Periodontol 1990;61:553.

51. Lipp M, Dick W, Daublander M, et al. Exogenous and endogenous plasma levels of epinephrine during dental treatment under local anesthesia. Reg Anesth 1993;18:6.

52. Replogle K, Reader A, Nist R, et al. Cardiovascular effects of intraosseous injections of 2 percent lidocaine with 1:100,000 epinephrine and 3 percent mepivacaine. J Am Dent Assoc 1999;130:649.

53. Pallasch TJ. Vasoconstrictors and the heart. Calif Dent Assoc J. 1998.

54. Hecht A, App GR. Blood volume loss during gingivectomy using two different anesthetic techniques. J Periodontol 1974;45:9.

55. Lindorf HH. Investigation of the vascular effects of newer local anesthetics and vasoconstrictors. Oral Surg 1979;48:292.

56. Cutright DE, Hunsuck, EE. Microcirculation of the perioral regions of the *Macaca Rhesus*. Oral Surg 1970;29:776.

57. Gutmann JL, Harrison JW. Posterior endodontic surgery: anatomical considerations and clinical techniques. Int Endod J 1985;18:8.

58. Castelli WA, Huelke DF. The arterial system of the head and neck of the rhesus monkey with emphasis on the external carotid system. Am J Anat 1965;116:149.
59. Davis WL. Oral histology: cell structure and function. Philadelphia:WB Saunders; 1986; p. 154.
60. Hooley JR, Whitacre RJ. A self-instructional guide to oral surgery in general dentistry. 2nd ed. Seattle: Stoma Press;1980.
61. Luebke RG, Ingle JI. Geometric nomenclature for mucoperiosteal flaps. Periodontics 1964;2:301.
62. Macphee R, Cowley G. Essentials of periodontology and periodontics. 3rd ed. Oxford: Blackwell Scientific Publications; 1981.
63. Velvart P, Ebner-Zimmermann U, Ebner JP. Comparison of long-term loss of papilla healing following sulcular full thickness flap and papilla base flap in endodontic surgery. Int Endod J 2004;37:687.
64. Harrison JW, Jurosky KA. Wound healing in the tissues of the periodontium following periradicular surgery. 1. The incisional wound. J Endod 1991;17:425.
65. Harrison JW, Jurosky KA. Wound healing in the tissues of the periodontium following periradicular surgery. 2. The dissectional wound. J Endod 1991;17:544.
66. Kohler CA, Ramfjord SP. Healing in gingival mucoperiosteal flaps. Oral Surg 1960;13:89.
67. Levine LH. Periodontal flap surgery with gingival fiber retention. J Periodontol 1972;43:91.
68. Tetsch P. Development of raised temperatures after osteotomies. J Maxillofac Surg 1974;21:141.
69. Eriksson AR, Albrektsson T. Heat induced bone tissue injury. Swed Dent J 1982;6:262.
70. Eriksson AR, Albrektsson T, Grane B, McQueen D. Thermal injury to bone. A vital-microscopic description of heat effects. Int J Oral Surg 1982;11:115.
71. Eriksson AR, Albrektsson T. Temperature threshold levels for heat-induced bone tissue injury: A vital-microscopic study in the rabbit. J Prosthet Dent 1984;50:101.
72. Eriksson AR, Albrektsson T. The effect of heat on bone regeneration: an experimental study in the rabbit. J Oral Maxillofac Surg 1984;42:705.
73. Boyne P. Histologic response of bone to sectioning by high-speed rotary instruments. J Dent Res 1966;45:270.
74. Moss R. Histopathologic reaction of bone to surgical cutting. Oral Surg 1964;17:405.
75. Argen E, Arwill T. High-speed or conventional dental equipment for the removal of bone in oral surgery. III: A histologic and micro radiographic study on bone repair in the rabbit. Acta Odontol Scand 1968;26:223.
76. Calderwood RG, Hera SS, Davis JR,Waite DE. A comparison of the cutting effect on bone after the production of defects by various rotary instruments. J Dent Res 1964;43:207.
77. Falomo OO. Surgical emphysema following root canal therapy: Report of a case. Oral Surg 1984;58:101.
78. Battrum DE, Gutmann JL. Implications, prevention and management of subcutaneous emphysema during endodontic treatment. Endod Dent Traumatol 1995;11:109.
79. Stockdale CR, Chandler NP. The nature of the periapical lesion–a review of 1108 cases. J Dent 1988;16:123.
80. Lin LM, Gaengler P, Langeland K. Periradicular curettage. Inter Endod J 1996;29:220.
81. el-Swiah JM, Walker RT. Reasons for apicectomies: a retrospective study. Endod Dent Traumatol 1996;12:185.
82. Ingle JI, Cummings RR, Frank AL, et al. Endodontic Surgery. In: Endodontics 4th ed. Ingle JI and Bakland LK editors. Baltimore, Williams and Wilkins, 1994; p. 723.
83. Gutmann JL, Pitt Ford TR. Management of the resected root end: a clinical review. Int Endod J 1993;26:273.
84. Nedderman TA, Hartwell GR, Portell FR. A comparison of root surfaces following apical root resection with various burs: scanning electron microscopic evaluation. J Endod 1988;14:423.
85. Morgan LA, Marshall JG. The topography of root ends resected with fissure burs and refined with two types of finishing burs. Oral Surg Oral Med Oral Pathol Oral Radiol Endod 1998;85:585.
86. Ebihara A, Wadachi R, Sekine Y, et al. Application of Er:YAG laser to apicoectomy, 6th International Congress on Lasers in Dentistry, 1998.
87. Komori T, Yokoyama K, Matsumoto Y, :YAG laser root resection of extracted human teeth. J Clin Laser Med Surg 1997;15:9.
88. Moritz A, Gutknecht N, Goharkhay K, et al. The carbon dioxide laser as an aid in apicoectomy: an *in vitro* study. J Clin Laser Med Surg 1997;15:185.
89. Maillet WA, Torneck CD, Friedman S. Connective tissue response to root surfaces resected with Nd:YAG laser or burs. Oral. Surg Oral Med Oral Pathol Oral Radiol Endod 1996;82:681.
90. Miserendino LJ. The laser apicoectomy: endodontic application of the CO_2 laser for periapical surgery. Oral Surg Oral Med Oral Pathol Oral Radiol Endod 1988;66:615.
91. Komori T, Yokoyama K, Takato T, Matsumoto K. Clinical application of the Erbium:YAG laser for apicoectomy. J Endod 1997;23:748.
92. Slaton CC, Loushine RJ, Weller RN, et al. Identification of resected root-end dentinal cracks: a comparative study of visual magnification. J Endod 2003;29:519.
93. Wright HM, Loushine RJ, Weller RN, et al. Identification of resected root-end dentinal cracks: a comparative study of transillumination and dyes. J Endod 2004;30:712.
94. Bellizzi R, Loushine R. A Clinical Atlas of Endodontic Surgery, Quintessence Publishing Co., 1991.

95. Arens DE, Adams WR, DeCastro RA. editors. Endodontic surgery, Philadelphia, Harper and Row, 1981.

96. Weine FS, Gerstein H. Periapical surgery. In: Weine FS, editor. Endodontic therapy, 4th ed., St. Louis, The CV Mosby Co., 1982.

97. Arens DE. Surgical Endodontics. In: Cohen S, Burns R, editors. Pathways of the pulp. 4th ed., St. Louis, The CV Mosby Co., 1987.

98. Gerstein H. Surgical Endodontics. In: Laskin DN, editor. Oral and maxillofacial Surgery, Vol. II, St. Louis, The CV Mosby Co., 1985.

99. Vertical RJ, Beatty RG. Apical leakage associated with retro fillings techniques: a dye study. J Endod 1986;12:331.

100. Cresco WR, Ellison RL, Corcoran JF, Krause DC. A spectrophotometer analysis of dentinal leakage in the resected root. J Endod 1991;17:503.

101. Beatty R. The effect of reverse filling preparation design on apical leakage. J Dent Res 1986;65:259 (Abstract #805).

102. Giuliani M, Tastier S, Molina R. Ultrasonic root-end preparation: influence of cutting angle on the apical seal. J Endod 1998;24:726.

103. Glean PA, Figwort D, Teas MJ. Apical dentin permeability and microleakage associated with root-end resection and retrograde filling. J Endod 1994;20:22.

104. Timers BG, Arrow smith MG. Dentinal tubules at the root ends of apiece teeth: a scanning electron microscopic study. Int Endod J 1989;22:184.

105. Alexander RE. Patient understanding of postsurgical instruction forms. Oral Surg 1999;87:153.

106. Carr GB, Bent over SK. Surgical Endodontics. In: 7th ed. Cohen S Burns R, editors. Pathways of the pulp. 1997; p. 619.

107. Scrota KS, Krakow AA. Retrograde instrumentation and obscuration of the root canal space. J Endod 1983;9:448.

108. von Arx T, Walker WA. Microsurgical instruments for root-end cavity preparation following apicoectomy: a literature review. Endod Dent Traumatol 2000;16:47.

109. Mehlhaff DS, Marshall JG, Baumgartner JC. Comparison of ultrasonic and high-speed-bur root-end preparations using bilaterally matched teeth. J Endod 1997;23:448.

110. Wuchenich G, Meadows D, Torabinejad M. A comparison between two root end preparation techniques in human cadavers. J Endod 1994;20:279.

111. Zuolo ML, Perin FR, Ferreira MOF, Faria FP. Ultrasonic root-end preparation with smooth and diamond-coated tips. Endod Dent Traumatol 1999;15:265.

112. Engel TK, Steiman HR. Preliminary investigation of ultrasonic root end preparation. J Endod 1995;21:443.

113. Gutmann JL, Saunders WP, Nguyen L, et al. Ultrasonic root-end preparation Part I. SEM analysis. Int Endod J 1994;27:318.

114. Gorman MC, Steiman HR, Gartner AH. Scanning electron microscopic evaluation of root-end preparations. J Endod 1995;21:113.

115. Navarre SW, Steiman HR. Root-end fracture during retropreparation: a comparison between zirconium nitride-coated and stainless steel microsurgical ultrasonic instruments. J Endod 2002;28:330.

116. Abedi HR, Van Mieilo BL, Wilder-Smith P, Torabinejad M. Effects of ultrasonic root-end cavity preparation on the root apex. Oral Surg Oral Med Oral Pathol Oral Radiol Endod 1995;80:207.

117. Frank RJ, Antrium DD, Bakland LK. Effect of retrograde cavity preparations on root apexes. Endod Dent Traumatol 1996;12:100.

118. Beling KL, Marshall JG, Morgan LA, Baumgartner JC. Evaluation for cracks associated with ultrasonic root-end preparation of gutta-percha filled canals. J Endod 1997;23:323.

119. Brent PD, Morgan LA, Marshall JG, Baumgartner JC. Evaluation of diamond-coated ultrasonic instruments for root-end preparation. J Endod 1999;25:672.

120. Rainwater A, Jeansonne BG, Sarkar N. Effects of ultrasonic root-end preparation on microcrack formation and leakage. J Endod 2000;26:72.

121. Calzonetti KJ, Iwanowski T, Komorowski R, Friedman S. Ultrasonic root-end cavity preparation assessed by an in situ impression technique. Oral Surg Oral Med Oral Pathol Oral Radiol Endod 1998;85:210.

122. Morgan LA, Marshall JG. A scanning electron microscopic study of in vivo ultrasonic root-end preparations. J Endod 1999;25:567.

123. Witherspoon DE, Gutmann JL. Haemostasis in periradicular surgery. Int Endod J 1996;29:135.

124. Horsley V. Antiseptic wax. Brit Med J 1892;1:1165.

125. Ibarrola JL, Bjorenson JE, Austin BP, Gerstein H. Osseous reactions to three hemostatic agents. J Endod 1985;11:75.

126. Aurelio J, Chenail B, Gerstein H. Foreign-body reaction to bone wax. Oral Surg Oral Med Oral Pathol Oral Radiol Endod 1984;58:98.

127. Finn MD, Schow SR, Schneiderman ED. Osseous regeneration in the presence of four hemostatic agents. J Oral Maxilofac Surg 1992;50:608.

128. Solheim E, Pinholt EM, Bang G, Sudmann E. Effect of local hemostatics on bone induction in rats: A comparative study of bone wax, fibrin-collagen paste and bioerodible polyorthoester with and without gentamicin. J Biomed Mat Res 1992;26:791.

129. von Arx T, Jensen SS, Hanni S, Schenk RK. Haemostatic agents used in periradicular surgery: an experimental study of their efficacy and tissue reaction. Int Endod J 2006;39:800.

130. Vickers FJ, Baumgartner JC, Marshall G. Hemostatic efficacy and cardiovascular effects of agents used during endodontic surgery. J Endod 2002;28:322.

131. Vy CH, Baumgartner JC, Marshall JG. Cardiovascular effects of a hemostatic agent in periradicular surgery. J Endod 2004;30:379.
132. Besner E. Systemic effects of racemic epinephrine when applied to the bony cavity during periapical surgery. Va Dent J 1972;49:9.
133. Lemon RR, Steele PJ, Jeansonne BG. Ferric sulfate hemostasis: effect on osseous wound healing. I. Left in situ for maximum exposure. J Endod 1993;19:170.
134. Jeansonne BG, Boggs WS, Lemon RR. Ferric sulfate hemostasis: effect on osseous wound healing. II. With curretage and irrigation. J Endod 1993;19:174.
135. Rossman JA, Rees TD. The use of hemostatic agents in dentistry. Postgrad Dent 1996;3:1.
136. Pecora G, Adreana S, Margarone JE, et al. Bone regeneration with a calcium sulfate barrier. Oral Surg Oral Med Oral Pathol Oral Radiol 1997;84:424.
137. Kim S, Rethnam S. Hemostasis in endodontic microsurgery. Dent Clin N Am 1997;41:499.
138. Boyes-Varley JG, Cleaton-Jones PE, Lownie JR. Effects of a topical drug combination on the early healing of extraction sockets in the vervet monkey. Int J Oral. Maxillofac Surg 1988;17:138.
139. Olson RAJ, Roberts DL, Osbon DB. A comparative study of polylactic acid, Gelfoam, and Surgicel in healing extraction sites. Oral Surg Oral Med Oral Pathol Oral Radiol Endod 1982;53:441.
140. Caen JP, Legrand Y, Sultan Y. Platelets: Collagen interactions. Thrombosis and Haemostasis 1970;40:181.
141. Mason RG, Read MS. Some effects of microcrystalline collagen preparations on blood. Haemostasis 1974;3:31.
142. Mattsson T, Anneroth G, Kondell PA, Nordenram A. ACP and Surgicel in bone hemostasis. Swed Dent J 1990;14:57.
143. Swan N. Textured collagen, a hemostatic agent. Oral Surg Oral Med Oral Pathol Oral Radiol Endod 1991;72:642.
144. Haasch GC, Gerstein H, Austin BP. Effect of two hemostatic agents on osseous healing. J Endod 1989;15:310.
145. Finn MD, Schow SR, Schneiderman ED. Osseous regeneration in the presence of four common hemostatic agents. J Oral Maxillofac Surg 1992;50:608.
146. Takeuchi H, Konaga E, Kashitani M. The usefulness of Avitene for the control of oozing in laparoscopic cholecystectomy. Surg Gynecol Obstet 1993;176:495.
147. Gartner AH, Dorn SO. Advances in endodontic surgery. Dent Clin North Am 1992;36:357.148 – Jou YT, Pertl C. Is there a best retrograde filling material. Dent Clin North Am 1997;41:555.
149. Owadally ID, Chong BS, Pitt Ford TR, Wilson RF. Biological properties of IRM with the addition of hydroxyapatite as a retrograde root filling material. Endod Dent Traumatol 1994;10:228.
150. Makkawy HM, Koka S, Lavin MT, Ewoldsen NO. Cytotoxicity of root perforation materials. J Endod 1998;24:477.
151. Chong BS, Owadally ID, Pitt Ford TR, Wilson RF. Cytotoxicity of potential retrograde root-filling materials. Endod Dent Traumatol 1994;10:129.
152. Zhu Q, Safavi E, Spangberg LSW. Cytotoxic evaluation of root-end filling materials in cultures of human osteoblast-like cells and periodontal ligament cells. J Endod 1999;25:410.
153. Harrison JW, Johnson SA. Excisional wound healing following the use of IRM as a root-end filling material. J Endod 1997;23:19.
154. Pitt Ford TR, Andreasen JO, Dorn SO, Kariyawasam SP. Effect of IRM root-end fillings on healing after replantation. J Endod 1994;20:381.
155. Pitt Ford TR, Andreasen JO, Dorn SO, Kariyawasam SP. Effect of Super-EBA as a root-end filling on healing after replantation. J Endod 1995;21:13.
156. Maeda H, Hashiguchi I, Nakamuta H, et al. Histological study of periapical tissue healing in the rat molar after retrofillings with various materials. J Endod 1999;25:38.
157. Torabinejad M, Hong CU, McDonald F, Pitt Ford T. Physical and chemical properties of a new root-end filling material. J Endod 1995;21:349.
158. Torabinejad M, Pitt Ford TR, Abedi HR, et al. Tissue reaction to implanted root-end filling materials. J Endod 1998;24:468.
159. Torabinejad M, Watson TF, Pitt Ford TR. Sealing ability of a mineral trioxide aggregate when used as a root-end filling material. J Endod 1993;19:591.
160. Torabinejad M, Higa RK, McKendry, DJ, Pitt Ford TR. Dye leakage of four root-end filling materials: effects of blood contamination. J Endod 1994;20:159.
161. Bates CF, Carnes DL, Del Rio CE. Longitudinal sealing ability of mineral trioxide aggregate as a root-end filling material. J Endod 1996;22:575.
162. Fischer EJ, Arens DE, Miller CH. Bacterial leakage of mineral trioxide aggregate as compared with zinc-free amalgam, intermediate restorative material, and Super-EBA as a root-end filling material. J Endod 1998;24:176.
163. Torabinejad M, Rastegar AF, Kettering JD, Pitt Ford TR. Bacterial leakage of mineral trioxide aggregate as a root-end filling material. J Endod 1995;21:109.
164. Torabinejad M, Smith PW, Kettering JD, Pitt Ford TR. Comparative investigation of marginal adaptation of mineral trioxide aggregate and other commonly used root-end filling materials. J Endod 1995;21:295.
165. Koh ET, McDonald R, Pitt Ford TR, Torabinejad M. Cellular response to mineral trioxide aggregate. J Endod 1998;24.
166. Torabinejad M, Hong CU, Pitt Ford TR, Kettering JD. Cytotoxicity of four root end filling material. J Endod 1995;21:489.
167. Kettering JD, Torabinejad M. Investigation of mutagenicity of mineral trioxide aggregate and other commonly used root-end filling materials. J Endod 1995;21:537.

168. Torabinejad M, Hong CU, Pitt Ford TR. Tissue reaction to implanted Super-EBA and mineral trioxide aggregate in the mandibles of guinea pigs: a preliminary report. J Endod 1995;21:569.

169. Torabinejad M, Hong CU, Lee SJ, et al. Investigation of mineral trioxide aggregate for root end filling in dogs. J Endod 1995;21:603.

170. Torabinejad M, Pitt Ford TR, McKendry DJ, et al. Histologic assessment of mineral trioxide aggregate as a root-end filling in monkeys. J Endod 1997;23:225.

171. Oynick J, Oynick T. A study of a new material for retrograde fillings. J Endod 1978;4:203.

172. Dorn SO, Gartner AH. Retrograde filling materials: a retrospective success-failure study of amalgam, EBA, and IRM. J Endod 1990;16:391.

173. Pantschev A, Carlsson AP, Andersson L. Retrograde root filling with EBA cement or amalgam. A comparative clinical study. Oral Surg 1994;78:101.

174. Rud J, Munksgaard EC, Andreasen JO, et al. Retrograde root fillings with composite and a dentin-bonding agent. Endod Dent Traumatol 1991;7(Pt 1):118.

175. Rud J, Munksgaard EC, Andreasen JO, Rud V. Retrograde root fillings with composite and a dentin-bonding agent. Endod Dent Traumatol 1991;7:126.

176. Rud J, Rud V, Munksgaard EC. Long-term evaluation of retrograde root fillings with dentin-bonded resin composite. J Endod 1996;22:90.

177. Rud J, Rud V, Munksgaard EC. Retrograde root filling with dentin-bonded modified resin composite. J Endod 1996;22:477.

178. Rud J, Rud V, Munksgaard EC. Effect of root canal contents on healing of teeth with dentin-bonded resin composite retrograde seal. J Endod 1997;23:535.

179. Michelich VJ, Schuster GS, Pashley DH. Bacterial penetration of human dentin in-vivo. J Dent Res 1980;59:1398.

180. Barkhordar RA, Watanabe LG, Marshall GW, Hussain MZ. Removal of intracanal smear layer by Doxycycline in vitro. Oral Surg 1997;84:420.

181. Craig KR, Harrison JW. Wound healing following demineralization of resected root ends in periradicular surgery. J Endod 1993;9:339.

182. Minabe M, Takeuchi K, Kumada H, Umemoto T. The effect of root conditioning with minocycline HCL in removing endotoxin from the roots of periodontally involved teeth. J Periodontol 1994;65:387.

183. Barkhordar RA, Russel T. Effect of Doxycycline on the apical seal of retrograde filling materials. J Calif Dent Assoc 1998.

184. Chong BS, Pitt Ford TR, Hudson MB. A prospective clinical study of mineral trioxide aggregate and IRM when used as root-end filling materials in endodontic surgery. Int Endod J 2003;36:520.

185. Holland R, de Souza V, Nery MJ, et al. Reaction of rat connective tissue to implanted dentin tubes filled with a white mineral trioxide aggregate. Braz Dent J 2002;13:23.

186. Fitzpatrick EL. Steiman HR. Scanning electron microscopic evaluation of finishing techniques on IRM and EBA retrofillings. J Endod 1997;23:423.

187. Forte SG, Hauser MJ, Hahn C, Hartwell GR. Microleakage of Super-EBA with and without finishing as determined by the fluid filtration method. J Endod 1998;24:799.

188. Eriksson L. Cyanoacrylate for closure of wounds in the oral mucosa in dogs. Odontol Rev 1976;27:19.

189. Javelet J, Torabinejad M, Danforth R, Isobutyl cyanoacrylate: a clinical and histological comparison with sutures in closing mucosal incisions in monkeys. Oral Surg 1985;59:91.

190. Vanholder R, Misotten A, Roels H, Matton G. Cyanoacrylate tissue adhesive for closing skin wounds: a double blind randomized comparison with sutures. Biomaterials 1993;14:737.

191. Simon HK, McLario KJ, Bruns TB, et al. Long-term appearance of lacerations repaired using a tissue adhesive. Pediatrics 1997;99:193.

192. Samuel PR, Roberts AC, Nigam A. The use of Indermil (n-butyl cyanoacrylate) in otorhinolaryngology and head and neck surgery. A preliminary report on the first 33 patients. J Laryngol Otol 1997;111:536.

193. Giray CB, Atasever A, Durgun B, Araz K. Clinical and electron microscopic comparison of silk sutures and n-butyl-2-cyanoacrylate in human mucosa. Aust Dent J 1997;42:255.

194. Grisdale J. The use of cyanoacrylate in periodontal therapy. J Can Dent Assoc 1998;64:632.

195. Lilly GE, Armstrong JH, Salem JE, Cutcher JL. Reaction of oral tissues to suture materials. Oral Surg 1968;26:592.

196. Lilly GE, Armstrong JH, Cutcher JL. Reaction of oral tissues to suture materials. Oral Surg 1969;26:432.

197. Lilly GE, Cutcher JL, Nones TC, Armstrong JH. Reaction of oral tissues to suture materials. Oral Surg 1972;33:152.

198. Ebert JR. Method for scanning electron microscopic study of plaque on periodontal suture material. J Dent Res 1974;53:1298.

199. Rakusin H, Harrison JW, Marker VA. Alteration of the manipulative properties of plain gut suture material by hydration. J Endod 1988;14:121.

200. Craig PH, Williams JA, Davis KW. A biologic comparison of polyglactin 910 and polyglycolic acid synthetic sutures. Surg Gynecol Obstet 1975;141:1.

201. Nelson EH, Junakoshi E, O'Leary TJ. A comparison of the continuous and interrupted suturing technique. J Periodontol 1977;48:273.

202. Ramfjord SP, Nissle RR. The modified Widman flap. J Periodontol 1974;45:601.

203. Guyton AC. Textbook of medical physiology. 7th ed. St Louis (MO): Mosby;1986. p. 860.
204. Seymour RA, Meedhan JG, Blair GS. Postoperative pain after apicoectomy. Int Endod J 1986;19:242.
205. Davis W, Oakley J, Smith E. Comparison of the effectiveness of etidocaine and lidocaine as local anesthetic agents during oral surgery. Anesth Prog 1984;31:159.
206. Dunsky J, Moore P. Long-acting local anesthetics: a comparison of bupivacaine and etidocaine in endodontics. J Endod 1984;10:6.
207. Weisman MI. Comfortable suture removal. J Endod 1981;7:186.
208. Weine FS. The case against intentional replantation. J Am Dent Assoc 1980;100:644.
209. Dean JW, Lenox RA, Lucas FL, et al. Evaluation of a combined surgical repair and guided tisssue regeneration technique to treat recent root canal perforations. J Endod 1997;23:525.
210. Kirchoff DA, Gerstein H. Presurgical crown contouring for root amputaion procedures. Oral Surg Oral Med Oral Pathol Oral Radiol Endod 1969;27:379.
211. Bergenholtz A. Radectomy of multirooted teeth. J Am Dent Assoc 1972;85:870.
212. Klanan B. Clinical observations following root amputation in maxillary molar teeth. J Periodont 1975;46:1.
213. Hamp SE, Nyman S, Lindhe J. Periodontal treatment of multirooted teeth. Results after 5 years. J Clin Periodont 1975;2:126.
214. Langer B, Stein SD, Wagenberg B. An evaluation of root resections. A ten-year study. J Periodont 1981;52:719.
215. Erpenstein H. A 3-year study of hemisected molars. J Clin Periodont 1983;10:1.
216. Buhler H. Evaluation of root-resected teeth. Results after 10 years. J Periodont 1988;59:805.
217. Carnevale G, Febo GD, Tonelli MP, et al. A retrospective analysis of the periodontal-prosthetic treatment of molars with interradicular lesions. Int J Periodont Rest Dent 1991;11:189.
218. Basten CHJ, Ammons WF, Persson R. Long-term evaluation of root-resected molars. A retrospective study. Int J Periodont Rest Dent 1996;16:207.
219. Blomlof L, Jansson L, Appelgren R, et al. Prognosis and mortality of root-resected molars. Int J Periodont Rest Dent 1997;17:191.
220. Carnevale G, Pontoriero R, di Fego G. Long-term effects of root-resective therapy in furcation-involved molars. A 10-year longitudinal study. J Clin Periodont 1998;25:209.
221. Anson D. Calcium sulfate: A 4-year observation of its use as a resorbable barrier in guided tissue regeneration of periodontal defects. Compend Cont Educ Dent 1996;17:895.
222. Bier SJ, Sininsky MC. The versatility of calcium sulfate: Resolving periodontal challenges. Compend Cont Educ Dent 199;20:655.
223. Gottlow J, Laurell L, Teiwik A, Genon. Guided tissue regeneration using a bioresorbable matrix barrier. Pract Perio Aesth Dent 1994;6:71.
224. Abramowitz PN, Rankow H, Trope M. Multidisciplinary approach to apical surgery in conjunction with the loss of buccal cortical plate. Oral Surg Oral Med Oral Pathol Oral Radiol Endod 1994;77:502.
225. Kellert M, Chalfin H, Solomon C. Guided tissue regeneration: An adjunct to endodontic surgery. J Am Dent Assoc 1994;125:1229.
226. Lundgren D, Mathisen T, Gottlow J. The development of a bioresorbable barrier for guided tissue regeneration. J Swed Dent Assoc 1994;86:741.
227. Pecora G, Kim S, Celletti R, Davarpanah M. The guided tissue regeneration principle in endodontic surgery: One-year postoperative results of large periapical lesions. Int Endod J 1995;28:41.
228. Rankow HJ, Krasner PR. Endodontic applications of guided tissue regeneration in endodontic surgery. J Endod 1996;22:34.
229. Uchin RA. Use of a bioresorbable guided tissue membranes as an adjunct to bony regeneration in cases requiring endodontic surgical intervention. J Endod 1996;22:94.
230. Tseng CC, Harn WM, Chen YH, et al. A new approach to the treatment of true-combined endodontic-periodontic lesions by the guided tissue regeneration technique. J Endod 1996;22:693.
231. Pecora G, Baek SH, Rethman S, Kim S. Barrier membrane techniques in endodontic microsurgery. Dent Clin N Am 1997;41:585.
232. Santamaria J, Garcia AM, de Vincente JC, et al. Bone regeneration after radicular cyst removal with and without guided bone regeneration. Int J Oral Maxillofac Surg 1998;27:118.
233. Douthitt JC, Gutmann JL, Witherspoon DE. Histologic assessment of healing after the use of a bioresorbable membrane in the management of buccal bone loss concomitant with periradicular surgery. J Endod 2001;27:404.
234. Grossman LI. Intentional replantation of teeth: A clinical evaluation. J Am Dent Assoc 1982;104:633.
235. Bender IB, Rossman LE. Intentional replantation of endodontically treated teeth. Oral Surg Oral Med Oral Pathol Oral Radiol Endod 1993;76:623.
236. Weinberger B. Introduction to the history of dentistry. Vol. 1. St. Louis, 1948, CV Mosby, p. 105.
237. Hammer H. Replantation and implantation of teeth. Int Dent J 1955;5:439.
238. Grossman L, Chacker F. Clinical evaluation and histologic study of intentionally replanted teeth. In: Grossman L. editor

Transactions of the Fourth International Conference on Endodontics. Philadelphia, University of Pennsylvania, 1968, p. 127.

239. Dryden JA, Arens DE. Intentional replantation: A viable alternative for selected cases. Dent Clin N Am 1994;38:325.

240. Kingsbury B, Weisenbaugh J. Intentional replantation of mandibular premolars and molars. J Am Dent Assoc 1971;83:1053.

241. Koenig K, Nguyen N, Barkholder. Intentional replantation: A report of 192 cases. Gen Dent 1988;36:327.

242. Raghoebar GM, Vissink A. Results of intentional replantation of molars. J Oral. Maxillofac Surg 1999;57:240.

243. Kratchman S. Intentional replantation. Dent Clin N Am 1997;41:603.

244. Nosonowitz D, Stanley H. Intentional replantation to prevent predictable endodontic failures. Oral Surg Oral Med Oral Pathol Oral Radiol Endod 1984;57:423.

245. Weine FS. The case against intentional replantation. J Am Dent Assoc 1980;100:664.

246. Orlay HG. Endodontic splinting treatment in periodontal disease. Brit Dent J 1960;108:118.

247. Frank AL. Improvement in the crown:root ratio by endodontic endosseous implants. J Am Dent Assoc 1967;74:451.

248. Frank AL. Endodontic endosseous implants and treatment of the wide-open apex. Dent Clin N Am 1967;11:675.

249. Frank AL, Abrams AM. Histologic evaluation of endodontic implants. J Am Dent Assoc 1969;78:520.

250. Weine FS, Frank AL. Survival of the endodontic endosseous implant. J Endod 1993;19:524.

251. Rud J, Andreasen JO, Jensen JEM. Radiographic criteria for the assessment of healing after endodontic surgery. Int J Oral Surg 1972;1:195.

252. Rud J, Andreasen JO, Jensen JEM. A follow-up study of 1,000 cases treated by endodontic surgery. Int J Oral Surg 1972;1:215.

253. Altonen M, Mattila K. Follow-up study of apicoectomized molars. Int J Oral Surg 1976;5:33.

254. Frank AL, Glick DH, Patterson SS, Weine FS. Long-term evaluation of surgically placed amalgam fillings. J Endod 1992;18:391.

255. Friedman S, Lustmann J, Shaharabany V. Treatment results of apical surgery in premolar and molar teeth. J Endod 1991;17:30.

256. Rapp EL, Brown CE, Newton CW. An analysis of success and failure of apicoectomies. J Endod 1991;17:508.

257. Rud J, Rud V, Munksgaard EC. Periapical healing of mandibular molars after root-end sealing with dentin-bonded composite. Int Endod J 2001;34:285.

258. Rubinstein RA, Kim S. Short-term observation of the results of endodontic surgery with the use of a surgical operation microscope and Super-EBA as root-end filling material. J Endod 1999;25:43.

259. Rubinstein RA, Kim S. Long-term follow-up of cases considered healed one year after apical microsurgery. J Endod 2002;28:378.

260. Maddalone M, Gagliani M. Periapical endodontic surgery: a 3-year follow-up study. Int Endod J 2003;36:193.

261. von Arx T, Jensen SS, Hanni S. Clinical and radiographic assessment of various predictors for healing outcome 1 year after periapical surgery. J Endod 2007;33:123.

262. Taschieri S, Del Fabbro M, Testori T, et al. Endodontic surgery with ultrasonic retrotips: one-year follow-up. Oral Surg Oral Med Oral Pathol Oral Radiol Endod 2005;100:380.

263. Lindeboom JAH, Frenken JWFH, Kroon FHM, van den Akker HP. A comparative prospective randomized clinical study of MTA and IRM as root-end filling materials in single-rooted teeth in endodontic surgery. Oral Surg Oral Med Oral Pathol Oral Radiol Endod 2005;100:495.

264. Peterson J, Gutmann JL. The outcome of endodontic resurgery: a systematic review. Int Endod J 2001;34:169.

265. Gagliani MM, Gorni FGM, Strohmenger L. Periapical resurgery versus periapical surgery: a 5-year longitudinal comparison. Int Endod J 2005;38:320.

Chapter 34

Osseointegrated Dental Implants

Jaime L. Lozada, Alejandro Kleinman

Implant Dentistry in the Endodontic Practice

One of the main objectives in dentistry is prevention of oral disease and the preservation of the natural dentition, frequently achieved by root canal treatment.[1] When this is not possible, osseointegrated implants can play a significant role in the rehabilitation of patients who have lost their teeth or have hopeless teeth because of periodontal or restorative concerns.[2] Implants are increasingly being used to replace missing teeth in a variety of situations, including the **missing single tooth.**

There is, however, considerable variation in treatment planning philosophy among clinicians encountering patients with pulpally involved teeth with a questionable prognosis.[3-7] The decision between retention of endodontically involved teeth versus extraction and implant placement is a clinical decision that requires careful evaluation of all of the factors influencing the outcome of the proposed treatment.[8,9]

The treatment decision depends on the following variables: the quality of the support the tooth will provide for planned restorations, predicted longevity, and its role in the overall rehabilitation, functionally, esthetically, and financially.[2,10] Before a definitive treatment decision is made, it is important to assess the quality of tooth support compared with that provided by implants.

Dental implants have by no means constituted the only significant recent advance in dentistry. In endodontics, for instance, the use of microscopes, nickel titanium files, electronic apex locators, and ultrasonic instruments are but a few of the developments enabling practitioners to perform endodontic treatment with greater precision and efficiency, fewer errors, and better success rates than ever before.[11] Of course, success in endodontic treatment is not solely dependent on instruments and technique. It is also affected by such factors as the level of disease progression (i.e., the presence of apical pathosis), case selection, restoration quality, iatrogenic errors, and, very importantly, postendodontic control of coronal microleakage.[12,13]

The determination of success is usually based on clinical parameters, including cessation of symptoms and complete repair of periapical tissues. Success for a patient, however, may simply be to have a tooth that is in function, one that may not be totally comfortable to chew on but otherwise is clinically sound. Endodontic therapy alone does not guarantee successful retention of a tooth or prevent its future loss as most failures associated with endodontically treated teeth are not endodontic in nature. Recurrent dental caries, root fractures, and periodontal disease, in conjunction with recurring apical periodontitis, have been associated with these failures.[9,14,15] These studies also suggest that such factors are indications for tooth extraction more frequently than endodontic failure itself. The loss of tooth structure is directly related to the ability of a tooth to resist fracture.[16] More specific data regarding the success and survival of endodontically treated teeth are described in Chapter 31, "Outcomes of Endodontic Treatment."

As with conventional endodontic therapy, the long-term success of implant-based treatment varies, depending on the experience of the clinician, implant location, surgical and prosthetic technique, and type of implants used.[17] However, long-term implant survival rates better than 90% are well supported by the literature.[14,18-21] Modern implant surfaces provide more predictable integration (measured by bone-implant contact, removal torque, and Resonance Frequency Analysis) at all time intervals, making implants a predictable treatment foundation for the long-term restoration of missing teeth.

When one compares the predictability of endodontically treated teeth versus implants as foundations for restorative dentistry, the literature provides some advantages for implants. This is most likely related to their obvious resistance to dental caries, periodontal disease, and structural deficiencies. The clinical literature reports survival rates up to and exceeding 97% depending on the location in the arch and bone density.[22–24]

Single-rooted teeth with structural integrity and **intact coronal structure** are the best candidates for traditional endodontic treatment, especially in instances in which the esthetic outcome is important to the patient. The loss of vitality in these teeth is often caused by trauma. In contrast, teeth requiring endodontic therapy that have a significant caries and restorative history end up with substantial loss of coronal structure. Most of these teeth require additional restorative care, and this further compromises the retained structure and periodontal and caries status. Correctly placed implants, positioned in idealized sites, with the use of appropriately timed provisional restorations to shape the surrounding soft tissue, can be associated with esthetic results comparable (and often superior) to fixed prosthodontic restoration on natural teeth.[25]

Extraction and immediate placement of dental implants to support replacements of single teeth, even in esthetic sites, are now very predictable.[26–28] Immediately placed implants have numerous advantages over delayed placement techniques, including maintenance of the existing gingival embrasure form, any marginal contour, preservation of the existing bone, reduced surgical procedures, and shorter treatment times.[28,29]

When the diagnosis of endodontic failure has been made,[30–33] three treatment options exist to resolve the problem: conservative retreatment, apical surgery, or extraction.[34] The literature indicates that the success of retreatment is higher than surgical treatment when access to the root canals is feasible.[30] Retreatment, however, should be avoided in teeth that cannot be satisfactorily restored (Figure 1). Additionally, in cases with periodontal involvement, the prognosis of combined therapy should be assessed before proceeding with the endodontic retreatment.[35] Several factors may dictate surgical endodontics as the treatment of choice. These factors include failure of conventional endodontic treatment, difficulties in performing conventional endodontic treatment, root fractures, root perforations, and endodontic-periodontal complications. A poor prognosis with an increased probability of failure may be associated with any of those factors.

When a tooth is considered to be in a hopeless condition, extraction is indicated. Immediate placement of an implant following extraction has been suggested by several investigators to take advantage of the present osseous dimensions and to minimize further osseous resorption.[29,36]

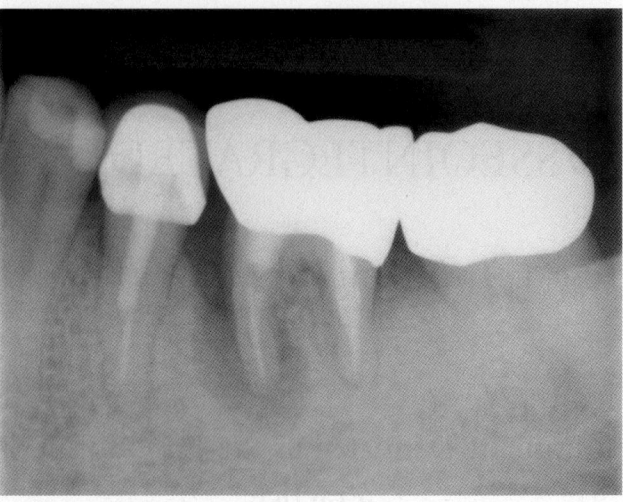

Figure 1 An endodontically treated tooth is failing because of vertical root fracture of the mesial root. This is a situation in which replacing the tooth with an implant is a good option.

Immediate placement has several advantages, including the following: decreased operatory time with less trauma to the tissues and less discomfort to the patient; easier implant orientation and better restorations can be achieved; crestal bone loss can be minimized; through the use of a longer implant, the long-term prognosis can be increased; and greater support can be obtained for guided bone regeneration procedures in cases of bone-implant deficiency to maintain or enhance the bone width and height.[36]

Contraindications to immediate implant placement include the presence of active infection, if bone regeneration is important, or if there is difficulty in obtaining primary closure.

Immediate implant placement is a predictable and a widely practiced procedure with demonstrated efficacy for long-term restoration of missing teeth. The clinician now has an additional choice of treatment in cases in which tooth extraction is inevitable. The decision to either maintain an endodontically involved tooth or do the extraction and place an implant can be a very complex issue and must be based on a number of factors, not the least of which is the long-term predictability of treatment outcome. According to Bader, there is no generic answer to this clinical issue, and every patient, indeed every site, must be examined and evaluated on an individual basis.[8]

Historical Background

Over the past 40 years, endosseous dental implantation has been established as a credible method of oral rehabilitation. The replacement of teeth by implantation techniques was started a long time ago by our ancestors. Skeletal remains from ancient Egyptian and South American cultures give evidence of these efforts.[37] Gold and ivory dental implants were used in the sixteenth and seventeenth centuries.[38] Since then, until the 1960s, multiple materials and surgical techniques were used without any major breakthroughs in replacing teeth.

Root replacement by allogenic tooth transplantation became popular in seventeenth century England, France, and the Americas and continued well into this century. Metal implant devices of gold, iridium, tantalum, stainless steel, and cobalt alloy were developed in the early twentieth century.[39]

Classic Dental Implant Devices

BLADE-FORM IMPLANTS

This type of implant also is known as a plate-form implant. It is a type of endosseous implant with the geometric shape of a rectangle, with a narrow buccal-lingual dimension designed, once inserted, to be restored and splinted to a natural tooth abutment (Figure 2).

The endosteal blade implant was introduced independently in 1967 by Leonard Linkow and by Ralph

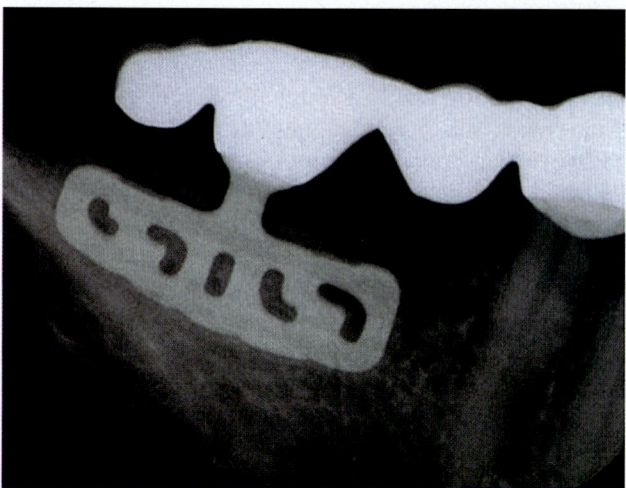

Figure 2 An example of a blade-form implant. These implants were typically splinted to natural teeth.

and Harold Roberts. In 1979, the National Institutes of Health Office of Medical Applications of Research (OMAR) scheduled a consensus development conference titled "Dental Implants: Benefits and Risks." For blade-form implants in the free end application that primarily involves bridges or one pontic and two or more natural abutments, the data suggested that the 5-year survival rate may have been as high as 90%. However, data presented at the meeting suggested a 5-year survival rate as low as 65%. The device is not as popular today as it was 20 years ago.[40]

SUBPERIOSTEAL IMPLANTS

One of the earliest designers of a subperiosteal implant was the Swedish practitioner Gustav Dahl, who placed his first subperiosteal implant in 1940.[41] Aaron Gershkoff and Norman Goldberg of Providence, Rhode Island, were leading American pioneers in subperiosteal implant designs and techniques. They brought the technique of Dahl to the United States and performed their first surgical placement in 1948. Their work consisted of making a complete mandibular impression of the soft tissues covering the edentulous jaw. They estimated the thickness and character of the mucosa using radiographs and palpation. They then scraped a cast to remove the appropriate amount of stone to reflect the tissue thickness. From the modified cast, they fabricated a vitallium casting. The tissues were then reflected, and the implant was fitted on the bone and held in place with screws.

Another American, Nicholas Berman of Seattle, Washington, altered Goldberg and Gershkoff's early technique. Recognizing that the bone must be exposed to accurately determine its morphology, Berman fabricated a stone cast from a modeling plastic impression of the mandible after the soft tissue had been reflected. Two or three weeks after the initial impression, he again uncovered the bone and fitted the meshwork under the periosteum and over the bone.[42]

In 1980, Philip Truit, a graduate student in implant dentistry at Loma Linda University School of Dentistry, using computed tomography (CT), produced a morphologic replication of the mandible. His work consisted of comparing actual measurements with CT measurements on dry skulls and subsequently on cadavers. Adequate accuracy was not obtained on the first attempt, and certain regions of the jaw were not accurately recorded when 18 separate anatomic landmarks were evaluated.[43]

Subsequent research and improvements produced frameworks that fit with gaps that were generally less

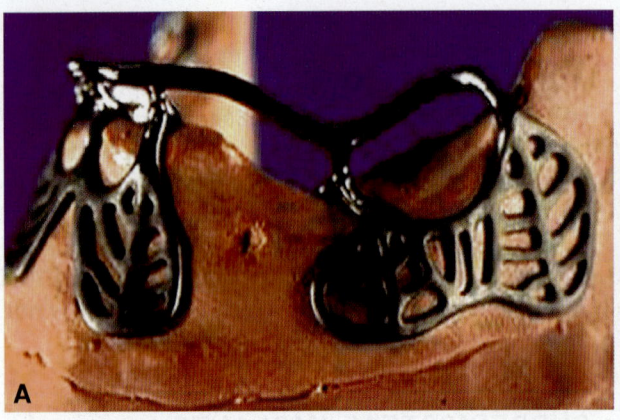
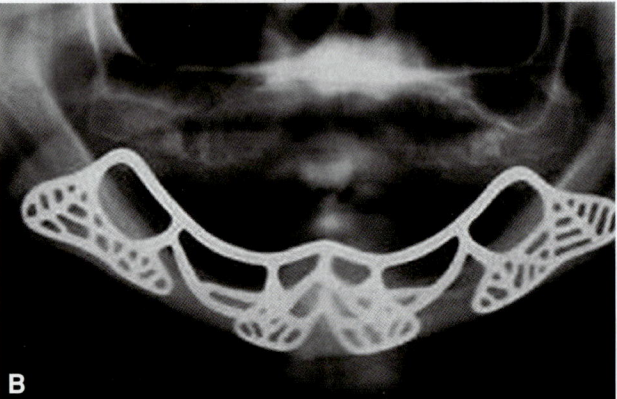

Figure 3 *A,* An example of a subperiosteal implant on a duplicate of the tridimensional model of a patient's alveolar arch. *B,* Panoramic radiograph of the subperiosteal implant in the patient's mouth.

than 0.5 mm. The results, using this process, showed sufficient accuracy to apply to clinical patient treatment. Over 200 subperiosteal implants were subsequently fabricated and placed at Loma Linda using the three-dimensional modeling protocol that eliminated the need for a bone impression (Figure 3).

ENDODONTIC IMPLANTS

The concept behind endodontic implants is that if a rigid implant can safely extend out through the apex of the tooth into sound bone, and by so doing stabilize a tooth with weakened support, the patient is well served and perhaps can avoid replacement for some time. Unfortunately, a high failure rate of endodontic implants developed, and the profession backed off from their use. Weine and Frank, however, retrospectively "revisited" their endodontic implant cases placed over a 10-year period.[44] While admitting to "many that did fail," they "noted some remarkable long-term successes with the technique." Their recommendation was that endodontic implants not be discarded totally but used only in carefully selected cases (Figure 4).

Orlay may have been among the first to use and advocate endodontic implants.[45] Frank is credited, however, with standardizing the technique, developing the proper instruments, and matching implants.[46,47] Frank and Abrams were also able to show that a properly placed endodontic implant was accepted by the apical tissues and that a narrow "collar" of healthy fibrous connective tissue, much like a circular periodontal ligament, surrounded the metal implant and separated it from the alveolar bone.[48]

Placing endodontic implants is a technique-sensitive procedure. A **perfectly round preparation** must be reamed out through the root apex and into the alveolar bone. Failure to accomplish this, results in leakage around the implant-dentin interface at the apex and eventual failure results.

ENDOSSEOUS ROOT FORM IMPLANTS

It has been proposed that the term *root-form implant* be avoided since it perpetuates a faulty concept that cylindrical implants resemble the roots of natural teeth. However, an alternate term that differentiates the endosseous implants approximating the form of a tooth from those that are plate-like in form has not emerged. Therefore, the term *endosseous root-form implant* continues to be widely used (Figure 5).

OSSEOINTEGRATION

In the 1950s and 1960s, Professor Per-Ingvar Brånemark and his colleagues completed experimental work that was started in 1952. Their research led to the development and introduction of titanium root-form implants.[49] His work revolutionized the approach to and acceptance of implants as a treatment modality. This type of endosseous root-form implant has become the most widely used implant in the world.

After the validation of osseointegration, which is now a clinical realty, the root-form implant once again has become implant dentistry's most dominant design. A multitude of solid and hollow screw and press-fit forms have been developed with and without

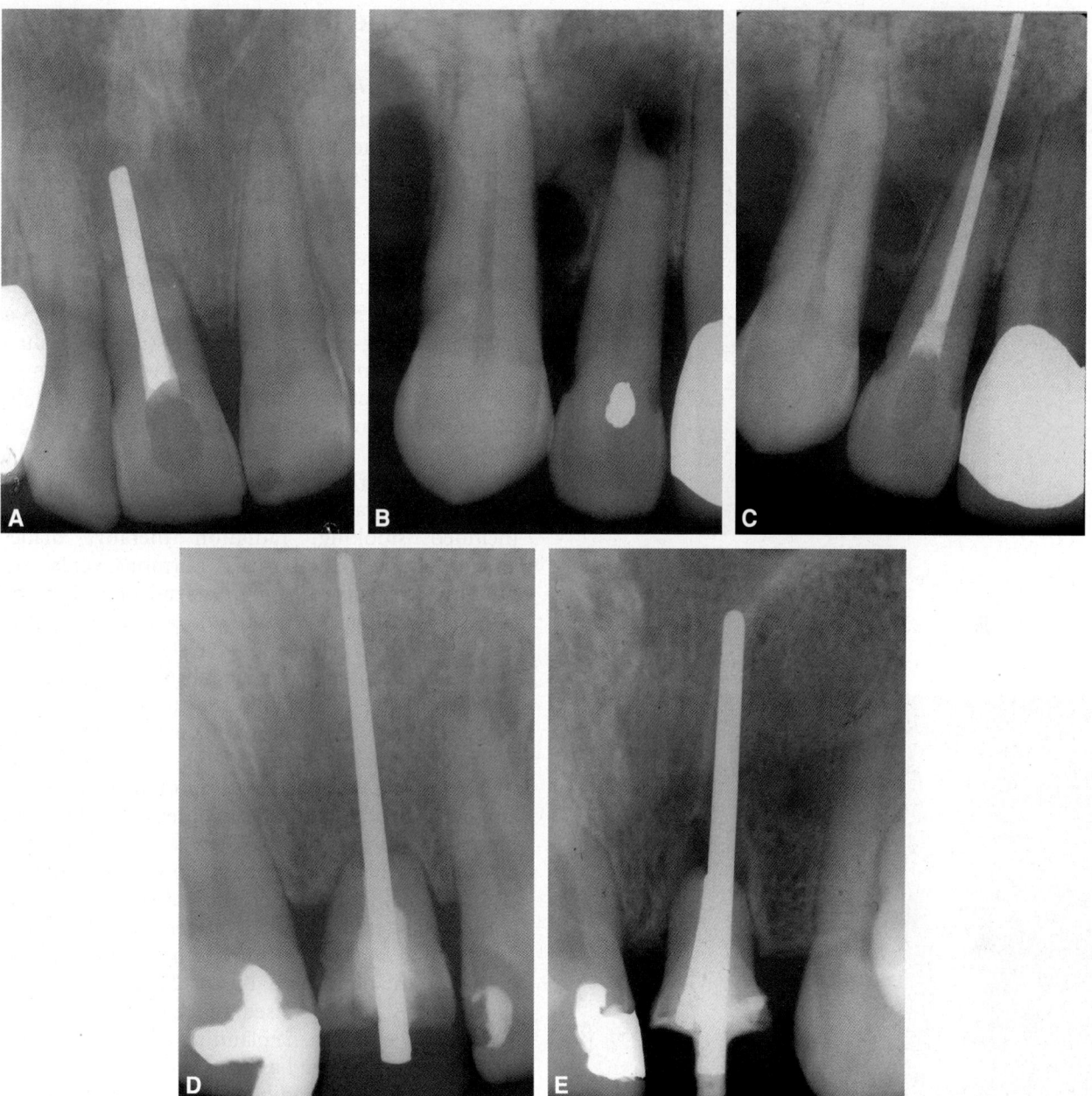

Figure 4 Examples of the use of endodontic implants. *A,* Eight-year follow-up of treatment of a tooth with an endodontic implant for a horizontal root fracture in which the apical segment had been removed. *B,* An example of a tooth with extensive periodontal bone loss, one of the indications for an endodontic implant. *C,* The tooth in *B* 2 years after implant placement. *D,* An endodontic implant after 6.5 years. *E,* An endodontic implant in place after 32 years. 3*D* and *E* are courtesy of Dr. Pabla Barrientos, Santiago, Chile.

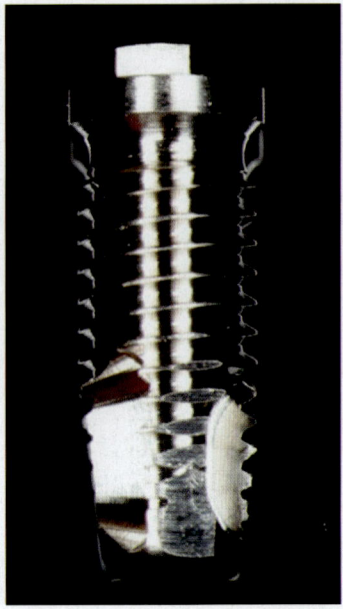

Figure 5 Brånemark Pure Ti machined implant (MKIII).

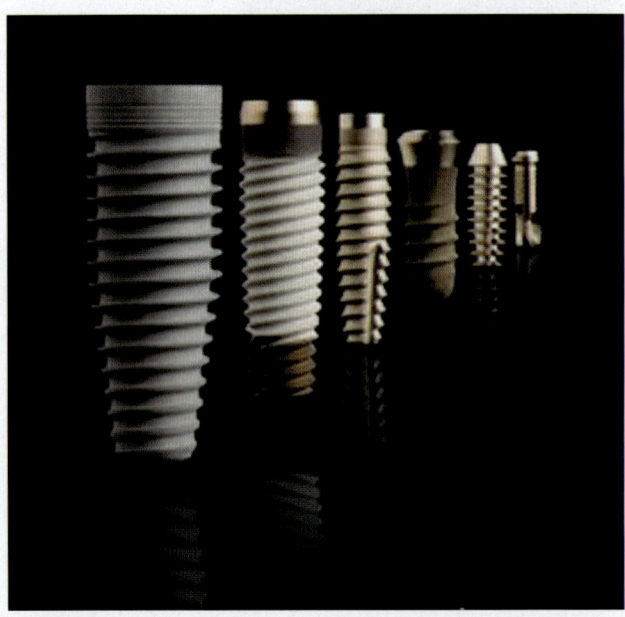

Figure 6 Various titanium implant surface designs and coatings.

titanium plasma spray, surface oxidation, and hydroxyapatite coatings (Figure 6).

Single-Implant Restorations

DIAGNOSIS AND TREATMENT PLAN

Endodontic clinicians repeatedly face decision making in providing the best form of treatment for compromised teeth. From endodontic retreatment, tooth extraction, and alveolar preservation to simultaneous dental implant placement, endodontists today are preparing themselves to be well equipped to provide all of these forms of treatment.

Several diseases, medications, treatments, and habits affecting implant success have been evaluated and reported in the literature. Some have been definitively correlated with increased implant failure rates; others have been evaluated, but no correlation with increased failure has been noted. Data about other factors are limited and do not permit conclusions to be drawn. These factors investigated have included smoking, radiation therapy, diabetes, chemotherapy, osteoporosis, hormone replacement therapy, scleroderma, Sjögren syndrome, Parkinson disease, multiple myeloma, and a human immunodeficiency virus (HIV)-positive status.[50]

An important part of diagnosis is determining if sufficient bone is available for the placement of an implant. When teeth approximate edentulous areas, it is important to determine if the teeth and bone are free from disease. It is also important to locate vital anatomic structures that can interfere with implant placement, such as the maxillary sinus, inferior alveolar canal, mental foramen, and approximating roots.

Radiographic images are necessary to assess available bone sites for implant placement. The number, angulation, and dimensions (length and width) of implants are dependent on available bone volume. Radiographs are also used to identify bone quality. To aid in the treatment planning of implant patients, a classification system has been developed for both the maxilla and the mandible related to the degree of resorption and morphology of the residual ridge. The bone quality noted radiographically has also been classified (Figure 7).

The faciolingual dimensions of residual bone have also been measured using bone sounding and ridge mapping. With bone sounding, a periodontal probe is pushed through anesthetized mucosa to locate the depth of the bone beneath the facial and lingual mucosa. Special bone calipers with sharp points have

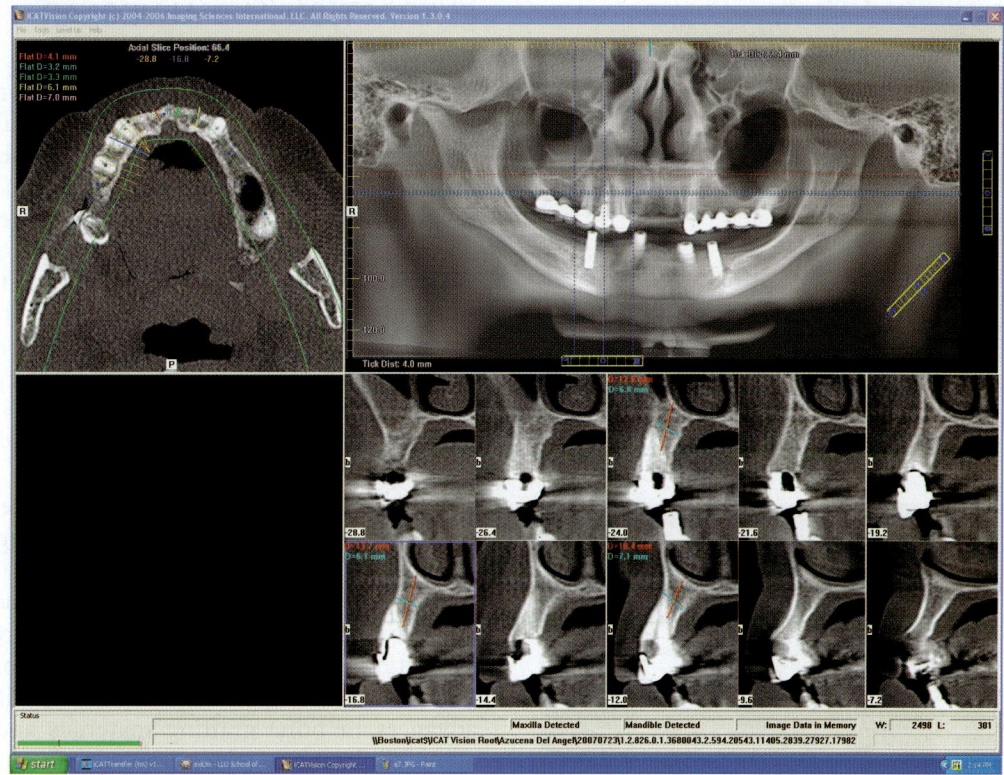

Figure 7 Bone quality can be measured and classified from the Cone Bean Computed Tomography.

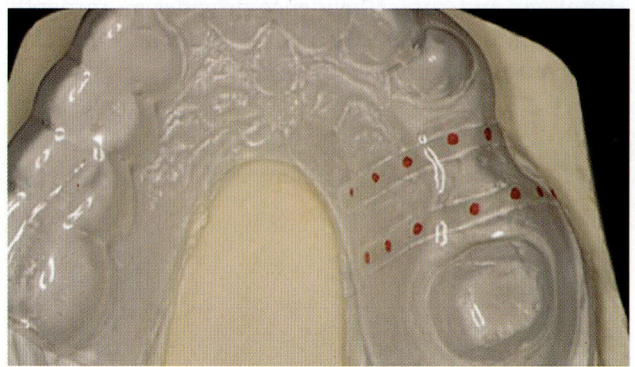

Figure 8 Template in the diagnostic model with buccal and lingual perforations to guide the bone sounding.

Figure 9 Probing in the buccal area of the alveolar ridge to locate the depth of the bone beneath the facial mucosa.

also been developed for this purpose (Figures 8 to 10). The points more easily penetrate the anesthetized mucosa, and a measurement scale identifies the bone thickness.[51]

Using a radiograph template, the selected radiograph is made and analyzed. Bone dimensions are measured, and the location of the bone, relative to the prosthetic teeth, can be analyzed. The cone beam tomogram

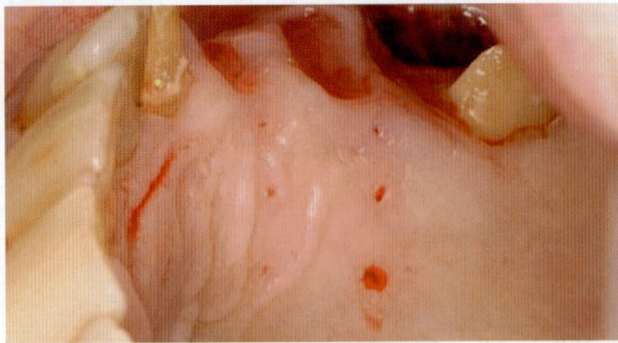

Figure 10 The points will transfer the information to the model, and a measurement scale identifies the bone thickness.

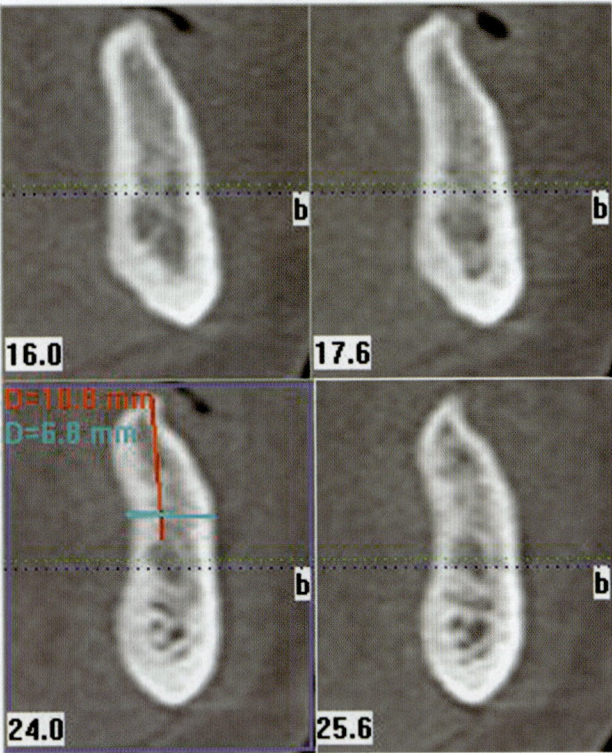

Figure 11 Bone quantity can be measured with accuracy using computed tomography.

and CT scan are the two most common types of advanced radiographs used in conjunction with implant dentistry.

The effectiveness and accuracy of cone beam CT have been validated, and articles have described the clinical use of linear tomography in presurgical planning.[52] The accuracy of cone beam CT has also been favorably compared with the accuracy of panoramic and periapical radiographs (Figure 11).

EXTRACTION AND ALVEOLAR PRESERVATION

The alveolar ridge, after dental extraction, undergoes resorption produced by a lack of stimulus. The stimulus is interrupted when exodontia is performed owing to the loss of periodontal ligament attached to surrounding bone. Maxillary ridge resorption occurs approximately four times more rapidly than mandibular ridge resorption; this is due to the loss of anatomic, mechanic, and biologic factors. The absence of stimulation of the alveolar bone plays an important role in the continuous resorption of the basilar cortical plates.[53]

In the 1980s, replacing vital roots with synthetic roots was highly recommended for the preservation of alveolar bone for complete denture wearers.[54] Synthetic hydroxyapatite roots were advantageous in preservation of the alveolar ridge. Recent publications demonstrate that immediately postextraction, maintenance of the alveolar ridge minimizes residual ridge resorption and, thus, allows placement of an implant that satisfies esthetic and functional criteria. Recent advances in bone grafting materials and techniques allow clinicians to place implants in sites that were considered compromised in the past. The focus is on the healing pattern of sockets, with and without the use of regenerative materials, and the rationale for **preserving the dimensions of the extraction socket.** Histologic and clinical evidence provides an in-depth understanding of the logic behind and value of socket preservation (Figures 12 to 16).[55]

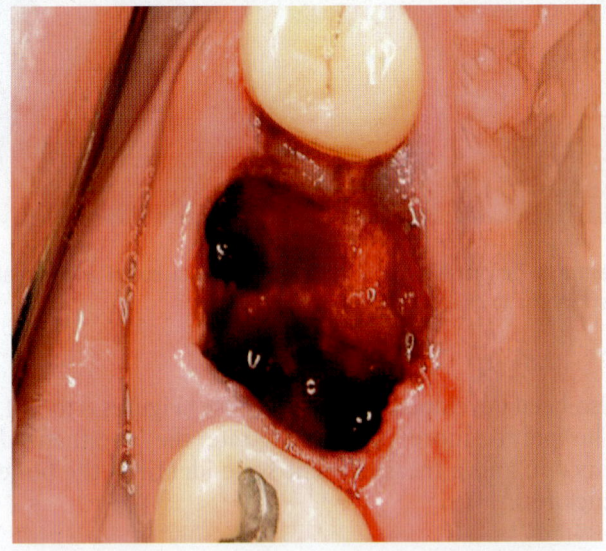

Figure 12 Atraumatic extraction to preserve all of the bone walls and septum.

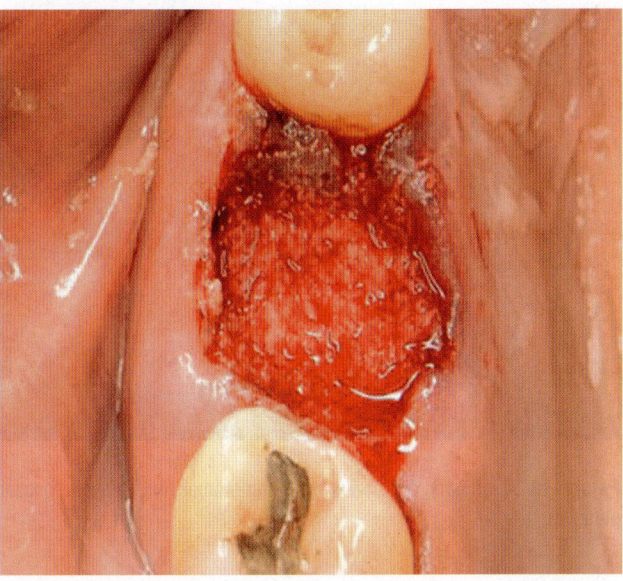

Figure 13 Socket filled with allograft hydroxyapatite to minimize residual ridge resorption.

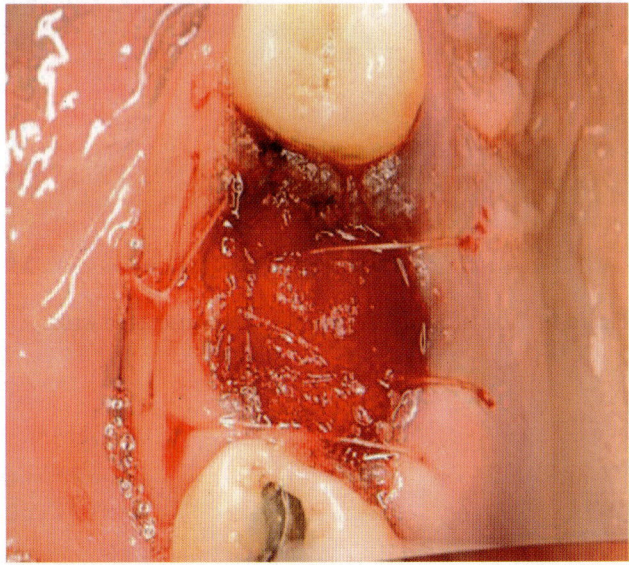

Figure 14 Graft material covered with a collagen membrane. The suture will hold the membrane in place.

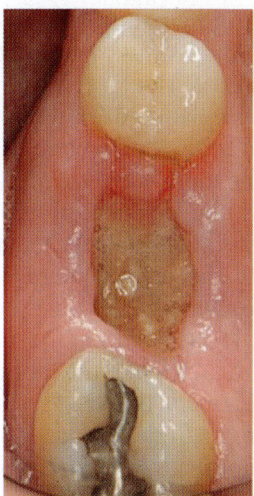

Figure 15 Healing wound 2 weeks after extraction at suture removal. The granulation tissue is growing, covering the membrane.

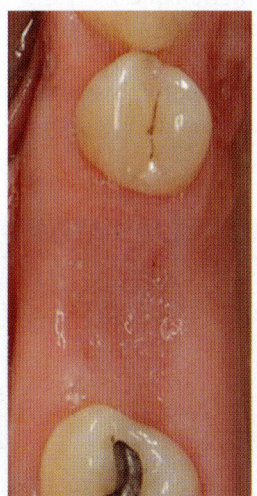

Figure 16 Four months later, ready for implant placement.

IMMEDIATE EXTRACTION AND IMMEDIATE IMPLANT PLACEMENT

When an implant is planned for an area currently occupied by a tooth that must be removed, it may be advantageous to immediately place the implant following tooth extraction. Immediate placement offers several potential advantages compared with extracting a tooth, allowing the bone to heal and then subsequently placing the implant:

1. The bone that originally surrounded the tooth is more likely to be preserved. Thin bone (such as the facial bone of maxillary teeth) and interproximal bone can rapidly disappear after tooth extraction. Placing an implant at the time the tooth is extracted helps preserve the remaining bone and decreases the need for subsequent ridge augmentation procedures. This bone preservation is important in conjunction with maxillary posterior roots encased in a thin bony housing that extends into the sinus. Months after extraction, implant placement might not be possible without

sinus bone augmentation surgery owing to rapid bone loss and sinus pneumatization, which occurs after extraction.
2. More ideal implant positioning is possible. For single-rooted teeth, the implant is positioned where the root of the tooth was located, which is advantageous unless the position of the tooth prior to extraction was undesirable. When implants are centered beneath the crowns, there is more favorable loading. Also, screw access holes are more likely to be centrally located within the peripheral crown dimensions that facilitate the fabrication process.
3. The total treatment time is decreased.
4. The number of surgical procedures is reduced.
5. There is a shorter time period when the patient is subjected to the challenges of being edentulous and wearing a provisional removable prosthesis.
6. The overall cost is reduced.
7. Soft tissue contours and height are better preserved in esthetic zones.
8. There is better acceptance of the treatment plan by the patient.
9. The opportunities for osseointegration are better owing to the healing potential of fresh extraction sockets (Figures 17 to 21).[56,57]

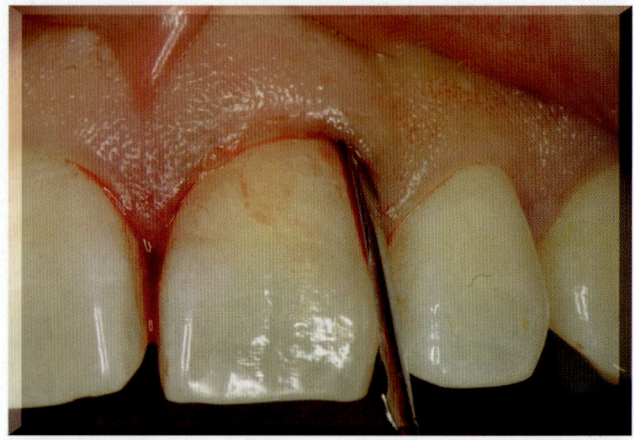

Figure 18 Atraumatic extraction with periotomes will prevent buccal plate fracture.

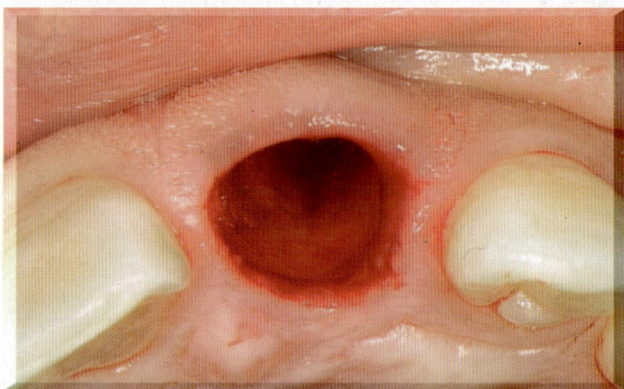

Figure 19 Occlusal view of the socket with the intact bone walls.

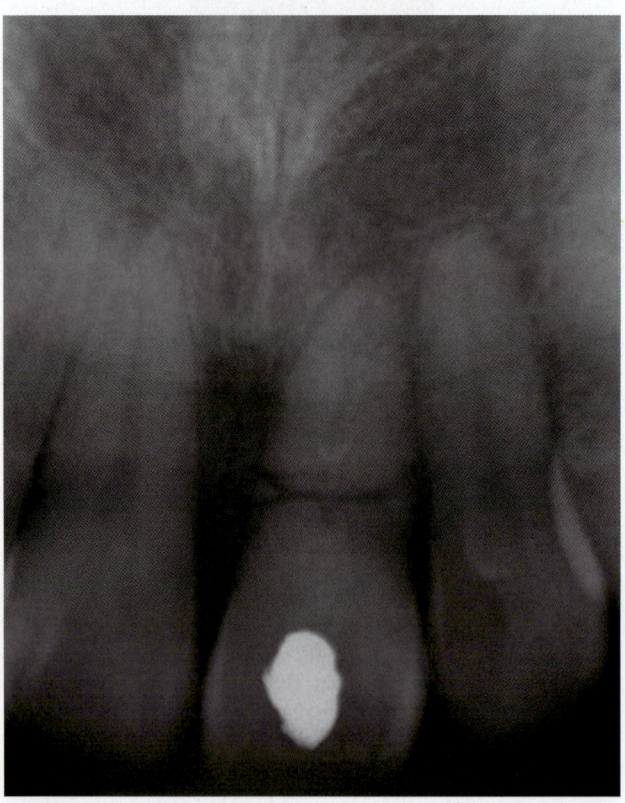

Figure 17 Hopeless tooth with horizontal root fracture.

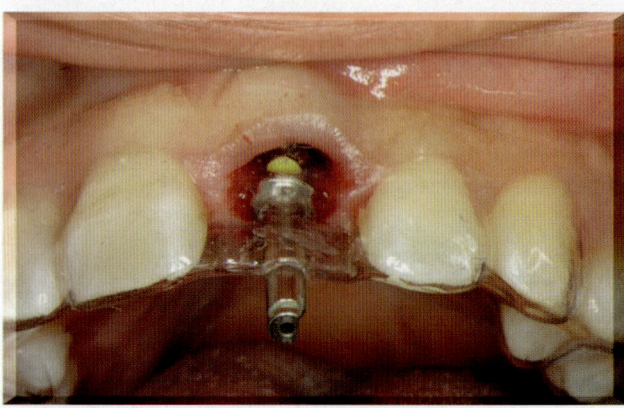

Figure 20 Final drill in position with the surgical template, to verify the correct direction of the osteotomy.

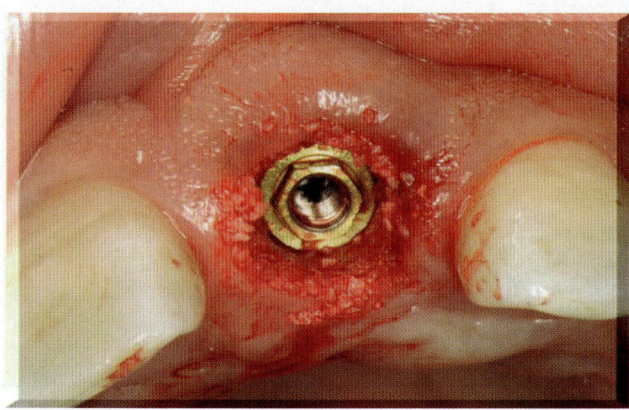

Figure 21 Immediate implant placement after grafting the gaps between the implant and the bone walls.

IMMEDIATE LOADING PROTOCOL

Immediate loading, by placing the prosthesis on the implant immediately after implant placement, was developed because of the desire to reduce treatment time and provide patients with a stable, esthetic replacement either the same day or within a very short time. For patients who have been wearing dentures, a few more months of wearing a removable prosthesis usually produces little concern. However, the standard protocol requires that they not wear any prosthesis for the first 10 days following surgery or that the prosthesis be relieved extensively to ensure that there is no contact with the soft tissue overlying the implants. Both of these options produce a challenge or inconvenience to patients.

There are also patients who are losing teeth and have never worn a removable prosthesis. These individuals can experience significant psychological and functional difficulties throughout the submerged healing time when they have to wear an interim removable prosthesis. Therefore, modifications to the original two-stage protocol were developed. Immediate loading has the following advantages:

1. The implant and crown or prosthesis are placed the same day, thereby providing the patient with an esthetic and stable replacement for the missing tooth or teeth in one appointment.
2. The number of surgical procedures is reduced.
3. The total treatment time is reduced.

Minimal surgical insertion torque values have been used as a means of determining if implants are suitable for immediate loading. It has been suggested that implants whose torque at placement was more than 40 Ncm are suitable for immediate loading, whereas those torqued to less than 27 Ncm should be submerged. Bicortical anchorage and primary implant stability up to a torque of 40 Ncm have been proposed as mandatory.[58] The minimum insertion torque for immediately loaded implants has been described as 32 Ncm (Figures 22 to 25).

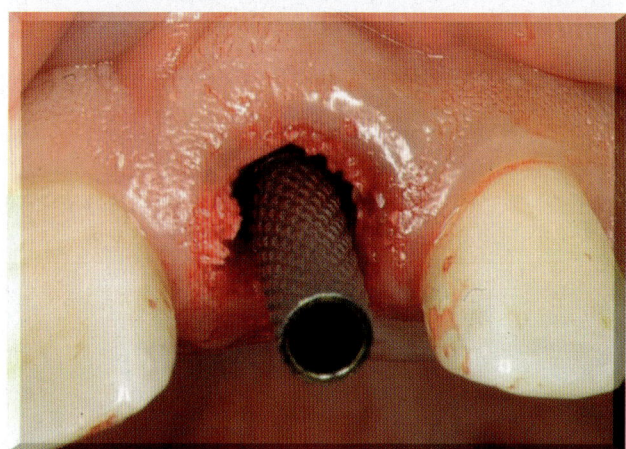

Figure 22 Provisional abutment fixed to the implant.

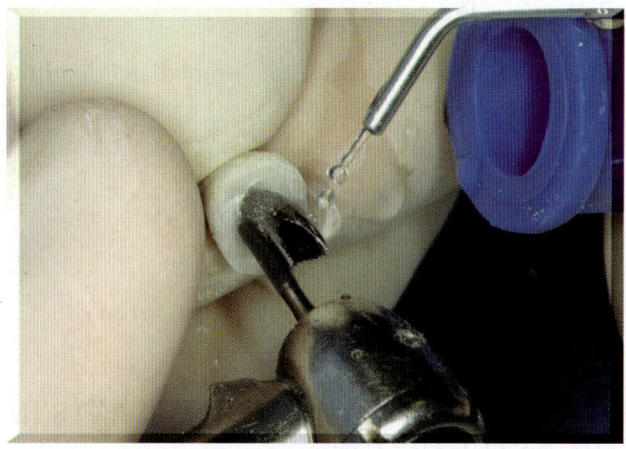

Figure 23 Shaping the customized cervical collar of the temporary abutment to guide soft tissue healing.

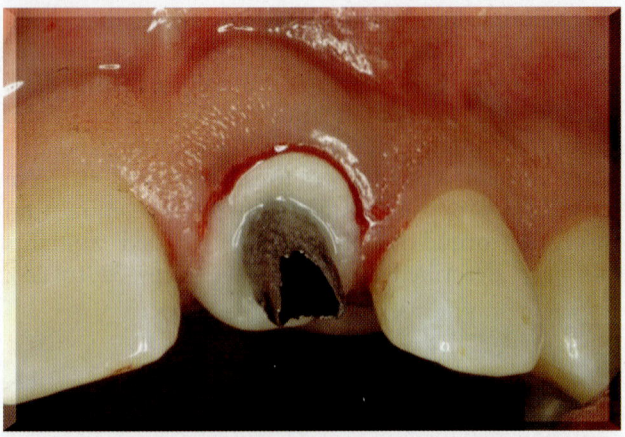

Figure 24 Temporary abutment finished in the patient's mouth.

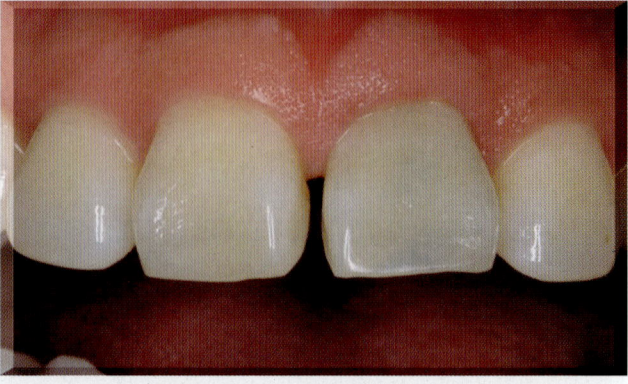

Figure 26 Clinical situations after complete implant osseointegration (6 months). The provisional crown can be removed, and the patient is ready for the final impression.

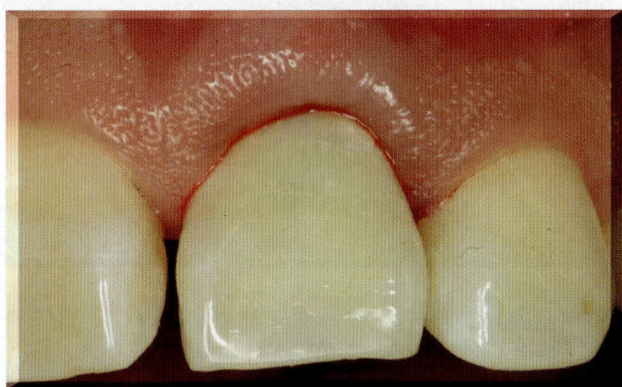

Figure 25 Provisional crown in place the same day as the surgery.

Additional requirements for immediate loading have been described as follows:[59]

- Provisional restoration and diet
- No centric occlusal contact
- No eccentric occlusal contact
- Liquid diet for 2 weeks after surgery
- Soft diet for 2 months after surgery
- Regular diet initiated 2 months after surgery

PROVISIONAL RESTORATIONS ON IMPLANTS AND DENTAL IMPLANTS IN THE ESTHETIC ZONE

Kan et al. proposed that immediate placement of a single implant into the anterior esthetic zone is most predictable when the prospective implant site possesses certain characteristics prior to tooth extraction.[58] They indicate the dentogingival complex dimensions (distance from free gingival crest to the osseous crest) should ideally be 3 mm on the facial surface of the tooth to be extracted and 4.5 mm on the interproximal surfaces of the adjacent teeth. Deviations from these dimensions will likely produce deficits in the soft tissue esthetics. The authors also reported a technique whereby the papilla can be retained between adjacent single implants. This interimplant papilla preservation involves alternate immediate implant placement and provisionalization, one following the bone integration period of the other. The process involves extracting one of the two teeth, immediately placing the implant, attaching a provisional metal abutment with resin added to create the proper emergence profile, and provisionalization with a resin crown. In this way, the soft tissue around the implant is preserved in its normal location. After 6 months, the procedure is repeated for the adjacent tooth, thereby preserving the interimplant papilla. The authors reported highly satisfactory esthetic results when treating consecutive patients in this manner (Figure 26).

Complications

Complications have been defined as secondary conditions that develop during or after implant surgery or prosthesis placement.[50] The occurrence of complication does not necessarily indicate that substandard dental care has been provided and also does not necessarily mean that clinical failure has occurred. Complications and failures in relation to dental implants with association of surgical and prosthetic stages are multifactorial, caused by inadequate planning, surgical insult, systemic factors, and early and late failures. Late failures occur during the prosthodontic and maintenance phases after initial successful osseointegration. Early failures may be due to undiagnosed systemic diseases, systemic factors such as traumatic surgical technique, bacterial contamination, smoking, infection, premature loading, or inadequate home care.

Improper implant placement location and angulation can be due to a lack of bone in the preferred location for the implant owing to bone resorption, disease, or trauma. It can also occur owing to a lack of planning, failure to evaluate the location, angulation identified by the surgical template, or inadequate surgical technique.[50]

HEMORRHAGE

Minor bleeding, hematomas, and ecchymosis are somewhat common surgical complications that are expected side effects associated with surgery. Lengthy surgeries or excessive trauma can lead to more hemorrhage-related complications, such as penetration of the lingual cortex, inadvertent bleeding on raising the buccal flap, intraosseous hemorrhage, and arteriovenous malformation.[50]

NEUROSENSORY DISTURBANCE

A modestly high percentage of paresthesia of the mental nerve follows placement of implants in the area of the mental foramen. If the surgery is without incident and the mental nerve exiting the foramen is well identified during the placement of implants, paresthesia can still result owing to inadvertent stretching of the mental nerve or to implants placed into the inferior canal; implants anterior to the mental nerve can also damage some incisive nerve branches, retard formation of reparative bone, and exert pressure from a removable prosthesis.[50]

ADJACENT TOOTH DEVITALIZATION

The pulps in adjacent teeth can be devitalized when an implant is placed too close to a tooth or invades the periodontal ligament space of adjacent teeth. It is best to place the implant so that the edge of the implant is greater than 1 mm away from the root of the adjacent tooth. The anatomy of an adjacent tooth root can often be visualized so that care is taken to avoid encroaching on this apical space. Periapical radiographs can be taken during surgery to assess the initial drill direction before completing the entire osteotomy.[50]

PERIAPICAL LESIONS ON ADJACENT TEETH

It has been noted that endodontic pathosis in teeth adjacent to recently placed titanium implants can lead to implant failure.[50]

PERIAPICAL LESION ON THE EXTRACTION SITE

Sites where teeth with apical lesions are to be extracted and implants immediately placed must be meticulously managed. After extraction, the socket must be carefully curetted and thoroughly rinsed with saline solution to ensure elimination of the lesion. The use of topical antibiotics may be indicated before implant placement, as well as the use of systemic antibiotics preoperatively and postoperatively.[50]

SINUS TRACTS

Sinus tracts have been noted when there are loose and/or fractured screws that attach a crown, prosthesis, or prosthetic component to an implant. Sinus tracts are commonly located at the level where the mechanical deficiency is present. Sinus tracts have also been noted around cemented crowns or prostheses when excess cement is retained subgingivally. The problem occurs when deep subgingival margins make removal of excess cement difficult. In situations in which two-stage surgery is used, insufficient tightening of the implant cover screw may result in its loosening and the development of a sinus tract within a few days of surgery.[50]

IMPLANT FRACTURE

Implant fractures have occurred owing to heavy occlusal forces and to the presence of substantial cantilevers on the crown or prosthesis. Fractures have also been found after improper surgical placement of root-form implants when excessive insertion torque is used, especially with small-diameter implants. When excessive force is used to insert an implant into dense bone that should have been tapped, the implants can fracture.[50]

ESTHETIC COMPLICATIONS

Esthetic complications have been reported in conjunction with fixed complete dentures, fixed partial dentures, and single crowns. Contour, shade, embrasure spaces, and gingival recession have been identified as sources of esthetic challenges that are related to malpositioning of implants. Bone resorption prior to implant placement, preventing the ideal placement of implants, can produce open cervical embrasures between single crowns. Achieving ideal soft tissue form and interdental papilla height can be a challenge when placing implants into highly visible edentulous areas. The marginal tissue may be thicker than the gingival margin present around adjacent teeth, interdental spaces may be present, the apical location of the soft tissue margin may not be at the same height as adjacent or contralateral natural teeth, interdental papilla may not possess the most desirable form or height, or recession of the soft tissue may lead to crown length variations. Placement of implants in the esthetic zone in the wrong position (mesiodistal, buccolingual) creates substantial problems that cannot be overcome. When existing bone dimensions permit, implants should be placed slightly facial to the faciolingual center of the edentulous area.[50]

Gingival recession can cause esthetic challenges; recession can continue for up to 1 year. Since most of the recession occurs within the first 3 months, a 3-month waiting period has been proposed, followed by abutment connection surgery, before making the definitive impression.[59] Currently, the tendency is to connect the final abutment at the time of implant placement and to build the temporary crown on top of this final abutment, thus avoiding the constant connection and reconnection of the different implant restoration components that produce an insult to the peri-implant tissues with esthetic consequences.[60]

References

1. DeVan MM. The nature of the partial denture foundation: suggestions for its preservation. J Prosthet Dent 1952;2:210–18.
2. Torabinejad M. Apples and oranges. J Endod 2003;29:541–2.
3. Henry PJ. Tooth loss and implant replacement. Aust Dent J 2000;45:150–72.
4. Lewis S. Treatment planning: teeth vs. implants. Int J Periodontics Restorative Dent 1996;16:366–77.
5. Rose LF, Weisgold AS. Teeth or implants: a 1990s dilemma. Compend Contin Educ Dent 1996;17:1151–9.
6. Davarpanah M, Martinez H, Tecucianu JF, et al. To conserve or implant: which choice of therapy? Int J Periodontics Restorative Dent 2000;20:412–22.
7. Spear F. When to restore, when to remove: the single debilitated tooth. Compend Contin Educ Dent 1999;20:316–18.
8. Bader HI. Treatment planning for implants vs. root canal therapy: a contemporary dilemma. Implant Dent 2002;11:217–23.
9. Caplan DJ, Weintraub JA. Factors related to loss of root canal filled teeth. J Public Health Dent 1997;57:31–9.
10. Kinsel RP, Lamb RE, Ho D. The treatment dilemma of the furcated molar: root resection versus single tooth implant restoration. A literature review. Int J Oral Maxillofac Implants 1998;13:322.
11. Kim S. Modern endodontic practice: instruments and techniques. Dent Clin North Am 2004;48:1–9.
12. Ray HA, Trope M. Periapical status of endodontically treated teeth in relation to the technical quality of the root feeling and the coronal restoration. Int Endod J 1995;28:12–18.
13. Wong R. Conventional endodontic failure and retreatment. Dent Clin North Am 2004;48:265–89.
14. Adell R, Lekholm U, Rockler B, et al. A 15 year study of osseointegrated implants in the treatment of the edentulous jaw. Int J Oral Surg 1981;10:387.
15. Sorensen JA, Martinoff JT. Endodontically treated teeth as abutments. J Prosthet Dent 1985;53:631.
16. Reeh ES, Messer HH, Douglas WH. Reduction in teeth stiffness as a result of endodontic and restorative procedures. J Endod 1989;15:512.
17. Esposito M, Hirsh JM, Lekholm U, et al. Biological factors contributing to failures of osseointegrated implants (II). Etiopathogenesis. Eur J Oral Sci 1998;106:721.
18. Gelb DA. Immediate implant surgery: three year retrospective evaluation of 50 consecutive cases. Int J Oral Maxillofac Implants 1993;8:388.
19. Parel SM, Triplett RG. Immediate fixture placement: a treatment planning alternative. Int J Oral Maxillofac Implants 1990;5:337.
20. Buser D, Mericske-Stern, Bernard JP, et al. Long-term evaluation of non-submerged ITI implants. Part I: 8 year life table analysis of a prospective multi-center study with 2,359 implants. Clin Oral Implant Res 1997;8:161.
21. Lekholm U, Gunne J, Henry P, et al. Survival of the Br{150}nemark implant in partially edentulous jaws: a 10 year prospective multicenter study. Int J Oral Maxillofac Implants 1999;14:639.
22. Iacono VJ. Committee on Resarch, Science and Therapy, the American Academy of Periodontology. Dental implants in periodontal therapy; position paper. J Periodontol 2000;71:1934–42.
23. Laney WR, Jemt T, Zarb GA. Osseointegrated implants for single-tooth replacement: progress report from a multicenter prospective study after three years. Int J Oral Maxillofac Implants 1994;9:49–54.
24. Albrektsson T, Zarb GA, Worthington P, et al. The long-term efficacy of currently used dental implants: a review and proposed criteria of success. Int J Oral Maxillofac Implants 1986;1:1–25.
25. Goodacre JC, Spolnik KJ. The prosthodontic management of endodontically treated teeth: a literature review. Part 1. Success and failure data, treatment concepts. J Prosthodont 1994;3:243.

26. Paolantonio M, Dolci M, Scarano A, et al. Immediate implantation in fresh extraction sockets. A controlled clinical and histologic study in man. J Periodontol 2001;72:1560–71.

27. Schwartz-Arad D, Chaushu G. Placement of implants into fresh extraction sites: 4 to 7 years retrospective evaluation of 95 immediate implants. J Periodontol 1997;68:1110.

28. Kan JYK, Rungcharassaeng K, Lozada J. Immediate placement and provisionalization of maxillary anterior single implants: 1-year prospective study. Int J Oral Maxillofac Implants 2003;18:31.

29. Lazzara R. Immediate implant placement into extraction sites: surgical and restorative advantages. Int J Periodontics Restorative Dent 1989;9:333–43.

30. Allen RK, Newton CW, Brown CE Jr. A statistical analysis of surgical and nonsurgical endodontic retreatment cases. J Endod 1989;15:261–6.

31. Paik S, Sechrist C, Torabinejad M. Level for evidence for the outcome of endodontic retreatment. J Endod 2004;37:745–50.

32. Wang Q, Cheung GS, Ng RP. Survival of surgical endodontic treatment performed in a dental teaching hospital: a cohort study. Int Endod J 2004;37:764–75.

33. Torbjörner A, Fransson B. Biomechanical aspects of prosthetic treatment of structurally compromise teeth. Int J Prosthodont 2004;17:135–41.

34. Lovdahl PE. Endodontic re-treatment. Dent Clin North Am 1992;36:473–90.

35. Friedman S, Stabholz A. Endodontic re-treatment—case selection and technique. Part I: criteria for case selection. J Endod 1986;12:28–33.

36. Block M, Kent J. Placement of endosseous implants into tooth extraction sites. J Oral Maxillofac Surg 1991;49:1269–76.

37. Marziani L. Gerustimplantae zu prosthetischen Zweckenl. Dtsch Zahnarztl Z 1955;10:1115.

38. Lemons J, Natiella J. Biomaterials, biocompatibility and peri-implant considerations. Dent Clin North Am 1986;30:4.

39. Shulman LB. Dental replantation and trasplantation. J Oral Maxillofac Surg 1985;2:132, 133, 136.

40. Schnitman PA, Shulman LB. Recommendations of the consensus development conference on dental implants. J Am Dent Assoc 1979;98:373–7.

41. Dahle E. Transplantation to osseointegration. A chronology of dental implants. Bull Hist Dent 1990;38:19–24.

42. Berman N. Implant technique for full lower denture. Washington Dent J. Dec 1950;19:15–17.

43. Truitt HP, James R, Boyne P. Noninvasive technique for mandibular subperiosteal implant: a preliminary report. J Prosthet Dent 1986;55:494–7.

44. Weine FS, Frank AL. Survival of the endodontic endosseous implant. J Endod 1993;19:524.

45. Orlay JG. Endodontic splinting treatment in periodontal disease. Br Dent J 1960;108:118.

46. Frank AL. Improvement in the crown:root ratio by endodontic endosseous implants. J Am Dent Assoc 1967;74:451.

47. Frank AL. Endodontic endosseous implants and treatment of the wide-open apex. Dent Clin North Am 1967;Nov;675–700.

48. Frank AL, Abrams AM. Histologic evaluation of endodontic implants. J Am Dent Assoc 1969;78:520.

49. Brånemark PI, Zarb GA, Albrektsson T. Tissue integrated prostheses. Chicago: Quintessence; 1985.

50. Goodacre CJ, Bernal G, Rungcharassaeng K, Kan JY. Clinical complications with implants and implant prostheses. J Prosthet Dent 2003;90:121–32.

51. Wilson DJ. Ridge mapping for determination of alveolar ridge width. Int J Oral Maxillofac Implants 1989;4:41–3.

52. Kassebaum DK, Nummikoski PV, Triplett RG, Langlais RP. Cross-sectional radiography for implant site assessment. Oral Surg Oral Med Oral Pathol Oral Radiol Endod 1990;70:674–8.

53. Atwood DA, Coy WA. Clinical, cephalometric, and densitometric study of reduction of residual ridges. J Prosthet Dent 1971;26:280–99.

54. Quinn, JH, Kent JN. Alveolar ridge maintenance with solid nonporous hydroxylapatite root implants. Oral Surg Oral Med Oral Pathol Oral Radiol Endod 1984;58:511–21.

55. Irinakis T. Rationale for socket preservation after extraction of a single-rooted tooth when planning for future implant placement. J Can Dent Assoc 2006;72:917–22.

56. Grunder U, Polizzi G, Goene R, et al. A 3-year prospective multicenter follow-up report on the immediate and delayed-immediate placement of implants. Int J Oral Maxillofac Implants 1999;14:210–6.

57. Schwartz-Arad D, Chaushu G. The ways and wherefores of immediate placement of implants into fresh extraction sites: a literature review. J Periodontol 1997;68:915–23.

58. Kan JY, Rungcharassaeng K, Lozada J. Immediate placement and provisionalization of maxillary anterior single implants: 1-year prospective study. Int J Oral Maxillofac Implants. 2003;18:31–9.

59. Small PN, Tarnow DP. Gingival recession around implants: a 1-year longitudinal prospective study. Int J Oral Maxillofac Implants 2000;15:527–32.

60. Cochran DL, Hermann JS, Schenk RK, et al. Biologic width around titanium implants: a histometric analysis of the implanto-gingival junction around unloaded and loaded non-submerged implants in the canine mandible. J Periodontol 1997;68:186–98.

RELATED ENDODONTIC TREATMENT

CHAPTER 35

VITAL PULP THERAPY

GEORGE BOGEN, NICHOLAS P. CHANDLER

Healing is a matter of time, but it is sometimes also a matter of opportunity.

—Hippocrates

Vital pulp therapy is broadly defined as treatment initiated to preserve and maintain pulp tissue in a healthy state, tissue that has been compromised by caries, trauma, or restorative procedures. The objective is to stimulate the formation of reparative dentin to retain the tooth as a functional unit. This is particularly important in the young adult tooth, where apical root development may be incomplete. This chapter describes advances in direct pulp capping and pulpotomy, where the treatment has been redefined by newly developed materials and protocols that are rapidly replacing long accepted strategies. The focus is directed toward the preservation of the pulpally involved **permanent tooth**, based on the premise that pulp tissue has an innate capacity for repair in the absence of microbial contamination.[1]

During the last decade, exceptional progress was made in the field of vital pulp therapy. Materials used in the past were both biologic and nonbiologic.[2] Since the concept of indirect pulp capping was first documented in the eighteenth century by Pierre Fauchard, clinicians have recognized the innate capacity of the pulp tissue to initiate repair after injury from trauma, caries, or mechanical exposure.[3] The first documented instance of vital pulp therapy is attributed to Phillip Pfaff, who placed gold foil against an exposed pulp with the intention to promote pulpal healing.[4] Since the beginning of modern dentistry, researchers have endeavored to better understand and expand their knowledge of pulp physiology, microbiology, and caries progression. This has coincided with the quest to identify bioactive materials and physiologic mediators that consistently stimulate reparative dentin formation and protect the pulp against microbial ingress.

There is a long-held perception that pulp exposures in a carious field have an unfavorable prognosis and that more aggressive treatment, such as pulpotomy or pulpectomy, should be considered.[5,6] These strategies are based on traditional treatment protocols and materials that did not provide a consistently suitable environment for pulpal repair and reparative bridge formation. Moreover, the diagnosis of the pulpal histologic condition is difficult to ascertain owing to the lack of a fundamental understanding of pulpal physiology, patient subjectivity, and the presence of inflammatory mediators that cannot be assessed clinically.[7] Proper case selection, based on a new understanding of inflammatory mechanisms responsible for producing irreversible changes in pulpal tissue, can help identify teeth with a greater likelihood for favorable outcomes.

The challenge is to identify a reliable pulp capping or pulpotomy agent and a suitable delivery technique. The introduction of mineral trioxide aggregate (MTA) has opened a new frontier in vital pulp therapy and changed the perception that pulp capping in carious exposed teeth is unpredictable and therefore contraindicated. The outcome of vital pulp therapy will depend on the age of the patient, the size of the pulp, bacterial contamination, the pulp capping material, and the quality of the final restoration. The importance of establishing a differential diagnosis and proper case selection cannot be overemphasized. The pulp status must be determined carefully, establishing a differential diagnosis using multiple tests. According to the American Academy of Pediatric Dentistry, "Teeth exhibiting provoked pain of short duration, that is relieved, upon the removal of the stimulus, with analgesics, or by brushing, without signs and symptoms of irreversible pulpitis, have a clinical diagnosis of reversible pulpitis and are candidates for vital pulp therapy."[8] The assessment of a definitive pulpal status prior to treatment is often difficult to establish; however, a diagnosis of reversible pulpitis increases the probability of a favorable outcome.[7] A negative patient report, that is subjective and variable, does not always indicate that the pulp capping or pulpotomy procedure cannot be successful. Moreover, pain associated with cold testing prior to treatment or a pulp exposure during caries excavation does not necessarily mandate a poor prognosis for the involved tooth.

The Vital Dental Pulp

The pulp is a highly vascular tissue that has the unique distinction of being encased within a rigid chamber composed of dentin, cementum, and enamel.[9] These hard tissues provide mechanical support and protection from the microorganisms associated with the oral cavity.[10] The tissue performs several important functions, including dentinogenesis, immune cell defense, and nutrition and proprioceptor cognizance. The retention and maintenance of the dental pulp are crucial to the long-term function of the tooth since during the life of the tooth, the healthy pulp produces reparative, secondary, and peritubular dentin in response to various biologic and pathologic stimuli.[11]

Since the vital pulp is capable of demonstrating competent immune defense mechanisms, it is desirable to preserve the vitality of an exposed pulp since its retention is crucial to the tooth's long-term survival. If the hard casing of the tooth is compromised and the pulp is subjected to microbial ingression, inflammatory changes can lead to pulp necrosis and further pathologic changes, including infection and its consequences.[12,13] Circulating immunocompetent cells limit microbial challenges, and functioning proprioceptors and pressoreceptors guard against excessive occlusal loading. By contrast, structurally compromised teeth that have been endodontically treated and restored with various post and core systems are more susceptible to fracture and failure owing to the loss of protective mechanisms. Although studies show that the loss of moisture from dentin after endodontic therapy is minimal,[14,15] cumulative loss of tooth structure is implicated in the failure of root-treated teeth.[16]

The dental pulp is composed of four distinct zones: a cell-rich zone, a core composed of major vessels and nerves, a cell-free zone, and the odontoblastic layer at the periphery. The major cell populations found in the pulp include fibroblasts, undifferentiated mesenchymal cells, odontoblasts, macrophages, and other immunocompetent cells. The odontoblasts have the distinction of forming a single layer lining the periphery of the pulp and feature odontoblastic processes extending into the dentin, sometimes to the dentoenamel junction.[17–19] When the dental pulp is injured by trauma or carious exposure, the mechanism of healing is similar to that observed in normal connective tissue (see Chapter 5, "Embryology, Histology, and Physiology of the Dentin-Pulp Complex").

Wound healing is a continuous process, and a sequence of four phases of healing overlap, including hemostasis, inflammation, proliferation, and remodeling.[20] After an injury, the tissue adjacent to the exposure is characterized by inflammatory cells, extravasated erythrocytes, and potentially necrotic tissue. An acute response is mounted, dominated by neutrophils in the presence of exudated fibrinogen and blood coagulation. Vascular permeability is altered when proinflammatory cytokines are released by immunocompetent cells in response to both trauma and bacterial by-products. Chemotactic signals prompt adhesion molecule interactions between leukocytes and endothelium, enabling transmigration of inflammatory cells. These cell interactions form an adhesion cascade mediated by chemoattractant/activator molecules interacting with sets of cell adhesion molecules.[21]

Reparative Dentin Formation

The reformation of a protective dentinal bridge by tertiary dentinogenesis is a primary goal of vital pulp therapy. The repair of pulpodentinal defects is orchestrated by the migration of granulation tissue to the site from the cell-rich and deep pulp subodontoblastic layers that differentiate into new odontoblast-like cells. Although these progenitor cells are most likely derived from undifferentiated mesenchymal cells, other cell populations migrating via the bloodstream, such as bone marrow stem cells and perivascular cells, have been proposed as possible precursors.[22]

The migration and proliferation of these cells were studied in nonhuman primates after direct pulp capping with calcium hydroxide ($Ca(OH)_2$).[23] At the calcium hydroxide–pulp interface, a continuous influx of newly differentiating odontoblast-type cells with initial matrix formation was observed as early as day 8. Labeled odontoblast-like cells showed differences in cell types and grain counts between zones, indicating that at least two deoxyribonucleic acid (DNA) replications had occurred between initial treatment and differentiation. Studies have suggested that the mineralization of dentin bridges is more dependent on the extracellular matrix than the pulp capping or pulpotomy material.[24–26]

In a transmission electron microscopic study by Hayashi, initial calcification during pulp healing, characterized by an abundance of extracellular matrix vesicles, was located between the amputated pulp surface and the forming cells that contained needle-like crystals and osmiophilic material.[27] After the disappearance of the vesicular membrane, a calcified front formed as crystals and aggregate accumulated. The presence of calcium and phosphate ions within the crystals suggested that they were produced during the calcification process, similar to the calcification in other biologically normal or diseased tissues. Dentin bridge formation can be seen after 1 month at the site of the surgical wound, although pulp healing defects can be associated with different pulp capping agents and include tunnel defects, operative debris, pulpal inflammatory cell activity, and bacterial microleakage.[28]

Techniques for Generating Reparative Dentin

DIRECT PULP CAPPING

The most widely used vital pulp therapy techniques for permanent teeth include direct and indirect pulp capping and partial or complete pulpotomy. **Direct pulp capping** is defined as the "treatment of an exposed vital pulp by sealing the pulpal wound with a dental material placed directly on a mechanical or traumatic exposure to facilitate the formation of reparative dentin and maintenance of the vital pulp."[29] The indications for direct pulp capping include exposures as a result of caries removal, tooth preparation, or trauma. Pulp tissue, jeopardized by a long-standing exposure to oral microorganisms and acute inflammation, may be unsuitable for direct pulp capping.[30] Direct pulp capping for carious exposures is discussed in detail later in this chapter.

INDIRECT PULP CAPPING

Indirect pulp capping is defined as "a procedure in which a material is placed on a thin partition of remaining carious dentin that, if removed, might expose the pulp in immature permanent teeth."[29] This technique shows some success in teeth with an absence of symptomatology and with no radiographic evidence of pathosis.[30] It has been controversial for decades.[31] The strategy involved various techniques in which caries removal was completed to a point near the pulp tissue without direct exposure. The potential for pulpal repair has been demonstrated in selected teeth with deep carious lesions where caries excavation was conservative and direct pulp exposures were avoided.[32,33] Indirect pulp caps are completed using either $Ca(OH)_2$ or zinc oxide–eugenol (ZOE) in a one- or two-stage procedure. The major difficulty with the procedure (one or two stage) is to determine at what point excavation is halted. Moreover, voids under the restorative material result during the remineralization process, in which the carious dentin dries out and loses volume. Another complication is restoration failure and rapid reactivation of a dormant lesion.[34] Indirect pulp capping is not recommended as a predictable treatment for permanent teeth.

PULPOTOMY

Pulpotomy is a more extensive procedure defined as "the surgical removal of the coronal portion of a vital pulp as a means of preserving the vitality of the remaining radicular portion."[29] After the complete removal of the coronal pulp, a material is placed over the canal orifices. A variety of dressing materials, with varying toxicity, have been used for this purpose. They include phenol, creosote, ferric sulfate, polycarboxylate cement, glutaraldehyde, ZOE, $Ca(OH)_2$, and formaldehyde, which mummifies the remaining tissue.[35] Although studies indicate that short-term success rates are favorable, this procedure is generally advocated for deciduous teeth. Pulpotomies in young adult teeth have been completed with formocresol, although the material has distinct disadvantages.[36] Aside from the issue of systemic sensitivity to the agent, experiments with primates have shown a high incidence of internal resorption.[37] Also, orthograde endodontic treatment can be difficult to complete owing to changes in the canal system apical to the formocresol.[38] In addition to pulpotomies performed on permanent teeth, recent studies have shown MTA to be a suitable replacement for formocresol in pulpotomy of primary molars.[39,40]

PARTIAL PULPOTOMY

Partial pulpotomy (Cvek pulpotomy) is defined as "the surgical removal of a small portion of the coronal portion of a vital pulp as a means of preserving the remaining coronal and radicular pulp."[29] In this instance, inflamed tissue is removed to expose deeper, healthy coronal pulp tissue.[41] Direct pulp capping and partial pulpotomy are considered similar procedures and differ only in the amount of undestroyed tissue remaining after treatment.

Indications for Vital Pulp Therapy

Vital pulp therapy is indicated whenever the remaining pulp exhibits reversible pulpitis and can be selectively induced to produce a reparative barrier that protects the tissue from microbial challenges. In particular, direct pulp capping can be performed for teeth with deep caries, mechanical exposures, and traumatic injuries to maximize pulpal preservation. The outcome of treatment for direct pulp capping or pulpotomy will be determined by the initial diagnosis, which includes radiographic evaluation, pulp testing, clinical evaluation, and patient history. The intention is to postpone more aggressive therapies that could eventually lower the long-term prognosis for tooth retention and function. Teeth undergoing orthograde root canal therapy and placement of posts and cores, followed by full coverage or cuspal coverage restorations, show lower long-term survival rates than teeth with vital pulps.[42–48]

Vital Pulp Therapy Materials

The search for the ideal vital pulp therapy material has led researchers to investigate many different materials. These include $Ca(OH)_2$ compounds,[49–52] zinc oxide, calcium phosphate, zinc phosphate and polycarboxylate cements, calcium-tetracycline chelate, antibiotic and growth factor combinations, calcium phosphate ceramics, Emdogain, Bioglass, cyanoacrylate, hydrophilic resins, hydroxyapatite, resin-modified glass ionomers, and, recently, MTA.[53–63] Other studies have included Ledermix, glycerrhetinic acid–antibiotic mix, potassium nitrate, and dimethyl isosorbide.[64] Innovative methods have also been used to eliminate caries progression and stimulate the repair of affected pulpal tissue and include ozone technology, lasers, and bioactive agents that activate pulpal defenses.[65–68] Favorable outcomes in direct pulp capping have varied depending on the techniques and materials, with human retrospective studies showing 30 to 85% success rates at 5 to 10 years.[49–52] Researchers have strived for decades to identify and produce a pulp capping material that, ideally, would exhibit the following characteristics:[69]

- Stimulate reparative dentin formation
- Maintain pulpal vitality
- Release fluoride to prevent secondary caries
- Bactericidal or bacteriostatic
- Adhere to dentin
- Adhere to restorative material
- Resist forces during restoration placement
- Must resist forces under restoration during lifetime of restoration
- Sterile
- Radiopaque
- Provide bacterial seal

CALCIUM HYDROXIDE

This material, long considered the "benchmark" for vital pulp therapy materials (Figure 1), has been shown to have some desirable properties, but long-term study outcomes have been variable.[51,52] Beneficial characteristics include a bactericidal component owing to its high alkaline pH and the irritation of pulp tissue that stimulates pulpal defense and repair.[70] Conversely, $Ca(OH)_2$ has been shown to be cytotoxic in cell cultures, does not exclusively stimulate reparative dentin formation, shows poor marginal adaptation to dentin, and induces pulp cell apoptosis.[71–73] The material can be associated with primary tooth resorption, it can degrade and dissolve beneath restorations, and it can also suffer interfacial failure upon amalgam condensation.[74–76] It produces a gap between the dentin interface when used with bonding resins.[77] Dentin bridges beneath $Ca(OH)_2$ are associated with tunnel defects, and the material fails to provide a long-term seal against microleakage when used as a pulp capping agent.[71,76] The disintegration of $Ca(OH)_2$ under restorations associated with defects in the dentinal bridge can provide microorganisms with a pathway for penetration into pulpal tissue and the subsequent stimulation of circulating immune cells, inducing pulpal irritation and potential pulpal calcification and canal obliteration.

ADHESIVE RESINS AND RESIN-MODIFIED GLASS IONOMERS

The use of adhesive systems for direct pulp capping was first introduced by Japanese researchers in the early 1980s.[78–80] Preliminary research with nonhuman primate models using ISO standards was encouraging.[81–85] Exposed pulps directly capped with various resins and

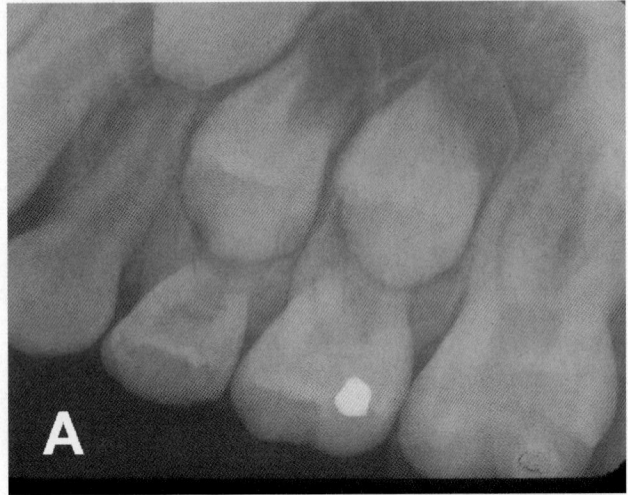
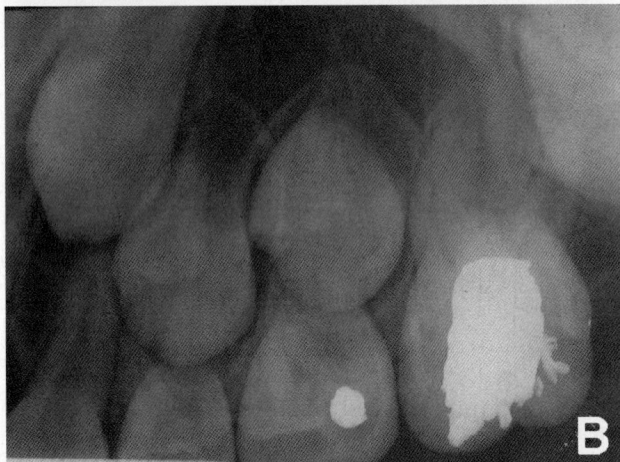
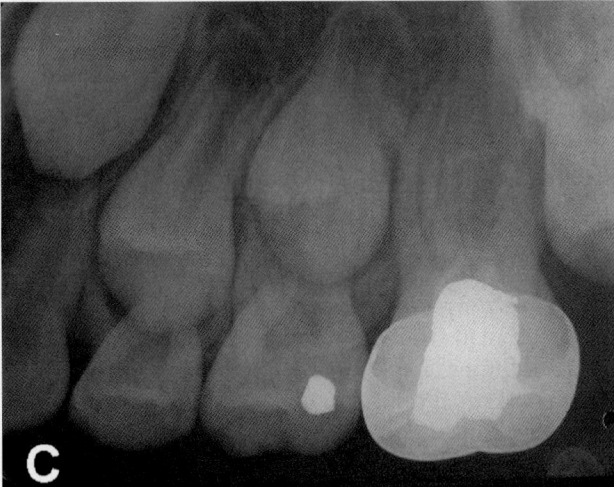

Figure 1 Pulpotomy with calcium hydroxide and amalgam. **A**, A 10-year-old boy with a deep carious lesion of the maxillary molar; clinical symptoms and examination indicated reversible pulpitis. **B**, Complete pulpotomy of the coronal pulp was done, followed by placement of a calcium hydroxide hard-setting paste and amalgam restoration. **C**, One-year follow-up shows additional placement of a stainless steel crown. The tooth was asymptomatic, and there were no radiographic changes. Courtesy, Dr. Leif K. Bakland.

evaluated histologically for pulpal reaction, microbial presence, and the formation of reparative dentin formation showed favorable biocompatibility. Although these favorable results were observed in nonhuman primates, the transition was not paralleled in human subjects.[86–90] Research by several investigators in humans showed unfavorable histologic reactions to the resins when placed directly against pulp tissue. Many histologic sections from these investigations were characterized by mononuclear inflammatory infiltrates, macrophages, polymorphonuclear leukocytes, multinuclear giant cells, and an absence of calcific bridge formation.[86,87,90]

Two clinical studies on human subjects compared direct pulp capping with either resin-modified glass ionomer cement or with a hydrophilic resin.[91,92] Histologic results showed that both Vitrebond (3M Espe Dental Products, St. Paul, MN) and Clearfil Liner Bond 2 (Kuraray Co., LTD, Osaka, Japan) resulted initially in a moderate to intense inflammatory response and did not stimulate reparative dentin formation at 300 days. Further investigations in nonhuman subjects have revealed the unpredictable nature of reparative dentin formation and the contamination of reparative dentin bridges by bacteria. In a study by Murray et al., in which the hierarchy of repair was measured against microbial contamination, 18.6% of resin-based composite, 22.2% of resin-modified glass ionomer, and 47.0% of $Ca(OH)_2$ specimens showed bacterial contamination of the reparative dentin bridge.[93] This is an indication that these pulp capping materials do not allow for predictable pulpal healing, nor do they provide a favorable environment for reparative dentin formation and the exclusion of microorganisms.[94,95] Repair should proceed successfully beneath the material when bacterial microleakage is precluded.

MINERAL TRIOXIDE AGGREGATE

MTA was introduced to endodontics by Lee et al. in the early 1990s.[96] This bioactive silicate cement was originally composed of tricalcium silicate, tricalcium aluminate, tricalcium oxide, silicate oxide, and other mineral oxides.[97] The product is currently marketed under several names around the world and in one form (ProRoot MTA, Tulsa/Dentsply, Tulsa, OK) has changed in composition since its introduction with the substitution of dicalcium silicate for tricalcium silicate and the addition of tertracalcium aluminoferrite, calcium sulfate dehydrate, and bismuth oxide; the latter was added to impart radiopacity.[98] Originally a gray powder, white MTA was produced for esthetic reasons with the reduction of ferrite (Fe_3O_3) with no detectable change in clinical performance.[98–101]

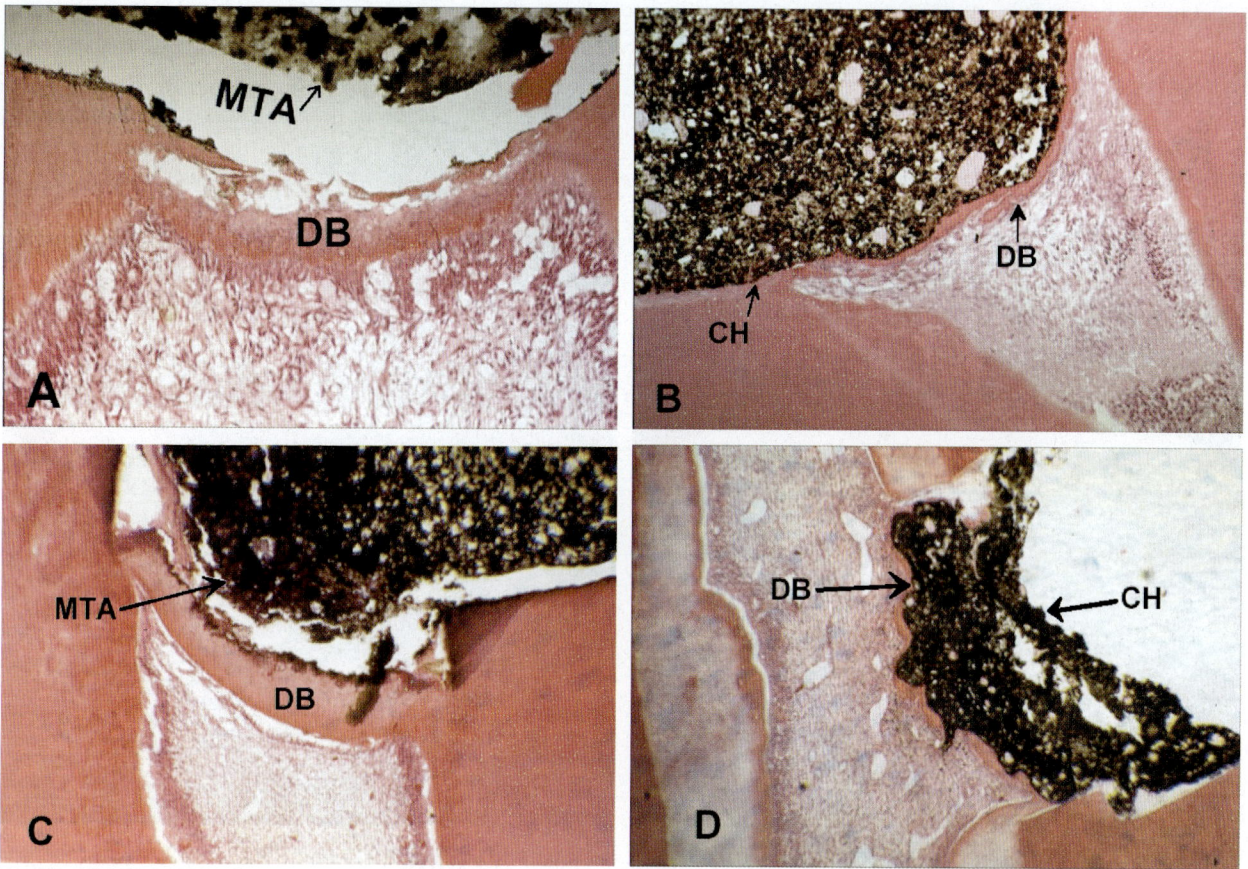

Figure 2 Comparison of dentin bridge formation using mineral trioxide aggregate (MTA) or calcium hydroxide in dog pulps. *A*, After 1 week, a noticeable bridge has formed subjacent to MTA. *B*, A comparable bridge under calcium hydroxide after 2 weeks. *C*, A 4-week specimen with MTA shows excellent bridge formation. *D*, Consistently, the bridge formation under calcium hydroxide lagged behind MTA; an example of bridge formation under calcium hydroxide after 8 weeks. CH = calcium hydroxide; DB = dentin bridge; MTA = mineral trioxide aggregate. Reproduced with permission from Junn DJ.[111]

The cement exhibits many favorable characteristics, which make it a superior material when used as a direct pulp capping material in adult teeth or as an agent in partial or complete pulpotomy in primary teeth.[102,103] MTA is structurally similar to Portland cement, which physiochemically allows the material to set in the presence of blood and moisture.[104] It exhibits a superior marginal adaptation and is nonabsorbabale, and when it cures in the presence of calcium ions and tissue fluids, it forms a reactionary layer at the dentin interface resembling hydroxyapatite in structure.[104–106] Other biocompatible characteristics include a sustained alkaline pH after curing, small particle size, and a slow release of calcium ions.[107] Studies have also demonstrated that MTA stimulates cytokine release, induces pulpal cell proliferation, and promotes hard tissue formation.[108,109] The high alkalinity of MTA and its calcium release and sustained pH at 12.5 is most likely responsible for preventing any further microbial growth of residual microorganisms left after caries excavation. The high pH also extracts growth factors from adjacent dentin thought to be responsible for promoting dentinal bridging.[108,110]

Direct pulp capping with MTA has proven to be effective in stimulating tertiary dentin formation in canine models (Figure 2) and primates.[60,111,112] Recent investigations have shown favorable short-term outcomes in humans when pulpotomies (partial or complete) (Figure 3) or direct pulp capping using MTA was examined.[113–117] According to Tomson et al., the bioactive properties of MTA that stimulate reparative bridge formation can be attributable to the material providing a biocompatible noncytotoxic antibacterial environment.[118] MTA also provides a favorable surface morphology for cell attachment and has the ability to form hydroxyapatite on its surface in the presence of tissue fluid. They hypothesized that soluble components of MTA during and after setting on the dentin interface may cause the release of growth factors

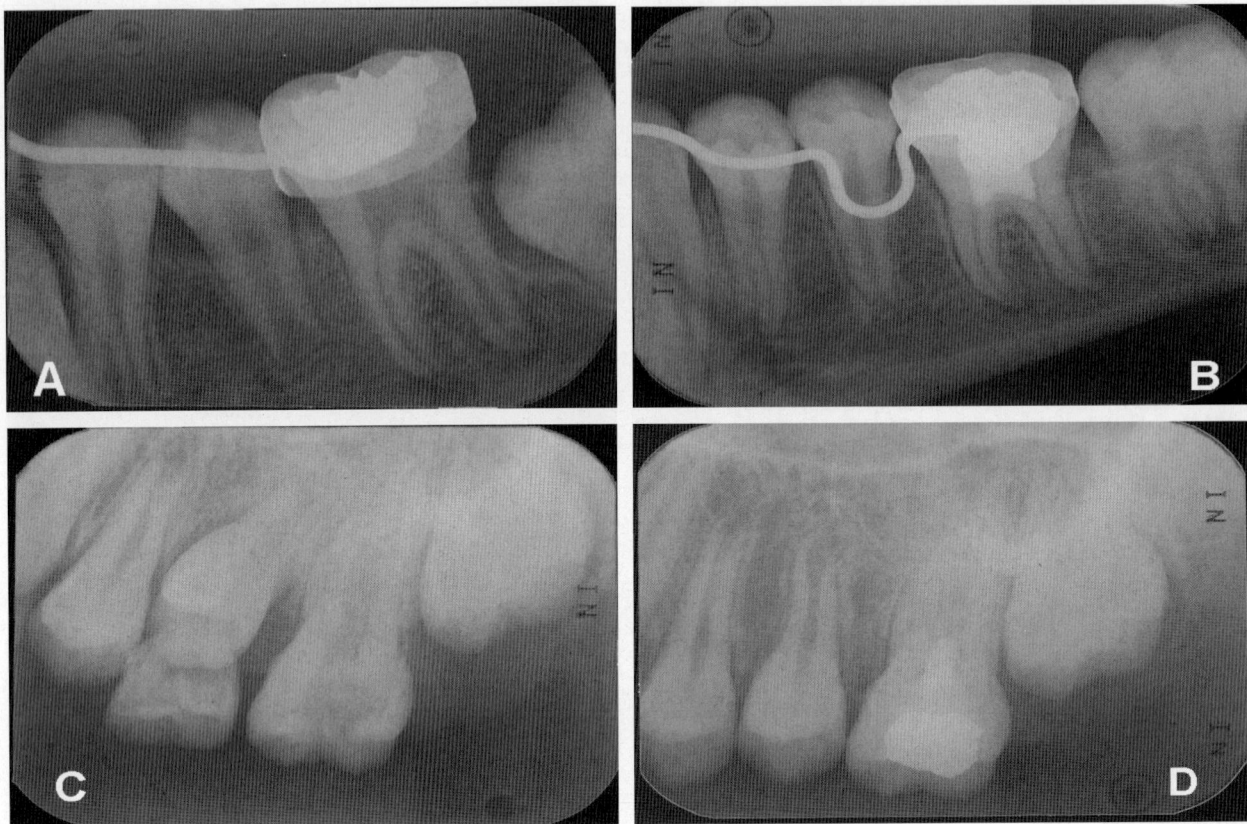

Figure 3 Pulpotomy on young immature permanent teeth using mineral trioxide aggregate (MTA). **A,** Recurrent decay under a previous restoration (amalgam and stainless steel crown); clinical symptoms and examination indicated reversible pulpitis. Complete pulpotomy of coronal pulp using MTA and amalgam was done. **B,** Follow-up evaluation 18 months later shows continued root formation, and the tooth is asymptomatic. **C,** Radiograph of a maxillary molar in a 10-year-old girl shows extensive caries involvement; based on clinical symptoms and examination, the pulp was determined to be reversibly involved. After caries excavation, the coronal pulp tissue was removed and MTA was placed followed by amalgam. **D,** The 18-month follow-up shows normal periapical tissues, and the tooth was asymptomatic. Reproduced with permission from Lauer HH. Vital pulp therapy with MTA: an outcomes study [thesis]. Loma Linda (CA): Loma Linda University; CA, 2005.

and other bioactive molecules, such as transforming growth factor beta (TGF-β_1) and adrenomedullin. The increased presence of these dentine extracellular proteins as the result of MTA culminates in dentin bridge formation after stimulating reparative dentinogenic mechanisms.

A current observational study examined MTA as a direct pulp capping agent using a two-visit protocol in permanent teeth in which cold testing determined a pulpal diagnosis no more severe than irreversible pulpitis.[119] Teeth were selected for treatment that exhibited no detectable pathosis based on radiographic evidence and no clinical signs of swelling, furcation defects, or sinus tracts. Teeth received caries removal under magnification using a caries detector dye. Hemostasis was provided by direct contact with 5.25 to 6.0% sodium hypochlorite (NaOCl) for periods of 5 to 10 minutes. MTA was placed over the exposure, and all surrounding dentin of the pulpal roof or axial wall and teeth received interim restorations with a moist cotton pellet and unbonded Photocore (Kuraray Co., LTD).

On a second visit, after 5 to 10 days, the teeth were permanently restored with a bonded composite (Clearfil LinerBond 2 and Clearfil AP-X composite, Kuraray Co.), but only after confirmation that the MTA had set and normal responses to vitality testing were elicited. Radiographic recalls were evaluated for reparative dentin formation, pulpal calcification, continued normal root development, and the absence of pathosis. Forty-nine teeth were observed for a 1- to 9-year period, with an average observation time of 3.94 years. Favorable outcomes, based on subjective symptomatology and cold testing, was 97.96%. Pulpal calcifications were seen in 10.6% (5 of 49) of cases, and all teeth (15 of 15) in younger patients showed complete root formation (apexogenesis) when open apices were present initially.[119]

The remarkable outcomes for direct pulp capping with MTA are attributable to distinctive properties inherent to the material. The sustained alkaline pH of the set cement is bactericidal and most likely contributes with NaOCl to the elimination of many residual microorganisms left at the dentin-pulpal interface after exposure. MTA is hygroscopic and sets in the presence of moisture, so direct contact with tissue fluids or blood does not affect the curing properties. The close adaptation of the silicate cement produces a virtually gap-free interface owing to the small particle size and precludes microleakage and bacterial ingression. MTA may also act to entomb residual microorganisms at the dentin interface. The slow release of calcium ions also allows the material to stimulate growth factors from the dental pulp and promote signaling molecules (TGF-β, interleukin [IL]-1α, IL-β, macrophage colony-stimulating factor (MCSF), that encourage hard tissue formation.[108] The compressive strength and surface texture of the set cement allow strong bonding with adhesive restorations and minimal compression under heavy loading when a final restoration is placed.

Diagnostic Criteria for Successful Outcome

Direct pulp capping and partial and complete pulpotomy are important treatment options for the immature permanent tooth. Whether the coronal pulp tissue is preserved in toto, partially removed, or removed to the base of the pulpal floor, the preservation of the radicular pulp tissue allows continuing development and apical maturation (apexogenesis) of teeth with open apices. Moreover, in cases of trauma, in which tooth development may be interrupted, induction of apexogenesis should be the clinician's primary goal, with the pulp protected and encouraged to remain vital.[120–122]

Before treatment can be initiated, the clinician must make a careful assessment of all available information. Important aspects of vital pulp therapy include a differential diagnosis based on medical history, radiographic evidence, patient report, percussion testing, and vitality testing. Clinical evaluation must also include assessment of mobility, periodontal probing, localized swelling, and the presence of sinus tracts. Radiographs (both periapical views and bitewings) must be assessed for the absence of periapical pathosis, furcation radiolucencies, internal or external resorption defects, and pulp calcification owing to previous restorations or trauma.

After the radiographic and clinical assessments indicate an absence of disease, subjective symptomatology must be considered. Although most patients with deep carious lesions can often experience sensitivity to heat, cold, and certain acidic or sweet foods, the subjective response to cold testing can be variable, and a short, lingering response (1–2 seconds) may not be an indication that the pulp is irreversibly involved. Studies have shown that cold testing responses in primary teeth are unpredictable, and testing may also be confounded in some individuals in immature permanent teeth.[123,124] Pain to percussion is most often associated with irreversible pulpitis. In teeth with open apices with irreversible pulpitis, pulpectomy is recommended using MTA as a root-end plug to promote root-end closure (apexogenesis).[122,125]

All teeth that have previous restorations, or a history of trauma, have a lower prognosis for repair and tertiary dentin formation than teeth with initial caries alone.[126,127] In mature permanent teeth receiving full coverage, only teeth with no previous history of restorative treatment should be considered for direct pulp capping. From a technical standpoint, pulp exposure on the occlusal surface of a full crown preparation may have the best prognosis. Pulp exposures on axial walls of full-coverage preparations are extremely difficult to treat clinically owing to the handling properties of MTA and the technical challenge of placing the material against an open vertical wall. In these cases, orthograde root canal therapy should be considered a more predictable and suitable treatment option.

The remaining tooth structure should also be considered when selecting an appropriate vital pulp treatment. In teeth exhibiting advanced caries and severe coronal breakdown, requiring full coverage, pulpotomy rather than direct pulp capping is recommended. In patients with rampant caries, pulpotomies are recommended rather than direct pulp capping since the majority of these patients will exhibit recurrent caries at a higher rate.[128–130] Young patients who exhibit initial caries on all first molars can still be considered excellent candidates for direct pulp capping if the differential diagnosis indicates reversible pulpitis in all teeth evaluated. It is also evident that a favorable prognosis for vital pulp therapy diminishes with the increasing age of the patient.[52,130]

The diagnosis can be further confirmed at the time of pulp exposure when the pulp is visualized and hemorrhage control is assessed. In cases without bleeding, then the tissue is most likely necrotic and should be removed to a point where bleeding is encountered. A partial pulpotomy is completed with a high-speed diamond round bur with direct placement of MTA against the entire wound after achieving hemostasis. In teeth with pulp exposures, where bleeding cannot be controlled with 3 to 6% NaOCl within a 10-minute contact period, the diagnosis must be changed to irreversible pulpitis, and pulpotomy or pulpectomy is recommended. The type of vital pulp therapy delivered is based on the option that will best benefit the patient and secure the optimum prognosis for the long-term retention of the tooth.

Pulp sizes are underestimated on radiographs, possibly leading to a greater risk of an unexpected and sizeable pulpal exposure.[131] The observation of Matsuo et al. that the size of an exposure has no influence on the outcome is important.[132] Erroneously, clinicians probably assume that larger exposures have a poorer prognosis and may include size in their decision making. In a recent study involving the examination of simulated exposures (0.5–0.9 mm), dentists without a ruler or previous calibration overestimated exposure size by a mean of 26%.[133] There may also be differences in some pulp dimensions between the genders and among racial groups.[134]

Caries Removal

Dental dam isolation, aided by a caries detector dye and optical magnification during caries removal may be critical implements in achieving favorable results for direct pulp capping. Fusayama et al. made considerable progress in caries research by redefining the carious process and presenting a technique for objectively removing infected tissue, thus contributing to pulpal protection and survival.[135,136] They indicated that gram-positive bacteria, whose main by-product is lactic acid, first break down hydroxyapatite and collagen in the outer carious layer but spare banded collagen in the second layer, where the intermolecular cross-links are still intact.[137,138] They also discovered that pulpal repair and preservation were possible in teeth sealed with bonded composites if the upper layer of two distinctive carious layers could be selectively stained and carefully removed.

Preservation of the second (caries affected) layer allowed for the exclusion of the majority of necrotic dentin and invading bacteria at the deepest point of microbial penetration, responsible for the production of proinflammatory mediators at the pulp-dentin interface. Moreover, since restoration placement was no longer dependent on retentive cavity preparations, more tooth structure could be spared, with less resultant trauma to the dental pulp.

The development of caries staining using a propylene glycol solution of Acid Red 52 dye (a common food and cosmetic coloring dye) provides visible differentiation of the two carious layers and is a selective method to remove the necrotic and infected dentin.[138] The retained caries-affected layer of dentin, which contains banded, intact collagen, allows for the remineralization of the altered tissue by calcium phosphate secreted from the pulp via the dentinal tubules. In the dentinal tubules, calcium and phosphate ions induce the formation of whitlockite crystals, which block the tubules. This remineralization of caries-affected dentin has been confirmed in canine and primate models.[139,140] Fusayama argued that conservative objective caries removal promotes pulpal preservation without injuring residual **caries-affected dentin** that is reparable and remineralizable when a bonded composite restoration is placed to prevent microbial leakage.[138] Although several studies have questioned the efficacy of caries removal using a caries detector dye, the material does allow the operator to visually inspect under magnification infected dentin that may have been overlooked and potentially compromise the outcome for direct pulp capping (Figure 4).[141–144]

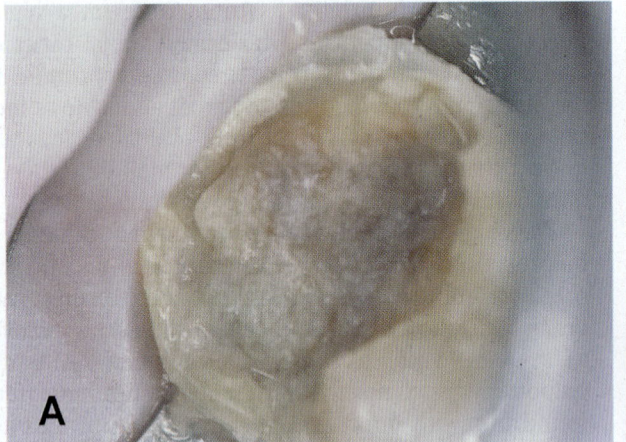 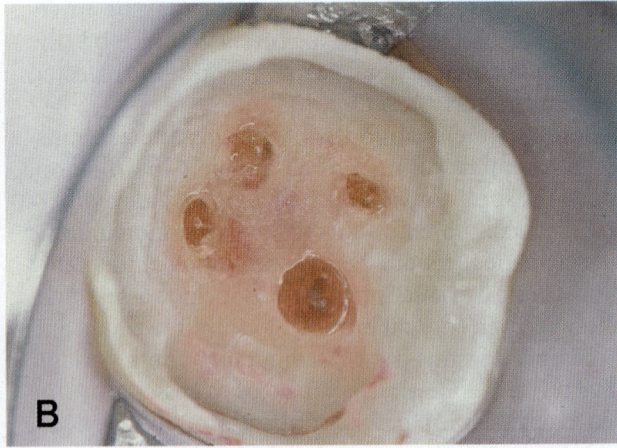

Figure 4 Caries removal procedure. **A,** Clinical appearance of a mandibular molar with extensive caries after dental dam placement. **B,** Occlusal view after caries removal, including the use of a caries detector dye, and hemostasis using 6.0% NaOCl for a 5-minute period. Note four pulp horn exposures ranging in size from 0.5 to 2.0 mm; hemorrhaging has stopped. Courtesy, Dr. George Bogan.

Hemostasis

Many different hemostatic agents and antimicrobial materials have been introduced into the field of vital pulp therapy. These include ferric sulfate, disinfectants such as Concepsis (Ultradent Products Inc., South Jordan, UT) and Tubulicid (Global Dental Products, North Bellmore, NY) epinephrine, and varying concentrations of hydrogen peroxide (H_2O_2) and NaOCl. The most commonly accepted technique has been direct pressure at the exposure site with cotton pellets moistened in sterile water or saline. Other techniques using electrosurgery and lasers have shown limited value in hemorrhage control.[145] NaOCl, widely regarded as the most effective antimicrobial irrigant in endodontic therapy during chemomechanical cleaning of the root canal system, has been advocated as an agent in direct pulp capping and pulpotomy since the early 1950s.[146,147] The main advantages of NaOCl not only include excellent hemostasis at the pulpal wound site, but the solution also allows for the clearance of most dentin chips, biofilm removal, chemical amputation of the blood clot and fibrin, disinfection of the cavity interface, and the removal of damaged cells from the mechanical or traumatic exposure.[145,148,149] The dissolving capacity of 5.25% to 6.0% NaOCl appears to affect only the peripheral pulp cells without impairing underlying pulp tissue.[150] Although concentrations of NaOCl greater than 0.025% have been shown to be adverse to wound healing as a fluid dressing in burn victims, the reaction to pulp tissue appears to be relatively benign.[151]

The importance of hemostasis in vital pulp therapy was demonstrated in an eloquent study by Matsuo et al., in which treatment outcomes revealed a 2-year success rate of 81.8%.[132] Teeth were directly pulp-capped with a fast-setting $Ca(OH)_2$ material after pulp exposures occurred during caries removal. Caries removal was completed under the guide of a caries detector dye, and hemorrhage control was completed with 10% NaOCl. Statistical analysis showed that the age of the patients, type of teeth, responses to thermal stimuli and percussion, and diameter of the pulpal exposure had no bearing on the success rate. The one significant measurable variable that predicted a favorable outcome was the degree to which bleeding could be arrested at the exposure site. This observation underscores the importance of proper hemostasis in the success of direct pulp capping and pulpotomy procedures.

It has been shown that higher levels of inflammatory mediators, including immunoglobulin (Ig)M, IgG, IgA, prostaglandin E_2, and elastase, are present in clinically inflamed pulps.[152] This suggests that greater levels of these mediators may affect the degree of intrapulpal pressure and the likelihood of securing pulpal hemostasis. In cases in which pulpal hemostasis cannot be achieved within 5 to 10 minutes, the diagnosis should be considered **irreversible pulpitis,** and pulpotomy or pulpectomy should be considered.

The use of undiluted NaOCl (5.25%) was investigated histologically in beagle dogs on vital pulp tissue exposed on freshly cut dentin prepared to a depth of 2 mm. After the cavities were sealed with Cavit, pulps examined at 1- and 4-week time periods were free of inflammatory cells. The use of NaOCl did not appear to cause any additional pulpal damage after the trauma of exposing dentin and vital dentinal tubules.[153] Similarly, NaOCl at varying concentrations did not affect positive outcomes in primates when pulps were capped directly with adhesive resins.[148,149]

In a clinical evaluation by Demir and Cehreli, 1.25% NaOCl was used for 60 seconds to ensure hemorrhage control in human primary teeth that were pulp-capped with either $Ca(OH)_2$ or various adhesive bonding agents.[154] The teeth were evaluated clinically and radiographically over a period of 24 months, and the outcome revealed a 93% survival rate when exfoliations were excluded. Sodium hypochlorite hemostasis did not seem to impair the biologic repair and subsequent tertiary dentinogenesis. This was reaffirmed in a study by Vargas et al. in which pulpotomies were compared using either NaOCl or ferric sulfate ($FeSO_4$) on primary teeth that were then restored with Intermediate restorative material (IRM) base/stainless steel crowns.[155] Short-term evaluation at 1 year showed a 100% retention rate of all teeth in the NaOCl group and 79% radiographic success, higher than the $FeSO_4$ group. Although $FeSO_4$ is effective as a hemostatic agent and recommended as a replacement for formocresol in pulpotomies on deciduous teeth, its use is not recommended if bonded restorations are used since it interferes with the bond strength of adhesive resins.[156]

In a study completed on human third molars, direct pulp caps were examined histologically at 30 and 90 days after pulp capping with either $Ca(OH)_2$ or a self-etching adhesive system after using 2.5% NaOCl for hemostasis.[157] Although $Ca(OH)_2$ appeared to perform better biologically, pulpal repair was not compromised by the use of NaOCl. When comparing hemostatic agents in healthy human pulp tissue, the exposure to 0.9% saline, 5.25% NaOCl, or 2% chlorhexidine digluconate did not incapacitate healing after direct pulp capping with $Ca(OH)_2$ at 90 days.[158] Clearly, the use of **NaOCl** in concentrations of 1.25 to 6.0% for direct pulpal exposures **can**

be recommended as a relatively safe and practical method to predictably achieve hemostasis in vital pulp therapy.[154,155,157,158]

Another emerging potential hemostatic agent is MTAD (Biopure, Tulsa/Dentsply), an irrigant and an antimicrobial agent introduced for removal of the smear layer during nonsurgical initial endodontic treatment and retreatment.[159] The solution is a mixture of tetracycline isomer (doxycycline), an acid (citric acid), and a detergent (Tween 80). The irrigant shows many desirable properties and may be a suitable replacement for ethylenediaminetetraacetic acid in conjunction with NaOCl. The solution shows an antimicrobial effect against some strains of *Enterococcus faecalis*, cleans the dentin–pulp tissue interface, and does not affect the flexural strength and modulus of elasticity of dentin.[160–162] Initial trials with MTAD indicate favorable results when used in direct pulp capping and partial pulpotomy (Dr. Mahmoud Torabinejad, personal communication, 2007).

Direct Pulp Capping

TREATMENT RECOMMENDATIONS

Recommended steps for direct pulp capping with MTA using a two-visit format (Figure 5):

1. Following diagnosis, the tooth has been identified as having either reversible pulpitis or a normal healthy pulp. After profound local anesthesia, the tooth is isolated with a dental dam, further sealed with an agent such as Oraseal (Ultradent Products Inc., South Jordan, UT) or a comparable product if required, and disinfected with either chlorhexidine or NaOCl. Working under magnification is highly recommended. The undermined enamel is removed with a diamond or carbide bur, and soft debris is removed with a spoon excavator.

2. After the carious dentin is air-dried, a caries detector dye is applied for 10 seconds, and the tooth is washed and dried. Caries removal is completed with slow-speed number 4–2 carbide round burs and spoon excavators until minimal (light pink) or no profound stained dentin is evident. The caries detector is again reapplied on air-dried dentin for 10 seconds, and the process is repeated carefully (possibly five to seven applications) until no or only light pink staining is evident.

3. If a pulpal exposure occurs during the caries removal, the bleeding can be controlled by the placement of a cotton pellet moistened with 3 to 6% NaOCl for 20 to 60 seconds, and the staining and removal process is continued carefully around the exposure site until little or no staining is visible.

4. After caries removal, the exposure(s) should be hemorrhaging to some degree. A cotton pellet moistened with 3% to 6% NaOCl is placed directly against the exposure(s) for a contact time of 1 to 10 minutes. If hemostasis is not achieved within 10 minutes, the diagnosis is changed to irreversible pulpitis and more aggressive treatment is indicated. Conversely, if bleeding is not evident after pulpal exposure, the tissue is most likely necrotic, and partial or complete pulpotomy or pulpectomy must be initiated using a high-speed diamond round bur. If, during the course of caries removal, the entire pulpal roof or axial wall is removed, a pulpotomy must be considered.

5. The MTA is mixed according to the manufacturer's instructions (3:1, MTA:H_2O) and will have the consistency of wet sand. The cement is brought to the site in bulk with either a hand instrument (Glick or spoon excavator) or an MTA carrier gun. The MTA should be placed directly over the exposed pulp tissue and all surrounding dentin. The material is gently patted down with a small moist cotton pellet or a dry pellet if the mixture is too wet, and when in place, it should be at least 1.5 mm thick. If MTA is pushed inadvertently into the pulp chamber, it will not impact the outcome negatively. A circumferential region of dentin and enamel measuring approximately 1.5 mm should be cleared around the MTA with a small (2 mm) moist cotton pellet placed at the end of an explorer. This will allow an adequate area for the future bonded restoration to provide an effective seal.

6. A custom-fabricated, flat (1–2 mm), moist cotton pellet is then placed over the entire area of the MTA. If the area involves a Class II preparation exposure including the axial wall, then the moist pellet may require placement in two sections. If the patient is willing to return within 4 hours, a large moist cotton pellet can be placed and the patient instructed not to eat or chew during the interim since this may disrupt the MTA placement.

7. After the cotton pellet placement, a strong interim restoration is provided, preferably an unbonded composite material that will facilitate removal during the second visit (e.g., Photocore, Kuraray). Unless amalgam is the designated restorative material, interim restorations such as

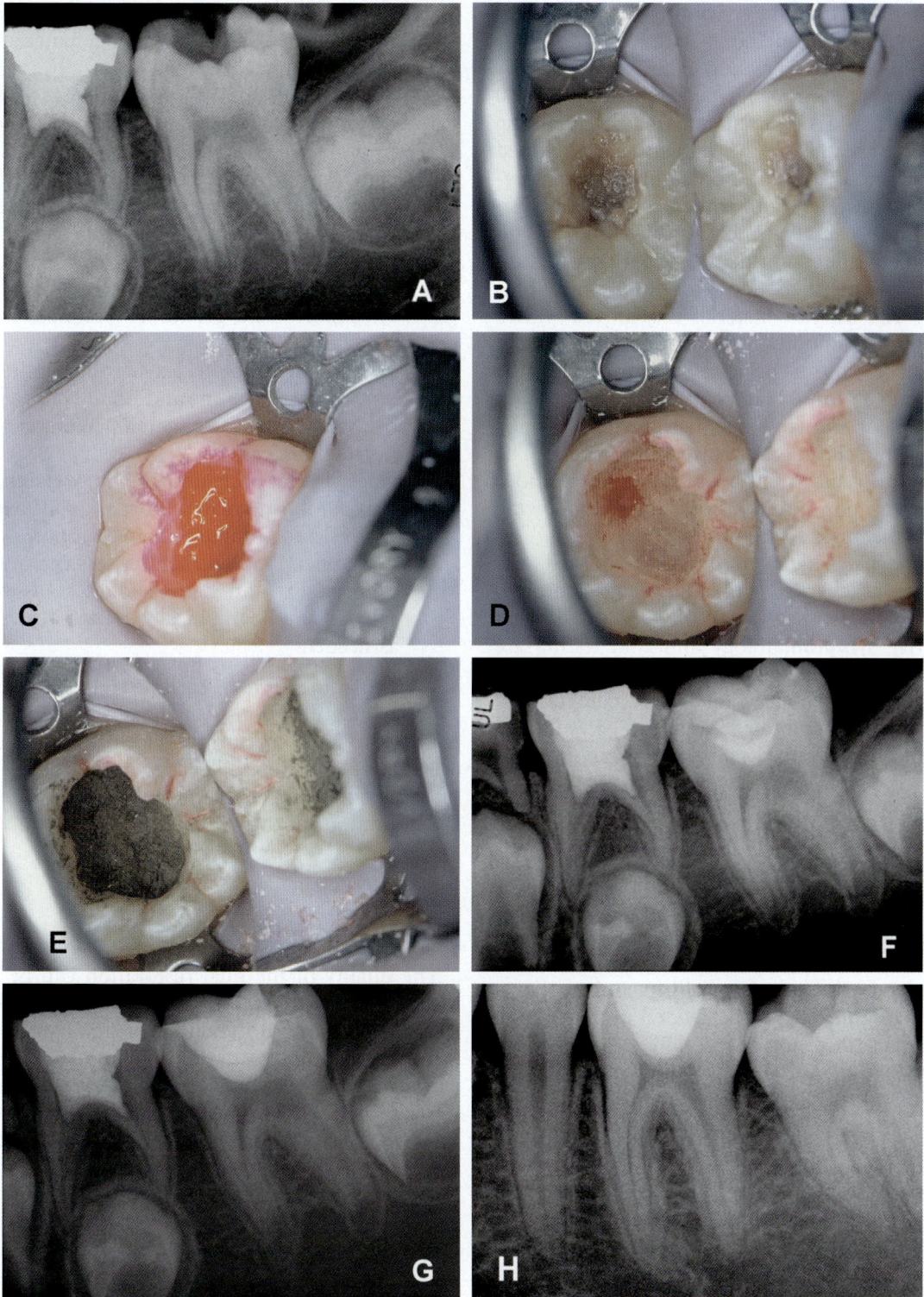

Figure 5 Radiographic and clinical sequence showing direct pulp capping of a mandibular left molar in a 7-year-old female patient. ***A,*** Pretreatment radiograph showing caries and the presence of immature apices. ***B,*** Clinical presentation following dental dam placement. ***C,*** Caries detector stain applied after removal of undermined enamel. ***D,*** Two-millimeter pulp exposure after caries removal and 5.25% NaOCl hemostasis. ***E,*** MTA of 2.5 mm thickness placed over the entire pulpal roof. ***F,*** Radiograph of MTA with a moist cotton pellet and unbonded Photocore as the interim restoration. ***G,*** Bonded composite restoration placed over cured MTA 10 days after direct pulp capping. ***H,*** Eight-year 4-month recall radiograph showing completed root formation. The tooth has a normal response to CO_2 ice testing. ***A, F,*** and ***G,*** reproduced with permission from Schmitt D et al.[102]

IRM or ZOE (that are eugenol based) will interfere with adhesion and bond strengths of adhesive resins and should be avoided.[163]

8. The second appointment can be scheduled 5 to 10 days after MTA placement. Before attaining profound anesthesia, the patient is questioned about sensitivity, mastication comfort, or the presence of pain. The tooth is then cold-tested (CO_2 ice or Endo-Ice, Hygienic Corp., Akron, OH) to confirm continued normal vitality. After injection of a local anesthetic, the tooth is isolated as before. The interim material is removed with a high-speed diamond or carbide bur under water spray. The cotton pellet is removed and the imbedded cotton fibers removed with a spoon excavator or similar hand instrument. Working with magnification is strongly recommended. The MTA is checked to ensure proper curing, and a bonded composite restoration is placed following the manufacturer's recommendations.

9. After the permanent restoration is placed, the occlusion is checked and adjusted as required. The patient is then recalled at 6 weeks, and subjective symptomatology and cold testing are evaluated. If it appears that the procedure was successful, radiographic follow-up, cold testing, and subjective symptomatology can be evaluated at 6 and 12 months. The patient can then be evaluated on a yearly basis thereafter.

ONE-STEP PULP CAPPING

According to the one manufacturer of MTA (ProRoot MTA), pulp capping can be completed in one visit. In some situations, treatment of the immature permanent tooth can be difficult, especially in young patients with challenging medical or behavioral problems that may require treatment under sedation. When one step is indicated, the manufacturer of MTA recommends the following protocol:[98]

1. Under a dental dam, a cavity preparation outline using high-speed burs under constant water cooling is completed.
2. If caries is present, excavate using a round bur in a handpiece at low speed or use hand instruments.
3. Rinse the cavity and exposure site(s) with 2.6% to 5% NaOCl. Heavy bleeding may be controlled with a cotton pellet moistened with sterile saline.
4. Prepare ProRoot MTA according to the listed instructions.
5. Using a small ball applicator or similar device, apply a small amount of the material over the exposure.
6. Remove excess moisture at the site with a moist cotton pellet.
7. Apply a small amount of Dyract Flow flowable compomer (Dentsply International, York, PA) (or an equivalent light-cured resin, glass ionomer liner) to cover the MTA and light-cure according to its instructions.
8. Etch the remaining cavity walls with 34% to 37% phosphoric acid gel for 15 seconds. Rinse thoroughly.
9. Dry the cavity gently, leaving the dentin moist but not wet. Apply Prime and Bond NT material or an equivalent bonding material. Cure according to its instructions.
10. Place TPH Spectrum (Dentsply/Caulk, Milford, DE) composite material or an equivalent composite resin to complete the restoration.
11. At the next appointment, assess the pulp vitality. Pulp vitality and status should be assessed clinically and radiographically every 3 to 6 months or as needed.

We recommend that caries removal be completed under magnification with the aid of a caries detector dye (step 2). Also, during MTA placement against the exposure site (step 5), a larger bulk of MTA should be placed that includes the majority of surrounding dentin at a thickness greater than 1.5 mm.

Final Restoration

The quality of the final restoration can be critical to the long-term maintenance of pulp vitality and sustained normal function of the pulp-capped or pulpotomized tooth. Pulp inflammation is directly associated with bacterial microleakage around restorations, and the frequency varies according to the material used.[164] In the absence of microleakage, the pulp will have the highest probability for wound repair and survival.[165–167] It has been suggested that leaking restorations may be more harmful to pulp tissue than cavity preparations that are unfilled and left open.[168] The clinician must determine an appropriate restorative material for each case that provides the best likelihood of a predictable seal against microleakage and deliver it with a high level of skill. Adhesive restorative materials are technique sensitive, and clinicians must execute treatment protocols following the manufacturer's guidelines. Specific composite materials should be matched with their respective and recommended bonding resins.[169]

Restorative procedures for immature permanent teeth include full-coverage restorations, composite resins, and bonded or unbonded amalgam restorations. The more conservative the restorative treatment, preserving the remaining healthy tooth structure, the higher the probability of pulp survival.[138] The age of the patient, the size and depth of the cavity preparation, and the choice of restorative material are all factors affecting repair mechanisms within pulp tissue.[170] Amalgam has proven to be a reliable material, inexpensive and relatively simple to place. It has disadvantages, which include esthetic concerns and potential health risks for dental providers. Restorations can be associated with coronal infractions or cuspal fracture, particularly if cusps are not protected.[171–173] Amalgam may exhibit less microleakage if placed in conjunction with a bonding resin or resin-modified glass ionomer liners.[164,174,175] Although retention rates of composite restorations are improving as technology advances,[176,177] amalgam restorations remain a reliable, safe, and predictable long-term treatment option.[178–182]

Postoperative Follow-Up

Clinical recall and radiographic evaluation are the most accurate predictors for measuring survival rates in vital pulp therapy. Recall compliance is generally more challenging with successful asymptomatic cases than teeth that become irreversibly inflamed or progress to acute apical periodontitis after treatment. The importance of follow-ups after vital pulp therapy cannot be overstated since the occurrence of recurrent caries, restoration failure, poor oral hygiene, or other conditions may be present, requiring attention. Compliance rates for follow-up with child patients can be mediocre as some parents lack basic oral health knowledge and do not practice preventive care.[183,184] The time sequence necessary for proper follow-up assessment is based on the common practice of the 6-month recall, usually related to the oral examination and oral prophylaxis and has recently come into question.[185] Optimal recall rates should be established individually, based on the patient's need, caries index, periodontal status, symptomatology, and the need for observation of craniofacial development in younger patients.[186]

In an investigation in which direct pulp capping was completed with $Ca(OH)_2$, it was determined that 3 months was an adequate time period for a tentative diagnosis of survivability.[132] The same study also showed that an observation period of 21 to 24 months was sufficient to establish a prognosis for long-term pulp survival. When MTA is used in the two-visit protocol (described earlier in this chapter), the clinician has the opportunity to examine the treated tooth at 5 to 10 days. If the treatment appears successful at that appointment, the provider can confidently schedule the next follow-up at 6 weeks if possible and then at 6 and 12 months.[119]

In direct pulp capping and pulpotomy, with **immature permanent teeth**, the most reliable prognostic indicator for success is the radiographic confirmation of root-end closure (apexogenesis). Apexogenesis of the immature adult tooth is one of the key objectives in vital pulp therapy. The process encourages physiologic development and formation of the root end and should advance successfully in healthy patients at the same rate after the application of MTA, whether direct pulp capping or pulpotomy was performed.[114,115,187,188]

In vital teeth, this natural succession of tooth development should follow a predictable pattern viewed chronologically and compared radiographically with contralateral teeth.[189] Following contralateral tooth development is an excellent way to observe the success of vital pulp therapy. In teeth that have suffered trauma, with necrotic pulps and periapical pathosis, teeth are treated to stimulate apical barrier formation (apexification). The time required to barrier formation can be variable, with times from 5 to 20 months.[190] Similarly, MTA, which has been shown to be a suitable replacement for $Ca(OH)_2$ in pulpotomy and direct pulp capping treatments, can be expected to provide apical maturation at comparable time periods.[191] The human pulp and surrounding tissue have extraordinary regenerative capacity when a **microbe-free environment** is provided.[169,192] MTA is the first of many new bioactive substances that will potentiate the ability of the dental pulp to heal, thereby retaining and maintaining its natural evolutionary function and purpose.

Acknowledgment

We wish to thank Dr. Rajneesh Roy for his contributions to this chapter.

References

1. Kakehashi S, Stanley HR, Fitzgerald RT. The effects of surgical exposures of dental pulps in germ-free and conventional laboratory rats. Oral Surg Oral Med Oral Pathol Oral Radiol Endod 1965;20:340–9.

2. Rutherford B, Fitzgerald M. A new biological approach to vital pulp therapy. Crit Rev Oral Biol Med 1995;6:218–29.

3. Dummet CO, Kopel MK. Pediatric endodontics. In: Ingle JI, Bakland LK, editors. Endodontics. 5th ed. Hamilton (ON): BC Decker; 2002. pp. 861–902.

4. Glass RL, Zander HA. Pulp healing. J Dent Res 1949;28:97–107.

5. Tronstad L, Mjör IA. Capping of the inflamed pulp. Oral Surg Oral Med Oral Pathol Oral Radiol Endod 1972;34:477–85.

6. Langeland K. Management of the inflamed pulp associated with deep carious lesion. J Endod 1981;7:169–81.

7. Hørsted P, Søndergaard B, Thylstrup A, et al. A retrospective study of direct pulp capping with calcium hydroxide compounds. Endod Dent Traumatol 1985;1:29–34.

8. Guideline on pulp therapy for primary and young permanent teeth. American Academy of Pediatric Dentistry Clinical Affairs Committee-Pulp Therapy Subcommitte: American Academy of Pediatric Dentistry Council on Clinical Affairs. Pediatr Dent 2005;27:130–4.

9. Yu C, Abbott PV. An overview of the dental pulp: its functions and responses to injury. Aust Dent J Suppl 2007;52:S4–16.

10. Leeson TS, Leeson CR, Paparo AA. The digestive system. In: Atlas of histology. Philadelphia (PA): WB Saunders; 1988. pp. 401–8.

11. Stockton LW. Vital pulp capping: a worthwhile procedure. J Can Dent Assoc 1999;65:328–31.

12. Brännström M, Lind PO. Pulpal response to early dental caries. J Dent Res 1965;44:1045–50.

13. Bjørndal L, Darvann T, Thylstrupt A. A quantitative light microscopic study of the odontoblast and subodontoblastic reactions to active and arrested enamel caries without cavitation. Caries Res 1998;32:59–69.

14. Helfer AR, Melnick S, Schilder H. Determination of the moisture content of vital and pulpless teeth. Oral Surg Oral Med Oral Pathol Oral Radiol Endod 1972;34:661–70.

15. Jameson MW, Hood JAA, Tidmarsh BG. The effects of dehydration and rehydration on some mechanical properties of human dentine. J Biomech 1993;26:1055–65.

16. Linn J, Messer HH. Effect of restorative procedures on the strength of endodontically treated molars. J Endod 1994;20:479–85.

17. Ten Cate AR. Dentin-pulp complex. In: Oral histology. 4th ed. RW Reinhardt, editor, St. Louis (MO): Mosby; 1994. p. 184.

18. Yamada T, Nakamura K, Iwaku M, Fusayama T. The extent of the odontoblast process in normal and carious human dentin. J Dent Res 1983;62:798–802.

19. Grötz KA, Duschner H, Reichert TE, et al. Histotomography of the ododontoblast processes at the dentine-enamel junction of permanent healthy human teeth in the confocal laser scanning microscope. Clin Oral Invest 1998;2:21–5.

20. Gottrup F, Andreasen JO. Wound healing subsequent to injury. In: Andreason JO, Andreason FM, editors. Textbook and color atlas of traumatic injuries to teeth. Copenhagen (Denmark): Munksgaard; 1994. pp. 13–76.

21. Albelda SM, Smith CW, Ward PA. Adhesion molecules and inflammatory injury. FASEB J 1994;8:504–12.

22. Tziafas D. Basic mechanisms of cytodifferentiation and dentinogenesis during dental pulp repair. Int J Dev Biol 1995;39:281–90.

23. Fitzgerald M, Chiego DJJ, Heys DR. Autoradiographic analysis of odontoblast replacement following pulp exposure in primate teeth. Arch Oral Biol 1990;35:707–15.

24. Oguntebi BR, Heaven T, Clark AE, Pink FE. Quantitative assessment of dentin bridge formation following pulp-capping in miniature swine. J Endod 1995;21:79–82.

25. Inoue H, Muneyuki H, Izumi T, et al. Electron microscopic study on nerve terminals during dentin bridge formation after pulpotomy in dog teeth. J Endod 1997;23:569–71.

26. Kitasako Y, Shibata S, Arakawa M, et al. A light and transmission microscopic study of mechanically exposed monkey pulps: dynamics of fiber elements during early dentin bridge formation. Oral Surg Oral Med Oral Pathol Oral Radiol Endod 2000;89:224–30.

27. Hayashi Y. Ultrastructure of initial calcification in wound healing following pulpotomy. J Oral Pathol 1982;11:174–80.

28. Kitasako Y, Murray PE, Tagami J, Smith AJ. Histomorphometric analysis of dentinal bridge formation and pulpal inflammation. Quintessence Int 2002;33:600–8.

29. Glossary of endodontic terms. 7th ed. American Association of Endodontists; Chicago, (IL): 2003.

30. Marchi JJ, de Araujo FB, Fröner AM, et al. Indirect pulp capping in the primary dentition: a 4 year follow-up study. J Clin Pediatr Dent 2006;31:68–71.

31. Mass E, Zilberman U, Fuks AB. Partial pulpotomy: another treatment option for cariously exposed permanent molars. J Dent Child 1995;62:342–5.

32. Hawes RR, Dimaggio JJ, Sayegh F. Evaluation of direct and indirect pulp capping [abstract]. J Dent Res 1964;43:808.

33. Jordan RE, Suzuki M. Conservative treatment of deep carious lesions. J Can Dent Assoc 1971;37:337–42.

34. Bjørndal L, Larsen T, Thylstrup A. A clinical and microbiological study of deep carious lesions during stepwise excavation using long treatment intervals. Caries Res 1997;31:411–17.

35. Ørstavik D, Pitt Ford TR. Essential endodontology: prevention and treatment of apical periodontitis. Oxford (UK): Blackwell Science; 1998.

36. Rothman MS. Formocresol pulpotomy: a practical procedure for permanent teeth. Gen Dent 1977;25:39–41.

37. Fuks AB, Bimstein E, Bruchim A. Radiographic and histologic evaluation of the effect of two concentrations of formocresol on pulpotomized primary and young permanent teeth in monkeys. Pediatr Dent 1983;5:9–13.

38. Rölling I, Hasselgren G, Tronstad L. Morphologic and enzyme histochemical observations on the pulp of human primary molars 3 to 5 years after formocresol treatment. Oral Surg Oral Med Oral Pathol Oral Radiol Endod 1976;42:518–28.

39. Holan G, Eidelman E, Fuks AB. Long-term evaluation of pulpotomy in primary molars using mineral trioxide aggregate or formocresol. Pediatr Dent 2005;27:129–36.

40. Caicedo R, Abbott PV, Alongi DJ, Alarcon MY. Clinical, radiographic and histological analysis of the effects of mineral trioxide aggregate used in direct pulp capping and pulpotomies of primary teeth. Aust Dent J 2006; 51:297–305.

41. Cvek M. A clinical report on partial pulpotomy and capping with calcium hydroxide in permanent incisors with complicated root fractures. J Endod 1978;4:232–7.

42. Randow K, Glantz PO. On cantilever loading of vital and non-vital teeth. An experimental clinical study. Acta Odontol Scand 1986;44:271–7.

43. Mentink AG, Meeuwissen R, Käyser AF, Mulder J. Survival rate and failure characteristics of the all metal post and core restoration. J Oral Rehabil 1993;20:455–61.

44. Torbjörner A, Karlsson S, Odman PA. Survival rate and failure characteristics for two post designs. J Prosthet Dent 1995;73:439–44.

45. Caplan DJ, Kolker J, Rivera EM, Walton RE. Relationship between number of proximal contacts and survival of root treated teeth. Int Endod J 2002;35:193–9.

46. Caplan DJ, Cai J, Yin G, White BA. Root canal filled versus non-root canal filled teeth: a retrospective comparison of survival times. J Public Health Dent 2005;65:90–6.

47. Wegner PK, Freitag S, Kern M. Survival rate of endodontically treated teeth with posts after prosthetic restoration. J Endod 2006;32:928–31.

48. De Backer H, van Maele G, Decock V, van den Berghe L. Long-term survival of complete crowns, fixed dental prostheses, and cantilever prostheses with post and cores on root-canal treated teeth. Int J Prosthodont 2007;20:229–34.

49. Haskell EW, Stanley HR, Chellemi J, Stringfellow H. Direct pulp capping treatment: a long-term follow-up. J Am Dent Assoc 1978;97:607–12.

50. Baume LJ, Holz J. Long term clinical assessment of direct pulp capping. Int Dent J 1981;31:251–60.

51. Barthel CR, Rosenkranz B, Leuenberg A, Roulet JF. Pulp capping of carious exposures treatment outcome after 5 and 10 years: a retrospective study. J Endod 2000;26:525–8.

52. Auschill TM, Arweiler NB, Hellwig E, et al. Success rate of direct pulp capping with calcium hydroxide. Schweiz Monatsschr Zahnmed 2003;113:946–52.

53. Beagrie GS, Main JH, Smith DC, Walshaw PR. Polycarboxylate cement as a pulp capping agent. Dent J 1974;40:378–83.

54. Sveen OB. Pulp capping of primary teeth with zinc oxide eugenol. Odontol Tidskr 1969;77:427–36.

55. Bhaskar SN, Beasley JD, Ward JP, Cutright DE. Human pulp capping with isobutyl cyanoacrylate. J Dent Res 1972;51:58–61.

56. Heller AL, Koenigs JF, Brilliant JD, et al. Direct pulp capping of permanent teeth in primates using a resorbable form of tricalcium phosphate ceramic. J Endod 1975;1:95–101.

57. Kashiwada T, Takagi M. New restoration and direct pulp capping systems using adhesive composite resin. Bull Tokyo Med Dent Univ 1991;38:45–52.

58. Higashi T, Okamoto H. Influence of particle size of hydroxyapatite as a capping agent on cell proliferation of cultured fibroblasts. J Endod 1996;22:236–9.

59. Yoshimine Y, Maeda K. Histologic evaluation of tetracalcium phosphate-based cement as a direct pulp-capping agent. Oral Surg Oral Med Oral Pathol Oral Radiol Endod 1995;79:351–8.

60. Pitt Ford TR, Torabinejad M, Abedi HR, et al. Using mineral trioxide aggregate as a pulp-capping material. J Am Dent Assoc 1996;127:1491–4.

61. Stanley HR, Clark AE, Pameijer CH, Louw NP. Pulp capping with a modified bioglass formula (#A68-modified). Am J Dent 2001;14:227–32.

62. Olsson H, Davies JR, Holst KE, et al. Dental pulp capping: effect of Emdogain Gel on experimentally exposed human pulps. Int Endod J 2005;38:186–94.

63. Zhang W, Walboomers XF, Jansen JA. The formation of tertiary dentin after pulp capping with a calcium phosphate cement, loaded with PLGA microparticles containing TGF-beta1. J Biomed Mater Res A 2007 [In press].

64. Miyashita H, Worthington HV, Qualtrough A, Plasschaert A. Pulp management for caries in adults: maintaining pulp vitality. Cochrane Database Syst Rev 2007;18:CD004484.

65. Moritz A, Schoop U, Goharkhay K, Sperr W. The CO_2 laser as an aid in direct pulp capping. J Endod 1998;24:248–51.

66. Goldberg M, Six N, Decup F, et al. Bioactive molecules and the future of pulp therapy. Am J Dent 2003;16:66–76.

67. Dähnhardt JE, Jaeqqi T, Lussi A. Treating open carious lesions in anxious children with ozone. A prospective controlled clinical study. Am J Dent 2006;19:267–70.

68. Olivi G, Genovese MD, Maturo P, Docimo R. Pulp capping: advantages of using laser technology. Eur J Paediatr Dent 2007;8:89–95.

69. Cohen BD, Combe EC. Development of new adhesive pulp capping materials. Dent Update 1994;21:57–62.

70. Cox CF, Sübay RK, Ostro E, Suzuki S, Suzuki SH. Tunnel defects in dentin bridges: Their formation following direct pulp capping. Oper Dent 1996;21:4–11.

71. Schröder U. Effect of calcium hydroxide-containing pulp capping agents on pulp cell migration, proliferation, and differentiation. J Dent Res 1985;66:1166–74.

72. Andelin WE, Shabahang S, Wright K, Torabinejad M. Identification of hard tissue after experimental pulp capping using dentin sialoprotein (DSP) as a marker. J Endod 2003;29:646–50.

73. Goldberg M, Lasfargues JJ, Legrand JM. Clinical testing of dental materials—histological considerations. J Dent 1994;22:S25–8.

74. Via W. Evaluation of deciduous molars by treated pulpotomy and calcium hydroxide. J Am Dent Assoc 1955;50:34–43.

75. Barnes IM, Kidd EA. Disappearing Dycal. Br Dent J 1979;147:111.

76. Cox CF, Suzuki S. Re-evaluating pulp protection: calcium hydroxide liners vs. cohesive hybridization. J Am Dent Assoc 1994;125:823–31.

77. Goracci G, Mori G. Scaning electron microscopic evaluation of resin-dentin and calcium hydroxide dentin-interface with resin composite restorations. Quintessence Int 1996;27:129–35.

78. Inokoshi S, Iwaku M, Fusayama T. Pulpal response to a new adhesive resin material. J Dent Res 1982;61:1014–19.

79. Yamani T, Yamashita A, Takeshita N, Nagai N. Histopathological evaluation of the effects of a new dental adhesive resin on dog dental pulps. J Jpn Prosth Soc 1986;30:671–8.

80. Matsuura T, Katsumata T, Matsuura T, et al. Histopathological study of pulpal irritation of dental adhesive resin. Part 1. Panavia EX. Nihon Hotetsu Shika Gakkai Zasshi 1987;31:104–15.

81. Tarmin B, Hafez AA, Cox CF. Pulpal response to a resin-modified glass-ionomer material on nonexposed and exposed monkey pulps. Quintessence Int 1998;29:535–42.

82. Cox CF, Hafez AA, Akimoto N, et al. Biocompatibility of primer, adhesive and resin composite systems on non-exposed and exposed pulps of non-human primate teeth. Am J Dent 1998;11:S55–63.

83. Akimoto N, Momoi Y, Kohno A, et al. Biocompatibility of Clearfil Liner Bond 2 and Clearfil AP-X system on nonexposed and exposed primate teeth. Quintessence Int 1998;29:177–88.

84. Tarim B, Hafez AA, Suzuki SH, et al. Biocompatibility of Optibond and XR-Bond adhesive systems in nonhuman primate teeth. Int J Periodontics Restorative Dent 1998;18:86–99.

85. Tarim B, Hafez AA, Suzuki SH, et al. Biocompatability of compomer restorative systems on nonexposed dental pulps of primate teeth. Oper Dent 1997;22:149–58.

86. Gwinnett J, Tay FR. Early and intermediate time response of the dental pulp to an acid etch technique in vivo. Am J Dent 1997;10:S35–44.

87. Hebling J, Giro EMA, deSouza Costa CA. Biocompatibility of an adhesive system applied to exposed human dental pulp. J Endod 1999;25:676–82.

88. Mjör IA. Pulp-dentin biology in restorative dentistry. Part 7: the exposed pulp. Quintessence Int 2002;33:113–35.

89. Hörsted-Bindslev P, Vilkinis V, Sidlauskas A. Direct capping of human pulps with a dentin bonding system or with calcium hydroxide cement. Oral Surg Oral Med Oral Pathol Oral Radiol Endod 2003;96:591–600.

90. Accorinte Mde L, Loguercio AD, Reis A, et al. Adverse effects of human pulps after direct pulp capping with different components from a total-etch, three-step adhesive system. Dent Mater 2005;21:599–607.

91. do Nascimento ABL, Fontana UF, Teixeira HM, de Souza Costa CA. Biocompatibility of a resin-modified glass-ionomer cement applied as pulp capping in human teeth. Am J Dent 2000;13:28–34.

92. de Souza Costa CA, Lopes do Nascimento AB, Teixeira HM, Fontana UF. Response of human pulps capped with a self-etching adhesive system. Dent Mater 2001;17:230–40.

93. Murray PE, Hafez AA, Smith AJ, Cox CF. Hierarchy of pulp capping and repair activities responsible for dentin bridge formation. Am J Dent 2002;15:236–43.

94. Murray PE, García-Godoy F. The incidence of pulp healing defects with direct capping materials. Am J Dent 2006;19:171–7.

95. Olsson H, Petersson K, Rohlin M. Formation of a hard tissue barrier after pulp capping in humans. A systematic review. Int Endod J 2006;39:429–42.

96. Lee SJ, Monsef M, Torabinejad M. The sealing ability of a mineral trioxide aggregate for repair of lateral root perforations. J Endod 1993;19:541–4.

97. Torabinejad M, Hong CU, McDonald F, Pitt Ford TR. Physical and chemical properties of a new root-end filling material. J Endod 1995;21:349–53.

98. Dentsply Tulsa Dental. ProRoot MTA [product literature].

99. Holland R, de Souza V, Nery MJ, et al. Reaction of rat connective tissue to implanted dentin tubes filled with a white mineral trioxide aggregate. Braz Dent J 2002;13:23–6.

100. Ferris DM, Baumgartner JC. Perforation repair comparing two types of mineral trioxide aggregate. J Endod 2004;30:422–4.

101. Menezes R, Bramante CM, Letra A, et al. Histologic evaluation of pulpotomies in dog using two types of mineral trioxide aggregate and regular and white Portland cements as wound dressings. Oral Surg Oral Med Oral Pathol Oral Radiol Endod 2004;98:376–9.

102. Schmitt D, Lee J, Bogen G. Multifaceted use of ProRoot MTA root canal repair material. Pediatr Dent 2001;23:326–30.

103. Torabinejad M, Chivian N. Clinical applications of mineral trioxide aggregate. J Endod 1999;25:197–205.

104. Torabinejad M, Higa RK, McKendry DJ, Pitt Ford TR. Dye leakage of four root-end filling materials: effects of blood contamination. J Endod 1994;20:159–63.

105. Torabinejad M, Smith PW, Kettering JD, Pitt Ford TR. Comparative investigation of marginal adaptation of mineral trioxide aggregate and other commonly used root-end filling materials. J Endod 1995;21:295–9.

106. Sarkar NK, Caicedo R, Ritwik P, et al. Physiochemical basis of the biologic properties of mineral trioxide aggregate. J Endod 2005;31:97–100.

107. Moghaddame-Jafari S, Mantellini MG, Botero M, et al. Effect of ProRoot MTA on pulp cell apoptosis and proliferation in vitro. J Endod 2005;31:387–91.

108. Koh ET, Pitt Ford TR, Torabinejad M, McDonald F. Mineral trioxide aggregate stimulates cytokine production in human osteoblasts. J Bone Miner Res 1995;10S:S406.

109. Andelin WE, Shabahang S, Wright K, Torabinejad M. Identification of hard tissue after experimental pulp capping using dentin sialoprotein (DSP) as a marker. J Endod 2003;29:646–50.

110. Tziafas D, Pantelidou O, Alvanou A, et al. The dentinogenic effect of mineral trioxide aggregate (MTA) in short-term capping experiments. Int Endod J 2002;35:245–54.

111. Junn DJ. Quantitative assessment of dentin bridge formation following pulp-capping with mineral trioxide aggregate [master's thesis]. Loma Linda (CA): Loma Linda University; 2000.

112. Faraco IM Jr, Holland R. Response of the pulp of dogs to capping with mineral trioxide aggregate or a calcium hydroxide cement. Dent Traumatol 2001;17:163–6.

113. Aeinehchi M, Eslami B, Ghanabriha M, Saffar AS. Mineral trioxide aggregate (MTA) and calcium hydroxide as pulp capping agents in human teeth: a preliminary report. Int Endod J 2003;36:225–31.

114. Witherspoon DE, Small JC, Harris GZ. Mineral trioxide aggregate pulpotomies: a case series outcome assessment. J Am Dent Assoc 2006;137:610–18.

115. Barrieshi-Nusair KM, Qudeimat MA. A prospective clinical study of mineral trioxide aggregate for partial pulpotomy in cariously exposed permanent teeth. J Endod 2006;32:731–5.

116. Iwamoto CE, Adachi E, Pameijer CH, et al. Clinical and histological evaluation of white ProRoot MTA in direct pulp capping. Am J Dent 2006;19:85–90.

117. Farsi N, Alamoudi N, Balto K, Mushayt A. Clinical assessment of mineral trioxide aggregate (MTA) as direct pulp capping in young permanent teeth. J Clin Pediatr Dent 2006;31:72–6.

118. Tomson PL, Grover LM, Lumley PJ, et al. Dissolution of bio-active dentine matrix components by mineral trioxide aggregate. J Dent 2007;35:636–42.

119. Bogen G, Kim JS, Bakland LK. Direct pulp capping with mineral trioxide aggregate: an observational study. [In press]

120. Gutmann JL, Heaton JF. Management of the open (immature) apex. 1. Vital teeth. Int Endod J 1981;14:166–72.

121. Fuks AB. Pulp therapy for the primary and young permanent dentitions. Dent Clin North Am 2000;44:571–96.

122. Shabahang S, Torabinejad M. Treatment of teeth with open apices using mineral trioxide aggregate. Pract Periodontics Aesthet Dent 2000;12:31.

123. Fulling HJ, Andreasen JO. Influence of maturation status and tooth type of permanent teeth upon electrometric and thermal pulp testing. Scand J Dent Res 1976;84:286–90.

124. Karibe H, Ohide Y, Kohno H, et al. Study on thermal pulp testing of immature permanent teeth. Shigaku 1989;77:1006–13.

125. Bortoluzzi EA, Souza EM, Reis JM, et al. Fracture strength of bovine incisors after intra-radicular treatment with MTA in an experimental immature tooth model. Int Endod J 2007;40:684–91.

126. Abou-Rass M. The stressed pulp condition: an endodontic-restorative diagnostic concept. J Prosthet Dent 1982;48:264–7.

127. Mjör IA. Pulp-dentin biology in restorative dentistry. Part 5: clinical management and tissue changes associated with wear and trauma. Quintessence Int 2001;32:771–88.

128. Brambilla E, García-Godoy F, Strohmenger L. Principles of diagnosis and treatment of high-caries-risk subjects. Dent Clin North Am 2000;44:507–40.

129. Tinanoff N, Douglass JM. Clinical decision making for caries management in children. Pediatr Dent 2002;24:386–92.

130. Camp J. Pediatric endodontic treatment. In: Cohen S, Burns RC, editors. Pathways of the pulp. 7th ed. St. Louis (MO): Mosby;1998. pp. 718–58.

131. Chandler NP, Pitt Ford TR, Monteith BD. Pulp size in molars: underestimation on radiographs. J Oral Rehabil 2004;31:764–9.

132. Matsuo T, Nakanishi T, Shimizu H, Ebisu S. A clinical study of direct pulp capping applied to carious-exposed pulps. J Endod 1996;22:551–6.

133. Gracia TB. Accuracy of size estimations by dentists of simulated pulp exposures and cavity preparations. MDS (endodontics) research report. Otago (New Zealand): University of Otago; 2006.

134. Chandler NP, Pitt Ford TR, Monteith BD. Coronal pulp size in molars: a study of bitewing radiographs. Int Endod J 2003;36:757–63.

135. Fusayama T, Okuse K, Hosoda H. Relationship between hardness, discoloration, and microbial invasion in carious dentin. J Dent Res 1966;45:1033–46.

136. Fusayama T, Kurosaki N. Structure and removal of carious dentin. Int Dent J 1972;22:401–11.

137. Sato Y, Fusayama T. Removal of dentin guided by Fuchsin staining. J Dent Res 1976;55:678–83.

138. Fusayama T. A simple pain-free adhesive restorative system by minimal reduction and total etching. St. Louis (MO): Ishiyaku EuroAmerica Publishing; 1993.

139. Kato S, Fusayama T. Recalcification of artificially decalcified dentin in vivo. J Dent Res 1970;49:1060–7.

140. Tatsumi T. Physiological remineralization of artificially decalcified monkey dentin under adhesive composite resin. J Stom Soc Jpn 1989;56:47–74.

141. Kidd EA, Joyston-Bechal S, Beighton D. The use of a caries detector dye during cavity preparation: a microbiological assessment. Br Dent J 1993;174:245–8.

142. Lennon AM, Attin T, Buchalla W. Quantity of remaining bacteria and cavity size after excavation with FACE, caries detector dye and conventional excavation in vitro. Oper Dent 2007;32:236–41.

143. Zacharia MA, Munshi AK. Microbiological assessment of dentin stained with a caries detector dye. J Clin Pediatr Dent 1995;19:111–15.

144. Yazici AR, Baseren M, Gokalp S. The in vitro performance of laser fluorescence and caries-detector dye for detecting residual carious dentin during tooth preparation. Quintessence Int 2005;36:417–22.

145. Garcia-Godoy F, Murray PE. Systemic evaluation of various haemostatic agents following local application prior to direct pulp capping. Braz J Oral Sci 2005;4:791–7.

146. Hirota K. A study on the partial pulp removal (pulpotomy) using four different tissue solvents. J Jpn Stomatol Soc 1959;26:1588–603.

147. Sudo C. A study on partial pulp removal (pulpotomy) using NaOCl (sodium hypochlorite). J Jpn Stomatol Soc 1959;26:1012–24.

148. Cox CF, Hafez AA, Akimoto N, et al. Biocompatibility of primer, adhesive and resin composite systems on non-exposed and exposed pulps of non-human primate teeth. Am J Dent 1998;11:S55–63.

149. Hafez AA, Cox CF, Tarim B, et al. An in vivo evaluation of hemorrhage control using sodium hypochlorite and direct capping with a one-or two-component adhesive system in exposed nonhuman primate pulps. Quintessence Int 2002;33:261–72.

150. Rosenfeld EF, James GA, Burch BS. Vital pulp tissue response to sodium hypochlorite. J Endod 1978;4:140–6.

151. Heggers JP, Sazy JA, Stenberg BD, et al. Bactericidal and wound-healing properties of sodium hypochlorite solutions: the 1991 Lindberg Award. J Burn Care Rehabil 1991;12:420–4.

152. Nakanishi T, Matsuo T, Ebishu S. Quantitative analysis of immunoglobulins and inflammatory factors in human pulpal blood from exposed pulps. J Endod 1995;21:131–6.

153. Tang HM, Nordbö H, Bakland LK. Pulpal response to prolonged dentinal exposure to sodium hypochlorite. Int Endod J 2000;33:505–8.

154. Demir T, Cehreli ZC. Clinical and radiographic evaluation of adhesive pulp capping in primary molars following hemostasis with 1.25% sodium hypochlorite: 2-year results. Am J Dent 2007;20:182–8.

155. Vargas KG, Packham B, Lowman D. Preliminary evaluation of sodium hypochlorite for pulpotomies in primary molars. Pediatr Dent 2006;28:511–17.

156. Salama FS. Influence of zinc-oxide eugenol, formocresol, and ferric sulfate on bond strength of dentin adhesives to primary teeth. J Contemp Dent Pract 2005;6:14–21.

157. Elias RV, Demarco FF, Tarquinio SB, Piva E. Pulp responses to the application of a self-etching adhesive in human pulps after controlling bleeding with sodium hypochlorite. Quintessence Int 2007;38:67–77.

158. Silva AF, Tarquinio SBC, Demarco FF, et al. The influence of haemostatic agents on healing of healthy human dental pulp tissue capped with calcium hydroxide. Int Endod J 2006;39:309–16.

159. Torabinejad M, Cho Y, Khademi AA, et al. The effect of various concentrations of sodium hypochlorite on the ability of MTAD to remove the smear layer. J Endod 2003;29:233–9.

160. Machnick TK, Torabinejad M, Munoz CA, Shabahang S. Effect of MTAD on flexural strength and modulus of elasticity of dentin. J Endod 2003;29:747–50.

161. Torabinejad M, Shabahang S, Aprecio RM, Kettering JD. The antimicrobial effect of MTAD: an in vitro investigation. J Endod 2003;29:400–3.

162. Shabahang S, Torabinejad M. Effect of MTAD on *Enterococcus faecalis*-contaminated root canals of extracted human teeth. J Endod 2003;29:576–9.

163. al-Wazzan KA, al-Harbi AA, Hammad IA. The effect of eugenol-containing temporary cement on the bond strength of two resin composite core materials to dentin. J Prosthodont 1997;6:37–42.

164. Murray PE, Hafez AA, Smith AJ, Cox CF. Bacterial microleakage and pulp inflammation associated with various restorative materials. Dent Mater 2002;18:470–8.

165. Bergenholtz G, Cox CF, Loesche WJ, Syed SA. Bacterial leakage around dental restorations: its effect on the dental pulp. J Oral Pathol 1982;11:439–50.

166. Cox CF, Keall CL, Keall HJ, et al. Biocompatibility of surface-sealed dental materials against exposed dental pulps. J Prosthet Dent 1987;57:1–8.

167. Pashley DH, Pashley EL, Carvalho RM, Tay FR. The effects of dentin permeability on restorative dentistry. Dent Clin North Am 2002;46:211–45.

168. Sasafuchi Y, Otsuki M, Inokoshi S, Tagami J. The effects on pulp tissue of microleakage in resin composite restorations. J Med Dent Sci 1999;46:155–64.

169. Murray PE, Smith AJ. Saving pulps—a biological basis. An overview. Prim Dent Care 2002;9:21–6.

170. Murray PE, About I, Lumley PJ, et al. Postoperative pulpal and repair responses. J Am Dent Assoc 2000;131:321–9.

171. Van Nieuwenhuysen JP, D'Hoore W, Carvalho J, Qvist V. Long-term evaluation of extensive restorations in permanent teeth. J Dent 2003;31:395–405.

172. Wahl MJ, Schmitt MM, Overton DA, Gordon MK. Prevalence of cusp fractures in teeth restored with amalgam and with resin-based composite. J Am Dent Assoc 2004;135:1127–32.

173. Halbach S, Vogt S, Köhler W, et al. Blood and urine mercury levels in adult amalgam patients of a randomized controlled trial: interaction of Hg species in erythrocytes. Environ Res 2007 [In press].

174. Marchiori S, Baratieri LN, de Andrada MA, et al. The use of liners under amalgam restorations: an in vitro study on marginal leakage. Quintessence Int 1998;29:637–42.

175. Luz MA deC, Ciaramicoli-Rodrigues MT, Garone Netto N, De Lima ACP. Long-term clinical evaluation of fracture and pulp injury following glass-ionomer cement or composite resin applied as a base filling in teeth restored with amalgam. J Oral Rehabil 2001;28:634–9.

176. Gaengler P, Hoyer I, Montag R. Clinical evaluation of posterior composite restorations: the 10-year report. J Adhes Dent 2001;3:185–94.

177. Gordan VV, Mondragon E, Watson RE, et al. A clinical evaluation of a self-etching primer and a giomer restorative material: results at eight years. J Am Dent Assoc 2007;138:621–7.

178. Collins CJ, Bryant RW, Hodge KLV. A clinical evaluation of posterior composite resin restorations: 8-year findings. J Dent 1998;26:311–17.

179. DeRouen TA, Martin MD, Leroux BG, et al. Neurobehavioral effects of dental amalgam in children: a randomized clinical trial. J Am Dent Assoc 2006;295:1784–92.

180. Martin MD, Woods JS. The safety of dental amalgam in children. Exp Opin Drug Saf 2006;5:773–81.

181. Bernardo M, Luis H, Martin MD, et al. Survival and reasons for failure of amalgam versus composite posterior restorations placed in a randomized clinical trial. J Am Dent Assoc 2007;138:775–83.

182. Soncini JA, Maserejian NN, Trachtenberg F, et al. The longevity of amalgam versus compomer/composite restorations in posterior primary and permanent teeth: findings from the New England Children's Amalgam Trial. J Am Dent Assoc 2007;138:763–72.

183. Jamieson WJ, Vargas K. Recall rates and caries experience of patients undergoing general anesthesia for dental treatment. Pediatr Dent 2007;29:253–7.

184. Primosch RE, Balsewich CM, Thomas CW. Outcomes assessment an intervention strategy to improve parental compliance to follow-up evaluations after treatment of early childhood caries using general anesthesia in a Medicaid population. ASDC J Dent Child 2001;68:102–8.

185. Mettes D. Insufficient evidence to support or refute the need for 6-monthly dental check-ups. What is the optimal recall frequency between dental checks? Evid Based Dent 2005;6:62–3.

186. Nikiforuk G. Optimal recall intervals in child dental care. J Can Dent Assoc 1997;63:618–24.

187. Weisleder R, Benitez CR. Maturogenesis: is it a new concept? J Endod 2003;29:776–8.

188. Patel R, Cohenca N. Maturogenesis of a cariously exposed immature permanent tooth using MTA for direct pulp capping: a case report. Dent Traumatol 2006;22:328–33.

189. Ballesio I, Marchetti E, Mummolo S, Marzo G. Radiographic appearance of apical closure in apexification: follow-up after 7–13 years. Eur J Paediatr Dent 2006;7:9–34.

190. Sheehy EC, Roberts GJ. Use of calcium hydroxide for apical barrier formation and healing in non-vital immature permanent teeth: a review. Br Dent J 1997;183:241–6.

191. El-Meligy OAS, Avery DR. Comparison of mineral trioxide aggregate and calcium hydroxide as pulpotomy agents in young permanent teeth (apexogenesis). Pediatr Dent 2006;28:399–404.

192. Chueh LH, Huang GT. Immature teeth with periradicular periodontitis or abscess undergoing apexogenesis: a paradigm shift. J Endod 2006;32:1205–13.

Chapter 36

Endodontic Considerations in Dental Trauma

Martin Trope

Traumatic injuries to the teeth result in damage to many dental and periradicular structures. Therefore, the management and consequences of these injuries are multifactorial, and knowledge of the interrelating healing patterns of these tissues is essential.

The focus of this chapter is the dental pulp and how damage to the dentinopulpal complex can contribute to complications after a traumatic injury and how correct diagnosis and treatment can result in favorable healing after an injury. More information on management of dental trauma can be obtained by going on the Web site of the International Association of Dental Traumatology: <http://www.iadt-dentaltrauma.org>.

Unique Aspects of Dental Trauma

Most dental trauma occurs in the 7- to 10-year-old age group owing to falls and accidents near home or school.[1,2] It occurs primarily in the anterior region of the mouth, affecting the maxilla more than the mandible.[3]

Thus, in many cases after a dental traumatic injury, endodontic therapy is provided to caries-free, single-rooted, **young** permanent teeth. Therefore, maintenance of the tooth is particularly important in these young individuals. Luckily, the potential for a successful endodontic outcome is very good if timely and correct treatment is provided soon after the injury.

Crown Fractures

The primary aim from an endodontic point of view is to **maintain pulp vitality** after fractures involving the crowns of teeth.

Crown Infractions—"Incomplete fracture or crack of enamel without loss of tooth structure"[4] and **Uncomplicated Crown Fractures**—"Fractures of the enamel only or enamel and dentin without pulp exposure"[4] are injuries that have little danger of resulting in pulp necrosis. In fact, the biggest danger to the health of the pulp is through iatrogenic causes during the esthetic restoration of these teeth. Therefore, meticulous follow-up over a 5-year period is an important endodontic preventive measure in these cases. Endodontic intervention should be considered at any follow-up time when reactions to sensitivity tests change, apical periodontitis develops, the root appears to have stopped development, or the pulp is obliterating.

COMPLICATED CROWN FRACTURES

By definition, complicated crown fractures involve enamel, dentin, and pulp[4] and occur in 0.9 to 13% of all dental injuries.[5–7] A crown fracture involving the pulp, if left untreated, will always result in pulp necrosis.[8] However, the manner and time sequence in which the pulp becomes necrotic allow a great deal of potential for successful intervention in maintaining pulp vitality. The first reaction after an injury is

Chapter 36 / Endodontic Considerations in Dental Trauma

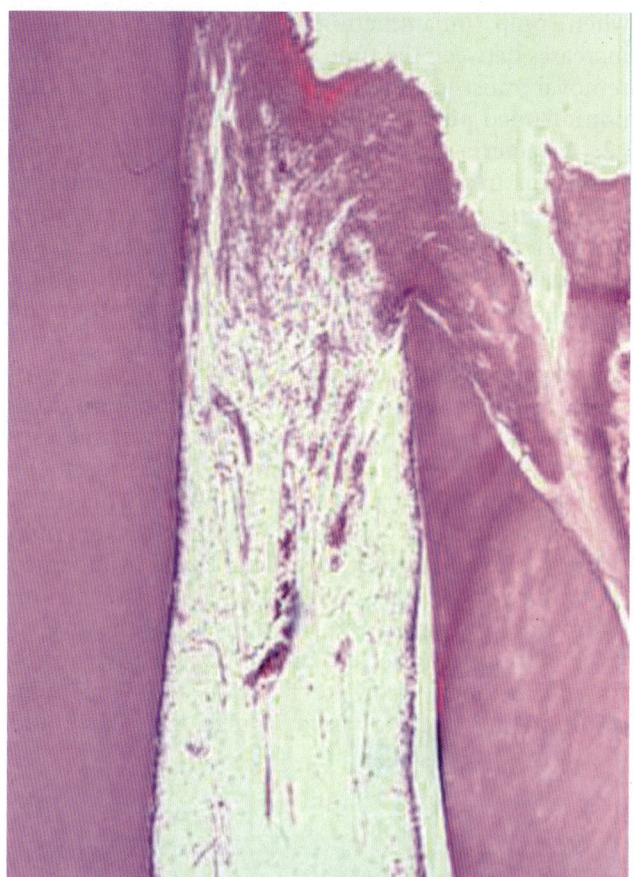

Figure 1 Histologic appearance of the pulp within 24 hours of a traumatic exposure. The pulp proliferates over the exposed dentinal tubules. There is approximately 1.5 mm of inflamed pulp below the surface of the fracture.

hemorrhage and local inflammation. Subsequent inflammatory changes are usually proliferative but can be destructive. A proliferative reaction is favored in traumatic injuries since the fractured surface is usually flat, allowing salivary rinsing with little chance of impaction of contaminated debris. Therefore, unless impaction of contaminated debris is obvious, it is expected that within the first 24 hours after the injury, a proliferative response with inflammation will extend no more than 2 mm into the pulp (Figure 1).[9–11] In time, however, bacterial infection will result in local pulp necrosis and a slow apical spread of pulpal inflammation.

TREATMENT

Treatment options are (1) **vital pulp therapy** comprising pulp capping, partial pulpotomy, and full pulpotomy or (2) **pulpectomy**. The choice of treatment depends on the stage of development of the tooth, time between the accident and treatment, concomitant periodontal injury, and the restorative treatment plan.

STAGE OF DEVELOPMENT OF THE TOOTH

Loss of vitality in an immature tooth can have catastrophic consequences. Root canal treatment on a tooth with a "blunderbuss" canal is time consuming and difficult. Of more importance, however, is the fact that necrosis of an immature tooth leaves it with thin dentinal walls that are susceptible to fracture both during and after an apexification procedure.[12] Therefore, every effort must be made to keep the pulp vital at least until the apex and cervical root have completed development. Pulpectomy in a mature tooth has a high success rate,[13] but vital pulp therapy (rather than removal) on a mature tooth performed under optimal conditions can also be carried out successfully.[14,15] Therefore, vital pulp therapy can be an option under certain circumstances, even though a pulpectomy is the treatment affording the most predictable success. **In an immature tooth, vital pulp therapy should be attempted, if at all feasible, because of the tremendous advantages of maintaining the vital pulp.**

TIME BETWEEN THE ACCIDENT AND TREATMENT

For 48 hours after a traumatic injury, the initial reaction of the pulp is proliferative, with a depth of no more than 2 mm of pulpal inflammation (see Figure 1). After 48 hours, chances of direct bacterial contamination of the pulp increase as the zone of inflammation progresses apically.[16] Thus, with time, the chance of success in maintaining a healthy pulp decreases.

CONCOMITANT ATTACHMENT DAMAGE

A concomitant periodontal injury will compromise the nutritional supply of the pulp. This fact is particularly important in mature teeth, in which the chance of pulp survival is not as good as for immature teeth.[17,18]

RESTORATIVE TREATMENT PLAN

In a mature tooth, pulpectomy is a viable treatment option, unlike an immature tooth, in which the benefits of maintaining vitality of the pulp are great. However, if performed under optimal conditions, vital pulp therapy after traumatic exposures can be successful. Thus, if the restorative treatment plan is simple, and a composite resin restoration will suffice as the permanent restoration, this treatment option should be given serious consideration. If a more complex restoration is to be placed (eg, a crown), pulpectomy would be the more predictable treatment method.

Vital Pulp Therapy for Traumatic Dental Injuries

REQUIREMENTS FOR SUCCESS

Vital pulp therapy in traumatically injured teeth has a very high success rate if the following requirements are adhered to:

1. **Treatment of a healthy pulp** has been shown to be an essential requirement for successful therapy.[19,20] Vital pulp therapy of the inflamed pulp, on the other hand, affords a lower success rate.[19,20] Therefore, the optimal time for treatment is within the first 24 hours, when pulp inflammation is superficial. As time increases between the time of injury and therapy, pulp removal must be extended apically to ensure that noninflamed pulp tissue has been reached.

2. **A bacteria-tight seal** is the most critical factor for successful treatment.[20] Challenge by bacteria during the healing phase will cause failure.[21] On the other hand, if the exposed pulp is effectively sealed from bacterial access, successful healing of the pulp with a hard tissue barrier will occur, independent of the dressing placed on the pulp.[21]

3. **A proper pulp dressing** is important, and, presently, calcium hydroxide is the most common dressing used for vital pulp therapy. Its advantages are that it is antibacterial[22,23] and will disinfect the superficial pulp. Pure calcium hydroxide (pH 12.5) will cause necrosis of about 1.5 mm of the pulp tissue[24,25] involving the superficial layers of inflamed pulp if present (Figure 2). The toxicity of the calcium hydroxide appears to be neutralized as the deeper layers of pulp are affected, causing coagulative necrosis at the junction of the necrotic and vital pulp, resulting in only a mild irritation. This mild

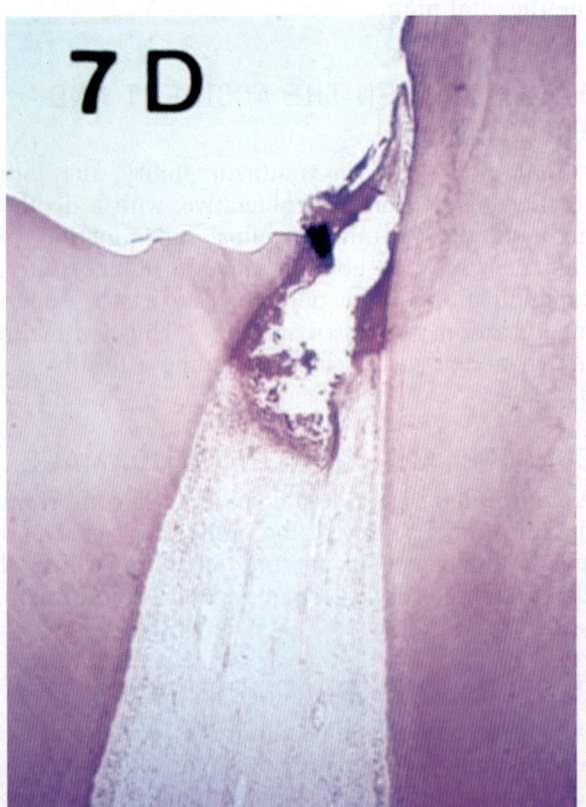 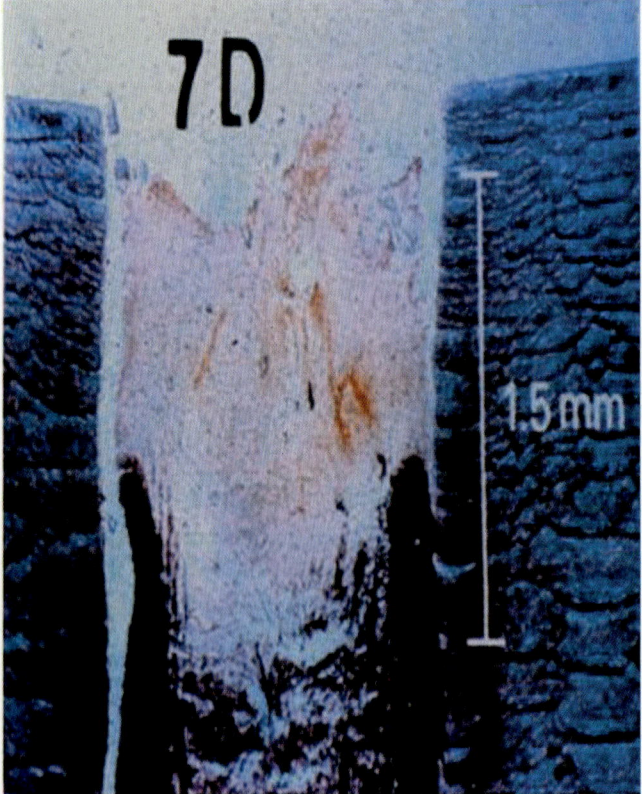

Figure 2 Pulp necrosis (1.5 mm) as a result of the high pH of calcium hydroxide.

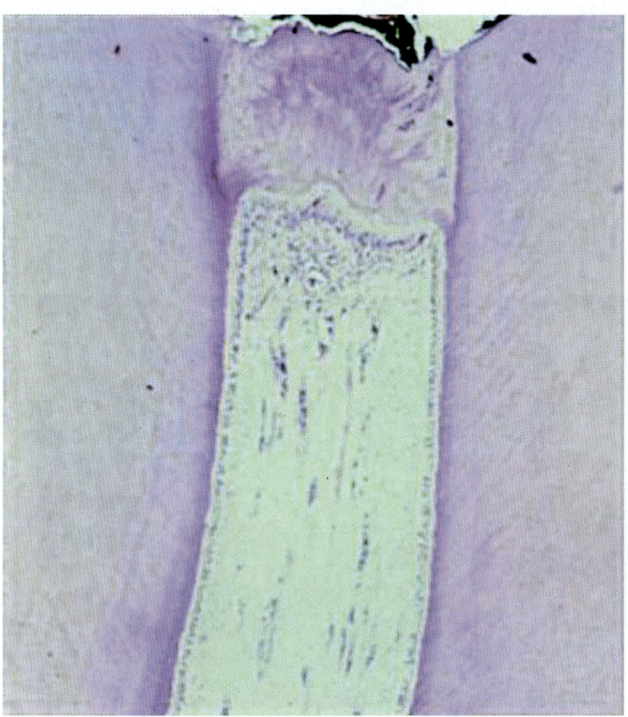

Figure 3 Hard tissue barrier developed after calcium hydroxide partial pulpotomy. Histologic appearance of replacement odontoblasts and a hard tissue barrier.

irritation will initiate an inflammatory response and in the absence of bacteria[24] will heal with a hard tissue barrier (Figure 3).[25,26] Hard-setting calcium hydroxide does not cause necrosis to the superficial layers of pulp but has been shown to initiate healing with a hard tissue barrier as well.[27,28] A major disadvantage of calcium hydroxide is that it does not seal the fractured surface. Therefore, an additional material must be used to ensure that the pulp is not challenged by bacteria, particularly during the critical healing phase.

Other materials, such as zinc oxide–eugenol,[20] tricalcium phosphate,[29] and composite resin,[30] have been proposed as materials for vital pulp therapy. They have not afforded the predictability of calcium hydroxide used in conjunction with a well-sealed coronal restoration.

Mineral trioxide aggregate (MTA) has been reported to show promise as a pulp capping agent.[31] It has a high pH, similar to calcium hydroxide, when unset[32] and after setting will create an excellent bacteria-tight seal.[33] It also sets hard enough to act as a base for a final restoration.[34] MTA has not as yet gained popularity as a pulp capping agent, probably because of its need for a moist environment for 6 hours to set. Thus, what is normally a one-step procedure for other medicaments becomes a two-step procedure with MTA since a wet cotton pellet should be placed over it until it is set, and then later the permanent restoration can be fabricated.

Treatment Methods

PULP CAPPING

Pulp capping implies placing a dressing directly onto the pulp exposure. As indicated by the success rate of this procedure (80%) compared with that of partial pulpotomy (95%),[34] it appears that a superficial pulp cap should not be considered after traumatic pulp exposures. The lower success rate is not difficult to understand since superficial inflammation develops soon after the traumatic exposure. Thus, if the treatment is at the superficial level, a number of inflamed (rather than healthy) pulps will be treated, lowering the potential for success. In addition, a bacteria-tight coronal seal is much more difficult to achieve in superficial pulp capping since there is no cavity depth to create this bacteria-tight seal, as there is with a partial pulpotomy.

PARTIAL PULPOTOMY

Partial pulpotomy implies the removal of coronal pulp tissue to the level of healthy pulp tissue. In traumatic injuries, this level can be accurately determined owing to the knowledge of the reaction of the pulp after a traumatic injury. This procedure is commonly called the "Cvek pulpotomy."

TECHNIQUE

Anesthesia, rubber dam placement, and superficial disinfection are performed. A 1 to 2 mm deep cavity is prepared into the pulp using a sterile diamond bur of appropriate size with copious water coolant

(Figure 4).[35] A slow-speed bur or spoon excavator should be avoided unless cooling of the high-speed bur is not possible. If bleeding is excessive, the pulp is amputated deeper until only moderate hemorrhage is seen. Excess blood is carefully removed by rinsing with sterile saline or anesthetic solution and dried with a sterile cotton pellet. Care must be taken not to allow a blood clot to develop as this will compromise the prognosis.[26,34] If the pulp is of sufficient size to allow 1 to 2 mm of additional pulp necrosis, a thin layer of pure calcium hydroxide is mixed with sterile saline or anesthetic solution and carefully placed. If

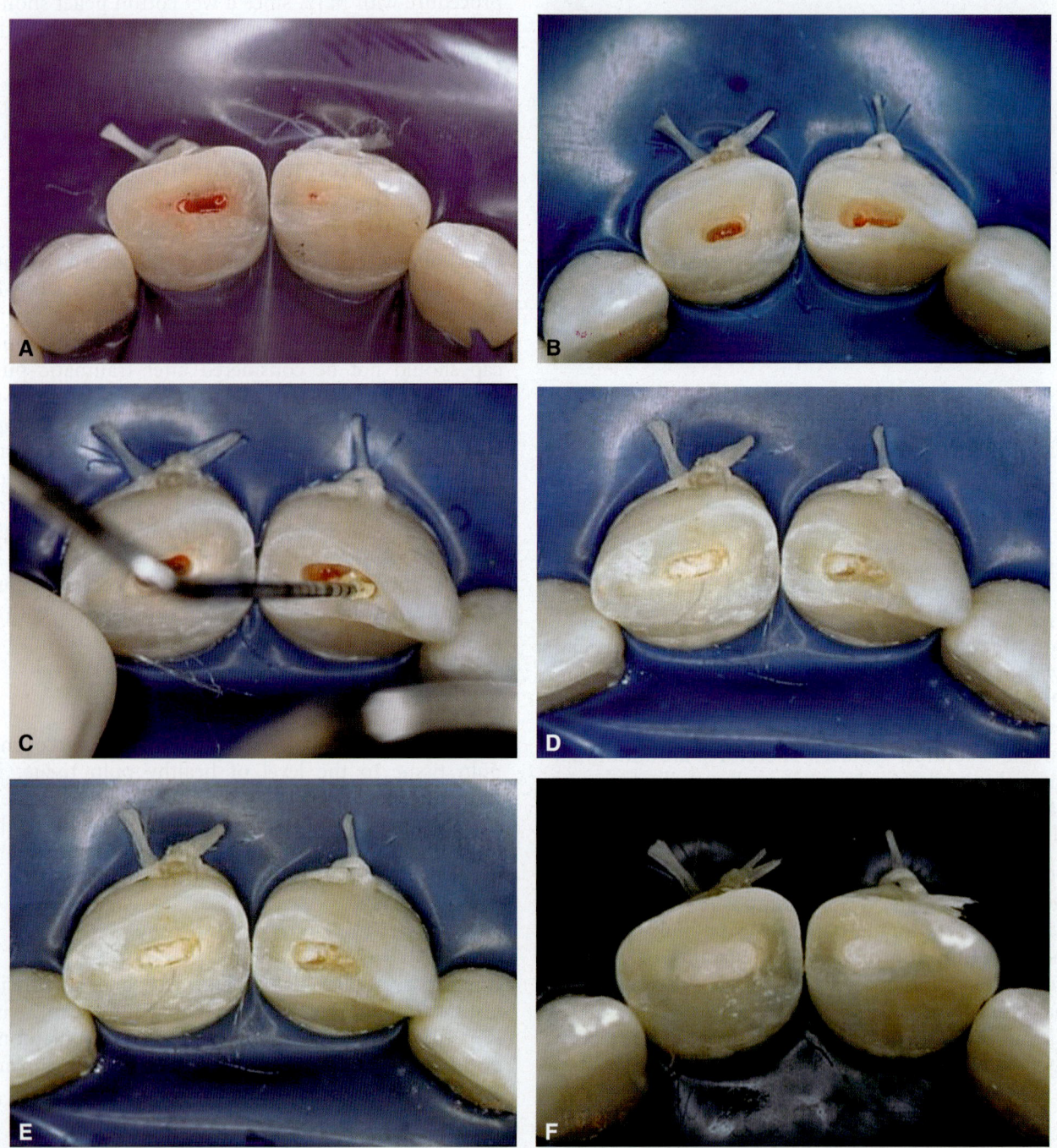

Figure 4 (Continued)

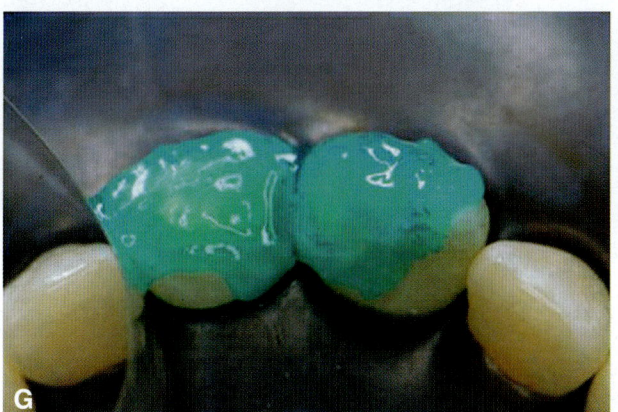
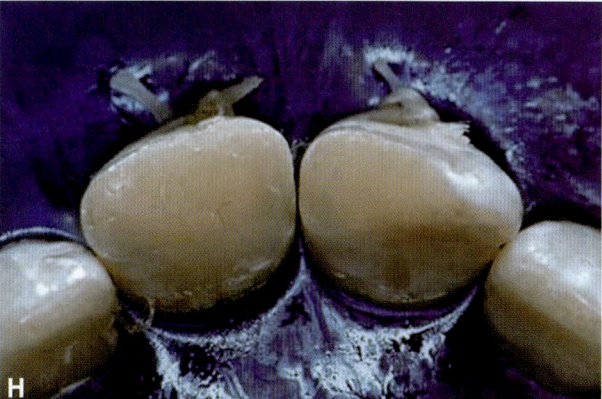
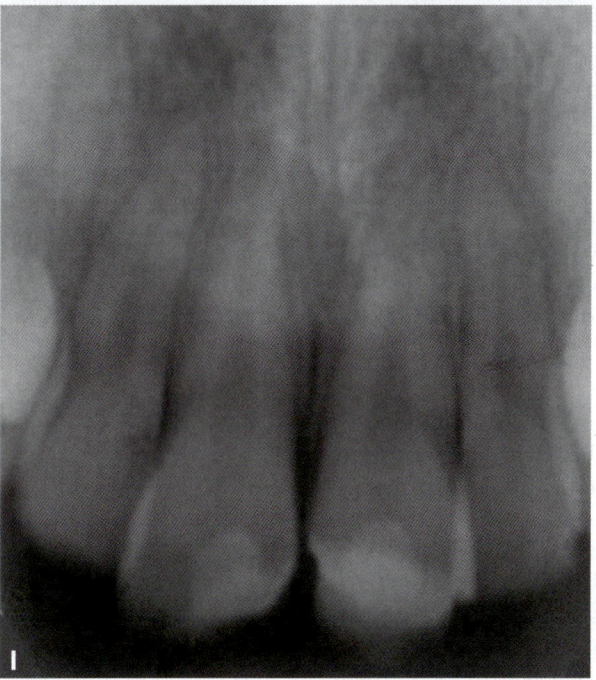

Figure 4 Cvek partial pulpotomy. **A,** The fractured teeth are cleaned and disinfected and a rubber dam is placed. **B,** Cavities are prepared at high speed with a round diamond bur that includes 1 to 2 mm of superficial pulp tissue. **C,** Calcium hydroxide is placed on a plugger and **D,** placed on the soft tissue of the pulp (only). **E,** Calcium hydroxide is removed from the walls of the cavities. **F,** The cavity preparations are filled with glass ionomer cement. **G,** The exposed dentin is etched, and **H,** the dentin is covered with composite resin. **I,** The radiograph taken 6 months later shows the formation of hard tissue barriers in both teeth. Courtesy of Dr. Allessandra Ritter.

the pulp size does not permit additional loss of pulp tissue, a commercial hard-setting calcium hydroxide can be used.[36] The prepared cavity is filled with a material with the best chance of a bacteria-tight seal (zinc oxide–eugenol or glass ionomer cement) to a level flush with the fractured surface. The material in the pulpal cavity, and all exposed dentinal tubules are covered with hard-setting calcium hydroxide. The enamel is then etched and restored with bonded composite resin, as in pulp capping. The use of MTA for pulp capping and pulpotomies is described in Chapter 35, "Vital Pulp Therapy."

Follow-up places the emphasis on maintenance of positive sensitivity tests and radiographic evidence of continued root development. Partial pulpotomy affords many advantages over pulp capping. Superficial inflamed pulp is removed in the preparation of the pulpal cavity. Calcium hydroxide disinfects dentin and pulp and removes additional pulpal inflammatory tissue. Most importantly, space is provided for a material that will provide a bacteria-tight seal to allow pulpal healing with hard tissue development under optimal conditions. Additionally, coronal pulp tissue remains that allows sensitivity testing to be carried out at the follow-up visits. The prognosis is excellent (94–96%).[34,37]

FULL PULPOTOMY

This procedure involves removal of the entire coronal pulp to the level of root orifices. This level of pulp amputation is chosen arbitrarily because of its anatomic convenience. Therefore, since the inflamed pulp sometimes extends past the canal orifices into the root pulp, many "mistakes" are made, resulting in treatment of an inflamed rather than a noninflamed pulp. This procedure is indicated when it is predicted that the pulp is inflamed to deeper levels of the coronal pulp. Traumatic exposures after 72 hours and a carious exposure are two examples in which this type of treatment may be indicated. Because of the fairly good chance that the dressing will be placed on an inflamed pulp, full pulpotomy is contraindicated in mature teeth. However, the benefits outweigh the risks for this treatment in immature teeth with incompletely formed apices and thin dentinal walls.

TECHNIQUE

Anesthesia, rubber dam placement, and superficial disinfection are done as described with pulp capping and partial pulpotomy. The coronal pulp is removed to the level of the root orifices. Calcium hydroxide dressing, a bacteria-tight seal, and coronal restoration are a part of the technique as described with partial pulpotomy. The follow-up is done as described with pulp capping and partial pulpotomy. A major disadvantage of this treatment method is that sensitivity testing is not possible owing to the loss of coronal pulp. Therefore, radiographic follow-up is extremely important to monitor for continuation of root formation and signs of apical periodontitis.

Since the cervical pulpotomy is performed on pulps that are expected to have deep inflammation, and the site of pulp amputation is arbitrary, more "mistakes" are made, leading to treatment of the inflamed pulp. Consequently, prognosis in the range of 75% is poorer than partial pulpotomy.[38] Because of the inability to evaluate pulp status after a full pulpotomy, some authors have recommended routine pulpectomy after the roots have fully formed (Figure 5). This philosophy is based on the fact that the pulpectomy procedure has a success rate in the range of 95%, whereas if apical periodontitis develops following pulpotomy, the prognosis of root canal treatment drops significantly to about 80%.[13,39]

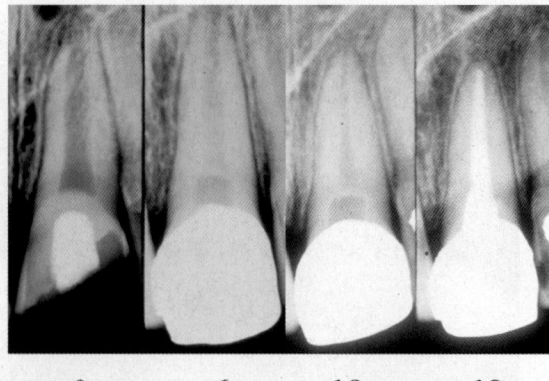

Time: 0   6m   18m   18m

Figure 5 Successful pulpotomy followed by a pulpectomy at 18 months. Courtesy of Dr. Leif Tronstad.

PULPECTOMY

Pulpectomy implies removal of the entire pulp to the level of the apical foramen. The indications are for complicated crown fracture of mature teeth (if conditions are not ideal for vital pulp therapy). This procedure is not different from root canal treatment of a vital, nontraumatized tooth.

Treatment of Nonvital Pulps

IMMATURE TOOTH: APEXIFICATION

Apexification is indicated for teeth with open apices and thin dentinal walls in which standard instrumentation techniques cannot create an apical stop to facilitate effective root canal filling.

BIOLOGIC CONSEQUENCES

A nonvital immature tooth presents a number of difficulties for adequate endodontic therapy. The canal is (often) wider apically than coronally, necessitating the use of a filling material that conforms to the shape of the apical part of the canal. Since the apex is extremely wide, no barrier exists to stop this material from moving into and traumatizing the apical periodontal tissues. Also, the lack of an apical stop and extrusion of material might result in a canal that is susceptible to leakage. An additional problem in immature teeth with thin dentinal walls is their susceptibility to fracture both during and after treatment. These problems are overcome by stimulating the formation of a hard tissue barrier to allow for optimal filling of the canal and reinforcing the weakened root against fracture both during and after apexification.[12,40]

TECHNIQUE

Since in the vast majority of nonvital teeth are infected,[41,42] the first phase of treatment is to disinfect the root canal system to ensure periapical healing.[16,22] The canal length is estimated with a parallel preoperative radiograph and confirmed radiographically with the first endodontic instrument. Preparation of the canal (owing to the thin dentinal walls) is performed **very lightly** and with **copious** irrigation using 0.5% sodium hypochlorite.[43,44] A lower strength and increased volume of NaOCl are used because of the increased danger of extruding sodium hypochlorite through the open apex in immature teeth. An irrigation needle that can passively reach close to the apical level is used in disinfecting the canals. The canal is dried with paper points, and a creamy mix of calcium hydroxide is spun into the canal with a lentulo-spiral. The calcium hydroxide is left in the canal for at least 1 week to be effective in accomplishing disinfection.[23] The continuation of treatment can take place any time after 1 week. Further treatment should not be delayed more than 1 month since the calcium hydroxide could be washed out by tissue fluids through the open apex, leaving the canal susceptible to reinfection.

Hard Tissue Apical Barrier

TRADITIONAL METHOD

The formation of a hard tissue barrier at the apex requires an environment similar to that required for hard tissue formation in vital pulp therapy, that is, a mild inflammatory stimulus, to initiate healing and a bacteria-free environment to ensure that inflammation is not progressive. As with vital pulp therapy, calcium hydroxide is used for this procedure.[45–47] Pure calcium hydroxide powder is mixed with sterile saline (or anesthetic solution) to a thick (powdery) consistency. Ready-mixed commercial calcium hydroxide can also be used. The calcium hydroxide is packed against the apical soft tissue with a plugger or thick point to initiate hard tissue formation. This step is followed by backfilling with calcium hydroxide to completely fill the canal, thus ensuring a bacteria-free canal with little chance of re-infection during the 6 to 18 months required for hard tissue formation at the apex. The calcium hydroxide is meticulously removed from the access cavity to the level of the root orifices, and a well-sealing temporary filling is placed in the access cavity. A radiograph is taken, and the canal should appear to have become calcified, indicating that the entire canal has been filled with the calcium hydroxide. Because calcium hydroxide washout is evaluated by its relative radiodensity in the canal, it is prudent to use a calcium hydroxide mixture without the addition of a specific material to enhance the radiopaque property of the medicament such as barium sulfate. These additives do not wash out as readily as calcium hydroxide, so if they are present in the canal, evaluation of washout is not possible.

At 3-month intervals, a radiograph is taken to evaluate whether a hard tissue barrier has formed and if the calcium hydroxide has washed out of the canal. This is assessed to have occurred if the canal can again be seen radiographically. If calcium hydroxide washout is seen, it is replaced as before. If no washout is evident, it can be left intact for another 3 months. Excessive calcium hydroxide dressing changes should be avoided if at all possible since the initial toxicity of the material is thought to delay healing.[48]

When completion of a hard tissue barrier is suspected, the calcium hydroxide should be washed out of the canal with sodium hypochlorite and a radiograph taken to evaluate the radiodensity of the apical stop. A file that can easily reach the apex can be used to gently probe for a stop at the apex. When a hard tissue barrier is indicated radiographically and can be probed with an instrument, the canal is ready for filling (Figure 6).

MTA BARRIER

The creation of a physiologic hard tissue barrier using calcium hydroxide, although quite predictable, takes anywhere from 3 to 18 months. The disadvantage of this long time period is that the patient is

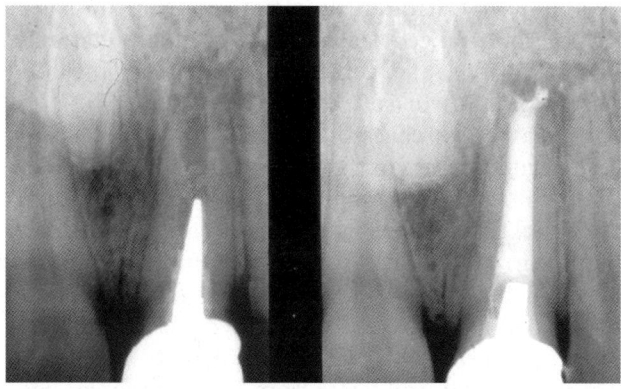

Figure 6 Successful apexification. The patient presented with an acute abscess. The canal was disinfected, and the wide apical lumen was closed with a long-term calcium hydroxide application. When a barrier was felt, the canal was filled with a permanent root filling.

required to present for treatment multiple times; also, the tooth may fracture during treatment, before the thin weak roots can be strengthened. In addition, one study has indicated that long-term treatment with calcium hydroxide may weaken the dentin of the roots and make them even more susceptible to fracture.[49]

MTA has been used to create a hard tissue barrier quickly after the disinfection of the canal. Calcium sulfate can be pushed through the apex to provide a resorbable extraradicular barrier against which to pack the MTA. The MTA is mixed and placed into the apical 3 to 4 mm of the canal in a manner similar to the placement of calcium hydroxide. A wet cotton pellet is placed against the MTA and left for at least 6 hours, and then the entire canal is filled with a root filling material. The filling can also be placed immediately since the tissue fluids of the open apex will probably provide enough moisture to ensure that the MTA will set sufficiently. The cervical canal is then reinforced with composite resin to below the marginal bone level as described below.

A number of case reports have been published using this MTA apical barrier technique,[50,51] and it has steadily gained popularity with clinicians. Presently, no prospective long-term outcome study is available comparing its success rate with the traditional calcium hydroxide technique.

FILLING OF THE ROOT CANAL

Since the apical diameter is larger than the coronal diameter in most of these canals, a softened filling technique is indicated. Care must be taken to avoid excessive lateral force during filling owing to the thin root walls. If the hard tissue barrier was "produced" by long-term calcium hydroxide therapy, it consists of irregularly arranged layers of coagulated soft tissue, calcified tissue, and cementum-like tissue. Included also are islands of soft connective tissue, giving the barrier a "Swiss cheese" consistency.[52,53] Because of the irregular nature of the barrier, it is not unusual for cement or softened filling material to be extruded into the apical tissues (see Figure 6). Formation of the hard tissue barrier may also be some distance short of the radiographic apex. This is because it forms wherever the calcium hydroxide comes in contact with vital tissue. In teeth with wide open apices, vital tissue can survive and proliferate from the periodontal ligament a few millimeters into the root canal. The root canal filling should be completed to the level of the hard tissue barrier and not forced toward the radiographic apex.

REINFORCEMENT OF THE THIN DENTINAL WALLS

The apexification procedure has become a predictably successful procedure. However, the thin dentinal walls present a clinical problem. Should secondary injuries occur, teeth with thin dentinal walls are more susceptible to fractures, rendering them nonrestorable.[54,55] It has been reported that approximately 30% of these teeth will fracture during or after endodontic treatment.[56] Consequently, some clinicians have questioned the advisability of the apexification procedure and have opted for more radical treatment procedures, including extraction followed by extensive restorative procedures such as dental implants. Recent studies have shown that intracoronal bonded restorations can internally strengthen endodontically treated teeth and increase their resistance to fracture.[12,57] Thus, after root filling, the material should be removed to below the marginal bone level and a bonded resin filling placed.

Routine follow-up evaluation should be performed to monitor the outcome. Restorative procedures should be assessed to ensure that they do not promote root fractures. Periapical healing and the formation of a hard tissue barrier occur predictably with long-term calcium hydroxide treatment (79–96%).[47,56] However, long-term survival is jeopardized by the fracture potential of the thin dentinal walls. It is expected that internal strengthening of teeth as described above will increase their long-term survivability.

Pulp Revascularization

Regeneration of a necrotic pulp has been considered possible only after avulsion of an immature permanent tooth. The advantages of pulp revascularization are the possibility of further root development, reinforcement of dentinal walls by deposition of hard tissue, and thus strengthening the root against fracture. After replantation of an avulsed immature tooth, a unique set of circumstances exists that allows regeneration to take place. The young tooth has an open apex and is short, which allows new tissue to grow into the pulp space relatively quickly. The pulp is necrotic but usually not degenerated and infected, so it will act as a matrix into which the new tissue can grow. It has been experimentally shown that the apical part of a pulp may remain vital and after replantation proliferate coronally, replacing the necrotized portion of the pulp.[58–60] In addition, the fact that, in most cases, the crown of the tooth is intact and caries free ensures that bacterial penetration into the pulp space through cracks[61] and defects will be a slow process. Thus, the race between the new tissue and infection of the pulp space favors the new tissue.

Regeneration of pulp tissue in a necrotic infected tooth with apical periodontitis has been thought until now to be impossible. However, if it were possible to create a similar environment as described above for the avulsed tooth, regeneration should occur. Thus, if the canal is effectively disinfected, a matrix into which new tissue could grow is provided, and the coronal access is effectively sealed, regeneration should occur as in an avulsed immature tooth. A report by Banchs and Trope reproduced results in cases reported by others that indicate that it may be possible to replicate the unique circumstances of an avulsed tooth so as to revascularize the pulp in infected necrotic immature roots[62] (Figure 7). The case presented describes the treatment of a maxillary central incisor with radiographic and clinical signs of apical periodontitis after a failed partial pulpotomy. The canal was disinfected without mechanical instrumentation but with copious irrigation with 5.25% sodium hypochlorite and the use of a mixture of antibiotics.[62] A blood clot was produced to the level of the cementoenamel junction to provide a matrix for the ingrowth of new tissue, followed by a deep coronal restoration to provide a bacteria-tight seal. Clinical and radiographic evidence of healing was seen after 6 months; the large radiolucency had disappeared, and at the 12-month follow-up, it was obvious that the root walls were thickening. Recent studies have confirmed the potent antibacterial properties of the triantibiotic paste used in this case,[63,64] and studies are under way to find a synthetic matrix that will act as a more predictable scaffold for new ingrowth of tissue than the blood clot used in these previous cases. The procedure described in this section can be attempted in most cases, and if after 3 months no signs of regeneration are present, the more traditional treatment methods should be initiated.

MATURE TEETH

Traumatized mature teeth are routinely treated endodontically in the same manner as non-traumatized teeth.

Crown-Root Fractures

These fractures are first treated periodontally to ensure that a good margin for restoration is possible. If the tooth can be maintained from a periodontal point of view, the pulp is treated as a crown fracture.

Horizontal Root Fractures

This injury implies fracture of the cementum, dentin, and pulp. They are relatively infrequent injuries, occurring in less than 3% of all dental injuries.[65] Incompletely formed roots with vital pulps rarely fracture horizontally.[66] When a root fractures horizontally, the coronal segment is displaced to a varying degree, but, generally, the apical segment is not displaced. Because the apical pulpal circulation is not disrupted, pulp necrosis in the apical segment is extremely rare. Pulp necrosis develops in the coronal segment owing to its displacement but occurs in only about 25% of cases.[67] The clinical presentation is similar to that of luxation injuries. The extent of displacement of the coronal segment is usually indicative of the location of the fracture and can vary from none, simulating a concussion injury (apical fracture), to severe, simulating extrusive luxation (cervical fracture). Radiographic examination for root fractures is extremely important. Since root fractures are usually oblique (facial to palatal), one periapical radiograph can easily miss its presence. It is imperative to take at least three angled radiographs (45, 90, and 110 degrees) so that at least at one angulation the x-ray beam will pass directly through the fracture line to make it visible on the radiograph (Figure 8).

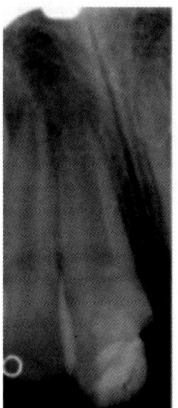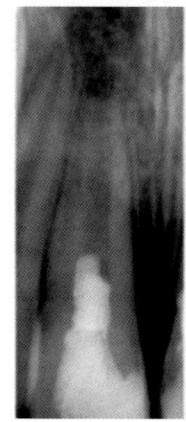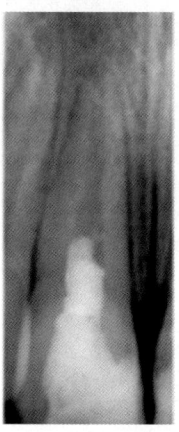

Figure 7 A, Immature tooth with a necrotic infected canal with apical periodontitis. The canal is disinfected with copious irrigation with sodium hypochlorite and triantibiotic paste. After 4 weeks, the antibiotic is removed and a blood clot is created in the canal space. The access is filled with a mineral trioxide aggregate (MTA) base and bonded resin above it. **B,** At 7 months, the patient is asymptomatic and the apex shows some signs of healing of the apical periodontitis and closure of the apex. **C,** At 12 months, apical healing is obvious and root wall thickening has occurred, indicating that the root canal has been revascularized with vital tissue. Courtesy of Dr. Blayne Thibodeau.

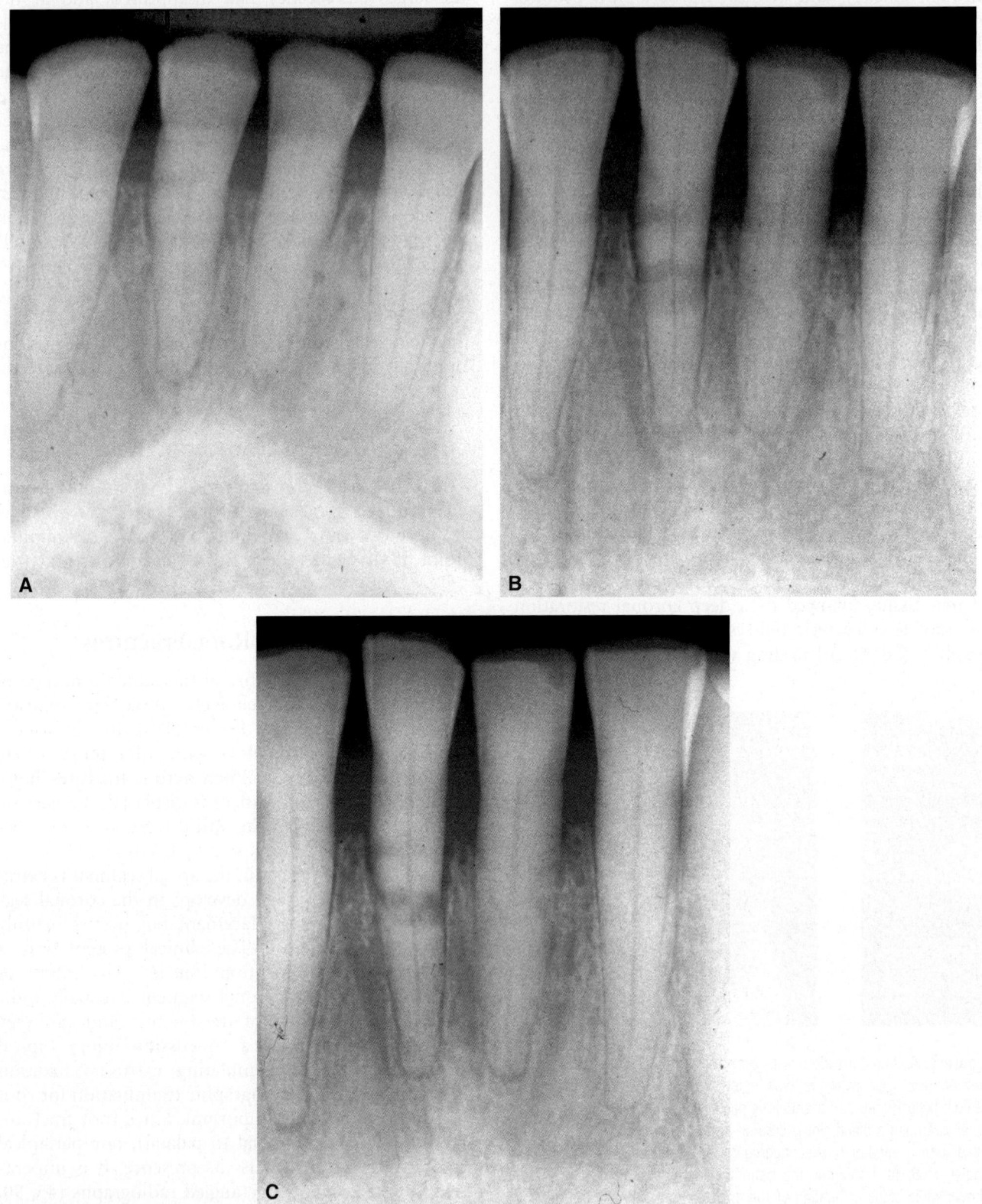

Figure 8 Radiographs showing the importance of an angled x-ray beam for diagnosis of root fracture. Three different vertical angled radiographs produce different radiographic images.

TREATMENT

Emergency treatment involves repositioning of the segments in as close proximity as possible and splinting to adjacent teeth for 2 to 4 weeks with a functional splint.[68] This splinting protocol has recently changed from the 2 to 4 months of rigid splinting that had been recommended for many years.[69] If a long time has elapsed between the injury and treatment, it will likely not be possible to reposition the segments close to their original position, compromising the long-term prognosis of the tooth.

Treatment of Root Fracture Complications

CORONAL ROOT FRACTURES

Historically, it had been thought that fractures in the cervical segment had a poor prognosis, and extraction of the coronal segment was recommended. Research does not support such treatment, and, in fact, if the coronal segment is below the attachment level and adequately splinted, the chances of healing do not differ from those of midroot or apical fractures.[67]

MIDROOT AND APICAL ROOT FRACTURES

Pulp necrosis occurs in 25% of root fractures.[67,70] In the vast majority of cases, the necrosis occurs in the coronal segment only with the apical segment remaining vital. Therefore, endodontic treatment is indicated in the coronal root segment only unless a periapical lesion is seen in the apical segment. In most cases, the canal lumen is wide at the apical extent of the coronal segment, so long-term calcium hydroxide treatment or an MTA apical plug is indicated. The coronal segment is root-filled after a hard tissue barrier has formed apically in the coronal segment and periapical healing has taken place (Figure 9). If MTA is used, the root filling will be placed before healing is seen, making follow-up visits essential in these cases.

In rare cases, when both the coronal and apical pulp areas are necrotic, treatment is more complicated. Endodontic treatment through the fracture is extremely difficult and should be avoided. Endodontic manipulations, medicaments, and filling materials all have a detrimental effect on healing of the fracture site. In more apical root fractures, necrotic apical segments can be surgically removed. This is a viable treatment if the remaining root is long enough to provide adequate periodontal support. Removal of the apical segment in midroot fractures leaves the coronal segment with a compromised attachment, and the crown to root ratio must be assessed before the decision to maintain the tooth is made.

After the splinting period is completed, follow-up is conducted at the same intervals as all dental traumatic injuries: at 3, 6, and 12 months and yearly thereafter.

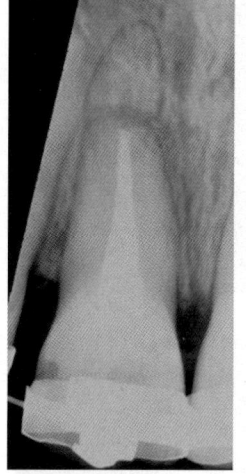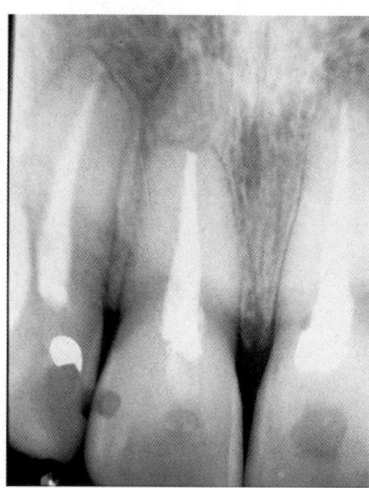

Figure 9 The coronal segment (only) is root-filled after a hard tissue barrier has formed at the most apical part of the coronal segment.

FACTORS INFLUENCING REPAIR

1. The degree of dislocation and mobility of the coronal fragment are extremely important in determining outcome.[71–73] Increased dislocation and coronal fragment mobility result in a decreased prognosis.
2. Immature teeth are seldom involved in root fractures, but when they are, the prognosis is good.[72,74]
3. Quality of treatment: prognosis increases with early treatment, close reduction of the root segments, and semi-rigid splinting for 2 to 4 weeks.[68]

Complications are as follows: (1) pulp necrosis that can be treated successfully[67,70] by treating the coronal segment with adequate disinfection and long-term calcium hydroxide or MTA and filling when a hard tissue barrier has formed; (2) root canal obliteration

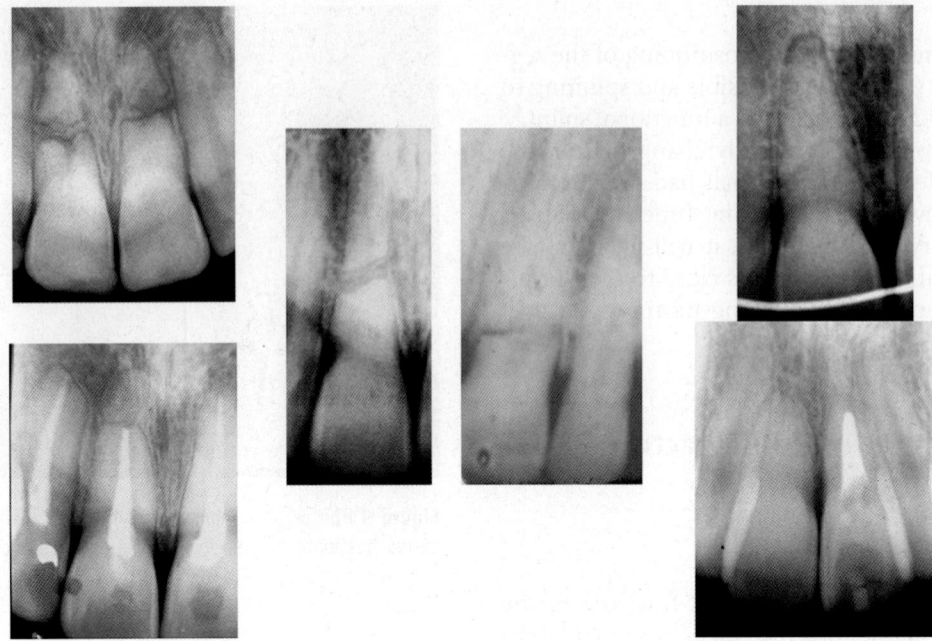

Figure 10 Examples of root canal obliteration in root-fractured teeth. It is common for the segments that maintain vitality to obliterate.

is not uncommon if the root segment (coronal or apical) remains vital (Figure 10).

ENDODONTIC ESSENTIALS

If the coronal segment is reduced quickly and a functional splint is placed for 2 to 4 weeks, pulp necrosis is remarkably low. It will occur only 25% of the time, and in the vast majority of cases, the necrosis will occur only in the coronal segment. Root canal obliteration of both segments is very common. When necrosis does occur, disinfection of the coronal segment only should be initiated, followed by initiation of a physiologic barrier with long-term calcium hydroxide or a physical barrier with MTA. Root canal obliteration is usually not treated endodontically.

Luxation Injuries

DEFINITIONS

1. **Concussion** implies no displacement, normal mobility, sensitivity to percussion.
2. **Subluxation** implies sensitivity to percussion, increased mobility, no displacement.
3. **Lateral luxation** implies displacement labially, lingually, distally, or incisally.
4. **Extrusive** luxation implies displacement in a coronal direction.
5. **Intrusive** luxation implies displacement apically into the alveolus.

Definitions 1 through 5 describe injuries of increasing magnitude in terms of the intensity of the injury and subsequent sequelae.

Luxation injuries result in damage to the attachment apparatus (periodontal ligament and cemental layer), the severity of which is dependent on the type of injury sustained (concussion least, intrusion most). The apical neurovascular supply to the pulp is also affected to varying degrees, resulting in altered or total loss of pulp vitality in the tooth. If the luxation injury is mild, the inflammatory response to the external root surface will be small and the pulp will maintain vitality. Inflammation owing to the trauma will thus be self-limiting, and cemental (favorable) healing will result.

If, on the other hand, the luxation injury is severe, the damage to the external root surface may be so diffuse that healing with new cementum alone may not be possible. If bone attaches directly to the root (ankylosis), the root will eventually be replaced by bone through physiologic resorption and apposition of the bone (osseous replacement). In addition and of special interest to the endodontist, with a severe luxation injury, the neurovasculature tissues of the pulp may be severed, resulting in a necrotic pulp. If this necrotic pulp becomes infected, the microbial toxins will pass through the tubules and the damaged cemental covering of the root, resulting in potentially catastrophic periradicular inflammation with bone and root resorption.

There are two types of trauma-related resorption in which the pulp plays an essential role:

1. In **external** inflammatory root resorption, the **necrotic, infected pulp** provides the stimulus for periodontal inflammation. If the cementum has been damaged and the intermediate cementum penetrated, as when the tooth undergoes a severe traumatic injury, the inflammatory stimulators in the pulp space are able to diffuse through the dentinal tubules and stimulate an inflammatory response over large areas of the periodontal ligament. Owing to the lack of cemental protection, periodontal inflammation will include root resorption and the expected bone resorption.
2. In **internal** inflammatory root resorption, the inflamed pulp is the tissue involved in resorbing the root structure. The pathogenesis of internal root resorption is not completely understood. It is believed that coronal necrotic infected pulp provides a stimulus for pulpal inflammation in the more apical parts of the pulp. If in "rare" cases, the inflamed pulp is adjacent to a root surface that has lost its predentin protection, internal root resorption will result. Thus, both the necrotic infected pulp and the inflamed pulp contribute to this type of root resorption.

Consequences of Apical Neurovascular Damage

PULP CANAL OBLITERATION
Pulp canal obliteration is common after luxation injuries, if not severe enough to sever the neurovascular supply apically. The frequency of pulp canal obliteration appears inversely proportional to that of pulp necrosis. The exact mechanism of pulp canal obliteration is not known. It is theorized that the sympathetic or parasympathetic control of blood flow to odontoblasts is altered, resulting in uncontrolled reparative dentin formation.[66,75] Another theory is that hemorrhage and blood clot formation in the pulp after injury are a nidus for subsequent calcification if the pulp remains vital.[66,75] Pulp canal obliteration can usually be diagnosed within the first year after injury[76] and was found to be more frequent in teeth with open apices (>0.7 mm radiographically), in teeth with extrusive and lateral luxation injuries, and in teeth that have been rigidly splinted.[76]

PULP NECROSIS
The factors most important for the development of pulp necrosis are the type of injury (concussion least, intrusion most) and the stage of root development (mature apex > immature apex).[77] Pulp necrosis can lead to infection of the root canal system, with external inflammatory root resorption as the consequence. To develop pulp space infection, the pulp must first become necrotic. In trauma, necrosis is usually due to displacement of the tooth, resulting in severing of the apical blood vessels. In mature teeth, pulp regeneration cannot occur, and usually by 3 weeks, the necrotic pulp will become infected. For details of the typical bacterial contents of a traumatized necrotic pulp, see Chapter 7, "Microbiology of Endodontic Disease." Because serious injury is required for pulp necrosis, it is usual that areas of cemental covering of the root are also affected, resulting in the loss of its protective (insulating) quality. Now microbial toxins can pass through the dentinal tubules and stimulate an inflammatory response in the corresponding periodontal ligament. The result is resorption of the root and bone. The periodontal infiltrate consists of granulation tissue with lymphocytes, plasma cells, and polymorphonuclear leukocytes. Multinucleated giant cells resorb the denuded root surface, and this continues until the stimulus (pulp space bacteria) is removed (Figure 11).[78] Radiographically, the resorption is

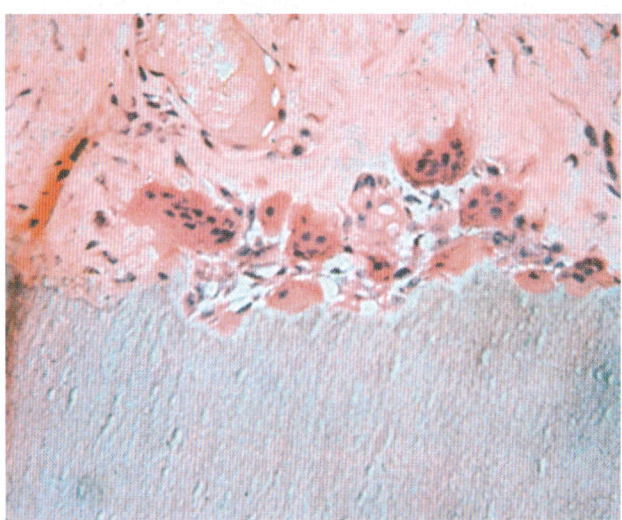

Figure 11 Histologic appearance of multinucleated osteoclasts (dentinoclasts) resorbing the dentin of the root.

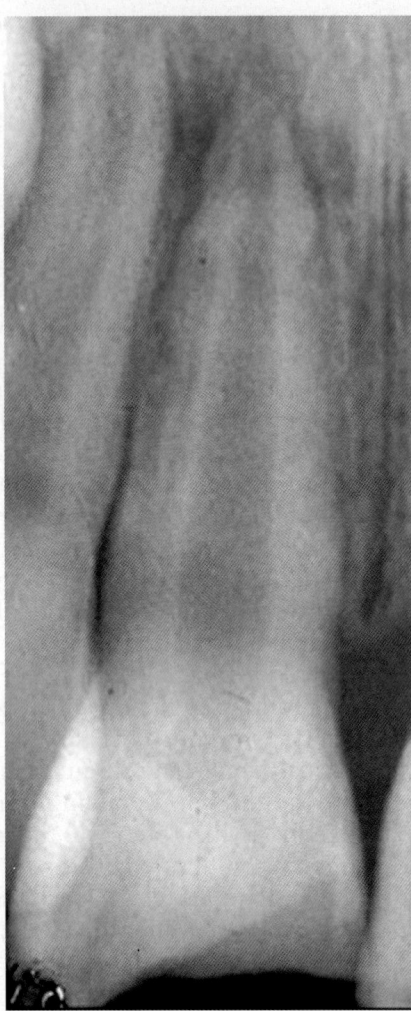

Figure 12 Inflammatory root resorption owing to pulp space infection. Note the radiolucencies in the root **and** surrounding bone. Courtesy of Dr. Fred Barnett.

observed as progressive radiolucent areas of the root and adjacent bone (Figure 12).

TREATMENT

The attachment damage owing to the traumatic injury is often the focus of an emergency visit that, unfortunately, rarely involves the endodontist. The clinician's attention to pulp space infection should ideally be within 7 to 10 days after the injury.[79,80] Root canal therapy either removes the necrotic pulp as a nidus for microbes or removes the stimulus (microbes already present) to the periapical inflammation. Without microbial stimulation, resorption will not occur or will heal.[33–35] In most cases, a new cemental attachment will form, but if a large area of root is affected, osseous replacement (ankylosis) can result by the mechanism already described. Treatment principles include prevention of pulp space infection or elimination of the bacteria if they are present in the pulp space.

1. **Prevention of pulp space infection**
   a) **Reestablish the vitality of the pulp.** If the pulp stays vital, the canal will be free of bacteria, and external inflammatory root resorption will not occur. In severe injuries in which vitality has been lost, it is possible under some circumstances to promote revascularization of the pulp. Revascularization is possible in young teeth with incompletely formed apices if the teeth are replaced in their original position within 60 minutes of the injury.[81,82] However, even under the best conditions, revascularization will fail to occur on many occasions. Thus, a diagnostic dilemma results. If the pulp revascularizes, external root resorption will not occur and the root will continue to develop and strengthen. However, if the pulp becomes necrotic and infected, the subsequent external inflammatory root resorption that develops could result in the loss of the tooth in a very short time. At present, the diagnostic tools available cannot detect a vital pulp in this situation before approximately 6 months after successful revascularization. This period of time is obviously unacceptable since by that time, the teeth not revascularized could be lost to the resorption process. Recently, the laser Doppler flowmeter has been shown to be an excellent diagnostic tool for the detection of revascularization in immature teeth (see Chapter 14C, "Laser Doppler Flowmetry"). These devices appear to accurately detect the presence of vital tissue in the pulp space by 4 weeks after the traumatic injury.[83]
   b) **Prevent root canal infection by root canal treatment at 7 to 10 days.** In teeth with closed apices, revascularization cannot occur. These teeth should be endodontically treated within 7 to 10 days of the injury before the ischemically necrosed pulp becomes infected.[79,80] This is also a convenient time because this is the time period in which the functional splint is removed and chemotherapeutic medicaments to limit the initial inflammatory response are stopped.[79] From a theoretical point of view, the teeth treated at this time can be considered equivalent to the treatment of a tooth with a vital pulp. Therefore, the endodontic treatment could be completed in one visit. However, efficient

treatment is extremely difficult so soon after a serious traumatic injury, and it is beneficial to start the endodontic treatment with pulpectomy and canal preparation followed by an intracanal dressing with a creamy mix of calcium hydroxide.[79,80] The practitioner can now fill the canal at his or her convenience, after periodontal healing of the injury is complete, approximately 1 month after the instrumentation visit. There appears to be no necessity for long-term calcium hydroxide treatment in cases in which the endodontic treatment is started within 10 days of the injury. Notwithstanding, in a compliant patient, the calcium hydroxide can be applied for a long term (up to 6 months) to ensure periodontal health prior to final root canal filling.[80]

2. **Elimination of pulp space infection**
When root canal treatment is initiated later than 10 days after the accident, or if active external inflammatory resorption is observed, the preferred antibacterial protocol consists of microbial control followed by a long-term dressing with densely packed calcium hydroxide.[80] Calcium hydroxide can affect an alkaline pH in the surrounding dentinal tubules, kill bacteria, and neutralize endotoxin, a potent inflammatory stimulator.

The first visit consists of the microbial control phase with instrumentation of the canal and placement with a lentulo-spiral of a creamy mix of calcium hydroxide as an intracanal antibacterial agent. The patient is seen in approximately 1 month, at which time, the canal is filled with a dense mix of calcium hydroxide. Once filled, the canal should appear radiographically to be calcified since the radiodensity of calcium hydroxide in the canal is usually similar to that of the surrounding dentin (Figure 13). A radiograph is then taken at 3-month intervals. At each visit, the tooth is tested for symptoms of periodontitis. In addition, healing of the resorptive process and the presence or absence of the calcium hydroxide (ie, calcium hydroxide washout) are assessed. Since the root surface is so radiodense as to make the assessment of healing difficult, the adjacent bone healing is assessed. If the adjacent bone has healed, it is assumed that the resorptive process has stopped in the root as well, and the canal can be permanently root-filled (Figure 14). If it is felt that additional healing would be beneficial before root filling, the need for replacing the calcium hydroxide in the canal is assessed. If the canal

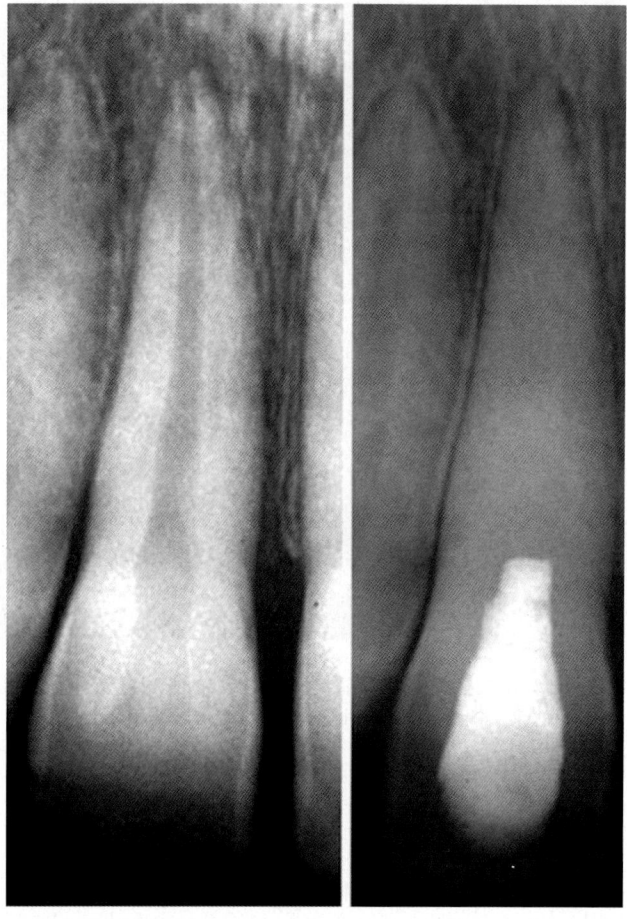

Figure 13 Root canal that "disappears" after placement of a thick mix of pure calcium hydroxide. Courtesy of Dr. Fred Barnett.

still appears calcified radiographically, there is no need to replace the calcium hydroxide. If, on the other hand, the canal has regained its lucent appearance, the calcium hydroxide should be repacked and reassessed in another 3 months.

Treatment of Established External Root Resorption in a Young Patient

Arresting external inflammatory root resorption owing to pulp space infection is achieved by disinfecting the pulp space. This is particularly difficult after a luxation injury since the cemental covering is also damaged. This results in the microbes and their by-products moving deep into the dentinal tubules to stimulate and maintain the inflammation in the surrounding periapical tissues.

Recently, a triantibiotic paste introduced by Hoshino et al.[84] has been used in the revascularization

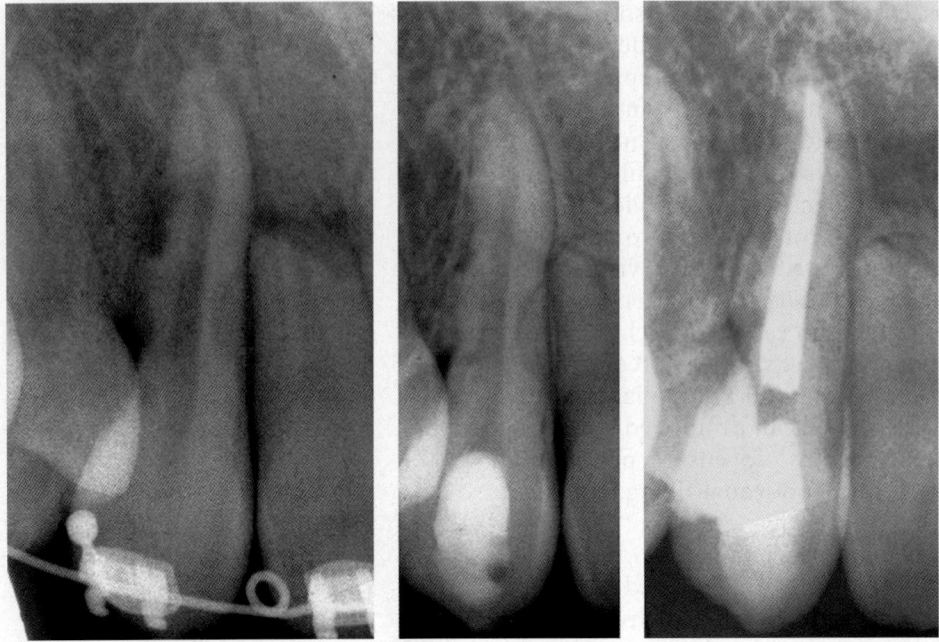

Figure 14 The root canal is filled when the adjacent bone has healed, indicating that root resorption has stopped. **Left,** Active root resorption with lucencies in the root and bone. **Middle,** After long-term calcium hydroxide treatment, the adjacent bone has healed. **Right,** The canal is now filled.

process of necrotic teeth with open apices and apical periodontitis.[85] The antibiotic paste comprising metronidazole, ciprofloxacin, and minocycline has been shown to have an excellent antimicrobial spectrum for pulp space microbes and an excellent ability to penetrate the dentinal tubules. Since many cases of external inflammatory resorption owing to pulp space infection occur in immature teeth or teeth with apical resorption, the same procedure for the healing of external resorption and revascularization should work in these cases also. With this antibacterial medicament, the potential exists to arrest the external inflammatory root resorption and revascularize the root canal (Figure 15).

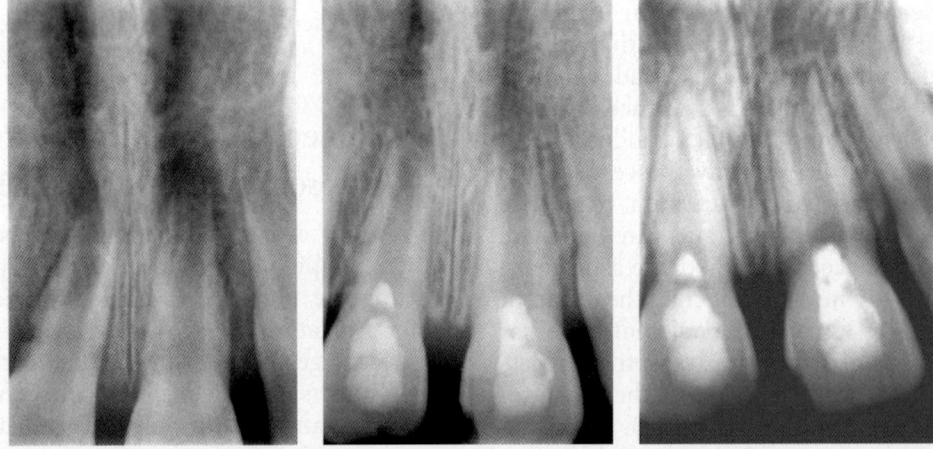

Figure 15 Immature tooth with a necrotic infected pulp, apical periodontitis, and external inflammatory root resorption. Treatment is as described in Figure 7. Note the healing of the external root resorption and the continued root development. Courtesy of Dr. Linda Levin.

The canal is disinfected without mechanical instrumentation but with copious irrigation with 5.25% sodium hypochlorite and the use of a mixture of antibiotics for at least 4 weeks.[64,85] A blood clot is produced by mechanically irritating the periradicular tissues to the level of the cementoenamel junction to provide a matrix for the ingrowth of new tissue followed by a deep coronal restoration to provide a bacteria-tight seal. The patient is followed every 3 months until evidence of healing of the external root resorption and thickening of the dentinal walls are seen (see Figures 7 and 15).

Recent studies have confirmed the potent antibacterial properties of the triantibiotic paste used in this case,[64] and studies are under way to find a synthetic matrix that will act as a more predictable scaffold for new ingrowth of tissue than the blood clot that was used in these previous cases. The procedure described here can be attempted in most cases, and if after 3 months no signs of resorption repair and regeneration are present, the more traditional treatment methods can be initiated.

Endodontic Essentials

CONCUSSION AND SUBLUXATION

Since both of these injuries imply no noticeable displacement of the tooth in its socket, pulp consequences should not be expected. However, baseline and follow-up diagnostic tests are essential to pick up late complications such as pulp canal obliteration (most likely) or pulp necrosis.

Teeth that give a positive pulp test response at the initial examination cannot be assumed to be healthy and continue to give a positive response over time. Teeth that yield a negative response or no response, however, cannot be assumed to have necrotic pulps because they may give a positive response at later follow-up visits. It has been demonstrated that it may take as long as 9 months for normal blood flow to return to the coronal pulp of a traumatized fully formed tooth. As circulation is restored, the responsiveness to pulp testing returns.[85]

The transition from a negative to a positive response at a subsequent test may be considered a sign of a healthy pulp. The repetitious finding of positive responses may also be taken as a sign of a healthy pulp. The transition from a positive to a negative response may be taken as an indication that the pulp is probably undergoing degeneration. The persistence of a negative response would suggest that the pulp has been irreversibly damaged, but even this is not absolute.[86] Thermal and electric pulp tests of all anterior teeth (canine to canine) of the maxillary and mandibular jaws should be performed at the time of the initial examination and carefully recorded to establish a baseline for comparison with subsequent repeated tests in later months. These tests should be repeated at 3 weeks; 3, 6, and 12 months; and yearly intervals following the accident. The purpose of the tests is to establish a trend as to the physiologic status of the pulps of these teeth. Particularly in traumatized teeth, carbon dioxide snow (-78°C) or dichlordifluoromethane (-40°C) placed on the incisal third of the facial surface gives more accurate responses than does a water ice pencil.[87,88] The intense cold seems to penetrate the tooth and splints or restorations and reach the deeper areas of the tooth. In addition, dry ice does not form ice water, which could disperse over adjacent teeth or gingiva to give a false-positive response. The electric pulp test relies on electric impulses directly stimulating the nerves of the pulp. These tests have limited value in young teeth but are useful in cases in which the dentinal tubules are closed and do not allow dentinal fluid to flow in them. This situation is typical of teeth in elderly patients or in traumatized teeth that are undergoing premature sclerosis. In these situations, the thermal tests that rely on fluid flow in the tubules cannot be used and the electric pulp test becomes important.

LATERAL LUXATION, EXTRUSIVE LUXATION

The tooth should be repositioned as soon as possible and a functional splint placed. The endodontic focus takes place at 7 to 10 days after the emergency visit. The endodontist must evaluate the potential for revascularization of the pulp and therefore not initiate root canal treatment, or if revascularization is not likely, root canal treatment should be initiated at this 7- to 10-day time period.

The potential for revascularization depends primarily on the width of the apical constriction at the time of repositioning. If the width is 1.0 mm or more, revascularization is considered a possibility. The wider the apical opening is, the higher the likelihood of revascularization.[89] If revascularization is considered possible, a regular follow-up regimen must be scheduled. Since pulp testing is so erratic in these types of teeth, radiographic follow-up at short intervals with similar angulations is undertaken. A small amount of radiographically appearing root resorption should be expected owing to the initial inflammation. This should be self-limiting and not increase in size after 3 weeks. If the radiographic resorption increases or any other signs of pulp infection are present, root canal therapy should be quickly initiated. If the apical opening is < 1 mm, root canal treatment should be started immediately. If the patient does not present to the clinician within 7 to 10 days postinjury, or if radiographic evidence of active external resorption is present, long-term calcium hydroxide treatment or a triantibiotic regimen should be initiated.

INTRUSIVE LUXATION

Intrusive luxation is the most destructive traumatic injury. Attachment damage is diffuse, and pulp survival is considered impossible. It is possible that in immature roots, spontaneous re-erupt and revascularization may occur, but in mature teeth, pulp necrosis is a certainty.[4] Thus, at the first chance of accessing the pulp space, root treatment should be initiated.

The Avulsed Tooth

The conditions at the emergency visit will have an important effect on the steps taken at the second visit. Ideally, the tooth should be replanted as soon as possible after the avulsion and functionally splinted. If unable to replant the tooth, it should be placed in a physiologic storage solution to allow for an extended extraoral time with fewer resorption complications after reimplantation. At the emergency visit, the root is prepared depending on the maturity of the tooth (open versus closed) and the extraoral **dry time.** A dry time of 60 minutes is considered the point at which survival is unlikely for periodontal ligament cells.

Extraoral Dry Time < 60 Minutes

CLOSED APEX

The root should be rinsed of debris with water or saline and replanted in as gentle a fashion as possible. If the tooth has a closed apex, revascularization is not possible,[89] but because the tooth was dry for less than 60 minutes (replanted or placed in appropriate medium), the chance for periodontal healing exists. Most importantly, the chance of a severe inflammatory response at the time of replantation is lessened. A dry time of less than 15 to 20 minutes is considered optimal where periodontal healing would be expected.[90–92]

A continuing challenge is the treatment of the tooth that has been dry for more than 20 minutes (periodontal cell survival is ensured) but less than 60 minutes (periodontal survival unlikely). In these cases, logic suggests that the root surface consist of some cells with the potential to regenerate and some that will act as inflammatory stimulators. Exciting new strategies are under investigation that may be extremely valuable in these cases. The use of Ledermix placed in the canal space at the emergency visit has been found to be valuable in cases that were considered hopeless in the past[93] (see below), and this medicament may prove extremely valuable in the 20- to 60-minute dry time period. Studies are ongoing to evaluate its potential.

OPEN APEX

Soak in doxycycline or cover with minocycline for 5 minutes, gently rinse off debris, and replant. In an open-apex tooth, revascularization of the pulp and continued root development are possible (Figure 16). Cvek et al.[94] found in monkeys that soaking the tooth in doxycycline (1 mg in approximately 20 mL of physiologic saline) for 5 minutes before replantation significantly enhanced revascularization. This result was confirmed in dogs by Yanpiset et al.[95] A recent study found that covering the root with minocycline that attaches to the root for approximately 15 days further increased the revascularization rate in dogs.[96] Although these animal studies do not provide us with a prediction of the rate of revascularization in humans, it is reasonable to expect that the same enhancement of revascularization that occurred in two animal species will occur in humans as well. As with the tooth with the closed apex, the open-apex tooth is then gently rinsed and replanted.

Exraoral Dry Time > 60 Minutes

CLOSED APEX

Remove the periodontal ligament by placing it in etching acid for 5 minutes, soak it in fluoride, and replant. When the root has been dry for 60 minutes or more, survival of the periodontal ligament cells is not expected.[90,97] In these cases, the root should be prepared to be as resistant to resorption as possible (attempting to slow the ankylotic osseous replacement process). These teeth should be soaked in an acid for 5 minutes to remove all remaining periodontal ligament

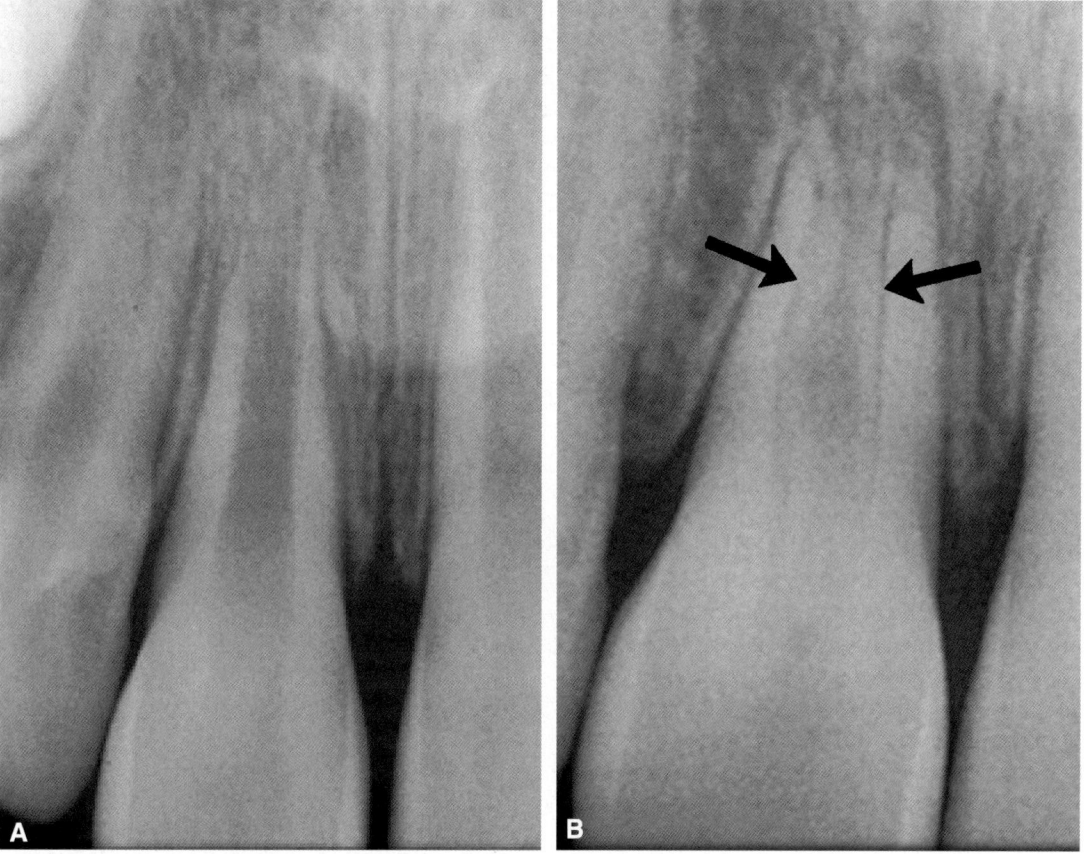

Figure 16 Revascularization of an immature root. A tooth with an open apex was replanted soon after the avulsion. The follow-up radiograph 1 year later confirmed that revascularization had taken place. In this case, it appears that new periodontal tissue has formed with a lamina dura within the pulp canal. Courtesy of Dr. Russell Stock.

and thus remove the tissue that will initiate the inflammatory response on replantation. The tooth should then be soaked in 2% stannous fluoride for 5 minutes and replanted.[98,99] Alendronate was found to have resorption slowing effects similar to those of fluoride when used topically,[100] but further studies need to be carried out to evaluate whether its effectiveness is superior to fluoride and if this justifies its added cost. Some studies have found that Emdogain (enamel matrix protein) may be beneficial in teeth with extended extraoral dry times, not only to make the root more resistant to resorption but also possibly to stimulate the formation of new periodontal ligament from the socket.[101,102] More recent studies have not confirmed the beneficial effect of Emdogain.[103]

If the tooth has been dry for more than 60 minutes and no consideration is given to preserving the periodontal ligament, the endodontics may be performed extraorally. In the case of a tooth with a closed apex, no advantage exists to this additional step at the emergency visit. However, in a tooth with an open apex, the endodontic treatment, if performed after replantation, involves a long-term apexification procedure. In these cases, completing the root canal treatment extraorally, where a seal in the "blunderbuss" apex is easier to achieve, may be advantageous. When endodontic treatment is performed extraorally, it must be performed aseptically with the utmost care to achieve a root canal system free of bacteria.

OPEN APEX

Replant? If yes, treat as described with a closed-apex tooth. Endodontic treatment may be performed out of the mouth. Since these teeth are in young patients in whom facial development is usually incomplete, many pediatric dentists consider the prognosis to be so poor and the potential complications of an ankylosed tooth so severe as to recommend that these teeth not be replanted. However, considerable debate exists as to whether it would be beneficial to replant the root even though it will inevitably be lost owing to osseous replacement. If the patients are followed carefully and the root is submerged at the appropriate time,[104,105] the height and, more importantly, the width of the alveolar bone will be maintained. This allows for easier permanent restoration, when the facial development of the child is complete. Studies are ongoing to evaluate whether the present recommendations should be changed.

Adjunctive Therapy

Systemic antibiotics given at the time of replantation and prior to endodontic treatment are effective in preventing bacterial invasion of the necrotic pulp and therefore subsequent inflammatory resorption.[106] Tetracycline has the additional benefit of decreasing root resorption by affecting the motility of the osteoclasts and reducing the effectiveness of collagenase.[107] The administration of system antibiotics is recommended beginning at the emergency visit and continuing until the splint is removed.[108] For patients not susceptible to tetracycline dentin staining, doxycycline twice daily for 7 days at an appropriate dose for patient age and weight[107,108] is the antibiotic of choice. Penicillin V 1,000 mg and 500 mg every 6 hours for 7 days has also been shown to be beneficial. The bacterial content of the sulcus also should be controlled during the healing phase. In addition to stressing to the patient the need for adequate oral hygiene, chlorhexidine rinses for 7 to 10 days are useful.

In a recent study by our group, great benefit was seen in removal of the pulp contents at the emergency visit and placing Ledermix (not available in the United States) into the root canal.[93] This product contains a tetracycline corticosteroid combination that has been shown to move through the dentinal tubules. Based on the results of the study, the use of the medicament was able to shut down the inflammatory response after replantation to allow for more favorable healing compared with those teeth that did not have the medicament.

The need for analgesics should be assessed on an individual case basis. Mild analgesics are usually adequate, or a nonsteroidal anti-inflammatory drug may be recommended. The patient should be sent to a physician for consultation regarding a tetanus booster within 48 hours of the initial visit.

SECOND VISIT

This visit should take place 7 to 10 days after the emergency visit. At the emergency visit, emphasis is placed on the preservation and healing of the attachment apparatus. The focus of this visit is the prevention or elimination of potential irritants from the root canal space. These irritants, if present, provide the stimulus for the progression of the inflammatory response and bone and root resorption. Also at this visit, the course of systemic antibiotics is completed, the chlorhexidine rinses can be stopped, and the splint is removed.

Endodontic Treatment

EXTRAORAL TIME < 60 MINUTES

Closed Apex.
Initiate endodontic treatment at 7 to 10 days. In cases in which endodontic treatment is delayed or signs of resorption are present, treat with calcium hydroxide until evidence of healing is present, such as redevelopment of the periodontal ligament space. The root canal can then be filled and the crown restored.

Open Apex
Avoid endodontic treatment and look for evidence of revascularization. At the first indication of an infected pulp, initiate the apexification procedure.

EXTRAORAL TIME > 60 MINUTES

Closed Apex
These teeth are treated endodontically in the same way as those teeth that had an extraoral time of < 60 minutes.

Open Apex
If endodontic treatment was not performed out of the mouth, initiate the apexification procedure. In these teeth, the chance of revascularization is extremely poor.[80,109] Therefore, no attempt is made to revitalize these teeth. An apexification procedure is initiated at the second visit if root canal treatment was not performed at the emergency visit. If a root canal filling was placed at the emergency visit, the second visit is a recall visit to assess initial healing only.

Temporary Restoration
Effectively sealing the coronal access is essential to prevent infection of the canal between visits. Recommended temporary restorations are reinforced zinc oxide–eugenol cement, acid-etch composite resin, or

glass ionomer cement. The depth of the temporary restoration is critical to its sealing ability. A depth of at least 4 mm is recommended and a cotton pellet need not be placed; the temporary restoration is placed directly onto the calcium hydroxide in the access cavity. Calcium hydroxide should first be removed from the walls of the access cavity because it is soluble and will wash out when it comes in contact with saliva, leaving a defective temporary restoration. After initiation of the root canal treatment, the splint is removed. If time does not permit complete removal of the splint at this visit, the resin tacks are smoothed so as not to irritate the soft tissues and the residual resin is removed at a later appointment. At this appointment, healing is usually sufficient to perform a detailed clinical examination on the teeth surrounding the avulsed tooth. The sensitivity tests, reaction to percussion and palpation, and periodontal probing measurements should be carefully recorded for reference at follow-up visits.

Root Filling Visit

The root canal can be filled at the practitioner's convenience or, in the case of long-term calcium hydroxide therapy, when an intact lamina dura can be traced. If the endodontic treatment was initiated 7 to 10 days after the avulsion and clinical and radiographic examinations do not indicate pathosis, filling of the root canal at this visit is acceptable, although the use of long-term calcium hydroxide is a proven option for these cases. On the other hand, if endodontic treatment was initiated more than 7 to 10 days after the avulsion or if active resorption is visible, the pulp space must first be disinfected before root filling. Traditionally, the reestablishment of a lamina dura (see Figure 14) is a radiographic sign that the canal bacteria have been controlled. When an intact lamina dura can be traced, root filling can take place. The canal is cleaned, shaped, and irrigated under strict asepsis. After completion of the instrumentation, the canal can be filled by any acceptable technique, with special attention to an aseptic technique and the best possible seal of the filling material.

PERMANENT RESTORATION

Much evidence exists that coronal leakage caused by defective temporary and permanent restorations results in a clinically relevant amount of bacterial contamination in the root canal after root filling.[110] Therefore, the tooth should receive a permanent restoration at or soon after the time of filling of the root canal. As with the temporary restoration, the depth of restoration is important for its seal; therefore, the deepest restoration possible should be made. A post should be avoided if possible. Because most avulsions occur in the anterior region of the mouth, where esthetics is important, composite resins with the addition of dentin bonding agents are usually recommended in these cases. They have the additional advantage of internally strengthening the tooth against fracture if another traumatic event should occur.

FOLLOW-UP CARE

Follow-up evaluations should take place at 3 months, at 6 months, and yearly for at least 5 years. If osseous replacement (ankylosis) is identified (Figure 17),

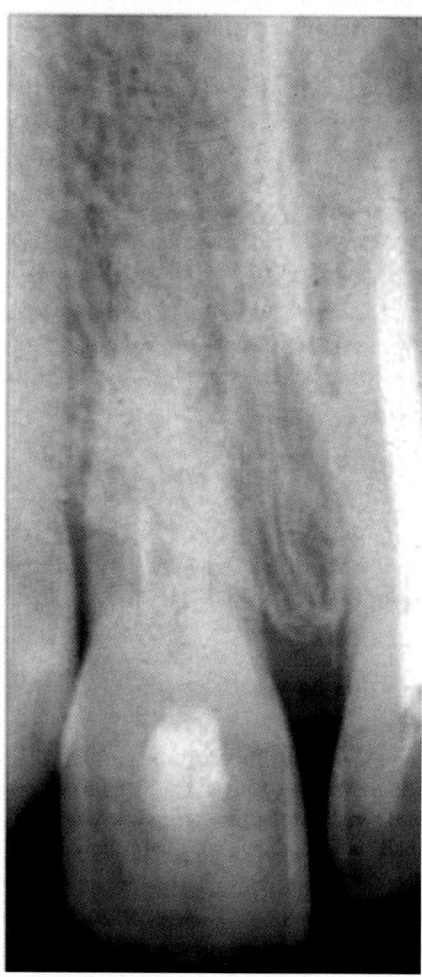

Figure 17 Radiographic appearance of osseous replacement. The root acquires the radiographic appearance of the surrounding bone (without a lamina dura). Note that radiolucencies typical of active inflammation are **not** present.

timely revision of the long-term treatment plan is indicated. In the case of inflammatory root resorption (see Figure 12), a new attempt at disinfection of the root canal space by standard retreatment can reverse the process. Teeth adjacent to and surrounding the avulsed tooth or teeth may show pathologic changes long after the initial accident. Therefore, these teeth should be tested at recall and the results compared with those collected soon after the accident.

Internal Root Resorption

Internal root resorption is **rare** in permanent teeth. Internal resorption is characterized by an oval-shaped enlargement of the root canal space.[4] External resorption, which is much more common, is often misdiagnosed as internal resorption. Internal root resorption is characterized by resorption of the internal aspect of the root by multinucleated giant cells adjacent to granulation tissue in the pulp. Chronic inflammatory tissue is common in the pulp but only rarely does it result in resorption. There are different theories on the origin of the pulpal granulation tissue involved in internal resorption. The most logical explanation is that it is pulp tissue that is inflamed owing to an infected coronal pulp space. Communication between the coronal necrotic tissue and the vital pulp is through appropriately oriented dentinal tubules.[78] In addition to the requirement of granulation tissue, root resorption takes place only if the odontoblastic layer and predentin are lost or altered.[78]

Reasons for the loss of predentin adjacent to the granulation tissue are not obvious. Trauma frequently has been suggested as a cause.[111,112] Some report that trauma may be recognized as an initiating factor in internal resorption.[113] They are divided into a transient type and a progressive type, the latter requiring continuous stimulation by infection. Another reason for the loss of predentin might be extreme heat produced when cutting on dentin without an adequate water spray. The heat presumably would destroy the predentin layer, and if later the coronal aspect of the pulp became infected, the bacterial products could initiate the typical inflammation in conjunction with resorbing giant cells in the vital pulp adjacent to the denuded root surface. Internal root resorption has been produced experimentally by the application of diathermy.[113]

Internal root resorption is usually asymptomatic and is first recognized clinically through routine

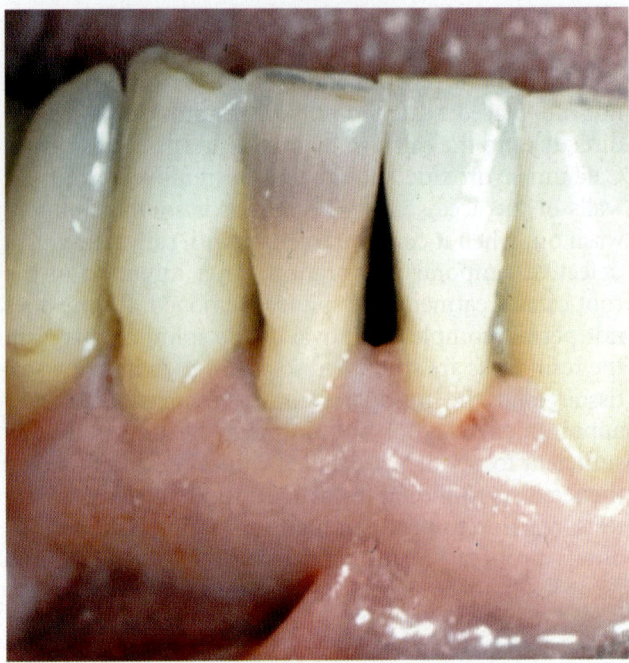

Figure 18 Pink spot associated with internal root resorption.

radiographs. Pain may be a presenting symptom if perforation of the crown occurs and the metaplastic tissue is exposed to the oral fluids. For internal resorption to be active, at least part of the pulp must be vital, so a positive response to pulp sensitivity testing is possible. The coronal portion of the pulp is often necrotic, whereas the apical pulp that includes the internal resorptive defect remains vital. Therefore, a negative sensitivity test result does not rule out active internal resorption. It is also possible that the pulp becomes nonvital after a period of active resorption, giving a negative sensitivity test, radiographic signs of internal resorption, and radiographic signs of apical inflammation. Traditionally, the pink tooth has been thought pathognomonic of internal root resorption. The pink color is due to the granulation tissue in the coronal dentin undermining the crown enamel (Figure 18). The pink tooth can also be a feature of cervical subepithelial external inflammatory root resorption that must be ruled out before a diagnosis of internal root resorption is made.

RADIOGRAPHIC APPEARANCE

The usual radiographic presentation of internal root resorption is a fairly uniform radiolucent enlargement of the pulp canal (Figure 19). Because the resorption is initiated in the root canal, the resorptive defect includes some part of the root canal space. Therefore, the original outline of the root canal is distorted. Only on rare occasions, when the internal resorptive defect penetrates the root and impacts the periodontal ligament, does the adjacent bone show radiographic changes.

HISTOLOGIC APPEARANCE

Similar to other inflammatory resorptive defects, the histologic picture of internal resorption is granulation tissue with multinucleated giant cells. An area of necroticpulp is found coronal to the granulation tissue. Dentinal tubules containing microorganisms and communicating between the necrotic zone and the granulation tissue can sometimes be seen.[78,80,113,114]

Unlike external root resorption, the adjacent bone is not affected with internal root resorption.

ENDODONTIC TREATMENT

Treatment of internal root resorption is conceptually very easy. Since the resorptive defect is the result of the inflamed pulp and the blood supply to the tissue is through the apical foramina, endodontic treatment that effectively removes the blood supply to the resorbing cells is the treatment approach. After adequate anesthesia is obtained, the canal apical to the internal defect is explored and a working length short of the radiographic apex is used. The apical canal is thoroughly instrumented to ensure that the blood supply to the tissue resorbing the root is cut off. **By completion of the root canal instrumentation, it should be possible to obtain a blood-free and dry canal with paper points.** Calcium hydroxide is spun into the canal to facilitate the removal of the tissue in the irregular defect at the next visit. At the second visit, the tooth and defect are filled with a soft root filling technique (Figure 20). With modern dental techniques, this treatment alternative should be weighed against the advantages of implant dentistry.

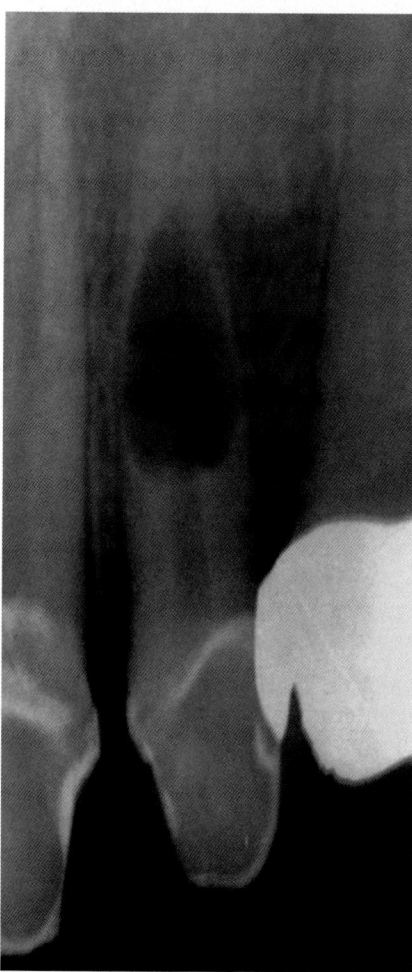

Figure 19 Uniform radiolucency observed in teeth with internal root resorption.

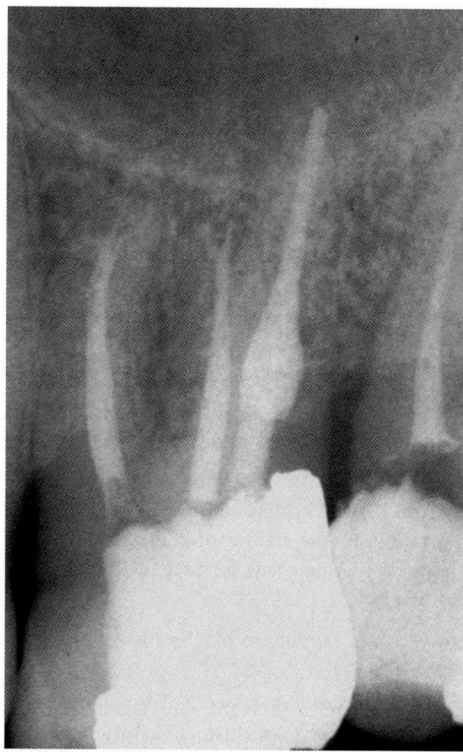

Figure 20 An internal root resorption defect is filled with a softened gutta-percha filling technique.

References

1. Andreasen JO, Ravn JJ. Epidemiology of traumatic dental injuries to primary and permanent teeth in a Danish population sample. Int J Oral Surg 1972;1:235.
2. Skaare AB, Jacobsen I. Dental injuries in Norwegians aged 7–18 years. Dent Traumatol 2003;19:67.
3. Bastone EB, Freer TJ, McNamara JR. Epidemiology of dental trauma: a review of the literature. Aust Dent J 2000;45:2.
4. Andreasen JO, Andreasen FM. Textbook and color atlas of traumatic injuries to the teeth. 3rd ed. Copenhagen and St. Louis: Munksgaard and CV Mosby; 1994.
5. Canakci V, Akgul HM, Akgul N, Canakci CF. Prevalence and handedness correlates of traumatic injuries to the permanent incisors in 13-17-year-old adolescents in Erzurum, Turkey. Dent Traumatol 2003;19:248.
6. Saroglu I, Sonmez H. The prevalence of traumatic injuries treated in the pedodontic clinic of Ankara University, Turkey, during 18 months. Dent Traumatol 2002;18:299.
7. Tapias MA, Jimenez-Garcia R, Lamas F, Gil AA. Prevalence of traumatic crown fractures to permanent incisors in a childhood population: Mostoles, Spain. Dent Traumatol 2003;19:119.
8. Kakehashi S, Stanley HR, Fitzgerald RJ. The effect of surgical exposures on dental pulps in germ-free and conventional laboratory rats. Oral Surg Oral Med Oral Pathol Oral Radiol Endod 1965;20:340.
9. Cvek M, Cleaton-Jones PE, Austin JC, Andreasen JO. Pulp reactions to exposure after experimental crown fractures or grinding in adult monkeys. J Endod 1982;8:391.
10. Cvek M. A clinical report on partial pulpotomy and capping with calcium hydroxide in permanent incisors with complicated crown fracture. J Endod 1978;4:232.
11. Heide S, Mjor IA. Pulp reactions to experimental exposures in young permanent monkey teeth. Int Endod J 1983;16:11.
12. Katebzadeh N, Dalton BC, Trope M. Strengthening immature teeth during and after apexification. J Endod 1998;24:256.
13. Sjogren U, Hagglund B, Sundqvist G, Wing K. Factors affecting the long-term results of endodontic treatment. J Endod 1990;16:498.
14. Masterton JB. The healing of wounds of the dental pulp. An investigation of the nature of the scar tissue and of the phenomena leading to its formation. Dent Pract Dent Rec 1966;16:325.
15. Weiss M. Pulp capping in older patients. N Y State Dent J 1966;32:451.
16. Cvek M, Hollender L, Nord CE. Treatment of non-vital permanent incisors with calcium hydroxide. VI. A clinical, microbiological and radiological evaluation of treatment in one sitting of teeth with mature or immature root. Odontol Revy 1976;27:93.
17. Andreasen JO. Luxation of permanent teeth due to trauma. A clinical and radiographic follow-up study of 189 injured teeth. Scand J Dent Res 1970;78:273.
18. Eklund G, Stalhane I, Hedegard B. A study of traumatized permanent teeth in children aged 7–15 years. Part III. A multivariate analysis of post-traumatic complications of subluxated and luxated teeth. Sven Tandlak Tidskr 1976;69:179.
19. Swift EJ Jr, Trope M. Treatment options for the exposed vital pulp. Pract Periodontics Aesthet Dent 1999;11:735.
20. Tronstad L, Mjor IA. Capping of the inflamed pulp. Oral Surg Oral Med Oral Pathol Oral Radiol Endod 1972;34:477.
21. Cox CF, Keall CL, Keall HJ, et al. Biocompatibility of surface-sealed dental materials against exposed pulps. J Prosthet Dent 1987;57:1.
22. Bystrom A, Claesson R, Sundqvist G. The antibacterial effect of camphorated paramonochlorophenol, camphorated phenol and calcium hydroxide in the treatment of infected root canals. Endod Dent Traumatol 1985;1:170.
23. Sjogren U, Figdor D, Spangberg L, Sundqvist G. The antimicrobial effect of calcium hydroxide as a short-term intracanal dressing. Int Endod J 1991;24:119.
24. Mejare I, Hasselgren G, Hammarstrom LE. Effect of formaldehyde-containing drugs on human dental pulp evaluated by enzyme histochemical technique. Scand J Dent Res 1976;84:29.
25. Schroder U, Granath LE. Early reaction of intact human teeth to calcium hydroxide following experimental pulpotomy and its significance to the development of hard tissue barrier. Odontol Revy 1971;22:379.
26. Schroder U. Reaction of human dental pulp to experimental pulpotomy and capping with calcium hydroxide [thesis]. Odont Revy 1973;24 Suppl 25:97.
27. Stanley HR, Lundy T. Dycal therapy for pulp exposures. Oral Surg Oral Med Oral Pathol Oral Radiol Endod 1972;34:818.
28. Tronstad L. Reaction of the exposed pulp to Dycal treatment. Oral Surg Oral Med Oral Pathol Oral Radiol Endod 1974;38:945.
29. Heller AL, Koenigs JF, Brilliant JD, et al. Direct pulp capping of permanent teeth in primates using a resorbable form of tricalcium phosphate ceramic. J Endod 1975;1:95.
30. Arakawa M, Kitasako Y, Otsuki M, Tagami J. Direct pulp capping with an auto-cured sealant resin and a self-etching primer. Am J Dent 2003;16:61.
31. Deutsch AS, Musikant BL, Cavallari J, et al. Root fracture during insertion of prefabricated posts related to root size. J Prosthet Dent 1985;53:786.
32. Torabinejad M, Hong CU, McDonald F, Pitt Ford TR. Physical and chemical properties of a new root-end filling material. J Endod 1995;21:349.

33. Torabinejad M, Rastegar AF, Kettering JD, Pitt Ford TR. Bacterial leakage of mineral trioxide aggregate as a root-end filling material. J Endod 1995;21:109.

34. Cvek M. A clinical report on partial pulpotomy and capping with calcium hydroxide in permanent incisors with complicated crown fracture. J Endod 1978;4:232.

35. Granath LE, Hagman G. Experimental pulpotomy in human bicuspids with reference to cutting technique. Acta Odontol Scand 1971;29:155.

36. Stanley HR, Lundy T. Dycal therapy for pulp exposures. Oral Surg Oral Med Oral Pathol Oral Radiol Endod 1972;34:818.

37. Fuks AB, Cosack A, Klein H, Eidelman E. Partial pulpotomy as a treatment alternative for exposed pulps in crown-fractured permanent incisors. Endod Dent Traumatol 1987;3:100.

38. Gelbier MJ, Winter GB. Traumatised incisors treated by vital pulpotomy: a retrospective study. Br Dent J 1988;164:319.

39. Seltzer S, Bender IB, Turkenkopf S. Factors affecting successful repair after root canal therapy. J Am Dent Assoc 1963;52:651.

40. Teixeira FB, Teixeira EC, Thompson JY, Trope M. Fracture resistance of roots endodontically treated with a new resin filling material. J Am Dent Assoc 2004;135:646.

41. Bergenholtz G. Micro-organisms from necrotic pulps of traumatized teeth. Odont Revy 1974;25:347–58.

42. Shuping G, {145}rstavik D, Sigurdsson A, Trope M. Reduction of intracanal bacteria using nickel-titanium rotary instrumentation and various medications. J Endod 2000;26:751–5.

43. Cvek M, Nord CE, Hollender L. Antimicrobial effect of root canal debridement in teeth with immature root. A clinical and microbiologic study. Odontol Revy 1976;27:1.

44. Spangberg L, Rutberg M, Rydinge E. Biologic effects of endodontic antimicrobial agents. J Endod 1979;5:166.

45. Heithersay GS. Calcium hydroxide in the treatment of pulpless teeth with associated pathology. J Br Endod Soc 1962;8:74.

46. Herforth A, Strassburg M. [Therapy of chronic apical periodontitis in traumatically injuring front teeth with ongoing root growth]. Dtsch Zahnarztl Z 1977;32:453.

47. Cvek M. Prognosis of luxated non-vital maxillary incisors treated with calcium hydroxide and filled with gutta-percha. A retrospective clinical study. Endod Dent Traumatol 1992;8:45.

48. Lengheden A, Blomlof L, Lindskog S. Effect of delayed calcium hydroxide treatment on periodontal healing in contaminated replanted teeth. Scand J Dent Res 1991;99:147.

49. Andreasen JO, Farik B, Munksgaard EC. Long-term calcium hydroxide as a root canal dressing may increase risk of root fracture. Dent Traumatol 2002;18:134.

50. Giuliani V, Baccetti T, Pace R, Pagavino G. The use of MTA in teeth with necrotic pulps and open apices. Dent Traumatol 2002;18:217.

51. Maroto M, Barberia E, Planells P, Vera V. Treatment of a non-vital immature incisor with mineral trioxide aggregate (MTA). Dent Traumatol 2003;19:165.

52. Binnie WH, Rowe AH. A histological study of the periapical tissues of incompletely formed pulpless teeth filled with calcium hydroxide. J Dent Res 1973;52:1110.

53. Cvek M. Treatment of non-vital permanent incisors with calcium hydroxide. IV. Periodontal healing and closure of the root canal in the coronal fragment of teeth with intraalveolar fracture and vital apical fragment. A follow-up. Odontol Revy 1974;25:239.

54. Trabert KC, Caput AA, Abou-Rass M, et al. A histological study of the periapical tissues of incompletely formed pulpless teeth filled with calcium hydroxide. J Dent Res 1973;52:1110.

55. Deutsch AS, Musikant BL, Cavallari J, et al. Root fracture during insertion of prefabricated posts related to root size. J Prosthet Dent 1985;53:786.

56. Kerekes K, Heide S, Jacobsen I. Follow-up examination of endodontic treatment in traumatized juvenile incisors. J Endod 1980;6:744.

57. Goldberg F, Kaplan A, Roitman M, et al. Reinforcing effect of a resin glass ionomer in the restoration of immature roots in vitro. Dent Traumatol 2002;18:70.

58. Barrett AP, Reade PC. Revascularization of mouse tooth isografts and allografts using autoradiography and carbon-perfusion. Arch Oral Biol 1981;26:541.

59. Ohman A. Healing and sensitivity to pain in young replanted human teeth. An experimental, clinical and histological study. Odontol Tidskr 1965;73:166.

60. Skoglund A, Tronstad L. Pulpal changes in replanted and autotransplanted immature teeth of dogs. J Endod 1981;7:309.

61. Love RM. Bacterial penetration of the root canal of intact incisor teeth after a simulated traumatic injury. Endod Dent Traumatol 1996;12:289.

62. Banchs F, Trope M. Revascularization of immature permanent teeth with apical periodontitis: new treatment protocol? J Endod 2004;30:196.

63. Thibodeau B, Teixeira F, Yamauchi M, et al. Pulp revascularization of immature dog teeth with apical periodontitis J Endod 2007;33:680–9.

64. Yanpiset K, Trope M. Pulp revascularization of replanted immature dog teeth after different treatment methods. Endod Dent Traumatol 2000;16:211–16.

65. Windley W III, Teixeira F, Levin L, et al. Disinfection of immature teeth with a triple antibiotic paste. J Endod 2005;31:439–43.

66. Zachrisson BU, Jacobsen I. Long-term prognosis of 66 permanent anterior teeth with root fracture. Scand J Dent Res 1975;83:345.

67. Andreasen FM. Pulpal healing after luxation injuries and root fracture in the permanent dentition. Endod Dent Traumatol 1989;5:111.

68. Jacobsen I, Kerekes K. Diagnosis and treatment of pulp necrosis in permanent anterior teeth with root fracture. Scand J Dent Res 1980;88:370.

69. Andreasen JO, Andreasen FM, Mejare I, Cvek M. Healing of 400 intra-alveolar root fractures. 2. Effect of treatment factors such as treatment delay, repositioning, splinting type and period and antibiotics. Dent Traumatol 2004;20:203.

70. Rabie G, Barnett F, Tronstad L. Long-term splinting of maxillary incisor with intra-alveolar root fracture. Endod Dent Traumatol 1988;4:99.

71. Cvek M. Treatment of non-vital permanent incisors with calcium hydroxide. IV. Periodontal healing and closure of the root canal in the coronal fragment of teeth with intra-alveolar fracture and vital apical fragment. A follow-up. Odontol Revy 1974;25:239.

72. Jacobsen I, Zachrisson BU. Repair characteristics of root fractures in permanent anterior teeth. Scand J Dent Res 1975;83:355.

73. Andreasen JO, Andreasen FM, Mejare I, Cvek M. Healing of 400 intra-alveolar root fractures. 1. Effect of pre-injury and injury factors such as sex, age, stage of root development, fracture type, location of fracture and severity of dislocation. Dent Traumatol 2004;20:192.

74. Andreasen FM. Pulpal healing after luxation injuries and root fracture in the permanent dentition. Endod Dent Traumatol 1989;5:111.

75. Jacobsen I. Root fractures in permanent anterior teeth with incomplete root formation. Scand J Dent Res 1976;84:210.

76. Andreasen JO. Review of root resorption systems and models. Etiology of root resorption and the homeostatic mechanisms of the periodontal ligament.

77. Andreasen FM, Zhijie Y, Thomsen BL, Andersen PK. Occurrence of pulp canal obliteration after luxation injuries in the permanent dentition. Endod Dent Traumatol 1987;3:103.

78. Andreasen FM, Pedersen BV. Prognosis of luxated permanent teeth—the development of pulp necrosis. Endod Dent Traumatol 1985;1:207.

79. Tronstad L. Root resorption—etiology, terminology and clinical manifestations. Endod Dent Traumatol 1988;4:241.

80. Trope M, Moshonov J, Nissan R, et al. Short vs. long-term calcium hydroxide treatment of established inflammatory root resorption in replanted dog teeth. Endod Dent Traumatol 1995;11:124.

81. Trope M, Yesilsoy C, Koren L, et al. Effect of different endodontic treatment protocols on periodontal repair and root resorption of replanted dog teeth. J Endod 1992;18:492.

82. Cvek M, Cleaton-Jones P, Austin J, et al. Effect of topical application of doxycycline on pulp revascularization and periodontal healing in reimplanted monkey incisors. Endod Dent Traumatol 1990;6:170.

83. Yanpiset K, Vongsavan N, Sigurdsson A, Trope M. Efficacy of laser Doppler flowmetry for the diagnosis of revascularization of reimplanted immature dog teeth. Dent Traumatol 2001;17:63.

84. Hoshino E, Kurihara-Ando N, Sato I, et al. In-vitro antibacterial susceptibility of bacteria taken from infected root dentine to a mixture of ciprofloxacin, metronidazole and minocycline. Int Endod J 1996;29:125–30.

85. Gazelius B, Olgart L, Edwall B. Restored vitality in luxated teeth assessed by laser Doppler flowmeter. Endod Dent Traumatol 1988;4:265.

86. Bhaskar SN, Rappaport HM. Dental vitality tests and pulp status. J Am Dent Assoc 1973;86:409.

87. Fulling HJ, Andreasen JO. Influence of maturation status and tooth type of permanent teeth upon electrometric and thermal pulp testing. Scand J Dent Res 1976;84:286.

88. Fuss Z, Trowbridge H, Bender IB, et al. Assessment of reliability of electrical and thermal pulp testing agents. J Endod 1986;12:301.

89. Kling M, Cvek M, Mejare I. Rate and predictability of pulp revascularization in therapeutically reimplanted permanent incisors. Endod Dent Traumatol 1986;2:83–9.

90. Soder PO, Otteskog P, Andreasen JO, Modeer T. Effect of drying on viability of periodontal membrane. Scand J Dent Res 1977;85:164.

91. Andreasen JO. Effect of extra-alveolar period and storage media upon periodontal and pulpal healing after replantation of mature permanent incisors in monkeys. Int J Oral Surg Oral Med Oral Pathol Oral Radiol Endod 1981;10:43.

92. Barrett EJ, Kenny DJ. Avulsed permanent teeth: a review of the literature and treatment guidelines. Endod Dent Traumatol 1997;13:153.

93. Bryson EC, Levin L, Banchs F, et al. Effect of immediate intracanal placement of Ledermix Paste® on healing of replanted dog teeth after extended dry times. Endod Dent Traumatol 2002;18:316–21.

94. Cvek M, et al. Effect of topical application of doxycycline on pulp revascularization and periodontal healing in reimplanted monkey incisors. Endod Dent Traumatol 1990;6:170–7.

95. Yanpiset K, Trope M. Pulp revascularization of replanted immature dog teeth after different treatment methods. Endod Dent Traumatol 2000;16:211–17.

96. Ritter AL, Ritter AV, Murrah V, et al. Pulp revascularization of replanted immature dog teeth after treatment with minocycline and doxycycline assessed by laser flowmetry, radiography and histology. Dent Traumatol 2004;5:75–84.

97. Andreasen JO, Kristerson L. The effect of limited drying or removal of the periodontal ligament. Periodontal healing after replantation of mature permanent incisors in monkeys. Acta Odontol Scand 1981;39:1.

98. Bjorvatn K, Selvig KA, Klinge B. Effect of tetracycline and SnF2 on root resorption in replanted incisors in dogs. Scand J Dent Res 1989;97:477.

99. Selvig KA, Zander HA. Chemical analysis and microradiography of cementum and dentin from periodontically diseased human teeth. J Periodont 1962;33:103.

100. Levin L, Bryson EC, Caplan D, Trope M. Effect of topical alendronate on root resorption of dried replanted dog teeth. Dent Traumatol 2001;17:120.

101. Filippi A, Pohl Y, von Arx T. Treatment of replacement resorption with Emdogain—preliminary results after 10 months. Dent Traumatol 2001;17:134.

102. Iqbal MK, Bamaas N. Effect of enamel matrix derivative (EMDOGAIN) upon periodontal healing after replantation of permanent incisors in beagle dogs. Dent Traumatol 2001;17:36.

103. Araujo M, Hayacibara R, Sonohara M, et al. Effect of enamel matrix proteins (Emdogain) on healing after re-implantation of "periodontally compromised" roots. An experimental study in the dog. J Clin Periodontol 2003;30:855–61.

104. Flores MT, Andersson L, Andreasen JO, et al. Guidelines for the management of traumatic dental injuries. II. Avulsion of permanent teeth. Dent Traumatol 2007;3:130–6.

105. Andersson L, Malmgren B. The problem of dentoalveolar ankylosis and subsequent replacement resorption in the growing patient. Aust Endod J 1999;25:57.

106. Hammarstrom L, Pierce A, Blomlof L, et al. Tooth avulsion and replantation—a review. Endod Dent Traumatol 1986;2:1.

107. Sae-Lim V, Wang CY, Choi GW, Trope M. The effect of systemic tetracycline on resorption of dried replanted dogs' teeth. Endod Dent Traumatol 1998;14:127.

108. Sae-Lim V, Wang CY, Trope M. Effect of systemic tetracycline and amoxicillin on inflammatory root resorption of replanted dogs' teeth. Endod Dent Traumatol 1998;14:216.

109. Trope M. Root resorption of dental and traumatic origin: classification based on etiology. Pract Periodontics Aesthet Dent 1998;10:515.

110. Ray HA, Trope M. Periapical status of endodontically treated teeth in relation to the technical quality of the root filling and the coronal restoration. Int Endod J 1995;28:12.

111. Seltzer S. Endodontology. Philadelphia: Lea & Febiger; 1988.

112. Wedenberg C, Zetterqvist L. Internal resorption in human teeth—a histological, scanning electron microscopic, and enzyme histochemical study. J Endod 1987;13:255.

113. Wedenberg C, Lindskog S. Experimental internal resorption in monkey teeth. Endod Dent Traumatol 1985;1:221.

114. Silverman S. The dental structures in primary hyperparathyroidism. Oral Surg Oral Med Oral Pathol Oral Radiol Endod 1962;15:426.

CHAPTER 37

PATHOLOGIC TOOTH RESORPTION

JENS OVE ANDREASEN, LEIF K. BAKLAND

The resorption of permanent teeth has been considered an unfortunate and unpredictable phenomenon. During the past 30 years, a wealth of new knowledge about the nature of osteoclasts, and more specifically how they behave in the oral environment, has provided more information about the previously mysterious osteoclastic attacks on roots.[1] This chapter describes the sequence of traumatic and pathologic events that may lead to root resorption; however, it may be of interest to consider why permanent teeth normally survive without succumbing to root resorption.

Homeostasis Phenomenon of Pulp and Periodontal Ligament Preventing Osteoclastic Attacks

It is a surprising fact that a permanent tooth throughout life is placed in an environment of alveolar bone surrounded by very active osteoblasts and osteoclasts without being approached by any of these two cell lines under normal conditions (Figure 1).[2] Several experimental studies indicate that this immunity possibly relates to the presence of intact cementoblast and odontoblast cell layers, and perhaps also adjacent cell layers.[2] In various animal experiments, it has been shown that physical and chemical insults to these cell layers can result in loss of protection, leading to active root resorption, both on the external root surface and in the root canal.[3,4]

To understand the full scope of tooth resorption, it is necessary to understand the nature of osteoclasts, a cell with multipotential behavior that plays at least five significant roles during adolescence and adult life.

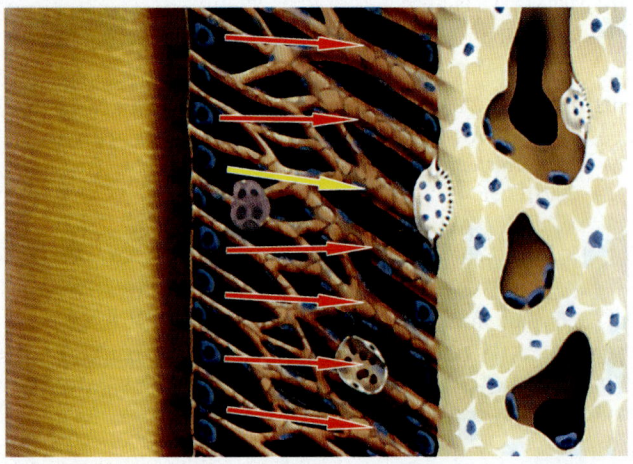

Figure 1 Antisorptive and antiosteogenesis signals released from cementoblasts, periodontal ligament cells, and Mallassez epithelial islands, creating a periodontal ligament space homeostasis. Reproduced with permission from Lindskog SF et al.[1]

Physiology of Osteoclasts

The osteoclasts represent a syncytium of stimulated macrophage progenitor cells. This stimulation is under the control of the RANK-RANKL-OPG system (RANK = receptor activator of nuclear factor; RANKL = receptor activator of nuclear factor ligand; OPG = osteoprotegerin).[1] It serves as an on-off system for osteoclast activity, where downregulating of the OPG system and upregulating of the RANKL system may favor differentiation of new osteoclasts and the opposite regulation may downregulate osteoclastic activity (Figures 2 and 3).

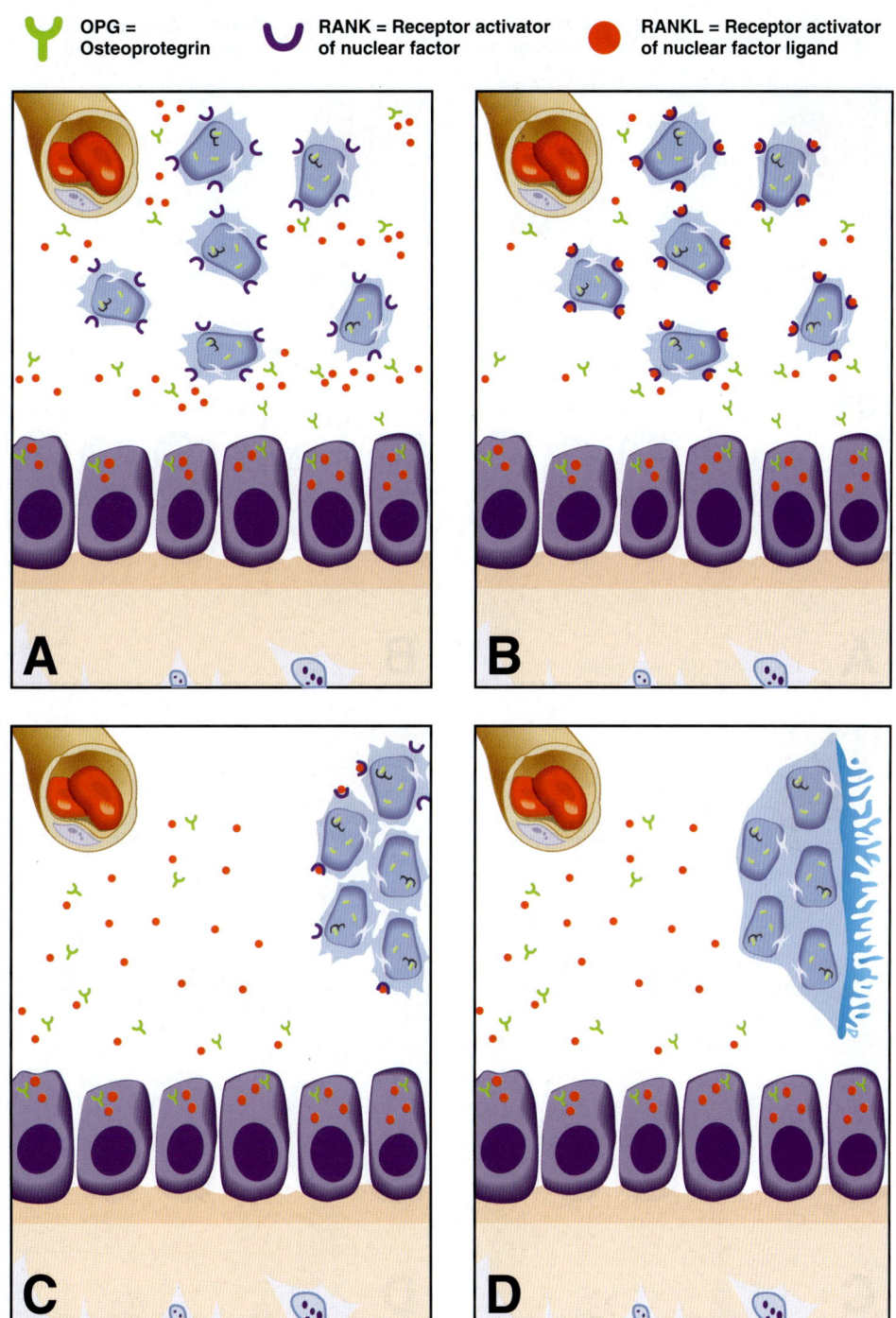

Figure 2 *A* and *B*, Activation of the RANK-RANKL-OPG system. Osteoclastogenesis is the result of differentiation of mononuclear/macrophage progenitor cells (MP) and fusion of these cells to become osteoclasts. The commitment of these cells to become osteoclasts depends on the activation of the RANK receptors on the surface of RANKL, which is produced by stroma cells and osteoblast (OB). *C,* RANKL is liberated into the tissue and attaches to the receptors of the mononuclear/macrophage progenitor cells. *D,* Mononuclear/macrophage cells aggregate, fuse, and form osteoclasts. Proresorptive factors are hormones and cytokines such as parathyroid hormone, 1,25dihydroxyvitamin D_3, interleukin-1, interleukin-6, tumor necrosis factor, leukemia inhibitory factor (LIF), and corticosteroids, which activate osteoblasts and stroma cells to produce RANKL and depress OPG. Reproduced with permission from Lindskog SF et al.[1]

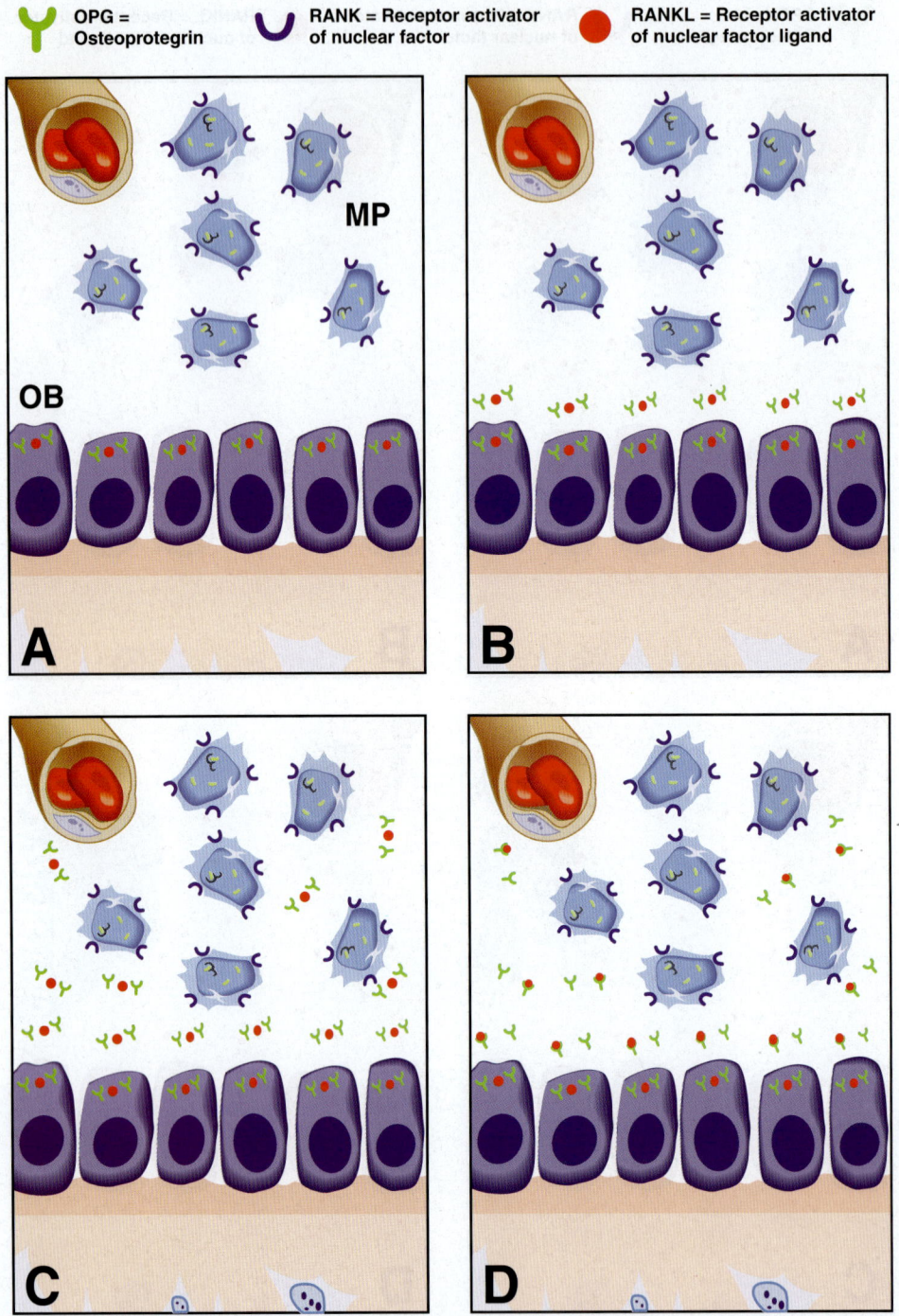

Figure 3 *A–C,* Inactivation of the RANK-RANKL-OPG system. Antiresorptive factors such as estrogens, calcitonin, bone morphogenetic protein, transforming growth factor {158}, interleukin-17, platelet-derived growth factor, and calcium depress RANKL production by osteoblasts and stroma cells and activate their OPG production. *D,* OPG binds and neutralizes RANKL, leading to a block in osteoclastogenesis and decreased survival of osteoclast. Reproduced with permission from Lindskog SF et al.[1]

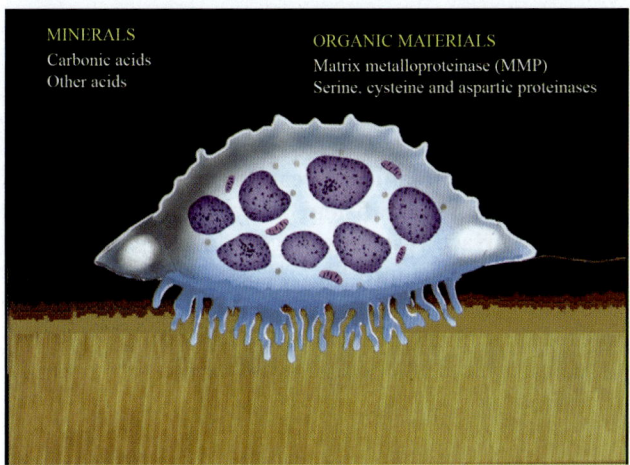

Figure 4 Physiology of an osteoclast: removal of inorganic material by acids (proton pump) and organic material by matrix metalloproteinases, serine, cysteine, and aspartic proteases.

Mechanism of Hard Tissue Deconstruction

After an osteoclast has been formed, it will start to resorb hard tissue (ie, cementum, dentin, enamel, or bone). The mechanism of hard tissue deconstruction is dissolution of inorganic material by acids associated with a breakdown of the organic structures (Figure 4).[1]

Osteoclast as a Cell Responsible for Tooth Eruption

The osteoclast plays a key role in the shedding of primary teeth (**physiologic resorption**). At a certain stage in the development of a permanent successor and the eruption process, the coronal part of the follicle induces a rim of osteoclasts that over a couple of years resorb the roots of the primary predecessor and the adjacent bone.[5–7] In the case of the ectopic position of a permanent tooth germ, **nonphysiologic root resorption** may affect adjacent permanent teeth.

ENDODONTIC IMPLICATIONS

In regard to physiologic resorption of primary teeth, it should be noted that chronic periapical inflammation from pulp necrosis in primary teeth accelerates shedding.[6,7] For example, with the ectopic eruption of a canine, resorption of the permanent lateral incisor may take place (Figure 5). If the lateral incisor has an intact pulp and if the ectopic eruption path

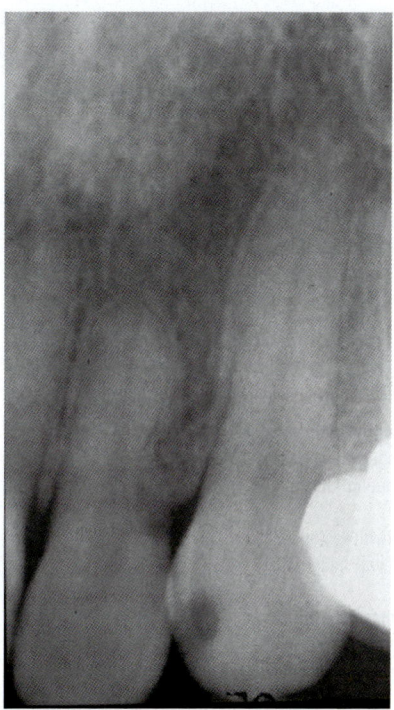

Figure 5 An example of lateral root resorption on a maxillary lateral incisor from the ectopic eruption of the adjacent canine.

changes to a normal path, or if the canine is removed, the resorption process of the lateral incisor will be arrested and the pulp should survive. Consequently, root canal treatment of such teeth is definitely not indicated.

Osteoclast as a Cell Involved in Alveolar Bone Growth and Maintenance

The alveolar bone structure is entirely dependent on a controlled symbiosis between osteoblastic and osteoclastic activity whereby a continuous turnover of bone takes place throughout life (Table 1). If there is a lack of equilibrium in the activity of these two cell types, either osteoporosis or osteosclerosis will occur.[1,6]

ENDODONTIC IMPLICATIONS

In case of a replacement resorption (ankylosis) of a tooth (external root surface or internal root canal), the tooth becomes part of the general bone remodeling system and continuous replacement of the root with bone takes place. Internal (root canal) replacement resorption leading to infraocclusion can be arrested by pulp extirpation and root filling. In case of external (root surface) replacement resorption, the condition

Table 1 Stimulatory and inhibitory factors associated with osteoclast activity. After Lindskog et al.[1]

Factors	Stimulatory	Inhibitory
Hormones		
Androgens		+
Calcitonin		+
Calcitonin gene-related peptide		+
Glucocorticoids	+	
Oestrogen		+
Parathyroid hormone	+	
PTHrP	+	
Thyroid hormone	+	
1,25(OH)$_2$vitamin D3	+	
Cytokines and growth factors		
Bone morphogenic proteins, BMP	+	
Colony stimulating factors, CSF-1	+	
Endothelin-1	+	
Epidermal growth factor, EGF	+	
Fibroblast growth factor, FGF	+	+
	+	
Granulocyte macrophage colony stimulating factor, GM-CSF		
Insulin-like growth factor, IGF-1	+	
Interferon		+
Interleukin	+	
Kinins	+	
Macrophage inflammatory protein 1-α, MIP-1α	+	
Nitric oxide		+
Platelet-derived growth factor, PDGF	+	
Prostaglandins	+	
Transforming growth factor alpha, TGF-α	+	
Tissue inhibitors of metalloproteinases, TIMP		+
Transforming growth factor β, TGF-β	+	
Tumour necrosis factor, TNF-α	+	
Tumour necrosis factor β, TNF-β	+	
Substance P	+	
Vasoactive intestinal peptide, VIP	+	
Pharmaceuticals		
Bisphosphonates		+
Corticosteroids		+

can, as a rule, not be successfully treated today, at least if the ankylosis has reached a certain extent. Endodontic interventions and placement of calcium hydroxide may slow, but not arrest, the ankylosis process. It also carries the risk of accelerating the process.[8]

Osteoclast as a Member of the Repair Team after Injury

In revascularization situations in bone and teeth, the osteoclast and ingrowing vessels work jointly together as part of the wound healing module,[2] the osteoclast having the role of creating space for the new vascular tissue to grow into narrow spaces (root canal). This is later reversed by apposition of new hard tissue (cementum or bone). This phenomenon has been termed **transient apical breakdown, transient marginal breakdown, transient ankylosis, and transient internal surface resorption** according to the location of the process (Figure 6).[2,9] These events are rather frequently seen after luxation injuries and root fractures with displacement, where avascular but sterile pulp tissue is replaced in conjunction with the revascularization process.

ENDODONTIC IMPLICATIONS
It is very important to consider that the radiographic signs of osteoclastic activity are not always signs of ongoing infection but may represent an actual healing process and therefore only require observation.

Osteoclast as a Defense Cell against Microbial Invasion

In the periodontal ligament (PDL) area, a constant fight takes place between microbial invasion in the cervical area owing to plaque accumulation and periodontal pocket formation and in the apical area owing to bacterial accumulation in the root canal. In both cases, a series of osteoclast-promoting signals are released by bacteria and inflammatory cells, stimulating osteoclast generation and accelerating osteoclast activities (Figure 7).[1,10] This typically results after some time in marginal or periapical bone loss. Likewise, if a combined injury has happened to the root surface and the pulp canal has become infected, the osteoclast may get a dual stimulation to resorb the root surface. In fact, the first tissue damage to the root surface initiates resorption, and after penetration of the cementum, the osteoclasts are triggered by bacterial toxins from the root canal through the dentinal tubules to continue to resorb dentin (see later).

ENDODONTIC IMPLICATIONS
When radiographic signs of apical or marginal breakdown or external root resorption become evident, an infection-related root resorption caused by necrotic and infected pulp tissue should be suspected (see

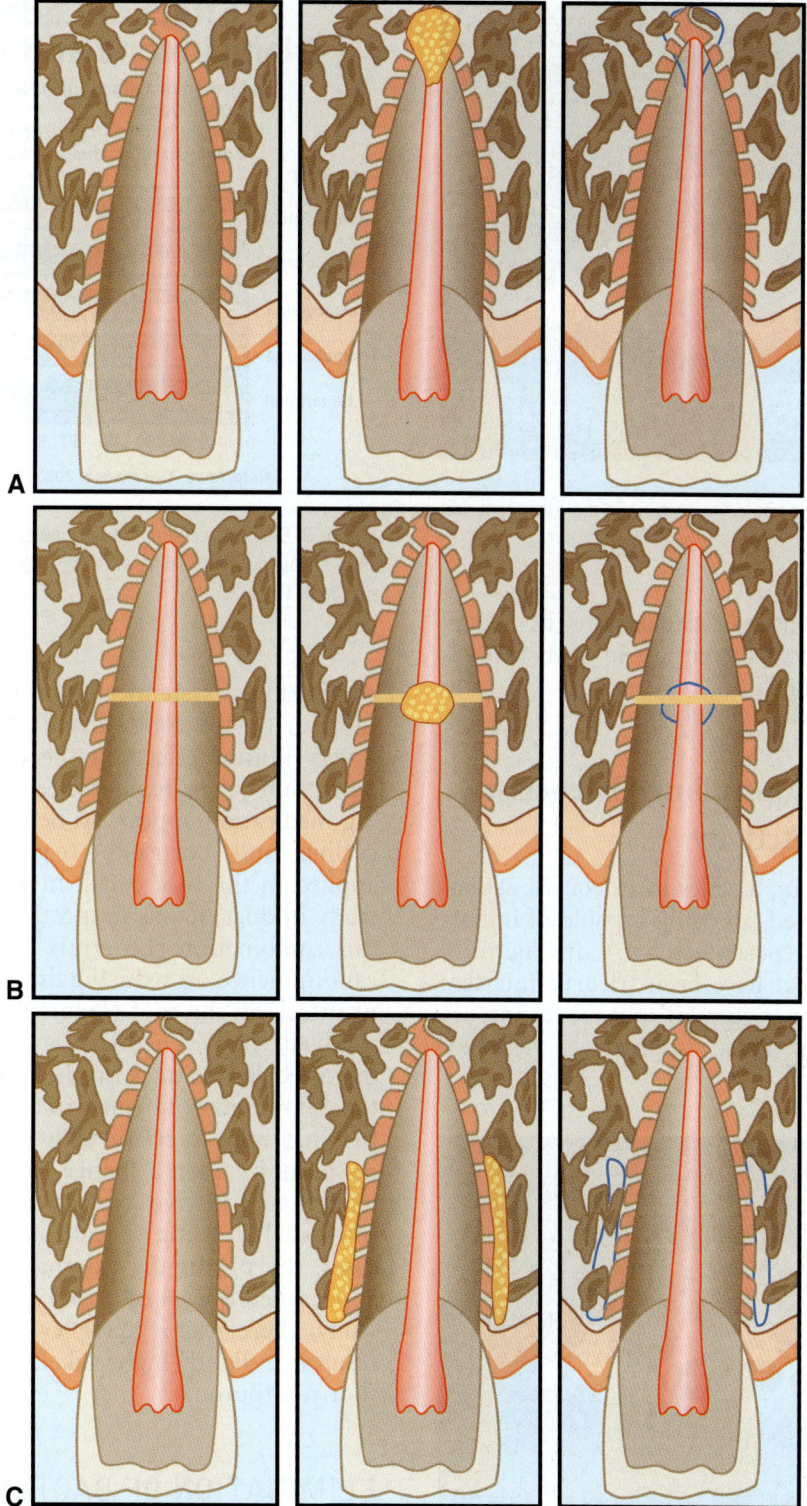

Figure 6 Examples of various transient pathologic events. ***A,*** Transient apical breakdown. ***B,*** Transient internal surface resorption. ***C,*** Transient marginal breakdown.

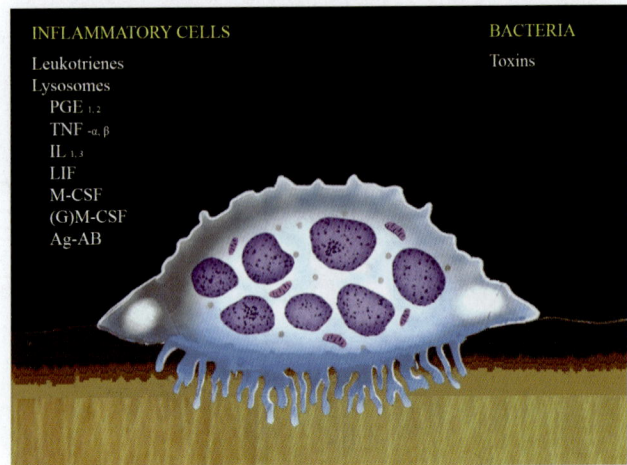

Figure 7 Osteoclast activators related to bacteria in the root canal and dentinal tubules.

Chapter 36, "Endodontic Considerations in Dental Trauma"). Endodontic intervention in such cases is indicated and most beneficial.

Methods for Controlling Osteoclast Activity

During the past century, a series of osteoclast activators have been identified, all being capable of initiating and activating osteoclast activity.[11] In Figure 8, some of the agents that have been tried to interfere with or inactivate these triggers of root resorption are shown.[2,11] (Figure 8). These approaches, whether

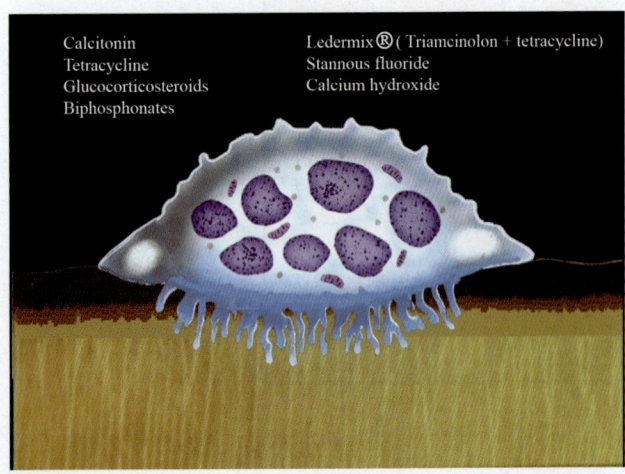

Figure 8 Example of various medicaments used to influence osteoclast activity.

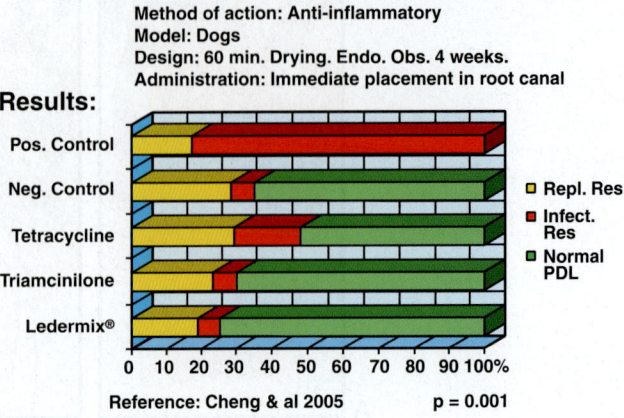

Figure 9 Effect of Ledermix (triamcinolone and tetracycline) on periodontal ligament (PDL) healing after replantation. Reproduced with permission from Chen H et al.[12]

administered systemically or topically (in the root canal or on the root surface), have had either no or a very limited effect on the osteoclastic activity on resorption-prone replanted teeth.[11] The most promising medication appears to be a combination of tetracycline and cortisone (e.g., Ledermix) topically applied in the root canal. In a detailed experimental study in dogs, it was found that the cortisone part of this combination (Ledermix®) had the most significant influence on reducing the extent of the osteoclastic attack on the root (Figure 9).[12]

An alternative chemical way of arresting or preventing osteoclastic attack on the root surface is to change the dentin environment from a neutral pH to a basic pH that may interfere with the osteoclast's mineral dissolution.[1] Such a change has been shown in several in vitro and in vivo experiments to be possible by an intracanal dressing of calcium hydroxide.[8] In these cases, the pH of the external portion of the dentin approached a level of 9 to 10 pH.[13,14] In one clinical study, there was a tendency for an elevated pH to result in a slightly higher likelihood of healing external root resorption.[8]

ELIMINATION OF BACTERIA RESPONSIBLE FOR INFECTION-RELATED RESORPTION

Only one clinical study has investigated the use of antibiotics for infection-related resorption, and it appears that short-term use of antibiotics (a mixture

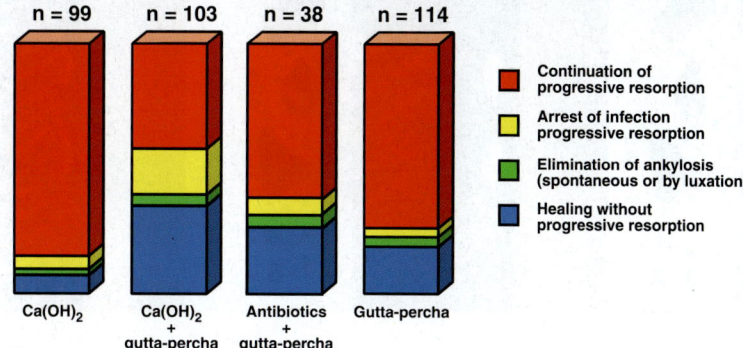

Figure 10 Efficacy of various endodontic procedures to reduce progressive root resorption after replantation in a clinical study of 334 replanted human teeth. Reproduced with permission from Andreasen JO et al.[8]

of neomycin and bacitracin) has almost the same capacity as short-term use of calcium hydroxide in reducing the extent of infection-related resorption in replanted human teeth (Figure 10).[8] Owing to the possible side effects of antibiotics (allergy), it seems inappropriate today to use antibiotics for these purposes. In the future, there might be an indication for disinfection of the root canal and dentin with antibiotics in cases in which pulp revascularization is the intent (see Chapter 36). Calcium hydroxide, however, is not able in all cases to eliminate bacteria in the root canal, which seems to be necessary for successful revascularization.

Types of Root Resorption

The following short, systematic synopsis presents the various root resorption types and how they relate to endodontic practice. The reader is also referred to a series of survey articles dealing with diagnosis and treatment of root resorption.[4,15–22]

External Surface Resorption (Repair-Related Resorption)

ETIOLOGY

This resorption entity represents the healing response to chronic and/or acute injury in the PDL, affecting the cells adjacent to the root surface. The typical situation in which **acute** repair-related resorption occurs appears to be after luxation injuries such as concussion, subluxation, and lateral luxation. It can also occur following intrusion and replantation of avulsed teeth, where it may affect all parts of a root, and in root fractures, where it is observed adjacent to the fracture line. This type of resorption also frequently occurs after **chronic** injury affecting the PDL and associated with orthodontic treatment, traumatic occlusion, and pressure from developing cysts or apical granulomas and ectopically erupting teeth. When the trauma and/or pressure has been discontinued, spontaneous healing

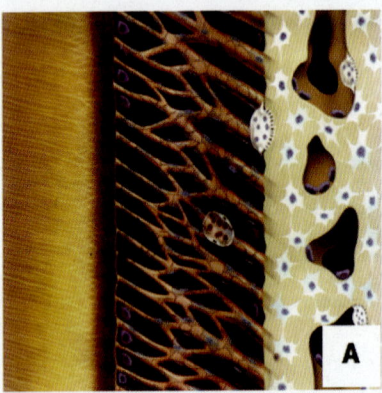 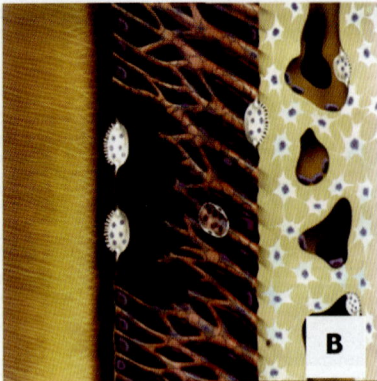 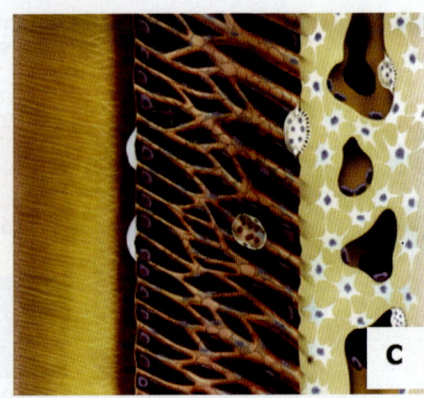

Figure 11 *A,* Pathogenesis of surface resorption (repair-related resorption): healing with minor injury to the periodontal ligament. *B,* The injury site is resorbed by macrophages and osteoclasts. The osteoclasts have exposed factors and other soluble molecules in dentin, such as insulin-like growth factor 1, transforming growth factor {158}, platelet-derived growth factor, bone morphogenetic proteins, fibroblast growth factor 2, and A4 (amelogenin gene splice products). These molecules may serve as stimulators for cementoblasts. *C,* Subsequent repair takes place by the formation of new cementum and insertion of Sharpey fibers. Reproduced with permission from Andreasen JO and Løwschall H.[2]

takes place, which is a typical feature of repair-related resorption.[2]

Pathogenesis

The injured tissue adjacent to the root and surface cementum are removed by macrophages and osteoclasts. These events take 2 to 4 weeks. Repair is by progenitor cells from the adjacent PDL. New cementum is formed with insertion of PDL fibers (Figure 11).[2]

RADIOGRAPHIC FINDINGS

After 2 to 4 weeks, a localized widening of the PDL space can be seen owing to loss of surface layers of the cementum and the bony alveolar socket. At this time, the radiographic images are similar to infection-related root surface resorption. Subsequently, however, healing takes place with reformation of the PDL and deposition of hard tissues. Radiographically, slight cavitations may be seen on the root surface.[16,23,24] However, most repair-related root surface resorptions have such a limited size that they cannot be recognized radiographically.[25,26]

ENDODONTIC IMPLICATIONS

Owing to their nature, being primarily related to a periodontal injury, endodontic intervention is not indicated for teeth with this type of root resorption. However, a diagnostic problem may exist since a progressing infection-related resorptive process may have an identical debut.

TREATMENT

If trauma and/or pressure are eliminated, there is almost 100% repair. If the root apex has been resorbed, excessive mobility becomes a problem if the root is shorter than 12 mm.[27]

External Infection-Related Resorption (Inflammatory Root Resorption)

ETIOLOGY

This resorption entity was described in a clinical and histologic study in 1965 of avulsed and replanted teeth.[23,24] Infection-related resorption represents a combined injury to the pulp and PDL and where bacteria, primarily located in the pulp space and in dentinal tubules, trigger osteoclastic activity on the root surface. This type of resorption can affect all parts of the root. Infection-related resorption is typically diagnosed 2 to 4 weeks after injury. The resorption is a rapidly progressing process that may result in total resorption of the root within a few months. It is almost exclusively related to acute trauma and is especially common after intrusion and replantation of avulsed teeth.[16]

PATHOGENESIS

In the event that the initial resorption has penetrated the cementum and exposed dentinal tubules, toxins from bacteria present in the dentinal tubules and/or the infected root canal can be diffused via the exposed

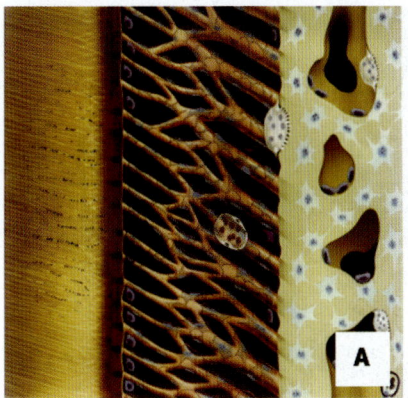 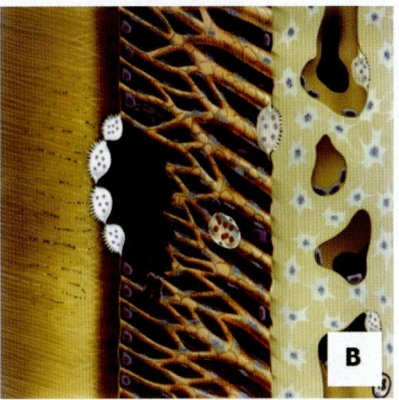 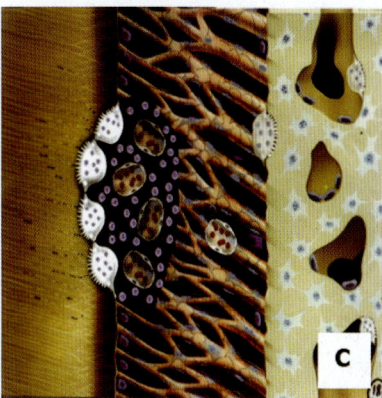

Figure 12 *A,* Pathogenesis of inflammatory resorption (infection-related resorption): healing with moderate or extensive injury to the periodontal ligament and associated infection in the pulp and/or dentinal tubules. *B,* The initial injury to the root surface triggers a macrophage and osteoclast attack on the root surface. *C,* Osteoclasts are exposed to toxins from bacteria located in the root canal and dentinal tubules, such as lipopolysaccharide, muramyl dipeptide, and lipoteichoic acid. These toxins serve as direct activators of osteoclastic activity. The resorption process is accelerated, and granulation tissue ultimately invades the root canal. Reproduced with permission from Andreasen JO and Løwschall H.[2]

tubules to the PDL (Figure 12).[2,28] This results in continuation of the osteoclastic process and an associated inflammation in the PDL, leading to resorption of adjacent alveolar bone. The process usually progresses, and root dentin is resorbed, until the root canal is exposed. If bacteria are eliminated from the root canal and dentinal tubules by endodontic therapy, the resorptive process will be arrested.[27–39] The resorption cavity will then be filled in with cementum or bone, according to the type of vital tissue found next to the resorption site (PDL or bone marrow–derived tissue).

CLINICAL FINDINGS

The tooth undergoing infection-related root resorption will have increased mobility and have a dull percussion tone. Sometimes the tooth may be extruded. Sensibility testing gives no response, and sometimes a sinus tract develops.

RADIOGRAPHIC FINDINGS

Infection-related resorption is typically diagnosed 2 to 4 weeks after injury and appears as progressive cavitations involving the root and adjacent alveolar bone. The resorption is a rapidly progressing event that may result in total loss of root structure after only a few months, particularly in young children (Figure 13).

ENDODONTIC IMPLICATIONS

This type of resorption represents a combined periodontal and pulpal injury and requires immediate endodontic treatment to control or remove the osteoclast-promoting factors (bacterial toxins from the root canal system).

TREATMENT

The treatment goal is to remove or destroy bacteria in the root canal and dentinal tubules to allow healing to take place in the entire periradicular space (root surface, PDL, and adjacent alveolar bone). The bacteria are best destroyed by using $Ca(OH)_2$ as an intracanal medicament. A side effect, however, of using $Ca(OH)_2$ for a long term (> 30 days) is weakening of the root structure in **immature** teeth; this may lead to cervical root fractures. This is a risk that has been found to be as high as 66 to 72% in two clinical studies.[31,32] In **mature** teeth, the problem apparently does not exist.[31] The endodontic technique therefore varies according to the maturity of the tooth (see Chapter 36).

MATURE TEETH

In fully developed teeth with infection-related resorption, endodontic treatment should include prophylactic extirpation of the pulp in replanted avulsed teeth. Biomechanical canal preparation should include the use of sodium hypochlorite and $Ca(OH)_2$. The latter can be expected to have accomplished its task of disinfection so that the canal can be filled 2 to 3 weeks after treatment.

IMMATURE TEETH

In situations in which the pulp becomes necrotic before the root is fully developed, the apical opening

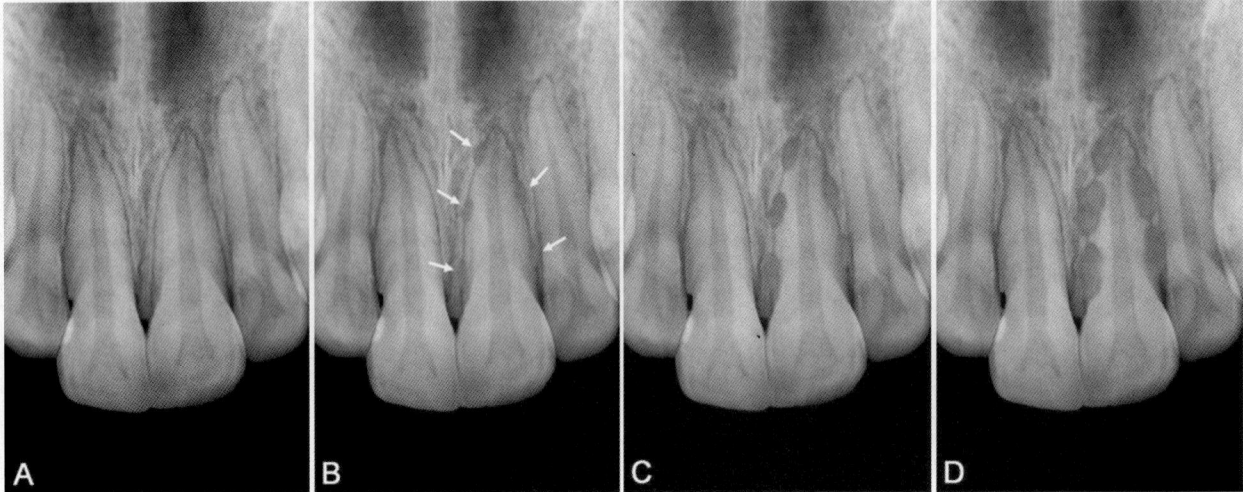

Figure 13 Progression of infection-related resorption. Reproduced with permission from Andreasen JO et al.[55] *A,* Replanted avulsed maxillary left central incisor. *B,* Beginning resorption from trauma-related inflammation in the periodontal ligament (arrows). *C,* Infected necrotic pulp tissue stimulates continuing resorption. *D,* Failure to control infection in the necrotic pulp can rapidly lead total tooth loss.

is often too large to create a resistance to retain the root canal filling. Apexification procedures using calcium hydroxide have been performed with good success. The disadvantage of using calcium hydroxide for apexification is that it takes many months to obtain enough of an apical barrier to allow placement of a root canal filling. Additionally, it appears that long-term use of Ca(OH)$_2$ can weaken dentin, possibly by dissolving its organic component and thereby resulting in cervical root fracture on even slight impacts or normal use.[33] By using mineral trioxide aggregate (MTA) as a physical barrier apically, a root canal filling can be placed immediately without waiting for a biologic response (Figure 14). Minimizing exposure of root dentin to calcium hydroxide results in less damage to the dentin.[34,35]

PROGNOSIS

It needs to be understood that dentin lost through resorption cannot be replaced by new dentin (at least with today's treatment approaches). Healing occurs by arresting the resorption process and replacement with either a layer of new cementum or bone and establishment of new PDL. The amount of healing has been found to be 88% in two clinical studies.[36,37]

External Trauma-Related Replacement Resorption (Ankylosis)

This PDL complication represents a sequel to a defect in or injury to the PDL cells, including the

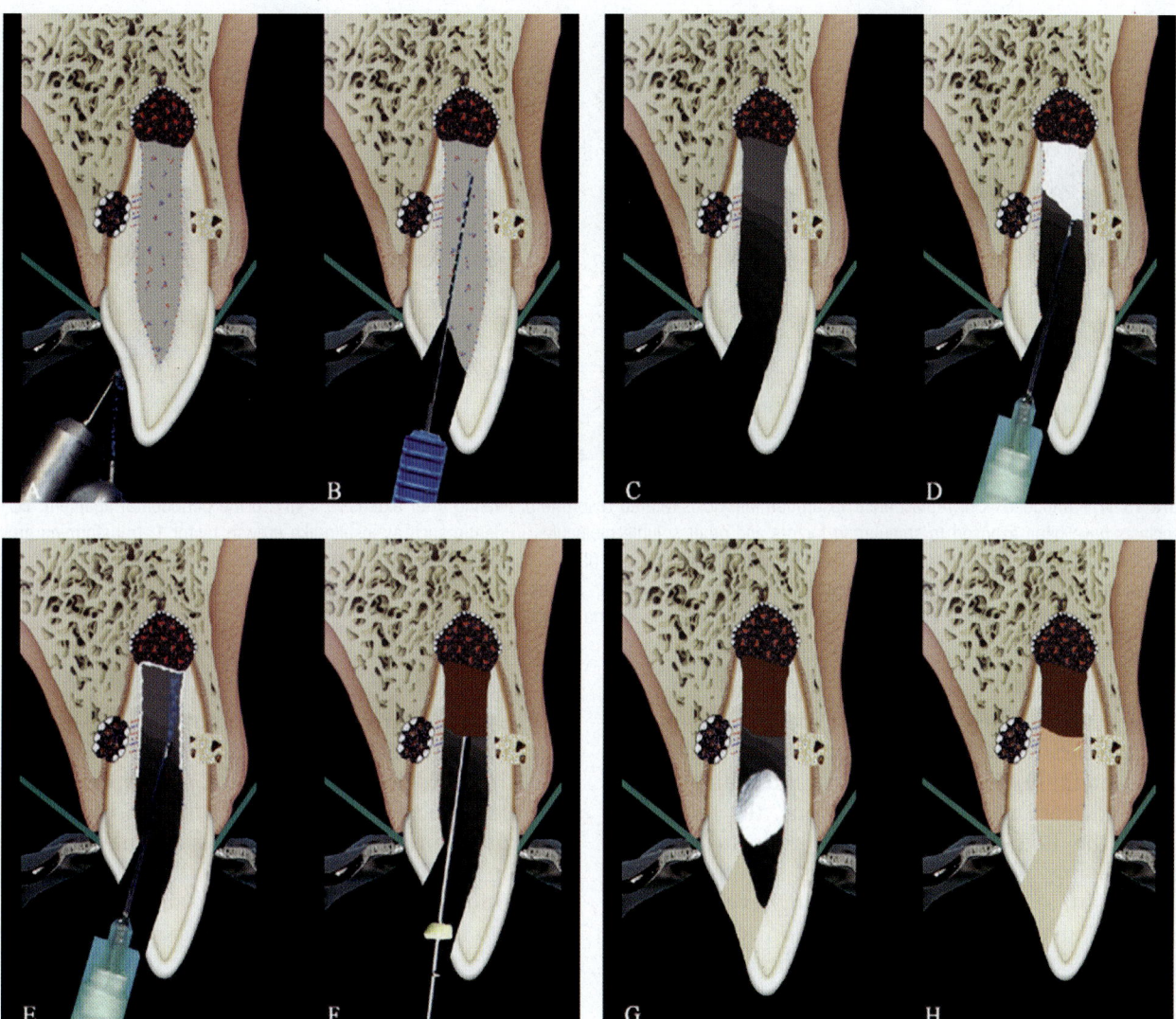

Figure 14 Combined calcium hydroxide and mineral trioxide aggregate (MTA) treatment of a traumatized permanent tooth with immature root formation. ***A,*** The tooth is isolated with rubber dam, the crown is disinfected, and an access cavity to the root canal is prepared. ***B,*** Extirpation of necrotic pulp tissue is done to a level apically, where fresh bleeding from healthy tissue is encountered. This can be anywhere from several millimeters from the apex to flush with the apical foramen. ***C,*** Root canal preparation in developing teeth requires a conservative approach so as to preserve as much root dentin as possible. Hence, minimal canal shaping is appropriate. ***D,*** Disinfection of the root canal with sodium hypochlorite is followed by short-term (approximately 2 to 4 weeks) interim dressing with calcium hydroxide. The use of calcium hydroxide allows acceptable disinfection of the root canal system and provides a dry root canal, free of seepage of apical exudates. The coronal access opening must be sealed with a dependable temporary restoration. ***E,*** At the next visit, the calcium hydroxide is removed and the canal is thoroughly irrigated with saline or sodium hypochlorite to obtain a debris-free canal. Small increments of the MTA-water mixture are introduced into the canal and gently condensed. Length can be controlled using a rubber stopper on a plugger. No harm is done, however, with slight overfilling. ***F,*** When properly condensed, the apical MTA plug should be at least 4 mm thick. The entire canal can be filled with MTA (to the cervical level), or the coronal part of the canal can later be filled with gutta-percha and sealer. ***G,*** To allow setting, a moistened (water) cotton pellet is placed in the access cavity, which is then sealed with a temporary filling material. Once set (usually within 4 to 6 hours), the canal can be conventionally filled. ***H,*** The temporary material and cotton pellet are removed, and the apical plug is checked for setting hardness; it should not be vigorously probed as the material can break. The canal is then irrigated, dried, and filled, followed by a bonded coronal composite restoration. Reproduced with permission from Bakland L.[35]

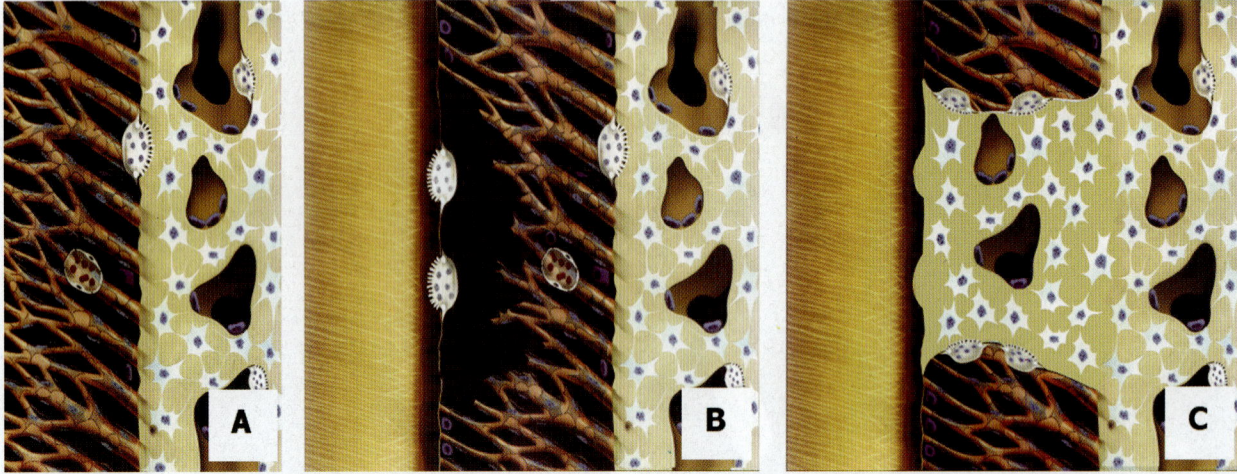

Figure 15 *A,* Pathogenesis of replacement resorption (ankylosis-related resorption): healing after extensive injury to the periodontal ligament. *B,* The osteoclasts have been exposed to stimulating factors and other soluble molecules in dentin such as insulin-like growth factor 1, transforming growth factor {158}, platelet-derived growth factor, bone morphogenetic proteins, fibroblast growth factor 2, and A4 (amelogenin gene splice products). These molecules may serve as stimulators for cementoblasts and/or osteoblasts.[2] *C,* Ankylosis is formed because healing occurs almost exclusively by cells from the alveolar wall. Reproduced with permission from Andreasen JO and Løwschall.[2]

cell layer next to the cementum.[2] The most frequent cause appears to be acute trauma (severe luxations such as lateral luxations, intrusions, and replantation of avulsed teeth).[2] In those situations, the homeostasis of the PDL is lacking. This leads to healing events taking place from adjacent healthy PDL, resulting in a normal PDL. Healing events from the bony alveolus result in creation of a bony bridge between the socket wall and the root surface (Figure 15).

In situations of moderately sized injuries (1–4 mm^2), an initial ankylosis forms. If the tooth is allowed functional mobility by the use of a nonrigid splint or no splinting, small areas of resorption can later be replaced with new cementum and PDL attachment (transient ankylosis).[22,38–42] In more extensive injuries (> 4 mm^2), a progressive ankylosis takes place. This implies that the tooth becomes an integral part of the bone remodeling system. The entire process includes osteoclastic resorption dependent on bone remodeling processes, parathyroid hormone–induced resorption, remodeling owing to function, and resorption owing to bacteria present in the gingival area and/or the root canal.[2] All of these processes are very active in children and lead to gradual infraocclusion and arrested development of the alveolar process.[43] As a result, this combination of resorption processes leads to loss of ankylosed teeth within 1 to 5 years. In older individuals, replacement resorption is significantly slower and often allows a tooth to function for much longer periods of time (ie, 5–20 years), and the position of the tooth in the arch remains the same (similar to an implant).[44]

CLINICAL FINDINGS

A tooth undergoing ankylosis-related root resorption appears very firm in its socket, eliciting a high metallic sound on percussion. This can be demonstrated 4 to 6 weeks post-trauma.[42,45]

RADIOGRAPHIC FINDINGS

The resorption process is in response to extensive damage to the layer of the PDL closest to the root surface. Owing to the predominant healing response from the bony socket wall, ankylosis takes place.

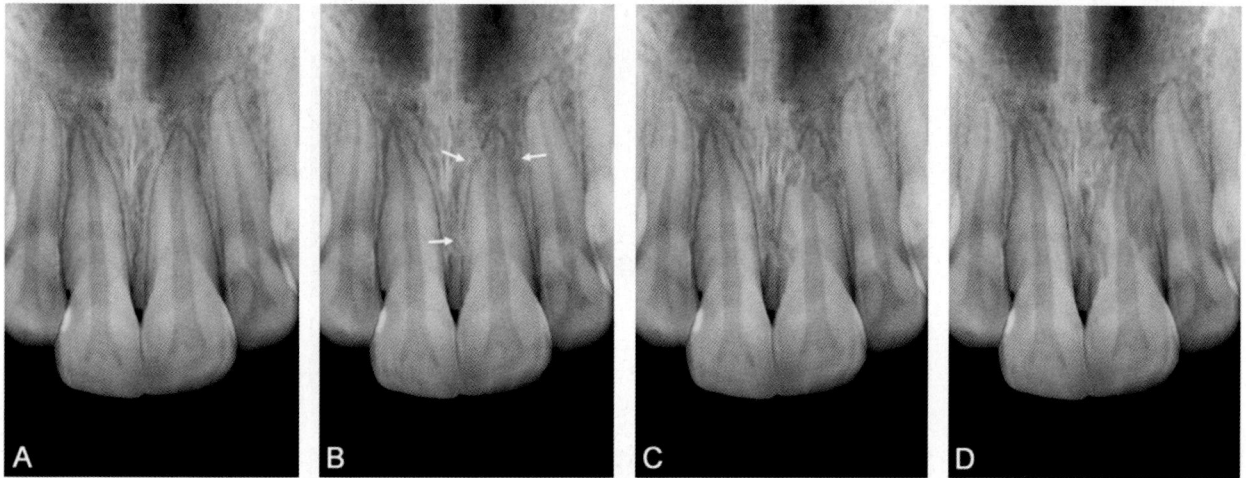

Figure 16 Progression of replacement resorption (ankylosis). Reproduced with permission from Andreasen JO et al.[55] **A,** Delayed replantation of maxillary left central incisor. **B,** Initial ankylosis-related resorption due to necrosis of the periodontal ligament cells. **C,** The root is gradually being replaced by bone. **D,** Eventually the entire root is replaced by bone.

Because of the normal remodeling characteristic of bone, the root structure is gradually replaced by bone (Figure 16). Ankylosis is a frequent occurrence after intrusion and replantation of avulsed teeth. It can usually be diagnosed radiographically within 2 months after injury and clinically within 1 month by a high percussion sound.[42,45]

ENDODONTIC IMPLICATIONS

Endodontic therapy cannot arrest the progressive ankylosis-related resorption process. If the pulp is vital, no endodontic procedures should be undertaken. In the case of an associated pulp necrosis, the treatment described for infection-related root resorption is applicable to control the progression of the process of replacement resorption.[8]

TREATMENT

In **adolescents,** the ankylosed tooth will fail to erupt and will gradually go into infraposition. The younger the age, the more pronounced is the infraposition (Figure 17).

Presently, there are five treatment approaches:

1. Decoronation (to maintain and augment the alveolar process)
2. Luxation of the tooth (breaking of ankylosis sites)
3. Vertical distraction
4. Prosthetic elongation
5. Acceptance of the resorbing tooth

Of the above approaches, the decoronation treatment is very suitable in children and adolescence, when significant remaining alveolar growth is

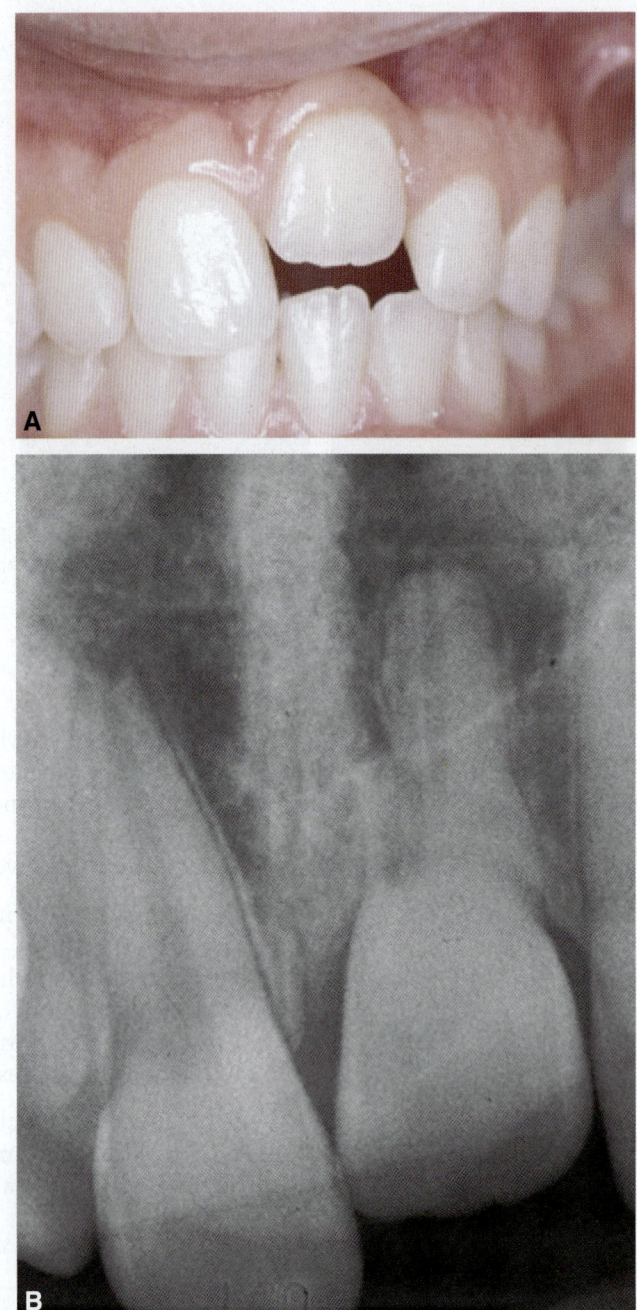

Figure 17 Infrapositioned maxillary central incisor initially intruded at the age of 9. *A*, A clinical photograph shows the position of the tooth at age 13 years. *B*, A radiograph shows the extent of ankylosis-related resorption. The pulp retained vitality, which is not unusual in teeth with ankylosis-related resorption.

expected. The procedure involves removal of the crown of the tooth (leaving what remains of the root), allowing continued vertical growth of the alveolus.[46–49] If the crown is surgically removed slightly below the cervical bone level and the root filling or pulp tissue is removed, the remaining root will maintain the labiolingual content of the alveolar process. The reformation of the interdental fibers, dentoperiosteal fibers, and periosteum will lead to a normalization of the bone level.[48] Owing to the ankylosis-related resorption of the remaining root with bone replacement, the alveolar structure will

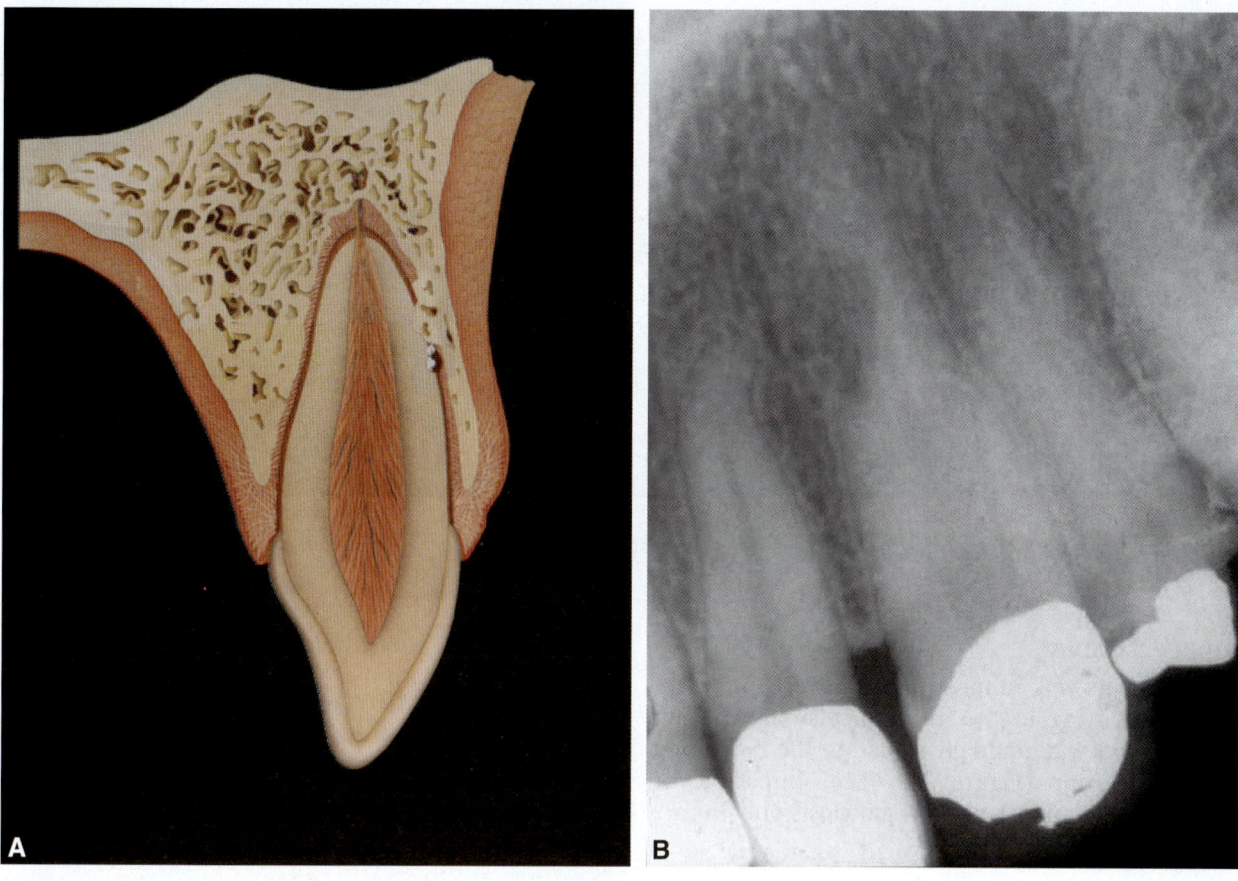

Figure 18 External spontaneous ankylosis resorption. ***A***, Graphic illustration of spontaneous ankylotic resorption. ***B***, Clinical example of such resorption.

be optimal for implants placed later when growth has been completed.[46–49]

External Spontaneous Ankylotic Resorption

ETIOLOGY
This type of ankylosis may affect one or a few primary or permanent teeth. The etiology is presently not known but is suspected to be related to the instability of the RANK-RANKL-OPG system (Figure 18).[2]

PATHOGENESIS
The ankylosis-related resorption process leads to infraposition of the involved teeth in young individuals and in all cases to gradual substitution of the root substance with bone.

CLINICAL FINDINGS

Primary Dentition
This resorption type especially affects the primary molars, and the mandibular second primary molar is most prone to be involved (20%).[50] Ankylosis leads to gradual infraposition and tilting of neighboring teeth.[50]

Permanent Dentition
The first and second permanent molars are most prone to show this type of resorption. These molars will, in young individuals, show a gradual infraposition, and the percussion tone is high and metallic.[6,7,51]

RADIOGRAPHIC FINDINGS

Primary Molars
The ankylosis process starts to affect the interdental area and gradually spreads to the remaining part of the root.

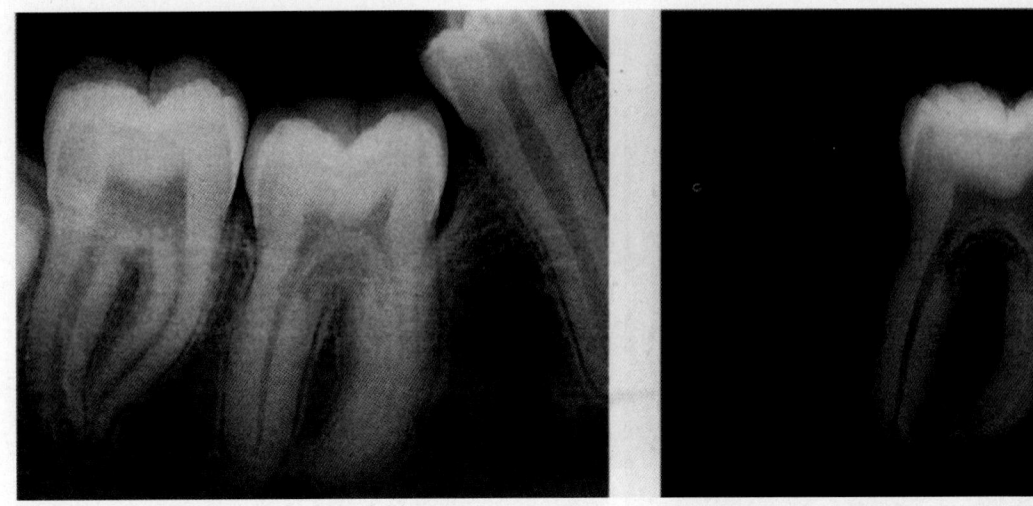

Figure 19 Spontaneous ankylosis affecting the interdental area of a first molar. Reproduced with permission from Andreasen JO, Kurol J.[51]

Permanent Molars

The first molars will, in most cases, show replacement resorption starting in the intraradicular area. From this location, it will gradually spread to the remaining part of the root (Figure 19). Semi-impacted or impacted third molars will show ankylosis only in rare cases.

ENDODONTIC IMPLICATIONS

This is primarily a PDL problem, and endodontic intervention may actually aggravate the aggressive nature of the ankylosis process.

TREATMENT

Primary Dentition

If diagnosed early, decoronation is a reasonable option. If diagnosed late in adolescence, the crown may be rebuilt to prevent overeruption of the antagonist.

Permanent Dentition

If diagnosed in early adolescence, the ankylosed tooth should be extracted. At later stages, the crown may be rebuilt with a restoration to achieve a functional occlusal level.

External Multiple Sites of Ankylosis- or Infection-Related Resorption

ETIOLOGY

These are very rare types of root resorptions; only a handful of new cases are reported each year in Denmark (6 million inhabitants). The etiology is suspected to be a defect in the RANK-RANKL-OPG system and a hereditary background is found in some cases.[2]

PATHOGENESIS

Any permanent tooth may become involved. The process takes place over 10 to 20 years. It usually affects a single group of teeth (premolars, molars) and gradually affects other groups of teeth.

RADIOGRAPHIC FINDINGS

The radiographic images will show cervical invasive resorption cavities that involve multiple teeth. The

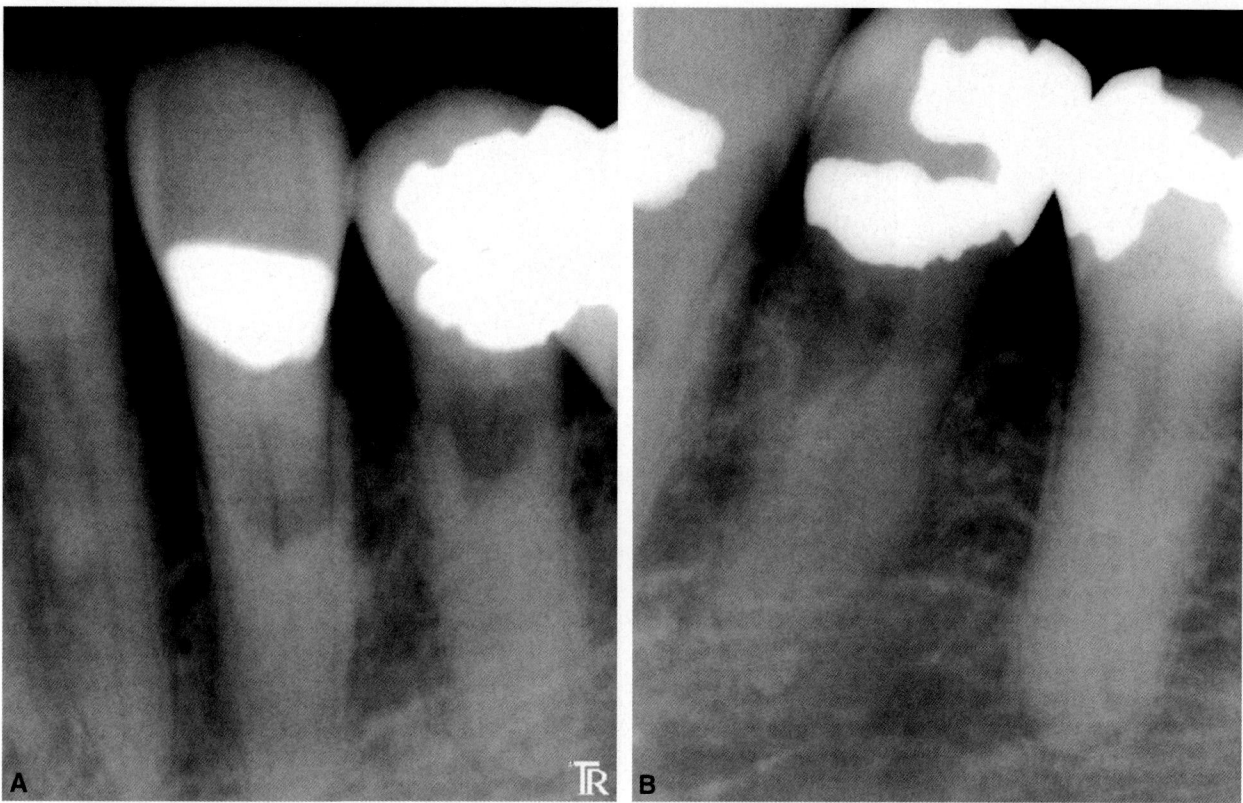

Figure 20 *A* and *B*, Multiple cervical invasive resorption cavities. This is sometimes referred to as idiopathic external root resorption because of uncertainty about etiology.

resorption process expands over time in all directions, resulting in the eventual breakdown of the involved teeth (Figure 20).

CLINICAL FINDINGS

In case of ankylosis, the tooth involved gives a high percussion tone. In case of inflammatory resorption, granulomatous tissue is found in the cervical region and is often recognized by a pink spot in that area of the crown.

ENDODONTIC IMPLICATIONS

Endodontic treatment may only promote the resorption process and is therefore not indicated.

TREATMENT

There is currently no predictable treatment available, so the gradual replacement of involved teeth with implants appears to be all that can be offered.

Cervical Invasive Resorption

ETIOLOGY

The cause of cervical invasive resorption may possibly be related to a defect in the cementoblast layer in its RANK-RANKL-OPG system.[2] In a large clinical study of 259 teeth with invasive cervical resorption, Heithersay found that 23% were related to orthodontic treatment, 15% to acute trauma, and 14% to a cervical restoration.[52]

PATHOGENESIS

The initial cervical resorption cavity gradually spreads and may progress in both an apical and a coronal direction, leading eventually to a tooth fracture.

CLINICAL FINDINGS

Often expansive lesions will show up as a "pink spot" next to the cervical margin (Figure 21C).

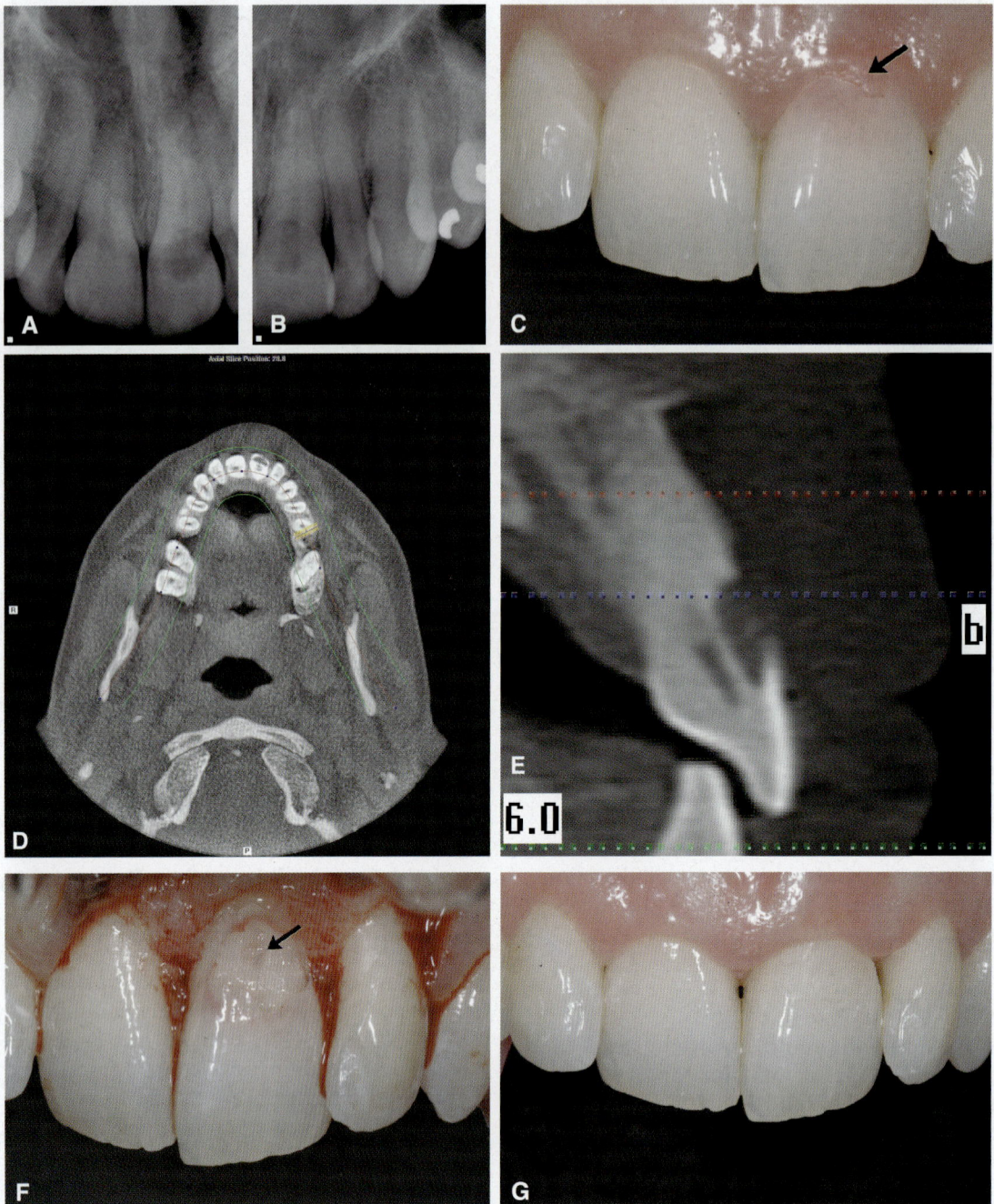

Figure 21 Maxillary central incisor with cervical invasive resorption. The tooth was intact, with no carious lesions. Possible history of trauma many years earlier. *A* and *B,* Periapical radiographs show two views of the well-delineated lesion. *C,* Clinical photograph shows the location of the resorptive lesion (*arrow*), giving the tooth a "pink tooth" appearance. *D* and *E,* Two views obtained with a cone beam three-dimensional imaging system (I-CAT, Imaging Science Int., Inc., Hatfield, PA). Note the ability to clearly determine the location and size of the lesion and relationship to the pulp. Cervical invasive resorptions do not invade the pulps directly, something that can be demonstrated with imaging of this nature. *F,* Removal of the granulation tissue in the resorptive lesion shows a thin layer of dentin covering the pulp (*arrow*). *G,* Appearance after restoration with dentin-bonded restoration. If pulpal symptoms develop, endodontic treatment is indicated. Reproduced with permission from the Endodontic Clinic, Loma Linda University, CA.

RADIOGRAPHIC FINDINGS

A cervical bowl-shaped lesion is the start of an invasive progression of resorption in coronal and apical directions. The pulp canal is not invaded in the initial phases (Figure 21A, B, D, and E).

Endodontic Implications

The pathology is entirely related to a PDL defect and therefore does not primarily imply endodontic considerations. However, the invasive nature of the resorption process will finally encroach on the pulp cavity, necessitating endodontic treatment.[53]

TREATMENT

A surgical flap can be raised to remove the granulation tissue and to place a dentin-bonded restoration (Figure 21F and G). The prognosis appears to be strongly related to the apical extension of the resorption process (Figure 22).[54]

Internal Surface Resorption

ETIOLOGY

Internal surface resorption can be found in areas where revascularization occurs, such as in fracture lines of root fractures and in the apical part of the root canal of a luxated tooth undergoing revascularization (see Figure 6B and Figure 23).[55]

PATHOGENESIS

Osteoclastic activity is part of the process, along with the formation of granulation tissue.

RADIOGRAPHIC FINDINGS

Radiographically, there appears to be a temporary widening of the root canal.

ENDODONTIC IMPLICATIONS

It is very important to consider that this resorption process is a sign of progressing pulp healing and that any endodontic intervention may arrest this process.

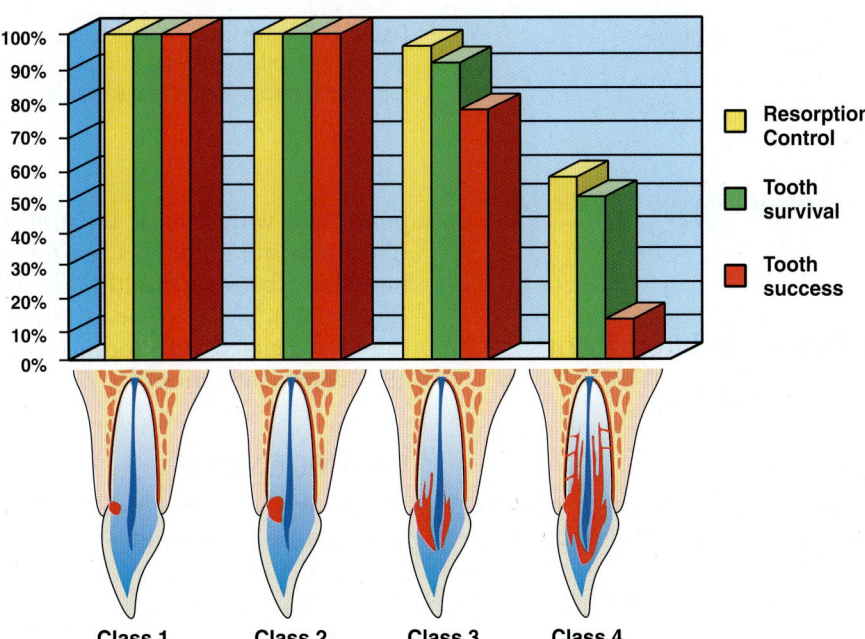

Figure 22 Prognosis of treatment related to the initial extent of cervical invasive resorption. Reproduced with permission from Heithersay GS.[53]

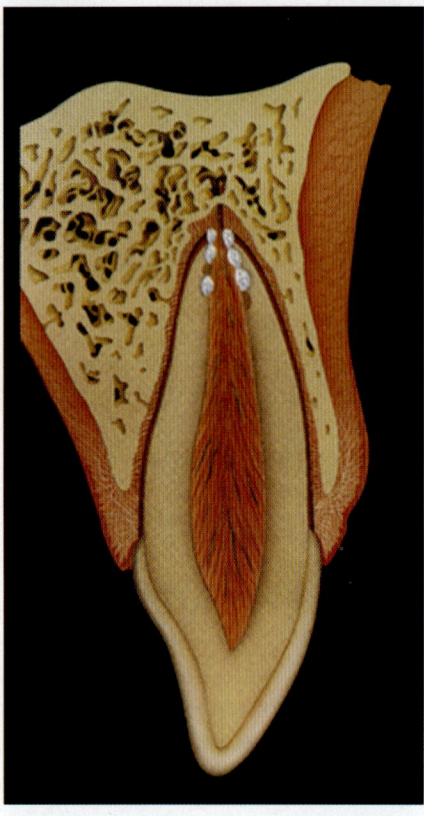

Figure 23 Internal (root canal) surface resorption.

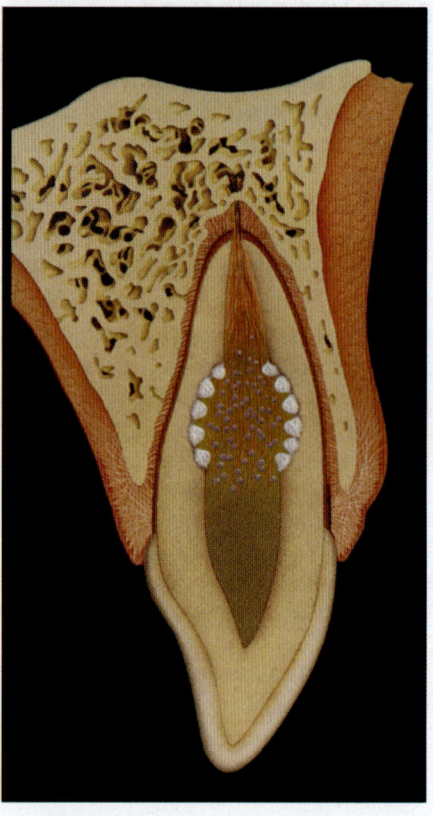

Figure 24 Internal infection-related root resorption. The resorption site represents resorbing granulation tissue interposed between vital (apically) and diseased (coronally) pulp tissue.

TREATMENT
No treatment is recommended except periodic observation.

Internal Infection-Related Root Resorption

ETIOLOGY
Coronal to the resorption site in the pulp, necrotic infected tissue (root canal and dentinal tubules or pulp tissue with chronic inflammation) is found. The resorption site represents resorbing granulation tissue interposed between healthy and diseased pulp tissue (Figure 24).[55] This type of resorption can also be found associated with tooth infractions (see Chapter 19, "Tooth Infractions").

PATHOGENESIS
The resorptive process will gradually expand, leading to a fracture of the root.

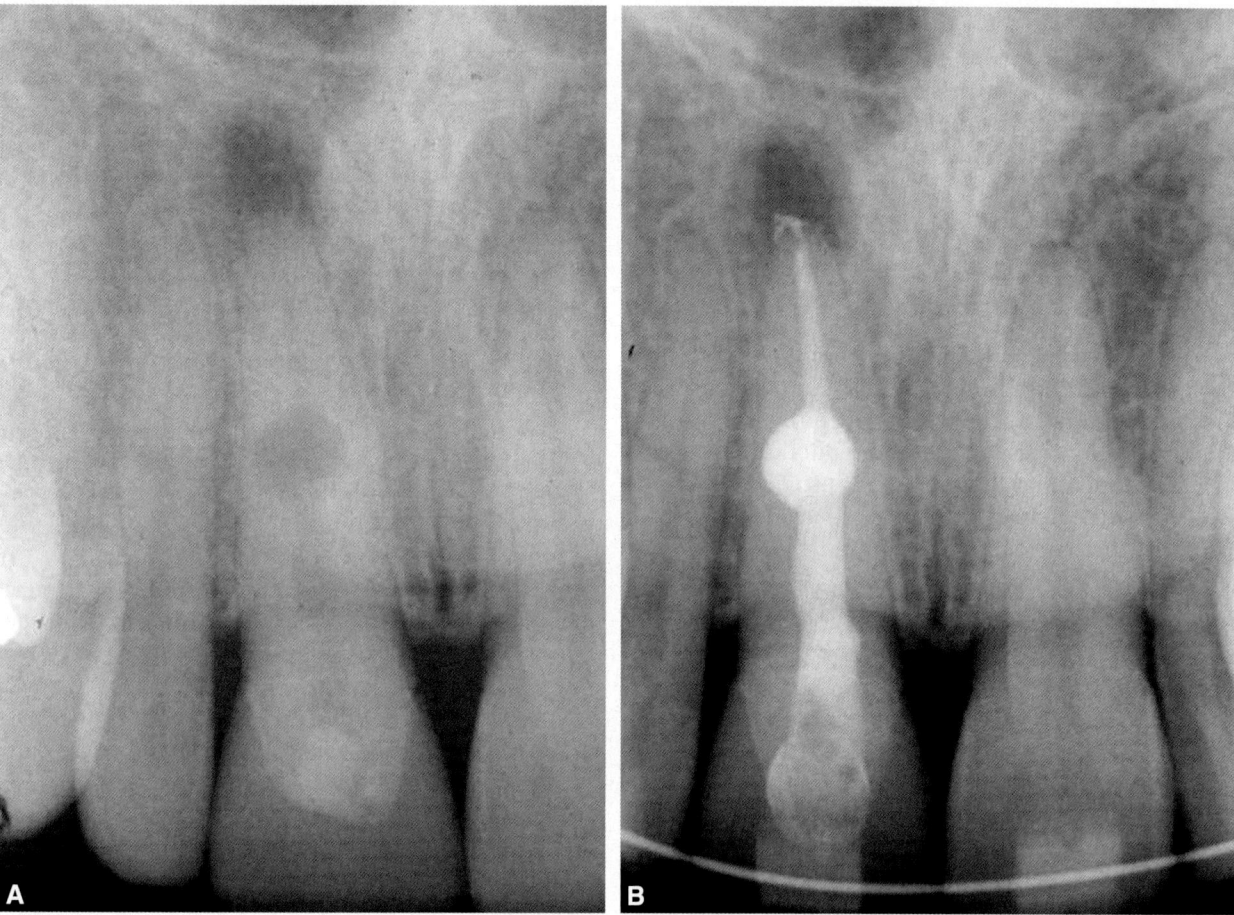

Figure 25 Teeth with internal root resorption can be treated successfully with any of the many endodontic techniques that allow filling material to be compacted into canal irregularities. ***A,*** Preoperative radiograph of a maxillary central incisor with internal resorption midroot. ***B,*** Radiograph after completion of the endodontic treatment procedure. Courtesy of Dr. Steve Morrow, Loma Linda University, CA.

TREATMENT

Endodontic treatment is appropriate and requires a technique that allows management of the resorbed area of the root canal (Figure 25).

Internal Replacement Resorption

ETIOLOGY

When damaged pulp tissue is replaced as part of a healing process, tissue metaplasia may take place, leading to formation of bone tissue in the pulp canal. The damage to the pulp tissue is usually related to trauma, and the damaged pulp tissue is replaced with an ingrowth of new tissue, which includes bone-derived cells.[54]

PATHOGENESIS

The root will gradually be replaced with bone. In some cases, the bone replacement will spontaneously arrest.

CLINICAL FINDINGS

The teeth are asymptomatic, but if ankylosis occurs, the teeth will gradually develop infraocclusion.

RADIOGRAPHIC FINDINGS

A dissecting resorptive area may be seen in the root canal; initially, the root canal appears intact. Mesiodistal and orthoradiographic exposures should verify the central location of the ankylosis site.

ENDODONTIC IMPLICATIONS

Since the eventual outcome of allowing this type of condition to continue is the loss of the tooth, it may be advantageous to treat the tooth endodontically, in spite of the fact that it may lead to a poor prognosis owing to the lack of root maturity.

Summary

With few exceptions, pathologic tooth resorptions have endodontic implications that knowledgeable clinicians can address. It is clear that most infection-related resorptions respond well to endodontic treatment. It is hoped that the future will provide avenues for successful management of ankylosis-related resorptions that currently are not available.

References

1. Lindskog SF, Dreyer CW, Pierce AM, et al. In: Andreasen JO, Andreasen FM, Andersson L, editors. Textbook and color atlas of traumatic injuries to the teeth. 4th ed. Oxford: Blackwell; 2007. pp. 137–71.
2. Andreasen JO, L{145}vschall H. Response of oral tissues to trauma. In: Andreasen JO, Andreasen FM, Andersson L, editors. Textbook and color atlas of traumatic injuries to the teeth. 4th ed. Copenhagen: Munksgaard; 2007. pp. 62–113.
3. Andreasen JO. Experimental dental traumatology: development of a model for external root resorption. Endod Dent Traumatol 1987;3:269–87.
4. Andreasen JO. Review of root resorption systems and models. Etiology of root resorption and the homeostatic mechanisms of the periodontal ligament. In: Davidovitch Z, editor. The biological mechanisms of tooth eruption and root resorption. Birmingham: EBSCO Media; 1988. pp. 9–21.
5. Marks SC, Svendsen H, Andreasen JO. Theories of tooth eruption. In: Andreasen JO, Kølsen Petersen J, Laskin DM, editors. Textbook and color atlas of tooth impactions. Copenhagen: Munksgaard; 1996. pp. 125–65.
6. Andreasen JO. Normal and abnormal tooth eruption in humans. In: Andreasen JO, Kølsen Petersen J, Laskin DM, editors. Textbook and color atlas of tooth impactions. Copenhagen: Munksgaard; 1996. pp. 49–64.
7. Andreasen JO. Treatment strategies for eruption disturbances. In: Andreasen JO, Kølsen Petersen J, Laskin DM, editors. Textbook and color atlas of tooth impactions. Copenhagen: Munksgaard;1996. pp. 66–86.
8. Andreasen JO, Borum MK, Loft Jacobsen H, Andreasen FM. Replantation of 400 traumatically avulsed permanent incisors. VI–Endodontic factors related to progression of root resorption. Dent Traumatol 2008. [Accepted]
9. Andreasen FM. Transient apical breakdown and its relation to color and sensibility changes after luxation injuries to teeth. Endod Dent Traumatol 1986;2:9–19.
10. Andreasen JO, Torabinejad M, Finkelman RD. Response of oral tissues to trauma and inflammation and mediators of hard tissue resorption. In: Andreasen JO, Andreasen FM, editors. Textbook and color atlas of traumatic injuries to the teeth. 3rd ed. Copenhagen: Munksgaard; 1993. pp. 77–133.
11. Trope M. Physical and chemical methods to optimize pulpal and periodontal healing after traumatic injuries. In: Andreasen JO, Andreasen FM, Andersson L, editors. Textbook and color atlas of traumatic injuries to the teeth. 4th ed. Oxford: Blackwell; 2007. pp. 172–96.
12. Chen H, Teixira FB, Ritter AL, et al. The effect of intracanal antiinflammatory medicaments on external root resorption of replanted dog teeth after extended extra-oral dry time [abstract]. J Endod 2005;31:233.
13. Nerwich A, Figdor D, Messer HH. pH changes in root dentin over 4-week period following root canal dressing with calcium hydroxide. J Endod 1993;19:302–6.
14. Tronstad L, Andreasen JO, Hasselgren G, et al. pH changes in dental tissues after root canal filling with calcium hydroxide. J Endod 1981;7:17–21.
15. Andreasen JO. External root resorption: its implications in dental traumatology, paedodontics, periodontics, orthodontics and endodontics. Int Endod J 1985;18:109–18.
16. Andreasen JO, Andreasen FM. Root resorption following traumatic dental injuries. Proc Finn Dent Soc 1991;88:95–114.
17. Tronstad L. Root resorption—etiology, terminology and clinical manifestations. Endod Dent Traumatol 1988;4:241–52.
18. Pierce AM. Experimental basis for the management of dental resorption. Endod Dent Traumatol 1989;5:255–65.
19. Heithersay GS. External root resorption. Ann R Australas Coll Dent Surg 1994;12:46–59.
20. Frank AL. Extracanal invasive resorption: an update. Compend Contin Educ Dent 1995;16:250–4.
21. Finucane D, Kinirons M. External inflammatory and replacement resorption of luxated, and avulsed replanted permanent incisors: a review and case presentation. Dental Traumatol 2003;19:170–4.
22. Andersson L, Bodin I, Sörensen S. Progression of root resorption following replantation of human teeth after extended extraoral storage. Endod Dent Traumatol 1989;5:38–47.

23. Andreasen JO, Hjörting-Hansen E. Replantation of teeth II. Histological study of 22 replanted anterior teeth in humans. Acta Odontol Scand 1966;24:287–306.

24. Andreasen JO, Hjörting-Hansen E. Replantation of teeth. Radiographic and clinical study of 110 human teeth replanted after accidental loss. Acta Odontol Scand 1966;24:263–86.

25. Andreasen FM, Sewerin I, Mandel U, Andreasen JO. Radiographic assessment of simulated root resorption cavities. Endod Dent Traumatol 1987;3:21–7.

26. Henry JL, Weinmann JP. The pattern of resorption and repair of human cementum. J Am Dent Assoc 1951;42:270–90.

27. Andreasen JO. Treatment of fractured and avulsed teeth. ASDC J Dent Child 1971;38:1–5.

28. Andreasen JO. Relationship between surface and inflammatory resorption and changes in the pulp after replantation of permanent incisors in monkeys. J Endod 1981;7:294–301.

29. Andreasen JO. The effect of pulp extirpation or root canal treatment on periodontal healing after replantation of permanent incisors in monkeys. J Endod 1981;7:245–52.

30. Andreasen JO, Kristerson L. The effect of extra-alveolar root filling with calcium hydroxide on periodontal healing after replantation of permanent incisors in monkeys. J Endod 1981;7:349–54.

31. Cvek M. Prognosis of luxated non-vital maxillary incisors treated with calcium hydroxite and filled with gutta-percha. Endod Dent Traumatol 1992;8:45–55.

32. Störmer K, Jacobsen I, Attramadal A. Hvor funktjonsdyktige bliver rottfylte unge permanente incisiver? Nordisk forening for pedodonti. Bergen: Aarsmöte; 1988.

33. Andreasen JO, Farik B, Munksgaard EC. Long-term calcium hydroxide as a root canal dressing may increase risk of root fracture. Dent Traumatol 2002;18:134–7.

34. Andreasen JO, Munksgaard EC, Bakland LK. Comparison of fracture resistance of immature sheep teeth after root canal calcium hydroxide or MTA. Dent Traumatol 2006;22:154–6.

35. Bakland L. New endodontic procedures using mineral trioxide aggregate (MTA) for teeth with traumatic injuries. In: Andreasen JO, Andreasen FM, Andersson L, editors. Textbook and color atlas of traumatic injuries to the teeth. 4th ed. Copenhagen: Munksgaard; 2007. pp. 658–68.

36. Abou Ameira G, Anand P, Ashley P, Gelbier M. Outcomes of non-vital traumatized incisors managed with MTA. Poster no 105; IAPD Congress; 2007; Hong Kong.

37. Chadwick BL, Hingston E, Hayes J, Hunter ML. An audit of MTA in immature permanent incisors. Poster no. 022; IAPD Congress; 2007; Hong Kong.

38. Andreasen JO. The effect of splinting upon periodontal healing after replantation of permanent incisors in monkeys. Acta Odontol Scand 1975;33:313–23.

39. Andersson L, Lindskog S, Blomlöf L, et al. Effect of masticatory stimulation on dentoalveolar ankylosis after experimental tooth replantation. Endod Dent Traumatol 1985; 1:13–16.

40. Andreasen JO. Periodontal healing after replantation of traumatically avulsed human teeth. Assessment by mobility testing and radiography. Acta Odont Scand 1975;33: 325–35.

41. Andreasen JO, Andreasen FM. Avulsions. In: Andreasen JO, Andreasen FM, Andersson L, editors. Textbook and color atlas of traumatic injuries to the teeth. 4th ed. Oxford: Blackwell; 2007. pp. 444–88.

42. Andreasen JO, Borum MK, Jacobsen HL, Andreasen FM. Replantation of 400 traumatically avulsed permanent incisors. 4. Factors related to periodontal ligament healing. Endod Dent Traumatol 1995;11:59–89.

43. Malmgren O, Malmgren B. Orthodontic management of the traumatized dentition. In: Andreasen JO, Andreasen FM, Andersson L, editors. Textbook and color atlas of traumatic injuries to the teeth. 4th ed. Copenhagen: Munksgaard; 2007. pp. 669–715.

44. Andreasen JO, Borum MK, Andreasen FM. Progression of root resorption after replantation of 400 avulsed human incisors. In: Davidovitch Z, editor. The biological mechanisms of tooth eruption, resorption and replacement by implants. Boston: Harvard Society for the Advancement of Orthodontics; 1994. pp. 577–82.

45. Andersson L, Blomlöf L, Lindskog S, et al. Tooth ankylosis. Clinical, radiographic and histological assessments. Int J Oral Surg 1984;13:423–31.

46. Malmgren B, Cvek M, Lundberg M, Frykholm A. Surgical treatment of ankylosed and infrapositioned reimplanted incisors in adolescents. Scand J Dent Res 1984;92: 391–9.

47. Malmgren B. Decoration: how, why, and when? J Calif Dent Assoc 2000;28:846–54.

48. Malmgren B, Malmgren O, Andreasen JO. How does decoronation after ankylosis maintain or augment the alveolar process? A theoretical explanation based on tooth eruption and bone biology. Endod Top 2007 [Accepted].

49. Andreasen JO, Malmgren B, Bakland L. Tooth avulsion in children: to replant or not. Endod Top 2007 [Accepted].

50. Kurol J. Infra-occlusion of primary molars. An epidemiologic, familial, longitudinal, clinical, and histological study. Swed Dent J Suppl 1984;21:1–67.

51. Andreasen JO, Kurol J. The impacted first and second molar. In: Andreasen JO, Kølsen Petersen J, Laskin DM, editors. Textbook and color atlas of tooth impactions. Copenhagen: Munksgaard; 1996. pp. 198–216.

52. Heithersay GS. Invasive cervical resorption: an analysis of potential predisposing factors. Quintessence Int 1999; 30:83–95.

53. Heithersay GS. Treatment of invasive cervical resorption: an analysis of results using topical application of trichoracetic acid, curettage, and restoration. Quintessence Int 1999;30:96–110.

54. Andreasen FM, Andreasen JO. Resorption and mineralization processes following root fracture of permanent incisors. Endod Dent Traum 1988;4:202–14.

55. Andreasen FM, Andreasen JO. Luxation injuries of permanent teeth: general findings. In: Andreasen JO, Andreasen FM, Andersson L, editors. Textbook and color atlas of traumatic injuries to the teeth. 4th ed. Oxford: Blackwell; 2007. pp. 372–403.

CHAPTER 38

Tooth Discoloration and Bleaching

Ilan Rotstein, Yiming Li

Tooth discoloration is a clinical problem in dental practice. Both intracoronal and extracoronal bleaching techniques have been used to correct tooth color.

Etiology of Tooth Discoloration

Tooth discoloration is defined as "any change in the hue, color, or translucency of a tooth due to any cause; restorative filling materials, drugs (both topical and systemic), pulpal necrosis, or hemorrhage may be responsible."[1] The discoloration may be induced by intrinsic stains incorporated in tooth structures and extrinsic stains deposited on tooth surfaces (Table 1). This can be due to patient- or dentist-related causes[2,3] as shown in Table 1.

PATIENT-RELATED CAUSES

Pulp Necrosis

Bacterial, mechanical, or chemical irritation to the pulp may result in tissue necrosis. Disintegration by-products penetrate the dentinal tubules and discolor the surrounding dentin. The degree of discoloration is directly related to how long the pulp has been necrotic. The longer the discoloring compounds are present in the pulp chamber, the greater is the discoloration. This type of discoloration can usually be bleached intracoronally (Figure 1).

Intrapulpal Hemorrhage

Intrapulpal hemorrhage and lysis of erythrocytes are common results of traumatic injury to a tooth. Blood disintegration products, mainly iron sulfides, flow into the tubules and discolor the surrounding dentin. If the pulp becomes necrotic, the discoloration persists and usually becomes more severe with time. If the pulp recovers, the discoloration may be reversed, with the tooth regaining its original shade. The severity of such discoloration is again time-dependent;

Table 1 Major Sources of Tooth Stains	
Extrinsic Stains	**Intrinsic Stains**
Foods	Aging
Beverages	Pulpal necrosis
Mouth rinses	Intrapulpal hemorrhage
Tobacco products	Calcific metamorphosis
Restorative materials	Drugs (e.g., tetracycline)
Chromogenic microorganisms	Diseases (e.g., porphyria, erythroblastosis fetalis)

intracoronal bleaching is usually quite effective in this type of discoloration.[4–6]

Calcific metamorphosis

Calcific metamorphosis is seen most frequently in the anterior teeth, and it is a pulpal response to trauma that is characterized by rapid deposition of hard tissue within the root canal space.[7] In certain traumatic injuries, a temporary disruption of blood supply occurs, followed by the destruction of odontoblasts. These are replaced by undifferentiated mesenchymal cells that rapidly form reparative dentin. As a result, the translucency of the crowns of such teeth gradually decreases, giving rise to a yellowish or a yellow-brown discoloration. Root canal therapy is often required, followed by intracoronal bleaching.

Age

Tooth color tends to become progressively darker with age, which is a physiological change resulting from dentin apposition and thinning of the enamel, and changes of optical properties of tooth structure. Cumulative extrinsic stains from food and beverages also contribute to this type of tooth discoloration, which becomes more pronounced in the elderly, owing to the inevitable cracking, crazing, and incisal

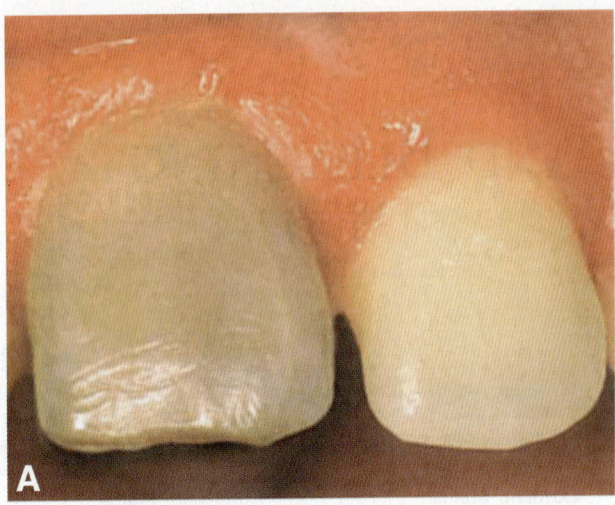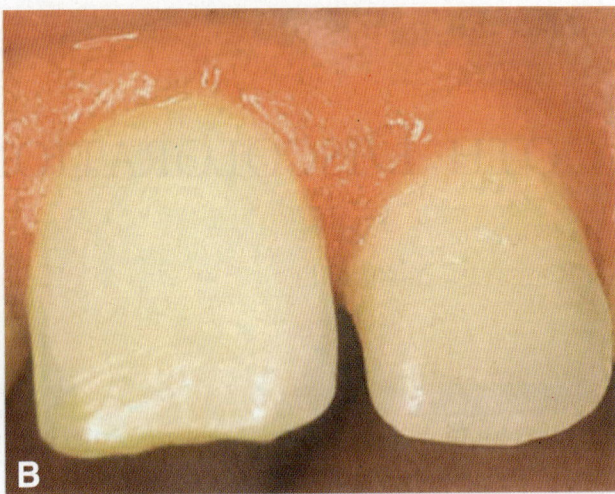

Figure 1 *A,* Posttraumatic discoloration of a maxillary central incisor caused by pulpal necrosis. *B,* A mixture of sodium perborate and distilled water, placed in the chamber two times for over 3 weeks, achieved lightening of the tooth to its natural color. Reproduced with permission from Claisse-Crinquette A, Endo Contact, Paris, France; 1999;2:16.

wear of the enamel and the underlying dentin. When indicated, extracoronal bleaching can be successful for many types of discolorations in elderly patients.

Developmental Defects in Tooth Structure

Discoloration may result from developmental defects during enamel and dentin formation, either hypocalcific or hypoplastic. Enamel *hypocalcification*, a distinct brownish or whitish area, is commonly found on the facial aspect of affected crowns. The enamel is well formed with an intact surface.

Enamel *hypoplasia* differs from hypocalcification in that the enamel is defective and porous. This condition may be hereditary, as in *amelogenesis imperfecta*, or hereditary hypophosphatemia, or a result of environmental factors such as infections, tumors, or trauma. Presumably, during enamel formation, the matrix is altered and does not mineralize properly. The defective enamel is porous and readily discolored by materials in the oral cavity. In such cases, bleaching effect may not be permanent, depending on the severity and extent of hypoplasia and the nature of discoloration.

Dental fluorosis, or mottled tooth, is a type of enamel hypoplasia. It is caused by the excessive exposure to fluoride during tooth formation, resulting in defects in mineralized structures, particularly in the enamel matrix. The severity of subsequent staining generally depends on the degree of hypoplasia that is directly related to the amount of fluoride exposure during odontogenesis.[8] The affected teeth are not discolored on eruption, but their porous surface attracts extrinsic stains present in the oral cavity. Discoloration is usually bilaterally symmetric. It presents as various degrees of intermittent white spotting, chalky or opaque areas, yellow or brown discoloration, and, in severe cases, surface pitting of the enamel. Discoloration of mild to moderate dental fluorosis can be bleached externally (Figure 2) however, restorative approaches should be considered for the cases of severe dental fluorosis.

Several systemic conditions may also cause tooth discoloration. *Erythroblastosis fetalis*, for example, may occur in the fetus or in a newborn because of Rh-incompatibility factors, resulting in the lysis of erythrocytes and incorporation of hemosiderin pigment in the forming dentin.[9] However, such discoloration is now uncommon. High fever during tooth formation may result in chronologic enamel hypoplasia that gives rise to banding-type surface discoloration. Porphyria, a metabolic disease, may also cause reddish or brownish discoloration of deciduous and permanent teeth. Thalassemia and sickle cell anemia may cause intrinsic blue, brown, or green discolorations. *Amelogenesis imperfecta* may result in yellow or brown discolorations. *Dentinogenesis imperfecta* causes brownish violet, yellowish, or gray discoloration. These conditions are usually not amenable to bleaching and correction by restorative means is preferred.

Tetracycline

Administration or ingestion of certain drugs during tooth formation may cause severe discoloration both

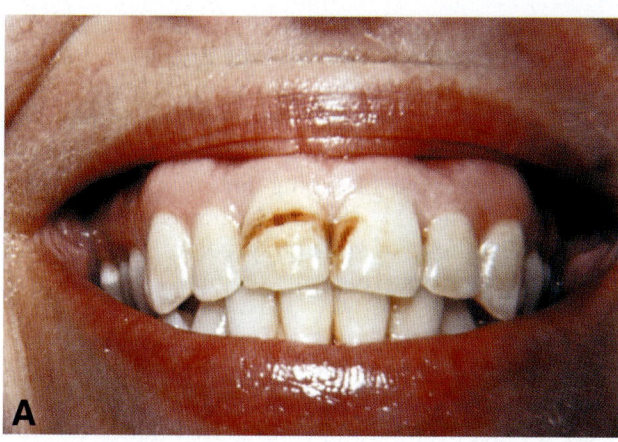 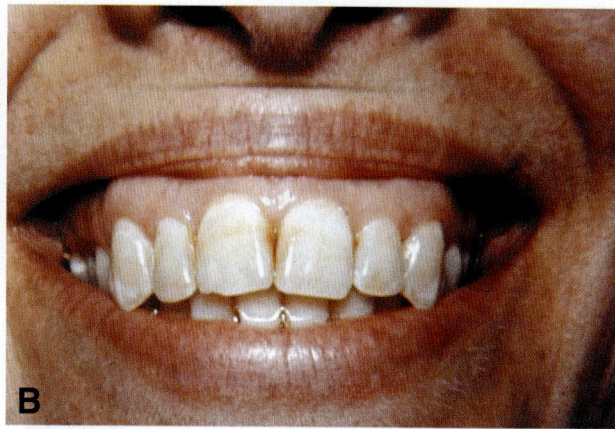

Figure 2 Fluorosis of central incisors treated by external bleaching. **A,** Before treatment. **B,** One month following external bleaching treatment. Reproduced with permission from Meyers, DL.

in enamel and dentin.[10–12] Tetracycline is an antibiotic that was used extensively during the 1950s and 1960s for prophylactic protection and for the treatment of chronic obstructive pulmonary disease, mycoplasma, and rickettsial infections. It was sometimes prescribed for long periods of time, years in some cases, and therefore was a common cause of tooth discoloration in children. While tetracycline is no longer prescribed for prolonged periods, dentists still face the residue of damage to the teeth appearance of the prior two generations.

Tooth shades can be yellow, yellow-brown, brown, dark gray, or blue depending on the type of tetracycline, dosage, duration of intake, and patient's age at the time of administration. Discoloration is usually bilateral, affecting multiple teeth in both arches. Deposition of tetracycline may be continuous or in stripes depending on whether the ingestion was continuous or interrupted (Figure 3).

The mechanism of tetracycline discoloration is not fully understood. Tetracycline bound to calcium is thought to be incorporated into the hydroxyapatite crystal of both enamel and dentin, but mostly found in dentin. The exposure of tetracycline-stained teeth to ultraviolet radiation leads to the formation of a reddish-purple oxidation by-product that discolors the teeth. In children, the anterior teeth often discolor first, whereas the less-exposed posterior teeth are discolored more slowly. In adults, natural photobleaching of the anterior teeth has been observed, particularly in individuals whose teeth are excessively exposed to sunlight owing to maxillary lip insufficiency.

Tetracycline discoloration has been classified into three groups according to severity.[13] First-degree discoloration is light yellow, light brown, or light gray and occurs uniformly throughout the crown, without banding. Second-degree discoloration is more intense and also without banding. Third-degree discoloration

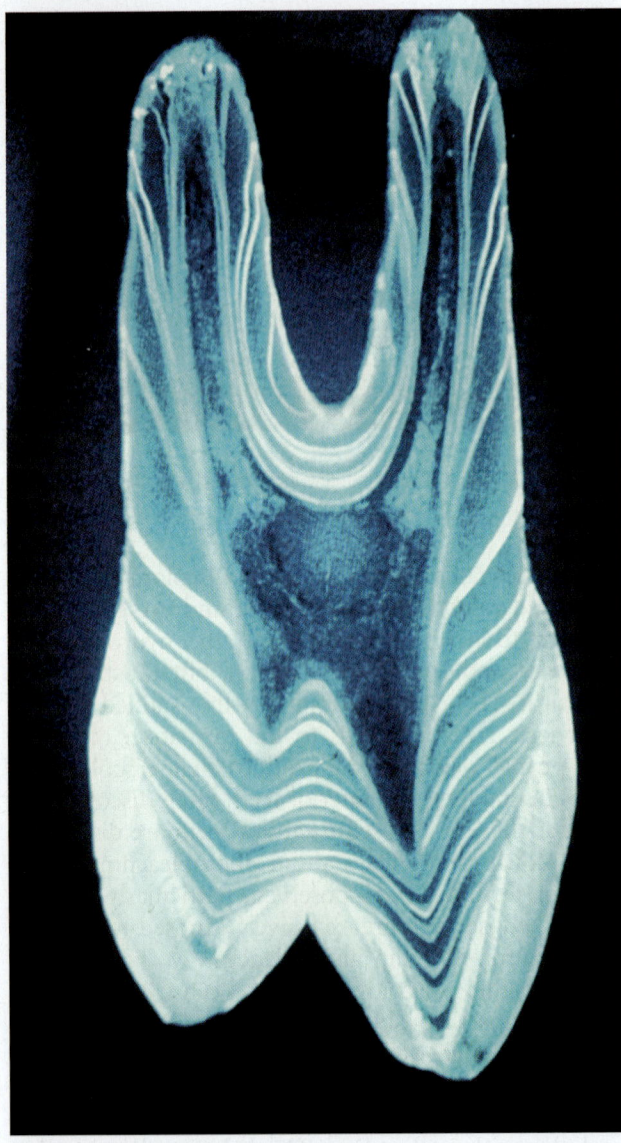

Figure 3 Fluorescent photomicrograph of tetracycline-discolored tooth. Tetracycline deposition is seen as stripes caused by start and stop ingestion. Reproduced with permission from Meyers, DL.

is very intense, and the clinical crown exhibits horizontal color banding. This type of discoloration usually predominates in the cervical regions.

Correction of tetracycline-stained teeth may pose a clinical challenge. For mild to certain moderate cases, repeated external bleaching for an extended period can be effective[14,15] (Figure 4); however, severe cases, especially those of dark gray color, should be corrected by restorative means.

DENTIST-RELATED CAUSES

Tooth discolorations caused by certain dental materials or inappropriate operating techniques do occur; such dentist-related discolorations are usually preventable and efforts should be made to avoid them.

Pulp Tissue Remnants

The tissue remaining in the pulp chamber disintegrates gradually and may cause discoloration. Therefore, pulp horns must always be included in the access cavity to ensure removal of pulpal remnants and to prevent retention of sealers at a later stage. Intracoronal bleaching in these cases is usually successful.

Intracanal Medicaments

Several intracanal medicaments can cause internal staining of dentin. Phenolics or iodoform-based medicaments sealed in the root canal and chamber are in direct contact with dentin, sometimes for long periods, allowing penetration and oxidation. These compounds have a tendency to discolor the dentin gradually. Intracoronal bleaching may be used to correct the problem.

Obturating materials

This is a frequent and severe cause of single tooth discoloration. Incomplete removal of obturating materials and sealer remnants from the pulp

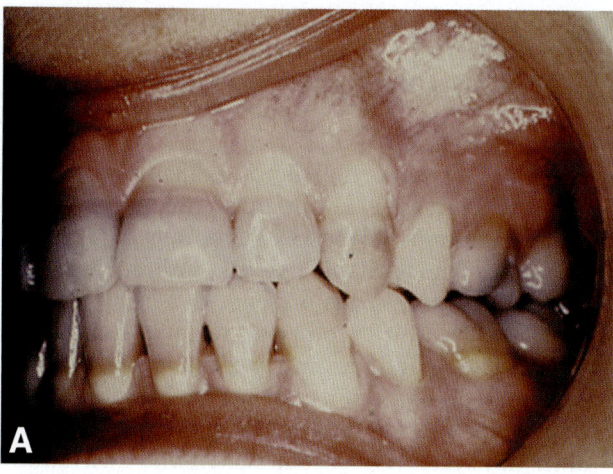
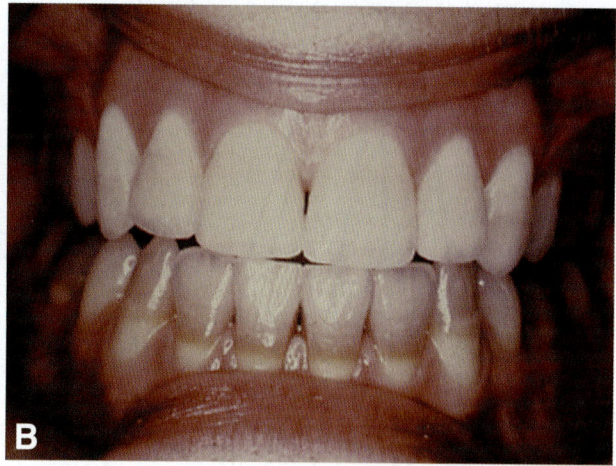

Figure 4 Extracoronal bleaching of tetracycline-discolored maxillary incisors. **A,** Before bleaching. **B,** After three sessions of heat-activated bleaching as compared to unbleached discolored mandibular incisors.

chamber, mainly those containing metallic components, often results in dark discoloration.[16–18] This can be easily prevented by removing all materials to a level just below the gingival margin (Figure 5). Intracoronal bleaching is the treatment of choice in addition to removing the obturating material; prognosis, however, depends on the type of sealer and the duration of discoloration.

Amalgams

Amalgams are frequently used to restore lingual access preparations or a developmental groove in anterior and premolar teeth. In addition to the inherent dark, metallic color of an amalgam restoration, amalgams degrade over time and corrosion products can cause tooth discoloration. Such discolorations are difficult to bleach and tend to rediscolor with time.

Sometimes the dark appearance of the crown is caused by an amalgam restoration that can be seen through the tooth structure. In such cases, replacing the amalgam with an esthetic restoration usually corrects the problem.

Pins and Posts

Metal pins and prefabricated posts have sometimes been used to reinforce a composite restoration in the anterior dentition. Discoloration from inappropriately placed pins and posts is caused by the metal seen through the composite or tooth structure. In such cases, coverage of the pins with a white cement or removal of the metal and replacement of the composite restoration is indicated.

Resin Composites

Microleakage around resin composite restorations attracts extrinsic stains. Open margins allow stains to enter the interface between the restoration and the tooth structure and discolor the underlying dentin. Resin composites may also become discolored with time, affecting the shade of the crown. These conditions are generally corrected by replacing the old composite restoration with a new, well-sealed one.

Tooth Bleaching

Bleaching is a treatment modality involving an oxidative chemical that alters the light-absorbing and/or light-reflecting nature of a material structure, thereby increasing its perception of whiteness. In-office tooth bleaching using peroxide compounds, both intracoronally and extracoronally, has been practiced in dentistry for more than a century.[19] At-home bleaching, however, was not widely available until 1989.[20]

BLEACHING MATERIALS

The active ingredient in tooth bleaching materials is peroxide compounds. While currently a variety of bleaching materials are available, the most commonly used peroxide compounds are hydrogen peroxide, sodium perborate, and carbamide peroxide. Bleaching materials for extracoronal bleaching mainly contain hydrogen peroxide and carbamide peroxide, whereas sodium perborate is used

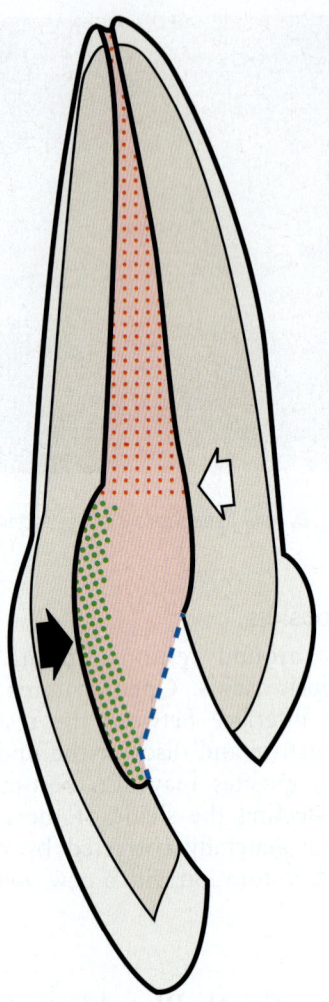

Figure 5 Gutta-percha, sealer, and dentin removal prior to bleaching. Green-dotted area represents gutta-percha filling that is removed to a level below the attached gingival (open arrow) along with the removal of dentin to eliminate heavy stain concentration and pulp horn material (black arrow).

for intracoronal bleaching. Both sodium perborate and carbamide peroxide decompose to release hydrogen peroxide in an aqueous medium.

Hydrogen Peroxide

Hydrogen peroxide (H_2O_2) is used in both in-office and at-home bleaching materials. In-office bleaching materials contain high concentrations of H_2O_2 (typically 25% to 38%), while the H_2O_2 concentration in at-home bleaching products usually range from 3% to 7.5%; however, there have been products containing up to 14% H_2O_2 for home use by patients.

H_2O_2 at high concentration, such as those in the in-office bleaching materials, is caustic and burns tissues on contact. These materials must be handled with care to avoid their contact with tissues during the handling and bleaching treatment.

Sodium Perborate

Sodium perborate ($NaBO_3$) is available in powdered form or as various commercial preparations. When fresh, it contains about 95% perborate, corresponding to 9.9% of the available oxygen. Sodium perborate is stable when dry. In the presence of acid, warm air, or water, however, it decomposes to form sodium metaborate, H_2O_2, and nascent oxygen.

Three types of sodium perborate preparations are available: monohydrate, trihydrate, and tetrahydrate. They differ in oxygen content that determines their bleaching efficacy.[21] Commonly used sodium perborate preparations are alkaline, and their pH depends on the amount of H_2O_2 released and the residual sodium metaborate.[22]

Sodium perborate is more easily controlled and is safer than concentrated H_2O_2. Therefore, it is the material of choice in most intracoronal bleaching procedures (Figure 6).

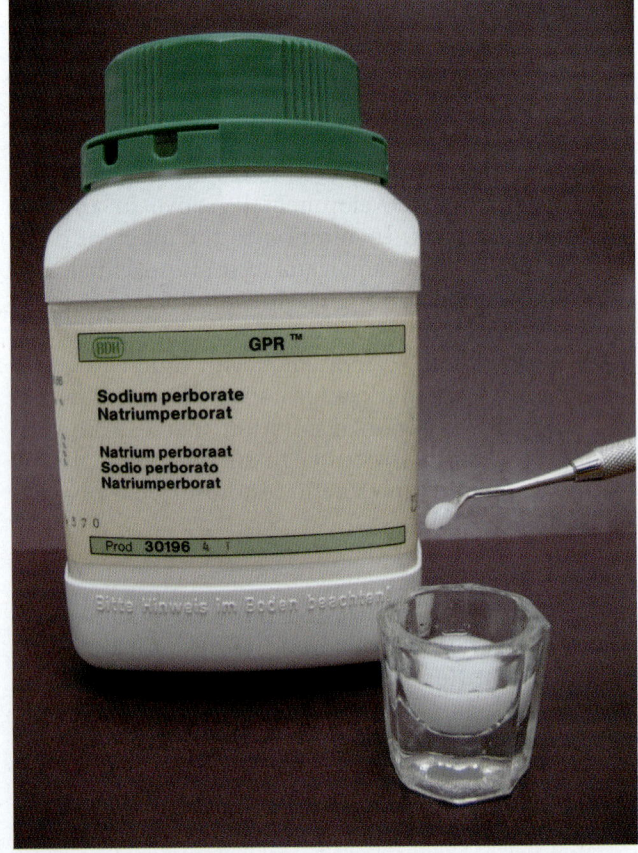

Figure 6 Sodium perborate powder and water are mixed to a thick consistency of wet sand.

Carbamide Peroxide

Carbamide peroxide ($CH_6N_2O_3$), also known as urea hydrogen peroxide, exists in the form of white crystals or as a crystallized powder containing approximately 35% H_2O_2. It forms H_2O_2 and urea in aqueous solution. It is mostly used in home-use bleaching materials with concentrations ranging from 10 to 30% (equivalent to approximately 3.5% to 8.6% H_2O_2); however, those containing 10% carbamide peroxide appear to be the most common.

Bleaching preparations containing carbamide peroxide usually also include glycerine or propylene glycol, sodium stannate, phosphoric or citric acid, and flavor additives. In some preparations, carbopol, a water-soluble polyacrylic acid polymer, is added as a thickening agent. Carbopol also prolongs the release of active peroxide and improves shelf life.

BLEACHING MECHANISMS

The mechanisms of tooth bleaching remain unclear at present; however, it is generally believed that free radicals produced by H_2O_2 may be responsible for bleaching effects, and they are similar to that in textile and paper bleaching. H_2O_2 diffuses through the enamel and dentin, producing free radicals that react with pigment molecules breaking their double bonds. The change in pigment molecule configuration and/or size may result in changes in their optical properties, and consequently, the perception of a lighter color by human eyes. This assumption also helps to explain the common observation of shade rebounding shortly after the bleaching treatment, probably due to the reformation of double bonds. In addition to the chemical effect, other possible mechanisms include cleansing of tooth surface, temporary dehydration of enamel during the bleaching process, and change of enamel surface.

A number of factors, relating to both the patient (e.g., age, gender, and initial tooth color), the bleaching material used (e.g., type of peroxide compound, peroxide concentration, other ingredients), and application method (e.g., contact time, application frequency, enamel prophylaxis prior to bleaching treatment), may contribute to the bleaching efficacy and the subsequent stability of the bleaching achieved. Among these factors, the contact time of the bleaching material to the enamel surface appears to be more influential than the others.[23]

INTRACORONAL BLEACHING OF ENDODONTICALLY TREATED TEETH

Intracoronal bleaching of endodontically treated teeth may be successfully carried out many years after root canal therapy and discoloration. A successful outcome depends mainly on the etiology, correct diagnosis, and proper selection of bleaching technique (Table 2).

The methods most commonly employed to bleach endodontically treated teeth are the "walking bleach" and the thermocatalytic techniques. Walking bleach is preferred since it requires less chair time and is safer and more comfortable for the patient.[24–27]

Table 2 Indications and Contraindications for Bleaching Endodontically Treated Teeth

Indications	Contraindications
Discolorations of pulp chamber	Superficial enamel discolorations
Dentin discolorations	Defective enamel formation
Discolorations not amenable to extracoronal bleaching	Severe dentin loss
	Presence of caries
	Discolored composites

Walking Bleach

The term *walking bleach* was first coined by Nutting and Poe[28] in 1961 referring to the bleaching action occurring between patients' visits. Since that time, the technique evolved and underwent few modifications, mainly by eliminating the use of Superoxol (H_2O_2, 30%) making it a very popular and safe technique.[27,29] The walking bleach technique should be attempted first in all cases requiring intracoronal bleaching. It involves the following steps:

1. Familiarize the patient with the possible causes of discoloration, the procedure to be followed, the expected outcome, and the possibility of future rediscoloration.
2. Radiographically assess the status of the periapical tissues and the quality of endodontic obturation. Endodontic failure or questionable obturation should always be retreated prior to bleaching.
3. Assess the quality and shade of any restoration present and replace it if defective. Tooth discoloration is frequently the result of leaking or discolored restorations. In such cases, cleaning the pulp chamber and replacing the defective restorations will usually suffice.
4. Evaluate tooth color with a shade guide and, if possible, take clinical photographs at the beginning of and throughout the procedure. These provide a point of reference for future comparison.
5. Isolate the tooth with a rubber dam. The dam must fit tightly at the cervical margin of the tooth

to prevent possible leakage of the bleaching agent onto the gingival tissue. Interproximal wedges and ligatures may also be used for better isolation.

6. Remove all restorative materials from the access cavity, expose the dentin, and refine the access. Verify that the pulp horns and other areas containing the pulp tissue are clean.
7. Remove all materials to a level just below the labial–gingival margin. Orange solvent, chloroform, or xylene on a cotton pellet may be used to dissolve sealer remnants. Etching the dentin with phosphoric acid is unnecessary and may not improve the prognosis.[30]
8. Apply a sufficiently thick layer, at least 2 mm, of a protective white cement barrier, such as polycarboxylate cement, zinc phosphate cement, glass ionomer, intermediate restorative material (IRM) (Dentsply/Caulk, York, PA), or Cavit (3M ESPE, St. Paul, MN,) to cover the endodontic obturation. The coronal height of the barrier should protect the dentinal tubules and conform to the external epithelial attachment.[31]
9. Prepare the walking bleach paste by mixing sodium perborate and an inert liquid, such as water, saline, or anesthetic solution, to a thick consistency of wet sand. Although sodium perborate plus 30% H_2O_2 mixture may bleach faster, in most cases, long-term results are similar to those with sodium perborate and water alone and therefore need not be used routinely.[5,6,29] With a plastic instrument, pack the pulp chamber with the paste. Remove excess liquid by tamping with a cotton pellet. This also compresses and pushes the paste into all areas of the pulp chamber.
10. Remove the excess bleaching paste from undercuts in the pulp horn and gingival area and apply a thick well-sealed temporary filling (preferably IRM) directly against the paste and into the undercuts. Carefully pack the temporary filling, at least 3 mm thick, to ensure a good seal.
11. Remove the rubber dam and inform the patient that bleaching agents work slowly and that significant lightening may not be evident for several days.
12. Evaluate the patient 2 weeks later and, if necessary, repeat the procedure several times.[27] Repeat treatments are similar to the first one.
13. As an optional procedure, if initial bleaching is not satisfactory, strengthen the walking bleach paste by mixing sodium perborate with gradually increasing concentrations of H_2O_2 (3% to 30%) instead of water. The more potent oxidizers may have an enhanced bleaching effect but are not used routinely because of the possibility of permeation into the tubules and damage to the cervical periodontium by these more caustic agents. In such cases, a protective cream, such as Orabase or Vaseline, must be applied to the surrounding gingival tissues prior to dam placement.
14. In most cases, discoloration will improve after 1 to 2 treatments. If after three attempts there is no significant improvement, reassess the case for correct diagnosis of the etiology of discoloration and treatment plan.

Thermocatalytic

This technique involves placement of the oxidizing chemical, generally 30% to 35% H_2O_2 (Superoxol), into the pulp chamber followed by heat application either by electric heating devices or specially designed lamps.[32] Care must be taken when using these heating devices to avoid overheating of the teeth and the surrounding tissues. Intermittent treatment with cooling breaks is preferred over a continuous session. In addition, the surrounding soft tissues should be protected with Vaseline, Orabase, or cocoa butter during treatment to avoid heat damage.

Potential damage by the thermocatalytic approach is external cervical root resorption caused by irritation to the cementum and the periodontal ligament. This is possibly attributable to the oxidizing agent combined with heating.[33,34] Therefore, application of highly concentrated H_2O_2 and heat during intracoronal bleaching is questionable and should not be carried out routinely.

Ultraviolet Photooxidation

This technique applies ultraviolet light to the labial surface of the tooth to be bleached. A 30% to 35% H_2O_2 solution is placed in the pulp chamber on a cotton pellet followed by a 2-minute exposure to ultraviolet light. Supposedly, this causes oxygen release, like the thermocatalytic bleaching technique.[35]

COMPLICATIONS AND ADVERSE EFFECTS FROM INTRACORONAL BLEACHING

External Root Resorption

Clinical reports[36–46] and histological studies[33,34,47] have shown that intracoronal bleaching may induce external cervical root resorption (Table 3) and (Figure 7). This is probably caused by the highly concentrated oxidizing agent, particularly 30 to 35% H_2O_2. The mechanism of bleaching-induced damage to the periodontium or the cementum is not completely clear. Presumably, the irritating chemical diffuses via unprotected dentinal tubules and cementum defects[48,49] and causes necrosis of the cementum, inflammation of the periodontal ligament, and, subsequently, root resorption. The process may be enhanced if heat is applied[50] or in the presence of bacteria.[51] Previous traumatic injury and age may act as predisposing factors.[36,52]

Chemical Burns

Superoxol (H_2O_2 at 30%) is highly caustic and causes chemical burns and sloughing of the gingiva. When using such solutions, the soft tissues should always be protected with Vaseline, Orabase, or cocoa butter.

Inhibition on Resin Polymerization and Bonding Strength

Oxygen inhibits resin polymerization; consequently, residual H_2O_2 in tooth structure after bleaching adversely affects the bonding strength of resin composites to enamel and dentin.[53,54] Scanning electron microscopy (SEM) examination has shown an increase in resin porosity.[55] This presents a clinical problem when immediate esthetic restoration of the bleached tooth is required. It is therefore recommended that residual H_2O_2 be totally eliminated prior to composite placement. One study reported that 3 minutes of catalase treatment effectively removed all of the residual H_2O_2 from the pulp chamber of human teeth.[56]

SUGGESTIONS FOR SAFE BLEACHING OF ENDODONTICALLY TREATED TEETH

- Isolate the tooth effectively. Intracoronal bleaching should always be carried out under rubber dam isolation. Interproximal wedges and ligatures may also be used for better protection.
- Protect the oral mucosa. Protective creams, such as Orabase or Vaseline, must be applied to the surrounding oral mucosa to prevent chemical burns by caustic oxidizers. Animal studies suggest that catalase applied to oral tissues prior to bleaching treatment totally prevents the associated tissue damage.[57]
- Verify adequate endodontic obturation. The quality of root canal obturation should always be assessed

Table 3 Clinical Reports of External Root Resorption Associated with Hydrogen Peroxide Bleaching								
			Previous Trauma		Heat Applied		Barrier Used	
Authors	No. of Cases	Age of Patients	Yes	No	Yes	No	Yes	No
Harrington and Natkin[36]	7	10–29	7	0	7	0	0	7
Lado et al[37]	1	50	0	1	1	0	0	1
Montgomery[38]	1	21	1	0	?	?	?	?
Shearer[39]	1	?	0	1	1	0	0	1
Cvek and Lindvall[40]	11	11–26	10	1	11	0	0	11
Latcham[41]	1	8	1	0	0	1	0	1
Goon et al[42]	1	15	?	?	0	1	0	1
Friedman et al[43]	4	18–24	0	4	3	1	0	4
Gimlin and Schindler[44]	1	13	1	0	1	0	0	1
Al-Nazhan[45]	1	27	0	1	1	0	0	1
Heithersay et al[46]	4	10–20	4	0	4	0	0	4

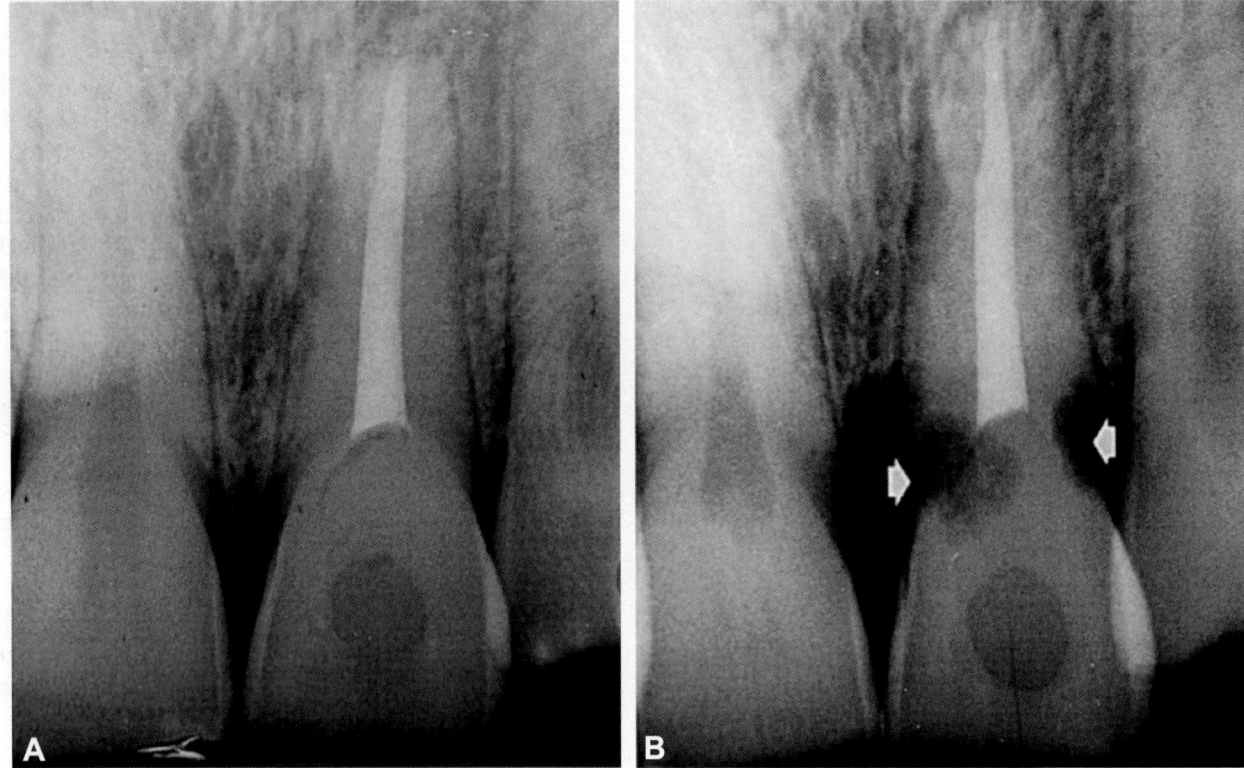

Figure 7 Postbleaching external root resorption. **A,** Nine-year recall radiograph of a central incisor devitalized by trauma and treated endodontically shortly thereafter. **B,** Radiograph taken 2 years following bleaching. Superoxol and heat were used first and followed by "walking bleach" with Superoxol and sodium perborate. Reproduced with permission from Steiner D, Harrington G.

clinically and radiographically prior to bleaching. Adequate obturation ensures a better overall prognosis of the treated tooth. It also provides an additional barrier against damage by oxidizers to the periodontal ligament and periapical tissues.
- Use protective barriers over the coronal extent of the root canal filling. This is essential to prevent leakage of bleaching agents that may infiltrate between gutta-percha and root canal walls, reaching the periodontal ligament via dentinal tubules, lateral canals, or the root apex. In none of the clinical reports of postbleaching root resorption was a protective barrier used. Various materials can be used for this purpose. Barrier thickness and its relationship to the cementoenamel junction are most important.[31,58] The ideal barrier should protect the dentinal tubules and conform to the external epithelial attachment (Figure 8).
- Avoid acid etching. It has been suggested that acid etching of dentin in the chamber to remove the smear layer and open the tubules would allow better penetration of the oxidizer. This procedure has not proved beneficial.[30] The use of caustic chemicals in the pulp chamber is undesirable as they may result in irritation to the periodontal ligament.
- Avoid strong oxidizers. Procedures and techniques applying strong oxidizers should be avoided if they are not essential for bleaching. Solutions of 30% to 35% H_2O_2, either alone or in combination with other agents, should not be used routinely for intracoronal bleaching. Sodium perborate is mild and quite safe, and usually no additional protection of the soft tissues is required. Generally, however, oxidizing agents should not be exposed to more of the pulp space and dentin than absolutely necessary to obtain a satisfactory clinical result.
- Avoid heat. Excessive heat may damage the cementum and the periodontal ligament as well as dentin and enamel, especially when combined with strong oxidizers.[33,34] Although no direct correlation has been established between heat application and external cervical root resorption, it should be limited during bleaching procedures.

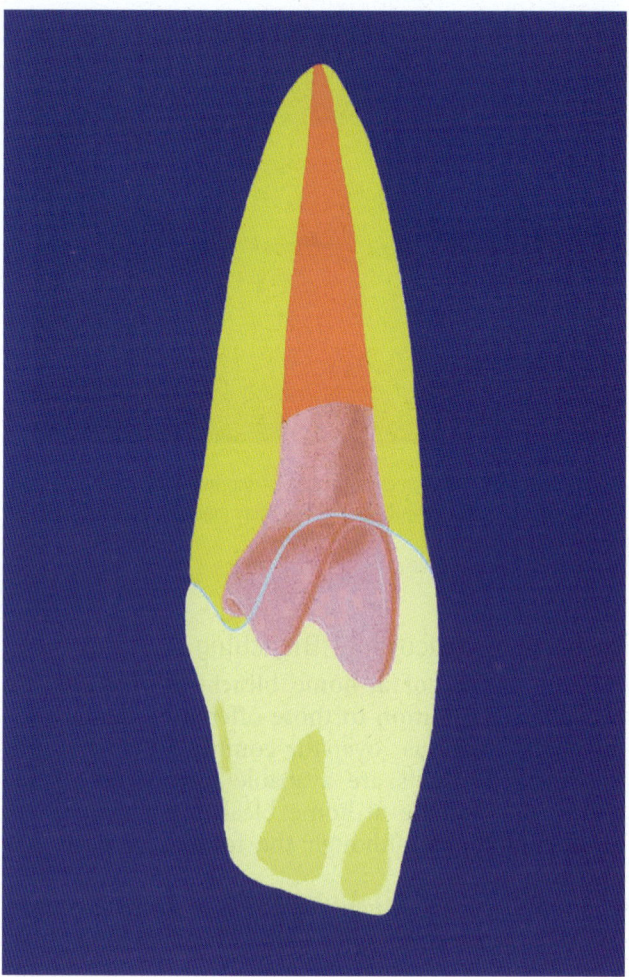

Figure 8 Schematic illustration of the intracoronal protective bleach barrier. The shape of the barrier matches the contour of the external epithelial attachment. Reproduced with permission from Steiner DR and West JD, J Endod 1994;20:304.

- Recall periodically. Bleached teeth should be frequently examined both clinically and radiographically. Root resorption may occasionally be detected as early as 6 months after bleaching. Early detection improves the prognosis since corrective therapy may still be applied.

RESTORATION OF INTRACORONALLY BLEACHED TEETH

Proper tooth restoration is essential for long-term successful bleaching results. Microleakage of lingual access restorations is a problem,[59] and a leaky restoration may again lead to tooth discoloration.

There is no ideal method for filling the chamber after intracoronal bleaching. The pulp chamber and the access cavity should be carefully restored with a light shade, light-cured, acid-etched composite resin. The composite material should be placed at a depth that seals the cavity and provides some incisal support. Light curing from the labial surface, rather than the lingual surface, is recommended since this results in the shrinkage of the composite resin toward the axial walls, reducing the rate of microleakage.[60] Placing white cement beneath the composite access restoration is recommended. Filling the chamber completely with composite may cause loss of translucency and difficulty in distinguishing between composite and tooth structure during rebleaching.[61]

As stated previously, residual H_2O_2 from bleaching treatment may adversely affect the bonding strength of composites.[53] Therefore, waiting for at least 7 days after bleaching, prior to restoring the tooth with resin composites, has been recommended. Catalase treatment at the final visit may enhance the removal of residual peroxides from the access cavity; however, this requires further clinical investigation.[56] Packing calcium hydroxide paste in the pulp chamber for a few weeks prior to the placement of final restoration, to counteract acidity caused by bleaching agents and to prevent root resorption, has also been suggested; this procedure, however, is unnecessary with walking bleach.[22]

EXTRACORONAL BLEACHING

Extracoronal bleaching may be used for whitening vital or nonvital teeth as well as a single tooth or whole arch. It has experienced a dramatic advancement in materials as well as techniques after at-home extracoronal bleaching was first introduced.[20,62] Research efforts and clinical advancements have also revolutionized the in-office extracoronal bleaching technology.

In-office Extracoronal Bleaching

Various materials and clinical procedures are available for in-office extracoronal bleaching, also called chairside bleaching or power bleaching. As indicated by the terms, the bleaching procedures are performed in the clinic by a dental professional.

Current commercial in-office bleaching materials are almost exclusively in the form of a gel, with 25% to 38% H_2O_2. It is not advisable to directly use high concentrations of aqueous H_2O_2 solutions for tooth bleaching as practiced in early years. Besides a higher risk of tissue contact due to its lack of proper viscosity, the high concentrations of aqueous H_2O_2 solutions are thermodynamically unstable and may explode unless properly stored in a dark container and kept refrigerated.

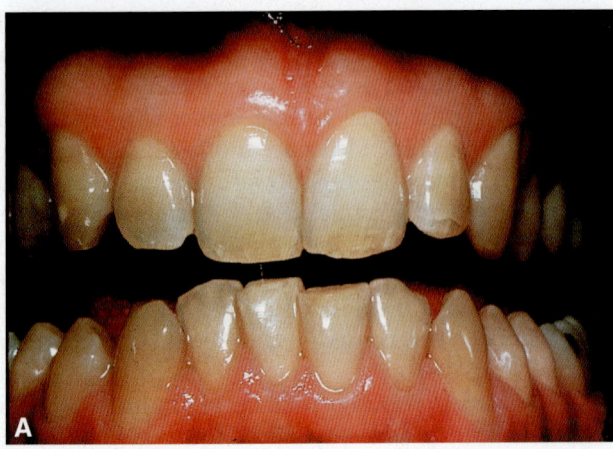 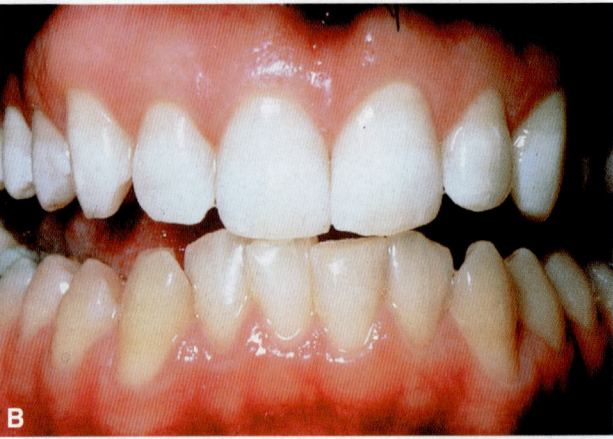

Figure 9 Extracoronal mouthguard bleaching with carbamide peroxide gel. ***A***, Before treatment. ***B***, Bleaching results of the maxillary teeth after two treatments. Discolored teeth that are not internally stained will respond to external bleaching. Subsequently, the patient may maintain the color with an occasional repeat of the procedure with the bleaching gel. Courtesy, Ultradent Products, Inc.

In-office extracoronal bleaching may be performed using a bleaching gel alone or a gel with a *light*. In early years of in-office bleaching, heat, electric current, and other chemicals such as ether were often applied with H_2O_2 solution in an attempt to enhance its bleaching efficacy.[19] While these approaches are rarely seen in current practice, various lights have been used during the in-office bleaching process; the light may be specialized for such procedure, or it can be a regular curing light for resin composites. The light source can be a laser (e.g., argon, CO_2), halogen, plasma arc, or light-emitting diodes (LED). The wavelength may range from high ultraviolet spectra, low visible blue light spectra, to invisible infrared spectra such as the CO_2 laser.[32,63] Studies have found no significant advantages of using laser lights for bleaching; consequently, laser bleaching has become less popular than other light systems.[32]

The light exposure is intended to enhance the bleaching efficacy by activating the bleaching gel, either through a specific catalyst or heat, to promote the decomposition process of H_2O_2. So far, however, the research on the efficacy of using the light for in-office bleaching has been limited, and the results have been controversial; several studies reported an enhancing effect, while others detected no differences between teeth bleached with and without a light.[32,63–65] In general, there may be a short-term effect of the light exposure depending on the in-office bleaching and light system. However, currently long-term studies are insufficient regarding the benefits of light-activated bleaching.

At-home Extracoronal Bleaching

A large variety of at-home bleaching products are available. In addition to those offered by dental professionals, various over-the-counter (OTC) tooth bleaching products are available directly to consumers. Most of the at-home bleaching products are gel formulations, although the form of a paste has also been used.

For *professional at-home bleaching*, custom tray technique is most commonly used. The bleaching gel is loaded in the tray, and the patient wears the tray for several hours up to overnight daily usually for 2 weeks or until a satisfactory tooth shade is achieved. Both H_2O_2 and carbamide peroxide are used as active ingredients for professional at-home bleaching products, mostly containing 3% to 7.5% H_2O_2 or 10 to 22% carbamide peroxide, with latter, especially those with 10% carbamide peroxide, being more popular (Figure 9). An H_2O_2-based professional bleaching strip is also available for at-home bleaching. As the application technique may vary, it is advisable that clinicians follow manufacturers' instructions for using such treatment modality.

While the majority of the *OTC at-home bleaching* materials are also gels, their application may use trays, strips, or brushes. In addition to the bleaching gel, some products offer prebleaching rinses and after-bleaching rubbing-on powders. The range of peroxide content in OTC bleaching products is comparable to that of the professional at-home bleaching materials; however, the quality of the OTC products may vary greatly. Their peroxide content may not be consistent and stable, and some products, including the pre-bleaching rinses, may come with an excessively low pH.

COMPLICATIONS AND ADVERSE EFFECTS FROM EXTRACORONAL BLEACHING

Extracoronal tooth bleaching can provide lighter tooth shade that is retained up to 10 years after the initial professional tray bleaching treatment.[66] However, there have been concerns with its safety since the introduction of at-home bleaching materials.[19,67–72] The safety concerns are mainly associated with potential toxicological effects of free radicals produced by the peroxides used in the bleaching materials. Free radicals are known to be capable of reacting with proteins, lipids, and nucleic acids, consequently causing cellular damage. Consequently, the topic of bleaching safety has been controversial. It appears, however, that no significant long-term oral or systemic health risks are associated with professional extracoronal bleaching with materials containing 10% carbamide peroxide. However, adverse effects may occur depending on the quality of the bleaching material, the techniques used, and the individual's response to the bleaching treatment.

Tooth Sensitivity

Tooth sensitivity to temperature changes is a commonly observed clinical side effect during or after extracoronal bleaching of vital teeth, with an incidence of up to 50%.[73] The sensitivity, usually mild to moderate and transient, often occurs during the early stages of treatment and usually persists for 2 to 3 days.[73–75] The development of tooth sensitivity does not appear to be related to the patient's age or sex, defective restorations, enamel–cementum abrasion, or the dental arch treated; however, the risk increases in patients who change the bleaching gel more than once a day.[73] If the patient develops significant sensitivity, shorter bleaching periods are recommended. Topical fluoride application and desensitizing toothpastes may also be used to alleviate the symptoms.

Tooth sensitivity has been suggested as an indication of possible pulpal inflammation.[71] Studies, most of which are used in vitro models, have shown that H_2O_2 in bleaching gel applied on the enamel surface is capable of penetrating through the enamel and dentin and reaching the pulp chamber.[76–82] Less than 30 μg of H_2O_2 may reach the dental pulp after application of gels with up to 12% H_2O_2 on the enamel surface for up to 7 hours. The amount of H_2O_2 detected in the pulp chamber tends to increase with time and H_2O_2 concentration in the gel, but not proportionally. It has been suggested that 50,000μg H_2O_2 is needed to inhibit pulpal enzymes, so that the detected amount of H_2O_2 penetrated into the pulp chamber from the at-home whiteners appears unlikely to cause significant damage to the pulp tissues. However, sufficient in vivo studies on this topic are lacking. Therefore, adequate cautions are advisable, and extracoronal bleaching should not be performed on teeth with caries, exposed dentin, or in close proximity to pulp horns. Defective restorations must be replaced prior to bleaching, and extra caution should be applied to children and adolescents.[83]

Enamel Damage

The effect of extracoronal bleaching on enamel has been conducted mainly using in vitro systems to examine changes in enamel surface microhardness and morphology.[84–93] Most SEM studies showed little or no morphological changes in the bleached enamel surface. On the other hand, several investigators reported alteration of enamel surfaces associated with bleaching treatments, including shallow depression, increased porosity, and slight erosion. In most cases, however, the observed alterations of enamel surface morphology varied among different products and were associated with products using acidic prerinse or gels of low pH. A 6-month clinical study reported that long-term use of a bleaching gel containing 10% carbamide peroxide did not adversely affect the surface morphology of human enamel.[93]

To date, no clinical evidence of adverse effects of the dentist-monitored at-home whiteners on enamel has been reported. However, there have been two clinical cases of significant damage on enamel associated with the use of OTC tooth-whitening products.[94,95]

Gingival Irritation

Gingival irritation is also a commonly observed clinical side effect in extracoronal bleaching, sometimes also associated with tooth sensitivity.[57,87,96–99] The gingival irritation is usually mild to moderate, occurring in 2 to 3 days of using the bleaching gel and then dissipating, and for most patients it is tolerable till the completion of treatment. When using the tray systems, an ill-fitted tray can cause irritation, and the gingival irritation usually resolves after proper trimming of the tray. For at-home bleaching, the risk of the gingival irritation appears to be related to the H_2O_2 concentration of the gel and the contact of the gel to the gingiva. Gingival irritation associated with in-office bleaching is mostly caused by a leaky or failed gingival barrier protection. Care must be taken to check the barrier for signs of leakage, usually indicated by air bubbles, and the patient's complaint of discomfort during the bleaching treatment. When tissue burn is detected, the surface should be extensively rinsed with water until the whiteness is reduced. In more severe cases, a topical anesthetic, limited movements, and a good oral hygiene aid healing. Application of protective creams such as Vaseline or cocoa butter can prevent most of these complications.

Mercury Release from Amalgam Restorations

Mercury release from amalgam restorations during and after extracoronal bleaching has been reported.[100–103] The amount of mercury release may vary, and the health implications of these mercury amounts require further investigation. It is not advisable to perform extracoronal bleaching for teeth with extensive amalgam restorations.

ROLE OF DENTAL PROFESSIONALS IN EXTRACORONAL BLEACHING TREATMENT

Dental professionals should be involved in tooth bleaching, including at-home bleaching. Initial evaluation and examination of tooth discoloration is necessary for proper diagnosis and treatment. Discoloration, particularly intrinsic stains, may not simply be an esthetic problem,[71] and at-home bleaching may not be the appropriate or the best choice for the treatment. For the tray-based at-home bleaching systems, professionally fabricated, custom-fit trays reduce the amount of gel needed for the whitening efficacy and minimize gel contact with oral soft tissues. In addition, routine monitoring of bleaching by dentists allows early detection of any possible complications and reduces the risk of using inferior bleaching products and inappropriate application procedures as well as any temptation to abuse the product.[94,95] For further information on extracoronal bleaching, the reader is encouraged to refer to additional publications.[104–111]

References

1. Jablonski S. Jablonski's dictionary of dentistry. Melbourne: Krieger Publishing Company; 1992. p. 253.
2. Rotstein I, Walton RE. Bleaching discolored teeth: Internal and external. In: Walton RE, Torabinejad M, editors. Principles and practice of endodontics. 3rd ed. Philadelphia, PA: W.B. Saunders; 2002. p. 405.
3. Shafer WG, Hine MK, Levy BM, Tomich CE. Textbook of oral pathology. 4th ed. Philadelphia, PA: W.B. Saunders; 1983. p. 766.
4. Freccia WF, Peters DD, Lorton L, Bernier WE. An in vitro comparison of non-vital bleaching techniques in the discolored tooth. J Endod 1982;8:70.
5. Rotstein I, Zalkind M, Mor C, et al. *In vitro* efficacy of sodium perborate preparations used for intracoronal bleaching of discolored non-vital teeth. Endod Dent Traumatol 1991;7:177.
6. Rotstein I, Mor C, Friedman S. Prognosis of intracoronal bleaching with sodium perborate preparations *in vitro*: 1 year study. J Endod 1993;19:10.
7. Glossary of Endodontic Terms. 7th ed. American Association of Endodontists;, 2003.
8. Driscoll WS, Horowitz HS, Meyers RJ, et al. Prevalence of dental caries and dental fluorosis in areas with optimal and above-optimal water fluoride concentrations. J Am Dent Assoc 1983;107:42.
9. Atasu M, Genc A, Ercalik S. Enamel hypoplasia and essential staining of teeth from erythroblastosis fetalis. J Clin Pediatr Dent 1998;22:249.
10. Lochary ME, Lockhart PB, Williams WT Jr. Doxycycline and staining of permanent teeth. Pediatr Infect Dis J 1998;17:429.
11. Livingston HM, Dellinger TM. Intrinsic staining of teeth secondary to tetracycline. Ann Pharmacother 1998;32:607.
12. Tredwin CJ, Scully C, Bagan-Sebastian JV. Drug-induced disorders of teeth. J Dent Res 2005;84:596.
13. Jordan RE, Boskman L. Conservative vital bleaching treatment of discolored dentition. Compend Contin Educ Dent 1984;5:803.
14. Arens DE, Rich JJ, Healey HJ. A practical method of bleaching tetracycline-stained teeth. Oral Surg Oral Med Oral Pathol Oral Radiol Endod 1972;34:812.
15. Seale N, Thrash W. Systematic assessment of color removal following vital bleaching of intrinsically stained teeth, J Dent Res 1985;64:457.
16. Van der Burgt TP, Plasschaert AJM. Bleaching of tooth discoloration caused by endodontic sealers. J Endod 1986;12:231.
17. Parsons JR, Walton RE, Ricks-Williamson L. *In vitro* longitudinal assessment of coronal discoloration from endodontic sealers. J Endod 2001;27:699.
18. Davis MC, Walton RE, Rivera EM. Sealer distribution in coronal dentin. J Endod 2002;28:464.
19. Li Y. Biological properties of peroxide-containing tooth whiteners. Food and Chem Toxicol 1996;34:887.
20. Haywood V B, Heymann H O. Nightguard vital bleaching. Quintessence Int 1989;20:173.

21. Weiger R, Kuhn A, Löst C. *In vitro* comparison of various types of sodium perborate used for intracoronal bleaching. J Endod 1994;20:338.
22. Rotstein I, Friedman S. pH variation among materials used for intracoronal bleaching. J Endod 1991;17:376.
23. Li Y, Lee S, Cartwright S, Wilson A. Comparison of clinical efficacy and safety of three professional at-home tooth whitening systems. Compendium 2003;24:357.
24. Spasser HF. A simple bleaching technique using sodium perborate. NY State Dent J 1961;27:332.
25. Jimenez-Rubio A, Segura JJ. The effect of the bleaching agent sodium perborate on macrophage adhesion *in vitro*: implications in external cervical root resorption. J Endod 1998;24:229.
26. Asfora KK, Santos Mdo, Montes MA, de Castro CN. Evaluation of biocompatibility of sodium perborate and 30% hydrogen peroxide using the analysis of the adherence capacity and morphology of macrophages. J Dent 2005;33:155.
27. Attin T, Paqué F, Ajam F, Lennon AM. Review of the current status of tooth whitening with the walking bleach technique. Int Endod J 2003;36:313.
28. Nutting EB, Poe GS. A new combination for bleaching teeth. J South Calif Dent Assoc 1963;31:289.
29. Holmstrup G, Palm AM, Lambjerg-Hansen H. Bleaching of discoloured root-filled teeth. Endod Dent Traumatol 1988;4:197.
30. Casey LJ, Schindler WG, Murata SM, Burgess JO. The use of dentinal etching with Endodontic bleaching procedures. J Endod 1989;15:535.
31. Steiner DR, West JD. A method to determine the location and shape of an intracoronal bleach barrier. J Endod 1994;20:304.
32. Buchalla W, Attin T. External bleaching therapy with activation by heat, light or laser-a systemic review. Dent Mater 2007;23:586.
33. Madison S, Walton RE. Cervical root resorption following bleaching of endodontically treated teeth. J Endod 1990; 16:570.
34. Rotstein I, Friedman S, Mor C, et al. Histological characterization of bleaching-induced external root resorption in dogs. J Endod 1991;17:436.
35. Lin LC, Pitts DL, Burgess LW. An investigation into the feasibility of photobleaching tetracycline-stained teeth. J Endod 1988;14:293.
36. Harrington GW, Natkin E. External resorption associated with bleaching of pulpless teeth. J Endod 1979;5:344.
37. Lado EA, Stanley HR, Weisman MI. Cervical resorption in bleached teeth. Oral Surg Oral Med Oral Pathol Oral Radiol Endod 1983;55:78.
38. Montgomery S. External cervical resorption after bleaching a pulpless tooth. Oral Surg Oral Med Oral Pathol Oral Radiol Endod 1984;57:203.
39. Shearer GJ. External resorption associated with bleaching of a non-vital tooth. Aust Endod Newslett 1984;10:16.
40. Cvek M, Lindvall AM. External root resorption following bleaching of pulpless teeth with oxygen peroxide. Endod Dent Traumatol 1985;1:56.
41. Latcham NL. Postbleaching cervical resorption. J Endod 1986;12:262.
42. Goon WWY, Cohen S, Borer RF. External cervical root resorption following bleaching. J Endod 1986;12:414.
43. Friedman S, Rotstein I, Libfeld H, et al. Incidence of external root resorption and esthetic results in 58 bleached pulpless teeth. Endod Dent Traumatol 1988;4:23.
44. Gimlin DR, Schindler WG. The management of postbleaching cervical resorption. J Endod 1990;16:292.
45. Al-Nazhan S. External root resorption after bleaching: a case report. Oral Surg Oral Med Oral Pathol Oral Radiol Endod 1991;72:607.
46. Heithersay GS, Dahlstrom SW, Marin PD. Incidence of invasive cervical resorption in bleached root-filled teeth. Aust Dent J 1994;39:82.
47. Heller D, Skriber J, Lin LM. Effect of intracoronal bleaching on external cervical root resorption. J Endod 1992;18:145.
48. Rotstein I, Torek Y, Misgav R. Effect of cementum defects on radicular penetration of 30% H_2O_2 during intracoronal bleaching. J Endod 1991;17:230.
49. Koulaouzidou E, Lambrianidis T, Beltes P, et al. Role of cementoenamel junction on the radicular penetration of 30% hydrogen peroxide during intracoronal bleaching *in vitro*. Endod Dent Traumatol 1996;12:146.
50. Rotstein I, Torek Y, Lewinstein I. Effect of bleaching time and temperature on the radicular penetration of hydrogen peroxide. Endod Dent Traumatol 1991;7:196.
51. Heling I, Parson A, Rotstein I. Effect of bleaching agents on dentin permeability to *Streptococcus faecalis*. J Endod 1995;21:540.
52. Tredwin CJ, Naik S, Lewis NJ, Scully C. Hydrogen peroxide tooth-whitening (bleaching) products: reviewof adverse effects and safety issues. Br Dent J 2006;200:371.
53. Titley KC, Torneck CD, Ruse ND, Krmec D. Adhesion of a resin composite to bleached and unbleached human enamel. J Endod 1993;19:112.
54. Attin T, Hannig C, Weigand A, Attin R. Effect of bleaching on restorative materials and restorations- a systematic review. Dent Mater 2004;20:852.
55. Titley KC, Torneck CD, Smith DC, et al. Scanning electron microscopy observations on the penetration and structure of resin tags in bleached and unbleached bovine enamel. J Endod 1991;17:71.
56. Rotstein I. Role of catalase in the elimination of residual hydrogen peroxide following tooth bleaching. J Endod 1993;19:567.

57. Rotstein I, Wesselink PR, Bab I. Catalase protection against hydrogen peroxide-induced injury in rat oral mucosa. Oral Surg Oral Med Oral Pathol Oral Radiol Endod 1993;75:744.

58. Rotstein I, Zyskind D, Lewinstein I, Bamberger N. Effect of different protective base materials on hydrogen peroxide leakage during intracoronal bleaching *in vitro*. J Endod 1992;18:114.

59. Wilcox LR, Diaz-Arnold A. Coronal microleakage of permanent lingual access restorations in endodontically treated anterior teeth. J Endod 1989;15:584.

60. Lemon R. Bleaching and restoring endodontically treated teeth. Curr Opin Dent 1991;1:754.

61. Freccia WF, Peters DD, Lorton L. An evaluation of various permanent restorative materials' effect on the shade of bleached teeth. J Endod 1982;8:265.

62. Joiner A. The bleaching of teeth: a review of the literature. J Dent 2006;25:101.

63. Reyto R. Laser tooth whitening. Dent Clin North Am 1998;42:755.

64. Kugel G, Papathanasiou A, Williams AJ, et al. Clinical evaluation of chemical and light-activated tooth whitening systems. Compend Contin Educ Dent. 2006;27:54.

65. Tavares M, Stultz J, Newman M, et al. Light augments tooth whitening with peroxide. J Am Dent Assoc. 2003;134:167.

66. Leonard RH. Long-term treatment results with nightguard vital bleaching. Compend Contin Educ Dent. 2003;24:364.

67. Haywood VB, Heymann HO. Nightguard vital bleaching: how safe is it? Quintessence Int 1991;22:515.

68. Li Y. Toxicological considerations of tooth bleaching using peroxide-containing agents. J Am Dent Assoc 1997;128:31S.

69. Li Y. Tooth bleaching using peroxide-containing agents: current status of safety issues. Compend Contin Educ Dent 1998;19:783.

70. Li Y. Peroxide-containing tooth whiteners: an update on safety. Compend Contin Educ Dent 2000;21(Suppl 28):S4.

71. Li Y. The safety of peroxide-containing at-home tooth whiteners. Compend Contin Educ Dent 2003;24:384.

72. Li Y. Common questions about the safety of tooth whitening. Inside Dentistry 2006;2:60.

73. Leonard RH, Haywood VB, Phillips C. Risk factors for developing tooth sensitivity and gingival irritation in nightguard vital bleaching. Quintessence Int 1997;28:527.

74. Jorgensen MG, Carroll WB. Incidence of tooth sensitivity after home whitening treatment. J Am Dent Assoc 2002;133:1076.

75. Pohjola RM, Browning WD, Hackman ST, et al. Sensitivity and tooth whitening agents. J Esthet Restor Dent 2002;14:85.

76. Bowles WH, Ugwuneri Z. Pulp chamber penetration of hydrogen peroxide following vital bleaching procedures. J Endodont 1987;8:875.

77. Cooper J, Bokmeyer T, Bowles W. Penetration of the pulp chamber by bleaching agents. J Endod 1992;18:315.

78. Thitinanthapan W, Satamanont P, Vongsavan N. In vitro penetration of the pulp chamber by three brands of carbamide peroxide. Esthet Dent 1999;11:259.

79. Gokay O, Yilmaz F, Akin S, et al. Penetration of the pulp chamber by bleaching agents in teeth restored with various restorative materials. J Endod 2000;26:92.

80. Slezak B, Santarpia P, Xu T, et al. Safety profile of a new liquid whitening gel. Compend Contin Educ Dent 2002;23(Suppl 1):4.

81. Benetti AR, Valera MC, Mancini MN, et al. *In vitro* penetration of bleaching agents into the pulp chamber. Int Endod J 2004;37:120.

82. Pugh G, Zaidel L, Lin N, et al. High levels of hydrogen peroxide in overnight tooth-whitening formulas: effects on enamel and pulp. J Esthet Restor Dent. 2005;17:40.

83. Lee SS, Zhang W, Lee DH, Li Y. Tooth whitening in children and adolescents: a literature review. Pediatr Dent 2005;27:362.

84. Rotstein I, Lehr T, Gedalia I. Effect of bleaching agents on inorganic components of human dentin and cementum. J Endod 1992;18:290.

85. Chng HK, Ramli HN, Yap AU, Lim CT. Effect of hydrogen peroxide on intertubular dentine. J Dent 2005;33:363.

86. Rotstein I, Dankner E, Goldman A, et al. Histochemical analysis of dental hard tissues following bleaching. J Endod 1996;22:23.

87. Leonard RH. Efficacy, longevity, side effects, and patient perceptions of nightguard vital bleaching. Compend Contin Educ Dent 1998;19:766.

88. Swift EJ, Perdigao J. Effects of Bleaching on teeth and restorations. Compend Contin Educ Dent 1998;19:815.

89. Bitter NC. A scanning electron microscope study of the long-term effect of bleaching agents on the enamel surface *in vivo*. Gen Dent 1998;46:84.

90. Potocnik I, Kosec L, Gaspersic D. Effect of 10% carbamide peroxide bleaching gel on enamel microhardness, microstructure, and mineral content. J Endod 2000;26:203.

91. White DJ, Kozak KM, Zoladz JR, et al. Peroxide interactions with hard tissues: effects on surface hardness and surface/subsurface ultrastructural properties. Compend Contin Educ Dent 2002;23:42.

92. Lopes GC, Bonissoni L, Baratieri LN, et al. Effect of bleaching agents on the hardness and morphology of enamel. J Esthet Restor Dent 2002;14:24.

93. Haywood VB, Leonard RH, Dickinson GL. Efficacy of six-months nightguard vital bleaching of tetracycline-stained teeth. J Esthet Dent 1997;9:13.

94. Cubbon T, Ore D. Hard tissue and home tooth whiteners. CDS Rev 1991;June:32.

95. Hammel S. Do-it-yourself tooth whitening is risky. US News World Rep 1998;April 2:66.

96. Schulte JR, Morrissette DB, Gasior EJ, Czajewski MV. Clinical changes in the gingiva as a result of at home bleaching. Compend Contin Educ Dent 1993;14:1362.

97. Kugel G, Aboushala A, Zhou X, et al. Daily use of whitening strips on tetracycline-stained teeth: comparative results after 2 months. Compend Contin Educ Dent 2002;23:29.

98. Gerlach RW, Zhou X. Comparative clinical efficacy of two professional bleaching systems. Compend Contin Educ Dent 2002;23:35.

99. Gerlach RW, Sagel PA, Jeffers ME, et al. Effect of peroxide concentration and brushing on whitening clinical response. Compend Contin Educ Dent 2002;23:16–21.

100. Rotstein I, Mor C, Arwaz JR. Changes in surface levels of mercury, silver, tin and copper of dental amalgam treated with carbamide peroxide and hydrogen peroxide. Oral Surg Oral Med Oral Pathol Oral Radiol Endod 1997;83:506.

101. Rotstein I, Dogan H, Avron Y, et al. Mercury release from dental amalgam following treatment with 10% carbamide peroxide in vitro. Oral Surg Oral Med Oral Pathol Oral Radiol Endod 2000;89:216.

102. Rotstein I, Avron Y, Shemesh H, et al. Factors affecting mercury release from dental amalgam exposed to carbamide peroxide bleaching agent. Am J Dent 2004;17:347.

103. Rotstein I, Dogan H, Avron Y, et al. Protective effect of Copalite surface coating on mercury release from dental amalgam following treatment with carbamide peroxide. Endod Dent Traumatol 2000;16:107.

104. Haywood VB. Bleaching vital teeth: current concepts. Quintessence Int 1997;28:424.

105. Haywood VB. Critical appraisal: at home bleaching. J Esthet Dent 1998;10:94.

106. Ritter AV, Leonard RH Jr, St Georges AJ, et al. Safety and stability of nightguard vital bleaching: 9 to 12 years post-treatment. J Esthet Restor Dent 2002;14:275.

107. Haywood VB. New bleaching considerations compared with at-home bleaching. J Esthet Restor Dent 2003;15:184.

108. de Silva GM, Brackett MG, Haywood VB. Number of in-office light-activated bleaching treatments needed to achieve patient satisfaction. Quintessence Int 2006;37:115.

109. Goldstein RE, Garber DA. Complete dental bleaching. Hanover Park, IL: Quintessence Publishing; 1995.

110. Greenwall L. Bleaching techniques in restorative dentistry, an illustrated guide. London: Martin Dunitz Ltd.; 2001.

111. Haywood VB. Tooth whitening: indications and outcomes of nightguard vital bleaching. Hanover Park, IL: Quintessence Publishing; 2007.

CHAPTER 39

ENDODONTIC THERAPY FOR PRIMARY TEETH

J. TODD MILLEDGE

Dedicated to the memory of Dr. Clifton Dummett Jr., 1944–2006, professor and chair of pediatric dentistry, Louisiana State University.

A dentist who provides emergency or restorative care for children will inevitably encounter a situation where a primary tooth has a pulp exposure. This could be from a traumatic injury or as the result of a mechanical or a carious pulp exposure. It is important that the practitioner understands the options available for proper treatment.

Dental treatment of primary teeth must satisfy different goals than treatment for permanent teeth. Primary teeth have a limited life span, and if the choice of dental care is properly matched to the needs of the patient's tooth, it is often possible to treat a primary tooth once. Treating primary teeth more than once in the tooth's life span wastes time and is costly. Primary teeth are very important for the child's smile, for proper chewing, and for maintaining space for the developing permanent dentition. Premature loss of a primary tooth can cause a number of problems including arch perimeter loss, supraeruption of opposing teeth, and changes in the patient's occlusion. There are situations where it is impossible to save a primary tooth and extraction of the tooth is indicated. In these cases a space maintainer needs to be placed and monitored to prevent negative changes in the patient's occlusion.

The main goal of endodontic therapy for primary teeth is to maintain an intact dental arch, a healthy periodontium, and vitality of the dental pulp when possible. In situations where a tooth's pulp becomes necrotic or irreversibly involved, a tooth can still be treated and maintained in a healthy state until exfoliation. In this chapter, there will be a number of references to a document entitled *Guideline on Pulp Therapy for Primary and Young Permanent Teeth* published by the American Academy of Pediatric Dentistry.[1] These guidelines are prepared by a committee of pediatric dentists to sum up the current recommendations from the Academy for dentists who provide dental care for children. Currently accepted endodontic therapy for primary teeth can be divided into two categories: vital pulp therapy and root canal therapy. Vital pulp therapy includes indirect pulp cap, direct pulp cap, and pulpotomy. Root canal therapy includes pulpectomy. This chapter is intended to provide information on endodontic therapy for primary teeth only. For information on pulp therapy for young permanent teeth, please see Chapter 35, "Vital Pulp Therapy".

A Comparison of Primary and Permanent Tooth Anatomy

The anatomical structure of primary teeth differs from permanent teeth in a number of ways. Compared to permanent teeth, primary teeth have thinner enamel and it is more consistent in thickness. The pulp space of primary teeth is very large in comparison to the overall size of the tooth. The dentin that separates the enamel and the pulp does not provide very much protection to the large pulp (Figure 1). Once a carious lesion begins in a primary tooth, it can quickly progress through the thin enamel, the thin dentin, and infect the pulp more quickly than in a permanent tooth (Figure 2).

In a study of the root canal anatomy of primary incisors and molars, Salama et al.[2] found that primary central incisor root canals have a fairly consistent length of 16 to 17 mm. Primary lateral incisors root canals are more varied, ranging from 14 to 16 mm. Incisors do not have any significant differentiation between the chamber and the root canal, and roots of incisors frequently curve facially in the apical third to half of the root. The cross-sectional shape of incisor root canals varies from round or oval to triangular. Apical foramina are generally associated with the

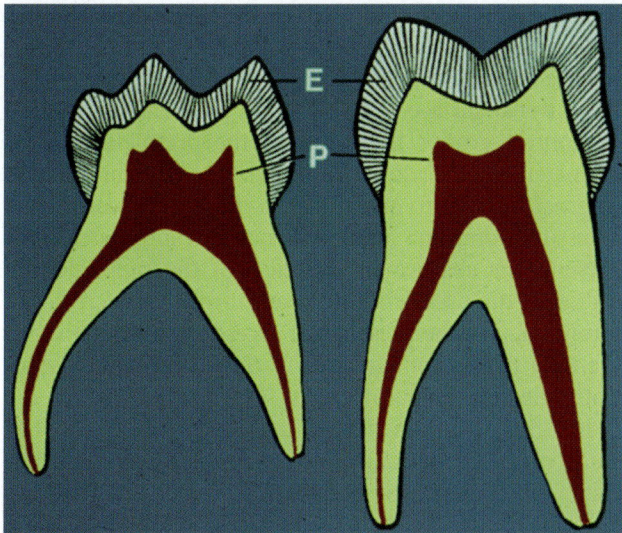

Figure 1 Contrasting primary (left) and permanent (right) tooth. Note large pulp space and thin dentin in the primary tooth.

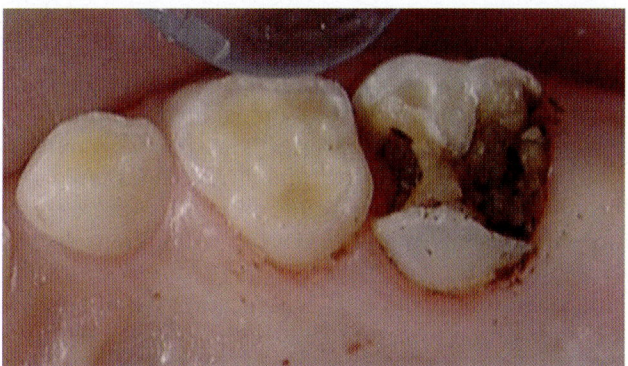

Figure 2 Severely cariously involved primary second molar.

anatomical apex of the root. Mandibular primary molars are found to have three to four root canals. The lengths of root canals in primary molars are more variable than in primary incisors with the mesiobuccal canal usually being the longest in mandibular primary molars. The cross-sectional shape of the canal in mandibular primary molars is usually oval and the mesial canals are wider buccolingually than the distal root canals. Maxillary primary molars were not included in the study.

Puddhikarant[3] did a radiographic study of pulp chambers of primary molars. Twenty primary molars were radiographed prior to any preparation of the teeth. The pulp chambers were outlined on the radiographs and the number of pulp horns were counted. The teeth were then sectioned at the cervix and filled with a radiopaque resin. Each of the teeth was sectioned mesiodistally and radiographed from the buccal side of the section. The radiographs were then projected onto a screen and a tracing was made for each specimen. The tracings were superimposed and analyzed.

The radiographs of the presectioned *mandibular second primary molars* demonstrated three to four pulp horns with the mesial pulp horn being the largest. The radiograph of the buccal section demonstrated three pulp horns with the mesiobuccal pulp horn being the largest. The lingual section demonstrated two pulp horns: a mesial and a distal. The mesial pulp horn was the largest.

Mandibular first primary molars demonstrated two pulp horns in the presectioned radiographs. The mesial pulp horn was the largest. The radiographs of the sectioned crowns demonstrated both a mesial and a distal pulp horn for both the buccal and lingual sections. The mesial pulp horns were larger than the distal for both sections.

Maxillary second primary molars showed two to four pulp horns in the presectioned radiographs. The mesial pulp horn was the largest. In the sectioned groups, the radiographs of the buccal and lingual sections showed pulp horns on both the mesial and the distal. The mesial pulp horns were larger than the distal.

The radiographs of the presectioned *maxillary first primary molars* demonstrated mesial and distal pulp horns. The buccal and lingual sections also revealed mesial and distal pulp horns with the mesial being the largest. The authors of this study made the following conclusions: Radiographs of extracted unsectioned primary molars showed two to five overlapped pulp horns. The radiographs of the sectioned buccal and lingual specimens showed that the lingual pulp horns were superimposed by the larger buccal pulp horns.

The clinical significance of this research is that pulp exposures can occur very easily in primary molars. Overextending an amalgam or a composite resin preparation, either axially or buccolingually, or over-reducing the occlusal reduction of a stainless steel crown preparation can very easily cause a pulp exposure in a primary molar tooth.

Another study of primary molars demonstrated that cervical pulp horns exist bilaterally in slightly over one-third of all molars. The average buccal extension of the pulp horns was one-quarter to one-third of a millimeter. It was speculated that pulpal sensitivity can occur when a primary molar with cervical pulp horns is prepared or overprepared in the cervical area.[4] It is interesting to note that instructions for the preparation of primary molar teeth in pediatric dental texts as well as crown manufacturers of stainless steel crowns do not routinely recommend reduction of the buccal surface of the tooth. Reduction of the buccal surface is recommended only in situations where there is an excessive buccal cervical bulge. It seems wise to avoid reducing or overreducing the buccal cervical area of primary molars when possible and to avoid causing irritation to the teeth with cervical pulp horns.

Numerous studies have been performed to determine the presence of accessory canals in primary molar furcations. In 1965, Moss[5] studied histologically the pulpal floor of primary molars. Fifty-six teeth were chosen because they had more than half of the root present and preextraction radiographs demonstrated that furcal radiolucencies were confined to the area directly below the furcation. The study was divided into two parts. First, to determine if pulpally infected primary molar teeth furcations were more porous than noninfected teeth. Second, to study the dental hard tissues of furcations of infected and noninfected molars to determine if there was any change in the infected teeth that allowed the formation of the interradicular radiolucencies noted in radiographs.

Overall findings of this study demonstrated that infected primary molar teeth furcations have an increase in porosity of the dentin and cementum. In addition, accessory canals were not always present in all primary molars and therefore could not be considered as the only pathway for the formation of an interradicular radiolucency. Finally, the dentin and cementum of the infected teeth had structural changes in the dentin and cementum.

Ringelstein[6] using dye penetration with the aid of vacuum suction, showed that 42.7% of primary molars in the study had foramina in the furcation region. Paras[7] used scanning electron microscopy (SEM) to ascertain the presence of accessory foramina in the internal and external furcation surfaces of primary molar teeth. Accessory foramina were present on 20% of internal surfaces and 50% of external surfaces. Wrbas[8] used light microscopy to study the furcation of 40 primary molars that were decalcified and embedded in paraffin, and then sectioned. The sections were studied sequentially. Channels were classified as an accessory canal if patency was evident from the pulp completely through to the periodontal ligament. Accessory foramina with a completely patent canal were present in approximately 30% of the maxillary and mandibular primary second molars.

Kramer[9] also performed an SEM study of the furcations of primary molar teeth. The teeth were taken from two groups: previously infected teeth and healthy unaffected teeth. He found that in the specimens studied, 53% of the teeth had accessory foramina in the external surface of the tooth and 25% had accessory foramina in the internal surface. There was no difference in the test or control groups in regard to the prevalence or the diameter of accessory foramina. He concluded that external furcation areas had a higher prevalence of accessory foramina than internal furcation areas, the presence or absence of infection of the pulp did not influence the prevalence or anatomical characteristics of foramina, and the presence of accessory foramina is not the only reason for furcation pathological bone resorption following pulpal necrosis.

In 2004, Dammaschke et al.[10] performed an SEM study on permanent and primary molar teeth to determine the presence of accessory foramina. Ninety-four percent of the primary molars were found to have accessory foramina with maxillary and mandibular molars having equal numbers. Primary molars had significantly more accessory foramina and foramina of larger diameter than the permanent molars studied. There was no attempt to determine if there was a patent canal connected to the foramina. The authors concluded that accessory canals might contribute to furcation bone resorption when molars have pulpal inflammation.

In conclusion, furcal bone resorption associated with primary molars with pulpal necrosis should not be considered to be the result only of the presence of accessory canals in the furcation. Alterations in the structure of the dental tissues in the furcation of the tooth could also allow communication from a necrotic pulp to the furcation.

Medical Factors in Determining if a Primary Tooth Should be Saved

A thorough medical history is an essential part of the patient's initial examination and can play an important part in the treatment planning process. Listed below are certain medical conditions that contraindicate endodontic therapy in the primary dentition.[11]

CONTRAINDICATIONS

- Patients with congenital cardiac defects
- Immunosuppressed patients
- Patients who do not heal well, that is, those with uncontrolled diabetes or patients being treated for cancer
- Patients with severe medical conditions who must be treated with general anesthesia in an operating room where the risk of treatment failure and the

need for a second general anesthetic must be minimized

There are also some medical conditions where it would be advisable to perform endodontic therapy in order to avoid extraction of a tooth.[11]
- Bleeding and coagulation disorders such as hemophilia
- Hypodontia in the permanent dentition, where a primary tooth is expected to remain as long as possible or for the life of the patient.

Diagnosis of Pulpal Pathosis in Children

The first question to ask in regard to a primary tooth with pulp exposure is: Should the tooth be retained or extracted? Other important questions include:[11]
- Is the tooth close to exfoliation?
- Does the tooth have excessive mobility?
- Is the extent of the infection severe enough to warrant extraction?
- Is the crown of the tooth restorable?
- Is there a permanent successor to the primary tooth? If not, the primary tooth may take on additional importance and may need to be treated similar to a permanent tooth with a conventional root canal treatment to extend the life of the tooth as long as possible (Figure 3).
- Is this tooth critical to the eruption of other teeth? It may be important to save a primary second molar prior to the eruption of a first permanent molar in order to prevent its mesial tipping or drifting. This could interfere with the patient's occlusion and prevent the second premolars from erupting correctly.

Aside from specific medical and dental indications and contraindications for endodontic therapy for primary teeth, there are some other real-life challenges that may influence the choice of care for a child's tooth. A dentist may technically be able to perform endodontic therapy for a child, but if the child cannot cooperate for the treatment or sit still for a long enough period of time, extraction may be the treatment of choice.

Once the dentist and the patient have decided to keep the tooth, a correct pulpal diagnosis must be made. The type of endodontic therapy chosen for a primary tooth must be based on the clinical diagnosis of normal pulp, reversible pulpitis, irreversible pulpitis, or necrotic pulp. The choice of treatment must also include evaluation of the following criteria:

1. Consideration of the patient's dental history, including any signs or symptoms the patient may have experienced.
2. A thorough clinical examination including any tests. Percussion and mobility are helpful but electric pulp testing is not reliable in children.
3. Periapical and bitewing radiographs

It is very important to discuss with the parent and the patient the types of signs or symptoms the patient has been experiencing. Provoked pain or pain that occurs only when the patient eats sweet, hot or cold foods or liquids, but resolves when the stimulus is removed, is usually indicative of reversible pulpitis. In these situations, vital pulp therapy is usually the appropriate treatment. Spontaneous or nocturnal pain usually indicates irreversible pulpitis or pulpal necrosis. Teeth that exhibit irreversible pulpitis or necrosis will usually have associated signs such as pathologic mobility, sinus tract, internal and/or external resorption, and furcal or periapical radiolucency.[1]

Treatment of Deep Caries: Indirect Pulp Therapy

Indirect pulp therapy can be performed when a tooth has a deep carious lesion that is very close to the pulp and it is anticipated that the pulp would be exposed when the caries is excavated. The tooth should not have any signs or symptoms of irreversible pulpitis. This treatment relies on the natural ability of teeth to

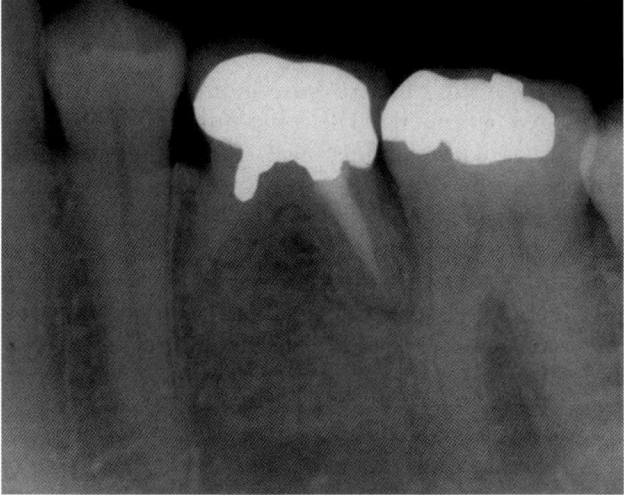

Figure 3 Primary second molar with no permanent successor has received root canal treatment with gutta-percha. Such teeth may last for many years.

form reparative dentin. In this treatment the caries is removed in all areas of the lesion except where there would be an exposure. The most infected portion of the caries is removed leaving less infected demineralized dentin. The remaining demineralized dentin is usually covered with a calcium hydroxide liner. The tooth is then restored to completely seal the tooth from the oral environment. When bacteria are excluded from the caries, the tooth can remineralize the dentin directly over the site where the exposure would have occurred. The patient should not experience any pain with this procedure.[1]

The literature concerning indirect pulp therapy contains some very interesting studies and results. In a study in 1966, Aponte et al.[12] studied 30 primary molars that received calcium hydroxide indirect pulp therapy, zinc phosphate bases, and amalgam restorations. These teeth were evaluated post operatively by removing the amalgam restoration and cement base with sterile burs and rubber dam isolation. The hardness of the dentin was checked and a culture of the remaining dentin was taken. The cultures were incubated and evaluated for bacterial growth. The cultures of 93% of the teeth were sterile. Two teeth were positive for lactobacilli and streptococci. The dentin was hard and shiny in appearance. They concluded that in 93% of the molars studied, the residual carious dentin was free of microorganisms 6 to 46 months after treatment. In addition there was radiographic evidence of reparative dentin formation in many of the postoperative radiographs. Some of the earlier studies, regarding indirect pulp therapy, were concerned about calcium hydroxide formulation. In a 1982 study, Sawusch[13] tested Dycal (Dentsply International, York, PA) and a newer formulation of Dycal. He demonstrated that both formulations of Dycal were acceptable for use in indirect pulp therapy, and the teeth that failed generally were associated with a faulty restoration. In similar studies, success rates have been about 94%.[14,15]

Coll et al.[16] performed a study comparing pulpotomy, indirect pulp therapy, and pulpectomy on primary incisors. In this study of 45 patients, 28 received pulpotomy, 26 were treated with indirect pulp therapy, and 27 received pulpectomy. These were compared with a control group of 58 teeth receiving no treatment. The teeth receiving the pulpotomy treatment met the following criteria: no medical contraindication, radiographic visible caries approximating the pulp with no contraindicating pathosis, no pathologic mobility, no history of traumatic dental injuries, presence of a carious pulp exposure after caries excavation, and appropriate hemorrhage in the pulp chamber after pulp amputation. Teeth treated with indirect pulp therapy had deep caries approximating the pulp, with no signs of irreversible pulpitis. Criteria for pulpectomy were based on clinical signs of pulp necrosis, total lack of hemorrhage in the canal, and 90% of the teeth had a sinus tract. The teeth were followed clinically and radiographically. The overall success rate for pulpotomy was 85.7% for teeth followed for a mean of 43.8 months. Teeth treated with indirect pulp therapy had a success rate of 92.3% at 42 months. The teeth treated with pulpectomy had a success rate of 77.7% at 45.5 months. They found, however, that when endodontically treated incisors exfoliated, in 73% of the cases, zinc oxide–eugenol (ZOE) cement remained in site. The researchers concluded that in a clinical situation where there was deep caries but no pulp exposure, indirect pulp therapy would be indicated. When there was a direct pulp exposure of an otherwise healthy pulp, pulpotomy should be the treatment of choice. They also concluded that because of the high incidence of retained ZOE, pulpectomy treatment should be chosen only if there is evidence of pulp necrosis.

Farooq et al.[17] performed a retrospective study comparing the success rates of formocresol pulpotomy and indirect pulp therapy for primary teeth. In this study, 133 primary molars with deep caries were treated with either indirect pulp therapy or formocresol pulpotomy. All of the indirect pulp therapy teeth were restored with stainless steel crowns. Sixty-one of the pulpotomized teeth received a stainless steel crown, 13 received a reinforced ZOE base, and 4 received an amalgam. The overall success for *indirect pulp therapy* was 93% compared to 74% for the *formocresol pulpotomized* teeth. Of the teeth treated with formocresol pulpotomy, 38% exfoliated prematurely while the teeth treated with indirect pulp therapy exfoliated normally. The pulpotomized teeth that had immediate stainless steel crowns had the best success rate of 82%, while the ZOE base-restored teeth had a success rate of only 39%. The conclusion was that indirect pulp therapy had a success rate that was much higher than formocresol pulpotomy. They also concluded that indirect pulp therapy can be performed as a one-step procedure, and restoring a pulpally treated tooth with a stainless steel crown immediately after the pulp therapy increases the chances of success.

In 2002, a study by Al-Zayer et al.[18] demonstrated that 187 posterior primary teeth treated with *indirect pulp treatment* had a success rate of 95%. All the teeth received a Dycal calcium hydroxide liner to cover the remaining carious dentin. Ninety-one of the teeth that received stainless steel crowns had cement bases and the crowns were cemented with ZOE cement. Eighteen additional teeth received a resin-modified glass ionomer material for base and for cementing the crowns. Sixty-eight teeth were restored with amalgam and 13 were restored with a composite resin. There are a number of interesting conclusions to this study. First primary molars were more likely to fail than second primary molars. Teeth restored with amalgam, after an indirect pulp treatment, are 7.7 times more likely to fail than teeth restored with a stainless steel crown. Teeth that had a base placed over the calcium hydroxide liner had a higher success rate than teeth that received no base.

Dentists today are more likely to restore teeth with adhesive restorations. Amalgam and stainless steel crowns are becoming less desirable to patients and their parents. A 2002 study by Falster et al.[19] compared indirect pulp treatment using an adhesive resin system and the traditional calcium hydroxide base. Forty-eight primary molar teeth, treatment planned for an occlusal resin restoration for deep caries, were divided into two groups and followed for 2 years depending on the type of pulpal protection used: calcium hydroxide (Dycal) and Scotchbond MultiPurpose (3M, St. Paul, MN). The researchers found that 83% of the teeth treated with calcium hydroxide and 96% of the teeth treated with Scotchbond MultiPurpose were found to be successful. They concluded that protection of the pulp, with indirect pulp treatment with an adhesive resin, is as effective as the use of a traditional calcium hydroxide liner when placed under a single surface resin restoration. In addition, they stated that after removing deep caries in a primary tooth and establishing a good seal, the tooth's innate healing abilities are more important to success than the use of calcium hydroxide.

In a recent study, Vij et al.[20] compared caries control procedures on the success rate of indirect pulp treatment and formocresol pulpotomy. Teeth with deep caries were treated with either formocresol pulpotomy or indirect pulp treatment. Seventy-eight of the teeth were treated with caries control 1 to 3 months prior to the actual procedure. Caries control is a procedure similar to alternative restorative treatment where a large part of the caries is removed and a reinforced ZOE or a glass ionomer base is placed. This is done to slow the progression of the caries and allow the tooth to heal itself by forming reparative dentin. The success rate of indirect pulp treatment after 3 years follow-up was 94%, whereas formocresol treatment attained a success rate of only 70%. Pulpotomized teeth that had only a reinforced ZOE base as the final restoration had a success rate of 39%. When these teeth were excluded from the total number of pulpotomized teeth, the success rate of the pulpotomies increased to 74%, still much lower than the 94% of the indirect pulp treatments. Thirty-six percent of the pulpotomized teeth but only 2% of the indirect pulp-treated teeth exfoliated early. Conclusions from this study include the following: long-term success rates of indirect pulp therapy was much better than the success rate for formocresol pulpotomy; glass ionomer caries control 1 to 3 months prior to the actual treatment increased the chances of success; vital pulp therapy in primary first molars was lower than primary second molars; and teeth with formocresol pulpotomy exfoliated earlier than teeth treated with indirect pulp therapy.

It seems that success with indirect pulp treatment depends on a number of important criteria: no symptoms or symptoms consistent with reversible pulpitis, absence of clinical or radiographic lesions such as internal or external resorption or furcation radiolucency, complete removal of caries on all of the walls of the preparation leaving only a small amount of caries in the area where there would be an exposure, and placement of a restoration that provides an excellent seal to prevent recontamination from bacteria. All these improve the tooth's innate capabilities to remineralize the dentin and heal the pulp.

Vital Pulp Therapy for Children: Direct Pulp Cap

Direct pulp cap is a treatment option for teeth with traumatic or mechanical pulp exposures. It should be attempted only when the pulp is vital and has not had any signs or symptoms of irreversible pulpitis. The exposed pulp and the adjacent dentin are covered with a base such as calcium hydroxide or Mineral Trioxide Aggregate (MTA) and the tooth receives a permanent restoration. The patient should not experience any pain and reparative dentin is expected to form. The tooth pulp should remain vital and free of any signs or symptoms of irreversible pulpitis.[1] In spite of the recommendation from the American Academy of Pediatric Dentistry, direct pulp capping is not a common procedure for most pediatric dentists. In the current editions of both of the most accepted pediatric dental textbooks,[21,22] the sections are very small and contain relatively few journal references. Both of these textbooks make the following recommendations regarding direct pulp cap for primary teeth. Direct pulp cap is indicated for pinpoint-sized mechanical or traumatic pulp exposures. Direct pulp capping of a carious pulp exposure is not recommended. There should be an absence of pain and no bleeding or only a small amount of bleeding consistent with a healthy pulp. The cap should be performed with the use of a rubber dam to prevent any contamination of the pulp. Calcium hydroxide remains the pulp capping agent of choice at this time.[21,22] Direct pulp capping should be performed in older children where the pulp capped tooth is not expected to last for more than a couple of years until normal exfoliation.

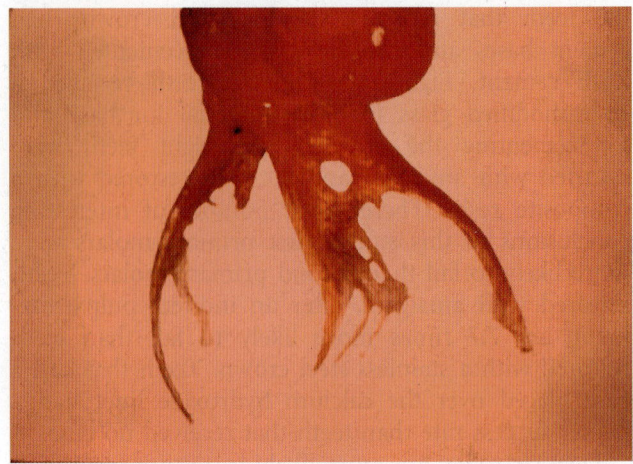

Figure 4 Root canal system of a primary molar (resin impression).

Pulpotomy

Pulpotomy is a procedure for teeth with healthy pulps or teeth with symptoms of reversible pulpitis and deep caries where carious pulp exposure is encountered. Radiographically, the tooth should not show signs of pathological resorption or radiolucency.[1]

Pulpotomy is also an alternative for a tooth with traumatic pulp exposure. The coronal pulp is amputated leaving an intact vital radicular pulp. The remaining radicular pulp is treated with an appropriate medicament, the chamber filled with a suitable base and the tooth is restored with a suitable restorative material.[1] Under ideal circumstances it may be preferable to do pulpectomy and root canal treatment for such teeth, but as described earlier, primary teeth have very unpredictable and tortuous root canal systems. It can be very difficult or impossible to clean and shape and properly obturate the root canals (Figure 4). In addition, primary teeth have thin enamel and large pulp chambers and caries can progress very quickly. Cooperation can be difficult for some children and behavior management can be difficult for the dentist who has to provide extensive restorative treatment. Pulpotomy seems to be a reasonable treatment option to meet these situations. By removing only the coronal pulp, the difficult root canal systems are avoided. A pulpotomy certainly requires less time than complete root canal treatment, solving the problem of keeping a child patient in the dental chair too long. It is recommended that all pulp therapies be performed with a rubber dam to protect the patient from accidental swallowing or aspiration and to prevent contamination of the tooth during treatment.[1] Clinical signs and symptoms should resolve within about 2 weeks. After this, the pulpotomized tooth should remain asymptomatic exhibiting no pathologic mobility, sensitivity, or pain.

Formocresol

Formocresol is the most common pulpotomy medicament used in pediatric dentistry today. It is the standard to which all other pulpotomy procedures are compared. For these two reasons, it is important to understand the history of formocresol in pediatric dentistry.

The use of formocresol as pulp medicament is attributed to Buckley from 1904 to 1906.[23,24] Buckley outlined the use of a mixture of formalin and cresol to treat necrotic or "putrescent" pulps. In the 1930s, Sweet[25–27] developed a multiappointment pulpotomy procedure that became very popular and is the predecessor for our current single-appointment pulpotomy. In his articles, he recommended a five-appointment procedure that he later modified to three appointments. Since then, formocresol has been the subject of a great deal of research. A modern formocresol pulpotomy generally involves removal

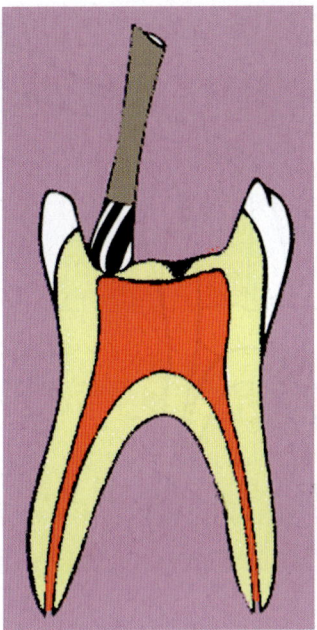

Figure 5 Caries removal.

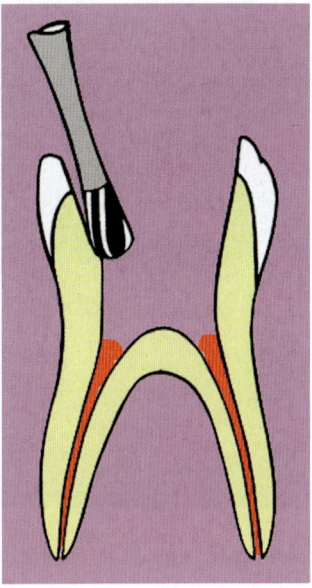

Figure 6 Removal of the roof of the pulp chamber.

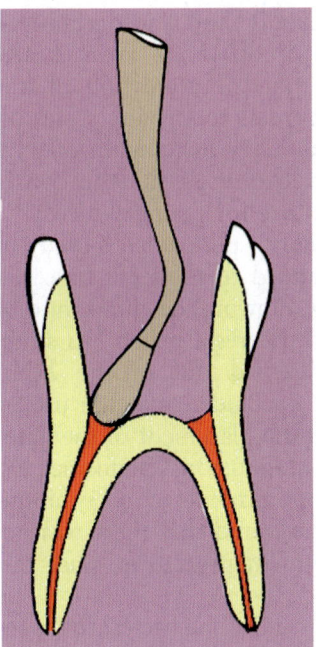

Figure 7 Removal of the coronal pulp with a spoon excavator.

of the carious tooth structure with a slow-speed round bur (Figure 5) followed by removal of the roof of the pulp chamber with a high-speed bur with water spray (Figure 6). The coronal pulp is then removed with a slow-speed round bur or an excavator (Figure 7). Hemostasis is obtained with sterile cotton pellets. After hemostasis, a medicated pellet with either full-strength or diluted formocresol is placed with slight pressure for 5 minutes (Figure 8), after which the medicated pellet is removed and the pulp is assessed for continued bleeding. When bleeding has been completely controlled, a ZOE base is placed (Figure 9), followed by a final restoration (Figure 10). Research reports are usually based on modifications of the above procedure. The following review of the literature follows a historical sequence. It is difficult to directly compare the studies since each one contains some variables that are different from the other studies. Therefore each study, and its conclusions, must be evaluated individually.

The first area considered will be overall success rates of formocresol pulpotomies. In 1975 to 1978, Rolling[28] studied formocresol pulpotomies for a period of up to

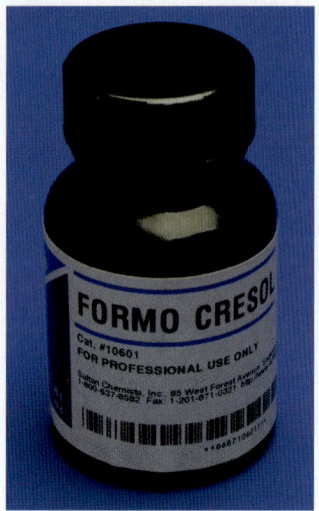

Figure 8 Formocresol used for pulpotomy in primary teeth.

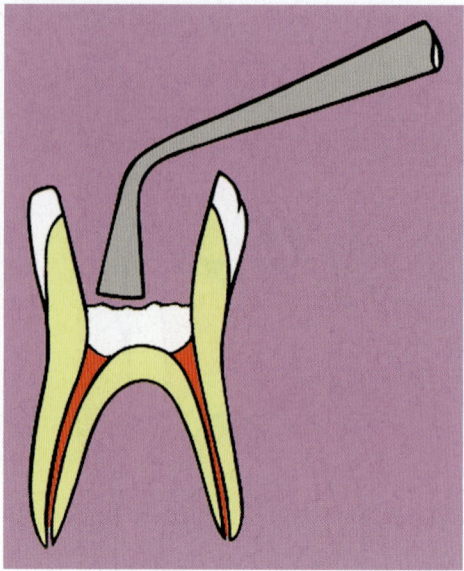

Figure 9 Placement of a zinc oxide–eugenol (ZOE) base.

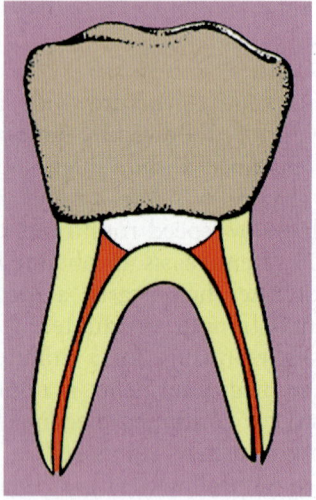

Figure 10 Primary molar with a stainless steel crown.

36 months. She used full-strength formocresol and also added formocresol to her ZOE base. The results of her study found that there was a success rate of 90% after 3 months and an overall success rate of 70% after 3 years. In a follow-up study, Rolling et al.[29] continued evaluation of the same group of teeth. They found that the pulp conditions, as evidenced by enzyme histochemical methods, varied from normal to total necrosis. They concluded that the formocresol procedure should be regarded only as a way to keep primary teeth with exposed pulps functioning for a short time. In a third study from 1978, Rolling et al.[30] examined histologically the pulps of primary molars treated with formocresol pulpotomy which were considered to be both clinically and radiographically successful for a period of up to 24 months after treatment. They found that the condition of the pulp varied from total necrosis to varying states of fixation and inflammation. They once again concluded that formocresol pulpotomy should be considered a temporary procedure for primary teeth.

In 1975, Ranly[31] performed a study to determine if formocresol added to the ZOE base was adequate to treat the pulp, allowing the clinician to skip the step of placing the formocresol pellet. His study showed that formocresol leached out of the ZOE in adequate amounts and concluded that the use of a medicated pellet prior to the placement of the base was unnecessary. In 1978, Magnusson[32] performed a study comparing a two-appointment to a 5-minute formocresol pulpotomy. He found that there was no advantage in a two-appointment procedure, since the success rates were similar.

Cox et al.[33] studied the bactericidal potential of materials used in primary tooth pulpotomies. They found that plain zinc oxide did not have any inhibitory effect on the bacteria tested. When eugenol was added, the growth of gram-positive organisms was retarded. Addition of zinc acetate as an accelerator to the cement inhibited both the gram-positive and the gram-negative bacteria. When formocresol or paraformaldehyde was added to the zinc oxide–eugenol–zinc acetate cement, there was an even greater inhibitory effect. They concluded that zinc oxide–eugenol–zinc acetate cement, with or without formocresol, was probably effective in eliminating bacteria from pulpotomized primary teeth. Adding highly cytotoxic materials to cement bases that remain active for long periods of time may not be necessary for successful treatment.

Mejare[34] studied mandibular primary molar pulpotomies on teeth with diagnosis either of clinically healthy or clinically inflamed root pulp, using full-strength formocresol ZOE base. She had a success rate of 63% and concluded that there was no statistical difference in the two groups. In 1982, Garcia-Godoy[35] published two studies. In the first, he compared the pulpal response of various application times to formocresol in dogs. He found that an application time of 1 minute produced less inflammation than 3 and 5 minutes. He also found that when formocresol was incorporated into the ZOE base, it produced a more intense inflammatory response. He concluded that the longer formocresol is in contact with the pulp tissue, the worse the tissue response. In addition, he stated that additional studies should compare 1- and 5-minute pulpotomy application times. In his second dog study, Garcia-Godoy[36] compared formocresol pulpotomy with two different bases, ZOE and polycarboxylate. He had two pulpotomy treatment groups, one without formocresol treatment and either a ZOE or polycarboxylate cement base, and the other group was treated with formocresol followed with either a ZOE or polycarboxylate cement. The polycarboxylate groups had similar amounts of inflammation. The ZOE-treated teeth that had not been treated previously with formocresol had more intense inflammatory responses than the teeth treated with formocresol. He concluded that formocresol seems to reduce the pulpal response to ZOE; probably the eugenol in the ZOE base is an irritant. He concluded that dentists should rethink the use of ZOE as a base in pulpotomies.

In 1986, van Amerongen et al.[37] compared formocresol pulpotomy treated teeth with their untreated contralateral teeth. They found that there was no significant difference in the life span between the formocresol-treated teeth and the control teeth concluding that formocresol pulpotomy is a reasonable treatment for primary teeth with pulp exposure. In 1986, Hicks et al.[38] performed a study in a pediatric dentist's practice and evaluated formocresol pulpotomized teeth radiographically. In this office, the dentists did not use a formocresol-treated cotton pellet after obtaining hemostasis, but instead they immediately placed a ZOE base that also contained formocresol. When they evaluated the radiographs, they found furcation radiolucency in 3.7% of the cases. When they classified the results as successful, questionable, or failure, the success rate was 89%. When they combined the successful with the radiographically questionable but clinically successful cases, the success rate jumped to 93.8%. Clinically, this is how most pediatric dentists deal with their patients.

There are certain clinical outcomes that would be definite failures and others that are questionable but tolerable. Most practitioners play a waiting game, hoping that these questionable teeth will exfoliate before they have a problem that requires extraction. Thompson et al.[39] studied the formocresol pulpotomy opting to delete the step that obtains hemostasis with dry sterile cotton pellets and instead they obtained hemostasis with the formocresol pellet that was placed over the amputated pulp. They studied 194 teeth for up to 38 months. The radiographic success rate was 87% with the most frequent radiographic problems being pulp canal obliteration and internal resorption. Overall clinical success rate was 98%. They concluded that skipping the step of obtaining hemostasis with a dry cotton pellet was an acceptable variation of the formocresol pulpotomy when hemostasis was obtained with the formocresol-treated pellet. Strange et al.,[40] using modified radiographic success and failure criteria, studied formocresol pulpotomies with a ZOE base incorporating formocresol instead of a formocresol-medicated cotton pellet. Traditionally, internal resorption has been considered a sign of failure. More recently, researchers have joined clinical dentists in excluding internal resorption as a sign of failure. A small area of internal resorption that does not perforate the root can be tolerated and probably indicates the pulp is still vital. In this study, Strange et al. studied 196 primary molars for up to 49 months. Using the traditional radiographic failure criteria, a success rate of 79% was obtained. When internal resorption was excluded, the radiographic success rate jumped to 99%. Overall clinical success rate was 99%. They concluded that incorporating formocresol into the ZOE base was a successful form of formocresol pulpotomy.

Holan et al.[41] compared the success rate of formocresol pulpotomy when restored with amalgam and stainless steel crowns. They concluded that formocresol pulpotomized teeth that were restored with two or more surface amalgams had a higher failure rate than formocresol pulpotomized teeth restored with a one-surface amalgam or a stainless steel crown. They concluded that pulpotomized primary molars can be successfully restored with a one-surface amalgam if the tooth is expected to naturally exfoliate in less than 2 years.

Guelmann et al.[42] evaluated the success of emergency pulpotomies on primary molars. They studied the records of 216 formocresol pulpotomies that were temporarily restored with a reinforced ZOE material. The outcome was determined at the time of placement of the permanent restoration. Sixty-four teeth were available for the study. A 53% success rate was obtained if the tooth was restored in the first 3 months after the pulpotomy and 31% success if the tooth was restored after 1 year. They concluded that the low success rate in the first 90 days was probably attributed to an undiagnosed pulpitis at the time of treatment and later failures were probably associated with microleakage of the ZOE material. Their second follow-up study revealed that when a stainless steel crown was placed immediately or very soon after the emergency pulpotomy, the success rate increased significantly.[43] Guelmann et al.[44] also studied the success of formocresol pulpotomized teeth that were restored with a resin. Fifty-nine teeth were included in the study with an average follow-up time of 21 months. Overall, pulpotomized teeth with a resin restoration had success rates that were inferior to the previously published success rates of stainless steel crowns. When the occlusal surface was the only surface restored, however, the success rate was 100%. Overall, formocresol pulpotomies have success rates that range from a low in the 50% range up into the mid 90% range. As one can see, there are many variables and techniques used, and it depends on whether clinical or radiographic or combined success rates are being considered.

A number of studies have questioned the postoperative effect of formocresol pulpotomy on the primary teeth, and also on the succedaneous premolars. It has been demonstrated in studies, and it is obvious to clinicians, that teeth treated with formocresol pulpotomy routinely demonstrate pulp canal calcification.[45,46] Conflicting information has been published regarding the effect of pulpotomized primary molars on their permanent successors. Some studies show that premolars, successors to pulpotomized primary molars, demonstrate no correlation.[47–50]

Early on, clinicians and researchers began to question Buckley's original formulation strength and wondered if a more dilute concentration would be just as effective as full strength. A number of in vitro and in vivo studies tested formocresol to determine the minimum effective concentration that would give the same or very similar benefit while reducing the negative effects.[51–60] From these studies, it is generally agreed that 20% dilution of the original Buckley's formulation is an effective concentration for clinical practice. Unfortunately, in spite of the science, pediatric dentists persist in using full-strength formocresol. In 2002, a survey of 422 pediatric dentists revealed that 84% of those who responded use formocresol for pulpotomies. Of that group, 69% use full-strength formocresol. Many unknowingly use full-strength formocresol and think they are using a diluted product. These latter dentists stated that they buy diluted formocresol even though it is not available commercially. It is unfortunate that a technique that is so widely used has so much confusion in practice.[61]

Formocresol has been found to be cytotoxic to pulp tissues. In studies, formocresol, formaldehyde, and cresol have been placed in contact with pulp cells. Formocresol and formaldehyde have been found to be more cytotoxic than cresol. The response of the pulp tissue appears to be time- and concentration-dependent. The more dilute the concentration of formocresol, the less intense the inflammatory response. In addition, the longer formocresol is in contact with the pulp tissue, the more intense the inflammatory response. The formocresol-treated pulp responds by forming a number of "zones" depending on the proximity of the tissue to the medicament. At the amputation site, and where the formocresol concentration is the highest, the tissue is fixed and eosinophilic. Below this fixed zone there is a pale zone with poor cellular definition that some have described as necrotic. Close to the apex, the tissue is chronically inflamed.[62–69]

Several researchers have performed studies that measured the systemic distribution of formocresol that is applied to the pulp in the pulpotomy technique. Meyers et al.[70] studied pulpotomies on monkey teeth and found that in a 5-minute pulpotomy with ^{14}C-formaldehyde, there was systemic absorption into the plasma of approximately 1% of the dose of the medicament placed in the tooth. A 2-hour exposure did not increase the absorption. Multiple pulpotomies performed sequentially caused a higher systemic absorption of the medicament. When ^{131}I was applied to a pulpotomy not previously treated with formocresol, it was absorbed systemically in large amounts. When ^{131}I was applied to a formocresol-treated pulp, it was absorbed only in moderate amounts. This indicates that formocresol compromises the circulation of the pulp and probably limits its systemic uptake. Timed urinalysis after treating the teeth with formocresol showed that formocresol was excreted and not protein-bound. In a follow-up study, researchers in the previous study wanted to determine where the absorbed formocresol was going. In a dog study, they confirmed their previous findings that formocresol was systemically absorbed. In addition, formocresol was found in the liver, lung, muscle, heart, spleen, kidney, and even in the cerebral spinal fluid. They found that formocresol could be metabolized and excreted through the lung, but the reaction was not very fast and certainly not quick enough to account for the total amount of the medicament. Tissue binding seems to account for most of the systemic absorption. The researchers concluded that formocresol is absorbed in small quantities and they did not think that the use of formocresol should be discontinued.[71] Block et al.[72] performed another dog study and found that ^{14}C-labeled paraformaldehyde incorporated within formocresol was systemically distributed in the blood, regional lymph nodes, kidney, and liver. They measured the radioactivity over time and found that it decreased. They concluded that formocresol should not be brought into contact with vital tissues.

Ranly[73] studied pulpotomies in rats, in response to the previous two studies, because he saw a possible clinical correlation for children receiving multiple pulpotomies during full mouth dental care under general anesthesia. They were concerned with the possible transient systemic morbidity associated with a larger than normal amount of systemically absorbed formocresol. In this rat model, Ranly determined that approximately 30% of the formaldehyde that was placed into the pulp chamber was absorbed systemically in 5 minutes. He concluded that with larger doses, comparable to multiple pulpotomies, the metabolic systems that break down the medicament were not overloaded or damaged. In part two of his study, Ranly[74] questioned the findings of two previous studies.[68,71] He found that the formaldehyde used in his study required higher levels than the formocresol used in the other studies to produce biochemical changes and seemed to infer that it would require a higher quantity of formaldehyde than had been suggested to cause morbidity.

All of these studies demonstrated that formocresol is distributed systemically. There is disagreement, however, about whether this distribution can be tolerated or whether there is some lasting damage.

Other researchers sought to determine the allergenic potential of formocresol. A human study on children who had received pulpotomy treatment 2 months to 8 years prior to a skin patch allergy test showed no positive test results for formaldehyde, eugenol, or cresol.[75] Another study presensitized guinea pigs with formaldehyde or cresol. The presensitized animals received an endodontic procedure using formocresol and subsequently skin tested. In the test, the researchers demonstrated a weak allergenic potential.[76] One study documents the embryotoxicity and teratogenicity of formocresol to chick embryos.[77] Additional journals articles thoroughly document the mutagenic and carcinogenic potential of formaldehyde and formocresol.[78–80]

In 2004, the International Agency for Research on Cancer concluded that formaldehyde is carcinogenic to humans. In addition, they state that there is strong but insufficient evidence that formaldehyde is a causative agent for leukemia.[81] It would seem that with such a strong statement by the World Health Organization, and the weight of the evidence from the dental and medical literature, formocresol would have been banned for use in humans. However, the debate still goes on regarding its safety and use in dentistry. In 2005 and 2006, two articles[82,83] present opposite sides of the formocresol debate demonstrating that the debate is not over. In conclusion, two excellent articles by Srinivasan et al.[84,85] did a great job of summarizing the use of formocresol for pulpotomies and discussing medicaments that may take its place.

Glutaraldehyde

In 1975 to 1976, 's-Gravenmade[86] and Dankert et al.[87] proposed that glutaraldehyde could be an alternative pulpotomy fixative medicament. They stated that glutaraldehyde would be less likely to diffuse out of the apical foramen and it has effective disinfecting properties. It was also found to have better fixative properties with true crosslinking. The property of glutaraldehyde not diffusing out of the apex of tooth has been confirmed in studies.[88,89] It has also been demonstrated that glutaraldehyde is absorbed into the systemic circulation after being applied to a pulpotomy site.[90–92] There was a low amount of tissue binding and the remainder of the glutaraldehyde was excreted in the urine or exhaled as carbon dioxide. It has further been shown that glutaraldehyde does not reach the nucleus of cells and its potential for mutagenicity is low.[92] Ranly et al.[93] demonstrated that buffering glutaraldehyde increased its concentration, and along with applying it for longer periods of time increased fixation. It was only when the concentration was made stronger that the glutaraldehyde penetrated deeper into the tissues.

In 1980, Kopel et al.[94] used 2% glutaraldehyde to perform pulpotomies on primary teeth. They found it to be a biologically acceptable pulp medicament capable of maintaining the vitality of the radicular pulp following pulpotomy. The remaining pulpal tissue did not resemble the tissues of teeth subjected to treatment with formocresol. Adjacent to the pulp dressing there is surface fixation where the pulp is amputated and treated. The remaining pulp appears normal.[95] Glutaraldehyde has been shown to be less cytotoxic than formocresol.[96]

A study by Ranly[97] demonstrated that glutaraldehyde produced less allergenic response than formocresol. Multiple studies have shown no damage to the erupted permanent teeth adjacent to the glutaraldehyde-treated primary teeth.[98,99] Numerous clinical studies have documented the clinical success of glutaraldehyde pulpotomies with ZOE base in the range of 74.1 to 100% with times ranging from 6 to 42 months.[100–106] It is important to note that the highest success rates were from studies that had shorter study periods, and that none of the studies had a study time longer than 3.5 years. Glutaraldehyde pulpotomies with calcium hydroxide base have a lower success rate than pulpotomies using a ZOE base.[107]

Ranly and Garcia-Godoy[108] found it not advisable to skip the step of applying the glutaraldehyde directly to the pulp stumps with medicated pellets for 5 minutes, instead of incorporating the medicament into the cement subbase. This modification of the pulpotomy procedure produced a failure rate of 48.6%. A potential drawback to using glutaraldehyde is its limited shelf life. Glutaraldehyde has been tested for many years now. It appears that this medicament is not the ideal material to replace formocresol. It has many of the same problems and concerns in regard to safety, and there are conflicting studies about clinical success rates.

Freeze-Dried Bone

Two studies were performed on monkeys using freeze-dried bone as a pulp capping agent.[109,110] In the first study, 15 primary teeth and 1 permanent tooth were treated with freeze-dried bone as the pulp capping material. The monkeys were sacrificed after 12 weeks and the teeth were evaluated histologically. The results showed that the teeth treated with freeze-dried bone demonstrated a complete or partial calcific barrier next to the pulp with normal odontoblastic cells. The researchers concluded that freeze-dried bone produced favorable results but that the material should be evaluated for longer periods of time and with a larger sample size. The same researchers performed a second study again using 15 primary teeth on monkeys. These teeth were followed for periods of 6 weeks to 6 months. In the 6-week samples, all of the pulps were vital and a dentin bridge formed in 87.5% of the teeth. In the samples evaluated after 6 months, 83.3% of the teeth had vital pulps and all of the samples had a dentin bridge. The researchers recommended clinical studies with freeze-dried bone on human teeth.

Electrosurgery/Electrofulguration

Numerous researchers have proposed electrosurgery or electrofulguration as an alternative to chemicals or cements for pulpotomies in primary teeth. In 1983, Ruemping et al.[111] performed electrosurgical pulpotomies on monkey teeth. After making access preparations, the pulps were amputated with sharp spoon excavators and hemostasis was obtained with dry cotton pellets. Then the pulp stumps were treated with the electrosurgical unit. They were careful to limit the amount of contact of the electrosurgery unit with the pulp, and when multiple treatments were needed, a 10-second delay was recommended to prevent overheating of the pulp tissue. A ZOE base was then placed. The teeth were followed for periods from 1 hour up to 2 months and evaluated histologically. In the 1-hour specimens, the electrosurgically treated specimens demonstrated tissue debris and coagulation necrosis on the surface and increased fibrosis in the coronal one-fourth of the pulp. There was no involvement of the furcation or at the tooth apex. The 1-week specimens again demonstrated coagulation necrosis at the electrosurgically treated surface and increased fibroblasts below. The apical four-fifths of the pulp as well as the furcation and the periapical areas was normal. The 2-month specimens demonstrated some chronic inflammation and fibroblasts oriented in the long axis of the tooth with some secondary dentin seen below this area. The remaining apical two-thirds of the pulp was normal to slightly fibrous, with no apical or furcation involvement noted. The researchers concluded that the electrosurgically treated teeth maintained vitality for up to 2 months with no evidence of periapical or furcation involvement.

In 1987, Morton, one of the researchers from the previous primate study, and Sheller[112] published a study pilot testing electrosurgical pulpotomies on humans. They tested 11 primary human canine teeth scheduled for extraction for orthodontic reasons. They used an Ellman 90 FFP Dento Surg unit (Ellman International, Inc., Oceanside, NY) at a setting of 3 (139.5V) and were careful not to overheat the pulp. Warm gutta-percha was gently condensed on top of the pulp and covered with Cavit (3M). Clinically, all patients were asymptomatic at 6 and 48 hours. One patient developed symptoms at 72 hours and the tooth had to be extracted. Histologically, the two teeth extracted 1 hour after treatment were free of acute inflammation. The teeth that were extracted after 6 days showed acute inflammation in the apical third and edema and necrosis in the remaining pulp. The 13-day posttreatment specimens varied in their responses to treatment. One tooth had necrotic pulp. Another tooth had acute and chronic inflammation with some necrosis in the apical two-thirds and pulp calcifications in the coronal third. The one tooth that was considered successful had limited necrosis at the pulp amputation site and the middle and apical thirds of the pulp were vital. The two 17-day posttreatment specimens were similar, with acute and chronic inflammation in the coronal third and secondary dentin on the walls of the coronal and middle thirds of the canal. One of the specimens had a pulp stone. The best results were obtained in the 70-day posttreatment specimens. Some acute and chronic inflammatory cells were visible in the coronal third of the pulp and secondary dentin and pulp stones were also present. In the 100-day posttreatment specimens, one of the teeth was considered successful, but had chronic inflammation and secondary dentin formation. The other tooth had acute inflammation in the remaining pulp and secondary dentin.

The conclusion of this pilot study was that electrosurgical pulpotomy could not be recommended as a pulpotomy technique superior to formocresol. Sheller and Morton from the previous two studies, as well as two other researchers, published another primate study later in 1987. In this study, they used a split-mouth design, performing equal numbers of electrosurgical and formocresol pulpotomies. The formocresol pulpotomy technique was a standard 5-minute pulpotomy and the electrosurgical pulpotomy was the same as described in their previous studies. The teeth were followed for up to 6 months. The teeth were evaluated histologically and revealed that the two techniques produced similar results, which can be summarized as acute and chronic inflammation in the coronal third of the pulp. Some teeth demonstrated reparative dentin, and a few had periapical or furcation pathosis. Most of the teeth had vital pulp tissue in the apical third of the root. They concluded that the next step should be well-designed studies of electrosurgical pulpotomies on humans.[113]

Shulman et al.[114] compared electrosurgical and formocresol pulpotomies in monkey teeth. They studied 80 primary teeth divided into treatment groups that included electrosurgery, ^{14}C-labeled full-strength formocresol in a ZOE base, and a combined technique of electrosurgery and formocresol. When performing these electrosurgical pulpotomies, the researchers did not mechanically remove the pulp first and then treat the remaining pulp with the electrosurgical current. Instead they used the electrosurgical unit to completely remove the coronal pulp and treat the radicular pulp. This appears to have been an important finding. They concluded that removing the coronal pulp with the electrosurgical unit probably produces too much lateral heat injuring the remaining pulp irreversibly and causing the treatment to fail. The conclusions of this study were that this particular electrosurgical technique produced periapical and furcation pathosis and root resorption, and using formocresol after the electrosurgical technique produced no better results than the electrosurgery alone.

Mack et al.[115] did a retrospective study of patients treated with electrosurgical pulpotomy with the dental tip of electrofulguration. All of the procedures were performed by the same operator on primary molars with carious pulp exposures. They followed 164 pulpotomies on children aged 18 months to 10 years old (mean age, 5 years 11 months), for up to 5 years 10 months (mean postoperative time, 2 years 3 months). Of the 164 teeth studied, 127 were considered normal at the last observation, 32 had exfoliated, 4 had an abnormality that was not considered a failure, and 1 tooth was considered a failure. The overall clinical and radiographic success rate was 99.4%.

Two studies comparing histological results of electrosurgical and formocresol pulpotomies on dog primary teeth were performed by two different groups. In the first study, they found that conventional formocresol pulpotomy was histologically superior to electrosurgical pulpotomy.[116] In the second study, they concluded the opposite, that electrosurgical pulpotomy exhibited less histopathological reaction than formocresol pulpotomy.[117] The two studies used different electrosurgical units and this may account for the different results.

Two other human studies using the Hyfrecator (ConMed Corporation, Utica, NY) to perform electrofulguration pulpotomies were performed by different research groups. In the first study, Fishman et al.[118] tested 47 primary molars for up to 6 months using two different bases, ZOE in one group and calcium hydroxide in the second group. Clinical and radiographic success rates were 77 and 55%, respectively, for the ZOE group and 81 and 57%, respectively, for the calcium hydroxide group. They concluded that when used with an electrofulguration pulpotomy, there was no statistical difference between ZOE and calcium hydroxide. In the second study,[119] formocresol and electrosurgical pulpotomy with the Hyfrecator were again compared. The formocresol-treated teeth received full-strength formocresol and both groups received a ZOE base. The teeth were followed for up to 5 months. Clinical and radiographic success rates for the formocresol were 100 and 92%, respectively, and 96 and 84%, respectively, for the electrosurgically treated teeth. The researchers concluded that there was no statistical difference in the success of the two techniques.

Sasaki et al.[120] tested calcium hydroxide pulpotomy with and without the use of an electrosurgical unit. Thirty-three primary molars were followed for a period of up to 34 months (mean, 12 months). Caries was removed with an excavator or a slow-speed bur. After carious exposure, a high-speed diamond was used to open the access preparation. The coronal pulp was amputated with a high-speed bur with continuous water spray. Cotton pellets were placed to obtain hemostasis. If hemostasis was achieved, a calcium hydroxide base was placed. If hemostasis was not obtained, the electrosurgical unit was used to stop the bleeding. This was followed by a calcium hydroxide base. The teeth were restored with a crown. Clinical and radiographic success rates were 93.8% and 93.8%, respectively, for the electrosurgical group and 94.1 and 88.2%, respectively, for the nonelectrosurgical group.

Rivera et al.[121] performed a clinical study on 80 primary molars comparing formocresol and electrosurgical pulpotomies on children aged 4 to 7. In order to be included in the study, the child had to have two molars requiring pulpotomy. In each child, one tooth received formocresol pulpotomy and the other tooth received electrosurgical pulpotomy. Both teeth received a ZOE base and were followed for up to 6 months. In both of the groups, 7.5% of the teeth failed. There were no statistically significant differences in the success of the two groups. The authors acknowledged that this was a fairly short observation period, but observed that, when comparing equal success rates of formocresol and electrosurgery, electrosurgery has distinct advantages. It is faster and there are no risks of formocresol side effects.

A common problem with dental research for electrosurgical pulpotomies is that there are different techniques, materials, and electrosurgical units among the various studies. This can produce vastly different results and makes it difficult to compare the studies. Dentists in private practice are left wondering which technique of electrosurgical pulpotomy is right.

Lasers

Lasers have been suggested for a number of procedures in dentistry including pulpotomy. Some of the earlier studies used CO_2, argon, and Nd:YAG lasers to perform pulpotomies on dogs and swine.[122–124] The results of these studies demonstrated that using a laser to perform pulpotomies was a viable option in animal models and should be attempted in humans.

Subsequent to these animal studies, six studies had been published on the use of lasers to perform pulpotomies in primary teeth. Liu et al.[125] published a case report of 23 teeth that received pulpotomy treatment with an Nd:YAG laser with the following settings, 2 W, 20 Hz, 100 mJ, and followed for 12 to 27 months. The teeth were anesthetized and isolated with a rubber dam. Caries was excavated and the roof of the chamber was removed with a high-speed bur. The coronal pulp was removed with a spoon excavator and hemorrhage control was obtained with dry sterile cotton. The laser was used to treat the pulp after the removal of the cotton, and IRM cement was used to fill the chamber. The teeth were restored with a composite resin or a stainless steel crown. All of the teeth were clinically successful with no signs or symptoms. One tooth showed signs of internal resorption at the 6-month recall visit. At 9 months, approximately half of the teeth show some canal calcification.

Elliott et al.[126] compared CO_2 laser pulpotomies with formocresol pulpotomies. In this study, the caries- and restoration-free primary canine teeth were anesthetized, isolated with a rubber dam, and cleaned with providine iodine and isopropyl alcohol. An access preparation was made on the lingual surface of each tooth and the coronal pulp was removed with a slow-speed round bur. A damp sterile cotton was placed for 5 minutes to obtain hemostasis. The teeth were treated with the laser or with formocresol, and both groups of teeth received a zinc oxide and eugenol base and an amalgam restoration. The settings on the laser were 6 W, 0.1 second, and a single impulse. The distance from the tip to the canal orifice was 1 to 1.5 mm. The laser was fired until there was a char layer and no more bleeding. The teeth received a periapical radiograph prior to extraction and were extracted at 28 or 90 days. The teeth were evaluated radiographically and histologically. These researchers concluded that on the basis of symptomatic, clinical, radiographic, and histological findings, the CO_2 laser compares favorably to formocresol pulpotomies.

A study was performed comparing a conventional formocresol–ZOE pulpotomy with a diode laser-MTA pulpotomy. In this study, the teeth were studied clinically and radiographically for a period of up to 15.7 months. The researchers concluded that the laser-MTA pulpotomy showed slightly reduced radiographic success rates compared to the formocresol–ZOE pulpotomy, but the results were not statistically significant. They recommended that a larger sample with a longer follow-up was needed to consider the laser-MTA as an alternative to the formocresol–ZOE pulpotomy.[127]

In a study by Huth et al.,[128] four pulpotomy techniques were compared: calcium hydroxide, Er:YAG, dilute formocresol, and ferric sulfate on a sample of 200 primary molars treated and followed for up to 24 months. The teeth were anesthetized and isolated with a rubber dam, and the caries was excavated and the roof of each pulp chamber removed with a diamond bur. The coronal pulp was removed with a slow-speed round bur and a spoon excavator. Hemostasis was obtained by placing wet cotton pellets with slight pressure in the chamber for 5 minutes. Formocresol-medicated cotton pellets were applied to the pulp for 5 minutes in the control group. In the laser group, the teeth were treated with an Er:YAG laser set at 2 Hz and 180 mJ per pulses without water cooling. The mean number of laser pulses per tooth was 31.5 ± 5.9. In the calcium hydroxide group, the teeth were dressed with aqueous calcium hydroxide and covered with calcium hydroxide cement. In the last group, the teeth were treated with cotton pellets wetted with ferric sulfate for 15 seconds. All of the teeth received an IRM base, followed by a glass ionomer cement and a stainless steel crown, or a composite resin. The teeth were followed clinically and radiographically for up to 24 months. After 24 months, the total (combined clinical and radiographic success rates) and clinical success rate percentages (in parenthesis) were as follows: formocresol 85 (96%), laser 78 (93%), calcium hydroxide 53 (87%), and ferric sulfate 86 (100%). The authors concluded that calcium hydroxide was significantly less effective than formocresol. They also pointed out that an increased sample size would be necessary before it could be definitively said that this laser technique or ferric sulfate was equal to, or better, than formocresol.

A study by Liu,[129] which was conducted similarly to his previously published case report, using an Nd:YAG laser with follow-up for up to 64 months demonstrated a 97% clinical success rate and a 94.1% radiographic success rate for the laser group that was compared to the 85.5% clinical success rate and a 78.3% radiographic success rate for the formocresol control group.

Odabas et al.[130] performed a clinical, radiographic, and histological study of Nd:YAG laser pulpotomies compared to formocresol pulpotomies on 42 primary teeth studied for a period of up to 12 months. This study was conducted nearly identically to the previous studies. The laser group had a clinical success rate of 85.71%, and a radiographic success rate of 71.42%, at 9 and 12 months. The formocresol group had a clinical success rate of 90.47% and a radiographic success rate of 90.47% at 9 and 12 months. These researchers conclude that the Nd:YAG laser may be considered as an alternative to formocresol for pulpotomies for primary teeth.

As lasers become more commonplace in dentistry, dentists who own a laser now have a body of research literature to justify the use of the laser to perform pulpotomies for children in their practices.

Ferric Sulfate

The use of ferric sulfate as a primary tooth pulpotomy medicament begins to appear in the literature in the late 1980s when Landau and Johnson[131] published an abstract describing the use of ferric sulfate as a pulp medicament in monkey's teeth. The sample size was small and followed for only 60 days. They noted secondary dentin formation and partial dentin bridging. They also described ferric sulfate as a "promising medicament for teeth indicated for pulpotomies." Subsequently, Fei et al.[132] presented the first clinical study of ferric sulfate as a pulpotomy medicament for primary teeth. In this study, 29 primary molars received ferric sulfate pulpotomies and 27 received 1:5 Buckley's formocresol pulpotomies. Both groups received a ZOE base and were followed over 12 months. Criteria for clinical success included no symptoms of pain, no tenderness to percussion, no swelling or fistula, and no pathological mobility. Criteria for radiographic success included normal periodontal ligament space, no pathological internal or external resorption, and no furcal or apical radiolucency. Results of the study showed that after 1 year, 28 of 29 of the ferric sulfate-treated teeth were considered successful while only 21 of 27 of the formocresol-treated teeth were considered successful. Combined overall success rates were 96.6% for the ferric sulfate group and 77.8% for the formocresol group. They raised some interesting points in their discussion. The use of ZOE as a base for formocresol pulpotomies is standard for this procedure. A ZOE base is also paired with ferric sulfate in order to standardize the two pulpotomy treatments. The authors suggested that ZOE is appropriate for formocresol because the pulp tissue is somewhat fixed from formocresol and would not react with the slightly irritating eugenol. Because ferric sulfate is not a tissue fixative, and probably leaves the tissue in a more vital state, using ZOE as a base introduces an irritant that may contribute to failure. They suggested that it would be advisable to continue to study ferric sulfate as a primary tooth pulp medicament for longer periods of time and with more inert base materials.

Additional animal studies on rat and baboon teeth have been performed to assess histologically the pulpal healing response after pulpotomy with ferric sulfate and dilute formocresol. In her study using rats, Cotes[133] had four test groups pairing ferric sulfate and dilute formocresol each with ZOE and polycarboxylate cements. She demonstrated that in the coronal third of the teeth tested, there was necrosis for all groups tested. In the middle third, there was a lesser degree of inflammation for the dilute formocresol–ZOE and ferric sulfate–polycarboxylate groups. In the apical third, the dilute formocresol–ZOE group showed the least inflammation. In addition, reparative dentin formation was noted in the apical third of the pulp in the ferric sulfate–ZOE group while it was not found in the other groups. Conclusions from this study include the following: dilute formocresol–ZOE produced the least inflammation, the use of polycarboxylate cement as a substitute for ZOE did not improve the pulpal response, and significant differences were not found regarding the pulpal inflammation between ZOE and polycarboxylate cements.

Fuks et al.[134] studied ferric sulfate and dilute formocresol pulpotomies in baboon teeth. Both medicaments produced similar degrees of pulpal inflammation and dentin bridging. Sixty percent of the teeth had normal pulps and the remaining 40% had severe inflammation. They recommended more clinical study of ferric sulfate. A number of clinical studies comparing ferric sulfate and formocresol pulpotomies have been performed. In 1997, Fuks et al.[135] performed dilute formocresol and ferric sulfate pulpotomies and evaluated the teeth for up to 34 months. They concluded that dilute formocresol and 15.5% ferric sulfate have similar success rates. Smith et al.[136] performed a retrospective study of clinical and radiographic data from the charts of patients who received ferric sulfate pulpotomies and ZOE base. They followed 242 teeth for 4 to 57 months (mean, 19 months). Their clinical success rate was 99% and the radiographic success rate was 74% to 80%. The longer the teeth were followed, the more failures were noted radiographically. The most common pathological radiographic observations were calcific metamorphosis and internal resorption (Figure 11). Ninety percent of the teeth survived after 3 years. They concluded that ferric sulfate has a success rate similar to dilute formocresol. In addition, if the radiographic changes are separated into dental and osseous categories, and the

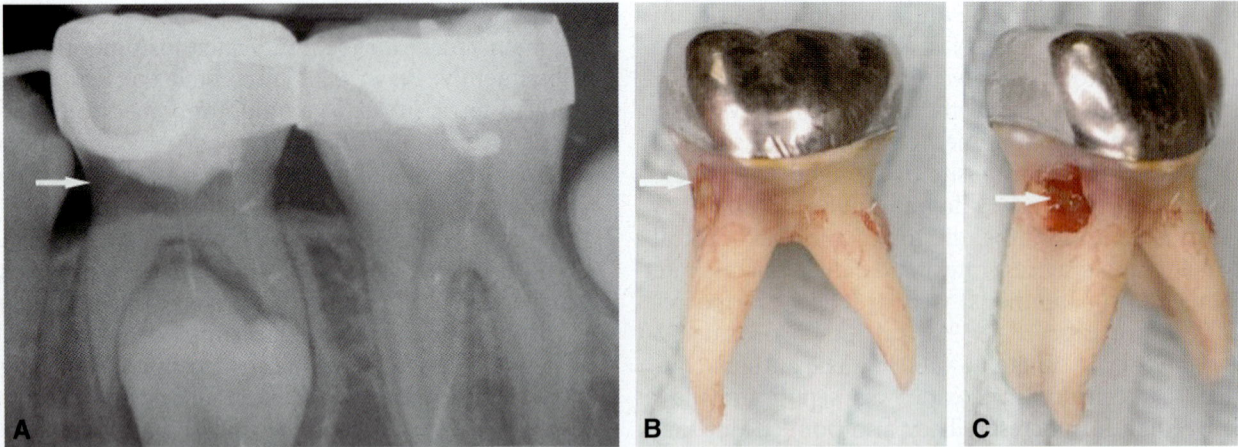

Figure 11 *A*, Radiograph showing internal resorption in a primary molar after ferric sulfate pulpotomy. *B*, Resorption resulted in perforation (arrow). *C*, Perforated area resulting from the resorptive process (arrow).

dental changes (internal resorption and calcific metamorphosis) are reclassified as acceptable variations of success, then the radiographic success rate would be 84% to 92%. The only radiographic changes that would be classified as failures were interradicular or periapical bone destruction and external resorption. These investigators also suggest that since the goal is to keep the pulpotomized tooth asymptomatic until exfoliation, some degree of dental changes is acceptable as long as it does not cause pain or any symptoms.

Additional clinical and retrospective studies and one evidence-based assessment conclude that ferric sulfate and dilute formocresol have similar clinical and radiographic rates of success.[137–139] Vargas[140] demonstrated that both ferric sulfate and formocresol pulpotomies can cause early exfoliation of the pulpotomized teeth with the subsequent need of space maintenance until the premolar erupts.

While most of the published studies on ferric sulfate compare it to formocresol pulpotomy, Casas et al.[141,142] took a different path, comparing it instead to primary tooth root canal therapy (pulpectomy). Root canal therapy with a plain ZOE obturation and ferric sulfate pulpotomy were found to have similar success rates up to about 2 years, but past 2 years, the root canal treatment had better success. They suggested that complete obturation of the canal rather than the partial treatment of the pulp is the best treatment for pulpally involved primary teeth. They did concede that it will be difficult to get the pediatric dental community to change because of the relatively high success rates of pulpotomy, because this was the treatment they learned as a student or a resident, and because pulpotomy is a simple treatment and some children are not cooperative enough to sit for a pulpectomy treatment (Figure 12).

Mineral Trioxide Aggregate

MTA has only recently been recommended as a pulp capping agent in primary teeth. The first published clinical trials in primary teeth began in 2001 and in animal studies occurred in 2003 to 2004 in rat and dog teeth.

A study involving rat first molars demonstrated that after 2 weeks the treated teeth responded well to MTA and were attempting to form dentinal bridges. In the 4-week samples, dentin bridges were completely formed at the pulp–MTA interface and the pulps appeared normal.[143] In the dog study, the researchers tested white and gray MTA as well as regular and white Portland cements as pulpotomy medicaments. Seventy-six teeth from mongrel dogs received pulpotomy treatments. The teeth were evaluated after 120 days and all four of the materials were found to have similar results. The pulps healed with dentin bridges that completely closed the pulpotomy access preparations and the pulps appeared normal. The researchers concluded that both MTA and Portland cement were good pulp capping agents, and they further suggested that Portland cement has the potential to be used as a less expensive material in endodontics.[144] They did not address the fact that Portland cement is not approved for human use.

A number of human studies using MTA as a pulp capping material in primary teeth have demonstrated that MTA performs as well or better than formocresol. Teeth in these studies were followed for periods of 6 to 74 months. Pulp canal obliteration was a common finding in teeth treated with MTA. Various authors conclude that MTA is a reasonable replacement for formocresol because of its high success rates and it lacks the undesirable side effects of formocresol.[145–150] Studies that tested both gray and white MTA concluded that the gray formulation produces better results than the white.[146,150] While MTA has shown excellent results as a pulp capping agent for primary teeth pulpotomies, the one factor that seems to keep it from becoming the new gold standard replacement for formocresol is the cost of the material. Only time will tell if MTA will replace formocresol as the most commonly used pulp capping material for primary teeth.

Nonvital Pulp Therapy for Children

In children, complete root canal treatment on primary teeth is often referred to as a pulpectomy procedure. While the term pulpectomy only infers removal of the pulp, this term in pediatric dentistry has come to mean removal of the caries and the inflamed or necrotic

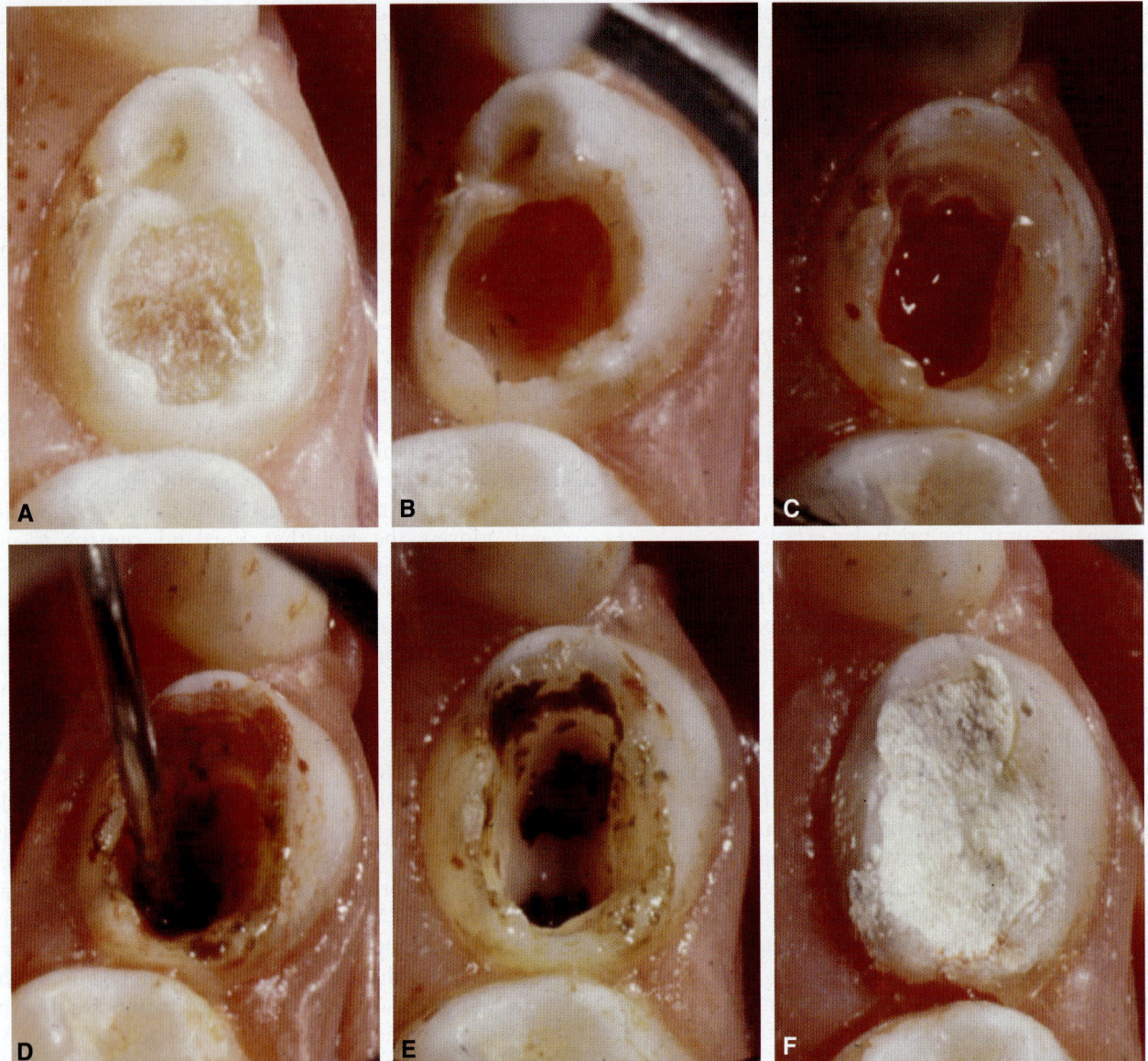

Figure 12 Pulpotomy technique. **A,** Primary molar with large carious lesion. **B,** Caries removed and pulp exposed. **C,** Pulp tissue removed from the chamber. **D,** Pulp space being treated with ferric sulfate. **E,** After treatment with ferric sulfate. **F,** ZOE base has been placed.

pulp, cleaning and shaping the root canals, and obturation of the tooth with a resorbable root filling material. Pulpectomy is indicated when a tooth has irreversible pulpitis or a necrotic pulp or when a tooth has been treatment planned for a pulpotomy and excessive hemorrhage (hyperemia) is encountered at the time of treatment.[1] Some pediatric dentists prefer pulpectomy procedure for primary anterior teeth even if the tooth could be a candidate for only a pulpotomy procedure or if the tooth has only reversible pulpitis symptoms because they believe a complete obturation of the canal is preferable to partial obturation whenever possible. A number of articles recommend pulpectomy as a substitute for all pulpotomies.[151–153]

Pulpectomy procedures for primary teeth must be done with a consideration for the subjacent succedaneous tooth (Figure 13). It begins with profound pulpal anesthesia followed by placement of a rubber dam.

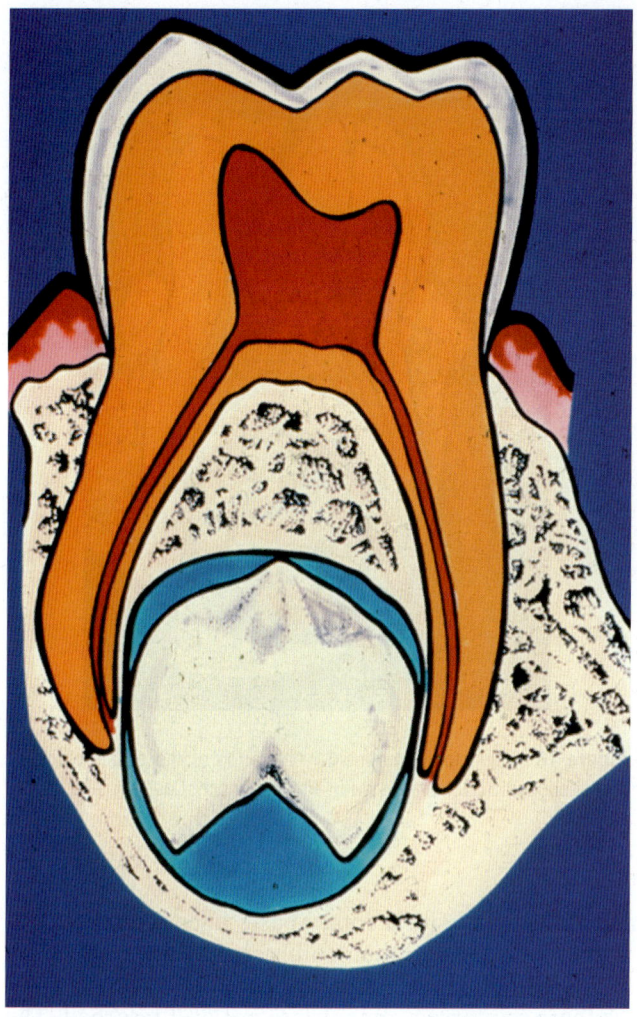

Figure 13 Illustration shows the proximity of primary molar roots to subjacent succedaneous tooth. Courtesy of Dr. A.C. Goerig.

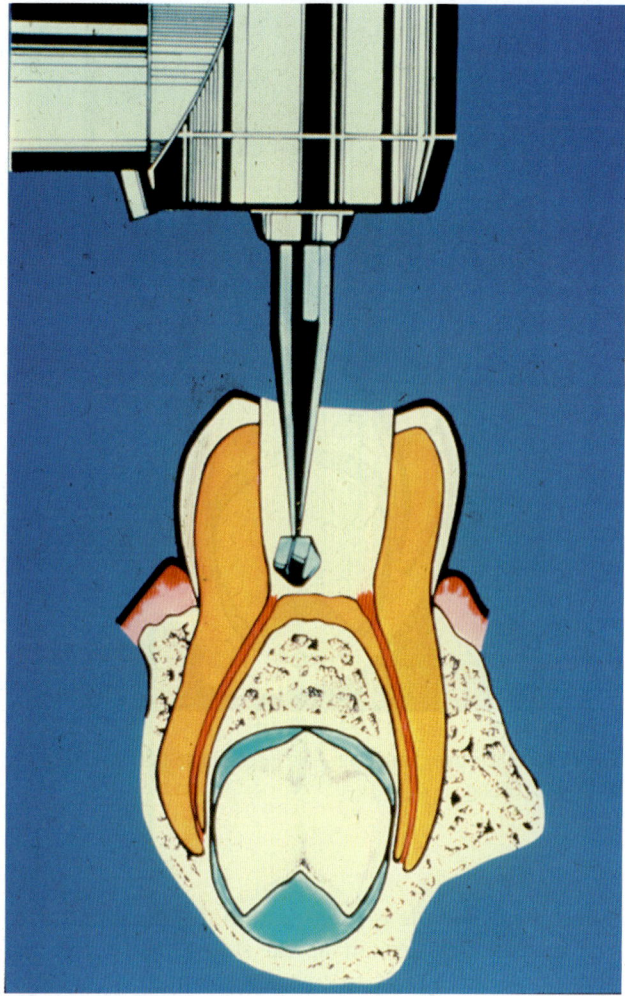

Figure 14 Removal of the roof of the chamber and coronal pulp. Courtesy of Dr. A.C. Goerig.

All caries are removed with a slow-speed round bur or a spoon excavator (Figure 14). From the point of the pulp exposure, an access preparation is made by connecting the pulp horns with the bur. This creates the outline of the access preparation. The roof of the chamber and the coronal pulp are removed. The access preparation is refined to make sure that access to all of the canals is possible. There should be slight flaring of the access to allow for ease of insertion of the files.

In clinical situations where a primary incisor has no caries but has been affected by dental trauma that caused a gray discoloration, the access can be performed from the facial. It is very similar to a lingual access, as it connects the pulp horns and makes a triangular-shaped preparation that is combined with a facial veneer preparation. Following pulpectomy, the tooth can be restored with a light composite resin in the pulp chamber to veneer the facial surface of the tooth to mask the discoloration.

To remove the radicular pulp in anterior teeth, a good technique is to insert two very small files (size 10 or 15) on either side of the pulp and twist the files removing the whole pulp in one motion. In posterior teeth, a barbed broach is used. The canals can be irrigated with sodium hypochlorite or sterile saline. It will be necessary to irrigate the canal several times throughout the procedure.

Files are measured 1 mm short of the apex by comparing them to the length of the tooth on a radiograph. This gives a preliminary working length. It is important to avoid extending instruments into the

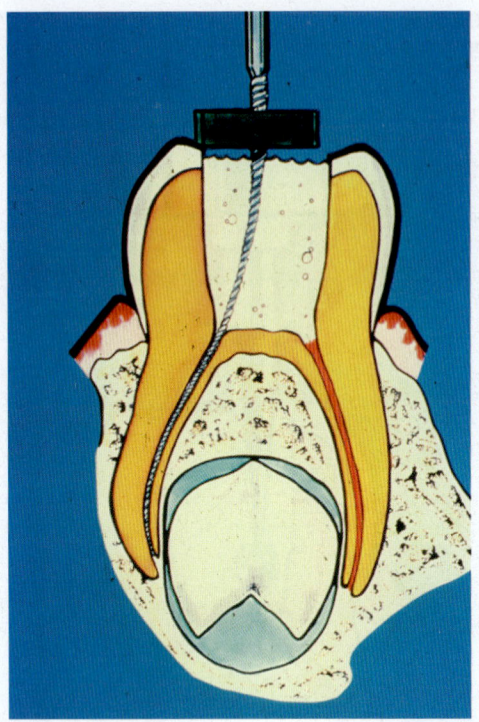

Figure 15 Pulpectomy treatment—file inserted into the canal. Courtesy of Dr. A.C. Goerig.

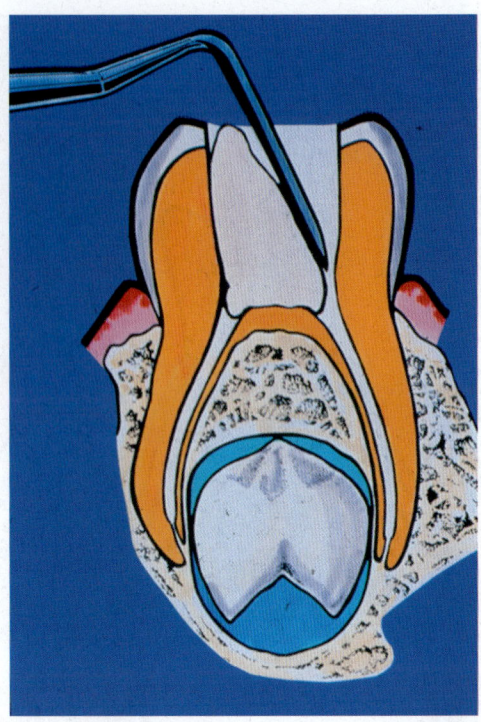

Figure 16 Pulpectomy treatment—obturation of the canals with zinc oxide–eugenol (ZOE) placed with an instrument. Courtesy of Dr. A.C. Goerig.

apical area. The file is inserted into the canal and with tactile sense felt for an apical stop (Figure 15). An alternative method is to insert a medium or a large-sized file (medium for molars and larger files for anterior teeth) into the canal of the tooth and feel for an apical stop. This measurement is then compared to the radiograph. After the correct length is established, smaller files are set to this length. Studies have shown that electronic apex locators can accurately be used when treating primary teeth.[154,155] Excessive cleaning and shaping of the canal should be avoided since that can damage the tooth and lead to extraction caused by perforation in the furcation or the lateral wall of a canal. The purpose of filing is to remove the pulp tissue and make room for the root canal filling material. After the canals are cleaned, they should be irrigated again and dried with appropriately sized sterile paper points.

There are a number of choices of root canal filling materials that can be used for primary teeth, and each of these materials has an appropriate obturation technique (Figure 16). Unreinforced zinc oxide and eugenol is a very common material and is easily placed into the canal with a rotary paste filler (Figure 17). It is very important that commercially prepared zinc oxide cements, with reinforcing fibers, *not* be used, as these reinforced cements are not well resorbed. The unreinforced ZOE is mixed into a thick paste. Large rotary spirals work well for maxillary anterior teeth, and small spirals are suited for molars and mandibular incisors. The rotary spiral is inserted into the canal while it is not turning and is used to search for the apical stop. The paste filler is then slightly removed so that it is short of the apical stop and the handpiece is revolved slowly. The dental assistant places the ZOE on the spatula next to the revolving paste filler that pulls the ZOE off the spatula and introduces the cement into the canal. The speed of the handpiece can be adjusted to cause the ZOE to completely fill the canal. When the dentist believes that the canal is completely filled, the paste filler is removed while still rotating. If the paste filler is removed after it has stopped, it will pull the ZOE from the canal.

A periapical radiograph is then exposed to determine the adequacy of the root canal filling. If the

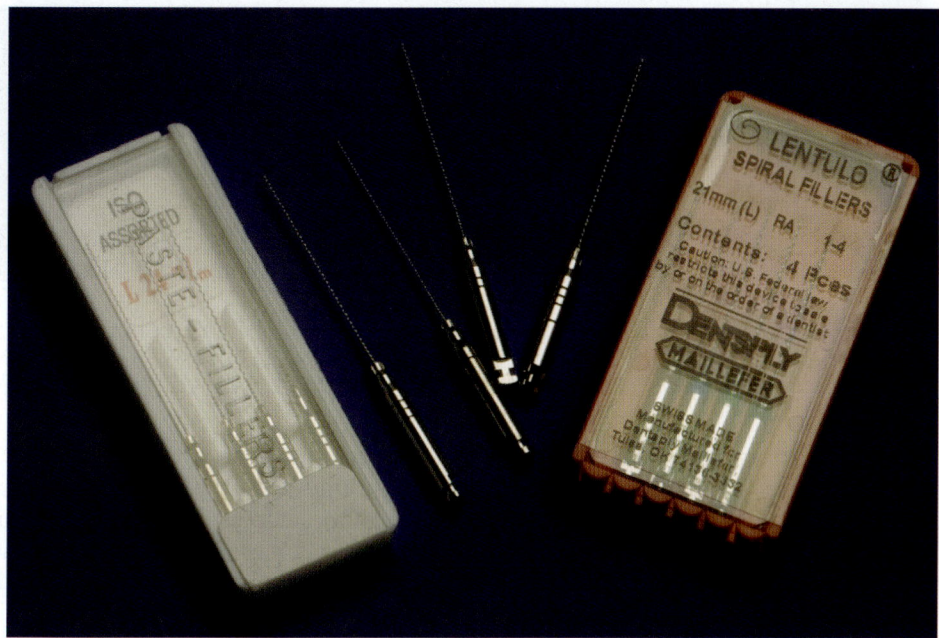

Figure 17 Examples of rotary paste fillers.

canal is not completely filled, the paste filler is reintroduced into the canal to achieve a better obturation. Small amounts of ZOE overfill can be expected to be resorbed uneventfully although it is better to have an underfill than an overfill. The tooth is then restored and monitored until it exfoliates[21,22,151,156] (Figures 18 and 19).

There have been many articles that quantify the success rate of pulpectomy and root canal treatments in primary teeth. In 1978, Jokinen et al.[157] studied 1,304 pulpectomies and found that only 53% were successful. Success rates in the mandible and maxilla were nearly equal. This study is of historical interest, but it is difficult to use these results in judging today's dental care because the technique was very different than the average pulpectomy that is performed today.

Flaitz et al.[158] followed 87 pulpectomies in primary incisors that were obturated with ZOE, with a drop of formocresol in the cement mixture, for a period of 37.4 months. They found a success rate of 84%. In a follow-up study of 62 patients over a period of 12 to 74 months, these same researchers demonstrated a success rate of 82.3% for primary molar pulpectomies with a ZOE filling material.[159] Yacobi[153] et al. performed ZOE pulpectomies on both primary incisors and molars on 51 children over a period of 12 months and found a success rate of 76% for the anterior teeth and a success rate of 84% for the posteriors. Payne et al.[160] studied primary 253 anterior and posterior primary teeth for up to 24 months. Their success rate for anterior teeth was

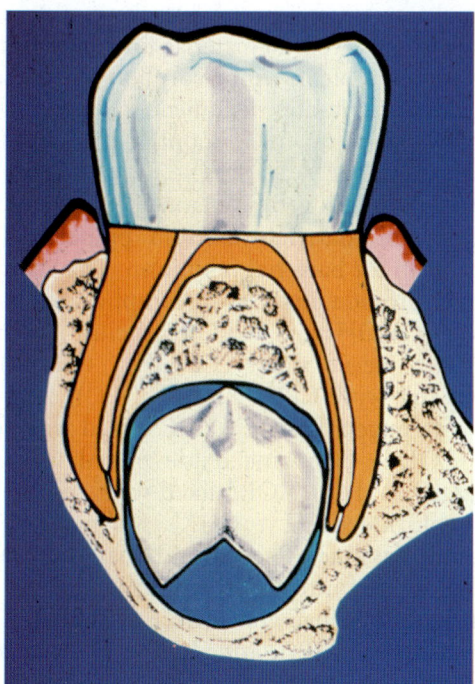

Figure 18 Pulpectomy treatment—tooth restored with a stainless steel crown. Courtesy of Dr. A.C. Goerig.

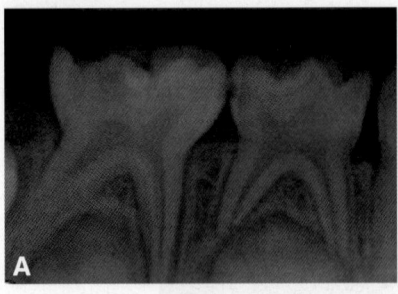 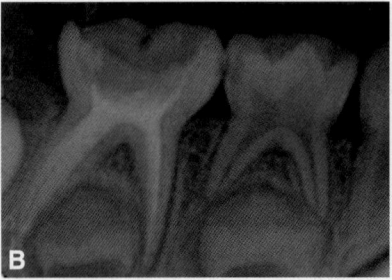 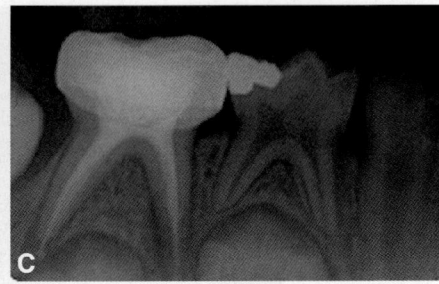

Figure 19 *A,* Primary molar with large caries lesion involving the pulp. *B,* Radiograph taken after pulpectomy and root canal filling. *C,* Evaluation 1 year later.

82.8% and 90.3% for posterior teeth. Coll et al.[161] followed 65 ZOE pulpectomies for a period of 90.8 months. The overall success rate was 77.7%. Two additional studies provide success rates of 76% and 78.5% for ZOE pulpectomies.[162,163]

Rifkin[164] used Kri Paste (a mixture of *p*-chlorophenol, camphor, menthol, and iodoform) to treat 45 primary teeth. The teeth were treated in either 1 or 2 appointments depending on the symptoms. After 1 year, 42 of the 45 teeth were asymptomatic. Garcia-Godoy[165] treated 55 primary teeth with multiple appointment pulpectomies, obturated with Kri Paste, and followed for up to 2 years. There were no clinical or radiographic signs or symptoms in 95.6% of the teeth. Coll et al.[166] compared 41 pulpectomies on primary teeth with pulp necrosis that were obturated with Kri Paste over a period of up to 6 years 10 months. The teeth had a success rate of over 80%. An additional study by Coll[167] confirmed this success rate. Another study by Reyes and Reina[168] with a similar technique documented a 100% success rate. Thomas et al.[169] studied 36 primary teeth for 3 months after pulpectomies and obturated with iodoform paste. They found a success rate of 94.4%. Holan and Fuks[170] compared ZOE- and Kri Paste-filled pulpectomies on primary molars evaluated for periods up to 48 months. They demonstrated a success rate of 84% for Kri Paste and 65% for ZOE. After a number of clinical studies using Kri Paste for pulpectomies, Wright et al.[171] performed an in vitro antimicrobial and cytotoxic study of Kri Paste and ZOE. In this study, they found that ZOE had better antimicrobial activity and that both materials had similar cytotoxicity.

Hendry[172] and his fellow researchers performed pulpectomies using calcium hydroxide and plain ZOE on mongrel dogs. They exposed the pulps of the dogs to produce inflamed pulps. The teeth were later instrumented and obturated with either calcium hydroxide or ZOE. Clinical, radiographic, and histological evaluations of both calcium hydroxide and ZOE found that the calcium hydroxide specimens were more successful in all areas. Another study by Mani et al.[173] compared 60 ZOE and calcium hydroxide pulpectomies. Combined clinical and radiographic success rates were 83.3% for the ZOE group and 86.7% for the calcium hydroxide group. Ozalp et al.[174] found a success rate of 80 to 90% for pulpectomies that were obturated with calcium hydroxide.

Vitapex (NeoDental International, Inc., Federal Way, WA) is a commercially prepared calcium hydroxide and iodoform mixture that is prepackaged in syringes specifically for pulpectomies. It has been tested by a number of researchers. A case report by Nurko et al.[175] recommends it as an excellent material for pulpectomies in spite of some problems with resorption of the material. Three additional studies document the use of Vitapex with follow-up of up to 22 months; the success rates approached 100%.[162,174,176]

One *in vitro* study by Tchaou et al.[177] compared various dental materials used in pulpectomies for primary teeth for bacterial inhibition. They compared calcium hydroxide mixed with camphorated *p*-chlorophenol ($Ca(OH)_2$ + CPC), calcium hydroxide mixed with sterile water ($Ca(OH)_2$ + H_2O), zinc oxide mixed with CPC (ZnO + CPC), zinc oxide mixed with eugenol (ZOE), ZOE mixed with formocresol (ZOE + FC), zinc oxide mixed with sterile water (ZnO + H_2O), ZOE mixed with chlorhexidine dihydrochloride (ZOE + CHX), Kri paste, Vitapex paste, and Vaseline. They found that the materials could be divided into three groups. Category I with the strongest antibacterial effect included ZnO + CPC, $Ca(OH)_2$ + CPC, and ZOE + FC. Category II with a medium bacterial effect included ZOE + CHX, Kri, ZOE, and ZnO + H_2O. Category III with no or minimal antibacterial effect included Vitapex, $Ca(OH)_2$ + H_2O, and Vaseline.

There are many articles that describe aspects of the pulpectomy technique and the instruments involved in the procedure. Once a primary molar begins to resorb, from physiological resorption or from pathosis, it can be difficult for the dentist to know if the canals of the tooth can be properly instrumented or even to obtain a correct working length. Rimondini and Baroni[178] studied 80 primary molars in children 4 to 12 years old, 75 of which were extracted because of pulpal involvement. The teeth were measured and the apices and areas of resorption were located. They found that roots that were longer than 10 mm were related to a curved root shape with no external resorption. Roots with length between 4 to 7 mm were associated with advanced root resorption. Roots that were shorter than 4 mm were associated with resorption and perforation of the furcation. They identified 4 mm as the limit of the length of a root that can be treated successfully.

Barr et al.[179] presented the use of rotary nickel–titanium files to prepare primary teeth for pulpectomy treatment. Advantages of this technique include ease of removal of tissue and debris, flexible design allowing access to canals, files prepare the canal in a funnel shape to ease obturation, and the files are available in 21 mm length. Disadvantages of the use of these files include cost of the equipment (handpiece), increased cost of the files, and the time required to learn the technique. An in vitro study was performed on three pulpectomy filling devices: Lentulo spiral (Dentsply International), NaviTip (Ultradent Products, Inc., South Jordan, UT), and Vitapex syringe (NeoDental International, Inc.). Seventy extracted primary teeth were prepared and mounted in acrylic blocks. The teeth were divided into three groups and pulpectomies were done followed by obturation with three different methods. The specimens were radiographed and evaluated and the conclusion was that the NaviTip produced the best quality fill.[180] Bawazir and Salama[181] studied two methods of obturating root canals with Lentulo spiral paste fillers. One technique was with the Lentulo mounted on a slow-speed handpiece and the other method was with a handheld Lentulo. They concluded that there was no difference in the two methods as far as the quality of the fill or in the success of the obturation.

Johnson et al.[182] performed an in vitro study using an apical resorbable collagen barrier to prevent overfill of the canal. The apices of the teeth were coated with wax and the teeth were embedded into acrylic. The canals were filed, rinsed, and dried. A resorbable collagen barrier was packed into some of the canals and the remainder of the teeth served as controls. The teeth were then obturated with Vitapex. Radiographs were evaluated for the presence of an overfill. In the test group, overfills were present in 16% of teeth. In the control group (no barrier), overfills were present in 42% of teeth. They suggest that resorbable collagen barriers can help prevent overfills. One problem that can be experienced with resorbable cements placed in root canals of primary teeth is overretention of the material in the alveolus after exfoliation of the primary tooth (Figure 20). Studies by Sadrian and Coll[183] and Coll et al.[166,167] have shown that ZOE cement was retained in the alveolus in 49.4% to 73.3% of the exfoliated teeth, and this material was still retained in 27.3% of the patients after 40.2 months. Short-filled pulpectomies were significantly less likely to overretain ZOE.[161] One of the two studies evaluated over 6,000 charts in a pediatric dentistry private practice.[183] Jerrell and Ronk[184] presented a case study of the arrest of eruption of a permanent premolar after ZOE material was extruded from the primary molar pulpectomy into the developing tooth bud. Fortunately in the case of this particular patient, premolar extraction was a part of the patient's orthodontic treatment plan, so the tooth was extracted. It is reassuring that studies have shown a low incidence of enamel hypoplasia in succedaneous teeth when the primary teeth have been treated with pulpectomy techniques.[161,166]

Educational Curricula and Attitudes of Pediatric Dentists

A study by Avran[185] in 1987 surveyed pediatric dentistry residencies in Canada and a number of dental schools worldwide. He found that in Canada among pediatric dental specialists, the preferred pulp medicament for 50% of the respondents was 1:5 formocresol and full-strength formocresol was preferred by 42.2%. In Canadian pediatric dental residency programs, full-strength formocresol was preferred by 40.8% of respondents and 1:5 formocresol was preferred by 36%. Seventy percent of respondents in Scandinavian dental schools preferred calcium hydroxide. This is not unexpected since much of the research on calcium hydroxide as a pulp medicament has been done there. When respondents were asked if they were considering a change to another medicament, many said they would consider glutaraldehyde.

A second study was published by Primosch[186] in 1997 based on a survey of the pediatric dental

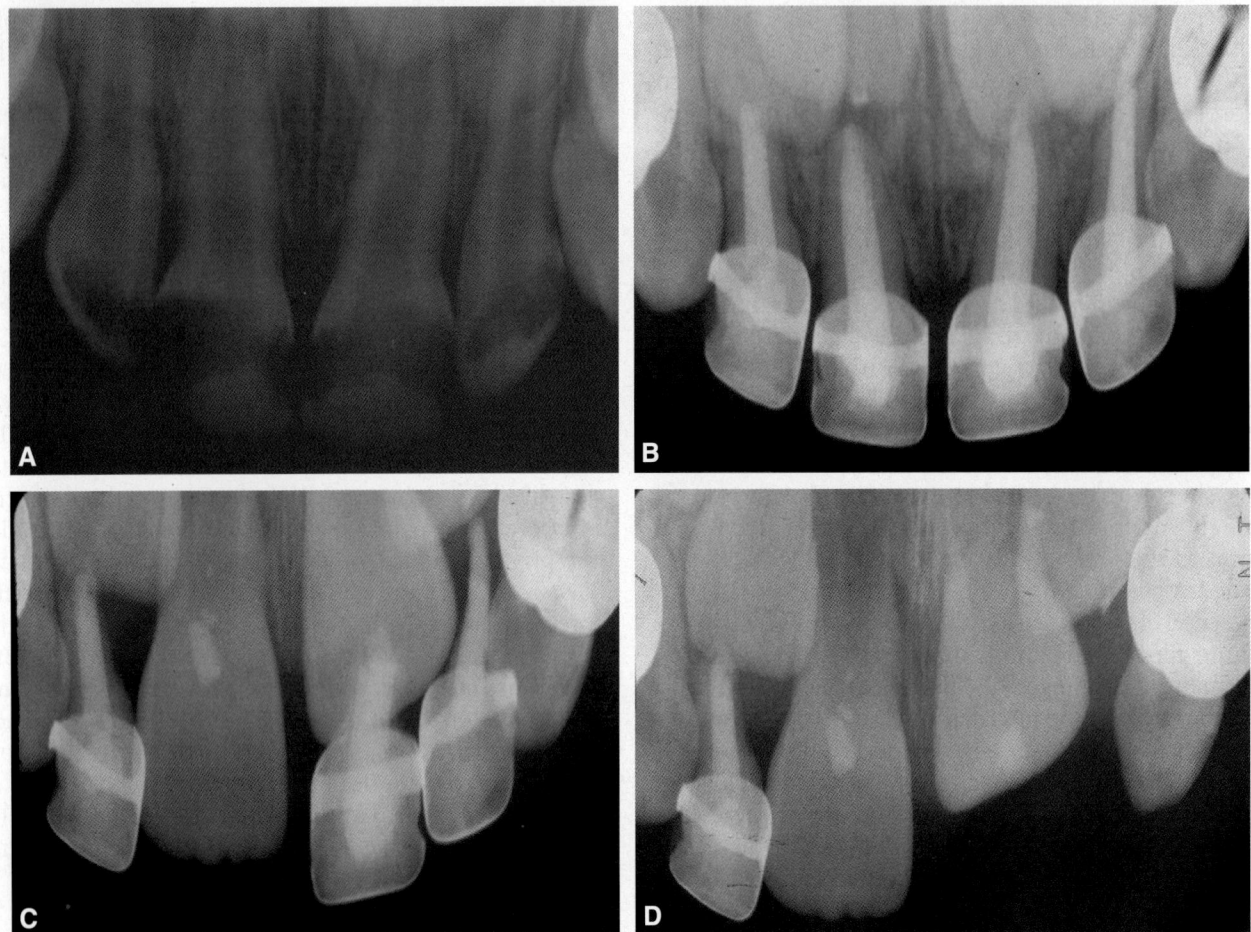

Figure 20 ***A,*** Large caries on primary incisors at the time of diagnosis. ***B,*** Approximately 3 years after endodontic treatment. ***C,*** Five and half years after treatment, the primary tooth is retained and deflecting permanent successor. ***D,*** The primary incisor has been extracted. Radiograph shows retained zinc oxide–eugenol (ZOE) material. The right primary incisor was subsequently extracted.

programs in the United States regarding curricula for pulp therapy in children. Calcium hydroxide was the preferred base for pulp capping. Most schools taught that after the first appointment of an indirect pulp cap, it would be necessary to reenter the tooth only if the patient experienced symptoms. A 1:5 dilution of formocresol was the most commonly (71.7%) recommended medicament for pulpotomy procedure, and it was left in the tooth for 5 minutes (94.3%). ZOE was the most commonly recommended base (92.4%). It is interesting to note that while some practitioners were considering changing from formocresol to glutaraldehyde in Avram's study in the 1980s, no US dental school included glutaraldehyde in the curriculum in the 1997 study. Further, the Primosh's study reported that 2 of 53 dental schools in 1997 were teaching ferric sulfate or 1:5 formocresol to their students. While interest in glutaraldehyde has decreased, interest and research on ferric sulfate has greatly increased.

In regard to pulpectomy procedure, 98% of US dental schools were teaching hand instrumentation of canals, with the majority of schools not recommending any enlargement of the canal. The most commonly recommended irrigants were sodium hypochlorite, sterile water or saline, and local anesthetic. Ninety percent of schools recommended zinc oxide and eugenol as the preferred filling for root canals. These two studies have now become outdated. So why include this information? These are only two journal articles that quantify what is being taught in dental schools. It is important to realize that formocresol has been advocated as a pulp medicament for a very long time, and it seems to be very entrenched in pediatric dental education. While it may have a number of problems, no substitute has been overwhelmingly advocated to take its place. It is certain that there is much room for research on new pulp medicaments to replace formocresol.

Conclusion

Endodontic therapy, from pulp capping, pulpotomy or to pulpectomy, is an excellent procedure to prevent the premature loss of primary teeth. When the appropriate treatment is selected for each situation, success and preservation of the tooth can be anticipated. Vital pulp therapy is indicated when the pulp has the potential for healing, and nonvital pulp therapy is indicated when irreversible pulpitis or necrosis exists. Preserving primary teeth keeps young smiles beautiful and dental arches intact preventing space loss and malocclusion.

References

1. Guideline of pulp therapy for primary and young permanent teeth. [Special Reference Manual] Pediatr Dent 2006–07; 28(7):144–8.
2. Salama FS, Anderson RW, McKnight-Hanes C, et al. Anatomy of primary incisor and molar teeth. Pediatr Dent 1992;14(2):117–18.
3. Puddhikarant P, Rapp R. Radiographic anatomy of pulpal chambers of primary molar. Pediatr Dent 1983;5(1):25–9.
4. Goto G, Zhang Y. Study of cervical pulp horns in human primary molars. J Clin Pediatr Dent 1995;20(1):41–4.
5. Moss SJ, Addelston H, Goldsmith ED. Histologic study of pulpal floor of deciduous molars. J Am Dent Assoc 1965;70:372–9.
6. Ringelstein D, Seow WK. The prevalence of furcation foramina in primary molars. Pediatr Dent 1989;11(3):198–202.
7. Paras LG, Rapp R, Piesco NP, et al. An investigation of accessory foramina in furcation areas of human primary molars: Part 1 SEM observations of frequency, size and location of accessory foramina in the internal and external furcation areas. J Clin Pediatr Dent 1993;17(2):65–9.
8. Wrbas K, Kielbassa AM, Hellwig E. Microscopic studies of accessory canals in primary molar furcations. ASCD J Dent Child 1997;64(2):118–22.
9. Kramer PF, Faraco IM Jr, Meira, R. A SEM investigation of accessory foramina in the furcation areas of primary molars. J Clin Pediatr Dent 2003;27(2):157–61.
10. Dammaschke T, Witt M, Ott K, Schafer E. Scanning electron microscopic investigation of incidence, location, and size of accessory foramina in primary and permanent molars. Quintessence Int 2004;35:699–705.
11. Kilpatrick N, Seow WK, Cameron A, Widmer R. Pulp therapy for primary and young permanent teeth. Handbook of pediatric dentistry. 2nd ed. Edinbergh: Mosby; 2003.
12. Aponte AJ, Hartsook JT, Crowley MC. Indirect pulp capping success verified. ASDC J Dent Child 1966;33:164–6.
13. Sawusch RH. Direct and indirect pulp capping with two new products. J Am Dent Assoc 1982;104:459–62.
14. Nirschl RF, Avery DR. Evaluation of a new pulp capping agent: a clinical investigation. [Special Issue A] J Dent Res 1980;March;59:362.
15. Nirschl RF, Avery DR. Evaluation of a new pulp capping agent in indirect pulp therapy. ASCD J Dent Child 1983; 50:25–30.
16. Coll JA, Josell S, Nassof S, et al. An evaluation of pulpal therapy in primary incisors. Pediatr Dent 1988;10(3):78–184.
17. Farooq NS, Coll JA, Kuwabara A, Shelton P. Success rates of formocresol pulpotomy and indirect pulp therapy in the treatment of deep dentinal caries in primary teeth. Pediatr Dent 2000;22(4):278–86.
18. Al-Zayer MA, Straffon LH, Feigal RJ, Welch KB. Indirect pulp treatment of primary posterior teeth: a retrospective study. Pediatr Dent 2002;25(1):29–36.
19. Falster CA, Auaujo FB, Straffon LH, Nor JE. Indirect pulp treatment: in vivo outcomes of an adhesive resin system vs. calcium hydroxide for protection of the dentin–pulp complex. Pediatr Dent 2002;24(3):241–8.
20. Vij R, Coll JA, Shelton P, Farooq NS. Caries control and other variables associated with success of primary molar vital pulp therapy. Pediatr Dent 2004;26(3):214–20.
21. Fuks AB. Pulp therapy for the primary dentition. In: Pinkham JR, editor. Pediatric dentistry: infancy through adolescence. 4th ed. St. Louis, MO: Elsevier Saunders; 2005.
22. McDonald RE, Avery DR, Dean JA. Treatment of deep caries, vital pulp exposure, and pulpless teeth. In: McDonald RE, editor. Dentistry for the child and adolescent. 8th ed. St. Louis, MO: Mosby; 2004.
23. Buckley JP. The chemistry of pulp decomposition, with a rationale treatment for this condition and its sequelae. J Am Dent Assoc 1904;3:764–71.
24. Buckley JP. The rational treatment of putrescent pulps and their sequelae. Dental Cosmos 1906;48:537–44.
25. Sweet CA. Procedure for treatment of exposed and pulpless deciduous teeth. J Am Dent Assoc 1930;17:1150–3.
26. Sweet CA. Treatment for deciduous teeth with exposed pulps. J Michigan Dent Soc 1937;19:3–16.
27. Sweet CA. Treatment of vital primary teeth with pulpal involvement. J Colo State Dent Assoc 1955;33:10–14.
28. Rolling I, Thylstrup A. A 3-year clinical follow-up study of pulpotomized primary molars treated with the formocresol technique. Scand J Dent Res 1975;83:47–53.
29. Rolling I, Hasselgren G, Tronstad L. Morphologic and enzyme histochemical observations of the pulp of human primary molars 3 to 5 years after formocresol treatment.

Oral Surg Oral Med Oral Pathol Oral Radiol Endod 1976; 42(4):518–28.

30. Rolling I, Lamberg-Hansen H. Pulp condition of successfully formocresol-treated primary molars. Scand J Dent Res 1978; 86:267–72.

31. Ranly DM, Montgomery EH, Pope HO. The loss of 3H-formaldehyde from zinc oxide–eugenol cement—an in vitro study. ASDC J Dent Child 1975;42(2):128–32.

32. Magnusson BO. Therapeutic pulpotomies in primary molars with the formocresol technique. Acta Odontol Scand 1978; 36:157–65.

33. Cox ST, Hembree JH, McKnight JP. The bactericidal potential of various endodontic materials for primary teeth. Oral Surg Oral Med Oral Pathol Oral Radiol Endod 1978;45(6): 947–54.

34. Mejare I. Pulpotomy of primary molars with coronal or total pulpitis using formocresol technique. Scand J Dent Res 1979;87:208–16.

35. Garcia-Godoy F. Pulpal response to different application times of formocresol. J Pedod 1982;6(2):176–93.

36. Garcia-Godoy F. A comparison between zinc oxide–eugenol and polycarboxylate cements on formocresol pulpotomies. J Pedod 1982;6(3):203–17.

37. van Amerongen WE, Mulder GR, Vingerling PA. Consequences of endodontic treatment in primary teeth. Part I: A clinical and radiographic study of the influence of formocresol pulpotomy on the lifespan of primary molars. ASCD J Dent Child 1986;53(5):364–70.

38. Hicks MJ, Barr ES, Flaitz CM. Formocresol pulpotomies in primary molars: a radiographic study in a pediatric dental practice. J Pedod 1986;10(4):331–9.

39. Thompson KS, Seale NS, Nunn ME, Huff G. Alternative method of hemorrhage in full strength formocresol pulpotomy. Pediatr Dent 2001;23(3):217–22.

40. Strange DM, Seale NS, Nunn ME, Strange M. Outcome of formocresol/ZOE sub-base pulpotomies utilizing alternative radiographic success criteria. Pediatr Dent 2001;23(3):331–6.

41. Holan G, Fuks AB, Keltz N. Success rate of formocresol pulpotomy in primary molars restored with stainless steel crown vs. amalgam. Pediatr Dent 2002;24(3):212–16.

42. Guelmann M, Fair J, Turner C, Courts FJ. The success of emergency pulpotomies in primary molars. Pediatr Dent 2002;24(3):217–20.

43. Guelmann M, Fair J, Bimstein E. Permanent versus temporary restorations after emergency pulpotomies in primary molars. Pediatr Dent 2005;27(6):478–81.

44. Guelmann M, McIlwain MF, Primosch RE. Radiographic assessment of primary molar pulpotomies restored with resin-based materials. Pediatr Dent 2005;27(1):24–7.

45. Willard RM. Radiographic changes following formocresol pulpotomy in primary molars. ASCD J Dent Child 1976; 43(6):414–15.

46. Garcia-Godoy F. Radiographic evaluation of root canal "calcification" following formocresol pulpotomy. ASCD J Dent Child 1983;50(6):430–2.

47. Pruhs RJ, Olen GA, Sharma PS. Relationship between formocresol pulpotomies on primary teeth and enamel defects on their permanent successors. J Am Dent Assoc 1977;94:698–700.

48. Mulder GR, van Amerongen WE, Vingerling PA. Consequences of endodontic treatment of primary teeth Part II. A clinical investigation into the influence of formocresol pulpotomy on the permanent successor. ASCD J Dent Child 1987;54(1):35–9.

49. Rolling I, Poulsen S. Formocresol pulpotomy of primary teeth and occurrence of enamel defects on the permanent successors. Acta Odontol Scand 1978;36:243–7.

50. Messer LB, Cline JT, Korf NW. Long term effects of primary molar pulpotomies on succedaneous bicuspids. J Dent Res 1980;59(2):116–23.

51. Straffon LH, Han SS. Effects of varying concentrations of formocresol on RNA synthesis of connective tissue in sponge implants. Oral Surg Oral Med Oral Pathol Oral Radiol Endod 1970;29:915–25.

52. Loos PJ, Han SS. An enzyme histochemical study of the effect of various concentrations of formocresol on connective tissue. Oral Surg Oral Med Oral Pathol Oral Radiol Endod 1971;31(4):571–85.

53. Loos PJ, Straffon LH, Han SS. Biological effects of formocresol. ASCD J Dent Child 1973;40:193–7.

54. Morawa AP, Straffon LH, Han SS, Corpron RE. Clinical evaluation of pulpotomies using dilute formocresol. ASDC J Dent Child. 1975;42:360–3.

55. Garcia-Godoy F. Penetration and pulpal response by two concentrations of formocresol using two methods of application. J Pedod 1981;5(2):102–35.

56. Fuks AB, Bimstein E. Clinical evaluation of diluted formocresol pulpotomies in primary teeth in school children. Pediatr Dent 1981;3(4):321–4.

57. Chiniwalla NP, Rapp R. The effect of pulpotomy using formocresol on blood vessel architecture in primary anterior teeth of Macaca rhesus monkeys. J Endod 1982;8(5):205–7.

58. Van Mullem PJ, Wijnbergen-Buijen Van Weelderen M. The pulpal effects of medicaments containing formaldehyde following pulpotomy in monkeys. Int Endod J 1983; 16:3–10.

59. Fuks AB, Bimstein E, Bruchim A. Radiographic and histologic evaluation of the effect of two concentrations of formocresol on pulpotomized primary and young permanent teeth in monkeys. Pediatr Dent 1983;5(1):9–13.

60. Verco PJ. Microbiological effectiveness of a reduced concentration of Buckley's formocresol. Pediatr Dent 1985; 7(2):130–3.

61. King SRA, McWhorter AG, Seale NS. Concentration of formocresol used by pediatric dentists in primary tooth pulpotomy. Pediatr Dent 2002;24(2):157–9.

62. Massler M, Mansukhani H. Effects of formocresol on the dental pulp. ASCD J Dent Child 1959;26:277.
63. Berger J. Pulp tissue reaction from formocresol and zinc oxide and eugenol. ASCD J Dent Child 1965;32:13–28.
64. Mejare I, Hasselgren G, Hammearstrom LE. Effect of formaldehyde-containing drugs on human pulp evaluated by enzyme histochemical technique. Scand J Dent Res 1976;84(1):29–36.
65. Ranly DM, Fulton R. An autoradiographic study of the response of rat molar pulp to formocresol using 3H-thymidine. Pediatr Dent 1983;5(1):20–4.
66. van Mullem PJ, van Weelderen MW. The pulpal effects of medicaments containing formaldehyde following pulpotomy in monkeys. Int Endod J 1983;16(1):3–10.
67. Russo MC, Holland R, Okamoto T, deMello W. In vivo fixative effect of formocresol on pulpotomized deciduous teeth of dogs. Oral Surg Oral Med Oral Pathol Oral Radiol Endod 1984;58(6):706–14.
68. Jeng HW, Feigal RJ, Messer HH. Comparison of the cytotoxicity of formocresol, formaldehyde, cresol, and glutaraldehyde using human pulp fibroblast cultures. Pediatr Dent 1987;9(4):295–300.
69. Sun HW, Feigal RJ, Messer HH. Cytotoxicity of glutaraldehyde and formocresol in relation to time of exposure and concentration. Pediatr Dent 1990; 12(5):303–7.
70. Meyers DR, Shoaf HK, Dirksen TR, et al. Distribution of 14C-formaldehyde after pulpotomy with formocresol. J Am Dent Assoc 1978;96(5):805–13.
71. Pashley EL, Myers DR, Pashley DH, Whitford GM. Systemic distribution of ^{14}C-formaldehyde from formocresol-treated pulpotomy sites. J Dent Res 1980; 59(3):603–8.
72. Block RM, Lewis RD, Hirsch J, et al. Systemic distribution of [14C]-labeled paraformaldehyde incorporated within formocresol following pulpotomies in dogs. J Endod 1983;9(5):176–89.
73. Ranly DM. Assessment of the systemic distribution and toxicity of formaldehyde following pulpotomy treatment: part one. ASCD J Dent Child 1985;52:431–4.
74. Ranly DM, Horn D. Assessment of the systemic distribution and toxicity of formaldehyde following pulpotomy treatment: part two. ASCD J Dent Child 1987;54:40–4.
75. Rolling I, Thulin H. Allergy tests against formaldehyde, cresol, and eugenol in children with formocresol pulpotomized primary teeth. Scand J Dent Res 1976;84:345–7.
76. van Mullem PJ, Simon M, Lamers AC. Formocresol: a root canal disinfectant provoking allergic skin reactions in pre-sensitized guinea pigs. J Endod 1983;9(1):25–9.
77. Friedberg BH, Gartner LP. Embryotoxicity and teratogenicity of formocresol on developing chick embryos. J Endod 1990;16(9):434–7.
78. Lewis BB, Chestner SB. Formaldehyde in dentistry: a review of mutagenic and carcinogenic potential. J Am Dent Assoc 1981;103:429–34.
79. Perera F, Petito C. Formaldehyde: a question of cancer policy. Science 1982;216:1285–91.
80. ZarZar PA, Rosenblatt A, Takahashi CS, et al. Formocresol mutagenicity following primary tooth pulp therapy: an in vivo study. J Dent 2003;31:479–85.
81. World Health Organization, International Agency for Research on Cancer. Press Release Number 153; June 16, 2004.
82. Casas MJ, Kenny DJ, Judd PL, Johnson DH. Do we still need formocresol in pediatric dentistry? J Can Dent Assoc 2005;71(10):749–51.
83. Milnes AR. Persuasive evidence that formocresol use in pediatric dentistry is safe. J Can Dent Assoc 2006;72(3):247–8.
84. Srinivasan V, Patchett CL, Waterhouse PJ. Is there life after Buckley's formocresol? Part I – A narrative review of alternative interventions and materials. Int J Paediatr Dent 2006;16:117–27.
85. Patchett CL, Srinivasan V, Waterhouse PJ. Is there life after Buckley's formocresol? Part II – Development of a protocol for the management of extensive caries in the primary molar. Int J Paediatr Dent 2006;16:199–206.
86. 's-Gravenmade EJ. Some biochemical considerations of fixation in endodontics. J Endod 1975;1(7):233–7.
87. Dankert J, 's-Gravenmade EJ, Wemes JC. Diffusion of formocresol and glutaraldehyde through dentin and cementum. J Endod 1976;2(2):42–6.
88. Leeka M, Hume WR, Wolinsky LE. Comparison between formaldehyde and glutaraldehyde diffusion through the root tissues of pulpotomy-treated teeth. J Pedod 1984;8(2):185–91.
89. Rusmah M, Rahim ZHA. Diffusion of buffered glutaraldehyde and formocresol from pulpotomized primary teeth. J Dent Child 1992;59(2):108–10.
90. Myers DR, Pashley DH, Lake FT, et al. Systemic absorption of 14C-glutaraldehyde-treated pulpotomy sites. Pediatr Dent 1986;8(2):134–8.
91. Ranly DM, Horn D, Hubbard GB. Assessment of the systemic distribution and toxicity of glutaraldehyde as a pulpotomy agent. Pediatr Dent 1989;11(1):8–13.
92. Ranly DM, Amstutz L, Horn D. Subcellular localization of glutaraldehyde. Endod Dent Traumatol 1990;6(6):251–4.
93. Ranly DM, Garcia-Godoy F, Horn D. Time, concentration, and pH parameters for the use of glutaraldehyde as a pulpotomy agent: an in vitro study. Pediatr Dent 1987;9(3):199–203.
94. Kopel HM, Bernick S, Zachrisson E. DeRomero SA. The effects of glutaraldehyde on primary pulp tissue following coronal amputation: an in vivo histologic study. J Dent Child 1980;47(6):425–30.
95. Rusmah M. Pulpal tissue reaction to buffered glutaraldehyde. J Clin Pediatr Dent 1992;16(2):101–6.
96. Hill SD, Berry CW, Seale NS, Kaga M. Comparison of antimicrobial and cytotoxic effects of glutaraldehyde and

formocresol. Oral Surg Oral Med Oral Pathol Oral Radiol Endod 1991;71(1):89–95.

97. Ranly DM, Horn D, Zislis T. The effect of alternatives to formocresol on antigenicity of proteins. J Dent Res 1985; 64(10):1225–8.

98. Tagger E, Tagger M, Sarnat H. Pulpal reactions to glutaraldehyde and paraformaldehyde pulpotomy dressings in monkey primary teeth. Endod Dent Traumatol 1986; 2(6):237–42.

99. Alacam A. Long term effects of primary teeth pulpotomies with formocresol, glutaraldehyde–calcium hydroxide and glutaraldehyde–zinc oxide eugenol on succudaneous teeth. J Pedod 1989;13(4):307–13.

100. Garcia-Godoy F. Clinical evaluation of glutaraldehyde pulpotomies in primary teeth. Acta Odontol Pediatr 1983;4(2):41–4.

101. Fuks AB, Binstein E, Klein H. Assessment of a 2% buffered glutaraldehyde solution in pulpotomized primary teeth of school children: A preliminary report. J Pedod 1986;10(4): 323–30.

102. Garcia-Godoy F. A 42 month clinical evaluation of glutaraldehyde pulpotomies in primary teeth. J Pedod 1986;10(2): 148–55.

103. Prakash C, Chandra S, Jaiswal JN. Formocresol and glutaraldehyde pulpotomies in primary teeth. J Pedod 1989;13(4): 314–22.

104. Fuks AB, Bimstein E, Guelmann M, Klein H. Assessment of a 2 percent buffered glutaraldehyde solution in pulpotomized primary teeth of schoolchildren. J Dent Child 1990;57(5): 371–5.

105. Tsai TP, Su HL, Tseng LH. Glutaraldehyde preparations and pulpotomy in primary molars. Oral Surg Oral Med Oral Pathol Oral Radiol Endod1993;76(3):346–50.

106. Shumayrikh NM, Adenubi JO. Clinical evaluation of glutaraldehyde with calcium hydroxide and glutaraldehyde with zinc oxide eugenol in pulpotomy of primary molars. Endod Dent Traumatol 1999;15(6):259–64.

107. Alacam A. Pulpal tissue changes following pulpotomies with formocresol, glutaraldehyde–calcium hydroxide, glutaraldehyde–zinc oxide eugenol pastes in primary teeth. J Pedod 1989;13(2):123–32.

108. Garcia-Godoy F, Ranly DM. Clinical evaluation of pulpotomies with ZOE as the vehicle for glutaraldehyde. Pediatr Dent 1987;9(2):144–6.

109. Fadavi S, Anderson AW, Punwani IC. Freeze-dried bone in pulpotomy procedures in Monkey. J Pedod 1989;13(2):108–21.

110. Fadavi S, Anderson AW. A comparison of the pulpal response to freeze-dried bone, calcium hydroxide, and zinc oxide-eugenol in primary teeth in two cynomolgus monkeys. Pediatr Dent 1996;18:52–6.

111. Ruemping DR, Morton TH Jr, Anderson MW. Electrosurgical pulpotomy in primates – a comparison with formocresol pulpotomy. Pediatr Dent 1983;5(1):14–18.

112. Sheller B, Morton TH Jr. Electrosurgical pulpotomy: a pilot study in humans. J Endod 1987;13(2):69–76.

113. Shaw DW, Sheller B, Barrus BD, Morton TH Jr. Electrosurgical Pulpotomy – A 6-month study in primates. J Endod 1987;13(10):500–5.

114. Shulman ER, McIver FT, Burkes EJ Jr. Comparison of electrosurgery and formocresol as pulpotomy techniques in monkey primary teeth. Pediatr Dent 1987;9(3):189–94.

115. Mack RB, Dean JA. Electrosurgical pulpotomy: a retrospective human study. ASCD J Dent Child 1993;60:107–14.

116. Oztas N, Ulusu T, Oygur T, Cokpekin F. Comparison of electrosurgical and formocresol as pulpotomy techniques in dog primary teeth. J Clin Pediatr Dent 1994;18(4): 285–9.

117. El-Meligy O, Abdalla M, El-Barawy S, et al. Histological evaluation of electrosurgery and formocresol pulpotomy techniques in primary teeth of dogs. J Clin Pediatr Dent 2001;26(1):81–5.

118. Fishman SA, Udin RD, Good DL, Rodef F. Success of electrofulguration pulpotomies covered by zinc oxide and eugenol or calcium hydroxide: a clinical study. Pediatr Dent 1996;18(5):385–90.

119. Dean JA, Mack RB, Fulkerson BT, Sanders BJ. Comparison of electrosurgical and formocresol pulpotomy procedures in children. Int J Pediatr Dent 2002;12:177–82.

120. Sasaki H, Ogawa T, Koreeda M, et al. Electrocoagulation extends the indication of calcium hydroxide pulpotomy in the primary dentition. J Clin Pediatr Dent 2002;26(3): 275–7.

121. Rivera N, Reyes E, Mazzaoui S, Moron A. Pulpal therapy for primary teeth: formocresol vs. electrosurgery: a clinical study. ASCD J Dent Child 2003;70:71–3.

122. Shoie S, Nakamura M, Houiuchi H. Histological changes in dental pulps irradiated by CO_2 laser: a preliminary report on laser pulpotomy. J Endod 1985; 11(9):379–84.

123. Wilderson MK, Hill SD, Arcoria CJ. Effects of the argon laser on primary tooth pulpotomies in swine. J Clin Laser Med Surg 1996;14(1):37–42.

124. Jukic S, Anic I, Koba K, et al. The effect of pulpotomy using CO_2 and Nd:YAG lasers on dental pulp tissues. Int Endod J 1997;30:175–80.

125. Liu JF, Chen LR, Chao SY. Laser pulpotomy of primary teeth. Pediatr Dent 1999;21(2):128–9.

126. Elliott RD, Roberts MW, Burkes J, Phillips C. Evaluation of the carbon dioxide laser on vital human primary pulp tissue. Pediatr Dent 1999;21(6):327–31.

127. Saltzman B, Sigal M, Clokie C, et al. Assessment of a novel alternative to conventional formocresol–zinc oxide eugenol pulpotomy for the treatment of pulpally involved human primary teeth: diode laser–mineral trioxide aggregate pulpotomy. Int J Paediatr Dent. 2005;15:437–47.

128. Huth KC, Paschos E, Hajek-Al-Khatar N, et al. Effectiveness of 4 pulpotomy techniques-randomized controlled trial. J Dent Res 2005;84(12):1144–8.

129. Liu, JF. Effects of Nd:YAG laser pulpotomy on human primary molars. J Endod 2006;32(5):404–7.

130. Odabas ME, Bodur H, Baris E, Demir C. Clinical, Radiographic, and Histopathologic evaluation of Nd:YAG laser pulpotomy on human primary teeth. J Endod 2007;33(4):415–21.

131. Landau MJ, Johnson DC. Pulpal response to ferric sulfate in monkeys. J Dent Res 1988;67:215.

132. Fei AL, Udin RD, Johnson R. A clinical study of ferric sulfate as a pulpotomy agent in primary teeth. Pediatr Dent 1977; 13:327–32.

133. Cotes O, Boj JR, Canalda C, Carreras M. Pulpal tissue reaction to formocresol vs. ferric sulfate in pulpotomized rat teeth. J Clin Pediatr Dent 1997;21(3):247–53.

134. Fuks AB, Eidelman E, Cleaton-Jones P, Michaeli Y. Pulp response to ferric sulfate, diluted formocresol, and IRM in pulpotomized primary baboon teeth. ASCD J Dent Child 1997;64(4):254–9.

135. Fuks AB, Holan G, Davis JM, Eidelman E. Ferric sulfate versus dilute formocresol in pulpotomized primary molars: long-term follow up. Pediatr Dent 1997;19(5):327–30.

136. Smith NL, Seale NS, Nunn ME. Ferric sulfate pulpotomy in primary molars: a retrospective study. Pediatr Dent 2000; 22(3):192–9.

137. Ibricevic H, Al-Jame Q. Ferric sulfate as pulpotomy agent in primary teeth: twenty month clinical follow-up. J Clin Pediatr Dent 2000;24(4):269–72.

138. Burnett S, Walker J. Comparison of ferric sulfate, formocresol, and a combination of ferric sulfate/formocresol in primary tooth vital pulpotomies: a retrospective radiographic survey. ASDC J Dent Child 2002;69:44–8.

139. Loh A, O'Hoy P, Tran X, et al. Evidence-based assessment: evaluation of the formocresol versus ferric sulfate primary molar pulpotomy. Pediatr Dent 2004;26(5):401–9.

140. Vargas KG, Packham B. Radiographic success of ferric sulfate and formocresol pulpotomies in relation to early exfoliation. Pediatr Dent 2005;27(3):233–7.

141. Casas MJ, Layug MA, Kenny DF, et al. Two-year outcomes of primary molar ferric sulfate pulpotomy and root canal therapy. Pediatr Dent 2003;25(2):97–102.

142. Casas MJ, Kenny DF, Johnson DH, Judd PL. Long-term outcomes of primary molar ferric sulfate pulpotomy and root canal therapy. Pediatr Dent 2004;26(1):44–8.

143. Salako N, Joseph B, Ritwik P, et al. Comparison of bioactive glass, mineral trioxide aggregate, ferric sulfate, and formocresol as pulpotomy agents in rat molar. Dent Traumatol 2003;19:314–20.

144. Menezes R, Bramante CM, Letra A, et al. Histologic evaluation of pulpotomies in dog using two types of mineral trioxide aggregate and regular and white Portland cements as wound dressings. Oral Surg Oral Med Oral Pathol Oral Radiol Endod 2004;98:376–9.

145. Eidelman E, Holan G, Fuks AB. Mineral trioxide aggregate vs. formocresol in pulpotomized primary molars: a preliminary report. Pediatr Dent 2001;23:15–18.

146. Agamy HA, Bakry NS, Mounir MMF, Avery DR. Comparison of mineral trioxide aggregate and formocresol as pulp-capping agents in pulpotomized primary teeth. Pediatr Dent 2004;26:302–9.

147. Holan G, Eidelman E, Fuks AB. Long-term evaluation of pulpotomy in primary molars using mineral trioxide aggregate or formocresol. Pediatr Dent 2005;27:129–36.

148. Farsi N, Alamoudi N, Balto K, Mushayt A. Success of mineral trioxide aggregate in pulpotomized primary molars. J Clin Pediatr Dent 2005;29(4):307–12.

149. Maroto M, Barberia E, Planells P, Garcia-Godoy F. Dentin bridge formation after mineral trioxide aggregate (MTA) pulpotomies in primary teeth. Am J Dent 2005;18:151–4.

150. Maroto M, Barberia E, Vera V, Garcia-Godoy F. Dentin bridge formation after white mineral trioxide aggregate (white MTA) pulpotomies in primary molars. Am Jf Dent 2006;19:75–9.

151. Judd P, Kenny D. Non-aldehyde pulpectomy technique for primary teeth. Ont Dent 1991;68(8):25–8, 32.

152. Payne RG, Kenny DJ, Johnson DH, Judd PL. Two-year outcome study of zinc oxide–eugenol root canal treatment for vital primary teeth. J Can Dent Assoc. 1993;59(6):528–30, 533–6.

153. Yacobi R, Kenny DJ, Judd PL, Johnson DH. Evolving primary pulp therapy techniques. J Am Dent Assoc 1991;122(2):83–5.

154. Subramaniam P, Konde S, Mandanna DK. An in vitro comparison of root canal measurement in primary teeth. J Indian Soc Pedod Prev Dent 2005;23(3):124–5.

155. Katz A, Mass E, Kaufman AY. Electronic apex locator: a useful tool for root canal treatment in the primary dentition. ASDC J Dent Child 1996;63(6):414–17.

156. Kopel HM. Root canal therapy for primary teeth. J Mich Dent Assoc 1970;52(2):28–33.

157. Jokinen MA, Kotilainen R, Poikkeus P, et al. Clinical and radiographic study of pulpectomy and root canal therapy. Scand J Dent Res 1978; 86:366–73.

158. Flaitz CM, Barr ES, Hicks MJ. Radiographic evaluation of pulpal therapy for primary anterior teeth. J Dent Child 1989;56(3):182–5.

159. Barr ES, Flaitz CM, Hicks MJ. A retrospective radiographic evaluation of primary molar pulpectomies. Pediatr Dent 1991;13(1):4–9.

160. Payne RG, Kenny DJ, Johnson DH, Judd PL. Two-year outcome study of zinc oxide-eugenol root canal treatment for vital primary teeth. J Can Dent Assoc 1993;59(6):528–36.

161. Coll JA, Sadrian R. Predicting pulpectomy success and its relationship to exfoliation and succedaneous dentition. Pediatr Dent 1996;18(1):57–63.

162. Mortazavi M, Mesbahi M. Comparison of zinc oxide and eugenol, and Vitapex for root canal treatment of necrotic teeth. Int J Paediatr Dent 2004;14(6):417–24.

163. Primosch RE, Ahmadi A, Setzer B, Guelmann M. A retrospective assessment of zinc oxide–eugenol pulpectomies in vital maxillary primary incisors successfully restored with composite resin crowns. Pediatr Dent 2005;27(6): 470–7.

164. Rifkin A. A simple, effective, safe technique for the root canal treatment of abscessed primary teeth. J Dent Child 1980;47(6):435–41.

165. Garcia-Godoy F. Evaluation of an iodoform paste in root canal therapy for infected primary teeth. J Dent Child 1987;54(1):30–4.

166. Coll JA, Josell S, Casper JS. Evaluation of a one-appointment formocresol pulpectomy technique for primary molars. Pediatr Dent 1985;7(2):123–9.

167. Coll JA, Josell S, Nassof S, et al. An evaluation of pulpal therapy in primary incisors. Pediatr Dent 1988;10(3):178–84.

168. Reyes AD, Reina ES. Root canal treatment in necrotic primary molars. J Pedod 1989;14(1):36–9.

169. Thomas AM, Chandra S, Chandra S, Pandey RK. Elimination of infection in pulpectomized deciduous teeth: a short-term study using iodoform paste. J Endod 1994;20(5):233–5.

170. Holan G, Fuks AB. A comparison of pulpectomies using ZOE and Kri paste in primary molars: a retrospective study. Pediatr Dent 1993;15(6):403–7.

171. Wright KJ, Barbosa SV, Araki K, Spangberg LSW. In vitro antimicrobial and cytotoxic effects of Kri 1 paste and zinc oxide–eugenol used in primary tooth pulpectomies. Pediatr Dent 1994;16(2):102–6.

172. Hendry JA, Jeansonne BG, Dummett CO, Burrell W. Comparison of calcium hydroxide and zinc oxide eugenol pulpectomies in primary teeth of dogs. Oral Surg Oral Med Oral Pathol Oral Radiol Endod 1982; 54(4):445–51.

173. Mani SA, Chawla HS, Tewari A, Goyal A. Evaluation of calcium hydroxide and zinc oxide eugenol as root canal filling materials in primary teeth. J Dent Child 2000; 67(2):142–7.

174. Ozalp N, Saroglu I, Sonmez H. Evaluation of various root canal filling materials in primary molar pulpectomies: an in vivo study. Am J Dent 2005;18(6):347–50.

175. Nurko C, Ranly DM, Garcia-Godoy F, Lakshmyya KN. Resorption of a calcium hydroxide/iodoform (Vitapex) in root canal therapy for primary teeth: a case report. Pediatr Dent 2000;22(6):517–20.

176. Nurco C, Garcia-Godoy F. Evaluation of a calcium hydroxide/iodoform paste (Vitapex) in root canal therapy for primary teeth. J Clin Pediatr Dent 1999; 23(4):289–94.

177. Tchaou WS, Turng BF, Minah GE, Coll JA. In vitro inhibition of bacteria from root canals of primary teeth by various dental materials. Pediatr Dent 1995;17(5):351–5.

178. Rimondini L, Baroni C. Morphologic criteria for root canal treatment of primary molars undergoing resorption. Endod Dent Traumatol 1995;11(3):136–41.

179. Barr ES, Kleier DJ, Barr NV. Use of nickel–titanium rotary files for root canal preparation in primary teeth. Pediatr Dent. 1999;21(7):453–4. Also reprinted in Pediatr Dent 2000;22(1):77–8.

180. Guelman M, McEachern M, Turner C. Pulpectomies in primary incisors using three delivery systems: an in vitro study. J Clin Pediatr Dent 2004;28(4):323–6.

181. Bawazir OA, Salama FS. Clinical evaluation of root canal obturation methods in primary teeth. Pediatr Dent 2006;28(1):39–47.

182. Johnson MS, Britto LR, Guelmann M. Impact of a biological barrier in pulpectomies of primary molars. Pediatr Dent 2006;28(6):506–10.

183. Sadrian R, Coll JA. A long-term follow-up on the retention rate of zinc oxide eugenol filler after primary tooth pulpectomy. Pediatr Dent 1993;15(4):249–53.

184. Jerrell RG, Ronk SL. Developmental arrest of a succedaneous tooth following pulpectomy in a primary tooth. J Pedod 1982;6(4):337–42.

185. Avran DC, Pulver F. Pulpotomy medicaments for vital primary teeth ASCD J Dent Child 1989;56(6):426–34.

186. Primosch RE, Glomb TA, Jerrell RG. Primary tooth pulp therapy as taught in predoctoral pediatric dental programs in the United States. Pediatr Dent 1997;19(2):118–22.

CHAPTER 40

Restoration of Endodontically Treated Teeth

Charles J. Goodacre, Nadim Z. Baba

Various methods of restoring pulpless teeth have been reported for more than 200 years. In 1747, Pierre Fauchard[1] described the process by which roots of maxillary anterior teeth were used for the restoration of single teeth and the replacement of multiple teeth (Figure 1). Posts were fabricated of gold or silver and held in the root canal space with a heat-softened adhesive called "mastic."[1,2] The longevity of restorations made using this technique was attested to by Fauchard: "Teeth and artificial dentures, fastened with posts and gold wire, hold better than all others. They sometimes last fifteen to twenty years and even more without displacement. Common thread and silk, used ordinarily to attach all kinds of teeth or artificial pieces, do not last long."[1]

The replacement crowns were made from bone, ivory, animal teeth, and sound natural tooth crowns. Gradually the use of these natural substances declined, to be slowly replaced by porcelain. A pivot (what is today termed a post) was used to retain the artificial porcelain crown into a root canal and the crown–post combination was termed a "pivot crown." Porcelain pivot crowns were described in the early 1800s by a well-known dentist of Paris, Dubois de Chemant.[2] Pivoting (posting) of artificial crowns to natural roots became the most common method of replacing artificial teeth and was reported as the "best that can be employed" by Chapin Harris in *The Dental Art* in 1839.[3]

Early pivot crowns in the United States used seasoned wood (white hickory) pivots.[4] The pivot was adapted to the inside of an all-ceramic crown and also into the root canal space. Moisture would swell the wood and retain the pivot in place.[2] Surprisingly, Prothero[2] reported removing two central incisor crowns with wooden pivots that had been successfully used for 18 years. Subsequently, pivot crowns were fabricated using wood/metal combinations and then more durable all-metal pivots were used. Metal pivot retention was achieved by various means such as threads, pins, surface roughening, and split designs that provided mechanical spring retention.[2]

Unfortunately, adequate cements were not available to these early practitioners, cements that would have enhanced post retention and decreased abrasion of the root caused by movement of metal posts within the canal. One of the best representations of a pivoted tooth appears in *Dental Physiology and Surgery*, written by Sir John Tomes in 1849 (Figure 2).[5] Tomes' post length and diameter conformed closely to today's principles in fabricating posts.

Endodontic therapy, by these dental pioneers, embraced only minimal efforts to clean, shape, and obturate the canal. Frequent use of the wooden posts in empty canals led to repeated episodes of swelling and pain. Wooden posts, however, did allow the escape of the so-called "morbid humors." A groove in the post or the root canal provided a pathway for continual suppuration from the periradicular tissues.[1]

Although many of the restorative techniques used today had their inception in the 1800s and early 1900s, proper endodontic treatment was neglected until years later. Today, both endodontic and prosthodontic aspects of treatment have advanced significantly, new materials and techniques have been developed, and a substantial body of scientific knowledge is available upon which to base clinical treatment decisions.

The purpose of this chapter is to answer questions frequently encountered when dental treatment involves endodontically treated teeth and to describe the techniques commonly employed when restoring these

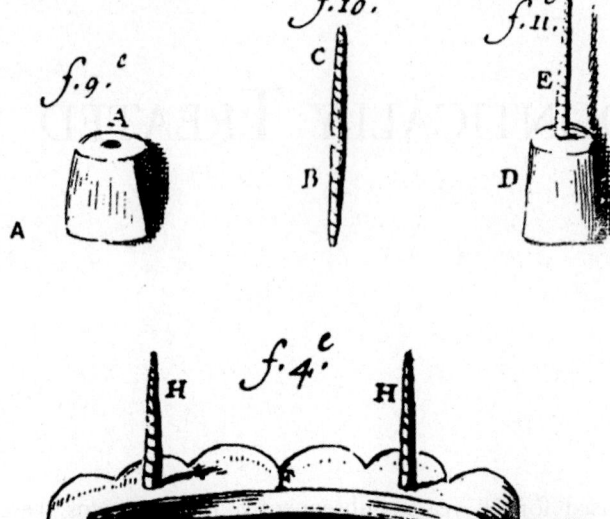

Figure 1 Early attempts to restore single or multiple units. ***A***, "Pivot tooth" consisting of crown, post, and assembled unit. ***B***, Six-unit anterior fixed partial dental prosthesis "pivoted" in lateral incisors with canines cantilevered. Crowns were fashioned from a diversity of materials. Human, hippopotamus, sea horse, and ox teeth were used, as well as ivory and oxen leg bones. Posts were usually made from precious metals and fastened to the crown and root by using a heated sticky "mastic" prepared by gum, lac, turpentine, and white coral powder.

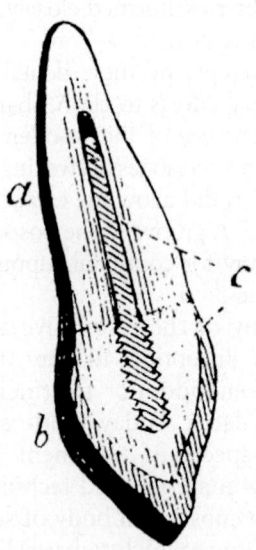

Figure 2 Principles used today in selecting post length and diameter were understood and taught by early practitioners during mid-1800s.

teeth. Whenever possible, the answers and discussion will be supported by scientific evidence. Conflicting results will be presented to provide a comprehensive understanding of the available evidence.

Should Crowns Be Placed on Endodontically Treated Teeth?

A retrospective study[6] of 1,273 teeth endodontically treated 1 to 25 years previously compared the clinical success of anterior and posterior teeth. Endodontically treated teeth with restorations that encompassed the tooth (onlays, partial or complete coverage metal crowns, and metal ceramic crowns) were compared with endodontically treated teeth with no coronal coverage restorations. It was determined that coronal coverage crowns did not significantly improve the success of endodontically treated anterior teeth. This finding supports the use of a conservative restoration such as an etched resin restoration in the access opening of otherwise intact or minimally restored anterior teeth. Crowns are indicated only on endodontically treated anterior teeth when they are structurally weakened by the presence of large and/or multiple coronal restorations or they require significant form/color changes that cannot be effected by bleaching, resin bonding, or porcelain laminate veneers. Scurria et al.[7] collected data from 30 insurance carriers in 45 states regarding the procedures 654 general dentists performed on endodontically treated teeth. The data indicated that 67% of endodontically treated anterior teeth were restored without a crown, supporting the concept that many anterior teeth are being satisfactorily restored without the use of a crown.

When endodontically treated *posterior teeth* (with and without coronal coverage restorations) were compared, a significant increase in the clinical success was noted when cuspal coverage crowns were placed on maxillary and mandibular molars and premolars.[6] In a study of 116 failed and extracted endodontically treated teeth, Vire[8] reported that teeth restored with crowns had greater longevity than uncrowned teeth. A strong association was found between crown placement and the survival of endodontically treated teeth. If long-term tooth survival is the primary goal, placing

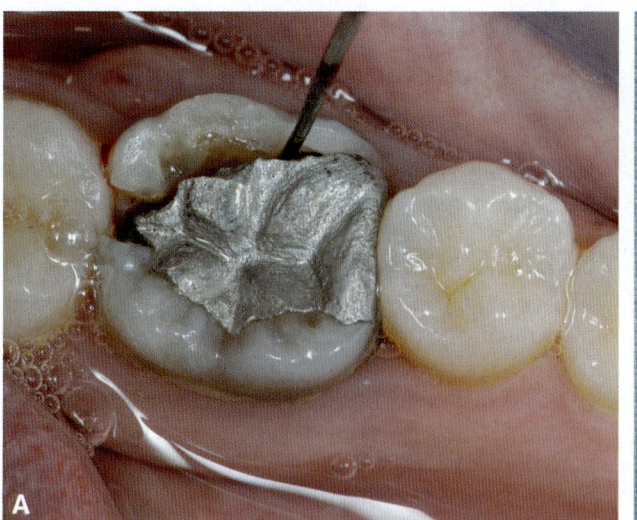
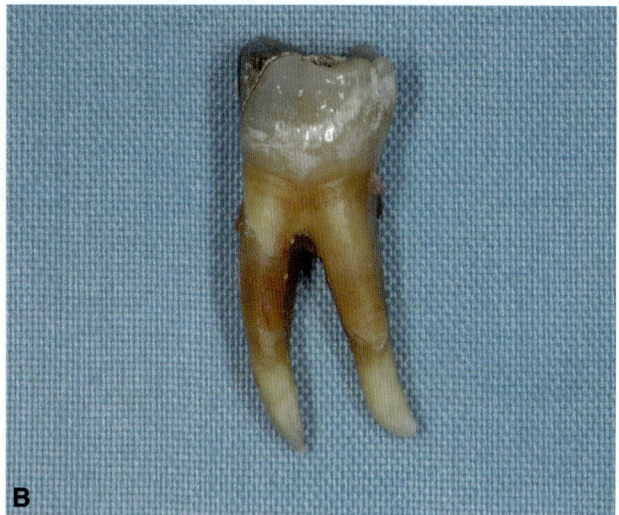

Figure 3 ***A,*** Occlusal view showing the fracture of the buccal cusp of an endodontically treated mandibular left first molar. ***B,*** Extracted tooth showing the fracture extending down both roots.

a crown on an endodontically treated posterior tooth enhances survival (Figure 3).[9] Therefore, restorations that encompass the cusps should be used on posterior teeth that have intercuspation with opposing teeth and thereby receive occlusal forces that push the cusps apart. The previously discussed insurance data[7] indicated that 37 to 40% of posterior endodontically treated teeth were restored by practitioners without a crown, a method of treatment not supported by the long-term clinical prognosis of posterior endodontically treated teeth that do not have cusp-encompassing crowns. There are, however, certain posterior teeth (not as high as 40%) that do not have substantive occlusal intercuspation or have an occlusal form that precludes intercuspation of a nature that attempts to separate the cusps (such as mandibular first premolars with small, poorly developed lingual cusps). When teeth are intact or minimally restored (small MO or DO restorations), they would be reasonable candidates for restoration of only the access opening without the use of a coronal coverage crown.[10]

In contrast to the above recommendations, a 3-year clinical study by Mannocci et al.[11] evaluated the clinical success rate of endodontically treated premolars restored with a post and direct composite resin restorations with and without complete crown coverage. They found that both had a similar success rate. Nagasiri et al.,[12] in a retrospective cohort study, indicated that when endodontically treated molars are completely intact except for a conservative access opening, they could be restored successfully by using composite resin restorations.

Multiple clinical studies of fixed partial dentures, many with long spans and cantilevers, have determined that endodontically treated abutments failed more often than vital teeth due to tooth fracture,[13–17] supporting the greater fragility of endodontically treated teeth and the need to design restorations that reduce the potential for both crown and root fractures when extensive fixed prosthodontic treatment is required.

Gutmann[18] reviewed the literature and presented an overview of several articles that identify what happens when teeth are endodontically treated. These articles provide background information important to an understanding of why coronal coverage crowns help prevent fractures of posterior teeth. Endodontically treated dog teeth have been found to have 9% less moisture than vital teeth.[19] In addition, it was found that dehydration increases stiffness and decreases the flexibility in teeth. However, dehydration by itself does not account for the physical property changes in dentin.[20] Also, with aging, greater amounts of peritubular dentin are formed, which decreases the amount of organic materials that may contain moisture. It has been shown that endodontic procedures reduce tooth stiffness by 5%, attributed primarily to the access opening.[21] Tidmarsh[22] described the structure of an intact tooth that permits deformation when loaded occlusally and elastic recovery after removal of the load. The direct relationship between tooth structure removed during tooth preparation and tooth deformation under load has been described.[23] Dentin from endodontically treated teeth has been shown to exhibit significantly lower shear strength and toughness when compared with vital dentin.[24] Rivera et al.[25] stated that the effort required to fracture dentin may be less when teeth are endodontically treated because of more immature (potentially weaker) collagen intermolecular cross-links. In a recent study, it was found that collagen fibrils degraded over time in teeth with zinc phosphate-cemented posts. Acid demineralization can also occur from bacteria and acid etching.[26]

CONCLUSIONS

Restorations that encompass the cusps of endodontically treated posterior teeth have been found to increase the clinical longevity of these teeth. Therefore, crowns should be placed on endodontically treated posterior teeth that have occlusal intercuspation with opposing teeth of the nature that places expansive forces on the cusps. Since crowns do not enhance the clinical success of anterior endodontically treated teeth, their use on relatively sound teeth should be limited to situations where esthetic and functional requirements cannot be adequately achieved by other more conservative restorations (Figure 4).

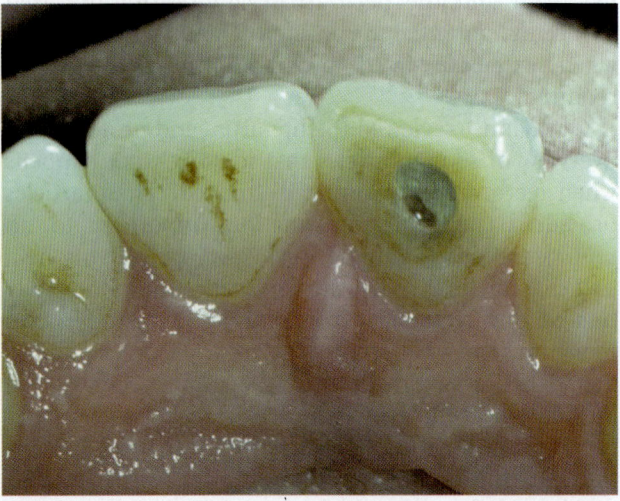

Figure 4 Traumatized tooth before endodontic procedure. Placement of a bonded resin restoration in the access opening after root canal treatment and whitening is the only treatment required since crowns do not enhance the longevity of anterior endodontically treated teeth. A crown will be indicated only when esthetic and functional needs cannot be achieved through more conservative treatments.

With Pulpless Teeth, Do Posts Improve Long-Term Clinical Prognosis or Enhance Strength?

Historically, the use of posts was based on the concept that a post reinforces the tooth.

LABORATORY DATA

Virtually all laboratory studies[27–37] have shown that placement of a post and core either fails to increase the fracture resistance of endodontically treated extracted teeth or decreases the fracture resistance of the tooth when a force is applied via a mechanical testing machine. Lovdahl and Nicholls[27] found that endodontically treated maxillary central incisors were stronger when the natural crown was intact except for the access opening than when they were restored with cast posts and cores or pin-retained silver amalgams. Lu[28] found that posts placed in intact endodontically treated central incisors did not lead to an increase in the force required to fracture the tooth or in the position and angulation of the fracture line. Pontius[29] found that maxillary incisors, without posts, resisted higher failure loads than the other groups with posts and crowns. Gluskin[30] found that mandibular incisors with intact natural crowns exhibited greater resistance to transverse loads compared with teeth with posts and cores. McDonald[31] found no difference in the impact fracture resistance of mandibular incisors with or without posts. Eshelman and Sayegh[32] reported similar results when posts were placed in extracted dog lateral incisors. Guzy and Nicholls[33] determined that there was no significant reinforcement achieved by cementing a post into an endodontically treated tooth that was intact except for the access opening. Leary et al.[34] measured the root deflection of endodontically treated teeth before and after posts of various lengths were cemented into prepared root canals. They found no significant differences in strength between the teeth with or without a post. Trope et al.[35] determined that preparing a post space weakened endodontically treated teeth compared with ones in which only an access opening was made, but no post space.

A potential situation where a post and core could strengthen a tooth was identified by Hunter et al.[36] using photoelastic stress analysis. They determined that removal of internal tooth structure during endodontic therapy is accompanied by a proportional increase in stress. They also determined that minimal root canal enlargement for a post does not substantially weaken a tooth but when excessive root canal enlargement has occurred, a post strengthens the tooth. Therefore, if the walls of a root canal are thin due to the removal of internal root caries or overinstrumentation during post preparation, then a post may potentially strengthen the tooth.

Two-dimensional finite element analysis was used in one study[37] to determine the effect of posts on dentin stress in pulpless teeth. When loaded vertically along the long axis, a post reduced maximal dentin stress by as much as 20%. However, only a small (3 to 8%) decrease in dentin stress was found when a tooth with a post was subjected to masticatory and traumatic loadings at 45° to the incisal edge. The authors proposed that the reinforcement effect of posts is doubtful for anterior teeth because they are subjected to angular forces.

CLINICAL DATA

Sorensen and Martinoff[38] evaluated endodontically treated teeth with and without posts and cores. Some of the teeth were restored with single crowns while others served as fixed partial denture abutments or removable partial denture abutments. Posts and cores significantly decreased the clinical success rate of teeth with single crowns, improved the clinical success of removable partial denture abutment teeth, and had little influence on the clinical success of fixed partial denture abutments. Eckerbom et al.[39] examined the radiographs of 200 consecutive patients and reexamined the patients radiographically 5 to 7 years later to determine the prevalence of apical periodontitis. Of the 636 endodontically treated teeth evaluated, 378 had posts and 258 did not have posts. At both examinations, apical periodontitis was significantly more common in teeth with posts than in endodontically treated teeth without posts. Morfis[40] evaluated the incidence of vertical root fracture in 460 endodontically treated teeth, 266 of which had posts. There were 17 teeth with root fracture after a time period of at least 3 years. Nine of the 17 fractured teeth had posts and 8 root fractures occurred in teeth without posts. Morfis[40] concluded that the endodontic technique can cause vertical root fracture. In an analysis of data from multiple clinical studies, Goodacre[41] found that 3% of teeth with posts fractured. None of these clinical data provide definitive support for the concept that posts and cores strengthen endodontically treated teeth or improve their long-term prognosis.

THE PURPOSE OF POSTS

Since clinical and laboratory data indicate that teeth are not strengthened by posts, their purpose is for retention of a core that will provide appropriate support for the definitive crown or prosthesis. Unfortunately, this primary purpose has not been completely recognized. Hussey[42] noted that 24% of general dental practitioners felt that a post strengthens teeth. A 1994 survey (with responses from 1066 practitioners and educators) revealed some interesting facts. Ten percent of the dentist respondents felt that every endodontically treated tooth should receive a post. It was determined that 62% of dentists over age 50 believed a post reinforces the tooth whereas only 41% of the dentists under age 41 believed in that concept. Thirty-nine percent of part-time faculty, 41% of full-time faculty, and 56% of nonfaculty practitioners felt that posts reinforce teeth.[43]

CONCLUSIONS

Both laboratory and clinical data fail to provide definitive support for the concept that posts strengthen endodontically treated teeth. Therefore, the purpose of a post is to provide retention for a core.

What Is the Clinical Failure Rate of Posts and Cores?

Several studies provide clinical data regarding the number of posts and cores that failed over certain time periods[44–55] (Table 1). When this number is divided by the total number of posts and cores placed, a failure

Table 1 Clinical Failure Rate of Posts and Cores

Lead Author	Study Length	Percentage of Clinical Failure
Turner (1982)*	5 years	9 (6 of 66)
Sorenson (1984)	1–25 years	9 (36 of 420)
Bergman (1989)*	6 years	9 (9 of 96)
Weine (1991)*	10 years or more	7 (9 of 138)
Hatzikyriakos (1992)*	3 years	11 (17 of 154)
Mentink (1993)*	1–10 years (mean 4.8)	8 (39 of 516)
Wallerstedt (1984)*	4–10 years (mean 7.8)	14 (8 of 56)
Torbjörner (1995)	4–5 years	9 (72 of 788)
Balkenhol (2006)	1–9 years (mean 2.1)	7 (50 of 802)
Valderhaug (1997)	1–25 years (mean 2.1)	10 (40 of 397)
Mean values§	8 years	9 (292 of 3433)

*Studies used to calculate mean study length.
§Calculation made by averaging numerical data from all studies.

percentage is determined. A 9% overall average for failure was calculated by averaging the failure percentages from 10 studies (an average study length of 6 years). In these studies, the failure percentage ranged from 7% to 14%.

A review of more specific details from the 10 studies provides insight into the length of each study and the number of posts and cores evaluated. The findings of a 5-year retrospective study of 66 posts and cores indicate there were 6 failures and a 9% failure rate.[44] Another study found that 17 of 154 posts failed after 3 years for an 11% failure rate.[45] A failure rate of 9% was found in three studies.[46–48] Two studies reported a 7% post and core failure rate after 9 years or more.[49,55] An 8% failure rate (39 of 516 posts and cores) was published when 516 posts and cores placed by senior dental students were retrospectively evaluated,[50] whereas another study recorded a 14% failure rate (8 failures in 56 posts and cores) from posts and cores placed by dental students.[51] A study of 397 posts followed for 25 years reported a 10% post and core failure rate after 25 years (40 of 397 posts failed).[54]

Kaplan-Meier survival statistics (percentage of survival over certain time periods) were presented or could be calculated from the data in nine studies[52] (Table 2). The survival rates ranged from a high of 99% after 10 years or more of follow-up to a 78% survival rate after a mean time of 5.2 years. The failure percentage per year has also been calculated and ranged from 1.56% per year[47] to 4.3% per year.[53]

CONCLUSIONS

Posts and cores had an average clinical failure rate of 9% (7 to 14% range) when the data from 10 studies were combined (average study length of 8 years).

What Are the Most Common Types of Post and Core Failures?

Eight studies indicate that post loosening is the most common cause of post and core failure[44,45,47,48,50,55–57] (Figure 5). Turner[44] reported on 100 failures of post-retained crowns and indicated that post loosening was the most common type of failure. Of the 100 failures, 59 were caused by post loosening. The next most common occurrences were 42 apical abscesses followed by 19 carious lesions. There were 10 root fractures and 6 post fractures. In another paper by Turner,[56] he reported the findings of a 5-year retrospective study of 52 post-retained crowns. Six posts had come loose, which was the most common failure. Lewis and Smith[57] presented data regarding 67 post and core failures after 4 years. Forty-seven of the failures resulted from post loosening, 8 from root fractures, 7 from caries, and 4 from bent or fractured posts. Bergman et al.[47] found 8 failures in 96 posts after 5 years. Six posts had loosened and 2 roots had fractured. Hatzikyriakos et al.[45] reported on 154 posts and cores after 3 years. Five posts had come loose, five crowns had come loose, four roots fractured, and caries caused three failures. Mentink[50] identified 30 post loosenings and 9 tooth fractures when evaluating 516 posts and cores over a 1- to 10-year time period (4.8 years mean study length). Torbjörner et al.[48] reported on the frequency of three technical failures (loss of retention, root fracture, and post fracture). They did not report biological failures. Loss of retention was the most frequent post failure, accounting for 45 of the 72 post and core failures. Root

Table 2 Kaplain–Meier Survival Data (%) of Posts and Cores

Lead Author	Study Length	Percentage of Survival
Robert (1970)	5.2 years mean	78
Wallerstedt (1984)	4–10 years range	86
Sorenson (1985)	1–25 years range	90
Weine (1991)	10 years or more	99
Hatzikyriakos (1992)	3 years	92
Mentink (1993)	1–10 years (mean 4.8)	82
Creugers (1993) (meta-analysis)	6 years	81 (threaded posts), 91 (cast posts)
Balkenhol (2006)	1–9 years range (mean 2.1)	89
Valderhaug (1997)	1–25 years range	80

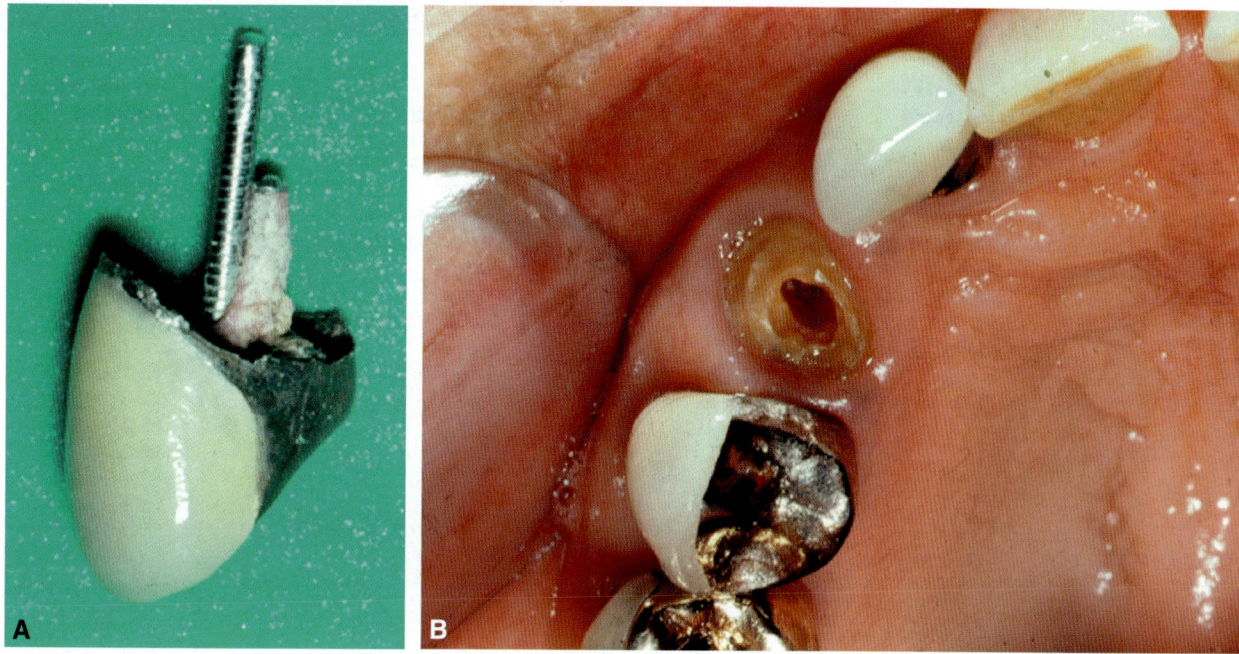

Figure 5 Post and crown loosened from maxillary canine a few years after placement. ***A,*** Both the post/core and the crown came off. ***B,*** Clinical photo shows very little cervical tooth structure for retention of the crown.

fracture (Figure 6) was the second most common failure cause followed by post fracture. Balkenhol et al.[55] reported on 802 posts and cores over a 10-year period.

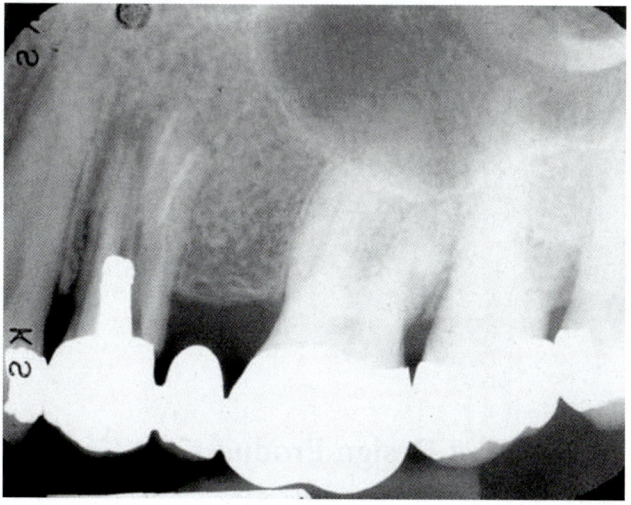

Figure 6 Radiograph of a fractured maxillary first premolar with a post with excessive diameter and insufficient length, two problems frequently seen in conjunction with fractured roots.

Thirty-nine posts had loosened, eight had longitudinal root fracture, and six had transverse root fracture.

In two studies, factors other than loss of retention were listed as the most common cause of failure.[46,49] Sorensen and Martinoff[46] evaluated 420 posts and cores and recorded 36 failures. Of the 36 failures, 8 were related to restorable tooth fractures, 12 to nonrestorable tooth fractures, 13 to loss of retention, and 3 were caused by root perforations. Weine et al.[49] found 9 failures in 138 cast posts and cores after 10 years or more. Three failures were caused by restorative procedures, two by endodontic treatment, two by periodontal problems, and two by root fractures. No posts failed due to loss of retention.

Four studies have provided data on the incidence of tooth fracture but no information regarding post loosening. Linde[58] reported that 3 of 42 teeth fractured, Ross[59] found no fractures with 86 posts, Morfis[40] found that 10 of 266 teeth fractured, and Wallerstedt[51] identified 2 fractures with 56 posts.

Loss of retention and tooth fracture (in that order of occurrence) are the 2 most common causes of failure when these studies are collectively analyzed by averaging the numerical data from all the studies. Five percent of the posts placed (144 of 2,980 posts)

Table 3 Clinical Loss of Retention Associated with Posts and Cores

Lead Author	Study Length	Percentage of Posts Placed that Loosened	Post Form	Percentage of Failures Owing to Loosening
Turner (1982)	5 years	9 (6 of 66)	Appeared to be tapered	*
Turner (1982)	1–5 years or more	*	Tapered	59 (59 of 100)
Sorensen (1984)	1–25 years	3 (13 of 420)	Tapered and parallel	36 (13 of 36)
Lewis (1988)	4 years	*	Threaded, tapered, and parallel	70 (47 of 67)
Bergman (1989)	6 years	6 (6 of 96)	Tapered	67 (6 of 9)
Weine (1991)	10 years or more	0 (0 of 138)	Tapered	0 (0 of 9)
Hatzikyriakos (1992)	3 years	3 (5 of 154)	Threaded, tapered, and parallel	29 (5 of 17)
Mentink (1993)	1–10 years (mean 4.8)	6 (30 of 516)	Tapered	77 (30 of 39)
Torbjörner (1995)	4–5 years	6 (45 of 788)	Tapered and parallel	63 (45 of 72)
Balkenhol (2006)	1–9 years (mean 2.1)	5 (39 of 802)	Tapered	43 (39 of 90)
Mean values§		5 (144 of 2980)		56 (244 post loosenings of 439 total failures)

*Data not available in publication.
§Calculation made by averaging numerical data from all studies.

Table 4 Clinical Tooth Fractures Associated with Posts and Cores

Lead Author	Study Length	Percentage of Teeth Restored with Posts that Fractured	Post Form(s) Studied	Percentage of Failures Owing to Fracture
Turner (1982)	5 years	0 (0 of 66)	Appeared to be tapered	*
Turner (1982)	1–5 years or more	*	Tapered, parallel, and threaded	10 (10 of 100)
Sorensen (1984)	1–25 years	3 (12 of 420)	Tapered and parallel	33 (12 of 36)
Linde (1984)	2–10 years (5 years, 8 months mean)	7 (3 of 42)	Threaded	38 (3 of 8)
Lewis (1988)	4 years	*	Threaded, tapered, and parallel	12 (8 of 67)
Bergman (1989)	6 years	3 (3 of 96)	Tapered	33 (3 of 9)
Ross (1980)	5 years or more	0 (0 of 86)	Tapered, parallel, and threaded	0 (0 of 86)
Morfis (1990)	3 years at least	4 (10 of 266)	Threaded and parallel	*
Weine (1991)	10 years or more	1 (2 of 138)	Tapered	50 (2 of 4)
Hatzikyriakos (1992)	3 years	3 (4 of 154)	Threaded, tapered, and parallel	3 (4 of 17)
Mentink (1993)	1–10 years (mean 4.8)	2 (9 of 516)	Tapered	23 (9 of 39)
Wallerstedt (1984)	4–10 years (mean 7.8)	4 (2 of 56)	Threaded	25 (2 of 8)
Torbjörner (1995)	4–5 years	3 (21 of 788)	Tapered and parallel	29 (21 of 72)
Balkenhol (2006)	1–9 years (mean 2.1)	2 (14 of 802)	Tapered	15 (14 of 90)
Valderhaug (1997)	1–25 years (mean 2.1)	1 (2 of 397)	Tapered	5 (2 of 40)
Mean values§		2 (82 of 3827)		16 (90 tooth fractures of 576 total failures)

*Data not available in publication.
§Calculation made by averaging numerical data from all studies.

experienced loss of retention (Table 3). Two percent of the posts placed (82 of 3,827 posts) failed via tooth fracture (Table 4).

CONCLUSIONS
Loss of retention and tooth fracture are the two most common causes of post and core failure.

Which Post Design Produces the Greatest Retention?

LABORATORY DATA
There have been many laboratory studies comparing the retention of various post designs. Threaded posts provide the greatest retention, followed by cemented,

parallel-sided posts. Tapered cemented posts are the least retentive. Cemented, parallel-sided posts with serrations are more retentive than cemented, smooth-sided parallel posts. These laboratory data are discussed below.

CLINICAL DATA

There is clinical support for these laboratory studies. Torbjörner et al.[48] reported significantly greater loss of retention with tapered posts (7%) compared with parallel posts (4%). Sorensen and Martinoff[46] determined that 4% of tapered posts failed by loss of retention whereas 1% of parallel posts failed in that manner. Turner[56] indicated that tapered posts loosened clinically more frequently than parallel-sided posts. Lewis and Smith[57] also found a higher loss of retention with smooth-walled tapered posts than parallel posts. Bergman et al.[47] and Mentink et al.[50] evaluated only tapered posts, and both studies reported that 6% of tapered posts failed via loss of retention, values higher than those recorded by Torbjörner et al.[48] and Sorensen and Martinoff[46] for parallel posts.

Contrasting results were reported by Weine et al.[49] They found no clinical failures from loss of retention with cast tapered posts. Hatzikyriakos et al.[45] studied tapered threaded posts, parallel cemented posts, and tapered cemented posts. The only posts that loosened from the root were parallel cemented posts.

CONCLUSIONS

Tapered posts are the least retentive and threaded posts the most retentive in laboratory studies. Most of the clinical data support the laboratory findings.

Is There a Relationship Between Post Form and the Potential for Root Fracture?

LABORATORY DATA

Using photoelastic stress analysis, Henry[60] determined that threaded posts produced undesirable levels of stress. Another study used strain gauges attached to the root and compared four parallel-sided threaded posts with one parallel-sided nonthreaded post.[59] Two of the threaded posts produced the highest strains, whereas two other threaded posts caused strains comparable to the nonthreaded post. Standlee et al.,[61] using photoelastic methods, indi-

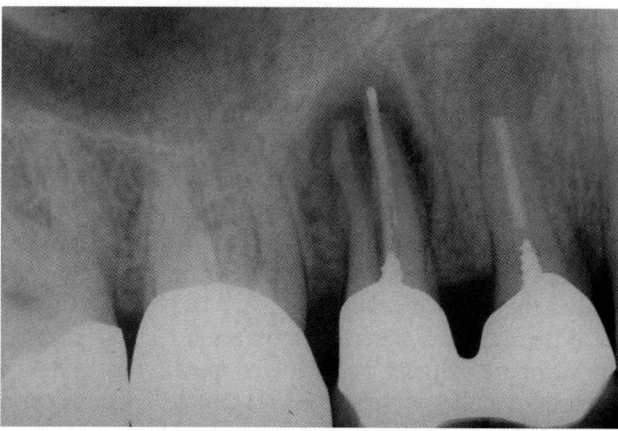

Figure 7 Radiograph showing a threaded post that may have caused root fracture in the second premolar.

cated that tapered, threaded posts were the worst stress producers. When three types of threaded posts were compared in extracted teeth, Deutsch et al.[62] found that tapered threaded posts increased root fracture by 20 times that of the parallel threaded posts (Figure 7).

Laboratory testing of split threaded posts has provided varying results, but more research groups have concluded that they do not reduce the stress associated with threaded posts. Thorsteinsson et al.[63] determined that split threaded posts did not reduce stress concentration during loading. In another study, split threaded posts were found to produce installation stresses comparable to other threaded posts.[64] Greater stress concentrations than those of some other threaded posts were reported under simulated functional loading.[65–67] Rolf et al.[68] found that a split threaded post produced comparable stress to one type of threaded post and less stress than a third threaded post design. Ross et al.[59] determined that a split threaded post produced less root strain than two other threaded posts and comparable strain to a third threaded post and a nonthreaded post. Another research group[69] concluded that the split threaded design reduced the stresses caused during cementation compared with a rigid threaded post design. Multiple photoelastic stress studies have concluded that posts designed for cementation produced less stress than threaded posts.[60,61,68]

When parallel-sided cemented posts were compared with tapered cemented posts, photoelastic stress testing results generally favored parallel-sided posts. Using this methodology, Henry[60] found that parallel-sided posts distribute stress more evenly to the root. Finite element analysis studies produced similar results.[70,71] Two additional photoelastic studies[63,66] concluded that parallel posts concentrate stress apically and tapered posts concentrate stress at the post–core junction. Also using photoelastic testing, Assif et al.[72] found that tapered posts showed equal stress distribution between the cementoenamel junction and the apex compared with parallel posts that concentrated the stress apically.

When fracture patterns in extracted teeth were used to compare parallel and tapered posts, the evidence favoring parallel posts was less favorable. Sorensen and Engelman[73] determined that tapered posts caused more extensive fractures than parallel-sided posts did, but the load required to create fracture was significantly higher with tapered posts. Lu,[28] also using extracted teeth, found no difference in the fracture location between prefabricated parallel posts and cast posts and cores. Assif et al.[74] tested the resistance of extracted teeth to fracture when the teeth were restored with either parallel or tapered posts and complete crowns. No significant differences were noted, and post design did not influence fracture resistance.

In analyzing the stress distribution of posts, it was noted that tapered posts generate the least cementation stress and should be considered for teeth that have thin root walls, are nearly perforated, or have perforation repairs.[66]

CLINICAL DATA

There are several clinical studies that provide data related to the incidence of root fracture associated with different post forms. Some of these studies provide a comparison of multiple post forms, whereas other studies evaluated only one type of post. Combining all the root fracture data for each post form from both types of studies reveals some interesting trends (Table 5). Five studies present data regarding root fractures and threaded posts,[40,46,51,58,75] four regarding fractures associated with parallel-sided cemented posts[40,46,48,75] and nine related to tapered cemented posts.[40,46–49,50,54,55,75] If the total number of threaded posts evaluated in the five studies is divided into the total number of fractures found with threaded posts, a percent value can be determined that represents the average incidence of tooth fracture associated with threaded posts in the five studies. The same data can be calculated for parallel cemented and tapered cemented posts, permitting a comparison of the root fracture incidences associated with these three post forms.

Table 5 Post Form and Tooth Fracture

Clinical Data (Percentage of Post and Cores Studied that Failed via Tooth Fracture)

Threaded Posts (Lead Author)	Parallel-Sided Posts (Lead Author)	Tapered Posts (Lead Author)
40 (2 of 5) (Sorensen)	0 (0 of 170) (Sorensen)	7 (18 of 245) (Sorensen)
0 (0 of 10) (Ross)	2 (5 of 332) (Torbjörner)	4 (16 of 456) (Torbjörner)
4 (2 of 56) (Wallerstedt)	0 (0 of 39) (Ross)	1 (2 of 138) (Weine)
7 (3 of 42) (Linde)	3 (4 of 146) (Morfis)	2 (9 of 516) (Mentink)
7 (4 of 56) (Morfis)		3 (3 of 96) (Bergman)
		0 (0 of 38) (Ross)
		3 (2 of 64) (Morfis)
		2 (14 of 802) (Balkenhol)
		1 (2 of 397) (Valderhaug)
7% Mean* (11 of 169)	1% Mean* (9 of 687)	2% Mean* (66 of 2752)

*Calculation made by averaging numerical data from all studies.

Combining the five studies that reported data relative to threaded posts produced a mean fracture rate of 7% (11 fractures from 169 posts). The four clinical studies that contain fracture data from parallel-sided cemented posts produced a mean fracture incidence of 1% (9 fractures from 687 posts). From the seven studies reporting root fracture with tapered posts, there is a mean fracture rate of 2% (66 root fractures from 2,752 posts). This combined study data support the previously cited photoelastic laboratory stress tests, indicating that the greatest incidence of root fractures occurred with threaded posts and that the lowest incidence of root fracture was associated with parallel cemented posts. In a meta-analysis of selected clinical studies, Creugers et al.[52] calculated a 91% tooth survival rate for cemented cast posts and cores and an 81% survival rate for threaded posts with resin cores.

While the combined data from all the studies for each type of post revealed certain trends, analysis of individual studies (where multiple post forms were compared in the same study) produced less conclusive results. One study of threaded posts and cemented posts determined that teeth with threaded posts were lost more frequently than teeth with cast posts.[39] In three other clinical comparisons of threaded and cemented posts, no tooth fracture differences were noted.[40,45,75] In addition to the comparisons of threaded and cemented posts, four clinical studies provide data comparing the tooth fracture incidences associated with parallel-sided and tapered posts. In comparing parallel and tapered posts by reviewing dental charting records, a higher failure rate was reported with tapered posts than with parallel posts in two studies, and the failures were judged to be more severe with tapered posts.[46,48] Two other clinical studies determined that there were no differences between tapered and parallel-sided posts.[48,75] Hatzikyriakos et al.[45] found no significant differences between 47 parallel cemented posts and 44 tapered cemented posts after three years of service. Ross[75] evaluated 86 teeth with posts and cores that had been restored at least five years previously. No fracture differences were found between 38 tapered cemented posts and 39 parallel cemented posts.

Unfortunately, the total number of clinical studies that compared multiple post forms in the same study is limited. Also, several factors may have affected the findings of available studies. Two of the papers that contained a comparison of multiple post forms covered sufficiently long time periods (10 to 25 years) that the tapered cemented posts may have been in place for much longer time periods than the parallel-sided cemented posts (due to the later introduction of parallel posts into the dental market).[46,48] The mean time since the placement of each post form was not identified in these studies. Also, both of these studies were based on reviews of patient records (rather than clinical examinations) and depended on the accuracy of dental charts in determining if and when posts failed as well as the cause of the failure. Another factor that affected the results of many of the referenced clinical studies was the length of the posts. For instance, in Sorensen and Martinoff's study,[46] 44% of the tapered cemented posts had a length that was half (or less than half) the incisocervical/occlusocervical dimension of the crown whereas only 4% of the parallel cemented posts were that short. Since short posts have been associated with higher root stresses in laboratory studies, the difference in post length may have affected their findings where tooth fractures occurred with 18 of 245 tapered posts compared with no fractures with 170 parallel posts.

CONCLUSIONS

When evaluating the relationship between post form and root fracture, laboratory tests generally indicate that all types of threaded posts produce the greatest potential for root fracture. When comparing tapered and parallel cemented posts by using photoelastic stress analysis, the results generally favor the parallel cemented posts. However, the evidence is mixed when the comparison between tapered and parallel posts is based on fracture patterns in extracted teeth created by applying a force via a mechanical testing machine.

When evaluating the combined data from multiple clinical studies, threaded posts generally produced the highest root fracture incidence (7%) compared with tapered cemented posts (2%) and parallel cemented posts (1%). Analysis of individual clinical studies as opposed to the combined data produces less conclusive results. Additional comparative clinical studies would be beneficial, including designs that have not yet been evaluated in comparative studies.

What Is the Proper Length for a Post?

A wide range of recommendations have been made regarding post length, which includes the following:

1. The post length should equal the incisocervical or occlusocervical dimension of the crown.[76-83]
2. The post should be longer than the crown.[84]
3. The post should be one-third of the crown length.[85]
4. The post should be half of the root length.[86,87]
5. The post should be two-thirds of the root length.[88-92]
6. The post should be four-fifths of the root length.[93]
7. The post should be terminated halfway between the crestal bone and the root apex.[94-96]
8. The post should be as long as possible without disturbing the apical seal.[60]

A review of scientific data provides the basis for differentiating between these varied guidelines.

While short posts have never been advocated, they have been frequently observed during radiographic examinations (Figures 8 and 9). Grieve and

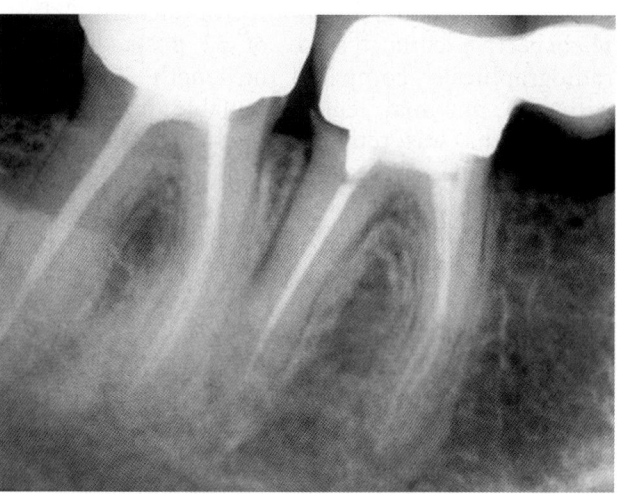

Figure 8 Radiograph displaying a very short post in the distal root of a first molar. The prosthesis has loosened.

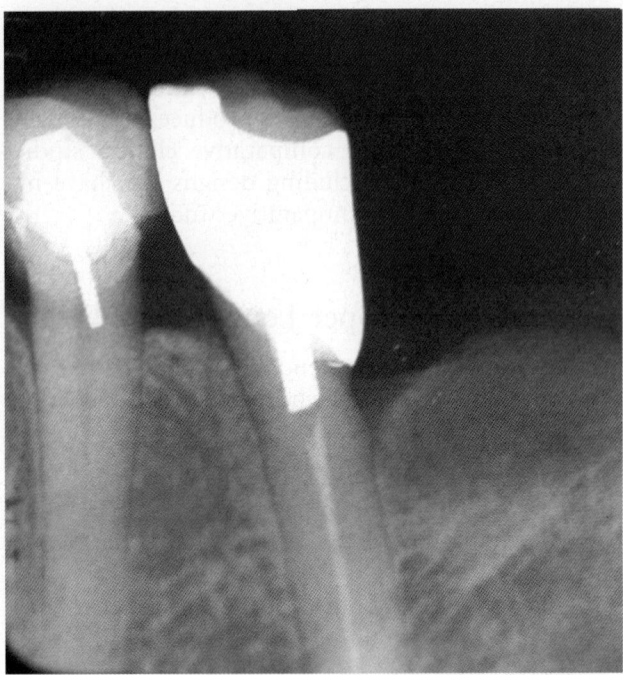

Figure 9 Radiograph of a second premolar with a very short post; the lack of adequate retention for the core can result in the prosthesis loosening.

McAndrew[97] found that only 34% of 327 posts were as long as the incisocervical length of the crown. In a clinical study of 200 endodontically treated teeth, Ross[75] determined that only 14% of posts were two-thirds or more of the root length and 49% of the posts were one-third or less of the root length. A radiographic study of 217 posts determined that only 5% of the posts were two-thirds to three-fourths of the root length.[98] In a retrospective clinical study of 52 posts, Turner[44] radiographically compared the length of the post with the maximal length available if 3 mm of gutta-percha was retained. Posts that came loose used only 59% of the ideal length and only 37% of the posts were longer than the proposed maximal length. Nine millimeters was proposed as the ideal length. Short posts have been associated with higher root stresses[36,64,66,70,71] and a greater tendency for root fracture to occur.

Sorensen and Martinoff[46] determined that the clinical success was markedly improved when the post was equal to or greater than that of the crown length. Johnson and Sakumura[99] determined that posts that were three-fourths or more of the root length were up to 30% more retentive than posts that were half of the root length or equal to the crown length. Leary et al.[100] indicated that posts with a length at least three-fourths of the root offered the greatest rigidity and least root bending.

These data indicate that post length would appropriately be three-fourths that of the root length. However, some interesting results occur when post length guidelines of two-thirds to three-fourths of the root length are applied to teeth with average, long, and short root lengths. It was determined that a post approaching this recommended length range is not possible without compromising the apical seal by retaining less than 5 mm of gutta-percha.[101] When post length was half that of the root, the apical seal was rarely compromised on average length roots. However, when posts were two-thirds of the root length, many of the average and short roots would have less than the optimal gutta-percha seal. Shillingburg et al.[102] also indicated that making the post length equal to the clinical crown length can cause the post to encroach on the 4-mm "safety zone" required for an apical seal.

Abou-Rass et al.[103] proposed a post length guideline for maxillary and mandibular molars based on the incidence of lateral root perforations when post preparations were made in 150 extracted teeth. They determined molar posts should not be extended more than 7 mm apical to the root canal orifice.

When teeth have diminished bone support, stresses increase dramatically and are concentrated in the dentin near the post apex.[104] A recent finite element model study established a relationship between post length and alveolar bone level.[105] To minimize stress in the dentin and in the post, the post should extend more than 4 mm apical to the bone.

CONCLUSIONS

Reasonable clinical guidelines for length include the following:

1. Make the post approximately three-fourths of the length of the root when treating long-rooted teeth.
2. When average root length is encountered, post length is dictated by retaining 5 mm of apical gutta-percha and extending the post to the gutta-percha (Figure 10).

3. Whenever possible, posts should extend at least 4 mm apical to the bone crest to decrease dentin stress.
4. Molar posts should not be extended more than 7 mm into the root canal apical to the base of the pulp chamber (Figure 11).

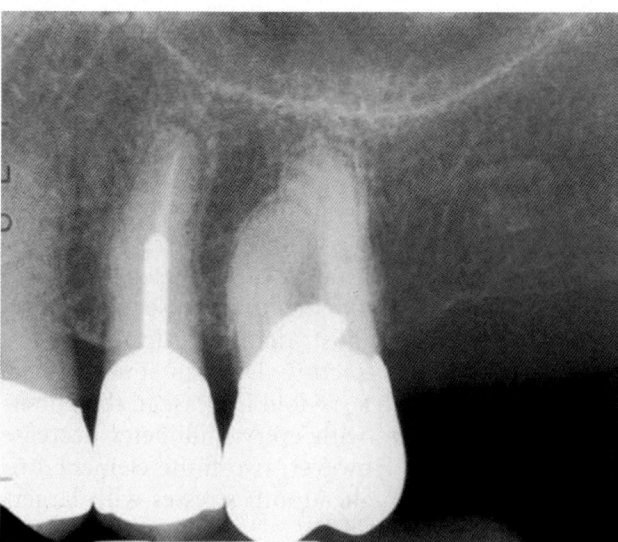

Figure 10 Five millimeters of gutta-percha was retained in the maxillary premolar and the post extended to that point.

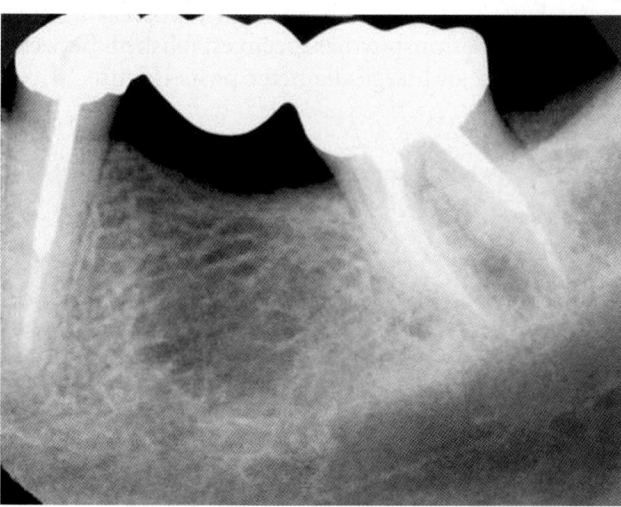

Figure 11 The post in the distal canal of the mandibular molar extends to a maximal length of 7 mm.

How Much Gutta-Percha Should Be Retained to Preserve the Apical Seal?

It has been determined that when 4 mm of gutta-percha was retained, only 1 of 89 specimens showed leakage, whereas 32 of 88 specimens leaked when only 2 mm of gutta-percha was retained.[106] Two studies found no leakage at 4 mm,[107,108] and two additional studies found little leakage at 4 mm.[106,109] Portell et al.[110] found that most specimens with only 3 mm of apical gutta-percha had some leakage. When the leakage associated with 3, 5, and 7 mm of gutta-percha was compared, Mattison et al.[111] found significant leakage differences between each of the dimensions. They proposed that at least 5 mm of gutta-percha is required for an adequate apical seal. Nixon et al.[112] compared the sealing capabilities of 3, 4, 5, 6, and 7 mm of apical gutta-percha using dye penetration. The greatest leakage occurred when only 3 mm was retained, and it was significantly different from the other groups. They also noted a significant decrease in leakage when 6 mm of gutta-percha remained. Raiden and Gendelman[113] cemented stainless steel posts with zinc phosphate cement in teeth with residual root canal fillings of 1, 2, 3, and 4 mm. They tested apical leakage using a passive dye system. They concluded that 4 mm of apical seal provided a leakage value of zero. Kvist et al.[114] examined radiographs from 852 clinical endodontic treatments. Posts were present in 424 of the teeth. Roots with posts in which the remaining root filling material was shorter than 3 mm showed a significantly higher frequency of periapical radiolucencies. Using a pressure-driven tracer assay, Wu et al.[115] and Abramovitz et al.[116] found that 4 or 5 mm of apical seal was inferior in their ability to prevent leakage, compared with an original full-length root canal filling. Similarly, Metzger et al.[117] compared the sealing capabilities of 3, 5, 7, and 9 mm of apical gutta-percha using a pressure-driven radioactive tracer assay. They concluded that the sealing is proportional to the length of the remaining filling and that original full-length root canal fillings have a superior seal compared with 3, 5, and 7 mm of apical gutta-percha.

CONCLUSIONS

Since there is greater leakage when only 2 to 3 mm of gutta-percha is present (Figure 12), 4 to 5 mm should be retained apically to ensure an adequate seal. Although studies indicate that 4 mm produces an adequate seal, stopping precisely at 4 mm is difficult and radiographic angulation errors could lead to retention of less than 4 mm. Therefore, 5 mm of gutta-percha should be retained apically. This seal is complemented by the seal provided by the post and core, and the overlying crown (Figure 11).

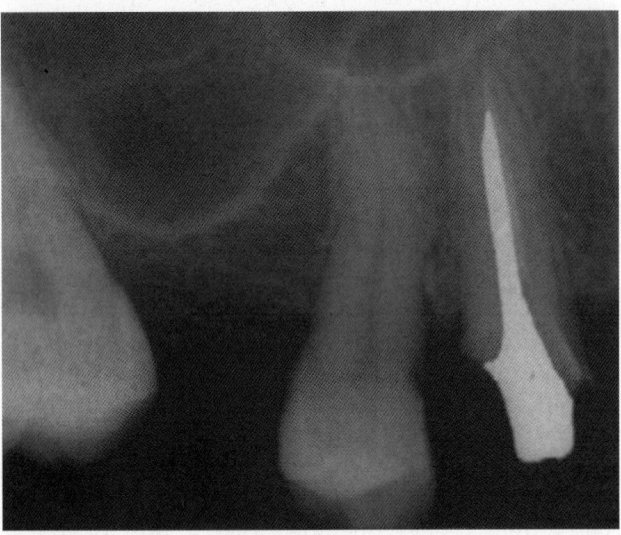

Figure 12 Less than 2 mm of gutta-percha remains in the maxillary first premolar apical to the cast post and core, increasing the risk of failure.

Does Post Diameter Affect Retention and the Potential for Tooth Fracture?

Studies relating post diameter to post retention have failed to establish a definitive relationship. Two studies determined that there was an increase in post retention as the diameter increased,[102,118] whereas three studies found no significant retention changes with diameter variations.[119,110,120] Krupp et al.[121] indicated that post length was the most important factor affecting retention and post diameter was a secondary factor.

A more definitive relationship has been established between post diameter and stress in the tooth. Mattison[122] found that as the post diameter increased, stress increased in the tooth. Trabert et al.[123] measured the impact resistance of extracted maxillary central incisors as post diameter increased and found that increasing the post diameter decreased the tooth's resistance to fracture. Deutsch et al.[62] determined that there was a six-fold increase in the potential for root fracture with every millimeter decrease in tooth diameter. However, two finite element studies failed to find higher tooth stresses with larger-diameter posts.[70,71]

CONCLUSIONS

Laboratory studies relating retention to post diameter have produced mixed results, whereas a more definitive relationship has been established between root fracture and large-diameter posts (Figure 13).

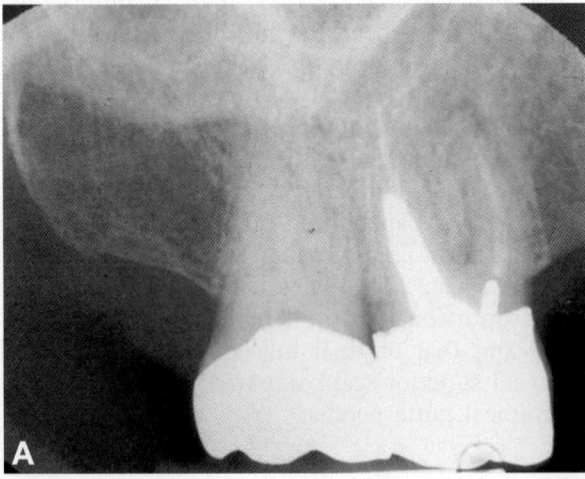 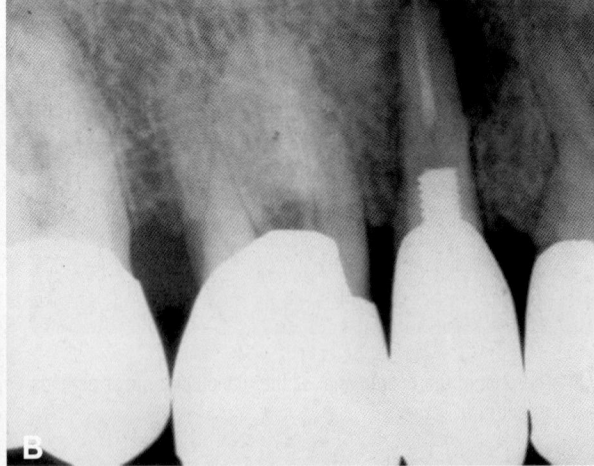

Figure 13 Excessive post diameters. **A,** Large-diameter post placed in the palatal root of the maxillary molar. **B,** Large-diameter threaded post caused fracture of the maxillary second premolar. The radiographic appearance of the bone is typical of a fractured root—a teardrop-shaped lesion with diffuse border.

What Is the Relationship Between Post Diameter and the Potential for Root Perforations?

In a literature review of guidelines associated with post diameter, Lloyd and Palik[124] indicated that there are three distinct philosophies of post space preparation. One group advocates the narrowest diameter for fabrication of a certain post length (the conservationists). Another group proposes a space with a diameter that does not exceed one-third of the root diameter (the proportionists). The third group advises leaving at least 1 mm of sound dentin surrounding the entire post (the preservationists).

Based on the proportional concept of one-third of the root diameter, three articles measured the root diameters of extracted teeth and proposed post diameters that would not exceed this proportion.[102,103,125] Tilk et al.[125] examined 1,500 roots. They measured the narrowest mesiodistal dimension at the apical, middle, and cervical one-thirds of the teeth except the palatal root of the maxillary first molar that was measured faciolingually. Based on the 95% confidence level that post width would not exceed one-third of the apical width of the root, they proposed the following post widths (Table 6): small teeth such as mandibular incisors (0.6 to 0.7 mm); large-diameter roots such as maxillary central incisors and the palatal root of the maxillary first molar (1.0 mm); and for the remaining teeth (0.8 to 0.9 mm).

Shillingburg et al.[102] measured 700 root dimensions to determine the post diameters that would minimize the risk of perforation. Also based on not exceeding one-third of the mesiodistal root width, they recommended the following post diameters (see Table 6): mandibular incisors (0.7 mm); maxillary central incisors or other large roots (1.7 mm—which was the maximal recommended dimension); post tip diameter (at least 1.5 mm less than the root diameter at that point); and post diameter at the middle of the root length (2.0 mm less than the root diameter).

Post spaces were prepared in 150 extracted maxillary and mandibular molars by using different instrument diameters and the resulting incidences of perforations were recorded.[103] The authors determined that the mesial roots of mandibular molars and the buccal roots of maxillary molars should not be used for posts due to the higher risk of perforation on the furcation side of the root. For the principal roots (mandibular distal and maxillary palatal), they determined that posts should not be extended more than 7 mm into the root canal (apical to the pulp chamber) due to the risk of perforation. Regarding instrument size, they concluded that post preparations can be safely completed by using a No. 2 Peeso instrument, but perforations are more likely when the larger Nos. 3 and 4 Peeso instruments are used.

Raiden et al.[126] evaluated several instrument diameters (0.7, 0.9, 1.1, 1.3, 1.5, and 1.7 mm) to determine which one(s) would preserve at least 1 mm of root wall thickness following post preparation in maxillary first premolars. They determined that instrument diameter must be small (0.7 mm or less) for maxillary first premolars with single canals because the mesial and distal developmental root depressions restrict the amount of available tooth structure in the centrally located single root canal. However, when there are dual canals, the instrument can be as large as 1.1 mm because the canals are located buccally and lingually into thicker areas of the roots.

CONCLUSIONS

Instruments used to prepare posts should be related in size to root dimensions to avoid excessive post diameters that lead to root perforation (Figure 14). Safe instrument diameters to use are 0.6 to 0.7 mm for small teeth such as mandibular incisors and 1 to

Table 6 Post Space Preparation Widths (in Millimeters)

	Maxillary		Mandibular	
	Tilk et al	Shillingburg et al	Tilk et al	Shillingburg et al
Central incisor	1.1	1.7	0.7	0.7
Lateral incisor	0.9	1.3	0.7	0.7
Canine	1.0	1.5	0.9	1.3
First premolar				
(B)	0.9	0.9		
(L)	0.9	0.9		
Second premolar	0.9	1.1	0.9	1.3
First molar				
(MB)	0.9	1.1	(MB) 0.9	1.1
(DB)	0.8	1.1	(ML) 0.8	0.9
(L)	1.0	1.3	(D) 0.9	1.1
Second molar				
(MB)	-	1.1	(MB) -	0.9
(DB)	-	0.9	(ML) -	0.9
(L)	-	1.3	(D) -	1.1

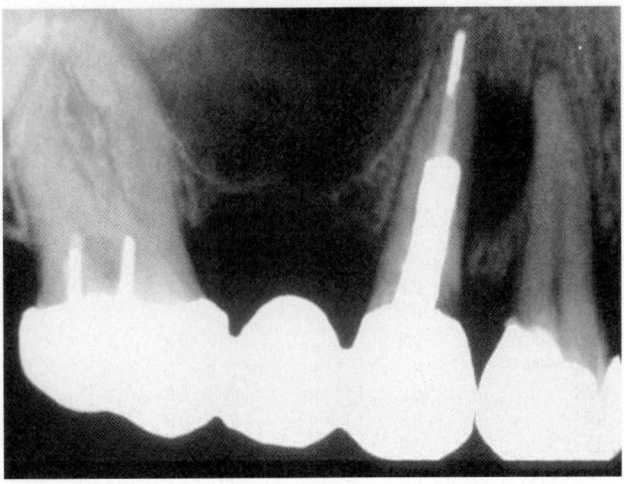

Figure 14 Excessive post diameter in the maxillary second premolar created a perforation in the mesial root concavity. Note the distinct border and round form of the radiolucent lesion, characteristics indicative of a root perforation.

1.2 mm for large-diameter roots such as the maxillary central incisors. Molar posts longer than 7 mm have an increased chance of perforations and therefore should be avoided even when using instruments of an appropriate diameter.

Can Gutta-Percha Be Removed Immediately after Endodontic Treatment and a Post Space Prepared?

Several studies indicate that there is no difference in the leakage of the root canal filling material when the post space is prepared immediately after completing endodontic therapy.[107,109,127,128] Bourgeois and Lemon[127] found no difference between immediate preparation of a post space and preparation 1 week later when 4 mm of gutta-percha were retained. Zmener[109] found no difference in dye penetration between gutta-percha removal after 5 minutes and 48 hours. Two sealers were tested and 4 mm of gutta-percha was retained apically. When lateral condensation of gutta-percha was used, Madison and Zakariasen[107] found no difference in the dye penetration between immediate removal and 48-hour removal. Using the chloropercha filling technique, Schnell[128] found no difference between immediate removal of gutta-percha and no removal of gutta-percha. By contrast, Dickey et al.[129] found significantly greater leakage with immediate gutta-percha removal.

Kwan and Harrington[130] tested the effect of immediate gutta-percha removal using both warm instruments and rotary instruments. There was no significant difference between the controls and immediate removal using warm pluggers and files. Compared with the controls, there was significantly less leakage with immediate removal of gutta-percha when using Gates Glidden drills.

Karapanou et al.[131] compared immediate and delayed removal of two sealers (a zinc oxide–eugenol-based sealer and a resin-based sealer). No difference between immediate and delayed removal was noted with the resin-based sealer, but delayed removal of the zinc oxide–eugenol-based sealer produced significantly greater leakage. Abramovitz et al.[116] compared immediate gutta-percha removal using hot pluggers and delayed gutta-percha removal (after 2 weeks) using Gates Glidden drills. They found no difference between the two methods.

Portell et al.[132] found that delayed gutta-percha removal (after 2 weeks) caused significantly more leakage than immediate removal when only 3 mm of gutta-percha was retained apically. Fan et al.[133] found more leakage from delayed removal of gutta-percha. Solano et al.[134] found a less significant difference in apical leakage between teeth whose post spaces were prepared at the time of the obturation and 1 week later using warm gutta-percha condensation and AH Plus sealer.

CONCLUSIONS

Adequately condensed gutta-percha can be safely removed immediately after endodontic treatment.

What Instruments Remove Gutta-Percha Without Disturbing the Apical Seal?

Three methods have been advocated for the removal of gutta-percha during preparation of a post space: chemical (oil of eucalyptus, oil of turpentine, and chloroform), thermal (electrical or heated instruments), and mechanical (Gates Glidden drills, Peeso reamers, etc.). The chemical removal of gutta-percha for post space preparation is not utilized for specific reasons (microleakage, inability to control removal).[111,127] However, thermal and mechanical techniques or a combination of both are routinely used.

Multiple studies have determined that there is no difference in leakage between removing gutta-percha with hot instruments and removing it with rotary instruments.[106,111,135] Suchina and Ludington[135] and Mattison et al.[111] found no difference between hot instrument removal and removal with Gates Glidden drills. Camp and Todd[106] found no difference between Peeso reamers, Gates Glidden drills, and hot instruments. Hiltner et al.[136] compared warm plugger removal with two types of rotary instruments (GPX burs and Peeso reamers). There were no significant differences in dye leakage between any of the groups. Contrasting results were found by Haddix et al.[137] They measured significantly less leakage when gutta-percha was removed with a heated plugger than when either a GPX instrument or Gates Glidden drills were used. DeCleen[138] found that it is desirable to remove gutta-percha using a heated instrument first, and then using a small Gates Glidden drill. Using a pressure-driven radioactive tracer assay, Abramovitz et al.[116] found no difference in apical leakage between hot pluggers and Gates Glidden drills. Balto et al.[139] compared two methods of gutta-percha removal and their impact on apical leakage. They found that removing gutta-percha with Peeso reamers showed less leakage compared with using a hot plugger.

CONCLUSIONS

Both rotary instruments and hot hand instruments can be safely used to remove adequately condensed gutta-percha when 5 mm is retained apically.

Can a Separated Instrument Be Removed During Post Space Preparation and Still Maintain the Apical Seal?

Following root canal therapy, the endodontically treated tooth could present with a separated instrument (files, rotary instruments, etc.) in any part of the canal. Attempts to remove these fragments prior to post space preparation could lead to loss of apical seal, perforations, ledge formation, and/or over enlargement of the canal. A decision to bypass or remove the fragment will depend on the type and position of the broken instrument and should be determined by an endodontist with the use of an operating microscope.

Bypassing fractured instruments seems to be the best approach. Hülsmann and Schinkel[140] reported an overall success rate of 68% when bypassing broken instruments from canals in vivo. Ward et al.[141] reported an overall success rate of 73%. Suter et al.[142] with the use of an dental operating microscope were able to achieve an overall success rate of 87% when removing broken instruments.

CONCLUSIONS

If a separated fragment of any instrument cannot be removed from the canal during post space preparation, it should be bypassed or left in the canal.

Can a Portion of a Silver Point Be Removed and Still Maintain the Apical Seal?

In one study, all the specimens leaked when 1 mm of a 5-mm long silver point was removed by using a round bur.[109] Neagley[108] found that removal of the filling material coronal to the silver point with a Peeso reamer caused no leakage. However, when all the filling materials and 1 mm of the silver point were removed, complete dye penetration occurred in eight of nine specimens.

CONCLUSIONS

The removal of a portion of a silver point during post preparation causes apical leakage.

How Soon should the Definitive Restoration Be Placed After Post Space Preparation?

ONE-PIECE PROVISIONAL RESTORATION

It is well established that a deficient root canal obturation and a poor coronal restoration will potentially allow endotoxins, bacteria, and saliva to penetrate the root canal causing periapical inflammation.[143–149]

Provisional restorations are mainly used to provide the patient with a functional and esthetic restoration. They also protect the hard and soft tissues prior to placement of the definitive restoration. However, provisional restorations are considered restorations with poor coronal seal. Several studies indicate that there is significant coronal leakage when the tooth is restored with a provisional restoration.[139,150–153] Demarchi et al.[150] found that a tooth restored with a temporary post–crown combination had significantly greater leakage than definitively cemented prefabricated posts and separate crowns. Similar results were found by Fox et al.[151] when they compared cast posts and cores cemented with zinc phosphate cement, prefabricated posts and composite resin cores cemented with resin cement, and provisional post–crowns cemented with zinc oxide–eugenol cement. In a 3-year retrospective clinical study, Lynch et al.[152] evaluated 176 endodontically treated teeth. They found that the loss of endodontically treated teeth occurred more often with those teeth restored with provisional restorations. Following these results, several studies[139,151] suggested that the definitive post and restoration should be cemented as soon as possible to prevent recontamination of the root canal. However, to minimize leakage and enhance long-term success, the definitive coronal restoration should be of superior quality.[147,154–157]

TEMPORARY CORONAL ACCESS FILLING

Balto et al.[139] compared the leakage of different provisional materials used in post-prepared root canals. They found that none of the provisional restorations tested (Cavit, IRM, and Temp Bond) prevented coronal leakage when left for a long period of time (30 days). Safavi et al.[153] evaluated the prognosis of endodontically treated teeth following delayed placement of the definitive coronal restoration. A total of 464 endodontically treated teeth were followed radiographically. They found a higher success rate when the definitive restorations (silver amalgam, composite resin, or definitive restoration with or without posts and cores) were placed as compared with teeth restored with provisional coronal access restorations (IRM or Cavit).

Torabinejad et al.[147] found that defective restorations could cause root canal system reinfection within 19 days. Ray and Trope[154] found that a combination of a poor coronal restoration and poor endodontic treatment resulted in a high failure rate of endodontically treated teeth. In a retrospective study, Iqbal et al.[155] found that a combination of good quality endodontic treatment and coronal restoration leads to a high success rate of endodontically treated teeth. Contrasting results were reported by Tronstad et al.[156] who found that the quality of the endodontic treatment was significantly more important than that of the coronal restoration.

CONCLUSIONS

Following endodontic treatment, post space preparation should be performed and a post definitively cemented as soon as possible: the same day for a prefabricated post, and as soon as possible for a custom-fabricated post and core. The prepared tooth should then be restored with a well-fitting provisional restoration (good marginal seal and occlusion) followed by cementation of the definitive crown in as short a time as possible.

Does the Use of a Cervical Ferrule that Engages Tooth Structure Help Prevent Tooth Fracture?

Survey data have been published that indicate the percentage of respondents who felt a ferrule (circumferential band of metal) increased a tooth's resistance to fracture.[43] Fifty-six percent of general dentists, 67% of prosthodontists, and 73% of board-certified prosthodontists felt that core ferrules increased a tooth's fracture resistance. To investigate this concept, several research studies have been performed. Some of the articles found ferrules are beneficial whereas others found no increase in fracture resistance.

The results appear indecisive until differences between study designs are analyzed. First, some of the studies tested ferrules that were part of a cast metal core (core ferrules),[158–162] whereas other studies evaluated the effectiveness of ferrules created by the overlying crown engaging tooth structure.[163–176] One study evaluated both core ferrules and crown ferrules.[177] Second, there were differences in the form of the ferrule, and therefore, the manner by which the metal engaged tooth structure (beveled sloping surface versus extension over relatively parallel prepared tooth structure). Third, there were variations in the amount of tooth structure encompassed by the

Table 7 Comparison of Studies and Effectiveness of Various Core and Crown Ferrules

Study	Ferrule Form	Was Ferrule Effective?	Materials/Type of Test
Barkhordar (1989)	2 mm parallel extension of core over the tooth	Yes	Extracted teeth/angular lingual force applied to p and c (no overlying crown)
Sorensen (1990)	1 mm wide 60° bevel at the tooth-core junction	No	Extracted teeth/angular lingual force applied to p and c (with overlying crown)
Tjan (1985)	60° bevel at the tooth-core junction	No	Extracted teeth/angular lingual force applied to p and c (no overlying crown)
Loney (1990)	1.5 mm parallel extension of core over the tooth	No	Photoelastic teeth/angular lingual force applied to p and c (no overlying crown)
Hemmings (1991)	45° bevel	Yes	Extracted teeth/torsional force applied to p and c (no overlying crown)
Saupe (1996)	2 mm parallel extension of core over *thin* dentin wall (0.5–0.75 mm thick)	No	Extracted teeth/angular lingual force applied to p and c (no overlying crown)
Sorensen (1990)	130° sloping finish line	No	Extracted teeth/p and c with crown
	1–2 mm of tooth grasped by crown	Yes	Extracted teeth/p and c with crown
Libman (1995)	0.5–1 mm of prepared tooth grasped by crown	No	Extracted teeth/p and c with crown/cyclic loading
	1.5–2 mm of prepared tooth grasped by crown	Yes	Extracted teeth/p and c with crown/cyclic loading
Milot (1992)	1 mm wide 60° bevel grasped by crown	Yes	Plastic analogues of teeth/p and c with crowns
Isidor (1999)	1.25 mm of prepared tooth grasped by crown	Yes	Bovine teeth/cyclic angular load/p and c with crown
	2.5 mm of prepared tooth grasped by crown	Yes, but more effective than 1.25 mm	Bovine teeth/cyclic angular load/p and c with crown
Hoag (1982)	1–2 mm of prepared tooth grasped by crown	Yes	Extracted teeth/p and c with crown
Gegauff (2000)	2 mm of prepared tooth grasped by crown; 0 mm of prepared tooth grasped by a crown	Yes	Composite teeth/p and c with crown

ferrules. Table 7 permits a comparison of the studies and the effectiveness of the various core and crown ferrules.

The data generally indicate that ferrules formed as part of the core are less effective than ferrules created when the overlying crown engages tooth structure. In four of the six core ferrule studies, they were found to be ineffective.[159,160,162,177] Also, in one of the two studies where the core ferrule was effective, the ferrule form was a 2-mm parallel extension of the core over tooth structure as opposed to a bevel.[158] In the other study where core ferrules were found to be effective, a torsional force was used as opposed to an angular lingual force.[161] In the crown ferrule studies, most of the ferrules effectively increased a tooth's resistance to fracture. Only when the crown ferrule was of minimal dimension or had a sloping form, it was found to be ineffective.[163,177] In support of these studies, Rosen and Partida-Rivera[178] found that a 2-mm cast gold collar (not part of the post and core) was very effective in preventing root fracture when a tapered screw post was intentionally threaded into roots so as to induce fracture. Assif et al.[179] found no difference in the tooth fracture patterns of parallel posts, tapered posts, and parallel posts with a tapered end when they were covered by a crown that grasped 2 mm of tooth structure. Akkayan et al.[170] found no significant difference between fiber-reinforced and zirconia dowels when the ferrule length was 2 mm.

The data also support the concept that ferrules that grasp larger amounts of tooth structure are more effective than those engaging only a small amount of tooth structure. In both the core and crown ferrule studies, the tooth's resistance to fracture was increased when a substantive amount of tooth structure was engaged (2 mm in the core ferrule studies and 1 to 2 mm in the crown ferrule studies). Libman and Nicholls[163] found the 0.5- to 1.0-mm crown ferrule to be ineffective whereas a 1.5- to 2.0-mm crown ferrule to be effective. Isidor et al.[165] determined that increasing the crown ferrule length significantly increased the number of cyclic cycles required to cause specimen failure. They compared no ferrule with 1.25 and 2.55 mm crown ferrules. They concluded that ferrule length was more important than post length in increasing a tooth's resistance to fracture under cyclic loading. Zhi-Yue and Yu-Xing[169] found that a 2-mm crown ferrule effectively enhanced the fracture strength of endodontically treated teeth when a cast post and core was used. Pereira et al.[176] compared the effect of no crown ferrule with 1, 2, and 3-mm crown ferrules. They found that a 3-mm crown ferrule significantly increased the fracture resistance of endodontically treated teeth compared with a 2-mm crown ferrule.

The form of the prepared ferrule also appears to affect a tooth's fracture resistance in the previously cited studies. Only one beveled/sloping ferrule was effective in enhancing a tooth's fracture resistance and that was when a torsional force was applied to the tooth. Tan et al.[172] compared a 2-mm uniform crown ferrule that extended around the entire crown circumference with a 2-mm nonuniform crown ferrule where the ferrule was only 0.5 mm on the proximal surfaces. The uniform ferrule produced significantly greater fracture resistance than a nonuniform ferrule. In an in vitro study, Naumann et al.[173] evaluated the effect of chewing simulation on the fracture resistance of maxillary endodontically treated teeth with incomplete crown ferrules. The greatest variation of failure load was associated with the absence of portions (facial, palatal, or interproximal) of the crown ferrule. Ng et al.[174] investigated the effect of limited residual axial tooth structure on the fracture resistance of maxillary anterior endodontically treated teeth. They found that in the absence of 360° of circumferential coronal tooth structure, the location of the remaining coronal tooth structure may be an important factor for determining the fracture resistance of endodontically treated teeth. The palatal axial wall was as effective as a 360° circumference in providing fracture resistance.

CONCLUSIONS

Differences of opinion exist regarding the effectiveness of ferrules in preventing tooth fracture. Ferrules have been tested when they are part of the core and also when the ferrule is created by the overlying crown engaging tooth structure. Most of the data indicate that a ferrule created by the crown encompassing tooth structure is more effective than a ferrule that is part of the post and core (Figure 15). Ferrule effectiveness is enhanced by grasping larger amounts of tooth structure. The amount of tooth structure engaged by the overlying crown appears to be more important than the length of the post in increasing a tooth's resistance to fracture. Ferrules are more effective when the crown encompasses relatively parallel prepared tooth structure than when it engages beveled/sloping tooth surfaces. Ferrules that encompass 2 mm of tooth structure around the entire circumference of a tooth are more effective than nonuniform ferrules.

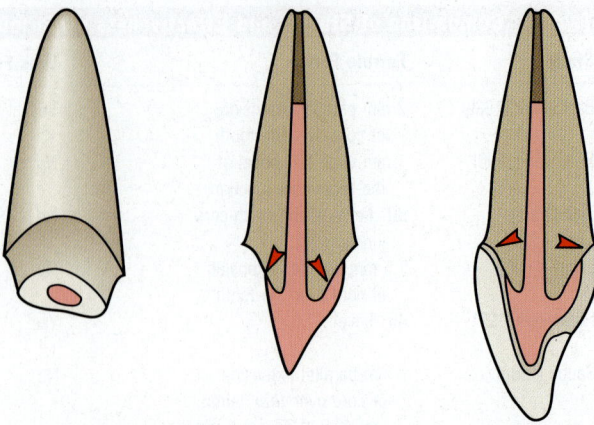

Figure 15 Types of ferrules. **A**, Tooth prepared for a post and core. **B**, Post and core has been cemented into the tooth. The arrows note how the core has created a ferrule around the tooth (note the reduction in the width of remaining coronal tooth structure to develop this core ferrule). **C**, A metal ceramic crown has been cemented over the core. The arrows show how the crown encompasses the tooth cervically, establishing a crown ferrule.

Post and Core Placement Techniques

PRETREATMENT DATA REVIEW

When it has been determined that a post and core is required to properly retain a definitive single crown or fixed partial denture, the following characteristics should be determined prior to beginning the clinical procedures associated with the fabrication of a post and core.

POST LENGTH

Since 5 mm of gutta-percha should be retained apically to ensure a favorable seal (as measured radiographically), posts should be extended to that length in all teeth except molars. With molars, posts should be placed in the primary roots (palatal root of maxillary molars and distal roots of mandibular molars) and should not be extended more than 7 mm apical to the origin of the root canal in the base of the pulp chamber (Figure 11). Extension beyond this length can lead to root perforation or only very thin areas of remaining tooth structure.

POST DIAMETER

A frequently used and clinically appropriate guideline for post diameter is not to exceed one-third of the root diameter. It has been determined that when a root canal is prepared for a post and the diameter is increased beyond one-third of the root diameter, the tooth becomes exponentially weaker. Each millimeter increase (beyond one-third of the root diameter) causes a six-fold increase in the potential for root fracture.[62] Based on measuring the root dimensions of 1,500 teeth (125 for each tooth) and using the guideline that the post should be one-third of the root diameter, optimal post diameter measurements have been determined to be approximately 0.6 mm for mandibular incisors, 1.0 mm for maxillary central incisors, maxillary and mandibular canines, and the palatal root of the maxillary first molar.[125] The recommended post diameter for the other teeth was 0.8 mm.[125] Another study of 700 teeth recommended that post diameter should range from 0.7 mm for mandibular incisors to a maximum of 1.7 mm for maxillary central incisors.[102]

ANATOMICAL/STRUCTURAL LIMITATIONS

The practitioner who completed the endodontic treatment is ideally suited to identify characteristics of the pulpal chamber, rooted canal(s) anatomy, and completed endodontic filling that should be reviewed before placing a post and core. These characteristics include the presence and the extent of dentinal craze lines, identification of teeth where further root preparation (beyond that needed to complete endodontic instrumentation) will result in less than 1 mm of remaining dentin or a post diameter greater than one-third of the root diameter area, information regarding areas where the remaining tooth structure is thin, and the point at which significant root curvature begins.

CRAZE LINES

Cracks in dentin are areas of weakness where further propagation may result in root fracture and tooth loss (see Chapter 19). The patient should be informed of their presence with appropriate chart documentation of crack location. It is prudent to avoid post placement, if possible, in favor of a restorative material core. If a post is required, it should passively fit the canal, and the definitive restoration should entirely encompass the cracked area, whenever possible, by forming a ferrule.

DENTIN THICKNESS AFTER ENDODONTIC TREATMENT

Following normal and appropriate endodontic instrumentation, teeth can possess less than 1 mm of dentin, indicating that there should be no further root preparation for the post. When these teeth are encountered, it is best to fabricate a post that fits into the existing morphological form and diameter rather than additionally preparing the root to accept a prefabricated type of post. This characteristic is one of the primary indications for the use of a custom cast post and core. One study determined that canines (maxillary and mandibular), maxillary central and lateral incisors, and the palatal root of maxillary first molars possessed more than 1 mm of dentin after endodontic cleaning and shaping.[181] All other teeth had roots with less than 1 mm of remaining dentin following endodontic treatment. With the goal of preserving 1 mm of remaining dentin lateral to posts, it has been determined that single-canal maxillary first premolars should have posts that are 0.7 mm in diameter or less.[126] Mandibular premolars with oval/ribbon-shaped canals should not be subjected to any preparation of the root canal for a post since it will result in less than 1 mm of dentin.[181] Preparation of the mesial root canals in mandibular molars and the facial root canals in maxillary molars can result in perforation or only thin areas of remaining dentin. Based on the measurements of residual dentin thickness, it is recommended that posts not be placed in these roots if possible.

ROOT CURVATURE

When root curvature is present, post length must be limited so as to preserve remaining dentin, thereby helping to prevent root fracture or perforation. Root curvature occurs most frequently in the apical 5 mm of the root. Therefore, if 5 mm of gutta-percha is retained apically, curved portions of the root are usually avoided. As discussed previously under post length, molar posts should not exceed 7 mm in the roots because of the potential for perforation due to root curvature and the presence of developmental root depressions. Molar roots are frequently curved and the post should terminate at the point where substantive curvature begins.

TYPE OF POST AND CORE

Custom Cast Post

For many years, custom cast posts and cores have been considered to be the standard of care when restoring endodontically treated teeth and have historically been made of metal. Gold, silver–palladium, and base metal alloys are the most commonly used metals. For economic reasons, base metal alloys were introduced as an alternative metal to high-noble alloys. The major disadvantages of base metal alloys are their manipulation (laboratory and clinical), their hardness, and their unstable chemical structure.[182] The degradation of base metal alloys releases substances that could be harmful to the patient.[182–184] Silver–palladium alloys were introduced as a replacement for gold and base metal alloys. They are relatively easy to manipulate and have many properties similar to those of gold casting alloys.[185] However, the castability of silver–palladium alloys was shown to be inferior to that of gold-based alloys.[182,186,187]

Cast posts and cores can be fabricated by using either a direct or an indirect technique, and several methods have been described for the intraoral fabrication of an acrylic resin pattern for a direct post and core.[188–192] Prefabricated plastic patterns are commonly used, and they are relined to fit the post space with an autopolymerizing acrylic resin (Figure 16). The coronal adaptation of the tooth is usually completed by using the same resin, and the core is contoured intraorally to the desired form. The only disadvantage of this direct technique is the amount of chairside time required to perform the procedure.

As an alternative, indirect techniques for the fabrication of cast posts and cores have been proposed.[193–195] However, this procedure requires meticulous attention to a defined protocol to ensure success. One technique uses a Lentulo spiral instrument to carry an impression material to the apical aspect of the prepared post space. Since a thin projection of a polymerized impression material can be distorted or torn upon removal from the mouth, reinforcement of the impression material is required. This reinforcement can be accomplished by using several materials such as a plastic pin or a metal wire. Care must be taken when using plastic pins to ensure that they are not slightly flexed by placement into a curved canal or through contact with the impression tray, thereby allowing a return to their original form upon impression removal with some resulting distortion. The use of a portion of a safety pin is an excellent material so long as it is made of spring steel, thereby preventing flexion. A bendable metal pin can be distorted upon impression removal. Complete seating of a section from a safety pin until it contacts the gutta-percha is recommended. Upon removal of the impression from the mouth, the presence of the metal pin at the apical extension of the impression

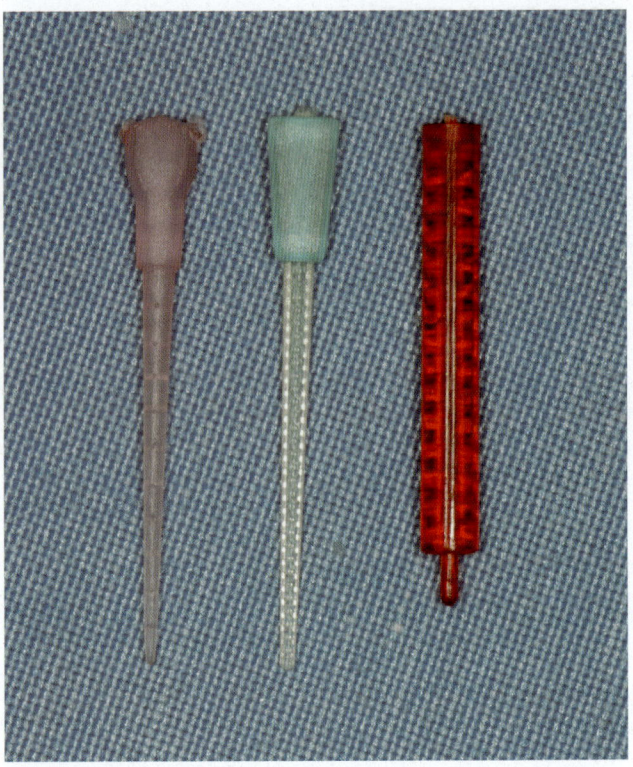

Figure 16 Prefabricated plastic patterns commonly used for the direct technique method for the intraoral fabrication of an acrylic resin pattern for a cast post and core.

material indicates that there was no elongation of the impression material upon removal.

To make the impression technique easier, prefabricated precision plastic dowels were introduced.[196,197] After the selection of the desired diameter for the dowel, a corresponding drill is used to prepare the post space at the appropriate length. The dowel is then inserted into the prepared canal, picked up in an impression, and transferred to the dental laboratory for fabrication.

A proposed advantage of cast posts and cores is their purported ease of removal in case of an endodontic retreatment.[198–200] In addition, several long-term clinical studies have reported high success rates with cast post and cores.[50,201]

Prefabricated Posts

Prefabricated posts have become quite popular and a wide variety of systems are available: parallel-sided or tapered, smooth or serrated, passive (cement/bonded) or active (threaded), or combinations of these.[202–204] Threaded posts depend primarily on engaging the tooth—either through threads formed in the dentin as

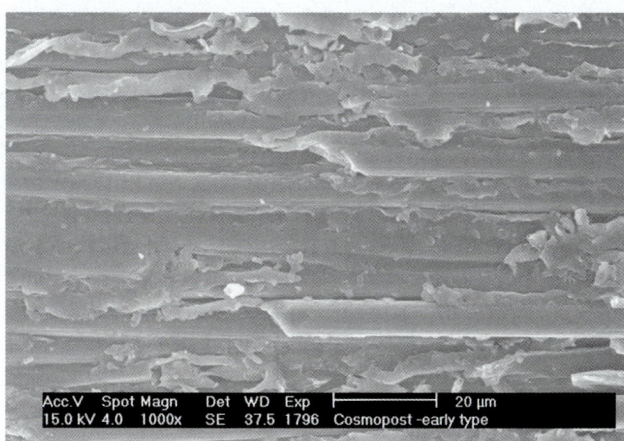

Figure 17 Surface texture of a carbon fiber-reinforced epoxy resin dowel (SEM magnification: ×1000).

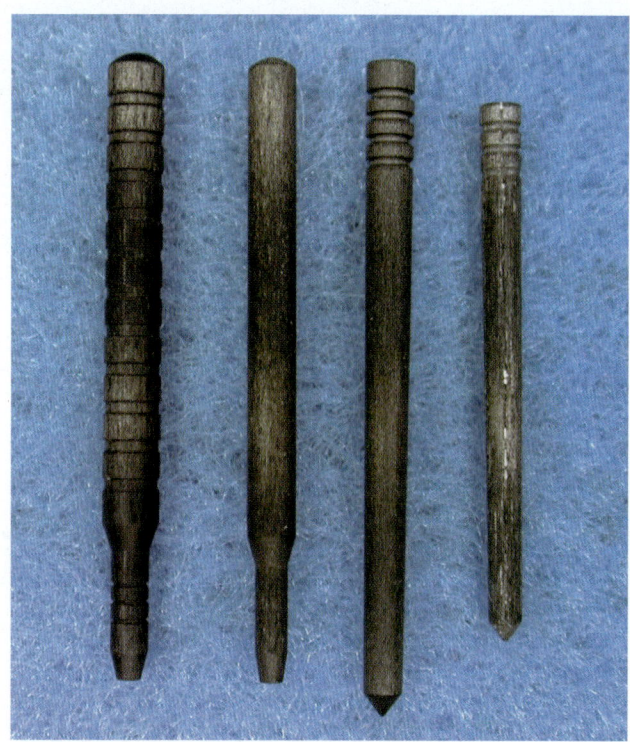

Figure 18 Available shapes of carbon fiber-reinforced epoxy resin posts.

the post is screwed into the root or through threads previously "tapped" into the dentin. The majority of these posts are metallic. Recently, in response to a need for tooth-colored posts, several nonmetallic posts such as carbon fiber epoxy resin, zirconia, glass fiber-reinforced (GFR) epoxy resin, and ultrahigh strength polyethylene fiber-reinforced (PFR) posts are available and early data indicates that they can be acceptable alternatives to metallic posts.

The *carbon fiber-reinforced (CFR) epoxy resin* post system was developed in France in 1988 by Duret and Renaud[205–207] and first introduced in Europe in the early 1990s.[208–210] The matrix for this post is an epoxy resin reinforced with unidirectional carbon fibers parallel to the long axis of the post. The fibers are 8 μm in diameter and uniformly embedded in the epoxy resin matrix. By weight, the fibers comprise 64% of the post and are stretched before injection of the resin matrix to maximize the physical properties of the post (Figure 17).[205,211,212] The post is reported to absorb applied stresses and distribute these stresses along the entire post channel.[213] The bulk of the carbon fibers is made from polyacrylonitrile by heating it in air at 200° to 250°C and then in an inert atmosphere at 1200°C. This process removes hydrogen, nitrogen, and oxygen, leaving a chain of carbon atoms and forming carbon fibers.[214]

The CFR post has been reported to exhibit high fatigue strength, high tensile strength, and a modulus of elasticity similar to dentin.[208,211,215–218] The post was originally radiolucent; however, a radiopaque post is now available. Radiopacity is produced by placing traces of barium sulfate and/or silicate inside the post. Mannocci et al.[219] examined radiographically five different types of fiber posts. They found that only Composipost and Snowpostposts had uniform radiopacity. Finger et al.[220] examined the radiopacity of seven fiber-reinforced resin posts compared with a titanium post. Compared to other posts, they found CFR posts had an acceptable radiopacity.

The posts are available in different shapes: double cylindrical with conical stabilization ledges or conical shapes (Figure 18). The surface texture of the post may be smooth or serrated. Studies have indicated that serrations increased mechanical retention although the smooth post also bonded well to adhesive dental resin.[217,221] The post has a surface roughness of 5 to 10 μm to enhance mechanical adhesion of the autopolymerizing luting material, and the post appears to be biocompatible based on cytotoxicity tests.[216,222]

Several studies indicate that CFR posts exhibit adequate physical properties compared to metal posts.[212,215,223,224] In a retrospective study over 4 years, Ferrari et al.[223] indicated that the Cosmopost system was superior to the conventional cast post and core system. King and Setchell[215] and Duret et al.[212] evaluated the physical properties (fracture resistance and modulus of elasticity) of CFR posts and both reported that these posts are stronger than prefabricated metal posts.

Contrasting results were reported by Sidoli et al.[225] in an in vitro study. They found that CFR posts exhibited inferior strength when compared with metallic posts. Similar results were also obtained by Purton and Love[226] and Asmussen et al.[227]

Martinez-Insua et al.[228] studied the fracture resistance of teeth restored with CFR posts and cast posts. They reported a significantly higher fracture threshold for cast post and cores. A clinical evaluation of CFR posts suggested that these posts did not perform as well as conventional cast post and cores.[229] However, the results of this study must be interpreted with caution because of the relatively small sample size (27 teeth) used in this study.

Multiple studies indicate that there is a decrease in the strength of CFR posts after thermocycling and cyclic loading.[230–233] In addition, contact of the post with oral fluids reduced their flexural strength values.[222–234]

In two studies, results indicated no significant difference among a CFR post, cast post and cores, and metal posts when restoring mandibular incisor teeth. No differences were noted in the mode or state of fracture observed.[235,236]

Multiple in-vitro studies have reported that CFR posts are less likely to cause fracture of the root at failure. The mode of failure of teeth restored with CFR posts in these studies was more favorable to the remaining tooth structure.[170,215,225,228,237–241]

However, despite all these advantageous properties, in vivo applications of the CFR post should be questioned. When the ferrule is small or absent in an endodontically treated tooth restored with a CFP post, loads may cause the post to flex causing a micromovement of the entire core. The cement seal at the margin of the crown can be compromised, accompanied by microleakage of oral bacteria and fluids. As a result, secondary caries may develop in the space and may not be easily detected.[241]

The short-term clinical studies of CFR posts appear promising but some of the longer-term studies report higher failure rates. Wennström[209] restored 173 teeth with CFR posts and reported two failures after a period of 3 to 4 years. A short-term retrospective study of 236 teeth treated 2 to 3 years previously reported no failures of the posts.[242] Ferrari et al.[223] studied 100 CFR posts and reported a failure rate of 3.2% after a mean time of 3.8 years of clinical service. In a prospective study of 59 CFR posts, Glazer et al.[243] indicated that these posts did not fracture and there was a 7.7% absolute failure rate. Another retrospective study[244] of 1,304 CFR posts followed from 1 to 6 years found a 3.2% failure rate that was attributed to debonding during removal of temporary crowns and periapical lesions. Hedlund et al.[245] studied the clinical performance of 65 CFR posts for an average of 2.3 years of clinical service and found a 3% failure rate. In a retrospective study of 64 CFR posts, Segerström et al.[246] found that nearly 50% of the CFR posts were lost after a mean time of 6.7 years.

Should fracture of a CFR post occur, a potential advantage is the relative ease of removal from the post space compared with metal posts. A removal kit has been suggested for this procedure and the latter is recommended as a single use only item.[247–251]

Glass fiber-reinforced epoxy resin posts The high demand for esthetic restorations and all-ceramic crowns led to the development of a variety of tooth-colored post systems as an alternative to metal and CFR posts.

The GFR epoxy resin post is made of glass or silica fibers (white or translucent). Glass fiber posts can be made of different types of glasses: electrical glass, high-strength glass, or quartz fibers (Figure 19).[233,252] The commonly used fibers are silica-based (50% to 70% SiO_2), in addition to other oxides.[253]

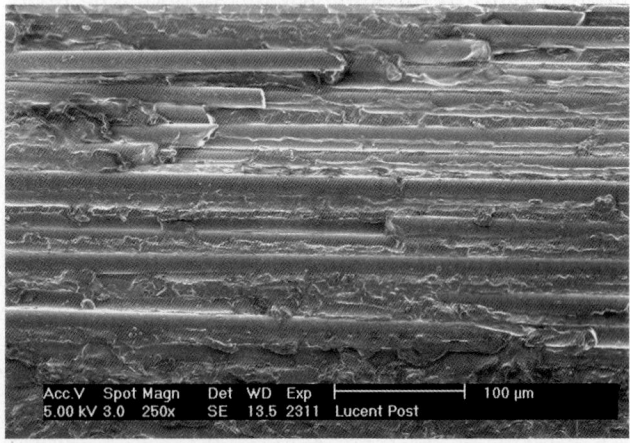

Figure 19 Surface texture of a glass fiber-reinforced epoxy resin post (SEM magnification: ×250).

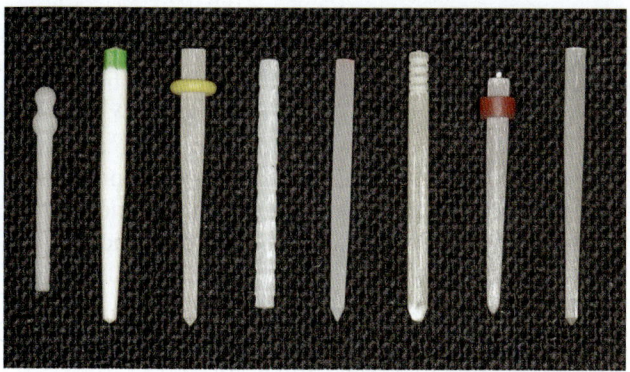

Figure 20 Available shapes and designs for glass fiber-reinforced epoxy resin posts.

The GFR post is available in different shapes: cylindrical, cylindroconical, or conical shape (Figure 20). An in vitro assessment of several GFR post systems indicated that parallel-sided GFR posts are more retentive than tapered GFR posts.[254]

The composition of the glass fibers in the matrix tends to play an important role in the strength of the post. Newman et al.[232] compared the fracture resistance of two GFR posts containing different weight percentages of glass fibers. They found that the higher content of glass fibers in the post contributed to the greater strength displayed by the tested post.

The GFR post has been reported to exhibit high fatigue strength, high tensile strength, and a modulus of elasticity closer to dentin than that of CFR posts.[218,227,255] The GFR post is as strong as the CFR post and approximately twice as rigid.[256]

The flexural strength of GFR posts is not related to the type of glass fiber used. Galhano et al.[218] evaluated the flexural strength of carbon fiber, quartz fiber, and glass fiber posts. They found that the posts behaved similarly because of the same concentration and type of the epoxy resin used to join the fibers together. Pfeiffer et al.[257] evaluated, in vitro, the yield strength of GFR post, titanium, and zirconia posts. They found that the yield strength was significantly higher for the zirconia and titanium posts when compared with GFR posts.

Several studies have determined that there is a decrease in the strength (about 40%) of GFR posts after thermocycling and cyclic loading. In addition, contact of the post with oral fluids (short- and long-term) reduced flexural strength.[230,233,258–260]

Two studies indicated that the tensile bond strength between the composite resin core material and the GFR post is less than that developed with a titanium post.[261,262] Other studies indicated that there was a good adhesive bond between the GFR post and composite resin cements.[261,263,264] The bonding of the core to the post can be improved by treating the post with airborne-particle abrasion.[265] Similar results were obtained by treating the surface of the post with hydrogen peroxide and silane or hydrofluoric acid and silane.[266,267] During fatigue loading, a composite resin core bonded to a GFR post provided significantly stronger crown retention than cast gold posts and cores and titanium posts with composite resin cores.[171]

Similar to CFR posts, multiple studies have shown that GFR posts are less likely to cause fracture of the root at failure.[232,268–270] The mode of failure of teeth restored with CFR posts in these studies was more favorable to the remaining tooth structure. However, studies have discussed the importance of the presence of a ferrule effect in achieving a high success rate.[170,173,174,271] Malferrari et al.[270] restored 180 teeth with GFR posts and reported no post, core, or root fracture after 30 months of service. Naumann et al.[272] found that the survival rate of parallel-sided and tapered GFR posts was similar.

Polyethylene fiber-reinforced posts (PFR) are made of ultrahigh molecular weight polyethylene-woven fiber ribbon (Ribbond, Ribbond Inc., Seattle, WA). They are not posts and cores in the traditional sense. The post is a polyethylene-woven fiber ribbon that is coated with a dentin bonding agent and packed into the canal, where it is then light polymerized in position.[273–275] The Ribbond material has a three-dimensional structure due to either a leno weave or a triaxial architectural design. These designs are composed of a great number of nodal intersections that prevent crack propagation and provide a mechanical retention for the composite resin cement. When PFR posts were compared with metal posts in the laboratory, the fiber-reinforced posts reduced the incidence of vertical root fracture. The addition of a small-size prefabricated post to the PFR post increased the strength of the post-and-core complex. However, the strength of the PFR post did not approach that of a cast metal post and core.[273]

When compared with other fiber-reinforced composite post systems, the PFR posts were also found to protect the remaining tooth structure.[232] These results may be attributed to the manufacturer's recommendations of not enlarging the root canals, not removing undercuts present in the root canal, and forming a 1.5 to 2mm crown ferrule. The presence of a large volume of core material and a sufficient dentin bonding area coronally seems to greatly affect the mean load-to-failure value of PFR posts.[232] Eskitascioglu et al.[276] evaluated two post and core systems using a fracture strength test and a finite element analysis. They found that stress accumulated along the cervical region of the tooth and along the buccal bone. Minimal stress was recorded within the PFR post system. They suggested that the PFR post could be advantageous for the restoration of teeth with apical resection.

Newman et al.[232] compared the effect of three fiber-reinforced composite post systems on the fracture resistance of endodontically treated teeth. They found that when PFR posts were placed in narrow canals, they performed better than GFR posts. They suggested the PFR post be formed to the shape of the canal.

The use of PFR posts to restore endodontically treated teeth appears to be a promising alternative to the stainless steel and zirconia dowel posts with respect to microleakage.[277] Usumez et al.[277] compared in vitro the microleakage of three esthetic, adhesively luted post systems with a conventional post system. They found that the PFR posts and the GFR posts exhibited less microleakage compared with zirconia posts.

Zirconia posts The trend toward the use of all-ceramic crowns has encouraged manufacturers to explore the development of all-ceramic posts.[278–281] A metal-free post avoids discoloration of tooth structure that can occur with metal posts and produces optical properties comparable to all-ceramic crowns.[282–285] One type of all-ceramic post is the zirconia post, composed of zirconium oxide (ZrO_2), an inert material used for a range of applications. Its high fracture toughness, high flexural strength, and excellent resistance to corrosion encouraged orthopedists to use it at articulation surfaces.[286] Studies have suggested that zirconia specimens transplanted in animals were very stable after long-term aging, and there was no apparent degradation of the specimens.[286,287–290]

Zirconia (tetragonal zirconium polycrystals, TZP) exhibits phase transformation. Low-temperature degradation of TZP is known to occur as a result of spontaneous phase transformation of tetragonal zirconia to monoclinic phase during ageing at 130° to 300°C possibly within a water environment. It has been reported that this degradation leads to a decrease in strength due to the formation of microcracks accompanying the phase transformation. To inhibit this phase transformation, certain oxides (magnesium, yttrium, or calcium oxide) are added to fully or partially stabilize the tetragonal phase of zirconia at room temperature. This mechanism is known as transformation toughening.[281,287,291–293]

The type of zirconia used for dental posts is composed of TZP with 3 mol% yttrium oxide (Y_2O_3) and is called YTZP (yttria-stabilized tetragonal polycrystalline zirconia).[281,294] YTZP is composed of a dense fine-grained structure (0.5 μm average diameter) that provides the post with toughness and a smooth surface.[292,294,295]

The zirconia post is extremely radiopaque, biocompatible, possesses high flexural strength and fracture toughness, and may act similar to steel.[287–291,296–304] In addition, the post has a low solubility[301] and is not affected by thermocycling.[230] The post is available in a cylindroconical shape (Figure 21).

The zirconia post has a smooth surface configuration with no grooves, serrations, or roughness to

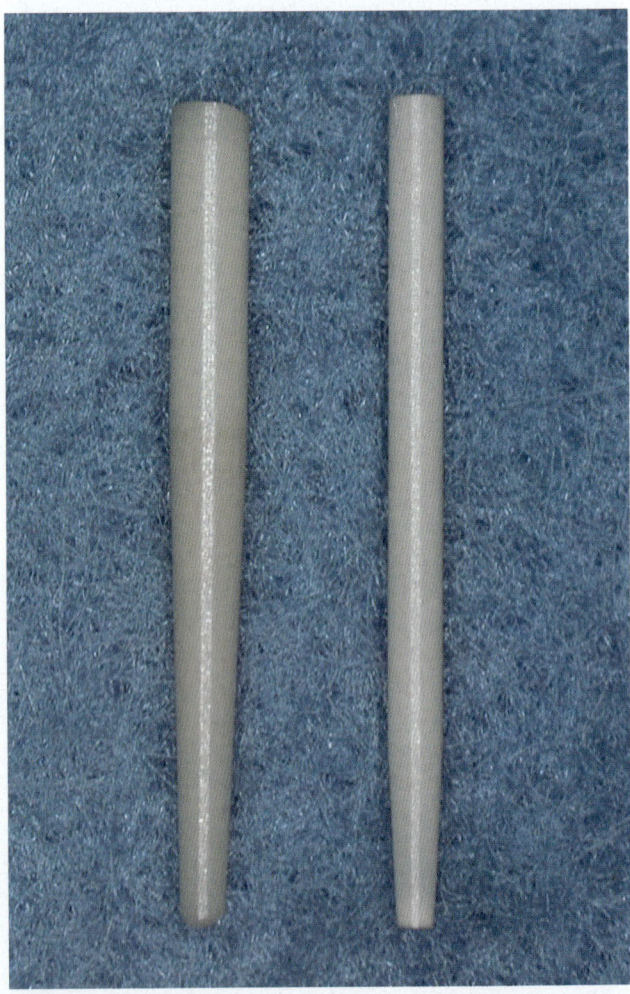

Figure 21 Available shapes and designs for zirconia posts.

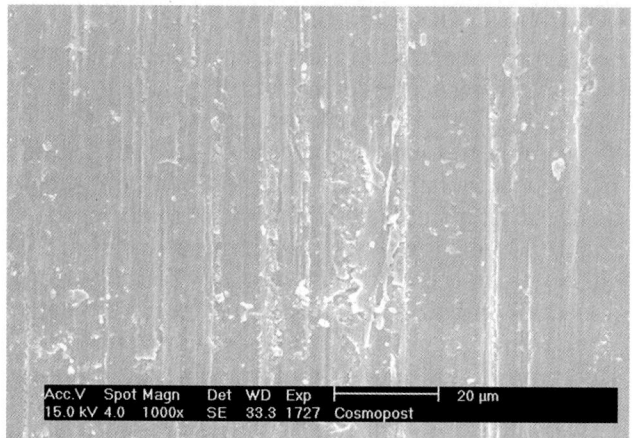

Figure 22 Surface texture of zirconia post (SEM magnification: ×1000).

enhance mechanical retention (Figure 22). As a result, the zirconia post does not bond well to composite resins and may not provide the best support for a brittle all-ceramic crown.[261,305–308] Dietschi et al.[307] found that these posts also have poor resin-bonding capabilities to dentin after dynamic loading and thermocycling due to the rigidity of the post. In a cyclic loading test performed in a wet environment, Mannocci et al.[239] found that the survival rate of zirconia posts compared with fiber posts was significantly lower.

In vitro studies[261,264,308,309] indicated that the smooth surface configuration of untreated zirconia posts leads to failure at the cement/post interface. The vast majority of the cement remained in the root and was not attached to the zirconia posts. Wegner and Kern[310] evaluated the bond strength of composite resin cement to zirconia posts. They found that the long-term bond strength of the resin composite cement to zirconia posts is weak. Several studies found that acid etching and silanization of zirconia posts does not improve the strength of the resin bond to the zirconia-based material because of the lack of or no silica content in the post.[310–313] However, tribochemical silica coating was found to increase the bond strength of the composite resin to the zirconia post.[314,315] Oblak et al.[316] compared the fracture resistance of prefabricated zirconia posts after different surface treatments. They found that airborne particle-abraded posts exhibited significantly higher resistance to fracture than posts that have been ground with a diamond instrument.

The use of heat-pressed glass to form the core instead of composite resin has been suggested.[201,299,300] This approach may improve the physical properties of the all-ceramic post and core.

When the mechanical properties of zirconia posts were evaluated, it was reported that these posts are very stiff and strong, with no plastic behavior.[227,298,299] Pfeiffer et al.[257] found that the zirconia post had a significantly higher yield strength compared with titanium and GFR posts.

Several studies indicated that many commonly used posts exhibit higher fracture resistance than zirconia posts.[238,297,317,318] In addition, once they fracture the, irretrievable posts will leave unrestorable roots.[170,318]

Nothdurft et al.[319] evaluated the clinical performance of 30 zirconia posts in a short-term retrospective study. They found no signs of failure of these posts. However, these results should be analyzed with caution because of the small sample size and a short follow-up time.

Root Selection for Multirooted Teeth

PREMOLARS
When posts and cores are needed in premolars, posts are best placed in the palatal root of the maxillary premolar and the straightest root of the mandibular premolar. The buccal root could be prepared to a depth of 1 to 2 mm and to serve as an antirotational lock, if needed.

MOLARS
When posts and cores are needed in molars, posts are best placed in roots that have the greatest dentin thickness and the smallest developmental root depressions. The most appropriate roots (the primary roots) in maxillary molars are the palatal roots and in

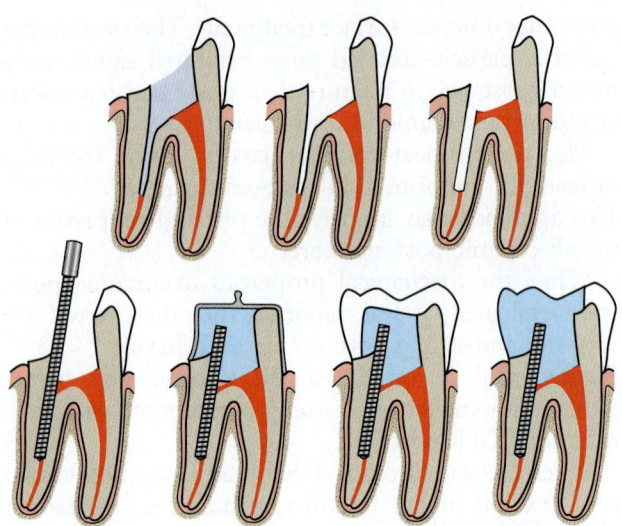

Figure 23 Placement of ParaPost and restorative material core in a molar. ***A***, Endodontic treatment completed. ***B***, Provisional restorative material in the pulpal chamber has been removed and gutta-percha removed from the distal root canal. ***C***, Post space formed with a drill. ***D***, Trial placement of the post. ***E***, The post has been shortened and cemented. A restorative material core has been formed. ***F***, The tooth with core has been prepared, an impression made, and the definitive crown cemented. ***G***, If there is an extended time delay between placement of the core and preparation of the tooth for a crown, the core can be built to full tooth contour to serve as the interim restoration.

mandibular molars are the distal roots (Figure 23). The facial roots of maxillary molars and the mesial root of mandibular molars should be avoided if at all possible. If these roots must be used in addition to the primary roots, then the post length should be short (3 to 4 mm) and a small-diameter instrument should be used (no larger than a No. 2 Peeso instrument that is 1.0 mm in diameter). When 7-mm long posts were placed in the mesial root of mandibular molars, 20 of the 75 tested teeth had only a thin layer of remaining dentin or were perforated.[90]

Type of Definitive Restoration

It is important to know the type of single crown or retainer (all-metal, all-ceramic, metal ceramic) that will be used as the definitive restoration for each endodontically treated tooth that requires a post and core. This knowledge permits the tooth to be reduced in accordance with the reduction depths and form recommended for each type of crown/retainer.

CORONAL TOOTH PREPARATION

Restoration of endodontically treated teeth must be a team effort between the endodontist and the dentist responsible for the coronal restoration, requiring two-way communication. If it can be co-coordinated, the first step in the fabrication of a post and core should ideally be preparation of the coronal tooth structure (Figure 24) for the type of definitive restoration that will be placed (all-metal crown, metal ceramic crown, all-ceramic crown). This procedure will help in determining the structure of the post–core fabrication. Each type of restoration requires different amounts of tooth reduction, and the form of the tooth preparation varies considerably. By preparing the coronal tooth structure first, the structural integrity of remaining dentin and enamel can be assessed. When the remaining peripheral tooth structure is very thin and would likely not possess sufficient strength to resist occlusal forces transmitted through the crown to the tooth, the thin structure is removed and replaced as part of the core. This order of procedure also establishes morphological borders that can be used to guide core fabrication so that it is confluent with the surrounding tooth structure and possesses the desired tooth preparation form.

PULPAL CHAMBER PREPARATION

Treatment materials present in the pulpal chamber following endodontic treatment (restorative materials

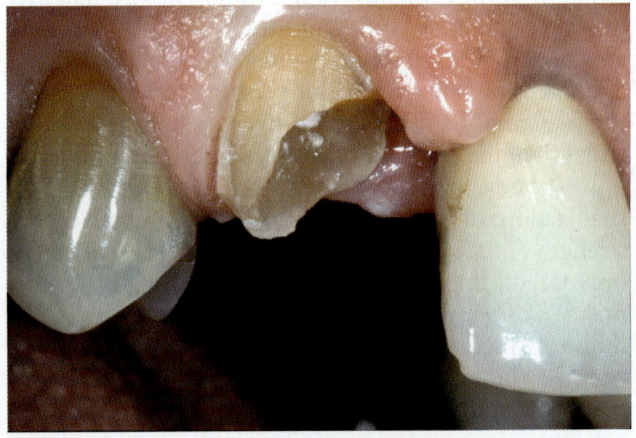

Figure 24 Coronal tooth preparation. The existing crown has been removed on an endodontically treated tooth. Initial reduction of the tooth has been completed to permit assessment of integrity of remaining coronal tooth structure.

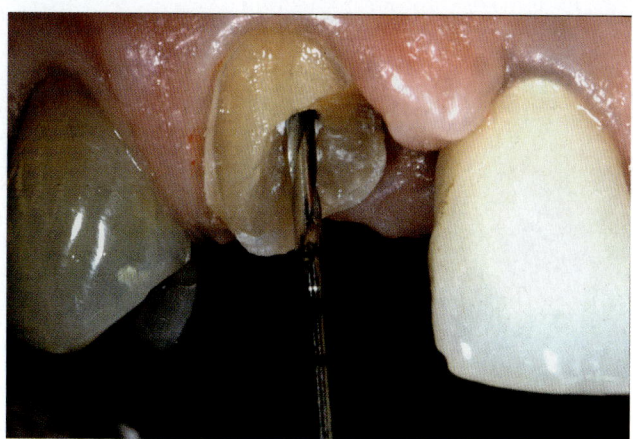

Figure 25 Pulp chamber preparation. Rotary instrument being used to remove provisional material.

sealing the coronal access and gutta-percha) are removed by using rotary instruments (Figure 25). If a prefabricated post is cemented into a root canal and a restorative material core built around the post, morphological undercuts present in the pulpal chamber should be retained for core retention. If a custom cast post and core is fabricated, then pulpal chamber undercuts must be either blocked out with a definitive cement or a restorative material that is bonded to the tooth or the undercut eliminated by removing the tooth structure. If removing the undercut through tooth preparation would result in substantive tooth structure removal that weakens the tooth, then blocking out the undercut is the treatment of choice.

ROOT CANAL PREPARATION

The individual who completed the root canal is ideally suited to prepare the root canal, being the one that is most knowledgeable regarding root curvatures and areas where no further root preparation should be performed because it will result in areas of thin residual dentin. For this reason, it may be prudent to prepare the root canal for a post as a continuation of the endodontic treatment.

If the canal has not been prepared for a post as part of the endodontic treatment process, it is necessary to remove the filling material using either a warm endodontic hand instrument or a slow-speed rotary instrument such as a Gates Glidden drill (Dentsply International, Tulsa, OK) or a Peeso instrument (Dentsply International). If a warm hand instrument is used, it is advisable to place a rubber dam so as to prevent aspiration or swallowing of the hand instrument should it be dropped.

Successful use of rotary instruments is related to initially using a small-diameter instrument (one that removes only the filling material without dentin removal). This small-diameter instrument is used to remove small vertical increments (1 to 2 mm) of the root canal filling material. After each vertical increment is removed, a visual inspection should be made to verify that the endodontic filling material is centered in the post preparation. The incremental root canal filling removal is continued until the appropriate length is established (Figure 26). Post preparation length is determined using a periodontal probe. Remaining gutta-percha length is evaluated by comparing periodontal probing depths with landmarks on the postendodontic radiograph and by making a radiograph of the prepared post space. After the length is established, any required increases to the post diameter are performed using incrementally larger rotary instruments or hand files.

Preparation for Overdentures

"The overdenture is a complete denture supported by retained teeth and the residual alveolar ridge."[320] Because the "retained teeth" are shortened, contoured,

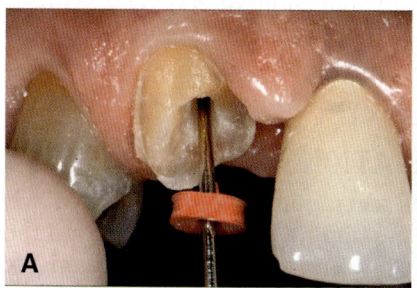 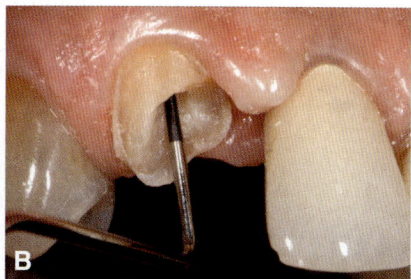 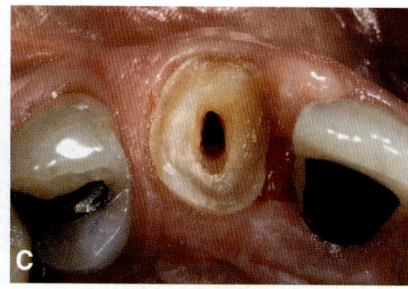

Figure 26 Root canal preparation. ***A***, Rotary instrument being used to prepare post space in the root canal. Note the rubber ring around the instrument to identify the appropriate apical extension of the post preparation. ***B***, Periodontal probe being used to measure post space depth. ***C***, Post space preparation completed.

and altered to be covered, root canal therapy is almost always required. In 1969, Lord and Teel[321] coined the term "overdenture" and described the combined endodontic–periodontic–prosthodontic technique applied thereto. As early as 1916, however, Prothero had referred to the use of root support, stating, "Oftentimes two or three widely separated roots or teeth can be utilized for supporting a denture."[322] It should also be noted that much earlier, in 1789, George Washington's first lower denture, constructed of ivory by John Greenwood, retained a mandibular left premolar.[323]

Retaining roots in the alveolar process is based on the proven observation that so long as the root remains, the bone surrounding it remains (Figure 27). This overcomes the age-old prosthetic problem of ridge resorption. Ideally, then, retaining four teeth, two molars, and two canines, one each at the four divergent points of an arch, should ensure prosthesis balance and long "life" to a complete overdenture (Figure 28). Unfortunately, patients requiring prostheses seldom present just these ideal conditions. Decisions regarding which teeth to retain usually focus on keeping some of the healthiest teeth located in strategic positions such as canines. One situation to be warned against, however, is the diagonal cross-arch arrangements, a molar abutment on one side, for example, and a canine on the opposite side. The rocking and torquing action set up by this arrangement often leads to problems and loss of one or both abutments. The molar abutment alone is preferable to the diagonal cross-arch situation.

If the selected abutment tooth is reduced to a short rounded or bullet-shaped structure and literally "tucking" the abutments inside the denture base, the crown–root ratio of the tooth is vastly improved, especially when periodontally involved teeth have lost some alveolar support. As a shortened tooth, however, it will serve admirably as an abutment for an overdenture.

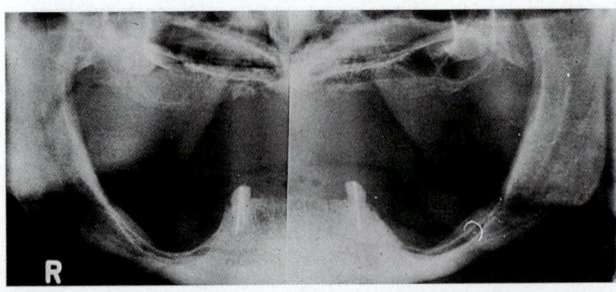

Figure 27 Dramatic demonstration of alveolar bone remaining around retained canines but badly resorbed under complete maxillary and posterior mandibular removable partial dentures.

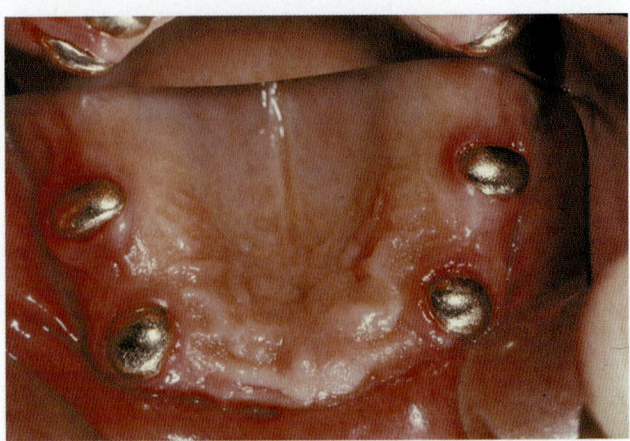

Figure 28 Mirror view of four retained abutments providing ideal support for an overdenture. Note the properly contoured and polished copings protecting the abutment teeth.

INDICATIONS AND ADVANTAGES

The indications for overdentures include the psychic support some patients receive from *not* being totally edentulous. Even more important are the preservation of the alveolar ridge and the shielding of the ridge from stress provided by firm abutment teeth. It should also be noted that occlusal vertical dimension is better preserved if ridge height is maintained. A bonus to all these advantages is the support, the stability, and retention derived from abutments. All these advantages are heightened in the young patient who must wear dentures for years to come.

Complete overdentures should be considered for virtually every patient for whom complete mouth extractions are being considered. Sometimes, certain teeth can be periodontally and endodontically treated and retained as abutments to support an overdenture. The overdenture better resists occlusal forces than the totally tissue-supported complete denture. Some attribute this resistance to the proprioceptive sensory mechanism derived from the retained roots under the overdenture. Application of the overdenture to removable partial denture support is also indicated, even if only one abutment is available.

CONTRAINDICATIONS

The overdenture technique is contraindicated when remaining alveolar support is so lacking that no tooth can be retained for very long. This condition often supports the use of endosseous root-form implants to support and retain a prosthesis. Overdentures are also contraindicated if the remaining natural teeth are adequate to restore the mouth with fixed partial dentures or removable partial dentures. The overdenture technique should be no pathway to expediency.

ABUTMENT TOOTH SELECTION

"A healthy abutment tooth for an overdenture must have minimal mobility, a manageable sulcus depth, and an adequate band of attached gingiva."[320] If these prerequisites are lacking, the pocket depth can be reduced and attached gingiva developed by using appropriate periodontal procedures.

ABUTMENT TOOTH LOCATION

Ideal teeth to retain are those whose occlusal forces wreak greatest destruction upon the ridges. Opposite a natural dentition, the canine teeth are ideal to retain. In edentulous patients, the anterior portion of the arches is particularly susceptible to resorption, so canines and premolars are again the first choice to be saved, with incisors the second choice. It is especially important to save mandibular teeth because of difficulties encountered in retaining mandibular dentures. Even saving a single tooth, a molar in particular, may contribute greatly to long-term denture success.

TECHNIQUE

After the selection of the most favorable abutment teeth, the key to successful overdenture fabrication is simplicity of technique (Figure 29). If an immediate denture is to be placed, the endodontic therapy, extractions, and periodontal treatment can sometimes be done at the denture placement appointment. The crowns of these teeth are amputated 3 to 4 mm above the gingival level and the endodontic procedure completed. The coronal 5 to 6 mm of the gutta-percha restoration is removed, the preparation is undercut, and a well-condensed amalgam filling is placed to restore and help seal the canal obturation.

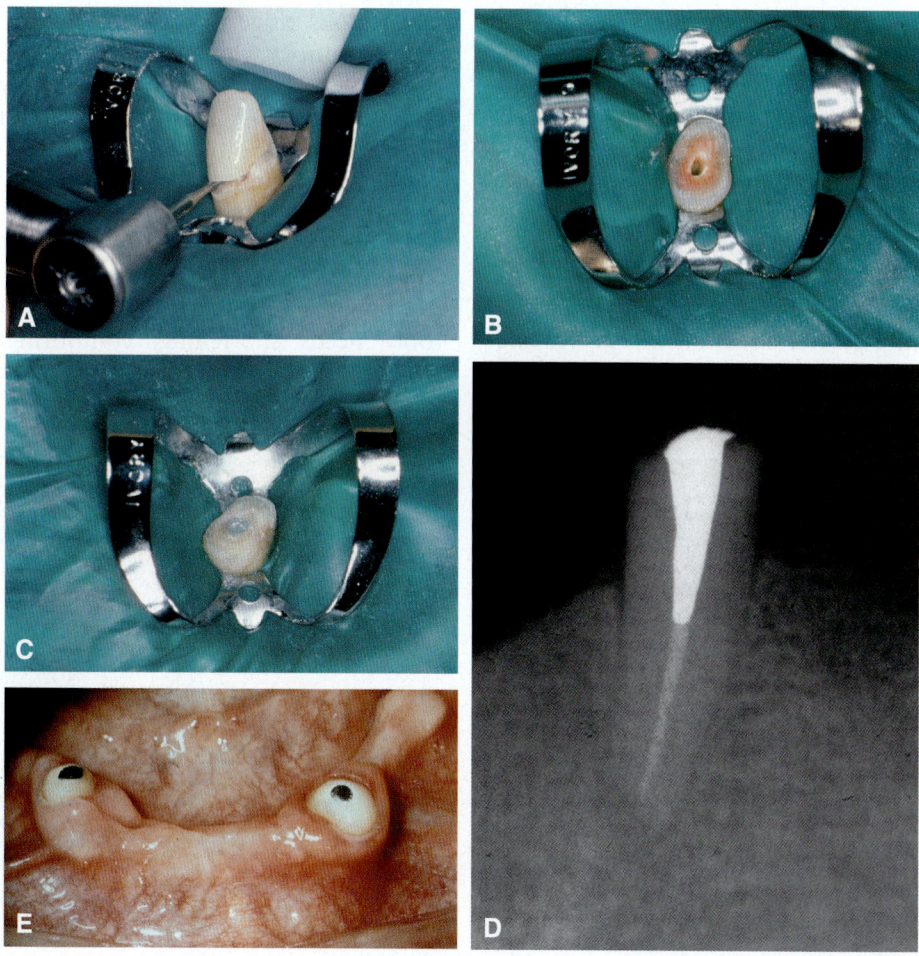

Figure 29 Preparing an overdenture abutment. **A,** The crown is amputated 3 to 4 mm above the gingival level. **B,** The endodontic procedure is started. **C** and **D,** An amalgam restoration is placed in the coronal 5 to 6 mm. **E,** In preparation for fitting the prosthesis, the abutments are shaped and polished.

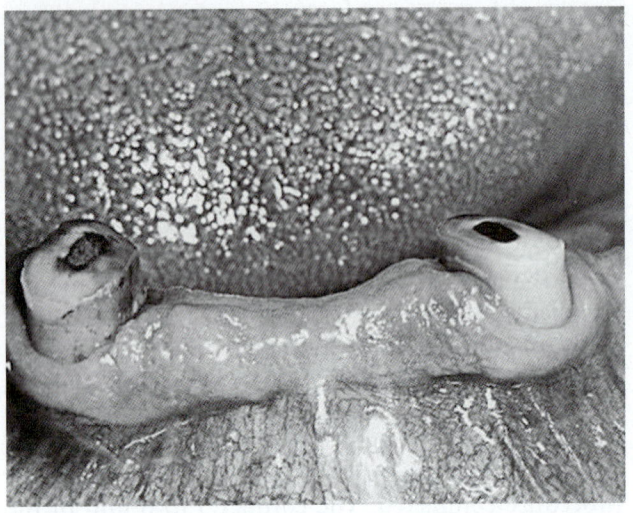

Figure 30 Improperly contoured overdenture abutments. Square edges invite grip by overdenture and torquing action. Prominent buccal contour and extra height comprise the contour of the overdenture. Courtesy of Dr. David H. Wands.

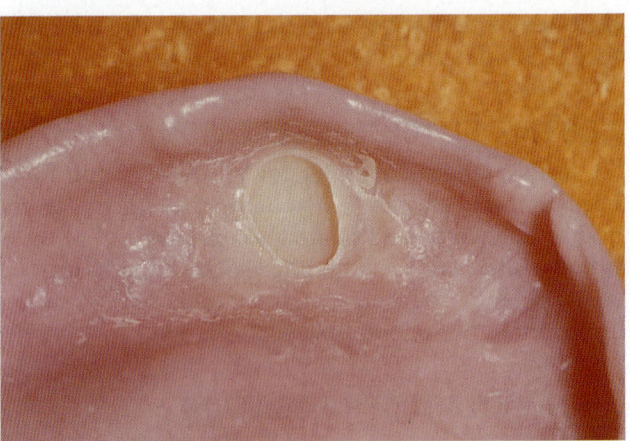

Figure 31 Soft, autopolymerizing acrylic resin fills the depression prepared in the denture to receive the abutment. This may be replaced whenever necessary.

At this time as well, the abutments should be shaped to rise 2 to 3 mm above the tissue, and be rounded or bullet-shaped with a slope back from the labial to accommodate the denture tooth to be set above it. They should then be highly polished. The abutments must not be too short or the tissue will grow over them as a "lawn grows over a sidewalk";[320] nor should they be too long, compromising the denture contour and placing greater stress on the supporting teeth (Figure 30).

The denture is relieved over the abutments and adaptation is achieved between the denture base and edentulous ridge tissues without touching the abutment teeth. It is then adapted to the abutment teeth by using a small amount of autopolymerizing acrylic resin (Figure 31). This proper relationship of denture to tissue and tooth is important for denture stability and to keep the stresses on the teeth within physiological limits.

Some overdenture abutment teeth may not need root canal therapy because they are so abraded that the pulp has receded to a level where the tooth only needs shortening, contouring, and polishing (Figure 32). This technique simplifies the treatment and reduces the cost to the patient.

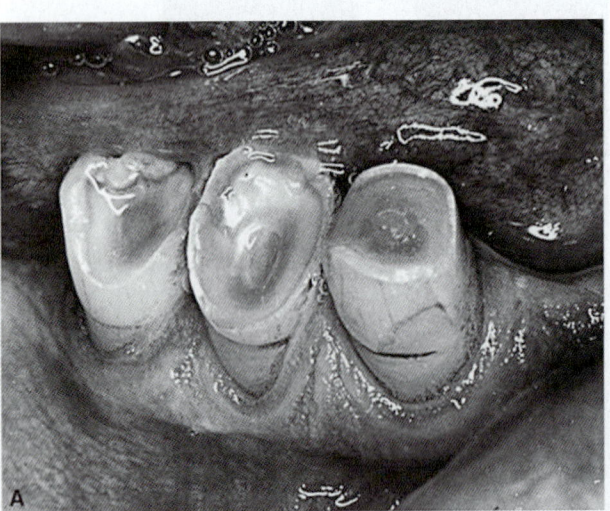
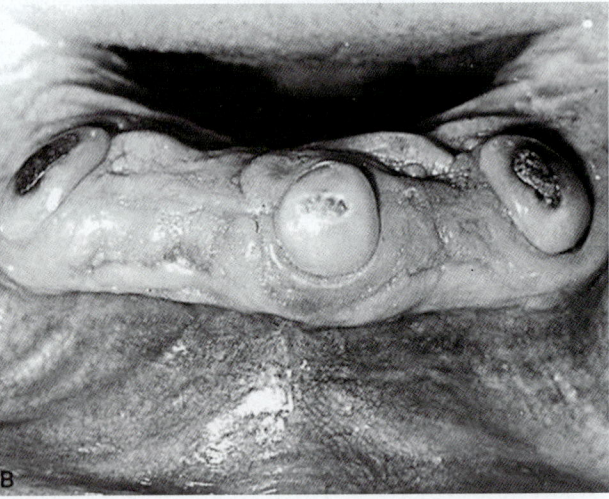

Figure 32 ***A,*** Teeth with vital, receded pulps but severe abrasion can be ideal overdenture abutments. ***B,*** Incisor overdenture abutment not requiring therapy owing to pulp recession. The calcified pulpal area should be carefully explored. Courtesy of Dr. David H. Wands.

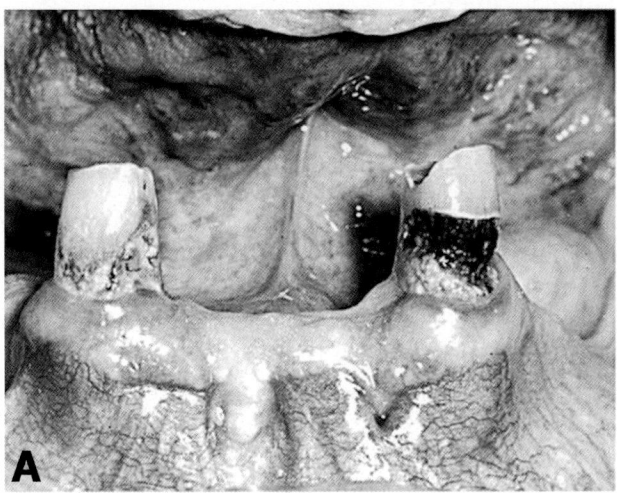
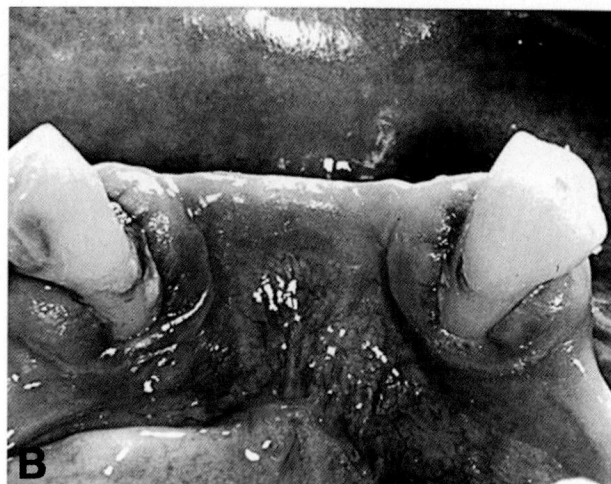

Figure 33 Rather typical neglect by many denture patients. ***A***, Caries and periodontal disease forecast probable lack of future patient cooperation. ***B***, Mirror view of lingual gingiva of two possible overdenture abutments. Because it is virtually impossible to develop attached gingiva in the lingual area, the use of these teeth as abutments is contraindicated. Courtesy of Dr. David H. Wands.

If the abutment teeth are periodontally involved or are not surrounded by a good collar of attached gingiva, periodontal therapy will be required to correct these aberrations.

PROBLEMS

A number of problems have arisen with overdentures, most of them related to poor patient selection and lack of patient cooperation. The most serious problems are associated with dental caries and periodontal disease. It must be remembered that throughout their lives, candidates for complete dentures are those who have usually been neglectful of their teeth and supporting structures and have a history of extensive dental disease (Figure 33). In recommending overdentures, there is some risk. The patients' habits must change and they must become motivated and adept at oral hygiene to retain the vestiges of their dentition. That some do not, should come as no surprise (Figure 34). The importance of good home care must be emphasized to the overdenture patient and is a critical factor in long-term success. In a longitudinal study, Ettinger and Qian[324,325] evaluated the differences in people who experienced postprocedural problems with overdentures and compared them with people who had no problems for the duration of the study. They found that most of the failures could have been prevented by better oral hygiene. The most common problem was the development of periradicular problems around endodontically treated teeth because of recurrent caries causing the loss of the restoration sealing the root canal. Other challenges related to the use of endodontically treated teeth included wear of the dentin and the need for auxiliary prosthesis retention.

POSSIBLE SOLUTIONS TO THE PROBLEMS

Quite naturally the prime solution to the caries–periodontal problem is better patient cooperation in home care. Fluoride gels should regularly be placed in the "well" of the dentin base where the abutments are located to remineralize the dentin.[326,327] This, of

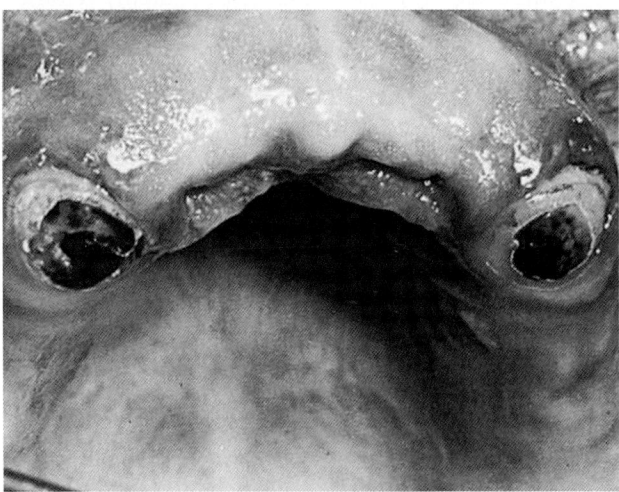

Figure 34 Two-year recall reveals advanced caries and periodontal disease of abutments. The patient did not remove the denture for days at a time. Courtesy of Dr. David H. Wands.

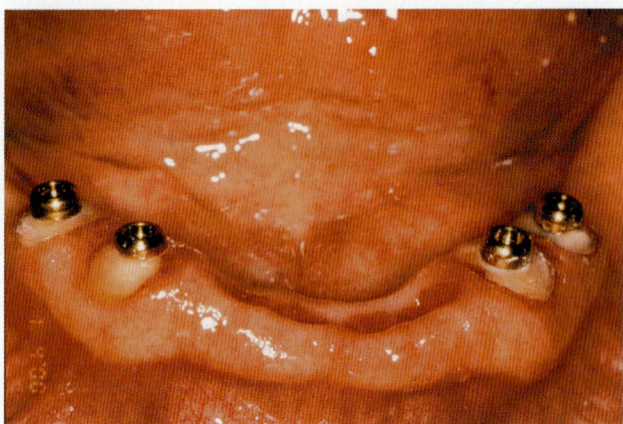

Figure 35 Four Locator overdenture attachments (Zest Anchors) ensure adequate retention for a mandibular complete denture.

course, will do nothing for periodontal disease, which can only be controlled by plaque removal and by proper and equal force placed on the abutments. More frequent denture relines may also be required.

Coverage of the dentinal surfaces is recommended for those situations where wear of the contacting dentinal surfaces is noticed. Bruxism is a principal etiological factor in producing wear. Even gold castings placed over the teeth may eventually be worn through, but it takes a much longer time.[328]

A possible solution to inadequate denture retention or to the rotational problem centering around a single anterior abutment tooth involves the use of mechanical attachments. There are a number of attachments on the market and they include ball and socket type of attachments, o-rings and magnets, frequently retained in the root through the use of a post (Figure 35).

References

1. Fauchard P. The surgeon dentist. 2nd ed. Vol. II. Birmingham, AL: Reprinted by the Classics of Dentistry Library; 1980. pp. 173–204.
2. Prothero JH. Prosthetic dentistry. 2nd ed. Chicago, IL: Medico-Dental Publishing Co.; 1916. pp. 1116:1152–62.
3. Harris CA. The dental art. Baltimore, MD: Armstrong and Berry; 1839. pp. 305–47.
4. Richardson J. A practical treatise on mechanical dentistry. Philadelphia, PA: Lindsay and Blakiston; 1880. pp. 148–9, 152–3.
5. Tomes J. Dental physiology and surgery. London: John W. Parker, West Strand; 1848. pp. 319–21.
6. Sorensen JA, Martinoff JT. Intracoronal reinforcement and coronal coverage: a study of endodontically treated teeth. J Prosthet Dent 1984;51:780–4.
7. Scurria MS, Shugars DA, Hayden WJ, Felton DA. General dentists' patterns of restoring endodontically treated teeth. J Am Dent Assoc 1995;126:775–9.
8. Vire DE. Failure of endodontically treated teeth: classification and evaluation. J Endod 1991;17:338–42.
9. Aquilino S, Caplan D. Relationship between crown placement and a survival of endodontically treated teeth. J Prosthet Dent 2002;87:256–63.
10. Hansen EK, Asmussen E, Christiansen NC. In vivo fractures of endodontically treated posterior teeth restored with amalgam. Endod Dent Traumatol 1990;6:49–55.
11. Mannocci F, Bertelli E, Sherriff M, et al. Three-year clinical comparison of survival of endodontically treated restored with either full cast coverage or with direct composite restoration. J Prosthet Dent 2002;88:297–301.
12. Nagasiri R, Chitmongkolsuk S. Long-term survival of endodontically treated molars without crown coverage: a retrospective cohort study. J Prosthet Dent 2005;93:164–70.
13. Reuter JE, Brose MO. Failures in full crown retained dental bridges. Br Dent J 1984;157:61–3.
14. Randow K, Glantz PO, Zöger B. Technical failures and some related clinical complications in extensive fixed prosthodontics: An epidemiological study of long-term clinical quality. Acta Odontol Scand 1986;44:241–55.
15. Karlsson S. A clinical evaluation of fixed bridges, 10 years following insertion. J Oral Rehab 1986;13:423–32.
16. Palmqvist S, Swartz B. Artificial crowns and fixed partial dentures 18 to 23 years after placement. Int J Prosthodont 1993;6:279–85.
17. Sundh B, Ödman P. A study of fixed prosthodontics performed at a university clinic 18 years after insertion. Int J Prosthodont 1997;10:513–19.
18. Gutmann JL. The Dentin-root complex: anatomic and biologic considerations in restoring endodontically treated teeth. J Prosthet Dent 1992;67:458–67.
19. Helfer AR, Melnick S, Schilder H. Determination of the moisture content of vital and pulpless teeth. Oral Surg 1972;34:661–70.
20. Huang TJ, Schilder H, Nathanson D. Effects of moisture content and endodontic treatment on some mechanical properties of human dentin. J Endod 1992;18:209–15.
21. Reeh ES, Messer HH, Douglas WH. Reduction in tooth stiffness as a result of endodontic and restorative procedures. J Endod 1989;15:512–16.
22. Tidmarsh BG. Restoration of endodontically treated posterior teeth. J Endod 1976;2:374–5.

23. Grimaldi J. Measurement of the lateral deformation of the tooth crown under axial compressive cuspal loading [thesis]. Dunedin, New Zealand: University of Otago; 1971.
24. Carter JM, Sorensen SE, Johnson RR, et al. Punch shear testing of extracted vital and endodontically treated teeth. J Biomech 1983;16:841–8.
25. Rivera E, Yamauchi G, Chandler G, Bergenholtz G. Dentin collagen cross-links of root-filled and normal teeth. J Endod 1988;14:195.
26. Ferrari M, Mason PN, Goracci C, et al. Collagen degradation in endodontically treated teeth after clinical function. J Dent Res 2004;83:414–19.
27. Lovdahl PE, Nicholls JI. Pin-retained amalgam cores vs. cast-gold dowel-cores. J Prosthet Dent 1977;38(5):507–14.
28. Lu YC. A comparative study of fracture resistance of pulpless teeth. Chin Dent J 1987;6(1):26–31.
29. Pontius O, Hutter JW. Survival rate and fracture strength of incisors restored with different post and core systems and endodontically treated incisors without coronoradicular reinforcement. J Endod 2002;28:710–15.
30. Gluskin AH, Radke RA, Frost SL, Watanabe LG. The mandibular incisor: rethinking guidelines for post and core design. J Endod 1995;21:33–7.
31. McDonald AV, King PA, Setchell DJ. In vitro study to compare impact fracture resistance of intact root-treated teeth. Int Endod J 1990;23:304–12.
32. Eshelman EG Jr, Sayegh FS. Dowel materials and root fracture. J Prosthet Dent 1983;50:342–4.
33. Guzy GE, Nicholls JI. In vitro comparison of intact endodontically treated teeth with and without endo-post reinforcement. J Prosthet Dent 1979;42:39–44.
34. Leary JM, Aquilino SA, Svare CW. An evaluation of post length within the elastic limits of dentin. J Prosthet Dent 1987;57:277–81.
35. Trope M, Maltz DO, Tronstad L. Resistance to fracture of restored endodontically treated teeth. Endod Dent Traumatol 1985;1:108–11.
36. Hunter AJ, Feiglin B, Williams JF. Effects of post placement on endodontically treated teeth. J Prosthet Dent 1989;62:166–72.
37. Ko CC, Chu CS, Chung KH, Lee MC. Effects of posts on dentin stress distribution in pulpless teeth. J Prosthet Dent 1992;68:421–7.
38. Sorensen JA, Martinoff JT. Endodontically treated teeth as abutments. J Prosthet Dent 1985;53:631–6.
39. Eckerbom M, Magnusson T, Martinsson T. Prevalence of apical periodontitis, crowned teeth and teeth with posts in a Swedish population. Endodont Dent Traumatol 1991;7:214–20.
40. Morfis AS. Vertical root fractures. Oral Surg Oral Med Oral Pathol Oral Radiol Endod 1990;69:631–5.
41. Goodacre CJ, Bernal G, Rungcharassaeng K, Kan JY. Clinical complications in fixed prosthodontics. J Prosthet Dent 2003;90:31–41.
42. Hussey DL, Killough SA. A survey of general dental practitioners' approach to the restoration of root-filled teeth. Int Endod J 1995;28:91–4.
43. Morgano SM, Hashem AF, Fotoohi K, Rose L. A nationwide survey of contemporary philosophies and techniques of restoring endodontically treated teeth. J Prosthet Dent 1994;72:259–67.
44. Turner CH. The utilization of roots to carry post-retained crowns. J Oral Rehab 1982;9:193–202.
45. Hatzikyriakos AH, Reisis GI, Tsingos N. A 3-year postoperative clinical evaluation of posts and cores beneath existing crowns. J Prosthet Dent 1992;67:454–8.
46. Sorensen JA, Martinoff JF. Clinically significant factors in dowel design. J Prosthet Dent 1984;52:28–35.
47. Bergman B, Lundquist P, Sjögren U, Sundquist G. Restorative and endodontic results after treatment with cast posts and cores. J Prosthet Dent 1989;61:10–15.
48. Torbjörner A, Karlsson S, Ödman PA. Survival rate and failure characteristics for two post designs. J Prosthet Dent 1995;73:439–44.
49. Weine FS, Wax AH, Wenckus CS. Retrospective study of tapered, smooth post systems in place for ten years or more. J Endod 1991;17:293–7.
50. Mentink AG, Meeuwissen R, Käyser AF, Mulder J. Survival rate and failure characteristics of the all metal post and core restoration. J Oral Rehabil 1993;20:455–61.
51. Wallerstedt D, Eliasson S, Sundström. A follow-up study of screwpost-retained amalgam crowns. Swed Dent J 1984;8:165–70.
52. Creugers NH, Mentink AG, Käyser AF. An analysis of durability data on post and core restorations. J Dent 1993;21:281–4.
53. Roberts DH. The failure of retainers in bridge prostheses. Br Dent 1970;128:117–24.
54. Valderhaug A, Jokstad A, Ambjornsen E, Norheim PW. Assessment of the periapical and clinical status of crowned teeth over 25 years. J Dent 1997;25:97–105.
55. Balkenhol M, Wöstmann B, Rein C, Ferger P. Survival time of cast post and cores: a 10-year retrospective study. J Dent 2007;35(1):50–8. Epub Jun 5, 2006.
56. Turner CH. Post-retained crown failure: a survey. Dent Update 1982;9:221–34.
57. Lewis R, Smith BG. A clinical survey of failed post retained crowns. Br Dent J 1988;165:95–7.
58. Linde LÅ. The use of composites as core material in root-filled teeth. II. Clinical investigation. Swed Dent J 1984;8:209–16.
59. Ross RS, Nicholls JI, Harrington GW. A comparison of strains generated during placement of five endodontic posts. J Endod 1991;17:450–6.

60. Henry PJ. Photoelastic analysis of post core restorations. Aust Dent J 1977;22:157–9.

61. Standlee JP, Caputo AA, Holcomb JP. The dentatus screw: comparative stress analysis with other endodontic dowel designs. J Oral Rehabil 1982;9:23–33.

62. Deutsch AS, Musikant BL, Cavallari J, et al. Root fracture during insertion of prefabricated posts related to root size. J Prosthet Dent 1985;53:786–9.

63. Thorsteinsson TS, Yaman P, Craig RG. Stress analyses of four prefabricated posts. J Prosthet Dent 1992;67:30–3.

64. Standlee JP, Caputo AA. The retentive and stress distributing properties of split threaded endodontic dowels. J Prosthet Dent 1992;68:436–42.

65. Standlee JP, Caputo AA, Holcomb J, Trabert KC. The retentive and stress-distributing properties of a threaded endodontic dowel. J Prosthet Dent 1980;44:398–404.

66. Standlee JP, Caputo AA, Collard EW, Pollack MH. Analysis of stress distribution by endodontic posts. Oral Surg Oral Med Oral Pathol Oral Radiol Endod 1972;33:952–60.

67. Caputo AA, Hokama SN. Stress and retention properties of a new threaded endodontic post. Quintessence Int 1987;18:431–5.

68. Rolf KC, Parker MW, Pelleu GB. Stress analysis of five prefabricated endodontic dowel designs: A photoelastic study. Oper Dent 1992;17:86–92.

69. Cohen BI, Musikant BL, Deutsch AS. Comparison of the photoelastic stress for a split-shank threaded post versus a threaded post. J Prosthodont 1994;3:53–5.

70. Davy DT, Dilley GL, Krejci RF. Determination of stress patterns in root-filled teeth incorporating various dowel designs. J Dent Res 1981;60:1301–10.

71. Peters MC, Poort HW, Farah JW, Craig RG. Stress analysis of a tooth restored with a post and core. J Dent Res 1983;62:760–3.

72. Assif D, Oren E, Marshak BL, Aviv I. Photoelastic analysis of stress transfer by endodontically treated teeth to the supporting structure using different restorative techniques. J Prosthet Dent 1989;61:535–43.

73. Sorensen JA, Engelman MJ. Effect of post adaptation on fracture resistance of endodontically treated teeth. J Prosthet Dent 1990;64:419–24.

74. Assif D, Bitenski A, Pilo R, Oren E. Effect of post design on resistance to fracture of endodontically treated teeth with complete crowns. J Prosthet Dent 1993;69:36–40.

75. Ross IF. Fracture susceptibility of endodontically treated teeth. J Endod 1980;6:560–5.

76. Harper RH, Lund MR. Treatment of the pulpless tooth during post and core construction. Oper Dent 1976;1:55–60.

77. Mondelli J, Piccino AC, Berbert A. An acrylic resin pattern for a cast dowel and core. J Prosthet Dent 1971;25:413–7.

78. Pickard HM. Variants of the post crown. Br Dent J 1964;117:517–26.

79. Blaukopf ER. Direct acrylic Davis crown technique. J Am Dent Assoc 1944;31:1270–1.

80. Sheets CE. Dowel and core foundations. J Prosthet Dent 1970;23:58–65.

81. Goldrich N. Construction of posts for teeth with existing restorations. J Prosthet Dent 1970;23:173–6.

82. Rosen H. Operative procedures on mutilated endodontically treated teeth. J Prosthet Dent 1961;11:973–86.

83. Rosenberg PA, Antonoff SJ. Gold posts. Common problems in preparation and technique for fabrication. NY St Dent J 1971;37:601–6.

84. Silverstein WH. Reinforcement of weakened pulpless teeth. J Prosthet Dent 1964;14:372–81.

85. Dooley BS. Preparation and construction of post retention crowns for anterior teeth. Aust Dent J 1967;12:544–50.

86. Baraban DJ. The restoration of pulpless teeth. Dent Clin North Am 1967;633–53.

87. Jacoby WE. Practical technique for the fabrication of a direct pattern for a post core restoration. J Prosthet Dent 1976;35:357–60.

88. Dewhirst RB, Fisher DW, Schillingburg HT. Dowel core fabrication. J South Calif Dent Assoc 1969;37:444–9.

89. Hamilton AI. Porcelain dowel crowns. J Prosthet Dent 1959;9:639–44.

90. Larato DC. Single unit cast post crown for pulpless anterior tooth roots. J Prosthet Dent 1966;16:145–9.

91. Christy JM, Pipko DJ. Fabrication of a dual post veneer crown. J Am Dent Assoc 1967;75:1419–25.

92. Bartlett SO. Construction of detached core crowns for pulpless teeth in only two sittings. J Am Dent Assoc 1968;77:843–5.

93. Burnell SC. Improved cast dowel and base for restoring endodontically treated teeth. J Am Dent Assoc 1964;68:39–45.

94. Perel ML, Muroff FI. Clinical criteria for posts and cores. J Prosthet Dent 1972;28:405–11.

95. Stern N, Hirshfeld Z. Principles of preparing endodontically treated teeth for dowel and core restorations. J Prosthet Dent 1973;30:162–5.

96. Hirschfeld Z, Stern N. Post and core—the biomechanical aspect. Aust Dent J 1972;17:467–8.

97. Grieve AR, McAndrew R. A radiographic study of post-retained crowns in patients attending a dental hospital. Br Dent J 1993;174:197–201.

98. Martin N, Jedynakiewicz N. A radiographic survey of endodontic post lengths. IADR Abstract No. 418. J Dent Res [Special Issue] 1989;68:919.

99. Johnson JK, Sakumura JS. Dowel form and tensile force. J Prosthet Dent 1978;40:645–9.
100. Leary JM, Aquilino SA, Svare CW. An evaluation of post length within the elastic limits of dentin. J Prosthet Dent 1987;57:277–81.
101. Zillich RM, Corcoran JF. Average maximum post lengths in endodontically treated teeth. J Prosthet Dent 1984;52:489–91.
102. Shillingburg HT, Kessler JC, Wilson EL. Root dimensions and dowel size. Calif Dent Assoc J 1982;10:43–9.
103. Abou-Rass M, Jann JM, Jobe D, Tsutsui F. Preparation of space for posting: effect on thickness of canal walls and incidence of perforation in molars. J Am Dent Assoc 1982;104:834–7.
104. Reinhardt RA, Krejci RF, Pao Y, Stannard JG. Dentin stresses in post-reconstructed teeth with diminishing bone support. J Dent Res 1983;62:1002–8.
105. Buranadham S, Aquilino SA, Stanford CM. Relation between dowel extension and bone level in anterior teeth. IADR Abstract No. 930. J Dent Res [Special Issue]1999;78:222.
106. Camp LR, Todd MJ. The effect of dowel preparation on the apical seal of three common obturation techniques. J Prosthet Dent 1983;50:664–6.
107. Madison S, Zakariasen KL. Linear and volumetric analysis of apical leakage in teeth prepared for posts. J Endod 1984;10:422–7.
108. Neagley RL. The effect of dowel preparation on the apical seal of endodontically treated teeth. Surg Oral Med Oral Pathol Oral Radiol Endod 1969;28:739–45.
109. Zmener O. Effect of dowel preparation on the apical seal of endodontically treated teeth. J Endod 1980;6:687–90.
110. Kurer HG, Combe EC, Grant AA. Factors influencing the retention of dowels. J Prosthet Dent 1977;38:515–25.
111. Mattison GD, Delivanis PD, Thacker RW, Hassell KJ. Effect of post preparation on the apical seal. J Prosthet Dent 1984;51:785–9.
112. Nixon C, Vertucci FJ, Swindle R. The effect of post space preparation on the apical seal of root canal obturated teeth. Todays FDA 1991;3:1–6C.
113. Raiden GC, Gendelman H. Effect of dowel space preparation on the apical seal of root canal fillings. Endod Dent Traumatol 1994;10:109–12.
114. Kvist T, Rydin E, Reit C. The relative frequency of periapical lesions in teeth with root canal-retained posts. J Endod 1989;15:578–80.
115. Wu MK, Pehlivan Y, Kontakiotis EG, Wesselink PR. Microleakage along apical root fillings and cemented posts. J Prosthet Dent 1998;79:264–9.
116. Abramovitz I, Tagger M, Tamse A, Metzger Z. The effect of immediate vs. delayed post space preparation on the apical seal of a root canal filling. A study in an increased-sensitivity pressure-driven system. J Endod 2000;26:435–9.
117. Metzger Z, Abramovitz R, Abramovitz I, Tagger M. Correlation between remaining length of root canal filling after immediate post space preparation and coronal leakage. J Endod 2000;26:724–8.
118. Turner CH, Willoughby AF. The retention of vented-cast dental posts. J Dent 1985;13:267–70.
119. Standlee JP, Caputo AA, Hanson EC. Retention of endodontic dowels: effects of cement, dowel length, diameter, and design. J Prosthet Dent 1978;39:401–5.
120. Hanson EC, Caputo AA. Cementing mediums and retentive characteristics of dowels. J Prosthet Dent 1974;32:551–7.
121. Krupp JD, Caputo AA, Trabert KC, Standlee JP. Dowel retention with glass-ionomer cement. J Prosthet Dent 1979;41:163–6.
122. Mattison GD. Photoelastic stress analysis of cast-gold endodontic posts. J Prosthet Dent 1982;48:407–11.
123. Trabert KC, Caputo AA, Abou-Rass M. Tooth fracture—a comparison of endodontic and restorative treatments. J Endod 1978;4:341–5.
124. Lloyd PM, Palik JF. The philosophies of dowel diameter preparation: a literature review. J Prosthet Dent 1993;69:32–6.
125. Tilk MA, Lommel TJ, Gerstein H. A study of mandibular and maxillary root widths to determine dowel size. J Endod 1979;5:79–82.
126. Raiden G, Costa L, Koss S, et al. Residual thickness of root in first maxillary premolars with post space preparation. J Endod 1999;25:502–5.
127. Bourgeois RS, Lemon RR. Dowel space preparation and apical leakage. J Endod 1981;7:66–9.
128. Schnell FJ. Effect of immediate dowel space preparation on the apical seal of endodontically filled teeth. Surg Oral Med Oral Pathol Oral Radiol Endod 1978;45:470–4.
129. Dickey DJ, Harris GZ, Lemon RR, Luebke RG. Effect of post space preparation on apical seal using solvent techniques and peeso reamers. J Endod 1982;8:351–4.
130. Kwan EH, Harrington GW. The effect of immediate post preparation on apical seal. J Endod 1981;7:325–9.
131. Karapanou V, Vera J, Cabrera P, et al. Effect of immediate and delayed post preparation on apical dye leakage using two different sealers. J Endod 1996;22:583–5.
132. Portell FR, Bernier WE, Lorton L, Peters DD. The effect of immediate versus delayed dowel space preparation on the integrity of the apical seal. J Endod 1982;8:154–60.
133. Fan B, Wu MK, Wesselink PR. Coronal leakage along apical root fillings after immediate and delayed post space preparation. Endod Dent Traumatol 1999;15:124–6.
134. Solano F, Hartwell G, Appelstein C. Comparison of apical seal leakage between immediate versus delayed post space preparation using AH Plus sealer. J Endod 2005;31:752–4.

135. Suchina JA, Ludington JR. Dowel space preparation and the apical seal. J Endod 1985;11:11–17.
136. Hiltner RS, Kulild JC, Weller RN. Effect of mechanical versus thermal removal of gutta-percha on the quality of the apical seal following post space preparation. J Endod 1992;18:451–4.
137. Haddix JE, Mattison GD, Shulman CA, Pink, FE. Post preparation techniques and their effect on the apical seal. J Prosthet Dent 1990;64:515–19.
138. DeCleen MJ. The relationship between the root canal filling and post space preparation. Int Endod J 1993;26:53–8.
139. Balto H, Al-Nazhan S, Al-Mansour K, et al. Microbial leakage of Cavit, IRM, and Temp Bond in post-prepared root canals using two methods of gutta-percha removal: an in vivo study. J Contemp Dent Pract 2005;6:53–61.
140. Hülsmann M, Schinkel I. Influence of several factors on the success or failure of removal of fractured instruments from the root canal. Endod Dent Traumatol 1999;15:252–8.
141. Ward JR, Parashos P, Messer HH. Evaluation of an ultrasonic technique to remove fractured rotary nickel–titanium endodontic instruments from root canals: an experimental study. J Endod 2003;29:756–63.
142. Suter B, Lussi A, Sequeria P. Probability of removing fractured instruments from root canals. Int Endod J 2005;38:112–23.
143. Saunder WP, Saunders EM. Coronal leakage as a cause of failure in root-canal therapy: a review. Endod Dent Traumatol 1994;10:105–8.
144. Heling I, Gorfil C, Slutzky H, et al. Endodontic failure caused by inadequate restorative procedures: review and treatment recommendations. J Prosthet Dent 2002;87:674–8.
145. Trope M, Chow E, Nissan R. In vitro endotoxin penetration of coronally unsealed endodontically treated teeth. Endod Dent Traumatol 1995;11:90–4.
146. Alves J, Walton R, Drake D. Coronal leakage: endotoxin penetration from mixed bacterial communities through obturated, post-prepared root canals. J Endod 1998;24:587–91.
147. Torabinejad M, Ung B, Kettering JD. In vitro bacterial penetration of coronally unsealed endodontically treated teeth. J Endod 1990;16:566–9.
148. Khayat A, Lee SJ, Torabinejad M. Human saliva penetration of coronally unsealed obturated root canals. J Endod 1993;19:458–61.
149. Swanson K, Madison S. An evaluation of coronal microleakage in endodontically treated teeth. Part I. Time periods. J Endod 1987;13:56–9.
150. Demarchi MG, Sato EF. Leakage of interim post and cores used during laboratory fabrication of custom posts. J Endod 2002;28:328–9.
151. Fox K, Gutteridge DL. An in vitro study of coronal microleakage in root-canal-treated teeth restored by the post and core technique. Int Endod J 1997;30:361–8.
152. Lynch CD, Burke FM, Ni Riordain R, Hannigan A. The influence of coronal restoration type on the survival of endodontically treated teeth. Eur J Prosthodont Restor Dent 2004;12:171–6.
153. Safavi KE, Dowen WE, Langeland K. Influence of delayed coronal permanent restoration on endodontic prognosis. Endod Dent Traumatol 1987;3:187–91.
154. Ray HA, Trope M. Periapical status of endodontically treated teeth in relation to the technical quality of the root filling and the coronal restoration. Int Endod J 1995;28:12–18.
155. Iqbal MK, Johansson AA, Akeel RF, et al. A retrospective analysis of factors associated with the periapical status of restored, endodontically treated teeth. Int J Prosthodont 2003;16:31–8.
156. Tronstad L, Asblornsen K, Doving L, et al. Influence of coronal restorations on the periapical health of endodontically treated teeth. Endod Dent Traumatol 2000;16:218–21.
157. Valderhaug J, Jokstad A, Ambjørnsen E, Norheim PW. Assessment of the periapical and clinical status of crowned teeth over 25 years. J Dent 1997;25:97–105.
158. Barkhordar RA, Radke R, Abbasi J. Effect of metal collars on resistance of endodontically treated teeth to root fracture. J Prosthet Dent 1989;61:676–8.
159. Tjan AH, Whang SB. Resistant to root fracture of dowel channels with various thicknesses of buccal dentin walls. J Prosthet Dent 1985;53:496–500.
160. Loney RW, Kotowicz WE, McDowell GC. Three-dimensional photoelastic stress analysis of the ferrule effect in cast post and cores. J Prosthet Dent 1990;63:506–12.
161. Hemmings KW, King PA, Setchell DJ. Resistance to torsional forces of various post and core designs. J Prosthet Dent 1991;66:325–9.
162. Saupe WA, Gluskin AH, Radke RA Jr. A comparative study of fracture resistance between morphologic dowel and cores and a resin-reinforced dowel system in the intraradicular restoration of structurally compromised roots. Quintessence Int 1996;27:483–91.
163. Libman WJ, Nicholls JI. Load fatigue of teeth restored with cast posts and cores and complete crowns. Int J Prosthodont 1995;8:155–61.
164. Milot P, Stein RS. Root fracture in endodontically treated teeth related to post selection and crown design. J Prosthet Dent 1992;68:428–35.
165. Isidor F, Brøndum K, Ravnholt G. The influence of post length and crown ferrule length on the resistance to cyclic loading of bovine teeth with prefabricated titanium posts. Int J Prosthodont 1999;12:78–82.
166. Hoag EP, Dwyer TG. A comparative evaluation of three post and core techniques. J Prosthet Dent 1982;47:177–81.
167. Gegauff AG. Effect of crown lengthening and ferrule placement on static load failure of cemented cast post–cores and crowns. J Prosthet Dent 2000;84:169–79.

168. Mezzomo E, Massa F, Libera SD. Fracture resistance of teeth restored with two different post-and-core designs cemented with two different cements: an in vitro study. Part I. Quintessence Int 2003;34:301–6.

169. Zhi-Yue L, Yu-Xing Z. Effects of post–core design and ferrule on fracture resistance of endodontically treated maxillary central incisors. J Prosthet Dent 2003;89:368–73.

170. Akkayan B. An in vitro study evaluating the effect of ferrule length on fracture resistance of endodontically treated teeth restored with fiber-reinforced and zirconia dowel systems. J Prosthet Dent 2004;92:155–62.

171. Goto Y, Nicholls JI, Phillips KM, Junge T. Fatigue resistance of endodontically treated teeth restored with three dowel-and-core systems. J Prosthet Dent 2005;93:45–50.

172. Tan PLB, Aquilino SA, Gratton DG, et al. In vitro fracture resistance of endodontically treated central incisors with varying ferrule heights and configurations. J Prosthet Dent 2005;93:331–6.

173. Naumann M, Preuss A, Rosentritt M. Effect of incomplete crown ferrules on load capacity of endodontically treated maxillary incisors restored with fiber posts, composite build-ups, and all ceramic crowns: An in vitro evaluation after chewing simulation. Acta Odontol Scand 2006;64:31–6.

174. Ng CCH, Dumbrigue HB, Al-Bayat MI, et al. Influence of remaining coronal tooth structure location on the fracture resistance of restored endodontically treated anterior teeth. J Prosthet Dent 2006;95:290–6.

175. Ichim I, Kuzmanovic DV, Love RM. A finite element analysis of the ferrule design on restoration resistance and distribution of stress within a root. Int Endod J 2006;39:443–52.

176. Pereira JR, de Ornelas F, Conti PC, do Valle AL. Effect of a crown ferrule on the fracture resistance of endodontically treated teeth restored with prefabricated posts. J Prosthet Dent 2006;95:50–4.

177. Sorensen JA, Engelman MJ. Ferrule design and fracture resistance of endodontically treated teeth. J Prosthet Dent 1990;63:529–36.

178. Rosen H, Partida-Rivera M. Iatrogenic fracture of roots reinforced with a cervical collar. Oper Dent 1986;11:46–50.

179. Assif D, Bitenski A, Pilo R, Oren E. Effect of post design on resistance to fracture of endodontically treated teeth with complete crowns. J Prosthet Dent 1993;69:36–40.

180. Ouzounian ZS, Schilder H. Remaining dentin thickness after endodontic cleaning and shaping before post space preparation. Oral Health 1991;81:13–15.

181. Pilo R, Tamse A. Residual dentin thickness in mandibular premolars prepared with Gates Glidden and ParaPost drills. J Prosthet Dent 2000;83:617–23.

182. Bessing C. Alternatives to high noble dental casting gold alloys type 3. An in vitro study. Swed Dent J Suppl 1988;53:1–56.

183. Can G, Akpinar G, Can A. Effects of base-metal casting alloys on cytoskeletal filaments in cultured human fibroblasts. Int J Prosthodont 2004;17:45–51.

184. Al-Hiyasat AS, Bashabsheh OM, Darmani H. An investigation of the cytotoxic effects of dental casting alloys. Int J Prosthodont 2003;16:8–12.

185. Nitkin DA, Asgar K. Evaluation of alternative alloys to type III gold for use in fixed prosthodontics. J Am Dent Assoc 1976;93:622–9.

186. Stokes AN, Hood JA. Influence of casting procedure on silver-palladium endodontic posts. J Dent 1989;17:305–7.

187. Oilo G, Holland RI, Johansen OA. Porosities in dental silver–palladium casting alloy. Acta Odontol Scand 1985;43:9–13.

188. Miller AW. Direct pattern technique for post and cores. J Prosthet Dent 1978;40:392.

189. Gentile D. Direct dowels for endodontically treated teeth. Dent Dig 1965;71:500–1.

190. Shadman H, Azermehr P. A direct technique for fabrication of posts and cores. J Prosthet Dent 1975;34:463–6.

191. Aquilino SA, Jordan RD, Turner KA, Leary JM. Multiple cast post and cores for severely worn anterior teeth. J Prosthet Dent 1986;55:430–3.

192. Bluche LR, Bluche PF, Morgano SM. Vacuum-formed matrix as a guide for fabrication of multiple direct patterns for cast post and cores. J Prosthet Dent 1997;77:326–7.

193. Sabbak SA. Indirect fabrication of multiple post-and-core patterns with vinyl polysiloxane matrix. J Prosthet Dent 2002;88:555–7.

194. Von Krammer R. A time-saving method for indirect fabrication of cast posts and cores. J Prosthet Dent 1996;76:209–11.

195. Emtiaz S, Carames JM, Guimaraes N, et al. Indirect impression technique for multiple cast dowel and cores facilitated with three putty indexes. Pract Proced Aesthet Dent 2005;17:201–8.

196. Rosenstiel E. Impression technique for cast core preparations. Br Dent J 1967;123:599–600.

197. Chiche GJ, Mikhail MG. Laminated single impression technique for cast posts and cores. J Prosthet Dent 1985;53:325–8.

198. Williams VD, Bjorndal AM. The Masserann technique for the removal of fractures posts in endodontically treated teeth. J Prosthet Dent 1983;49:46–8.

199. Warren SR, Gutmann JL. Simplified method for removing intraradicular posts. J Prosthet Dent 1979;42:353–6.

200. Machtou P, Sarfati P, Cohen AG. Post removal prior to retreatment. J Endod 1989;15:552–4.

201. Butz F, Lennon AM, Heydecke G, Strub JR. Survival rate and fracture strength of endodontically treated maxillary incisors

201. with moderate defects restored with different post-and-core systems: an in vitro study. Int J Prosthodont 2001;14:58–64.
202. Kurer PF. The Kurer anchor system for the post crown restoration. J Ont Dent Assoc 1968;45:57–97.
203. Baraban DJ. A simplified method for making post and core. J Prosthet Dent 1970;24:287–97.
204. Musikant BL. A new prefabricated post and core system. J Prosthet Dent 1984;52:631–4.
205. Duret B, Renaud M, Duret F. Un nouveau concept de reconstitution corono-radiculaire: Le Composipost (1). Chir Dent Fr 1990;60:131–41.
206. Duret B, Renaud M, Duret F. Un nouveau concept de reconstitution corono-radiculaire: Le Composipost (2). Chir Dent Fr 1990;60:69–77.
207. Duret B, Renaud M, Duret F. Intérêt des matériaux à structure unidirectionnelle dans les reconstitutions corono-radiculaires. J Biomater dent 1992;7:45–57.
208. Rovatti L, Mason PN, Dallari A. New research on endodontic carbon-fiber posts. Minerva Stomatol 1994;43:557–63.
209. Wennström J. The C-Post system. Compend Contin Educ Dent 1996;Suppl 20:S80–5.
210. Trushkowsky RD. Coronoradicular rehabilitation with a carbon-fiber post. Compend Contin Educ Dent 1996;Suppl 20:S74–9.
211. Viguie G, Malquarti G, Vincent B, Bourgeois D. Epoxy/carbon composite resins in dentistry: mechanical properties related to fiber reinforcements. J Prosthet Dent 1994;72:245–9.
212. Duret B, Duret F, Renaud M. Long-life physical property preservation and postendodontic rehabilitation with Composipost. Compend Contin Educ Dent 1996;Suppl 20:S50–60.
213. Dallari A, Rovatti L. Six years of in vitro/in vivo experience with Composipost. Compend Contin Educ Dent 1996;Suppl 20:S57–63.
214. Yazdanie N, Mahood M. Carbon fiber acrylic resin composite: an investigation of transverse strength. J Prosthet Dent 1985;54:543–7.
215. King PA, Setchell DJ. An in vitro evaluation of a prototype CFRC prefabricated post developed for the restoration of pulpless teeth. J Oral Rehabil 1990;17:599–609.
216. Malquarti G, Berruet RG, Bois D. Prosthetic use of carbon fiber-reinforced epoxy resin for esthetic crowns and fixed partial dentures. J Prosthet Dent 1990;63:251–7.
217. Purton DE, Payne JA. Comparison of carbon fiber and stainless steel root canal posts. Quintessence Int 1996;27:93–7.
218. Galhano GA, Valandro LF, de Melo RM, et al. Evaluation of the flexural strength of carbon fiber, quartz fiber, and glass fiber-based posts. J Endod 2005;31:209–11.
219. Mannocci F, Sherriff M, Watson TF. Three-point bending test of fiber posts. J Endod 2001;27:758–61.
220. Finger WJ, Ahlstrand WM. Fritz UB. Radiopacity of fiber-reinforced resin posts. Am J Dent 2002;15:81–4.
221. Love RM, Purton DG. The effect of serrations on carbon fiber posts-retention within the root canal, core retention, and post rigidity. Int J Prosthodont 1996;9:484–8.
222. Torbjörner A, Karlsson S, Syverud M, Hensten-Pettersen A. Carbon fiber reinforced root canal posts: mechanical and cytotoxic properties. Eur J Oral Sci 1996;104:605–11.
223. Ferrari M, Vichi A, Garcia-Godoy F. Clinical evaluation of fiber-reinforced epoxy resin posts and cast post and cores. Am J Dent 2000;13(Spec. No.):15–18B.
224. Ottl P, Hahn L, Lauer H, Fay M. Fracture characteristics of carbon fibre, ceramic and non-palladium endodontic post systems at monotonously increasing loads. J Oral Rehabil 2002;29:175–83.
225. Sidoli GE, King PA, Setchell DJ. An in vitro evaluation of carbon fiber-based post and core system. J Prosthet Dent 1997;78:5–9.
226. Purton DG, Love RM. Rigidity and retention of carbon fiber versus stainless steel root canal posts. Int J Endod 1996;29:262–5.
227. Asmussen E, Peutzfeldt A, Heitmann T. Stiffness, elastic limit, and strength of newer types of endodontic posts. J Dent Res 1999;27:275–8.
228. Martinez-Insua A, da Silva L, Rilo B, Santana U. Comparison of the fracture resistance of pulpless teeth restored with a cast post and core or carbon-fiber post with a composite core. J Prosthet Dent 1998;80:527–32.
229. King PA, Setchell DJ, Rees JS. Clinical evaluation of a carbon fiber reinforced endodontic post. J Oral Rehabil 2003;30:785–9.
230. Drummond JL, Bapna MS. Static and cyclic loading of fiber-reinforced dental resin. Dent Mater 2003;19:226–31.
231. Drummond JL, Toepke TR, King TJ. Thermal and cyclic loading of endodontic posts. Eur J Oral Sci 1999;107:220–4.
232. Newman MP, Yaman P, Dennison J, et al. Fracture resistance of endodontically treated teeth restored with composite posts. J Prosthet Dent 2003;89:360–7.
233. Lassila LV, Tanner J, Le Bell AM, et al. Flexural properties of fiber reinforced root canal posts. Dent Mater 2004;20:29–36.
234. McDonald AV, King PA, Setchell DJ. In vitro study to compare impact fracture resistance of intact root-treated teeth. Int Endod J 1990;23:304–12.
235. Raygot CG, Chai J, Jameson DL. Fracture resistance and primary failure mode of endodontically treated teeth restored with carbon fiber-reinforced resin post system in vitro. Int J Prosthodont 2001;14:141–5.
236. Isidor F, Ödman P, Brøndum K. Intermittent loading of teeth restored using prefabricated carbon fiber posts. Int J Prosthodont 1996;9:131–6.

237. Dean JP, Jeansonne BG, Sarkar N. In vitro evaluation of a carbon fiber post. J Endod 1998;24:807–10.

238. Cormier CJ, Burns DR, Moon P. In vitro comparison of fracture resistance and failure mode of fiber, ceramic, and conventional post systems at various stages of restoration. J Prosthodont 2001;10:26–36.

239. Mannocci F, Ferrari M, Watson TF. Intermittent loading of teeth restored using quartz fiber, carbon-quartz fiber, and zirconium dioxide ceramic root canal posts. J Adhes Dent 1999;1:153–8.

240. Fokkinga WA, Kreulen CM, Vallittu PK, Creugers NH. A structured analysis of in vitro failure loads and failure modes of fiber, metal, and ceramic post-and-core systems. Int J Prosthodont 2004;17:476–82.

241. Mannocci F, Qualtrough AJ, Worthington HV, et al. Randomized clinical comparison of endodontically treated teeth restored with amalgam or with fiber posts and resin composite: five-year results. Oper Dent 2005;30(1):9–15.

242. Fredriksson M, Astbäck J, Pamenius M, Arvidson K. A retrospective study of 236 patients with teeth restored by carbon fiber-reinforced epoxy resin posts. J Prosthet Dent 1998;80:151–7.

243. Glazer B. Restoration of endodontically treated teeth with carbon fiber posts- a prospective study. J Can Dent Assoc 2000;66:613–18.

244. Ferrari M, Vichi A, Mannocci F, Mason PN. Retrospective study of the clinical performance of fiber posts. Am J Dent 2000;13(Spec. No.):9B–13B.

245. Hedlund SO, Johansson NG, Sjögren G. A retrospective study of pre-fabricated carbon fiber root canal posts. J Oral Rehabil 2003;30:1036–40.

246. Segerström S, Astback J, Ekstrand KD. A retrospective long term study of teeth restored with prefabricated carbon fiber reinforced epoxy resin posts. Swed Dent J 2006;30:1–8.

247. Gesi A, Magnolfi S, Goracci C, Ferrari M. Comparison of two techniques for removing fiber posts. J Endod 2003;29(9):580–2.

248. De Rijk WG. Removal of fiber posts from endodontically treated teeth. Am J Dent 2000;13 (Spec. No.):19B–21B.

249. Sakkal S. Carbon-fiber post removal technique. Compend Contin Educ Dent 1996;20:586

250. Peters SB, Canby FL, Miller DA. Removal of a carbon fiber post system. J Endod 1996;22:215.

251. Abbott PV. Incidence of root fractures and methods used for post removal. Int Endod J 2002;35:63–7.

252. Murphy J. Reinforced plastics handbook. Oxford: Elsevier; 1988.

253. Chawla KK. Composite materials: science and engineering. 2nd ed. New York: Springer-Verlag; 1998.

254. Teixeira ECN, Teixeira FB, Piasick JR, Thompson JY. An in vitro assessment of prefabricated fiber post systems. J Am Dent Assoc 2006;137:1006–12.

255. Bae JM, Kim KN, Hattori M, et al. The flexural properties of fiber-reinforced composite with light-polymerized polymer matrix. Int J Prosthodont 2001;14:33–9.

256. Triolo PT, Trajtenberg C, Powers JM. Flexural properties and bond strength of an esthetic post. [abstract 3538] J Dent Res 1999;78:548.

257. Pfeiffer P, Schulz A, Nergiz I, Schmage P. Yield strength of zirconia and glass fibre-reinforced posts. J Oral Rehabil 2006;33:70–4.

258. Vallittu P. Effect of 180-week water storage on the flexural properties of E-glass and silica fiber acrylic resin composite. Int J Prosthodont 2000;13:334–9.

259. Lassila LVJ, Nohrström T, Vallitu P. The influence of short-term water storage on the flexural properties of unidirectional glass fiber-reinforced composites. Biomaterials 2002;23:2221–9.

260. Grant T, Bradley W. In-situ observations in SEM of degradation of graphite/epoxy composite materials due to seawater immersion. J Compos Mater 1995;29:852–67.

261. Al-harbi F, Nathanson D. In vitro assessment of retention of four esthetic dowels to resin core foundation and teeth. J Prosthet Dent 2003;90:547–55.

262. Coelho Santos G Jr, El-Mowafy O, Henrique Rubo J. Diametral tensile strength of a resin composite core with non-metallic prefabricated posts: an in vitro study. J Prosthet Dent 2004;91:335–41.

263. Le Bell AM, Lassila LVJ, Kangasniemi I, Vallittu PK. Bonding of fibre-reinforced composite post to root canal dentin. J Dent 2005;33:533–9.

264. Hedlund SO, Johansson NG, Sjögren G. Retention of prefabricated and individually cast root canal posts in vitro. Br Dent J 2003;195:155–8.

265. Balbosh A, Kern M. Effect of surface treatment on retention of glass-fiber endodontic posts. J Prosthet Dent 2006;95:218–23.

266. Vano M, Goracci C, Monticelli F, et al. The adhesion between fibre posts and composite resin core: the evaluation of microtensile bond strength following various surface chemical treatments to posts. Int Endod J 2006;39:31–9.

267. Monticelli F, Toledano M, Tay FR, et al. Post-surface conditioning improves interfacial adhesion in post/core restorations. Dent Mater 2006;22:602–9.

268. Stricker EJ, Göhring TN. Influence of different posts and cores on marginal adaptation, fracture resistance, and fracture mode of composite resin crowns on human mandibular premolars. An in vitro study. J Dent 2006;34:326–35.

269. Hu S, Osada T, Shimizu T, et al. Resistance to cyclic fatigue and fracture of structurally compromised root restored with different post and core restorations. Dent Mater J 2005;24:225–31.

270. Malferrari S, Monaco C, Scotti R. Clinical evaluation of teeth restored with quartz fiber-reinforced epoxy resin posts. Int J Prosthodont 2003;16:39–44.

271. Naumann M, Preuss A, Frankenberger R. Reinforcement effect of adhesively luted fiber reinforced composite versus titanium posts. Dent Mater 2007; 23 (2):138–44.

272. Naumann M, Blankenstein F, Dietrich T. Survival of glass fiber reinforced composite post restorations after 2 years—an observational clinical study. J Dent 2005;33:305–12.

273. Sirimai S, Riis DN, Morgano SM. An in vitro study of the fracture resistance and the incidence of vertical root fracture of pulpless teeth restored with six post-and-core systems. J Prosthet Dent 1999;81:262–9.

274. Deliperi S, Bardwell DN, Coiana C. Reconstruction of devital teeth using direct fiber-reinforced composite resins: a case report. J Adhes Dent 2005;7:165–71.

275. Eskitascioglu G, Belli S. The use of bondable reinforcement fiber for post-and-core buildup in an endodontically treated tooth: a case report. Quintessence Int 2002;33:549–51.

276. Eskitascioglu G, Belli S, Kalkan M. Evaluation of two post core systems using two different methods (fracture strength test and a finite element analysis). J Endod 2002;28:629–33.

277. Usumez A, Cobankara FK, Ozturk N, et al. Microleakage of endodontically treated teeth with different dowel systems. J Prosthet Dent 2004;92:163–9.

278. Meyenberg KH, Lüthy H, Schärer P. Zirconia posts: a new all-ceramic concept for non-vital abutment teeth. J Esthet Dent 1995;7:73–80.

279. Zalkind M, Hochman N. Esthetic considerations in restoring endodontically treated teeth with posts and cores. J Prosthet Dent 1998;79:702–5.

280. Zalkind M, Hochman N. Direct core buildup using a preformed crown and prefabricated zirconium oxide post. J Prosthet Dent 1998;80:730–2.

281. Ahmad I. Yttrium-partially stabilized zirconium dioxide posts: an approach to restoring coronally compromised teeth. Int J Periodont Restor Dent 1998;18:454–65.

282. Sorensen JA, Mito WT. Rationale and clinical technique for esthetic restoration of endodontically treated teeth with Cosmopost and IPS Empress post system. QDT 1998;81–90.

283. Michalakis KX, Hirayama H, Sfolkos J, Sfolkos K. Light transmission of posts and cores used for the anterior esthetic region. Int J Periodont Restor Dent 2004;24:462–9.

284. Carossa S, Lombardo S, Pera P, et al. Influence of posts and cores on light transmission through different all-ceramic crowns: spectrophotometric and clinical evaluation. Int J Prosthodont 2001;14:9–14.

285. Ottl P, Hahn L, Lauer HCh, Fay M. Fracture characteristics of carbon fibre, ceramic and non-palladium endodontic post systems at monotonously increasing loads. J Oral Rehabil 2002 Feb;29(2):175–83.

286. Cales B, Stefani Y, Lilley E. Long-term in vivo and in vitro aging of a zirconia ceramic used in orthopaedy. J Biomed Mater Res 1994;28:619–24.

287. Christel P, Meunier A, Heller M, et al. Mechanical properties and short-term in vivo evaluation of yttrium-oxide-partially-stabilized zirconia. J Biomed Mater Res 1989;23:45–61.

288. Ichikawa Y, Akagawa Y, Nikai H, Tsuru H. Tissue compatibility and stability of a new zirconia ceramic in vivo. J Prosthet Dent 1992;68:322–6.

289. Purton DG, Love RM, Chandler NP. Rigidity and retention of ceramic root canal posts. Oper Dent 2000;25:223–7.

290. Drouin JM, Cales B, Chevalier J, Fantozzi G. Fatigue behavior of zirconia hip joint heads: experimental results and finite element analysis. J Biomed Mater Res 1997;34:149–55.

291. Porter DL, Heuer AH. Mechanism of toughening partially stabilized zirconia ceramics (PSZ). J Am Ceram Soc 1977;60:183–4.

292. Gubta TK, Lange FF, Bechtold JH. Effect of stress-induced phase transformation on the metastable tetragonal phase. J Mater Sci 1978;13:1464–70.

293. Guazzato M, Albakry M, Ringer SP, Swain MV. Strength, fracture toughness and microstructure of a selection of all-ceramic materials. Part II. Zirconia-based dental ceramics. Dent Mater 2004;20:449–56.

294. Schweiger M, Frank M, Rheinburger V, Holand W. New sintered glass-ceramics based on apatite and zirconia endosseous implant in initial bone healing. J Prosthet Dent 1993;69:599–604.

295. Hulbert TK, Lange FF, Bechtold JH. Effect of stress-induced phase transformation on the metastable tetragonal phase. J Mater Sci 1978;13:1464–70.

296. Soares CJ, Mitsui FH, Neto FH, et al. Radiodensity evaluation of seven root post systems. Am J Dent 2005 Feb;18(1):57–60.

297. Rosentritt M, Fürer C, Behr M, et al. Comparison of in vitro fracture strength of metallic and tooth-coloured posts and cores. J Oral Rehabil 2000;27:595–601.

298. Taira M, Nomura Y, Wakasa K, et al. Studies on fracture toughness of dental ceramics. J Oral Rehabil 1990;17:551–63.

299. Hochman N, Zalkind M. New all-ceramic indirect post-and-core system. J Prosthet Dent 1999;81:625–9.

300. Dilmener FT, Sipahi C, Dalkiz M. Resistance of three new esthetic post-and-core systems to compressive loading. J Prosthet Dent 2006;95:130–6.

301. Piconi C, Maccauro G. Zirconia as a ceramic biomaterial. Biomaterials 1999;20:1–25.

302. Kakehashi Y, Luthy H, Naef R, et al. A new all-ceramic post and core system: clinical, technical, and in vitro results. Int J Periodont Restor Dent 1998;18:586–93.

303. Koutayas SO, Kern M. All-ceramic posts and cores: the state of the art. Quintessence Int 1999;30:383–92.

304. Heydecke G, Butz F, Hussein A, Strub JR. Fracture strength after dynamic loading of endodontically treated teeth

restored with different post-and-core systems. J Prosthet Dent 2002;87:438–45.

305. Perdigao J, Geraldeli S, Lee IK. Push-out bond strength of tooth-colored posts bonded with different adhesive systems. Am J Dent 2004;17:422–6.

306. Cohen BI, Pagnillo MK, Newman I, et al. Retention of core material supported by three post head designs. J Prosthet Dent 2000;83:624–8.

307. Dietschi D, Romelli M, Goretti A. Adaptation of adhesive posts and cores to dentin after fatigue testing. Int J Prosthodont 1997;10:498–507.

308. Baba NZ. The effect of eugenol and non-eugenol endodontic sealers on the retention of three prefabricated posts cemented with a resin composite cement [thesis]. Boston, MA: Boston University; 2000.

309. Gernhardt CR, Bekes K, Schaller HG. Short-term retentive values of zirconium oxide posts cemented with glass ionomer and resin cement: an in vitro study and a case report. Quintessence Int 2005;36:593–601.

310. Wegner SM, Kern M. Long-term resin bond strength to zirconia ceramic. J Adhes Dent 2000;2:139–47.

311. Madani M, Chu FCS, McDonald AV, Smales RJ. Effects of surface treatments on shear bond strengths between a resin cement and an alumina core. J Prosthet Dent 2000;83:644–7.

312. Blixt M, Adamczak E, Linden L, et al. Bonding to densely sintered alumina surfaces: effect of sandblasting and silica coating on shear bond strength of luting cements. Int J Prosthodont 2000;13:221–6.

313. Ozcan M, Alkumru HN, Gemalmaz D. The effect of the surface treatment on the shear bond strength of luting cement to glass-infiltrated alumina ceramic. Int J Prosthodont 2001;14:335–9.

314. Matinlinna JP, Lassila LV, Ozcan M, et al. An introduction to silanes and their clinical applications in dentistry. Int J Prosthodont 2004;17:155–64.

315. Xible AA, de Jesus Tavares RR, de Araujo Cdos R, Bonachela WC. Effect of silica coating and silanization on flexural and composite-resin bond strength of zirconia posts: an in vitro study. J Prosthet Dent 2006;95:224–9.

316. Oblak C, Jevnikar P, Kosmac T, et al. Fracture resistance and reliability of new zirconia posts. J Prosthet Dent 2004;91:342–8.

317. Mitsui FH, Marchi GM, Pimenta LA, Ferraresi PM. In vitro study of fracture resistance of bovine roots using different intraradicular post systems. Quintessence Int 2004;35:612–16.

318. Akkayan B, Gülmez T. Resistance to fracture of endodontically treated teeth restored with different post systems. J Prosthet Dent 2002;87:431–7.

319. Nothdurft FP, Pospiech PR. Clinical evaluation of pulpless teeth restored with conventionally cemented zirconia posts: a pilot study. J Prosthet Dent 2006;95:311–14.

320. Lord JL, Teel S. The overdenture: Patient selection, use of copings, and follow-up evaluation. J Prosthet Dent 1974;32:41–51.

321. Lord JL, Teel S. The overdenture. Dent Clin North Am 1969;13:871.

322. Prothero JH. Prosthetic dentistry. 2nd ed. Chicago, IL: Medicodental Publishing Co.; 1916. pp. 476, 519.

323. Sognnaes RF. America's most famous teeth. Smithsonian 1973;3:47.

324. Ettinger RL, Qian F. Postprocedural problems in an overdenture population: a longitudinal study. J Endod 2004;30(5):310–14.

325. Ettinger RL, Qian F. Abutment tooth loss in patients with overdentures. J Am Dent Assoc 2004;135(6):739–46.

326. Shannon IL. Chemical preventive dentistry for overdenture patients. In: Brewer AA, Morrow RM, editors. Overdentures. 2nd ed. St. Louis, MO: CV Mosby Co; 1980. pp. 322–40.

327. Key MC. Topical fluoride treatment of overdenture abutments. Gen Dent 1980;28:58.

328. Brewer AA, Morrow RM. Overdenture problems. In: Brewer AA, Morrow RM, editors. Overdentures. 2nd ed. St. Louis, MO: CV Mosby Co; 1980. p. 345.

Chapter 41

Operations Management in Endodontic Practice

Martin D. Levin

The establishment of any professional practice should include the development of a vision that promotes excellence in both clinical application and performance. With the advent of new technologies such as in-office cone beam computed tomography, the emergence of molecular dentistry and medicine, new pharmacogenomics, increased dissemination of knowledge on the Internet, and improved electronic communications, we are at the threshold of a new era in patient care. Concurrently, these new technologies, improved relationships, and continual improvements in clinical and experiential performance require good management strategies and, ultimately, financial success to create and maintain an outstanding practice. To accomplish sustainable success, we must not only have mastery of the clinical tools of our profession, but also possess the skills necessary to run a successful business.

To remain successful, this vision must include the possibility that your practice will have to undergo both planned changes to implement new procedures and the need to respond to developments over which the organization will have little or no control. In fact, it has been postulated that today "more than half of the economic value of dental care is derived from procedures that were not available just 20 years ago."[1]

To train practitioners and employees, upgrade technology, and improve client service continually, the practice of dentistry requires entrepreneurial training. Dr. Harold Slavkin, former director of the National Institute of Dental and Craniofacial Research (NIDCR), recognized the need for business training when he proposed increasing "the education and training of our student learners in the field of leadership and management of dental practices."[2] Today's endodontist must be a clinician, infection control expert, entrepreneur, insurance and financial manager, and human resource (HR) authority.[3]

Clinical excellence is the hallmark of every true world-class practice. What really matters is adopting an ethical and philosophical level of quality that will enable each practice to do the right thing every time. Basically, we are in the people business, and people naturally align with organizations that value integrity, compassion, quality of care, and high standards of behavior. Only by viewing your organization as a collection of interdependent systems and processes that ultimately depend on each employee to reach his or her full potential will your practice reach the desired result. As outlined by Abraham Maslow[4] over 50 years ago, successful organizations are the ones that genuinely encourage self-actualization to ensure that people identify and pursue their own unique personal potential.

To this end, this chapter will highlight operational strategies that focus on creating a vision that will fund sustainable success by building a *brand-driven culture* within your organization that is supported by high-performance human systems.

Choosing How You Want to Practice

The healthcare industry is a services profession, and as such has different characteristics than companies producing physical goods.[5] According to Leonard Berry,[6] Distinguished Professor of Marketing at the Mays Business School at Texas A&M University, "marketing a performance [e.g., medical services] is not the same as marketing an object... In packaged goods the emphasis is on differentiating tangibles through imagery; in services the emphasis is tangibilizing the intangible." To truly understand the medical services world, Berry spent his sabbatical at the Mayo Clinic, immersed in day-to-day hospital procedures and interactions. He came away with a new appreciation for the importance of reliability as the basis of services marketing excellence. What he is saying, essentially, is that you have to do the job right the first time, every time because "who wants to travel on an airline whose pilots are *usually* dependable, [or] be operated on by a surgeon who *usually* remembers where on the body the surgery is to be done?"

As a services profession, the delivery of dental care requires both the provider and the consumer to be present at the same time. This one-on-one relationship gives rise to the potential of real-time customization, one of the most powerful tools available to healthcare providers. When you and the patient are working together to create an agreed-upon result, you can decide how much, or if any, customization will occur, and even whether that customization will occur in the front office, the back office, or both. This consultative function should be managed to create value that satisfies patient and referrer needs. From a customer-centered perspective, it means providing what both the patient and referring doctor want, on their terms, when and how they want it.[7]

Organizations need to establish a strategic framework in order to reach their full potential. This framework consists of (1) a vision for the future, (2) a mission that defines what you are doing now, (3) a step-by-step strategy to clarify your individual situation and develop a program to achieve future objectives, (4) goals and action plans that guide day-to-day decision making,[8] and (5) feedback to see what really works.

VISION AND MISSION STATEMENTS

A vision statement is a clearly articulated, future-oriented declaration that articulates what your organization wants to become. Vision statements range in length from a couple of words to several pages; shorter vision statements tend to be easier to recall and use.

This statement should resonate with all members of the practice and help them feel proud, excited, and part of something larger than themselves. A vision should stretch the organization's capabilities and image of itself. It should give clarity, shape, and direction to the organization's future. Do you want to be the most technologically advanced specialist in your community? Do you want to achieve a high return on your investment? Do you want to be a thought leader, a fee leader, or both? Answers to these and other questions will help you create a vision for your practice.

A mission statement is a succinct proclamation of the practice's purpose for existence. It should include measurable criteria and address such concepts as image, customer demographics, target market, and expectations for growth and profitability. Mission statements should be broad enough to incorporate every service provided and should include the practice's moral and ethical position, geographic and demographic domain, and the expectations as well as hopes for growth and profitability.

Once a mission statement is adopted by the organization, everyone must subscribe to its precepts or its usefulness will diminish. It is critical that you align your practice with your mission so that every interaction between employees and patients builds value. Unfortunately, the Workplace 2000 Employee Insight Survey, conducted by Tom Terez, author of "22 Keys to Creating a Meaningful Workplace,"[9] found that only 23% of US workers say that their company's mission statement has become a way of doing business.

Visions and missions are usually linked to strategies and goals that are specific, measurable, and short term. Once a vision and mission statement has been adopted and becomes part of the fabric of your practice, you can develop an implementation strategy and a list of annual goals. Finally, adding deadlines and a system of measurement will allow you to continually gauge your progress.

STRATEGIC PLANNING

What is a strategy? The word comes from the Greek word *strategia*, meaning "generalship." While it is difficult to find agreement on an exact definition of strategy because it includes "thoughts, ideas, insights, experiences, goals, expertise, memories, perceptions and expectations,"[10] almost everyone can agree that it is about the means to reach an end, not what those aims are or how they are established. In most successful practices, the leadership alone is responsible for assuring that the office's policies are legitimate and ethical. Strategy, on the other hand, is the province of both leadership and management, while tactics are the responsibility of management alone. In other words, determining the goals of an enterprise is mainly a governance issue, while employment of resources is the job of management. Keep in mind that strategy is a changing perspective of what is required to obtain the ends that have been specified in policies, and is dependent on the actual results as measured by business performance. So strategy and tactics actually bridge the gap between resources and policy.

Two useful techniques to evaluate your future practice's potential for success are the SWOT (Strengths, Weaknesses, Opportunities, and Threats) and PEST

Table 1 SWOT (Strengths, Weaknesses, Opportunities, and Threats) Anaylsis	
Strengths: What you do better than the competition	**Weaknesses:** Things that the competition does better than you
Opportunities: Trends, changes, and characteristics of your market that may offer opportunities for your business now or in the future	**Threats:** Trends and changes associated with your market that may present your business with problems either now or in the future
This SWOT analysis form measures a business proposition or idea by assessing core issues. Most practices can apply the ideas developed here to understand their current position and help plan future initiatives.	

(Political, Economic, Social, and Technological) analyses. A SWOT analysis measures a business proposition or idea. Long-range strategic planners often use SWOT analysis to assess core issues and develop a plan based on current perceptions (Table 1). Practices can also benefit by completing a SWOT analysis to evaluate a competitor.

A PEST analysis helps to measure the external macro-environment that affects all businesses. The most useful analysis for a dental practice will be the social and technological analysis portion. The social section is where patients' and referrers' demographics, class structure, education, culture, and attitudes about healthcare are considered. Technological analysis looks at recent technological developments, their impact on the value-chain structure, cost, and efficiency. For example, should you consider purchasing or leasing a cone beam computed tomography scanner, panoramic device, or refer patients needing advanced evaluation to a center with these capabilities? PEST analysis allows for proactive marketing and business development assessment.

SETTING GOALS

Goals are plain language statements that describe priorities or actions to be accomplished. Practices should have a number of goals, each describing a desired result toward which your efforts should be directed. Goals set priorities for management and staff and establish measurement parameters for evaluating success. Goals serve to keep an organization focused on success and away from activities that tend to distract and drain resources. If the goals are accomplished, then the business should be a success.

Practice goals are generally derived from mission statements and describe how the mission will be accomplished, while mission statements describe exactly what needs to be accomplished. A goal should be simple, clearly written, state the conditions that will exist if the goal is accomplished, and set action-oriented tasks that you want to accomplish in 1 to 3 years. Some business goals will have a 1-year time frame, while others may have longer or shorter time frame. It is not unusual for a practice to have a mix of business goals starting and ending at different times. Most importantly, a goal needs to be achievable and challenge the people responsible for its accomplishment.

As more employees understand and commit to your vision for the practice, it is the job of leadership to continually reaffirm it through every available channel of communication, such as staff meetings, or when conversing with co-therapists, and so on. According to Lionel Urwick's[11] classic *Harvard Business Review* article, 1956, "There is nothing which rots morale more quickly and more completely than...the feeling that those in authority do not know their own minds." Once the plan is created, be ready to change it. Strategic plans are dynamic, living documents that are not a once-a-year project, but can be modified repeatedly as it needs warrant. Strategic planning is one of the key activities that forces organizations to focus on the right priorities to foster growth. In the end, all strategic planning models are goal-based and rely on clearly defined, understood, and communicated action steps. A strategy is not useful, however, if it is not realized. A Fortune Magazine study has shown that 7 out of 10 CEOs fail because of poor execution, not because of bad strategy.[12]

PRACTICE MODELS

Unlike the practice of medicine, which is becoming increasingly complex and business-like, Marjorie Jeffcoat,[13] the Morton Amsterdam Dean at the School of Dental Medicine, University of Pennsylvania, says that "dentistry has remained a profession dominated by small, independent practices." In fact, Kathleen Roth, president of the American Dental Association (ADA), in a 2007 address to the Small Business Committee of the U.S. Congress, reported that over 90% of practicing dentists are in the private sector and 85% of those practitioners operate independent solo practices.[14] But the need to investigate organizational alternatives is becoming more urgent with the expectation that there will be a sea change in the way health care is organized and funded in the future. While dentists may continue to practice independently, other dental practice models will show strong growth and evolve as business entities.

Armstrong et al.[15] have postulated that some practices adhere to the "service factory model," where low cost and standardization predominates, delivering consistent but standardized service. Conversely, other practices act as "service theaters," or niche practices, where a select clientele undergo premium-priced procedures that are individualized and scripted for maximum effect. Patients choose this type of practice if price is no object. They want a high-tech approach, presented with personal attention in an office that rivals the ambiance of a fine hotel. Employees are not just hired here; they are trained to serve as members of a team that values a high-touch, patient-centered experience.

Other attempts to categorize practice models have been proposed by the Dental Trade Alliance (DTA). Jeffery Lavers,[16] Marketing Director of 3M ESPE, says that continual change in the dental marketplace is certain and will be influenced by demographics, technology, disease patterns, patient behavior, and service choices and dental workforce. Providers of dental care, for example, will be reduced from their current level of 130,000 full-time equivalent practicing U.S. dentists by more women providers practicing fewer hours and lower numbers of dental school graduates than in the past. These factors and an associated increase in the U.S. population will continue to decrease the dentist/population ratio.

The DTA has proposed the following emerging practice models, which it predicts will provide over 60% of all dental services by 2010 (reproduced by permission of the DTA):

Ready Access Model—High-process standardization, convenience-oriented, highly flexible operating systems, focused on a dynamic "retail" service experience

Tech Station Model—High level of technical resources, procedural leading edge, "gee-whiz" experience backed by relatively high-touch patient communication

Small Group Model—Well-integrated staff with broad range of scope, seamless teamwork of staff geared to provide service efficiency and throughput

Cosmetic Center Model—A variation on the conventional practice with heavy emphasis on elective care in personal aesthetics and restorative services

Super Norm Model—Emphasis on high-touch, service-intensive patient experience, customer intimacy, and high-margin work with demanding patients

Armstrong's service theater approach is similar to the "super-norm model" proposed by the DTA's description of emerging practice models, with an emphasis on a customer-centered approach that treats demanding patients and produces high-margin work. Practice models will continue to evolve, and some practices will incorporate elements of several business forms. One practice model may use technology while also providing cosmetic procedures based on personal aesthetics and high-end customer service. What does all of this have to do with your endodontic practice? Simply put, running a successful practice requires a powerful vision of where you want to go.

Starting a new practice, associating with an established endodontic practice, or choosing a hybrid format is the first of many decisions that every endodontist will have to make when beginning his or her career. What follows is a short primer on the risks and benefits of three employment options.

NEW PRACTICE

What are the benefits of starting your own practice? You will have complete autonomy in setting practice policies and making decisions. Every decision, that is, the selection of particular equipment and designing treatment protocols, as well as the selection of employees, will be yours to make. When it is your business, you dictate the way things are done. The scheduling of employee and your own vacations is at your discretion. Then there is personal fulfillment. Owning and running your own business can be more satisfying than working for someone else, and many practitioners enjoy the respect they earn from their peers for having the courage to go out on their own. When you own your own practice, you may have to forgo a regular paycheck, but the upside earnings potential may be greater than any other alternative. If these aspects have strong appeal, then starting your own practice should be considered.

There are formidable risks to starting your own practice, and a careful analysis is critical. As a sole practitioner, you must spend the time to research all decisions yourself or engage advisors to assist you in this process. Solo practice will require an emergency coverage arrangement with another practitioner when you are out of town. You will have no immediate peer consultation to explore the treatment of difficult cases. And you will face a greater risk of losing your investment. Although relatively rare, some practitioners just cannot earn sufficient income to remain profitable. This may occur as a result of choosing a poor location, competing unsuccessfully with established neighboring practices, or assuming too much debt. Finally, opening your own business can come at a high personal cost. It will take a lot of energy and personal sacrifice to get going, likely necessitating working at night and on weekends, infringing on personal time.

ASSOCIATE-EMPLOYEE OR ASSOCIATE-INDEPENDENT CONTRACTOR

For a recent graduate with little or no prior practice experience, the benefits afforded by having a transitional period with an established practice can be priceless. Serving as an associate-employee allows the new practitioner to assume the reputation of the other member(s) of the practice, and by inference, more quickly establish a good professional reputation of his or her own. Other benefits include practice ownership opportunities, no initial financial investment, immediate patient flow, peer clinical consultation, shared emergency coverage, and the freedom to move easily to another locale if a change is desired.

Risks of the associate-employee and associate-independent contractor path include the lack of total control over the practice, loss of individuality, and the legal constraint of practicing with a restrictive covenant. A restrictive covenant is a contractual agreement usually between an associate and his or her employer that prevents the associate from practicing in a certain geographic area for a specified time period after termination of employment. These agreements are used by employers to protect their investment in start-up costs associated with bringing on an associate and their referral network from competition. Most contracts will include a restrictive covenant, also known as a non-compete agreement. Generally, courts have held that restrictive covenants are enforceable, but not in all states or under all conditions, so get good legal advice.

Associate-independent contractors are independent practitioners who provide services to a dental practice on a contractual basis. This form of practice must be carefully structured to remain in compliance with Internal Revenue Service (IRS) guidelines. Under current IRS rules, the practice owner cannot control both the means of work and the results of the independent contractor's efforts. No benefits, retirement plans, or employment taxes are paid by the practice for the associate-independent contractor. Additionally, the practice owner cannot furnish supplies, equipment and instruments, impose safety precautions, plan work to be done, control office hours, or assume liability stemming from the independent contractor's performance. The associate-independent contractor relationship must be properly constructed to avoid incurring significant taxes, interest charges, and penalties. This is the province of an attorney with experience in such transactions.

HYBRID

A hybrid form of employment may include any combination of the following part-time schemes: (1) serving as an associate-employee or associate-independent contractor in an established endodontic practice, (2) starting your own practice, and (3) serving as an independent contractor in one or more general dentists offices. The latter will not likely result in a stable long-term practice situation, and should be viewed as a temporary solution, at best. The value of this arrangement is that it can serve as an interim step that can financially sustain the new endodontist until he or she builds a referral base.

Winning Management Practices

Forming and operating an endodontic practice is a complex and nuanced undertaking. The notion that we are simply a profession and not also a business seeking financial success is to miss the opportunity to generate fair compensation for your knowledge and professional skills. Generating a healthy revenue stream is the only way to ensure that you can continue to provide the most advanced care available. In fact, Joe Blaes, editor of *Dental Economics*, states that "it is impossible for you to stay in practice without a reasonable profit."[17] How do you learn the basics of practice profitability? By studying other businesses to gain insights about operations management and best practices.

What really works in the business world? In the landmark Evergreen Project, 50 leading academics, led by William Joyce, Professor of Strategy and Organizational Theory at Dartmouth College's Tuck School of Business, and Nitin Nohria, the Richard P. Chapman Professor of Business Administration at the Harvard Business School,[18] looked at 40 narrowly defined industries with $100 million to $6 billion in gross revenue and determined that winning companies adopted four primary management practices and two of four secondary management practices. Adapting this scheme to endodontic practice, the following sections summarize the study's findings:

PRIMARY MANAGEMENT PRACTICES

1. Strategy: Develop a step-wise plan to clarify your individual situation and develop a program to achieve future goals:
   a. A clear value proposition: What patients and referrers want most are *results* and *process quality*. That the endodontic treatment works and the patient can maintain their dentition and the treatment meets or exceeds the specifications of the referring doctor is only the "results" part of the equation. "Process quality" measures how the patient was treated. This is the experiential piece, and endodontic treatment is usually defined by patients in these terms. At the end of the day, when patients ask the question "How was I treated?," they are actually assessing process quality. Remember, there is no reasonable way for patients to easily understand the five points of the technical side of treatment.
   b. "Outside-In": To put this concept in perspective for our profession, it means understanding what your patients and referring doctors want and creating systems to satisfy those needs, from their perspective. Finding out exactly what patients and referrers deeply value and how to deliver it with passion is the holy grail of practice excellence.
   c. Continually measure and refine: Practice metrics can be an important indicator of your success. Understanding the referral process, measuring new patient referrals, and tracking "fading referrals" are examples of ways to measure the success of your efforts (Sidebar 1).

MEASURING CUSTOMER DEFECTIONS

In today's competitive marketplace, success in a referral-based business like endodontics is all about building relationships. According to Frederick Reichheld,[105] a business consultant and author of *The Loyalty Effect*, a business invests in customers, and premature customer (e.g., referring doctor) defections will ultimately result in diminished profitability.

Reducing defections (also referred to as "fading referrals") begins with measuring the rate of defection. According to Reichheld,[106] in another article in the *Harvard Business Review*, "customer defection is one of the most illuminating metrics in business." Some defections are normal in any business and in rare cases they can even be welcomed. A percentage of referring doctors will never be loyal and can even diminish morale and increase stress if they continue to send patients. But, such welcomed defections are few and far between. In most instances, it is important to preserve and encourage continued referrals. So, what action should you take if a referral begins to fade? The best approach is to contact the individual who has stopped making referrals and find out why. Always avoid getting defensive, practice active listening, and no matter what you hear, thank them for their time and candor. You may not get these referrers back in the fold, but you may learn how to keep others from defecting in the future.

Once you loose a referrer, replacing him or her will not be easy nor inexpensive. In fact, Reichheld's survey of 100 companies in 24 industries found that longer customer retention led to increased profits. No surprise here. Many companies make the mistake of not even keeping track of customer defections because they are unaware of the cost to replace them. And many business owners find that customer defections are hard to track, especially when referrals are based on business cycles and sometimes involve only partial defections. Measuring defections can be unpleasant and remedial action is often difficult to accomplish. Even so, it is important to quantify such defections and set goals to improve those relationships.

Measuring referrals is a necessary part of operating a referral-based practice. Look for practice management software that analyzes referral trends within a given time period. It should take just a few mouse clicks to get the information. Some industries report that reducing defections "by as little as five points...can double profits,"[106] and monitoring the "fading referral" to measure declining business will yield valuable insights that need to be addressed immediately.

The most profitable companies champion customers, recognizing that the longer a company keeps its customers, the more successful it will be. Loyal customers result in more profits, because loyal customers buy more, take less of a company's resources and are willing to pay a price premium. Why? Because they do not want to start with new people either. Best of all, loyal referrers and patients are more likely to refer new patients.

Table 2 The Focusing Matrix

What you do best	"Stop"	"Go"
What you do not do best	"Stop"	"Go with Partners"
	What your patients do not value	What your patients value

The Focusing Matrix demonstrates the convergence of what you do best and what your patients and referring doctors value most. For example, take one-visit endodontic procedures. These are valued by your patients and referrers and are more efficient for your office to perform. Put them in the "Go" category. If a procedure falls in the "Stop" category, consider a change.

   d. Keep focused: Understand your core business and focus on the convergence of what you do best and most profitably with what your patients really want. Consider a focusing matrix showing the relationship between what you do best and what your patient's value most (Table 2). When the two converge, you have a winner!

2. Execution: Deliver products and services that consistently meet patient expectations. Every business tries to set their customer's expectations. This research project has demonstrated that consistently satisfying customer expectations is far more important than exceeding expectations in one or more areas and falling below the grade in another. The customer will judge and remember the worst performing parameter or interaction, and his or her negative experience will overshadow any exceptional service provided. Another way to improve is to eliminate waste and increase productivity by constantly evaluating operations and making changes that improve the bottom line.

3. Culture: Inspire to do your best. Every office employee looks to the doctor(s) and office administrators for leadership. We must continually refine and measure our care and motivate the members of our office team to strive for excellence. Rewarding achievement with acknowledgement and remuneration based on performance will create a fulfilling workplace.

4. Structure: Simplify. Placing the best employee(s) close to the customer is another way top businesses achieve outstanding results. While most businesses promote the highest achievers to the next level in a vertically structured organization, this action usually takes the best and brightest and moves them away from the customers who interact with the company. So consider this action carefully when reorganizing your staff. Keeping the vertical structure will simplify administration and will allow the staff with the best people skills to stay closest to those they serve.

SECONDARY MANAGEMENT PRACTICES

The Evergreen study also found a correlation between any two of the following four secondary attributes:

1. Talent: The value of developing and keeping great employees cannot be underestimated; most winning companies reward exemplary employees to keep them motivated. These rewards can take many forms, among them salary, benefits, vacation, and probably most importantly a safe and inspiring working environment that drives personal achievement.

2. Innovation: Advanced services and technologies are critical to your success. Working with sophisticated practice management software, advanced communications between the office and co-therapists, and treatment technologies such as microscopes and digital radiographic are increasingly important and expected.

3. Leadership: Trust and confidence in top leadership is one of the single most reliable predictors of employee satisfaction. Leaders help employees understand the organization's overall business strategy and how they can contribute to achieving key business objectives. Sharing information and communicating about performance in a small office environment by non-professional HR managers/doctors can be challenging. To improve overall performance, rewarding individual employees and managers for leadership and creativity is a must.

4. Mergers and partnerships: Partnering with another practice to maximize the value of diverse talents is often overlooked in cottage industries and small businesses. Strategic alliances and mergers of individual practices to provide better coverage and economies of scale can produce benefits. This can take the form of an alliance between several endodontic practices or the combining of an endodontic practice with a periodontal practice, and so on. Establishing a solo group where two or more endodontists practice in the same facility with shared common areas and administration but separate practice entities is another possibility to economize and protect against the consequences of disability or death.

How to Get Started

Opening a new office for the practice of endodontics will require many months of planning. The project should begin with identifying your objectives. Do you want to establish a boutique or niche practice or a more traditional practice? Will you accept insurance assignment or participate with a preferred provider network or health maintenance organization? To succeed, you will need to make sure your practice will be appropriate to the needs and expectations of your community.

Begin by creating a business plan, develop a timeline, and establish an office location that will accommodate the unique requirements of an endodontic practice. Because endodontic offices require special planning, the time needed for construction and installation will far exceed the time and expense required for a typical non-healthcare facility. Ranking variables like location, parking, home-office travel times, amenities, and proximity to other medical and dental practitioners are necessary parts of the decision-making process. To get this right, you will need the services of an attorney, accountant, banker, commercial real estate broker, architect, interior designer, dental equipment supplier(s), and computer and telephone system engineers.

FIRST THINGS FIRST: CREATING A BUSINESS PLAN

The two essential elements of a good business plan are a winning vision and a clear path to profitability. To borrow money, carefully design the plan to "sell" your vision to a skeptical bank loan officer. The business plan should include the following:

1. A persuasive introduction to describe your planned practice, including features and benefits, and a request for funds.
2. A statement of the purpose.
3. A detailed description of how an endodontic practice works, office location overview, whether you will have employees, and who will provide your equipment and supplies.
4. An analysis of your market demographics (who are your patients?).
5. An evaluation of your main competitors.
6. A description of your brand strategy and how you will use marketing to drive your brand to top-of-mind-status (see "Branding: Enabling Your Practice Success").
7. A resume setting forth your educational and professional accomplishments.
8. Detailed financial information, including your best estimates of start-up costs, revenues and expenses, and your ability to make a profit.

Help in designing a business plan is available from the U.S. Small Business Administration (SBA) and online software guides like Business Plan Pro (Palo Alto Software, Eugene, OR). Focus on creating a polished plan that can be presented to several bankers and their loan boards for consideration. The better it looks, the more likely you will get a favorable loan offer. If you are self-financing, concentrate on financial projections, because the cost of services, sales revenue, and profit will all figure prominently in how much you will have to invest. Remember that starting a new professional business will require money to market the practice. Very few offices today, especially in crowded urban markets, can just hang out a shingle and expect to be busy. Good planning requires making educated guesses about income and spending, based on the following projections:

1. A break-even analysis to determine if you will make money:
   a. Projected collections
   b. Fixed and variable costs (estimate)
   c. Gross profit
   d. Break-even revenue
2. A start-up cost estimate to evaluate the amount of money needed just to open the door on the first day of practice.
3. A profit-and-loss analysis to refine the month-to-month projection of profits for the first year of practice.
4. A cash flow projection to ensure that even if your business is profitable, there is enough money on hand to operate from month to month.

No business plan would be complete without consideration of what business structure the practice will take. Keep in mind that this decision will affect your personal liability as well as the amount of tax you and your organization will pay. Whether you choose a "C" or "S" corporation, a limited liability company (LLC), limited liability partnership (LLP), general partnership, or sole proprietorship, your attorney and accountant will need to provide advice.

CHOOSING AN OFFICE LOCATION

Choosing where to practice is one of the most important decisions a new practitioner will make. Family considerations, personal preferences, weather, career opportunities for your spouse, and lifestyle issues are among some of the considerations that should govern your decision. Establishing a successful endodontic practice will require a location that will provide enough new patients to support the practice's expenses and result in the best opportunity for you to utilize your skills. Because the number of dentists in postdoctoral endodontic programs continues to increase faster than any other dental specialty,[19] practice location will prove to be a key predictor of success. Studies by Wright,[20] and Solomon and Glickman,[21] using sophisticated statistical analysis, clearly establish the relationship between the location of general dentists and the location of endodontic offices. Because endodontic practice is referral-based, the proximity of a referral network, followed by adequate population and other criteria such as socio-economic characteristics, are all variables that will affect the economics of your practice.

The economic potential of your proposed office location should be appraised to determine its professional desirability. People living in similar neighborhoods generally exhibit similar lifestyle and spending profiles. One of the easiest ways to learn about your clientele is to understand their geodemographical classifications. These data, available from vendors like Business Information Solutions (ESRI BIS, an internationally recognized provider of information services), will allow analysis of clinic site locations by creating a visual depiction of data which is spatially referenced to the earth, also known as geographic information systems (GIS) mapping. GIS-generated information will greatly improve your business planning and allow you to base location and growth decisions on the best available information. A new type of classification introduced by ESRI BIS, called the "Community Tapestry" segmentation system, provides an accurate, detailed description of America's neighborhoods. U.S. residential areas are divided into 65 segments based on demographic variables such as age, income, home value, occupation, household type, education, and other consumer behavior characteristics. ESRI BIS offers market surveys that provide a detailed look at data within various radii around a given geographical address. This is called a "Market Profile Report" and is based on the updated U.S. Census, including 5-year projections. Reports can also be ordered with specific filters, such as a plot of all general and specialty practices in the zones of interest. You can find them on the Web at http://www.esribis.com. Also, ESRI BIS offers a free Web-based lookup of demographic data based on ZIP codes, but ZIP codes will not provide adequate specificity for making a final decision.

Further analysis can be performed by purchasing a list from your state dental society in Excel format, and then using a program such as Microsoft MapPoint to plot the data. Of course, there is no guarantee of success with any particular location, but a poor choice may lead to economic hardship. It is critical that you create a comprehensive plan to assure that your proposed site is architecturally and financially sound. Plan on specifying about 400 to 500 square feet per operatory in your new office.[22]

According to Gregory L. Morgan,[23] Managing Director of Sperry Van Ness – Morgan Realty Advisors, specify your geographic parameters, space requirements, parking availability, modes of access, and street exposure if applicable. Then engage an experienced commercial real estate leasing professional to canvas your prospective area and match your requirements with properties using real estate databases, brokerage relationships, publications, and the Internet. Comparing the economics and qualitative differences between properties and market information is where a commercial real estate leasing professional will provide essential guidance. Hopefully, you will have several options to review, creating a competitive atmosphere where multiple landlords are competing for your business. As you will learn early on, the effective rent can be based on one of several formulas, and extending these costs over many years can add up to a significant difference. Even if you are especially focused on one of these locations, it is important to go through the exercise of requesting proposals from several property owners and managers. Some landlords will offer concessions in areas where others will not, helping you to identify the most important considerations for your business: property location, economics, and functionality. Analyzing the proposals will then help you request aggressive but fair economic concessions from the finalists based on what other competing landlords have offered.

The next step is to decide on the number of operatories and what supporting facilities will be required. Engage an architect or dental office designer to draw basic floor plans and confirm that adequate plumbing and electrical infrastructure needs are met. Now, with several lease proposals in hand, you should meet with a real estate attorney for further analysis.

According to leasing attorney Charles J. Levin,[24] some of the attributes of a successful commercial lease are summarized as follows: (1) lease terms and conditions are expressed in a complete written lease with no oral agreements and understandings; (2) all contingencies are considered and resolved; (3) lease terms and conditions are aligned with your needs; (4) the leased premises suits your needs; (5) you have protected yourself from operating expense charges that are not customary and you understand what to expect with those that are passed through; (6) there are no defects like possible noise, odor, vibration, or other similar problems; (7) you have warranties protecting you from issues such as zoning, water quality, mold, asbestos, Americans with Disability Act (AwDA), and so on; (8) you have thoroughly reviewed the build-out letter with your architect and contractor and included all necessary details in the lease; (9) you have expressly excluded certain types of objectionable tenants from being in the building or on your floor (e.g., music school, barbeque restaurant, and social security office); (10) you have flexibility to renew, expand, and terminate; (11) you have option to purchase, if appropriate; (12) other tenants have no major complaints; (13) you have looked into the future and considered all of the possibilities with respect to issues such as fire and casualty, condemnation, changes in governmental requirements, assignment and subletting, and the many other issues that can arise; and (14) you, your commercial real estate leasing professional, attorney, and architect have all reviewed your office selection. Lastly, create a ticker file in your office management software as a reminder of notification dates memorialized in your lease.

Levin further emphasizes the importance of you being engaged in all aspects of the negotiations and that you understand the significance of each and every provision of the lease as it is being negotiated. It is a mistake to hand the lease to your attorney for negotiation and expect that your interests are being protected without your involvement. There are many aspects of the lease that combine both business and legal issues that will have a profound effect upon the success of the practice. The selection of an experienced commercial real estate leasing professional and real estate attorney cannot be overemphasized because of the complex and nuanced nature of leasing space and the long-term and potentially devastating implications of getting it wrong.

Once the lease is executed, the next step is contacting the telephone company to obtain a telephone number and secure a listing in the local phone directory. Many telephone providers will allow you to select a unique telephone number without charge or for a small fee. Generally, it is only necessary to secure one number, which will serve as your main trunk line. Additional numbers can be secured at a later time for use with multi-line phone systems, to avoid paying for reserving hidden numbers prior to the opening of the office. Today, most offices will have a choice between several trunk line providers and systems, such as copper wire or fiber optic. Use of Internet phone services over fiber-optic connections, such as Voice over IP, is becoming more popular, and packaged with Internet connectivity and television services, may prove a viable alternative to traditional service.

After securing a telephone number and phone book listing, order the practice management software and a computer workstation which will become the front desk system. Once setup, this workstation can be located off-site to configure your practice management software and allow training of new employees. Every endodontic practice, including a de novo practice, must have practice management software to manage appointments, prescriptions, reports, and other communications with referrers, not to mention the financial aspects of treatment and insurance.

CREATING A WINNING OFFICE DESIGN

Although building a new office from an empty shell is a daunting challenge, it provides the opportunity to set up the office to your specifications, within budget and space constrains. A key element to insuring success is the early involvement of your design team—and the design team starts with your architect or dental design firm. Try to choose an architect who is familiar with the design of medical facilities, the AwDA (Americans with Disabilities Act)[25] standards, hygiene requirements, and your local building codes. By helping you define the building project, architects can provide meaningful guidance for the contractor and other construction professionals. They can conduct site studies, help secure planning and zoning approvals, perform a variety of other pre-design tasks. Evaluate for handicapped patients, transportation, parking, and general convenience. When experienced architects are involved at the earliest planning stage, they gain opportunities to understand your business, develop creative solutions, and propose ways to reduce costs. The long-term result is a facility that adds to the productivity and image of the practice. Specialty architects who design just dental or healthcare facilities are also an excellent option, and the more endodontic offices they have designed, the better probability that all details will be considered. The American Institute of Architects[26] provides good resources on their Web site and lists numerous standard agreement forms that can be tailored to the types of services that are required.

Steven Covey's[27] maxim "begin with the end in mind," plays a large part in creating your desired outcome. What do you want your office to look like? How will patients and referring doctors be best served? Of course, ownership of your space in either a condominium or a stand-alone building that you are purchasing or building will require special considerations.

After the plans are approved by the building owner, your architect and/or dental designer will be responsible for meeting with you and any interested contractors to explain the scope of the project and solicit a quote for construction. The following architectural drawings and specifications will need to be available: (1) site plan; (2) demolition plan, if applicable; (3) reflected ceiling plan; (4) mechanical plan, for example, smoke/fire detectors and fire annunciators, sprinkler system, heating, and cooling; (5) electrical plan, for example, power, telephone, and computer installation; (6) plumbing plan; (7) millwork; and (8) finish schedule, for example, flooring, wall coverings, and paint. The contactor will generally be responsible for getting approval from local building officials to begin construction.

Designing the office for new and even future technologies will require some coordination between the various planners of your space. The wires and cables must be installed and integrated for the practice management system, digital radiography, entertainment, power, fire and smoke annunciators, security systems, and climatic systems.

Design Aesthetics

According to Schmitt and Simonson,[28] "aesthetics is one of the major satisfiers in consumers' experiential worlds." They state that intangibles like experiences become key selling points when services are perceived as the same across an industry.

How can Starbucks charge over $4 for a cup of coffee? It is because they provide experiences that customers can see, hear, touch, and feel—experiences that add value and allow for premium pricing. In the same way, your practice will become identified with certain traits that create a practice image, requiring "a careful mapping of a strategic vision to create sensory stimuli and communications that evoke that vision – that instantiate the identity".[29] It is important to establish a style that is consistent throughout everything your practice does, from your Web site, to your brochure, to the design of the office interior. Bloch,[30] in his research to conceptualize consumer reactions to a product's design, says there are three basic consumer responses, namely, "cognitive, affective and behavioral". He goes on to state that product form—or in this case office aesthetics—influences behavioral responses through cognitive and affective responses and are based on individual tastes and preferences.

Research in the organizational sciences has shown a direct relationship between office design and impression management. The physical environment will convey social messages to your patients. Consider designing with positive visual impact, such as added accent lighting, dry-wall soffits in key areas, upgraded ceilings, an enhanced level of detail and color balance, pleasant artwork and furnishings, and fabrics to further establish your desired image. Keep in mind that some businesses, such as Starbucks, have left the traditional marketing to their competitors, differentiating themselves through the inviting "look" of their hip aesthetic that evokes a satisfying experience.[30] Some of the "don'ts" when it comes to office design are creating physiological barriers, that is, sliding glass enclosures between patients and the patient coordinator, showcasing your hobbies; unclean, inexpensive, or misarranged furniture; and off-putting signs in the reception area [a big no-no, with the exception of a Health Insurance Portability and Accountability Act (HIPAA) notice, if applicable]. Signs that tell patients about office policies, in general, are unwelcome reminders of what your office personnel should have advised either verbally, or in the office's literature or Web site in the first place.

Branding: Enabling Your Practice Success

Dental practice begins as a journey after dental school with little or no training in the business aspects of practice. Unfortunately, talent and education alone are not enough to ensure success in our increasingly competitive healthcare marketplace. Getting and keeping patients in our endodontic practices will undoubtedly become more challenging, especially in mature urban settings. In order to develop long-term, directed growth, we must learn to manage our practice building efforts through trial and error, intuition, reading, continuing education, and use of management consultantancies.

Before we address the ins and outs of practice operations, we should first explore the case for concern, the meaning of branding, and ultimately how to build a brand-driven culture within your organization. At the end of the day, building your brand in a way that energizes all referrers, patients, vendors, and employees must become the mantra of your operational strategy.

THE CASE FOR INCREASED CONCERN

In the United States, we are facing many new challenges in private endodontic practice. Endodontics is one of the smaller clinical specialties in dentistry, with about

4,000 practicing clinicians in 2007, and a population to endodontist ratio of about 75,000 individuals per endodontist. However, with our population projected at 340 million in 2035, and with endodontists graduating and leaving practice at approximately the same rate as today, we are projected to have approximately 6,580 active clinicians or a population to endodontist ratio of 54,270 individuals per endodontist. At current graduation rates, the number of dentists completing endodontic residency programs has been increasing faster than the number of general practitioners, and as a consequence, the practitioner to endodontist ratio has also been declining. The vast majority of endodontists practice in the Northeast and West Coast areas, and if misdistribution trends continue, the number of over-served areas will continue to increase with resultant case-load challenges. Other factors, such as the higher relative failure rates in restorative materials like resins, general dentist busyness, and increased productivity among all practitioners will continue to be some of the issues affecting the profession.[31] A report by the DTA concluded that up to 40% of all practices are not reaching their full production. By the year 2010, it has been postulated that less than 40% of all dental care will be provided by non-owner doctors rather that more traditional practice models.[32] The competitive landscape will continue to change, according to Eric Solomon,[33] Professor of Public Health Sciences at the Baylor College of Dentistry, in his *Dental Economics* article "The Future of Dentistry." He predicts that the number of specialists in dentistry will increase from the current level of 20% to 27% by the year 2020," leading to an increasingly competitive marketplace for the new specialist. The days of opening a new office in a major metropolitan area and instantly generating a sustainable financial model are becoming increasingly rare.

Increasing competition, demographic shifts, market saturation, bunching of endodontic practices in already crowded urban centers, insurance company control, and an insidious lack of customer loyalty will always challenge endodontic practices in the most desirable markets. Central to meeting these challenges is creating a brand identity that consistently conveys our special skills to referring doctors and patients. What follows is a summary of branding basics, with an emphasis on the connection between best business practices and the dental profession.

UNDERSTANDING YOUR BRAND

What is a brand? A brand is simply a *promise*—the expectations that exist in each customer's mind about a product or service. According to John Hagel,[34] a business strategy consultant, in the past, a brand used to say, "If you buy this product or buy from my company, you can rely on me because of the attributes attached to the brand." He goes on to state that we are seeing "a new kind of branding emerge, a much more customer-centric branding, where the promise is, 'I know you as an individual customer better than anyone else, and you can trust me to assemble the right products or services to meet your individual needs.'" Brands are imbedded in our minds and used in our daily lives, like "FedEx that photo to San Francisco." Your brand is your personality; brands are the reason that companies exist, and they are based on multiple experiences over time. These experiences, from the patient intake process through treatment and post-treatment interactions, need to be delivered with consistency and be perceived as unequaled relative to the competition. In short, your patient's and referrer's experiences need to result in deep, trust-based relationships which generate loyalty. Your brand should reflect a high level of education, proficiency, and confidence that you are offering the best care.

While brands speak to the mind, brand identity or brandmark is the sensory expression of a brand. You can touch it, hear it, feel it, and it increases the customer's consciousness and builds loyalty. Your brandmark can include a name, design, or symbol that visually represents the value of your practice beyond its functional purpose. The velocity of life in the future will inevitably demand that brands leverage the power of symbols. Whether it is a photograph, mark, graphic, or typographical image, which can be as simple as the practice name written in an artful font, symbols can trigger recall and stimulate emotion. A brand identity helps to manage perceptions of your practice and differentiates it from other practices.

Offices must deliver their services to create value that relies on understanding results and process quality from the referrer's and patient's perspective. When it comes to understanding your clients, according to Marty Neumeier,[35] a branding consultant, "Brand is not what you say it is. It is what they say it is." Although branding is a simple concept, it is not that easy to accomplish. It takes a long-term commitment and hard work.

In the early 1990s, brands were a series of marketing tactics like the advertising icons made famous by Nike, Alka Seltzer, and even KFC. Brands now have strategic importance, brands result in deep, trust-based relationships which in turn garners customer's loyalty. Products and services need to be delivered with consistently high level of quality and value, perceived to be unparalleled relative to the competition.

Adopting this brand-driven approach, "where making the brand the central focus of the organization clarifies what is 'on-brand and what is off-brand'".[36] Then the entire organization needs to adopt this brand-driven approach to guide critical business decisions as well as determine appropriate staff behaviors. Building a brand-based culture is simply not a quick fix program. It requires a solid dedication to the organization's brand vision and an understanding that branding cannot be overemphasized an overall strategy.

As we learned in the beginning of this section, a brand is a promise that defines a patients' value proposition that both their treatment and their experience will be as expected or better than expected. "It has meaning, prestige, and presence, and it helps confirm what is expected".[37] The treatment performed must be unrivaled and the patient and referrer experience must be unequalled. According to Prophets 2002 Best Practices Study,[38] there are three main goals of any branding strategy: (1) increasing customer loyalty, (2) differentiating your organization from the competition, and (3) establishing market leadership. Let us look at each of these goals and how they affect practice success.

1. Increasing customer loyalty: A classic study by Xerox in the 1990s (Figure 1) looked at satisfaction and found that highly satisfied customers were six times more likely to repurchase a Xerox product than a merely satisfied customer.[39] This means that every highly satisfied patient will demonstrate repeat behavior and require much less effort on your part to maintain their loyalty than patients who are just along for the ride. Even more important, a patient who repeats their behavior is much more likely to continue repeating it, becoming more profitable as time goes on. For example, it takes the average credit card company 3 to 4 years of marketing effort to attract a new customer, or 7 to 10 times the cost of merely maintaining an existing customer. An increase in customer loyalty of just 2% will equal the equivalent of a 10% cost reduction program, and an increase of 5% in loyal customers can deliver 95% greater profitability over the lifetime of that customer.[40] Even more striking is that 50% of customers will try a new product or service from a preferred brand because of the implied endorsement, credibility, and trust.[41] According to Robinette et al.[42] of Hallmark Cards, Inc, "increased customer loyalty is the single most important driver of long-term profit-

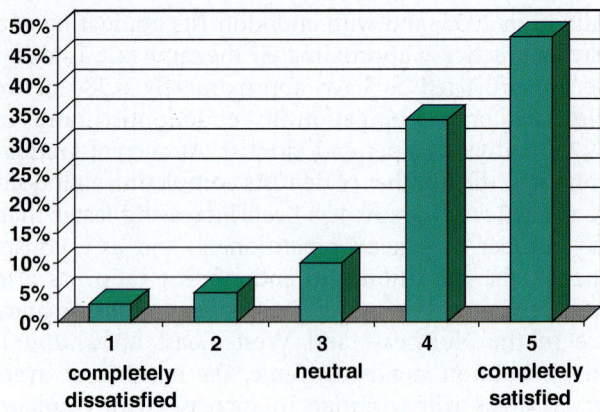

Figure 1 Customer Satisfaction Index. In this typical customer satisfaction index, completely satisfied customers, rated 5, were six times more likely to repurchase a product or service over the next 18 months than just merely satisfied customers, rated 4.[40]

ability." If we look at the lifetime value (LTV) of a top-tier referring doctor whose career spans 35 years, revenue generated will easily exceed $1.5 million. While calculating LTV is complex because of varying costs to acquire and maintain each customer, there is no doubt that looking at the "customer back" will allow formulation of strategies for each customer segment. Customer loyalty rules!

2. Differentiating your organization from the competition: If a customer cannot tell the difference between your service and another, they will buy on price. A practice needs to invest in the things that highlight a unique benefit to the customer and deliver it with skill and finesse, like a concierge at a fine hotel. Identify and build on the qualities or characteristics which make your practice distinctive.[43] Every customer, whether purchasing a car, hospital services, or endodontic care usually has a choice. Your job is to wind up in the referrers' final consideration set and then be chosen because of your unique capabilities. It can range from a high-tech approach using a Web based patient intake process to digital radiography and microscopic imaging to non-surgical revision therapy to diagnosing a difficult case. Remember that technology implementation costs money, so do not market your practice as the best in town and then price it low, because you are sending a mixed message and wasting some of your marketing dollars. Learn what characteristics

make you office distinctive. If you are going to be a brand, you must be inexorably focused on what you do that adds value.

3. Establishing market leadership: First and foremost, communicate that you are a specialist. Make sure that patients understand that you have undergone extensive post-graduate training. Use verbal and written communication to focus attention on continually improving outcomes with the latest science by using evidence-based treatment that leads to a painless procedure with the highest level of success possible. Reveal the hidden by using models, drawings, and microscopic/radiographic imaging to increase the patient's understanding of the procedure. For example, drawing a scaled diagram for each patient at the end of their visit will demonstrate your special skills. Be sure to let patients know that treatment you perform through the microscope is reflected through a mirror, so that every hand movement is reversed. Use technology to create a value proposition for all stakeholders—defined by modern management science as everyone with an interest in what the organization does, such as clients, employees, and vendors. Demonstrate your proficiency both singly and as a team, reaffirm the patient's choice of endodontic treatment over extraction by addressing the benefits of decreasing dental disease to improve overall health, show sensitivity to patient's mental and physical comfort, provide impeccable service, and offer superb facilities.[44]

One of the best ways to establish market leadership is to use state-of-the-art technology to create value in the referrer's and patient's mind that they can see and understand. Every patient treatment communication should reflect your technological competence. Digital radiographs and photographic images along with cogent narratives of treatment should reflect your commitment to the latest technology and help operationalize your brand. Performing a state-of-the-art procedure and then communicating the results by sending a film-based image and a few handwritten notes misses the opportunity to maximize your image as technologically sophisticated. This leads us to the next section about how to develop brand-building programs that are the most cost efficient, effective, and credible.

There are many ways to help define a brand. Volunteerism and community outreach programs are valuable ways to "give back" and also help your stakeholders understand your brand philosophy. The list of opportunities to partner with other professionals or community organizations is endless. Here are a few examples: (1) teaching at a dental school, (2) getting involved in philanthropic and civic organizations, (3) providing continuing education, (4) sponsoring a blood drive with the American Red Cross (Sidebar 2), and (5) partnering with another dental office to benefit a community program like a soup kitchen, food bank, and so on.

USING TECHNOLOGY TO OPERATIONALIZE YOUR BRAND

Although all endodontic practices provide basic specialty services to patients and referring doctors, it is the value-added services that can help differentiate your practice from competing practices. Research continues to link business success and professional achievement with developing long-term appeal and credibility. And adopting proven technologies is one of the most visible and reliable ways to create a positive impression and to continually engage patients, referrers, and staff, to say nothing of the clinical advantages.

Patients expect a high-tech approach to treatment. In fact, the National Health Information Infrastructure (NHII) is establishing a national electronic information network for heath care. The NHII proposes to implement a computer-based patient record for most Americans by 2014.[45] So how will your practice measure up? With the expanding use of technology in every aspect of life, patients expect their healthcare encounters to include the newest technologies. Use of the Internet to improve patient intake, receiving electronic receipt of patient pre-treatment radiographs and information, digital radiography, computerized charting, microscopes with imaging capability, instant communication of your treatment reports by email, online pharmacology information at the chairside, and music and entertainment options are all ways that your office can project a technologically advanced practice image. The list goes on and on, but the importance of differentiating your practice cannot be overestimated, and one of the best ways is with useful and visible technology.

"A brand strategy is a statement of the brand's sustainable competitive advantage, usually consisting of a demographic and psychographic description of the intended customers and the benefits they get from the brand.".[46] A brand-driven approach will create customer loyalty that will ultimately translate into a competitive advantage and increased profitability. Modern management science defines everyone with

OFFICE DESIGN

Appealing to consumer needs has defined marketing for the past one hundred years. According to Abraham Maslow[107] in his book *Motivation and Personality*, once basic consumer needs like survival and safety are satisfied, higher order needs like experiential and aesthetic needs become increasingly important. A simplified version of his thesis depicts a pyramid with experiential and aesthetic needs at the top, which leads to the false conclusion that aesthetics is a luxury that humans care about only when they are wealthy. To the contrary, Virginia Postrel,[108] in her book *The Substance of Style*, states that "aesthetics is not a luxury, but a universal human desire." She contends that humans do not wait for all of their lower order needs to be satisfied before wanting aesthetic environments and products. She goes on to say that "there is no pyramid of needs, where each layer depends on what we already have," but rather we make important decisions every day based on our sensory experiences. These experiences are based on the precept that appearance counts and that aesthetic value is real and gaining even more importance in the twenty-first century. According to Postrel, we have entered the "Age of Aesthetics" when beauty and style are found everywhere in market economies. Simply put, increasingly sophisticated consumers demand "an enticing, stimulating, diverse and beautiful world."[109] To this end, a coordinated and appropriate office aesthetic is important, and color, texture, sounds, lighting, and artwork will all lead to an identity that will satisfy patients experiential and aesthetic needs.

Creating positive attitudes and beliefs about your organization and its services will be influenced by how you deal with your brand identity. The overall impression of your practice will often depend on the management of the themes inherent in individual identity elements that must be coordinated and designed to convey your brand characteristics.[110] Themes are an expression of your organization's core values or mission and are typically created by graphic designers, interior designers, architects, and marketing experts.

The level of finishes you choose should follow a consistent design theme and may include (1) lighting accent fixtures; (2) dry-wall soffits and upgraded ceilings; (3) color balanced walls and carpets; (4) coordinated artwork and furnishings; and (5) harmonized vinyl, fabrics, and custom finishes. Items that may cause negative visual impact include (1) showcasing your outside interests; (2) inexpensive furnishings and artwork; (3) unclean and misarranged furniture; and (4) signage that gives information that could be reasonably explained by the office staff. I hate reception area signs!

When designing or renovating your office, strongly consider what the patient sees and design with them in mind. An office design that resonates with patients is an important factor in establishing a patient's trust and helps them measure the quality of your treatment. Design themes should be repeated and coordinated to express a close association that increases recall and puts your practice in "top-of-mind status."

an interest in what the organization does, such as clients, employees, and vendors are called stakeholders. And each interaction with a stakeholder must be understood and prioritized along the entire treatment cycle.

How important are employees to the branding process? The success of any branding strategy depends on engaging employees around your brand in a way that encourages ownership of the brand. We have all experienced the exceptional employee who understands the brand's unique character and communicates it to all of the practice's patients, for example, patients, referring doctors, and fellow staff members. Employees who are engaged around the brand confirm that the patient, referrer, and the brand are the things to focus on. It facilitates recruiting and retention of employees and improves morale, aligning each team member with your brand promise. All employees need to think, speak, and behave in ways that create the kind of patient and referring doctor experience that has lasting impact. Assimilating your brand among the employees of your organization will ensure that all employees understand and embrace your brand and can translate this into actionable behavior. This way employees become brand advocates that understand how his or her impact can affect satisfaction and ultimately loyalty.

EMPLOYEE MOTIVATION AND MORALE

Every business relies on its organizational values to deliver on its brand promise. Employee attitudes and retention rely on a cohesive and upbeat culture. In order to develop brand advocates among all of your employees, your practice must first generate excitement about what it does. If each employee understands the benefits of modern endodontic treatment, it will reinforce their choice of employment. It can foster a sense of belonging to a profession they are passionately proud of. Employees need a leader who clearly understands the mission of the practice and can communicate his or her vision to each employee, patient, and referring doctor.

Brand-driven behaviors are enhanced by establishing a strong brand-based culture that is constantly fed and nurtured. It is crucial that your brand commitment is evident from the top down. If employees think that the practice leadership believes brand building is a priority, they will embrace it with the same passion. Each endodontist in the practice must communicate their endorsement of the practices' brand vision so that every employee experiences appropriate modeling at every level of stake holder interaction. Without leadership support and willingness to lead by example, the old Russian proverb "the fish always stinks from the head downwards," will resonate loudly.

Successful brand strategies require a clearly articulated vision of what your organization's brand stands for and how to link it to your overall business strategy. For example, if employees are to bring the brand to life, a strategic foundation must be established. One important first step is to establish well-defined roles for your most important asset—your employees. The notion that your patient coordinator can just answer the phone, assign appointment times, and have customers fill out forms in the reception area will not lead to a patient-centered practice model that will generate a loyal following. There needs to be a conversation between the patient, referring doctor's office, and your staff that is welcoming, informative, and nurturing. It is clear from the work of Silversen and the Werthlen Group that the better prepared a patient is before treatment, the more positive their treatment experience will be.[47] Of course, our treatment must conform to the best available practices of the day, but also must provide the key satisfiers of the patient experience. In Bernick's[48] *Harvard Business Review* article about corporate culture, Alberto-Culver was able to boost sales 50% by creating a more customer-centered approach. It embraced a management culture that listened to its employees, celebrating events like birthdays and anniversaries, and creating passionate advocates of their brand. Without brand advocates, your practice will just muddle along, reducing the likelihood of reaching your desired future.

BECOMING A LEARNING ORGANIZATION

When you go to a barber shop or a salon to get a haircut, you tell the barber or hair stylist exactly how you want your hair done. After a few visits to the same person, he or she will probably know just how to shampoo, cut and, blow-dry your hair. You have invested time and energy to tell them how you want it, and they will have likewise invested in learning your preferences. In fact, the more you tell them about what you want, the more likely you will revisit the same hair stylist, because, after all, you have invested in them to create a mutual relationship. We have all experienced this kind of service and will tend to frequent the same establishment time and again because they have established a learning relationship. If you were to switch to another barber or stylist, you would have to make that investment all over again. According to Pine et al.[49] in an article in the *Harvard Business Review*, customers "want exactly what they want – when, where and how they want it." And a company that aspires to give customers exactly what they want must establish a learning relationship that ensures that all stakeholders collaborate. Developing learning relationships with referrers is critically important. The more you know about how they want it (new patients sent right over for consultation, one-visit treatment whenever possible, etc.), the greater chance that this referrer will continue to use your services. If you think about the cost of replacing one referrer with another, consider their lifetime value (LTV). LTV is the sum of the stream of profits attributable to this referrer. Take the average value of referrals in a year and multiply it by the projected number of years you intend to practice and you will see how important each referrer is to the bottom line.

New paradigms of patient care are emerging as the relationship between oral disease and systemic heath become clearer. Developing a learning relationship with physicians is an emerging area that can enhance your professional image with non-dental sources of referral. In order to continually differentiate your practice, consider practice-building strategies that incorporate the latest research in endodontics or health care in general. Liaising with other healthcare providers is a good way to promote improved health and communicate your brand identity. Study clubs, continuing education opportunities, one-on-one meetings, Web sites, and publications can create valuable brand advocates.

BRAND ASSIMILATION: PUTTING THE PROGRAM INTO ACTION

The most successful organizations divide brand assimilation into three phases: strategic development, foundation building, and implementation. First, develop a strategic plan that defines the scope and objectives of your program so that the right people and systems are identified to carry out your program. The second phase is foundation building, the process of aligning all employees around the central theme of your branding initiative through office workshops and reading. This is where each employee segment (e.g., chairside assistants and patient coordinators) learns about your brand initiatives and their role in communicating your message. The idea here is to guide behaviors that foster participation and allow all employees to understand the benefits of your key objectives. Implementation, the final phase, is where a range of tactics are employed to create key materials and talk about successes that will change employee behavior throughout the practice. As always, it is important to monitor the responses to your program and make changes as necessary.

Establishing a brand assimilation program will lead to a number of changes, but at what cost? How do you measure success? The first hurdle is to make sure that your employees understand your brand initiative. They have to be invested in developing significant relationships with your patients. When your employees assimilate your brand, you can begin to implement an action plan that markets your brand. One effective program can be an orientation luncheon for a referring office. Have all of the referrer's office staff join your staff for a catered luncheon, conduct a brief office tour, and present a short program to let them know how you welcome new patients and how good communication between your offices can build patient confidence. The practice should strive to highlight the ways that both practices can work together.

Changes in organizational culture do not happen quickly. It takes a considerable amount of leadership and vision to promote meaningful changes to employee behavior. But the payoff will be a strong brand that will resonate with patients and referrers and help excite employees. This will ultimately result in increased loyalty.

While the detailed application of these disciplines is beyond the scope of this chapter, it is instructive to look at the relationship between providing services and recognizing the link between loyalty and profitability. The service-profit chain provides just such a model for operating in the medical environment. This is where leadership develops a dedicated team that provides superb service to patients that go on to develop loyalty to your organization.

When customers are highly loyal, there are minimal considerations of other brands. In the Xerox study quoted earlier, a survey of 430,000 customers revealed that highly satisfied customers were six times more likely to repurchase a Xerox product than merely satisfied customers.[50] What is the take-home from this study? Simply put, the key to business success is to create as many loyal referrers and patients as possible. Then to market your practice in a way that not only maintains your most loyal referrers and patients, but attempts to increase their ranks by "marketing below the gold." In other words, spend the bulk of your energy and precious marketing dollars taking a *merely* satisfied referrer and elevate them to the *extremely* satisfied category.

What are the benefits of loyalty? Patients will recommend your office to others. Hearing about how great your brand is from someone else will clearly be much more effective than self-promotion. Loyal patients are more accepting of new services, will say "no" to substitutes, and will pay a premium price for you to treat them. According to Passikoff,[51] over 50% of customers would pay a premium of 20 to 25% before they would switch to another brand. The benefits of developing loyal patients cannot be overemphasized. It takes 7 to 10 times the cost to gain a new customer than to keep an existing customer. So do whatever it takes to retain your current patients. Remember that a service needs to do what is expected, as expected, for as long as expected throughout the customer experience.

Build on what differentiates you from the competition. If a patient cannot tell the difference between one service and another, they will buy on price. A practice needs to invest in the things that highlight a unique benefit to the patient and referrer and deliver it with skill and finesse, like a concierge does in a fine hotel. After all, patients and referrers really want just two things: *results* and *process quality*. The results part of the equation applies to a great diagnosis or root canal procedure, where the patient feels that he or she received caring service and state-of-the-art care and the referrer feels confident to complete their restoration. Process quality is how the referrer and patient were treated. Was the patient seen on a timely basis? Was the referral handled seamlessly? Was their treatment compassionate, respectful, and safe? Did the procedure make the referring clinician seem like everyone was on the same team?

Today's consumers are increasingly brand-centric, and developing a brand identity is an important element in differentiating your services.[52] The problem is how to get started so that you can deliver your brand across every touchpoint and every stakeholder. Begin by formulating a brand strategy that creates visibility and recognition, unaided recall, top-of-mind status, deep customer relationships, and build differentiation.

Does this seem impossible? Collins and Porras[53] ask the question of how to use words that are not meaningless. All McDonald's corporate strategies are still guided by Ray Crock, McDonald's late founder's acronym, QSVC (Quality, Service, Cleanliness, and Value). Social psychology research indicates that when people publicly espouse a particular point of view, they become more likely to behave in a manner consistent with that point of view, even if they did not previously hold that belief. "Passion is a pretty fool proof test of whether a value is a core value," says Mike Moser,[54] an advertising and marketing expert. "It will help you include your heart in the decision-making process instead of just your head. Passion is what creates an emotional connection that transcends ads, public relations, brochures, or any other crafted messages that a company puts out."

The brand–customer relationship remains one of the most underleveraged and yet potentially powerful ways to drive sustainable, profitable, and long-term value back to your practice. First, determine your practice's core values. "Visionary companies tend to have only a few core values, usually 3 to 6...only a few values can be truly core values so fundamental and deeply held" that they will rarely change.[55]

Every office has a personality, so maximizing the benefits of your practice by showing genuine warmth and sincere concern for the patient's comfort are part of a thoughtful brand approach. Simple things like offering a warm, moist towel after treatment, providing appropriate music or video entertainment, and always using the most current technology are critical to establishing your brand personality.[56] Always make sure your brand personality is appropriate for your audience. Is it predominately male or female, blue collar, white collar, or service workers? Demographic studies have shown that endodontic patients are 60% female, average 48 years old, with 69% older than 40 years old.[57]

BRAND TOUCHPOINT OVERVIEW

Like most world-class businesses, the best endodontic practices operate with a clear vision to ensure peak performance. Just like an Olympic hurdler who mentally previews his or her performance before an event, from leaving the starting block to breaking the finish line, each element in the patient's visit must be carefully planned to ensure that patients feel they are in right place. Every staff member contributes to a successful visit by interacting with patients in a professional and caring way. It is useful here to visualize the patient and referring doctor experience as a continuum that begins with the introduction of endodontic therapy and only ends when the patient no longer needs your services. Dividing these interactions into three brand life-cycle stages, pre-treatment, treatment, and post-treatment procedures, each interaction can be choreographed to create a value chain that consistently fulfills the patient's clinical and experiential needs. These steps are really brand touchpoints, or the different ways your services interact with patients, referrers, and fellow staff members. The members of your staff have to serve as brand ambassadors, and each interaction with patients and referring doctors must be consistent to ensure the best experience.

In order to be truly successful, every functional area in your organization must be responsible for bringing the brand promise to life. There must be total alignment between your organization and your brand strategy, so that you control the critical interactions your patients and referrers, or stakeholders, have with your brand. What are all the touchpoints that exist between your brand and a current or potential stakeholder? How can you create a brand-driven organization? Outlined below are 10 brand touchpoints commonly found in endodontic practices. Please note that only 5 of the 10 involve the practitioner, and only one of these involves the practitioner alone. The importance of selecting an outstanding staff and taking control of all patient and referring doctor touchpoints cannot be overemphasized.

1. Patient is informed that they need endodontic treatment: The process begins when the patient is advised that he or she needs an endodontic consultation. Providing each referrer with a kit that contains your office brochure, referral forms, appointment cards, business reply envelopes, and Web site information will help introduce patients to your practice. According to Jack Silversin,[58] in his American Association of Endodontists-funded study to learn about the endodontist–patient relationship, the more your patients know about their treatment in advance, the better their treatment experience will be.
2. Patient calls for their first appointment: When a new patient calls for an appointment, complete a written telephone intake form or software-based pre-registration form, and set up an initial appointment. The telephone intake form should be designed with a sequenced set of questions in order to get efficiently critical information and document that all pre-treatment instructions were given.

Telephones are an essential part of the new patient experience, so make sure that proper telephone etiquette is practiced at all times. According to Albert Mehrabian,[59] a pioneer in communications research, there are three elements to any face-to-face communication: words, tone of voice, and body language. When it comes to feelings and attitudes, approximately 7% of meaning is in the words that are spoken, 38% of meaning is paralinguistic (the way that the words are said, like smiling on the phone), and 55% of meaning is in facial expression. The telephone creates an immediate communication gap because facial expression is not apparent, so the words and paralinguistic attributes take on added importance.

New patients should be queried about their status, because patients in pain and/or swelling are interested in immediate treatment and will generally accept scheduling at the convenience of the office. These patients will ideally need to be appointed the same day they call. Patients who have no discomfort or mild discomfort will generally be interested in convenience.

There are several methods available to provide pre-treatment information. Invite new patients to view your office Web site, where they can complete a secure patient registration and health history form. Web sites are necessary, if not a necessity, in today's healthcare environment. According to Harris Interactive, in a poll of 1,015 US adults conducted in 2005, 72% search the Internet for health-related information.[60] Almost 58% report looking for information often search the Internet for health topics and only 14% say that they hardly ever search health topics. Even more remarkable, 85% of those who have ever searched the Internet for health-related information did so in the last month of the study, and now averages seven searches each month per patient. What does this mean to the endodontic practitioner? Today, patients expect to meet their prospective practitioner on the Internet. Mailing, faxing, or emailing a "welcome kit" to patients with a welcome letter, brochure, procedure explanation, doctor biography, financial policy, registration, health history form, and map are also valuable ways to streamline new patient intake. Creating a Web site to provide patient education opportunities, contact information, and referral materials will further enhance pre-treatment preparation and provide the most convenient and cost-effective solution. While society is becoming more accustomed to automation and the advantages it provides, "dentists must be careful not to allow technology to interfere with the relationship between patient and doctor and the patient and staff."[61]

If the office must meet the requirements of HIPAA, all online transactions, as well as the office network, must be secure. If the office uses a wireless network, appropriate security measures are required.[62]

3. Patient arrives for first visit: When patients arrive for their initial visit, be prepared and give them a warm and sincere welcome. Patients can complete their registration on a reception area computer kiosk connected to the practice's network or the Internet, or fill out paper-based forms and view educational materials while in the reception area. This is the time for scanning any film-based radiographs or appending digitally transmitted images into your radiographic database, if applicable. Some endodontic software can allow front office personnel to indicate the patient's status from their arrival at the office and transitioning through treatment and finally discharge. Besides depicting the status of each patient in the office, recording the chair time for each type of procedure will allow create metrics that can be used to measure profitability.

4. Patient is escorted to operatory: Escorting patients to the operatory is an opportunity to connect staff and patient. Employee name badges and a policy of each staff member introducing himself or herself to the patient by name should be practiced at all times. Also, chance encounters in the office where a patient is within five feet should prompt a "hello" greeting.

When the patient is seated in the dental chair, the patient's individual record should appear on the chairside computer screen in the operatory, maintaining HIPAA compliance, and assuring the patient that your efforts will be focused on them. Once seated, the assistant should confirm that the patient has followed all pre-treatment instructions, including their antibiotic pre-medication regimen if any, other pre-treatment medications, and have eaten breakfast or lunch to ensure a normal blood glucose level, whichever is appropriate. Of course, staff should confirm that all prescribed medications have been taken on schedule, and if sedation is contemplated, an escort is present to accompany the patient after treatment completion. This is the time for your staff to tell the patient what comes next and set their expectations for their visit. Assuring that their comfort is of utmost importance, offering a blanket or pillow, describing what treatment will be performed, length of the visit, and so on are all important. Acknowledge and reassure the patient that his or her concerns will be addressed. This is also the time to project a safe practice image. Sanitize your hands in front of the patient or let them know you are leaving the operatory to wash. Wear proper clothing and limit masks, gloves, and other protective gear to the clinical areas of the office. It is incumbent on the endodontic practitioner to convey a sense of safety throughout each visit.[63]

This is the time for the dental auxiliary to record the chief complaint, history of present illness, medical history and review all current medications. Once the general area of interest is determined, the auxiliary should expose dental radiographs, record photographic images, take vital signs, answer questions, and, most importantly, comfort the patient. Each staff member should be dressed and groomed appropriately, scripted for this interaction, with the best answers to commonly asked questions to promote consistency and accuracy. Of course, all medications should be recorded in the patient's database so new prescriptions can be automatically checked for advised interactions and cautions.

5. Doctor consults with patient: After introduction by the dental assistant, you should establish eye contact, make sure the patient is comfortable, listen attentively without interrupting, and according to MaryJo Ludwig[64] Clinical Faculty, Department of Family Medicine at the University of Washington Hospital, "acknowledge and legitimize feelings, explain and reassure during examinations, and ask explicitly if there are other areas of concern." First impressions are important, and your first contact with the patient is no exception. Psychiatrists Leonard and Natalie Zunin,[65] stated in their book "Contact: The First Four Minutes," that, on average, there is only a short moment in time, a 4-minute window, "to grab someone's attention and establish credibility and rapport." These first impressions demonstrate our compassion, care, intelligence, attention to detail, and pride. Be sure to limit the time you spend with the computer at the expense of eye contact and personal interaction with the patient. Once the patient's dental needs and intake data are reviewed, the initial oral exam is completed, a discussion and informed consent can take place. According to Peter Sfikas,[66] chief legal counsel of the ADA, the ADA's Code of Professional Conduct requires dentists to "inform patients of proposed treatment and any reasonable alternatives in a manner that allows the patient to become involved in the treatment decision." Every dentist should understand the requirements of their state practice laws with regard to informed consent. In this regard, states differ greatly. In Pennsylvania, for example, a court ruling held that orthograde endodontic treatment was a surgical procedure requiring written informed consent, while treatment considered non-surgical in nature does not require informed consent. Conversely, courts in New Jersey require dentists to provide informed consent even for non-invasive procedures. Also, a patient's refusal of recommended treatment should be documented in writing to ensure that the patient comprehends the possible consequences of refusing treatment. After the discussion and informed consent processes are completed, any additional pre-operative issues should addressed. Any patient who has not eaten a timely meal and will receive local anesthetic should receive an appropriate nutrient supplement to avoid syncope from low blood glucose levels. Ensure® and Glucerna® are lactose-free drinks designed for occasional meal replacement and intended for non-diabetic and diabetic patients, respectively. If non-steroidal anti-inflammatory drugs or antibiotics are indicated, they can be dispensed at this time.

6. Doctor treats patient: Every effort should be made to include the patient in the treatment process. Confirm that all of the patient's questions are answered. Then treatment can be initiated along with documentation of the visit. If digital scheduling is available, patients can be reappointed while still in the operatory and their insurance information can be sent to the office financial coordinator via the network or directly to the insurance company, if the office LAN integrates with the Internet.

7. Doctor discharges patient: Once the treatment is completed, the final 4 minutes should focus on the patient and their post-operative instructions. Communicate that you are a specialist by drawing a scaled diagram for each patient at the end of their visit that explains the intricacy of your procedures. Use technology to create a value proposition for all patients. In the end, be sure to take every opportunity to complement the patient on their cooperative attitude. Medications can now be dispensed, as necessary, and prescriptions selected and sent to the printer.

8. Patient is escorted to front desk: Patients are then escorted to the office departure station and reintroduced by their escorting assistant to the patient coordinator. Sit-down departure stations at the front desk will serve to increase patient comfort and to better accommodate disabled patients. In some endodontic offices, advanced practice management software will allow the clinician or assisting staff to forward all pertinent billing statements and post-operative instructions to the front desk computer with a few mouse clicks.

9. Patient is checked out: Once the patient is brought to the departure station, they are asked the "1, 2, 3 questions": (1) The patient coordinator asks the

patient how they are feeling; (2) Next, the patient receives customized instructions, which outline their post-operative instructions and an explanation of check-up recommendations. Patients are then appointed for their next visit and receive any prescriptions and a patient satisfaction survey with a business reply form centered on the reverse side for mailing convenience; (3) Lastly, patients are asked to satisfy their financial obligation.

A business reply permit can be obtained from your local post office at a nominal cost. Patients can either fill out the form immediately (highest response rate) or return it by mail. If patients are invited to fill out the form in the office, a box should be available for the completed survey. Because people often feel awkward expressing their real views, this anonymity will improve compliance.

Measuring patient satisfaction will provide two main benefits: (1) it will allow patients to vent about issues that will ultimately affect their loyalty and their likelihood to return for additional treatment, and (2) surveys present valuable feedback about what really works and what doesn't. All too often, we are providing what we want to and not what the patient deeply values. In a recent 2-year examination linking customer satisfaction with purchasing behavior, and ultimately with company growth, Reichheld[67] concluded that the likelihood of a customer recommending your services to a colleague or friend was directly related to increased growth.

Patient treatment reports and other correspondence can be created by the front desk or assisting staff, reviewed by the practitioner, and then transmitted to a printer and/or email client for distribution to referrers. It is important for the patient to list all of their co-therapists during registration, so they will automatically receive the final treatment reports.

10. Doctor telephones patient in evening: The last touchpoint is the evening phone call by the practitioner to the patient. The value of this call cannot be overemphasized, as it is one of the most appreciated services reported by patients on their satisfaction surveys.

Remember that patients want to be treated in a clean and welcoming office environment. They evaluate your office on a continual basis, and educating your patients about the safety precautions you take will add value. Always assure patients that their comfort and safety are major objectives of their treatment. Try to explain the procedure, with permission, to the patient in terms they can understand. Use every opportunity to further establish your technological leadership by making them a partner in their treatment. The relevance of your brand involves reverse thinking. You need to "move out of your world and into theirs."[68] It is not what you are selling; it is what they are buying, that counts!

DEVELOPING A CULTURE OF EXCELLENCE AROUND YOUR BRAND

The operation of the practice can be managed by asking a key question: How can I be excellent? And the answer is by designing systems that allow you to do the job right the first time. Creating a strategy to achieve success requires five basic steps, each dependent on the preceding step to accomplish your goals.

1. Step 1: Identify which patients you really want. Begin with a clear understanding of who your patients are and which ones you want to serve.
2. Step 2: Identify what your targeted referrers and patients deeply value. All purchasers of services or products want *results* and *process quality*. Finishing treatment with a pain-free and fully functioning tooth is the results part. And having a positive experience where respect, timeliness, courtesy and treatment with all needs (in the mind of the patient or referrer) met on a consistent basis is the process quality part of the equation.
3. Step 3: Develop a "customer-centered focus." Learn to manage the convergence between what your patients deeply value and the things that you do best. This means that the core procedures are performed in a caring and expert manner. Focus on the routine procedures that lend themselves to the highest levels of success with the most profit.
4. Step 4: Make "creating a customer-centered focus" your mission. Your mission is your "compass" in an increasingly challenging practice environment. This means understanding your mission and how each stakeholder will support and interact with the mission. Everyone needs a program that they can own, but be ready to change on a routine basis.
5. Step 5: Create an organization-wide obsession with your mission. To become consistent and successful, communicate your mission to your staff, your referring doctors, and patients.[69] In fact, brands demand consistency. According to Straine and Straine,[70] "If your receptionist is rude, if your office manager is unhelpful when a patient needs financing, if your policies are always changing, the negative impact on your brand" will destroy your efforts to achieve clinical excellence.

"QUALITY IN FACT" AND "QUALITY IN KIND"

Another important concept that will help the empathize with patients and referring doctors is the concept of treatment quality as viewed from the patient perspective. In a look at quality, former Malcolm Baldridge Award examiner Patrick Townsend[71] defines *quality in fact* as goods or services that measure up to the specifications of the provider. For example, when an endodontic procedure is completed, does it meet all of the desired specifications as defined by the practitioner? Are all of the canals identified, cleaned, shaped, and obturated to completely seal the root canal system? If so, then the procedure meets the specifications of the provider and satisfies the criteria of a satisfactory case. But that is only half of the story. The other half is defined by the authors as *quality in kind*, or the way that the patient perceives the procedure—from their viewpoint. For patients, a successful visit will hinge on how the patient was treated, because the success of the procedure will be judged on the subjective quality as the patient sees it, or the experiential aspects of their visit. And do not short change the importance of the physical environment of the office. If the office looks tired, patients will respond in kind, because patients will "judge the book by its cover." There is no way for most customers to even begin to assess the quality of the endodontic treatment they receive, they can only judge by how they were treated, the appearance of the office, and other non-technical aspects of their treatment. Take a quick mental journey through your office, reception area, front desk area, hallways, sterilization area, and operatories. Do they reflect your intended practice image? Are they modern, clean, efficient, organized, and calm? Does it send the message that your practice is up-to-date? Pay attention to the details—your patients and referrers are. Remember, you do not get a second chance to make a great first impression.

UNDERSTANDING SATISFACTION

A typical business customer satisfaction index is shown in Figure 1. If the satisfied and completely satisfied patients total 81%, should the directors of this company be content? Should a business concentrate its resources on increasing the satisfaction of the very dissatisfied patients or try to raise the merely satisfied customer to a completely satisfied level?

Studies have shown that it is far cheaper to raise the customer with a satisfaction index of from between 3.5 and 4.5 to a 5 than move a very dissatisfied customer to a higher level.[72] Many businesses spend a disproportionate amount of resources on a small percentage of customers who are almost impossible to please. Pursuing these customers also may hurt company morale and will disparage the company to other potential patients.

What impact will this have on an endodontic practice? Referring doctors and patients who enjoy complete satisfaction with your services are more likely to be loyal "apostles" of the office than those who are just satisfied.

Professor James Hasket[73] of the Harvard Business School, in his ground-breaking research on the "satisfaction-loyalty link," states that "if employee performance and loyalty is good within an organization, then that organization's customers will be more likely to repurchase a product or service." One way to measure the satisfaction of your referring doctors and customers is to use a satisfaction survey. This tool, outlined in more detail above, can point out areas that you can improve, such as front desk operations, office hours, parking, and so on.

Once you have identified areas that need corrective action, be prepared to create an action plan to fix the problem. Remember, a problem exists if a referring doctor or a patient perceives a problem. Problems can be fixed and loyalty maintained if the problem is fixed quickly. It has been shown that 95% of customers will repurchase a product or service if the problem is fixed on the spot, and 78% of customers will repurchase if the problem is fixed within 24 hours.

Every patient and referring doctor should receive the basic elements they expect, like a professionally performed and technologically advanced procedure. Everyone receives the basic support services that include instructions, assistance with financial arrangements, and insurance filing. Everyone gets the basic recovery help that includes an apology for an appointment delay or correction of a billing error. But only certain referrers will get extraordinary services that excel in meeting their personal preference that make the service seem customized. An example of the extraordinary services you might provide to a core referrer might be treating a patient for his or her convenience on a Saturday for non-emergent treatment when you normally do not conduct business on a weekend.

PATIENT SATISFACTION SURVEYS

Patient questionnaires seek explicit information that can be analyzed and trended over time. Patient opinion surveys can help determine satisfaction with office personnel, procedures, or other aspects of the practice which may ultimately affect patient and referring doctor loyalty. Opinion surveys can be customized to fit the needs of each practice and allow customers to vent if there are problems.

Several options are available, each of which can be integrated into broader Total Quality Management (TQM) initiatives or performance assessment strategies. Surveys can be short in-office questionnaires, with each patient filling out a form while in the office, or longer take-home questionnaires. Anonymity may prompt patients to be more honest with their feedback. If identity is disclosed, the surveys can include call-backs to patients after they have returned home. They can even involve focus groups to investigate very specific questions about programs, services, and staff. Other forms of surveys include mail and email surveys, sent to a random selection of patients. These survey channels may give the patient more time to complete the survey, which may result in a more in-depth response.

The most personal way to conduct a satisfaction survey is in person or by telephone. You can have a staff member or research professional perform the survey. Patients can more easily elaborate on their responses, but these types of surveys can be expensive.

In recent research published by Press Ganey Associates[74] to evaluate heathcare satisfaction, patients rated the courtesy, friendliness, and professionalism of the dental assistant as more important than that of the dentist! Infection control and cleanliness was rated second. While the dentist's skill was important, the dentist's attention to patient anxiety and concerns were directly related to patient loyalty and their potential to refer other patients. Patients also rated the amount of time spent with a patient and explanation of treatment options as important indicators of practice quality.

Installation of a bulletin board at your office to allow clinicians and staff to read each survey is an easy way to share comments and build a consensus. Many surveys reinforce employee behavior, especially if they mention a staff member by name. Each survey is an opportunity for your organization to improve.

CREATING A WEB SITE, STATIONARY, AND BROCHURE

One of the most often neglected parts of an office branding program is the production of Internet resources and coordinated office publications. Internet technology is advancing at a record pace. In every field, including dentistry, entrepreneurs are using it to devise new and better ways to develop business and lower costs. To ensure brand awareness in the future, endodontists must acknowledge the enormous potential of this technology and develop sound strategies for harnessing all its capabilities. In the larger context, an Internet site can be part of your overall identity management program that ties together all marketing materials to communicate your practices vision. Using a professional design firm to create your Web site, stationary, and brochures will ensure a coordinated look that will be more powerful than unmatched pieces. Internet technology can enable your practice to broaden the scope of patient relations and increase communications with patients, referring doctors, and study clubs. Over the last few years, the Internet has become a unique medium for the endodontist to promote innovative and technically sophisticated treatment.

Getting started on a Web site can be a challenging because there is a tendency to keep changing, and the possibilities are virtually limitless. Here are some pointers to help you get started:

1. The best way to begin is to visit other medical and dental provider's Web sites. Learn how to navigate their site, what elements are required and if you want to include programs with more high-end graphic effects. Simple is better, but patients and referring doctors will want to see some "eye candy" and learn on each visit. Video segments featuring you and your staff are becoming more commonplace as video technology over the Internet improves.
2. Decide on your goals. Is it to generate referrals via Internet search engines, develop links to sites that market dentists, or serve as a resource for your patients and referring doctors?
3. Work with Web site professionals to create a design for your site. Remember that the design of the site should complement the image you are trying to project. Also, consider employing search engine optimization techniques to make your site more prominent.
4. Outline your proposed site and create a storyboard that includes navigation possibilities for your audience. Design every page on a separate piece of paper and test your ideas with friends, selected patients, and referring doctors.
5. Choose a Uniform Resource Locator (URL) so that Internet address can be easily remembered and entered in a browser with a minimum of effort and confusion. The URL should tie into your desired image.
6. Then just fill in the blanks with copy, photographs, and an appealing style that projects your vision. Keep it fresh. If you want repeat visitors,

continually update the site and make sure your links are relevant and functional.

Human Resources

Organizational success in endodontic practice requires a high-performance staff.[75] After all, your employees are your brand. They must understand what your brand stands for and how to deliver on your brand promise. Pfeffer and Veiga[76] observe that "there is a substantial and rapidly expanding body of evidence, some of it quite methodologically sophisticated, that speaks to the strong connection between how firms manage their people and the economic results achieved." Exactly how important is marinating a well-trained and dedicated staff? Recent studies looked at 968 firms representing all major industries and found that just a 7% decrease in employee turnover resulted in a per employee increase of $27,044 more in sales and $18,641 more in market value.[77] It is clear that any business, including an endodontic practice, can benefit by adopting employee-related best practices to ensure financial success and ultimately clinical excellence.

According to Pfeffer and Veiga,[78] the most important elements of a successful HR management program are (1) providing long-term job security to assure that employee efforts will be rewarded; (2) recruiting and hiring the right people from the beginning; (3) creating self-managed project teams of peers to increase their sense of responsibility and accountability; (4) providing high compensation that is contingent on performance; (5) investing in extensive training for all employees; (6) reducing status differences between employees to improve idea generation from all employees; and (7) teaching information sharing to create a high-trust organization that allows inclusiveness.

JOB DESCRIPTION

The largest cost items for most endodontic practices is employee wages and benefits.[79] The plethora of regulations, such as equal employment opportunity (EEO) legislation enacted by local, state, and federal governments, has made job analysis a mandatory part of HR management. One of the most useful products of comprehensive job analysis is the job description, an Americans with Disability Act (AwDA) compliant narrative of the major responsibilities and duties associated with each job. While most job descriptions are limited to a single type of service or project, many endodontic offices require the use of cross-functional team members to complete certain tasks or to fill-in for a vacationing employee.

A good starting point is to consult O*NET, a US Department of Labor (DOL)-sponsored comprehensive source for continually updated information on occupational characteristics. Based on the most current version of the Standard Occupational Classification System, each O*NET occupational title and code includes descriptors for skills, abilities, knowledge, tasks, work activities, work context, experience levels required, job interests, and work values.[80] A partial sample of O*NET's listed tasks, knowledge, and abilities section for dental assistants (code 31-9091.00) are summarized in Table 3.

THE STANDARD OPERATING PROCEDURE

Often overlooked but extremely valuable, the standard operating procedure (SOP) is a written practices and procedures reference, which is designed to ensure that key procedures are performed in a safe and compliant manner. The SOP is typically written by the current job holder and edited by the practice administrator.[81] SOPs force employees to think through a procedure

Table 3 Tasks, Knowledge, and Ability Tasks

Importance	Category	Tasks
99	Core	Prepare patient, sterilize and disinfect instruments, set up instrument trays, prepare materials, and assist dentist during dental procedures
92	Core	Expose dental diagnostic X-rays (certification may be required)
90	Core	Record treatment information in patient records
88	Core	Take and record medical and dental histories and vital signs of patients
88	Core	Provide post-operative instructions prescribed by dentist
87	Core	Assist dentist in management of medical and dental emergencies
77	Core	Instruct patients in oral hygiene and plaque control programs
79	Supplemental	Apply protective coating of fluoride to teeth
76	Supplemental	Schedule appointments, prepare bills and receive payment for dental services, complete insurance forms, and maintain records, manually or using computer

Importance	Knowledge
87	Medicine and Dentistry—Knowledge of the information and techniques needed to diagnose and treat human injuries, diseases, and deformities. This includes symptoms, treatment alternatives, drug properties and interactions, and preventive healthcare measures
73	Customer and Personal Service—Knowledge of principles and processes for providing customer and personal services. This includes customer needs assessment, meeting quality standards for services, and evaluation of customer satisfaction
64	English Language—Knowledge of the structure and content of the English language including the meaning and spelling of words, rules of composition, and grammar
59	Clerical—Knowledge of administrative and clerical procedures and systems such as word processing, managing files and records, stenography and transcription, designing forms, and other office procedures and terminology
51	Chemistry—Knowledge of the chemical composition, structure, and properties of substances and of the chemical processes and transformations that they undergo. This includes uses of chemicals and their interactions, danger signs, production techniques, and disposal methods
42	Computers and Electronics—Knowledge of circuit boards, processors, chips, electronic equipment, and computer hardware and software, including applications and programming
40	Psychology—Knowledge of human behavior and performance; individual differences in ability, personality, and interests; learning and motivation; psychological research methods; and the assessment and treatment of behavioral and affective disorders
40	Public Safety and Security—Knowledge of relevant equipment, policies, procedures, and strategies to promote effective local, state, or national security operations for the protection of people, data, property, and institutions
36	Mechanical—Knowledge of machines and tools, including their designs, uses, repair, and maintenance

Importance	Ability
78	Oral Expression—The ability to communicate information and ideas in speaking so others will understand
75	Oral Comprehension—The ability to listen to and understand information and ideas presented through spoken words and sentences
72	Near Vision—The ability to see details at close range (within a few feet of the observer)
72	Written Expression—The ability to communicate information and ideas in writing so others will understand
66	Information Ordering—The ability to arrange things or actions in a certain order or pattern according to a specific rule or set of rules (e.g., patterns of numbers, letters, words, pictures, and mathematical operations)
66	Speech Clarity—The ability to speak clearly so others can understand you
62	Arm-Hand Steadiness—The ability to keep your hand and arm steady while moving your arm or while holding your arm and hand in one position
60	Speech Recognition—The ability to identify and understand the speech of another person
56	Finger Dexterity—The ability to make precisely coordinated movements of the fingers of one or both hands to grasp, manipulate, or assemble very small objects
56	Problem Sensitivity—The ability to tell when something is wrong or is likely to go wrong. It does not involve solving the problem, only recognizing there is a problem
56	Selective Attention—The ability to concentrate on a task over a period of time without being distracted
56	Written Comprehension—The ability to read and understand information and ideas presented in writing
53	Flexibility of Closure—The ability to identify or detect a known pattern (a figure, object, word, or sound) that is hidden in other distracting material
53	Manual Dexterity—The ability to quickly move your hand, your hand together with your arm, or your two hands to grasp, manipulate, or assemble objects

Table 3 continued on page 1499

Table 3 continued from page 1498

53	■■■■	Time Sharing—The ability to shift back and forth between two or more activities or sources of information (such as speech, sounds, touch, or other sources)
50	■■■■	Category Flexibility — The ability to generate or use different sets of rules for combining or grouping things in different ways
50	■■■■	Control Precision—The ability to quickly and repeatedly adjust the controls of a machine or a vehicle to exact positions
50	■■■■	Deductive Reasoning—The ability to apply general rules to specific problems to produce answers that make sense

National wage and employment trends

Category	Occupation information
Employment (2004)	267,000 employees
Projected growth (2004–2014)	■■■■ Much faster than average (36+ %)
Projected need (2004–2014)	189,000 additional employees

A partial list of the tasks, knowledge, and ability associated with dental assisting is reproduced above. Adapted from O*NET Web site http://online.onetcenter.org/link/details/31-9091.00, accessed May 1, 2007. O*NET is a service of the U.S. Department of Labor and acts as a comprehensive source of ranked descriptors for more than 900 occupations.

step by step and are in themselves useful training tools. More complex tasks lend themselves to the SOP structure for training new employees and modifying procedures to improve efficiency and safety. While SOPs work well for procedures that require safety and standardization, they may limit creativity where imagination is warranted. The best approach is to be concise and make the document as dynamic as possible. SOPs should be easily accessible to all employees via the practice's computer network and at a minimum should be updated on an annual basis.

Each SOP should have a header with the title, original issue date, revision dates, number of pages, the author of the SOP, and "approved by" signature plus the following basic elements (Table 4):

1. Desired outcome
2. Definitions
3. Measurement
4. General information
5. Step-by-step procedure with identification of critical information
6. Attachments and forms to be used, if any

CREATING THE EMPLOYEE HANDBOOK

Employee handbooks help to establish the employer's expectations and can prevent misunderstandings that may reduce the risk of litigation. Because most employees want to be successful, they will generally welcome a description of expectations, procedures for obtaining a promotion or raise, policies on dress, leave requests, work hours, disciplinary issues, and other important guidelines. The process involved in creating a handbook can also help you think through and establish your own unique policies. To aid in the process, consider getting professional advice from your attorney, accountant, or a personnel advisory firm, so that personnel procedures are documented before contentious issues arise. Personnel advisory firms can provide comprehensive and cost-effective help and implementation, providing excellent handbooks, supporting resource manuals, and technical assistance. The ADA also sells a hand-book resource manual with step-by-step guidance.

Courts generally view both verbal and written policies as a contract. However, unwritten policies may pose more risk than written policies, because verbal policies either can be implied or given by someone with no authority. Written handbooks help avoid conflict by reducing the chances of a dispute between you and employee, especially in the most litigious areas of firing and discipline. It is critical that your handbook is properly vetted by knowledgeable advisors, because, as Peter Sfikas,[82] ADA general council notes, courts "have determined that manuals, handbooks and booklets can create implied employment contracts, subjecting the employer and employee to additional terms and conditions of employment." In the interest of both the employer and the employee, written handbooks that clearly state the policies of the practice serve to minimize the risk of litigation, and well-drafted disclaimers may help to maintain the "at will" status of employees. Generally, a clear statement at the beginning of the handbook stating that the handbook is not a contract and that the policies therein can change at any time without advanced notice will provide some measure of protection.

According to the U.S. SBA,[83] an employee handbook should include the following:

1. Overview of practice philosophy and history
2. Equal opportunity statement that hiring, promotion, pay, and benefits are not related to employee's

Table 4 Standard Operating Procedures: Computers

<u>Desired Outcome:</u> All computer equipment in the Practice will operate efficiently to create and store all radiographic and visible light images, clinical charts, patient financial transactions, appointments, protected health information (PHI), and other materials related to the Practice. Patient confidentiality will be maintained in accordance with the Practice's current Health Insurance Portability, and Accountability Act (HIPAA) Manual and office policies.

<u>Definitions:</u> Information technology (IT) refers to the use of computers and computer software to manage office information.

<u>Measurement:</u> Evaluation of internal and external customer satisfaction by "Employee Evaluation of Office" and "Patient Satisfaction Survey." Internal customers will experience infrequent computer down time, undergo adequate training, and use programs that do the intended job right the first time.

<u>Introduction:</u> All computer systems in the office are critical to the success of the Practice. The Practice stores all clinical and administrative data on the office computer system. Therefore, the Practice's computers and networks are to be used for Practice-related work only.

No expectation of privacy: In the course of operation and maintenance activities, use of computers and networks may be monitored to ensure the continuing effectiveness and integrity of the Practice's IT resources. Email, Web logs and data, and other files created or received while using the Practice's computers are neither private nor confidential. The Practice reserves the right to access and disclose all messages sent by its computers and networks, as well as any data created, received, or stored on them.

Computer security and access to files and email: Although the Practice intends to convey no expectation of privacy, its business communications must be protected from unauthorized access. At no time may any employee remove or transfer any data to computers outside of the office by any means, including disks, jump-drives, CD-ROMs, or the Internet for any reason.

Employees are not to give any computer information to anyone on the telephone who calls our office without specific permission from Dr. Levin or Dr. Lee. The only exception is our IT services company.

No disks, CD-ROMS, or other material of any kind can be brought from the home of an employee and placed on the Practice's computer systems at any time.

Patient confidentiality: see HIPAA Manual and office policies as published periodically.

Internet use: No employee is allowed to use the computer system for personal use at any time.

Web: When using the Web, only the approved Internet browser is permitted. Approved sites include only those directly related to the business of the Practice.

Email: Only MS Outlook, Google, and Yahoo are approved for email use. Any email messages generated or viewed at the office are the property of the Practice.

Virus protection: We use McAfee Enterprise virus protection, which automatically updates all of our workstations every night via the McAfee Web site and our LAN. All computers will be running McAfee virus protection at all times. This will protect our system from virus destruction and other potentially harmful computer intrusions. Confirm that this software is active at start-up and remains active at all times.

Firewall protection: We are protected from hackers through our Internet switch called WatchGuard "Firebox." Make sure this equipment is on at all times.

Backup: We use a tape backup system, located in the server. Each business day, a numbered tape is placed in the server and noted on the "Backup Log" by the operator's initials. Every Friday, the cleaning tape is placed in the tape drive, allowed to complete one cycle that takes approximately 1 minute, and is removed from the drive. On Monday, the Friday night tape is placed on Dr. Levin's laptop bag for off-site storage.

Passwords: Each employee will be issued a discrete user name and password to log into EndoVision. As there are nine levels of security, some codes will not allow every user to perform all tasks.

SQL: EndoVision (EV) and Schick (CDR) use their own database engines that reside on the server. This SQL database software must be active on the server to allow workstation access to EV and CDR. Both of these SQL database engines will be running on the "Taskbar" of the server. If you cannot login from any workstation for either EV or CDR, check the server to see if their individual SQL database engines (icons in the taskbar) are active.

PC software and hardware controls: Users may not download, purchase, or install software or hardware on office computers unless it is approved by Dr. Levin or Dr. Lee. Copyrighted and licensed materials may not be used on a PC or the Internet unless legally owned or otherwise in compliance with intellectual property laws.

Critical information is italicized.

---

race, color, religion, sex, age, disability, or national origin.

3. Work hours should be defined, including time for lunch and conditions that could require late hours, such as treating after-hours emergencies.
4. Wage policies should include general information about when paychecks will be issued, how and when promotions are handled, classification of part-time, full–time, and on-call employees, overtime, loans, and leaves without pay.
5. The performance review section should describe how and when employees will be evaluated; unscheduled evaluations may be made at any time to advise employees of unsatisfactory work.
6. Paid holidays and all types of leave, including family (maternity, adoption, and elder care), medical, dental, funeral, personal, jury, and military should be listed.
7. A termination section should inform employees about causes that will trigger firing, including criminal activity, insubordination, absenteeism, and poor work performance.
8. All forms should be included, such as sample requests for vacation, medical leave, hepatitis vaccination declination, and so on.

9. Acknowledgement of receipt and reading of handbook by employees should be required by the practice and kept in the employee's personnel folder or other secure location.

Employee handbooks should be written by a lawyer specializing in employment law or by consultants who provide HR advice. A poorly written handbook may contain legal pitfalls that can lead to litigation. The following suggestions may help avoid some common errors:

1. A statement that conforms to your state's "employment-at-will" doctrine, which specifies that employment can be terminated at any time, for any reason, or no reason at all, will generally provide some measure of protection against successful litigation. Good advice here is critical, because construction of the document, obtaining written acknowledgement by the employee, public policy exceptions, situations where an expressed or implied employment contract exists, and "situations where an implicit duty of good faith exists in the employment relationship" can lead to confusion and ultimately to litigation.[84]
2. Announcing a "probationary period" of employment may wrongly imply that employees are entitled to continuing employment after the probation period is over.
3. Employee manuals should not include benefit plan documents, but simply point employees toward other documentation.
4. Do not outline specific pre-firing procedures, because courts have held employers liable for "wrongful termination when those steps were not followed."[85]
5. Generally, paychecks must be paid within a specified time limit, so be sure to specify these guidelines in accordance with local wage and hour laws.
6. Ensure that employees sign an acknowledgement that they have received, read, and agreed to the provisions of the handbook. Otherwise, an employee may claim that he or she never received the manual.
7. Limitations on employee–employee communications about wages or benefits are not allowed.

The employee handbook should be a positive tool for promoting better communication and improving morale. Be sure to review the handbook at least annually to be sure it is consistent with office policies. Also, annualizing employee performance reviews, raises and updating state and federal withholding forms to coincide with the date of hire for each employee, will help improve compliance by the practice.

EMPLOYEE SELECTION CRITERIA

What are the predictors of the best job performance? In an article reviewing 85 years of the practical and theoretical implications of personnel psychology, researchers Schmidt and Hunter[86] have shown that, on average, intelligence or general mental ability (GMA) is the most useful primary personnel measure for hiring decisions when compared to all other attributes, including conscientiousness. The positive economic effects of assessing an applicant's intelligence and hiring only the top performers cannot be overestimated. Furthermore, this study states that performance in a skilled job will benefit more from a higher GMA than performance in a semi-skilled job. It turns out that people with a high GMA scientifically correlate with conscientiousness, agreeableness, and emotional stability.[87] Other studies have demonstrated that while intelligence is the best single predictor of performance, screening employees for how well their values fit with their employer's values (value fit) is also a predictor of employee satisfaction and retention. However, when interdependent tasks were measured against non-interdependent tasks, value fit predicted only better citizenship behaviors, not higher performance.[88]

Of course, the success of your practice will depend, in part, on the people you hire. Ritz-Carlton hotels use an elaborate system for assessing job candidates, and the qualities the company believes are crucial to its success. When Paul Hemp,[89] a senior editor at the *Harvard Business Review*, spent a week at the hotel as a room-service waiter, he went through the new employee interview to see if he was the kind of candidate the Ritz was looking for. He said that "even after fudging my answers to a few questions, I got only ten points out of a possible fifteen in the composite hospitality assessment." The interviewer told Hemp that a score of 10 was not bad, but they wanted someone with a score of 12. He later found that just taking care of his sister in a time of need was not an extraordinary example of caring, but if he had given her his house for a month, he would have earned a higher score. Using scientifically based criteria, the Ritz has managed to reduce its annual employee turnover from the industry average of 55 to 28%!

Surveys that rank the importance of pay is another area of interest for the endodontic practice. Research has shown that self-reports of pay significance are likely to "underestimate its importance due to norms that view money as a somewhat crass source of motivation."[90] But money speaks, and getting the right combination of remuneration and benefits will positively impact your practice.

However, be certain to have any pre-employment exams or surveys thoroughly reviewed by an attorney or HR consultancy in order to ensure that it does not unintentionally skew results that disfavor applicants based on their protected EEO classes.

HIRING THE BEST PERSON FOR THE JOB

The hiring process should begin only after creating a set of job descriptions and an employee handbook. Once these documents are created, the next step is placing a job announcement in the print or online media or contracting with an employment agency. Typically, the Internet will produce same-day results and can be placed free of charge or on fee-based sites. An example of a job announcement for a Patient Coordinator written for Craig's List, a popular online listing service follows:

Dental specialty office has immediate opening for a Patient Coordinator with a friendly attitude. If you share our vision of a customer-centered focus with a high-tech approach, this is the job for you! We are looking for someone who is a team player and enthusiastic (someone who likes to smile). You will need excellent telephone and customer service skills. Proficiency with MS Word and Excel is required. Responsibilities include answering the phones, scheduling, and welcoming new patients, billing, and organizing practice promotion activities.

This position requires some schedule flexibility as patient appointments may occasionally extend the workday. Our usual hours of operation are Monday to Friday 8:15 am until 5:15 pm. Employee handbook and complete benefits package including medical and parking await the right candidate. Please email your resume without attachments (cut and paste into body of email).

When candidates respond to the job announcement, a pre-interview screening of the applications by the person in charge of personnel can help in choosing the best qualified candidates. Ideally, the screener should review the applications for basic objective criteria and reject those that do not possess the minimum education, experience, or skills set. Having a formal intermediary step in the screening process may help insulate against litigation because it will interject an objectively neutral perspective into the hiring process that can mitigate any claims of bias.

It may also be helpful for you to conduct brief telephone interview with each of the remaining candidates. Asking a few open-ended questions like "Tell me about your recent job experience" may help to identify those applicants you deem worthy of further consideration and will provide an opportunity for the candidate to ask questions to determine whether they believe the job is right for them. After a positive phone conversation, invite the candidate for a face-to-face interview.

Have a job application form ready for the new candidate and make sure it includes appropriate language authorizing reference checks. Notifying the candidate of your intention to check references gives the candidate time to alert contacts to expect your inquiry. If you want to know what the prospective employee is really like, contacting his or her former employers may be the best way to find out. Many companies check references as the final part of their hiring process, and sometimes extend job offers with the condition that references check out. Using a reference request form with a waiver signed by the prospective hire is a good way to safely get the information. Try contacting former employers et al. at more than one company, if possible, to get the broadest picture of the candidate. It is best to restrict questions to those that relate to education, training, experience, qualifications, job performance, professional conduct, and reason for termination.

Check with your attorney or HR consultancy to make sure that you are in compliance with state employment laws. To ensure that the information exchanged is from a legitimate former employer, try using fax or mail to verify the information. To help make the process a little less litigious, many states have enacted legislation providing some immunity from civil liability for providing information about the employee. Also, many employers have their own policies regarding reference checks on current and former employees that restrict the information they divulge to position title and dates of employment. If you encounter such a response, do not automatically assume that the applicant had a negative employment experience with their previous employer.

The purpose of the initial interview is to form an impression of how the candidate will fit into the practice culture, confirm his or her technical skills, and narrow down the field of applicants. Keep a record of the conversation, with each question and answer documented for future reference. Always meet candidates at your office during regular business hours with other staff on premises during the entire meeting to preclude any chance of allegations of inappropriate behavior. Unfortunately, many interviewers are improperly trained or uninterested in meeting with applicants. Nonetheless, endodontic practices, like other small businesses, need to adhere to good hiring practices or hire employees through employment agencies. Because many questions can open the door to non-job-related information that may be illegal, try to formulate behavioral questions guided by the job description. Having this list of questions ready will ensure that you get the precise information you need every time. Examples of good questions to ask are the following:

1. Tell me about a time when your teamwork with a co-worker helped you meet a patient's needs.
2. Give me an example of a mistake you made while carrying out your job duties. What happened? How did you correct the mistake?
3. Tell me the procedures used for sterilizing a treatment setup.
4. What steps do you take to ensure patient and operator safety when working with a patient?

Asking the right questions allows you to control the interview and helps to make certain that the interview is legally compliant.[91] It is important that you ask the same questions for each candidate during the hiring process to ensure that each applicant is treated equally.

Remember that there are areas where caution should be used in making pre-employment inquiries. Whether asked on an application form or in an interview, the EEO Commission and state Departments of Labor will consider some questions as evidence of discrimination, unless the employer is able to show that the inquiries are job-related or that there is a documented business-related necessity for asking the question. Partial list of subject areas to avoid during interviews:[92]

1. Arrest records
2. Garnishment records
3. Marital status
4. Child-care provisions
5. Contraceptive practices
6. Pregnancy and future childbearing plans
7. Physical or mental disabilities
8. Age, height, and weight
9. Nationality, race, or ancestry
10. Other areas of potential discrimination include certain limiting physical requirements, availability for weekend work, appearance standards, and fluency of the English language

Always avoid asking about the applicant's immigration or citizenship status. Although it will be necessary for the applicant to establish that they are lawfully permitted work in the United States, questions regarding the specific immigration status of the applicant can give rise to national origin discrimination claims. It is permissible to ask the applicant the yes or no question "are you lawfully permitted to work in the United States?"

Interviewers should avoid any assurances related to job security. Assuring the interviewee that they will "have their job for as long as they do a good job" is fraught with risk. If the applicant accepts the job and 6 months later is laid off, a breach of contract claim could be filed, where the employee asserts that he or she cannot be terminated unless they did not do a good job.

Once an offer of employment has been extended and the candidate has accepted the offer, a welcome packet of office information should be presented. This packet can include a welcome letter, employee handbook, a listing of compensation and benefits, employee roster, hepatitis vaccination verification or declination form (if applicable), health insurance application, payment options, retirement plans (if applicable), and any other information deemed important for the new employee. In addition, federal and state withholding forms, along with the Department of Homeland Security, U.S. Citizenship and Immigration Services' Employment Eligibility Verification form must be completed within 3 business days of the employment commencement date.[93]

POSTING OF EMPLOYEE NOTICES

The US DOL[94] and all states including the District of Columbia require that notices be provided to employees and/or posted in the workplace where employees can readily observe them.[95] Designating a wall area in the employee locker room or break room will provide an ideal place for a bulletin board to post periodic notices to staff and federal and state posters. DOL provides free electronic and printed copies of these required notices and posters at the "elaws® Poster Advisor" on the DOL Web site.[96] State posting requirements can be determined by contacting your state DOL through the links page located on the DOL Web site. In addition, some states, like California, require distribution of pamphlets, such as the State Disability Insurance and Paid Family Leave pamphlets, to employees under certain circumstances.[97]

EMPLOYEE BENEFIT AND SALARY ADMINISTRATION

Compliance with statutory wage and hour requirements is one of the areas that endodontic practices may find confusing, that is, hourly versus salaried compensation or complying with wage and hour requirements for staff travel to and attendance at continuing education meetings. Be sure to check with your HR advisors to determine the best policy.

Many practices use outside services for payroll processing and tax filing (i.e., W-2 and 1099 annual filing), reducing the chance of errors and incorrect filing of federal and state taxes. According to a recent study, the average small business that "ran payroll in-house and filed and paid quarterly taxes manually spent more than 250 hours away from customers... doing these tasks."[98] Offering direct deposit of wages to each employee's own bank account is an additional way to improve security and encourage staff members to maintain individual privacy and avoid salary comparisons. Direct deposit has the added advantage of ensuring that wages are available to employees as quickly as possible. No one benefits by stressed-out staff members leaving the office during the business day to deposit their payroll checks. Check your state wage and hour laws to determine if you can require direct deposit before mandating this service. Some new endodontic practice management software even includes timesheets with biometric fingerprint identification technology.

Additional information is available from the American Dental Assistants Association, ADA, Dental Assisting National Board, Inc. and the DOL, Bureau of Labor Statistics, on the national estimates for dental assistant wages, including industry and metropolitan area profiles for this occupation (Table 5).

There are several important laws governing salary and benefits compensation packages. The Fair Labor Standards Act (FLSA), the Employee Retirement Income Security Act (ERISA), and the (HIPAA) impose a myriad of complicated rules and regulations governing retirement plans, health insurance, cafeteria plans, and other benefits of employment. It is important that you seek guidance from a plan benefits advisor and attorney or HR consultant in deciding how to structure your employee salary and benefits packages.

TERMINATION

Few practice owners or managers want to face the emotionally charged process of firing people. Terminating employees in a way that preserves their dignity while preventing costly mistakes will benefit both the employee and the practice. The actual termination process will stay in everyone's mind for a long time and speak volumes about the practice. At best, a successful termination can make the employee a friend of the practice and in the worst scenario can result in a costly legal process. A termination will also affect co-workers if not handled properly, even if the employee is not well liked. Remember that in most jurisdictions, employees have the right to claim unemployment benefits which will often raise the practice's tax rate. The burden of proof is almost always on the practice to prove the reason for the separation in unemployment claims cases.

Even after carefully vetting new employees, he or she may not meet your expectations or may even act illegally. As soon as performance or discipline problems become apparent, start documenting your communications with the employee in question. Before terminating an employee, review your

Table 5 Dental Assistant Wages

Employment	Employment RSE	Mean Hourly Wage	Mean Annual Wage	Wage RSE	
270,720	1.3%	$14.41	$29,970	0.6%	
Percentile wage estimates for this occupation					
Percentile	10%	25%	50% (Median)	75%	90%
Hourly Wage	$9.46	$11.53	$14.19	$16.92	$20.21
Annual Wage	$19,680	$23,980	$29,520	$35,190	$42,030

Employment estimate and mean wage estimates for all categories of dental assistants, (31-9091) for May 2005 (Adapted from http://www.bls.gov/oes/current/oes319091.htm, accessed March 2, 2007). According to the Dental Assisting National Board, certified dental assistants earn higher wages than those who are not certified (Adapted from http://www.dentalassisting.com, accessed March 2, 2007).

employment offer letters, company policies, handbooks, and performance reviews to assure compliance with the practice's policies. If an employee performance review was conducted, exercising special care will help reduce the chances of litigation in the following situations: (1) when firing someone who has filed prior complaints about harassment or Occupational Safety and Health Act (OSHA) violations; (2) is older than 40 and covered by the Age Discrimination in Employment Act (ADEA); (3) is a member of a minority group because of race, color, gender, religion, or national origin; (4) has an employment contract; (5) has been promised job security or long tenure; and (6) if you are laying off more than one employee at once. In all cases, every employee must be treated even-handedly.

In determining whether to discipline or terminate an employee, it may be helpful to consider various factors to preserve objectivity. Consider the following:

1. The nature and seriousness of the offense and its relation to the employee's duties, position, and responsibilities, including whether the offense was intentional, technical, inadvertent, malicious, for personal gain, or was frequently repeated.
2. The employee's job level and type of employment, including supervisory or fiduciary role and contacts with customers.
3. The employee's past disciplinary record.
4. The employee's past work record, including length of service, performance on the job, ability to get along with fellow workers, and dependability.
5. The effect of the offense upon the employee's ability to perform at a satisfactory level and its effect upon supervisors' confidence in the employee's work ability to perform assigned duties.
6. Consistency of the penalty with those imposed upon other employees for the same or similar offenses.
7. The notoriety of the offense or its impact upon the reputation of the practice.
8. The clarity with which the employee was on notice of any rules that were violated in committing the offense or had been warned about the conduct in question.
9. The potential for the employee's rehabilitation.
10. Mitigating circumstances surrounding the offense such as unusual job tensions, personality problems, mental impairment, harassment, or bad faith, malice or provocation on the part of others involved in the matter.
11. The adequacy and effectiveness of alternative sanctions to deter such conduct in the future by the employee or others.

Although this list is not complete, it is a good starting point to consider when dealing with employee misconduct.

In sensitive firing situations or if terminating an employee is new to you, consult with an experienced employment lawyer or labor advisor ahead of time to prepare what to say, understand state laws that govern termination, and have all paperwork, salary checks, and severance pay ready to give to the employee. Always keep all discussions confidential and document the termination to aid in future communications with any state or federal agencies. Be prepared to answer the employee's questions about their schedule, severance pay, references, what will co-workers be told, medical and other insurance benefits, keys and security cards, profit sharing plan, if any, and eligibility for unemployment insurance.

Conducting an exit interview is another way to improve the work environment for the practice. Exit interviews should be conducted separately from the termination meeting and in small practices can be a simple survey to be mailed back or a phone conversation. Explain that the purpose of the interview is to gather information about the employee's experience at the practice and how it treats employees. Be sure to set the right tone, stay objective, and listen without providing opinions or becoming defensive.

EMPLOYMENT LAW

Many dentists assume that as they are practicing in an "at-will" state, they can discharge employees at anytime without problems. In certain circumstances, other issues can supersede the "at-will" prerogative, like violating an employee's civil rights. For example, the practice cannot discriminate against an employee who belongs to a protected class, where issues regarding age, sex, race, color, religion, disability, or national origin may play a role. Get the advice of legal council or your HR advisory firm if you plan to discharge an employee whose dismissal may trigger other issues.

It is best to administer your employment practices in a fair, equal, and consistent manner by counseling and documenting disciplinary and performance problems in written form. Include specific comments (i.e., reason for counseling, nature of disciplinary action, corrective action expected, consequences of non-compliance, and employee and employer comments) that are dated and signed by the administrator, employee, and a neutral witness, if possible. Never include an employee's co-workers or peers in the termination process.[99]

The following suggestions may help avoid common legal pitfalls

1. Maintain two types of personnel files for each employee, regular and confidential. The I-9 form should be kept in the confidential file and should not be given to anyone for inspection without legal advice. The I-9 form should be kept for 3 years from date of hire or 1 year from termination, which ever is longer.
2. Have an established protocol to follow when an employee or former employee or their attorney asks to review his or her personnel file.
3. Have a signed employment handbook with each employee.
4. Prohibiting employees from talking about their wages or benefits is not allowed under the National Labor Relations Act which specifies the right of employees at all workplaces, unionized or not, to engage in collective bargaining.
5. To protect the privacy of employees, keep all employee files locked or off-site. Records in many states can only be disposed of by destruction, modification, or other reasonable action to protect personal information.[99]
6. Employee records must be maintained on the following schedule.[100] OSHA: OSHA requires that records of job-related injuries and illnesses be kept for 5 years. Employers are also required to fill out and post an annual summary. Any exposure to toxic substances and blood-borne pathogens along with any records related to medical exams must be retained for 30 years after termination of employment. FLSA: Under the FLSA, the record-keeping requirements are 3 years to cover both supplementary basic records and payroll records. Civil Rights Act of 1964, Title VII, ADEA and the Americans with Disabilities Act (AwDA): Under the Civil Rights Act of 1964, Title VII, and the AwDA, employers with at least 15 employees must retain applications and other personnel records relating to hires, rehires, tests used in employment, promotion, transfers, demotions, selection for training, layoff, recall, terminations of discharge, for 1 year from making the record or taking the personnel action. The ADEA requires the retention of the same records for 1 year for employers with 20 or more employees. Title VII and the AwDA require that basic employee demographic data, pay rates, and weekly compensation records be retained for at least 1 year.
7. Family and Medical Leave Act (FMLA): The FMLA requires the retention of certain records for 3 years with respect to payroll and demographic information as well as information related to the individual employee's leave of absence.
8. IRS: IRS rules require keeping copies of employment tax records (Social Security documents) for 4 years after the due date of the tax. If a claimant files a claim, the retention period should extend for 4 years after the date of the filing. (26 CFR 31.6001).

Other employment law issues to be aware of include the following:

1. The Uniformed Services Employment and Reemployment Rights Act (USERRA): USERRA requires employers to hold available the position of employees who are active reservists called for duty. This includes short-term assignments for training which may only require a few days of leave, or long-term active duty in times of conflict. Additional guidance may be found at the DOL Web site at http://www.dol.gov/elaws/userra.htm.
2. The Pregnancy Discrimination Act: An amendment to Title VII of the Civil Rights Act of 1964, the Pregnancy Discrimination Act prohibits an employer from treating an employee who becomes pregnant differently than any other employee with a serious medical condition. For example, if your practice grants extended leave (either paid or unpaid) to an employee recovering from a heart attack, you must grant the same consideration to a pregnant employee. Keep in mind, that pregnant employees may also have additional rights under the Family Medical Leave Act.
3. Sexual Harassment: It is imperative that your practice have a strongly worded written policy stating that sexual harassment will not be tolerated. It should include a provision that employees who report sexual harassment will not be retaliated against and notify them of a confidential process for reporting any instances of harassment. You should take prompt and remedial action in addressing any allegations of harassment including investigating the claims, separating the person who reported the harassment from the alleged harasser, and taking any necessary disciplinary actions. For more information, please refer to the U.S. Equal Employment Opportunities Commission (EEOC) guidance at http://www.eeoc.gov/policy/docs/harassment.html.
4. Local Laws: Local laws may expand or modify Federal employment statues, so it is necessary that

you consult with an attorney or HR consultancy to become aware of any additional requirements. For example, some jurisdictions also prohibit discrimination on the bases of sexual orientation and/or political affiliation.

CONFIDENTIALITY AND NON-COMPETITION COVENANTS

Some employers require employees to sign non-compete covenants and confidentiality clauses. Generally, non-competition covenants with administrative or clerical staff will be held invalid. Some firms may legitimately enter into non-competition clauses with associates or other professional staff within their practice so long as they are for a limited duration (1 or 2 years); not overly restrictive (limited to a specialty practice and not the entire medical or dental profession); and of a limited geographic scope (a few mile radius of the current practice location). Keep in mind state laws and professional ethics rules may bar any non-compete covenants.

Contrary to covenants not to compete, confidentiality clauses can be enforced so long as they pertain to proprietary procedures or information and patient medical information. Consult with an attorney if you are considering either covenant.

EMPLOYMENT LIABILITY PRACTICES INSURANCE

Liability arising from employment practices continues an upward trend that shows no signs of abating. Unlike comprehensive general liability (CGL) policies, which insure against claims for tangible damages, for example, property damage, employment practices liability insurance (EPLI) insures against claims arising from employment practices. CGL policies differ from EPLI policies by excluding intentional acts and bodily injury that might occur while working. Also, CGL policies cover claims made while the policy is in effect, even if the claim is brought years later, whereas EPLI will cover only claims made during the coverage period or claims that the employer knew about or should have known about during the coverage period.

Many EPLI policies include wording that requires the insurance carrier to defend the employer against claims, even if the deductible has not been met. However, these clauses allow the carrier to choose the attorney who will defend the employer against the claim. Some policies also contain a provision that allows the carrier to settle the case, and if the employer rejects the settlement offer, the carrier can limit its liability to the amount offered in settlement or require arbitration. Before purchasing coverage, carefully review limitations and exclusions to make sure the policy fits your needs, as follows: (1) find out what is covered in addition to wrongful termination, harassment, and discrimination, such as invasion of privacy, negligent supervision, and hiring issues; (2) check to see if the policy will cover claims made by current part-time or temporary employees, independent contractors, and the EEOC; (3) confirm that you can choose your legal defense team; and (4) choose a carrier that has a solid track record in the field.

WORKERS' COMPENSATION

Workers' compensation provides wage replacement benefits, medical treatment, vocational rehabilitation, and other benefits to certain workers or their dependents that experience work-related injury or an occupationally related disease. Workers' compensation claims can be minimized by ensuring a safe workplace and making sure employees are capable of performing their jobs before they are hired. Employers cannot ask about a prospective employee's Workers' compensation history before a job offer is made.

Whenever a work-related injury occurs, make sure that an accident report is completed and a notification is provided to your Workers' compensation insurance provider. Any work-related injury that occurs over a period of time, like carpal tunnel syndrome or hearing loss, must be reported by the employee as soon as he or she learns that it is work-related.

STAFF MEETINGS AND PEAK PERFORMANCE

As the U.S. demographic picture continues to change, and the population/dentist ratio exacerbates healthcare manpower shortages, especially in rural and underserved areas, there has never been a greater need for the dental team to work more efficiently. Dental practices must not only "provide optimum patient care, but also must operate as a profit-making business"[101] to ensure the ability to upgrade facilities and acquire new technologies and training

Along with hiring the right people, using meetings to enhance peak performance and improve service quality are the hallmarks of a well run office. The "morning huddle," a 10- to 15-minute briefing, facilitated by the patient coordinator, is a valuable way to keep up-to-date on patients, procedures, scheduling, upcoming events, and miscellaneous matters. As a group, determining the best place to schedule emergency patients and share suggestions about how to fill appointment openings will improve efficiency and reduce stress. The agenda should include a brief review of production and collections from the previous day, expected for the current day, and the month, along with some time to discuss operational issues that need attention. Try to end on a positive note, adding a birthday or anniversary acknowledgement, a joke or a complement.[102]

Regular staff meetings are another way that practices stay ahead. Start by creating a file for staff to place suggestions and complaints between meetings (a word processing file accessible to all computers on the network will be helpful). Make the meetings a safe environment for all to be heard, take minutes, and create a written action plan that gets reviewed in 48 hours to measure progress.[103] Hotel chains like the Ritz-Carlton, home of legendary customer service excellence and two-time winner of the Malcolm Baldridge Award, have pioneered many innovations in customer service. Believing that employees are one of the keys to success, the Ritz-Carlton hotels "win the hearts and minds of its employees by making them feel part of a proud heritage."[104] Success in dental practice, and any profession for that matter, involves the construction of organizational processes and capabilities necessary to achieve performance through people delivering results and process quality.

Lastly, and all too often, organizations reach their goals and start planning new initiatives while forgetting to celebrate their accomplishments. Take time to acknowledge practice accomplishments by scheduling events, sending letters of praise, and giving out bonuses that say "Thank You!"

Acknowledgements

Thank you to the following experts who reviewed sections of the manuscript for this project: Gregory L. Morgan, Managing Director, Sperry Van Ness—Morgan Realty Advisors, Inc.; Robert S. Rubin, Ph.D., Assistant Professor of Management, DePaul University; Frank Hotchkiss, Operations Manager, Bent Ericksen & Associates; Janet L. Cornfeld, Ph.D., Clinical Psychologist; Charles J. Levin, Esq., Landlord Attorney; Kevin L. Owen, Esq., Labor and Employment Attorney; and Susan D. Levin, my wife and CFO.

Disclaimer: The information in this chapter should not be construed as legal advice or a standard of care. Readers should not act upon any information unless they consult with an attorney as management advice must be tailored to the specific circumstances of each case. Nothing provided herein should be used as a substitute for individual endodontic or dental management advice. Laws vary considerably from jurisdiction to jurisdiction, and even within jurisdictions. Therefore, some information may not be correct for a jurisdiction or locale.

References

1. Lavers JR. Market trends in dentistry. Dent Econ 2002;92:64–72.
2. Dentistry Today. The future of dentistry: Interview with Harold C. Slavkin. Dent Today 2006;10:90–2.
3. McGuigan PJ, Eisner AB. Marketing the dental practice: Eight steps toward success. J Am Dent Assoc 2006;137:1426–33.
4. Maslow AH. A theory of human motivation. Psychological Review 1943;50:370–96.
5. Berry LL. Services marketing is different. Business 1980;30:24–30.
6. Berry LL, Parasuraman A. Marketing services: competing through quality. Free Press;New York:2004.
7. Armstrong J, Pitt L, Berthon P. From production to performance: Solving the positioning dilemma in dental practice. J Am Dent Assoc 2006;137:1283–8.
8. Porter ME. What is strategy? Harv Bus Rev 1996;75:156–7.
9. Terez T. Workplace 2000 Employee Insight Survey. http://www.betterworkplacenow.com/insightsurvey/index.html (accessed May 3, 2007).
10. Nickols F. Strategy, definitions and meanings. http://home.att.net/~discon/strategy_definitions.pdf (accessed May 1, 2007).
11. Urwick LE. The manager's span of control. Harv Bus Rev 1956;34:39–47.
12. Charan R, Colvin G. Why CEOs fail. Fortune 1999;139:69.
13. Jeffcoat MK. Entrepreneur or employee: Right-sizing the dental practice. J Am Dent Assoc 2003;134:1302–3.
14. Roth K. Statement of the American Dental Association to the Small Business Committee, U. S. House of Representatives. http://www.ada.org/prof/advocacy/issues/incentives_testimony_070308.pdf (accessed May 3, 2007).
15. Armstrong J, Pitt L, Berthon P. From production to performance: Solving the positioning dilemma in dental practice. J Am Dent Assoc 2006;137:1283–8.
16. Lavers JR. Market trends in dentistry. Dent Econ 2002;92:64–72.
17. Blaes J. 2006 dental practice survey. Dent Econ 2006;96:64–73.

18. Nohria N, Joyce W, Robertson B. What really works. Harv Bus Rev 2003;81:42–52.
19. American Association of Endodontists. The economics of endodontics. Available from: <http://www.aae.org/NR/rdonlyres/1B54A2D9-4BA8-4AB9-BFB4-ED8AA9B59D2B/0/EconomicsofEndodontics.pdf (accessed May 10, 2007).
20. Wright S. The spatial distribution and geographic analysis of endodontic office locations at the national level. J of Endod 1994;20:500–5.
21. Solomon ES, Glickman GN. Demographic characteristics of endodontic practice sites in the United States. J Endod 2006;32:924–7.
22. Crafton BC, Lofft AH. Opening a new office: The dentist's personal frontier. J Am Dent Assoc 2006;137:81–5.
23. Morgan, GL. Personal communication, November 5, 2006.
24. Levin, CJ. Florida legal guide for non-residential property managers and leasing professionals. Tampa:Levin; 2006.
25. U.S. Department of Justice. ADA standards for accessible design. Code of Federal Regulations, Washington, DC: GPO; 1994.
26. American Institute of Architects. Document synopses. http://aia.org/docs2_template.cfm?pagename=docs%5Fsynopses (accessed May 3, 2007).
27. Covey, S. The seven habits of highly successful people. New York: Simon & Schuster; 1989.
28. Schmit B, Simonson A. Marketing aesthetics. New York: Simon & Schuster; 1997.
29. Bloch PH. Seeking the ideal form: Product design and consumer response. J Marketing. 1995;59:16–29.
30. Schmit B, Simonson A. Marketing aesthetics. New York: Simon & Schuster; 1997.
31. Johns BA, Brown LJ, Nash KD, Warren M. The endodontic workforce. J Endod 2006;32:838–46.
32. Lavers JR. What's a super norm model? Dent Econ 2003;93:26.
33. Solomon E. The future of dentistry. Dent Econ 2005;95:132–6.
34. Hagel J, Singer M. Net worth: Shaping markets when customers make the rules. Boston: Harvard Business School Press; 1999.
35. Neumeier M. The brand gap. Indianapolis: New Riders; 2003.
36. Davis SM, Dunn M. Building the brand-driven business. San Francisco: Jossey-Bass;2002.
37. Elliscu AT. How branding can position your practice for success. Physicians Marketing & Management, Sept 1997.
38. Association of National Advertisers. 2002 Best practices for operationalizing your brand. San Francisco:Prophet;2002.
39. Jones TO, Sasser WE. Why satisfied customers defect. Harv Bus Rev 1995;73:88–91.
40. Passikoff R. Predicting market success New York: John Wiley & Sons; 2006.
41. Davis SM. Brand asset management: How businesses can profit from the power of brand. J of Consumer Marketing 2002;19:351–8.
42. Robinette S, Brand C, Lenz V. Emotion marketing. New York: McGraw-Hill; 2001.
43. Peters T, The brand called you. Fast Company Aug/Sept 1997.
44. American Association of Endodontists. Patient focus group, factors associated with value. Chicago, IL: American Association of Endodontists; 1993.
45. Schleyer TKL. Should dentistry be part of the National Health Information Infrastructure? J Am Dent Assoc 2004; 135:1687–95.
46. Levit Partners. Branding. http://www.newyorkadvertisingagency.com/ConferenceRoom/Branding/branding.html (accessed May 12, 2007).
47. American Association of Endodontists. Patient focus group, factors associated with value. Chicago, IL: American Association of Endodontists; 1993.
48. Bernick CL. When your culture needs a makeover. Harv Bus Rev 2001;79:53–61.
49. Pine BJ, Peppers D, Rogers M. Do you want to keep your customers forever? Harv Bus Rev 1995;73:103–14.
50. Haskett J, Sasser E, Schlesinger L. The service profit chain, New York:Free Press; 1997.
51. Passikoff R. Predicing market success. New York: John Wiley & Sons; 2006.
52. Hotels. When two or three or four names are better than one. Hotels 2004;38:20–20.
53. Collins JC, Porras JI. Built to last: Successful habits of visionary companies. New York: Harper Business;1997.
54. Moser M. United we brand: How to create a cohesive brand that's seen, heard and remembered. Boston: Harvard Business School Press;2003;21–21.
55. Collins JC, Porras, JI. Built to last: successful habits of visionary companies. New York: Harper Business;1994.
56. Aaker, DA. Building strong brands. New York: Simon & Schuster; 1996.
57. Nash KD, Brown LJ, Hicks ML. Private practicing endodontists: production of endodontic services and implications for workforce policy. J Endod 2002;28:699–705.
58. Silversin J. Building relationships. Video Workshop. Chicago, IL: American Association of Endodontists; 1993.
59. Mehrabian A. Silent messages: Implicit communication of emotions and attitudes. 2nd ed., Belmont, CA Wadsworth; 1981.
60. Harris Interactive. Number of "cyberchondriacs" – U.S. adults who go online for health information – increases to estimated

61. Anderson HL. Integrated office technology: How technology can help improve office efficiency., J Am Dent Assoc 2004;135:185–225.
62. NetMotion Wireless. HIPAA Security for Wireless Networks. White Paper. http://wireless.ittoolbox.com/pub/MM020102.pdf (accessed May 10, 2007).
63. Eklund KJ, Bednarsh H, Haaland CO. OSAP Interact infection control and safety training system. Brunswick:InVision;1999.
64. Ludwig MJ. Physician-Patient Relationship, http://depts.washington.edu/bioethx/topics/physpt.html (accessed May 10, 2007).
65. Zunin LM, Zunin N. Contact: the first four minutes. Los Angeles: Nash;1972.
66. Sfikas PM. A duty to disclose, J Am Dent Assoc 2003;134:1329–33.
67. Reichheld, FF. The one number you need to grow. Harv Bus Rev 2003;81:46–54.
68. McNally D, Speak KD. Be your own brand. San Francisco: Berrett-Koehler Publishers; 2002.
69. Whiteley R, Hessan D. Customer centered growth: Five proven strategies for building competitive advantage. Boston: Addison-Wesley; 1997.
70. Straine OM, Straine KK. Success simply isn't enough…you can experience significance! Dent Today 2003;9:118–21.
71. Townsend PG. Commit to quality. New York: John Wiley & Sons; 1986.
72. Haskett JL, Jones TO, Loveman GW, et al. Putting the service-profit chain to work. Harv Bus Rev 1994;72:164–70.
73. Haskett JL, Sasser WE, Schlesinger LA. The sevice profit chain: How leading companies link profit and growth to loyalty, satisfaction and value. New York: The Free Press; 1997.
74. Leddy, K, Williams A. 2005 Health care satisfaction report. South Bend, IN: Press Ganey Associates; 2005.
75. Becker B, Gerhart B. The impact of human resource management on organizational performance. Acad Man J 1996;39:779–801.
76. Pfeffer J, Veiga JF. Putting people first for organizational success. Acad Man Exec 1999;13:37–48.
77. Huselid MA. The impact of human resource management practices on turnover, productivity, and corporate financial performance. Acad Man J 1995;38:635–72.
78. Pfeffer J, Veiga JF. Putting people first for organizational success. Acad Man Exec 1999;13:37–48.
79. Lindner J. Writing job descriptions for small businesses. Community Development Fact Sheet, Misc. Pub 93-9. Piketon Research and Extension Center, Piketon, Ohio: The Ohio State University;1995.
80. U.S. Department of Labor, Employment & Training Administration. O NET – beyond information. http://www.doleta.gov/Programs/onet/– intelligence (accessed May 1, 2007).
81. Sondalini, M. Employee training and development with SOP. http://www.bin95.com/ebooks/sop_training.htm (accessed May 7, 2007).
82. Sfikas PM. What dentists need to know about employment law. J Am Dent Assoc 1996;127:394–5.
83. U.S. Small Business Administration. www.sba.gov/gopher/Business-Development/Success-Series/Vol10/handbook.txt (accessed Oct 1, 2006).
84. Sfikas PM. What dentists need to know about employment law. J Am Dent Assoc 1996; 127:394–5.
85. Sfikas PM. What dentists need to know about employment law. J Am Dent Assoc 1996;127:394–5.
86. Schmidt FL, Hunter IE. The validity and utility of selection methods in personnel psychology: Practical and theoretical implications of 85 years of research findings. Psy Bull 1998; 124:262–74.
87. Goff M, Ackerman PL. Personality-intelligence relations: Assessment of typical intellectual engagement. J Ed Psy 1992;84:537–52.
88. Lauver K, Kristof-Brown A. Distinguishing between employees' perceptions of person-job and person-organization fit. J Voc Beh 2001;59:454–70.
89. Hemp P. My week as a room-service waiter at the Ritz. Harv Bus Rev 2002;80:50–62.
90. Rynes SL, Brown, KG, Colbert, AE. Seven common misconceptions about human resource practices: research findings versus practitioner beliefs. Acad Man Exe 2002; 16:92–103.
91. Half R. Robert Half on hiring. New York: Penguin; 1985.
92. State of Idaho. www.cl.idaho.gov/lawintvw3.htm#_Toc426425143 (accessed Oct 10, 2006).
93. U.S. Department of Homeland Security, U. S. Citizenship and Immigration Services. http://www.uscis.gov/files/form/i-9.pdf (accessed May 5, 2007).
94. U.S. Department of Labor, Office of Small Business Programs. http://www.dol.gov/osbp/statemap.htm (accessed May 5, 2007).
95. U.S. Department of Labor. http://www.dol.gov/compliance/topics/posters.htm#overview (accessed May 5, 2007).
96. U.S. Department of Labor. http://www.dol.gov/elaws/posters.htm (accessed May 5, 2007).

97. U.S. Department of Labor, Employment Standards Administration, Wage and Hour Division. http://www.dol.gov/esa/programs/whd/state/state.htm (accessed May 5, 2007).

98. American Dental Association. Thinking of changing payroll providers? ADA News. http://www.ada.org/prof/resources/pubs/adanews/adanewsarticle.asp?articleid=2219 (accessed May 10, 2007).

99. Ericksen B, Twigg T. Case study: Documentation. Dent Econ 2006;96:48.

100. Eskridge GL. How long must employers retain employee records? http://library.findlaw.com/2000/Oct/1/131863.html (accessed Feb 3, 2007).

101. Garganta KT. Steps for staff meeting success. Dent Econ 1995;85:31–2.

102. Ousborne AL. Morning meetings that matter. Dent Econ 2003;34:34.

103. Rose, KA. Personal communication, Jan 8, 2007.

104. Hemp P. My week as a room-service waiter at the Ritz. Harv Bus Rev 2002;80:50–62.

105. Reichheld FF. The loyalty effect. Boston: Harvard Business School Press; 1996.

106. Reichheld FF. Learning from customer defections. Harv Bus Rev 1996:74:56–69.

107. Maslow AH. Motivation and personality. New York: Harper & Row; 1970.

108. Postrel V. The substance of style: How the rise of aesthetic value is remaking commerce, culture and consciousness. New York: HarperCollins, 2003; 34–47.

109. Postrel V. The substance of style: How the rise of aesthetic value is remaking commerce, culture and consciousness. New York: HarperCollins, 2003; 4–5.

110. Schmit B, Simonson A. Marketing aesthetics. New York: Simon & Schuster; 1997.

INDEX

Page numbers followed by "f" indicate figures; page numbers followed by "t" indicate tables.

A

AAE. *See* Association of Endodontists (AAE)
Abscess theory, 313, 506
Abutment tooth selection technique, 1461
Access cavity, 894, 1127
  magnified view, 1098f
  preparation, 877
    effect on structural integrity, 1033
    finding pulp chamber, 895
    increased susceptibility to fracture, 918f
    obtaining SLA, 894
    obtain uniform contact of file, 861
    penetration through occlusal surface, 896
    sequence of steps, 927f
    unroofing dentin, 886
    types of designs, 943
    varying according to degree of curvature, 887
Actinomyces, 258
Actinomyces israelii, 500
Activated pathways during inflammatory response, 353f
Acute inflammation, 345, 473–474
  histologic evidence, inflammation in underlying pulp, 473f
  polymorphonuclear leukocytes, early inflammation, 474f
Acute inflammatory process, 381
Acute rhinosinusitis, 628. *See also* Chronic rhinosinusitis; Subacute rhinosinusitis

ADA. *See* American Dental Association (ADA)
Adaptive immunity, cells of
  regulatory T lymphocytes, 351f
  subpopulations of T cells, 349t
  T cells and Naïve CD4 T cells, 349–350
  T cytotoxic and B cells, 348–357
  Th3 cells, 349
  Treg and Tr1 cells, 350
A-δ fibers, 664
Adjunctive procedures, root canal treatment, 113
Adjunctive therapy, 1350
Adrenal suppression and long-term steroid use, 770
Adverse effects, drugs combination
  coumadin with quinolone, 784
  digoxin–tetracycline, 784
  macrolide–quinolone combination, 784
  methotrexate with penicillin, 780
AEL. *See* Electronic apex locator (AEL)
AH 26 (thermaseal), 1071–1072
  fluid conductance model, 1071f
ALARA, 574, 584
Allergy to materials used in endodontic therapy, 770, 771f
Alveolar bone, 13
Amalgam
  perforation repair, 1156
Ameloblastoma, 616f
  desmoplastic type, 617f
  growth/removal, 101f
American Association of Endodontists (AAE), 86, 93, 103, 266, 660

American Dental Association (ADA), 4, 87, 88, 113, 709, 748, 814, 1476
American Endodontic Society, 1066
American National Standards Institute (ANSI), 814, 1036
American Society of Anesthesiologists (ASA), 749
  categories and classifications, 755–758
Anaerobic bacteriologic techniques, 24
Anatomic apex, 25
Anesthetics and drugs, 786t
ANSI. *See* American National Standards Institute (ANSI)
Anterior cingulated cortex (ACC), 398
Antibacterial/microbial activity, 992
  CHX, 1005–1010
  EDTA, citric acid and other acids, 990–1015
  hydrogen peroxide, 1002
  NaOCl, 994–997
Antibiotic prophylaxis regimens for patients with total joint replacement, 768f
Antibiotics, 775
  and analgesics, 772–776
  and effects on oral contraceptives, 751
Anticoagulant therapy and bleeding disorders
  discontinuing aspirin prior to proposed surgery, 760
  modification of anticoagulant therapy, 760

Antigen-presenting cells (APCs), 497
Antimicrobial peptides,
  β-defensins, 360
Anxiety/fear problem, endodontics
  management, 741
  recognition, 748–749
APCs. *See* Antigen-presenting cells
  (APCs)
APEXIT, 1070
Apical cholesteatoma, 325
Apical constriction, 25, 930
  lost, 930
Apical dental cyst, 584f
Apical diagnosis
  acute apical abscess, 529
  acute/chronic apical abscess, 529
  apical scar, 529
  asymptomatic apical
    periodontitis, 529
  cellulitis, 529
  condensing osteitis, 529
  normal periapical tissues, 529
  prognosis and informed consent,
    530–531
  symptomatic apical
    periodontitis, 529
Apical foramen, 25, 640
Apical lamina dura
  resorption/remodeling of, 602,
    602f
  surgical endodontic, 602
Apical leakage, 1068
  delayed filling and, 1098, 1079f
  and lasers, 1073
  mean leakage values of sealers,
    1071f
  microleakage and its evaluation,
    1068–1069
  smear layer and, 1073
Apical neurovascular damage,
  consequences
  prevention of pulp space
    infection, treatment,
    1343–1344
  pulp canal obliteration, 1343
    multinucleated osteoclasts,
      appearance of, 1343,
      1343f
  pulp necrosis, 1348
  root canal disappearance,
    placement of thick
    calcium hydroxide, 1345,
    1345f

Apical patency/preparation, 28–29
Apical perforation management,
  1133
Apical periodontitis, 2, 311, 603,
  604, 887, 1092
  causage, 936
  cholesterol and, 324
    crystals and cystic condition
      of, 325f
  clinical relevance of cysts,
    322–324
  condensing at distal root, 603f
  cone beam CT, 606f
  criteria for assessing healing of,
    919
  cystic, 311f
  diagnoses, 597
    echographic examinations, 598
    endodontic orthograde
      treatment, 597
  etiology of refractory, after
    treatment, 1901–1903
  giant cell granuloma mimicking,
    614f
  healing of, 607, 607f
  lesions, 318f, 321f
    prevalence of cysts in post
      treatment, 324t
  microbial etiology of refractory,
    1192
  molar with canal in mesiobuccal
    root unfilled and with,
    605f
  more frequent, 930
  origin of cyst epithelium, 344
  persistence or recurrence of, 1193
  per-treatment variables
    apical enlargement, 1201
    bacterial culture before root
      filling, 1197
    complications, 1209
    flare-up during treatment,
      1198
    length of canal preparation
      and filling, 1195–1199
    materials and techniques, 1207
    number of treatment sessions,
      1198
  post-treatment variables
    restoration, 1209–1211
  prevalence of
    radicular cysts, 312t
    in 35–45 year-olds, 622f

  radiographic
    aspects of, 605
    and histological appearance
      of, 534f
  reversal/regression in healing of,
    1189f
  success and failure of endodontic
    treatment, 617–618
  teeth treated with associated, 1198
    dynamics of healing, 1191
    functional teeth, 1191
    healed teeth, 1198–1199
    healing in progress, 1191
  teeth treated without associated
    dynamics of developing
      disease, 1184–1187
    functional teeth, 1184
    healed teeth, 1191
Apical scar, progressive
  development of, 1164
Apical sizes and preparation
  diameter of, 886
  larger sizes, 944
  measured diameters and
    suggested size for, 932t
  pre- and postoperative canal
    diameters, 933f
Apical surgery, 324, 337
  follow-up studies reporting on
    outcome, 1212t
  laser in endodontics, 868
  outcome assessment of multi-
    rooted tooth after, 1173f
  potential for healing and retained
    function after, 1201
  dynamics of healing, 1191
  functional teeth, 1191
  healed teeth, 1199–1192
  healing in progress, 1191
  recurrence of disease, 1211f
Apical surgery, factors influencing
  healing after, 1210
  post-treatment variable
    dynamics of resorption, 1211
    endodontic treatment,
      outcome, 1222–1224
    potential for healing and
      function after
      replantation, 1119–1121
    results of biopsy, 1209
  pretreatment variables
    age, gender, and systemic
      health of patient, 1212

apparent quality of previous root filling, 1195
clinical signs and symptoms, 1202
restoration, 1213
size of radiolucency, 1202
supporting bone loss, 1202
tooth location, 1201–1204
second-time surgery, pretreatment variables, 1202–1207
antibiotics, 1214
barriers and bone grafting substances, 1209
complications, 1209
hemostasis, 1214
laser irradiation, 1209
level of apical resection and degree of beveling, 1204
magnification and illumination, 1208
operator's skill, 1209
presence or absence of root-end filling, 1214
quality and depth of root-end filling, 1205
retrograde root canal re-treatment, 1208
root-end cavity design, 1205
root-end filling material, 1214–1215
surgical and orthograde treatment, 1208
Apical surgery, persistent infection after, 1203–1204
healing after
endodontic treatment, 1201
nonsurgical treatment, 1201
pretreatment variables
age and gender of patient, 1201–1204
apparent quality of previous root filling (in re-treatment), 1202
clinical signs and symptoms, 1202
elapsed time after previous treatment (in re-treatment), 1195
periodontal support, 1194–1195
presence/absence, radiolucency, 1205

previous perforation (in re-treatment), 1195
pulp vitality or necrosis (in initial treatment), 1194
size of radiolucency, 1202
systemic health, 1201–1205
tooth location, 1201
Apicalterminus/cleaning, apical patency, 25–28
Apical transportation, managing
Type I transportation, 1124
Type II transportation, 1124–1125
clinical steps for, 1126f
MTA as barrier for choice of, 1133–1135
Type III transportation, 1125
Apical true cysts, 313
Apicoectomy. See Root-end resections
Applications of LDF, dentistry
clinical dentistry, 551
dental trauma, 551
Appropriateness, Care and Quality Assurance Guidelines
AAE, 88
Arachidonic acid, prostaglandins/ leukotrienes, 395
Armamentarium, clinical, 885
accessory instruments, 895–896
Stropko Irrigator, 885–896
burs, 888
examples, 890f
rotary instruments, 885
Arrhythmias and cardiac pacemakers, 761
Arteriovenous anastomosis (AVA), 131
and "U"-turn loops blood flow, regulation of, 132, 133f
Association of Endodontists (AAE), 809
guidelines of, 56
Assorted gutta-percha points, 1022f
Asthma, 763
Atherosclerosis, 324
high level of cholesterol, 324
Automatic Exposure Compensation (AEC), 573, 586
Autotransplantation of human teeth, 31

Avulsed tooth
open/closed apex, 1339–1152
dry time, 1356
replant, 1357

B

Bacteria
coccal forms of, 225f
cultured/identified from root canals of teeth with apical radiolucencies, 227t
in dentin repair, 224f
influencing the outcome, 242–243
persistence after intracanal disinfection procedures, 242t
intracanal disinfection procedures, 241
invasion of pulp cavity, 225
one visit versus two visits, 240–241
post-instrumentation/ post-medication/ post-obturation samples, 240–241
Bacterial biofilms, 268–273
characteristics, 270
communication/exchange genetic materials/acquiring new traits, 271, 271f
criteria, 268
dentistry, 277–278
development, 271
co-aggregation/co-adhesion, 273f
factors influencing initial bacteria–substrate interaction, 272f
stages, 273f
nutrient trapping/establishment of metabolic cooperativity, 270
organized internal compartmentalization, 270–271
protection from environmental threats, 270
resistance of microbes, antimicrobials, 281-3, 273–274
ultrastructure, 277–278, 269f

Bacterial elimination in periapical
lesions
  apical periodontitis, pain,
      501–502
    SRIF, 501–502
  athymic animals, studies in,
      503–504
  bacteria in periapical
      lesions, 499
    extraradicular infection, 499
  B cells/plasma cells/
      immunoglobulin
      production
    antigen-presenting cells
        (APCs), 497
  bone-resorbing cytokines,
      cellular sources, 503–510
  bone resorption in periapical
      lesions, 502–503
    NSAIDs, 502
  cells/immunoglobulins/
      cytokines, periapical
      lesions, 495
  complement activation (chain
      reaction), 494
  diapedesis, 494
  equilibrium, bacteria and host,
      500–501
  flare-ups in periapical lesions,
      immunobiological view,
      500–501
  immunobiological concept of
      periapical lesions,
      evolution, 495–496
  local activation, nociceptors in
      apical granuloma, 501f
  macrophage presence, kinetics
      of, 499
  macrophages in periapical
      granuloma, 511–512, 505f
  osteoclast activation
    osteoprotegerin ligand,
        functions, 504
  PMNs, 494
  protective function of T
      lymphocytes in periapical
      granuloma
    T lymphocytes, role of,
        508–509, 505f
  T lymphocytes, periapical
      granuloma, 497–498
Bacterial factors, flare-ups,
    707–708

Bacterial plaque, 318f
Bacteriostatic, 995
Bacteroides melaninogenicus, 237
BBHI-2. *See* Brief Battery for
    Health Improvement
    (BBHI)
B-cell antigen receptor (BCRs), 348
Behavioral factors, pain behaviors,
    403
Benzodiazepine
  and all drugs, 783t
Biofilm, 999
Biomaterial-centered infection
    (BCI), 285–286
BioPure. *See* MTAD
Bisphosphonate-associated
    osteonecrosis of jaws, 766
Bisphosphonates, 967
Bleaching of discolored dentin/
    enamel, causes, 70
Bleeding
  increased risk of, 755
Blood flow rate, 133f
"Blunderbuss" canal, 27
BMS. *See* Burning mouth
    syndrome (BMS)
Bone loss, fenestration type of, 679,
    679f
Bone marrow and solid organ
    transplantation
  hematopoietic stem cell
      transplantation, 766–767
Bone resorption, mechanisms of
  mediators promote or inhibit, 364t
  regulations of osteoclast
      differentiation and key
      cytokines, 365f
Brief Battery for Health
    Improvement (BBHI), 406
Brynolf's interpretation, 26f
Buccal cusp, occlusal view, 1433f
Bull-like teeth. *See* Taurodontism
Burning mouth syndrome (BMS),
    453, 454–455

C

Calciobiotic root canal sealer, 1035
Calcitonin gene-related peptide
    (CGRP), 395, 461
  and substance P (SP receptors),
      120, 120f

Calcitonin gene-related peptide-
    immunoreactive
    (CGRP-IR), 138f
  immunohistochemical staining of
      nerve fibers in rat dental
      pulp, 138f
  nerve fibers, 138f, 139f
Calcium hydroxide, 992–912,
    1067–1069
  for perforation repair, 1129
  periapical repair following
      application of, 1968f
Calcium hydroxide disinfection, 24
Calcium phosphate cement (CPC),
    1066–1067
Calcium sulfate
  as perforation barrier material,
      1142
Campylobacter gracilis, 237
Campylobacter rectus, 237
Canal(s)
  accessory, 154
  curvature, observing
      radiographically, 886
  managing blocked, lubrication,
      1133
  shaping procedures, 907
    effect of, anatomy, 961
  surface modification, 970–971
    appearance after shaping, 933f
    irrigation dynamics, 967
    photodynamic therapy, 970
    smear layer removal, 966t
  surfaces, 969
  systems to prepare canal, 966t
  in tooth, identification of, 581
  transportation, 961
  types
    Sert and Bayirli's, 154f
    Vertucci classification, 154f, 155f
  variations
    factors contributing to,
        151–152t
    in number of, 153
Canal, preparation
  anticurvature filing, 939
  balanced force, 940–946
    description, 943
    principles of the, 965f
  cross sections before and after
      preparation, 958f
  crown-down pressureless, 942–943
    sequence of instruments in, 960f

devices for powered, 951
    motors for rotary instrumentation, 951–953
    sonic canal instrumentation, 954
    ultrasonic canal instrumentation, 953–954
double flare, 943
handpieces with continuous rotation, 961
instruments
    cutting blade design, 961
    instrument shaft design, 961
    k-files, 963
    prevalence of instruments fracture, studies on, 983
    relationship of torque during and fracture load, 953f
root canal
    aseptic techniques and disinfectant, 1057, 1058f
    filling/vertical root fracture, 959f
    preparation, 959f
sequential mechanical enlargement, 960f
standardized, 936–937
step-back (telescopic technique), 937
    sequence of instruments, 938f
step-down, 945–946
    procedure itself, 938f
    purpose, 945
    shaping coronal aspect, 938f, 945
ultrasonic inserts fracturing, 955f
Canal Finder system, 951
Cancer chemotherapy and radiation therapy, 765–767
Ca(OH)$_2$. *See* Calcium hydroxide
Capillary loops, 132f
Capset. *See* Calcium sulfate
Carbon fiber-reinforced (CFR) epoxy resin post, 1453–1454, 1453f
Caries removal, vital pulp therapy
    caries affected dentin, 1318
    rubber dam isolation, 1391
Catonella morbi, 237
Causalgic pains
    sympathetically maintained pains (SMPs), 443–444

Cavit, 1042
    endodontic perforation repair, 1128
Cavity
    cleansing, 481
    crown preparation, 480
Cavity preparation
    access, 886–889
        improper angulations and, 882f
        standard hand instruments, 884
    coronal access, 877
CBVCT. *See* Cone-Beam Computed Tomography (CBCT)
Cellulose granuloma, 334
    paper-point granuloma affecting root-canal-treated human tooth, 335f
Cemental apposition, healing, 62f
Cementodentinal junction, 26
Cemento-enamel junction (CEJ), 638, 883–884
    centered pulp chamber, 891f
Cements and pastes (filling materials)
    calcium hydroxide, 1067–1068
    calcium phosphate cement, 1066–1067
    dentin chip apical obturation, 1067–1068
    N2/Sargenti paste, 1066
    resin cements, 1067
Central incisors fluorosis, treated by external bleaching, 1385
Central mechanisms, 384
    alternative hypotheses, 385f
    sensitization, 384
Central nervous system (CNS), 393
    definition, 764
    depressants, 743t
Central trigeminal pain system, organization and function of, 379
Cervical root resorption, 602f, 603f
    progress, apical, 603f
CGRP. *See* Calcitonin gene-related peptide (CGRP)
Charge-Coupled Device (CCD), 573, 577, 581
Chemokines
    adhesion molecules, tissue distribution and ligands, 353t

CC chemokines, 352
    common chemokines, receptors and cells, 352t
CXC chemokines, 352
Children, treatment for
    educational curricula and attitudes of pediatric dentists, 1423–1425
    nonvital pulp therapy, 1417–1418
    pulpal pathosis in children, diagnosis of, 1403
Chlorhexidine digluconate (CHX), 1002–1006, 1010–1011
Choice of practice, operations management, 1474
    associate-employee/independent contractor, 1478
        Internal Revenue Service (IRS) guidelines, 1478
    part-time schemes, combination, 1478
    hybrid, 1478
    new practice, 1477–1478
    practice models, 1476–1477
        ADA, 1476–1477
        DTA, proposed model, 1477
        service factory model, 1477
        service theaters, 1477
        super-norm model/Armstrong's service theater approach, 1477
    setting goals, 1476
        practice goals, 1476–1477
    strategic planning, 1475–1476
    vision and mission statements, 1475
        "22 Keys to Creating a Meaningful Workplace," 1475
    mission, definitions, 1475
    PEST analysis, 1476
    SWOT analysis, 1476t
Cholesterol, 324
    apical periodontitis, 324–325
    crystals, accumulation of, 325
    cyclopentanoperhydrophenanthrine, 324f
    in disease, 324
    Teflon cage model, 325
    tissue reaction to, 325, 326f, 327f
Chronic apical periodontitis, 1099
Chronic inflammation, 345, 474–475
    granuloma, 475

pulpal abscess, 475
  beneath deep cavity preparation, 486f
Chronic obstructive pulmonary disease (COPD), 752
Chronic rhinosinusitis, 628, 634
Claims against, endodontists, 87t
Clark's rule of horizontal angulation, 560, 561f, 929. *See also* Ingle's MBD rule
Cleaning/disinfecting, root canal system (laser), 860–861
Cleaning/shaping, instruments, 813–838
  basics. *See* Endodontic instruments
  Nickel-Titanium. *See* Ni-Ti endodontic instruments
  rotary. *See* Rotary instruments
Clinical examination, endodontics, 524
  vital signs, 524
    blood pressure/temperature/cancer screen, 524–525
    coronal evaluation, 525
    extra/intra oral examination, 525
Clinical guidelines, preoperative, 886
  assessing complicating factors, 886
  assessing occlusal/external root form, 886
  determining point of penetration, 886
  radiographic assessment and measurement, 886
CMOS-APS, 573, 577–578
CNS. *See* Central nervous system (CNS)
Codes of Ethics, ADA, 88, 102
Collagen, 129–130
  as perforation barrier material, 1130
Color power Doppler (CPD), 592
  application to echography, 593
  confirming information, 593
  picture representing the echo, 608f
Complementary Metal Oxide Semiconductor (CMOS), 573, 577, 580f
Complement cascade, 354f
Composite resins, 1042
Computed Dental Radiography (CDR), 573, 586

Cone-Beam Computed Tomography (CBCT), 573
  demonstrating apical dental cyst, 600f
Cone positioning, endodontic radiography, 559
  horizontal cone angulations. *See* Horizontal cone angulations
  long cone, 557
  short cone, 557
  teeth, 559f
Congestive heart failure, 761–762
  New York Heart Association's classification system, 762f
Coronal access cavity preparation, 877
Coronal disassembly devices
  active instruments, 1096–1097, 1097f
  grasping instruments, 1096
  percussive instruments, 1096
Coronal evaluation
  intraorifice barrier, 1042
Coronal leakage, 645, 1091
  barrier, 645
  closure materials and variations in, 1076, 1077f
  evaluation methods, 1056
  leak proof amalgam, 1078f
Coronal leakage and prognosis for healing, 1091–1093
  armamentaria and missed canals, 1097–1100
  coronal disassembly, 1095
  coronal disassembly devices. *See* Coronal disassembly devices
  factors influencing restorative removal, 1095–1096
  non-surgical *versus* surgical retreatment, 1095
  technology of retreatment, 1094–1095
  temporary coronal restorations, 1093–1094
Coronal pulp, 131f
Coronal restorations, temporary, 1093–1094
Coronal restorative procedures, 71
  root canal space/coronal access openings, involvement, 71

Coronal tooth preparation, 1458, 1458f
Corrective surgery
  bicuspidization, definition, 1281
  curved periodontal probe, 1279f
  definition, 1274
  hemisection, 1279–1281
    completed on mandibular second molar with fracture, 1299f
  periodontal regenerative procedures/contraindications, 1281
  periradicular repair, 1295–1296
  replantation, intentional, 1281–1284
  root amputation, 1277–1279
    nonsurgical root canal therapy, 1277
    root canal therapy, completed, 1298f
  traumatic root fracture repair, 1277
Cracked tooth, 660
Crown fractures
  complicated, 1330–1331
    histologic appearance, pulp within 24 hours of traumatic exposure, 1353f
  concomitant attachment damage, 1331
  restorative treatment plan, 1331–1332
  root
    horizontal, 1304f, 1339
    treatment, 1341
  time between accident/treatment, 1331
  tooth development, stage of "blunderbuss," 1331
  treatment, 1331
  vital pulp therapy, 1313
C-shaped canals, 915
Cuspal fracture odontalgia
  identification problem, 663
Cyclopentanoperhydrophenanthrine, 324f
Cyst, 311, 321
  bay cyst, 313
  nonsurgical root canal therapy, 322
  radicular cyst, 323f
    apical pocket cysts, 315f, 316
    apical true cysts, 313

Cystic apical periodontitis, 311f
cysts and periapical healing,
321–322
diagnosis of periapical cysts,
309–310
foreign bodies, 328–332
genesis of pocket cysts, 316–321
genesis of true cysts, 313–316
oral pulse granuloma, 332–334
periapical cysts
histopathology of, 312–313
incidence of, 309
Cystic lesions, 320–321
ciliated columnar epithelial cells
(CEP) lining of, 312f
Cyst luminal wall, 317f
Cyst management, 60f
Cyst *versus* granulomas, 597
differential diagnosis, 595
Cytokines
origin and actions of, 356–357t
roles of cytokines in
periradicular bone
resorption, 366
systemic effects of, 358

D

Decayed-missing-filled (DMF), 10
Decimated dentition, 15f
Deep caries, treatment of,
1403–1405
pulpotomy treatment and
indirect pulp therapy,
1403–1405
success rate of, studies,
1404–1405
Definitive restoration, type of
coronal tooth preparation, 1458
DEJ. *See* Dentin-enamel junction
(DEJ)
Dens evaginatus, 165, 201
Dens invaginatus, 165
type 1, 162
type 2, 162
type 3, 160f, 161f, 158–165
radicular-form of, 165f
Dental claims, frequency, 87t
Dental implants
on endodontics, effects of, 108
provisional restorations,
1296–1306

Dental materials, 482
Dental pulp, 37, 119, 119f, 126. *See also* Vital dental pulp
chronology of discoveries
histology, 37t–38t
pulpodentinal histology, 37
layers in, 126f
photos, 39f
sensory and sympathetic nerves
to, 137f
Dental Trade Alliance (DTA), 1477
Dental trauma, treatment methods
Cvek partial pulpotomy, 1335f
full pulpotomy, 1336
partial pulpotomy, 1333
"Cvek pulpotomy," 1333
pulp capping, 1333
pulpectomy, 1336
technique, 1333–1337
Dental treatment
level of compliance, 750
modification of, 749
need for modification
MD-RAM, 752, 753f
physical examination prior to, 751
previous dental, 751
recommendations for
modification of, 752
stress of, 751
Dentin, 121
permeability, 121f
and pulp, balance between, 123f
and pulp complex, structure of,
118
sensitivity, theories of, 124
tubules, 121
Dentinal hypersensitivity, 386
Dentinal tubules
exposed, as communication
pathways between pulp
and periodontal ligament,
638, 608f
scanning electron micrograph of
open, 639
Dentin chip apical obturation, 1067
root canal plug after 3 months,
1068f
Dentin-enamel junction (DEJ), 481
Dentin–pulp complex, 118
embryology, 118–121
nerves in pulp
classification of nerves,
136–137, 137t

distribution, 137–139
function, 139–141
neuropeptides, 137
neurophysiology, 142–143
receptors, 141–142
structures and functions
arteriovenous anastomosis and
"U"-turn loops, 131–132,
132f
cellular structures, 127
dental pulp, 125–126
dental–pulp complex, 121
dentin permeability, 121–123
dentin sensitivity, 124–125
dentin structure, 121
extracellular matrix, 129
fibers, 129–130
fibroblast, 127
ground substance, 130
immunocompetent cells, 129
interstitial fluid, 125–127
low-compliance system theory,
134–135
lymph vessels, 136
odontoblasts, 127–129
pulpal microvasculatures,
130–131
pulp reaction to permeating
substances, 123–124
regulation of pulpal blood
flow, 132–134
stealing theory, 134
transcapillary fluid flow, 135
Dentin thickness, after endodontic
treatment
post/core, type of
prefabricated, 1452–1457
Dentistry, initial suggestions,
549–550
Design aesthetics, operations
management, 1484
branding, 1484–1485
assimilation, program in
action, 1489–1490
brand–customer relationship,
1491
customer relationship, 1491
developing culture of excellence,
basic steps, 1494
enabling successful practice,
1484
increased concern, case,
1484–1485

office personality, 1488
strategic development, 1489–1490
strategic development/ foundation building/ implementation, 1489–1490
technology to operationalize, use of, 1487–1488
touchpoint overview, 1491–1494
understanding, 1494–1495
creating a web site/stationary/ brochure
web site, starting pointers, 1506
customer satisfaction index, 1486, 1486f
employee motivation and morale, 1488–1489
attitudes/retention, 1492
brand-driven behaviors, 1489
goals, branding strategy, 1486
HIPAA, 1492
learning organization, existence, 1489
NHII, 1487
office design, 1483t
patient satisfaction surveys, 1495–1496
TQM, 1496
"quality in fact"/"quality in kind," 1495
understanding satisfaction, 1495
Diabetes, 762–763
Diagnosis
case history, 407
classification, 407
clinical classification of craniofacial pain, 407t
extracranial/intracranial pathema, 408
history
chronic paroxysmal hemicrania (CPH), 409
general inspection, 410
myofascial TrP pain, 409
past medical, 410
PHN, 408
social, 410
temporal patterns, 408
operant pain (pain behavior)
somatization/malingering/ munchausen syndrome, 414

physical examination
cranial nerve examination, 411, 411t
inspection, 411, 423t
local pathosis of extracranial structures, 413t
myofascial TrP examination, 411
psychogenic pain, 413
Diagnostician, requirements
curiosity, 521
interest, 520, 521
intuition, 521
knowledge, 521
patience, 521
Diagnostic studies, 412, 412t
Diagnostic testing
anesthetic test, 542
infiltration, 542
dyes, 542–543
caries indicator solutions, 543f
electric pulp testing. *See* Electric pulp test (EPT)
magnification, 542
mobility, 539
Miller Index, 539
palpation, 539–540
crown of tooth with crack located transilluminator, 553f
toris mandibularis, 540
PDL injection, 542
percussion, 539
periodontal probing, 541
double-ended instruments, 541
Glickman classification system, 541
methylene blue dye, 541f
vertical root fracture (VRF), 541
pulpal blood flow, measurement, 544
system B hot pulp test tip, 537
test cavity, 541–542
thermal tests, 533–537
carbon dioxide snow, 535
cold response, 534
false negative, definition, 534
solid CO_2, applied on tooth/ tank, 536f
warm/cold, 535–538
warm thermal technique, 537
tooth surface temperatures, measurement, 543–544

electronic thermography, 543
Hughes Probeye 4300 thermal video system, 543
transillumination, 540
fiberoptic illumination, 541
ultraviolet light, 544
visual oral examination/review of systems. *See* Visual oral examination, diagnostic testing
Diaket, 1070
Dialister invisus, 237
Dialister pneumosintes, 237
Differential scanning calorimetry (DSC), 802–807, 804f, 805f, 827
Digital Imaging and Communication in Medicine (DICOM), 573, 576, 579
Digital intraoral radiography, endodontic roots of, 574
Direct pulp cap, 1405
treatment recommendations, 1320–1322
vital pulp therapy
of mandibular left molar, radiographic/clinical sequence, 1322
one-step pulp capping, 1322
Discoloration, 11
Doctor-Patient Relationship (DPR), 86
Dog pulp, 118f
Doppler technique, 134
Drainage through coronal access opening, 706
complex diagnoses, 707
instrumentation, 707
magnification/illumination, enhanced, 707
trephination, 707
Drug administration, comparison of routes, 747t
Drug–drug interactions
antibiotics and effects on oral contraceptives, 781
effect of oral contraceptives, 781
effects of combination of drugs, 781
patient's response to, 780
problems with higher levels of combination of drugs, 782

serious drug reactions with macrolides, 782
unexpected effects of new drugs, 781
Drug interactions
 change in reactions, 781
  by combination of drugs, 781
  increased/decreased effects, 781
 with food and herbals, decrease/increase effects of
  Ginkgo biloba, 787
  Kava, 787
  Khat, 787
  Licorice, 788
  orange juice, 788
  other drugs, 787
Drug interactions and laboratory tests
 with food and herbals, 787–788
  drugs prescribed by dentist that may interact with herbal medicines, 802t
  lab tests of potential importance in endodontics, 788–789
Drugs, banned, 781
Drugs prescribed by dentists interact with warfarin anticoagulant, 787f
DSC. *See* Differential scanning calorimetry (DSC)
DSC heating (lower)/cooling (upper) curves, 803f, 804f, 805f
D-speed film radiographs *versus* TACT, 582–583
DTA. *See* Dental Trade Alliance (DTA)

E

Echography, 309
The Economics of Endodontics, 4
Edentulism, 10
Educational curricula and attitudes of pediatric dentists, 1423–1425
 caries on primary incisors, 1424f
EEO. *See* Equal employment opportunity (EEO)
Eikenella corrodens, 237
Electric foramen locator, 929

Electric pulp test (EPT), 630
 Analytic Technology pulp tester, 538, 538f
 Electrocardiogram (EKG), 538
 patient placing finger lightly on metal part of the probe handle, 538f
Electric pulp tester, 534, 547, 713
Electronic apex locator (AEL)
 accuracy, 844
  dual-frequency electronic apex locators, 851–852
  high/low frequency apex locators, 851
  multiple-frequency electronic apex locators, 852–853
  resistance-based electronic apex locators, 849–850
  voltage gradient apex locators, 851
 generations, first to fifth, 849
 parameters for use, 853
Electrosurgery/electrofulguration, 1412–1414
 comparing studies, 1413–1417
Emergency surgical procedures
 radiographic interpretation, 1285
Emphysema, 1146
 radiograph of lower left canine, 1147f
 swollen tissues, 1146, 1147f
Employee Retirement Income Security Act (ERISA), 1504
Enamel knot, 119
Endodontics, 3–4, 12f
 access
  clinical methods, 153
  laboratory methods, 153
 anxiety/fear problem
  management, 738
  recognition, 737–738
  regulation, 739–740
 areas, 37
 chronology, developments, 51t–52t
 clinical symptoms and lesions of, origin, 1097f
 defined, 1
 definition, 37
 DPR. *See* Doctor-Patient Relationship (DPR)
 ethics/morals, 86–88

  ethical basis for standard of care, 88
  moral behavior, 88
 factors deciding retreatment, 1100
 fractured premolar restoration, 12f
 frequency of claims, 86–87
 future of, 74
 historical stalwarts, 73–74
 informed consent, 87–94
  AAE, 93
  definition, 92
  objective standard, 92
 length determination
  controversies in, 1139–1140
 malpractice, common elements, 86t
 miracle cures/pastes/mystery, 73
  anesthetics, 74
  irrigants, 73
  medicaments, 73
  obturation materials/techniques, 74
  surgical materials/instruments/techniques, 74
 non-surgical treatment, root canal systems, 48–53
 periapical origin
  differential diagnosis/treatment, oral pain in pulp, 43–46
  etiology/diagnosis/prevention/treatment, pulp disease, 40–43
  morphology/physiology/human dental pulp, pathology/periapical tissues, 37–40
 periapical pathosis, surgical removal, 53–66
 record keeping, 98–100
  SOAP format, 98
 referrals, 100–103
  four general categories, 102
  subsequent radiograph, 100
 scopes, 65
 standard of care, 88–91
  controversy, 89
  definition, 88
  endodontic instrument, 89f
  informed/uninformed, consent, 91

instrument breakage, 89
legal claims, role of, 88
paresthesia, 91
root canal filling, 89
vital pulp therapy, 46–48
Endodontic abscesses/cellulitis, treatment of, 692
  acrylic stint in place for decompression, 699f
  antibiotics, 692–698
    in endodontics, 693–695
  aspirate from abscess/cellulitis, 693f
  biopsy from window consistent with radicular cyst, 699f
  capillary/penrose/rubber dam, drain, 693f
  collection of a microbial sample, 696
  conditions not requiring, adjunctive antibiotics, 694t
  cortical trephination, 696–697, 699f
  decompression, aspiration and irrigation, 697–701
    nasogastric tubing in cyst for decompression., 700f
  drain sutured in place, 692f
  healed surgical window, 699f
  incision for drainage, 692–693
  needle aspiration, 692–694
  prophylactic antibiotics for medically compromised patients
    AHA, 695
  surgical window into cyst, 699f
Endodontically treated teeth
  risks associated with post-retained restorations of, 1200
Endodontic biofilms, 278–279
Endodontic considerations in dental trauma
  adjunctive therapy, 1350
  apical neurovascular damage, effects, 1343–1345
  avulsed tooth, 1348–1352
  crown fracture, 1330–1332
  dental trauma, unique aspects, 1330
  endodontic essentials/treatment. See Endodontics, essentials
  hard tissue apical barrier, 1337–1338
  internal root resorption, 1352–1353
  luxation injury, 1347–1348
  pulp revascularization, 1338–1339
    mature teeth, 1339
  root filling visit, 1351
  treatment. See also Dental trauma, treatment methods
    established external root resorption, 1345–1347
    nonvital pulps. See Nonvital pulps treatment
    root fracture complications. See Root fracture complications, treatment of
  vital pulp therapy. See Vital pulp therapy, traumatic dental injuries
Endodontic disease, microbiology
  actinomyces, 262–263
  bacterial biofilms, 268–269
    adoption of resistance, phenotype, 276–277
    BCI. See Biomaterial-centered infection (BCI)
    characteristics, 270
    communicate, exchange genetic materials/acquire new traits, 271
    in dentistry, 277–278
    development, 271–273
    endodontic, 278–279
    extracellular polymeric matrix, resistance, 276
    extraradicular microbial, 283–284
    growth rate/nutrient availability, resistance, 276
    intracanal microbial, 279–283
    microbes to antimicrobials, resistance, 273–275
    organized internal compartmentalization, 270–271
    periapical microbial, 284–285
    protection from environmental threats, 270
    ultrastructure, 269–270
  diagnostic techniques, microbiological, 227–228
  culture, advantages/limitations, 234–236, 230t
  endodontic flare-ups, 266
    specific bacteria, endodontic symptoms/associations, 267–269
  intracanal disinfection procedures, 241
  microbes, association, 224–227
  outcome, bacterial influence, 241–243
  primary intraradicular infections, 236–238
Endodontic disease, primary endodontic therapy, 626
  in mandibular first molar with necrotic pulp, 648f
  osseous repair, following trauma, 648f
Endodontic endosseous implants, 69–70
Endodontic examination
  apical diagnosis. See Apical diagnosis
  clinical examination. See Clinical examination, endodontics
  diagnostician, requirements of, 520
  history
    chief complaint, 523
    medical history form, 521, 522t
    present dental illness, 523–525
  pulpal diagnosis, 526
Endodontic failure, 309, 1296, 1296f
  cause, 1125
Endodontic flare-ups
  age of patient, 701
  anatomic location, 701–702
  anxiety, 702
  gender, 701
  glossary, endodontic terms, 700
  inter-appointment pain, causes of, 702
  mechanical/chemical injuries, 702
  obturation, 704
  preoperative history, tooth, 702
  pulp/periapical status, 702
  re-treatment cases, 703
    swelling associated with flare-up following revision, 703f
  systemic conditions, 701

treatment of teeth, vital/non-vital pulps, 702–703
treatment visits, number of, 702
working length, 703–704
Endodontic flare-ups, treatment of diagnosis and definitive treatment, 705–706
Endodontic implants, 1298, 1299f
Endodontic infections, 223–224
  anachoresis, 225
  colonization, 223
  control of
    host defense system, 992
    instrumentation and irrigation, 992
    intracanal medicaments, 1009
    permanent root filling, 992, 1003
  interaction and characteristics, 1089f
  microorganisms, 238–240
    archaea, 238
    fungi, 238
    virus, 238–240
  missed canals, finding, 1100
  and MSDO, 631–635
  pathogenicity, 224
  polymicrobial interactions/ nutritional requirements, 225–226
  pulpal/periapical pathoses, 224
  virulence factors, 245–249
Endodontic instruments, 2, 89f, 814
  AAE, 814
  ADA, 814
  ANSI, 814
  barbed broaches, 823–824, 823f
  cutting blades, 814
  endodontic instrument standardization
    autoclaving, 814
      K-style modification, 815–816
      unused instruments, condition of (comparisons), 815f
  files, 816–820
    competing brands for cutting ability, comparison, 817
    instrument breakages, Sotokawa's classification of instrument damage, 819f
    instrument fracture, cracks and deformation, 820f
    fracture mechanisms, 943
    gates glidden modification, 823
    hand instrument conclusions, 823
    hedstrom files, retraction, 821–822
    H-style file modification, 822
    Quantec 'files,' 823
    reamers, 816
    tip modification, 820–821
      H-style instruments, 821f
    U-file, 822
      cross-sectional view, 822f
      lightspeed instrument, unusual, 822f
      marketed names, 820–821
Endodontic panacea. *See* Calcium hydroxide
Endodontic patient, medically complex, management of
  adrenal suppression and long-term steroid use, 770
  allergy to materials in endodontic therapy
    antibiotics and analgesics, 772–773
    intracanal medications, cements, and filling materials, 773–774
    irrigating solutions, 773
    latex, 772
    local anesthetics, 770–772
  assessing need for treatment modifications
    multidimensional risk assessment model (MD-RAM), 752–754
  bone marrow and solid organ transplantation
    hematopoietic stem cell transplantation, 766–767
    solid organ transplantation, 767
  cancer chemotherapy and radiation therapy, 765–766
  bisphosphonate-associated osteonecrosis of jaws, 766
  cardiovascular disease
    anticoagulant therapy and bleeding disorders, 761
    arrhythmias and cardiac pacemakers, 761
    congestive heart failure, 762–763
    diabetes, 762–763
    heart murmurs and valvular disease, 757–760
    hypertension, 754–757
    ischemic heart disease, 756–767
    vasoconstrictor use in patients with cardiovascular disease, 755–756
  central nervous system, 764–765
  human immunodeficiency virus, 768–769
  liver disease, 769
  medical consultations, 752
  medical history and patient interview, 749–750
  medications and allergies, 750–751
  physical exam: vital signs, 751
  physical health status, 751–752
  pregnancy, 768
  previous dental treatment, 751
  prosthetic joints and other prosthetic devices, 767–768
  pulmonary disorders: asthma, COPD, and tuberculosis, 763–764
  relative stress of planned procedure and behavioral considerations, 751
  renal disease and dialysis, 765
  sickle cell anemia, 769
Endodontic–periodontal diseases, 654, 654f
  communication, main pathways, 638
  diagnosis for treatment and prognosis, 647
    primary endodontic disease, 647
    primary periodontal disease, 647
    secondary periodontal involvement, 647–650
  endodontic and periodontal, 638
  in mandibular first molar, 655f
  presence and prevalence of fungi, 643–644
  role of bacteria, 641–644
Endodontic–periodontal interrelationships
  communication, 638

apical foramen, 640
dentinal tubules, 638
lateral and accessory canals, 638–640
contributing factors, 644
coronal leakage, 645
developmental malformations, 646–647
inadequate endodontic treatment, 644
root perforations, 646
traumatic injuries, 645–646
dentin exposure, importance in progression, 638
differential diagnosis, 647
primary endodontic disease, 647
with secondary periodontal involvement, 647–650
primary periodontal disease, 647
secondary endodontic involvement, 650–653
prognosis, 654–656
true combined diseases, 653–654
etiological factors, 641
bacteria, 641–643
fungi, 643–644
viruses, 644
pulpal–periodontal interrelationship, 640–641
Endodontic-periodontal lesion, 608f
Endodontic procedures, nonsurgical
confined to root canal, 930
Endodontic radiography, 554
application of radiography to endodontics, 554–556
limitations of radiographs, 556
technology systems, 556–557
cone positioning, 559
diagnostic radiographs, 558
extraoral film placement, 570
film, 557
horizontal angulation, 560
horizontal cone angulations. *See* Horizontal cone angulations
intraoral film placement, 557–558
long cone, 557

processing, 570
rapid-processing solutions, 570–571
short cone, 557
table-top developing, 571
traditional machines, 557
vertical angulation, 560
working radiographs, 558–559
Endodontic retreatment
preoperative radiograph of non-healing maxillary central incisor, 1094f
special concerns in, 1090
Endodontics, digital imaging for, 573–574
digital intraoral X-ray imaging options
digital radiography, 576–577
using secondary capture of analog film images, 574–576
radiation dose, 583–587
working principles of digital systems
advantages of digital X-ray imaging, 579
conventional *versus* digital, 581
detection of periapical lesions, 581–582
detection of root canal anatomy, 582–583
digital subtraction radiography, 583
evaluation of assessment of root canal length, 582
examples of digital images used in endodontics, 579–580
solid-state systems, 577–578
storage phosphor detectors, 578–579
Endodontics, essentials, 1348
concussion/subluxation, 1347
extrusive/intrusive/lateral luxation, 1347–1348
treatment, 1350–1351
Endodontic sealers, 1068
APEXIT, 1070
bonding to gutta-percha and dentin, 1072f
calciobiotic root canal sealer, 1069

kerr pulp canal sealer EWT, 1069
rationale for use of sealers, 1068–1069
roth's 801, 1069
SealApex, 1069–1070
VITAPEX, 1070
Endodontics mode, 878
accessing through crown, disadvantages, 878
areas in, use of lasers, 962–963
existing restorations, advantages, 878
Endodontic specialists, 3, 5f, 6f, 7f
Endodontic studies
acceptable, relevant procedures, 1178
categories, 1171
evidence-based practice, 1171
minimizing bias in studies, 1171
research design, 1170
confounding effects of different variables, 1179–1181
considerations specific to, 1179
treatment differences in studies on apical surgery, 1190
variation in treatment procedures, 1175–1177
Endodontic surgery
anatomical considerations, 1235–1237
anesthesia and hemostasis, 1237–1239
adrenergic receptors in tissues, 1238
beta-adrenergic effect, 1239
objectives, 919
osteotomy on mandibular molar, 1238f
periradicular surgery, 1244
vasoconstrictor, 1249
vasopressor agents, 1237
corrective surgery. *See* Corrective surgery
emergency procedures. *See* Emergency surgical procedures
flap design and soft tissue management. *See* Soft tissue management and flap design
greater palatine foramen, opening of, 1235f

historical perspectives
  microsurgical endodontics, 1233
  specific indications, 1234
horizontal/vertical sulcular incisions, 1241, 1241f
implant surgery. See Implant surgery
indications/contraindications/ classification
  endodontic surgery, contemporary classification of, 1234
palatal flap reflected and sutured, 1244f
periradicular surgery/treatment. See Periradicular surgery, treatment planning
rectangular flap to perform periapical surgery on maxillary central and lateral incisors, 1242f
resection, root-end. See Root-end resections
scar (arrow) in gingival tissues resulting from use of semilunar flap for periapical surgery, 1243f
soft tissue lesion, 1250
submarginal flap at time of suture placement, 1244f
surgical outcomes. See Surgical outcomes
tissue management
  hard, curettage. See Hard tissue management and curettage
  soft, suturing/postoperative care. See Soft tissue management, suturing and postoperative care; Soft tissue management and flap design
topical/local, hemostasis. See Hemostasis, topical/local
triangular flap to perform periapical surgery
  distobuccal root of maxillary molar, 1241f
  mandibular second premolar, 1241f
Endodontic techniques
  aspects of, 1198–1199

Endodontic therapy
  allergy to materials used in, 770, 771f
  anticipating the future, 29
  case representation, 10–12
    considerations, 16
    indications, 12–15
    oral conditions, 16–21
  change
    attitudes, 4
    endodontics, 3–4
    instrument design/ standardization, 2–3
    nomenclature, 1–2
  endodontics, controversies
    apical patency and its preparation, 28–29
    apicalterminus and cleaning apical patency, 25–28
    postoperative pain, 23
    single-appointment therapy, 21–23
    success versus failure, 23–25
  factors influencing post removal and heat transfer, 1136–1138
  future, as speciality, 4–10
  inadequate radiograph of mandibular first molar with crown, screw post, 1115f
  mishaps and serious complications of
    factors influencing post removal and heat transfer, 1135–1137
    thermal injury with use of ultrasonics, 1135–1136
  past/present, future prologue, 29–30
  post insufficient, 1097f
  thermal injury with use of ultrasonics, 1135–1136
  transforming advances
    saliva, diagnostic/informative fluid, 30
    tissue engineering, 30
    tooth regeneration, 30–31
Endodontic therapy, primary teeth
  comparison of primary and permanent tooth anatomy, 1400–1402
  diagnosis of pulpal pathosis in children, 1416

  educational curricula and attitudes of pediatric dentists, 1423–1425
  electrosurgery/electrofulguration, 1412–1414
  ferric sulfate, 1259–1260
  formocresol, 1406–1411
  freeze-dried bone, 1412
  glutaraldehyde, 1411–1412
  lasers, 1414–1415
  medical factors in determining if a primary tooth should be saved
    contraindications, 1460–1461
  mineral trioxide aggregate, 1030
  nonvital pulp therapy for children, 1417–1423
  pulpotomy, 1406
  treatment of deep caries: indirect pulp therapy, 1403–1405
  vital pulp therapy for children: direct pulp cap, 1332–1333
Endodontic therapy and mishap management, retreatment of non-healing, 1088
  air emphysema, 1146
  blocks, ledges, and apical transportations, 1122
    techniques for managing apical transportations, 1123–1125
    techniques for managing blocked canals, 1122–1123
    techniques for managing canal ledges, 1123
  carrier-based gutta-percha, 1141
  coronal leakage and prognosis for healing, 1091–1093
    armamentaria and techniques associated with missed canals, 1097–1100
    coronal disassembly, 1095
    coronal disassembly devices. See Coronal disassembly devices
    factors influencing restorative removal, 1095–1096
    non-surgical versus surgical retreatment, 1095
    technology of retreatment, 1094–1095
    temporary coronal restorations, 1093–1094

damage to neurovascular
  anatomy: causes and
  outcomes, 1141–1142
 diagnosis and management of
  inferior alveolar nerve
  injury, 1142–1143
 management of inferior
  alveolar nerve injuries,
  1143–1144
 fractured instrument removal,
  1114–1115
  coronal and radicular access
   for, 1116–1117
  creating a staging platform,
   1117
  factors influencing, 1136–1137
  removal using microtube
   system, 1120–1121
  techniques for, 1122
  ultrasonic techniques for,
   1117–1119
 length determination
  controversies in
  endodontics, 1139–1140
 mishaps and serious
  complications of
  endodontic therapy
  factors influencing post
   removal and heat transfer,
   1136–1138
  thermal injury with use of
   ultrasonics, 1135–1136
 NaOCl accident, 1145
  causes of NAOCL accident,
   1145
  management, 1145–1146
  prevention, 1146
 obturation and irrigation
  mishaps, 1137–1138
  anatomic and imaging
   characteristics of inferior
   alveolar canal, 1138–1139
  anatomic and imaging
   characteristics of
   maxillary sinus, 1138
  importance of accurate
   radiographic imaging, 1138
 perforation and prognosis for
  healing, 1125
  barrier materials for perforation
   repair, 1130–1131
  clinical considerations
   influencing perforation
   repair based on evidence,
   1129
  esthetics and perforation
   repair, 1130
  hemostatics for perforation
   repair, 1130
  location of perforation,
   1127–1128
  MTA for perforation repair,
   1129
  perforation repair materials,
   1128
  periodontal condition and
   perforation repair,
   1129–1130
  restorative materials in
   perforation repair, 1131
  size of perforation, 1128
  techniques for perforation
   repair, 1131–1135
  timing of perforation repair,
   1125–1127
  treatment sequence for
   perforation repair, 1130
  vision and perforation repair,
   1130
 post removal, 1110
  factors influencing, 1110
  mechanical devices,
   1112–1114
  techniques for, 1110–1112
 post-treatment infection of root
  canal system
  disease factors, 1088–1089
  previous root canal treatment,
   1089
 prevention of obturation
  mishaps, 1144–1145
 removal of obturation materials,
  1100
  gutta-percha, 1131,
   1138–1389. *See also*
   Gutta-percha (filling
   material), removal of
  microtube removal options,
   1105–1107
  paste removal, 1108–1110
  Resilon, 1103
  silver points, 1065
 risks *versus* benefits, 1089
  benefits, 1089–1090
  patient considerations,
   1090–1091
  risks, 1090
  special concerns in endodontic
   retreatment, 1090
  techniques for obturation control
   when neurovascular
   proximity exists, 1140
  thermoplasticized gutta-percha
   and effects of heat,
   1140–1141
Endodontic treatment
 aim and asymptomatic function,
  1165
 consent, 530–531
  ameloblastoma, 100f
 disinfecting agents
  Ca(OH)$_2$, 1009
  CHX, 1002
  hydrogen peroxide, 1388
  NaOCl, 997–1002
 and increased susceptibility
  fracture, 920f
 internal resorption, 601f
 local contraindications, 48f
 non-surgical, 643f
 persistent disease after
  re-treatment, 1174f
 replacing pulp tissue, 921
 re-treatment in conjunction with
  internal perforation
  repair, 1196f
 role of radiograph, 574
 root-end management with
  bonded composite resin,
  1177f
 success of, 573
Endodontic treatment failure,
  microbes, 257–258
Endodontic treatment outcome,
  1173
 ambiguity of outcome definition,
  1162–1165
 consequences of using terms
  "success" and "failure,"
  1163–1165
 lenient definition of "success,"
  1163
 outcome definition as
  "uncertain,"
  "questionable,"
  "doubtful," or
  "improved," 1163
 strict definition of "success,"
  1163

antibacterial efficacy of intra-
    canal procedures, 1200
apical enlargement, 1201
dressing with medication,
    1200–1201
factors influencing healing
    after apical surgery, 1201
irrigation, 1200
apical periodontitis, teeth
    treated with associated,
    1187
dynamics of healing,
    1199–201
functional teeth, 1184
healed teeth, 1184–1189
healing in progress, 1188
apical periodontitis, teeth treated
    without associated
dynamics of developing
    disease, 1184–1187
functional teeth, 1188
healed teeth, 1190
apical surgery, potential for
    healing and retained
    function after, 1190
dynamics of healing, 1191
functional teeth, 1191
healed teeth, 1187–1188
healing in progress, 1188
appraisal of endodontic outcome
    studies, 1171–1181
exposure (treatment,
    intervention), 1175–1178
outcome assessment,
    1187–1179
reporting of data and analysis,
    1179–1181
appraisal of studies, 1171–1175
appraisal of studies, general
    considerations, 1170–1171
dynamics of developing disease,
    1184–1187
evidence-base for outcome of
    endodontic treatment,
    1165–1170
radiographic outcome
    assessment, 1162
selected studies comprising
    "best" evidence, 1181
potential for healing and
    function after
    nonsurgical treatment,
    1192–1194

teeth treated without
    associated apical
    periodontitis, 1181–1183
Endogenous opioid system, 382
pain modulation
    endogenous opioid peptides,
    398
pain suppression, 398
Endo-Rez, 1072
Endoscope visual system (EVS), 873f
Endoscopic sinus surgery
    rhinosinusitis, 629
Endosseous root form implants,
    1298
Endotoxin, 1103
Enterococcus, 258–260
prevalence in endodontic
    infections, 259t
Enterococcus faecalis
cells, 999f
samples of, 996f
Enterococcus faecalis, 227
Enzyme-linked immunosorbent
    assay (ELISA), 1028
Epinephrine
containing local anesthetics and
    all drugs, 786t
Epiphany, 1073
sealer, 1028f
Epoxy resin sealers, 1035–1037
Epstein–Barr virus (EBV), 238
EPT. *See* Electric pulp test (EPT)
Equal employment opportunity
    (EEO), 1497
Equipment, rubber dam, 791
adjuncts to rubber dam
    placement, 796
plastic/cement instrument/
    dental floss, 796
clamps, 795
variety, 795f
winged clamp/wedjets cord,
    796f
dam material, 791–792
forceps, 795–796
rubber dam clamp selection,
    795t
frame/dam combinations, 794f
frames, 792–795
hinged rubber dam frame, 794f
latex-free barrier/U-shaped
    Young's rubber dams, 793f
punch, 792

swallowed endodontic file in
    appendix resulting in
    acute appendicitis, 792f
Erbium:YAG laser
removal of debris, effective, 963,
    964f
ERISA. *See* Employee Retirement
    Income Security Act
    (ERISA)
Escherichia coli, 232
Ethylenediaminetetraacetic acid
    (EDTA), 1075
citric acid and other acids,
    1000–1002
Etiological factor of apical
    periodontitis, bacteria,
    990
Eubacterium, 226
Extracellular matrix (ECM), 127,
    129
Extraction/alveolar preservation
allograft hydroxyapatite, 1303f
atraumatic extraction, 1302f
Extraction/implant placement,
    immediate
atraumatic extraction, 1302f
final drill, surgical template,
    1304f
grafting the gaps, implant/bone
    walls, 1305f
horizontal root fracture, 1304f
Extraradicular infections,
    endodontics, 243–244
apical actinomycosis, 243
Extraradicular microbial biofilms,
    283–284, 283f

F

Fair Labor Standards Act (FLSA),
    1504
Federation Dentaire Internationale
    (FDI), 1036
Ferric sulfate
comparing with formocresol
    pulpotomies and
    inference, 1429–1430
internal resorption in a primary
    molar, 1416f
Fiber optic endoscope (orascope),
    873, 873f, 874f
fogging, 873

Fibrefill, 1073
Fibroblast, 127
Fibronectin, 355
Filifactor alocis, 237
Filling
   gutta-percha *versus* Resilon, 1065f
   lateral canal, significance of, 1075, 1075f
   success/failure of root canal therapy, 1056t
   with and without radiography, clinical success of, 1055t
Film, X-ray machine, 559
   film placement
     extraoral film placement, 571
     intraoral film placement, 557–558
     teeth, 568f
   hemostat, 558f
     advantages, 561
   holder, 558f
   processing, 571
     rapid-processing solutions, 570–571
     table-top developing, 571
"Finger-powered" instruments, 3
First molar, 14f
Fixed partial denture (FPD), 105–106
Flaring apex, 22
FLSA. *See* Fair Labor Standards Act (FLSA)
Focal infection theory, 221–223
Food–drug interactions, 775
Foreign body reaction
   nonmicrobial aspects of disease
     accumulation of cholesterol crystals, 325
     cystic lesions, 320–321
     root canal filling, 328
     scar tissue healing, 336–337
Formocresol, 1417
   caries removal, 1407f
   placement of zinc oxide, 1408f
   primary molar with stainless steel crown, 1408f
   pulpotomy in primary teeth, 1408f
   removal of roof of pulp chamber and coronal pulp, 1407f
   studies on, 1421–1424
Fractured instrument removal, 1115–1116

challenge to remove broken Ni-Ti file, 1130
coronal and radicular access for instrument removal, 1116–1117
factors influencing fractured instrument removal, 1115–1116
File Adapter, 1119
   staging platform, 1118
     Gates Glidden drills, 1117f
     graphic representation of, 1117f
techniques, 1128
   Titanium instruments, 1117–1119, 1118f
   ultrasonic preparation, 1118
   ultrasonic techniques, 1117–1120
     design of, 1128–1129
     direct contact with obstruction and activation, 1118
     use of piezoelectric ultrasonic, 1128
   using a microtube system, 1120–1121
     creating potential for instrument retrieval, 1120f
Freeze-dried bone inference, 1478
Furcation perforation, 1127
Fusobacterium nucleatum, 237
Fusobacterium periodonticum, 237

G

Galilean optics, 871f
Gates Glidden (GG) burs, 880, 1117f
General mental ability (GMA), 1501
General practitioners (GPs), 113
Gene-targeting experiments, 119
Genetic polymorphism, 343
Gene transfer systems, 249
   antibiotic resistance/virulence, with plasmids, 252
   horizontal gene pool, 249–252
   pheromone-initiated conjugative transfer of plasmids, 252
GFR. *See* Glass fiber-reinforced epoxy resin (GFR)

Giant cell granuloma, 615f
Ginkgo biloba, 749
Glass fiber-reinforced epoxy resin (GFR), 1453–1455, 1454–1455f
Glass ionomer repair
   perforation repair, 1128
Glass ionomers, 1042
Glickman classification system, periodontal probing, 541
Glutaraldehyde, 1411–1412
GMA. *See* General mental ability (GMA)
Granulomas, 595–597
Grossman's sealer, 1038, 1069, 1072. *See also* Zinc oxide–eugenol-containing sealers
Growth factor
   bone regeneration, 361
   classifications, 360t
Guarded enthusiasm, 31
Gutta-balata, 1028. *See also* Gutta-percha
Gutta-percha delivery system, thermoplasticized
   Calamus system, 1024–1025, 1025f
   elements system, 1024f
   UltraFil system, 1025
Gutta-percha (filling material), 1066
   biological objectives, 933
   carrier-based, 1025–1027, 1141
     Densfil, 1025
     errors in technique, 1141
     removal, techniques used for, 1100–1107
     SimpliFil, 1027, 1027f
     SuccessFil, 107
   chlorhexidine, 1021
   composition, 1020t
   design objectives for cases to be filled with, 932
   disintegrated, 329f
   enterococcus faecalis, 1021
   giant cells within apical periodontitis, 332f
   inject-R fill, 1062
   lateral/vertical compaction of, 1062
   undesirable stress concentration, 1063

nickel–titanium *versus* stainless steel spreaders, 1058
observation in lateral grooves, 1075f
perforation repair with phosphate cement, 1131
plastic-embedded semithin of apical area, 331f
properties, 1027–1028
removal of, 1111–1112
   carrier-based, 1107–1108
   heat and instrument, 1102
   paper point and chemical removal, 1102–1103
   rotary instrumentation, 1100–1102, 1108f
   ultrasonic, 1102
versus Resilon, 1064f
root-filled and periapically affected left central maxillary incisor, 330f
root filling in split tooth model with straight and round canal, 1062f
sodium hypochlorite, structural effects, 1023
stereochemical structure, 1021f
system B plugger technique, 1061–1062
thermomechanical compaction, 1025
   MicroSeal System, 1022–1025
thermomechanical compaction of, 1060
thermomechanical solid core, 1060
thermoplasticized, 1023–1024
   and effects of heat, 1140–1141
   injectable, 1061
tissue reaction to, 328f
ultrasonic plasticized, 1060–1061
vertical *versus* lateral, 1062–1063
Gutta-percha point, 90f

H

Hard tissue apical barrier
  crown-root fractures, 1339
  filling of root canal, 1338
    "Swiss cheese" consistency, 1338
  horizontal root fractures, 1339
  treatment, 1341

MTA barrier, 1337–1338
  apexification, successful, 1337f
pulp revascularization, 1338–1339
  immature tooth, necrotic infected canal with apical periodontitis, 1346f
reinforcement of thin dentinal walls, 1338
traditional method, 1337
Hard tissue deconstruction, mechanism of, 1361
Hard tissue management and curettage
  bony window of adequate size to perform periapical surgery on mandibular premolar, 1250f
  bur, shape, 1249f
  curettage of inflammatory soft tissue, 1251
  curettage of soft tissue lesion allows for visualization of mesiobuccal root apex, 1251f
  osseous tissue response, surgical removal, 1249
  root end located following careful osseous removal, 1249f
  root surface distinguis, 1253
HBD. *See* Hypophosphatemic bone disease (HBD)
H&D curve, 585, 586, 586f
Healing, perforation and prognosis for, 1125
  barrier materials for perforation repair, 1130–1131
  clinical considerations influencing perforation repair based on evidence, 1129
  esthetics and perforation repair, 1130
  hemostatics for perforation repair, 1130
  location of perforation, 1127–1128
  MTA for perforation repair, 1129
  perforation repair materials, 1128

periodontal condition and perforation repair, 1129–1130
restorative materials in perforation repair, 1131
size of perforation, 1128
techniques for perforation repair, 1131–1135
timing of perforation repair, 1125–1127
treatment sequence for perforation repair, 1130
vision and perforation repair, 1130
Health Insurance Portability and Accountability Act (HIPAA), 1488
Heart murmurs and valvular disease, 757–760
  antibiotic prophylaxis for dental procedures, 759f
  antibiotic prophylaxis recommended, 758f
  increased risk for infective endocarditis, 757
  risk of dental procedures, 758f
Hematogenous total joint infection, 767f
Hematopoiesis of immune cells, 344
Hemostasis, topical/local, 1258
  bone wax, 1258
  calcium sulfate, 1260
  collagen products, 1260
  ferric sulfate, 1259
  gelfoam/spongostan, 1260
  microfibrillar collagen hemostat, 1260–1261
  racellet container and pellets, 1258
  root-end filling materials, 1261–1266
  surgicel, 1261
  thrombin, 1260
  vasoconstrictor-impregnated cotton pellets/sponges, 1258–1259
Hemostasis, vital pulp therapy, 1319–1320
  enterococcus, faecalis, 1320
  evaluation, clinical/short-term, 1319
  importance, 1319

irreversible pulpitis, 1319
NaOCl
  advantages of, 1319
  recommendations, 1320
Hemostat, straight, 558, 558f
  advantages, 559
Herbal medicine–drug interactions, 780
Hermetic, 1053. *See also* Impermeable seal
Heterogenous nature of dentin tubular, 122f
HIPAA. *See* Health Insurance Portability and Accountability Act (HIPAA)
Histopathology of periapical lesions of endodontic origin
  "abscess theory," 506
  acute apical abscess, 500, 508
    apical granuloma, 501f
      epithelial strands in apical granuloma, 505f
  apical cyst, 506, 506f
  apical scar, 508–509
  asymptomatic apical periodontitis, 507
  cellulitis, 508
  chronic apical abscess, 508
  condensing osteitis, 508
  normal periapical tissues, 507
  nutritional deficiency theory, 506
  symptomatic apical periodontitis, 507
  true cysts, 506
Historical stalwarts, endodontics, 73–74
Homeostasis phenomenon of pulp, periodontal ligament preventing osteoclastic attacks, 1358
Horizontal cone angulations, 560
  mandibular anterior teeth, 568–569
  mandibular molars, 560–565
  mandibular premolars, 565–566
  maxillary anterior teeth, 569–570
  maxillary molars, 566–567
  maxillary premolars, 567–568
Host defense, 1011
Human cytomegalovirus (HCMV), 238–240

Human immunodeficiency virus, 768–769
Human pulp, 126f
Human resources, operations management in endodontics
  confidentiality/non-competition covenants, 1507
  dental assistant wages, 1504t
  EEO, 1497
  employee benefit and salary administration
    ERISA, 1504
    FLSA, 1504
    HIPAA, 1504
  employee handbook, suggestions for creation, 1499–1501
    standard operating procedures: computers, 1500t
  employee notices, posting, 1503
  employee selection criteria, 1501–1502
    GMA, 1501
  employment law, 1505–1507
    law issues, 1506
    suggestions, avoid common legal pitfalls, 1506
  employment liability practices insurance, 1507
  hiring best person for job, 1502–1503
    areas to avoid, interviews, 1503
  job description, 1497
  management program, elements, 1497
  staff meetings and peak performance, 1507–1508
  standard operating procedure (SOP), 1497–1499
  tasks/knowledge/ability tasks, 1498t–1499t
  termination, 1504–1505
    factors, preserve objectivity, 1505
  workers' compensation, 1507
Hurter and Driffield curve. *See* H&D curve
Hydrogen peroxide, 1002
Hygroscopy, desiccation by, 483
Hyperparathyreoidism, primary, 616f

Hypersensitivity reactions
  innate, 368
  types, 367–368
Hypertension, 754–755
  blood pressure classification, 755f
Hypophosphatemic bone disease (HBD), 487

I

IASP. *See* International Association for the Study of Pain (IASP)
Iatrogenic effects, dental pulp, 479–482
  "blushing," 480
  cavity cleansing, 481
    dentin-enamel junction (DEJ), 481
    etching dentin/smear layer, 481
  cavity/crown preparation
    heat
      cutting dentin, 480
      experimental observations, 480
      laser beams, 481
    tooth structure, safe preparation, 481
  crown cementation, 482
  dental materials, 482
    desiccation by hygroscopy, 483
    heat upon setting, 482
    microleakage/cytotoxicity, 482
  impressions and temporary crowns, microleakage, 482
  local anesthetics, 479
  pins, 481
Iatrogenic perforations
  management, 1144
  setting of MTA and required treatment, 1124f
Idiopathic osteosclerosis, 608
IHS. *See* International Headache Society (IHS)
Imaging Plate, 573–579
Immune complex reactions, 367–368
Immunological methods, 230
Immunologic reactions, 367

Impermeable seal, 1053
Implant fracture, esthetic, 1307
Implant surgery
　endodontic endosseous implants, 1294
　osseointegrated implants, 1295
Incisive canal cyst, 613f
Indirect pulp therapy, 1425
Inferior alveolar nerve (IAN), 714
Inflamed dental pulp
　acute inflammatory process, 381
Inflammation, 344
Inflammation and immunological responses
　β-defensins, 348
　cells of adaptive immunity, 348–351
　cells of innate immunity, 344–348
　cytokines
　　proinflammatory cytokines, 356–358
　　systemic effects of, 358
　growth factors, 360–361
　hypersensitivity reactions, 367–368
　inflammation-induced bone resorption
　　inhibition of bone resorption by bisphosphonates, 366
　　mechanisms of bone resorption, 364–365
　　microbial role in pathogenesis of periradicular lesion, 363
　　role of immune cells in periapical lesion formation, 364
　　roles of cytokines in periradicular bone resorption, 366–367
　innate and adaptive immune systems, 344–345
　MHC and antigen presentation, 351–352
　molecular mediators of anti-inflammatory reactions
　　anti-inflammatory cytokines: IL-10, TGF-β, IL-4, and IL0-0, 362
　　membrane phospholipids/ arachidonic acid metabolic pathways, 361–362
　　NF-kB and NF-kB-activating pathways, 362–363
　molecular mediators of proinflammatory response
　　adhesion molecules, 352
　　chemokines, 352
　　plasma proteases, 353
　　　coagulation cascade and fibrinolytic systems, 354
　　　complement system, 354
　　　kinin system: bradykinin, 353
　　　matrix metalloproteinases, 354–355
　　　neutrophil elastase, 355
　　　platelet-activating factor, 352
　　neuropeptides, 358–359
　　nitric oxide, 355
　　oxygen-derived free radicals, 355–356
　　toll-like receptors, 359–360
Inflammatory mediators, 383
Inflammatory response, 343, 352, 353, 353f, 357, 358, 468
Infraorbital nerve block injection, 721
Ingle's MBD rule, 561, 564, 935
Inhibition of bone resorption by bisphosphonates
　mechanism of bisphosphonate (BP)-induced, osteoclast apoptosis, 366, 365f
Innate immune system, 344
　phagocytosis, 345
Innate immunity, cells of
　comparison of mast cells and basophils, 347t
　dendritic cells (DCs) and NK cells, 347–348
　eosinophils and basophils, 347
　odontoblasts, 348
　PMNs and macrophages, 346–347
Instrumentation and irrigation, 242
Instrumented and uninstrumented root canal wall after irrigation, 1000f, 1001f, 1007f
Instrument Removal System (iRS), 1107, 1108f, 1120, 1121
　clinical case utilizing, 1120f
Insular cortex (IC), 398
Intact coronal structure, 1296
Intentional replantation, 1220–1221
Intentional teeth replantation, 67–69
Interactions, microorganisms, 249–257
　antibiotic resistance and virulence associated with plasmids, 252
　cooperative/antagonistic, 253–254
　extra-chromosomal DNA, horizontal gene pool, 249–252
　gene transfer systems, 249
　pheromone-initiated conjugative transfer of plasmids, 252
　plasmids in oral and endodontic microflora, 253
　species-specific interactions, microorganisms in root canal infections, 254–256
International Association for the Study of Pain (IASP), 393
International Headache Society (IHS), 426
International Standards Organization, 573
Interradicular periodontal lesions, 69
Intracanal disinfection procedures, 241
Intracanal irrigation, 696
Intracanal medicaments containing antibiotics, 1011
Intracanal medications, cements, and filling materials, 772–773
Intracanal microbial biofilms, 279–283, 279f
Intranasal drug (IN drug), 746
Intraoral X-ray sensors, diversity of, 575f
Intravenous conscious sedation, 743–745
Iodine potassium iodide, 1006
IRM, 1043
Irrigants and intracanal medicaments, 992
　alternatives for interappointment medicaments
　　intracanal medicaments containing antibiotics, 1011
　　phenol compounds, 1011

developments in root canal disinfection, 1009
effect of instrumentation on root canal microbes, 993–994
elimination of microbes in root canal system, 992–993
goal of endodontic treatment, 993
infection control in human body, 992
instrumentation of root canal, 985
intracanal interappointment medicaments
   $Ca(OH)_2$, 1006–1007
   CHX, 1002–1006
physical means of canal cleaning and disinfection
   lasers, 1008–1009
   ultrasonic cleaning, 1007–1008
root canal disinfection by chemical means
   antibacterial irrigating solutions, 997
   CHX, 995–1003
   EDTA, citric acid and other acids, 1000–1002
   hydrogen peroxide, 1002
   iodine potassium iodide, 1006
   NaOCl, 997–1001
antibiotic-containing irrigation solutions
   MTAD and tetraclean, 1006–1007
   challenges, 994
   ex vivo and in vivo models, 995–997
   in vitro models, 994–995
Irrigating solutions, 771
Irrigation dynamics, 967–968
   effect of sizes and canal diameters needle position, 967f
   irrigation performance and size of needle, 968
Ischemic heart disease, 756–758
   treatment modification, 757

J

Japanese
   and one appointment therapy, 21
Journal of Endodontia, 36

K

Kava, 787
Kerr Broach, 2f
Kerr pulp canal sealer EWT, 1069
Ketac-endo, 1071
Khat, 787

L

Lactobacillus casei, 245
Lamina dura, 564–566
Laser-assisted canal preparation, 962–964
   limitations of, 964
   removal of debris using erbium:YAG laser, 989f
   effective, 990f
   shaping of single rooted teeth, 989f
   use in endodontics, 968
Laser beam, 857–861
Laser doppler flowmetry (LDF), 859
   applications. *See* Applications of LDF, dentistry
   laser Doppler setup, example, 548f
   potential modalities, 551–552
   technology, development and principle, 547
      Fast Fourier Transform (FFT) analysis, 548
      laser Doppler machine, readout, 563f
   use and development, 552
Laser in endodontics
   apical surgery, 865–866
      preparation of apical cavities, Er:YAG laser/ultrasonics, 866
   cleaning/disinfecting, root canal system, 860–864
      intra-canal use of lasers, limitations, 861
   endodontic retreatment, 865
   laser interactions, basic types, 874f
   laser irradiation, 878f
   obturation, root canal system, 864–865
      thermoplasticized compaction, concept, 864
   parameters, while operating laser, 874f
   principles of operation
      LASER beam, 857–859
      "surgical" beam, 857
   pulpal diagnosis, 859
      LDF, 859
   pulp capping/pulpotomy, 859–860
      mineral trioxide aggregate (MTA), 1030–1033
   radiograph, vertical root fracture, 879f
   schematic diagram of laser, 873f
   wavelengths, laser types according to emission spectra, 873f
Lasers, 1428
   compared with four pulpotomy techniques, 1415
   in endodontics, 1005–1006
Lasers in Endodontics, 857
Lateral canals
   clinical aids for identification, 640
   detection, 640
   vessels, 131f
Latex, use of, 770
LDF. *See* Laser Doppler Flowmetry (LDF)
LDF technology, development/principle, 547–549
Licorice, 787
LightSpeed (LSX), 944
Lightspeed NiTi rotary instrument, 805
Limited liability company (LLC), 1481
Limited liability partnership (LLP), 1481
Lipopolysaccharide (LPS), 224, 245–246, 468
Lipotechoic acid (LTA), 246–247, 468
Liver disease, 769
LLC. *See* Limited liability company (LLC)
LLP. *See* Limited liability partnership (LLP)
Loading protocol, immediate additional requirement, 1306
   advantages, 1315
Local anesthetics, 768

and all drugs, 783
EPT, 714
preliminary factors, clinical trial literature, 713
Loupes, visual enhancement
single/multi lens loupes, 870
Low-compliance system theory, 135
LPS. *See* Lipopolysaccharide (LPS)
LPS-binding protein (LBP), 346
LTA. *See* Lipotechoic acid (LTA)
Luxation injuries
definitions
concussion, 1347
direction, 1342
extrusive, 1342
lateral luxation, 1347
subluxation, 1353
trauma, types, 1354
external/internal inflammatory root resorption, 1343

M

Macrolides
potential reactions between macrolide antibiotics and all drugs, 783t
Macrophage colony-stimulating factor (MCSF), 365
Macrophages, 327
activation and function, 346f
Macrophages release somatostatin (SRIF), 502
Major histocompatibility complex (MHC), type II, 470
Malignant tumors in jaws, 617
Malpractice/negligence, common elements, 86t
Management (winning) practices, operations management in endodontic practice
focusing matrix, 480t
measuring customer defections, 1479t
primary, 1479–1480
secondary, 1480
Mandibular anesthesia, 714–716
adverse effects, 722
articaine, 715
bidirectional rotation method, 716

IAN block injections, 716
factors, for success, 717
lack of success, 716
reasons, lack of success, 716
intraligamentary injection, supplemental, 717–718
effects, potential adverse, 717
intraosseous
anesthesia delivery system X-tip, 737f
characteristics, 718–720
stabident system, 718
intrapulpal injection, 720
long-acting local anesthetics, 715
mepivacaine, 715
prolonged pain control, 715
ropivacaine, 716
time-response curve, development of pulpal anesthesia, 712f
VGSC, 716
Mandibular anterior teeth
horizontal cone angulations, 560–570
horizontal X-ray projections, 583f
projecting directly through canine, 584f
Mandibular canines
anatomy and morphology, 909–913
versus mandibular incisors, 912
canal system, 188, 188t
clinical, 913–914
external root morphology, 191–192
labial and mesial view, 194f
mesial curvature of root in apical third, 196f
1 root and 1 wide canal, 195f
root cross-sections, 195f
labial, mesial, and incisal views, 933f
root number and form, 193, 193t
similarity to maxillary incisors, 930f
treatment sequence of two canals in, 934f
variations and anomalies, 197
dens invaginatus, 197, 198f
fusion, 191
gemination, 197, 198f
presence of two canals, 191

radicular third root bifurcation, 196f
two canals and two roots, 194
Mandibular central incisor
canal system, 181–183
number of canals and apices, 179
shape, 184
external root morphology, 184
labial and mesial view, 185f
root cross-sections, 185f
length of, 184
versus mandibular lateral incisors
exihibiting fusion, 188f
number of canals, 183t
root number and form, 184
1 root and 1 canal, 186f
two canals
connecting apical third web-canal and one apical foramen, 187f
and one apex, 187f
two separate apical foramina, 188f
variations and anomalies, 186
dens invaginatus, 184
fusion, 188f
gemination, 188–189, 189f
Mandibular first molars
achieving SLA, 939f
anatomical variations in, 940f
anatomy and morphology, 915–916
canal system, 210
three-rooted, 205t
two-rooted, 209t
clinical, 919–921
distal canal, 915
external root morphology, 205–206
buccal and mesial, 209f, 210f
root cross-sections, 210f
2 roots and 3 canals, 210f, 211f
length of, 206
with periapical lesion, 1165f
presence and impact of furcation canals, discussion, 915
root and root canal anatomy
of distal root, 932t
of mesial root, 932t
root number and form, 209–210
Mongoloid *versus* non-Mongoloid, 206–208

number of roots, 208t
searching middle mesial canals, 939, 940f
variations and anomalies, 209–210
extra canal, 213f
supernumerary roots and canals, 213f, 214f
taurodontism, 214f
Mandibular first premolars
anatomy and morphology, 909
bifurcated teeth, 193
buccal, mesial, and occlusal views, 935f
canal system, 201–202
number of canals and apices, 204t
clinical, 915
external root morphology, 191–193
buccal and mesial view of, 199f
root cross-sections, 200f
length of, 198
versus mandibular second premolar
number of canals and apices, 204t
separate canals, 209
removal of more buccal cusp than lingual, access cavity, 936f
root and root canal anatomy, 912t
root number and form, 203
main buccal and vestigial mid-root lingual root, 195f
single root and single canal, 194f, 195f
Tome's root, 193
two root canals, incidence, 199–200
variations and anomalies, 200
rare three-rooted, 202f
three canals and two roots, 196, 196f
three canals in single root, 196, 196f
Mandibular incisors
anatomy and morphology, 909
buccal and lingual canals with separate apical foramina, 916f
clinical, 909

fin or groove with pulp tissue between them, 928f, 910
labial, mesial, and incisal views, 890f, 905f
root and root canal anatomy, 912t
Mandibular lateral incisors
canal system, 191t
shape, 191
two canals and one apical foramen, 192f
external root morphology, 187
labial and mesial view, 188f
root cross-sections, 189f
length of, 187
root number and form, 187–188, 190t
1 root and 1 canal, 190f
1 root and 1 canal with multiple lateral canals, 190f
separation of single canal into 2 canals, 190f
variations and anomalies, 191
dens invaginatus, 191
fusion, 192, 193f
gemination, 192, 193f
Mandibular molars
access preparations, 918f, 938f
moderate/severe root curvature, 937f
buccal mesial occlusal views, 936f
four canals, 578f
horizontal cone angulations, 560–570
hourglass-shaped canal, 579f
and lamina dura, 565–566
lingual and mesial inclination of, 880
"opening up" roots, 571f
root canal-treated, 928f
standard horizontal X-ray projection, 561f
Mandibular premolars
first premolar, 580f
horizontal cone angulations, 560–570
Mandibular second molars, 209
anatomy and morphology, 915
canal system, 213–215
two-rooted teeth, 216, 209t
clinical, 921

C-shaped canals, 915
external root morphology, 205
buccal and mesial view, 214f
root cross-sections, 215f
2 roots and 3 canals, 215f, 216f
length of, 216
root number and form, 206, 208t
variations and anomalies, 209–210
additional canals, 218f
C-shaped canal, 216
fused or single roots, 209, 210f
two canals, 210f
variations in anatomy, 926f
Mandibular second premolars
anatomy and morphology, 915
buccal, mesial, and occlusal views, 928f
canal system, 208–209, 208t
incidence of two or more canals, 200
clinical, 915
external root morphology, 202–203
buccal and mesial view, 205f
root cross-sections, 205f
single root and single canal, 194f
length of, 203, 205
root number and form, 205t, 206
variations and anomalies, 205
dens evaginatus, 200, 200f
two canals, 200, 201f
two roots, 208
Mandibular third molars
anatomy and morphology, 915–916
clinical, 922
Master apical file (MAF), 880
Matrix database elements, diagnostic software (AEL), 850f
Matrix metalloproteinase (MMP), 127, 354, 355t
Maxillary anesthesia
anterior middle superior alveolar (AMSA), 721
infraorbital nerve block injection, 721
palatalanterior superior alveolar (P-ASA) injection, 721
Maxillary anterior teeth
horizontal cone angulations, 560–561

radiographs of extracted teeth, 570f
Maxillary canines
  anatomy and morphology, 901–903
  canal system, 162–169
    accessory foramina, 165
    two canals canines, 167, 169t
  clinical, 900
  external root morphology, 163
    root shape, 166
  labial, mesial, and incisal views, 905f
  left canine
    exhibiting radicular-form of dens invaginatus type 3 labial and mesial view, 164f
    large lateral canal on mesial aspect midroot, 165f
    mesial and apical lateral canal in apical third, 164f
    numerous lateral canals on mesial aspect of root, 164f
    root cross-sections, 163f
  length, 165
  root number and form, 164t, 167
  variations and anomalies, 165
Maxillary central incisors
  anatomy and morphology, 895
  canal system, 158–160, 156t
    two and three mesial lateral canals, 157f
  clinical, 895–897
  cross-sectional root anatomy, 156f
    labial and mesial view, 156f
  external root morphology, 156
  impact of initial entry, 891
  length of, 156
  root number and form, 156, 156t
  showing labial, mesial, and incisal views, 907f
  variations and anomalies, 158
    dens invaginatus Type 3, 158f, 159f
    incidence of radicular grooves, 161t
    prevalence of fusion and germination, 158t
Maxillary first molar
  anatomy and morphology, 903
  buccal, mesial palatal and occlusal views, 912f

canal system, 176
  3 canals, 176f
  6 canals, 176f
  mesial view, 153f
  mesiobuccal view, 152f
  number of canals and apices, 175
  single/one canal, 174
  two canals, 174
clinical, 902–907
external root morphology, 172–174
  buccal and mesial view, 172f
  root cross-sections of, 172f
mesiobuccal root canal system
  laboratory studies *versus* clinical studies, 174
mesiobuccal view of canal system, 152f
root and root canal anatomy of, studies
  distobuccal root, 897t
  mesiobuccal root, 902t
  palatal root, 902f, 903t
root canal-treated, 945f
root number and form, 177–179
  C-chaped roots, 174
  fused roots, 174
  number of roots, 171
  3 roots and 3 canals, 173f, 178
  3 roots and 4 canals, 178f
  4 roots and 4 canals, 176f
variations and anomalies, 175–177
  second mesiobuccal canal (MB2), 175
variations in anatomy of mesiobuccal root canal system, radiographs, 901f
Maxillary first premolars
  anatomy and morphology, 901–903
  buccal, mesial, and occlusal views, 909f
  canal system, 169–170
    number of canals, 169t
  clinical, 902
  endodontically treated canals of, 910f
  external root morphology, 166–167
    buccal and mesial, 166, 167
    prominent root concavities, 166
    root anatomy, 166–167
    root cross-sections, 166

length of, 167
root and root canal anatomy, studies, 912t
root number and form, 167–168
  number of roots, 169, 170t
  three roots, 170f, 171f
variations and anomalies, 169
Maxillary lateral incisors
  anatomy and morphology, 896
  canal system, 160–161, 161t
  design of access into, 892f
  external root morphology, 159–160
    cross-sectional root anatomy, 159
  left incisor, 160
  length of, 160
  with necrotic pulp, 640f
  right incisor
    labial and mesial view, 163f
    root cross-sections, 163f
  root number and form, 160–161, 161t
  variations and anomalies, 161–163
    communication between groove and pulp, 161
    lingual view of periodontal failure left incisor, 164f
    radicular grooves, 157, 158t
Maxillary molars
  cross section of, 1085f
  difficulty to radiograph, 567
  horizontal cone angulations, 560–570
    moved zygomatic process, 567
  mesial inclination of, 907f
  mesiobuccal root, 582f
  mesiobuccal root second canal. *See* MB2
Maxillary premolars
  horizontal cone angulations, 560–570
  periapical radiographs of, before orthodontic treatment, 604
  single canal image, 583f
Maxillary rhinosinusitis
  need for effective diagnosis of, 626
  rhinosinusitis, 645f
Maxillary second molars

anatomy and morphology, 904–906
canal system, 181
  C-shaped canals, 179
  number of canals and apices, 169t
clinical, 903
external root morphology, 177
  root cross-sections, 178f
length of, 181
occlusal view, 908
root and root canal anatomy of, 903t
root number and form, 181
  number of roots, 163t
  root fusion, 160t
  3 roots and 4 canals, 174f, 178f
  3 roots and 3 canals
    distal curved MB and DB roots, 178f
    s-shaped distobuccal root, 178f
variations and anomalies, 179–181
  conical C-shaped root, 183–184
Maxillary second premolars, 170
  anatomy and morphology, 901–903
  buccal, mesial, and occlusal views, 909f
  with buccal and lingual root, 172
  canal system, 170
    number of canals and apices, 175t
  cross-sectional root anatomy, 169
  external root morphology, 169–172
    buccal and mesial view of, 170f
    root cross-sections, 170f
  length of, 170
  root number and form, 171t, 174
    number of roots, 170
    single root and single canal, 170f
  variations and anomalies, 171
    presence of three roots and three canals, 173f
    presence of two roots and three canals, 172f
Maxillary sinusitis of dental origin (MSDO), 631, 633f, 634f
  challenges faced, 626
  and endodontic infections, 632
  periapical osteoperiositis, 632f
  symptoms of, 632
Maxillary sinus pain, 629, 631f
  left maxillary sinus, 635f
Maxillary third molars
  anatomy and morphology, 903
  clinical, 903–904
Maximum recommended therapeutic dose (MRTD), 739
Mazer wood. *See* Gutta-percha
MB1, 900f
MB2, 573, 583
MCSF. *See* Macrophage colony-stimulating factor (MCSF)
Medical condition, patients
  ASA health classification system and treatment modification, 750f
Medical Dictionary, Dorland, 392
Medical history, endodontic examination, 523–524
  form, 535t, 523
Medicated gutta-percha (MGP), 1020–1021
Medullary dorsal horn
  components of, 380–381
Members Insurance (MI), 87
Membrane phospholipids, pathways of lipid mediator production from, 361f
Mesial view of canal system, maxillary first molar, 153f
Mesiobuccal canal
  first (MB1), 898f
    isthmus between two mesiobuccal canals, 899f
  second (MB2), 904
    location, 899, 900f
    three mesiobuccal canal orifices, 900f
  variations in access cavity shapes, f
Mesiobuccal view of canal system, maxillary first molar, 152f
MetaSEAL, 1073
Metastatic breast carcinoma in mandible, 617, 619f
Methacrylate resin sealers
  Endo-Rez, 1072
  Epiphany, 1073
  Fibrefill, 1073
  MetaSEAL, 1073
Metronidazole (Flagyl) and all drugs, 78t
MFP, myofascial pain, 445
MHC. *See* Major histocompatibility complex (MHC), type II
MHC and antigen presentation
  cells and molecules in, 351f
  class I MHC, 351
  class II MHC, 351
Microbes/unsuccessful endodontic treatment, 257–258
Microbial irritants, 344, 345, 347
Microbiological diagnostic techniques, endodontics, 227–228
  culture, definition, 228
  culture dependent techniques, 228–231
    advantages/limitations of culture method, 230t
    difficulties, 229–230
  immunological methods, 230
  microscopy, 230
  molecular biology methods, 230–231
Microleakage, 1069
  evaluation of, 1069
Micromonas micros, 237
Microorganisms, 244
  host, interactions, 244
Microscopes, visual enhancement
  Endoscope visual system (EVS), 873f
  hemostasis, 866
  rod–lens endoscope, 874f
  SOM benefits, 871–872
  surgical operating microscope, 871f, 872f
Microscopy, 230
Microtube removal options, 1105–1106, 1106f
Mineral trioxide aggregate (MTA), 867, 1051–1052, 1124f, 1148, 1329, 1339
  as capping agent, 1417
  for perforation repair, 1
Minimum bactericidal concentration (MBC), 273
Minimum inhibitory concentration (MIC), 273

Minnesota Multiphasic Personality
    Inventory (MMPI/
    MMPI-II), 406
MMPI/MMPI-II. *See* Minnesota
    Multiphasic Personality
    Inventory (MMPI/
    MMPI-II)
Modifying pain, physiological
    mechanisms
  physiological factors, 403
    affective variables, 403
    cognitive/affective factors, 403
    illness, definition, 403
  physiological mechanisms
    autonomic factors, 402
    sensitization, 402
    spreading muscle spasm, 402
Molecular biology methods,
    233–234
  "dead-cell" issue, 235–236
  DNA-DNA hybridization,
    233–234
  drawbacks, advantages/
    limitations, 234, 234t
  FISH, 234
  PCR method, 231–233
  "too-high sensitivity" issue,
    234–235
MSDO. *See* Maxillary sinusitis of
    dental origin (MSDO)
MTA. *See* Mineral trioxide
    aggregate (MTA)
MTAD, 967
  and tetraclean, 1003–1004
MTwo, 943, 945
Multidimension Risk Assessment
    Model (MD-RAM), 752,
    753
  behavioral scale-patient's self-
    reported dental anxiety,
    754f
  estimating procedural stress, 754f
  interpretation of, 753f
Multi-lens optic system, 870
Multirooted teeth, root selection
    for, 1457
Muscle palpation for myofascial
    trigger points (TrPs), 451f
Muscular pains, 428–429, 429t
  local myalgia, unclassified, 445
  macrotrauma or cumulative
    microtrauma, 446
  myofascial pain, 445–452

  coexisting migraine/tension-
    type headache, 452
  headaches, tension-type, 452
  multiple TrPs, 449–450
  palpable nodule, 448
  referred pain site, 446f, 447f,
    448f
  spray and stretch, sequence of
    steps, 450, 452f
  systematic fingertip
    examination, 450
  "tension headaches," 448f
  trigger point (TrP) complex,
    449
  systematic fingertip
    examination, 448
  myositis, 445
  myospasm, 444–445
  SEA, 447
  secondary myofascial TrPs, 446
  unclassifiable pains/atypical
    facial pains, 452, 453t
    atypical odontalgia,
      deafferentation, 453–456
    burning mouth syndrome
      (BMS), 453, 454–455
Myofascial trigger points (TrPs),
    399

N

NaOCl, 997–1000
NaOCl accident, 1145
  after several hours, 1145f
  causes of, 1152
  management, 1155–1157
  prevention, 1150
  symptoms, 1145
Narcotics and all drugs, 785t
National Health and Nutrition
    Examination Survey
    (NHANES), 10
National Health Information
    Infrastructure (NHII),
    1487
National Institute of Dental and
    Craniofacial Research
    (NIDCR), 10, 1474
National standard of care, 88
Nd:YAG, 963
  to clean root canal, 963
  laser pulpotomy, effects, 860

  process of melting and
    recrystallizing root canal
    surfaces, 963
Necrosis, 345
Nerve-derived neuropeptide Y
    (NPY), 120
Nerve growth factor (NGF), 355,
    476
  administration of, 383f
Neuroanatomic model, new
    receptive fields apperance,
    400f
Neuropeptides, 137, 354
  calcitonin gene-related peptide
    (CGRP), 120
  effects of, 139f
  neurokinin A (NKA), 137
  neuropeptide Y (NPY), 358
  origins including actions and
    specific receptors, 141
  quantification of, 142f
  substance P (SP receptors), 120
  vasoactive intestinal peptide
    (VIP), 137
Neuropeptide Y-immunoreactive
    (NPY-IR) fibers in
    inflamed dental pulp, 141
Neurophysiology, pain
  acute pain pathways, 393. *See
    also* Arachidonic acid
  allodynia, normally
    nonpainful stimuli, 395,
    397f
  allodynia and central
    sensitization, 397
  axon reflex, 396
  behavioral factors. *See* Pain
  central sensitization, 397
  CGRP, 395
  chronic pain
    "crazy"/"malingering," 402
  cutaneous nerve, components,
    394
  descending inhibitory, 398
  exaggerated response to
    noxious stimuli (primary
    hyperalgesia), 395
  inflammatory mediators, 386
  "inflammatory soup," 395, 396f
  modulation, definition, 395f,
    398. *See also* Endogenous
    opioid system, pain
    modulation

neural structures, pain relevant, 395f
NMDAr, 397
nociceptors, silent/afferent, 394
norepinephrine, 395
perception, 398
physiological mechanisms modifying pain, 402–403
referred pain. *See* Referred pain, acute pain pathways
"secondary mechanical hyperalgesia," 397
sympathetic nerve terminal, 395
"temporal summation," 397
transduction, 394
transmission, definition, 395
trigeminal system. *See* Trigeminal system, acute pain pathways
"wind-up," 397
pain assessment tools, 404
Neurosensory disturbance, 1307
Neurovascular anatomy, damage to: causes and outcomes, 1141–1142
diagnosis and management of inferior alveolar nerve injury, 1142–1143
management of inferior alveolar nerve injuries, 1154–1155
overfill of N2 and similar paraformaldehyde pastes, 1141
Neutrophils, 319f
New drugs, change in reactions of, 781
New York Heart Association's classification system, 762f
NGF. *See* Nerve growth factor (NGF)
NHANES. *See* National Health and Nutrition Examination Survey (NHANES)
NHII. *See* National Health Information Infrastructure (NHII)
Nickel–titanium alloy to endodontics, introduction of
DSC to study Nickel–Titanium alloys, use of, 798–801
SEM photograph of cutting tip for LightSpeed instrument, 802f
failure of Nickel–Titanium instruments/mechanisms, 802–804
SEM photograph of clinically fractured ProTaper instrument, 807f
SEM photomicrograph of in vitro fracture surface, NiTi Gates Glidden drill, 809f
heat sterilization effects, properties of Nickel–Titanium instruments, 806–807
improved Nickel–Titanium instruments, strategies, 809–812
heat treatment, 806
physical vapor deposition (PVD) process, 809
mechanical behavior/NiTi phases, Nickel–Titanium alloys, 800–802
"Nitinol," 800
superelastic/nonsuperelastic NiTi orthodontic wires, comparison, 801, 801f
Nickel–titanium (NiTi) rotaries, 880
Nickel–titanium spreader, 1029
gutta-percha *versus* Resilon, 1047
NIDCR. *See* National Institute of Dental and Craniofacial Research (NIDCR)
NiTi. *See* NiTi, Nickel-Titanium
Ni–Ti, Nickel–Titanium, 801–802
Ni–Ti endodontic instruments, 828–829
canal cleanliness, 830–831
comparisons, 789
HERO 642, 827
Mtwo system, 830
canal shape, 816
comparative studies, 826–827
engine-driven instruments, 832
slower handpiece, 833
fatigue and flexibility of rotary Nickel–Titanium files, 820
lubrication, 824
ProTaper/ProFile instrument, comparison, 818
forces, encountered, 825
irrigants and sterilization, 829
manufacture, 828
Ni–Ti spreaders, 832
precautions/prevention, 825
reciprocating handpiece, 833
Endo-Gripper, 834
Giromatic handpiece, 834
Kerr M4, 834
M4 Safety handpiece, 833f
rotary contra-angle handpiece instruments, 833
rotary Nickel–Titanium files, 820
separation and distortion, 828–829
super elasticity, 824
surface treatment, 829
torsional strength and separation, 824
ANSI/ADA specification, 822
K-type/U-type, comparison, 818
vertical stroke handpiece, 830
NMDAr. *See* N-methyl-D-aspartate receptor
N-methyl-D-aspartate receptor, 397
Nociceptive processing, 381
Nociceptors, 382
function of peripheral, 382
Noninstrumentation technique, 964
application of, 965f
cleansing of root canal system, 970
Nonmicrobial endodontic disease
cystic apical periodontitis, 311
body cells and inelimination of cholesterol crystals, 327–328
cellulose granuloma, 334
cholesterol and apical periodontitis, 324
cholesterol in apical periodontitis, 330
cholesterol in disease, 324
clinical relevance of cysts in primary and posttreatment apical periodontitis, 322–324
cysts and periapical healing, 321–322
diagnosis of periapical cysts, 309

foreign bodies, 328–332
genesis of pocket cysts, 316
genesis of true cysts, 313–315
histopathology of periapical cysts, 312–313
incidence of periapical cysts, 310
oral pulse granuloma, 332–334
origin of cyst epithelium, 310
other foreign materials, 334–337
prevalence of cysts in periapical lesions, 310–312
tissue reaction to cholesterol, 325–327
Nonodontogenic toothache and chronic head and neck pains
causalgic pains, 442–444
diagnosis, 427
modifying pain, 402–403
muscular pains, 444–444t
neurophysiology, pain, 403
pain, specifics of broad categories, 414
pain experience, quantification, 403
Nonsteroid anti-inflammatory drugs (NSAIDs), 502
and other drugs, 787t
Nonsurgical root canal therapy, 322
Nonsurgical root canal treatment (NS RCT), 532
Nontraditional techniques, 962
Nonvital pulps treatment
biologic consequences, 1336
immature tooth, apexification, 1336
technique, 1338
Nonvital pulp therapy for children, 1417–1420
examples of rotary paste fillers, 1421f
primary molar with large caries lesion, 1422f
proximity of primary molar roots to succedaneous tooth, 1419f
pulpectomy treatment, 1420–1421f
pulpotomy technique, 1418f

removal of roof of chamber and coronal pulp, 1419f
NSAIDs. *See* Nonsteroid anti-inflammatory drugs (NSAIDs)
NSAIDS and acetaminophen, 705. *See also* Pharmacologic strategies, flare-ups
N2/Sargenti paste, 1066
severe inflammation of pulp, 1067f
NS RCT. *See* Nonsurgical root canal treatment (NS RCT)
Nucleus caudalis, 379
Nutritional deficiency theory, 313

O

Obtura system, 1023–1024, 1024f
Obturation
compaction
hand-lateral *versus* ultrasonic, 1061f
lateral, 1038
vertical, 1034
without sealer, 1060f
dentin chip apical, 1048
root canal plug after 3 months, 1068f
and irrigation mishaps, 1137–1138
anatomic and imaging characteristics of inferior alveolar canal, 1138–1139
anatomic and imaging characteristics of maxillary sinus, 1138
extreme overfill, 1138f
importance of accurate radiographic imaging, 1138
microleakage, 1058
mishaps, prevention of, 1155–1156
radicular space, 1053–1054, 1054f
root canal system, 857–860
techniques for control when neurovascular proximity exists, 1140
tissue toxicity in, 1056

Obturation, rationale of
desired properties of obturating materials, 1055
historical perspective, 1053
objective of obturation, 1053
obturating canal, 1053–1055
Obturation materials
paste removal, 1108–1109
heat for, 1109
micro-debriders, 1109–1110
rotary instruments, 1109
solvents and paper points, 1109
ultrasonic energy, 1109
removal of, 1111
gutta-percha, 1100, 1107–1109. *See also* Gutta-percha (filling material), removal of
microtube removal options, 1105–1107
paste removal, 1108–1109
Resilon, 1103
silver points, 1103
Odontalgia *versus* sinus pain, symptoms of, 629–630
Odontoblast, 127
electron microscopic study, 128f
odontoblastic process, 128
pseudostratified appearance of, 127f
Odontogenic and non-odontogenic pain, mechanisms
central mechanisms, 384–386
alternative hypotheses of mechanical allodynia, 385f
mechanical pain thresholds, 386f
dentinal hypersensitivity, 386–387
inflamed dental pulp, 381
innervation of pulp–dentin complex
human dental pulp, 378f
organization and function
of central trigeminal pain system, 379–381
WDR projection neuron, 380f
of peripheral trigeminal pain system, 376–378
peripheral pain mechanisms, 381–384

effect of pretreatment with epinephrine or vehicle, 382f
expression of receptors and ion channel on peripheral nociceptors, 382f
transcription-dependent changes, 386
trigeminal pain system, overview of, 376
Operations management in endodontic practice
brand-driven culture, 1474
design aesthetics. *See* Design aesthetics, operations management
human resource. *See* Human resources, operations management in endodontics
NIDCR, 1474
office, opening. *See* Operations management in endodontic practice, new offices
practice, choice. *See* Choice of practice, operations management
strategic framework, 1475
Operations management in endodontic practice, new offices
choosing office location, 1481–1483
commercial lease, 1482–1483
"Community Tapestry," 1482
geographic information systems (GIS), 1482
creating winning office design
architectural drawings/specifications, 1483–1484
design aesthetics. *See* Design aesthetics, operations management
first things first: creating a business plan
LLC, 1481
LLP, 1481
Small Business Administration (SBA), 1481
management (winning) practices. *See* Management (winning) practices,
operations management in endodontic practice
"Market Profile Report," 1482
Opioid analgesics, 726–727
Optical definitions
convergence angle, 870
depth of field, 870
field of view, 870
viewing angle, 870
working distance, 870
Oral conscious sedation (OCS), 742–743
Oral contraceptives, 781
antibiotics and effects on, 781
Oral pulse granuloma
intact birefringent body, 333f
Orange juice, 763, 788
Orascope, 869–870
Orthodontic misalignment, 17–18
Orthodontics. *See* Pulp pathosis
Orthograde re-treatment, follow-up studies on outcome of, 1187t
Osseointegration, 1298–1300
provisional crown, 1306f
Osseointegration, dental implants
background, 1297
complications, 1316–1317
dental implant devices (classic)
blade-form implants, 1297
endodontic implants, 1298, 1298f
endosseous root form implants, 1298
implant dentistry, 1295–1296
Osseous (cemental) dysplasia, 631f
Ossifying fibroma, 618f
Osteoclast activity, methods for controlling
bacteria elimination, infection-related resorption, 1375–1376
Osteolytic endodontic lesions, 590
Osteomyelitis, 609f
Osteoradionecrosis, 611f
Overdenture(s), 12
abutment, 1461, 1461f
attachments, 12f
preparation, 1459–1460, 1459f
abutment tooth selection, 1461
contraindications, 1460–1461
indications/advantages, 1460
problems, 1463
possible solutions, 1463–1464
retained abutments, 1460f

P

Pain
assessment tools, 404
behavioral factors, 403–404
learned pain behaviors, 403–404
pain/well behaviors, 403
behaviors, 403
components, 392
definitions
Dorland's, 392
Field's, 392
IASP, 393
Pain, specifics of broad categories
ankylosis/osteoarthritis, 419, 419t
congenital or developmental disorders, 419
continuous neuralgias, 440
anesthesia dolorosa, 442
postherpetic neuralgia, 440–442
posttraumatic neuralgias, 442
disk derangement disorder, 419, 419t
headaches, abuse/withdrawalsubstances/metabolic disorders
neuropathic pains, 435–436, 436t
headaches associated with vascular disorders, 418
carotid or vertebral artery pain, hypertension, 429t
giant cell arteritis (temporal arteritis), 434
headaches unassociated with structural lesion, 434
inflammatory disorders of the joint, 419–421
internal derangement, 419
intraoral/extraoral source structures, 416–418
osteoarthritis (noninflammatory), 423
paroxysmal neuralgias
glossopharyngeal neuralgia, 416

laryngeal neuralgia, superior, 437
nervus intermedius neuralgia, 437
neuromas, 439–440
occipital neuralgia, 437, 438
trigeminal neuralgia and pretrigeminal neuralgia, 436
referred pain from remote pathological sites
Angina Pectoris, 424–425
aura (with/without), migraine, 430–431
benign thyroid tumor, 426f
carotid artery, 426–427
carotid artery/carotidynia, 426–427
cervical joint dysfunction, 427–428
cervical spine, 427
IHS, 426
intracranial pathosis, 429, 434
migraine, vascular head ache types, 430–431, 430t
myocardial infarction, 425–426
neurovascular pains, 429–430, 429t
thyroid, 426
temporomandibular joint articular disorders, 418–419, 419t
temporomandibular joint dislocation, 423
ankylosis, 424
trigeminal autonomic cephalagias, 432
chronic paroxysmal hemicrania (CPH), 433
cluster headaches, 434
Paradental cyst, 612f
Paranasal sinuses, 643, 644f
Partial pulpectomy, 27, 27f
Paste fillers, 1100
Paste removal, 1108
heat for, 1109
micro-debriders, 1109–1110
rotary instruments, 1109
solvents and paper points, 1110
Endosolv R and Endosolv E, 1109f
ultrasonic energy, 1109

Pathologic tooth resorption, 1369
activation of OPG/RANK/RANKL system, 1360
cervical invasive resorption, 1375–1377
external infection-related resorption, 1366–1368
external multiple sites of ankylosis/infection-related resorption, 1374–1375
spontaneous ankylosis affecting interdental area of first molar, 1373f
external spontaneous ankylotic resorption, 1373–1374
external surface resorption (repair-related resorption), 1365–1366
etiology, acute repair-related resorption, 1365–1366
external trauma-related replacement resorption (ankylosis)
external spontaneous ankylosis resorption, 1373, 1373f
infrapositioned maxillary central incisor initially intruded at age of 9, 1372f
internal infection-related root resorption, 1378–1379
internal replacement resorption, 1379
internal surface resorption, 1377
lateral root resorption, 1361f
osteoclast activity, methods for controlling, 1364–1365
osteoclast as cell involved in alveolar bone growth/maintenance
endodontic implications, 1366–1367
osteoclast as cell responsible for tooth eruption, 1361
endodontic implications, 1361–1362
osteoclast as defense cell against microbial invasion
endodontic implications, 1362–1364
osteoclast as member of repair team after injury
endodontic implications, 1363

pathogenesis of surface resorption, 1366f
physiology of osteoclasts, 1358, 1359f
progression of replacement resorption (ankylosis), 1371f
types of root resorption, 1365–1366
Patient records, 7–9
Patient-related causes, tooth discoloration. See Tooth discoloration, etiology of
Pattern recognition receptors (PRR), 344
PCR and derivatives, 231
broad-range PCR, 232–233
T-RFLP, 233
PCR-based microbial typing, 231–232
real-time PCR, 232
reverse transcriptase PCR, 231–232
touchdown PCR, 231
PDL. See Periodontal ligament (PDL)
Penicillin or cephalosporin and all drugs, 783t
Peptidoglycan (PG), 244
Peptococcus, 226
Peptostreptococcus, 226
Percussion sensitivity, 669
Perforation, dental, 1140–1141
characteristics complicating treatment outcome, 1140
endodontic, 1124
furcation, 1124
location, 1126–1127
apical, 1127
midroot, 1127
subgingival, 1127
periodontal condition, 1129–1130
post space, 1125
size of, 1128
Perforation repair
barrier materials for, 1130–1131
absorbable, 1130–1131
non-absorbable, 1131
clinical considerations influencing, 1129
esthetics and, 1130
hemostatics for, 1130

material, 1128
MTA, 1124
periodontal condition, 1129–1130
restorative materials, 1131
techniques for, 1131
   cleaning, shaping and obturation following, 1094f
   coronal one-third and furcal perforations, 1131–1133
   middle one third, perforations in, 1133
   selection of appropriate barrier and restorative, 1131
timing, 1125–1127
treatment sequence, 1130
vision and, 1130
Periapical Actinomyces infection, 642f
Periapical bone resorption, 507
Periapical cyst, 309
   diagnostic methods, 309–310
   frequency of, 309
   histopathology of, 312–313
   nonsurgical root canal therapy, 322
   pocket cyst, 320f
   prevalence of, 309–311
   true cyst, 314f
      phases, 313
Periapical disease, 2
Periapical index (PAI) scoring system, 622
   monitor and compare healing of apical periodontitis, 621f
   monitor healing, 621f
   prevalence of apical periodontitis in 35–45 year-olds, 622
   scores, 930
Periapical lesion
   detection, 495
   electron micrograph of nucleus of macrophage, 644
   fungi in, 646f
   and mechanically created lesions, 581
Periapical lesions, endodontic origin
   bacterial elimination. *See* Bacterial elimination in periapical lesions
   histopathology. *See* Histopathology of periapical lesions of endodontic origin
   polymorphonuclear leukocytes (PMNs), 494
   traditional concepts *versus* futuristic view, 509–510
Periapically affected central maxillary incisor, 323f, 330f
Periapical microbial biofilms, 284–285, 284f
Periapical mucositis, 630, 630f, 631f
Periapical osteoperiositis and MSDO, 632f
Periapical pathosis
   relationship between length of fill and presence and absence of, 923f
   short fills not resulting in, examples, 922f
Periapical tissues
   diseases, 44–58
Periodontal cyst, lateral, 610f
Periodontal disease, primary, 641
   healing with endodontic treatment, 654, 639f
   in mandibular second molar, 649f
   in maxillary first premolar, 651f
   on pulp, effect of, 731
   pulp tests, 649f
   radiographic appearance of, 602f, 657
   and root perforations, 1128–1129
   with secondary endodontic involvement, 650–654
      endodontic and periodontal treatment, 654
      in maxillary premolar, 681
      simulating endodontic lesion, 650f
   treatment complications, 653
Periodontal lesions, 16, 17
Periodontal ligament (PDL), 121, 130, 143, 529, 539, 677–680
   cause, 676
   fracture line within, 601–603
   periapical radiograph of mandibular premolar, 680
Periodontal therapy, 110
Peripheral pain mechanisms, 379, 381

Peripheral trigeminal pain system
   classification of peripheral neurons, 377t
   conceptual model, 377f
   detection of, 377–379
   perception, 377–391
   processing, 377–391
Periradicular curettage, 62f
Periradicular inflammation, 362
Periradicular lesion, 363
Periradicular region, 358
Periradicular surgery, treatment planning, 1244–1245, 1250
   concepts/principles, 1235
   patient communication, 1235
PEST. *See* Political Economical Social Technological (PEST) analysis
Phagocytosis, 345–347
   formation of phagosome, 346f
   oxidative burst reactions, 346f
Pharmacodynamic drug interactions, 780
Pharmacokinetic drug interactions, 780
Pharmacological management, endodontic pain
   acetaminophen, 723
   anesthesia
      comparison of local anesthetics for inferior alveolar nerve anesthesia, 715t
      local. *See* Local anesthetics
      mandibular. *See* Mandibular anesthesia
      maxillary. *See* Maxillary anesthesia
   non-narcotic analgesics, nonsteroidal anti-inflammatory/acetaminophen, 721–723
   meta-analysis of non-narcotic analgesics for relief of postoperative pain, 722–723, 722t
   opioid analgesics, 726, 773
      combinations, 726t
   steroids
      intraoral injection, preferred, 728
      necrosis/radiolucency, 726

Pharmacologic strategies, flare-ups
 antibiotics, 705
 long-acting local anesthetics, 705, 715
 NSAIDS and acetominophen, 705
Phenol compounds, 1011
PHN. See Postherpetic neuralgia (PHN)
Photodynamic therapy, 975–977
 EndoVac system (Discus Dental) for apical negative pressure irrigation, 970f
 use of lasers, 969
 use of photoactivated disinfection, 971f
Photostimulable phosphor, 573, 574, 577f, 578f, 581
 image formation, 578f
 imaging plate, 578f
 laser scanner, 578f
Piezoelectric ultrasonics, 1098
Plastic- and resin-based sealers
 AH 26 (thermaseal), 1071
 Diaket, 1071
 Ketac-endo, 1071–1073
 Roeko-seal automix, 1072
 Sealer 26, 1072
Pocelain fused to metal (PFM), removal, 1097f
Political Economical Social Technological (PEST) analysis, 1476
Polyethylene fiber-reinforced posts (PFR), 1455
 transformation toughening, 1456
Polymerase chain reaction (PCR), 222
Polymorphonuclear leukocytes (PMNs). See Neutrophils
Porphyromonas endodontalis, 227, 235, 1041
Porphyromonas gingivalis, 235
Porphyromonas sp., 632
Post-endodontic disease
 use of photoactivated disinfection, 971f
Postherpetic neuralgia (PHN), 408
Postoperative pain, 23
Post placement techniques
 anatomical/structural limitations, 1451
 diameter, 1467
 post length, 1450

Post removal, 1126
 factors influencing, 1115
 and heat transfer, 1136
 maximize energy transfer, 1111, 1111f
 mechanical devices, 1112
  post-engaged tubular tap, 1112f, 1114
  protective rubber cushion, 1112f, 1114
  PRS clinicians with alternative method, 1112f, 1114
  transmetal bur, 1114, 1114f
  trephine and machined down coronal, 1114f, 1125
  tubular tap, 1144f, 1114
 strongly anchored, 1114, 1115f
 system kit, 1106
 techniques for, 1122–1123
  rotosonic vibration, 1111
  ultrasonic energy, 1125
 techniques for access for, 1110
  ultrasonic instruments, 1104f, 1121
  water port technology in non-surgical ultrasonic instruments, 1111
 ultrasonic energy
  decreasing heat buildup, 1112f, 1137
  heat as by-product of, 1111, 1112f
  posts safely and successfully removed, 1111, 1112f
  successful and safe removal, 1111, 1112f
Posts
 apical seal, 1467
 cement, 1448
 clinical failure rate, 1435–1436, 1435t
 clinical tooth fractures associated with, 1438
 design of, 1440
 diameter, 1451, 1467
 distal canal, 1443f
 failure, types, 1436
  crown loosened from maxillary canine, and, 1437f
  fractured maxillary first premolar, radiograph, 1437f

 loss of retention, clinical, 1438t
 tooth fractures, clinical, 1438t
 gutta-percha, 1443f
 Kaplain–Meier survival data, 1436t
 length, 1465–1469
 long-term prognosis, 1435
 mandibular molars, 1451, 1458
 parallel cement, 1453–1455
 placement techniques, 1450
 post space preparation, 1467
 preparation of post space, without disturbing apical seal, 1467, 1468
 proper length, 1441
 purpose, 1449
 radiograph displaying, 1441f
 reasonable clinical guidelines, length, 1442
 relationship, form/potential for root fracture, 1451, 1455
 short post, second premolar radiograph, 1442f
 tooth fracture, prevention, 1450
 two-dimensional finite element analysis, 1435
Post space perforation, 1125
Posttraumatic discoloration of maxillary central incisor caused by pulpal necrosis, 1384f
Post-treatment variable
 comments on case selection, 1213
 outcome of apical surgery, 1214–1215t
  prevalence of apical periodontitis and inadequate root fillings in root-filled teeth, 1216t
 dynamics of resorption, 1211
 potential for healing and function after intentional replantation, 1221
 intentional replantation, 1210f
 optimal conditions for, 1211
 realistic outcome of endodontic treatment in population, 1211
 outcome of initial root canal treatment, 1212f
 outcome of orthograde retreatment, 1213f
 results of biopsy, 1209

Potential role of enterococci, unsuccessful root canal, 260
Praxis Concept theory, 1090
Precussion sensitivity, 669
Prefrontal cortex (PFC), 398
Pregnancy, 768
Pretreatment variables
   age, gender, and systemic health of patient, 1201
   antibiotics, 1209
   apparent quality of previous root filling, 1202
   barriers and bone grafting substances, 1209
   clinical signs and symptoms, 1202
   complications, 1209
   concurrent surgical and orthograde treatment, 1208
   hemostasis, 1214
   laser irradiation, 1208
   level of apical resection and degree of beveling, 1204
      patent dentinal tubules at cut apical root surface, 1205f
   magnification and illumination, 1208
   operator's skill, 1209
   persistent disease after apical surgery, 1203f
   presence or absence of a root-end filling1204
      suspected extra-radicular infection, 1206f
   quality and depth of root-end filling, 1205
   repeat surgery, 1204f
   restoration, 1199
   retrograde root canal re-treatment, 1208
   root-end cavity design, 1205
   root-end filling material, 1207, 1214
      efficacy of, 1207f
   second-time surgery, 1204
      versus first-time surgery, 1219
   size of radiolucency, 1202
   supporting bone loss, 1202
   tooth location, 1201
Preventive strategies, flare-ups anxiety reduction, 704

behavioral intervention, 704
occlusal reduction, 704, 711
Prevotella baroniae, 237
Prevotella denticola, 237, 227
Prevotella intermedia, 226, 237
Prevotella multissacharivorax, 237
Prevotella nigrescens, 227, 236, 237
Prevotella tannerae, 227, 237
Primary intraradicular infections, endodontics, 236–238, 241
   candidate endodontic pathogen, 236–238
Primary molars, 1410
   primary and permanent tooth, 1401f
   primary second molar, cariously involved, 1401f
   root canal system, 1406f
   with stainless steel crown, 1408f
Primary teeth
   anatomical structure of1400
      mandibular first and second primary molars, 1237
      maxillary first and second primary molars, 1236
   dental treatment of
      premature loss of primary tooth, 1400
      root canal therapy, 1417
   and permanent tooth anatomy, 1400
   root canal anatomy of, 1400
   studies of, 1409–1413
Procosol. *See* Zinc oxide–eugenol-containing sealers
Proliferative periostitis of Garré, 610f
Propionibacterium, 263–264
Propionibacterium propionicum, 237
Prosthetic joints and other prosthetic devices
   antibiotic prophylaxis for patients with total joint replacement, 758f
   hematogenous total joint infection, 767f
ProTaper, 943, 961, 968, 974
   mandibular canine shaped with, 967f
Pseudoramibacter alactolyticus, 237
Pulp
   capping/pulpotomy, 857

conditions, 31, 57, 108
differential diagnosis of inflammatory diseases, 44t
diseases, 44
exposure in a rodent molar, 345f
involvement of incisors, 15
Pulpal chamber preparation, 1458–1459, 1459f
Pulpal diagnosis, 857
   irreversible pulpitis, 528
   normal pulp, 528
   previously initiated therapy, 526, 529
   previously treated, 529
   pulpalgia, 526
   pulp necrosis, 528
   reversible pulpitis, 528
Pulpalgia, irreversible/advance, 1
Pulpal inflammation, vicious cycle of, 124f
Pulpal microvascular units, 131f
Pulpal necrosis, 106f
Pulpal pain
   differential diagnosis/treatment, 43–44
Pulpal pathosis
   in children, diagnosis of, 1417
   proven etiological factors, 887
Pulpal pathosis/tooth structures, 53
   resectioradicis, 55
   root-end resections
      evaluation and technique, 56–58, 65
      problems, 59
Pulpal/periodontal diseases, interrelationships, 69
Pulpal vasculature, characteristics of, 132f
Pulp–dentin complex, innervation of, 378
Pulpectomy, 1425
   technique, 1418f
   treatment, 1420f
Pulpitis, 1, 992, 994
Pulpotomy, 46, 1418
   treatment, 1405, 1406, 1426
Pulp pathosis
   dental caries, response of pulp. *See* Pulp response, dental caries
   iatrogenic effects on dental pulp. *See* Iatrogenic effects, dental pulp

orthodontics
    removal of orthodontic brackets, 465
    tooth movement, 485
polishing restorations, 484
postrestorative hypersensitivity, 484
specific materials
    amalgam, 484
    glass ionomer cements, 483
    polycarboxylate cement, 483
    restorative resins, 483
    zinc oxide–eugenol, 483
    zinc phosphate cement, 483
systemic factor
    hereditary hypophosphatemia, 486
ultrasonic scaling, 485
unusual pulp dystrophy in hereditary hypophosphatemia, 486f
vitality testing, 484
vital tooth bleaching, 484
Pulp response, dental caries
    antigen recognition, dental pulp, 470
    area of inflammation in pulp, 470f
    B cells, 471
    dendritic cell
        confocal miscroscope image, 472
        odontoblast layer/blood vessels/area of inflammation, 470f
        types/T-helper cell (Tc), 471f
    macrophages, 470
    major histocompatibility complex (MHC), type II, 470
    occasional T cells, 471
    odontoblasts, 472
    process of, 473
    toll-like receptors (green), bacterial components on odontoblasts, 473f
    anti-inflammatory/anti-nociceptive mechanisms, dental pulp mechanisms, 498
    odontogenic and nonodontogenic pain, mechanisms, 477

bacteria by-products reaching pulp, other sources, 469
anomalous crown morphology/fractures/cracks, 469
blood stream (anachoresis), 469
periodontal disease, 469
bacteria in dentinal tubules, 468f
calcification and resorption, 477
    Ehlers–Danlos syndrome, 477, 489
    internal resorption, 477f
    multiple pulp stones, pulp chamber of molar, 477f
carious attack at early stages, nonspecific immune response (acute inflammation), 488. See also Acute inflammation
carious attack at later stages, nonspecific immune response (chronic inflammation), 474. See also Chronic inflammation
dental caries, source of bacteria
    cariogenic bacteria, products formed, 469, 473
    porphyromonas endodontalis, 468
    products released, death of bacteria (LPS/LTA), 468
encouraging successful response, 479
    pulp polyp, hyperplastic pulpitis, 479f
    pulp polyp, structure/hyperplastic pulpitis, 479f
factors limiting pulp's response, 479
hemodynamic changes in pulp, during caries, 475–476
    blood flow, 481
    interstitial fluid pressure 475–476
immune response, dental pulp, 469–470
neural changes, pulpal inflammation, 476
neuropeptides, release of substance P/CGRP, 476
pulpal injury, 476

pulpal disease, responsiblity of bacteria, 468
repair and regeneration, 477
    reactionary (tertiary) dentin (Rc) beneath deep cavity preparation, 478f

Q

Quantifying pain experience
    Brief Battery for Health Improvement (BBHI-2)
        dimensions of pain, 406
    classification, 407
    diagnostic studies, 385
    history, 408–410
    making diagnosis, 407
    Mcgill pain questionnaire, 405–406, 405t
    MMPI/MMPI-II, 406
    operant pain (pain behavior), 413
    physical examination, 410–411
    psychogenic pain, 413
    psychological assessment
        making diagnosis, 407
        psychological/physical diagnosis, 406
    visual analog scales, 404, 404f
Quinolone
    antibiotics and all drugs, 784t

R

Radicular/coronal spaces, preparations, 887, 933, 977–979
    access cavity preparation, 886, 889
    canal surface modification, 965, 970
        irrigation dynamics, 967, 968
        photodynamic therapy, 969
    clinical armamentarium, 884
        accessory instruments, 885
        burs, 884
        rotary instruments, 885
    clinical determination of working length, 928
        working width, 930
    clinical determination of working

length, 934–935
width, 930
clinical guidelines
  preoperative clinical guidelines, 886
coronal access cavity preparation, 887
devices for powered canal preparation, 951
  motors for rotary instrumentation, 951
  sonic canal instrumentation, 953, 954
  ultrasonic canal instrumentation, 953, 954
effect of access cavity preparation on structural integrity, 917
evaluation of canal preparation techniques, 955
evidence and strategies for shaping the root canal system, 921
general principles
  assessment of restorability, 878
  confirmation of etiology of pulpal pathosis, 877
  external root surface as guide, 881–883
  knowledge of percentages for number of canals within root, 883
  magnification/microscope, 884
  mindful practice/avoid harming, 877
  mindset, 884
  straight-line access, 878
  three-dimensional position of teeth in jaws, 880
histological *versus* clinical material, 919, 920f
instrument movements while shaping
  filing, 938
  potential shapes, 935
  reaming, 935
  rotary movements, 941
  watch-winding, 934
mandibular canines
  anatomy and morphology, 904
  clinical, 915
mandibular central and lateral incisors
  anatomy and morphology, 909
  clinical, 915
mandibular first molars
  anatomy and morphology, 896
  clinical, 896
mandibular first premolars
  anatomy and morphology, 894
  clinical, 895
mandibular second molars
  anatomy and morphology, 901
  clinical, 909
mandibular second premolar
  anatomy and morphology, 909
  clinical, 909
mandibular third molars
  anatomy and morphology, 915
  clinical, 915
maxillary canines
  anatomy and morphology, 893
  clinical, 894
maxillary central incisors
  anatomy and morphology, 904
  clinical, 904
maxillary first molar
  anatomy and morphology, 894
  clinical, 895
maxillary first premolars
  anatomy and morphology, 895
  clinical, 896
maxillary lateral incisors
  anatomy and morphology, 891
maxillary second molars
  anatomy and morphology, 901
  clinical, 902
maxillary second premolar
  anatomy and morphology, 909
maxillary third molars
  anatomy and morphology, 903
  clinical, 903
means for radicular shaping, 933
methodological considerations, 925
nontraditional techniques, 962
  laser-assisted canal preparation, 962
  noninstrumentation technique, 964
objectives, 1475
preparation size and elimination of bacteria, 921f
preparation techniques
  anticurvature filing, 939
  balanced force, 940–942
  crown-down pressureless, 942
  double flare, 943
  standardized, 943
  step-back, 943, 944
  step-down, 940
procedural mishaps, 916
  overextension, 917
  underextension, 917
radicular preparations, 919
requirements for, 935, 936f
rotary instrumentation, 951
shaping root canal system, 922
working length, determination of, 928
  anatomical apex, 926
  apical constriction, 924f
Radicular cyst, 312f
  apical pocket cysts, 323, 315f
Radicular dentin removal, principles, 937
Radicular dentin tubules, 638
Radicular space, obturation, 1053
  cements and pastes as root canal filling materials
    calcium hydroxide, 1067
    calcium phosphate cement, 1066–1067
    dentin chip apical obturation, 1067
    N2/Sargenti paste, 1066
    resin cements, 1067
  coronal protection of obturation
    methods of evaluating coronal leakage, 1076
    permanent coronal closure materials, 1076
    rationale for coronal seal, 1076
    temporary coronal closure materials, 1076
  criteria for evaluation of obturating materials and sealers, 1056
    tissue toxicity, 1056
    voids in obturating materials, 1056
  endodontic sealers and apical leakage, 1068
    APEXIT, 1070
    calciobiotic root canal sealer, 1069
    kerr pulp canal sealer EWT, 1069
    microleakage and its evaluation, 1069

rationale for use of sealers, 1068
roth's 801, 1069
SealApex, 1069
VITAPEX, 1070
zinc oxide–eugenol-containing sealers, 1069
filling lateral and accessory canals, 1075–1076
influence of post space preparation on obturation, 1078–1079
lasers and apical microleakage, 1073
methacrylate resin sealers
  Endo-Rez, 1072
  Epiphany, 1073
  Fibrefill, 1073
  MetaSEAL, 1073
plastic- and resin-based sealers
  AH 26 (thermaseal), 1071–1072
  Diaket, 1071
  Ketac-endo, 1071
  Roeko-seal automix, 1072
  Sealer 26, 1072
rationale of obturation
  desired properties of obturating materials, 1055
  historical perspective, 1053
  objective of obturation, 1053
  obturating canal, 1054
smear layer and apical leakage, 1073
solid core carriers with manual placement techniques, 1063
  effect of heat on periapical tissues, 1064
  Resilon, 1064–1065
  silver points, 1065–1066
  Thermafil, 1063–1064
techniques of obturation, 1056–1057
  condensation forces: vertical *versus* lateral, 1062–1063
  inject-R fill, 1062
  lateral compaction, 1057–1059
  lateral/vertical compaction of warm gutta-percha hybrid technique, 1062
  system B plugger technique, 1061–1062
  thermomechanical compaction of gutta-percha, 1060
  thermomechanical solid core gutta-percha obturation, 1060
  thermoplasticized injectable gutta-percha, 1061
  ultrasonic plasticized gutta-percha, 1060–1061
  vertical compaction, 1059–1060
Radioallergosorbent test (RAST), 1028
Radiographic apex, 25
Radiographic approaches, 556
  digital radiography, advantages and disadvantages, 556
Radiographic data, digital quantification of, 621
  areas to be monitored during healing, 622f
  healing after treatment of apical periodontitis, 621t
Radiographic interpretation, 600
  advanced multiplanar imaging, 604–606
  biological processes related to radiographic diagnosis, 600
  caries, 600
  pathological reactions of tooth structure, 601–602
  periapical changes, 602–603
  periapical radiology, endodontic applications of, 603
  pulpal changes, 600–601
periapical diagnosis, 603–604
periapical radiographs in clinical and epidemiological endodontic research, 617
  applications to clinical research, 622
  digital quantification of radiographic data, 621
  epidemiology, 621–622
  periapical index scoring system, 618–621
  probability assessments, 618
  radiography in future of endodontics, 623
  specificity and sensitivity, reproducibility, 617
  success and failure, 617–618
problems and potentials
  anatomical limitations, 607
  differential diagnosis, 608–617
  healing of apical periodontitis, 607
  incipient changes, 607
Radiographic parallelism, 558f
Radiograph(s), 554
  diagnostic radiographs, 560
  discovery and use, 554
  essential functions in endodontics, 554
    disclosing and locating canals, 555f
  importance of, 600
  limitations of, 607
RadioVisioGraphy (RVG), 573, 574, 583
  commercial version of, 575f
  components, 575f
  endodontic evaluations using, 580f
  first clinical RVG image, 575f
Rampant decay, 16
Randomized controlled trial (RCT), 112
Rash, 11f
RC2B. *See* N2/Sargenti paste
  massive overextension, 90f
RCT. *See* Root canal treatment (RCT)
Real Seal. *See* Methacrylate resin sealers
Reamers, 816
Recalcitrant asymptomatic radiolucencies, biological factors, 1088–1091
Record keeping, endodontic treatment, 98–100
  medical history, elements, 99t
  SOAP record documentation, 99t
  typical contents, 99t
Referred pain, acute pain pathways
  convergence-facilitation theory, 398
    myofascial trigger points (TrPs), 399
  convergence-projection theory, 398–399, 399f
  mechanism of, 399
Renal disease and dialysis, 765

Reparative dentin, techniques for
    generating
  direct/indirect pulp capping
    definition/recommondations,
      1320
    formation, 1323
  partial pulpotomy, definition,
    1313
  pulpotomy, calcium hydroxide
    and amalgam, 1312, 1314f
Resilon, 1064–1065
  adhesive strength of
    methacrylate-based sealer
    versus, 1065
  gaps along canal walls and apical
    leakage, 1064f
  versus gutta-percha, 1064f
  removal of, 1110
Resin cements, 1067
Restoration, endodontically treated
    teeth
  clinical longevity, increase, 1435
  coverage crowns, 1432
  dentin, 1433
  posterior teeth, 1432–1433
  traumatized tooth, 1434
Restorative materials, 1102
  factors influencing removal of,
    1110–1111
  microleakage associated with,
    1131
  permanent, 1107–1108
  and post removal, 1110
Retirement Plans (RP), 87
Retreatment
  endodontic surgery as primary
    approach, 1095f
  non-surgical endodontic, 1094,
    1095
  non-surgical (NSRT) versus
    surgical (SRT), 1095
  risks versus benefits, 1089
    benefits, 1089–1090
    concerns in endodontic
      retreatment, 1090
    patient considerations,
      1090–1091
    risks, 1190
  technology, 1094–1095
Retreatment preference score
  (RPS), 1091f
Revascularization, immature root,
  1349f

Reversible incipient pulpalgia, 1
Rhinosinusitis, 626
  acute rhinosinusitis, 628
  and endodontic disease
    distinguishing differences
      between symptoms of
      odontalgia and sinus pain,
      629–630
    maxillary rhinosinusitis as
      source of dental pain, 626
    maxillary sinusitis of dental
      origin, 631–635
    maxillary sinus pain to teeth,
      referral of, 629
    paranasal sinuses: anatomy
      and function, 626–627
    periapical mucositis, 630–631
    rhinosinusitis: etiology,
      epidemiology, symptoms,
      and treatment, 627–627
  endoscopic sinus surgery, 629
  maxillary rhinosinusitis, 628f
  resistant to antibiotic, 628–629
  treatment for, 628–629
Rod–lens endoscope, 872–873
Roeko-seal automix, 1072
Root apices, 26f
  and anatomical landmarks, 926f
  stereomicroscopic, 158
Root canal, 4
  evaluation/comparison of
    sealers, 1038–1039
Root canal disinfection, new
    developments in
  bioactive glass, 1009
Root canal filling, 328
  radiograph, 101f
Root canal filling materials
  gutta-percha
    carrier-based, 1025–1026
    thermomechanical, 1025
    thermoplasticized, 1023–1025
  mineral trioxide aggregate,
    1030–1033
  newer solid-core, 1028–1030
  paraformaldehyde pastes,
    1033–1034
  paste filling materials, 1030
  requirements, 1019
  semisolid-core filling materials,
    1020–1023
  solid-core filling materials,
    1019–1020

Root canal instruments
  overextension, 28f
Root canal preparation, 1459f
Root canal sealer
  calcium hydroxide-containing,
    1035
  evaluation/comparison, 1038–1039
  glass ionomer-based sealers, 1037
  paraformaldehyde-containing,
    1038
  paraformaldehyde pastes,
    1033–1034
    AAE, 1033–1034
    Endomethasone, 1040
    Riebler's paste, 1034
  requirements, 1034
  resin sealers, 1035–1037
    epoxy resin sealers, 1035–1036
  silicone-based sealers, 1037
  solubility of, 1041
  solvent-based sealers, 1037
  urethane methacrylate sealers,
    1037–1038
  zinc oxide-containing, 1034–1035
Root canal shapes after
    preparation, schematic
    diagrams of potential,
    962–964, 964f
Root canal system
  anatomy of, 933
    schematic diagram of typical,
      947f
  ending of root canal, 927–939
  evidence and strategies for
    shaping, 921–923
  example of root canal-treated
    tooth with fracture prior
    to restoration, 928f
  filled teeth not following
    principles for optimized
    shape, 935f
  flexible endodontic files, 960f
  fracture of, instrument, 961
  host–microbe interactions, 245
  obturation, 848
  potential role of enterococci,
    260–261
  preparation, prerequisite for
    success, 919f
  relationship between cross
    sections of roots and, 922f
  removal of microorganisms in
    instrumentation, 965

sequence of instruments to safely enlarge
and shape apical two-thirds of curved, 948f
and shape coronal part of, 946f
species-specific interactions, 254–256
straight instruments
argument against, 949
Root canal systems (non-surgical/surgical), 48–53, 70
toothache, cure, 48
cardisus spinosimus, 51
treatment procedures, 53f
Root canal therapy, 3, 14, 108, 109f
Root canal treatment (RCT), 8f, 16, 112–113, 112f, 155, 338, 1433. *See also* Periodontal therapy
access cavity in mandibular first molar four orifices, 1098f
adjunctive procedures, 113
alternative treatment, 113
assessing outcome of, 920f
clinically successful despite short fills, 922f
cost of treatment, 113
indications for, 1233
infection of
disease factors, 1088–1089
previous root canal treatment, 1089
maxillary premolar with paste material, 1109f
maximized endodontic prognosis, 1109
outcomes, 1178
follow-up studies, 1212t
postoperative radiograph of completed, 1121f
previous, 1187
pulpectomy, 1406
technical aspects of, 1479
Root-end resections
angle of root-end resection, 1254
bur/laser selection, 1252–1254
evaluation, 57–58
extent of root-end resection, 1261–1266
factors to be considered, 1262
Farrar's diagram, 65f
indications, 1233

methylene blue dye, stained PDL of resected root end, 1256f
performance, 64–65
plain fissure/multi-purpose bur, 1252f
preop digital image of mandibular molar following nonsurgical retreatment, 1263
pretreatment radiograph of maxillary right second molar, 1255
root-end filling materials
filling, types, 1274
MTA, 1133
placement into preparation, 1141
tetracyclines, properties, 1264
in vitro cytotoxicity and biocompatibility studies, 1262
root-end preparation, 1266–1268
filled with root-end filling material, 1276
gauze sponge moistened with saline and applied to flap both
before/after, suturing, 1266f
using ultrasonic tips, 1265
technique, 1269
ultrasonic root-end preparation illustration, 1266f
vital pulp procedure, teeth1310
Root filling, 994, 997
periapically extruded, 1197f
Root filling visit, 1351
osseous replacement, radiographic appearance, 1342f
permanent restoration, 1351–1352
Root fracture complications, treatment of
coronal root fractures, 1341
endodontic essentials, 1342
factors influencing repair, 1341–1342
complications, 1199
midroot/apical root fractures, 1341
root canal obliteration in root-fractured teeth, 1342f

Root fractures
difficulty in diagnosing, 602
oblique-vertical, 608f
two days after trauma, 601f
Root repair procedures, 66–67
treatment modalities, 67
Root resorption, 71
internal
defect filled with softened gutta-percha filling technique, 1353f
endodontic treatment, 1188
histologic appearance, 1353
loss of predentin, reasons, 1358
radiographic appearance, 1363–1364
uniform radiolucency observed in teeth with internal root resorption, 1353f
internal chronic inflammatory tissue, 1366
Root selection, multirooted teeth, 1457
Rotary instrumentation, 951, 953
apical enlargement, 944
calcification, 949
occurring apically and WL, 950f
crown-down approach, 943
current designs, 961
different paradigms for use of, 945
motors for, 957–959
NiTi alloy, 943
use of, 944
reduce incidence of file fracture, 962
straight instrument, argument against using, 962
flexible endodontic files, 949f
taper lock when canal taper approaches, 944f
torque-control motors
requirement of minimum torque to work against friction, 953f
simplified WL control and, 951, 952f
types of contra-angle handpieces, 951

Rotary instruments
  automated devices, comparative conclusion of, 971–973
  efficacy/safety, automated canal preparation devices, comparisons in, 1109
    Micro Mega Sonic Air system, Rispi and Shaper, 833
    Peeso reamer (Dentsply/Maillefer), 823
    sonic handpieces, 830–832
      choices, 831
      instruments used with Micro Mega 1500, 836f
  ultrasonic/sonic handpieces, 951
Roth's 1021
Rubber dam, application
  equipment. *See* Equipment, rubber dam
  purposes, 786
  techniques
    bridge abutments/splints/orthodontics with wires, 799
    calcified pulp chamber/canal tooth, 799
    dam, removal of, 883
    double motion technique, 797
    insufficient tooth structure/porcelain crowns of veneers, 798–799
    multiple adjacent teeth, extreme mobility, 798
    partially erupted first molar clamped, 797f
    routine techniques, 796, 797
    single motion technique, 797
    terminal tooth with insufficient tooth structure, 878
    tooth, calcified pulp chamber/canal, 799

S

Saliva as diagnostic and informative fluid, 30
Salvizol, 966
SBA. *See* Small Business Administration (SBA)
Scar tissue healing, 529–530
  periapical scar (SC) of root canal (RC)-treated tooth, 336f
SEA. *See* Spontaneous electrical activity (SEA)
SealApex, 1032
Sealer 1030
Sealer, use of, 1068
Sedation
  analgesia, levels, 738t
  conscious, 738t, 739
  deep, 741
  iatrosedation: nondrug techniques, 741
  inhalation, 740
  N_2O-O_2, 739
  intravenous conscious, 743–745
    NPO status, 744–5 747, 748
  minimal, 757
  oral conscious, 742–743
  pharmacosedation: drug techniques, 741
Seizures, 737
Shunts, 765
Sickle cell anemia, 769
Signal-to-Noise Ratio (SNR), 573–574
Silver points, 1019, 1020, 1065–1056
  access to, 833
  drawback, 848
  files, solvents, and chelators to remove, 967
  placement into canals, 1105
  pliers to remove, 1103–1105
  removal of, 1114
Simple bone cyst, 613f
Single-appointment therapy, 21–23
Single-implant restorations, 1300–1302
Single nucleotide polymorphism (SNP), 344
Single-tooth implants, indications, 107
Single-visit endodontics, 22–23
Sinus tracts, 1307
SLOB rule (Same Lingual, Opposite Buccal). *See* Clark's rule of horizontal angulation
Small Business Administration (SBA), 1499
Smear layer
  removal, 1006
    after instrumentation, 1000f
    citric acid, 1001
    by irrigation, 1001f
    MTAD, 1006–1007
    solutions and pastes for, 966t
  removal and importance, 1074f
Sodium hypochlorite with chlorhexidine, 1005f
Soft tissue anatomy, 556
  periodontal biotype, 556
Soft tissue management, suturing and postoperative care
  bleeding and swelling, 1271, 1271
    supportive therapy, additional, 1282
  collagen, 1272
  gut, 1268
  interrupted loop (interdental) suture, 1269
  interrupted suture, single, 1269
  needle selection (conventional/reverse), 1268
  oral hygiene, 1323
  PGA, 1268
  postoperative care, 1270, 1271
  postsurgical pain control, 1283
  principles/guidelines, 1273
  repositioning and compression, 1266
  sample instructions, postoperative care following endodontic surgery, 1266t
  silk, advantage, 1267f
  silk suture, high power view of, 1267f
  single interrupted sutures, horizontal/vertical incision, 1269f
  sling suture, single, 1269
  surgeons' knot, modification, 1271f
  suturing, 1266, 1266f
  suturing technique, 1269
    single interrupted sutures, 1269
    sling, 1270, 1271f
    vertical mattress suture, 1270, 1270f
Soft tissue management and flap design, 1269–1278. *See also* Endodontic surgery
  endodontic tissue retractors, 1248f

flap
  reflection, 1279
  retraction, 1248
initial elevation of flap, 1247f
neurovascular bundle exiting from mental foramen, 1247f
surgical flaps, classification of, 1241t
Solid organ transplantation, 765
Solid-state systems, digital systems
  charge-coupled device, 573
  complimentary metal oxide semiconductor active pixel technology (CMOS-APS), 573
SOM. See Surgical operating microscope (SOM)
Sonic canal instrumentation, 826
  canal segments after passive ultrasonic irrigation, 926f
  effect of ultrasonic activation on intracanal temperature, 927f
Spontaneous electrical activity (SEA), 447
SRIF. See Macrophages release somatostatin (SRIF)
Staphylococcus epidermidis, 273, 274f
Stealing theory, 134, 134f
Stem cells, 30
Stereomicroscopic images of human cleared roots, 1057f
Steroids, 723–726
Straight-line access (SLA), 878–880, 892f
  reaching apex with minimal deflection, 906f
Streptococcus, 261–262
Streptococcus gordonii, 237
Streptococcus mitisi, 237
Streptococcusmutans, 245
Streptococcus sanguinis, 237
Streptococcus viridans, 42
Stroke, 764–765
Stropko Irrigator, 885–886
Subacute rhinosinusitis, 628
Subperiosteal implants, 1297–1298
Superoxol, internal bleaching treatment, 22f
Surgical operating microscope (SOM), 153

Surgical outcomes
  failure, 1285
  healing
    complete, 1285–1286
    incomplete, 1285
Surgical root-end filling materials/procedures, 72–73
super-EBA root-end filling, 72
SWOT (Strengths, Weaknesses, Opportunities, and Threats) Analysis, 1475–1476
Sybron Elements Diagnostic Unit, 850f
Sympathetic nerves on teeth, effects of, 143f
Sympathetic nerve terminal, 395
Symptomatic infections, 240
Symptomatic teeth
  non-surgical management, 73
Systemic epinephrine, avoiding, 781

T

Tannerella forsythia, 235, 237
Taurodontism, 180
T-cell antigen receptors (TCRs), 348
Teeth
  cracked
    tooth infractions, 662
    VRFs, 662
  discoloring due enamel fracture, 660f
  morphology and root canal systems, 151–155
  multiple craze lines in, 660f
  three-dimensional position of, 880–881
Teeth, traumatic injuries to, 645–646
  surgical exposure, 667f
Teeth radiography, film placement and cone positioning for, 571f
Teflon cage model, 325
Temperature-modulated DSC (TMDSC), 827
Temporary filling coronal materials, 1043–1044
Terminal capillary networks (TCN), 131

Tetracycline
  and all drugs, 786t
Tetragonal zirconium polycrystals (TZP) post, 1456–1457, 1456f
Tetrodotoxin-resistant (TTXr), 713–714
Therapeutics, definition, 40
Thermafil, 1063–1064, 1063f
ThermaFil Plus Obturator, 1025f
Thermal Tests, diagnostic testing, 533–537
Thermaseal. See AH 26 (thermaseal)
Tissue engineering, 30
Tissue tolerance, 1039–1040
Toll-like receptors (TLRs), 359
  examples of, 359t
Tomography, juvenile rheumatoid arthritic temporomandibular joint, 420f
Toothace in World War II, 1
Tooth bleaching
  complications/adverse effects from intracoronal bleaching
    chemical burns, 1391
    external root resorption, 1391
    inhibition on resin polymerization and bonding strength, 1391
  complications and adverse effects from extracoronal bleaching
    enamel damage, 1395
    gingival irritation, 1395
    mercury release from amalgam restorations, 1396
    tooth sensitivity, 1395
  definitions, 1342
  extracoronal bleaching, 1393
    at-home, 1394–1395
    in-office, 1393–1394
  gutta-percha/sealer/dentin removal prior to bleaching, 1388f
  indications/contraindications for bleaching endodontically treated teeth, 1389t
  intracoronal bleaching of endodontically treated teeth

thermocatalytic, 1389
ultraviolet photooxidation, 1390
walking bleach, 1389
materials, 1388
mechanisms, 1389
postbleaching external root resorption, 1392f
restoration of intracoronally bleached teeth, 1393
role of dental professionals, 1389
extracoronal bleaching treatment, 1396
safe bleaching of endodontically treated teeth, suggestions, 1391–1393
schematic illustration of intracoronal protective bleach barrier, 1393
Tooth development, human, 118–119
ectoderm and neural crest cells, 119
formation of tooth, 119
stages, 119
Tooth discoloration, etiology of
dentist-related causes
amalgams, 1387
extracoronal bleaching of tetracycline-discolored maxillary incisors, 1387f
fluorescent photomicrograph of tetracycline-discolored tooth, 1386f
intracanal medicaments, 1386
obturating materials, 1386–1387
pulp tissue remnants, 1386
resin composites, 1387
patient-related causes
age, 1383–1384
amelogenesis imperfecta, 1384
calcific metamorphosis, 1383
dental fluorosis, 1384
dentinogenesis imperfecta, 1384
enamel hypoplasia, 1384
erythroblastosis fetalis, 1384
hypocalcification, 1384
intrapulpal hemorrhage, 1383
pulp necrosis, 1383
tetracycline, 1384–1386
tooth structure, developmental defects, 1384

Tooth fractures
cracked teeth, 660, 660f
craze lines, 660f
crown–root, 660
cuspal fracture, 660, 661f
root fractures, 660
split tooth, 660, 662f
trauma-related crown, 660
vertical root fractures (VRF), 660, 662f
Tooth infractions, 660–662
accidental biting, 666
acute trauma, 666, 667f
characteristics of
distribution, 663
etiology, 665–667
pain characteristics, 663–665
problems in diagnosis, 663
clinical test for, 664f
biting test, 668
cold stimulus application and electric pulp testing, 669
tooth slooth, 668–669, 669f
use of fiber optic light source, 668f
defined, 660–662
diagnosis of, 667
clinical examination, 668–670
future, 670
radiographic examination, 670
symptoms, 667–668
incidence of, 663
initial treatment to determine pulpal involvement, 671f
long-term follow-up of endodontically treated, 673f
maxillary molar with, radiography of, 670f
not responding to treatment, 672
pain
chewing pain, 672
confounding, 665
"relief" pain, 664
temperature change or coldness, 664, 672
percussion sensitivity, 669
periodontal probing, 669, 669f
prevention, 673–674
radiograph with internal resorption, 670f
and restored teeth, 682
removal of restoration and dye highlighting, 668f

use of pins, 665, 666f
treatment, 670–672
prognosis, 672–673
types, 662
Tooth regeneration, 30–31
Tooth replantation procedure, 67–69
abulcasis, 68
Tooth resorption, 71–72
Tooth stains, sources of, 1383t
Total Quality Management (TQM), 1496
TQM. *See* Total Quality Management (TQM)
Traditional concepts *versus* a futuristic view
alveolar osteoporosis associated with bruxism, 512–513, 512f
apexum device/procedure/ healing, 511f
endodontic treatment, 509
local sustained delivery, 510
methods used, achievement, 509
potential pharmacological modulation, healing of apical granuloma, 510f
Transcription-dependent changes, 386
Transcription factors and signals (tooth development), 120f
Transcriptome, 30
Treatment of endodontic infections/cysts/flare-ups
abscesses/cellulitis. *See* Endodontic abscesses/ cellulitis, treatment of
bacterial factors associated with flare-ups, 707–708
coronal access opening, drainage. *See* Drainage through coronal access opening
flare-ups. *See* Endodontic flare-ups
pharmacologic strategies. *See* Pharmacologic strategies, flare-ups
spaces
buccal/submasseteric/ pterygomandibular/ parapharyngeal/ pretracheal/prevertebral/ danger, 691f

mental/submental/sublingual, 690f
submandibular/sublingual, 691f
strategies to prevent flare-ups. *See* Preventive strategies, flare-ups
treatment of endodontic flare-ups, 705
Treatment of established external root resorption in young patient, 1345–1347, 1346f
Treatment outcomes, 113–114, 1177
  assessment, 1178
    criteria inconsistency, 1179
    radiographs interpretation, 1178–1179
  disease, 1184, 1189f
  functional, 1200f
  healed, 1184, 1180f
  healing, 1184, 1180f
  varied outcomes, 1187
Treatment planning for prosthodontics/ periodontics/endodontics, effects of dental implants
  alternative treatments, root canal, 114
  cost of treatment, 113
  dental implants on endodontics/ periodontics, effects of, 107–108
    paradigm shift, 107
    treatment, benefits of, 108
  dental implants on prosthodontics, effects of, 106–107
  endodontic treatment, 106f
  outcomes, root canal treatment, 112–113
  patient-related factors
    biologic environmental considerations, 109–110
    pulp/periodontal conditions, 108–109
    soft tissue anatomy, 110
    systemic/local health factors, 108
    teeth with unique color characteristics, 110
  root canal therapy, 109f
  single-tooth implants, 109f

treatment-related factors
  adjunctive procedures, required, 113
  ethical considerations, 110–112
  patient comfort/perceptions, 112
  procedural complications (root canal treatment), 112–113
Treponema spp., 243
Trigeminal nerve, primary afferent nociceptive fibers, 401f
Trigeminal neuralgia, 665
Trigeminal system, acute pain pathways
  cervical pain disorders, 402
  neuroanatomic model, appearance of new receptive fields, 400f
  trigeminal nerve, primary afferent nociceptive fibers, 401f
  trigeminal nociceptive fibers, arrangement, 401f
TrPs. *See* Myofascial trigger points (TrPs)
Tuberculosis (TB), 764
Tuned Aperture Computed Tomography (TACT), 573, 582–583

U

Ultrasonic canal instrumentation, 953–954
  effect of ultrasonic activation on intracanal temperature, 956f
Ultrasonic cleaning, 1007
Ultrasonic energy, sources, 1137
Ultrasonic imaging, 590
  anechoic and dishomogeneous echo, 592
  basic principles of, 590–593
  follow-up of endodontic treatment, 597
  lesion of endodontic origin
    in mandible, 610f
    in maxilla, 611f
  monitoring inflammatory changes in diseased bone, 597
  piezoelectric effect, 590

  schematic representation of sending, 590f
  in study of periapical lesions, 593–597
  two different lesions in jaws, 608f
Ultrasonic instruments, 1099
  in intraradicular obstruction removal, 1137
  monitoring usage intervals to assess overheating, 1136f
Ultrasonic irrigation, 954
  varying effect of ultrasonic activation, 955
Ultrasound technical equipment, 591f

V

Valvular disease
  antibiotic prophylaxis for dental procedures, 758f
  recommendations for antibiotic prophylaxis based on risk stratification for infective endocarditis, 768f
  risk of dental procedures, 768f
Vasoactive intestinal peptide (VIP), 137
Vasoconstriction, 133
Vasoconstrictor use in patients with cardiovascular disease, 755–756
  and anesthetics, 755
  choice of local anesthetic, 756
  limitations for, 756
  restricted to cardiovascular disease, 755–756
Veillonella parvula, 237
Vertical root fractures of endodontically treated teeth, 670
  in buccal and lingual roots of maxillary bifurcated premolar, 684f
  clinical diagnosis, 677–680
    diagnostic difficulty, 677
  etiology, 682–685
  iatrogenic etiological factors, 685–686
  prevention, 686
  radiographic diagnosis, 680–682
  treatment, 686

Vertical root fractures (VRFs), 662, 676
  bifurcation radiolucency, 682
    bony periradicular radiolucencies in mandibular molars, 683f
  bone loss associated with, 673f
  with bone resorption, 608f
  complete fracture in mandibular premolar, 676f
  deep osseous defect, 677, 677f
  endodontically treated maxillary premolars, 685f
  etiology, 676, 682–683
    iatrogenic factors, 685–686
  exploratory surgery, 680
  frequent feature, 681–682
  "halo" radiolucency, 682
    apical and mesial aspects, 682f
    isolated lateral radiolucency, 682f
    mesial and distal aspects, 682f
  incomplete fracture in maxillary premolar, 682f
  late diagnosis of, 678f
  lingual aspect of tooth with, 680
  mandibular premolar suspected of, 677f
  minimizing risk of, 683
  predisposing factor/reason for susceptiblity
    anatomical entities, 683
    biochemical properties of dentin, 684
    canal and root shape, 683
    missing tooth structure due to caries or trauma, 684
  prevention, accomplishing, 686
  radiographically detecting endodontically treated tooth
    hair-like fracture line radiolucency, 681f
    separation of root segments, 681f
  relationship between location, clinical, and radiographic appearance, 659f
  tomography to detect, 682
  treatment, 686
    constant ingress of bacteria, 686
VGSC. See Voltage-gated sodium channels (VGSC)

VIP-immunoreactive (VIP-IR), 138
Virulence factors, endodontic infections, 245–249
  capsules, 247
  exotoxins, 248
  extracellular proteins, 248
  extracellular vesicles, 247
  fimbriae, 247
  LPS. See Lipopolysaccharide (LPS)
  LTA. See Lipoteichoic acid (LTA)
  pathogens and, 246t
  PG. See Peptidoglycan (PG)
  polyamines, 248–249
  short-chain fatty acids, 248
  superoxide anions, 249
Visual enhancement
  definitions. See Optical definitions
  loupes, 870–871
  magnification versus differentiation
    definition, 874–875
  microscope–endoscope combination, 874, 875f
  microscopes. See Microscopes, visual enhancement
  microsurgery, 870
  orascope. See Fiber optic endoscope (orascope)
Visual oral examination, diagnostic testing
  diagnostic grid for recording pulp testing results, 533t
  "tunnel vision," 533
Vital dental pulp
  chemotactic signals, 1311
  immune defense mechanisms, 1311
Vital pulp therapy, 1425. See also Vital dental pulp
  apexogenesis, 46
  caries removal. See Caries removal, vital pulp therapy
  for children, 1405
  dentin bridge formation using MTA/calcium hydroxide in dog pulps, comparison, 1315f
  diagnostic criteria for successful outcome, 1317–1318
  pulp sizes, 1318

  direct pulp cap, 1405–1406
  final restoration
    restorative procedures, immature permanent teeth, 1323
  hemostasis. See Hemostasis, vital pulp therapy
  indications, 1313
  indirect pulp cap, 1424
  materials. See Vital pulp therapy materials
  MTA, 1314–1317
  permanent tooth (pulpally involved), preservation of, 1310
  postoperative follow-up, 1323
  pulp capping, 46–48
    direct, 1333. See also Direct pulp cap, vital pulp therapy
  pulpotomy, 47, 1418f
  reparative dentin
    formation, 1323
    techniques for generating, 1312
  vital dental pulp, 1311
Vital pulp therapy, traumatic dental injuries
  requirements for success, 1332–1333
    bacteria-tight seal, 1332
    healthy pulp, treatment of, 1332
    MTA, 1333
    proper pulp dressing, 1332
    pulp necrosis, 1332f
Vital pulp therapy materials
  adhesive resins/resin-modified glass ionomers, 1313–1314
  calcium hydroxide, 1313
  characteristics, ideal, 1313
  MCSF, 1317
  mineral trioxide aggregate
    direct pulp capping, effectiveness, 1320–1322
    outcomes, direct pulp capping with MTA, 1315–1316
    two-visit protocol, permanent teeth, 1316
  pulpotomy on young immature permanent teeth using mineral MTA, 1316f

VITAPEX, 1070
Voltage-gated sodium channels (VGSC), 716

W

Walking bleach, 1389
Weight loss products, harms, 750–751
Weine's recommendations, 27f
Working length (WL), 923
    comparison of radiographic and histological aspects of, 925f
    radiographic determination, 929
    radiographic estimation, 928
    reliable means of determining using paper, 929–930
    sequence of steps in determination of, 927f
        precise apex locators, 929
        using electric foramen locator, 929
        watch-winding movement to reach, 934

X

XLH. *See* X-linked hypophosphatemia (XLH)
X-linked hypophosphatemia (XLH), 487
X-ray diffraction (XRD), 827
X-ray films, intraoral digital, 574
    disadvantages of analog, 574
    solid-state X-ray sensor, 577f
    technologies used, 576
X-ray imaging, digital
    advantages and potential disadvantages, 579
    examples of digital images, 579, 580f
X-ray machine, 557
    cone positioning, 558f, 559
    horizontal and vertical angulation, 560
    film. *See* Film, X-ray machine
    film placement, 557–558
    long cone, 557
    short cone, 557

Y

Yeast, role in endodontics, 264–265

Z

Zinc oxide–eugenol-containing sealers, 1069–1072. *See also* Kerr pulp canal sealer EWT
    extruded into mental foramen from canal of mandibular second premolar, 1144
perforation repair, 1128